KU-712-737

Textbook of Pain

For Churchill Livingstone:

Commissioning Editor: Michael J Houston
Project Editor: Deborah Russell
Project Manager: Nora Naughton
Designer: Charles Simpson
Page Make-up: Gerard Heyburn

The publisher's policy is to use paper manufactured from sustainable forests

Textbook of Pain

EDITED BY

Patrick D Wall FRS DM FRCP

Division of Physiology, St Thomas' Hospital, London, UK

Ronald Melzack OC FRSC PhD

Department of Psychology, McGill University, Montreal,
Quebec, Canada

FOURTH EDITION

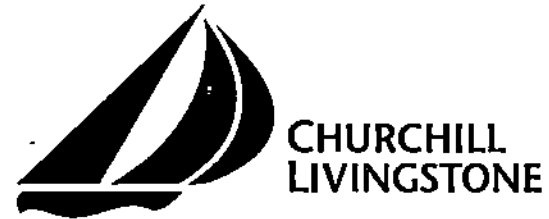

EDINBURGH LONDON NEW YORK OXFORD PHILADELPHIA ST LOUIS SYDNEY TORONTO 1999

CHURCHILL LIVINGSTONE
An imprint of Elsevier Science Limited

First edition 1984
Second edition 1989
Third edition 1994
Fourth edition 1999
Reprinted 2000, 2002, 2003

ISBN 0443 06252 8

British Library Cataloguing in Publication Data
A catalogue record for this book is available from the British Library.

Library of Congress Cataloging in Publication Data
A catalog record for this book is available from the Library of Congress.

Note
Medical knowledge is constantly changing. As new information becomes available, changes in treatment, procedures, equipment and the use of drugs become necessary. The authors and the publishers have, as far as it is possible, taken care to ensure that the information given in this text is accurate and up to date. However, readers are strongly advised to confirm that the information, especially with regard to drug usage, complies with the latest legislation and standards of practice.

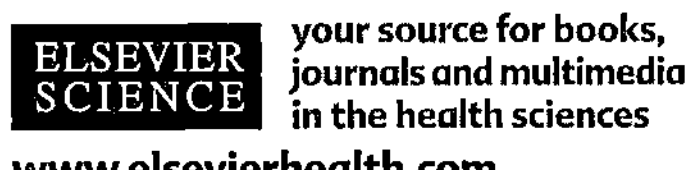

Printed in China
C/04

Contents

SECTION 2 - CLINICAL STATES

Soft tissue, joints and bones

Deep and visceral pain

Head

Nerve and root damage

Central nervous system

Special cases

SECTION 3 - THERAPEUTIC ASPECTS

Pharmacology

Contributors

Ralf Baron
Dept of Neurology
Klinik für Neurologie
Christian-Albrechts-Universität
Kiel, Germany

Allan I Basbaum PhD
Dept of Anatomy
University of California, San Francisco
School of Medicine
San Francisco, USA

David LH Bennet MB PhD
Research Fellow
St Thomas' Hospital, UK

Robert M Bennet MD
Dept of Medicine
Oregon Health Sciences University
Portland, USA

Charles B Berde MD PhD
Pain Treatment Service
Children's Hospital
Boston, USA

Aleksandar Berić MD DSc
Associate Professor of Neurology
Dept of Neurology
Hospital for Joint Diseases
NYU School of Medicine
New York, USA

Karen J Berkley PhD
McKenzie Professor
Program in Neuroscience
Florida State University
Tallahassee, USA

Stuart J Bevan BSc PhD
Novartis Institute for Medical Research
London, UK

Laurence M Blendis MD
Dept of Gastroenterology
Tel-Aviv Sourasky Medical Center
Tel-Aviv, Israel

Jörgen Boivie MD PhD
Dept of Neurology
University Hospital
Linköping, Sweden

William Breitbart MD
Chief of Psychiatric Services
Dept of Psychiatry and Behavioral Sciences
Memorial Sloan-Kettering Cancer Center
New York, USA

Kay Brune MD
Institute of Pharmacology & Toxicology
University of Erlangen-Nuremberg
Erlangen, Germany

Arthur L Burnett MD
Associate Professor of Urology
Johns Hopkins University School of Medicine
The James Buchanan Brady Urological Institute, Baltimore, USA

James N Campbell
Dept of Neurosurgery
Johns Hopkins University
Baltimore, USA

Nathan I Cherny MB BS FRACD M.D
Director, Cancer Pain and Palliative Care
Dept of Medical Oncology
Shaare Zedek Medical Center
Jerusalem, Israel

John J Collins MB BS PhD FRACP
Vicent Fairfax Pain Unit
New Children's Hospital
Westmead, NSW 2145, Australia

Michael Cousins AM MBBS MD
University of Sydney
Dept of Anaesthesia and Pain Management
Royal North Shore Hospital, Australia

AD Craig PhD
Atkinson Pain Research Scientist
Division of Neurosurgery
Barrow Neurological Institute
Phoenix, USA

Kenneth D Craig
Dept of Psychology
University of British Columbia
School of Medicine, Vancouver
British Columbia, Canada

Paul Creamer MD MRCP
Consultant Rheumatologist and Senior Lecturer, North Bristol NHS Trust,
Bristol, UK

Amanda Claire de C Williams PhD
Consultant Clinical Psychologist
INPUT Pain Management Unit
Guy's & St Thomas' NHS Trust
London, UK

Barbara J de Lateur
Dept of Rehabilitation Medicine
University of Washington School of Medicine, Seattle, USA

Marshall Devor PhD
Dept of Cell & Animal Biology

Institute of Life Sciences
Hebrew University of Jerusalem, Israel

Jonathan O Dostrovsky PhD
Professor, Dept of Physiology
Director of Program in Neuroscience
University of Toronto, Toronto, Canada

Timothy P Doubell PhD
Research Fellow
University Laboratory of Physiology
Oxford University, Oxford, UK

Ronald Dubner DDS PhD
Professor and Chair
Dept of Oral and Craniofacial Biological Sciences, University of Maryland Dental School, Baltimore, Maryland, USA

David Dubuisson MD PhD
Dept of Surgery, Beth Israel Hospital, Boston, USA

Howard L Fields MD PhD
Dept of Neurology
University of California San Francisco School of Medicine, San Francisco, USA

Maria Fitzgerald PhD
Dept of Anatomy & Developmental Biology, University College London
London, UK

Lucy Gagliese PhD
Dept of Psychology
The Toronto Hospital, General Division
Toronto, Canada

Richard H Gracely PhD
Pain and Neurosensory Mechanisms Branch, National Institute of Dental and Craniofacial Research
National Institutes of Health
Bethesda, Maryland, USA

Jan M Gybels MD PhD
Laboratory of Experimental Neurosurgery/Neuroanatomy
Katholieke University/Provisorium 1, Leuvenn, Belgium

Scott Haldeman DC MD PhD FRCP(C)
1125 17th St. West, Suite W-127
Santa Ana, USA

Per Hansson MD PhD DDS
Neurogenic Pain Center
Dept of Rehabilitation Medicine
Karolinska Hospital, Sweden

Raymond G Hill B Pharm PhD
Executive Director
Pharmacology and Analgesia Research
Merck Sharp & Dohme Research Laboratories, Neuroscience Research Centre, Essex, UK

Anita Holdcroft MD FRCA
Reader in Anaesthesia
Dept of Anaesthesia and Intensive Care
Hammersmith Hospital and Imperial College of Science, Technology and Medicine, London, UK

Paul Hooper DC
Chair, Department of Principles and Practice, Los Angeles College of Chiropractic, Whittier, California, USA

Jen-Chuen Hsieh MD PhD
Assoc Prof & Project Coordinator,
Integrated Brain Research Unit
Veterans General Hospital – Taipei
Taiwan

Martin Ingvar MD PhD
Dept of Radiology
Karolinska Hospital
Sweden

Malcolm IV Jayson MD FRCP
Consultant Rheumatologist and Emeritus Professor of Rheumatology
Rheumatic Diseases Centre
University of Manchester
Salford, UK

Troels Staehelin Jensen MD PhD
Professor, Dept of Neurology
Danish Pain Research Center
Aarhus University Hospital
Denmark

Joel Katz PhD C Psych.
Dept of Psychology
The Toronto Hospital, University of Toronto, Toronto, Canada

Francis J Keefe PhD
Professor, Health Psychology Program
Dept of Psychology
Ohio University
Athens, Ohio, USA

John C Lefebvre PhD
Assistant Research Professor
Health Psychology Program
Dept of Psychology
Ohio University
Athens, Ohio, USA

Justus F Lehmann MD
Dept of Rehabilitation Medicine
University of Washington School of Medicine, Seattle, USA

Jon Levine MD PhD
NIH University of California San Francisco Pain Center,
San Francisco, USA

Steven James Linton PhD
Psychologist
Program for Behavioral Medicine
Dept of Occupational and Environmental Medicine, Örebro Medical Center
Örebro, Sweden

Donlin M Long MD PhD
Dept of Neurosurgery
Johns Hopkins Hospital
Baltimore, USA

Thomas Lundeberg MD PhD
Dept of Rehabilitation Medicine
Karolinska Hospital, Sweden

Richard J Mannion PhD
Research Fellow
Dept of Anatomy and Developmental Biology, University College London
London, UK

Marco Maresca MD
Researcher, Pain Center
University of Florence
Florence, Italy

Bruce Masek PhD
Dept of Psychiatry
Harvard Medical School
Boston, MA, USA

John S McDonald MD
Depat of Anesthesiology
Ohio State University Hospital
Columbus, USA

Patrick J McGrath PhD
Professor of Psychology
Pediatrics and Psychiatry
Dalhousie University and IWK Grace Health Centre, Nova Scotia, Canada

Robert F McLain MD
Dept of Orthopedic Surgery
The Cleveland Clinic Foundation
Cleveland, Ohio, USA

Stephen B McMahon BSc PhD
Sherrington Professor of Physiology

King's College London
UK

H J McQuay DM
Clinical Reader in Pain Relief
Pain Research
Nuffield Dept of Anaesthetics
Oxford Radcliffe Hospital
Oxford, UK

Ronald Melzack OC FRSC PhD
Dept of Psychology
McGill University, Montreal
Quebec, Canada

Harold Merskey DM FRCP FRCPSYCH
Professor Emeritus of Psychiatry
University of Western Ontario
London Health Sciences Campus
Ontario, Canada

Richard A Meyer
Johns Hopkins Applied Physics
Laboratory, Johns Hopkins University
Baltimore, USA

Kerry Raphael Mills PhD FRCP
Professor of Clinical Neurophysiology
Guy's, King's & St Thomas' Medical
School, University of London
London, UK

Richard C Monks MD
Geriatric Psychiatrist
Upper Island Geriatric Research Team
Courtenay, Canada

RA Moore DSc
Honorary Consultant Biochemist
Pain Research
Nuffield Dept of Anaesthetics
Oxford Radcliffe Hospital
Oxford, UK

Rajesh Munglani DA DCH FRCA
Director – Pain Relief Service
Unit of Anaesthesia
Addenbrookes Hospital
Cambridge, UK

Dianne Jane Newham MSCP MPhil PhD
Professor of Physiotherapy
School of Biomedical Sciences
King's College London
Guy's Campus, London, UK

Lone Nickolajsen MD PhD
Dept of Anesthesiology
Danish Pain Research Center
Aarhus University Hospital
Denmark

Akiko Okifuji PhD
Research Assistant Professor
Dept of Anesthesiology
University of Washington
Seattle, Washington, USA

Steven D Passik PhD
Director, Oncology Symptom Control
and Research
Community Cancer Care, Inc
Indianapolis, Indiana, USA

Michael Platt
Dept of Anesthetics
St. Mary's Hospital
London, UK

Russell K Portenoy MD
Chairman, Dept of Pain Medicine
and Palliative Care
Beth Israel Medical Center
New York, USA

Ian Power MB CHB Bsc (Hons) MD FRCA
Associate Professor
University of Sydney at the Royal North
Shore Hospital, Australia

Paolo Procacci MD
Professor of Internal Medicine
Director of the Pain Center
University of Florence
Florence, Italy

Srinivasa N Raja
Dept of Anesthesiology and Critical Care
Medicine, Division of Pain Medicine
Johns Hopkins Hospital
Baltimore, USA

Andrea J Rapkin MD
Professor of Obstetrics and Gynecology
UCLA School of Medicine
Los Angeles, California, USA

David B Reichling PhD
NIH Pain Center
University of California, San Francisco
San Francisco, California, USA

Ke Ren MD PhD
Assistant Professor
Dept of Oral and Craniofacial Biological
Sciences, University of Maryland Dental
School, Baltimore, USA

Matthias Ringkamp
Dept of Neurosurgery
Johns Hopkins University
Baltimore, USA

Barry D Rosenfeld PhD
Dept of Psychology
Long Island University
New York, USA

Michael C Rowbotham
Dept of Anesthesiology
University of California, San Francisco
School of Medicine, San Francisco, USA

Peter S Sándor MD
Neurology Department
University Hospitals Zurich
Switzerland

Cicely M Saunders OM DBE FRCP
St. Christopher's Hospice
London, UK

John W Scadding BSc MD FRCP
Consultant Neurologist
The National Hospital for Neurology &
Neurosurgery, London, UK

Jean Schoenen MD PhD
Professor of Neuroanatomy
Dept of Neurology and Neuroanatomy
University of Liège, Belgium

Ze'ev Seltzer
Physiology Branch
Hebrew University
Hadassah Schol of Dentistry
Jerusalem, Israel

Yair Sharav DMD MS
Professor of Oral Medicine
Chairman, Dept of Oral Diagnosis,
Oral Medicine and Radiology
School of Dental Medicine
Hebrew University-Hadassah
Jerusalem, Israel

Charles E Short DVM, PhD DACVA,
DECVA
Professor of Anesthesiology and Pain
Management, College of Veterinary
Medicine, Cornell University
Ithaca New York, USA

Brian A Simpson MA MD FRCS
Dept of Neurosurgery
University Hospital of Wales
Cardiff, UK

Anders E Sola MD MS
Clinical Assistant Professor
Dept of Anesthesiology and Pain Service
University of Washington School of
Medicine, Seattle, Washington, USA

Erik Spangfort MD PhD
Associate Professor of Orthopaedic Surgery, Karolinska Institute
Stockholm, Sweden

Ronald R Tasker MD
Professor Emeritus Surgery
University of Toronto
Neurosurgical Division
Toronto Hospital
Toronto, Canada

Dennis C Turk PhD
John and Emma Bonica Professor of Anesthesiology & Pain Research
Dept of Anesthesiology
University of Washington School of Medicine, Seattle Washington, USA

Robert G Twycross DM
Sir Michael Sobell House
Churchill Hospital
Oxford, UK

Anita M Unruh BScOT MSW PhD
Associate Professor of Occupational Therapy, Dalhousie University
Halifax, Nova Scotia, Canada

Patrick D Wall FRS DM FRCP
Division of Physiology, St Thomas' Hospital, London, UK

James N Weinstein DO MSc
Professor of Orthopedics and Community and Family Medicine
Dartmouth Medical School
Hanover, New Hampshire, USA

Matisyohu Weisenberg PhD
Dept of Psychology
Bar-Ilan University
Ramat Gan, Israel

Ursula Wesselmann MD
Assistant Professor of Neurology, Neurological Surgery and Biomedical Engineering
Johns Hopkins University School of Medicine, Dept of Neurology
Baltimore, USA

Clifford J Woolf MD PhD
Richard J Kitz Professor of Anesthesia Research, Harvard Medical School
Director, Neural Plasticity Research Group
Dept of Anesthesia and Critical Care
Massachusetts General Hospital-East
Charlestown, USA

Tony L Yaksh PhD
Dept of Anesthesiology/0818
University of California, San Diego
School of Medicine, La Jolla
USA

Joanna M Zakrzewska FDSRCS FFD RCSI
Head of Dept of Oral Medicine
Senior Lecturer/Honorary Consultant
St. Bartholomew's and The Royal London, School of Medicine and Dentistry, London, UK

Hanns Ulrich Zeilhofer MD
Institute of Experimental and Clinical Pharmacology and Toxicology
University of Erlangen-Nuremberg
Erlangen, Germany

Massimo Zoppi M.D
Associate Professor of Rheumatology
University of Florence
Florence, Italy

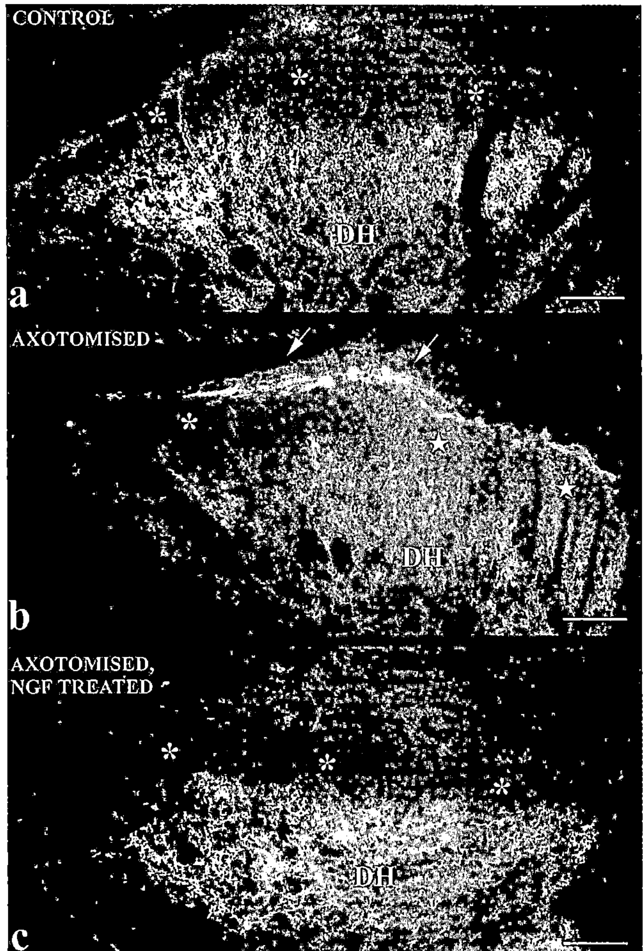

Fig. 4.5 Anatomical reorganization of primary afferent terminals after peripheral axotomy is blocked by NGF. Double-stained transverse sections of rat lumbar spinal cord, showing CGRP staining in red and labelling of myelinated afferent fibre terminals (following anterograde transport of Cholera B into sciatic nerve) in green. **a** The staining pattern obtained in normal animals. Note there is very little overlap: the myelinated staining stops at the lamina II/III border and the CGRP staining is dorsal to this (lamina II is denoted by asterisks). After sciatic axotomy (**b**), CGRP is lost in the medial part of the cord and in this region myelinated fibres sprout, evidenced by the presence of cholera B staining throughout the medial superficial dorsal horn, sprouting also occurs in lamina I, demonstrated by an arrow. In animals treated with intrathecal NGF and subjected to sciatic nerve section (**c**) the expected downregulation of CGRP and the sprouting of myelinated fibres is prevented. (Reproduced from Bennett et al 1996a.) (see p 115)

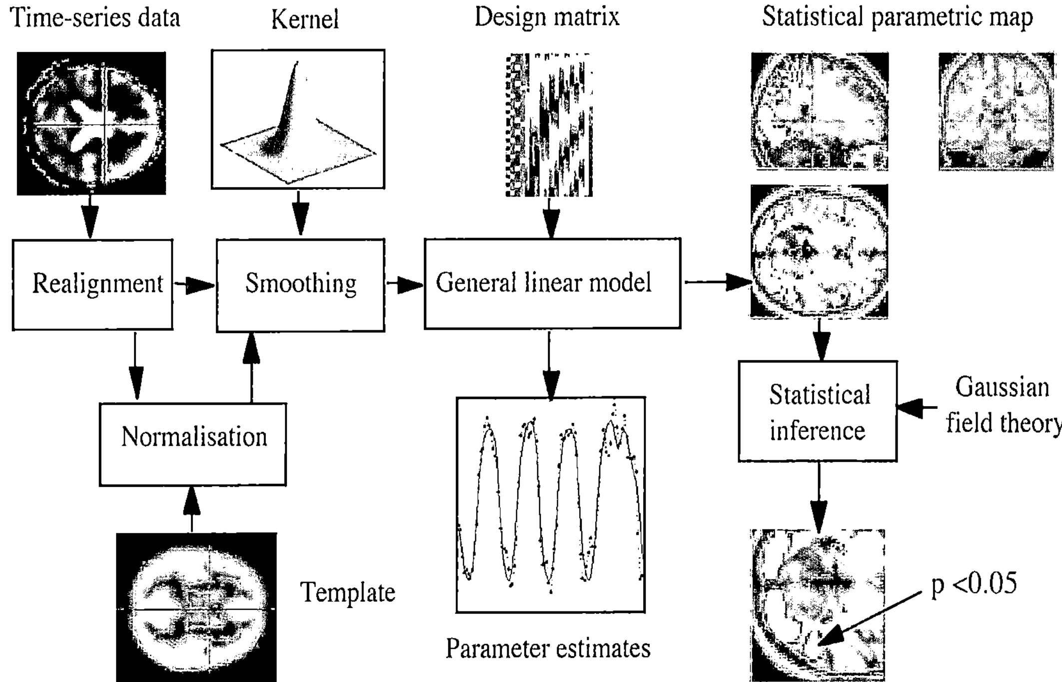

Fig. 8.3 A schematic presentation of the different steps of post processing of image data from PET/fMRI. The realignment step checks for movement-related artefacts. Normalization is an optional step where all images are transformed to a common anatomical space, smoothing is used to handle high-frequency noise in the image. Following this a statistical model is applied and then maps are created which depict the results. (Courtesy of Karl Friston 1998, see further http://www.fil.ion.ucl.ac.uk/spm/course/notes.html.) (see p 218)

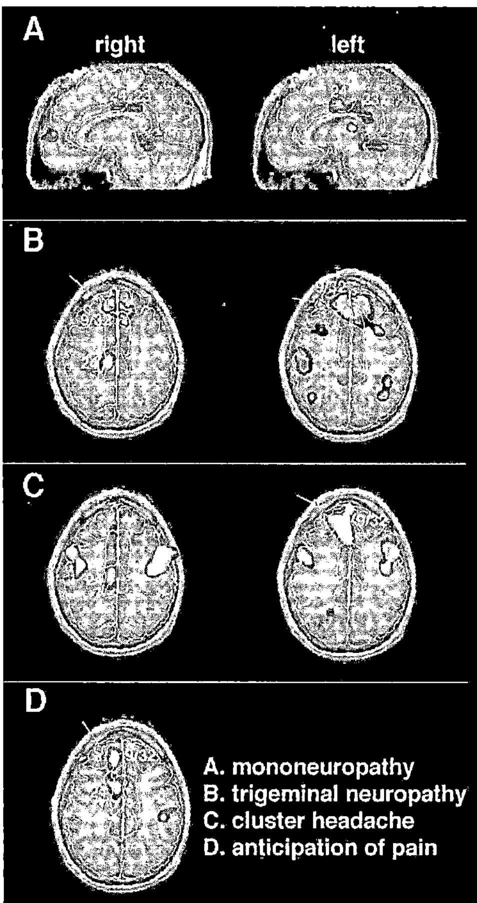

Fig. 8.5 The omnibus significance maps (thresholded at $P < 0.01$) were superimposed on a transformed MRI image and were colour coded into four levels defined by $0.001 \leq P < 0.01$ (increase = red; decrease = blue) and $P < 0.001$ (increase = yellow; decrease = light blue). In peripheral neuropathy (**A**), both right-sided and left-sided affliction lead to a right-sided activation in the ACC. Data for trigeminal neuropathy (**B**) and cluster headache (**C**) were pooled in the respective groups irrespective of the side of painful input to identify, on a system level, the regions consistently engaged in central pain processing (for data treatment see Bottini et al 1995, Hsieh et al 1995, 1996a). The right hemisphere is on the reader's left. Area 24 & 9/32 are indicated with blue arrows. (see p 227)

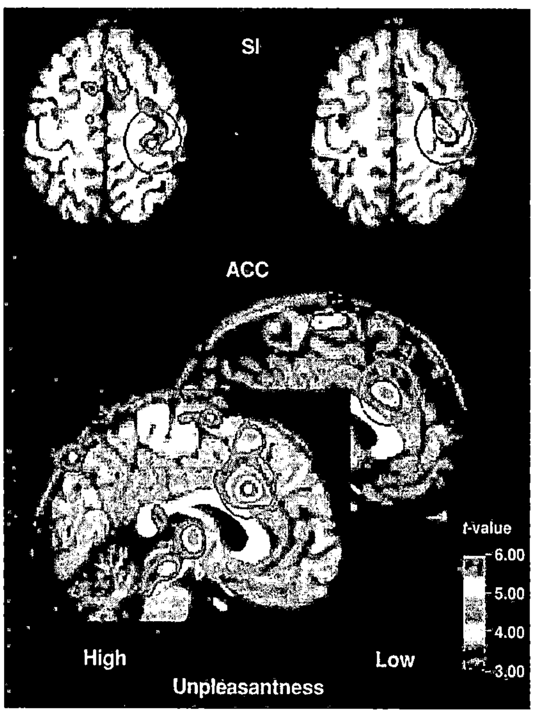

Fig. 57.11 Changes in pain-related activity associated with hypnotic suggestions of high and low unpleasantness (left and right images, respectively) are revealed by subtracting PET data recorded during the neutral/hypnosis control condition from those of the painfully hot/-UNP and painfully hot/-UNP conditions. PET data, averaged across 11 experimental sessions, are illustrated against an MRI from one person; horizontal and saggittal slices through S1 and ACC, respectively, are centred at the activation peaks observed during the relevant suggestion conditions; red circles indicate the location and size of VOIs used to analyse activation levels across the two conditions. UNP = hypnotic suggestion for increased (+) or decreased (–) unpleasantness; VOI = volume of interest. (Reproduced from Rainville et al 1997 with permission.) (see p 1332)

Introduction to the fourth edition

PATRICK D. WALL

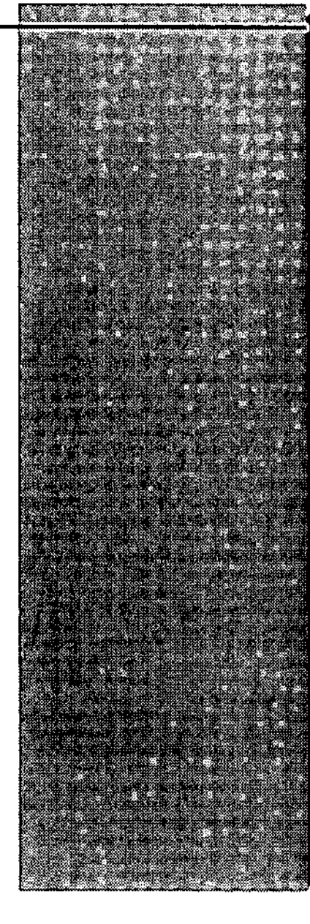

The chapters in this book express the independent views of the selected authors. Everyone writing on pain has in mind a plan of how pain mechanisms operate. There are many different plans and some are complementary rather than contradictory. The editors have made no attempt to unify these concepts because we would rather leave the reader with the opportunity to select between the various widely held views. There are those who still believe pain can be adequately described as the result of activity in a dedicated pathway originating in peripheral nociceptors. Others propose a more complex approach which takes into account the plasticity of all the conduction pathways and the nature of pattern detection by parallel processing and the active participation of the brain in perception. The traditional scheme starts with a stimulus and follows the consequences through to a sensory-emotional response. In this introduction, I propose a way to bring all the chapters together by a search beginning with the perception of pain.

ATTENTION

No conscious awareness of anything is possible until it has captured our attention. Our sense organs in the eyes, ears, nose and body are in continuous action, day and night, awake or asleep. The central nervous system is receiving steady reports of all the events these sense organs are capable of detecting. Obviously, it would be a disaster of excess if we were continuously aware of the entire mass of arriving information. We completely ignore most of the information most of the time. And yet any fraction of this inflow is capable of rivetting attention. For this to happen, there has to be a selective attention mechanism which must have a set of rules. Those rules are not arbitrary. Every species displays their rules which incorporate a selection of those events that are important to survival and well-being. Some rules seem to be built in. Large, sudden novel events have precedence in their attention-grabbing ability. And, I would propose, that the arrival in the nervous system of messages signalling tissue damage is another of these built-in high-priority events.

There is a learned component of our selective attention mechanism. The bored radar operator sits staring at the screen which is a snow storm of random blinking dots. Let one of these dots begin to move in a consistent line and attention locks onto that dot to the exclusion of all the others. Let the classical migraine sufferer detect a small twinkling area in the visual field and his attention is rivetted on this trivial event because he has learned that the aura on his oncoming migraine attack begins with just such a scintillating area.

In social animals, subtle triggers of attention can be shared. In West Africa, two species of monkeys feed together in flocks but eat different fruits. Their main enemy is the monkey eagle and one species is quicker to spot arriving eagles so that both species benefit from the alarm of one. In Australia, a grouse selects her ground nest close to a tree containing a hawk nest, because the hawk's superior height and eyesight detects distant predators long before the earth-bound grouse. And so it is with humans, where attention is infectious.

The attention mechanism must be continuously scanning the available information in the incoming messages and assigning a priority to the biological importance of the message. There are examples of 'thoughtless' decision, as in the switch of attention in the car driver in conversation with a passenger while engaged in 'unconscious' skilled driving until some fool cuts in front of her, whereupon attention promptly switches from conversation to avoidance. This brings out the second rule of selective attention, which is that only one target at a time is permitted. Obviously it is possible to switch attention back and forth quite rapidly. However, at any one instant, only one collection of information is available for conscious sensory analysis. This one object can itself be preset. An example is the detection of the mention of your name in the random buzz of cocktail party conversation. It is possible to scan a long list of names and detect the one you seek with no recall of any of the other names.

It is not intuitively obvious that attention can only be directed to one subject at any one time. It would seem a rather ridiculous limitation in a mental process which clearly has freedom to rove over vast areas; 'shoes and ships and sealing-wax, cabbages and kings'. An explanation for this strict limit on attention could be that sensory events are analysed in terms of the action which might be appropriate to the event. If the aim of attention relates to appropriate action, then it follows that a fundamental requirement of nature is that only one action at a time is permitted. It is not possible to move forwards and backwards simultaneously. You must 'make up your mind'. The explanation for the singleness of momentary attention would then derive from the purpose of attention, which is to assemble and highlight those aspects of the sensory input that would be relevant to carrying out one act.

Of course, rival sensory events may compete for attention. The myth of the ass who starves to death when placed equidistant between two bales of hay is indeed a myth which would never happen. There may be many events occurring simultaneously each demanding attention. They are rank ordered into a hierarchy in terms of biological importance. The practical consequence of this ordering is the apparent paradox of the painless injury. Each of these victims was involved in a situation where some action, other than attending to their wound, had top priority. Getting out of a burning aircraft is more urgent than attending to a broken leg. The attention does not oscillate between the two demands. One is assigned complete domination until safety is achieved. Only then is the alternate assigned the top position, attention shifts and pain occurs. The workman in the course of a skilled task and the tackled footballer about to score a goal carry on to complete the task with engrossed attention in spite of the conflicting demands of their coincidental injury. Only when the conditions of the top priority fade, there is a reassessment of the next most urgent priority. In conditions of complete 'emergency analgesia', pain emerges as the dominant fact when the emergency is over. The priority ranking of importance of what deserves attention is partly built in and partly learned from personal experience and partly a component of culture.

From the first positron emission tomographic (PET) images of people in pain, intense activity was detected in the anterior cingulate. It is even apparent in patients with very chronic pain associated with a single nerve neuropathy and, even more surprising, it is only present on the right side irrespective of which side the pain is on. However, this general area is also active in many other situations, including directed visual or auditory attention, precise eye and hand movements, and even during complex speech. The suggestion that this zone is involved in attention mechanisms fits with the results of surgical destruction of the area as a treatment of obsessional melancholic depression which I take to be a disorder of attention.

Therapy based on a moulding of attention is effective. It is called distraction. When a toddler trips, smacks into the pavement and howls, what does a parent do? Pick it up, dance about, coo, oo and ah, kiss it better. These are distractions. Because you can only attend to one thing at a time, it follows that you can only have one pain at a time. This fact led to many excellent folk remedies; hot poultices, horse linaments and mustard plasters. They are called counterstimulants. When pain really sets in, attention is utterly monopolized and nothing else exists in the world but the pain. Many therapies attempt to intrude on this fixation. The distraction that is effective may be simple but it will depend on established priorities. A game of cards, letting the cat out or the sight of a hated neighbour can provide a brief interlude in pain. Some victims discover this for themselves and prolong their brief holidays from pain by inventing distractions, while others get professional help in occupational therapy. In another distraction therapy given the pretentious title of cognitive therapy, the victim learns to day dream where they play out an internal fantasy. It may be that they are on a warm sunny beach or at a football match or in their favourite bar. Some people can become very skilled at these distractions and give themselves longer and longer respites from their miserable pain.

ALERTING, ORIENTATION AND EXPLORATION

As attention shifts to pain, alertness appears. There is something wrong. Alarm bells. Action stations. Muscles tense and the body stiffens to a ramrod. Unknown to the victim, these overt changes are part of a massive reorganization of many parts of the body. The heart and vascular system get ready for action. The hormone system mobilizes sugar and alerts the immune system. The gut becomes stationary. Sleep as an option is cancelled.

The eyes, head and neck turn to inspect where the pain seems located. The hands explore the area. Muscles are contracted to learn what makes the pain worse and what eases it and to seek a comfortable position and then hold it. The end result is a body fixed in an overall pain posture. Muscles are in steady contraction and, as time goes by, some muscles grow while joints and tendons deteriorate because this frozen posture itself sets off local changes. The vascular and endocrine systems hold their emergency state if pain is prolonged and these systems are not evolved to cope with this prolonged stress state. The quiet gut demonstrates its inactivity as constipation. Perhaps worst of all, sleep is impossible and chronic pain patients become completely exhausted. Even intermittent sleep deprivation drives the strongest of us into pretty peculiar ways of thinking, as any doctor on night duty knows and as any parent with a new baby knows. Chronic pain patients get to their wits end as their grim experience is prolonged.

Clearly this state of affairs needs therapeutic attack. The key word is relaxation and much ingenuity has been used. The problem is to override a natural defense mechanism which has a protective role in brief emergencies but which becomes maladaptive when prolonged. Drugs to inhibit the overactive muscle are commonly prescribed but they are sedative and intellectually flattening. After a while, patients refuse them or become zombies. Physiotherapists have many ways of relaxing muscles and of re-establishing movement in frozen zones. First they have to overcome the patient's natural fear that movement which produces pain does not necessarily increase the injury and that lack of movement which seemed at first to prevent pain eventually plays a role in prolonging the pain. Yoga and the Alexander technique are examples of posture training. Relaxation is not easy and training methods are needed. One successful version, 'bio-feedback' training, provides the patient with an electronic indicator of the amount of contraction in a muscle and allows the patient to judge second by second his success in relaxation. The patient has to learn how to relax and how to prolong the effect into real life outside the training sessions. Sleep follows relaxation but it may need additional help until the patient can sleep on his own.

THE SENSATION OF PAIN ITSELF

We are used to discussing sensation as the consequence of stimulation in a series of boxes: firstly injury generates an announcement of its presence in sensory nerves; secondly the attention mechanism selects the incoming message as worthy of entry; thirdly the brain generates the sensation of pain. Now the question is 'how does the brain interpret the input?' The classical theory is that the brain analyses the sensory input to determine what has happened and presents the answer as a pure sensation. I propose an alternate theory that the brain analyses the input in terms of what action would be appropriate.

Let us explore the alternate theory as it has practical consequences for pain. If the classical theory were true, the first action of the brain is to identify the nature of the events which generated the sensory input. This should produce the first sensation of injury as pure pain. The next stage of the classical theory is that different parts of the brain perceive the pure sensation and generate an assessment of affect, that is to say 'is the pure pain miserable, dangerous, frightening and so on?' My first reaction, on introspection, is that I have never felt a pure pain. Pain for me arrives as a complete package. A particular pain is at the same time painful and miserable and disturbing and so on. I have never heard a patient speak of pain isolated from its companion affect. Because classical theory assigns different parts of the brain to the task of the primary sensory analysis and others for the task of adding affect, one would expect some disease to separate pain from misery. No such disease is known. During neurosurgical operations, very small areas of brain can be stimulated and some cause pain. There has never been a report of pain evoked which was not accompanied by fear or misery or other strong affects. Finally there are parts of brain, the primary sensory cortex, which have been classically assigned the role of primary sensory analysis and yet, in the imaging studies, these areas are often reported as silent while the subject reports pain. Even for the sympathetic pain on hearing of the death of a friend, the sensation is inseparable from the sadness and loneliness.

Therefore let us explore the alternative, which is that the brain analyses its sensory input in terms of the possible action which would be appropriate to the event which triggered the whole process. There is in this absolutely no suggestion that any action need actually take place. Trained subjects and stoics may receive a clearly painful stimulus with no overt movement even though they can later report the nature of the pain they felt. There are elaborate and extensive areas of our brain concerned with motor planning as distinct from motor movement itself. It is precisely these areas that are most obviously active when the brain is imaged in subjects who are in pain but who are quite stationary with no movement. Chapter 8 by Ingvar describes the areas found to be active while the subjects feel pain. The first area of surprise to be reported was the anterior cingulate which becomes active in any act of attention and this is exactly what is expected given the evidence that attention is a prerequisite of pain. The other areas consistently reported as active by many investigators are the premotor cortex, the frontal lobes, basal ganglia and cerebellum. All of the last hundred years of neurology have assigned these areas a role in the preparation for skilled planned movement.

Because I am proposing a quite new hypothesis here, one should explore widely to see if there are facts which support the possibility that sensory analysis is carried on in terms of motor action which would be appropriate to the input. Of the many imaging studies carried out on normal subjects or on patients in pain, some have shown no activation of the primary sensory cortex and even in those showing such activation, the area extends rostrally into the motor area in spite of the fact that no overt motor movement is detected. The marked activation of the cerebellum is a great surprise because classical opinion assigned no sensory role to the cerebellum. However, more recent work has clearly shown that the cerebellum plays a role in the analysis of sensory input in the course of establishing conditioned responses. Similarly the basal ganglia, putamen and globus pallidus were classically only given a function in overt movement and yet show marked activation in subjects in pain who show no signs of movement. However, muscle ache is a common prodromal sign of parkinsonism and responds to L-DOPA, which is reported to reduce neuropathic pain.

Sometimes the detection of a sensory input is demonstrated by motor movement. Mimicry is an example. The earliest sign that a baby is detecting complex visual stimuli is its mimicry of facial expression; opening the mouth, smiling, etc. Cells in monkey cortex in the inferior precental area have been detected which respond when the animal carries out a complex hand movement such as grasping but astonishingly these same cells also become active when the animal observes someone else making the same movement even though the animal makes no such movement. The acquisition of bird song has been studied in great detail in the zebra finch and necessarily involves the motor system during the learning phase. Even in human speech, Chomsky and Halle described a form of recognition which they termed analysis by synthesis. Here the correct detection of a sound pattern is confirmed by imitation. In these examples, the brain is showing and proving that it has detected a sensory input and checks the correctness of its analysis by producing an imitative movement. Now we ask if the movement is necessary. The nature of the stimulus must also be represented in the premotor system which preceded the movement of mimicry.

Evidence for this is seen in the firing of single cells in the posterior parietal areas when the animal is presented with visual targets on which it will fixate. In a classical sensory system, the target would first be located in a visual space after which the motor system would decide what would be the appropriate movement. What is found in fact is that the cells respond from the beginning in terms of the appropriate movement. Another example is observed in the best studied auditory cortex which is that of bats. The animal locates its prey by analysing return echoes. If this was a classical sensory system, the brain would analyse the echoes in order to locate the target's position when the sound bounced off the target. In fact the cortex also analyses the speed and vectors of target and the outcome is the collision course on where the target will be when the bat gets there. This is analogous to the display in modern aeroplanes on auto-pilot which show not primarily the position of the plane but the course to the chosen destination and at the same time the courses to all the alternate airports in range. The sensory information from the inertial navigation equipment is displayed in terms of appropriate action.

The most dramatic example in man is the unilateral neglect syndrome seen in patients with inferior parietal lobe destruction. If the lesion is on the right side, no visual or auditory or somatic stimuli on the left side are detected or identified. If such patients are asked to draw a clock face, they number correctly the hours 12–6 but fail completely on the left side. On classical theory, these patients have a hole smashed in their sensory map. Recently a new dimension of this large sensory deficit has been observed by a number of groups and has been imaged by PET scanning. If the vestibular system is stimulated by cooling one external ear canal, the patient has a nystagmus and experiences spinning in one direction. While this is going on, the neglect of the left sensory input disappears completely. There are three conclusions: (1) the sensory analysis mechanism had not been destroyed by the lesion; (2) sensory analysis is only possible in a predetermined frame of motor response; and (3) one of the factors determining the location of that sensory frame is the vestibular system. The vestibular system determines the posture of appropriate motor action and evidently of sensory analysis. I propose that these are one and the same mechanism.

What would be the consequences of following the hypothesis that sensory events are analysed in terms of the appropriate potential motor responses? It would provide a more satisfactory explanation of the paradoxes produced by the classical hypothesis and the beginning of understanding of the facts just described. What are the appropriate motor responses to the arrival of injury signals? They attempt to: (1) remove the stimulus; (2) adopt a posture to limit further injury and optimize recovery; and (3) seek safety and relief and cure. The youngest most inexperienced animal may attempt a series of these responses triggered by built-in mechanisms. As the animal grows in experience, the reactions will become more subtle, elaborate and sophisticated. If the sequence is frustrated at any stage, the sensation-posture remain fixed.

Humans develop and elaborate the three-stage response from the moment of birth. Until about 10 years ago, pain in the newborn was neglected and even denied by professionals for two reasons. The first was that the human brain was seen as a hierarchy of levels – the spinal cord, the brainstem and the cortex. This view had been introduced by Hughlings Jackson in the nineteenth century. Each level was believed to dominate and control the level below. The hierarchy of levels was believed to be an evolutionary development and to be repeated in the development of each individual. The ability to feel pain, misery and suffering was assigned as a property unique to the cortex. All reactions to injury in the absence of cortex were called simple reflexes and thought to be mechanical and free of sensation or emotion. This view led Descartes to deny mind to lower creatures and was perpetuated in post-Darwinian neurology which assigned sensation and emotion to recently evolved structures such as the forebrain and cortex. It is true that we have a poorly developed cortex at birth. It takes 2 years for the major motor outflow from the cortex to establish control over the spinal cord. The second line of reasoning by professionals was that because babies could not feel pain, there was no point in giving them potentially dangerous analgesic drugs.

Fortunately, thinking has changed and pain in babies and children has become a major focus of attention. The chapters in this book by Fitzgerald and by Berde demonstrate the progress (see Chs 9 and 42). Turning away from endless inconsequential philosophy on whether a baby feels pain, they and others turned to practical objective measures. The first question was whether a baby who must be operated on soon after birth prospers better if treated with the full battery of analgesics which would be given an adult. The answer was a powerful yes and the result has been a marked change in neonatal anaesthesia and in survival. The second question was to ask if the injuries commonly suffered by babies, especially premature ones, produce a long-term shift of behaviour. Again the answer is yes. Fitzgerald showed that even the act of taking a blood sample without anaesthesia changed the motor behaviour of premature babies. This has focused new studies on long-term effects. Most surprising is a Swedish study confirmed in Canada where a large group of boys who had been circumcised soon after birth were compared with similar boys who were not circumcised. These children were observed 6 months later when they received their standard immunization injections. The circumcised boys struggled, shouted and cried far more than the others. Subtle controls showed that it was indeed the circumcision which had engendered the abnormal reaction to subsequent minor injury. In the child and the adult, there is a continuous development of the way in which the victim moves through the three stages of reaction. Experience teaches skills. Society adds its methods of help and its prohibitions. Expectation becomes tuned.

Finally, we need to re-examine the alternative either that pain signals the presence of a stimulus or that it signals the stage reached in a sequence of possible actions. Obviously the placebo phenomenon represents a profound challenge to these alternatives. The placebo by definition is not active and therefore cannot change the signal produced by the stimulus. It can hardly be categorized as a distraction of attention. Someone who has received placebo treatment for pain does not actively switch attention to some alternate target. On the contrary, they await passively the onset of the beneficial effect of the placebo while continuing the active monitoring of the level of pain. If, however, the sensation of pain is associated with a series of potential actions – remove the stimulus, change posture, seek safety and relief – eventually the appropriate action is to apply therapy. If the person's experience has taught them that a particular action is followed by relief, then they respond if they believe the action has occurred. In this scheme of thinking, the placebo is not a stimulus but an appropriate action. As such the placebo terminates and cancels the sense of pain by fulfilling the expectation that appropriate action has been taken.

WHEN PAIN PERSISTS

THE DISEASE DEVELOPS

In chapters in this book, repeated examples are given where damage to tissue is followed by inflammation. The quality of the pain and what to do about it changes. In postoperative pain, the initial acts of tissue damage were carried out under anaesthesia and the patient wakes up to sense only the later stages where the body attempts repair. In slow-onset diseases such as arthritis, pain escalates as the disease process extends. Pain may grow in sudden jumps as in some cancer pains where the tumour has expanded into new territory and blocks the normal flow of blood or the intestines or urine or nerve impulses. Intermittent pains can grow with each episode. Someone of my age walking up hill may be struck by a chest pain. Stop walking and the pain goes. This is angina of effort where the heart is announcing that it can no longer pump enough blood around in response to the energy demand of walking up hill. As time goes by, the arteries continue to clog and their maximum blood flow drops. As this proceeds, the steepness of the hill which can be climbed drops, the amount of exercise which pain permits drops and rest periods prolong. Eventually, if untreated, the angina forbids even standing up. These are the expected reasons why pain may persist or escalate which it may be possible to attack at source. However, there are a series of quite different changes that accompany pain which we must now examine because they play an important role in pain intensity.

FEAR AND ANXIETY

Anyone who senses an unexpected new pain and does not feel fear is not normal. There is a natural fear of the unknown in all of us and this is coupled with a fear of the consequent future. As part of the innate urge to explore, there is an immediate urge to know what is going on. We fear the cause and its meaning. When a patient goes to the doctor with bad pain and tenderness in the abdomen, the doctor may diagnose appendicitis or cancer or an ulcer or constipation and so on. The patient may laugh with relief if the diagnosis is appendicitis because she has learnt to believe that this is cured with a minor operation. This is a socially educated twentieth-century response since 200 years ago it might have been the worst of all the diagnoses because many patients with this disorder were in rapid decline and dead within days.

Quite obviously the amount of fear and the target of the fear will depend crucially on the person and their experience and their situation. A middle-aged man from a family where all the men died of heart attacks in their fifties and sixties has good reason to blanche with terror at the first twinge of chest pain. There are those with reason to fear cancer who develop an obsessed phobia and become crippled by their inability to accept medical assurance that they do not have cancer. The fear may become the disease.

Fear of consequences can be even more widespread and wild and personally eccentric and therefore hidden to the witnesses. 'Who is going to marry me now' said an Israeli woman officer with the amputated leg. 'What a fool they will think of me to have let this happen' said a machine shop foreman with an accidentally amputated foot. Fears do not often relate to death but very frequently to the manner of the death. Fears relate to jobs, to sports, to sex and to all manner of personal needs. There is a type of macho tough-guy who has 'never had a day's illness in his life' who falls apart at the seams with his first experience of pain and fear which breaks into his accustomed absolute self-control. There is every reason for each person to identify fears of cause or of consequence.

Fear generates anxiety and anxiety focuses the attention. The more attention is locked, the worse the pain. Therefore there is a marked correlation between pain and anxiety. The anxiety may focus on the pain or it may be of the free-floating variety with a feeling of general disquiet that something is wrong that cannot be identified. The anxiety of pain is generated by the unknown and grows worse as the pain persists and short-term expectations of relief fail to be fulfilled.

Therefore a major aim of therapy should be to identify, understand and treat the anxiety. This may need to start immediately after an accident. A type of very distressed patient can be seen in any emergency room who is agitated by the scare of the rough and tumble of what they have just been through although pain is their complaint. Of course, the pain should be treated but they respond best if they also get care to help them calm down. Unfortunately, most chronic pain patients have settled into a rather steady state of fear and anxiety which becomes progressively harder and harder to shift. This by itself is justification for early treatment. A very good example is the effect on postoperative pain produced by a quite brief talk with the anaesthestist before the operation. The aim is to educate the patient with a step-by-step explanation of the stages to be expected. The expectation allows the patient to face the progressive stages of her recovery with familiarity and therefore with less tension and anxiety. This points to the value of education in decreasing anxiety by illuminating the unknown. Well-designed programmes for the relief of chronic pain teach as much as the patient wishes to understand of her own pain problems. It is always surprising to me what a revelation such courses are to the patient who has been carrying a load of magical mumbo-jumbo myths which nourish their anxiety. A crucial example which hinders recovery guided by physiotherapy is the myth that no movement is permitted which increases pain because that movement would increase injury. This myth helps freeze the patient into narrower and narrower ranges of movement. Ignorance is never blessed. Any knowledge which brings the patient into a clearer appreciation of her condition thereby decreases anxiety. For that reason, this book is written. It is true that there is a well-recognized type of patient who sits in front of the doctor and says in effect 'Cure me' with the unspoken coda that they are totally passive and expect curative action to be impressed on them by others. One's heart sinks especially when you recognize that you are the twentieth doctor who has been invited to cure this patient. As I have presented pain as an active process involved with the brain's analysis of appropriate behaviour, I would prefer to see the patient as an active member of the patient's own treatment team. Anxiety has been a traditional subject for psychiatrists and psychologists and it is most encouraging that they are beginning to apply their skills to the specific anxiety component of pain.

FAILURE AND DEPRESSION

If pain persists and treatment fails, it is not surprising that depression sets in. Some patients plod sadly on, convinced that somewhere in the world a therapist exists with the answer. For some, it is a variation of the same answer but administered by a therapist with the right stuff. More than 10 repeated operations on the same painful back are well known in affluent countries. Surgeons are nothing if not high in confidence and not above hinting to the patient that they had been unlucky to encounter incompetent butchers before they reached the right one. Early in his career, the Canadian neurosurgeon Wilder Penfield learned that his sister had a brain tumour and said 'She must be operated on by the best neurosurgeon in the world. Me!' Sometimes these charismatic fireworks are associated with success and sometimes not. The higher the patient scales the ladder of more and more distinguished therapists, the harder the fall. Frustration and anger are added to depression. Depression is a progressive certainty in a miserable future. Attention scans every detail of the pain to confirm that no change for the better has occurred and that it is in fact even worse than suspected. Every small change becomes a catastrophe for some.

This grim picture of anxiety and depression, phobia and fatalism are so commonly seen in chronic pain patients that there are those who claim that these conditions become the primary cause of the pain rather than being secondary to the pain which caused the anxiety and depression in the first instance. Needless to say this view is popular among doctors committed to some therapy which has failed a particular patient. Such doctors believe they have given the appropriate therapy to the patient and if the patient fails to respond it must be the fault of the patient. There are, of course, psychologists of the 'mind over matter' psychosomatic school who are happy to support doctors who claim that the apparent body fault must be produced by faulty thinking because the patient has failed to respond to therapy. One important school of behaviour therapy believes that one can condition the patient out of his pain by ignoring any sign or word associated with pain and by rewarding and encouraging any sign or word associated with non-painful activity. Needless to say, smart patients soon learn what the therapists want and shut up about their pains. They are considered successes.

I have not seen a scrap of convincing evidence that the mood and attitude create the pain. A recent new successful therapy provides clear evidence that the pain drives the attitude. A rare urological disease, 'flank pain with haematuria', is characterized by intense pain, no known pathology and no known therapy. The patients are anxious, depressed, heavy users of narcotics and at their wits end. The treatment consists of flushing the affected kidney under anaesthesia with capsaicin, a specific nerve poison. The patients become pain free and at the same time their anxious depressed personalities return into the normal range. These are not anxious depressed personalities liable to create or exaggerate kidney pain. However, there is no doubt that the pain-produced anxiety, fear, depression and obsession feeds back onto attention and posture and makes pain and living with pain harder to bear. Therefore every effort made to treat these helps the patient. Rehabilitation programmes focusing on education and movement and relief of fear, depression and anxiety do not cure pains but give the patients a freer lifestyle which persists.

COPING

Some fortunate patients can learn to cope with their ongoing pain. Coping is not ignoring. In fact, it is the opposite. These people have learned to live with their pain in a realistic context. The pain persists but no longer demands emergency responses. Pain is not necessarily a catastrophe, signalling impending anihilation. Patients obviously need help to reach this conclusion. It is the beginning of a series of steps which gives a sense of understanding and of a type of control. Berde's chapter on pain in children (see Ch. 42), lists characteristics of young people in prolonged pain of neuropathic origin which is demolishing their lives. They tend to be depressed, anxious, in wheelchairs or on crutches, missing school, stressed, with a distorted body image, with eating disorders and in awful relations with their parents and siblings. This gruesome picture contrasts with children of the same age with a painful disorder with obvious disease, rheumatoid arthritis, who have the example of fellow sufferers and learn to cope. I recommend going to talk with a Second World War amputee who has been in severe pain for 50 years. Give him a chance to talk and he will describe precisely his pain now and the misery of the early days after his injury. Somehow with the help of his comrades, he learned to ignore the fool doctors who dismissed his pain and to weave a life around the pain. He will also tell you that some of those comrades coped by killing themselves with bullets or booze. Coping is clearly a skill which may be learned with help. There is no chance of coping if attention is monopolized by fear, anxiety and depression. There is no chance of coping while passively awaiting death or the invention of a cure. Coping is an active process directed at everything other than the pain itself. It needs inspiration and inspired help to live with pain.

FINALLY

This book is about the many challenges of the many pains.

Inevitably the authors and the readers have repeatedly turned to tackle the urgent practical question of how to control pains. Beyond that question, there are deeper ones and the practical question will not be answered satisfactorily until we understand more of the context in which pain resides. Pain is one facet of the sensory world in which we live. It is inherently ridiculuous to consider pain as an isolated entity although many do exactly that. Our understanding brains steadily combine all available information from the outside world and from within our own bodies and from our personal histories and our genetic histories. The outcomes are decisions of the tactics and strategies which could be appropriate to respond to the situation. We use the word pain as shorthand for one of these groupings of relevant response tactics and strategies.

SECTION 1

BASIC ASPECTS

- Peripheral & Central
- Psychology
- Measurement

Peripheral neural mechanisms of nociception

1

SRINIVASA N. RAJA, RICHARD A. MEYER, MATTHIAS RINGKAMP & JAMES N. CAMPBELL

One of the vital functions of the nervous system is to provide information about the occurrence or threat of injury. The sensation of pain, by its inherent aversive nature, contributes to this function. This chapter considers the peripheral neural apparatus that responds to noxious (injurious or potentially injurious) stimuli and thus provides a signal to alert the organism of potential injury. This apparatus must respond to the multiple energy forms that produce injury (such as heat, mechanical and chemical stimuli) and provide information to the central nervous system (CNS) regarding the location and intensity of noxious stimuli.

First the nociceptive apparatus associated with skin is considered, because skin has been the most extensively studied tissue. Investigators have studied cutaneous sensibility by recording from single nerve fibres in different species, including man. Stimuli are applied to the receptive field (i.e., area of the tissue responsive to the applied stimulus) of single fibres, and the characteristics of the neural response are noted. This analysis is particularly powerful when combined with correlative psychophysical studies, in which identical stimuli are rated by human subjects.

Highly specialized sensory fibres, alone or in concert with other specialized fibres, provide information to the CNS not only about the environment, but also about the state of the organism itself. In the case of the sensory capacity of the skin, cutaneous stimuli may evoke a sense of cooling, warmth or touch. Accordingly, there are sensory fibres that are selectively sensitive to these stimuli. Warm fibres, which are predominately unmyelinated fibres, are exquisitely sensitive to gentle warming of their punctate receptive fields. These fibres have been shown to signal exclusively the quality and intensity of warmth sensation (Konietzny & Hensel 1975, Darian-Smith et al 1979a,b, Johnson et al 1979). Similar types of studies have shown that a subpopulation of the thinly myelinated Aδ fibres respond selectively to gentle cooling stimuli and encode the sense of cooling (Darian-Smith et al 1973). For the sense of touch there are different classes of mechanoreceptive afferent fibres that are exquisitely sensitive to deformations of the skin. These low-threshold mechanoreceptors encode such features as texture and shape.

The remaining class of cutaneous receptors is distinguished by a relatively high threshold to the adequate stimulus, be it heat, mechanical or cooling stimuli. Because these receptors respond preferentially to noxious stimuli, they are termed nociceptors (Sherrington 1906). Nociceptors are subclassified with respect to three criteria:

1. Unmyelinated, C-fibre afferents (conduction velocity < 2 m/s) versus myelinated, A-fibre afferents (conduction velocity > 2 m/s).
2. Modalities of stimulation that evoke a response.
3. Response characteristics.

The properties of cutaneous nociceptors will be considered, and then how their function is thought to relate to the sensation of pain will be reviewed.

Tissue damage results in a cascade of events that leads to enhanced pain to natural stimuli, termed hyperalgesia. A corresponding increase in the responsiveness of nociceptors, called sensitization, occurs. The characteristics of hyperalgesia and its neurophysiological counterpart, sensitization, will be discussed in a later section in this chapter.

PROPERTIES OF NOCICEPTORS IN UNINJURED SKIN

Unlike other types of cutaneous receptors, many nociceptors respond to multiple stimulus modalities, including mechanical, heat, cold and chemical stimuli (Bessou & Perl 1969, Beck & Handwerker 1974, Van Hees & Gybels 1981). Nature might have designed nociceptors such that each had the capacity to respond to the full complement of stimulus energy forms that pose potential risks to the organism (thermal, mechanical and chemical). What nature has adopted instead is a mixed strategy whereby many nociceptors respond to multiple stimulus modalities (polymodal) and others have more specialized response properties. These specialized response properties probably at least in part account for different aspects of nociceptive sensory function (e.g., itch, burning, aching, pricking, prickle). As will be delineated later, nociceptors have distal effector functions as well, and specialization may also play a role here. The end result of this is that nociceptors have a complex biology and heterogeneous properties. Nociceptors thus represent a fertile topic for scientific inquiry.

The receptive field of a nociceptor is often first localized by the use of mechanical stimuli. Various other stimulus modalities are then applied to this receptive field. In most early studies of nociceptors, only heat and mechanical stimuli were used to study the nociceptors. Therefore the nomenclature of CMH and AMH is often used to refer to C-fibre mechano-heat-sensitive nociceptors and A-fibre mechano-heat-sensitive nociceptors, respectively. A later study in primates (Davis et al 1993) has shown that if a fibre responds to heat and mechanical stimuli, the fibre will in most cases respond to chemical stimuli as well. Thus, CMHs and AMHs may also be referred to as *polymodal* nociceptors.

The issue of whether a given nociceptor responds to a particular stimulus modality is perilous because the presumed lack of response to a given modality may in fact represent failure to apply the stimulus with sufficient intensity. The problem with the application of high-intensity stimuli is that the stimulus may alter the properties of the nociceptor in an enduring manner. A selection bias occurs: nociceptors with lower thresholds are more likely to be studied. The easiest way to find a nociceptor for electrophysiological study is to apply squeezing (mechanical) stimuli to the skin and thus identify the receptive field. This selection process identifies what are termed '*mechanically sensitive afferents*' (*MSAs*). In time it has become apparent that selection bias from this approach has led to an oversight of an important class of nociceptors: '*mechanically insensitive afferents*' (*MIAs*). Because these fibres by definition have high mechanical thresholds, finding the mechanical receptive field of these fibres is difficult. An alternative technique described by Meyer et al (1991) has been to apply electrical stimuli to the skin to identify the putative receptive field. With this technique it turns out that about half of the Aδ-fibre nociceptors and 30% of the C-fibre nociceptors are MIAs, whereas MIAs are defined as afferents that have very high mechanical thresholds (> 6 bar = 600 KPa = 60 g/mm^2) or are unresponsive to mechanical stimuli (Handwerker et al 1991b, Meyer et al 1991, Kress et al 1992, Schmidt et al 1995). MIAs have also been reported in knee joint (Schaible & Schmidt 1985), viscera (Häbler et al 1988) and cornea (Tanelian 1991). As will be seen, this MIA–MSA distinction is of significance when distinguishing nociceptors types. From the perspective of nomenclature it should be emphasized that MIAs are not defined as fibres that have no response to mechanical stimuli, but rather as fibres that have a very high threshold (or no sensitivity at all), such that demonstration of a response to mechanical stimuli in electrophysiological studies is difficult.

C-FIBRE MECHANO-HEAT NOCICEPTORS

The C-fibre mechano-heat nociceptor (CMH) is a commonly encountered cutaneous afferent and activity in these fibres of sufficient magnitude is thought to evoke a burning pain sensation. The receptive field size appears to scale with the size of the animal. Typical values for monkey are between 15 and 20 mm^2 (LaMotte & Campbell 1978) and for humans are near 100 mm^2 (Schmidt et al 1997). There are often discrete areas of mechanical sensitivity (hot spots) within the receptive field (Kenins 1988), but in many fibres the areas of mechanical responsiveness tend to fuse over the region of the receptive field. Most CMHs respond to chemical stimuli (though not as well as A-fibre nociceptors; Davis et al 1993) and can therefore be considered polymodal.

Responses to heat stimuli have been studied in considerable detail. The response of a typical CMH to a random sequence of heat stimuli ranging from 41 to 49°C is shown in Figure 1.1. It can be seen that the response increases monotonically with stimulus intensity over this temperature range which encompasses the pain threshold in humans.

Thermal modelling studies combined with electrophysiological analysis have indicated that:

1. The heat threshold of CMHs depends on the temperature at the depth of the receptor and not the rate of temperature increase.
2. The transduction of heat stimuli (conversion of heat energy to action potentials) occurs at different skin depths for different CMHs (Tillman et al 1995b).
3. The suprathreshold responses of CMHs vary directly with the rate of temperature increase (Yarnitsky et al 1992, Tillman et al 1995b).

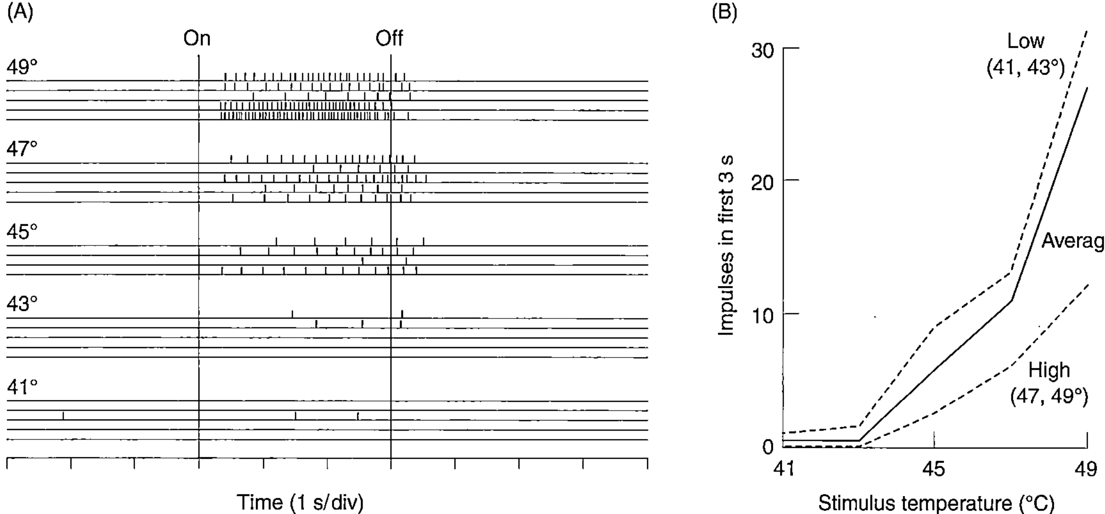

Fig. 1.1 Response of a typical C-fibre nociceptor to heat stimuli. Three-second duration heat stimuli, ranging from 41 to 49°C, were presented at 25-s interstimulus intervals to the glabrous skin of the monkey hand. Each stimulus occurred with equal frequency and was preceded by every other stimulus an equal number of times. Within these constraints, the order of stimulus presentation was randomized. Base temperature was 38°C. **A** Replicas of the response. Each horizontal line corresponds to one trial, and the trials are grouped by stimulus temperature. Each vertical tic corresponds to an action potential. **B** Stimulus–response function for this nociceptor. The solid line represents the total response to a given temperature averaged across all presentations. The dotted lines represent the stimulus–response functions obtained when the preceding temperature was of low (41 and 43°C) or high (47 and 49°C) intensity. (Reproduced from LaMotte & Campbell 1978 with permission.)

The depth of the heat-responsive terminals of CMHs varies quite widely (range from 20 to 570 μm, Tillman et al 1995a). When a stepped temperature stimulus is applied to the skin, the temperature increases at the subsurface levels more slowly because of thermal inertia. The disparity in the surface temperature compared to the temperature at the level of the receptor varies directly with depth and indirectly with time. Given that the depth of CMH terminals varies widely, the true heat thresholds are obtained when the rate of temperature increase is very gradual or when stimulus duration is very long. Although the literature reflects a wide range of heat thresholds for CMHs, when tested with these types of heat stimuli, the heat threshold of the majority of CMHs is between a remarkably narrow range from 39 to 41°C (Tillman et al 1995a).

The response of CMHs is also strongly influenced by the stimulus history. Both fatigue and sensitization are observed. One example of fatigue is the observation that the response to the second of two identical heat stimuli is substantially less than the response to the first stimulus (Fig. 1.2). This fatigue is dependent on the time between stimuli, with full recovery taking more than 10 min (Tillman 1992). A similar reduction in the pain intensity of repeated heat stimuli is observed in human subjects (LaMotte & Campbell 1978). Fatigue is also apparent in Figure 1.1B, where the response to a given stimulus varied inversely with the intensity of the preceding stimulus. The enhanced response, or sensitization, that may occur in CMHs after tissue injury will be described below in the section on hyperalgesia.

Responses to mechanical stimuli will be covered in more detail below. As with heat stimuli, CMHs usually display a slowly adapting response to mechanical stimuli of a given force. As will be noted later, MSA–CMHs have a graded response to punctate stimuli, but their stimulus response functions saturate at levels substantially below the threshold for pain. MIA–C-fibre nociceptors are heterogeneous with regard to responses to chemical and heat stimuli and some respond only to mechanical stimuli (but of course with a very high mechanical threshold). The sensitivity to mechanical stimuli has no obvious correlation to heat threshold (Davis et al 1993).

Low-threshold C-fibre mechanoreceptors which do not respond to heat have been described in the cat (Bessou & Perl 1969) and the rabbit (Shea & Perl 1985b). In primates, including man, these fibres tend to occur in proximal areas of the body and not in the distal extremities (Kumazawa & Perl 1977b, Nordin 1990). The role of these fibres in sensation is unclear.

A-FIBRE NOCICEPTORS

A-fibre nociceptors are thought to evoke pricking pain, sharpness and perhaps aching pain. As a general rule species

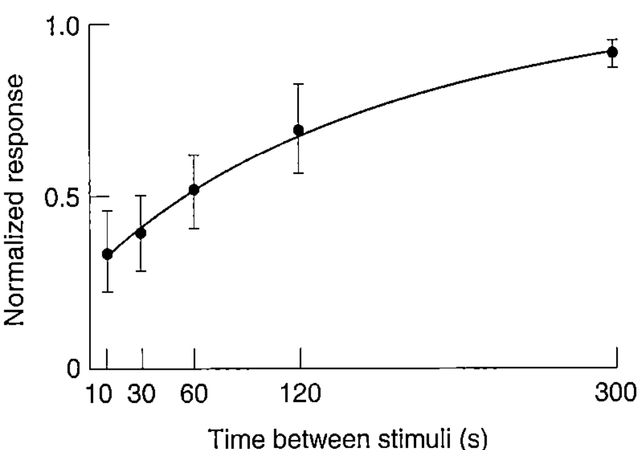

Fig. 1.2 Fatigue of response of C-fibre nociceptors to repeated heat stimuli depends on the time interval between stimuli. The response to the second stimulus is expressed as a fraction of the response to the first stimulus. Fatigue was greatest at the short interstimulus intervals ($n = 13$, mean ± SD). (Adapted from Tillman 1992 with permission.)

of A-fibre nociceptors do what C-fibre nociceptors do, but they do it more robustly. They respond with higher discharge frequencies, and provide more discriminative information to the CNS (e.g., see Fig. 1.8).

One would have to do much 'hair splitting' to distinguish distinct classes of C-fibre nociceptors, but with A-fibre nociceptors two clear types are apparent (Dubner et al 1977, Campbell & Meyer 1986, Treede et al 1998). A summary of their properties is shown in Table 1.1. Type I fibres are typically responsive to heat, mechanical and chemical stimuli and may therefore be referred to as A-fibre mechano-heat nociceptors (AMHs) or polymodal nociceptors. Because with short duration stimuli the heat thresholds are high (typically >53°C), the responsiveness of these fibres to heat has been overlooked in some studies. Consequently, these fibres have been called high-threshold mechanoreceptors (HTMs) by many investigators (Burgess & Perl 1967, Burgess et al 1968, Perl 1968). When heat thresholds are determined with long-duration temperature stimuli, however, the thresholds are in the mid 40–50°C range (Treede et al 1998). Type I AMHs are seen in hairy and glabrous skin (Campbell et al 1979) and have also been described in cat and rabbit (Fitzgerald & Lynn 1977, Roberts & Elardo 1985a). The mean conduction velocity for type I AMHs in monkey is 25 m/s and extends as high as 55 m/s. Thus, by conduction velocity criteria, type I AMHs fall into a category between that of Aδ and Aβ fibres. Nearly all type I AMHs are MSAs. Their receptive field size is similar to that of CMHs, but the presence of 'hot spots' to mechanical stimuli is much more obvious.

Type II A-fibre nociceptors were encountered only infrequently in early studies. This is because the thresholds to mechanical stimuli place the majority of these fibres in the MIA category. Many have no demonstrable response to mechanical stimuli. When an unbiased electrical search stimulus is used however, the prevalence of type I and type II A-fibre nociceptors in hairy skin of the primate is similar. They do not occur on the glabrous skin of hand (where type I AMHs are prevalent). The mean conduction velocity, 15 m/s, is also lower than that of type I AMHs. The responses to heat resemble CMHs. Responses to chemical stimuli resemble that seen with type I A-fibre nociceptors (Davis et al 1993).

Examples of the differing responses of the two types of A-fibre nociceptors to a heat stimulus are shown in Figure 1.3. Type I fibres have a distinctive gradually increasing response to heat. They sensitize to burn and chemical injury and are likely to play a role in the development of hyperalgesia. Type II fibres respond to heat in a similar fashion to CMHs: early peak frequency and a slowly adapting response (Treede et al 1995). As will be noted later,

Table 1.1 Comparison of type I and type II A-fibre nociceptors

Characteristic	*Type I*	*Type II*
Heat threshold to short stimuli	High	Low
Heat threshold to long stimuli	Low	Low
Response to intense heat	Slowly increasing	Adapting
Response latency to intense heat	Long	Short
Time to peak frequency	Late	Early
Mechanical threshold	Most are MSAs	Most are MIAs
Conduction velocity	Aδ and Aβ fibres	Aδ fibres
Sensitization to heat injury	Yes	No
Location	Hairy and glabrous skin	Hairy skin

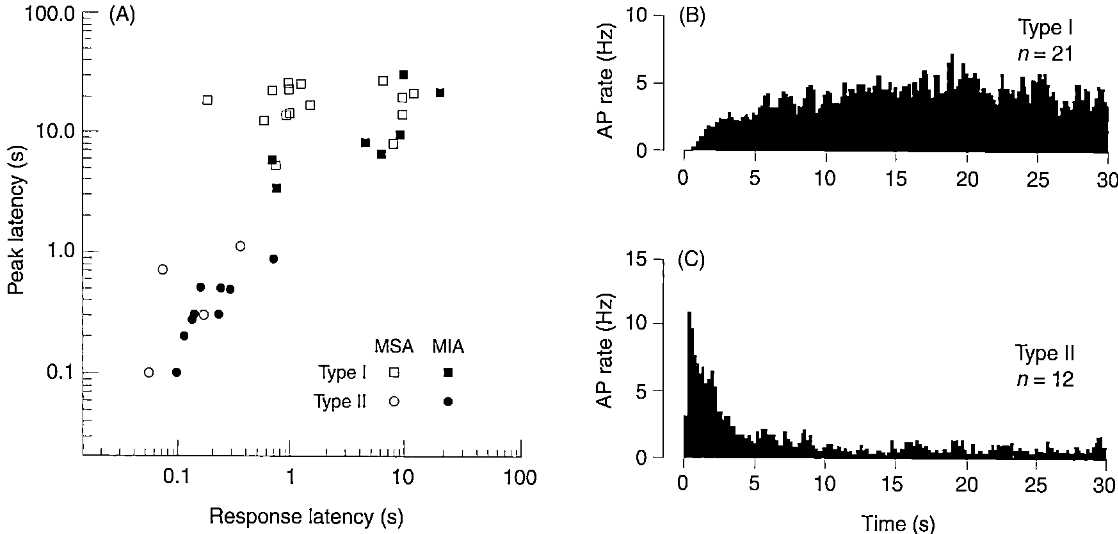

Fig. 1.3 Response of the A-fibre nociceptor population to a 53°C, 30-s heat stimulus. **A** Scatter plot of peak discharge latency versus response latency for mechanically insensitive afferents (MIA: black symbols, n=16) and mechanically sensitive afferents (MSA: open symbols, n=19). Mechanical sensitivity was classified according to previously published operational criteria (Meyer et al 1991). Receptors that had a long peak discharge latency were considered to have a type I heat response (squares). Receptors that had a short response latency and a peak discharge near the stimulus onset were considered to have a type II heat response (circles). The type II heat response was found more frequently in the MIA group ($P \leq 0.05$, χ^2 test). **B** Average peristimulus frequency histogram (obtained with 0.2-s bin width) of the response to the 53°C, 30-s stimulus for A-fibre nociceptors that had a type I heat response (n = 21). **C** Average peristimulus frequency histogram for A-fibre nociceptors that had a type II heat response (n=12). (Reproduced from Treede et al 1998 with permission.)

type II A-fibre nociceptors are thought to signal first pain sensation to heat. Recent evidence suggests that type II fibres may contribute to the pain following the application of capsaicin to the skin (Ringkamp et al 1997).

COUPLING BETWEEN C-FIBRE NOCICEPTORS

The activation of one fibre from action potential activity in another is referred to as coupling. Coupling of action potential activity occurs between C fibres in the normal peripheral nerve of monkey (Meyer et al 1985b). Coupling frequently involves conventional CMHs. The coupling is eliminated by injection of small amounts of local anaesthetic at the receptive field of the CMH, indicating that the site of coupling is near the receptor. Collision studies indicate that the coupling is bidirectional. Sympathetic fibres appear not to be involved in this coupling, as demonstrated by experiments where the sympathetic chain is stimulated or ablated (Meyer & Campbell 1987). The role of coupling is unknown, but it may relate to the flare response or other efferent functions of nociceptors (see below). Coupling between peripheral nerve fibres is also one of the pathological changes associated with nerve injury (Wall & Gutnick 1974, Seltzer & Devor 1979, Blumberg & Jänig 1982, Meyer et al 1985b,c). In this case, coupling occurs at the site of axotomy.

ANATOMICAL STUDIES OF CUTANEOUS NOCICEPTORS

Immunostaining for protein gene product 9.5 (PGP), a carboxy-terminal ubiquitin hydrolase, has proved particularly sensitive in identifying small-diameter afferents in the skin (Hsieh et al 1996). Rich numbers of unmyelinated fibres can be traced far into the epidermal layer (Fig. 1.4). These fibres are likely to be sensory and serve sensations of pain and temperature. The parent axons of these unmyelinated terminals are probably both myelinated and unmyelinated. Some of these fibres contain substance P (SP) or calcitonin gene-related peptide (CGRP) (Gibbins et al 1987). In small-fibre neuropathies where patients have pain and deficits in cutaneous pain sensibility, these axonal terminals stained by PGP are markedly diminished (Holland et al 1998). Vertical sections reveal that epidermal axons emerge from superficial dermal nerve plexuses running beneath the epidermis. Schwann cells encase the axons at the dermal level, but as the axons rise into the epidermis between keratinocytes, the Schwann cell encasements are lost

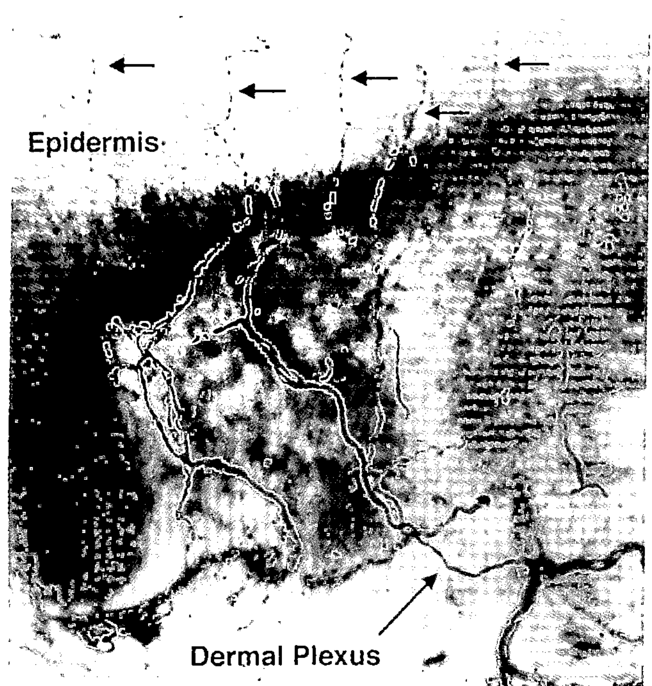

Fig. 1.4 Cutaneous innervation of human back. Arrows indicate epidermal axons which may represent the terminals of nociceptors in this vertical section of skin. The skin was immunocytochemically stained with the antibody against protein gene product 9.5. (Photograph graciously provided by JC McArthur and JW Griffin, Department of Neurology, Johns Hopkins University.)

(Kruger et al 1981). Both clear round and large dense core vesicles are noted at the epidermal penetration site. The vesicles are similar morphologically to vesicles present in other cells involved in hormone and neurotransmitter secretion. It is presumed that these vesicles secrete their contents into the tissues upon activation (see 'Efferent functions of nociceptors' below). Some of these fibres appear to innervate Langerhans cells.

THE RELATIONSHIP OF NOCICEPTOR ACTIVITY TO PAIN SENSATIONS

CMHs SIGNAL PAIN FROM HEAT STIMULI TO GLABROUS SKIN

The evidence that CMHs signal pain will now be examined. In glabrous skin of the hand, two types of fibres, CMHs (not AMHs) and warm fibres, respond to short-duration heat stimuli (≤5 s) at temperatures near the pain threshold in humans (i.e., around 45°C). It is of interest, therefore, to compare how warm fibres and CMHs encode information about noxious heat stimuli. Warm fibres respond vigorously to gentle warming of the skin and are thought to signal the sensation of warmth (Konietzny & Hensel 1975, Darian-Smith et al 1979b). An example of the response of a warm fibre to stimuli in the noxious heat range is shown in Figure 1.5. The response of warm fibres is not monotonic over this temperature range. In the example shown in Figure 1.5, the total evoked response at 49°C was less than that at 45°C. Psychophysical studies carried out in man demonstrate that pain increases monotonically with stimulus intensities between 40 and 50°C (LaMotte & Campbell 1978). Because the responses of CMHs increase monotonically over this temperature range (Fig. 1.1), and the responses of warm fibres do not (Fig. 1.5), it follows that CMHs are likely to signal the sensation of heat pain to the glabrous skin of the hand (LaMotte & Campbell 1978).

Other evidence in support of a role of CMHs in pain sensation includes:

1. Human judgments of pain to stimuli over the range of 41–49°C correlate well with the activity of CMH nociceptors over this range (Fig. 1.6; Meyer & Campbell 1981b).
2. Selective A-fibre ischaemic blocks or C-fibre (local anaesthetic) blocks indicate that C-fibre function is necessary for thermal pain perception near the pain threshold (Sinclair & Hinshaw 1950, Torebjörk & Hallin 1973).
3. Stimulus interaction effects observed in psychophysical experiments (LaMotte & Campbell 1978) are also observed in recordings from CMHs (Figs 1.1, 1.2).
4. The latency to pain sensation on glabrous skin following step temperature changes is long and consistent with input from CMHs (Campbell & LaMotte 1983).
5. In patients with congenital insensitivity to pain, microscopic examination of the peripheral nerves indicates an absence of C fibres (Bischoff 1979).

HUMAN MICRONEUROGRAPHIC RECORDINGS

Microneurography has been used to record from nociceptive afferents in awake humans and allows correlations between the discharge of afferents and the reported sensations of the subject. The technique involves percutaneous insertion of a microelectrode into fascicles of nerves such as the superficial radial nerve at the wrist. These studies have demonstrated that the properties of nociceptors in man and monkey are similar (Ochoa & Torebjörk 1983, Schmidt et al 1997). In some experiments, the microelectrode is also used to stimulate the identified, single nerve fibre in awake human subjects, evoking specific sensations. With stimulation of

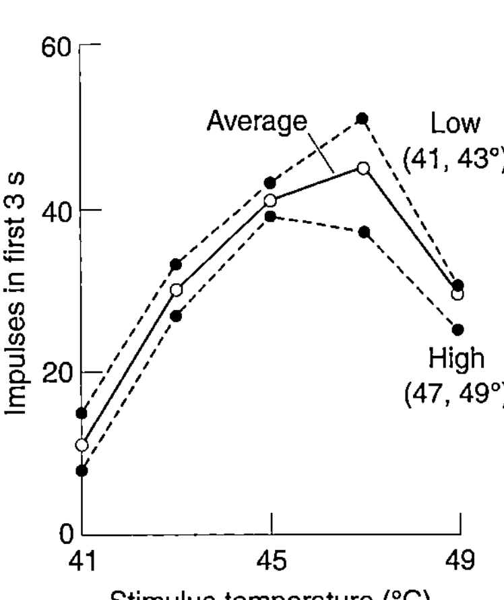

Fig. 1.5 Non-monotonic response of a warm fibre to heat stimuli in the noxious range. The stimulus presentation paradigm is the same as for Figure 1.1. The total response during the 3-s stimulus interval is plotted as a function of stimulus temperature. (Reproduced from LaMotte & Campbell 1978 with permission.)

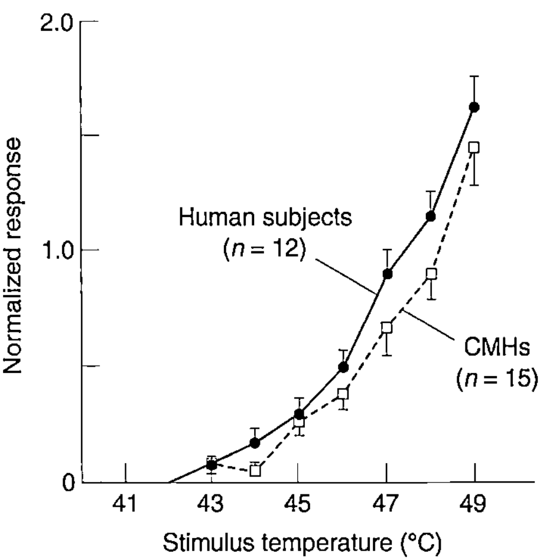

Fig. 1.6 Correlation of response of C-fibre nociceptors in monkey with pain ratings of human subjects. The close match between the curves supports a role of C-fibre nociceptors in heat pain sensation from the glabrous skin. The first stimulus of the heat sequence was always 45°C. The remaining nine stimuli ranged from 41 to 49°C in 1°C increments and were presented in random order. Human judgements of pain were measured with a magnitude-estimation technique: subjects assigned an arbitrary number (the modulus) to the magnitude of pain evoked by the first 45°C stimulus and judged the painfulness of all subsequent stimuli as a ratio of this modulus. The response to a given stimulus was normalized by dividing by the modulus for each human subject or by the average response to the first 45°C stimulus for the CMHs. (Reproduced from Meyer & Campbell 1981 with permission.)

CMHs, subjects report pain (or sometimes itch, see below). Some argue that the size of the stimulating electrode is too large to stimulate individual units (Wall & McMahon 1985). Given this reservation the following evidence from microneurographic studies in humans points to the capacity of activity in CMHs to evoke pain:

1. Intraneural electrical stimulation of presumed single identified CMHs in humans elicits pain (Torebjörk & Ochoa 1980).
2. The heat threshold for activation of CMHs recorded in awake humans is just below the pain threshold (Gybels et al 1979, Van Hees & Gybels 1981).
3. A linear relationship exists between responses of CMHs recorded in awake humans and ratings of pain over the temperature range 39–51°C (Torebjörk et al 1984).

CORRELATIONS BETWEEN PSYCHOPHYSICAL MEASURES OF HEAT PAIN THRESHOLD AND NEUROPHYSIOLOGICAL RESULTS

It is noted above that the heat threshold of CMHs is dependent on the temperature at the level of the receptor and is independent of the rate of temperature change. At the same time when threshold temperature is measured at the surface of the skin, CMHs have a lower threshold when the rate of temperature increase is slow. As discussed above, the reason for this relates to thermal inertia.

Human pain thresholds are sometimes measured as the temperature that corresponds to the first report of pain as skin temperature is increased linearly (Marstock technique). Investigators have noted that faster rates of change in temperature lead to lower estimates of heat pain threshold (Yarnitsky & Ochoa 1990, Tillman et al 1995a). This is the opposite of the situation with the surface temperature threshold of CMHs, but fits with the finding that suprathreshold responses of CMHs vary directly with the rate of temperature increase. Thus it is *unlikely* that the threshold responses of CMHs are responsible for heat pain thresholds. Rather, current evidence indicates that nociceptors must reach a certain discharge frequency (about 0.5 impulses/s) for pain to be perceived (Van Hees 1976, Bromm & Treede 1984, Yarnitsky et al 1992, Tillman et al 1995a).

A-FIBRE NOCICEPTORS AND PAIN

As shown in Figure 1.7, a long-duration heat stimulus applied to the glabrous skin of the hand in human subjects evokes substantial pain for the duration of the stimulus. CMHs have a prominent discharge during the early phase of the stimulus, but this response adapts within seconds to a low level. In contrast, type I AMHs are initially unresponsive, but then discharge vigorously. Therefore, type I AMHs are likely to contribute to the pain during a

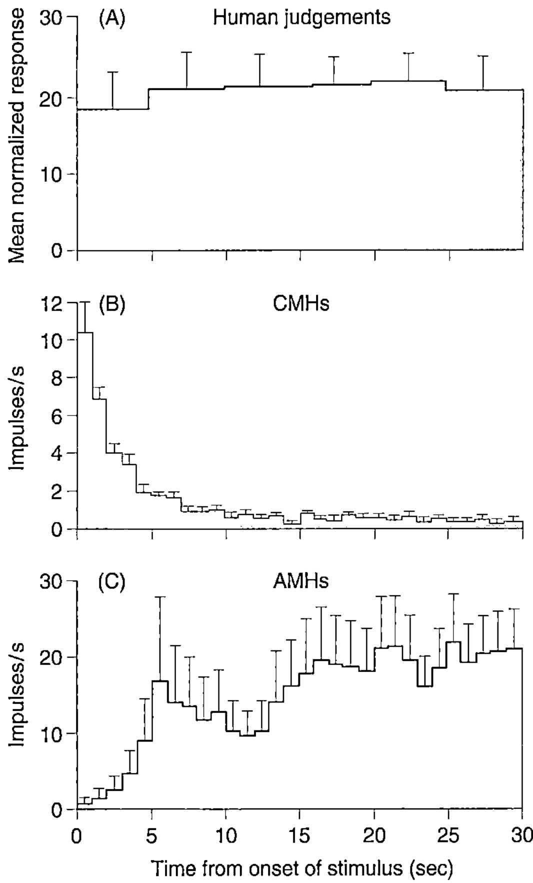

Fig. 1.7 Ratings of pain by human subjects during a long-duration, intense heat stimulus (53°C, 30 s) applied to the glabrous hand are compared with responses of CMHs and Type I AMHs. **A** Pain was intense throughout the stimulus (*n* = 8). **B** The brisk response of the CMHs at the beginning of the stimulus changed to a low rate of discharge after 5 s (*n* = 15). **C** The response of the AMHs increased during the first 5 s and remained high throughout the stimulus (*n* = 14). (Reproduced from Meyer & Campbell 1981a with permission.)

sustained high-intensity heat stimulus (Meyer & Campbell 1981a).

In the hairy skin, stepped heat stimuli evoke a double pain sensation (Lewis & Pochin 1937, Campbell & LaMotte 1983). The first perception is a sharp pricking sensation, and the second sensation is a burning feeling that occurs after a momentary lull during which little if anything is felt. Myelinated afferent fibres must signal the first pain, because the latency of response to first pain is too quick to be carried by slowly conducting C fibres (Campbell & LaMotte 1983). Type II A-fibre nociceptors (Fig. 1.3) are ideally suited to signal this first pain sensation:

1. The thermal threshold is near the threshold temperature for first pain (Dubner et al 1977).
2. The receptor utilization time (time between stimulus onset and receptor activation) is short (Meyer et al 1985c, Treede et al 1998).
3. The burst of activity at the onset of the heat stimulus is consistent with the percept of a momentary pricking sensation.

The absence of a first pain sensation to heat stimuli applied to the glabrous skin of the human hand (Campbell & LaMotte 1983) correlates with the failure to find type II A-fibre nociceptors on the glabrous skin of the hand in monkey.

The preceding discussion indicates that nociceptors may signal pain to heat stimuli. However, two caveats are in order:

1. This does not mean that activity in nociceptors always signals pain. It is clear that low-level discharge rates in nociceptors do not always lead to sensation (e.g., Van Hees & Gybels 1981, Adriaensen et al 1984, Cervero 1993). Central mechanisms for attention quite obviously play a crucial role in whether and how much nociceptor activity leads to the perception of pain.
2. It is probable that receptors other than nociceptors signal pain in certain circumstances. For example, the pain to light touch which occurs after certain nerve injuries or with tissue injury appears to be signalled by activity in low-threshold mechanoreceptors (see below).

NOCICEPTOR RESPONSES TO CONTROLLED MECHANICAL STIMULI

The study of response properties of nociceptors to mechanical stimuli has proved to be more difficult than for heat. Particularly in A-fibre nociceptors, the areas within the receptive field responsive to mechanical stimuli are discrete punctate regions separated by unresponsive regions. Thus slight movement of the stimulus may substantially affect the response properties (Slugg et al 1995). Also more intense mechanical stimuli may indent the skin in an enduring fashion, and thus affect mechanical transmission properties for subsequent stimuli. Nevertheless, some understanding of mechanical response has emerged.

The area of the receptive field that responds to mechanical stimuli has been also found to respond to heat stimuli (Treede et al 1990a). However, the transducer elements that account for mechanosensitivity are likely to be different from those responsible for heat. Analgesia to heat but not mechanical stimuli was observed following the application of capsaicin to the skin of humans (Simone & Ochoa 1991, Davis et al 1995). Similarly, when capsaicin was administered to

C-fibre polymodal nociceptors in the cornea, their response to heat and chemical stimuli was eliminated, but they still responded to mechanical stimuli (Belmonte et al 1991). This suggests that the mechanical and heat transducer mechanisms are different.

Much has been learned about the features of a mechanical stimulus that determine the response of nociceptors to mechanical stimuli. The discharge of nociceptors increases with force and with pressure, but these functions vary depending on probe size (Fig. 1.8; Garell et al 1996). If the intensity of the stimulus is calculated based on force per length of the perimeter, then the discharge as a function of stimulus intensity overlaps regardless of probe size. This suggests that the stress/strain maximum that occurs at the edge of the stimulus is the critical locus of stimulus transmission to the nociceptor terminals.

Nociceptive afferents are often vigorously activated by mechanical stimuli which are reported to be non-painful (Gybels et al 1979, Van Hees & Gybels 1981). In fact, the responses of MSA–CMHs saturate at stimulus intensities that, when applied to human skin, are non-painful. Garell et al (1996) studied populations of feline cutaneous nociceptors to graded force stimuli with probes of different diameter (Fig. 1.8). Four groups of fibres were studied: A-fibre MSAs and MIAs, and C-fibre MSAs and MIAs. Five main ideas emerge from these data:

1. The response increases as a function of stimulus intensity.
2. Small probes evoke more discharge for a given force than large probes.
3. A-fibre MSAs discharge more than C-fibre MSAs and differentially respond to different probe sizes better than the C-fibre MSAs.
4. As expected, MSAs respond more than MIAs.
5. A-fibre MIAs distinguish probe size and stimulus intensity the best.

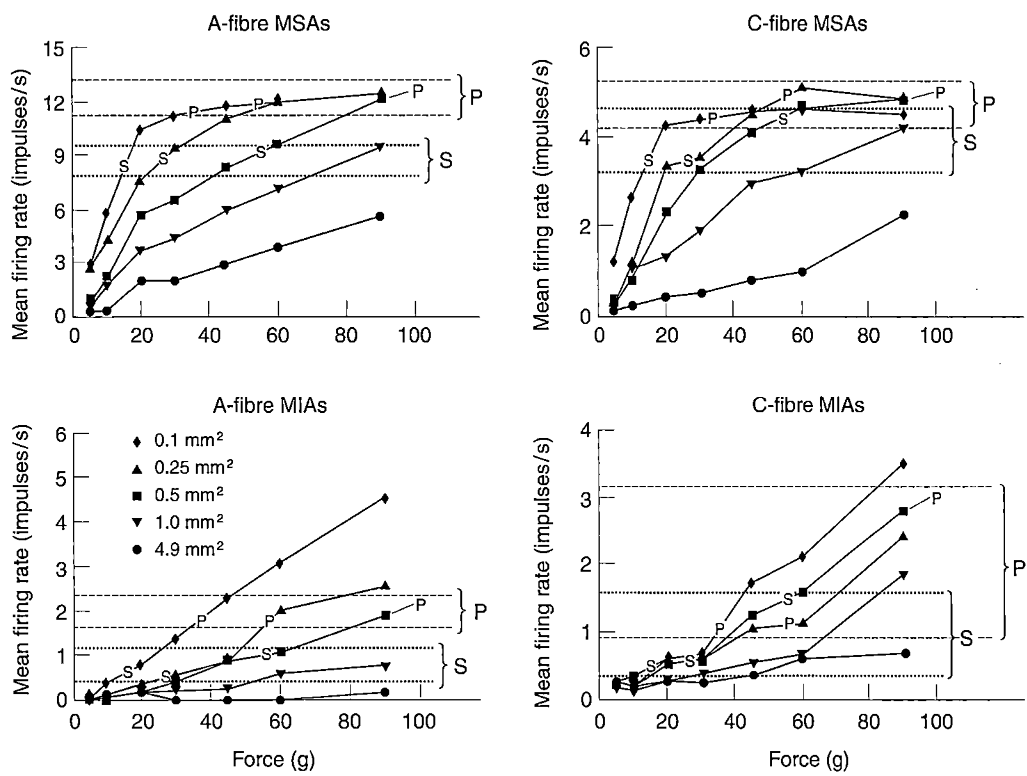

Fig. 1.8 Responses of nociceptors to mechanical stimuli. Average response rates of A-fibre (left) and C-fibre (right) nociceptors are plotted as a function of stimulus strength. Controlled force stimuli were delivered with the use of cylindrical probes with tip areas ranging from 0.1 to 4.9 mm². The response of the mechanically sensitive afferents (MSAs, top panel) tended to saturate at the higher force levels, whereas the response of the mechanically insensitive afferents (MIAs, bottom panel) increased monotonically with force. The range in psychophysical thresholds for sharpness (S) and pain (P) for the three smallest probes are indicated by the horizontal dashed lines. The A-fibre nociceptors show a greater separation in response rates associated with sharpness and pain threshold compared with the C-fibre nociceptors. (Reprinted from Garell et al 1996 with permission.)

The results were correlated with prior psychophysical studies in humans using identical stimuli (Greenspan & McGillis 1994). Garell et al (1996) argue that A-fibre MSAs (which should correspond mainly to type I A-fibre nociceptors in primates) are well suited to signal the sensation of sharpness, whereas the A-fibre MIAs (the majority of which would be classified as type II A-fibre nociceptors in primates) are best suited to signal pain to mechanical stimuli. Other interpretations are possible. Although the MSAs show saturated stimulus-response functions in the pain range when stimuli are applied directly to the 'hot spots', this may not be the case when stimuli are delivered to the area adjacent to the hot spot. Thus as stimulus intensity is increased, input from more MSAs is likely to be recruited. Thus intensity may be encoded through the recruitment (spatial summation) of a larger population of MSAs (Slugg et al 1995). MIAs may discriminate high-intensity mechanical stimuli better than MSAs, but A-fibre MIAs respond much less vigorously than A-fibre MSAs. This paucity of response could detract from the role that MIAs play. Given these arguments, the relative roles of MIAs and MSAs in signalling pain from mechanical stimuli remain unresolved.

A paradox with mechanically induced pain is that a mechanical stimulus that evokes the same level of activity in C-fibre nociceptors as a heat stimulus evokes less pain than the heat stimulus (e.g., Van Hees & Gybels 1981). Again, however, this apparent discrepancy could be a result of spatial summation (i.e., recruitment of more nociceptors). Heat stimuli are applied over a larger area and thus will activate a larger population of nociceptors than mechanical stimuli applied to a punctate area. Even if large-diameter probes were used to deliver mechanical stimuli, the actual relevant stimulus feature is likely to be the edge of the stimulus. Thus, the disparity in pain from mechanical and heat stimuli is likely to be a function of the difference in the number of nociceptors stimulated by each stimulus. Van Hees and Gybels (1981) suggested, alternatively, that coactivation of low-threshold mechanoreceptors with the mechanical, but not the heat, stimuli could result in the suppression of pain through central inhibitory mechanisms.

For long-duration mechanical stimuli, the response of nociceptors to suprathreshold stimuli adapts with time. By contrast, when similar long-duration mechanical stimuli are applied to human subjects, pain increases throughout the stimulus (Adriaensen et al 1984). Reeh et al (1987) postulated that the recruitment of activity in nociceptors that innervate nearby skin might explain the increased pain with time. When a stimulus was applied outside the receptive field of A-fibre nociceptors, the evoked response began several seconds after the stimulus onset and did not adapt. A similar delayed response of C-fibre nociceptors has been demonstrated for long-duration mechanical stimuli which are initially below threshold (White et al 1991).

NOCICEPTORS AND COLD PAIN SENSATION

Just as the sensation of warmth is served by a specific set of primary afferents (predominantly C fibres), the sense of cooling is served by a specific set of primary afferents (viz. cold fibres). Cold fibres are predominantly of the Aδ type. Stimuli that induce cold pain are not encoded well by these cold fibres. Thus there has long been a suspicion that nociceptors must somehow signal cold pain. While the majority of nociceptors have some response to ice stimuli applied to the skin, Simone and Kajander (1997) showed that all A-fibre nociceptors respond to cold stimuli below 0°C. C-fibre nociceptors may play a role in signalling cold pain sensation as well (LaMotte & Thalhammer 1982). Klement and Arndt (1992) demonstrated that cold pain could be evoked by cold stimuli applied within the veins of human subjects. A local anaesthetic applied within the vein, but not in the overlying skin, abolished cold pain sensibility. It is therefore possible that cold pain is served by vascular receptors.

HYPERALGESIA: ROLE OF NOCICEPTORS AND OTHER AFFERENT FIBRES

To understand the peripheral neural mechanisms of pain to noxious stimuli is to understand only one aspect of pain sensibility. There is, in fact, a dynamic plasticity that relates stimulus intensity and sensation. Of great biological importance in this regard is the phenomenon of hyperalgesia. *Hyperalgesia* is defined as a *leftward shift of the stimulus–response function that relates the magnitude of pain to stimulus intensity.* An example of this is seen in Figure 1.9A, which shows human judgements of pain to heat stimuli before and after a burn. It is evident that the threshold for pain is lowered and pain to suprathreshold stimuli is enhanced.

Hyperalgesia is a consistent feature of somatic and visceral tissue injury and inflammation. Pharyngitis is associated with hyperalgesia in the pharyngeal tissues, such that merely swallowing induces pain. Micturition in the presence of a urinary tract infection is painful, again reflecting the presence of hyperalgesia. In arthritis, slight motion of the joint leads to pain. Ironically, with most diseases we think in terms of loss of function, whereas neuropathic conditions

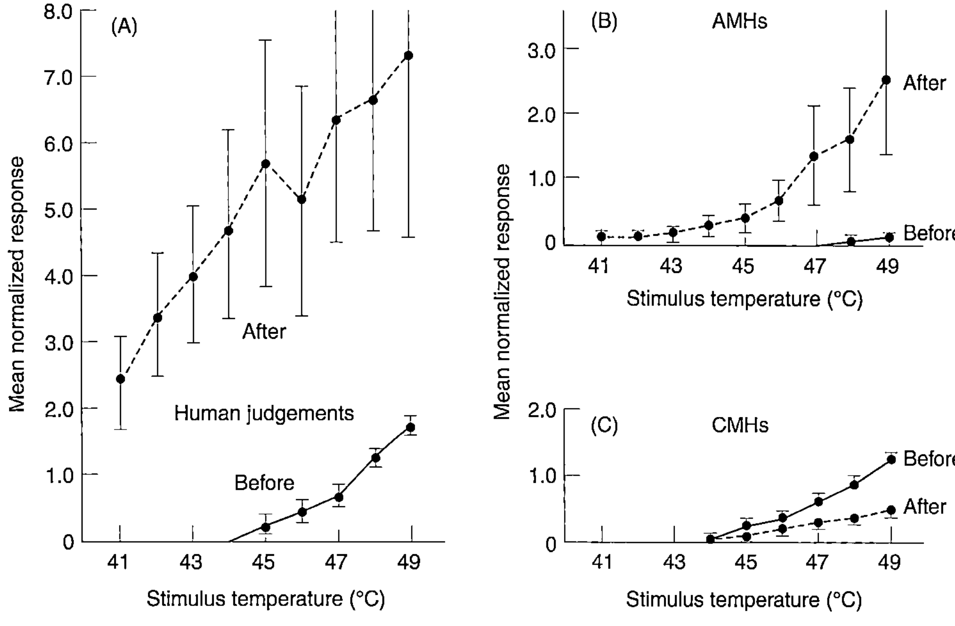

Fig. 1.9 Hyperalgesia and nociceptor sensitization after a cutaneous burn injury. Responses to heat stimuli were obtained 5 min before and 10 min after a 53°C 30-s burn to the glabrous skin of the hand. The burn resulted in increases in the magnitude of pain (hyperalgesia) in human subjects, which were matched by enhanced responses (sensitization) in type I AMHs in monkey. By contrast, CMHs exhibited decreased sensitivity after the burn. **A** Human judgments of pain (n = 8). **B** Responses of A-fibre nociceptive afferents (type I AMHs) in monkeys (n = 14). **C** Responses of C-fibre nociceptive afferents (CMHs) in monkeys (n = 15). The same type of random heat sequence and normalization described in Figure 1.6 was used. Because the AMHs did not respond to the 45°C stimulus before the burn, the AMH data were normalized by dividing by the response to the first 45°C after the burn. (Reproduced from Meyer & Campbell 1981a with permission.)

sometimes lead to enhanced function, i.e., hyperalgesia. Hyperalgesia may be prominent in neuropathic conditions such as postherpetic neuralgia, certain cases of diabetic neuropathy and certain cases of traumatic nerve injury.

The peripheral neural mechanisms of hyperalgesia have been studied in various tissues, including the joint, cornea, testicle, gastrointestinal tract and bladder. Much of the theoretical work on hyperalgesia, however, has evolved from studies of the skin, and it is this work that will receive attention here. Neural mechanisms in other tissues will be discussed in later sections.

Hyperalgesia occurs not only at the site of injury but also in the surrounding uninjured area. Hyperalgesia at the site of injury is termed *primary hyperalgesia*, while hyperalgesia in the uninjured skin surrounding the injury is termed *secondary hyperalgesia* (Lewis 1935, 1942). As we will see, the neural mechanisms for primary and secondary hyperalgesia differ.

In discussing hyperalgesia, it is useful to consider the following variables: (i) energy form of the *injury*; (ii) type of *tissue* involved; (iii) energy form of the *test stimulus*; and (iv) *location of the testing* relative to the area injured. These variables interact in complex ways. For example, it will be shown that nociceptors will sensitize to mechanical stimuli (the energy form of the test stimulus), but only after certain forms of injury (viz., injection of inflammatory mediators).

An experimental design frequently used for the study of the neural mechanisms of hyperalgesia is to characterize the response properties of a given fibre, then apply a manipulation which under usual circumstances would produce hyperalgesia, and finally assess whether this manipulation has altered the response properties of the fibre in question. Cutaneous hyperalgesia has been studied after thermal injuries (burn or freeze lesions) and chemical injuries induced by capsaicin or mustard oil. As shown in Figure 1.10, the relative locations of the injury site, the test site and the receptive field of the sensory neuron being studied dictate whether the experiment provides information about the mechanisms of primary or secondary hyperalgesia (Treede et al 1992). These three variables may interact in any of six ways. As shown in Figure 1.10, when the injury and the test site coincide (Fig. 1.10 A, B), the study has provided a basis by which to consider the mechanism for primary hyperalgesia, whereas when the test site and the

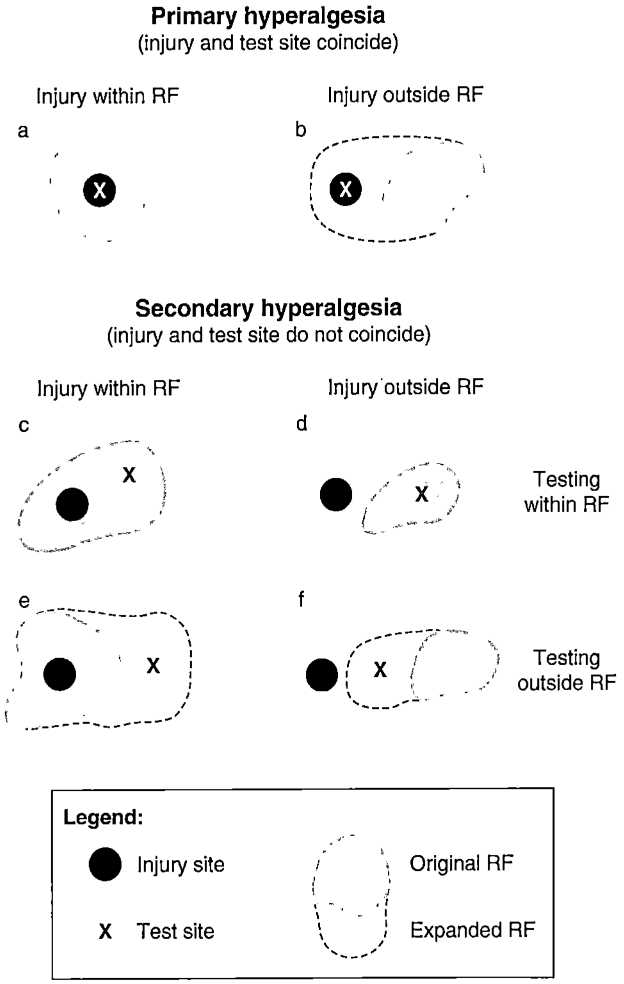

Fig. 1.10 Experimental configurations for testing the neural mechanisms of primary and secondary hyperalgesia. To study primary hyperalgesia, the site of injury (indicated by filled circle) and the site of testing (indicated by the X) must coincide. Alterations of the stimulus–response functions from stimuli applied to the original receptive field (RF) (**a**) or expansion of the receptive field towards the injury site (**b**) are substrates for primary hyperalgesia. To study secondary hyperalgesia, the site of injury and the site of testing must not coincide (**c–d**). A sensitization of the stimulus–response function revealed by testing within the original receptive field may occur following injuries within (**c**) or outside (**d**) the receptive field. An expansion of the receptive field to include a test site outside the original receptive field may occur for injuries within (**e**) or outside (**f**) the receptive field. (Reproduced from Treede et al 1992 with permission.)

injury site diverge (Fig. 1.10C–F), the study has provided a basis by which to account for secondary hyperalgesia.

When the paradigms shown in Figure 1.10A and B are used, it is found that, under certain circumstances, nociceptors have an increased response to the test stimulus. Thus peripheral neural mechanisms are likely to account for at least some aspects of primary hyperalgesia. In contrast, nociceptors do not develop an enhanced response to the test stimulus when the paradigms shown in Figure 1.10C–F are investigated. By default, therefore, the mechanism for secondary hyperalgesia must reside within the CNS.

PRIMARY HYPERALGESIA

Hyperalgesia to heat stimuli

The situation where a burn injury is applied to the skin, where the test stimulus is heat that is applied to the location of the burn injury, is considered first. When a burn is applied to the glabrous skin of the hand, marked hyperalgesia to heat develops as shown in Figure 1.9A (Meyer & Campbell 1981a). The hyperalgesia is manifest as a leftward shift of the stimulus–response function that relates magnitude of pain to stimulus intensity. For example, the 41°C stimulus after injury was as painful as the 49°C stimulus prior to injury.

Peripheral sensitization as a mechanism for primary hyperalgesia to heat stimuli

Substantial evidence favours the concept that the primary hyperalgesia to heat stimuli that develops at the site of a burn injury is mediated by sensitization of nociceptors (Meyer & Campbell 1981b, LaMotte et al 1982). *Sensitization* is defined as a *leftward shift of the stimulus–response function that relates magnitude of the neural response to stimulus intensity.* Sensitization is characterized by a decrease in threshold, an augmented response to suprathreshold stimuli and ongoing spontaneous activity (Bessou & Perl 1969, Beck et al 1974, Beitel & Dubner 1976). These properties correspond to the properties of hyperalgesia (Table 1.2).

To explain the hyperalgesia that occurs with a burn to the glabrous skin of the hand, a correlative analysis of subjective ratings of pain in humans with responses of nociceptors (CMHs and type I AMHs) in anaesthetized monkeys was performed (Meyer & Campbell 1981a). Test heat stimuli were applied to the glabrous skin of the hand before and after a 53°C, 30-s burn. The burn led to prominent

Table 1.2 Comparison of characteristics of hyperalgesia and sensitization

Hyperalgesia (subject response)	*Sensitization (fibre response)*
Decreased pain threshold	Decreased threshold for response
Increased pain to suprathreshold stimuli	Increased response to suprathreshold stimuli
Spontaneous pain	Spontaneous activity

hyperalgesia in the human subjects (Fig. 1.9A). The CMHs showed a decreased response following the burn (Fig. 1.9C), whereas the type I AMHs were markedly sensitized (Fig. 1.9B). Thus, it is likely that, for thermal injuries to the glabrous skin of the hand, AMHs, not CMHs, code for the heat hyperalgesia.

Sensitization is not a uniform property of nociceptors. Tissue type and the nature of the injury are important variables. For example, CMHs that innervate the glabrous skin of the hand do not sensitize to a burn injury, whereas CMHs that innervate hairy skin do (Campbell & Meyer 1983b). Thus, CMHs appear to play a role in accounting for hyperalgesia to heat stimuli on hairy skin (LaMotte et al 1983, Torebjörk et al 1984). These data support the conclusion that the hyperalgesia to heat stimuli that occurs at the site of an injury results from sensitization of primary afferent nociceptors.

Hyperalgesia to mechanical stimuli

In some respects, distinguishing hyperalgesia to mechanical stimuli in the primary and secondary zone may be incorrect. There is evidence that the mechanism for hyperalgesia in the two zones may have some common elements. The mechanisms discussed in this section, however, will be limited to those which may be applicable to the primary zone.

Different forms of mechanical hyperalgesia have been characterized. One form of mechanical hyperalgesia is evident when the skin is gently stroked with a cotton swab and may be called *stroking hyperalgesia*, dynamic hyperalgesia or allodynia. The second form of hyperalgesia is evident when punctuate stimuli, such as von Frey probes, are applied, and accordingly has been termed *punctate hyperalgesia.* Hyperalgesia to tonic stimulation with a blunt probe called *pressure hyperalgesia*, and *impact hyperalgesia* to shooting small bullets against the skin with controlled velocities, have also been described in the primary hyperalgesic zone (Kilo et al 1994). As will be discussed in the section on secondary hyperalgesia, the mechanism for these different forms of mechanical hyperalgesia is likely different. Stroking hyperalgesia is thought to be signalled by low-threshold mechanoreceptors, while punctate hyperalgesia persists during an A-fibre block, suggesting that it is mediated at least in part by C fibres (Kilo et al 1994). Pressure hyperalgesia and impact hyperalgesia are probably mediated by sensitized C fibres. More recently, another form of mechanical hyperalgesia termed 'progressive tactile hypersensitivity', which may contribute to the allodynia associated with inflammation, has been described (Ma & Woolf 1996).

Nociceptor sensitization as a mechanism for mechanical hyperalgesia in the primary zone

It was initially presumed that sensitization of nociceptors accounts for mechanical hyperalgesia, particularly in the area of primary hyperalgesia. However, within the original receptive field, thresholds to mechanical stimulation of either CMHs or AMHs recorded in primates or humans, as measured with von Frey hairs (a punctate stimulus), are not changed by heat and/or mechanical injury (Campbell et al 1979, 1988a, Thalhammer & LaMotte 1982, Schmelz et al 1996). Although threshold is not altered, responses to suprathreshold stimuli may be augmented (Cooper et al 1991, D Andrew & JD Greenspan, personal communication).

Expansion of the receptive field of a nociceptor into an adjacent area of injury is an alternate peripheral mechanism which may account for primary hyperalgesia to mechanical, as well as heat, stimuli. The receptive fields of AMH fibres, as well as some CMH fibres, expand modestly into the area of an adjacent heat (Thalhammer & LaMotte 1982) or mechanical (Reeh et al 1987) injury. As a result of this expansion, heat or mechanical stimuli delivered after the injury will activate a greater number of fibres. This spatial summation would be expected to induce more pain. The physiological basis of this expansion is unknown. Because the mechanical thresholds within the expansion areas are similar to those in the original receptive fields (Thalhammer & LaMotte 1982), this form of sensitization is not likely to account for the significant decrease in threshold associated with stroking hyperalgesia.

Loss of central inhibition as a mechanism of mechanical hyperalgesia in the primary zone

Under usual circumstances, the production of pain from the activation of nociceptors with mechanical stimuli is inhibited in the CNS by the concurrent activation of low-threshold mechanoreceptors (Noordenbos 1959, Van Hees & Gybels 1981, Bini et al 1984). There is evidence that injury decreases the responsiveness of low-threshold mechanoreceptors. A decrease in the responsiveness of low-threshold mechanoreceptors in the cat footpad was observed when the receptive field was heated to noxious temperatures (Beck et al 1974). In addition, slowly adapting, low-threshold mechanoreceptors in the primate have a reduced response to mechanical stimuli after a burn to their receptive field (AA Khan, RA Meyer & JN Campbell, unpublished observations). Hyperalgesia to mechanical stimuli in the primary zone could therefore be due to injury to low-threshold mechanoreceptors, which would lead to a central disinhibition of nociceptor input, and thus result in enhanced pain (viz., hyperalgesia).

Nociceptor sensitization after exposure to chemicals

Inflammatory mediators may sensitize nociceptors to mechanical and/or heat stimuli (Martin et al 1987, Davis et al 1993). Figure 1.11 shows the response of an Aδ-fibre MIA to mechanical stimuli before and after exposure to a mixture of algesic inflammatory mediators (bradykinin, histamine, serotonin and prostaglandin E_1).

Cellular and molecular basis of transduction and sensitization

A number of recent studies using isolated dorsal root ganglion neurons in culture have shed light on the cellular and molecular properties of nociceptors. The small sensory neurons in culture share many of the properties of nociceptive nerve terminals such as expression of neuropeptides (e.g., SP and CGRP), response to bradykinin and capsaicin, and excitation by heat stimuli in the noxious range (for a review see Cesare & McNaughton 1997). An ion current activated specifically by noxious heat has been characterized (Cesare & McNaughton 1996). In addition, nociceptor-specific ATP- and proton-gated channels, and a non-selective cation channel activated by heat and capsaicin (the capsaicin receptor), have been cloned (Bevan & Geppetti 1994, Chen et al 1995, Waldmann et al 1997, Caterina et al 1998). Two distinct mechanisms for the sensitization of nociceptors have been identified. Inflammatory mediators such as prostaglandins modify a voltage-sensitive tetrodotoxin-resistant Na^+ current specific to nociceptors, increase intracellular cAMP levels and the excitability of the sensory neuron (England et al 1996, Gold et al 1996). An additional mechanism specific to the heat-activated current involves activation of protein kinase C by inflammatory mediators such as bradykinin and a resultant sensitization of the response to heat (Cesare & McNaughton 1996; see also Chapter 3).

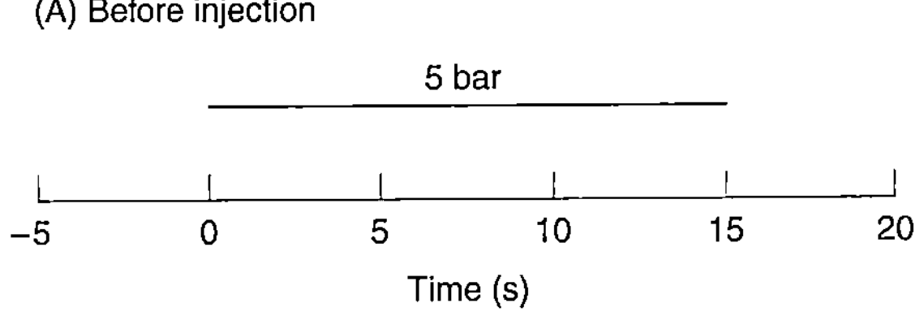

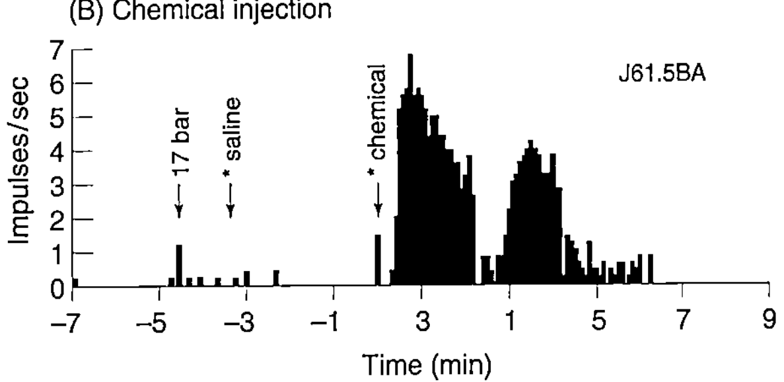

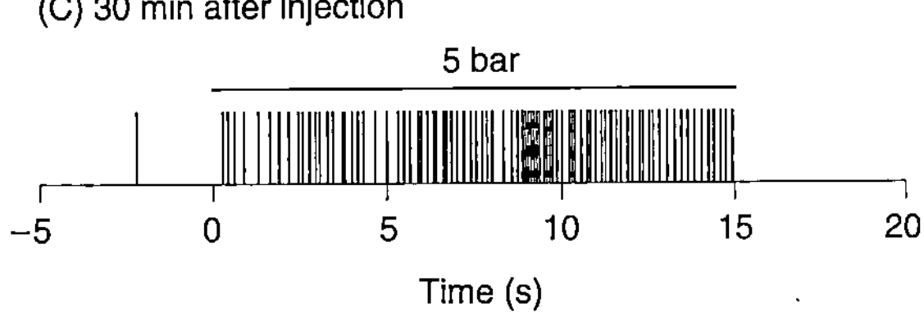

Fig. 1.11 Example of sensitization to mechanical stimuli following a chemical injection for an AS-fibre nociceptor. **A** The fibre did not respond to application of a 5-bar stimulus for 15 s to the most sensitive area within its receptive field. The initial mechanical threshold for this fibre was 10 bar and therefore it was a mechanically insensitive afferent (MIA). **B** This MIA responded vigorously to a 10-µl intradermal injection of a chemical mixture containing 10 nmol bradykinin, 0.3 nmol prostaglandin E_1, 30 nmol serotonin and 30 nmol histamine. (Each asterisk indicates time of needle insertion; bin size = 5 s.) **C** Sensitization to mechanical stimuli was demonstrated in this fibre 30 min after the chemical injection. The fibre now responded to application of the 5-bar stimulus. Each vertical tic corresponds to the time of occurrence of an action potential. The von Frey threshold decreased (from 10 bar to 4 bar) and the receptive field area increased (from 9 mm² to 88 mm²). No response to heat was observed either before or after the injection. (Reproduced from Davis et al 1993 with permission.)

SECONDARY HYPERALGESIA

An understanding of secondary hyperalgesia is important not only in understanding the neural mechanisms of inflammatory pain, but also in understanding many aspects of chronic pain. This section considers the nature of secondary hyperalgesia and its possible peripheral and central mechanisms.

Secondary hyperalgesia to mechanical but not heat stimuli

Primary hyperalgesia is characterized by the presence of enhanced pain to heat *and* mechanical stimuli, whereas secondary hyperalgesia is characterized by enhanced pain to *only* mechanical stimuli (Raja et al 1984, Dahl et al 1993, Ali et al 1996, Warncke et al 1997). In one study that compared the sensory changes which occur in the zones of primary and secondary hyperalgesia (Raja et al 1984), burn injuries were induced in two locations on the glabrous skin of the hand in human subjects (Fig. 1.12A). Within minutes of the injury, lightly touching the skin at the site of the two burns, as well as in a large area surrounding the burns, caused pain. The decrease in the pain threshold to von Frey hairs in the primary (injured) zone was similar to that in the area of secondary hyperalgesia (Fig. 1.12B). Marked

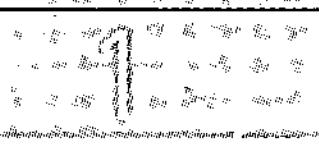

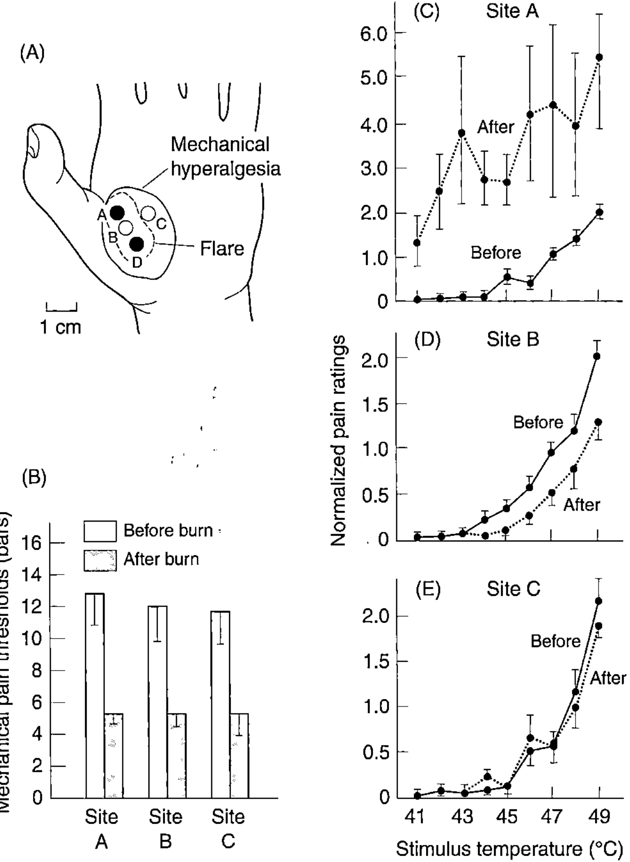

Fig. 1.12 Hyperalgesia to mechanical and heat stimuli develops at the site of injury (zone of primary hyperalgesia), whereas hyperalgesia to mechanical, but not heat, stimuli develops in the uninjured area surrounding an injury (zone of secondary hyperalgesia). **A** Two burns (53°C, 30 s) were applied to the glabrous skin of the hand (sites A and D). Mechanical thresholds for pain and ratings of pain to heat stimuli were recorded before and after the burns at one of the injury sites (site A), in the uninjured skin between the two burns (site B) and at an adjacent site (site C). The areas of flare and mechanical hyperalgesia following the burns in one subject are also shown. In all subjects, the area of mechanical hyperalgesia was larger than the area of flare. Mechanical hyperalgesia was present even after the flare disappeared. **B** Mean mechanical thresholds for pain before and after burns are shown for seven subjects. The mechanical threshold for pain was significantly decreased following the burn. The mechanical hyperalgesia was of similar magnitude at each of the three test spots (A, B, C). **C–E** Mean normalized ratings of painfulness of heat stimuli (same as described in Fig. 1.6) before and after burns are shown. **C** At burn site A, all the characteristics of heat hyperalgesia (i.e. decrease in pain threshold, increase in pain to suprathreshold stimuli and spontaneous pain) were observed after the burns (n = 8). **D** In the uninjured area between the two burns (site B), pain ratings decreased after the burns. Thus, heat *hyp*algesia was observed (n = 9). **E** At site C, pain ratings before and after the burns were not significantly different (n = 8). (Reproduced from Raja et al 1984 with permission.)

hyperalgesia to heat was observed in the area of primary hyperalgesia (site A, the injury site; Fig. 1.12C). In the uninjured region between the two burns, however, the painfulness of the heat stimuli actually decreased (Fig. 1.12D). Notably, the area between the burns was *hyp*algesic to heat, while being *hyper*algesic to mechanical stimuli. At site C, remote from the burn injury, pain ratings to the thermal stimuli before and after the burns were similar (Fig. 1.12E).

Spreading sensitization of nociceptors does not occur

Activation of nociceptors leads to a flare response. This response is neurogenic in the sense that it depends on intact innervation of the skin by nociceptors. The flare response extends well outside the area of initial injury. One explanation of the flare response is that it involves a spreading activation of nociceptors. Activation of one nociceptor leads to release of chemicals that activate neighbouring nociceptors, leading to further release of chemicals and activation of additional nociceptors. Lewis (1942) believed that a similar mechanism, which he termed 'spreading sensitization', accounted for secondary hyperalgesia. Activation and sensitization of one nociceptor leads to spread of this sensitization to another nociceptor, possibly as a result of the effects of a sensitizing substance released from the nociceptor initially activated.

Several lines of evidence indicate that spreading sensitization does not occur:

1. A heat injury to one half of the receptive field of nociceptors does not alter sensitivity of the other half to heat stimuli (Thalhammer & LaMotte 1983).
2. A mechanical injury adjacent to the receptive field of nociceptors fails to alter the responses of CMHs in monkey (Campbell et al 1988a) and rat (Reeh et al 1986).
3. Antidromic stimulation of nociceptive fibres in monkey (Meyer et al 1988) and rat (Reeh et al 1986) does not cause sensitization.
4. Application of mustard oil to one part of the receptive field of C-fibre nociceptors in human does not lead to sensitization of other parts of the receptive field (Schmelz et al 1996).

Other differences exist between flare and secondary hyperalgesia:

1. The zone of secondary hyperalgesia is generally larger than the zone of flare (Raja et al 1984, LaMotte et al 1991, Koltzenburg et al 1992b, Ali et al 1996).
2. Flare can be induced without inducing secondary hyperalgesia (e.g., with histamine), and secondary hyperalgesia can be induced without a flare response (LaMotte et al 1991).

3. Secondary hyperalgesia does not spread beyond the body's midline, whereas the flare response does (LaMotte et al 1991).

Central mechanisms of secondary hyperalgesia

If peripheral sensitization does not account for secondary hyperalgesia, the mechanisms noted in Figure 10C–F should be examined in the CNS. Indeed, it has been relatively easy to demonstrate enhanced responsiveness of the CNS neurons to mechanical stimuli after cutaneous injury (e.g., Simone et al 1991b). Substantial evidence favours this important tenet: *the peripheral signal for pain does not reside exclusively with nociceptors. Under pathological circumstances, other receptor types, which are normally associated with the sensation of touch, acquire the capacity to evoke pain.* This principle applies not only to secondary hyperalgesia, but also to neuropathic pain states in general. This condition arises through augmentation of responsiveness of central pain-signalling neurons to input from low-threshold mechanoreceptors, a phenomenon often termed 'central sensitization'.

Many of the insights acquired about secondary hyperalgesia have been gained from studies with capsaicin, the active ingredient in hot peppers. Investigators have been drawn to the use of capsaicin as the 'injury' stimulus for several reasons:

1. Capsaicin selectively activates nociceptors (Szolcsányi 1990).
2. Capsaicin causes intense pain and a large zone of secondary hyperalgesia when applied topically, or intradermally, to the skin (Simone et al 1989).
3. Injection of capsaicin into the skin does not produce any apparent tissue injury.
4. The characteristics of hyperalgesia resemble those for heat or cut injuries.

Immediately around the injection site, heat and mechanical hyperalgesia are present. Outside this area of primary hyperalgesia is a large zone of secondary hyperalgesia which is characterized by mechanical hyperalgesia but not heat hyperalgesia (Ali et al 1996).

LaMotte and colleagues performed a number of pivotal experiments to determine the relative importance of peripheral and central sensitization in secondary hyperalgesia (LaMotte et al 1991). To test whether peripheral nerve fibres are sensitized, capsaicin was administered under conditions of a proximal nerve block, and the magnitude of hyperalgesia was determined after the effects of the anaesthetic had dissipated. When the relevant nerve is blocked proximal to the capsaicin injection site, the CNS is spared the nociceptive input generated at the time of injection. The peripheral nervous system effects of the capsaicin are not affected, because the nerve block is proximal to the area of capsaicin application. Figure 1.13 shows the results of this experiment in one subject. No hyperalgesia was present after the block had worn off. Thus, when the CNS is spared the input of nociceptors at the time of the acute insult, the

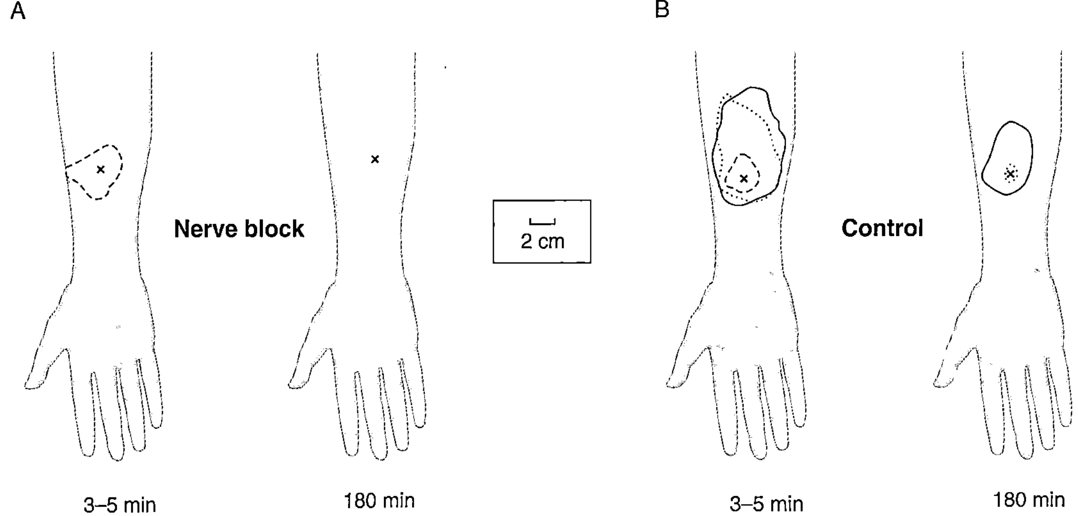

Fig. 1.13 A proximal nerve block prevents the development of secondary hyperalgesia. **A** After blockade of the lateral antebrachial nerve with 1% xylocaine, capsaicin (100 μg in 10 μl) was injected into the anaesthetic skin. A flare (dashed line) developed within 5 min. No hyperalgesia was present 180 min after the capsaicin injection when the local anaesthetic block had recovered. **B** On the control arm, normal flare and hyperalgesia to stroking (dotted line) and punctate (solid line) stimuli developed within 5 min, and hyperalgesia to punctate stimuli was still present 180 min after the capsaicin injection. (Reproduced from LaMotte et al 1991 with permission.)

hyperalgesia does not develop (LaMotte et al 1991, Pedersen et al 1996). In addition, secondary hyperalgesia following the injection of capsaicin within the territory of a given nerve spreads into the territory of an adjacent nerve (Sang et al 1996). Thus, central sensitization, not peripheral sensitization, plays a major role in secondary hyperalgesia.

Different mechanisms for stroking and punctate hyperalgesia

Two distinct forms of mechanical hyperalgesia are observed in the zone of secondary hyperalgesia, punctate hyperalgesia and stroking hyperalgesia. Hyperalgesia to blunt pressure is not observed in the secondary zone (Koltzenburg et al 1992b). First, stroking hyperalgesia (allodynia) is considered. Stroking hyperalgesia appears to be mediated by activity in low-threshold mechanoreceptors. When a pressure cuff was used to selectively block myelinated fibres, the pain to stroking disappeared at a time when touch sensation was lost, but when heat and cold sensation were still present (LaMotte et al 1991, Koltzenburg et al 1992b). This is also true for patients with stroking hyperalgesia from neuropathic pain (Campbell et al 1988b). In another series of experiments, Torebjörk and colleagues performed intraneural microstimulation in awake human subjects (Torebjörk et al 1992). As shown in Figure 1.14, the stimulation of primary afferent fibres normally concerned with tactile sensibility evoked pain when (but not before) secondary hyperalgesia was produced.

Whereas stroking hyperalgesia appears to be mediated by activity in low-threshold mechanoreceptors, several lines of evidence indicate that punctate hyperalgesia has a different neural mechanism and is mediated by activity in nociceptors:

1. The area of punctate hyperalgesia is consistently larger than that of stroking hyperalgesia.
2. Stroking hyperalgesia after capsaicin injection lasts 1–2 h, whereas punctate hyperalgesia lasts more than 12 h (LaMotte et al 1991).
3. Punctate hyperalgesia, not stroking hyperalgesia, developed after intradermal capsaicin injection into the arm of a patient with a severe large-fibre neuropathy (Treede & Cole 1993). This evidence suggests that punctate hyperalgesia is mediated by small-diameter (presumably nociceptive) fibres.
4. The pain produced by touching the skin with different wool fabrics was greatly increased in the region of secondary hyperalgesia (Cervero et al 1993). The pain was proportional to the prickliness of the fabrics. Because nociceptors, and not low-threshold mechanoreceptors, exhibit a differential response to different wool fabrics (Garnsworthy et al 1988), activity in nociceptors is likely to contribute to this form of secondary hyperalgesia to wool fabrics.

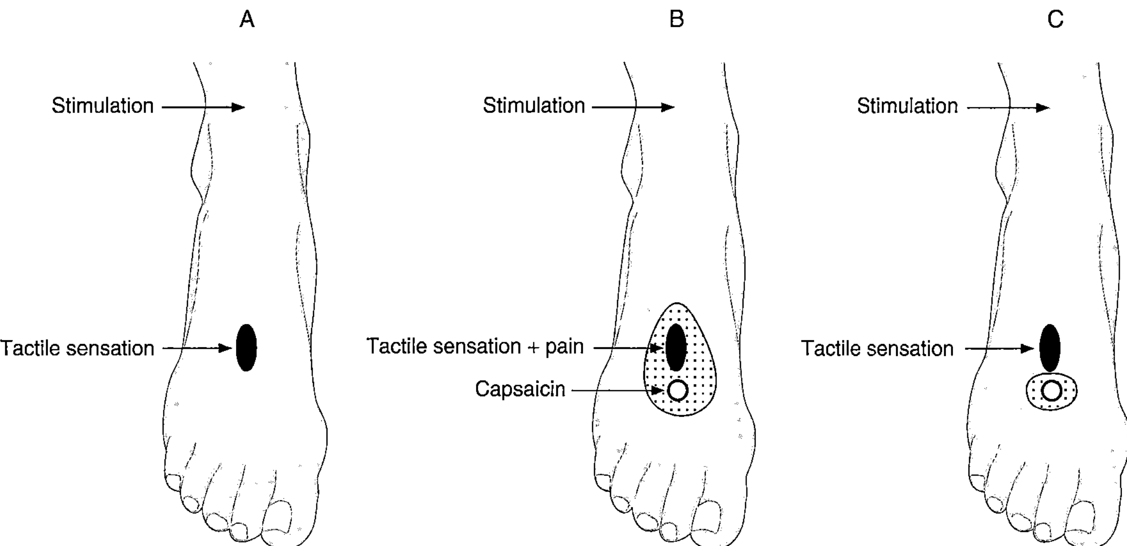

Fig. 1.14 Microneurographic evidence that large-diameter myelinated fibres are involved in the pain observed in the zone of secondary hyperalgesia. **A** Intraneural electrical stimulation of the superficial peroneal nerve at a fixed intensity and frequency evoked a purely tactile (non-painful) sensation projected to a small skin area on the dorsum of the foot (black area). **B** After intradermal injection of capsaicin (100 μg in 10 μl) adjacent to the projected zone (at the site indicated by the open circle), a zone of secondary hyperalgesia developed that overlapped the sensory projection field. Now, intraneural stimulation at the same intensity and frequency as in **A** was perceived as a tactile sensation accompanied by pain. **C** When the zone of secondary hyperalgesia no longer overlapped the sensory projection field, the intraneural stimulation was again perceived as purely tactile, without any pain component. (Reproduced from Torebjörk et al 1992 with permission.)

When the area of primary hyperalgesia is anaesthetized or cooled, stroking hyperalgesia is eliminated, whereas punctate hyperalgesia persists (LaMotte et al 1991, Andersen et al 1995). Therefore, stroking hyperalgesia has continuing dependence on inputs from the sensitized area, whereas punctate hyperalgesia is more enduring and less dependent on continuing discharge from the sensitized area.

Huang et al (1997) recently reported that the pain to a controlled punctate stimulus did not vary significantly across the zone of secondary hyperalgesia but decreased precipitously at the border. This suggests that the sensitization responsible for secondary hyperalgesia is an all-or-nothing phenomenon. In addition, subjects were able to grade the magnitude of pain from stimuli of different intensities (LaMotte et al 1991, Huang et al 1997). Interestingly, the threshold for pain to punctate stimuli decreases in the zone of secondary hyperalgesia (LaMotte et al 1991, Huang et al 1997, Magerl et al 1998), but the threshold for touch detection increases (W Magerl & R-D Treede, personal communication).

Model for stroking hyperalgesia

Secondary hyperalgesia to stroking stimuli appears to be due to a central sensitization such that input from low-threshold mechanoreceptors gains access to the pain system. Cervero and Laird (1996a,b) recently proposed a model for stroking hyperalgesia in which Aβ mechanoreceptors gain access to the nociceptive neurons by means of a presynaptic link (Fig. 1.15). Activation of low-threshold mechanoreceptors from normal skin leads to primary afferent depolarization (PAD) of nociceptive neurons (Fig. 1.15, top). According to their model, the afferent barrage in nociceptors during tissue injury leads to a sensitization of the interneurons associated with PAD. As a consequence, activation of low-threshold mechanoreceptors produces a very intense PAD which is capable of generating spike activity in nociceptive afferents (Fig. 1.15, bottom). This spike activity is propagated antidromically in the form of dorsal root reflexes (e.g., Rees et al 1995, Sluka et al 1995a) and is conducted orthodromically leading to activation of second-order neurons in the pain-signalling pathway. Thus, light touching of the skin becomes painful.

Models for punctate hyperalgesia

Punctate hyperalgesia appears to be mediated by central sensitization to nociceptor input. However, most nociceptors respond to heat stimuli. Why is there not hyperalgesia to heat stimuli in the secondary hyperalgesic zone? Two possible explanations for this apparent paradox are shown in Figure 1.16. One possibility is that this central sensitization involves a mechano-specific channel (Fig. 1.16A). In this model, punctate hyperalgesia is mediated by mechano-specific primary afferent which project, via sensitized mechano-specific interneurons, to central pain signalling neurons (CPSNs). A sensitized interneuron is missing for input from the heat-sensitive C-fibre nociceptors. Support for this mechano-specific hypothesis has come from recent

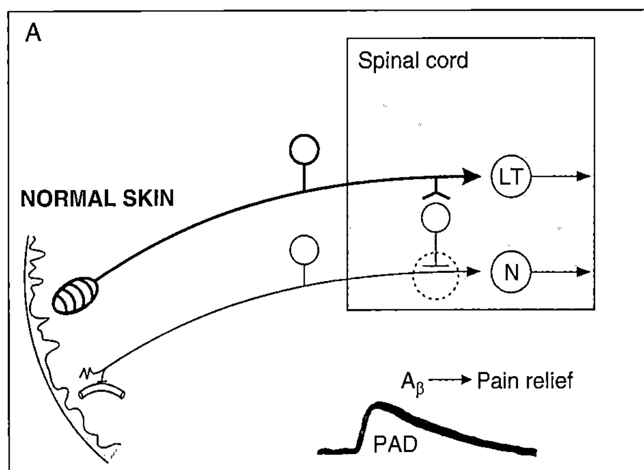

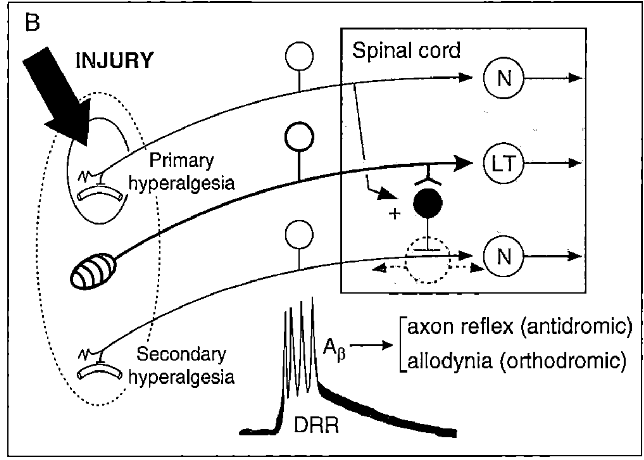

Fig. 1.15. Model to explain touch-evoked pain in the zone of secondary hyperalgesia. **A** In normal skin, stimulation of Aβ low-threshold mechanoreceptors evokes primary afferent depolarization (PAD) in small-diameter nociceptive fibres. **B** Following an injury, the interneurons associated with PAD are sensitized by the nociceptive barrage during the tissue injury (black neuron). Now stimulation of low-threshold mechanoreceptors leads to a PAD that is sufficient to generate action potentials in the nociceptive afferents. These action potentials propagate to second-order nociceptive neurons (N) and account for the pain to light touch. LT = Low threshold neuron, DRR = dorsal root reflex (Reprinted from Cervero & Laird 1996b with permission.)

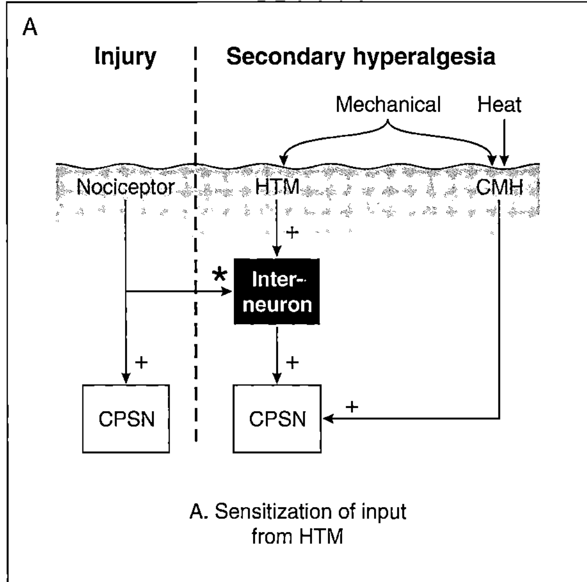

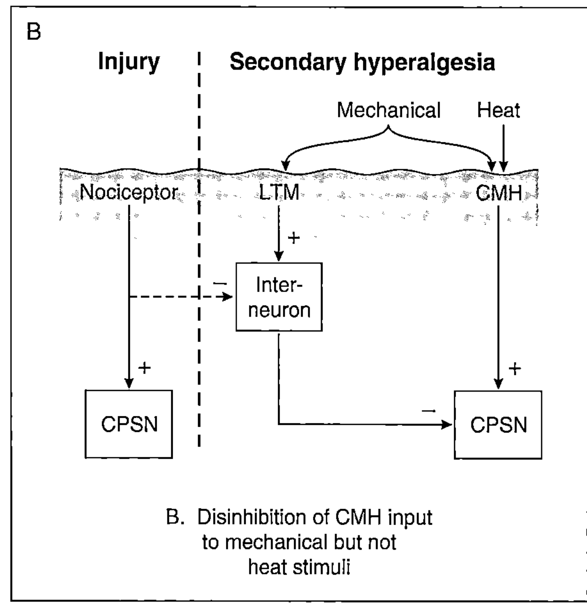

Fig. 1.16 Two possible models to account for the lack of heat hyperalgesia in the zone of secondary hyperalgesic to punctuate stimuli. **A** Sensitization of a mechano-specific sensory channel. An injury or capsaicin injection sensitizes (*) mechano-sensitive dorsal horn interneurons which receive input from afferents that innervate the skin surrounding the injury site. Responses to mechanical stimulation of the skin surrounding the injection site are conveyed to sensitized mechano-sensitive dorsal horn neurons by high-threshold mechanoreceptive nociceptors (HTMs), resulting in a zone of secondary mechanical hyperalgesia. Heat-sensitive primary afferents (CMH) project to non-sensitized central pain signalling neurons (CPSN) so that there is no corresponding zone of heat hyperalgesia. **B** Disinhibition by low-threshold mechanoreceptors. CPSNs receive both excitatory (+) and inhibitory (–) inputs. High-intensity mechanical stimulation coactivates both low-threshold mechanoreceptors (LTMs) and CMHs, while radiant heat activates only CMHs. Activity in LTMs (+) normally activates inhibitory interneurons in the dorsal horn, tempering the effects of mechanical stimulation of CMHs. Injury or capsaicin injection removes the inhibitory influences of the dorsal horn interneurons that innervate the skin surrounding the injection site, resulting in a zone of mechanical hyperalgesia surrounding the injection site. (Adapted from Ali et al 1996a with permission.)

experiments in which secondary hyperalgesia to punctate stimuli was found to be present in skin that had been desensitized to heat by the topical application of capsaicin (Meyer et al 1998). A second possibility is that this central sensitization involves a disinhibition of mechanical input from CMHs (Fig. 1.16B). According to this model, low-threshold mechanoreceptor input normally leads to an inhibition of central neurons associated with pain. The nociceptor barrage associated with the injury leads to a removal of this inhibitory influence.

One well-studied form of central sensitization, termed wind-up, is characterized by a slowly increasing response of central neurons to repeated C-fibre stimulation at rates greater than 0.3 Hz (Mendell & Wall 1965, Price 1972, Cervero et al 1984). The perceptual correlate of wind-up is temporal summation (Price et al 1977). The finding that temporal summation does not change in the zone of secondary hyperalgesia argues against wind-up as a mechanism for secondary hyperalgesia (Woolf 1996, Magerl et al 1998, Pedersen et al 1998).

NOCICEPTORS AND THE SYMPATHETIC NERVOUS SYSTEM

Activity in nociceptors induces an increase in sympathetic discharge. Under usual circumstances, the converse is not true: sympathetic activity does not impact on the discharge of nociceptive neurons. In certain patients with pain, however, nociceptors appear to be under the influence of the sympathetic nervous system. Pain dependent on activity in the sympathetic nervous system is referred to as sympathetically maintained pain (SMP).

SMP can be manifest in a variety of situations. For example, pain that arises in a subset of patients with chronic arthritis, acute herpes zoster, soft-tissue trauma, metabolic neuropathies, complex regional pain syndromes (reflex sympathetic dystrophy and causalgia), as well as other conditions, may be based on activity in the sympathetic nervous system (for reviews see Jänig et al 1996, Jänig & Stanton-Hicks 1996).

ROLE OF THE SYMPATHETIC NERVOUS SYSTEM IN INFLAMMATION

Nociceptors normally do not respond to sympathetic stimulation (Shea & Perl 1985a; Roberts & Elardo 1985a,b, Barasi & Lynn 1986). In addition, sympathectomy and depletion of catecholamine stores with reserpine have no effect on acute inflammation (Lam & Ferrell 1991, Sluka et al 1994b). In contrast, sympathectomy reduces the severity of injury in chronic adjuvant-induced arthritis (Levine et al 1986a). Inflammation may lead to catechol sensitization of cutaneous nociceptors (Hu & Zhu 1989; see also Chapter 2). Sympathetic stimulation and close arterial injection of norepinephrine also excite 35–40% of C-polymodal nociceptors in chronically inflamed rats (Sato et al 1993a). This adrenergic activation of nociceptors was blocked by α_2, but not α_1, adrenergic antagonists. Sympathetic efferent fibres are also considered to play a role in neurogenic inflammation (Levine et al 1988).

In human skin sensitized by the topical application of capsaicin, hyperalgesia persists longer at sites where exogenous norepinephrine was administered, and this α-adrenoceptor-mediated effect was independent of the vasoconstrictor response (Drummond 1995, 1996). Additionally, the local administration of an α-adrenergic antagonist reduced the spontaneous pain and hyperalgesia resulting from the intradermal injection of capsaicin (Liu et al 1996, Kinnman et al 1997). These observations suggest that sympathetic efferent activity might increase the pain associated with cutaneous injury and inflammation.

ROLE OF THE SYMPATHETIC NERVOUS SYSTEM IN NEUROPATHIC PAIN

Clinical studies support the concept that nociceptors may develop catechol sensitivity after partial nerve injury. For example, intraoperative stimulation of the sympathetic chain induces pain in patients with causalgia (Walker & Nulson 1948, White & Sweet 1969). The injection of noradrenaline around stump neuromas or skin in patients with postherpetic neuralgia induces an increase in spontaneous pain (Chabal et al 1992, Choi & Rowbotham 1997, Raja et al 1998). In SMP, anaesthetic blockade of the sympathetic nervous system relieves pain and hyperalgesia; intradermal injection of noradrenaline into the previously hyperalgesic area induces pain (Wallin et al 1976, Davis et al 1991). Noradrenaline injected into normal subjects evokes no pain. This suggests that SMP does not arise from too much adrenaline but rather from the presence of adrenergic receptors in the skin that are coupled to nociceptors. Therefore, in SMP, noradrenaline that normally is released from the sympathetic terminals acquires the capacity to evoke pain.

This production of pain is mediated through activation of α receptors. Phentolamine, an α-adrenergic antagonist, relieves pain when given to patients with SMP (Arner 1991, Raja et al 1991). Clonidine, an α_2-adrenergic agonist, also relieves pain when applied topically in patients with SMP (Davis et al 1991). The activation of α_2-adrenergic receptors, located on sympathetic terminals, blocks norepinephrine release. Thus, clonidine appears to relieve pain by blocking norepinephrine release. When phenylephrine, a selective α_1-adrenergic agonist, was applied to the clonidine-treated area, pain was rekindled in patients with SMP (Davis et al 1991). Thus, clinical data suggests that the α_1-adrenergic receptor plays a pivotal role in SMP. This leads to the hypothesis that nociceptors develop sensitivity to norepinephrine through the expression of α_1 receptors. This may involve a phenotypic change in nociceptors, such that nociceptors acquire an abnormal sensitivity to norepinephrine. Alternatively, an increase in the density of α_1 adrenoceptors may also contribute to the mechanism of SMP, or receptors normally present but inactive may be rendered functional as a result of injury. Quantitative autoradiographic studies indicate that the density of α_1 adrenoceptors in the epidermis of hyperalgesic skin of patients with reflex sympathetic dystrophy is increased compared to pain-free skin and normal controls (Drummond et al 1996).

Certain nerve lesions in animals produce a state that resembles neuropathic pain in man and is reported to be eliminated by a sympathectomy (Kim & Chung 1991, Neil et al 1991, Shir & Seltzer 1991, Kinnman & Levine 1995). The sympathetic dependence of the pain behaviour, however, appears to be influenced by the species of the animal (Chung et al 1997). After axotomy, interactions between somatic afferent fibres and sympathetic efferent fibres may develop at multiple sites. One such site is the neuroma that develops at the site of nerve injury. Some fibres that innervate the resulting neuroma respond to local catechol application and to sympathetic stimulation (Wall & Gutnick 1974, Devor & Jänig 1981, Scadding 1981, Häbler et al 1987; see also Chapter 5). Another potential site of interaction between the sensory and sympathetic systems is at the periphery distal to the site of the nerve lesion. After partial nerve section, many of the remaining intact nociceptive fibres develop sensitivity to sympathetic stimulation (Sato & Perl 1991). Notably, these effects are antagonized by the α_2 antagonists, yohimbine and rauwolscine. Recent in vitro studies in skin from primates with a spinal nerve injury indicate that the uninjured cutaneous afferents develop sensitivity to α_1- and α_2-adrenergic agonists (Ali et al 1999). These observations are in agreement with the above clinical observations that the sympathetic-adrenergic interactions are mediated via an α receptor. Another possible site of interaction between the sympathetic fibres and the somatosensory system may be within the dorsal root ganglia (Devor et al 1994, Chen et al 1996, Michaelis et al 1996, Petersen et al 1996). Further work will be necessary to determine the mechanism for catechol sensitization and to determine the receptor subtype responsible for this interaction.

In contrast to the direct coupling mechanisms discussed above, other investigators believe that the coupling between sympathetic efferent and primary afferent fibres is indirect, mediated by non-adrenergic chemicals released by sympathetic postganglionic terminals (Tracey et al 1995, Levine et al 1986b). However, recent studies suggest that injured afferents can maintain their adrenosensitivity despite the absence of sympathetic postganglionic endings (Rubin et al 1997).

One model that explains SMP is shown in Figure 1.17. In SMP, nociceptors are thought to develop an α-adrenergic sensitivity, probably as the result of the expression of α-adrenergic receptors on their terminals. In this pathological situation, sympathetic efferent activity leads to low-grade ongoing activity in the nociceptors. This ongoing activity in the nociceptors maintains the central pain-signalling neurons in a sensitized state so that input from low-threshold mechanoreceptors and cold receptors produces mechanical and cold allodynia (Koltzenburg 1996). The continuing nociceptor activity probably also contributes to the continuing pain perceived by the patients.

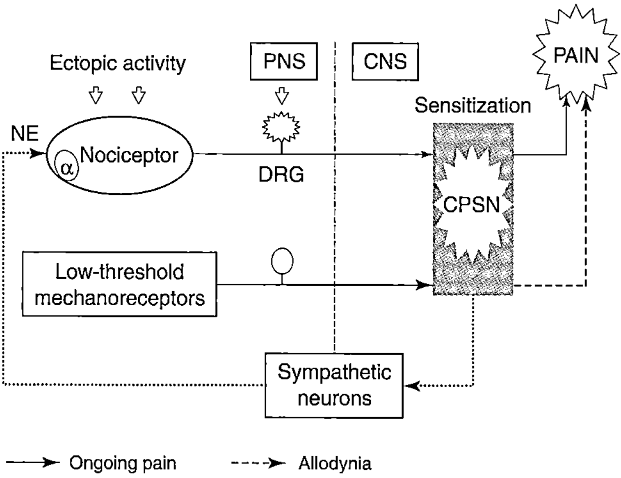

Fig. 1.17 Model to explain the hyperalgesia that develops in sympathetically maintained pain (SMP). In SMP, nociceptors develop α-adrenergic sensitivity, such that the release of noradrenaline by the sympathetic nervous system produces spontaneous activity in the nociceptors. This spontaneous activity maintains the CNS in a sensitized state. Pain to light touch (allodynia) is signalled by activity in low-threshold mechanoreceptors in the presence of a sensitized central pain-signalling neuron (CPSN). Nerve injury or inflammation can also lead to the development of ectopic activity in primary afferent fibres as well as in the neurons in the dorsal root ganglia (DRG). CNS= central nervous system; PNS = peripheral nervous system.

Therapeutic measures that are aimed at eliminating the continuing activity in the nociceptors should lead to relief of the continuing pain and the pain to light touch. For SMP, procedures that reduce or eliminate the excitation of the α receptors will be successful. An anaesthetic block of the sympathetic ganglia is effective because it eliminates the efferent drive. Topical application of clonidine is effective because it activates the α_2 autoreceptor which reduces the release of noradrenaline from the sympathetic terminals. Systemic phentolamine, phenoxybenzamine and prazosin are α-adrenergic receptor antagonists and therefore block the activation of the nociceptors. Intravenous regional guanethidine eliminates the norepinephrine stores in the sympathetic terminals.

CHEMICAL SENSITIVITY OF NOCICEPTORS

Injury results in the local release of numerous chemicals which mediate or facilitate the inflammatory process, including bradykinin, prostaglandins, leukotrienes, serotonin, histamine, substance P, thromboxanes, platelet activating factor, protons and free radicals. Cytokines, such as interleukins and tumour necrosis factor, and neurotrophins, especially nerve growth factor (NGF), are also generated during inflammation. Recent evidence suggests that NGF is not only necessary for the survival of nociceptors during development, but also plays an important role during inflammatory processes in adult animals (for review see: McMahon et al 1997; Chapter 4). Some of these agents can directly activate nociceptors, while others act indirectly via inflammatory cells, which in turn release algogenic agents. Other mediators lead to a sensitization of the nociceptor response to natural stimuli and therefore play a role in primary hyperalgesia. The variety of chemical mediators released during inflammation can have a synergistic effect in potentiating nociceptor responses.

A variety of receptors, including purinergic and glutaminergic receptors, have been identified on dorsal root ganglion cells and on peripheral terminals of nociceptive afferent fibres (Fig. 1.18). However, for some of these receptors it is questionable if binding of the specific ligand

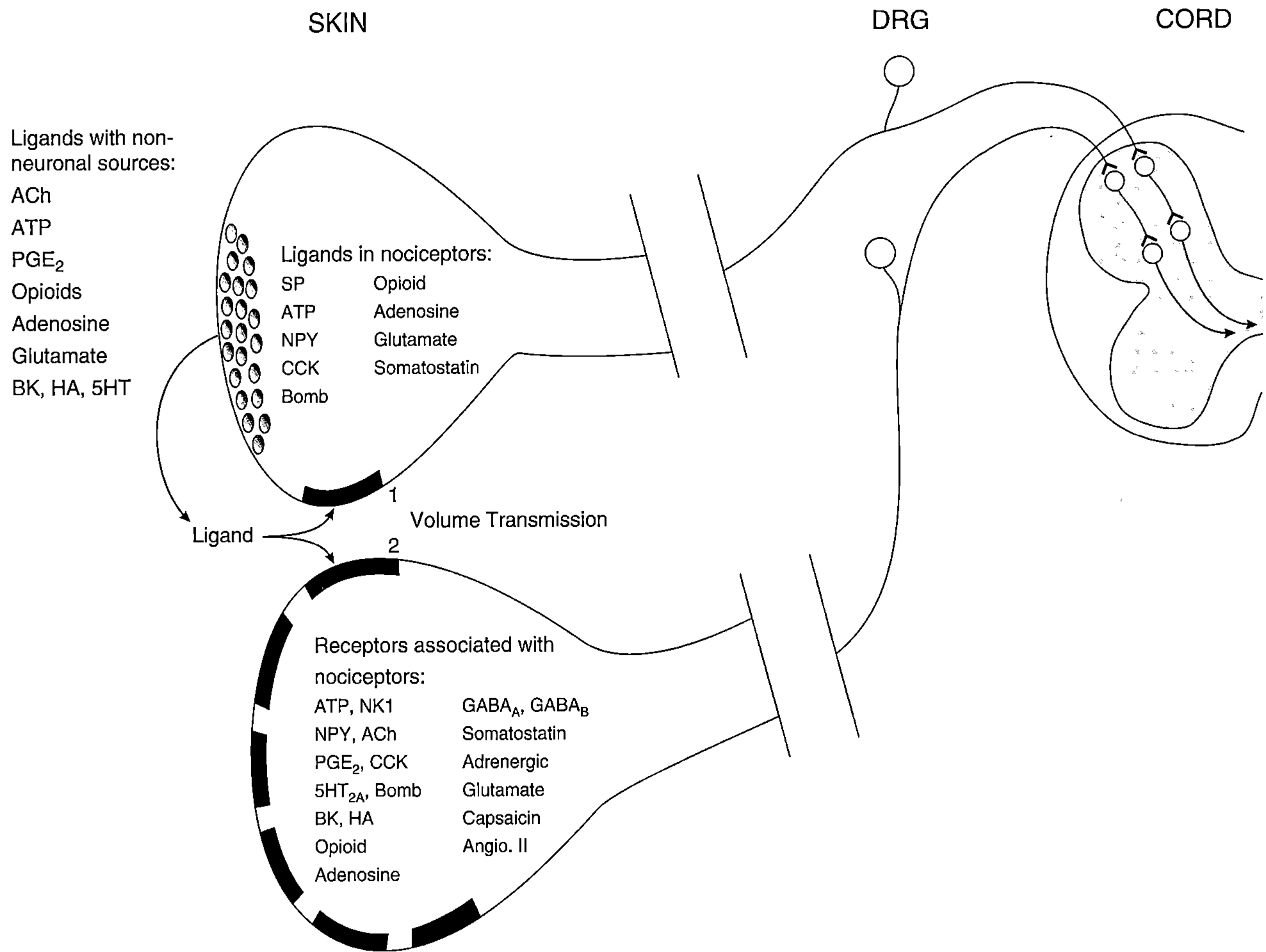

Fig. 1.18 Schematic summary of ligands and receptors present on peripheral terminals of nociceptive afferent nerve fibres. Cutaneous peripheral terminals are disproportionately enlarged for clarity. Dorsal root ganglion (DRG) and spinal cord (CORD) are depicted at the right side. Evidence for the presence of ligands/receptors on peripheral terminals is from anatomical, electrophysiological and pharmacological studies. Ligands can be classified by their origin as (a) ligands from a non-neuronal source (e.g., skin, vessels, inflammatory cells) and (b) those that can be released from peripheral nerve terminals (upper terminal). Receptors on nerve terminals are shown in the lower terminal. Receptors on peripheral nerve terminals can be activated by ligands from non-neuronal sources or by those released from a neighbouring fibre in an autocrine (1) or paracrine (2) fashion. ACh= acetylcholine; ATP= adenosine triphosphate; Angio. II= angiotensin II; Bomb= bombesin; BK= bradykinin; CCK= cholecystokinin; HA= histamine; NK1= neurokinin 1; NPY= neuropeptide Y; PGE= prostaglandin E; 5HT= serotonin; SP= substance P. (Reproduced from Carlton & Coggeshall 1998 with permission.)

results in excitation of nociceptive fibres (Vyklický & Knotková-Urbancová 1996, Reeh & Kress 1998). Alternatively, activation of these receptors may modulate the sensitivity of the peripheral nociceptors to exogenous stimuli (Carlton & Coggeshall 1998).

BRADYKININ

Bradykinin is released upon tissue injury (e.g., from plasma) and is present in inflammatory exudates (Rocha e Silva & Rosenthal 1961, Melmon et al 1967, DiRosa et al 1971). Bradykinin has been shown to produce pain in man when given intradermally, intra-arterially, intravenously or intraperitoneally (Cormia & Dougherty 1960, Guzman et al 1962, Coffman 1966, Lim et al 1967, Ferreira et al 1971, Ferreira 1983, Manning et al 1991, Kindgen-Milles et al 1994).

The administration of bradykinin in the region of the receptive field of unmyelinated and myelinated nociceptors results in an evoked response in the fibres (Beck & Handwerker 1974, Handwerker 1976a,b, Lang et al 1990, Mizumura et al 1990, Khan et al 1992). A pronounced tachyphylaxis of the evoked response is observed following repeated presentations of bradykinin. Bradykinin administration leads to a transient sensitization of the response of nociceptors to heat stimuli (Kumazawa et al 1991, Khan et al 1992, Koltzenburg et al 1992a) which correlates with the transient hyperalgesia to heat observed in humans (Manning et al 1991). In contrast to its effect on evoked response, bradykinin-induced sensitization (Reeh & Sauer 1997) and hyperalgesia to heat do not undergo tachyphylaxis (Manning et al 1991). Sensitization and excitation appear to be predominantly mediated via the B2 receptor, although in some fibres a B1 receptor-mediated effect has been observed (Reeh & Sauer 1997). Responses to bradykinin can be enhanced by a strong heat stimulus (Mizumura et al 1992).

PROTONS

The low pH levels found in inflamed tissues have led to the hypothesis that local acidosis may contribute to the pain and hyperalgesia associated with inflammation. Continuous administration of low pH solutions in humans causes pain and hyperalgesia to mechanical stimuli (Steen & Reeh 1993). This correlates with the observation that protons selectively activate nociceptors (Fig. 1.19) and produce a sensitization of nociceptors to mechanical stimuli (Steen et al 1992). The excitation of nociceptors by protons does not undergo tachyphylaxis or adaptation (Steen et al 1992, 1995b), and a synergistic excitatory effect of protons and a combination of inflammatory mediators has been reported (Steen et al 1995a, 1996).

SEROTONIN

Mast cells, upon degranulation, release platelet activating factor, which in turn leads to serotonin release from platelets. Serotonin causes pain when applied to a human blister base (Richardson & Engel 1986) and can activate nociceptors (Fock & Mense 1976, Lang et al 1990). Serotonin can also potentiate the pain induced by bradykinin (Sicuteri et al 1965, Fock & Mense 1976, Richardson & Engel 1986) and enhance the response of nociceptors to bradykinin (Fjallbrant & Iggo 1961, Hiss & Mense 1976, Nakano & Taira 1976, Mense 1981, Lang et al 1990).

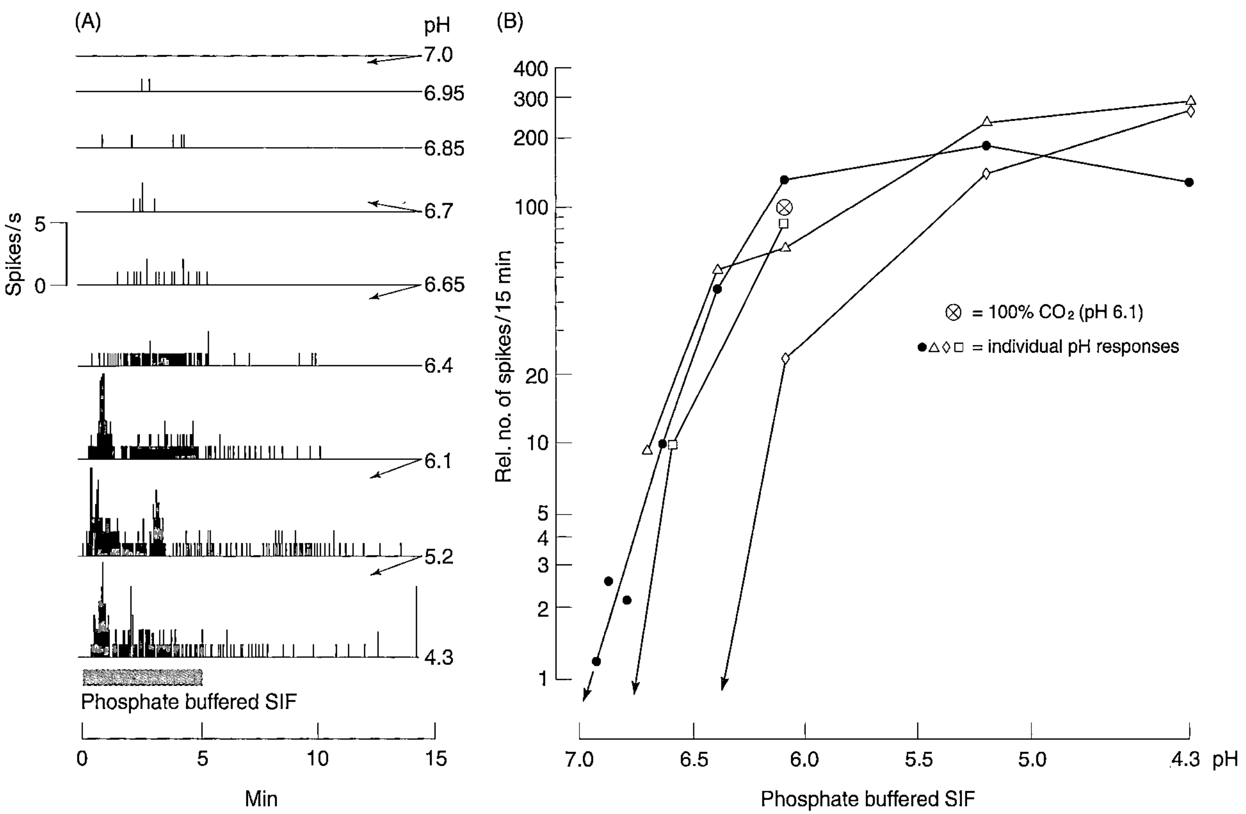

Fig. 1.19 Excitation of cutaneous polymodal C-fibre nociceptive afferents by protons in an in vitro skin-nerve preparation. **A** Example of in vitro recordings of a CMH whose receptive field was consecutively exposed to synthetic interstitial fluid (SIF) of different pH for 5 min. The response increased as the pH decreased. **B** Individual dose–response curves for four polymodal C-fibres exposed to SIF of varying pH. The responses were normalized to the response to SIF bubbled with 100% CO_2 (pH 6.1). Filled circles represent responses of the same fibre as in **A**. (Reprinted from Steen et al 1992 with permission.)

HISTAMINE

Substance P released from nociceptor terminals can cause the release of histamine from mast cells. Histamine can lead to a variety of responses, including vasodilatation and oedema. The role of histamine in pain sensation is less clear, because application of exogenous histamine to the skin produces itch and not pain sensations (Simone et al 1991a). Histamine excites polymodal visceral nociceptors, especially when applied in high concentrations (Koda et al 1996), and potentiates the responses of nociceptors to bradykinin and heat (Mizumura et al 1994, 1995, Koda et al 1996). Mechanosensitive cutaneous nociceptors in rats and humans respond only weakly to histamine (Lang et al 1990, Handwerker et al 1991a, Koppert et al 1993). However, a subpopulation of mechanoinsensitive C-fibres was vigorously excited by histamine (Schmelz et al 1997).

ARACHIDONIC ACID METABOLITES

The prostaglandins, thromboxanes and leukotrienes are a large family of arachidonic acid metabolites collectively known as eicosanoids. The eicosanoids are generally considered not to activate nociceptors directly, but rather to sensitize the nociceptors in skin and viscera to natural stimuli and other endogenous chemicals (Ferreira et al 1974, Mizumura et al 1987, 1991, Rueff & Dray 1993, Kumazawa et al 1996). A sensitizing and a direct excitatory effect for PGE_2 and PGI_2, however, has been demonstrated in afferents innervating joints (Schaible & Schmidt 1988a, Birrell et al 1991, 1993, Schepelmann et al 1992). Of the different prostaglandins, PGI_2, PGE_1, PGE_2 and PGD_2 are most likely to have a role in inflammatory pain and hyperalgesia.

Of the leukotrienes (metabolites of the lipoxygenase pathway), LTD_4 and LTB_4 have been suggested to play a role in hyperalgesia (Levine et al 1984b, Bisgaard & Kristensen 1985, Denzlinger et al 1985) and in sensitization to mechanical stimuli (Martin et al 1987).

ADENOSINE AND ADENOSINE PHOSPHATES

During inflammation and tissue injury, adenosine and its mono- or polyphospate derivates (AMP, ADP, ATP) may be released or leak into the extracellular space and activate nociceptors (Burnstock 1996, 1997). Adenosine and its phosphates have been reported to induce pain in humans (Bleehen et al 1976, Bleehen & Keele 1977). Intra-arterial or intradermal injection of adenosine causes pain (Sylvén et al 1988, Pappagallo et al 1993) and intravenous/intracoronary infusion of adenosine induces angina-like symptoms (Sylvén et al 1986a,b, Crea et al 1990, 1992, Gaspardone et al 1994, 1995). In animals, adenosine enhances the response to formalin, presumably via the A2 receptor (Taiwo & Levin 1990, Karlsten et al 1992, Doak & Sawynok 1995). Animals lacking the adenosine A2a receptor are hypoalgesic to heat stimuli (Ledent et al 1997).

Adenosine triphosphate (ATP) presumably activates nociceptive neurons via the $P2X_3$ receptor and the heteromeric $P2X_2/P2X_3$ receptor (Chen et al 1995a, Lewis et al 1995, Cook et al 1997). Messenger RNA for the $P2X_3$ receptor and the receptor protein have been found in small-diameter neurons in the dorsal root ganglia (Chen et al 1995a, Cook et al 1997, Vulchanova et al 1997). Local intradermal injection of agents activating P2X receptors results in pain behaviour in animals (Bland-Ward & Humphrey 1997) and enhances the pain behaviour to formalin (Sawynok & Reid 1997). However, intradermal injections of ATP in humans are not painful (Reeh & Kress 1998).

CYTOKINES

During inflammation cytokines (e.g., interleukin 1β, IL-1β; tumour necrosis factor α, TNFα; interleukin 6, IL-6) are released by a variety of cells (e.g., macrophages) and regulate the inflammatory response (Arai et al 1990, Kuby 1994). Clinical studies showed that TNFα levels in synovial fluid were increased in painful joints (Shafer et al 1994). Treatment with antibodies against TNFα has been reported to improve the symptoms accompanying rheumatoid arthritis, including pain (Elliott et al 1994). Studies in animals have demonstrated mechanical and thermal hyperalgesia after systemic or local injection of IL-1β, IL-6 and TNFα (Ferreira et al 1988, Cunha et al 1992, Watkins et al 1994, 1995, Ferreira et al 1997). Additionally, treatment with antiserum against TNFα is able to inhibit or delay the onset of hyperalgesia in experimental models of inflammation (Cunha et al 1992, Woolf et al 1997). A direct excitation and sensitization to thermal and mechanical stimuli of nociceptive afferent fibres have been shown for IL-1β and TNFα (Fukuoka et al 1994, Sorkin et al 1997). When applied along the peripheral nerve, TNFα induces ectopic activity in nociceptive afferent fibres (Sorkin et al 1997). Blocking TNF receptor 1 or decreasing the level of endoneurial TNFα was found to attenuate thermal and mechanical hyperalgesia in animals with a chronic constriction injury of the sciatic nerve (Sommer et al 1997, 1998). These findings, together with the observation that TNFα can be released by macrophages as well as Schwann cells, suggest that TNFα may play a role in hyperalgesia accompanying peripheral neuropathy.

EXCITATORY AMINO ACIDS

Glutamate receptors are expressed in dorsal root ganglion cells (Sato et al 1993b) and have also been identified on peripheral terminals of cutaneous nociceptors (Carlton et al 1995). The peripheral application of glutamate activates nociceptors (Ault & Hildebrand 1993) and the peripheral administration of ligands binding to glutamate receptors induces pain behaviours in animals (Zhou et al 1996). An involvement of peripheral glutamate receptors in formalin-induced pain behaviours has been demonstrated (Davidson et al 1997). Intra-articular injection of excitatory amino acids and inflammatory agents results in signs of hyperalgesia that are reversed by glutamate receptor antagonists (Lawand et al 1997). However, the peripheral algogenic action of glutamate is unclear, as it failed to excite nociceptors and it does not induce pain when injected into human skin (Vyklický & Knotková-Urbancová 1996).

OPIOIDS

Besides its central analgesic action, morphine and other opioids produce analgesia in inflamed tissues by a peripheral mechanism (Stein et al 1988, 1989). Opioid receptors have been demonstrated on peripheral terminals of afferent fibres (Stein et al 1990, Coggeshall et al 1997) and axonal transport of these receptors is enhanced during inflammation (Hassan et al 1993). Peripheral analgesia by opioids appears to be part of a physiological antinociceptive system, because increased amounts of endogenous opioids have been found in inflamed tissues (Stein et al 1990). Inflammatory cells such as macrophages, monocytes and lymphocytes contain opioid peptides (Przewlocki et al 1992). The release of endogenous opioids and antinociception can be induced by interleukin 1β and corticotropin-releasing hormone originating from the inflamed tissue (Schäfer et al 1994, 1996).

EFFERENT FUNCTIONS OF NOCICEPTORS

Nociceptors, apart from signalling pain, serve regulatory and trophic functions (Kruger 1988, McMahon & Koltzenburg 1990). This might explain the finding that small-diameter fibres outnumber large-diameter fibres by a factor of 4 (Ochoa & Mair 1969). An efferent role for nociceptors was suggested by several investigators almost a century ago (for a historical review see Lynn 1996; Lewis 1937). Two efferent cutaneous phenomena have been identified that depend on the integrity of afferent nociceptive fibres and are part of the so-called neurogenic inflammation (Jansco et al 1967, 1968): vasodilatation, which becomes visible as a flare surrounding a site of injury, and plasma extravasation, which may become apparent as a wheal at the site of injury. Both phenomena are mediated by vasoactive neuropeptides (SP, CGRP) that are released from peripheral terminals of nociceptors upon activation. SP and CGRP also play a role in immunological processes (e.g., the migration of leucocytes at sites of tissue injury (Nilsson et al 1985, Kjartansson et al 1987), and they stimulate the epidermal cells (e.g., keratinocytes and Langerhans cells) which are necessary for the maintenance and repair of skin integrity (Hsieh et al 1996, Kruger 1996). Afferent fibres are also considered to play a role in the regulation of activity of autonomic ganglia and visceral smooth muscles (for reviews see Maggi & Meli 1988, Lynn 1996, Szolcsanyi 1996, Holzer 1998). Afferent fibres therefore serve a trophic efferent function in somatic and visceral tissues (for review see Kruger 1996).

The principal lines of evidence indicating that afferent neurons are involved in neurogenic inflammation are:

1. The responses are abolished by surgical or chemical ablation (e.g., capsaicin) of the sensory innervation of the involved tissues (Jansco et al 1977, Lembeck & Holzer 1979, Gamse et al 1980, Carpenter & Lynn 1981, Pinter & Szolcsanyi 1995).
2. The responses occur independent of the autonomic nervous system (Couture et al 1985, Blumberg & Wallin 1987).

The fibres involved in the reflex vasodilatation are polymodal nociceptive C fibres that are capsaicin sensitive (Jansco et al 1967, 1968). Stimulation of Aδ fibres may also result in a flare response (Jänig & Lisney 1989, Kolston & Lisney 1993).

Flare is thought to be caused by a peripheral axon reflex. The activation of one branch of a nociceptor by a noxious stimulus results in the antidromic invasion of action potentials into adjacent branches of the nociceptor which, in turn, causes the release of vasoactive substances from the terminals of the nociceptor. However, the extent of the flare far exceeds the size of the receptive fields of conventional nociceptors (Beitel & Dubner 1976, Kumazawa & Perl 1977a,b, Campbell & Meyer 1983, Raja et al 1984, Treede et al 1990b). Possible explanations for this discrepancy might include:

1. Flare is mediated by a subpopulation of chemosensitive nociceptive fibres with large receptive fields (Lewis 1937). Some C fibres with large, complex receptive fields have been reported (Meyer et al 1991, Schmelz et al 1997).

2. Flare results from spreading depolarization along adjacent nociceptive terminals via a daisy-chain cascade mechanism (Lembeck & Gamse 1982).
3. Axo-axonal coupling between small fibres may be responsible for the spread of the flare reaction (Mathews 1976, Meyer et al 1985b).

Several lines of evidence indicate that the neural substrates for vasodilatation and the perception of pain are different.

1. The magnitude of vasodilatation induced by a noxious stimulus does not always increase with the intensity of pain (Koltzenburg & Handwerker 1994).
2. Low activity (<1 Hz) in C fibres can generate significant vasodilatation (Lynn & Shakhanbeh 1988) which, in man, does not cause any conscious sensation (Gybels et al 1979).
3. Histamine can produce a large flare with little or no pain (Treede 1992).

Possible explanations include: (i) different discharge patterns are needed for pain versus flare in a given fibre population or (ii) certain classes of afferents are better designed for flare than pain and vice versa.

Recent evidence suggests that the antidromic activity involved in the effector responses can originate from the spinal cord. A series of studies in a model of acute arthritis indicates that primary afferent input to the spinal cord activates multisynaptic central neuronal pathways that in turn influence the development of neurogenic inflammation (Sluka and Westlund 1993, Sluka et al 1994a,b, for review see Sluka et al 1995b). The activation of primary afferent fibres may result in depolarization of the central terminals of other afferent fibres (PAD). If the PAD is large enough (e.g., under peripheral inflammatory conditions), the depolarization can be sufficient to initiate action potentials at the central terminals that are conducted antidromically in the primary afferent fibres (dorsal root reflexes, DRRs). It is postulated that the antidromic impulses (DRRs) triggered by PAD result in release of neuropeptides in the joint from peripheral terminals of the afferents and contribute to the inflammatory process. DRRs have been recorded in C-, Aδ- and Aβ-fibre types in rat models of acute arthritis (Rees et al 1995, Sluka et al 1995a). The joint inflammation and the DRRs were attenuated by prior dorsal rhizotomy (Sluka et al 1994b, Rees et al 1995). The increase in blood flow that has been measured in response to painful stroking stimuli applied to the zone of secondary hyperalgesia appears to be a human correlate of the dorsal root reflex (Cervero & Laird 1996a).

Anatomical, immunological and histochemical studies have revealed the presence of several peptides in sensory neurons and their peripheral and central projections. These peptides include substance P and other tachykinins such as neurokinins A and K, CGRP, somatostatin and vasoactive intestinal polypeptide (Lembeck & Gamse 1982, Holzer 1988, Micevych & Kruger 1992). The presence and release of neuropeptides from capsaicin-sensitive sensory nerve endings, their ability to induce many of the signs of acute inflammation, including vasodilatation and plasma extravasation, and the inhibition of neurogenic vasodilatation by selective neuropeptide antagonists indicate that they are the principal mediators of neurogenic inflammation and axon reflexive flare (Saria 1984, Helme et al 1986, Lembeck & Donnerer 1992, Escott & Brain 1993). The vasodilatation induced by substance P may, at least in part, be an indirect effect related to histamine release from mast cells (Hagermark et al 1978, Barnes et al 1986, Ebertz et al 1987). CGRP also has potent and prolonged vasodilator properties in humans and may be one of the mediators of neurogenic vasodilatation, possibly playing a role in the long-term vascular responses to injury (Brain et al 1985, 1986, Piotrowski & Foreman 1986, Pedersen-Bjergaard et al 1991. Other efferent actions of nociceptors that are mimicked by vasoactive neuropeptides are contraction of smooth muscles, stimulation of mucous secretion from airways and leucocyte adhesion (Lundberg 1993, Smith et al 1993, Ramnarine et al 1994). Some efferent functions of nociceptors and the chemical mediators involved in cutaneous and visceral tissues are shown in Figure 1.20.

Substance P, neurokinin A and CGRP are also released from trigeminovascular axons in the pial and dural circulations, resulting in vasodilatation and plasma extravasation (Moskowitz et al 1983, 1989). This release of vasoactive neuropeptides from perivascular sensory nerves via axon reflex-like mechanisms may play an important role in the pathophysiology of vascular headache and cerebral hyperperfusion syndromes (MacFarlane et al 1991, Moskowitz 1991). Other diseases in which a neurogenic component is suspected include rheumatoid arthritis, asthma, inflammatory diseases of the gastrointestinal tract and ocular inflammatory disease (see Maggi et al 1993).

NEURAL MECHANISMS OF ITCH

Itch is the common sensory phenomenon associated with the desire to scratch. Like pain, itch can be produced by chemical, mechanical, thermal or electrical stimuli. However, itch differs from pain in that itch can be evoked only from the superficial layers of skin, mucosa and

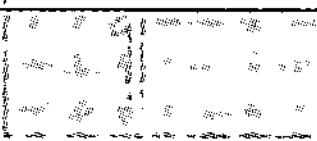

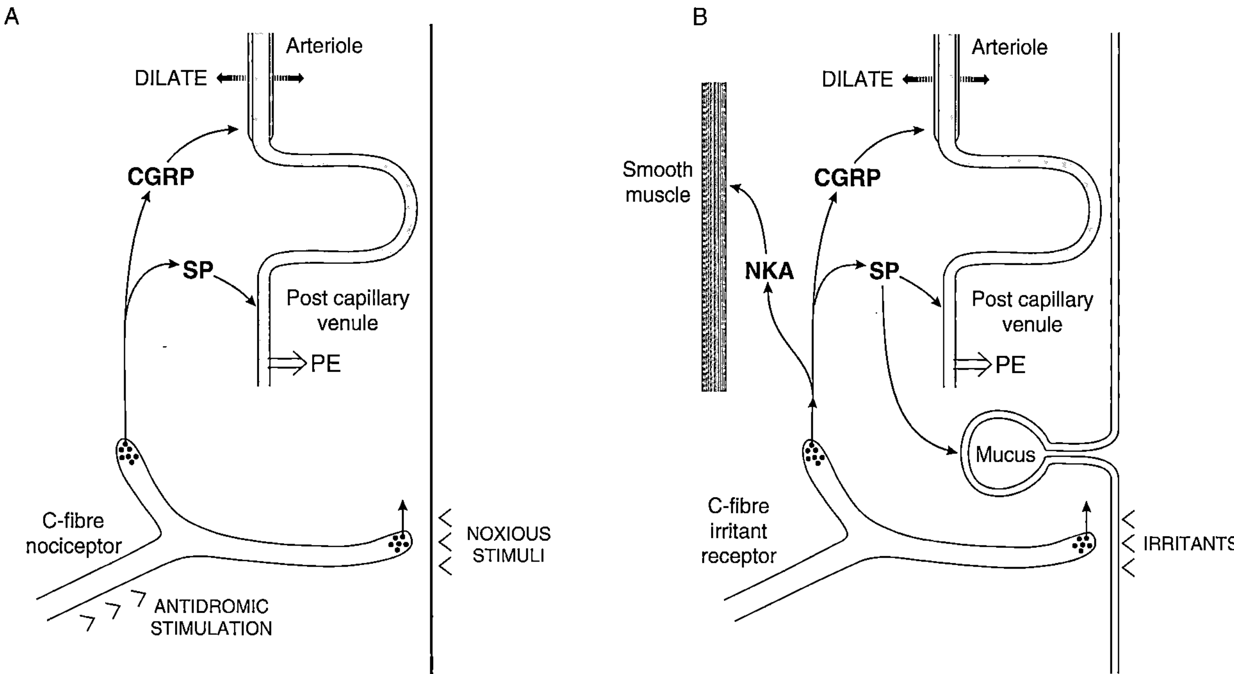

Fig. 1.20 Schematic representation of some efferent actions of nociceptors in skin (**A**) and airways (**B**). **A** Antidromic stimulation of nociceptors leads to the release of neuropeptides, such as substance P (SP) and calcitonin gene-related peptide (CGRP), which induce arteriolar and veno-dilatation and plasma extravasation (PE). **B** In viscera such as the airways, activation of nociceptors by irritants leads to similar vasodilatation and plasma extravasation. In addition, neurokinin A (NKA) and SP can also cause contraction of smooth muscle and stimulation of mucous secretion in the airways. (Reprinted from Lynn 1996 with permission.)

conjunctiva, and not from deep tissues. In addition, itch and pain usually do not occur simultaneously from the same skin region, and, in fact, mild painful stimuli (e.g., scratching) are effective in abolishing itch.

Itch appears to be signalled in the periphery by activity in unmyelinated and perhaps thinly myelinated fibres:

1. Itch persists during a selective block of A-fibre function (Bickford 1938, Handwerker et al 1987).
2. Electrical stimulation of itch spots produces itch at a long latency consistent with conduction in C fibres (Arthur & Shelley 1959).
3. Intraneural microstimulation of identified C-fibre receptors leads to the perception of itch (Torebjörk & Ochoa 1981).
4. Topical application of capsaicin, which desensitizes receptors of unmyelinated fibres, leads to a decrease in itch sensitivity (Toth-Kasa et al 1986, Handwerker et al 1987, Simone & Ochoa 1991).

The neural basis for itch sensation is not well understood. A number of different theories have been proposed, including the three summarized below (McMahon & Koltzenburg 1992, Ekblom 1995, Greaves & Wall 1996, Teofoli et al 1996).

1. Specificity theory

According to the specificity theory, a group of afferents exists that respond specifically to pruritic substances. Activation of this labelled line then leads to itch sensation. A small percentage of C-fibre receptors respond to pruritic substances such as histamine (Khan et al 1987, Handwerker 1992). However, these histamine-sensitive receptors also respond to algesic substances (e.g., mustard oil) and other noxious stimuli (Tuckett & Wei 1987, Handwerker et al 1991a) and, thus, are polymodal receptors similar to typical nociceptors described above. Because itch can be produced by mechanical, heat and chemical stimuli, it is reasonable to expect that the 'itch receptor' is polymodal in nature.

Schmelz et al (1997) recently reported that a subpopulation of C-fibre afferents which are mechanically insensitive may be selectively sensitive to pruritic substances. As shown in Figure 1.21, iontophoresis of histamine into the receptive field of a C-fibre MIA in humans led to a vigorous response with a time course that matched the magnitude of itch perception.

2. Pattern theory

According to the pattern theory, the temporal pattern of neural activity in nociceptors is used to distinguish between

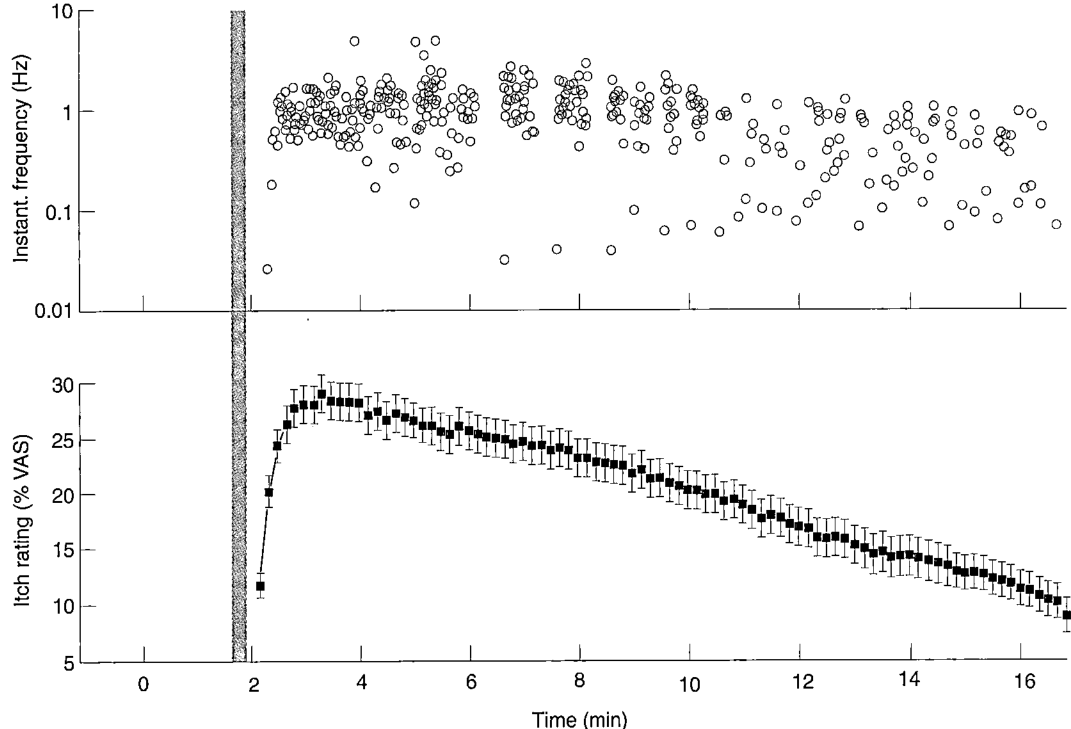

Fig. 1.21 Histamine iontophoresis into the receptive field of a mechanically insensitive afferent led to a vigorous discharge whose time course matched the perception of itch. Top panel: Instantaneous discharge frequency of a C-fibre nociceptor (MIA) recorded from the superficial peroneal nerve of a human subject using microneurographic techniques. The afferent was not spontaneously active initially but developed a long-lasting response after the histamine iontophoresis (vertical grey bar). Bottom panel: Average itch magnitude ratings of a group of 21 healthy volunteers after an identical histamine stimulus. The visual-analogue scale (VAS) had end-point labels of no itch and unbearable itch. (Adapted with permission from Schmelz et al 1997.)

itch and pain. One possibility is that itch is perceived at low levels of nociceptor activity and pain is perceived at higher levels of nociceptor activity. However, this possibility seems unlikely because electrical stimulation of itch spots produces itch at a low stimulation frequency which becomes intense itch, but not pain, at higher frequencies of stimulation (Tuckett 1982). Similarly, intrafascicular electrical stimulation of presumed single C-fibre afferents in humans could produce pure itch sensation which did not become pain at higher stimulus frequencies (Torebjörk & Ochoa 1981).

3. Central processing theory

According to this theory, pruritic and noxious stimuli excite a largely overlapping population of primary afferent nociceptors, and the perception of itch or pain depends on central processing. One possibility is that pruritic stimuli result in activation of one subpopulation of central neurons, whereas pain-producing stimuli activate another. Another possibility is that noxious stimuli result in an inhibition of activity in the subpopulation that is activated by pruritic stimuli.

Pruritic stimuli may also lead to 'itchy skin' in the region surrounding the stimulus site where mechanical stimuli elicit the sensation of itch (Bickford 1938). This is analogous to the region of secondary hyperalgesia to mechanical stimuli that surrounds a noxious stimulus. This area of itchy skin appears to be due to an alteration in central processing, such that tactile stimuli are able to activate central neurons responsible for itch (Simone et al 1991, LaMotte 1992).

The sense of prickle is often confused with itch, but unlike itch, prickle does not produce the urge to scratch. Prickle also appears to be signalled by activity in nociceptors. When wool fabrics that were rated by human subjects as slightly prickly to very prickly were applied to the receptive fields of primary afferents, the response of nociceptors increased with the prickliness of the fabric, whereas the response of low-threshold mechanoreceptors was independent of the prickliness of the fabric (Garnsworthy et al 1988).

NOCICEPTORS IN TISSUES OTHER THAN SKIN

As an understanding of nociception has advanced in studies of the skin, increased attention has turned to other organs.

Psychophysical correlations with physiological studies, however, have proved more difficult. The demonstration that a receptor has a high threshold does not mean that it necessarily signals pain. Receptive properties of afferents are dependent on the properties of the tissues in which they are embedded. Differences in receptor sensitivity reflect in part variations in the position of the transducing element within the tissue with respect to the experimental stimulus.

For many tissues (i.e. tooth pulp and cornea), only pain sensations can be evoked. Thus, the afferent fibres signal pain. For other deep tissues such as muscle, fascia, joints, bone, vascular structures and viscera, more multifarious perceptual possibilities complicate analysis. Some afferent fibres may be important in normal organ function and not involved in conscious sensation. Others may be involved in sensations other than pain.

While studies on somatic afferents have provided considerable support for a specificity theory of pain mechanisms, the mode of encoding noxious events by visceral efferents has remained controversial (Cervero & Jänig 1992, Cervero 1996). Behavioural and clinical studies indicate that there are important differences between cutaneous and deep pain. For example, unlike cutaneous pain, deep pain is diffuse and poorly localized. Deep pain may be associated with strong autonomic responses such as sweating, changes in heart rate, blood pressure and respiration, and may be produced by stimuli that are not tissue damaging, for example, distention of bowel and bladder (Ness & Gebhart 1990, Dubner 1991). In addition, visceral pains may be associated with referred pain as well as cutaneous and deep tissue hyperalgesia. Evidence from these neurophysiological studies indicates that a population of sensory receptors with a high threshold for activation and an encoding range within noxious levels exists in many viscera. Two other populations of visceral afferents which may contribute to visceral pain have also been described. These include a group of 'silent' nociceptors that are sensitized by inflammation and a population of intensity-encoding 'wide-dynamic range' visceral afferents (Cervero 1996). The latter group consists of afferents that respond to a wide range of stimulus intensities, ranging from innocuous to noxious.

CORNEA

Although the threshold for activation serves as a reasonable criterion to distinguish nociceptors from other afferent fibre types in the skin, the cornea illustrates the problem with use of this criterion alone for other tissue types. The mean threshold for activation of primary afferent fibres that innervate the cornea is comparable to the threshold for activation of low-threshold mechanoreceptors in skin (Belmonte & Giraldez 1981, Tanelian & Beuerman 1984). It is likely, however, that mild stimuli may injure the cornea, and it certainly is clear that low-intensity stimuli to the cornea induce pain. Thus, it is reasonable to label the afferent fibres that innervate the cornea nociceptors, because, in the spirit of Sherrington's original usage, these receptors are concerned with the detection of injury.

Although pain is generally thought to be the only sensation that can be elicited from stimulation of the cornea, some studies have suggested that thermal and mechanical stimuli can be differentiated (Lele & Weddell 1959, Kenshalo et al 1960, Beuerman & Tanelian 1979). There are no obvious specialized sense organs. Sensory terminals end in the intraepithelial tissue as unmyelinated fibres. The innervation density is 300–600 times that of the skin (Rozsa & Beuerman 1982). The mechanical receptive fields of the nociceptors are uniformly sensitive and broad, covering as much as 20% of the corneal surface. The majority of fibres innervating the cornea are thinly myelinated and unmyelinated fibres sensitive to mechanical, heat and chemical stimuli, that is they represent polymodal nociceptors (Belmonte et al 1991, Gallar et al 1993). Like cutaneous nociceptors, nociceptors in the cornea can be activated by capsaicin, protons, bradykinin and a combination of inflammatory mediators (Belmonte et al 1991, Gallar et al 1993, Belmonte et al 1994, Chen et al 1995b, Belmonte & Gallar 1996, Chen et al 1997).

Nociceptors in the cornea are also sensitized to heat by repetitive heat stimulation (Belmonte & Giraldez 1981, Gallar et al 1993) and they develop spontaneous activity after corneal injury (Belmonte & Giraldez 1981, Belmonte & Gallar 1996).

TOOTH PULP AND PERIODONTAL LIGAMENT

Although it is disputed whether pain is the only sensation evoked by stimulation of the tooth pulp, certainly pain is the predominant sensation. The tooth pulp and dentine are innervated by Aδ and C fibres (Harris & Griffin 1968, Byers 1984), which form an interlacing network, the subodontoblastic plexus. From this plexus, nerve fibres extend to the odontoblastic layer, predentine and dentine, and terminate as free nerve endings. Human premolars receive about 2300 axons at the root apex; 87% of these fibres are unmyelinated (Nair 1995). The sensory receptors respond to chemical, thermal and mechanical stimuli and thus are polymodal (Funakoshi & Zotterman 1963, Haegerstam et al 1975, Mathews 1977, Dubner 1978). Single-fibre recordings suggest that CGRP-containing Aδ fibres with receptive fields located at the pulpal periphery and inner dentine, but not C fibres, respond to stimuli associated with cavity preparation, such as drilling, desiccation or scraping of dentine (Närhi et al 1982, Byers 1994). The resultant sensation is a short, well-localized, sharp pain (Ahlquist & Franzen 1994). Pulpal C fibres respond to gradual warming of the tooth to noxious temperatures. Impulses in the C fibres are perceived as dull, poorly localized and lingering pain. Thus, it appears that Aδ fibres are responsible for dentinal pain, whereas C fibres may respond to pain originating from the pulp (Närhi 1985a,b, Trowbridge 1985). Studies indicate that periodontal C fibres are predominantly nociceptive, and the polymodal response characteristics of most of these fibres are similar to the response characteristics of pulpal C fibres (Jyväsjärvi & Kniffki 1989, Mengel et al 1992).

MUSCLE

Muscle pain is a frequently experienced sensation, and occurs after strenuous exercise, direct trauma, inflammation and during sustained muscular contractions (for recent reviews see Mense 1996). Torebjörk et al (1984) demonstrated with electrical stimulation of nerve fascicles in awake humans that deep muscle pain is dependent on the activation of small-diameter afferent fibres. It has been observed that pain can be produced by noxious stimulation of muscle, facia and tendons. The many free nerve endings found in the connective tissue of the muscle, between muscle fibres, in blood vessel walls and in tendons are thought to be the receptors for the muscle's nociceptive afferent fibres.

The small myelinated afferent fibres found in muscle are labelled group III fibres and have conduction velocities from 2.5 to 20 m/s (Paintal 1960). The unmyelinated fibres are termed group IV fibres and have conduction velocities less than 2.5 m/s (Mense & Schmidt 1974, Fock & Mense 1976, Hiss & Mense 1976). Of all of the group III and IV fibres, 40% are thought to be nociceptors. Another 20% are contraction sensitive and are thought to be involved in the cardiopulmonary adjustments that occur during exercise (Hnik et al 1969, McCloskey & Mitchell 1972). Approximately 30% are low-threshold mechanoreceptors and may signal deep pressure sensations. The final 10% are thermally responsive and may be involved in thermoregulation (Mense & Meyer 1985).

In several species, the group III and IV muscle afferent fibres have been characterized by their vigorous response to endogenous substances such as bradykinin, serotonin, histamine and potassium. In contrast, muscle spindles and tendon organs do not exhibit comparable responses (Paintal 1960, Kumazawa & Mizumura 1976, Mense 1977). Fibres responsive to bradykinin have also been observed to be selectively sensitive to high-intensity mechanical stimuli (Paintal 1961). In addition, muscle nociceptors may be sensitized by catecholamines (Kieschke et al 1988) and by changes in the biochemical environment resulting from hypoxia and impaired metabolism. Sensitization of muscle nociceptors by the release of endogenous chemicals may explain the local tenderness often associated with muscle trauma or unaccustomed exercise.

JOINT

Much of what is known about joint afferent fibres is based on studies in the cat (for review see Schmidt 1996). Nerve fibre counts in the articular nerves of the knee reveal that the afferent fibres are predominately group III (thinly myelinated) and group IV (unmyelinated) (Skoglund 1956, Freeman & Wyke 1967, Langford & Schmidt 1983). Nociceptors in the joint are located in the joint capsule and ligaments, bone, periosteum, articular fat pads and perivascular sites, but probably not in the joint cartilage. The sensory endings of the group III and IV nerve fibres lack a myelin sheath and are not surrounded by perineurium. The branched, terminal tree of these fibres has a string-of-beads appearance which may represent multiple receptive sites in the nerve endings (Heppelmann et al 1990). At the sites of the axonal beads, a large proportion of the axolemma is devoid of a Schwann cell covering, and the axon fibre has a number of vesicles (Fig. 1.22).

Based on their sensitivities to pressure and joint movements, afferent fibres of the knee joint have been classified under five categories:

1. and 2. Low-threshold units that are excited strongly or weakly, respectively, by innocuous pressure and movements of the knee joint.
3. High-threshold units that are activated only by noxious pressure or movements exceeding the working range of the joint.
4. Units that respond to strong pressure to the knee, but not to movement.
5. Units that do not react to any mechanical stimulus to the normal joint, referred to as 'silent nociceptors' (Schaible & Schmidt 1988a).

It is suggested that, in the normal joint, the high-threshold units signal pain evoked by extreme joint movement (Schaible & Schmidt 1983a,b, Grigg et al 1986).

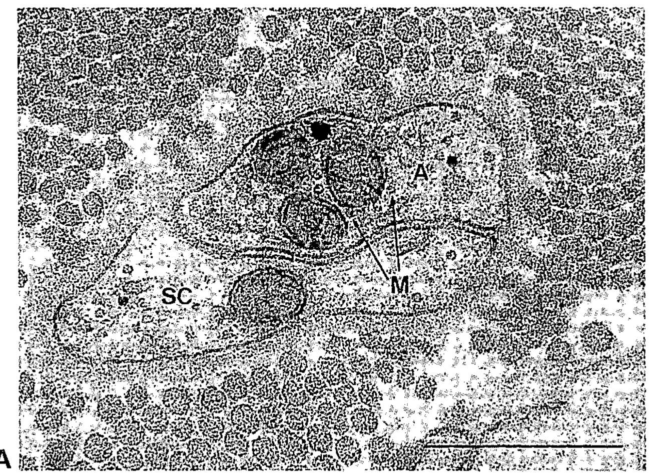

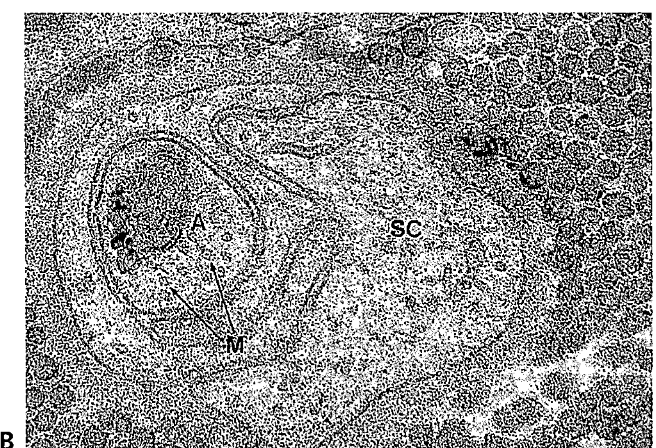

Fig. 1.22 Electron micrographs of sensory endings of group IV nerve endings in the knee joint capsule. **A** Cross-section of the nerve fibre at the site of an axonal bead showing mitochondria, glycogen particles and vesicles. The major part of the axolemma is devoid of Schwann cell covering and directly abuts the basal lamina. **B** Section close to a waist-like region of the nerve fibre about 47 μm distant from the top section. At this level the axon is completely wrapped by Schwann cell lamellae. A= sensory axon; M= microtubules; SC= Schwann cell. × 93 000; Scale bar = 0.5 μm. (Reprinted from Heppelmann et al 1990 with permission.)

Experimentally induced arthritis is associated with dramatic changes in the response properties of joint afferents (Heppelmann et al 1985, 1987, Schaible & Schmidt 1985). Sensitization is observed in all types of afferent fibres. This sensitization may take the form of afferent activation by movements in the working range, activation by pressure, and induction or increase in resting discharges. Of particular interest is the sensitization of fibres in categories 4 and 5 that were initially insensitive to joint movements. Sensitization in these fibres occurs in the second to third hour after injection of the inflammatory compounds, a time course that matches the behavioural changes in test animals (Neugebauer & Schaible 1988, Schaible & Schmidt 1988b). Chemical mediators of inflammation, such as bradykinin, prostaglandins, leukotrienes, potassium ions, serotonin and, possibly, interleukins are considered to play an important role in the sensitization of joint afferent fibres (Heppelmann et al 1985, Schaible & Schmidt 1988a, Herbert & Schmidt 1992). This inflammation-induced sensitization of articular afferents is likely to contribute to the enhanced pain that accompanies arthritis. Studies by Levine and coworkers have suggested that substances such as substance P released from the peripheral terminals of small-diameter afferent fibres (see 'Efferent functions of nociceptors' above) may contribute to the severity of joint injury (Levine et al 1984a, 1985). Articular tissues are also innervated by sympathetic efferents, and a modulatory role for these fibres via a prostaglandin-mediated mechanism has been suggested in arthritis (for review see Basbaum & Levine 1991).

THE RESPIRATORY SYSTEM

A large percentage of mucosal sensory fibres have the characteristic attributes of cutaneous polymodal nociceptors. These Aδ and C fibres respond not only to mechanical and thermal stimuli but also to chemonociceptive stimuli such as high CO_2 concentrations, intranasally applied irritants such as mustard oil and air-borne stimuli (Peppel & Anton 1993). Most of the myelinated laryngeal afferent fibres are pressure sensitive and respond to irritant gases. Their role in sensation is not known. Unmyelinated afferent fibres that innervate the larynx have not been well studied (for reviews see Coleridge & Coleridge 1984, Paintal 1986, Widdicombe 1986, Martling 1987).

Three main groups of receptors which innervate the tracheobronchial tree and lungs have been characterized:

1. Slowly adapting stretch receptors are localized in airway smooth muscle and are involved in reflexes. Their activity does not appear to reach consciousness.
2. The rapidly adapting 'irritant' stretch receptors respond to inflation and deflation of the airways and lungs. They are also sensitive to inhaled dusts and irritant chemicals. Like cutaneous polymodal receptors, these receptors are also stimulated by a number of chemical mediators such as histamine, serotonin and acetylcholine. Prostaglandin $F_2\alpha$ and E_2 potentiate mechanical responsiveness (Paintal 1986, Sant' Ambragio 1987). The discharge and sensitivity of these receptors is increased in a number of pathological conditions.
3. The C-fibre receptors first studied by Paintal (1955) and termed J receptors have many properties in common with the rapidly adapting mechanoreceptors.

They have little tonic discharge normally, and are stimulated or sensitized in a variety of lung conditions such as congestion, lung oedema and pneumonia. These receptors are activated by a variety of chemicals, such as bradykinin, prostaglandins, serotonin, histamine, acetylcholine and capsaicin, and are also activated by some inhaled gases. The burning sensation produced by an endotracheal/bronchial catheter can be abolished by vagal block (Klassen et al 1951). Certain conditions, such as pulmonary congestion, intravascular injection of lobeline (nicotinic ganglionic agonist) and rigorous physical exercise, strongly excite lung C-fibre receptors in animals. It has been suggested that these receptors play a role in the generation of dyspnoeic sensations during pulmonary oedema (Paintal 1986). A subpopulation of afferent fibres in the lung that are activated by capsaicin contain neuropeptides of the tachykinin family (substance P, neurokinin A and neuropeptide K) as well as CGRP (Lundberg & Saria 1987). The release of the neuropeptides induces protein extravasation, increases local blood flow and causes bronchoconstriction (Martling 1987).

THE CARDIOVASCULAR SYSTEM

Puncture of the arterial wall in humans induces pain. The neural apparatus for this effect probably resides in the nervi vasorum, but to date these receptors have been little studied. Psychophysical studies (Arndt & Klement 1991) have been performed by applying noxious stimuli to isolated vein segments in human subjects. Osmotic, stretching, cold and heat stimuli evoke similar sensations. This suggests that the venous wall has polymodal nociceptive fibres.

The heart has an intrinsic nervous system that contains both afferent and efferent neurons. Cardiac afferent receptors are connected to cell bodies in dorsal root and nodose ganglia. Pain from endogenous or exogenous stimulation of the heart usually occurs only under certain pathological conditions such as myocardial ischaemia. It is unclear whether pain from the heart is signalled by sympathetic afferent fibres or the parasympathetic afferent fibres in the vagus nerve (Baker et al 1980, Coleridge & Coleridge 1980, 1981, Kaufman et al 1980, Malliani et al 1986). Traditionally, the sympathetic afferents are considered to be solely responsible for signalling pain arising from the heart. Based on an extensive review of the literature, Meller and Gebhart (1992) propose that vagal afferents may also contribute to the pain associated with myocardial ischaemia. Many sympathetic afferent nerve fibres innervating the heart respond to bradykinin (Baker et al 1980, Lombardi et al 1981). However, there is conflicting evidence as to whether bradykinin causes pain when injected into coronary arteries (Malliani et al 1984, Pagani et al 1985). Other chemical mediators of cardiac pain may include serotonin (Takahashi 1985, James et al 1988), adenosine (Sylvén et al 1986a,b, Crea et al 1990), histamine (Guzman et al 1962), prostaglandins, lactate and potassium (for reviews see Meller & Gebhart 1992, Sylvén 1993). During myocardial ischaemia, large quantities of adenosine are released into the interstitial space. Adenosine evokes angina-like pain in the absence of ECG signs of ischaemia in healthy volunteers and patients with ischaemic heart disease (Sylvén 1993).

THE DIGESTIVE SYSTEM

Progress in understanding visceral pain from the gastrointestinal tract has been limited by the lack of an agreement on an adequate noxious, visceral stimulus. Colorectal distension is a reliable noxious visceral stimulus that induces pain in humans (Ness & Gebhart 1988, 1990).

Afferent fibres in the digestive system can be subdivided into those with specific properties, such as digestive chemoreceptors, thermoreceptors and low-threshold mechanoreceptors, and those with polymodal sensitivity. Afferent fibres that serve the digestive system are, as with the heart, found in conjunction with the motor fibres of both the sympathetic and parasympathetic systems.

Clinically, visceral pain of reflux oesophagitis may mimic angina pectoris as the pain is often referred to the same somatic regions (Lee et al 1985, Richter et al 1989). A likely explanation for the above clinical phenomenon is the observation that the somatic input from the upper thoracic dermatomes and the visceral inputs from the distal oesophagus and the heart converge on the same spinal neurons (Garrison et al 1992).

Afferent fibres that course with the vagus nerve are known to be responsible for nociceptive reactions to stimuli applied to the upper oesophagus and for certain forms of gastrointestinal discomfort associated with ulcers (Mei 1983). Pain of lower oesophageal and intestinal origin is usually signalled by afferent fibres in the thoracic sympathetic chain or the splanchnic nerves (Sengupta et al 1990). Visceral afferents from the lower oesophagus are either rapidly adapting, slowly adapting or have a slow adaptation with an afterdischarge to a sustained distension, and fibres have been classified as low-threshold mechanoreceptors, wide-dynamic-range mechanonociceptors or high-threshold mechanonociceptors (Sengupta et al 1990, 1992). The last two classes are also responsive to the systemic administration of bradykinin (Sengupta et al 1992). Studies on the distal oesophagus indicate that the inflamed gut is more sensitive to distension than a non-inflamed viscera (Garrison et al 1992).

Cervero (1982, 1983) identified a group of units in the ferret that innervate the bile duct and which respond preferentially to high luminal pressure. These fibres were therefore classified as nociceptors and it seems likely that such afferents mediate the pain that accompanies the passage of gallstones.

Afferent fibres from the vagus nerve and fibres in the thoracic sympathetic chain also innervate stomach, duodenum or jejunum. Sympathetic afferent fibres unresponsive to ischaemia can also be activated by innocuous mechanical distension, whereas ischaemia-sensitive afferents have a high mechanical threshold for activation. Both classes could be activated by bradykinin (Pan & Longhurst 1996). Fibres sensitive to ischaemia can also be activated by prostaglandins, lactic acid, oxygen-derived free radicals and lypoxygenase products (Longhurst & Dittman 1987, Stahl & Longhurst 1992, Stahl et al 1993, Pan et al 1995).

The majority of the visceral afferent fibres from the colon and rectum are Aδ and C fibres that course with the parasympathetic nerves (Vera & Nadelhaft 1990b). Many afferent fibres respond to non-noxious stimulation and also have a monotonically increasing response to stimuli in the noxious range (Blumberg et al 1983, Cervero & Sharkey 1988, Jänig & Koltzenburg 1991a,b, Sengupta & Gebhart 1994a). Besides this class of fibres activated by low-threshold stimuli, a second group characterized by a high mechanical threshold for activation has been described (Sengupta & Gebhart 1994a). A third group of afferent fibres innervating the colon does not respond to innocuous and noxious mechanical stimulation (Jänig & Koltzenburg 1991a,b, Sengupta & Gebhart 1994b). It has been speculated that these fibres are the visceral counterparts of the 'silent nociceptors' described in somatic structures (Jänig & Koltzenburg 1991a,b). Haupt et al (1983) demonstrated that ischaemia of the colon excites afferent fibres that also respond to distension and to bradykinin. During inflammation, spontaneous activity in afferent fibres innervating the colon increases and they become sensitized to mechanical stimuli (Fig. 1.23) (Su et al 1997a). Responses to noxious colorectal distension could be inhibited by κ-opioid agonists, whereas agonists directed against other opioid receptors were ineffective (Sengupta et al 1996, Su et al 1997a).

THE UROGENITAL SYSTEM

The differences between mechanisms of nociception in the skin and viscera are emphasized by studies on the response properties of visceral afferents from the urinary tract (for review see Gebhart 1996). There is ongoing controversy as to whether visceral pain is mediated by a specific subgroup of nociceptive fibres (specificity theory) or by the spatial and temporal patterns of discharges in non-specific afferent fibres (pattern theory) (Jänig & Morrison 1986, Cervero & Jänig 1992, Cervero 1996). Two distinct groups of afferent fibres capable of signalling noxious stimuli have been identified from the urinary bladder. Visceral afferents from the urinary bladder are either unmyelinated C fibres or myelinated Aδ fibres (Vera & Nadelhaft 1990a, Su et al 1997b). The majority of visceral primary afferents from the bladder, urethra, and reproductive and other pelvic organs encode for both noxious and non-noxious stimuli (Bahns et al 1986, 1987, Berkley et al 1990, Häbler et al 1990). These low-threshold fibres respond to peristaltic contractions and are thought to be involved in the regulatory functions of the viscera (Sengupta et al 1990, Hammer et al 1993). A subset (20–30%) of the unmyelinated, pelvic nerve afferent fibres projecting to the sacral spinal cord accurately encode intravesical pressure changes in the noxious range (Häbler et al 1990, Sengupta & Gebhart 1994b, Su et al 1997b). The high-threshold fibres generally have lower rates of spontaneous activity, a lower maximum response to the same distension pressures than the low-threshold fibres and do not respond to peristaltic contractions (Sengupta & Gebhart 1994b). These high-threshold, mechanosensitive afferent fibres are considered to be visceral nociceptors (Cervero 1994). In addition, a subpopulation of C-fibre visceral afferents has been identified which is not mechanically sensitive, but is excited by chemical irritants (Koltzenburg & McMahon 1986, Häbler et al 1988, 1990). Reflexes and responses of the visceral afferent fibres evoked by urinary bladder distension in rats are increased by mucosal inflammation. Thus, pain originating from the bladder may be intensified by the presence of inflammation (McMahon & Abel 1987, McMahon 1988, Häbler et al 1988, 1990). Peripherally administered kappa, but not mu or delta, opioid receptor agonists attenuate the responses to noxious urinary bladder distension following inflammation (Su et al 1997b). In contrast to afferents from the urinary bladder, almost 90% of ureteric afferent fibres respond only to high distension pressures (Cervero & Sann 1989, Hammer et al 1993). These ureteric nociceptors also respond to hypoxia of the ureteric mucosa and intraluminal applications of bradykinin, potassium and capsaicin.

Studies indicate that uterine afferent fibres are present both in the hypogastric and pelvic nerves. These fibres are capable of signalling information about temporal and spatial aspects of mechanical and chemical stimulation of the uterus (Floyd et al 1977, Berkley et al 1988, 1990, Berkley

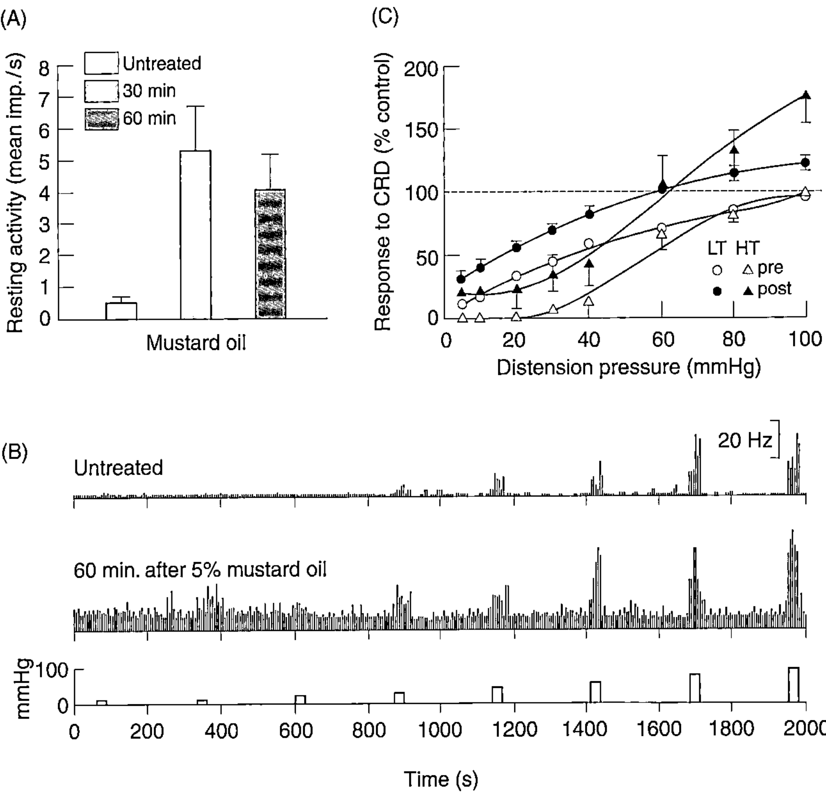

Fig. 1.23 Response of afferent fibres innervating the colon to colorectal distension before and after an application of mustard oil (5%) for 15 min which resulted in an inflammation. **A** Increase in spontaneous activity was observed in 16/17 fibres 30 and 60 min after the induction of the inflammation. **B** Specimen recording showing the effect of mustard oil-induced inflammation on the responses of a high threshold pelvic nerve afferent to colorectal distension. Top trace: Responses before the application of mustard oil; middle trace: responses 60 min after the instillation of mustard oil; lower trace: distension pressures applied. Note the increase in resting activity and the sensitization to colorectal distension during inflammation. **C** Population stimulus–response function for low-threshold (circles, $n = 14$) and high-threshold afferents (triangles, $n = 3$) before (open symbols) and after (filled symbols) the instillation of mustard oil. Inflammation induced a leftward shift in the stimulus–response function, representing lowering in activation threshold and increased responses to suprathreshold stimuli. (Reproduced from Su et al 1997a with permission.)

1993). The afferents are mostly C fibres, although Aδ fibres are also present. The high-threshold afferent fibres had lower thresholds to mechanical stimulation of the uterus during oestrus than in non-oestrus cycles. The hypogastric afferents are activated by chemicals such as bradykinin, 5-HT, KCl and high doses of CO_2 (Berkley et al 1988, Berkley 1993).

Free nerve endings derived from Aδ or C fibres are abundant throughout the glans penis (Johnson & Halata 1991). The two fibre types associated with these endings appear to be slowly adapting, low-threshold stretch receptors and high-threshold mechanoreceptors (Kitchell et al 1982, Johnson & Kitchell 1987).

Kumazawa and colleagues (1986) have characterized the response properties of visceral afferent fibres that innervate the testes of the dog. More than 95% of the fibres of the superior spermatic nerve are unmyelinated, with the great majority having polymodal properties (i.e. responding to mechanical, chemical and thermal stimuli). Responses of the polymodal receptor are augmented by application of prostaglandins E_2 and I_2 (Mizumura et al 1991) and of bradykinin acting via a B2 receptor (Mizumura et al 1990). The prostaglandins are less potent in their ability to excite nociceptors as compared to their efficacy as potentiators of the response to bradykinin (Mizumura et al 1991). Sensitization of the bradykinin response is mediated via EP_3

receptors, while the heat response is sensitized by the activation of the EP_2-receptor subtype (Kumazawa 1993, Kumazawa et al 1996). Activation of the EP_2 receptor stimulates adenylyl cyclase and increases intracellular cAMP, while activation of the EP_3 subtype suppresses cAMP production (Mizumura et al 1996). Thus, the heat and the bradykinin responses have differential effects on intracellular cAMP responses. The effects of algesic substances on the testicular polymodal nociceptors may also result from Ca^{2+}-dependent membrane surface potential changes (Sato et al 1989). A series of studies by Kumazawa and colleagues indicates that interaction of intracellular messenger pathways between themselves and with ion channels are responsible for the sensitizing actions of inflammatory mediators (for review see Kumazawa et al 1996).

BRAIN AND MENINGES

Clinically, headache and visceral pain have several common features. Both are diffuse, poorly localized, and are often associated with intense autonomic responses. Considerable experimental evidence indicates that nociceptive information from cranial blood vessels, in particular the vessels within the dura mater and the leptomeninges, play an important role in headache (for reviews see Moskowitz 1991, Moskowitz & Macfarlane 1993, Zagami 1994). The meningeal blood vessels are surrounded by a dense plexus of sensory axons emanating from the cells in the trigeminal ganglia and from the upper cervical dorsal root ganglia (Mayberg et al 1981, Arbab et al 1986). Each ganglion cell has divergent axon collaterals that innervate multiple large vessels supplying both brain parenchyma and the overlying dura mater (Arbab et al 1986, O'Connor & van der Kooy 1986). The trigeminovascular nerves are predominantly C fibres that have 'naked' nerve endings with vesicles. The vesicles contain several polypeptides, including substance P, neurokinin A, CGRP and galanin. The neurophysiological properties of afferents innervating the superior sagittal sinus and the surrounding dura have been recently characterized (Bove & Moskowitz 1997). Most axons had conduction velocities in the unmyelinated range and were polymodal nociceptors that were activated by capsaicin, inflammatory mediators, acidic buffer, and heat and cold stimuli. Electrical stimulation of the trigeminal ganglia or activation of intracranial parasympathetic fibres by stimulation of the sphenopalatine ganglion, or infusion of tachykinins results in vasodilatation and plasma protein leakage in rat dura mater (Markowitz et al 1987, Delepine & Aubineau 1997). Recent neurophysiological studies of primary afferent trigeminal neurons indicate that chemical sensitization of the receptive field of dural nociceptors leads to activation and sensitization of the cells' response to mechanical stimuli (Strassman et al 1996). In addition, the trigeminal neurons exhibited an enhanced response to cutaneous thermal and mechanical stimuli (Burstein et al 1998). The latter phenomenon may explain the extracranial cutaneous hypersensitivity that often accompanies headaches. Ergot alkaloids, which are therapeutically useful in the management of vascular headaches, may act by blockade of the small-fibre-mediated neurogenic inflammation in the dura mater (Saito et al 1988). Physiological studies also indicate that the trigeminovascular axons within the dura have prejunctional $5HT_{1B/D}$-like receptors and agonists of this receptor, for example sumatriptan, block neurogenic plasma extravasation and are clinically useful in the management of vascular headaches (Buzzi & Moskowitz 1990).

Anatomical studies have demonstrated that the pia mater covering the spinal cord and its roots have considerable unmyelinated fibre innervation. Little is known about the physiology of these primary afferent fibres innervating the spinal meninges. A recent report indicates that a subpopulation of unmyelinated fibres in the ventral root serve as primary afferent fibres innervating the root proper or its sheath (Jänig & Koltzenburg 1991b). These pial afferents have no resting discharges and appear to be maximally activated by noxious stimuli.

Acknowledgements

We appreciate the assistance of S. J. Horasek and T. V. Hartke. This research was supported by NIH grants NS-14447, NS-26363 and NS-32386.

REFERENCES

Adriaensen H, Gybels J, Handwerker HO, Van Hees J 1984 Nociceptor discharges and sensations due to prolonged noxious mechanical stimulation – a paradox. Human Neurobiology 3: 53–58

Ahlquist ML, Franzen OG 1994 Encoding of the subjective intensity of sharp dental pain. Endodontics and Dental Traumatology 10(4): 153–166

Ali Z, Meyer RA, Campbell JN 1996 Secondary hyperalgesia to mechanical but not heat stimuli following a capsaicin injection in hairy skin. Pain 68: 401–411

Ali Z, Ringkamp M, Hartke TV, Chien HF, Flavahan NA, Campbell JN, Meyer RA 1999 Uninjured C-fibernociceptors develop spontaneous activity and alpha adrenergic sensitivity following L6 spinal nerve ligation in the monkey. Journal of Neurophysiology 81 (in press)

Andersen OK, Gracely RH, Arendt-Nielsen L 1995 Facilitation of the human nociceptive reflex by stimulation of Aβ-fibres in a secondary hyperalgesic area sustained by nociceptive input from the primary hyperalgesic area. Acta Physiologica Scandinavica 155: 87–97

Arai K, Lee F, Miyajima A, Miyatake N, Arai N, Yokota T 1990 Cytokines: coordinators of immune and inflammatory responses. Annual Review of Biochemistry 59: 783–836

Arbab MAR, Wiklund L, Svengaard ND 1986 The distribution of cerebral vascular innervation from superior cervical, trigeminal, and spinal ganglia investigated with retrograde and anterograde WGA-HRP tracing in the rat. Neuroscience 19: 695–708

Arndt JO, Klement W 1991 Pain evoked by polymodal stimulation of hand veins in humans. Journal of Physiology (London) 440: 467–478

Arner S 1991 Intravenous phentolamine test: diagnostic and prognostic use in reflex sympathetic dystrophy. Pain 46: 17–22

Arthur RP, Shelley WB 1959 The peripheral mechanisms of itch in man. In: Wolstenholme GEW, O'Connor M (eds) Pain and itch: nervous mechanisms. Little, Brown and Co, Boston

Ault B, Hildebrand LM 1993 L-glutamate activates peripheral nociceptors. Agents and Actions 39: C142–C144

Bahns E, Ernsberger U, Jänig W, Nelke A 1986 Functional characteristics of lumbar visceral afferent fibres from the urinary bladder and the urethra in the cat. Pflugers Archiv 407: 510–518

Bahns E, Halsband U, Jänig W 1987 Functional characteristics of sacral afferent fibres from the urinary bladder, urethra, colon, and anus. Pflugers Archiv 410: 296–303

Baker DG, Coleridge HM, Coleridge JCG, Nerdrum T 1980 Search for a cardiac nociceptor: stimulation by bradykinin of sympathetic afferent nerve endings in the heart of the cat. Journal of Physiology (London) 306: 519–536

Barasi S, Lynn B 1986 Effects of sympathetic stimulation on mechanoreceptive and nociceptive afferent units from the rabbit pinna. Brain Research 378: 21–27

Barnes PJ, Brown MJ, Dollery CT, Fuller RW, Heavey DJ, Ind PW 1986 Histamine is released from skin by substance P but does not act as the final vasodilator in the axon reflex. British Journal of Pharmacology 88: 741–745

Basbaum AI, Levine JD 1991 The contribution of the nervous system to inflammation and inflammatory disease. Canadian Journal of Physiology and Pharmacology 69: 647–651

Beck PW, Handwerker HO 1974 Bradykinin and serotonin effects on various types of cutaneous nerve fibers. Pflugers Archiv 347: 209–222

Beck PW, Handwerker HO, Zimmermann M 1974 Nervous outflow from the cat's foot during noxious radiant heat stimulation. Brain Research 67: 373–386

Beitel RE, Dubner R 1976 Response of unmyelinated (C) polymodal nociceptors to thermal stimuli applied to monkey's face. Journal of Neurophysiology 39: 1160–1175

Belmonte C, Gallar J 1996 Corneal nociceptors. In: Belmonte C, Cervero F (eds) Neurobiology of nociceptors. Oxford University Press, Oxford, pp 146–183

Belmonte C, Giraldez F 1981 Responses of cat corneal sensory receptors to mechanical and thermal stimulation. Journal of Physiology (London) 321: 355–368

Belmonte C, Gallar J, Pozo MA, Rebollo I 1991 Excitation by irritant chemical substances of sensory afferent units in the cat's cornea. Journal of Physiology (London) 437: 709–725

Belmonte C, Gallar J, Lopez-Briones LG, Pozo MA, 1994 Polymodality in nociceptive neurons: experimental models of chemotransduction In: Urban L (ed) Cellular mechanisms of sensory processing. Nato ASI Series. H79. Springer-Verlag, Berlin, pp 87–117

Berkley KJ 1993 Functional differences between afferent fibers in the hypogastric and pelvic nerves innervating female reproductive organs in the rat. Journal of Neurophysiology 69: 533–544

Berkley KJ, Robbins A, Sato Y 1988 Afferent fibers supplying the uterus in the rat. Journal of Neurophysiology 59: 142–163

Berkley KJ, Hotta H, Robbins A, Sato Y 1990 Functional properties of afferent fibers supplying reproductive and other pelvic organs in pelvic nerve of female rat. Journal of Neurophysiology 63: 256–272

Bessou P, Perl ER 1969 Response of cutaneous sensory units with unmyelinated fibers to noxious stimuli. Journal of Neurophysiology 32: 1025–1043

Beuerman RW, Tanelian DL 1979 Corneal pain evoked by thermal stimulation. Pain 7: 1–14

Bevan S, Geppetti P 1994 Protons: small stimulants of capsaicin-sensitive sensory nerves. Trends in Neurosciences 17: 509–512

Bickford RG 1938 Experiments relating to the itch sensation, its peripheral mechanism and central pathways. Clinical Science 3: 377–386

Bini G, Crucci G, Hagbarth KE, Schady W, Torebjörk E 1984 Analgesic effect of vibration and cooling on pain induced by intraneural electrical stimulation. Pain 18: 239–248

Birrell GJ, McQueen DS, Iggo A, Coleman RA, Grubb BD 1991 PGI_2-induced activation and sensitization of articular mechanonociceptors. Neuroscience Letters 124: 5–8

Birrell GJ, McQueen DS, Iggo A, Grubb BD 1993 Prostanoid-induced potentiation of the excitatory and sensitizing effects of bradykinin on articular mechanonociceptors in the rat ankle joint. Neuroscience 54: 537–544

Bischoff A 1979 Congenital insensitivity to pain with anhidrosis. A morphometric study of sural nerve and cutaneous receptors in the human prepuce. In: Bonica JJ, Liebeskind JC, Albe-Fessard DG (eds) Advances in pain research and therapy. 3. Raven Press, New York, pp 53–65

Bisgaard H, Kristensen JK 1985 Leukotriene B produces hyperalgesia in humans. Prostaglandins 30: 791–797

Bland-Ward PA, Humphrey PPA 1997 Acute nociception mediated by hindpaw P2X receptor activation in the rat. British Journal of Pharmacology 122: 365–371

Bleehen T, Keele CA 1977 Observations on the algogenic actions of adenosine compounds on the human blister base preparation. Pain 3: 367–377

Bleehen T, Hobbiger F, Keele CA 1976 Identification of algogenic substances in human erythrocytes. Journal of Physiology (London) 262: 131–149

Blumberg H, Jänig W 1982 Activation of fibers via experimentally produced stump neuromas of skin nerves: ephaptic transmission or retrograde sprouting. Experimental Neurology 76: 468–482

Blumberg H, Wallin BG 1987 Direct evidence of neurally mediated vasodilatation in hairy skin of the human foot. Journal of Physiology (London) 382: 105–121

Blumberg H, Haupt P, Jänig W, Kohler W 1983 Encoding of visceral noxious stimuli in the discharge patterns of visceral afferent fibres from the colon. Pflugers Archiv 398: 33–40

Bove GM, Moskowitz MA 1997 Primary afferent neurons innervating guinea pig dura. Journal of Neurophysiology 77: 299–308

Brain SD, Williams TJ, Tippins JR, Morris HR, MacIntyre I 1985 Calcitonin gene related peptide is a potent vasodilator. Nature 313: 54–56

Brain SD, Tippins JR, Morris HR, MacIntyre I, Williams T 1986 Potent vasodilator activity of calcitonin gene-related peptide in human skin. Journal of Investigative Dermatology 87: 533–536

Bromm B, Treede R-D 1984 Nerve fibre discharges, cerebral potentials and sensations induced by CO_2 laser stimulation. Human Neurobiology 3: 33–40

Burgess PR, Perl ER 1967 Myelinated afferent fibres responding specifically to noxious stimulation of the skin. Journal of Physiology (London) 190: 541–562

Burgess PR, Petit D, Warren RM 1968 Receptor types in cat hairy skin supplied by myelinated fibers. Journal of Neurophysiology 31: 833–848

Burnstock G 1996 A unifying purinergic hypothesis for the initiation of pain. Lancet 347: 1604–1605

Burnstock G 1997 The past, present and future of purine nucleotides as signaling molecules. Neuropharmacology 36: 1127–1139

Burstein R, Yamamura H, Malick A, Strassman A 1998 Chemical stimulation of the intracranial dura induces enhanced responses to facial stimulation in brain stem trigeminal neurons. Journal of Neurophysiology 79: 964–982

Buzzi MG, Moscowitz MA 1990 The antimigraine drug, sumatriptan (GR43175), selectively blocks neurogenic plasma extravasation from blood vessels in dura mater. British Journal of Pharmacology 99: 202–206

Byers MR 1984 Dental sensory receptors. International Review of Neurobiology 25: 39–94

Byers MR 1994 Dynamic plasticity of dental sensory nerve structure and cytochemistry. Archives of Oral Biology 39: 12S–21S

Campbell JN, LaMotte RH 1983 Latency to detection of first pain. Brain Research 266: 203–208

Campbell JN, Meyer RA 1983 Sensitization of unmyelinated nociceptive afferents in the monkey varies with skin type. Journal of Neurophysiology 49: 98–110

Campbell JN, Meyer RA 1986 Primary afferents and hyperalgesia. In: Yaksh TL (ed) Spinal afferent processing. Plenum, New York, pp 59–81

Campbell JN, Meyer RA, LaMotte RH 1979 Sensitization of myelinated nociceptive afferents that innervate monkey hand. Journal of Neurophysiology 42: 1669–1679

Campbell JN, Khan AA, Meyer RA, Raja SN 1988a Responses to heat of C-fiber nociceptors in monkey are altered by injury in the receptive field but not by adjacent injury. Pain 32: 327–332

Campbell JN, Raja SN, Meyer RA, Mackinnon SE 1988b Myelinated afferents signal the hyperalgesia associated with nerve injury. Pain 32: 89–94

Carlton SM, Coggeshall RE 1998 Nociceptive integration: does it have a peripheral component? Pain Forum 7: 71–78

Carlton SM, Hargett GL, Coggeshall RE 1995 Localization and activation of glutamate receptors in unmyelinated axons of rat glabrous skin. Neuroscience Letters 197: 25–28

Carpenter SE, Lynn B 1981 Vascular and sensory responses of human skin to mild injury after topical treatment with capsaicin. British Journal of Pharmacology 73: 755–758

Caterina MJ, Schumacher MA, Tominaga M, Rosen TA, Levine JD, Julius D 1998 The capsaicin receptor: a heat-activated ion channel in the pain pathway. Nature 389: 816–824

Cervero F 1982 Afferent activity evoked by natural stimulation of the biliary system in the ferret. Pain 13: 137–151

Cervero F 1983 Mechanisms of visceral pain. In: Lipton S, Miles J (eds) Persistent pain. Academic, London, pp 1–19

Cervero F 1994 Sensory innervation of the viscera: peripheral basis of visceral pain. Physiological Reviews 74: 95–138

Cervero F 1996 Visceral nociceptors. In: Belmonte C, Cervero F (eds) Neurobiology of nociceptors. Oxford University Press, Oxford, pp 220–240

Cervero F, Jänig W 1992 Visceral nociceptors: a new world order. Trends in Neurosciences 15: 374–378

Cervero F, Laird JMA 1996a Mechanisms of allodynia: interactions between sensitive mechanoreceptors and nociceptors. Neuroreport 7: 526–528

Cervero F, Laird JMA 1996b Mechanisms of touch-evoked pain (allodynia): a new model. Pain 68: 13–23

Cervero F, Sann H 1989 Mechanically evoked responses of afferent fibres innervating the guinea-pigs ureter an in vitro study. Journal of Physiology (London) 412: 245–266

Cervero F, Sharkey KA 1988 An electrophysical and anatomical study of intestinal afferent fibres in the rat. Journal of Physiology (London) 401: 381–397

Cervero F, Shouenborg J, Sjolund BH, Waddell PJ 1984 Cutaneous inputs to dorsal horn neurones in adult rats treated at birth with capsaicin. Brain Research 301: 47–57

Cervero F, Gilbert R, Hammond RGE, Tanner J 1993 Development of secondary hyperalgesia following non-painful thermal stimulation of the skin: a psychophysical study in man. Pain 54: 181–189

Cervero F, Meyer RA, Campbell JN 1994 A psychophysical study of secondary hyperalgesia: evidence for increased pain to input from nociceptors. Pain 58: 21–28

Cesare P, McNaughton P 1996 A novel heat-activated current in nociceptive neurons and its sensitization by bradykinin. Proceedings of the National Academy of Sciences USA 93: 15435–15439

Cesare P, McNaughton P 1997 Peripheral pain mechanisms. Current Opinion in Neurobiology 7: 493–499

Chabal C, Jacobson L, Russell LC, Burchiel KJ 1992 Pain response to perineuromal injection of normal saline, epinephrine, and lidocaine in humans. Pain 49: 9–12

Chen CC, Sivilotti LG, Colquhoun D, Burnstock G, Wood JN 1995a A P2X purinoceptor expressed by a subset of sensory neurons. Nature 377: 428–431

Chen X, Gallar J, Pozo MA, Baeza M, Belmonte C 1995b CO_2 stimulation of the cornea: a comparison between human sensation and nerve activity in polymodal nociceptive afferents of the cat. European Journal of Neuroscience 7: 1154–1163

Chen Y, Michaelis M, Janig W, Devor M 1996 Adrenoreceptor subtype mediating sympathetic-sensory coupling in injured sensory neurons. Journal of Neurophysiology 76: 3721–3730

Chen X, Belmonte C, Rang HP 1997 Capsaicin and carbon dioxide act by distinct mechanisms on sensory nerve terminals in the cat cornea. Pain 70: 23–29

Choi B, Rowbotham MC 1997 Effect of adrenergic receptor activation on post-herpetic neuralgia pain and sensory disturbances. Pain 69: 55–63

Chung JM, Lee DH, Chung K 1997 Strain differences in sympathetic dependency of neuropathic pain in a rat model. Society for Neuroscience Abstracts 23: 2356 (abstract)

Coffman JD 1966 The effect of aspirin on pain and hand flow responses to intra-arterial injection of bradykinin in man. Clinical Pharmacology and Therapeutics 7: 26–37

Coggeshall RE, Zhou ST, Carlton SM 1997 Opioid receptors on peripheral sensory axons. Brain Research 764: 126–132

Coleridge HM, Coleridge JCG 1980 Cardiovascular afferents involved in regulation of peripheral vessels. Annual Review of Physiology 42: 413–427

Coleridge HM, Coleridge JCG 1981 Afferent fibres involved in defence reflexes from the respiratory tract. In: Hutas I, Debreczeni LA (eds) Advances in physiological sciences. Pergamon, Budapest, pp 467–477

Coleridge JCG, Coleridge HM 1984 Afferent vagal C-fibre innervation of the lungs and airways and its functional significance. Review of Physiology Biochemistry and Pharmacology 99: 1–110

Cook SP, Vulchanova L, Hargreaves KM, Elde R, McCleskey EW 1997 Distinct ATP receptors on pain-sensing and stretch-sensing neurons. Nature 387: 505–508

Cooper B, Ahlquist M, Friedman RM, Labanc J 1991 Properties of high-threshold mechanoreceptors in the goat oral mucosa. II. Dynamic and static reactivity in carrageenan-inflamed mucosa. Journal of Neurophysiology 66: 1280–1290

Cormia FE, Dougherty JW 1960 Proteolytic activity in development of pain and itching: cutaneous reactions to bradykinin and kallikrein. Journal of Investigative Dermatology 35: 21–26

Couture R, Cuello AC, Henry JL 1985 Trigeminal antidromic vasodilation and plasma extravasation in the rat: effects of sensory, autonomic, and motor denervation. Brain Research 346: 108–114

Crea FM, Giuseppe P, Galassi AR et al 1990 A role of adenosine in pathogenesis of anginal pain. Circulation 81: 164–172

Crea F, Gaspardone A, Kaski JC, Davies G, Maseri A 1992 Relation between stimulation site of cardiac afferent nerves by adenosine and distribution of cardiac pain: results of a study in patients with stable angina. Journal of the American College of Cardiology 20: 1498–1502

Cunha FQ, Poole S, Lorenzetti BB, Ferreira SH 1992 The pivotal role of tumour necrosis factor α in the development of inflammatory hyperalgesia. British Journal of Pharmacology 107: 660–664

Dahl JB, Brennum J, Arendt-Nielsen L, Jensen TS, Kehlet H 1993 The effect of pre- versus postinjury infiltration with lidocaine on thermal and mechanical hyperalgesia after heat injury to the skin. Pain 53: 43–51

Darian-Smith I, Johnson KO, Dykes R 1973 'Cold' fiber population innervating palmar and digital skin of the monkey: responses to cooling pulses. Journal of Neurophysiology 36: 325–346

Darian-Smith I, Johnson KO, LaMotte C, Kenins P, Shigenaga Y, Ming VC 1979a Coding of incremental changes in skin temperature by single warm fibers in the monkey. Journal of Neurophysiology 42: 1316–1331

Darian-Smith I, Johnson KO, LaMotte C, Shigenaga Y, Kenins P, Champness P 1979b Warm fibers innervating palmar and digital skin of the monkey: responses to thermal stimuli. Journal of Neurophysiology 42: 1297–1315

Davidson EM, Coggeshall RE, Carlton SM 1997 Peripheral NMDA and non-NMDA glutamate receptors contribute to nociceptive behaviors in the rat formalin test. Neuroreport 8: 941–946

Davis KD, Treede R-D, Raja SN, Meyer RA, Campbell JN 1991 Topical application of clonidine relieves hyperalgesia in patients with sympathetically-maintained pain. Pain 47: 309–317

Davis KD, Meyer RA, Campbell JN 1993 Chemosensitivity and sensitization of nociceptive afferents that innervate the hairy skin of monkey. Journal of Neurophysiology 69: 1071–1081

Davis KD, Meyer RA, Turnquist JL, Filloon TG, Pappagallo M, Campbell JN 1995 Cutaneous injection of the capsaicin analogue, NE-21610, produces analgesia to heat but not to mechanical stimuli in man. Pain 61: 17–26

Delepine L, Aubineau P 1997 Plasma protein extravasation induced in the rat dura mater by stimulation of the parasympathetic sphenopalatine ganglion. Experimental Neurology 147: 389–400

Denzlinger C, Rapp S, Hagmann W, Keppler D 1985 Leukotrienes as mediators in tissue trauma. Science 230: 330–332

Devor M, Jänig W 1981 Activation of myelinated afferents ending in a neuroma by stimulation of the sympathetic supply in the rat. Neuroscience Letters 24: 43–47

Devor M, Jänig W, Michaelis M 1994 Modulation of activity in dorsal root ganglion neurons by sympathetic activation in nerve-injured rats. Journal of Neurophysiology 71: 38–47

DiRosa M, Giroud JP, Willoughby DA 1971 Studies of the mediators of the acute inflammatory response induced in rats in different sites by carrageenan and turpentine. Journal of Pathology 104: 15–29

Doak GJ, Sawynok J 1995 Complex role of peripheral adenosine in the genesis of the response to subcutaneous formalin in the rat. European Journal of Pharmacology 281: 311–318

Drummond PD 1995 Noradrenaline increases hyperalgesia to heat in skin sensitized by capsaicin. Pain 60: 311–315

Drummond PD 1996 Independent effects of ischaemia and noradrenaline on thermal hyperalgesia in capsaicin-treated skin. Pain 67: 129–133

Drummond PD, Skipworth S, Finch PM 1996 α_1-Andrenoceptors in normal and hyperalgesic human skin. Clinical Science 91: 73–77

Dubner R 1978 Neurophysiology of pain. Dental Clinics of North America 22: 11–30

Dubner R 1991 I. Introductory remarks: basic mechanisms of pain associated with deep tissues. Canadian Journal of Physiology and Pharmacology 69: 607–609

Dubner R, Hu JW 1977 Myelinated (A-delta) nociceptive afferents innervating the monkey's face. Journal of Dental Research 56: A167

Dubner R, Price DD, Beitel RE, Hu JW 1977 Peripheral neural correlates of behavior in monkey and human related to sensory-discriminative aspects of pain. In: Anderson DJ, Mathews B (eds) Pain in the trigeminal region. Elsevier North Holland, Amsterdam, pp 57–66

Ebertz JM, Hirshman CA, Kettelkamp NS, Uno H, Hanifin JM 1987 Substance P-induced histamine release in human cutaneous mast cells. Journal of Investigative Dermatology 88: 682–685

Ekblom A 1995 Some neurophysiological aspects of itch. Seminars in Dermatology 14: 262–270

Elliott MJ, Maini RN, Feldmann M et al 1994 Randomised double-blind comparison of chimeric monoclonal antibody to tumour necrosis factor α (cA2) versus placebo in rheumatoid arthritis. Lancet 344: 1105–1110

England S, Bevan S, Docherty RJ 1996 PGE_2 modulates the tetrodotoxin-resistant sodium current in neonatal rat dorsal root ganglion neurones via the cyclic AMP-protein kinase A cascade. Journal of Physiology 495: 429–440

Escott KJ, Brain SD 1993 Effect of a calcitionin gene-related peptide antagonist (CGRP8-37) on skin vasodilatation and oedema induced by stimulation of the rat saphenous nerve. British Journal of Pharmacology 110: 772–776

Ferreira SH 1983 Peripheral and central analgesia. In: Bonica JJ, Lindblom U, Iggo A (eds) Advances in pain research and therapy, vol 5. Raven, New York, pp 627–634

Ferreira SH, Moncada S, Vane JR 1971 Indomethacin and aspirin abolish prostaglandin release from the spleen. Nature 231: 237–239

Ferreira SH, Moncada S, Vane JR 1974 Proceedings: potentiation by prostaglandins of the nociceptive activity of bradykinin in the dog knee joint. British Journal of Pharmacology 50: 461P

Ferreira SH, Lorenzetti BB, Bristow AF, Poole S 1988 Interleukin-1β as a potent hyperalgesic agent antagonized by a tripeptide analogue. Nature 334: 698–700

Ferreira SH, Cunha FQ, Lorenzetti BB et al 1997 Role of lipocortin-1 in the antihyperalgesic actions of dexamethasone. British Journal of Pharmacology 121: 883–888

Fitzgerald M, Lynn B 1977 The sensitization of high threshold mechanoreceptors with myelinated axons by repeated heating. Journal of Physiology 265: 549–563

Fjallbrant N, Iggo A 1961 The effect of histamine, 5-hydroxytryptamine and acetylcholine on cutaneous afferent fibres. Journal of Physiology 156: 578–590

Floyd K, Hick VE, Morrison JFB 1977 Mechanosensitive afferent units in the hypogastric nerve of the cat. Journal of Physiology (London) 259: 457–471

Fock S, Mense S 1976 Excitatory effects of 5-hydroxytryptamine, histamine and potassium ions on muscular group IV afferent units: a comparison with bradykinin. Brain Research 105: 459–469

Freeman MAR, Wyke B 1967 The innervation of the knee joint. An anatomical and histological study in the cat. Journal of Anatomy 101: 505–532

Fukuoka H, Kawatani M, Hisamitsu T, Takeshige C 1994 Cutaneous hyperalgesia induced by peripheral injection of interleukin-1β in the rat. Brain Research 657: 133–140

Funakoshi M, Zotterman Y 1963 A study in the excitation of dental nerve fibers. In: Anderson DJ (ed) Sensory mechanism in dentine. Pergamon, Oxford

Gallar J, Pozo MA, Tuckett RP, Belmonte C 1993 Response of sensory units with unmyelinated fibres to mechanical, thermal and chemical stimulation of the cat's cornea. Journal of Physiology 468: 609–622

Gamse R, Holzer P, Lembeck F 1980 Decrease of substance P in primary afferent neurones and impairment of neurogenic plasma extravasation by capsaicin. British Journal of Pharmacology 68: 207–213

Garell PC, McGillis SLB, Greenspan JD 1996 Mechanical response properties of nociceptors innervating feline hairy skin. Journal of Neurophysiology 75: 1177–1189

Garnsworthy RK, Gully RL, Kenins P, Mayfield RJ, Westerman RA 1988 Identification of the physical stimulus and the neural basis of fabric-evoked prickle. Journal of Neurophysiology 59: 1083–1097

Garrison DW, Chandler MJ, Foreman RD 1992 Viscerosomatic convergence onto feline spinal neurons from esophagus, heart and somatic fields: effects of inflammation. Pain 49: 373–382

Gaspardone A, Crea F, Tomai F et al 1994 Substance P potentiates the algogenic effects of intraarterial infusion of adenosine. Journal of the American College of Cardiology 24: 477–482

Gaspardone A, Crea F, Tomai F et al 1995 Muscular and cardiac adenosine-induced pain is mediated by α_1 receptors. Journal of the American College of Cardiology 25: 251–257

Gebhart GF 1996 Visceral polymodal receptors. In: Kumazawa T, Kruger L, Mizumura K (eds) Progress in Brain Research. Elsevier, British Vancouver, pp 101–112

Gibbins IL, Wattchow D, Coventry B 1987 Two immunohistochemically identified populations of calcitonin gene-related peptide (CGRP)-immunoreactive axons in human skin. Brain Research 414: 143–148

Gold MS, Reichling DB, Shuster MJ, Levine JD 1996 Hyperalgesic agents increase a tetrodotoxin-resistant Na^+ current in nociceptors. Proceedings of the National Academy of Sciences USA 93: 1108–1112

Greaves MW, Wall PD 1996 Pathophysiology of itching. Lancet 348: 938–940

Greenspan JD, McGillis SLB 1994 Thresholds for the perception of pressure, sharpness, and mechanically evoked cutaneous pain: effects of laterality and repeated testing. Somatosensory and Motor Research 11: 311–317

Grigg P, Schaible HG, Schmidt RI 1986 Mechanical sensitivity of group III and IV afferents from posterior articular nerve in normal and inflamed cat knee. Journal of Neurophysiology 55: 635–643

Guzman F, Braun C, Lim RKS 1962 Visceral pain and the pseudaffective response to intra-arterial injection of bradykinin and other algesic agents. Archives of International Pharmacodynamics 136: 353–384

Gybels J, Handwerker HO, Van Hees J 1979 A comparison between the discharges of human nociceptive nerve fibers and the subjects ratings of his sensations. Journal of Physiology (London) 292: 193–206

Häbler H-J, Jänig W, Koltzenburg M 1987 Activation of unmyelinated afferents in chronically lesioned nerves by adrenaline and excitation of sympathetic efferents in the cat. Neuroscience Letters 82: 35–40

Häbler H-J, Jänig W, Koltzenburg M 1988 A novel type of unmyelinated chemosensitive nociceptor in the acutely inflamed urinary bladder. Agents and Actions 25: 219–221

Häbler H-J, Jänig W, Koltzenburg M 1990 Activation of unmyelinated afferent fibres by mechanical stimuli and inflammation of the urinary bladder in the cat. Journal of Physiology (London) 425: 545–562

Haegerstam G, Olgart L, Edwall L 1975 The excitatory action of acetylcholine on intradental sensory units. Acta Physiologica Scandinavica 93: 113–118

Hagbarth KE, Vallbo AB 1967 Mechanoreceptor activity recorded percutaneously with semimicroelectrodes in human peripheral nerves. Acta Physiologica Scandinavica 69: 121–122

Hagermark O, Hokfelt T, Pernow B 1978 Flare and itch induced by substance P in human skin. Journal of Investigative Dermatology 71: 233–235

Hammer K, Sann H, Pierau FK 1993 Functional properties of mechanosensitive units from the chicken ureter in vitro. Pflugers Archiv 425: 353–361

Handwerker HO 1976a Influences of algogenic substances and prostaglandins on the discharges of unmyelinated cutaneous nerve fibers identified as nociceptors. In: Bonica JJ, Albe-Fessard D (eds) Advances in pain research and therapy, vol 1. Raven, New York, pp 41–45

Handwerker HO 1976b Pharmacological modulation of the discharge of nociceptive C fibers. In: Zotterman Y (ed) Sensory functions of the skin in primates. Pergamon, Oxford, pp 427–439

Handwerker HO 1992 Pain and allodynia, itch and alloknesis: an alternative hypothesis. American Pain Society Journal 1: 135–138

Handwerker HO, Forster C, Kirchhoff C 1991a Discharge patterns of human C-fibers induced by itching and burning stimuli. Journal of Neurophysiology 66: 307–315

Handwerker HO, Kilo S, Reeh PW 1991b Unresponsive afferent nerve fibres in the sural nerve of the rat. Journal of Physiology 435: 229–242

Handwerker HO, Magerl W, Klemm F, Lang E, Westerman RA 1987 Quantitative evaluation of itch sensation. In: Schmidt RF, Schaible HG, Vahle-Hinz C (eds) Fine afferent nerve fibers and pain. Weinheim, New York, pp 461–473

Harris R, Griffin CJ 1968 Fine structure of nerve endings in the human dental pulp. Archives of Oral Biology 13: 773–778

Hassan AHS, Ableitner A, Stein C, Herz A 1993 Inflammation of the rat paw enhances axonal transport of opioid in the sciatic nerve and increases their density in the inflamed tissue. Neuroscience 55: 185–195

Haupt P, Jänig W, Kohler W 1983 Response pattern of visceral afferent fibres, supplying the colon, upon chemical and mechanical stimuli. Pflugers Archiv 398: 41–47

Helme RD, Koschorke GM, Zimmermann M 1986 Immunoreactive substance P release from skin nerves in the rat by noxious thermal stimulation. Neuroscience Letters 63: 295–299

Heppelmann B, Schaible HG, Schmidt RF 1985 Effects of prostaglandins E1 and E2 on the mechanosensitivity of group III afferents from normal and inflamed cat knee joints. In: Fields HL, Dubner R, Cervero F (eds) Advances in pain research and therapy, vol 9. Raven, New York, pp 91–102

Heppelmann B, Herbert MK, Schaible HG, Schmidt RF 1987 Morphological and physiological characteristics of the innervation of cats normal and arthritic knee joint. In: Pubols LS, Sessle BJ, Liss AR (eds) Effects of injury in trigeminal and spinal somatosensory system. Alan R Liss, New York, pp 19–27

Heppelmann B, Messlinger K, Neiss WF, Schmidt RF 1990 Ultrastructural three-dimensional reconstruction of group III and group IV sensory nerve endings ('free nerve endings') in the knee joint capsule of the cat: evidence for multiple receptive sites. Journal of Comparative Neurology 292: 103–116

Herbert MK, Schmidt RF 1992 Activation of normal and inflamed fine articular afferent units by serotonin. Pain 50: 79–80

Hiss E, Mense S 1976 Evidence for the existence of different receptor sites for algesic agents at the endings of muscular group IV afferent units. European Journal of Physiology 362: 141–146

Hnik P, Hudlicka O, Kuchera J, Payne R 1969 Activation of muscle afferents by nonproprioceptive stimuli. American Journal of Physiology 217: 1451–1458

Holland NR, Crawford TO, Hauer P, Cornblath DR, Griffin JW, McArthur JC 1998 Small-fiber sensory neuropathies: clinical course and neuropathology of idiopathic cases. Annals of Neurology 44: 47–59

Holzer P 1988 Local effector functions of capsaicin-sensitive sensory nerve endings: involvement of tachykinins, calcitonin gene-related peptide and other neuropeptides. Neuroscience 24: 739–768

Holzer P 1998 Neurogenic vasodilatation and plasma leakage in the skin. General Pharmacology 30: 5–11

Hsieh ST, Choi S, Lin W-M, Chang Y-C, McArthur JC, Griffin JW 1996 Epidermal denervation and its effects on keratinocytes and Langerhans cells. Journal of Neurocytology 25: 513–524

Hu S, Zhu J 1989 Sympathetic facilitation of sustained discharges of polymodal nociceptors. Pain 38: 85–90

Huang JH, Ali Z, Campbell JN, Meyer RA 1997 Pain ratings to punctate mechanical stimuli are similar through-out the zone of secondary hyperalgesia. Society for Neuroscience Abstracts 23: 1258

James TN, Rossi L, Hagerman GR 1988 On the pathogenesis of angina pectoris. Annals of Thoracic Surgery 41: 572–578

Jancso G, Kiraly E, Jansco-Gabor A 1977 Pharmacologically induced selective degeneration of chemosensitive primary sensory neurones. Nature 270: 741–743

Jancso N, Jansco-Gabor A, Szolcsányi J 1967 Direct evidence for neurogenic inflammation and its prevention by denervation and by pretreatment with capsaicin. British Journal of Pharmacology 31: 138–151

Jancso N, Jansco-Gabor A, Szolcsányi J 1968 The role of sensory nerve endings in neurogenic inflammation induced in human skin and in the eye and paw of the rat. British Journal of Pharmacology 32: 32–41

Jänig W, Koltzenburg M 1991a Receptive properties of pial afferents. Pain 45: 77–85

Jänig W, Koltzenburg M 1991b Receptive properties of sacral primary afferent neurons supplying the colon. Journal of Neurophysiology 65: 1067–1077

Jänig W, Lisney JW 1989 Small diameter myelinated afferents produce vasodilation but not plasma extravasation in rat skin. Journal of Physiology 415: 477–486

Jänig W, Morrison JFB 1986 Functional properties of spinal visceral afferents supplying abdominal and pelvic organs, with special emphasis on visceral nociception. In: Cervero F, Morrison JFB (eds) Progress in brain research: visceral sensation. Elsevier, Amsterdam, pp 87–114

Jänig W, Stanton-Hicks M (eds) 1996 Reflex sympathetic dystrophy – a reappraisal. ISAP, Seattle,

Jänig W, Levine JD, Michaelis M 1996 Interactions of sympathetic and primary afferent neurons following nerve injury and tissue trauma. In: Kumazawa T, Kruger L, Mizumura K (eds) The polymodal receptors Gateway to Pathological pain. Elsevier Science, Amsterdam pp 161–184

Johnson RD, Halata Z 1991 Topography and ultrastructure of sensory nerve endings in the glans penis of the rat. Journal of Comparative Neurology 312: 299–310

Johnson RD, Kitchell RL 1987 Mechanoreceptor response to mechanical and thermal stimuli in the glans penis of the dog. Journal of Neurophysiology 57: 1813–1836

Johnson KO, Darian-Smith I, LaMotte C, Johnson B, Oldfield S 1979 Coding of incremental changes in skin temperature by a monkey: correlation with intensity discrimination in man. Journal of Neurophysiology 42: 1332–1353

Jyväsjärvi E, Kniffki K-D 1989 Afferent C fibre innervation of cat tooth pulp: confirmation by electrophysiological methods. Journal of Physiology 411: 663–675

Karlsten R, Gordh T, Post C 1992 Local antinociceptive and hyperalgesic effects in the formalin test after peripheral administration of adenosine analogues in mice. Pharmacology and Toxicology 70: 434–438

Kaufman MP, Baker DG, Coleridge HM, Coleridge JC 1980 Stimulation by bradykinin of afferent vagal C-fibers with chemosensitive endings in the heart and aorta of the dog. Circulation Research 46: 476–484

Kenins P 1988 The functional anatomy of the receptive fields of rabbit C polymodal nociceptors. Journal of Neurophysiology 59: 1098–1115

Kenshalo DR, Childers BP, Webb R 1960 Comparison of thermal sensitivity of the forehead, lip, conjunctiva, and cornea. Journal of Applied Physiology 15: 987–991

Khan AA, Meyer RA, Campbell JN 1987 Responses of unmyelinated nociceptive afferents to histamine. Society for Neuroscience Abstracts 13: 214.10 (abstract)

Khan AA, Raja SN, Manning DC, Campbell JN, Meyer RA 1992 The effects of bradykinin and sequence-related analogs on the response properties of cutaneous nociceptors in monkeys. Somatosensory Motor Research 9: 97–106

Kieschke J, Mense S, Prabhakar NR 1988 Influence of adrenaline and hypoxia on rat muscle receptors in vitro. In: Hamann W, Iggo A (eds) Progress in brain research, vol 74. Elsevier Science Publishers, British Vancouver, pp 91–97

Kilo S, Schmelz M, Koltzenburg M, Handwerker HO 1994 Different patterns of hyperalgesia induced by experimental inflammation in human skin. Brain 117: 385–396

Kim SH, Chung JM 1991 Sympathectomy alleviates mechanical allodynia in an experimental animal model for neuropathy in the rat. Neuroscience Letters 134: 131–134

Kindgen-Milles D, Klement W, Arndt JO (1994) The nociceptive systems of skin, paravascular tissue and hand veins of humans and their sensitivity to bradykinin. Neuroscience Letters 181: 39–42

Kinnman E, Levine JD 1995 Sensory and sympathetic contributions to nerve injury-induced sensory abnormalities in the rat. Neuroscience 64: 751–767

Kinnman E, Nygårds EB, Hansson P 1997 Peripheral α-adrenoreceptors are involved in the development of capsaicin induced ongoing and stimulus evoked pain in humans. Pain 69: 79–85

Kitchell RL, Gilanpour H, Johnson RD 1982 Electrophysiologic studies of penile mechanoreceptors in the rats. Experimental Neurology 75: 229–244

Kjartansson J, Dalsgaard CJ, Jonsson CE 1987 Decreased survival of experimental critical flaps in rats after sensory denervation with capsaicin. Plastic and Reconstructive Surgery 79: 218–221

Klassen KP, Morton DR, Curtis GM 1951 The clinical physiology of the human bronchi. III. The effect of the vagus section on the cough reflex, bronchial caliber and clearance of bronchial secretions. Surgery 29: 483–490

Klement W, Arndt JO 1992 The role of nociceptors of cutaneous veins in the mediation of cold pain in man. Journal of Physiology (London) 449: 73–83

Koda H, Minagawa M, Si-Hong L, Mizumura K, Kumazawa T 1996 H_1-receptor-mediated excitation and facilitation of the heat response by histamine in canine visceral polymodal receptors studied in vitro. Journal of Neurophysiology 76: 1396–1404

Kolston J, Lisney SJW 1993 A study of vasodilator responses evoked by antidromic stimulation of A delta afferent fibers supplying normal and reinnervated rat skin. Microvascular Research 46: 143–147

Koltzenburg M 1996 Afferent mechanisms mediating pain and hyperalgesias in neuralgia. In: Janig W, Stanton-Hicks M (eds) Reflex sympathetic dystrophy – a reappraisal. ISAP Hicks, Seattle, pp 123–150

Koltzenburg M, Handwerker HO 1994 Differential ability of human cutaneous nociceptors to signal mechanical pain and to produce vasodilatation. Journal of Neuroscience 14: 1756–1765

Koltzenburg M, Kress M, Reeh PW 1992a The nociceptor sensitization by bradykinin does not depend on sympathetic neurons. Neuroscience 46: 465–473

Koltzenburg M, Lundberg LER, Torebjörk HE 1992b Dynamic and static components of mechanical hyperalgesia in human hairy skin. Pain 51: 207–219

Koltzenburg M, McMahon SB 1986 Plasma extravasation in the rat urinary bladder following mechanical, electrical and chemical stimuli: evidence for a new population of chemosensitive primary sensory afferents. Neuroscience Letters 72: 352–356

Konietzny F, Hensel H 1975 Warm fiber activity in human skin nerves. European Journal of Physiology 359: 265–267

Koppert W, Reeh PW, Handwerker HO 1993 Conditioning of histamine by bradykinin alters responses of rat nociceptor and human itch sensation. Neuroscience Letters 152: 117–120

Kress M, Koltzenburg M, Reeh PW, Handwerker HO 1992 Responsiveness and functional attributes of electrically localized terminals of cutaneous C-fibers in vivo and in vitro. Journal of Neurophysiology 68: 581–595

Kruger L 1988 Morphological features of thin sensory afferent fibers: a new interpretation of 'nociceptor' function. In: Hamann W, Iggo A (eds) Progress in brain research, vol 74. Elsevier Science Publishers, British Vancouver, pp 253–257

Kruger L 1996 The functional morphology of thin sensory axons: some principles and problems. In: Kumazawa T, Kruger L, Mizumura K (eds) The polymodal receptor: a gateway to pathological pain. Elsevier, Amsterdam, pp 255–272

Kruger L, Perl ER, Sedivec MJ 1981 Fine structure of myelinated mechanical nociceptor endings in cat hairy skin. Journal of Comparative Neurology 198: 137–154

Kuby J 1994 Immunology. In: Kuby J (ed) Immunology, 2nd edn. WH Freeman, New York, pp 297–322

Kumazawa T 1993 Involvement of EP_3 subtype of prostaglandin E receptors in PGE_2 induced enhancement of the bradykinin response of nociceptors. Brain Research 632: 321–324

Kumazawa T, Mizumura K 1976 The polymodal C-fiber receptor in the muscle of the dog. Brain Research 101: 589–593

Kumazawa T, Perl ER 1977a Primate cutaneous receptors with unmyelinated (C) fibres and their projection to the substantia gelatinosa. Journal of Physiology (Paris) 73: 287–304

Kumazawa T, Perl ER 1977b Primate cutaneous sensory units with unmyelinated (C) afferent fibers. Journal of Neurophysiology 40: 1325–1338

Kumazawa T, Mizumura K, Minagawa M, Tsujii Y 1991 Sensitizing effects of bradykinin on the heat responses of the visceral nociceptor. Journal of Neurophysiology 66: 1819–1824

Kumazawa T, Mizumura K, Koda H, Fukusako H 1996 EP receptor subtypes implicated in the PGE_2-induced sensitization of polymodal receptors in response to bradykinin and heat. Journal of Neurophysiology 75: 2361–2368

Lam FY, Ferrell WR 1991 Specific neurokinin receptors mediate plasma extravasation in the rat knee joint. British Journal of Pharmacology 103: 1263–1267

LaMotte RH 1992 Subpopulations of 'nocifensor neurons' contributing to pain and allodynia, itch and alloknesis. American Pain Society Journal 2: 115–126

LaMotte RH, Campbell JN 1978 Comparison of responses of warm and nociceptive C-fiber afferents in monkey with human judgements of thermal pain. Journal of Neurophysiology 41: 509–528

LaMotte RH, Thalhammer JG 1982 Response properties of high-threshold cutaneous cold receptors in the primate. Brain Research 244: 279–287

LaMotte RH, Thalhammer JG, Torebjörk HE, Robinson CJ 1982 Peripheral neural mechanisms of cutaneous hyperalgesia following mild injury by heat. Journal of Neuroscience 2: 765–781

LaMotte RH, Thalhammer JG, Robinson CJ 1983 Peripheral neural correlates of magnitude of cutaneous pain and hyperalgesia: a comparison of neural events in monkey with sensory judgements in human. Journal of Neurophysiology 50: 1–26

LaMotte RH, Shain CN, Simone DA, Tsai E-FP 1991 Neurogenic hyperalgesia: psychophysical studies of underlying mechanisms. Journal of Neurophysiology 66: 190–211

Lang E, Novak A, Reeh PW, Handwerker HO 1990 Chemosensitivity of fine afferents from rat skin in vitro. Journal of Neurophysiology 63: 887–901

Langford LA, Schmidt RF 1983 Afferent and efferent axons in the medial and posterior articular nerves of the cat. Anatomical Record 206: 71–78

Lawand NB, Willis WD, Westlund KN 1997 Excitatory amino acid receptor involvement in peripheral nociceptive transmission in rats. European Journal of Pharmacology 324: 169–177

Ledent C, Vaugeois J-M, Schiffmann SN et al 1997 Aggressiveness, hypoalgesia and high blood pressure in mice lacking the adenosine A_{2a} receptor. Nature 388: 674–678

Lee MG, Sullivan SN, Watson WC, Melendez L 1985 Chest pain – esophageal disease. Gastroenterology 29: 719–743

Lele PP, Weddell G 1959 Sensory nerves of the cornea and cutaneous sensibility. Experimental Neurology 1: 334–359

Lembeck F, Donnerer J 1992 The non-peptide tachykinin antagonist, CP-96,345, is a potent inhibitor of neurogenic inflammation. British Journal of Pharmacology 105: 527–530

Lembeck F, Gamse R 1982 Substance P in peripheral sensory processes. CIBA Foundation Symposium 91: 35–54

Lembeck F, Holzer P 1979 Sustance P as neurogenic mediator of antidromic vasodilation and neurogenic plasma extravasation. Naunyn-Schmiedebergs Archives of Pharmacology 310: 175–183

Levine JD, Clark R, Devor M, Helms C, Moskowitz MA, Basbaum AI 1984a Intraneuronal substance P contributes to the severity of experimental arthritis. Science 226: 547–549

Levine JD, Lau W, Kwiat G, Goetzl EJ 1984b Leukotriene B4 produces hyperalgesia that is dependent on polymorphonuclear leukocytes. Science 225: 743–745

Levine JD, Dardick SJ, Basbaum AI, Scipio E 1985 Reflex neurogenic inflammation. I. Contribution of the peripheral nervous system to spatially remote inflammatory responses that follow injury. Journal of Neuroscience 5: 1380–1386

Levine JD, Dardick SJ, Roizen MF, Helms C, Basbaum AI 1986a Contribution of sensory afferents and sympathetic efferents to joint injury in experimental arthritis. Journal of Neuroscience 6: 3423–3429

Levine JD, Taiwo YO, Collins SD, Tam JK 1986b Noradrenaline hyperalgesia is mediated through interaction with sympathetic postganglionic neurone terminals rather than activation of primary afferent nociceptors. Nature 323: 158–160

Levine JD, Coderre TJ, Basbaum AI 1988 The peripheral nervous system and the inflammatory process. In: Dubner R, Gebhart GF, Bond MR (eds) Pain research and clinical management, vol 3. Elsevier, Amsterdam, pp 33–43

Lewis C, Neidhart S, Holy C, North RA, Buell G, Surprenant A 1995 Coexpression of $P2X_2$ and $P2X_3$ receptor subunits can account for ATP-gated currents in sensory neurons. Nature 377: 432–435

Lewis T 1935 Experiments relating to cutaneous hyperalgesia and its spread through somatic fibres. Clinical Science 2: 373–423

Lewis T 1937 The nocifensor system of nerves and its reactions. British Medical Journal 431–435

Lewis T 1942 Pain. Macmillan, New York

Lewis T, Pochin EE 1937 The double pain response of the human skin to a single stimulus. Clinical Science 3: 67–76

Lim RKS, Miller DG, Guzman F et al 1967 Pain and analgesia evaluated by intraperitoneal bradykinin-evoked pain method in man. Clinical Pharmacology and Therapeutics 8: 521–542

Liu M, Parada S, Rowan JS, Bennett GJ 1996 The sympathetic nervous system contributes to capsaicin-evoked mechanical allodynia but not pinprick hyperalgesia in humans. Journal of Neuroscience 16: 7331–7335

Lombardi F, Della BP, Casati R, Malliani A 1981 Effects of intracoronary administration of bradykinin on the impulse activity of afferent sympathetic unmyelinated fibers with left ventricular endings in the cat. Circulation Research 48: 69–75

Longhurst JC, Dittman LE 1987 Hypoxia, bradykinin, and prostaglandins stimulate ischemically sensitive visceral afferents. American Journal of Physiology 253: H556–H567

Lunberg JM 1993 Capsaicin-sensitive nerves in the airways – implications for protective reflexes and disease. In: Wood JN (ed) Neuroscience perspectives: capsaicin in the study of pain. Academic, London, pp 219–227

Lundberg JM, Saria A 1987 Polypeptide-containing neurons in airway smooth muscle. Annual Review of Physiology 49: 557–572

Lynn B 1996 Efferent function of nociceptors. In: Belmonte C, Cervero F (eds) Neurobiology of nociceptors. Oxford University Press, Oxford, pp 418–438

Lynn B, Shakhanbeh J 1988 Neurogenic inflammation in the skin of the rabbit. Agents and Actions 25: 228–230

Ma QP, Woolf CJ 1996 Progressive tactile hypersensitivity: an inflammation-induced incremental increase in the excitability of the spinal cord. Pain 67: 97–106

Macfarlane R, Moskowitz MA, Sakas DE, Tasdemiroglu E, Wei EP, Kontos HA 1991 The role of neuroeffector mechanisms in cerebral hyperfusion syndromes. Journal of Neurosurgery 75: 845–855

Magerl W, Wilk SH, Treede R-D 1998 Secondary hyperalgesia and perceptual wind-up following intradermal injection of capsaicin in humans. Pain 74: 257–268

Maggi CA, Meli A 1988 The sensory-efferent function of capsaicin-sensitive sensory neurons. General Pharmacology 19: 1–43

Maggi CA, Patacchini R, Rovero P, Giachetti A 1993 Tachykinin receptors and tachykinin receptor antagonists. Journal of Autonomic Pharmacology 13: 23–93

Malliani A, Pagani M, Lombardi F 1984 Visceral versus somatic mechanisms. In: Wall PD, Melzack R (eds) Textbook of pain. Churchill Livingstone, Edinburgh, pp 100–109

Malliani A, Lombardi F, Pagani M 1986 Sensory innervation of the heart. In: Cervero F, Morrison JFB (eds) Progress in brain research: visceral sensation. Elsevier, Amsterdam, pp 39–48

Manning DC, Raja SN, Meyer RA, Campbell JN 1991 Pain and hyperalgesia after intradermal injection of bradykinin in humans. Clinical Pharmacology and Therapy 50: 721–729

Markowitz S, Saito K, Moskowitz MA 1987 Neurogenically mediated leakage of plasma proteins occurs from blood vessels of dura mater in the rat brain. Journal of Neuroscience 7: 4129–4136

Martin HA, Basbaum AI, Kwiat GC, Goetzl EJ, Levine JD 1987 Leukotriene and prostaglandin sensitization of cutaneous high-threshold C- and A-delta mechanonociceptors in the hairy skin of rat hindlimbs. Neuroscience 22: 651–659

Martling CR 1987 Sensory nerves containing tachykinins and CGRP in the lower airways. Functional implications for bronchoconstriction, vasodilatation and protein extravasation. Acta Physiologica Scandinavica Supplement 563: 1–57

Mathews B 1976 Coupling between cutaneous nerves. Journal of Physiology 254: 37P–38P

Mathews B 1977 Responses of intradental nerves to electrical and thermal stimulation of teeth in dogs. Journal of Physiology (London) 264: 641–664

Mayberg M, Langer RS, Zervas NT, Moskowitz MA 1981 Perivascular meningeal projections from cat trigeminal ganglia: possible pathway for vascular headaches in man. Science 213: 228–230

McCloskey DI, Mitchell JH 1972 Reflex cardiovascular and respiratory responses originating in exercising muscle. Journal of Physiology (London) 224: 173–186

McMahon SB, 1988 Neuronal and behavioural consequences of chemical inflammation of rat urinary bladder. Agents and Actions 25: 231–233

McMahon SB, Abel C 1987 A model for the study of visceral pain states: chronic inflammation of the chronic decerebrate rat urinary bladder by irritant chemicals. Pain 28: 109–127

McMahon S, Koltzenburg M 1990 The changing role of primary afferent neurones in pain. Pain 43: 269–272

McMahon SB, Koltzenburg M 1992 Itching for an explanation. Trends in Neuroscience 15: 497–501

McMahon SB, Bennett DLH, Koltzenburg M 1997 The biological effects of nerve growth factor on primary sensory neurons. In: Borsook D (ed) Molecular neurobiology of pain, vol 9. ISAP Press, Seattle, pp 59–78

Mei N 1983 Sensory structures in the viscera. In: Ottoson D (ed) Sensory physiology 4. Springer-Verlag, New York, pp 2–42

Meller ST, Gebhart GF 1992 A critical review of the afferent pathways and the potential chemical mediators involved in cardiac pain. Neuroscience 48: 501–524

Melmon KL, Webster ME, Goldfinger SE, Seegmiller JE 1967 The presence of a kinin in inflammatory synovial effusion from arthritides of varying etiologies. Arthritis and Rheumatism 10: 13–20

Mendell LM, Wall P 1965 Responses of single dorsal cord cells to peripheral cutaneous unmyelinated fibres. Nature 206: 97–99

Mengel MKC, Jyväsjärvi E, Kniffki K-D 1992 Identification and characterization of afferent periodontal C fibres in the cat. Pain 48: 413–420

Mense S 1977 Muscular nociceptors. Journal of Physiology 73: 233–240

Mense S 1981 Sensitization of group IV muscle receptors to bradykinin by 5-hydroxytryptamine and prostaglandin E2. Brain Research 225: 95–105

Mense S 1996 Nociceptors in skeletal muscle and their reaction to pathological tissue changes. In: Belmonte C, Cervero F (eds) Neurobiology of nociceptors. Oxford University Press, Oxford, pp 184–201

Mense S, Meyer H 1985 Different types of slowly conducting afferent units in cat skeletal muscle and tendon. Journal of Physiology (London) 363: 403–417

Mense S, Schmidt RF 1974 Activation of group IV afferent units from muscle by algesic agents. Brain Research 72: 305–310

Meyer RA, Campbell JN 1981a Myelinated nociceptive afferents account for the hyperalgesia that follows a burn to the hand. Science 213: 1527–1529

Meyer RA, Campbell JN 1981b Peripheral neural coding of pain sensation. Johns Hopkins APL Technical Digest 2: 164–171

Meyer RA, Campbell JN 1987 Coupling between unmyelinated peripheral nerve fibers does not involve sympathetic efferent fibers. Brain Research 437: 181–182

Meyer RA, Campbell JN, Raja SN 1985a Peripheral neural mechanisms of cutaneous hyperalgesia. In: Fields HL, Dubner R, Cervero F (eds) Advances in pain research and therapy, vol 9. Raven, New York, pp 53–71

Meyer RA, Raja SN, Campbell JN 1985b Coupling of action potential activity between unmyelinated fibers in the peripheral nerve of monkey. Science 227: 184–187

Meyer RA, Raja SN, Campbell JN, Mackinnon SE, Dellon AL 1985c Neural activity originating from a neuroma in the baboon. Brain Research 325: 255–260

Meyer RA, Campbell JN, Raja SN 1988 Antidromic nerve stimulation in monkey does not sensitize unmyelinated nociceptors to heat. Brain Research 441: 168–172

Meyer RA, Davis KD, Cohen RH, Treede R-D, Campbell JN 1991 Mechanically insensitive afferents (MIAs) in cutaneous nerves of monkey. Brain Research 561: 252–261

Meyer RA, Magerl W, Campbell JN, Fuchs PN 1998 Normal punctate hyperalgesia in capsaicin desensitized skin. Society for Neuroscience Abstracts 24: 2086

Micevych PE, Kruger L 1992 The status of calcitonin gene-related peptide as an effector peptide. Annals of the New York Academy of Sciences 657: 379–396

Michaelis M, Devor M, Jänig W 1996 Sympathetic modulation of activity in rat dorsal root ganglion neurons changes over time following peripheral nerve injury. Journal of Neurophysiology 76: 753–763

Mizumura K, Sato J, Kumazawa T 1987 Effects of prostaglandins and other putative chemical intermediaries on the activity of canine testicular polymodal receptors studied in vitro. Pflugers Archiv 408: 565–572

Mizumura K, Minagawa M, Tsujii Y, Kumazawa T 1990 The effects of bradykinin agonists and antagonists on visceral polymodal receptor activities. Pain 40: 221–227

Mizumura K, Sato J, Kumazawa T 1991 Comparison of the effects of prostaglandins E_2 and I_2 on testicular nociceptor activities studied in vitro. Naunyn-Schmiedebergs Archives of Pharmacology 344: 368–376

Mizumura K, Sato J, Kumazawa T 1992 Strong heat stimulation sensitizes the heat response as well as the bradykinin response of visceral polymodal receptors. Journal of Neurophysiology 68: 1209–1215

Mizumura K, Minagawa M, Koda H, Kumazawa T 1994 Histamine-induced sensitization of the heat response of canine visceral polymodal receptors. Neuroscience Letters 168: 93–96

Mizumura K, Minagawa M, Koda H, Kumazawa T 1995 Influence of histamine on the bradykinin response of canine testicular polymodal receptors in vitro. Inflammation Research 44: 376–378

Mizumura K, Koda H, Kumazawa T 1996 Opposite effects of increased intracellular cyclic AMP on the heat and bradykinin responses of canine visceral polymodal receptors in vitro. Neuroscience Research 25: 335–341

Moskowitz MA 1991 The visceral organ brain: implications for the pathophysiology of vascular head pain. Neurology 41: 182–186

Moskowitz MA, Macfarlane R 1993 Neurovascular and molecular mechanisms in migraine headaches. Cerebrovascular and Brain Metabolism Reviews 5: 159–177

Moskowitz MA, Brody M, Liu-Chen L-Y 1983 In vitro release of immuno-reactive substance P from putative afferent nerve endings in bovine pia-arachnoid. Neuroscience 9: 809–814

Moskowitz MA, Buzzi MG, Sakas DE, Linnik MD 1989 Pain mechanisms underlying vascular headaches. Revue Neurologique (Paris) 145: 181–193

Nair PN 1995 Neural elements in dental pulp and dentin. Oral Surgery, Oral Medicine, Oral Radiology and Endodentics 80: 710–719

Nakano T, Taira N 1976 5-Hydroxytryptamine as a sensitizer of somatic nociceptors for pain-producing substances. European Journal of Pharmacology 38: 23–29

Närhi MVO 1985a Dentin sensitivity: a review. Journal de Biologie Buccale 13: 75–96

Närhi MVO 1985b The characteristics of intradental sensory units and their responses to stimulation. Journal of Dental Research 64 (special issue): 564–571

Närhi MVO, Jyväsjärvi E, Hirvonen T, Huopaniemi T 1982 Activation of heat-sensitive nerve fibers in the dental pulp of the cat. Pain 14: 317–326

Neil A, Attal N, Guilbaud G 1991 Effects of guanethidine on sensitization to natural stimuli and self-mutilating behaviour in rats with a peripheral neuropathy. Brain Research 565: 237–246

Ness TJ, Gebhart GF 1988 Colorectal distension as a noxious visceral stimulus: physiologic and pharmacologic characterization of pseudaffective reflexes in the rat. Brain Research 450: 153–169

Ness TJ, Gebhart GF 1990 Visceral pain: a review of experimental studies. Pain 41: 167–234

Neugebauer V, Schaible H-G 1988 Peripheral and spinal components of the sensitization of spinal neurons during an acute experimental arthritis. Agents and Actions 25: 234–236

Nilsson J, von Euler AM, Dalsgaard C-J 1985 Stimulation of connective tissue cell growth by substance P and substance K. Nature 315: 61–63

Noordenbos W 1959 Pain. Elsevier, Amsterdam, pp 1–182

Nordin M 1990 Low-threshold mechanoreceptive and nociceptive units with unmyelinated (C) fibres in the human supraorbital nerve. Journal of Physiology (London) 426: 229–240

O'Connor TP, van der Kooy D 1986 Pattern of intracranial and extracranial projections of trigeminal ganglion cells. Journal of Neuroscience 6: 2200–2207

Ochoa J, Mair WGP 1969 The normal sural nerve in man. I. Ultrastructure and numbers of fibers and cells. Acta Neuropathologica (Berlin) 13: 197–216

Ochoa JL, Torebjörk HE 1983 Sensations evoked by intraneural microstimulation of single mechanoreceptor units innervating the human hand. Journal of Physiology (London) 342: 633–654

Pagani M, Pizzinelli P, Furlan R et al 1985 Analysis of the pressor sympathetic reflex produced by intracoronary injections of bradykinin in conscious dogs. Circulation Research 56: 175–183

Paintal AS 1955 Impulses in vagal afferent fibres from specific pulmonary deflation receptors. The response of these receptors to phenyl diguanide, potato starch, 5-hydroxytryptamine and nicotine, and their role in respiratory and cardiovascular reflexes. Quarterly Journal of Experimental Physiology 40: 89–111

Paintal AS 1960 Functional analysis of group III afferent fibers of mammalian muscle. Journal of Physiology (London) 152: 250–270

Paintal AS 1961 Participation by pressure-pain receptors of mammalian muscles in the flexion reflex. Journal of Physiology (London) 156: 498–514

Paintal AS 1986 The visceral sensations – some basic mechanisms. Progress in Brain Research 67: 3–19

Pan HL, Longhurst JC 1996 Ischaemia-sensitive sympathetic afferents innervating the gastrointestinal tract function as nociceptors in cats. Journal of Physiology 492: 841–850

Pan HL, Stahl GL, Longhurst JC 1995 Differential effect of 5- and 15-lipoxygenase products on ischemically sensitive abdominal visceral afferents. American Journal of Physiology 269: H96–H105

Pappagallo M, Gaspardone A, Tomai F, Iamele M, Crea F, Gioffre PA 1993 Analgesic effect of bamiphylline on pain induced by intradermal injection of adenosine. Pain: 199–204

Pedersen-Bjergaard U, Nielsen LB, Jensen K, Edvinsson L, Jansen I, Olesen J 1991 Calcitonin gene-related peptide, neurokinin A and substance P: effects on nociception and neurogenic inflammation in human skin and temporal muscle. Peptides 12: 333–337

Pedersen JL, Crawford ME, Dahl JB, Brennum J, Kehlet H 1996 Effect of preemptive nerve block on inflammation and hyperalgesia after human thermal injury. Anesthesiology 84: 1020–1026

Pedersen J, Andersen OK, Arendt-Nielsen L, Kehlet H 1998 Hyperalgesia and temporal summation of pain after heat injury in man. Pain 74: 189–197

Peppel P, Anton F 1993 Responses of rat medullary dorsal horn neurons following intranasal noxious chemical stimulation: effects of stimulus intensity, duration, and interstimulus interval. Journal of Neurophysiology 70: 2260–2275

Perl ER 1968 Myelinated afferent fibres innervating the primate skin and their response to noxious stimuli. Journal of Physiology (London) 197: 593–615

Petersen M, Zhang J, Zhang JM, LaMotte RH 1996 Abnormal spontaneous activity and responses to norepinephrine in dissociated dorsal root ganglion cells after chronic nerve constriction. Pain 67: 391–397

Pinter E, Szolcsanyi J 1995 Plasma extravasation in the skin and pelvic organs evoked by antidromic stimulation of the lumbosacral dorsal roots of the rat. Neuroscience 68: 603–614

Piotrowski W, Foreman JC 1986 Some effects of calcitonin gene-related peptide in human skin and on histamine release. British Journal of Dermatology 114: 37–46

Price DD 1972 Characteristics of second pain and flexion reflexes indicative of prolonged central summation. Experimental Neurology 37: 371–387

Price DD, Hu JW, Dubner R, Gracely RH 1977 Peripheral suppression of first pain and central summation of second pain evoked by noxious heat pulses. Pain 3: 57–68

Przewlocki R, Hassan AHS, Lason W, Epplen C, Herz A, Stein C 1992 Gene expression and localization of opioid peptides in immune cells of inflamed tissue: functional role in antinociception. Neuroscience 48: 491–500

Raja SN, Abatzis V, Hocasek SJ, Frank S 1998 Role of α-adrenoceptors in neuroma pain in amputees. American Society of Anesthesiology 89(3A):.A1082
Raja SN, Campbell JN, Meyer RA 1984 Evidence for different mechanisms of primary and secondary hyperalgesia following heat injury to the glabrous skin. Brain 107: 1179–1188
Raja SN, Treede R-D, Davis KD, Campbell JN 1991 Systemic alpha-adrenergic blockade with phentolamine: a diagnostic test for sympathetically maintained pain. Anesthesiology 74: 691–698
Ramnarine SI, Hirayama Y, Barnes PJ, Rogers DF 1994 'Sensory-efferent' neural control of mucus secretion: characterization using tachykinin receptor antagonists in ferret trachea in vitro. British Journal of Pharmacology 113: 1183–1190
Reeh PW, Kress M 1998 Boole's algebra and the gordian knot in peripheral nociception. Pain Forum 7: 84–86
Reeh PW, Sauer SK 1997 Chronic aspects in peripheral nociception. In: Jensen TS, Turner JA, Wiesenfeld-Hallin Z (eds) Progress in pain research and management, 8. IASP, Seattle, pp 115–131
Reeh PW, Kocher L, Jung S 1986 Does neurogenic inflammation alter the sensitivity of unmyelinated nociceptors in the rat? Brain Research 384: 42–50
Reeh PW, Bayer J, Kocher L, Handwerker HO 1987 Sensitization of nociceptive cutaneous nerve fibers from the rat tail by noxious mechanical stimulation. Experimental Brain Research 65: 505–512
Rees H, Sluka KA, Westlund KN, Willis WD 1995 The role of glutamate and GABA receptors in the generation of dorsal root reflexes by acute arthritis in the anaesthetized rat. Journal of Physiology (London) 484: 437–446
Richardson BP, Engel G 1986 The pharmacology and function of 5-HT3 receptors. Trends in Neurosciences 9: 424–427
Richter JE, Bradley LA, Castell DO 1989 Esophageal chest pain: current controversies in pathogenesis, diagnosis, and therapy. Annals of Internal Medicine 110: 66–78
Ringkamp M, Peng YB, Campbell JN, Meyer RA 1997 Intradermal capsaicin produces a vigorous discharge in mechanically-insensitive A-fiber nociceptors of the monkey. Society for Neuroscience Abstracts 23: 1258
Roberts WJ, Elardo SM 1985a Sympathetic activation of A-delta nociceptors. Somatosensory Research 3: 33–44
Roberts WJ, Elardo SM 1985b Sympathetic activation of unmyelinated mechanoreceptors in cat skin. Brain Research 339: 123–125
Rocha e Silva M, Rosenthal SR 1961 Release of pharmacologically active substances from the rat skin in vivo following thermal injury. Journal of Pharmacology and Experimental Therapeutics 132: 110–116
Rozsa AJ, Beuerman RW 1982 Density and organization of free nerve endings in the corneal epithelium of the rabbit. Pain 14: 105–120
Rubin G, Kaspi T, Rappaport ZH et al 1997 Adrenosensitivity of injured afferent neurons does not require the presence of postganglionic sympathetic terminals. Pain 72: 183–191 (abstract)
Rueff A, Dray A 1993 Sensitization of peripheral afferent fibres in the in vitro neonatal rat spinal cord-tail by bradykinin and prostaglandins. Neuroscience 54: 527–535
Saito K, Markowitz S, Moskowitz MA 1988 Ergot alkaloids block neurogenic extravasation in dura mater: proposed action in vascular headaches. Annals of Neurology 24: 732–737
Sang CN, Gracely RH, Max MB, Bennett GJ 1996 Capsaicin-evoked mechanical allodynia and hyperalgesia cross nerve territories – evidence for a central mechanism. Anesthesiology 85: 491–496
Sant'Ambrogio G 1987 Nervous receptors of the tracheobronchial tree. Annual Review of Physiology 49: 611–627
Saria A 1984 Substance P in sensory nerve fibres contributes to the development of oedema in the rat hind paw after thermal injury. British Journal of Pharmacology 82: 217–222
Sato J, Perl ER 1991 Adrenergic exitation of cutaneous pain receptors induced by peripheral nerve injury. Science 251: 1608–1610
Sato J, Mizumura K, Kumazawa T 1989 Effects of ionic calcium on the responses of canine testicular polymodal receptors to algesic substances. Journal of Neurophysiology 62: 119–125
Sato J, Suzuki S, Iseki T, Kumazawa T 1993a Adrenergic excitation of cutaneous nociceptors in chronically inflamed rats. Neuroscience Letters 164: 225–228
Sato K, Kiyama H, Park HT, Tohyama M 1993b AMPA, KA, and NMDA receptors are expressed in the rat DRG neurones. Neuroreport 4: 1263–1265
Sawynok J, Reid A 1997 Peripheral adenosine 5′-triphosphate enhances nociception in the formalin test via activation of a purinergic p_{2x} receptor. European Journal of Pharmacology 330: 115–121
Scadding JW 1981 Development of ongoing activity, mechanosensitivity and adrenaline sensitivity in severed peripheral nerve axons. Experimental Neurology 73: 345–364
Schafer M, Carter L, Stein C 1994 Interleukin 1β and corticotropin-releasing factor inhibit pain by releasing opioids from immune cells in inflamed tissue. Proceedings of the National Academy of Sciences USA 91: 4219–4223
Schafer M, Mousa SA, Zhang Q, Carter L, Stein C 1996 Expression of corticotropin-releasing factor in inflamed tissue is required for intrinsic peripheral opioid analgesia. Proceedings of the National Academy of Sciences USA 93: 6096–6100
Schaible HG, Schmidt RF 1983a Activation of groups III and IV sensory units in medial articular nerve by local mechanical stimulation of knee joint. Journal of Neurophysiology 49: 35–44
Schaible HG, Schmidt RF 1983b Responses of fine medial articular nerve afferents to passive movements of knee joint. Journal of Neurophysiology 49: 1118–1126
Schaible HG, Schmidt RF 1985 Effects of an experimental arthritis on the sensory properties of fine articular afferent units. Journal of Neurophysiology 54: 1109–1122
Schaible H-G, Schmidt RF 1988a Excitation and sensitization of fine articular afferents from cat's knee joint by prostaglandin E_2. Journal of Physiology (London) 403: 91–104
Schaible H-G, Schmidt RF 1988b Time course of mechanosensitivity changes in articular afferents during a developing experimental arthritis. Journal of Neurophysiology 60: 2180–2195
Schepelmann K, Messlinger K, Schaible H-G, Schmidt RF 1992 Inflammatory mediators and nociception in the joint: excitation and sensitization of slowly conducting afferent fibers of cat's knee by prostaglandin I_2. Neuroscience 50: 237–247
Schmelz M, Schmidt R, Ringkamp M, Forster C, Handwerker HO, Torebjörk HE 1996 Limitation of sensitization to injured parts of receptive fields in human skin C-nociceptors. Experimental Brain Research 109: 141–147
Schmelz M, Schmidt R, Bickel A, Handwerker HO, Torebjork HE 1997 Specific C-receptors for itch in human skin. Journal of Neuroscience 17: 8003–8008
Schmidt R, Schmelz M, Forster C, Ringkamp M, Torebjörk E, Handwerker H 1995 Novel classes of responsive and unresponsive C nociceptors in human skin. Journal of Neuroscience 15: 333–341
Schmidt R, Schmelz M, Ringkamp M, Handwerker HO, Torebjork HE 1997 Innervation territories of mechanically activated C nociceptor units in human skin. Journal of Neurophysiology 78: 2641–2648
Schmidt RF 1996 The articular polymodal nociceptor in health and disease. In: Kumazawa T, Kruger L, Mizumura K (eds) Progress in brain research, 113. Elsevier Science, British Vancouver, pp 53–81
Seltzer Z, Devor M 1979 Ephatic transmission in chronically damaged peripheral nerves. Neurology 29: 1061–1064
Sengupta JN, Gebhart GF 1994a Characterization of mechanosensitive pelvic nerve afferent fibers innervating the colon of the rat. Journal of Neurophysiology 71: 2046–2060

Sengupta JN, Gebhart GF 1994b Mechanosensitive properties of pelvic nerve afferent fibers innervating the urinary bladder of the rat. Journal of Neurophysiology 72: 2420–2430

Sengupta JN, Saha JK, Goyal RK 1990 Stimulus-response function studies of esophageal mechanosensitive nociceptors in sympathetic afferents of opossum. Journal of Neurophysiology 64: 796–812

Sengupta JN, Saha JK, Goyal RK 1992 Differential sensitivity to bradykinin of esophageal distension-sensitive mechanoreceptors in vagal and sympathetic afferents of the opossum. Journal of Neurophysiology 68: 1053–1067

Sengupta JN, Su X, Gebhart GF 1996 κ, but not μ or σ, opioids attenuate responses to distention of afferent fibers innervating the rat colon. Gastroenterology 111: 968–980

Shafer DM, Assael L, White LB, Rossomando EF 1994 Tumor necrosis factor-α as a biochemical marker of pain and outcome in temporomandibular joints with internal derangements. Journal of Oral and Maxillofacial Surgery 52: 786–791

Shea VK, Perl ER 1985a Failure of sympathetic stimulation to affect responsiveness of rabbit polymodal nociceptors. Journal of Neurophysiology 54: 513–519

Shea VK, Perl ER 1985b Sensory receptors with unmyelinated (C) fibers innervating the skin of the rabbit's ear. Journal of Neurophysiology 54: 491–501

Sherrington CS 1906 The integrative action of the nervous system. Scribner, New York

Shir Y, Seltzer Z 1991 Effects of sympathectomy in a model of causalgiform pain produced by partial sciatic nerve injury rats Pain 45: 309–320

Sicuteri F, Fanciullacci M, Franchi G, Del Bianco PL 1965 Serotonin-bradykinin potentiation on the pain receptors in man. Life Sciences 4: 309–316

Simone DA, Kajander KC 1997 Responses of cutaneous A-fiber nociceptors to noxious cold. Journal of Neurophysiology 77: 2049–2060

Simone DA, Ochoa J 1991 Early and late effects of prolonged topical capsaicin on cutaneous sensibility and neurogenic vasodilatation in humans. Pain 47: 285–294

Simone DA, Baumann TK, LaMotte RH 1989 Dose-dependent pain and mechanical hyperalgesia in humans after intradermal injection of capsaicin. Pain 38: 99–107

Simone DA, Alreja M, LaMotte RH 1991a Psychophysical studies of the itch sensation and itchy skin ('Alloknesis') produced by intracutaneous injection of histamine. Somatosensory and Motor Research 8: 271–279

Simone DA, Sorkin LS, Oh U et al 1991b Neurogenic hyperalgesia: central neural correlates in responses of spinothalamic tract neurons. Journal of Neurophysiology 66: 228–246

Sinclair DC, Hinshaw JR 1950 A comparison of the sensory dissociation produced by procaine and by limb compression. Brain 73: 480–498

Skoglund S 1956 Anatomical and physiological studies of knee joint innervation in the cat. Acta Physiologica Scandinavica (suppl) 124: 1–101

Slugg RM, Meyer RA, Campbell JN 1995 Mechanical receptive field structure for cutaneous C-fiber and A-fiber nociceptors in the monkey determined with graded intensity stimuli. Society for Neuroscience Abstracts 21: 1161

Sluka KA, Westlund KN 1993 Centrally administered non-NMDA but not NMDA receptor antagonists block peripheral knee joint inflammation. Pain 55: 217–225

Sluka KA, Jordan HH, Westlund KN 1994a Reduction in joint swelling and hyperalgesia following post- treatment with a non-NMDA glutamate receptor antagonist. Pain 59: 95–100

Sluka KA, Lawand NB, Westlund KN 1994b Joint inflammation is reduced by dorsal rhizotomy and not by sympathectomy or spinal cord transection. Annals of the Rheumatic Diseases 53: 309–314

Sluka KA, Rees H, Westlund KN, Willis WD 1995a Fiber types contributing to dorsal root reflexes induced by joint inflammation in cats and monkeys. Journal of Neurophysiology 74: 981–989

Sluka KA, Willis WD, Westlund KN 1995b The role of dorsal root reflexes in neurogenic inflammation. Pain Forum 4: 141–149

Smith CH, Barker J, Morris RW, MacDonald DM, Lee TH 1993 Neuropeptides induce rapid expression of endothelial cell adhesion molecules and elicit infiltration in human skin. Journal of Immunology 151: 3274–3282

Sommer C, Schmidt C, George A, Toyka KV 1997 A metalloprotease-inhibitor reduces pain associated behavior in mice with experimental neuropathy. Neuroscience Letters 237: 45–48

Sommer C, Schmidt C, George A 1998 Hyperalgesia in experimental neuropathy is dependent on the TNF receptor 1. Experimental Neurology 151: 138–142

Sorkin LS, Xiao W-H, Wagner R, Myers RR 1997 Tumour necrosis factor-α induces ectopic activity in nociceptive primary afferent fibres. Neuroscience 81: 255–262

Stahl GL, Longhurst JC 1992 Ischemically sensitive visceral afferents: importance of H^+ derived from latic acid and hypercapnia. American Journal of Physiology 262: H748–H753

Stahl GL, Pan HL, Longhurst JC 1993 Activation of ischemia- and reperfusion-sensitive abdominal visceral c fiber afferent. Role of hydrogen peroxide and hydroxyl radicals. Circulation Research 72: 1266–1275

Steen KH, Reeh PW 1993 Sustained graded pain and hyperalgesia from harmless experimental tissue acidosis in human skin. Neuroscience Letters 154: 113–116

Steen KH, Reeh PW, Anton F, Handwerker HO 1992 Protons selectively induce long lasting excitation and sensitization to mechanical stimulation of nociceptors in rat skin, in vitro. Journal of Neuroscience 12: 86–95

Steen KH, Steen AE, Reeh PW 1995a A dominant role of acid pH in inflammatory excitation and sensitization of nociceptors in rat skin, in vitro. Journal of Neuroscience 15: 3982–3989

Steen KH, Issberner U, Reeh PW 1995b Pain due to experimental acidosis in human skin: evidence for non-adapting nociceptor excitation. Neuroscience Letters 199: 29–32

Steen KH, Steen AE, Kreysel HW, Reeh PW 1996 Inflammatory mediators potentiate pain induced by experimental tissue acidosis. Pain 66: 163–170

Stein C, Millan MJ, Yassouridis A, Herz A 1988 Antinociceptive effects of mμ- and kappa-agonists in inflammation are enhanced by a peripheral opioid receptor-specific mechanism. European Journal of Pharmacology 155: 255–264

Stein C, Millan MJ, Shippenberg TS, Peter K, Herz A 1989 Peripheral opioid receptors mediating antinociception in inflammation. Evidence for involvement of mu, delta and kappa receptors. Journal of Pharmacology and Experimental Therapeutics 248: 1269–1275

Stein C, Hassan AHS, Przewlocki R, Gramsch C, Peter K, Herz A 1990 Opioids from immunocytes interact with receptors on sensory nerves to inhibit nociception in inflammation. Proceedings of the National Academy of Sciences USA 87: 5935–5939

Strassman AM, Raymond SA, Burstein R 1996 Sensitization of meningeal sensory neurons and the origin of headaches. Nature 384: 560–564

Su X, Sengupta JN, Gebhart GF 1997a Effects of kappa opioid receptor-selective agonists on responses of pelvic nerve afferents to noxious colorectal distension. Journal of Neurophysiology 78: 1003–1012

Su X, Sengupta JN, Gebhart GF 1997b Effects of opioids on mechanosensitive pelvic nerve afferent fibers innervating the urinary bladder of the rat. Journal of Neurophysiology 77: 1566–1580

Sylvén C 1993 Mechanisms of pain in angia pectoris – a critical review of the adenosine hypothesis. Cardiovascular Drugs and Therapy 7: 745–759

Sylvén C, Beermann B, Jonzon B, Brandt R 1986a Angina pectoris-like pain provoked by intravenous adenosine in healthy volunteers. British Medical Journal 293: 227–230

Sylvén C, Edlund A, Brandt R, Beermann B, Jonzon B 1986b Angina pectoris-like pains provoked by intravenous adenosine. British Medical Journal 293: 1027–1028

Sylvén C, Jonzon B, Fredholm BB, Kaijers L 1988 Adenosine injection into the brachial artery produces ischaemia like pain or discomfort in the forearm. Cardiovascular Research 22: 674–678

Szolcsányi J 1990 Capsaicin, irritation, and desensitization: neurophysiological basis and future perspectives. In: Green BG, Mason JR, Kare MR (eds) Chemical senses: vol 2 – irritation. Marcel Dekker, New York, pp 141–169

Szolcsányi J 1996 Capsaicin-sensitive sensory nerve terminals with local and systemic efferent functions: facts and scopes of an unorthodox neuroregulatory mechanism. Progress in Brain Research 113: 343–359

Taiwo YO, Levine JD 1990 Direct cutaneous hyperalgesia induced by adenosine. Neuroscience 38: 757–762

Takahashi H 1985 Cardiovascular and sympathetic responses to intracarotid and intravenous injections of serotonin in rats. Naunyn-Schmiedebergs Archives of Pharmacology 329: 222–226

Tanelian DL 1991 Cholinergic activation of a population of corneal afferent nerves. Experimental Brain Research 86: 414–420

Tanelian DL, Beuerman RW 1984 Responses of rabbit corneal nociceptors to mechanical and thermal stimulation. Experimental Neurology 84: 165–178

Teofoli P, Procacci P, Maresca M, Lotti T 1996 Itch and pain. International Journal of Dermatology 35: 159–166

Thalhammer JG, LaMotte RH 1982 Spatial properties of nociceptor sensitization following heat injury of the skin. Brain Research 231: 257–265

Thalhammer JG, LaMotte RH 1983 Heat sensitization of one-half of a cutaneous nociceptor's receptive field does not alter the sensitivity of the other half. In: Bonica JJ, Lindblom U, Iggo A (eds) Advances in pain research and therapy, vol 5. Raven, New York, pp 71–75

Tillman DB 1992 Heat response properties of unmyelinated nociceptors PhD Dissertation, The Johns Hopkins University, pp 1–187

Tillman DB, Treede R-D, Meyer RA, Campbell JN 1995a Response of C fibre nociceptors in the anaesthetized monkey to heat stimuli: correlation with pain threshold in humans. Journal of Physiology 485: 767–774

Tillman DB, Treede R-D, Meyer RA, Campbell JN 1995b Response of C fibre nociceptors in the anaesthetized monkey to heat stimuli: estimates of receptor depth and threshold. Journal of Physiology 485: 753–765

Torebjörk E, Ochoa J 1980 Specific sensations evoked by activity in single identified sensory units in man. Acta Physiologica Scandinavica 110: 445–447

Torebjörk HE, Ochoa JL 1981 Pain and itch from C-fiber stimulation. Society for Neuroscience Abstracts 7: 228

Torebjörk HE, Hallin RG 1973 Perceptual changes accompanying controlled preferential blocking of A and C fibre responses in intact human skin nerves. Experimental Brain Research 16: 321–332

Torebjörk HE, LaMotte RH, Robinson CJ 1984 Peripheral neural correlates of magnitude of cutaneous pain and hyperalgesia: simultaneous recordings in humans of sensory judgments of pain and evoked responses in nociceptors with C-fibers. Journal of Neurophysiology 51: 325–339

Torebjörk HE, Lundberg LER, LaMotte RH 1992 Central changes in processing of mechanoreceptive input in capsaicin-induced secondary hyperalgesia in humans. Journal of Physiology (London) 448: 765–780

Toth-Kasa I, Jancso G, Bognar A, Husz S, Obal F Jr 1986 Capsaicin prevents histamine-induced itching. International Journal of Clinical Pharmacology and Research 6: 163–169

Tracey DJ, Cunningham JE, Romm MA 1995 Peripheral hyperalgesia in experimental neuropathy: mediation by α_2- adrenoreceptors on post-ganglionic sympathetic terminals. Pain 60: 317–327

Treede R-D 1992 Vasodilator flare due to activation of superficial cutaneous afferents in humans: heat-sensitive versus histamine-sensitive fibers. Neuroscience Letters 141: 169–172

Treede R-D, Cole JD 1993 Dissociated secondary hyperalgesia in a subject with large fibre sensory neuropathy. Pain 53: 169–174

Treede R-D, Meyer RA, Campbell JN 1990a Comparison of heat and mechanical receptive fields of cutaneous C-fiber nociceptors in monkey. Journal of Neurophysiology 64: 1502–1513

Treede R-D, Meyer RA, Davis KD, Campbell JN 1990b Intradermal injections of bradykinin or histamine cause a flare-like vasodilatation in monkey. Evidence from laser Doppler studies. Neuroscience Letters 115: 201–206

Treede R-D, Meyer RA, Raja SN, Campbell JN 1992 Peripheral and central mechanisms of cutaneous hyperalgesia. Progress in Neurobiology 38: 397–421

Treede R-D, Meyer RA, Raja SN, Campbell JN 1995 Evidence for two different heat transduction mechanisms in nociceptive primary afferents innervating monkey skin. Journal of Physiology 483: 747–758

Treede R-D, Campbell JN, Meyer RA 1998 Myelinated mechanically-insensitive afferents from monkey hairy skin: heat response properties. Journal of Neurophysiology 82: 1082–1093

Trowbridge HO 1985 Intradental sensory units: physiological and clinical considerations. Journal of Endodontics 11: 489–498

Tuckett RP 1982 Itch evoked by electrical stimulation of the skin. Journal of Investigative Dermatology 79: 368–373

Tuckett RP, Wei JY 1987 Response to an itch-producing substance in cat.I. Cutaneous receptor populations with myelinated axons. Brain Research 413: 87–94

Van Hees J 1976 Human C-fiber input during painful and nonpainful skin stimulation with radiant heat. In: Bonica JJ, Albe-Fessard DG (eds) Advances in pain research and therapy, vol 1. Raven, New York, pp 35–40

Van Hees J, Gybels JC 1981 C nociceptor activity in human nerve during painful and nonpainful skin stimulation. Journal of Neurology, Neurosurgery and Psychiatry 44: 600–607

Vera PL, Nadelhaft I 1990a Conduction velocity distribution of afferent fibers innervating the rat urinary bladder. Brain Research 520: 83–89

Vera PL, Nadelhaft I 1990b The conduction velocity and segmental distribution of afferent fibers in the rectal nerves of the female rat. Brain Research 526: 342–354

Vulchanova L, Riedl MS, Shuster SJ et al Immunohistochemical study of the $P2X_2$ and $P2X_3$ receptor subunits in rat and monkey sensory neurons and their central terminals. Neuropharmacology 36: 1229–1242

Vyklický L, Knotková-Urbancová H 1996 Can sensory neurones in culture serve as a model of nociception? Physiological Research 45: 1–9

Waldmann R, Champigny G, Bassilana F, Heurteaux C, Lazdunski M 1997 A proton-gated cation channel involved in acid sensing. Nature 386: 173–177

Walker AE, Nulson F 1948 Electrical stimulation of the upper thoracic portion of the sympathetic chain in man. Archives of Neurology and Psychiatry 59: 559–560

Wall PD, Gutnick M 1974 Ongoing activity in peripheral nerves: the physiology and pharmacology of impulses originating from a neuroma. Experimental Neurology 43: 580–593

Wall PD, McMahon SB 1985 Microneuronography and its relation to perceived sensation. A critical review. Pain 21: 209–229

Wallin BG, Torebjörk E, Hallin RG 1976 Preliminary observations on the pathophysiology of hyperalgesia in the causalgic pain syndrome. In:

Zotterman Y (ed) Sensory functions of the skin of primates with special reference to man. Pergamon, Oxford, pp 489–499

Warncke T, Stubhaug A, Jorum E 1997 Ketamine, an NMDA receptor antagonist, supresses spatial and temporal properties of burn-induced secondary hyperalgesia in man: a double-blind, cross-over comparison with morphine and placebo. Pain 72: 99–106

Watkins LR, Wiertelak EP, Goehler LE, Smith KP, Martin D, Maier SF 1994 Characterization of cytokine-induced hyperalgesia. Brain Research 654: 15–26

Watkins LR, Goehler LE, Relton J, Brewer MT, Maier SF 1995 Mechanisms of tumor necrosis factor-α (TNF-α) hyperalgesia. Brain Research 692: 244–250

White DM, Taiwo YO, Coderre TJ, Levine JD 1991 Delayed activation of nociceptors: correlation with delayed pain sensations induced by sustained stimuli. Journal of Neurophysiology 66: 729–734

White JC, Sweet WH 1969 Pain and the neurosurgeon: a forty year experience. Charles C Thomas, Springfield

Widdicombe J 1986 The neural reflexes in the airways. European Journal of Respiratory Diseases 144 (suppl): 1–33

Woolf CJ 1996 Windup and central sensitization are not equivalent. Pain 66: 105–108

Woolf CJ, Allchorne A, Safieh-Garabedian B, Poole S 1997 Cytokines, nerve growth factor and inflammatory hyperalgesia: the contribution of tumour necrosis factor α. British Journal of Pharmacology 121: 417–424

Yarnitsky D, Ochoa JL 1990 Studies of heat pain sensation in man: perception thresholds, rate of stimulus rise and reaction time. Pain 40: 85–91

Yarnitsky D, Simone DA, Dotson RM, Cline MA, Ochoa JL 1992 Single C nociceptor responses and psychophysical parameters of evoked pain: effect of rate of rise of heat stimuli in humans. Journal of Physiology (London) 450: 581–592

Zagami AS 1994 Pathophysiology of migraine and tension-type headache. Current Opinion in Neurobiology 7: 272–277

Zhou ST, Bonasera L, Carlton SM 1996 Peripheral administration of NMDA, AMPA or KA results in pain behaviors in rats. Neuroreport 7: 895–900

Peripheral mechanisms of inflammatory pain

JON D. LEVINE & DAVID B. REICHLING

2

INTRODUCTION

Inflammation is the single greatest cause of pain. Inflammatory diseases (identified by the suffix '-itis') can afflict any organ system in the body (identified by prefix, e.g., 'card-', 'col-', 'neur-', 'myos-', and 'arthr-'). This chapter describes mechanisms by which inflammatory mediators cause the increased activity in nociceptive primary afferent nerve fibres that underlies inflammatory pain. Also, while mechanisms of neuropathic pain are not discussed in detail, it is important to note that inflammatory mechanisms play an important role in pain induced by nerve injury (Richardson & Lu 1994, Tracey & Walker 1995, Wagner et al 1998). Inflammatory pain involves sensitization of spinal circuitry that is initiated, and possibly maintained, by the inflammation-induced increase in activity of primary afferent nerve fibres (Cook et al 1987, Laird & Cervero 1989, Simone et al 1989, Schaible & Schmidt 1996) (see Ch. 5).

THE INFLAMMATORY PROCESS

Inflammation is a critical protective reaction to irritation, injury, or infection, characterized by redness (rubor), heat (calor), swelling (tumor), loss of function (functio lasea) and pain (dolor) (Gallin et al 1992). Redness and heat are the result of an increase in blood flow, swelling is the result of increased vascular permeability, and pain is the result of activation and sensitization of primary afferent nerve fibres. Under normal conditions these changes in inflamed tissue serve to isolate the effects of the insult and thereby limit the threat to the organism. The process of inflammation leads to removal of injured tissue and repair of the injury site. The role of inflammatory pain in this protective process is to prevent further trauma to the already injured tissue. Inflammatory mediators, including bradykinin, platelet-activating factor, prostaglandins, leukotrienes, amines, purines, cytokines and chemokines, act on specific targets (e.g., microvasculature) (Robinson 1989, Armstrong et al 1991, Colditz 1991), cause the local release of other mediators from leucocytes (e.g., mast cells and basophils) (Kaliner 1989, Brunner et al 1993) and attract other leucocytes to the site of inflammation (e.g., neutrophils) (Borish & Joseph 1992, Harbuz et al 1993). In summary, inflammation involves a complex cascade of events that functions to insure a rapid response to injury.

Although pain is a major complaint of patients with ongoing inflammation, the majority of such patients do not experience continuous 'spontaneous' pain. Rather, pain is experienced predominantly and most severely when the inflamed site is mechanically stimulated by being moved or touched. This 'tenderness', or lowered threshold for stimulation-induced pain, is referred to as 'hyperalgesia'. Inflammatory hyperalgesia is thought to be produced by inflammatory mediators released from circulating leucocytes and platelets, vascular endothelial cells, immune cells resident in tissue (including mast cells), and sensory and sympathetic nerve fibres. The first inflammatory mediator recognized to have potent hyperalgesic properties was bradykinin (Armstrong et al 1953). Since then, a host of inflammatory mediators have been identified which can produce hyperalgesia, including prostaglandins, leukotrienes, serotonin, adenosine, histamine, interleukin 1, interleukin 8 and nerve growth factor.

INTRODUCTION: DEVELOPMENTAL NEUROBIOLOGY OF PAIN

An important mechanism of inflammatory mediator-induced hyperalgesia is an increase in the excitability of sensory nerve fibres. Various techniques have been useful in studying mechanisms by which inflammatory mediators lower nociceptive thresholds and cause inflammatory pain. The technique of microneurography for obtaining recordings from nerve fibres in awake humans has allowed a direct correlation between discharges from these nociceptors and the report of pain, but is limited by practical considerations. In animal studies, both behavioural techniques employing nociceptive reflex tests and electrophysiological recordings from single sensory nerve fibres have been employed extensively to study the mechanisms underlying inflammatory pain (Bessou & Perl 1969, Beck & Handwerker 1974, Mense & Schmidt 1974, Meyer & Campbell 1981, LaMotte et al 1982, Torebjörk et al 1984, Reeh et al 1987, Mense & Meyer 1988, Schaible & Schmidt 1988, Neugebauer et al 1989, Cohen & Perl 1990, Habler et al 1990, Kirchhoff et al 1990, White et al 1990, Cooper et al 1991, Kumazawa et al 1991, Koltzenburg et al 1992).

Sensory neurons responding to stimuli capable of producing tissue damage (termed 'nociceptors') have either myelinated small-diameter (Aδ) or unmyelinated (C) fibre axons (Torebjörk & Hallin 1974, Handwerker 1976). In primates, C fibres account for most of the identified primary afferent nociceptors (Kumazawa & Perl 1997a,b). Activity is induced in C fibres by noxious heat (>44°C), intense mechanical pressure or chemical mediators of inflammation, such as bradykinin, serotonin and elevated hydrogen ion concentration (Gilfort & Klanni 1965, Beck & Handwerker 1974, Richardson & Engel 1986, Dray & Perkins 1988, Bevan & Yeats 1991, Kumazawa et al 1991). A subset of C fibres called 'silent' fibres has been described which are apparently non-responsive to mechanical stimuli, although some have been described to be chemosensitive and may develop a response to mechanical stimuli after exposure to inflammatory mediators (see Chs 1, 7).

In the presence of inflammation, individual nociceptors become sensitized, that is, they are activated by stimuli that previously would not be intense enough to cause activation; at the same time, a previously noxious stimulus produces an even greater sensation of pain (Cervero 1995, Perl 1996). The electrophysiological correlates of this altered pain response include a lowered threshold for nociceptor activation, increased spontaneous activity, and an increased frequency of firing in response to a suprathreshold stimulus (Fig. 2.1). Nociceptors have been shown to develop a lowered threshold at inflammatory sites and also after administration of inflammatory mediators by various routes (intradermal, intra-arterial and intra-articular).

Increased activity in the primary afferent neuron also contributes to inflammation (Lembeck & Holzer 1979). Neurotransmitters, including calcitonin gene-related peptide (CGRP) and substance P, can be released from the peripheral endings of nociceptive primary afferents, and exert pro-inflammatory effects in peripheral tissues (Holzer et al 1995, Maggi 1997). This positive feedback phenomenon is known as neurogenic inflammation (Lynn 1996).

Activity in large-diameter non-nociceptive afferent fibres may also contribute to the generation of inflammatory pain (see Chs 1, 7). For example, in secondary hyperalgesia and chronic pain states, input via small-diameter afferents to the

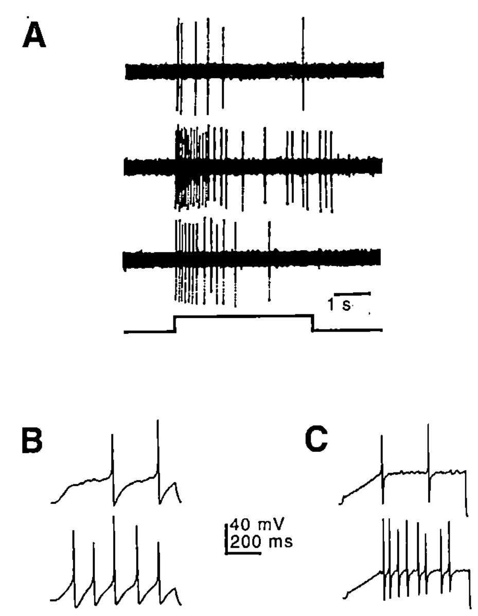

Fig. 2.1 Primary afferent sensitization demonstrated in vivo and in vitro. **A** Sensitization of a C-fibre nociceptive sensory nerve fibre by the inflammatory mediator bradykinin. The top trace shows the response to a threshold-level von Frey hair mechanical stimulus (3.6 g). After intradermal injection of bradykinin this fibre shows an enhanced response to the same 3.6-g stimulus (middle trace). After bradykinin injection, the fibre can respond to a stimulus (1.48 g) that was previously below threshold. The time course of the stimulus is indicated below the bottom trace, and the scale bar represents 1 s. **B** Sensitization of a cultured dorsal root ganglion neuron by PGE_2 in vitro. Action potentials were evoked in these current-clamped neurons by a 250-ms ramped current. Before PGE_2 application two action potentials were evoked (upper trace); after the application of 1 μM PGE_2 the same current ramp evoked five action potentials. In addition to the increase in the number of action potentials generated, a decrease in threshold is also evident as a shorter latency to the first action potential during the ramped stimulus. **C** Example of a neuron in which PGE_2 induced a change only in the number of action potentials. (Adapted from Gold et al 1996a.)

spinal cord results in pain caused by stimulation of large-diameter fibres in the area of sensitization (Torebjörk et al 1992, Treede et al 1992, Woolf & Doubell 1994). Furthermore, inflammatory hyperalgesia might involve a phenotypic switch in some myelinated primary sensory neurons that causes them to express characteristics of unmyelinated nociceptors (Neumann et al 1996).

INDIRECT EFFECTS OF INFLAMMATORY MEDIATORS ON NOCICEPTORS VIA OTHER CELL TYPES

SYMPATHETIC NEURON-DEPENDENT HYPERALGESIA

While activity in the sympathetic nervous system alone rarely if ever causes pain under physiological conditions, following tissue or nerve injury the activity of nociceptors can be modulated by catecholamines (Jänig et al 1996). This phenomenon may play an important role in the development of certain pain syndromes, including reflex sympathetic dystrophy, causalgia and some types of headache (White & Sweet 1969, Stanton-Hicks et al 1995, Appenzeller & Oribe 1997). Several inflammatory mediators require the postganglionic sympathetic neuron terminal for full expression of hyperalgesia (Fig. 2.2).

Bradykinin

Bradykinin is a nonapeptide cleaved from plasma α_2-globulins by kallikreins that circulate in the plasma and are activated at sites of tissue injury (Garrison 1996) (Fig. 2.3). Therefore, bradykinin is present in relatively high concentrations at sites of inflammation (Rocha et al 1961, Melmon et al 1967, Di Rosa et al 1971). Bradykinin sensitizes nociceptors to produce hyperalgesia (Beck & Handwerker 1974, Handwerker 1976, Mense & Meyer 1988, Neugebauer et al 1989) and lowers behavioural nociceptive thresholds (Levine et al 1986c, Taiwo & Levine 1988a). Mechanical and thermal sensitization appear to use two different mechanisms. Bradykinin-induced sensitization of primary afferent neurons and mechanical hyperalgesia have been shown to depend on the production of prostaglandins via phospholipase A_2 in sympathetic postganglionic neurons (Lembeck et al 1976, Levine et al 1986c, Taiwo & Levine 1988b, Taiwo et al 1990, Kumazawa et al 1991). By contrast, thermal sensitization by bradykinin (Koltzenburg

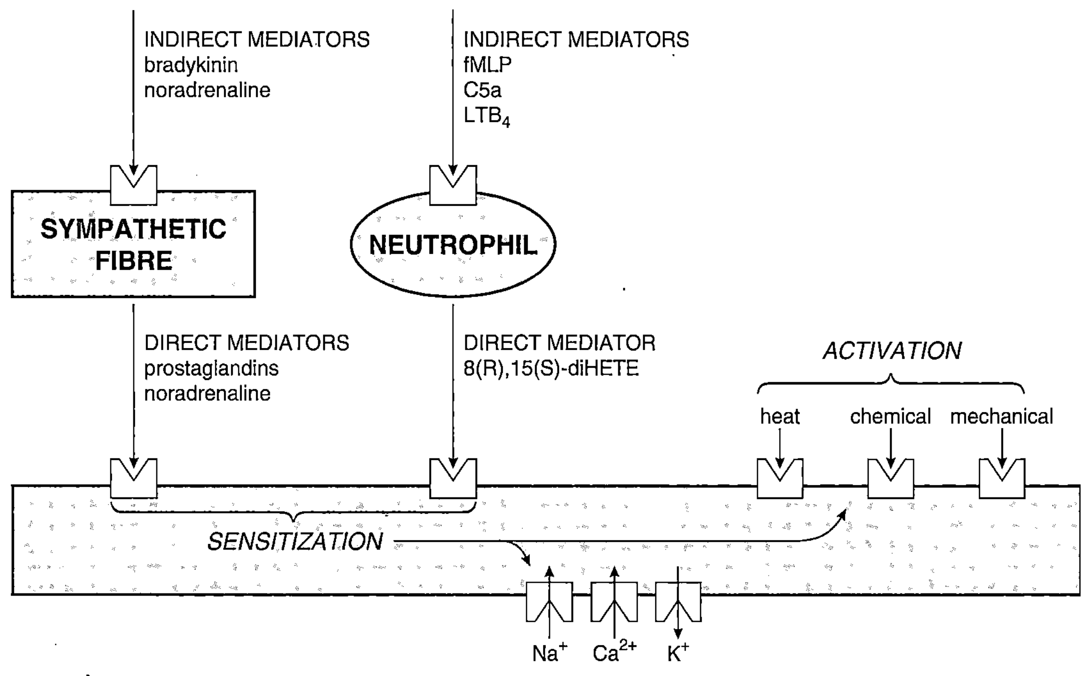

Fig. 2.2 Direct and indirect mechanisms by which inflammatory mediators sensitize primary afferent nociceptors.

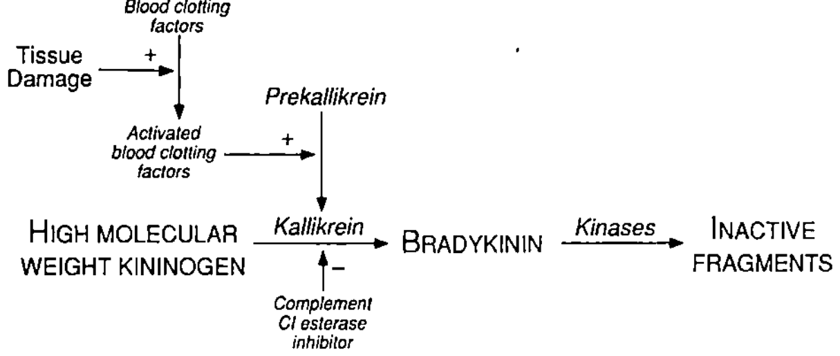

Fig. 2.3 Biochemical pathway of bradykinin production in inflamed tissues. A series of steps after tissue injury leads to liberation of the inflammatory mediator bradykinin, which is both a primary afferent activator and sensitizer. Circulating clotting factors, an α_2-globulin (high molecular kininogen) and activated enzymes (kallikreins) are involved. Bradykinin is rapidly inactivated by kinases present at sites of inflammation. The production of bradykinin can be inhibited by endogenous substances (e.g., by complement C1 esterase inhibitor).

& McMahon 1991, Kumazawa et al 1991), which also depends on prostaglandin synthesis, is not affected by surgical sympathectomy (Kumazawa et al 1991, Koltzenburg et al 1992).

In normal rats the administration of bradykinin induces hyperalgesia by an action at B_2 bradykinin receptors. Recent evidence suggests that in the setting of chronic inflammation, bradykinin-induced hyperalgesia is mediated by both B_{12}- and B_2-receptor subtypes (Dray & Perkins 1993, Khasar et al 1995, Rupniak et al 1997). Thus, prolonged inflammatory states can apparently induce a novel B_2-receptor-dependent mechanism of hyperalgesia.

Noradrenaline

Sympathectomy attenuates noradrenaline hyperalgesia (Levine et al 1986c), and it has been hypothesized that noradrenaline acts on the sympathetic postganglionic neuron to stimulate the production of hyperalgesic prostaglandins (Gonzales et al 1989). Consistent with this idea is the clinical observation that cutaneous application of noradrenaline can aggravate pain in patients with sympathetically maintained pain syndromes (Torebjörk et al 1995). Noradrenaline-induced mechanical hyperalgesia in rats appears to depend on the production of prostaglandin I_2 via phospholipase C in sympathetic postganglionic neurons (Taiwo et al 1990).

Early studies of experimentally induced neuromas lead to the suggestion that noradrenaline produces hyperalgesia via upregulation of α-adrenergic receptors on injured primary afferent nociceptors (Wall & Gutnick 1974, Devor & Jänig 1981, Devor 1983, Blumberg & Jänig 1984). However such upregulation of α-adrenergic receptors on primary afferents and coupling to nociceptive mechanisms remains to be demonstrated.

Nerve growth factor

Levels of nerve growth factor (NGF) are elevated at sites of inflammation (Halliday et al 1998). NGF production is induced by the inflammatory mediator interleukin 1β which can be upregulated by tumour necrosis factor α (Woolf et al 1997). Consistent with a contribution of NGF to inflammatory pain (McMahon 1996), NGF administration causes hyperalgesia (Amann et al 1996), and antagonism of NGF action reduces inflammatory hyperalgesia (Woolf et al 1994, Dmitrieva et al 1997, Ma & Woolf 1997). NGF can sensitize primary afferent nerve fibres. This effect is mediated, at least in part by sympathetic neurons (Dmitrieva & McMahon 1996, Rueff & Mendell 1996). Specifically, thermal hyperalgesia induced by intradermal injection of NGF requires, in part, sympathetic postganglionic neurons (Lewin et al 1994, Andreev et al 1995). The induction of mechanical hyperalgesia by NGF and an inflammatory stimulus involves a transient contribution of sympathetic neurons (Lewin et al 1994, Woolf et al 1996).

LEUCOCYTE-DEPENDENT HYPERALGESIA

Neutrophils

The polymorphonuclear leucocyte (neutrophil) is a principal effector cell in inflammatory reactions. It accumulates at sites of inflammation primarily to destroy and evacuate antigenic material. The accumulation of neutrophils is commonly associated with marked hyperalgesia as, for example, in rheumatoid arthritis (Pillinger & Abramson 1995) and gout (Matsukawa et al 1998).

Leukotriene B_4

A specific inflammatory mediator, leukotriene B_4 (LTB_4), which is a potent neutrophil attractant (Ford-Hutchinson 1985), has been shown to produce hyperalgesia both in humans (Bisgaard & Kristensen 1985) and in animals (Rackham & Ford-Hutchinson 1983, Levine et al 1984, 1985, 1986b). The hyperalgesia induced by intradermal injection of leukotriene B_4 in rats is dependent on the presence of circulating neutrophils (Levine et al 1984).

Leukotriene B_4-induced hyperalgesia appears to be mediated by the attraction and activation of neutrophils and their release of a hyperalgesic product of the leukotriene pathway of arachidonic acid metabolism, 8(R),15(S)-

dihydroxyeicosatetraenoic acid (8(R),15(S)-diHETE), which directly sensitizes primary afferent nociceptors (Levine et al 1984, 1986b) (Fig. 2.2). In addition, cytokines are produced by leucocytes in response to exposure to bacterial toxins or to inflammatory mediators (Dinarello 1989). The cytokines, interleukin 1β and interleukin 1α, produce hyperalgesia, although interleukin 1β is a thousand-fold more potent (Ferreira et al 1988). Like bradykinin and noradrenaline, interleukin 1 has been shown to induce E-type prostaglandin production in non-neuronal cells (Dayer et al 1986), and interleukin 1 hyperalgesia is probably also mediated by prostaglandins. Interleukin 8 has also been found to produce a sympathetic-dependent hyperalgesia which does not appear to be mediated by prostaglandins (Cunha et al 1991).

Two other substances that attract and activate neutrophils – C_{5a}, the anaphylactoid fragment of the fifth component of the complement cascade, and formyl methionyl-leucylphenylalanine (fMLP), a bacterial cell wall fragment peptide – have been shown to produce neutrophil-dependent hyperalgesia, by eliciting the production of 8(R),15(S)-diHETE (Levine et al 1985).

Substance P

Substance P, an undecapeptide located in one-tenth to one- third of dorsal root ganglion neurons and transported to the peripheral primary afferent terminals (Brimijoin et al 1980, Harmar & Keen 1982), is released peripherally after afferent activation (Bill et al 1979, Brodin et al 1981, Moskowitz et al 1983, White & Helme 1985). While electrophysiological experiments suggest that substance P does not directly sensitize cutaneous nociceptors (Cohen & Perl 1990), it may contribute to hyperalgesia indirectly via its numerous pro-inflammatory effects. Substance P contributes to the inflammatory response by causing vasodilatation and increased vascular permeability (Lembeck & Holzer 1979, Saria 1984), increased production and release of lysosomal enzymes (Johnson & Erdos 1973), release of prostaglandin E_2, for example from synoviocytes (Lotz et al 1987), and release of interleukin 1 and the neutrophil chemoattractant interleukin 6 (Lotz et al 1988).

Mast cells

Mast-cell degranulation and release of histamine and serotonin can cause hyperalgesia (Coelho et al 1998), and inhibition of mast-cell degranulation reduces inflammatory hyperalgesia (Mazzari et al 1996).

Nerve growth factor

An important aspect of NGF action in inflammation is its interaction with mast cells (Levi-Montalcini et al 1996). Hyperalgesia induced by NGF depends on the presence of mast cells (Lewin et al 1994, Rueff & Mendell 1996, Woolf et al 1996). NGF-induced degranulation of mast cells (Tal & Liberman 1997) and release of histamine and serotonin (Ferjan et al 1997) occurs at sites of inflammation (Aloe et al 1995).

Adenosine

Activation of peripheral adenosine A_3 receptors produces hyperalgesia indirectly by stimulating the release of serotonin and histamine from mast cells (Sawynok et al 1997).

Macrophages

While the role of the macrophage in inflammatory pain has only recently begun to be explored (Chou et al 1998), this immunocompetent cell has been implicated in various models of neuropathic pain (Myers et al 1996, Wagner et al 1998). The contribution of macrophages to neuropathic pain is thought to be mediated by its release of the inflammatory mediator tumour necrosis factor α (TNFα) (Wagner et al 1998), which has been linked to the pathogenesis of arthritis (Matsukawa et al 1998) as well as to neuropathic pain (Chou et al 1998). The contribution of TNFα to nociception may be dependent on its ability to regulate the production of NGF and interleukin 1 at sites of inflammation (Woolf et al 1997).

DIRECT ACTION OF INFLAMMATORY MEDIATORS ON PRIMARY AFFERENT NOCICEPTORS

Inflammatory mediators act on primary afferent nociceptors to cause pain by either inducing activity in nociceptors (activation) or increasing nociceptor responses evoked by other stimuli (sensitization). Direct action of a hyperalgesic inflammatory mediator on primary afferent nociceptors can be suggested by in vivo experiments showing short latency to onset of hyperalgesia induced by injection of the mediator, and by insensitivity of such hyperalgesia to elimination of known indirect pathways (Taiwo et al 1987, Taiwo & Levine 1989b, 1990, 1992). However, the most conclusive evidence that a mediator can act directly on sensory neurons is obtained by in vitro demonstration that it activates or sensitizes isolated sensory neurons in culture. Putative nociceptors can be identified in vitro by their co-expression of a variety of properties that are characteristic of nociceptors in vivo (Gold et al 1996a, Vyklicky & Knotkova-Urbancova 1996) (Fig. 2.4).

INFLAMMATORY MEDIATORS THAT DIRECTLY ACTIVATE PRIMARY AFFERENT NOCICEPTORS

Bradykinin

In addition to sensitizing nociceptors and producing hyperalgesia by sympathetic-dependent mechanisms (see above), bradykinin can itself produce pain in humans (Cormia & Dougherty 1960, Lim et al 1967, Ferreira et al 1971, Whalley et al 1989). Bradykinin activates primary afferent nerve fibres in vivo (Dray & Perkins 1988, Haley et al 1989, Kumazawa et al 1991) and in vitro, and directly excites sensory neurons in culture (Baccaglini & Hogan 1983, Kitakoga & Kuba 1993, Kano et al 1994, Noda et al 1997). Sensory neurons can express both B_1 and B_2 bradykinin receptor subtypes (Davis et al 1996, Segond von Banchet et al 1996). It has been suggested that bradykinin-induced activation of nociceptors involves the generation of diacyl glycerol and the activation of protein kinase C (PKC), leading to an increase in sodium conductance (Dray & Perkins 1988, Burgess et al 1989, Morell et al 1991). However, more recent evidence suggests that PKC plays a non-essential role (Dunn & Rang 1990, McGuirk & Dolphin 1992) in modulating bradykinin-induced activation which is mediated by cGMP (McGehee et al 1992, Bauer et al 1995).

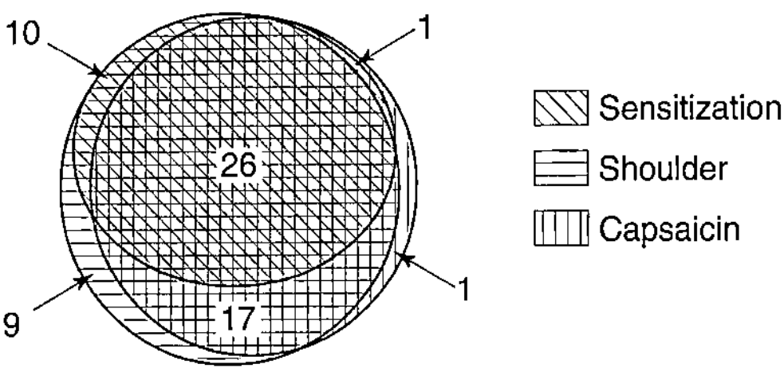

Fig. 2.4 Coexpression of some nociceptor properties among dorsal root ganglion neurons isolated in culture. This Venn diagram illustrates the number of dorsal root ganglion neurons in a sample of 64 that, in whole-cell patch-clamp recordings, coexpress the following electrophysiological properties which are characteristic of primary afferent nociceptors: sensitization in response to 1 μM PGE_2 (Sensitization), a 'shoulder' on the action potential waveform (Shoulder) and responsiveness to capsaicin (Capsaicin). Numbers indicate the number of cells that express each combination of properties; areas in the diagram are not exactly proportional to the numbers. (Adapted from Gold et al 1996a.)

Serotonin

Serotonin (5HT), released from activated platelets (and in some species from mast cells), is elevated in inflammatory exudates and has been reported to cause pain in humans, probably by acting at $5HT_3$ receptors to activate primary afferent nerve fibres (Fozard 1984, Richardson et al 1985, Richardson & Engel 1986, Giordano & Dyche 1989, Giordano & Rogers 1989). Serotonin is implicated in the aetiology of migraine (Fozard 1995) and other inflammatory pain states (Morteau et al 1994, Harbuz et al 1996, Pierce et al 1996b). Although dorsal root ganglion neurons may express as many as nine 5HT receptor subtypes (Pierce et al 1996a, 1997), potential roles of most of these in nociception remain to be elucidated.

Excitatory amino acids

Glutamate is present at peripheral sites of inflammation (Nordlind et al 1993, Omote et al 1998), and activation of peripheral *N*-methyl-D-aspartate (NMDA) and non-NMDA glutamate receptors contributes to inflammatory hyperalgesia (Jackson et al 1995, Davidson et al 1997). Furthermore, glutamate injection in the skin causes mechanical and thermal hyperalgesia (Carlton et al 1995, 1998b, Davidson et al 1997). Glutamate may cause pain, in part, by exacerbating the inflammatory process (Sluka et al 1994) via actions on non-sensory cells, including postganglionic sympathetic fibres (Carlton et al 1998a). However, it is likely that glutamate also acts directly upon primary afferent nociceptors, because these sensory fibres express NMDA, kainate, AMPA and metabotropic glutamate receptors (Agrawal & Evans 1986, Huettner 1990, Liu et al 1994, Carlton et al 1995, Crawford et al 1997, Li et al 1997) and are activated by glutamate in vitro (Lovinger & Weight 1988, Ault & Hildebrand 1993). Although glutamate is produced by a variety of non-neuronal cells in inflammation, including macrophages (Newsholme & Calder 1997), it is also released by peripheral primary afferent nerve fibres themselves (Westlund et al 1989, Juranek & Lembeck 1997) and this source of glutamate is enhanced in inflammation (Westlund et al 1992). This raises the possibility that glutamate acts at autoreceptors on primary afferent nerve endings in inflamed tissues, causing a positive-feedback enhancement of nociceptor excitability. This would be analogous to the presynaptic action of glutamate on primary afferent terminals in the spinal cord

(Ferreira & Lorenzetti 1994, Liu et al 1997) that is thought to contribute to excitatory amino acid-mediated sensitization of spinal sensory circuitry (Dougherty et al 1992, Coderre 1993, Meller & Gebhart 1994, Urban et al 1994, Dickenson et al 1997, Baranauskas & Nistri 1998).

Hydrogen ions

Acidic pH (which is an increased concentration of hydrogen ions/protons) produces pain in normal tissues (Steen et al 1995a, Issberner et al 1996), and a pH as low as 5.4 has been reported in inflamed tissues (Jacobus et al 1977). Exposure of nociceptors to solutions with a pH of approximately 6 or lower activates a subpopulation of C and Aδ fibres, and repeated exposure to low pH produces sensitization to mechanical stimuli (Steen et al 1992, Bevan & Geppetti 1994). Activation by low pH is mediated by a non-selective cation-permeable channel that is activated by hydrogen ions (Bevan & Yeats 1991). Because NGF regulates the proton-gated current in dorsal root ganglion neurons, NGF produced in inflammation might enhance pain caused by the acidosis of inflamed tissues (Bevan & Winter 1995). Recent evidence suggests an alternative mechanism by which hydrogen ions might activate nociceptors: acidic pH enables a mixture of other inflammatory mediators to activate capsaicin receptors on sensory neurons (Vyklicky et al 1998). The recent cloning of a dorsal root ganglion-specific acid-sensing ion channel (DRASIC), a member of the amiloride-sensitive sodium channel/degenerin family of ion channels (Waldmann et al 1997a,b) and of a capsaicin receptor (Caterina et al 1997), will facilitate studies to investigate mechanisms by which acid pH contributes to inflammatory pain.

INFLAMMATORY MEDIATORS THAT DIRECTLY SENSITIZE PRIMARY AFFERENT NOCICEPTORS

Prostaglandins

Prostaglandins are considered prototypic sensitizing agents. Their administration does not elicit overt pain (Crunkhorn & Willis 1971), yet they decrease nociceptive threshold in behavioural tests in animals (Ferreira & Nakamura 1979, Taiwo et al 1987, Taiwo & Levine 1989b) and produce tenderness in humans (Ferreira 1972). In electrophysiological studies in animals, prostaglandin E_2 sensitizes high-threshold somatic and visceral afferents when administered systemically (Juan & Lembeck 1974, Handwerker 1976, Fowler et al 1985a) or when injected directly into the receptive field of a nociceptive afferent (Pateromichelakis & Rood 1982, Martin et al 1987).

The rapid onset of hyperalgesia following intradermal injection of the arachidonic acid metabolites (Taiwo et al 1987), and the persistence of this hyperalgesia following the elimination of inflammatory cells (Taiwo & Levine 1989b) or the sympathetic postganglionic neuron, suggest a direct action on the primary afferent (Taiwo et al 1987, Taiwo & Levine 1989b). The most convincing evidence that prostaglandins act directly on the primary afferent nociceptor and do not require intermediary cells, derives from studies performed in vitro (Baccaglini & Hogan 1983, England et al 1996, Gold et al 1996b). Whole cell patch clamp electrophysiology recordings performed on isolated dorsal root ganglion neurons expressing nociceptor properties demonstrate that prostaglandin E_2 and prostaglandin I_2 (prostacyclin) increase the electrical excitability of sensory neurons (Gold et al 1996a, Noda et al 1997).

Prostaglandins are not stored; rather, in response to an inflammatory mediator or to trauma they are synthesized de novo from arachidonic acid released from membrane phospholipids (Kunze & Vogt 1971, Irvine 1982, O'Flaherty 1987) (Fig. 2.5). Free arachidonic acid is metabolized to prostanoids by the cyclooxygenase (COX) pathway (Samuelsson 1972, 1983) or to leukotrienes by the lipoxygenase pathway (Roth & Siok 1978, Mizuno et al 1982). Prostaglandin E_2 and prostaglandin I_2 have been found to mediate bradykinin- and noradrenaline-induced hyperalgesias, respectively (Taiwo et al 1990). (8(R), 15(S)-diHETE) has been found to mediate the neutrophil-dependent hyperalgesia induced by leukotriene B_4. Prostaglandin $F_{2\alpha}$, prostaglandin D_2, 12(S) hydroxyheptadecatrienoic acid and thromboxane B_2 appear not to be hyperalgesic, although there is a report of prostaglandin D_2-induced hyperalgesia (Ohkubo et al 1983). The analgesic properties of aspirin, indomethacin and other non-steroidal anti-inflammatory analgesics (NSAIDs), which inhibit the COX pathway (Smith & Willis 1971, Vane 1971, Ferreira et al 1973), emphasize the clinical importance of prostaglandin hyperalgesia.

8(R),15(S)-dihydroxyeicosatetraenoic acid

In its role as mediator of leukotriene B_4 induced neutrophil-dependent hyperalgesia, described above, 8(R),15(S)-diHETE appears to act directly at a receptor on the primary afferent itself (Levine et al 1986b, Taiwo et al 1987). This effect is antagonized by the stereoisomer 8(S),15(S)-diHETE, and is therefore not mediated by action at prostaglandin receptors (Levine et al 1986b, White et al 1990).

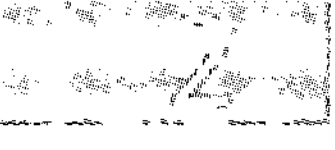

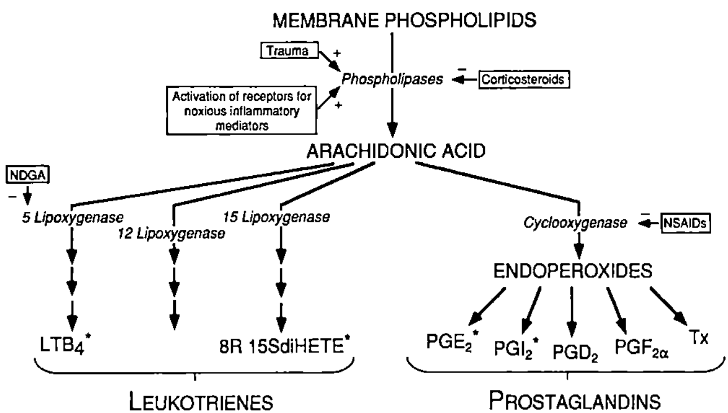

Fig. 2.5 Cascade for the production of hyperalgesic leukotrienes and prostaglandins from arachadonic acid in response to inflammatory stimuli. Membrane phospholipases are activated in response to trauma or inflammatory mediators. The cascade can be modulated at several points by corticosteroids, non-steroidal anti-inflammatory agents (NSAIDs) and nordihydroguaiaretic acid (NDGA). Metabolites that have been shown to cause hyperalgesia are marked by an asterisk. LTB_4 = leukotriene B_4; (8R 15SdiHETE = 8(R), 15(S)-dihydroxyeicosatetraenoic acid; PGE_2 = prostaglandin E_2; PGI_2 = prostaglandin I_2; PGD_2 = prostaglandin D_2; $PGF_{2\alpha}$ = prostaglandin $F_{2\alpha}$; Tx = thromboxane.

Serotonin

In addition to activating primary afferent nerve fibres via $5HT_3$ receptors, serotonin produces mechanical hyperalgesia by acting at a different receptor in the periphery, most likely the $5HT_{1A}$-receptor subtype (Taiwo et al 1992) (with possible contributions from the $5HT_{1C}$- (Bervoets et al 1990) and $5HT_7$- (Eglen et al 1997) receptor subtypes. Direct action of serotonin upon primary afferent nerve fibres in vivo is suggested by the extremely short latency to onset of serotonin-induced hyperalgesia, as well as by its independence from sympathetic postganglionic neurons, neutrophils and prostaglandin synthesis (Taiwo & Levine 1992). The ability of serotonin to directly sensitize primary afferent neurons has been verified in vitro by patch clamp electrophysiological studies (Cardenas et al 1997).

Noradrenaline

The catecholamine noradrenaline has been reported to produce hyperalgesia but, interestingly, only in the presence of tissue injury, such as exists during inflammation (Taiwo et al 1990). Electrophysiological observations seem to parallel this finding in that inflammation induces novel noradrenaline excitability in primary afferent nerve fibres (Sato et al 1993) that is not blocked by sympathectomy (Sato et al 1994). Increases in intracellular calcium may play a role in the induction of noradrenaline sensitivity (Taiwo et al 1990). That the effect of noradrenaline could be mediated by direct action on the primary afferent is suggested by the observation of nerve injury-induced noradrenaline-induced activation in dorsal root ganglion neurons in vitro (Petersen et al 1996). The potential involvement of other catecholamines, including adrenaline, in inflammatory pain remains to be examined.

Adenosine

Adenosine, which is generated during inflammatory tissue hypoxia (Edlund et al 1983), has been shown to activate unmyelinated afferents (Katholi et al 1985, Monteiro & Ribeiro 1987, Runold et al 1990), to produce pain in humans (Bleehen & Keele 1977, Sylven et al 1988), and to elicit nociceptive behaviour in animals (Collier et al 1966). In addition to activating nociceptors, adenosine also induces hyperalgesia, mediated by adenosine A_2 receptors (Sawynok & Reid 1997) apparently located on the primary afferent itself (Taiwo & Levine 1990). Consistent with a role for A_2 receptors, mice lacking the A_{2A} receptor exhibit hypoalgesia (Ledent et al 1997). By contrast, the action of adenosine at an A_1 receptor in the periphery is antihyperalgesic (Taiwo & Levine 1990).

Adenosine 5′-triphosphate

The discovery that P2X receptors for adenosine 5′-triphosphate (ATP) are expressed in cell bodies and sensory nerve endings of the subpopulation of small-diameter dorsal root ganglion neurons (Chen et al 1995, Cook et al 1997, Vulchanova et al 1997), stimulated interest in its potential contribution to nociception (Burnstock 1996, Burnstock & Wood 1996). ATP has been shown to produce pain (Bland-Ward & Humphrey 1997) and to enhance nociception in the formalin test (Sawynok & Reid 1997).

Nitric oxide

Nitric oxide (NO) and other reactive oxygen species are produced by a variety of cell types in peripheral tissues during the oxidative stress of inflammation (Bruch-Gerharz et al 1998). NO appears to exert peripheral pro-nociceptive effects. For example, the peripheral administration of NO precursors produces pain and hyperalgesia in animals and humans (Corrado & Ballejo 1992, Kawabata et al 1994, Alm et al 1995, Kindgen-Milles & Arndt 1996, Aley et al 1998), and the inhibition of NO synthase in peripheral tissues can specifically reduce inflammatory pain (Lawand et al 1997). Because NO produced within sensory neurons acts as a second messenger mediating nociceptor sensitization, its direct effects on nociceptor excitability are discussed in greater detail in the section concerning second messengers below. Other reactive oxygen species such as peroxide, superoxide anion and hydroxyl can induce a painful inflammatory state (Ridger et al 1997), and antioxidative therapy may relieve inflammatory pain (Aaseth et al 1998). However, these oxygen radicals do not appear to play a specific role in nociceptor sensitization (Kress et al 1995). Finally, it is noteworthy that in addition to its role in peripheral mechanisms of inflammatory pain, the production of NO in the spinal cord also appears to contribute to spinal mechanisms of inflammatory pain (Yonehara et al 1997, Wu et al 1998).

Nerve growth factor

Although the high-affinity nerve growth factor (NGF) receptor, TrkA, is expressed by primary afferent nociceptors (McMahon 1996), direct sensitization of dorsal root ganglion neurons in vitro by NGF has not been reported. NGF does, however, appear to act directly on primary afferent neurons to alter their pattern of gene expression of mRNA encoding a large variety of peptides that may affect their excitability including, for example, bradykinin receptors (Petersen et al 1998), sodium channels (Zur et al 1995, Black et al 1997, Oyelese et al 1997), calcium channels (Fitzgerald & Dolphin 1997), nitric oxide synthase (Thippeswamy & Morris 1997) and brain-derived neurotrophic factor (BDNF) (Apfel et al 1996, Michael et al 1997). Such altered gene expression is likely to contribute to inflammatory hyperalgesia (Woolf 1996). A variety of observations suggest that peripheral inflammation, specifically, induces NGF-mediated increases in the expression of: calcitonin gene-related peptide (Donaldson et al 1992), BDNF (Cho et al 1997), growth-associated protein 43 and preprotachykinin (Leslie et al 1995, Cho et al 1996), capsaicin receptor (Hu-Tsai et al 1996), and the transcription factors, Oct-2 and AP2 (Donaldson et al 1995, Ensor et al 1996), in dorsal root ganglion neurons.

INTERACTIONS AMONG INFLAMMATORY MEDIATORS

Investigations of the actions of inflammatory mediators in which they are applied in isolation, are an experimental simplification of the inflammatory process which induces the release of a variety of mediators in concert. Interactions among those mediators undoubtedly gives rise to effects different from those induced by single mediators acting alone (Kessler et al 1992). For example, prostaglandins can enhance the response of nociceptors to other inflammatory mediators including amines and kininis (Fock & Mense 1976, Nicol & Cui 1994, Stucky et al 1996). Serotonin potentiates pain induced by other inflammatory mediators (Douglas & Ritchie 1957, Fjallbrant & Iggo 1961, Sicuteri et al 1965, Beck & Handwerker 1974, Fock & Mense 1976, Hiss & Mense 1976, Nakano & Taira 1976, Neto 1978, Mense 1981, Richardson et al 1985, Hong & Abbott 1994, Abbott et al 1996). Bradykinin enhances responses to hydrogen ions (Stucky et al 1998), and this enhancement is augmented in the presence of serotonin, prostaglandin E_2 and histamine (Kress et al 1997). Hydrogen ions enhance ATP-induced excitation of sensory neurons (Li et al 1996), attenuate tachyphylaxis of the response to combinations of inflammatory mediators (Steen et al 1995b) and, acting in synergy with other inflammatory mediators, may be able to activate the vanilloid receptor (Vyklicky et al 1998). Inflammatory mediators may act to enhance the effects of protons (Steen et al 1996). Investigation of the biochemical and molecular bases for such interactions is becoming an important area of investigation (Cui & Nicol 1995).

INTRACELLULAR SECOND-MESSENGER MECHANISMS OF NOCICEPTOR SENSITIZATION

CYCLIC ADENOSINE MONOPHOSPHATE

The identification of a diverse group of inflammatory mediators producing hyperalgesia by action at different G-protein-coupled cell-surface receptors on the primary afferent nociceptor prompted a search for a common second messenger. Prostaglandins (Hamprecht & Schultz 1973, Collier & Roy 1974), adenosine (Sattin & Rall 1970, Daly 1977, Daly et al 1983, Snyder 1985) and serotonin (Neufeld et al 1982) have been shown to elevate intracellular cyclic adenosine monophosphate (cAMP) in numerous tissues. Coupling of receptors located on the primary afferent nociceptor to adenylyl cyclase activity appears to be via a stimulatory guanine nucleotide regulatory protein (G_s) (Taiwo & Levine 1989a). Analogues of cAMP and forskolin, which directly activates adenylyl cyclase, produce hyperalgesia (Taiwo et al 1989). In addition, inhibitors of the enzyme that degrades cAMP, phosphodiesterase, significantly prolong hyperalgesia induced by 8-bromo cAMP or other directly acting agents (Taiwo et al 1989, 1992, Taiwo

& Levine 1990). The idea that the cAMP second messenger system plays a critical role in nociceptor sensitization is supported by patch clamp electrophysiology observations that cAMP analogues mimic, and antagonists inhibit, the sensitizing effects of prostaglandin E_2 in cultured dorsal root ganglion neurons (Fock & Mense 1976, England et al 1996, Lopshire & Nicol 1998). Agents which activate inhibitory guanine nucleotide regulatory protein (G_i), such as opioids and adenosine acting at the A_1 receptor (Levine & Taiwo 1989, Taiwo & Levine 1990, 1991b), inhibit hyperalgesia.

The hyperalgesic effect of cAMP is thought to be largely mediated by cAMP-dependent protein kinase (PKA). Consistent with this idea, PKA antagonists reduce hyperalgesia (Taiwo & Levine 1991a), nociceptor sensitization (Lynn & O'shea 1998) and enhancement of depolarizing currents in dorsal root ganglion neurons (England et al 1996). Furthermore, the observation that mice with a null mutation in the PKA regulatory subunit exhibit decreased inflammation-induced pain behaviour suggests that PKA activity is an important second messenger mediator of inflammatory pain, specifically (Malmberg et al 1997a). A diagram representing the role of the cAMP second messenger system in inflammatory hyperalgesia and its modulation is shown in Figure 2.6.

Another mechanism by which cAMP could potentially alter nociceptor excitability is regulation of gene transcription via the cAMP-responsive element binding protein (CREB) in dorsal root ganglion neurons (Fields et al 1997). CREB has been shown to be upregulated in dorsal root ganglion neurons following nerve injury (Herdegen et al 1992), although, as yet, its role in inflammatory pain has not been investigated.

NITRIC OXIDE

Neural nitric oxide synthase (nNOS), is present in dorsal root ganglion and trigeminal ganglion neurons (Morris et al 1992, Aoki et al 1993, Terenghi et al 1993, Jarrett et al 1994, Steel et al 1994, Vizzard et al 1994, Zhang et al 1996). That nociceptors, in particular, express NOS is suggested by the observations that nNOS is present in small- and medium-diameter dorsal root ganglion neurons (Zhang et al 1993, Qian et al 1996) and in dorsal root

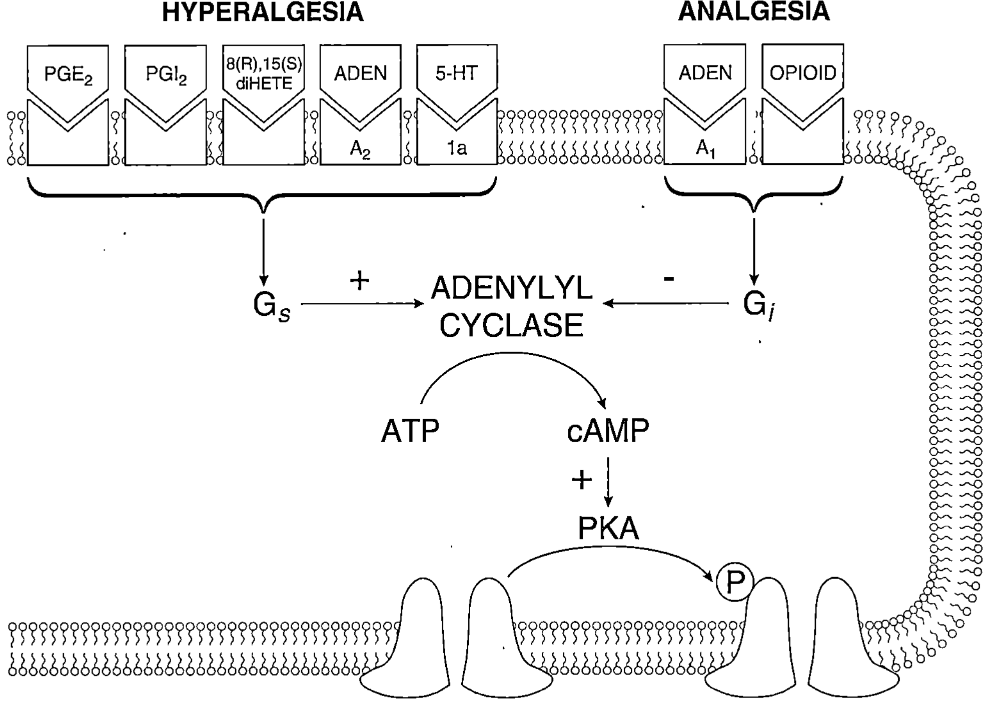

Fig. 2.6 The cAMP second-messenger system mediates hyperalgesia via a stimulatory G-protein, adenylyl cyclase. PKA and ultimately modulation of ion channels, e.g., the TTX-resistant sodium channel. Activation of an inhibitory G-protein can antagonize hyperalgesia. Aden = adenosine; 5-HT = serotonin; (8R) 15SdiHETE = 8(R), 15(S)-dihydroxyeicosatetraenoic acid; G_s = stimulatory G-protein; G_i = inhibitory G-protein; PGE_2 = prostaglandin E_2; PGI_2 = prostaglandin I_2.

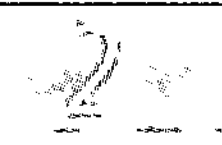

ganglion neurons that contain substance P and calcitonin gene-related peptide (CGRP) (Zhang et al 1993, Majewski et al 1995, Vanhatalo et al 1996), and nNOS immunoreactivity is greatly reduced in dorsal root ganglion neurons in neonatally capsaicin-treated rats (Ren & Ruda 1995). Furthermore, nNOS immunoreactivity in lumbar dorsal root ganglion neurons is increased by noxious irritation of the bladder (Vizzard et al 1996), noxious stimulation with capsaicin (Farkas-Szallasi et al 1995, Vizzard et al 1995), sciatic nerve of lumbar dorsal roots (Choi et al 1996) or nerves (Beesley 1995).

NO can affect nociceptor function, and this is suggested by the observations that sodium nitroprusside (a donor of NO) enhances the release of substance P and CGRP from slices of rat spinal cord dorsal horn (Dymshitz & Vasko 1994, Garry et al 1994), and that inhibition of NOS suppresses activity in lumbar dorsal rootlets originating from a sciatic neuroma (Wiesenfeld-Hallin et al 1993).

It has recently been shown that peripheral administration of NOS inhibitor attenuates PGE_2-induced hyperalgesia (Aley et al 1998). This interaction of NO with the cAMP second messenger pathway apparently occurs at a point before the action of PKA (Aley et al 1998). Although NO produces many of its effects by activation of guanylyl cyclase (Jaffrey & Snyder 1995), this effect on PGE_2-induced hyperalgesia is independent of guanylyl cyclase (Aley et al 1998). In addition to this guanylyl cyclase-independent enhancement of hyperalgesia produced via the cAMP/PKA pathway, NO itself can induce hyperalgesia via guanylyl cyclase-dependent mechanisms (Aley et al 1998). Therefore, NO may contribute to inflammatory hyperalgesia by sensitizing primary afferent nociceptors via both guanylyl cyclase-dependent and -independent mechanisms.

PROTEIN KINASE C

While there is less evidence for a role of protein kinase C (PKC) in inflammatory pain, numerous observations indicate that activation of PKC (by phorbol ester or by the potent inflammatory mediator, bradykinin) can not only activate primary afferent neurons (Dray & Perkins 1988, Rang & Ritchie 1988, Burgess et al 1989, Schepelmann et al 1993), but also increase their excitability. For example:

1. PKC activation sensitizes nociceptors to thermal (Leng et al 1996) and mechanical stimuli (Schepelmann et al 1993)
2. hyperalgesia and C-fibre sensitization in diabetes is mediated, in part, by PKC (Ahlgren & Levine 1994)
3. in cultured dorsal root ganglion neurons, PKC activation sensitizes responses to thermal stimuli (Cesare & McNaughton 1996), enhances calcium currents (Zong & Lux 1994, Hall et al 1995) and increases CGRP expression and release (Supowit et al 1995)
4. also, in vitro, inhibition of PKC reduces hyperexcitability of dorsal root ganglion neurons caused by bradykinin or by GTPγS (McGuirk & Dolphin 1992).

PKC occurs in at least 12 isoforms that are classified in three groups. 'Conventional' isoforms (α, β_I, β_{II} and γ) are activated by calcium and phorbol esters, 'novel' isoforms (δ, ε, θ, η and μ) are activated by phorbol esters, but calcium-independent and 'atypical' isoforms (ζ, λ and τ) are calcium and phorbol insensitive (Jaken 1996). PKCγ in the spinal cord has been implicated in CNS mechanisms of neuropathic pain (Mao et al 1995, Malmberg et al 1997b). However, at present little is known about PKC isoforms within dorsal root ganglion neurons and their contribution to sensitization of primary afferent nociceptors. Resiniferatoxin and capsaicin cause translocation of PKC in rat dorsal root ganglion neurons (Harvey et al 1995), and rat dorsal root ganglion neurons, including small-diameter neurons, are labelled by antibodies to PKC ∂ isoform (Roivainen et al 1993, Molliver et al 1995).

MOLECULAR TARGETS OF MODULATION BY SECOND MESSENGERS IN SENSITIZATION

The excitability of neurons is controlled by transmembrane ionic conductances, and ion channels are presumably the ultimate downstream targets of second-messenger mechanisms that sensitize primary afferent nociceptors in inflammation. Consistent with this idea, recent investigations have revealed second-messenger mechanisms of ion channel modulation that alter the excitability of primary afferent neurons.

TETRODOTOXIN-RESISTANT SODIUM CHANNEL

Although voltage-gated sodium currents in most neurons are potently blocked by the puffer fish toxin, tetrodotoxin (TTX), many neurons that exhibit nociceptor properties express a TTX-resistant sodium current (TTX-R I_{Na}) (Caffrey et al 1992, Campbell 1992, Roy & Narahashi

1992, Elliott & Elliott 1993, Ogata & Tatebayashi 1993, Jeftinija 1994, Pearce & Duchen 1994, Rizzo et al 1994, Arbuckle & Docherty 1995, Akopian et al 1996, Gold et al 1996b, Sangameswaran et al 1996, Yoshimura et al 1996, Souslova et al 1997). The inflammatory mediators, prostaglandin E_2, adenosine, and serotonin enhance TTX-R I_{Na} in cultured dorsal root ganglion neurons at least in part via the cAMP/PKA pathway (England et al 1996, Gold et al 1996b, Cardenas et al 1997), and the prostaglandin E_2-induced enhancement is inhibited by pretreatment with μ-opioid (Gold & Levine 1996) (Figs 2.6, 2.7). Theoretical studies suggest that even small increases in sodium currents can dramatically increase excitability (Matzner & Devor 1994).

In addition to the relatively rapid modulation of pre-existing sodium channels by inflammatory mediators, changes in the ratio of expression of TTX-sensitive to TTX-resistant sodium currents can also alter the activity of primary afferent nociceptors (Schild & Kunze 1997). Although inflammation does not cause an increase in the overall level of TTX-R I_{Na} expression in the dorsal root ganglion (Okuse et al 1997), treatment with the inflammatory mediator NGF increases the proportion of cultured dorsal root ganglion neurons that express TTX-R I_{Na} (Oyelese et al 1997), and expression of TTX-R I_{Na} is increased in dorsal root ganglion neurons innervating inflamed tissue (Tanaka et al 1998).

POTASSIUM CHANNELS

Voltage-activated potassium channels

Voltage-activated potassium currents that might modulate threshold, resting potential or firing pattern include the:

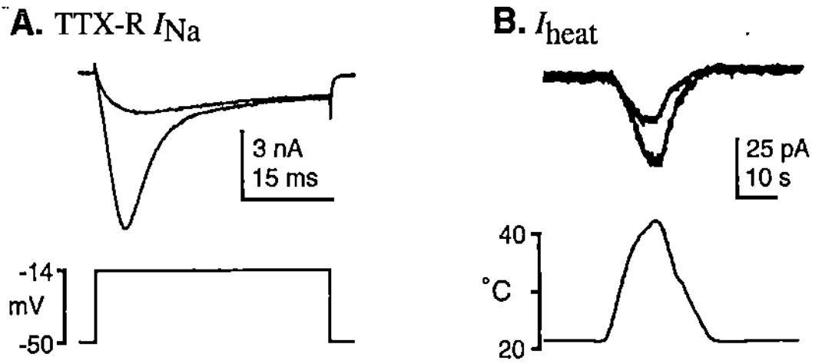

Fig. 2.7 PGE_2 enhances nociception-related excitatory currents in voltage-clamped dorsal root ganglion neurons isolated in vitro. **A** TTX-R I_{Na} was evoked by a voltage step (lower trace) from a holding potential of −50 mV to −14 mV in the presence of TTX. Two TTX-R I_{Na} currents (upper traces) are overlain, a smaller control current evoked before PGE_2 application and a larger current evoked after application of 1 μM PGE_2. **B** In a different neuron, I_{heat} was evoked by transiently heating the bath solution to a peak temperature of 43°C (lower trace). Two I_{heat} currents (upper traces) are overlain, a smaller control current evoked before PGE_2 application and a larger current evoked after application of 10 nM PGE_2. (Adapted from Gold et al 1996b and Reichling & Levine 1997.)

'S' (Shuster et al 1985), 'M' (Brown & Adams 1980), slowly inactivating (I_{AS}) (Stansfeld et al 1986), rapidly inactivating (I_{AF}) (Connor & Stevens 1971), delayed rectifier (I_K) (Perozo et al 1989) and anomalous rectifier (I_H) (Kostyuk et al 1981) currents. In rodent sensory neurons I_{AF}, I_{AS}, I_K and an anomalous rectifying cation current ($I_{K/Na}$) (Kostyuk et al 1981, Mayer & Westbrook 1983, Mayer & Sugiyama 1988, McFarlane & Cooper 1991) have been described. Prostaglandin-induced inhibition of voltage-gated potassium currents in sensory neurons (England et al 1996, Nicol et al 1997) might contribute to a decreased threshold for activation of nociceptive nerve fibres.

Calcium-activated potassium channels

Dorsal root ganglion neurons contain two calcium-activated potassium currents (I_{KCa}): *BK* (Distasi et al 1995) and *SK* (Fowler et al 1985b). *BK* is a large, rapidly activating, rapidly inactivating current sensitive to charybdotoxin (ChTx) (Blatz & Magleby 1987). *SK* is a slowly activating, slowly inactivating current blocked by apamin (Blatz & Magleby 1987). A current with characteristics similar to those described for *SK* is known to be modulated by hyperalgesic agents in visceral sensory neurons (Fowler et al 1985b, Weinreich & Wonderlin 1987, Weinreich et al 1995), and the slow afterhyperpolarization carried by *SK* may modulate accommodation (Blatz & Magleby 1987). However, whether activity in these visceral neurons produces pain has not been established.

CALCIUM CHANNELS

Voltage-activated calcium currents (VACCs) also are well-described targets of modulation. Four VACCS have been described in mammalian sensory neurons, including the T, L, N and P currents, specifically blocked by amiloride, dihydropyridines, ω-conotoxin and ω-agatoxin, respectively (Scroggs & Fox 1992). In addition, a fifth calcium current may exist in dorsal root ganglion which is resistant to these blockers (Scroggs & Fox 1992). Calcium currents in rat dorsal root ganglion neurons can be modulated in a use-dependent manner (Tatebayashi & Ogata 1992) or by neurotransmitters (Gross & Macdonald 1987). Such modulation may be mediated by both PKA- (Gross et al 1990) and PKC-dependent (Werz & Macdonald 1987, Gross & MacDonald 1989) pathways. In chick dorsal root ganglion neurons the L-current is modulated by PGE_2 (Nicol et al 1992). T-currents may underlie bursting firing patterns in adult rat dorsal root ganglion neurons (White et al 1989),

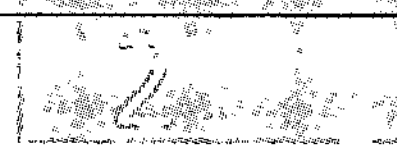

although the magnitude of this current is relatively small in capsaicin-sensitive neurons of adult rat dorsal root ganglion (Petersen & LaMotte 1991). On the other hand, pharmacological manipulation of N- and L-currents can alter the amount of transmitter released by cultured dorsal root ganglion neurons (Maggi et al 1989, Yu et al 1992), and it is possible that such effects on transmitter secretion might contribute to hyperalgesia that involves changes in primary afferent transmission in the spinal cord (Hingtgen et al 1995). VACCs depolarize the membrane and indirectly activate calcium-activated potassium and chloride currents to produce membrane hyperpolarization. Therefore, if calcium currents are involved in PGE_2-induced sensitization, it is difficult to predict whether they would be increased or decreased.

HYPERPOLARIZATION-INDUCED NON-SELECTIVE CATION CHANNEL

A hyperpolarization-induced inward current, termed 'I_H', is expressed in dorsal root ganglion neurons. Although the current is most pronounced in large-diameter neurons, it also occurs in small-diameter neurons exhibiting electrophysiological properties of A-type neurons, but not C-type neurons (Pearce & Duchen 1994, Scroggs et al 1994). Therefore, I_H might influence the excitability of Aδ nociceptors. Prostaglandin E_2 can enhance I_H in cultured dorsal root ganglion neurons, apparently via the cAMP/PKA pathway (Ingram & Williams 1996, Raes et al 1997). Such enhancement of I_H could potentially reduce hyperpolarization of the membrane and thereby contribute to activation and sensitization of myelinated Aδ nociceptors in inflammation. Also consistent with a role of I_H in inflammatory hyperalgesia is the observation that opioids reverse the cAMP-dependent enhancement of the current (Ingram & Williams 1994).

HEAT-ACTIVATED CHANNELS

Recent investigations have begun to explore the cellular mechanisms of heat transduction in primary afferent neurons. Although the relationship among the reported heat-activated currents is not yet resolved, they share some characteristics. In general, they are non-selective cation currents (Cesare & McNaughton 1996, Caterina et al 1997, Reichling et al 1997, Reichling & Levine 1997), resulting from the opening of ion channels (Caterina et al 1997, Reichling & Levine 1997), that are preferentially expressed in small-diameter sensory neurons (Caterina et al 1997, Kirschstein et al 1997, Reichling & Levine 1997), and may be calcium dependent (Reichling et al 1997, Reichling & Levine 1997), and at least one is also a capsaicin receptor (Caterina et al 1997, Kirschstein et al 1997). Heat-activated currents may be enhanced by the inflammatory mediators prostaglandin E_2 via the cAMP second-messenger cascade (Reichling & Levine 1997, Lopshire & Nicol 1998) (Fig. 2.7) and by bradykinin via the PKC cascade (Cesare & McNaughton 1996). These data suggest that the enhancement of heat-transducing currents in primary afferent nociceptors might contribute to inflammation-induced thermal hyperalgesia.

MECHANICALLY ACTIVATED CHANNELS

Our knowledge of the mechanisms of mechanical transduction, although critical to an understanding of inflammatory pain, has lagged considerably behind our knowledge of chemical and thermal transduction in somatosensory neurons. The aminoglycoside, gentamicin, a blocker of some mechano-gated ion channels, blocks the initial burst of C-fibre nociceptor activity evoked by mechanical stimuli (White & Levine 1991), and another aminoglycoside, neomycin, blocks the slowly adapting activity of mechanoreceptors (Baumann et al 1988). A mechanically activated ion channel underlies these effects, which is supported by the observation of stretch-activated single channels in dorsal root ganglion neurons (Yang et al 1986), and by genetic evidence of touch-cell-specific ion channels in the nematode *Caenorhabditis elegans* (Herman 1996) and of a related ion channel in presumptive mechanoreceptive neurons in *Drosophila melanogaster* (Darboux et al 1998). The investigation of mechanical transduction is likely to become a much more active area of pain research in coming years.

PHARMACOTHERAPY FOR INFLAMMATORY PAIN

NON-STEROIDAL ANTI-INFLAMMATORY DRUGS

Non-steroidal anti-inflammatory drugs (NSAIDs), the most commonly used analgesics, are potent agents for the treatment of inflammatory pain. Their primary analgesic action appears to be the inhibition of prostaglandin synthesis at peripheral sites of inflammation (Lim et al 1964, Ferreira et al 1971, Ferreira 1972). However, there is mounting evidence that they may also alter nociception by acting on prostaglandin production within the CNS where they can modulate neurotransmitter release (Ferreira et al 1978, Yaksh 1982, Devoghel 1983, Taiwo & Levine 1988b). At sites of inflammation, the inhibition of prostaglandin synthesis not only eliminates the direct hyperalgesic action of these mediators, but also results in a decrease in the sensitizing effects of other inflammatory mediators (Fock & Mense 1976). NSAIDs are useful for a variety of mild to moderate inflammatory pains and also for severe pains, such as ureteral and biliary colic and severe dysmenorrhoea, subsequent to the introduction of injectable and rectal suppository NSAIDs that allow higher doses to be better tolerated (Thornell et al 1979, Marsala 1980). NSAIDs have been remarkably successful in preventing postoperative pain, when administered prophylactically (Dionne & Cooper 1978). Nevertheless, despite these successes, a variety of inflammatory pain states remain poorly managed by NSAIDs. This is probably due, in part, to the multiplicity of inflammatory mediators that are apable of directly sensitizing the primary afferent and, in part, to adverse effects arising from inhibition of prostaglandin production in other tissues (e.g., gastrointestinal ulcer and bleeding, and renal failure).

The key enzyme in the production of prostaglandins, COX, is now known to occur as two isoforms: COX1, which is constitutively active, and COX2, which is inducible by stimuli including pro-inflammatory cytokines (Vane et al 1998). The currently available NSAIDs inhibit both COX1 and COX2 (Cryer & Feldman 1998, Vane et al 1998). Because the protective effects of prostaglandins on gastrointestinal and kidney functions are mediated by COX1, inhibitors of COX2 are being developed as analgesics. COX2 inhibitors might also be useful for reducing pro-nociceptive effects of prostaglandins in the CNS because COX2 expression in the spinal cord is increased by chronic inflammation (Goppelt-Struebe & Beiche 1997).

CORTICOSTEROIDS

Corticosteroids have been used to control pain, particularly in clinical syndromes that are recalcitrant to NSAIDs. The success of corticosteroids can be understood in view of their potent inhibition of phospholipase A2 and, therefore, to prevent the release of arachidonic acid, thereby attenuating the synthesis of both hyperalgesic prostaglandins and leukotrienes (Levine et al 1984, 1985, 1986b). Glucocorticoids are also potent inhibitors of COX2, which may explain their anti-inflammatory effect (Seibert et al 1997). The use of corticosteroids is quite limited, however, by their significant systemic side effects, especially with chronic use.

SYMPATHOLYTIC THERAPY

Although the mechanism by which sympathetic postganglionic neuron terminals contribute to pain is incompletely understood (Koltzenburg & McMahon 1991), a number of diverse painful clinical conditions can be effectively relieved by sympathetic ablation (Loh & Nathan 1978, Glynn et al 1981, Levine et al 1986a), especially those characterized by an altered autonomic control in effector organs. The necessary contribution of the sympathetic nervous system to the action of various hyperalgesic inflammatory mediators, including bradykinin, noradrenaline, interleukin 1β and NGF, may help to explain the efficacy of sympatholysis in inflammatory pain states.

ANTAGONISTS OF OTHER INFLAMMATORY MEDIATORS

The identification of inflammatory mediators, present in inflammatory and neuropathic pain states, that alter pain sensation has also led to interest in the possible development of specific mediator receptor antagonists. To this end, antagonists of prostaglandin receptors (Sanner 1969, Rakovska & Milenov 1984), bradykinin (particularly B_2 receptors (Whalley et al 1989)), interleukin 1β (Ferreira et al 1988) and neurokinins, including substance P (Garret et al 1993), are in various stages of development as analgesic agents. The enhanced selectivity of action of these agents may also reduce side effects.

Another approach to selective inhibition of inflammatory mediator action is the development of inhibitors of the specific enzymes involved in mediator synthesis. Enzyme targets under investigation include phospholipases, lipoxygenases and kallikreins.

The elucidation of the cAMP second messenger system as a common mediator of primary afferent hyperalgesia allows the possibility of another novel approach to the treatment of inflammatory pain, namely antagonism of the cAMP second-messenger system. Agents inhibiting stimulatory G-protein activity or activating inhibitory G-proteins would be potential analgesics and might allow single-agent analgesia. Although the second-messenger pathways mediating pain are present in virtually every cell of the body, the identification of molecular isoforms (e.g., for adenylyl cyclase, protein kinase A, protein kinase C and nitric oxide synthase) may allow the development of novel analgesics with minimal adverse effects.

Interestingly, δ- and κ-receptor-specific opioid agonists have also been shown to produce antinociception in inflamed tissue (Stein et al 1988b, 1989). They do not inhibit direct hyperalgesia, such as that of prostaglandin E_2 (Levine & Taiwo 1989), but inhibit sympathetic postganglionic neuron-dependent hyperalgesia (Taiwo & Levine 1991b), probably by acting on δ- and κ-opioid receptors known to be present on sympathetic postganglionic neuron terminals (Hughes et al 1975, Illes et al 1985, Berzetei et al 1988).

Finally, other specific antagonists, for example those directed at inhibiting receptor action of substance P, interleukin and bradykinin, are all potential agents for the treatment of inflammatory pain and hyperalgesia. Advances in the understanding of inflammatory pain, including the discovery of as yet unknown mediator actions as well as better understanding of the mechanism in the primary afferent to produce sensitization and activation, will undoubtedly suggest even more approaches to the treatment of inflammatory pain.

PERIPHERAL OPIOID ANALGESIA

μ-opioids, which are known to activate inhibitory G-proteins and decrease intracellular cAMP (Sharma et al 1975, Law et al 1981, Childers & LaRiviere 1984, Makman et al 1988), have been shown to produce naloxone-antagonizable analgesia when injected into sites of inflammation (Joris et al 1987, Stein et al 1988a, Stein et al 1988b, 1989, 1990, Levine & Taiwo 1989, Stein 1995). However, the rapid development of tolerance to the peripheral actions of opioids might limit their clinical usefulness (Aley & Levine 1997).

INFLAMMATION AND THE CENTRAL NERVOUS SYSTEM

Although this chapter has focused on the hyperalgesic effects of inflammatory mediators in peripheral tissues, a recent series of studies has revealed that prostaglandins can also exert hyperalgesic actions in the spinal cord (Taiwo & Levine 1988b, Minami et al 1995, Saito et al 1995, Ferreira & Lorenzetti 1996). Peripheral inflammatory stimuli can cause increased levels of prostaglandin E_2 in the spinal cord (Malmberg & Yaksh 1995, Yang et al 1996, Scheuren et al 1997), at least in part by upregulation of COX-2 (Goppelt-Struebe & Beiche 1997, Hay & de Belleroche 1997), and COX-2 activity (Yamamoto & Nozaki-Taguchi 1997, Dirig et al 1998) and prostaglandin receptors (Malmberg et al 1994) contribute to hyperalgesia induced by peripheral inflammation. This spinal hyperalgesic effect of prostaglandins is thought to involve facilitation of transmitter release from spinal terminals of primary afferent nociceptors (Vasko 1995, White 1996). As a result of this line of research, spinal COX is becoming recognized as a potentially important new target of anti-inflammatory analgesic drug therapy (McCormack 1994a, 1994b, Bannwarth et al 1995, Bjorkman 1995).

CONCLUSION

The study of inflammatory pain has been one of the most rapidly advancing and expanding areas of pain research in recent years. Some emerging subjects were not covered in this chapter but are likely to grow in prominence in the near future. One concept that is likely to become increasingly influential in our understanding of nociceptor physiology is the parallelism between the central and peripheral endings of primary afferent nerve fibres. These antipodal endings perform distinctive functions: synaptic transmitter release versus stimulus transduction. However, there is growing recognition that these two endings share many physiological characteristics. For example, most, if not all receptor molecules are transported bidirectionally from the soma to both nerve endings. Evidence of this is the observations (described above) that the spinally acting opioid analgesics can also produce analgesia by acting on peripheral nerve endings, and that the peripherally acting nonsteroidal anti-inflammatory agents may also exert analgesic actions on spinal cord circuitry. Another topic growing in importance is the influence of sex hormones on primary afferent nociceptor function. Thus, dorsal root ganglion neurons express sex hormone receptors (Sohrabji et al 1994, Papka et al 1997), and this might contribute to gender-dependent differences in inflammation (Da Silva et al 1994). Finally, the physiological basis of the differences between acute and chronic pain are only beginning to be explored. Future investigations in these emerging subject areas may lead to important insights that will guide the development of therapeutic approaches to the treatment of inflammatory pain.

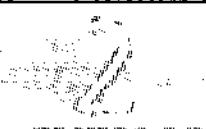

REFERENCES

Aaseth J, Haugen M, Forre O 1998 Rheumatoid arthritis and metal compounds – perspectives on the role of oxygen radical detoxification. Analyst 123: 3–6

Abbott F V, Hong Y, Blier P 1996 Activation of 5-HT2_A receptors potentiates pain produced by inflammatory mediators. Neuropharmacology 35: 99–110

Agrawal S G, Evans R H 1986 The primary afferent depolarizing action of kainate in the rat. British Journal of Pharmacology 87: 345–355

Ahlgren S C, Levine J D 1994 Protein kinase C inhibitors decrease hyperalgesia and C-fiber hyperexcitability in the streptozotocin-diabetic rat. Journal of Neurophysiology 72: 684–692

Akopian A N, Sivilotti L, Wood J N 1996 A tetrodotoxin-resistant voltage-gated sodium channel expressed by sensory neurons. Nature 379: 257–262

Aley K O, Levine J D 1997 Dissociation of tolerance and dependence for opioid peripheral antinociception in rats. Journal of Neuroscience 17: 3907–3912

Aley K O, McCarter G, Levine J D 1998 NO signalling in pain and nociceptor sensitization in the rat. Journal of Neuroscience 18: 7008–7014

Alm P, Uvelius B, Ekstrom J, Holmqvist B, Larsson B, Andersson K E 1995 Nitric oxide synthase-containing neurons in rat parasympathetic, sympathetic and sensory ganglia: a comparative study. Histochemical Journal 27: 819–831

Aloe L, Probert L, Kollias G, Micera A, Tirassa P 1995 Effect of NGF antibodies on mast cell distribution, histamine and substance P levels in the knee joint of TNF-arthritic transgenic mice. Rheumatology International 14: 249–252

Amann R, Schuligoi R, Herzeg G, Donnerer J 1996 Intraplantar injection of nerve growth factor into the rat hind paw: local edema and effects on thermal nociceptive threshold. Pain 64: 323–329

Andreev N, Dimitrieva N, Koltzenburg M, McMahon S B 1995 Peripheral administration of nerve growth factor in the adult rat produces a thermal hyperalgesia that requires the presence of sympathetic post-ganglionic neurones. Pain 63: 109–115

Aoki E, Takeuchi I K, Shoji R, Semba R 1993 Localization of nitric oxide-related substances in the peripheral nervous tissues. Brain Research 620: 142–145

Apfel S C, Wright D E, Wiideman A M, Dormia C, Snider W D, Kessler J A 1996 Nerve growth factor regulates the expression of brain-derived neurotrophic factor mRNA in the peripheral nervous system. Molecular and Cellular Neurosciences 7: 134–142

Appenzeller O, Oribe E 1997 The autonomic nervous system: an introduction to basic and clinical concepts. Elsevier, Amsterdam

Arbuckle J B, Docherty R J 1995 Expression of tetrodotoxin-resistant sodium channels in capsaicin-sensitive dorsal root ganglion neurons of adult rats. Neuroscience Letters 185: 70–73

Armstrong D, Dry R M L, Keele C A, Markham J W 1953 Observations on chemical excitant of cutaneous pain in man. Journal of Physiology (London) 120: 326–351

Armstrong R A, Matthews J S, Jones R L, Wilson N H 1991 Characterization of PGE_2 receptors mediating increased vascular permeability in inflammation. In: Samuelsson B, Ramwell P W, Paoletti G, Folco R, Granstrom R (eds) Prostaglandins and related compounds. Seventh International Conference, Florence, Italy. Raven Press, New York, pp 375–378

Ault B, Hildebrand L M 1993 L-glutamate activates peripheral nociceptors. Agents Actions 39: C142–144

Babe K S Jr, Serafin W E 1996 Histamine, bradykinin and their antagonists. In: Hardman J G, Limbird L E, Molinoff P B, Ruddon R W, Goodman Gilman A (ed) Goodman & Gilman's The pharmacological basis of therapeutics. McGraw-Hill, New York, pp 581–600

Baccaglini P I, Hogan P G 1983 Some rat sensory neurons in culture express characteristics of differentiated pain sensory cells. Proceedings of the National Academy of Sciences USA 80: 594–598

Bannwarth B, Demotes-Mainard F, Schaeverbeke T, Labat L, Dehais J 1995 Central analgesic effects of aspirin-like drugs. Fundamental and Clinical Pharmacology 9: 1–7

Baranauskas G, Nistri A 1998 Sensitization of pain pathways in the spinal cord: cellular mechanisms. Progress in Neurobiology 54: 349–365

Bauer M B, Murphy S, Gebhart G F 1995 Stimulation of cyclic GMP production via a nitrosyl factor in sensory neuronal cultures by algesic or inflammatory agents. Journal of Neurochemistry 65: 363–372

Baumann K I, Hamann W, Leung M S 1988 Responsiveness of slowly adapting cutaneous mechanoreceptors after close arterial infusion of neomycin in cats. Progress in Brain Research 74: 43–49

Beck P W, Handwerker H O 1974 Bradykinin and serotonin effects on various types of cutaneous nerve fibers. Pflügers Archiv (European Journal of Physiology) 347: 209–222

Beesley J E 1995 Histochemical methods for detecting nitric oxide synthase. Histochemical Journal 27: 757–769

Bervoets K, Millan M J, Colpaert F C 1990 Agonist action at 5-HT_{1C} receptors facilitates 5-HT_{1A} receptor-mediated spontaneous tail-flicks in the rat. European Journal of Pharmacology 191: 185–195

Berzetei I P, Fong A, Yamamura H I, Duckles S P 1988 Characterization of kappa opioid receptors in the rabbit ear artery. European Journal of Pharmacology 151: 449–455

Bessou P, Perl E R 1969 Response of cutaneous sensory units with unmyelinated fibers to noxious stimuli. Journal of Neurophysiology 32: 1025–1043

Bevan S, Geppetti P 1994 Protons: small stimulants of capsaicin-sensitive sensory nerves. Trends in Neuroscience 17: 509–512

Bevan S, Winter J 1995 Nerve growth factor (NGF) differentially regulates the chemosensitivity of adult rat cultured sensory neurons. Journal of Neuroscience 15: 4918–4926

Bevan S, Yeats J 1991 Protons activate a cation conductance in a sub-population of rat dorsal root ganglion neurones. Journal of Physiology (London) 433: 145–161

Bill A, Stjernschantz J, Mandahl A, Brodin E, Nilsson G 1979 Substance P: release on trigeminal nerve stimulation, effects in the eye. Acta Physiologica Scandinavica 106: 371–373

Bisgaard H, Kristensen J K 1985 Leukotriene B4 produces hyperalgesia in humans. Prostaglandins 30: 791–797

Bjorkman R 1995 Central antinociceptive effects of non-steroidal anti-inflammatory drugs and paracetamol. Experimental studies in the rat. Acta Anaesthesiologica Scandinavica. Supplementum 103: 1–44

Black J A, Langworthy K, Hinson A W, Dib-Hajj S D, Waxman S G 1997 NGF has opposing effects on Na^+ channel III and SNS gene expression in spinal sensory neurons. Neuroreport 8: 2331–2335

Bland-Ward P A, Humphrey PP 1997 Acute nociception mediated by hindpaw P2X receptor activation in the rat. British Journal of Pharmacology 122: 365–371

Blatz A L, Magleby K L 1987 Calcium-activated potassium channels. Trends in Neuroscience 10: 463–467

Bleehen T, Keele C A 1977 Observations on the algogenic actions of adenosine compounds on the human blister base preparation. Pain 3: 367–377

Blumberg H, Jänig W 1984 Discharge pattern of afferent fibers from a neuroma. Pain 20: 335–353

Borish L, Joseph B Z 1992 Inflammation and the allergic response. Medical Clinics of North America 76: 765–787

Brimijoin S, Lundberg J M, Brodin E, Hokfelt T, Nilsson G 1980 Axonal transport of substance P in the vagus and sciatic nerves of the guinea pig. Brain Research 191: 443–457

Brodin E, Gazelius B, Olgart L, Nilsson G 1981 Tissue concentration and release of substance P-like immunoreactivity in the dental pulp. Acta Physiologica Scandinavica 111: 141–149

Brown D A, Adams P R 1980 Muscarinic suppression of a novel voltage-sensitive K^+ current in a vertebrate neurone. Nature 283: 673–676

Bruch-Gerharz D, Ruzicka T, Kolb-Bachofen V 1998 Nitric oxide in human skin: current status and future prospects. Journal of Investigative Dermatology 110: 1–7

Brunner T, Heusser C H, Dahinden C A 1993 Human peripheral blood basophils primed by interleukin 3 (IL-3) produce IL-4 in response to immunoglobulin E receptor stimulation. Journal of Experimental Medicine 177: 605–611

Burgess G M, Mullaney I, McNeill M, Dunn P M, Rang H P 1989 Second messengers involved in the mechanism of action of bradykinin in sensory neurons in culture. Journal of Neuroscience 9: 3314–3325

Burnstock G 1996 A unifying purinergic hypothesis for the initiation of pain. Lancet 347: 1604–1605

Burnstock G, Wood J N 1996 Purinergic receptors: their role in nociception and primary afferent neurotransmission. Current Opinion in Neurobiology 6: 526–532

Caffrey J M, Eng D L, Black J A, Waxman S G, Kocsis J D 1992 Three types of sodium channels in adult rat dorsal root ganglion neurons. Brain Research 592: 283–297

Campbell D T 1992 Large and small vertebrate sensory neurons express different Na and K channel subtypes. Proceedings of the National Academy of Sciences USA 89: 9569–9573

Cardenas C G, Del Mar L P, Cooper B Y, Scroggs R S 1997 $5HT_4$ receptors couple positively to tetrodotoxin-insensitive sodium channels in a subpopulation of capsaicin-sensitive rat sensory neurons. Journal of Neuroscience 17: 7181–7189

Carlton S M, Hargett G L, Coggeshall R E 1995 Localization and activation of glutamate receptors in unmyelinated axons of rat glabrous skin. Neuroscience Letters 197: 25–28

Carlton S M, Chung K, Ding Z, Coggeshall R E 1998a Glutamate receptors on postganglionic sympathetic axons. Neuroscience 83: 601–605

Carlton S M, Zhou S, Coggeshall R E 1998b Evidence for the interaction of glutamate and NK1 receptors in the periphery. Brain Research 790: 160–169

Caterina M J, Schumacher M A, Tominaga M, Rosen T A, Levine J D, Julius D 1997 The capsaicin receptor: a heat-activated ion channel in the pain pathway. Nature 389: 816–824

Cervero F 1995 Visceral pain: mechanisms of peripheral and central sensitization. Annals of Medicine 27: 235–239

Cesare P, McNaughton P 1996 A novel heat-activated current in nociceptive neurons and its sensitization by bradykinin. Proceedings of the National Academy of Sciences USA 93: 15435–15439

Chen C C, Akopian A N, Sivilotti L, Colquhoun D, Burnstock G, Wood J N 1995 A P2X purinoceptor expressed by a subset of sensory neurons. Nature 377: 428–431

Childers S R, LaRiviere G 1984 Modification of guanine nucleotide-regulatory components in brain membranes. II. Relationship of guanosine 5′-triphosphate effects on opiate receptor binding and coupling receptors with adenylate cyclase. Journal of Neuroscience 4: 2764–2771

Cho H J, Park E H, Bae M A, Kim J K 1996 Expression of mRNAs for preprotachykinin and nerve growth factor receptors in the dorsal root-ganglion following peripheral inflammation. Brain Research 716: 197–201

Cho H J, Kim J K, Zhou X F, Rush R A 1997 Increased brain-derived neurotrophic factor immunoreactivity in rat dorsal root ganglia and spinal cord following peripheral inflammation. Brain Research 764: 269–272

Choi Y, Raja S N, Moore L C, Tobin J R 1996 Neuropathic pain in rats is associated with altered nitric oxide synthase activity in neural tissue. Journal of the Neurological Sciences 138: 14–20

Chou R C, Dong X L, Noble B K, Knight P R, Spengler R N 1998 Adrenergic regulation of macrophage-derived tumor necrosis factor-alpha generation during a chronic polyarthritis pain model. Journal of Neuroimmunology 82: 140–148

Coderre T J 1993 The role of excitatory amino acid receptors and intracellular messengers in persistent nociception after tissue injury in rats. Molecular Neurobiology 7: 229–246

Coelho A M, Fioramonti J, Bueno L 1998 Mast cell degranulation induces delayed rectal allodynia in rats: role of histamine and 5-HT. Digestive Diseases and Sciences 43: 727–737

Cohen R H, Perl E R 1990 Contributions of arachidonic acid derivatives and substance P to the sensitization of cutaneous nociceptors. Journal of Neurophysiology 64: 457–464

Colditz I G 1991 The induction of plasma leakage in skin by histamine, bradykinin, activated complement, platelet-activating factor and serotonin. Immunology and Cell Biology 69: 215–219

Collier H O, Roy A C 1974 Morphine-like drugs inhibit the stimulation of E prostaglandins of cyclic AMP formation by rat brain homogenate. Nature 248: 24–27

Collier H O, James G W, Schneider C 1966 Antagonism by aspirin and fenamates of bronchoconstriction and nociception induced by adenosine-5′-triphosphate. Nature 212: 411–412

Connor J A, Stevens C F 1971 Prediction of repetitive firing behaviour from voltage clamp data on an isolated neurone soma. Journal of Physiology (London) 213: 31–53

Cook A J, Woolf C J, Wall P D, McMahon S B 1987 Dynamic receptive field plasticity in rat spinal cord dorsal horn following C-primary afferent input. Nature 325: 151–153

Cook S P, Vulchanova L, Hargreaves K M, Elde R, McCleskey E W 1997 Distinct ATP receptors on pain-sensing and stretch-sensing neurons. Nature 387: 505–508

Cooper B, Ahlquist M, Friedman R M, Labanc J 1991 Properties of high-threshold mechanoreceptors in the goat oral mucosa. II. Dynamic and static reactivity in carrageenan-inflamed mucosa. Journal of Neurophysiology 66: 1280–1290

Cormia F E, Dougherty J W 1960 Proteolytic activity in development of pain and itching: cutaneous reactions to bradykinin and kallikrein. Journal of Investigative Dermatology 35: 21–26

Corrado A P, Ballejo G 1992 Is guanylate cyclase activation through the release of nitric oxide or a related compound involved in bradykinin-induced perivascular primary afferent excitation? Agents and Actions 36: 238–250

Crawford J H, Wootton J F, Seabrook G R, Scott R H 1997 Activation of Ca^{2+}-dependent currents in dorsal root ganglion neurons by metabotropic glutamate receptors and cyclic ADP-ribose precursors. Journal of Neurophysiology 77: 2573–2584

Crunkhorn P, Willis A L 1971 Cutaneous reactions to intradermal prostaglandins. British Journal of Pharmacology 41: 49–56

Cryer B, Feldman M 1998 Cyclooxygenase-1 and cyclooxygenase-2 selectivity of widely used nonsteroidal anti-inflammatory drugs. American Journal of Medicine 104: 413–421

Cui M, Nicol G D 1995 Cyclic AMP mediates the prostaglandin E_2-induced potentiation of bradykinin excitation in rat sensory neurons. Neuroscience 66: 459–466

Cunha F Q, Lorenzetti B B, Poole S, Ferreira S H 1991 Interleukin-8 as a mediator of sympathetic pain. British Journal of Pharmacology 104: 765–767

Da Silva J A, Larbre J P, Seed M P et al 1994 Sex differences in inflammation induced cartilage damage in rodents. The influence of sex steroids. Journal of Rheumatology 21: 330–337

Daly J W 1977 Cyclic nucleotides in the nervous system. Plenum Press, New York

Daly J W, Butts-Lamb P, Padgett W 1983 Subclasses of adenosine receptors in the central nervous system: interaction with caffeine and related methylxanthines. Cellular and Molecular Neurobiology 3: 69–80

Darboux I, Lingueglia E, Pauron D, Barbry P, Lazdunski M 1998 A new member of the amiloride-sensitive sodium channel family in *Drosophila melanogaster* peripheral nervous system. Biochemical and Biophysical Research Communication 246: 210–216

Davidson E M, Coggeshall R E, Carlton S M 1997 Peripheral NMDA and non-NMDA glutamate receptors contribute to nociceptive behaviors in the rat formalin test. Neuroreport 8: 941–946

Davis C L, Naeem S, Phagoo S B, Campbell E A, Urban L, Burgess G M 1996 B_1 bradykinin receptors and sensory neurones. British Journal of Pharmacology 118: 1469–1476

Dayer J M, de Rochemonteix B, Burrus B, Demczuk S, Dinarello C A 1986 Human recombinant interleukin 1 stimulates collagenase and prostaglandin E_2 production by human synovial cells. Journal of Clinical Investigation 77: 645–648

Devoghel J C 1983 Small intrathecal doses of lysine-acetylsalicylate relieve intractable pain in man. Journal of International Medical Research 11: 90–91

Devor M 1983 Nerve pathophysiology and mechanisms of pain in causalgia. Journal of the Autonomic Nervous System 7: 371–384

Devor M, Jänig W 1981 Activation of myelinated afferents ending in a neuroma by stimulation of the sympathetic supply in the rat. Neuroscience Letters 24: 43–47

Di Rosa M, Giroud J P, Willoughby D A 1971 Studies on the mediators of the acute inflammatory response induced in rats in different sites by carrageenan and turpentine. Journal of Pathology 104: 15–29

Dickenson A H, Chapman V, Green G M 1997 The pharmacology of excitatory and inhibitory amino acid-mediated events in the transmission and modulation of pain in the spinal cord. General Pharmacology 28: 633–638

Dinarello C A 1989 Interleukin-1 and other growth factors. In: Kelley W M, Harris E D, Ruddy S, Sledge C B (eds) Textbook of rheumatology. Saunders, Philadelphia, pp 285–299

Dionne R A, Cooper S A 1978 Evaluation of preoperative ibuprofen for postoperative pain after removal of third molars. Oral Surgery Oral Medicine Oral Pathology 45: 851–856

Dirig D M, Isakson P C, Yaksh T L 1998 Effect of COX-1 and COX-2 inhibition on induction and maintenance of carrageenan-evoked thermal hyperalgesia in rats. Journal of Pharmacology and Experimental Therapeutics 285: 1031–1038

Distasi C, Munaron L, Laezza F, Lovisolo D 1995 Basic fibroblast growth factor opens calcium-permeable channels in quail mesencephalic neural crest neurons. European Journal of Neuroscience 7: 516–520

Dmitrieva N, McMahon S B 1996 Sensitisation of visceral afferents by nerve growth factor in the adult rat. Pain 66: 87–97

Dmitrieva N, Shelton D, Rice A S, McMahon S B 1997 The role of nerve growth factor in a model of visceral inflammation. Neuroscience 78: 449–459

Donaldson L F, Harmar A J, McQueen D S, Seckl J R 1992 Increased expression of preprotachykinin, calcitonin gene-related peptide, but not vasoactive intestinal peptide messenger RNA in dorsal root ganglia during the development of adjuvant monoarthritis in the rat. Brain Research. Molecular Brain Research 16: 143–149

Donaldson L F, McQueen D S, Seckl J R 1995 Induction of transcription factor AP2 mRNA expression in rat primary afferent neurons during acute inflammation. Neuroscience Letters 196: 181–184

Dougherty P M, Palecek J, Paleckova V, Sorkin L S, Willis W D 1992 The role of NMDA and non-NMDA excitatory amino acid receptors in the excitation of primate spinothalamic tract neurons by mechanical, chemical, thermal, and electrical stimuli. Journal of Neuroscience 12: 3025–3041

Douglas W W, Ritchie J M 1957 On excitation of non-medullated afferent fibers in the vagus and aortic nerves by pharmacological agents. Journal of Physiology (London) 138: 31–43

Dray A, Perkins M N 1988 Bradykinin activates peripheral capsaicin-sensitive fibres via a second messenger system. Agents and Actions 25: 214–215

Dray A, Perkins M 1993 Bradykinin and inflammatory pain. Trends in Neuroscience 16: 99–104

Dunn P M, Rang H P 1990 Bradykinin-induced depolarization of primary afferent nerve terminals in the neonatal rat spinal cord in vitro. British Journal of Pharmacology 100: 656–660

Dymshitz J, Vasko M R 1994 Nitric oxide and cyclic guanosine 3′, 5′-monophosphate do not alter neuropeptide release from rat sensory neurons grown in culture. Neuroscience 62: 1279–1286

Edlund A, Fredholm B B, Patrignani P, Patrono C, Wennmalm A, Wennmalm M 1983 Release of two vasodilators, adenosine and prostacyclin, from isolated rabbit hearts during controlled hypoxia. Journal of Physiology (London) 340: 487–501

Eglen R M, Jasper J R, Chang D J, Martin G R 1997 The 5-HT_7 receptor: orphan found. Trends in Pharmacological Sciences 18: 104–107

Elliott A A, Elliott J R 1993 Characterization of TTX-sensitive and TTX-resistant sodium currents in small cells from adult rat dorsal root ganglia. Journal of Physiology (London) 463: 39–56

England S, Bevan S, Docherty R J 1996 PGE_2 modulates the tetrodotoxin-resistant sodium current in neonatal rat dorsal root ganglion neurones via the cyclic AMP-protein kinase A cascade. Journal of Physiology 495: 429–440

Ensor E, Kendall G, Allchorne A, Woolf C J, Latchman D S 1996 Induction of the Oct-2 transcription factor in primary sensory neurons during inflammation is nerve growth factor-dependent. Neuroscience Letters 204: 29–32

Farkas-Szallasi T, Lundberg J M, Wiesenfeld H Z, Hokfelt T, Szallasi A 1995 Increased levels of GMAP, VIP and nitric oxide synthase, and their mRNAs, in lumbar dorsal root ganglia of the rat following systemic resiniferatoxin treatment. Neuroreport 6: 2230–2234

Ferjan I, Carman-Krzan M, Erjavec F 1997 Comparison of histamine and serotonin release from rat peritoneal mast cells induced by nerve growth factor and compound 48/80. Inflammation Research 46(suppl 1): S23–24

Ferreira S H 1972 Prostaglandins, aspirin-like drugs and analgesia. Nature New Biology 240: 200–203

Ferreira S H, Lorenzetti B B 1994 Glutamate spinal retrograde sensitization of primary sensory neurons associated with nociception. Neuropharmacology 33: 1479–1485

Ferreira S H, Lorenzetti B B 1996 Intrathecal administration of prostaglandin E_2 causes sensitization of the primary afferent neuron via the spinal release of glutamate. Inflammation Research 45: 499–502

Ferreira S H, Moncada S, Vane J R 1971 Indomethacin and aspirin abolish prostaglandin release from the spleen. Nature New Biology 231: 237–239

Ferreira S H, Moncada S, Vane J R 1973 Prostaglandins and the mechanism of analgesia produced by aspirin-like drugs. British Journal of Pharmacology 49: 86–97

Ferreira S H, Lorenzetti B B, Correa F M 1978 Central and peripheral antialgesic action of aspirin-like drugs. European Journal of Pharmacology 53: 39–48

Ferreira S H, Nakamura M 1979 I – Prostaglandin hyperalgesia, a cAMP/Ca^{2+} dependent process. Prostaglandins 18: 179–190

Ferreira S H, Lorenzetti B B, Bristow A F, Poole S 1988 Interleukin-1 beta as a potent hyperalgesic agent antagonized by a tripeptide analogue. Nature 334: 698–700

Fiallos-Estrada C E, Kummer W, Mayer B, Bravo R, Zimmermann M, Herdegen T 1993 Long-lasting increase of nitric oxide synthase immunoreactivity, NADPH-diaphorase reaction and c-JUN co-expression in rat dorsal root ganglion neurons following sciatic nerve transection. Neuroscience Letters 150: 169–173

Fields R D, Eshete F, Stevens B, Itoh K 1997 Action potential-dependent regulation of gene expression: temporal specificity in Ca^{2+}, cAMP-responsive element binding proteins, and mitogen-activated protein kinase signaling. Journal of Neuroscience 17: 7252–7266

Fitzgerald E M, Dolphin A C 1997 Regulation of rat neuronal voltage-dependent calcium channels by endogenous p21-ras. European Journal of Neuroscience 9: 1252–1261

Fjallbrant N, Iggo A 1961 The effect of histamine, 5-hydroxytryptamine and acetylcholine on cutaneous afferent fibers. Journal of Physiology (London) 156: 578–590

Fock S, Mense S 1976 Excitatory effects of 5-hydroxytryptamine, histamine and potassium ions on muscular group IV afferent units: a comparison with bradykinin. Brain Research 105: 459–469

Ford-Hutchinson A W 1985 Leukotrienes: their formation and role as inflammatory mediators. Federation Proceedings 44: 25–29

Fowler J C, Greene R, Weinreich D 1985a Two calcium-sensitive spike after-hyperpolarizations in visceral sensory neurones of the rabbit. Journal of Physiology (London) 365: 59–75

Fowler J C, Wonderlin W F, Weinreich D 1985b Prostaglandins block a Ca^{2+}-dependent slow spike afterhyperpolarization independent of effects on Ca^{2+} influx in visceral afferent neurons. Brain Research 345: 345–349

Fozard J R 1984 Neuronal 5-HT receptors in the periphery. Neuropharmacology 23: 1473–1486

Fozard J R 1995 The 5-hydroxytryptamine-nitric oxide connection: the key link in the initiation of migraine? Archives Internationales de Pharmacodynamie et de Therapie 329: 111–119

Gallin J I, Goldstein I M, Snyderman R 1992 Inflammation: basic principles and clinical correlates, 2nd edn. Raven, New York

Garret C, Carruette A, Fardin V et al 1993 Antinociceptive properties and inhibition of neurogenic inflammation with potent SP antagonists belonging to perhydroisoindolones. Regulatory Peptides 46: 24–30

Garry M G, Richardson J D, Hargreaves K M 1994 Sodium nitroprusside evokes the release of immunoreactive calcitonin gene-related peptide and substance P from dorsal horn slices via nitric oxide-dependent and nitric oxide-independent mechanisms. Journal of Neuroscience 14: 4329–4337

Gilfort T M, Klanni I 1965 5-Hydroxytryptamine, bradykinin and histamine as mediators of inflammatory hyperesthesia. Journal of Physiology (London) 208: 867–876

Giordano J, Dyche J 1989 Differential analgesic actions of serotonin 5-HT_3 receptor antagonists in the mouse. Neuropharmacology 28: 423–427

Giordano J, Rogers L V 1989 Peripherally administered serotonin 5-HT_3 receptor antagonists reduce inflammatory pain in rats. European Journal of Pharmacology 170: 83–86

Glynn C J, Basedow R W, Walsh J A 1981 Pain relief following post-ganglionic sympathetic blockade with I.V. guanethidine. British Journal of Anaesthesia 53: 1297–1302

Gold M S, Levine J D 1996 DAMGO inhibits prostaglandin E_2-induced potentiation of a TTX-resistant Na^+ current in rat sensory neurons in vitro. Neuroscience Letters 212: 83–86

Gold M S, Dastmalchi S, Levine J D 1996a Co-expression of nociceptor properties in dorsal root ganglion neurons from the adult rat in vitro. Neuroscience 71: 265–275

Gold M S, Reichling D B, Shuster M J, Levine J D 1996b Hyperalgesic agents increase a tetrodotoxin-resistant Na^+ current in nociceptors. Proceedings of the National Academy of Sciences USA 93: 1108–1112

Gonzales R, Goldyne M E, Taiwo Y O, Levine J D 1989 Production of hyperalgesic prostaglandins by sympathetic postganglionic neurons. Journal of Neurochemistry 53: 1595–1598

Goppelt-Struebe M, Beiche F 1997 Cyclooxygenase-2 in the spinal cord: localization and regulation after a peripheral inflammatory stimulus. Advances in Experimental Medicine and Biology 433: 213–216

Gross R A, Macdonald R L 1987 Dynorphin A selectively reduces a large transient (N-type) calcium current of mouse dorsal root ganglion neurons in cell culture. Proceedings of the National Academy of Sciences USA 84: 5469–5473

Gross R A, MacDonald R L 1989 Activators of protein kinase C selectively enhance inactivation of a calcium current component of cultured sensory neurons in a pertussis toxin-sensitive manner. Journal of Neurophysiology 61: 1259–1269

Gross R A, Moises H C, Uhler M D, Macdonald R L 1990 Dynorphin A and cAMP-dependent protein kinase independently regulate neuronal calcium currents. Proceedings of the National Academy of Sciences USA 87: 7025–7029

Habler H J, Jänig W, Koltzenburg M 1990 Activation of unmyelinated afferent fibres by mechanical stimuli and inflammation of the urinary bladder in the cat. Journal of Physiology (London) 425: 545–562

Haley J E, Dickenson A H, Schachter M 1989 Electrophysiological evidence for a role of bradykinin in chemical nociception in the rat. Neuroscience Letters 97: 198–202

Hall K E, Browning M D, Dudek E M, Macdonald R L 1995 Enhancement of high threshold calcium currents in rat primary afferent neurons by constitutively active protein kinase C. Journal of Neuroscience 15: 6069–6076

Halliday D A, Zettler C, Rush R A, Scicchitano R, McNeil J D 1998 Elevated nerve growth factor levels in the synovial fluid of patients with inflammatory joint disease. Neurochemical Research 23: 919–922

Hamprecht B, Schultz J 1973 Stimulation by prostaglandin E_1 of adenosine 3′: 5′-cyclic monophosphate formation in neuroblastoma cells in the presence of phosphodiesterase inhibitors. FEBS Letters 34: 85–89

Handwerker H O 1976 Influences of algogenic substances and prostaglandins on the discharges of unmyelinated cutaneous nerve fibers identified as nociceptors. In: Bonica J J (ed) Advances in pain research and therapy. Raven Press, New York, pp 41–45

Harbuz M S, Rees R G, Lightman S L 1993 HPA axis responses to acute stress and adrenalectomy during adjuvant-induced arthritis in the rat. American Journal of Physiology 264: R179–185

Harbuz M S, Perveen-Gill Z, Lalies M D, Jessop D S, Lightman S L, Chowdrey H S 1996 The role of endogenous serotonin in adjuvant-induced arthritis in the rat. British Journal of Rheumatology 35: 112–116

Harmar A, Keen P 1982 Synthesis, and central and peripheral axonal transport of substance P in a dorsal root ganglion-nerve preparation in vitro. Brain Research 231: 379–385

Harvey J S, Davis C, James I F, Burgess G M 1995 Activation of protein kinase C by the capsaicin analogue resiniferatoxin in sensory neurones. Journal of Neurochemistry 65: 1309–1317

Hay C, de Belleroche J 1997 Carrageenan-induced hyperalgesia is associated with increased cyclo-oxygenase-2 expression in spinal cord. Neuroreport 8: 1249–1251

Herdegen T, Fiallos-Estrada C E, Schmid W, Bravo R, Zimmermann M 1992 The transcription factors c-JUN, JUN D and CREB, but not FOS and KROX- 24, are differentially regulated in axotomized neurons following transection of rat sciatic nerve. Brain Research. Molecular Brain Research 14: 155–165

Herman R K 1996 Touch sensation in *Caenorhabditis elegans.* BioEssays 18: 199–206

Hingtgen C M, Waite K J, Vasko M R 1995 Prostaglandins facilitate peptide release from rat sensory neurons by activating the adenosine 3′,5′-cyclic monophosphate transduction cascade. Journal of Neuroscience 15: 5411–5419

Hiss E, Mense S 1976 Evidence for the existence of different receptor sites for algesic agents at the endings of muscular group IV afferent units. Pflugers Archiv (European Journal of Physiology) 362: 141–146

Holzer P, Wachter C, Heinemann A, Jocic M, Lippe I T, Herbert M K 1995 Sensory nerves, nitric oxide and NANC vasodilatation.

Archives Internationales de Pharmacodynamie et de Therapie 329: 67–79
Hong Y, Abbott F V 1994 Behavioural effects of intraplantar injection of inflammatory mediators in the rat. Neuroscience 63: 827–836
Hu-Tsai M, Woolf C, Winter J 1996 Influence of inflammation or disconnection from peripheral target tissue on the capsaicin sensitivity of rat dorsal root ganglion sensory neurones. Neuroscience Letters 203: 119–122
Huettner J E 1990 Glutamate receptor channels in rat DRG neurons: activation by kainate and quisqualate and blockade of desensitization by Con A. Neuron 5: 255–266
Hughes J, Kosterlitz H W, Leslie F M 1975 Effect of morphine on adrenergic transmission in the mouse vas deferens. Assessment of agonist and antogonist potencies of narcotic analgesics. British Journal of Pharmacology 53: 371–381
Illes P, Pfeiffer N, von Kugelgen I, Starke K 1985 Presynaptic opioid receptor subtypes in the rabbit ear artery. Journal of Pharmacology and Experimental Therapeutics 232: 526–533
Ingram S L, Williams J T 1994 Opioid inhibition of Ih via adenylyl cyclase. Neuron 13: 179–186
Ingram S L, Williams J T 1996 Modulation of the hyperpolarization-activated current (I_h) by cyclic nucleotides in guinea-pig primary afferent neurons. Journal of Physiology (London) 492: 97–106
Irvine R F 1982 How is the level of free arachidonic acid controlled in mammalian cells? Biochemical Journal 204: 3–16
Issberner U, Reeh P W, Steen K H 1996 Pain due to tissue acidosis: a mechanism for inflammatory and ischemic myalgia? Neuroscience Letters 208: 191–194
Jackson D L, Graff C B, Richardson J D, Hargreaves K M 1995 Glutamate participates in the peripheral modulation of thermal hyperalgesia in rats. European Journal of Pharmacology 284: 321–325
Jacobus W E, Taylor G J T, Hollis D P, Nunnally R L 1977 Phosphorus nuclear magnetic resonance of perfused working rat hearts. Nature 265: 756–758
Jaffrey S R, Snyder S H 1995 Nitric oxide: a neural messenger. Annual Review of Cell and Developmental Biology 11: 417–440
Jaken S 1996 Protein kinase C isozymes and substrates. Current Opinion in Cell Biology 8: 168–173
Jänig W, Levine J D, Michaelis M 1996 Interactions of sympathetic and primary afferent neurons following nerve injury and tissue trauma. Progress in Brain Research 113: 161–184
Jarrett W A, Price G T, Lynn V J, Burden H W 1994 NADPH-diaphorase-positive neurons innervating the rat ovary. Neuroscience Letters 177: 47–49
Jeftinija S 1994 The role of tetrodotoxin-resistant sodium channels of small primary afferent fibers. Brain Research 639: 125–134
Johnson A R, Erdos E G 1973 Release of histamine from mast cells by vasoactive peptides. Proceedings of the Society for Experimental Biology and Medicine 142: 1252–1256
Joris J L, Dubner R, Hargreaves K M 1987 Opioid analgesia at peripheral sites: a target for opioids released during stress and inflammation? Anesthesia and Analgesia 66: 1277–1281
Juan H, Lembeck F 1974 Action of peptides and other algesic agents on paravascular pain receptors of the isolated perfused rabbit ear. Naunyn-Schmiedebergs Archives of Pharmacology 283: 151–164
Juranek I, Lembeck F 1997 Afferent C-fibres release substance P and glutamate. Canadian Journal of Physiology and Pharmacology 75: 661–664
Kaliner M 1989 Asthma and mast cell activation. Journal of Allergy and Clinical Immunology 83: 510–520
Kano M, Kawakami T, Hikawa N, Hori H, Takenaka T, Gotoh H 1994 Bradykinin-responsive cells of dorsal root ganglia in culture: cell size, firing, cytosolic calcium, and substance P. Cellular and Molecular Neurobiology 14: 49–57
Katholi R E, McCann W P, Woods W T 1985 Intrarenal adenosine produces hypertension via renal nerves in the one-kidney, one clip rat. Hypertension 7: 88–93
Kawabata A, Manabe S, Manabe Y, Takagi H 1994 Effect of topical administration of L-arginine on formalin-induced nociception in the mouse: a dual role of peripherally formed NO in pain modulation. British Journal of Pharmacology 112: 547–550
Kessler W, Kirchhoff C, Reeh P W, Handwerker H O 1992 Excitation of cutaneous afferent nerve endings in vitro by a combination of inflammatory mediators and conditioning effect of substance P. Experimental Brain Research 91: 467–476
Khasar S G, Miao F J, Levine J D 1995 Inflammation modulates the contribution of receptor-subtypes to bradykinin-induced hyperalgesia in the rat. Neuroscience 69: 685–690
Kindgen-Milles D, Arndt J O 1996 Nitric oxide as a chemical link in the generation of pain from veins in humans. Pain 64: 139–142
Kirchhoff C, Jung S, Reeh P W, Handwerker H O 1990 Carrageenan inflammation increases bradykinin sensitivity of rat cutaneous nociceptors. Neuroscience Letters 111: 206–210
Kirschstein T, Busselberg D, Treede R D 1997 Coexpression of heat-evoked and capsaicin-evoked inward currents in acutely dissociated rat dorsal root ganglion neurons. Neuroscience Letters 231: 33–36
Kitakoga O, Kuba K 1993 Bradykinin-induced ion currents in cultured rat trigeminal ganglion cells. Neuroscience Research 16: 79–93
Koltzenburg M, McMahon S B 1991 The enigmatic role of the sympathetic nervous system in chronic pain. Trends in Pharmacological Sciences 12: 399–402
Koltzenburg M, Kress M, Reeh P W 1992 The nociceptor sensitization by bradykinin does not depend on sympathetic neurons. Neuroscience 46: 465–473
Kostyuk P G, Veselovsky N S, Fedulova S A, Tsyndrenko A Y 1981 Ionic currents in the somatic membrane of rat dorsal root ganglion neurons-III. Potassium currents. Neuroscience 6: 2439–2444
Kress M, Riedl B, Reeh P W 1995 Effects of oxygen radicals on nociceptive afferents in the rat skin in vitro. Pain 62: 87–94
Kress M, Reeh P W, Vyklicky L 1997 An interaction of inflammatory mediators and protons in small diameter dorsal root ganglion neurons of the rat. Neuroscience Letters 224: 37–40
Kumazawa T, Mizumura K, Minagawa M, Tsujii Y 1991 Sensitizing effects of bradykinin on the heat responses of the visceral nociceptor. Journal of Neurophysiology 66: 1819–1824
Kumazawa T, Perl E R 1977a Primate cutaneous receptors with unmyelinated (C) fibres and their projection to the substantia gelatinosa. Journal of Physiology (Paris) 73: 287–304
Kumazawa T, Perl E R 1977b Primate cutaneous sensory units with unmyelinated (C) afferent fibers. Journal of Neurophysiology 40: 1325–1338
Kunze H, Vogt W 1971 Significance of phospholipase A for prostaglandin formation. Annals of the New York Academy of Sciences 180: 123–125
Laird J M, Cervero F 1989 A comparative study of the changes in receptive-field properties of multireceptive and nocireceptive rat dorsal horn neurons following noxious mechanical stimulation. Journal of Neurophysiology 62: 854–863
LaMotte R H, Thalhammer J G, Torebjork H E, Robinson C J 1982 Peripheral neural mechanisms of cutaneous hyperalgesia following mild injury by heat. Journal of Neuroscience 2: 765–781
Law P Y, Wu J, Koehler J E, Loh H H 1981 Demonstration and characterization of opiate inhibition of the striatal adenylate cyclase. Journal of Neurochemistry 36: 1834–1846
Lawand N B, Willis W D, Westlund K N 1997 Blockade of joint inflammation and secondary hyperalgesia by L-NAME, a nitric oxide synthase inhibitor. Neuroreport 8: 895–899
Ledent C, Vaugeois J M, Schiffmann S N et al 1997 Aggressiveness,

hypoalgesia and high blood pressure in mice lacking the adenosine A_{2a} receptor. Nature 388: 674–678

Lembeck F, Holzer P 1979 Substance P as neurogenic mediator of antidromic vasodilation and neurogenic plasma extravasation. Naunyn-Schmiedebergs Archives of Pharmacology 310: 175–183

Lembeck F, Popper H, Juan H 1976 Release of prostaglandins by bradykinin as an intrinsic mechanism of its algesic effect. Naunyn-Schmiedebergs Archives of Pharmacology 294: 69–73

Leng S, Mizumura K, Koda H, Kumazawa T 1996 Excitation and sensitization of the heat response induced by a phorbol ester in canine visceral polymodal receptors studied in vitro. Neuroscience Letters 206: 13–16

Leslie T A, Emson P C, Dowd P M, Woolf C J 1995 Nerve growth factor contributes to the up-regulation of growth-associated protein 43 and preprotachykinin A messenger RNAs in primary sensory neurons following peripheral inflammation. Neuroscience 67: 753–761

Levi-Montalcini R, Skaper S D, Dal Toso R, Petrelli L, Leon A 1996 Nerve growth factor: from neurotrophin to neurokine. Trends in Neuroscience 19: 514–520

Levine J D, Taiwo Y O 1989 Involvement of the mu-opiate receptor in peripheral analgesia. Neuroscience 32: 571–575

Levine J D, Lau W, Kwiat G, Goetzl E J 1984 Leukotriene B_4 produces hyperalgesia that is dependent on polymorphonuclear leukocytes. Science 225: 743–745

Levine J D, Gooding J, Donatoni P, Borden L, Goetzl E J 1985 The role of the polymorphonuclear leukocyte in hyperalgesia. Journal of Neuroscience 5: 3025–3029

Levine J D, Fye K, Heller P, Basbaum A I, Whiting-O'Keefe Q 1986a Clinical response to regional intravenous guanethidine in patients with rheumatoid arthritis. Journal of Rheumatology 13: 1040–1043

Levine J D, Lam D, Taiwo Y O, Donatoni P, Goetzl E J 1986b Hyperalgesic properties of 15-lipoxygenase products of arachidonic acid. Proceedings of the National Academy of Sciences USA 83: 5331–5334

Levine J D, Taiwo Y O, Collins S D, Tam J K 1986c Noradrenaline hyperalgesia is mediated through interaction with sympathetic postganglionic neurone terminals rather than activation of primary afferent nociceptors. Nature 323: 158–160

Lewin G R, Rueff A, Mendell L M 1994 Peripheral and central mechanisms of NGF-induced hyperalgesia. European Journal of Neuroscience 6: 1903–1912

Li C, Peoples R W, Weight F F 1996 Acid pH augments excitatory action of ATP on a dissociated mammalian sensory neuron. Neuroreport 7: 2151–2154

Li H, Ohishi H, Kinoshita A, Shigemoto R, Nomura S, Mizuno N 1997 Localization of a metabotropic glutamate receptor, mGluR7, in axon terminals of presumed nociceptive, primary afferent fibers in the superficial layers of the spinal dorsal horn: an electron microscope study in the rat. Neuroscience Letters 223: 153–156

Lim R K, Guzman F, Roders D W 1964 Site of action of narcotic and non-narcotic analgesics determined by blocking bradykinin evoked visceral pain. Archives Internationales de Pharmacodynamie et de Therapie 152: 25–58

Lim R K, Miller D G, Guzman F et al 1967 Pain and analgesia evaluated by the intraperitoneal bradykinin-evoked pain method in man. Clinical Pharmacology and Therapeutics 8: 521–542

Liu H, Wang H, Sheng M, Jan L Y, Jan Y N, Basbaum A I 1994 Evidence for presynaptic *N*-methyl-D-aspartate autoreceptors in the spinal cord dorsal horn. Proceedings of the National Academy of Sciences USA 91: 8383–8387

Liu H, Mantyh P W, Basbaum A I 1997 NMDA-receptor regulation of substance P release from primary afferent nociceptors. Nature 386: 721–724

Loh L, Nathan P W 1978 Painful peripheral states and sympathetic blocks. Journal of Neurology, Neurosurgery and Psychiatry 41: 664–671

Lopshire J C, Nicol G D 1998 The cAMP transduction cascade mediates the prostaglandin E_2 enhancement of the capsaicin-elicited current in rat sensory neurons: whole-cell and single-channel studies. Journal of Neuroscience 18: 6081–6092

Lotz M, Carson D A, Vaughan J H 1987 Substance P activation of rheumatoid synoviocytes: neural pathway in pathogenesis of arthritis. Science 235: 893–895

Lotz M, Vaughan J H, Carson D A 1988 Effect of neuropeptides on production of inflammatory cytokines by human monocytes. Science 241: 1218–1221

Lovinger D M, Weight F F 1988 Glutamate induces a depolarization of adult rat dorsal root ganglion neurons that is mediated predominantly by NMDA receptors. Neuroscience Letters 94: 314–320

Lynn B 1996 Neurogenic inflammation caused by cutaneous polymodal receptors. Progress in Brain Research 113: 361–368

Lynn B, O'Shea N R 1998 Inhibition of forskolin-induced sensitisation of frog skin nociceptors by the cyclic AMP-dependent protein kinase A antagonist H-89. Brain Research 780: 360–362

Ma Q P, Woolf C J 1997 The progressive tactile hyperalgesia induced by peripheral inflammation is nerve growth factor dependent. Neuroreport 8: 807–810

McCormack K 1994a Non-steroidal anti-inflammatory drugs and spinal nociceptive processing. Pain 59: 9–43

McCormack K 1994b The spinal actions of nonsteroidal anti-inflammatory drugs and the dissociation between their anti-inflammatory and analgesic effects. Drugs 47: 28–45

McFarlane S, Cooper E 1991 Kinetics and voltage dependence of A-type currents on neonatal rat sensory neurons. Journal of Neurophysiology 66: 1380–1391

McGehee D S, Goy M F, Oxford G S 1992 Involvement of the nitric oxide-cyclic GMP pathway in the desensitization of bradykinin responses of cultured rat sensory neurons. Neuron 9: 315–324

McGuirk S M, Dolphin A C 1992 G-protein mediation in nociceptive signal transduction: an investigation into the excitatory action of bradykinin in a subpopulation of cultured rat sensory neurons. Neuroscience 49: 117–128

McMahon S B 1996 NGF as a mediator of inflammatory pain. Philosophical Transactions of the Royal Society of London. Series B: Biological Sciences 351: 431–440

Maggi C A 1997 The effects of tachykinins on inflammatory and immune cells. Regulatory Peptides 70: 75–90

Maggi C A, Patacchini R, Santicioli P et al 1989 Multiple mechanisms in the motor responses of the guinea-pig isolated urinary bladder to bradykinin. British Journal of Pharmacology 98: 619–629

Majewski M, Sienkiewicz W, Kaleczyc J, Mayer B, Czaja K, Lakomy M 1995 The distribution and co-localization of immunoreactivity to nitric oxide synthase, vasoactive intestinal polypeptide and substance P within nerve fibres supplying bovine and porcine female genital organs. Cell and Tissue Research 281: 445–464

Makman M H, Dvorkin B, Crain S M 1988 Modulation of adenylate cyclase activity of mouse spinal cord-ganglion explants by opioids, serotonin and pertussis toxin. Brain Research 445: 303–313

Malmberg A B, Yaksh T L 1995 Cyclooxygenase inhibition and the spinal release of prostaglandin E_2 and amino acids evoked by paw formalin injection: a microdialysis study in unanesthetized rats. Journal of Neuroscience 15: 2768–2776

Malmberg A B, Brandon E P, Idzerda R L, Liu H, McKnight G S, Basbaum A I 1997a Diminished inflammation and nociceptive pain with preservation of neuropathic pain in mice with a targeted mutation of the type I regulatory subunit of cAMP-dependent protein kinase. Journal of Neuroscience 17: 7462–7470

Malmberg A B, Chen C, Tonegawa S, Basbaum A I 1997b Preserved acute pain and reduced neuropathic pain in mice lacking PKC_{gamma}. Science 278: 279–283

Malmberg A B, Rafferty M F, Yaksh T L 1994 Antinociceptive effect of spinally delivered prostaglandin E receptor antagonists in the formalin test on the rat. Neuroscience Letters 173: 193–196

Mao J, Price D D, Phillips L L, Lu J, Mayer D J 1995 Increases in protein kinase C gamma immunoreactivity in the spinal cord dorsal horn of rats with painful mononeuropathy. Neuroscience Letters 198: 75–78

Marsala F 1980 Treatment of ureteral and biliary pain with an injectable salt of indomethacin. Pharmatherapeutica 2: 357–362

Martin H A, Basbaum A I, Kwiat G C, Goetzl E J, Levine J D 1987 Leukotriene and prostaglandin sensitization of cutaneous high-threshold C- and A-delta mechanonociceptors in the hairy skin of rat hindlimbs. Neuroscience 22: 651–659

Matsukawa A, Yoshimura T, Maeda T, Takahashi T, Ohkawara S, Yoshinaga M 1998 Analysis of the cytokine network among tumor necrosis factor alpha, interleukin-1beta, interleukin-8, and interleukin-1 receptor antagonist in monosodium urate crystal-induced rabbit arthritis. Laboratory Investigation 78: 559–569

Matzner O, Devor M 1994 Hyperexcitability at sites of nerve injury depends on voltage-sensitive Na^+ channels. Journal of Neurophysiology 72: 349–359

Mayer M L, Sugiyama K 1988 A modulatory action of divalent cations on transient outward current in cultured rat sensory neurones. Journal of Physiology (London) 396: 417–433

Mayer M L, Westbrook G L 1983 A voltage-clamp analysis of inward (anomalous) rectification in mouse spinal sensory ganglion neurones. Journal of Physiology (London) 340: 19–45

Mazzari S, Canella R, Petrelli L, Marcolongo G, Leon A 1996 *N*-(2-hydroxyethyl) hexadecanamide is orally active in reducing edema formation and inflammatory hyperalgesia by down-modulating mast cell activation. European Journal of Pharmacology 300: 227–236

Meller S T, Gebhart G F 1994 Spinal mediators of hyperalgesia. Drugs 5: 10–20

Melmon K L, Webster M E, Goldfinger S E, Seegmiller J E 1967 The presence of a kinin in inflammatory synovial effusion from arthritides of varying etiologies. Arthritis and Rheumatism 10: 13–20

Mense S 1981 Sensitization of group IV muscle receptors to bradykinin by 5-hydroxytryptamine and prostaglandin E_2. Brain Research 225: 95–105

Mense S, Schmidt R F 1974 Activation of group IV afferent units from muscle by algesic agents. Brain Research 72: 305–310

Mense S, Meyer H 1988 Bradykinin-induced modulation of the response behaviour of different types of feline group III and IV muscle receptors. Journal of Physiology (London) 398: 49–63

Meyer R A, Campbell J N 1981 Myelinated nociceptive afferents account for the hyperalgesia that follows a burn to the hand. Science 213: 1527–1529

Michael G J, Averill S, Nitkunan A et al 1997 Nerve growth factor treatment increases brain-derived neurotrophic factor selectively in TrkA-expressing dorsal root ganglion cells and in their central terminations within the spinal cord. Journal of Neuroscience 17: 8476–8490

Minami T, Nishihara I, Ito S, Sakamoto K, Hyodo M, Hayaishi O 1995 Nitric oxide mediates allodynia induced by intrathecal administration of prostaglandin E_2 or prostaglandin F_2 alpha in conscious mice. Pain 61: 285–290

Mizuno K, Yamamoto S, Lands W E 1982 Effects of non-steroidal anti-inflammatory drugs on fatty acid cyclooxygenase and prostaglandin hydroperoxidase activities. Prostaglandins 23: 743–757

Molliver D C, Radeke M J, Feinstein S C, Snider W D 1995 Presence or absence of TrkA protein distinguishes subsets of small sensory neurons with unique cytochemical characteristics and dorsal horn projections. Journal of Comparative Neurology 361: 404–416

Monteiro E C, Ribeiro J A 1987 Ventilatory effects of adenosine mediated by carotid body chemoreceptors in the rat. Naunyn-Schmiedebergs Archives of Pharmacology 335: 143–148

Morell P, Allen A C, Gammon C M, Lyons S A 1991 Arachidonate release consequent to bradykinin-stimulated phospholipid metabolism in dorsal root ganglion cells. Biochemical Society Transactions 19: 411–416

Morris R, Southam E, Braid D J, Garthwaite J 1992 Nitric oxide may act as a messenger between dorsal root ganglion neurones and their satellite cells. Neuroscience Letters 137: 29–32

Morteau O, Julia V, Eeckhout C, Bueno L 1994 Influence of 5-HT_3 receptor antagonists in visceromotor and nociceptive responses to rectal distension before and during experimental colitis in rats. Fundamental and Clinical Pharmacology 8: 553–562

Moskowitz M A, Brody M, Liu-Chen L Y 1983 In vitro release of immunoreactive substance P from putative afferent nerve endings in bovine pia arachnoid. Neuroscience 9: 809–814

Myers R R, Heckman H M, Rodriguez M 1996 Reduced hyperalgesia in nerve-injured WLD mice: relationship to nerve fiber phagocytosis, axonal degeneration, and regeneration in normal mice. Experimental Neurology 141: 94–101

Nakano T, Taira N 1976 5-Hydroxytryptamine as a sensitizer of somatic nociceptors for pain-producing substances. European Journal of Pharmacology 38: 23–29

Neto F R 1978 The depolarizing action of 5-HT on mammalian nonmyelinated nerve fibers. European Journal of Pharmacology 49: 351–356

Neufeld A H, Ledgard S E, Jumblatt M M, Klyce S D 1982 Serotonin-stimulated cyclic AMP synthesis in the rabbit corneal epithelium. Investigative Ophthalmology and Visual Science 23: 193–198

Neugebauer V, Schaible H G, Schmidt R F 1989 Sensitization of articular afferents to mechanical stimuli by bradykinin. Pflugers Archiv (European Journal of Physiology) 415: 330–335

Neumann S, Doubell T P, Leslie T, Woolf C J 1996 Inflammatory pain hypersensitivity mediated by phenotypic switch in myelinated primary sensory neurons. Nature 384: 360–364

Newsholme E A, Calder P C 1997 The proposed role of glutamine in some cells of the immune system and speculative consequences for the whole animal. Nutrition 13: 728–730

Nicol G D, Cui M 1994 Enhancement by prostaglandin E_2 of bradykinin activation of embryonic rat sensory neurones. Journal of Physiology (London) 480: 485–492

Nicol G D, Klingberg D K, Vasko M R 1992 Prostaglandin E_2 increases calcium conductance and stimulates release of substance P in avian sensory neurons. Journal of Neuroscience 12: 1917–1927

Nicol G D, Vasko M R, Evans A R 1997 Prostaglandins suppress an outward potassium current in embryonic rat sensory neurons. Journal of Neurophysiology 77: 167–176

Noda K, Ueda Y, Suzuki K, Yoda K 1997 Excitatory effects of algesic compounds on neuronal processes in murine dorsal root ganglion cell culture. Brain Research 751: 348–351

Nordlind K, Johansson O, Liden S, Hokfelt T 1993 Glutamate- and aspartate-like immunoreactivities in human normal and inflamed skin. Virchows Archiv. B. Cell Pathology including Molecular Pathology 64: 75–82

O'Flaherty J T 1987 Phospholipid metabolism and stimulus-response coupling. Biochemical Pharmacology 36: 407–412

Ogata N, Tatebayashi H 1993 Kinetic analysis of two types of Na^+ channels in rat dorsal root ganglia. Journal of Physiology (London) 466: 9–37

Ohkubo T, Shibata M, Takahashi H, Inoki R 1983 Effect of prostaglandin D_2 on pain and inflammation. Japanese Journal of Pharmacology 33: 264–266

Okuse K, Chaplan S R, McMahon S B et al 1997 Regulation of expression of the sensory neuron-specific sodium channel SNS in inflammatory and neuropathic pain. Molecular and Cellular Neurosciences 10: 196–207

Omote K, Kawamata T, Kawamata M, Namiki A 1998 Formalin-induced release of excitatory amino acids in the skin of the rat hindpaw. Brain Research 787: 161–164

Oyelese A A, Rizzo M A, Waxman S G, Kocsis J D 1997 Differential effects of NGF and BDNF on axotomy-induced changes in GABA(A)-receptor-mediated conductance and sodium currents in cutaneous afferent neurons. Journal of Neurophysiology 78: 31–42

Papka R E, Srinivasan B, Miller K E, Hayashi S 1997 Localization of estrogen receptor protein and estrogen receptor messenger RNA in peripheral autonomic and sensory neurons. Neuroscience 79: 1153–1163

Pateromichelakis S, Rood J P 1982 Prostaglandin E_1-induced sensitization of A delta moderate pressure mechanoreceptors. Brain Research 232: 89–96

Pearce R J, Duchen M R 1994 Differential expression of membrane currents in dissociated mouse primary sensory neurons. Neuroscience 63: 1041–1056

Perl E R 1996 Cutaneous polymodal receptors: characteristics and plasticity. Progress in Brain Research 113: 21–37

Perozo E, Bezanilla F, Dipolo R 1989 Modulation of K channels in dialyzed squid axons. ATP-mediated phosphorylation. Journal of General Physiology 93: 1195–1218

Petersen M, LaMotte R H 1991 Relationships between capsaicin sensitivity of mammalian sensory neurons, cell size and type of voltage gated Ca-currents. Brain Research 561: 20–26

Petersen M, Zhang J, Zhang J M, LaMotte R H 1996 Abnormal spontaneous activity and responses to norepinephrine in dissociated dorsal root ganglion cells after chronic nerve constriction. Pain 67: 391–397

Petersen M, Segond von Banchet G, Heppelmann B, Koltzenburg M 1998 Nerve growth factor regulates the expression of bradykinin binding sites on adult sensory neurons via the neurotrophin receptor p75. Neuroscience 83: 161–168

Pierce P A, Xie G X, Levine J D, Peroutka S J 1996a 5-Hydroxytryptamine receptor subtype messenger RNAs in rat peripheral sensory and sympathetic ganglia: a polymerase chain reaction study. Neuroscience 70: 553–559

Pierce P A, Xie G X, Peroutka S J, Levine J D 1996b Dual effect of the serotonin agonist, sumatriptan, on peripheral neurogenic inflammation. Regional Anesthesia 21: 219–225

Pierce P A, Xie G X, Meuser T, Peroutka S J 1997 5-Hydroxytryptamine receptor subtype messenger RNAs in human dorsal root ganglia: a polymerase chain reaction study. Neuroscience 81: 813–819

Pillinger M H, Abramson S B 1995 The neutrophil in rheumatoid arthritis. Rheumatic Diseases Clinics of North America 21: 691–714

Qian Y, Chao D S, Santillano D R et al 1996 cGMP-dependent protein kinase in dorsal root ganglion: relationship with nitric oxide synthase and nociceptive neurons. Journal of Neuroscience 16: 3130–3138

Rackham A, Ford-Hutchinson A W 1983 Inflammation and pain sensitivity: effects of leukotrienes D_4, B_4 and prostaglandin E_1 in the rat paw. Prostaglandins 25: 193–203

Raes A, Wang Z, van den Berg R J, Goethals M, Van de Vijver G, van Bogaert P P 1997 Effect of cAMP and ATP on the hyperpolarization-activated current in mouse dorsal root ganglion neurons. Pflugers Archiv (European Journal of Physiology) 434: 543–550

Rakovska A, Milenov K 1984 Antagonistic effect of SC-19220 on the responses of guinea-pig gastric muscles to prostaglandins E_1, E_2 and F_2 alpha. Archives Internationales de Pharmacodynamie et de Therapie 268: 59–69

Rang H P, Ritchie J M 1988 Depolarization of nonmyelinated fibers of the rat vagus nerve produced by activation of protein kinase C. Journal of Neuroscience 8: 2606–2617

Reeh P W, Bayer J, Kocher L, Handwerker H O 1987 Sensitization of nociceptive cutaneous nerve fibers from the rat's tail by noxious mechanical stimulation. Experimental Brain Research 65: 505–512

Reichling D B, Levine J D 1997 Heat transduction in rat sensory neurons by calcium-dependent activation of a cation channel. Proceedings of the National Academy of Sciences of the United States of America 94: 7006–7011

Reichling D B, Barratt L, Levine J D 1997 Heat-induced cobalt entry: an assay for heat transduction in cultured rat dorsal root ganglion neurons. Neuroscience 77: 291–294

Ren K, Ruda M A 1995 Nitric oxide synthase-containing neurons in sensory ganglia of the rat are susceptible to capsaicin-induced cytotoxicity. Neuroscience 65: 505–511

Richardson B P, Engel G 1986 The pharmacology and function of 5-HT_3 receptors. Trends in Neurosciences 9: 424–428

Richardson B P, Engel G, Donatsch P, Stadler P A 1985 Identification of serotonin M-receptor subtypes and their specific blockade by a new class of drugs. Nature 316: 126–131

Richardson P M, Lu X 1994 Inflammation and axonal regeneration. Journal of Neurology 242: S57–60

Ridger V C, Greenacre S A, Handy R L et al 1997 Effect of peroxynitrite on plasma extravasation, microvascular blood flow and nociception in the rat. British Journal of Pharmacology 122: 1083–1088

Rizzo M A, Kocsis J D, Waxman S G 1994 Slow sodium conductances of dorsal root ganglion neurons: intraneuronal homogeneity and interneuronal heterogeneity. Journal of Neurophysiology 72: 2796–2815

Robinson D R 1989 Eicosanoids, inflammation, and anti-inflammatory drugs. Clinical and Experimental Rheumatology 7(suppl 3): S155–161

Rocha E, Silver M, Rosenthal S R 1961 Release of pharmacologically active substances from the rat skin in vivo following thermal injury. Journal of Pharmacology and Experimental Therapeutics 132: 110–116

Roivainen R, Nikkari S T, Iadarola M J, Koistinaho J 1993 Co-localization of the beta-subtype of protein kinase C and phosphorylation-dependent immunoreactivity of neurofilaments in intact, decentralized and axotomized rat peripheral neurons. Journal of Neurocytology 22: 154–163

Roth G J, Siok C J 1978 Acetylation of the NH_2-terminal serine of prostaglandin synthetase by aspirin. Journal of Biological Chemistry 253: 3782–3784

Roy M L, Narahashi T 1992 Differential properties of tetrodotoxin-sensitive and tetrodotoxin-resistant sodium channels in rat dorsal root ganglion neurons. Journal of Neuroscience 12: 2104–2111

Rueff A, Mendell L M 1996 Nerve growth factor NT-5 induce increased thermal sensitivity of cutaneous nociceptors in vitro. Journal of Neurophysiology 76: 3593– 3596

Runold M, Cherniack N S, Prabhakar N R 1990 Effect of adenosine on chemosensory activity of the cat aortic body. Respiration Physiology 80: 299–306

Rupniak N M, Boyce S, Webb J K et al 1997 Effects of the bradykinin B1 receptor antagonist des-Arg9[Leu8]bradykinin and genetic disruption of the B2 receptor on nociception in rats and mice. Pain 71: 89–97

Saito Y, Kaneko M, Kirihara Y, Kosaka Y, Collins J G 1995 Intrathecal prostaglandin E1 produces a long-lasting allodynic state. Pain 63: 303–311

Samuelsson B 1972 Biosynthesis of prostaglandins. Federation Proceedings 31: 1442–1450

Samuelsson B 1983 Leukotrienes: mediators of immediate hypersensitivity reactions and inflammation. Science 220: 568–575

Sangameswaran L, Delgado S G, Fish L M et al 1996 Structure and function of a novel voltage-gated, tetrodotoxin-resistant sodium channel specific to sensory neurons. Journal of Biological Chemistry 271: 5953–5956

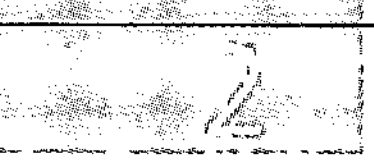

Sanner J H 1969 Antagonism of prostaglandin E_2 by 1-acetyl-2-(8-chloro-10,11-dihydrodibenz (b,f) (1,4) oxazepine-10-carbonyl) hydrazine (SC-19220). Archives Internationales de Pharmacodynamie et de Therapie 180: 46–56

Saria A 1984 Substance P in sensory nerve fibres contributes to the development of oedema in the rat hind paw after thermal injury. British Journal of Pharmacology 82: 217–222

Sato J, Suzuki S, Iseki T, Kumazawa T 1993 Adrenergic excitation of cutaneous nociceptors in chronically inflamed rats. Neuroscience Letters 164: 225–228

Sato J, Suzuki S, Tamura R, Kumazawa T 1994 Norepinephrine excitation of cutaneous nociceptors in adjuvant-induced inflamed rats does not depend on sympathetic neurons. Neuroscience Letters 177: 135–138

Sattin A, Rall T W 1970 The effect of adenosine and adenine nucleotides on the cyclic adenosine 3′, 5′-phosphate content of guinea pig cerebral cortex slices. Molecular Pharmacology 6: 13–23

Sawynok J, Reid A 1997 Peripheral adenosine 5′-triphosphate enhances nociception in the formalin test via activation of a purinergic p2X receptor. European Journal of Pharmacology 330: 115–121

Sawynok J, Zarrindast M R, Reid A R, Doak G J 1997 Adenosine A3 receptor activation produces nociceptive behaviour and edema by release of histamine and 5-hydroxytryptamine. European Journal of Pharmacology 333: 1–7

Schaible H G, Schmidt R F 1988 Excitation and sensitization of fine articular afferents from cat's knee joint by prostaglandin E_2. Journal of Physiology (London) 403: 91–104

Schaible H G, Schmidt R F 1996 Neurophysiology of chronic inflammatory pain: electrophysiological recordings from spinal cord neurons in rats with prolonged acute and chronic unilateral inflammation at the ankle. Progress in Brain Research 110: 167–176

Schepelmann K, Messlinger K, Schmidt R F 1993 The effects of phorbol ester on slowly conducting afferents of the cat's knee joint. Experimental Brain Research 92: 391–398

Scheuren N, Neupert W, Ionac M, Neuhuber W, Brune K, Geisslinger G 1997 Peripheral noxious stimulation releases spinal PGE_2 during the first phase in the formalin assay of the rat. Life Sciences 60: 295–300

Schild J H, Kunze D L 1997 Experimental and modeling study of Na^+ current heterogeneity in rat nodose neurons and its impact on neuronal discharge. Journal of Neurophysiology 78: 3198–3209

Scroggs R S, Fox A P 1992 Calcium current variation between acutely isolated adult rat dorsal root ganglion neurons of different size. Journal of Physiology (London) 445: 639–658

Scroggs R S, Todorovic S M, Anderson E G, Fox A P 1994 Variation in I_H, I_{IR}, and I_{LEAK} between acutely isolated adult rat dorsal root ganglion neurons of different size. Journal of Neurophysiology 71: 271–279

Segond von Banchet G, Petersen M, Heppelmann B 1996 Bradykinin receptors in cultured rat dorsal root ganglion cells: influence of length of time in culture. Neuroscience 75: 1211–1218

Seibert K, Zhang Y, Leahy K, Hauser S, Masferrer J, Isakson P 1997 Distribution of COX-1 and COX-2 in normal and inflamed tissues. Advances in Experimental Medicine and Biology 400A: 167–170

Sharma S K, Nirenberg M, Klee W A 1975 Morphine receptors as regulators of adenylate cyclase activity. Proceedings of the National Academy of Sciences USA 72: 590–594

Shuster M J, Camardo J S, Siegelbaum S A, Kandel E R 1985 Cyclic AMP-dependent protein kinase closes the serotonin-sensitive K^+ channels of Aplysia sensory neurones in cell-free membrane patches. Nature 313: 392–395

Sicuteri F, Franciullacci M, Franchi G, Del Bianco P L 1965 Serotonin-bradykinin potentiation on the pain receptors in man. Life Sciences 4: 309–316

Simone D A, Baumann T K, Collins J G, LaMotte R H 1989 Sensitization of cat dorsal horn neurons to innocuous mechanical stimulation after intradermal injection of capsaicin. Brain Research 486: 185–189

Sluka K A, Jordan H H, Westlund K N 1994 Reduction in joint swelling and hyperalgesia following post-treatment with a non-NMDA glutamate receptor antagonist. Pain 59: 95–100

Smith J B, Willis A L 1971 Aspirin selectively inhibits prostaglandin production in human platelets. Nature New Biology 231: 235–237

Snyder S H 1985 Adenosine as a neuromodulator. Annual Review of Neuroscience 8: 103–124

Sohrabji F, Miranda R, Toran-Allerand C 1994 Estrogen differentially regulates estrogen and nerve growth factor receptor mRNAs in adult sensory neurons. Journal of Neuroscience 14: 459–471

Souslova V A, Fox M, Wood J N, Akopian A N 1997 Cloning and characterization of a mouse sensory neuron tetrodotoxin- resistant voltage-gated sodium channel gene, Scn10a. Genomics 41: 201–209

Stansfeld C E, Marsh S J, Halliwell J V, Brown D A 1986 4-Aminopyridine and dendrotoxin induce repetitive firing in rat visceral sensory neurones by blocking a slowly inactivating outward current. Neuroscience Letters 64: 299–304

Stanton-Hicks M, Janig W, Hassenbusch S, Haddox J D, Boas R, Wilson P 1995 Reflex sympathetic dystrophy: changing concepts and taxonomy. Pain 63: 127–133

Steel J H, Terenghi G, Chung J M, Na H S, Carlton S M, Polak J M 1994 Increased nitric oxide synthase immunoreactivity in rat dorsal root ganglia in a neuropathic pain model. Neuroscience Letters 169: 81–84

Steen K H, Reeh P W, Anton F, Handwerker H O 1992 Protons selectively induce lasting excitation and sensitization to mechanical stimulation of nociceptors in rat skin, in vitro. Journal of Neuroscience 12: 86–95

Steen K H, Steen A E, Kreysel H W, Reeh P W 1996 Inflammatory mediators potentiate pain induced by experimental tissue acidosis. Pain 66: 163–170

Steen K H, Issberner U, Reeh P W 1995a Pain due to experimental acidosis in human skin: evidence for non-adapting nociceptor excitation. Neuroscience Letters 199: 29–32

Steen K H, Steen A E, Reeh P W 1995b A dominant role of acid pH in inflammatory excitation and sensitization of nociceptors in rat skin, in vitro. Journal of Neuroscience 15: 3982–3989

Stein C 1995 The control of pain in peripheral tissue by opioids. New England Journal of Medicine 332: 1685–1690

Stein C, Millan M J, Shippenberg T S, Herz A 1988a Peripheral effect of fentanyl upon nociception in inflamed tissue of the rat. Neuroscience Letters 84: 225–228

Stein C, Millan M J, Yassouridis A, Herz A 1988b Antinociceptive effects of mu- and kappa-agonists in inflammation are enhanced by a peripheral opioid receptor-specific mechanism. European Journal of Pharmacology 155: 255–264

Stein C, Millan M J, Shippenberg T S, Peter K, Herz A 1989 Peripheral opioid receptors mediating antinociception in inflammation. Evidence for involvement of mu, delta and kappa receptors. Journal of Pharmacology and Experimental Therapeutics 248: 1269–1275

Stein C, Hassan A H, Przewlocki R, Gramsch C, Peter K, Herz A 1990 Opioids from immunocytes interact with receptors on sensory nerves to inhibit nociception in inflammation. Proceedings of the National Academy of Sciences USA 87: 5935–5939

Stucky C L, Thayer S A, Seybold V S 1996 Prostaglandin E_2 increases the proportion of neonatal rat dorsal root ganglion neurons that respond to bradykinin. Neuroscience 74: 1111–1123

Stucky C L, Abrahams L G, Seybold V S 1998 Bradykinin increases the proportion of neonatal rat dorsal root ganglion neurons that respond to capsaicin and protons. Neuroscience 84: 1257–1265

Supowit S C, Christensen M D, Westlund K N, Hallman D M, DiPette D J 1995 Dexamethasone and activators of the protein kinase A and

C signal transduction pathways regulate neuronal calcitonin gene-related peptide expression and release. Brain Research 686: 77–86

Sylven C, Jonzon B, Fredholm B B, Kaijser L 1988 Adenosine injection into the brachial artery produces ischaemia like pain or discomfort in the forearm. Cardiovascular Research 22: 674–678

Taiwo Y O, Levine J D 1988a Characterization of the arachidonic acid metabolites mediating bradykinin and noradrenaline hyperalgesia. Brain Research 458: 402–406

Taiwo Y O, Levine J D 1988b Prostaglandins inhibit endogenous pain control mechanisms by blocking transmission at spinal noradrenergic synapses. Journal of Neuroscience 8: 1346–1349

Taiwo Y O, Levine J D 1989a Contribution of guanine nucleotide regulatory proteins to prostaglandin hyperalgesia in the rat. Brain Research 492: 400–403

Taiwo Y O, Levine J D 1989b Prostaglandin effects after elimination of indirect hyperalgesic mechanisms in the skin of the rat. Brain Research 492: 397–399

Taiwo Y O, Levine J D 1990 Direct cutaneous hyperalgesia induced by adenosine. Neuroscience 38: 757–762

Taiwo Y O, Levine J D 1991a Further confirmation of the role of adenyl cyclase and of cAMP-dependent protein kinase in primary afferent hyperalgesia. Neuroscience 44: 131–135

Taiwo Y O, Levine J D 1991b Kappa- and delta-opioids block sympathetically dependent hyperalgesia. Journal of Neuroscience 11: 928–932

Taiwo Y O, Levine J D 1992 Serotonin is a directly-acting hyperalgesic agent in the rat. Neuroscience 48: 485–490

Taiwo Y O, Goetzl E J, Levine J D 1987 Hyperalgesia onset latency suggests a hierarchy of action. Brain Research 423: 333–337

Taiwo Y O, Bjerknes L K, Goetzl E J, Levine J D 1989 Mediation of primary afferent peripheral hyperalgesia by the cAMP second messenger system. Neuroscience 32: 577–580

Taiwo Y O, Heller P H, Levine J D 1992 Mediation of serotonin hyperalgesia by the cAMP second messenger system. Neuroscience 48: 479–483

Taiwo Y O, Heller P H, Levine J D 1990 Characterization of distinct phospholipases mediating bradykinin and noradrenaline hyperalgesia. Neuroscience 39: 523–531

Tal M, Liberman R 1997 Local injection of nerve growth factor (NGF) triggers degranulation of mast cells in rat paw. Neuroscience Letters 221: 129–132

Tanaka M, Cummins T R, Ishikawa K, Dib-Hajj S D, Black J A, Waxman S G 1998 SNS Na^+ channel expression increases in dorsal root ganglion neurons in the carrageenan inflammatory pain model. Neuroreport 9: 967–972

Tatebayashi H, Ogata N 1992 Use-dependent facilitation of L-like Ca^{2+} channels counteracts $GABA_B$-mediated inhibition of N-like Ca^{2+} channels in rat sensory neurons. Neuroscience Letters 137: 49–52

Terenghi G, Riveros M V, Hudson L D, Ibrahim N B, Polak J M 1993 Immunohistochemistry of nitric oxide synthase demonstrates immunoreactive neurons in spinal cord and dorsal root ganglia of man and rat. Journal of the Neurological Sciences 118: 34–37

Thippeswamy T, Morris R 1997 Nerve growth factor inhibits the expression of nitric oxide synthase in neurones in dissociated cultures of rat dorsal root ganglia. Neuroscience Letters 230: 9–12

Thornell E, Jansson R, Kral J G, Svanvik J 1979 Inhibition of prostaglandin synthesis as a treatment for biliary pain. Lancet 1i: 584

Torebjörk H E, Hallin R G 1974 Identification of afferent C units in intact human skin nerves. Brain Research 67: 387–403

Torebjörk H E, LaMotte R H, Robinson C J 1984 Peripheral neural correlates of magnitude of cutaneous pain and hyperalgesia: simultaneous recordings in humans of sensory judgments of pain and evoked responses in nociceptors with C-fibers. Journal of Neurophysiology 51: 325–339

Torebjörk H E, Lundberg L E, LaMotte R H 1992 Central changes in processing of mechanoreceptive input in capsaicin-induced secondary hyperalgesia in humans. Journal of Physiology (London) 448: 765–780

Torebjork E, Wahren L, Wallin G, Hallin R, Koltzenburg M 1995 Noradrenaline-evoked pain in neuralgia. Pain 63: 11–20

Tracey D J, Walker J S 1995 Pain due to nerve damage: are inflammatory mediators involved? Inflammation Research 44: 407–411

Treede R D, Meyer R A, Raja S N, Campbell J N 1992 Peripheral and central mechanisms of cutaneous hyperalgesia. Progress in Neurobiology 38: 397–421

Urban L, Thompson S W, Dray A 1994 Modulation of spinal excitability: co-operation between neurokinin and excitatory amino acid neurotransmitters. Trends in Neuroscience 17: 432–438

Vane J R 1971 Inhibition of prostaglandin synthesis as a mechanism of action for aspirin-like drugs. Nature New Biology 231: 232–235

Vane J R, Bakhle Y S, Botting R M 1998 Cyclooygenase 1 and 2. Annual Review of Pharmacology and Toxicology 38: 97–120

Vanhatalo S, Klinge E, Sjostrand N O, Soinila S 1996 Nitric oxide-synthesizing neurons originating at several different levels innervate rat penis. Neuroscience 75: 891–899

Vasko M R 1995 Prostaglandin-induced neuropeptide release from spinal cord. Progress in Brain Research 104: 367–380

Vizzard M A, Erdman S L, Erickson V L, Stewart R J, Roppolo J R, De Groat W C 1994 Localization of NADPH diaphorase in the lumbosacral spinal cord and dorsal root ganglia of the cat. Journal of Comparative Neurology 339: 62–75

Vizzard M A, Erdman S L, de Groat W C 1995 Increased expression of neuronal nitric oxide synthase in dorsal root ganglion neurons after systemic capsaicin administration. Neuroscience 67: 1–5

Vizzard M A, Erdman S L, de Groat W C 1996 Increased expression of neuronal nitric oxide synthase in bladder afferent pathways following chronic bladder irritation. Journal of Comparative Neurology 370: 191–202

Vulchanova L, Riedl M S, Shuster S J et al 1997 Immunohistochemical study of the P2X2 and P2X3 receptor subunits in rat and monkey sensory neurons and their central terminals. Neuropharmacology 36: 1229–1242

Vyklicky L, Knotkova-Urbancova H 1996 Can sensory neurones in culture serve as a model of nociception? Physiological Research 45: 1–9

Vyklicky L, Knotkova-Urbancova H, Vitaskova Z, Vlachova V, Kress M, Reeh P W 1998 Inflammatory mediators at acidic pH activate capsaicin receptors in cultured sensory neurons from newborn rats. Journal of Neurophysiology 79: 670–676

Wagner R, Janjigian M, Myers R R 1998 Anti-inflammatory interleukin-10 therapy in CCI neuropathy decreases thermal hyperalgesia, macrophage recruitment, and endoneurial TNF-alpha expression. Pain 74: 35–42

Waldmann R, Bassilana F, de Weille J, Champigny G, Heurteaux C, Lazdunski M 1997a Molecular cloning of a non-inactivating proton-gated Na^+ channel specific for sensory neurons. Journal of Biological Chemistry 272: 20975–20978

Waldmann R, Champigny G, Bassilana F, Heurteaux C, Lazdunski M 1997b A proton-gated cation channel involved in acid-sensing. Nature 386: 173–177

Wall P D, Gutnick M 1974 Ongoing activity in peripheral nerves: the physiology and pharmacology of impulses originating from a neuroma. Experimental Neurology 43: 580–593

Weinreich D, Wonderlin W F 1987 Inhibition of calcium-dependent spike after-hyperpolarization increases excitability of rabbit visceral sensory neurones. Journal of Physiology (London) 394: 415–427

Weinreich D, Koschorke G M, Undem B J, Taylor G E 1995 Prevention of the excitatory actions of bradykinin by inhibition of PGI_2 formation in nodose neurones of the guinea-pig. Journal of Physiology (London) 483: 735–746

Werz M A, Macdonald R L 1987 Phorbol esters: voltage-dependent effects on calcium-dependent action potentials of mouse central and peripheral neurons in cell culture. Journal of Neuroscience 7: 1639–1647

Westlund K N, McNeill D L, Coggeshall R E 1989 Glutamate immunoreactivity in rat dorsal root axons. Neuroscience Letters 96: 13–17

Westlund K N, Sun Y C, Sluka K A, Dougherty P M, Sorkin L S, Willis W D 1992 Neural changes in acute arthritis in monkeys. II. Increased glutamate immunoreactivity in the medial articular nerve. Brain Research. Brain Research Reviews 17: 15–27

Whalley E T, Clegg S, Stewart J M, Vavrek R J 1989 Antagonism of the algesic action of bradykinin on the human blister base. Advances in Experimental Medicine and Biology 247A: 261–268

White D M 1996 Mechanism of prostaglandin E_2-induced substance P release from cultured sensory neurons. Neuroscience 70: 561–565

White D M, Helme R D 1985 Release of substance P from peripheral nerve terminals following electrical stimulation of the sciatic nerve. Brain Research 336: 27–31

White D M, Levine J D 1991 Different mechanical transduction mechanisms for the immediate and delayed responses of rat C-fiber nociceptors. Journal of Neurophysiology 66: 363–368

White J C, Sweet W H 1969 Pain and the neurosurgeon: a forty year experience. Thomas, Springfield

White G, Lovinger D M, Weight F F 1989 Transient low-threshold Ca^{2+} current triggers burst firing through an afterdepolarizing potential in an adult mammalian neuron. Proceedings of the National Academy of Sciences USA 86: 6802–6806

White D M, Basbaum A I, Goetzl E J, Levine J D 1990 The 15-lipoxygenase product, 8R, 15S-diHETE, stereospecifically sensitizes C-fiber mechanoheat nociceptors in hairy skin of rat. Journal of Neurophysiology 63: 966–970

Wiesenfeld-Hallin Z, Hao J X, Xu X J, Hokfelt T 1993 Nitric oxide mediates ongoing discharges in dorsal root ganglion cells after peripheral nerve injury. Journal of Neurophysiology 70: 2350–2353

Woolf C J 1996 Phenotypic modification of primary sensory neurons: the role of nerve growth factor in the production of persistent pain. Philosophical Transactions of the Royal Society of London. Series B: Biological Sciences 351: 441–448

Woolf C J, Doubell T P 1994 The pathophysiology of chronic pain – increased sensitivity to low threshold A beta-fibre inputs. Current Opinion in Neurobiology 4: 525–534

Woolf C J, Safieh-Garabedian B, Ma Q P, Crilly P, Winter J 1994 Nerve growth factor contributes to the generation of inflammatory sensory hypersensitivity. Neuroscience 62: 327–331

Woolf C J, Ma Q P, Allchorne A, Poole S 1996 Peripheral cell types contributing to the hyperalgesic action of nerve growth factor in inflammation. Journal of Neuroscience 16: 2716–2723

Woolf C J, Allchorne A, Safieh-Garabedian B, Poole S 1997 Cytokines, nerve growth factor and inflammatory hyperalgesia: the contribution of tumour necrosis factor alpha. British Journal of Pharmacology 121: 417–424

Wu J, Lin Q, Lu Y, Willis W D, Westlund K N 1998 Changes in nitric oxide synthase isoforms in the spinal cord of rat following induction of chronic arthritis. Experimental Brain Research 118: 457–465

Yaksh T L 1982 Central and peripheral mechanisms for the analgesic action of acetylsalicylic acid. In: Barnett H J M, Mustard J F (eds) Acetylsalicylic acid: new uses for an old drug. Raven Press, New York, pp 137–151

Yamamoto T, Nozaki-Taguchi N 1997 Role of spinal cyclooxygenase (COX)-2 on thermal hyperalgesia evoked by carageenan injection in the rat. Neuroreport 8: 2179–2182

Yang L C, Marsala M, Yaksh T L 1996 Characterization of time course of spinal amino acids, citrulline and PGE_2 release after carrageenan/kaolin-induced knee joint inflammation: a chronic microdialysis study. Pain 67: 345–354

Yang X C, Guharay F, Sachs F 1986 Mechanotransducing ion channels: ionic selectivity and coupling to viscoelastic components of the cytoskeleton. Biophysical Journal 49: 373a

Yonehara N, Takemura M, Yoshimura M et al 1997 Nitric oxide in the rat spinal cord in Freund's adjuvant-induced hyperalgesia. Japanese Journal of Pharmacology 75: 327–335

Yoshimura N, White G, Weight F F, de Groat W C 1996 Different types of Na^+ and A-type K^+ currents in dorsal root ganglion neurones innervating the rat urinary bladder. Journal of Physiology (London) 494: 1–16

Yu C, Lin P X, Fitzgerald S, Nelson P 1992 Heterogeneous calcium currents and transmitter release in cultured mouse spinal cord and dorsal root ganglion neurons. Journal of Neurophysiology 67: 561–575

Zhang X, Verge V, Wiesenfeld-Hallin Z et al 1993 Nitric oxide synthase-like immunoreactivity in lumbar dorsal root ganglia and spinal cord of rat and monkey and effect of peripheral axotomy. Journal of Comparative Neurology 335: 563–575

Zhang X, Ji R R, Arvidsson J et al 1996 Expression of peptides, nitric oxide synthase and NPY receptor in trigeminal and nodose ganglia after nerve lesions. Experimental Brain Research 111: 393–404

Zong X, Lux H D 1994 Augmentation of calcium channel currents in response to G protein activation by GTP gamma S in chick sensory neurons. Journal of Neuroscience 14: 4847–4853

Zur K B, Oh Y, Waxman S G, Black J A 1995 Differential up-regulation of sodium channel alpha- and beta 1-subunit mRNAs in cultured embryonic DRG neurons following exposure to NGF. Brain Research. Molecular Brain Research 30: 97–105

Nociceptive peripheral neurons: cellular properties

STUART BEVAN

INTRODUCTION

Nociception involves the transduction of specific noxious signals and the generation of action potentials by the peripheral terminals of small-diameter sensory neurons. These action potentials are propagated to the spinal cord where they stimulate the release of fast neurotransmitters and slower acting mediators from the central afferent terminals located in the dorsal horn. Nociceptive neurons can also have a peripheral effector role mediating responses associated with neurogenic inflammation (vasodilatation, vascular leakage) and neuroimmune regulation. In addition they can influence smooth muscle contraction and glandular secretion in organs, such as the airways, gastrointestinal and urinary tracts (Maggi 1996).

Nociceptive afferent neurons are sensitive to different kinds of noxious stimuli (thermal, mechanical, chemical) and some fibres, the polymodal nociceptors, are sensitive to all three modalities. A considerable amount of information has been accumulated about the mechanisms underlying the chemosensitivity of nociceptive afferent neurons. The available information indicates that mediators released during inflammation can excitate and sensitize nociceptive afferents by acting on ligand-gated ion channels, G-protein-coupled receptors or tyrosine kinase-linked receptors. Furthermore, some of the sensitizing effects of inflammatory agents may be mediated indirectly by effects on voltage-gated ion channels. The mechanisms of thermotransduction are also becoming better understood, but there has been relatively little progress in our understanding of the processes of mechanotransduction in nociceptive neurons.

The properties of nociceptive afferent neurons are subject to environmental influences. Short-term changes, such as sensitization, are generally associated with activation of intracellular second messenger systems and modifications to the phosphorylation levels of key membrane proteins. The phenotypic properties of these neurons are not fixed and undergo dramatic longer-term changes in response to inflammatory mediators and to nerve damage.

This chapter will focus on the cellular characteristics of nociceptive afferent neurons, their ion channels and signal transduction pathways, and discuss the ways in which they contribute to the function of these cells under normal and pathological circumstances.

ION CHANNELS OF SENSORY NEURONS

Studies on the cell soma membrane of dorsal root ganglion neurons show that sensory neurons display the same types of ion channels as other excitable cells (Scott 1992). However, it is unclear whether the properties of the nerve terminal membrane, where the processes of transduction and encoding take place, are the same as those of the somal membrane.

In general activation of inward (depolarizing) membrane currents, or inactivation of outward currents, will lead to increased excitability of the membrane, whereas the opposite changes will inhibit the cell from firing. It is convenient to divide membrane ion channels into those that are gated by changes in membrane potential and those that are gated by chemical ligands.

VOLTAGE-GATED ION CHANNELS

The main channels responsible for inward membrane currents in nociceptive afferent neurons are the voltage-activated sodium and calcium channels, while outward current is carried mainly by potassium ions (Nowycky 1992). For each of these principal ions, there are several distinct types of voltage-gated channels. The excitability of neurons can be controlled either by regulating ion channel expression or by modulating the activity of one or more channel types.

Sodium channels

Sodium (Na) channels open rapidly and transiently when the membrane is depolarized beyond about −60 to −40 mV and are responsible in most neurons for action potential generation and conduction. C cells, which have unmyelinated axons, and correspond mainly to the physiologically defined polymodal nociceptive neurons, usually have slow action potentials, with a clearly defined inflection on the falling phase. They can be distinguished from A cells, which have myelinated axons and much faster action potentials, though there is some overlap between the thinly myelinated Aδ- and C-cell populations (Koerber & Mendell 1992). One difference between the action potentials in A and C cells is their sensitivity to blockade by tetrodotoxin (TTX). The action potentials and Na currents of C cells are largely resistant to block by tetrodotoxin (TTX), because they possess a distinct population of TTX-resistant (TTX-R) Na channels. These channels activate more slowly than the TTX-sensitive (TTX-S) channels which predominate in A cells (Koerber & Mendell 1992, Arbuckle & Docherty 1995). Molecular cloning has identified one type of channel (SNS) responsible for the expression of TTX-R currents (Akopian et al 1996, Sangameswaran et al 1996). mRNAs encoding several types of TTX-S channels have been reported in spinal sensory neurons but the relationship between these mRNAs and the physiologically identifiable TTX-S current has not been established.

Sodium channel properties

The biophysical properties of the TTX-S and TTX-R currents show important differences (Kostyuk et al 1981a, Ogata & Tatebayashi 1993, Roy & Narahashi 1992, Elliott & Elliot 1993). In addition to their slower time course, the TTX-R currents are activated at more depolarized membrane potentials than the TTX-S currents: the potential for activation of half of the channels in the cell is in the range −25 to −40 mV for TTX-S and −9 to −16 mV for TTX-R. A similar difference in voltage sensitivity for inactivation is seen and the half inactivation potential for TTX-S channels (about −65 mV) is sufficiently negative that a substantial proportion of the channels are inactivated at the resting potential. By contrast, the half inactivation potential for TTX-R channels (−30 to −40 mV) ensures that they are fully available at normal resting potentials. A further difference between TTX-R and TTX-S channels is the faster rate of recovery from inactivation of the TTX-R subtype. These differences mean that C cells have a higher depolarization threshold for action potential generation, and are also less liable than A cells to become refractory during a sustained depolarization. Thus TTX-R Na currents are ideally suited to generating sustained bursts of action potentials in response to a prolonged depolarizing noxious stimulus (Elliott & Elliot 1993, Elliott 1997).

Sodium channel expression

The mRNAs for at least six functional Na channels are expressed by dorsal root ganglion (DRG) neurons. The pattern of expression is shown in Table 3.1, where it can be seen that the type I and II channels are expressed under all conditions while the type III channel, which is found in developing DRG neurons and is essentially absent from the neurons in the adult rat, appears to be strongly expressed after nerve injury (Waxman et al 1994). Conversely, expression of the TTX-R channel, SNS, is downregulated after axotomy (Cummins & Waxman 1997, Dib-Hajj et al 1998), although not in an experimental partial nerve injury (chronic constriction injury, CCI) model (Novakovic et al 1998). A possible basis for the downregulation of SNS expression following axotomy is control of SNS gene expression by growth factors such as nerve growth factor (NGF), which are produced by target tissues in the periphery and

Table 3.1 Expression of sodium channel α subunits in rat DRG neurons estimated by in situ hybridization signal or RT-PCR. The effects of axotomy were studied in adult rat DRG and NGF effects studied in neonatal animals exposed to NGF for 4 days in vitro. For the TTX-R SNS/PN3 channel changes in expression have also been studied electrophysiologically. In addition the TTX sensitivity of the expressed cloned channels is shown

mRNA	*TTX sensitive*	*Expression in adult*	*Effect of axotomy*	*NGF effects*
I	Yes	++	↑	↑
II	Yes	+	↑	↑
III	Yes	0/+	↑↑	
SNS/PN3	No	++	↓	↓
NaCh6	Yes	++		
PN1	Yes	++		

Data from Black & Waxman 1996, Waxman et al 1994, Dib-Hajj et al 1996, 1998, Black et al 1996, Akopian et al 1996.

transported retrogradely to the cell soma. Nerve section interrupts the supply of NGF and results in a downregulation of functional TTX-R channel expression (Cummins & Waxman 1997, Zhang et al 1997), which can be reversed if NGF is applied to the damaged nerve endings (Dib-Hajj et al 1998). The significance of these induced changes in the expression of different Na-channel subtypes has not yet been elucidated, although an increased expression of the TTX-R channels induced by an increased production and supply of NGF during inflammation (see Ch. 4) may facilitate the generation of prolonged bursts of action potentials. In general, an increase in Na-channel density at any region of the neuron will facilitate action potential generation at that site. Few physiological correlates of the observed changes in the mRNA expression for Na-channel subtypes have been reported, although the finding that TTX-S currents in axotomized DRG neurons recover faster from inactivation than in control neurons may reflect a change in channel subtype expression possibly related to the appearance of type III channels (Cummins & Waxman 1997).

Na channels have several amino acid residues that can be phosphorylated by specific protein kinases (Numann et al 1991, Li et al 1992) and there is now good evidence that the properties of at least one type of DRG sodium channel, TTX-R, are modified by inflammatory mediators acting through a cAMP–protein kinase A (PKA) pathway such that the channels open in response to smaller depolarizing stimuli (see below).

In addition to regulation by cAMP- and PKA-linked pathways, Na channels also have amino acid residues that are substrates for protein kinase C (PKC)-mediated phosphorylation. Phorbol esters which activate PKC directly can shift Na-channel activation to more hyperpolarized potentials, thereby promoting channel opening by any given stimulus (Numann et al 1991).

Sodium channels as therapeutic targets

Spontaneous action potential discharge occurs in sensory nerves after nerve damage, originating at or near the sites of injury and in the region of the soma (e.g. see Xie et al 1995), and may account for the pain associated with such lesions (see Ch. 5). It is possible that the accumulation of additional Na channels in the axonal membrane proximal to the site of nerve transection (Devor et al 1993, England et al 1996a, Novakovic et al 1998) is a factor in this altered membrane behaviour. The addition of extra Na channels will facilitate action potential discharge by lowering the threshold potential but may not be the only factor required to elicit spontaneous activity. It is possible that, as in other types of spontaneously active neurons (Hille 1992), there is a 'pacemaker' current which depolarizes the sensory neurons towards the threshold potential. The spontaneous membrane potential fluctuations that can evoke action potentials in axotomized, but not control, DRG neurons (Study & Kral 1996) may reflect the presence of such a pacemaker current.

The observation that Na-channel expression in DRG neurons is regulated and can be modified by axotomy or inflammatory agents such as NGF raises the possibility that the Na channels underlying the excitability of nociceptive neurons in chronic pain conditions are pharmacologically distinct from those expressed normally by sensory neurons or most other neurons. Such a difference offers the prospect of new therapeutic approaches to neuropathic pain. The precise molecular target for such a development is unclear, although the observation that ectopic activity can be blocked by local application of TTX (Omana-Zapata et al 1997) suggests that one or more of the TTX-S channels are likely substrates. A differential blockade of Na-channel subtypes may underlie the clinical observation that some Na-channel blocking agents, such as phenytoin, carbamazepine and tocainide, may be efficaceous analgesics in neuropathic pain (Tanelian & Brose 1991), although it is not known whether this is due to an action on sensory neuron excitability.

Potassium channels

The opening and closing of potassium (K) channels is an important regulatory process for cell excitability and is reflected in a great heterogeneity of K-channel subtypes. A variety of voltage-gated K channels are found in sensory neurons (Nowycky 1992, Cardenas et al 1995, Gold et al 1996b, Safranov et al 1996), which parallels the observed heterogeneity of molecularly defined K-channel subunits that are expressed in these neurons (Beckh & Pongs 1990).

Several delayed rectifier type K channels (I_k) have been described in small, as well as larger, diameter DRG neurons (Gold et al 1996b, Safranov et al 1996). These channels open in response to depolarization and are largely responsible for the rapid repolarization of the membrane that terminates the action potential. In general I_k determines the action potential configuration and has little effect on the firing pattern although some subtypes activate near the resting membrane potential and can influence membrane excitability (Safranov et al 1996).

A second major type of K current (I_A) activates more rapidly in response to depolarization, but also inactivates if the membrane remains even slightly depolarized. These currents effectively oppose the rapidly activating Na current needed to generate an action potential. Thus when I_A is inactivated by a small resting depolarization of the membrane, the Na current is effectively unopposed, and membrane excitability is increased. The rapid switch-on of I_A during an action potential means that the K conductance of the membrane is high immediately afterwards, so the neuron cannot fire again until I_A has subsided. I_A is therefore regarded as one of the main factors regulating the maximum firing frequency of neurons (Connor & Stevens 1971). Many studies have reported A channels in sensory neurons (e.g. Kostyuk et al 1981b, McFarlane & Cooper 1991) and recent reports have shown that I_A is expressed by small diameter, capsaicin-sensitive neurons (Cardenas et al 1995, Gold et al 1996b). Any suppression of the A current could, in principle, contribute to the type of spontaneous activity associated with damage to nociceptive peripheral sensory neurons.

Calcium-activated potassium channels

Calcium-activated K channels ($I_{K(Ca)}$) occur in many types of neurons and are responsible for the later phases of the afterhyperpolarization (AHP) that follows an action potential. Calcium-activated K channels impose a period of reduced excitability after each action potential, and are thus important in regulating the firing pattern of the neuron (Hille 1992). The channels are opened by the influx of calcium through voltage-activated Ca channels which open during the action potential (see below). Sensory neurons show two distinct types of spike AHP, with different time courses (Higashi et al 1984, Fowler et al 1985), which are associated with the activation of two types of calcium-activated channel. The fast AHP, which decays within a few milliseconds, is mainly due to the rapid opening of the 'big' conductance (BK) channels, and occurs in all sensory neurons. More interesting is the very prolonged AHP, lasting for several seconds, which is seen in a subpopulation of C neurons, but not in A neurons, from both nodose (Fowler et al 1985) and spinal (Akins & McCleskey 1993, Gold et al 1996c) ganglia. This current is associated with the opening of 'small' conductance (SK) channels, and has a major influence on the ability of the neuron to fire repetitively in response to a maintained depolarization (Weinreich & Wonderlin 1987). The slow AHP is susceptible to an inhibition by inflammatory mediators, such as prostaglandins (Weinreich & Wonderlin 1987, Gold et al 1996c), bradykinin (Weinreich 1986), 5-hydroxytryptamine (Christian et al 1989) and histamine (Jafri et al 1997), which promotes repetitive firing.

Inwardly rectifying channels

Sensory neurons express two types of voltage-dependent inwardly rectifying channels, I_h and I_{IR}, both of which are activated by membrane hyperpolarization. I_{IR} channels are permeable to potassium ions and activate almost instantaneously when the membrane is hyperpolarized. These channels are thought to be important in maintaining the resting potential near the potassium reversal potential (E_K) (Hille 1992). The I_{IR} channels close down when the membrane depolarizes and thereby allow the potential to change more easily in response to a stimulus. Generally I_{IR} currents are thought to be important in allowing more prolonged depolarizing responses in other cell types (Hille 1992), although the finding that expression of this current is confined largely to medium-diameter DRG neurons, with little expression in large- or small-diameter cells (Scroggs et al 1994), raises questions about its role in shaping nociceptive responses.

I_h channels are permeable to both sodium and potassium ions and are slowly activated when the membrane is hyperpolarized beyond its normal resting potential of about −70 mV (Mayer & Westbrook 1983). Among sensory neurons, I_h is largely confined to A cells (Nowycky 1992, Scroggs et al 1994), although some C cells do express this current (Scroggs et al 1994, Cardenas et al 1995, Ingram & Williams 1996). In other cell types, including heart muscle, I_h contributes to pacemaking or repetitive firing by influencing the rate of repolarization following an hyperpolarization. I_h is activated by the hyperpolarizing phase of an action potential and generates a depolarizing inward current that speeds the repolarization towards the threshold potential. The physiological role of I_h in sensory neurons is unclear. I_h in trigeminal and nodose ganglion neurons is, however, potentiated by prostaglandin E_2, which may lead to a more rapid repolarization after an action potential and facilitation of repetitive firing (Ingram & Williams 1996).

Calcium channels

At least five major types of voltage-activated calcium channels are expressed in sensory neurons (L, N, P/Q, T and R). They can be distinguished on the basis of the degree of membrane depolarization needed to activate the currents (activation threshold), their inactivation characteristics and their pharmacological properties. T channels, sometimes referred to as LVA (low voltage-activated) channels, form a well-defined class, characterized by a low threshold for activation. The currents activated at more depolarized membrane potentials can be distinguished pharmacologically on the basis of their sensitivity to block by dihydropyridine calcium channel antagonists (L) and their sensitivity (N,P/Q) or resistance (R) to various snail toxins (e.g. see Dunlap et al 1995). Collectively these channels have been termed HVA (high voltage-activated). The expression of the channel subtypes can vary between DRG neurons. For example, T channels are absent in large-diameter neurons (presumably A cells), very abundant in medium-diameter neurons, and present at lower abundance in small-diameter, capsaicin-sensitive, neurons (Scroggs & Fox 1992).

Calcium entry through voltage-gated Ca channels can affect many cellular processes, including activation of other membrane channels, release of transmitters, and regulation of many enzymes (especially kinases and phosphatases) and can initiate a variety of short- and long-term cellular effects. The inward current contributes directly to membrane depolarization, and the characteristic 'hump' on the falling phase of the C-cell action potential is due to a Ca current. The HVA currents in DRG neurons are inhibited by many agents (e.g., baclofen, noradrenaline, dopamine, somatostatin, opiates) via the actions of G-protein-coupled receptors. These Ca-channel modifications are usually mediated by the direct interaction of the βγ subunits of G-proteins with the Ca channels (Hille 1994, Dolphin 1995). Although modulation of the various Ca-channel subtypes has not been fully investigated for all ligands, the available data suggest that the properties of both N- and P/Q-type channels can be modified. In many neurons, transmitter release is mediated via N and P/Q channels (Reuter 1996) and the data from sensory neuron preparations conform to this general pattern. For example, neuropeptide release is relatively insensitive to block by dihydropyridines but is sensitive to ω-conotoxin (Evans et al 1966, Santicioli et al 1992), suggesting that N channels are important routes of Ca entry for the release process. Modulation of HVA-channel properties by various agents is therefore an important regulatory mechanism for transmitter and neuropeptide release.

Calcium entry through T channels appears to be involved mainly in the control of neuronal firing patterns (Huguenard 1996), partly on account of the depolarizing inward current itself, and partly through the opening of various calcium-activated ion channels.

CHEMICAL EXCITATION AND SENSITIZATION OF SENSORY NEURONS

Excitation of sensory nerves requires depolarization of the membrane at some region of the nerve to the threshold potential for action potential initiation. This occurs at peripheral nerve terminals either by opening ion channels that have a high permeability for sodium and, in some cases, calcium ions, or by closing potassium permeable ion channels that are open in the 'resting' membrane. Neuronal firing will also depend on the properties of the voltage-gated ion channels responsible for action potential initiation, which can be modified by phosphorylation of key amino acid residues on the channels. Transmitters or inflammatory mediators can, therefore, influence the probability of neuronal firing not only by depolarizing the membrane but also by modifying the voltage-gated Na and K channels.

Ion channels and G-protein-coupled receptors

Ion channels are opened, either by a ligand binding to and directly gating a receptor–ion channel complex, or by activation of G-protein-coupled receptors that stimulate the production of intracellular messengers (Fig. 3.1). Direct ion channel activation is rapid and usually operates in the millisecond time scale, while G-protein-coupled receptor events operate over a time scale of seconds or minutes. Table 3.2 illustrates the major physiological effects of transmitters and mediators that act on sensory neurons.

Many mediators produced during inflammation, such as bradykinin, 5HT and prostaglandins, act via G-protein-coupled receptors. These receptors have seven transmembrane domains and a cytoplasmic domain that interacts with a heterotrimeric G-protein to elicit a specific biochemical response which depends on the type of G-protein that is activated. The G-proteins activated in sensory neurons can be classified on the basis of their α-subunit composition. G_s stimulates adenylate cyclase to raise the concentration of cAMP in the neuron, while G_i inhibits the activity of this enzyme to lower cAMP levels. Stimulation of G_q activates phospholipases, notably phospholipase C (PLC), which generates inositol 1,4,5-trisphosphate (IP_3) and diacylglycerol (DAG) from a membrane lipid precursor. G_q activation can also stimulate phospholipase A_2 (PLA_2), which in turn produces the prostaglandin precursor, arachidonic acid. G-protein control of cellular function can also involve a direct action of βγ subunits on ion channels and enzymes, such as PLA_2 (Clapham & Neer 1997).

The various signalling pathways can interact and mediators that raise the level of cAMP in the neuron may alter the activity of ligand-gated channels by phosphorylation. There is also evidence that G-protein pathways can influence the activity of tyrosine kinase receptor-linked pathways, which are important for the transduction of growth factor signals.

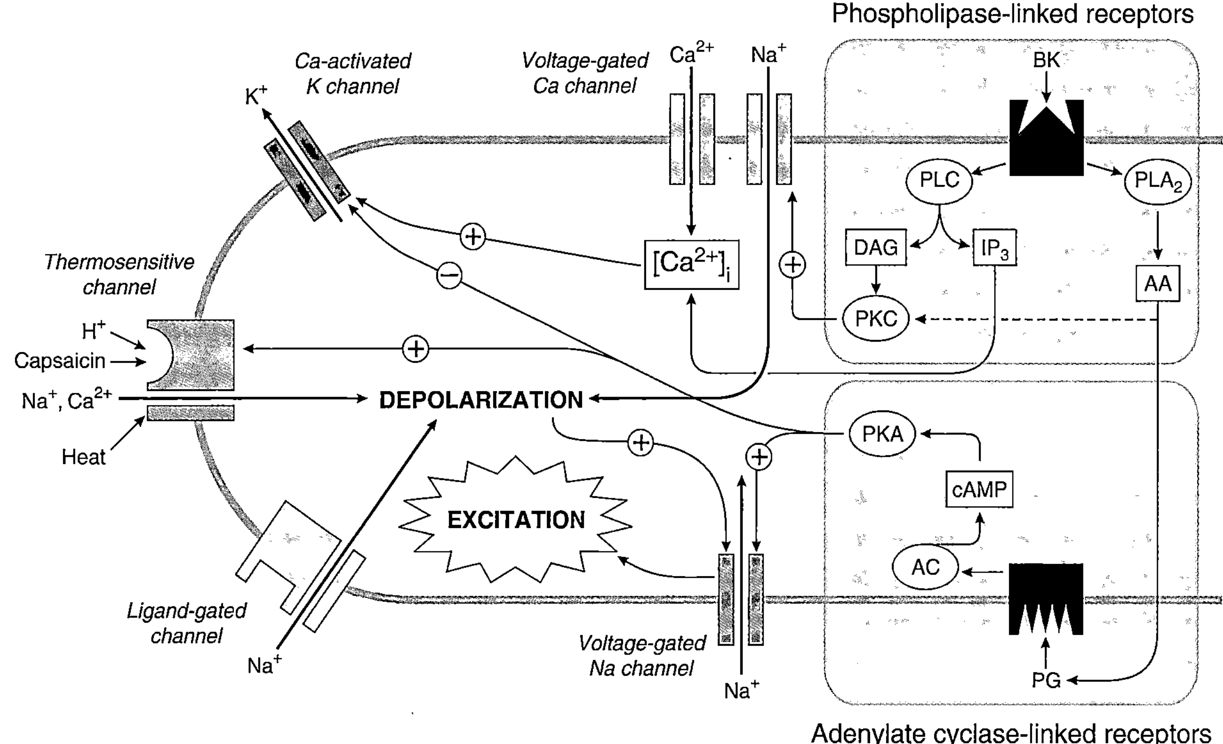

Fig. 3.1 Simplified scheme illustrating some of the molecular events that control the excitability of nociceptive peripheral neurons. Note not all interactions are shown (e.g., PKC regulation of heat responses). PLC = phospholipase C; PLA_2 = phospholipase A_2; DAG = diacylglycerol; IP_3 = inositol-1,4,5-trisphosphate; PKC = protein kinase C; AA = arachidonic acid; PG = prostaglandin; AC = adenylate cyclase; cAMP = cyclic adenosine monophosphate; PKA = cAMP-dependent protein kinase; BK = bradykinin.

Table 3.2. Different receptor types on sensory neurons and their cellular effects

Transduction mechanism	*Example*	*Cellular effect*
Ligand-gated channel	Capsaicin – heat H^+ 5HT ($5HT_3$) ATP (P_{2X}) Gluamate GABA ($GABA_A$)	Excitation
G-protein linked	GABA ($GABA_B$) Somatostatin Opiates Adenosine Adrenoreceptors Neuropeptide Y 5HT ($5HT_{1B/D}$)	Inhibition of transmitter and peptide release: Presynaptic inhibition
	Bradykinin (B_2) 5HT ($5HT_{1A/2}$) Histamine (H_1) Adrenoreceptors (α_2) PGE_2	Excitation and/or sensitization
Tyrosine kinase linked	NGF (Trk A)	Control of gene expression

Intracellular messengers

Nociceptive neurons use a range of intracellular mediators: the cyclic nucleotides (cAMP and cGMP), inositol trisphosphate, calcium ions, nitric oxide and the cyclooxygenase and lipoxygenase products of arachidonic acid metabolism. A change in the level of phosphorylation of specific proteins is often a key step in cell signalling, and many of these second messengers regulate phosphorylation (via protein kinases) or dephosphorylation (via protein phosphatases) of channels, receptors and enzymes. Some mediators can also stimulate other biochemical processes, such as methylation and the production of ceramide, which may operate in nociceptive neurons.

LIGAND-GATED CHANNELS

A number of transmitters and mediators act directly on receptor/ion channel complexes in DRG neurons. Receptor activation by 5HT, ATP, acetylcholine, glutamate (via a kainate-type receptor), protons and the algogen capsaicin stimulates sensory neurons by opening ion channels that have a high permeability for sodium ions. GABA also acts directly on $GABA_A$ receptors to increase the permeability of the membrane to chloride ions, and this presynaptic action is an important regulator of central afferent terminal function.

The significance of these receptor activations is not clear for glutamate and acetylcholine, but the available evidence indicates an excitatory (patho)physiological role for 5HT, ATP and protons associated with tissue damage or inflammation. 5HT is released from platelets and mast cells during tissue damage and can stimulate sensory neurons by activation of $5HT_3$ ligand-gated receptors found on small-diameter, capsaicin-sensitive sensory neurons (Bevan & Robertson 1991, Fozard 1994). This may be the major mechanism of excitation by 5HT, as the pain produced by application of 5HT to a human blister base can be inhibited by a specific $5HT_3$ antagonist (Richardson et al 1985).

ATP is released when cells are damaged and can also be co-released with noradrenaline and neuropeptide Y (NPY) from sympathetic nerves (Burnstock 1996). ATP activates sensory nerves when, for example, applied to a blister base (Bleehen & Keele 1977). The stimulatory effects of ATP appear to be mediated by activation of cation channel-linked P_{2x} receptors in which a sensory neuron specific subunit ($P_{2\times3}$ is probably a major component (Burnstock & Wood 1996). P_{2x} receptors differ structurally from most other types of ligand-gated ion channel as they are constructed of subunits with only two transmembrane domains (Brake et al 1994, Valera et al 1994).

The pH of the extracellular environment is known to fall in a number of pathophysiological conditions such as hypoxia/anoxia as well as in inflammation (Jacobus et al 1977, Corbe & Poole-Wilson 1980). Low pH solutions evoke a prolonged activation of sensory nerves (Steen et al 1992) and produce a sharp stinging pain in humans (Lindahl 1962, Steen & Reeh 1993). Prolonged activation of sensory nerves is probably mediated by the opening of non-selective cation-permeable channels that are activated when the extracellular pH falls below about pH 6.5 (Bevan & Yeats 1991). The observations that capsaicin and proton sensitivity are co-expressed in small-diameter DRG neurons (Bevan & Docherty 1993) and that expression of both chemosensitivities is regulated by NGF (Bevan & Winter 1995), together with the finding that the properties of the single-channel currents evoked by either stimulus are essentially identical (Bevan et al 1993), led to the hypothesis that protons and capsaicin activate the same ion channels. The important finding that the cloned capsaicin-activated ion channel, VR1, is thermosensitive (see below) suggests that protons and noxious temperatures could interact to activate ion channels in a synergistic manner.

PHOSPHOLIPASE-LINKED G PROTEIN-COUPLED RECEPTORS

Bradykinin B_2 receptors

Signalling via phospholipase-linked receptors has been well documented for bradykinin (BK) and the related peptide kallidin (Lys^0-BK) acting through the B_2-receptor subtype, which is expressed constituitively by nociceptive sensory nerves as well as other, non-neuronal cell types. The intracellular events evoked by B_2 receptor activation are illustrated in Figure 3.2. BK excites sensory neurons mainly through the activation of a pertussis toxin-sensitive G-protein which stimulates a phosphatidylinositol specific phospholipase C (PLC). PLC cleaves the substrate membrane lipids to generate two intracellular messengers, DAG and IP_3 (Thayer et al 1988, Burgess et al 1989a, Gammon et al 1989).

The excitation of sensory neurons is mainly through the actions of DAG, which stimulates PKC to phosphorylate various cellular proteins including membrane receptors and ion channels (Shearman et al 1989). PKC depolarizes the neurons by opening a cation (Na^+, K^+) permeable ion channel (Burgess et al 1989a, McGehee & Oxford 1991). The responses of sensory neurons to BK are inhibited by a relatively specific PKC inhibitor, staurosporine (Burgess et al 1989a), which also attenuates the responses of skin afferents (Dray et al 1992). Phorbol esters, which bind to and activate PKC, also mimic the BK-induced membrane currents, depolarization and calcium entry in sensory nerves. Furthermore, the bradykinin responses of many, but not all, neurons are reduced or abolished when PKC activity is down regulated by prolonged exposure to phorbol esters (Rang & Ritchie 1988, Burgess et al 1989a). The failure to inhibit the responsiveness of all sensory neurons with staurosporine or prolonged exposure to phorbolesters suggests that excitation can be mediated by another pathway. Activation of such a pathway may underlie the finding that staurosporine does not inhibit the BK-evoked depolarization of dorsal roots in a rat spinal cord preparation (Dunn & Rang 1990).

BK activation of sensory neurons raises the concentration of free intracellular calcium ($[Ca^{2+}]_i$) in two ways. Depolarization activates voltage-gated Ca channels, and IP_3 production stimulates the release of calcium from intracellular stores (Thayer et al 1988, Burgess et al 1989a). In some other neuronal cell types, elevation of $[Ca^{2+}$ $_i$ opens calcium-activated K channels, but this is not an obvious feature of DRG neurons, perhaps because the channels in DRG neurons have a lower sensitivity to calcium ions (Naruse et al 1992). The calcium that enters through voltage-gated Ca channels stimulates the production of cGMP,

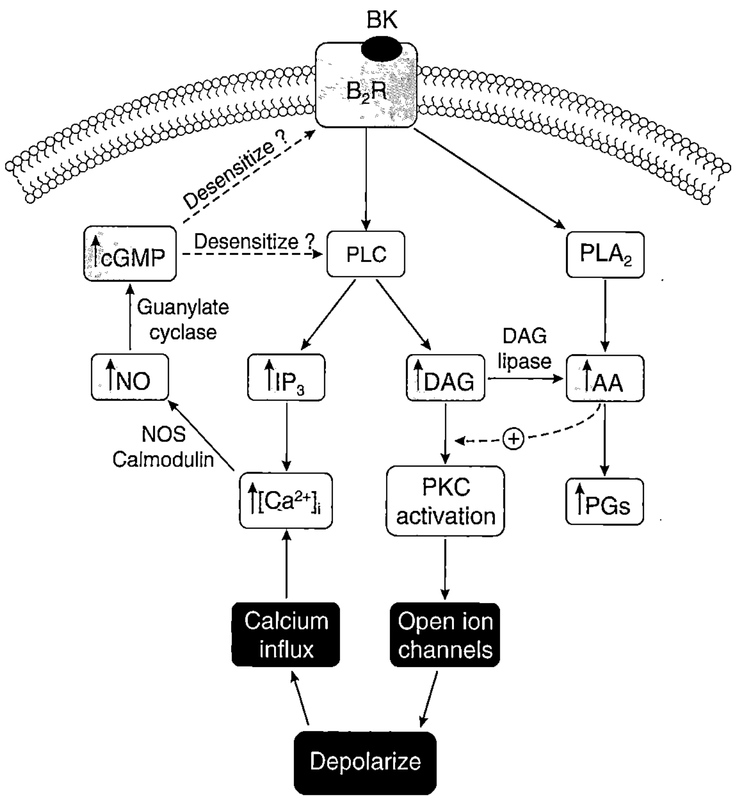

Fig. 3.2 Scheme illustrating the actions of bradykinin on sensory neurons mediated by B_2 receptors. Abbreviations as in Figure 3.2, plus NOS = nitric oxide synthase; NO = nitric oxide; cGMP = cyclic guanosine monophosphate.

although this is not evoked by the IP_3 -induced release of intracellular calcium (Burgess et al 1989b). The likely mechanism for cGMP production is stimulation of calmodulin by calcium ions, followed by calmodulin activation of nitric oxide synthase and a consequent generation of nitric oxide which stimulates guanylate cyclase. cGMP appears to be an important regulator of B_2-receptor function, as it acts to attenuate the response at a step after BK binding. The likely sites of action are receptor desensitization or inhibition of the G-protein or PLC (Burgess et al 1989b, McGhee et al 1992).

BK can generate arachidonic acid and prostanoids in neural tissues either by activation of PLC (Gammon et al 1989, Allen et al 1992) or more directly by activation of PLA_2 (Farmer & Burch 1992). Most of the available evidence, however, suggests that mammalian sensory nerves produce little or no prostaglandins and that the majority of the prostanoids (PGE_2, PGD_2, PGI_2) generated in sensory nerve preparations are produced by non-neuronal cells. Although prostaglandins may mediate some of the excitatory effects of BK (Geppetti et al 1991, Hua & Yaksh 1993, Rueff & Dray 1993), their major action is to sensitize sensory neurons.

Bradykinin B_1 receptors

Des-Arg[9]-BK and des-Arg[10]-kallidin, which are degradation products of BK and kallidin, are biologically active and exert their effects via a second type of G-protein-coupled receptor, the B_1 receptor. The B_1 receptor transduction mechanisms are very similar to those for B_2 receptors (Smith et al 1995). B_1 receptors are not normally expressed in tissues but their expression is induced by tissue injury when they contribute significantly to inflammatory hyperalgesia (Dray & Perkins 1993, Perkins et al 1993, Davis & Perkins 1994). The weight of evidence suggests that functional B_1 receptors are not expressed on sensory nerves and that the effects of B_1 agonists are mediated via non-neuronal cells (Davis et al 1996, Seabrook et al 1997), although the expression of neuronal B_1 receptors cannot be discounted (Petersen et al 1988, Seabrook et al 1997). B_1-receptor activation evokes the release of PGE_2 and PGI_2 (D'Orleans-Juste et al 1989, Lerner & Modeer 1991), nitric oxide (D'Orleans-Juste et al 1989) and various cytokines (D'Orleans-Juste et al 1989, Tiffany & Burch 1989) from non-neuronal cells, and these inflammatory mediators are probably responsible for the hyperalgesia induced by B_1-receptor agonists.

Monoamine receptors

Although the ability of histamine to evoke the sensations of itch and, at higher concentrations, pain by activation of small-diameter afferents is well documented (e.g. see Simone et al 1991, Handwerker et al 1991, Koda et al 1996), the underlying mechanisms are poorly understood. Pharmacological experiments indicate that the excitation (and sensitization) of afferents is mediated by H_1 and not by H_2 or H_3 receptors (Tani et al 1990, Hutcheon et al 1993, Koda et al 1996), and H_1-receptor expression has been detected in small-diameter DRG neurons by autoradiography (Ninkovic & Hunt 1985) and in situ hybridization (Senba & Kashiba 1996). H_1 receptors are usually coupled to DAG/IP_3 production, but the involvement of these mediators in the excitation induced by histamine has not been shown. Histamine depolarizes some trigeminal and nodose ganglion neurons but usually does not elicit action potentials (Hutcheon et al 1993, Undem & Weinrich 1993). The depolarizations are associated with variable changes (increases and decreases) in membrane conductance which suggests multiple effects on ion channels. The sensitizing effects of histamine are mediated by the same (H_1) receptor subtype and probably involve the actions of prostanoids.

Although many of the excitatory actions of 5HT have been ascribed to the ligand gated $5HT_3$ receptor, there is good evidence that 5HT can activate and sensitize nociceptors by actions on G-protein-coupled receptors. In some cases the observed hyperalgesia is mediated via adenylate cyclase (see below). In other experiments, the evidence indicates a thermal hyperalgesia induced by an action on peripheral $5HT_2$ receptors (Rueff & Dray 1992, Abbott et al 1996, Tokunaga et al 1998). The cellular mechanisms responsible for these effects are unclear. $5HT_2$ receptors are usually linked to the PLC pathway. Activation of $5HT_2$ receptors depolarizes capsaicin-sensitive DRG neurons by reducing a resting potassium conductance (Todorovic & Anderson 1990), and such an effect could contribute to both excitation and sensitization of nociceptive peripheral neurons.

ADENYLATE CYCLASE-LINKED G-PROTEIN-COUPLED RECEPTORS

5-Hydroxytryptamine receptors

5HT released from platelets and mast cells can influence the activity of adenylate cyclase via two receptor subtypes, although the precise distribution of these receptors on different classes of sensory neurons is unknown. $5HT_4$ receptors are positively coupled to adenylate cyclase and receptor activation stimulates cAMP production, while $5HT_1$ receptors are negatively coupled to the enzyme and will inhibit cAMP formation.

The activation of a subtype of $5HT_1$ receptors ($5HT_{1B/D}$) is of considerable clinical significance, as these receptors are associated with trigeminal afferents innervating the dura mater. $5HT_{1B/D}$ receptors are located on the terminals of these sensory afferents and activation inhibits adenylate cyclase via activation of $G_{i/o}$ proteins. Drugs of the triptan class act in this way to inhibit neuropeptide release from the terminals of these afferents.

5HT has also been reported to produce a peripherally mediated mechanical hyperalgesia by an action on $5HT_{1A}$ receptors (Taiwo & Levine 1992). The findings that this effect can be blocked by a PKA inhibitor, Rp-cAMP, and augmented by a phosphodiesterase inhibitor which should raise cAMP levels (Taiwo et al 1992) could be explained if the $5HT_{1A}$ receptors were unusually coupled to a mechanism that increased cAMP production. The observation that $5HT_{1A}$ receptor activation hyperpolarizes DRG neurons (Todorovic & Anderson 1992) is not consistent with the cited behavioural data. The mechanisms associated with peripheral $5HT_{1A}$ activation clearly need further investigation.

Adenosine

Intravenous administration of adenosine produces pain in human volunteers (Sylven 1989) and sensitizes cat myelinated and unmyelinated vagal afferents (Cherniak et al 1987). Local application of adenosine in the rat has also been reported to produce a mechanical hyperalgesia in some (Taiwo & Levine 1990), but not all (Ashgar et al 1992), experiments. The pharmacological characteristics of the induced hyperalgesia in the rat suggest an action on afferent adenosine A_2 receptors (Taiwo & Levine 1990), which are usually positively coupled to adenylate cyclase. Conversely, adenosine A_1-receptor activation, which typically inhibits adenylate cyclase activity, antagonizes the hyperalgesic effects of both A_2 agonists and PGE_2 (Taiwo & Levine 1990). These findings are consistent with the hypothesis that adenosine-mediated mechanical hyperalgesia is linked to the production of cAMP. Curiously the pain-enhancing actions of adenosine administered intra-arterially, intramuscularly or intradermally in humans appear to be mediated by A_1 receptors (Pappagallo et al 1993, Gaspardone et al 1995). The basis for the discrepancy between rat and humans studies is not clear (Sawynok 1997) but, as in the case of

$5HT_{1A}$ receptors noted above, would suggest that receptors that usually couple negatively to adenylate cyclase can, in some way, induce pain and hyperalgesia.

Noradrenaline

An excitatory effect of noradrenaline on intact as well as damaged sensory neurons is seen after nerve injury (see Ch. 5). The precise mechanisms that underlie the effect, notably the site of action (sensory afferent or sympathetic neurons), are contentious but the pharmacology is typical of an action at α_2 receptors, which normally act by inhibiting adenylate cyclase or by modulating ion channels via direct G-protein interactions. The anatomical evidence demonstrates that α_2 receptors are expressed by some sensory neurons and that their expression is upregulated after nerve injury (Nicholas et al 1993, Perl 1994).

NITRIC OXIDE AND cGMP

Nitric oxide (NO) is an important intercellular mediator and is produced by many cells that have a close physical association with sensory neurons. NO is formed from l-arginine following the activation of the enzyme nitric oxide synthase (NOS) by calcium and other co-factors including calmodulin. NO diffuses to its site of action where it stimulates guanylate cyclase to produce cGMP. NO can also act in other ways, for example by activating cyclooxygenase enzymes and by S-nitrosylation of proteins (Bredt & Snyder 1994).

The physiological actions of NO in nociceptive neurons are unclear. Intradermal injections of NO evokes a concentration dependent pain in human volunteers (Holthusen & Arndt 1994) and sodium nitroprusside (SNP), which generates NO, evokes substance P and CGRP release from sensory nerves in spinal cord slices through an NO-dependent mechanism (Garry et al 1994). In contrast, SNP has no obvious stimulatory effect on isolated DRG neurons although it enhances BK desensitization in the same neurons (McGehee et al 1992).

The NOS inhibitor, L-NAME, inhibits the spontaneous firing of damaged afferents but is without effect on normal nerve activity (Wiesenfeld-Hallin et al 1993). NOS is found in some DRG neurons under normal conditions and the expression of this enzyme is increased following nerve section (Verge et al 1992) or partial nerve ligation (Steel et al 1994). One possibility is that the upregulation of NOS is associated with an enhanced NO production that increases excitability. The effects of NO may involve cGMP-mediated modification of ion channels, such as K channels (Cohen et al 1994). NO can also activate cyclooxygenase enzymes to stimulate the production of prostaglandins (Salvemini et al 1993), and this may be an important mechanism for nociceptive sensory neurons. Further studies are required to see whether NO has major, physiologically relevant effects on nociceptors and to elucidate the cellular mechanisms.

INTRACELLULAR MESSENGERS AND SENSITIZATION

Although many agents act to sensitize nociceptive afferents, there is good evidence that the sensitization process often involves a common step; namely a rise in neuronal cAMP levels. Some mediators such as adenosine (via A_2 receptors) raise cAMP levels directly (see above) but others, whose receptors are not coupled positively to adenylate cyclase, often act by generating prostanoids.

Nociceptor sensitization by BK involves the production of arachidonic acid, which can occur via two pathways (Fig. 3.3). One mechanism that occurs in sensory neurons is activation of PLC to generate DAG followed by hydrolysis of the DAG by the enzyme DAG lipase to form monoacylglycerol and arachidonic acid (Gammon et al 1989, Allen et al 1992). Activation of PLA_2 is responsible for arachidonic acid production in non-neuronal cells (Burch & Axelrod 1987, Conklin et al 1988). In both cases, arachidonic acid is hydrolysed by cyclooxygenase enzymes to generate prostanoids.

Histamine sensitizes polymodal nociceptive afferents to heat stimuli via H_1-receptor activation (Mizimura et al 1994, Koda et al 1996). As prostaglandins are released from some tissues in response to histamine (Falus & Merety 1992), it is possible that the sensitizing effects are mediated, in part, by prostanoid production, although this has not been established and the process may involve an action of PKC (see below).

Prostaglandins

Prostaglandins (PGs), such as PGE_2, PGD_2 and PGI_2, are produced during inflammation and act with some specificity on different prostanoid receptors, termed EP, DP and IP, respectively. Each of the prostanoid receptors has distinct coupling to G-proteins and the pattern of coupling determines the biochemical consequence of receptor activation. Four major types of EP receptors (EP_{1-4}) have been described and splice variants of the EP_3 subclass have also been identified, which probably explains the multiplicity of transduction pathways that have been associated with this receptor. In situ hybridization studies have shown the presence of mRNAs for IP, EP_1, EP_3 and EP_4 receptors in DRG neurons. About half of the neurons express EP_3 receptor mRNA, 40% IP mRNA, 30% EP_1 mRNA and 20% EP_4 mRNA with some degree of co-expression (Sugimoto et al 1994, Oida et al 1995). Of these EP_1, EP_4, IP and some splice variants of EP_3 receptors (EP_{3B} and EP_{3C}) couple positively via G_s to stimulate adenylate cyclase and raise cAMP levels. Activation of EP_1 receptors raises intracellular calcium, possibly by activating a calcium-permeable channel in some way (see Narumiya 1996).

A major effect of the prostaglandins PGE_2 and PGI_2 is to sensitize afferent neurons to noxious chemical, thermal and mechanical stimuli (e.g. see Mizimura et al 1987, Schaible & Schmidt 1988, Birrell et al 1991), although PGD_2 shows little or no such activity (Rueff & Dray 1993). The ability of prostanoids to sensitize nociceptors also depends on the modality of the noxious stimulus. For example, PGE_2 sensitizes afferents to the effects of BK but much higher concentrations are required to sensitize nociceptors to either heat or mechanical stimuli (Schaible & Schmidt 1988, Grubb et al 1991, Mizimura et al 1993). This disparity suggests that sensitization can involve differential regulation of distinct transduction pathways. Much of the available evidence, however, indicates that PGE_2 and PGI_2 sensitize nociceptive neurons by elevating cAMP levels.

Sensitization by cAMP

There is ample evidence that agents and procedures that raise cAMP levels in cells elicit hyperalgesia by a direct action on peripheral neurons (Taiwo et al 1989, Taiwo & Levine 1991), probably by phosphorylation of a variety of receptors, ion channels and other cellular targets. Sensitization of nociceptors, irrespective of modality, can be achieved by modifying the voltage-gated ion channels that either control action potential initiation or control firing frequence. The activity of TTX-R Na channels expressed in nociceptors is regulated by inflammatory mediators, including PGE_2 (England et al 1996b, Gold et al 1996a), adenosine (Gold et al 1996a) and 5HT acting via $5HT_4$ receptors (Cardenas et al 1997). Activation of these receptors raises cAMP levels and the available evidence indicates that the raised cAMP levels activate PKA which, in turn, phosphorylates the channels (England et al 1996b). This modification shifts the activation curve for TTX-R channels to less depolarized levels and therefore increases the probability that a membrane depolarization will evoke an action potential Figure 3.3. Voltage-gated K currents are also inhibited by PGE_2 (Nicol et al 1997). The net effect is a lowered threshold for action potential initiation and repetitive firing (Fig. 3.3A).

Prostaglandins can also regulate the amplitude of receptor-operated responses. For example, PGE_2 and PGI_2 augment the membrane response to capsaicin and this effect can be mimicked by agents that elevate cAMP levels (Pitchford & Levine 1991, Lopshire & Nicol 1997). Conversely, loss of capsaicin sensitivity, evoked by repeated agonist application, is inhibited by treatments that inhibit protein phosphatase 2B (calcineurin) activity (Docherty et al 1996). These findings suggest that the activity of the capsaicin receptor/ion channel is regulated by the degree of phosphorylation. The discovery that the capsaicin-sensitive VR1 channel is a noxious thermoreceptor suggests that sensitization to noxious heat responses is likely to involve the same mechanisms contolling protein phosphorylation.

Another mechanism of sensitization that has been well documented for visceral (nodose) ganglion neurons is inhibition of the slow AHP which follows each action potential and limits the firing that can be evoked by a given depolarizing stimulus. Prostaglandins, 5HT, inhibitors of NOS, histamine and bradykinin (via prostanoid production) all inhibit the slow AHP and allow the cell to fire repetitively in response to an excitatory stimulus (see above). This effect is probably mediated by a variety of underlying mechanisms some, but not all, involving cAMP and channel phosphorylation.

Other mechanisms of sensitization

Sensitization of nociceptive afferent neurons can also be elicited by agents and transduction pathways which do not normally link positively to cAMP production. At least some of the mechanisms involve protein phosphorylation mediated via PKC. For example, the bradykinin-induced sensitization of the noxious heat-evoked current in DRG neurons is mimicked by a phorbol ester (PMA), which activates PKC, and is inhibited by a kinase inhibitor, staurosporine (Cesare & McNaughton 1996). A similar sensitization of the heat response is evoked by bradykinin, histamine (via H_1 receptors) and a phorbol ester in testicular polymodal nociceptors (Koda et al 1996, Leng et al 1996).

Activation of ligand-gated ion channels, such as the $5HT_3$ receptor, can also sensitize nociceptors (Richardson et al 1985). The mechanisms for such a sensitization have not been elucidated but could involve calcium entry through the activated channels followed by a calcium-

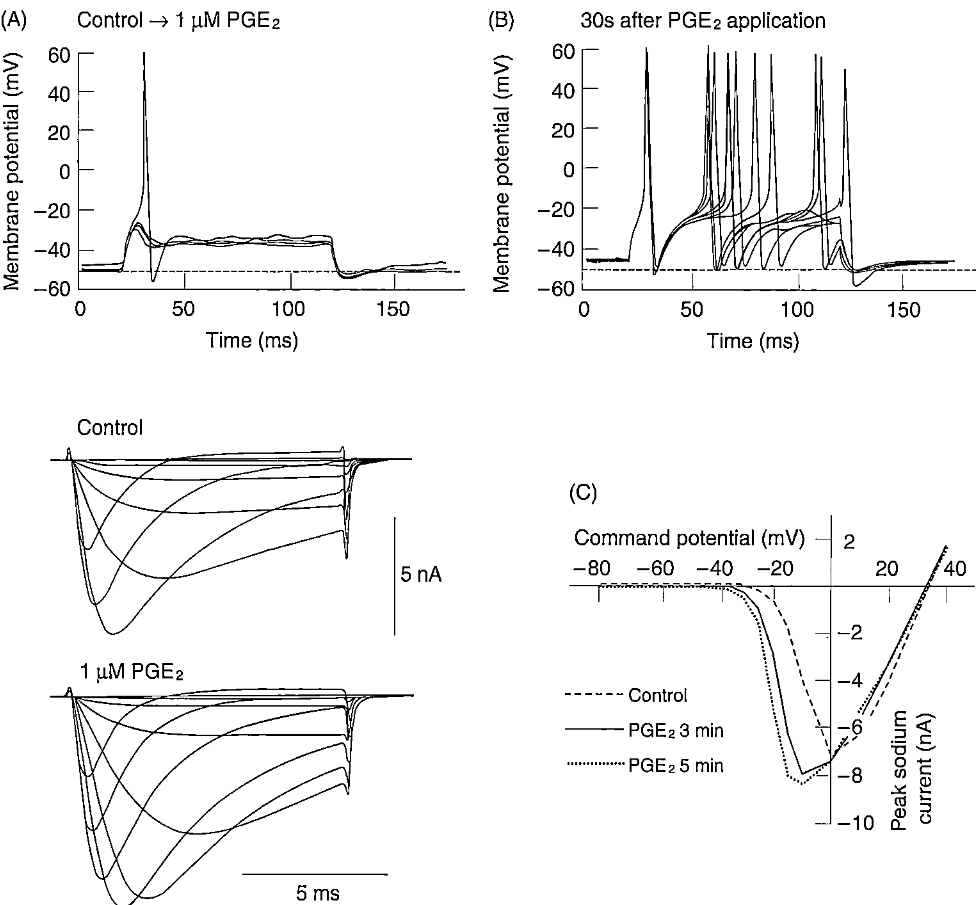

Fig. 3.3 Effect of PGE_2 on action potentials and TTX-R sodium currents in rat DRG neurons. TTX is present throughout. **A** *Left*: A normally subthreshold current pulse evokes an action potential soon after PGE_2 application. *Right*: Repetitive firing with same depolarizing current in presence of PGE_2. **B** TTX-R Na currents evoked at different potentials before and during PGE_2 application. **C** Current voltage curves from neuron in **B** show the shift in channel activation to lower membrane potentials. (Reproduced from England et al 1996b.)

mediated elevation of cGMP (Reiser & Hamprecht 1989) possibly mediated by calcium-calmodulin-stimulated NOS activity.

MECHANOTRANSDUCTION

Both C polymodal nociceptive fibres and a subpopulation of Aδ fibres are responsive to noxious mechanical stimuli and the sensitivity of both classes of neurons increases during inflammation (e.g. see Grubb et al 1991). Products of both cyclo-oxygenase and lipoxygenase pathways of arachidonic acid metabolism are responsible for an increase in mechanosensitivity, although the extent to which this reflects an effect on the primary transduction mechanism rather than action potential discharge is unknown. Mechanical factors may also be important in some conditions; for example, intra-articular pressure may increase during joint inflammation.

The mechanisms that underlie the initial steps in mechanotransduction of mammalian primary afferents are unknown. A genetic analysis of behavioural mutants of the nematode *Caenorhabditis elegans* has revealed candidate molecules for mechanotransduction, degenerins (García-Añoveros & Corey 1997). These ion channels show the same structural motif as the mammalian purinoceptor P_{2x} channel and epithelial Na^+ channels with two transmembrane segments. Structurally related channels are found in DRG and other neurons where they are can be activated by acidification of the external medium (Krishtal & Pidoplichko 1980, Bevan & Yeats 1991, Waldmann et al 1997). Whether molecules of this class are responsible for mechanotransduction of noxious and/or non-noxious stimuli in nociceptors remains to be investigated.

THERMOTRANSDUCTION – A ROLE FOR CAPSAICIN-SENSITIVE ION CHANNELS

Skin afferents show several types of thermal responses. C fibres in primate skin rapidly respond to a noxious heat stimulus with a median threshold temperature of 41°C. By contrast, A fibres show two distinct response patterns. One class responds rapidly to the heat stimulus with a median threshold temperature of 46°C, while the other class responds relatively slowly with a higher median threshold temperature (>53°C) (Treede et al 1995, Campbell & Meyer 1996). Experiments on isolated DRG neurons have begun to reveal the ionic mechanisms responsible for thermoreception. Some thermoresponsive currents are activated within the physiological range (Cesare & McNaughton 1996, Reichling & Levine 1997) and probably play no role in noxious thermal transduction. Noxious temperatures (>43°C) activate another type of current in a subset of DRG neurons (Fig. 3.4) and ion substitution experiments have shown that the activated ion channels discriminate relatively poorly between sodium, caesium and calcium ions (Cesare & McNaughton 1996, Nagy & Rang 1998a).

There is a correlation between capsaicin sensitivity and noxious heat sensitivity in DRG neurons (Kirschstein et al 1997), which suggests some link between the two sensitivities. The amplitude and ion selectivity of noxious heat-operated ion channels in DRG neurons also show a striking resemblance to those of capsaicin-activated channels (Vlachová & Vyklicky 1993, Bevan & Docherty 1996, Oh et al 1996, Nagy & Rang 1998b). The definitive evidence that capsaicin-operated ion channels are thermotransducers was, however, obtained when a functional capsaicin (vanilloid) receptor (VR1) was cloned and expressed in an heterologous system (Caterina et al 1997). Expression of VR1 confers not only capsaicin sensitivity but also a thermosensitivity restricted to noxious (48°C) temperatures (Fig. 3.5). The data are, therefore, consistent with the hypothesis that VR1 channels are responsible for noxious thermal transduction, although the available data do not rule out the possibility that other types of noxious thermosensitive channels may exist.

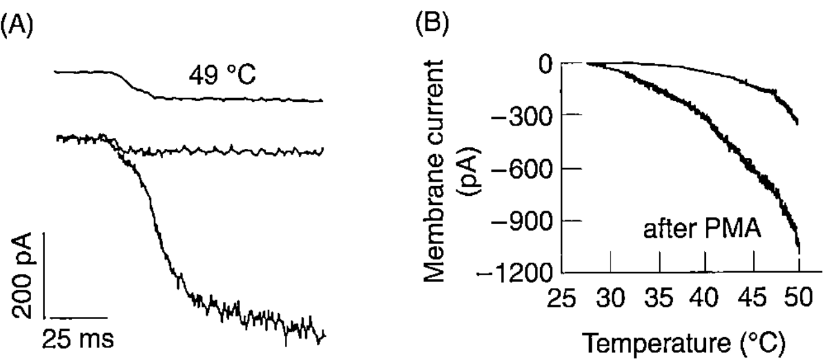

Fig. 3.4 **A** A noxious heat stimulus (top trace, 25°C to 49°C) evokes a depolarizing current response in a heat-sensitive (bottom trace) but not in a heat-insensitive (middle trace) neuron. The top trace shows the temperature dependence of the noxious heat-evoked current. **B** After application of a phorbol ester (PMA), the current is augmented and the activation is shifted to lower temperatures. (Reproduced from Cesare & McNaughton 1996.)

LONGER-TERM REGULATION – SIGNALLING VIA TYROSINE KINASE RECEPTORS

The properties of nociceptors can be regulated by environmental factors such as the supply of growth factors to the neurons. Of these, the actions of nerve growth factor (NGF) have been studied most intensively. The roles of NGF in modifying the neuronal phenotype and the functional importance of these changes for hyperalgesia are discussed in Chapter 4. This account will illustrate the general signal transduction pathways that are thought to operate in sensory neurons (Ganju et al 1998, see Fig. 3.6), although many details of the signalling pathways have been inferred from studies in other cell types (Heumann 1994).

Most of the known effects of NGF are mediated by the high-affinity TrkA receptor, which has intrinsic tyrosine kinase activity. NGF cross links two adjacent receptors. This triggers each TrkA molecule to phosphorylate tyrosine residues on the cytoplasmic domain of its cross-linked neighbour. Phosphorylation causes conformational changes which expose binding sites for proteins with domains of about 100 amino acids (SH2 domains) that have a high affinity for phosphorylated tyrosine residues. A PLC subtype (PLC-γ1) and phosphoinositol-3-kinase are two such

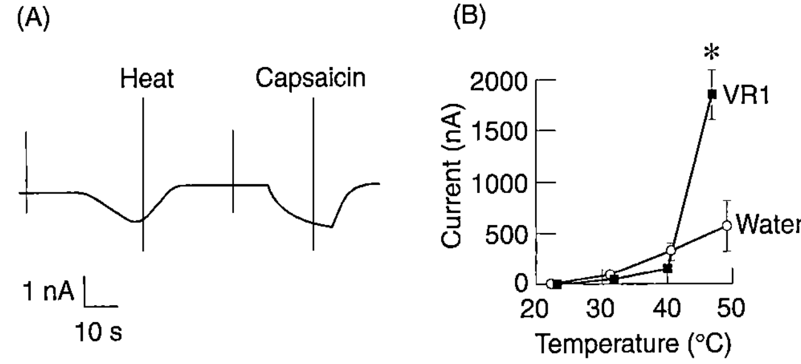

Fig. 3.5 **A** HEK293 cells transfected with VR1 (capsaicin-receptor) cDNA are responsive to both noxious heat (48°C) and capsaicin. **B** Xenopus oocytes injected with VR1 cRNA respond to noxious heat unlike control (water-injected) oocytes. (Reproduced from Caterina et al 1997.)

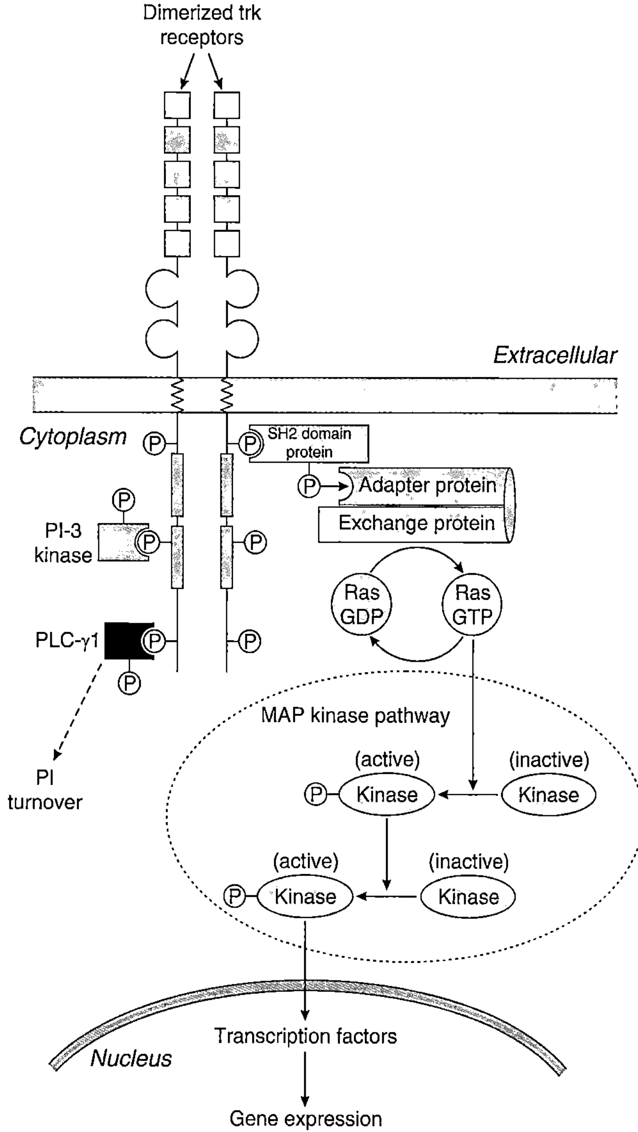

Fig. 3.6 Simplified scheme showing signalling via the high-affinity (TrkA) NGF receptor.

SH2 domain proteins and these are phosphorylated and activated by direct binding to TrkA. Activation of PLC-γ1 may result in a rise in $[Ca^{2+}]_i$ via IP_3 formation.

A major pathway activated by TrkA stimulates the activity of a small GTP-binding protein, p21-Ras, which leads to a cascade of protein phosphorylations involving mitogen-activated protein kinases (MAP kinases). The result of MAP kinase activation is a regulation of gene transcription which underlies many of the longer-term events evoked by exposure to NGF, such as an increase in substance P expression and capsaicin sensitivity, as well as neurite outgrowth and cell survival.

A second signalling pathway, which probably operates in DRG neurons, is signalling via the low-affinity NGF receptor p75. NGF can act via this receptor to stimulate a sphingomyelin-specific PLC (sphingomyelinase) to breakdown the membrane lipid, sphingomyelin, to yield ceramide. Although the functions of ceramide in sensory neurons are unclear, it stimulates the activity of protein phosphatases in other cells (Liscovitch & Cantley 1994).

NEUROCHEMISTRY OF SENSORY NEURONS

Sensory neurons synthesize a variety of substances (amino acids, neuropeptides, etc.) which perform a multiplicity of functions (neurotransmitter, neuroeffector, neurotrophic) by acting on central or peripheral tissues. Glutamate released from the central terminals of nociceptive and non-nociceptive afferents acts as the fast transmitter in the dorsal horn. Some, but not all, nociceptive afferents also synthesize a range of neuropeptides, notably substance P which is released by intense noxious stimuli and has an important role in nociceptive signalling in the dorsal horn.

A multitude of neuropeptides have been identified in small sensory neurons (Lawson 1992, 1996) and their expression may be changed in inflammation and experimental arthritis (e.g., Calzà et al 1997) or after damage to the peripheral axons (Hökfelt & Wiesenfeld-Hallin 1994). Transection or damage to peripheral afferents leads to a reduction in the content of neurokinins, calcitonin gene-related peptide (CGRP) and their respective mRNAs in sensory ganglia. On the other hand such injuries provoke an expression of neuropeptide Y, not normally detected in sensory neurons, and an increase in the expression of galanin. Table 3.3 illustrates the expression pattern of neuropeptides in DRG neurons and the changes seen with peripheral axotomy. Inflammation also modifies neuropeptide expression and increases the mRNA levels encoding neurokinins and CGRP as well as raising the respective peptide levels. These observations illustrate the longer-term adaptive responses of sensory neurons, and suggest that the cell phenotype and peptide synthesis can be regulated by the supply of neurotrophic factors from target organs, or by other environmental factors that change with nerve injury and inflammation. The mechanisms and functional consequences of such changes are discussed elsewhere in this volume.

 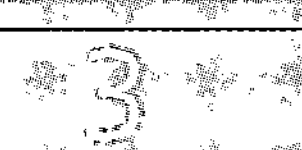

Table 3.3 Expression of neuropeptides in sensory neurons and changes with peripheral axotomy.

Peptide	*% Neurons**	*Cell Sizes*	*After axotomy*	
Substance P	12–38	S m	↓	
CGRP	28–60	S M 1	↓	
Somatostatin	5–15	S	↓	
VIP †	0–5	S m	↑	95% S M L
Galanin †	0–5	S	↑	34% S M
Bombesin †	0–8	S	↑	
CCK	0		↑	30% S
NPY	0–rare		↑	~25% s M L
Dynorphin	0–3	S		

*Percentage range illustrates the variability in expression between species and at various spinal cord levels.
Immunocytochemical and (+) in situ hybridization Data from Lawson (1992, 1996).
S=small; M=medium; L=large: lower case indicates a few neurons in this range.

REFERENCES

Abbott FV, Hong Y, Blier P 1996 Activation of 5-HT$-_{2A}$ receptors potentiates pain produced by inflammatory mediators. Neuropharmacology 35: 99–110

Akins PT, McCleskey EW 1993 Characterization of potassium currents in adult rat sensory neurons and modulation by opioids and cyclic AMP. Neuroscience 56: 759–769

Akopian AN, Sivilotti L, Wood JN 1996 A tetrodotoxin-resistant voltage-gated sodium channel expressed by sensory neurons. Nature 379: 257–262

Allen AC, Gammon CM, Ousley AH, McCarthy KD, Morell P 1992 Bradykinin stimulates arachidonic acid release through the sequential actions of an sn-1 diacylglycerol lipase and a monoacylglycerol lipase. Journal of Neurochemistry 58: 1130–1139

Arbuckle JB, Docherty RJ 1995 Expression of tetrodotoxin-resistant sodium channels in capsaicin-sensitive dorsal root ganglion neurons of adult rats. Neuroscience Letters 185: 70–73

Asghar AUR, McQueen DS, Macdonald AE 1992 Absence of effect of adenosine on the discharge of articular mechanoreceptors in normal and arthritic rats. British Journal of Pharmacology 105: 309P

Beckh S, Pongs O 1990 Members of the RCK potassium channel family are differentially expressed in the rat nervous system. EMBO Journal 9: 777–782

Bevan S, Docherty RJ 1993 Cellular mechanisms of the action of capsaicin. In: Wood J (ed) Capsaicin in the study of pain. Academic, London, pp 27–44

Bevan S, Docherty RJ 1996 The ionic basis of capsaicin-evoked responses. In: Geppetti P, Holzer P (eds) Neurogenic inflammation. CRC Press, Boca Raton, pp 63–67

Bevan S, Robertson B 1991 Properties of 5-hydroxytryptamine, receptor-gated currents in adult rat dorsal root ganglion neurones. British Journal of Pharmacology 102: 272–276

Bevan S, Winter J 1995 Nerve growth factor (NGF) differentially regulates the chemosensitivity of adult rat cultured sensory neurons. Journal of Neuroscience 15: 4916–4926

Bevan S, Yeats J 1991 Protons activate a cation conductance in a sub-population of rat dorsal root ganglion neurones. Journal of Physiology 433: 145–161

Bevan S, Forbes CA, Winter J 1993 Protons and capsaicin activate the same ion channels in rat isolated dorsal root ganglion neurones. Journal of Physiology 459: 401P

Birrell GJ, McQueen DS, Iggo A, Coleman RA, Grubb BD 1991 PGI_2-induced activation and sensitization of articular mechanonociceptors. Neuroscience Letters 124: 5–8

Black JA, Waxman SG 1996 Sodium channel expression: a dynamic process in neurons and non-neuronal cells. Developmental Neuroscience 18: 139–152

Black JA, Dib-Hajj S, McNabola K et al 1996 Spinal sensory neurons express multiple sodium channel α-subunit mRNAs. Molecular Brain Research 43: 117–131

Bleehen T, Keele CA 1977 Observations on the algogenic actions of adenosine compounds on the human blister base preparation. Pain 3: 367–377

Brake AJ, Wagenbach MJ, Julius D 1994 New structural motif for ligand-gated ion channels defined by an ionotropic ATP receptor. Nature 371: 519–523

Bredt DS, Snyder SH 1994 Nitric oxide: a physiologic messenger molecule. Annual Reviews of Biochemistry 63: 175–195

Burch RM, Axelrod J 1987 Dissociation of bradykinin-induced prostaglandin formation from phosphoinositol turnover in Swiss 3T3 fibroblasts: evidence for G protein regulation of Phospholipase A_2. Proceedings of the National Academy of Sciences USA 84: 6372–6378

Burgess GM, Mullaney J, McNeil M, Dunn P, Rang HP 1989a Second messengers involved in the action of bradykinin on cultured sensory neurones. Journal of Neuroscience 9: 3314–3325

Burgess GM, Mullaney I, McNeil M, Coote PR, Minhas A, Wood JN 1989b Activation of guanylate cyclase by bradykinin in rat sensory neurones is mediated by calcium influx: possible role of the increase in cyclic GMP. Journal of Neurochemistry 53: 1212–1218

Burnstock G 1996 A unifying prinergic hypothesis for the initiation of pain. Lancet 347: 1604–1605

Burnstock G, Wood JN 1996 Purinergic receptors: their role in nociception and primary afferent neurotransmission. Current Opinion in Neurobiology 6: 526–532

Calzà L, Pozza M, Zanni M, Manzinin CU, Manzinin E, Hökfelt T 1997 Peptide plastivity in primary sensory neurons and spinal cord during adjuvant-induced arthritis in the rat: an immunocytochemical and in situ hybridization study. Neuroscience 82: 575–589

Campbell JN, Meyer RA 1996 Cutaneous nociceptors. In: Belmonte C, Cervero F (eds) Neurobiology of nociceptors. Oxford University Press, Oxford, pp 117–145

Cardenas CG, Del Mar LP, Scroggs RS 1995 Variation in serotonergic inhibition of calcium currents in four types of rat sensory neurons differentiated by membrane properties. Journal of Neurophysiology 74: 1870–1879

Cardenas CG, Del Mar LP, Cooper BY, Scroggs RS 1997 $5HT_4$ receptors couple positively to tetrodotoxin-insensitive sodium channels in a subpopulation of capsaicin-sensory neurons. Journal of Neuroscience 17: 7181–7189

Caternia MJ, Schumacher MA, Tominga M, Rosen TA, Levine JD, Julius D 1997 The capsaicin receptor: a heat-activated ion channel in the pain pathway. Nature 389: 816–824

Cesare P, McNaughton P 1996 A novel heat-activated current in nociceptive neurons and its sensitization by bradykinin. Proceedings of the National Academy of Sciences USA 93: 15435–15439

Cherniak NS, Runold M, Prabhakar NR, Mitra J 1987 Effect of adenosine on vagal sensory pulmonary afferents. Federation Proceedings 46: 825

Christian EP, Taylor GE, Weinreich D 1989 Serotonin increases excitability of rabbit C-fibre neurons by two distinct mechanisms. Journal of Applied Physiology 67: 584–591

Clapham DE, Neer EJ 1997 G protein $\beta\gamma$ subunits. Annual Review of Pharmacology and Toxicology 37: 167–203

Cohen AS, Weinrich D, Kao JPY 1994 Nitric oxide regulates spike frequency accommodation in nodose neurons of the rabbit. Neuroscience Letters 173: 17–20

Conklin BR, Burch RM, Steranka LR, Axelrod J 1988 Distinct bradykinin receptors mediate stimulation of prostaglandin synthesis by endothelial cells and fibroblasts. Journal of Pharmacology and Experimental Therapeutics 244: 646–649

Connor JA, Stevens CF 1971 Prediction of repetitive firing behaviour from voltage clamp data on an isolated neurone soma. Journal of Physiology 213: 31–52

Corbe SM, Poole-Wilson PA 1980 The time of onset and severity of acidosis in myocardial ischaemia. Journal of Molecular and Cellular Cardiology 12: 745–760

Cummins TR, Waxman SG 1997 Downregulation of tetrodotoxin-resistant sodium currents and upregulation of a rapidly repriming tetrodotoxin-sensitive sodium current in small spinal sensory neurons after injury. Journal of Neuroscience 17: 3503–3514

Davis AJ, Perkins MN 1994 Induction of B1 receptors in vivo in a model of persistent inflammatory mechanical hyperalgesia in the rat. Neuropharmacology 33: 127–133

Davis CL, Naeem S, Phagoo SB, Campbell EA, Urban L, Burgess GM 1996 B1 bradykinin receptors and sensory neurones. British Journal of Pharmacology 118: 1496–1476

Devor M, Govrin-Lippmann R, Angelides K 1993 Na^+ channel immunolocalization in peripheral mammalian axons and changes following nerve injury and neuroma formation. Journal of Neuroscience 13: 1966–1992

Dib-Hajj SD, Black JA, Felts P, Waxman SG 1996 Down-regulation of transcripts for Na channel α-SNS in spinal sensory neurons following axotomy. Proceedings of the National Academy of Sciences USA 93: 14950–14954

Dib-Hajj SD, Black JA, Cummins TR, Kenney AM, Kocsis JD, Waxman SG 1998 Rescue of α-SNS sodium channel expression in small dorsal root ganglion neurons after axotomy by nerve growth factor in vivo. Journal of Neurophysiology 79: 2668–2676

Docherty RJ, Yeats JC, Bevan S, Boddeke HW 1996 Inhibition of calcineurin inhibits the desensitization of capsaicin-evoked currents in cultured dorsal root ganglion neurons from adult rats. Pflugers Archiv 431: 828–837

Dolphin A 1995 Voltage-dependent calcium channels and their modulation by neurotransmitters and G proteins. Experimental Physiology 80: 1–36

D'Orleans-Juste P, de Nucci G, Vane JR 1989 Kinins act on B_1 and B_2 receptors to release conjointly endothelium-derived relaxing factor and prostacyclin from bovine aortic endothelial cells. British Journal of Pharmacology 96: 920–926

Dray A, Perkins M 1993 Bradykinin and inflammatory pain. Trends in Neurosciences 16: 99–104

Dray A, Patel IA, Perkins MN, Rueff A 1992 Bradykinin-induced activation of nociceptors: receptor and mechanistic studies on the neonatal rat spinal cord-tail preparation in vitro. British Journal of Pharmacology 107: 1129–1134

Dunlap K, Luebbke JI, Turner TJ 1995 Exocytotic Ca^{2+} channels in mammalian central neurons. Trends in Neurosciences 18: 89–98

Dunn PM, Rang HP 1990 Bradykinin-induced depolarisation of primary afferent nerve terminals in the neonatal rat spinal cord in vitro. British Journal of Pharmacology 100: 656–660

Elliott JR 1997 Slow Na^+ channel inactivation and bursting discharge in a simple model axon: implications for neuropathic pain. Brain Research 754: 221–226

Elliott AA, Elliott JR 1993 Characterization of TTX-sensitive and TTX-resistant sodium currents in small cells from adult rat dorsal root ganglia. Journal of Physiology 463: 39–56

England JD, Happel LT, Kline DG et al 1996a Sodium channel accumulation in humans with painful neuromas. Neurology 47: 272–276

England S, Bevan S, Docherty RJ 1996b PGE_2 modulates the tetrodotoxin-resistant sodium current in neonatal rat dorsal root ganglion neurones via the cyclic AMP-protein kinase A cascade. Journal of Physiology 495: 429–440

Evans AR, Nicole GD, Vasko MR 1996 Differential regulation of evoked peptide release by voltage-sensitive calcium channels in rat sensory neurons. Brain Research 712: 265–273

Falus A, Meretey K 1992 Histamine: an early messenger in inflammatory and immune reactions. Immunology Today 13: 154–156

Farmer SG, Burch RM 1992 Biochemical and molecular pharmacology of kinin receptors. Annual Review of Pharmacology 32: 511–536

Fowler JC, Greene R, Weinreich D 1985 Two calcium-sensitive spike after-hyperpolarization in visceral sensory neurones of the rabbit. Journal of Physiology 365: 59–75

Fozard JR 1994 Role of $5\text{-}HT_3$ receptors in nociception. In: King FD, Jones BJ, Sanger GJ (eds) 5-Hydroxytryptamine receptor antagonists. CRC Press, Boca Raton, pp 241–253

Gammon CM, Allen AC, Morell P 1989 Bradykinin stimulates phosphoinositide hydrolysis and mobilisation of arachidonic acid in dorsal root ganglion neurons. Journal of Neurochemistry 53: 95–101

Ganju P, O'Bryan JP, Der C, Winter J, James IF 1998 Differential regulation of SHC proteins by nerve growth factor in sensory neurons and PC12 cells. European Journal of Neuroscience 10: 1995–2008

García-Añoveros J, Corey DP 1997 The molecules of sensation. Annual Review of Neuroscience 20: 567–594

Garry MG, Richardson JD, Hargreaves KM 1994 Sodium nitroprusside evokes the release of immunoreactive calcitonin gene-related peptide and substance P from dorsal horn slices via nitric oxide-dependant and nitric oxide-independent mechanisms. Journal of Neuroscience 14: 4329–4337

Gaspardone A, Crea F, Tomao F et al 1995 Muscular and cardiac adenosine-induced pain is mediated by A_1 receptors. Journal of the American College of Cardiology 24: 477–482

Geppetti P, Del Bianco E, Tramontana M et al 1991 Arachidonic acid and bradykinin share a common pathway to release neuropeptide from capsaicin-sensitive sensory nerve fibers of the guinea pig heart. Journal of Pharmacology and Experimental Therapeutics 259: 759–765

Gold MS, Reichling DB, Shuster MJ, Levine JD 1996a Hyperalgesic agents increase a tetrodotoxin-resistant Na^+ current in nociceptors. Proceeding of the National Academy of Sciences USA 93: 1108–1112

Gold MS, Shuster MJ, Levine JD 1996b Characterization of six voltage-gated K^+ currents in adult rat sensory neurons. Journal of Neurophysiology 75: 2629–2646

Gold MS, Shuster MJ, Levine JD 1996c Role of a Ca^{2+} dependant slow after hyperpolarization in prostaglandin E_2-induced sensitization of cultures rat sensory neurons. Neuroscience Letters 205: 161–164

Grubb BD, Birrell GJ, McQueen DS, Iggo A 1991 The role of PGE_2 in the sensitization of mechanoreceptors in normal and inflamed ankle joints of the rat. Experimental Brain Research 84: 383–392

Handwerker HO, Forster C, Kirchoff C 1991 Discharge patterns of human C-fibres induced by itching and burning stimuli. Journal of Physiology 66: 307–315

Heumann R 1994 Neurotrophin signalling. Current Opinion in Neurobiology 4: 668–679

Higashi H, Morita K, North RA 1984 Calcium-dependant after potentials in visceral afferent neurones of the rabbit. Journal of Physiology 355: 479–492

Hille B 1992 Ionic channels of excitable membranes. Sinauer, Sunderland, MA

Hille B 1994 Modulation of ion-channal function by G-protein coupled receptors. Trends in Neurosciences 17: 531–536

Hökfelt T, Wiesenfeld-Hallin Z 1994 Messenger plasticity in primary sensory neurons following axotomy and its functional implications. Trends in Neurosciences 17: 22–30

Holthusen H, Arndt JO 1994 Nitric oxide evokes pain in humans on intracutaneous injection. Neuroscience Letters 165: 71–74

Hua X-Y, Yasksh TL 1993 Pharmacology of the effects of bradykinin, serotonin and histamine on the release of calcitonin gene-related peptide in the rat trachea. Journal of Neuroscience 13: 1947–1953

Huguenard JR 1996 Low-threshold calcium currents in central nervous system neurons. Annual Reviews of Physiology 58: 329–348

Hutcheon B, Puil E, Spigelman I 1993 Histamine actions and comparisons with substance P effects in trigeminal neurons. Neuroscience 55: 521–529

Ingram SL, Williams JT 1996 Modulation of the hyperpolarization-activated current (I_h) by cyclic nucleotides in guinea-pig primary afferent neurons. Journal of Physiology 429: 97–106

Jacobus WE, Taylor GJ, Hollis DP, Nunally RL 1977 Phosphorus magnetic resonance of perfused working rat heart. Nature 265: 756–758

Jafri MS, Moore KA, Taylor GE, Weinrich D 1997 Histamine H1 receptor activation blocks two classes of potassium current,$IK_{(est)}$ and I_{AHP}, to excite ferret vagal afferents. Journal of Physiology 503: 533–546

Kirschstein T, Büsselberg D, Treede R-D 1997 Coexpression of heat-evoked and capsaicin-evoked inward currents in acutely dissociated rat dorsal root ganglion neurons. Neuroscience Letters 231: 33–36

Koda H, Minagawa M, Leng S-H, Mizimura K, Kumazawa T 1996 H1 receptor mediated excitation and facilitation of the heat response by histamine in canine visceral polymodal receptors studied in vitro. Journal of Neurophysiology 76: 1396–1404

Koerber HR, Mendell LM 1992 Functional heterogeneity of dorsal root ganglion cells. In: Scott SA (ed) Sensory neurons: diversity, development and plasticity. Oxford University Press, New York, pp 77–96

Kostyuk PG, Veselovsky NS, Tsyndrenko AY 1981a Ionic currents in the somatic membrane of rat dorsal root ganglion neurons. I. Sodium currents. Neuroscience 6: 2423–2430

Kostyuk PG, Veselovsky NS, Fedulova SA, Tsyndrenko AY 1981b Ionic currents in the somatic membrane of rat dorsal root ganglion neurons. III. Potassium currents. Neuroscience 6: 2439–2444

Krishtal OA, Pidoplichko VI 1980 A receptor for protons in the membrane of sensory neurons. Neuroscience 5: 2325–2357

Lawson SN 1992 Morphological and biochemical cell types of sensory neurons. In: Scott SA (ed) Sensor neurons: diversity, development and plasticity. Oxford University Press, New York, pp 27–59

Lawson SN 1996 Neurochemistry of cutaneous nociceptors. In: Belmonte C, Cervero F (eds) Neurobiology of nociceptors. Oxford University Press, Oxford, pp 72–91

Leng S, Mizimura K, Koda H, Kumazawa T 1996 Excitation and sensitization of the heat response induced by a phorbol ester in canine visceral polymodal receptors studied in vitro. Neuroscience Letters 206: 13–16

Lerner UH, Modeer T 1991 Bradykinin B1 and B2 agonists synergistically potentiate interleukin-1-induced prostaglandin biosynthesis in human gingival fibroblasts. Inflammation 15: 427–436

Li M, West JW, Scheuer T, Catterall WA 1992 Functional modulation of brain sodium channels by cAMP-dependent phosphorylation. Neuron 8: 1151–1159

Lindahl O 1962 Pain: a chemical explanation. Acta Rheumatologica Scandinavica 8: 161–169

Liscovitch M, Cantley LC 1994 Lipid second messengers. Cell 77: 329–334

Lopshire JC, Nicol GD 1997 Activation and recovery of the PGE2-mediated sensitization of the capsaicin in rat sensory neurons. Journal of Neurophysiology 78: 3154–3164

Maggi 1996 Pharmacology of the efferent function of primary afferent sensory neurons. In: Geppetti P, Holzer P (eds) Neurogenic inflammation. CRC Press, Boca Raton, pp 81–90

Mayer ML, Westbrook GL 1983 A voltage-clamp analysis of inward (anomalous) rectification in mouse spinal sensory ganglion neurones. Journal of Physiology 340: 19–45

McFarlane S, Cooper E 1991 Kinetics and voltage dependence of A-type currents in neonatal rat sensory neurons. Journal of Neurophysiology 66: 1380–1391

McGhee DS, Oxford GS 1991 Bradykinin modulates the electrophysiology of cultured rat sensory neurons through a pertussis toxin-insensitive G protein. Molecular Cellular Neuroscience 2: 21–30

McGhee DS, Goy MF, Oxford GS 1992 Involvement of the nitric oxide-cyclic GMP pathway in the desensitization of bradykinin responses of cultured ray sensory neurons. Neuron 9: 315–324

Mizumura K, Sato J, Kumazawa T 1987 Effects of prostagladins and other putative chemical intermediaries on the activity of canine testicular polymodal receptors studied in vitro. Pflugers Archiv 408: 565–572

Mizumura K, Minagawa M, Tsujii Y, Kumazawa T 1993 Prostaglandin E_2-induced sensitization of the heat response of canine visceral polymodal receptors in vitro. Neuroscience Letters 161: 117–119

Mizumura K, Minagawa M, Koda H, Kumazawa T 1994 Histamine-induced sensitization of the heat response of canine visceral polymodal receptors. Neuroscience Letters 168: 93–96

Nagy I, Rang HP 1998a Noxious heat-activated currents in rat dorsal root ganglion neurons. Journal of Physiology 506: 153P

Nagy I, Rang HP 1998b Noxious heat-activated microscopic currents in rat dorsal root ganglion neurons. Journal of Physiology 507: 29P

Narumiya S 1993 Prostanoid receptors and signal transduction. Progress in Brain Research 113: 231–241

Naruse K, McGhee DS, Oxford GS 1992 Differential responses of Ca-activated K channels to bradykinin in sensory neurons and F-11 cells. American Journal of Physiology 262: C453–C460

Nicholas AP, Pieribone V, Hokfelt T 1993 Distribution of mRNAs for alpha-2 adrenergic receptor subtypes in rat brain: an in situ hybridization study. Journal of Comparative Neurology 328: 575–594

Nicol GD, Vasko MR, Evans AR 1997 Prostaglandins suppress an outward potassium current in embryonic rat sensory neurones. Journal of Physiology 77: 167–176

Ninkovic M, Hunt SP 1985 Opiate and histamine H1 receptors are present on some substance P-containing dorsal root ganglion cells. Neuroscience Letters 53: 133–137

Novakovic SD, Tzoumaka E, McGivern JG et al 1998 Distribution of tetrodotoxin-resistant sodium channel PN3 in rat sensory neurons in normal and neuropathic conditions. Journal of Neuroscience 18: 2174–2187

Nowycky M 1992 Voltage-gated ion channels in dorsal root ganglion neurons. In: Scott AS (ed) Sensory neurons: diversity, development and plasticity. Oxford University Press, New York, pp 97–115

Numann R, Caterall WA, Scheuer T 1991 Functional modulation of brain sodium channels by protein kinase. C phosphorylation. Science 254: 115–118

Ogata N, Tatebayashi H 1993 Kinetic analysis of two types of Na^+ channels in rat dorsal root ganglia. Journal of Physiology 466: 9–37

Oh U, Hwang SW, Kim D 1996 Capsaicin activates a nonselective cation channel in cultured neonatal rat dorsal ganglion neurons. Journal of Neuroscience 16: 1659–1667

Oida H, Namba T, Sugimoto Y et al 1995 In situ hybridization studies of prostacyclin receptor mRNA expression in various mouse organs. British Journal of Pharmacology 116: 2828–2837

Omana-Zapata I, Khabbaz MA, Hunter JC, Clarke DE, Blev KR 1997 Tetrodotoxin inhibits neuropathic ectopic activity in neuromas, dorsal root ganglia and dorsal horn neurons. Pain 7: 41–49

Papagallo M, Gaspardone A, Tomai F, Iamele M, Crea F, Cioffre 1993 Analgesic effect of bamiphylline on pain induced by intradermal injection of adenosine. Pain 53: 199–204

Perkins MN, Campbell E, Dray A 1993 Anti-nociceptive activity of the B1 and B2 receptor antagonists desArg9Leu9Bk and HOE 140, in two models of persistent hyperalgesia in the rat. Pain 53: 191–197

Perl ER 1994 A reevaluation of the mechanisms leading to sympathetically related pain. In: Fields HL, Liebeskind JC (eds) Pharmacological approaches to the treatment of chronic pain: new concepts and critical issues. IASP Press, Seattle, pp 129–150

Petersen M, Eckert AS, Segon von Banchet G, Heppelmann B, Klush A, Kniffi KD 1988 Plasticity in the expression of bradykinin binding sites in sensory neurons after mechanical nerve injury. Neuroscience 83: 949–959

Pitchford S, Levine JD 1991 Prostaglandins sensitize nociceptors in cell culture. Neuroscience Letters 132: 105–108

Rang HP, Ritchie JM 1988 Depolarization of nonmyelinated fibers of the rat vagus nerve produced by activation of protein kinase C. Journal of Neuroscience 8: 2606–2617

Reichling DB, Levine JD 1997 Heat transduction in rat sensory neurons by calcium-dependent activation of a cationic channel. Proceedings of the National Academy of Sciences USA 94: 7006–7011

Reiser G, Hamprecht B 1989 Serotonin raises the cyclic GMP level in a neuronal cell line via 5-HT3 receptors. European Journal of Pharmacology 172: 195–198

Reuter H 1996 Diversity and function of presynaptic calcium channels in the brain. Current Opinions in Neurobiology 6: 331–337

Richardson BP, Engel G, Fonatsch P, Stadler PA 1985 Identification of serotonin M-receptor subtypes and their specific blockade by a new class of drugs. Nature 316: 126–131

Roy ML, Narahashi T 1992 Differential properties of tetrodotoxin-sensitive and tetrodotoxin-resistant channels in rat dorsal root ganglion neurons. Journal of Neuroscience 12: 2104–2111

Rueff A, Dray A 1992 5-hydroxytryptamine-induced sensitization and activation of peripheral fibers in the neonatal rat are mediated via different 5-hydroxytryptamine receptors. Neuroscience 50: 899–905

Rueff A, Dray A 1993 Sensitization of peripheral afferent fibres in the in vitro rat spinal cord-tail by bradykinin and prostaglandins. Neuroscience 54: 527–535

Safranov BV, Bischoff U, Vogel W 1996 Single voltage-gated K^+ channels and their functions in small dorsal root ganglion neurones of the rat. Journal of Physiology 493: 393–408

Salvemini D, Misko TP, Masferrer JL, Seibert K, Currie MG, Needleman P 1993 Nitric oxide activates cyclooxygenase enzymes. Proceedings of the National Academy of Sciences USA 90: 7240–7244

Sangameswaran L, Delgado SG, Fish LM et al 1996 Structure and function of a novel voltage-gated tetrodotoxin-resistant sodium channel specific to sensory neurons. Journal of Biological Chemistry 271: 5953–5956

Santicioli P, Del Biamco E, Tranmontana M, Geppetti P, Maggi CA 1992 Release of calcitonin gene-related peptide-like immunoreactivity induced by electric field stimulation from rat spinal afferents is mediated by conotoxin-sensitive calcium channels. Neuroscience Letters 136: 161–164

Sawynok J 1997 Purines and nociception. In: Jacobson KA, Jarvis MF (eds) Purinergic approaches in experimental therapeutics. Wiley-Liss, New York, pp 495–513

Schaible H-G, Schmidt RF 1988 Excitation and sensitization of fine articular afferents from cat's knee joint by prostaglandin E2. Journal of Physiology 403: 91–104

Scott SA 1992 Sensory neurones diversity, development and plasticity. Oxford University Press, New York

Scroggs RS, Fox AP 1992 Calcium current variation between acutely isolated adult rat dorsal root ganglion neurons of different sizes. Journal of Physiology 445: 639–658

Scroggs RS, Todorovic SM, Andersen EG, Fox AP 1994 Variation in Ih, IIR and ILEAK between acutely isolated adult rat dorsal root ganglion neurons of different size. Journal of Neurophysiology 71: 271–279

Seabrook GR, Bowery BJ, Heavens R et al 1997 Expression of B1 and B2 bradykinin receptor mRNA and their functional roles in synpathetic ganglia and sensory dorsal root ganglia from wild-type and B2 receptor knockout mice. Neuropharmacology 36: 1009–1017

Senba E, Kashiba H 1996 Sensory afferent processing in muli-responsive DRG neurons. Progress in Brain Research 113: 387–410

Shearman MS, Sekiguchi K, Nishizuka Y 1989 Modulation of ion channel activity: a key function of the protein kinase C enzyme family. Pharmacological Review 41: 211–237

Simone DA, Alrejo M, LaMotte RH 1991 Psychophysical studies of the itch sensation and itchy skin ('allokinesis') produced by intracutaneous injection of histamine. Somatosensory and Motor Research 8: 271–279

Smith JAM, Webb C, Holford J, Burgess GM 1995 Signal transduction pathways for B1 and B2 bradykinin receptors in bovine pulmonary artery endothelial cells. Molecular Pharmacology 47: 525–534

Steel JH, Terenghi G, Chung JM, Na HS, Carlton SM, Polak JM 1994 Increased nitric oxide synthase immunoreactivity in rat dorsal root ganglia in a neuropathic pain mode. Neuroscience Letters 169: 81–84

Steen KH, Reeh PW 1993 Sustained graded pain and hyperalgesia from harmless experimental tissue acidosis in human skin. Neuroscience Letters 154: 113–116

Steen KH, Reeh PW, Anton F, Handweker HO 1992 Protons selectively induce lasting excitation and sensitization to mechanical stimuli of nociceptors in rat skin, in vivo. Journal of Neuroscience 12: 86–95

Study RE, Kral M 1996 Spontaneous action potential activity in isolated dorsal root ganglion neurons from rats with a painful neuropathy. Pain 65: 235–242

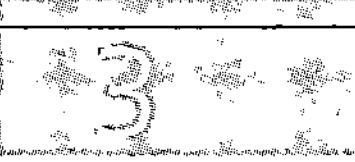

Sugimoto Y, Shigemoto R, Namba T et al 1994 Distribution of the messenger RNA for the prostaglandin E receptor subtype EP3 in the mouse nervous system. Neuroscience 62: 919–928

Sylven C 1989 Angina pectoris. Clinical characteristics, neurophysiological and molecular mechanisms. Pain 36: 145–167

Taiwo YO, Levine JD 1990 Direct cutaneous hyperalgesia induced by adenosine. Neuroscience 38: 757–762

Taiwo YO, Levine JD 1991 Further confirmation of the role of adenyl cyclase and of cAMP-dependent protein kinase in primary afferent hyperalgesia. Neuroscience 44: 131–135

Taiwo YO, Levine JD 1992 Serotonin is a directly-acting hyperalgesia agent in the rat. Neuroscience 48: 485–590

Taiwo YO, Bjerknes LK, Goetzl EJ, Levine D 1989 Mediation of primary afferent hyperalgesia by the cAMP second messenger system. Neuroscience 32: 577–580

Taiwo YO, Heller PH, Levine JD 1992 Mediation of serotonin hyperalgesia by the cAMP second messenger system. Neuroscience 48: 479–483

Tanelian DL, Brose WG 1991 Neuropathic pain can be relieved by drugs that are use-dependent sodium channel blockers: lidocaine, carbamazepine and mexilitine. Anesthesiology 74: 949–951

Tani E, Shiosaka S, Sato M, Ishikawa T, Tohyama M 1990 Histamine acts directly on calcitonin gene-related peptide- and substance P-containing trigeminal ganglion neurons as assessed by calcium influx and immunocytochemistry. Neuroscience Letters 115: 171–176

Thayer SA, Perney TM, Miller RJ 1988 Regulation of calcium homeostasis in sensory neurons by bradykinin. Journal of Neuroscience 8: 4089–4097

Tiffany CW, Burch RM 1989 Bradykinin stimulates tumor necrosis factor and interleukin 1 release from macrophages. FEBS Letters 247: 189–192

Todorovic S, Anderson EG 1990 5-HT2 and 5-HT3 receptors mediate two distinct depolarizing responses in rat dorsal root ganglion neurons. Brain Research 511: 71–79

Todorovic S, Anderson EG 1992 Serotonin preferentially hyperpolarizes capsaicin-sensitive C type sensory neurons by activating 5-HT1A receptor. Brain Research 585: 212–218

Tokunaga A, Saika M, Senba E 1998 5-HT2A receptor subtype is involved in thermal hyperalgesia mechanism of serotonin in the periphery. Pain 76: 349–355

Treede RD, Meyer RA, Raja SN, Campbell JN 1995 Evidence for two different heat transduction mechanisms in nociceptive primary afferents innervating monkey skin. Journal of Physiology 483: 747–758

Undem B, Weinrich D 1993 Electrophysiological properties and chemosensitivity of guinea pig ganglion neurons in vitro. Journal of the Autonomic Nervous System 44: 17–33

Valera S, Hussy N, Evans RJ et al 1994 Cloning and expression of the P2X receptor for extracellular ATP reveals a new class of ligand-gated ion channel. Nature 371: 516–519

Verge VMK, Xu XJ, Wiesenfeld-Hallin Z, Hokfelt T 1992 Marked increase in nitric oxide synthase mRNA in rat dorsal root ganglion after peripheral axotomy; in situ hybridization and functional studies. Proceedings of the National Academy of Sciences USA 89: 11617–11621

Vlachová V, Vyklický L 1993 Capsaicin-induced membrane currents in cultured sensory neurons of the rat. Physiological Research 42: 301–311

Waldmann R, Champigny G, Bassilana F, Heurteaux C, Lazdunski M 1997 A proton-gated channel involved in acid sensing. Nature 386: 173–177

Waxman SG, Kocsis JD, Black JA 1994 Type III sodium channel mRNA is expressed in embryonic but not adult spinal sensory neurones and is reexpressed following axotomy. Journal of Neurophysiology 72: 466–470

Weinrich D 1986 Bradykinin inhibits a slow spike after-hyperpolarization in visceral sensory neurons. European Journal of Pharmacology 132: 61–63

Weinrich D, Wonderlin WF 1987 Inhibition of calcium-dependent spike after-hyperpolarization increases excitability of rabbit visceral sensory neurones. Journal of Physiology 394: 415–427

Wiesenfeld-Hallin Z, Hao j-X, Xu X-J, Hokfelt T 1993 Nitric oxide mediates ongoing discharges in dorsal root ganglion cells after peripheral nerve injury. Journal of Neurophysiology 70: 2350–2535

Xie Y-K, Zhang J-M, Petersen M, LaMotte RH 1995 Functional changes in dorsal root ganglion cells after chronic nerve constriction in the rat. Journal of Neurophysiology 73: 1811–1820

Zhang J-M, Donnelly DF, Song X-J, LaMotte RH 1997 Axotomy increases the excitability of dorsal ganglion cells with unmyelinated axons. Journal of Neurophysiology 78: 2790–2794

Trophic factors and pain

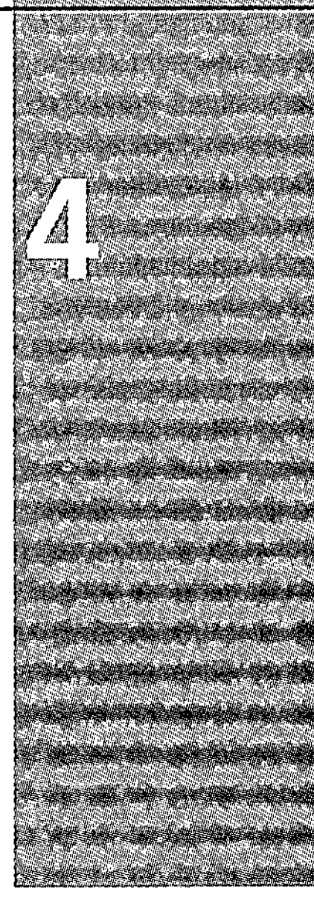

STEPHEN B. MCMAHON & DAVID L. H. BENNETT

INTRODUCTION

In 1996 a study was published on the genetic basis of the congenital insensitivity to pain observed in a single family (Indo et al 1996). A mutation was identified in the gene encoding a tyrosine kinase receptor known as trkA. This protein is known to be the high-affinity receptor for a single trophic factor, nerve growth factor (NGF, see below), and the mutation disrupts the normal signalling of NGF. This single example provides a startling example of the potential importance of trophic factors in general and NGF in particular for normal nociceptive functioning. We now have a good (if incomplete) understanding of the mechanisms by which NGF interacts with pain signalling systems, and this is reviewed in this chapter. It has also become apparent that NGF is only one of several growth factors that affect these systems. In general, different factors have distinct rather than common actions.

Neurotrophic factors can be defined as factors which regulate the long-term survival, growth or differentiated function of discrete populations of nerve cells. This definition is less than ideal because a very wide variety of agents could in the extreme fall within it. However, in the context of the adult nervous system, it is preferable to the more narrow definition often used by developmental biologists, which emphasizes the survival-promoting effects of agents. The reason is that several factors which are essential for the survival of particular neuronal subpopulations in the developing animal (such as NGF itself) are no longer essential in the adult animal, although they continue to exert profound effects on the phenotype of the same cells (see below).

Cell biologists, particularly those interested in development, have long recognized the importance and potency of neurotrophic factors. Indeed, much of our current understanding of the range and mode of action of these factors, and their identity, has emerged from these studies. One fact to emerge is that there are many neurotrophic factors. It is also apparent that multiple factors can affect a single population of neurons. For instance, a recent review (Oppenheim 1996) described more than 20 factors capable of regulating the survival of one cell type, spinal motoneurons. Nonetheless, there is an emerging order in this complexity. It transpires that many trophic factors fall into a smaller number of families, in which members are related by high levels of structural homology or by the common or related receptors they use in exerting biological actions. The number of factors identified as affecting sensory processing is much more limited. Most of the data is related to just two families of factors, the neurotrophin family and the GDNF-related family (GDNF – glial cell line-derived neurotrophic factor). It is clear that these will not be the only significant factors, but our knowledge of others is currently much more limited. This review will consider primarily the members of these two families. For each factor, a brief overview of signalling systems that are utilized and the developmental role of the factor, and a fuller account of the biological effects and functional roles in pain signalling in the adult, will be provided. The former issues are considered in greater detail in a number of recent reviews, and the developmental role of factors is also considered elsewhere in this volume (see Ch. 9).

Sensory neuron heterogeneity

Sensory neurons can be divided into a number of broad subgroups based on their anatomical, histochemical and physiological properties (Lawson 1992). One theme that has arisen from work on trophic factors and sensory neurons, both during development and in the adult animal, is that particular subpopulations of sensory neurons have a selective sensitivity to certain trophic factors. There is a 'large light' population (30% of dorsal root ganglion, DRG cells) which can be identified using anti-neurofilament antibodies (Lawson et al 1984). These have myelinated axons and a large cell diameter. These DRG cells respond principally to low-threshold stimuli and include large muscle afferents which terminate in the ventral horn of the spinal cord and cutaneous afferents which terminate in laminae I,III–VI of the dorsal horn. The classical 'small dark' population of DRG cells which have a small cell diameter, unmyelinated axons and which are nociceptors or thermoceptors can be subdivided into two roughly equal groups. One subgroup (40% of total DRG cells) constitutively synthesize neuropeptides and a good marker for these cells is calcitonin gene-related peptide (CGRP). These cells have terminations principally in laminae I and IIo of the dorsal horn. The other subgroup (30% of DRG cells) are non-peptidergic, they possess cell surface glycoconjugates which can be identified by binding of the lectin IB4 (Silverman & Kruger 1988) and express the enzyme activities fluoride-resistant acid phosphatase (FRAP) and thiamine monophosphatase (TMP). These neurons terminate principally in lamina IIi of the dorsal horn.

THE NEUROTROPHIN FAMILY (NGF, BDNF, NT3 AND NT4/5)

The prototypical neurotrophic factor is NGF, first purified from mouse submandibular gland by Levi-Montalcini, Booker and Cohen (for review see Levi-Montalcini 1987). Other members of the family include: brain-derived neurotrophic factor (BDNF), neurotrophin-3 (NT3), neurotrophin-4/5 (NT4/5) and neurotrophin-6 (NT6) which is only present in teleost fish (Lindsay 1996, Gotz et al 1994). The neurotrophins are expressed as preproprecursors which when processed yield highly basic mature proteins of around 13 kDa (120 amino acids). There is around 50% amino acid homology between family members and at physiological concentrations the neurotrophins exist as homodimers. Gene deletion studies have demonstrated widespread and important functions of the neurotrophins in the development of the nervous system (Snider 1994) and it is now clear that they also exert important actions in the adult animal.

NEUROTROPHIN RECEPTORS

Binding studies have demonstrated the presence of high- and low-affinity binding sites for NGF on responsive cell lines (Bothwell 1995). Two different classes of neurotrophin receptor have now been characterized (for reviews see Barbacid 1995, Chao & Hempstead 1995). The first to be cloned was the p75 or low-affinity nerve growth factor receptor, LNGFR, which binds all the neurotrophins equally with relatively low affinity (Chao et al 1986). Additionally there is a family of high-affinity receptors, trks, which are tyrosine kinase receptors (Kaplan et al 1991).

The p75 receptor contains a single transmembrane segment flanked by extracellular and intracellular domains. The exact role of the p75 receptor, and the question as to whether the trk receptors can form high-affinity binding sites in the absence of p75, are points of contention. The p75 receptor may well interact with the trk receptors and modulate the specificity and sensitivity of their interaction with the neurotrophins.

There are three known members of the trk family of receptors, termed trkA, trkB and trkC, which show different specificities for the neurotrophins. NGF is the preferred ligand for trkA, BDNF and NT4/5 the preferred ligands for trkB, and NT3 the preferred ligand for trkC (Ip et al 1993). NT3 has a reputation as being more 'promiscuous' than the other neurotrophins as *in vitro* it can activate all of the trk receptors (albeit with different potencies), although whether this is significant *in vivo* is still unclear. A schematic illustration of the neurotrophin interactions of the trk receptors is shown in Figure 4.1.

Most of the information about signal transduction following trk activation comes from studying events following activation of trk by NGF in PC12 cells. Following NGF binding, receptor dimerization occurs. This appears critical for receptor activation (Clary et al 1994). The tyrosine-kinase domain of the receptor is activated and a number of substrates are phosphorylated and autophosphorylation of the receptor also occurs. Proteins which contain an SH2 domain are recruited to the phosphorylated residues on the receptor (Schlessinger 1994). After this interaction has occurred, a wide number of intracellular pathways become activated (Marshall 1995). More information is now available about events that occur following NGF binding to p75. It has recently been demonstrated in cultured Schwann cells that NGF could induce activation of the transcription factor NFκB and this was dependent on the presence of the p75 receptor (Carter et al 1996).

 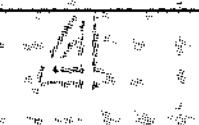

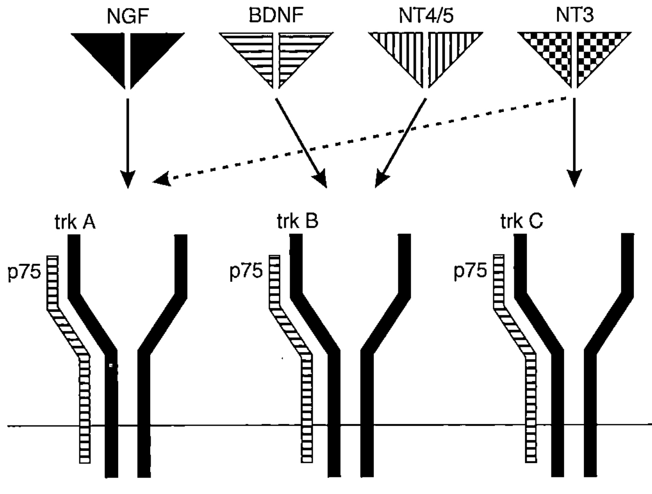

Fig. 4.1 A schematic illustration of the neurotrophin interactions of the trk receptors. NGF is the preferred ligand for trkA, NT4/5 and BDNF are the preferred ligands at the trkB receptor and NT3 is the preferred ligand at the trkC receptor, although it will bind to all the trk receptors albeit with different potencies. All the neurotrophins bind the p75 receptor with equal affinity.

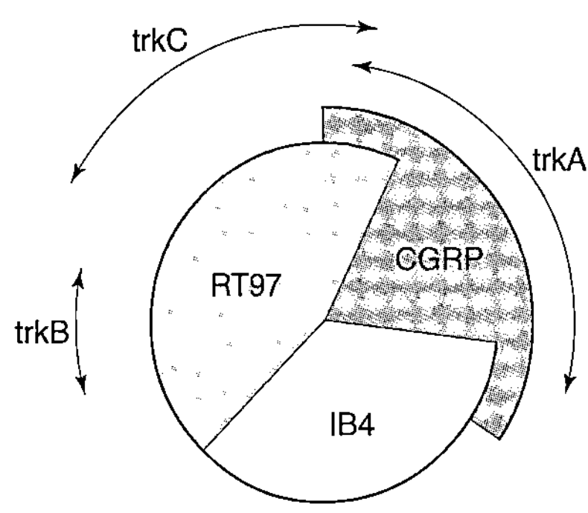

Fig. 4.2 Pie chart relating the distribution of neurotrophin receptors to neurochemically defined DRG subclasses. trkA is expressed principally in the 'small dark' population of DRG cells which contain neuropeptides, the best marker for which is CGRP. trkC is expressed principally in the 'large light' population of DRG cells which can be identified with the neurofilament antibody RT97. trkB expression cannot be related simply to any one class of DRG cells. Note the population of non-peptidergic IB4-binding DRG cells appear to represent a class of DRG cells which do not express trk receptors of any type and hence may not respond to neurotrophins under normal circumstances. See text for further details.

NEUROTROPHIN RECEPTOR EXPRESSION WITHIN ADULT SENSORY NEURONS

There is now a large body of evidence demonstrating that neurotrophin receptors are expressed in specific populations of DRG cells. Using double labelling techniques it has been possible to relate receptor expression to different functional classes of DRG cells (Fig. 4.2). Multiple approaches have demonstrated that approximately 40% of DRG cells express the NGF receptor trkA (Table 4.1; Verge et al 1989, 1992, McMahon et al 1994, Averill et al 1995, Kashiba et al 1995, Molliver et al 1995, Wetmore & Olson 1995), and those cells which express trkA are principally of small cell diameter. TrkA is principally expressed in the peptidergic population of small-diameter DRG cells, whilst very few non-peptidergic (IB4 binding) small-diameter DRG cells express trkA (Averill et al 1995, Molliver et al 1995). A few of the myelinated DRG cells (i.e. those which express RT 97) do express trkA (around 20%). TrkA immunoreactive terminals within the spinal cord are present within lamina I and IIo. TrkA is therefore expressed in small-diameter DRG cells which express CGRP and project to the superficial laminae of the spinal cord. These are all characteristic of nociceptive afferents.

Accounts of the proportion of adult lumbar DRG cells which express full-length trkB vary from 5 to 27% (Table 4.1). TrkB is present within DRG cells of both small and large cell diameter (McMahon et al 1994) and there does not appear to be any simple relationship between trkB expression and the different histochemical or functional subgroups of DRG cells.

Around 20% of DRG cells express trkC (see Table 4.1 for references) and it is clear that in contrast to trkA, trkC is

Table 4.1 The percentage of adult DRG cells expressing trkA, B, C, p75 or no known trk as shown by studies using in situ hybridization (in situ), binding of iodinated NGF to sections (binding) or immunocytochemistry (immuno) in lumbar (L) or thoracic (T) dorsal root ganglia

	McMahon et al (1994) In-situ L	*Wetmore & Olson. (1995) In-situ L*	*Kashiba et al (1995) in-situ L*	*Verge et al (1989, 1992) Binding L*	*Averill et al (1995) Immuno L*	*Molliver et al (1995) Immuno T*
TrkA	44	45	40	40–50	40	47
TrkB	27	26	5	—	—	—
TrkC	17	21	20	—	—	—
no trk	34	—	—	—	—	—
p75	—	74	45	—	—	—

expressed almost exclusively in large-diameter afferents. This is consistent with observations that proprioceptive afferents whose development is critically dependent on NT3 have myelinated axons and a large cell diameter.

Except for a few trkC-expressing cells, all DRG cells expressing a trk also express the p75 receptor, and p75 is never expressed independently of a trk receptor (Wright & Snider 1995). In general, trk expression defines distinct populations of DRG cells and most DRG cells would be expected to respond to only one neurotrophin.

Interestingly there is a population of adult DRG cells that do not express any known trk. Estimates of the size of this population vary from 26 to 34% of DRG cells (McMahon et al 1994, Wright & Snider 1995). Studies using in situ hybridization combined with immunocytochemistry have demonstrated that this population comprises principally IB4-binding DRG cells (G.J. Michael and J.V. Priestley, unpublished observations). It has, in fact, become recently apparent that it is this population of DRG cells which are GDNF sensitive.

NERVE GROWTH FACTOR

DEVELOPMENTAL ROLE

Early studies on the role of NGF in the sympathetic and sensory nervous system gave rise to the neurotrophic concept. The tissue to be innervated by a particular group of neurons produces a limiting amount of a trophic factor, which, at a critical stage during target innervation, binds to receptors on the innervating neurons and is internalized and retrogradely transported by these neurons. The essence of the hypothesis is that the retrograde transport of neurotrophin is critical for the survival and differentiated function of the responsive neurons. Hence, a selection process would ensure an appropriate innervation density and the elimination of inaccurate projections. Studies of transgenic animals with null mutations of the neurotrophin genes or their receptors have provided perhaps the most compelling evidence for the neurotrophic hypothesis as applied to neurons of the peripheral sensory nervous system. It appears that functionally distinct groups of sensory neurons depend on different neurotrophins for survival during development.

Animals with a gene deletion of either NGF or trkA are born with DRG lacking virtually all small-diameter primary sensory neurons, including the peptidergic neurons expressing CGRP and substance P, which have been associated with nociceptive function (Crowley et al 1994). Primary afferent projections to laminae I and II of the dorsal horn, the primary site of nociceptive processing, are lost, although projections to deep dorsal horn are spared (Smeyne et al 1994). These animals are, as expected, profoundly hypoalgesic. *In utero* deprivation of NGF, achieved by antibody treatment, produces similar effects (Johnson et al 1980, Ruit et al 1992). The effects of deletion of the low-affinity receptor $p75^{NTR}$ are more subtle: they include decreased cutaneous innervation by peptidergic sensory neurons, decreased noxious thermal and mechanical sensitivity, and a loss of all major subclasses of DRG cells (Lee et al 1992, Bergman et al 1996). Consistent with a role in modulating trkA function, sensory neurons from these $p75^{NTR}$ mutants display a decreased sensitivity to NGF at the peak of naturally occurring cell death (Davies et al 1993).

The role of NGF during development is not limited to its survival-promoting effects during embryogenesis. During the postnatal period NGF is important in the phenotypic specification of sensory neurons, for instance the Aδ high-threshold mechanoreceptor fails to develop if animals are deprived of NGF during a critical postnatal period (Ritter et al, 1991). Changes in NGF sensitivity also occur postnatally. In NGF knock-out animals, the non-peptidergic IB4 binding population of DRG cells fail to develop (Silos-Santiago et al 1995). IB4 DRG cells are therefore sensitive to NGF during embryogenesis and yet, as described above, these neurons fail to express trkA receptors in the adult. In fact, the IB4 binding population downregulate their expression of trkA during the postnatal period (Bennett et al 1996c, Molliver & Snider 1997) and it appears that at the same time they become sensitive to another trophic factor, GDNF (Molliver et al 1997, Bennett et al 1998b).

BIOLOGICAL ACTIONS

Actions on cultured sensory neurons

The developmental dependence of nociceptors on NGF for survival is lost in the postnatal period, some time before the second week of life in the rat. However, NGF continues to exert profound effects on adult nociceptors. Adult DRG neurons can be cultured in the absence of added trophic factors (Lindsay 1988). If NGF is then added to these cultures, it promotes extensive neurite outgrowth of trkA-expressing cells. NGF in these cultures also regulates the expression of the neuropeptides substance P and CGRP (Lindsay & Harmar 1989). In addition, NGF regulates the chemical sensitivity of cultured sensory neurons. The sensitivity of cultured sensory neurons to the potent algogen capsaicin is increased by NGF, as is their sensitivity to protons and to GABA (Winter et al 1988, Bevan & Winter

1995). Recently the expression of bradykinin binding sites in cultured sensory neurons has also been shown to be regulated by NGF (Petersen et al 1998). This is dependent on the presence of the p75 receptor, as antibodies to p75 prevent the upregulation of bradykinin binding sites in the presence of NGF. This marked regulation of the chemosensitivity of cultured sensory neurons by NGF is interesting in relation to the association between NGF and inflammatory pain which will be discussed later.

More recently, the effects of NGF have been studied *in vivo*. The effects of NGF extend from the peripheral to central terminals of sensory neurons, and many are mediated via altered gene expression in neurons expressing trkA (these effects are summarized in Fig. 4.3).

Actions at peripheral terminals

The administration of small doses of NGF to adult animals and man can produce pain and hyperalgesia. In rodents, a thermal hyperalgesia is present within 30 min of systemic NGF administration and both a thermal and a mechanical hyperalgesia after a couple of hours (Lewin et al 1993). Subcutaneous injections of NGF also produce both thermal and mechanical hyperalgesia at the injection site. In

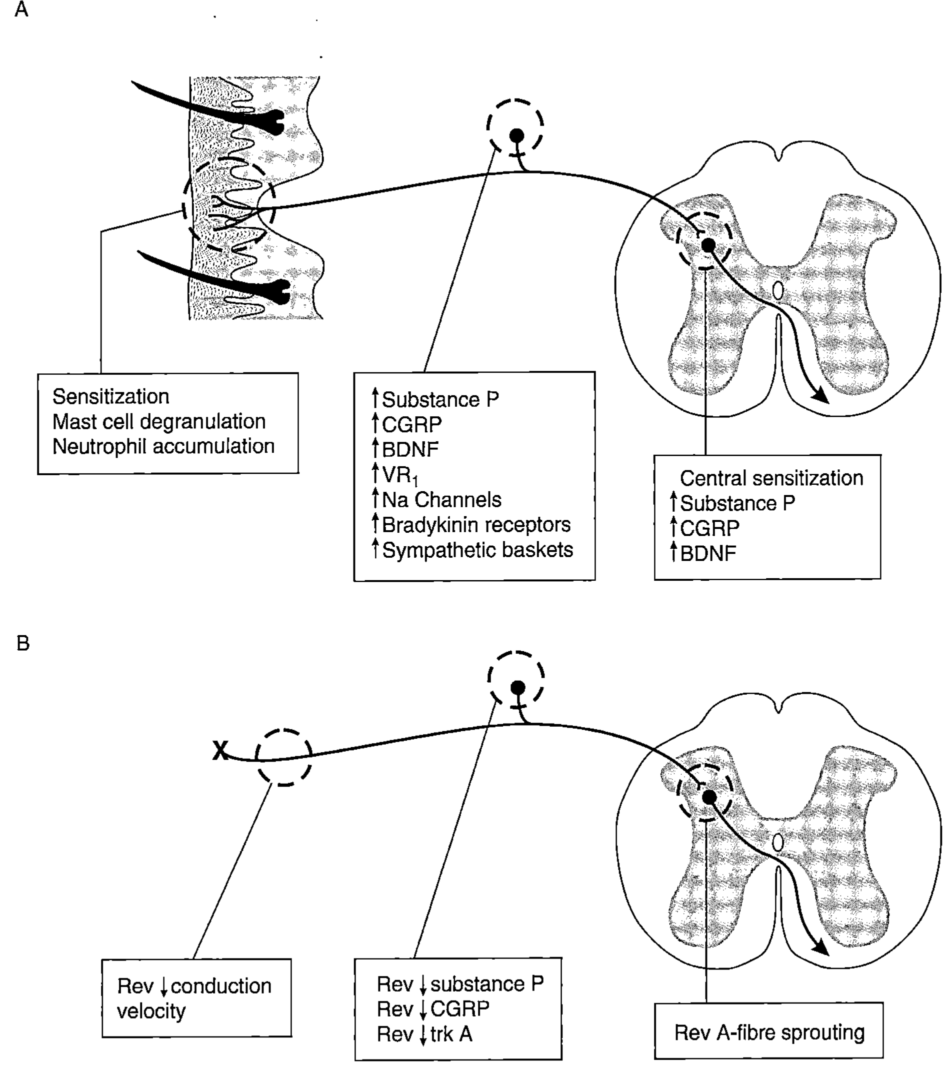

Fig. 4.3 Summary of the biological effects of exogenous NGF on pain-signalling systems, in both normal animals (**A**) and animals with nerve injury (**B**). In the normal animal, NGF causes a peripheral sensitization of some nociceptors, much of it is apparently an indirect effect. It also regulates the expression of many genes in trkA-expressing neurons, ranging from transmitters/modulators, ion channels and receptors. In the spinal cord, NGF produces central sensitization, via altered expression of putative neuromodulators, particularly BDNF. After nerve injury, NGF can reverse many of the changes normally seen in damaged neurons. See text for fuller description.

humans, intravenous injections of very low doses of NGF produce widespread aching pains in deep tissues and hyperalgesia at the injection site (Petty et al 1994). The rapid onset of some of these effects, and their localization to the injection site, strongly suggests that they arise at least in part from a local effect on the peripheral terminals of nociceptors. This has been substantiated by the observation that acute administration of NGF can sensitize nociceptive afferents to thermal and chemical stimuli (Rueff et al, 1996). Interestingly, it does not induce spontaneous activity in cutaneous nociceptors. NGF may achieve this sensitization by a direct action on primary afferent nociceptors: many nociceptive afferents express trkA receptors and receptor activation will lead to tyrosine phosphorylation of intracellular targets such as ion channels. It has been shown that neurotrophins can have rapid actions on synaptic action and neuronal excitability (Thoenen 1995).

Because cellular elements other than nociceptors in peripheral tissues express trkA, the sensitization of nociceptors by NGF may arise indirectly. Mast cells contain a number of inflammatory mediators known to excite primary afferents, including histamine and serotonin (Leon et al 1994). Some types of mast cells express trkA receptors (Horigome et al 1994). NGF can produce mast cell degranulation (Mazurek et al 1986, Horigome et al 1994) and increase the proliferation of mast cells resident in tissue. In peritoneal mast cell cultures, NGF induces the expression of a number of cytokines in mast cells, namely IL-3 (interleukin 3), IL-4, IL-10, TNFα (tumour necrosis factorα) and GM-CSF (granulocyte) macrophage colony-stimulating factor) (Bullock & Johnson 1996). Mast cell degranulators and serotonin antagonists have both been demonstrated to partially prevent the thermal but not the mechanical hyperalgesia (Lewin et al 1994, Woolf et al 1996) that occurs in response to NGF. Mast cell degranulators can significantly reduce hyperalgesia (both thermal and mechanical) and the upregulation of NGF expression induced by complete Freund's adjuvant (Woolf et al 1996).

In skin, NGF may also affect keratinocytes, some of which express p75 receptors. NGF increases the proliferation of keratinocytes in culture (Paus et al 1994, Fantini et al 1995). This effect may contribute to tissue remodelling after inflammation. In addition, NGF may also target eosinophils, converting circulating eosinophils into tissue-type eosinophils (Hamada et al 1996), and has been reported to increase B- and T-cell proliferation (Otten et al 1989), suggesting a role of NGF as an immunoregulatory factor.

There may be an interaction between NGF and sympathetic neurons during inflammation. Sympathetic efferents also possess the trkA receptor (Smeyne et al 1994). Surgical or chemical sympathectomy can reduce the short latency thermal and mechanical hyperalgesia evoked by NGF (Andreev et al 1995, Woolf et al 1996). The production of eicosanoids by sympathetic efferents within the skin has been suggested to contribute to hyperalgesia under some inflammatory conditions (Levine et al 1986). A role for eicosanoids is not supported by the observation that NGF-induced hyperalgesia is unaffected by the non-steroidal anti inflammatory drug indomethacin (which inhibits cyclooxygenase) (Amann et al 1996b).

It has also recently been shown that NGF may produce peripheral sensitization via activation of the 5-lipoxgenase pathway (Amann et al 1996a, Bennett et al 1998e). The enzyme 5-lipoxygenase converts arachidonic acid into leukotrienes. Leukotriene B_4 (LTB_4) has been demonstrated to sensitize nociceptive afferents to thermal and mechanical stimuli (Martin et al 1988). NGF can stimulate the production of LTB_4 in skin and inhibitors of the 5-lipoxygenase enzyme prevent the development of thermal hyperalgesia following intraplantar NGF injection (Amann et al 1996a). The leukotrienes are powerful chemotactic factors for neutrophils and indeed the hyperalgesia induced by LTB_4 has been shown to be leucocyte dependent (Levine et al 1984). Intraplantar injection of NGF results in local neutrophil accumulation within 3 h of injection and this accumulation is lipoxygenase dependent. Animals in which neutrophils have been depleted do not show a thermal hyperalgesia in response to NGF, indicating that neutrophil accumulation may be critical for the sensitizing actions of NGF (Bennett et al 1998e). The hyperalgesia evoked by LTB_4 is not prevented by indomethacin, whereas inhibition of lipoxygenase is effective in preventing the sensitizing effects of NGF. This pharmacology may prove useful in the future for the development of novel drugs for the treatment of inflammatory pain or as a means of preventing the unwanted hyperalgesia that accompanies the therapeutic use of NGF (Apfel et al 1996a).

It should be pointed out that not all of the algogenic and hyperalgesic effects of NGF can be readily explained by peripheral processes. As we discuss below, it is likely that many aspects of NGF actions are centrally mediated, via altered gene expression in nociceptors.

The effects of NGF on gene expression and the phenotypic properties of sensory neurons

There appear to be a group of peptides which are constitutively expressed in trkA cells and whose expression is controlled mainly by NGF, increasing following NGF supplementation and decreasing following NGF depletion (resulting from peripheral axotomy). CGRP and substance P belong to this group (Goedert et al 1981, Otten et al 1984, Verge et al 1995). Based on NGF's ability to reverse some axotomy-induced peptide increases (see below), it would appear that there is also a group of peptides whose production is partly inhibited by neurotrophins: vasoactive intestinal peptide (VIP), cholecystokinin (CCK), neuropeptide Y (NPY) and galanin belong to this group. Direct inhibition has not yet been demonstrated in intact neurons *in vivo*: it is possible that *in vivo* other factors may act as positive regulators (e.g. exogenous LIF increases galanin expression; Thompson et al 1998b). In addition to an effect on substance P and CGRP, NGF has recently been shown to produce a dramatic upregulation of BDNF mRNA and protein in trkA-expressing DRG cells (Apfel et al 1996b, Michael et al 1997). There is now growing evidence that BDNF may serve as a central regulator of excitability, as discussed below.

NGF also regulates the expression of some of the receptors expressed by nociceptors. Capsaicin sensitivity is increased *in vivo* by NGF. The recent cloning of the capsaicin receptor, VR1, has allowed the expression of receptor mRNA and protein to be directly studied. NGF-sensitive nociceptors (i.e. those expressing trkA) have the highest levels of VR1 (Tominaga et al 1998). Because the VR1 receptor is sensitive to heat and, at body temperature apparently also to protons, this regulation by NGF is likely to have profound consequences for the responsiveness of nociceptors to noxious stimuli. Finally, there are several suggestions that ion channel expression, notably several kinds of sodium channel, might be regulated by NGF (Black & Waxman 1996). However, the degree of regulation is less clear (Okuse et al 1997).

Actions on spinal processing of nociceptive information: central sensitization

NGF given systemically fails to penetrate into the spinal cord. There is also little trkA expression in the spinal cord, with the receptor largely restricted to the terminals of primary afferent nociceptors (Averill et al 1995). One might therefore imagine that exogenously administered NGF would have little effect on spinal nociceptive processes. However, several of the biological effects of NGF described above are capable of leading to secondary effects on the spinal cord. Firstly, the activation and sensitization of primary afferent nociceptors may lead to sufficient afferent activity to trigger central changes. Peripheral NGF administration to some visceral structures results in a somatotopically appropriate induction of c-*fos* in the dorsal horn (Dmitrieva et al 1996). Secondly, the altered chemistry of afferent neurons produced by NGF (see above) may lead to increased neurotransmitter/neuromodulator release from nociceptive afferent terminals (Malcangio et al 1997). The release of some sensory neuropeptides are well-recognized triggers for the induction of central sensitization (McMahon et al 1993). One might therefore expect that peripheral NGF treatment could lead to the induction of central sensitization. It has been shown that several hours after systemic NGF treatment, C-fibre stimulation produced greater than normal amounts of central sensitization, seen as wind-up of ventral root reflexes (Thompson et al 1995). A fibres also develop the novel ability to produce wind-up. Such changes in the central processing of nociceptive information may occur during inflammation secondary to SP expression within A fibres (Neumann et al 1996). As we discuss in some detail below, there is now evidence accumulating that the ability of NGF to upregulate BDNF expression in some nociceptors may prove to be the most significant mechanism by which NGF regulates the sensitivity of spinal processing of noxious stimuli.

Neuroprotective effects

Following nerve injury, sensory neurons become disconnected from their targets and hence the normal retrograde supply of trophic factor is interrupted. After nerve injury the retrograde transport of NGF to sensory neurons is reduced (Heuman et al 1987, Raivich et al 1991). There is a compensatory response which occurs in the distal nerve stump whereby non-neuronal cells express NGF mRNA. There are two phases of increased NGF expression, one rapid (over 1 day) and one long (over a week). The second peak of expression is mediated by the invasion of macrophages and the release of IL-1(Heumann et al 1987), although the magnitude of this effect is inadequate to compensate for lost target-derived NGF. Given this reduced transport, one might expect that the provision of exogenous NGF would have a neuroprotective role on these neurons and this is indeed the case.

Nerve injury results in marked phenotypic changes within sensory neurons, ranging from changes in their neurochemistry to their functional properties. After axotomy, cell death has been reported to occur in around 30% of DRG cells (Arvidsson et al 1986, Rich et al 1987). There has recently been some re-assessment of the degree and timing of cell death following axotomy (Coggeshall et al 1997). However, local administration of exogenous NGF to the site of axotomy is reported to prevent the cell death of primary sensory neurons which normally occurs (Rich et al 1987).

There are marked changes in gene expression within sensory neurons following nerve injury. Expression of the immediate early gene c-*jun* increases in sensory neurons after axotomy – this may be upstream to a number of the other changes in gene expression that occur in sensory neurons (Mulderry & Dobson 1996), for instance the increased expression of VIP (discussed more fully below). The increased expression of c-*jun* after axotomy can be prevented in small-diameter sensory neurons by treatment with NGF (Gold et al 1993). There are also marked changes in neuropeptide expression in injured DRG cells (Hokfelt et al 1994), which may have an important impact on the spinal processing of sensory information in the dorsal horn. There is a reduction in the levels of one group of peptides including Substance P and CGRP, and increased expression in another group, including VIP and galanin. The administration of exogenous NGF can prevent the reduction in Substance P and CGRP expression that occurs in primary afferents following axotomy (Fitzgerald et al 1985, Wong & Oblinger 1991, Verge et al 1995) and can also partially prevent the upregulation of galanin and VIP (Verge et al 1995). After axotomy there is an increase in GAP-43 expression in DRG cells (Woolf et al 1990). GAP-43 is a phosphoprotein thought to be important in the development and plasticity of the nervous system. The role of NGF in regulating GAP-43 expression is unclear (Hu-Tsai et al 1994), (Mohiuddin et al 1995). Following nerve injury there is a reduction in neurofilament expression, axon diameter and conduction velocity. NGF can partially reverse all of these changes particularly in small-diameter DRG cells (Verge et al 1990, Gold et al 1991, Bennett et al 1998b).

The majority of experimental studies have used axotomy as the model of nerve injury. The most common clinical neuropathy is that associated with diabetes, which is typically seen as a distal polyneuropathy, occurring as a consequence of 'dying back' of nerve terminals. A decrement of thermosensation and nociception highlights the involvement of small-diameter DRG cells in this neuropathy. NGF has been demonstrated to reverse a number of the changes of diabetic neuropathy in animals (McMahon & Priestley 1995) and clinical trials are in progress in humans. Such trials indicate that NGF can indeed improve small-fibre function in people (Apfel et al 1996a).

In summary, administration of exogenous NGF can reverse many of the changes associated with nerve injury within small-diameter DRG cells.

FUNCTIONAL ROLE

The dramatic effects of exogenously administered NGF on pain signalling systems does not reveal the role of endogenous NGF. In order to ascertain if any of the 'pharmacological' effects of NGF truly reflect those of endogenous NGF, one must perform experiments in which the biological actions of endogenous NGF are somehow blocked. This has been achieved by two major experimental approaches: targeted recombination in embryonic stem cells to selectively 'knock out' either NGF or its receptor trkA, and the administration of proteins which inhibit the bioactivity of NGF. Each of these techniques has advantages and disadvantages, but studies using them largely confirm an important role for endogenous NGF in regulating pain sensitivity. The knock-out approach has provided information particularly regarding the developmental role of NGF and has confirmed that essentially all spinal nociceptive afferents require this factor for survival in the perinatal period, as discussed above.

Because mice with NGF or trkA deletions rarely survive past the first postnatal week, most of what we know about endogenous NGF function in the adult has been determined by the use of blocking agents. There are a number of studies using autoimmune models of NGF deprivation or infusions of NGF antisera to study the effects of NGF in normal adult animals. These studies are difficult to perform and interpret, as this approach leads to a different dose of NGF antisera being present in each animal. The infusion of exogenous antiserum to NGF also frequently leads to a large immune response in the host animals. Some of these difficulties can be avoided by the use of a chimeric protein consisting of the extracellular domain of trkA fused to the Fc tail of human immunoglobulin (trkA-IgG). This molecule binds to NGF and blocks its activity, but is incapable of binding to NGF when the NGF is bound to either trkA or p75 receptors. In addition, the Fc used does not fix complement. These two properties allow the unambiguous interpretation of data obtained *in vivo*. Local infusion of trkA-IgG into the rat hindpaw leads to thermal hypoalgesia and a decrease in CGRP content in those DRG neurons projecting to the infused area (McMahon et al 1995). These changes take several days to develop. In addition, there is a decrease in the thermal and chemical sensitivity of nociceptors projecting to the area and a decrease in the epidermal innervation density (Bennett et al 1998c). These results provide strong evidence that NGF continues to play an important role in regulating the function of the small, peptidergic sensory neurons in the adult.

NGF acts as an inflammatory mediator

By far the most extensively studied area of endogenous NGF function in the adult is in relatively acute models of inflammatory pain (lasting up to several days). NGF is found in many cell types in tissues subject to inflammatory insult, and much evidence now supports the hypothesis that upregulation of NGF levels is a common component of the inflammatory response that relates to hyperalgesia (see above). Elevated NGF levels have been found in a variety of inflammatory states in humans including in the bladder of patients with cystitis (Lowe et al 1997) and increased levels in synovial fluid from patients with arthritis (Aloe et al 1992). In animal studies, NGF is found in the exudate produced during blistering of the skin (Weskamp & Otten 1987) and is elevated in skin after inflammation induced by complete Freund's adjuvant (Donnerer et al 1992, Woolf et al 1994), IL-1 (Safieh-Garabedian et al 1995), ultraviolet light (Gillardon et al 1995) or TNFα (Woolf et al 1997).

Given the increased NGF levels during inflammation and the marked sensitizing actions of this factor on nociceptive systems, it appears logical to ask whether it acts as a key inflammatory mediator. While there are some slight discrepancies in the details, there is now widespread agreement that blocking NGF bioactivity (either systemically or locally) largely blocks the effects of inflammation on sensory nerve function (Table 4.2). For instance, intraplantar injection of carrageenan produces an acute inflammatory reaction, which has previously been widely used in the study of the analgesic effects of non-steroidal inflammatory drugs (NSAIDs). When the trkA-IgG molecule was coadministered with carrageenan, it could almost completely prevent the development of the thermal hyperalgesia that normally develops (McMahon et al 1995) (Fig. 4.4). The properties of nociceptive afferents innervating carrageenan-inflamed skin were also studied. Following carrageenan inflammation there was a marked increase in spontaneous activity in these afferents and an increased thermal and chemical sensitivity

Table 4.2 Experimental manipulations (mostly experimental inflammation) in which anti-NGF strategies have been reported to modify (reduce or prevent) the listed biological effects. (Reproduced from Bennett et al 1999)

Inflammatory agent	*Site*	*Effect*	*Reference*
Freund's	Hindpaw	Neuropeptide upregulation	Donnerer et al 1992
Freund's	Hindpaw	Behavioural hyperalgesia	Lewin et al 1994
Freund's	Hindpaw	Neuropeptide upregulation	Woolf et al 1994
Freund's	Hindpaw	Behavioural hyperalgesia	Woolf et al 1994
Carrageenan	Hindpaw	Behavioural hyperalgesia	McMahon et al 1995
Turpentine	Urinary bladder	Hyperreflexia	Dmitrieva et al 1997
Turpentine	Urinary bladder	*c-fos* induction in dorsal horn	Dmitrieva et al 1996
Freund's	Hindpaw	Oct-2 transcription factor induction	Kendall et al 1995
Freund's	Hindpaw	GAP-43 induction	Leslie et al 1995
Freund's	Hindpaw	Neuropeptide induction	Leslie et al 1995
Carrageenan	Forelimb skeletal muscle	grip strength	Kehl et al 1998
Incision	Hindpaw	Behavioural hyperalgesia	Brennan et al 1998
Carrageenan	Hindpaw	Primary afferent sensitisation	Bennett et al 1996b
Freund's	Hindpaw	Progressive tactile hyperalgesia	Ma & Woolf 1997
Freund's	Hindpaw	Neuropeptide upregulation	Safieh-Garabedian et al 1995
IL-1β	Hindpaw	Behavioural hyperalgesia	Safieh-Garabedian et al 1995
TNF-α	Hindpaw	Behavioural hyperalgesia	Woolf et al 1997

(Fig. 4.4). This probably represents the multiple peripheral actions of NGF described earlier. Administration of the trkA-IgG molecule could largely prevent these changes (Bennett et al 1996b). Similar results have now been found in a number of different inflammatory models (Table 4.2).

Increased NGF levels observed after inflammatory stimuli result from increased synthesis and release of NGF from cells in the affected tissue. Studies in cell culture suggest that a large number of stimuli can alter NGF production. Many growth factors and cytokines can increase NGF secretion and NGF mRNA levels, including: IL-1, IL-4, IL-5, TNFα, transforming growth factor β (TGFβ), platelet-derived growth factor (PDGF), acidic and basic fibroblast growth factors (FGF-1, FGF-2) and epidermal growth factor (EGF), particularly potent agents being IL-1 and PDGF (see Bennett et al 1998d for discussion). Adrenergic receptor agonists and reactive oxygen species also enhance NGF gene expression or secretion in cell lines, and these processes may be important in inflammation. Some agents consistently decrease NGF mRNA levels or secretion, these include glucocorticoids and the interferons. The effects of various agents differ according to the cell types studied. These differences are most likely to be due to the complement of receptors expressed by various cell types. IL-1β and TNFα have been shown to mediate changes in NGF expression during inflammation *in vivo* and the hyperalgesia produced by these cytokines can be prevented by NGF antagonism (Table 4.2).

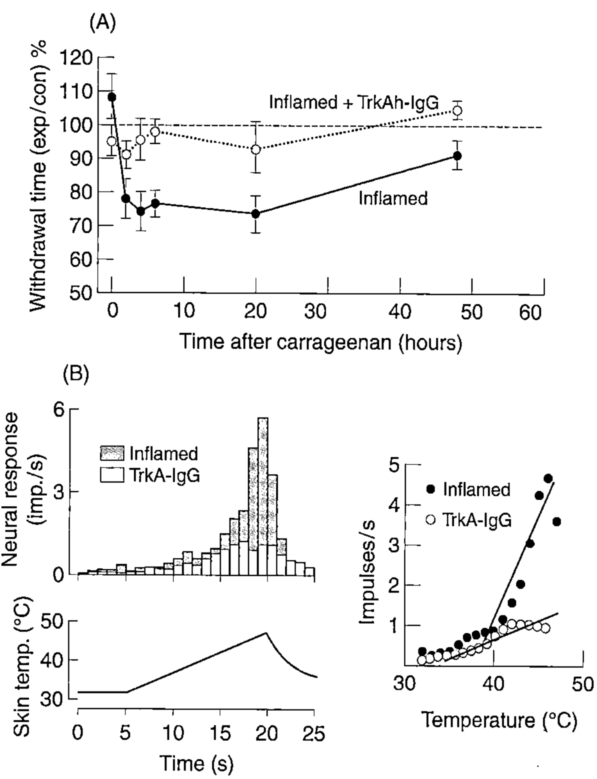

Fig. 4.4 The role of NGF in inflammation revealed by the use of the NGF-sequestering protein trkA-IgG. **A** The thermal hyperalgesia that develops in rats in the hours following intraplantar carrageenan. The ordinate plots the ratio of the withdrawal times to radiant noxious heat applied to the inflamed and the un-inflamed contralateral paw. Animals inflamed and concurrently treated with trkA-IgG fail to develop most of the expected thermal hyperalgesia. **B** The effects of carrageenan inflammation on the properties of primary afferent nociceptors. Recordings were made from an isolated skin-nerve preparation a few hours after the inflammatory stimulus was given in vivo, and afferents tested for their responses to a ramp increase in skin temperature. In inflamed skin, some nociceptors develop spontaneous activity and show a thermal sensitization. In animals inflamed with carrageenan and concurrently treated with trkA-IgG, the thermal sensitization of nociceptors is completely blocked. The insert on the right shows the average stimulus–response functions for nociceptors in these groups. (Modified from McMahon et al (1995) and M. Koltzenburg, D.L.H. Bennett and S.B. McMahon, unpublished observations.)

NGF and the evolution of neuropathic pain

NGF now has a clear role as an inflammatory mediator. However, its possible involvement in the evolution of neuropathic pain is much less defined. As described earlier, axotomy results in reduced retrograde transport of NGF to DRG cell bodies. It appears, however, that different models of nerve injury have differing effects on NGF levels. For instance chronic constriction injury (CCI) results in increased NGF levels (Herzberg et al 1997), while spinal nerve ligation results in a transient reduction in NGF levels (Lee et al 1998). It seems intuitively true that normalizing NGF levels may help prevent the evolution of neuropathic pain. Certainly, as described earlier NGF has powerful neuroprotective effects, especially on small-diameter DRG cells. Some of the changes seen following axotomy that are reversed by exogenous NGF (e.g. cell death, altered neurochemistry) may be important in the development of chronic pain states. It has also recently become clear that following nerve injury there are alterations in synaptic connectivity within the sensory nervous system and NGF may also have a role in these changes.

An important effect of axotomy and many other neuropathic conditions is the development of an abnormal connectivity between the sympathetic and sensory nervous systems, in which sympathetic activity can actually maintain the pain state (Janig 1995). This has been repeatedly demonstrated both in human and animal studies. Sensory neurons become responsive to adrenergic agonists after nerve injury, these may act directly on sensory neurons or possibly indirectly via eicosanoids (Levine et al 1986). The interaction between sympathetic and sensory neurons may not only occur at the level of the nerve terminal but also at the cell body. One manifestation of this is the formation of abnormal basket-like terminations of postganglionic sympathetic neurons around sensory neurons within the dorsal root ganglion (McLachlan et al 1993). It has recently been demonstrated that animals which actually overexpress NGF in the periphery also possess these abnormal sympathetic terminations within the DRG (Davis et al 1994), and these animals are also hyperalgesic (Davis et al 1993). The administration of exogenous NGF to adult animals promotes basket formation (Jones et al 1998) and conversely the administration of NGF antiserum can prevent sympathetic sprouting into the DRG in the CCI model (Ramer & Bisby 1998). This is a different situation to axotomy where the retrograde supply of NGF is reduced but demonstrates that an imbalance in NGF distribution can result in the development of this abnormal connectivity between the sympathetic and sensory nervous systems.

Alterations of connectivity also occur within the dorsal horn of the spinal cord following nerve injury. Normally, unmyelinated afferents (C fibres) terminate within the superficial laminae (laminae I and II) of the dorsal horn. Conversely, myelinated afferents (A fibres) terminate within lamina I and laminae III–V, importantly A-fibre terminals are excluded from lamina II. After axotomy, there is a profuse sprouting of myelinated afferents into lamina IIo, demonstrated by both bulk labelling of A fibres (Woolf et al 1992) and fills of single A fibres (Woolf et al 1992, Shortland & Woolf 1993). This finding is not restricted to axotomy but extends also to other models of neuropathic pain, including spinal nerve ligation (Lekan et al 1996) and CCI (Shortland et al 1995). Therefore, after nerve injury, lamina II (which normally only receives an input from unmyelinated, principally nociceptive afferents) now also receives an input from myelinated, low-threshold afferents. Clearly, the novel connectivity of A fibres might contribute to touch-evoked pain, a frequent component of neuropathies. Nerve injury results in a transganglionic degenerative atrophy of the central terminals of C fibres (Knyihar-Csillik et al 1987), which may result in an increase in synaptic space within the superficial laminae of the dorsal horn. Injury to C fibres appears to be critical for the development of A-fibre sprouting (Mannion et al 1996) and deafferentation alone is insufficient to promote this phenomenon (Mannion et al 1998). Two studies have now shown that the administration of NGF following axotomy can prevent the A-fibre sprouting (Bennett et al 1996a, Eriksson et al 1997) (Fig. 4.5). The mechanism whereby NGF prevents sprouting is likely to be secondary to the neuroprotective action of NGF on peptidergic small-diameter DRG cells.

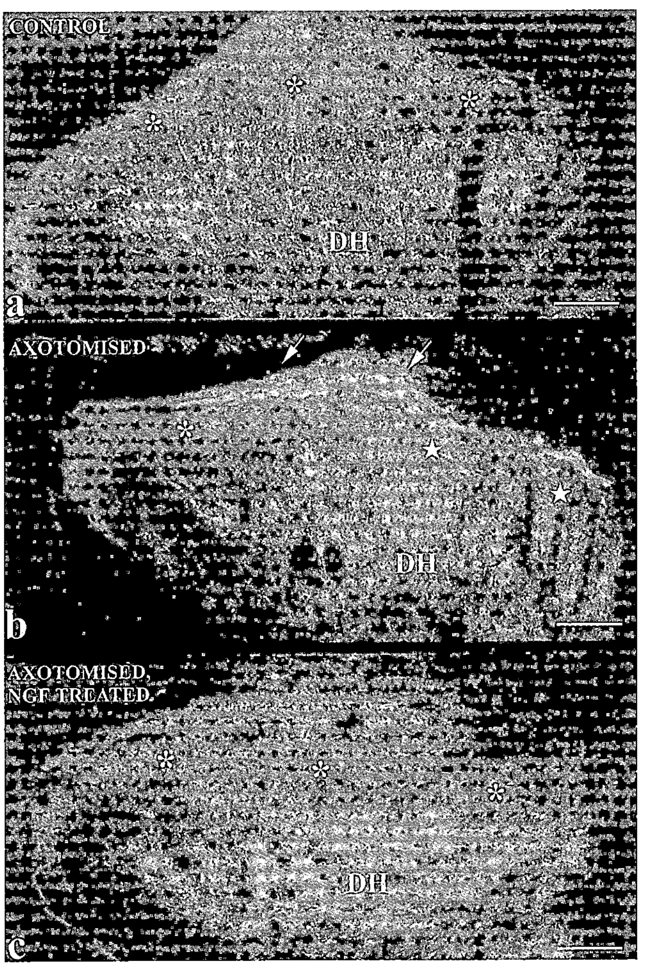

Fig. 4.5 Anatomical reorganization of primary afferent terminals after peripheral axotomy is blocked by NGF. Double-stained transverse sections of rat lumbar spinal cord, showing CGRP staining in red and labelling of myelinated afferent fibre terminals (following anterograde transport of Cholera B into sciatic nerve) in green. **a** The staining pattern obtained in normal animals. Note there is very little overlap: the myelinated staining stops at the lamina II/III border and the CGRP staining is dorsal to this (lamina II is denoted by asterisks). After sciatic axotomy (**b**), CGRP is lost in the medial part of the cord and in this region myelinated fibres sprout, evidenced by the presence of cholera B staining throughout the medial superficial dorsal horn, sprouting also occurs in lamina I, demonstrated by an arrow. In animals treated with intrathecal NGF and subjected to sciatic nerve section (**c**) the expected downregulation of CGRP and the sprouting of myelinated fibres is prevented. (Reproduced from Bennett et al 1996a.) (see colour plate)

NGF therefore has a powerful neuroprotective effect on small-diameter DRG cells following nerve injury, and altered NGF levels are implicated in a number of the alterations in connectivity that occur following nerve injury. The confusion over exactly what happens to NGF levels following various models of nerve injury is reflected in somewhat conflicting results when studying the effects of NGF supplementation or antagonism on pain-related behaviour following nerve injury. For instance, one study has shown that the administration of exogenous NGF onto a ligated nerve (in the CCI model) abolishes the thermal and mechanical hyperalgesia that normally occurs (Ren et al 1995), and yet another study has shown that administration of NGF antiserum has the same effect (Ramer & Bisby 1998). One possible explanation may be that the development of neuropathic pain is likely to be a multifactorial process and that NGF may have opposing effects on a number of the different mechanisms underlying this phenomenon.

Summary of the functional role of NGF in persistent pain states

Findings from the sequestration of endogenous NGF and the administration of exogenous NGF suggest that this factor is important in modulating the sensitivity of the sensory nervous system to noxious stimuli. The evidence that NGF levels increase during inflammation and results from studies using NGF antagonism make a strong case for NGF being a critical mediator of inflammatory pain. NGF clearly has a powerful neuroprotective effect on small-diameter sensory neurons and NGF levels have been shown to change in a number of models of nerve injury. However, its exact role in the development of neuropathic pain is at present unclear.

BRAIN-DERIVED NEUROTROPHIC FACTOR

BDNF was the second member of the neurotrophin family to be identified. Its name reflects the fact that it was originally purified from brain, but it is now clear that its expression is not restricted to this organ. The role of BDNF is less well defined than that of NGF. Developmentally, it appears to act as a target-derived factor for some neurons. Thus, BDNF or trkB knock-out mice show a very pronounced loss of placode-derived sensory neurons such as those located in the nodose ganglion and projecting through the vagal nerve (Klein et al 1993, Ernfors et al 1994b, Jones et al 1994). However, for spinal sensory neurons (that is, those with their cell bodies in the DRG) there is very limited, if any, cell death in these knock-outs (Snider & Silos-Santiago 1996), despite the fact that a significant subpopulation of spinal afferents express trkB receptors (see below). It has been suggested that BDNF serves to regulate the functional properties of these afferents during development. In particular, the mechanosensitivity of many developing cutaneous afferents is found to be reduced in the BDNF knock-out animal (Carroll et al 1998), suggesting this may be one important developmental function of this neurotrophin.

BIOLOGICAL ACTIONS

BDNF promotes neurite outgrowth of cultured nodose ganglion afferents. Its effects on adult spinal sensory neurons appear, in this respect, to be quite modest, perhaps reflecting the limited number of cells with trkB receptors, or perhaps a different role for BDNF. However, it has recently emerged that BDNF may have a completely different role in nociceptive systems. One key observation is that unlike NGF which is retrogradely transported from sensory neuronal targets, DRG cells themselves synthesize BDNF (Schecterson & Bothwell 1992, Apfel et al 1996b, Michael et al 1997). One function of this BDNF may be to act as an autocrine or paracrine survival factor for DRG cells (Acheson et al 1995), but this synthesis of BDNF may also have important implications for nociceptive signalling. In normal animals, a modest proportion of small cells contain the protein. Interestingly, these cells virtually all express trkA (Michael et al 1997). That is, they are sensitive to NGF and exogenous NGF greatly promotes the expression of BDNF in these cells (Apfel et al 1996b, Michael et al 1997) (Fig. 4.6). It has also been found that inflammatory stimuli (that are themselves known to result in increased NGF production) also increase BDNF expression in small sensory neurons (Cho et al 1997a,b). The BDNF that is produced in sensory neurons is transported anterogradely out of the cell bodies and towards the spinal cord (Fig. 4.6). In the terminals of nociceptors in the superficial dorsal horn, BDNF is found in dense core vesicles. This BDNF is lost following dorsal rhizotomy, demonstrating its location in afferent terminals. Together, then, these localization data raise the possibility that BDNF might be released with

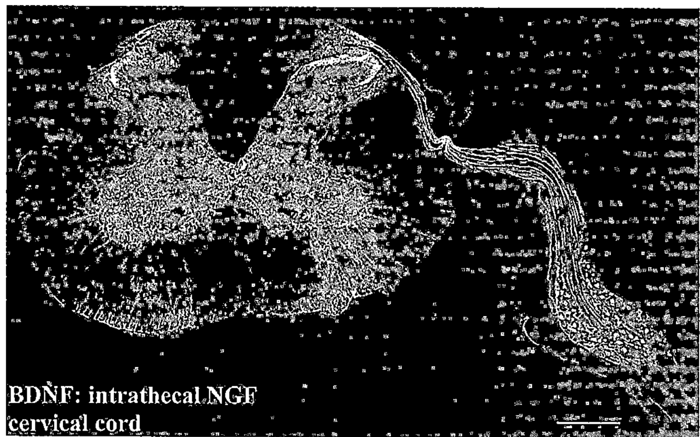

Fig. 4.6 Transverse section of spinal cord and attached root and DRG at cervical level, stained for BDNF immunoreactivity. The animal had received intrathecal NGF 24 h previously, which increases the expression of BDNF so that virtually all trkA expressing DRG cells (about 40% of all DRG cells) now express the protein. It is shipped anterogradely to the central terminals of these small afferents. (Reproduced from Michael et al 1997.)

activity from nociceptive terminals and serve as a neurotransmitter or neuromodulator within the superficial dorsal horn.

The postsynaptic effects of BDNF are only now beginning to be examined. There is a compelling body of data that in another brain region, the hippocampus, BDNF serves as a modulator of neuronal excitability. Thus, several forms of long-term potentiation depend upon activity-induced release of BDNF (Kang & Schuman 1995, Akaneya et al 1997). Hippocampal long-term potentiation is reduced in the BDNF knock-out animal and in normal animals by BDNF blocking reagents (Korte et al 1995, Patterson et al 1996). Analogous data is now accumulating for the spinal cord. It has been demonstrated both in an *in vitro* spinal cord preparation and *in vivo* that application of exogenous BDNF could cause a facilitation of the flexor reflex (Dassan et al 1998, Mannion et al 1999) (Fig. 4.7). The mechanism of action is likely to be on postsynaptic dorsal horn neurons which are known to express the receptor for BDNF (trkB). Activation of trkB can lead to phosphorylation of the NMDA receptor (Levine et al 1998, Lin et al 1998) and, of course, NMDA receptors have been implicated in the evolution of many forms of central hyperexcitable states (McMahon et al 1993). The hippocampal

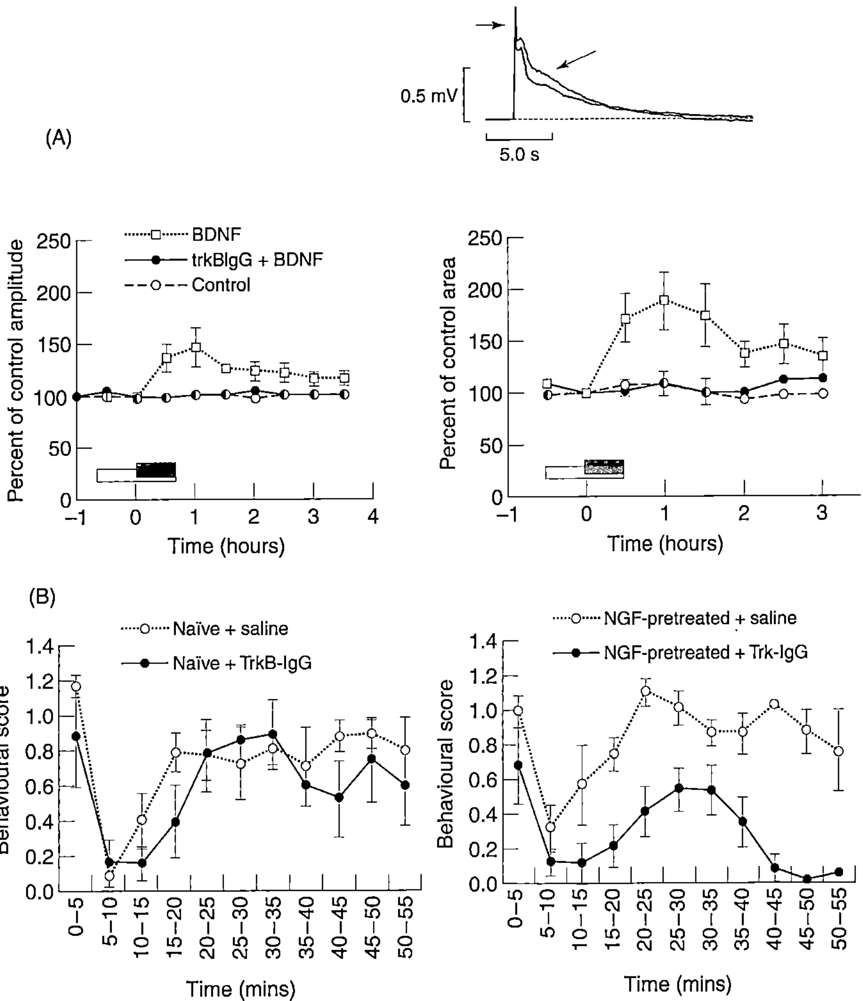

Fig. 4.7 Evidence supporting the role of BDNF as a neuromodulator released from nociceptors and regulating excitability of spinal cord sensory processing. **A** The effects of exogenous BDNF on ventral reflexes elicited by noxious stimulation in an isolated spinal cord preparation studied *in vitro*. BDNF was included in the perfusate (at 200 ng/ml) for the time period indicated by the open bar. It caused a small transient increase in the magnitude of short latency (low-threshold) responses (left) and a larger, more persistent increase in long latency (high-threshold) latencies (right). When the BDNF was administered with trkB-IgG (timings shown by open bar), the increases in reflexes were not seen. **B** Pain-related behaviour in animals given a standard formalin test. In normal animals (left), intrathecal trkB-IgG (1 h before the test) had no effect on pain-related behaviour triggered by formalin. When animals were pretreated with NGF, however, the second phase of the formalin test was increased somewhat, and this phase was largely attenuated by the intrathecal trkB-IgG treatment. The data suggest that spinally acting BDNF plays a critical role in this persistent pain behaviour. (Modified from Dassan et al 1998.)

effects of BDNF are also believed to depend on increases in postsynaptic calcium levels. Intrathecal BDNF treatment in rats results in a rapid induction of c-*fos* in some superficial dorsal horn neurons (Dassan et al 1998), another indication of its ability to produce altered dorsal horn function.

The expression of BDNF is altered in a most interesting way in another pathophysiological state, that associated with peripheral nerve injury. After sciatic axotomy BDNF is upregulated in large-diameter DRG cells and anterograde transport to the dorsal horn of the spinal cord increases (Tonra et al 1998, Michael et al 1999). Thus, BDNF expression switches from nociceptors to large neurons, known normally to be connected mostly to innocuous mechanoreceptors in the periphery. The signal for the novel expression in large cells is not yet known. Possibly, it could be the reduced retrograde transport of NT3 by large cells (see below). It is tempting to speculate that this BDNF may also have similar postsynaptic effects to those proposed above. Of course, in this case any such effects are likely to be found in deeper dorsal horn laminae, the known normal termination sites of large afferents.

FUNCTIONAL ROLE

The phenomena described above suggest that BDNF might mediate altered states of spinal excitability. One can imagine that BDNF would be released from small-diameter afferent terminals, particularly in conditions of inflammation, and from large-diameter terminals in some neuropathic states. One can further imagine that the BDNF released might trigger postsynaptic changes in excitability, as described above, contributing to the abnormal pain states frequently seen in these pathophysiological conditions.

Is there any evidence that this in fact happens? Pharmacological 'antagonism' of BDNF can alter spinal sensory processing (Dassan et al 1998, Mannion et al 1999) (Fig. 4.7). The tool used is a synthetic fusion protein, trkB-IgG, a recombinantly produced protein consisting of the extracellular domain of the trkB receptor coupled to the fc region of an IgG. This stable molecule is capable of binding BDNF with a high affinity and specificity (Shelton et al 1995) thereby leading to its sequestration. Following inflammation or NGF treatment there is an enhanced excitability of C-fibre reflexes within the spinal cord. This can be largely reversed by administration of the trkB-IgG molecule (Fig. 4.7). Furthermore, BDNF sequestration can prevent some of the pain-related behaviour associated with either inflammation or NGF treatment (Fig. 4.7).

Together, these initial reports are consistent with the notion that BDNF may prove an important centrally acting modulator of persistent pain states. Clearly, several other molecules have been implicated in this process of central sensitization, most notably the tackykinin substance P and the NMDA glutamate receptor (see Ch. 6). It is possible that BDNF is simply one of a series of modulators capable of triggering postsynaptic change, perhaps via a common mechanism of NMDA receptor phosphorylation. It is interesting that the substance P is itself regulated in a very similar fashion to that described above for BDNF. That is, it is upregulated in trkA-expressing cells by exogenous NGF, or by inflammatory stimuli in an NGF-dependent fashion. Moreover, its expression falls in these cells after peripheral axotomy, but the same stimulus apparently can induce expression in some large neurons. The clear effects of trkB-IgG coupled with the rather modest phenotype of substance P and NK1 null-mutant animals (Woolf et al 1998) may indicate that BDNF is a more important mediator of these central changes and antagonism of this molecule may provide a novel therapeutic target.

NT3 AND NT4/5

NT3 is critically required for the development of a group of large-diameter DRG cells, particularly Ia afferents (Ernfors et al 1994a, Klein et al 1994, Farinas et al 1994). Its developmental role is complicated by the fact that it may stimulate proliferation of neuronal precursors (Elshamy & Ernfors 1996). The development of D-hair afferents is dependent on NT4/5 (Stucky et al 1998). The development of nociceptive afferents, however, appears to be largely independent of these factors.

In the adult animal, there are a few reports that administration of these factors may be able to produce a hyperalgesia (Malcangio et al 1997, Shu et al 1998), although this is much less marked than that evoked by NGF. These effects are probably caused by these ligands acting at their non-preferred receptors. For instance, the preferred receptor for NT4/5 is trkB. However, appropriate concentrations of NT4/5 have also been reported to activate trkA receptors. Perhaps it is not so surprising then that some cutaneous nociceptors are found to show thermal sensitization after exposure to NGF or NT4/5 (Shu et al 1998).

Similarly, the preferred receptor for NT3 is trkC, although it is clear that this molecule can also activate other neurotrophin receptors, notably trkA. In this respect, it is again perhaps not surprising that NT3 can induce hyperalgesia when given systemically (Malcangio et al 1997). However, some of the effects of NT3 acting at trkC receptors may be relevant to pain states. TrkC receptors are expressed selectively by large-diameter DRG cells (McMahon et al 1994). These cells are known, for the most part, to possess myelinated axons which form innocuous mechanoreceptive endings in skin and deeper tissue. The trkC null-mutant animal has a selective loss of this peripheral fibre type and abnormal proprioceptive capacities. Most NT3 available to these sensory neurons appears to be target derived. Following peripheral nerve injury a series of changes are found in these large sensory neurons which include altered expression of ion channels, receptors and neuromodulators, as well as some anatomical rearrangement of afferent terminals. Several of these changes have been proposed to contribute to sensory abnormalities often found after peripheral nerve damage. Treatment of damaged nerves with NT3 can ameliorate some of these axotomy-induced changes (Ohara et al 1995, Munson et al 1998), although not the central sprouting of A-fibres (discussed above). Thus, it is possible that this factor will be protective against some of the features of neuropathic pain, although such a role has not been tested experimentally.

THE GDNF FAMILY OF TROPHIC FACTORS (GDNF, NTN AND PSP)

Recently a novel family of trophic factors has been characterized which in a similar fashion to the neurotrophins are likely to be important both in the development of the sensory nervous system and in adult sensory function. This family belongs to the TGFβ superfamily, of which glial cell line-derived neurotrophic factor (GDNF) was the first member to be characterized (Lin et al 1993). The family also includes neurturin (NTN) (Kotzbauer et al 1996) and persephin (PSP) (Milbrandt et al 1998). There are differences between these factors in their survival-promoting activities on neurons of the peripheral nervous system. NTN and GDNF promote the survival of enteric, sympathetic (superior cervical) and sensory (trigeminal, nodose, and DRG) neurons (Buj-Bello et al 1995, Kotzbauer et al 1996), PSP does not have any survival-promoting effect on these populations (Milbrandt et al 1998).

RECEPTORS FOR THE GDNF FAMILY

Members of the GDNF family signal via a receptor complex. This consists of RET, a tyrosine kinase receptor which acts as a signal transducing domain and a member of the GFRα family of GPI-linked receptors (GFRα1–4) which act as ligand binding domains (Durbec et al 1996, Jing et al 1996, Treanor et al 1996, Baloh et al 1997, Buj-Bello et al 1997, Creedon et al 1997, Jing et al 1997, Klein et al 1997, Sanicola et al 1997, Baloh et al 1998, Naveilhan et al 1998, Thompson et al 1998a, Worby et al 1998). Either GFRα-1 or GFRα-2 in conjunction with RET can mediate GDNF or NTN signalling, although GDNF is thought to bind preferentially to GFRα-1 and NTN to GFRα-2. The fact there is significant cross-talk between GDNF/NTN and their respective GFRα receptors was recently demonstrated by findings from GFRα-1-deficient mice. Results from GDNF-, RET- and GFRα-1-deficient mice indicate these are all essential for the development of the kidney and enteric nervous system (Schuchardt et al 1994, Moore et al 1996, Pichel et al 1996, Sanchez et al 1996, Cacalano et al 1998, Enomoto et al 1998). However, although RET and GDNF are required for the development of a number of peripheral ganglia (cervical and nodose), these are virtually unaffected in GFRα-1-deficient mice, indicating that GDNF must be acting via another receptor component (GFRα-2) in supporting these populations. The receptor components via which PSP acts are as yet unknown. Fibroblasts transfected with RET in combination with GFRα-1 or GFRα-2 did not respond to PSP (Milbrandt et al 1998), suggesting that this factor uses either different or additional receptor components. The ligands acting at GFRα-3 and GFRα-4 are also as yet unknown. A schematic illustration of the interaction of members of the GDNF family with their receptors is shown in Figure 4.8.

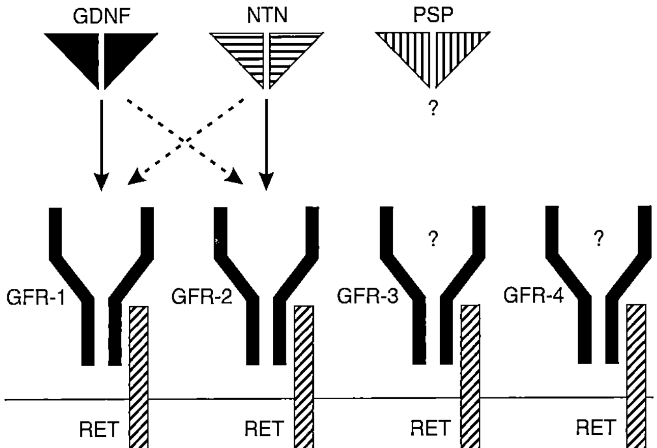

Fig. 4.8 Schematic illustration of the interaction of the GDNF family with their receptors. Members of the GDNF family signal via a receptor complex. This consists of RET, a tyrosine kinase receptor, which acts as a signal transducing domain and a member of the GFRα family of GPI-linked receptors (GFRα 1–4) which act as ligand binding domains. GDNF is thought to bind preferentially to GFRα-1 and NTN to GFRα-2, although there is some 'cross-talk' in this interaction. The receptor for PSP is unknown and the ligand-binding specificities of GFRα3 and 4 are also unknown.

THE GDNF FAMILY AND SENSORY NEURON DEVELOPMENT

GDNF can support the survival of a population of embryonic sensory neurons *in vitro* and, interestingly, the size of this population increases as development proceeds (Buj-Bello et al 1995). A physiological role for GDNF during sensory neuron development is supported by the fact that at P0 there is already a significant (20%) loss of DRG cells in GDNF-deficient mice (Moore et al 1996). Whether this loss occurs in a specific subset of sensory neurons is not known.

RET is the signal-transducing domain of the GDNF receptor and is expressed by DRG cells early in development (E11.5 in the mouse (Molliver et al 1997)). RET is initially expressed in large-diameter DRG cells which innervate hair follicles and which terminate in deep laminae of the spinal cord. As development proceeds (and through the postnatal period) the small-diameter IB4 binding DRG cells begin to express RET, exactly during the period when the same cells are losing their NGF sensitivity by downregulating trkA expression (Bennett et al 1996c). With emerging RET expression these neurons become sensitive to GDNF, as demonstrated by the fact that GDNF promotes the survival of IB4 binding neurons *in vitro* (Molliver et al 1997). The postnatal period therefore represents a period when IB4 binding DRG cells switch from NGF to GDNF dependence. It should be noted that a significant proportion of large-diameter DRG cells express RET and therefore would be expected to be GDNF sensitive. The developmental role of GDNF on these neurons is as yet unknown.

NTN is expressed in a number of peripheral tissues and can support a population of embryonic sensory neurons *in vitro* (Kotzbauer et al 1996). However, whether this represents a specific population (for instance IB4 binding) of DRG cells is unknown. A NTN knockout would provide more information on the developmental role of this protein. PSP (unlike GDNF and NTN) does not have survival promoting effects on embryonic sensory neurons *in vitro* (Milbrandt et al 1998). It is also expressed at extremely low levels in the periphery and is inefficiently spliced. In summary, there is growing evidence that GDNF and NTN play a role in sensory neuron development but a detailed analysis of knock-out animals will be required for a full description of their actions.

THE EXPRESSION OF RET AND GFRα RECEPTORS IN ADULT SENSORY NEURONS

RET is expressed by 60% of DRG cells, both of small and large cell diameter (Molliver et al 1997, Bennett et al 1998b). The relationship of GDNF receptor expression to different subgroups of sensory neurons has now been studied (Fig. 4.9). The pattern of RET expression in small-diameter DRG cells is interesting, as it is expressed in virtually all IB4-binding DRG cells but very few CGRP-expressing DRG cells. GFRα-1 is expressed by 40% of DRG cells, again of both small and large cell diameter. It is highly co-expressed with RET and like RET is expressed by a large proportion of IB4 binding DRG cells. GFRα-2 is expressed by 30% of DRG cells which are principally of small cell diameter and again is selectively expressed by IB4-binding DRG cells. GFRα-3 is also expressed in DRG cells but its pattern of expression has not yet been fully characterized. As has been previously described with the receptors for other trophic factors, there appears to be a high degree of plasticity in GDNF receptor expression following nerve injury. Interestingly, different receptor components are differentially regulated (Bennett et al 1998a). Following axotomy there is an increase in the proportion of DRG cells that express RET and GFR-1 (to 75 and 70% of DRG cells, respectively), so that virtually all large-diameter DRG cells express these receptors. There is also an increase in the expression of GFRα-3 in small-diameter DRG cells but a reduction in the expression of GFRα-2.

In summary, GDNF receptor components are expressed in a population of both small- and large-diameter DRG cells. Within small-diameter DRG cells they are expressed

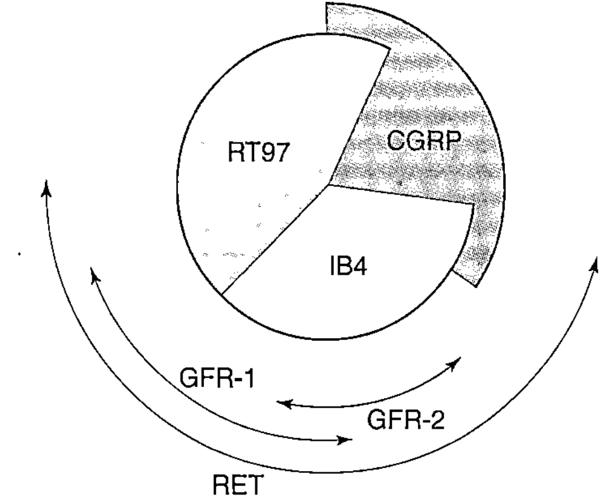

Fig. 4.9 Pie chart relating the distribution of GDNF family receptor components to neurochemically defined DRG subclasses. RET and GFRα-1 are expressed both in the IB4 binding non-peptidergic population of small-diameter DRG cells and in some of the 'large light' population of DRG cells which can be identified by the neurofilament antibody RT97. GFRα-2 is expressed principally in the IB4 binding population. Receptors for GDNF are therefore expressed selectively in the IB4 binding population of small-diameter DRG cells and not in the CGRP expressing population. The expression of GFRα-3 and GFRα-4 has not yet been related to the different DRG subclasses of sensory neurons. One would predict that the lectin-binding group of nociceptors would be sensitive to GDNF and NTN, while the peptidergic nociceptors would not. See text for further details.

by a population of neurons which are non-peptidergic, IB4 binding and which do not express trk receptors and hence are unresponsive to the neurotrophins. Plasticity in receptor component expression following nerve injury implies that the sensitivity of sensory neurons to different members of the GDNF/NTN/PSP family will change (i.e. there will be increased sensitivity to GDNF and reduced sensitivity to NTN).

THE BIOLOGICAL EFFECTS OF GDNF ON ADULT SENSORY NEURONS

The high level of expression of GDNF receptor components within IB4-binding DRG cells is reflected in the fact that this factor has potent biological actions on these neurons. *In vitro* GDNF has been demonstrated to selectively enhance the outgrowth of IB4-stained neurites from DRG explants (Leclere et al 1998). *In vivo* GDNF also has selective trophic effects on this population of sensory neurons (Bennett et al 1998b). There is marked plasticity in the expression of many neurochemical markers within sensory neurons following nerve injury (as described earlier). In the IB4 binding population of small-diameter DRG cells there is a reduction in IB4 binding and a reduced activity of the enzyme TMP following axotomy. These changes are seen both at the level of the cell body and within the dorsal horn of the spinal cord, and can be reversed by administration of GDNF (Fig. 4.10). It has also recently been shown that IB4-binding DRG cells selectively express the purinergic receptor $P2X_3$(Bradbury et al 1998). Expression of this receptor falls following axotomy and again this can be restored by administration of GDNF. GDNF, however, has no rescue effect on the peptidergic (CGRP expressing) population of small-diameter DRG cells. Following axotomy, these histochemical changes are accompanied by a conduction velocity slowing within sensory neurons. This conduction velocity slowing could be partially reversed within a population of C fibres following GDNF administration. GDNF can therefore restore many different properties of neuronal function within the IB4-binding population of DRG cells following nerve injury. The efficacy of NTN on this population of sensory neurons has yet to be assessed.

Another consequence of axotomy is that large-diameter Aβ fibres sprout inappropriately into lamina II of the dorsal horn, a region of the spinal cord which does not normally receive an input from these afferents (discussed above). GDNF administration can prevent this change. The mechanism for this effect is unclear. However there is growing evidence that A-fibre sprouting occurs secondarily to injury to C fibres and hence the rescue effect of GDNF on the IB4-binding population of C fibres may prevent this phenomenon.

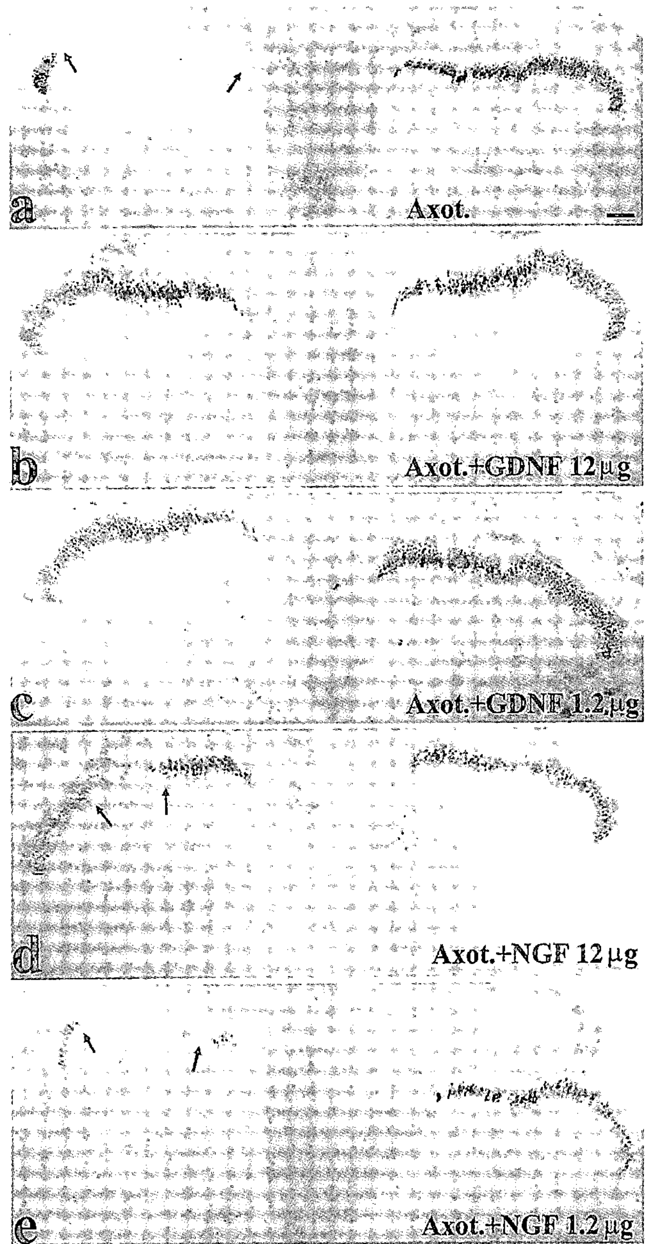

Fig. 4.10 The downregulation of TMP activity in primary sensory neurons is fully reversed by GDNF treatment but only partially reversed by NGF. Each panel shows a transverse section of rat lumbar spinal cord stained for activity of the enzyme TMP (present in only about one-half of C-fibres). After sciatic axotomy (**a**), TMP activity is lost from the terminals of sciatic afferents (between the arrows). However, sciatic axotomy combined with intrathecal GDNF fully reverses this affect at 12 µg/day (**b**) and partially at 1.2 µg/day (**c**). NGF at the same doses (**d,e**, respectively) is much less effective. Reproduced from Bennett et al, 1998b.

FUNCTIONAL IMPORTANCE OF GDNF

Studying the effects of exogenous GDNF is obviously very different from understanding the physiological role of the endogenous protein. To study the role of endogenous GDNF some kind of pharmacological antagonism is required, which is as yet unavailable. As discussed above, there is evidence that GDNF can prevent a number of changes in IB4-binding DRG cells and also the A-fibre sprouting that occurs following axotomy. What functional importance may this have? These changes may be important in the evolution of neuropathic pain. We have found that administration of GDNF can greatly reduce the mechanical allodynia and thermal hyperalgesia associated with the Seltzer model of nerve injury (T. Boucher et al, unpublished observations). We have also found that, unlike NGF, the acute or chronic administration of GDNF has no effect on sensory thresholds (unpublished observations). So although GDNF can exert important trophic effects on the IB4-binding population of sensory neurons (for instance following nerve injury), it does not appear to have acute sensitizing actions on these neurons. It remains to be seen if GDNF has more subtle effects on sensory function, for example in modulating ATP sensitivity. It is clear, however, that small-diameter DRG cells can be divided into two roughly equal populations: a group of peptidergic, trkA-expressing neurons which are NGF sensitive and a group of non-peptidergic (IB4-binding) neurons which express RET and GFRα-1 and which are GDNF sensitive.

LEUKAEMIA INHIBITORY FACTOR

Leukaemia inhibitory factor (LIF) is one of a family of neuropoeitic cytokines defined by their binding to the common receptor gp130. Other members include IL-6, IL-11, ciliary-derived neurotrophic factor (CNTF), oncostatin M and cardiotrophin-1 (CT-1). LIF signals via a receptor complex of LIFR-β and gp 130 and is retrogradely transported by a population of small-diameter DRG cells (Thompson et al 1997). Levels of LIF are normally very low. However following nerve injury LIF expression increases at the site of injury (Banner & Patterson 1994). Nerve injury also results in a large increase in the expression of the neuropeptide galanin within sensory neurons. Evidence from both animals deficient in LIF (Sun & Zigmond 1996) and the administration of exogenous LIF (Thompson et al 1998b) indicates that LIF is responsible for this upregulation. LIF may also be implicated in the sprouting of postganglionic sympathetic neurons which occurs around DRG cell bodies following nerve injury (Thompson & Majithia 1998).

The actions of LIF are not restricted to nerve injury but also extend to inflammatory conditions (Banner et al 1998). LIF levels increase during inflammation. In LIF knock-out mice there is an enhanced inflammatory reaction. Conversely, the administration of exogenous LIF can attenuate both the hyperalgesia and the increased NGF expression which normally occurs during inflammation. Confusingly, the effects of exogenous LIF may be dose dependent, as another study has found that administration of this factor to naive animals may itself produce a hyperalgesia (Thompson et al 1996). Endogenous LIF, however, appears to have an interesting role as a mediator, which suppresses the inflammatory reaction possibly at an early stage by negatively regulating the expression of IL-1β and NGF. A role for other members of this cytokine family within the sensory nervous system has yet to be established.

CONCLUSIONS

This chapter has discussed the biological effects and roles of a small series of neurotrophic factors. Of course, other families and many other individual factors have not been discussed here, many of which exert potent biological effects on sensory neurons in culture. It seems likely, if presently untested, that at least several other factors will be found to exert important roles in regulating the function of the nociceptive system. On the other hand, many of the properties of, in particular, peripheral pain signalling systems, appear to be regulated by the factors that have been discussed here. Thus, the plastic changes that are observed in the functional properties of nociceptors, including changes in neurotransmitter, ion channel and receptor expression under conditions of inflammation and nerve damage, are apparently well explained by altered availability of two factors, NGF and GDNF. Indeed, cutaneous nociceptors projecting to the spinal cord form two minimally overlapping groups: peptidergic (CGRP-expressing) and non-peptidergic (IB4-binding) neurons which are NGF and GDNF sensitive respectively. As summarized in Figure 4.11, these two groups are distinguished by many other features extending beyond chemical phenotype to include distinct anatomical terminations in the superficial dorsal horn. It is not yet clear whether these two groups exhibit differences in peripheral target innervation.

One obvious question, to which there is currently no clear answer, is whether these two groups of nociceptors

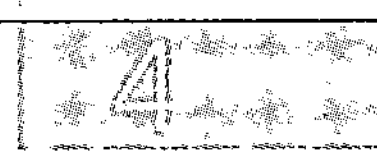

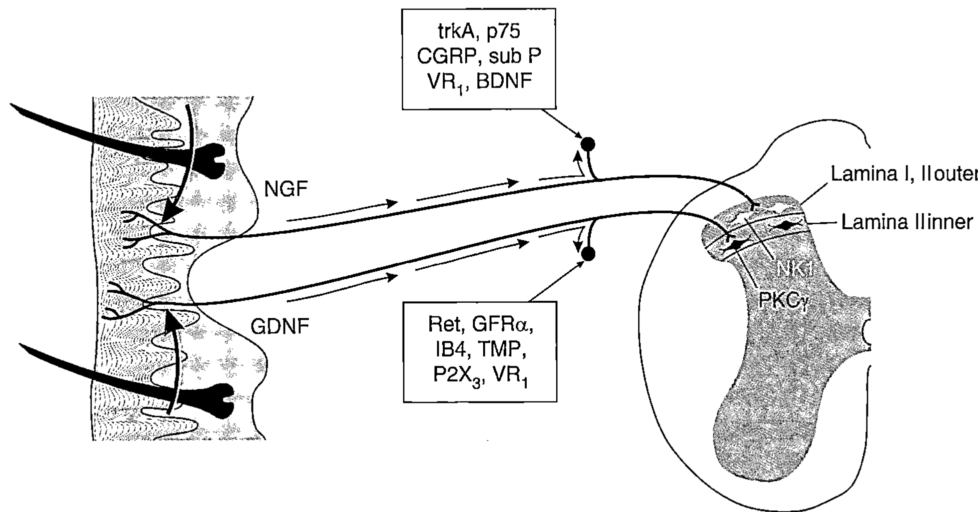

Fig. 4.11 Two distinct subgroups of cutaneous C fibres can be recognized, one sensitive to NGF and the other to GDNF. These two groups differ in many ways, including the expression of neuromodulators and receptors and in their anatomical terminations in the dorsal horn. It is not yet clear if these two groups have distinct physiological responsiveness or if they might have different functional roles in chronic pain states. (Modified from Snider & McMahon 1998.)

have different functional properties. The presence of mRNA encoding the capsaicin receptor VR1 in both groups suggests they may be responsive to noxious heat, although interestingly VR1 appears more strongly localized in the peptidergic NGF-sensitive population of nociceptors. The presence of one purinoreceptor $P2X_3$ on one subpopulation indicates the two groups may have different chemical sensitivities. Whether or not these two groups have different sensitivities to mechanical stimuli is currently unknown. Another distinguishing feature of these two populations is that the NGF-sensitive population of DRG cells actually synthesizes BDNF, which is anterogradely transported to the dorsal horn of the spinal cord. BDNF expression is regulated by NGF and increases in inflammatory conditions. This BDNF may be released and potentiate the transmission of nociceptive information at the level of the dorsal horn of the spinal cord.

The existence of two groups of nociceptors with distinct trophic requirements raises the intriguing possibility that they may play very different roles in persistent pain states. Work on trophic factors and sensory neurons has certainly produced insights into the development and function of the sensory nervous system. Perhaps in the future new analgesic targets will be identified based on these findings.

REFERENCES

Acheson A, Conover JC, Fandl JP et al 1995 A BDNF autocrine loop in adult sensory neurons prevents cell death [see comments]. Nature 374: 450–453

Akaneya Y, Tsumoto T, Kinoshita S, Hatanaka H 1997 Brain-derived neurotrophic factor enhances long-term potentiation in rat visual cortex. Journal of Neuroscience 17: 6707–6716

Aloe L, Tuveri MA, Carcassi U, Levi-Montalcini R 1992 Nerve growth factor in the synovial fluid of patients with chronic arthritis. Arthritis and Rheumatism 35: 351–355

Amann R, Schuligoi R, Lanz I, Bernhard A, Peskar A 1996a Effect of 5-lipoxygenase inhibitor on nerve growth factor-induced thermal hyperalgesia in the rat. European Journal of Pharmacology 306: 89–91

Amann R, Schuligoi R, Herzeg G, Donnerer J 1996b Intraplantar injection of nerve growth factor into the rat hind paw: local edema and effects on thermal nociceptive threshold. Pain 64: 323–329

Andreev NY, Dimitrieva N, Koltzenburg M, McMahon SB 1995 Peripheral administration of nerve growth factor in the adult rat produces a thermal hyperalgesia that requires the presence of sympathetic post-ganglionic neurons. Pain 63: 109–115

Apfel SC, Adornato BT, Dyck PJ et al 1996a Results of a double blind, placebo controlled trial of recombinant human nerve growth factor in diabetic polyneuropathy, Annals of Neurology 40(3): 194

Apfel SC, Wright DE, Wiideman AM, Dormia C, Snider WD, Kessler JA 1996b Nerve growth factor regulates the expression of brain-derived neurotrophic factor mRNA in the peripheral nervous system. Molecular and Cellular Neurosciences 7: 134–142

Arvidsson J, Ygge J, Grant G 1986 Cell loss in lumbar dorsal root ganglia and transganglionic degeneration after sciatic nerve resection in the rat. Brain Research 373: 15–21

Averill S, McMahon SB, Clary DO, Reichardt LF, Priestley JV 1995 Immunocytochemical localization of trkA receptors in chemically identified subgroups of adult rat sensory neurons. European Journal of Neuroscience 7: 1484–1494

Baloh RH, Tansey MG, Golden JP et al 1997 TrnR2, a novel receptor that mediates neurturin and GDNF signaling through Ret. Neuron 18: 793–802

Baloh RH, Gorodinsky A, Golden JP et al 1998 GFRalpha3 is an orphan member of the GDNF/neurturin/persephin receptor family. Proceedings of the National Academy of Sciences USA 95: 5801–5806

Banner LR, Patterson PH 1994 Major changes in the expression of the messenger-RNAS for cholinergic differentiation factor leukemia inhibitory factor and its receptor after injury to adult peripheral-nerves and ganglia. Proceedings of the National Academy of Sciences USA 91: 7109–7113

Banner LR, Patterson PH, Allchorne A, Poole S, Woolf CJ 1998 Leukemia inhibitory factor is an anti-inflammatory and analgesic cytokine. Journal of Neuroscience 18: 5456–5462

Barbacid M 1995 Neurotrophic factors and their receptors [review]. Current Opinion in Cell Biology 7: 148–155

Bennett DLH, French J, Priestley JVP, McMahon SB 1996a NGF but not NT-3 or BDNF prevents the A fiber sprouting into lamina II of the spinal cord that occurs following axotomy. Molecular and Cellular Neurosciences 8: 211–220

Bennett DLH, McMahon SB, Shelton D, Koltzenburg M 1996b NGF sequestration using a trkA-IgG fusion molecule prevents primary afferent sensitisation to carrageenin inflammation. 8th World Congress on Pain 35: 120

Bennett DLH, Averill S, Clary DO, Priestley JV, McMahon SB 1996c Postnatal changes in the expression of the trkA high affinity NGF receptor in primary sensory neurons. European Journal of Neuroscience 8: 2204–2208

Bennett DLH, Boucher T, Armanini MP, Phillips HS, McMahon SB, Shelton DL 1998a RET, GFRα-1,2 and 3 expression within sensory neurons innervating different targets and the response to nerve injury. Society of Neuroscience Abstracts 24: 1545

Bennett DLH, Michael GJ, Ramachandran N et al 1998b. A distinct subgroup of small DRG cells express GDNF receptor components and GDNF is protective for these neurons after nerve injury. Journal of Neuroscience 18: 3059–3072

Bennett DLH, Koltzenburg M, Priestley JV, Shelton DL, McMahon SB 1998c Endogenous nerve growth factor regulates the sensitivity of nociceptors in the adult rat. European Journal of Neuroscience 10: 1282–1291

Bennett DLH, McMahon SB, Rattray M, Shelton D 1998d Nerve growth factor and sensory nerve function. In: Brain SD, Moore PK, (eds) Pain and neurogenic inflammation Birkhauser

Bennett G, Al-Rashed S, Hoult JRS, Brain SD 1998e Nerve growth factor induced hyperalgesia in the rat hind paw is dependent on circulating neutrophils. Pain (in press)

Bergman I, Priestley JV, McMahon SB, Brocker EB, Toyka KV, Koltzenbürg M 1996 Analysis of cutaneous sensory neurons in transgenic mice lacking the low affinity neurotrophin receptor p75. European Journal of Neuroscience 9: 18–28

Bevan S, Winter J 1995 Nerve growth factor (NGF) differentially regulates the chemosensitivity of adult rat cultured sensory neurons. Journal of Neuroscience 15: 4918–4926

Black JA, Waxman SG 1996 Sodium channel expression: a dynamic process in neurons and non-neuronal cells [review]. Developmental Neuroscience 18: 139–152

Bothwell M 1995 Functional interactions of neurotrophins and neurotrophin receptors. Annual Review of Neuroscience 18: 223–253

Bradbury EJ, Burnstock G, McMahon SB 1998 The expression of $P2X_3$ purinoceptors in sensory neurons: effects of axotomy and glial-derived neurotrophic factor (GDNF). Molecular and Cellular Neurosciences 12: 256–268

Brennan TJ, Barr MT, Zhan PK, Shelton DL 1998 Role of nerve growth factor in a rat model of postoperative pain. Society of Neuroscience Abstracts 24: 880 (abstract)

Buj-Bello A, Buchman VL, Horton A, Rosenthal A, Davies AM 1995 GDNF is an age-specific survival factor for sensory and autonomic neurons. Neuron 15: 821–828

Buj-Bello A, Adu J, Pinon LGP et al 1997 Neurturin responsiveness requires a GPI-linked receptor and Ret receptor tyrosine kinase. Nature 387: 721–724

Bullock ED, Johnson EM Jr 1996 Nerve growth factor induces the expression of certain cytokine genes and bcl-2 in mast cells. Potential role in survival promotion. Journal of Biological Chemistry 271: 27500–27508

Cacalano G, Farinas I, Wang LC et al 1998 GFRα-1 is an essential receptor component for GDNF in the developing nervous system and kidney. Neuron 21: 53–62

Carroll P, Lewin GR, Koltzenburg M, Toyka V, Thoenen H 1998 A role of BDNF in mechanosensation. Nature Neuroscience 1: 42–46

Carter BD, Kaltschmidt C, Kaltschmidt B et al 1996 Selective activation of NF-kappa B by nerve growth factor through the neurotrophin receptor p75. Science 272: 542–545

Chao MV, Hempstead BL 1995 p75 and trk: a two-receptor system. Trends in Neurosciences 18: 321–326

Chao MV, Bothwell MA, Ross AH, Koprowski H, Lanahan AA, Buck CR 1986 Gene transfer and molecular cloning of the human NGF receptor. Science 232: 518–521

Cho HJ, Kim JK, Zhou XF, Rush RA 1997a Increased brain-derived neurotrophic factor immunoreactivity in rat dorsal root ganglia and spinal cord following peripheral inflammation. Brain Research 764: 269–272

Cho HJ, Kim SY, Park MJ, Kim DS, Kim JK, Chu MY 1997b Expression of mRNA for brain-derived neurotrophic factor in the dorsal root ganglion following peripheral inflammation. Brain Research 749: 358–362

Clary DO, Weskamp G, Austin LR, Reichardt LF 1994 TrkA cross-linking mimics neuronal responses to nerve growth factor. Molecular Biology of the Cell 5: 549–563

Coggeshall RE, Lekan HA, Doubell TP, Allchorne A, Woolf CJ 1997 Central changes in primary afferent fibers following peripheral nerve lesions. Neuroscience 77: 1115–1122

Creedon DJ, Tansey MG, Baloh RH et al 1997 Neurturin shares receptors and signal transduction pathways with glial cell line-derived neurotrophic factor in sympathetic neurons. Proceedings of the National Academy of Sciences USA 94: 7018–7023

Crowley C, Spencer SD, Nishimura MC et al 1994 Mice lacking nerve growth factor display perinatal loss of sensory and sympathetic neurons yet develop basal forebrain cholinergic neurons. Cell 76: 1001–1011

Dassan P, Trevedi P, McMahon SB et al 1998 BDNF induces prolonged increases in spinal reflex activity in vitro. Society for Neuroscience Abstracts 24(154.13): 394

Davies AM, Lee KF, Jaenisch R 1993 p75-deficient trigeminal sensory neurons have an altered response to NGF but not to other neurotrophins. Neuron 11: 565–574

Davis BM, Lewin GR, Mendell LM, Jones ME, Albers KM 1993 Altered expression of nerve growth factor in the skin of transgenic mice leads to changes in response to mechanical stimuli. Neuroscience 56: 789–792

Davis BM, Albers KM, Seroogy KB, Katz DM 1994 Overexpression of nerve growth factor in transgenic mice induces novel sympathetic projections to primary sensory neurons. Journal of Comparative Neurology 349: 464–474

Dmitrieva N, Iqbal R, Shelton DL, McMahon SB 1996 c-fos induction in a rat model of cystiris: role of NGF. Society of Neuroscience Abstracts 22: 751

Dmitrieva N, Shelton D, Rice ASC, McMahon SB 1997 The role of nerve growth factor in a model of visceral inflammation. Neuroscience 78: 449–459

Donnerer J, Schuligoi R, Stein C 1992 Increased content and transport of substance P and calcitonin gene-related peptide in sensory nerves innervating inflamed tissue: evidence for a regulatory function of nerve growth factor in vivo. Neuroscience 49: 693–698

Durbec P, Marcos-Gutierrez CV, Kilkenny C et al 1996 GDNF signalling through the Ret receptor tyrosine kinase. Nature 381: 789–793

Elshamy WM, Ernfors P 1996 Requirement of neurotrophin-3 for the survival of proliferating trigeminal ganglion progenitor cells. Development 122: 2405–2414

Enomoto H, Araki A, Jackman A et al 1998 GFRα1-deficient mice have deficits in the enteric nervous system and kidneys. Neuron 21: 317–324

Eriksson NP, Aldskogius H, Grant G, Lindsay RM, Rivero-Melian C 1997 Effects of nerve growth factor, brain-derived neurotrophic factor and neurotrophin-3 on the laminar distribution of transganglionically transported choleragenoid in the spinal cord dorsal horn following transection of the sciatic nerve in the adult rat. Neuroscience 78: 863–872

Ernfors P, Lee KF, Kucera J, Jaenisch R 1994a Lack of neurotrophin-3 leads to deficiencies in the peripheral nervous system and loss of limb proprioceptive afferents. Cell 77: 503–512

Ernfors P, Lee KF, Jaenisch R 1994b Mice lacking brain-derived neurotrophic factor develop with sensory deficits. Nature 368: 147–150

Fantini F, Giannetti A, Benassi L, Cattaneo V, Magnoni C, Pincelli C 1995 Nerve growth factor receptor and neurochemical markers in human oral mucosa: an immunohistochemical study. Dermatology 190: 186–191

Farinas I, Jones KR, Backus C, Wang XY, Reichardt LF 1994 Severe sensory and sympathetic deficits in mice lacking neurotrophin-3. Nature 369: 658–661

Fitzgerald M, Wall PD, Goedert M, Emson PC 1985 Nerve growth factor counteracts the neurophysiological and neurochemical effects of chronic sciatic nerve section. Brain Research 332: 131–141

Gillardon F, Eschenfelder C, Rush RA, Zimmerman M 1995 Increase in neuronal Jun immunoreactivity and epidermal NGF levels following UV exposure of rat skin. Neuroreport 6: 1322–1324

Goedert M, Stoeckel K, Otten U 1981 Biological importance of the retrograde axonal transport of nerve growth factor in sensory neurons. Proceedings of the National Academy of Sciences USA 78: 5895–5898

Gold BG, Mobley WC, Matheson SF 1991 Regulation of axonal caliber, neurofilament content, and nuclear localization in mature sensory neurons by nerve growth factor. Journal of Neuroscience 11: 943–955

Gold BG, Storm-Dickerson T, Austin DR 1993 Regulation of the transcription factor c-JUN by nerve growth factor in adult sensory neurons. Neuroscience Letters 154: 129–133

Gotz R, Koster R, Winkler C, Raulf F, Lottspeich F, Schartl M 1994 Neurotrophin-6 is a new member of the nerve growth factor family. Nature 372: 266–269

Hamada A, Watanabe N, Ohtomo H, Matsuda H 1996 Nerve growth factor enhances survival and cytotoxic activity of human eosinophils. British Journal of Haematology 93: 299–302

Herzberg U, Eliav E, Dorsey JM, Gracely RH, Kopin IJ 1997 NGF involvement in pain induced by chronic constriction injury of the rat sciatic nerve. Neuroreport 8: 1613–1618

Heumann R, Korsching S, Bandtlow C, Thoenen H 1987 Changes of nerve growth factor synthesis in nonneuronal cells in response to sciatic nerve transection. Journal of Cell Biology 104: 1623–1631

Hokfelt T, Zhang X, Wiesenfeld-Hallin Z 1994 Messenger plasticity in primary sensory neurons following axotomy and its functional implications. Trends in Neurosciences 17: 22–30

Horigome K, Bullock ED, Johnson EM Jr 1994 Effects of nerve growth factor on rat peritoneal mast cells. Survival promotion and immediate-early gene induction. Journal of Biological Chemistry 269: 2695–2702

Hu-Tsai M, Winter J, Emson PC, Woolf CJ 1994 Neurite outgrowth and GAP-43 mRNA expression in cultured adult rat dorsal root ganglion neurons: effects of NGF or prior peripheral axotomy. Journal of Neuroscience Research 39: 634–645

Indo Y, Tsuruta M, Hayashida Y et al 1996 Mutations in the TRKA/NGF receptor gene in patients with congenital insensitivity to pain with anhidrosis. Nature Genetics 13: 485–488

Ip NY, Stitt TN, Tapley P et al 1993 Similarities and differences in the way neurotrophins interact with the Trk receptors in neuronal and nonneuronal cells. Neuron 10: 137–149

Janig W 1995 The sympathetic nervous system in pain [review]. European Journal of Anaesthesiology – Supplement 10: 53–60

Jing S, Wen D, Yu Y et al 1996 GDNF-induced activation of the ret protein tyrosine kinase is mediated by GDNFR-alpha, a novel receptor for GDNF. Cell 85: 1113–1124

Jing S, Yu Y, Fang M et al 1997 GFRalpha-2 and GFRalpha-3 are two new receptors for ligands of the GDNF family. Journal of Biological Chemistry 272: 33111–33117

Johnson EM Jr, Gorin PD, Brandeis LD, Pearson J 1980 Dorsal root ganglion neurons are destroyed by exposure in utero to maternal antibody to nerve growth factor. Science 210: 916–918

Jones KR, Farinas I, Backus C, Reichardt LF 1994 Targeted disruption of the BDNF gene perturbs brain and sensory neuron development but not motor neuron development. Cell 76: 989–999

Jones MG, Munson JB, Thompson SWN 1998 A role for nerve growth factor in sympathetic sprouting in rat dorsal root ganglia. Pain 79: 21–29

Kang H, Schuman EM 1995 Long-lasting neurotrophin-induced enhancement of synaptic transmission in the adult hippocampus. Science 267: 1658–1662

Kaplan DR, Hempstead BL, Martin-Zanca D, Chao MV, Parada LF 1991 The trk proto-oncogene product: a signal transducing receptor for nerve growth factor. Science 252: 554–558

Kashiba H, Noguchi K, Ueda Y, Senba E 1995 Coexpression of trk family members and low-affinity neurotrophin receptors in rat dorsal root ganglion neurons. Brain Research. Molecular Brain Research 30: 158–164

Kehl IJ, Trempe TM, Shelton DL, Hargreaves KM 1998 Exogenous and endogenous NGF modulate carrageenan-evoked muscle hyperalgesia. Journal of Dental Research 77: 1271

Kendall G, Brar-Rai A, Ensor E, Winter J, Wood JN, Latchman DS 1995 Nerve growth factor induces the Oct-2 transcription factor in sensory neurons with the kinetics of an immediate-early gene. Journal of Neuroscience Research 40: 169–176

Kerr BJ, Bradbury EJ, Trivedi PM et al 1999 Brain Derived Neurotrophic Factor (BDNF) is a prolonged modulator of spinal synaptic excitability. (submitted)

Klein R, Smeyne RJ, Wurst W et al 1993 Targeted disruption of the trkB neurotrophin receptor gene results in nervous system lesions and neonatal death. Cell 75: 113–122

Klein R, Silos-Santiago I, Smeyne RJ et al 1994 Disruption of the neurotrophin-3 receptor gene trkC eliminates la muscle afferents and results in abnormal movements. Nature 368: 249–251

Klein RD, Sherman D, Ho WH et al 1997 A GPI-linked protein that interacts with Ret to form a candidate neurturin receptor. Nature 387: 717–721

Knyihar-Csillik E, Rakic P, Csillik B 1987 Transganglionic degenerative atrophy in the substantia gelatinosa of the spinal cord after peripheral nerve transection in rhesus monkeys. Cell and Tissue Research 247: 599–604

Korte M, Carroll P, Wolf E, Brem G, Thoenen H, Bonhoeffer T 1995 Hippocampal long-term potentiation is impaired in mice lacking brain-derived neurotrophic factor. Proceedings of the National Academy of Sciences USA 92: 8856–8860

Kotzbauer PT, Lampe PA, Heuckeroth RO et al 1996 Neurturin, a relative of glial-cell-line-derived neurotrophic factor. Nature 384: 467–470

Lawson SN 1992 Morphological and biochemical cell types of sensory neurons. In: Scott SA (ed) Sensory neurons. Oxford University Press, New York, pp 27–59

Lawson SN, Harper AA, Harper EI, Garson JA, Anderton BH 1984 A monoclonal antibody against neurofilament protein specifically labels a subpopulation of rat sensory neurones. Journal of Comparative Neurology 228: 263–272

Leclere PG, Ekstrom P, Edstrom A, Priestley JV, Averill S, Tonge DA 1998 Effects of glial cell line-derived neurotrophic factor on axonal growth and apoptosis in adult mammalian sensory neurons in vitro. Neuroscience 82: 545–558

Lee KF, Li E, Huber LJ, Landis SC et al 1992 Targeted mutation of the gene encoding the low affinity NGF receptor p75 leads to deficits in the peripheral sensory nervous system. Cell 69: 737–749

Lee SE, Shen H, Tagliatela G, Chung JM, Chung K 1998 Expression of nerve growth factor in the dorsal root ganglion after peripheral nerve injury. Brain Research 796: 99–106

Lekan HA, Carlton SM, Coggeshall RE 1996 Sprouting of A beta fibres into lamina II of the rat dorsal horn in peripheral neuropathy. Neuroscience Letters 208: 147–150

Leon A, Buriani A, Dal Toso R et al 1994 Mast cells synthesize, store, and release nerve growth factor. Proceedings of the National Academy of Sciences USA 91: 3739–3743

Leslie TA, Emson PC, Dowd PM, Woolf CJ 1995 Nerve growth factor contributes to the up-regulation of growth-associated protein 43 and preprotachykinin A messenger RNAs in primary sensory neurons following peripheral inflammation. Neuroscience 54: 753–762

Levi-Montalcini R 1987 The nerve growth factor: thirty-five years later. Bioscience Reports 7: 681–699

Levine ES, Crozier RA, Black IB, Lummer MR 1998 Brain-derived neurotrophic factor modulates hippocampal synaptic transmission by increasing *N*-methyl-D-aspartic acid receptor activity. Proceedings of the National Academy of Science USA 95: 10235–10239

Levine JD, Lau W, Kwiat G, Goetzl EJ 1984 Leukotriene B4 produces hyperalgesia that is dependent on polymorphonuclear leukocytes. Science 225: 743–745

Levine JD, Taiwo YO, Collins SD, Tam JK 1986 Noradrenaline hyperalgesia is mediated through interaction with sympathetic postganglionic neurone terminals rather than activation of primary afferent nociceptors. Nature 323: 158–160

Lewin GR, Ritter AM, Mendell LM 1993 Nerve growth factor-induced hyperalgesia in the neonatal and adult rat. Journal of Neuroscience 13: 2136–2148

Lewin GR, Rueff A, Mendell LM 1994 Peripheral and central mechanisms of NGF-induced hyperalgesia. European Journal of Neuroscience 6: 1903–1912

Lin LF, Doherty DH, Lile JD, Bektesh S, Collins F 1993 GDNF: a glial cell line-derived neurotrophic factor for midbrain dopaminergic neurons [see comments]. Science 260: 1130–1132

Lin SY, Wu K, Levine ES, Mount HTJ, Suen PC, Black IB 1998 BDNF acutely increases tyrosine phosphorylation of the NMDA receptor subunit 2B in cortical and hippocampal postsynaptic densities. Molecular Brain Research 55: 20–27

Lindsay RM 1988 Nerve growth factors (NGF, BDNF) enhance axonal regeneration but are not required for survival of adult sensory neurons. Journal of Neuroscience 8: 2394–2405

Lindsay RM 1996 Role of neurotrophins and trk receptors in the development and maintenance of sensory neurons: an overview. Philosophical Transactions of the Royal Society of London. Series B 351: 365–373

Lindsay RM, Harmar AJ 1989 Nerve growth factor regulates expression of neuropeptide genes in adult sensory neurons. Nature 337: 362–364

Lowe EM, Anand P, Terenghi G et al 1997 Increased nerve growth factor levels in the urinary bladder of women with idiopathic sensory urgency and interstitial cystitis. British Journal of Urology 79: 572–577

Ma QP, Woolf CJ 1997 The progressive tactile hyperalgesia induced by peripheral inflammation is nerve growth factor dependent. Neuroreport 8: 807–810

Malcangio M, Garrett NE, Cruwys S, Tomlinson DR 1997 Nerve growth factor- and neurotrophin-3-induced changes in nocciceptive threshold and the release of substance P from the rat isolated spinal cord. Journal of Neuroscience 17: 8459–8467

Mannion RJ, Doubell TP, Coggeshall RE, Woolf CJ 1996 Collateral sprouting of uninjured primary afferent A-fibers into the superficial dorsal horn of the adult rat spinal cord after topical capsaicin treatment of the sciatic nerve. Journal of Neuroscience 16: 5189–5195

Mannion RJ, Doubell TP, Gill H, Woolf CJ 1998 Deafferentation is insufficient to induce sprouting of A-fibre central terminals in the rat dorsal horn. Journal of Comparative Neurology 393: 135–144

Mannion RJ, Costigan M, Ma QP et al 1999 Brain-derived neurotrophic factor-a centrally acting pain modulator (in press)

Marshall CJ 1995 Specificity of receptor tyrosine kinase signaling: transient versus sustained extracellular signal-regulated kinase activation. Cell 80: 179–185

Martin HA, Basbaum AI, Goetzl EJ, Levine JD 1988 Leukotriene B4 decreases the mechanical and thermal thresholds of C-fiber nociceptors in the hairy skin of the rat. Journal of Neurophysiology 60: 438–445

Mazurek N, Weskamp G, Erne P, Otten U 1986 Nerve growth factor induces mast cell degranulation without changing intracellular calcium levels. FEBS Letters 198: 315–320

McLachlan EM, Jang W, Devor M, Michaelis M 1993 Peripheral nerve injury triggers noradrenergic sprouting within dorsal root ganglia. Nature 363: 543–546

McMahon SB, Lewin GR, Wall PD 1993 Central hyperexcitability triggered by noxious inputs. Current Opinion in Neurobiology 3: 602–610

McMahon SB, Priestley JV 1995 Peripheral neuropathies and neurotrophic factors: animal models and clinical perspectives. Current Opinion in Neurobiology 5: 616–624

McMahon SB, Armanini MP, Ling LH, Phillips HS 1994 Expression and coexpression of Trk receptors in subpopulations of adult primary sensory neurons projecting to identified peripheral targets. Neuron 12: 1161–1171

McMahon SB, Bennett DLH, Priestley JV, Shelton DL 1995 The biological effects of endogenous NGF in adult sensory neurons revealed by a trkA-IgG fusion molecule. Nature Medicine 1(8): 774–780

Michael GJ, Averill S, Nitkunan A et al 1997 Nerve growth factor treatment increases brain-derived neurotrophic factor selectively in TrkA-expressing dorsal root ganglion cells and in their central terminations within the spinal cord. Journal of Neuroscience 17: 8476–8490

Michael GJ, Averill S, Shortland PJ, Yan Q, Priestley JV 1999 Axotomy results in major changes in BDNF expression by dorsal root ganglion cells: BDNF expression in large trkB and trkC cells, in pericellular baskets, and in projections to deep dorsal horn and dorsal column nuclei (submitted).

Milbrandt J, De Sauvage FJ, Fahrner TJ et al 1998 Persephin, a novel neurotrophic factor related to GDNF and neurturin. Neuron 20: 245–253

Mohiuddin L, Fernyhough P, Tomlinson DR 1995 Reduced levels of mRNA encoding endoskeletal and growth-associated proteins in sensory ganglia in experimental diabetes. Diabetes 44: 25–30
Molliver DC, Snider WD 1997 Nerve growth factor receptor TrkA is down-regulated during postnatal development by a subset of dorsal root ganglion neurons. Journal of Comparative Neurology 381: 428–438
Molliver DC, Radeke MJ, Feinstein SC, Snider WD 1995 Presence or absence of trkA protein distinguishes subsets of small sensory neurons with unique cytochemical characteristics and dorsal horn projections. Journal of Comparative Neurology 361: 404–416
Molliver DC, Wright DE, Leitner ML et al 1997 IB4-binding DRG neurons switch from NGF to GDNF dependence in early postnatal life. Neuron 19: 849–861
Moore MW, Klein RD, Farinas I et al 1996 Renal and neuronal abnormalities in mice lacking GDNF. Nature 382: 76–79
Mulderry PK, Dobson SP 1996 Regulation of VIP and other neuropeptides by c-Jun in sensory neurons: implications for the neuropeptide response to axotomy. European Journal of Neurosciences 8: 2479–2491
Munson JB, Shelton DL, McMahon SB 1998 Adult mammalian sensory and motor neurons: roles of endogenous neurotrophins and rescue by exogenous neurotrophins after axotomy. Journal of Neuroscience 17: 470–476
Naveilhan P, Baudet C, Mikaels A, Shen L, Westphal H, Ernfors P 1998 Expression and regulation of GFRalpha3, a glial cell line-derived neurotrophic factor family receptor. Proceedings of the National Academy of Sciences USA 95: 1295–1300
Neumann S, Doubell TP, Leslie T, Woolf CJ 1996 Inflammatory pain hypersensitivity mediated by phenotypic switch in myelinated primary sensory neurons. Nature 384: 360–364
Ohara S, Tantuwaya V, Distefano PS, Schmidt RE 1995 Exogenous NT-3 mitigates the transganglionic neuropeptide Y response to sciatic nerve injury. Brain Research 699: 143–148
Okuse K, Chaplan SR, McMahon SB et al 1997 Regulation of expression of the sensory neuron-specific sodium channel SNS in inflammatory and neuropathic pain. Molecular and Cellular Neurosciences 10: 196–207
Oppenheim RW 1996 Neurotrophic survival molecules for motoneurons: an embarrassment of riches. Neuron 17: 195–197
Otten U, Baumann JB, Girard J 1984 Nerve growth factor induces plasma extravasation in rat skin. European Journal of Pharmacology 106: 199–201
Otten U, Ehrhard P, Peck R 1989 Nerve growth factor induces growth and differentiation of human B lymphocytes. Proceedings of the National Academy of Sciences USA 86: 10059–10063
Patterson SL, Abel T, Deuel TA, Martin KC, Rose JC, Kandel ER 1996 Recombinant BDNF rescues deficits in basal synaptic transmission and hippocampal LTP in BDNF knockout mice. Neuron 16: 1137–1145
Paus R, Luftl M, Czarnetzki BM 1994 Nerve growth factor modulates keratinocyte proliferation in murine skin organ culture. British Journal of Dermatology 130: 174–180
Petersen M, Segond VB, Heppelmann B, Koltzenburg M 1998 Nerve growth factor regulates the expression of bradykinin binding sites on adult sensory neurons via the neurotrophin receptor p75. Neuroscience 83: 161–168
Petty BG, Cornblath DR, Adornato BT et al 1994 The effect of systemically administered recombinant human nerve growth factor in healthy human subjects. Annals of Neurology 36: 244–246
Pichel JG, Shen L, Sheng HZ et al 1996 Defects in enteric innervation and kidney development in mice lacking GDNF. Nature 382: 73–76
Raivich G, Hellweg R, Kreutzberg GW 1991 NGF receptor-mediated reduction in axonal NGF uptake and retrograde transport following sciatic nerve injury and during regeneration. Neuron 7: 151–164
Ramer MS, Bisby MA 1999 Adrenergic innervation of rat sensory ganglia following proximal or distal painful sciatic neuropathy: distinct mechanisms revealed by anti-NGF treatment Eve J. Neuro Science. (1999) 11: 837–846
Ren K, Thomas DA, Dubner R 1995 Nerve growth factor alleviates a painful peripheral neuropathy in rats. Brain Research 699: 286–292
Rich KM, Luszczynski JR, Osborne PA, Johnson EM Jr 1987 Nerve growth factor protects adult sensory neurons from cell death and atrophy caused by nerve injury. Journal of Neurocytology 16: 261–268
Ritter AM, Lewin GR, Kremer NE, Mendell LM. 1991. Requirement of nerve growth factor in the development of myelinated nociceptors in vivo. Nature 350: 500–502.
Rueff A, and Mendell LM 1996. Nerve growth-factor and NT-5 induce increased thermal sensitivity of cutaneous nociceptors in vitro. Journal of Neurophysiology 76: 3593–3596.
Ruit KG, Elliott JL, Osborne PA, Yan Q, Snider WD 1992 Selective dependence of mammalian dorsal root ganglion neurons on nerve growth factor during embryonic development. Neuron 8: 573–587
Safieh-Garabedian B, Poole S, Allchorne A, Winter J, Woolf CJ 1995 Contribution of interleukin-1 beta to the inflammation-induced increase in nerve growth factor levels and inflammatory hyperalgesia. British Journal of Pharmacology 115: 1265–1275
Sanchez MP, Silos-Santiago I, Frisen J, He B, Lira SA, Barbacid M 1996 Renal agenesis and the absence of enteric neurons in mice lacking GDNF. Nature 382: 70–73
Sanicola M, Hession C, Worley D et al 1997 Glial cell line-derived neurotrophic factor-dependent RET activation can be mediated by two different cell-surface accessory proteins. Proceedings of the National Academy of Sciences USA 94: 6238–6243
Schecterson LC, Bothwell M 1992 Novel roles for neurotrophins are suggested by BDNF and NT-3 mRNA expression in developing neurons. Neuron 9: 449–463
Schlessinger J 1994 SH2/SH3 signaling proteins. Current Opinion in Genetics and Development 4: 25–30
Schuchardt A, D'Agati V, Larsson-Blomberg L, Constantini F, Pachnis V 1994 Defects in the kidney and enteric nervous system of mice lacking the tyrosine kinase receptor Ret. Nature 367: 380–383
Shelton DL, Sutherland J, Gripp J et al 1995 Human trks: molecular cloning, tissue distribution, and expression of extracellular domain immunoadhesins. Journal of Neuroscience 15: 477–491
Shortland P, Woolf CJ 1993 Chronic peripheral nerve section results in a rearrangement of the central axonal arborizations of axotomized A beta primary afferent neurons in the rat spinal cord. Journal of Comparative Neurology 330: 65–82
Shortland P, Yu LC, Lundeberg T, Molander C 1995 Neuropathic nerve injury induces sprouting of A fibre primary afferents into substantia gelatinosa of the adult rat spinal cord. Society of Neuroscience Abstracts 21: 356
Shu XQ, Llinas A, Mendell LM 1998 Effects of trkB and trkC neurotrophin receptor agonists on thermal nociception: a behavioural and electrophysiological study. Pain [In press]
Silos-Santiago I, Molliver DC, Ozaki S et al 1995 Non-TrkA-expressing small DRG neurons are lost in TrkA deficient mice. Journal of Neuroscience 15: 5929–5942
Silverman JD, Kruger L 1988 Lectin and neuropeptide labeling of separate populations of dorsal root ganglion neurons and associated 'nociceptor' thin axons in rat testis and cornea whole-mount preparations. Somatosensory Research 5: 259–267
Smeyne RJ, Klein R, Schnapp A et al 1994 Severe sensory and sympathetic neuropathies in mice carrying a disrupted Trk/NGF receptor gene. Nature 368: 246–249
Snider WD 1994 Functions of the neurotrophins during nervous system development: what the knockouts are teaching us. Cell 77: 627–638

Snider WD, McMahon SB 1998 Tackling pain at the source: new ideas about nociceptors. Neuron 20: 629–632
Snider WD, Silos-Santiago I 1996 Dorsal root ganglion neurons require functional neurotrophin receptors for survival during development [review]. Philosophical Transactions of the Royal Society of London. Series B 351: 395–403
Stucky CL, Dechiara TM, Lindsay RM, Yancopoulos GD, Koltzenburg M 1998 Neurotrophin 4 is required for the survival of a subclass of hair follicle receptors. Journal of Neuroscience 18: 7040–7046
Sun Y, Zigmond RE 1996 Leukaemia inhibitory factor induced in the sciatic nerve after axotomy is involved in the induction of galanin in sensory neurons. European Journal of Neuroscience 8: 2213–2220
Thoenen H 1995 Neurotrophins and neuronal plasticity [review]. Science 270: 593–598
Thompson J, Doxakis E, Pinon LG et al 1998a GFRalpha-4, a new GDNF family receptor. Molecular and Cellular Neurosciences 11: 117–126
Thompson SW, Majithia AA 1998 Leukemia inhibitory factor induces sympathetic sprouting in intact dorsal root ganglia in the adult rat in vivo. Journal of Physiology 506: 809–816
Thompson SW, Dray A, Urban L 1996 Leukemia inhibitory factor induces mechanical allodynia but not thermal hyperalgesia in the juvenile rat. Neuroscience 71: 1091–1094
Thompson SWN, Dray A, McCarson KE, Krause JE, Urban L 1995 Nerve growth factor induces mechanical allodynia associated with novel A fibre-evoked spinal reflex activity and enhanced neurokinin-1 receptor activation in the rat. Pain 62: 219–231
Thompson SW, Vernallis AB, Heath JK, Priestley JV 1997 Leukaemia inhibitory factor is retrogradely transported by a distinct population of adult rat sensory neurons: co-localization with trkA and other neurochemical markers. European Journal of Neuroscience 9: 1244–1251
Thompson SW, Priestley JV, Southall A 1998b gp130 cytokines, leukemia inhibitory factor and interleukin-6, induce neuropeptide expression in intact adult rat sensory neurons in vivo: time-course, specificity and comparison with sciatic nerve axotomy. Neuroscience 84: 1247–1255
Tominaga M, Caterina MJ, Malmberg AB et al 1998 The cloned capsaicin receptor integrates multiple pain-prducing stimuli. Neuron 21: 531–543
Tonra JR, Curtis R, Wong V et al 1998 Axotomy upregulates the anterograde transport and expression of brain-derived neurotrophic factor by sensory neurons. Journal of Neuroscience 18: 4374–4383
Treanor JJ, Goodman L, De Sauvage F et al 1996 Characterization of a multicomponent receptor for GDNF. Nature 382: 80–83
Verge VM, Richardson PM, Benoit R, Riopelle RJ 1989 Histochemical characterization of sensory neurons with high-affinity receptors for nerve growth factor. Journal of Neurocytology 18: 583–591
Verge VM, Tetzlaff W, Bisby MA, Richardson PM 1990 Influence of nerve growth factor on neurofilament gene expression in mature primary sensory neurons. Journal of Neuroscience 10: 2018–2025
Verge VM, Merlio JP, Grondin J et al 1992 Colocalization of NGF binding sites, trk mRNA, and low-affinity NGF receptor mRNA in primary sensory neurons: responses to injury and infusion of NGF. Journal of Neuroscience 12: 4011–4022
Verge VM, Richardson PM, Wiesenfeld-Hallin Z, Hokfelt T 1995 Differential influence of nerve growth factor on neuropeptide expression in vitro: a novel role in peptide suppression in adult sensory neurons. Journal of Neuroscience 15: 2081–2096
Weskamp G, Otten U 1987 An enzyme-linked immunoassay for nerve growth factor (NGF): a tool for studying regulatory mechanisms involved in NGF production in brain and in peripheral tissues. Journal of Neurochemistry 48: 1779–1786
Wetmore C, Olson L 1995 Neuronal and nonneuronal expression of neurotrophins and their receptors in sensory and sympathetic ganglia suggest new intercellular trophic interactions. Journal of Comparative Neurology 353: 143–159
Winter J, Forbes CA, Sternberg J, Lindsay RM 1988 Nerve growth factor (NGF) regulates adult rat cultured dorsal root ganglion neuron responses to the excitotoxin capsaicin. Neuron 1: 973–981
Wong J, Oblinger MM 1991 NGF rescues substance P expression but not neurofilament or tubulin gene expression in axotomized sensory neurons. Journal of Neuroscience 11: 543–552
Woolf CJ, Reynolds ML, Molander C, O'Brien C, Lindsay RM, Benowitz LI 1990 The growth-associated protein GAP-43 appears in dorsal root ganglion cells and in the dorsal horn of the rat spinal cord following peripheral nerve injury. Neuroscience 34: 465–478
Woolf CJ, Safieh-Garabedian B, Ma QP, Crilly P, Winter J 1994 Nerve growth factor contributes to the generation of inflammatory sensory hypersensitivity. Neuroscience 62: 327–331
Woolf CJ, Shortland P, Coggeshall RE 1992 Peripheral nerve injury triggers central sprouting of myelinated afferents. Nature 355: 75–78
Woolf CJ, Ma QP, Allchorne A, Poole S 1996 Peripheral cell types contributing to the hyperalgesic action of nerve growth factor in inflammation. Journal of Neuroscience 16: 2716–2723
Woolf CJ, Allchorne A, Safieh-Garabedian B, Poole S 1997 Cytokines, nerve growth factor and inflammatory hyperalgesia: the contribution of tumour necrosis factor alpha. British Journal of Pharmacology 121: 417–424
Woolf CJ, Mannion RJ, Neumann S 1998 Null mutations lacking substance: elucidating pain mechanisms by genetic pharmacology. Neuron 20: 1063–1066
Worby CA, Vega QC, Chao HH, Seasholtz AF, Thompson RC, Dixon JE 1998 Identification and characterization of GFRalpha-3, a novel Co-receptor belonging to the glial cell line-derived neurotrophic receptor family. Journal of Biological Chemistry 273: 3502–3508
Wright DE, Snider WD 1995 Neurotrophin receptor mRNA expression defines distinct populations of neurons in rat dorsal root ganglia. Journal of Comparative Neurology 351: 329–338

Pathophysiology of damaged nerves in relation to chronic pain

MARSHALL DEVOR & ZE'EV SELTZER

INTRODUCTION

Trauma or disease affecting peripheral nerves frequently results in the development of chronic, often intractable, pain. The clinical importance of these 'neuropathic' pain syndromes provides a strong incentive for understanding the underlying pathophysiological mechanisms. There is a general consensus today that both peripheral and central nervous system (PNS, CNS) processes play a role. The aim of this chapter is to summarize the state of knowledge on PNS pathophysiology associated with neuropathic pain, with special emphasis on processes relevant to clinical symptomatology.

THE PARADOX OF NEUROPATHIC PAIN

Chronic pain following nerve injury is a paradox. Just as cutting a telephone wire leaves the line dead, cutting axons should deaden sensation. Why then is nerve injury and disease frequently associated with:

1. spontaneous paraesthesias, dysaesthesia and frank pain
2. pain evoked by movement
3. tenderness of the partly denervated body part?

Moreover, why are the sensations associated with nerve injury so often peculiar? For example, why is neuropathic pain often paroxysmal, electric shock-like, tingling, shooting or burning? And how do we account for 'hyperpathia', the fact that pain sometimes persists after the stimulus has ended, spreads from the site of stimulation or starts dull but winds up to an intense crescendo on repeated touching (Noordenbos 1959)? Although uncertainties remain, recent animal and clinical research has begun to provide cogent answers to these questions.

CHRONIC PAIN DEPENDS ON THE BEHAVIOUR OF NEURONS

Although it may seem trivially obvious, it is emphasized at the outset that skin, muscle, bone and viscera cannot give rise to a sensation of pain except inasmuch as they contribute to the initiation of electrical impulses in nerve fibres. On the other hand, impulses that arise directly in nerves or the CNS evoke sensations that are felt in (i.e. 'referred to') the corresponding peripheral tissues. Sensation, including pain, is the domain of the nervous system. To understand neuropathic pain, we must know how injury and disease affect the generation of afferent (i.e. sensory) signals, how they affect the transmission of afferent signals to the CNS and how they affect central processing of these signals.

'NORMAL', 'NOCICEPTIVE', 'INFLAMMATORY', 'PATHOPHYSIOLOGICAL' AND 'NEUROPATHIC' PAIN

Normally, pain is felt when impulses reach a conscious brain along thinly myelinated (Aδ) and/or unmyelinated (C) nociceptive afferents. Examples are pinprick or a stubbed toe. Due to the high threshold of most Aδ- and C-afferent endings, noxious stimuli are required to activate them. The resulting sensation (pain) matches the stimulus (noxious). This is 'normal' ('nociceptive') pain.

Minor tissue injuries, including burns, abrasions and infections, often cause a reduction in the threshold of nociceptor endings, sensitizing them. This change is caused by chemical inflammatory mediators released in the tissue (see Ch. 2). Certain irritant chemicals applied to skin or deep tissue can trigger such 'peripheral sensitization' directly. Once sensitized, nociceptors respond to weak, non-noxious stimuli. The resulting tenderness is termed primary 'allodynia'. In addition, noxious stimuli typically evoke more pain than normal ('primary hyperalgesia'; Merskey & Bogduk 1994). The sensation (pain) no longer matches the stimulus in the normal way.

In addition to peripheral sensitization, allodynia and hyperalgesia can also result from abnormal signal amplification in the CNS, a process called 'central sensitization' (Hardy et al 1952, Woolf 1991, Devor et al 1991). There is now good evidence that in the presence of central sensitization peripheral input entering the CNS along non-nociceptive, thickly myelinated, Aβ touch afferents may evoke pain (e.g., Cook et al 1987, Campbell et al 1988, Woolf 1991, Torebjork et al 1992, Koltzenburg et al 1994b). This is a clear violation of the classical dogma that pain is derived exclusively by Aδ and C afferents, and constitutes a revolution in our understanding of the pain system.

The one condition known to reliably trigger central sensitization is strong nociceptive input. Central sensitization is transient, fading in minutes or hours, but it may be maintained indefinitely if nociceptor input persists. Consider the aftermath of a mild burn or abrasion. The initial noxious event triggers central sensitization, while inflamed peripherally sensitized nociceptors may maintain it for days. So long as central sensitization is present, Aβ touch input from the affected tissue and its immediate surrounds adds to the pain ('secondary hyperalgesia'). The bottom line is that nociceptors and Aβ touch afferents both contribute to everyday inflammatory pain. It should be pointed out that a host of neurochemical and structural changes are evoked in the spinal cord by nerve injury and intense noxious input (Devor 1988, Dubner & Ruda 1992, Hokfelt et al 1997), most of which are not connected in any obvious way to the transient central sensitization mechanism noted (e.g., Munglani et al 1996). One or more of these could subserve prolonged 'centralization' of pain, a quite different process. The evidence for 'centralization', however, remains tentative (see below and Ch. 6).

Peripheral and central sensitization should not be thought of as disease states. They probably evolved as useful adaptations intended to augment pain, and hence protective behaviours, in the event of everyday tissue injuries. Because pain of this sort involves temporarily elevated sensitivity of the pain system, and usually tissue injury and inflammation, we consider it to be 'pathophysiological'. Others call inflammatory pain 'nociceptive', seeing it as a type of 'normal' pain (Fig. 5.1).

Pain may also result from injuries and disease that affect the nervous system directly. This is 'neuropathic' pain (Merskey & Bogduk 1994). Neuropathic pain is thought to result when sensory neurons in the PNS generate impulses at abnormal (ectopic) locations, for example at sites of nerve injury. In addition to firing spontaneously, these ectopic pacemaker sites are often excited by mechanical forces applied to them during movement. The result is spontaneous and movement-evoked pain. The term neuropathic also includes pain associated with damage to spinal roots ('radiculopathic' pain) and to the CNS proper ('central pain'). Stroke or CNS trauma, for example, may cause ectopic firing of central origin, or render brain circuits hyperexcitable, abnormally amplifying input from the periphery. The processes underlying ectopic impulse generation and mechanosensitivity are discussed in detail below.

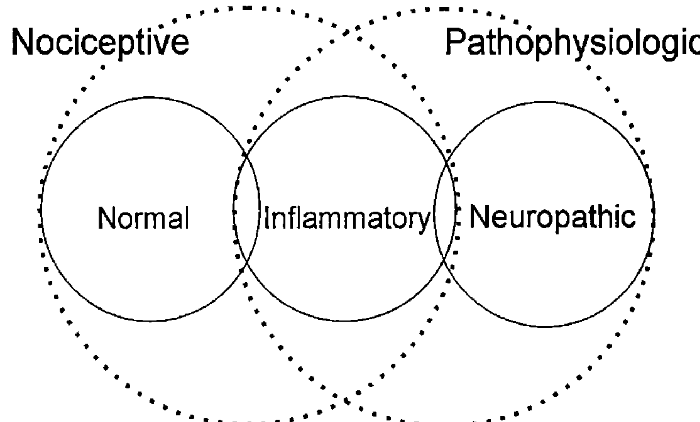

Fig. 5.1 Pain terms. 'Nociceptive pain' refers to the normal, acute pain sensation evoked by noxious stimuli in intact tissue, in the absence of peripheral or central sensitization. Some authors include in this category the subacute spontaneous pain and hypersensitivity that arises in inflamed tissue when nociceptor endings have undergoine peripheral sensitization (central sensitization may also be present). We, on the other hand, prefer to group inflammatory and neuropathic pain under the heading 'pathophysiological', as both involve sensitization of the pain system, due to tissue or nerve pathology, respectively.

A ROLE FOR CENTRAL SENSITIZATION IN NEUROPATHIC PAIN

Nociceptor input triggers and maintains central sensitization whether it arises from inflamed tissue, or from ectopic neuropathic sources. In the case of neuropathic pain, central sensitization has two effects. First, it renders ectopic Aβ input painful, augmenting spontaneous and movement-evoked pain. Second, it renders input from residual uninjured Aβ touch afferents painful. This is thought to be a major cause of allodynia and hyperalgesia in neuropathic pain states.

Such a sequence is illustrated in Figure 5.2. In this study, Sheen and Chung (1993) severed the L5 (or L5+6) spinal nerve, thus injuring about half of the afferents in the sciatic

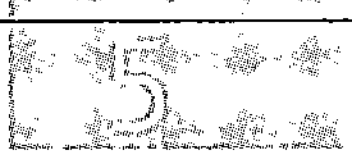

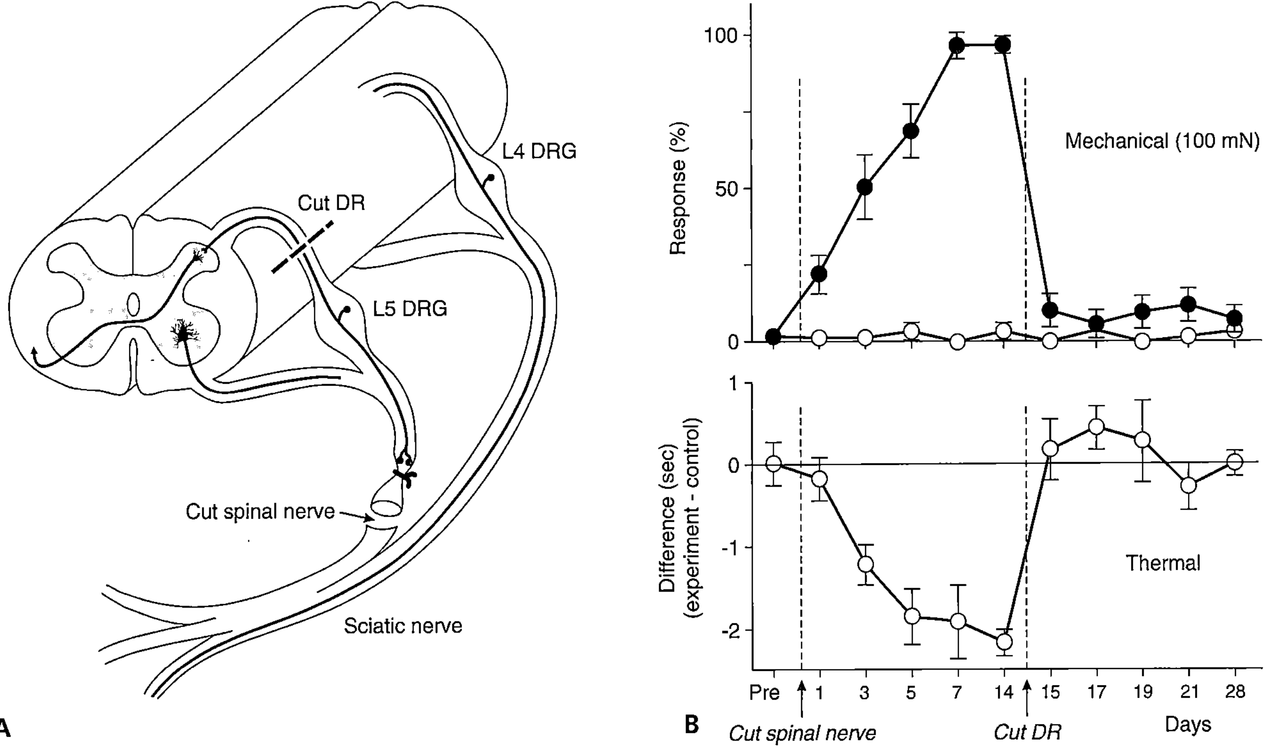

Fig. 5.2 Ectopic discharge originating at sites of nerve injury and associated DRGs contributes to cutaneous hypersensitivity. **A** Primary sensory neurons in lumbar DRGs L4 and L5. Each sends an axonal branch out along a peripheral nerve, and a second through the dorsal root (DR) into the spinal cord. Cutting spinal nerve L5 (arrow, and L6) lead to mechanical and thermal (heat) allodynia on the hindpaw. This is shown in the graphs (**B**) which plot (upper) the percentage of rats tested showing paw withdrawal to gentle mechanical probing (-○- intact side; -●- operated side), and (lower) the time difference (operated – intact) to elicit withdrawal from radiant heating of the paw. Preoperatively (pre) the feet were symmetrical. Allodynia was subsequently eliminated by cutting the L5 DR. This prevented the ectopic discharge from reaching the CNS, allowing central sensitization to dissipate. (See text for further explanation; data from Sheen & Chung 1993).

nerve. This created a source of spontaneous ectopic discharge, and resulted in behavioural signs of spontaneous pain, including licking and protective postures. In addition, however, the ipsilateral hindpaw became abnormally tender to touch and heat stimuli. This is the *opposite* of what might reasonably have been expected from partial denervation, an example of the neuropathic pain paradox. When the investigators later prevented the ectopic firing from gaining access to the CNS by cutting the L5 dorsal root, the spontaneous discomfort was eliminated, as expected. Remarkably, however, the cut also eliminated the hindpaw allodynia. The interpretation is that allodynia in the hindpaw was due to spinal amplification of sensory input arising in the residual undamaged L4 afferents still serving the hindlimb. When the ectopic activity was prevented from reaching the spinal cord, the central sensitization faded and with it the cutaneous allodynia (Sheen & Chung 1993, Yoon et al 1996). Corresponding observations have been reported in humans with neuropathic pain as a result of ectopic pacemaker activity (Gracely et al 1992, Rowbotham & Fields 1996).

IS NEUROPATHIC PAIN A UNITARY PHENOMENON? SPLITTERS VERSUS LUMPERS

Clinical discussions of neuropathic pain frequently point out the dramatic differences among the various neuropathic pain states: differences in aetiology, differences in symptomatology and differences in response to treatment. The implication, stated or implied, is that conditions such as postherpetic neuralgia, intercostal neuralgia and trigeminal neuralgia are fundamentally different diseases. Our thesis is that from the point of view of underlying mechanism the neuropathic pain syndromes have much in common; that many of the apparent differences will turn out to reflect subtleties of the ectopic firing process. For example, sympathetic related pain conditions may be distinguished by excess ectopic adrenosensitivity, while trigeminal neuralgia is distinguished by excess ectopic cross-excitation (see below).

This chapter will deal only in passing with the mechanisms of peripheral and central sensitization. These subjects are discussed in detail elsewhere in this textbook (see Chs 2 and 6).

Rather, it focuses on pathophysiological changes in injured peripheral nerve, ectopic impulse generation ('ectopia') in particular. Because ectopia constitutes a direct nociceptive drive as well as evoking and maintaining central sensitization, its elimination should relieve both the spontaneous and the evoked aspects of neuropathic pain, thus killing two birds with one stone. The reader is encouraged to reflect on the striking parallels between the abnormal electrogenic (i.e. impulse-generating) behaviour of injured sensory neurons and the sensory peculiarities characteristic of various clinical pain syndromes. This resemblance supports the hypothesis that the pathophysiological changes in injured nerves constitute the principal cause of chronic neuropathic pain.

EXCITABILITY: MECHANISMS OF IMPULSE GENERATION (ELECTROGENESIS)

To understand the abnormal electrogenesis that underlies pathophysiological pain one needs to be fluent with the fundamentals of electrogenesis in *normal* sensory neurons. What follows is a brief and qualitative refresher. For a detailed, quantitative discussion the reader is referred to Loewenstein (1971), Jack et al (1983), Sachs (1986) and Hille (1992a). Later in this chapter we will discuss how neural injury and disease pervert normal electrogenesis.

THE PRIMARY AFFERENT NEURON

Afferent axons run uninterrupted from their sensory ending in innervated peripheral tissue to their central synaptic endings in the CNS. The cell body lies along this path in the dorsal root ganglia (DRGs) near the spine (Fig. 5.2), or the cranial nerve ganglia at the base of the skull. Normally, each neuron constitutes an independent sensory communication channel. The main role of the cell body is to provide metabolic support for the axon, i.e. to manufacture all of the various molecules required by the axon to carry out its functions. The axon, in turn, has three distinct functions: to *encode*, to *conduct* and to *relay* sensory messages. Each of these functions imposes particular design demands in response to which evolution has provided the axon with a high degree of regional specialization (Fig. 5.3; Lieberman 1976, Waxman et al 1995). Consider, for example, a myelinated afferent innervating skin of the fingertip. The distal few tens of microns are specialized for translating (transducing and encoding) a mechanical, thermal or chemical stimulus into a propagated impulse train. The mid-axon part, which may be a metre or more in length, is specialized for conducting this signal rapidly and accurately without missing impulses or adding extra ones. The central terminal arbor, with its synaptic endings, is specialized for relaying the sensory message into the CNS.

The diverse electrical properties of the three parts of the axon must be closely regulated. If sensory endings underwent uncontrolled changes in their sensitivity, for example, the CNS would have no way of telling from the incoming impulse train what the original stimulus really was. This regulation is not trivial. Indeed, it is hard to conceive of how stability is maintained year after year, especially in nociceptors, which are rarely if ever activated. Disruption of the normal regulation of regional properties of the sensory neuron by injury or disease contributes significantly to chronic pain.

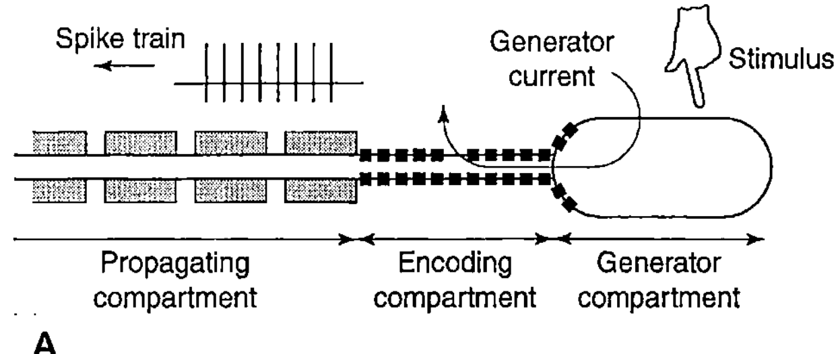

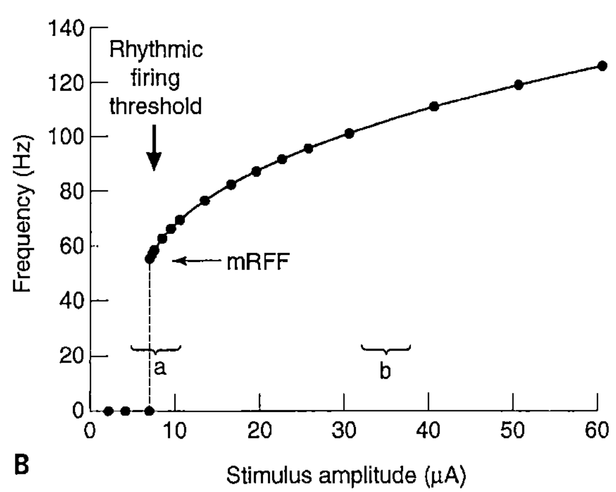

Fig. 5.3 Principles of rhythmic firing. **A** Sketch of a sensory ending showing generator, encoding and propagating compartments. Generator and encoding compartments might be combined in neuroma endbulbs. **B** Frequency–stimulus relationship (encoding function) in response to a prolonged depolarizing generator current (computer simulation). At threshold, the firing rate jumps from zero to the fibre's minimum rhythmic firing frequency (mRFF). A small change in stimulus strength around threshold (region a) has a much larger effect on firing frequency than the same change in region b. (Reproduced from Matzner & Devor 1992.)

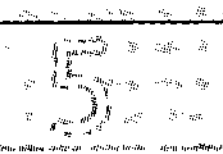

TRANSDUCTION AND ENCODING

Sensory impulse generation typically begins when a stimulus causes an increase in the permeability of the membrane of sensory endings to various ions, particularly Na^+. In mechanoreceptors, stretching triggers the opening of the transmembrane pore of specific transducer proteins called 'stretch-activated channels' (SA channels; Sachs 1986, Hamill & McBride 1994, Nakamura & Strittmatter 1996, Garcia-Anoveros & Corey 1997). Ions then flow through these channels following their electrical and concentration gradient (the generator current), producing partial depolarization of the sensory ending (the generator potential, Fig. 5.3). Likewise, thermal transduction depends on channels whose ionic conductance varies with temperature, and response to chemicals (e.g. bee-sting toxins or capsaicin) depends on generator currents formed when the chemical binds to corresponding receptors (e.g., Caterina et al 1997).

In addition to these transducer molecules, sensory endings contain voltage-sensitive ion-channels. These proteins respond to transmembrane voltage rather than to stretch etc. At rest, the most important of these, the voltage-sensitive Na^+ channels, are closed. Stimulation (mechanical, thermal or chemical) induces a slow generator depolarization which triggers the most sensitive Na^+ channels to open. This lets in a stream of Na^+ ions, adding to the generator depolarization. The now augmented depolarization, in turn, opens still more Na^+ channels, letting in still more Na^+ ions and so forth. The rapidly cascading activation of voltage-sensitive channels causes a depolarizatory explosion, the action potential (also called the nerve impulse, or 'spike'). Note the dual process: a slow ramp depolarization due to transduction channels triggers an explosive action potential due to voltage-sensitive ion channels.

Having opened, Na^+ channels rapidly close again, and the membrane potential drifts back towards its initial resting level. This repolarization may be accelerated by the transient opening of K^+-selective channels. When prolonged, the opening of K^+ channels produces hyperpolarization, delaying recovery to rest. If the stimulus-evoked generator current is still present after the first spike is completed, the spike initiation sequence may repeat itself, yielding a train of action potentials, 'repetitive firing'. By controlling the *rate* of repolarization, K^+ channels act in concert with transducer and voltage-sensitive Na^+ channels to control firing frequency. The translation of the generator potential into a spike train is the 'encoding' process (Fig. 5.3).

THRESHOLD FOR IMPULSE INITIATION AND FOR REPETITIVE FIRING

It is obviously inappropriate to have nerve impulses set off by infinitesimally small stimuli, and this does not happen. The reason is straightforward. When the sensory ending starts to be depolarized, K^+ ions start to flow outward. This K^+ current is hyperpolarizatory and tends to neutralize the depolarizatory generator current, suppressing further depolarization. Only if the generator current (i.e. the stimulus) is large enough to overpower the outward K^+ current will a spike be set off. If it is too small, the depolarization will simply damp out. This establishes a 'threshold' for impulse initiation. Note that the threshold is not a fixed value. Rather, it is a dynamic equilibrium between inward and outward ion currents.

Although the individual action potential is the basic unit of neural signalling, sensory communication, and certainly chronic pain, depends on *sustained* firing. Some cells will not fire more than a few spikes even with intense maintained depolarization. Others fire rapidly with minimal sustained depolarization. Interestingly, in sensory neurons capable of firing repetitively, the threshold for generating repetitive discharge tends to be much higher than the threshold for eliciting a single spike.

Repetitive firing capability ('pacemaker' capability) is a specialized property of the encoding compartment of some sensory endings. It does not normally exist away from the sensory ending. Try applying pressure over the median nerve in your forearm. This does not evoke impulses in the mid-axon portion of the median nerve afferents where the pressure is applied. If it did, you would feel tingling in the medial part of your hand. Injury can bring about a change in the regional repetitive firing properties of the mid-nerve axon. If there had been a neuroma or a patch of demyelination along the course of your median nerve, applying pressure there would have produced a referred sensation in the hand, perhaps even a painful one (Tinel sign). Increased electrical excitability of sensory neurons following injury and disease, and particularly the emergence of ectopic pacemaker capability, appears to be a fundamental substrate of neuropathic pain. The mechanisms that control repetitive firing are therefore important for understanding chronic pain.

REPETITIVE FIRING CAPABILITY

There are two quite different repetitive firing processes. The first is the classical Hodgkin–Huxley (H–H) process described above, whereby a persistent generator potential repeatedly draws the neuronal membrane toward threshold following each spike. The second pacemaker process, which is different from the H–H process, depends on intrinsic reverberatory properties of the neuronal membrane. Specifically, we recently found that some sensory neurons, many following nerve injury, exhibit spontaneous subthreshold oscillations of their membrane potential. When a depolarizing (generator) potential is applied, the peaks of these oscillations reach threshold and initiate high-frequency repetitive firing (Fig. 5.4B, Amir et al 1998). Often, additional ionic conductances modulate repetitive firing on a slower timescale, yielding bursting, accommodation and adaptation.

Both repetitive firing processes, H–H and subthreshold oscillations, feature an interesting non-linearity in the relation of firing frequency to stimulus intensity (encoding or f-I curve; Stein 1967, Matzner & Devor 1992). Below a threshold generator potential the neuron is silent. However once threshold is reached, sustained firing begins with a sudden jump to a relatively high 'minimum rhythmic firing frequency' (mRFF, Fig. 5.3B). The pronounced non-linear jump in the f-I curve at the rhythmic firing threshold yields amplification, and is important for discharge patterning, as described below. In principle, hyperalgesic agents and neuropathy could act by reducing repetitive firing threshold, or enhancing subthreshold oscillations, rather than by augmenting the generator potential as is usually assumed.

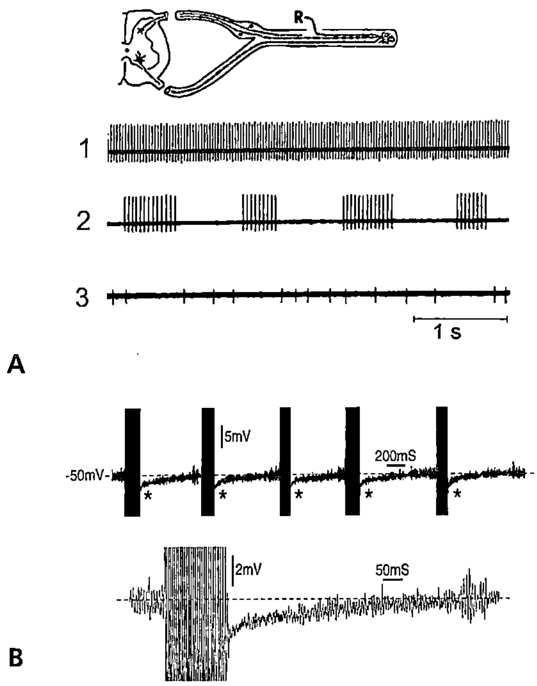

Fig. 5.4 Patterns of spontaneous ectopic discharge recorded from sensory axons ending in a neuroma. **A** Fine axon bundles were microdissected from an injured nerve and placed on a recording electrode (R). Spontaneously active fibres fire tonically (1), in bursts (2) or irregularly (3). **B** Intracellular recording from a DRG neuron with ectopic burst discharge (asterisks, spike height is truncated). One burst is shown in detail below. Bursts are triggered when ongoing membrane potential oscillations reach threshold. The burst initiates a hyperpolarizing shift which stops firing and re-sets the oscillations. (Reproduced from Amir & Devor 1997.)

ECTOPIC REPETITIVE FIRING IN INJURED PERIPHERAL NERVES

NERVE INJURY AND DISEASE, REGENERATION AND NEUROMA FORMATION

When an axon is severed by trauma or as a result of disease, the proximal stump, the part still connected to the cell body, seals off and forms a terminal swelling or 'endbulb'. It may also die back for up to a few millimetres and the myelin sheath near the cut end is invariably disrupted (Cajal 1928, Morris et al 1972, Fawcett & Keynes 1990, Fried et al 1991). In neonates most axotomized cells die, but in adults the majority survive. Within hours or days numerous fine processes start to grow out from the proximal cut end of the axon. Under optimal conditions one of these regenerating 'sprouts' reaches peripheral target tissue and establishes a functional receptor ending. Excess sprouts are then culled. When forward growth is blocked, terminal endbulbs persist, and sprouts either turn back on themselves or form a tangled mass. This structure is a 'neuroma'.

Regeneration is often ideal if the nerve has undergone blunt compression or freezing. But whenever the nerve sheath (perineurium) is breached, disrupting endoneurial/basal lamina tubes, a neuroma is created. 'Nerve-end neuromas', for example, *always* form after limb amputation. If the ends of a cut nerve are reapproximated, some fibres cross the gap and proceed to elongate. Even in the most favourable cases, however, many fibres are trapped near the suture line in a 'neuroma-in-continuity', or begin to elongate but get caught up subsequently, forming disseminated 'microneuromas' scattered along the distal nerve trunk, its branches and its target tissue.

ENDBULBS AND SPROUTS GENERATE ECTOPIC REPETITIVE FIRING

In 1974 Wall and Gutnick reported the presence of massive spontaneous impulse discharges in lower lumbar dorsal roots in rats in which an experimental neuroma had been made by cutting the sciatic nerve. Firing was also affected

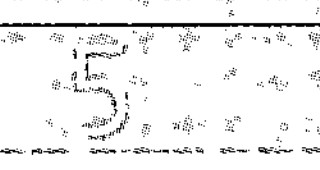

by mechanical and chemical stimulation of the neuroma. This supported suggestions, based on behavioural indicators, that abnormal neural activity generated at ectopic locations in the PNS can trigger neuropathic dysaesthesias and pain (Kugelberg 1946, Konoski & Lubinska 1946).

It was clear from Wall and Gutnick's study that many abnormal impulses originated ectopically in the neuroma, because pressing on it augmented the discharge and anaesthetizing it reduced the discharge. However, because the active roots also contained afferents from nerves that had not been cut, some of the recorded activity undoubtedly originated in intact, spontaneously active proprioceptive and thermosensitive fibres, and in sensory cell somata in the DRG (see below). This ambiguity was resolved when Govrin-Lippmann and Devor (1978), and later a number of other groups, observed ectopic firing of myelinated (A) and unmyelinated (C) axons in recordings made from the nerve itself, just proximal to the neuroma (Fig. 5.4A; e.g. Wiesenfeld & Lindblom 1980, Scadding 1981, Blumberg & Janig 1984, Burchiel 1984a, Brewart & Gentle 1985, Meyer et al 1985, Welk et al 1990, Pinault 1995, Bongenhielm & Robinson 1996). Subsequent experiments showed that ectopic firing likewise originates at neuromas-in-continuity, disseminated microneuromas, sites of nerve compression and regenerating sprouts (e.g. Xie et al 1993, Amir & Devor 1993, Koltzenburg et al 1994a, Pinault 1995, Tal & Eliav 1996, Bongenhielm & Robinson 1998, Chen & Devor 1998), and that, as expected, this ectopic PNS discharge activates second- and higher-order neurons in the CNS (Mao et al 1992, Palecek et al 1992, Laird & Bennett 1993, Sotgiu et al 1994, 1996, Pertovaara et al 1997).

MECHANOSENSITIVITY, THERMOSENSITIVITY AND CHEMOSENSITIVITY

From the earliest reports it was clear that spontaneous ectopic firing is often associated with abnormal response to a range of applied stimuli (hyperexcitability). Such stimuli may enhance ongoing firing or elicit firing in previously silent afferents.

Mechanosensitivity

By exploring the nerve surface in the region of injury with fine probes, it is possible to locate tiny mechanosensitive 'hotspots'. In neuromas, these are clustered close to the cut nerve end. This zone is rich in neuroma endbulbs and sprouts, the structures implicated as the source of the ectopia (Fig. 5.5; Fried et al 1991, Chen & Devor 1998). Mechanosensitive 'hotspots' likewise occur in areas of nerve

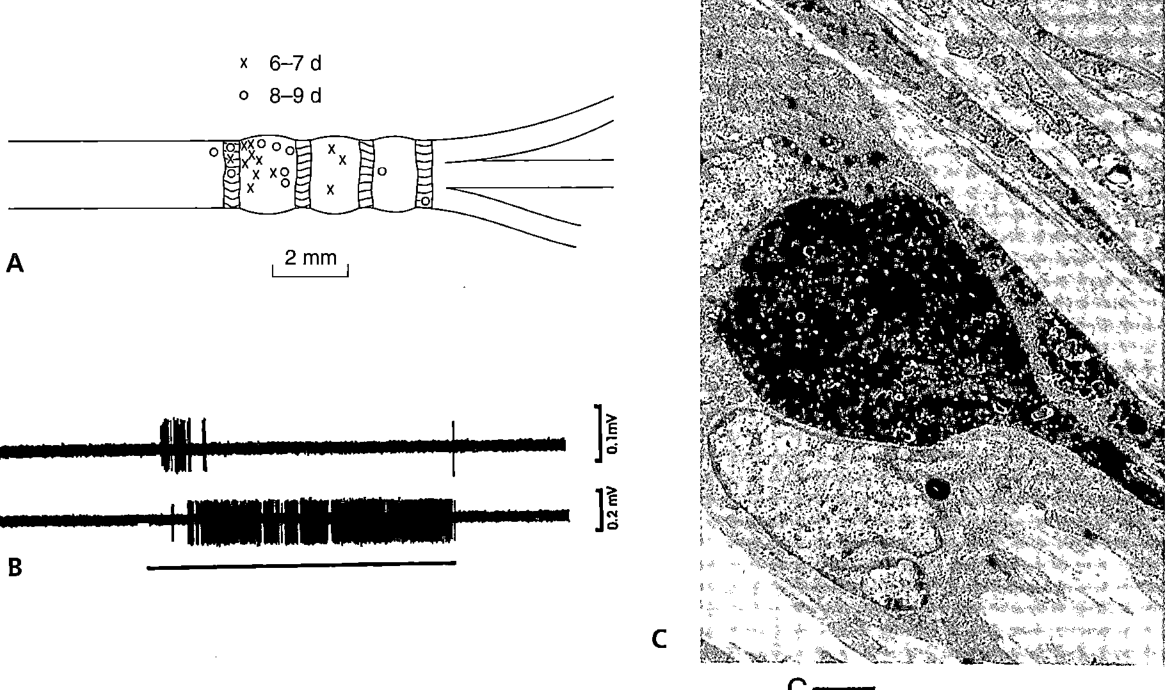

Fig. 5.5 Punctate mechanosensitive 'hotspots' in an injured nerve. **A** Hotspots recorded from the sciatic nerve 6–9 days after chronic constriction injury (CCI, distal tributaries of the nerve are to the right). **B** Traces show rapidly adapting (above) and slowly adapting (below) responses. (Reproduced from Chen & Devor 1998.) **C** A neuroma endbulb, 7 days postinjury, visualized by anterograde filling with WGA-HRP/DAB reaction product. This is the probable appearance of a mechanosensitive hotspot. Scale bar = 3 μm. (Reproduced from Fried et al 1991.) Scalebar (c) 3μm

constriction, and at the outgrowing front in regenerating nerve, where their presence is responsible for the Tinel sign (e.g. Konorski & Lubinska 1946, Tal & Eliav 1996, Chen & Devor 1998). Locations where nerves run adjacent to tendon and bone (e.g., the carpal tunnel), or where small branches cross over tough fascial planes (in low back pain, in fibromyalgia?), are particularly at risk of developing consistently located mechanosensitive triggerpoints (Travell & Simons 1984, Bennett 1990). Hyperexcitable neuroma endbulbs and sprouts are easily missed in routine nerve pathology, but can be visualized using special preparative techniques (Fig. 5.5c).

We have recently shown that spontaneous ectopic firing and ectopic mechanosensitivity originate at the same site, or at least in very close proximity (Chen & Devor 1998). This means that the mechanosensitive hotspots are also the *spontaneous* pacemaker sites. Many injured axons show both abnormalities, although mechanosensitivity can occur without spontaneous firing, and spontaneous firing can occur without mechanosensitivity. Mechanically evoked ectopic discharge is sometimes limited to a short burst at the moment of stimulus onset and/or release (rapid adaptation), or it may last for the duration of force application (Fig. 5.5, slow adaption). Sometimes it continues well after the end of the stimulus (Fig. 5.6A). Such 'afterdischarge' may contribute to the persistence of sensation common in neuropathic pain states (hyperpathia).

Exacerbation of ectopic discharge by temperature and by chemical mediators

Temperature has a paradoxical effect on chronic neuroma endings. In myelinated fibres, the rate of spontaneous discharge increases with warming and additional, previously silent, fibres are recruited. Cooling suppresses firing. Unmyelinated axons, by contrast, tend to be suppressed by warming and excited by cooling (Matzner & Devor 1987). This behaviour may be related to 'cold-intolerance' in amputees.

Metabolic and chemical factors that influence membrane potential can also excite ectopic discharge and exacerbate pain. Examples include tissue ischaemia and anoxia, changes in blood gases and ion concentrations, and numerous endogenous neuroactive substances including catecholamines, peptides, cytokines, neurotrophins, histamine, bradykinin, prostaglandins and a range of other inflammatory mediators (e.g., Wall & Gutnick 1974, Korenman & Devor 1981, Scadding 1981, Devor 1983a, Blumberg & Janig 1984, Low 1985, Zimmermann et al 1987, Devor et al 1992b, Tracey & Walker 1995, Noda et al 1997, Michaelis et al 1998b). Among these, catecholamines and inflammatory mediators appear to play particularly important roles. Anomalous sensitivity to circulating adrenaline, and to noradrenaline released from sympathetic efferent axons, forms the basis for 'sympathetic–sensory coupling', a phenomenon thought to underlie sympathetic-dependent chronic pain. As for inflammatory mediators, damaged nerve fibres come into contact with these substances both at the injury site and during regeneration into injured and inflamed tissue (Rotshenker 1997). Both of these issues are discussed in more detail below.

EVIDENCE OF ECTOPIC FIRING IN PAINFUL NERVE INJURIES IN MAN

The method of percutaneous microneurographic recording from single nerve fibres in awake humans (Vallbo et al 1979) provides a means of verifying the clinical relevance of the animal data on ectopic hyperexcitability. Although practitioners have been justifiably reluctant to insert microelectrodes into problematical nerves in humans for essentially

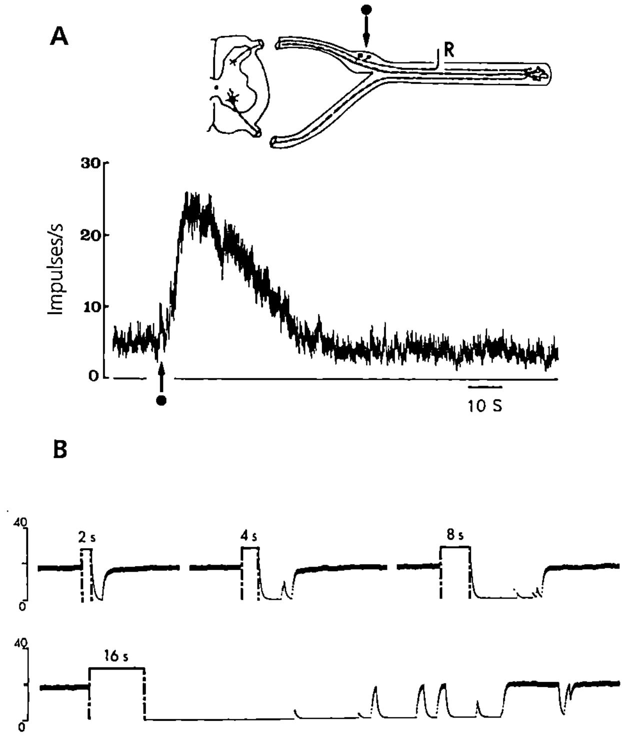

Fig. 5.6 A Afterdischarge originating in a DRG neuron following momentary (0.5-s) application of a 150-mg stimulus to the DRG surface (arrow). The sciatic nerve had been cut 11 days previously. **B** This neuroma ending fired spontaneously at about 20 imp/s (experimental setup as sketch in Fig. 5.4). Stimulation of the nerve central to the injury site (100 Hz) silenced the firing for periods which increased with increasing stimulation duration.

experimental purposes, a small number of such studies has appeared (Torebjork et al 1979, Ochoa & Torebjork 1980, Nystrom & Hagbarth 1981, Ochoa et al 1982, Nordin et al 1984, Cline et al 1989, Mackel 1985, Campers et al 1998). In each, ectopia was observed much as in the animal preparations. Moreover, the authors found a striking correlation between observed ectopic discharges, and felt neuropathic paraesthesias and pain.

For example, Nystrom and Hagbarth (1981) documented ongoing firing in the peroneal nerve in a lower extremity amputee. The patient had ongoing phantom foot pain which was augmented by percussion of the neuroma. The same percussion elicited an intense burst of spike activity, mostly in slowly conducting axons. These bursts were eliminated, along with the evoked pain, by local anaesthetic block of the neuroma. Interestingly, much of the ongoing discharge persisted. Clearly it did not originate in the neuroma, but rather in another ectopic location, central to the recording site. Based on recent animal studies, the most likely location is the DRG (see below). In a related study dysaesthesias referred to the foot were triggered by straight-leg lifting (Lasegue's sign) in a patient with radicular pain related to surgery for disc herniation (Nordin et al 1984). This manoeuvre evoked ectopic bursts in the sural nerve, the intensity of which waxed and waned in close correlation with the abnormal sensation. Nerve blocks indicated that the ectopic source was in the injured spinal root or DRG. Corresponding data were obtained in patients with positive sensory signs (dysaesthesias and pain) associated with entrapment neuropathy. One final case in this series deserves note. This was a patient with multiple sclerosis, in whom positive sensory signs, and impulse activity in the median nerve, were evoked by neck flexion (Lhermitte's sign). The interpretation is that ectopic discharge was generated in a demyelination plaque in the dorsal columns (CNS). Impulses ran centrally causing pain, and antidromically in the same axons, out along the median nerve to where they were picked up by the recording microelectrode.

An additional line of clinical evidence is sensory change evoked by the injection of test substances into foci of neuropathic pain. Animal studies, for example, predict that adrenaline, or K^+-channel blockers injected into a neuroma should augment ectopia and evoke pain, while the injection of Na^+-channel blockers (e.g. lidocaine) should suppress it. These predictions have been verified in man (Chabal et al 1989b, 1992).

RESIDUAL INTACT AFFERENTS MAY ALSO BECOME HYPEREXCITABLE

At the same time that injured axons undergo changes in their excitability, residual uninjured axons in the same nerve, and axons in neighbouring intact nerves, are also affected. The response of residual intact axons is easiest to understand in situations where two nerves have a common border of cutaneous innervation, and one is injured. This triggers endings of the second nerve to start growing. Specifically, nociceptive afferents emit outgrowing sprouts which invade the neighbouring denervated territory and at least partially restore sensation (Fig. 5.7A; Weddell et al 1941, Devor et al 1979). This phenomenon, 'collateral sprouting', appears to be triggered at least in part by local release of nerve growth factor (NGF) from reactive cells in the skin (macrophages, keratinocytes, fibroblasts and replicating Schwann cells (Diamond et al 1987, Rotshenker 1997, Gallo & Letourneau 1998)). The same mechanism no doubt also triggers sprouting of residual intact axons in the centre of the territory served by a nerve that has been partly damaged (Fig. 5.7B). NGF and related neurokines are also known to induce afferent sensitization. Sprouting and sensitization may account for the observation of spontaneous firing and abnormal responses in spared afferents in partially denervated skin (Levine et al 1990, Na et al 1993, Koltzenburg et al 1994a, Ali et al 1999). Likewise, they presumably contribute to pain in borderline and partly denervated skin, along with central sensitization (see below).

Collateral sprouting across a border

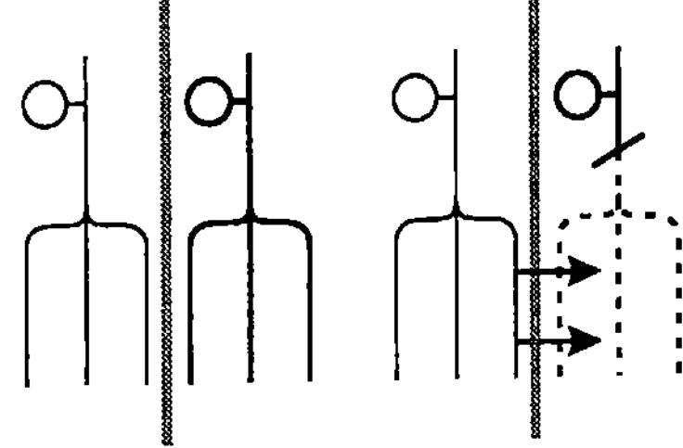

Sprouting within a field of partial denervation

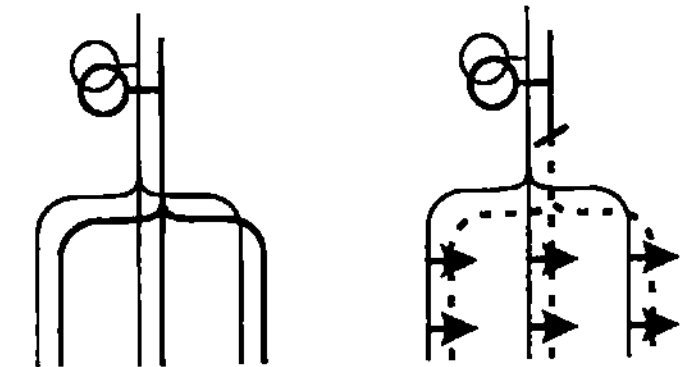

Fig. 5.7 Anterograde degeneration of afferent axons distal to a nerve injury (broken lines) promotes sprouting of residual intact neighbouring afferents. Such sprouting is well documented in the case of nerves sharing a common border (collateral sprouting), and very likely occurs also within the field of innervation of a single nerve following incomplete nerve damage. In each sketch, the sensory cell somata in the DRG are indicated at the top, and afferent innervation fields in the skin are indicated at the bottom.

ECTOPIC ELECTROGENESIS AFTER DEMYELINATION AND IN PERIPHERAL NEUROPATHIES

Trauma and disease that cause focal demyelination may lead to ectopic firing even when the injury is not severe enough to produce frank axonal degeneration (e.g. Calvin et al 1977, Rasminsky 1978, Smith & McDonald 1980, Burchiel 1980, Calvin et al 1982, Baker & Bostock 1992). Indeed, part of the ectopia in neuromas is no doubt generated in the region of dysmyelination invariably present just central to the injury site. A priori, myelin loss is expected to reduce fibre excitability and block axonal conduction. This is a major cause of morbidity in demyelinating diseases. However, secondary remodelling of membrane electrical properties (see below) can induce ectopia and associated positive sensory symptoms, including pain. Multiple sclerosis, nerve entrapment syndromes such as carpal tunnel and occupationally related 'repetitive strain injuries' are examples (e.g. Rasminsky 1981, Nordin et al 1984). Sciatica and trigeminal neuralgia may share this aetiology (see below). Interestingly, while demyelination in the CNS leads to ectopic hyperexcitability (Smith & McDonald 1980), severing CNS axons may not (Papir-Kricheli & Devor 1988).

Dyck and others (see Dyck et al 1993) carried out extensive quantitative histopathological studies of a wide range of peripheral neuropathies. Aetiologies studied include trauma, metabolic failure, toxins including heavy metals, autoimmune attack, etc. In most of these conditions there is clear histological evidence of demyelination and disseminated axonal interruption and sprouting, and a diversity of positive sensory symptoms including pain. Unfortunately, this work yielded no obvious correlation between the degree or type of axonal damage, and the sensory symptoms. As a fallback position, Dyck et al (1976) postulated that the histopathological correlate of pain may be the *dynamics* of degeneration and regeneration, i.e. the *rate* at which these processes occur. We posit that the functional link is not histopathology per se, but the membrane remodelling and ectopic hyperexcitability that develop in consequence. Specifically, it is hypothesized that any pathological condition which undermines the integrity of sensory axons or their myelin sheath might trigger electrical hyperexcitability, ectopic firing and pain. Supporting evidence includes the observation of abnormal neural activity in experimental models of diabetic polyneuropathy (Burchiel et al 1985, Ahlgren et al 1992), postherpetic neuralgia (Mayer et al 1986) and methylmercury intoxication (Delio et al 1992). Many other experimental models, and clinical conditions, remain to be tested (e.g. Martini 1997). Diseases in which there is massive histopathology, but few positive neuropathic symptoms, may be particularly informative. One such condition is Hanson's disease (leprosy; Anand 1996).

DORSAL ROOT GANGLIA ARE YET ANOTHER SOURCE OF ECTOPIC DISCHARGE

Axotomized sensory cell somata in dorsal root ganglia (DRGs) contribute to the ectopic neuropathic barrage in traumatized nerves. The first indication of this is due to Kirk (1974). Motivated by evidence of important sensory differences between axotomy peripheral versus central to the DRG (Kirk & Denny-Brown 1970), Kirk (1974) recorded from dorsal roots in animals with spinal nerve injury and found high levels of ongoing impulse discharge. This activity was attributed to the DRG, although an origin at the nerve injury site was not convincingly ruled out. Definitive evidence that the DRG proper is a major ectopic source following nerve trauma of various sorts was obtained only a decade later (De Santis & Duckworth 1982, Wall & Devor 1983, Burchiel 1984b, Kajander et al 1992, Rizzo et al 1995, Xie et al 1995, Study & Kral 1996, Zhang et al 1997). Interestingly, a small number of DRG neurons fire spontaneously even in the absence of nerve injury (Wall & Devor 1983). When neuropathic paraesthesias and pain persist despite nerve block, an ectopic source in the DRG must be considered. For example, ectopia originating in DRGs may explain cases in which local anaesthetic block of stump neuromas fails to relieve phantom limb pain.

Ectopic firing of DRG neurons is exacerbated by many of the same factors as neuromas. Among these mechanosensitivity is particularly salient, as it probably plays a major role in movement-evoked pain in disorders of the vertebral column (Howe et al 1977, Wall & Devor 1983). Kuslich et al (1991), for example, exposed the spinal nerves and DRGs in patients with sciatica using a local anaesthetic technique which permitted them to talk to the patient during the procedure. Mechanical stimulation on the spinal nerve and DRG capsule consistently provoked the patients' sciatica pain, while probing the local fascia, annulus, periosteum, etc. produced only local sensations. The nerve root and DRG is subject to considerable tensile stress during everyday movement and during manoeuvres such as straight-leg lifting (Breig 1978, Nowicki et al 1996). Normally this has no effect. But if there is ectopic mechanosensitivity due to radiculopathy or hyperexcitability of the DRG, these stresses are translated directly into ectopic impulse discharge and pain (e.g., Nordin et al 1984).

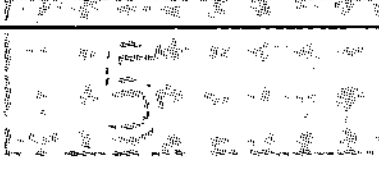

The very existence of repetitive firing capability in DRGs deserves comment. Protected from mechanical stimulation in its bony foramen, and containing virtually no synapses, the DRG has always been assumed to be a nutritive depot for the sensory axon, with no direct involvement in signal generation or processing (Lieberman 1976). Why, then, are DRG neurons capable of generating impulses at all, and why do some fire spontaneously even in the absence of nerve injury? Consider two possibilities. First, DRG excitability may have no adaptive purpose. It may simply reflect a biophysical design quirk required to insure against conduction failure as nerve impulses propagate through the DRG (Devor & Obermeyer 1984, Luscher et al 1994). A second, and more speculative possibility is that DRG electrogenesis serves some hitherto unsuspected function in the intact organism. Possible roles include the provision of a sensory 'background' to the CNS body schema. For example, when all nerves to a limb are blocked in healthy subjects, most feel a 'normal phantom', rather than absence of the limb (Melzack & Bromage 1973). Alternatively, the DRG might serve some previously unsuspected chemosensory function. Hints of this include the facts that DRG somata express a large variety of chemoreceptor molecules (references in Shinder & Devor 1994), and that unlike the rest of the PNS, the DRG lacks a blood–nerve barrier (Jacobs et al 1976, Allen & Kiernan 1994, Wadhwani & Rapoport 1994). Holes in the blood–brain barrier, such as in the area postrema and the circumventricular organs, are thought to mark specialized chemosensory areas (Gross 1987).

ECTOPIA AND THE SENSORY PECULIARITY OF NEUROPATHIC PAIN

Sensation in neuropathic conditions, both ongoing sensation and response to stimuli, is usually distinctive and sometimes bizarre. For example, causalgia (chronic regional pain syndrome, CRPS2), a chronic pain syndrome associated with bullet wounds with near-miss of a nerve trunk, was named for its characteristic burning pain (*caustos* = burnt in Greek). Neuropathic pains are often described in terms of natural stimuli: stabbing, crushing, intense cold, etc. A logical inference is that these sensations derive from ectopic activity in corresponding afferent types (e.g., thermonociceptors in the case of burning pain). It is more difficult to understand sensations that do not correspond to particular receptor types. Examples are 'pins-and-needles', electric shock-like paroxysms and hyperpathia (defined in the 'Introduction'). Sometimes patients are frustrated by an inability to find words that convey exactly what they are feeling. Mechanisms of sensory paroxysms, hyperpathia and related sensory peculiarities are discussed below. In general, neuropathic sensation is probably a direct reflection of the particular chorus of ectopic firing generated in the periphery, and modulated by the CNS. Ultimately one wants to compare sensation with ectopia in conscious humans. In the meanwhile, peculiarities of the ectopic firing in animal preparations provide suggestive hints.

ECTOPIA: TYPES OF FIBRES, PREVALENCE AND PATTERNS OF DISCHARGE

The prevalence of axons that show ectopic activity after nerve injury (per cent of axons sampled) can be determined with some accuracy (Devor 1999). Unfortunately, information about the *types* of afferents that preferentially generate ectopic firing is much more difficult to obtain. The problem is that axotomy disconnects the receptor ending from the rest of the axon, and then it takes additional hours or days for ectopia to develop (Govrin-Lippman & Devor 1978, Koschorke et al 1991, Michaelis et al 1995). Heroic efforts are required to obtain direct information about afferent type in recordings from chronic nerve injury sites. Nonetheless, partial information can be obtained from conduction velocity, by comparing recordings from dorsal *versus* ventral roots, and from examination of cutaneous nerves *versus* nerves serving muscle, etc.

Studies of this sort have indicated that, in rodents at least, the great bulk of spontaneous ectopic activity is generated in sensory, rather than motor fibres. Aβ- and Aδ-afferents are represented roughly according to their numbers in the nerve, with activity very prominent during the first two weeks postinjury, and then fading. Afferent C fibres are underrepresented in the ectopic barrage at short postinjury times and over-represented in chronic preparations (Fig. 5.8). As for receptor type, slowly adapting afferents, particularly proprioceptors, make up the bulk of the spontaneous A-fibre discharge in mixed nerves. Cutaneous afferents show mechanosensitivity, but relatively little spontaneous activity (Johnson & Munson 1991, Proske et al 1995, Tal & Devor 1999). These and other observations suggest that neuroma endbulbs and sprouts develop the same types of sensitivities that the neuron had originally, before the nerve injury (Devor et al 1990, Koschorke et al 1991, Michaelis et al 1998a). This speculation is attractive since the transduction properties of an afferent are mostly determined by the types of transducer, receptor and chan-

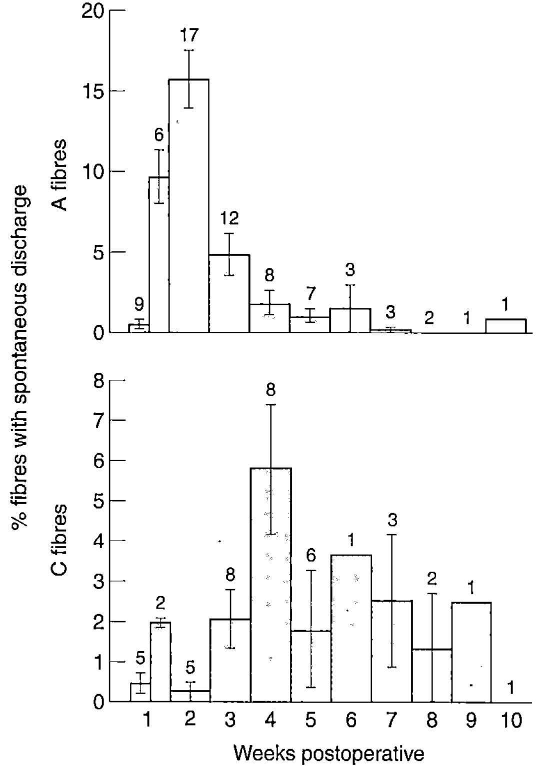

Fig. 5.8 The incidence (mean ± SD) of spontaneous ectopic firing in myelinated (A) and unmyelinated (C) fibres in experimental sciatic nerve neuromas with time postinjury. The value atop each column is the number of animals studied within the time window indicated. (Reproduced from Govrin-Lippmann & Devor 1978, Devor & Govrin-Lippmann 1985.)

nel proteins produced in the cell soma and transported down to the axon end (see below).

Ectopic firing in A afferents, no matter what the type of nerve injury, is usually rhythmic. That is, the interval between adjacent impulses within a train is highly regular (Fig. 5.4A). Interspike interval in spontaneously active fibres usually falls within the range of 65–35 ms, which translates to an instantaneous discharge rate in the range of 15–30 Hz. Such rates represent a substantial sensory stimulus. In about a third of neuroma afferents, spontaneous rhythmic discharge is interrupted by silent pauses, resulting in a 'bursty', on–off pattern ('interrupted autorhythmicity'; Fig. 5.3A). The remaining A fibres, and most C fibres, fire in a slow, irregular pattern (0.1–10 Hz).

Despite efforts to standardize experimental conditions, many authors report finding considerable variability in ectopic afferent firing from one experiment to the next. Following clues based on animal-to-animal variation in neuropathic pain behaviour (autotomy, see below), we examined neuromas of different rat strains. In Lewis rats, a strain that expresses very low levels of autotomy, we found much less ectopic neuroma activity than in Sabra-strain rats, which have high levels of autotomy (Devor et al 1982, also see Hao & Wiesenfeld-Hallin 1994). Moreover, first-generation offspring of Sabra × Lewis parents revealed low levels of activity resembling the Lewis parent. These observations, together with related behavioural data discussed below, suggest that susceptibility to neuropathic sensory abnormalities may be in part heritable. This conclusion has obvious implications for the gross variability of neuropathic symptoms in human patient populations.

SYMPATHETIC–SENSORY COUPLING EXACERBATES ECTOPIC FIRING

In some patients neuropathic pain is exacerbated by sympathetic efferent activity and relieved by sympathetic block (Bonica 1990, Janig & Stanton-Hicks 1997). Conditions in which sympathetic involvement is suspected include causalgia (CRPS2) and reflex sympathetic dystrophy (RSD, CRPS1). Because of the availability of sympathectomy as a therapeutic option, effective prognosis, based on an understanding of the nature of sympathetic–sensory coupling in peripheral nerves, is an important priority (Arner 1991, Raja et al 1991).

It was once assumed that RSD/causalgia/CRPS results from excess sympathetic drive. But recent evidence has shown that sympathetic efferent activity is, if anything, *decreased* in sympathetically related pain states (Drummond et al 1991; reviewed in Janig & Stanton-Hicks 1997). Moreover, even if it were increased, normal nociceptive afferents respond only minimally to sympathetic stimulation. It is unlikely, therefore, that pain in CRPS is due to increased sympathetic output. Rather, the weight of evidence points to sympathetic–sensory coupling being caused primarily by increased responsiveness of altered sensory neurons. For example, experimentally injured A and C afferents respond to circulating adrenaline, and to noradrenaline released from postganglionic sympathetic endings. Spike activity can also be evoked in axotomized DRG neurons and in partly denervated skin (Wall & Gutnick 1974, Korenman & Devor 1981, Devor & Janig 1981, Burchiel 1984b, Habler et al 1987, Sato & Perl 1991, Devor et al 1994a, Tracey et al 1995, Ali et al 1998). Corresponding clinical indicators of abnormal adrenosensitivity are discussed below. Changes on the efferent side, however, may nonetheless play a role. Specifically, nerve injury induces sprouting of sympathetic fibres at the injury site, within affected DRGs (Fig. 5.9), and probably also in partially denervated skin (Goldstein et al 1989, Small et al 1996, McLachlan et al 1993). This is expected to increase

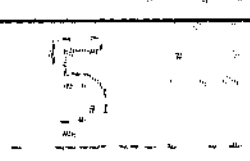

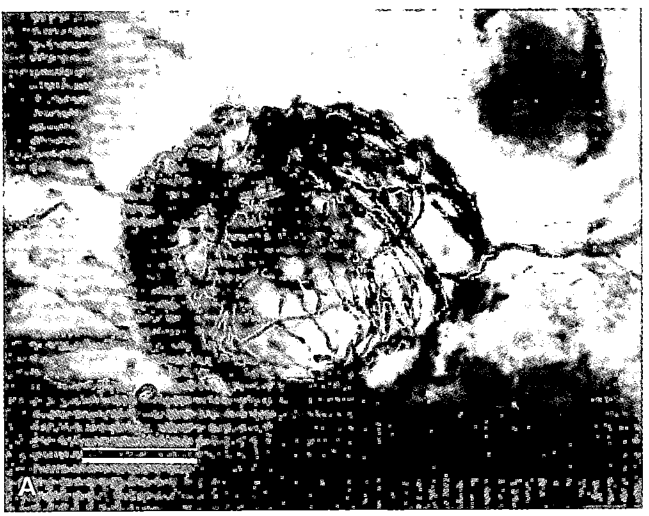

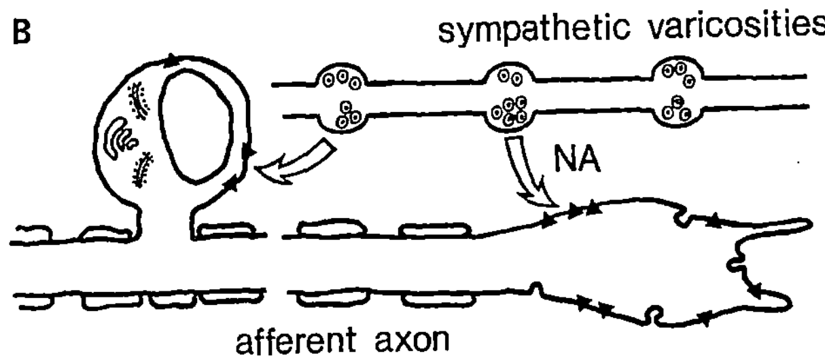

Fig. 5.9 Sympathetic–sensory coupling at sites of nerve injury and associated DRGs results from noradrenaline (NA), released from sympathetic postganglionic axons, binding to adrenoreceptors (triangles) on the membrane of injured hyperexcitable sensory neurons (**B**). The photomicrograph (**A**) shows sympathetic axons forming a basket-like skein around an axotomized DRG neuron. Tyrosine hydroxylase immunocytochemistry; scale bar = 20 μm.

the amount of sympathetically released noradrenaline, and to enhance its access to hypersensitive afferent neurons and their axonal endings, even if the sympathetic efferent barrage remains unchanged.

The use of receptor-selective pharmacological agents has shown that sympathetic–sensory coupling is mediated primarily by adrenoreceptors of the α_2 type, with a minor role played by α_1 adrenoreceptors (Sato & Perl 1991, Xie et al 1995, Chen et al 1996). Specifically, circulating or released adrenergic agonists reach adrenosensitive sites on injured sensory neurons by diffusion, bind to α adrenoreceptors on the cell membrane and initiate ectopic firing (Devor 1983b). The coupling appears not to be due to vasoconstriction-induced ischaemia or other indirect processes (Korenman & Devor 1981, Levine et al 1986), but rather to a direct action of α agonists on neuronal adrenoreceptors (Sato et al 1993, Petersen et al 1996, Rubin et al 1997). Are α adrenoreceptors normally present on sensory neurons, or does their appearance depend on de novo receptor synthesis? There is now abundant evidence that many intact, uninjured DRG neurons express α-adrenoreceptor mRNA and protein (Pieribone et al 1994, Devor et al 1995, Gold et al 1997). De novo synthesis can therefore be ruled out. There is tentative evidence of receptor upregulation following axotomy (Perl 1994, Davar et al 1996), but this remains uncertain and is probably not a necessary condition for the emergence of sympathetic–sensory coupling. Rather, α adrenoreceptors normally expressed by DRG neurons might yield suprathreshold responses following nerve injury simply due to the electrical hyperexcitability of axotomized sensory neurons.

The sympathetic–sensory coupling hypothesis provides a rationale for those cases of RSD/causalgia/CRPS and related conditions in which chemical and surgical sympathectomy is effective. It is consistent with the observation that direct electrical stimulation of sympathetic efferent fibres in man evokes pain, but only in patients with RSD (Walker & Nulsen 1948, White & Sweet 1969). Likewise, the hypothesis accounts for the observation that α-adrenoreceptor agonists evoke pain when injected into the skin in RSD patients whose hyperalgesia was previously relieved by treatments which reduce endogenous sympathetic drive (Wallin et al 1976, Davis et al 1991, Torebjork et al 1995).

Sustained ectopic firing, particularly when it originates in mid-nerve axons or the DRG, may be responsible for the oedema, and 'trophic' changes in skin, nails and bone that characterize longstanding RSD/CRPS2 (Bonica 1990, Janig & Stanton-Hicks 1997). When intact nerves are activated experimentally in midcourse, impulses travel antidromically out into the periphery, as well as toward the CNS. Antidromic impulses in C fibres are known to trigger the release of various vasoactive peptides from peripheral nociceptor endings, notably substance P. This causes local vasodilatation (hence warming and reddening of the skin), and plasma extravasation from postcapillary venules (hence oedema). These are the signs of 'neurogenic inflammation' (Ninian Bruce 1913, Lembeck & Holzer 1979, Lotz et al 1988). If neurogenic inflammation persisted for long periods of time, tissue integrity and growth patterns might be compromised.

ENDOGENOUS AMPLIFICATION MECHANISMS

Self-sustained discharge, aftersuppression and spike bursting

Sensory receptor endings respond to applied stimuli and then rapidly return to rest. Ectopic pacemaker sites, by contrast, can sometimes be 'turned on' by stimuli, continuing to fire for a time as if they were spontaneously active. If, as is often the case, an ectopic pacemaker site is at rest just below the repetitive firing threshold, weak depolarizing stimuli that bring it to threshold will trigger a disproportionate jump in firing frequency (Fig. 5.3 bottom). This property yields signal amplification. Furthermore, once brought into the rhythmic firing domain, the discharge may persist (Lisney & Devor 1987). The DRG neuron in Figure 5.6A, for example, responded to momentary mechanical stimuli with afterdischarge lasting more than 30 s and including about 500 extra spikes. Much longer responses have also been observed. Several factors can contribute to such self-sustained firing. For example, spikes in some sensory neurons are followed by a brief depolarizing afterpotential (DAP, Raymond 1979). The DAP following one spike triggers a second, the second a third, and so on. Alternatively, K^+ ions released during firing can generate a prolonged depolarization, maintaining discharge (e.g. Kapoor et al 1993). Self-sustained discharge is a likely explanation of hyperpathic aftersensations and mechanical 'triggerpoints', e.g. in fibromyalgia and spinal column disorders.

Episodes of high frequency firing, no matter what the cause, often trigger endogenous suppression mechanisms. In Figure 5.6B, for example, a few seconds of excitation by electrical pulses was followed by a period of silence before baseline firing resumed. The suppression appears to work as follows (Amir & Devor 1997). During spike activity, Ca^{2+} ions enter the neuron, activating Ca^{2+}-dependent K^+ channels. The resulting outward K^+ current hyperpolarizes the pacemaker site, suppressing firing. An alternative hyperpolarizing mechanism is activation of the Na^+ pump by repetitive spike activity (Na^+–K^+ATPase; Rang & Ritchie 1968). If the stimulus (generator current) that caused the self-sustained discharge in the first place is still present when the activity-evoked suppression dissipates, a second and then a third burst will occur. Such on–off firing (bursting) can go on indefinitely (Fig. 5.4B).

A likely clinical expression of activity-evoked suppression is the 'refractory period' that follows individual pain paroxysms in trigeminal neuralgia (Kugelberg & Lindblom 1959, Rappaport & Devor 1994). During the refractory period it is difficult or impossible to trigger another burst. Likewise, activity-dependent hyperpolarization, rather than gate control, may be the mechanism of pain relief during dorsal column and transcutaneous electrical nerve stimulation (TENS).

Amplification by 'extra spikes'

Calvin et al (1977) proposed an additional type of afterdischarge. They pointed out that if the duration of a propagating action potential were to increase, it might outlast the absolute refractory period of the axon, re-excite the membrane it had just passed over, and thus generate an extra spike. Knowing that demyelination has just such an impulse broadening effect, the authors sought and found extra spike production in experimentally demyelinated axons. Production of the occasional extra spike does not, in itself, yield important afterdischarge amplification. However, if there were multiple sites of demyelination along a single axon, a brief stimulus might trigger reverberating cascades of extra spikes.

CROSSTALK AMONG SENSORY NEURONS: A GENERATOR OF PAIN PAROXYSMS?

Each primary sensory neuron normally constitutes an independent signal conduction pathway. In the event of neural injury, however, excitatory interactions develop among neurons. These amplify and spread sensory signals. Cross-excitation in the PNS may underlie the hyperpathia, pain paroxysms and shock-like sensations that are so characteristic of neuropathies.

Ephaptic crosstalk

The most widely known, if not necessarily the most important, form of PNS cross-excitation is ephaptic (i.e. electrical) crosstalk. In the mid 1940s Granit and Skoglund (1945) discovered that acute nerve transection short-circuits the insulation between neighbouring axons permitting current from the cut end of one fibre to directly excite neighbours. This acute coupling decays and vanishes within minutes of injury and is therefore unlikely to be of much functional significance. However, several weeks later ephaptic crosstalk develops again, now in an enduring form (Seltzer & Devor 1979, Blumberg & Janig 1982, Lisney & Pover 1983, Kocsis et al 1984, Meyer et al 1985).

Ephapsis in a neuroma is illustrated in Figure 5.10. Similar crosstalk occurs in regenerating nerve distal to the site of injury (Seltzer & Devor 1979), and in patches of demyelination (Rasminsky 1978). It is thought to result from close apposition between adjacent axons in the absence of the normal glial insulation (Fig. 5.11; Rasminsky 1978, Fried et al 1993). Because coupled fibres are frequently of different types, ephaptic crosstalk could cause nociceptors to be driven by activity in low-threshold afferents or even efferents. Ephapsis does not occur in DRGs following nerve injury (Devor & Wall 1990). However, the observation of ephaptic coupling among DRG neurons after infection by

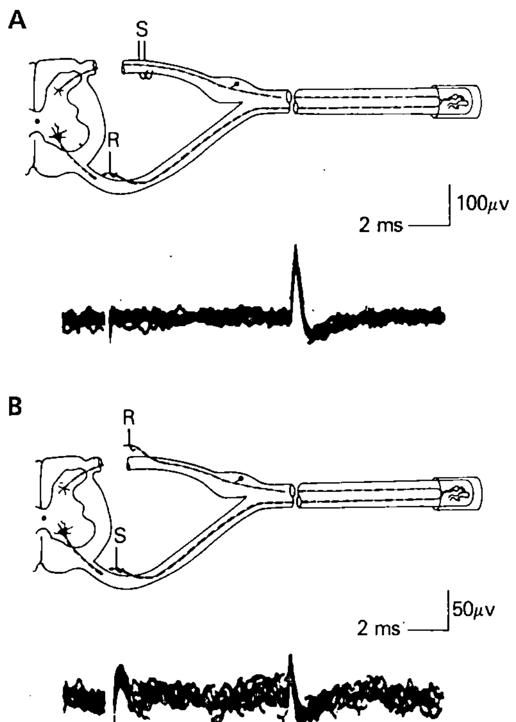

Fig. 5.10 Bidirectional ephaptic crosstalk between a pair of fibres ending in an experimental nerve-end neuroma. **A** First, a fibre was found in the L5 ventral root that responded (R) at fixed latency to electrical stimulation (S) of ipsilateral dorsal roots (DRs). **B** Then, stimuli were applied to the fibre, and fixed-latency responses were sought in the DRs. One responding fibre was found in the L4DR. Note that response latency for conduction in the two directions is identical. (Modified from Seltzer & Devor 1979.)

certain strains of herpes simplex virus implicates the process in the pain of postherpetic neuralgia (Mayer et al 1986).

Non-ephaptic cross-excitation

Lisney and Devor (1987) discovered a very different type of cross-excitation termed 'crossed afterdischarge' (also see Amir & Devor 1992). It is probably more important than ephapsis because it develops more rapidly, and affects a much larger proportion of afferents. Unlike ephapsis, single impulses have no effect. However, repetitive stimulation excites passive, non-stimulated, neighbours to self-sustained discharge. Crossed afterdischarge also occurs prominently in DRGs, a fact that may have considerable functional significance.

Consider the experiment illustrated in Figure 5.12, in which ectopic discharge originating from a DRG neuron that had been disconnected from the periphery was recorded (Devor & Wall 1990). The nerve was partially damaged, but natural stroking of the skin activated residual intact axons and sent sensory impulses centrally along the nerve and into the spinal cord. As these impulses traversed the DRG they cross-excited the recorded neuron and increased its firing rate. Most sensory neurons are subject to such cross-excitation, even in intact DRGs (Utzschneider et al 1992). However, the contribution to ectopic firing is negligible except when the neurons are hyperexcitable. Crossed afterdischarge in the DRG is therefore a potential cause of hyperalgesia following partial nerve injury, a mechanism for 'winding up' ectopic discharge on repeated stimulation, and a means for spreading abnormal activity across a dermatome. These are all symptoms of hyperpathia.

Crossed-afterdischarge is chemically, not electrically, mediated

The signature of ephaptic crosstalk is high safety-factor, bidirectional coupling: a single impulse in an active fibre evokes a single impulse in its coupled neighbour (Fig. 5.10). Non-ephaptic cross-excitation works differently. Single impulses do little. Repetitive spiking, however, causes both an increase in extracellular K^+ concentration, and (non-synaptic) release of a still undefined neurotransmitter substance(s) from the stimulated neurons. These chemicals accumulate in the extracellular space during stimulation, diffuse toward neighbouring neurons, and excite them (Shinder & Devor 1994, Amir & Devor 1996). Excitation by K^+ results from Nernstian depolarization. Excitation by the neurotransmitter(s) modulates membrane ion channels causing excitation by depolarization combined with decreased membrane conductance (Utzschneider et al 1992, Amir & Devor 1996).

Cross-excitation and pain paroxysms

The combination of neuronal hyperexcitability and cross-excitation sets the stage for a remarkable process that could, in principle at least, lead to the electric shock-like pain paroxysms common in neuropathic pain conditions, notably trigeminal neuralgia (Rappaport & Devor 1994). Electric shock stimuli are distinct from natural ones such as touch, heat and cold in that they activate the different types of afferents indiscriminately and synchronously. Imagine that a small cluster of neurons in a hyperexcitable nerve, root or sensory ganglion becomes active, perhaps due to movement, a cutaneous trigger stimulus, or spontaneously. Coupling now causes passive neighbours to start firing. This recruits more neighbours and they recruit still more. The resulting positive feedback 'chain-reaction' can culminate in an 'explosion' of discharge involving many neurons

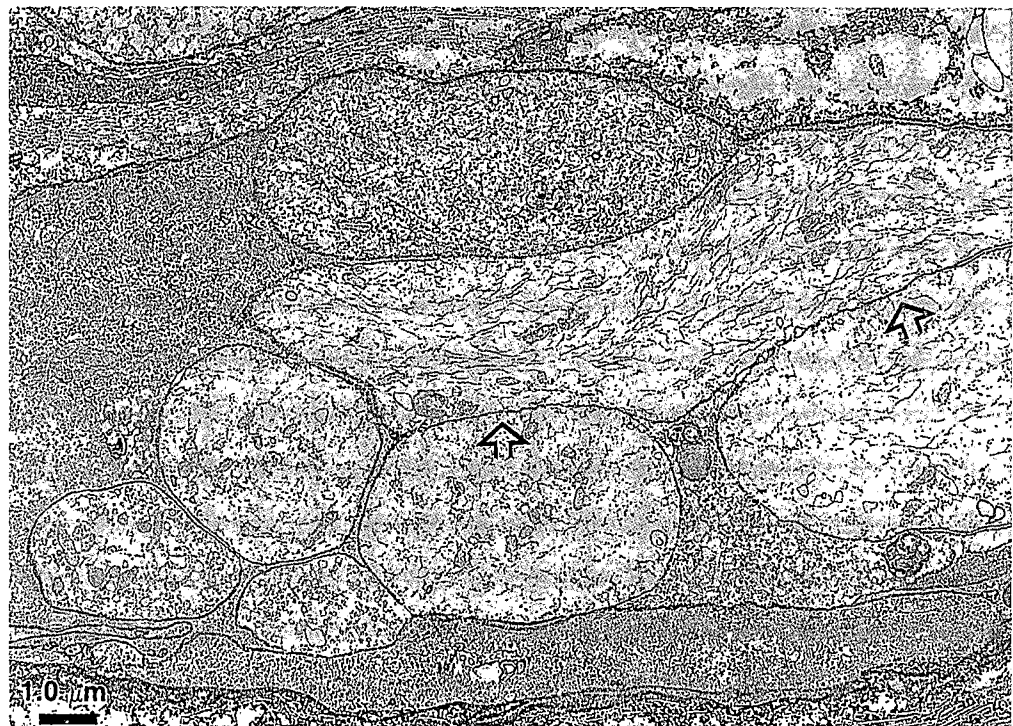

Fig. 5.11 Arrows show regions of close apposition between neighbouring demyelinated axons, in the absence of an intervening glial (Schwann cell) process. Other axons are compartmentalized by (dark) Schwann cell cytoplasm as in normal nerves (lower left). Rat sciatic nerve neuroma 25 days postinjury (see Fried et al 1991). Scale bar = 1 µm.

of all types – a shock-like 'epileptic seizure' of the nerve or DRG. In time the activity-evoked hyperpolarizing process described above kicks in. This suppresses the sensory 'explosion', establishes a period of refractoriness, and then resets the system until the next paroxysm. This mechanism is expected to be sensitive to drugs that reduce membrane hyperexcitability, such as carbamazepine (Tegretol) and diphenylhydantoin (Dilantin, see below). Indeed, this is the therapeutic spectrum in trigeminal neuralgia.

ANIMAL MODELS OF NEUROPATHIC PAIN

EXPERIMENTAL ASSAYS OF NOCICEPTION

Behavioural studies of pain in animals contribute essential information on clinical pain conditions which cannot be obtained in any other way. Non-human mammals clearly feel pain. This inference is based on observation of behavioural responses to noxious stimuli: withdrawal, escape, defence/attack postures and movements, alarm and distress vocalization, writhing, autonomic and endocrine responses, protective postures, mouthing of the affected limb, sleep fragmentation, avoidance learning and so forth. Such behavioural signs of pain are termed 'nocifensive' behaviours (Lewis 1942). The denial that animals have mental states including pain was common among investigators of the Behaviourist School some decades ago, but among most current investigators agree that this view reflects an extraordinary obtuseness. That is not to say that inferring pain from observations of behaviour is trivial or without uncertainty. We recognize behaviours as nocifensive because they occur in the context of noxious stimuli, because they are adaptive, and because we can empathize. The more distant a species from human in terms of habitat, lifestyle and evolutionary history, the less confident we can be about interpreting a particular behavioural pattern as nocifensive.

Over the years investigators have selected specific instinctive nocifensive responses as laboratory measures of pain, often for screening candidate analgesics (Seltzer 1995; for more details see Ch. 14). Most such work is done with rats and mice. Until recently, nociceptive assays employed acute and subacute noxious stimuli exclusively. These include mechanical pressure (e.g., Randall Selitto, von Frey filaments), heat and cold (e.g., hotplate, coldplate, tailflick, tail immersion, Hargreaves test, CO_2 laser pulses) or noxious chemicals (e.g., writhing in response to intraperitoneal injection of acetic acid or $MgSO_4$, or intradermal injection

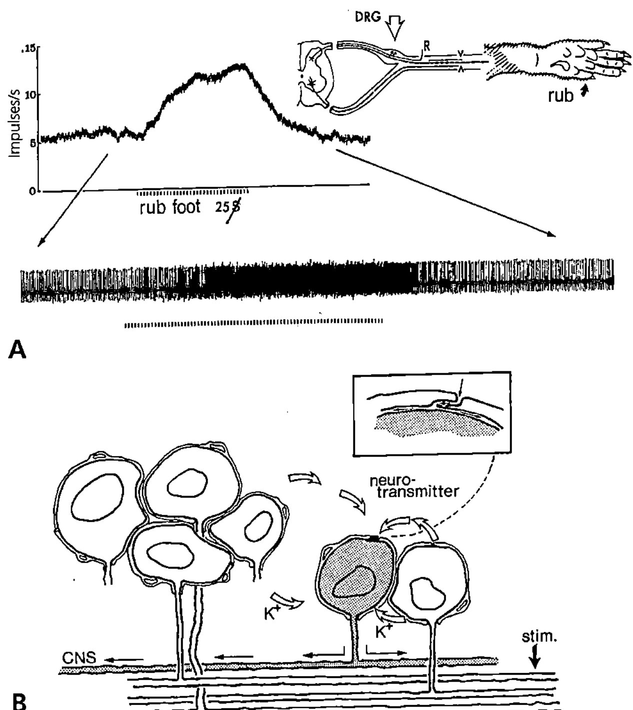

Fig. 5.12 Non-ephaptic, chemically mediated cross-excitation within a DRG. **A** The sciatic nerve was partially injured and ectopic firing originating in the DRG was recorded as shown in the sketch. Rubbing the rat's foot increased the baseline spontaneous firing of this neuron due to DRG crossed afterdischarge (from Devor & Wall 1990). **B** The presumed mechanism: active neurons (white) release K^+ ions and a neurotransmitter(s) into the extracellular space within the DRG. These access and excite passive (i.e. non-stimulated) neighbours (grey). (See Amir & Devor 1996.)

of dilute formalin or bee venom). The approach is either to gradually increase stimulus intensity and define a threshold for evoking a predetermined nocifensive endpoint, or to use a fixed suprathreshold stimulus and measure the intensity of the emitted response (e.g., Zeltser & Seltzer 1994). Ethical guidelines must be followed, of course (Zimmerman 1983). Such assays are intuitive and easy to apply. However, skill and attention to detail is essential to avoid pitfalls. For example, animals tend to change their response with stimulus repetition, anxiety (e.g., in novel environments), and with the circadian clock. Stimulus control is also essential. For example, the effect of a fixed thermal stimulus on thermoreceptor endings deep in the skin depends on baseline skin surface temperature and tissue perfusion (Hole & Tjolsen 1993). Likewise, response to mechanical probing with a fixed-force von Frey filament depends on such details as the kinetics of force application, and whether the filament tip has a sharp spur. Even the choice of housing cage affects cutaneous sensitivity (Mizisin et al 1998).

BEHAVIOURAL MODELS OF PATHOLOGY AND DISEASE: RATIONALE

Chronic pain involves distinct pathophysiological mechanisms, and is not simply acute pain extended in time. This realization has encouraged the development of rodent 'models' for use as research surrogates for human patients. Two focuses have been painful rheumatic disease (e.g., arthritis evoked by injection of carrageenan or Freund's adjuvant) and neuropathic pain. In models, animals are usually subjected to clinically relevant lesions or disease-causing agents, the effects of which are then evaluated over time using one or more behavioural endpoint selected from the list of nociceptive assays noted above. All animal models face the inevitable critique that they are not identical to the corresponding human condition. Humans, for example, do not have a tail to flick. However, such critiques do not address the fact that most of the experiments that need to be done cannot be done in humans. Ultimately, the relevance of a particular animal surrogate depends not on its identity to a clinical condition, but on whether it usefully predicts drug efficacy, or provides insights into mechanism. Animal models are preludes to clinical trials, not substitutes.

In recent years there has been a virtual explosion of neuropathic pain models, each employing a particular lesion and nociceptive endpoint. For comprehensive reviews see Zeltser and Seltzer (1994), Bennett (1994) and Seltzer (1995). The first step is usually to validate the model, for example by showing responsiveness to treatment modalities effective in humans. Having done so, the hope is to go beyond existing knowledge.

AUTOTOMY: MODELLING SPONTANEOUS PARAESTHESIAS, DYSAESTHESIAS AND PAIN

The first neuropathic pain model to be widely adopted is autotomy. Animals, rodents to primates, that have suffered nerve section, or dorsal root section or avulsion, tend to lick, scratch and bite at their denervated and anaesthetic limb. The resulting tissue injury is 'autotomy'. Basbaum (1974) and Wall and collaborators (Wall et al 1979a) were the first to propose that autotomy behaviour, scored on a standard scale over time post surgery, is a measure of the unpleasantness of phantom limb sensation felt by the animal, i.e. that autotomy is a model of anaesthesia dolorosa or brachial plexus avulsion pain. The fact that autotomy is a spontaneously emitted behaviour, and that human socialization usually intervenes before self-mutilation occurs in patients with similar injuries (but not always, see Levitt 1985, Albe-Fessard et al 1990, Procacci & Maresca 1990, Winchel & Stanley 1991, Mailis 1996), has made this interpretation controversial. Moreover, there are rare reports of directed self-injurious behaviour in humans in the apparent absence of pain (Sweet 1981). In principle, autotomy could reflect numb anaesthesia (Rodin & Kruger 1984). This alternative, however, does not consider the facts that autotomy in animals occurs only in the context of neuropathy (psychiatric disturbance, in particular, is excluded), that autotomy is responsive to clinically appropriate therapies, and that the autotomy model has generated many new clinically relevant observations and ideas (see below). Evidence that autotomy indeed occurs in response to neuropathic sensation includes:

1. *Relation to ectopic input.* There is a highly suggestive correlation between autotomy and ectopic afferent discharge, particularly in peripheral C fibres, across many experimental variables (e.g. Wall et al 1979a, Wiesenfeld & Lindblom 1980, Devor et al 1982, Levitt 1985, Coderre et al 1986, Albe-Fessard et al 1990, Asada et al 1996). Indeed, the original idea that autotomy reflects positive sensation emerged from the observation of ectopic discharge in animals performing autotomy. Resecting neuromas delays autotomy until a new neuroma forms (Seltzer et al 1985, 1991a, Barbera et al 1988). Correspondingly, permanent destruction of peripheral C fibres by neonatal capsaicin treatment suppresses autotomy (Devor et al 1982).
2. *Type of nerve injury matters.* Different forms of nerve section (cut, freeze, cautery, crush, etc.) produce identical anaesthesia, but yield different degrees of autotomy, apparently because of differences in the resulting ectopic input or injury discharge emitted at the time of nerve injury (e.g., Wall et al 1979a, Wiesenfeld & Lindblom 1980, Yamamoto et al 1983). Autotomy is *not* directed towards a limb numbed by sustained local anaesthetic block (Blumenkopf & Lipman 1991).
3. *Response to analgesic drugs.* Autotomy is suppressed in a dose-dependent manner by drugs that reduce ectopic firing and/or relieve neuropathic pain in humans. These include anticonvulsants (phenytoin and carbamazepine), topical and systemic local anaesthetics, glycerol, tricyclics (amitriptyline), guanethidine, GABA agonists (diazepam), NMDA receptor antagonists (MK801, 5APV, HU211) and (intrathecal) amines and peptides (e.g. Duckrow & Taub 1977, Wall et al 1979b, Seltzer et al. 1987, 1989, 1991a,b,c, Coderre et al 1986, Gonzales-Darder et al 1986, Kauppila & Pertovaara 1991, Puke & Wiesenfeld-Hallin 1993, Banos et al 1994, Colado et al 1994, Sanchez et al 1995). By contrast, daily injection of NSAIDs and (systemic) morphine, which are relatively ineffective for neuropathic pain clinically, do not suppress autotomy (Seltzer et al 1989, Yamamoto & Mizuguchi 1991, Xu et al. 1993), although morphine injected intrathecally may be effective (Wiesenfeld-Hallin 1984).
4. *Evoked autotomy.* Spinal injection of irritants that almost certainly cause pain induce scratching and biting of the corresponding limb, and sometimes frank autotomy. Such compounds include strychnine, tetanus toxin, alumina cream, penicillin and substance P (Kennard 1950, Kryzhanovsky 1976, Hylden & Wilcox 1981, Coderre et al 1986). Likewise, blockade of the descending antinociceptive control by appropriate brainstem or spinal tract lesions augments autotomy (Coderre et al 1986, Saade et al 1993), while midbrain or dorsal column stimulation, and dorsal root entry zone (DREZ) lesions, suppress it (Albe-Fessard et al 1990, Rossitch et al 1993, Gao et al 1996).
5. *Exacerbating factors.* Palpating neuromas in rats evokes distress vocalization and struggling. Autotomy is accompanied by other behavioural signs of pain such as paw guarding, protective gait, sleep disturbances, sometimes weight loss, and stress-related increase in plasma corticosterone levels (Coderre et al 1986, Seltzer et al 1987, Albe-Fessard et al 1990). It is also augmented by stressful conditions such as isolation and cold stress, and reduced by taming and social contact (Wiesenfeld & Hallin 1981, Berman & Rodin 1982, Coderre et al 1986, Kauppila & Pertovaara 1991).

PARTIAL NERVE INJURY MODELS: SPONTANEOUS PAIN COMBINED WITH EVOKED ALLODYNIA AND HYPERALGESIA

Autotomy rarely occurs except in areas rendered anaesthetic by complete transection of a major nerve, or in anaesthetic islands created following partial nerve injury (Wall et al 1979a, Bennett & Xie 1988, Neil et al 1991). With even partial residual innervation, the very act of biting is painful, providing protective sensory cover. However, areas bordering anaesthetic zones, and partly denervated skin, often show allodynia and hyperalgesia (Rivers & Head 1908, Trotter & Davis 1909, Sunderland 1978, Bonica 1990). Animal models that exhibit such cutaneous hypersensibility sidestep the uncertainties of autotomy.

The first descriptions of neuropathic allodynia came from studies of major nerve and root transection in which sensibility was tested in borderline skin still innervated by neighbouring intact nerves (Kirk & Denny-Brown 1970, Markus et al 1984, Kingery & Vallin 1989, Vallin &

Kingery 1991). Allodynia due to afferent input travelling through neighbouring intact nerves has likewise been demonstrated in the partial nerve injury models described below (Ro & Jacobs 1993, Kingery et al 1993, Tracey & Cunningham 1993, Attal et al 1994, Tal & Bennett 1994a). However, since major nerve transection also triggers autotomy, there is a clear advantage to using partial lesion models that do not render any part of the limb entirely anaesthetic.

In the first such partial nerve injury model, a surrogate for entrapment neuropathy, Bennett and Xie (1988) reported the effects of chronic constriction injury (CCI) using loosely applied chromic gut ligatures. Rats with CCI of the sciatic nerve show indications of spontaneous pain (paw-protecting postures), allodynia to mechanical and thermal stimuli (using various of the assays noted above) and reduced grooming, resulting in excessive nail growth, for example. These indicators of neuropathic pain emerge gradually over the first 2–5 days following the lesion, and persist for up to 2 months. Structurally, CCI causes the nerve to slowly swell and strangulate under the ligatures. This results in degeneration of essentially all A fibres, and many but not all C fibres (Basbaum et al 1991, Carlton et al 1991). When the suture material begins to resorb and the swelling subsides, the injured fibres regenerate and sensation normalizes. Electrophysiological recordings in CCI reveal massive ectopic firing originating at the nerve injury site and the associated DRGs, much as in neuromas (Fig. 5.5; Xie & Xiao 1990, Kajander et al 1992, Xie et al 1995, Study & Kral 1996, Tal & Eliav 1996, Chen & Devor 1998). CCI of other nerves yields similar behavioural indicators of pain, appropriate to the peripheral structures affected. These include CCI-like damage to spinal nerves, DRGs or dorsal roots (Kawakami et al 1994, Cavanaugh 1995) and CCI of the infraorbital nerve in the face (Vos et al 1994, Imamura et al 1997).

A more direct model of partial nerve injury, intended to simulate trauma rather than entrapment, was reported by Seltzer et al (1990). Here, a tight silk ligature was placed through the sciatic nerve in the upper thigh, severing A and C fibres in one-third to one-half of the nerve, but leaving the remaining axons intact. A variant of this procedure was developed by Kim and Chung (1992; also see Choi et al 1994). They moved centrally along the sciatic nerve to a point where it naturally splits into its component spinal nerves at spinal segments L4, L5 and L6, and tightly ligated and/or cut L5 (or L5+6; Fig. 5.2 left). Both of these partial nerve section models yielded indicators of spontaneous pain, and both mechanical and thermal allodynia and hyperalgesia on the effected hindpaw (Fig. 5.2, right). Like the CCI model, the model of Kim & Chung (1992) has been adapted to other nerves to similar effect (e.g. Na et al 1994).

The models of Seltzer et al (1990) and Kim & Chung (1992), in their various forms, involve ligation and transection of nerves in a manner identical to the autotomy model. In each case a neuroma is formed, and ectopic firing arises from the injury site, sprouts and the DRG. As noted above, the same is true in the CCI model, and no doubt also in several additional neuropathic pain models in which peripheral nerves are partially damaged in one way or another (e.g. Willenbring et al 1995, Kupers et al 1998). Autotomy is generally avoided in these models because sensory cover of the hindlimb is preserved. Behavioural evidence of ongoing dysaesthesias, however, is routinely reported. We believe that ectopia, directly and in conjunction with central sensitization, is the proximate cause of the nocifensive behaviour in all of these models.

The partial nerve injury models, collectively, enjoy intuitive a priori validity as surrogates for the corresponding clinical pain conditions, with allowances, of course, for the obvious differences involved. In addition, like the autotomy model, they have been experimentally validated using a wide range of drugs and procedures that reduce ectopia and/or central sensitization, and that have proven therapeutic efficacy in humans (e.g., Yamamoto & Yaksh 1992, Ardid & Guilbaud 1992, Lee et al 1995, Meyerson et al 1995, Ollat & Cesaro 1995, Chaplan et al 1995, Jett et al 1997, Hunter et al 1997, Chapman et al 1998).

It should be pointed out that although similar to one another, the partial nerve injury models probably do not yield identical symptoms. Significant differences have been reported in specific nocifensive parameters such as time-course and modality selectivity (reviewed by Zeltser & Seltzer 1994, Seltzer 1995, Coyle 1996, Kim et al 1997a, b), and in the response to therapeutic modalities such as sympathectomy (see below).

AVENUES OF DISCOVERY BASED ON BEHAVIOURAL MODELS OF NEUROPATHIC PAIN

The validation of the neuropathic pain models based on existing therapeutic modalities means that these models can be used with some confidence as screening tools in the discovery of therapeutic compounds and procedures not previously proven in man. The first major example is the NMDA receptor-antagonists. Their promise in the relief of neuropathic pain was first established in the autotomy and partial nerve injury models (Seltzer et al 1991b,c Davar et al 1991, Tal & Bennett 1994b, Banos et al 1994, Danilova et al 1997, Kim et al 1997b, Malcangio & Tomlinson 1998) and has since become the focus of an extensive series of clinical drug trials. Additional examples include the efforts to develop analgesics based on cannabinoid receptor agonists (Seltzer et al 1991d, Herzberg et al 1997), Ca^{2+}-channel antagonists (Xiao & Bennett 1995) and intrathecally implanted bovine chromaffin cells (Ginzburg & Seltzer 1990, Hama & Sagen 1994, Decosterd et al 1998, Siegan & Sagen 1998).

Beyond drug screening, the animal surrogates provide unique opportunities for the discovery of novel mechanisms, including those inaccessible to clinical research. Examples include:

1. *Genetic factors underlying neuropathic pain.* An outstanding feature of neuropathic pains as manifest clinically is the variability seen from individual to individual, even when the lesion is essentially identical. Is there a heritable component to this variability, or is it all due to socialization? Research using inbred strains of mice and rats, where variability is due almost exclusively to genotype, has revealed dramatic across-strain differences on assays of basal nociception, and in models of inflammation and neuropathic pain (Mogil et al 1999, Devor et al 1982, Wiesenfeld & Hallin 1981). Such differences permit one to determine which measures correlate with one another, and which are independent. Moreover, they permit the identification of the genetic polymorphisms responsible for phenotypic variability (quantitative trait loci, QTLs; Mogil et al 1996). In a related approach, Devor and Raber (1990), using selective breeding, derived rat lines that consistently exhibited high (HA) versus low (LA) levels of autotomy (Fig. 5.13). This proves that the trait is heritable. Subsequent hybridization and backcross experiments indicated that autotomy is a Mendelian trait, transmitted primarily by a single autosomal recessive gene with minor modifiers (Devor & Raber 1990).

   The genetic approach differs fundamentally from the like-sounding gene knock-out and knock-in methods (Mogil & Grisel 1998). The latter are used to test whether the protein products of particular identified genes play a role in nociception. Candidates for testing usually come from knowledge of pain physiology and pharmacology ... opioid, peptide or NMDA receptors, for example. The former, by contrast, makes no prior assumptions, attempting rather to identify those genes that in fact make a difference. The hope is that unimagined aspects of pain physiology may be discovered in this way.

2. *Effects of nutrition and diet.* There is an emerging body of literature indicating that nutrients consumed by animals perioperatively and postoperatively affect nociceptive measures at baseline and in neuropathic pain models (Abbott & Young 1991, Yehuda & Carasso 1987, 1993, Shir et al 1997, 1998). For example, autotomy following complete nerve injury is suppressed, while allodynia and hyperalgesia following partial nerve injury is enhanced, in rats fed a diet in which casein is the sole source of protein (Shir et al 1997, 1998). Soy suppresses neuropathic hypersensibility.
3. *Sympathetic–sensory coupling.* Can the study of animal models break the impass in understanding why some chronic pains are dependent on an intact sympathetic nervous system while others are sympathetically independent? Autotomy, for example, is augmented by the mono-amine oxidase inhibitor pargyline, and by adrenaline, and suppressed by sympatholysis (Wall et al 1979b, Coderre et al 1986). Likewise, sympathetic agonists enhance cutaneous allodynia in several partial nerve transection models, while sympathectomy relieves it (Shir & Seltzer 1990, Kim & Chung 1991, Kim et al 1993, Tracey et al 1995, Kinnaman & Levine 1995, Ali et al 1998; but see Ringkamp et al 1998). In the CCI model, by contrast, mechanical allodynia appears to be unaffected by sympathectomy, although thermal (especially cold) allodynia is reduced (Neil et al 1991, Perrot et al 1993, Desmeules et al 1995). A caveat here is that sympathectomy may reduce the nerve swelling required to produce the CCI lesion in the first place. Allodynia in

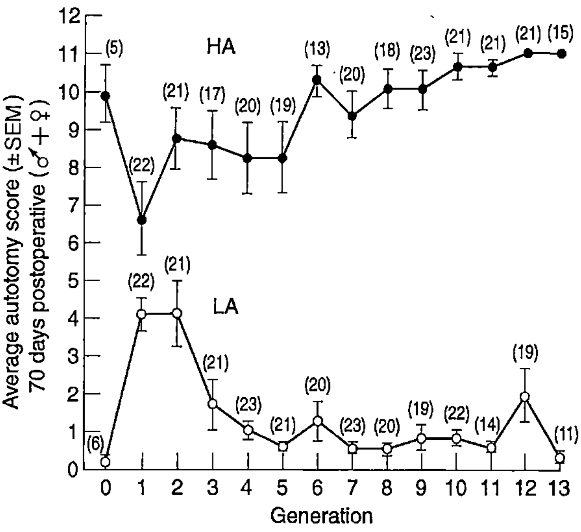

Fig. 5.13 Genetic selection for rats with high (HA) versus low (LA) levels of autotomy. Numbers in parentheses are the number of animals tested in each generation. (Reproduced from Devor & Raber 1990.)

borderline skin, and in streptozotocin-induced diabetic neuropathy, is apparently sympathetically independent (Vallin & Kingery 1991, Ahlgren & Levine 1993). Details of the lesion, testing modality, genetic background, etc. may ultimately account for the variability.

4. *Acute injury effects and pre-emptive analgesia.* Acute noxious input triggers transient allodynia by initiating central sensitization (see above). If such input were particularly intense or prolonged, might it leave a lasting trace (Katz & Melzack 1990)? The 'injury discharge' that occurs on acute nerve injury (Wall et al 1974, Blenk et al 1996) might be such a stimulus. A number of animal studies have shown that the prevention of injury discharge using local anaesthetic block can reduce the later development of autotomy and allodynia (Gonzales-Darder et al 1986, Seltzer et al 1991b, Dougherty et al 1992, Yamamoto et al 1993 Seltzer 1995). Such observations led to the suggestion that if one were to prevent the intense noxious input associated with presurgical morbidity or with surgery itself, one might reduce postsurgical pain, and perhaps even avoid the later development of chronic pain. A torrent of clinical trials of this 'pre-emptive analgesia' approach have yielded mixed results, at best (Niv & Devor 1996, Nikolajsen et al 1998). Enthusiasm remains, however, at least in some quarters.

CELLULAR AND MOLECULAR MECHANISMS OF ECTOPIC HYPEREXCITABILITY

The functional importance of ectopic afferent discharge as a primary source of spontaneous neuropathic pain, and as a factor that triggers and maintains central sensitization and hence neuropathic hypersensibility, motivates investigation of the underlying mechanisms.

MEMBRANE REMODELLING

Repetitive firing (pacemaker) capability depends on the distribution and gating properties of specific transmembrane ion channels. Although many details remain to be worked out, there is steadily increasingly support for a general picture of how nerve injury leads to the remodelling of the neuronal membrane and to ectopic hyperexcitability (Devor 1983b). This model is based on the processes that regulate neuronal excitability in normal, uninjured sensory neurons (Fig. 5.14). Briefly the proteins responsible for afferent hyperexcitability, noteably voltage-sensitive Na^+, K^+ and Ca^{2+} channels, transducer molecules (e.g., SA channels) and receptor molecules of various sorts, are synthesized on ribosomes in the DRG cell soma. They are then loaded into the membrane of intracytoplasmic transport vesicles, and vectorially transported down the axon along with the rest of the axoplasmic freight. When these proteins arrive at their intended address, they are inserted into the local membrane in the process of vesicle exocytosis.

In normal neurons this process is closely regulated so that the correct molecules arrive at their correct addresses in appropriate numbers. The regulation is dynamic. That is, a constant flow and insertion of freshly synthesized channel, transducer and receptor molecules is balanced by reuptake and degradation of previously inserted molecules. The turnover half-life of Na^+ channels, for example, is 1–3 days (Schmidt & Catterall 1986, Brismar & Gilly 1987). The precise control of this process is understood only sketchily, but it clearly involves a complex and delicately balanced system of signals within and among the sensory neurons themselves, and associated non-neuronal cells such as glia and Merkel cells. Nerve injury causes failure of regulation, with resultant remodelling of the afferents' membrane electrical properties. Dysregulation and remodelling involves at least the three interrelated processes, described below.

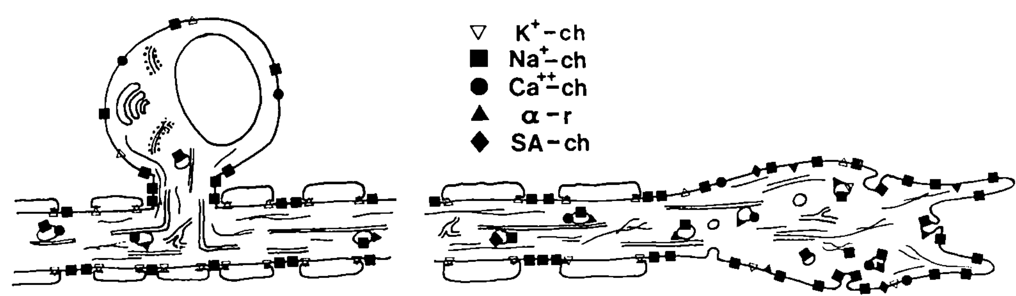

Fig. 5.14 The neural mechanism of hyperexcitability in injured afferent neurons (working hypothesis). Various ion channels, transducer molecules and receptors are synthesized in the cell soma (left), transported along the axon, and incorporated in excess into the axon membrane of endbulbs and sprouts associated with the injury. K^+-ch = potassium channels; Na^+-ch = sodium channels; Ca^{++}-ch = calcium channels; α-r = α adrenoreceptor; SA-ch = stretch-activated transducer channel. (Modified from Devor 1983b.)

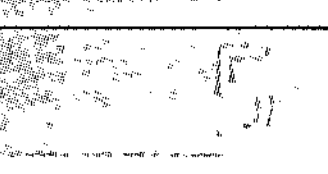

1. Ion channel accumulation

The first process is failure in the regulation of vectorial transport and membrane insertion of voltage-sensitive channels. For example, Na^+ channels are known to accumulate in excess numbers in the axonal membrane at neuroma endbulbs, in patches of demyelination, and in aborted and regenerating sprouts (Fig. 5.15; Lombet et al 1985, Devor et al 1989, 1993, Gilly et al 1990, Black et al 1991, England et al 1991, 1996a, Novakovic et al 1998). Na^+-channel accumulation renders these ectopic pacemaker sites hyperexcitable (Matzner & Devor 1992, 1994, Devor et al 1994b, Omana-Zapata et al 1997). Although the evidence is still fragmentary, it is likely that other channels, and transducer and receptor molecules, likewise accumulate and for the same reasons. This might contribute to abnormal mechanosensitivity, thermosensitivity and chemosensitivity. Partial axoplasmic transport block reduces spontaneous firing and mechanosensitivity in neuromas (Devor & Govrin-Lippmann 1983, Koschorke et al 1994). Ca^{2+}-channel accumulation probably plays only a minor role, as topical application of various Ca^{2+}-channel blockers does not much affect ectopic neuroma discharge (Matzner & Devor 1994; but see Xie et al 1993).

Functional remodelling of the axonal membrane by channel accumulation does not require a de novo process, only a quantitative shift in the normal equilibrium of channel insertion and reuptake. Both permissive and promotional factors appear to be involved. Axonal membrane under myelin normally contains a very low density of Na^+ channels, presumably because myelin prevents their insertion into subjacent axolemma (Waxman & Ritchie 1985). Injury-induced myelin stripping, sprouting and endbulb formation eliminate this suppression. Axotomy also *promotes* membrane remodelling. Normally, the large amount of Na^+-channel protein transported down the axon supports rapid turnover at downstream nodes of Ranvier, internodal membrane and sensory endings. Following axotomy, these targets no longer exist. In-transit channels are therefore shunted into whatever competent membrane sites remain, notably endbulbs and sprouts (Fig. 5.15). Sites far upstream of the injury might also receive some of the now excess channel protein. If this includes the cell soma (Gilly & Brismar 1989), it could contribute to the hyperexcitability of axotomized DRGs.

2. Upregulation of the molecules of excitability

The excitability of a particular neuronal type depends on the particular ensemble of channels, transducers and receptors synthesized in the cell soma. This ensemble changes following nerve injury. A simple calculation reveals that in sensory neurons serving the extremities >99% of the cells' cytoplasmic mass is in the axon. It is therefore no surprise that axonal injury in mid-nerve has major metabolic consequences, including those for the molecules of excitability. It has been known for decades that the synthesis of many different proteins in DRG neurons is either increased (upregu-

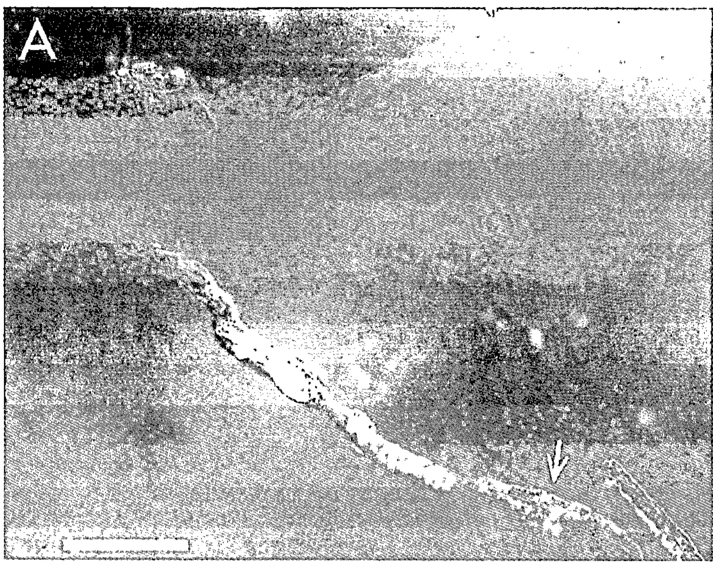

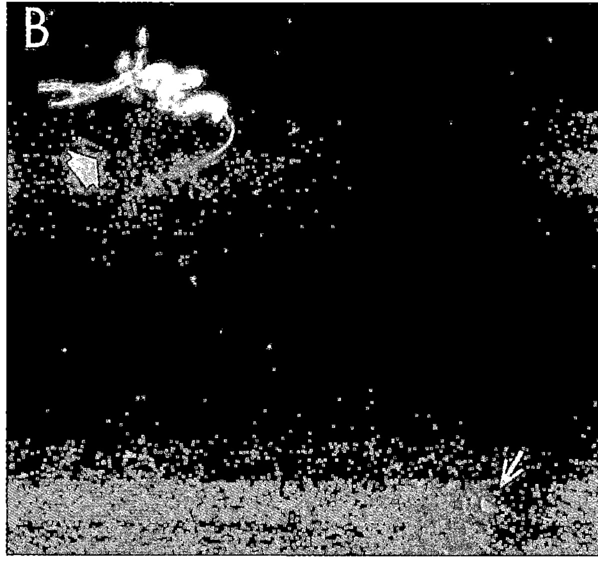

Fig. 5.15 Evidence for Na^+ channel accumulation on neuroma endbulbs. **A** Nomarski differential interference contrast micrograph of a chronically injured afferent axon endbulb with sprouts. Myelin is present until about 250 μm from the axon end. The thin arrow marks the location of a node of Ranvier. **B** The same axon immunofluorescently labelled using an antibody that recognizes voltage-sensitive Na^+ channels. Note the accumulation of label on the demyelinated distal portion of the axon, and on the endbulb and sprouts (thick arrow). Scale bar = 100 μm. (Reproduced from Devor et al 1989.)

lated), or decreased (downregulated), following axotomy (Brattgard et al 1957, Grafstein & McQuarrie 1978). This conclusion has been extended to many more molecules using modern hybridization methods (e.g., Nahin et al 1994, Hokfelt et al 1997). A traditional rule-of-thumb holds that structural molecules are upregulated following axotomy, and neurotransmitter-related molecules downregulated, all in the service of regeneration (Grafstein & McQuarrie 1978). However, this scheme is frequently violated. At present there is no reliable way to predict how regulation of a particular molecule will change following axotomy; each must be checked empirically. On the other hand, the functional effect of increasing or decreasing the density of a particular channel can often be predicted using computer models and drugs which enhance or block channel function. For example, simulation of increased Na^+ conductance (fast or slow) predicts a modest reduction in single-spike threshold, and dramatic facilitation of repetitive spiking (Fig. 5.16A). Likewise, a decrease in the delayed rectifier K^+ conductance is expected to yield hyperexcitability (Fig. 5.16B; Matzner & Devor 1992, Devor et al 1994b, Elliott 1997, Schild & Kunze 1997). Both predictions are consistent with results of drug application (e.g., Devor 1983a, Burchiel & Russell 1985, Matzner & Devor 1994, Omana-Zapata et al 1997).

The empirical evaluation of changes in expression of the molecules of excitability following various forms of nerve injury has only just begun. It is complicated by the fact that all of the ion channels, transducer molecules and receptors that determine the excitability of sensory neurons probably occur in a variety of subtypes, coded by different genes (and their mRNA transcripts), and/or result from differential post-transcriptional processing. For example, at the time of writing a family of 11 genes has been identified that code for the main (α) subunit of Na^+ channels in mammalian cells, and several have splice variants. Others code for accessory ($\beta 1$ and $\beta 2$) subunits of the Na^+ channel. At least seven α subunits are known to be expressed in sensory neurons (Catterall 1992, Black et al 1996, Dib-Hajj et al 1998b, Plummer & Meisler 1999).

With respect to ectopic firing, perhaps the most interesting observation to date is that the brain type III Na^+-channel subtype is considerably upregulated beginning a few days after axotomy (Waxman et al 1994, Cummins & Waxman 1997). This change could be responsible for the net increase in Na^+ current generated in axotomized DRG neurons (Rizzo et al 1995, Zhang et al 1997) and for its accelerated kinetics (Cummins & Waxman 1997), changes that contribute to the overall electrical hyperexcitability of these neurons. However, the fact that the concerto of excitability is played by so many molecular types and subtypes, each differentially regulated, means that things may soon become very complicated. For example, while type III Na^+ channels are upregulated following axotomy, the PN3/SNS and NaN/SN52 Na^+ channel subtypes are ***down-regulated*** (Cummins & Waxman 1997, Oaklander & Belzberg 1997, Dib-Hajj et al 1998b; Tate et al 1998 but see Novakovic et al 1998). Ultimately, changes in all the key molecular players are integrated. The net effect on cell excitability is likely to vary with the type of afferent, the type of nerve injury, the time post injury, the age, the genetic background and all of the other factors that contribute to the variability of neuropathic pain symptomatology. Interestingly, even if expression of a particular channel type is unchanged or downregulated, it could nonetheless contribute to functional *hyper*excitability. For example, the mRNA for the PN3/SNS Na^+ channel is probably downregulated in the cell soma, but its protein product accumulates in neuroma endings (Novakovic et al 1998).

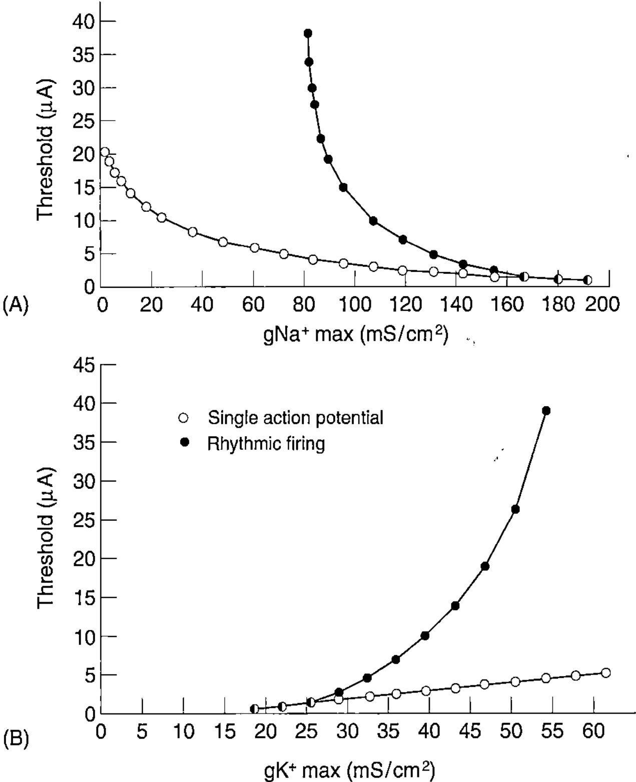

Fig. 5.16 The threshold for repetitive firing is highly sensitive to the density of Na^+ and K^+ channels in the encoding zone of the afferent axon end. **A** Computer simulation of the threshold for evoking a single spike (-○-), and for evoking rhythmic firing (-●-), as the maximal Na^+ current (gNa+max) is varied. (Based on the H-H model of the squid giant axon (Matzner & Devor 1992). **B** Same type of simulation as above, but keeping gNa+max constant and varying gK+max. (Reproduced from Devor et al 1994a.)

Downregulation of K^+ channels is also expected to yield hyperexcitability (Fig. 5.16B; Everill & Kocsis 1998).

Important information on channel regulation, including therapeutic opportunities, is likely to come from knowledge of the mechanism by which axotomy triggers altered channel expression. There is accumulating evidence that nerve growth factor (NGF) and related neurotrophic molecules are important mediators. NGF has been recognized since the 1950s as being essential for the survival and differentiation of many DRG neurons during development (Levi-Montalcini & Angeletti 1968). It is now known that it, along with related neurokines such as fibroblast growth factor (FGF), interleukin (IL-6) and leukaemia inhibitory factor (LIF), also plays a key role in adulthood as regulators of gene expression and hence function ('phenotype') in DRG neurons that bear the corresponding receptors (Pollock et al 1990, Lewin & Mendell 1993, Ji et al 1996, Lesser et al 1997, McMahon et al 1997). NGF provided in vitro triggers the upregulation of Na^+-channel synthesis in many cell types, including DRG neurons (Aguayo & White 1992, Zur et al 1995). This suggests that loss of NGF normally supplied by retrograde transport from the periphery may be the signal that triggers upregulation of type III Na^+-channel expression, and downregulation of PN3/SNS and NaN/SNS 2 Na^+ channels following axotomy. Indeed, provision of excess NGF to the cut nerve end in vivo partially prevents many of the retrograde effects of axotomy, including the changes in Na^+-(and K^+-) channel expression (Oyelese et al 1997, Dib-Hajj et al 1998a). It should be kept in mind, however, that glial proliferation and immune cell recruitment triggered by nerve injury results in the local release of large quantities of neurotrophins at and distal to the injury site, and in the DRG (e.g., Heumann et al 1987, Sebert & Shooter 1993, Rotshenker 1997). Pathways for the regulation of excitability are further complicated by the fact that different neurotrophins affect Na^+-channel subtypes differentially (Friedel et al 1997, Lesser et al 1997).

3. Control of the functional parameters of ion channels

The third process that contributes to the remodelling of membrane excitability is direct control of the functional properties of ion channel, transducer and receptor molecules (in contrast to control of their density). For example, enzymatic addition of a phosphate group to the Na^+-channel molecule reduces Na^+ current, while dephosphorylation returns it to normal (e.g., Li et al 1992). Because certain hormones, trophic factors, neuromodulatory peptides and inflammatory mediators can activate phosphorylating enzymes including protein kinase A and C (PKA, PKC), they are well positioned to affect afferent excitability. As noted above, many such hyperalgesic agents are present at sites of nerve injury and they contribute to ectopia. The alteration of Na^+- and K^+-channel kinetics is probably a contributing mechanism (Gold et al 1996, England et al 1996b, Nicol et al 1997). Some neurons are thought to contain latent channels which only become active in the presence of appropriate mediators (e.g., Cohan et al 1985). At the level of the whole cell, there are afferents that do not respond to any stimuli until they are sensitized by inflammatory mediators (Schmidt et al 1994).

While cytokines and growth factors affect afferent excitability by controlling channel expression and function, the reader should not conclude that each such regulatory molecule has these two effects. Regulatory molecules can have numerous effects (pleiotropy) which, together, reorder the entire physiological agenda of the cell. For example, β-adrenergic stimulation of cardiac cells simultaneously affects ion pumps, metabolic enzymes, the cytoskeleton, many ion channels and gene expression (see Hille 1992b). Likewise, serotonin leads to the phosphorylation of at least 17 cytoplasmic proteins in *Aplysia* sensory neurons (Sweatt & Kandel 1989). As noted above, nerve injury probably alters more proteins in axotomized DRG neurons than it leaves unchanged. The challenge is to determine *which* of the changes play an important role in the development of neuropathic pain.

A RELATION BETWEEN NEUROPATHIC PAIN PROCESSES AND INFLAMMATION?

It is traditional to think of inflammatory and neuropathic pain as two distinct entities. Advances in our understanding of cellular and molecular mechanisms are rapidly changing this conception. First, central sensitization is an important cause of allodynia in both inflammatory and neuropathic pain states; the transient central sensitization mechanism is engaged whether the nociceptive input that triggers and maintains it comes from inflamed, peripherally sensitized nociceptors or from ectopic neuropathic sources. Second, channel, transducer and receptor redistribution, upregulation and modulation apply to both, and involve the same families of mediator molecules (e.g., Gould et al 1998, Tanaka et al 1998; see Ch. 2).

An interesting example of the increasingly fuzzy border between neuropathic and inflammatory pain comes from recent experiments using the CCI model of neuropathic pain in rats (see above). At least part of the pain in this model appears to be due to local inflammation generated by the chromic gut suture material used to constrict the nerve

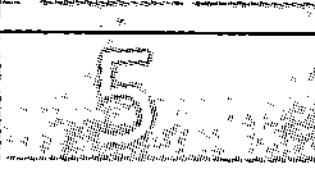

(Maves et al 1993). Nociceptor axons traumatized by the constriction develop ectopic sensitivity to mediator molecules released by inflammatory cells recruited to the CCI site (Zimmermann et al 1987, Devor et al 1992b, Tracey & Walker 1995, Noda et al 1997, Michaelis et al 1998b). It has even been proposed that one inflammatory mediator, TNFα, can evoke ectopic firing in mid-nerve axons that have *not* undergone trauma (Sorkin et al 1997).

These considerations have led to a novel hybrid hypothesis concerning the origins of low back pain and sciatica, a hypothesis that might be equally applicable to other chronic musculoskeletal pain conditions (Kawakami et al 1994, 1996, Cavanaugh 1995, Olmarker & Myers 1998 Devor 1996). Briefly, it is proposed that the herniation of an intervertebral disc causes mechanical trauma to axons and/or somata of sensory neurons. This renders them spontaneously active, and hyperexcitable to mechanical stimulation and to chemical mediators as discussed above. In addition, however, rupture of the annulus fibrosus during disc herniation leads to the release of inflammatory mediators from the nucleus pulposus, and from inflammatory/immune cells recruited to the site. These mediators exacerbate the ectopia and the resulting pain.

AVENUES FOR THE MEDICAL CONTROL OF ECTOPIC NEURAL DISCHARGE

The ultimate test of the ectopic pacemaker hypothesis is the extent to which it can explain clinical manifestations and therapeutic efficacy, and predict novel treatment approaches. In the discussion above, many examples were given in which the abnormal discharge properties of injured afferents account well for neuropathic symptomatology. In this section the relation of ectopia to treatment modalities is discussed.

MEMBRANE STABILIZATION VERSUS SYNAPTIC BLOCKADE

Ectopic discharge originating in the PNS feeds into the CNS, providing a primary neuropathic signal, and maintaining elevated central amplification (central sensitization) and hence allodynia. The CNS components of the pain system include ascending transmission, descending control and signal processing networks that extend from the spinal cord to the highest levels of cognitive function. Each CNS component invites particular therapeutic approaches. For example, opiates activate descending control circuits, and there is hope that NMDA-receptor antagonists may control abnormal signal amplification in the spinal cord. Such drugs modulate *synaptic transmission.* The ectopic pacemaker hypothesis points to a different approach, the targeting of ***membrane excitability.***

MODERATING MEMBRANE HYPEREXCITABILITY

The research to date points to vectorial redistribution, upregulation and functional modulation of Na^+ channels as the main culprits in neuropathic membrane hyperexcitability. Many drugs that block Na^+ channels are available for clinical use. The most widely used are the local anaesthetics. Lidocaine and bupivicaine, of course, are routinely employed for blocking nerve conduction. For the relatively brief duration of their action they are highly effective at relieving pain whose source is distal to the block. This is so for pain signals of nociceptive as well as neuropathic origin (see Ch. 52). However, it would be lethal to administer systemically the concentrations of local anaesthetics required to block nerve conduction (2% lidocaine = 20 mg/ml). Nonetheless, intravenous lidocaine at low concentrations (2–4 µg/ml plasma, 3–5 mg/kg IV over 30 min; see Wallace et al 1996) has been used for many years, with proven efficacy in double-blind placebo controlled trials involving a range of different neuropathic pain states (Glazer & Portnoy 1991, Fields et al 1997, Kalso et al 1998). The classic mystery of how lidocaine concentrations which are far too low to block nerve conduction can, nonetheless, relieve neuropathic pain is resolved by the observation that 5 mg/kg is more than enough to suppress ectopic neuroma and DRG discharge (Fig. 5.17; Devor et al 1992a, Matzner & Devor 1994, Chaplan et al 1995, Omana-Zapata et al 1997).

While systemic lidocaine has a place in neuropathic pain control, its utility is limited by its short serum half-life, the need to administer intravenously and adverse side effects. The first two problems are solved by certain anticonvulsants (notably carbamazepine, phenytoin and lamotrigine) and antiarrhythmics (mexiletine) whose mode of action is Na^+-channel blockade (Catterall 1987, Macdonald & Greenfield 1997). Each suppresses ectopic firing (e.g., Yaari & Devor 1985, Burchiel 1988, Chabal et al 1989a) and offers relief from neuropathic pain (McQuay et al 1995, Fields et al 1997, Kalso et al 1998). Indeed, response to intravenous lidocaine predicts their efficacy (Galer et al 1996). Together, these 'adjuvants' (i.e. drugs developed for other indications) constitute one of today's two frontline therapeutic options in the treatment of neuropathic pain. It is noteworthy that *synaptically* acting anticonvulsants like barbiturates are relatively ineffective as analgesics.

The second frontline therapeutic option is low-dose antidepressants, notably amitriptyline (McQuay et al 1996).

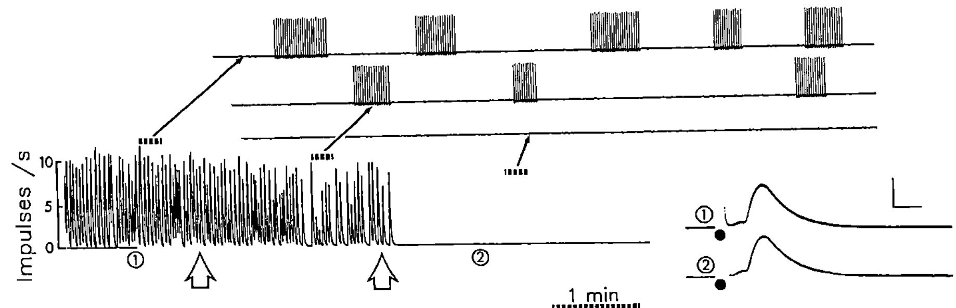

Fig. 5.17 Systemic lidocaine silences ectopia without blocking the ability of axons to conduct impulses. The recording shows spontaneous burst discharge originating in an experimental nerve-end neuroma (8 days post operation, experimental setup as in the sketch in Fig. 5.4). A first injection of lidocaine (left open arrow, 100 μl 1% lidocaine) slowed the rate of bursting. A second injection stopped the firing altogether (right open arrow). The continued response of the axon to electrical stimulation just central to the neuroma (lower right) proves that axonal conduction was *not* blocked. Action potentials were evoked at times 1 and 2. Calibration = 1.5 mV, 0.5 ms. (Reproduced from Devor et al 1992a.)

The mechanism of action of amitriptyline in pain control is uncertain, but the recent discovery that it, too, blocks Na^+ channels (Pancrazio et al 1998) and suppresses ectopic neuroma discharge (M Devor, unpublished) provides a possible answer. Corticosteroids also have membrane-stabilizing properties, in addition to their better known anti-inflammatory actions. The suppression of ectopia may contribute significantly to the efficacy of depot-form corticosteriods when injected into painful trigger points (Travell & Simons 1984, Devor et al 1985).

The practical limitation on systemically delivered Na^+-channel blockers, the reason that higher and presumably more effective doses cannot be reached, is their adverse side effects. These include vertigo, nausea and somnolence, and at very high dose convulsions. Interestingly, cardiac side effects are rarely a problem. The dose-limiting effects result from CNS suppression; all of these drugs are lipophilic and enter the brain. The excitability of CNS neurons also depends on Na^+ channels. Indeed CNS suppression may contribute to the analgesic effect of systemic Na^+-channel blockers (Woolf & Wiesenfeld-Hallin 1985, Sotgiu et al 1994).

The avoidance of adverse CNS side effects requires selective drug delivery. Several potential solutions present themselves. An approach that has attracted particular attention recently is the hope of developing blockers selective for Na^+-channel types that occur only in the PNS. The lead targets today are the PN3/SNS and the NaN/SN52 Na^+ channel subtypes because of their selective expression in (small diameter) DRG neurons. Even though downregulated following nerve injury, they may still make a significant contribution to the overall excitability of nociceptors, especially in neuroma endings (Dib-Hajj et al 1998a,b, Novakovic et al 1998). Another approach is the development of lidocaine-like drugs with preserved PNS action that fail to cross the blood–brain barrier. Although not trivial, potential approaches exist. Likewise, one might improve the delivery of conventional Na^+-channel blockers to sites of ectopic electrogenesis, including the DRG. Finally, therapeutic targets might be found among the various processes that regulate Na^+ channels, and among the other channel, transducer and receptor molecules responsible for neuronal hyperexcitability.

SOURCES OF VARIABILITY: WHY DO SO MANY THINGS NOT WORK?

It is instructive to consider therapeutic approaches that ought to work, but do not (e.g., Sherman et al 1980). First, reamputation. It seems logical that if neuromas are an important source of painful ectopic discharge, that resecting neuromas ought to bring relief. The problem here is that beginning hours after the resection (Koschorke et al 1991, Michaelis et al 1995) the same pathophysiological processes are engaged as before, and a new source of ectopia is created. Resection is expected to be effective only if it removes the neuroma from influences that exacerbate ectopic firing, such as mechanical compression.

Nerve block is often effective, but safely maintaining the block for long periods of time is not trivial (e.g., Byers et al 1973). Furthermore, ectopic sources central to the block, particularly the DRG and spinal roots, must be considered. Nerve blocks sometimes provide pain relief for much longer than expected (e.g., Arner et al 1990). This may be due to the bistable nature of the repetitive firing process and residual low tissue levels of the local anaesthetic (Fig. 5.3B). However, nothing about the ectopic pacemaker hypothesis predicts that one or a series of local anaesthetic blocks should have permanent effects.

As noted above, adrenergic agonists and sympathetic stimulation activate a high proportion of ectopic pacemaker sites, and injection of adrenaline into a neuroma is consistently painful. Why, then, is sympatholysis effective only infrequently? It must be recalled that in each neuropathic pain syndrome ectopic firing appears to be sustained by an idiosyncratic ensemble of stimulating factors. Only if adrenosensitivity is the major factor in a particular patient is sympathectomy expected to bring dramatic improvement. This is the main advantage of suppressing the Na^+-channel-dependent encoding (pacemaker) process; all of the various contributions to the generator current are funnelled through it (Fig. 5.3A).

The question of individual differences, of course, goes beyond the issue of sympathetic–sensory coupling. Why, for example, does a particular grade of injury, say below the knee amputation, result in sustained pain in one individual and not in another? The fact that reamputation is usually not an effective option, that another 'roll of the dice' tends to yield the same result as before, indicates that the source of variability lies with the individual and not with the surgeon. The evidence, drawn from animal models, that susceptibility to neuropathic pain is a heritable trait was discussed above. This may hold for humans as well. We can only guess at which level(s) of the pain system, peripheral nerve, spinal cord, brain or consciousness, neuropathic pain genes express themselves.

SUMMARY

When a telephone cable is cut across, the signal at both ends falls silent. Damaged nerves behave differently. Axonal injury triggers a range of metabolic and functional responses in the sensory cell soma that are ultimately responsible for positive sensory symptoms including chronic neuropathic pain. The most important pathophysiological change is that injured sensory neurons tend to become electrically hyperexcitable, and generate ectopic impulse discharge. Ectopia involves spontaneous firing in some neurons, and abnormal responsiveness to mechanical, thermal and chemical stimuli in many more. Sources of ectopic firing include neuroma endbulbs, regenerating sprouts, the cell soma in the DRG, patches of demyelination and even neighbouring uninjured axons. Moreover, ectopia is associated with distorting and amplifying mechanisms such as afterdischarge, and neuron-to-neuron cross-excitation. The cellular/molecular mechanism which appears to underlie ectopic hyperexcitability is the remodelling of the voltage-sensitive ion channels, transducer molecules and receptors in the cell membrane. Na^+ channels appear to be the main culprits, as they are the most directly involved in neuronal hyperexcitability. Na^+ channels accumulate in the membrane at sites of nerve injury and demyelination, some subtypes are upregulated, and their responsiveness is increased by hyperalgesic mediators. Ectopic discharge is thought to contribute to neuropathic pain in two ways. First, it constitutes a direct afferent signal. This is felt as ongoing pain and pain on movement. In addition, it can trigger and maintain central sensitization. The result is allodynia in borderline skin and zones of partial denervation. The new information currently available on mechanisms of neuropathic pain suggests specific new avenues for the development of more effective treatment options.

Acknowledgements

We thank R. Amir, J. Kocsis and C-N. Liu for their helpful comments. The support of the United States–Israel Binational Science Foundation, the Fritz Thyssen Stiftung, the Israel Science Foundation and the Hebrew University Center for Research on Pain is gratefully acknowledged.

REFERENCES

Abbott F, Young SN 1991 The effect of tryptophan supplementation on autotomy induced by nerve lesions in rats. Physiology, Biochemistry and Behavior 40: 301–304

Aguayo LG, White G 1992 Effects of nerve growth factor on TTX- and capsaicin-sensitivity in adult rat sensory neurons. Brain Research 570: 61–67

Ahlgren SC, Levine JC 1993 Mechanical hyperalgesia in streptozotocin-diabetic rats is not sympathetically maintained. Brain Research 18: 5403–5414

Ahlgren SC, White DM, Levine JD 1992 Increased responsiveness of sensory neurons in the saphenous nerve of the streptozotocin-diabetic rat. Journal of Neurophysiology 68: 2077–2085

Albe-Fessard D, Giamberardino A, Rampin O 1990 Comparison of different models of chronic pain. Advances in Pain Research and Therapy 13: 11–27

Ali Z, Ringkamp M, Hartke TV, Chien HF, Flavahan NA, Campbell JN, Meyer RA 1999 Uninjured cutaneous C-fiber nociceptors develop spontaneous activity and alpha adrenergic sensitivity following L6 spinal nerve ligation in the monkey. Journal of Neurophysiology 81: 455–467

Allen DT, Kiernan JA 1994 Permeation of proteins from the blood into peripheral nerves and ganglia. Neuroscience 59: 755–764

Amir R, Devor M 1992 Axonal cross-excitation in nerve-end neuromas: comparison of A- and C-fibers. Journal of Neurophysiology 68: 1160–1166

Amir R, Devor M 1993 Ongoing activity in neuroma afferents bearing retrograde sprouts. Brain Research 630: 283–288

Amir R, Devor M 1996 Chemically-mediated cross-excitation in rat dorsal root ganglia. Journal of Neuroscience 16: 4733–4741

Amir R, Devor M 1997 Spike-evoked suppression and burst patterning in dorsal root ganglion neurons. Journal of Physiology 501: 183–196

Amir M, Michaelis M and Devor M 1998 Membrane potential oscillations trigger the ectopic discharge that underlies neuropathic pain. Neuroscience Lett suppl. 51, St

Anand P 1996 Neurotrophins and peripheral neuropathy. Philosophical Transactions of the Royal Society of London. Series B 351: 449–454

Ardid D, Guilbaud G 1992 Antinociceptive effects of acute and 'chronic' injections of tricyclic antidepressant drugs in a new model of mononeuropathy in rats. Pain 49: 277–285

Arner S 1991 Intravenous phentolamine test: diagnostic and prognostic use in reflex sympathetic dystrophy. Pain 46: 17–22

Arner S, Lindblom U, Meyerson BA, Molander C 1990 Prolonged relief of neuralgia after regional anesthetic blocks. A call for further experimental and systematic clinical studies. Pain 43: 287–297

Asada H, Yamaguchi Y, Tsunoda S, Fukuda Y 1996 Relation of abnormal burst activity of spinal neurons to the recurrence of autotomy in rats. Neuroscience Letters 213: 99–102

Attal N, Filliatreu G, Perrot S, Jazat F, diGiamberardino L, Guilbaud G 1994 Behavioural pain-related disorders and contribution of the saphenous nerve in crush and chronic constriction injury of the rat sciatic nerve. Pain 59: 301–312

Baker M, Bostock H 1992 Ectopic activity in demyelinated spinal root axons of the rat. Journal of Physiology (London) 451: 539–552

Banos JE, Verdu E, Buti M, Navarro X 1994 Effects of dizocilpine on autotomy behavior after nerve section in mice. Brain Research 636: 107–110

Barbera J, Garcia G, Lopez-Orta A, Gil-Salu JL 1988 The role of the neuroma in autotomy following sciatic nerve section in rats. Pain 33: 373–378

Basbaum AI 1974 Effects of central lesions on disorders produced by multiple dorsal rhizotomy in rats. Experimental Neurology 42: 490–501

Basbaum AI, Gautron M, Jazat F, Mayes M, Guilbaud G 1991 The spectrum of fiber loss in a model of neuropathic pain in the rat: an electron microscopic study. Pain 47: 359–367

Bennett GJ 1994 Animal models of neuropathic pain. In: Gebhart GF, Hammond DL, Jensen TS (eds) Proceedings of the 7th world congress on pain, progress in pain research and management, vol 2. IASP Press, Seattle, pp 495–510

Bennett GJ, Xie Y-K 1988 A peripheral mononeuropathy in rat that produces disorders of pain sensation like those seen in man. Pain 33: 87–107

Bennett RM 1990 Myofascial pain syndromes and the fibromyalgia syndrome: a comparative analysis. In: Friction JR, Awad E (eds) Myofascial pain and fibromyalgia; Advances in pain research and therapy, vol 17, Raven, New York, pp 43–65

Berman D, Rodin BE 1982 The influence of housing conditions on autotomy following dorsal rhizotomy in rats. Pain 13: 307–311

Black JA, Felts P, Smith KJ, Kocsis JD, Waxman SG 1991 Distribution of sodium channels in chronically demyelinated spinal cord axons: immuno-ultrastructural localization and electro-physiological observations. Brain Research 544: 59–70

Black JA, Dib-Hajj S, McNabola K et al 1996 Spinal sensory neurons express multiple sodium channel α-subunit mRNAs. Molecular Brain Research 43: 117–131

Blenk K-H, Janig W, Michaelis M, Vogel C 1996 Prolonged injury discharge in unmyelinated nerve fibres following transection of the sural nerve in rats. Neuroscience Letters 215: 185–188

Blumberg H, Janig W 1982 Activation of fibers via experimentally produced stump neuromas of skin nerves: ephaptic transmission or retrograde sprouting? Experimental Neurology 76: 468–482

Blumberg H, Janig W 1984 Discharge pattern of afferent fibers from a neuroma. Pain 20: 335–353

Blumenkopf B, Lipman JJ 1991 Studies in autotomy: its pathophysiology and usefulness as a model of chronic pain. Pain 45: 203–210

Bongenhielm U, Robinson PP 1996 Spontaneous and mechanically evoked afferent activity originating from myelinated fibres in ferret inferior alveolar nerve neuromas. Pain 67: 399–406

Bongenhielm U, Robinson PP 1998 Afferent activity from myelinated inferior alveolar nerve fibres in ferrets after constriction or section and regeneration. Pain 74: 123–132

Bonica JJ 1990 Causalgia and other reflex sympathetic dystrophies. In: Bonica JJ (ed) The management of pain. Lea and Febinger, Philadelphia, pp 220–243

Brattgard SO, Hyden H, Sjostrand J 1957 The chemical changes in regenerating neurons. Neurochemistry 1: 316–325

Breig A 1978 Adverse mechanical tension in the central nervous system. Almqvist and Wiksell, Stockholm

Brewart J, Gentle MJ 1985 Neuroma formation and abnormal afferent discharges after partial beak amputation (beak trimming) in poultry. Experientia 41: 1132–1134

Brismar T, Gilly WF 1987 Synthesis of sodium channels in the cell bodies of squid giant axons. Proceedings of the National Academy of Sciences USA 84: 1459–1463

Burchiel KJ 1980 Ectopic impulse generation in focally demyelinated trigeminal nerve. Experimental Neurology 69: 423–429

Burchiel KJ 1984a Effects of electrical and mechanical stimulation on two foci of spontaneous activity which develop in primary afferent neurons after peripheral axotomy. Pain 18: 249–265

Burchiel KJ 1984b Spontaneous impulse generation in normal and denervated dorsal root ganglia: sensitivity to alpha-adrenergic stimulation and hypoxia. Experimental Neurology 85: 257–272

Burchiel KJ 1988 Carbamazepine inhibits spontaneous activity in experimental neuromas. Experimental Neurology 102: 249–253

Burchiel KJ, Russell LC 1985 Effects of potassium channel blocking agents on spontaneous discharge from neuromas in rats. Journal of Neurosurgery 63: 243–249

Burchiel KJ, Russell LC Lee RP, Sima AA 1985 Spontaneous activity of primary afferent neurons in diabetic BB/Wistar rats: a possible mechanism of chronic diabetic neuropathic pain. Diabetes 34: 1210–1213

Byers MR, Fink BR, Kennedy RD, Middaugh ME, Hendrickson AE 1973 Effects of lidocaine on axonal morphology, microtubules, and rapid transport in rabbit vagus nerve in vitro. Journal of Neurobiology 4: 125–143

Cajal S, Ramon Y 1928 Degeneration and regeneration of the nervous system. Hafner, New York. [Translated by RM May 1968]

Calvin WH, Howe JF, Loeser JD 1977 Ectopic repetitive firing in focally demyelinated axons and some implications for trigeminal neuralgia. In: Anderson D, Matthews B (eds) Pain in the trigeminal region. Elsevier, Amsterdam, pp 125–136

Calvin WH, Devor M, Howe J 1982 Can neuralgias arise from minor demyelination? Spontaneous firing, mechanosensitivity and after-discharge from conducting axons. Experimental Neurology 75: 755–763

Campbell JN, Raja SN, Meyer RA, MacKinnon SE 1988 Myelinated afferents signal the hyperalgesia associated with nerve injury. Pain 32: 89–94

Carlton SM, Dougherty M, Pover CM, Coggeshall RE 1991 Neuroma formation and numbers of axons in a rat model of experimental peripheral neuropathy. Neuroscience Letters 131: 88–92

Caterina MJ, Schumacher MA, Tominaga M, Rosen TA, Levine JD, Julius D 1997 The capsaicin receptor: a heat-activated ion channel in the pain pathway. Nature 389: 816–824

Catterall WA 1987 Common modes of drug action on Na^+ channels: local anaesthetics, antiarrhythmics and anticonvulsants. Trends in Pharmacological Sciences 8: 57–65

Catterall WA 1992 Cellular and molecular biology of voltage-gated sodium channels. Physiological Reviews 72: 15–48

Cavanaugh JM 1995 Neural mechanisms of lumbar pain. Spine 20: 1804–1809

Chabal C, Russell LC, Burchiel KJ 1989a The effect of intravenous lidocaine, tocainide, and mexiletine on spontaneously active fibers originating in rat sciatic neuromas. Pain 38: 333–338

Chabal C, Jacobson L, Burchiel KJ 1989 Pain responses to perineuromal injection of normal saline, gallamine, and lidocaine in humans. Pain 36: 321–325

Chabal C, Jacobson L, Russell LC, Burchiel KJ 1992 Pain responses to perineuromal injection of normal saline, epinephrine, and lidocaine in humans. Pain 49: 9–12

Chaplan SR, Bach FW, Shafer SL, Yaksh TL 1995 Prolonged alleviation of tactile allodynia by intravenous lidocaine in neuropathic rats. Anesthesiology 83: 775–785

Chapman V, Suzuki R, Chamarette HL, Rygh LJ, Dickenson AH 1998 Effects of systemic carbamazepine and gabapentin on spinal neuronal responses in spinal nerve ligated rats. Pain 75: 261–272

Chen Y, Devor M 1998 Ectopic mechanosensitivity in injured sensory axons arises from the site of spontaneous electrogenesis. European Journal of Pain 2: 165–178

Chen Y, Michaelis M, Janig W, Devor M 1996 Adrenoreceptor subtype mediating sympathetic-sensory coupling in injured sensory neurons. Journal of Neurophysiology 76: 3721–3730

Choi Y, Yoon YW, Na HS, Kim SH, Chung JM 1994 Behavioral signs of ongoing pain and cold allodynia in a rat model of neuropathic pain. Pain 59: 369–376

Cline MA, Ochoa J, Torebjork HE 1989 Chronic hyperalgesia and skin warming caused by sensitized C nociceptors. Brain 112: 621–647

Coderre TJ, Grimes RW, Melzack R 1986 Deafferentation and chronic pain in animals: an evaluation of evidence suggesting autotomy is related to pain. Pain 26: 61–84

Cohan CS, Haydon PG, Kater SB 1985 Single channel activity differs in growing and nongrowing growth cones of isolated identified neurons of Helisoma. Journal of Neuroscience Research 13: 285–300

Colado MI, Del Rio J, Peralta E 1994 Neonatal guanethidine sympathectomy suppresses autotomy and prevents changes in spinal and supraspinal monoamine levels induced by peripheral deafferentation in rats. Pain 56: 3–8

Cook AJ, Woolf CJ, Wall PD, McMahon SB 1987 Dynamic receptive field plasticity in rat spinal cord dorsal horn following C-primary afferent input. Nature (London) 325: 151–153

Coyle D 1996 Efficacy of animal models for neuropathic pain. PSNS SIG Newsletter (IASP) Spring: 2–7

Cummins TR, Waxman SG 1997 Downregulation of tetrodotoxin-resistant sodium currents and upregulation of a rapidly repriming tetrodotoxin-sensitive sodium current in small spinal sensory neurons after nerve injury. Journal of Neuroscience 17: 3503–3514

Danilova EI, Grafova VN, Reshetniak VK 1997 The role of the NMDA-receptor blocker and stimulator ketamine and glycine in the development of a neuropathic pain syndrome. Experimental and Clinical Pharmacology 60: 10–13

Davar G, Fareed M, Lee DH, Noh HR, Chung JM 1996 Identification and increased expression of a novel alpha 2-adrenoreceptor mRNA in dorsal root ganglia in a rat model of experimental painful neuropathy. In: IASP Abstracts, vol 8. IASP Press, Seattle, p 29

Davar G, Hama A, Deykin A, Vos B, Maciewicz R 1991 MK-801 blocks the development of thermal hyperalgesia in a rat model of experimental painful neuropathy. Brain Research 553: 327–330

Davis KD, Treede RD, Raja SN, Meyer RA, Campbell JN 1991 Topical application of clonidine relieves hyperalgesia in patients with sympathetically maintained pain. Pain 47: 309–317

De Santis M, Duckworth JW 1982 Properties of primary afferent neurons from muscles which are spontaneously active after a lesion of their peripheral process. Experimental Neurology 75: 261–274

Decosterd I, Buchser E, Gilliard N, Saydoff J, Zurn AD, Aebischer P 1998 Intrathecal implants of bovine chromaffin cells alleviate mechanical allodynia in a rat model of neuropathic pain. Pain 76: 159–166

Delio DA, Reuhl KR, Lowndes HE 1992 Ectopic impulse generation in dorsal root ganglion neurons during methylmercury intoxication: an electrophysiological and morphological study. Neurotoxicology 13: 527–540

Desmeules JA, Kayser V, Weil-Fuggaza J, Bertrand A, Guilbaud G 1995 Influence of the sympathetic nervous system in the development of abnormal pain-related behaviours in a rat model of neuropathic pain. Neuroscience 67: 941–951

Devor M 1983a Potassium channels moderate ectopic excitability of nerve-end neuromas in rats. Neuroscience Letters 40: 181–186

Devor M 1983b Nerve pathophysiology and mechanisms of pain in causalgia. Journal of the Autonomic Nervous System 7: 371–384

Devor M 1988 Central changes mediating neuropathic pain. In: Dubner R, Gebhart GF, Bond MR (eds) Pain research and clinical management, vol 3. Proceedings of the Vth World Congress on Pain. Elsevier, Amsterdam, pp 114–128

Devor M 1996 Pain arising from nerve roots and the DRG. In: Weinstein J, Gordon S (eds) Low back pain: a scientific and clinical overview. American Academy of Orthopaedic Surgery, Rosemont, IL, pp 187–208

Devor M 1999 Teased-fiber recording from peripheral nerves and spinal roots. In: Kocsis J (ed) Electrophysiological methods for the study of the mammalian nervous system. Appleton and Lange, New York (in press)

Devor M, Govrin-Lippmann R 1983 Axoplasmic transport block reduces ectopic impulse generation in injured peripheral nerves. Pain 16: 73–85

Devor M, Govrin-Lippmann R 1985 Spontaneous neural discharge in neuroma C-fibers in rat sciatic nerve. Neuroscience Letters Supplement 22: S32

Devor M, Janig W 1981 Activation of myelinated afferents ending in a neuroma by stimulation of the sympathetic supply in the rat. Neuroscience Letters 24: 43–47

Devor M, Obermeyer M-L 1984 Membrane differentiation in rat dorsal root ganglia and possible consequences for back pain. Neuroscience Letters 51: 341–346

Devor M, Raber P 1990 Heritability of symptoms in an experimental model of neuropathic pain. Pain 42: 51–67

Devor M, Wall PD 1990 Cross excitation among dorsal root ganglion neurons in nerve injured and intact rats. Journal of Neurophysiology 64: 1733–1746

Devor M, Schonfeld D, Seltzer Z, Wall PD 1979 Two modes of cutaneous reinnervation following peripheral nerve injury. Journal of Comparative Neurology 185: 211–220

Devor M, Inbal R, Govrin-Lippmann R 1982 Genetic factors in the development of chronic pain. In: Lieblich, I (ed) Genetics of the brain. Elsevier, Amsterdam, pp 273–296

Devor M, Govrin-Lippmann R, Raber P 1985 Corticosteroids suppress ectopic neuronal discharge originating in experimental neuromas. Pain 22: 127–137

Devor M, Keller CH, Deerinck TJ, Ellisman MH 1989 Na^+ channel accumulation on axolemma of afferent endings in nerve end neuromas in *Apteronotus*. Neuroscience Letters 102: 149–154

Devor M, Keller CH, Ellisman MH 1990 Spontaneous discharge of afferents in a neuroma reflects original receptor tuning. Brain Research 517: 245–250

Devor M, Basbaum AI, Bennett GJ et al 1991 Group Report: mechanisms of neuropathic pain following peripheral injury. In: Basbaum AI, Besson J-M (eds) Towards a new pharmacotherapy of pain. Dahlem Konferenzen, Wiley, Chichester, pp 417–440

Devor M, Wall PD, Catalan N 1992a Systemic lidocaine silences ectopic neuroma and DRG discharge without blocking nerve conduction. Pain 48: 261–268

Devor M, White DM, Goetzl EJ, Levine JD 1992b Eicosanoids, but not tachykinins, excite C-fibre endings in rat sciatic nerve-end neuromas. Neuroreport 3: 21–24

Devor M, Govrin-Lippmann R, Angelides K 1993 Na+ channel immunolocalization in peripheral mammalian axons and changes following nerve injury and neuroma formation. Journal of Neuroscience 13: 1976–1992

Devor M, Janig W, Michaelis M 1994a Modulation of activity in dorsal root ganglion (DRG) neurons by sympathetic activation in nerve-injured rats. Journal of Neurophysiology 71: 38–47

Devor M, Lomazov P, Matzner O 1994b Na+ channel accumulation in injured axons as a substrate for neuropathic pain. In: Boivie J, Hansson P, Lindblom U (eds) Touch, temperature and pain in health and disease. Wenner-Gren Center Foundation Symposia. IASP Press, Seattle, pp 207–230

Devor M, Shinder V, Govrin-Lippmann R 1995 Sympathetic sprouting in axotomized rat DRG: ultrastructure. Society for Neuroscience Abstracts 21: 894

Diamond J, Coughlin M, MacIntyre L, Holmes M, Visheau 1987 Evidence that endogenous β nerve growth factor is responsible for the collateral sprouting, but not the regeneration, of nociceptive axons in adult rats. Proceedings of the National Academy of Sciences USA 84: 6596–6600

Dib-Hajj SD, Black JA, Cummins TR, Kenney AM, Kocsis JD, Waxman SG 1998a Rescue of α-SNS sodium channel expression in small dorsal root ganglion neurons after axotomy by nerve growth factor in vivo. Journal of Neurophysiology 79: 2668–2676

Dib-Hajj SD, Tyrrell L, Black JA, Waxman SG 1998b NaN, a novel voltage-gated Na+ channel preferentially in peripheral sensory neurons and down-regulated after axotomy. Proceedings of the National Academy of Sciences USA 95: 8963–8968

Dougherty PM, Garrison CJ, Carlton SM 1992 Differential influence of local anesthetic upon two models of experimentally induced peripheral mononeuropathy in the rat. Brain Research 570: 109–115

Drummond PD, Finch PM, Smythe A 1991 Reflex sympathetic dystrophy: the significance of differing plasma catecholamine concentrations in affected and unaffected limbs. Brain 114: 2025–2036.

Dubner R, Ruda MA 1992 Activity-dependent neuronal plasticity following tissue injury and inflammation. Trends in Neuroscience 15: 96–103

Duckrow RB, Taub A 1977 The effects of diphenylhydantoin inflammation on self-mutilation in rats produced by unilateral multiple dorsal rhizotomy. Experimental Neurology 54: 33–41

Dyck PJ, Lambert EH, O'Brien PC 1976 Pain in peripheral neuropathy related to rate and kind of fibre degeneration. Neurology 26: 466–471

Dyck PJ, Thomas PK, Griffin JW, Low PA, Podulso JF 1993 Peripheral neuropathy, 3rd edn. Saunders, Philadelphia

Elliott JR 1997 Slow Na+ channel inactivation and bursting discharge in a simple model axon: implications for neuropathic pain. Brain Research 754: 221–226

England JD, Gamboni F, Levinson SR 1991 Increased numbers of sodium channels form along demyelinated axons. Brain Research 548: 334–337

England JD, Happel LT, Kline DG et al 1996a Sodium channel accumulation in humans with painful neuromas. Neurology 47: 272–276

England S, Bevan S, Docherty RJ 1996b PGE2 modulates the TTX-resistant sodium current in neonatal rat DRG neurons via the cAMP-protein kinase A cascade. Journal of Physiology 495: 429–440

Everill B, Kocsis JD 1998 Effect of nerve growth factor on potassium conductance after nerve injury in adult cutaneous afferent dorsal root ganglion neurons. Society of Neuroscience Abstracts 24: 1332

Fawcett JW, Keynes RJ 1990 Peripheral nerve regeneration. Annual Review of Neuroscience 13: 43–60

Fields HL, Rowbotham MC, Devor M 1997 Excitability blockers: anticonvulsants and low concentration local anesthetics in the treatment of chronic pain. In: Dickenson AH, Besson J-M (eds) Handbook of experimental pharmacology, the pharmacology of pain. Springer Verlag, Heidelberg, pp 93–116

Fried K, Govrin-Lippmann R, Rosenthal F, Ellisman M, Devor M 1991 Ultrastructure of afferent axon endings in a neuroma. Journal of Neurocytology 20: 682–701

Fried K, Govrin-Lippmann R, Devor M 1993 Close apposition among neighbouring axonal endings in a neuroma. Journal of Neurocytology 22: 663–681

Friedel RH, Schnurch H, Stubbusch J, Barde Y-A 1997 Identification of genes differentially expresses by nerve growth factor and neurotrophin-3-dependent sensory neurons. Proceedings of the National Academy of Sciences USA 94: 12670–12675

Galer BS, Harle J, Rowbotham MC 1996 Response to intravenous lidocaine predicts subsequent response to oral mexiletine: a prospective study. Journal of Pain and Symptom Management 12: 161–167

Gao XX, Ren B, Linderoth B, Meyerson BA 1996 Daily spinal cord stimulation suppresses autotomy behavior in rats following peripheral deafferentation. Neuroscience 75: 463–470

Gallo G, Letourneau PC 1998 Localized sources of neurotrophins initiate axon collateral sprouting. Journal of Neuroscience 18: 5403–5414

Garcia-Anoveros J, Corey DP 1997 The molecules of mechanoreception. Annual Reviews in Neuroscience 20: 567–594

Gilly WF, Brismar T 1989 Properties of appropriately and inappropriately expressed sodium channels in squid giant axon and its soma. Journal of Neuroscience 9: 1362–1374

Gilly WF, Lucero MT, Horrigan FT 1990 Control of the spatial distribution of sodium channels in giant fiber lobe neurons of the squid. Neuron 5: 663–674

Ginzburg R, Seltzer Z 1990 Subdural spinal cord transplantation of adrenal medulla suppresses chronic pain behavior in rats. Brain Research 523: 147–150

Glazer S, Portnoy RK 1991 Systemic local anesthetics in pain control. Journal of Pain and Symptom Management 6: 30–39

Gold MS, Reichling DB, Shuster MJ, Levine JD 1996 Hyperalgesic agents increase a tetrodotoxin-resistant Na+ current in nociceptors. Proceedings of the National Academy of Sciences USA 93: 1108–1112.

Gold MS, Dastmalchi S, Levine JD 1997 α_2-Adrenergic receptor subtypes in rat dorsal root and superior cervical ganglion neurons. Pain 69: 179–190

Goldstein RS, Raber P, Govrin-Lippmann R, Devor M 1989 Timecourse of catecholamine histofluorescence in experimental nerve-end neuromas in the rat. Neuroscience Letters 94: 58–62

Gonzales-Darder JM, Barbera J, Abellan MJ 1986 Effect of prior anaesthesia on autotomy following sciatic transection in rats. Pain 24: 87–91

Gould HJ III, England JD, Liu ZP, Levinson SR 1998 Rapid sodium channel augmentation in response to inflammation induced by complete Freund's adjuvant. Brain Research 802: 69–75

Govrin-Lippmann R, Devor M 1978 Ongoing activity in severed nerves: source and variation with time. Brain Research 159: 406–410

Gracely RH, Lynch SA, Bennett GJ 1992 Painful neuropathy: altered central processing, maintained dynamically by peripheral input. Pain 51: 175–194

Grafstein B, McQuarrie IG 1978 The role of the nerve cell body in axonal regeneration. In: CW Cotman (ed) Neuronal plasticity. Raven, New York, pp 155–195

Granit R, Skoglund CR 1945 Facilitation, inhibition and depression at

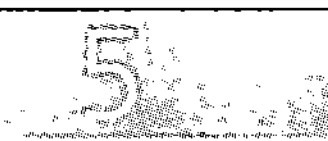

the 'artificial synapse' formed by the cut end of a mammalian nerve. Journal of Physiology (London) 103: 435–448

Gross PM 1987 Circumventricular organs and body fluids, vols I,II,III. CRC Press, Boca Raton.

Habler H-J, Janig W, Koltzenburg M 1987 Activation of unmyelinated afferents in chronically lesioned nerves by adrenaline and excitation of sympathetic efferents in the cat. Neuroscience Letters 82: 35–40

Hama AT, Sagen J 1994 Alleviation of neuropathic pain symptoms by xenogeneic chromaffin cell grafts in the spinal subarachnoid space. Brain Research 651: 183–193

Hamill OP, McBride DW 1994 The cloning of a mechano-gated membrane ion channel. Trends in Neuroscience 17: 439–443

Hao J-X, Wiesenfeld-Hallin Z 1994 Variability in the occurrence of ongoing discharges in primary afferents originating in the neuroma after peripheral nerve section in different strains of rats. Neuroscience Letters 169: 119–121

Hardy JD, Wolf HG, Goodell H 1952 Pain sensations and reactions. William and Wilkins, New York

Herzberg U, Eliav E, Bennett GJ, Kopin IJ 1997 The analgesic effects of R(+)-WIN 55,212-2 mesylate, a high affinity cannabinoid agonist, in a rat model of neuropathic pain. Neuroscience Letters 221: 157–160

Heumann R, Korsching S, Bandtlow C, Thoenen H 1987 Changes of nerve growth factor synthesis in non-neuronal cells in response to sciatic nerve transection. Journal of Cell Biology 104: 1623–1631

Hille B 1992a Ionic channels of excitable membranes, 2nd edn. Sinauer and Sunderland, Massachussets

Hille B 1992b G protein-coupled mechanisms and nervous signaling. Neuron 9: 187–195

Hokfelt T, Zhang X, Xu Z-Q et al 1997 Phenotype regulation in dorsal root ganglion neurons after nerve injury: focus on peptides and their receptors. In: Borsook D (ed) Molecular neurobiology of pain. IASP Press, Seattle

Hole K, Tjolsen A 1993 The tail-flick and formalin tests in rodents: changes in skin temperature as a confounding factor. Pain 53: 247–254

Howe JF, Loeser JD, Calvin WH 1977 Mechanosensitivity of dorsal root ganglia and chronically injured axons: a physiological basis for radicular pain of nerve root compression. Pain 3: 25–41

Hunter JC, Gogas KR, Hedley LR et al 1997 The effect of novel anti-epileptic drugs in rat experimental models of acute and chronic pain. European Journal of Pharmacology 324: 153–160

Hylden JLK, Wilcox GL 1981 Intrathecal substance P elicits a caudally-directed biting and scratching behavior in mice. Brain Research 217: 212–215

Imamura Y, Kawamoto H, Nakanishi O 1997 Characterization of heat-hyperalgesia in an experimental trigeminal neuropathy in rats. Experimental Brain Research 116: 97–103

Jack JJB, Noble D, Tiens RW 1983 Electric current flow in excitable cells. Clarendon, Oxford

Jacobs JM, MacFarland RM, Cavanagh JB 1976 Vascular leakage in the dorsal root ganglia of the rat studied with horseradish peroxidase. Journal of the Neurological Sciences 29: 95–107

Janig W, Stanton-Hicks MD (eds) 1997 Reflex sympathetic dystrophy: a reappraisal. Progress in pain research and management, vol 6. IASP Press, Seattle

Jett MF, McGuirk J, Waligora D, Hunter JC 1997 The effects of mexiletine, desipramine and fluoxetine in rat models involving central sensitization. Pain 69: 161–169

Ji R-R, Zhang Q, Pettersson RF, Hokfelt T 1996 aFGF, bFGF and NGF, differentially regulate neuropeptide expression in dorsal root ganglion after axotomy and induced autotomy. Regulatory Peptides 66: 179–189

Johnson RD, Munson JB 1991 Regenerating sprouts of axotomized cat muscle afferents express characteristic firing patterns to mechanical stimulation. Journal of Neurophysiology 66: 2155–2158

Kajander KC, Wakisaka S, Bennett GJ 1992 Spontaneous discharge originates in the dorsal root ganglion at the onset of a painful peripheral neuropathy in the rat. Neuroscience Letters 138: 225–228

Kalso E, Tramer MR, McQuay HJ, Moore RA 1998 Systemic local-anaesthetic-type drugs in chronic pain: a systematic review. European Journal of Pain 2: 3–14

Kapoor R, Smith KJ, Felts PA, Davies M 1993 Internodal potassium currents can generate ectopic impulses in mammalian myelinated axons. Brain Research 611: 165–169

Katz J, Melzack R 1990 Pain 'memories' in phantom limbs: review and clinical observations. Pain 43: 319–336

Kauppila T, Pertovaara A 1991 Effects of different sensory and behavioral manipulations on autotomy caused by a sciatic lesion in rats. Experimental Neurology 111: 128–130

Kawakami M, Weinstein JN, Chatani K-I, Spratt KF, Meller ST, Gebhart GF 1994 Experimental lumbar radiculopathy: behavioral and histologic changes in a model of radicular pain after spinal nerve root irritation with chromic gut ligatures in the rat. Spine 19: 1795–1802

Kawakami M, Tamaki T, Weinstein JN, Hashizume H, Nishi H, Meller ST 1996 Pathomechanism of pain-related behavior produced by allografted disc in the rat. Spine 18: 2101–2107

Kennard MA 1950 Chronic focal hyper-irritability of sensory nervous system in cats. Journal of Neurophysiology 13: 215–222.

Kim SH, Chung JM 1991 Sympathectomy alleviates mechanical allodynia in an experimental model for neuropathy in the rat. Neuroscience Letters 134: 131–134

Kim SH, Chung JM 1992 An experimental model for peripheral neuropathy produced by segmental spinal nerve ligation in the rat. Pain 50: 355–363

Kim SH, Na HS, Sheen K, Chung JM 1993 Effects of sympathectomy on a rat model of peripheral neuropathy. Pain 155: 85–92

Kim KJ, Yoon YW, Chung JM 1997a Comparison of three rodent neuropathic pain models. Experimental Brain Research 113: 200–206

Kim YI, Na HS, Yoon YW, Han HC, Ko KH, Hong SK 1997b NMDA receptors are important for both mechanical and thermal allodynia from peripheral nerve injury in rats. Neuroreport 8: 2149–2153

Kingery WS, Vallin JA 1989 The development of chronic mechanical hyperalgesia, autotomy and collateral sprouting following sciatic nerve section in rat. Pain 38: 321–332

Kingery WS, Castellote JM, Wang EE 1993 A loose ligature-induced mononeuropathy produces hyperalgesias mediated by both the injured sciatic nerve and the adjacent saphenous nerve. Pain 55: 297–304

Kinnman E, Levine JD 1995 Sensory and sympathetic contributions to nerve injury-induced sensory abnormalities in the rat. Neuroscience 64: 751–767

Kirk EJ 1974 Impulses in dorsal spinal nerve rootlets in cats and rabbits arising from dorsal root ganglia isolated from the periphery. Journal of Comparative Neurology 2: 165–176

Kirk EJ, Denny-Brown D 1970 Functional variation in dermatomes in the macaque monkey following dorsal root lesions. Journal of Comparative Neurology 139: 307–320

Kocsis JD, Preston RJ, Targ EF 1984 Retrograde impulse activity and horseradish peroxidase tracing of nerve fibers entering a neuroma studied in vitro. Experimental Neurology 85: 400–412

Koltzenburg M, Kees S, Budweiser S, Ochs G, Toyka KV 1994a The properties of unmyelinated nociceptive afferents change in a painful chronic constriction neuropathy. In: Gebhart GF, Hammond DL, Jensen TS (eds) Progress in pain research and management, vol 2. IASP Press, Seattle, pp 511–521

Koltzenburg M, Torebjork HE, Wahren LK 1994b Nociceptor modulated central sensitization causes mechanical hyperalgesia in acute chemogenic and chronic neuropathic pain. Brain 117: 579–591

Konorski J, Lubinska L 1946 Mechanical excitability of regenerating nerve-fibers. Lancet 250: 609–610

Korenman EMD, Devor M 1981 Ectopic adrenergic sensitivity in damaged peripheral nerve axons in the rat. Experimental Neurology 72: 63–81

Koschorke GM, Meyer RA, Tillman DB, Campbell JN 1991 Ectopic excitability of injured nerves in monkey: entrained responses to vibratory stimuli. Journal of Neurophysiology 65: 693–701

Koschorke GM, Meyer RA, Campbell JN 1994 Cellular components necessary for mechanoelectrical transduction are conveyed to primary afferent terminals by fast axonal transport. Brain Research 641: 99–104

Kryzhanovsky GN 1976 Experimental central pain and itch syndromes: modeling and general theory. In: Bonica JJ, Albe-Fessard D (eds) Advances in pain research and therapy, vol 1. Raven, New York, pp 225–230

Kugelberg E 1946 'Injury activity' and 'trigger zones' in human nerves. Brain 69: 310–324

Kugelberg E, Lindblom U 1959 The mechanism of the pain in trigeminal neuralgia. Journal of Neurology, Neurosurgery and Psychiatry 22: 36–43

Kupers R, Yu W, Person JKE, Xu X-J, Wiesenfeld-Hallin Z 1998 Photochemically-induced ischemia of the rat sciatic nerve produces a dose-dependent and highly reproducible mechanical, heat and cold allodynia, and signs of spontaneous pain. Pain 76: 45–59

Kuslich SD, Ulstro CL, Michael CJ 1991 The tissue origin of low back pain and sciatica. Orthopaedic Clinics of North America 22: 181–187

Laird JMA, Bennett GJ 1993 An electrophysiological study of dorsal horn neurons in the spinal cord of rats with an experimental peripheral neuropathy. Journal of Neurophysiology 69: 2072–2085

Lee Y-W, Chaplan SR, Yaksh TL 1995 Systemic and supraspinal, but not spinal, opiates suppress allodynia in a rat neuropathic pain model. Neuroscience Letters 186: 111–114

Lembeck F, Holzer P 1979 Substance P as neurogenic mediator of antidromic vasodilation and neurogenic plasma extravasation. Archives of Pharmacology 310: 175–183

Lesser SS, Sherwood NT, Lo DC 1997 Neurotrophins differentially regulate voltage-gated ion channels. Molecular and Cellular Neuroscience 10: 173–183

Levi-Montalcini R, Angeletti PU 1968 Nerve growth factor. Physiological Reviews 48: 534–569

Levine JD, Taiwo YO, Collins SD, Tam JK 1986 Noradrenalin hyperalgesia is mediated through interaction with sympathetic postganglionic neurone terminals rather than activation of primary afferent nociceptors. Nature (London) 323: 158–169

Levine JD, Coderre TJ, White DM, Finkbeiner WE, Basbaum AI 1990 Denervation-induced inflammation in the rat. Neuroscience Letters 119: 37–40

Levitt M 1985 Dysesthesias and self-mutilation in humans and subhumans: a review of clinical evidence and experimental studies. Brain Research Reviews 10: 247–290

Lewin GR, Mendell LM 1993 Nerve growth factor and nociception. Trends in Neuroscience 16: 353–359

Lewis T 1942 Pain. MacMillan, New York

Li M, West JW, Lai Y, Scheuer Y, Catterall WA 1992 Functional modulation of brain sodium channels by cAMP-dependent phosphorylation. Neuron 8: 1151–1159

Lieberman AR 1976 Sensory ganglia. In: London DN (ed) The peripheral nerve. Chapman and Hall, London, pp 188–278

Lisney SJW, Devor M 1987 Afterdischarge and interactions among fibers in damaged peripheral nerve in the rat. Brain Research 415: 122–136

Lisney SJW, Pover CM 1983 Coupling between fibers involved in sensory nerve neuromata in cats. Journal of the Neurological Sciences 59: 255–264

Loewenstein WR 1971 Mechano-electric transduction in Pacinian corpuscle. Initiation of sensory impulses in mechanoreceptors. In: Iggo A (ed) Handbook of sensory physiology, vol I. Springer, New York, pp 267–290

Lombet A, Laduron P, Mourre C, Jacomet Y, Lazdunski M 1985 Axonal transport of the voltage-dependent Na^+ channel protein identified by its tetrodotoxin binding site in rat sciatic nerves. Brain Research 345: 153–158

Lotz M, Vaughn JH, Carson DA 1988 Effect of neuropeptides on production of inflammatory cytokines by human monocytes. Science 241: 1218–1221

Low PA 1985 Endoneurial potassium is increased and enhances spontaneous activity in regenerating mammalian nerve fibers – implications for neuropathic positive symptoms. Muscle and Nerve 8: 27–33

Luscher C, Streit J, Lipp P, Luscher H-R 1994 Action potential propagation through embryonic dorsal root ganglion cells in culture. II Decrease of conduction reliability during repetitive stimulation. Journal of Neurophysiology 72: 634–643

Macdonald RL, Greenfield LJ Jr 1997 Mechanisms of action of new antiepileptic drugs. Current Opinion in Neurology 10: 121–128

Mackel R 1985 Human cutaneous mechanoreceptors during regeneration: physiology and interpretation. Annals of Neurology 18: 165–172

Mailis A 1996 Compulsive targeted self-injurious behaviour in humans with neuropathic pain: a counterpart of animal autotomy? Four case reports and literature review. Pain 64: 569–578

Malcangio M, Tomlinson DR 1998 A pharmacologic analysis of mechanical hyperalgesia in streptozotocin/diabetic rats. Pain 76: 151–157

Mao J, Price DD, Coghill RC, Mayer DJ, Hayes RL 1992 Spatial patterns of spinal cord metabolic activity in a rodent model of peripheral mononeuropathy. Pain 50: 89–100

Markus H, Pomerantz B, Krushelnycky D 1984 Spread of saphenous somatotopic projection map in spinal cord and hypersensitivity of the foot after chronic sciatic denervation in adult rat. Brain Research 296: 27–39

Martini R 1997 Animal models for inherited peripheral neuropathies. Journal of Anatomy 191: 321–336

Matzner O, Devor M 1987 Contrasting thermal sensitivity of spontaneously active A- and C-fibers in experimental nerve-end neuromas. Pain 30: 373–384

Matzner O, Devor M 1992 Na^+ conductance and the threshold for repetitive neuronal firing. Brain Research 597: 92–98

Matzner O, Devor M 1994 Hyperexcitability at sites of nerve injury depends on voltage-sensitive Na^+ channels. Journal of Neurophysiology 72: 349–357

Maves TJ, Pechman PS, Gebhart GF, Meller ST 1993 Possible chemical contribution from chromic gut sutures produces disorders of pain sensation like those seen in man. Pain 54: 57–69

Mayer ML, James MH, Russell RJ, Kelly JS, Pasternak CA 1986 Changes in excitability induced by herpes simplex viruses in rat dorsal root ganglion neurons. Journal of Neuroscience 6: 391–402

McLachlan EM, Janig W, Devor M, Michaelis M 1993 Peripheral nerve injury triggers noradrenergic sprouting within dorsal root ganglia. Nature 363: 543–546

McMahon SB, Bennett DLH, Koltzenburg M 1997 The biological effects of nerve growth factor on primary sensory neurons. In: Borsook D (ed) Molecular neurobiology of pain. IASP Press, Seattle

McQuay H, Carroll D, Jadad AR, Wiffen P, Moore RA 1995 Anticonvulsant drugs for management of pain: a systematic review. British Medical Journal 311: 1047–1052

McQuay H, Tramer M, Nye BA, Carroll D, Wiffen P, Moore RA 1996 A systematic review of antidepressants in neuropathic pain. Pain 68: 217–227

Melzack R, Bromage PR 1973 Experimental phantom limbs. Experimental Neurology 39: 261–269

Merskey H, Bogduk N (eds) 1994 Classification of chronic pain. Descriptions of chronic pain syndromes and definitions of pain terms, 2nd edn. IASP Press, Seattle, pp 40–43

Meyer RA, Raja SN, Campbell JN, Mackinnon SE, Dellon AL 1985 Neural activity originating from a neuroma in the baboon. Brain Research 325: 255–260

Michaelis M, Blenk K-H, Janig W, Vogel C 1995 Development of spontaneous activity and mechanosensitivity in axotomized afferent nerve fibers during the first hours after nerve transection in rats. Journal of Neurophysiology 74: 1020–1027

Michaelis M, Blenk K-H, Vogel C, Janig W 1998a Distinct response types are specifically distributed among axotomized cutaneous afferents. Pflugers Archives 435(suppl): R154

Michaelis M, Vogel C, Blenk K-H, Arnarson A, Janig W 1998b Inflammatory mediators sensitize acutely axotomized nerve fibers to mechanical stimulation in the rat. Journal of Neuroscience 18: 7581–7587

Mizisin AP, Kalichman MW, Garrett RS, Dines KC 1998 Tactile hyperesthesia, altered epidermal innervation and plantar nerve injury in the hindfeet of rats housed on wire grates. Brain Research 788: 13–19

Mogil JS, Grisel JE 1998 Transgenic studies of pain. Pain 77: 107–128

Mogil JS, Sternberg WF, Marek P, Sadowski B, Belknap JK, Liebeskind JC 1996 The genetics of pain and pain inhibition. Proceedings of the National Academy of Sciences USA 93: 3048–3055

Mogil JS, Wilson SG, Bon K et al 1999 Heritability of nociception. I. Responses of eleven inbred mouse strains on twelve measures of nociception pain

Morris JH, Hudson AR, Weddell GA 1972 A study of degeneration and regeneration in the divided rat sciatic nerve based on electron microscopy. I, II, III, IV. Zeitschrift fur Zellforschung und Microskopische Anatomie 124: 76–203

Munglani R, Harrison SM, Smith GD et al 1996 Neuropeptide changes persist in spinal cord despite resolving hyperalgesia in a rat model of mononeuropathy. Brain Research 743: 102–108

Myerson BA, Ren B, Herregodts P, Linderoth B 1995 Spinal cord stimulation in animal models of mononeuropathy: effects on the withdrawal response and the flexor reflex. Pain 61: 229–243

Na HS, Leem JW, Chung JM 1993 Abnormalities of mechanoreceptors in a rat model of neuropathic pain: possible involvement in mediating mechanical allodynia. Journal of Neurophysiology 70: 522–528

Na HS, Han JS, Ko KH, Hong SK 1994 A behavioral model for peripheral neuropathy produced in rat's tail by inferior caudal trunk injury. Neuroscience Letters 177: 50–52

Nahin RL, Ren K, de Leon M, Ruda M 1994 Primary sensory neurons exhibit altered gene expression in a rat model of neuropathic pain. Pain 58: 95–108

Nakamura F, Strittmatter SM 1996 P2Y1 purinergic receptors in sensory neurons: contribution to touch-induced impulse generation. Proceedings of the National Academy of Sciences USA 93: 10465–10470

Neil A, Attal N, Guilbaud G 1991 Effects of guanethidine on sensitization to natural stimuli and self-mutilating behavior in rats with a peripheral neuropathy. Brain Research 565: 237–246

Nicol GD, Vasko MR, Evans AR 1997 Prostaglandins suppress an outward potassium current in embryonic rat sensory neurons. Journal of Neurophysiology 77: 167–176

Nikolajsen L, Ilkjaere S, Christensen JH, Kroner K, Jensen TS 1998 Randomized trial of epidural bupivicaine and morphine in prevention of stump and phantom pain in lower-limb amputees. Lancet 350: 1353–1357

Ninian Bruce A 1913 Vaso-dilator axon-reflexes. Quarterly Journal of Experimental Physiology 6: 339–354

Niv D, Devor M 1996 Preemptive analgesia in the relief of postoperative pain. Current Reviews on Pain 1: 79–92

Noda K, Ueda Y, Suzuki K, Yoda K 1997 Excitatory effects of algesic compounds on neuronal processes in murine dorsal root ganglion cell culture. Brain Research 751: 348–351

Noordenbos W 1959 Pain. Elsevier, Amsterdam, pp 1–176

Nordin M, Nystrom B, Wallin U, Hagbarth K-E 1984 Ectopic sensory discharges and paresthesiae in patients with disorders of peripheral nerves, dorsal roots and dorsal columns. Pain 20: 231–245

Novakovic SD, Tzoumaka E, McGivern JC et al 1998 Distribution of the tetrodotoxin-resistant sodium channel PN3 in rat sensory neurons in normal and neuropathic conditions. Journal of Neuroscience 18: 2174–2187

Nowicki BH, Haughton VM, Schmidt TA et al 1996 Occult lumbar lateral spinal stenosis in neural foramen subjected to physiologic loading. American Journal of Neuroradiology 17: 1605–1614.

Nystrom B, Hagbarth KE 1981 Microelectrode recordings from transected nerves in amputees with phantom limb pain. Neuroscience Letters 27: 211–216

Oaklander AL, Belzberg A 1997 Unilateral nerve injury down-regulates mRNA for Na^+ channel SCN10A bilaterally in rat dorsal root ganglion. Molecular Brain Research 52: 162–165

Ochoa J, Torebjork HE 1980 Paraesthesiae from ectopic impulse generation in human sensory nerves. Brain 103: 835–854

Ochoa J, Torebjork HE, Culp WL, Schady W 1982 Abnormal spontaneous activity in single sensory nerve fibers in humans. Muscle and Nerve 5: 574–577

Ochoa JL 1998 Ectopic impulse generation and autoexcitation in single myelinated afferent fibers in patients with peripheral neuropathy and positive sensory symptoms. Muscle and Nerve 21: 1661–1667.

Ollat H, Cesaro P 1995 Pharmacology of neuropathic pain. Clinical Neuropharmacology 18: 391–404

Olmarker K, Myers RR 1998 Pathogenesis of sciatic pain: role of herniated nucleus pulposus and deformation of spinal nerve root and DRG. Spine Pain 78: 99–105

Omana-Zapata I, Khabbaz MA, Hunter JC, Clarke DE, Bley KR 1997 Tetrodotoxin inhibits neuropathic ectopic activity in neuromas, dorsal root ganglia and dorsal horn neurons. Pain 72: 41–49

Oyelese AA, Rizzo MA, Waxman SG, Kocsis JD 1997 Differential effects of NGF and BDNF on axotomy-induced changes in $GABA_A$ receptor-mediated conductances and sodium currents in cutaneous afferent neurons. Journal of Neurophysiology 78: 31–41

Palacek J, Paleckova V, Dougherty PM, Carlton SM, Willis WD 1992 Responses of spinothalamic tract cells to mechanical and thermal stimulation of skin in rats with experimental peripheral neuropathy. Journal of Neurophysiology 67: 1562–1573

Pancrazio JJ, Kamatchi GL, Roscoe AK, Lynch C III 1998 Inhibition of neuronal Na^+ channels by antidepressant drugs. Journal of Pharmacology and Experimental Therapeutics 284: 208–214

Papir-Kricheli D, Devor M 1988 Abnormal impulse discharge in primary afferent axons injured in the peripheral versus the central nervous system. Somatosensory and Motor Research 6: 63–77

Perl ER 1994 A reevaluation of mechanisms leading to sympathetically related pain. In: Fields HI, Liebeskind JC (eds) Pharmacological approaches to the treatment of chronic pain: new concepts and critical issues. IASP Press, Seattle, pp 129–150

Perrot S, Attal N, Ardid D, Guilbaud G 1993 Are mechanical and cold allodynia in mononeuropathic and arthritic rats relieved by systemic treatment with calcitonin or guanethidine? Pain 52: 41–47

Pertovaara A, Kontinen VK, Kalso EA 1997 Chronic spinal nerve ligation induces changes in response characteristics of nociceptive spinal dorsal horn neurons and in their descending regulation originating in the periaqueductal gray in the rat. Experimental Neurology 147: 428–436

Petersen M, Zhang J, Zhang J-M, La Motte R 1996 Abnormal spontaneous activity and responses to norepinephrine in dissociated dorsal root ganglion cells after chronic nerve constriction. Pain 67: 391–397

Pieribone V, Nicholas AP, Dagerlind A, Hokfelt T 1994 Distribution of α_1 adreno-receptors in rat brain by in situ hybridization experiments using subtype-specific probes. Journal of Neuroscience 14: 4252–4268

Pinault D 1995 Backpropagation of action potentials generated at ectopic axonal loci: hypothesis that axon terminals integrate local environmental signals. Brain Research Reviews 21: 42–92

Plummer NW, Meister MH. 1999 Evolution and diversity of mammalian sodium channel genes. Genomics 57: 323-331

Pollock JD, Krempin M, Rudy B 1990 Differential effects of NGF, FGF, EGF, cCAMP and dexamethasone on neurite outgrowth and sodium channel expression in PC12 cells. Journal of Neuroscience 10: 2626–2637

Procacci P, Maresca M 1990 Autotomy. Pain 43: 394

Proske U, Iggo A, Luff AR 1995 Mechanical sensitivity of regenerating myelinated skin and muscle afferents in the cat. Experimental Brain Research 104: 89–98

Puke MJ, Wiesenfeld-Hallin Z 1993 The differential effects of morphine and the alpha 2-adrenoceptor agonists clonidine and dexmedetomidine on the prevention and treatment of experimental neuropathic pain. Anesthesia and Analgesia 77: 104–109

Raja SN, Treede R-D, Davis KD, Campbell JN 1991 Systemic alpha-adrenergic blockade with phentolamine: a diagnostic test for sympathetically maintained pain. Anesthesiology 74: 691–698

Rang HP, Ritchie JM 1968 On the electrogenic sodium pump in mammalian non-myelinated nerve fibers and its activation by various external cations. Journal of Physiology (London) 196: 183–221

Rappaport ZH, Devor M 1994 Trigeminal neuralgia: the role of self-sustaining discharge in the trigeminal ganglion (TRG). Pain 56: 127–138

Rappaport ZH, Seltzer Z, Zagzag D 1986 The effect of glycerol on autotomy. An experimental model of neuralgia pain. Pain 26: 85–91

Rasminsky M 1978 Ectopic generation of impulses and cross-talk in spinal nerve roots of 'dystrophic' mice. Annals of Neurology 3: 351–357

Rasminsky M 1981 Hyperexcitability of pathologically myelinated axons and positive symptoms in multiple sclerosis. In: Waxman SG, Ritchie JM (eds) Demyelinating diseases: basic and clinical electrophysiology. Raven Press, New York, pp 289–297

Raymond SA 1979 Effects of nerve impulses on threshold of frog sciatic nerve fibers. Journal of Physiology (London) 290: 273–303

Ringkamp M, Eschenfelder S, Grethel E et al 1998 Lumbar sympathectomy failed to reverse mechanical allodynia- and hyperalgesia-like behavior in rats with L5 spinal nerve injury. Pain 79: 143–153

Rivers WHR, Head H 1908 A human experiment in nerve division. Brain 70: 145

Rizzo MA, Kocsis JD, Waxman SG 1995 Selective loss of slow and enhancement of fast Na^+ currents in cutaneous afferent dorsal root ganglion neurones following axotomy. Neurobiology of Disease 2: 87–96

Ro L-S, Jacobs JM 1993 The role of the saphenous nerve in experimental sciatic nerve mononeuropathy produced by loose ligatures: a behavioral study. Pain 52: 359–369

Rodin BE, Kruger L 1984 Deafferentation in animals as a model for the study of pain: an alternative hypothesis. Brain Research Reviews 7: 213–228

Rossitch E Jr, Abdulhak M, Olvelmen-Levitt J, Levitt M, Nashold BS Jr 1993 The expression of deafferentation dysesthesias reduced by dorsal root entry zone lesions in the rat. Journal of Neurosurgery 78: 598–602

Rotshenker S 1997 The cytokine network of Wallerian degeneration. Current Topics in Neurochemistry 1: 147–156

Rowbotham MC, Fields HL 1996 The relation of pain, allodynia and thermal sensation in post-herpetic neuralgia. Brain 119: 347–354

Rubin G, Kaspi T, Rappaport ZH, Cohen S et al 1997 Adrenosensitivity of injured afferent neurons does not require the presence of postganglionic sympathetic terminals. Pain 72: 183–191

Saade NE, Ibrahim MZM, Atweh SF, Jabbur SJ 1993 Explosive autotomy induced by simultaneous dorsal column lesion and limb denervation: a possible model for acute deafferentation pain. Experimental Neurology 119: 272–279

Sachs F 1986 Biophysics of mechanoreception. Membrane Biochemistry 6: 173–192

Sanchez A, Niedbala B, Feria M 1995 Modulation of neuropathic pain in rats by intrathecally injected serotonergic agonists. Neuroreport 6: 2585–2588.

Sato J, Perl ER 1991 Adrenergic excitation of cutaneous pain receptors induced by peripheral nerve injury. Science 251: 1608–1610

Sato J, Suzuki S, Iseki T, Kumazawa T 1993 Adrenergic excitation of cutaneous nociceptors in chronically inflamed rats. Neuroscience Letters 164: 225–228

Scadding JW 1981 Development of ongoing activity, mechanosensitivity, and adrenalin sensitivity in severed peripheral nerve axons. Experimental Neurology 73: 345–364

Schild JH, Kunze DL 1997 Experimental and modeling study of Na^+ current heterogeneity in rat nodose neurons and its impact on neuronal discharge. Journal of Neurophysiology 78: 3198–3209

Schmidt JW, Catterall WA 1986 Biosynthesis and processing of the α subunit of the voltage-sensitive sodium channel in rat brain neurons. Cell 46: 437–445

Schmidt RF, Schaible H-G, Meslinger K, Heppelmann B, Hanesch U, Pawalak M 1994 Silent and active nociceptors: structure, function, and clinical implications. In: Gebhart GF, Hammond DL, Jensen TS (eds) Progress in pain research and management, vol 2. IASP Press, Seattle, pp 13–25

Sebert ME, Shooter EM 1993 Expression of mRNA for neurotrophic factors and their receptors in the rat dorsal root ganglion and sciatic nerve following nerve injury. Journal of Neuroscience Research 36: 357–367

Seltzer Z 1995 The relevance of animal neuropathy models for chronic pain in humans. Seminars in Neuroscience 7: 31–39

Seltzer Z, Devor M 1979 Ephaptic transmission in chronically damaged peripheral nerves. Neurology 29: 1061–1064

Seltzer Z, Rappaport ZH, Zagzag D 1985 A pharmaco-behavioral assay of the efficacy of drugs topically applied to a nerve-end neuroma in a chronic pain model. Journal of Neuroscience Methods 33: 223–229

Seltzer Z, Herzberg R, Rozin M, Adziashvili L 1987 Further evidence correlating autotomy with chronic pain in peripherally deafferented rats: postoperative alterations in plasma corticosterone levels. Neuroscience 22: S321

Seltzer Z, Tal M, Sharav Y 1989 Suppression of autotomy following peripheral nerve injury in rats by amitriptyline and diazepam. Pain 37: 245–252

Seltzer Z, Dubner R, Shir Y 1990 A novel behavioral model of neuropathic pain disorders produced in rats by partial sciatic nerve injury. Pain 43: 205–218

Seltzer Z, Paran Y, Eisen A, Ginzburg R 1991a Neuropathic pain behavior in rats depends on the afferent input from nerve-end neuroma including histamine-sensitive C-fibers. Neuroscience Letters 128: 203–206

Seltzer Z, Beilin B, Ginzburg R, Paran Y, Shimko T 1991b The role of injury discharge in the induction of neuropathic pain behavior in rats. Pain 46: 327–336

Seltzer Z, Cohn S, Ginzburg R, Beilin B 1991c Modulation of neuropathic pain behavior in rats by spinal disinhibition and NMDA receptor blockade of injury discharge. Pain 45: 69–75

Seltzer Z, Zeltser R, Eisen A, Feigenbaum J, Mechoulam R 1991d Suppression of neuropathic pain in rats by a synthetic cannabinoids with NMDA receptor blocking properties. Pain 47: 95–103

Sheen K, Chung JM 1993 Signs of neuropathic pain depend on signals from injured fibers in a rat model. Brain Research 610: 62–68

Sherman R, Sherman CJ, Gall NG 1980 A survey of current phantom limb pain treatment in the United States. Pain 8: 85–99

Shinder V, Devor M 1994 Structural basis of neuron-to-neuron cross-excitation in dorsal root ganglia. Journal of Neurocytology 23: 515–531

Shir Y, Seltzer Z 1990 Effects of sympathectomy in a model of causalgiform pain produced by partial sciatic nerve injury in rats. Pain 45: 309–320

Shir Y, Ratner A, Seltzer Z 1997 Diet can modify autotomy behavior in rats following peripheral neurectomy. Neuroscience Letters 236: 71–74

Shir Y, Ratner A, Raja SN, Campbell JN, Seltzer Z 1998 Neuropathic pain following partial nerve injury in rats is suppressed by dietary soy. Neuroscience Letters 240: 73–76

Siegan JB, Sagen J 1998 Adrenal medullary transplants attenuate sensorimotor dysfunction in rats with peripheral neuropathy. Pharmacology Biochemistry and Behavior 59: 97–104

Small JR, Scadding JW, Landon DN 1996 Ultrastructural localization of sympathetic axons in experimental rat sciatic nerve neuromas. Journal of Neurocytology 25: 573-582

Smith KJ, McDonald WI 1980 Spontaneous and mechanically evoked activity due to a central demyelinating lesion. Nature (London) 286: 154–156

Sorkin LS, Xiao W-H, Wagner R, Myers RR 1997 Tumor necrosis factor-alpha induces ectopic activity in nociceptive primary afferent fibers. Neuroscience 81: 255–262

Sotgiu ML, Biella G, Castagna A, Lacerenza M, Marchettini P 1994 Differential time-course of i.v. lidocaine effects on ganglionic and spinal units in neuropathic rats. Neuroreport 5: 873–876

Sotgiu ML, Biella G, Lacerenza M 1996 Injured nerve block alters adjacent nerves spinal interaction in neuropathic rats. Neuroreport 7: 1385–1388

Stein RB 1967 The frequency of nerve action potentials generated by applied currents. Proceedings of the Royal Society of London. Series B 167: 64–86

Study RE, Kral MG 1996 Spontaneous action potential activity in isolated dorsal root ganglion neurons from rats with a painful neuropathy. Pain 65: 235–242

Sunderland S 1978 Nerves and nerve injuries, 2nd edn. Churchill Livingstone, London

Sweatt JD, Kandel ER 1989 Persistent transcriptionally-dependent increase in protein phosphorylation in long-term facilitation of Aplysia sensory neurons. Nature 339: 51–54

Sweet WH 1981 Animal models of chronic pain: their possible validation from human experience with posterior rhizotomy and congenital analgesia. Pain 10: 275–295

Tal M, Bennett GJ 1994a Extra-territorial pain in rats with a peripheral mononeuropathy: mechano-hyperalgesia and mechano-allodynia in the territory of an uninjured nerve. Pain 57: 375–382

Tal M, Bennett GJ 1994b Neuropathic pain sensations are differentially sensitive to dextrophan. Neuroreport 5: 1438–1440

Tal M, Wall PD Devor M 1999 Myelinated afferent fiber types that become spontaneously active and mechanosensitive following nerve transection in the rat. Brain Research 824: 218–223

Tal M, Eliav E 1996 Abnormal discharge originates at the site of nerve injury in experimental constriction neuropathy (CCI) in the rat. Pain 64: 511–518

Tanaka M, Cummins TR, Ishikawa K, Dib-Hajj SD, Black JA, Waxman SG 1998 SNS Na^+ channel expression increases in dorsal root ganglion neurons in the carrageenan inflammatory pain model. Neuroreport 9: 967–972

Tate S, Benn S, Hick C Trezise D, John V, Manion RJ et al 1998 Two sodium channels contribute to the TTX-R sodium current in primary sensory neurons Nature Neuroscience 1: 653-655

Torebjork HE, Ochoa JL, McCann FV 1979 Paraesthesiae: abnormal impulse generation in sensory nerve fibers in man. Acta Physiologica Scandinavica 105: 518–520

Torebjork HE, Lundberg LER, LaMotte RH 1992 Central changes in processing of mechanoreceptive input in capsaicin-induced secondary hyperalgesia in humans. Journal of Physiology (London) 448: 765–780

Torebjork E, Wahren I, Wallin G, Hallin R, Koltzenburg M 1995 Noradrenaline-evoked pain in neuralgia. Pain 63: 11–20

Tracey DJ, Cunningham JE 1993 The role of the saphenous nerve in experimental sciatic nerve mononeuropathy produced by loose ligatures: comment. Pain 55: 128

Tracey DJ, Walker JS 1995 Pain due to nerve damage: are inflammatory mediators involved? Inflammation Research 44: 407–411

Tracey DJ, Cunningham JE, Romm MA 1995 Peripheral hyperalgesia in experimental neuropathy: mediation by α_2-adrenoreceptors on post-ganglionic sympathetic terminals. Pain 60: 317–327

Travell JG, Simons DG 1984 Myofacial pain and dysfunction: the trigger point manual. Williams and Wilkins, Baltimore

Trotter WB, Davis HM 1909 Experimental studies in the innervation of the skin. Journal of Physiology (London) 38: 134–246

Utzschneider D, Kocsis J, Devor M 1992 Mutual excitation among dorsal root ganglion neurons in the rat. Neuroscience Letters 146: 53–56

Vallbo AB, Hagbarth KE, Torebjork HE, Wallin BG 1979 Somatosensory, proprioceptive, and sympathetic activity in human peripheral nerves. Physiological Review 59: 919–957

Vallin JA, Kingery WS 1991 Adjacent neuropathic hyperalgesia in rats: a model for sympathetic independent pain. Neuroscience Letters 133: 241–244

Vos BP, Strassman AM, Maciewicz RJ 1994 Behavioral eidence of trigeminal neuropathic pain following chronic constriction injury to the rat's infraorbital nerve. Journal of Neuroscience 14: 2708–2723

Wadhwani KC, Rapoport SI 1987 Transport properties of vertebrate blood-nerve barrier: comparison with blood-nerve barrier. Progress in Neurobiology 43: 235–279

Walker AE, Nulsen F 1948 Electrical stimulation of the upper thoracic portion of the sympathetic chain in man. Archives of Neurology and Psychiatry (Chicago) 59: 559–560

Wall PD, Devor M 1983 Sensory afferent impulses originate from dorsal root ganglia as well as from the periphery in normal and nerve-injured rats. Pain 17: 321–339

Wall PD, Gutnick M 1974 Ongoing activity in peripheral nerves: the physiology and pharmacology of impulses originating from a neuroma. Experimental Neurology 43: 580–593

Wall PD, Waxman S, Basbaum AI 1974 Ongoing activity in peripheral nerve: injury discharge. Experimental Neurology 45: 576–589

Wall P, Devor M, Inbal FR, Scadding JW, Schonfeld D, Seltzer Z, Tomkiewicz MM 1979a Autotomy following peripheral nerve lesions: experimental anaesthesia dolorosa. Pain 7: 103–113

Wall PD, Scadding JW, Tomkiewitz MM 1979b The production and prevention of experimental anaesthesia dolorosa. Pain 6: 175–185

Wallace MS, Dyck JB, Rossi SS, Yaksh TL 1996 Computer-controlled lidocaine infusion for the evaluation of neuropathic pain after peripheral nerve injury. Pain 66: 69–77

Wallin G, Torebjork E, Hallin R 1976 Preliminary observations on the pathophysiology of hyperalgesia in the causalgic pain syndrome. In: Zotterman Y (ed) Sensory functions of the skin in primates. Pergamon, New York, pp 489–502

Waxman SG, Ritchie JM 1985 Organization of ion channels in the myelinated nerve fiber. Science 228: 1502–1507
Waxman SG, Kocsis JD, Black JA 1994 Type III sodium channel mRNA is expressed in embryonic but not in adult spinal sensory neurons, and is reexpressed following axotomy. Journal of Neurophysiology 72: 466–470
Waxman SL, Kocsis J, Stys PK (eds) 1995 The axon. Oxford University Press, London
Weddell G, Guttmann L, Gutmann 1941 The local extension of nerve fibers into denervated areas of skin. Journal of Neurological Psychiatry 4: 206–225
Welk E, Leah JD, Zimmerman M, Reichling DB 1990 Characteristics of A- and C-fibers ending in a sensory nerve neuroma in the rat. Journal of Neurophysiology 63: 759–766
White JC, Sweet WH 1969 Pain and the neurosurgeon. Thomas, Springfield
Wiesenfeld-Hallin Z 1984 The effects of intrathecal morphine and naltrexone on autotomy in sciatic nerve sectioned rats. Pain 18: 267–268
Wiesenfeld Z, Hallin RG 1981 Influence of nerve lesions, strain differences and continuous cold stress on chronic pain behavior in rats. Physiology and Behavior 27: 735–740
Wiesenfeld Z, Lindblom U 1980 Behavioural and electrophysiological effects of various types of peripheral nerve lesions in the rat: a comparison of possible models for chronic pain. Pain 8: 285–298
Willenbring S, Beauprie I, Deleo JA 1995 Sciatic cryoneurolysis in rats: a model of sympathetically independent pain. Part 1: Effects of sympathectomy. Anesthesia and Analgesia 81: 544–548
Winchel RM, Stanley M 1991 Self-injurious behaviour: a review of the behaviour and biology of self-mutilation. American Journal of Psychiatry 148: 306–317
Woolf CJ 1991 Excitability changes in central neurons following peripheral damage. In: Willis WD Jr (ed) Hyperalgesia and allodynia. Raven, New York, pp 221–243
Woolf CJ, Wiesenfeld-Hallin Z 1985 The systemic administration of local anesthetics produces a selective depression of C-afferent fibre evoked activity in the spinal cord. Pain 23: 361–374
Xiao W-H, Bennett GJ 1995 Synthetic ω-conopeptides applied to the site of nerve injury suppress neuropathic pains in rats. Journal of Pharmacology and Experimental Therapeutics 274: 666–672
Xie Y, Zhang J, Petersen M, LaMotte RH 1995 Functional changes in dorsal root ganglion cells after chronic nerve constriction in the rat. Journal of Neurophysiology 73: 1811–1820
Xie Y-K, Xiao W-H 1990 Electrophysiological evidence for hyperalgesia in the peripheral neuropathy. Science in China (B) 33: 663–667
Xie Y-K, Xiao W-H, Li H-Q 1993 The relationship between new ion channels and ectopic discharges from a region of nerve injury. Science in China (B) 36: 68–74
Xu XJ, Puke MJ, Verge VM, Wiesenfeld-Hallin Z, Hughes J, Hokfelt T 1993 Up-regulation of cholecystokinin in primary sensory neurons is associated with morphine insensitivity in experimental neuropathic pain in the rat. Neuroscience Letters 152: 129–132
Yaari Y, Devor M 1985 Phenytoin suppresses spontaneous ectopic discharge in rat sciatic nerve neuromas. Neuroscience Letters 58: 117–122
Yamamoto T, Mizuguchi T 1991 The effects of oral morphine and buprenorphine on autotomy following brachial nerve sections in rat. Pain 47: 353–358
Yamamoto T, Yaksh TL 1992 Spinal pharmacology of thermal hyperesthesia induced by constriction injury of sciatic nerve. Excitatory amino acid antagonists. Pain 49: 121–128
Yamamoto T, Shimoyama N, Mizuguchi T 1993 Role of injury discharge in the development of thermal hyperesthesia after sciatic nerve constriction injury in the rat. Anesthesiology 79: 993–1002
Yehuda S, Carasso RL 1987 Effects of dietary fats on learning, pain threshold, thermoregulation, and motor activity in rats: interaction with the length of the feeding period. International Journal of Neuroscience 32: 919–925
Yehuda S, Carasso RL 1993 Modulation of learning, pain thresholds, and thermoregulation in the rat by preparations of free purified α-linolenic and linoleic acids: determination of optimal n-3 to n-6 ratio. Proceedings of the National Academy of Sciences USA 90: 10345–10349
Yoon YW, Na HS, Chung JM 1996 Contributions of injured and intact afferents to neuropathic pain in an experimental rat model. Pain 64: 27–36
Zeltser R, Ginzburg R, Beilin B, Seltzer Z 1998 Comparison of neuropathic pain induced in rats by various clinically-used neurectomy methods. Pain (in press)
Zhang J-M, Donnelly DF, Song X-J, LaMotte RH 1997 Axotomy increases the excitability of dorsal root ganglion cells with unmyelinated axons. Journal of Neurophysiology 78: 2790–2794
Zimmermann M 1983 Ethical guidelines for investigations of experimental pain in conscious animals. Pain 16: 109–110
Zimmermann M, Koschorke G-M, Sanders K 1987 Response characteristics of fibers in regenerating and regenerated cutaneous nerves in cat and rat. In: Pubols S M, Sessle B J (eds) Effects of injury on trigeminal and spinal somatosensory systems. Liss, New York, pp 93–106
Zur KB, Oh Y, Waxman SG, Black JA 1995 Differential up-regulation of sodium channel α- and β1-subunit mRNAs in cultured embryonic DRG neurons following exposure to NGF. Molecular Brain Research 30: 97–103

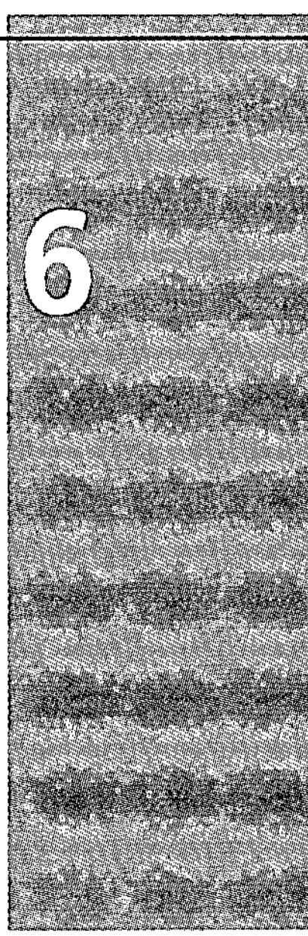

The dorsal horn: state-dependent sensory processing, plasticity and the generation of pain

TIMOTHY P. DOUBELL, RICHARD J. MANNION & CLIFFORD J. WOOLF

Our sensory experiences, including that of pain, are determined both by the capacity of our nervous systems to extract particular features from the stimuli that impinge upon our bodies and by the active processing of the neural input. Feature extraction is initiated by the highly specialized transduction properties of primary sensory neurons; sensory processing is performed by neurons within the central nervous system (CNS), the first stage of which occurs for the somatosensory system in the dorsal horn of the spinal cord or its homologue in the medulla, the spinal nucleus of the trigeminal. The dorsal horn essentially consists of the central terminals of primary sensory neurons, intrinsic dorsal horn neurons and inputs from and outputs to the rest of the CNS arranged in a pattern of bewildering complexity. Although considerable effort has been devoted to the study of the structure and function of the dorsal horn, we do not yet fully understand the principles of its organization in terms of what specific neural elements operate together to form functional processing units, transferring particular types of afferent input to particular output elements of the system. However, an enormous amount of information is available on the morphology of primary afferent central terminals, dorsal horn neurons and descending systems, together with their chemical neuroanatomy, synaptic arrangements, transmitter systems and functional properties. In addition, we now understand some of its major processing functions and how they relate to different clinical pain states. This chapter will be devoted to a general analysis of the roles of the dorsal horn in nociception and pain and not to a detailed analysis of its structure or of the functional properties of its elements.

The key to understanding the role of the dorsal horn in pain mechanisms has been the appreciation that the sensory response generated by the somatosensory system to a defined input is not fixed or static but dynamic. A stimulus that generates an innocuous sensation on one occasion may produce pain on another; similarly, a noxious stimulus does not always elicit pain. The reason for this is that the somatosensory system operates in a number of distinct states or modes. One state is that which is present when non-injurious stimuli are applied to healthy tissue, the situation that holds under what we could call normal or physiological situations. Another state occurs when similar stimuli are applied to inflamed or damaged tissue, and a third when peripheral stimuli are applied in the presence of damage to some component of the somatosensory system itself. Changes in the functional, chemical and structural properties of primary sensory neurons, neurons in the dorsal horn and brain are responsible for the dynamic switching between states in the somatosensory system. This neuronal modifiability, – or plasticity, represents an essential aspect of the state dependency of sensory perception, and clinical pain is a manifestation of this modifiability. It is simply not valid to assume that the sensory mechanisms that operate in the normal situation are the same as those operating in chronic pain syndromes. Our sensory experiences are instead state dependent and the challenge now is to elucidate the mechanisms that operate to change the system from one state to another and target our treatment strategies accordingly.

STATE-DEPENDENT SENSORY PROCESSING

A highly simplified analysis of the different states of the somatosensory system is presented in Table 6.1 and Figures 6.1–6.4.

Table 6.1 State-dependent sensory processing in the dorsal horn

Mode	*Stimulus*	*Primary afferent*	*Sensation*	*Clinical syndrome*	*Physiological change*
1. Normal Normal transmission	LI HI	Aβ Aδ/C	Innocuous sensation Nociceptive pain	Physiological sensibility	Normal transmission Normal transmission
2. Suppressed Reduced pain sensibility	HI	Aδ/C	Innocuous sensation	Hyposensibility	Reduced excitation Increased inhibition
3. Sensitized Increased pain sensibility (transient)	LI HI	Aβ Aδ/C	Allodynia Hyperalgesia	Post-injury hypersensibility Inflammatory pain Neuropathic pain	Increased excitation Reduced inhibition
4. Reorganized Increased pain sensibility (persistent)	LI HI	Aβ Aδ/C	Allodynia Hyperalgesia	Peripheral neuropathic pain Central neuropathic pain	Structural reorganization

LI = low intensity; HI = high intensity.

In the normal state, Mode 1 or normal sensibility, a low-intensity stimulus, of sufficient energy to only activate low-threshold primary afferent neurons, will produce a sensation which is always interpreted as being innocuous; and a high-intensity stimulus sufficient to activate high-threshold primary afferent nociceptors, but not produce tissue injury, produces a transient localized pain (Fig. 6.1). In Mode 1, low-intensity stimuli evoke innocuous sensations such as touch, vibration, pressure, warmth and cool, and high-intensity stimuli pain. This normal sensibility is the consequence of the activation of distinct neural substrates specialized to encode the different kinds of stimuli and provides information on the intensity, duration and location of the stimuli as well as their modality. This state operates in healthy individuals and enables a clear distinction to be made between damaging and non-damaging stimuli. The reaction to noxious stimulation, including the elicitation of an unpleasant sensation, is a key physiological protective mechanism warning of impending tissue damage and eliciting reflex and behavioural avoidance responses.

Mode 2 represents that situation where transmission in the somatosensory system is suppressed as a result of the activation of segmental and descending inhibitory mechanisms operating on the spinal cord (Fig. 6.2). Under these conditions a high-intensity stimulus, although activating nociceptors, fails to result in the sensation of pain. This hyposensibility can have a tremendous survival value, enabling flight or fight reactions in the presence of substantial injury. Inhibitory mechanisms can be activated by diverse peripheral inputs as well as higher order brain function, and contribute to the analgesia produced by transcutaneous electrical nerve stimulation (TENS), counter-irritation, including acupuncture, as well as the analgesic actions of placebo, suggestion, hypnosis, distraction and cognition. Moreover, endogenous inhibitory mechanisms can be mimicked pharmacologically with agents such as opiates and α-adrenergic agonists.

Mode 3 is that state where dorsal horn excitability is increased, and as a consequence its response to sensory input is facilitated or sensitized (Fig. 6.3). A low-intensity stimulus acting via low-threshold afferents now generates pain, the phenomenon of allodynia; and noxious inputs result in a pain response that is augmented in amplitude and duration (hyperalgesia). This mode needs to be differentiated from the situation which operates when the transduction properties of the peripheral terminals of high-threshold primary afferents are changed so that their threshold falls (peripheral sensitization), which contributes to altered sensibility limited to the site of tissue injury (see Ch. 1). The sensitization of the dorsal horn is initiated following peripheral tissue injury, peripheral inflammation and damage to the peripheral and central nervous systems. Mode 3 essentially represents an increase in the gain of the dorsal horn exaggerating pain responses, in contrast to Mode 2, which reflects a decrease in gain diminishing pain.

Like Mode 2, Mode 3 also can have survival value. Central sensitization, which increases the gain of dorsal horn neurons, is triggered by the nociceptor afferent input which occurs with tissue damage and peripheral inflammation. A state of excessive sensitivity, such that low-intensity stimuli begin to initiate pain, can potentially help to protect injured body parts from further injury while recuperation or healing occurs. The survival advantages of the activity-dependent facilitation of the pain system is such that it is present early in evolution including invertebrates (Woolf & Walters 1991). Central sensitization also contributes to the

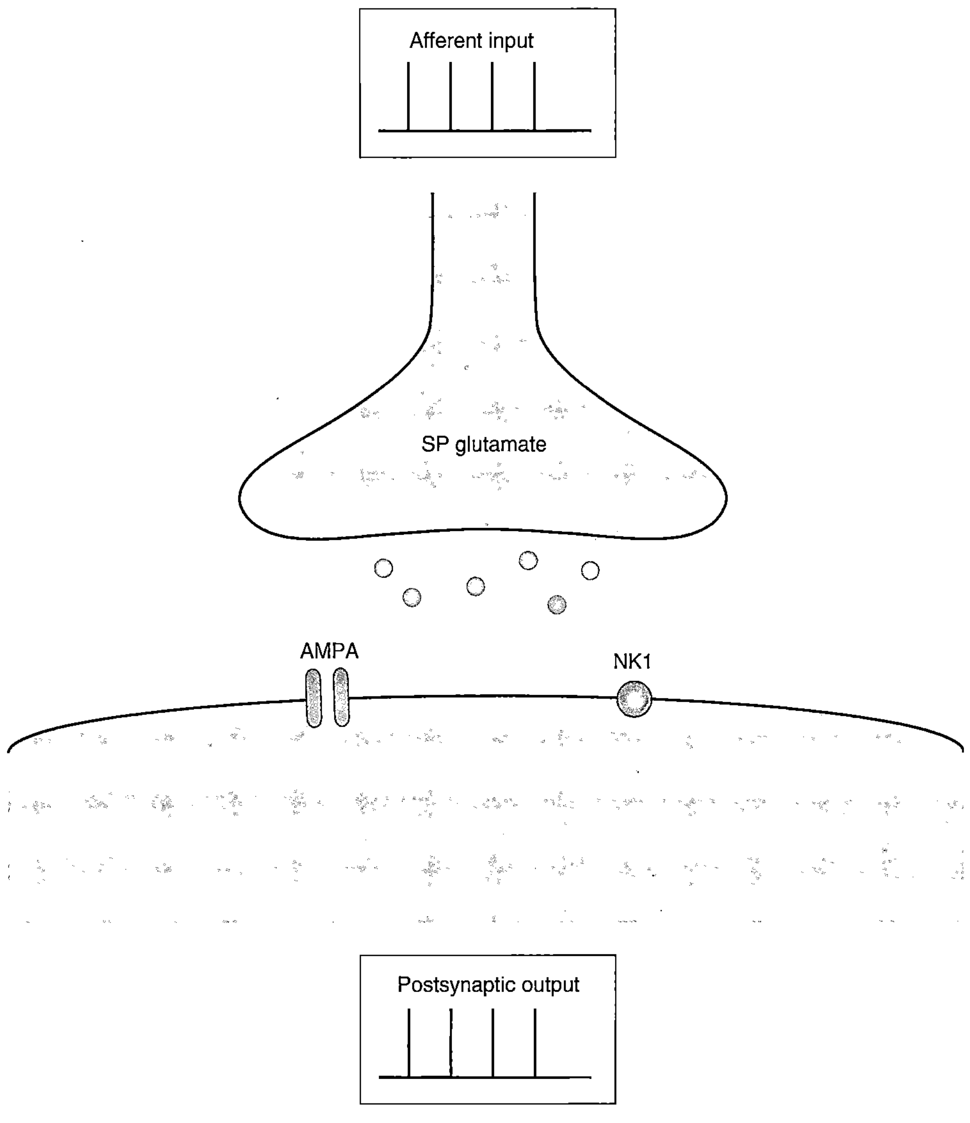

Fig. 6.1 A simple model illustrating key features of Mode 1. A generalized C-primary afferent terminal makes contact with the dendrite of a dorsal horn neuron. Following a noxious stimulus a standard amount of presynaptic activity (see afferent input) will be generated in the primary afferent as a result of the specialized transducing functions of the afferent peripheral terminal. This activity will be conducted to the central terminal in the dorsal horn and will induce synaptic vesicle fusion and excitatory amino acid and neuropeptide release resulting in postsynaptic depolarization via activation of glutamate α-amino-3-hydroxy-5-methyl-4-isoxazole propionic acid (AMPA) and substance P neurokinin 1 (NK1) receptors. If enough transmitter is released to depolarize the dorsal horn neuron to threshold, then the primary afferent activity will result in postsynaptic activity (postsynaptic output). During Mode 1 operation, low-intensity and high-intensity stimulation result in innocuous and noxious sensations respectively i.e. normal sensibility. SP = substance P.

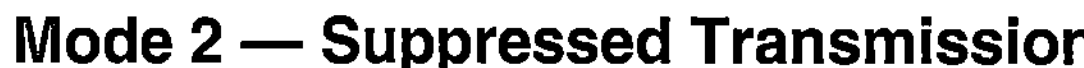

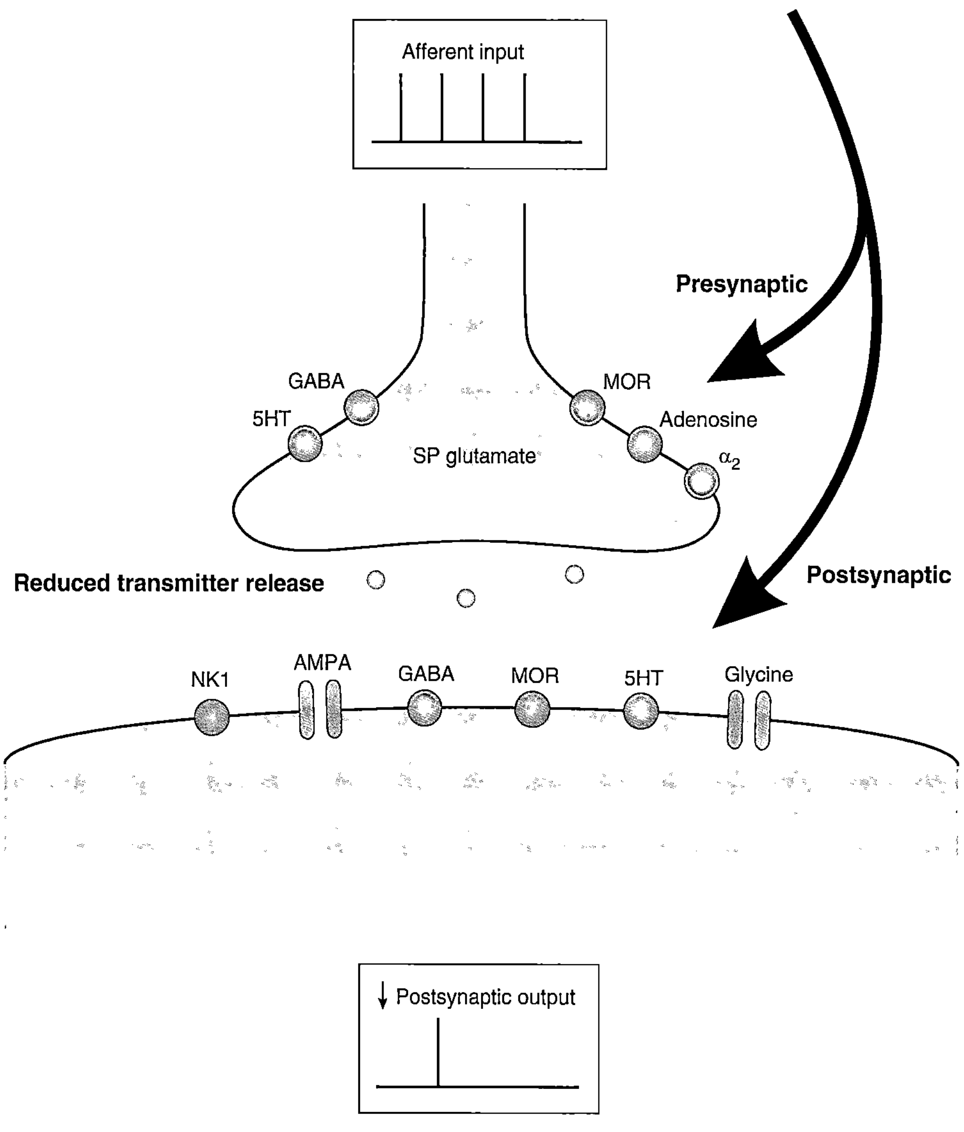

Fig. 6.2 A simple model of sensory processing in Mode 2. Activation of segmental and descending inhibitory systems, via pre- and postinhibitory synapses mediated by GABA, glycine, noradrenaline, enkephalin and adenosine and their specific receptors, reduce transmitter release and postsynaptic depolarization, and thereby reduce the dorsal horn activity evoked by a standard input in primary afferents and consequently pain sensibility. AMPA = α-amino-3-hydroxy-5-methyl-4-isoxazole propionic acid; GABA = gamma-amino butyric acid; 5HT = Serotonin; NK1= neurokinin 1; MOR = mu opiod receptor.

pain sensitivity in patients with nerve injury. However, in this situation the plasticity and the pain it produces have no survival advantage.

The transitions between Modes 1, 2 and 3 are due to the capacity of the nervous system for functional plasticity, from normal to suppressed to hypersensitive states, and in this way determines what sensation will be produced by defined stimuli (Fig. 6.5, Table 6.1). Mode 4 is, however, qualitatively quite different: here there is a structural reorganization of the synaptic circuitry of the system (Fig. 6.4).

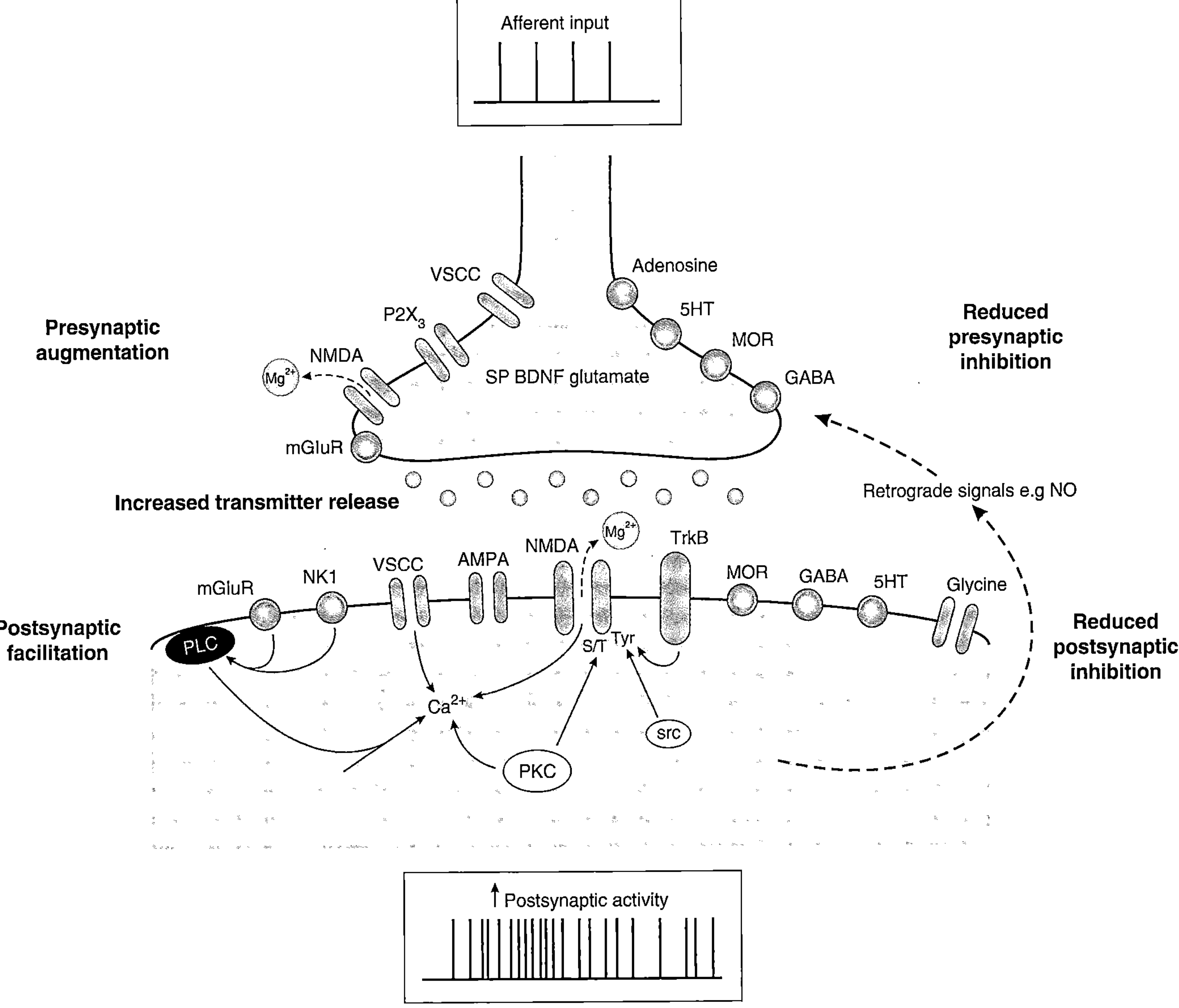

Fig. 6.3 In Mode 3 synaptic transmission between primary afferents and dorsal horn neurons are facilitated through two mechanisms; increased excitation and reduced inhibition. In this situation a standard amount of primary afferent activity gives rise to much more postsynaptic activity than in Mode 1 or 2. The induction of central sensitization is associated with multiple mechanisms:

1. *Enhanced transmitter release* from primary afferent terminals because of: (i) decreased inhibition via presynaptically located receptors (adenosine, 5HT, μ-opiate receptor, $GABA_{A/B}$; (ii) presynaptic facilitation via positive feedback autoreceptors (NMDA, $P2X_3$, mGluR); (iii) retrograde messengers like nitric oxide (NO) released from postsynaptic dendrites diffusing into the presynaptic axon terminal and induce increased transmitter release; and (iv) augmentation of voltage-sensitive calcium channels (VSCC).
2. *Increased postsynaptic depolarization mediated by* excitatory transmitters which will the remove the voltage-dependent magnesium blockade of NMDA and enhance postsynaptic activity.
3. *Post-translational changes in receptors* mediated by the activation of metabotropic receptors (mGluR, NK1), voltage-sensitive ion channels and ionotropic NMDA receptors which leads to increases in intracellular calcium, which in turn activates protein kinase C (PKC), stimulating phosphorylation of the NMDA receptor, thereby removing its magnesium blockade at resting membrane potentials. Activation of tyrosine kinases, e.g. TrkB and src, will phosphorylate the NMDA receptor and increase its channel open time.
4. Lastly postsynaptic efficacy can be increased by the *increased expression of excitatory receptors* following gene upregulation.
   AMPA = α-amino-3-hydroxy-5-methyl-4-isoxazole propionic acid; GABA = gamma-amino butyric acid; mGluR = metabotropic glutamate receptor; 5HT = Serotonin; MOR = mu opiod receptor; NK1 = neurokinin 1; NMDA = *N*-methyl-D aspartate; P2X3 = purinoreceptor type 2X3; TrkB-turosine kinase B.

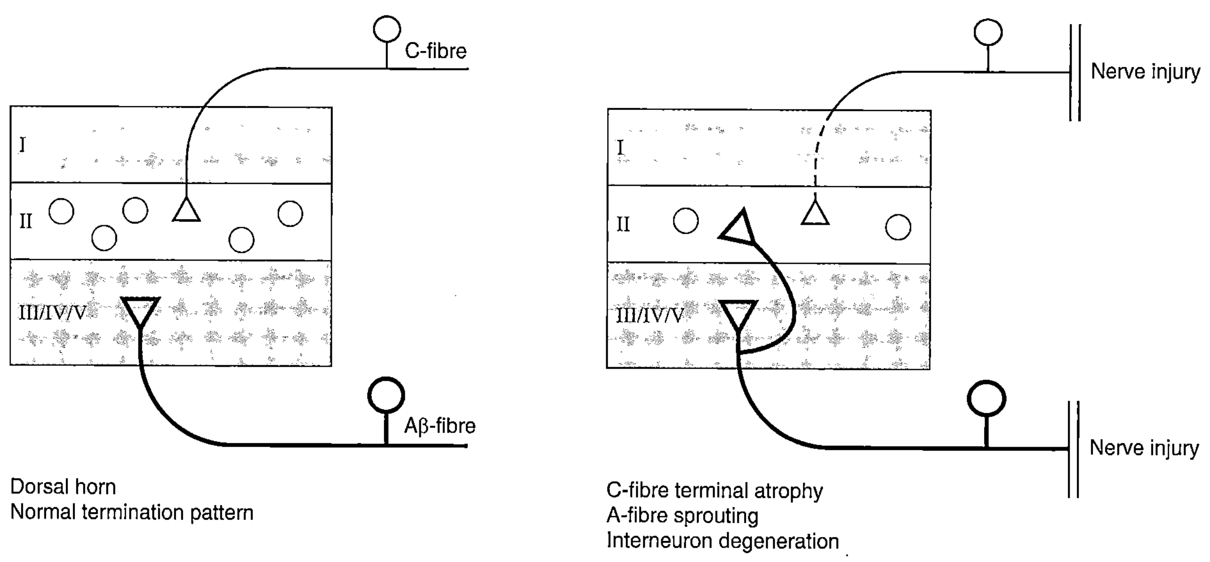

Fig. 6.4 A schematic diagram of primary afferent A-fibre and C-fibre terminals in the dorsal horn. After nerve injury the central terminals of C fibres atrophy creating vacant synaptic sites, allowing A fibres to sprout and form novel synapses in lamina II which create inappropriate functional connections leading to persistent hypersensibility.

Cells die, axon terminals degenerate or atrophy, new axon terminals appear, and the structural contact between cells at the synapses may be considerably modified. Such changes occur after injury to the nervous system, both peripheral and central, and contribute to a range of sensory abnormalities including neuropathic pain. Unlike Modes 2 and 3, which tend to be transient, structural reorganization within the dorsal horn and its functional sequelae can last long after the initial injury has healed, representing a persistent change in dorsal horn sensory processing. These changes are always maladaptive and are the expression of pathological changes in the nervous system.

The rationale for analysing the dorsal horn in the context of its ability to operate in different modes or states is that treating a sensory disorder on the basis of the sensation experienced is simply not sufficient – the underlying mechanism is the ultimate target for treatment rather than the associated symptoms. The mechanisms that produce different dorsal horn states, and subsequently clinical pain, have to be understood. To be effective pain therapy needs to be more than symptom management. To highlight this, Table 6.1 shows how pain can be experienced in a number of quite different states by low- as well as high-intensity stimuli. In the same way that a sensation can not by itself be used to establish the neural mechanisms that produced it, a particular stimulus can clearly not be used as a predictor of the sensation that will be elicited without knowing what mode the system is in. Appropriate treatment requires an understanding of the underlying mechanisms; the mode must be known, as must the mechanisms involved in the transition from one mode to another. Optimal treatment will often be that which restores normal sensitivity, resetting the system to Mode 1; normalization of sensibility rather than creating analgesia, the elimination of pain reactivity. The rest of this chapter will briefly survey the sensory processing that occurs in the different modes and the mechanisms involved in their transitions.

DORSAL HORN – ANATOMY AND PHYSIOLOGY

PRIMARY AFFERENT INPUT

In Mode 1, low-intensity stimuli never normally produce pain while a readily detectable pain threshold to intense mechanical and thermal stimuli can be measured. Increasing stimulus strength results in a progressive increase in primary afferent firing which correlates with the pain experienced until tissue damage is produced. In general terms there is a very good correlation in this mode between sensation and the functional specialization of primary afferents, particularly for low-threshold afferents (Torebjork et al 1987).

The cell bodies of primary sensory neurons are located in the dorsal root/cranial ganglia and give rise to a single axon which bifurcates into a peripheral branch innervating a receptor (mechanoreceptor, thermoreceptor, proprioreceptor, nociceptor and chemoreceptor) located in the target organ, and a central branch which enters and synapses in the dorsal horn (Fig. 6.1). Anatomically the primary afferent input to the dorsal horn can be broadly divided into large fast-conducting myelinated Aβ axons carrying signals about non-noxious stimuli and smaller slowly conducting thinly myelinated Aδ and unmyelinated C fibres carrying information about thermal and noxious stimuli. Individual afferents within these classes have different particular properties of modality sensitivity, adaptation and activation thresholds, but all encode stimulus intensity with action potential firing.

The central terminals of primary afferents occupy highly ordered spatial locations in the dorsal horn. In the dorsoventral (laminar) plane this order reflects the threshold sensitivity of the afferents, with specific termination sites for functionally distinct afferent types (Fig. 6.6). From the perspective of nociception, high-threshold C and Aδ nociceptors terminate predominantly in laminae I and II with some contribution to lamina V, while low-threshold Aβ mechanoreceptors terminate in deeper laminae. The rostrocaudal and mediolateral location of the central terminals of primary afferents in the dorsal horn encodes the location of the afferents' peripheral receptive field, generating a somatotopic map of the body surface in the horizontal plane of the dorsal horn. At the level of individual nerve territories the map is organized such that neighbouring peripheral fields occupy contiguous parts of the spinal cord (Swett & Woolf 1985, Maslany et al 1992).

Intra-axonal staining of individual fibres has enabled the central terminal axon of primary afferents to be studied in exquisite detail. What has become apparent is that different afferents possess distinct morphological patterns of central terminals, which have been particularly well described for the large myelinated mechanoreceptor (Brown et al 1977, Semba et al 1985) (Woolf 1987). The number of Aδ and C fibres labelled in this way has been limited because of the technical difficulty (Light et al 1979, Sugiura et al 1989). Beyond the precisely mapped somatotopically organized terminals, some myelinated afferents extend long branches for many segments outside the normal termination site (Shortland & Wall 1992).

Using electron microscopy combined with intra-axonal labelling, the structure of synaptic boutons of identified primary afferents has begun to be studied (Maxwell & Rethelyi 1987, Alvarez et al 1992). This has enabled detailed observation of synaptic terminations and transmitter content of the central terminals of identified primary afferents. These kind of ultrastructural details reveal that different functional classes of primary afferent have specialized central axon arbor morphology and that their termination zones within the dorsal horn are largely segregated into different laminae.

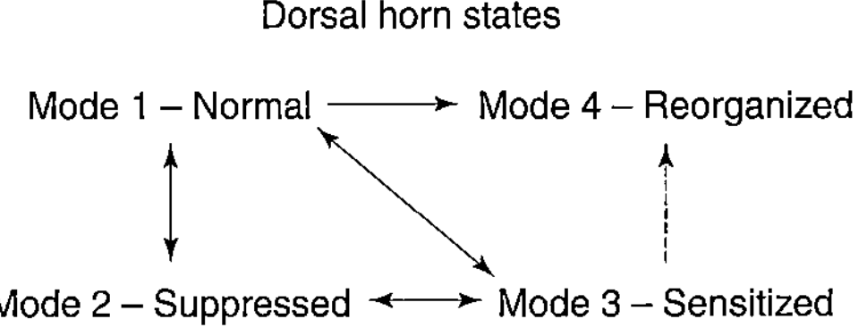

Fig. 6.5 A flow diagram showing possible transitions between different modes of the dorsal horn. The dotted line indicates the possibility that the sensitized state (Mode 3) could lead to permanent structural changes (i.e. to Mode 4). Switches into Mode 4 producing structural changes are unidirectional.

DORSAL HORN NEURONS

Based on the projection of their axons, dorsal horn neurons can be divided into three classes: projecting neurons, propriospinal neurons and local interneurons (Fig. 6.6). Although the projecting neurons transfer sensory information from the spinal cord to the brain, they represent only a tiny minority of the total number of cells (Chung et al 1984). Apart from transferring information to those higher brain centres involved in perception, attention, learned behaviour, emotional and autonomic responses, projection neurons are also involved in the activation of descending control systems, which in turn control the gain of dorsal

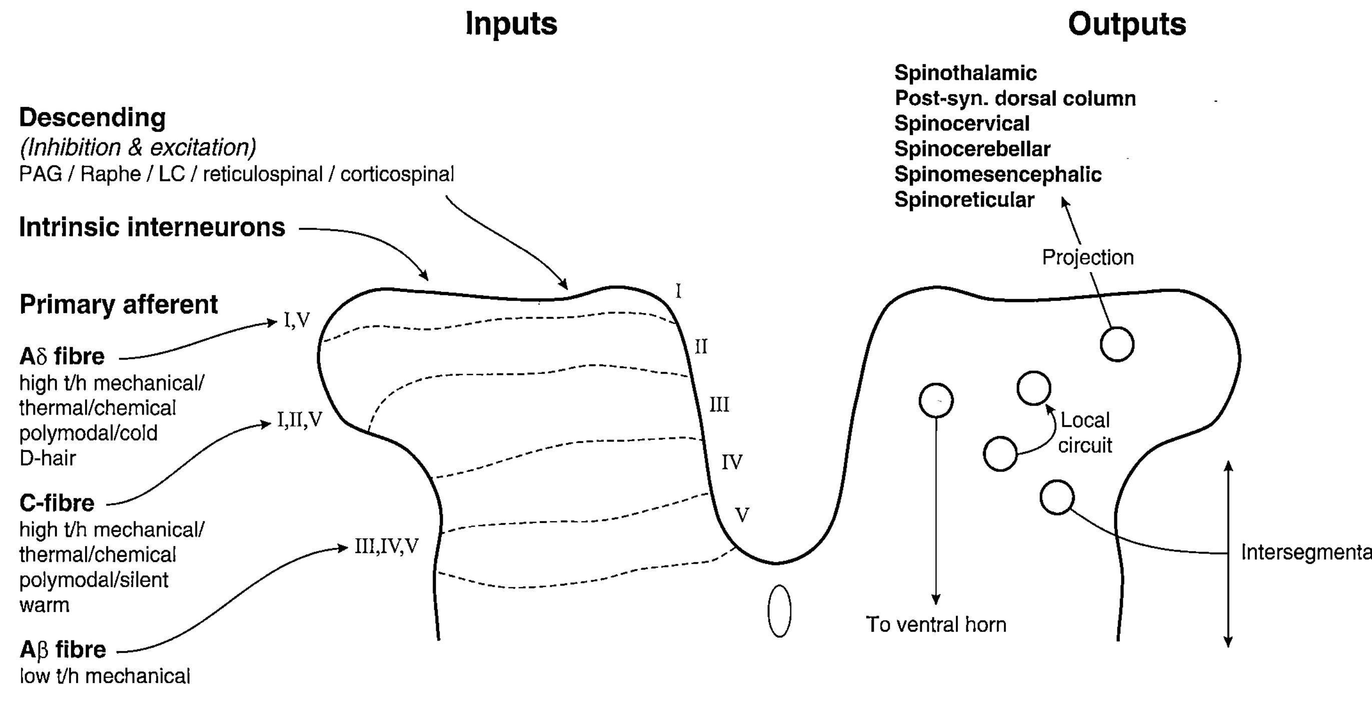

Fig. 6.6 A schematic diagram showing the major sources of inputs into and outputs from the dorsal horn.

horn neurons through excitatory and inhibitory mechanisms (Schaible et al 1991).

Propriospinal neurons transfer inputs from one segment of the spinal cord to another; their role in nociception is poorly understood but they appear to be able to act as a multisynaptic pathway that transfers information to the brain in some circumstances. The vast majority of intrinsic dorsal horn neurons are, however, local interneurons, which send their axons for only a short distance within the spinal cord.

Inhibitory interneurons containing gamma-aminobutyric acid (GABA) and/or glycine as neurotransmitters synapse both presynaptically on primary afferent endings and postsynaptically on dorsal horn neurons. Presynaptic inhibition decreases transmitter release from primary afferent terminals while postsynaptic inhibition reduces simultaneously active excitatory input. Because many inhibitory interneurons are also excited by primary afferent stimulation and from midbrain descending projections, there exists a phasic inhibitory feedback preventing overstimulation. Furthermore, many interneurons are spontaneously active and maintain an ongoing tonic inhibitory control over dorsal horn processing.

One way in which inhibition might directly modulate dorsal horn neuron responses is by modulating the amount of synaptic input that reaches threshold. Both inhibitory and excitatory interneurons play homeostatic roles in maintaining and defining the receptive fields of dorsal horn neurons. Activity in some primary afferent synapses and interneuron synapses onto dorsal horn neurons can induce excitatory postsynaptic potentials (EPSPs) that do not depolarize the cell sufficiently to reach threshold. These subthreshold synaptic inputs are a potential store of excitatory drive to the dorsal horn that can be accessed when sensory transmission needs to be increased. This could theoretically occur in two ways: by increasing synaptic efficacy at excitatory synapses (primary afferent facilitation or heterosynaptic interneuron facilitation) or by decreasing inhibitory synaptic activity (changes in descending or segmental inhibition).

While there are suggestions that a particular ascending spinothalamic pathway comprising modality specific high threshold-only cells exists for nociception, projecting from lamina I and terminating in a specific thalamic nucleus (Craig et al 1994), the specific contribution that these and other ascending pathways make to pain sensibility, including autonomic, emotional or perceptional components of pain, is simply not known. In fact, it has also been suggested that it is dorsal horn cells that respond both to low- and high-threshold inputs rather than those cells that are activated solely by intense or damaging peripheral stimuli, which are likely to be responsible for the conscious appreciation of pain (Dubner et al 1989). As a caveat, it must be noted that classifying the functional class of a cell in terms of its receptive field is difficult, however, when a considerable part of its response may normally be subthreshold. Fundamental questions remain as to why do multiconvergent cells in the normal state appear to contribute to the generation of pain, when low-intensity stimuli which activate the cells only produce innocuous sensations (Le Bars et al 1986).

It is important to recognize that single dorsal horn cells are unlikely by themselves to carry information that would lead directly to any sensation. From the study of cortical sensory neurons, an alternative hypothesis for coding of sensory information has been proposed involving the concerted/synchronized firing of groups of neurons (deCharms & Merzenich 1996). In this situation, the collective responses of an ensemble of neurons correlates better with a certain stimulus feature than the response of a single neuron. Changes in correlated activity in dorsal horn neurons could be accomplished without affecting the overall action potential firing rate, simply by alterations in the relative timing or pattern of action potential firing. Although dorsal horn neurons can show highly synchronized action potential firing patterns, it still remains to be tested whether population coding is involved in nociception or chronic pain states (Eblen-Zajjur & Sandkuhler 1997).

SYNAPTIC TRANSMISSION IN THE DORSAL HORN

Synaptic transfer of information is governed by the nature and amount of the transmitter released by different primary afferents, the density and identity of postsynaptic receptors (ionotropic and metabotropic), the kinetics of receptor activation and ion-channel opening and closing, and the factors responsible for the removal or breakdown of the transmitter. Each of these factors is subject to pre- and postsynaptic modulatory influences. The main synaptic transmitter present in all types of primary afferent is glutamate. The bulk of transmission between primary afferents and dorsal horn neurons occurs through postsynaptically located ionotropic α-amino-3-hydroxyl-5-methyl-4-isoxazole propionic acid (AMPA) receptors with a smaller *N*-methyl-D-aspartate (NMDA) component (Yoshimura & Nishi 1993). In addition to neurotransmitters, there are though a growing number of substances in the spinal cord which can modulate synaptic transmission, such as brain-derived neurotrophic factor (BDNF), prostaglandins and ATP. NMDA receptors, the metabotropic GluR and the P2X purinergic receptor are also present presynaptically on primary C-fibre terminals, where they may act as autoreceptors (Kato et al 1994), modulating the release of transmitters such as substance P (Gu & MacDermott 1997, Liu et al 1997).

Synaptic transmission occurs in a time range from tens of milliseconds for fast transmitters (e.g., glutamate acting on AMPA receptors), hundreds of milliseconds (e.g., glutamate acting on NMDA receptors) (Gerber & Randic 1989a,b), to tens of seconds (e.g., tachykinins acting on neurokinin receptors or glutamate on metabotropic mGluR receptors). Simultaneous release of glutamate and neuropeptides from the same afferent means that both fast and slow synaptic currents are generated concurrently in dorsal horn neurons. The former seem to be responsible for signalling information related to the location, intensity and duration of peripheral stimuli by reflecting the information content in the trains of action potentials arriving at the axon terminal, while the latter provide the opportunity for integrating input both temporally and spatially (Thompson et al 1990). The actions of transmitters may not be limited to the site of release and may spread through the extracellular space to distant neurons (volume transmission); this appears to be particularly true for neuropeptides.

Following noxious stimulation capable of releasing SP from nociceptor terminals, SP binds to tachykinin NK1 receptors on dorsal horn neurons in lamina I which are endocytosed into the cytoplasm, and this may explain receptor desensitization. Immunocytochemical localization of the internalized receptor has also been used to map the spatial extent of SP release (Allen et al 1997), while a targeted ablation of dorsal horn neurons expressing the NK1 receptor can be achieved using SP conjugated to saporin toxin, which binds to NK1 receptors and is internalized, leaving rats behaviourally unresponsive to intense noxious stimuli (Mantyh et al 1997).

Synaptic efficacy may be modulated by activated dorsal horn neurons that signal back to primary afferent terminals via a retrograde messenger. Postsynaptic activation of dorsal horn neurons by activating second-messenger systems may result in the synthesis and release of diffusible messengers such as nitric oxide, which could feedback onto the presynaptic terminals and modulate transmitter release (Meller & Gebhart 1993).

Modulation of synaptic efficacy in the dorsal horn is of fundamental importance for its operation. The strength of a synaptic contact may vary from, at one extreme, a failure to produce any postsynaptic response (known as an ineffective or silent synapse) to a situation where a single excitatory postsynaptic current is sufficient to reach threshold and generate an action potential in the target neuron. It is likely that under normal circumstances most synapses operate to produce subthreshold responses of varying amplitude and action potentials in postsynaptic cells are generated by multiple inputs (Woolf & King 1989, 1990). This offers the possibility of increasing or decreasing the strength of synaptic inputs in a range of different ways. By exploiting these features, the state of the spinal cord sensory processing can be rapidly changed (transitions between the Modes 1, 2 and 3) depending on the pattern of segmental and descending inputs to the dorsal horn and the transmitter/receptor systems they use.

MODE OR STATE TRANSITION

The dorsal horn in Mode 1, the control or physiological state, is stable in the sense that the processing of information (stimulus–response function) normally occurs in a highly reproducible and predictable way within a range of stimuli below that which produces tissue damage. The state of the dorsal horn can, however, shift dramatically, such that its response to defined inputs becomes fundamentally altered (Fig. 6.5). A key issue then is what is responsible for such mode shifts. It is clear that mode transitions are not simply a threshold phenomenon, where certain defined inputs exceed a set threshold value and increase the response output of the system. The transitions represent instead a non-linear transformation of the properties of the system from one stable condition to another quite different but also stable state. The capacity for such mode transitions implies a programmed instability in the overall design of the system such that when a certain input is achieved the system flips into a new state and mechanisms are brought into operation which stabilize the system in its current mode. The mode transitions are shifts in the properties of the whole system rather than just in some component part. Nevertheless, a deterministic approach to mode transitions is possible, and the cellular and molecular changes that contribute to the transitions, i.e. the mechanisms of neural plasticity in the dorsal horn, are analysed below.

SHIFTING FROM MODE 1 TO MODE 2: SUPPRESSING SENSORY TRANSMISSION

One explanation for the generation of pain is that activity in the spinothalamic tract or similar neurons above a certain critical threshold level, both in terms of frequency and number of cells active, leads to the sensation of pain. According to such a theory, low-intensity stimuli activating low-threshold mechanoreceptors do not drive the projection neurons sufficiently to ever cross this threshold, but activity generated in nociceptors by high-intensity stimuli can. If, however, the activity elicited in the dorsal horn by high-intensity stimuli is suppressed by inhibitory mechanisms so that insufficient output is generated by the projection neurons to exceed a critical threshold, then pain will not be experienced (Fig. 6.2). A great deal of information is now known about endogenous pain control mechanisms in terms of their anatomy and pharmacology (see Ch. 11). What is less well understood are the precise ways in which such endogenous control mechanisms are activated and exactly how they suppress the sensation of pain. Dorsal horn transmission is under the control of inhibitory mechanisms driven by midbrain descending projections and segmental projections which synapse directly or indirectly onto primary afferent terminals, dorsal horn projection neurons and interneurons which can presynaptically reduce transmitter release from primary afferent terminals or hyperpolarize dorsal horn neurons. Both of these actions reduce the likelihood of dorsal horn neuron firing. These inhibitory pathways may be activated by peripheral sensory stimulation or cortical and subcortical inputs, mediating the pain-suppressing effects of counterirritation, stress, suggestion, emotion and learned behaviour. Mimicking these inhibitory mechanisms either pharmacologically by the administration of drugs such as opioids or α_2-adrenergic agonists, or by attempting to directly activate the control mechanisms with peripheral or central stimulation, remains a valuable therapeutic approach.

SHIFTING FROM MODE 1 TO MODE 3: THE GENERATION OF CENTRAL SENSITIZATION

It has been unequivocally demonstrated in recent years that the hyperalgesia and allodynia following peripheral tissue injury has a central component. A number of laboratories have demonstrated repeatedly that dorsal horn neurons, including spinothalamic tract neurons, are 'sensitized' following brief bursts of activity in nociceptors. Central sensitization manifests in three main ways: (i) as a reduction in the threshold; (ii) as an increase in the responsiveness of dorsal horn neurons; (iii) as the expansion of the extent and the recruitment of novel inputs to receptive fields (Woolf 1983, Cook et al 1987, Hoheisel & Mense 1989, Hylden et al 1989, Neugebauer & Schaible 1990, Woolf & King 1990, Simone et al 1991, Hu et al 1992). The changes in receptive field properties are due to the recruitment of previously subthreshold components of the receptive field as a result either of increased synaptic output or increased excitability of the postsynaptic cell (Woolf 1991).

Underlying this functional plasticity are activity-dependent changes in synaptic efficacy within the dorsal horn. The key regulator of synaptic efficacy is the NMDA glutamate recep-

 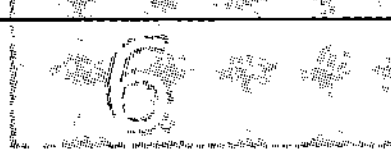

tor which, at normal resting membrane potentials, contributes relatively little to the primary afferent evoked synaptic currents in dorsal horn neurons, which are mostly dependent on glutamate acting on AMPA receptors (Yoshimura & Nishi 1993). This is because, at resting membrane potentials, the NMDA receptor ion channel is blocked by a magnesium ion, and therefore when glutamate binds to the NMDA receptor at resting membrane potentials no response is elicited because no current can be carried by the passage of sodium or calcium ions through the channel. When the membrane is depolarized, the magnesium blockade is lost. Central sensitization at the molecular level is essentially about either the removal of the magnesium block in the NMDA receptor ion channel or a change in the channel kinetics augmenting the NMDA response. This occurs as a result of post-translational changes mediated by the phosphorylation of the receptor either on its serine/threonine or tyrosine residues. Central sensitization is induced or initiated by stimuli that ultimately result in the activation of protein kinase C (PKC) or tyrosine kinases in the postsynaptic neuron which mediate the phosphorylation of the NMDA receptor. PKC is highly calcium sensitive, and any stimulus which increases intracellular calcium in those dorsal horn neuron which contains this enzyme (Malmberg et al 1997) will activate it. This may be via calcium entry into the cell through ionotropic ion channels, particularly the NMDA receptor itself, and via the activation of voltage-gated calcium channels. In both cases the initial activation of AMPA, metabotropic glutamate receptor (mGluR) and neurokinin 1 (NK1) receptors on dorsal horn neurons will produce slow synaptic potentials in response to C-fibre primary afferent activity. Such slow synaptic potentials are elicited only by C and not A fibres, and summate temporally on repeated C-fibre input, and spatially with the simultaneous activation of different C fibres. The summation of these potentials leads to a progressively more depolarized membrane which results in the loss of the magnesium block of the NMDA receptors, enabling synaptically released glutamate on binding the receptors to generate an inward current, which includes calcium entry into the cell which will act on PKC. The depolarization will also activate voltage-sensitive calcium ion channels, allowing further calcium entry. Intracellular calcium can also be increased by release of calcium from intracellular stores. This occurs in response to the activation of G-protein-coupled metabotropic receptors, including mGluR and NK1 receptors. Phosphorylation of NMDA receptors on its serine/threonine residues via PKC decreases the magnesium block at resting membrane potentials and produces long-lasting increases in synaptic efficacy (Chen & Huang 1992). Inhibitors of PKC have been shown to reduce central sensitization of spinothalamic neurons and reduce hyperalgesia (Coderre et al 1993, Lin et al 1996) and a PKC knockout animal has reduced pain behavior (Malmberg et al 1997). Phosphorylation of the NMDA receptor on its tyrosine residues via the activation of tyrosine kinases produces different effects, prolonged channel open time and increased burst clusters which will also increase excitability (Yu et al 1997). One tyrosine kinase that may be very important is TrkB, the high affinity receptor for BDNF.

While multiple mechanisms can induce central sensitization provided they lead to the phosphorylation of the NMDA receptor, its maintenance appears to be largely if not exclusively through the persistence of these post-translational changes of the NMDA receptor. This has important implications for therapy. NMDA receptor or neurokinin antagonists prevent the establishment of central sensitization, but only NMDA antagonists reverse established central sensitization (Woolf & Thompson 1991, Ma & Woolf 1995, Traub 1996).

Normally, only C-fibre input can initiate central sensitization and this can be easily detected in human volunteers following the application of C-fibre irritants like capsaicin or mustard oil (Koltzenburg et al 1992) which results in an Aβ-fibre-mediated tactile allodynia. Following both nerve injury and peripheral inflammation, however, the propensity of primary afferent to induce central sensitization increases because some A fibres switch chemical phenotype and begin to express substance P and other modulators including BDNF, such that low-intensity stimulation begins to induce prolonged excitability changes in dorsal horn neurons which never normally occur in the naive animal (Noguchi et al 1995, Neumann et al 1996, Abbadie et al 1997). The behavioural manifestation of this is progressive tactile allodynia, a centrally mediated progressive increase in pain sensitivity initiated by repeated touch stimulation of inflamed skin (Ma and Woolf 1996, Ma and Woolf 1998).

Acute tissue damage and inflammatory states will directly and indirectly lead to the activation of nociceptors which will induce central sensitization. On recovery from the damage or inflammation, the source of the input during the central changes is removed and the hyperalgesia and allodynia commonly disappear within several hours or days. Neuropathic pain, in contrast, is typically persistent and intractable. One explanation may be that following nerve injury axotomized primary afferent neurons become spontaneously active and generate ectopic actions potentials which create a constant drive of input maintaining central sensitization. However a major component may also arise from gene transcription changes in dorsal horn neurons in response to the increased primary afferent activity following tissue injury. Following injury novel transcription factors c-*fos* and CREB are rapidly induced in the dorsal horn (Hunt et al 1987, Ji & Rupp 1997), which may regulate the expression of neurotransmitters/receptors, which are also altered (Dubner & Ruda 1992), and may be responsible for the long-term facilitation of dorsal horn neuron excitability in chronic disease states.

The recognition that the dorsal horn can shift from its normal state (Mode 1) to a hyperexcitable state (Mode 3) has enormous implications for therapy, both in terms of the development of potentially new analgesics such as NMDA or neurokinin receptor antagonists, and by the appreciation that the prevention of the establishment of central sensitization may substantially reduce pain hypersensitivity following surgery. One outcome of central sensitization and an indication of its importance in the pathogenesis of clinical pain has been the development of the strategy of pre-emptive analgesia (Woolf & Chong 1993). Because the afferent input following tissue damage sensitizes the dorsal horn into a hyperexcitable state, then a treatment which blocks sensory input into the CNS or its transmission through the CNS during surgery should decrease the level of sensitization, and subsequently the hyperalgesia and analgesics required by patients following surgery. Pre-emptive analgesia has been shown now in a number of double-blind clinical trials both to reduce the acute postoperative pain and the risk of patients developing chronic pain after surgery (Selby et al 1987, Richmond et al 1993, Eide et al 1994, Breivik et al 1996, Choe et al 1997, Stubhaug et al 1997, Gottschalk et al 1998).

Although considerable work has demonstrated increases in dorsal horn excitability following conditioning primary afferent input in nociceptors, similar changes may potentially occur by the blockade of inhibitory mechanisms. For example, disinhibition as a result of the administration of GABA or glycine antagonists can produce touch-evoked allodynia (Yaksh 1989, Sivilotti & Woolf 1994). Peripheral nerve damage certainly results in a decrease in segmental inhibition (Devor and Wall 1981, Woolf & Wall 1982), which may be due to a number of factors – reduction in inhibitory transmitter, for example GABA or its receptors, due to transcriptional downregulation or loss of inhibitory interneurons. Cell death occurs in the dorsal horn after nerve injury possibly due to excitotoxic actions and if these are indeed inhibitory interneurons the overall effect would be to disinhibit surviving dorsal horn neurons (Castro-Lopes et al 1993, Oliveira et al 1997). The net effect of this would be to exaggerate the synaptic responses to afferent input. Spinal cord injury, stroke and a number of central lesions may also alter sensory processing in the spinal cord by removing some of the descending influences originating from the brainstem that control the gain of the system. If such changes resulted in a removal of a descending inhibitory input, the consequence might be a form of sustained central sensitization due to disinhibition.

SHIFTING FROM MODE 1 TO MODE 4: STRUCTURAL REORGANIZATION OF THE DORSAL HORN

If the highly ordered structure of the dorsal horn is modified this will naturally have implications for sensory processing within the dorsal horn (Fig. 6.4). Peripheral nerve injury, for example, results in the withdrawal of C-fibre central axon terminals form lamina (Castro-Lopes et al 1990), degenerative changes in some of the remaining afferent terminals (Aldskogius et al 1985, Knyihar-Csillik et al 1987, 1990) and, after a long time, dorsal root ganglion cell death (Coggeshall et al 1997). While this will result in the direct uncoupling of some afferent input to dorsal horn neurons, other changes occur which result in modifications other than just a reduction in synaptic drive.

It has recently become apparent that degeneration is not the only consequence of peripheral nerve injury – regenerative changes also occur. As part of the induction of an injured primary sensory neuron into a growth mode, to permit peripheral regeneration, developmentally regulated growth associated proteins are expressed (Skene 1989). These are also distributed to the central terminals of axotomized primary afferents (Woolf et al 1990, Coggeshall et al 1991), where the combination of vacant synaptic sites and axon terminals controlling the molecular machinery necessary for growth leads to the 'regenerative growth' of at least some of the central axonal terminals. Of particular interest is the finding that large myelinated afferent fibres, which normally terminate in the deeper laminae of the dorsal horn, grow into lamina II, the site of C-fibre terminals (Fig. 6.4) and (Woolf et al 1992, Koerber et al 1994, 1995), and do not need to be injured to do so (Mannion et al 1996, Doubell et al 1997). Prevention of C-fibres atrophy by supply of exogenous NGF or GDNF can prevent A-fibre sprouting (Bennett et al 1996, 1998, Eriksson et al 1997). When A-fibre sprouting occurs it is highly directionally specific, only occurring in the dorsal-ventral plane into areas of lamina II. Possible cellular mechanisms involved in A-fibre sprouting are not only likely to involving the creation of vacant synaptic sites, but also intrinsic attractant/repellent guidance factors and trophic signals within the dorsal root

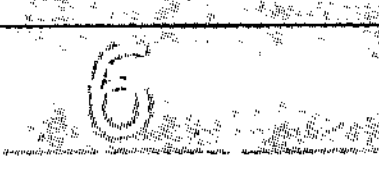

ganglion. Sprouting A fibres send collaterals into lamina II which form novel and ectopic synapses within 2 weeks after nerve injury (Woolf et al 1992, Doubell & Woolf 1997), dramatically altering the central processing of low-threshold mechanoreceptive input (Fig. 6.4). Recordings from lamina II neurons never normally show a monosynaptic excitatory postsynaptic potential (EPSC) in response to Aβ primary stimulation; after nerve injury, however, monosynaptic EPSCs begin to be elicited (Okamoto et al 1996). Peripheral neuropathic pain may be an expression in part, therefore, of an alteration in the circuitry of the spinal cord as well as of changes due to the induction and maintenance of central sensitization by an increased nociceptor drive.

CLINICAL IMPLICATIONS OF MODE TRANSITIONS

Pain therapy can be seen as having three distinct aims when defined in the context of the different possible sensory processing modes of the somatosensory system. The first is to *normalize* sensibility; that is to return the system from a state of hypo- or hypersensibility to one where the response to defined low- or high-intensity stimuli is an innocuous or painful sensation respectively (i.e., convert established Modes 2, 3 or 4 back to Mode 1). The second is to *prevent* a transition from normal to abnormal sensibility (i.e., maintain the system in Mode 1 in the face of stimuli which might be expected to change the mode). The final aim is, under particular circumstances such as surgery or acute trauma, to uncouple the response between a noxious stimulus and the painful sensation it normally elicits (i.e., shift the system into Mode 2).

For any pain therapy to be maximally effective it needs to be targeted at the specific mechanisms responsible for the maintenance and transition of the different modes, as discussed earlier in the chapter.

ESTABLISHING MODE 2

In order to establish Mode 2 in a patient, i.e. a state of true analgesia, two general approaches are possible, either to mimic the body's endogenous inhibitory systems or specifically interrupt nociceptive sensory transfer. The prime example of the first approach is the use of opiates, which have multiple actions on opiate receptors, whose natural ligands are the enkephalins and endorphins, and which are located on the peripheral and central terminals of nociceptors, as well as on dorsal horn and brain neurons. This represents the prototypic example of a pharmacologically controlled mode transition, albeit with significant side effects. The best developed approach to interrupt nociceptive sensory transfer is the use of sodium channel blockers at doses that block action potential conduction in sensory fibres. These can be delivered in the periphery, regionally or epidurally/intraspinally, but at present lack specificity – all conduction is interrupted. The recent discovery of sodium channels uniquely expressed on nociceptor neurons in the dorsal root ganglion offers the possibility that conduction block in particular subsets of sensory neurons is a realistic possibility.

PREVENTING MODE TRANSITIONS

In order to prevent mode transitions, therapy targeted at interrupting the chain of events that lead to the establishment of a new mode is necessary. This has two major requirements: treatment in anticipation of a possible mode transition i.e. pre-emptive treatment, and an understanding of the mechanisms that operate to produce the transitions. Most progress in this area has come from the development of strategies for pre-emptive analgesia to prevent the establishment of central sensitization (or Mode 3) after elective surgery. From the substantial understanding that has now been accrued about how central sensitization is initiated, rational therapy can be designed to interrupt this process and thereby prevent postinjury hypersensibility. At present, though, practical clinical approaches are limited by the restricted number of interventions currently available; sodium channel blockers to prevent nociceptor input entering the CNS, opiates to suppress C-fibre evoked central excitation, and NMDA-receptor antagonists, blocking this key excitatory amino acid receptor that mediates most of the central excitability changes that constitute central sensitization. Unfortunately, all the available drugs have major limitations, the sodium channel blockers are not modality specific, the opiates have many peripheral and central side effects which limit their usefulness and NMDA antagonists, such as ketamine, dextrophan or memantine, lack specificity and potency as well as exhibiting undesirable psychotropic side effects. A number of drugs that have exciting potential for use as antihypersensitivity agents are in various stages of development by the pharmaceutical industry. However, in spite of the limitations of the approaches now available, it is possible to make a clinically useful impact in pre-emptive analgesia for elective surgery as a number of recent double-blind trials have demonstrated unequivocally.

Much less is known about the sequence of events which may result after damage to the nervous system, the transition to Mode 4. In addition, there are no good diagnostic tools available to determine the presence in patients of Mode 4. While there are anecdotal reports that early intensive therapy of patients with neuropathic pain may abort or retard the development of intractable pain, this has not been formally examined. A number of trials have attempted to prevent the development of phantom limb pain, which may or may not be an expression of Mode 4, by pre-amputation epidural local anaesthesia and opioids, but with limited or no success (Nikolajsen et al 1997). This is not too surprising, because the mechanisms that produce structural reorganization of synaptic circuitry are unlikely to be blocked by such therapy. What may be required is neurotrophin replacement and other therapy directed at those events that determine the formation of novel connections in the dorsal horn.

NORMALIZING ABNORMAL SENSITIVITY

The greatest challenge clinically is to return the somatosensory system from an abnormal state of established hypersensibility back to normal sensibility. Pre-emptive approaches, even if available, are simply not possible in most patients with persistent pain who only present well after the initial transition phase is over. The appropriate strategy for such patients requires knowledge both of which mode their nervous system is operating in and what interventions can convert the system back to Mode 1. At present both the diagnostic tools and the treatment options are limited. In a given patient with a complex mixture of spontaneous and stimulus-provoked pain, neither the disease that produced the symptoms (e.g., post herpetic neuralgia, low back pain or diabetic neuropathy) nor the symptoms themselves (burning pain, tactile allodynia) define what mechanisms/modes are operating (ectopic discharge in injured sensory fibres, central sensitization or novel connectivity). As a consequence, treatment tends to be empirical and often unsatisfactory. It is here that the unmet need is greatest. Nevertheless, the pace of progress in our understanding of the different modes of operation in the spinal cord and their transitions, and the opportunities this provides for the development of new therapeutic approaches, makes it very likely that pain management is about to be revolutionized by the application of truly rational rather than empirical therapy.

CONCLUSION

The dorsal horn has the capacity to operate in three modes: a control mode, a suppressed mode and a sensitized mode. These alterations in the functional performance of the cord will alter sensory processing and are likely to account both for the failure to react to tissue damage on some occasions and the generation of pain in reaction to low-intensity stimuli in others. Understanding the factors controlling or determining which mode the spinal cord is in is essential in order to understand the pathogenesis of pain. The circuitry of the dorsal horn can, however, also be permanently altered or reorganized following peripheral or CNS damage. This may result in irreversible changes in sensory processing, with persistent clinical sensory disorders.

REFERENCES

Abbadie C, Trafton J, Liu H, Mantyh PW, Basbaum AI 1997 Inflammation increases the distribution of dorsal horn neurons that internalize the neurokinin-1 receptor in response to noxious and non-noxious stimulation. Journal of Neuroscience 17: 8049–6060

Aldskogius H, Arvidsson J, Grant G 1985 The reactions of primary sensory neurons to peripheral nerve injury. Brain Research 373: 15–21

Allen BJ, Rogers SD, Ghilardi JR et al 1997 Noxious cutaneous thermal stimuli induce a graded release of endogenous substance P in the spinal cord: imaging peptide action in vivo. Journal of Neuroscience 17: 5921–5927

Alvarez FJ, Kavookjian AM, Light AR 1992 Synaptic interactions between GABA-immunoreactive profiles and the terminals of functionally defined myelinated nociceptors in the monkey and cat spinal cord. Journal of Neuroscience 12: 2901–2917

Bennett DL, Michael GJ, Ramachandran N et al 1998 A distinct subgroup of small DRG cells express GDNF receptor components and GDNF is protective for these neurons after nerve injury. Journal of Neuroscience 18: 3059–3072

Bennett DLH, French J, Priestley JV, McMahon SB 1996 NGF but not NT-3 or BDNF prevents the A fiber sprouting into lamina II of the spinal cord that occurs following axotomy. Molecular and Cellular Neuroscience 8: 211–220

Breivik H, Breivik EK, Stubhaug A 1996 Clinical aspects of pre-emptive analgesia: prevention of post-operative pain by pretreatment and continued optimal treatment. Pain Reviews 3: 63–78

Brown AG, Rose PK, Snow PJ 1977 The morphology of hair follicle afferent fibre collaterals in the spinal cord of the cat. Journal of Physiology (London) 272: 779–797

Castro-Lopes JM, Coimbra A, Grant G, Arvidsson J 1990 Ultrastructural changes of the central scalloped (C1) primary afferent endings of synaptic glomeruli in the substantia gelatinosa Rolandi of the rat after peripheral neurotomy. Journal of Neurocytology 19: 329–337

Castro-Lopes JM, Tavares I, Coimbra A 1993 GABA decreases in the spinal cord dorsal horn after peripheral neurectomy. Brain Research 620: 287–291

Chen L, Huang L-YM 1992 Protein kinase C reduces Mg^{2+} block of NMDA-receptor channels as a mechanism of modulation. Nature 356: 521–523

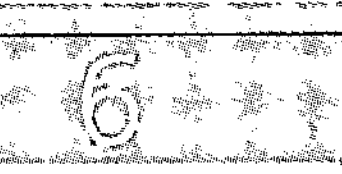

Choe H, Choi YS, Kim YH et al 1997 Epidural morphine plus ketamine for upper abdominal surgery: improved analgesia from preincisional versus postincisional administration. Anesthesia and Analgesia 84: 560–563

Chung K, Kevetter GA, Willis WD, Coggeshall RE 1984 An estimate of the ratio of the propriospinal to long tract neurons in the sacral spinal cord of the rat. Neuroscience Letters 44: 173–177

Coderre TJ, Katz J, Vaccarino AL, Melzack R 1993 Contribution of central neuroplasticity to pathological pain: review of clinical and experimental evidence. Pain 52: 259–285

Coggeshall RE, Reynolds ML, Woolf CJ 1991 Distribution of the growth associated protein GAP-43 in the central processes of axotomized primary afferents in the adult rat spinal cord; presence of growth cone-like structures. Neuroscience Letters 131: 37–41

Coggeshall RE, Lekan HA, Doubell TP, Allchorne A, Woolf CJ 1997 Central changes in primary afferent fibers following peripheral nerve lesions. Neuroscience 77: 1115–1122

Cook AJ, Woolf CJ, Wall PD, McMahon SB 1987 Dynamic receptive field plasticity in rat spinal cord dorsal horn following C primary afferent input. Nature 325: 151–153

Craig AD, Bushnell MC, Zhang ET, Blomqvist A 1994 A thalamic nucleus specific for pain and temperature sensation. Nature 372: 770–773

Dahl JB, Hansen BL, Hjortoso NC 1992 Influence of timing on the effect of continuous extradural analgesia with bupivacaine and morphine after major abdominal surgery. British Journal of Anaesthesiology 69: 4–8

deCharms RC, Merzenich MM 1996 Primary cortical representation of sounds by the coordination of action-potential timing. Nature 381: 610–613

Devor M, Wall PD 1981 Plasticity in the spinal cord sensory map following peripheral nerve injury in rats. Journal of Neuroscience 1: 679–684

Doubell TP, Woolf CJ 1997 Growth-associated protein 43 immunoreactivity in the superficial dorsal horn of the rat spinal cord is localized in atrophic C-fiber, and not in sprouted A-fiber, central terminals after peripheral nerve injury. Journal of Comparative Neurology 386: 111–118

Doubell TP, Mannion RJ, Woolf CJ 1997 Intact sciatic myelinated primary afferent terminals collaterally sprout in the adult rat dorsal horn following section of a neighbouring peripheral nerve. Journal of Comparative Neurology 380: 95–104

Dubner R, Ruda MA 1992 Activity-dependent neuronal plasticity following tissue injury and inflammation. Trends in Neurosciences 15(3): 96–103

Dubner R, Kenshalo DR Jr, Maixner W, Bushnell MC, Oliveras J-L 1989 The correlation of monkey medullary dorsal horn neural activity and the perceived intensity of noxious heat stimuli. Journal of Neurophysiology 62: 450–457

Eblen-Zajjur AA, Sandkuhler J 1997 Synchronicity of nociceptive and non-nociceptive adjacent neurons in the spinal dorsal horn of the rat: stimulus-induced plasticity. Neuroscience 76: 39–54

Eide PK, Jorum E, Stubhaug A, Bremmes J, Breivik H 1994 Relief of post-herpetic neuralgia with the *N*-methyl-D-aspartic acid receptor antagonist ketamine: a double-blind, cross-over comparison with morphine and placebo. Pain 58: 347–354

Eriksson NP, Aldskogius H, Grant G, Lindsay RM, Rivero-Melian C 1997 The effects of nerve growth factor, brain-derived neurotrophic factor and neurotrophin-3 on the laminar distribution of transganglionically transported choleragenoid in the spinal cord dorsal horn following transection of the sciatic nerve in the adult rat. Neuroscience 78: 863–872

Gerber G, Randic M 1989a Excitatory amino acid mediated components of synaptically evoked input from dorsal roots to deep dorsal horn neurons in the rat spinal cord slice. Neuroscience Letters 106: 211–219

Gerber G, Randic M 1989b Participation of excitatory amino acid receptors in the slow excitatory synaptic transmission in the rat spinal dorsal horn in vitro. Neuroscience Letters 106: 220–228

Gottschalk A, Smith DS, Jobes DR et al 1998 Preemptive epidural analgesia and recovery from radical prostatectomy: a randomized controlled trial. Journal of the American Medical Association 279: 1076–1082

Gu JG, MacDermott AB 1997 Activation of ATP P2X receptors elicits glutamate release from sensory neuron synapses. Nature 389: 749–753

Hoheisel U, Mense S 1989 Long-term changes in discharge behaviour of cat dorsal horn neurones following noxious stimulation of deep tissues. Pain 36: 239–247

Hori Y, Endo K, Takahashi T 1992 Presynaptic inhibitory action of enkephalin on excitatory transmission in superficial dorsal horn of rat spinal cord. Journal of Physiology (London) 450: 673–685

Hu JW, Sessle BJ, Raboisson P, Dallel R, Woda A 1992 Stimulation of craniofacial muscle afferents induces prolonged facilitatory effects in trigeminal nociceptive brain-stem neurones. Pain 48: 53–60

Hunt SP, Pini A, Evan G 1987 Induction of c-*fos*-like protein in spinal cord neurones following sensory stimulation. Nature 328: 632–634

Hylden JLK, Nahin RL, Traub RJ, Dubner R 1989 Expansion of receptive fields of spinal lamina I projection neurons in rats with unilateral adjuvant-induced inflammation: the contribution of dorsal horn mechanisms. Pain 37: 239–243

Ji RR, Rupp F 1997 Phosphorylation of transcription factor CREB in rat spinal cord after formalin-induced hyperalgesia: relationship to c-*fos* induction. Journal of Neuroscience 17: 1776–1785

Kato H, Liu Y, Kogure K, Kato K 1994 Induction of 27-kDa heat shock protein following cerebral ischemia in a rat model of ischemic tolerance. Brain Research 634: 235–244

Knyihar-Csillik E, Rakic P, Csillik B 1987 Transganglionic degenerative atrophy in the substantia gelatinosa of the spinal cord after peripheral nerve transection in rhesus monkeys. Cell and Tissue Research 247: 599–604

Knyihar-Csillik E, Torok A, Csillik B 1990 Primary afferent origin of substance P-containing axons in the superficial dorsal horn of the rat spinal cord: depletion, regeneration and replenishment of presumed nociceptive central terminals. Journal of Comparative Neurology 297: 594–612

Koerber HR, Mirnics K, Brown PB, Mendell LM 1994 Central sprouting and functional plasticity of regenerated primary afferents. Journal of Neuroscience 14: 3655–3671

Koerber HR, Mimics K, Mendell LM 1995 Properties of regenerated primary afferents and their functional connections. Journal of Neurophysiology 73: 693–702

Koltzenburg M, Lundberg LER, Torebjork HE 1992 Dynamic and static components of mechanical hyperalgesia in human hairy skin. Pain 51: 207–220

Le Bars D, Dickenson AH, Besson JM, Villanueva L 1986 Aspects of sensory processing through convergent neurones. In: Yaksh TL (ed) Spinal afferent processing. Plenum, New York, pp 467–504

Light AR, Trevino DL, Perl ER 1979 Morphological features of functionally defined neurons in the marginal zone and substantia gelatinosa of the spinal dorsal horn. Journal of Comparative Neurology 186: 151–172

Lin Q, Peng YB, Willis WD 1996 Possible role of protein kinase C in the sensitization of primate spinothalamic tract neurons. Journal of Neuroscience 16: 3026–3034

Liu H, Mantyh PW, Basbaum AI 1997 NMDA-receptor regulation of substance P release from primary afferent nociceptors. Nature 386: 721–724

Ma Q-P, Woolf CJ 1995 Involvement of neurokinin receptors in the induction but not the maintenance of mechanical allodynia in the rat

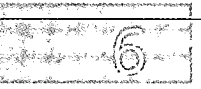

flexor motoneurones. Journal of Physiology (London) 486: 769–777
Ma Q-P, Woolf CJ 1996 Progressive tactile hypersensitivity: an inflammation-induced incremental increase in the excitability of the spinal cord. Pain: 67 97–106
Ma Q-P, Woolf CJ 1998 Morphine, the NMDA receptor antagonist MK 801 and the tachykinin NK1 receptor antagonist RP67580 attenuate the development of inflammation-induced progressive tactile hypersensitivity. Pain 77: 49–57
Malmberg AB, Chen C, Tonegawa S, Basbaum AI 1997 Preserved acute pain and reduced neuropathic pain in mice lacking PKC gamma. Science 278: 279–283
Mannion RJ, Doubell TP, Coggeshall RE, Woolf CJ 1996 Collateral sprouting of injured primary afferent A-fibers into the superficial dorsal horn of the adult rat spinal cord after topical capsaicin treatment to the sciatic nerve. Journal of Neuroscience 16: 5189–5195
Mantyh PW, Rogers SD, Honore P et al 1997 Inhibition of hyperalgesia by ablation of lamina I spinal neurons expressing the substance P receptor. Science 278: 275–279
Maslany S, Crockett DP, Egger MD 1992 Organization of cutaneous primary afferent fibers projecting to the dorsal horn in the rat: WGA-HRP versus B-HRP. Brain Research 569: 123–135
Maxwell DJ, Rethelyi M 1987 Ultrastructure and synaptic connections of cutaneous afferent fibers in the spinal cord. Trends Neuroscience 10: 117–122
Meller ST, Gebhart GF 1993 Nitric oxide (NO) and nociceptive processing in the spinal cord. Pain 52: 127–136
Neugebauer V, Schaible H-G 1990 Evidence for a central component in the sensitization of spinal neurons with joint input during development of acute arthritis in cat's knee. Journal of Neurophysiology 64: 299–311
Neumann S, Doubell TP, Leslie TA, Woolf CJ 1996 Inflammatory pain hypersensitivity mediated by phenotypic switch in myelinated primary sensory neurones. Nature 384: 360–364
Nikolajsen L, Ilkjaer S, Christensen JH, Kroner K, Jensen TS 1997 Randomised trial of epidural bupivacaine and morphine in prevention of stump and phantom pain in lower-limb amputation. Lancet 350: 1353–1357
Noguchi K, Kawai Y, Fukuoka T, Senba E, Miki K 1995 Substance P induced by peripheral nerve injury in primary afferent sensory neurons and its effect on dorsal column nucleus neurons. Journal of Neuroscience 15: 7633–7643
Okamoto M, Yoshimura M, Baba H, Higashi H, Shimoji K 1996 Synaptic plasticity of substantia gelatinosa neurons in the chronic pain model rat. Japanese Journal of Physiology 46:
Oliveira AL, Risling M, Deckner M, Lindholm T, Langone F, Cullheim S 1997 Neonatal sciatic nerve transection induces TUNEL labeling of neurons in the rat spinal cord and DRG. Neuroreport 8: 2837–2840
Richmond CE, Bromley LM, Woolf CJ 1993 Preoperative morphine pre-empts postoperative pain. Lancet 342: 73–75
Schaible H-G, Neugebauer V, Cervero FA, Schmidt RF 1991 Changes in tonic descending inhibition of spinal neurons with articular input during the development of acute arthritis in the cat. Journal of Neurophysiology 66: 1021–1032
Selby MJ, Edwards R, Sharp F, Rutter WJ 1987 Mouse nerve growth factor gene: structure and expression. Molecular and Cellular Biology 7: 3057–3064
Semba K, Masarachia P, Malamed S et al 1985 An electron microscopic study of terminals of rapidly adapting mechanoreceptive afferent fibers in the cat spinal cord. Journal of Comparative Neurology 232: 229–240
Shortland P, Wall PD 1992 Long range afferents in the spinal cord. 2. Afferents which penetrate grey matter. Philosophical Transaction of the Royal Society of London et al 337: 445–455
Simone DA, Sorkin LS, Oh U et al 1991 Neurogenic hyperalgesia: central neural correlates in responses of spinothalamic tract neurons. Journal of Neurophysiology 66: 228–246
Sivilotti LG, Woolf CJ 1994 The contribution of $GABA_A$ and glycine receptors to central sensitization: disinhibition and touch-evoked allodynia in the spinal cord. Journal of Neurophysiology 72: 169–179
Skene JHP 1989 Axonal growth associated proteins. Annual Review of Neuroscience 12: 127–156
Stubhaug A, Breivik H, Eide PK, Kreunen M, Foss A 1997 Mapping of punctuate hyperalgesia around a surgical incision demonstrate that ketamine is a powerful suppressor of central sensitization to pain following surgery. Acta Anaesthesiologica Scandinavica 41: 1124–1132
Sugiura Y, Terui N, Hosoya Y, Aanonsen LM 1989 Difference in distribution of central terminals between visceral and somatic unmyelinated (C) primary afferent fibers. Journal of Neurophysiology 62: 834–840
Swett JE, Woolf CJ 1985 Somatotopic organization of primary afferent terminals in the superficial dorsal horn of the rat spinal cord. Journal of Comparative Neurology 231: 66–71
Thompson SWN, King AE, Woolf CJ 1990 Activity-dependent changes in rat ventral horn neurones in vitro: summation of prolonged afferent evoked postsynaptic depolarizations produce a D-APV sensitive windup. European Journal of Neuroscience 2: 638–649
Torebjork HE, Vallbo AB, Ochoa JL 1987 Intraneural microstimulation in man. Its relation to specificity of tactile sensations. Brain 110: 1509–1529
Traub RJ 1996 The spinal contribution of substance P to the generation and maintenance of inflammatory hyperalgesia in the rat. Pain 67: 151–161
Woolf CJ 1983 Evidence for a central component of post-injury pain hypersensitivity. Nature 306: 686–688
Woolf CJ 1987 Central terminations of cutaneous mechanoreceptive afferents in the rat lumbar spinal cord. Journal of Comparative Neurology 261: 105–119
Woolf CJ 1991 Central mechanisms of acute pain. In: Bond MR, Charlton JE, Woolf CJ (eds) Proceedings of the 6th World Congress on Pain. Elsevier, Amsterdam pp 25–34
Woolf CJ, Chong MS 1993 Pre-emptive analgesia – treating postoperative pain by preventing the establishment of central sensitization. Anesthesia and Analgesia 77: 1–18
Woolf CJ, King AE 1989 Subthreshold components of the cutaneous mechanoreceptive fields of dorsal horn neurons in the rat lumbar spinal cord. Journal of Neurophysiology 62: 907–916
Woolf CJ, King AE 1990 Dynamic alterations in the cutaneous mechanoreceptive fields of dorsal horn neurons in the rat spinal cord. Journal of Neuroscience 10: 2717–2726
Woolf CJ, Thompson SWN 1991 The induction and maintenance of central sensitization is dependent on *N*-methyl-D-aspartic acid receptor activation; implications for the treatment of post-injury pain hypersensitivity states. Pain 44: 293–299
Woolf CJ, Wall PD 1982 Chronic peripheral nerve section diminishes the primary afferent A-fibre mediated inhibition of rat dorsal horn neurones. Brain Research 242: 77–85
Woolf CJ, Walters ET 1991 Common patterns of plasticity contributing to nociceptive sensitization in mammals and aplysia. Trends in Neurosciences 14(2): 74–78
Woolf CJ, Reynolds ML, Molander C, O'Brien C, Lindsay RM, Benowitz LI 1990 GAP-43 a growth associated protein, appears in dorsal root ganglion cells and in the dorsal horn of the rat spinal cord following peripheral nerve injury. Neuroscience 34: 465–478
Woolf CJ, Shortland P, Coggeshall RE 1992 Peripheral nerve injury triggers central sprouting of myelinated afferents. Nature 355: 75–77

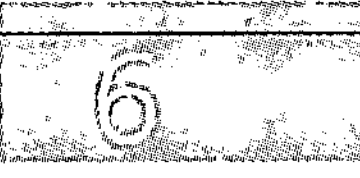

Yaksh TL 1989 Behavioural and autonomic correlates of the tactile evoked allodynia produced by spinal glycine inhibition: effect of modulatory receptor systems and excitatory amino acid antagonists. Pain 37: 111–123

Yoshimura M, Nishi S 1993 Blind patch-clamp recordings from substantia gelatinosa neurons in adult rat spinal cord slices: pharmacological properties of synaptic currents. Neuroscience 53: 519–526

Yu XM, Askalan R, Keil GJ, Salter MW 1997 NMDA channel regulation by channel-associated protein tyrosine kinase Src. Science 275: 674–678

Medulla to thalamus

A. D. CRAIG & J. O. DOSTROVSKY

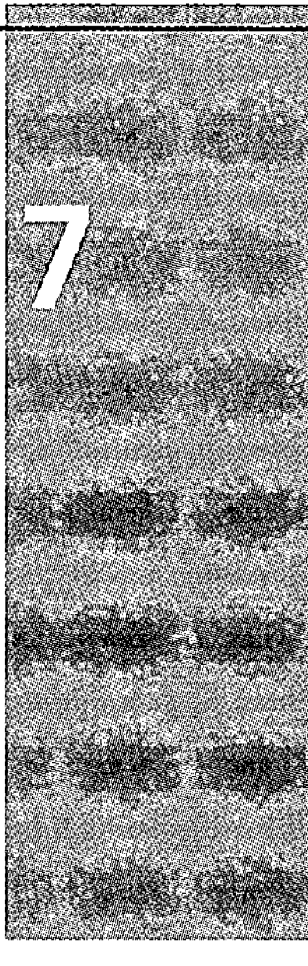

INTRODUCTION

The importance of the thalamus in the higher level processing of nociceptive inputs and the perception of pain has been recognized since the turn of the century (see below). However the complexity of the thalamus and its reciprocal connections with cortex and the technical difficulties associated with studying this region of the brain have greatly impeded progress in gaining a clear understanding of its role in pain. This chapter reviews and synthesizes our current knowledge of thalamic function in pain. Also highlighted is a critical review of the ascending pathways involved in pain with respect to their clinical importance and relevance in interpreting the function of their brainstem and thalamic targets. The possible function of brainstem sites involved in nociceptive processing and several cortical sites that are targets of thalamic regions implicated in pain are briefly discussed. A short review of the processing of craniofacial nociceptive inputs in the trigeminal brainstem complex (TBC) is included for completeness.

ASCENDING NOCICEPTIVE PATHWAYS

Stimuli that can cause pain activate various populations of spinal neurons that project via ascending pathways to brainstem and thalamic sites. These pathways can be associated with pain based on the afferent and efferent connectivity of the source and target regions, the response properties of the projecting cells and of their target regions, and the effects observed when these pathways or their terminal regions are stimulated or blocked in behaving animals or in patients. Not all ascending pathways from the spinal cord that can be activated by somato-visceral stimuli need to be considered here, for example, the various spinocerebellar projections or the spinal input to certain motor-related brainstem sites, such as the lateral reticular nucleus or the inferior olive. The ascending pathways of primary importance with respect to central nociceptive processing or the sensation of pain are:

1. The direct projections to the thalamus (the spinothalamic tract (STT)).
2. The direct projections to the reticular and homeostatic control regions of the medulla and brainstem, i.e. spinobulbar (spinoreticular (SRT) and spinomesencephalic (SMT) tracts) projections.
3. The direct projections to the hypothalamus and ventral forebrain (spinohypothalamic tract (SHT)).

In addition, indirect ascending pathways are integrated and relayed by intermediate stations, viz., the postsynaptic dorsal column (PSDC) system, the spinocervicothalamic (SCT) pathway and the spinoparabrachial pathways. These pathways ascend from the spinal cord and carry activity from the postcranial body, and similar pathways also originate from the trigeminal sensory nuclei in the medulla and represent facial structures (see below). The functional anatomical characteristics of each of these ascending pathways, that is the connectivity and functional characteristics of their cells of origin, the locations of their ascending axons and the distribution of their terminations, are described below. Several reviews may be consulted for more comprehensive literature references (Brodal 1981, Albe-Fessard et al 1985, Willis 1985, 1987, Fields 1987, Lenz & Dougherty 1997).

SPINOTHALAMIC PROJECTIONS

The direct spinothalamic (and trigeminothalamic) projection is classically most closely associated with pain and temperature sensation, because it has been recognized since the beginning of the twentieth century that lesions of this pathway (at spinal, medullary or mesencephalic levels) result clinically in the loss of pain and temperature sensations, that is, analgesia or hypalgesia and thermanaesthesia (see below) (Thiele & Horsley 1901, May 1906, Foerster & Gagel 1932, Kuru 1949, White & Sweet 1969, Perl 1984a, Willis 1985, Craig 1991a). The characteristics of this pathway are consistent with this seminal finding, and considerable information is now available regarding the components of this pathway.

Cells of origin

STT cells have been identified in various experimental mammals with anatomical tracers that label the neuronal cell bodies by retrograde transport from their axonal termination sites in the thalamus (Carstens & Trevino 1978, Willis et al 1979, Giesler et al 1981, Jones et al 1987, Craig et al 1989, Apkarian & Hodge 1989a, Burstein et al 1990, Zhang & Craig 1997). Comparable evidence was obtained in humans by examination of chromatolytic spinal cells in autopsy material following cordotomies in terminal patients by Kuru (1949). STT cells are found primarily in three regions of the spinal grey matter (Fig. 7.1):

1. The most superficial aspect of the dorsal horn, which is called the marginal zone, or lamina I.
2. The lateral portion of the neck of the dorsal horn, or laminae IV–V (or equivalently, the deep dorsal horn).
3. The intermediate zone and medial ventral horn, or laminae VII–VIII.

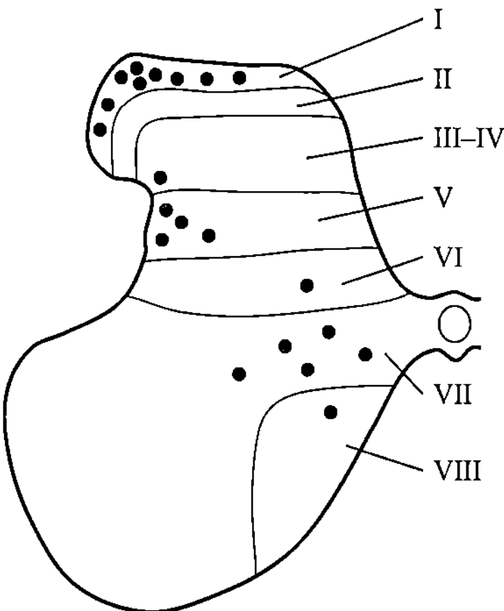

Fig. 7.1 Schematic diagram summarizing the locations of the three concentrations of STT cells in mammals, i.e. the marginal zone (lamina I), the neck of the dorsal horn (laminae IV–V), and the intermediate zone and ventral horn (laminae VII–VIII).

Although there are minor differences between species, approximately one-half of STT cells are located in lamina I, about one-quarter are found in laminae IV–V and another quarter are in laminae VII–VIII. Following a large injection of tracer in the thalamus on one side, about 85–90% of the labelled spinal cells are found on the contralateral side, and about 10–15% are on the ipsilateral side. The contralateral STT cells that project to thalamus on one side number in the order of 10 000 cells. Concentrations of STT cells are located in the cervical and lumbosacral enlargements, and an additional, large population of STT cells is located bilaterally throughout the C1–2 spinal grey matter.

Each of the main three populations of spinal cord neurons is dominated by afferent input from a different constellation of primary afferent fibres (Perl 1984a, Willis 1985, Fields 1987, Light 1992, Craig 1996). Briefly, lamina I neurons, which are small cells that arborize in the horizontal plane, receive small-diameter (Aδ and C) primary afferent terminations from fibres originating in all tissues of the body, including skin, muscle, joint and viscera (and also specialized trigeminal structures). Laminae IV–V neurons, which are large cells with dorsally and mediolaterally radiating dendrites, receive input from large-diameter (Aβ) fibres from skin, and they may also receive direct input from small-diameter Aδ fibres (and polysynaptic input from C fibres) from skin, muscle or viscera. Laminae VII–VIII cells, whose somata have not been well characterized, generally receive convergent input from large-diameter skin and deep (muscle, joint) inputs and also other (polysynaptic) inputs. Cells in the most medial intermediate zone, near the central canal (lamina X), may also receive small-diameter visceral input.

Accordingly, each of these spinal cell populations displays a different pattern of functional activity. Physiological experiments have characterized several basic types of STT cells, based on single-unit microelectrode recordings and identification by antidromic activation from their termination sites in the thalamus. Each population of STT cells is dominated by particular types of cells.

Lamina I STT cells

Lamina I contains three major classes of STT cells (Christensen & Perl 1970, Gobel 1978, Perl 1984a, Craig 1996, Han et al 1998). There are nociceptive-specific (NS) cells that respond within a small cutaneous receptive field to noxious mechanical or noxious thermal stimuli or both, but not to innocuous stimulation. There are polymodal nociceptive (HPC) cells that respond to noxious heat, pinch or cold. These are dominated by C-fibre input. Either of these types of nociceptive cells may also respond to noxious stimulation of muscle, joint or viscera. In addition, lamina I contains thermoreceptive-specific (COLD) cells that are excited by innocuous cooling and inhibited by warming of the skin (warm-responsive STT cells are very rare) (Dostrovsky & Hellon 1978, Craig & Hunsley 1991, Dostrovsky & Craig 1996a). Thus, lamina I STT cells are modality selective and their activity is specifically related to pain and temperature stimulation. Each of these distinct classes has a particular somatodendritic morphology (Han et al 1998); NS cells are fusiform neurons (with unmyelinated axons), HPC cells are multipolar neurons and COLD cells are pyramidal neurons. These subsets each form about one-third of the population of lamina I STT cells, although the NS cells predominate. HPC and COLD cells are concentrated in the cervical and lumbosacral enlargements (Zhang & Craig 1997). The fundamental role of lamina I may be to distribute modality selective afferent activity related to the physiological status and maintenance of the tissues of the body, including specific activity related to pain and temperature sensations.

Laminae IV–V STT cells

Laminae IV–V contain two major types of STT cells. Some are low-threshold (LT) cells that respond only to non-noxious mechanical cutaneous stimulation (Willis et al 1974). These may respond to brushing (hair) or to both brushing and graded pressure. Others are so-called 'wide dynamic range' (WDR) nociceptive cells that respond to both innocuous and noxious stimuli over a fairly large cutaneous receptive field in a graded manner (Willis 1985, Price 1988, Dubner et al 1989, Maixner et al 1989). That is, they respond to brushing and pressure, and are maximally activated by pinch or noxious heat. Some receive only Aβ and Aδ input, whereas others receive strong (polysynaptic) C-fibre input, and their responses to C-fibre activation typically 'wind up', meaning they increase with repetitive stimulation at rates faster than 0.3 Hz (Mendell & Wall 1965). Lamina V cells often receive convergent deep and visceral input (Foreman et al 1979, Tattersall et al 1986, Ness & Gebhart 1990, Chandler et al 1991). These cells may serve as cumulative integrators of the entire spectrum of somatic afferent inflow.

Laminae VII–VIII STT cells

Laminae VII–VIII STT cells are generally complex cells that respond to innocuous or noxious stimulation within large, bilateral or widely separated somatic regions. They can have large inhibitory fields and can respond differently to different modes of stimulation, often including proprioceptive or visceral inputs (Giesler et al 1981, Milne et al 1982, Menetrey et al 1984). These cells may serve to integrate somatic and motoric afferent with spinal interneuronal activity.

The correspondence between laminar location and cell type is not absolute, that is, there are a few lamina I cells that are WDR cells (in the monkey), and some lamina V cells may be NS cells with respect to cutaneous input. Noxious stimulation of deep (muscle, joint) tissues or visceral tissues can activate some cells in all of these locations. Nociceptive cells that are activated by visceral or deep stimulation usually, but not always (Craig & Kniffki 1985b, Ness & Gebhart 1990), receive cutaneous input as well.

Physiological support for the involvement of WDR STT cells (in laminae I and V) in pain sensation is provided by the close correlations observed between their discharge activity and simultaneously observed, operant aversive responses of awake, behaviourally trained monkeys to noxious heat stimuli (see below) (Price 1988, Dubner et al 1989, Maixner et al 1989). The discharge activity of lamina I NS neurons is also correlated with aversive responses (Bushnell et al 1984). In addition, the activity of lamina V WDR cells can be enhanced by stimuli that produce hyperalgesia in humans, such as intradermal capsaicin or intramuscular irritation, in parallel with psychophysical results (Simone et al 1991, Palecek et al 1992, Hoheisel et al 1993). The activity of lamina I HPC STT cells corresponds uniquely with the sensation evoked by the thermal grill illusion of pain (in which burning, ice-like pain is elicited by interlaced cool and warm stimuli) (Craig & Bushnell 1994). Lamina I COLD STT cells are the only type of ascending thermoreceptive-specific neurons known, and their activity can be associated directly with human thermal sensibility (Dostrovsky & Hellon 1978, Poulos 1981, Davies et al 1983, Craig & Bushnell 1994, Craig 1996).

Organization of ascending STT axons

Ascending axons of STT cells generally cross in the dorsal or ventral commissure to the contralateral ventrolateral spinal white matter within one to two segments rostral to the cell of origin. The ascending STT axons are concentrated in two locations: the middle of the lateral funiculus (the classical 'lateral' spinothalamic tract) and the middle of the anterior (ventral) funiculus (the classical 'anterior' spinothalamic tract) (May 1906, Kuru 1949, Craig 1991a). (These have also been called the 'dorsal' or 'dorsolateral' STT and the 'ventral' STT (Jones et al 1987, Apkarian &

Hodge 1989b, Ralston III & Ralston 1992).) These bundles were originally observed using silver stains for degenerating fibres in human autopsy material and in primates following spinal hemisections (Thiele & Horsley 1901, May 1906, Kuru 1949). Recent anterograde and retrograde labelling studies have confirmed that the axons in the lateral STT originate predominantly from lamina I cells, whereas the ascending axons in the anterior STT originate generally from deeper laminae V and VII cells (Stevens et al 1989, Apkarian & Hodge 1989b, Craig 1991a). The lateral STT can also be visualized with immunohistochemical labelling for calbindin, which labels lamina I cells as well as their terminations in the thalamus (Aronin et al 1991, Craig et al 1994, 1998). There is, nonetheless, considerable dispersion and individual variability from this general pattern. Within the ascending tract, there is a crude somatotopic organization. The crossing fibres displace ascending axons laterally, with the result that axons from caudal body regions tend to be located more superficially in the white matter, whereas those from rostral body regions tend to be located more medially (proximal to midline). At the spinomedullary junction the two ascending STT bundles coalesce in the ventrolateral aspect of the medulla (Mehler et al 1960, Westlund & Craig 1996). Trigemino-thalamic axons intermingle with the medial aspect of the STT at this level. At the caudal end of the pons the STT shifts dorsally to pass along the lateral aspect of the parabrachial region and then occupies a position ventrolateral to the inferior colliculus, near its brachium. The STT ascends in this region through the lateral aspect of the mesencephalon to the thalamus.

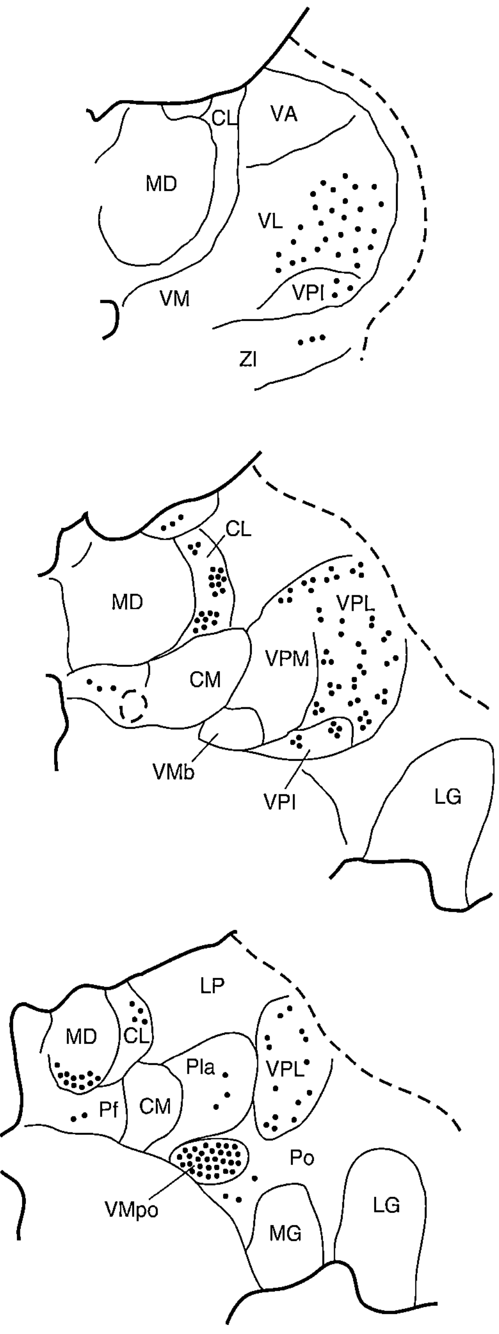

Fig. 7.2 Schematic diagram summarizing the distribution and relative density of STT terminations in the macaque monkey at three frontal levels, from caudal to rostral. Abbreviations of thalamic nuclei: CL=central lateral; CM=centre median; LG=lateral geniculate; LP=lateral posterior; MD=medial dorsal; MG=medial geniculate; Pf=parafascicular; Pla=anterior pulvinar; Po=posterior; VA=ventral anterior; VL=ventral lateral; VMb=basal part of the ventral medial; VM=ventral medial; VMpo=posterior part of the ventral medial; VPI=ventral, posterior inferior; VPL=ventral posterior lateral; VPM=ventral posterior medial; ZI=zona incerta.

STT projection sites

Based on the results of anterograde tracing experiments in primates and silver-stained degeneration material following cordotomies in humans, it is known that the STT terminates in six distinct regions of the thalamus, which are indicated in Figure 7.2 (Bowsher 1961, Mehler 1969, Boivie 1979, Berkley 1980, Burton & Craig 1983, Albe-Fessard et al 1985, Apkarian & Hodge 1989c, Craig 1995b):

1. The ventral posterior nuclei (VPL, VPM, and VPI).
2. The posterior portion of the ventral medial n. (VMpo).
3. The ventral lateral n. (VL).
4. The central lateral n. (CL).
5. The parafascicular n. (Pf).
6. The ventral caudal portion of the medial dorsal n. (MDvc).

These regions are generally named similarly in the human, but some atlases vary significantly (Olszewski 1952, Mehler 1966, Hassler 1970, Jones 1985, 1997, Hirai & Jones 1989a). In the human, the VPM and VPL nuclei have been called the ventral caudal internal and external nuclei, and VPI has been called the parvicellular part of the ventral caudal nuclei. The posterior inferior portion of somatosensory thalamus that contains VMpo is anatomically part of the suprageniculate/posterior complex in earlier works (Olszewski 1952, Jones 1985, Ralston III & Ralston 1992, Craig et al 1994), and it is probably equivalent to the caudal VP of Mehler (1966) and the limitans portae or VC portae of Hassler (1970).

Ventral posterior nuclei

There are pronounced clusters of STT terminations (classically termed 'pleides' or 'archipelago') scattered throughout the VP nuclei, which historically were the first STT terminations observed (Clark & Gros 1936, Walker 1940, Mehler 1969, Albe-Fessard et al 1985, Jones 1985). These clusters are particularly dense in the dorsal rostral portion and the ventral caudal portion of VP and near the fibre laminae that subdivide VP (Burton & Craig 1983). They are topographically organized in the mediolateral direction in parallel with the precise somatopic lamellae of VP; trigeminothalamic cells project to VPM, cervical STT cells project to medial VPL and lumbar STT cells project to lateral VPL. The STT terminations in VP originate primarily from cells in laminae IV–V (Boivie 1979, Apkarian & Hodge 1989c, Craig 1995b). These terminations are associated with VP cells immunopositive for calbindin, whereas lemniscal inputs (from the dorsal column nuclei and the principal trigeminal nucleus) are associated with VP cells that are immunoreactive for parvalbumin (Rausell & Jones 1991). Although the significance of this distinction is not appreciated, it emphasizes the likelihood that these tracts are associated with neuronal systems with a distinguishable pharmacology and biochemistry. Similarly, it has been reported that STT terminations on VP cell dendrites differ from lemniscal terminations in that they have less involvement with GABAergic presynaptic dendrites (Ralston III & Ralston 1994). A few STT axons that terminate in VP have a collateral in CL (Applebaum et al 1979, Giesler et al 1979, 1981, Craig et al 1989, Stevens et al 1989). STT-recipient VP cells project to the primary somatosensory cortex (SI), possibly to its superficial layers only (Gingold et al 1991, Rausell & Jones 1991). The nucleus VPI, a cell-sparse region which lies at the ventral medial aspect of VPL and ventral to VPM, receives a separate STT input that originates from lamina I and lamina IV–V STT cells (Burton & Craig 1983, Apkarian et al 1991, Ralston III & Ralston 1992, Craig 1995b); this nucleus projects to the region of the second somatosensory cortex in the lateral sulcus (Friedman & Murray 1986a, Stevens et al 1993). STT input to VP presumably subserves aspects of discriminative pain, as described below.

Ventral medial nucleus

The densest STT termination field is in VMpo, which lies immediately posterior to VMb and VPM. VMpo is the primary projection target of lamina I STT cells in the primate (Ralston III & Ralston 1992, Craig et al 1994, Craig 1995b), which are nearly the exclusive source of its ascending input. This projection is organized topographically in the anteroposterior direction, with lumbar input found most posterior and with cervical and trigeminal input found successively more anterior. VMpo thus serves as a dedicated thalamocortical relay nucleus for lamina I STT cells (as described physiologically below). This lamina I STT termination site is characterized by a dense field of fibres (not cells) immunoreactive for calbindin, reflecting the strong calbindin immunoreactivity of lamina I cells (Aronin et al 1991). This feature has been used to identify VMpo in the human thalamus (Craig et al 1994), which corresponds with the region of dense STT terminations demonstrated with silver stains following cordotomy. This nucleus is present only in primates, and in humans it is particularly large (approximately 2×4×4 mm). Ultrastructural findings indicate that the lamina I STT terminations in VMpo are glutamatergic and form triadic arrangements with relay cell dendrites and GABAergic presynaptic dendrites, assuring high synaptic and temporal fidelity in a lemniscal fashion (Blomqvist et al 1996). VMpo projects topographically to the dorsal sulcal margin of the anterior insular cortex buried in the lateral sulcus (Burton & Jones 1976, Friedman & Murray 1986, Craig 1995b). Together with the adjacent insular projection of visceral afferents related to vagal and gustatory (parasympathetic) input via VMb, the VMpo projection to insular cortex forms the basis for a sensory representation of the physiological condition of the body (Craig 1996), reflecting the general association of the insula with autonomic sensorimotor activity and with integration of somatosensory and limbic activity (Mufson & Mesulam 1984, Friedman et al 1986, Allen et al 1991, Yasui et al 1991).

Ventral lateral nucleus

There is moderately dense STT input to VL, rostral to VP, which overlaps with projections from the deep cerebellar nuclei (Berkley 1980, Asanuma et al 1983, Burton & Craig 1983). It probably originates from STT cells in lamina V and particularly lamina VII. It provides the basis for some somatosensory responsiveness in this region (Mackel et al 1992). VL projects to the motor cortex (Jones 1985), and this STT component is likely to be associated with somatomotor integration.

Central lateral nucleus

There is dense STT input to particular segments of CL, particularly its caudal portion. This projection arises primarily from lamina VII STT cells (Applebaum et al 1979, Giesler et al 1979, 1981, Apkarian & Hodge 1989b, Craig et al 1989, Stevens et al 1989, Huber et al 1994). This projection does not appear to have a simple topography; rather, several individual clusters of CL cells may receive STT input from different portions of the spinal cord (Craig & Burton 1985). CL also receives dense input from the cerebellum, the substantia nigra, the tectum, the globus pallidus, the mesencephalic tegmentum and motor cortex. The majority of cells in this portion of the intralaminar thalamus project to the basal ganglia, and others project to the superficial and deep layers of motor and posterior parietal cortices (Jones 1985, Royce et al 1989). This STT component is likely to be involved in somatomotor integration and the control of orientation.

Parafascicular nucleus

There is a weak STT projection to Pf that originates from lamina I and lamina V cells. The centre median (CM) was once thought to receive STT input, but modern evidence indicates it does not. The connections of Pf and CM are generally motor related. Cells in Pf project to the basal ganglia or to the motor cortex (Jones 1985, Royce et al 1989, François et al 1991, Sadikot et al 1992).

Medial dorsal nucleus

It has recently been recognized that there is a moderately dense STT projection to the ventral caudal part of the medial dorsal nucleus (MDvc). It has an anteroposterior topography, with trigeminal input located most posterior (Ganchrow 1978, Burton & Craig 1983, Apkarian & Hodge 1989c). This STT projection originates from lamina I cells (Albe-Fessard et al 1975, Craig et al 1994, Craig 1995b). Cells in MDvc project to area 24c in the cortex at the fundus of the anterior cingulate sulcus, rather than to the orbitofrontal and prefrontal cortex where most of MD projects (Ray & Price 1993, Craig & Zhang 1996). Imaging studies indicate that this STT component must be particularly important for pain (see below).

Species differences

Anatomical studies have been carried out in a variety of mammalian species, and there are several distinguishable species differences in STT terminations. These differences are presently not well understood, but as more sophisticated insights are acquired such comparative anatomical differences may provide important clues to the association of different projections with different functions.

In the cat (Berkley 1980, Albe-Fessard et al 1985, Craig & Burton 1985) the major STT termination sites are the caudal posterior complex, the ventral aspect of VP (including VPI), the ventral aspect of the basal part of the ventral medial n. (VMb), Pf, CL, VL and nucleus submedius (Sm) in the medial thalamus. There are few STT terminations within VP in the cat, in stark contrast to the monkey. The moderately dense and weakly topographic lamina I and lamina V STT terminations that occur along the ventral aspect of VP and ventral VMb (Craig & Burton 1985, Craig 1996a) may form a primordial homologue of the lamina I STT projection to VMpo in the primate; a strong projection to the insular cortex originates from ventral VMb (Clascá et al 1997). However, this termination region in the cat is characterized by immunoreactivity for substance P as well as calbindin (Battaglia et al 1992). As in the monkey, the STT projections to VL and CL originate from laminae V and VII cells, and the projection to Pf is sparse. Dense, topographic terminations in Sm originate almost exclusively from lamina I STT cells (Craig & Burton 1981); this region may be analogous to the lamina I projection to MDvc in the primate, because Sm is a developmental offshoot of the pronucleus of MD. However, Sm in the cat (and the rat) projects to ventral lateral orbital (VLO) cortex (Craig et al 1982, Coffield et al 1992, Yoshida et al 1992), and STT input to the anterior cingulate in the cat passes instead through the ventral aspect of VP (Musil & Olson 1988, Yasui et al 1988).

STT terminations in the rat differ from both monkey and cat (Mehler 1969, Peschanski 1984, Cliffer et al 1991, Iwata et al 1992); the major targets are VP, ventral VMb (usually called VPpc in this species), CL, Sm and Pf. The STT terminations occur throughout VP, and STT cells from laminae I, V and VII all project to VP in the rat, which may reflect the broad overlap of the somatosensory and motor cortices in this species. The sources of STT input to Sm differ from the cat; trigeminal cells are found in the most rostral part of n. caudalis, as well as in lamina I, and also in interpolaris, whereas lumbar STT cells that project to Sm are located predominantly in lamina VI (Dado & Giesler 1990, Yoshida et al 1991, 1992).

SPINOHYPOTHALAMIC PATHWAY

Recent retrograde labelling evidence indicates that there is a massive spinal projection to the anterior and lateral portions of the hypothalamus in the rat (Burstein & Potrebic 1993, Burstein et al 1996). This spinohypothalamic tract (SHT) appears to originate bilaterally from cells in laminae I, V, VII and X over the entire length of the cord, with concentrations at C1–2 and S1–3. It consists of thousands of cells, about as many as in the STT of the rat (Dado et al 1994b). Physiological evidence indicates that these cells include nociceptive neurons. Extensive antidromic mapping studies have revealed that SHT axons are often collaterals of STT axons, and that they can pursue a tortuous course, ascending through the contralateral thalamus and hypothalamus to decussate in the optic chiasm and then descending through the ipsilateral hypothalamus. There may be separate components to the medial and lateral hypothalamus. In addition, there are minor projections to various other ventral forebrain regions, such as the nucleus accumbens, the septal nuclei and the pallidum; these have also been seen in the squirrel monkey (Burstein & Potrebic 1993, Newman et al 1996). The possibilities for a role of the SHT in autonomic, neuroendocrine, and emotional aspects of pain seem numerous. However, the terminations of SHT axons have not been clearly defined either electrophysiologically or with anatomical anterograde labelling (Cliffer et al 1991, Iwata et al 1992, Dado et al 1994a). Only a weak projection has been reported in the cat, which originates nearly entirely from the sacral spinal segments (Katter et al 1991), and its extent in the primate remains to be established.

SPINOBULBAR PROJECTIONS

Spinobulbar nociceptive projections are important for the integration of nociceptive activity with the homeostatic processes that are subserved in the brainstem. In addition, there may be indirect projections of nociceptive activity to the forebrain that pass via brainstem neurons, as well as modulatory influences on forebrain function activated by spinobulbar inputs that may be important for the forebrain integration of the sensory experience of pain.

Cells of origin

Retrograde identification of the cells of origin of spinal projections to the brainstem is still complicated by the technical difficulty imposed by the ascending STT fibres of passage, which overlap with the location of spinobulbar axons and their terminations. Present data indicate that the distribution of spinobulbar (spinoreticular and spinomesencephalic) cells is quite similar to the distribution of STT cells. They are found in laminae I, V and VII in monkey, cat and rat (Kevetter et al 1982, Wiberg & Blomqvist 1984, Panneton & Burton 1985, Wiberg et al 1987, Yezierski 1988, Menétrey & de Pommery 1991, Yezierski & Mendez 1991). In addition, the same physiological response categories as STT cells have been described (Fields et al 1977, Menetrey et al 1980, 1984, Hylden et al 1986, Yezierski & Schwartz 1986, Yezierski et al 1987, Ammons 1987, Light et al 1993), with the exception that few thermoreceptive spinobulbar cells have yet been identified (Light et al 1993). These similarities might suggest that STT and spinobulbar projections could originate from the same populations of cells; however, few STT cells have been identified by means of retrograde double labelling, or by antidromic activation that have collateral projections to regions in the brainstem (Kevetter & Willis 1983, Hylden et al 1985, Panneton & Burton 1985, Yezierski 1988, Hylden et al 1989, Zhang et al 1990, Light et al 1993). It is likely that these pathways originate largely (80–90%) from different spinal neurons, which provides the nervous system with the significant capacity to differentially control the activity of spinal ascending projections to different rostral targets that have different functions (Jasmin et al 1994). Whereas spinal input to the thalamus is contralateral, spinal projections to the medulla are bilateral and those to the pons and mesencephalon have a contralateral dominance.

Spinobulbar terminations

Anatomical evidence indicates that ascending spinobulbar terminations are concentrated in four major areas of the brainstem, as indicated in Figure 7.3 (Mehler et al 1960, Mehler 1969, Wiberg & Blomqvist 1984, Wiberg et al 1987, Craig 1995a, Westlund & Craig 1996):

1. The regions containing the brainstem catecholamine cell groups, i.e., the ventrolateral medulla (A1, C1, A5), the nucleus of the solitary tract (A2), the locus coeruleus (A6) and the subcoerulear and Kölliker–Füse regions in the dorsolateral pons (A7).
2. The parabrachial n. (PB).
3. The periaqueductal grey (PAG).
4. The brainstem reticular formation.

Tracer studies indicate that lamina I cell terminations occur in the first three sites, but not in the reticular formation (Burton et al 1979, Blomqvist & Craig 1991, Craig 1995a, Westlund & Craig 1996). The evidence indicates that the terminations of spinal laminae V and VII cells

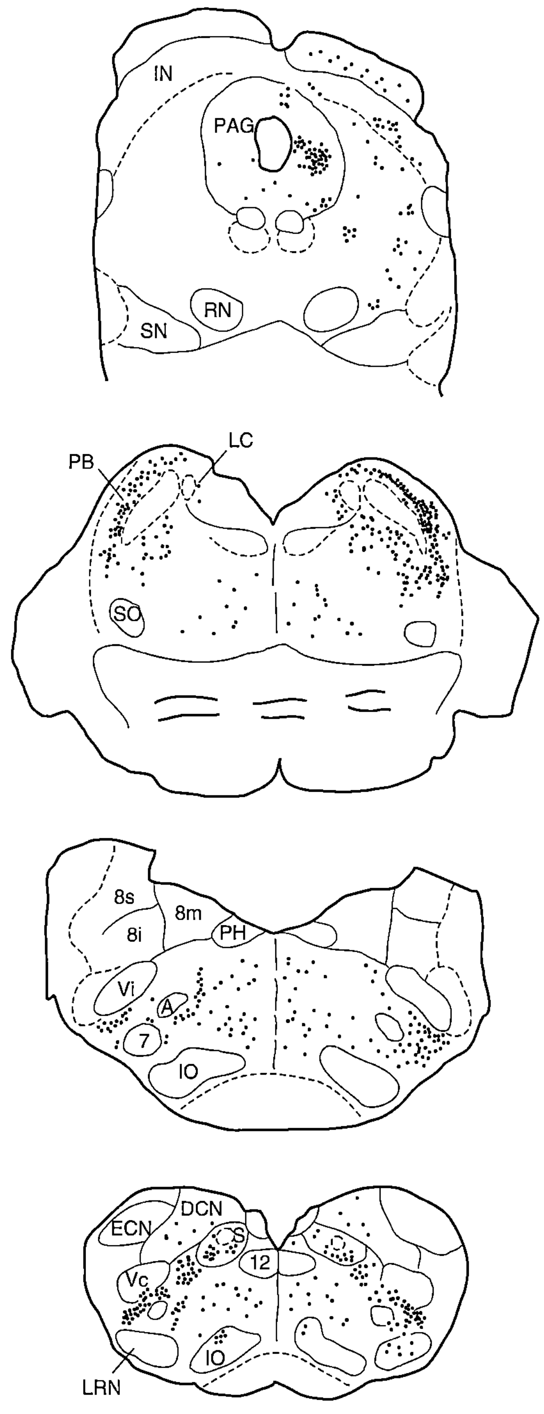

Fig. 7.3 Schematic diagram summarizing the distribution and relative density of spinobulbar terminations in the macaque monkey at four tranverse levels, from caudal to rostral. Abbreviations of brainstem nuclei: A=ambiguus; DCN=dorsal column nuclei; ECN=external cuneate; IN=intercollicular; IO=inferior olive; LC=locus coeruleus; LRN=lateral reticular; PAG=periaqueductal grey; PB=parabrachial; PH=praepositus hypoglossi; RN=red nucleus; S=solitary complex; SN=substantia nigra; SO=superior olive; Vc=trigeminal nucleus caudalis; Vi=trigeminal nucleus interpolaris; 7=facial; 8i=inferior vestibular; 8m=medial vestibular; 8s=superior vestibular; 12= hypoglossal.

probably occur in the reticular formation and the solitary n., with relatively minor projections to PB and to the region surrounding the PAG (Kevetter et al 1982, Cechetto et al 1985, Menetrey & Basbaum 1987, Yezierski 1988, Menétrey & de Pommery 1991, Kitamura et al 1993).

Catecholamine cell groups

There is moderately dense spinal input to all brainstem catecholamine cell groups. These are well-known integration sites for cardiorespiratory and homeostatic function, and contain pre-autonomic bulbospinal neurons that drive sympathetic outflow (Loewy & Spyer 1990). Spinal input to the solitary complex may provide a pathway for brainstem activity due to visceral inflammation (Menétrey & de Pommery 1991). Spinal input to the catecholamine cell groups in the ventrolateral medulla presumably are involved in integrative cardiorespiratory and other autonomic functions, including spino-bulbo-spinal somato-autonomic reflex arcs (Sato & Schmidt 1973), as well as descending antinociceptive mechanisms. Lamina I terminations are especially dense in the caudal ventrolateral medulla around cells of the A1 cell group, whose projection to the hypothalamus is responsible for the release of ACTH and vasopressin in response to noxious stimulation (Day & Sibbald 1990; for other references see Craig 1995a). Terminations in the rostral ventrolateral medulla (C1, subretrofacial n.) may engage adrenergic cells that give rise to descending projections to the thoracolumbar sympathetic region (Morrison & Reis 1989). Lamina I input to cells in the A6 and A7 groups in the dorsolateral pons is of particular interest, because the catecholamine A7 cells appear to provide the major source of descending noradrenergic modulation of nociceptive dorsal horn activity (Basbaum & Fields 1978, Westlund et al 1984, Clark & Proudfit 1991, Young et al 1992). These neurons are activated by noxious stimuli (Hermanson & Blomqvist 1997), and they are involved in the 'diving reflex' activated by cold stimulation (Panneton & Yavari 1995). Descending enkephalinergic bulbospinal cells in this region may also receive direct spinal input (Blomqvist et al 1994, Hermanson & Blomqvist 1995). Projections from the locus coeruleus (A6) include the entire neuraxis, in accordance with its putative role in vigilance and attention, and lamina I spinobulbar input to this nucleus may activate such processes (Craig 1992, Westlund & Craig 1996).

Parabrachial nucleus

PB receives a dense spinal input that is concentrated in its lateral part but that overlaps partially in the medial and dorsal parts with general visceral afferent input from the solitary n. (Mehler 1969, Burton et al 1979, Fulwiler & Saper 1984, Cechetto et al 1985, Panneton & Burton 1985, Blomquvist et al 1989, Berkley & Scofield 1990, Craig 1995a). It originates primarily, but not exclusively, from lamina I. The terminations are weakly organized topographically (Feil & Herbert 1995). PB has numerous interconnections with cell groups in the pontine and medullary reticular formation (including the catecholamine cell groups) appropriate for its role in homeostasis and cardiovascular integration (Holstege 1988, Gang et al 1990, Herbert et al 1990, Chamberlin & Saper 1992). It also projects to the anterior and lateral hypothalamus, to the central nucleus of the amygdala, to Sm (in rats), and to a portion of the ventrobasal thalamus (the basal portion of VM, included in VPpc in rats) that serves as a relay to the insular cortex for general and special visceral sensory activity (Saper & Loewy 1980, Cechetto & Saper 1987, Bernard et al 1991, Halsell 1992, Yoshida et al 1992, Bernard et al 1993). This pathway is strongly associated with several peptides, most notably CGRP (Mantyh & Hunt 1984, Yasui et al 1989). Nociceptive neurons recorded in PB (Fig. 7.4) have been antidromically activated from the amygdala or from the hypothalamus (Bernard & Besson 1990). Their response characteristics are similar to those of lamina I neurons, including both nociceptive and thermoreceptive sensitivity. The lamina I input to PB thus serves as an indirect pathway for nociceptive activity to reach the forebrain, as well as a substrate for integration of physiological activity regarding tissue status, including nociception, with general visceral and homeostatic mechanisms.

Periaqueductal grey

The PAG is a major integration site for homeostatic control and limbic motor output, and it has both ascending and descending projections. Spinal input to the PAG is moderately dense and is concentrated in its lateral and ventrolateral (caudal) portions. It originates primarily, but not exclusively, from lamina I (Blomqvist & Craig 1991, Yezierski & Mendez 1991). It is topographically organized rostrocaudally in a trigeminal, cervical, lumbar progression within the lateral PAG (Wiberg et al 1987, Blomqvist & Craig 1991), but not in the ventrolateral PAG. The ventrolateral PAG also receives bilateral input from cells in the intermediate zone and ventral horn of the C1–2 segments (Keay et al 1997). Stimulation of either of these portions of the PAG can simultaneously elicit aversive behaviours, cardiovascular changes and antinociceptive modulation. These efferent actions appear to be topographically organized in parallel with the topography of spinal and trigeminal inputs, and in a manner appropriate for different behavioural states (Bandler et al 1991, Depaulis et al 1992). Thus, spinal input to the PAG may be integrated with descending antinociceptive modulation of the spinal cord, which involves projections to the raphe magnus, the ventromedial reticular formation, the dorsolateral pons and the ventrolateral medulla (Basbaum & Fields 1978, Fields 1987, Cameron et al 1995). Notably, the same portions of the PAG that receive spinal input also have ascending projections to the hypothalamus and to the thalamus (Mantyh 1983, Rinvik & Wiberg 1990, Meller & Dennis 1991, Reichling & Basbaum 1991), specifically to the thalamic reticular n., to Pf, and to the centre median (CM). Thus, spinal input to the PAG may also influence brainstem modulation of forebrain processing. The spino-bulbo-PAG-diencephalic pathway could also provide an indirect alternative pathway for nociceptive sensory activity to affect the thalamus.

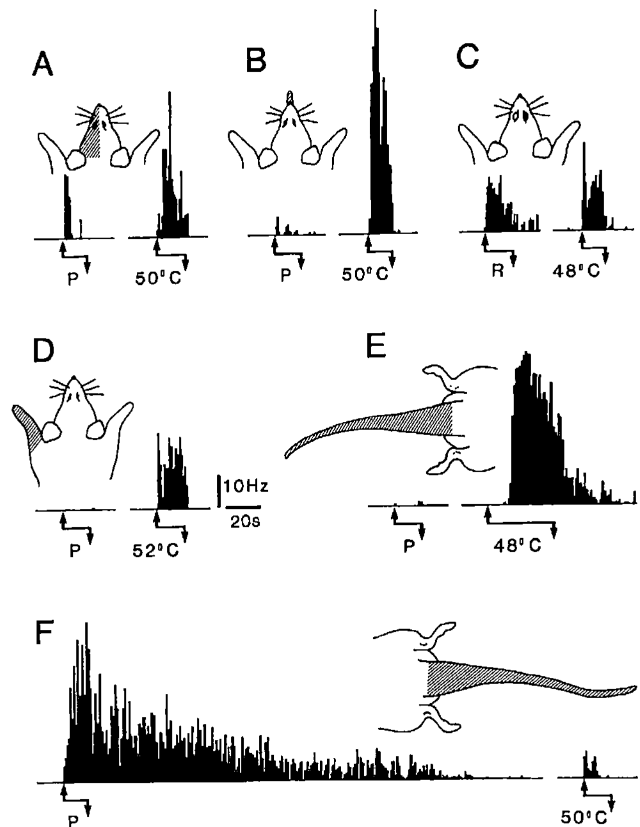

Fig. 7.4 A–F Examples of six NS neurons recorded in the parabrachial nucleus and antidromically activated from the amygdalla. Each example shows the location of the receptive field, and firing rate histograms showing responses to noxious mechanical (P=pinch; R=rubbing cornea) and thermal stimuli. (Reproduced from Bernard & Besson 1990 with permission.)

Reticular formation

There is scattered spinal input to the reticular formation that has been observed with silver degeneration techniques (Thiele & Horsley 1901, Mehler et al 1960, Mehler 1969), but which has not been well examined with more modern methods. There are nociceptive neurons in the reticular formation, some of which apparently project back to the spinal cord and could modulate sensory or motor activity. Many neurons in the brainstem core, particularly rostrally, project to the thalamus, so the possibility exists that some of these might relay nociceptive activity to the thalamus. A so-called 'spinoreticulothalamic' pathway has long been hypothesized as a multi-synaptic route which might provide an alternative pathway for pain-related activity to reach the forebrain and to serve the motivational aspect of pain (Bishop 1959, Melzack & Casey 1968, Bowsher 1975, Bonica 1990). However, the distribution of brainstem neurons that project to the thalamus shows little overlap with the distribution of spinal input to the brainstem (Mehler 1969, Carstens et al 1990, Blomqvist & Berkley 1992), suggesting that the spinal inputs to the PAG and to PB are the major routes for indirect ascending access to the thalamus via the brainstem. Nonetheless, recent evidence indicates that neurons in the dorsomedial reticular formation in the caudal medulla (the so-called subnucleus reticularis dorsalis, or SRD) receive direct input from spinal laminae I and V cells, display nociceptive response characteristics within large receptive fields, and project to the thalamus or back to the spinal cord (Bernard et al 1990, Villanueva et al 1991, 1998, Roy et al 1992). The role of such cells in pain has not been determined.

OTHER INDIRECT PATHWAYS

There are two other indirect pathways for pain-related activity to reach the forebrain that relay in the spinal cord itself (Brodal 1981, Willis 1985). These are the post-synaptic dorsal column (PSDC) system and the spino-cervico-thalamic pathway (SCTP). The PSDC originates from second-order cells in the spinal dorsal horn, primarily in laminae IV–V. Their axons project via the base of the dorsal columns and the superficial aspect of the dorsolateral funiculus to the dorsal column nuclei (gracile and cuneate). These axons terminate within the ventral and rostral portions of the dorsal column nuclei, where GABAergic interneurons are located and from which projections to motor-related portions of the brainstem and the thalamus originate (Berkley et al 1986). Accordingly, one role of this pathway may be to engage inhibitory interneurons that reduce activity in mechanoreceptive dorsal column nuclear cells. The SCTP originates from a similar, overlapping population of second-order cells in laminae IV–V of the spinal dorsal horn that project via the dorsolateral funiculus to the lateral cervical nucleus in C1–2 (Boivie 1983). This pathway is large in carnivores (cat, raccoon), but much smaller in primates. Lateral cervical neurons project to VP in the thalamus via the medial lemniscus. Activity in both of these pathways is dominated by low-threshold mechanoreceptor stimulation, but nociceptive neurons have been recorded in both the PSDC and SCTP pathways (Kajander & Giesler 1987, Downie et al 1988, Ferrington et al 1988, Craig et al 1992). There is new evidence that PSDC input to gracilothalamic neurons may be an important pathway for sacral visceral nociceptive activity in the rat, and recent studies have begun to examine this possibility in the monkey (Al-Chaer et al 1997, 1998, Zhang et al 1997).

TRIGEMINAL BRAINSTEM COMPLEX AND NOCICEPTION

The craniofacial region contains several unique structures of particular interest in pain research: the tooth pulp, the cerebrovasculature, nasal mucosa and the cornea. Pain is the primary or exclusive sensation evoked from these structures and the former two are frequent sources of pain. The sensory afferents that innervate the craniofacial region terminate primarily within the trigeminal brainstem complex, which consists of the main or principal sensory nucleus and the spinal tract nucleus, the latter comprising the subnuclei oralis, interpolaris and caudalis. The caudalmost region, subnucleus caudalis (SNC), is structurally and functionally very similar to the spinal dorsal horn with which it merges in the upper cervical cord, and it is frequently termed also the medullary dorsal horn (e.g. see Dubner et al 1978, Gobel et al 1981, Hu et al 1981, Dubner & Bennett 1983, Sessle 1987). SNC is the major termination site for small-diameter trigeminal primary afferents (Jacquin et al 1986, Light 1992), contains many nociceptive neurons in the superficial and deep layers and has a major projection to thalamus (e.g. see Dubner et al 1978, Gobel et al 1981, Hu et al 1981, Dubner & Bennett 1983, Sessle 1987, Yoshida et al 1991, Guilbaud et al 1994, Craig & Dostrovsky 1997). Noxious orofacial stimulation results in considerable C-*fos* expression in SNC (e.g. Coimbra & Coimbra 1994, Strassman et al 1994, Hathaway et al 1995). For these and other reasons SNC has long been considered as the main brainstem site responsible for processing and relaying nociceptive inputs from the craniofacial region. Consistent with this notion are the well-established reports demonstrating that lesions of the afferent inputs to SNC at the level of the obex (trigeminal tractotomy procedure and Wallenberg's syndrome) or disruption of SNC processing result in loss of pain and temperature sensation in the facial region and disruption of nociceptive behaviours (e.g. Sjoqvist 1938, Rosenfeld et al 1983, Young & Perryman 1984, Luccarini et al 1995, Duale et al 1996, Oliveras et al 1996, Sessle 1996).

As in the spinal cord there is a differential distribution of neurons in the different layers of SNC. In laminae I and II are located primarily NS and thermoreceptive specific neurons, whereas lamina V contains many WDR neurons as well as some NS and LTM neurons (Price et al 1976, Yokota & Nishikawa 1980, Hu et al 1981, Amano et al 1986, Craig & Dostrovsky 1991, Hutchison et al 1997). Many of the nociceptive neurons in SNC receive inputs from non-cutaneous tissues including muscle, temporomandibular joint, intranasal mucosa, cornea, tooth-pulp and intracranial blood vessels (Nagano et al 1975, Amano et al 1986, Sessle et al 1986, Strassman et al 1986, Broton et al 1988, Davis & Dostrovsky 1988, Dostrovsky et al 1991, Meng et al 1997). These neurons also have cutaneous receptive fields and these are likely to play an important role in the common referral of pain arising from some of these deep structures.

The ascending projections from the SNC are in many ways similar to those from the spinal cord. A major termination site is in VPM but, like the spinothalamic tract, there are also projections to POm, VMpo, submedius, MDvc and CL. Projections from lamina I to the brainstem are also very similar to those reported for spinal lamina I neurons, with a prominent projection to the parabrachial region, and in the rat at least, also a projection to hypothalamus (see above and reviews in Dubner et al 1978, Sessle 1987, Sessle 1996).

Although SNC is the major region implicated in pain, there is also evidence that the more rostral subnuclei of the spinal tract nucleus are involved, especially for inputs arising from intraoral and perioral regions. For example, following tractotomy at the obex level there is partial sparing of pain sensation from the intraoral and perioral region (Kunc 1970, Young 1982). Behavioural responsiveness to noxious orofacial stimuli may persist following tractotomy or SNC lesions in animals (Vyklicky et al 1977, Broton & Rosenfeld 1986), and lesions of oralis may interfere with nociceptive behaviour (e.g. Sessle & Greenwood 1976, Vyklicky et al 1977, Rosenfeld et al 1983, Young & Perryman 1984, Dallel et al 1988, 1989, Graham et al 1988, Luccarini et al 1995). In support of these findings are reports of the existence of nociceptive neurons in interpolaris and oralis (Eisenman et al 1963, Sessle & Greenwood 1976, Azerad et al 1982, Jacquin et al 1989, Dallel et al 1990, Hu et al 1992), including neurons that receive convergent inputs from tooth pulp, muscle or dura (Hayashi et al 1984, Davis & Dostrovsky 1988). Most of the neurons found in oralis, both nociceptive and non-nociceptive, have receptive fields that include the intraoral and perioral region. Furthermore, disruption of the rostral components of the V brainstem complex including oralis has been reported to interfere with thalamocortical neuronal activity evoked by noxious facial and pulpal stimulation (e.g. Keller et al 1974, Dong & Chudler 1985).

FUNCTIONAL ROLE OF ANTEROLATERAL TRACT AXONS

Early clinical investigators of pain sensation concluded that the two ascending bundles of STT fibres are associated with different functions, based for some on small sequential lesions of the spinal white matter made in awake pain patients under local anaesthesia (May 1906, Foerster & Gagel 1932, Kuru 1949). They associated the lateral STT with pain and temperature sensation, and the anterior STT with crude touch and movement sensation. Modern clinical findings have verified that cordotomy lesions in the middle of the lateral funiculus, just anterior to the level of the denticulate ligament and at the level of the central canal, are critical for the production of contralateral analgesia and thermanaesthesia that begins within two segments caudal to the lesion (Nathan & Smith 1979, Norrsell 1989) (Fig. 7.5). Similar findings have been obtained in monkeys (with the consideration that the smaller corticospinal tract in monkeys causes less anterior displacement of the ascending STT fibres) (Vierck et al 1986). This location corresponds with the location of ascending lamina I STT fibres (Craig 1991a, Ralston, III & Ralston 1992, Craig et al 1998), indicating that they have a critical role in specific pain and temperature sensations. This conclusion is consistent with the functional characteristics of lamina I STT cells and of their main terminus in thalamus, VMpo, and also with the one-to-one correspondence between the thalamocortical targets of ascending lamina I STT projections (Fig. 7.6) and the four cortical sites activated by pain in human imaging studies (see below).

The role of ascending STT fibres in pain is further supported by the direct production of burning pain sensations by electrical stimulation of the anterolateral quadrant during cordotomies, and with the correlation of lesions made at such sites with the successful production of analgesia

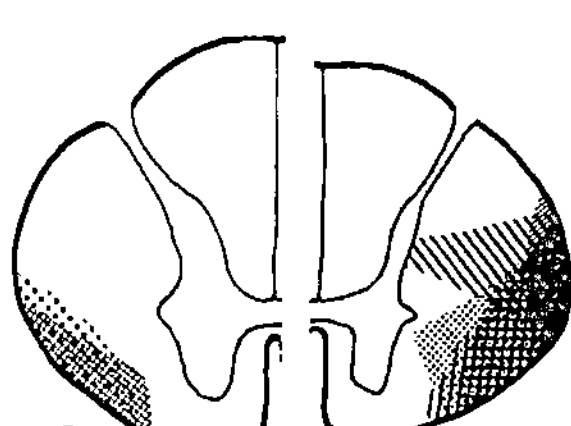

Fig. 7.5 Diagram showing locations of cordotomy incisions that caused dense analgesia in a limited region of the body. C=cervical cord; T=thoracic cord. Each case of cordotomy has the lesion illustrated by a different form of cross-hatching. (Reproduced from Nathan & Smith 1979 with permission.)

(Gildenberg 1972, Mayer et al 1975). In addition, Noordenboos and Wall observed that contralateral pain sensation and some touch sensibility was preserved in a patient who suffered a nearly complete spinal transection, except for the anterolateral quadrant (Noordenbos & Wall 1976).

However, the available evidence suggests that the sensation of pain involves more than this critical pathway. Considerable experience with cordotomies has led neurosurgeons to conclude that, if performed, cordotomies should be made through the entire anterolateral quadrant, and only for terminal cancer patients, because even if initially successful, the pain can return or a central pain syndrome can develop following a variable delay (White & Sweet 1969, Gybels & Sweet 1989, Vierck et al 1990). Similarly, in the patient examined by Noordenboos and Wall, although basically only one anterolateral quadrant remained, the patient had bilateral pain sensibility. Other clinical examples support the inference that the biological representation of pain in man must be redundant, variable and plastic, and suggest the idea that there may be ascending pathways with substantial involvement in pain in addition to the lateral STT lamina I pathway (White & Sweet 1969, Bonica 1990).

Ample evidence indicates a probable role in pain processing for WDR lamina V STT cells whose axons ascend largely in the anterior STT (Price 1988) (Fig. 7.7). Their discharge properties are closely correlated with the discriminative responses of awake, behaviourally trained monkeys to noxious heat stimuli applied to the face (Bushnell et al 1984, Dubner et al 1989, Maixner et al 1989). Their responses are augmented by a tonic noxious stimulus (capsaicin or repetitive C-fibre stimulation) in a manner that closely correlates with the hyperalgesia experienced by humans following such a stimulus (Simone et al 1991, Palecek et al 1992). Further, a comparative study of stimulation of anterolateral quadrant fibres has shown that the

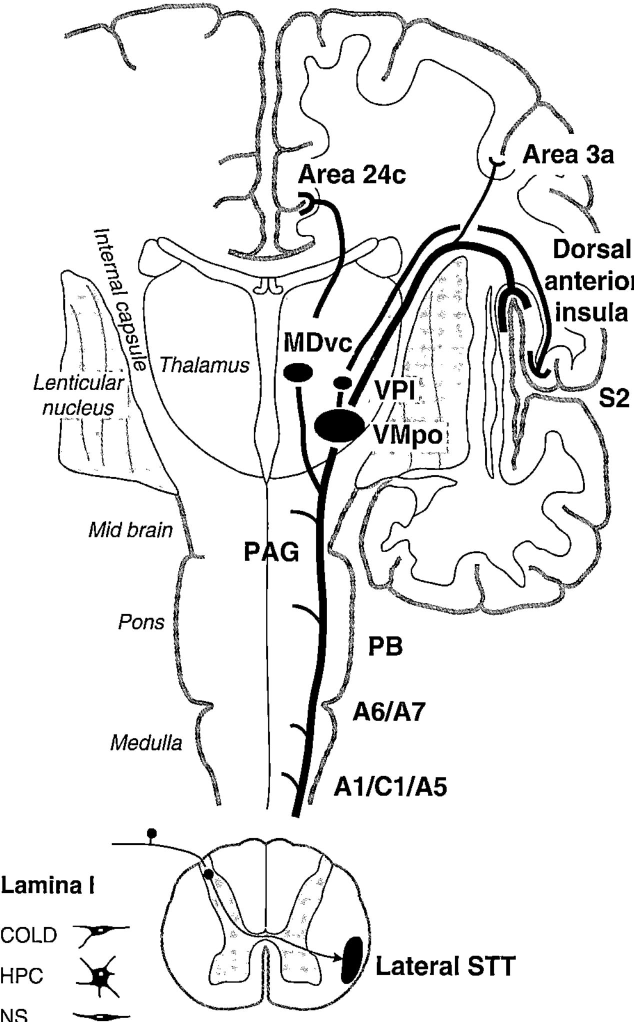

Fig. 7.6 Schematic diagram summarizing the ascending projections of lamina I cells in the macaque monkey. The three major classes of lamina I cells (COLD, HPC and NS) are indicated. Their axons decussate and ascend in the lateral STT. Terminations occur in the brainstem in the ventrolateral medulla (A1/C1/A5), the dorsolateral pons (A6/A7), the parabrachial nucleus (PB) and the periaqueductal grey (PAG). In the thalamus, lamina I STT terminations occur in VMpo, VPI and MDvc, whose cortical projections are shown.

refractory period of WDR lamina V STT axons in monkeys corresponds with the interpulse intervals at which human chronic pain patients reported an increase of pain (upon stimulation with a percutaneous spinal electrode with a 2-mm tip), albeit with an unknown relationship to their pathology (Mayer et al 1975). This study also reported a similar increase in pain at short inter-pulse intervals that could have activated thin lamina I STT axons by latent addition, that is, by exceeding their chronaxie. It has also been argued that the activity of WDR lamina V cells may be most important for tonic pain stimuli, to which they display

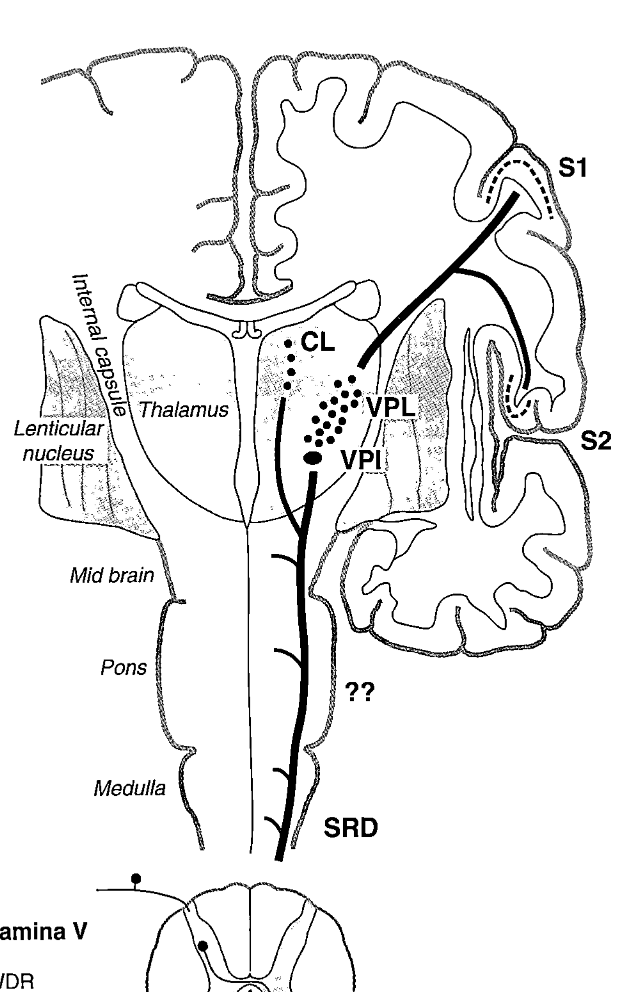

Fig. 7.7 Schematic diagram summarizing the ascending projections of laminae IV–V cells in the macaque monkey. The axons of both low-threshold (LT) and wide dynamic range (WDR) cell types decussate and ascend in the anterior STT. Terminations occur in the brainstem in the subnucleus reticularis dorsalis (SRD) and other sites, probably including the reticular core. In the thalamus, laminae IV–V STT terminations occur in VPI, in VPL and in CL.

a maintained discharge, similar to the evoked pain sensation, while the discharge of NS cells adapts to a lower level, similar to the responses of C-fibre and Type I Aδ nociceptors (Coghill et al 1993, Mao et al 1993). An alternative role for WDR lamina V cells that has been suggested is that they function as cumulative integrators of somatosensory activity which subserve inhibitory gain setting functions at supraspinal sites (Perl 1984b). This idea is supported by recent evidence for deep dorsal horn inhibition of dorsal column nuclear cells (Dykes & Craig 1998) and for the inhibition of mechanosensory activity in cortical area 3b by noxious heat (Tommerdahl et al 1996). Ultimately, the generation of pain by the central effects of WDR lamina V STT cells clearly requires integration with other populations of neurons, because their activity is modality-ambiguous.

Thus, the most parsimonious and prospective view is that the activity of all of these ascending pathways must be integrated in the forebrain in the context of current conditions and past experience in order for all aspects of the sensation of pain to be generated. Elimination of a portion of this system or a given pathway, such as by a partial lesion in the periphery, the spinal cord or the forebrain, could cause an imbalance that might have variable effects on integrated sensation. For example, it may result in pain without a noxious stimulus has in phantom pain (Flor et al 1995, Davis et al 1998) or in central pain (Craig 1998) (see below). These considerations emphasize the complexity of the spinal and supraspinal interconnections involved in the experience of pain that remain to be identified.

FUNCTIONAL CHARACTERISTICS OF THALAMIC NOCICEPTIVE NEURONS

The following sections summarize the functional evidence related to pain processing that is available for several thalamic regions, with primary emphasis on primates and humans. This evidence includes both physiological recordings and the effects of stimulation or reduction of activity. All of these thalamic regions receive ascending STT projections, and some also receive nociceptive input from other ascending pathways, as described above.

VENTRAL POSTERIOR NUCLEI

These are the main somatosensory relay nuclei of the thalamus, which contain a somatotopic representation of the cutaneous mechanoreceptive surface and which relay lemniscal input from the dorsal column nuclei and the principal trigeminal nucleus to the main somatosensory (S1) cortex, areas 3b and 1. The face is represented medially in VPM and the forelimb and hindlimb are represented successively more laterally in the medial and lateral parts of VPL, and distal cutaneous surfaces are represented ventrally and proximal (posterior) surfaces dorsally (Poggio & Mountcastle 1960, Jones 1985). The most dorsal and rostral portion of VP (called the anterior or oral subdivision) relays low-threshold proprioceptive (muscle and joint) activity to areas 3a and 2 (Kaas et al 1984, Jones 1990). The main input to the several components of the second somatosensory cortical region arises from VPI and parts of VP (Krubitzer et al 1995).

Nociceptive neurons are scattered among the many low-threshold neurons in VP in the anaesthetized or awake monkey, and they amount to about 10% of VP neurons (Willis 1997). Their receptive fields are generally in register with the somatotopography of VP, but they are concentrated in the posterior dorsomedial aspect of VPM, and in VPL they are found caudoventrally and also near the major fibre laminae (Kenshalo et al 1980, Casey & Morrow 1983, Chung et al 1986, Bushnell et al 1993). These locations correspond to the concentrations of STT terminations, and these neurons apparently receive direct STT input (Applebaum et al 1979, Boivie 1979, Burton & Craig 1983, Apkarian & Hodge 1989c, Gingold et al 1991). Nearly all of these nociceptive VP neurons are WDR neurons that respond to graded low-threshold mechanical stimuli and discharge maximally to noxious mechanical and sometimes noxious heat stimuli (Fig. 7.8). Some also respond physically to innocuous cooling (Bushnell et al 1993). These cells tend to have receptive fields of moderate size, similar to lamina V STT cells; that is, they may respond to stimuli over a third to half or even the entire face or hand or arm. The stimulus-response functions of these cells are consistent with the discriminative operant escape responses of behaviourally trained monkeys (Bushnell et al 1993).

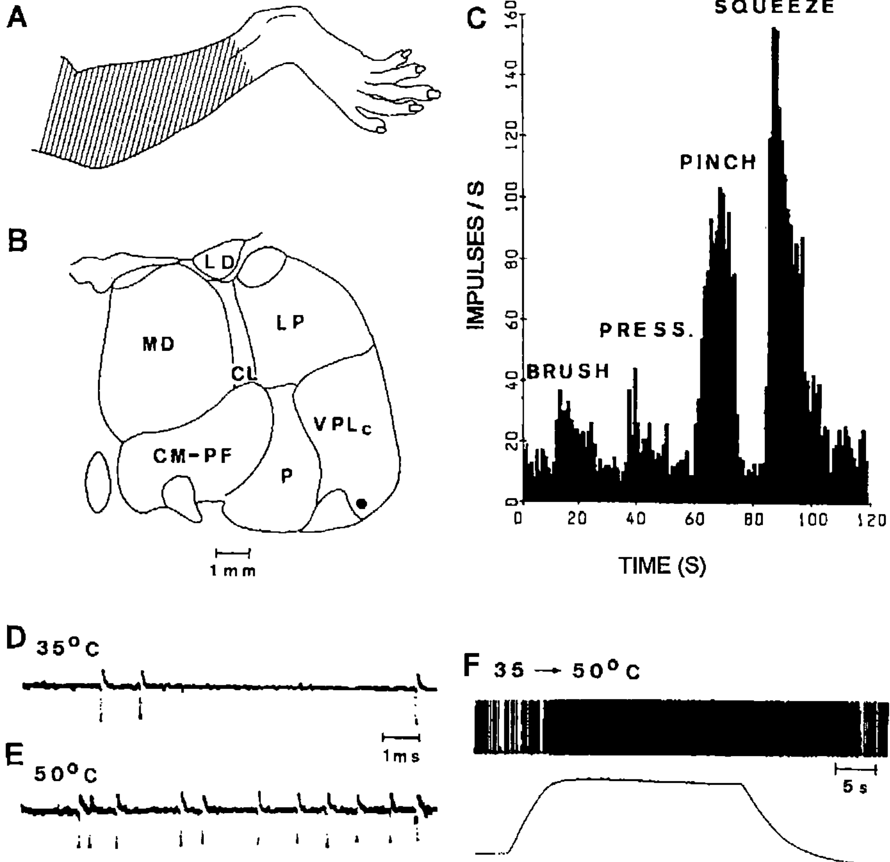

Fig. 7.8 Responses of a nociceptive neuron in the VPL nucleus of a monkey. The receptive field is shown in **A**. The location of the neuron is indicated by the filled circle in **B**. Responses to graded mechanical stimuli applied to the receptive field are shown in **C**. The stimuli included brush (repeated strokes of camel hair brush), press (application of a large arterial clip to the skin; this was near pain threshold when applied to human subjects), pinch (application of a small arterial clip to the skin; painful but not damaging), and squeeze (damaging compression of the skin with serrated forceps). The background activity is shown in **D** when the skin was held at an adapting temperature of 35°C. The firing rate increases considerably when a noxious heat pulse of 50°C is applied. The pen recorder record in **F** shows the time course of the change in discharge and the temperature of the skin. Abbreviations of thalamic nuclei: CL=central lateral; CM-PF=centre median-parafascicular; LD=lateral dorsal; LP=lateral posterior; MD=medial dorsal; P=pulvinar; VPL_c=ventral posterolateral, pars caudalis. (Reproduced from Kenshalo et al 1980 with permission.)

Their responses can be affected by the state of arousal (Morrow & Casey 1992). Some WDR cells in VP have been antidromically activated from areas 3b and 1 in the primary somatosensory cortex (Kenshalo et al 1980). Visceral noxious stimuli can activate some of these cells but also other low-threshold VP cells, with inconsistent evidence of topographic order (Chandler et al 1992, Brüggemann et al 1994a, Al-Chaer et al 1998).

Both WDR and NS (nociceptive-specific) cells have been recorded in VPI (Apkarian et al 1991). There appears to be a separate topographic representation of the body in this nucleus. These neurons tend to have larger receptive fields than the nociceptive neurons in VP (Fig. 7.9).

Electrical microstimulation within VP in awake humans, performed during stereotactic neurosurgical procedures for movement disorders, generally evokes reports of topographically well-localized paraesthesia and only rarely a report of a painful sensation, in contrast to the region immediately posterior to VP described below (Fig. 7.10) (Hassler & Riechert 1959, Halliday & Logue 1972, Tasker 1984, Lenz et al 1993b, Lenz & Dougherty 1997). Reports of pain are significantly more common in response to VP stimulation in patients with chronic pain (Davis et al 1996). In pain patients with deafferentation syndromes, VP neurons without peripheral input display calcium spike bursting activity that could be related to their chronic pain (Lenz & Dougherty 1997), but there is no direct evidence of a correlation. By contrast, electrical stimulation of VP through chronically implanted electrodes can be very effective in alleviating deafferentation and other pain conditions (Siegfried 1987, Gybels & Sweet 1989, Kupers & Gybels 1993). In the awake, behaving monkey, lidocaine injections

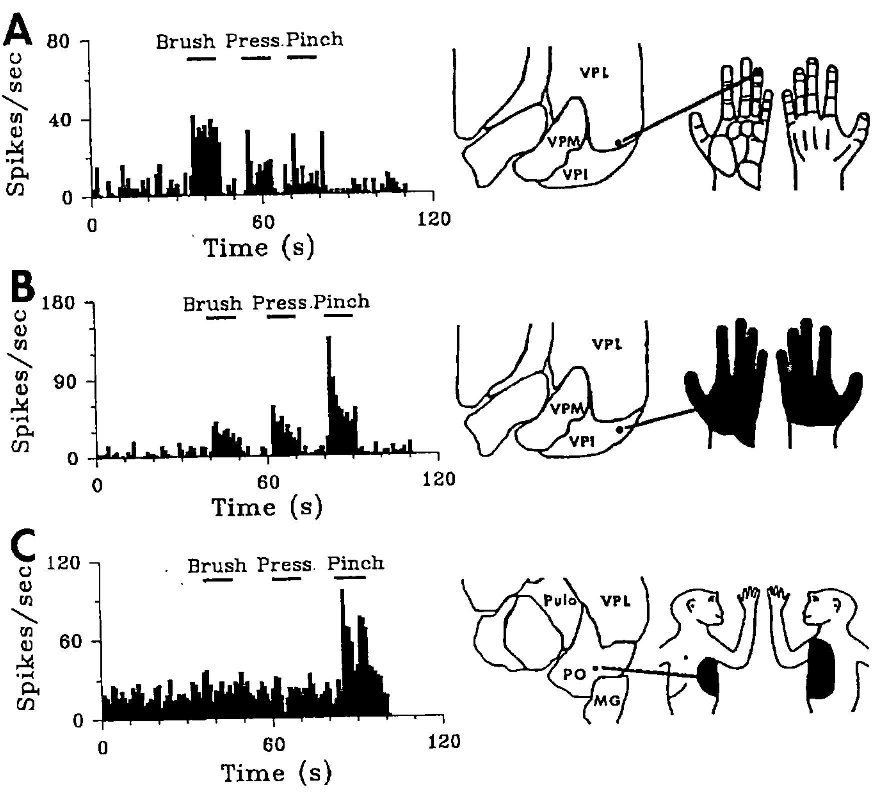

Fig. 7.9 Peristimulus time histograms of responses of thalamic neurons during mechanical stimulation, recording locations and receptive fields are shown for three neurons. **A** A neuron, classified as non-nociceptive, had a receptive filed at the tip of digit 4, and was located just above the ventral border of the ventral posterolateral nucleus (VPL). This unit had a brisk response to brushing of the skin and reduced response to pressure and pinch. **B** A neuron, classified as wide dynamic range (WDR), had a receptive field that covered the whole contralateral hand and was located in the ventral posterior inferior nucleus (VPI). The unit activity increased with increasing the intensity of the stimulation from brushing to innocuous pressure to noxious pinching. **C** A neuron classified as a nociceptive-specific cell (NS) had a receptive field that covered contralateral chest and back and was located in the posterior region. The unit activity increased only during noxious pinching. MG = Medial geniculate; VPM = ventral posterior medial nucleus. (Reproduced from Apkarian & Shi 1994 with permission.)

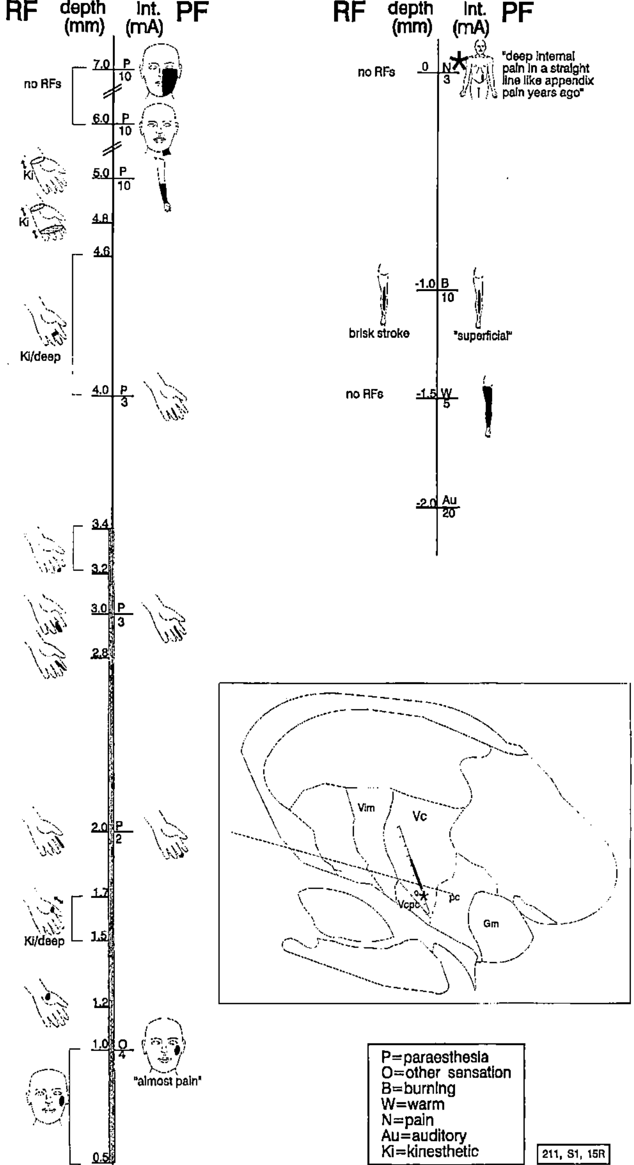

Fig. 7.10 Reconstruction of the data obtained during an electrode trajectory through the lateral thalamus in a patient with essential tremor. The receptive fields (RF) of neurons encountered during the penetration are shown to the left of the vertical line. The stimulus intensity (Int.) and evoked sensation and projected fields (PF) are shown to the right of the vertical line. The patient's description of certain evoked sensations are indicated in quotes. The shaded bar indicates the presumed tactile region of the ventral caudal nucleus (Vc) based on neuronal responses to tactile stimuli. The inset shows the thalamic map determined by the patient's anterior and posterior commissures and presumed location of the trajectory based on stereotactic coordinates. The asterisk indicates the site where stimulation evoked a visceral pain response. Gm=medial geniculate nucleus; pc = posterior commissure; Vcpc=parvocellular ventrocaudal nucleus; Vim = ventral intermediate nucleus. (Reproduced from Davis et al 1995a with permission.)

into VPM can impair behavioural discrimination of noxious heat and innocuous cool stimuli, particularly if a sufficiently large region is injected, probably including the region posterior and inferior to VP described below (Duncan et al 1993).

In other experimental species, the organization of nociceptive neurons in the ventrobasal thalamus differs markedly. There are almost no nociceptive cells within VP in the cat. Instead, they are found in the dorsal and ventral aspects of VP, including VPI and the ventral aspect of VMb (Honda et al 1983, Kniffki & Mizumura 1983, Kniffki & Craig 1985, Yokota et al 1988, Horie et al 1991). These neurons include NS and WDR cells that can encode stimulus intensity in the noxious range. They are crudely topographically organized, with trigeminal cells located medially, and cervical and lumbar cells located successively more laterally, but they are not in register with the adjoining VP. They can be activated by stimulation of skin, muscle, tooth pulp, viscera or cranial vasculature (Kniffki & Mizumura 1983, Davis & Dostrovsky 1988, Asato & Yokota 1989, Horie & Yokota 1990, Brüggemann et al 1994b). Some of these cells project to the somatosensory cortex (area 3a or the S2 region) or the anterior cingulate cortex (Kniffki & Craig 1985, Yasui et al 1988). Lesions of the VPM that also encompass Sm (see below) in the cat can produce hypalgesia to tooth pulp stimulation (Kaelber et al 1975). In the rat, nociceptive cells are found throughout VP intermixed (in topographic register) with low-threshold neurons (Guilbaud et al 1977, 1980, Peschanski et al 1980). Both NS and WDR cells have been reported that encode stimulus intensity and that generally have large, often bilateral, receptive fields (Fig. 7.11). Visceral convergence has been reported (Guilbaud et al 1993b). In rats with experimentally induced arthritis or neuropathies, many more WDR cells are reported in VP that project to the somatosensory cortex (Guilbaud et al 1990). Modulation by electrical stimulation of the PAG or the raphe or by infusion of analgesic compounds has been described (Horie et al 1991, Koyama & Yokota 1993).

POSTERIOR REGION

This region was formerly regarded as undifferentiated, primordial thalamus, but recent evidence has demonstrated that in primates it contains a distinct nucleus, VMpo, that is a dedicated lamina I STT thalamocortical relay. The functional evidence is consistent with the role of VMpo as a specific sensory relay nucleus for pain and temperature (Craig et al 1994). Almost all neurons in VMpo in the anaesthetized monkey are nociceptive-specific or thermoreceptive-specific neurons (Fig. 7.12), and the two modalities are segregated mediolaterally. The nociceptive neurons have

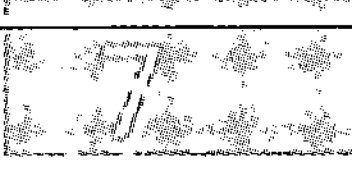

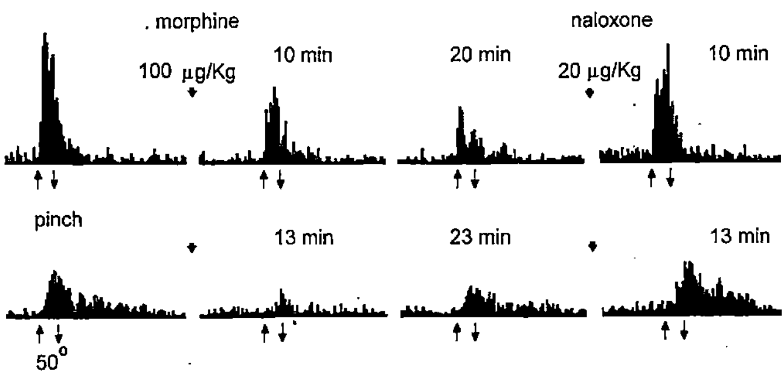

Fig. 7.11 Firing rate histograms showing depressive effect of systemic morphine upon responses in rat ventral caudal nerve elicited in the same neuron by pinch and noxious heat and reversal by naloxone. (Reproduced from Benoist et al 1983 with permission.)

steeply graded stimulus-response functions to noxious pinch and/or heat stimuli, like those of lamina I STT cells. Their receptive fields are similarly small, and they are topographically organized rostrocaudally, corresponding with the anatomical findings for the lamina I STT terminations in VMpo. Nociceptive-specific neurons have also been observed in this region in the squirrel monkey and the owl monkey (Apkarian et al 1991, Blomquvist et al 1995).

In the awake human, recordings have recently been reported from nociceptive-specific and thermoreceptive-specific neurons in the comparable region, posterior and inferior to the main somatosensory representation (Lenz et al 1993, Dostrovsky et al 1996, Lenz & Dougherty 1998). Modern evidence shows that electrical microstimulation in this region in humans produces discrete reports of well-localized pain or cold sensations (see Figs. 7.10, 7.13) (Lenz et al 1993b, Davis et al 1996, Dostrovsky et al 1996) confirming the early demonstration by Hassler (Hassler & Riechert 1959). By contrast, stimulation caudal to VMpo (where ascending STT fibres would be involved) produces mostly reports of warmth (Tasker 1984, Lenz & Dougherty 1997). Stimulation in the region of VMpo in humans has also produced reports of visceral pain (Davis et al 1995a, Lenz et al 1995).

Lidocaine injections in awake monkeys into VPM that probably spread posteriorly into this region can reduce behavioural responses to noxious heat or to innocuous cold stimuli (Duncan et al 1993). Infarcts or surgical lesions of the region of VMpo in humans can produce analgesia and thermanaesthesia (Head & Holmes 1911, Hassler & Riechert 1959, Hassler 1970, Tasker 1984, Boivie & Leijon 1991). In about half of such cases, however, a central pain syndrome develops, in which burning, dysaesthetic pain is referred to deep tissue in the analgesic region (see below) (Dejerine & Roussy 1906, Pagni 1976, Boivie & Leijon 1991, Bowsher 1996, Craig 1998).

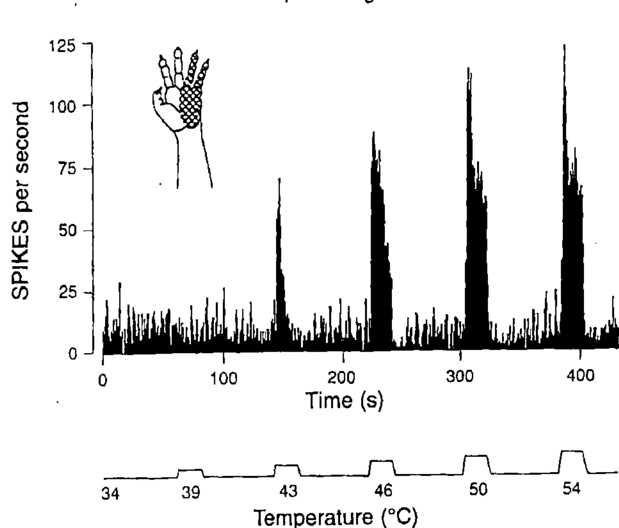

Fig. 7.12 Examples of the responses of neuronsin the posterior part of the ventral medial nucleus (VMpo). The clustered thermoreceptive-specific neurons (top) had ongoing activity that was inhibited by radiant warming, and they were excited by cooling (application of wet ice cube) and by no other stimuli from a receptive field on the contralateral tongue. The histogram (bottom) shows the graded responses of a single nociceptive-specific neuron to noxious heat pulses applied with a thermoelectric stimulator to the receptive field on the contralateral ulnar hand. (Reproduced from Craig et al 1994 with permission.)

In the cat, an early study indicated that many cells in the posterior complex were nociceptive units with very large receptive fields, but subsequent evidence is conflicting (Poggio & Mountcastle 1960, Curry 1972, Brinkhus et al 1979, Carstens & Yokota 1980). The portion of PO found dorsal to VP in the cat differs from the portion found caudal to VP, because it projects to area 5a (Jones 1985), but it also seems to contain nociceptive cells (Kniffki & Craig 1985, Hutchison et al 1992, Nomura et al 1992, Brüggemann et al 1994b). In the rat, PO receives convergent descending input from VP via the somatosensory cortex (Diamond et al 1992), and accordingly, it contains neurons responsive to noxious stimulation as well. A recent

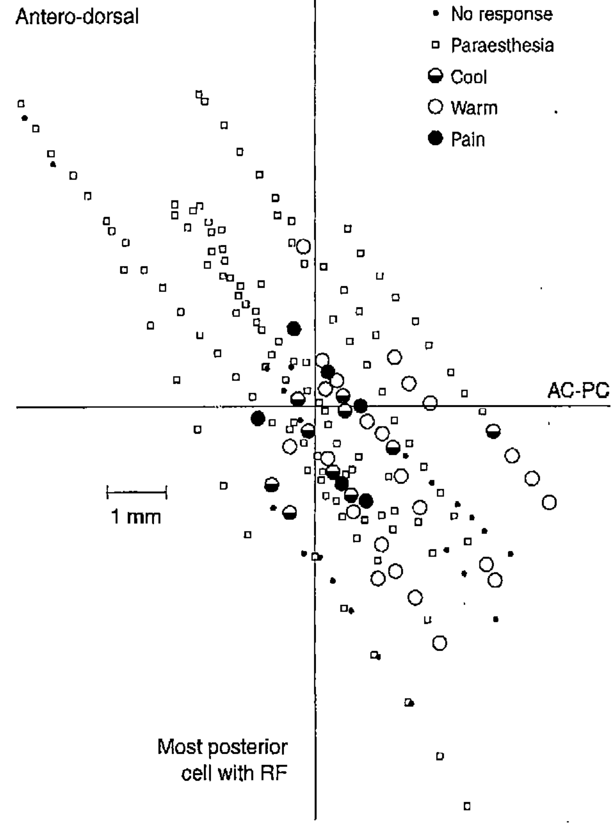

Fig. 7.13 Locations of sites in the thalamus of awake human patients where paraesthetic or thermal/pain sensations were evoked. The quality of the evoked sensation is as listed in the key. The sites are shown relative to the anterior commissure–posterior commissure line (AC-PC, horizontal line) and a vertical line defined as the anteroposterior location of the most posterior cell responding to innocuous somatosensory stimulation. Therefore the region located posterior to the vertical line is the postero-inferior region. (Reproduced from Lenz et al 1993b with permission.)

study in the rat indicates that nociceptive cells with visceral input are located not only within VP but also on its borders (Berkley et al 1993). In both cat and rat, a region along the ventral aspect of VMb appears to be analogous to the primate's VMpo, in that the region contains both nociceptive and visceroceptive neurons and projects to the insular cortex (Yasui et al 1991, Clascá et al 1997). However, this small region seems to be primordial in comparison to the large, well-developed nucleus that appears in primates (Craig 1996).

INTRALAMINAR NUCLEI

In the awake or the anaesthetized monkey, nociceptive neurons have been recorded in most areas of the medial thalamus, though with a concentration in posterior CL and Pf (Casey 1966, Bushnell & Duncan 1989). Most such cells have large receptive fields, and the stimulus encoding properties of these neurons have not been well studied, but some show clearly graded responses to noxious heat. The response of these cells can be affected by attention (Fig. 7.14). Many CL neurons discharge with eye movements (Schlag & Schlag-Rey 1986), consistent with the dominant ascending inputs to CL from the cerebellum and the superior colliculus and a putative role in gaze orientation (Jones 1985, 1990). Nociceptive neurons have also been recorded in the human medial thalamus (Sano 1979; for other references see Lenz & Dougherty 1997); in pain patients, cells with bursting properties have been reported (Jeanmonod et al 1994), but the significance of this for pain is unknown. Electrical stimulation in humans can cause reports of pain from the posterior aspect of medial thalamus (Sano 1979, Jeanmonod et al 1994). These sites may have included CL or Pf or even MDvc.

Lesions have been made in the medial thalamus in chronic pain patients with mixed success (Tasker 1984, Lenz & Dougherty 1997); large lesions could have involved both VMpo and MDvc. Lesions in the medial thalamus reportedly do not cause thalamic pain syndrome (Bogousslavsky et al 1988).

In the cat and the rat, a large number of studies have reported nociceptive neurons in the intralaminar nuclei and other medial thalamic sites (Albe-Fessard & Kruger 1962, Dong et al 1978, Peschanski et al 1981, Dostrovsky & Guilbaud 1988, Olausson et al 1992, Sugiyama et al 1992). Most of these investigations relied on responses to strong electrical stimuli, but some responses to natural noxious stimulation have been reported (Peschanski et al 1981, Dostrovsky & Guilbaud 1990). The data indicate that such neurons are widely scattered throughout the medial thalamus, with no apparent localization; similar findings were obtained using c-*fos* activation (Bullitt 1990). Some neurons with graded responses have been observed, and modulation by stimulation of various brain regions, primarily motor related, has been reported (Sugiyama et al 1992).

MEDIAL DORSAL NUCLEUS

The presence of lamina I STT input to the ventral caudal part of MD (MDvc) and its projection to the anterior cingulate cortex indicate an important role in pain (Craig & Zhang 1996). It is noteworthy that many of the neurosurgical lesions made in the medial thalamus (directed toward the CM-Pf region) for the purpose of alleviating chronic pain could have involved MDvc (Richardson 1967, Rinaldi et al 1991, Jeanmonod et al 1994, Craig 1995b, Lenz & Dougherty 1997), but whether this might explain the variable success of such lesions is unknown.

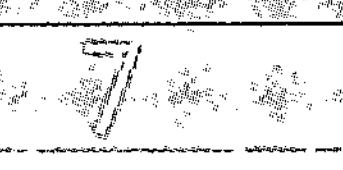

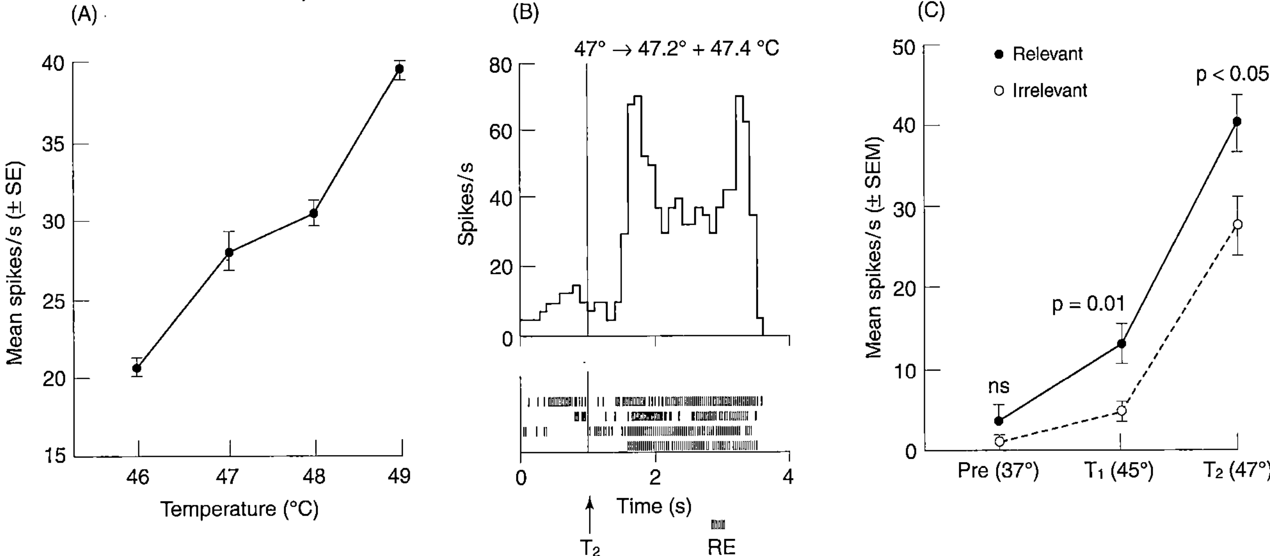

Fig. 7.14 Responses of a neuron in the medial thalamus (dorsomedial centre median) of an awake monkey to noxious thermal stimuli to the face. **A** The mean firing rate to increasing temperatures. **B** A peristimulus histogram with associated dot raster display showing the increased firing when the temperature increased from 47°C to 47.2 or 47.4°C. In this particular example the monkey did not respond until the end of the trial (RE=button release). **C** The neuron responded more intensely during a task in which the monkey was rewarded for detecting a 47°C stimulus (T2; solid line, *n*=10) compared to a task in which the monkey was rewarded for ignoring the thermal stimulus and waiting for a later change in a visual stimulus (dashed line *n*=5). (Reproduced from Bushnell & Duncan 1989 with permission.)

Recordings in awake monkeys of nociceptive neurons in the medial thalamus ascribed to CM, Pf and CL may have included cells in MDvc (Fig. 7.14) (Bushnell & Duncan 1989). New evidence in barbiturate-anaesthetized monkeys indicates that MDvc contains a concentration of nociceptive-specific neurons with large, sometimes bilateral receptive fields (Craig 1998). Their ongoing activity can often be inhibited by innocuous thermal (cool, warm) stimuli, consistent with a role in the cold-induced inhibition of pain and in the thermal grill illusion of pain (see below). It has also been proposed that this region is important for the development of the central pain syndrome following loss of the lateral pain and temperature pathway through VMpo (Craig 1998). Lesions in the medial thalamus never cause central pain (Pagni 1976, Bogousslavsky et al 1988, Boivie & Leijon 1991).

The medial thalamic nucleus submedius (Sm) in the cat and the rat receives lamina I input, just as MDvc does, and it may be functionally similar, although it projects to the ventral lateral orbital cortex rather than to the anterior cingulate. Nociceptive-specific neurons have been recorded in Sm in the cat (Craig 1990), and primarily nociceptive but also a few low-threshold cells have been found there in the rat (Dostrovsky & Guilbaud 1988, Miletic & Coffield 1989, Kawakita et al 1993). Inputs from cutaneous and deep tissues has also been recorded in the rat. In the cat, both nociceptive and thermoreceptive lamina I STT cells project to Sm (Craig & Dostrovsky 1991), but no cells excited by cold have been observed there, consistent with the possibility that cold-induced inhibition of nociceptive processing could occur there, as in MDvc of the primate. Ultrastructural observations of differential lamina I terminations on GABAergic interneurons in Sm support this possibility (Ericson et al 1996). In the arthritic rat, many Sm cells are responsive to innocuous joint movements (Dostrovsky & Guilbaud 1988). Noxious stimulation can produce increased gene transduction (c-*fos* activity) in Sm in the rat (Bullitt 1990). Lesion and stimulation studies in behaving rats suggest that Sm may be involved in the activation of descending antinociceptive controls (Roberts & Dong 1994). It should also be noted that several studies have focused on the possibility that the habenula (adjacent to MD) may be involved in pain modulation (Mahieux & Benabid 1987, Terenzi & Prado 1990, Rinaldi et al 1991, Cohen & Melzack 1993), but the significance of this is unclear because of the hippocampal and limbic connections of this nucleus.

OTHER STRUCTURES

Amygdala

Nociceptive neurons have been identified in the central nucleus of the amygdala in the rat; these studies confirm the efficacy of the nociceptive PB neurons that project there (Bernard et al 1992). Lesions of the amygdala in primates can cause memory deficits, but effects on pain sensibility apparently have not been reported clinically. Increased glucose metabolism in the amygdala has been observed in a neuropathic pain model in the rat (Mao et al 1993). The amygdala may be significant for the analgesic effects of systemic morphine and for fear-conditioned descending antinociception (Helmstetter & Bellgowan 1993, Helmstetter et al 1993).

Basal ganglia

Nociceptive neurons have been recorded in these presumably sensorimotor-related structures in the rat (Bernard et al 1992, Chudler et al 1993), but not in the cat or the primate. Nociceptive responses have also been obtained in the substantia nigra that are sensitive to systemic morphine. Clinical lesions of the basal ganglia and diseases that affect these structures (e.g. Parkinson's or Huntington's) may have some effect on pain perception (Chudler & Dong 1995).

Hypothalamus

Nociceptive neurons have not been well studied in the hypothalamus, but cells that respond to visceral or tooth pulp stimulation have been recorded in the rat (Hamba et al 1990). In humans, lesions of the periventricular grey, involving the posterior hypothalamus, have been used to alleviate pain (Sano 1979, Sweet 1982, Gybels & Sweet 1989).

PHARMACOLOGICAL CHARACTERISTICS OF THALAMIC NOCICEPTIVE NEURONS

Our knowledge of the pharmacology of thalamic nociceptive neurons is very limited; however, it is likely that many of their properties are similar to those of other thalamocortical neurons about which more is known and which are reviewed in greater detail by McCormick (1992), Craig & Dostrovsky (1997) and Steriade et al (1997). The two most important thalamic neurotransmitters are undoubtedly glutamate and GABA.

There is good evidence that excitatory amino acids, probably glutamate, are the excitatory transmitters released by the terminals of the ascending spinal afferents, including those of lamina I STT cells onto brainstem and thalamocortical neurons (Magnusson et al 1987, Ericson et al 1995, Blomqvist et al 1996). Not surprisingly both NMDA and non-NMDA glutamate receptors are involved in mediating these excitatory responses. Responses of rat Vc nociceptive neurons have been shown to be largely due to activation of NMDA receptors with a contribution from metabotropic glutamate receptors (Eaton & Salt 1990, Eaton et al 1993). Thalamic cells receive a massive excitatory cortical projection which is mediated by the release of excitatory amino acids acting at NMDA, non-NMDA and metabotropic glutamate receptors (Rustioni et al 1983, Jones 1987, Deschenes & Hu 1990, Eaton & Salt 1995). There is also evidence that thalamocortical neurons release glutamate at their cortical terminals and that AMPA receptors are involved in this excitation (Kharazia & Weinberg 1994, Pirot et al 1994).

GABA is the major inhibitory neurotransmitter in the thalamus. The thalamus of cats and primates contains many GABAergic interneurons. In all species there is also an extensive reciprocal and topographic innervation by the GABAergic neurons of the thalamic reticular nucleus (TRN)(Steriade et al 1997, Houser et al 1980, Rustioni et al 1983, Jones 1985). Studies on non-nociceptive thalamic neurons have shown that the GABA antagonist bicuculline increases the duration of excitatory responses and reduces inhibition of thalamic neurons. Short latency IPSPs resulting from TRN activation are mediated primarily by $GABA_A$ receptors, whereas longer latency inhibition is mediated by $GABA_B$ receptors (Lee et al 1994). Interestingly release of GABA from TRN terminals is depressed by presynaptic glutamate metabotropic receptors (Salt & Eaton 1995). Although there have been no direct studies involving nociceptive neurons, it is known that Sm, which contains many nociceptive neurons, receives a dense projection from the TRN, and it is likely that these nociceptive neurons receive GABAergic inhibitory inputs. Furthermore, GABA has been shown to inhibit nociceptive neurons in rat Pf (Reyes-Vazquez & Dafny 1993). It has been proposed that deafferentation pain may be mediated by reduced GABAergic inhibition at the thalamic level (Roberts et al 1992). Consistent with this proposal, it has been shown that there is a downregulation of thalamic $GABA_A$ receptors following chronic cervical rhizotomy in primates (Rausell et al 1992).

The thalamus also receives inputs from brainstem serotoninergic, noradrenergic and cholinergic afferents, and the corresponding receptors are present on thalamic neurons (see reviews by McCormick 1992, Steriade et al 1997). Although they clearly have an important modulatory function, their role in nociception is not known. A number of neuropeptides have also been identified in thalamic afferents and neurons. Some of these are presumed to be colocalized with excitatory amino acids. Tachykinins, cholecystokinin and enkephalins have been identified in spinothalamic fibres ending in the rat and human thalamus (Coffield & Miletic 1987, Gall et al 1987, Hirai & Jones 1989b, Battaglia et al 1992, Nishiyama et al 1995).

Although it is generally accepted that the analgesia produced by opiates results from an action at the spinal and brainstem levels, the existence of opiate receptors and enkephalinergic terminals in thalamus (Mansour et al 1987, Miletic & Coffield 1988) raises the possibility that depression of thalamic nociceptive neurons by systemic opiates may contribute to the analgesia. Not surprisingly systemic morphine inhibits thalamic nociceptive neurons (e.g., Benoist et al 1983; Fig. 7.11). Of more interest are a few studies that have shown that local application of opioid agents can depress the responses of thalamic nociceptive neurons (He et al 1991, Coffield & Miletic 1993), thus suggesting that the analgesic action of opioid agents may reflect in part an action at the thalamic level.

THALAMUS AND PAIN

The critical role of the thalamus in pain sensation was first given serious consideration by Head and Holmes (Head & Holmes 1911), who in 1911 reported their careful analysis of 23 patients with the Dejerine–Roussy thalamic pain syndrome (Dejerine & Roussy 1906). Known today as central pain (Boivie & Leijon 1991, Craig 1991b, 1998, Bowsher 1996), this syndrome causes patients to experience ongoing pain that is often described as burning and that is referred to an area of the body (face, arm, hemi-body) in which they have a paradoxical loss of cutaneous pain sensitivity (analgesia), accompanied virtually always by thermanaesthesia. Head and Holmes thought that the characteristic infarct in the posterolateral thalamus found in many such patients had destroyed a specific sensory substrate for pain, and that this had released (disinhibited) activity in an emotional centre (the medial thalamus, they presumed) that was experienced as pain. They thought that the cortex had only a modulatory role in pain sensation, because lesions of the somatosensory cortex rarely produce analgesia (White & Sweet 1969, Sweet 1982; but see Russell 1945, Perl 1984a), and they speculated about pathways for central irritation that might explain the exacerbated pain that such patients experience in response to cold or weak mechanical stimuli (allodynia).

Their ideas led many to teach that pain sensation occurs in the thalamus, ignoring its intimate relationship with the cerebral cortex. Their ideas also led to the suggestion that a 'spinoreticulthalamic' pathway must be responsible for pain after a lesion of the specific lateral STT pain pathway (Bishop 1959, Bowsher 1975, Bonica 1990), and they originated the enduring notion that the lateral thalamus is involved in the discriminative sensory aspects of pain and the medial thalamus in the emotional, motivational aspects of pain (see especially Melzack & Casey 1968). This latter idea has been used to explain certain subsequent findings, such as alleviation of pain suffering by destruction of the frontal cortex or cingulate cortex (White & Sweet 1969, Sweet 1982, Gybels & Sweet 1989).

The functional anatomy of ascending pain pathways and their terminations, as summarized above, indicate that painful stimuli activate multiple pathways and thereby multiple regions of the forebrain that must be integrated with past experience and present context to result in the complete, multidimensional pain experience. Although particular pathways and regions may have a predominant contribution to one or another aspect of the pain experience, it is the constellation of activity in all these areas that forms the basis for the conscious experience.

Accordingly, modern functional imaging studies (PET, fMRI) of the forebrain have shown that several areas are activated by noxious stimulation (Jones et al 1991, Talbot et al 1991, Casey et al 1992, Davis et al 1995b, Craig et al 1996). Noxious heat and noxious cold stimuli activate four main cortical sites: the region of the central sulcus (referred to as S1), the region of the lateral operculum (referred to as S2), the insula and the anterior cingulate cortex. Physiological studies of laser-evoked pain EEG potentials are consistent with these findings (Bromm & Treede 1987). In addition, PET activation of particular subcortical sites has been reported, such as the periaqueductal grey, the hypothalamus, the amygdala and the cerebellum. All of these regions (including the cerebellum) receive ascending nociceptive activity, as described above.

The nociceptive cells in VP thalamus apparently project to the supragranular layers of S1 and S2. Nociceptive cells have been recorded in monkeys in areas 3b and 1 of S1, in S2, and in area 7 of lateral parietal cortex (Kenshalo & Isensee 1983, Dong et al 1994, Willis 1997). These are primarily WDR neurons, and consistent with the recordings in VP, their activity can be directly correlated with discriminative aversive behaviour in monkeys (Kenshalo et al 1989). Nociceptive neurons have also been recorded in rat S1 (Guilbaud et al 1992, 1993a). Nonetheless, recent optical imaging evidence in the monkey indicates that noxious heat activates area 3a (which receives input from VMpo) and inhibits mechanically evoked activity in area 3b (Tommerdahl et al 1996). Clusters of nociceptive neurons were also recorded in area 3a. Lesions of area 3b and 1 may affect discriminative pain behaviour in monkeys, but lesions of the postcentral gyrus clinically have minimal effects on pain sensation, and similar to VP, electrical stimulation there rarely causes pain in humans (Perl 1984a).

The specific thalamic pain and temperature relay nucleus, VMpo, projects topographically to the insular cortex, and nociceptive-specific neurons have recently been recorded there in anaesthetized monkeys (Craig 1995b, Dostrovsky & Craig 1996b). The insula is strongly activated in PET studies by noxious heat and noxious cold stimuli, and by innocuous cool and warm stimuli as well (Coghill et al 1994, Craig et al 1996). This is consistent with the concept that this spino-thalamo-cortical pathway serves as a representation of the physiological status of the body tissues, including specific pain and temperature (Craig 1996). Clinically, lesions of the parieto-insular cortex or the underlying internal capsule have been associated with hypalgesia, thermanaesthesia, central pain syndrome and pain asymbolia (Biemond 1956, Berthier et al 1988, Boivie & Leijon 1991, Greenspan & Winfield 1992). The buried location of this cortex, which would not be affected by superficial cortical wounds, may partially exonerate the early belief that the cortex had little involvement in pain sensation. The posterior insula may also provide a pathway for somatosensory cortical information to reach the amygdala and hippocampus (Friedman et al 1986).

The nociceptive region of medial thalamus in primates, MDvc, projects to area 24c in the fundus of the anterior cingulate sulcus, just anterior to the cingulate motor areas (Craig & Zhang 1996). This region is strongly activated in PET and fMRI studies by noxious heat and noxious cold (Talbot et al 1991, Craig et al 1996, Davis et al 1997), but not at all by innocuous stimuli, and late EEG potentials have been localized there with laser heat stimulation (Bromm & Treede 1987, Lenz et al 1998). Activation of the anterior cingulate is uniquely associated with the sensation of burning, ice-like pain elicited by the thermal grill illusion of pain (Craig et al 1996), and it is strongly correlated with hypnotic modulation of pain affect ('unpleasantness') (Rainville et al 1997). A few nociceptive neurons have been recorded in anterior cingulate cortex in humans (Hutchison et al 1993), and comparable recordings have been obtained in the rat and the rabbit, although these are perhaps not homologous (Sikes & Vogt 1992). Clinically, lesions of the anterior cingulate can have significant but variable effects on pain; however, the localization of such lesions has not been well controlled (Sweet 1982, Davis et al 1994). In cat and rat, noxious stimuli selectively activate the ventrolateral orbital cortex (VLO), which receives input from Sm (Tsubokawa et al 1981, Backonja & Miletic 1991, Snow et al 1992).

Thus, the cortical projection targets of each of these regions of thalamus that receive nociceptive input and contain nociceptive neurons are associated with pain. In particular, it is interesting that there is a one-to-one correspondence between the cortical projection targets of the lateral STT lamina I pathway and the sites activated in PET studies. This further substantiates the critical role of this pathway in pain sensation.

The divergence of this pathway at the thalamic level may be related to the different functional roles of these different cortical regions in pain. That is, the activation of area 3a in the postcentral sulcus may be related to the discriminative and motoric aspects of pain sensation, the activation of insular and opercular cortices may be related to the distinct sensory quality of pain and its homeostatic functions, and the activation of anterior cingulate cortex may be related to the motivational aspect of pain. However, these areas are interrelated with subcortical sites, such as the amygdala, the hypothalamus and the periaqueductal grey, that are also involved in the experience of pain, and these interrelationships may be crucial for the forebrain processing of pain.

The importance of these interrelationships is emphasized by the phenomenon of the central (thalamic) pain syndrome, mentioned above. The occurrence of central pain is directly correlated with lesions that interrupt the critical ascending pathway for pain, the lateral STT lamina I pathway through VMpo to the insula (Pagni 1976, Boivie & Leijon 1991, Bowsher 1996). Such lesions can produce analgesia, but in half of such cases this disruption results, after a variable delay, in the appearance of ongoing pain in the deafferented region. This must result from an imbalance among the forebrain regions involved in pain sensation, due to the disruption of their interactions at cortical and subcortical levels. One of these interactions is the effect of thermosensory (and thermoregulatory) integration on pain, that is, the inhibition of pain induced by cold, and it has recently been proposed that the interruption of this particular interaction may be one of the possible causes of central pain, based on similarities with the thermal grill illusion of pain (Craig 1998). Future research on the interactions between the multiple sites of forebrain pain activity and the multiple ascending pathways activated by noxious stimuli will hopefully provide further illumination of the complex representation of pain in the forebrain.

REFERENCES

Al-Chaer ED, Westlund KN, Willis WD 1997 Nucleus gracilis: an integrator for visceral and somatic information. Journal of Neurophysiology 78: 521–527

Al-Chaer ED, Feng Y, Willis WD 1998 A role for the dorsal column in nociceptive visceral input into the thalamus of primates. Journal of Neurophysiology 79: 3143–3150

Albe-Fessard D, Kruger L 1962 Duality of unit discharges from cat centrum medianum in response to natural and electrical stimulation. Journal of Neurophysiology 25: 3–20

Albe-Fessard D, Boivie J, Grant G, Levante A 1975 Labelling of cells in the medulla oblongata of the monkey after injections of horseradish peroxidase in the thalamus. Neuroscience Letters 1: 75–80

Albe-Fessard D, Berkley KJ, Kruger L, Ralston HJ, III, Willis WD Jr. 1985 Diencephalic mechanisms of pain sensation. Brain Research Review 9: 217–296

Allen GV, Saper CB, Hurley KM, Cechetto DF 1991 Organization of visceral and limbic connections in the insular cortex of the rat. Journal of Comparative Neurology 311: 1–16

Amano N, Hu JW, Sessle BJ 1986 Responses of neurons in feline trigeminal subnucleus caudalis (medullary dorsal horn) to cutaneous, intraoral, and muscle afferent stimuli. Journal of Neurophysiology 55: 227–243

Ammons WS 1987 Characteristics of spinoreticular and spinothalamic neurons with renal input. Journal of Neurophysiology 58: 480–495

Apkarian AV, Hodge CJ 1989a Primate spinothalamic pathways: I. A quantitative study of the cells of origin of the spinothalamic pathway. Journal of Comparative Neurology 288: 447–473

Apkarian AV, Hodge CJ 1989b Primate spinothalamic pathways: II. The cells of origin of the dorsolateral and ventral spinothalamic pathways. Journal of Comparative Neurology 288: 474–492

Apkarian AV, Hodge CJ 1989c Primate spinothalamic pathways: III. Thalamic terminations of the dorsolateral and ventral spinothalamic pathways. Journal of Comparative Neurology 288: 493–511

Apkarian AV, Shi T 1994, Squirrel monkey lateral thalamus. I. Somatic nociresponsive neurons and their relation to spinothalamic terminals. Journal of Neuroscience 14: 6779–6790

Apkarian AV, Shi T, Stevens RT, Kniffki K-D, Hodge CJ 1991 Properties of nociceptive neurons in the lateral thalamus of the squirrel monkey. Society for Neuroscience Abstracts 17: 838

Applebaum AE, Leonard RB, Kenshalo DR Jr, Martin RF, Willis WD 1979 Nuclei in which functionally identified spinothalamic tract neurons terminate. Journal of Comparative Neurology 188: 575–586

Aronin N, Chase K, Folsom R, Christakos S, DiFiglia M 1991 Immunoreactive calcium-binding protein (calbindin-D_{28k}) in interneurons and trigeminothalamic neurons of the rat nucleus caudalis localized with peroxidase and immunogold methods. Synapse 7: 106–113

Asanuma C, Thach WT, Jones EG 1983 Distribution of cerebellar terminations and their relation to other afferent terminations in the ventral lateral thalamic region of the monkey. Brain Research Reviews 5: 237–265

Asato F, Yokota T 1989 Responses of neurons in nucleus ventralis posterolateralis of the cat thalamus to hypogastric inputs. Brain Research 488: 135–142

Azerad J, Woda A, Albe-Fessard D 1982 Physiological properties of neurons in different parts of the cat trigeminal sensory complex. Brain Research 246: 7–21

Backonja M, Miletic V 1991 Responses of neurons in the rat ventrolateral orbital cortex to phasic and tonic nociceptive stimulation. Brain Research 557: 353–355

Bandler R, Carrive P, Zhang SP 1991 Integration of somatic and autonomic reactions within the midbrain periaqueductal grey: viscerotopic, somatotopic and functional organization. In: Holstege G (ed) Progress in brain research, vol 87. Elsevier, New York, pp 269–305

Basbaum AI, Fields HL 1978 Endogenous pain control mechanisms: review and hypothesis. Annals of Neurology 4: 451–462

Battaglia G, Spreafico R, Rustioni A 1992 Substance P innervation of the rat and cat thalamus. I. Distribution and relation to ascending spinal pathways. Journal of Comparative Neurology 315: 457–472

Benoist JM, Kayser V, Gautron M, Guilbaud G 1983 Low dose of morphine strongly depresses responses of specific nociceptive neurones in the ventrobasal complex of the rat. Pain 15: 333–344

Berkley KJ 1980 Spatial relationships between the terminations of somatic sensory and motor pathways in the rostral brainstem of cats and monkeys. I. Ascending somatic sensory inputs to lateral diencephalon. Journal of Comparative Neurology 193: 283–317

Berkley KJ, Scofield SL 1990 Relays from the spinal cord and solitary nucleus through the parabrachial nucleus to the forebrain in the cat. Brain Research 529: 333–338

Berkley KJ, Budell RJ, Blomqvist A, Bull M 1986 Output systems of the dorsal column nuclei in the cat. Brain Research Bulletin 11: 199–225

Berkley KJ, Guilbaud G, Benoist J-M, Gautron M 1993 Responses of neurons in and near the thalamic ventrobasal complex of the rat to stimulation of uterus, cervix, vagina, colon, and skin. Journal of Neurophysiology 69: 557–568

Bernard JF, Besson JM 1990 The spino(trigemino)pontoamygdaloid pathway: electrophysiological evidence for an involvement in pain processes. Journal of Neurophysiology 63: 473–490

Bernard JF, Alden M, Besson JM 1993 The organization of the efferent projections from the pontine parabrachial area to the amygdaloid complex: *a Phaseolus vulgaris* leucoagglutinin (PHA-L) study in the rat. Journal of Comparative Neurology 329: 201–229

Bernard JF, Villanueva L, Carroué J, Le Bars D 1990 Efferent projections from the subnucleus reticularis dorsalis (SRD): a *Phaseolus vulgaris* leucoagglutinin study in the rat. Neuroscience Letters 116: 257–262

Bernard JF, Carroué J, Besson JM 1991 Efferent projections from the external parabrachial area to the forebrain: a *Phaseolus vulgaris* leucoagglutinin study in the rat. Neuroscience Letters 122: 257–260

Bernard JF, Huang GF, Besson JM 1992 Nucleus centralis of the amygdala and the globus pallidus ventralis: electrophysiological evidence for an involvement in pain processes. Journal of Neurophysiology 68: 551–569

Berthier ML, Starkstein SE, Leiguarda RC 1988 Asymbolia for pain: a sensory-limbic disconnection syndrome. Annals of Neurology 24: 41–49

Biemond A 1956 The conduction of pain above the level of the thalamus opticus. Archives of Neurology and Psychiatry 75: 231–244

Bishop GH 1959 The relation between nerve fiber size and sensory modality: phylogenetic implications of the afferent innervation of cortex. Journal of Nervous and Mental Disease 128: 89–114

Blomqvist A, Berkley KJ 1992 A re-examination of the spino-reticulo-diencephalic pathway in the cat. Brain Research 579: 17–31

Blomqvist A, Craig AD 1991 Organization of spinal and trigeminal input to the PAG. In: Depaulis A, Bandler R (eds) The midbrain periaqueductal gray matter. Plenum, New York, pp 345–363

Blomqvist A, Ma W, Berkley KJ 1989 Spinal input to the parabrachial nucleus in the cat. Brain Research 480: 29–36

Blomqvist A, Hermanson O, Ericson H, Larhammar D 1994 Activation of a bulbospinal opioidergic projection by pain stimuli in the awake rat. NeuroReport 5: 461–464

Blomqvist A, Zhang E-T, Craig AD 1995 A thermoreceptive sub-region of lamina I in n. caudalis of the owl monkey. Society for Neuroscience Abstracts 21: 108

Blomqvist A, Ericson AC, Craig AD, Broman J 1996 Evidence for glutamate as a neurotransmitter in spinothalamic tract terminals in the posterior region of owl monkeys. Experimental Brain Research 108: 33–44

Bogousslavsky J, Regli F, Uske A 1988 Thalamic infarcts: clinical syndromes, etiology, and prognosis. Neurology 38: 837–848

Boivie J 1979 An anatomical reinvestigation of the termination of the spinothalamic tract in the monkey. Journal of Comparative Neurology 186: 343–370

Boivie J 1983 Anatomic and physiologic features of the spino-cervico-thalamic pathway. In: Macchi G, Rustioni A, Spreafico R (eds) Somatosensory integration in the thalamus. Elsevier, Amsterdam, pp 63–106

Boivie J, Leijon G 1991 Clinical findings in patients with central poststroke pain. In: Casey KL (ed) Pain and central nervous system disease: the central pain syndromes. Raven, New York, pp 65–76

Bonica JJ 1990 Anatomic and physiologic basis of nociception and pain. In: Bonica JJ (ed) The management of pain. Lea, Fibiger, Philadelphia, pp 28–95

Bowsher D 1961 The termination of secondary somatosensory neurons within the thalamus of *Macaca mulatta*: an experimental degeneration study. Journal of Comparative Neurology 117: 213–227

Bowsher D 1975 Diencephalic projections from the midbrain reticular formation. Brain Research 95: 211–220

Bowsher D 1996 Central pain: clinical and physiological characteristics. Journal of Neurology, Neurosurgery and Psychiatry 61: 62–69

Brinkhus HB, Carstens E, Zimmerman M 1979 Encoding of graded noxious skin heating by neurons in posterior thalamus and adjacent areas in the cat. Neuroscience Letters 15: 37–42

Brodal A 1981 Neurological anatomy. Oxford University Press, New York

Bromm B, Treede RD 1987 Human cerebral potentials evoked by CO_2 laser stimuli causing pain. Experimental Brain Research 67: 153–162

Broton JG, Rosenfeld P 1986 Cutting rostral trigeminal complex projections preferentially affects perioral nociception in the rat. Brain Research 397: 1–8

Broton JG, Hu JW, Sessle BJ 1988 Effects of temporomandibular joint stimulation on nociceptive and nonnociceptive neurons of the cat's trigeminal subnucleus caudalis (medullary dorsal horn). Journal of Neurophysiology 59: 1575–1589

Brüggemann J, Shi T, Apkarian AV 1994a Squirrel monkey lateral thalamus. II. Viscerosomatic convergent representation of urinary bladder, colon, and esophagus. Journal of Neuroscience 14: 6796–6814

Brüggemann J, Vahle-Hinz C, Kniffki K-D 1994b Projections from the pelvic nerve to the periphery of the cat's thalamic ventral posterolateral nucleus and adjacent regions of the posterior complex. Journal of Neurophysiology 72: 2237–2245

Bullitt E 1990 Expression of C-*fos*-like protein as a marker for neuronal activity following noxious stimulation in the rat. Journal of Comparative Neurology 296: 517–530

Burstein R, Potrebic S 1993 Retrograde labeling of neurons in the spinal cord that project directly to the amygdala or the orbital cortex in the rat. Journal of Comparative Neurology 335: 469–485

Burstein R, Dado RJ, Giesler GJ Jr 1990 The cells of origin of the spinothalamic tract of the rat: a quantitative reexamination. Brain Research 511: 329–337

Burstein R, Falkowsky O, Borsook D, Strassman A 1996 Distinct lateral and medial projections of the spinohypothalamic tract of the rat. Journal of Comparative Neurology 373: 549–574

Burton H, Craig AD Jr 1983 Spinothalamic projections in cat, raccoon and monkey: a study based on anterograde transport of horseradish peroxidase. In: Macchi G, Rustioni A, Spreafico R (eds) Somatosensory integration in the thalamus. Elsevier, New York, pp 17–41

Burton H, Jones EG 1976 The posterior thalamic region and its cortical projection in new world and old world monkeys. Journal of Comparative Neurology 168: 249–302

Burton H, Craig AD Jr, Poulos DA, Molt J 1979 Efferent projections from temperature sensitive recording loci within the marginal zone of the nucleus caudalis of the spinal trigeminal complex in the cat. Journal of Comparative Neurology 183: 753–788

Bushnell MC, Duncan GH 1989 Sensory and affective aspects of pain perception: is medial thalamus restricted to emotional issues. Experimental Brain Research 78: 415–418

Bushnell MC, Duncan GH, Dubner R, He LF 1984 Activity of trigeminothalamic neurons in medullary dorsal horn of awake monkeys trained in a thermal discrimination task. Journal of Neurophysiology 52: 170–187

Bushnell MC, Duncan GH, Tremblay N 1993 Thalamic VPM nucleus in the behaving monkey. I. Multimodal and discriminative properties of thermosensitive neurons. Journal of Neurophysiology 69: 739–752

Cameron AA, Khan IA, Westlund KN, Willis WD 1995 The efferent projections of the periaqueductal gray in the rat: a *Phaseolus vulgaris*-leucoagglutinin study. II. Descending projections. Journal of Comparative Neurology 351: 585–601

Carstens E, Trevino DL 1978 Laminar origins of spinothalamic projections in the cat as determined by the retrograde transport of horseradish peroxidase. Journal of Comparative Neurology 182: 151–166

Carstens E, Yokota T 1980 Viscerosomatic convergence and responses to intestinal distension of neurons at the junction of midbrain and posterior thalamus in the cat. Experimental Neurology 70: 392–402

Carstens E, Leah J, Lechner J, Zimmermann M 1990 Demonstration of extensive brainstem projections to medial and lateral thalamus and hypothalamus in the rat. Neuroscience 35: 609–626

Casey KL 1966 Unit analysis of nociceptive mechanisms in the thalamus of the awake squirrel monkey. Journal of Neurophysiology 29: 727–750

Casey KL, Morrow TJ 1983 Ventral posterior thalamic neurons differentially responsive to noxious stimulation of the awake monkey. Science 221: 675–677

Casey KL, Minoshima S, Berger KL, Koeppe RA, Morrow TJ, Frey KA 1992 PET analysis of brain structures differentially activated by noxious thermal stimuli. Society for Neuroscience Abstracts 18: 833–836

Cechetto DF, Saper CB 1987 Evidence for a viscerotopic sensory representation in the cortex and thalamus in the rat. Journal of Comparative Neurology 262: 27–45

Cechetto DF, Standaert DG, Saper CB 1985 Spinal and trigeminal dorsal horn projections to the parabrachial nucleus in the rat. Journal of Comparative Neurology 240: 153–160

Chamberlin NL, Saper CB 1992 Topographic organization of cardiovascular responses to electrical and glutamate microstimulation of the parabrachial nucleus in the rat. Journal of Comparative Neurology 326: 245–262

Chandler MJ, Hobbs SF, Bolser DC, Foreman RD 1991 Effects of vagal afferent stimulation on cervical spinothalamic tract neurons in monkeys. Pain 44: 81–87

Chandler MJ, Hobbs SF, Fu Q-G, Kenshalo DR Jr, Blair RW, Foreman RD 1992 Responses of neurons in ventroposterolateral nucleus of primate thalamus to urinary bladder distension. Brain Research 571: 26–34

Christensen BN, Perl ER 1970 Spinal neurons specifically excited by noxious or thermal stimuli: marginal zone of the dorsal horn. Journal of Neurophysiology 33: 293–307

Chudler EH, Dong WK 1995 The role of the basal ganglia in nociception and pain. Pain 60: 3–38

Chudler EH, Sugiyama K, Dong WK 1993 Nociceptive responses in the neostriatum and globus pallidus of the anesthetized rat. Journal of Neurophysiology 69: 1890–1903

Chung JM, Lee KH, Surmeier DJ, Sorkin LS, Kim J, Willis WD 1986 Response characteristics of neurons in the ventral posterior lateral nucleus of the monkey thalamus. Journal of Neurophysiology 56: 370–390

Clark FM, Proudfit HK 1991 The projection of noradrenergic neurons in the A7 catecholamine cell group to the spinal cord in the rat demonstrated by anterograde tracing combined with immunocytochemistry. Brain Research 547: 279–288

Clark WE, Gros LE 1936 The termination of ascending tracts in the thalamus of the macaque monkey. Journal of Anatomy 71: 7–40

Clascá F, Llamas A, Reinoso-Suárez F 1997 Insular cortex and neighboring fields in the cat: a redefinition based on cortical microarchitecture and connections with the thalamus. Journal of Comparative Neurology 384: 456–482

Cliffer KD, Burstein R, Giesler GJ Jr 1991 Distributions of spinothalamic, spinohypothalamic, and spinotelencephalic fibers revealed by anterograde transport of PHA-L in rats. Journal of Neuroscience 11: 852–868

Coffield JA, Miletic V 1987 Immunoreactive enkephalin is contained within some trigeminal and spinal neurons projecting to the rat medial thalamus. Brain Research 425: 380–383

Coffield JA, Miletic V 1993 Responses of rat nucleus submedius neurons to enkephalins applied with micropressure. Brain Research 630: 252–261

Coffield JA, Bowen KK, Miletic V 1992 Retrograde tracing of projections between the nucleus submedius, the ventrolateral orbital cortex, and the midbrain in the rat. Journal of Comparative Neurology 321: 488–499

Coghill RC, Mayer DJ, Price DD 1993 Wide dynamic range but not nociceptive-specific neurons encode multidimensional features of prolonged repetitive heat pain. Journal of Neurophysiology 69: 703–716

Coghill RC, Talbot JD, Evans AC et al 1994 Distributed processing of pain and vibration by the human brain. Journal of Neuroscience 14: 4095–4108

Cohen SR, Melzack R 1993 The habenula and pain: Repeated electrical stimulation produces prolonged analgesia but lesions have no effect on formalin pain or morphine analgesia. Behavioural Brain Research 54: 171–178

Coimbra F, Coimbra A 1994 Dental noxious input reaches the subnucleus caudalis of the trigeminal complex in the rat, as shown by c-*fos* expression upon thermal or mechanical stimulation. Neuroscience Letters 173: 201–204

Craig AD 1990 Nociceptive neurons in the nucleus submedius (Sm) in the medial thalamus of the cat. Pain, Supplement 5: S492

Craig AD 1991a Spinal distribution of ascending lamina I axons anterogradely labeled with *Phaseolus vulgaris* leucoagglutinin (PHA-L) in the cat. Journal of Comparative Neurology 313: 377–393

Craig AD 1991b Supraspinal pathways and mechanisms relevant to central pain. In: Casey KL (ed) Pain and central nervous system disease: the central pain syndromes. Raven, New York, pp 157–170

Craig AD 1992 Spinal and trigeminal lamina I input to the locus coeruleus anterogradely labeled with *Phaseolus vulgaris* leucoagglutinin (PHA-L) in the cat and the monkey. Brain Research 584: 325–328

Craig AD 1995a Distribution of brainstem projections from spinal lamina I neurons in the cat and the monkey. Journal of Comparative Neurology 361: 225–248

Craig AD 1995b Supraspinal projections of lamina I neurons. In: Besson J-M (ed) Forebrain processing of pain. John Libbey, Paris, pp 13–25

Craig AD 1996 Pain, temperature, and the sense of the body. In: Franzen O, Johansson R, Terenius L (eds) Somesthesis and the neurobiology of the somatosensory cortex. Birkhäuser Verlag, Basel, pp 27–39

Craig AD 1998 A new version of the thalamic disinhibition hypothesis of central pain. Pain Forum 7: 1–14

Craig AD Jr, Burton H 1981 Spinal and medullary lamina I projection to nucleus submedius in medial thalamus: a possible pain center. Journal of Neurophysiology 45: 443–466

Craig AD Jr, Burton H 1985 The distribution and topographical organization in the thalamus of anterogradely-transported horseradish peroxidase after spinal injections in cat and raccoon. Experimental Brain Research 58: 227–254

Craig AD, Bushnell MC 1994 The thermal grill illusion: unmasking the burn of cold pain. Science 265: 252–255

Craig AD, Dostrovsky JO 1991 Thermoreceptive lamina I trigeminothalamic neurons project to the nucleus submedius in the cat. Experimental Brain Research 85: 470–474

Craig AD, Dostrovsky JO 1997 Processing of nociceptive information at supraspinal levels. In: Yaksh TL (ed) Anesthesia: biologic foundations. Lippincott–Raven, Philadelphia, pp 625–642

Craig AD, Hunsley SJ 1991 Morphine enhances the activity of thermoreceptive cold-specific lamina I spinothalamic neurons in the cat. Brain Research 558: 93–97

Craig AD Jr, Kniffki K-D 1985b Spinothalamic lumbosacral lamina I cells responsive to skin and muscle stimulation in the cat. Journal of Physiology (London) 365: 197–221

Craig AD, Zhang E-T 1996 Anterior cingulate projection from MDvc (a lamina I spinothalamic target in the medial thalamus of the monkey). Society for Neuroscience Abstracts 22: 111

Craig AD Jr, Wiegand SJ, Price JL 1982 The thalamocortical projection of nucleus submedius in the cat. Journal of Comparative Neurology 206: 28–48

Craig AD Jr, Linington AJ, Kniffki K-D 1989 Cells of origin of spinothalamic tract projections to the medial and lateral thalamus in the cat. Journal of Comparative Neurology 289: 568–585

Craig AD, Broman J, Blomqvist A 1992 Lamina I spinocervical tract terminations in the medial part of the lateral cervical nucleus in the cat. Journal of Comparative Neurology 322: 99–110

Craig AD, Bushnell MC, Zhang E-T, Blomqvist A 1994 A thalamic nucleus specific for pain and temperature sensation. Nature 372: 770–773

Craig AD, Reiman EM, Evans A, Bushnell MC 1996 Functional imaging of an illusion of pain. Nature 384: 258–260

Craig AD, Zhang E-T, Blomqvist A 1998 Immunohistochemical identification of ascending lamina I axons in the lateral spinothalamic tract. Society for Neuroscience Abstracts 24: 387

Curry MJ 1972 The exteroceptive properties of neurones in the somatic part of the posterior group (PO). Brain Research 44: 439–462

Dado RJ, Giesler GJ Jr 1990 Afferent input to nucleus submedius in rats: retrograde labeling of neurons in the spinal cord and caudal medulla. Journal of Neuroscience 10: 2672–2686

Dado RJ, Katter JT, Giesler GJ Jr 1994a Spinothalamic and spinohypothalamic tract neurons in the cervical enlargement of rats. I. Locations of antidromically identified axons in the thalamus and hypothalamus. Journal of Neurophysiology 71: 959–980

Dado RJ, Katter JT, Giesler GJ Jr 1994b Spinothalamic and spinohypothalamic tract neurons in the cervical enlargement of rats. II. Responses to innocuous and noxious mechanical and thermal stimuli. Journal of Neurophysiology 71: 981–1002

Dallel R, Raboisson P, Auroy P, Woda A 1988 The rostral part of the trigeminal sensory complex is involved in orofacial nociception. Brain Research 448: 7–19

Dallel R, Clavelou P, Woda A 1989 Effects of tracetotomy on nociceptive reactions induced by tooth pulp stimulation in the rat. Experimental Neurology 106: 78–84

Dallel R, Raboisson P, Woda A, Sessle BJ 1990 Properties of nociceptive and non-nociceptive neurons in trigeminal subnucleus oralis of the rat. Brain Research 521: 95–106

Davies SN, Goldsmith GE, Hellon RF, Mitchell D 1983 Facial sensitivity to rates of temperature change: neurophysiological and psychophysical evidence from cats and humans. Journal of Physiology (London) 344: 161–175

Davis KD, Dostrovsky JO 1988 Responses of feline trigeminal spinal tract nucleus neurons to stimulation of the middle meningeal artery and sagittal sinus. Journal of Neurophysiology 59: 648–666

Davis KD, Hutchison WD, Lozano AM, Dostrovsky JO 1994 Altered pain and temperature perception following cingulotomy and capsulotomy in a patient with schizoaffective disorder. Pain 59: 189–199

Davis KD, Kiss ZHT, Tasker RR, Dostrovsky JO 1996 Thalamic stimulation-evoked sensation in chronic pain patients and in nonpain (movement disorder) patients. Journal of Neurophysiology 75: 1026–1037

Davis KD, Tasker RR, Kiss ZHT, Hutchison WD, Dostrovsky JO 1995a Visceral pain evoked by thalamic microstimulation in humans. NeuroReport 6: 369–374

Davis KD, Wood ML, Crawley AP, Mikulis DJ 1995b fMRI of human somatosensory and cingulate cortex during painful electrical nerve stimulation. NeuroReport 7: 321–325

Davis KD, Taylor SJ, Crawley AP, Wood ML, Mikulis DJ 1997 Functional MRI of pain- and attention-related activations in the human cingulate cortex. Journal of Neurophysiology 77: 3370–3380

Davis KD, Kiss ZHT, Luo L, Tasker RR, Lozano AM, Dostrovsky JO 1998 Phantom sensations generated by thalamic microstimulation. Nature 391: 385–387

Day TA, Sibbald JR 1990 Noxious somatic stimuli excite neurosecretory vasopressin cells via A1 cell group. American Journal of Physiology 258: R1516–R1520

Dejerine J, Roussy G 1906 La syndrome thalamique. Revue Neurologique 14: 521–532

Depaulis A, Keay KA, Bandler R 1992 Longitudinal neuronal organization of defensive reactions in the midbrain periaqueductal gray region of the rat. Experimental Brain Research 90: 307–318

Deschenes M, Hu B 1990 Electrophysiology and pharmacology of the corticothalamic input to lateral thalamic nuclei: an intracellular study in the cat. European Journal of Neuroscience 2: 140–152

Diamond ME, Armstrong-James M, Budway MJ, Ebner FF 1992 Somatic sensory responses in the rostral sector of the posterior group (POm) and in the ventral posterior medial nucleus (VPM) of the rat thalamus: dependence on the barrel field cortex. Journal of Comparative Neurology 319: 66–84

Dong WK, Chudler EH 1985 Origins of tooth pulp-evoked far-field and early near-field potentials in the cat. Journal of Neurophysiology 51: 859–889

Dong WK, Ryu H, Wagman IH 1978 Nociceptive responses of neurons in medial thalamus and their relationship to spinothalamic pathways. Journal of Neurophysiology 41: 1592–1613

Dong WK, Chudler EH, Sugiyama K, Roberts VJ, Hayashi T 1994 Somatosensory, multisensory, and task-related neurons in cortical area 7b (PF) of unanesthetized monkeys. Journal of Neurophysiology 72: 542–564

Dostrovsky JO, Craig AD 1996a Cooling-specific spinothalamic neurons in the monkey. Journal of Neurophysiology 76: 3656–3665

Dostrovsky JO, Craig AD 1996b Nociceptive neurons in primate insular cortex. Society for Neuroscience Abstracts 22: 111.

Dostrovsky JO, Guilbaud G 1988 Noxious stimuli excite neurons in nucleus submedius of the normal and arthritic rat. Brain Research 460: 269–280

Dostrovsky JO, Guilbaud G 1990 Nociceptive responses in medial thalamus of the normal and arthritic rat. Pain 40: 93–104

Dostrovsky JO, Hellon RF 1978 The representation of facial temperature in the caudal trigeminal nucleus of the cat. Journal of Physiology (London) 277: 29–47

Dostrovsky JO, Davis KD, Kawakita K 1991 Central mechanisms of vascular headaches. Canadian Journal of Physiology and Pharmacology 69: 652–658

Dostrovsky JO, Wells FEB, Tasker RR 1992 Pain sensations evoked by stimulation in human thalamus. In: Inoka R, Shigenaga Y, Tohyama M (eds) Processing and inhibition of nociceptive information, International Congress Series 989. Excerpta Medica, Amsterdam, pp 115–120

Dostrovsky JO, Davis KD, Kiss ZHT, Junn F, Lozano AM 1996 Evidence for a specific temperature relay site in human thalamus. In: Abstracts: 8th World Congress on Pain. IASP press, Seattle, p 440

Downie JW, Ferrington DG, Sorkin LS, Willis WD, Jr 1988 The primate spinocervicothalamic pathway: responses of cells of the lateral cervical nucleus and spinocervical tract to innocuous and noxious stimuli. Journal of Neurophysiology 59: 861–885

Duale C, Luccarini P, Cadet R, Woda A 1996 Effects of morphine microinjections into the trigeminal sensory complex on the formalin test in the rat. Experimental Neurology 142: 331–339

Dubner R, Bennett GJ 1983 Spinal and trigeminal mechanisms of nociception. Annual Review of Neuroscience 6: 381–418

Dubner R, Sessle BJ, Storey AT 1978 The neural basis of oral and facial function. Plenum, New York

Dubner R, Kenshalo DR Jr, Maixner W, Bushnell MC, Oliveras J-L 1989 The correlation of monkey medullary dorsal horn neuronal activity and the perceived intensity of noxious heat stimuli. Journal of Neurophysiology 62: 450–457

Duncan GH, Bushnell MC, Oliveras J-L, Bastrash N, Tremblay N 1993 Thalamic VPM nucleus in the behaving monkey. III. Effects of reversible inactivation by lidocaine on thermal and mechanical discrimination. Journal of Neurophysiology 70: 2086–2096

Dykes RW, Craig AD 1998 Control of size and excitability of mechanosensory receptive fields in dorsal column nuclei by homolateral dorsal horn neurons. Journal of Neurophysiology 80: 120–129

Eaton SA, Salt TE 1990 Thalamic NMDA receptors and nociceptive sensory synaptic transmission. Neuroscience Letters 110: 297–302

Eaton SA, Salt TE 1995 The role of excitatory amino acid receptors in thalamic nociception. In: Besson J-M, Guilbaud G, Ollat H (eds) Pain in forebrain areas. John Libbey Eurotext, Paris, pp 131–141

Eaton SA, Birse EF, Wharton B, Udvarhelyi PM, Watkins JC, Salt TE 1993 Mediation of thalamic sensory responses in vivo by ACPD-activated excitatory amino acid receptors. European Journal of Neuroscience 5: 186–189

Eisenman J, Landgren S, Novin D 1963 Functional organization in the main sensory trigeminal nucleus and in the rostral subdivision of the nucleus of the spinal trigeminal tract in the cat. Acta Physiologica Scandinavica. Supplement 59 214: 5–44

Ericson A-C, Blomqvist A, Craig AD, Ottersen OP, Broman J 1995 Evidence for glutamate as neurotransmitter in trigemino- and spinothalamic tract terminals in the nucleus submedius of cats. European Journal of Neuroscience 7: 305–317

Ericson AC, Blomqvist A, Krout K, Craig AD 1996 Fine structural organization of spinothalamic and trigeminothalamic lamina I terminations in the nucleus submedius of the cat. Journal of Comparative Neurology 371: 497–512

Feil K, Herbert H 1995 Topographic organization of spinal and trigeminal somatosensory pathways to the rat parabrachial and Kölliker-Fuse nuclei. Journal of Comparative Neurology 353: 506–528

Ferrington DG, Downie JW, Willis WD Jr 1988 Primate nucleus gracilis neurons: responses to innocuous and noxious stimuli. Journal of Neurophysiology 59: 886–907

Fields HL 1987 Pain. McGraw-Hill, New York

Fields HL, Clanton CH, Anderson SD 1977 Somatosensory properties of spinoreticular neurons in the cat. Brain Research 120: 49–66

Flor H, Elbert T, Knecht S et al 1995 Phantom-limb pain as a perceptual correlate of cortical reorganization following arm amputation. Nature 375: 482–484

Foerster O, Gagel O 1932 Die Vorderseitenstrangdurchschneidung beim Menschen. Eine klinisch-patho-physiologisch-anatomische Studie. Zentralblatt fur die Gesamte Neurologie und Psychiatrie 138: 1–92

Foreman RD, Schmidt RF, Willis WD 1979 Effects of mechanical and chemical stimulation of fine muscle afferents upon primate spinothalamic tract cells. Journal of Physiology (London) 286: 215–231

François C, Percheron G, Parent A, Sadikot AF, Fenelon G, Yelnik J 1991 Topography of the projection from the central complex of the thalamus to the sensorimotor striatal territory in monkeys. Journal of Comparative Neurology 305: 17–34

Friedman DP, Murray EA 1986 Thalamic connectivity of the second somatosensory area and neighboring somatosensory fields of the lateral sulcus of the macaque. Journal of Comparative Neurology 252: 348–373

Friedman DP, Murray EA, O'Neill JB, Mishkin M 1986 Cortical connections of the somatosensory fields of the lateral sulcus of macaques: evidence for a corticolimbic pathway for touch. Journal of Comparative Neurology 252: 323–347

Fulwiler CE, Saper CB 1984 Subnuclear organization of the efferent connections of the parabrachial nucleus in the rat. Brain Research Reviews 7: 229–259

Gall C, Lauterborn J, Burks D, Seroogy K 1987 Co-localization of enkephalin and cholecystokinin in discrete areas of rat brain. Brain Research 403: 403–408

Ganchrow D 1978 Intratrigeminal and thalamic projections of nucleus caudalis in the squirrel monkey (*Saimiri sciureus*): a degeneration and autoradiographic study. Journal of Comparative Neurology 178: 281–312

Gang S, Mizuguchi A, Kobayashi N, Aoki M 1990 Descending axonal projections from the medial parabrachial and Kölliker-Fuse nuclear complex to the nucleus raphe magnus in cats. Neuroscience Letters 118: 273–275

Giesler GJ Jr, Menetrey D, Basbaum AI 1979 Differential origins of spinothalamic tract projections to medial and lateral thalamus in the rat. Journal of Comparative Neurology 184: 107–126

Giesler GJ Jr, Yezierski RP, Gerhart KD, Willis WD 1981 Spinothalamic tract neurons that project to medial and/or lateral thalamic nuclei: evidence for a physiologically novel population of spinal cord neurons. Journal of Neurophysiology 46: 1285–1308

Gildenberg PL 1972 Physiologic observations concerned with percutaneous cordotomy. In: Somjen G (ed) Neurophysiology studied in man. Elsevier, Amsterdam, pp 231–236

Gingold SI, Greenspan JD, Apkarian AV 1991 Anatomic evidence of nociceptive inputs to primary somatosensory cortex: relationship between spinothalamic terminals and thalamocortical cells in squirrel monkeys. Journal of Comparative Neurology 308: 467–490

Gobel S 1978 Golgi studies of the neurons in layer I of the dorsal horn of the medulla (trigeminal nucleus caudalis). Journal of Comparative Neurology 180: 375–394

Gobel S, Hockfield S, Ruda MA 1981 An anatomical analysis of the similarities between medullary and spinal dorsal horns. In: Kawamura Y, Dubner R (eds) Oral-facial sensory and motor mechanisms. Quintessence, Tokyo, pp 211–223

Graham SH, Sharp FR, Dillon W 1988 Intraoral sensation in patients with brainstem lesions: role of the rostral spinal trigeminal nuclei in pons. Neurology 38: 1529–1533

Greenspan JD, Winfield JA 1992 Reversible pain and tactile deficits associated with a cerebral tumor compressing the posterior insula and parietal operculum. Pain 50: 29–39

Guilbaud G, Caille D, Besson JM, Benelli G 1977 Single units activities in ventral posterior and posterior group thalamic nuclei during nociceptive and non-nociceptive stimulations in the cat. Archives Italiennes de Biologie 115: 38–56

Guilbaud G, Peschanski M, Gautron M, Binder D 1980 Neurones responding to noxious stimulation in VB complex and caudal adjacent regions in the thalamus of the rat. Pain 8: 303–318

Guilbaud G, Benoist JM, Jazat F, Gautron M 1990 Neuronal responsiveness in the ventrobasal thalamic complex of rats with an experimental peripheral mononeuropathy. Journal of Neurophysiology 64: 1537–1554

Guilbaud G, Benoist JM, Levante A, Gautron M, Willer JC 1992 Primary somatosensory cortex in rats with pain-related behaviours due to a peripheral mononeuropathy after moderate ligation of one sciatic nerve: Neuronal responsivity to somatic stimulation. Experimental Brain Research 92: 227–245

Guilbaud G, Benoist JM, Condes-Lara M, Gautron M 1993a Further evidence for the involvement of SmI cortical neurons in nociception: their responsiveness at 24 hr after carrageenin-induced hyperalgesic inflammation in the rat. Somatosensory and Moter Research 10: 229–244

Guilbaud G, Berkley KJ, Benoist J-M, Gautron M 1993b Responses of neurons in thalamic ventrobasal complex of rats to graded distension of uterus and vagina and to uterine suprafusion with bradykinin and prostaglandin $F_{2\alpha}$. Brain Research 614: 285–290

Guilbaud G, Bernard JF, Besson JM 1994 Brain areas involved in nociception and pain. In: Wall PD, Melzack R (eds) Textbook of pain. Churchill Livingstone, Edinburgh, pp 113–128

Gybels JM, Sweet WH 1989 Neurosurgical treatment of persistent pain. Physiological and pathological mechanisms of human pain and headache, vol 11. Karger, Basel

Halliday AM, Logue V 1972 Painful sensations evoked by electrical stimulation in the thalamus. In: Somjen GG (ed) Neurophysiology studied in man. Excerpta Medica, Amsterdam, pp 221–230

Halsell CB 1992 Organization of parabrachial nucleus efferents to the thalamus and amygdala in the golden hamster. Journal of Comparative Neurology 317: 57–78

Hamba M, Hisamitsu H, Muro M 1990 Nociceptive projection from tooth pulp to the lateral hypothalamus in rats. Brain Research Bulletin 25: 355–364

Han Z-S, Zhang E-T, Craig AD 1998 Nociceptive and thermoreceptive lamina I neurons are anatomically distinct. Nature Neuroscience 1: 218–225

Hassler R 1970 Dichotomy of facial pain conduction in the diencephalon. In: Hassler R, Walker AE (eds) Trigeminal neuralgia. Sanders, Philadelphia, pp 123–138

Hassler R, Riechert T 1959 Klinische und anatomische Befunde bei stereotaktischen Schmerzoperationen im thalamus. Archiv fur Psychiatrie und Nervenkrankheiten (Berlin) 200: 93–122

Hathaway CB, Hu JW, Bereiter DA 1995 Distribution of Fos-like immunoreactivity in the caudal brainstem of the rat following noxious chemical stimulation of the temporomandibular joint. Journal of Comparative Neurology 356: 444–456

Hayashi H, Sumino R, Sessle BJ 1984 Functional organization of trigeminal subnucleus interpolaris: nociceptive and innocuous afferent inputs, projections to thalamus, cerebellum, and spinal cord, and descending modulation from periaqueductal gray. Journal of Neurophysiology 51: 890–905

He L, Dong W, Wang M 1991 Effects of iontophoretic etorphine and naloxone, and electroacupuncture on nociceptive responses from thalamic neurones in rabbits. Pain 44: 89–95

Head H, Holmes G 1911 Sensory disturbances from cerebral lesions. Brain 34: 102–254

Helmstetter FJ, Bellgowan PS 1993 Lesions of the amygdala block conditional hypoalgesia on the tail flick test. Brain Research 612: 253–257

Helmstetter FJ, Bellgowan PS, Tershner SA 1993 Inhibition of the tail flick reflex following microinjection of morphine into the amygdala. NeuroReport 4: 471–474

Herbert H, Moga MM, Saper CB 1990 Connections of the parabrachial nucleus with the nucleus of the solitary tract and the medullary reticular formation in the rat. Journal of Comparative Neurology 293: 540–580

Hermanson O, Blomqvist A 1995 Enkephalinergic and catecholaminergic neurons constitute separate populations in the rat Kölliker-Fuse/A7 region. Neuroscience Letters 190: 57–60

Hermanson O, Blomqvist A 1997 Subnuclear localization of FOS-like immunoreactivity in the parabrachial nucleus after orofacial nociceptive stimulation of the awake rat. Journal of Comparative Neurology 387: 114–123

Hirai T, Jones EG 1989a A new parcellation of the human thalamus on the basis of histochemical staining. Brain Research Reviews 14: 1–34

Hirai T, Jones EG 1989b Distribution of tachykinin- and enkephalin-immunoreactive fibers in the human thalamus. Brain Research Reviews 14: 35–52

Hoheisel U, Mense S, Simons DG, Yu X-M 1993 Appearance of new receptive fields in rat dorsal horn neurons following noxious stimulation of skeletal muscle: A model for referral of muscle pain. Neuroscience Letters 153: 9–12

Holstege G 1988 Anatomical evidence for a strong ventral parabrachial projection to nucleus raphe magnus and adjacent tegmental field. Brain Research 447: 154–158

Honda CN, Mense S, and Perl ER 1983 Neurons in ventrobasal region of cat thalamus selectively responsive to noxious mechanical stimulation. Journal of Neurophysiology 49: 662–673

Horie H, Yokota T 1990 Responses of nociceptive VPL neurons to intracardiac injection of bradykinin in the cat. Brain Research 516: 161–164

Horie H, Pamplin PJ, Yokota T 1991 Inhibition of nociceptive neurons in the shell region of nucleus ventralis posterolateralis following conditioning stimulation of the periaqueductal grey of the cat. Evidence for an ascending inhibitory pathway. Brain Research 561: 35–42

Houser CR, Vaughn JE, Barber RP, Roberts E 1980 GABA neurons are the major cell type of the nucleus reticularis thalami. Brain Research 200: 341–347

Hu JW, Dostrovsky JO, Sessle BJ 1981 Functional properties of neurons in cat trigeminal subnucleus caudalis (medullary dorsal horn). I. Response to oral-facial noxious and nonnoxious stimuli and projections to thalamus and subnucleus oralis. Journal of Neurophysiology 45: 173–192

Hu JW, Sessle BJ, Raboisson P, Dallel R, Woda A 1992 Stimulation of craniofacial muscle afferents induces prolonged facilitatory effects in trigeminal nociceptive brain-stem neurones. Pain 48: 53–60

Huber J, Grottel K, Celichowski J 1994 Dual projections of the ventromedial lamina VI and the medial lamina VII neurones in the second sacral spinal cord segment to the thalamus and the cerebellum in the cat. Neuroscience Research 21: 51–57

Hutchison WD, Lühn MAB, Schmidt RF 1992 Knee joint input into the peripheral region of the ventral posterior lateral nucleus of cat thalamus. Journal of Neurophysiology 67: 1092–1104

Hutchison WD, Dostrovsky JO, Davis KD, Lozano AM 1993 Single unit responses and microstimulation effects in cingulate cortex of an awake patient. In: Abstracts—7th World Congress on Pain IASP, Seattle, pp 461–461

Hutchison WD, Tsoukatos J, Dostrovsky JO 1997 Quantitative analysis of orofacial thermoreceptive neurons in the superficial medullary dorsal horn of the rat. Journal of Neurophysiology 77: 3252–3266

Hylden JLK, Hayashi H, Bennett GJ, Dubner R 1985 Spinal lamina I neurons projecting to the parabrachial area of the cat midbrain. Brain Research 336: 195–198

Hylden JLK, Hayashi H, Dubner R, Bennett GJ 1986 Physiology and morphology of the lamina I spinomesencephalic projection. Journal of Comparative Neurology 247: 505–515

Hylden JLK, Anton F, Nahin RL 1989 Spinal lamina I projection neurons in the rat: collateral innervation of parabrachial area and thalamus. Neuroscience 28: 27–37

Iwata K, Kenshalo DR Jr, Dubner R, Nahin RL 1992 Diencephalic projections from the superficial and deep laminae of the medullary dorsal horn in the rat. Journal of Comparative Neurology 321: 404–420

Jacquin MF, Renehan WE, Mooney RD, Rhoades RW 1986 Structure–function relationships in rat medullary and cervical dorsal horns. I. Trigeminal primary afferents. Journal of Neurophysiology 55: 1153–1186

Jacquin MF, Barcia M, Rhoades RW 1989 Structure–function relationships in rat brainstem subnucleus interpolaris: IV. Projection neurons. Journal of Comparative Neurology 282: 45–62

Jasmin L, Wang H, Tarczy-Hornoch K, Levine JD, Basbaum AI 1994 Differential effects of morphine on noxious stimulus-evoked Fos-like immunoreactivity in subpopulations of spinoparabrachial neurons. Journal of Neuroscience 14: 7252–7260

Jeanmonod D, Magnin M, Morel A 1994 A thalamic concept of neurogenic pain. Proceedings of the 7th Congress on Pain 2: 767–787

Jones AKP, Brown WD, Friston KJ, Qi LY, Frackowiak RSJ 1991 Cortical and subcortical localization of response to pain in man using positron emission tomography. Proceedings of the Royal Society for London [Biology] 244: 39–44

Jones EG 1985 The thalamus. Plenum, New York

Jones EG 1987 Immunocytochemical studies on thalamic afferent transmitters. In: Besson JM, Guilbaud G, Peschanski M (eds) Thalamus and pain. Excerpta Medica, Amsterdam, pp 83–109

Jones EG 1990 Correlation and revised nomenclature of ventral nuclei in the thalamus of human and monkey. Stereotactic and Functional Neurosurgery 54–55: 1–20

Jones EG 1997 A description of the human thalamus. In: Steriade M, Jones EG, McCormick DA (eds) Thalamus, vol II, Experimental and clinical aspects. Elsevier, Amsterdam, pp 425–500

Jones MW, Apkarian AV, Stevens RT, Hodge CJ Jr 1987 The spinothalamic tract: an examination of the cells of origin of the dorsolateral and ventral spinothalamic pathways in cats. Journal of Comparative Neurology 260: 349–361

Kaas JH, Nelson RJ, Sur M, Dykes RW, Merzenich MM 1984 The somatotopic organization of the ventroposterior thalamus of the squirrel monkey, *Saimiri sciureus*. Journal of Comparative Neurology 226: 111–140

Kaelber WW, Mitchell CL, Yarmat AJ, Afifi AK, Lorens SA 1975 Centrum medianum-parafascicularis lesions and reactivity to noxious and non-noxious stimuli. Experimental Neurology 46: 282–290

Kajander KC, Giesler GJ Jr 1987 Responses of neurons in the lateral cervical nucleus of the cat to noxious cutaneous stimulation. Journal of Neurophysiology 57: 1686–1704

Katter JT, Burstein R, Giesler GJ Jr 1991 The cells of origin of the spinohypothalamic tract in cats. Journal of Comparative Neurology 303: 101–112

Kawakita K, Dostrovsky JO, Tang JS, Chiang CY 1993 Responses of neurons in the rat thalamic nucleus submedius to cutaneous, muscle and visceral nociceptive stimuli. Pain 55: 327–338

Keay KA, Feil K, Gordon BD, Herbert H, Bandler R 1997 Spinal afferents to functionally distinct periaqueductal gray columns in the rat: an anterograde and retrograde tracing study. Journal of Comparative Neurology 385: 207–229

Keller O, Butkhuzi SM, Vyklicky L, Brozek G 1974 Cortical responses evoked by stimulation of tooth pulp afferents in the cat. Physiologia Bohemoslovaca 23: 45–53

Kenshalo DR Jr, Giesler GJ Jr, Leonard RB, Willis WD 1980 Responses of neurons in primate ventral posterior lateral nucleus to noxious stimuli. Journal of Neurophysiology 43: 1594–1614

Kenshalo DR Jr, Isensee O 1983 Responses of primate SI cortical neurons to noxious stimuli. Journal of Neurophysiology 50: 1479–1496

Kenshalo DR Jr, Anton F, Dubner R 1989 The detection and perceived intensity of noxious thermal stimuli in monkey and in human. Journal of Neurophysiology 62: 429–436

Kevetter GA, Willis WD 1983 Collaterals of spinothalamic cells in the rat. Journal of Comparative Neurology 215: 453–464

Kevetter GA, Haber LH, Yezierski RP, Chung JM, Martin RF, Willis WD 1982 Cells of origin of the spinoreticular tract in the monkey. Journal of Comparative Neurology 207: 61–74

Kharazia VN, Weinberg RJ 1994 Glutamate in thalamic fibers terminating in layer IV of primary sensory cortex. Journal of Neuroscience 14: 6021–6032

Kitamura T, Yamada J, Sato H, Yamashita K 1993 Cells of origin of the spinoparabrachial fibers in the rat: a study with fast blue and WGA-HRP. Journal of Comparative Neurology 328: 449–461

Kniffki K-D, Craig AD Jr 1985 The distribution of nociceptive neurons in the cat's lateral thalamus: the dorsal and ventral periphery of VPL. In: Rowe M, Willis WD (eds) Development, organization and processing in somatosensory pathways. Alan Liss, New York, pp 375–382

Kniffki K-D, Mizumura K 1983 Responses of neurons in VPL and VPL-VL regions of the cat to algesic stimulation of muscle and tendon. Journal of Neurophysiology 49: 649–661

Koyama N, Yokota T 1993 Ascending inhibition of nociceptive neurons in the nucleus ventralis posterolateralis following conditioning stimulation of the nucleus raphe magnus. Brain Research 609: 298–306

Krubitzer L, Clarey J, Tweedale R, Elston G, Calford M 1995 A redefinition of somatosensory areas in the lateral sulcus of macaque monkeys. Journal of Neuroscience 15: 3821–3839

Kunc Z 1970 Significant factors pertaining to the results of trigeminal tractotomy. In: Hassler R, Walker AE (eds) Trigeminal neuralgia. WB Saunders, Philadelphia, pp 90–98

Kupers RC, Gybels JM 1993 Electrical stimulation of the ventroposterolateral thalamic nucleus (VPL) reduces mechanical allodynia in a rat model of neuropathic pain. Neuroscience Letters 150: 95–98

Kuru M 1949 The sensory paths in the spinal cord and brain stem of man. Sogensya, Tokyo

Lee SM, Friedberg MH, Ebner FF 1994 The role of GABA-mediated inhibition in the rat ventral posterior medial thalamus. II. Differential effects of $GABA_A$ and $GABA_B$ receptor antagonists on responses of VPM neurons. Journal of Neurophysiology 71: 1716–1726

Lenz FA, Dougherty PM 1997 Pain processing in the human thalamus. In: Steriade M, Jones EG, McCormick DA (eds) Thalamus, vol II, Experimental and clinical aspects. Elsevier, Amsterdam, pp 617–652

Lenz FA, Dougherty PM 1998 Neurons in the human thalamic somatosensory nucleus (ventralis caudalis) respond to innocuous cool and mechanical stimuli. Journal of Neurophysiology 79: 2227–2230

Lenz FA, Seike M, Lin YC et al 1993a Neurons in the area of human thalamic nucleus ventralis caudalis respond to painful heat stimuli. Brain Research 623: 235–240

Lenz FA, Seike M, Richardson RT et al 1993b Thermal and pain sensations evoked by microstimulation in the area of human ventrocaudal nucleus. Journal of Neurophysiology 70: 200–212

Lenz FA, Gracely RH, Romanoski AJ, Hope EJ, Rowaland LH, Dougherty PM 1995 Stimulation in the human somatosensory thalamus can reproduce both the affective and sensory dimensions of previously experienced pain. Nature Medicine 1: 910–913

Lenz FA, Rios M, Zirh A, Chau D, Krauss G, Lesser RP 1998 Painful stimuli evoke potentials recorded over the human anterior cingulate gyrus. Journal of Neurophysiology 79: 2231–2234

Light AR 1992 The initial processing of pain and its descending control: spinal and trigeminal systems. Karger, Basel

Light AR, Sedivec MJ, Casale EJ, Jones SL 1993 Physiological and morphological characteristics of spinal neurons projecting to the parabrachial region of the cat. Somatosensory and Motor Research 10: 309–325

Loewy AD, Spyer KM 1990 Central regulation of autonomic functions. Oxford University Press, New York

Luccarini P, Cadet R, Saade M, Woda A 1995 Antinociceptive effect of morphine microinjections into the spinal trigeminal subnucleus oralis. NeuroReport 6: 365–368

Mackel R, Iriki A, Brink EE 1992 Spinal input to thalamic VL neurons: evidence for direct spinothalamic effects. Journal of Neurophysiology 67: 132–144

Magnusson KR, Clements JR, Larson AA, Mandl JE, Beitz AJ 1987 Localization of glutamate in trigeminothalamic projection neurons: a combination retrograde transport immunohistochemical study. Somatosensory and Motor Research 4: 177–190

Mahieux G, Benabid AL 1987 Naloxone-reversible analgesia induced by electrical stimulation of the habenula in the rat. Brain Research 406: 118–129

Maixner W, Dubner R, Kenshalo DR Jr, Bushnell MC, Oliveras J-L 1989 Responses of monkey medullary dorsal horn neurons during the detection of noxious heat stimuli. Journal of Neurophysiology 62: 437–449

Mansour A, Khachatourian H, Lewis ME, Akil H, Watson SJ 1987 Autoradiographic differentiation of mu, delta, and kappa opioid receptors in rat forebrain and midbrain. Journal of Neurosurgery 7: 2445–2464

Mantyh PW 1983 Connections of midbrain periaqueductal gray in the monkey. I ascending efferent projections. Journal of Neurophysiology 49: 567–581

Mantyh PW, Hunt SP 1984 Neuropeptides are present in projection neurones at all levels in visceral and taste pathways: from periphery to sensory cortex. Brain Research 299: 297–311

Mao J, Mayer DJ, Price DD 1993 Patterns of increased brain activity indicative of pain in a rat model of peripheral mononeuropathy. Journal of Neuroscience 13: 2689–2702

May WP 1906 The afferent path. Brain 29: 742–803

Mayer DJ, Price DD, Becker DP 1975 Neurophysiological characterization of the anterolateral spinal cord neurons contributing to pain perception in man. Pain 1: 51–58

McCormick DA 1992 Neurotransmitter actions in the thalamus and cerebral cortex and their role in neuromodulation of thalamocortical activity. Progress in Neurobiology 39: 337–388

Mehler WR 1966 The posterior thalamic region in man. Confinia Neurologica 27: 18–29

Mehler WR 1969 Some neurological species differences – a posteriori. Annals of the New York Academy of Science 167: 424–468

Mehler WR, Feferman ME, Nauta WJH 1960 Ascending axon degeneration following anterolateral cordotomy. An experimental study in the monkey. Brain 83: 718–750

Meller ST, Dennis BJ 1991 Efferent projections of the periaqueductal gray in the rabbit. Neuroscience 40: 191–216

Melzack R, Casey KL 1968 Sensory, motivational, and central control determinants of pain. In: Kenshalo DR (ed) The skin senses. Thomas, Springfield, pp 423–443

Mendell LM, Wall PD 1965 Responses of single dorsal cord cells to peripheral cutaneous unmyelinated fibres. Nature 206: 97–99

Meng ID, Hu JW, Benetti AP, Bereiter DA 1997 Encoding of corneal input in two distinct regions of the spinal trigeminal nucleus in the rat: cutaneous receptive field properties, responses to thermal and chemical stimulation, modulation by diffuse noxious inhibitory controls, and projections to the parabrachial area. Journal of Neurophysiology 77: 43–56

Menetrey D, Basbaum AI 1987 Spinal and trigeminal projections to the nucleus of the solitary tract: a possible substrate for somatovisceral and viscerovisceral reflex activation. Journal of Comparative Neurology 255: 439–450

Menétrey D, de Pommery J 1991 Origins of spinal ascending pathways that reach central areas involved in visceroception and visceronociception in the rat. European Journal of Neuroscience 3: 249–259

Menetrey D, Chaouch A, Besson JM 1980 Location and properties of dorsal horn neurons at origin of spinoreticular tract in lumbar enlargement of the rat. Journal of Neurophysiology 44: 862–877

Menetrey D, de Pommery J, Roudier F 1984 Properties of deep spinothalamic tract cells in the rat, with special reference to ventromedial zone of lumbar dorsal horn. Journal of Neurophysiology 52: 612–624

Miletic V, Coffield JA 1988 Enkephalin-like immunoreactivity in the nucleus submedius of the cat and rat thalamus. Somatosensory and Motor Research 5: 325–334

Miletic V, Coffield JA 1989 Responses of neurons in the rat nucleus submedius to noxious and innocuous mechanical cutaneous stimulation. Somatosensory and Motor Research 6: 567–588

Milne RJ, Foreman RD, Willis WD 1982 Responses of primate spinothalamic neurons located in the sacral intermediomedial gray (Stilling's nucleus) to proprioceptive input from the tail. Brain Research 234: 227–236

Morrison SF, Reis DJ 1989 Reticulospinal vasomotor neurons in the RVL mediate the somatosympathetic reflex. American Journal of Physiology 256: R1084–R1097

Morrow TJ, Casey KL 1992 State-related modulation of thalamic somatosensory responses in the awake monkey. Journal of Neurophysiology 67: 305–317

Mufson EJ, Mesulam MM 1984 Thalamic connections of the insula in the Rhesus monkey and comments on the paralimbic connectivity of the medial pulvinar nucleus. Journal of Comparative Neurology 227: 109–120

Musil SY, Olson CR 1988 Organization of cortical and subcortical projections to anterior cingulate cortex in the cat. Journal of Comparative Neurology 272: 203–218

Nagano S, Myers JA, Hall RD 1975 Representation of the cornea in the brain stem of the rat. Experimental Neurology 49: 653–670

Nathan PW, Smith MC 1979 Clinico-anatomical correlation in anterolateral cordotomy. In: Bonica JJ (ed) Advances in pain research and therapy, vol 3. Raven, New York, pp 921–926

Ness TJ, Gebhart GF 1990 Visceral pain: a review of experimental studies. Pain 41: 167–234

Newman HM, Stevens RT, Apkarian AV 1996 Direct spinal projections to limbic and striatal areas: anterograde transport studies from the upper cervical spinal cord and the cervical enlargement in squirrel monkey and rat. Journal of Comparative Neurology 365: 640–658

Nishiyama K, Kwak S, Murayama S, Kanazawa I 1995 Substance P is a possible neurotransmitter in the rat spinothalamic tract. Neuroscience Research 21: 261–266

Nomura T, Nishikawa N, Yokota T 1992 Intracellular HRP study of nociceptive neurons within the ventrobasal complex of the cat thalamus. Brain Research 570: 323–332

Noordenbos W, Wall PD 1976 Diverse sensory functions with an almost totally divided spinal cord. A case of spinal cord transection with preservation of part of one anterolateral quadrant. Pain 2: 185–195

Norrsell U 1989 Behavioural thermosensitivity after unilateral, partial lesions of the lateral funiculus in the cervical spinal cord of the cat. Experimental Brain Research 78: 369–373

Olausson B, Shyu B-C, Rydenhag B, Andersson S 1992 Thalamic nociceptive mechanisms in cats, influenced by central conditioning stimuli. Acta Physiologica Scandinavica 146: 49–59

Oliveras J-L, Maixner W, Dubner R 1996 Medullary dorsal horn: a target for expression of opiates effects upon the perceived intensity of noxious heat. Journal of Neuroscience 6: 3086–3093

Olszewski J 1952 The thalamus of the *Macaca mulatta*: an atlas for use with the stereotaxic instrument. Karger, Basel

Pagni CA 1976 Central pain and painful anesthesia. Progress in Neurological Surgery 8: 132–257

Palecek J, Dougherty PM, Kim SH et al 1992 Responses of spinothalamic tract neurons to mechanical and thermal stimuli in an experimental model of peripheral neuropathy in primates. Journal of Neurophysiology 68: 1951–1966

Panneton WM, Burton H 1985 Projections from the paratrigeminal nucleus and the medullary and spinal dorsal horns to the peribrachial area in the cat. Neuroscience 15: 779–797

Panneton WM, Yavari P 1995 A medullary dorsal horn relay for the cardiorespiratory responses evoked by stimulation of the nasal mucosa in the muskrat *Ondatra zibethicus*: evidence for excitatory amino acid transmission. Brain Research 691: 37–45

Perl ER 1984a Pain and nociception. In: Darian-Smith I (ed) Handbook of physiology, Section 1, The nervous system, vol III, Sensory processes. American Physiological Society, Bethesda, pp 915–975

Perl ER 1984b Why are selectively responsive and multireceptive neurons both present in somatosensory pathways? In: Ottoson D (ed) Somatosensory mechanisms. Plenum, New York, pp 141–161

Peschanski M 1984 Trigeminal afferents to the diencephalon in the rat. Neuroscience 12: 465–487

Peschanski M, Guilbaud G, Gautron M, Besson J-M 1980 Encoding of noxious heat messages in neurons of the ventrobasal thalamic complex of the rat. Brain Research 197: 401–413

Peschanski M, Guilbaud G, Gautron M 1981 Posterior intralaminar region in rat: neuronal responses to noxious and non-noxious cutaneous stimuli. Experimental Neurology 72: 226–238

Pirot S, Jay TM, Glowinski J, Thierry A-M 1994 Anatomical and electrophysiological evidence for an excitatory amino acid pathway from the thalamic mediodorsal nucleus to the prefrontal cortex in the rat. European Journal of Neuroscience 6: 1225–1234

Poggio GF, Mountcastle VB 1960 A study of the functional contributions of the lemniscal and spinothalamic systems to somatic sensibility. Bulletin of the Johns Hopkins Hospital 106: 266–316

Poulos DA 1981 Central processing of cutaneous temperature information. Federation Proceedings 40: 2825–2829

Price DD 1988 Psychological and neural mechanisms of pain. Raven, New York

Price DD, Dubner R, Hu JW 1976 Trigeminothalamic neurons in nucleus caudalis responsive to tactile, thermal, and nociceptive stimulation of monkey's face. Journal of Neurophysiology 39: 936–953

Rainville P, Duncan GH, Price DD, Carrier B, Bushnell MC 1997 Pain affect encoded in human anterior cingulate but not somatosensory cortex. Science 277: 968–971

Ralston HJ, III, Ralston DD 1992 The primate dorsal spinothalamic tract: evidence for a specific termination in the posterior nuclei (Po/SG) of the thalamus. Pain 48: 107–118

Ralston HJ, III, Ralston DD 1994 Medial lemniscal and spinal projections to the macaque thalamus: an electron microscopic study of differing GABAergic circuitry serving thalamic somatosensory mechanisms. Journal of Neuroscience 14: 2485–2502

Rausell E, Jones EG 1991 Chemically distinct compartments of the thalamic VPM nucleus in monkeys relay principal and spinal trigeminal pathways to different layers of the somatosensory cortex. Journal of Neuroscience 11: 226–237

Rausell E, Cusick CG, Taub E, Jones EG 1992 Chronic deafferentation in monkeys differentially affects nociceptive and nonnociceptive pathways distinguished by specific calcium-binding proteins and down-regulates gamma-aminobutyric acid type A receptors at thalamic levels. Proceedings of the National Academy of Sciences USA 89: 2571–2575

Ray JP, Price JL 1993 The organization of projections from the mediodorsal nucleus of the thalamus to orbital and medial prefrontal cortex in macaque monkeys. Journal of Comparative Neurology 337: 1–31

Reichling DB, Basbaum AI 1991 Collateralization of periaqueductal gray neurons to forebrain or diencephalon and to the medullary nucleus raphe magnus in the rat. Neuroscience 42: 183–200

Reyes-Vazquez C, Dafny N 1993 Microiontophoretically applied THIP effects upon nociceptive responses of neurons in medial thalamus. Applied Neurophysiology 46: 254–260

Richardson DE 1967 Thalamotomy for intractable pain. Confinia Neurologica 29: 139–145

Rinaldi PC, Young RF, Albe-Fessard D, Chodakiewitz J 1991 Spontaneous neuronal hyperactivity in the medial and intralaminar thalamic nuclei of patients with deafferentation pain. Journal of Neurosurgery 74: 415–421

Rinvik E, Wiberg M 1990 Demonstration of a reciprocal connection between the periaqueductal gray matter and the reticular nucleus of the thalamus. Anatomy and Embryology 181: 577–584

Roberts VJ, Dong WK 1994 The effect of thalamic nucleus submedius lesions on nociceptive responding in rats. Pain 57: 341–349

Roberts WA, Eaton SA, Salt TE 1992 Widely distributed GABA-mediated afferent inhibition processes within the ventrobasal thalamus of rat and their possible relevance to pathological pain states and somatotopic plasticity. Experimental Brain Research 89: 363–372

Rosenfeld JP, Pickrel C, Broton JG 1983 Analgesia for orofacial nociception produced by morphine microinjection into the spinal trigeminal complex. Pain 15: 145–155

Roy J-C, Bing Z, Villanueva L, Le Bars D 1992 Convergence of visceral and somatic inputs onto subnucleus reticularis dorsalis neurones in the rat medulla. Journal of Physiology (London) 458: 235–246

Royce GJ, Bromley S, Gracco C, Beckstead RM 1989 Thalamocortical connections of the rostral intralaminar nuclei: an autoradiographic analysis in the cat. Journal of Comparative Neurology 288: 555–582

Russell WR 1945 Transient disturbances following gunshot wounds of the head. Brain 68: 79–97

Rustioni A, Schmechel DE, Spreafico R, Cheema S, Cuenod M 1983 Excitatory and inhibitory amino acid putative neurotransmitters in the ventralis posterior complex: an autoradiographic and immunocytochemical study in rats and cats. In: Machhi G, Rustioni A, Spreafico R (eds) Somatosensory integration in the thalamus. Elsevier, Amsterdam, pp 365–383

Sadikot AF, Parent A, François C 1992 Efferent connections of the centromedian and parafascicular thalamic nuclei in the squirrel monkey: A PHA-L study of subcortical projections. Journal of Comparative Neurology 315: 137–159

Salt TE, Eaton SA 1995 Distinct presynaptic metabotropic receptors for L-AP4 and CCG1 on GABAergic terminals: pharmacological evidence using novel α-methyl derivative mGluR antagonists, MAP4 and MCCG, in the rat thalamus in vivo. Neuroscience 65: 5–13

Sano K 1979 Stereotaxic thalamolaminotomy and posteromedial hypothalamotomy for the relief of intractable pain. In: Bonica JJ, Ventafridda V (eds) Advances in pain research and therapy. Raven, New York, pp 475–485

Saper CB, Loewy AD 1980 Efferent connections of the parabrachial nucleus in the rat. Brain Research 197: 291–317

Sato A, Schmidt RF 1973 Somatosympathetic reflexes: afferent fibers, central pathways, discharge characteristics. Physiological Reviews 53: 916–947

Schlag J, Schlag-Rey M 1986 Role of the central thalamus in gaze control. Progress in Brain Research 64: 191–201

Sessle BJ 1987 The neurobiology of facial and dental pain: present knowledge, future directions. Journal of Dental Research 66: 962–981

Sessle BJ 1996 Craniofacial pain: brainstem mechanisms. Pain Research, Management 1: 111–118

Sessle BJ, Greenwood LF 1976 Inputs to trigeminal brain stem neurones from facial, oral, tooth pulp and pharyngolaryngeal tissues: I. Responses to innocuous and noxious stimuli. Brain Research 117: 211–226

Sessle BJ, Hu JW, Amano N, Zhong G 1986 Convergence of cutaneous, tooth pulp, visceral, neck and muscle afferents onto nociceptive and non-nociceptive neurones in trigeminal subnucleus caudalis (medullary dorsal horn) and its implications for referred pain. Pain 27: 219–235

Siegfried J 1987 Stimulation of thalamic nuclei in human: sensory and therapeutical aspects. In: Besson J-M, Guilbaud G, Peschanski M (eds) Thalamus and pain. Excerpta Medica, Amsterdam, pp 271–278

Sikes RW, Vogt BA 1992 Nociceptive neurons in area 24 of rabbit cingulate cortex. Journal of Neurophysiology 68: 1720–1732

Simone DA, Sorkin LS, Oh U et al 1991 Neurogenic hyperalgesia: central neural correlates in responses of spinothalamic tract neurons. Journal of Neurophysiology 66: 228–246

Sjoqvist O 1938 Studies on pain conduction in the trigeminal nerve. A contribution to the surgical treatment of facial pain. Acta Psychiatrica Scandinavica 17(suppl): 1–139

Snow PJ, Lumb BM, Cervero F 1992 The representation of prolonged and intense, noxious somatic and visceral stimuli in the ventrolateral orbital cortex of the cat. Pain 48: 89–99

Steriade M, Jones EG, McCormick DA 1997 Thalamus. Elsevier Science, Oxford

Stevens RT, Hodge CJ Jr, Apkarian AV 1989 Medial, intralaminar and lateral terminations of lumbar spinothalamic tract neurons: a fluorescent double-label study. Somatosensory Research 6: 285–308

Stevens RT, London SM, Apkarian AV 1993 Spinothalamocortical projections to the secondary somatosensory cortex (SII) in squirrel monkey. Brain Research 631: 241–246

Strassman A, Mason P, Moskowitz M, Maciewicz R 1986 Response of brainstem trigeminal neurons to electrical stimulation of the dura. Brain Research 379: 242–250

Strassman AM, Mineta Y, Vos BP 1994 Distribution of fos-like immunoreactivity in the medullary and upper cervical dorsal horn produced by stimulation of dural blood vessels in the rat. Journal of Neuroscience 14: 3725–3735

Sugiyama K, Ryu H, Uemura K 1992 Identification of nociceptive neurons in the medial thalamus: morphological studies of nociceptive neurons with intracellular injection of horseradish peroxidase. Brain Research 586: 36–43

Sweet WH 1982 Cerebral localization of pain. In: Thompson RA, Green JR (eds) New perspectives in cerebral localization. Raven, New York, pp 205–242

Talbot JD, Marrett S, Evans AC, Meyer E, Bushnell MC, Duncan GH 1991 Multiple representations of pain in human cerebral cortex. Science 251: 1355–1358

Tasker RR 1984 Stereotaxic surgery. In: Wall PD, Melzack R (eds) Textbook of pain. Churchill Livingstone, Edinburgh, pp 639–655

Tattersall JEH, Cervero F, Lumb BM 1986 Viscerosomatic neurons in lower thoracic spinal cord of the cat: excitations and inhibitions evoked by splanchnic and somatic nerve volleys and by stimulation of brain stem nuclei. Journal of Neurophysiology 56: 1411–1424

Terenzi MG, Prado WA 1990 Antinociception elicited by electrical or chemical stimulation of the rat habenular complex and its sensitivity to systemic antagonists. Brain Research 535: 18–24

Thiele FH, Horsley V 1901 A study of the degenerations observed in the central nervous system in a case of fracture dislocation of the spine. Brain 24: 519–531

Tommerdahl M, Delemos KA, Vierck CJ Jr, Favorov OV, Whitsel BL 1996 Anterior parietal cortical response to tactile and skin-heating stimuli applied to the same skin site. Journal of Neurophysiology 75: 2662–2670

Tsubokawa T, Katayama Y, Ueno Y, Moriyasu N 1981 Evidence for the involvement of frontal cortex in pain-related cerebral events in cats: increase in local cerebral blood flow by noxious stimuli. Brain Research 217: 179–185

Vierck CJ Jr, Greenspan JD, Ritz LA, Yeomans DC 1986 The spinal pathways contributing to the ascending conduction and the descending modulation of pain sensations and reactions. In: Yaksh TL (ed) Spinal afferent processing. Plenum, New York, pp 275–329

Vierck CJ Jr, Greenspan JD, Ritz LA 1990 Long-term changes in purposive and reflexive responses to nociceptive stimulation following anterolateral chordotomy. Journal of Neuroscience 10: 2077–2095

Villanueva L, de Pommery J, Menetrey D, Le Bars D 1991 Spinal afferent projections to subnucleus reticularis dorsalis in the rat. Neuroscience Letters 134: 98–102

Villanueva L, Desbois C, Le Bars D, Bernard JF 1998 Organization of diencephalic projections from the medullary subnucleus reticularis dorsalis and the adjacent cuneate nucleus: a retrograde and anterograde tracer study in the rat. Journal of Comparative Neurology 390: 133–160

Vyklicky L, Keller O, Jastreboff P, Vyklicky L Jr, Butkhuzi S 1977 Spinal trigeminal tractotomy and nociceptive reactions evoked by tooth pulp stimulation in the cat. Journal of Physiology (Paris) 73: 379–386

Walker AE 1940 The spinothalamic tract in man. Archives of Neurology and Psychiatry 43: 284–298

Westlund KN, Craig AD 1996 Association of spinal lamina I projections with brainstem catecholamine neurons in the monkey. Experimental Brain Research 110: 151–162

Westlund KN, Bowker RM, Ziegler MG, Coulter JD 1984 Origins and terminations of descending noradrenergic projections to the spinal cord of monkey. Brain Research 292: 1–16

White JC, Sweet WH 1969 Pain and the neurosurgeon: a forty-year experience. Thomas, Springfield

Wiberg M, Blomqvist A 1984 The spinomesencephalic tract in the cat: its cells of origin and termination pattern as demonstrated by the intraaxonal transport method. Brain Research 291: 1–18

Wiberg M, Westman J, Blomqvist A 1987 Somatosensory projection to the mesencephalon: an anatomical study in the monkey. Journal of Comparative Neurology 264: 92–117

Willis WD 1985 The pain system. Karger, Basel

Willis WD 1997 Nociceptive functions of thalamic neurons. In: Steriade M, Jones EG, McCormick DA (eds) Thalamus, vol II, Experimental and clinical aspects. Elsevier, Amsterdam, pp 373–424

Willis WD, Trevino DL, Coulter JD, Maunz RA 1974 Responses of primate spinothalamic tract neurons to natural stimulation of hindlimb. Journal of Neurophysiology 37: 358–372

Willis WD, Kenshalo DR Jr, Leonard RB 1979 The cells of origin of the primate spinothalamic tract. Journal of Comparative Neurology 188: 543–574

Woods AH 1913 Segmental distribution of spinal root nucleus of the trigeminal nerve. Journal of Nervous and Mental Disease 40: 91–101

Yasui Y, Itoh K, Kamiya H, Ino T, Mizuno N 1988 Cingulate gyrus of the cat receives projection fibers from the thalamic region ventral to the ventral border of the ventrobasal complex. Journal of Comparative Neurology 274: 91–100

Yasui Y, Saper CB, Cechetto DF 1989 Calcitonin gene-related peptide immunoreactivity in the visceral sensory cortex, thalamus, and related pathways in the rat. Journal of Comparative Neurology 290: 487–501

Yasui Y, Breder CD, Saper CB, Cechetto DF 1991 Autonomic responses and efferent pathways from the insular cortex in the rat. Journal of Comparative Neurology 303: 355–374

Yezierski RP 1988 Spinomesencephalic tract: projections from the lumbosacral spinal cord of the rat, cat, and monkey. Journal of Comparative Neurology 267: 131–146

Yezierski RP, Mendez CM 1991 Spinal distribution and collateral projections of rat spinomesencephalic tract cells. Neuroscience 44: 113–130

Yezierski RP, Schwartz RH 1986 Response and receptive-field properties of spinomesencephalic tract cells in the cat. Journal of Neurophysiology 55: 76–96

Yezierski RP, Sorkin LS, Willis WD 1987 Response properties of spinal neurons projecting to midbrain or midbrain-thalamus in the monkey. Brain Research 437: 165–170

Yokota T, Nishikawa N 1980 Reappraisal of somatotopic tactile representation within trigeminal subnucleus caudalis. Journal of Neurophysiology 43: 700–712

Yokota T, Asato F, Koyama N, Masuda T, Taguchi H 1988 Nociceptive body representation in nucleus ventralis posterolateralis of cat thalamus. Journal of Neurophysiology 60: 1714–1727

Yoshida A, Dostrovsky JO, Sessle BJ, Chiang CY 1991 Trigeminal projections to the nucleus submedius of the thalamus in the rat. Journal of Comparative Neurology 307: 609–625

Yoshida A, Dostrovsky JO, Chiang CY 1992 The afferent and efferent connections of the nucleus submedius in the rat. Journal of Comparative Neurology 324: 115–133

Young RF 1982 Effect of trigeminal tractotomy on dental sensation in humans. Journal of Neurosurgery 56: 812–818

Young RF, Perryman KM 1984 Pathways for orofacial pain sensation in trigeminal brain-stem nucleus complex of macaque monkey. Journal of Neurophysiology 61: 536–568

Young RF, Tronnier V, Rinaldi PC 1992 Chronic stimulation of the Kölliker-Fuse nucleus region for relief of intractable pain in humans. Journal of Neurosurgery 76: 979–985

Zhang ET, Craig AD 1997 Morphology and distribution of spinothalamic lamina I neurons in the monkey. Journal of Neuroscience 17: 3274–3284

Zhang D, Carlton SM, Sorkin LS, Willis WD 1990 Collaterals of primate spinothalamic tract neurons to the periaqueductal gray. Journal of Comparative Neurology 296: 277–290

Zhang JH, Chandler MJ, Miller KE, Foreman RD 1997 Cardiopulmonary sympathetic afferent input does not require dorsal column pathways to excite C_1–C_3 spinal cells in rats. Brain Research 771: 25–30

The image of pain

MARTIN INGVAR & JEN-CHUEN HSIEH

A picture says more than a thousand words
– and that is just the problem.

The development of experimental models possibly mimicking various clinical pain syndromes has provided a better view of the supraspinal mechanisms of pain (for a review see Bennett 1994). While it is possible to understand the rational for the development of animal models of nociception, such models are notoriously difficult to use when other aspects of pain are investigated. The human pain experience is a complex biopsychosocial event and a multidimensional experience manifesting sensory-discriminative, cognitive-evaluative and affective-motivational components (Melzack and Casey 1968). Functional neuroimaging of the pain experience provides a unique instrument for better understanding of this multifaceted entity, as can be seen in several chapters in this book. The technical complexity of brain imaging, but also the complexity in terms of the methods used for statistical characterization of the data, warrants scrutiny of some of the basic principles in order to correctly appraise what brain imaging can offer in furthering the knowledge on pain processing. Some of the imaging literature may appear difficult to reconcile with information from other sources. Also, the significant amount of variation in the results from imaging studies may be accounted for by differences in experimental paradigms and imaging technology/statistics.

Pain is an unpleasant experience that involves the conscious awareness of noxious sensations, hurting and aversive feelings associated with actual or potential tissue damage (IASP 1994). This wide definition recognizes that the experience of pain is modulated by a complex set of emotional, environmental and psychophysiological variables (Price 1988; Feuerstein 1989). Pain can therefore be expected to influence brain processing on many levels. This influence is not only expressed in terms of pain processing proper, but also by competition for central mechanisms of consciousness such as attention, information selection, learning and anticipation. This complexity represents a challenge in that most neuroimaging today has a modular approach where isolation of singular cognitive components are sought. The experience of pain like any conscious experience is multifaceted and modified by many mechanisms, and hence isolation of singular processing components is at best difficult. Great care has to be taken in the design in order to achieve interpretable results. The aim of this chapter is to provide enough background in imaging in order to correctly appreciate the flood of imaging literature on pain.

METHODOLOGICAL CONSIDERATIONS

Functional imaging data presents a mixture of morphological and functional information. Some entities are more apt to generate data on morphology whereas other often sacrifice resolution when gaining information that is related to function in the time domain. Since generalization of the data obtained is important when building knowledge, a central goal is to limit the impact of morphological differences between the subjects. The development of imaging with increasing resolution makes it even more difficult to reach this goal. Figure 8.1 illustrates the temporal and spatial resolution of current methods in functional imaging.

General limitations of different imaging tools

Our understanding of the brain's functional organization constrains and informs the way in which functional

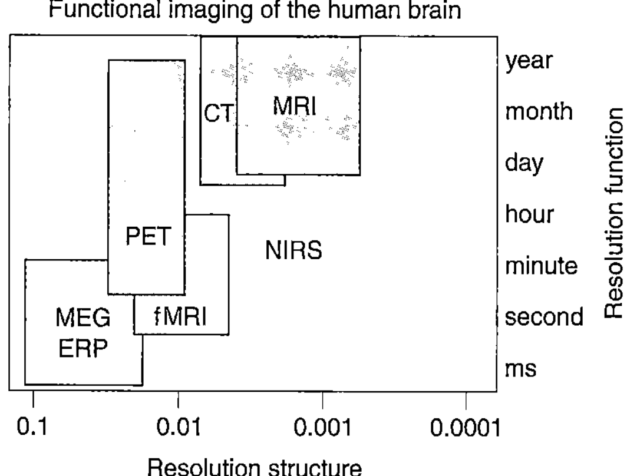

Fig. 8.1 Depiction of the temporal and spatial resolution of the currently used methods for functional neuroimaging in the intact human brain. (Freely adapted from Posner & Raichle 1994).

neuroimaging data are analysed and therefore also affects the results. Functional neuroimaging provides unique tools for such studies, as these methods allow the study of the whole brain either continuously or at discrete time points. Functional neuroimaging often rests on the haemodynamic response following a change in neuronal activity. The regional cerebral blood flow (rCBF) is increased following increased metabolic demand in the aftermath of increased neuronal traffic. Given that the energy reserve is very limited in the brain, the only way to increase the supply of oxygen and glucose is by increasing the rCBF. Even after a very brief and well-defined event this vascular response is late (≈5 s following the event) and biphasic, as it contains an early positive response followed by an undershoot that last up to 30 seconds. The relative tardiness of the response function has to be taken into account when designing experiments.

Resolution in time: single-events versus functional state changes

Our interpretation of functional imaging studies relies on many different models. Some are explicit (e.g., the general linear model used in statistical analysis) and some are of a more implicit nature (e.g., functional specialization when inferring the nature of activations or pure insertion in cognitive subtraction). These models embody the assumptions that are required to make sense of the data. Any assumption has a certain degree of uncertainty. Hence, the validity of the assumptions must be assured and, above all, one must be aware of what assumptions underlie any presented data.

Experimentally induced changes in brain activity which last considerably longer than the initiation of the vascular response can be considered as steady-state changes when imaged. If the studied event is shorter than the time resolution of the employed imaging method, often pseudo-steady-state changes are induced by repetition of the event at a known frequency. These study designs have an implication on how the imaging data may be interpreted, as frequency of repetition has an influence on the magnitude of response.

Transient changes elicited by brief stimuli can be detected as event-related signals with both electrophysiological and rCBF based methods (Friston et al 1998a,b). In most cases it seems important to perform repeated sampling in order to characterize the response. Such repetitions of stimulus are not trivial from the experimental point of view (see below). Event-related responses are characterized in their synchrony with the eliciting event. However, as most readers are aware, with each processing step, the response becomes less and less synchronous to the initial event and hence loose in detectability as a result of background noise.

Brain function is often described as organized as parallel distributed processes (Rumelhart & McClelland 1986) and the brain is normally not characterized by a serial mode of operation, rather it represents a parallel mode of working on many levels with feed-forwards and backwards mechanisms amply represented (Carpenter & Grossberg 1989). Hence, event-related methods have a limited application for events other than those that are well defined in time. In general terms, this implies events that are related to brain input or output because with input and output the phase determination for the recording can be made accurately. The neuronal response to repeated touch or painful events can therefore be well characterized with ERP methods, whereas higher order cortical events are more difficult to investigate with such methods.

Resolution and precision in space

Spatial resolution is an important issue in all imaging because it limits the information that it is possible to extract from the material. On many occasions the concept of resolution is misinterpreted for that of spatial precision. Resolution of an instrument is defined as FWHM (full width, half maximum), which is the distance between two equally strong point sources needed in order to diminish the value between them to half of that read in the maxima. It is often more appropriate to discuss the effective resolution, i.e. the resolution following all imaging processing steps, because realignment, reformatting and filtering of the images influence the final resolution. Post hoc estimation of the effective resolution is one way to account for the combination of method and biologically based autocorrelations (Friston et al 1991).

Spatial precision is critical when it comes to the anatomical interpretation of the results. Poor resolution of the imaging method adds complexity, because poor intrinsic resolution decreases the recovery of the true signal. The amount of filtering in the post processing must be determined thoughtfully. A filter is often applied for statistical reasons but too much filtering will decrease the signal (Fig. 8.2).

The trade-off between resolution and statistical power

In imaging each element of resolution is effectively assigned one null hypothesis. Multiple non-independent statistical processes necessitate correction for multiple comparisons (Fig. 8.3). A very conservative method for doing this would be to use Bonferroni-type correction (Friston et al 1991). However, such a procedure would, in many situations, be overly conservative and hence not a productive route. Several methods have been published in which different approaches have been developed to handle the problem of the error estimation and some of these have been severely criticized for being too liberal and thereby lacking specificity (Roland et al 1993, Frackowiak et al 1996, Roland & Gulyas 1996). The statistical methods have developed rapidly over the last years and several sophisticated means of determining differences within or between groups have been developed. It is noteworthy that the sample sizes in imaging studies have grown over the last years, with a general awareness of the instability of results with low numbers of observations.

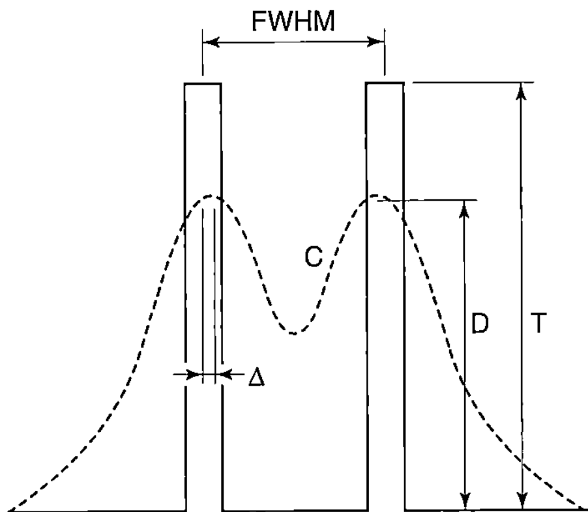

Fig. 8.2 Two point sources with equal signal (T) are detected with a signal strength (D) due to limited recovery of original signal. The resolution (FWHM) may be described as the distance between two sources that is necessary to decrease the signal strength by 50% (C). The spatial precision for the determination of the location of a point source is often better than the FWHM. Note that adjacent sources slightly dislocate the detected point of maxima by a distance Δ.

Adjacent pixels (picture elements) are correlated in that it is more likely that a pixel covaries with a chosen pixel than if the pixel is at a distance from the chosen one. This interdependency reduces the number of effective elements that can be resolved and thereby reduces the number of hypotheses that are tested. In this context it should be noted that a major difference between positron emission tomography (PET) and functional magnetic resonance imaging (fMRI) is that this correlation between observations also holds true for the time dimension in fMRI, making it even more complex to correctly estimate the levels of significance (Friston et al. 1995b,c, Worsley & Friston 1995).

Each pixel contains information on location and function. Hence, the more fine grained the morphological information, the higher the risk of contaminating the functional information with artefacts stemming from the morphology, especially if group/intergroup studies are performed. Most analysis approaches therefore contain a registering step in which differences in morphology between subjects are minimized by reformatting the images to a common stereotactical space. Mostly, global algorithms are used, i.e. algorithms that bend, skew, scale and twist the whole slice or image volume (Friston et al 1991, Greitz et al 1991, Friston et al 1995a). However lately algorithms that reformat the image locally have been introduced, but most of these have yet to prove improvements in specificity and sensitivity in the end result.

METHODS BASED ON THE CEREBROVASCULAR RESPONSE

Kety and Schmidt published the first paper on the quantitative measurement of cerebral blood flow and rapidly became aware of the fact that only course manipulations with the physiology (e.g. CO_2 and insulin coma) would induce changes in global CBF. They speculated that regional changes would be more expressed in normal variations of, for example, mental activity. A decade and a half later the method for measurement of rCBF in cortex based on injection of ^{133}Xe intracarotidly was published. The first conclusion was that indeed the regional variations in blood flow were more expressed than the global variations. Also, for the first time it was possible to study regional blood flow in conjunction with behaviour and different sensory stimuli and mental activity (Ingvar 1975, 1976). A drawback of the method is that it was not localizing the activity in 3D and a remaining unresolved difference between the results

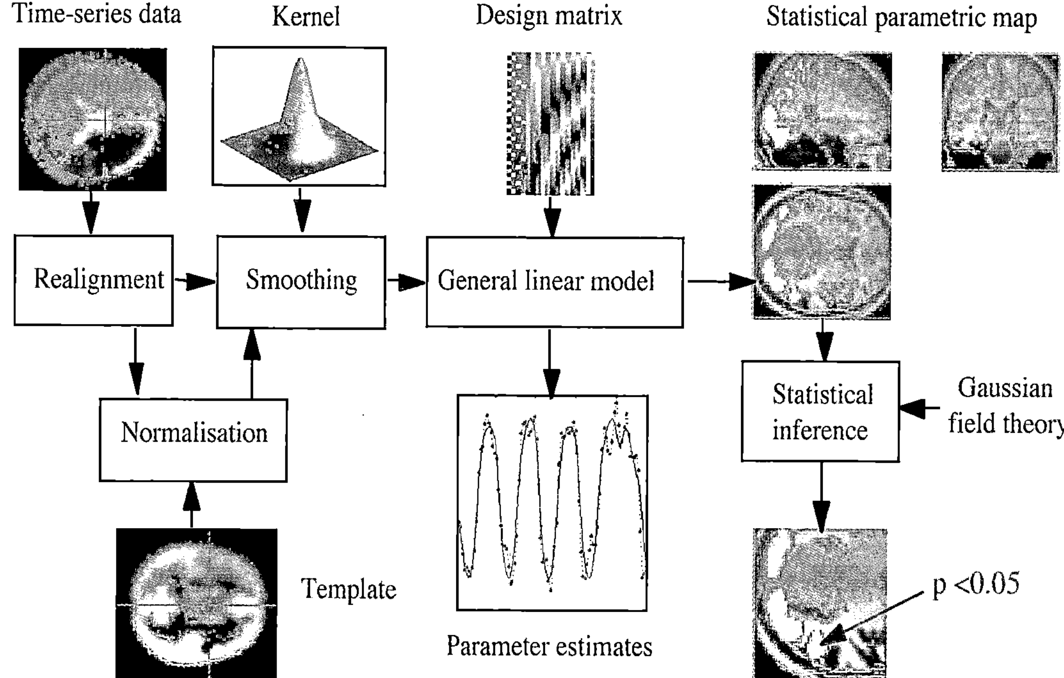

Fig. 8.3 A schematic presentation of the different steps of post processing of image data from PET/fMRI. The realignment step checks for movement-related artefacts. Normalization is an optional step where all images are transformed to a common anatomical space, smoothing is used to handle high-frequency noise in the image. Following this a statistical model is applied and then maps are created which depict the results. (Courtesy of Karl Friston 1998, see further http://www.fil.ion.ucl.ac.uk/spm/course/notes.html.) (see colour plate)

obtained with these methods and results from PET seems to be the 'hyperfrontal pattern' reported during undisturbed rest condition (Ingvar & Philipson 1977, Ingvar 1979). A full account of the nature of the resting state seems pertinent, because the resting state is not a passive state and rather stereotype changes in brain activity seem to occur when comparing the resting state with practically any state that requires attention to the outside world (Ghatan et al 1995, Shulman et al 1997, Ingvar et al 1998).

The two major methods presently used for functional imaging are PET and fMRI. They seem to reveal results that correlate closely albeit the signal response in fMRI is somewhat lower (Dettmers et al 1996).

PET rCBF

There are several excellent reviews and books available covering PET methodology in general (Frackowiak et al 1997, Raichle 1997). PET rCBF measurements have improved our knowledge to a great extent about the general principles of brain function and behaviour. The early limitations of the instrumentation are today much less of a problem with the advent of 3D acquisition and reconstruction of images. This technological step allowed a better use of the injected radioactivity and hence today 12 scans in one individual yields less than half of an absorbed dose of an ordinary clinical CT.

PET methodology rests on the intravenous injection of a tracer that is distributed in proportion to the blood flow. Well-established principles for the kinetic behaviour of the tracer are used (Lassen & Perl 1979). The injections can be made as a fast bolus injection but many laboratories have implemented a more protracted injection scheme in order to obtain a higher total radioactive count and thereby better image statistics. A measurement of the input function (the amount of radioactivity available for the brain) is necessary for the full quantification of the regional cerebral blood flow. However, this is seldom done because either normalization or covariance procedures can be used in order to account for variations in the global blood flow (Fox & Mintum 1989, Friston et al 1990, Ingvar et al 1994). The most common tracer is radioactive water ($[^{15}O]H_2O$), a tracer which has some diffusion limitation resulting in a slight underestimation at high levels of flow caused by loss of tracer in the tissue. On the other hand, $[^{15}O]$butanol, which avoids this problem and seems to allow for a proper quantification of the rCBF (Herzog et al 1996), only improves the detected signals slightly when applying the non-quantitative methods.

 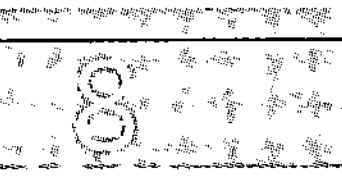

SPECT rCBF

Single photon emission computed tomography (SPECT) has been successfully used in pain imaging in a few instances. Limitations in resolution and in the number of studies that can be performed in the same subject (and especially in voluntary subjects) limits the ability to use SPECT in the collection of large data sets. The systematic differences between rCBF determined with PET and SPECT seems to be limited, in spite of the differences in the characteristics of the tracer substances (Jonsson et al 1998). The ability to extend the observation time for collection of the blood flow data and the possibility of performing the injection in a non-camera environment with later scanning may to some extent provide experimental advantages for this method.

fMRI

It is probable that the rapid developments within fMRI will improve our possibilities of achieving 3D functional imaging on an individual basis. The reasons are several. Firstly, imaging may be performed on regular clinically used instruments at 1.5 T (Schad et al 1995) which are present in many sites. Seemingly successful studies have even been reported at 1.0 T (Jones et al 1998). However, the trend is clear that several groups are taking advantage of higher field magnets in the urge to improve signal-to-noise characteristics of fMRI (Menon et al 1993). Secondly, fMRI has the advantage over PET that large amounts of data may be collected in each subject and essentially it is only the time in the camera and changes of response over time (habituation, learning, tiredness, etc.) which limits the time of study. Lastly, it is possible to successfully use fMRI to study the vascular response following single (but repeated) events (Buckner et al 1998, Friston et al 1998b, Rosen et al 1998).

In contrast to PET, the fMRI environment embodies physical constraints which may restrict the stimulus presentation and subject's response. It should be noted that access of the experimenter to the subject during the experiment is limited, as the subject needs to be placed completely inside the bore of the magnet. The most common fMRI methods rest on blood oxygen level detection (BOLD signal). This is essentially an intra- and perivascular signal. The advantage is that rapid repeated estimations of the BOLD signal can be made (semicontinuous measurements) during protracted sessions. The intravascular nature represents a problem in that it is non-stable and may move along the venous drainage. The lag of the blood flow response from time of stimulus onset combined with the poststimulus undershoot of the BOLD signal presents a special problem in that it directly interferes with the allowed design (e.g., rate of repetition).

Of special importance in pain studies are problems with paradigm-synchronous movements. Prestimulus apprehension seems to induce slight movements and must be avoided even if parts can be removed in the post processing by image realignment. A danger with this approach is in the event of stimulus correlated motion, where true signal correlations are removed from the time series. Also, physiological noise from respiration and circulation must be accounted for as it provides a significant interference with the interpretation of results. Most fMRI studies to date have been performed using a boxcar design with alternating epochs of rest and a single activation task of about 30 s. This ensures that activations of interest and physiological noise are confounded as little as possible. Lately, several groups have developed event-related fMRI (see below). Those approaches tend to minimize the noise from physiological variables, as the stimuli may be administered randomly in the time domain.

Increases and decreases in rCBF

Functional neuroimaging is heavily leaning on the idea that cerebral work leads to increased energy metabolism and a disproportional augmentation of cerebral blood flow (Fox & Raichle 1986). Hence, the signal does not separate primary excitatory and inhibitory neural firing. The cerebrovascular response only detects state-dependent changes in compounded activity of inhibitory and excitatory neurons. While increases in activity have been readily accepted as an expression of increased brain work, curiously, decreases have been less readily accepted as an index of the opposite. There is experimental data suggesting that an active inhibitory process may take place at the site of reduced rCBF (Freund & Antal 1988, Tsen & Haberly 1988, Seitz & Roland 1992, Ghatan et al 1995). Because the rCBF changes are tightly coupled to the levels of regional neuronal activity (Raichle 1987), the increase and decrease in rCBF accordingly indicate either an increased or a diminished net neuronal activity, respectively, and therefore physiologically imply a paradigm-specific (compared to the reference sate), functional activation or inhibition/disengagement of the involved brain regions (Haxby et al 1994, Drevets et al 1995, Ghatan et al 1998). It is therefore justifiable to base the interpretation of rCBF-based data on this operational interpretation.

METHODS BASED ON EVENT-RELATED RESPONSES

For obvious reasons recordings of the electrophysiological responses seem to be the ideal method in the quest for understanding the organization of the brain work. The unsurpassed resolution in time combined with increasing accuracy of models for 3D localization of activity makes these methods attractive candidates for the future (Hari & Kaukoranta 1985, Huttunen et al 1986, Fukushima et al 1994, Tarkka et al 1995, Thatcher 1995, Hari et al 1997). There still exist major problems in that the models of detection of multiple sources create problems for the investigation. Modern algorithms together with a multitude of squids show great promise, especially in the detection of cortically located pain responses, and reports on at least semiquantitive response evaluations have occurred (Hari et al 1997). Also, the impressive resolution in time makes it possible to enlighten the mechanisms underlying laterality in response to unilateral stimulation. Magnetoencephalography (MEG) data suggest that SII seems to receive bilateral input and respond synchronously to elicited pain (Kakigi et al 1995).

EEG-based methods have now improved a lot with the use of multielectrode arrays. The combination of different imaging methods shows a great promise (Rosler et al 1995). Realistic head models may provide further improvements and allow more than surface modelling of brain activity with spatial reliability (Babiloni et al 1997).

The combination of electrophysiology with fMRI has great promise for the future in improving the description of brain events in the spatial and temporal domain (Menon et al 1997). The importance of event-related fMRI is not only in the ability to time different events but also to reduce or even eliminate the problems with low-frequency physiological noise, because stimulus presentation can be randomized in the time domain (Friston et al 1998a,b). It is foreseeable that such approaches will dominate further developments in fMRI (Rosen et al 1998).

METHODS BASED ON CHEMICAL/PHARMACOLOGICAL RESPONSE

Receptor mapping studies

Studies of different brain receptor systems during pain are theoretically very appealing. Basic studies of pain-relevant receptor systems' anatomy can be obtained with PET (Jones et al 1991b). It would be of great interest to demonstrate changes in response to, for example, chronic pain. Indeed some successful trials have been reported demonstrating changes using diprenorphine as the probe. A group of four patients with rheumatoid arthritis were examined to test the hypothesis that there is a change in the endogenous opioid system in the brain during inflammatory pain. Regional cerebral opioid receptor binding was quantified using the opioid receptor antagonist [^{11}C]diprenorphine and positron emission tomography (PET). In the four patients studied in and out of pain, significant increases in [^{11}C]diprenorphine binding were seen in association with a reduction in pain. Increases were seen in most of the areas of the brain that were sampled apart from the occipital cortex. These findings suggest increases in occupancy by endogenous opioid peptides during inflammatory pain. (Jones et al 1994)

A major difficulty is the contamination of the blood flow signal when extracting the information about binding potential and also the more sophisticated receptor parameters when comparing receptor function in different brain states such as pain/pain free states (Jones et al 1991b) or rest versus mental activity (Koepp et al 1998). Kinetic methods seem to be especially prone to such a confounding and steady-state methods seem to be a solution for those who attempt such studies (Lassen 1992).

Future developments in this area seems to be in the serotonergic, dopaminergic and adenosinergic system. All these systems now have developed ligands for use in PET with medium affinity to the target area.

STATISTICAL CONSIDERATIONS

Cerebral functional imaging generates an abundance of data. The statistical treatment of the data is by no means trivial and global searches are notoriously insensitive. Data from subtraction analyses are sometimes difficult to interpret because the proper analysis rests on the ability to control all experimental details in such a way that only relevant details differ between the studied states (Friston et al 1996). However, in well-designed studies with properly formed hypotheses there are several strategies at hand to improve both specificity and sensitivity.

If the search volume is restricted to a few well-defined regions that can be anatomically described, then the effect of correcting for multiple comparisons becomes negligible, in other words if the study is made with the aim to understand one mechanism, then test only for that. A limitation of the anatomical search volume can also be made by inferring the result from another source (e.g., data from other scans in different or same subjects) by a masking and conjunction approach (Price & Friston 1997). Following restricted searches a global search of an exploratory nature can be performed.

Correlation with psychophysical measures and subjective rating

The approach of using external parameters regressing the rCBF can be used to estimate the relative involvement of

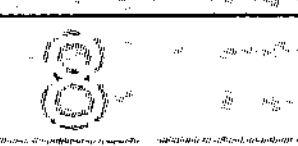

different cortical areas for the different aspects of a task (Grasby et al 1994), and is a method that seems well suited for the study of different aspects of pain perception such as pain affect.

Recently, it was demonstrated that hypnotic suggestions could alter selectively the unpleasantness of noxious stimuli, without changing the perceived intensity. PET revealed significant changes in pain-evoked activity within the anterior cingulate cortex, consistent with the encoding of perceived unpleasantness, whereas primary somatosensory cortex activation was unaltered (Rainville et al 1997). This study elegantly demonstrated that it is possible to separate the functional anatomy of the different axis of pain perception. Along these lines it has been shown that cognitive loading may reduce both the perceived pain intensity and also the level of activation due to experimentally induced pain (Hsieh et al 1998, Petrovic et al 1998a).

Principal component analyses and other non-explicitly hypothesis-driven statistical approaches

Functional integration is mediated by the interactions between functionally segregated areas. One way of characterizing these interactions is in terms of functional or effective connectivity. In the analysis of neuroimaging time series functional connectivity may be defined as the temporal correlations between spatially remote neurophysiological events (Friston et al 1993b). The alternative is to refer explicitly to effective connectivity (i.e., the influence one neuronal system exerts over another) (Friston et al 1993a). Principal component analysis could be viewed as an exploratory method for finding inherent structure in the imaging data. Such analyses could be interpreted in terms of functional connectivity, defined as the temporal correlation of a neurophysiological index measured in different brain areas. There are however no methods to date to allow a determination of what could be considered a good result. Hence, these approaches illustrate the learning paradox which states that if we do not understand something, we cannot set about learning it, because we do not know about how to begin (Plato, The dialogue Meno).

IMAGING THE CENTRAL PAIN MATRIX

Indeed methods other than functional neuroimaging have provided the basic information regarding the supraspinal organization of the pain systems. Advanced anatomical tracing techniques and delicate electrophysiological methods have not only allowed better mapping of the classical pathways but also revealed numerous novel ascending tracts and nociresponsive supraspinal structures (Apkarian & Shi 1994, Brüggemann et al 1994, Craig et al 1994, Guilbaud et al 1994).

For long it was debated to what extent the cerebral cortex was necessary for the experience of pain. The thalamus is the relay centre for afferent input to the brain and can be broadly characterized into medial (paleo-)thalamus and lateral (neo-)thalamus. Only the lateral systems seem to be somatotopically organized and project mainly to the sensory cortices (SI and SII). The medial thalamus receives input from multiple ascending systems of the spinal cord and the reticular formation. Pathways from the medial thalamus project diffusely to wide areas of the cortex and together comprise the 'medial pain system'. The supraspinal structures participating in processing nociceptive information include the reticular formation including the periaqueductal grey (PAG), the hypothalamus (HT), the thalamus, the limbic system and several areas in the cortex (for a review see Bonica 1990). To date a large number of imaging studies have been performed. In spite of sometimes very disparate study paradigms, a striking consistency seems to prevail about the functional neuroanatomy of the central pain matrix when examining main effects in subtraction designs (pain vs non-pain state). An anatomically stratified review of some of the most important structures will follow.

LATERAL AND MEDIAL PAIN SYSTEMS

The anterior cingulate cortex (BA 24/32):

The anterior cingulate cortex (ACC) is the cortical region that is activated in almost every study of elicited pain starting with the first studies of PET and pain (Jones et al 1991a, Talbot et al 1991). The ACC is a large structure that is functionally segregated in several parts, and the loci of activation in the ACC varies between studies based on the construction of the imaging paradigm. Previous studies have shown that the ACC is involved in nociceptive processing and that lesions in the ACC reduce the reaction to nociceptive input (Vaccarino & Melzack 1989). The rostral section (perigenual) will be activated in almost any study where differences in the level of attention has not been balanced between the different states, which is analogous to the ACC activation in studies of executive attention (Pardo et al 1990, Bench et al 1992, Ghatan et al 1995). In paradigms that are more balanced for attention the pain-elicited activation is generally more caudal and more confined to the Broddman area 24 (Hsieh et al 1995, Davis et al 1997). Thus, it seems that the general stratification of the ACC into subregions of visceromotor, skeletomotor control cortex and nociceptive cortex that was developed from animal studies and sparse human lesion data (Devinsky et al 1995) has been confirmed by functional imaging data. This general conclusion is however not undisputed. Vogt et al have argued that activations in the perigenual ACC represent affective components of pain, whereas the caudally situated activation is more representative of response selection like 'nocifensive reflex inhibition' (Vogt et al 1996). In a subsequent paper by Derbyshire and colleagues, an attempt was made to stratify the different components of the anterior cingulate cortex by using paradigms of either pain stimulus or challenge of attention mechanisms by means of the Stroop colour word interference test. The design was that of separate experiments in the same individuals and individual analysis suggested a separation of the functional anatomical representation for the two paradigms (Derbyshire et al 1998). This conclusion was based on observations from the different contrast rather than by calculation from a factorial design, and hence a firm conclusion on this matter remains tentative. In contrast to the studies on phasic pain, tonic stimuli of heat or cold seems less efficient in evoking rCBF changes in the ACC (Coghill et al 1993, DiPiero et al 1994). However with intense tonic stimuli there seems to be no difficulty in provoking ACC activations (Casey et al 1996).

ACC is part of the medial pain system and the functional significance of the caudal ACC activation seems to be in the affective-evaluative dimension (Vogt et al 1993). Robust activations are seen here in experimental conditions where acute pain is elicited (Talbot et al 1991; Guilbaud et al 1994, Tarkka & Treede 1994, Kakigi et al 1995, Davis et al 1997). This seems also to be true for visceral pain (Aziz et al 1997). In chronic pain states with habitual pain the activity is reduced upon pain alleviation (Hsieh et al 1995) (Fig. 8.4). In the study of Rainville and colleagues hypnotic suggestions were used to alter selectively the unpleasantness of noxious stimuli, without changing the perceived intensity. The pain-evoked activity within the ACC was significantly reduced by this manipulation, whereas primary somatosensory cortex activation was unaltered which indicates the selectivity of the ACC response (Rainville et al 1997). Reciprocally, it was possible by the experimental set-up of the thermal grill illusion to produce activation in the ACC. The illusion was created by touching warm and cool bars that were spatially interlaced and this produced a painful burning sensation resembling that caused by intense, noxious cold. The same area was also activated by noxious heat or cold but not by warm and cold stimuli (Craig et al 1996).

As mentioned, in chronic pain states with habitual pain the ACC is chronically activated (Hsieh et al 1995). In peripheral mononeuropathy where ongoing pain was present provocation of mechanical allodynia ('pain on pain') did not provoke an ACC activation, a finding that was interpreted as a different role of the ACC in chronic pain states (Peyron et al 1998). Given the presence of the spontaneous pain in the studied group of patients the variability in the ACC activity would be expected to be high, explaining the absence of significant activation. In a study of patients with mechanical allodynia we instead correlated the ACC activity to the reported pain intensity, thereby accounting for the presence of different levels of spontaneous and elicited pain, and found an activation in the ACC. Hence, our data do not support an altered correlation between the suffering component of pain and activity in the ACC in chronic pain (Petrovic et al 1998b).

Thalamus

The thalamus is the relay centre for afferent input to the brain and can be broadly characterized into medial (paleothalamus and lateral (neo-)thalamus. The former, which includes the medial and intralaminar nuclei, is not somato-

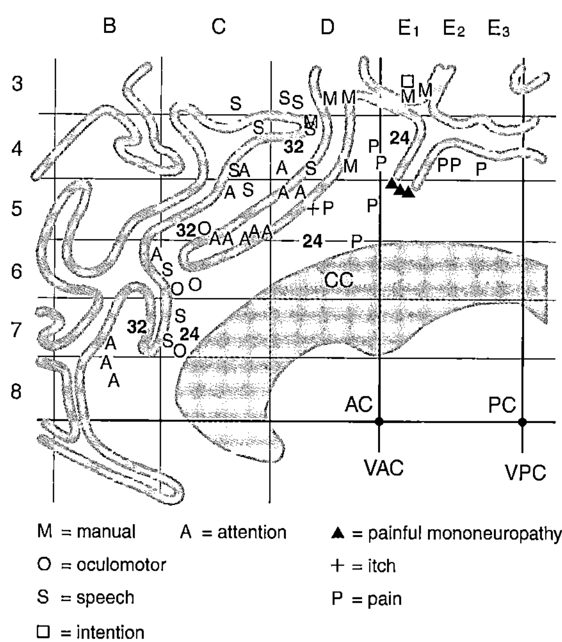

Fig. 8.4 Sagittal projection view of the foci of anterior cingulate activation/inhibition. The displayed sagittal view is a zoomed scope of the anterior cingulate cortex (BA 24, 32) sectioned at x = 5 mm (Talairach & Tournoux 1988). AC = anterior commissure; CC = corpus callosum; PC = posterior commissure; VAC = vertical anterior commissure line; VPC = vertical posterior commissure line. (Reproduced from Hsieh et al 1995 with permission.)

topically organized. It receives input from multiple ascending systems of the spinal cord and the reticular formation. Pathways from the medial thalamus project diffusely to wide areas of the cortex and together comprise the 'medial pain system'. On the hand, the ventrobasal thalamus is somatotopically highly organized. It receives input from a somatotopically organized ascending tract and sends fibres to the primary (SI) and secondary (SII) somatosensory areas of the cerebral cortex, where refined localization and discrimination of stimuli occur. These areas comprise the 'lateral pain system'. The activations of the thalamus elicited in experimental conditions seems less consistent than in the ACC. This could partly be explained by anatomical variations in a heterogeneous and complex structure, where the actual representation of pain-elicited activity appears only in circumscribed areas (Craig et al 1994). However, intraindividual direct comparison showed that a pain stimulus and not vibratory stimulation activated the thalamus (Coghill et al 1994, Disbrow et al 1998). In experimental allodynia based on the model of capsaicin preinjection the thalamus was also activated. The activation was attributed to the sensory-perceptual components of pain (Iadarola et al 1998). Given the anatomical connections of the limbic thalamus to the ACC (Vogt et al 1993), this does not seem to be a self-evident interpretation because the ACC and the lateral pain system were both activated in the same contrasts.

Several studies of clinical pain entities have shown an increased flow in the thalamus in response, correlating with increased pain of a localized nature (DiPiero et al 1997). In chronic ongoing pain due to mononeuropathy, alleviation of the ailment by local injection of xylocain leads to pain relief and in parallel increases in rCBF (Hsieh et al 1995). This suggestion of a regulation of the thalamic activity in chronic pain was corroborated by a study in which the contralateral thalamus was shown to have a decreased blood flow in patients with chronic neuropathic pain (Iadarola et al 1995).

SI and SII

The role of SI and SII in the perception of chronic pain has been discussed. Surgical extirpation of these areas in humans provides little or no relief from chronic, intractable pain (Head & Holmes 1911). Electrical stimulation of SI failed to evoke painful responses in neurosurgical patients nor did ablation of SII cause detectable sensory deficits (Penfield & Jasper 1954). However, recent clinical (Young & Blume 1983, Greenspan & Winfield 1992), physiological (Kenshalo et al 1988, Chudler et al 1990, Kenshalo & Willis 1991) and functional brain imaging studies (Talbot et al 1991, Casey et al 1994, 1996, Coghill et al 1994) suggest that the somatosensory cortex may participate not only in the discriminative aspects of nociception but also in a possible elaboration of the sensory experience of pain itself.

Accumulating evidence points to an important role of SI and SII in pain (Chudler et al 1990). Currently, it is accepted that the medial pain system is mainly involved in motivational and affective aspects of pain, while the lateral pain system is presumed to process and transmit discriminative aspects of noxious stimuli (Craig et al 1994). Although it seems generally accepted that the localizing components of a pain stimulus are coded in these regions, the question remains to what extent other pain components are represented here. Intensity coding seems to be part of the SI response. Early imaging studies were inconclusive. In studies on experimental tonic pain, rCBF in SI has been shown to increase, remain unaltered or vary individually (Coghill et al 1993, Derbyshire et al 1993, DiPiero et al 1994). Some studies even reported decreases in contralateral SI in response to pain stimulus (Apkarian et al 1992). By using the chemogenic algesic agent, capsaicin, where possible tactile components of the pain stimuli could be avoided, an activation in SI has been found (Iadarola et al 1993, 1998). The activity in the SI was also found to be correlated to the intensity of tonic (heat) painful input (Duncan et al 1994). Very intense pain stimuli seems to activate the SI consistently (Hsieh et al 1996b). The SI and MI (primary motor cortex) have been demonstrated to be coactivated (either confluently or discretely) in recent imaging studies on sustained high-intensity (visual analogue scale (VAS) ≥ 80%) tonic cold pain (DiPiero et al 1994), and acute phasic heat pain (using fMRI) (Gelnar et al 1994). The activity in these two regions could also be correlated to the pain intensity (tonic heat pain) (Duncan et al 1994). Thus the confluent activation of SI/MI may conform to the hypothesis that the pre- and postcentral areas often function in concert (Libet 1973). It may also at least in part be explained by the urge to move due to the pain stimulus (Hsieh et al 1994, Petrovic et al 1998b)

Taking into account the paucity of nociceptive neurons with bilateral and not-well-demarcated receptive fields (Dong et al 1989), the SII may not subserve the functions of precise spatial localization and intensity encoding. However, there is data suggesting that it is possible to detect a somatotopy in the pain response in SII with the foot region more posteriorily located than the hand (Andersson et al 1997, Petrovic et al 1998b). Also, the responses in SII seem often to be bilateral in response to a unilateral stimulus, but this trait is common to sensory stimuli that also are bilaterally represented in this region (Tarkka & Treede 1994).

The absence of significant cortical rCBF changes in SI and SII in chronic peripheral neuropathic pain (Hsieh et al 1995) does not refute cortical responses below the sensitivity of this technique, taking into account the conspicuous paucity of nociceptive neurons in the somatosensory cortex. The lack of detectable response may reside in the adaptive/learning mechanism that a familiarized mental task/workload does not require the same degree of neuronal activity (magnitude of change and the amount of neurons) as in the naive and acute situation (Jenkins et al 1994, Petersson et al 1997, Raichle 1997).

In cluster headache and visceral pain there seems to be less involvement of the SI region, in line with the feature of poor spatial localization for these two entities of clinical pain syndromes (Rosen et al 1994, Hsieh et al 1996a). However the paper by Azis and coworkers is at variance with this contention (Aziz et al 1997), because their model of oesophageal distension gave rise to a bilateral increase of the activity in SI and the authors speculate that the activation may hint at a possible mechanism for referred pain from the oesophagus.

Motor co-activations

The SI and MI have been demonstrated to be coactivated (either confluent or discrete) in several imaging studies on sustained high-intensity (VAS ≥ 80%) painful electrostimulation (Hsieh 1995), tonic cold pain (using SPECT) (DiPiero et al 1994) and acute phasic heat pain (using fMRI) (Gelnar et al 1994). The activity in these two regions could also be correlated to the pain intensity (tonic heat pain) (Duncan et al 1994). Thus the confluent activation of SI/MI may conform to the hypothesis that the pre- and postcentral areas often function in concert (Penfield & Jasper 1954, Libet 1973). In fact earlier rCBF studies noted the dominance of sensory activations in some motor paradigms and called this the sensory-motor paradox (Ingvar 1975). It is therefore not a trivial task in any high-intensity pain paradigm to determine the factors that activate the motor and sensory cortices. If an intensive pain stimulus leads to the urge to move (withdraw) the stimulated limb and the subject is asked to be still during the scan, major parts may be due to cortical overriding of otherwise automatic movements initiated as lower-level events.

Brain defence system

There is direct nociceptive input from spinal pathways to the limbic system and hypothalamic centres such as the autonomic and neuroendocrine control centres that mediate diverse neuroendocrine responses characterized by the 'stress response' (Kupfermann 1993). The fact that the hypothalamic neurons have substantial reciprocal connections with other limbic regions suggests that they may play a significant role in producing emotional responses to painful stimuli. The hypothalamus has large, direct projections to almost all areas in the CNS that are involved in the autonomic control of visceral organs, including prominent direct projections to preganglionic neurons in the brainstem and the spinal cord (Swanson 1987). The PAG subserves various functions of the defensive behaviour and modulates the nociceptive transmission and integrates together with the hypothalamus many endocrine and autonomic responses associated with aggressive-defensive behaviours (Bandler & Shipley 1994). The term brain defence system (BDS) has been used to describe the concerted function of these anatomical structures and the amygdala.

This system is commonly not activated in well-controlled experimental pain experiments where the subjects are well informed and actual tissue damage is avoided. When acute pain was instigated based on a minimal skin lesion, the BDS was activated (Hsieh et al 1996b). We suggest that the brain may recruit different operational mechanisms in processing a potential or actual traumatic painful event versus non-traumatic painful challenge with a low level of affective response. It may also represent the function of this region in the descending inhibitory system, which seems to be important in the regulation of the pain input to the brain.

A damaging stimulus, being threatening to the living organism, often produces changes in affect or mood, and causes a host of somatic and autonomic reflexive responses (Cousins 1994). In a study of angina pectoris (visceral pain) which signals cardiac ischaemia and thereby threat of tissue injury the BDS was also activated (Rosen et al 1994). In induced cluster headache attacks it was shown that there was an activation in the hypothalamus that was not present in control subjects where the same provocation with nitroglycerine was instigated (May et al 1998).

Anterior insula

The activation of the insula, a polymodal convergence area, has been consistently demonstrated in all studies of experimentally induced pain and throughout our studies (Hsieh et al 1995, Casey et al 1996, Andersson et al 1997, 1996a,b). Anterior-ventral insula has more extensive connections with orbitofrontal, temporopolar, anterior cingulate, olfactory, gustatory and autonomic structures, whereas the posterior-dorsal insular is more closely connected to somesthetic, auditory, motor and high-order association areas (Mesulam & Mufson 1985).

Direct comparison between vibrotactile stimulus and painful stimulation showed that whereas both these stimuli activated the SI/SII region, painful stimulus was significantly more effective in activating the anterior insula (Coghill et al 1994). In the interpretation of these authors: 'such connections may provide one route through which nociceptive input may be integrated with memory in order to allow a full appreciation of the meaning and dangers of painful stimuli'. Chronic pain where the localizing and discriminatory dimensions are less evident and the affective/evaluative component seem to dominate activate the anterior insular region bilaterally (Hsieh et al 1995).

Prefrontal cortex

Converging evidence suggests the 'supervisory' and 'regulatory' role of the prefrontal cortex, because damage here leads to impairments in planning, personality, behavioural control, affective attachment, motor programming and directed/sustained attention (Shallice 1982). Planning or suppressing a behaviour or maintaining a cortically controlled behaviour entails sequencing, i.e. maintaining a protocol of the planned behaviour. Such protocols are sensitive to disturbance and critically reliant on patent mechanisms of attention. In our limited space of consciousness pain makes its way by attention mechanisms which in turn rely both on acute localization phenomena (domination for the lateral pain system) and means of emotional mechanisms (medial pain system). Emotion entails complex, organized psychophysiological reactions consisting of cognitive appraisals, action impulses and patterned somatic reactions (Folkman & Lazarus 1991). Thus, being able to assess pain and feel unpleasantness reflect conscious awareness (LeDoux 1984).

The dorsolateral prefrontal cortex seems essential for the creation of willed acts (Ingvar 1985) and the ACC involvement in behavioural control depends critically on a close interaction with the prefrontal cortex (PFC) (Paus et al 1993). Also, the PFC is part of feedback arrangements pertaining to attention, cognitive evaluation and self-awareness (Cohen 1993). Nociresponsive neurons have also been demonstrated to exist in the PFC in animals (Snow et al 1992), suggesting also a direct association of the PFC with pain processing. Psychosurgery to disconnect the frontal and the limbic cortex (PFC, ACC, etc.) has been performed successfully for relieving intractable pain (Bouckoms 1994).

Pain stimuli elicits reactions of different complexity from reflexes to intention-driven behaviours, as well as changes in mood levels. It is therefore not surprising that experimental pain often leads to changes in activity in the frontal cortices (Derbyshire et al 1993, 1998, DiPiero et al 1994, Hsieh 1995, Hsieh et al 1995, 1996a, b). The activation foci in the right dorsolateral prefrontal cortical region (Broddman areas 9, 10, 46) seems more related to acutely elicited pain with its preponderance for withdrawal and motor behaviours. These regions are involved in planned motor behaviours and representation of delayed responses (Goldman-Rakic 1987). It was possible to provoke activations in this region by provoking itch sensation and asking the subjects not to move. This was understood as the urge to move elicited motor planning awaiting the possibility to scratch (Hsieh et al 1994).

The inferior lateral prefrontal cortex seems to be involved in cognitive emotional process and integrative regulation (Ketter et al 1993, George et al 1994). Chronic pain, with its impact on mood and emotion, seems to affect orbitofrontal cortices more (Hsieh 1995, Hsieh et al 1996a, b, Gyulai et al 1997, Peyron et al 1998). The ventromedial prefrontal cortex (BA 12), in conjunction with the ACC (BA 24′, 32), may exert inhibitory control on the pain-relevant affective signals from the limbic system (Davis et al 1997, Peyron et al 1998). The complexity of the activation patterns in the frontal cortex that are associated with pain make it very important in the future to design more specific paradigms that will address the precise roles of the many prefrontal cortical subregions in pain processing.

Posterior parietal cortex

The functions of the parietal lobes are many and diverse and they are regarded as a polymodal association area. It has not yet been established to what extent there are anatomical and functional homologies between the human parietal lobe and that of other primates. The posterior parietal cortex contains spatial representations (intrapersonal and extrapersonal space) (Deiber et al 1991, Grafton et al 1992), including a body scheme through which humans establish a physical sense of the self (Andersen 1987). Patients with lesions in the posterior parietal cortex (PPC), especially the right side, have severe attentional disturbances, designated as sensory neglect syndrome (Heilman & Watson 1977).

The PPC has nociceptive neurons with bilateral receptive fields, neurons that are also represented bilaterally in SII (Dong et al 1989). It has been demonstrated to be activated in either experimental pain (Coghill et al 1994, Derbyshire et al 1994), traumatic nociceptive pain (Hsieh et al 1996b) or chronic neuropathic pain (Hsieh et al

1995). A prominent activation has also been demonstrated in unpleasant itch (Hsieh et al 1994), a situation with no pain but where the urge to scratch invokes body coordination. As part of the posterior attentional system which has close anatomical connections to the anterior attentional networks and to the arousal/vigilance systems, the PPC may participate in orienting subjects to the sensory input (Posner & Raichle 1994). Given the complexity of activation patterns by using different cognitive and perceptual tasks as documented in the functional brain imaging literature, more specific paradigms are needed to delineate the subdominant regions of the PPC, if any, in response to pain.

CLINICAL VERSUS EXPERIMENTAL STUDIES

A critical factor in the quality of imaging studies is the sample size. While it is often necessary to limit the studies of clinical entities due to limited patient access, it is difficult today to accept experimental studies because the methods for studies have become standard (Frackowiak et al 1997). In clinical studies often the strategy of predefining the search volume (see 'Statistical considerations' above) can be used with success. There seem to be differences in the brain processes of chronic pathological pain and experimentally induced acute pain. The brain activation pattern in chronic pain emphasizes the emotional aspect whereas acutely elicited pain seem to include more expressed localization/discrimination components. In painful mononeuropathy the ACC is activated in the habitual pain state with no concurrent activation of the lateral pain system (Hsieh et al 1995), whereas acute pain exacerbation in allodynia leads to strong coactivations in the lateral pain system (Petrovic et al 1998a).

Tonic pain stimulation with cold pressor test of each hand in chronic cluster headache patients outside of the active headache period showed a differential response depending on the side of stimulation. Stimulation of the contralateral side of the headache affliction led to a more expressed activation in the thalamus than ipsilateral stimulation (DiPiero et al 1997). Aberrant pain processing in chronic pain seems plausible and more studies in this area are warranted.

Headache/migraine

The vascular nature of different headaches has made it natural to use rCBF methods in the search for pathophysiological mechanisms (Hachinski et al 1977, Olesen et al 1990, Friberg et al 1994). In migraine there is to date no consensus on the pathophysiological significance of the changes in CBF that have been demonstrated.

Using a PET study it was shown recently that in migraine without aura certain areas in the brainstem were activated during the headache state, but not in the headache-free interval (Weiller et al 1995). It was suggested that this brainstem activation is inherent to the migraine attack itself and represents the so called 'migraine generator'. The same authors performed an experimental pain study in seven healthy volunteers, using the same positioning in the PET scanner as in the migraine patients. A small amount of capsaicin was administered subcutaneously in the right forehead to evoke a burning painful sensation in the area of the first division of the trigeminal nerve. Increases in regional cerebral blood flow (rCBF) were found bilaterally in the insula, in the anterior cingulate cortex, the cavernous sinus and the cerebellum. No brainstem activation was found in the acute pain state (May et al 1998).

Provoking cluster headache has been shown in PET and it was demonstrated that not only is there an activation of the central pain systems (both lateral and medial) but also the activation in the ACC was right sided irrespective of the afflicted side (Hsieh et al 1996b). Also there was a prominent increase in isotope presence in the cavernous sinus, possibly mirroring the vascular origin of the disorder. However, this contention was argued against by May et al, because they found a similar activity in the cavernous sinus when injecting capsaicin in the forehead skin and suggested that this structure is more likely to be involved in trigeminal transmitted pain as such, rather than in a specific type of headache as was suggested for cluster headache (May et al 1998). May and colleagues have published a paper in which they studied nitroglycerine-provoked cluster headache. With the reasoning that the prominent circadian rhythmicity of the symptom occurrence did not indicate a vascular origin, they speculated on an intracerebral mechanism as a trigger. They used the subgroup of chronic cluster headache patients. Patients not in bout were used as controls. As previously demonstrated in acute severe experimental pain (Hsieh et al 1996a,b), an increased activity was noted in the hypothalamus during the painful events. However, the control group did not have such an activation. The authors gave the interpretation that this represented 'the primum movens' in the pathophysiology in this disorder. In the first PET study of provoked cluster headaches that was published, there was no similar finding of hypothalamic activation (Hsieh et al 1996b). The literature on possible vascular origin of the cluster headache, where correlations of vascular diameters and pain seem well established, and therefore the finding of May et al (1998), may need replication before their interpretation can reach general acceptance.

LATERALIZATION OF THE PAIN RESPONSE

There is evidence that the right hemisphere is more involved in emotional evaluation than the left (Gainotti et al 1993). In line with this are the suggestions from experimental and clinical studies that pain sensitivity is lateralized in humans, with the non-dominant hemisphere manifesting a relatively higher response than the dominant hemisphere. Studies examining pain threshold or pain tolerance by means of various experimental pain-inducing procedures have revealed a lower pain threshold or pain tolerance when noxious stimuli are applied to the left side of the body in right-handers (Heilman & Watson 1977). In several of the studies from our group (Hsieh 1995, Hsieh et al 1995, 1996a,b) we demonstrated a preferential activation of the right ACC, regardless of the side of the painful input. Other authors have made this finding but have not commented upon it (Weiller et al 1995). It may be regarded as difficult to judge what side of the ACC is activated the most, but the numerous findings of the right-sided preference suggest it is not a spurious finding (Fig. 8.5). This is seen as emphasizing the right lateralized mechanism for negative emotion relevant to a sustained aversive painful condition. The lateralization is not confined to the ACC but rather is both frontal and SII (Hari et al 1997). Also in the frontal lobe there is a lateralization, as chronic pain seems to activate the right side preferentially. Chronic pain means a constant interaction with previous pain experiences, and this pain response pattern is therefore not surprising as basic memory functions support a preferential role for the right frontal lobe in the recall of memories (Buckner 1996, Nyberg et al 1996).

MODULATORY INFLUENCES ON THE EXPERIENCE OF PAIN

Anticipatory events

Hierarchical processing is a purposeful organization because it allows processes to be handled without competing for the limited space on consciousness (Posner 1990). In the establishment of priorities of cerebral processing it is also of clear computational value to preprocess information in order to prepare behaviour. Itch is defined as the urge to scratch, and hence if itch is induced combined with the instruction 'do not move', imaging the brain will be an image of the urge to scratch, i.e. the network combined of sensory and motor regions necessary to perform the purposeful behaviour at a later stage (Hsieh et al 1994). This is a significant finding in pain imaging, because most studies of experimental pain instigate a pain stimulus concurrently with the instruction of avoiding movements. This is an important potential confounder for many studies in the interpretation of the results, because actual movements and suppressed movements activate the same mechanisms in the cerebellum (Ito 1993) and the rest of the motor system.

The expectancy of a pure sensory event invoked a decrease of activity in SI/SII ipsilaterally to the site of

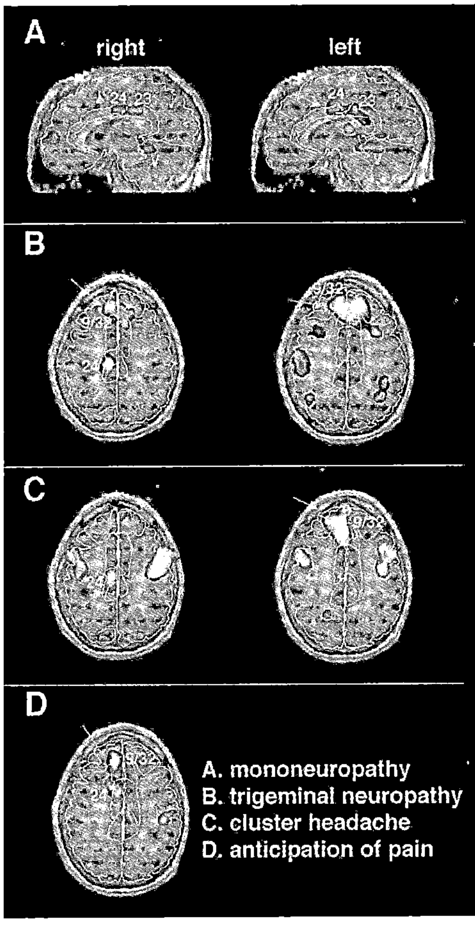

Fig. 8.5 The omnibus significance maps (thresholded at $P < 0.01$) were superimposed on a transformed MRI image and were colour coded into four levels defined by $0.001 \leq P < 0.01$ (increase = red; decrease = blue) and $P < 0.001$ (increase = yellow; decrease = light blue). In peripheral neuropathy (**A**), both right-sided and left-sided affliction lead to a right-sided activation in the ACC. Data for trigeminal neuropathy (**B**) and cluster headache (**C**) were pooled in the respective groups irrespective of the side of painful input to identify, on a system level, the regions consistently engaged in central pain processing (for data treatment see Bottini et al 1995, Hsieh et al 1995, 1996a). The right hemisphere is on the reader's left. Area 24 & 9/32 are indicated with blue arrows. (see colour plate)

stimulation. Additionally, in the anticipatory states the SI displayed decreases contralaterally to the site of stimulation outside the primary projection area for the stimulus (Drevets et al 1995, Hsieh 1995). Such an inhibition may function as a gating mechanism and could facilitate focusing and localizing the somatic stimulus (Drevets et al 1995, Hsieh 1995). Thus, the activity in the SI/SII can be modulated by attentional mechanisms, a phenomenon documented for other primary sensory cortices, for example the primary visual cortex (Corbetta et al 1991), and has been termed top-down modulation of primary cortices (Shulman et al 1997, Ghatan et al 1998).

A warning beforehand of a potential harm is a powerful adaptational tool. The cognitive evaluation, referred to as appraisal, is a dynamic process which changes according to the person's perception of the consequences of an event (Folkman & Lazarus 1991). The anticipation of a harmful encounter involves cognitive appraisal and thereby anticipatory coping (Folkman & Lazarus 1991). Thus the anticipation, or expectation, of pain can trigger the same emotional response as pain itself. By imaging the pre-pain cerebral activity during anticipation of a painful encounter (Hsieh 1995), we charted a neurophysiological process underlying the affective modulation of attention according to the cognitive appraisal of pain.

The ACC and the ventromedial prefrontal cortex constitute a bridge between the autonomic nervous system, the limbic system and the prefrontal cortex (Vogt et al 1993, Tranel & Damasio 1994). The integration of emotion/cognition/attention is dependent on these structures (Devinsky et al 1995). There are clinical observations that limbic forebrain surgery (e.g. cingulotomy, frontolobotomy) alleviates the affective impact, attention and cognitive appraisal of intractable pain while preserving the perception of pain (Bouckoms 1994). Anticipation of pain should therefore modulate the activity in these mentioned areas.

An experiment in which subjects anticipated either an unknown (but per instruction not dangerous) painful event or a pre-trained known but unavoidable event was carried out (Hsieh 1995). On the behavioural level this experimental difference induces different responses. The unknown stimulus leads to apprehension whereas the other invokes avoidance. In line with this, the subjects self-reported that they promptly attended to the anticipated pain of unknown character or intentionally diverged attention from the source of distress when the upcoming stimulus was known. The unknown stimulus increased the activity in the prefrontal cortex, ACC and PAG. On the other hand, the anticipation of the known pain stimulus leads to decreases in the same regions. Hence, the anticipatory phase imposed changes in brain activity compliant with the two different reported reactions to the upcoming pain stimulus, reflecting either the vigilant (directing attention to the encounter) or avoidant strategies (diverting attention from the source of distress), respectively (Lazarus 1991).

Cognitive modulation of the pain response

As mentioned above anticipation of pain is not a unitary reaction scheme. The same variability can be seen in the actual response to pain, both at the behavioural and the physiological level. It is an everyday experience that it is possible to modify the experience of pain by means of attentional mechanisms. By actively disengaging the thoughts on the suffering component of pain it may become more bearable. Petrovic et al have tested this with a factorial design by exposing subjects to experimental pain (cold pressor test – left hand in ice cold water) with and without cognitive loading. Indeed, the pain-evoked activations in the lateral pain system were less expressed during cognitive performance and the pain-evoked decreases in the basal forebrain were less expressed (Petrovic et al 1998a). In a similar design where the pain provocation was more expressed Hsieh et al demonstrated that also the activity in the medial pain system could be damped by cognitive loading (Hsieh et al 1998). Pharmacological manipulations also demonstrate that the blood flow increase in the medial pain system and the reciprocal decrease in the basal forebrain parallel the reported level of pain discomfort (Gyulai et al 1997). Hence, intentional diversion of attention from the pain stimulus decreases the intensity of the pain experience and this is paralleled by less expressed activations in the central pain systems.

Decreases in activity in areas outside a process relevant network is a common finding in imaging studies (Ghatan et al 1995). This has been questioned if it represents a real finding or rather if it reflects a top-down regulatory measure of attention mechanisms. Challenging these concepts it was recently shown that process relevant information handling coinciding with suppression of processing of potentially disturbing information were present concurrently (Ghatan et al 1998). Decreases in the medial temporal lobe in intense pain paradigms have been reported from some studies (Hsieh 1995, Hsieh et al 1996b, Petrovic et al 1998b). It may be suggested that this represents a meaningful suppression of memory encoding during the ongoing pain, as pain is known to interfere with memory function. However, the critical experiment remains to be done to prove that this represents an active suppression.

FINAL REMARKS

Imaging of pain has improved our knowledge of the central pain mechanisms in many aspects. The rapid development of the imaging methods has over the last years led to a decrease in the variability in the description of the central pain matrix between different studies and led to a definition of a central pain matrix in man. The future will yield studies elucidating the interaction of the central pain systems and attention, cognition and emotional regulation.

Acknowledgements

Studies were supported by the Swedish Bank Tercentennial Foundation, Medical Research Council (8246) and the Knut and Alice Wallenberg Foundation. The authors are grateful to all subjects participating in the studies mentioned.

REFERENCES

Andersen RA 1987 Inferior parietal lobule function in spatial perception and visuomotor integration. In: Mountcastle VB, Plum F, Geiger SR (eds) Handbook of physiology. Section 1; The Nervous system, vol V, Higher functions of the brain, part 2. American Physiological Society, Bethesda, pp 483–518

Andersson JL, Lilja A, Hartvig P et al 1997 Somatotopic organization along the central sulcus, for pain localization in humans, as revealed by positron emission tomography. Experimental Brain Research 117: 192–199

Apkarian AV, Shi T 1994 Squirrel monkey lateral thalamus. I. Somatic nociresponsive neurons and their relation to spinothalamic terminals. Journal of Neuroscience 14: 6779–6795

Apkarian AV, Stea RA, Manglos SH, Szeverenyi NM, King RB, Thomas FD 1992 Persistent pain inhibits contralateral somatosensory cortical activity in humans. Neuroscience Letters 140: 141–147

Aziz Q, Andersson JL, Valind S et al 1997 Identification of human brain loci processing esophageal sensation using positron emission tomography. Gastroenterology 113: 50–59

Babiloni F, Babiloni C, Carducci F, Del Gaudio M, Onorati P, Urbano A 1997 A high resolution EEG method based on the correction of the surface Laplacian estimate for the subject's variable scalp thickness. Electroencephalography and Clinical Neurophysiology 103: 486–492

Bandler R, Shipley MT 1994 Columnar organization in the midbrain periaqueductal gray: modules for emotional expression? Trends in Neurosciences 17: 379–389

Bench CJ, Friston KJ, Brown RG et al 1992 The anatomy of melancholia – focal abnormalities of cerebral blood flow in major depression. Psychological Medicine 22: 607–615

Bennett GJ 1994 Animal models of neuropathic pain. In: Gebhart GF, Hammond DL, Jensen TS (eds) Proceedings of the 7th World Congress on Pain. IASP Press, Seattle, pp 495–510

Bonica JJ 1990 Anatomic and physiologic basis of nociception and pain. In: Bonica JJ (ed) The management of pain. Lea & Febiger, Philadelphia, pp 28–94

Bottini G, Corcoran R, Sterzi R et al 1995 The role of the right hemisphere in the interpretation of figurative aspects of language: a positron emission tomography activation study. Brain 117: 1241–1253

Bouckoms AJ 1994 Limbic surgery for pain. In: Wall PD, Melzack R (eds) Textbook of pain. Churchill Livingstone, Edinburgh, pp 1171–1187

Brüggemann J, Shi T, Apkarian AV 1994 Squirrel monkey lateral thalamus. II. Viscerosomatic convergent representation of urinary bladder, colon and esophagus. Journal of Neuroscience 14: 6796–6814

Buckner RL 1996 Beyond HERA: contributions of specific prefrontal brain areas to long-term memory retrieval. Psychonomic Bulletin Review 3: 149–158

Buckner RL, Koutstaal W, Schacter DL, Dale AM, Rotte M, Rosen BR 1998 Functional–anatomic study of episodic retrieval. II. Selective averaging of event-related fMRI trials to test the retrieval success hypothesis. Neuroimage 7: 163–175

Carpenter GA, Grossberg S 1989 Self-organizing neural network architectures for real time adaptive pattern recognition. In: Zornetzer SF, Davis JL, Lau C (eds) An introduction to neural and electronic networks. Academic, London, pp 455–478

Casey KL, Minoshima S, Berger KL, Koeppe RA, Morrow TJ, Frey KA 1994 Positron emission tomography analysis of cerebral structures activated specifically by repetitive noxious heat stimuli. Journal of Neurophysiology 2: 802–807

Casey KL, Minoshima S, Morrow TJ, Koeppe RA 1996 Comparison of human cerebral activation pattern during cutaneous warmth, heat pain, and deep cold pain. Journal of Neurophysiology 76: 571–581

Chudler EH, Anton F, Dubner R, Kenshalo DRJ 1990 Responses of nociceptive SI neurons in monkeys and pain sensation in humans elicited by noxious thermal stimulation: effect of interstimulus interval. Journal of Neurophysiology 63: 559–569

Coghill RC, Morin C, Evans AC et al 1993 Cerebral blood flow (CBF) during tonic pain in man. Society of Neuroscience Abstracts 19: 1573

Coghill RC, Talbot JD, Evans AC et al 1994 Distributed processing of pain and vibration by the human brain. Journal of Neuroscience 14: 4095–4108

Cohen RA 1993 Consciousness and self-directed attention. In: The neurophychology of attention. Plenum, London, pp 353–359

Corbetta M, Miezin FM, Shulman GL, Petersen SE 1991 Selective attention modulates extrastriate visual regions in humans during visual feature discrimination and recognition, exploring brain functional anatomy with positron tomography. In: Chedwick DJ, Whelan J (eds) Ciba Foundation Symposium 163. John Wiley, Chichester, pp 165–180

Cousins M 1994 Acute and postoperative pain. In: Wall PD, Melzack R (eds) Textbook of pain, 3rd edn. Churchill Livingstone, Edinburgh, pp 357–385

Craig AD, Bushnell MC, Zhang E-T, Blomqvist A 1994 A thalamic nucleus specific for pain and temperature sensation. Nature 372: 770–773

Craig AD, Reiman EM, Evans A, Bushnell MC 1996 Functional imaging of an illusion of pain [see comments]. Nature 384: 258–260

Davis KD, Taylor SJ, Crawley AP, Wood ML, Mikulis DJ 1997 Functional MRI of pain- and attention-related activations in the human cingulate cortex. Journal of Neurophysiology 77: 3370–3380

Deiber M-P, Passingham RE, Colebatch JG et al 1991 Cortical areas and the selection of movement: a study with positron emission tomography. Experimental Brain Research 84: 393–402

Derbyshire SW, Vogt BA, Jones AK 1998 Pain and stroop interference tasks activate separate processing modules in anterior cingulate cortex. Experimental Brain Research 118: 52–60

Derbyshire SWG, Jones AKP, Brown WD et al 1993 Cortical and subcortical responses to pain in male and female volunteers. Journal of Cerebral Blood Flow and Metabolism 13 (suppl 1): S546

Derbyshire SWG, Jones AKP, Devani P et al 1994 Cerebral responses to pain in patients with atypical facial pain measured by positron emission tomography. Journal of Neurology, Neurosurgery and Psychiatry 57: 1166–1172

Dettmers C, Connelly A, Stephan KM et al 1996 Quantitative comparison of functional magnetic resonance imaging with positron emission tomography using a force-related paradigm. Neuroimage 4: 201–209

Devinsky O, Morrell MJ, Vogt BA 1995 Contributions of anterior cingulate cortex to behaviour. Brain 118: 279–306

DiPiero V, Ferracuti S, Sabatini U, Pantano P, Cruccu G, Lenzi GL 1994 A cerebral blood flow study on tonic pain activation in man. Pain 56: 167–173

DiPiero V, Fiacco F, Tombari D, Pantano P 1997 Tonic pain: a SPET study in normal subjects and cluster headache patients. Pain 70: 185–191

Disbrow E, Buoncore M, Antognini J, Carstens E, Rowley H 1998 Somatosensory cortex; a comparison of the response to noxious thermal, mechanical, and electric stimuli using functional magnetic resonance imaging. Human Brain Mapping 6: 150–159

Dong WK, Salonen LD, Kawakami Y, Shiwaku T, Kaukoranta EM, Martin RF 1989 Nociceptive responses of trigeminal neurons in SII-7b cortex of awake monkeys. Brain Research 484: 314–324

Drevets WC, Burton H, Videen TO, Snyder AZ JRS Jr, Raichle ME 1995 Blood flow changes in human somatosensory cortex during anticipated stimulation. Nature 373: 249–252

Duncan GH, Morin C, Coghill RC, Evans A, Worsley KJ, Bushnell MC 1994 Using psychophysical ratings to map the human brain: regression of regional cerebral blood flow (rCBF) to tonic pain perception. Society of Neuroscience Abstracts 20: 1672

Feuerstein M 1989 Definitions of pain. In: Tollison CD, Tollison JW, Trent GG (eds) Handbook of chronic pain management. Silliams & Wilkins, London, pp 1–714

Folkman S, Lazarus RS 1991 Coping and emotion. In: Monat A, Lazarus RS (eds) Stress and coping. Columbia University Press, New York, pp 207–227

Fox P, Mintum M 1989 Noninvasive functional brain mapping by change-distribution analysis of averaged PET images of H215O tissue activity. Journal of Nuclear Medicine 30: 141–149

Fox PT, Raichle ME 1986 Focal physiological uncoupling of cerebral blood flow and oxidative metabolism during somatosensory stimulation in human subjects. Proceedings of the National Academy of Sciences USA 83: 1140–1144

Frackowiak R, Friston K, Frith C, Dolan R, Mazziotta J 1997 Human brain function. Academic, London

Frackowiak RSJ, Zeki S, Poline J-B, Friston KJ 1996 A critique of a new analysis proposed for functional neuroimaging. European Journal of Neuroscience 8: 2229–2231

Freund TF, Antal M 1988 GABA-containing neurons in the septum control inhibitory interneurons in the hippocampus. Nature 336: 170–173

Friberg L, Olesen J, Lassen NA, Olsen TS, Karle A 1994 Cerebral oxygen extraction, oxygen consumption, and regional cerebral blood flow during the aura phase of migraine. Stroke 25: 974–979

Friston K, Frith C, Frackowiak R 1993a Time-dependent changes in effective connectivity measured with PET. Human Brain Mapping 1: 69–80

Friston K, Frith C, Liddle P, Frackowiak R 1993b Functional connectivity: the principal component analysis of large (PET) data sets. Journal of Cerebral Blood Flow and Metabolism 13: 5–14

Friston KJ, Frith CD, Liddle PF, Dolan RJ, Lammertsma AA, Frackowiak RS 1990 The relationship between global and local changes in PET scans. Journal of Cerebral Blood Flow and Metabolism 10: 458–466 [see comments]

Friston KJ, Frith CD, Liddle PF, Frackowiak RSJ 1991 Comparing functional (PET) images: the assessment of significant change. Journal of Cerebral Blood Flow and Metabolism 11: 690–699

Friston KJ, Frith CD, Turner R, Frackowiak RS 1995a Characterizing evoked hemodynamics with fMRI [In Process Citation], Neuroimage 2: 157–65

Friston KJ, Holmes AP, Poline JB et al 1995b Analysis of fMRI time-series revisited. Neuroimage 2: 45–53 [see comments]

Friston KJ, Holmes AP, Worsley KJ, Poline J-P, Frackowiak RSJ 1995c Stastistical parametric maps in functional imaging: a general linear approach. Human Brain Mapping 2: 189–210

Friston KJ, Price CJ, Fletcher P, Moore C, Frackowiak RS, Dolan RJ 1996 The trouble with cognitive subtraction. Neuroimage 4: 97–104

Friston KJ, Josephs O, Rees G, Turner R 1998a Nonlinear event-related responses in fMRI. Magnetic Resonance Medicine 39: 41–52

Friston KJ, Fletcher P, Josephs O, Holmes A, Rugg MD, Turner R 1998b Event-related fMRI: characterizing differential responses. Neuroimage 7: 30–40

Fukushima T, Ikeda T, Uyama E, Uchino M, Okabe H, Ando M 1994 Cognitive event-related potentials and brain magnetic resonance imaging in HTLV-1 associated myelopathy (HAM). Journal of the Neurological Sciences 126: 30–39

Gainotti G, Caltagirone C, Zoccolotti P 1993 Left/right and cortical/subcortical dichotomies in the neuropsychological study of human emotions. Cognition and Emotion 7: 71–93

Gelnar PA, Szeverenyi NM, Apkarian AV 1994 SII has the most robust response of the multiple cortical areas activated during painful thermal stimuli in humans. Society of Neuroscience Abstracts 20: 1572

George MS, Ketter TA, Parekh PI et al 1994 Regional brain activity with selecting a response despite interference: an H215O. PET study of the stroop and an emotional stroop. Human Brain Mapping 1: 194–209

Ghatan PH, Hsieh JC, Wirsen-Meurling A et al 1995 Brain activation induced by the perceptual maze test: a PET study of cognitive performance. Neuroimage 2: 112–124

Ghatan PH, Hsieh JC, Petersson KM, Stone-Elander S, Ingvar M 1998 Coexistence of attention-based facilitation and inhibition in the human cortex. Neuroimage 7: 23–29

Goldman-Rakic PS 1987 Circuitry of primate prefrontal cortex and regulation of behavior by representational memory. In: Mountcastle VB, Plum F, Geiger SR (eds) Handbook of physiology. Section 1; The nervous system, vol V, Higher functions of the brain, part 1. American Physiological Society, Bethesda, pp 373–417

Grafton ST, Mazziota JC, Woods RP, Phelps ME 1992 Human functional anatomy of visually guided finger movements. Brain 115: 565–587

Grasby PM, Frith CD, Friston KJ, Simpson J et al 1994 A graded task approach to the functional mapping of brain areas implicated in auditory-verbal memory. Brain 117: 1271–1282

Greenspan JD, Winfield JA 1992 Reversible pain and tactile deficits associated with a cerebral tumor compressing the posterior insula and parietal operculum. Pain 58: 29–39

Greitz T, Bohm C, Holte S, Eriksson L 1991 A computerized brain atlas: construction, anatomical content and some applications. Journal of Computer Assisted Tomography 15: 26–38

Guilbaud G, Bernard JF, Besson JM 1994 Brain areas involved in nociception and pain. In: Wall PD, Melzack R (eds) Textbook of pain, 3rd edn. Churchill Livingstone, Edinburgh, pp 113–128

Gyulai FE, Firestone LL, Mintun MA, Winter PM 1997 In vivo imaging of nitrous oxide-induced changes in cerebral activation during noxious heat stimuli. Anesthesiology 86: 538–548

Hachinski VC, Olesen J, Norris JW, Larsen B, Enevoldsen E, Lassen NA 1977 Cerebral hemodynamics in migraine. Canadian Journal of Neurological Sciences 4: 245–249

Hari R, Kaukoranta E 1985 Neuromagnetic studies of somatosensory system: principles and examples. Progress in Neurobiology 24: 233–256

Hari R, Portin K, Kettenmann B, Jousmaki V, Kobal G 1997 Right-hemisphere preponderance of responses to painful CO_2 stimulation of the human nasal mucosa. Pain 72: 145–151

Haxby JV, Horwitz B, Ungerleider LG, Maisog JM, Pietrini P, Grady CL 1994 The functional organization of human extrastriate cortex: a PET-rCBF study of selective attention to faces and locations. Journal of Neuroscience 14: 6336–6353

Head H, Holmes G 1911 Sensory disturbances from cerebral lesions. Brain 34: 102–254

Heilman KM, Watson RT 1977 The neglect syndrome—a unilateral defect of the orienting response. In: Harnad S, Doty RW, Goldstein L, Jaynes J, Krauthamer G (eds) Lateralization in the nervous system. Academic, New York, pp 1–537

Herzog H, Seitz RJ, Tellmann L et al 1996 Quantitation of regional cerebral blood flow with ^{15}O-butanol and positron emission tomography in humans. Journal of Cerebral Blood Flow and Metabolism 16: 645–649

Hsieh J 1995 Central processing of pain: functional imaging studies of pain, Thesis, Karolinska Institut, Stockholm, pp 1–128

Hsieh J-C, Hägermark Ö, Ståhle-Bäckdahl M et al 1994 The urge to scratch represented in the human cerebral cortex during itch. Journal of Neurophysiology 72: 3004–3008

Hsieh JC, Belfrage M, Stone-Elander S, Hansson P, Ingvar M 1995 Central representation of chronic ongoing neuropathic pain studied by positron emission tomography. Pain 63: 225–236

Hsieh JC, Hannerz J, Ingvar M 1996a Right-lateralised central processing for pain of nitroglycerin-induced cluster headache. Pain 67: 59–68

Hsieh J-C, Ståhle-Bäckdahl M, Hägermark Ö, Stone-Elander S, Rosenquist G, Ingvar M 1996b Traumatic nociceptive pain activates the hypothalamus and the periaqueductal grey: a positron emission tomography study. Pain 64: 303–314

Hsieh J, Tu C, Tsai J et al 1998 Effective cognitive coping modulates the central processing of pain: a PET study. NeuroImage 7: S438

Huttunen J, Kobal G, Kaukoranta E, Hari R 1986 Cortical responses to painful CO_2 stimulation of nasal mucosa; a magnetoencephalographic study in man. Electroencephalography and Clinical Neurophysiology 64: 347–349

Iadarola MJ, Berman KF, Byas-Smith M et al 1993 Positron Emission Tomography (PET) studies of pain and allodynia in normals and patients with chronic neuropathic pain. Society of Neuroscience Abstracts 19: 1074

Iadarola MJ, Max MB, Berman KF et al 1995 Unilateral decrease in thalamic activity observed with positron emission tomography in patients with chronic neuropathic pain. Pain 63: 55–64

Iadarola MJ, Berman KF, Zeffiro TA et al 1998 Neural activation during acute capsaicin-evoked pain and allodynia assessed with PET. Brain 121: 931–947

IASP 1994 Classification of chronic pain: descriptions of chronic pain syndromes and definitions of pain terms. Task force on taxonomy, suppl 3. IASP Press, Seattle, S217 pp.

Ingvar DH 1975 Patterns of brain activity revealed by measurements of regional cerebral blood flow. In: Ingvar DH, Lassen NA (ed) Brain work: the coupling of function metabolism and blood flow in the brain. Munksgaard, Copenhagen, pp 397–413

Ingvar DH 1976 Functional landscapes of the dominant hemisphere. Brain Research 107: 181–197

Ingvar DH, Philipson L 1977 Distribution of cerebral blood flow in the dominant hemisphere during motor ideation and motor performance. Annals of Neurology 2: 230–237

Ingvar DH 1979 'Hyperfrontal' distribution of the cerebral grey matter flow in resting wakefulness; on the functional anatomy of the conscious state. Acta Neurologica Scandinavica 60: 12–25

Ingvar DH 1985 'Memory of the future': an essay on the temporal organization of conscious awareness. Human Neurobiology 4: 127–136

Ingvar M, Eriksson L, Greitz T et al 1994 Methodological aspects of brain activation studies: cerebral blood flow determined with [^{15}O]butanol and positron emission tomography. Journal of Cerebral Blood Flow and Metabolism 14: 628–638

Ingvar M, Ghatan PH, Wirsen-Meurling A et al 1998 Alcohol activates the cerebral reward system in man [In Process Citation]. Journal of Studies in Alcohol 59: 258–269

Ito M 1993 Movement and thought: identical control mechanisms by the cerebellum. Trends in Neurosciences 16: 448–450

Jenkins IH, Brooks DJ, Nixon PD, Frackowiak RSJ, Passingham RE 1994 Motor sequence learning: a study with positron emission tomography. Journal of Neurosciences 14: 3775–3790

Jones AK, Brown WD, Friston KJ, Qi LY, Frackowiak RS 1991a Cortical and subcortical localization of response to pain in man using positron emission tomography. Proceedings of the Royal Society of London. Series B: Biological Sciences 244: 39–44

Jones AK, Liyi Q, Cunningham VV et al 1991b Endogenous opiate response to pain in rheumatoid arthritis and cortical and subcortical response to pain in normal volunteers using positron emission tomography. International Journal of Clinical Pharmacology and Research 11: 261–266

Jones AK, Cunningham VJ, Ha-Kawa S et al 1994 Changes in central opioid receptor binding in relation to inflammation and pain in patients with rheumatoid arthritis. British Journal of Rheumatology 33: 909–916

Jones AP, Hughes DG, Brettle DS et al 1998 Experiences with functional magnetic resonance imaging at 1 tesla. British Journal of Radiology 71: 160–166

Jonsson C, Pagani M, Ingvar M et al 1998 Resting state rCBF mapping with single-photon emission tomography and positron emission tomography: magnitude and origin of differences. European Journal of Nuclear Medicine 25: 157–165

Kakigi R, Koyama S, Hoshiyama M, Kitamura Y, Shimojo M, Watanabe S 1995 Pain-related magnetic fields following painful CO_2 laser stimulation in man. Neuroscience Letters 192: 45–48

Kenshalo DRJ, Willis WDJ 1991 The role of the cerebral cortex in pain sensation. In: Peters A, Jones EG (eds) Cerebral cortex, vol 9. Plenum, New York, pp 153–212

Kenshalo DRJ, Chudler EH, Anton F, Dubner R 1988 SI nociceptive neurons participate in the encoding process by which monkeys perceive the intensity of noxious thermal stimulation. Brain Research 454: 378–382

Ketter TA, Andreason PJ, George MS, Herscovitch P, Post RM 1993 Paralimbic rCBF increases during procaine-induced psychosensory and emotional experiences. Biological Psychiatry 33: 66A

Koepp M, Gunn R, Lawrence A et al 1998 Evidence for endogenous dopamine release induced by behavioural manipulation. NeuroImage 7: A51

Kupfermann I 1993 Localization of higher cognitive and affective functions: the association cortices. In: Kandel ER, Schwartz JH, Jessell TM (eds) Principles of neural science. Elsevier, New York, pp 823–838

Lassen N, Perl W 1979 Tracer kinetic methods in medical physiology. Raven Press, New York

Lassen NA 1992 Neuroreceptor quantitation in vivo by the steady-state principle using constant infusion or bolus injection of radioactive

tracers. Journal of Cerebral Blood Flow and Metabolism 12: 709–716
Lazarus RS 1991 Emotion and adaptation. Oxford University Press, New York
LeDoux JE 1984 Cognition and emotion. In: Gazzaniga MS, (ed) Handbook of cognitive neuroscience. Plenum, London, pp 357–368
Libet B 1973 Electrical stimulation of cortex in human subjects and conscious sensory aspects. In: Iggo A (ed) Handbook of sensory physiology, vol 2. Springer, Berlin, pp 744–790
May A, Bahra A, Buchel C, Frackowiak R, Goadsby P 1998a Hypothalamic activation in cluster headache attacks. *Lancet* 352: 275–278
May A, Kaube H, Buchel C et al 1998b Experimental cranial pain elicited by capsaicin: a PET study. Pain 74: 61–66
Melzack R, Casey KL 1968 Sensory, motivational, and central control determinants of pain. In: Kenshalo DR (ed) The skin senses. CC Thomas, Springfield, pp 423–439
Menon R, Ogawa S, Tank D, Ugurbil K 1993–4 Tesla gradient recalled echo characteristics of photic stimulation induced signal changes in the human primary visual cortex. Magnetic Resonance in Medicine 30: 380–386
Menon V, Ford JM, Lim KO, Glover GH, Pfefferbaum A 1997 Combined event-related fMRI and EEG evidence for temporal-parietal cortex activation during target detection. NeuroReport 8: 3029–3037
Mesulam MM, Mufson EF 1985 The insula of Reil in man and monkey. Architectonics, connectivity and function. In: Peters A, Jones EG (eds) Cerebral cortex, vol 4. Plenum, New York, pp 179–226
Nyberg L, Cabeza R, Tulving E 1996 PET studies of encoding and retrieval: the HERA model. Psychonomic Bulletin Review 3: 135–148
Olesen J, Friberg L, Olsen TS et al 1990 Timing and topography of cerebral blood flow, aura, and headache during migraine attacks. Annals of Neurology 28: 791–798
Pardo JV, Pardo PJ, Janer KW, Raichle ME 1990 The anterior cingulate cortex mediates processing selection in the Stroop attentional conflict paradigm. Proceedings of the National Academy of Sciences USA 87: 256–259
Paus T, Petrides M, Evans AC, Meyer E 1993 Role of the human anterior cingulate cortex in the control of oculomotor, manual, and speech responses: a positron emission tomography study. Journal of Neurophysiology 70: 453–469
Penfield W, Jasper H 1954 Epilepsy and the functional anatomy of the human brain. Little Brown, Boston, 895 pp.
Petersson KM, Elfgren C, Ingvar M 1997 A dynamic role of the medial temporal lobe during retrieval of declarative memory in man. Neuroimage 6: 1–11
Petrovic P, Ghatan P, Petersson K, Ingvar M 1998a Cognition alters pain related activity in the lateral pain system. NeuroImage 7: S437
Petrovic P, Ingvar M, Petersson K, Stone-Elander S, Hansson P 1998b A PET activation study of dynamic mechanical allodynia. NeuroImage 7: S428
Peyron R, Garcia-Larrea L, Gregoire MC et al 1998 Allodynia after lateral-medullary (Wallenberg) infarct. A PET study. Brain 121: 345–356
Posner MI 1990 Hierarchical distributed networks in the neuroposychology of selective attention. In: A. Caramazza A (ed) Cognitive neuropsychology and neurolinguistics: advances in models of cognitive function and impairement. Plenum, New York, pp 187–210
Posner MI, Raichle ME 1994 Images of mind. Scientific American Library, New York, pp 153–180
Price CJ, Friston KJ 1997 Cognitive conjunction: a new approach to brain activation experiments. Neuroimage 5: 261–270
Price DD 1988 Psychological and neural mechanisms of pain. Raven, New York
Raichle ME 1987 Circulatory and metabolic correlates of brain function in normal humans. In: Mountcastle VB, Plum F, Geiger SR (eds) Handbook of physiology. Section 1; The nervous system, vol V, Higher functions of the brain, Part 2. American Physiology Society, pp 643–673
Raichle ME 1997 Food for thought. The metabolic and circulatory requirements of cognition. Annals of the New York Academy of Sciences 835: 373–385
Rainville P, Duncan GH, Price DD, Carrier B, Bushnell MC 1997 Pain affect encoded in human anterior cingulate but not somatosensory cortex. Science 277: 968–971
Roland PE, Gulyas B 1996 Assumptions and validations of statistical tests for functional neuroimaging. European Journal of Neurosciences 8: 2232–2235
Roland PE, Levin B, Kawashima R, Åkerman S 1993 Three-dimensional analysis of clustered voxels in 15-O-butanol brain activation images. Human Brain Mapping 1: 3–19
Rosen SD, Paulesu E, Frith CD et al 1994 Central nervous pathways mediating angina pectoris. Lancet 344: 147–150
Rosen BR, Buckner RL, Dale AM 1998 Event-related functional MRI: past, present, and future. Proceedings of the National Academy of Sciences USA 95: 773–780
Rosler F, Heil M, Hennighausen E 1995 Exploring memory, functions by means of brain electrical topography: a review. Brain Topography 7: 301–313
Rumelhart D, McClelland J 1986 Parallel distributed processing: explorations in the microstructures of cognition. MIT Press, Cambridge, MA
Schad LR, Wiener E, Baudendistel KT, Muller E, Lorenz WJ 1995 Event-related functional MR imaging of visual cortex stimulation at high temporal resolution using a standard 1.5 T imager. Magnetic Resonance Imaging 13: 899–901
Seitz RJ, Roland PE 1992 Vibratory stimulation increases and decrease the regional cerebral blood flow and oxidative metabolism: a positron emission tomography (PET) study. Acta Neurologica Scandinavica 86: 60–67
Shallice T 1982 Specific impairments of planning in frontal lobe damage. Philosophical Transactions of the Royal Society of London. Series B: Biological Sciences 298: 199–209
Shulman GL, Corbetta M, Buckner RL et al 1997 Top-down modulation of early sensory cortex. Cerebral Cortex 7: 193–206
Snow PJ, Lumb BM, Cervero F 1992 The representation of prolonged and intense, noxious somatic and visceral stimuli in the ventrolateral orbital cortex of the cat. Pain 48: 89–99
Swanson LW 1987 The hypothalamus. In: Björklund A, Hökfelt T, Swanson LW (eds) Handbook of chemical neuroanatomy. Elsevier Science, New York, pp 1–459
Talairach J, Tournoux P 1988 Co-planar stereotaxic atlas of the human brain. George Thieme Verlag, Stuttgart
Talbot JD, Marrett S, Evans AC, Meyer E, Bushnell MC, Duncan GH 1991 Multiple representations of pain in human cerebral cortex. Science 251: 1355–1358
Tarkka IM, Treede RD 1994 Distributed processing of pain and vibration by the human brain. Journal of Neuroscience 14: 4095–4108
Tarkka IM, Stokic DS, Basile LF, Papanicolaou AC 1995 Electric source localization of the auditory P300 agrees with magnetic source localization. Electroencephalography and Clinical Neurophysiology 96: 538–545
Thatcher RW 1995 Tomographic electroencephalography/magnetoencephalography. Dynamics of human neural network switching. Journal of Neuroïmaging 5: 35–45
Tranel D, Damasio H 1994 Neuroanatomical correlates of electrodermal skin conductance responses. Psychophysiology 31: 427–438

Tsen GF, Haberly LB 1988 Characterization of synaptically mediated fast and slow inhibitory processes in piriform cortex in and in vitro slice preparation. Journal of Neurophysiology 59: 1352–1376

Vaccarino AL, Melzack R 1989 Analgesia produced by injection of lidocaine into the anterior cingulum bundle of the rat. Pain 39: 213–219

Vogt BA, Sikes RW, Vogt LJ 1993 Anterior cingulate cortex and the medial pain system. In: Vogt BA, Gabriel M (eds) Neurobiology of cingulate cortex and limbic thalamus. Birkhäuser, Boston, pp 313–344

Vogt BA, Derbyshire S, Jones AK 1996 Pain processing in four regions of human cingulate cortex localized with co-registered PET and MR imaging. European Journal of Neuroscience 8: 1461–1473

Weiller C, May A, Limmroth V et al 1995 Brain stem activation in spontaneous human migraine attacks. Nature Medicine 1: 658–660

Worsley KJ, Friston KJ 1995 Analysis of fMRI time-series revisited – again. Neuroimage 2: 173–181 [comment]

Young GB, Blume WT 1983 Painful epileptic seizures. Brain 106: 537–554

Developmental neurobiology of pain

MARIA FITZGERALD

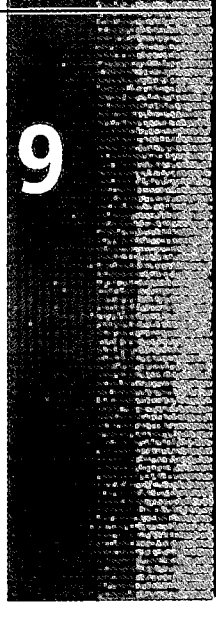

INTRODUCTION

Increasing recognition of the importance of pain in infancy and childhood has focused attention on the basic neurobiology of developing pain pathways. Advances in the general field of developmental neuroscience, particularly at the level of brain organization, have shown that the infant nervous system is not simply an immature adult nervous system undergoing step-by-step construction. Complex changes at the molecular, cellular and organizational levels result in a series of transient functional stages throughout development until the adult pattern is achieved. To understand the development of pain processing we must therefore appreciate the changing nature of the fetal and neonatal central nervous system (CNS).

THE DEVELOPMENT OF PAIN BEHAVIOUR

The development of pain behaviour requires a nervous system that can not only react to sensory stimuli but also distinguish between different modalities of stimuli, for example tactile versus noxious, to produce different reflex responses. These responses are not evidence of pain perception, of 'feeling' pain as such, but do provide information about the sensitivity and selectivity of the fetal and neonatal nervous system to nociceptive stimuli.

Reflex responses to somatic stimuli begin at 7.5 weeks in the human fetus (Bradley & Mistretta 1975) and 15 days (E15, where gestation is 21.5 days) in the rat fetus (Narayanan et al 1971). The first area to become sensitive is the perioral region. In the human, the palms of the hands are sensitive to stroking at 10.5 weeks; at E16 the rat forepaws are similarly sensitive. By 13.5–14 weeks in the human and E17 in the rat, the sensitive area has spread over the body and down to the hindlimbs. The feet and tail regions are the last to become responsive at E18–19. At the same time as the onset of evoked reflexes, the fetus begins to move spontaneously in the absence of any obvious external stimulation. Real-time ultrasound recording of human fetuses in utero has revealed a complex variety of movements including stretching, hand-to-face contact, startle and sucking which build up over 7.5–15 weeks' gestation and continue into postnatal life (De Vries et al 1982). Analogous spontaneous movements begin in the rat at E15 (Narayanan et al 1971).

It is important to emphasize that movements evoked at this stage are of a reflex or spontaneous nature only, even if they involve extensive body regions and therefore intersegmental and brainstem connections. They occur, albeit in abnormal patterns, in anencephalic fetuses of 16–35 weeks, even in severe cases where only parts of the spinal cord are intact (Visser et al 1985). The cortex is not a functional unit at this stage (see 'Development of peripheral and central connections related to pain' below) and therefore any discussion of 'perception' or of 'conscious' reaction to stimuli is inappropriate (Prechtl 1985).

Early reflexes are evoked by tactile stimulation or light pressure to the body surface and are not necessarily nociceptive. In fact, small-diameter afferents known to subserve nociception have still not penetrated the human fetal spinal cord at 19 weeks' gestational age (Konstantinidou et al 1995). However, by 26 weeks' gestational age even very low birth weight infants show a clear and measurable flexion withdrawal reflex to noxious stimulation, suggesting that nociceptive afferent input to the spinal cord is now present (Andrews & Fitzgerald 1994). In addition, infants of 26–31 weeks' gestational age show coordinated facial actions in response to noxious stimuli from a heel prick (Craig et al 1993). In contrast to spinal cord reflex responses, younger gestational age is associated with less reactivity in facial expression to heel lance, suggesting that the youngest infants are less able to display more complex affective reactions to pain (Stevens et al 1994), infants from 23 weeks' gestational age are capable of mounting a hormonal response when needles are inserted into the innervated intrahepatic vein (Giannakoulopoulos et al 1994), although the link between reported levels of pain and such stress response in adults is unpredictable and increasingly questioned (Wolf 1993).

POSTNATAL PAIN BEHAVIOUR

Fetal somatosensory reflexes are still prominent at birth but change considerably over the postnatal period. In the neonate a prick on the hind foot may bring about 'a whole body movement' involving wriggling, rolling, and simultaneous responses from fore and hindlimbs, but as it matures the response becomes more individuated and restricted to an isolated leg or foot movement. Isolated responses can be observed from birth however and, even late in life, intensely painful stimuli can still bring about chaotic responses. The individuation of movements seem not to be achieved through disintegration or breaking up of the total patterns, but by an inhibitory process, whereby they go into the background and remain in a seemingly dormant stage, but from which they may be aroused at any time later on appropriate stimulation (Angulo y Gonzalez 1932). The appropriate stimulation may well be a noxious one such as in inflammation or nerve damage, which lead to central sensitization and hypersensitive behaviour in adults which have many features in common with the newborn animal (Woolf 1994, Woolf & Doubell 1994).

A feature of individual cutaneous reflexes in the newborn rat, kitten and human is that they are exaggerated compared to the adult (Ekholm 1967, Stelzner 1971, Issler & Stephens 1983, Fitzgerald & Gibson 1984, Andrews & Fitzgerald 1994). Thresholds are lower and the reflex muscle contractions more synchronized and long lasting. Repeated skin stimulation results in considerable hyperexcitability or sensitization with generalized movements of all limbs. Ekholm (1967) detected that in young kittens the elicitation of a flexor reflex response often did not require a painful stimulus as in the adult but only light touch and this has been confirmed in newborn human infants and rat pups (Fitzgerald et al 1988). Flexor reflex thresholds are very low in preterm infants and newborn rat pups but increase with postconceptional age (PCA). Furthermore, the sensitization caused by repeated stimulation is found to be present in both species but becomes much less pronounced after 29–35 weeks PCA in the human and postnatal day 8 (P8) in the rat (Andrews & Fitzgerald 1994). Thresholds for withdrawal from heat stimuli are also lower in younger animals (Lewin et al 1993, Falcon et al 1996, Hu et al 1997, Marsh et al 1998b). The response to formalin has a ten-fold higher sensitivity in neonatal rats compared to weanlings (Teng & Abbott 1998), although up until day 10, the responses are predominantly 'non-specific' whole-body movements, while the 'specific' flexion reflex and shaking and licking the paw predominates from then on. Interestingly, the biphasic behavioural response to formalin is not apparent until P15, coinciding with the overall depression in the response (Guy & Abbot 1992). In contrast to the formalin response, the hyperalgesia or drop in mechanical threshold that follows carrageenan injection (Marsh et al 1998b) and mustard oil application (Jiang & Gebhart 1998) is clear in neonates but smaller in amplitude than in older animals.

SUMMARY AND CONCLUSIONS

The immature rat pup and human infant display clear reflex responses to noxious cutaneous stimuli in fetal life which continue into the postnatal period. While these are often generalized, whole-body movements in the very young pup, localized isolated reflexes are also present, becoming predominant as the animal matures. Immature cutaneous reflexes are generally exaggerated and the flexor reflex can be evoked to a lesser extent by non-noxious as well as noxious stimulation. The emergence of specific nociceptive responses that cannot be evoked by low-intensity stimuli occurs postnatally, coinciding with a depression of the overall response. While providing important information as to how the immature nervous system reacts to noxious stimulation, reflex responses cannot be equated with true pain experience, which requires functional maturation of higher brain centres. Stronger reflexes do not necessarily mean more pain but are likely to reflect the absence of the normal inhibitory control or 'dampening' influences that higher brain structures normally exert at more mature stages.

DEVELOPMENT OF PERIPHERAL AND CENTRAL CONNECTIONS RELATED TO PAIN

PERIPHERAL CONNECTIONS

The majority of lumbar dorsal root ganglion (DRG) cells in the rat are born between E11 and E18 (Altman & Bayer

1984, Coggeshall et al 1994). Cell death overlaps with cell division so that DRG cell numbers rise until E15 and then level off until birth, with a small 19% loss over the first postnatal 10 days (Coggeshall et al 1994). In addition there is loss of nearly 50% of axons from peripheral nerves from birth to adulthood which cannot be explained by neuron cell death (Jenq et al 1986). Peripheral nerves reach the base of the rat hindlimb bud by embryonic day E13 and the toes by E19 (Reynolds et al 1991). Skin innervation appears to occur in advance of muscle innervation, beginning at E14 in the proximal thigh and the toes at E21. Despite the fact that large, light dorsal root ganglion cells giving rise to future A fibres are born in advance of small dark cells giving rise to C fibres (Lawson et al 1974, Kitao et al 1996) and are the first group to grow central projections into the spinal cord grey matter (Fitzgerald 1987b), both populations appear to innervate the skin at the same time (Jackman & Fitzgerald 1998). The cues used by cutaneous afferents to reach their appropriate skin targets is a subject of some research and molecules capable of axon guidance through inhibitory or growth cone collapsing activity, such as semaphorin III, play an important role in directing normal peripheral nerve outgrowth (Behar et al 1996).

Before the appearance or innervation of specific terminal end organs, the sensory axons in the rat form a dense and organized terminal plexus that penetrates right to the surface of the fetal epidermis at E17–18 in the rat hindlimb (Fitzgerald 1966, Jackman & Fitzgerald 1998). The terminal plexus gradually withdraws as end organs appear and the epidermis becomes thinner, leaving a major subepidermal plexus, with a few axons penetrating up into the epidermis as seen in the adult (Fitzgerald 1966, Reynolds et al 1991, Jackman et al 1998). In the rat hindlimb, these changes take place in the late fetal and early neonatal period. Merkel cells begin to appear and are innervated at birth in the rat (English et al 1980), whereas hindlimb hair follicle innervation does not begin until postnatal day 7 (28 weeks in humans) (Payne et al 1991) and a few days earlier in mystacial skin (Munger & Rice 1986). Meissner's corpuscles do not appear in the rat until P8 (Zelena et al 1990) and early in the third trimester in primates (Renehan & Munger 1990).

Despite the lack of anatomically distinct sensory endings, in vivo electrophysiological recordings from individual embryonic rat DRG cells reveal clearly defined cutaneous receptive fields on the hindfoot from the onset of innervation at E17 (Fitzgerald 1987a, Fitzgerald & Fulton 1992). Frequency of firing and total number of impulses per stimulus are low compared to the adult, but increase with embryonic age. At this early stage, afferents fall into two clear categories, rapidly adapting pressure units and slowly adapting higher-threshold units. Examples of both receptor types are found that respond to noxious heating and chemical stimulation. One day later, at E18, a third category of low-threshold, rapidly adapting mechanoreceptor emerges, responding to light touch or brushing the skin, analogous to adult hair or touch mechanoreceptors. These do not respond to thermal or chemical stimuli. Fetal pressure receptors are still prominent in both fast and slow conduction groups at birth, but gradually disappear by P14 (Fitzgerald 1987c). They may represent a transient population of afferents functional only during early development or, alternatively, simply be immature low-threshold mechanoreceptors.

All the broad functional cutaneous afferent types found in the adult rat are found in the rat hindlimb at birth, although their maturity depends on receptor type (Fitzgerald 1987c, Fitzgerald & Fulton 1992). Polymodal nociceptors are fully mature in their thresholds, pattern and frequency of firing at birth. High-threshold Aδ mechanoreceptors can also be distinguished, but their peak firing frequencies are lower than in adults. Low-threshold mechanoreceptors are, relatively, the most immature at birth, with low frequencies of firing and amplitude of response.

The role of neurotrophic factors in the survival and maintenance of sensory neurons has been the subject of considerable recent research (Snider 1994, McMahon et al 1996). Nerve growth factor (NGF), produced in the skin and other target cells for example, is critically important for the survival of small nociceptor peptidergic C neurons (Ruit et al 1992). However, neurotrophic factors also play an important role in the development of receptor phenotype. Neonatal anti-NGF treatment leads to the conversion of myelinated nociceptors into low-threshold D-hairs and the remaining nociceptors have elevated mechanical thresholds (Ritter et al 1991). In addition, C-mechanoheat receptors are converted to a low-threshold mechanical pressure receptor by neonatal anti-NGF (Lewin & Mendell 1994). On the other hand, systemic neonatal NGF treatment leads to mechanical hyperalgesia and an increase in the proportion of C-heat nociceptors (Lewin et al 1993). BDNF-deficient mutant mice show a profound reduction in slowly adapting mechanoceptor sensitivity which is restored by brain-derived neurotrophic factor (BDNF) treatment (Carroll et al 1998).

DEVELOPMENT OF SPINAL CORD CONNECTIONS

Primary afferent central terminals

In the rat lumbar cord, large-diameter dorsal root afferents arrive at the spinal cord from E12 onwards but do not penetrate the grey matter for some days. Instead they travel rostocaudally in the bundle of His until E15, when the first main wave of collaterals begin to grow into the dorsal grey (Smith 1983, Fitzgerald et al 1991). It seems likely that the growth of collaterals into the grey matter is triggered by the innervation of the skin and other targets in the periphery (Fitzgerald et al 1991, Jackman et al 1998). Cutaneous afferents grow directly into the dorsal horn avoiding the ventral horn, probably due to release of an inhibitory factor, semaphorin III, from that area (Fitzgerald et al 1993a, Messersmith et al 1995, Puschel et al 1996) and terminal elaboration and characteristic U-shaped collaterals of hair-follicle afferents can be seen at E19 (Beal et al 1988, Fitzgerald et al 1994, Mirnics & Koerber 1995). Some central synapses with interneurons leading to cutaneous reflex responses are clearly made as early as E15.5 (see below), but the first Ia afferents reach the motoneuron pool at E17 coinciding with the onset of a Ia reflex (Ziskind-Conhaim 1990). C fibres grow into the spinal cord considerably later than A fibres, at E19 onwards (Fitzgerald 1987b), and many chemical markers associated with C fibres are not apparent in the spinal cord until the perinatal period (Coimbra et al 1986). C-type afferent terminals within synaptic glomeruli are not observed at EM level until P5 (Pignatelli et al 1989).

The growth of both A and C fibres into the cord is somatotopically precise (Fitzgerald & Swett 1983, Fitzgerald 1987b), presumably following from early fetal organization within the DRG themselves (Wessels et al 1990). This is not true of the laminar organization, however. While in the adult, Aβ afferents are restricted to laminae III and IV, in the fetus and neonate their terminals extend dorsally right up into laminae II and I to reach the surface of the grey matter (Fitzgerald et al 1994, Mirnics & Koerber 1995) where they can be seen to form synaptic connections at EM level (Coggeshall et al 1994). This is followed by a gradual withdrawal from the superficial laminae over the first 3 postnatal weeks (Fitzgerald et al 1994). C fibres, on the other hand, grow specifically to laminae I and II and for a considerable postnatal period these laminae are occupied by both A- and C-fibre terminals (Fitzgerald et al 1994). The presence of C fibres is an important factor in the withdrawal of A fibres from laminae I and II, because administration of neonatal capsaicin, which destroys the majority of C fibres, leaves A-fibre terminals located more superficially than in normal animals (Shortland et al 1990).

Development of functional connections within the dorsal horn

The spinal cord develops ventrodorsally: motoneurons are born first, followed by intermediate neurons, deep dorsal horn neurons and, finally, neurons of substantia gelatinosa (laminae I & II) (Nornes & Das 1974, Altman & Bayer 1984). There are also indications that axon outgrowth and synapses mature in the same direction; the first synapses occurring between interneurons and motoneurons followed by primary afferents and interneurons (Vaughn & Grieshaber 1973, Fitzgerald et al 1991). This retrograde development is by no means absolute and after the early stages of neurogenesis and axon outgrowth, cord maturation becomes highly complex and not obviously polarized.

Within the dorsal horn itself, projection neurons develop in advance of local interneurons (Bicknell & Beal 1984), and this is consistent with functional evidence suggesting that some inhibitory mechanisms commonly attributed to interneuronal activity in the dorsal horn are absent in the newborn (see below). Projection neurons such as the spinocerebellar and spinothalamic tract neurons are generated as distinct populations at E13–15 (Beal & Bice 1994), and those with the longest axons are generated first independent of target site (Nandi et al 1993). Synaptogenesis in the dorsal horn is at its maximum in the first postnatal weeks.

Prenatal cutaneous evoked activity must arise from A fibres because C fibres have not yet grown into the spinal cord. Low-threshold A fibres rapidly form synaptic connections prenatally and evoke brisk mono- and polysynaptic responses that can be recorded in the dorsal horn and from the ventral root soon after they grow into the spinal cord (Fitzgerald 1991a, b). Stimulation of the L4 dorsal root in the embryonic rat spinal cord in vitro begins to produce long-latency (presumably polysynaptic) reflexes in the L4 ventral root (Saito 1979, Kudo & Yamada 1987) and long-latency excitatory postsynaptic potentials (EPSPs) in L4 motoneurons (Ziskind-Conhaim 1990) between E15.5 and E16. Neither presumptive monosynaptic reflexes nor Ia EPSPs are observed until E17.5–18.5.

In vivo recording of cutaneous evoked activity of lumbar dorsal horn cells in rat embryos (Fitzgerald 1991a) shows that while synchronous input provided by electrical stimulation evokes spikes in dorsal horn cells at E17, it is several days before cutaneous afferents are capable of producing suprathreshold excitation under physiological conditions. Natural stimulation of the hindpaw evokes a spike discharge in dorsal horn cells at E19, initially by high-intensity skin stimulation only, but by E20 low-intensity brush and touch of the skin also excites dorsal horn cells.

In the newborn, the synaptic linkage between afferents and dorsal horn cells is still weak and electrical stimulation often evokes only a few spikes at long and variable latencies (Fitzgerald 1985a, Jennings & Fitzgerald 1998), but natural stimulation of receptive fields can often evoke long-lasting excitation lasting minutes and which which may lower the threshold to subsequent stimuli. Repeated low-intensity mechanical or A-fibre stimulation can lead to sensitization of dorsal horn cell responses beyond the period of stimulation (Jennings and Fitzgerald 1998). Furthermore, the receptive fields of the dorsal horn cells are larger in the newborn and gradually diminish over the first 2 postnatal weeks (Fitzgerald 1985a). The result of these properties is that otherwise weak cutaneous inputs are made more effective centrally and may underlie the exaggerated low-threshold cutaneous reflexes observed in the neonatal rat and human. The excitatory influence of A fibres may be a result of their synaptic connections within SG at this time. The expression of c-fos in SG neurons, which in adults is evoked by noxious and Aδ- and C-fibre inputs only, can also be evoked by innocuous inputs and A fibres in the newborn (Jennings & Fitzgerald 1996). The lack of inhibitory control at this age (see below) is also likely to be a factor.

The postnatal maturation of synaptic connections between afferent C fibres and SG cells takes place over a prolonged period. C-fibre activation is unable to evoke spike activity in the spinal cord until the second postnatal week (Fitzgerald & Gibson 1984, Fitzgerald 1988, Jennings & Fitzgerald 1998). Consistent with this is the absence of a long latency burst of activity on the ventral root after stimulation of C fibres in the dorsal root or cutaneous nerve during the first postnatal week (Fitzgerald et al 1987, Hori & Watanabe 1987). However, stimulation of a dorsal root at C-fibre intensities or noxious stimulation of the tail produces a long-latency (2–5 s), long-lasting (30 s) potential that can be recorded from the ventral root (Akagi et al 1983). It is blocked by substance P antagonists, the C-fibre neurotoxin capsaicin, and is reduced by morphine and other opioids in a naloxone-reversible manner (Yanagisawa et al 1985). This slow potential is particularly prominent in the newborn rat and can be evoked from many neighbouring dorsal roots. It appears to result from a widespread depolarization of spinal cord cells in response to the release of substance P and other neurochemicals from C-fibre terminals, rather than a specific synaptically mediated C-fibre evoked excitation. The widespread substance P receptor distribution within the spinal cord of the newborn rat (see 'Developmental pharmacology of pain' below) may also be responsible (Charlton & Helke 1986). Responses to noxious mechanical stimulation or non-specific chemical irritants, such as formalin, both of which have an A-fibre component, produce clear reflex activity and c-fos induction from birth (Fitzgerald & Gibson 1984, Williams et al 1990), but responses to pure C-fibre inputs remain subthreshold or low amplitude for a considerable period postnatally (Fitzgerald 1991b, Soyguder et al 1994, Jiang & Gebhart 1998).

SEGMENTAL AND DESCENDING INHIBITION

Gradual suppression or inhibition of neural connections is a feature of the developing somatosensory system and has an important influence on the postnatal organization of pain responses and the gradual diminution of behavioural reflexes and dorsal horn cell excitability over the postnatal period. Not all segmental inhibition is absent in the newborn rat cord. Renshaw cell inhibition (Naka 1984) and some contralateral inhibitory mechanisms (Fitzgerald 1985a) are well developed at birth. Nevertheless the maturation of interneurons in substantia gelatinosa, which appear to be particularly important for control of sensory processing, is largely postnatal (Bicknell & Beal 1984). Interestingly, this coincides with the arrival of afferent C fibres in the dorsal horn and the two events may be causally linked. Animals treated at birth with the neurotoxin capsaicin, which destroys afferent C fibres, retain large receptive fields in the dorsal horn and cortex perhaps due to inadequate interneurone function (Fitzgerald 1983).

Descending inhibitory controls are immature at birth (Fitzgerald 1991c). Animals given a midthoracic spinal cord transection before P15 are markedly less affected than those transected at older ages (Weber & Stelzner 1977). In spinalized rats below 15 days of age, tactile and noxious stimuli continue to evoke withdrawal responses that are similar to those observed in intact rats. Older animals show severely depressed responses for several days and then recover flexor responses to cutaneous stimuli with decreased duration. The slow maturation of descending inhibitory pathways travelling from the brainstem via the dorsolateral funiculus of the spinal cord to the dorsal horn is particularly relevant to pain processing. Although descending axons from brainstem projection neurons grow down the spinal cord early in fetal life, they do not extend collateral branches into the dorsal horn for some time and do not become functionally effective until postnatal day 10 in the rat (Fitzgerald & Koltzenburg 1986). This may be due in part to deficiency of neurotransmitters, in this case 5HT (serotonin) and noradrenaline, but it may also be due to delayed maturation of crucial interneurons. It has been suggested that the maturation of descending inhibition is dependent upon afferent C-fibre activity, because rats treated with capsaicin as adults have reduced inhibitory controls (Cervero & Plenderleith 1985) and mutant mice lacking the NK-1 receptor gene (and consequently altered C-fibre activity) have high dorsal horn cell firing rates (De Felipe et al 1998). The lack of descending inhibition in the neonatal dorsal horn means that there is no endogenous analgesic system to 'dampen' noxious inputs as they enter the CNS and their effects may therefore be more profound than in the adult. It also explains why stimulus-produced analgesia from the periacqueductal grey is not effective until P21 in rats (van Praag & Frenk 1991).

DEVELOPMENT OF CONNECTIONS IN HIGHER CENTRES

Despite the usefulness of the flexion reflex in understanding spinal cord pain mechanisms, it would be a mistake to equate it with true pain experience which must involve the cortex and develop postnatally along with memory, anxiety and other cognitive brain functions. A better idea of this may be obtained from behavioural investigations of infant pain such as facial actions (Grunau & Craig 1987, Johnston et al 1993), cry characteristics (Grunau et al 1990) and body movements and posture (Stevens et al 1994), all of which have shown that there are particular facial expressions, body actions or patterns of cry associated with tissue insult. Behavioural state and severity of illness influenced these responses (Stevens et al 1994), but even very low birth weight infants between 26 and 31 weeks' gestational age show a significantly different maximum heart rate and upper facial action response to painful heel prick versus sham (Johnston et al 1995). In contrast to spinal cord reflex responses, younger gestational age is associated with less reactivity in facial expression to heel lance (Johnston et al 1995). This may be a reflection of immature motor control which is likely to affect the more complex activity patterns of facial motoneurons more than those of lumbar spinal motoneurons, or alternatively it may show that sensory events at spinal cord level do not always reflect activity at higher brain levels. Much less is known of the maturation of projection pathways, thalamic and cortical connections in relation to pain processing compared to events in the periphery and spinal cord.

In the rat, dorsal horn projection cells begin to grow axons prenatally (Bicknell & Beal 1984, Fitzgerald et al 1991) and afferents reach the thalamus at E19. The earliest thalamic axons reach the cortical plate also at E19 (22–34 weeks in the human), and by P0 there is a plexus of growth-cone-tipped axons in the cortical plate and a few thalamic axons have reached the marginal zone (Mrzljak et al 1988, Erzurumlu & Jhaveri 1990). At postnatal days 2–5, many thalamocortical synapses are silent, consisting of NMDA receptors only, and are converted to functional synapses (NMDA and AMPA receptors) by activity dependent mechanisms at day 8–9. These findings correlate well with functional studies showing that evoked potentials from the forepaw in the rat somatosensory cortex reach maturity by P12 (Thairu 1971) and the onset of equivalent potentials in humans is at 29 weeks' gestation (Klimach & Cooke 1988). Electrophysiological analysis of cortical cells at P7 shows them to be organized in columns as in the adult but to have larger receptive fields, suggesting a lack of inhibition as discussed above for the spinal cord (Armstrong-James 1975). The delayed maturation of inhibitory processes occurring several weeks after excitatory connections have been established has been observed in the neonatal rat hippocampus (Michelson & Lothman 1989) and may be a general pattern in developing cortex. The rodent cortex remains immature for up to 6 weeks after birth and the human cortex for many years. The complex developmental processes taking place over this period are beyond the scope of this chapter. The development of attention and memory, and the many important cognitive factors contributing to the cortical perception of pain in infants and children, are reviewed elsewhere (Gaffney 1993).

SUMMARY AND CONCLUSIONS

By the time a rat is born, the basic sensory connections in the periphery and spinal cord are in place. Nevertheless, enormous changes take place over the early postnatal period coinciding with the final trimester and early neonatal period in man. The maturation of A- and C-fibre synaptic connections in the dorsal horn, interneuronal development in substantia gelatinosa and functional development of descending inhibition from the brainstem all take place postnatally in the rat. These important parts of the pain pathway display late maturation compared to the basic excitatory connections from low-threshold inputs. The effect of this is that while the newborn nervous system does mount a clear response to painful stimuli, this response is not always predictable or organized. Lack of inhibition means that responses to all sensory inputs, low and high threshold, are exaggerated and generalized and specific pain responses may require convergent inputs building up over time to become apparent.

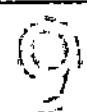

DEVELOPMENTAL PHARMACOLOGY OF PAIN

EXCITATORY PATHWAYS: I. GLUTAMATE

The role of glutamate in excitatory pathways related to pain is well established (see Ch. 10). Glutamate-NMDA activity takes on a further interesting dimension here in view of its general role in development and plasticity of connections in the immature CNS (Garthwaite 1989, Hofer & Constantine-Paton 1994).

NMDA receptors

The neonatal spinal cord has a higher concentration of NMDA receptors in the grey matter than that observed in older animals (Gonzalez et al 1993). All laminae in the dorsal horn are uniformly labelled with NMDA-sensitive [^{3}H]glutamate until days 10–12, when higher densities gradually appear in substantia gelatinosa so that by P30 binding is similar to that in the adult. Furthermore, the affinity of the receptors for NMDA decreases with postnatal age (Hori & Kanda 1994). In the immature hippocampus, where similar high densities are found, NMDA-evoked excitatory postsynaptic potentials (EPSPs) are much greater in amplitude and less sensitive to Mg^{2+} than in the adult (Morrisett et al 1990), and the antagonist activity of D-AP5 to the NMDA-evoked response is two to three times greater during this period (Brady et al 1994). The situation is similar in the neonatal dorsal horn where NMDA-evoked calcium efflux in rat substantia gelatinosa is very high in the first postnatal week and then declines (Hori & Kanda 1994). This is delayed by neonatal capsaicin treatment, suggesting that C-fibre afferent activity regulates the postnatal maturation of NMDA receptors (Hori & Kanda 1994). The developmental regulation of NMDA receptor function in neonatal pain transmission has not been directly investigated, although NMDA-dependent C-fibre-evoked depolarization of spinal cord cells and 'wind-up' of cells to repeated C-fibre stimulation has been demonstrated in the young (8–14-day) spinal cord in vitro (Thompson et al 1992, King & Lopez-Garcia 1993, Sivilotti et al 1995).

The different NMDA receptor channel subunits are independently regulated. Of particular interest are the NR2 subunits, which are modulatory because their expression alters properties such as voltage-dependent Mg^{2+} block and deactivation kinetics of NMDA receptors. The subunit composition of the NMDA channel complex undergoes considerable rearrangement during spinal cord development (Watanabe et al 1994), which appears to be activity dependent (Audinat et al 1994). The change in NMDA receptor properties is thought to reflect its different roles during development from survival, migration and neurite growth, which may require tonic activation by glutamate at extrasynaptic receptors, to neurotransmission involving phasic activation of receptors at synapses. Important changes in the sharpening and fine tuning of synapses have been observed in the developing visual system following chronic NMDA blockade (for a review see Hofer & Constantine-Paton 1994), and daily doses of MK-801 to embryonic chick disrupts the somatotopic organization of cutaneous nerve projections in the chick spinal cord (Mendelson 1994).

AMPA receptors

AMPA receptor expression in the neonatal spinal cord shows a wider distribution than in the adult, which decreases over the first postnatal 3 weeks (Jakovec et al 1995a). The Glu Rl, 2 and 4 subunits are generally more abundant in the neonatal compared to the adult cord, although the ratio of Glu2 to Glul, 3 and 4 is lower. As Glu2 does not allow Ca^{2+} flux, there will be relatively more non-NMDA-dependent Ca^{2+} influx in neonates. There are also changes in the distribution of the flip-flop variants with postnatal age. The functional importance of this lies in the fact that different combinations of subunits will affect desensitization, ionic permeability and current/voltage relationships. The flip variants are generally more sensitive to agonists than the flop, resulting in higher levels of depolarization from glutamate release. If the AMPA and NMDA receptors are co-localized this could lead to enhanced NMDA receptor activation (Jakowec et al 1995b).

Little is known about the functional role of immature AMPA receptors in neonatal pain, but at postnatal days 10–14 in the rat the AMPA antagonist, CNQX, abolishes dorsal horn cell firing to both low- and high-threshold inputs in vitro (King & Lopez-Garcia 1993).

Metabotropic receptors

Metabotropic glutamate receptors in the spinal cord are also differentially regulated during development. Autoradiographic studies show that there are large numbers of low-affinity quisqualate binding sites at birth and fewer high affinity ones. In situ studies of the subtypes, mGluR 1–5, show that mGluR, R2 and R4 are generally low at birth and increase to adult levels, whereas mGluR3 and R5 are high at birth and decrease to adult levels (Catania et al

1994). Signal transduction pathways mediated by mGluRs show opposing developmental patterns: phosphoinositide hydrolysis is very high in the first postnatal week and then decreases, whereas inhibition of cAMP formation is only accomplished in the adult (Nicoletti et al 1986, Casabona et al 1992).

Functional studies of these changes in metabotropic receptors in the dorsal horn have not been undertaken, but the NMDA-dependent, long-duration, C-fibre-evoked slow ventral root potentials and their wind-up on repeated stimulation are unaffected by the metabotropic antagonist, L-AP3, in 8–12 day cord (Thompson et al 1992).

EXCITATORY PATHWAYS: II. NEUROPEPTIDES

The importance of substance P and NK-1 receptors in pain processing is well established (Cao et al 1998, De Felipe et al 1998). Substance P containing primary afferent terminals first appear in the substantia gelatinosa of the rat at E18–19 and at 11 weeks in the human fetus (Senba et al 1982, Marti et al 1987). Calcitonin gene-related peptide (CGRP) and somatostatin appear at about the same time. Cell bodies positive for these peptides are apparent in the dorsal root ganglia from E17 onwards. Vasoactive intestinal peptide (VIP) immunoreactivity is detected much later than other primary afferent associated peptides in both rat, chick and human (Charnay et al 1985, New & Mudge 1986, Marti et al 1987). Despite the early appearance of these peptides, levels are very low at first and increase throughout fetal life, showing a marked increase perinatally to approach adult levels by P14.

Immunostaining of neonatal lumbar cord shows that the adult pattern of distribution of substance P and CGRP are present by P4 but adult staining intensities are not achieved until P10 (Reynolds & Fitzgerald 1992). This is also true of somatostatin and galanin (Marti et al 1987). Neuropeptides and their mRNAs are not expressed in DRG until their axons connect with their peripheral target, which appears to be an important trigger and modulatory influence on chemical phenotype (Hall et al 1997).

Substance P receptor density is maximal in the first two postnatal weeks – at P60, the cord has one-sixth of the binding sites present at P11. Furthermore, in the newborn there is the inverse receptor distribution of the adult. The superficial laminae have very few substance P receptors and the high density observed in the adult substantia gelatinosa is not apparent until the second week of life (Charlton & Helke 1986, Kar & Quirion 1995). Recent analysis in 12–20-day rats shows that the NK_1 receptors in substantia gelatinosa are not on the neurons themselves but on laminae III and IV cell dendrites that run through lamina II and terminate in lamina I (Bleazard et al 1994). Only 10% of the neurons in substantia gelatinosa respond to a selective NK_1-receptor agonist, compared to 48% in deeper laminae. It seems likely, therefore, that the lack of these receptors in neonatal substantia gelatinosa reflects the lack of dendritic growth of laminae III and IV cells at this age. Other neuropeptide receptors, for VIP, SOM, CGRP, neurotensin, galanin and neurokinin 3 (NK3), are also overexpressed in the immature spinal cord but all to different extents and some, like galanin, show a clear concentration in substantia gelatinosa from birth (Kar & Quirion 1995). Vasopressin receptors are transiently expressed in the immature cord and physiological studies show them to be functionally active in the neonate (Tribollet et al 1991), although they are lost in the adult.

Despite low levels, substance P can be released on stimulation of central C-fibre terminals to produce a long-lasting ventral root potential that is blocked by substance P antagonists (Akagi et al 1993). At P12, both NK_1 and NK_2 receptors are involved in C-fibre-evoked slow potentials (Nagy et al 1994). On the other hand substance P is not apparently released in sufficient quantities from peripheral C-fibre terminals to produce neurogenic extravasation, which cannot be observed until P10 (Fitzgerald & Gibson 1984), although exogenously applied substance P can produce extravasation before this age (Gonzales et al 1991).

INHIBITORY PATHWAYS: I. GABA

GABA

Gamma-aminobutyric acid (GABA) is transiently overexpressed in developing spinal cord and during the first 2 postnatal weeks, 50% of neurons are GABA positive compared to 20% in the third postnatal week (Schaffner et al 1993). At birth, cells expressing two forms of γ-aminobutyric acid decarboxylase (GAD) mRNA, GAD65 and GAD67, are widely distributed in all laminae, except in motoneurons of the spinal cord. This is followed by an overall decrease in the number of GAD mRNA-labelled cells in all layers, particularly within ventral portions of the spinal cord, a transient increase in expression between P7 and P14, and then a marked decline to adult (Ma et al 1994, Somogyi et al 1995).

In the adult spinal cord GABA is an inhibitory amino-acid transmitter that produces membrane hyperpolarization through the activation of postsynaptic $GABA_A$ and $GABA_B$ receptors and depresses transmitter release acting through presynaptic $GABA_B$ receptors, playing a crucial role in preventing the spread of excitatory glutamatergic activity. Recently, it has become clear that, during early stages of development, GABA mediates most of the *excitatory* drive in the hippocampal CA3 region (Ben-Ari et al 1994, Strata & Cherubini 1994). The activation of $GABA_A$ receptors induces a depolarization and excitation of immature CA3 pyramidal neurons and increases intracellular Ca^{2+} ($[Ca^{2+}{}_i]_i$) during the first postnatal week of life. This presumably arises from higher intracellular CL^- in immature neurons, perhaps due to immature co-transport mechanisms (Ben-Ari et al 1994). During the same developmental period, the postsynaptic $GABA_B$-mediated inhibition is poorly developed. By contrast, the presynaptic $GABA_B$-mediated inhibition is well developed at birth and plays a crucial role in modulating the postsynaptic activity by depressing transmitter release at early postnatal stages (Gaiarsa et al 1995a,b). A similar situation occurs in the neonatal dorsal horn where, in 90% of E15–16 dorsal horn neurons cultured for more than a week, both GABA- and glycine-induced increased $[Ca^{2+}{}_i]$ and depolarization (Reichling et al 1994). The depolarization and entry of Ca^{2+} through voltage-gated channels by bicuculline-sensitive GABA receptors and strychnine-sensitive glycine receptors decreases with age in culture and is gone by 30 days (Wang et al 1994).

GABA is another example of a classic neurotransmitter acting as a developmental signal. Transient increases in GAD mRNA expression during the early postnatal period coincide with, and may be linked to, synapse formation and synapse elimination of the developing spinal cord (Ma et al 1994).

INHIBITORY PATHWAYS: II. OPIOIDS

The developmental pharmacology of opioid analgesia and its role in paediatric pain management has been recently reviewed (Marsh et al 1998c).

Opioid peptides appear in the rat brain before their receptors. β-endorphin, met-enkephalin and dynorphin are all found at E11.5, followed by μ-receptor binding at E12.5, κ-receptor binding at E14.5 and δ-receptor binding at P0 (Rius et al 1991). High-affinity opioid receptor binding increases three-fold in the first 2 postnatal weeks, correlating with a 40-fold increase in opioid analgesic properties (Zhang & Pasternak 1981). At brainstem and spinal levels, however, enkephalin is not expressed in dorsal horn neurons, midbrain raphe or reticular formation until E20–P1 (Pickel et al 1982, Senba 1982, Marti et al 1987). Both μ- and κ-receptor binding sites appear in the rat spinal cord early in fetal life (E15), whereas δ-receptor sites do not appear until after birth (Attali et al 1990). Autoradiographic studies show a higher proportion of μ-receptor binding in the newborn dorsal horn compared to the adult (Rahman et al 1998). μ-receptor binding sites are concentrated in the superficial laminae of the dorsal horn in the adult, but at P1 the deeper layers share this relatively high density, with a marked change in distribution occurring with development (Kar & Quirion 1995). The relative proportion of κ-receptors is also higher in the newborn, while δ-receptor binding is absent until the end of the first postnatal week (Rahman et al 1998).

There is ample evidence that these endogenous opioid systems contribute to functioning analgesic mechanisms in the early postnatal period, although there has been some disagreement in the literature. Morphine analgesia to thermal nociception has been shown to increase with age in neonatal rat pups, progressing to a 40-fold analgesic potency at P14 compared to P3 (Zhang & Pasternak 1981, Barr et al 1986, Giordano & Barr 1987, Fanselow & Cramer 1988), and was without any detectable effect in a tail-flick nociceptive test until P12 (Barr et al 1986). Whereas morphine was more potent than ketocyclazocine (a kappa agonist) in producing analgesia to thermal nociception, ketocyclazocine was more effective at producing analgesia to a mechanical stimulus in younger animals (Barr et al 1986). However, more recent studies emphasize the antinociceptive effects of morphine soon after birth. Morphine (0.5–4.0 mg/kg) produces a dose-related increase in hindlimb withdrawal latency to a hot-plate from day 2 with maximum sensitivity at day 6 (Blass et al 1993), and the pain responses induced by the formalin inflammatory model is suppressed by 1–2 mg/kg morphine in 3-day-old rats (McLaughlin et al 1990). These discrepancies may arise from the central effects of opioids, especially those related to decreased respiration, because brainstem μ receptors are also postnatally developmentally regulated (Murphey & Olsen 1995). Also, early studies have warned of the susceptibility of neonates to the CNS-depressant effects of opioids, but a comparison of the sedative and analgesic effects of systemic morphine and pentobarbital in infant rats have shown that morphine produces analgesia to an intraplantar injection of formalin at all ages, which is qualitatively different from the sedative effects of pentobarbitone 10 mg/kg (Abbott & Guy 1995). Epidural application of morphine in neonatal rats is far more effective at raising mechanical flexion reflex thresholds in the newborn than in older animals, as are κ agonists and to a lesser extent delta agonists. These effects were upon low-threshold mechanoreceptive reflexes and contrast with effects in adults where these intrathecal opioids act relatively selectively on nociceptive or C-fibre-evoked activity (Dickenson & Sullivan 1986, Dickenson et al 1987, Sullivan & Dickenson 1991). The in vivo data here also contrasts with findings in isolated neonatal spinal cord preparations where the effects of opioid agonists are also restricted to C-fibre-evoked responses (Hori & Watanabe 1987, Sivilotti et al 1995). The effects of opioids upon mechanical thresholds in vivo may be due to the different distribution of μ, κ and δ receptors in neonates, perhaps on the A-fibre presynaptic terminals or on a different set of postsynaptic cells.

In contrast to the effects on mechanical thresholds, morphine is less effective on nociceptive heat thresholds in younger animals and increases its analgesic potency with age in these tests (Giordano & Barr 1987, Marsh et al 1998a). The heat-evoked flexion reflex is likely to be mediated by Aδ and C fibres and the low efficacy of morphine in these tests may reflect the immaturity of C fibres in the newborn (Fitzgerald 1988). Interestingly, the developmental profile of the κ agonist on heat nociception is almost the mirror image of morphine, being more effective at early ages and gradually decreasing in efficacy. In the adult, κ agonists are relatively devoid of activity on thermal tests (Yaksh & Stevens 1984). The δ-receptor agonist does not show the marked developmental changes observed in μ and κ agonists. In nociceptive heat tests, it is weakly analgesic at all ages.

The hyperalgesia produced by subcutaneous injection of carrageenan is also blocked by low doses of all three agonists at all ages, relative effectiveness varying with age but comparison with potencies in acute tests (Marsh et al 1998a) show that opioid potency is significantly greater in the presence of carrageenan inflammation at all ages (Marsh et al 1998b).

INHIBITORY PATHWAYS: III. MONOAMINES

Noradrenaline-containing terminals first appear in the rat dorsal horn at P4 and achieve the adult pattern by the second to third postnatal week, although they appear in the ventral horn well before that (Commission 1983). Peak noradrenergic receptor development in rat spinal cord occurs at around P12; this is consistent with the analgesic effects of intrathecal noradrenaline and the α_2 agonist, clonidine, in P10 rat pups (Hughes & Barr 1988). 5-hydroxy-tryptamine (5HT) develops considerably later than other neurotransmitters. It has not been detected at all in fetal or neonatal spinal cord in humans and is thought to develop some time after the first 6 postnatal weeks (Marti et al 1987). While 5HT is clearly involved in spinal analgesia, the multiple receptor makes its mode of action obscure (Lucas & Hen 1995). However, the onset of expression of both 5HT and its receptors precedes their specific functions in the spinal cord, suggesting that they, like glutamate, may play a trophic role during development (Rajaofetra et al 1992, Ziskind-Conhaim et al 1993).

5HT projections grow into the rat ventral horn between days 16 and 18 (Ziskind-Conhaim et al 1993), but are not present in the dorsal horn until day 0. A laminar distribution is apparant at day 5 but the adult distribution and density is not achieved until the end of the second week (Marti et al 1987, Wang et al 1991). There is also evidence of a transient overexpression of 5HT in the spinal cord at P14 (Bregman 1987). Levels of 5HT are not apparently sufficient for effective function of descending inhibitory pathways to the spinal cord from the brainstem until the second or third postnatal week (Fitzgerald & Koltzenburg 1986, van Praag & Frenk 1991). D-amphetamine (2 mg/kg) at doses that would enhance release of all three monoamines does not begin to affect pain behaviour before 10 days of age, suggesting that these monoamines are not fully functional in the pain pathways before that time (Abbot & Guy 1995).

Noradrenergic (NA) axons invade the spinal cord at E16, beginning in the ventral cord and reaching the dorsal horn by P0. The pattern of innervation in the dorsal horn is like that of the adult at P7, but adult density is not reached until P30 (Rajaofetra et al 1992). Peak noradrenergic receptor development in rat spinal cord occurs at around P12, consistent with the analgesic effects of intrathecal noradrenaline and the α_2 agonist, clonidine, in P10 rat pups (Hughes & Barr 1988). Noradrenaline-containing terminals first appear in the dorsal horn at P4 and achieve the adult pattern by 14–21 days (Commission 1983).

SUMMARY AND CONCLUSIONS

Many neurotransmitters and signalling molecules involved in pain pathways are expressed early in the developing nervous system but do not reach adult levels for a considerable period. More importantly, receptors are frequently transiently overexpressed or expressed in areas during development where they are not seen in the adult and may have a different functional profile. Low levels of neurotransmitter may reduce transmission, but widespread, high-density receptors with greater ligand responsiveness may compensate for this and also lead to important functional differences between the neonate and adult. This will have consequences on pain behaviour in the newborn and the effects of analgesics in controlling infant pain.

DEVELOPMENT OF CHRONIC PAIN MECHANISMS

NEONATAL RESPONSE TO INFLAMMATION AND TISSUE INJURY

Peripheral tissue injury in newborn infants results in a fall in the flexor reflex threshold and a hyperalgesic state results. In premature infants the cutaneous flexor reflex threshold in an area of local tissue damage created by repeated heel lances is half the value of that on the intact contralateral heel (Fitzgerald et al 1988). The 'tenderness' is established for days and weeks in the presence of tissue damage (Fitzgerald et al 1989).

In the adult this hyperalgesia is produced by the peripheral activation of C afferents which modifies the functional response of the spinal cord to other inputs applied long after the conditioning input (Woolf 1994). However little is known of this process in the neonatal CNS, occurring as it does against an existing background of high neuronal excitability. The two transmitter systems involved in the adult hypersensitivity generated by inflammation are glutamate acting on NMDA receptors and tachykinins operating on NK_1 and NK_2 neurokinin receptors, and the changing properties of these systems during development have already been described above. The activation of intracellular enzymes, protein kinase C and nitric oxide synthase may also differ in the neonate. C-fibre activation by mustard oil does not induce nitric oxide synthase (NOS) in the dorsal horn in the first postnatal week (Soyguder et al 1994).

Established pain following injury in the newborn may also have a peripheral component. Cutaneous sensory neurons undergo considerable growth and reorganization in the postnatal period (Reynolds et al 1991) and the growth-associated protein GAP-43 mRNA continues to be expressed in these neurons until P10 (Chong et al 1992). Neonatal cutaneous terminals are also capable of terminal sprouting following partial denervation (Kinnman & Aldskogius 1986, Diamond et al 1987, Payne & Fitzgerald 1998). Tissue damage in the early postnatal period causes a profound and lasting sprouting response of the local sensory nerve terminals, leaving an area of hyperinnervation in the wounded area that lasts into adulthood (Reynolds & Fitzgerald 1995). Behavioural studies show long-lasting hypersensitivity and a lowered mechanical threshold in the injured region. The sprouting response is clearly greatest when the wound is performed at birth and declines with age at wounding. The response to adult wounds is weak and transient in comparison, resulting in a temporary hyperinnervation that recovers after a few weeks. Both myelinated A fibres and unmyelinated C fibres, but not sympathetic fibres, contribute to the sprouting response (Reynolds et al 1991) and it is unaffected by local anaesthetic block of the sensory nerve during wounding (De Lima et al 1998). The substantial A-fibre contribution is in contrast to collateral sprouting which appears, in adults, to be largely restricted to small-diameter afferents (Horsch 1981, Jackson & Diamond 1983), although there is some evidence that myelinated fibres may be involved at an early postnatal age (Kinnman & Aldskogius 1986, Jackson & Diamond 1984, Shortland & Fitzgerald 1994, Payne & Fitzgerald 1998). One possibility, then, is that while C fibres retain the ability to sprout into adulthood, A-fibre sprouting is only possible within a critical developmental period. It seems likely that the sprouting results from the release of neurotrophic factors from the damaged region. The sprouts are all oriented towards the wound margin exactly as if attracted to the wound site by a specific signal. Skin wounding at birth results in a substantial upregulation of NGF (Constantinou et al 1994) that decreases with increasing age, but this is unlikely to be the main cause of sprouting because anti-NGF treatment fails to prevent neurite outgrowth towards injured skin in an in vitro co-culture model (Reynolds et al 1997). Nevertheless, upregulation of NGF at the site of injury may lead to changes in receptor function (see 'Peripheral Connections' above). BDNF, NT-3 and NT-4 are also all expressed in the skin during development (Ernfors et al 1992) and may be upregulated following skin wounds along with other growth factors (Whitby & Fergusson 1991). Furthermore the immune cytokines, released after tissue injury from macrophages or even neurons and glia, may directly affect neurite outgrowth (Heumann et al 1987, Schwartz et al 1991) via a mechanism not involving NGF as an intermediary (Jonakait 1993).

These findings have important implications for the consequences of injury and tissue trauma in the newborn infant, where hyperinnervation resulting in pain or hypersensitivity at the site of the injury occurs long after the original wound has healed.

NERVE DAMAGE

The developing nervous system is much more vulnerable to peripheral injury than the adult. This is especially well demonstrated in the neurons of the dorsal root ganglion where section/ligation of the sciatic nerve results in more rapid and extensive death of 75% of axotomized neurons in newborn rats compared to 30% in adult rats (Himes & Tessler 1989). As a result of the death of dorsal root ganglion cells the central dorsal root terminals of nearby intact nerves sprout in the spinal cord to occupy areas normally exclusively devoted to the sectioned nerve (Fitzgerald 1985, Fitzgerald & Vrbova 1985, Reynolds & Fitzgerald 1992). These new sprouts form inappropriate functional connections with dorsal horn cells in areas far outside their normal termination area (Shortland & Fitzgerald 1991). This means that the nervous system becomes permanently distorted with a greater proportion than normal devoted to inputs surrounding the denervated skin. Although in the short term this could be a useful compensatory device to restore sensory input from an area of the body surface in which it has been lost, the long-term effects of a permanent alteration in the sensory mapping of the body may be detrimental. The effects are not confined to primary afferent nerves, but spread to postsynaptic dorsal horn cells (Fitzgerald & Shortland 1988) and from these to higher levels of the nervous system including the cortex (Kaas et al 1983, Killackey & Dawson 1989). The extensive depletion of neuropeptides in the dorsal horn that follow nerve injury in the adult is not observed in the first postnatal week. Substance P and CGRP levels show remarkable plasticity to nerve section in the newborn, which can only be partially explained by collateral sprouting (Reynolds & Fitzgerald 1992).

The epidemiology of neuropathic pain in infants and children is not well established (Olsson & Berde 1993). Infants suffering traction on their brachial plexus on delivery have not been reported to suffer allodynia or hyperalgesia, but no systematic testing of their sensory receptive fields adjacent to the area of sensory loss has been undertaken. The widely accepted belief that children do not experience phantom limb pain is incorrect and young rats display much more vigorous behavioural signs of mechanical allodynia and ongoing pain following nerve injury than either mature or old rats (Chung et al 1994).

SUMMARY AND CONCLUSIONS

Experimental laboratory evidence points to the long-term consequences upon the somatosensory nervous system of local peripheral nerve damage or tissue injury in infancy. The clinical implications of these findings, if true in man, are extremely important.

It has been reported that children with birth weights under 750 g but without overt neurological damage are still at high risk for neurobehavioural dysfunction and poor school performance and early sensory experiences in intensive care may be an important factor here (Hack 1994). Infants born at less than 1000 g when assessed at 18 months of age are found to have significantly lower pain sensitivity compared to controls (Grunau et al 1994a,b). Neonatal circumcision in the absence of analgesia results in increased pain responses during subsequent routine vaccination, months later (Taddio et al 1997). In view of the changing nature of neonatal somatosensory and pain pathways and the vulnerability of the developing nervous system to alterations in sensory stimulation, it is important to ask to what extent early pain and tissue trauma can determine future pain processing in the adult.

REFERENCES

Abbott FV, Guy ER 1995 Effects of morphine, pentobarbital and amphetamine on formalin-induced behaviours in infant rats: sedation versus specific suppression of pain. Pain 62: 303–312

Akagi H, Konishi S, Yanagisawa M, Otsuka M 1983 Effects of capsaicin and a substance P antagonist on a slow reflex in the isolated rat spinal cord. Neurochemical Research 8: 795–796

Altman J, Bayer SA 1984 The development of the rat spinal cord. Advances in Anatomy, Embryology and Cell Biology 85: 1–166

Andrews K, Fitzgerald M 1994 The cutaneous withdrawal reflex in human neonates: sensitization, receptive fields, and the effects of contralateral stimulation. Pain 56: 95–101

Angulo y Gonzalez AW 1932 The prenatal development of behaviour in the albino rat. Journal of Comparative Neurology 55: 395–442

Armstrong-James M 1975 The functional status and columnar organization of single cells responding to cutaneous stimulation in neonatal rat somatosensory cortex SI. Journal of Physiology 246: 501–538

Attali B, Saya D, Vogel Z 1990 Pre- and postnatal development of opiate receptor subtypes in rat spinal cord. Developmental Brain Research 53: 97–102

Audinat E, Lambolez B, Rossier J, Crepel F 1994 Activity-dependent regulation of *N*-methyl-D-asparate receptor subunit expression in rat cerebellar granule cells. European Journal of Neuroscience 6: 1792–1800

Barr GA, Paredes W, Erickson KL et al 1986 κ-opioid receptor mediated analgesia in the developing rat. Developmental Brain Research 29: 145–152

Beal JA, Bice TN 1994 Neurogenesis of spinothalamic and spinocerebellar tract neurons in the lumbar spinal cord of the rat. Brain Research Development Brain Research 78(1): 49–56

Beal JA, Knight DS, Nandi KN 1988 Structure and development of central arborizations of hair follicle primary afferent fibers. Anatomy and Embryology 178: 271–279

Behar-O, Golden-JA, Mashimo-H, Schoen-FJ, Fishman-MC 1996

Semaphorin III is needed for normal patterning and growth of nerves, bones and heart. Nature 383: 525–528

Ben-Ari Y, Tseeb V, Raggozzino D, Khazipov R, Gaiarsa JL 1994 Gamma-aminobutyric acid (GABA): a fast excitatory transmitter which may regulate the development of hippocampal neurones in early postnatal life. Progress in Brain Research 102: 261–273

Bicknell HR, Beal JA 1984 Axonal and dendritic development of substantia gelatinosa neurons in the lumbosacral spinal cord of the rat. Journal of Comparative Neurology 226: 508–522

Blass EM, Cramer CP, Fanselow MS 1993 The development of morphine induced antinociception in neonatal rats: a comparison of forepaw, hindpaw and tail retraction from a thermal stimulus. Pharmacology, Biochemistry Behavior 44: 643–649

Bleazard L, Hill RG, Morris R 1994 The correlation between the distribution of the NK_1 receptor and the actions of tachykinin agonists in the dorsal horn of the rat indicates that substance P does not have a functional role on substantia gelatinosa (lamina II) neurons. Journal of Neuroscience 14: 7655–7664

Bradley RM, Mistretta CM 1975 Fetal sensory receptors. Physiological Reviews 55: 352–382

Brady RJ, Gorter JA, Monroe MT, Swann JW 1994 Developmental alterations in the sensitivity of hippocampal NMDA receptors to AP5. Developmental Brain Research 83: 190–196

Bregman BS 1987 Development of serotonin immunoreactivity in the rat spinal cord and its plasticity after neonatal spinal cord lesions. Developmental Brain Research 34: 245–263

Cao YQ, Mantyh PW, Carlson EJ, Gillespie A-M, Epstein CJ, Basbaum AI 1998 Primary afferent tachykinins are required to experience moderate to intense pain. Nature 392: 390–394

Carroll P, Lewin GR, Koltzenburg M, Toyka K, Thoenen H 1998 A role for BDNF in mechanosensation. Nature Neuroscience 1: 42–46

Casabona G, Genazzi AA, Di SM, Sortino MA, Nicoletti F 1992 Developmental changes in the modulation of cyclic AMP formation by the metabotropic glutamate receptor agonist 15, 3R aminocyclopentane-1,3 dicarboxylicacid in brain slices. Journal of Neurochemistry 89: 1161–1163

Catania MV, Landwehrmeyer GB, Testa CM, Standaert DG, Penney JB Jr, Young AB 1994 Metabotropic glutamate receptors are differentially regulated during development. Neuroscience 61: 481–495

Cervero F, Plenderleith MB 1985 C-fibre excitation and tonic descending inhibition of dorsal horn neurones in adult rats treated at birth with capsaicin. Journal of Physiology 365: 223–237

Charlton CG, Helke CJ 1986 Ontogeny of substance P receptors in rat spinal cord: quantitative changes in receptor number and differential expression in specific loci. Developmental Brain Research 29: 81–91

Charnay Y, Chayvaille J-A, Said SI et al 1985 Localization of vasoactive intestinal peptide immunoreactivity in human foetus and newborn infant spinal cord. Neuroscience 14: 195–205

Chong MS, Fitzgerald M, Winter J et al 1992 GAP-43 mRNA in rat spinal cord and dorsal root ganglia neurons: developmental changes and re-expression following peripheral nerve injury. European Journal of Neurology 4: 883–895

Chung JM, Choi Y, Yoon YW, Na HS 1994 Effects of age on behavioural signs of neuropathic pain in an experimental rat model. Neuroscience Letters 183: 54–57

Coggeshall RE, Pover CM, Fitzgerald M 1994 Dorsal root ganglion cell death and surviving cell numbers in relation to the development of sensory innervation in the rat hindlimb. Developmental Brain Research 82: 193–212

Coimbra A, Ribeiro-da-Silva A, Pignatelli D 1986 Rexed's laminae and the FRAP-band in the spinal cord of the neonatal rat. Neuroscience Letters 71: 131–137

Commission JW 1983 The development of catecholaminergic nerves in the spinal cord of the rat. II. regional development. Developmental Brain Research 11: 75–92

Constantinou J, Reynolds ML, Woolf CJ, Safieh-Garabedian B, Fitzgerald M 1994 Nerve growth factor levels in developing rat skin: upregulation following skin wounding. Neuroreport 5: 2281–2284

Craig KD, Whitfield MF, Grunau RVE, Linton J, Hadjistavropoulos HD 1993 Pain in the preterm neonate: behavioural and physiological indices. Pain 287–299

De Felipe C, Herreo JF, O'Brien JA et al 1998 Altered nociception, analgesia and aggression in mice lacking the receptor for substance P. Nature 392: 394–397

De Lima J, Alvares D, Reynolds M, Fitzgerald M 1998 Sensory hyperinnervation following neonatal skin wounding: the effect of bupivicaine sciatic nerve blockade. European Journal of Neuroscience 10(suppl 10): 79

De Vries JIP, Visser GHA, Prechtl HFR 1982 The emergence of foetal behaviour. I. Qualitative aspects. Early Human Development 12: 301–322

Diamond J, Coughlin MD, MacIntyre L, Holmes M, Visheau B 1987 Evidence that endogenous NGF is responsible for the collateral sprouting, but not regeneration, of nociceptive axons in adult rats. Proceeding of the National Academy of Sciences USA 84: 6596–6600

Dickenson AH, Sullivan AF 1986 Electrophysiological studies on the effects of intrathecal morphine on nociceptive neurons in the rat dorsal horn. Pain 24: 211–222

Dickenson AH, Sullivan AF, Knox R, Zajac JM, Roques BP 1987 Opioid receptor subtypes in the rat spinal cord: electrophysiological studies with μ- and δ-opioid receptor agonists in the control of nociception. Brain Research 413: 36–44

Ekholm J 1967 Postnatal changes in cutaneous reflexes and in the discharge pattern of cutaneous and articular sense organs. Acta Physiologica Scandinavica. Supplement 297: 1–130

English KB, Burgess PR, Van Norman KD 1980 Development of rat Merkel cells. Journal of Comparative Neurology 194: 475–496

Ernfors P, Wetmore C, Olson L, Persson H 1992 Cells expressing mRNA for neurotrophins and their receptors during embryonic rat development. European Journal of Neuroscience 4: 1140–1158

Erzurumlu RS, Jhaveri S 1990 Thalamic axons confer a blueprint of the sensory periphery onto the developing rat somatosensory cortex. Developmental Brain Research 56: 229–234

Falcon M, Guendellman D, Stolberg A, Frenk H, Urca G 1996 Development of thermal nociception in rats. Pain 67: 203–208

Fanselow MS, Cramer CP 1988 The ontogeny of opiate tolerance and withdrawal in infant rats. Pharmacology, Biochemistry and Behavior 31: 431–438

Fitzgerald M, Shortland P 1988 The effect of neonatal peripheral nerve section on the somdendritic growth of sensory projection cells in the rat spinal cord. Developmental Brain Research 41: 129–136

Fitzgerald M, Koltzenburg M 1986 The functional development of descending inhibitory pathways in the dorsolateral funiculus of the newborn rat spinal cord. Developmental Brain Research 24: 261–270

Fitzgerald M 1983 Capsaicin and sensory neurones – a review. Pain 15: 109–130

Fitzgerald M 1985a The postnatal development of cutaneous afferent fibre input and receptive field organization in the rat dorsal horn. Journal of Physiology 364: 1–18

Fitzgerald M 1985b The sprouting of saphenous nerve terminals in the spinal cord following early postnatal sciatic nerve section in the rat. Journal of Comparative Neurology 240: 407–413

Fitzgerald M 1987a Spontaneous and evoked activity of fetal primary afferents 'in vivo'. Nature 326: 603–605

Fitzgerald M 1987b Prenatal growth of fine-diameter primary afferents into the rat spinal cord: a transganglionic tracer study. Journal of Comparative Neurology 261: 98–104

Fitzgerald M 1987c Cutaneous primary afferent properties in the hindlimb of the neonatal rat. Journal of Physiology 383: 79–92
Fitzgerald M 1988 The development of activity evoked by fine diameter cutaneous fibres in the spinal cord of the newborn rat. Neuroscience Letters 86: 161–166
Fitzgerald M 1991a A physiological study of the prenatal development of cutaneous sensory inputs to dorsal horn cells in the rat. Journal of Physiology 432: 473–482
Fitzgerald M 1991b The developmental neurobiology of pain. In: Bond MR, Charlton JE, Woolf CJ (eds) Proceedings of VIth World Congress on Pain, 1991. Elsevier, Amsterdam, pp 253–261
Fitzgerald M 1991c The development of descending brainstem control of spinal cord sensory processing. In: Hanson M (ed) Fetal and neonatal brainstem: developmental and clinical issues. Cambridge University Press, Cambridge, pp 127–136
Fitzgerald M, Fulton B 1992 The physiological properties of developing sensory neurons. In: Sheryl Scott (ed) Sensory neurons. Oxford University Press, Oxford, pp 287–306
Fitzgerald M, Gibson S 1984 The physiological and neurochemical development of peripheral sensory C fibers. Neuroscience 13: 933–944
Fitzgerald M, King AE, Thompson SWN, Woolf CJ 1987 The postnatal development of the ventral root reflex in the rat: a comparative 'in vivo' and 'in vitro' study. Neuroscience Letters 78: 41–45
Fitzgerald M, Koltzenburg M 1986 The functional development of descending inhibitory pathways in the dorsolateral funiculus of the newborn rat spinal cord. Developmental Brain Research 24: 261–270
Fitzgerald M, Swett JW 1983 The termination pattern of sciatic nerve afferent in the substantia gelatinosa of neonatal rats. Neuroscience Letters 43: 149–154
Fitzgerald M, Vrbova G 1985 Plasticity of acid phosphatase (FRAP) afferent terminal fields and of dorsal horn cell growth in the neonatal rat. Journal of Comparative Neurology 240: 414–422
Fitzgerald M, Shaw A, McIntosh N 1988 Postnatal development of the cutaneous flexor reflex: comparative study of preterm infants and newborn rat pups. Developmental Medicine and Child Neurology 30: 520–526
Fitzgerald M, Millard C, MacIntosh N 1989 Cutaneous hypersensitivity following peripheral tissue damage in newborn infants and its reversal with topical anaesthesia. Pain 39: 31–36
Fitzgerald M, Reynolds ML, Benowitz LI 1991 GAP-43 expression in the developing rat lumbar spinal cord. Neuroscience 14: 187–199
Fitzgerald M, Kwiat G, Middleton JM, Pini A 1993a Ventral spinal cord inhibition of neurite outgrowth from embryonic rat dorsal root ganglia. Development 117: 1377–1384
Fitzgerald M, Butcher T, Shortland P 1994 Developmental changes in the laminar termination of A fibre cutaneous sensory afferents in the rat spinal cord dorsal horn. Journal of Comparative Neurology 348: 225–233
Fitzgerald MJT 1966 Perinatal changes in epidermal innervation in rat and mouse. Journal of Comparative Neurology 126: 37–42
Gaffney A 1993 Cognitive developmental aspects of pain in school-age children. In: Schechter N, Berde C, Yaster M (eds) Pain in infants, children and adolescents. Williams & Wilkins, Baltimore, pp 75–86
Gaiarsa JI, McLean H, Congar P et al 1995a Postnatal maturation of gamma-aminobutyric acid A and B-mediated inhibition in the CA3 hippocampal region of the rat. Journal of Neurobiology 26: 339–349
Gaiarsa JL, Tseeb V, Ben-Ari Y 1995b Postnatal development of pre- and post-synaptic GABAB-mediated inhibitions in the CA3 hippocampal region of the rat. Journal of Neurophysiology 73: 246–255
Garthwiate 1989 NMDA receptors, neuronal development and neurodegeneration. In: Watkins JC, Collinridge GL (eds) The NMDA receptor. IRL Press, Oxford, pp 187–205
Giannkopoulos X, Sepulveda W, Kourkis P, Glover V, Fisk NM 1994 Fetal plasma cortisol and b-endorphin response to intrauterine needling. Lancet 344: 77–81
Giordano J, Barr GA 1987 Morphine- and ketocyclazocine-induced analgesia in the developing rat: differences due to type of noxious stimulus and body topography. Developmental Brain Research 32: 247–253
Gonzales R, Coderre TJ, Sherbourne CD, Levine JD 1991 Postnatal development of neurogenic in the rat. Neuroscience Letters 127: 25–27
Gonzalez DL, Fuchs JL, Droge MH 1993 Distribution of NMDA receptor binding in developing mouse spinal cord. Neuroscience Letters 151: 134–137
Grunau RVE, Craig KD 1987 Pain expression in neonates: facial action and cry. Pain 28: 395–410
Grunau RVE, Johnston CC, Craig KD 1990 Neonatal facial action and cry responses to invasive and non-invasive procedures. Pain 42: 295–305
Grunau RVE, Whitfield MF, Petrie JH, Fryer EL 1994a Early pain experience, child and family factors, as precursors of somatization: a prospective study of extremely premature and fullterm children. Pain 56: 353–359
Grunau RVE, Whitfield MF, Petrie JH 1994b Pain sensitivity and temperament in extremely low birth weight premature toddlers and preterm and full term controls. Pain 58: 341–346
Guy ER, Abbott FV 1992 The behavioural response to formalin pain in preweanling rats. Pain 51: 81–90
Hack MB 1994 School age outcomes in children with birth weights under 750 g. New England Journal of Medicine 331: 753–759
Hall AK, Ai X, Hickman GE, MacPhedraen SE, Nduaguba CO, Robertson CP et al 1997 The generation of neuronal heterogeneity in a rat sensory ganglion. Journal of Neuroscience 17: 6069–6076
Heumann R, Korsching S, Bandtlow C, Thoenen H 1987 Changes of nerve growth factor synthesis in nonneuronal cells in response to sciatic nerve transection. Journal of Cell Biology 104: 1623–1631
Himes BT, Tessler A 1989 Death of some DRG neurons and plasticity of others following sciatic nerve section in adult and neonatal rats. Journal of Comparative Neurology 284: 215–230
Hofer M, Constantine-Paton M 1994 Regulation of N-methyl-D-aspartate (NMDA) receptor function during the rearrangement of developing neuronal connections. Progress in Brain Research 102: 277–285
Hori Y, Kanda K 1994 Developmental alterations in NMDA receptor-mediated $[Ca^{2+}]_i$ elevation in substantia gelatinosa neurons of neonatal rat spinal cord. Developmental Brain Research 80: 141–148
Hori Y, Watanabe S 1987 Morphine sensitive late components of the flexion reflex in the neonatal rat. Neuroscience Letters 78: 91–96
Horsch K 1981 Absence of functional collateral sprouting of mechanoreceptor axons into denervated areas of mammalian skin. Experimental Neurology 74: 313–318
Hu-D, Hu-R, Berde-CB 1997 Neurologic evaluation of infant and adult rats before and after sciatic nerve blockade. Anesthesiology 957–965
Hughes HE, Barr GA 1988 Analgesic effects of intrathecally applied noradrenergic compounds in the developing rat: differences due to thermal vs mechanical nociception. Developmental Brain Research 41: 109–120
Issler H, Stephens JA 1983 The maturation of cutaneous reflexes studied in the upper limb in man. Journal of Physiology 335: 643–654
Jackman A, Fitzgerald M 1998 The development of cutaneous sensory innervation of the limb by different subpopulations of sensory neurons. (Unpublished observations)
Jackson PC, Diamond J 1983 Failure of intact cutaneous mechano-sensory axons to sprout functional collaterals in skin of adult rabbits. Brain Research 273: 277–283

Jackson PC, Diamond J 1984 Temporal and spatial constraints on the collateral sprouting of low threshold mechanosensory nerves in the skin of rats. Journal of Comparative Neurology 226: 336–345

Jakowec MW, Fox AJ, Martin CJ, Kalb RG 1995a Quantitative and qualitative changes in AMPA receptor expression during spinal cord development. Neuroscience 67: 893–907

Jakowec MW, Yen L, Kalb RG 1995b In situ hybridization analysis of AMPA receptor subunit gene expression in the developing rat spinal cord. Neuroscience 67: 909–920

Jennings E, Fitzgerald M 1996 C-Fos can be induced in the neonatal rat spinal cord by both noxious and innocuous peripheral stimulation. Pain 68: 301–306

Jennings E, Fitzgerald M 1998 Postnatal changes in responses of rat dorsal horn cells to afferent stimulation: A fibre induced sensitization. Journal of Physiology 509: 859–867

Jenq C-B, Chung K, Coggeshall RE 1986 Postnatal loss of axons in normal rat sciatic nerve. Journal of Comparative Neurology 244: 445–450

Jiang MC, Gebhart GF 1998 Development of mustard oil-induced hyperalgesia in rats. Pain 77: 305–313

Johnston CC, Stevens BJ, Craig KD, Grunau RVE 1993 Development changes in pain expression in premature, fullterm, two and four month-old infants. Pain 52: 201–228

Johnston CC, Stevens BJ, Yang F, Horton L 1995 Differential response to pain by very premature neonates. Pain 61: 471–479

Jonakait GM 1993 Neural–immune interactions in sympathetic ganglia. trends in Neuroscience 16: 419–423

Kaas JH, Merzenich MM, Killackey HP 1983 The reorganization of somatosensory cortex following peripheral nerve damage in adult and developing mammals. Annual Review of Neuroscience 6: 325–356

Kar S, Quirion R 1995 Neuropeptide receptors in developing and adult rat spinal cord: an in vitro quantitative autoradiography study of calcitonin gene-related peptide, neurokinins, μ-opioid, galanin, somatostatin, neurotensin and vasoactive intestinal polypeptide receptors. Journal of Comparative Neurology 354: 253–281

Killackey HP, Dawson DR 1989 Expansion of the central hindpaw representation following fetal forelimb removal in the rat. European Journal of Neuroscience 1: 210–221

King AE, Lopez-Garcia JA 1993 Excitatory amino acid receptor mediated neurotransmission from cutaneous afferents in rat dorsal horn 'in vitro'. Journal of Physiology (London) 472: 443–457

Kinnman E, Aldskogius H 1986 Collateral sprouting of sensory axons in the glabrous skin of the hindpaw after chronic sciatic lesion in adult and neonatal rats: a morphological study. Brain Research 377: 73–82

Kitao Y, Robertson B, Kudo M, Grant G et al 1996 Neurogenesis of subpopulations of rat lumbar dorsal root ganglion neurons including neurons projecting to the dorsal column nuclei. Journal of Comparative Neurology 371: 249–257

Klimach VJ, Cooke RWI 1988 Mutaration of the neonatal somatosensory evoked response in preterm infants. Developmental Medicine and Child Neurology 30: 208–214

Konstantinidou AD, Silos-Santiago I, Flaris N, Snider WD 1995 Development of primary afferent projection in human spinal cord. Journal of Comparative Neurology 354: 1–12

Kudo N, Yamada T 1987 Morphological and physiological studies of the development of the monosynaptic reflex pathway in the rat lumbar spinal cord. Journal of Physiology 389: 441–459

Lawson SN, Caddy KWT, Biscoe TJ 1974 Development of rat dorsal root ganglion neurones. Cell and Tissue Research 153: 399–413

Lewin GR, Mendell LM 1994 Regulation of cutaneous C-fibre heat nociceptors by nerve growth factor in the developing rat. Journal of Neurophysiology 71: 941–949

Lewin GR, Ritter AM, Mendell LM 1993 Nerve growth factor-induced hyperalgesia in the neonatal and adult rat. Journal of Neuroscience 13: 2136–2148

Loizu LA 1972 The postnatal ontogeny of monoamine albino containing neurones in the central nervous system of the rat. Brain Research 40: 395–418

Lucas JJ, Hen R 1995 New players in the 5-HT receptor field: genes and knockouts. Trends in Pharmacological Science 16: 217–252

Ma W, Behar T, Chang L, Barker JL 1994 Transient increase in expression of GAD65 and GAD67 mRNAs during development of rat spinal cord. Journal of Comparative Neurology 346: 151–160

McLaughlin CR, Lichtman AH, Fanselow MS, Cramer CP 1990 Tonic nociception in neonatal rats. Pharmacology, Biochemistry and Behavior 36: 859–862

McLaughlin CR, Dewy WL 1994 Comparison of the antinociceptive effects of opioid agonists in neonatal and adult rats in phasic and tonic nociceptive tests. Pharmacology, Biochemistry and Behavior 49: 1017–1023

McMahon SB et al (eds) 1996 Neurotrophins and sensory neurons: role in development, maintenance and injury. Philosophical Transactions of the Royal Society of London. Series B 351: 405–411

Marsh D, Dickenson AH, Hatch D, Fitzgerald M 1998a Epidural opioid analgesia in infant rats: mechanical and heat responses. Pain (submitted)

Marsh D, Dickenson AH, Hatch D, Fitzgerald M 1998b Epidural opioid analgesia in infant rats: II: responses to carageenan and capsaicin. Pain (submitted)

Marsh DF, Hatch DJ, Fitzgerald M 1998c Opioid systems and the newborn. British Journal of Anaesthesia 79: 787–795

Marti E, Gibson SJ, Polak JM et al 1987 Ontogeny of peptide- and amine-containing neurones in motor, sensory and autonomic regions of rat and human spinal cord, dorsal root ganglia and rat skin. Journal of Comparative Neurology 266: 332–359

Mendelson B 1994 Chronic embryonic MK-801 exposure disrupts the somatotopic organization of cutaneous nerve projections in the chick spinal cord. Developmental Brain Research 82: 152–166

Messersmith EK, Leonardo ED, Shatz CJ, Tessier-Lavigne M, Goodman CS, Kolodkin AL 1995 Semaphorin III can function as a selective chemorepellent to pattern sensory projections in the spinal cord. Neuron 14: 949–959

Michelson AB, Lothman EW 1989 An in vivo electrophysiological study of the ontogeny of excitatory and inhibitory processes in the rat hippocampus. Developmental Brain Research 47: 113–122

Mirnics K, Koerber HR 1995 Prenatal development of rat primary afferent fibres: II Central projections. Journal of Comparative Neurology 355: 601–614

Morrisett RA, Mott DD, Lewis DV et al 1990 Reduced sensitivity of the *N*-methyl-D-aspartate component of synaptic transmission to magnesium in hippocampal slices from immature rats. Developmental Brain Research 56: 257–262

Mrzljak L, Uylings HBM, Kostovic I, van Eden CG 1988 Prenatal development of neurons in prefrontal cortex: a qualitative Golgi study. Journal of Comparative Neurology 271: 355–386

Munger BL, Rice FL 1986 Successive waves of differentiation of cutaneous afferents in rat mystacial skin. Journal of Comparative Neurology 252: 404–414

Murphey LJ, Olsen GD 1995 Developmental change of mu receptors in neonatal guinea pig brain stem. Developmental Brain Research 85: 146–148

Nagy I, Miller BA, Woolf CJ 1994 NK_1 and NK_2 receptors contribute to C-fibre evoked slow potentials in the rat spinal cord. Neuroreport 5: 2105–2108

Naka KI 1984 Electrophysiology of the fetal spinal cord. II. Interaction among peripheral inputs and recurrent inhibition. Journal of General Physiology 47: 1023–1038

Nandi KN, Knight DS, Beal JA 1993 Spinal neurogenesis and axon projection: a correlative study in the rat. Journal of Comparative Neurology 328(2): 252–262

Narayanan CH, Fox MV, Hamburger V 1971 Prenatal development of spontaneous and evoked activity in the rat. Behaviour 40: 100–134

New HV, Mudge AW 1986 Distribution and ontogeny of P, CGRP, SOM and VIP in chick sensory and sympathetic ganglia. Developmental Biology 116: 337–346

Nicoletti F, Iadotola MJ, Wroblewski JT, Costa E 1986 Excitatory amino acid recognition sites coupled with inositol phospholipid metabolism: developmental changes and interaction with α_1-adrenoreceptors. Proceedings of the National Academy of Sciences USA 83: 1931–1935

Nornes HO, Das GH 1974 Temporal pattern of neurogenesis in spinal cord of rat. I. An autoradiographic study-time and sites of origin and migration and settling patterns of neuroblasts. Brain Research 73: 121–138

Olsson G, Berde C 1993 Neuropathic pain in children and adolescents. In: Schecter N, Berde C, Yaster M (eds) Pain in infants, children and adolescents. Williams and Wilkins, Baltimore, pp 473–493

Payne J, Middleton JM, Fitzgerald M 1991 The pattern and timing of cutaneous hair follicle innervation in the rat pup and human fetus. Developmental Brain Research 61: 173–182

Pickel VM, Sumal KK, Miller RJ 1982 Early prenatal development of Substance P and enkephalin containing neurons in the rat. Journal of Comparative Neurology 210: 411–422

Pignatelli D, Ribeiro-da-Silva A, Coimbra A 1989 Postnatal maturation of primary afferent terminations in the substantia gelatinosa of the rat spinal cord. An electron microscope study. Brain Research 491: 33–44

Prechtl HFR 1985 Ultrasound studies of human foetal behaviour. Early Human Development 12: 91–98

Puschel AW, Adams RH, Betz H 1996 The sensory innervation of the mouse spinal cord may be patterned by differential responsiveness to semaphorins. Molecular and Cellular Neuroscience 7: 419–431

Rahman W, Dashwood MR, Fitzgerald M, Aynsley-Green A, Dickenson AH 1998 Postnatal development of multiple opioid receptors in the spinal cord and development of spinal morphine analgesia. Developmental Brain Research 108: 239–254

Rajaofetra N, Poulat P, Marlier L, Geffard M, Privat A 1992 Pre- and post-natal development of noradrenergic projections to the rat spinal cord: an immunocytochemical study. Developmental Brain Research 67: 237–246

Reichling DB, Kyrozis A, Wang J, McDermott AB 1994 Mechanisms of GABA and glycine depolarization-induced calcium transients in rat dorsal horn neurons. Journal of Physiology (Lond) 476: 411–421

Renehan WE, Munger BL 1990 The development of Meissner corpuscles in primate digital skin. Developmental Brain Research 51: 35–44

Reynolds ML, Fitzgerald M 1992 Neonatal sciatic nerve section results in TMP but not P or CGRP depletion from the terminal field in the dorsal horn of the rat: the role of collateral sprouting. Neuroscience 51: 191–202

Reynolds M, Fitzgerald M 1995 Long term sensory hyperinnervation following neonatal skin wounds. Journal of Comparative Neurology 358: 487–498

Reynolds ML, Fitzgerald M, Benowitz LI 1991 GAP-43 expression in developing cutaneous and muscle nerves in the rat hindlimb. Neuroscience 41: 201–211

Reynolds ML, Alvares D, Middleton J, Fitzgerald M 1997 Neonatally wounded skin induces NGF-independent sensory neurite outgrowth in vitro. Developmental Brain Research 102: 275–283

Ritter AM, Lewin GR, Kremer NE, Mendell LM 1991 Requirement for nerve growth factor in the development of myelinated nociceptors in vivo. Nature 350: 500–502

Rius RA, Barg J, Bern WT et al 1991 The prenatal developmental profile of expression of opioid peptides and receptors in the mouse brain. Developmental Brain Research 58: 237–241

Ruit KG, Elliot JL, Osborne PA, Yan Q, Snider WD 1992 Selective dependence of mammalian dorsal root ganglion neurons on nerve growth factor during embryonic development. Neuron 8: 573–587

Saito K 1979 Development of spinal reflexes in the rat fetus studied in vitro. Journal of Physiology 294: 581–594

Schaffner AE, Behar T, Nadi S, Barker JL 1993 Quantitative analysis of transient GABA expression in embryonic and early postnatal rat spinal neurons. Developmental Brain Research 72: 265–276

Schwartz M, Solomon A, Lavie V, Bengassat S, Belkin M, Cohen A 1991 Tumour-necrosis factor facilitates regeneration of injured central nervous system axons. Brain Research 545: 334–338

Semba E, Shiosaka S, Hara Y 1982 Ontogeny of the peptidergic system in the rat spinal cord. Journal of Comparative Neurology 208: 54–66

Shortland P, Fitzgerald M 1991 Functional connections formed by saphenous nerve terminal sprouts in the dorsal horn following neonatal nerve section. European Journal of Neuroscience 3: 383–396

Shortland P, Fitzgerald M 1994 Neonatal sciatic nerve section results in a rearrangement of the central terminals of saphenous and axotomized sciatic nerve afferents in the dorsal horn of the spinal cord of the adult rat. European Journal of Neuroscience 6: 75–83

Shortland P, Molander C, Woolf CJ, Fitzgerald M 1990 Neonatal capsaicin treatment induces invasion of the substantia gelatinosa by the terminal arborizations of hair follicle afferents in the rat dorsal horn. Journal of Comparative Neurology 296: 23–31

Sivilotti LG, Gerber G, Rawat B, Woolf CJ 1995 Morphine selectively depresses the slowest, NMDA-dependent component of C-fibre evoked synaptic activity in the rat spinal cord 'in vitro'. European Journal of Neuroscience 7: 12–18

Smith CL 1983 The development and postnatal organization of primary afferent projections to the rat thoracic spinal cord. Journal of Comparative Neurology 220: 29–43

Snider WD 1994 Functions of neurotrophins during nervous system development: what the knockouts are teaching us. Cell 77: 627–638

Somogyi R, Wen X, Ma W, Barker JL 1995 Developmental kinetics of GAD family mRNAs parallel neurogenesis in the rat spinal cord. Journal of Neuroscience 15: 2575–2591

Soyguder Z, Schmidt HHHW, Morris R 1994 Postnatal development of nitric oxide synthase type I expression in the lumbar spinal cord of the rat: a comparison of c-fos in response to peripheral application of mustard oil. Neuroscience Letters 180: 188–192

Stelzner DJ 1971 The normal postnatal development of synaptic end-feet in the lumbosacral spinal cord and of responses in the hindlimbs of the albino rat. Experimental Neurology 31: 337–357

Stevens BJ, Johnston CC, Horton L 1994 Factors that influence the pain response of premature infants. Pain 59: 101–109

Strata F, Cherubini E 1994 Transient expression of a novel type of GABA response in rat CA3 hippocampal neurones during development. Journal of Physiology (London) 480: 493–503

Sullivan AF, Dickenson AH 1991 Electrophysiologic studies on the spinal antinociceptive action of opioid agonists in the adult and 21-day-old rat. Journal of Pharmacology and Experimental Therapy 256: 1119–1125

Taddio A, Katz J, Ilersich AL, Koren G 1997 Effect of neonatal circumcision on pain response during subsequent routine vaccination. Lancet 349: 599–603

Teng CJ, Abbott FV 1998 The formalin test: a dose-response analysis at three developmental stages. Pain 76: 337–347

Thairu BK 1971 Postnatal changes in the somaesthetic evoked potentials in the albino rat. Nature 231: 30–31

Thompson SWN, Gerber G, Sivilotti LG, Woolf CJ 1992 Long duration ventral root potentials in the neonatal rat spinal cord 'in vitro', the effects of ionotropic and metabotropic excitatory amino acid receptor antagonists. Brain Research 595: 87–97

Tribollet E, Goumaz M, Raggenbas M, Dubois-Dauphin M, Dreifuss J-J 1991 Early appearance and transient expression of vasopressin receptors in the brain of rat fetus and infant. An autoradiographical and electrophysiological study. Developmental Brain Research 58: 13–24

van Praag H, Frenk H 1991 The development of stimulation-produced analgesia (SPA) in the rat. Developmental Brain Research 64: 71–76

Vaughn JE, Grieshaber JA 1973 A morphological investigation of an early reflex pathway in developing rat spinal cord. Journal of Comparative Neurology 220: 29–43

Visser GHA, Laurini RN, de Vries JIP, Bekendam DJ, Prechtl HFR 1985 Abnormal motor behaviours in anencephalic fetuses. Early Human Development 12: 173–182

Wang SD, Goldberger ME, Murray M 1991 Normal development and the effects of early rhizotomy on spinal systems in the rat. Developmental Brain Research 64: 57–69

Wang J, Reichling DB, Kyrozis A, MacDermott AB 1994 Developmental loss of GABA- and glycine-induced depolarization and Ca^{2+} transients in embryonic rat dorsal horn neurons in culture. European Journal of Neurosciences 6: 1275–1280

Watanabe M, Mishina M, Inoue Y 1994 Distinct spatiotemporal distributions of the *N*-methy-o-D-aspartate receptor channel subunit mRNAs in the mouse cervical cord. Journal of Comparative Neurology 345: 314–319

Weber ED, Stelzner DJ 1977 Behavioural effects of spinal cord transection in the developing rat. Brain Research 125: 241–255

Wessels WJT, Feirabend HKP, Marani E 1990 Evidence for a rostrocaudal organization in dorsal root ganglia during development as demonstrated by intra-uterine WGA-HRP injections into the hindlimb of rat fetuses. Developmental Brain Research 54: 273–281

Whitby DJ, Fergusson MWJ 1991 Immunohistochemical localization of growth factors in fetal wound healing. Developmental Biology 147: 207–215

Williams S, Evan G, Hunt SP 1990 Spinal c-*fos* induction by sensory stimulation in neonatal rats. Neuroscience Letters 109: 309–314

Wolf AR 1993 Treat the babies not their stress responses. Lancet 319: 342

Woolf CJ 1994 A new strategy for the treatment of inflammatory pain: prevention or elimination of central sensitization. Drugs 47: 1–9

Woolf CJ, Doubell TP 1994 The pathophysiology of chronic pain-increased sensitivity to low threshold Aβ-fibre inputs. Current Opinion in Neurobiology 4: 525–534

Woolf CJ, King AE 1987 Physiology and morphology of multireceptive neurons with C afferent fibre inputs in the deep dorsal horn of the rat lumbar spinal cord. Journal of Neurophysiology 58: 463–479

Yaksh TL, Stevens CW 1988 Properties of the modulation of spinal nociceptive transmission by receptor-selective agents. Pain Research Clinical Management 3: 3417–3435

Yanagisawa M, Murakoshi T, Tamai S, Otsuka M 1985 Tail pinch method in vitro and the effects of some antinociceptive compounds. European Journal of Pharmacology 106: 231–239

Zelena J, Jirmanova I, Nitatori T 1990 Enforcement and regeneration of tactile lamellar corpuscles of rat after postnatal crush. Neuroscience 39: 513–522

Zhang AZ, Pasternak GW 1981 Ontogeny of opioid pharmacology and receptors: high and low affinity site differences. European Journal of Pharmacology 73: 29–40

Ziskind-Conhaim L 1990 NMDA receptors mediate poly- and monosynaptic potentials in motoneurones of rat embryos. Journal of Neuroscience 10: 125–135

Ziskind-Conhaim L, Seebach BS, Gao BX 1993 Changes in serotonin-induced potentials during spinal cord development. Journal of Neurophysiology 69: 1338–1349

Central pharmacology of nociceptive transmission

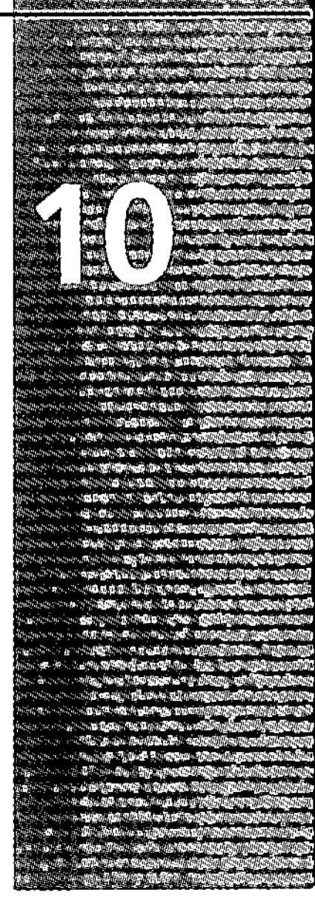

TONY L. YAKSH

INTRODUCTION

NOCICEPTION AND THE PAIN STATE

'Stimuli become adequate as excitants of pain when they are of such an intensity as threatens damage to the skin' (Sherrington 1906). This statement summarizes the construct that refers to the organized physiological response of the organism to a strong, noxious stimulus, wherein noxious is defined as representing a stimulus that is potentially tissue injuring. In the context of the Sherrintonian view, this reflects upon the construct of 'nociception'. Melzack and Casey (1968), considering the phenomena from the perspective of the human experience, noted that the individual may respond to a strong, noxious stimulus by reporting its intensity, location and, to some degree, modality. This was referred to as the sensory-discriminative component, and it mechanistically parallels the Sherringtonian construct of nociception. In addition, Melzack and Casey considered that at higher levels of function, humans will address the physical stimulus in the context provided by their prior experience (learning and memory). They referred to this component as the affective-motivational component and it is this functional counterpart to nociception that defines the pain state. This chapter aims to review the organization of the systems that underlie these components in the context of the pharmacology of the neural systems that mediate expression of the sensory-discriminative and the affective-motivational dimensions. Perhaps not surprisingly, given the complexity of the behavioural elements, we know a great deal about the former and comparatively little about the latter.

The acute stimulus and nociception

Thermal or mechanical stimuli, or molecules elaborated by such stimuli from damaged tissue applied acutely to the skin, muscle or viscera of the animal, will evoke a constellation of well-defined behaviours and characteristic changes in autonomic function that may be defined as indicating nociception. The composition of the behavioural syndrome may vary with the species or age, but will typically include signs of agitation (vocalization), coordinated efforts to escape (lifting or withdrawal of the paw) or attenuate the magnitude of the stimulus (i.e., lick the paw). For example, placing a rat on a surface with a temperature greater than approximately 46°C reveals an initial increase in behavioural activity, a shifting of the weight back and forth between the hind paws and, within a short period of time, a characteristic licking of the hind paw. If the rat is left for longer periods on the surface, it will display other components, including high-pitched vocalization, efforts to jump or other adaptive behaviours. Similarly, delivery of an irritant such as formalin or an acidic solution into the paw will quickly evoke grooming/licking and a shaking/flinching of the injected paw. All of the above described tests employ an acute, unconditioned stimulus and form the basis for investigating the behavioural components of the animal's response to an acute potential injurious stimulus (Yaksh 1997a).

The dynamic response properties of sensory processing

In recent years it has become increasingly appreciated that, in addition to the acute component, a persistent activation of small afferents can evoke pronounced changes in pain behaviour, suggesting an augmented processing of the nociceptive response, i.e., a hyperalgesic state. Thus, the injection of an irritant into the skin or the induction of local inflammation will lead to an acute barrage followed by a protracted ongoing low level of C-fibre activity in the skin (Heapy et al 1987, Puig & Sorkin 1996) and joints (Schaible & Schmidt 1996, Raja et al 1997). Under these circumstances, a multiphase component of licking and flinching behaviour is observed, followed, after a brief period of quiescence, by an intense second phase of agitation (Dubuisson and Dennis 1977, Wheeler-Aceto et al 1990). The high level of activity in the second phase appears exaggerated given the relatively modest afferent input. Similarly, a mild thermal injury to the paw leads to the development of a state in which the latency to an escape response to thermal stimulus applied to the injured site is significantly reduced, while the response to a light tactile stimulus applied to a non-injured site on the foot results in a vigorous withdrawal, indicating a state of thermal hyperalgesia and tactile allodynia, respectively (Jun & Yaksh 1998, Nozaki-Taguchi and Yaksh 1998). Importantly, blocking the acute input generated by the initial injury can significantly reduce the magnitude of the exaggerated phase.

In humans, corresponding to the increased activity in the afferent, the psychophysics of the pain state is such that the reported pain is increased as a function of the intensity of an acute thermal or mechanical stimulus, or the concentration of certain agents such as bradykinin or K^+ (Raja et al 1997). Yet, like the animal models, it is evident that the pain state induced by a relatively brief afferent barrage evoked by an irritant stimulus (such as intradermal capsaicin) will lead to a pronounced and relatively long lasting state of secondary hyperalgesia and hyperesthaesia. This hyperesthaesia is referred to a skin area that is considerably greater than the area originally affected by the stimulus (LaMotte et al 1992, Torebjörk et al 1992). It would seem reasonable that these states of secondary hyperalgesia may constitute an important component of most postinjury pain states in humans, and the management of clinical pain will reflect the properties governing the origin and maintenance of such states of facilitated processing. Such observations suggest that the initial stimulus serves to initiate a cascade of events that subserve an exaggerated state of afferent processing. The comments of Sherrington thus reflect that while stimuli which threaten injury to the skin are adequate nociceptive stimuli, the definition must be broadened to include the notion that changes in function generated by tissue (or nerve) injury may lead to states where the adequate stimulus for a pain state may be less than that which threatens tissue injury.

Nociception versus the pain state

The preceding section discussed the activation of specific populations of afferents that evoke physiological responses that serve to attenuate the impact of the stimulus upon the body. This system level of organization explicitly defines the construct of nociception as defined by Sherrington.

Melzack and Casey (1968) emphasized that the human can attach a constellation of meaning to the noxious stimulus. This means the stimulus will evoke behavioural consequences that are distinctively altered because of prior experiences (memory), expectations and motivations. This additional component represents the 'affective-motivational' component of the pain state. As noted above, the mechanisms underlying the sensory-discriminative component can be modelled closely by systems that mediate the state of nociception. Here the system must provide a substrate for the encoding of the characteristics of the strong stimulus. The affective-motivational component, on the other hand, will be mediated by substrates that are not necessarily specific for the information generated by a strong stimulus and will be highly dependent upon prior experiences and learning. At its simplest, the emotional component of a behaviour can be classically conditioned, so the response that is naturally evoked by a strong stimulus can be associated with stimulus events that are not sufficient to evoke a state of nociception.

STRATEGIES FOR DEFINING THE PHARMACOLOGY OF SYSTEMS UNDERLYING THE PAIN STATE

An essential goal is to understand the mechanisms that mediate these behavioural phenomena. It is known that the behaviour evoked by the appropriate physical stimulus reflects the activation of specific populations of sensory afferents, which in turn serves to induce activity in a complex of dorsal horn neurons that project an excitatory outflow via long tracts, typically in the ventrolateral quadrant into the brainstem and diencephalon. The forward flow of information and the tracts by which such information flow occurs have been reviewed in detail elsewhere in this book. Equally important in assessing the functional organization of these projection systems is that the movement of excitatory input through the dorsal horn and into the brainstem is regulated by local circuits which, by actions pre- and postsynaptic to the afferent pathway, regulate the excitability of the synapse and the postsynaptic neurons. As noted above, the behavioural data clearly suggests that sensitivity to afferent input may be augmented or reduced.

An important insight into the understanding of the processing of this afferent traffic within the central nervous system is the identification of the pharmacology of these systems. Advances in histochemistry and receptor autoradiography, coupled with increasingly sophisticated pharmacological tools, make it possible to define the receptors and transmitters of pathways which are directly activated by the respective afferent stimulus and the role of these systems in regulating information flow in general. A common strategy in such investigations involves aspects of the following:

- Anatomical characterization of the transmitter system and its local receptors.
- Demonstrating activation of terminal systems containing 'X', showing the release of 'X' when the terminals are stimulated and the properties governing that release.
- Demonstration of the role of synaptic activity induced by 'X' by application of 'X' to the cell body/terminals postsynaptic to the cell containing 'X'.
- Demonstrating that the release of 'X' mediates the synaptic action produced when terminals containing 'X' are activated. This is accomplished by determining whether: (i) the local application of exogenous 'X' is an appropriate response with characteristics similar to those observed when the neuron containing 'X' is stimulated, and (ii) the effects of 'X' and the physiological actions produced when the neuronal system containing agent 'X' is activated are blocked by the local application of antagonists for 'X'.

Such a conceptual approach provides a powerful tool for identifying the transmitters and the systems relevant to a given function. In the present context, combining this strategy with bioassays of nociception, the pharmacology of nociceptive processing can be addressed.

BIOASSAYS OF NOCICEPTION AND ANTINOCICEPTION

Investigations related to the pharmacology of nociceptive processing must consider several methodological issues.

Firstly, an important caveat to the interpretation of the data generated by electrophysiological and biochemical studies is the relevance of these observations to pain processing. Such interpretation presumes that we know the functional significance of the activity evoked in that cell by noxious stimulation. This implies consideration of the effect of that stimulus in the context of the behaviour of the intact and unanaesthetized animal model. It is now clear that the bioassay of the nociceptive state may reflect upon the manifestation of different components of pain-processing systems. An acute, high-intensity stimulus may yield a reliable escape response with no evident changes in the subsequent responsiveness of these systems. Tests such as the hot plate or paw pressure tests define substrates that are activated by an acute, high-intensity stimulus. On the other hand, protracted afferent input, as generated by an injury state, may lead to a prominent hyperalgesia. Models such as the formalin test, or threshold responses following inflammation, appear to define systems that are brought into play by such ongoing afferent input. Finally, injury to the nerve may lead to persistent alterations in processing in which otherwise innocuous stimuli are responded to with characteristics indicating the nociceptive nature of the stimulus. Table 10.1 summarizes some of these characteristics.

Secondly, to define the role of a receptor in the dorsal horn in modulating the 'pain state', we must ultimately assess the role of manipulation of the respective systems in the bioassay which defines a pain state, i.e., the behaviour of the unanaesthetized and intact animal. Thus, by combining the various pain states induced by specific and well-defined stimuli with specific efforts to assess the pharmacology of the receptors that exist in the terminal regions of the links in the tracts through which information generated by such high-intensity stimuli project, the behavioural relevance of those systems to pain processing can be defined. Such focal pharmacological manipulation in the intact and unanaesthetized animal is achieved through the delivery of drugs in a reliable, delimited manner into specific regions of the CNS. In the brain, the placement of intracerebroventricular cannulae permit assessment of a central action, but there is little ability to define the drug effect in specific brain regions. The stereotaxic placement of microinjection cannulae and the concurrent use of small injection volumes permit a local influence on anatomically limited volumes of brain tissue. Spinal drug delivery using chronic catheters or acute injections has permitted the examination of the pharmacology of spinal systems that alter nociceptive transmission (Yaksh & Malkmus 1998). Factors governing the degree of localization of drug action after intracerebral or intrathecal delivery have been intensively reviewed elsewhere (Herz & Teschemacher 1971, Yaksh & Rudy 1978, Yaksh et al 1988b).

EXCITATORY TRANSMITTERS IN THE AFFERENT COMPONENTS OF NOCICEPTIVE PROCESSING

Consideration of the connectivity of the central systems activated by high-threshold afferent stimuli suggests that an

Table 10.1 Mechanistic components of preclinical models of nociception

Pain state (models)	*Stimulus*	*Time course*	*Input*	*Spinal system*
Acute • Hot plate • Tail flick • Paw pressure	High intensity Thermal/mech Chemical	Acute (mSec to Sec)	A∂/C	• Dorsal horn: nociceptive specific and wide dynamic range neurons • Response proportional to frequency and class of afferent input
Post tissue injury • Formalin (Ph 2) • Inflamed knee joint • Inflamed paw • Focal burn	High intensity Thermal/mech Chemical	Ongoing afferent input (Min to Hrs to Days)	A∂/C	• Dorsal horn: nociceptive specific and wide dynamic range neurones • Response proportional to frequency and fibre class of afferent input
	Low intensity Thermal/mech	Ongoing afferent input (Min to Hrs to Days)	Aβ/A∂/C	• Response to afferent input enhanced by conditioning stimuli
	1° Hyperalgesia 2° Allodynia			• Induction of reorganization of biochemistry of dorsal horn receptors, channels transmitters/enzymes
Post-nerve injury • Sciatic, loose lig (Bennett model) • Sciatic, partial lig (Shir & Seltzer) • Sciatic, freeze\ • L5/L6 nerve lig (Chung model) • Diabetic rat • IT strychnine • IV vincristine	Low intensity Thermal/mech	Ongoing afferent input (Hrs to Days) (Days to Wks)	Aβ/A∂/C	• Changes in central transport of trophic factor • Central sprouting of large afferents into lamina II • Peripheral terminal sprouting • DRG changes -> persistent spon activity • Transynaptic degeneration • Changes in terminal transmitter/receptor synthesis • Sympathetic sprouting into neuroma/DRG

For references regarding preclinical models see Yaksh 1997a.

important component of the organization is the primary afferent projections into the dorsal horn and the subsequent projections via crossed and uncrossed tracts into the brainstem and diencephalon. The following sections will consider the pharmacology of the systems that subserve the rostral flow of information generated by small afferent input.

PRIMARY AFFERENTS

Postsynaptic effects of primary afferents

Two principal properties characterize the nature of the neurotransmitters that are involved in the sensory afferent. Firstly, single unit recording has indicated that stimulation of the primary afferent will result in a powerful excitation of dorsal horn neurons. Dating from some of the earliest systematic studies (Hongo et al 1968), there has been no reported evidence that primary afferents induce a monosynaptic inhibition in the dorsal horn (e.g. see reviews of dorsal horn function by Willis & Coggeshall 1991, Light 1992). This property suggests that putative afferent transmitters should largely be characterized by their ability to evoke EPSPs in the second-order dorsal horn neurons. Secondly, stimulation of nerve filaments at intensities that activate small, slowly conducting afferents typically reveals the existence of at least two populations of EPSPs which are believed to be monosynaptic: (i) fast and of brief duration, and (ii) delayed and of extended duration (Urban & Randic 1984, King et al 1988, Schneider & Perl 1988, Gerber and Randic 1989a, Yoshimura & Jessell 1989). While the presence of different EPSPs on the same membrane may reflect monosynaptic input from two different families of axons and/or the presence of interneurons contributing to the slow EPSP, such multiple EPSP morphologies may also reflect the presence of at least two distinct classes of neurotransmitters acting on the dorsal horn neuron including excitatory amino acids (Jessell et al 1986, Schneider & Perl 1988, Gerber & Randic 1989a,b) and peptides (Ryu et al 1988, Murase et al 1989).

Transmitter pharmacology of primary afferents

At present, histochemical analysis of the marginal layers and gelatinosa of the dorsal horn (regions where small afferents are known to terminate) and the small ganglion cells of the dorsal root (considered to be the cells of origin of small, unmyelinated afferent axons) has revealed the presence of a large number of possible transmitter candidates. The properties of these agents, where examined, are summarized in Table 10.2.

Peptide

Neurokinins

Substance P (SP) was the first peptide defined to be specific for small sensory afferents and remains the best characterized. It is widely distributed among dorsal root ganglion neurons along with several sequence-similar peptides (e.g., NKA) (Zhang et al 1993). Based on the measured conduction velocity of identified axons, about half of the C fibres and 20% of Aδ fibres contain SP (McCarthy & Lawson 1989); SP release from the spinal cord has been shown secondary to direct stimulation of central C-fibre terminals by capsaicin (Jhamandas et al 1984), acute activation of C fibres (Yaksh et al 1980, Go & Yaksh 1987), and noxious mechanical (Oku et al 1987, Kuraishi et al 1989) and cold stimuli (Tiseo et al 1990). Using antibody-coated microelectrodes, SP and NKA have been shown to be released in the superficial dorsal horn in response to noxious thermal, mechanical and

Table 10.2 Summary of receptor-mediated effects of afferent transmitter candidates on spinal function

Candidate	*Receptor classes*	*DRG type*	*Location (binding or immunoreactivity)*	*Membrane effects*	*IT agonist (in vivo)*	*IT antagonist (in vivo)*
Tachykinins	NK1	small[1]	D>V[1]	SD[2,3]	PB, HY[4,5]	BHY[6]
	NK2	small[1]	D>V[1]	SD[2]	PB, HY[4,5]	?
	NK3	small[1]	D>V[1]	?	NE[5], BAP[4]	?
CGRP		small & medium[8]	D>V[8]	SD[9]	HY[5]	?
Bombesin		small[10]	D>V[11,12]	HP[13]	PB[11]	?
Somatostatin		small[14]	D>V[14]	HP[15]	NE[16], BAP[17]	BHY[18]
VIP		small & medium[19]	D>V[12]	SD[20]	NE[21]	?
Glutamate	NMDA	small[22]	D>V[23]	SD[24]	PB[25], HY[5,25]	BHY[26]
	Kainate		D>V[23]	FD[24]	PB[25], NE[5]	?
	AMPA		D>V[23]	FD[24]	PB[25], NE[5]	NE[5], BHY[27]
Nitric oxide (NO)	(activate guanylate cyclase)	medium[28] (No synthase)	D>V[29]	?	?	BHY[30,31] (enzyme inhibition)

Abbreviations: SD = slow depolarization; FD = fast depolarization; HP= hyperpolarization; ? = unknown; PB= evokes pain behaviour (i.e., scratching/biting); HY= evokes hyperalgesia (i.e., reduced nociceptive thresholds or response latencies); NE= produces of effect; BAP = blocks acute pain bevaviour (e.g., thermal such as hot plate, tail flick); BHY= blocks hyperalgesia as evoked by peripheral injection of irritants (i.e., formalin test, phase 2).

References:[1]Helke et al 1990; [2]Urban & Randic 1984; [3]L Fisher et al 1994; [4]Laneuville et al 1988; [5]Coderre & Melzack 1991; [6]Yamamoto & Yaksh 1991a; [7]Pohl et al 1990; [8]Kar and Quirion 1995; [9]Woodley & Kendig 1991; [10]Panula et al 1983; [11]O'Donohue et al 1984; [12]Yaksh et al 1989b; [13]De Koninck & Henry 1989; [14]Hökfelt et al 1976; [15]Murase et al 1982; [16]Gauman et al 1989; [17]Mollenholt et al 1988; [18]Ohkubo et al 1990; [19]Gibson et al 1984; [20]Jeftinija et al 1982; [21]Seybold et al 1982; [22]Battaglia & Rustioni 1988; [23]Jansen et al 1990; Mitchell & Anderson 1991; [24]Davies & Watkins 1983; [25]Aanonsen & Wilcox 1987; [26]Yamamoto & Yaksh 1992a; [27]A.B. Malmberg, unpublished observation; [28]Aimi et al 1991; [29]Mizukawa et al 1989 [30]Meller et al 1992; [31]Malmberg & Yaksh 1993a.

chemical stimuli (Diez Guerra et al 1988, Duggan et al 1988, 1990, 1995).

The spinal delivery of neurokinins, particularly SP has been shown to:

1. Evoke activity in nociceptive dorsal horn neurons (Salter & Henry 1991).
2. Produce a mild agitation (Hylden & Wilcox 1981, Seybold et al 1982).
3. Induce a potent hyperalgesia (Yashpal et al 1982, Papir-Kricheli et al 1987, Malmberg & Yaksh 1992a) and mild agitated behaviour in unanaesthetized animals.

Several classes of NK receptors have been identified, but many of the effects produced by SP are diminished by antagonists for the NK-1 receptor. NK-1 receptors are densely distributed on superficial dorsal horn neurons and, to a lesser degree, in the deeper dorsal horn (Stucky et al 1993). Using internalization of the NK-1 receptors as an index of synaptic activity, Mantyh and colleagues have indeed demonstrated that SP release and NK-1 receptor activation occurs after peripheral noxious stimuli (Mantyh et al 1995).

At several tachykinin sites, it appears that, based on the effects of agonists and antagonist studies, NK-1 and NK-2 receptors are most important in nociception (Fleetwood-Walker et al 1988a, Laneuville et al 1988). Spinal NK-1 receptor antagonists reduce afterdischarge in dorsal horn neurons evoked by noxious stimulus (Radhakrishnan & Henry 1991, Neugebauer et al 1994). Behavioural studies have emphasized that the spinal delivery of NK-1 antagonists fails to alter acute nociceptive behaviour (e.g., hot plate), but diminishes the hyperalgesic state induced by persistent stimuli (Yamamoto & Yaksh 1991a, Yashpal et al 1993, Smith et al 1994, Sakurada et al 1995).

Calcitonin gene-related peptide (CGRP) CGRP-like immunoreactivity is expressed in approximately 45–70% of lumbar DRG neurons (McCarthy & Lawson 1990, Verge et al 1993). Based on conduction velocity in identified neurons, the majority of CGRP-containing neurons could be classified as nociceptive (e.g., CGRP = 46% of the C fibres, 33% of the Aδ fibres and 17% of the Aβ fibres) (McCarthy & Lawson 1990). CGRP is released from the spinal terminals of primary afferent neurons by high-intensity mechanical thermal stimuli as well as by the injection of local irritants (Morton & Hutchison 1989, Garry & Hargreaves 1992, Hanesch et al 1995).

Somatostatin (SOM) SOM immunoreactivity is limited to populations of small cells in the dorsal root ganglion (O'Brien et al 1989, Zhang et al 1993). Differential release of SOM in the spinal cord is in response to noxious thermal but no noxious mechanical stimuli have been reported (Kuraishi et al 1985a, Morton et al 1989, Tiseo et al 1990).

Vasoactive intestinal polypeptide (VIP) Sensory axons arising from the thoracic, sacral and trigeminal systems innervating the viscera show a significant expression of VIP (Kuo et al 1985, Kawatani et al 1986, Yaksh et al 1988b). Afferent stimulation, but not spinal capsaicin, releases VIP from the spinal cord (Yaksh et al 1982, Takano et al 1993).

Galanin Expression of galanin occurs primarily in small cells, but neither the calibre of the fibres associated with galanin-positive neurons (Lawson et al 1993) nor the stimuli to which they respond have been characterized. The physiological stimuli that evoke the release of galanin in the spinal cord of normal animals has not been defined; however, the peptide is not released in response to noxious, thermal or mechanical stimulation (Morton & Hutchison 1989). Intrathecal galanin facilitates at low doses and enhances at higher doses the flexor reflex in response to noxious stimulation (Wiesenfeld-Hallin et al 1988).

Amino acids

Glutamate and aspartate are observed in approximately half of the dorsal root ganglia cells (Battaglia & Rustioni 1988, Tracey et al 1991). Most sensory neurons exhibiting glutamate immunoreactivity have small perikarya which link them to small primary afferents. Activation of small afferent terminals with capsaicin evokes glutamate release from primary afferent neurons (Jeftinija et al 1991). The concentrations of excitatory amino acids in spinal microdialysates increases after the peripheral injection of irritants (Skilling et al 1988, Sorkin et al 1992, Marsala et al 1995, Malmberg & Yaksh 1995).

The excitatory amino acids work three principle classes of receptors: (i) AMPA/kainate (ionotrophic); (ii) NMDA (ionotrophic), and (iii) metabotrophic. While beyond the scope of the present discussion, it should be stressed that all of these receptors are composed of a variety of subunits, and different combinations of subunits have been identified in the dorsal horn (Hollman & Heinemann 1994) which is likely to constitute the basis for complex drug effect profiles.

AMPA receptors are found in laminae I–II and are believed to be located on neurons postsynaptic to the primary afferent and on postsynaptic neurons in the dorsal horn. Their activation leads to a potent depolarization of the dorsal horn neuron. Conversely, a blockade of AMPA receptors attenuates synaptic activation of dorsal horn neurons by noxious and non-noxious stimuli (Dougherty et al 1992).

Spinal NMDA receptors are localized in the superficial dorsal horn as well as in deeper laminae. Distributional studies have shown that NMDA receptors may be located on both the terminals on the primary afferent as well on membranes that are postsynaptic to the primary afferent (Liu et al 1994). Electrophysiologically, NMDA results in potent excitation of dorsal horn nociceptors (Aanonsen et al 1990, Dougherty & Willis 1991a,b, Dougherty et al 1992). Of particular importance, it has been emphasized that activation of spinal NMDA receptors can induce a local state of facilitated processing secondary to small afferent stimulation that otherwise leads to an enhanced receptive field size and an increased response to low- and high-threshold stimulation (e.g., 'windup', Mendell & Wall 1965). Thus, spinal delivery of NMDA antagonists has little effect upon acute activation, but blocks the windup and receptive field size increase induced by C-fibre stimulation (Dickenson & Sullivan 1987, Lodge & Davies 1987, Thompson et al 1990). In parallel with the electrophysiological results, intrathecal delivery of NMDA will result in potent algogenic behaviour and a well-defined thermal hyperalgesia and tactile allodynia (Aanonsen & Wilcox 1987, Sun & Larson 1991, Coderre & Melzack 1992, Malmberg & Yaksh 1992a). Intrathecal NMDA antagonists have been shown to diminish the facilitated states that arise from repetitive, small afferent input, which are secondary to tissue injury and inflammation (Coderre & Melzack 1992, Dougherty & Willis 1992, Ren et al 1992, Coderre 1993, Coderre & Empel 1994, Zahn et al 1998, Chaplan et al 1997).

Metabotropic receptors for glutamate (mGluR) are present on the dendrites and soma of dorsal horn neurons (Ohishi et al 1993, Vidnyanszky et al 1994). As with the other glutamate receptors, there are multiple subtypes. Importantly, several of these subtypes have a net excitatory effect (Palecek et al 1994, Young et al 1994). On the other hand, subtypes of metabotrophic receptors couple via G_i-protein to inhibit adenylyl cyclase and increase potassium conductance. Therefore, the actions of non-selective agonists at the metabotrophic sites are likely to be complex, with both excitatory and inhibitory components (Jane et al 1994). Spinal delivery of metabotrophic glutamate receptor agonists evoke pain behaviour and a hyperalgesic state. Metabotrophic receptor antagonists have been shown to diminish the facilitated state observed following peripheral injury and inflammation (Neugebauer et al 1994, Young et al 1997). A variety of metabotrophic receptor antagonists given intrathecally have been shown to have no effect upon acute nociceptive processing (Nozaki-Taguchi and Yaksh, unpublished). Intrathecal delivery of antibodies for several components of metabotrophic receptors also suggested that these receptors play only a small role in acute processing, but may become particularly relevant in the hyperalgesia observed after nerve injury (Fundytus et al 1998).

Co-containment and joint postsynaptic effects

Electron microscopy has shown the presence of morphologically distinct (small open versus large dense core) populations of vesicles in the dorsal horn (Ju et al 1987, Hökfelt 1991). Such distinction is consistent with the broader appreciation in neurobiology that multiple vesicle morphologies reflect upon co-containment of different classes of neurotransmitters within the same terminal (De Biasi & Rustiani 1988). Examination of the distribution of glutamate indicates that it is probably contained in the small open core vesicles, while dense core vesicles are believed to contain peptides (Hökfelt 1991). With regard to the dense core vesicles, it is certain that distinct populations of afferents may be defined on the basis of peptide contents. Thus, histochemical analysis of dorsal root ganglion cells has revealed that 50% contain CGRP and 30% contain SP, and 96% of the CGRP-positive cells also showed SP immunoreactivity (Ju et al 1987). The role of such distinctive populations of phenotypically definable terminals remains to be determined, but suggests an important mechanism of afferent encodement. An important characteristic of these agents is their ability to be released into the extracellular milieu following depolarization of the primary afferent terminals. In vivo, following activation of C-fibre afferents, the release of SP (Yaksh et al 1980, Kuraishi et al 1989), CGRP (Saria et al 1986, Morton & Hutchinson 1990), VIP (Yaksh et al 1982), somatostatin (Morton et al 1988) and glutamate (Skilling et al 1988) has been shown.

Co-containment and release may have several possible manifestations. Consider the interaction between the potential dorsal horn actions of SP and glutamate release into the same dendritic field:

1. Given the acute release of glutamate, the initial depolarization evoked by AMPA/kainate receptor occupancy would serve to remove the magnesium block on the NMDA receptor and enhance the gating of the Ca current mediated by the NMDA receptor (Mayer & Westbrook 1987).
2. As noted above, peptides such as SP typically produce a long, slow depolarization. This would also lead to a

local membrane depolarization and removal of the magnesium block at the NMDA site.
3. NK-1 receptors may increase the phosphorylated state of the NMDA ionophore (Chen & Huang 1992, Rusin et al 1993) and thereby regulate (enhance) the NMDA-mediated excitable receptors (Randic et al 1990, Dougherty & Willis 1991a).
4. NMDA receptors located preterminally on primary afferents (see above) would serve to initiate a positive feedback loop driven by the effects of locally released glutamate. That would lead to an enhanced release of terminal contents (e.g., SP/CGRP) (Liu et al 1997) and an increase in excitation.
5. As noted, subtypes of metabotrophic receptors couple via G_i to inhibit adenylyl cyclase and increase potassium conductance leading to a local inhibition (Jane et al 1994).

In short, it is clear that the nature of the encoding evoked by local release of primary afferent transmitters is potentially very complicated, with a number of processes that, at the level of the afferent terminal, alter the encoding process. Importantly, the spinal manipulation of these systems by the use of selective antagonists supports the differential role of these systems in the encoding of acute nociception and facilitated states (see below).

Primary afferent transmitters and the encoding process.

Using electrophysiology, it has been shown that afferent traffic is able to encode location, intensity and modality.

Localization of the body map into the spinal cord is likely a function in part of the hard-wired projections at the segmental levels. This does not exclude excitatory input from extrasegmental sites that would serve to increase the size of the receptive field of the given spinal neuron.

Intensity is likely to be translated in terms of frequency of firing, corresponding to the increase in transmitter release in that afferent. In addition, as noted above, the magnitude of the response to the afferent drive in the face of persistent, small afferent stimulation is exaggerated by the combined release of amino acids and peptides. Thus, the intensity–response relationship would be enhanced by concurrent transmitter release.

With respect to modality, the association of terminal specificity appears intuitively important. However, while a relationship with nocisponsive afferents has been observed with CGRP (Hoheisel et al 1994), SP and somatostatin (Leah et al 1985), it is clear these peptides are not limited to primary afferent neurons with nociceptive properties. For example:

1. CGRP is found in Aβ fibres.
2. SP and somatostatin are in dorsal root ganglion neurons activated by low-intensity thermal and mechanical stimuli (Leah et al 1985).

Target organ associations have been reported. Several examples include:

1. VIP is present principally in visceral afferents.
2. CGRP and SP are expressed in relatively high fractions of visceral afferents and comparatively smaller fractions fibres that innervate the skin (O'Brien et al 1989, Lawson et al 1993).
3. Somatostatin containing neurons project to the skin with minimal projections to the muscle and viscera (O'Brien et al 1989).

Dynamic nature of the primary afferent transmitter phenotype

There is strong evidence that the expression of transmitters in the primary afferent (as in all neurons) is subject to change as a function of activity and the terminal milieu. This emphasizes the likelihood that the encoding process may be subject to alteration. Two examples will be cited:

1. SP, CGRP and galanin expression in dorsal root ganglia and axons may show an initial decline during the days after evocation of peripheral inflammation. Over intervals of weeks, expression of one or more of these peptides may be enhanced (Donnerer et al 1992, Hanesch et al 1995, Calza et al 1998).
2. SP and CGRP in afferent axons decreases after axotomy (Noguchi et al 1990), with increases in the cells that normally express the peptide.

Aside from an increased expression of transmitter, inflammation and nerve injury may alter the phenotype of the afferent. Thus, galanin is upregulated after axotomy in small as well as medium and large dorsal root ganglion neurons (Noguchi et al 1993, Zhang et al 1993), and peptides not normally present in sensory axons, cholecystokinin-8 and neuropeptide Y, appear following nerve injury (Wakisaka et al 1992, Verge et al 1993, Calza et al 1998). With regard to CGRP and galanin, after nerve injury, medium-to-large dorsal root ganglion neurons express α-CGRP messenger RNA and there is a corresponding increase in CGRP immunoreactivity in the gracile nucleus (the projection target of large myelinated axons that travel in the dorsal columns) and in laminae III–IV of the spinal dorsal horn (where large afferents terminate) (Ma & Bisby

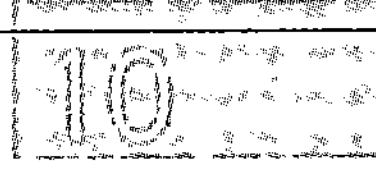

1997, Miki et al 1998). It is clear that changes in the milieu can influence the nature and levels of transmitter expression.

CENTRIFUGAL PROJECTIONS

The ascending projections by which sensory information is carried have been intensively reviewed elsewhere (Craig & Dostrovsky 1997, Sorkin & Carlton 1997. These projections may be broadly defined as:

1. Spinofugal projections to the brainstem or the diencephalon (spinobulbar: spinoreticular/spinothalamic).
2. Dorsal column to thalamus (lemniscal).
3. Thalamocortical.

It is appropriate to consider the transmitter systems that may be relevant to these components.

Postsynaptic effects of ascending tracts

As reviewed elsewhere in this text, the intervening links between the spinal cord and higher-order (supraspinal) processing are the long tracts which project into the brainstem and diencephalon. Single-unit recording suggests that the primary monosynaptic (or short latency) effect of spinobulbar activity is excitation (e.g., see Chung et al 1986, Sinclair et al 1991). Transmitter systems that mediate the effects of these spinofugal projections are characterized by:

1. Presence in the cell bodies of projecting neurons, and in their terminals.
2. Mimicry by the exogenous receptor agonist when applied in the terminal region.
3. A comparable antagonist pharmacology for the physiological stimulus and for the exogenous agonist.

Transmitter pharmacology in ascending projections

Excitatory amino acids

Spinobulbar projections Excitatory amino acids are believed to function in a variety of supraspinal projections. Thus, spinal neurons projecting supraspinally have been identified as containing glutamate and/or glutamate-synthesizing enzymes (Ericson et al 1995, Magnusson et al 1987, Blomqvist et al 1996). Glutamate has also been identified in trigemino-thalamic projections, suggesting the probable role of that excitatory amino acid (Magnusson et al 1987).

Of particular interest is the spinal projection to the n. submedius in the cat (medialis dorsalis pars caudalis in human). This system has been shown to receive spinal projections arising from lamina I trigemino and spinothalamic neurons. Histochemical track tracing work has indicated that these projections provide a strong glutamatergic input (Ericson et al 1995).

Lemniscal projections Anterograde labelling studies in the ventroposterolateral nucleus (VPL) demonstrated that lemniscal projections displayed strong glutamate immunoreactivity (De Biasi et al 1994).

Thalamocortical projections Glutamate release has been demonstrated from their cortico-petal terminals (Kharazia & Weinberg 1994, Pirot et al 1994). Cortical neurons excited by this input are mediated in part through AMPA receptors (Pirot et al 1994). Corticothalamic neurons also utilize glutamate and aspartate (Jones 1987) and the excitation evoked by activity in that system is mediated by both NMDA and non-NMDA receptors (Deschênes & Hu 1990). Glutamate-containing terminals in the n. submedius are known to arise in part from cortical projections (Ericson et al 1995).

EAA receptors Systematic studies have demonstrated that GluR2/3 (AMPA) and NMDAR1 (NMDA) immunolabelled neurons are present in the ventral posterior lateral nucleus (VPL) (Liu 1997). Of the GluR2/3 and NMDAR1 labelled synapses in the VPL, approximately one-third were lemniscal, while two-thirds were corticothalamic. The presence of non-NMDA (AMPA) receptors in the submedius has been supported by immunohistochemical mapping with selective antibodies (Hamlin et al 1996). In addition to the possible role of the ionotropic glutamate receptors, the synaptic response to noxious stimulation also appears to have a pharmacology suggesting the role of group I metabotropic glutamate receptors (Salt & Eaton 1995).

The iontophoresis of excitatory amino acids into the terminal regions of the spinofugal projections has shown that both NMDA and non-NMDA receptors mediate somatosensory inputs (Salt 1986, Salt & Eaton 1989, Eaton & Salt 1996). Responses of ventrobasal nociceptive neurons are blocked by NMDA but not non-NMDA receptor antagonists (Eaton & Salt 1990, however, see Vahle-Hinz et al 1994). Temporal coding of afferent input appears to be important. Stimuli of brief duration activate primarily non-NMDA receptors, whereas prolonged stimuli lead to the activation of NMDA receptors (Salt & Eaton 1989, Schwarz & Block 1994).

In the cortex, in slice preparations, thalamocortical projections were shown to induce excitation that was mediated by both NMDA and non-NMDA receptors (Gil & Amitai 1996).

Peptide projections

Spinobulbar projections Immunohistochemical investigations examining the content of dorsal horn neurons, which are labelled after the injection of retrogradely transported label into various brainstem sites, have demonstrated spinal projection neurons containing several peptides. Cholecystokinin-like immunoreactivity (LI), dynorphin 1–8, SOM, bombesin, VIPs and SP, have been shown to project into the bulbar reticular formation (Nahin 1987, 1988, Leah et al 1988). Spinofugal cells containing cholecystokinin and dynorphin-LI labelling have been found to project in and around the central canal.

Ascending tract cells located in lamina I, projecting into the spinomesencephalic pathways, were shown to contain dynorphin and VIP, while lamina V cells projecting in a spinoreticular component contained SOM (Leah et al 1988).

SP-labelled cells are sparsely found within the dorsal horn. SP-positive neurons or neurons containing messages for preprotachykinin projecting into the thalamus were found to originate in laminae I and V and around the central canal (Battaglia & Rustioni 1992, Battaglia et al 1992, Noguchi & Ruda 1992). SP-containing fibres arising from brainstem sites have been shown to project to the parafascicular and central medial nuclei of the thalamus (Sim & Joseph 1992).

Lemniscal projections Immunohistochemical studies have shown that projection into the ventroposterolateral thalamus arising from the dorsal column nucleus contains preprocholecystokinin messenger RNA, indicating that cholecystokinin may be involved in the transmission of tactile input to the thalamus (Farnebo et al 1997).

Thalamocortical projections Given the importance of these extraspinal terminals, the relative absence of precise information currently available on the transmitters in spinofugal pathways projecting to specific supraspinal regions is surprising. Future studies are likely to provide important insights on the identity of the long tract spinofugal systems and thus the supraspinal organization of the afferent input.

Effects of focally injected transmitter agonists and antagonists

The presence of projecting neurons containing these materials gives rise to the likelihood that they may serve as neurotransmitters released into the supraspinal projection regions of these cells. Given the importance of this ascending linkage, there is surprisingly little information on the nature of the unconditioned pain behaviour evoked by the microinjection of these agonists into the vicinity of these terminals. In unanaesthetized animals, the microinjection of glutamate in the vicinity of the terminals of ascending pathways, notably within the mesencephalic central grey, evoked spontaneous pain-like behaviour with vocalization and vigorous efforts to escape. Examination of the pharmacology of these effects revealed the ordering of activity to be: NMDA = kainate > quisqualate ≥ D-glutamate. The effects of NMDA were reversed by MK-801 and 2-amino-5 phosphonovalorate, emphasizing the presence of at least an NMDA site mediating the behavioural effects produced by NMDA in this region (Jensen & Yaksh 1992). The effects of local glutamate in generating a pain behaviour are consistent with the extensive literature, which indicates that stimulation in the central grey can evoke signs of significant agitation (e.g. Schmitt & Karli 1974, Kiser et al 1978, Fardin et al 1984). The failure to observe significant pain behaviour following injection of glutamate into either the thalamus or, modestly, the medulla, is surprising in view of early work emphasizing that electrical stimulation in this area is able to evoke prominent escape behaviour (Casey 1971, see Bowsher 1976 for a review of early literature), and given that afferent-evoked excitation of thalamic cells is inhibited by NMDA and non-NMDA antagonists (Salt 1986).

It should be emphasized that studies examining the behavioural effects arising from the direct activation of supraspinal systems must consider the possibility that complex species-specific behavioural patterns, not necessarily related to pain-evoked behaviour, are activated. Many of the complex behaviour patterns evoked by focal activation, for example within the mesencephalon, have substantial parallels with activities associated with operationally defined states of fear and anxiety in the so-called defence reaction (for a review see Bandler et al 1991). As discussed below, states of emotionality impact upon pain behaviour evoked by a noxious stimulus. In the context of the work discussed above, this raises the complication of attempting to define the link between the afferent pathways that process nociceptive information and those that govern the unconditioned behaviour of the animal in a given environment. This subtlety is likely to be an important feature of future studies in the behavioural syndromes associated with the pain state in animal models.

Supraspinal regulatory interactions

There is a significant amount of literature which emphasizes that the supraspinal component of sensory processing is regulated by complex circuitries. In many instances, the current literature often reflects principally on processes that deal with the encoding of tactile stimuli. Nevertheless, it seems certain that while data relating to large afferent input (e.g., lemniscal and spinobulbar) may not be relevant to nociception, generated by high-threshold afferents, the system-level interactions that control the spontaneous activity and evoked a response in neurons in the ventroposterolateral nucleus, for example, provides suggestions for future direction of understanding the pharmacology of supraspinal processes that encode nociceptive information. Two examples will be noted:

1. A cutaneous stimulus evokes a short latency excitatory response in VPL, followed by a period of inhibition, which is superimposed on the oscillatory background firing of both cell populations. This inhibition may then be followed by an interval of increased activity.
2. Local delivery of glutamate in the thalamic reticular nucleus (RTN) results in tonic excitation and this is accompanied by a corresponding decrease in VPL neuronal activity. RTN neurons fire tonically during aroused states, whereas during slow-wave sleep they fire at a high frequency (Warren & Jones 1994).

An important organizing principle appears to be the presynaptic localization of glutamate terminals on GABAergic neurons (Ericson et al 1995, Liu 1997, see Broman 1994).

MODULATION OF AFFERENT ENCODING OF ACTIVITY EVOKED BY HIGH-INTENSITY STIMULI

It is a useful simplification to consider the pharmacology of the transmitters and receptors that subserve the forward movement of excitatory information to rostral centres, as was done in the preceding section. However, a dominant principle of the organization of this excitatory drive evoked by the release of excitatory transmitters is that, at all levels, it is subject to pharmacological influences which enhance or diminish these excitatory influences. Psychophysical studies have shown that the reported intensity of a given physical stimulus can be significantly increased or decreased, producing a state of hyperalgesia or hypoalgesia, respectively. In the following sections, components of the spinal and supraspinal systems that underlie such regulatory influences will be considered.

SPINAL DORSAL HORN RECEPTOR SYSTEMS

Characteristics of modulation of afferent-evoked excitation of dorsal horn neurons

Several lines of investigation show evidence that the response properties of the dorsal horn neuron are not simply defined by the nature of the local excitatory afferent input, but reflect a series of active encoding events. An example of this is the ability to modify the response characteristics of a common class of spinal neurons: the wide dynamic range neuron that lies within the dorsal horn and receives strong monosynaptic excitatory input from large (AB, low-threshold tactile) and small (C, high-threshold polymodal nociceptor) primary afferents projecting to the respective segment (for a general review see Light 1992). The receptive field of these cells is typically complex, with dermatomal regions responding to low-threshold input overlapping with regions where the effective stimulus is a high-intensity thermal or mechanical stimulus. The response properties of such cells are not simply defined by the nature of the afferent connectivity, but also by the influence of a number of pharmacologically distinct neuronal systems, which serve to modify the reaction of the cell to its afferent input. Two examples of the response properties of these cells that are regulated in both a positive and negative fashion by convergent neuronal influences will be considered below.

Neuronal receptive field size

It has long been appreciated that the measured receptive field of a dorsal horn cell is not invariant. Sectioning of the lateral Lissauer tract (an intrasegmental projection system arising in part from the substantia gelatinosa) or the topical application of strychnine (a glycine receptor antagonist) will increase the size of the dermatome in the primate (Denny-Brown et al 1973). Prior iontophoretic delivery of glycine and GABA antagonists will similarly increase the receptive field size of dorsal horn neurons (Zieglgänsberger & Herz 1971, Lin et al 1996, Sorkin & Puig 1996). Repetitive activation of high-threshold afferent input will lead to a significant increase in the size of the receptive field of a given dorsal horn neuron and lead to a nociceptive component to input generated by otherwise low-threshold afferent input (Yaksh 1987). By contrast, other systems may serve to decrease the size or components of the receptive field of a given dorsal horn neuron. μ-opioid agonists diminish the size of the high-threshold (C-fibre) component of the receptive field, but have little or no effect upon the low-threshold component (Dickenson et al 1997).

Neuronal response to afferent input

The magnitude of the response to a given noxious stimulus may be altered in the absence of a change in the magnitude of the stimulus. Thus, as noted above, repetitive activation of C fibres will lead to an augmented response to subsequent C-fibre input, a phenomena referred to as 'windup' (Mendell 1966). Conversely, the activation of bulbospinal pathways has been shown to diminish the slope of the response (frequency of discharge) versus stimulus intensity curve of dorsal horn neurons, as well as shift the 'X' intercept of the stimulus–response curve to the left, indicating a reduction in the threshold stimulus intensity necessary to evoke activity in the cell (Gebhart et al 1983, 1984). As will be reviewed below, considerable evidence points to a complex set of modulatory substrates, some intrinsic to the spinal cord and some which are part of bulbospinal systems, typically shown to contain and release monoamines such as noradrenaline and serotonin. Based on the effects of receptor-selective agonists, it can be shown that certain receptor classes such as those for the μ and δ opioids, α_2 and the 5HT receptor will produce a powerful suppression of the excitation of those cells produced by the activation of populations of small afferents (Table 10.2). In addition to modifying the magnitude of the response to a given noxious stimulus, the local application of glycine or GABA antagonists will prominently augment the response of the dorsal horn wide dynamic range neuron to low threshold (AB) afferent input (Khayyat et al 1975, Yokota et al 1979, De Koninck & Henry 1994, Lin et al 1996, Sorkin & Puig 1996).

Facilitation of excitatory efficacy of afferent input

As noted above, the encoding of afferent input is subject to influences that may exaggerate the response of the processing system to a given stimulus. In the following section, two examples of such modulatory substrates will be considered.

Afferent-evoked facilitation

Repetitive C- but not A-fibre input will yield a highly augmented response to a subsequent C-fibre stimulus (Mendell & Wall 1965, Mendell 1966, Woolf & King 1987). This windup has been shown to be mediated in part by a glutamate receptor of the *N*-methyl-D-aspartate (NMDA) subtype (Davies & Lodge 1987, Dickenson & Sullivan 1990, Woolf & Thompson 1991). Electrophysiological studies indicate that NMDA antagonists cannot block the monosynaptic afferent-evoked activity in dorsal horn neurons. It has been suggested that the NMDA sites do not lie immediately on postsynaptic sites to the primary afferent and may reflect upon the intervening role of a glutamate-releasing interneuron (Davies & Watkins 1983), which is activated by the primary afferent excitatory input. Similarly, the administration of antagonists for the NK-1 tachykinin receptor has been shown to block the initiation of windup (De Koninck & Henry 1991).

The behavioural effects of activating these systems suggest they may play a role in facilitating the organized response of the animal to a given noxious stimulus. Thus, direct activation of spinal glutamate and tachykinin receptors with intrathecal agonists will induce an augmented response to a noxious thermal stimulus (i.e., a hyperalgesia: Moochhala & Sawynok 1984, Cridland & Henry 1986, Aanonsen & Wilcox 1987, Malmberg & Yaksh 1992a). Conversely, the exaggerated activation of dorsal horn neurons by repetitive small afferent stimulation has been shown to have behavioural correlates. The injection of an irritant such as formalin into the paw will result in an initial burst of small afferent activity, followed by a prolonged low level of afferent discharge (Heapy et al 1987). Behaviourally, the animal displays an initial transient phase of flinching and licking of the injected paw (phase 1), followed after a brief period of quiescence by a second prolonged phase of licking and flinching of the injected paw. Significantly, the spinal delivery of NMDA and NK-1 antagonists has little effect on the first phase, but will significantly diminish the magnitude of the second-phase response (Yamamoto & Yaksh 1991, 1992, Coderre & Melzack 1992). Physiological parallels to this behaviour have been observed where NMDA antagonists seem to have little effect upon acute excitation of dorsal horn neurons (Headley et al 1987, Sher & Mitchell 1990), but will significantly reduce the elevated ongoing activity evoked by the induction of a peripheral injury state (Haley et al 1990, Sher & Mitchell 1990, Schaible et al 1991).

Of equal importance, delivery of NMDA and NK-1 antagonists *after* the first phase of the formalin test results in a loss of their ability to alter the second-phase response (Yamamoto & Yaksh 1991a, 1992a,b, Coderre & Melzack 1992). These observations indicate that the magnitude of the second-phase response is dependent on processes which were initiated by the activation of NMDA and NK-1 sites during the first minutes after the injection of formalin, but these sites are not required for the sustenance of the second-phase activity and occur independently of these sites.

The mechanisms of this augmented responsiveness induced by repetitive C-fibre input and the activation of

NMDA and SP is not completely understood. However, several intervening mechanisms have been identified. It is presently believed that depolarization of the neurons and/or the activation of the NMDA receptor will lead to an increase in intracellular Ca^{2+} (MacDermott et al 1986). This initiates a cascade of biochemical events that alter the responsivity of the cell to subsequent depolarizing stimuli. Two elements of this cascade are considered below.

Prostaglandins One result of increased intracellular Ca^{2+} is the activation of phospholipase A_2, leading to increases in intracellular arachidonic acid and the subsequent formation of cyclooxygenase and lipoxygenase products (Leslie & Watkins 1985). Perfusion studies have shown that afferent stimulation or the direct activation of spinal neurons with NMDA will result in an increase in the extracellular levels of prostanoids in spinal cord (Ramwell et al 1966, Coderre et al 1990, Sorkin 1992). These extracellular lipidic acids can then exert powerful effects on adjacent neuronal elements.

Prostaglandins have been shown to increase Ca^{2+} conductance in dorsal root ganglion cells and increase the secretion of primary afferent peptides such as SP (Nicol et al 1992). Such a scenario leads to an augmented release in response to subsequent stimulation. Intrathecal prostaglandins delivered in the unanaesthetized rat evoke behavioural hyperalgesia (Yaksh 1982, Taiwo and Levine 1986, Uda et al 1990), while spinal cyclooxygenase inhibitors suppress the thermal hyperalgesia induced by spinally injected SP or NMDA (Malmberg & Yaksh 1992a), and the behavioural hyperalgesia resulting from peripheral tissue injury (Malmberg & Yaksh 1992b).

The spinal delivery of agents that block subclasses of E-type prostaglandin receptors (EP) will diminish the flinching evoked by subcutaneous formalin (Malmberg et al 1994). Activation of EP_2 receptors by locally applied PGE_2 evokes nociceptive neurotransmitter release from primary afferent fibres. This activation occurs by a G_s-mediated activation of adenylyl cyclase, and protein kinase A. Activation of EP_3 receptors by $PGF_{2\alpha}$ increases postsynaptic responsiveness via G_q-mediated activation of Phospholipase C PLC, production of diacylglycerol and activation of Protein Kinase C (PKC) (Minami et al 1994).

These observations suggest that there is a role for cyclooxygenase products in the regulation of spinal nociceptive processing, leading to a centrally mediated hyperalgesia, and that cyclooxygenase inhibitors exert a role in the modulation of hyperalgesia by a spinal site of action (Brune & Yaksh 1997).

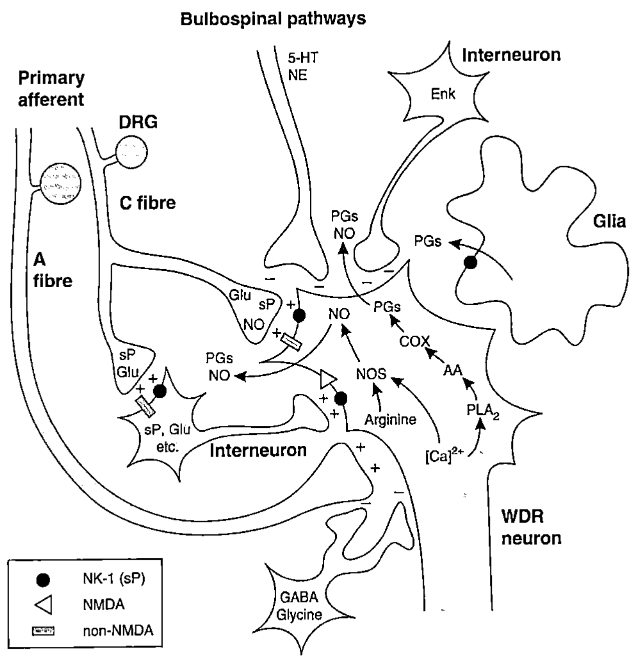

Fig. 10.1 Summary of the functional organization of elements in the dorsal horn discussed in the text which impact upon the processing of afferent input. Such an organization reflects the response to acute stimulation, development of the hyperalgesic state induced by repetitive small afferent stimulation and the development of anomalous pain states secondary to large afferent stimulation. See text for details and references.

1. The primary afferent C fibres contain and release both peptide (e.g., sP/CGRP/etc.) and excitatory amino acid (Glu) products. Small dorsal root ganglion cells (DRG) as well as postsynaptic elements are diaphorase positive, suggesting that they contain NO synthase (NOS) and are thus able upon depolarization to synthesize and release NO.
2. These peptides and excitatory amino acids, acting transynaptically, can evoke excitation in second-order neurons. For glutamate, it is believed that the excitation is mediated by non-NMDA receptors.
3. Under the appropriate circumstances, interneurons excited by the afferent barrage evokes excitation in the second-order neuron by an action mediated by an NMDA receptor. This leads to a marked increase in intracellular Ca^{2+} and the activation of a number of kinases and phosphorylating enzymes. In this scenario, based on the effects of various enzyme inhibitors, it is believed that cyclooxygenase (COX) products (prostaglandins = PGs) and NO are formed and released. These agents move extracellularly to subsequently facilitate transmitter release from primary and non-primary afferent terminals.
4. Intervening products, such as the prostanoids, may arise from non-neuronal structures, such as glia, by the action of sP (Marriott et al 1990).
5. In certain instances, second-order neurons also receive excitatory input from large afferents. Based on the effects of various inhibitory amino acid antagonists, it appears that the excitatory effects of large afferents is under a GABA-A/glycine modulatory control, removal of which results in an allodynea.
6. Interneurons containing peptides such as enkephalin, or bulbospinal pathways containing monoamines (noradrenaline, serotonin) and peptides (enkephalin, NPY), may be activated by afferent input and 'reflexly' exert a modulatory influence upon the release of C-fibre peptides and postsynaptically to hyperpolarize projection neurons.

Nitric oxide synthase A second event known to occur in certain neuronal systems secondary to increased intracellular Ca^{2+} is the synthesis of a novel second messenger, nitric oxide (NO). In the hippocampus, this increase has been demonstrated to be induced by NMDA receptor-mediated increases in Ca^{2+} (Garthwaite et al 1988). As indicated above, activation of spinal NMDA receptors can augment nociceptive processing and produce a hyperalgesic state. This hyperalgesia can be blocked by spinal injection of an inhibitor of NO synthesis (NOS) (Meller et al 1992, Malmberg & Yaksh 1993a). Spinal NOS inhibition reduces the response to iontophoretically applied NMDA and SP (Radhakrishnan & Henry 1993, Budai et al 1995). Importantly, peripheral injection of an irritant such as formalin produces a behaviourally defined hyperalgesia and, electrophysiologically, a prolonged discharge in wide dynamic range (WDR) neurons, both of which can be suppressed by spinal NO synthesis inhibition (Haley et al 1992, Malmberg & Yaksh 1993a). NO synthase, the enzyme responsible for NO synthesis, has been found to occur in areas important for nociceptive transmission, such as the dorsal horn (Mizukawa et al 1989, Anderson 1992) and in dorsal root ganglion cells (diaphorase-positive type B ganglion cells: Aimi et al 1991, Morris et al 1992). Because NO has the ability to readily penetrate cell membranes, it has been proposed as a likely candidate for a retrogradely acting messenger on presynaptic terminals (O'Dell et al 1991, Schuman & Madison 1991).

Suppression of the spinal excitatory efficacy of afferent input

A number of spinal systems, some with cell bodies intrinsic to the spinal cord and some originating from supraspinal sources, can reduce afferent-evoked excitation. Several of these systems are summarized in Table 10.2. In most cases, agonists for such agents applied by iontophoresis, topically to the surface of the spinal cord, or by systemic delivery in spinally transected animals, serve to reduce the magnitude of the response evoked by high-threshold afferent stimulation. In agents such as opiates, considerable data emphasizes that these agents serve to reduce the slope of the intensity–response curve (Yaksh 1997b) and diminish the magnitude of the response evoked by small high-threshold afferent input, with minimal effects upon the excitation produced by low-threshold afferents (see Table 10.2 for references).

The mechanisms of this reduction in the response evoked by high-intensity stimulation are multiple. However, examination of the data offers some common insights. Firstly, where examined, the majority of these agents shows predominance in binding in the dorsal horn of the spinal cord. As indicated in Table 10.2, for several families of receptor systems, this binding appears to be in part located on primary afferents in view of the significant reduction that is induced by rhizotomy. In specific instances, as with the opioids, treatment with capsaicin is known to be neurotoxic to small, unmyelinated primary afferents. The reduction in binding under such circumstances leads to the conclusion that a proportion of those sites are located on the terminals of the C fibre. Physiologically, those agents with receptors thought to be located preterminally on C fibres have been shown to reduce the depolarization-evoked release of peptides thought to be contained in these unmyelinated fibre systems. Such a correlation has been demonstrated, for example, with μ, δ, and α_2 receptors (see Table 10.2 for references). Some agents such as baclofen have been shown to have presynaptic binding, but fail to significantly alter the release of peptides such as SP (Go & Yaksh 1987, Sawynok et al 1982). This suggests that this binding may be on terminals that do not contain the respective transmitter. In addition to the afferent terminal actions of some classes of agents, virtually all of the compounds listed have been shown to have potent effects on the excitation evoked by the local application of an excitatory amino acid such as glutamate. Such postsynaptic effects have been described for μ, δ, κ, GABA-B, adenosine, and several serotonin sites. The mechanism of this postsynaptic inhibition has not been defined for all agents. However, for receptors such as those of the μ and α_2 type, intracellular studies of several neuronal systems have emphasized that they may hyperpolarize the membrane by a G-protein-coupled increase in K^+ conductance (North et al 1987, Holz et al 1989, Campbell et al 1993, Grundt & Williams 1994).

Influence of intrinsic modulatory systems on pain behaviour

Processing of high-intensity stimuli

The extensive presence of endogenous systems that regulate afferent-evoked excitation (see Table 10.2 and discussions above) leads to the speculation that several of these systems may serve to regulate, in a tonic fashion, the ongoing processing of nociceptive afferent input. Consider, for example, that opioids and adrenoceptor agonists have been shown to exert powerful effects upon pain behaviour. Receptors and the endogenous ligands for these systems are found within the dorsal horn (see Table 10.2). Measurement of release indicated these systems, following direct stimulation as in the activation of bulbospinal pathways (Hammond et al 1985, Sorkin et al 1992), or local depolarization as with enkephalin (Yaksh & Elde 1981, Cesselin et al 1984), will result in increases in the spinal extracellular levels of these agents. Under normal conditions, these levels are typically low but measurable. However, it has been shown that consequent to the activation of high-threshold (C afferents), but not low (A afferents) input, there is a reflexly evoked increase in the release of these agents: enkephalin (Yaksh & Elde 1981, Cesselin et al 1982, Le Bars et al 1987), noradrenaline and serotonin (Tyce & Yaksh 1981).

The potential role of such endogenous activity in regulating afferent processing can be assessed by the examination of the effects on pain behaviour produced by antagonists of the respective receptor and alterations in the disposition of endogenous agents through alterations in metabolism or reuptake. Table 10.3 summarizes the effects of antagonizing several spinal receptor systems on the thermally evoked spinal reflex (tail flick) and the responses to light, tactile stimulus applied to the lower back of the unanaesthetized rat. As indicated, these observations suggest that, aside from the opioid receptor (naloxone) and the α_2 adrenoceptor (yohimbine), there is little effect of antagonizing the receptors of a variety of spinal receptor systems on the thermally evoked nociceptive response. These data, although representing the results obtained in a single laboratory, typically parallel the relatively modest changes in baseline response latencies observed across several laboratories (e.g. see references cited in Table 10.3, viz. the respective agonists). The results suggest that, at best, these receptor systems, although clearly able to modify pain behaviour following their activation by spinal agonists (Table 10.3), exert a relatively modest ongoing modulation of nociceptive processing. Such observations do not exclude the possibility that other stimulus conditions might lead to an increasing activation of these several systems. Thus, vaginal probing has been shown to elevate the nociceptive threshold (Komisaruk & Whipple 1986). Cervical probing alone will elevate the release of noradrenaline and serotonin from the spinal cord in an anaesthetized rat, and the antinociceptive effects are diminished by intrathecal adrenoceptor and serotonin antagonism (Steinman et al 1983). Similarly, there is extensive literature on a variety of stressors, including cold water swim and foot shock (for reviews see Watkins & Mayer 1986, Bodnar 1991), showing potent effects on pain behaviour mediated by the activation of endogenous monoamine and opioid receptor systems. Foot shock-evoked antinociception in rats is reversed in part by spinal noradrenergic and serotonergic antagonists (Watkins et al 1984). Histamine has been shown to play a role in supraspinal regulation of pain behaviour (see below), and histamine antagonists have been shown to reverse both opioid and opioid-mediated stress-induced antinociception (Robertson et al 1988).

If these systems play a role in modulating endogenous nociceptive processing, reducing their clearance by altering their respective antagonism should result in an augmentation of their endogenous modulation.

Metabolism of enkephalin High-intensity stimulation has been shown to enhance the release of enkephalin from the brainstem and spinal cord (Yaksh & Elde 1981). The pentapeptides are rapidly degraded by a variety of endopeptidases. Blocking these peptidases has been shown to increase the levels of enkephalin released from spinal cord (Yaksh & Chipkin 1989, Suh & Tseng 1990, Yaksh et al 1991) and depress the firing of dorsal horn neurons (Dickenson et al 1988). The systemic, intracerebral and intrathecal injections of enkephalinase inhibitors have been shown to increase the response latency on thermal nociceptive endpoints (Dickenson et al 1988, Al-Rodhan et al 1990, Oshita et al 1990, Suh & Tseng 1990). These effects are typically reversed by naloxone, emphasizing an opioid receptor-mediated physiological effect. Consistent with the likelihood that stress may lead to a naloxone-sensitive change in the nociceptive threshold, enkephalinase inhibitors have been shown to enhance stress-induced antinociceptive states (Jayaram et al 1995, Stevens et al 1995).

Monoamines The administration of amine uptake blockers or monoamine oxidase inhibitors have been shown to increase in an acute, dose-dependent fashion, nociceptive response latencies and threshold in animals (Spiegel et al 1983, Bodnar et al 1985, Ardid et al 1991, Ardid & Guilbaud 1992), depress spontaneous pain behaviour in animals (Seltzer et al 1989). In humans, these agents have been shown to reduce nociceptive evoked reflexes (Coquoz et al 1991), and potentiate the antinociceptive effects of opiates (Kellstein et al 1988, Fialip et al 1989, Ventafridda et al 1990). Addition of uptake inhibitors indeed act to increase the morphine-evoked release of spinal serotonin, an effect consistent with the potentiation of opiate induced analgesia by these agents (Puig et al 1991).

Acetylcholine In nociceptive tests on animals, the inhibition of spinal cholinesterase has been shown to produce an acute dose-dependent increase in response latencies (Zhuo & Gebhart 1991, 1992, Naguib & Yaksh 1994), and these effects are antagonized by muscarinic antagonists (Naguib & Yaksh 1997), indicating an augmentation in the activation of muscarinic receptors. The intrathecal delivery of

Table 10.3 Summary of non-afferent spinal receptor systems which can modulate nociceptive processing

Endogenous ligand/origin	*Receptor*	*Location of spinal binding*		*Spinal effects SP release/WDR*		*Prototypical Agonist/antagonist*
Opioid						
Enkephalin	μ	Pre/Post[1,2]	D>V[3]	⇓[4]	⇓[5,6]	Morphine/naloxone
(Intrinsic BS project)						Sufentanil/CTAP
	δ	Pre/Post[1,2]	D>V[3]	⇓[4]	⇓[5,6]	DPDPE/naltrindole
						DADL/ICI174816
Dynorphin	κ	Pre/Post[1,2]	D>V[3]	⇔[4]	⇓[5,6]	U50488H/norBNI
(Intrinsic)						
Adrenergic						
Noradrenaline	α_1	?	?	⇔[4]	⇔[10]	Methoxamine/prazocin
(BS projections)	α_2	Pre/Post[7]	D>V[8]	⇓[4,9]	⇓[10]	Clonidine/yohimbine
						(nonA?) ST-91/prazocin
Dopamine	D_2	?	D>V[11]		⇓[12]	Dopamine/sulpiride
Serotonin						
Serotonin	5HT			⇔[4]	⇓[15]	5HT
(BS project)	$5HT_{1A}$	Pre/Post[12]	D>V[13,14]	?	⇓[15]	8-OH-DPAT/methiothepin
$5HT_{1B}$	?	D>V[14]		?	⇓[15]	RU-24969, DOI/ketanserin
	$5HT_2$	?	D>V[16]	?	⇔[15]	a-methyl-5HT/
	$5HT_3$	Pre/Post[16]	D>V[17]	⇑[18]	⇓[19]	2-methyl-5HT/
Adenosine	A_1/A_2	Post[20]	D>V[21]	⇔[22]	⇓[23]	L-PIA/theophylline
(Intrinsic, PA)						
GABA						
GABA	A	Pre/Post;	D>V[24]	⇓[4]	⇓[19]	Muscimol, THIP/bicuculine
(Intrinsic)	B	Pre/Post;	D>V[25]	⇔[4]	⇓[26]	Baclofen/phaclofen
Cholinergic						
ACh	M_1/M_2	Pre/Post[27]	D≈V[28]	?	⇓[29]	Oxotremorine/atropine
(BS project)	Nicotinic	?	D≈V[28]			
Neuropeptide Y						
NPY1–36		Pre/Post;	D>V[30]	⇓[31]	?	NPY 1–36, NPY 18–36
(BS project; PA)						
Neurotensin						
NT1–13		?	D>V[32]	⇑[33]		NT 1–13/
(Intrinsic)						
Glutamate						
Glutamate	NMDA	? (Post[34])	D>V[35]	?	⇑[36]	NMDA/MK-801
(BS project; non-NMDA						AMPA/CNQX
PA; DH neurons)						Kainate

Abbreviations: Origin of ligand: Intrinsic = cell bodies in the spinal cord; PA = primary afferents; BS project = spinopetal pathways originating in the brainstem. Location of binding in spinal cord: D = dorsal; V = ventral horn; Pre = binding presynaptic on primary afferent; Post = binding postsynaptic (not on primary afferent). Spinal effect (SP release) = ⇓ = depression; ⇑ = increase; ⇔ = no effect by agonist of the release of substance P from spinal cord. Spital effect (WDR): ⇓ = agonist depresses; ?⇑ = facilitates; ⇔ = does not change the discharge of wide dynamic range (WDR) neuron in spinal dorsal horn. Agonist/antagonist: representative competitive agonists and antagonists of the receptor.

References: [1]LaMotte et al 1976, Arvidsson et al 1995a; [2]Gamse et al 1979, Arvidsson et al 1995b; [3]Morris & Herz 1987, Arvidsson et al 1995c; [4]Go & Yaksh 1987; [5]Fleetwood-Walker et al 1988a; [6]Hope et al 1990; [7]Howe et al 1987; [8]Pascual et al 1992; [9]Ono et al 1991; [10]Fleetwood-Walker et al 1985; [11]Wamsley et al 1989; [12]Fleetwood-Walker et al 1988b; [13]Daval et al 1987; [14]Pazos & Palacios 1985; [15]El-Yassir et al 1988; [16]Pazos et al 1985; [17]Hamon et al 1989; [18]Saria et al 1990; [19]Alhaider et al 1991; [20]Geiger et al 1984; [21]Braas et al 1986; [22]Vasko et al 1986; [23]Salter & Henry 1987; [24]Todd & McKenzie 1989; [25]Price et al 1987; [26]Dickenson et al 1985; [27]Gillberg & Wiksten 1986; [28]Gillberg et al 1988; [29]Myslinski & Randic 1977; [30]Kar & Quirion 1992; [31]Duggan et al 1991; [32]Faull et al 1989; [33]Miletic & Randic 1979; [34]Davies & Watkins 1983; [35]Mitchell & Anderson 1991; [36]Schnieder & Perl 1985.

muscarinic agonists has been shown to block nociceptive responses (Yaksh et al 1985).

After spinal delivery, nicotinic agonists have been shown to be potent excitants of dorsal horn systems, leading to spontaneous pain behaviour and the release of excitatory amino acids (Khan et al 1994, 1996). There are, however, several nicotinic receptor subtypes (Lloyd et al 1998) and antinociception has been reported (Bannon et al 1998) after several nicotinic agonists. This may reflect a direct desensitization of spinal excitatory terminals (see Table 10.7). Alternatively, there are data to indicate that nicotinic receptors at the brainstem level may serve to activate bulbospinal modulatory projections (Hamann & Martin 1992, Bitner et al 1998)

Adenosine The spinal delivery of adenosine will produce a potent antinociception, particularly in models of facilitated processing that are believed to be mediated by an action at an adenosine A1 receptor (Sawynok et al 1986, Sosnowski & Yaksh 1989a,b, Fastbom & Fredholm 1990, Yamamoto & Yaksh 1991b, Lee & Yaksh 1996). Excitation evoked by low-threshold afferents, facilitated processing secondary to spinal GABA-A inhibition and the windup produced by repetitive small afferent stimulation are attenuated by adenosine A1 agonists (Salter & Henry 1987, DeKoninck & Henry 1992, Reeve & Dickenson 1995, Reeve et al 1998).

While the mechanisms of these actions are not fully understood, investigation of the pharmacology of the effects observed in different models has provided data suggesting that the actions reflect a reduction in the local release of glutamate. Adenosine agonists diminish glutamate release in the hippocampus (Corradetti et al 1984, Manzoni et al 1994). Importantly, it has been shown that spinal NMDA receptor activation in the brain and spinal cord will enhance extracellular adenosine levels (Hoehn & White 1990, Cerne et al 1993, Manzoni et al 1994, Conway et al 1997). These observations suggest that adenosine release may occur as a part of normal sensory processing. Spinal adenosine kinase inhibition increases endogenous adenosine release in vitro in the brain and spinal cord (Pak et al 1994, Golembiowska et al 1996) and in vivo in the spinal cord (Conway, Marsala and Yaksh, unpublished observations). Importantly, these adenosine kinase inhibitors given alone produce significant antinociceptive effects in mice (Keil & DeLander 1992) and rats (Poon & Sawynok 1995, 1998).

Importantly, it might be anticipated that those systems in which altering metabolism results in an analgesic action would be the systems in which the antagonist alone would yield an exaggerated response. In one case where virtually all of the systems were examined, it was shown that the classes of receptor-preferring antagonists have minimal effects at best on the response to acute pain stimuli in the normal animal. Such observations suggest that the effects of endogenous acetylcholine (for example) do not represent a particularly active endogenous 'anti-pain system'. By contrast, it seems probable, based on the observation that protracted afferent stimulation results in pronounced system activation (see above), that these systems may display a significant regulatory activity in models where there is an ongoing stimulus. As will be discussed below, for input generated by low-threshold input, a surprisingly effective moment-by-moment encoding of the afferent message seems to be in effect.

Processing of low-intensity stimuli

While several of these systems appear to be at least modestly influential in modifying the processing evoked by acute high-intensity thermal input, studies such as those shown in Table 10.3 indicate that low-threshold afferent stimuli, typically ineffective in producing evidence of escape behaviour, in fact was able to evoke a powerful pain behaviour after the spinal antagonism of GABA and glycine receptors (Yaksh 1989, Sherman & Loomis 1995, Onaka et al 1996). These observations are in concert with studies on the activity of trigeminal single units, where the local application of strychnine was shown to induce a powerful facilitation of the response of wide dynamic range neurons to low thresholds, otherwise innocuous mechanical stimuli (Khayyat et al 1975, Yokota et al 1979, Sivilotti & Woolf 1994, Sherman & Loomis 1996, Sorkin & Puig 1996). Conversely, iontophoretic delivery of glycine and GABA are able to diminish the size of the cutaneous receptive field (Zieglgansberger & Herz 1971). Such observations, although limited in scope, raise the likelihood that the encoding of low-threshold mechanical stimuli as innocuous depends completely on the presence of a tonic activation of intrinsic glycine and/or GABAergic neurons that are known to exist within the spinal dorsal horn (Todd & Sullivan 1990, Carlton et al 1992) and the presence of high levels of glycine (Zarbin et al 1981, Basbaum 1988) and GABA (Singer & Placheta 1980) binding in the dorsal horn. Importantly, these GABA-containing terminals are frequently presynaptic to the large central afferent terminal complexes and form reciprocal synapses (Barber et al 1978, Carlton & Hayes 1990). GABAergic axosomatic connections on spinothalamic cells have also been identified (Carlton et al 1992).

Several lines of evidence substantiate the relevance of these dorsal horn inhibitory amino acids in regulating the behaviour generated by low-threshold afferent transmission. Thus, genetic variants such as the poll Hereford calf (Gundlach et al 1988) and the spastic mouse (White & Heller 1982) have been shown to display a particular sensitivity to modest stimulation and these models show up to a 10-fold decrease in glycine binding. In humans, strychnine intoxication is characterized by a hypersensitivity to light touch (Arena 1970), and the role of such interneurons in the encoding of afferent input has been suggested as an important mechanism involved in the allodynia and hyperaesthesia evoked following spinal cord ischaemia (Hao et al 1992a,b, Marsala & Yaksh 1992) and peripheral nerve injury (Yaksh et al 1992).

SUPRASPINAL RECEPTOR SYSTEMS

In the preceding section, it was noted that significant regulation of the processing of afferent input occurred at the spinal cord level. In this section, the focus will be on certain supraspinal aspects of systems that regulate the animal's response to noxious stimuli. The integrated nature of these systems makes it difficult to extract a single system out of context. However, considerable evidence has evolved related to the mechanisms of actions of certain neurotransmitter receptor systems located in specific brain regions that exert a powerful influence upon the organized response of the unanaesthetized animal.

Because of the extensive insights garnered on the role of the opioid receptor, the following section is principally focused on the organization of the supraspinal systems with which they are affiliated.

SUPRASPINAL OPIOID RECEPTOR SYSTEMS

In the preceding section, it was indicated that opioids acting at spinal μ, ∂ and κ receptors can suppress the excitation otherwise evoked by small afferent input, and this effect is associated with an antinociceptive effect as assessed by a variety of electrophysiological and behavioural endpoints. Systematic studies have emphasized that opioids in addition may exert a powerful effect upon pain behaviour by a supraspinal action. The following sections will review those sites, their pharmacology and the mechanisms considered.

Sites of opioid action

Microinjection mapping of the brain in animals prepared with stereotaxically placed guide cannulae has revealed that opioid receptors are functionally coupled to the regulation of the animal's response to strong and otherwise noxious mechanical, thermal and chemical stimuli, which excites small primary afferents. The following will summarize several of the characteristics of sites that have been principally identified. Table 10.5 summarizes several of the characteristics of the sites of actions as they have been identified in the rat.

Mesencephalic central grey The early studies of Tsou and Jiang revealed in 1964 that the local action of morphine in the periventricular grey would block thermally evoked hind limb reflexes in the unanaesthetized rabbit. Subsequent work revealed a similar potent effect in the rat (Sharpe et al 1974, Jacquet & Lajtha 1976, Yaksh et al 1976, Lewis & Gebhart 1977, Jensen & Yaksh 1986c), mouse (Criswell 1976), cat (Ossipov et al 1984), dog (Wettstein et al 1982) and primate (Pert & Yaksh 1974, 1975; see below). Importantly, these effects were routinely reversed by low doses of naloxone given either systemically or into the microinjection site. These studies confirmed the generality of this site of opiate action across a wide range of species. As indicated in Table 10.4, the effects of periaqueductal grey (PAG) morphine are manifested in both spinal reflexes and supraspinally organized responses. Also of interest is the observation that the unilateral injection of morphine into the PAG results in antinociceptive effects which are somatotopically organized. Yaksh et al (1976) noted a rostral caudal distribution such that sites in the caudal PAG evoked a whole-body reduction in the pinch response, while those located rostrally tended to effect the fore paw and face. A somatotopic organization to the response evoked by PAG morphine has also been reported by Kasman and Rosenfeld (1986).

The pharmacology of the actions of opioids in the PAG have been systematically examined. As indicated in Table 10.4, based on the relative activity of several receptor agonists and antagonists, the effects appear to be mediated by μ or κ classes of receptors, but not δ_1 or δ_2. Thus, agents such as DAMGO, sufentanil and morphine are able to produce a powerful, dose-dependent antinociception with the ordering of potency being: sufentanil (μ) ≥ DAGO (μ) > morphine (μ) >> U50488 (κ) >>> DPDPE (δ) (see Yaksh 1987, 1997c, Ossipov et al 1995). In addition, binding studies focusing on the PAG have identified a single high-affinity μ site for which δ and κ agonists have low affinity and which is coupled to a G-protein (Fednyshyn et al 1989, Fednyshyn & Lee 1989).

Mesecephalic reticular formation Microinjection studies have shown that bilateral injection of morphine into the mesencephalic reticular formation (adjacent anatomically to active regions of the PAG) are able to significantly increase hot plate response latency with relatively modest effects upon spinal reflexes (Haiger & Spring 1978).

The pharmacology of these systems has not been systematically addressed, although the action of morphine clearly implicates a μ site.

Medulla Microinjection mapping studies have suggested that there are two distinct distributions of opiate-sensitive sites within the caudal medulla medial sites overlapping the region of the cell bodies of the nucleus raphe (Dickenson et al 1979, Levy & Proudfit 1979, Prado & Roberts 1984, Jensen & Yaksh 1986a), and lateral sites which correspond grossly to the region of the nucleus gigantocellularis (Takagi et al 1977, 1978, Akaike et al 1978, Azami et al 1982, Satoh et al 1983, Jensen & Yaksh 1986a). Microinjections of opiates into the medulla will increase in a dose-dependent fashion the response latencies on both spinally and supraspinally mediated endpoints (Table 10.4).

The pharmacology of these systems has been examined in some detail. Based on structure–activity relationships attained after intracerebral injection, it appears that both μ and δ sites exist within the caudal medulla (Takagi et al 1977, 1978, Jensen & Yaksh 1986c). Consideration of the δ pharmacology in the medulla has indicated that the medullary effects are mediated by δ_2 opioid receptors (Ossipov et al 1995).

Substantia nigra Baumeister and colleagues have demonstrated in rats that the bilateral microinjection of opioids into the substantia nigra will evoke a dose-dependent, naloxone-reversible increase in the tail flick and hot plate response latencies without evidence of significant motor impairment or change in the response to non-noxious stimuli (Baumeister et al 1987, 1990). Unilateral injections failed to alter spinal reflex responses, but following unilateral injection, rats were more likely to lick the contralateral paw.

Examination of the agonist and antagonist pharmacology of this nigral action reveals the role of μ, but not δ or κ receptors (Baumeister 1991).

The mechanisms of this opioid nigral effect are not clear. However, more than half of the cells in the pars compacta and reticularis respond complexly to noxious stimuli (Pay & Barasi 1982, Schultz & Romo 1987), while others display an inhibition (Tsai et al 1980). Electrical stimulation of the substantia nigra inhibits the response of dorsal horn nociceptors to peripheral stimulation (Barnes et al 1979). Alternately, while the effect of nigral opiates appears limited to the noxious component, catecholamine lesions of the nigra striatal pathways have been shown to produce an ipsilateral sensory inattention (Siegfried & Bures 1978), and this effect is mimicked by the nigral injection of a GABA A agonist (Houston et al 1980). The role of such changes in sensory-evoked awareness remains to be determined.

Nucleus accumbens/ventral forebrain In rats and rabbits, the injection of morphine into the ventral forebrain, notably the nucleus accumbens, preoptic and arcuate nuclei, has been shown to be able to block spinal nociceptive reflexes (Ma & Han 1992, Tseng & Wang 1992).

The pharmacology of these systems appears regionally complex. In rats, Tseng and colleagues have shown that in the preoptic and arcuate region, both β-endorphin and morphine yield a dose-dependent, naloxone-reversible increase in tail flick latencies. In the nucleus accumbens, β-endorphin displays significant activity but morphine does not. The likelihood that morphine and β-endorphin act in this model on discriminable subclasses of receptors (μ and ε, respectively) is hypothesized on the basis of the observation that morphine's actions are reversed by β-endorphin 1–27, a reported antagonist of the epsilon site, while the effects of morphine are reversed by D-Phe-Cys-Tyr-D-Tyr-Orn-Thr-Pen-Thr-NH_2, a μ-preferring antagonist (Tseng & Wang 1992).

Amygdala Early studies emphasized the effects of morphine given into the basolateral amygdala in altering hot plate, but not tail flick, response latencies (Yaksh et al 1976, Rodgers 1977). Changes in the response appear to depend upon concurrent bilateral opioid agonist activity. Recent work has reported a significant effect on spinal reflexes after injections into the basolateral amygdala (Helmstetter et al 1995, Pavlovic & Bodnar 1998). All reported effects are typically reversed by naloxone (Yaksh et al 1976, Rodgers 1977), and studies with specific agonists have indicated that the actions are mediated by μ, but not κ or δ receptors (Helmstetter et al 1995).

Other regions While in several microinjection mapping studies of opiate action there was no activity observed following thalamic injections (Pert & Yaksh 1974, Yaksh et al 1977), Prado (1989) reported that microinjection of morphine into the anterior pretectal region of the rat but not adjacent nuclei resulted in an inhibition of the tail flick.

Mechanisms of antinociception following supraspinal opioid action

Based on the microinjection studies, it is clear that opiates can exert an antinociceptive effect by acting at several dis-

Table 10.4 Effects of spinal agents upon tail-flick response latency and agitation response evoked by light touch in the unanaesthetized rat

Receptor class	*Spinal antagonist (dose)*	*Behavior Tail flick*	*Touch-evoked agitation*
Opioid[1]	Naloxone (30 μg)	⇓	0
Adrenergic[1]			
α_1	Prazocine (30 μg)	0	0
α_2	Yohimbine (30 μg)	⇓	0
β	Propranolol (30 μg)	0	0
Serotonin[2]			
$5HT_{1A}$	Methiothepin (30 μg)	0	0
$5HT_{1B}$	RU-24969 (30 μg)	0	0
$5HT_2$	Methysergide (15 μg)	0	0
Adenosine[3]			
A_1/A_2	Theophylline (20 μg)	0	0
Cholinergic[4]			
Muscarinic	Atropine (30 μg)	0	0
Nicotinic	Mecamylamine (30 μg)	0	0
GABA[1,5]			
A	Bicuculine (5 μg)	↓	⇑⇑
B	Phaclofen (30 μg)	0	0
Glycine[1]	Strychnine (5 μg)	↓	⇑⇑

Abbreviations: 0 = No change; ↓ = less than 10% decrease in baseline latency; ⇓ = greater than 10% decrease in baseline latency; ⇑ = incidence of tactile evoked hyperesthaesia (allodynia, see Yaksh 1989).
References: [1]Yaksh 1977; [2]K.R. Ware and T.L. Yaksh, unpublished; [3]Sosnowski & Yaksh 1989; [4]M. Naguib and T.L. Yaksh, unpublished; [5]T.L. Yaksh, unpublished.

crete sites. The question now is through which mechanisms do opiate receptors coupled to these systems act to alter nociceptive processing?

Bulbospinal projections In the initial studies with opiate microinjection, it was shown that the action of morphine in the brainstem was able to inhibit or increase the latency of spinal nociceptive reflexes. Similarly, microinjection of morphine into the PAG, the locus coeruleus/subcoeruleus region and raphe magnus will significantly reduce the increase in dorsal horn neuronal activity otherwise evoked by noxious stimuli (Bennet & Mayer 1979, Gebhart et al 1984, Gebhart & Jones 1988). These effects are in accord with a variety of studies in which pharmacological enhancement of spinal monoamine activity will lead to an inhibition of the magnitude of flexor reflex evoked ventral root reflex activity (Anden et al 1966). The linkage between the PAG and the RVM has been carefully investigated (Heinreicher 1997).

Support for the probable role of bulbospinal pathways in controlling spinal sensory processing in general, and for their role in the actions of opioid receptor linked systems in particular, is based on four sets of observations:

1. Supraspinal activation of bulbospinal terminals. The microinjection of morphine into the brainstem, notably the PAG or medulla, will increase the release or turnover of 5HT and/or noradrenaline at the spinal cord level (Takagi et al 1979, Yaksh & Tyce 1979). These observations are in accord with the effects produced when the bulbospinal pathways are directly stimulated (Hammond et al 1985), and emphasize that the actions of morphine in the PAG are in fact associated with an increase in spinofugal outflow (i.e., as opposed to a reduction in a descending excitatory drive). Considerable data has shown the presence of bulbospinal aminergic pathways in a variety of species, including primates (Helke et al 1990, Carlton et al 1991, Proudfit & Clark 1991).
2. Reversal at the spinal level of supraspinal actions. The effects of morphine given into the brainstem on spinal reflexes should be reversed by the spinal delivery of the

appropriate receptor antagonists. Thus, the spinal delivery of phentolamine and/or methysergide is able to produce a significant reversal of the inhibition of the nociceptive reflex otherwise evoked by the microinjection of morphine into the periaqueductal grey (Yaksh 1979, Camarata & Yaksh 1985). Importantly, the antagonist pharmacology appears to be similar for the spinal reflex inhibition evoked by morphine within the PAG, the direct stimulation with an excitatory amino acid (Jensen & Yaksh 1984a) and the focal electrical stimulation (Hammond & Yaksh 1984), again emphasizing that the effects of supraspinal morphine evoke a net increase in spinopetal outflow.

3. Physiological mimicry by exogenous spinal agonists. If bulbospinal pathways serve to regulate different facets of spinal nociceptive processing, the direct activation of those receptors by the spinal delivery of the respective agonists should provide a mimicry of that supraspinal action of morphine. As indicated in Table 10.7, the intrathecal injection of α_2-adrenoceptor agonists, 5HT, dopamine (apomorphine) and muscarinic agonists can produce a powerful, dose-dependent regulation of pain behaviour in several species. Of particular interest, these observations of the pharmacology of spinal regulatory systems provide insights on the possible utility of these systems in humans. Thus, the spinal delivery of clonidine, an α_2-adrenoceptor agonist, has been shown to exert a powerful analgesic effect on postoperative and chronic cancer pain in humans (e.g. see Eisenach et al 1989a,b).
4. Comparison of spinal antagonist pharmacology between the supraspinal stimulus versus exogenous agonist. If the effects of bulbospinal pathways activated by the supraspinal action of morphine are mediated by specific receptors that are acted upon by the respective exogenous agonists, the antagonist pharmacology of the effects of supraspinal morphine and the spinally delivered exogenous agonists should be the same. As noted above, in a variety of studies employing brainstem stimulation, glutamate and morphine, the effects of intrathecal 5HT are reversed by methysergide and the effects of noradrenaline are reversed by phentolamine and yohimbine, suggesting that there is a potential role for $5HT_2$ and α_2-adrenoceptor agonists, respectively. Importantly, the effects of supraspinal morphine are readily antagonized by prazocine (Camarata & Yaksh 1985). While this agent is typically considered to be an α_1 antagonist, it has been argued more recently that it may be an antagonist at an α_2 non-A subclass of site. Recent studies on the pharmacology of the adrenoceptor system have shown the possibility that α_2 non-A sites may play a role in spinal cord-mediated analgesia (Takano & Yaksh 1992, Takano et al 1992).

Several points should be considered with regard to the role of bulbospinal systems. Firstly, it seems apparent that the net effects of supraspinal opioids on spinal pathways must reflect a net activation of an inhibition (as opposed to the withdrawal of a facilitation). This is emphasized by several observations.

1. Supraspinal opioids increase the release of transmitters at the spinal cord level.
2. The effects of morphine in the PAG and medulla are mimicked by electrical stimulation and/or by the microinjection of glutamate (Hammond & Yaksh 1984, Jensen & Yaksh 1984a).

In general, such observations are consistent with the notion that opioid receptor occupancy may, through the respective circuitry, induce an excitatory outflow from the mesencephalic central grey to both the hindbrain (to be discussed below) and the forebrain. Similarly, other sites of opiate action such as the medulla appear to induce activation of bulbospinal projections by intermediate projections to cell systems possessing the appropriate neurotransmitter (such as noradrenaline: Clark & Proudfit 1991). In addition, the bulbospinal system activated by supraspinal opiates may not lead to net inhibition. Thus, opiates injected into the nucleus of the solitary tract serve to increase somatosympathetic reflexes and enhance C-fibre-evoked activity (Li et al 1996).

Secondly, based on the pharmacology of the spinal antagonists, it appears that several systems are involved in the spinal modulation induced by brainstem opioids. As summarized in Table 10.5, the mesencephalic and medullary sites of action may both serve to activate a variety of bulbospinal systems that regulate spinal reflex activities. Moreover, it appears likely that these descending mechanisms may be accessed by more rostral systems, such as the nucleus accumbens (Yu & Han 1989) or the amygdala (Helmstetter et al 1995).

Thirdly, it is clear that a variety of sites may be involved in the mechanisms that activate bulbospinal pathways. As noted in Table 10.4, the actions of opioids in regions as diverse as the medulla, the PAG, the mesencephalon and the forebrain are able to alter spinal nociceptive reflexes. While naloxone-sensitive excitatory effects of opiates have been reported (Huang 1992) in the brainstem, opioids have largely been shown to exert a suppressive effect upon neuronal function (Gebhart 1982). As suggested in earlier years (Yaksh et al 1976), it seems reasonable that the net outflow evoked by morphine from any given region must

Table 10.5 Summary of characteristics of actions of intracerebral opiates given into various sites in the unanaesthetized rat

Microinjection sites	Antinociceptive actions Tail flick/jaw jerk	hot plate/paw pressure	Pharmacology (opioid receptor type)	References
Forebrain / diencephalon				
Amygdala (corticomedial)	(–)	II-B	μ?	1
Nucleus accumbens	I		μ?/ε	2
Mesencephalon				
Periaqueductal grey	I	I	μ >> δ = κ = 0	3
Mesecephalic reticular formation	II-B	II-B	μ ?	4
Substantia nigra	II-B	II-B	μ >> δ = κ = 0	4
Lower brainstem				
Medial medulla	II	II	μ = δ > 0	5
Spinal cord	I	I	μ = δ > κ > 0	6

Abbreviations: Dose range for morphine sulphate to produce a comparable near maximum effect in the rat: B= Bilateral injection. Effective dose range: I, 1–5 μg; II, 5–15 μg; III, >15 μg; (–), inactive or prominent side effects occur at the dose.
References: [1]Rodgers 1977, Helmstetter et al 1995, 1998, Yaksh et al 1976; [2]Tseng & Wang 1992; [3]Jensen & Yaksh 1986c, Smith et al 1988, Sanchez-Blazquez & Garzon 1989; [4]Haigler & Spring 1978; [5]Jensen & Yaksh 1986c, Bodnar et al 1988; [6]Jensen & Yaksh 1986c, Bodnar et al 1988; [7] Drower et al 1991, Malmberg & Yaksh 1992c, Yaksh et al 1986, Schmauss & Yaksh 1984.

reflect an inhibition of an inhibition. The powerful role of GABAergic neurons within the medulla (Drower & Hammond 1988, Heinricher & Kaplan 1991) and the antinociceptive effects generated by the injection of GABA antagonists into the PAG (Moreau & Fields 1987) provide some insight into this system. Intracellular unit recording in ex vivo brainstem slices reveals that GABA A receptor antagonism will evoke significant depolarization of PAG neurons (Behbehani et al 1990). (For a detailed discussion of the microcircuitry involved in the brainstem actions of opiates, see Fields et al 1991. Pharmacological studies have implicated the role of excitatory amino acids (Aimone & Gebhart 1986, 1988), serotonin (Aimone & Gebhart 1988), neurotensin (Fang et al 1987) and α_1 receptors (Hammond et al 1980, Haws et al 1990) in mediating the excitatory interlink between the outflow of the regions where opiates are thought to act and the monoaminergic projection neurons.

Fourthly, it is possible that all of the structures may channel into a single spinopetal system that modulates small afferent input. As will be noted below, there are strong reciprocal relations between the PAG and the forebrain, as well as the more caudal brainstem from which these bulbospinal fibre systems originate. If activity in a particular region were to inhibit spinal processing in a manner that was pharmacologically distinct from a second, it could be argued that these two systems may not be serially organized. There are two examples which suggest such *non-serial* bulbospinal linkages.

1. van Praag and Frenk (1990) reported that the effects of morphine on tail flick in the rat were prevented by the microinjection of non-NMDA glutamate receptor antagonists into the raphe magnus. However, the effects of excitatory amino acids given into the PAG were not, suggesting alternative linkages through the caudal brainstem.
2. Tseng and colleagues have shown that the effects of β-endorphin in the accumbens will block spinal reflexes. This is reversed by the spinal release of enkephalin and, accordingly, the effects upon spinal reflexes are reversed by the spinal delivery of naloxone (Tseng & Fujimoto 1985, Tseng and Tang 1990, Tseng et al 1990, Tseng & Wang 1992). As noted in Table 10.5, the effects of receptor occupancy by morphine in the PAG are sensitive to spinal monoamine antagonists but not to naloxone.

Finally, as emphasized above, intrathecal antagonism of these bulbospinal systems will significantly diminish the antireflexive effects of supraspinal morphine. However, concurrent examination of the supraspinally mediated response reveals that the animal typically continues to display a clear analgesia as defined by both the hot plate response latency and the response to pinch (supraspinally organized responses; Yaksh 1979, Camarata & Yaksh 1985). Similarly, lesions made just caudal to the PAG significantly diminished the effects of PAG electrical stimulation on the tail flick (a spinal reflex), but not the hot plate test (a supraspinally organized endpoint (Morgan et al 1989). Such observations emphasize that other systems must be superimposed on the descending modulation to account for the effects of supraspinal opiates on the organized response to a strong cutaneous stimulus. At the extreme, these observations show the possibility that bulbospinal inhibition may play only a minor role in modulating the animal's supraspinally organized response to a strong stimulus following supraspinal opiate receptor occupancy. It should be emphasized that several laboratories failed to see a significant inhibitory influence of opiates given into the PAG on the evoked response of dorsal horn nociceptive neurons (Clarke et al 1983, Dickenson & Le Bars 1987).

Brainstem–brainstem indirect inhibition of afferent traffic Spinomedullary and spinal mesencephalic projections have been described and are thought to play a role in the generation of the message evoked by high-threshold stimuli. While not systemically examined, previous work has shown that stimulation within the PAG can result in an inhibition of neurons in the nucleus reticulogigantocellularis (Mohrland & Gebhart 1980). Fields and colleagues have shown powerful mesencephalic influences upon medullary cell populations. It seems probable, based on known effect projections of these systems, that some of the cells may represent projection neurons that contribute to the rostral movement of nociceptive information (Fields et al 1991). Thus, 'local' descending control of input through the linkages in these regions, inhibiting activity in projection neurons, could modify the content of the ascending message generated by a high-intensity stimulus.

Direct inhibition of brainstem afferent traffic In contrast to indirect modulation of afferent processing, it is believed that opiates in the brainstem may directly alter the excitatory input into the brainstem core. This possibility is based on several observations. Firstly, it is known that many spinobulbar neurons are directly sensitive to opioids delivered in the spinal cord (see above). Based on the likelihood that receptors synthesized in the cell body will be transported to the distal terminals (e.g. see Atweh et al 1978, Laduron 1984), opioid sites would be presynaptic on the brainstem terminals of spinobulbar neurons. Secondly, and more direct, it has been shown that cervical hemisection will result in a significant reduction in the levels of 3H dihydromorphine in the medulla and PAG/MRF ipsilateral to the cord hemisection (Ramberg & Yaksh 1989). Significantly, many of the regions in which opioids exert their effects, particularly within the mesencephalon and medulla, are known to receive significant input, either from direct spinobulbar projections or collaterals from spinodiencephalic projections (e.g. see Boive 1971, Kerr & Lippman 1974, Zhang et al 1990a. These observations thus support the hypothesis that locally administered opiates may alter nociceptive processing through a presynaptic action on the spinofugal terminals, thereby reducing the excitation otherwise evoked by the spinofugal projections in brainstem systems relevant to the organization of the response to the noxious event (e.g. see Bowsher 1976, Zemlan & Behbehani 1988).

It is interesting to note that populations of cell bodies in the substantia gelatinosa have been shown to project into the ventrolateral reticular formation (Lima & Coimbra 1991). Given that significant numbers of gelatinosa neurons contain glycine and GABA (see above), these observations raise the possibility that outflow from the dorsal horn generated by afferent input may result in inhibitory projections into the regions receiving afferent input. Further studies of such intrinsically organized systems are clearly required.

Forebrain mechanisms modulating afferent input While there is ample evidence suggesting opiates may interact with the mesencephalon to alter input by a variety of direct and indirect systems, the behavioural sequelae of opioids possess a significant component that reflects upon the affective component of the organism's response to the pain state. As will be discussed below, several forebrain sites may well reflect that component of the action of the opioid agonists. Nevertheless, there are significant rostral projections that connect the PAG with forebrain systems that are known to influence motivational and affective components of behaviour. Thus, while current interest has focused on the role of caudally projecting 5HT and noradrenergic systems, the raphe dorsalis lying in proximity to the ventral medial PAG sends 5HT projections rostrally to a variety of rostral sites, including the n. accumbens, amygdala and lateral thalamus (Westlund et al 1990, Ma et al 1991, Ma & Han 1992). Similarly, the locus coeruleus has ample projections into the limbic forebrain and thalamus (Amaral & Sinnamon 1977, Westlund et al 1990). Dialysis studies have shown that morphine, probably by an action in or near the dorsal raphe, will enhance the release of serotonin in several forebrain structures known to receive dorsal raphe projections, including the nucleus accumbens, amygdala, frontal cortex, striatum thalamus, hypothalamus and ventral hippocampus (Tao & Auerbach 1995). Both 5HT and noradrenergic systems have been implicated in emotionality and maintenance of consciousness. Early work with lesions of the raphe dorsalis revealed a significant diminution of the antinociceptive effects of morphine (Samanin et al 1970, Yaksh et al 1977). Depletion of serotonin by treatment with *p*-chlorphenylalanine, for example, has been classically known to produce rats that were particularly irritable (Tenen 1968).

More recent studies have emphasized the probable role of a forebrain circuit which can alter the nociceptive responsiveness. Thus, the microinjection of morphine into the accumbens can alter nociception and this effect is reported to be blocked by lesions of the arcuate nucleus or by the injection of naloxone or β-endorphin antisera into the PAG (Yu & Han 1989). Conversely, microinjections of morphine into the PAG evoked an increase in the release of β-endorphin and met-enkephalin-like immunoreactivity in the nucleus accumbens. Although there are differences, Tseng and colleagues have similarly emphasized the probable role of forebrain to brainstem projections modulating afferent transmission through input into the mesencephalic central grey (Tseng & Wang 1992). The organization of these caudally projecting systems is not clear. Behbehani et al (1988) have shown that glutamate microinjected into the lateral hypothalamus will increase firing in the PAG (and elevate spinal reflex latencies). Whether the excitatory effects of such forebrain stimulation are direct is unknown. Thus, opiocortin containing projections from the ventral forebrain, particularly the arcuate nucleus, have been demonstrated (Sim & Joseph 1989). The injection of NMDA receptor agonists into the arcuate evokes a significant increase in the release of β-endorphin-like immunoreactivity into ventriculocisternal perfusates (Bach & Yaksh 1992). The likelihood of an inhibition into the vicinity of the raphe might suggest a feedback inhibition on raphe fugal cells or, conversely, as in the PAG, these opioid inputs may mediate an inhibition of activity in GABA-containing interneurons and thus serve to increase raphe outflow (note the effects of GABA agonists/antagonists in the caudal brainstem: Drower & Hammond 1988).

Other systems In addition to those systems outlined above, substantial evidence has evolved to suggest that opiates may act through a number of neurochemical systems to alter pain behaviour. The mechanisms of such interactions are not clear.

Hough and colleagues have shown in a line of studies that brain systems releasing histamine may serve to mediate the processing of nociceptive information (for a review see Hough 1988). Thus, morphine has been shown to increase histamine release from the PAG (Barke & Hough 1992), and the effects of systemic morphine can be attenuated by the systemic or PAG injection of histamine antagonists, particularly of the H_2 type (Gogas et al 1989, Hough & Nalwalk 1992).

Sawynok and colleagues have characterized the role of adenosine in a number of spinal and supraspinal systems that modulate nociceptive processing (see Sawynok and Sweeny 1989). Their work suggests that many of the opioid effects could have as a common mechanism the release of a purine.

At the spinal cord level, morphine has been shown to increase the release of adenosine, which is mediated by a pertussis toxin-sensitive mechanism (Sawynok et al 1990). Based on the effects of prior treatment with capsaicin, it is believed that the adenosine release originates from primary afferent terminals (Sweeney et al 1989). Intrathecal adenosine has been shown to increase the nociceptive threshold (Sawynok et al 1986, 1991a, Sosnowski et al 1989).

In the brain, the antinociceptive effects of morphine in the PAG are antagonized by the adenosine receptor antagonist, 8-phenyltheophylline. The role of bulbospinal projections in this action is suggested by the observation that intraventricular morphine will release adenosine in the spinal cord (Sweeney et al 1991). The role of bulbospinal pathways in this effect is consistent with the observation that serotonin will release adenosine in the spinal cord (Sweeney et al 1990).

INTERACTIONS BETWEEN SUPRASPINAL AND SPINAL OPIOID REGULATED SYSTEMS

Based on a cursory analysis of the preceding section, it is evident that multiple entities can alter afferent processing with a diversity of mechanisms. It is of interest to consider the linearity with which these systems may interact. In fact, only a few of the many potential combinations have been considered and yet fewer have been systematically studied. In the following section, several representative anatomically linked examples will be considered.

Forebrain–brainstem

Concurrent microinjection of inactive doses of morphine into the amygdala and the central grey displays a synergic interaction as measured on a jump model, but not in the tail-flick test (Pavlovic & Bodnar 1998).

Brainstem–brainstem

As reviewed in the previous sections, it is clear that there are multiple points at which receptor occupancy may induce a potent antinociceptive effect. However, relatively few studies have investigated the interaction that may occur between these links. Two efforts that have been reported are considered briefly below.

Periaqueductal grey and locus coeruleus

Bodnar and colleagues (1991) have examined the effects of concurrent actions of microinjections into the PAG and locus coeruleus. Although systematic examinations were not performed, ethyketocyclazocine, reported to have μ agonist properties, did not effect either one when administered alone at different doses. Concurrent delivery at doses which together were less than injected in either site alone produced a significant, naloxone-reversible increase in response latency. These observations were argued to reflect a synergic interaction between the two anatomically distinct systems.

Periaqueductal grey and rostroventral medulla

Xia and colleagues (1992) examined the effects of concurrent delivery of met-enkephalin into the PAG and into the n. reticularis gigantocellularis of the medulla. In these studies, single-unit activity in the trigeminal nucleus was examined along with the response to noxious stimulation. Injection in both regions depressed escape behaviour and evoked neuronal activity. Conjoint delivery appeared to have only a simple additive interaction.

Brainstem–spinal cord

Opiates given systemically can produce a powerful and selective effect upon pain behaviour. As outlined above, opioids with an action limited to the spinal cord and to the brainstem are able to produce a powerful alteration in nociceptive processing. Yet, in early studies, it was shown that the delivery of an opioid antagonist into the cerebral ventricles (Tsou 1963, Vigouret et al 1973) or into the lumbar intrathecal space (Yaksh & Rudy 1978) could produce a complete antagonism of the effects of the systemic opioid agonist. This led to the hypothesis that the effects of opiate receptor occupancy in the brain must synergize with the effects produced by the concurrent occupancy of spinal receptors (Yaksh & Rudy 1978). With high occupancy (as produced when the drugs are delivered focally), the systems were able to independently produce a significant change in pain processing. Yeung and Rudy (1980) first demonstrated the validity of the hypothesis by showing that the concurrent administration of morphine both spinally and supraspinally would lead to a prominent synergy, as indicated by hyperbolic isobolograms. Similar results have been observed in mice (Roerig & Fujimoto 1989; see Tallarida et al 1989 for a discussion of analysis of synergic interactions).

Spinal cord–spinal cord

Consistent with the powerful non-linear interaction between spinal and supraspinal opiates, and the possible role of bulbospinal systems in mediating some of the supraspinal actions of opiates, it has been shown that the concurrent spinal delivery of α_2 and opioid agonists would also reveal a powerful synergy (Table 10.6).

The mechanism of this synergy is not known. It may be significant that one class of agents that routinely appears to show a non-linear interaction at the spinal level interacts presynaptically with primary afferents to diminish release (e.g., μ, δ and α_2) (Table 10.2). Based on our current understanding of mechanisms, neither adenosine nor kappa agonists are thought to have a potent effect on the release of afferent transmitters (Table 10.2). A second class of agents that appears to show significant spinal synergy with the opioids are the cyclooxygenase inhibitors. Given the presumed role outlined in preceding sections for the release of prostaglandins by afferent input and the probable role played by cyclooxygenase products in evoking a facilitated state of spinal processing, the synergy observed in the formalin test could be anticipated. A potent synergy has in fact been shown between these two classes of agents (Table 10.6; see Malmberg & Yaksh 1993b for a further discussion).

Aside from the synergic interactions that may occur between several receptor systems, there is increasing evidence that certain endogenous systems may serve to diminish the activity of receptor systems that modulate nociceptive transmission. Two examples of this interaction are considered.

Cholecystokinin

A number of groups have reported that cholecystokinin, particularly the octapeptide (CCK-8), may diminish the antinociceptive effects of morphine (Faris et al 1983, Wiertelak et al 1992) and reverse the inhibition of dorsal horn neurons produced by morphine (Kellstein et al 1991).

Table 10.6 Ability of intrathecal antagonists to reverse the effects of morphine given into several brainstem sites on spinal reflex activity

Receptor	*Spinal antagonist*	*Microinjection site (morphine)* *Periaqueductal grey*	*Raphe magnus*	*Medullary reticular form*	
α	Phentolamine	⇓[1–3]	⇓[2]	⇓[2]	
α_1	Corynanthine	0[1]			
α_2	Yohimbine	⇓[1]			
$\alpha_2$nonA	(Prazocin)	⇓[1]			
β	Propranolol	0[1]			
Dopamine	*cis*-flupentixol	0[1]	0[2]	0[2]	
	Haloperidol				
Opioid	Naloxone	0[1]	↓[2]	↓[2]	
$5HT_2$	Methysergide		⇓[1–3]	⇓[2]	0[2]

Abbreviations: ⇓ = significant reversal of tail flick inhibition; ↓ = modest reversal of tail flick; 0 = reversal of tail flick.
References: [1]Camarata & Yaksh 1985; [2]Jensen & Yaksh 1986b; [3]Yaksh 1979.

Given the presence and release of CCK from the spinal cord (Yaksh et al 1982a), this peptide could serve as an endogenous opioid antagonist. This hypothesis is supported by the observation that CCK antagonists (particularly of the A-type) can augment the effects of morphine (O'Neill et al 1989, Kellstein et al 1991). The nature and specificity of this interaction remain to be defined (for a review see Baber et al 1989). Thus, Tseng and Collins (1992) reported that intrathecal CCK would antagonize the effects of intraventricular β-endorphin.

Dynorphin

Fujimoto and colleagues have demonstrated that spinal dynorphin (Dyn 1–17) in low doses is able to antagonize the effects of intrathecal opiates (Fujimoto et al 1990). This effect does not appear to be produced by other dynorphin analogues (Rady et al 1991) and is not mediated by a κ receptor. Again, the presence of dynorphin in the spinal neurons, as well as its upregulation following inflammation (Iadarola et al 1988), provide evidence for its possible role as an endogenous 'anti-algesic' agent.

ROLE OF MODULATORY SUBSTRATES IN PAIN BEHAVIOUR

The above sections emphasize that the output of the spinal cord in response to a strong stimulus is subject to a pronounced modulation by a variety of neurotransmitter/receptor systems in the spinal cord. Given the reasonable presumption that the content of the message transmitted to higher centres by long tracts in part defines the sensory-discriminative component of the pain state, these intrinsic systems as outlined provide mechanisms whereby the content of the projected message may be associated with a potential response which is greater than would be anticipated for a given stimulus, inappropriate for the stimulus which generates the message or less than would be anticipated given the magnitude of the physical stimulus. These three conditions intuitively correspond to the behavioural states of hyperalgesia, hyperaesthesia (or allodynia) and hypoalgesia (analgesia). These states and aspects of the central pharmacology that may underlie these states of altered afferent encoding will be considered below.

STATES OF ALTERED PAIN PROCESSING

Hyperalgesia

Hyperalgesia indicates a pain behaviour that exceeds in magnitude the pain behaviour anticipated for a stimulus evoking a given afferent barrage. This might be evidenced by a decrease in response latency or increase in response magnitude otherwise evoked by a given aversive stimulus. As noted above, the generation of a modestly protracted afferent barrage by the injection of an irritant into the skin or the generation of a state of inflammation will evoke an acute pain state, followed by a profound hyperalgesia. Models such as the formalin test in the rat have been shown to be associated with a two-phased response, with the magnitude of the second phase behaviour being in excess of that anticipated on the basis of the afferent activity measured in the peripheral afferent at the corresponding time points (Heapy et al 1987, Wheeler-Aceto et al 1990, Puig & Sorkin 1996).

Similarly, other models of hyperalgesia involving chronic inflammatory states may well be involved in such states of facilitated processing. If the increased pain behaviour reflects a greater sensitivity of the peripheral nerve to the stimulus, this hyperalgesia might reflect a model mediated by a peripheral mechanism. The spinal delivery of certain afferent transmitters such as SP or NMDA will evoke a prominent decrease in the thermal nociceptive threshold of the unanaesthetized rat, corresponding to the presumed mechanisms set into play by repetitive afferent input (Table 10.2). In humans, the focal activation of cutaneous C fibres by the subcutaneous injection of capsaicin results in prominent, acute pain behaviour, followed by profound hyperalgesia over an area of skin that greatly exceeds the focal site of the original stimulus. Importantly, this secondary hyperalgesia appears to be centrally mediated, because as in the formalin test, if the acute afferent barrage is blocked by a local anaesthetic, the secondary phase does not occur (Torebjörk et al 1992, Kinnman et al 1997, Wallace et al 1997, Iadarola et al 1998). In addition, the distribution of the allodynia after a focal capsaicin stimulus appears in multiple dermatomes, emphasizing a central mechanism (Sang et al 1996).

Hyperaesthesia

The evocation of pain behaviour in response to light touch, referred to as allodynia, can be induced by the intrathecal delivery of low doses of glycine and GABA-A antagonists (Yaksh 1989). Importantly, this effect does not appear to be a simple exaggeration of all input, as the single-unit response to noxious stimuli or small afferents (Sherman & Loomis 1996, Sorkin & Puig 1996) or the response latency to noxious thermal stimuli (Yaksh 1989, Yamamoto & Yaksh 1993) is little affected. These behavioural effects produced by spinal amino acid antagonists correspond to the prominent hypersensitivity that is associated with genetic models where low levels of spinal glycine binding have been observed, such as in the poll Hereford calf (Gundlach et al 1988) and spastic mouse (White 1985). In humans, strychnine intoxication is reportedly associated with prominent hypersensitivity to innocuous stimuli (Arena 1979). Similarly, tactile allodynia has been reported in models of focal (Hao et al 1991) and global (Marsala & Yaksh 1992) spinal ischaemia. Animal models of chronic peripheral nerve compression (Bennett & Xie 1988, Shir & Seltzer 1990, Kim & Chung 1992) have shown the development of allodynia. The allodynic state in humans following nerve and spinal cord injury is well described. While the mechanisms of these hyperaesthetic states are not well defined, both peripheral nerve injury and incomplete spinal ischaemia is typically associated with prominent changes in the morphology of small interneurons (Kapadia & La Motte 1987), presumably similar to those which have been identified in the spinal dorsal horn and known to contain glycine and GABA (Todd & Sullivan 1990). Nerve injury has indeed been shown to reduce dorsal horn levels of GABA (Ibuki et al 1997).

Hypoalgesia

A reduction in the magnitude of pain generated by a given stimulus is the goal sought in the management of ongoing pain states. If there is no facilitated state of processing, we can precisely define such a hypoalgesia as analgesia, i.e., the animal's threshold for evocation of a response is elevated to above that which we would normally encounter in an untreated, unconditioned population of animals. As normoalgesia is a state which must be defined by exclusion of other states, it seems reasonable that analgesia would be reflected by the increased intensity required to produce a given response to an acute stimulus. Thus, in the absence of inflammation or injury, an animal exposed to a given thermal or mechanical stimulus will display escape behaviour within a certain latency or threshold. Agents which interact with a variety of specific receptors have been shown to produce a potent dose-dependent increase in the response latency. If a mechanism yielding augmented or altered processing is brought into play, an agent may yield a state of normoalgesia and thus be antihyperalgesic or antihyperaesthetic.

CLASSES OF RECEPTORS WHICH YIELD A STATE OF NORMOALGESIA AND ANALGESIA

Based on the commentary in the preceding section, it is reasonable to presume that agents may reduce the response evoked by a given noxious stimulus (and thus be an analgesic) or serve to normalize the pain behaviour evoked by an otherwise non-noxious (i.e., antihyperaesthetic) or noxious (antihyperalgesic) stimulus. Table 10.7 presents a summary of data (including literature references) on the spinal actions of a number of classes of agents which have been implicated in the modulation of spinal function. Based on these results, several points may be extracted.

Hypoalgesia and acutely evoked pain behaviour

In acute pain tests such as the hot plate, tail flick and visceral stimulation tests, intrathecal agents such as μ and δ opioids, α_2 adrenoceptor agonists, and NPY, typically produce an increase in the response latency or the threshold stimulus intensity. At the stimulus intensities typically employed, these agents can produce, in a dose-dependent, naloxone-reversible fashion, an elevation in the measured nociceptive endpoint to the maximum measurable effect, and this blockade is achieved in the absence of motor dysfunction. The selective antinociceptive effects of opiates have in fact been demonstrated across a wide range of species, including the frog (Stevens 1991), mouse (Hylden & Wilcox 1983a,b), rat (Yaksh & Rudy 1976a,b), rabbit (Yaksh & Rudy 1976), cat (Yaksh 1978b, Tung & Yaksh 1982), dog (Sabbe et al 1994) and non-human primate (Yaksh & Reddy 1981).

In contrast to the selective analgesia across a wide range of stimuli and doses, agonists such as those for adenosine, GABA-A or -B receptors appear to produce only modest effects at doses that do not produce motor impairment (Table 10.7). As reviewed above, the first group of agents are thought to exert their effects upon spinal nociceptive processing by producing a concurrent, presynaptic effect upon C-fibre transmitter release and postsynaptic effect upon wide dynamic range (WDR) neurons. Thus, even though they may exert an effect in the ventral horn (based on single-unit studies and the presence of the respective binding in the ventral horn), these agents, by their joint presynaptic effects upon C afferent input and a hyperpolarization of the postsynaptic neurons, exert a powerful effect upon nocisponsive behaviour at doses which only modestly influence motor horn function (or the excitation evoked in dorsal horn neurons by large afferents which presumably do not possess significant opioid receptor binding).

In contrast, GABA-B and adenosine agonists may act to inhibit the firing of WDR neurons, most likely through an increase in K^+ conductance (North et al 1987). These agents, however, do not appear to exert an effect on C-fibre transmitter release (Table 10.2). Therefore, we suspect that at concentrations that induce hyperpolarization of WDR neurons there are concurrent direct effects within the motor horn and this results in a low therapeutic ratio.

The failure of cyclooxygenase and nitric oxide (NO) synthase inhibitors to alter the acutely evoked behaviours indicate that these systems are not brought into play by such acute stimulation. Similarly, while glutamate and SP may be neurotransmitters released by the action of high-threshold afferents, the inability of NMDA, non-NMDA or NK-1 antagonists to effect the acute evoked responses suggests that they alone mediate the transfer of information relevant to the response evoked by these acute stimuli (Table 10.7).

Hyperalgesic behavioural states

Activity-dependent hyperalgesia

In the formalin test, agents which serve to block C-fibre evoked windup such as NMDA and NK-1 antagonists (Dickenson & Sullivan 1987, Haley et al 1990, Budai & Larson 1996) fail to have a significant action on phase 1, but significantly reduce the magnitude of phase 2 (Yamamoto & Yaksh 1991a, 1992a, Coderre & Melzack 1992, Chaplan et al 1997). The effect upon the second phase, while dose dependent, displays a plateau effect. In this model of hyperalgesia, the inhibition of spinal cyclooxygenase or NO synthase will similarly produce a dose-dependent but incomplete reduction in the magnitude of the second-phase response (Malmberg & Yaksh 1992b, 1993a,b, Meller & Gebhart 1993). These results are consistent with the hypothesis that the acute afferent barrage generated by formalin will evoke an initial pain state, and this barrage will subsequently evoke the release of NO and prostanoids in part by an NMDA- and NK-1-sensitive mechanism (Malmberg & Yaksh 1992a, 1993a). The failure of NMDA or NK-1 antagonists to significantly alter phase 1 is consistent with the failure of these agents to act in acute pain tests. The observation that NK-1 and NMDA antagonists given between phase 1 and phase 2 has little effect on phase 2 supports the idea that these receptor systems serve to initiate but not sustain the facilitated component of the second phase (Coderre & Melzack 1991, 1992, Yamamoto & Yaksh 1991a, 1992a). These agents as described serve as antihyperalgesics and, to the degree that a pain state is augmented by these processes, those classes of agents will normalize the facilitated pain state.

By contrast, agents such as the opioids in the formalin test serve as analgesics by blocking the afferent input responsible for evoking behaviour (as in phase 1 of the formalin test and the acute response on the hot plate or tail flick test). In addition, it is possible that because such agents block the afferent input, presumably by diminishing the release of the appropriate neurotransmitters, they may also block the development of the hyperalgesic state. Supporting evidence for this arises from studies in which it has been shown that pretreatment with intrathecal morphine will block phase 1. The injection of naloxone between phases 1 and 2 in an animal pretreated with morphine will continue to display a highly significant reduction in the phase 2 response (Abram & Yaksh 1993). Systemic infusion of a short-lasting opioid (remifentanil) during phase 1 will delay phase 2 (Taylor et al 1997). This may reflect the ability of the μ agonists to block the release of materials that lead to the hyperalgesic state manifested during the phase 2 response. Importantly, it is conceivable that agents that act postsynaptic to the primary afferent might suppress the appearance of behaviour, i.e., agents may be analgesic, but may not be able to correspondingly block the initiation of the hyperalgesic state. Thus, rats that are anaesthetized with a volatile anaesthetic during phase 1 and allowed to awaken during phase 2 will continue to show a significant phase 2 response (Abram & Yaksh 1993). Failure of the general anaesthetic to block the evolution of the hyperalgesic state in the formalin test is consistent with the fact that most studies examining the electrophysiology of windup or the release of neurotransmitters from the spinal cord have been carried out under a general anaesthetic regimen (e.g. Fraser et al 1992, Go & Yaksh 1987, respectively).

Nerve injury-evoked hyperalgesia

With regard to the thermal hyperalgesia induced by peripheral nerve compression (Bennett & Xie 1988), intrathecal injection of μ and α_2 agonists has been shown to produce a dose-dependent elevation in the thermally evoked withdrawal response of both the normal and the hind paw rendered hyperalgesic with a surgical compression of the ipsilateral sciatic nerve (Table 10.7). The dose–response curve for the hyperalgesic paw is displaced in a parallel fashion to the right, as compared to the curve obtained with the normal paw, with the maximum latency allowed being achieved with both normal and hyperalgesic paws with these agents. By contrast, intrathecal agents such as NMDA antagonists have no effect on the normal paw latency, but will produce a dose-dependent increase in the latency of the hyperalgesic paw to the normal (non-hyperalgesic) response latencies. In this sense, as with those agents which block in a limited, but dose-dependent, fashion the phase 2 of the formalin test, such agents might also be classified as being antihyperalgesic.

Comparability of hyperalgesic pain states

While there are certain parallels between the systems which underlie the mechanisms of the hyperalgesia observed in the formalin test and that in nerve injury, consideration of Table 10.7 emphasizes that the pharmacology of these two measured endpoints are not the same. Thus, for the nerve injury-evoked hyperalgesia, NK-1 antagonists and cyclooxygenase inhibitors are not active. Moreover, it is unknown if the spinal substrates through which the NMDA antagonists act to alter the two hyperalgesic states are the same. Heterogeneous spinal mechanisms may be involved in the different pain states, but at present it is not clear if all agents that block the hyperalgesic component observed following nerve lesion will block the facilitated component of phase 2 of the formalin test.

Hyperaesthetic pain states

In the strychnine model of tactile allodynia, intrathecal opiates and α_2 agonists appear to be only modestly active and not significantly different from baclofen. By contrast, NMDA antagonists are extremely effective in diminishing this allodynic state. While speculative, it has been suggested that this differentiation shows that allodynia is mediated by low-threshold mechanoreceptors (Yaksh 1989). Based on the binding studies and on the failure of the analgesic agents which C-fibre release to be particularly effective, it is believed that C-fibre input lacks a role in this pain state. Importantly, in deafferentation syndromes, dorsal horn neurons, some that are likely to represent projection neurons that were originally activated by high-threshold input, become spontaneously active. Under normal circumstances these cells have a low spontaneous activity and the nociceptive-evoked activity is readily suppressed by morphine. The increased spontaneous activity occurring in the differentiated states is considerably less sensitive to the actions of morphine, supporting the conclusion that the inhibition of the firing of these cells occurs normally by an effect upon afferent input and an effect postsynaptic to the primary afferent (Lombard & Besson 1989). The potent actions of the NMDA receptor antagonists clearly indicate an important intermediate role for generating this exaggerated state. These observations, excluding the role of C-fibres in the facilitated state, is further emphasized by the failure of the NK-1 antagonists to alter the strychnine-evoked allodynia. The particular activity of spinal adenosine receptor agonists is believed to reflect the ability of adenosine acting at A-1 receptors to block the release of glutamate (for references see above and Sosnowski & Yaksh 1989).

ANALGESIC ACTIONS OF CENTRALLY DELIVERED DRUGS IN PRIMATES AND HUMANS

In the preceding sections, it has been shown that a variety of spinal manipulations can serve to alter pain behaviour. Because the majority of these studies have been carried out in rodents, it is important to consider to what degree the pharmacology as outlined in the rodent model is representative of more complex pain models, notably those in non-human and human primates.

Table 10.7 Summary of the characteristics of the interaction of different classes of receptor agonists following intrathecal delivery

Spinal agonist pairing[a]	*Species*	*Test*	*Interaction*[b]	*References*
μ–δ	Rat	HP	Synergistic	Malmberg & Yaksh 1992c
	Rat	TF	Synergistic	Larson et al 1980
	Mouse	TF	Additive	Porreca et al 1987
μ–α_2	Rat	HP	Synergistic	Monasky et al 1990
	Rat	HP	Additive	Ossipov et al 1990a
	Rat	TF	Synergistic	Ossipov et al 1990a,b
μ–local anaesthetics	Rat	TF	Synergistic	Maves & Gebhart 1992
	Rat	HP	Synergistic	Penning & Yaksh 1992
μ–cyclooxygenase inhibitor	Rat	FOR	Synergistic	Malmberg & Yaksh 1993b
δ–α_2	Rat	TF	Synergistic	Ossipov et al 1990b
κ–α_2	Rat	TF	Synergistic	Ossipov et al 1990b
κ–cyclooxygenase inhibitor	Rat	FOR	Additive	Malmberg & Yaksh 1993b
α_2–cyclooxygenase inhibitor	Rat	FOR	Synergistic	Malmberg & Yaksh 1993b
L-PIA–cyclooxygenase inhibitor	Rat	FOR	Additive	Malmberg & Yaksh 1993b
NMDA antagonist–cyclooxygenase	Rat	FOR	Additive	S.E. Abram & T.L. Yaksh, unpublished

[a] All analysis employed either an isobolographic analysis or multiple dose combinations with a fixed additive dose (Tallarida et al 1989).
[b] Synergistic indicates that isobologram deviated significantly from linearity or that the left shift in the dose–response curve observed in the presence of the added drug was statistically greater than that predicted on the basis of simple effects-additivity.
Abbreviations: HP = hot plate; TF= Tail flick; FOR = formalin test.

Opioids

Spinally delivered opioids

Systematic studies in the primate have emphasized that several classes of spinally administered opiates can produce a powerful dose-dependent analgesia as measured in a number of endpoints, including the operant-controlled shock titration and the thermal escape threshold evoked by tail dip (Yaksh 1983, 1997a,b). The microinjection of opiates into the medullary dorsal horn of the trigeminal nucleus is similarly able to increase the thermal escape threshold in the unanaesthetized primate (Oliveras et al 1986a,b).

The pharmacology of these effects has been systematically examined in the shock titration endpoints, as well as thermal escape paradigms. In these models, as outlined in Table 10.8, the ordering of activity has been shown to be μ > δ >> κ (i.e., DAMGO, morphine, sufentanil > DPDPE >> U-50488 = 0) (Table 10.9). The effects of DAMGO and morphine are reversed by naloxone but not the δ-preferring antagonist naltrindole. In contrast, the effects of DPDPE are reversed by both naloxone and naltrindole (T.L. Yaksh 1997c). Such observations emphasize spinal μ and δ opioid receptors. Such observations are consistent with the absence of cross-tolerance between morphine and the δ-preferring agent DADL in animals made tolerant to morphine (Yaksh 1983).

In humans, the delivery of opioids by the intrathecal or epidural routes produces a powerful analgesia in a variety of acute postoperative (Abboud 1988, Sandler 1990, Tobias et al 1990, Shafer et al 1991) and chronic pain states (Payne 1987, Arner et al 1988, Iacono et al 1988). While there are few systematic studies on the pharmacology of the spinally administered opioids, considerable clinical experience (Table 10.8) has indicated involvement of a μ-opioid site as defined by the relative potency of the agents (lofentanil > sufentanil > morphine > meperidine). With regard to other receptors, limited experience has shown that the δ-preferring agonist DADL is efficacious following spinal delivery (Moulin et al 1985), suggesting that a δ receptor may also be present. Butorphanol is reputed to have κ-preferring activity and has been shown to have a mild action following epidural delivery. With regard to antagonism, relatively low doses of naloxone (10 μg/kg/h) produced approximately a

Table 10.8. Antinociceptive effects of spinally delivered receptor selective agents in the rat[a]

	Antinociceptive measure						
	HP[a]	*TF[b]*	*Visceral[c]*	*Formalin test[d]* Phase 1	Phase 2	*ThermalHy[e]* (nerve comp.)	*NMDA/Stry[f]* (allodynea)
Agonists							
Opioid							
μ	++[1]	++[1]	++[2]	++[3]	++[3]	+[4]	(+)[5]
δ	++[1]	++[1]	++[2]	?	++[6]	+[4]	(+)[5]
κ	(+)[1]	(+)[1]	?	0[7]	+[7]	0[4]	0[5]
α adrenergic							
$2_{A/non-A}$	++[8]	++[9]	++[10]	++[7]	++[7]	+[4]	0[5]
Serotonin							
$5HT_{1A}$	+[11]	+[12]	++[14]	?	?	?	?
$5HT_{1B}$	+[11]	+[12]	++[14]	?	?	?	?
$5HT_2$	0/+?[11]	+[12,13]	++[14]	?	?	?	?
$5HT_3$	+[15]	+[15]	++[14]	?	?	?	?
Adenosine							
A_1	+[16]	+[16]	+[16]	0[7]	+[7]	+[4]	++[17]
GABA							
A	0[18]	0[18]	?	?	+[38]	+	++[4]
B	+[19]	+[19]	?	?	+[38]	++[4]	+[5]
Benzodiazepine	+[20,21]						
Gabapentin	0[39]	0[40]	?	0	+[41]	+	+[42]
Cholinergic							
M	++[22]	++[23]	?	?	?	?	?
N							
Dopamine							
D_2	++[24]	++[25]	?	?	?	?	?
Neuropeptide Y	++[26]	?	?	?	?	?	?

	HP[a]	*TF[b]*	*Visceral[c]*	*Formalin test[d]* Phase 1	Phase 2	*ThermalHy[e]* (nerve comp.)	*NMDA/Stry[f]* (allodynea)
Antagonists							
Glutamate							
NMDA	0[27]	0[27]	?	+	+[3]	++[4]	++[5]
non-NMDA	+[27]	+[27]	?	+	+[27,28]	0[4]	+[5]
Tachykinin							
NK-1	0[29]	0[29]	?	+	+[30]	?	?
NK-2	+[31]	+[31]	?	?	?	?	?
Enzyme inhibitors							
Cholinesterase	++[32]	+[33]	?	?	?	?	?
Cyclooxygenase	0[34,35]	0[35]	?	(+)[34]	+[34]	0[29]	?
NO synthase	0[36]	?	?	(+)[36]	+[36]	?	?
Enkephalinase	+[37]	+[37]	?	?	?	?	?

Symbols: Antinociceptive effects of spinal agents: 0: No effect at doses that do not produce motor dysfunction; +mild effect; ++ moderate effect and +++: complete blockade of behavioural end point at doses that do not produce over-riding motor or behavioural side effects. ? = no information available.

[a] The confidence with which any receptor is affiliated with the specific changes in pain behaviour depends upon the use of receptor preferring agonists and antagonists. For the case of agents such as NPY, specific antagonists do not at present exist, or for the 5HT antagonists, there is controversy as to the selectivity of the agonists/antagonists and specific receptor designations must be considered as tentative. In the case of agents such as cholinesterase and enkephalinase inhibitors, the use of selective antagonists are used to define the site acted upon by the augmented levels of endogenous transmitter produced by the enzyme inhibitors.

[b] Distention of the bowel with balloon, examination of the behavioural or blood pressure response.

[c] Injection of dilute formalin into one hindpaw; assessment of licking/flinching during the first phase 5–10 min or second phase 10–60 min after formalin.

[d] Loose or partial compression of the sciatic nerve and examination of the thermal response latency.

[e] Intrathecal injection of the glycine antagonist strychnine evoked tactile evoked agitation (allodynea) or increase in blood pressure.

Abbreviations: HP = 52.5°C hot plate; TF = tail flick.

References: [1] Schmauss & Yaksh 1984; [2] Ness & Gebhart 1988; [3] Yamamoto & Yaksh 1992a; [4] Yamamoto & Yaksh 1991a; [5] Yaksh 1989; [6] Murray & Cowan 1991; [7] Malmberg & Yaksh 1993b; [8] Takano & Yaksh 1992; [9] and [10] Danzebrink & Gebhart 1990; [11] K.R. Ware & T.L. Yaksh, unpublished; [12] Eide & Hole 1991; [13] Solomon & Gebhart 1988; [14] Danzebrink & Gebhart 1991; [15] Glaum et al 1990; [16] Sosnowski et al 1989; [17] Sosnowski & Yaksh 1989; [18] Hammond & Drower 1984; [19] Aran & Hammond 1991; [20] Yanez et al 1990; [21] Edwards et al 1990; [22] Yaksh et al 1985; [23] Gillberg et al 1989; [24] Jensen & Yaksh 1984b; [25] Liu et al 1992; [26] Hua et al 1991; [27] Nässtrom et al 1992; [28] Malmberg and Yaksh, unpublished; [29] T. Yamamoto and Yaksh, unpublished; [30] Yamamoto and Yaksh 1991a; [31] Fleetwood-Walker et al 1990; [32] Naguib and Yaksh, unpublished; [33] Gordh et al 1989; [34] Malmberg & Yaksh 1992b; [35] Yaksh 1982; [36] Malmberg & Yaksh 1993a; [37] Oshita et al 1990; [38] Dirig & Yaksh 1995; [39] Jun & Yaksh 1998; [40] Field et al 1997; [41] Shimoyama et al 1997; [42] Partridge et al 1998.

Table 10.9. Effects of agents on pain behaviour in preclinical models and human pain states

Drug classes	*Animal models*	*Human pain states*	*Human drugs*	*Route (s)*	*Reference*
μ-opioid agonists	A/P	Post operative Cancer	Meperidine Methadone Morphine Alfentanil β-endorphin Sufentanil Buprenorphine Lofentanil	PO/IV Epidural/ Intrathecal	1 2 3 4 5 6 7 8
δ-opioid agonist		Cancer	DADL	Intrathecal	9
κ-opioid agonist		Post operative	Butorphanol	Epidural	10
α_2 agonist	A/P/N	Post operative Cancer Neuropathic	Clonidine	Epidural	11
AChase inhibitor	A/P	Post operative Cancer	Neostigmine	Intrathecal	12
Cyclooxygenase (COX) inhibitors (COX 2)	P	Post operative Cancer	Lysine ASA Ketorolac Celebrex Meloxicam	PO Epidural/ Intrathecal	13
Adenosine A-1 agonist	P/N	Neuropathic	R-PIA Adenosine	Intrathecal	14
GABApentin (?)	P/N	Neuropathic	GABApentin	PO	15
Sodium channel blocker	P/N	Cancer Neuropathic	Lidocaine Mexilethine	IV PO	16
Spinal N-type channel blocker	P/N	Cancer	SNX-111	Intrathecal	17
NMDA antagonist	P/N	Post operative Neuropathic	Ketamine CPP (spinal)	Epidural/ Intrathecal	18
AMPA/kainate antag	P/N	Experimental hyperalgesia	LY293558	IV	19

See Table 10.8 and text for further details regarding drug action.
Abbreviations: A = acute pain models (hot plate/tail flick); P= persistent pain states (formalin, inflamed knee joint/paw); N= neuropathic pain models (Bennett/Chung models).
References: [1] Perriss et al 1990; [2] Martin et al 1990; [3] Pybus & Torda 1982; Nordberg 1984; [4] Chauvin et al 1985; [5] Oyama et al 1982; [6] Whiting et al 1988; Graf et al 1991; Dottrens et al 1992; [7] Simpson et al 1988; [9] Onofrio and Yaksh 1983; Moulin 1985; [10] Lawhorn et al 1991; Palacios et al 1991; [11] Eisenach et al 1996; [12] Hood et al 1995; Laureti and Lima 1996; [13] Pace 1995; Lipsky and Isakson 1997; Devoghel 1983; Lauretti et al 1998; [14] Karlsten & Gordh 1995; Sollevi 1997; [15] Mellick and Mellick 1997; Backonja et al 1998; [16] Wallace et al 1996; Jarvis and Coukell 1998; [17] Brose et al 1997; [18] Abdel Ghaffar et al 1998; Takahashi et al 1998; Kristensen et al 1992; [19] Sang et al 1998.

50% reduction in the antinociceptive effects of epidural morphine (Rawal et al 1986). These data offer support for the presence of a μ-opioid site and are suggestive of the presence of a δ- and κ-opioid site. Clearly, further work is required to define the pharmacology of the human spinal cord.

Supraspinal opiate action in primates and humans

Systematic microinjection studies on primates examining the effects on the supraspinally organized operant shock titration response have revealed a distribution of sites which correspond closely with those systems that have been reported in the rodent. Active sites were distributed in at least two discriminable loci. The first was found to correspond to the periventricular/periaquaductal grey axis of the mesencephalon. The second showed that sites were distributed more caudally in the lower brainstem and corresponded to the medial and lateral aspects of the medulla (Pert & Yaksh 1974, 1975, Yaksh et al 1988b). Noticeably inactive was the thalamus, although a distribution of sites lying along the dorsal aspect of the periventricular grey and ventral aspect of the thalamus was described. The lateral distribution appears to correspond to those identified in the lateral aspects of the medullary reticular formation in the rat. There is, unfortunately, little comparative data on the pharmacology of these sites. In the primate, all that can be said is that the effects were readily antagonized by naloxone and were stereospecific (Pert & Yaksh 1974).

Microinjection studies have not been carried out in humans. However, intracerebroventricular injection of opioids such as morphine and β-endorphin have been shown to produce a powerful analgesic effect in patients suffering from pain secondary to head and neck cancer (Lazorthes 1988, Lee et al 1990, Sandouk et al 1991, Schulteis et al 1992). Given that the effects of morphine are potent in the regions immediately surrounding the periaqueductal grey in all models including primates, it is reasonable to hypothesize that a similar site of action explains the potent analgesia resulting from the actions of opiates delivered intracranially in humans.

While there are important parallels between the preclinical literature on primates and rodents, it should be stressed that the mechanisms of the effects in humans can only be hypothesized. For example, the prominent role of bulbospinal pathways defined in the rodent can be indirectly inferred on the basis of the action of adrenoceptor agonists in both human and non-human primates. On the other hand, the important observation that supraspinal morphine blocks spinal reflexes has not been reported in either primate model.

Non-opioids

The information in Tables 10.1, 10.8 and 10.9 emphasizes that activity in the rat on acute nociceptive endpoints (such as in the hot plate and tail flick tests) will predict the ability of classes of agents to display efficacy in a human postinjury pain state (e.g., postoperative/trauma/cancer). Based on the presumed mechanism of the actions of several classes of agents (e.g., opioids, α_2 adrenoceptor agonists), this appears to be a logical consequence of reducing activity evoked in dorsal horn projection neurons by small afferent input. By contrast, as indicated in Table 10.9, it is shown that agents that were active in postinjury pain models (e.g., formalin) were frequently noted to be effective in the postoperative state and in other tissue injury states. This incidence of activity of agents such as cycloxygenase inhibitors, NMDA antagonists and several channel blockers (e.g., N-type calcium channel blockers) is a likely indicator of the role routinely played by facilitated processing after injury. Finally, the efficacy of agents in neuropathic pain (e.g., using the Bennett or Chung models) appears to predict the efficacy of several classes of agents in human neuropathic pain states. Noteworthy in this regard are IV sodium channel blockers, systemic gabapentin and spinally delivered α_2-agonists, NMDA antagonists and N-type Ca-channel blockers. It is interesting that the preclinical studies have uniformly provided strong evidence that for the agents that are given systemically in humans, the preclinical work has emphasized the probability of a spinal site of action.

This ability to predict human antinociceptive activity suggests several important points. Firstly, these results suggest that the preclinical models of nociception (Table 10.1) engage certain mechanisms that are mediated by distinct but overlapping spinal pharmacologies. Secondly, the multiple mechanisms posited to play a role in pain processing in animal models also appear to apply to the human clinical condition. As such, these investigations shed light on novel mechanisms underlying clinical pain and point the way for the rational development of novel antinociceptive agents. It seems certain that complex human clinical conditions, such as those related to cancer or trauma, represent multiple mechanisms. Accordingly, efficacious interventions require polypharmacy. Finally, the convergence of spinal drug delivery studies carried out in humans and animals emphasizes that the encoding of input generated by tissue and peripheral nerve injury leading to a 'pain state' can occur at the segmental level. Accordingly, potent and selective regulation of pain may be achieved by targeting drug delivery at this level.

PHARMACOLOGY OF AFFECTIVE COMPONENTS OF PAIN BEHAVIOUR

THE INFLUENCE OF AFFECTIVE VARIABLES IN PAIN BEHAVIOUR

As reviewed in the introductory section of this chapter, the pain state can be defined in terms of the stimulus and the afferent traffic induced by the stimulus and by the syndrome of response and states induced by potentially tissue damaging stimuli. In the simplest construct, the pain state is defined by the observed responses that reflect characteristic motor patterns, which serve to remove the stimulus from the organism. At a more complex level, as with other stimulus modalities, the stimulus evokes patterns of associated memories that provide a context for the stimulus and serves to tailor the response evoked by that stimulus. This higher-order function provides the substrate for perception. As noted, the recognition that occasionally a less aversive or innocuous stimuli or no obvious stimulus can generate a pain state, reflecting hyperalgesia, allodynia or spontaneous dysaesthesias, or where an adequate noxious stimulus fails to evoke a response at all, emphasizes that there is no obligatory linkage between the nature of the stimulus and the measured response. Such changes in the response to a given stimulus can arise because of changes in the encoding process; or, depending on the level of organization, changes in the response function. At the motor level, such changes may occur by altering the excitability of the motor neuron pool (e.g., as in a Sherringtonian reflex). At higher levels of organization, changes in the context of the stimulus might alter the perception of the encoded stimulus leading to changes in the observed response. This context is established by processes that arise from linkages between memories, establishing prior stimulus response consequences, and provides the construct for emotion. In the preceding sections, emphasis has been on systems that can alter the encoding of high-intensity afferent input. In the following sections we will consider issues that impact upon the relationship between higher-order perceptual processes providing the context for the pain state.

Affect and human pain

There is a wide recognition that situational and environmental variables that do not impact upon the sensory message generated by a high-intensity stimulus can induce changes in the response evoked by that stimulus. In humans, the affective-motivational component of the pain state is widely appreciated (Melzack & Casey 1968, Melzack & Wall 1973. These perceptual components can alter the response to a given noxious stimulus. Significant depression (Kremer et al 1983, Turner & Romano 1984, Romano & Turner 1985), or anxiety (Beecher 1969, Katon 1984) can significantly enhance pain states. Positive mood states diminish the reported severity of a pain condition. Conversely, negative mood factors such as depression or aversion may augment the reported severity of the state (Chapman 1985) and correlate with lower indices of satisfaction and higher indices of the pain state (e.g. see Chapman 1985, Taenzer et al 1986).

Problems in mechanistic studies on the contribution of affect to the pain state

Great strides have been made in defining the mechanisms that alter afferent processing. When we have focused on spinal encoding, there is less appreciation of the mechanisms whereby supraspinal systems impact the affective components related to pain. Mechanistic studies that focus on the role of affect face at least four considerations:

1. In non-verbal animals, we are committed to the assessment of the pain behaviour generated by characteristic stimuli. As at the level of the spinal cord, we must query whether a manipulation serves to alter the observed behaviour because it actually makes the pain state more or less intense or whether it produces competing behaviours. Thus stressors result in freezing behaviour. The absence of a response in the face of a stressor does not necessarily indicate that the animal is without sensation. Failure to observe a response in an animal with lower motor neuron hyperpolarization and unable to move is not an indication of analgesia.
2. If noxious stimulation is increased, we anticipate an increasing output and an index of increasing pain behaviour. In the case of an issue related to affect, it would be naive to believe that stessors induce monotonic changes. It is probable, for example, that stressors cause a change in the affective state of the organism, represented definitionally as fear or anxiety. These affective states may enhance the response of the animal to a given stimulus by altering the organized response of the animal to the stimulus and may result in alteration of the myriad of modulatory systems that are found within the CNS to directly reduce the afferent input. This is clearly the case in several models of conditioned hypoalgesia.
3. With respect to drug action, if an agent is given systemically and serves to reduce the response measure, the effect may be related to a change in the afferent encoding process such that the afferent message is consistent with one that is generated by a lesser stimulus (e.g., as morphine is believed to do at the spinal level), or it may in fact alter the bias of the organized response such that a lesser response is produced in the face of an unaltered afferent message. This is not an insurmountable problem, but it will require the development of relatively sophisticated animal models which permit dissection of an effect upon afferent input as opposed to an effect upon the organization of higher-order functions related to pain encoding. In this regard, the action of agents that block hyperalgesia can only be

defined in the presence of a state of facilitated processing. Similarly, drugs which theoretically alter pain by altering a perceptual state will only be considered active when that state is present and is relevant to the pain state being examined. Typically, if a given class of agents alters the reported pain state in humans or a component of stimulus-evoked behaviour in animals, the role of a higher-order mechanism underlying these changes has not been well characterized with the current methods available for behavioural assessment. Thus, an agent may serve to alter the affective state of the organism (such as antidepressants or psychostimulants), but in many cases the action of these agents may also directly alter afferent traffic. The ability of higher-order systems to alter afferent processing can be supported by the observation that in animal paradigms of conditioned hypoalgesia, the state is associated with (i) a reduction in spinal nociceptive reflexes (Bellgowan & Helmstetter 1998) and (ii) reduced c-*fos* expression otherwise evoked by formalin (Harris et al 1995). Such observations emphasize that conditioned stimuli acting at higher centres can indeed attenuate spinofugal nociceptive transmission.

4. Finally, while we may intuit that 'affect' impacts upon pain perception and the manifested response, it is not evident how this concept plays out in terms of constructs which can be studied. To study affects we must operationally define the elements that constitute the 'affect variable'. Focusing on the major functional classes of drugs, we might consider that drugs that fall in the class of anxiolytics, antidepressants and stimulants exert actions that produce changes in affect and emotionality in the verbal and non-verbal animal. In the preclinical model, such major dimensions are operationally defined in terms of specific animal models that show activity in families of drugs that impact on human behaviour which are in accord with accepted psychiatric definitions. Interpretation of the role played by a particular system in affect is governed by our understanding of what experimentally constitutes 'affect' in preclinical (non-verbal) models.

The behavioural literature has provided models that have face validity and in turn serve to screen agents that can alter human states of depression and mania (e.g., the antidepressants and antipsychotics). This suggests that such models may reflect upon a correlate of human affective states (Eison 1984, Jesberger & Richardson 1985, Musty et al 1990, Detke et al 1997, Hansen et al 1997, Kelly et al 1997, Vaugeois et al 1997). Thus, anxiolytic actions are typically predicted in models using aversive contingencies wherein the drug either (i) attenuates increased behaviours, (ii) restores suppressed behaviours or (iii) reverses a pharmacologically induced anxiety. Agents such as benzodiazepines and agonists at 5HT1A receptors are typically effective in such models (Miczek et al 1995). Situational paradigms involving inescapable stressors such as aversive shock or forced swimming (Connor et al 1997, Amat et al 1998), or surgical manipulations such as olfactory bulbectomy (Kelly et al 1997), will induce persistent changes in function which are markedly influenced by a variety of agents that display antidepressant activity in humans (Kelly et al 1997, Leonard 1997).

NEURAL SUBSTRATES ASSOCIATED WITH AFFECT AND PAIN

There is not enough space here to permit a detailed review of the literature related to the assessment of anatomical structures that define the affective state and their potential role in the regulation of pain behaviour. However, several components may be noted.

Role of forebrain structures

Our intuition that affect is a component of higher-order function (supratentorial) is likely correct. In the early decades of this century, after the development of surgical procedures used in prefrontal lobotomy, we began to understand more clearly how the brain functions when a subject endures a painful stimulus. The patients would display minimal concern and were not troubled by the state, although they reported that the severity of the painful sensation remained (Freeman & Watts 1942, 1946). This dissociation provides clear parallels to the position that forebrain connections were important for the development of an affective component to the nociception induced by the stimulus.

This effect of forebrain lesions on the psychological consequence of nociception is paralleled by the observation that nociceptive stimuli can evoke prominent activity in forebrain systems that are not considered to be components of the somatosensory pathways that encode sensory traffic (e.g., somatotopically organized projections by WDR neuron projections to the ventrobasal thalamus and the somatosensory cortex). Aside from a large number of electrophysiological studies (Craig & Dostrovsky 1997), the nature of such higher level interconnections may be appreciated in the light of studies in which local cerebral blood flow or metabolism were assessed in brainstem and forebrain structures after local noxious stimulation. In rats, the injection of formalin into the paw resulted in increased activity in the somatosensory cortex. In addition to such anticipated somatosensory mapping of activity, there was significant increases in blood flow in the brainstem (interpeduncular nucleus and the periaqueductal grey) and bilaterally in several forebrain limbic structures, including the anterior dorsal nucleus and the retrosplenial cortex. In humans, local noxious thermal stimuli stimulated activity in the anticipated somatosensory areas, but in addition provided significant activation in the anterior cingulate (Rainville et al 1997). As reviewed above, the anterior cingulate receives projections from the n. submedius which is a primary recipient of input from lamina I nociceptive neurons.

As noted above, placing the animal in a contingency situation wherein prior experience pairs (the situation the conditioning stimulus) with a noxious stimulus (the unconditioned stimulus) can lead to a conditioned state believed to define the state of anxiety or fear. It can be shown that such complex associations can subsequently evoke, in the absence of the conditioning pain state, activation of specific forebrain structures. Using the induction of the immediate early gene c-*fos* as a marker of neuronal activation, limbic forebrain regions (cingulate, infralimbic and perirhinal cortex, nucleus accumbens, lateral septum, dorsal endopiriform nucleus and ventral segmental area) displayed significant induction after the subsequent presentation of the conditioned stimulus.

While important and provocative, such models alone cannot define whether the parallel drug effects reflect mechanistic identity or corollary phenomena (e.g., where ability of opiates to block the contraction of the guinea pig ileum will predict the analgesic activity of the agents).

A corollary of the preceding consideration is that lesion studies of the medial frontal cortex (Frysztak & Neafsey 1991, 1994), septum (Decker et al 1995) and amygdala (Ono et al 1995, Angrilli et al 1996) have suggested that the respective cell system plays a role in the expression of affect, as defined by behavioural effects in surrogate models. It has not been clearly defined which component(s) of the respective system function are related to the changes in affect. As an example, recent reviews emphasize the role of the amygdala in the long-term acquisition of stimulus–affect relationships. In effect it displays a comparator function which permits evaluation by the organism of the significance of a given stimulus on the basis of previously acquired memories (Ono et al 1995, Pitkanen et al 1997).

Brainstem

As noted previously, the organizational role of brainstem systems such as the periaqueductal grey is complicated. Opiates exert a local effect, increasing hot plate response latencies and thermal and shock titration escape thresholds, while the local injection of glutamate may evoke pain behaviour. This suggests there is an acute regulation of the afferent message generated by an unconditioned stimulus. In addition, it is now thought that the mesencephalic central grey plays a role in emotive constituents of the behaviour. It is significant that pathways traditionally considered to be related to changes in affective behaviour are being shown to exert correlated effects upon the organized response of the animal to an ongoing painful stimulus (Franklin 1989, Bandler et al 1991, Bandler & Shipley 1994, Bandler & Keay 1996, Bellgowan & Helmstetter 1998).

CLASSES OF MOOD-ALTERING DRUGS AND THEIR EFFECTS UPON PAIN STATES

A variety of agents may be considered as a function of their respective pharmacology. In the following sections, several major classes of agents which have been implicated in altering mood will be briefly considered in the context of their impact upon pain state expression.

Opioids

The current emphasis is on the mechanisms of opioid action and their ability to activate modulatory substrates. The perceptual and anxiolytic effects of the agents after systemic administration is widely appreciated as an important component of their clinical action (Lasagna et al 1955, Kaiko et al 1981). Early thinking pointed to the parallels between the effect of opiates and the effects of prefrontal lobectomies on affect in chronic pain states (Wikler 1950).

The complexity of the probable effects upon higher-order functioning, which may be relevant to the organization of the pain state, can be appreciated by considering the effects of opiates in complex behavioural tasks mediated by forebrain structures.

Conditioned place preference

Such behavioural systems are believed to define the rewarding nature of a treatment by associating a spatial location with the presence or absence of a treatment. In conditioned place preference studies, microinjections of morphine into the ventral segmental area or periaqueductal grey produced place preferences but not into the striatum; frontal cortex, hippocampus, amygdala, pedunculopontine segmental nucleus, hypothalamus or nucleus accumbens (Olmstead & Franklin 1997).

Conditioning to a noxious stimulus

Pairing of a noxious shock with an innocuous stimulus can lead to a learned association of the shock and the environment with the stimulus, providing a surrogate model for conditioned fear and anxiety. Microinjection of morphine into the amygdala reduced the expression of fear and impaired fear conditioning to a shock-paired stimulus and to the context where the shock occurred. Injection into the n. accumbens had no effect upon the fear conditioning, but did block the conditioning to the context in which the shock was applied. The results support a role for opioid mechanisms in the amygdala in the acquisition of stimulus/context–response associations that reflect fear (Good & Westbrook 1995, Westbrook et al 1997).

Antidepressants

Antidepressants form a complex class of agents that, with few exceptions, may be classified in terms of their ability to enhance the extracellular levels of catecholamines such as noradrenaline and dopamine (e.g., amitryptylline; Richelson & Pfenning 1984) and indoleamines such as serotonin (e.g., fluoxetine; Stark et al 1985) by blocking their reuptake. Tricyclic antidepressants, particularly those characterized as blocking noradrenergic reuptake, have been shown to be effective in a variety of persistent pain conditions (Bryson & Wilde 1996, Sindrup 1997). The mechanism or site of this action is not fully understood. Several lines of evidence suggest that the actions of the agents may not be related to their anti depressant actions. Some of the antinociceptive effects of these agents may result from a direct effect upon the processing of sensory information by enhancing the efficacy of bulbospinal monoaminergic transmission by increasing extracellular amine levels (see above; Ardid et al 1995). Systematic clinical trials have shown that a number of tricyclic antidepressants relieve the pain in normal and depressed patients secondary to neuropathies (Max et al 1991, Sindrup et al 1990b) and arthritis (Frank et al 1988). In addition, the antinociceptive effects appear more quickly than the antidepressant action (Sindrup et al 1990a), and lower doses are required to obtain pain relief than for antidepressant activity (Sindrup et al 1990c). These effects may appear in depressed as well as non-depressed patients (Max et al 1987, 1991, 1992).

Monoamine pathways arising from brainstem nuclei project to limbic forebrain structures and are known to modulate the response of the animal to the stimulus environment (Bandler et al 1985, 1991, Franklin 1989). The raphe dorsalis gives rise to 5HT projections to rostral sites, including the n. accumbens, amygdala and lateral thalamus (Westlund et al 1990, Ma et al 1991, Ma & Han 1992). The locus coeruleus also has strong noradrenergic projections into the limbic forebrain and thalamus (Westlund et al 1990).

As reviewed above, forebrain dopamine, serotonergic and noradrenergic systems have been broadly implicated in the manifestation of emotionality and maintenance of consciousness (Graeff et al 1997, Mongeau et al 1997, Onaka & Yagi 1998). Among the earliest studies, depletion of serotonin by *p*-chlorphenylalanine produces rats that were particularly irritable (Tenen 1968). Systematic microdialysis studies have emphasized that stress can increase forebrain release of these amines (Goldstein et al 1994, Finlay et al 1995). While the interaction between supraspinal activity generated specifically by small afferent input and the forebrain systems receiving monoamine input is at present modestly uncharacterized, Milne et al (1996) observed that the allodynia induced by the intrathecal delivery of strychnine was associated with a prominent stimulus-dependent increase in the activation of locus coeruleus neurons. Accordingly, such activation of forebrain noradrenergic projections could gain access to limbic structures that play an important role in the affective motivational component that contributes to pain behaviour (Derryberry & Tucker 1992, Frysztak & Neafsey 1994).

Benzodiazepines

Benzodiazepines produce potent anxiolytic actions in humans and in a variety of animal models. At the membrane, benzodiazepines can act at several binding sites to augment the actions of GABA at GABA-A receptors, leading to an enhancement of opening of the Clionophore (Korpi et al 1997). Binding sites for benzodiazepines are located throughout the brain, with particularly high densities in limbic system (Fernandez-Lopez et al 1997).

In humans, and animals, the ability of benzodiazepines to alter pain behaviour is complicated. In humans experimental models such as the cold pressor test, midazolam had no effect upon thresholds nor did they alter the antinociceptive effects of an opiate (Zacny et al 1996). In clinical studies, benzodiazepines have been widely recognized as adjuncts to opioid analgesics in burn, trauma and critical care (Vinik 1995, Murray et al 1995, Pal et al 1997, Patterson et al 1997).

In animal models, spinally delivered benzodiazepines augment opioid analgesia. In contrast, after intracranial delivery, these agents have been reported to antagonize the effects of morphine (an effect consistent with the presumed role of GABAergic interneurones in controlling PAG outflow exciting bulbospinal projections (see above) (Luger et al 1995, Feng and Kendig 1996, Gear et al 1997).

After chronic systemic delivery, benzodiazepines can be shown to exert a potent effect upon limbic circuitry (e.g., the Papez circuit), the nucleus accumbens and the basolateral amygdala (Pratt et al 1998). Midazolam administered by microinjection into the basolateral amygdala prior to exposure to noxious stimulus in a conditioned fear paradigm, reduced the conditioned fear acquisition. This effect of midazolam was reversed by the benzodiazepine receptor antagonist flumazenil. The results suggest that benzodiazepines acting within the amygdala produce a retrieval deficit in linkages which link the stimulus with the context (e.g., fear conditioning) (Harris & Westbrook 1995a,b). As noted above, forebrain catecholamine levels may be augmented by stress and by activation of rostrally projecting systems. Importantly, it has been shown that this forebrain release of dopamine is reduced by diazepam and by 5HT1a agonists (Finlay et al 1995, Wedzony et al 1996).

Psychomotor stimulants

A variety of psychomotor stimulants have been shown to augment the analgesic effects of opioids in man (Forrest et al 1977, Kaiko et al 1987, Bonica et al 1990, Reich & Razavi 1996). Interestingly, caffeine represents a widely used adjuvant in man and has been shown to modestly, but significantly, facilitate the analgesic effects of a variety of classes of agents, including opiates and non-steroidal anti-inflammatory agents (for a review see Sawynok & Yaksh 1993). In humans caffeine resembles the effects seen after other psychomotor stimulants, including amphetamine and fenfluramine (Chait et al 1987, Chait & Johanson 1988), inducing at low doses, mildly positive mood states and stimulant-like effects (Chait & Johanson 1988, Griffiths & Woodson 1988 a,b,c). Given the positive impact of caffeine on mood, it is a reasonable speculation that caffeine may contribute to analgesia (as opposed to an antinociceptive) by virtue of these positive changes in the affective state. The importance of such psychological variables to the behavioural syndrome observed in the presence of an ongoing pain state (as opposed to a reflex function) remains, however, to be systematically examined in a well-defined animal model. Mechanistically, a variety of studies have implicated the mesolimbic dopamine system in psychomotor stimulation by centrally active agents (Swerdlow et al 1986). Depletion of brain catecholamines reduces stimulation of motor activity by caffeine (Finn et al 1990). Lesions to the nucleus accumbens inhibit motor stimulation by amphetamine, cocaine and methylphenidate (Kelly & Iversen 1976). Such lesions, however, do not alter the effect of caffeine (Joyce & Koob 1981). Thus, while catecholamine systems are implicated in the stimulant action of caffeine, the neurotransmitters and specific pathways involved remain to be determined (for a review see Sawynok & Yaksh 1993).

CONCLUDING COMMENTS

This chapter has sought to adhere to four organizing principles. Firstly, our understanding of the mechanisms underlying pain processing requires convergence between behaviour and the properties predicted by the hypothesized mechanisms. Thus, for exaggerated spinal processing or a particular receptor to be related to pain, the properties of hyperalgesia must display similar characteristics. Secondly, the mechanisms for which we search must include those related to our ability to report location, quality and intensity as well as the affective correlates that such stimuli may generate, for example the sensory discriminative and the affective-motivational dimensions. It is clear that such a dichotomy is a useful tool but is likely to be artificial. Thus, the afferent message can drive the emotional components and the affective attributes arising from the context of the stimulus can modify the response not only by altering the interpretation of the stimulus in that context, but can feed back into systems that regulate the nature of the encoding process at the segmental level.

Given the above considerations, it is clear that considerable advances have been made since the first edition of this text in our appreciation of the pharmacology of the systems that process nociceptive information. The systematic characterization of the pharmacology of CNS systems that are involved in regulating the organism's response to a strong stimulus has provided insight into the complexity of the systems that are involved in controlling the throughput of such information. The appreciation that specific systems are activated by acute, unconditioned, high-intensity stimuli has been an important observation. However, the current appreciation that repetitive input can in fact generate profound changes in afferent processing makes it possible now to define behavioural states of hyperalgesia, hyperaesthesia and allodynia in terms of distinct receptor substrates and associated anatomical systems. The differential pharmacology that reflects upon these pain states emphasizes that the facilitated state of processing is a phenomena that is evoked by, but is distinct from, the pain state generated by the acute stimulus. The appreciation that florid changes in the response to light touch are induced by the mere blockade of a single class of inhibitory amino acids (glycine or GABA) not only suggests that these may be targets for degenerative processes that occur following nerve injuries leading to allodynic states, but also, from a theoretical perspective, that light touch itself possesses a non-noxious characteristic, only because of a very effective ongoing inhibition.

The final section of this review, although brief, represents in part the next important advances in our understanding of the processing of nociceptive information. Supraspinal components that reflect upon the affective state of the animal are clearly of theoretical and practical relevance. The interpretation of the powerful effect of opiates on perceptual processes is in part complicated because of the complicated and efficacious mechanisms by which this family of agents also control afferent processing. Perhaps will provide the simple drug caffeine more insight to the future of the classes of agents, as this drug seems to have little effect upon pain processing per se, but appears to exert its effects through subtle changes in affect. One would anticipate that as we extend our ability to ask increasingly subtle questions of the animal models, the pharmacology and mechanisms of the affective components of pain processing will acquire an importance equal to that which we place on the systems that modulate the afferent message.

Lastly, these advances in our understanding of the pharmacology of systems which normally process non-noxious and noxious information are ultimately important, as they provide the direct venue by which the various pain conditions may be differentially diagnosed. Selective modulation of various components of afferent processing, by the use of specific agents targeted at the relevant receptor and anatomical systems, promises to provide the essential tools for the management of the human pain state.

REFERENCES

Aanonsen LM, Wilcox GL 1987 Nociceptive action of excitatory amino acids in the mouse: effects of spinally administered opioids, phencyclidine and sigma agonists. Journal of Pharmacology and Experimental Therapeutics 243: 9–19

Aanonsen LM, Lei S, Wilcox GL 1990 Excitatory amino acid receptors and nociceptive neurotransmission in rat spinal cord. Pain 41: 309–321

Abboud TK 1988 Epidural and intrathecal administration of opioids in obstetrics. Acute Care 12(suppl 1): 17–21

Abdel-Ghaffar ME, Abdulatif MA, al-Ghamdi A, Mowafi H, Anwar A 1998 Epidural ketamine reduces post-operative epidural PCA consumption of fentanyl/bupivacaine. Canadian Journal of Anaesthesia 45:103–109

Abram SE, Yaksh TL 1993 Morphine, but not inhalation anesthesia, blocks post-injury facilitation. The role of preemptive suppression of afferent transmission. Anesthesiology 78: 713–721

Aimi Y, Fujimura M, Vincent SR, Kimura H 1991 Localization of NADPH-diaphorase-containing neurons in sensory ganglia of the rat. Journal of Comparative Neurology 306: 382–392

Aimone LD, Gebhart GF 1986 Stimulation produced spinal inhibition from the brainstem in the rat is mediated by an excitatory amino acid transmitter in the medial medulla. Journal of Neuroscience 6: 1803–1813

Aimone LD, Gebhart GF 1988 Serotonin and/or an excitatory amino acid in the medial medulla mediates stimulation-produced antinociception from the lateral hypothalamus in the rat. Brain Research 450: 170–180

Akaike A, Shibata T, Satoh M, Takagi H 1978 Analgesia induced by microinjection of morphine into and electrical stimulation of the nucleus reticularis gigantocellularis of rat medulla oblingata. Neuropharmacology 17: 775–778

Al-Rodhan N, Chipkin R, Yaksh TL 1990 The antinociceptive effects of SCH-32615, a neutral endopeptidase (enkephalinase) inhibitor, microinjected into the periaqueductal, ventral medulla and amygdala. Brain Research 520: 123–130

Alhaider AA, Kitto KF, Wilcox GL 1990 Nociceptive modulation by intrathecally administered 5-HT_{1A} and 5-HT_{1B} agonists in mice. Federation of American Societies for Experimental Biology Journal 4:A988

Alhaider AA, Lei SZ, Wilcox GL 1991 Spinal 5-HT_3 receptor-mediated antinociception: possible release of GABA. Journal of Neuroscience 11: 1881–1888

Amaral DG, Sinnamon HM 1977 The locus coereuleus: neurobiology of a central noradrenergic nucleus. Progress in Neurobiology 9: 147–196

Amat J, Matus-Amat P, Watkins LR, Maier SF 1998 Escapable and inescapable stress differentially and selectively alter extracellular levels of 5-HT in the ventral hippocampus and dorsal periaqueductal gray of the rat. Brain Research 797: 12–22

Anden N-E, Jukes GM, Lundberg A, Vyklicky L 1966 The effects of L-DOPA on the spinal cord. Acta Physiologica Scandinavica 67: 373–386

Anderson CR 1992 NADPH diaphorase-positive neurons in the rat spinal cord include a subpopulation of autonomic preganglionic neurons. Neuroscience Letters 139: 280–284

Angrilli A, Mauri A, Palomba D et al 1996 Startle reflex and emotion modulation impairment after a right amygdala lesion. Brain 119(pt 6): 1991–2000

Aran S, Hammond DL 1991 Antagonism of baclofen-induced antinociception by intrathecal administration of phaclofen or 2-hydroxy-saclofen, but not delta-aminovaleric acid in the rat. Journal of Pharmacology and Experimental Therapeutics 257: 360–368

Ardid D, Guilbaud G 1992 Antinociceptive effects of acute and 'chronic' injections of tricyclic antidepressant drugs in a new model of mononeuropathy in rats. Pain 49: 279–287

Ardid D, Eschalier A, Lavarenne J 1991 Evidence for a central but not a peripheral analgesic effect of clomipramine in rats. Pain 45: 95–100

Ardid D, Jourdan D, Mestre C, Villanueva L, Le Bars D, Eschalier A

1995 Involvement of bulbospinal pathways in the antinociceptive effect of clomipramine in the rat. Brain Research 695: 253–256

Arena JM 1970 Poisoning: toxicology, symptoms, treatments, 4th edn. Charles C Thomas, Springfield, IL

Arena JM 1979 Poisoning: toxicology, symptoms, treatment, 4th edn. Charles C Thomas, Springfield, pp 177–179

Arner S, Rawal N, Gustafsson LL 1988 Clinical experience of long-term treatment with epidural and intrathecal opioids – a nationwide survey. Acta Anaesthesiologica Scandinavica 32: 253–259

Arvidsson U, Riedl M, Chakrabarti S et al 1995a Distribution and targeting of a μ-opioid receptor (MOR1) in brain and spinal cord. Journal of Neuroscience 15: 3328–3341

Arvidsson U, Dado RJ, Riedl M et al 1995b Delta-opioid receptor immunoreactivity: distribution in brain stem and spinal cord and relationship to biogenic amines and enkephalin. Journal of Neuroscience 15: 1215–1235

Arvidsson U, Riedl M, Chakrabarti S et al 1995c The kappa-opioid receptor is primarily postsynaptic: combined immunohistochemical localization of the receptor and endogenous opioids. Proceedings of the National Academy of Sciences USA 92: 5062–5066

Atweh SF, Murrin LC, Kuhar MJ 1978 Presynaptic localization of opiate receptors in the vagal and accessory optic system: an autoradiographic study. Neuropharmacology 17: 65–71

Azami J, Llewelyn MB, Roberts MHT 1982 The contribution of nucleus reticularis gigantocellularis and nucleus raphe magnus to the analgesia produced by systematically administered morphine investigated with the microinjectior technique. Pain 12: 229–246

Baber NS, Dourish CT, Hill DR 1989 The role of CCK caerulein, and CCK antagonists in nociception. Pain 39: 307–328

Bach FW, Yaksh TL 1992 Release of β-endorphin-IR from brain is regulated by a hypothalamic NMDA receptor. Anesthesiology 77(suppl): A733

Bandler R, Keay KA 1996 Columnar organization in the midbrain periaqueductal gray and the integration of emotional expression. Progress in Brain Research 107: 285–300

Bandler R, Shipley MT 1994 Columnar organization in the midbrain periaqueductal gray: modules for emotional expression? Trends in Neurosciences 17: 379–389

Bandler R, McCulloch T, McDougall A, Prineas S, Dampney R 1985 Midbrain neural mechanisms mediating emotional behaviour. International Journal of Neurology 19: 40–58

Bandler R, Carrive P, Zhang SP 1991 Integration of somatic and autonomic reactions within the midbrain periaqueductal grey, viscerotopic, somatotopic and functional organization. Progress in Brain Research 87: 269–305

Bannon AW, Decker MW, Holladay MW et al 1998 Broad-spectrum, non-opioid analgesic activity by selective modulation of neuronal nicotinic acetylcholine receptors. Science 279: 77–81

Barber RP, Vaughn JE, Saito K, McLaughlin BJ, Roberts E 1978 GABAergic terminals are presynaptic to primary afferent terminals in the substantia gelatinosa of the rat spinal cord. Brain Research 141: 35–55

Barke KE, Hough LB 1992 Morphine-induced increases of extracellular histamine levels in the periaqueductal grey in vivo: a microdialysis study. Brain Research 572: 146–153

Barnes CD, Fung SJ, Adams WL 1979 Inhibitory effects of substantia nigra on impulse transmission from nociceptors. Pain 6: 207–215

Basbaum AI 1988 Distribution of glycine receptor immunoreactivity in the spinal cord of the rat: cystochemical evidence for a differential glycinergic control, of Lamina I and Lamina V neurons. Journal of Comparative Neurology 278: 330–336

Battaglia G, Rustioni A 1988 Coexistence of glutamate and substance P in dorsal root ganglion neurons of the rat and monkey. Journal of Comparative Neurology 277: 302–312

Battaglia G, Rustioni A 1992 Substance P innervation of the rat and cat thalamus. II. Cells of origin in the spinal cord. Journal of Comparative Neurology 315: 473–486

Battaglia G, Spreafico R, Rustioni A 1992 Substance P innervation of the rat and cat thalamus. I. Distribution and relation to ascending spinal pathways. Journal of Comparative Neurology 315: 457–472

Baumeister AA 1991 The effects of bilateral intranigral microinjection of selective opioid agonists on behavioral responses to noxious thermal stimuli. Brain Research 557: 136–145

Baumeister AA, Hawkins MF, Anticich TG et al 1987 Bilateral intranigral microinjection of morphine and opioid peptides produces antinociception in rats. Brain Research 411: 183–186

Baumeister AA, Nagy M, Hebert G, Hawkins MF, Vaughn A, Chatellier MO 1990 Further studies of the effects of intranigral morphine on behavioral responses to noxious stimuli. Brain Research 525: 115–125

Beecher HK 1969 Anxiety and pain. Journal of the American Medical Association 209: 1080–1083

Behbehani MM, Park MR, Clement ME 1988 Interactions between the lateral hypothalamus and the periaqueductal gray. Journal of Neuroscience 8: 2780–2787

Behbehani MM, Jiang MR, Chandler SD, Ennis M 1990 The effect of GABA and its antagonists on midbrain periaqueductal gray neurons in the rat. Pain 40: 195–204

Bellgowan PS, Helmstetter FJ 1998 The role of mu and kappa opioid receptors within the periaqueductal gray in the expression of conditional hypoalgesia. Brain Research 791: 83–89

Bennett GJ, Mayer DJ 1979 Inhibition of spinal cord interneurons by narcotic micro injection and focal electrical stimulation in the periaqueductal gray matter. Brain Research 172: 243–257

Bennett GJ, Xie YK 1988 A peripheral mononeuropathy in rat that produces disorders of pain sensation like those seen in man. Pain 33: 87–107

Bitner RS, Nikkel AL, Curzon P, Arneric SP, Bannon AW, Decker MW 1998 Role of the nucleus raphe magnus in antinociception produced by ABT-594: immediate early gene responses possibly linked to neuronal nicotinic acetylcholine receptors on serotonergic neurons. Journal of Neuroscience 18: 5426–5432

Blomqvist A, Ericson A-C, Craig AD, Broman J 1996 Evidence for glutamate as a neurotransmitter in spinothalamic tract terminals in the posterior region of owl monkeys. Experimental Brain Research 108: 33–44

Bodnar RJ 1991 Effects of opioid peptides on peripheral stimulation and 'stress'-induced analgesia in animals. Critical Reviews in Neurobiology 6: 39–49

Bodnar RJ, Mann PE, Stone EA 1985 Potentiation of cold-water swim analgesia by acute, but not chronic desipramine administration. Pharmacology, Biochemistry and Behavior 23: 749–752

Bodnar RJ, Williams CL, Lee SJ, Pasternak GW 1988 Role of mu 1-opiate receptors in supraspinal opiate analgesia: a microinjection study. Brain Research 447: 25–34

Bodnar R, Paul D, Pasternak GW 1991 Synergistic analgesic interactions between the periaqueductal gray and the locus coeruleus. Brain Research 558: 224–230

Boive J 1971 The termination of the spinothalamic tract in the cat. An experimental study with silver impregnation methods. Experimental Brain Research 12: 331–353

Bonica JJ, Ventafridda V, Twycross RG 1990 Cancer pain. In: Bonica JJ (ed) The management of pain. Lea and Febiger, Philadelphia, pp 400–460

Bowsher D 1976 Role of the reticular formation in response to noxious stimuli. Pain 2: 361–378

Braas KM, Newby AC, Wilson VS, Snyder SH 1986 Adenosine-containing neurons in the brain localized by immunocytochemistry. Journal of Neuroscience 6: 1952–1961

Broman J 1994 Neurotransmitters in subcortical somatosensory pathways. Anatomy and Embryology 189: 181–214

Brose WG, Gutlove DP, Luther RR, Bowersox SS, McGuire D 1997 Use of intrathecal SNX-111, a novel, N-type, voltage-sensitive, calcium channel blocker, in the management of intractable brachial plexus avulsion pain. Clinical Journal of Pain 13: 256–259

Brune K, Yaksh TL 1997 Antipyretic-analgesic drugs. In: Yaksh TL, Lynch III C, Zapol WM, Maze M, Biebuyck JF, Saidman LJ (eds) Anesthesia: biologic foundations. Lippincott–Raven, Philadelphia, pp 953–968

Bryson HM, Wilde MI 1996 Amitriptyline. A review of its pharmacological properties and therapeutic use in chronic pain states. Drugs and Aging 8: 459–476

Budai D, Larson AA 1996 Role of substance P in the modulation of C-fiber-evoked responses of spinal dorsal horn neurons. Brain Research 710: 197–203

Budai D, Wilcox GL, Larson AA 1995 Effects of nitric oxide availability on responses of spinal wide dynamic range neurons to excitatory amino acids. European Journal of Pharmacology 278: 39–47

Calza L, Pozza M, Zanni M, Manzini CU, Manzini E, Hokfelt T 1998 Peptide plasticity in primary sensory neurons and spinal cord during adjuvant-induced arthritis in the rat: an immunocytochemical and in situ hybridization study. Neuroscience 82: 575–589

Camarata PJ, Yaksh TL 1985 Characterization of the spinal adrenergic receptors mediating the spinal effects produced by the microinjection of morphine into the periaqueductal gray. Brain Research 336: 133–142

Campbell V, Berrow N, Dolphin AC 1993 $GABA_B$ receptor modulation of Ca^{2+} currents in rat sensory neurones by the G protein G(0): antisense oligonucleotide studies. Journal of Physiology 470: 1–11

Carlton SM, Hayes ES 1990 Light microscopic and ultrastructural analysis of GABA immunoreactive profiles in the monkey spinal cord. Journal of Comparative Neurology 300: 162–182

Carlton SM, Honda CN, Willcockson WS et al 1991 Descending adrenergic input to the primate spinal cord and its possible role in modulation of spinothalamic cells. Brain Research 543: 77–90

Carlton SM, Westlund KN, Zhang D, Willis WD 1992 GABA-immunoreactive terminals synapse on primate spinothalamic tract cells. Journal of Comparative Neurology 322: 528–537

Casey KL 1971 Escape elicited by bulbospinal stimulation in the cat. International Journal of Neuroscience 2: 29–34

Cerne R, Rusin KI, Randic M 1993 Enhancement of the *N*-methyl-D-aspartate response in spinal dorsal horn neurons by cAMP-dependent protein kinase. Neuroscience Letters 161: 124–128

Cesselin F, Oliveras JL, Bourgoin S et al 1982 Increased levels of met-enkephalin-like material in the CSF of anaesthetized cats after tooth pulp stimulation. Brain Research 237: 325

Cesselin F, Bourgoin S, Artaud F, Hamon M 1984 Basic and regulatory mechanisms of in vitro release of met-enkephalin from the dorsal zone of the rat spinal cord. Journal of Neurochemistry 43: 763

Chait LD, Johanson CE 1988 Discriminative stimulus effects of caffeine and benzphetamine in amphetamine-trained volunteers. Psychopharmacology 96: 302–308

Chait LD, Uhlenhuth EH, Johanson CE 1987 Reinforcing and subjective effects of several anorectics in normal human volunteers. Journal of Pharmacology and Experimental Therapeutics 242: 777–783

Chaplan SR, Malmberg AB, Yaksh TL 1997 Efficacy of spinal NMDA receptor antagonism in formalin hyperalgesia and nerve injury evoked allodynia in the rat. Journal of Pharmacology and Experimental Therapeutics 280: 829–838

Chapman CR 1985 Psychological factors in postoperative pain and their treatment. In: Smith G, Covino BG (eds) Acute pain. Butterworths, London, pp 121–146

Chauvin M, Salbaing J, Perrin D, Levron JC, Viars P 1985 Clinical assessment and plasma pharmacokinetics associated with intramuscular or extradural alfentanil. British Journal of Anaesthesia 57: 886–891

Chen L, Huang LY 1992 Protein kinase C reduces Mg^{2+} block of NMDA-receptor channels as a mechanism of modulation. Nature 356: 521–523

Chung JM, Lee KH, Surmeier DJ, Sorkin LS, Kim J, Willis WD 1986 Response characteristics of neurons in the ventral posterior lateral nucleus of the monkey thalamus. Journal of Neurophysiology 56: 370–390

Clark FM, Proudfit HK 1991 Projections of neurons in the ventromedial medulla to pontine catecholamine cell groups involved in the modulation of nociception. Brain Research 540: 105–115

Clarke SL, Edeson RO, Ryall, RW 1983 The relative significance of spinal supraspinal actions in the antinociceptive effect of morphine in the dorsal horn: an evaluation of the microinjection technique. British Journal of Pharmacology 79: 807–818

Coderre TJ 1993 The role of excitatory amino acid receptors and intracellular messengers in persistent nociception after tissue injury in rats [Review]. Molecular Neurobiology 7: 229–246

Coderre TJ, Empel IV 1994 The utility of excitatory amino acid (EAA) antagonists as analgesic agents. 2. Assessment of the antinociceptive activity of combinations of competitive and non-competitive NMDA antagonists with agents acting at allosteric-glycine and polyamine receptor sites. Pain 59: 353–359

Coderre TJ, Melzack R 1991 Central neural mediators of secondary hyperalgesia following heat injury in rats: neuropeptides and excitatory amino acids. Neuroscience Letters 131: 71–74

Coderre TJ, Melzack R 1992 The contribution of excitatory amino acids to central sensitization and persistent nociception after formalin-induced tissue injury. Journal of Neuroscience 12: 3665–3670

Coderre TJ, Gonzales R, Goldyne ME, West ME, Levine JD 1990 Noxious stimulus-induced increase in spinal prostaglandin E2 is noradrenergic terminal dependent. Neuroscience Letters 115: 253–258

Connor TJ, Kelly JP, Leonard BE 1997 Forced swim test-induced neurochemical endocrine, and immune changes in the rat. Pharmacology, Biochemistry and Behavior 58:961–967

Conway CM, Marsala M, Yaksh TL 1997 In vivo NMDA-induced release of spinal adenosine and amino acids. Anesthesiology 87: A655

Coquoz D, Porchet HC, Dayer P 1991 [Central analgesic effects of antidepressant drugs with various mechanisms of action: desipramine, fluvoxamine and moclobemide.] Schweizerische Medizinische Wochenschrift. Journal Suisse de Medecine 121: 1843–1845

Corradetti R, Lo Conte G, Moroni F, Passani MB, Pepeu G 1984 Adenosine decrease aspartate and glutamate release from rat hippocampal slices. European Journal of Pharmacology 104: 19–26

Craig AD, Dostrovsky JO 1997 Processing of nociceptive information at supraspinal levels. In: Yaksh TL, Lynch III C, Zapol WM, Maze M, Biebuyck JB, Saidman LJ (eds) Anesthesia: biologic foundations. Lippincott–Raven, Philadelphia, pp 625–642

Cridland RA, Henry JL 1986 Comparison of the effects of substance P, Neurokinin A, Physalaemin and Eledoisin in facilitating a nociceptive reflex in the rat. Brain Research 381: 93–99

Criswell HD 1976 Analgesia and hyperreactivity following morphine microinjections into mouse brain. Pharmacology, Biochemistry and Behavior 4: 23–26

Danzebrink RM, Gebhart GF 1990 Antinociceptive effects of intrathecal adrenoceptor agonists in a rat model of visceral nociception. Journal of Pharmacology and Experimental Therapeutics 253: 698–705

Danzebrink RM, Gebhart GF 1991 Evidence that spinal $5\text{-}HT_1$, $5\text{-}HT_2$ and $5\text{-}HT_3$ receptor subtypes modulate responses to noxious colorectal distention in the rat. Brain Research 538: 64–75

Daval G, Verge D, Basbaum AI, Bouroin S, Hamon M 1987 Autoradiographic evidence of serotonin-1 binding sites on primary

afferent fibers in dorsal horn of the rat spinal cord. Neuroscience Letters 83: 71–81
Davies SN, Lodge D 1987 Evidence for involvement of *N*-methylaspartate receptors in 'wind-up' of class 2 neurons in the dorsal horn of the rat. Brain Research 424: 402–406
Davies J, Watkins JC 1983 Role of excitatory amino acids receptors in mono- and polysynaptic excitation in the cat spinal cord. Experimental Brain Research 49: 280–290
De Biasi S, Rustioni A 1988 Glutamate and substance P coexist in primary afferent terminals in the superficial laminae of spinal cord. Proceedings of the National Academic of Science USA 85: 7820–7824
De Biasi S, Amadeo A, Spreafico R, Rustioni A 1994 Enrichment of glutamate immunoreactivity in lemniscal terminals in the ventropostero lateral thalamic nucleus of the rat: an immunogold and WGA-HRP study. Anatomical Record 240: 131–140
De Koninck Y, Henry JL 1989 Bombesin, neuromedin B and neuromedin C selectively depress superficial dorsal horn neurones in the cat spinal cord. Brain Research 498:105–117
De Koninck Y, Henry JL 1991 Substance P-mediated slow excitatory postsynaptic potential elicited in dorsal horn neurons in vivo by noxious stimulation. Proceeding of the National Academy of Sciences USA 88: 11344–11348
De Koninck Y, Henry JL 1992 Peripheral vibration causes an adenosine-mediated postsynaptic inhibitory potential in dorsal horn neurons of the cat spinal cord. Neuroscience 50: 435–443
De Koninck Y, Henry JL 1994 Prolonged $GABA_A$-mediated inhibition following single hair afferent input to single spinal dorsal horn neurones in cats. Journal of Physiology 476: 89–100
Decker MW, Curzon P, Brioni JD 1995 Influence of separate and combined septal and amygdala lesions on memory, acoustic startle, anxiety, and locomotor activity in rats. Neurobiology of Learning and Memory 64: 156–168
Denny-Brown D, Kirk EJ, Yanagisawa N 1973 The tract of lissauer in relations to sensory transmission in the dorsal horn of spinal cord in the Macaque monkey. Journal of Comparative Neurology 151: 175–200
Derryberry D, Tucker DM 1992 Neural mechanisms of emotion. Journal of Consulting and Clinical Psychology 60: 329–338
Deschnes M, Hu B 1990 Electrophysiology and pharmacology of the corticothalamic input to lateral thalamic nuclei: an intracellular study in the cat. European Journal of Neuroscience 2: 140–152
Detke MJ, Johnson J, Lucki I 1997 Acute and chronic antidepressant drug treatment in the rat forced swimming test model of depression. Experimental and Clinical Psychopharmacology 5: 107–112
Devoghel JC 1983 Small intrathecal doses of lysine-acetylsalicylate relieve intractable pain in man. Journal of International Medical Research 11: 90–1
Dickenson AH, Le Bars D 1987 Supraspinal morphine and descending inhibitions acting on the dorsal horn of the rat. Journal of Physiology 384: 81–107
Dickenson AH, Sullivan AF 1987 Evidence for a role of the NMDA receptor in the frequency dependent potentiation of deep rat dorsal horn nociceptive neurons following C fiber stimulation. Neuropharmacology 26: 1235–1238
Dickenson AH, Sullivan AF 1990 Differential effects of excitatory amino acid antagonists on dorsal horn nociceptive neurons in the rat. Brain Research 505: 31–39
Dickenson AH, Oliveras J-L, Besson J-M 1979 Role of the nucleus raphe magnus in opiate analgesia as studied by the microinjection technique in the rat. Brain Research 170: 95–111
Dickenson AH, Brewer CM, Hayes NA 1985 Effects of topical baclofen on c fibre-evoked neuronal activity in the rat dorsal horn. Neuroscience 14: 557–562
Dickenson AH, Sullivan AF, Roques BP 1988 Evidence that endogenous enkephalins and a delta opioid receptor agonist have a common site of action in spinal antinociception. European Journal of Pharmacology 148: 437–439
Dickenson AH, Stanfa LC, Chapman V, Yaksh TL 1997 Response properties of dorsal horn neurons: pharmacology of the dorsal horn. In: Yaksh TL, Lynch III C, Zapol WM, Maze M, Biebuyck JF, Saidman LJ (eds) Anesthesia: biologic foundations. Lippincott–Raven, Philadelphia, pp 611–624
Diez Guerra FJ, Zaidi M, Bevis P, MacIntyre I, Emson PC 1988 Evidence for release of calcitonin gene-related peptide and neurokinin A from sensory nerve endings in vivo. Neuroscience 25: 839–846
Donnerer J, Schuligoi R, Stein C 1992 Increased content and transport of substance P and calcitonin gene-related peptide in sensory nerves innervating inflamed tissue: evidence for a regulatory function of nerve growth factor in vivo. Neuroscience 49: 693–698
Dottrens M, Rifat K, Morel DR 1992 Comparison of extradural administration of sufentanil, morphine and sufentanil–morphine combination after caesarean section. British Journal of Anaesthesia 69: 9–12
Dougherty PM, Willis WD 1991a Enhancement of spinothalamic neuron responses to chemical and mechanical stimuli following combined micro-iontophoretic application of *N*-methyl-D-aspartic acid and substance P. Pain 47: 85–93
Dougherty PM, Willis WD 1991b Modification of the responses of primate spinothalamic neurons to mechanical stimulation by excitatory amino acids and an *N*-methyl-D-aspartate antagonist. Brain Research 542: 15–22
Dougherty PM, Willis WD 1992 Enhanced responses of spinothalamic tract neurons to excitatory amino acids accompany capsaicin-induced sensitization in the monkey. Journal of Neuroscience 12: 883–894
Dougherty PM, Palecek J, Paleckova V, Sorkin LS, Willis WD 1992 The role of NMDA and non-NMDA excitatory amino acid receptors in the excitation of primate spinothalamic tract neurons by mechanical, chemical, thermal, and electrical stimuli. Journal of Neuroscience 12: 3025–3041
Drower EJ, Hammond DL 1988 GABAergic modulation of nociceptive threshold: effects of THIP and bicuculline microinjected in the ventral medulla of the rat. Brain Research 450: 316–324
Drower EJ, Stapelfeld A, Rafferty MF, de Costa BR, Rice KC, Hammond DL 1991 Selective antagonism by naltrindole of the antinociceptive effects of the delta opioid agonist cyclic [D-penicillamine2-D-penicillamine5] enkephalin in the rat. Journal of Pharmacology and Experimental Therapeutics 259: 725–731
Dubuisson D, Dennis SG 1977 The formalin test: a quantitative study of the analgesic effects of morphine, meperidin, and brain stem stimulation in rats and cat. Pain 4: 161–174
Duggan AW, Hendry IA, Morton CR, Hutchison WD, Zhao ZQ 1988 Cutaneous stimuli releasing immunoreactive substance P in the dorsal horn of the cat. Brain Research 451: 261–273
Duggan AW, Hope PJ, Jarrott B, Schaible H-G, Fleetwood-Walker SM 1990 Release, spread and persistence of immunoreactive neurokinin A in the dorsal horn of the cat following noxious cutaneous stimulation. Studies with antibody microprobes. Neuroscience 35: 195–202
Duggan AW, Hope PJ, Lang CW 1991 Microinjection of neuropeptide Y into the superficial dorsal horn reduces stimulus-evoked release of immunoreactive substance P in the anaesthetized car. Neuroscience 44: 733–740
Duggan AW, Riley RC, Mark MA, MacMillan SJ, Schaible HG 1995 Afferent volley patterns and the spinal release of immunoreactive substance P in the dorsal horn of the anaesthetized spinal cat. Neuroscience 65: 849–858
Eaton SA, Salt TE 1990 Thalamic NMDA receptors and nociceptive sensory synaptic transmission. Neuroscience Letters 110: 297–302

Eaton SA, Salt TE 1996 The role of excitatory amino acid receptors in thalamic nociception. In: Besson JM (ed) Pain in forebrain areas. John Libbey Eurotext, Paris pp 286–302

Edwards M, Serrano JM, Gent JP, Goodchild CS 1990 On the mechanism by which midazolam causes spinally mediated analgesia. Anesthesiology 73: 273–277

Eide PK, Hole K 1991 Different role of 5-HT_{1A} and 5-H_{T2} receptors in spinal cord in the control of nociceptive responsiveness. Neuropharmacology 30: 727–731

Eide PK, Joly NM, Hole K 1990 The role of spinal cord 5-$HT_{1A}$and 5-HT_{1B} receptors in the modulation of a spinal nociceptive reflex. Brain Research 536: 195–200

Eisenach JC, Lysak SZ, Viscomi CM 1989a Epidural clonidine analgesia following surgery: phase I. Anesthesiology 71: 640–646

Eisenach JC, Rauck RL, Buzzanell C, Lysak SZ 1989b Epidural clonidine analgesia for intractable cancer pain: phase I. Anesthesiology 71: 647–652

Eisenach JC, De Kock M, Klimscha W 1996 Alpha (2)-adrenergic agonists for regional anesthesia. A clinical review of clonidine (1984–1995). Anesthesiology 8: 655–674

Eison MS 1984 Use of animal models: toward anxioselective drugs. Psychopathology 17 (suppl 1): 37–44

El-Yassir N, Fleetwood-Walker SM, Mitchell R 1988 Heterogeneous effects of serotonin in the dorsal horn of the rat: the involvement of 5-HT1 receptors subtypes. Brain Research 456: 147–158

Ericson AC, Blomqvist A, Craig AD, Ottersen OP Broman J 1995 Evidence for glutamate as neurotransmitter in trigemino- and spinothalamic tract terminals in the nucleus submedius of cats. European Journal of Neuroscience 7: 305–317

Fang FG, Moreau JL, Fields HL 1987 Dose dependent antinociceptive action of neurotensin microinjected into the rostroventral medulla of the rat. Brain Research 420: 171–174

Fardin V, Oliveras JL, Besson JM 1984 A re-investigation of the analgesic effects induced by stimulation of the periaqueductal gray matter in the rat. II. Differential characteristics of the analgesia induced by ventral and dorsal PAG stimulation. Brain Research 306: 125–139

Faris PL, Komisaruk B, Watkins LR, Mayer DL 1983 Evidence for the neuropeptide cholecstokinin as an antagonists of opiate analgesia. Science 219: 310–312

Farnebo S, Hermanson O, Blomqvist A 1997 Thalamic-projecting preprocholecystokinin messenger RNA-expressing neurons in the dorsal column nuclei of the rat. Neuroscience 78: 1051–1057

Fastbom J, Fredholm BB 1990 Antinociceptive effects and spinal distribution of two adenosine receptor agonists after intrathecal administration. Pharmacology and Toxicology 66: 69–72

Faull RL, Villiger JW, Dragunow M 1989 Neurotensin receptors in the human spinal cord: a quantitative autoradiographic study. Neuroscience 29: 603–613

Fedynyshyn JP, Lee NM 1989 Mu type opioid receptors in rat periaqueductal gray-enriched P2 membrane are coupled to G-protein-mediated inhibition of adenylyl cyclase. FEBS Letters 253: 23–27

Fedynyshyn JP, Kwiat G, Lee N 1989 Characterization of high affinity opioid binding sites in rat periaqueductal gray P2 membrane. European Journal of Pharmacology 159: 83–88

Feng J, Kendig JJ 1996 Synergistic interactions between midazolam and alfentanil in isolated neonatal rat spinal cord. British Journal of Anaesthesia 77: 375–380

Fernandez-Lopez A, Chinchetru MA, Calvo Fernandez P 1997 The autoradiographic perspective of central benzodiazepine receptors; a short review. General Pharmacology 29: 173–180

Field MJ, Oles RJ, Lewis AS, McCleary S, Hughes J, Singh L 1997 Gabapentin (neurontin) and *S*-(+)-3-isobutylgaba represent a novel class of selective antihyperalgesic agents. British Journal of Pharmacology 121: 1513–1522

Fields HL, Heinricher MM, Mason P 1991 Neurotransmitters in nociceptive modulatory circuits. Annual Review of Neuroscience 14: 219–245

Finlay JM, Zigmond MJ, Abercrombie ED 1995 Increased dopamine and norepinephrine release in medial prefrontal cortex induced by acute and chronic stress: effects of diazepam. Neuroscience 64: 619–628

Finn IB, Iuvone PM, Holtzman SG 1990 Depletion of catecholamines in the brain of rats differentially affects stimulation of locomotor activity by caffeine, D-amphetamine, and methylphenidate. Neuropharmacology 29: 625–631

Fleetwood-Walker SM, Mitchell R, Hope PJ, Molony V, Iggo A 1985 An $alpha_2$ receptor mediates the selective inhibition by noradrenaline of nociceptive responses of identified dorsal horn neurones. Brain Research 334: 243–254

Fleetwood-Walker SM, Hope PJ, Mitchell R, El-Yassir N, Molony V 1988a The influence of opioid receptor subtypes on the processing of nociceptive inputs in the spinal dorsal horn of the cat. Brain Research 451: 213–226

Fleetwood-Walker SM, Hope PJ, Mitchell R 1988b Antinociceptive actions of descending dopaminergic tracts on cat and rat dorsal horn somatosensory neurones. Journal of Physiology 399: 335–348

Fleetwood-Walker SM, Mitchell R, Hope PJ, El-Yassir N, Molony V, Bladon CM 1990 The involvement of neurokinin receptor subtypes in somatosensory processing in the superficial dorsal horn of the cat. Brain Research 519: 169–182

Forrest WH, Byron BW, Brown CR et al 1977 Dextroamphetamine with morphine for the treatment of postoperative pain. New England Journal of Medicine 296: 712–715

Frank RG, Kashani JH, Parker JC, Beck NC, Brownlee-Duffeck M, Elliot TR, Haut AE, Atwood C, Smith E, Kay DR 1988 Antidepressant analgesia in rheumatoid arthritis. Journal of Rheumatology 15:1632–1638

Franklin KBJ 1989 Analgesia and the neural substrate of reward. Neuroscience and Biobehavioral Reviews 13: 149–154

Fraser HM, Chapman V, Dickenson AH 1992 Spinal local anaesthetic actions on afferent evoked responses and wind-up of nociceptive neurones in the rat spina cord: combination with morphine produces marked potentiation of antinociception. Pain: 33–41

Freeman W, Watts JW 1942 Psychosurgery, intelligence, emotion and social behavior following prefrontal lobotomy for mental disorders. Charles C. Thomas, Springfield

Freeman W, Watts JW 1946 Pain of organic disease relieved by prefrontal lobotomy. Proceedings of the Royal Academy of Medicine 39: 44–447

Frysztak RJ, Neafsey EJ 1991 The effect of medial frontal cortex lesions on respiration, 'freezing', and ultrasonic vocalizations during conditioned emotional responses in rats. Cerebral Cortex 1: 418–425

Frysztak RJ, Neafsey EJ 1994 The effect of medial frontal cortex lesions on cardiovascular conditioned emotional responses in the rat. Brain Research 643: 181–193

Fujimoto JM, Arts KS, Rady JJ, Tseng LF 1990 Spinal dynorphin A (1–17): possible mediator of antianalgesic action. Neuropharmacology 29: 609–617

Fundytus ME, Fisher K, Dray A, Henry JL, Coderre TJ 1998 In vivo antinociceptive activity of anti-rat mGluR1 and mGluR5 antibodies in rats. Neuroreport 9(4): 731–735

Gamse R, Holzer P, Lembeck F 1979 Indirect evidence for presynaptic location of opiate receptors in chemosensitive primary sensory neurones. Neaunyn-Schmiedberg's Archives of Pharmacology 308: 281–285

Garry MG, Hargreaves KM 1992 Enhanced release of immunoreactive CGRP and substance P from spinal dorsal horn slices occurs during carrageenan inflammation. Brain Research 582: 139–142

Garthwaite J, Charles SL, Chess-Williams R 1988 Endothelium-derived relaxing factor release on activation of NMDA receptors suggests role as intracellular messengers in the brain. Nature 336: 385–388

Gaumann DM, Yaksh TL, Post C, Wilcox GL, Rodriguez M 1989 Intrathecal somatostatin in cat and mouse – studies on pain, motor behavior, and histopathology. Anesthesia and Analgesia 68: 623–632
Gear RW, Miaskowski C, Heller PH, Paul SM, Gordon NC, Levine JD 1997 Benzodiazepine mediated antagonism of opioid analgesia. Pain 71: 25–29
Gebhart GF 1982 Opiate and opioid peptide effects on brain stem neurons: relevance to nociception and antinociceptive mechanisms. Pain 12: 93–140
Gebhart GF, Jones SL 1988 Effects of morphine given in the brainstem on the activity of dorsal horn nociceptive neurons. Progress in Brain Research 77: 229–243
Gebhart GF, Sandkuhler J, Thalhammer JG, Zimmermann M 1983 Quantitative comparison of inhibition in spinal cord of nociceptive information by stimulation in periaqueductal gray or nucleus raphe magnus of the cat. Journal of Neurophysiology 50: 1433–1444
Gebhart GF, Sandkuhler J, Thalhammer J, Zimmerman M 1984 Inhibition in spinal cord of nociceptive information by electrical stimulation and morphine microinjections at identical sites in midbrain of the cat. Journal of Neurophysiology 51: 75–89
Geiger JD, Labella FS, Nagy JI 1984 Characterization and localization of adenosine receptors in rat spinal cord. Journal of Neuroscience 4: 2303–2310
Gerber G, Randic M 1989a Excitatory amino acid-mediated components of synaptically evoked input from dorsal roots to deep dorsal horn neurons in the rat spinal cord slice. Neuroscience Letters 106: 211–219
Gerber G, Randic M 1989b Participation of excitatory amino acid receptors in the slow excitatory synaptic transmission in the rat spinal dorsal horn in vitro. Neuroscience Letters 106: 220–228
Gibson SJ, Polak JM, Anand P et al 1984 The distribution and origin of VIP in the spinal cord of six mammalian species. Peptides 5: 201–207
Gil Z, Amitai Y 1996 Adult thalamocortical transmission involves both NMDA and non-NMDA receptors. Journal of Neurophysiology 76: 2547–2554
Gillberg P-G, Wiksten B 1986 Effects of spinal cord lesions and rhizotomies or cholinergic and opiate receptor binding sites in rat spinal cord. Acta Physiologica Scandinavica 126: 575–582
Gillberg P-G, d'Argy R, Aquilonius SM 1988 Autoradiographic distribution of 3H-acetylcholine binding sites in the cervical spinal cord of man and some other species. Neuroscience Letters 90: 197–202
Gillberg P-G, Gordh T Jr, Hartvig P, Jansson I, Pettersson J, Post C 1989 Characterization of the antinociception induced by intrathecally administered carbachol. Pharmacology and Toxicology 64: 340–343
Glaum SR, Proudfit HK, Anderson EG 1990 5-HT3 receptors modulate spinal nociceptive reflexes. Brain Research 510: 12–16
Go VLW, Yaksh TL 1987 Release of substance P from the cat spinal cord. Journal of Physiology 391: 141–167
Gogas KR, Hough LB, Eberle NB et al 1989 A role for histamine and H_2-receptors in opioid antinociception. Journal of Pharmacology and Experimental Therapeutics 250: 476–484
Goldstein LE, Rasmusson AM, Bunney BS, Roth RH 1994 The NMDA glycine site antagonist (+)-HA-966 selectively regulates conditioned stress-induced metabolic activation of the mesoprefrontal cortical dopamine but not serotonin systems: a behavioral, neuroendocrine, and neurochemical study in the rat. Journal of Neuroscience 14: 4937–4950
Golembiowska K, White TD, Sawynok J 1996 Adenosine kinase inhibitors augment release of adenosine from spinal cord slices. European Journal of Pharmacology 307: 157–162
Good AJ, Westbrook RF 1995 Effects of a microinjection of morphine into the amygdala on the acquisition and expression of conditioned fear and hypoalgesia in rats. Behavioral Neuroscience 109: 631–641
Gordh T, Jansson I, Hartvig P, Gillberg PG, Post C 1989 Interactions between noradrenergic and cholinergic mechanisms involved in spinal nociceptive processing. Acta Anesthesiologica Scandinavica 33: 39–47
Graeff FG, Viana MB, Mora PO 1997 Dual role of 5-HT in defense and anxiety. Neuroscience and Biobehavioral Reviews 21: 791–799
Graf G, Sinatra R, Chung J, Frasca A, Silverman DG 1991 Epidural sufentanil for postoperative analgesia: dose-response in patients recovering from major gynecologic surgery. Anesthesia and Analgesia 73: 405–409
Griffiths RR, Woodson PP 1988a Reinforcing effects of caffeine in humans. Journal of Pharmacology and Experimental Therapeutics 246: 21–29
Griffiths RR, Woodson PP 1988b Reinforcing properties of caffeine: studies in humans and laboratory animals. Pharmacology, Biochemistry and Behavior 29: 419–427
Griffiths RR, Woodson PP 1988c Caffeine physical dependence: a review of human and laboratory animal studies. Psychopharmacology 94: 437–451
Grundt TJ, Williams JT 1994 mu-Opioid agonists inhibit spinal trigeminal substantia gelatinosa neurons in guinea pig and rat. Journal of Neuroscience 14 (3 pt 2): 1646–1654
Gundlach AL, Dodd PR, Grabara Watson WEJ et al 1988 Deficits of spinal cord glycine/strychnine receptors in inherited myoclonius of poll Hereford calves. Science 241: 1807–1810
Haigler HJ, Spring DD 1978 A comparison of the analgesic and behavioral effects of [D-Ala2] met-enkephalinamide and morphine in the mesencephalic reticular formation of rats. Life Sciences 23: 1229–1240
Haley JE, Sullivan AF, Dickenson AH 1990 Evidence for spinal *N*-methyl-D-aspartate receptor involvement in prolonged chemical nociception in the rat. Brain Research 518: 218–226
Haley JE, Dickenson AH, Schachter M 1992 Electrophysiological evidence for a role of nitric oxide in prolonged chemical nociception in the rat. Neuropharmacology 31: 251–258
Hamann SR, Martin WR 1992 Opioid and nicotinic analgesic and hyperalgesic loci in the rat brain stem. Journal of Pharmacology and Experimental Therapeutics 261: 707–715
Hamlin L, Mackerlova L, Blomqvist A, Ericson AC 1996 AMPA-selective glutamate receptor subunits and their relation to glutamate- and GABA-like immunoreactive terminals in the nucleus submedius of the rat. Neuroscience Letters 217: 149–152
Hammond DL, Drower EJ 1984 Effects of intrathecally administered THIP, Baclofen and Muscimol on nociceptive threshold. European Journal of Pharmacology 103: 121–125
Hammond DL, Yaksh TL 1984 Antagonism of stimulation-produced antinociceptior by intrathecal administration of methysergide or phentolamine. Brain Research 298: 329–337
Hammond DL, Levy RA, Proudfit HK 1980 Hypoalgesia following microinjection of noradrenergic antagonists in the nucleus raphe magnus. Pain 9: 85–101
Hammond DL, Tyce GM, Yaksh TL 1985 Efflux of 5-hydroxytryptamine and noradrenaline into spinal cord superfusates during stimulation of the rat medulla. Journal of Physiology 359: 151–162
Hamon M, Gallissot MC, Menard F, Gozlan H, Bourgoin S, Verge D 1989 5-HT_3 receptor binding sites are on capsaicin-sensitive fibres in the rat spinal cord. European Journal of Pharmacology 164: 315–322
Hanesch U, Blecher F, Stiller RU, Emson PC, Schaible HG, Heppelmann B 1995 The effect of a unilateral inflammation at the rat's ankle joint on the expression of preprotachykinin-A mRNA and preprosomatostatin mRNA in dorsal root ganglion cells – a study using non-radioactive in situ hybridization. Brain Research 700: 279–284
Hansen HH, Sanchez C, Meier E 1997 Neonatal administration of the

selective serotonin reuptake inhibitor Lu 10-134-C increases forced swimming-induced immobility in adult rats: putative animal model of depression? Journal of Pharmacology and Experimental Therapeutics 283: 1333–1341
Hao JX, Xu XJ, Aldskogius H, Seiger A, Wiesenfeld-Hallin Z 1991 Allodynia-like effects in rat after ischaemic spinal cord injury photochemically induced by laser irradiation. Pain 45: 175–185
Hao JX, Xu XJ, Yu YX, Seiger A, Wiesenfeld-Hallin Z 1992a Transient spinal cord ischemia induces temporary hypersensitivity of dorsal horn wide dynamic range neurons to myelinated, but not unmyelinated, fiber input. Journal of Neurophysiology 68: 384–391
Hao JX, Xu XJ, Yu YX, Seiger A, Wiesenfeld-Hallin 1992b Baclofen reverses the hypersensitivity of dorsal horn wide dynamic range neurons to mechanical stimulation after transient spinal cord ischemia, implications for a tonic GABAergic inhibitory control of myelinated fiber input. Journal of Neurophysiology 68: 392–396
Harris JA, Westbrook RF 1995a Effects of benzodiazepine microinjection into the amygdala or periaqueductal gray on the expression of conditioned fear and hypoalgesia in rats. Behavioral Neuroscience 109: 295–304
Harris JA, Westbrook RF, Duffield TQ, Bentivoglio M 1995b Fos expression in the spinal cord is suppressed in rats displaying conditioned hypoalgesia. Behavioral Neuroscience 109: 320–328
Haws CM, Heinricher MM, Fields HL 1990 Alpha-adrenergic receptor agonists, but not antagonists, alter the tail-flick latency when microinjected into the rostral ventromedial medulla of the lightly anesthetized rat. Brain Research 533: 192–195
Headley PM, Parson CG, West DC 1987 The role of *N*-methylaspartate receptors in mediating responses of rats and cat neurones to defined sensory stimuli. Journal of Physiology 385: 169–188
Heapy CG, Jamieson A, Russell NJW 1987 Afferent C-fiber and A-delta activity in models of inflammation. British Journal of Pharmacology 90: 164P
Heinreicher M 1997 Organizational characteristics of supraspinally mediated responses to nociceptive input. In: Yaksh TL, Lynch III C, Zapol WM, Maze M, Biebuyck JF, Saidman LJ (eds) Anesthesia: biologic foundations. Lippincott–Raven, Philadelphia, pp 643–662
Heinricher MM, Kaplan HJ 1991 GABA-mediated inhibition in rostral ventromedial medulla: role in nociceptive modulation in the lightly anesthetized rat. Pain 47: 105–113
Helke CJ, Krause JE, Mantyh PW, Couture R, Bannon MJ 1990 Diversity in mammalian tachykinin peptidergic neurons: multiple peptides, receptors, and regulatory mechanisms. FASEB Journal 4: 1606–1615
Helmstetter FJ, Bellgowan PS, Poore LH 1995 Microinfusion of mu but not delta or kappa opioid agonists into the basolateral amygdala results in inhibition of the tail flick reflex in pentobarbital-anesthetized rats. Journal of Pharmacology and Experimental Therapeutics 275: 381–388
Helmstetter FJ, Tershner SA, Poore LH, Bellgowan PS 1998 Antinociception following opiod stimulation of the basolateral amygdala is expressed through the periaqueductal gray and rostral ventromedial medulla. Brain Research 779: 104–118
Herz A, Teschemacher H 1971 Activities and sites of adrinociceptive action of morphine-like analgesics and kinetics of distribution following intravenous, intracerebral and intraventricular application. Advances in Drug Research 6: 79–119
Hoehn K, WhiteTD 1990 N-methyl-D-aspartate, kainate and quisqualate release endogenous adenosine from rat cortical slices. Neuroscience 39:441–450
Hoheisel U, Mense S, Scherotzke R 1994 Calcitonin gene-related peptide-immunoreactivity in functionally identified primary afferent neurons in the rat. Anatomy and Embryology 189: 41–49
Høkfelt T 1991 Neuropeptides in perspective. Neuron 7: 867–879
Hollman M, Heinemann S 1994 Cloned glutamate receptors. Annual Review of Neuroscience 17: 31–108
Holz GG, Kream RM, Spiegel A, Dunlap K 1989 G proteins couple alpha-adrenergic and GABA-B receptors to inhibition of peptide secretion from peripheral sensory neurons. Journal of Neuroscience 9: 657–666
Hongo T, Jankowska E, Lundberg A 1968 Post synaptic excitation and inhibition from primary afferents in neurones of the spinocervical tract. Journal of Physiology (London) 199: 569–592
Hood DD, Eisenach JC, Tuttle R 1995 Phase I safety assessment of intrathecal neostigmine methylsulfate in humans. Anesthesiology 82: 331–343
Hope PJ, Fleetwood-Walker SM, Mitchell R 1990 Distinct antinociceptive actions mediated by different opioid receptors in the region of lamina I and laminae III–V of the dorsal horn of the rat. British Journal of Pharmacology 101: 477–483
Hough LB 1988 Cellular localization and possible functions for brain histamine: recent progress. Progress in Neurobiology 30: 469–505
Hough LB, Nalwalk JW 1992 Modulation of morphine antinociception by antagonism of H_2 receptors in the periaqueductal gray. Brain Research 588: 58–66
Houston JP, Nef B, Papadoupolous G, Welzl H 1980 Activation and lateralization of sensorimotor field and perioral biting reflex by intranigral GABA agonist and by systemic apomorphine in the rat. Brain Research Bulletin 5: 745–749
Howe JR, Yaksh TL, Go VLW 1987 The effect of unilateral dorsal root ganglionectomies or ventral rhizotomies on alpha$_2$-adrenoceptor binding to, and the substance P, enkephalin, and neurotensin content of, the cat lumbar spinal cord. Neuroscience 21: 385–394
Hua X-Y, Boublik JH, Spicer MA, Rivier JE, Brown MR, Yaksh TL 1991 The antinociceptive effects of spinally administered neuropeptide Y in the rat: systematic studies on structure-activity relationship. Journal of Pharmacology and Experimental Therapeutics 258: 243–248
Huang L-YM 1992 The excitatory effects of opioids. Neurochemistry International 20: 463–468
Hylden JLK, Wilcox GL 1981 Intrathecal substance P elicits a caudally-directed biting and scratching behavior in mice. Brain Research 217: 212–215
Iacono RP, Linford J, Sandyk R, Consroe P, Ryan MR, Bamford CR 1988 Intraspinal opiates for treatment of intractable pain in the terminally ill cancer patient. International Journal of Neuroscience 38: 111–119
Iadarola MJ, Brady LS, Draisci G, Dubner R 1988 Enhancement of dynorphin gene expression in spinal cord following experimental inflammation: stimulus specificity, behavioral parameters and opioid receptor binding. Pain 35: 313–326
Iadarola MJ, Berman KF, Zeffiro TA et al 1998 Neural activation during acute capsaicin-evoked pain and allodynia assessed with PET. Brain 121(pt 5): 931–947
Ibuki T, Hama AT, Wang XT, Pappas GD, Sagen J 1997 Loss of GABA-immunoreactivity in the spinal dorsal horn of rats with peripheral nerve injury and promotion of recovery by adrenal medullary grafts. Neuroscience 76:845–858
Jacquet YF, Lajtha A 1976 The periaqueductal gray site of morphine analgesia and tolerance as shown by 2-way cross-tolerance between systemic and intracerebral injections. Brain Research 103: 501–513
Jane DE, Jones PL, Pook PC, Tse HW, Watkins JC 1994 Actions of two new antagonists showing selectivity for different sub-types of metabotropic glutamate receptor in the neonatal rat spinal cord. British Journal of Pharmacology 112: 809–816
Jansen KLR, Faull RLM, Dragunow M, Waldvogel H 1990 Autoradiographic localization of NMDA, quisqualate and kainic acid receptors in human spinal cord. Neuroscience Letters 108: 53–57
Jarvis B, Coukell AJ 1998 Mexiletine A review of its therapeutic use in painful diabetic neuropathy. Drugs 56:691–707

Jayaram A, Singh P, Carp HM 1995 An enkephalinase inhibitor, SCH 32615, augments analgesia induced by surgery in mice. Anesthesiology 82:1283–1287

Jeftinija S, Murase K, Nedeljkov V, Randic M 1982 Vasoactive intestinal polypeptide excites mammalian dorsal horn neurons both in vivo and in vitro. Brain Research 243: 158–164

Jeftinija S, Jeftinija K, Liu F, Skilling SR, Smullin DH, Larson AA 1991 Excitatory amino acids are released from rat primary afferent neurons in vitro. Neuroscience Letters 125: 191–194

Jensen TS, Yaksh TL 1984a Spinal monoamine and opiate system pathways mediate the antinociceptive effects produced by glutamate at brainstem sites. Brain Research 321: 287–297

Jensen TS, Yaksh TL 1984b Effects of an intrathecal dopamine agonist, apomorphine, on thermal and chemical evoked noxious responses in rats. Brain Research 296: 285–293

Jensen TS, Yaksh TL 1986a I. Comparison of antinociceptive action of morphine in the periaqueductal gray, medial and paramedial medulla in rat. Brain Research 363: 99–113

Jensen TS, Yaksh TL 1986b II. Examination of spinal monoamine receptors through which brain stem opiate-sensitive systems act in the rat. Brain Research 363: 114–127

Jensen TS, Yaksh TL 1986c III. Comparison of the antinociceptive action of mu and delta opioid receptor ligands in the periaqueductal gray matter, medial and paramedial ventral medulla in the rat as studied by the microinjection technique. Brain Research 372: 301–312

Jensen TS, Yaksh TL 1992 Brainstem excitatory amino acid receptors in nociception: microinjection mapping and pharmacological characterization of glutamate-sensitive sites in the brainstem associated with algogenic behavior. Neuroscience 46: 535–547

Jesberger JA, Richardson JS 1985 Animal models of depression: parallels and correlates to severe depression in humans. Biological Psychiatry 20: 764–784

Jessell TM, Yoshioka K, Jahr CE 1986 Amino acids receptor mediated transmission at primary afferent synapses in rat spinal cord. Journal of Experimental Biology 124: 239–258

Jhamandas K, Yaksh TL, Harty G, Szolcsanyi J, Go VLW 1984 Action of intrathecal capsaicin and its structural analogues on the content and release of spinal substance P: Selectivity of action and relationship to analgesia. Brain Research 306: 215–225

Jones EG 1987 Immunocytochemical studies on thalamic afferent transmitters. In: Besson JM, Guilbaud G, Peschanski M (eds) Thalamus and pain. Amsterdam:Excerpta Medica, Amsterdam, pp 83–109

Joyce EM, Koob GF 1981 Amphetamine-, scopolamine- and caffeine-induced locomotor activity following 6-hydroxydopamine lesions in the mesolimbic dopamine system. Psychopharmacology 73: 311–313

Ju G, Høkfelt T, Brodin E, Fahrenkrug J et al 1987 Primary sensory neurons of the rat showing calcitonin gene-related peptide immunoreactivity and their relation to substance P-, somatostatin-, galanin-, vasoactive intestinal polypeptide- and cholecystokinin-immunoreactive ganglion cells. Cell and Tissue Research 247: 417–431

Jun JH, Yaksh TL 1998 The effect of intrathecal gabapentin and 3-isobutyl γ-aminobutyric acid on the hyperalgesia observed after thermal injury in the rat. Anesthesia and Analgesia 86: 348–354

Kaiko RF, Wallenstein SL, Rogers AG, Grabinski PY, Houde RW 1981 Analgesic and mood effects of heroin and morphine in cancer patients with postoperative pain. New England Journal of Medicine 304: 1501–1505

Kaiko RF, Kanner R, Foley KM et al 1987 Cocaine and morphine interaction in acute and chronic cancer pain. Pain 31: 35–45

Kapadia SE, LaMotte CC 1987 Deafferentation-induced alterations in rat dorsal horn: I Comparison of peripheral nerve injury vs rhizotomy effects on presynaptic, post-synaptic and glial processes. Journal of Comparative Neurology 266: 183–197

Kar S, Quirion R 1995 Neuropeptide receptors in developing and adult rat spinal cord: an in vitro quantitative autoradiography study of calcitonin gene-related peptide, neurokinins, mu-opioid, galanin, somatostatin, neurotensin and vasoactive intestinal polypeptide receptors. Journal of Comparative Neurology 354: 253–281

Kar S, Quirion R 1992 Quantitative autoradiographic localization of [^{125}I] neuropeptide Y receptor binding sites in rat spinal cord and the effects of neonatal capsaicin, dorsal rhizotomy and peripheral axotomy. Brain Research 574: 333–337

Karlsten R, Gordh T Jr 1995 An A1-selective adenosine agonist abolishes allodynia elicited by vibration and touch after intrathecal injection. Anesthesia and Analgesia 80: 844–847

Kasman GS, Rosenfeld JP 1986 Opiate microinjections into midbrain do not affect the aversiveness of caudal trigeminal stimulation but produce somatotopically organized peripheral hypoalgesia. Brain Research 383: 271–278

Katon W 1984 Panic disorder and somatization. Review of 55 cases. American Journal of Medicine 77: 101–106

Kawatani M, Nagel J, DeGroat WC 1986 Identification of neuropeptides in pelvic viscera and pudendal nerve afferent pathways to the sacral spinal cord of the cat. Journal of Comparative Neurology 249: 117–132

Keil II GJ, DeLander GE 1992 Spinally-mediated antinociception is induced in mice by an adenosine kinase-, but not by an adenosine deaminase-, inhibitor. Life Science 51: 171–176

Kellstein DE, Price DD, Mayer DJ 1991 Cholecystokinin and its antagonist lorglumide respectively attenuate and facilitate morphine-induced inhibition of C-fiber evoked discharges of dorsal horn nociceptive neurons. Brain Research 540: 302–306

Kelly JP, Wrynn AS, Leonard BE 1997 The olfactory bulbectomized rat as a model of depression: an update. Pharmacology and Therapeutics 74: 299–316

Kelly PH, Iversen SD 1976 Selective 6-OHDA induced destruction of mesolimbic dopamine neurons: abolition of psychostimulant induced locomotor activity in rats. European Journal of Pharmacology 40: 45–56

Kerr FWL, Lippman HH 1974 The primate spinothalamic tract as demonstrated by anterolateral cordotomy and commisural myelotomy. Advances in Neurology 4: 147–156

Khan IM, Taylor P, Yaksh TL 1994 Stimulatory pathways and sites of action of intrathecally administered nicotinic agents. Journal of Pharmacology and Experimental Therapy 271: 1550–1557

Khan IM, Marsala M, Printz MP, Taylor P, Yaksh TL 1996 Intrathecal nicotinic agonist-elicited release of excitatory amino acids as measured by in vivo spinal microdialysis in rats. Journal of Pharmacology and Experimental Therapy 278: 97–106

Kharazia VN, Weinberg RJ 1994 Glutamate in thalamic fibers terminating in layer IV of primary sensory cortex. Journal of Neuroscience 14: 6021–6032

Khayyat GF, Yu YJ, King RB 1975 Response patterns to noxious and non-noxious stimuli in rostral trigeminal relay nuclei. Brain Research 97: 47–60

Kim SH, Chung JM 1992 An experimental model for peripheral neuropathy produced by segmental spinal nerve ligation in the rat. Pain 50: 355–363

King AE, Thompson SW, Urban L, Woolf CJ 1988 An intracellular analysis of amino acid induced excitations of deep dorsal horn neurones in the rat spinal cord slice. Neuroscience Letters 89: 286–292

Kinnman E, Nygards EB, Hansson P 1997 Effects of dextromethorphan in clinical doses on capsaicin-induced ongoing pain and mechanical hypersensitivity. Journal of Pain and Symptom Management 14: 195–201

Kiser RS, Leibowitz RM, German DC 1978 Anatomic and pharmacological differences between two types of aversive midbrain stimulation. Brain Research 155: 331–342

Komisaruk BR, Whipple B 1986 Vaginal stimulation-produced analgesia in rats and women. Annals of the New York Academy of Sciences 467: 30–39

Korpi ER, Mattila MJ, Wisden W, Luddens H 1997 GABA(A)-receptor subtypes: clinical efficacy and selectivity of benzodiazepine site ligands. Annals of Medicine 29: 275–282

Kremer EF, Block A, Atkinson JH 1983 Assessment of pain behavior: factors that distort self-report. In: Melzack R (ed) Pain management and assessment. Raven, New York, pp 165–171

Kristensen JD, Svensson B, Gordh T Jr 1992 The NMDA-receptor antagonist CPP abolishes neurogenic 'wind-up pain' after intrathecal administration in humans. Pain 51: 249–253

Kuo DC, Kawatani M, De Groat WC 1985 Vasoactive intestinal polypeptide identified in the thoracic dorsal root ganglia of the cat. Brain Research 330: 178–182

Kuraishi Y, Hirota N, Sato Y, Hino Y, Satoh M, Takagi H 1985a Evidence that substance P and somatostatin transmit separate information related to pain in the spinal dorsal horn. Brain Research 325: 294–298

Kuraishi Y, Hirota N, Sato Y, Kaneko S, Satoh M, Takagi H 1985b Noradrenergic inhibition of the release of substance P from the primary afferents in the rabbit spinal dorsal horn. Brain Research 359: 177–182

Kuraishi Y, Hirota N, Sato Y, Hanashima N, Takagi H, Satoh M 1989 Stimulus specificity of peripherally evoked substance P release from the rabbit dorsal horn in situ. Neuroscience 30: 241–205

Laduron PM 1984 Axonal transport of opiate receptors in capsaicin-sensitive neurones. Brain Research 294: 157–160

LaMotte C, Pert CB, Snyder SH 1976 Opiate receptor binding in primate spinal cord: distribution and changes after dorsal root section. Brain Research 112: 407–412

LaMotte RH, Lundberg LE, Torebjörk HE 1992 Pain, hyperalgesia and activity in nociceptive C units in humans after intradermal injection of capsaicin. Journal of Physiology 448: 749–764

Laneuville O, Dorais J, Couture R 1988 Characterization of the effects produced by neurokinins and three agonists selective for neurokinin receptor subtypes in a spinal nociceptive reflex of the rat. Life Sciences 42: 1295–1305

Larson AA, Vaught JL, Takemori AE 1980 The potentiation of spinal analgesia by leukine enkephalin. European Journal of Pharmacology 61: 381–383

Lasagna L, Von Felsinger JM, Beecher HK 1955 Drug-induced mood changes in man. I. Observations on healthy subjects, chronically ill patients, and postaddicts. Journal of the American Medical Association 157: 1006–1020

Lauretti GR, Lima IC. The effects of intrathecal neostigmine on somatic and visceral pain: improvement by association with a peripheral anticholinergic. Anesthesia and Analgesia 82: 617–620

Lauretti GR, Reis MP, Mattos AL, Gomes JM, Oliveira AP, Pereira NL 1998 Epidural nonsteroidal antiinflammatory drugs for cancer pain. Anesthesia and Analgesia 86: 117–118

Lawson SN, Perry MJ, Prabhakar E, McCarthy PW 1993 Primary sensory neurones: neurofilament, neuropeptides, and conduction velocity. Brain Research Bulletin 30: 239–243

Lazorthes Y 1988 Intracerebroventricular administration of morphine for control of irreducible cancer pain. Annals of the New York Academy of Sciences 531: 123–132

Le Bars D, Bourgoin S, Clot AM, Hamon M, Cesselin F 1987 Noxious mechanical stimuli increase the release of met-enkephalin-like material heterosegmentally in the rat spinal cord. Brain Research 402: 188–192

Leah JD, Cameron AA, Snow PJ 1985 Neuropeptides in physiologically identified mammalian sensory neurons. Neuroscience Letters 56: 257–263

Leah J, Menetrey D, de Pommery J 1988 Neuropeptides in long ascending spinal tract cells in the rat: evidence for parallel processing of ascending information. Neuroscience 24: 195–207

Lee TL, Kumar A, Baratham G 1990 Intraventricular morphine for intractable craniofacial pain. Singapore Medical Journal 31: 273–276

Lee YW, Yaksh TL. Pharmacology of the spinal adenosine receptor which mediates the antiallodynic action of intrathecal adenosine agonists. Journal of Pharmacology and Experimental Therapy 277: 1642–1648

Leonard BE 1997 Noradrenaline in basic models of depression. European Neuropsychopharmacology (suppl 1): S11–16

Leslie JB, Watkins WD 1985 Eicosanoids in the central nervous system. Journal of Neurosurgery 63: 659–668

Levy RA, Proudfit HK 1979 Analgesia produced by microinjection of baclofen and morphine at brainstem sites. European Journal of Pharmacology 57: 43–55

Lewis VA, Gebhart GF 1977 Evaluation of the periaqueductal central gray (PAG) as a morphine specific locus of action and examination of morphine-induced and stimulation produced analgesia at coincident PAG loci. Brain Research 124: 283–303

Li WM, Sato A, Sato Y, Schmidt RF 1996 Morphine microinjected into the nucleus tractus solitarius and rostral ventrolateral medullary nucleus enhances somatosympathetic A- and C-reflexes in anesthetized rats. Neuroscience Letters 221: 53–56

Light AR 1992 The organization of nociceptive neurons in the spinal grey matter. In: Light AL (ed) The initial processing of pain and its descending control: spinal and trigeminal system. Karger, Basel, pp 109–168

Lima D, Coimbra A 1991 Neurons in the substantia gelatinosa rolandi (Lamina II) project to the caudal ventrolateral reticular formation of the medulla oblonga in the rat. Neuroscience Letters 132: 16–18

Lin Q, Peng YB, Willis WD 1996 Role of GABA receptor subtypes in inhibition of primate spinothalamic tract neurons: difference between spinal and periaqueductal gray inhibition. Journal of Neurophysiology 75: 109–123

Liu H, Wang H, Sheng M, Jan LY, Jan YN, Basbaum AI 1994 Evidence for presynaptic *N*-methyl-D-aspartate autoreceptors in the spinal cord dorsal horn. Proceedings of the National Academy of Sciences USA 91: 8383–8387

Liu H, Mantyh PW, Basbaum AI 1997 NMDA-receptor regulation of substance P release from primary afferent nociceptors. Nature 386: 721–724

Liu QS, Qiao JT, Dafny N 1992 D2 dopamine receptor involvement in spinal dopamine-produced antinociception. Life Sciences 51: 1485–1492

Liu XB 1997 Subcellular distribution of AMPA and NMDA receptor subunit immunoreactivity in ventral posterior and reticular nuclei of rat and cat thalamus. Journal of Comparative Neurology 388: 587–602

Lloyd GK, Menzaghi F, Bontempi BK et al 1998 The potential of subtype-selective neuronal nicotinic acetylcholine receptor agonists as therapeutic agents. Life Sciences 62: 1601–1606

Lodge D, Davies S 1987 Evidence for involvement of *N*-methylaspartate receptors in 'wind-up' of class 2 neurons in the dorsal horn of the rat. Brain Research 424: 402–406

Lombard MC, Besson JM 1989 Attempts to gauge the relative importance of pre- and postsynaptic effects of morphine on the transmission of noxious messages in the dorsal horn of the rat spinal cord. Pain 37: 335–435

Luger TJ, Hayashi T, Weiss CG, Hill HF 1995 The spinal potentiating effect and the supraspinal inhibitory effect of midazolam on opioid-induced analgesia in rats. European Journal of Pharmacology 275: 153–162

Ma QP, Han JS 1992 Neurochemical and morphological evidence of an antinociceptive neural pathway from nucleus raphe dorsalis to nucleus accumbens in the rabbit. Brain Research Bulletin 28: 931–936

Ma QP, Yin GF, Ai MK, Han JS 1991 Serotonergic projections from the nucleus raphe dorsalis to the amygdala in the rat. Neuroscience Letters 134: 21–24

Ma W, Bisby MA 1997 Differential expression of galanin immunoreactivities in the primary sensory neurons following partial and complete sciatic nerve injuries. Neuroscience 79: 1183–1195

McCarthy PW, Lawson SN 1989 Cell type and conduction velocity of rat primary sensory neurons with substance P-like immunoreactivity. Neuroscience 28: 745–753

MacDermott AB, Mayer ML, Westbrook GI, Smith SJ, Barker JL 1986 NMDA-receptor activation increases cytoplasmic calcium concentrations in cultured spinal cord neurones. Nature 321: 519–522

Magnusson KR, Clements JR, Larson AA, Madl JE, Beitz AJ 1987 Localization of glutamate in trigeminothalamic projection neurons: a combined retrograde transport – immunohistochemical study. Somatosensory Research 4: 177–190

Malmberg AB, Yaksh TL 1992a Hyperalgesia mediated by spinal glutamate or SP receptor blocked by spinal cyclooxygenase inhibition. Science 257: 1276–1279

Malmberg AB, Yaksh TL 1992b Antinociceptive actions of spinal non-steroidal anti-inflammatory agents on the formalin test in the rat. Journal of Pharmacology and Experimental Therapeutics 263: 136–146

Malmberg AB, Yaksh TL 1992c Isobolographic and dose response analyses of the interaction between intrathecal mu and delta agonists: effects of naltrindole and its benzofuran analog NTB. Journal of Pharmacology and Experimental Therapeutics 263: 264–275

Malmberg AB, Yaksh TL 1993a Pharmacology of the spinal action of ketorolac, morphine, ST-91, U50488H and L-PIA on the formalin test and an isobolographic analysis of the NSAID interaction. Anesthesiology 79: 270–281

Malmberg AB, Yaksh TL 1993b Spinal nitric oxide synthesis inhibition blocks NMDA-induced thermal hyperalgesia and produces antinociception in the formalin test in rats. Pain 54: 291–300

Malmberg AB, Yaksh TL 1995 Cyclooxygenase inhibition and the spinal release of prostaglandin E2 and amino acids evoked by paw formalin injection: a microdialysis study in anesthetized rats. Journal of Neuroscience 15: 2768–2776

Malmberg AB, Rafferty MF, Yaksh TL 1994 Antinociceptive effect of spinally delivered prostaglandin E receptor antagonists in the formalin test in the rat. Neuroscience Letters 173: 193–196

Mantyh PW, DeMaster E, Malhotra A et al 1995 Receptor endocytosis and dendrite reshaping in spinal neurons after somatosensory stimulation. Science 268: 1629–1632

Manzoni OJ, Manabe T, Nicoll RA 1994 Release of adenosine by activation of NMDA receptors in the hippocampus. Science 265–2101

Marsala M, Yaksh TL 1992 Reversible aortic occlusion in rats: post-reflow hyperesthesia and motor effects blocked by spinal NMDA antagonism. Anesthesiology 77 (suppl): A664

Marsala M, Malmberg AB, Yaksh TL 1995 The spinal loop dialysis catheter: characterization of use in the unanesthetized rat. Journal of Neuroscience Methods 62: 43–53

Martin CS, McGrady EM, Colquhoun A, Thorburn J 1990 Extradural methadone and bupivacaine in labour. British Journal of Anaesthesia 65: 330–332

Maves TJ, Gebhart GF 1992 Antinociceptive synergy between intrathecal morphine and lidocaine during visceral and somatic nociception in the rat. Anesthesiology 76: 91–99

Mayer ML, Westbrook GL 1987 The physiology of excitatory amino acids in the vertebrate central nervous system. Progress in Neurobiology 28: 197–276

Max MB, Culnane M, Schafer SC, Gracely RH, Walther DJ, Smoller B, Dubner R 1987 Amitriptyline relieves diabetic neuropathy pain in patients with normal or depressed mood. Neurology 37: 589–596

Max MB, Kishor-Kumar R, Schafer SC, Meister B, Gracely RH, Smoller B, Dubner R 1991 Efficacy of desiprammine in painful diabetic neuropathy: a placebo-controlled trail. Pain 45:3–9

Max MB, Lynch SA, Muir J, Shoaf SE, Smoller B, Dubner R 1992 Effects of desipramine, amitriptyline, and fluoxetine on pain in diabetic neuropathy. New England Journal of Medicine 326:1250–1256

Max MB, Schafer SC, Culnane M, Smoller B, Dubner R, Gracely RH 1998 Amitriptyline, but not lorazepam, relieves postherpetic neuralgia. Neurology 38:1427–1432

Meller ST, Gebhart GF 1993 Nitric oxide (NO) and nociceptive processing in the spinal cord. Pain 52: 127–136

Meller ST, Dykstra C, Gebhart GF 1992 Production of endogenous nitric oxide and activation of soluble guanylate cyclase are required for *N*-methyl-D-aspartate-produced facilitation of the nociceptive tail-flick reflex. European Journal of Pharmacology 214: 93–96

Melzack R, Casey KL 1968 Sensory, motivational, and central control determinants of pain: a new conceptual model. In: Kenshalo D (ed) The skin senses. Charles C Thomas, Springfield, IL, pp 423–443

Melzack R, Wall PD 1973 The puzzle of pain. Basic Books, New York

Mendell LM 1966 Physiological properties of unmyelinated fiber projections to the spinal cord. Experimental Neurology 16: 316–332

Mendell LM, Wall PD 1965 Responses of single dorsal cord cells to peripheral cutaneous unmyelinated fibers. Nature 206: 97–99

Miczek KA, Weerts EM, Vivian JA, Barros HM 1995 Aggression, anxiety and vocalizations in animals: GABAA and 5-HT anxiolytics. Psychopharmacology 121: 38–56

Miki K, Fukuoka T, Tokunaga A, Noguchi K 1998 Calcitonin gene-related peptide increase in the rat spinal dorsal horn and dorsal column nucleus following peripheral nerve injury: up-regulation in a subpopulation of primary afferent sensory neurons. Neuroscience 82: 1243–1252

Miletic V, Randic M 1979 Neurotensin excites cat spinal neurones located in laminae I-III. Brain Research 169: 600–604

Milne B, Duggan S, Jhamandas K, Loomis C 1996 Innocuous hair deflection evokes a nociceptive-like activation of catechol oxidation in the rat locus coeruleus following intrathecal strychnine: a biochemical index of allodynia using in vivo voltammetry. Brain Research 718: 198–202

Minami T, Uda R, Horiguchi S, Ito S, Hyodo M, Hayaishi O 1994 Allodynia evoked by intrathecal administration of prostaglandin E2 to conscious mice. Pain 57: 217–223

Mitchell JJ, Anderson KJ 1991 Quantitative autoradiographic analysis of excitatory amino acid receptors in the cat spinal cord. Neuroscience Letters 124: 269–272

Mizukawa K, Vincent SR, McGeer PL, McGeer EG 1989 Distribution of reduced-nicotinamide-adenine-dinucleotide-phosphate diaphorase-positive cells and fibers in the cat central nervous system. Journal of Comparative Neurology 279: 281–311

Mohrland S, Gebhart G 1980 Effects of focal electrical stimulation and morphine microinjection in the periaqueductal gray of the rat mesencephalon on neuronal activity in the medullary reticular formation. Brain Research 201: 23–37

Mollenholt P, Post C, Rawal N, Freedman J, Høkfelt T, Paulsson I 1988 Antinociceptive and 'neurotoxic' actions of somatostatin in rat spinal cord after intrathecal administration. Pain 32: 95–105

Monasky MS, Zinsmeister AR, Stevens CW, Yaksh TL 1990 Interaction of intrathecal morphine and ST-91 on antinociception in the rat: dose–response analysis, antagonism and clearance. Journal of Pharmacology and Experimental Therapeutics 254: 383–392

Mongeau R, Blier P, de Montigny C 1997 The serotonergic and noradrenergic systems of the hippocampus: their interactions and the effects of antidepressant treatments. Brain Research Reviews 23: 145–195

Moochhala SM, Sawynok J 1984 Hyperalgesia produced by intrathecal substance P and related peptides: desensitization and cross desensitization. British Journal of Pharmacology 82: 381–388
Moreau J-L, Fields HL 1987 Evidence for GABA involvement in midbrain control of medullary neurons that modulate nociceptive transmission. Brain Research 397: 37–46
Morgan MM, Sohn JH, Liebeskind JC 1989 Stimulation of the periaqueductal gray matter inhibits nociception at the supraspinal as well as spinal level. Brain Research 502: 61–66
Morris BJ, Herz A 1987 Distinct distribution of opioid receptor types in rat lumbar spinal cord. Naunyn-Schmiedeberg's Archives of Pharmacology 336: 240–243
Morris R, Southam E, Braid DJ, Gathwaite J 1992 Nitric oxide may act as a messenger between dorsal root ganglion neurones and their satellite cells. Neuroscience Letters 137: 29–32
Morton CR, Hutchison WD 1989 Release of sensory neuropeptides in the spinal cord: Studies with calcitonin gene-related peptide and galanin. Neuroscience 31: 807–815
Morton CR, Hutchinson WD 1990 Morphine does not reduce the intraspinal release of calcitonin gene-related peptide in the cat. Neuroscience Letters 117: 319–324
Morton CR, Hutchinson WD, Hendry IA 1988 Release of immunoreactive somatostatin in the spinal dorsal horn of the cat. Neuropeptides 12: 189–197
Morton CR, Hutchison WD, Hendry IA, Duggan AW 1989 Somatostatin: evidence for a role in thermal nociception. Brain Research 488: 89–96
Moulin DE, Max MB, Kaiko RF et al 1985 The analgesic efficacy of intrathecal D-Ala^2-D-Leu^5-enkephalin in cancer patients with chronic pain. Pain 23: 213–221
Murase K, Nedeljkov V, Randic M 1982 The actions of neuropeptides on dorsal horn neurons in the rat spinal cord slice preparation: an intracellular study. Brain Research 234: 170–176
Murase K, Ryu PD, Randic M 1989 Tachykinins modulate multiple ionic conductances in voltage-clamped rat spinal dorsal horn neurons. Journal of Neurophysiology 61: 854–865
Murray CW, Cowan A 1991 Tonic pain perception in the mouse: differential modulation by three receptor-selective opioid agonists. Journal of Pharmacology and Experimental Therapeutics 257: 335–341
Musty RE, Jordan MP, Lenox RH 1990 Criterion for learned helplessness in the rat: a redefinition. Pharmacology, Biochemistry and Behavior 36: 739–744
Myslinski NR, Randic M 1977 Responses of identified spinal neurones to acetylcholine applied by micro-electrophoresis. Journal of Physiology 269: 195–219
Naguib M, Yaskh TL 1994 Antinociceptive effects of spinal cholinesterase inhibition an isobolographic analysis of the interaction with mu and alpha 2 receptor systems. Anaesthesiology 80:1338–1348
Naguib M, Yaksh TL 1997 Characterization of muscarinic receptor subtypes that mediate antinociception in the rat spinal cord. Anesthesia and Analgesia 85: 847–853
Nahin RL 1987 Immunocytochemical identification of long ascending peptidergic neurons contributing to the spino reticular tract in the rat. Neuroscience 23: 859–869
Nahin RL 1988 Immunocytochemical identification of long ascending peptidergic lumbar spinal neurons terminating in either the medial or lateral thalamus in the rat. Brain Research 443: 345–349
Näsström J, Karlsson U, Post C 1992 Antinociceptive actions of different classes of excitatory amino acid receptor antagonists in mice. European Journal of Pharmacology 212: 21–29
Ness TJ, Gebhart GF 1988 Colorectal distention as a noxious visceral stimulus: physiologic and pharmacologic characterization of pseudoaffective reflexes in the rat. Brain Research 450: 153–169
Neugebauer V, Lucke T, Schaible HG 1994a Requirement of metabotropic glutamate receptors for the generation of inflammation-evoked hyperexcitability in rat spinal cord neurons. European Journal of Neuroscience 6: 1179–1186
Neugebauer V, Schaible HG, Weiretter F, Freudenberger U 1994b The involvement of substance P and neurokinin-1 receptors in the responses of rat dorsal horn neurons to noxious but not to innocuous mechanical stimuli applied to the knee joint. Brain Research 666: 207–215
Nicol GD, Klingberg DK, Vasko MR 1992 Prostaglandin E2 increases calcium conductance and stimulates release of substance P in Avian sensory neurons. Journal of Neuroscience 12: 1917–1927
Noguchi K, Ruda MA 1992 Gene regulation in an ascending nociceptive pathway: inflammation-induced increase in preprotachykinin mRNA in rat lamina I spinal projection neurons. Journal of Neuroscience 12: 2563–2572
Noguchi K, Senba E, Morita Y, Sato M, Tohyama M 1990 a-CGRP and b-CGRP mRNAs are differently regulated in the rat spinal cord and dorsal root ganglion. Molecular Brain Research 7: 299–304
Noguchi K, De León, M, Nahin RL, Senba E, Ruda MA 1993 Quantification of axotomy-induced alteration of neuropeptide mRNAs in dorsal root ganglion neurons with special reference to neuropeptide Y mRNA and the effects of neonatal capsaicin treatment. Journal of Neuroscience Research 35: 54–66
Nordberg G 1984 Pharmacokinetic aspects of spinal morphine analgesia. Acta Physiologica Scandinavica 79 (suppl): 7–37
North RA, Williams JT, Suprenant A, Christie MJ 1987 μ and δ receptors belong to a family of receptors that are coupled to potassium channels. Proceedings of the National Academy of Sciences USA 84: 5487–5491
Nozoki-Taguchi N, Yaksh TL 1998 A novel model of primary and secondary hyperalgesi after mild thermal injury in the rat. Neuroscience Letters 254:25–28
Nozoki-Taguchi N, Yaksh TL (Unpublished)
O'Brien C, Woolf CJ, Fitzgerald M, Lindsay RM, Molander C 1989 Differences in the chemical expression of rat primary afferent neurons which innervate skin, muscle or joint. Neuroscience 32: 493–502
O'Dell TJ, Hawkins RD, Kandel ER, Arancio O 1991 Tests of the roles of two diffusible substances in long-term potentiation: evidence for nitric oxide as a possible early retrograde messenger. Proceeding of the National Academy of Sciences USA 88: 11285–11289
O'Donohue TL, Massari VJ, Pazoles CJ et al 1984 A role for bombesin in sensory processing in the spinal cord. Journal of Neuroscience 4: 2956–2962
O'Neill MF, Dourish CT, Iversen SD 1989 Morphine induced analgesia in the rat paw pressure test is blocked by CCK and enhanced by the CCK antagonists MK-329. Neuropharmacology 28: 243–248
Ohishi H, Shigemoto R, Nakanishi S, Mizuno N 1993 Distribution of the mRNA for a metabotropic glutamate receptor (mGluR3) in the rat brain: an in situ hybridization study. Journal of Comparative Neurology 335: 252–266
Ohkubo T, Shibata M, Takahashi H, Inoki R 1990 Roles of substance P and somatostatin on spinal transmission of nociceptive information induced by formalin in spinal cord. Journal of Pharmacology and Experimental Therapeutics 252: 1261–1268
Oku R, Satih M, Takagi H 1987 Release of substance P from the spinal dorsal horn is enhanced in polyarthritic rats. Neuroscience Letters 74: 315–319
Oliveras J-L, Maixner W, Dubner R et al 1986a Dorsal horn opiate administration attenuated the perceived intensity of noxious heat stimulation in the behaving monkey. Brain Research 371: 368–371
Oliveras J-L, Maixner W, Dubner R et al 1986b The medullary dorsal horn: a target for the expression of opiates effects upon the perceived intensity of noxious heat. Journal of Neuroscience 6: 3086–3093

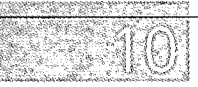

Olmstead MC, Franklin KB 1997 The development of a conditioned place preference to morphine: effects of microinjections into various CNS sites. Behavioral Neuroscience 111: 1324–1334

Onaka T, Yagi K 1998 Role of noradrenergic projections to the bed nucleus of the stria terminalis in neuroendocrine and behavioral responses to fear-related stimuli in rats. Brain Research 788: 287–293

Onaka M, Minami T, Nishihara I, Ito S 1996 Involvement of glutamate receptors in strychnine- and bicuculline-induced allodynia in conscious mice. Anesthesiology 84: 1215–1222

Ono H, Mishima A, Ono S, Fukuda H, Vasko MR 1991 Inhibitory effects of clonidine and tizanidine on release of substance P from slices of rat spinal cord and antagonism by alpha-adrenergic receptor antagonists. Neuropharmacology 30: 585–589

Ono T, Nishijo H, Uwano T 1995 Amygdala role in conditioned associative learning. Progress in Neurobiology 46: 401–422

Oshita S, Yaksh TL, Chipkin R 1990 The antinociceptive effects of intrathecally administered SCH32615, an enkephalinase inhibitor in the rat. Brain Research 515: 143–148

Ossipov MH, Goldstein FJ, Malseed RT 1984 Feline analgesia following central administration of opioids. Neuropharmacology 23: 925–929

Ossipov MH, Harris S, Lloyd P, Messineo E, Lin BS, Bagley J 1990a Antinociceptive interaction between opioids and medetomidine: systemic additivity and spinal synergy. Anesthesiology 73: 1227–1235

Ossipov MH, Lozito R, Messineo E, Green J, Harris S, Lloyd P 1990b Spinal antinociceptive synergy between clonidine and morphine, U69593, and DPDPE: isobolographic analysis. Life Sciences 47: 71–76

Ossipov MH, Kovelowski CJ, Nichols ML, Hruby VJ, Porreca F 1995 Characterization of supraspinal antinociceptive actions of opioid delta agonists in the rat. Pain 62: 287–293

Oyama T, Fukushi S, Jin T 1982 Epidural B-endorphin in treatment of pain. Canadian Anaesthetists Society Journal 29: 24–26

Pak MA, Haas HL, Decking UKM, Schrader J 1994 Inhibition of adenosine kinase increases endogenous adenosine and depresses neuronal activity in hippocampal slices. Neuropharmacology 33: 1049–1053

Palecek J, Paleckova V, Dougherty PM, Willis WD 1994 The effect of trans-ACPD, a metabotropic excitatory amino acid receptor agonist, on the responses of primate spinothalamic tract neurons. Pain 56: 261–269

Panula P, Hadjiconstantinou M, Yang H-YT, Costa E 1983 Immunohistochemical localization of bombesin/gastrin-releasing peptide and substance P in primary sensory neurons. Journal of Neuroscience 3: 2021–2029

Papir-Kricheli D, Frey J, Laufer R et al 1987 Behavioral effects of receptor-specific substance P agonists. Pain 31: 263–276

Partridge BJ, Chaplan SR, Sakamoto E, Yaksh TL 1998 Characterization of the effects of gabapentin and 3-isobutyl-gamma-aminobutyric acid on substance P-induced thermal hyperalgesia. Anesthesiology 88: 196–205

Pascual J, del Arco C, Gonzalez AM, Pazos A 1992 Quantitative light microscopic autoradiographic localization of alpha 2-receptors in the human brain. Brain Research 585: 116–127

Pavlovic ZW, Bodnar RJ 1998 Opioid supraspinal analgesic synergy between the amygdala and periaqueductal gray in rats. Brain Research 779: 158–169

Pay S, Barasi S 1982 A study of the connections of nociceptive substantia nigra neurons. Pain 12: 75–89

Payne R 1987 Role of epidural and intrathecal narcotics and peptides in the management of cancer pain. Medical Clinics of North America 71: 313–327

Pazos A, Palacios JM 1985 Quantitative autoradiographic mapping of serotonin receptors in the rat brain. I. Serotonin-1 receptors. Brain Research 346: 205–230

Pazos A, Cortés R, Palacios JM 1985 Quantitative autoradiographic mapping of serotonin receptors in the rat brain. II. Serotonin-2 receptors. Brain Research 346: 231–249

Penning J, Yaskh TL 1992 Interaction of intrathecal morphine with bupivacaine and lidocaine in the rat. Anaesthesiology 77:1186–1200

Perriss BW, Latham BV, Wilson IH 1990 Analgesia following extradural and i.m. pethidine in post-caesarean section patients. British Journal of Anaesthesia 3: 355–357

Pert A, Yaksh TL 1974 Sites of morphine induced analgesia in the primate brain: relation to pain pathways. Brain Research 80: 135–140

Pert A, Yaksh TL 1975 Localization of the antinociceptive action of morphine in primate brain. Pharmacology, Biochemistry and Behavior 3: 133–138

Pirot S, Jay TM, Glowinski J, Thierry A-M 1994 Anatomical and electrophysiological evidence for an excitatory amino acid pathway from the thalamic mediodorsal nucleus to the prefrontal cortex in the rat. European Journal of Neuroscience 6: 1225–1234

Pitkanen A, Savander V, LeDoux JE 1997 Organization of intra-amygdaloid circuitries in the rat: an emerging framework for understanding functions of the amygdala. Trends in Neurosciences 20: 517–523

Pohl M, Benoliel JJ, Bourgoin S et al 1990 Regional distribution of calcitonin gene-related peptide-, substance P-, cholecystokinin-, met5-enkephalin-, and dynorphin A (1–8)-like material in the spinal cord and dorsal root ganglia of adult rats: Effects of dorsal rhizotomy and neonatal capsaicin. Journal of Neurochemistry 55: 1122–1130

Poon A, Sawynok J 1995 Antinociception by adenosine analogs and an adenosine kinase inhibitor: dependence on formalin concentration. European Journal of Pharmacology 286: 177–184

Poon A, Sawynok J 1998 Antinociception by adenosine analogs and inhibitors of adenosine metabolism in an inflammatory thermal hyperalgesia model in the rat. Pain 74: 235–245

Porreca F, Heyman JS, Mosberg HI, Omnaas JR, Vaught JL 1987 Role of mu and delta receptors in the supraspinal and spinal analgesic effects of [D-Pen2, D-Pen5] enkephalin in the mouse. Journal of Pharmacology and Experimental Therapeutics 241: 393–400

Prado WA 1989 Antinociceptive effect of agonists microinjected into the anterior pretectal nucleus of the rat. Brain Research 493: 145–154

Prado WA, Roberts MHT 1984 Antinociception from a stereospecific action of morphine microinjected into the brainstem: a local or distant site of action. British Journal of Pharmacology 82: 877–882

Pratt JA, Brett RR, Laurie DJ 1998 Benzodiazepine dependence: from neural circuits to gene expression. Pharmacology, Biochemistry and Behavior 59: 925–934

Price GW, Kelly JS, Bowery NG 1987 The location of $GABA_B$ receptor binding sites in mammalian spinal cord. Synapse 1: 530–538

Proudfit HK, Clark FM 1991 The projections of locus coeruleus neurons to the spinal cord. Progress in Brain Research 88: 123–141

Puig S, Sorkin LS 1996 Formalin evoked activity in identified primary afferent fibers: Systemic lidocaine suppresses phase 2 activity. Pain 64: 345–355

Puig S, Rivot JP, Besson JM 1991 In vivo electrochemical evidence that the tricyclic antidepressant femoxetine potentiates the morphine-induced increase in 5-HT metabolism in the medullary dorsal horn of freely moving rats. Brain Research 553: 222–228

Pybus DA, Torda TA 1982 Dose effect relationships of extradural morphine. British Journal of Anaesthesiology 54: 1259–1262

Radhakrishnan V, Henry JL 1991 Novel Substance-P antagonist, CP-96, 345 blocks responses of cat spinal dorsal horn neurons to noxious cutaneous stimuli and to substance P. Neuroscience Letters 132: 39–43

Radhakrishnan V, Henry JL 1993 L-NAME blocks responses to NMDA,

Substance-P and noxious cutaneous stimuli in cat dorsal horn. Neuroreport 4: 323–326

Rady JJ, Fujimoto JM, Tseng LF 1991 Dynorphins other than dynorphin A(1–17) lack spinal antianalgesic activity but do act on dynorphin A(1–17) receptors. Journal of Pharmacology and Experimental Therapeutics 259: 1073–1080

Rainville P, Duncan GH, Price DD, Carrier B, Bushnell MC 1997 Pain affect encoded in human anterior cingulate but not somatosensory cortex. Science 277: 968–971

Raja SN, Meyer RA, Campbell JN 1997 Transduction properties of the sensory afferent fibers. In: Yaksh TL, Lynch III C, Zapol WM, Maze M, Biebuyck JF, Saidman LJ (eds) Anesthesia: biologic foundations. Lippincott–Raven, Philadelphia, pp 515–530

Ramberg DA, Yaksh TL 1989 Effects of cervical spinal hemisection of dihydromorphine binding in brainstem and spinal cord in cat. Brain Research 483: 61–67

Ramwell PW, Shaw JE, Jessup R 1966 Spontaneous and evoked release of prostaglandins from frog spinal cord. American Journal of Physiology 211: 998–1004

Randic M, Hecimovic H, Ryu PD 1990 Substance P modulates glutamate-induced currents in acutely isolated rat spinal dorsal horn neurones. Neuroscience Letters 117: 74–80

Rawal N, Schott U, Dahlström B et al 1986 Influence of naloxone infusion on analgesia and respiratory depression following epidural morphine. Anesthesiology 64: 194–201

Reeve AJ, Dickenson AH 1995 Electrophysiological study on spinal antinociceptive interactions between adenosine and morphine in the dorsal horn of the rat. Neuroscience Letters 194: 81–84

Reeve AJ, Dickenson AH, Kerr NC 1998 Spinal effects of bicuculline: modulation of an allodynia-like state by an A1-receptor agonist, morphine, and an NMDA-receptor antagonist. Journal of Neurophysiology 79: 1494–1507

Reich MG, Razavi D 19-96 [Role of amphetamines in cancerology: a review of the literature.] Bulletin du Cancer 83: 891–900

Ren K, Williams GM, Hylden JL, Ruda MA, Dubner R 1992 The intrathecal administration of excitatory amino acid receptor antagonists selectively attenuated carrageenan-induced behavioral hyperalgesia in rats. European Journal of Pharmacology 219: 235–243

Richelson E, Pfenning M 1984 Blockade by antidepressants and related compounds of biogenic amine uptake into rat brain synaptosomes. Most antidepressants selectively block norepinephrine uptake. European Journal of Pharmacology 104:227–286

Robertson JA, Hough LB, Bodnar RJ 1988 Potentiation of opioid and nonopioid forms of swim analgesia by cimetidine. Pharmacology, Biochemistry and Behavior 31: 107–112

Rodgers RJ 1977 Elevation of aversive threshold in rats by intraamygdaloid injection of morphine sulfate. Pharmacology, Biochemistry and Behavior 6: 385–390

Roerig SC, Fujimoto JM 1989 Multiplicative interaction between intrathecally and intracerebroventricularly administered mu opioid agonists but limited interactions between delta and kappa agonists for antinociception in mice. Journal of Pharmacology and Experimental Therapeutics 249: 762–768

Romano JM, Turner JA 1985 Chronic pain and depression: does the evidence support a relationship? Psychopharmacology Bulletin 97: 18–26

Rusin KI, Jiang MC, Cerne R, Randic M 1993 Interactions between excitatory amino acids and tachykinins in the rat spinal dorsal horn. Research Bulletin 30: 329–338

Ryu PD, Gerber G, Murase K, Randic M 1988 Actions of calcitonin gene-related peptide on rat spinal dorsal horn neurons. Brain Research 441: 357–361

Sabbe MB, Grafe MR, Mjanger E, Tiseo PJ, Hill HF, Yaksh TL 1994 Spinal delivery of sufentanil, alfentanil, and morphine in dogs. Physiologic and toxicologic investigations. Anesthesiology 81: 899–920

Sakurada T, Katsumata K, Yogo H et al 1995 The neurokinin-1 receptor antagonist, sendide, exhibits antinociceptive activity in the formalin test. Pain 60: 175–180

Salt TE 1986 Mediation of thalamic sensory input by both NMDA receptors and non-NMDA receptors. Nature 322: 263–265

Salt TE, Eaton SA 1989 Function of non-NMDA receptors and NMDA receptors in synaptic responses to natural somatosensory stimulation in the ventrobasal thalamus. Experimental Brain Research 77: 646–652

Salt TE, Eaton SA 1995 Distinct presynaptic metabotropic receptors for L-AP4 and CCG1 on GABAergic terminals: pharmacological evidence using novel alpha-methyl derivative mGluR antagonists, MAP4 and MCCG, in the rat thalamus in vivo. Neuroscience 65: 5–13

Salter MW, Henry JL 1987 Evidence that adenosine mediates the depression of spinal dorsal horn induced by peripheral vibration in the cat. Neuroscience 22: 631–650

Salter MW, Henry JL 1991 Responses of functionally identified neurones in the dorsal horn of the cat spinal cord to substance P, neurokinin A and physalaemin. Neuroscience 4: 601–610

Salter MW, Hicks JL 1994 ATP-evoked increases in intracellular calcium in neurons and glia from the dorsal spinal cord. Journal of Neuroscience 14: 1563–1575

Samanin R, Gumulka W, Valzelli L 1970 Reduced effect of morphine in midbrain raphe lesioned rats. European Journal of Pharmacology 10: 339

Sanchez-Blazquez P, Garzon J 1989 Evaluation of delta receptor mediation of supraspinal opioid analgesia by in vivo protection against the beta-funaltrexamine antagonist effect. European Journal of Pharmacology 159: 9–23

Sandler AN 1990 Epidural opiate analgesia for acute pain relief. Canadian Journal of Anaesthesia 3733–3739

Sandouk P, Serrie A, Urtizberea M, Debray M, Got P, Scherrmann JM 1991 Morphine pharmacokinetics and pain assessment after intracerebroventricular administration in patients with terminal cancer. Clinical Pharmacology and Therapeutics 49: 442–448

Sang CN, Gracely RH, Max MB, Bennett GJ 1996 Capsaicin-evoked mechanical allodynia and hyperalgesia cross nerve territories. Evidence for a central mechanism. Anesthesiology 85: 491–496

Saria A, Gamse R, Petermann J, Fischer JA, Theodorsson-Norheim E, Lundberg JM 1986 Simultaneous release of several tachykinins and calcitonin gene-related peptide from rat spinal cord slices. Neuroscience Letters 63: 310–314

Saria A, Javorsky F, Humpel C, Gamse R 1990 5-HT receptor antagonism inhibit sensory neuropeptide release from the rat spinal cord. Neuroreport 1: 104–106

Satoh M, Oku R, Akaike A 1983 Analgesia produced by microinjection of L-glutamate into the rostral ventromedial bulbar nuclei of the rat and its inhibition by intrathecal a-adrenergic blocking agents. Brain Research 261: 361–364

Sawynok J, Sweeney MI 1989 The role of purines in nociception. Neuroscience 32: 557–569

Sawynok J, Yaksh TL 1993 Caffeine as an analgesic adjuvant, a review of pharmacology and mechanisms of action. Pharmacological Reviews 45: 43–85

Sawynok J, Kato N, Navilicek V, Labella FS 1982 Lack of effect of baclofen on substance P and somatostatin release from the spinal cord in vitro. Naunyn-Schiemedberg's Archives of Pharmacology 319: 78–81

Sawynok J, Sweeney MI, White TD 1986 Classification of adenosine receptors mediating antinociception in the rat spinal cord. British Journal of Pharmacology 88: 923–930

Sawynok J, Sweeney M, Nicholson D, White T 1990 Pertussis toxin inhibits morphine-induced release of adenosine from the spinal cord. Progress in Clinical and Biological Research 328: 397–400

Sawynok J, Reid A, Nance D 1991a Spinal antinociception by adenosine analogs and morphine after intrathecal administration of the neurotoxins capsaicin, 6-hydroxydopamine and 5, 7-dihydroxytryptamine. Journal of Pharmacology and Experimental Therapeutics 258: 370–380

Sawynok J, Espey MJ, Reid A 1991b 8-Phenyltheophylline reverses the antinociceptive action of morphine in the periaqueductal gray. Neuropharmacology 30: 871–877

Schaible HG Schmidt RF 1996 Neurophysiology of chronic inflammatory pain: electrophysiological recordings from spinal cord neurons in rats with prolonged acute and chronic unilateral inflammation at the ankle. Progress in Brain Research 110: 167–176

Schaible HG, Grubb BD, Neugebauer V, Oppmann M 1991 The effects of NMDA antagonists on neuronal activity in cat spinal cord evoked by acute inflammation in the knee joint. European Journal of Neuroscience 3: 981–991

Schmauss C, Yaksh TL 1984 In vivo studies on spinal opiate receptor systems mediating antinociception. II. Pharmacological profiles suggesting a differential association of mu, delta and kappa receptors with visceral chemical and cutaneous thermal stimuli in the rat. Journal of Pharmacology and Experimental Therapeutics 228: 1–12

Schmitt P, Karli FEP 1974 Etudes des systemes de reforcement negatif et de reforsement positiv au niveau de la substance grise centrale chez le rat. Physiology and Behavior 12: 271–279

Schneider SP, Perl ER 1985 Selective excitation of neurones in the mammalian spinal dorsal horn by aspartate and glutamate in vitro: correlation with location and excitatory input. Brain Research 360: 339–343

Schneider SP, Perl ER 1988 Comparison of primary afferent and glutamate excitation of neurons in the mammalian spinal dorsal horn. Journal of Neuroscience 8: 2062–2073

Schultheiss R, Schramm J, Neidhardt J 1992 Dose changes in long- and medium-term intrathecal morphine therapy of cancer pain. Neurosurgery 31: 664–669

Schultz W, Romo R 1987 Response of nigro striatal dopamine neurons to high intensity somatosensory stimulation in the anesthetized monkey. Journal of Neurophysiology 57: 210–217

Schuman EM, Madison DV 1991 A requirement for the intracellular messenger nitric oxide in long-term potentiation. Science 254: 1503–1506

Schwarz M, Block F 1994 Visual and somatosensory evoked potentials are mediated by excitatory amino acid receptors in the thalamus. Electroencephalography and Clinical Neurophysiology 91: 392–398

Seybold VS, Hylden JLK, Wilcox GL 1982 Intrathecal substance P and somatostatin in rats: behaviors indicative of sensation. Peptides 3: 49–54

Shafer AL, Donnelly AJ 1991 Management of postoperative pain by continuous epidural infusion of analgesics. Clinical Pharmacy 10: 745–764

Sharpe LG, Garnett JE, Cicero TJ 1974 Analgesia and hyperreactivity produced by intracranial microinjections of morphine into the periaqueductal gray matter of the rat. Behavioral Biology 11: 303–313

Sher G, Mitchell D 1990 *N*-methyl-*d*-aspartate mediates responses of rat dorsal horn neurons to hind limb ischemia. Brain Research 522: 55–62

Sherman SE, Loomis CW 1995 Strychnine-dependent allodynia in the urethane-anesthetized rat is segmentally distributed and prevented by intrathecal glycine and betaine. Canadian Journal of Physiology and Pharmacology 73: 1698–1705

Sherman SE, Loomis CW 1996 Strychnine-sensitive modulation is selective for non-noxious somatosensory input in the spinal cord of the rat. Pain 66: 321–330

Sherrington C 1906 The integrative action of the nervous system. London

Shimoyama N, Shimoyama M, Davis AM, Inturrisi CE, Elliott KJ 1997 Spinal gabapentin is antinociceptive in the rat formalin test. Neuroscience Letters 222: 65–67

Shir Y, Seltzer Z 1990 A-fibers mediate mechanical hyperesthesia and allodynia and C-fibers mediate thermal hyperalgesia in a new model of causalgia from pain disorders in rats. Neuroscience Letters 115: 62–67

Siegfried B, Bures BJ 1978 Asymmetry of EEG arousal in rats with unilateral 6-hydroxydopamine lesions of substantia nigra: quantification of neglect. Experimental Neurology 62: 173–190

Sim LJ, Joseph SA 1989 Opiocortin and catecholamine projections to raphe nuclei. Peptides 10: 1019–1025

Simpson KH, Madej TH, McDowell JM, MacDonald R, Lyons G 1988 Comparison of extradural buprenorphine and extradural morphine after caesarean section. British Journal of Anaesthesia 60: 627–631

Sinclair RJ, Sathain K, Burton H 1991 Neuronal responses in ventroposterolateral nucleus of thalamus in monkeys (*Macaca mulatta*) during active touch of gratings. Somatosensory and Motor Research 8: 293–300

Sindrup SH 1997 Antidepressants as analgesics. In: Yaksh TL, Lynch III C, Zapol WM, Maze M, Biebuyck JF, Saidman LJ (eds) Anesthesia: biologic foundations. Lippincott–Raven, Philadelphia, pp 987–997

Sindrup SH, Gram LF, Skjold T, Grodum E, Brøsin K, Bech-Nielsen H 1990a Clomipramine vs. desipramine in the treatment of diabetic neuropathy symptoms. A double-blind cross-over study. British Journal of Clinical Pharmacology 30:683–691

Sindrup SH, Gram LF, Brøsen K, Eshøj O, Mogense EF 1990b The selective serotonin reuptake inhibitor paroxetine is effective in the treatment of diabetic neuropathy symptoms. Pain 42:135–144

Sindrup SH, Gram LF, Skjold T, Frøland A, Beck-Nielsen H 1990c Concentration-response relationship in imipramine treatment of diabetic neuropathy symptom. Clinical Pharmacology and Therapy 47:509–515

Singer E, Placheta P 1980 Reduction of 3H-muscimol binding sites in rat dorsal spinal cord after neonatal capsaicin treatment. Brain Research 202: 484–487

Sivilotti L, Woolf CJ 1994 The contribution of $GABA_A$ and glycine receptors to central sensitization: disinhibition and touch-evoked allodynia in the spinal cord. Journal of Neurophysiology 72: 169–179

Skilling SR, Smulling DH, Beitz AJ, Larson AA 1988 Extracellular amino acid concentrations in the dorsal spinal cord of freely moving rats following veratridine and nociceptive stimulation. Journal of Neurochemistry 51: 127–132

Smith DJ, Perrotti JM, Crisp T, Cabral ME, Long JT, Scalzitti JM 1988 The mu opiate receptor is responsible for descending pain inhibition originating in the periaqueductal gray region of the rat brain. European Journal of Pharmacology 156: 47–54

Smith G, Harrison S, Bowers J, Wiseman J, Birch P 1994 Non-specific effects of the tachykinin NK1 receptor antagonist, CP-99, 994, in antinociceptive tests in rat mouse and gerbil. European Journal of Pharmacology 271: 481–487

Sollevi A 1997 Adenosine for pain control. Acta Anaesthesiologica Scandinavica. Supplementum 110: 135–136

Solomon RE, Gebhart GF 1988 Mechanisms of effects of intrathecal serotonin on nociception and blood pressure in rats. Journal of Pharmacology and Experimental Therapeutics 245: 905–912

Sorkin LS 1992 Release of amino acids and PGE_2 into the spinal cord of lightly anesthetized rats during development of an experimental arthritis: enhancement of C-fiber evoked release. Society of Neuroscience Abstracts 429: 10

Sorkin LS, Carlton S 1997 Spinal anatomy and pharmacology of afferent processing. In: Yaksh TL, Lynch III C, Zapol WM, Maze M, Biebuyck JF, Saidmar LJ (eds) Anesthesia: biologic foundations. Lippincott–Raven, Philadelphia, pp 577–610

Sorkin LS, Puig S 1996 Neuronal model of tactile allodynia produced by spinal strychnine: effects of excitatory amino acid receptor antagonists and a mu-opiate opiate receptor agonist. Pain 68: 283–292

Sorkin LS, McAdoo DJ, Willis WD 1992a Stimulation in the ventral posterior lateral nucleus of the primate thalamus leads to release of serotonin in the lumbar spinal cord. Brain Research 581: 307–310

Sorkin LS, Westlund KN, Sluka KA, Dougherty PM, Willis WD 1992b Neural changes in acute arthritis in monkeys. IV. Time-course of amino acid release into the lumbar dorsal horn. Brain Research. Brain Research Reviews 17: 39–50

Sosnowski M, Yaksh TL 1989 Role of spinal adenosine receptors in modulating the hyperesthesia produced by spinal glycine receptor antagonism. Anesthesia and Analgesia 69: 587–592

Sosnowski M, Stevens CW, Yaksh TL 1989 Assessment of the role of A1/A2 adenosine receptors mediating the purine antinociception, motor and autonomic function in the rat spinal cord. Journal of Pharmacology and Experimental Therapeutics 250: 915–922

Spiegel K, Kalb R, Pasternak W 1983 Analgesic activity of tricyclic antidepressants. Annals of Neurology 13: 462–465

Stark P, Fuller RW, Wong DT 1985 The pharmacologic profile of fluoxetine. Journal of Clinical Psychiatry 46:7–13

Steinman JL, Komisaruk BR, Yaksh TL, Tyce GM 1983 Spinal cord monoamines mediate the antinociceptive effects of vaginal stimulation in rats. Pain 16: 156–166

Stevens CW 1991 Intraspinal opioids in frogs: a new behavioral model for the assessment of opioid action. Nida Research Monograph 105: 561–562

Stevens CW, Sangha S, Ogg BG 1995 Analgesia produced by immobilization stress and an enkephalinase inhibitor in amphibians. Pharmacology, Biochemistry and Behavior 51: 675–680

Stucky CL, Galeazza MT, Seybold VS 1993 Time-dependent changes in Bolton-Hunter-labeled ^{125}I-substance P binding in rat spinal cord following unilateral adjuvant-induced peripheral inflammation. Neuroscience 57: 397–409

Suh HH, Tseng LL 1990 Intrathecal administration of thiorphan and bestatin enhances the antinociception and release of Met-enkephalin induced by beta-endorphin intraventricularly in anesthetized rats. Neuropeptides 16: 91–96

Sun X, Larson AA 1991 Behavioral sensitization to kainic acid and quisqualic acid in mice: comparison to NMDA and substance P responses. Journal of Neuroscience 11: 3111–3123

Sweeney MI, White TD, Sawynok J 1989 Morphine, capsaicin and K^+ release purines from capsaicin-sensitive primary afferent nerve terminals in the spinal cord. Journal of Pharmacology and Experimental Therapeutics 248: 447–454

Sweeney MI, White TD, Sawynok J 1990 5-Hydroxytryptamine releases adenosine and cyclic AMP from primary afferent nerve terminals in the spinal cord in vivo. Brain Research 528: 55–61

Sweeney MI, White TD, Sawynok J 1991 Intracerebroventricular morphine releases adenosine and adenosine 3′, 5′-cyclic monophosphate from the spinal cord via a serotonergic mechanism. Journal of Pharmacology and Experimental Therapeutics 259: 1008–1013

Swerdlow NR, Vaccarino FJ, Amalric M, Koob GF 1986 The neural substrates for the motor activating properties of psychostimulants: a review of recent findings. Pharmacology Biochemistry and Behavior 25: 233–248

Taenzer P, Melzack R, Jeans ME 1986 Influence of psychological factors on postoperative pain, mood and analgesic requirements. Pain 24: 331–342

Taiwo YO, Levine JD 1986 Indomethacin blocks central nociceptive effects of PGF2a. Brain Research 373: 81–84

Takagi H, Satoh M, Akaike A, Shibata T, Kuraishi Y 1977 The nucleus reticularis gigantocellularis of the medulla oblongata is a highly sensitive site in the production of morphine analgesia in the rat. European Journal of Pharmacology 45: 91–92

Takagi H, Satoh M, Akaike A, Shibata T, Yajima H, Ogawa H 1978 Analgesia by enkephalins injected into the nucleus reticularis gigantocellularis of rat medulla oblongata. European Journal of Pharmacology 49: 113–116

Takagi H, Shiomi H, Kuraishi Y, Fukui K, Ueda H 1979 Pain and the bulbospinal noradrenergic system: pain-induced increase in normetanephrine content in the spinal cord and its modification by morphine. European Journal of Pharmacology 54: 99–107

Takahashi H, Miyazaki M, Nanbu T, Yanagida H, Morita S 1998 The NMDA-receptor antagonist ketamine abolishes neuropathic pain after epidural administration in a clinical case. Pain 75: 391–394

Takano Y, Yaksh TL 1992 Characterization of the pharmacology of intrathecally administered alpha-2 agonists and antagonist in rats. Journal of Pharmacology and Experimental Therapeutics 261: 764–772

Takano Y, Takano M, Yaksh TL 1992 The effect of intrathecally administered imiloxan and WB4101: possible role of a2-adrenoceptor subtypes in the spinal cord. European Journal of Pharmacology 219: 465–468

Takano M, Takano Y, Yaksh TL 1993 Release of calcitonin gene-related peptide (CGRP), substance P (SP), and vasoactive intestinal polypeptide (VIP) from rat spinal cord: modulation by α2 agonists. Peptides 14: 371–378

Tallarida RJ, Porreca F, Cowan A 1989 Statistical analysis of drug-drug and site-site interactions with isobolograms. Life Sciences 45: 947–961

Tao R, Auerbach SB 1995 Involvement of the dorsal raphe but not median raphe nucleus in morphine-induced increases in serotonin release in the rat forebrain. Neuroscience 68: 553–561

Taylor BK, Peterson MA, Basbaum AI 1997 Early nociceptive events influence the temporal profile, but not the magnitude, of the tonic response to subcutaneous formalin: effects with remifentanil. Journal of Pharmacology and Experimental Therapeutics 280: 876–883

Tenen SS 1968 Antagonism of the analgesic effect of morphine and other drugs by p-chlorophenylalanine, a serotonin depletor. Psychopharmacology 12: 278–285

Thompson SWN, King AE, Woolf CJ 1990 Activity dependent changes in rat ventral horn neurons in vitro: summation of prolonged afferent evoked postsynaptic depolarizations produce a D-APV sensitive windup. European Journal of Neuroscience 2: 638–649

Tiseo PJ, Adler MW, Liu-Chen L-Y 1990 Differential release of substance P and somatostatin in the rat spinal cord in response to noxious cold and heat; effect of dynorphin A(1–17). Journal of Pharmacology and Experimental Therapeutics 252: 539–545

Tobias JD, Deshpande JK, Wetzel RC, Facker J, Maxwell LG, Solca M 1990 Postoperative analgesia. Use of intrathecal morphine in children. Clinical Pediatrics 29: 44–48

Todd AJ, McKenzie J 1989 GABA-immunoreactive neurons in the dorsal horn of the spinal cord. Neuroscience 31: 799–806

Todd AJ, Sullivan AC 1990 Light microscopic study of the coexistence of GABA-like and glycine-like immunoreactivities in the spinal cord of the rat. Journal of Comparative Neurology 296: 496–505

Torebjörk HE, Lundberg LE, LaMotte RH 1992 Central changes in processing of mechanoreceptive input in capsaicin-induced secondary hyperalgesia in humans. Journal of Physiology 448: 765–780

Tracey DJ, De Biasi S, Phend K, Rustioni A 1991 Aspartate-like immunoreactivity in primary afferent neurons. Neuroscience 40: 673–686

Tsai C, Nakamura S, Iwama K 1980 Inhibition of neuronal activity of the substantia nigra by noxious stimuli and its modification by the caudate nucleus. Brain Research 195: 299–311

Tseng LF, Collins KA 1992 Cholecystokinin administered intrathecally selectively antagonizes intracerebroventricular beta-endorphin-induced tail-flick inhibition in the mouse. Journal of Pharmacology and Experimental Therapeutics 260: 1086–1092

Tseng LF, Fujimoto JM 1985 Differential actions of intrathecal naloxone on blocking the tail flick inhibition induced by intraventricular B-endorphin and morphine in the rats. Journal of Pharmacology and Experimental Therapeutics 232: 74–79

Tseng LF, Tang R 1990 Different mechanisms mediate beta-endorphin- and morphine-induced inhibition of the tail-flick response in rats. Journal of Pharmacology and Experimental Therapeutics 252: 546–551

Tseng LF, Wang Q 1992 Forebrain sites differentially sensitive to beta-endorphin and morphine for analgesia and release of Met-enkephalin in the pentobarbital-anesthetized rat. Journal of Pharmacology and Experimental Therapeutics 261: 1028–1036

Tseng LL, Tang R, Stackman R, Camara A, Fujimoto JM 1990 Brainstem sites differentially sensitive to beta-endorphin and morphine for analgesia and release of met-enkephalin in anesthetized rats. Journal of Pharmacology and Experimental Therapeutics 253: 930–937

Tsou K 1963 Antagonism of morphine analgesia by the intracerebral microinjection of nalorphine. Acta Physiologica Sinica 26: 332–337

Tung AS, Yaksh TL 1982 The antinociceptive effects of epidural opiates in the cat: studies on the pharmacology and the effects of lipophilicity in spinal analgesia. Pain 12: 343–356

Turner JA, Romano JM 1984 Review of prevalence of coexisting chronic pain and depression. In: Benedetti C, Moricca G, Chapman CR (eds) Advances in pain research and therapy. Raven, New York, pp 123–130

Tyce GM, Yaksh TL 1981 Monoamine release from cat spinal cord by somatic stimuli: an intrinsic modulatory system. Journal of Physiology (London) 314: 513–529

Uda R, Horiguchi S, Ito SM, Hayaishi O 1990 Nociceptive effects by intrathecal administration of prostaglandin D2, E2 or F2a to conscious mice. Brain Research 510: 26–32

Urban L, Randic M 1984 Slow excitatory transmission in rat dorsal horn: possible mediation by peptides. Brain Research 290: 336–341

Vahle-Hinz C, Hicks TP, Gottschaldt KM 1994 Amino acids modify thalamo-cortical response transformation expressed by neurons of the ventrobasal complex. Brain Research 637: 139–155

van Praag H, Frenk H 1990 The role of glutamate in opiate descending inhibition of nociceptive reflexes. Brain Research 524: 101–105

Vasko MR, Cartwright S, Ono H 1986 Adenosine agonists do not inhibit the K^+ stimulated release of substance P from rat spinal cord slices. Society of Neuroscience Abstracts 12: 799

Vaugeois JM, Passera G, Zuccaro F, Costentin J 1997 Individual differences in response to imipramine in the mouse tail suspension test. Psychopharmacology 134: 387–391

Verge VMK, Wiesenfeld-Hallin Z, Høkfelt T 1993 Cholecystokinin in mammalian primary sensory neurons and spinal cord: In situ hybridization studies in rat and monkey. European Journal of Neuroscience 5: 240–250

Vidnyanszky Z, Hamori J, Negyessy L et al 1994 Cellular and subcellular localization of the mGluR5a metabotropic glutamate receptor in rat spinal cord. Neuroreport 6: 209–213

Vigouret J, Teschemacher H, Albus K, Herz A 1973 Differentiation between spinal and supraspinal sites of action of morphine when inhibiting the hind limb flexor reflex in rabbits. Neuropharmacology 12: 111–121

Vinik HR 1995 Intravenous anaesthetic drug interactions: practical applications. European Journal of Anaesthesiology 12 (suppl): 13–19

Wakisaka S, Kajander KC, Bennett GJ 1992 Effects of peripheral nerve injuries and tissue inflammation on the levels of neuropeptide Y-like immunoreactivity in rat primary afferent neurons. Brain Research 598: 349–352

Walker MW, Ewald DA, Perney TM, Miller RJ 1988 Neuropeptide Y Modulates neurotransmitter release and Ca^{2+} currents in rat sensory neurons. Journal of Neuroscience 8:2438–2446

Wallace MS, Laitin S, Licht D, Yaksh TL 1997 Concentration–effect relations for intravenous lidocaine infusions in human volunteers: effects on acute sensory thresholds and capsaicin-evoked hyperpathia. Anesthesiology 86: 1262–1272

Wamsley JK, Gehlert DR, Filloux FM, Dawson TM 1989 Comparison of the distribution of D-1 and D-2 dopamine receptors in the rat brain. Journal of Chemical Neuroanatomy 2: 119–137

Warren RA, Jones EG 1994 Glutamate activation of cat thalamic reticular nucleus: effects on response properties of ventroposterior neurons. Experimental Brain Research 100(2): 215–226

Watkins LR, Mayer DJ 1986 Multiple endogenous opiate and non-opiate analgesia systems: evidence of their existence and clinical implications. Annals of the New York Academy of Sciences 467:273–299

Watkins LR, Johannessen JN, Kinscheck IB, Mayer DJ 1984 The neurochemical basis of footshock analgesia: the role of spinal cord serotonin and norepinephrine. Brain Research 290: 107–171

Wedzony K, Mackowiak M, Fijal K, Golembiowska K 1996 Evidence that conditioned stress enhances outflow of dopamine in rat prefrontal cortex: a search for the influence of diazepam and 5-HT1A agonists. Synapse 24: 240–247

Westbrook RF, Good AJ, Kiernan MJ 1997 Microinjection of morphine into the nucleus accumbens impairs contextual learning in rats. Behavioral Neuroscience 111: 996–1013

Westlund KN, Sorkin LS, Ferrington DG, Carlton SM, Willcockson HH, Willis WD 1990 Serotoninergic and noradrenergic projections to the ventral posterolateral nucleus of the monkey thalamus. Journal of Comparative Neurology 295: 197–207

Wettstein JG, Kamerling SG, Martin WR 1982 Effects of microinjections of opioids into and electrical stimulation (ES) of the canine periaqueductal gray (PAG) on electrogenesis (EEG), heart rate (HR), pupil diameter (OPD), behavior and analgesia. Neuroscience Abstract 8: 229

Wheeler-Aceto H, Porreca F, Cowan A 1990 The rat paw formalin test: comparison of noxious agents. Pain 40: 229–238

White WF 1985 The glycine receptor in the mutant mouse spastic (spa): strychnine binding characteristics and pharmacology. Brain Research 329: 1–6

White WF, Heller AH 1982 Glycine receptor alteration in the mutant mouse spastic. Nature 298: 655–657

Whiting WC, Sandler AN, Lau LC et al 1988 Analgesic and respiratory effects of epidural sufentanil in patients following thoracotomy. Anesthesiology 69: 36–43

Wiertelak EP, Maier SF, Watkins LR 1992 Cholecystokinin antianalgesia: safety cues abolish morphine analgesia. Science 256: 830–833

Wiesenfeld-Hallin Z, Villar MJ, Høkfelt T 1988 Intrathecal galanin at low doses increases spinal reflex excitability in rats more to thermal than mechanical stimuli. Experimental Brain Research 71: 663–666

Wikler A 1950 Sites and mechanisms of action of morphine and related drugs in the central nervous system. Pharmacological Reviews 2: 435–506

Willis WD, Coggeshall RE 1991 Sensory mechanisms of the spinal cord, 2nd edn. Plenum, New York

Woodley SJ, Kendig JJ 1991 Substance P and NMDA receptors mediate a slow nociceptive ventral root potential in neonatal rat spinal cord. Brain Research 559: 17–21

Woolf CJ, King AE 1987 Physiology and morphology of multireceptive neurons with C-afferent fiber inputs in the deep dorsal horn of the rat lumbar spinal cord. Journal of Neurophysiology 58: 460–479

Woolf CJ, Thompson WN 1991 The induction and maintenance of central sensitization is dependent on *N*-methyl D-aspartic acid receptor activation, implications for the treatment of post-injury pain hypersensitivity states. Pain 44: 293–299

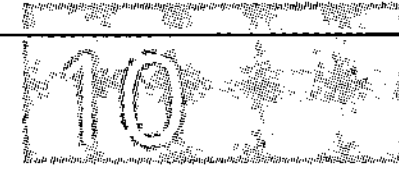

Xia LY, Huang KH, Rosenfeld JP 1992 Behavioral and trigeminal neuronal effects of rat brainstem-nanoinjected opiates. Physiology and Behavior 52: 65–73

Yaksh TL 1978a Inhibition by etorphine of the discharge of dorsal horn neurons: effects upon the neuronal response to both high- and low-threshold sensory input in the decerebrate spinal cat. Experimental Neurology 60: 23–40

Yaksh TL 1978b Analgetic actions of intrathecal opiates in cat and primate. Brain Research 153: 205–210

Yaksh TL 1979 Direct evidence that spinal serotonin and noradrenaline terminals mediate the spinal antinociceptive effects of morphine in the periaqueductal gray. Brain Research 160: 180–185

Yaksh TL 1982 Central and peripheral mechanisms for the analgesic action of acetylsalicylic acid. In: Barett HJM, Hirsh J, Mustard JF (eds) Acetylsalicylic acid: new uses for an old drug. Raven, New York, pp 137–151

Yaksh TL 1983 In vivo studies on spinal opiate receptor systems mediating antinociception. Mu and delta receptor profiles in the primate. Journal of Pharmacology and Experimental Therapeutics 226: 303–316

Yaksh TL 1987 Spinal opiates: a review of their effect on spinal function with emphasis on pain processing. Acta Anaesthesiologica Scandinavica 31: 25–37

Yaksh TL 1989 Behavioral and autonomic correlates of the tactile evoked allodynia produced by spinal glycine inhibition: effects of modulatory receptor systems and excitatory amino acid antagonists. Pain 37: 111–123

Yaksh TL 1997a Preclinical models of nociception. In: Yaksh TL, Lynch III C, Zapol WM, Maze M, Biebuyck JF, Saidman LJ (eds) Anesthesia: Biologic Foundations. Lippincott–Raven, Philadelphia, pp 685–718

Yaksh TL 1997b Pharmacology and mechanisms of opioid analgesic activity. In: Yaksh TL, Lynch III C, Zapol WM, Maze M, Biebuyck JF, Saidman LJ (eds) Anesthesia: biologic foundations. Lippincott–Raven, Philadelphia, pp 921–934

Yaksh TL 1997c Pharmacology and mechanisms of opioid analgesic activity. Acta Anaesthesiol Scand 41: 94–111

Yaksh TL, Chipkin RE 1989 Studies on the effect of SCH-34826 and thiorphan on [Met5] enkephalin levels and release in rat spinal cord. European Journal of Pharmacology 167: 367–373

Yaksh TL, Elde RP 1981 Factors governing release of methionine enkephalin-like immunoreactivity from mesencephalon and spinal cord of the cat in vivo. Neurophysiology 46: 1056–1075

Yaksh TL, Malkmus SA 1998 Animal models of intrathecal and epidural drug delivery. In: Yaksh TL (ed) Spinal drug delivery. Elsevier, Amsterdam, ch 13

Yaksh TL, Reddy SVR 1981 Studies in the primate on the analgetic effects associated with intrathecal actions of opiate, α-adrenergic agonists and baclofen. Anesthesiology 54: 451–467

Yaksh TL, Rudy TA 1976a Analgesia mediated by a direct spinal action of narcotics. Science 192: 1357–1358

Yaksh TL, Rudy TA 1976b Chronic catheterization of the spinal subarachnoid space. Physiology and Behavior 17: 1031–1036

Yaksh TL, Rudy TA 1977 Studies on the direct spinal action of narcotics in the production of analgesia in the rat. Journal of Pharmacology and Experimental Therapy 202:411–428

Yaksh TL, Rudy TA 1978 Narcotic analgesics: CNS sites and mechanisms of action as revealed by intracerebral injection techniques. Pain 4: 299–359

Yaksh TL, Tyce GM 1979 Microinjection of morphine into the periaqueductal gray evokes the release of serotonin from spinal cord. Brain Research 171: 176–181

Yaksh TL, Yeung JC, Rudy TA 1976 Systematic examination in the rat of brain sites sensitive to the direct application of morphine: observation of differential effect within the periaqueductal gray. Brain Research 114: 83–103

Yaksh TL, Plant RL, Rudy TA 1977 Studies on the antagonism by raphe lesions of the antinociceptive actions of systemic morphine. European Journal of Pharmacology 41: 399–408

Yaksh TL, Jessell TM, Gamse R, Mudge R, Leeman SE 1980 Intrathecal morphine inhibits substance P release from mammalian spinal cord in vivo. Nature 286: 155–156

Yaksh TL, Abay EO, Go VLW 1982a Studies on the location and release of cholecystokinin and vasoactive intestinal peptide in the rat and cat spinal cord. Brain Research 242: 279–290

Yaksh TL, Gross KE, Li CH 1982b Studies in the intrathecal effect of β-endorphin in primate. Brain Research 241: 261–269

Yaksh TL, Dirksen R, Harty GJ 1985 Antinociceptive effects of intrathecally injected cholinomimetic drugs in the rat and cat. European Journal of Pharmacology 117: 81–88

Yaksh TL, Noueihed RY, Durant PAC 1986 Studies of the pharmacology and pathology of intrathecally administered 4-anilinopiperidine analogues and morphine in rat and cat. Anesthesiology 64: 54–66

Yaksh TL, Michener SR, Bailey JE et al 1988a Survey of distribution of substance P, vasoactive intestinal polypeptide, cholecystokinin, neurotensin, met-enkephalin, bombesin and PHI in the spinal cord of cat, dog, sloth and monkey. Peptides 9: 357–372

Yaksh TL, Al-Rodhan NRF, Jensen TS 1988b Sites of action of opiates in production of analgesia. Progress in Brain Research 77: 371–394

Yaksh TL, Sabbe MB, Lucas D, Mjanger E, Chipkin RE 1991 Effects of [*N*-(L-(1-carboxy-2-phenyl) ethyl]-L-phenylalanyl-β-alanine (SCH32615), a neutral endopeptidase (enkephalinase) inhibitor, on levels of enkephalin, encrypted enkephalins and substance P in cerebrospinal fluid and plasma of primates. Journal of Pharmacology and Experimental Therapeutics 256: 1033–1041

Yaksh TL, Yamamoto T, Myers RR 1992 Pharmacology of nerve compression-evoked hyperesthesia. In: Willis WD (ed) Hyperalgesia and allodynia. Raven, New York, pp 245–258

Yamamoto T, Yaksh TL 1991a Stereospecific effects of a nonpeptidic NKl selective antagonist, CP, 96–345: antinociception in the absence of motor dysfunction. Life Sciences 49: 1955–1963

Yamamoto T, Yaksh TL 1991b Spinal pharmacology of thermal hyperesthesia induced by incomplete ligation of sciatic nerve. I. Opioid and nonopioid receptors. Anesthesiology 75: 817–826

Yamamoto T, Yaksh TL 1992a Comparison of the antinociceptive effects of pre and post treatment with intrathecal morphine and MK801, an NMDA antagonist on the formalin test in the rat. Anesthesiology 77: 757–763

Yamamoto T, Yaksh TL 1992b Effects of intrathecal capsaicin and an NK-1 antagonist, CP, 96–345, on the thermal hyperalgesia observed following unilateral constriction of the sciatic-nerve in the rat. Pain 51: 329–334

Yamamoto T, Yaksh L 1993 Effects of intrathecal strychnine and bicuculline on nerve compression-induced thermal hyperesthesia and selective antagonism by MK801. Pain 54: 79–84

Yanez A, Sabbe MB, Stevens CW, Yaksh TL 1990 Interaction of midazolam and morphine in the spinal cord of the rat. Neuropharmacology 29: 359–364

Yashpal K, Radhakrishnan V, Coderre TJ, Henry JL 1993 CP-96, 345 but not its stereoisomer, CP-96 344, blocks the nociceptive responses to intrathecally administered Substance-P and to noxious thermal and chemical stimuli in the rat. Neuroscience 52:1039–1047

Yashpal K, Wright DM, Henry JL 1982 Substance P reduces tail flick latency: implication for chronic pain syndromes. Pain 15: 155–167

Yeung JC, Rudy TA 1980 Multiplicative interaction between narcotic agonism expressed at spinal and supraspinal sites of antinociceptive action as revealed by concurrent intrathecal and intracerebroventricular injections of morphine. Journal of Pharmacology and Experimental Therapeutics 215: 633–642

Yokota T, Nishikawa N, Nishikawa Y 1979 Effects of strychnine upon different classes of trigeminal subnucleus caudalis neurons. Brain Research 168: 430–434

Yoshimura M, Jessell TM 1989 Primary afferent evoked synaptic response and slow potential generation in rat substantia gelatinosa neurons in vitro. Journal of Neurophysiology 622: 96–108

Young MR, Fleetwood-Walker SM, Dickinson T et al 1997 Behavioural and electrophysiological evidence supporting a role for group I metabotropic glutamate receptors in the mediation of nociceptive inputs to the rat spinal cord. Brain Research 777: 161–169

Young MR, Fleetwood-Walker SM, Mitchell R, Munro FE 1994 Evidence for a role of metabotropic glutamate receptors in sustained nociceptive inputs to rat dorsal horn neurons. Neuropharmacology 33: 141–144

Yu LC, Han JS 1989 Involvement of arcuate nucleus of hypothalamus in the descending pathway from nucleus accumbens to periaqueductal grey subserving an antinociceptive effect. International Journal of Neuroscience 48: 71–78

Zacny JP, Coalson DW, Klafta JM et al 1996 Midazolam does not influence intravenous fentanyl-induced analgesia in healthy volunteers. Pharmacology, Biochemistry and Behavior 55: 275–280

Zahn PK, Umali E, Brennan TJ 1998 Intrathecal non-NMDA excitatory amino acid receptor antagonists inhibit pain behaviors in a rat model of postoperative pain. Pain 74: 213–223

Zarbin MA, Wamsley JK, Kuhar MJ 1981 Glycine receptor: light microscopic autoradiographic localization with [3H] strychnine. Journal of Neuroscience 1: 532–547

Zemlan FP, Behbehani MM 1988 Nucleus cuneiformis and pain modulation: anatomy and behavioral pharmacology. Brain Research 453: 89–102

Zhang DX, Carlton SM, Sorkin LS, Willis WD 1990a Collaterals of primate spinothalamic tract neurons to the periaqueductal gray. Journal of Comparative Neurology 296: 277–290

Zhang SP, Bandler R, Carrive P 1990b Flight and immobility evoked by excitatory amino acid microinjection within distinct parts of the subtentorial midbrain periaqueductal gray of the cat. Brain Research 520: 73–82

Zhang X, Ju G, Elde R, Høkfelt T 1993 Effect of peripheral nerve cut on neuropeptides in dorsal root ganglia and the spinal cord of monkey with special reference to galanin. Journal Neurocytology 22: 342–381

Zhang X, Wiesenfeld-Hallin Z, Høkfelt T 1994 Effect of peripheral axotomy on expression of neuropeptide Y receptor mRNA in rat lumbar dorsal root ganglia. European Journal of Neuroscience 6: 43–57

Zhuo M, Gebhart GF 1991 Tonic cholinergic inhibition of spinal mechanical transmission. Pain 46: 211–222

Zhuo M, Gebhart GF 1992 Inhibition of a cutaneous nociceptive reflex by a noxious visceral stimulus is mediated by spinal cholinergic and descending serotonergic systems in the rat. Brain Research 585: 7–18

Zieglgänsberger W, Herz A 1971 Changes of cutaneous receptive fields of spino-cervical-tract neurones and other dorsal horn neurons by microelectrophoretically administered amino acids. Experimental Brain Research 13: 111–126

Central nervous system mechanisms of pain modulation

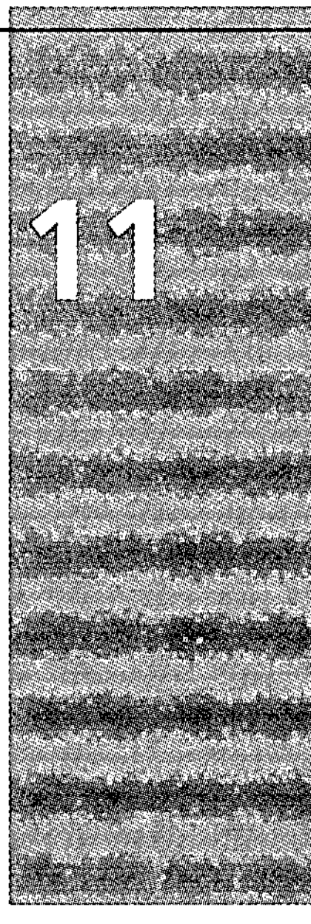

HOWARD L. FIELDS & ALLAN I. BASBAUM

INTRODUCTION

The relationship between reported pain intensity and the peripheral stimulus that evokes it depends on several factors, including arousal, attention and expectation. These psychological factors in turn are influenced by contextual cues that establish the significance of the stimulus and help determine an appropriate response to it. For example, traumatic injuries sustained during athletic competitions or combat are often initially reported as being relatively painless (Melzack & Wall 1982). In other circumstances, these same injuries can be extremely painful (Beecher 1959). The alteration of neural, behavioural and subjective pain responses by arousal, attention and expectation result from the action of central nervous system (CNS) networks that modulate the transmission of nociceptive messages. Presumably, pain-modulating circuits exist because the ability to suppress reflexes or pain behaviours, for example to facilitate escape in the face of threat, can enhance the survival of the individual.

The study of pain-modulating networks is challenging. Factors such as arousal and attention, which engage pain-modulatory networks, can only be studied in awake behaving animals (Duncan et al 1987, Oliveras et al 1990). Nonetheless, significant progress has been made; anatomically distinct and physiologically selective CNS pain-modulating networks have been identified and their pharmacology elucidated. One of these networks has links in the amygdala, hypothalamus and brainstem, controls nociresponsive dorsal horn neurons and is sensitive to opioids. This is the most extensively studied and will be the primary focus of this chapter.

DESCENDING MODULATORY CONTROL

As early as 1911 Head & Holmes explicitly postulated modulatory influences on pain. They proposed that the thalamus is the centre for the perception of pain and that the neocortex, the discriminative perception centre, continuously modulates the responses of the thalamus to noxious stimuli. According to their hypothesis, modulation of pain is a necessary part of the on-going process of discriminative sensation. Clearcut examples of descending modulation of sensory transmission were subsequently described. Hagbarth & Kerr (1954) provided the first direct evidence that supraspinal sites control ascending (presumably sensory) pathways and Carpenter et al (1965) demonstrated descending control of sensory input to ascending pathways. The existence of a specific *pain* modulatory system was, however, first clearly articulated in 1965 by Melzack & Wall in 'the Gate Control Theory' of pain. Supraspinal influences on the 'gate' were proposed but there was limited evidence for descending control of nociception. In 1967, Wall demonstrated that structures in the brainstem tonically inhibit nociresponsive neurons in the spinal cord.

The midbrain periaqueductal grey and stimulation-produced analgesia

Evidence that descending systems can *selectively* modulate pain was first provided by the discovery of stimulation-produced analgesia (SPA) (Reynolds 1969, Mayer et al 1971, Mayer & Price 1976). SPA is a highly specific suppression of behavioural responses to noxious stimuli produced by electrical stimulation of discrete brain sites. SPA was first elicited by electrical stimulation of the midbrain periaqueductal grey (PAG). During SPA, animals remain alert and active and, although their responses to most environmental stimuli are unchanged, their responses to noxious stimuli such as orientation, vocalization and escape are absent. Thus, in animals, SPA is both highly selective and robust.

An SPA-like effect can also be produced in humans (Boivie & Meyerson 1982, Baskin et al 1986). In patients with chronic pain, SPA is produced without eliciting any movement or consistent subjective sensation. As in rodents, SPA in humans is elicited by electrical stimulation of the PAG. Although this procedure is rarely performed at the present time, the specificity of the analgesic effect and the fact that it is consistently elicited from discrete brain sites that are homologous in a variety of species is important evidence that there is a pain-selective modulating system in humans.

The discovery of the pain-modulating effect of the PAG was a critical advance in understanding the mechanism of pain modulation. Subsequent research demonstrated that the PAG is part of a CNS circuit that controls nociceptive transmission at the level of the spinal cord (Mayer & Price 1976, Basbaum & Fields 1978, Fields 1988) (Fig. 11.1). In animals, SPA is associated with the inhibition of noxious stimulus-evoked reflexes, such as the tail flick, which are mediated by intraspinal connections. Furthermore, nociceptive neurons in the spinal cord dorsal horn are selectively inhibited by PAG stimulation and lesions of the spinal cord dorsolateral funiculus (DLF) block the brainstem inhibition of both nociceptive dorsal horn neurons and reflex responses to noxious stimuli (Basbaum et al 1976).

The PAG integrates inputs from the limbic forebrain and diencephalon with ascending nociceptive input from the dorsal horn (Bandler & Keay 1996). There are direct projections to the PAG from medial prefrontal and insular cortex (Hardy & Leichnetz 1981, Bandler & Shipley 1994). A major diencephalic source of afferents to the PAG is the hypothalamus (Beitz 1982a, Reichling & Basbaum 1990), and electrical stimulation or opioid microinjection in certain hypothalamic regions produces analgesia (Rhodes & Liebeskind 1978, Manning et al 1994).

The amygdala, which receives massive input from both the hippocampus and neocortex, is another major source of afferents to the PAG (Amaral et al 1992, Gray & Magnuson 1992). Analgesia resulting from microinjection of opioid agonists into the amygdala is blocked by lidocaine inactivation of (Helmstetter et al 1998) or opioid antagonist injection into the PAG (Pavlovic et al 1996).

Major brainstem inputs to the PAG arise from the adjacent nucleus cuneiformis, the pontomedullary reticular formation, the locus coeruleus and other brainstem catecholaminergic nuclei (Herbert & Saper 1992). The PAG is reciprocally connected with the rostral ventromedial medulla (see below). Finally, the PAG and adjacent nucleus cuneiformis receive a significant projection from spinal lamina I nociceptive neurons (Menétrey et al 1982, Hylden et al 1986).

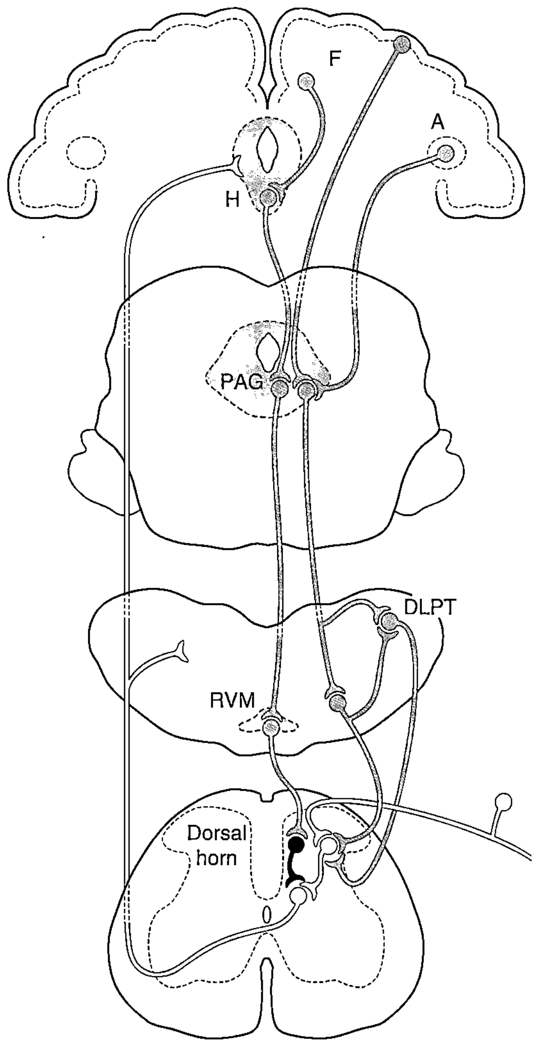

Fig. 11.1 Diagram of a major pain modulating pathway with major links in the midbrain periaqueductal gray (PAG) and rostral ventromedial medulla (RVM). Regions of the frontal lobe (F) and amygdala (A) project directly and via the hypothalamus to the PAG. The PAG in turn controls spinal nociceptive neurons through relays in the RVM and the dorsolateral pontine tegmentum (DLPT). The RVM, which projects directly and via the DLPT to the dorsal horn, exerts bidirectional control over nociceptive transmission. The control by RVM and DLPT involves both inhibitory (filled) and excitatory (unfilled) interneurons.

The PAG is cytoarchitectonically and chemically heterogeneous and has subdivisions which differ in their contribution to analgesia and autonomic control (Cannon et al 1982, Lovick 1993, Bandler & Shipley 1994, Keay et al 1994). For example, the major descending outflow from the *ventrolateral* PAG is to the nucleus raphe magnus (see below). By contrast, the *dorsolateral* PAG projects primarily to the dorsolateral pons (including the A5 noradrenergic cell group) and the ventrolateral medulla (Van Bockstaele et al 1991, Cameron et al 1995), areas which have been

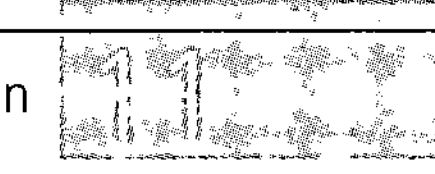

implicated in autonomic control. The PAG also projects rostrally to the medial thalamus and orbital frontal cortex, raising the possibility of ascending control of nociception (Coffield et al 1992).

The rostral ventromedial medulla

The rostral ventromedial medulla (RVM) includes the midline nucleus raphe magnus (NRM) and the adjacent reticular formation that lies ventral to the nucleus reticularis gigantocellularis. Electrical stimulation or microinjection of opioids or excitatory amino acids into the RVM produces analgesia and inhibits spinal dorsal horn neuronal responses to noxious stimulation (Basbaum & Fields 1984, Fields et al 1991).

The PAG and the adjacent nucleus cuneiformis are the major source of inputs to the RVM. Although the PAG contains a large number of enkephalin, substance P (SP) and gamma-aminobutyric acid containing (GABAergic) neurons (Hökfelt et al 1977a,b, Moss et al 1983), few of these neurons project to the RVM (Prichard & Beitz 1981, Ramírez & Vanegas 1989). The RVM does, however, receive an input from serotonin (5HT)-containing neurons of the dorsal raphe (Beitz 1982a) and there is a neurotensinergic connection between the PAG and the RVM (Beitz 1982a, Urban & Smith 1993, 1994a). The RVM also receives a major direct projection from the medial preoptic region of the hypothalamus (Shipley et al 1996). Direct spinal projections to the RVM are sparse but the RVM may receive spinal input indirectly from the PAG and nucleus cuneiformis. Another indirect route for spinal input is from the adjacent medullary nucleus reticularis gigantocellularis which has a large projection from nociceptive spinoreticular neurons and projects massively to the RVM (Fields et al 1977a). The RVM also receives noradrenergic input from the A5 and A7 cell groups of the dorsolateral pontomesencephalic tegmentum (Clark & Proudfit 1991a).

The PAG–RVM connection is critical for pain modulation. The PAG projects only minimally to the spinal cord dorsal horn and the pain-modulating action of the PAG upon the spinal cord is relayed largely, if not exclusively, through the RVM. Thus, anatomical lesions, reversible inactivation with lidocaine or microinjection of excitatory amino acid receptor antagonists into the RVM abolish the analgesia produced by stimulation of the PAG (Behbehani & Fields 1979, Aimone & Gebhart 1986, Urban & Smith 1994b).

The RVM is the major brainstem source of axons that project to the spinal cord dorsal horn. Electrical stimulation of the RVM selectively inhibits nociceptive dorsal horn neurons, an effect that is blocked by DLF lesions (Fields et al 1977b, 1991, Willis et al 1977, Basbaum & Fields 1978). The spinal terminals of RVM descending axons are most dense in dorsal horn laminae I, II (the substantia gelatinosa) and V (Basbaum et al 1978). These laminae are targets of nociceptive primary afferents and their constituent neurons respond maximally to stimuli that are noxious (Willis & Coggeshill 1991; and see Chapter 6). Most lamina II neurons are excitatory interneurons that relay inputs from primary afferents to marginal layer neurons (Bennett et al 1979). Other interneurons in laminae I and II contain inhibitory neurotransmitters (e.g. GABA and enkephalin; Todd et al 1992) and are a likely source of the inhibitory transmitters in terminals on projection neurons (see below).

The dorsolateral pontomesencephalic tegmentum

The dorsolateral area of the pontine and midbrain tegmentum also plays a critical role in the pain-modulating actions of the PAG and RVM (Haws et al 1989). The dorsolateral pontomesencephalic tegmentum (DLPT) includes the nucleus cuneiformis which is adjacent to the ventrolateral PAG (vlPAG) and shares many of its anatomical features, including an input from lamina I of the dorsal horn and a major projection to the RVM. Because its anatomical connections are similar to the vlPAG and because electrical stimulation of the nucleus cuneiformis inhibits dorsal horn nociceptive transmission via the RVM, it is reasonable to think of the RVM-projecting neurons of the vlPAG and the nucleus cuneiformis as a functional entity. Other regions within the DLPT, including the subcoerulear and parabrachial nuclei, also project to the RVM, to the spinal cord dorsal horn or both (Proudfit 1988, Clark & Proudfit 1991b, Kwiat & Basbaum 1992).

Brainstem noradrenergic neurons

Spinally-projecting brainstem noradrenergic neurons contribute significantly to pain modulation (Proudfit 1988). The DLPT includes all of the noradrenergic neurons that project to the RVM and spinal cord (Fig. 11.2). The locus coeruleus (LC) and the A5 and A7 group of noradrenaline (NA)-containing neurons are the major source of noradrenergic projections to the dorsal horn (Clark & Proudfit 1991b, Kwiat & Basbaum 1992). Electrical stimulation of all three sites inhibits spinal withdrawal reflexes and dorsal horn nociceptive neurons (Carstens et al 1980, Proudfit 1988, Haws et al 1989). Furthermore, electrical stimulation of the DLPT is reported to relieve clinically significant

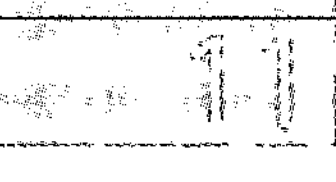

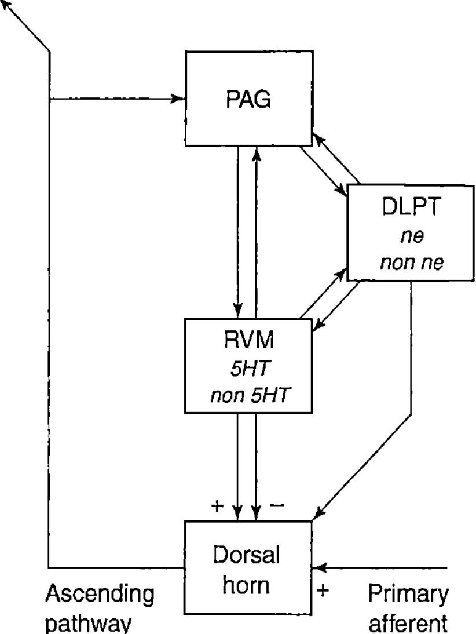

Fig. 11.2 Brainstem connections relevant to the pain modulating system illustrated in Figure 11.1. The RVM contains both serotonergic (5HT) and non-serotonergic projections to the dorsal horn. The DLPT provides the noradrenergic (ne) innervation of the dorsal horn.

chronic pain in people (Young et al 1992). Lesions of the LC exacerbate the allodynia associated with acute inflammation, which suggests that inhibitory controls are activated under these conditions (Tsuruoka & Willis 1996). Furthermore, destruction of the LC to spinal cord noradrenergic projection enhances the hyperalgesia of opioid abstinence (Rohde & Basbaum 1998). In general, noradrenergic inhibitory controls are mediated at the spinal level by the α_2 adrenoceptor (Yeomans et al 1992, Peng et al 1996). The importance of the spinal α_2 adrenoceptor to analgesia is strongly supported by clinical reports that intrathecal injection of α_2-adrenergic agonists produces significant analgesia (Glynn et al 1988, Curatolo et al 1997; and see Chapter 10).

Noradrenergic neurons in the DLPT provide an indirect relay for RVM actions on spinal cord nociceptive transmission. Electrical stimulation of the RVM evokes the release of NA in the spinal cord cerebrospinal fluid (CSF) (Hammond et al 1985). In addition, the inhibition of spinal withdrawal reflexes and nociceptive dorsal horn neurons by activation of the RVM is partially blocked by noradrenergic antagonists (Yaksh 1979, Barbaro et al 1985). The A7 region is a critical relay for RVM noradrenergic actions at spinal levels. The A7 is reciprocally connected to the RVM (Clark & Proudfit 1991a, Drolet et al 1992). Substance P-containing RVM neurons project to A7 (Yeomans et al 1990) and substance P microinjected into A7 produces a spinal antinociceptive effect that is blocked by intrathecal α-adrenergic antagonists (Yeomans et al 1992).

Opioid receptors and the endogenous opioid peptides

Morphine produces an analgesic effect when microinjected into the PAG, RVM and the amygdala (Yaksh & Rudy 1978, Fields et al 1991, Manning et al 1994; and see Chapter 10). Furthermore, inactivation of or microinjection of opioid antagonists into these sites reduces the analgesic effect of systemically administered opioids (Calvino et al 1982, Yaksh & Noueihed 1985, Manning & Mayer 1995, Manning & Franklin 1998). With the cloning of the three currently known opioid receptors (μ (MOR), δ (DOR) and κ (KOR)) and the generation of antibodies that selectively recognize them, it became possible to accurately map their CNS distribution. Each is present in the amygdala, hypothalamus, PAG, DLPT and RVM (Kuhar et al 1973, Atweh & Kuhar 1977, Mansour et al 1995). A neocortical area, the rostral anterior insular cortex, also has a high concentration of MOR and MOR agonists microinjected into this area produce analgesia (Burkey et al 1996).

The development of agonists and antagonists that are highly selective for the different opioid receptors and the study of mice with receptor gene knockouts has begun to clarify the contribution of each to pain modulation. Mu opioid receptor (MOR) agonists are the most effective analgesics, whether given systemically or by microinjection into the component nuclei of the pain-modulating circuit described above. Furthermore, in MOR knockout mice, morphine is completely ineffective, despite the fact that it has some affinity for both DOR and KOR (Goldstein & Naidu 1989, Akil et al 1997). It is intriguing that the analgesic effect of DOR agonists is markedly reduced in MOR knockout mice (Sora et al 1997). This raises the possibility that DOR agonists can elicit the release of endogenous opioid peptides acting at MOR.

At spinal sites, ligands for each of the three receptors can produce an analgesic effect, in part by reducing transmitter release from the dorsal horn terminals of primary afferent nociceptors. In vitro studies indicate that both MOR and DOR agonists block excitatory amino acid release from primary afferents (Glaum et al 1994, Grudt & Williams 1994). There is also evidence that opioids inhibit neuropeptide release from primary afferents Jessell & Iversen 1977, Suarez-Roca et al 1992). However, to what extent each receptor is found on primary afferents of a particular physiological class or on a subpopulation that contains a specific neuropeptide (e.g., substance P) is unclear.

At supraspinal sites, the effect of ligands selective for each opioid receptor is site dependent. For example, KOR agonists can produce an analgesic effect when injected into the third ventricle (Gogas et al 1995) but have an *anti-analgesic* effect when microinjected into the RVM (Pan et al 1997). DOR agonists have a modest analgesic effect when microinjected into the PAG (Rossi et al 1994) and RVM (Thorat & Hammond 1997).

Endogenous opioid peptides

The importance of endogenous opioid peptides to pain modulation was first suggested by reports that SPA in animals and humans is reduced by the narcotic antagonist naloxone (Akil et al 1976, Watkins & Mayer 1982). Hughes and his colleagues (Hughes et al 1975) isolated the first endogenous opioid peptides: the pentapeptides leucine (leu)- and methionine (met)-enkephalin (enk). In addition to the enkephalins, several other opioid peptides have been characterized (Miller 1981, Akil et al 1997) (Table 11.1). These include β-endorphin (BE), a 31-amino-acid peptide, the N-terminal of which is identical to met-enkephalin, and peptides with an N-terminal leu-enkephalin, which include dynorphin, a 17-amino-acid peptide, and the decapeptide α-neoendorphin (Table 11.1) (Goldstein et al 1979, Weber et al 1981). A fourth family of endogenous opioids, the endomorphins, has recently been discovered (Zadina et al 1997) (see below).

Peptide transmitters and hormones are derived by the cleavage of larger, usually inactive, precursor polypeptides. Met- and leu-enk are derived from a common precursor, preproenkephalin, each molecule of which generates multiple copies of met-enk and one of leu-enk (Comb et al 1982). BE is cleaved from a larger precursor protein, pro-opiomelanocortin, which also gives rise to adrenocorticotropic hormone (ACTH) and several copies of melanocyte-stimulating hormone (MSH) (Mains et al 1977). Two copies of dynorphin (A and B) and α-neoendorphin are generated from a third endogenous opioid precursor molecule (preprodynorphin).

Table 11.1 Sequences of endogenous opioid peptides involved in pain modulation

Leucine-enkephalin	Tyr-Gly-Gly-Phe-Leu-OH
Methionine-enkephalin	Tyr-Gly-Gly-Phe-Met-OH
β-endorphin	*Tyr-Gly-Gly-Phe-Met*-Thr-Ser-Glu-Lys-Ser-Gln-Thr-Pro-Leu-Val-Thr-Leu-Phe-Lys-Asn-Ala-Ile-Val-Lys-Asn-Ala-His-Lys-Gly-Gln-OH
Dynorphin	*Tyr-Gly-Gly-Phe-Leu*-Arg-Arg-Ile-Arg-Pro-Lys-Leu-Lys-Tyr-Asp-Asn-Gln-OH
Endomorphin I	Phe-Trp-Pro-Tyr-OH
Endomorphin II	Phe-Phe-Pro-Tyr-OH

There are discrete populations of BE-containing neurons in the ventromedial hypothalamus (Watson & Akil 1980). BE-containing neurons in the hypothalamus project to the PAG and have been implicated in the production of stimulation-produced and stress-induced analgesia (Millan et al 1986, 1987, Bach & Yaksh 1995). By contrast, the density of BE terminal fields in RVM is quite low. Met- and leu-enk are found in numerous cell groups throughout the neuraxis. Consistent with their having a common precursor, leu- and met-enk have completely overlapping distributions. Although the distribution of met- and leu-enk is not restricted to pain-modulating circuits, all of the CNS structures involved in opioid analgesia and pain modulation have significant levels of met- and leu-enk (Bloom et al 1978, Miller 1981, Khachaturian et al 1982, 1983, 1993, Moss et al 1983, Akil et al 1997). This includes the amygdala, hypothalamus, PAG, DLPT, RVM and superficial dorsal horn. The prodynorphin-derived peptides have a terminal distribution which roughly overlaps that of the enkephalins. Unlike BE, which derives exclusively from cells in the hypothalamus, enkephalin- and dynorphin-containing cell bodies are intrinsic to the PAG and RVM.

It is unclear which of the endogenous opioids act at which receptor, although anatomical studies indicate that the enkephalins are released in proximity to both MOR and DOR (Arvidsson et al 1995, Cheng et al 1996). In fact, both leu-enk and met-enk have somewhat higher affinity for DOR than MOR and both have very low affinity for KOR (Goldstein & Naidu 1989, Akil et al 1997). Dynorphins have a relatively high affinity for KOR and there is general agreement that dynorphins are the endogenous ligand for KOR. Like met-enk, BE has approximately equal affinity for DOR and MOR and much lower affinity for KOR.

The problem of matching an endogenous opioid with a particular receptor is complicated by several problems. First, there is the issue of which peptide fragment is actually released from the opioid terminal. This is not straightforward because in different tissues the precursor molecule can be cleaved into different fragments and these different fragments have different relative affinities for the three opioid receptors. For example, some of the longer proenkephalin-derived peptide fragments, which have higher affinity for MOR, also have high affinity for KOR (Akil et al 1997). Recently, endogenous peptides with high selectivity for MOR have been discovered (Zadina et al 1997). These peptides, termed endomorphin-1 (Tyr-Pro-Trp-Phe-NH_2) and endomorphin-2 (Tyr-Pro-Phe-Phe-NH_2), do not share the Tyr-Gly-Gly-Phe sequence common to the N-terminal of all the other known endogenous opioids. This implies that the endomorphin precursor molecule is distinct from that of the other three endogenous opioid families (Martin-Schild et al 1997, Schreff et al 1998). The endomorphins have over a thousand-fold selectivity for MOR versus KOR and DOR, inhibit C-fibre evoked responses of dorsal horn neurons (Chapman et al 1997) and have analgesic sites of action and potency similar to morphine (Stone et al 1997, Goldberg et al 1998). Consistent with the idea that endomorphins produce an analgesic effect through an action at MOR, endomorphin-2 is concentrated in many, but not all regions that express MOR, including the hypothalamus, amygdala, PAG, locus coeruleus and dorsal horn (Schreff et al 1998).

In summary, there are several distinct populations of opioid-peptide synthesizing cells and there are three opioid receptors. Both endogenous opioids and opioid receptors are distributed throughout the pain-modulating circuit described above. Although dynorphin appears to be the ligand for KOR, and the endomorphins show high selectivity for MOR, it is unclear whether met-enk, leu-enk or BE act exclusively at a single receptor type.

PHYSIOLOGY OF PAIN-MODULATING NETWORKS

Brainstem pain-modulating neurons

In addition to inhibition, pain-modulating networks can also facilitate nociceptive transmission (Fields 1992, Zhuo & Gebhart 1992, Urban & Gebhart 1997). It is likely that inhibitory and facilitatory controls are produced by different pain-modulating neurons. There are three classes of neuron in RVM: those that discharge beginning just prior to the occurrence of withdrawal from noxious heat (on-cells), those that shut off just prior to a withdrawal reflex (off-cells) and those that show no consistent changes in activity when withdrawal reflexes occur (neutral-cells) (Fields & Heinricher 1985, Fields et al 1991). Figure 11.3 illustrates the firing patterns of on- and off-cells. On-cells are consistently excited by noxious stimuli over much of the body surface. Most off-cells are inhibited by the same stimuli. Neutral-cells show variable responses or are unresponsive to noxious stimuli. A significant proportion of neurons of each class of RVM cell projects to the spinal cord. On- and off-cells project to laminae I, II and V of the dorsal horn (Fields et al 1995). Both on- and off-cells are excited by electrical stimulation of PAG; however, only the off-cell is excited by morphine (Fields et al 1991). Thus, activity of the off-cell is most consistently related to suppression of nociceptive transmission.

On-cells are inhibited by systemic, PAG or RVM opioid administration (Fields et al 1991, Heinricher et al 1992). Conversely, RVM on-cell activity increases during acute opioid abstinence. This increase in RVM on cell activity correlates with an enhancement of spinal withdrawal reflexes (Bederson et al 1990, Kim et al 1990) that can be blocked by inactivation of the RVM (Kaplan & Fields 1991). Thus it is likely that on-cells facilitate nociceptive transmission at the level of the dorsal horn. In addition to the RVM, these three classes of neurons are also present in the PAG (Heinricher et al 1987) and the DLPT (Haws et al 1989), which suggests that a common neural mechanism for opioid antinociception exists in these sites.

It is worth emphasizing that putative pain-modulating neurons in RVM, PAG and the DLPT have very large, virtually total body 'receptive fields' (RFs). In awake unrestrained rats, RVM neurons that resemble on-cells respond briskly to light touch and to sudden sound (Oliveras et al 1990). Individual RVM neurons project diffusely to the trigeminal dorsal horn and to multiple spinal levels. Furthermore, many RVM neurons have axons that are highly collateralized within the RVM itself (Mason & Fields 1989) and, at least in anaesthetized rats, cells of the same physiological class tend to fire at the same time (Heinricher et al 1989). This organization suggests that the neurons of each physiological class function as a unit that exerts global, rather than topographically discrete control over pain transmission.

Opioid actions in the RVM

Clearly, supraspinal opioid administration activates descending antinociceptive controls. How do opioids produce this effect? Is it by a direct action on pain-modulatory neurons? Our knowledge of the local circuitry underlying opioid analgesia is most extensive for the RVM. As described above, RVM off-cells are activated, on-cells inhibited and neutral-cells unaffected by opioids. Since off-cells inhibit and on-cells facilitate nociceptive transmission, opioid actions on these two classes of RVM neuron are likely to contribute to analgesia. There are at least two direct actions of opioid ligands upon neurons: one, a hyperpolarization due to increased potassium conductance and, two, reduced transmitter release secondary to inhibition of a voltage-dependent calcium conductance. Local iontophoretic application of morphine directly inhibits on-cells (Heinricher et al 1992) but has no effect on off- or neutral-cells. In vitro, μ opioids directly hyperpolarize a subset of RVM neurons (presumably on-cells) through an increase in K^+ conductance and they reduce a GABAergic inhibitory

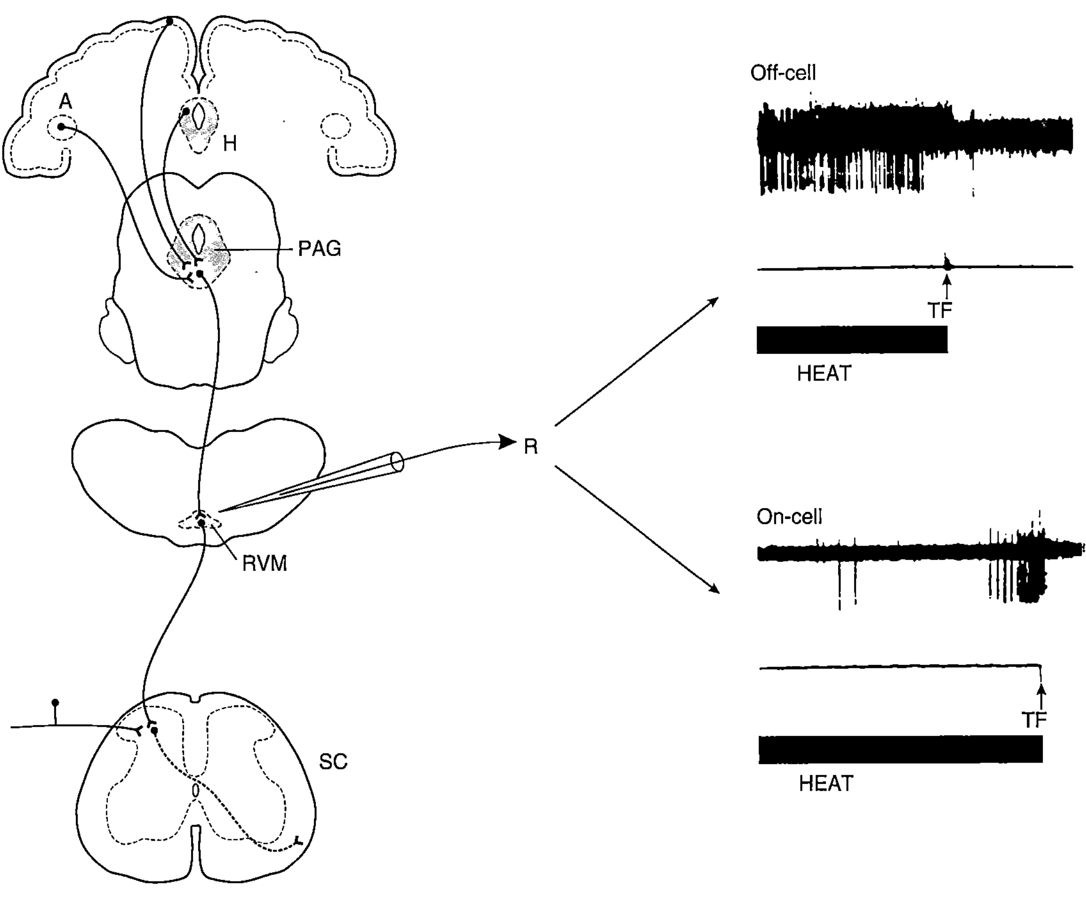

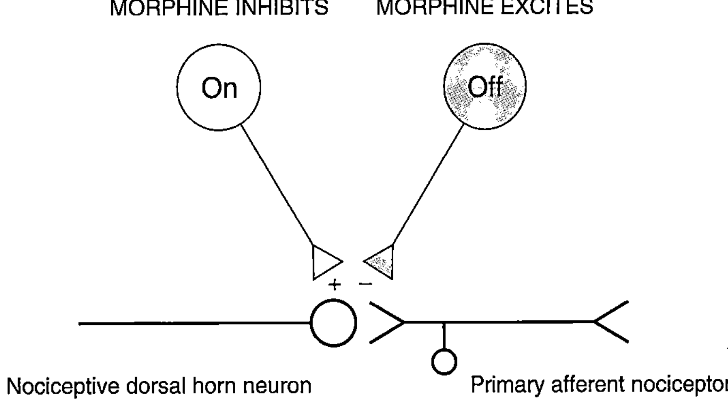

Fig. 11.3 Properties of proposed medullary pain modulating neurons. Upper left: microelectrode placement in the RVM for single unit extracellular recording. Upper right: top trace, a single oscilloscope sweep showing the off-cell pause occurring just prior to the tail flick reflex (middle trace: a force transducer showing movement) in response to noxious heat (bottom trace). Lower traces illustrate the typical on-cell firing pattern, which is a burst beginning before the tail flick. Bottom diagram illustrates that both on- and off-cells project to the spinal cord where they exert bidirectional control over nociceptive dorsal horn neurons. On-cells are inhibited and off-cells excited by morphine.

postsynaptic potential on a different subset of RVM neurons (presumably off-cells) (Pan et al 1990). These findings indicate that activation of off-cells by μ opioids is an indirect effect, secondary to inhibition of an inhibitory input. In fact, off-cells receive a direct GABAergic input (Skinner et al 1997b) and μ opioids inhibit the GABAergic pause of off-cells (Heinricher et al 1991, 1992). The simplest circuit that can account for these observations is illustrated in Figure 11.4.

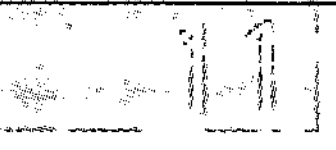

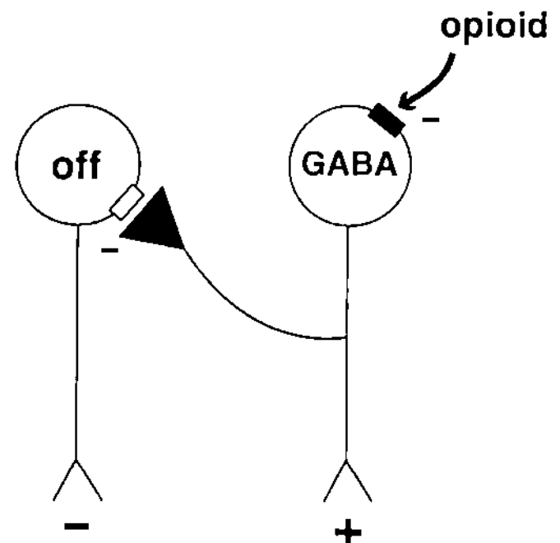

Fig. 11.4 Disinhibition model for opioid action in the RVM. The direct actions of opioids on neurons are predominantly inhibitory, yet when given systemically or locally by microinjection they excite RVM off-cells. This figure illustrates our proposed model in which opioids excite the off-cell indirectly by inhibiting a GABAergic inhibitory neuron that contacts the off-cell. The simplest arrangement is that the inhibitory input to off-cells derives from a subset of GABAergic on-cells.

According to this model, μ opioids inhibit a subset of GABAergic on-cells leading to disinhibition of off-cells. A similar microcircuit is probably also present in the PAG. Thus, both the MOR-selective agonist DAMGO and the $GABA_A$ receptor antagonist, bicuculline, have antinociceptive actions when microinjected into either the PAG (Moreau & Fields 1986, Depaulis et al 1987, Pan et al 1997) or the RVM (Drower & Hammond 1988, Heinricher et al 1991, 1994).

There is evidence that an endogenous opioid, presumably enkephalin, acting on this MOR-mediated local circuit in RVM provides a necessary link for the PAG–RVM–spinal cord pain-modulating pathway. RVM on-cells receive an enkephalinergic input (Mason et al 1992) and an enkephalinase inhibitor injected into the RVM produces analgesia (Al-Rodhan et al 1990). Furthermore, microinjecting naloxone or the MOR-selective antagonist CTOP into RVM blocks the inhibition of the tail flick produced by PAG bicuculline (BIC) or morphine (Kiefel et al 1993, Roychowdhury & Fields 1996), and the inhibition of RVM on-cells by PAG morphine or BIC is reversed by local iontophoresis of naloxone (Pan & Fields 1996). Figure 11.5 illustrates this enkephalin link in the RVM relay from PAG to the spinal cord dorsal horn.

Other opioid agonists differ in their actions on these circuits. In contrast to MOR agonists, KOR agonists have an *anti-analgesic* action in RVM. Our in vitro studies indicate that neurons with KOR represent a subpopulation of RVM neurons (presumably including off-cells) distinct from those bearing MOR (i.e. on-cells) (Fig. 11.5). Thus, in contrast to MOR agonists (but similar to MOR antagonists), KOR *agonists* microinjected into the RVM block the

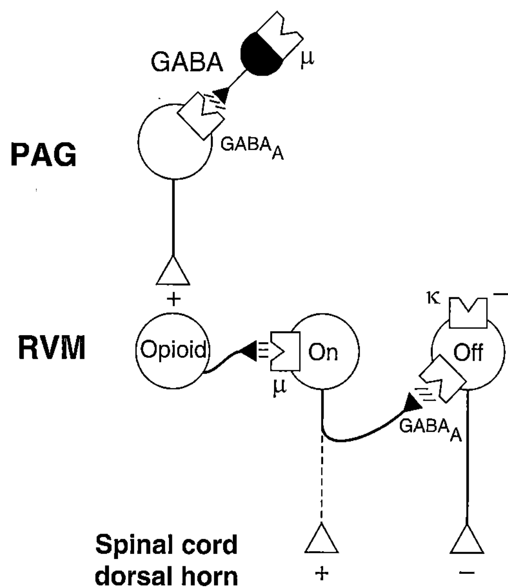

Fig. 11.5 Diagram of intrinsic opioid mediated brainstem connectivity. PAG neurons, disinhibited by opioids or GABA-A receptor antagonists, activate an opioid (presumably enkephalinergic) interneuron in the RVM. This endogenous opioid inhibits mu (μ) opioid receptor bearing on-cells. The inhibition of the on-cell disinhibits the off-cell which inhibits nociceptive transmission at the level of the dorsal horn.

analgesic effect of DAMGO microinjected into the PAG (Pan et al 1997).

Orphanin and nocistatin: opposing actions on pain modulation

Nociceptin, or orphanin FQ (OFQ), is a 17-amino-acid peptide, similar to dynorphin but missing an N-terminal Tyr residue. OFQ is an endogenous ligand for a receptor that has high amino acid sequence homology with the μ, κ and δ opioid receptors (termed LC132 or opioid receptor-$like_1$ (ORL_1) receptor (Bunzow et al 1994). ORL_1 has cellular actions indistinguishable from those of the opioid receptors (Connor et al 1996a, b, Vaughn et al 1997). At spinal levels, OFQ has an antinociceptive action (Stanfa et al 1996, King et al 1997, Yamamoto et al 1997). However, the behavioural effects of supraspinal OFQ are inconsistent (Darland et al 1998). The first studies reported pronociceptive effects (hence the name nociceptin) after intracerebroventricular injection. Furthermore, injection of nociceptin antisense, to block its synthesis, reduced nociception (Meunier et al 1995, 1997). Heinricher and colleagues (1997) have demonstrated that OFQ inhibits all three classes of RVM neuron. Thus, it would be expected to block antinociceptive actions that involve activation of

RVM off-cells. This would be consistent with the finding that supraspinal OFQ blocks stress-induced analgesia (Mogil et al 1996). The effect of OFQ in RVM will depend upon which class of neuron is active. For example, OFQ would also be expected to reduce a hyperalgesic state generated by increased RVM on-cell activity.

Cleavage of the pronociceptin precursor protein can also give rise to another peptide, *nocistatin*, which blocks the allodynia and hyperalgesia evoked by intrathecal nociceptin (Okuda-Ashitaka et al 1998; for review see Martin et al 1998). Importantly, nocistatin binds a receptor that is distinct from ORL1; thus the mechanism through which it counteracts nociceptin's effects remains to be determined. Intrathecal nocistatin, by itself, has no effect, which indicates that it is not an analgesic per se, but rather specifically counteracts exacerbated pain states. Furthermore, injection of antisense for nocistatin mRNA lowers the dose of nociceptin required to produce allodynia. This is probably one of the first examples in vertebrates in which peptides with opposing actions derive from the same precursor protein.

Cholecystokinin: an anti-opioid peptide

Our knowledge of other pairs of peptides having opposing effects on pain modulation is growing. For example, cholecystokinin (CCK) agonists, acting in the CNS at the CCK_B receptor, are well established as anti-opioid agents (Faris et al 1983; Crawley & Corwin 1994). CCK_B agonists have cellular actions opposite to those typically produced by opioids: they decrease K^+ conductance (Cox et al 1995) and increase GABA release (Miller et al 1997). There is a dense concentration of CCK-immunoreactive nerve terminals in the ventrocaudal PAG and the RVM, coextensive with that of enkephalin-immunoreactive terminal fields (Skinner et al 1997a) and CCK_B agonists, microinjected into RVM, block the antinociceptive effect of systemic and PAG opioids (Mitchell et al 1998). Conversely, CCK_B *antagonists* potentiate the analgesic effect of systemic enkephalinase inhibitors (Valverde et al 1994) and PAG DAMGO (H. Fields and S. Tershner, unpublished data). This indicates that endogenously released CCK acts as a functional antagonist for MOR-mediated antinociceptive actions of endogenous opioids in the RVM.

RVM neutral-cells and the role of serotonin in descending modulation of pain transmission

Serotonergic neurons comprise about 20% of the total RVM population (Moore 1981) and the vast majority of 5HT-containing RVM neurons are neutral-cells (Potrebic et al 1994). Because RVM serotonergic neurons are not affected by opioids or by electrical stimulation of the PAG (Gao et al 1997, 1998) they must have different afferent connections from those of RVM on- and off-cells. The conditions under which serotonergic RVM cells come into play is uncertain. Nevertheless, there is an extensive literature supporting a role for 5HT in descending modulation of pain transmission (Le Bars 1988, Mason & Gao 1998).

Electrical stimulation of the RVM evokes the release of 5HT in the spinal cord cerebrospinal fluid (CSF) and the analgesia produced by this stimulation is reduced by non-selective 5HT antagonists (Yaksh & Wilson 1979, Schmauss et al 1983, Barbaro et al 1985, Le Bars 1988, Alhaider et al 1991). Iontophoresis of 5HT inhibits the response of dorsal horn neurons to noxious stimulation (Randic & Yu 1976, Headley et al 1978, Jordan et al 1979) and 5HT applied directly to the spinal cord inhibits nociceptive transmission (Hylden & Wilcox 1983, Schmauss et al 1983, Solomon & Gebhart 1988). Although systemic opioids do not consistently evoke release of 5HT from the spinal cord (Matos et al 1992), the analgesia produced by intracerebral morphine can be partially blocked by intrathecal methysergide, a non-selective 5HT antagonist (Yaksh 1979). Furthermore, the analgesic action of systemic opiates can be at least transiently reduced by depletion of 5HT (Tenen 1968) or by neurotoxic destruction of spinal 5HT terminals (Vogt 1974, Roberts 1988). Because the RVM is the exclusive source of dorsal horn 5HT and because RVM serotonergic neurons have a slow tonic discharge, Mason (1997) has proposed that serotonergic RVM neurons tonically release 5HT at the level of the dorsal horn and this modulates the action of other descending systems (Mason & Gao 1998). For example, the activity of serotonergic RVM neurons is determined by the animal's behavioural state (i.e. level of arousal, stage of sleep) (Fornal et al 1985), and Mason proposes that this activity tonically modulates the effect of RVM on- and off-cells at spinal levels.

Nicotinic cholinergic actions in the RVM

Nicotinic acetylcholine receptors (nAChR) in RVM also contribute to pain modulation. Nicotinic agonists microinjected into the RVM inhibit hot-plate and tail-flick responses to noxious heat (Iwamoto et al 1991) as well as the formalin response (Bannon et al 1997). Furthermore, iontophoretic (Willcockson et al 1983) or systemic (Bitner et al 1998) administration of a nicotinic agonist produces a dose-related activation of RVM neurons. The pain-modulating actions of nicotinic agonists in RVM depend on serotonergic neurons and the nAChR receptor is, in fact, located predominantly on serotonergic neurons of the RVM (Bitner et al 1998). Furthermore, RVM injection of a serotonin-selective neurotoxin (5, 7-dihydroxytryptamine) markedly reduces the antinociceptive effect of systemic nicotinic agonists (Bannon et al 1998).

Actions of putative brainstem pain modulatory neurons upon spinal circuitry

Microinjection of opioids into either the PAG or the RVM produces behavioural antinociception. There is a significant correlation between suppression of pain behaviour by opioids and suppression of *Fos* staining in dorsal horn laminae containing nociresponsive neurons (Presley et al 1990, Tölle et al 1990, Gogas et al 1991, Hammond et al 1992). Consistent with the hypothesis that the analgesia produced by opioids involves the activation of descending inhibitory controls, injection of D-Ala, N-Me-Phe[4], Gly[5]-ol-enkephalin (DAMGO), a MOR-selective agonist, into the third ventricle, inhibits both pain behaviour and *Fos* expression in awake rats (Gogas et al 1991).

Direct inhibition of projection neurons

There are several possible circuits through which activation of RVM neurons could inhibit nociceptive transmission in the dorsal horn. One possibility is that brainstem neurons directly inhibit rostrally-projecting nociceptive dorsal horn cells (Fig. 11.6). In fact, electrical stimulation in RVM produces a monosynaptic inhibitory postsynaptic potential in spinothalamic tract (STT) neurons (Giesler et al 1981). Furthermore, because the RVM is the primary source of 5HT terminals in the dorsal horn, the demonstration that STT neurons receive a large 5HT input provides a substrate for direct postsynaptic control by brainstem neurons. Similarly, there is a direct catecholaminergic innervation of primate STT neurons which derives from brainstem neurons (Westlund et al 1990).

Activation of inhibitory interneurons

There is a subset of neurons in the superficial laminae of the dorsal horn that is excited by antinociceptive PAG stimulation

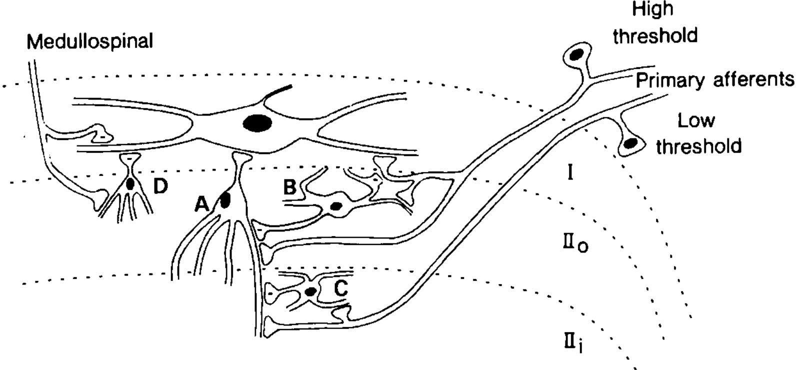

Fig. 11.6 Local circuitry in the superficial dorsal horn. Schematic illustration of afferent terminals and local circuitry within the superficial dorsal horn of the spinal cord. Nociceptive inputs, transmitted via high-threshold, primary afferent fibres, excite the nociceptive projection neurons of the marginal zone, lamina I. The same afferents excite dendrites of stalk cell excitatory interneurons (A) and inhibitory islet interneurons (B) of lamina IIo. The stalk cell input results in further excitatory drive on to marginal projection neurons; the input to the islet cell interneuron (B) in lamina IIo provides a circuit that generates an inhibitory, feedforward control of marginal neurons by nociceptive inputs.

Low-threshold primary afferent fibres provide a non-nociceptive input to marginal neurons via their excitatory connections with dendrites of stalk cell (A) in lamina IIi. By contrast, the non-nociceptive input to islet cell interneurons of lamina IIi (C) may contribute to the inhibitory control of nociceptive marginal neurons.

The schema also illustrates some possible descending control mechanisms. These may be exerted directly upon dorsal horn projection neurons. Alternatively, descending bulbospinal axons (some of which are 5HT-containing) may excite inhibitory interneurons (e.g. enkephalin-containing stalk (D) or islet cells), which in turn postsynaptically control the nociceptive projection neurons. Another possibility, not illustrated, is that the descending systems inhibit the excitatory stalk cell (A).

(Millar & Williams 1989). Many of the neurons in these laminae contain the inhibitory neurotransmitters GABA (Ruda et al 1986, Magoul et al 1987, Todd & McKenzie 1989), glycine and enkephalin (Glazer & Basbaum 1981, Ruda et al 1986). Furthermore, glycine is released into the spinal cord dorsal horn by stimulation in the RVM that inhibits the firing of nociceptive neurons (Sorkin et al 1993). These results suggest that inhibitory amino acids that are released from dorsal horn interneurons contribute to descending controls.

In view of the dense projection of RVM serotonergic neurons to the superficial dorsal horn and of the evidence implicating 5HT in pain modulation (Le Bars 1988), it is also important that there is a population of superficial dorsal horn neurons that is excited by iontophoresis of 5HT (Todd & Millar 1983b). Furthermore, the inhibition of dorsal horn neurons produced by 5HT agonists acting at the excitatory $5HT_3$ receptor is blocked by a $GABA_A$ receptor antagonist, suggesting that the 5HT 'inhibition' is mediated via a GABAergic inhibitory interneuron (Alhaider et al 1991).

The vast majority of opioid terminals in the dorsal horn derive from local interneurons (Hökfelt et al 1979). Enkephalin terminals and cells are present in superficial dorsal horn (Glazer & Basbaum 1981, Cruz & Basbaum 1985), as are dense concentrations of MOR (Besse et al 1992, Arvidsson et al 1995). Spinal application of opioids produces analgesia (see Chapter 10) and opioid iontophoresis inhibits dorsal horn nociceptive neurons (Duggan & North 1984, Fleetwood-Walker et al 1988). Intrathecal naloxone reduces the antinociceptive action of electrical stimulation of RVM (Zorman et al 1982, Aimone et al 1987) or supraspinal opioid administration (Levine et al 1982). Furthermore, intrathecal administration of drugs that block enkephalin-degrading enzymes produces behavioural antinociception (Oshita et al 1990) and inhibits nociceptive dorsal horn neurons (Dickenson et al 1987).

Activation of PAG neurons inhibits the response of sacral dorsal horn neurons to noxious heat, an effect that is blocked by local iontophoresis of MOR-selective antagonists (Budai & Fields 1998). Activation of these same dorsal horn neurons by iontophoretically applied excitatory amino acids is not blocked by PAG bicuculline, indicating that the endogenous opioid effect is exerted either on the terminals of afferents to the recorded dorsal horn cells or upon nearby excitatory interneurons.

Inhibition of primary afferents and excitatory interneurons

As described above, opioids inhibit the release of neurotransmitters from primary afferents. They have also been shown to directly inhibit lamina II interneurons. Lamina II interneurons provide a major excitatory input from C fibres to lamina I projection cells. Furthermore, some lamina II interneurons make asymmetric, presumably excitatory, synapses onto neurones in deeper laminae of the dorsal horn. In vitro studies have shown that MOR agonists hyperpolarize neurons in lamina II that are excited by dorsal root stimulation (Grudt & Williams 1994), and both MOR and DOR agonists presynaptically inhibit excitatory input to these neurons (Glaum et al 1994, Grudt & Williams 1994). In favour of a role in pain modulation for supraspinal inhibition of lamina II excitatory interneurons, Light and colleagues (1988) have described a population of nociceptive lamina II cells which is inhibited by RVM stimulation.

In summary, there is evidence that descending pain-modulatory neurons in RVM and DLPT inhibit nociceptive transmission by several mechanisms: direct inhibition of projection neurons, inhibition of transmitter release from primary afferents, excitation of inhibitory interneurons and inhibition of excitatory interneurons.

PHYSIOLOGICAL FUNCTION OF PAIN-MODULATING NETWORKS

The evidence outlined in this chapter demonstrates that there are networks that control nociceptive transmission, that brainstem to spinal cord projections are crucial to their operation, that the control is bidirectional and that endogenous opioid peptides are involved in their function. Despite these advances in our understanding, it has been difficult to identify how the system functions on a moment-to-moment basis in awake unrestrained animals or even to understand how pain modulatory systems contribute to survival.

Does pain inhibit pain? Multiple pain-modulating networks

Following the discovery of the PAG–RVM–dorsal horn modulatory pathway we proposed that noxious stimuli activate descending inhibitory controls, providing a negative feedback mechanism to dampen the nociceptive transmission at the level of the spinal cord (Basbaum & Fields 1984). Consistent with this idea, noxious stimuli in one part of the body inhibit dorsal horn nociceptive neurons in spinal segments innervating distant body parts. For example, primate STT neurons excited by noxious stimuli of one foot can be inhibited by noxious stimuli of the face or of the contralateral foot (Gerhart et al 1981). Furthermore, although naloxone does not induce pain in the absence of an imposed stimulus, when administered in the setting of injury, it can exacerbate pain. This suggested that endogenous opioid-mediated inhibitory controls are activated by nociceptive signals, and indeed noxious stimuli evoke the release of enkephalins at supraspinal and spinal levels (Yaksh & Elde 1981).

On the other hand, cutaneous noxious stimuli activate on-cells and inhibit off-cells. Because RVM neurons have total body receptive fields and because on-cells facilitate and off-cells inhibit nociceptive transmission, one would expect noxious stimuli in one part of the body to *enhance* nociceptive transmission in other parts of the body. Although this may occur under some circumstances (Ramírez & Vanegas 1989), noxious input more often activates systems that produce analgesia. In fact, acupuncture and many other traditional pain therapies based on counterirritation may operate through such a mechanism (Le Bars et al 1979a,b). Thus, biting your lip, banging your head against the wall, mustard plasters, cupping and other manipulations have been proposed to work by activation of pain-modulating systems (Melzack 1975).

In a thoughtful analysis of the interaction of nociceptive transmission systems, Le Bars and colleagues (1979a,b) have proposed a theoretical basis for understanding the inhibitory controls activated by noxious stimuli: the diffuse noxious inhibitory controls or DNIC. According to the DNIC hypothesis, noxious stimuli activate a 'surround' inhibition that sharpens contrast between the stimulus zone and adjacent areas. This sharpened contrast would actually have a net *enhancing* effect on the perceived intensity of pain. However, outside the stimulated zone there would be a net analgesic effect. It is this surround analgesia that has been used to explain various counterirritation mechanisms for producing pain relief, including acupuncture.

Because the PAG–RVM–dorsal horn pathway had been proposed as the efferent loop in a negative feedback circuit, it was surprising when the Le Bars group found that lesions of the nucleus raphe magnus were *without* effect on DNIC (Bouhassira et al 1993). They subsequently identified a group of neurons in the caudal medulla, the nucleus reticularis dorsalis (NRD), which receives nociceptive input from the spinal dorsal horn and in turn inhibits dorsal horn neurons. The SRD is not only another source of powerful descending inhibitory control, it also transmits nociceptive messages to several thalamic nuclei (Villaneuva et al 1996, Villaneuva 1998) as part of the spinoreticular–thalamic pathway.

In addition to this evidence that the NRD is a major source of spino-bulbo-spinal inhibitory controls, it also appears to be a source of descending *facilitatory* control. There are direct synaptic contacts of NRD axons upon lamina I neurons, which in turn project to the NRD, providing a reciprocal circuit (Almeida et al 1993). Bilateral lesions of NRD neurons result in increased latencies in the tail-flick and hot-plate tests, i.e. supporting the idea of a positive feedback circuit involving the NRD (Almeida et al 1996). By contrast, glutamate injections, to activate NRD neurons, shortened tail-flick latencies. Thus the NRD receives nociceptive inputs from dorsal horn neurons and, via the reciprocal projection, it increases the excitability of spinal cord lamina I neurons.

These studies emphasize that depending on the test used, one can reveal a complex mix of excitatory and inhibitory controls arising from brainstem sites. Just as the RVM contains neurons which can either increase or decrease the activity and excitability of dorsal horn neurons (and thus influence nociceptive processing), there appears to be a subtle interplay of facilitatory and inhibitory controls which are concurrently exerted by the NRD upon dorsal horn nociresponsive neurons. Thus, reducing the outflow from the spinal cord (and presumably reducing nociceptive processing) can be achieved not only by increasing descending inhibitory controls, but also by reducing the facilitatory influences that are activated in the setting of acute and persistent injury. It follows that the magnitude of central excitability that occurs in the setting of injury or inflammation is influenced by the balance of excitatory and inhibitory descending controls that are engaged. These results provide further evidence that the output of spinal nociresponsive neurons (and the pain that is ultimately produced) is a function of far more than just the direct effect of primary afferent input to them; the descending modulatory controls that are brought into play by these same stimuli must also be taken into account. Interestingly, recent studies of the activation of descending controls in the setting of persistent injury (rather than in response to an acute noxious stimulus) also provide evidence for both inhibitory and facilitatory descending effects (Herrero & Cervero 1996, Ren & Dubner 1996, Ren & Ruda 1996, Wei et al 1998).

These results also help to explain the paradox that noxious stimuli, which activate pain-facilitating on-cells, often inhibit neural and behavioural responses to noxious stimulation (Watkins & Mayer 1982, Watkins et al 1983, Morgan et al 1994). Thus noxious stimuli activate multiple CNS networks, some of which have an antinociceptive effect while others are pronociceptive. Whether responses to noxious stimuli are enhanced or suppressed will depend on stimulus location, duration, the environment in which the stimulus is applied and the behavioural state of the animal (Watkins et al 1982). In anaesthetized rats the diffuse inhibitory effect produced by noxious somatic stimuli (which does not involve the RVM) appears to override the potential facilitatory action on wide dynamic range neurons by RVM on-cells that are activated by the same stimulus (Bouhassira et al 1993, Morgan et al 1994).

Cytokines, hyperalgesia and pain-modulating networks

In addition to the evidence implicating RVM to spinal cord projections in the hyperalgesic effect of noxious cutaneous stimulation and inflammation, brainstem facilitatory influences appear to be a major contributor to the hyperalgesia that is observed following immune activation by cytokines and in certain types of localized inflammation and nerve injury. For example, intraperitoneal injection of lipopolysaccharides, which induce interleukin-1 in rodents, produces a syndrome of illness behaviour that includes fever, increased sleep, inactivity, decreased food and water intake and cutaneous hyperalgesia (Watkins et al 1995). This type of hyperalgesia depends on vagal afferents, which activate the nucleus raphe magnus via the nucleus of the solitary tract. The lipopolysaccharide-evoked hyperalgesia is blocked by lesions of the RVM or its outflow pathway to the dorsal horn, the dorsolateral funiculus.

What signals activate the endogenous opioid-mediated pain-modulating network? Noxious stimuli, stress-induced analgesia and conditioned fear

Under certain circumstances, a noxious stimulus can lead to an opioid-mediated analgesic effect that clearly involves the PAG–RVM network. For example, using relatively brief (90-s) shock, Watkins and Mayer (1983) and Watkins et al (1982, 1998) showed that forepaw shock analgesia is completely blocked by naloxone and by RVM lesions.

When placed in threatening situations such as proximity to a predator, many animals freeze and become unresponsive to noxious stimulation (Fanselow 1991). These responses are part of a repertoire of 'fear' behaviours that presumably promote survival by helping the animal escape detection. Similar responses can be learned. Thus analgesia can be conditioned either to a light or tone contingently paired with foot shock or to the environment in which the foot shock is received. The analgesia that accompanies these 'fear' situations is blocked by lesions of the amygdala as well as of the RVM and DLF (Watkins & Mayer 1982, dow 1991, Helmstetter 1992, Helmstetter et al 1994). It is also blocked by naloxone administered systemically or into the PAG (Watkins et al 1982, Helmstetter & Landeira-Fernandez 1990).

In addition to the analgesia associated with conditioned fear, it is possible to condition an ***anti-analgesic*** effect (Watkins et al 1998). When rats exposed to inescapable shock in a given context receive a light signal at the termination of the shock the light becomes a 'safety signal'. When the rats are returned to the context in which they received the shock, illuminating the light prevents expression of conditioned fear behaviours, including analgesia (Watkins et al 1992). The safety signal has a potent and generalized anti-opioid effect in that it blocks the analgesic effect of systemic or spinal morphine. This anti-analgesic effect is blocked by lesions of the midbrain dorsal raphe nucleus and the RVM. Furthermore, spinal intrathecal injection of a CCK antagonist restores the potency of spinal morphine, which indicates that the anti-opioid effect is mediated by the release of CCK at the level of the spinal cord. These experiments on conditioned analgesia and anti-analgesia are particularly interesting and valuable because they link antinociceptive actions to specific, biologically relevant environmental conditions and to specific neural networks and transmitter systems.

Expectation, attention and learning

That expectation and attentional factors can reliably alter perceived pain intensity is well established. For example, Miron and colleagues (1989) trained human subjects to make either a visual or noxious thermal discrimination. Prior to each discrimination trial they received a cue indicating whether they would be required to make a visual or noxious thermal discrimination. They consistently rated the noxious thermal stimulus as less intense when they received an 'incorrect' cue indicating that they would be required to make a visual discrimination. In monkeys, the responses of nociceptive dorsal horn neurons to the same noxious thermal stimulus was greater during the performance of a noxious thermal discrimination task than when the monkey was carrying out a visual discrimination (Hayes et al 1981). Furthermore, under conditions of correct cuing of a thermal discrimination task, monkeys have shorter response latencies for signalling their detection of the increase in skin temperature, from which it was inferred that they perceive the stimulus as more intense (Bushnell et al 1985). These studies suggest that there is a centrally generated component to the 'response' of dorsal horn neurons to noxious thermal stimulation and that this centrally generated increment adds to the perceived intensity of pain.

With learning, neutral contextual cues acquire the power to either increase or decrease the activity of nociceptive dorsal horn neurons *in the absence of a noxious stimulus.* Duncan et al (1987) recorded the activity of nociceptive trigeminal dorsal horn neurons, including some that project to the thalamus. These primates were trained to press a button in response to a light cue. Pressing the button initiated a trial during which the animal had to discriminate between two noxious thermal stimuli. Some neurons underwent abrupt increase or decreases in their activity that were time locked to the light cue or the button press. Importantly, these 'task-related' changes in activity occurred *prior to the onset of the thermal stimulus.* These experiments show that the activity of dorsal horn nociceptive neurons can be increased or decreased by a context-specific modulatory signal that originates in the CNS. The presence of facilitatory modulation of dorsal horn nociresponsive neurons raises the intriguing possibility that pain can be produced by centrally originating drive of dorsal horn nociceptive neurons, without activation of primary afferent nociceptors.

What is the evidence that an endogenous opioid-mediated pain-modulatory system exists in humans?

Unfortunately, it is difficult to directly test a specific neural circuit hypothesis underlying a complex human behaviour such as psychogenic pain or analgesia. At present, we must rely primarily upon indirect evidence to support the idea that the circuits we have been discussing in this chapter play a significant role in determining the variability of human pain perception. In fact, there is evidence that humans have similar pain-modulating circuitry. The brainstem-to-spinal cord circuitry implicated in conditioned analgesia is highly conserved in a variety of mammalian species, including rodents, carnivores, primates and marsupials. Importantly, the distribution of neurotransmitters, including opioid peptides, in this pathway is also conserved across species, including humans (Emson et al 1984, Pittius et al 1984). Furthermore, the MOR agonists that relieve clinically significant pain in patients inhibit withdrawal and escape behaviours in animals through the amygdala–PAG–RVM–spinal cord circuitry. Finally, as discussed above, the idea that homologous circuitry can produce analgesia in humans is strongly supported by the remarkable observation that patients with chronic pain report relief during stimulation of specific sites in the human midbrain. This observation in humans represents a critical extension of animal work, because it supports the idea that the behavioural antinociception produced by midbrain stimulation in animals is accompanied by subjective pain relief. In summary, several independent lines of evidence support the assumption that humans have neural circuitry homologous to that which mediates conditioned analgesia and which contributes to opioid analgesia in animals.

When is this opioid-mediated pain-modulating circuit activated in humans? The evidence on this issue comes largely from studies using the opioid antagonist naloxone. If this circuit is activated in humans, it should be possible to find situations in which endogenous opioids reduce pain, and under those circumstances naloxone should block the analgesia. Levine et al (1978a) were the first to clearly demonstrate that, compared with placebo, naloxone significantly worsens postoperative pain. Naloxone is an excellent drug to use in studies of subjective phenomena because, at the doses used to block endogenous opioids (10 mg), it is virtually non-psychoactive when used in opioid-naive, pain-free subjects (Grevert et al 1983b, Wolkowitz et al 1985). Thus, it can be given in a true double blind fashion. Naloxone hyperalgesia has been replicated in studies using both clinical and experimental pains (Grevert & Goldstein 1985). The significance of these naloxone studies is twofold. Firstly, they demonstrate, under controlled conditions, that an endogenous pain-modulating system in humans can be reproducibly activated. Secondly, the hyperalgesic response to naloxone suggests that the pain-modulating system has opioid links. One obvious possibility is that it is the pain-modulating circuit described above.

Placebo analgesia

One of the most fascinating phenomena in medical practice is placebo analgesia, i.e. pain relief in response to cues that suggest an effective treatment. In the quest to establish naloxone hyperalgesia, the question arose as to whether placebo analgesia is produced through the action of the opioid-mediated circuit described above (see Ch. 51). Several studies have addressed this question. In the first study (Levine et al 1978b), dental postoperative pain patients were given a placebo and then randomized to receive either a second placebo or naloxone. Naloxone increased pain in placebo responders but had no effect on non-responders. A subsequent study (Levine & Gordon 1984) used identical methods but included a natural history group that received hidden infusions of either naloxone or vehicle. In the later study, naloxone had no effect upon patients who had had no overt treatment. Together, these studies demonstrated that placebo analgesia can have a major naloxone-reversible component. Using tourniquet ischaemic pain as a model, it is possible to demonstrate a significant placebo analgesic effect. While naloxone (10 mg) does not affect pain in subjects who have not been given a placebo, it does significantly reduce placebo analgesia (Amanzio & Benedetti 1999, Grevert & Goldstein 1985). Furthermore, Lipman et al (1990) have reported endogenous opioid-like material in the CSF of chronic pain patients whose pain level dropped following placebo administration. Recently, Benedetti has demonstrated not only a reduction of placebo analgesia by naloxone but an *enhancement* by the CCK antagonist proglumide (Benedetti 1996). Although placebo analgesia can, under some conditions, have a significant non-opioid component (Grevert et al 1983a, Gracely et al 1983), the weight of current evidence supports a role for endogenous opioids and this provides a link between the placebo analgesia and specific pain-modulating circuitry.

SUMMARY AND CONCLUSIONS

This chapter has presented an overview of pain modulation with an emphasis on a specific network. Neurons in this network exert bidirectional control over dorsal horn nociceptive transmission neurons. Endogenous opioid peptides are present in neural somata and/or terminal fields in several component nuclei of this network, and each site within the network is sensitive to the antinociceptive actions of exogenous opioids. There is good evidence that this network is reliably activated in situations characterized by threat of injury. Furthermore, endogenous opioids contribute to placebo analgesia, an observation that implicates this network in pain control that is induced by psychological factors. There are clearly other CNS pathways without opioid links that can produce antinociceptive actions. Their behavioural significance and the neurotransmitter systems that underlie their action are presently unknown.

The discovery of pain-modulatory systems, the behavioural triggers and somatosensory stimuli that activate them and the neurotransmitters that mediate their action has provided us with a preliminary mechanistic understanding of the variability of pain. This greater understanding offers the promise of rationally developed treatments based on the manipulation of psychological variables, counterirritation and new, more selective drugs or drug combinations. These improvements in treatment will depend on further progress in elucidating the neural circuits involved in pain modulation.

REFERENCES

Aimone LD, Gebhart GF 1986 Stimulation-produced spinal inhibition from the midbrain in the rat is mediated by an excitatory amino acid neurotransmitter in the medial medulla. Journal of Neuroscience 6: 1803–1813

Aimone LD, Jones SL, Gebhart GF 1987 Stimulation-produced descending inhibition from the periaqueductal gray and nucleus raphe magnus in the rat: mediation by spinal monoamines but not opioids. Pain 31: 123–136

Akil H, Mayer DJ, Liebeskind JC 1976 Antagonism of stimulation-produced analgesia by naloxone, a narcotic antagonist. Science 191: 961–962

Akil H, Meng F, Devine DP, Watson SJ 1997 Molecular and neuroanatomical properties of the endogenous opioid system: implications for treatment of opiate addiction. Seminars in Neuroscience 9: 70–83

Alhaider AA, Lei, SZ, Wilcox GL 1991 Spinal 5-HT_3 receptor-mediated antinociception: possible release of GABA. Journal of Neuroscience 11: 1881–1888

Almeida A, Tavares I, Lima D, Coimbra A 1993 Descending projections from the medullary dorsal reticular nucleus make synaptic contacts with spinal cord lamina I cells projecting to that nucleus: an electron microscopic tracer study in the rat. Neuroscience 55: 1093–1106

Almeida A, Tjolsen A, Lima D, Coimbra A, Hole K 1996 The medullary dorsal reticular nucleus facilitates acute nociception in the rat. Brain Research Bulletin 39: 7–15

Al-Rodhan N, Chipkin R, Yaksh TL 1990 The antinociceptive effects of SCH-32615, a neutral endopeptidase (enkephalinase) inhibitor, microinjected into the periaqueductal, ventral medulla and amygdala. Brain Research 520: 123–130

Amaral DG, Price JL, Pitkanen A, Carmichael ST 1992 Anatomical organization of the primate amygaloid complex. In: Aggleton JP (ed) The amygdala. Wiley-Liss, New York, pp 1–66

Amanzio M, Benedetti F 1999 Neuropharmacological dissection of placebo analgesia: expectation-activated opioid systems versus conditioning-activated specific sub-systems. Journal of Neuroscience 19: 484–494

Arvidsson U, Riedl M, Chakrabarti S et al 1995 Distribution and targeting of a μ-opioid receptor (MOR1) in brain and spinal cord. Journal of Neuroscience 15: 3328–3341

Atweh SF, Kuhar MJ 1977 Autoradiographic localization of opiate receptors in rat brain. I. Spinal cord and lower medulla. Brain Research 124: 53–67

Bach FW, Yaksh TL 1995 Release of beta-endorphin immunoreactivity from brain by activation of a hypothalmic *N*-methyl-D-aspartate receptor. Neuroscience 65: 775–783

Bandler R, Keay KA 1996 Columnar organization in the midbrain periaqueductal gray and the integration of emotional expression. In: Holstege G, Bandler R, Saper C (eds) Progress in brain research vol 107. Elsevier, Amsterdam, pp 285–300

Bandler R, Shipley MT 1994 Columnar organization in the midbrain periaqueductal gray: Modules for emotional expression? Trends in Neuroscience 17: 379–389

Bannon AW, Decker MW, Holladay MW et al 1997 Broad-spectrum, non-opioid analgesic activity by selective modulation of neuronal nicotinic acetylcholine receptors. Science 279: 77–81

Barbaro NM, Hammond DL, Fields HL 1985 Effects of intrathecally administered methysergide and yohimbine on microstimulation-produced antinociception in the rat. Brain Research 343: 223–229

Basbaum AI, Fields HL 1978 Endogenous pain control mechanisms: review and hypothesis. Annals of Neurology 4: 451–462

Basbaum AI, Fields HL 1984 Endogenous pain control systems: brainstem spinal pathways and endorphin circuitry. Annual Review Neuroscience 7: 309–338

Basbaum AI, Clanton CH, Fields HL 1976 Opiate and stimulus-produced analgesia: functional anatomy of a medullospinal pathway. Proceedings of the National Academy of Sciences USA 73: 4685–4688

Basbaum AI, Clanton CH, Fields HL 1978 Three bulbospinal pathways from the rostral medulla of the cat: an autoradiographic study of pain modulating systems. Journal of Comparative Neurology 178: 209–224

Baskin DS, Mehler WR, Hosobuchi Y, Richardson DE, Adams JE, Flitter MA 1986 Autopsy analysis of the safety, efficacy and cartography of electrical stimulation of the central gray in humans. Brain Research 371: 231–236

Bederson JB, Fields HL, Barbaro NM 1990 Hyperalgesia during naloxone-precipitated withdrawal from morphine is associated with increased on-cell activity in the rostral ventromedial medulla. Somatosensory Motor Research 7: 185–203

Beecher HK 1959 The measurement of subjective responses. Oxford University Press, Oxford

Behbehani MM, Fields HL 1979 Evidence that an excitatory connection between the periaqueductal grey and nucleus raphe magnus mediates stimulation produced analgesia. Brain Research 170: 85–93

Beitz AJ 1982a The sites of origin of brainstem neurotensin and serotonin projections to the rodent nucleus raphe magnus. Journal of Neuroscience 2: 829–842

Benedetti F 1996 The opposite effects of the opiate antagonist naloxone and the cholecystokinin antagonist proglumide on placebo analgesia. Pain 64: 535–543

Bennett GJ, Hayashi H, Abdelmoumene M, Dubner R 1979 Physiological properties of stalked cells of the substantia gelatinosa intracellularly stained with horseradish peroxidase. Brain Research 164: 285–289

Besse D, Lombard MC, Besson JM 1992 Time related decreases in mu and delta opioid receptors in the superficial dorsal horn of the rat spinal cord following a large unilateral dorsal rhizotomy. Brain Research 578: 115–121

Bitner RS, Nikkel AL, Curzon P, Arneric SP, Bannon AW, Decker MW 1998 Role of the nucleus raphe magnus in antinociception produced by ABT-594: immediate early gene responses possibly linked to neuronal nicotinic acetylcholine receptors on serotonergic neurons. Journal of Neuroscience 18: 5426–5432

Bloom F, Battenberg E, Rossier J, Ling N, Guillemin R 1978 Neurons containing beta-endorphin in rat brain exist separately from those containing enkephalin: immunocytochemical studies. Proceedings of the National Academy of Sciences USA 75: 1591–1595

Boivie J, Meyerson BA 1982 A correlative anatomical and clinical study of pain suppression by deep brain stimulation. Pain 13: 113–126

Bouhassira D, Bing Z, Le Bars D 1993 Studies of brain structures involved in diffuse noxious inhibitory controls in the rat: the rostral ventromedial medulla. Journal of Physiology 463: 667–687

Budai D, Fields HL 1998 Endogenous opioid peptides acting at μ-opioid receptors in the dorsal horn contribute to midbrain modulation of spinal nociceptive neurons. Journal of Neuroscience 79: 677–687

Bunzow JR, Saez C, Mortrud M et al 1994 Molecular cloning and tissue distribution of a putative member of the rat opioid receptor gene family that is not a mu, delta or kappa opioid receptor type. FEBS Letters 347: 284–288

Burkey AR, Carstens E, Wenniger JJ, Tang J, Jasmin L 1996 An opioidergic cortical antinociception triggering site in the agranular insular cortex of the rat that contributes to morphine antinociception. Journal of Neuroscience 16: 6612–6623

Bushnell MC, Duncan GH, Dubner R, Jones RL, Maixner W 1985 Attentional influences on noxious and innocuous cutaneous heat detection in humans and monkeys. Journal of Neuroscience 5: 1103–1110

Calvino B, Levesque G, Besson J-M 1982 Possible involvement of the amygdaloid complex in morphine analgesia as studied by electrolytic lesions in rats. Brain Research 233: 221–226

Cameron AA, Kahn IA, Westlund KN, Willis WD 1995 The efferent projections of the periaqueductal gray in the rat: a *Phaseolus vulgaris*-leucoagglutinin study. II Descending projections. Journal of Comparative Neurology 351: 585–601

Cannon JT, Prieto GJ, Lee A, Liebeskind JC 1982 Evidence for opioid and non-opioid forms of stimulation-produced analgesia in the rat. Brain Research 243: 315–321

Carpenter D, Engberg I, Lundberg A 1965 Differential supraspinal control of inhibitory and excitatory actions from the FRA to ascending spinal pathways. Acta Physiologica Scandinavica 63: 103–110

Carstens E, Klumpp D, Zimmerman M 1980 Differential inhibitory effects of medial and lateral midbrain stimulation on spinal neuronal discharges to noxious skin heating in the cat. Journal of Neurophysiology 43: 332–342

Chapman V, Diaz A, Dickenson AH 1997 Distinct inhibitory effects of spinal endomorphin-1 and endomorphin-2 on evoked dorsal horn neuronal responses in the rat. British Journal of Pharmacology 122: 1537–1539

Cheng PY, Moriwaki A, Wang JB, Uhl GR, Pickel VM 1996 Ultrastructural localization of mu-opioid receptors in the superficial layers of the rat cervical spinal cord: extrasynaptic localization and proximity to Leu5-enkephalin. Brain Research 731: 141–154

Clark FM, Proudfit HK 1991a Projections of neurons in the ventromedial medulla to pontine catecholamine cell groups involved in the modulation of nociception. Brain Research 540: 105–115

Clark FM, Proudfit HK 1991b The projection of noradrenergic neurons in the A7 catecholamine cell group to the spinal cord in the rat demonstrated by anterograde tracing combined with immunocytochemistry. Brain Research 547: 279–288

Coffield JA, Bowen KK, Miletic V 1992 Retrograde tracing of projections between the nucleus submedius, the ventrolateral orbital cortex, and the midbrain in the rat. Journal of Comparative Neurology 321: 488–499

Comb M, Seeburg PH, Adelman J, Eiden L, Herbert E 1982 Primary structure of the human met- and leu-enkephalin precursor and its mRNA. Nature 295: 663–666

Connor M, Vaughn CW, Chieng B, Christie MJ 1996a Nociceptin receptor coupling to a potassium conductance in rat locus coeruleus neurones in vitro. British Journal of Pharmacology 119: 1614–1618

Connor M, Yeo A, Henderson G 1996b The effect of nociceptin on Ca^{2+} channel current and intracellular Ca^{2+} in the SH-SY5Y human neuroblastoma cell line. British Journal of Pharmacology 118: 205–207

Cox CL, Hugenard JR, Prince DA 1995 Cholecystokinin depolarizes rat thalamic reticular neurons by suppressing a κ+ conductance. Journal of Neurophysiology 74: 990–1000

Crawley JN, Corwin RL 1994 Biological actions of cholecystokinin. Peptides 15: 731–755

Cruz L, Basbaum AI 1985 Multiple opioid peptides and the modulation of pain: immunohistochemical analysis of dynorphin and enkephalin in the trigeminal nucleus caudalis and spinal cord of the cat. Journal of Comparative Neurology 240: 331–348

Curatolo M, Petersen-Felix S, Arendt-Nielsen L, Zbinden AM 1997 Epidural epinephrine and clonidine: segmental analgesia and effects on different pain modalities. Anesthesiology 87: 785–794

Darland T, Heinricher MM, Grandy DK 1998 Orphanin FQ/nociceptin: a role in pain and analgesia, but so much more. Trends in Neuroscience 21: 215–221

Depaulis A, Morgan MM, Liebeskind JC 1987 GABAergic modulation of the analgesic effects of morphine microinjected in the ventral periaqueductal gray matter of the rat. Brain Research 436: 223–228

Dickenson AH, Sullivan AF, Fournie-Zaluski MC, Roques BP 1987 Prevention of degradation of endogenous enkephalins produces inhibition of nociceptive neurones in rat spinal cord. Brain Research 408: 185–191

Drolet G, Van Bockstaele EJ, Aston-Jones G 1992 Robust enkephalin innervation of the locus coeruleus from the rostral medulla. Journal of Neuroscience 12: 3162–3174

Drower EJ, Hammond DL 1988 GABAergic modulation of nociceptive threshold: effects of THIP and bicuculline microinjected in the ventral medulla of the rat. Brain Research 450: 316–324

Duggan AW, North RA 1984 Electrophysiology of opioids. Pharmacological Reviews 35: 219–281

Duncan GH, Bushnell MC, Bates R, Dubner R 1987 Task-related responses of monkey medullary dorsal horn neurons. Journal of Neurophysiology 57: 289–310

Emson PC, Corder R, Ratter SJ et al Regional distribution of pro-opiomelanocortin-derived peptides in the human brain. Neuroendocrinology 38: 45–50

Fanselow MS In: Depaulis A, Bandler R, (eds) The midbrain periaqueductal gray matter. Plenum Press, New York, pp 151–173

Faris PL, Komisaruk BR, Watkins LR, Mayer DJ 1983 Evidence for the neuropeptide cholecystokinin as an antagonist of opiate analgesia. Science 219: 310–312

Fields HL 1992 Is there a facilitating component to central pain modulation? APS Journal 1: 139–141

Fields HL 1988 Sources of variability in the sensation of pain. Pain 33: 195–200

Fields HL, Heinricher MM 1985 Anatomy and physiology of a nociceptive modulatory system. Philosophical Transactions of the Royal Society of London B 308: 361–374

Fields HL, Basbaum AI, Clanton CH, Anderson SD 1977b Nucleus raphe magnus inhibition of spinal cord dorsal horn neurons. Brain Research 126: 441–453

Fields HL, Clanton CH, Anderson SD 1977a Somatosensory properties of spinoreticular neurons in the cat. Brain Research 120: 49–66

Fields HL, Heinricher MM, Mason P 1991 Neurotransmitters in nociceptive modulatory circuits. Annual Review of Neuroscience 14: 219–245

Fields HL, Malick A, Burstein R 1995 Dorsal horn projection targets of on and off cells in the rostral ventromedial medulla. Journal of Neurophysiology 74: 1742–1759

Fleetwood-Walker SM, Hope PJ, Mitchell R, El-Yassir N, Molony V 1988 The influence of opioid receptor subtypes on the processing of nociceptive inputs in the spinal dorsal horn of the cat. Brain Research 451: 213–226

Fornal C, Auerbach S, Jacobs BL 1985 Activity of serotonin-containing neurons in nucleus raphe magnus in freely moving cats. Experimental Neurology 88: 590–608

Gao K, Kim YH, Mason P 1997 Serotonergic pontomedullary neurons are not activated by antinociceptive stimulation in the periaqueductal gray. Journal of Neuroscience 17: 3285–3292

Gao K, Chen DO, Genzen JR, Mason P 1998 Activation of serotonergic neurons in the raphe magnus is not necessary for morphine analgesia. Journal of Neuroscience 18: 1860–1868

Gerhart KD, Yezierski RP, Giesler GJ 1981 Inhibitory receptive fields of primate spinothalmic tract cells. Journal of Neurophysiology 46: 1309–1325

Giesler GJ, Gerhart KD, Yezierski RP, Wilcox TK, Willis WD 1981 Postsynaptic inhibition of primate spinothalamic neurons by stimulation in nucleus raphe magnus. Brain Research 204: 184–188

Glaum SR, Miller RJ, Hammond DL 1994 Inhibitory actions of δ_1 δ_2, and μ-opioid receptor agonists on excitatory transmission in Lamina II neurons of adult rat spinal cord. Journal of Neuroscience 14: 4965–4971

Glazer EJ, Basbaum AI 1981 Immunohistochemical localization of leucine-enkephalin in the spinal cord of the cat: enkephalin-containing marginal neurons and pain modulation. Journal of Comparative Neurology 196: 377–390

Glynn C, Dawson D, Sanders R 1988 A double-blind comparison between epidural morphine and epidural clonidine in patients with chronic non-cancer pain. Pain 34: 123–128

Gogas KR, Presley RW, Levine JD, Basbaum AI 1991 The antinociceptive action of supraspinal opioids results from an increase in descending inhibitory control: correlation of nociceptive behavior and c-*fos* expression. Neuroscience 42: 617–628

Gogas KR, Levine JD, Basbaum AI 1995 Differential contribution of descending controls to the antinociceptive actions of kappa and mu opioids: an analysis of formalin-evoked fos expression. Journal of Pharmacology and Experimental Therapeutics (in press)

Goldberg IE, Rossi GC, Letchworth SR et al 1998 Pharmacological characterization of endomorphin-1 and endomorphin-2 in mouse brain. Journal of Pharmacology and Experimental Therapeutics 286: 1007–1013

Goldstein A, Naidu A 1989 Multiple opioid receptors: ligand selectivity profiles and binding site signatures. Molecular Pharmacology 36: 265–272

Goldstein A, Tachibana S, Lowney LI, Hunkapiller M, Hood L 1979 Dynorphin-(1–13), an extraordinarily potent opioid peptide. Proceedings of the National Academy of Science USA 16: 6666–6670

Gracely RH, Dubner R, Wolskee PJ, Deeter WR 1983 Placebo and naloxone can alter post-surgical pain by separate mechanisms. Nature 306: 264–265

Gray TS, Magnuson DJ 1992 Peptide immunoreactive neurons in the amygdala and the bed nucleus of the stria terminalis project to the midbrain central gray in the rat. Peptides 13: 451–460

Grevert P, Albert LH, Goldstein A 1983a Partial antagonism of placebo analgesia by naloxone. Pain 16: 129–143

Grevert P, Albert LH, Goldstein A 1983b Effects of eight-hour naloxone infusions on human subjects. Biological Psychology 18: 1375–1392

Grevert P, Goldstein A 1985 In: White L, Tursky B, Shwartz GE (eds) Placebo: theory, research and mechanisms. The Guilford Press, New York, pp 332–350

Grudt TJ, Williams JT 1994 μ-opioid agonists inhibit spinal trigeminal substantia gelatinosa neurons in guinea pig and rat. Journal of Neuroscience 14: 1646–1654

Hagbarth KE, Kerr DIB 1954 Central influences on spinal afferent conduction. Journal of Neurophysiology 17: 295–307

Hammond DL, Tyce GM, Yaksh TL 1985 Efflux of 5-hydroxytryptamine and noradrenaline into spinal cord superfusates during stimulation of the rat medulla. Journal of Physiology 359: 151–162

Hammond DL, Presley R, Gogas KR, Basbaum AI 1992 Morphine or U-50,488 suppresses Fos protein-like immunoreactivity in the spinal cord and nucleus tractus solitarii evoked by a noxious visceral stimulus in the rat. Journal of Comparative Neurology 315: 244–253

Hardy SGP, Leichnetz GR 1981 Cortical projections to the periaqueductal gray in the monkey: a retrograde and orthograde horseradish peroxidase study. Neuroscience Letters 22: 97–101

Haws CM, Williamson AM, Fields HL 1989 Putative nociceptive modulatory neurons in the dorsolateral pontomesencephalic reticular formation. Brain Research 483: 272–282

Hayes RL, Price DD, Ruda MA, Dubner R 1981 Neuronal activity in medullary dorsal horn of awake monkeys trained in a thermal discrimination task. II. Behavioral modulation of responses to thermal and mechanical stimuli. Journal of Neurophysiology 46: 428–443

Head H, Holmes G 1911 Sensory disturbances from cerebral lesions. Brain 34: 102–254

Headley PM, Duggan AW, Griersmith BT 1978 Selective reduction by noradrenaline and 5HT of nociceptive responses of cat dorsal horn neurons. Brain Research 145: 185–189

Heinricher MM, Cheng Z, Fields HL 1987 Evidence for two classes of nociceptive modulating neurons in the periaqueductal gray. Journal of Neuroscience 7: 271–278

Heinricher MM, Barbaro NM, Fields HL 1989 Putative nociceptive modulating neurons in the rostral ventromedial medulla of the rat: firing of on- and off-cells is related to nociceptive responsiveness. Somatosensory and Motor Research 6: 427–439

Heinricher MM, Haws CM, Fields HL 1991 Evidence for GABA-mediated control of putative nociceptive modulating neurons in the rostral ventromedial medulla: ionotophoresis of bicuculine eliminates the off-cell pause. Somatosensory and Motor Research 8: 215–225

Heinricher MM, Morgan MM, Fields HL 1992 Direct and indirect action of morphine on medullary neurons that modulate nociception. Neuroscience 48: 533–543

Heinricher MM, Morgan MM, Tortorici V, Fields HL 1994 Disinhibition of off-cells and antinociception produced by an opioid action within the rostral ventromedial medulla. Neuroscience 63: 279–288

Heinricher MM, McGaraughty S, Grandy DK 1997 Circuitry underlying antiopioid actions of orphanin FQ in the rostral ventromedial medulla. Journal of Neurophysiology 78: 3351–3358

Helmstetter FJ 1992 The amygdala is essential for the expression of conditioned hypoalgesia. Behavioral Neuroscience 106: 518–528

Helmstetter FJ, Landeira-Fernandez J 1990 Conditional hypoalgesia is attenuated by naltrexone applied to the periaqueductal gray. Brain Research 537: 88–92

Helmstetter FJ, Tershner SA 1994 Lesions of the periaqueductal gray and rostral ventromedial medulla disrupt antinociceptive but not cardiovascular aversive conditional responses. Journal of Neuroscience 14: 7099–7108

Helmstetter FJ, Tershner SA, Poore LH, Bellgowan PSF 1998 Antinociception following opioid stimulation of the basolateral amygdala is expressed through the periaquaductal gray and rostal ventromedial medulla. Brain Research 119: 104–118

Herbert H, Saper CB 1992 Organization of medullary adrenergic and noradrenergic projections to the periaqueductal gray matter in the rat. Journal of Comparative Neurology 315: 34–52

Herrero JF, Cervero F 1996 Supraspinal influences on the facilitation of rat nociceptive reflexes induced by carrageenan monoarthritis. Neuroscience Letters 209: 21–24

Hökfelt T, Elde R, Johansson O, Terenius L, Stein L 1977a The distribution of enkephalin-immunoreactive cell bodies in the rat central nervous system. Neuroscience Letters 5: 25–31

Hökfelt T, Ljungdahl A, Terenius LRE, Nilsson G 1977b Immunohistochemical analysis of peptide pathways possibly related to pain and analgesia: enkephalin and substance P. Proceedings of the National Academy of Sciences USA 74: 3081–3085

Hökfelt T, Terenius T, Kuypers HGJM, Dann O 1979 Evidence for enkephalin immunoreactive neurons in the medulla oblongata projecting to the spinal cord. Neuroscience Letters 14: 55–60

Hughes J, Smith TW, Kosterlitz HW, Fothergill LA, Morgan BA, Morris HR 1975 Identication of two related pentapeptides from the brain with potent opiate agonist activity. Nature 258: 577–579

Hylden JL, Hayashi H, Dubner R, Bennett GJ 1986 Physiology and morphology of the lamina I spinomesencephalic projection. Journal of Comparative Neurology 247: 505–515

Hylden JLK, Wilcox GL 1983 Intrathecal serotonin in mice: analgesia and inhibition of a spinal action of substance P. Life Sciences 33: 789–795

Iwamoto ET 1991 Characterization of the antinociception induced by nicotine in the pedunculopontine tegmental nucleus and the nucleus raphe magnus. Journal of Pharmacology and Experimental Therapeutics 257: 120–133

Jessell TM, Iversen LL 1977 Opiate analgesics inhibit substance P release from rat trigeminal nucleus. Nature (London) 268: 549–551

Jordan LM, Kenshalo DRJ, Martin RT, Willis WD 1979 Two populations of spinothalamic tract neurons with opposite responses to 5HT. Brain Research 164: 342–346

Kaplan H, Fields HL 1991 Hyperalgesia during acute opioid abstinence: evidence for a nociceptive facilitating function of the rostral ventromedial medulla. Journal of Neuroscience 11: 1433–1439

Keay KA, Clement CI, Owler B, Depaulis A, Bandler R 1994 Convergence of deep somatic and visceral nociceptive information onto a discrete ventrolateral midbrain periaqueductal gray region. Neuroscience 61: 727–732

Khachaturian H, Watson SJ, Lewis ME, Coy D, Goldstein A, Akil H 1982 Dynorphin immunocytochemistry in the rat central nervous system. Peptides 3: 941–954

Khachaturian H, Lewis ME, Watson SJ 1983 Enkephalin systems in diencephalon and brainstem of the rat. Journal of Comparative Neurology 220: 310–320

Khachaturian H, Schafer MKH, Lewis ME 1993 In: Herz A (ed) Handbook of experimental pharmacology, opioids I. Springer, Berlin, pp 471–497

Kiefel JM, Rossi GC, Bodnar RJ 1993 Medullary μ and δ opioid receptors modulate mesencephalic morphine analgesia in rats. Brain Research 624: 151–161

Kim DH, Fields HL, Barbaro NM 1990 Morphine analgesia and acute physical dependence: rapid onset of two opposing, dose-related processes. Brain Research 516: 37–40

Kuhar MJ, Pert CB, Snyder SH 1973 Regional distribution of opiate receptor binding in monkey and human brains. Nature 245: 447–450

Kwiat GC, Basbaum AI 1992 The origin of brainstem noradrenergic and serotonergic projections to the spinal cord dorsal horn in the rat. Somatsensory and Motor Research 9: 157–173

Le Bars D 1988 Serotonin and pain. In: Osborne NN, Hamon M (eds) Neuronal secretion. John Wiley, New York, pp 171–226

Le Bars D, Dickenson AH, Besson JM 1979a Diffuse noxious inhibitory controls (DNIC). I. Effects on dorsal horn convergent neurones in the rat. Pain 6: 283–304

Le Bars D, Dickenson AH, Besson JM 1979b Diffuse noxious inhibitory controls (DNIC). II. Lack of effect on non-convergent neurones, supraspinal involvement and theoretical implications. Pain 6: 305–327

Levine JD, Gordon NC 1984 Influence of the method of drug administration on analgesic response. Nature 312: 755–756

Levine JD, Gordon NC, Jones RT, Fields HL 1978a The narcotic antagonist naloxone enhances clinical pain. Nature 272: 826–827

Levine JD, Gordon NC, Fields HL 1978b The mechanism of placebo analgesia. Lancet ii: 654–657

Levine JD, Lane SR, Gordon NC, Fields HL 1982 A spinal opioid synapse mediates the interaction of spinal and brain stem sites in morphine analgesia. Brain Research 236: 85–91

Light AR, Kavookjian AM 1988 Morphology and ultrastructure of physiologically identified substantia gelatinosa (Lamina II) neurons with axons that terminate in deeper dorsal horn laminae (III–V). Journal of Comparative Neurology 267: 172–189

Lipman JJ, Miller BE, Mays KS, Miller MN, North WC, Byrne WL 1990 Peak B endorphin concentration in cerebrospinal fluid: reduced in chronic pain patients and increased during the placebo response. Psychopharmacology 102: 112–116

Lovick TA 1993 Integrated activity of cardiovascular and pain regulatory systems. Progress in Neurobiology 40: 631–644

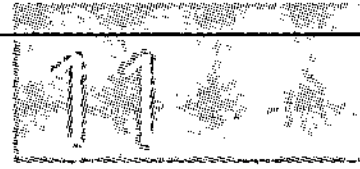

Magoul R, Onteniente B, Geffard M, Calas A 1987 Anatomical distribution and ultrastructural organization of the gabaergic system in the rat spinal cord. An immunocytochemical study using anti-GABA antibodies. Neuroscience 20: 1001–1009

Mains RE, Eipper BA, Ling N 1977 Common precursor to corticotrophin and endorphins. Proceedings of the National Academy of Sciences USA 74: 3014–3018

Manning BH, Franklin KBJ 1998 Morphine analgesia in the formalin test: reversal by microinjection of quaternary naloxone into the posterior hypothalamic area or periaqueductal gray. Behavioral Brain Research 92: 97–102

Manning BH, Mayer DJ 1995 The central nucleus of the amygdala contributes to the production of morphine antinociception in the rat tail-flick test. Journal of Neuroscience 15: 8199–8213

Manning BH, Morgan MJ, Franklin KBJ 1994 Morphine analgesia in the formalin test: evidence for forebrain and midbrain sites of action. Neuroscience 63: 289–294

Mansour A, Fox CA, Watson SJ 1995 Opioid-receptor mRNA expression in the rat CNS: anatomical and functional implications. Trends in Neuroscience 18: 22–29

Martin WJ, Malmberg AB, Basbaum AI 1998 Nocistatin spells relief. Current Biology 8: R525–527

Martin-Schild S, Zadina JE, Gerall AA, Vigh S, Kastin AJ 1997 Localization of endomorphin-2-like immunoreactivity in the rat medulla and spinal cord. Peptides 18: 1641–1649

Mason P 1997 Physiological identification of pontomedullary serotonergic neurons in the rat. Journal of Neurophysiology 77: 1087–1098

Mason P, Fields HL 1989 Axonal trajectories and terminations of on- and off-cells in the cat lower brainstem. Journal of Comparative Neurology 288: 185–207

Mason P, Gao K 1998 Raphe magnus serotonergic neurons tonically modulate nociceptive transmission. Pain Forum (in press)

Mason P, Back SA, Fields HL 1992 A confocal laser microscopic study of enkephalin-immunoreactive appositions onto physiologically identified neurons in the rostral ventromedial medulla. Journal of Neuroscience 12: 4023–4036

Matos FF, Rollema H, Brown JL, Basbaum AI 1992 Do opioids evoke the release of serotonin in the spinal cord? An in vivo microdialysis study of the regulation of extracellular serotonin in the rat. Pain 48: 439–447

Mayer DJ, Price DD 1976 Central nervous system mechanisms of analgesia. Pain 2: 379–404

Mayer DJ, Wolfe TL, Akil H, Carder B, Liebeskind JC 1971 Analgesia from electrical stimulation in the brain stem of the rat. Science 174: 1351–1354

Melzack R 1975 Prolonged relief of pain by brief, intense transcutaneous somatic stimulation. Pain 1: 357–373

Melzack R, Wall PD 1982 Acute pain in an emergency clinic: latency of onset and descriptor patterns related to different injuries. Pain 14: 33–43

Melzack R, Wall PD 1965 Pain mechanisms: a new theory. Science 150: 971–999

Menetrey DA, Chaouch A, Binder D, Besson JM 1982 The origin of the spinomesencephalic tract in the rat: an anatomical study using the retrograde transport of horseradish peroxidase. Journal of Comparative Neurology 206: 193–207

Meunier JC 1997 Nociceptin/orphanin FQ and the opioid receptor-like ORL1 receptor. European Journal of Pharmacology 340: 1–15

Meunier JC, Mollereau C, Tol L et al 1995 Isolation and structure of the endogenous agonist of opioid receptor-like ORL1 receptor. Nature (London) 377: 532–535

Millan MH, Millan MJ, Herz A 1986 Depletion of central β-endorphin blocks midbrain stimulation-produced analgesia in the freely-moving rat. Neuroscience 18: 641–649

Millan MJ, Czlonkowski A, Millan MH, Herz A 1987 Activation of periaqueductal grey pools of beta-endorphin by analgetic electrical stimulation in freely moving rats. Brain Research 407: 199–203

Millar J, Williams GV 1989 Effects of iontophoresis of noradrenaline and stimulation of the periaqueductal gray on single-unit activity in the rat superficial dorsal horn. Journal of Comparative Neurology 287: 119–133

Miller KK, Hoffer A, Svoboda KR, Lupica CR 1997 Cholecystokinin increases GABA release by inhibiting a resting κ+ conductance in hippocampal interneurons. Journal of Neuroscience 17: 4994–5003

Miller RJ 1981 Peptides as neurotransmitters: focus on the enkephalins and endorphins. Pharmaceutical Therapy 12: 73–108

Miron D, Duncan GH, Bushnell MC 1989 Effects of attention on the intensity and unpleasantness of thermal pain. Pain 39: 345–352

Mitchell JM, Lowe D, Fields HL 1998 The contribution of the rostral ventromedial medulla to the antinociceptive effects of systemic morphine in restrained and unrestrained rats. Neuroscience 87: 123–133

Mogil JS, Grisel JE, Reinscheid R, Civelli O, Belknap JK, Grandy DK 1996 Orphanin FQ is a functional anti-opioid peptide. Neuroscience 75: 333–337

Moore RY 1981 In: Jacobs BL, Gelperin A (eds) Serotonin neurotransmission and behavior. MIT Press, Cambridge, MA, pp 35–71

Moreau J-L, Fields HL 1986 Evidence for GABA involvement in midbrain control of medullary neurons that modulate nociceptive transmission. Brain Research 397: 37–46

Morgan MM, Heinricher MM, Fields HL 1994 Inhibition and facilitation of different nocifensor reflexes by spatially remote noxious thermal stimuli. Journal of Neurophysiology 72: 1152–1160

Moss MS, Glazer EJ, Basbaum AI 1983 The peptidergic organization of the cat periaqueductal gray. I. The distribution of immunoreactive enkephalin-containing neurons and terminals. Journal of Neuroscience 3: 603–616

Okuda-Ashitaka E, Minami T, Tachibana S et al 1998 Nocistatin, a peptide that blocks nociceptin action in pain transmission. Nature (London) 392: 286–289

Oliveras J-L, Martin G, Montagne J, Vos B 1990 Single unit activity at ventromedial medulla level in the awake, freely moving rat: effects of noxious heat and light tactile stimuli onto convergent neurons. Brain Research 506: 19–30

Oshita S, Yaksh TL, Chipkin R 1990 The antinociceptive effects of intrathecally administered SCH32615, an enkephalinase inhibitor, in the rat. Brain Research 515: 143–148

Pan ZZ, Fields HL 1996 Endogenous opioid-mediated inhibition of putative pain-modulating neurons in rat rostral ventromedial medulla. Neuroscience 74: 855–862

Pan ZZ, Williams JT, Osborne PB 1990 Opioid actions on single nucleus raphe magnus neurons from rat and guinea-pig in vitro. Journal of Physiology (London) 427: 519–532

Pan ZZ, Tershner SA, Fields HL 1997 Cellular mechanism for anti-analgesic action of agonists of the k-opioid receptor. Nature 389: 382–385

Pavlovic Z, Cooper M, Bodnar R 1996 Opioid antagonists in the periaqueductal gray inhibit morphine and betendorphin analgesia elicited from the amygdala of rats. Brain Research 741: 13–26

Peng YB, Lin Q, Willis WD 1996 Involvement of alpha-2 adrenoceptors in the periaqueductal gray-induced inhibition of dorsal horn activity in rats. Journal of Pharmacology and Experimental Therapeutics 278: 125–135

Pittius CW, Seizinger BR, Pasi A, Mehraein P, Herz A 1984 Distribution and characterization of opioid peptides derived from proenkephalin A in human and rat central nervous system. Brain Research 304: 127–136

Potrebic S, Fields HL, Mason P 1994 Serotonin immunocytochemistry is contained in one physiological cell class in the rat rostral ventromedial medulla. Journal of Neuroscience 14: 1655–1665

Presley RW, Menetrey D, Levine JD, Basbaum AI 1990 Systemic morphine suppresses noxious stimulus-evoked fos protein-like immunoreactivity in the rat spinal cord. Journal of Neuroscience 10: 323–335

Prichard SM, Beitz AJ 1981 The localisation of brainstem enkephalinergic and substance P neurons which project to the rodent nucleus raphe magnus. Society of Neuroscience Abstracts 7: 59

Proudfit HK In: Fields HL, Besson JM (eds) Progress in brain research, vol 77. Elsevier Science, pp 357–370

Ramírez F, Vanegas H 1989 Tooth pulp stimulation advances both medullary off-cell pause and tail flick. Neuroscience Letters 100: 153–156

Randic M, Yu HH 1976 Effects of 5-hydroxytryptamine and bradykinin in cat dorsal horn neurones activated by noxious stimuli. Brain Research 111: 197–203

Reichling DB, Basbaum AI 1990 Contribution of brainstem GABAergic circuitry to descending antinociceptive controls: I. GABA-immunoreactive projection neurons in the periaqueductal gray and nucleus raphe magnus. Journal of Comparative Neurology 302: 302–377

Ren K, Dubner R 1996 Enhanced descending modulation of nociception in rats with persistent hindpaw inflammation. Journal of Neurophysiology 76: 3025–3037

Ren K, Ruda MA 1996 Descending modulation of Fos expression after persistent peripheral inflammation. Neuroreport 7: 2186–2190

Reynolds DV 1969 Surgery in the rat during electrical analgesia by focal brain stimulation. Science 164: 444–445

Rhodes DL, Liebeskind JC 1978 Analgesia from rostral brain stem stimulation in the rat. Brain Research 143: 521–532

Roberts MHT 1989 Pharmacology of putative neurotransmitters and receptors: 5-hydroxytryptamine. In: Fields HL (ed) Pain modulation. Elsevier, Amsterdam, pp 329–338

Rohde DS, Basbaum AI 1998 Activation of coeruleospinal noradrenergic inhibitory controls during withdrawal from morphine in the rat. Journal of Neuroscience 18: 4393–4402

Rossi G, Pasternak G, Bodnar R 1994 Mu and delta opioid synergy between the periaquaductal gray and the rosro-ventral medulla. Brain Research 665: 85–93

Roychowdhury SM, Fields HL 1996 Endogenous opioids acting at a medullary μ-opioid receptor contribute to the behavioral antinociception produced by GABA antagonism in the midbrain periaqueductal gray. Neuroscience 74: 863–872

Ruda MA, Bennett GJ, Dubner R 1986 Neurochemistry and neural circuitry in the dorsal horn. Progress in Brain Research 66: 219–268

Schmauss C, Hammond DL, Ochi JW, Yaksh TL 1983 Pharmacological antagonism of the antinociceptive effects of serotonin in the rat and spinal cord. European Journal of Pharmacology 90: 349–357

Schreff M, Schulz S, Wiborny D, Höllt V 1998 Immunofluorescent identification of endomorphin-2-containing nerve fibers and terminals in the rat brain and spinal cord. Neuroreport 9: 1031–1034

Shipley MT, Murphy AZ, Rizvi TA, Ennis M, Behbehani MM 1996 In: Holstege R, Bandler R, Saper CB (eds) Progress in brain research, vol 107. Elsevier, New York, pp 355–377

Skinner K, Basbaum AI, Fields HL 1997a Cholecystokinin and enkephalin in brain stem pain modulating circuits. Neuroreport 8: 2995–2998

Skinner K, Fields HL, Basbaum AI, Mason P 1997b GABA-immunoreactive boutons contact identified OFF and ON cells in the nucleus raphe magnus. Journal of Comparative Neurology 378: 196–204

Solomon RE, Gebhart GF 1988 Mechanisms of effects of intrathecal serotonin on nociception and blood pressure in rats. Journal of Pharmacology and Experimental Therapeutics 245: 905–912

Sora I, Takahashi N, Funada M et al 1997 Opiate receptor knockout mice define mu receptor roles in endogenous nociceptive responses and morphine-induced analgesia. Proceedings of the National Academy of Sciences USA 94: 1544–1549

Sorkin LS, McAdoo DJ, Willis WD 1993 Raphe magnus stimulation-induced antinociception in the cat is associated with release of amino acids as well as serotonin in the lumbar dorsal horn. Brain Research 618: 95–108

Stanfa LC, Chapman V, Kerr N, Dickenson AH 1996 Inhibitory action of nociceptin on spinal dorsal horn neurones of the rat, in vivo. British Journal of Pharmacology 118: 1875–1877

Stone LS, Fairbanks CA, Laughlin TM et al 1997 Spinal analgesic actions of the new endogenous opioid peptides endomorphin-1 and -2. NeuroReport 8: 3131–3135

Suarez-Roca H, Abdullah L, Zuniga J, Madison S, Maixner W 1992 Multiphasic effect of morphine on the release of substance P from rat trigeminal nucleus slices. Brain Research 579: 187–194

Tenen SS 1968 Antagonism of the analgesic effect of morphine and other drugs by p-chlorophenylalanine, a serotonin depletor. Psychopharmacologia 12: 278–285

Thorat SN, Hammond DL 1997 Role of medullary delta-1 or delta-2 opioid receptors in antinociception: studies with subtype selective antagonists. Journal of Pharmacology and Experimental Therapeutics 283: 1185–1192

Todd AJ, McKenzie J 1989 GABA-immunoreactive neurons in the dorsal horn of the rat spinal cord. Neuroscience 31: 799–806

Todd AJ, Millar J 1983b Receptive fields and responses to iontophoretically applied noradrenaline and 5-hydroxytryptamine of units recorded in laminae I-III of cat dorsal horn. Brain Research 288: 159–167

Todd AJ, Spike RC, Johnston HM 1992 Immunohistochemical evidence that Met-enkephalin and GABA coexist in some neurons in rat dorsal horn. Brain Research 584: 149–156

Tölle TR, Castro LJ, Coimbra A, Zieglgänsberger W 1990 Opiates modify induction of c-*fos* proto-oncogene in the spinal cord of the rat following noxious stimulation. Neuroscience Letters 111: 46–51

Tsuruoka M, Willis WD 1996 Descending modulation from the region of the locus coeruleus on nociceptive sensitivity in rat model of inflammatory hyperalgesia. Brain Research 743: 86–92

Urban MO, Gebhart GF 1997 Characterization of biphasic modulation of spinal nociceptive transmission by neurotensin in the rat rostral ventromedial medulla. Journal of Neurophysiology 78: 1550–1562

Urban MO, Smith DJ 1993 Role of neurotensin in the nucleus raphe magnus in opioid induced antinociception from the periaqueductal gray. Journal of Pharmacology and Experimental Therapeutics 265: 580–586

Urban MO, Smith DJ 1994a Localization of the antinociceptive and antianalgesic effects of neurotensin within the rostral ventromedial medulla. Neuroscience Letters 174: 21–25

Urban MO, Smith DJ 1994b Nuclei within the rostral ventromedial medulla mediating morphine antinociception from the periaqueductal gray. Brain Research 652: 9–16

Valverde O, Maldonado R, Fournie-Zaluski MC, Roques BP 1994 Cholecystokinin B antagonists strongly potentiate antinociception mediated by endogenous enkephalins. Journal of Pharmacology and Experimental Therapeutics 270: 77–88

Van Bockstaele EJ, Aston-Jones G, Pieribone VA, Ennis M, Shipley MT 1991 Subregions of the periaqueductal gray topographically innervate the rostral ventral medulla in the rat. Journal of Comparative Neurology 309: 305–327

Vaughn CW, Ingram SL, Christie MJ 1997 Actions of the ORL receptor ligand nociceptin on membrane properties of rat periaqueductal gray neurons in vitro. Journal of Neuroscience 17: 996–1003

Villaneuva L 1998 Organization of diencephalic projections from the medullary subnucleus reticularis dorsalis and the adjacent cuneate nucleus: a retrograde and anterograde tracer study in the rat. Journal of Comparative Neurology 390: 133–160

Villaneuva L, Bourhassira D, Le Bars D 1996 The medullary subnucleus reticularis dorsalis (SRD) as a key link in both the transmission and modulation of pain signals. Pain 67: 231–240

Vogt M 1974 The effect of lowering the 5-hydroxytryptamine content of the rat spinal cord on analgesia produced by morphine. Journal of Physiology 236: 483–498

Wall PD 1967 The laminar organisation of dorsal horn and effects of descending impulses. Journal of Physiology 188: 403–423

Watkins LR, Cobelli DA, Mayer DJ 1982 Classical conditioning of front paw and hind paw footshock induced analgesia (FSIA): naloxone reversibility and descending pathways. Brain Research 243: 119–132

Watkins LR, Mayer DJ 1982 Organization of endogenous opiate and nonopiate pain control systems. Science 216: 1185–1192

Watkins LR, Maier SF, Goehler LE 1995 Immune activation: the role of pro-inflammatory cytokines in inflammation, illness responses and pathological pain states. Pain 63: 289–302

Watkins LR, Young EG, Kinscheck IB, Mayer JD 1983 The neural basis of footshock analgesia: the role of specific ventral medullary nuclei. Brain Research 276: 305–315

Watkins LR, Wiertelak EP, McGorry M et al 1998 Neurocircuitry of conditioned inhibition of analgesia: effects of amygdala, dorsal raphe, ventral medullary, and spinal cord lesions on antianalgesia in the rat. Behavioral Neuroscience 112: 360–378

Watson SJ, Akil H 1980 Alpha-MSH in rat brain: occurrence within and outside of beta-endorphin neurons. Brain Research 182: 217–223

Weber E, Roth KA, Barchas JD 1981 Colocalisation of alpha-neo-endorphin and dynorphin immunoreactivity in hypothalamic neurons. Biophysical Communications 103: 951–958

Wei F, Ren K, Dubner R 1998 Inflammation-induced Fos protein expression in the rat spinal cord is enhanced following dorsolateral or ventrolateral funiculus lesions. Brain Research 782: 136–141

Westlund KN, Carlton SM, Zhang D, Willis WD 1990 Direct catecholaminergic innervation of primate spinothalamic tract neurons. Journal of Comparative Neurology 299: 178–186

Wiertelak EP, Maier SF, Watkins LR 1992 Cholecystokinin antianalgesia: safety cues abolish morphine analgesia. Science 256: 830–833

Willcockson WS, Gerhart KD, Cargill CL, Willis WD 1983 Effects of biogenic amines on raphe-spinal tract cells. Journal of Pharmacology and Experimental Therapeutics 225: 637

Willis WD, Coggeshall RE 1991 Sensory mechanisms of the spinal cord, 2nd edn Plenum Press, New York, p 575

Willis WD, Haber LH, Martin RF 1977 Inhibition of spinothalamic tract cells and interneurons by brain stem stimulation in the monkey. Journal of Neurophysiology 40: 968–981

Wolkowitz OM, Tinklenberg JR 1985 Naloxone's effects on cognitive functioning in drug-free and diazepam-treated normal humans. Psychopharmacology 85: 221–223

Yaksh TL 1979 Direct evidence that spinal serotonin and noradrenaline terminals mediate the spinal antinociceptive effects of morphine in the periaqueductal grey. Brain Research 160: 180–185

Yaksh TL, Elde RP 1981 Factors governing release of methionine-enkephalin-like immunoreactivity from mesencephalon and spinal cord of cat in vivo. Journal of Neurophysiology 46: 1056–1075

Yaksh TL, Noueihed R 1985 The physiology and pharmacology of spinal opiates. Annual Review of Pharmacology and Toxicology 243: 433–462

Yaksh TL, Rudy TA 1978 Narcotic analgetics: CNS sites and mechanisms of action as revealed by intracerebral injection techniques. Pain 4: 299–359

Yaksh TL, Wilson PR 1979 Spinal serotonin system mediates antinociception. Journal of Pharmacology and Experimental Therapeutics 208: 446–453

Yamamoto T, Nozaki-Taguchi N, Kimura S 1997 Analgesic effect of intrathecally administered nociceptin, an opioid receptor-like 1 receptor agonist, in the rat formalin test. Neuroscience 81: 249–254

Yeomans DC, Clark FM, Paice JA, Proudfit HK 1992 Antinociception induced by electrical stimulation of spinally projecting noradrenergic neurons in the A7 catecholamine cell group of the rat. Pain 48: 449–461

Yeomans DC, Proudfit HK 1990 Projections of substance P-immunoreactive neurons located in the ventromedial medulla to the A7 noradrenergic nucleus of the rat demonstrated using retrograde tracing combined with immunocytochemistry. Brain Research 532: 329–332

Young RF, Tronnier V, Rinaldi PC 1992 Chronic stimulation of the Kolliker–Fuse nucleus region for relief of intractable pain in humans. Journal of Neurosurgery 76: 979–985

Zadina JE, Hackler L, Ge L, Kastin AJ 1997 A potent and selective endogenous agonist for the μ-opiate receptor. Nature 499–501

Zhuo M, Gebhart GF 1992 Characterization of descending facilitation and inhibition of spinal nociceptive transmission from the nuclei reticularis gigantocellularis and gigantocellularis pars alpha in the rat. Journal of Neurophysiology 67: 1599–1614

Zorman G, Belcher G, Adams JE, Fields HL 1982 Lumbar intrathecal naloxone blocks analgesia produced by microstimulation of the ventromedial medulla in the rat. Brain Research 236: 77–84

Emotions and psychobiology

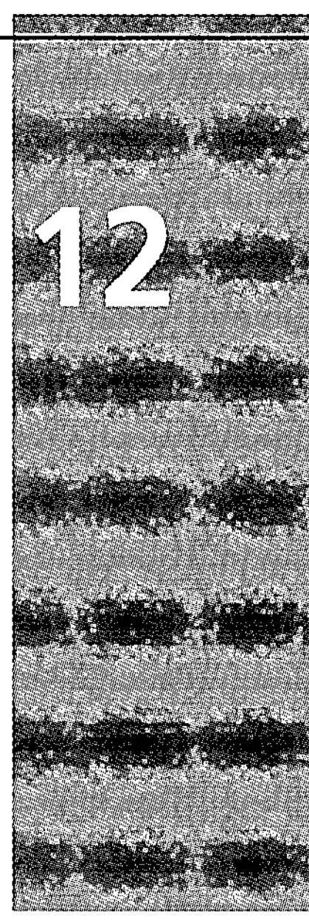

KENNETH D. CRAIG

SUMMARY

Emotional distress is the most undesirable feature of painful experiences. The many forms of pain are associated with varying severities and qualities of emotional distress, primarily fear, anxiety, anger and depression. While recognizing the importance of affect, most scientists and clinicians continue to focus upon 'pain sensation' rather than 'pain affect', despite the clinical importance of controlling the latter. An emerging literature describes central nervous system transmission systems for the affective-motivational components of pain, focusing upon spinoreticular pathways. Links with the biological substrates for the sensory-discriminative qualities of pain and cortical mechanisms are contributing to the broader perspective of pain that emphasizes affective and cognitive as well as sensory mechanisms. This broader model is reflected in the numerous behaviourally based studies examining anticipatory fear and avoidance of pain, the emotional consequences of pain, emotional distress as a source of pain, and investigations of concurrent psychological disorders. Greater integration of biological and behavioural perspectives is needed.

INTRODUCTION

The emotional distress arising from painful injuries and diseases is the most disruptive and undesirable feature of the usually tumultuous, dynamic flow of sensations, feelings, thoughts and images that pain can provoke. Most often one observes fear, anxiety, anger and depression, but frustration, guilt, disgust and subservience are not unusual. In the absence of negative affect and related fearful beliefs and apprehensions of physical threat, mutilation or death, people in pain could not reasonably be described as 'suffering'. In fact, the 'cold' information value of the sensory input alone can be construed as of considerable benefit because of its warning function. But the evolved reality is otherwise. Subjective experiences also have a 'hot' side. Through processes of selective adaptation, humans became equipped with a capacity to experience qualities of pain that are not only highly informative about threats to biological safety but also instigate states of distress varying from those that are tolerable to those that incite despair and terrible suffering.

The central role of emotional distress is recognized in the widely accepted and influential definition of pain promulgated by the International Association for the Study of Pain. It states that pain is 'an unpleasant sensory and emotional experience associated with actual or potential tissue damage, or described in terms of such damage' (Merskey & Bogduk 1994). The definition resonates with peoples' personal experiences and has substantial empirical support in both psychological studies of the subjective experience of pain and in our understanding of biological mechanisms that mediate the experience.

Dominant, comprehensive, theoretical models of pain also recognize affective qualities as integral and essential to the experience. The influence of the gate control theory of pain (Melzack & Wall 1965) can be attributed in part to its recognition that tissue stress concurrently activates both affective-motivational and sensory-discriminative components of pain (Melzack & Casey 1968). The sensory-discriminative information maps the nature of the stimulus (thermal, mechanical, or chemical) and the bodily location, intensity and temporal aspects of the experience. The affective-motivational features comprise the emotions of concern here, as well as their arousing, compelling and directive nature as they evoke action in the form of reflexes or complex behaviour leading to escape and avoidance. Both sensory and affective qualities combine with memories of earlier experiences to generate meaning and assist in evaluation of the experience.

While the profound role of affective discomfort is widely recognized, the focus of both practitioners and scientists has been on sensory-discriminative features. It seems surprisingly easy to ignore or subordinate the importance of the affective qualities of the pain experience. It is commonplace to talk about 'pain sensation', not 'pain affect'. A health professional's query of a patient, 'How is your pain', ordinarily evokes a response in terms of intensity or severity, with some qualitative terms perhaps added. However, these emotional qualities should not serve as mere overtones. They play a crucial role in the experience of the patient and knowledge of them can and should dictate diagnosis and treatment. Unfortunately, they are less easily described, unless explicit attention is attracted to them, perhaps in the form of questions prompting attention to them and supplying response alternatives (e.g., the McGill Pain Questionnaire; Melzack 1983).

Substantially greater advances have been made in understanding biological mechanisms subserving the sensory-discriminative features of nociception than the affective-motivational processes. It could be argued that the ease with which one can instigate and measure sensory-discriminative features of pain makes a focus upon sensory qualities inevitable. In the laboratory, one can control, with a high degree of precision, the sensory input instigating pain in both non-human and human species. In the clinic, it is also easier to determine the nature of physical damage or disease instigating sensory input than it is to assess the nature and determinants of emotional reactions. Likewise, response parameters reflecting sensory input are not difficult to construct and use, irrespective of the animal being studied. With non-human species, escape and other behavioural measures can be constructed somewhat readily, usually to examine pain sensation. For example, the investigations of Vierck et al (1989) examining pain sensitivity, as inferred from complex behaviours in laboratory animals, focuses on differentiating sensory, motor or attentional mechanisms, as well as the distinctions between reflexive and operant reactions and those between nociceptive and non-nociceptive sensations, rather than the emotions inferable from indices of escape and avoidance conditioning.

With humans, self-report methods are available for identifying both sensory-discriminative and affective-motivational qualities of their experiences and a considerable literature is available. However, the psychobiology of these experiences is not well understood. Humans are rarely studied experimentally when the biological substrates of pain are being examined. Bromm (1989) notes, 'Everything we know about the anatomy of the dorsal horn, the synaptic projections, the mechanisms of spatial and temporal summation, the interactions with other afferent and efferent systems, and the transmissions in ascending or descending pathways was learned from the laboratory animal' (p. 117). One cannot learn through self report from animals if they are suffering from feelings of fear, sadness, irritability, hopelessness, worthlessness or contemplating death or suicide. Thus, the pragmatics of investigating the biological substrates of these emotional experiences, to say nothing of the complex ethical considerations, are likely to delay the development of a solid knowledge base. Even when there are efforts to examine biological substrates of pain in humans, there seem to be subtle biases to remain focused upon sensory experiences. Even common speech habits can be problematic. Chapman notes that our habit of referring to pain as a sensation implies that it is a transient event. He argues that we should construe pain 'as a state of the organism that has as its primary defining feature awareness of and homeostatic adjustment to tissue trauma (p. 287)', and emphasizes that it is 'a state of discomfort and distress' (p. 298).

Pursuing both instigators and measures of affective qualities of pain is a particularly difficult task. What drives emotional reactions to painful events? The individual variability in response to painful tissue damage is well known, indeed almost infamous. Major variation undoubtedly derives from appraisal of the context of painful events. Measuring affective reactions is also challenging. Self-report methods are available (Jensen 1997) to provide at least partial access to subjective experiences, and measures are available for at least anxiety and depression (Craig & Dobson 1995). However these methods are limited by requirements for candid self report, the potential for situational biases, and needs to validate and establish the reliability of measurement tools and strategies.

Despite issues of experimental feasibility, we require a better understanding of biological mechanisms controlling affective responses to pain. Willis (1995) emphasizes the importance of understanding affective-motivational components of the biological pain system with the observation that 'Clinically, this may well be the most relevant component of human pain, and so deserves more experimental attention than it has received' (p. 7).

BIOLOGICAL SUBSTRATES OF AFFECTIVE COMPONENTS OF PAIN

Biological and psychological aspects of emotional aspects of pain must be understood, with each representing different, but complementary, levels of analysis. Each describes the same phenomenon but from different perspectives, with both necessary for comprehensive understanding in the interests of developing more effective treatments (Engel 1977, 1980). The reductionistic, biological perspective on emotional processes establishes how experience is encoded in fundamental structures and operating systems. While potentially progressively microanalytical in approach, ultimately biological explanations must be as system oriented as explanations at the psychological level because of the interconnectedness of perceptual, emotional, cognitive and behavioural phenomena. The biological systems represent fundamental constraints on experience, but these are not fixed or rigid. They were designed to permit adaptation to an extraordinary range of environments and situations and are capable of considerable plasticity. This is demonstrable through analysis of the memory and learning capabilities of organisms and at the level of biological plasticity.

We presently have a good understanding of the ascending pathways that convey nociceptive information from peripheral nociceptors to higher levels of the central nervous system, as well as descending pathways that modulate the pain system. Ascending neurons in the spinothalamic tract, the thalamus and the primary somatosensory cortex are responsible primarily for the sensory-discriminative features of pain. Affective-motivational qualities are transmitted and processed in the same pathways as well as in diencephalic and telencephalic structures, including the medial thalamus, hypothalamus, amygdala and limbic cortex (Willis 1995). The focus here is on those biological substrates responsible for the unpleasant and emotional subjective qualities of pain and is based on the rich literature on the neurobiology of emotion (Derryberry & Tucker 1992, Chapman 1995).

A variety of nociceptors innervate the skin, joints, muscles and viscera, with activation of different types of nociceptors resulting in particular qualities of pain. What the person perceives is determined not by the uniquely specialized fibre, but by the brain abstracting the spatial and temporal pattern of the afferent barrage (Wall & McMahon 1985). Even at the level of primary instigation of the noxious afferent signal, distinctions can be made between afferents primarily engaged in transmitting sensory-discriminative information and those associated with affective-discomfort. A common distinction in the qualities of an acute pain experience is made between first and second pain. The first represents the immediate sharp, 'bright' or pricking burst of awareness of acute trauma and is conveyed by Aδ fibres, while the second, conveyed in part by C fibres, represents the slower, more persistent burning pain or dull awareness of tissue damage. The former may serve as a warning of physical threat and the latter as a continuing reminder. People suffering acute pain do not usually make the distinction, although it becomes apparent when attention is directed to it. Bromm (1989) notes that volunteers usually spontaneously report first pain, but can be trained to perceive the second.

The potential for differentiation of sensory and affective processing of afferent input becomes evident in the dorsal horn of the spinal cord, with transmission of sensory-discriminative features primarily utilizing spinothalamic pathways and affective-motivational input ascending along spinoreticular pathways, although both transmit information about tissue injury. Price and Dubner (1977) carefully develop lines of evidence for identifying specific neurons and tracts as subserving sensory-discriminative functions. In addressing the question as to whether there is evidence for a distinct motivational-affective pain system that is activated separately and in parallel with sensory-discriminative systems, they express doubt that it would serve pain alone. They note that the neural structures proposed as part of this system are accessed by other modalities, for example bad tastes and smells.

Melzack and Casey (1968) inspired considerable interest in affective-motivational substrates of pain, noting that the reticular core of the brainstem, the medial thalamus, and parts of the limbic brain are responsible for the affective component of pain that drives the individual to seek relief. It is noteworthy that the limbic system is implicated in all emotional processes (Chapman 1996). Wall (1996) questions the validity of the argument that there are two anatomically distinct systems responsible for the sensory and emotional qualities of the experience, emphasizing the intimate association between the two. Nevertheless, he agrees with the general strategy of isolating pain affect for specific consideration.

Chapman (1995) describes how processing of nociceptive signals produces affect in multiple pathways that project from the thalamus to the cortex. Noradrenergic, serotonergic, dopaminergic and acetylcholinergic fibres are involved. Drawing upon an extensive literature on the biology of emotion (e.g., Gray 1987), noradrenergic pathways are recognized as linked most closely to negative emotional states. Of particular note are nociceptive afferent systems operating and transmitting through limbic brain mechanisms (in particular, the locus coeruleus, the dorsal noradrenergic bundle, the ventral noradrenergic bundle and the hypothalamo–pituitary–adrenocortical axis) that are not specific in their activation to nociception, but are also responsive to non-nociceptive, aversive emotional states. These systems are recognized as fostering survival by allowing biological vigilance to threatening and harmful stimuli, both external and internal. A succession of studies has demonstrated the important role of the limbic system in the affective-motivational component of pain. Injection of local anaesthetic into limbic structures, such as the lateral hypothalamus (Tasker et al 1987), the cingulum bundle (Vaccarino & Melzack 1989) and the dentate nucleus of the hippocampal formation (McKenna & Melzack 1992), temporarily blocks neural activity and may induce significant analgesia during late tonic pain perception. For example, Vaccarino and Melzack (1989) reported that rats subjected to intense, tonic pain, relative to rats suffering brief, phasic pain, displayed attenuated responses when lidocaine was injected into the cingulum, a major link between limbic structures and the cortex.

Cortical mechanisms of affective processing also have received attention. Kenshalo and Douglass (1995) provide evidence from both clinical observations and animal studies that the anterior cingulate cortex is involved in the affective-motivational aspects of pain. Medial thalamic neurons project to limbic cortices, including the anterior cingulate cortex. Surgical lesions of the cingulate cortex and/or the cingulum bundle are described as able to alleviate chronic pain. For example, Corkin and Hebbin (1981) reported that cingulotomy reduced the emotional but not the sensory component of chronic pain. The effects of cingulotomies apparently are more substantial among patients suffering anxiety and depression (Vaccarino & Melzack 1989, Kenshalo & Douglass 1995). As well, the lack of somatotopic organization and the convergence of cutaneous, visceral, and joint-related information suggest that the ventrolateral orbital cortex plays a role in affective-motivational components of pain. Kenshalo and Douglass (1995) suggest that activation of this area may be responsible for the unpleasant experience that causes organisms to attempt escape from prolonged painful stimulation.

New brain imaging techniques provide novel opportunities to study neurobiological correlates of human pain. Studies using positron-emission tomography (PET) to image brain response to painful heat stimuli applied to the arm of human subjects indicated activation of both the somatosensory cortex and the anterior cingulate gyrus (Talbot et al 1991). Rainville et al (1997) recently observed that pain affect is encoded in the anterior cingulate but not in the somatosensory cortex. Casey et al (1995) concluded, on the strength of PET scan images, that activation of structures associated with autonomic and limbic-system functions, such as the insula and anterior cingulate cortex, may reflect the affective aspect of pain experience. Morrow et al (1998), using PET scan with rats exposed to tonic pain, demonstrate further the role of limbic connection and their association with classical sensory projection systems.

In delineating biological mechanisms associated with the affective-motivational aspects of pain, one cannot consider only central nervous system structures. Contributing to the experience will be the afferent input from somatic reflexes, autonomic and visceral changes, and endocrine system involvement. Recognition of these mechanisms attracts attention to the role of emotions as constituting the psychological correlates of biological changes and adaptive regulatory systems designed to restore physiological balance or homeostasis. Conscious awareness of emotional distress in adult humans perhaps signals an integration of more primitive biological emotions with a capacity to think and reason to find solutions to personal harm and threat. One can bring to bear on our understanding of pain the extensive literatures on the neurophysiology and endocrinology of stress because of its significant participation in response to painful events.

PSYCHOLOGICAL PARAMETERS OF EMOTIONAL COMPONENTS OF PAIN

Behavioural manifestations of pain provide a valuable window on the psychobiology of pain perception, but difficult problems arise. Questions emerge concerning the validity of both verbal and non-verbal communication channels for accessing subjective experiences (Sullivan 1995). The dynamic, often turbulent, flow of feelings, images and thoughts is not readily reduced to descriptive language. Lewis (1942) observed that 'pain, like similar subjective feelings, is known to us by experience and described by illustration'. Melzack and Dennis (1980) note the vague and diffuse feelings associated with pain in observing that 'The affective dimension is difficult to express – words such as exhausting, sickening, terrifying, cruel, vicious and killing come close but are often inadequate descriptions of the affective experience of the pain of causalgia or cancer.'

Non-verbal expression provides complementary information. The experience and expression of emotion are intimately connected, with current concepts of non-verbal activity emphasizing its communicative functions (Prkachin & Craig 1995, Bavelas & Chovil 1997). For example, a bioevolutionary perspective on facial activity (Fridlund 1994), when extrapolated to pain, suggests that facial displays serve the purpose of conveying information about threats to safety to caretaking others who can provide protection. One can derive considerable information about others through attending to facial activity, gestures, body posture and actions, and other subtle non-verbal cues (e.g., Ekman & Rosenberg 1997). Using explicit and a priori criteria for facial displays of pain and a range of emotions, Hale and Hadjistavropoulos (1997) were able to identify among patients being subjected to venipuncture not only a display of pain but also the emotions of disgust, fear, and anger.

While judgements of the experiences of others can use multiple information channels, questions about the credibility of these sources are often raised. While verbal and non-verbal indexes of pain may agree, they often are discordant (Keefe & Dunsmore 1992). Sometimes this may represent purposeful misrepresentation of experience (Craig et al 1999). Patients not only have difficulty describing painful experiences, but they may also be unwilling, reluctant or incapable of confiding feelings of distress. Both clinicians and others in the non-clinical social environment are usually sensitively attuned to the facial and bodily activity of people in pain and often attach greater importance to non-verbal messages than to verbal report because it appears less vulnerable to purposeful misrepresentation (Craig 1992).

Thus, the task of understanding subtle qualities of another person's subjective distress rivals in complexity only the demands of reporting on the experience itself. Numerous, often idiosyncratic, sources of information must be integrated, including multiple cues from the suffering person, along with the observer's formal understanding of pain memories of personal experiences and contacts with other people experiencing similar distress. Clinicians and others find it difficult to genuinely understand or empathize with another person's painful distress and biased judgements are not uncommon (Hadjistavropoulos et al 1996).

There should be a concerted effort to assess all patients' emotional distress, whether they display organic pathology or not, with many strategies for assessing emotional processes readily available (Turk & Melzack 1992). Many patients experiencing pain with a substantial organic basis suffer serious psychological distress. Benjamin et al (1988) found that pain patients with diagnosable organic diseases had significantly higher ratings for the severity of psychiatric symptoms and they rejected the assumption that there is a simple dichotomy between patients with physical and mental illnesses.

While emotional aspects of pain may be difficult for patients to describe, they can be discriminated from sensory qualities at the level of experience and self-report (Gracely et al 1978, Price et al 1987, Wade et al 1990). They also are differentially sensitive to social and therapeutic influences (Fernandez & Turk 1992). This is consistent with the observations noted above that they have at least partially separate neuroanatomical substrates. As well, the emotional qualities tend to differ dramatically across different forms of clinical pain and within individuals over time quite independently of sensory qualities (Price et al 1987, Katz 1995). Anger, fear and sadness were predictive of the affective component of self-report measures of chronic pain (Fernandez & Milburn 1994).

INTERACTIONS BETWEEN EMOTIONAL DISTRESS AND PAIN

Emotional distress serves not only as a component of pain, but it may also be an issue because of its presence in anticipation of pain, as a consequence of pain, a cause of pain or represent a concurrent problem with independent sources. These distinctions have not always been made clear and there has been debate and confusion concerning, in particular, whether emotional processes should be conceptualized as causes or consequences of pain (Beutler et al 1986). The challenge is important because there are many chronic pain patients who can be characterized as 'dysfunctional' because of a consistent pattern of high levels of pain severity, affective distress, life interference and low levels of life control and activity (Turk & Rudy 1990). Clarification is to be found in conceptualizing both pain and emotion as multidimensional and sometimes overlapping processes with reciprocal influences on each other. Gamsa (1990) provides a critical literature review and a study of chronic pain patients, indicating that pain is more likely to cause emotional disturbances than be precipitated by them. Given the common psychobiological systems operating in pain and non-noxious emotional distress, synchronous arousal would be expected to facilitate each other. One could consider, for example, the emotional distress provoked by a diagnosis of cancer. Cancer is a highly feared condition. It is seen as a potentially lethal disease and there are expectancies that the pain associated with it is inevitable, untreatable and will become unbearable (Turk et al 1998). In this instance, the fear likely will have been established in advance of any painful symptomatology.

EMOTIONAL DISTRESS IN ANTICIPATION OF PAIN

Emotional distress appears most conspicuous when renewed or increased pain is anticipated. Impending harm can precipitate serious distress in the form of disorganized, hysterical behaviour, inappropriate avoidance strategies and substantial physiological arousal. Many people genuinely dread the prospect of pain and take desperate measures to avoid it, often refusing dental care or seeking medical consultation because of their fears. Bond (1980) has suggested that western cultures err in promoting the belief that medicine can make lives pain free. Asmundson et al (1999) review substantial evidence demonstrating that strong tendencies among chronic pain patients to avoid (or 'disuse') social and physical activities associated with pain represent a major component of their problem and are associated with poorer treatment outcome. This 'disuse' syndrome is associated with physical deconditioning, dysphoric affect and preoccupation with somatic symptoms. Pain behaviour and associated fear of work may also persist because it allows avoidance of feared responsibilities (Waddell et al 1993) and social anxiety may diminish through reduced social responsibility attached to work avoidance (Asmundson et al 1996). Taken to the extreme, it has been suggested that cognitive, physiological and behavioural responses to pain may in some instances represent a phobic response (McCracken et al 1992).

Anticipatory distress can have advantages provided it leads to problem-solving behaviour, for example inspiring use of healthcare. Moderate preoperative fear based on foreknowledge can trigger the use of coping skills that reduce postoperative distress. A variety of preparatory procedures for patients confronting painful medical and dental care have been developed (Melamed & Siegel 1980). By contrast, unreasonable apprehension of severe pain can have serious debilitating effects. For example, a pattern of 'catastrophizing' (Sullivan et al 1995), or excessive self-alarming thoughts, has been observed in patients with unrestrained pain displays, substantial emotional behaviour, somatic preoccupation, dependency on the healthcare system and behavioural disorganization (Rosenstiel & Keefe 1983, Reesor & Craig 1988, Sullivan & D'Eon 1990). The relationship between emotional distress and pain-related behaviour appears curvilinear. Lesser levels mobilize attention towards threat and lead to effective action. Increases beyond some optimal level lead to disorganized, inefficient action.

EMOTIONAL DISTRESS AS A CONSEQUENCE OF PAIN

Consideration of the temporal qualities of pain suggests that three different forms of pain can be distinguished (Melzack & Dennis 1980). Distinct affective states appear to be associated with each.

Phasic pain

Short-duration phasic pain reflects the immediate impact of the onset of injury. With some exceptions, traumatic injuries such as lacerations or burns provoke vigorous reflexive withdrawal, protective movements, and stereotyped patterns of verbal and non-verbal expressive behaviour recognizable as pain to onlookers (Craig et al 1992). The non-verbal pattern is evident even in a range of non-verbal populations. Both preterm and full-term newborns subjected to heel lancing to provide a blood sample (Grunau & Craig 1987, Craig et al 1993) and full-term neonates during circumcision (Taddio et al 1997) display it. Similarly the frail elderly suffering cognitive deficits (Hadjistavropoulos et al 1998) and persons with intellectual deficits (LaChapelle et al 1998) display the pattern, despite lack of a capacity to self-report pain, indicating that the emotional distress attached to pain exists independent of the cognitive facility to report pain.

Pain may not be the inevitable, immediate consequence of traumatic injury. Substantial numbers of people who sustain injuries report that pain emerged some time after the injury itself (Wall 1979). The most common sources of persistent pain arising from motor vehicle accidents, soft-tissue neck and low-back injuries, only infrequently provoke immediate pain. When it is reported, clinicians suspect earlier injuries or that the patient is exaggerating.

The primary biological function of pain may be to trigger recuperative behaviour rather than to signal physical threat or danger. Wall (1979) proposed that pain promotes actions directed at healing rather than defensive avoidance behaviour. Bolles and Fanselow (1980) similarly hypothesized that perception of traumatic threat, including physical pain, motivates fear and concerted defensive, self-preservative efforts. At the moment of injury, pain-instigated recuperative activity in the form of passivity and rest would be maladaptive; hence fear rather than pain would be the more adaptive reaction to injury. After the danger has passed and fear has dissipated, recuperative behaviours such as resting and immobilization would be appropriate. Anecdotal evidence is strong that people involved in activities that would be disrupted by pain sustain injuries without complaints. Wounds and injuries are often ignored, as exemplified by soldiers on the battlefield, athletes on the playing field, people engaged in masochistic erotic activities, and even the weekend gardener who ignores a blistered thumb. Thus, even the immediate reaction to physical insult is subject to modulation contingent upon the biological, physical and social context in which it occurs.

Acute pain

Acute pain is provoked by tissue damage and comprises both phasic pain and a tonic state, which persists for a variable period of time until healing takes place. The perception of traumatic injury or the precipitous onset of disease tends to provoke fear and anxious concern for one's well-being. Often, as a result of fear of pain, the anticipation may be more severe than the experience itself (Arntz et al 1991, Gross 1992) and the fear is capable of persisting after tissue damage has healed. The clinical observation that the greater the anxiety the greater the perception of events as painful appears warranted. Postoperative pain that is more severe than anticipated and reduced patient satisfaction are predicted by high anxiety about risks and problems (Thomas et al 1998). Postoperative anxiolytics are frequently prescribed because clinicians perceive their patients to be in emotional distress as well as suffering from pain (Taenzer 1983). In addition, anxiety disorders in children and adults are accompanied by an increased incidence of somatic symptoms and pain complaints (Beidel et al 1991).

Nevertheless, a clear empirical basis for the simple proposition that anxiety increases pain is not available. Arntz et al (1991) reviewed studies that varyingly indicated that anxiety enhances, relieves or has no impact on pain. Similarly, once phasic pain and the immediate perception of life-threatening danger have passed, acute pain may not be associated with high levels of anxiety, as in the case of acute back pain patients (Philips & Grant 1991).

Contradictions in findings concerning the relationship between pain and anxiety may reflect: (i) difficulties in clearly defining and measuring both pain and anxiety, (ii) response biases as people vary in their willingness to complain of pain when anxious (Malow et al 1989), and (iii) the moderating role that attention has on both anxiety and pain (Arntz et al 1991, Crombez et al 1998). There is also the issue of the direction of causality. Pain and anxiety can contribute to each other and to further deterioration in a vicious cycle, including physical decompensation and psychophysiological disorders.

While anxiety has conventionally been associated with acute pain, it is also recognized as a component of the constellation of emotional reactions to chronic pain. Thus, depression, somatic anxiety and anger frequently interact with each other in chronic pain syndromes (Blumer & Heilbronn 1982) and anxious chronic pain patients can be distinguished from those who are depressed (Krishnan et al 1985, Chaturvedi 1987, Hadjistavropoulos & Craig 1994). Chronic back pain patients displaying high levels of fear and avoidance are more likely to be behaviourally dysfunctional (Asmundson et al 1997)

Chronic pain

The psychological impact and behavioural course of painful conditions vary. The injury or the onset of disease alone may create emotional turmoil. Many pain patients display substantial emotional, behavioural and social disruption during the earliest stages of their illness. For many chronic pain patients, the long-term problem may be best conceptualized as persistence of this acute presentation (Philips & Grant 1991). Persistence of pain also can have a profoundly debilitating effect. In any of its recurrent, persistent or progressive forms, pain may dramatically impair the individual's social, vocational and psychological well-being (International Association for the Study of Pain 1986, Bonica 1990). There may be deprivation from customary roles at work, in the family or in social and leisure settings. This may be accompanied by the realization that neither one's own best efforts to promote healing nor the highly respected, best interventions of healthcare professionals have been effective. Challenges to the legitimacy of complaints can also represent a major source of stress. Recognition that pain and a disrupted lifestyle may have to be long endured takes its toll and despondency and a sense of hopelessness become likely outcomes. The emotional and behavioural disturbances provoked by chronic pain have been well documented (Bonica 1979, Sternbach 1986a), but they can be missed during diagnostic assessments when the focus is on pain and pathophysiological processes rather than on psychological well-being (Doan & Wadden 1989).

Deterioration over time is not inevitable. A follow-up study of chronic pain patients from family practice and specialty pain clinic settings indicated that, over 2 years, a substantial proportion no longer experienced pain. For those who continued to experience pain, it had become intermittent. As well, both emotional distress and demands on the healthcare system had strikingly diminished (Crook et al 1989). Many patients can expect the pain to disappear or become intermittent, despite treatment inefficacy.

Chronic pain is frequently associated with depression, which may be minor or severe. The common diagnostic criteria for depression include depressed mood, loss of pleasure or interest, appetite disturbance, sleep disturbance, loss of energy, concentration difficulties and suicidal ideation (Sullivan et al 1992). Depression appears to intensify pain. Affleck et al (1991) found that depression predicted pain severity in rheumatoid arthritis patients over a long sequence of days, independent of disease activity or disability. Doan and Wadden (1989) found that the severity of depressive symptoms predicted the number and severity of pain complaints. The depression may have lethal consequences. The lifetime prevalence of suicidality (thoughts about death, wishes to die, thoughts of committing suicide and suicide attempts) is substantially increased in people with chronic abdominal pain relative to those without (Magni et al 1998).

Estimates of the prevalence of mood disorders in chronic pain patients vary considerably, reflecting both the shortcomings of the measures used and variations in the populations studied (Romano & Turner 1985). Only a small proportion of chronic pain patients display debilitating depression. Magni et al (1990) supported this low prevalence rate on the basis of a large-scale population-based survey of pain and depression in the USA. Only 18% of people suffering from chronic pain could be classified as depressed using a stringent psychiatric criterion, whereas 8% of the population who did not suffer chronic pain satisfied this criterion. The latter indicates that pre-existing conditions or co-morbidity may be responsible for depression in many pain patients. Sullivan et al (1992) concluded that the prevalence of major depression in patients suffering chronic low back pain was approximately three to four times higher than in the general population, with highest incidence in specialty pain clinics. It is noteworthy that most people with chronic pain are not depressed. Chronic pain and depression exist as separate phenomena and they are best seen as independent processes. However, there is a possibility for mutual influence. A substantial proportion of chronic low back patients experience untoward life events and ongoing difficulties (Romano & Turner 1985, Atkinson et al 1988) that would be expected to produce stress and exacerbate pain. As well, the destructive life consequences of chronic pain would set the circumstances for depression.

There have been numerous attempts to untangle the causal relationship between pain and depression (Romano & Turner 1985). Crisson and Keefe (1988) found that depression was the consequence of the extent to which increases in pain severity interfered with important life activities, thereby limiting social rewards and reducing the patient's sense of self control or personal mastery. Brown's (1990) study of depression in rheumatoid arthritis patients provided support for a causal model in which pain predicts depression, but only after an extended period of time (1 year in this study). Certain recursive, vicious cycles are possible. Pain, by increasing unpleasant affect, promotes access to memories of unpleasant events. The negative memories and thoughts, in turn, intensify the unpleasant affect and help perpetuate pain (Eich et al 1990).

From a psychodynamic perspective, chronic pain patients and depressed patients share an inability to modulate or express intense, unacceptable feelings (Beutler et al 1986). This position would also be consistent with findings that adults and children frequently moralize about the meaning of pain, experiencing guilt and construing pain as punishment (Eisendrath et al 1986, Gaffney & Dunne 1987). Biomedical theories derive from the observation that pain and depression have common biological systems that subserve both processes (Beutler et al 1986, Magni 1987). Evidence based on meta-analyses of randomized, placebo-controlled studies of antidepressant treatment of chronic non-malignant pain (Onghena & Van Houdenhove 1992) and neuropathic pain (McQuay et al 1996) demonstrates clear analgesic effects. Often overlooked is the possibility that commonplace treatment recommendations for patients with persistent pain may have depressive effects; withdrawal from work and other activities, prolonged bed-rest, lapsing into the dependent sick role, and analgesics and medications may provoke or exacerbate depression. Aronoff et al (1986) reviewed evidence that benzodiazepines can increase depression, hostility, anger and pain.

While some patients display distress and depression, others maintain a dispassionate attitude and do not become heavy consumers of healthcare services (Zitman et al 1992). Well-adjusted patients with chronic pain appear to have either strong personal or social resources or the pain disorder provides a focus in life that enables them to ignore stressful life challenges, thereby controlling depression or resentment. In this paradoxical manner, pain can provide a means of coping with an unsatisfactory existence. Patients who voluntarily inflict self injury in the interests of instigating medical care and hospitalization, or to escape an intolerable setting (e.g., prison or marital distress), provide extreme illustrations.

A small portion of chronic pain patients becomes angry, demanding and manipulative in the course of their illness. Wade et al (1990) found that pain patients reported higher levels of frustration than any other negative emotion. Anxiety and frustration predicted the overall unpleasantness of pain, and anger was an important concomitant of the depression that pain patients experienced. Fernandez and Turk (1995) suggest that clinicians are inclined to underestimate anger because of patient denial, even though it has compounding effects on pain, depression and psychosocial functioning. Kerns et al (1994) found that inhibiting angry feelings was a good predictor of reports of pain intensity, pain behaviour and activity level. Clinicians should specifically assess for anger and, when warranted, target it for intervention.

EMOTIONAL DISTRESS AS A CAUSE OF PAIN

Evidence supporting the argument that severe emotional distress can trigger new pain or reinstigate old pain in the absence of physical pathology does not extend beyond clinicians' reports. Nevertheless, complaints of pain may be precipitated or exacerbated by emotional and social crises rather than tissue insult. The International Association for the Study of Pain description of chronic pain syndromes and definitions of pain terms (1986) acknowledges pain of psychological origin that may be attributed to specific delusional or hallucinatory causes. These syndromes are estimated to have a prevalence of less than 2% in patients with chronic pain without lesions.

Blumer and Heilbronn (1982) proposed that chronic pain without an identified organic basis is a variant of affective disorder and is best conceptualized as a syndrome within the spectrum of depressive disorders. The hypothesis suggests that an affective disorder underlies chronic pain even when there is no manifest evidence of depression. However, an empirical basis for this concept does not exist (Turk & Salovey 1984, Romano & Turner 1985, Ahles et al 1987).

Emotional stress may increase pain by precipitating activity in psychophysiological systems that are also activated by noxious events. Anxiety, depression, anger and other emotions provoke substantial autonomic, visceral and skeletal activity. The interactions among these biological systems are well illustrated by the 'pain–anxiety–tension' cycle that has been proposed to account for some forms of acute and chronic pain. This vicious cycle has frequently been observed in disorders involving the musculoskeletal system. Pain provokes anxiety, which in turn induces prolonged muscle spasm at the pain location and at trigger points, as well as vasoconstriction, ischaemia and release of pain-producing substances (Keefe & Gil 1986). The cycle may then repeat itself (Dolce & Racynski 1985). Flor et al (1985) found accelerated lumbar electromyogram (EMG) reactivity in chronic back pain patients when they discussed personal stress. Tension headaches have been assumed to be the result of sustained contraction of muscles of the face, scalp and neck in the absence of permanent structural change, usually as a reaction to life stress. However, Philips (1982) has observed that diagnoses of tension headache are most often made on the basis of exclusion of other diagnostic possibilities rather than by demonstrating excessive tension in head and neck muscles. Numerous studies now suggest that patients with tension headaches do not always display sustained or elevated levels of EMG activity (Philips 1982). Similarly, pain during labour contractions in childbirth is reported to be magnified by skeletal muscle tension and self-induced relaxation is assumed to interrupt vicious cycles of tension and pain. Again, the model lacks empirical support and is probably oversimplistic. For example, women's concerns about their ability to bear the child and the baby's health all contribute to the distress experienced (Beck & Siegel 1980). In general, more support is needed for the proposition that muscle tension provides a basis for chronic pain.

Emotional distress may produce disease with lesions that are painful themselves. The autonomic and neuroendocrine changes provoked by psychological stress have been associated with diseases in cardiovascular, digestive, respiratory and eliminative systems (Selye 1976). Distressing events are capable of contributing to the initiation and exacerbation of a large number of painful diseases, including angina pectoris, painful menstruation, rheumatoid arthritis, gastric ulcer, duodenal ulcer, regional enteritis and ulcerative colitis. Furthermore, recent evidence indicates that stress may inhibit the capacity of the immune system to deal with pathogens that lead to painful diseases (Beutler et al 1986).

EMOTIONAL DISTURBANCES CONCURRENT WITH PAIN PROBLEMS

Pain symptoms have been identified as generally prevalent in psychiatric patients, particularly among those suffering anxiety disorders and exogenous depression. Merskey (1986) found pain to be less frequently associated with schizophrenia or endogenous depression. About 50% of all patients with pain and depression develop the two disorders simultaneously (Romano & Turner 1985). Philips and Hunter (1982) found tension headaches to be no more prevalent in psychiatric than in general practice populations, but reported pain intensity in the psychiatric population to be substantially higher. Unfortunately, physical diagnoses in psychiatric populations are difficult to make because these patients tend to use pain language in a relatively indiscriminate and diffuse manner. Atkinson et al (1982) concluded that pain language is not accurate for medical diagnoses in patients who suffer affective disturbances.

COGNITIVE APPRAISAL AND EMOTIONAL ASPECTS OF PAIN

Emotional qualities of pain are influenced by the individual's appraisal of the event (Weisenberg 1977, Turk et al 1983). A vigorous search for information is usually dictated by the onset of pain because it may determine efforts to avoid pain. A variety of cognitive factors contribute to the severity of emotional distress that is experienced. Enhanced somatic awareness in the form of attention to symptoms can enhance distress. In turn, 'catastrophizing' thinking styles can amplify somatosensory information and prime fear mechanisms (Crombez et al 1998). People who 'catastrophize' or self-alarm by focusing negatively on their distress are the most disabled and benefit the least from conventional medical care (Sullivan et al 1995). Depressed chronic low back pain patients have also been found to misinterpret or distort the nature and significance of their dilemma (Lefebvre 1981). Cognitive errors of catastrophizing, overgeneralization (assuming similar outcomes of different experiences) and selective abstraction (selectively attending to negative aspects of experience) are particularly prominent when depressed low back pain patients focus on their disorder. Smith et al (1986) found that the pattern of cognitive distortion in depressed chronic low back patients was stronger in those who display general distress than in those who somatize their distress.

The availability of personal or external resources to control pain influences its emotional impact. Substantial individual differences exist in the coping strategies people use to modulate pain. In children, coping strategy use, perceived self efficacy and frequency of catastrophizing thoughts significantly predict postoperative pain, affective distress and physical recovery (Bennett-Branson & Craig 1993). The broad categories of attentional diversion, cognitive restructuring and self-relaxation serve as coping strategies for some people (Turk et al 1983, Lawson et al 1990). Distraction alone appears insufficient as an analgesic technique, probably also requiring substantive changes in mood or the meaning of the experience (Leventhal 1992, McCaul et al 1992). People's judgement of self efficacy or their ability to use self-control strategies (Bandura et al 1987) determines whether these strategies are actually applied to clinical pain (Manning & Wright 1983, Holroyd et al 1984). Loss of control is undoubtedly important in chronic pain. As patients pursue successive health practitioners, failure to find lasting relief contributes to feelings of hopelessness, helplessness, despair and pessimism. Patients with strong feelings of helplessness have higher levels of psychological distress (Keefe et al 1990). It is exceedingly difficult for people to abandon efforts to achieve control over chronic pain and the risks of vicious circles are considerable. Anxiety about pain directs attention to pain, which leads to stronger pain responses (Arntz et al 1991). Thus, ever more desperate measures carry the risk of compounding the initial problem.

INTEGRATION OF PSYCHOBIOLOGICAL CONSTRUCTS

It is evident that further integration of the psychosocially oriented and the biologically oriented perspectives is needed. Greater integration of these fields should generate new treatments, both psychosocially and pharmacologically based.

REFERENCES

Affleck G, Tennen H, Urrows S, Higgins P 1991 Individual differences in the day-to-day experience of chronic pain: a prospective daily study of rheumatoid arthritis patients. Health Psychology 10: 419–426

Ahles TA, Yunus MB, Masi AT 1987 Is chronic pain a variant of depressive disease? Pain 29: 105–112

American Psychiatric Association 1987 Diagnostic and statistical manual of mental disorders, 3rd edn (Revised). American Psychiatric Association, Washington, DC

Arntz A, Dreessen L, Merckelbach H 1991 Attention, not anxiety, influences pain. Behaviour Research and Therapy 29: 41–50

Aronoff GM, Wagner JM, Spangler AS 1986 Chemical interventions for pain. Journal of Consulting and Clinical Psychology 54: 769–775

Asmundson GJG, Jacobson SJ, Allerdings MD, Norton GR 1996 Social phobia in disabled workers with chronic musculoskeletal pain. Behaviour Research and Therapy 33: 49–53

Asmundson GJG, Norton PJ, Allerdings MD 1997 Fear and avoidance in dysfunctional chronic back pain patients. Pain 69: 231–236

Asmundson GJG, Norton PJ, Norton GR 1999 Beyond pain: the role of fear and avoidance in chronicity. Clinical Psychology Review 19: 97–119

Atkinson JH, Kremer EF, Ignelzi RJ 1982 Diffusion of pain language with affective disturbance confounds differential diagnosis. Pain 12: 375–384

Atkinson JH, Slater MA, Grant I, Patterson TL, Garfin SR 1988 Depressed mood in chronic low back pain: relationship with stressful life events. Pain 35: 47–55

Bandura A, O'Leary A, Taylor CB, Gauthier J, Gossard D 1987 Perceived self-efficacy and pain control: opioid and nonopioid mechanisms. Journal of Personality and Social Psychology 53: 563–571

Bavelas JB, Chovil N 1997 Faces in dialogue. In: Russell JA, Fernandez-Dols JM (eds) The psychology of facial expression. Cambridge University Press, Paris, pp 334–348

Beck NC, Siegel LJ 1980 Preparation for childbirth and contemporary research on pain, anxiety and stress reduction: a review and critique. Journal of Psychosomatic Research 24: 429–447

Beidel DC, Christ MAG, Long PJ 1991 Somatic complaints in anxious children. Journal of Abnormal Child Psychology 19: 659–670

Benjamin S, Barnes D, Berger S, Clarke I, Jeacock J 1988 The relationship of chronic pain, mental illness and organic disorders. Pain 32: 185–195

Bennett-Branson SM, Craig KD 1993 Postoperative pain in children: developmental and family influences on spontaneous coping strategies. Canadian Journal of Behavioural Science 25: 355–383

Beutler LE, Engle D, Oro-Beutler ME, Daldrup R, Meredith K 1986 Inability to express intense affect: a common link between depression and pain. Journal of Consulting and Clinical Psychology 54: 752–759

Blumer D, Heilbronn M 1982 Chronic pain as a variant of depressive disease. Journal of Nervous and Mental Disease 170: 381–414

Bolles RC, Fanselow MS 1980 A perceptual–defensive–recuperative model of fear and pain. Behavioural and Brain Sciences 3: 291–323

Bond MR 1980 The suffering of severe intractable pain. In: Kosterlitz HW, Terenius LY (eds) Pain and Society. Verlag Chemie, Weinheim, p 53

Bonica JJ 1979 Important clinical aspects of acute and chronic pain. In: Beers RE, Bassett EC (eds) Mechanisms of pain and analgesic compounds. Raven, New York, p 183

Bonica JJ (ed) 1990 The management of pain, 2 edn. Philadelphia, Lea & Febiger

Bromm B 1989 Laboratory animal and human volunteer in assessment of analgesic efficacy. In: Chapman CR, Loeser JD (eds) Issues in pain management. Raven, New York, pp 117–144

Brown GKA 1990 Causal analysis of chronic pain and depression. Journal of Abnormal Psychology 99: 127–137

Casey KM, Minoshima S, Morrow TJ, Koeppe RA, Frey KA 1995 Imaging the brain in pain: potentials, limitations, and implications. In: Bromm B, Desmedt JE (eds) Advances in pain research and therapy, vol 22. Raven, New York pp 201–212

Chapman CR 1995 The affective dimension of pain: a model. In: Advances in pain research and therapy, vol 22, Pain and the brain: from nociception to cognition. Raven, New York, pp 283–302

Chapman CR 1996 Limbic processes and the affective dimension of pain. Progress in Brain Research 110: 63–81

Chaturvedi SK 1987 A comparison of depressed and anxious chronic pain patients. General Hospital Psychiatry 9: 383–386

Corkin, S, Hebben N 1981 Subjective estimates of chronic pain before and after psychosurgery or treatment in a pain unit. Pain Supplement 1: S150

Craig KD 1992 The facial expression of pain: better than a thousand words? American Pain Society Journal 1: 153–162

Craig KD, Dobson KS (eds) 1995 Anxiety and depression in adults and children. Sage, Thousand Oaks, CA

Craig KD, Prkachin KM, Grunau RVE 1992 The facial expression of pain. In: Turk DC, Melzack R (eds) Handbook of pain assessment. Guilford Press, New York, pp 255–274

Craig KD, Whitfield MF, Grunau RVE, Linton J, Hadjistavropoulos HD 1993 Pain in the preterm neonate: behavioural and physiological indices. Pain 52: 287–299

Craig KD, Hill ML, McMurtry B 1999 Detecting deception and malingering. In: Block AR, Kremer EF, Fernandez E (eds) Handbook of chronic pain syndromes. Lawrence Erlbaum, New York pp 41–58

Crisson JE, Keefe FJ 1988 The relationship of locus of control to pain coping strategies and psychological distress in chronic pain patients. Pain 35: 147–154

Crombez G, Eccleston C, Baeyens F, Eelen P 1998 When somatic information threatens, catastrophic thinking enhances attentional interference. Pain 75: 187–198

Crook J, Weir R, Tunks E 1989 An epidemiological follow-up survey of persistent pain sufferers in a group family practice and specialty pain clinic. Pain 36: 49–61

Derryberry D, Tucker DM 1992 Neural mechanisms of emotion. Journal of Consulting and Clinical Psychology 60: 329–338

Doan BD, Wadden NP 1989 Relationship between depressive symptoms and descriptions of chronic pain. Pain 36: 75–84

Dolce JJ, Raczynski JM 1985 Neuromuscular activity and electromyography in painful backs: psychological and biomechanical models in assessment and treatment. Psychological Bulletin 97: 502–520

Eich E, Rachman S, Lopatka C 1990 Affect, pain, and autobiographical memory. Journal of Abnormal Psychology 99: 174–178

Eisendrath SJ, Way LW, Ostroff JW, Johanson CA 1986 Identification of psychogenic abdominal pain. Psychosomatics 27: 705–712

Ekman P, Rosenberg EL 1997 What the face reveals: basic and applied studies of spontaneous expression using the Facial Action Coding System (FACS). Oxford University Press, Oxford

Engel GL 1977 The need for a new medical model: a challenge for biomedicine. Science 196: 129–136

Engel GL 1980 The clinical application of the biopsychosocial model. American Journal of Psychiatry 137: 535–544

Fernandez E, Milburn TW 1994 Sensory and affective predictors of overall pain and emotions associated with affective pain. Clinical Journal of Pain 10: 3–9

Fernandez E, Turk DC 1992 Sensory and affective components of pain: separation and synthesis. Psychological Bulletin 112: 205–217

Fernandez E, Turk DC 1995 The scope and significance of anger in the experience of chronic pain. Pain 61: 165–175

Flor H, Turk DC, Birbaumer N 1985 Assessment of stress-related psychophysiological reactions in chronic back pain patients. Journal of Consulting and Clinical Psychology 53: 354–364

Fridlund A 1994 Human facial expression: an evolutionary view. Academic, Santa Barbara, CA

Gaffney A, Dunne EA 1987 Children's understanding of the causality of pain. Pain 29: 91–104

Gamsa A 1990 Is emotional disturbance a precipitator or a consequence of chronic pain. Pain 42: 183–195

Gracely RH, McGrath P, Dubner R 1978 Validity and sensitivity of ratio scales of sensory and affective verbal pain descriptors. Pain 5: 19–29

Gray, JA 1987 The psychology of fear and stress, 2nd edn. Cambridge, Cambridge University Press

Gross PR 1992 Is pain sensitivity associated with dental avoidance. Behaviour Research and Therapy 30: 7–13

Grunau RVE, Craig KD 1987 Pain expression in neonates: facial action and cry. Pain 28: 395–410

Hadjistavropoulos HD, Craig KD 1994 Acute and chronic low back pain: cognitive, affective and behavioural dimensions. Journal of Consulting and Clinical Psychology 62: 341–349

Hadjistavropoulos T, McMurtry B, Craig KD 1996 Beautiful faces in pain: biases and accuracy in the perception of pain signals. Psychology and Health 11: 411–420

Hadjistavropoulos T, LaChapelle D, MacLeod F, Hale C, O'Rourke N, Craig KD 1998 Cognitive functioning and pain reactions in hospitalized elders. Pain Research and Management 145–151

Hale CJ, Hadjistavropoulos T 1997 Emotional components of pain. Pain Research and Management 2: 217–225

Holroyd KA, Penzien DB, Hursey KG et al 1984 Change mechanisms, in EMG biofeedback training: cognitive changes underlying improvements in tension headache. Journal of Consulting and Clinical Psychology 52: 1039–1053

International Association for the Study of Pain 1986 Classification of chronic pain: descriptions of chronic pain syndromes and definitions, of pain terms. Pain (suppl 3): 1–222

Jensen MP 1997 Validity of self-report and observation measures. In: Jensen RS, Turner JA, Weisenfeld-Halleb Z (eds) Proceedings of the 8th World Congress on Pain. IASP Press, Seattle, pp 637–661

Katz J 1995 Pain in public and private places. Pain Forum 4: 19–22

Keefe FJ, Dunsmore J 1992 Pain behavior: concepts and controversies. American Pain Society Journal 1: 92–100

Keefe FJ, Gil KM 1986 Behavioral concepts in the analysis of chronic pain syndromes. Journal of Consulting and Clinical Psychology 54: 776–783

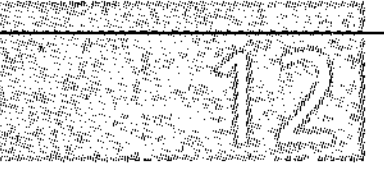

Keefe FJ, Crisson J, Urban BJ, Williams DA 1990 Analyzing chronic low back pain: the relative contribution of pain coping strategies. Pain 40: 293–301

Kenshalo DR, Douglass DK 1995 The role of the cerebral cortex in the experience of pain. In: Bromm B, Desmedt JE (eds) Advances in pain research and therapy, vol 22. Raven, New York, pp 21–34

Kerns RD, Rosenberg R, Jacob MC 1994 Anger expression and chronic pain. Journal of Behavioral Medicine 17: 57–70

Krishnan KRR, France RD, Pelton S, McCann UD, Davidson J, Urban BJ 1985 Chronic pain and depression. II. Symptoms of anxiety in chronic low back pain patients and their relationship to subtypes of depression. Pain 22: 289–294

LaChapelle D, Hadjistavropoulos T, Craig KD 1998 Pain measurement in persons with intellectual disabilities. Clinical Journal of Pain (in press)

Lawson K, Ressor KA, Keefe FJ, Turner JA 1990 Dimensions of pain related cognitive coping: cross-validation of the factor structure of the Coping Strategy Questionnaire. Pain 43: 195–204

Lefebvre MF 1981 Cognitive distortion and cognitive factors in depressed psychiatric and low back pain patients. Journal of Consulting and Clinical Psychology 49: 517–525

Leventhal H 1992 I know distraction works even though it doesn't. Health Psychology 11: 208–209

Lewis T 1942 Pain. MacMillan, London

McCaul KD, Monson N, Maki RH 1992 Does distraction reduce pain-produced distress among college students? Health Psychology 11: 210–217

McCracken LM, Zayfert C, Gross RT 1992 The Pain Anxiety Symptoms Scale: development and validation of a scale to measure fear of pain. Pain 50: 67–73

McKenna JE, Melzack R 1992 Analgesia produced by lidocaine microinjection into the dentate nucleus. Pain 49: 105–112

McQuay HJ, Tramer M, Nye BA, Carroll D, Wiffen PJ, Moore RA 1996 A systematic review of antidepressants in neuropathic pain. Pain 68: 217–227

Magni G 1987 On the relationship between chronic pain and depression when there is no organic lesion. Pain 31: 1–21

Magni C, Caldieron C, Rigatti-Luchini S, Merskey H 1990 Chronic musculoskeletal pain and depressive symptoms in the general population. An analysis of the first National Health and Nutrition Examination Survey data. Pain 43: 299–307

Magni G, Rigatti-Luchini S, Fracca F, Merskey H 1998 Suicidality in chronic abdominal pain: an analysis of the Hispanic Health and Nutrition Examination Survey (HHANES). Pain 76: 137–144

Malow RM, West JA, Sutker PB 1989 Anxiety and pain response changes across treatment: sensory decision analysis. Pain 38: 35–44

Manning MM, Wright TL 1983 Self-efficacy expectancies, outcome expectancies, and persistence of pain control in childbirth. Journal of Personality and Social Psychology 45: 421–431

Melamed BG, Siegel LJ 1980 Behavioural medicine: practical applications in health care. Springer, New York

Melzack R 1983. The McGill pain questionnaire. In: Melzack R (ed) Pain measurement and assessment. Raven, New York, pp 41–48

Melzack R, Casey KL 1968 Sensory, motivational and central control determinants of pain: a new conceptual model. In: Kenshalo DL (ed) The skin senses. CC Thomas, Springfield, IL, p 423

Melzack R, Dennis SG 1980 Phylogenetic evolution of pain expression in animals. In: Kosterlitz HW, Terenius LY (eds) Pain and society. Verlag Chemie, Weinheim, p 13

Melzack R, Wall PD 1965 Pain and mechanisms: a new theory. Science 150: 971–979

Merskey H 1986 Psychiatry and pain. In: Sternbach RA (ed) The psychology of pain. Raven, New York, pp 97–120

Merskey H, Bogduk N (eds) 1994 Classification of chronic pain. Descriptions of chronic pain syndromes and definitions of pain terms. International Association for the Study of Pain. Elsevier, New York

Morrow TJ, Paulson PE, Danneman PJ, Casey KL 1998 Regional changes in forebrain activation during the early and late phase of formalin nociception: analysis using cerebral blood flow in the rat. Pain 75: 355–365

Onghena P, Van Houdenhove B 1992 Antidepressant-induced analgesia in chronic nonmalignant pain: a meta-analysis of 39 placebo-controlled studies. Pain 49: 205–219

Philips C 1982 The nature and treatment of chronic tension headache. In: Craig KD, McMahon R J (eds) Advances in clinical behaviour therapy. Brunner/Mazel, New York, pp 211–231

Philips HC, Grant L 1991 The evolution of chronic back pain problems: a longitudinal study. Behaviour Research and Therapy 29: 435–441

Philips HC, Hunter M 1982 Headache in a psychophysical population. Journal of Nervous and Mental Disease 170: 1–12

Price DD, Dubner R 1977 Neurons that subserve the sensory-discriminative aspects of pain. Pain 4: 307–338

Price DD, Harkins SW, Baker C 1987 Sensory–affective relationships among different types of clinical and experimental pain. Pain 28: 297–308

Prkachin KM, Craig KD 1995 Expressing pain: the communication and interpretation of facial pain signals. Journal of Nonverbal Behavior 19: 191–205

Rainville P, Duncan GH, Price DD, Carrier B, Bushnell C 1997 Pain affect encoded in human anterior cingulate but not somatosensory cortex. Science 277: 968–971

Reesor KA, Craig KD 1988 Medically incongruent back pain: physical restriction, suffering, and ineffective coping. Pain 32: 35–45

Romano JM, Turner JA 1985 Chronic pain and depression: does the evidence support a relationship? Psychological Bulletin 97: 18–34

Rosensteil A, Keefe FJ 1983 The use of coping strategies in chronic low back pain patients: relationship to patient characteristics and adjustment. Pain 17: 33–43

Selye H 1976 The stress of life. McGraw-Hill, New York

Smith TW, Aberger EW, Follick M. J, Ahern DK 1986 Cognitive distortion and psychological distress in chronic low back pain. Journal of Consulting and Clinical Psychology 54: 573–575

Sternbach RA 1986a Clinical aspects of pain. In: Sternbach RA (ed) The psychology of pain, 2nd edn. Raven, New York, pp 223–239

Sullivan MD 1995 Pain in language: From sentience to sapience. Pain Forum 4: 3–14

Sullivan MJL, D'Eon JL 1990 Relation between catastrophizing and depression in chronic pain patients. Journal of Abnormal Psychology 99: 260–263

Sullivan MJL, Reesor K, Mikail S, Fisher R 1992 The treatment of depression in chronic low back pain: review; and recommendations. Pain 50: 5–13

Sullivan MJL, Bishop SR, Pivak J 1995 The pain catastrophizing scale: development and validation. Psychological Assessment 7: 524–532

Taddio A, Stevens B, Craig KD et al 1997 Efficacy and safety of lidocaine-prilocaine cream for pain during circumcision. New England Journal of Medicine 336: 1197–1201

Taenzer P 1983 Postoperative pain: relationships among measures of pain, mood and narcotic requirements. In: Melzack R (ed) Pain measurement and assessment. Raven, New York, pp 1–118

Talbot JD, Marrett S, Evans AC, Meyer E, Bushnell MC, Duncan JH 1991 Multiple representations of pain in human cerebral cortex. Science 251: 1355–1358

Tasker RAR, Choiniere M, Libman SM, Melzack R 1987 Analgesia produced by injection of lidocaine into the lateral hypothalamus. Pain 31: 237–248

Thomas T, Robinson C, Champion D, McKell M, Pell M 1998 Prediction and assessment of the severity of post-operative pain and of satisfaction with management. Pain 75: 177–185

Turk DC, Melzack R 1992 Handbook of pain assessment. Guilford, New York
Turk DC, Rudy TE 1990 The robustness of an empirically derived taxonomy of chronic pain patients. Pain 43: 27–35
Turk DC, Salovey P 1984 'Chronic pain as a variant of depressive disease': a critical reappraisal. Journal of Nervous and Mental Disorders 1972: 398–404
Turk DC, Meichenbaum DH, Genest M 1983 Pain and behavioural medicine: theory, research and clinical guide. Guilford, New York
Turk DC, Sist TC, Okifuji A et al 1998 Adaptation to metastic cancer pain, regional/local cancer pain and non-cancer pain: role of psychological and behavioral factors. Pain 74: 247–256
Vaccarino AL, Melzack R 1989 Analgesia produced by injection of lidocaine into the anterior cingulum bundle of the rat. Pain 39: 213–220
Vierck CJ, Cooper BY, Ritz LA, Greenspan JD 1989 Inference of pain sensitivity from complex behaviors of laboratory animals. In: Chapman CR, Loeser JD (eds) Issues in pain measurement. Raven, New York, pp 93–116
Waddell G, Newton M, Henderson I, Sommerville D, Main CJ 1993 A fear-avoidance beliefs questionnaire (FABQ) and the role of fear-avoidance beliefs in chronic low back pain and disability. Pain 52: 157–168
Wade JB, Price DD, Hamer RM, Schwartz SM, Hart RP 1990 An emotional component analysis of chronic pain. Pain 40: 303–310
Wall PD 1979 On the relation of injury to pain. Pain 6: 253–264
Wall PD 1996 Comments after 30 years of the gate control theory. Pain Forum 5: 12–22
Wall PD, McMahon SB 1985 Microneurography and its relation to perceived sensation: a critical review. Pain 21: 209–229
Weisenberg M 1977 Pain and pain control. Psychological Bulletin 84: 1008–1044
Willis WD 1995 From nociceptor to cortical activity. In: Bromm B, Desmedt JE (eds) Advances in pain research and therapy, vol 22 Raven, New York, pp 1–19
Zitman FG, Linssen CG, Van HRL 1992 Chronic pain beyond patienthood. Journal of Nervous and Mental Disease 180: 97–100

Cognitive aspects of pain

13

MATISYOHU WEISENBERG

SUMMARY

Cognitive approaches to pain have expanded to many areas of application. Examples include cancer, low-back pain, burns, rheumatoid arthritis, and abdominal pain in children. Often the cognitive intervention is part of a more comprehensive approach to treatment. As used in most research and treatment, cognitive approaches are concerned with the way the people perceive, interpret and relate to their pain rather than with the elimination of the pain per se. This chapter reviews some of the origins of cognitive theory and pain theory, as well as examples of the techniques used and the research support for the approach. Special emphasis is given to self-efficacy, catastrophizing, perceived control and stress inoculation therapy. There is also discussion of some of the limitations of the cognitive approach. The overall conclusion is that the cognitive approach is powerful and effective for pain control despite its limitations.

INTRODUCTION

Cognitive techniques and cognitive theory have continued to grow. Since the last edition of this text the major change has been the ever-increasing application of the cognitive approach in clinical settings for the treatment of pain. Cognition is 'a generic term embracing the quality of knowing, which includes perceiving, recognizing, conceiving, judging, sensing, reasoning and imagining' (Stedman's Medical Dictionary 1976). Often, cognitive interventions are part of a total multidisciplinary package offered by pain clinics. Examples of the problems to which the cognitive or cognitive-behavioural approach has been applied include low back pain (Nicholas et al 1992), rheumatoid arthritis (Young et al 1995), cancer pain (Syrjala et al 1995), bone marrow aspiration and lumbar puncture, headache in children (Ellis & Spanos 1994), abdominal pain in children (Sanders et al 1994, Ter Kuile et al 1995), temporomandibular joint dysfunction (Wilson et al 1992), preparation for treatment (Kessler & Dane 1996), pain of the upper limbs (Spence 1991), burns (Patterson & Sharar 1997–98), burning mouth syndrome (Bergdhal et al 1995), neck and shoulder pain (Jensen et al 1995) and as part of a multidisciplinary programme (Peters & Large 1990).

As used in most research and treatment, cognitive approaches are concerned with the way the person perceives, interprets and relates to the pain rather than with the elimination of the pain per se. Because pain patients often suffer from stress, anxiety or depression, it is likely that cognitive interventions affect pain directly as well as indirectly, by reducing the stress or the emotional disturbance (Sternbach 1986, Malone & Strube 1988, Rudy et al 1988, Tyrer et al 1989, Gamsa & Vikis-Freibergs 1991, Dworkin et al 1992).

This chapter reviews the theoretical and experimental bases of cognitive approaches to pain control. The applied aspects are found in other chapters.

COGNITIVE THEORIES: COPING AND BELIEVING

Theoretically, the basic cognitive concepts can be traced to Ellis (1962), Beck et al (1979, 1985, 1990), Roskies & Lazarus (1980), Lazarus & Folkman (1984), Meichenbaum (1977, 1985), Bandura (1977, 1984, 1989), Freeman et al (1990) and Kendall et al (1991). Applications to pain control also can be traced to Chaves & Barber (1974) as well as to Turk and his colleagues

(Meichenbaum & Turk 1976, Turk 1978, Turk & Rudy 1992).

Cognitive therapeutic techniques are designed to help people identify and correct distorted conceptualizations. Patients are taught how to monitor negative, automatic thoughts, to recognize the connections between cognition, affect and behaviour, to examine evidence for and against their distorted automatic thoughts, to substitute reality-oriented interpretations and to recognize dysfunctional or irrational beliefs that predispose them to distort experiences (Ellis 1962, Meichenbaum 1977, 1985, Beck et al 1979, 1985, 1990). Some of the more recent cognitive techniques and clinical approaches have not yet had much impact in the pain control literature (cf. Beck 1995, Haaga 1997). These include an emphasis on what is called schemes or core beliefs which usually lead the therapist to go back to childhood experiences of the patient, thus bringing the cognitive approach closer to classical psychodynamic techniques. As used in the majority of instances most pain interventions involve changing patients' thoughts, moods or behaviour. In pain control there are also times when cognitive distortions are purposely introduced, for example use of dissociation of a painful part of the body.

Coping has been conceptualized as 'the person's cognitive and behavioural efforts to manage (reduce, minimize, master or tolerate) the internal and external demands of the person–environment transaction that is appraised as taxing or exceeding the person's resources' (Folkman et al 1986a). According to Roskies and Lazarus (1980) and Lazarus and Folkman (1984), the way people cope with stressful situations depends on their view of the situation. This cognitive evaluation, referred to as appraisal, is a dynamic process which changes according to individuals' perception of the consequences of an event, its importance to their well-being, and the resources they have to cope with the threat. The appraisal process also changes as events change (Folkman et al 1986b).

Coping has been classified according to the mode of action used (direct action, action inhibition, information search, intrapsychic processes) as well as the function it serves: problem-oriented (or problem-focused) coping or palliative regulation of the emotional response (that is, emotion-focused coping). Most individuals use both modes of coping (problem-focused or emotion-focused) at various times. However, there are circumstances where one or the other mode is preferable. For example, Forsythe and Compas (1987) examined the relationships among individuals' appraisal of a situation as controllable or not, the mode of coping used and the psychological distress. Problem-focused coping was associated with lower levels of distress in situations perceived as controllable, and higher distress in situations perceived as uncontrollable. The opposite results were obtained with emotion-focused coping.

In general, cognitive-behavioural techniques are used as part of a more comprehensive approach to teach the relationship between thoughts, feelings, behaviour, environmental stimuli and pain. Patients are taught to become actively involved in their treatment. Patients with chronic pain, for example, may have negative expectations regarding their ability to exert any control over their pain and may see themselves as helpless. This could lead to demoralization, inactivity and a tendency to overreact to pain. If the pain is interpreted as caused by increasing tissue damage or a life-threatening situation, it could produce greater suffering than pain of the same or even higher intensity. In the cognitive approach, there is an emphasis on replacing helplessness and hopelessness with resourcefulness and hope. Patients also are taught a variety of coping strategies and skills to deal with the pain and the circumstances surrounding it. These include relaxation, imagery, cognitive restructuring, self-statements and attention diversion (Turk et al 1983, Turk & Fernandez 1990, Turk & Rudy 1992).

COGNITIVE COPING STRATEGIES

Earlier work on the use of cognitive techniques was designed to identify the basic strategies (see Weisenberg 1984, 1989). The basic coping techniques have been categorized. Wack and Turk (1984) demonstrated the use of latent structure analysis as a means of classifying the interrelationship of coping strategies as used in dealing with cold-pressor pain. Fernandez and Turk (1989) used a six-category classification to examine study outcomes via meta-analysis. The six groups included:

1. External focus of attention, such as slides of landscapes.
2. Neutral imagery, i.e. imagery that was neither pleasant or unpleasant.
3. Dramatized coping, involving reconstructing the context of the nociception such as a football game.
4. Rhythmic cognitive activity, which refers to cognitive activity of a repetitive or systematized nature, such as counting backwards from 100 by three.
5. Pain acknowledging, which involves a reappraisal of the nociception in terms of objective sensations.
6. Pleasant imagery, such as imagining oneself sitting comfortably and listening to music.

The meta-analysis, based on 51 studies, showed a significant advantage to the cognitive strategies as compared to the control groups or to placebo expectancy groups. No significant differences were obtained for the relative advantage of one strategy over the other. However, it seems that imagery strategies were most effective, while the repetitive cognitions or acknowledgement of sensations were least effective.

SOME CAUTIONS AND LIMITATIONS

The accumulated studies of the cognitive control of pain demonstrated that changing how a person thinks about the pain stimulus and the way the person attends to the pain stimulus can lead to an increase in pain tolerance. Several points would be worth noting. As mentioned in earlier articles (Weisenberg 1984, 1989, 1994), choosing a specific strategy must fit the context and the person. What can be acceptable and relaxing to one person can be aversive to another. It is also important to emphasize, as stated earlier, that motivational processes can be a vital key to determining the effectiveness of a given strategy and the willingness of the person to use the recommended strategy. Cognitive strategies have not always been effective with stimuli to which the person has had prior exposure before learning the strategy (Berntzen 1987) nor necessarily has there been generalization from one situation to another (Hackett et al 1979, Klepac et al 1981). Several studies also have shown that specifying a given time limit for the pain ('tolerate this for 15 minutes', as opposed to 'last as long as you can') has increased the pain tolerance and the effectiveness of the cognitive strategies (Williams & Thorn 1986, Thorn & Williams 1989).

It is also worth noting that cognitive techniques are not always successful for all sorts of problems, nor are they always the only approach possible in dealing with the pain. Thus, Keefe and Van Horn (1993) in a review of studies of cognitive therapy with rheumatoid arthritis patients showed that some patients were able to maintain and successfully use the cognitive techniques while others were not able to do so. Wilhelmsen et al (1994) reported that cognitive psychotherapy was ineffective for ulcer patients. Syrjala et al (1995) reported that for patients undergoing bone marrow transplants, relaxation and imagery training alone were as effective as a whole package of cognitive therapy skills that included relaxation and imagery. Similarly, for non-malignant pain, Pilowsky et al (1995) did not find any difference in the outcomes if the treatment was cognitive-behavioural plus amitriptyline or supportive therapy plus amitriptyline.

When using distraction, McCaul and Malott (1984) reviewed evidence showing that the more the distraction can gain the person's attention, the more effective it is. Distraction was found to be more effective for stimuli of low intensity while sensation redefinition was more effective for intense pain. The issue of distraction versus focus of attention on the pain stimulus is still not settled (Ecclestorn 1995). Leventhal (1992) has argued on the basis of his studies with women in labour that focusing on the pain is more effective. By contrast, distraction has been shown to be an important coping technique for patients suffering from rheumatoid arthritis (Affleck et al 1992a, b). It has been suggested that apart from stimulus intensity, there are individual differences that must be taken into account. Thus, Logan et al (1995) reported on the effectiveness of focusing on the pain while undergoing root canal therapy for patients who were classified as having a high desire for control and low perceived control. In a similar vein, Shilo (1997) reported that individual differences between women in their desire to cope or avoid, determined the perceived benefits obtained from watching the fetal monitor during labour pains.

Individual differences in coping preferences have been shown to affect coping success. Heyneman et al (1990) assessed the untrained, preferred-coping behaviours of subjects undergoing cold-pressor stimulation. During this baseline trial, subjects were asked to verbalize their thoughts while experiencing cold-pressor pain. Subjects were then classified as catastrophizers (use of a large number of negative self-statements or negative thoughts about the future) or non-catastrophizers. After random assignment, subjects were trained in either self-statement, self-instructional training (SI) or attention diversion (AD) coping strategies. The training more closely matched or mismatched the subject's untrained, preferred way of reacting to cold-pressor pain. Non-catastrophizers showed higher pain tolerance under AD than SI, while catastrophizers showed a greater increase in tolerance under SI than under AD. Interventions that matched the spontaneous preferences were more successful. In a similar fashion, Rokke and Absi (1992) were able to demonstrate the effectiveness for coping with cold-pressor pain by matching intervention strategy with the preferred mode of coping, as determined by means of a standardized coping questionnaire, the Cognitive Coping Strategy Inventory. The emphasis on and the importance of identifying coping strategies have led to the development of a number of measures, which will be discussed later.

According to Beck et al (1979, 1985, 1990), coping involves what individuals do as well as what they think and say to themselves. Cognitive processes and structures (schemata) include the assumptions, beliefs, commitments and meanings that influence the way individuals perceive and react to the world. These processes and structures help them to identify stimuli quickly, categorize them, fill in missing information, select a strategy for obtaining more information, solve a problem or reach a goal. Stressful events can trigger schemata that prime the individuals to respond in a given way. Distorted underlying assumptions and errors in information processing can serve to maintain emotional disturbance.

STRESS-INOCULATION THERAPY

Meichenbaum and Turk (1976) and Meichenbaum (1977, 1985) developed a technique called stress-inoculation training. It involves three basic phases of treatment (Meichenbaum 1985): the educational reconceptualization of pain, acquisition of skills and practice of what is taught. The coping strategies often include such things as relaxation, deep breathing, use of pleasant images, use of positive self-statements and self-reinforcement for having coped. Subjects were provided with self-instructional training (Meichenbaum 1977, 1985) consisting of coping statements. Subjects were taught self-talk for four stages of stimulus presentation:

1. Preparing for the stressor.
2. Confronting the pain.
3. Dealing with feelings at critical moments.
4. Self-reinforcement for having successfully coped.

A total of 81 female subjects were tested using cold-pressor pain. Results indicated that relaxation training produced an increased pain tolerance, while the distraction and imagery training resulted in a higher threshold score. Self-statements did not result in any significant effect and in fact reduced the effectiveness of distraction and imagery use. The failure of the self-statement group may have been a result of its lack of subject acceptance or outcome expectancies as a method to reduce pain.

In the Meichenbaum and Turk study using ischaemic pain, compared to a pretest duration of 17 minutes, post-training tolerance increased to 32 minutes.

Work in recent years has been characterized by more clinical than laboratory studies in assessing the application of cognitive-behavioural treatment of pain. Clinically, stress-inoculation has been applied successfully to such areas as pain in adult burn patients (Wernick et al 1981) as well as to pain in burns of children aged 5–12 years (Elliott & Olson 1983), preparation for surgery (Wells et al 1986), headaches (Newton & Barbaree 1987) and chronic pelvic pain (Kames et al 1990).

The effectiveness of stress-inoculation often requires the presence of the therapist (Elliott & Olson 1983, Hayes & Wolf 1984). Another important point demonstrated by D'Eon and Perry (1984) is that the type of coping strategy was less important than providing the subjects with the choice of strategy. A recent study by Miller and Bowers (1993) compared stress-inoculation and hypnosis. Although both techniques were successful in reducing pain, the hypnosis was more successful. Hypnosis also apparently required less cognitive effort than stress-inoculation. In general, it appears that stress-inoculation training can be beneficial in tolerating the stress of pain. However, as with other cognitive procedures it is still not clear exactly what the critical ingredients are and which of them are absolutely essential (Horan et al 1977, Vallis 1984, Moses & Holandsworth 1985, Kendall et al 1991).

INDIVIDUAL DIFFERENCES

It is clear that the various cognitive aspects of pain have a strong association with the reactions to pain. After reviewing the literature on coping with chronic pain, Jensen et al (1991a) concluded that beliefs and coping have a strong relationship to adjustment to chronic pain. Patients who believe they can control their pain, who avoid catastrophizing, and who believe that they are not severely disabled function better than those who do not. It is important, however, to note that much of the current data are correlational. As Kendall et al (1991) point out about cognitive theories in general, many of the beliefs measured at different stages of treatment may reflect a state of mind rather than a personality trait. Cause and effect are not always clear.

The Cognitive Strategies Questionnaire (CSQ) is a 42-item measure of different strategies used by pain patients which includes diverting attention, coping self-statements, praying or hoping, increased behavioural activities, reinterpretation of pain sensations, ignoring pain sensations and catastrophizing (Rosenstiel & Keefe 1983, Lawson et al 1990). Turner and Clancy (1986) used the CSQ to assess a cognitive or behavioural intervention for low back pain. They reported that increased use of praying and hoping strategies and less catastrophizing were associated with lower pain intensity. Keefe et al (1990) using the CSQ found that the helplessness factor accounted for 50% of the variance in psychological distress and 46% of the depression among chronic low back pain patients.

CATASTROPHIZING

Catastrophizing as it relates to pain refers to negative self-statements and overly negative thoughts and ideas about the present and/or the future (Rosenstiel & Keefe 1983, Heyneman et al 1990, Lawson et al 1990, Sullivan et al 1995). Examples of items from the CSQ used to measure catastrophizing include 'I feel my life isn't worth living', 'Its terrible and I feel its never going to get any better'. A future oriented example from the study of Heyneman et al (1990) includes the statement 'I'll get frostbite'. The Pain Catastrophizing Scale (PCS) of Sullivan et al (1995) includes three factors:

1. Rumination, 'I can't seem to keep it out of my mind'.
2. Magnification, 'I become afraid that the pain may get worse'.
3. Helplessness, 'I feel I can't stand it anymore'.

The scale is based on the work of Rosenstiel and Keefe (1983), Spanos et al (1979) and Chaves and Brown (1987). The reports of catastrophizing are undoubtedly related to some of the negative thinking described earlier, even though different terminology is used. Several researchers have suggested that the reduction of negative thoughts may be more important for adaptive coping than enhancing positive thoughts (Kendall 1985, Chaves & Brown 1987, Turk & Rudy 1992), or the increased use of coping strategies (Newton & Barbaree 1987). The authors postulate that the reduction in negative appraisal was the key change mechanism. It is worth noting that some authors do not include all of the dimensions of catastrophizing mentioned earlier. Thus, Chaves & Brown (1987) place emphasis on exaggerated fear or worry about the situation without necessarily including a future dimension. Other researchers have questioned whether or not catastrophizing is not simply an aspect of depressive phenomena (Sullivan & D'Eon 1990). Still other researchers used other names to describe similar phenomena. Thus, Asmundson and Norton (1995) speak of anxiety-sensitive low-back-pain patients who exhibit greater fear of pain and the negative consequenses of pain. In a recent study it was demonstrated that catastrophizers are hypervigilant to threatening somatic information. They appear unable to ignore somatic threats (Crombez et al 1998).

Catastrophizing has been singled out in several studies and reviews as particularly important in predicting reaction to pain and treatment, even though Lawson et al (1990) reported that it appears to be separate from other factors on the CSQ and has been viewed as a belief rather than a method of coping (Jensen et al 1991). For example, Keefe et al (1997) were able to predict 6 months later the pain intensity and functional impairment of 223 rheumatoid arthritis patients as found on the Arthritis Impact Measurement Scale (Meean et al 1984) on the basis of prior scores on the Catastrophizing Scale of the CSQ. Zautra and Manne (1992), after reviewing 10 years of coping research among rheumatoid arthritis patients, concluded that catastrophizing and wishful thinking were associated with poorer outcomes, while attempts to restructure thoughts to be more positive were associated with positive outcomes. Keefe et al (1997) reported that catastrophizing was associated with lower self-efficacy for the pain and for the arthritis symptoms. Reesor and Craig (1988) found more catastrophizing and less of a sense of control to typify chronic low back patients for whom the symptomatology was not congruent with the physical findings, had poorer outcomes to treatment and rehabilitation, and used healthcare resources excessively. Hill (1993) reported that catastrophizing explained the largest amount of variance in patient reports of phantom limb pain. Catastrophizing has also been found related to neuroticism. Rheumatoid arthritis patients who scored high on neuroticism also tended to use catastrophizing more (Affleck et al 1992b).

SELF-EFFICACY

It is important to emphasize that effective coping depends on individuals' assessment of their competence. It is not enough to possess the relevant skills. Individuals must *believe* that they have the skills and that they are capable of applying them as needed. This concept has been labelled 'self-efficacy' by Bandura (Bandura 1977, Maddux 1995). Individuals' beliefs in their own effectiveness determine whether they try to cope with or avoid a situation that is viewed as beyond their abilities. Efficacy expectations can also determine how much effort individuals will invest and how long they will persist in the face of aversive experiences. Lack of perceived self-efficacy leading to faulty appraisal of coping abilities can produce anxiety and behavioural dysfunction. Perceived self-efficacy is seen as influencing how individuals will behave, think and react emotionally in a challenging or stressful situation. Recent research has even shown that perceived self-efficacy could affect the body's endogenous opiate and immune systems (Bandura et al 1987, 1988, Wiedenfeld et al 1990). It is important to note that perceived self-efficacy is a changeable commodity.

Bandura (1977) has referred to four major sources by which self-efficacy can be influenced. They are performance experiences, vicarious experiences, verbal or social persuasion and emotional or physiological arousal. One of the most potent influences on self-efficacy is the mastery experience acquired through actual performance. In the pain area, self-efficacy has been shown to be a basic concept both in laboratory and clinical studies. Subjects who possess higher self-efficacy are willing to tolerate higher levels of pain (cf., Lin & Ward 1996, Weisenberg et al 1996, Kashikar-Zuck et al 1997, Keefe et al 1997). Manipulation of self-efficacy also appears to be causally related to the outcome (Vallis & Bucher 1986, Litt 1988).

In the laboratory, Dolce et al (1986a) found that self-efficacy expectancies were the best predictors of cold-pressor pain tolerance. They also found that setting of quotas contributed to increased pain tolerance, perhaps via the raising of self-efficacy expectations. In their clinical application and study, Dolce et al (1986b) utilized a quota system for exercise with chronic pain patients. After three baseline sessions, exercises were introduced on an increasing quota basis. Patients demonstrated an increase in self-efficacy for the physical activity. The authors conceptualize the approach as a desensitization of the avoidance behaviour associated with the faulty belief that activity is associated with harm and pain increase. Self-efficacy was increased at the same time as worry and concern over activity decreased.

The success of cognitive strategies depends to a great extent on motivational factors (Weisenberg 1984, 1989, 1994, Turk & Rudy 1990, 1991). Self-efficacy as used in pain control often refers to willingness or behavioural intention, rather than a judgment of ability (Kirsch 1995). Self-efficacy has been found to play a key motivational role in a person's life (Karoly & Ruehlman 1996, Karoly & Lecci 1997). For example, Holroyd et al (1984) told a group of patients that they had achieved high control over tension by relaxation of frontalis muscles in order to induce a high sense of self-efficacy that they could abort or reduce headache intensity. The actual amount of physiological change was found to be unrelated to headache activity. Perceived self-efficacy was the determining factor. Several studies with chronic pain patients have since reported that a key predictor of patient success at the conclusion of treatment was perceived self-efficacy (Council et al 1988, Kores et al 1990, Jensen et al 1991b, O'Leary & Brown 1995).

PERCEIVED CONTROL

Control as a variable has been shown to be important in both clinical and laboratory settings for both acute and chronic pain (Thompson 1981, Chapman & Turner 1986). Attribution of control to internal rather than to external factors has become a key factor in the clinical treatment of pain, especially for chronic pain (cf. Jensen et al 1991a). Patients with chronic pain often exhibit learned helplessness as a result of their disability, which tends to become reinforced by frequent medication and dependency on others. Patients, therefore, are taught self-regulation rather than drug regulation for dealing with their problems as part of a comprehensive treatment programme (cf. McArthur et al 1987). Several studies have shown that an internal locus of control was associated with better coping with pain while a chance, external orientation to control of pain was associated with maladaptive coping (cf. Crisson & Keefe 1988, Harkapaa et al 1991). The locus of control measure assesses the individual's perception that things are under a person's control (not that the person giving the rating necessarily can exert that control) rather than due to chance or luck. Spinhoven and Linssen (1991), reporting on their low-back-pain sample, suggested that at 6-month treatment follow-up the perception of control may be more important for pain reduction than the specific coping strategy used. In a recent study, Elliot (1992) reported that perceived ineffective personal control, a measure that reflects the extent to which the individual can regulate emotional reactions when problem-solving, was associated with higher levels of premenstrual and menstrual pain. Jensen and Karoly (1991) found in chronic patients that the patients' belief in control over pain, as well as the cognitive strategies used, were related to well-being and to activity level. In some instances this was valid only for a low level of pain severity. Affleck et al (1987) reported that patients' perceived control over the course of treatment for rheumatoid arthritis was associated with positive mood and global adjustment.

Clinically, patient controlled analgesia (PCA) has obtained much praise. A substantial number of studies have been performed to assess the use of PCA. The general conclusion is that it is safe, efficient, does not lead always to better levels of pain control but is often preferred by patients. Some of the areas for which PCA has been used successfully include postoperative pain, bone marrow transplantation (Hill et al 1990, Zucker et al 1998) and cancer patients (Bruera et al 1991).

Numerous laboratory studies have indicated that providing subjects with some degree of control over pain stimulation can reduce stress and increase pain tolerance (Weisenberg 1984, 1989). Control and predictability can be separated from each other (Miller 1980). Controllability refers to what the person can do about the event. Control can refer to changing the aversive stimulus itself or to changing one's response to the stimulus. The expectation of control can lead to improve performance even under conditions of learned helplessness (Mikulincer 1986).

When predictability is kept constant, Miller (1980) has suggested the minimax hypothesis to account for the effects of perceived control. This hypothesis views control as based upon an internal, stable attribution, for example the person's own response. When the situation is not controllable by the person himself, external attributions must be considered, for example the experimenter, chance, etc. The external factor may or may not be able to guarantee the low maximum level of aversiveness the person would be willing to have. Miller has suggested, with some empirical support, that individuals would be willing to hand over control to someone else when they doubt their own abilities to perform a given action in dealing with a threat, when the action to reduce the threat is unclear or when individuals perceive another to have more skill or expertise in dealing with the threat. Weisenberg et al (1985), in a laboratory study, found unexpectedly that a condition in which the experimenter exerted control yielded the lowest pain reaction among subjects with high perceived self-efficacy for pain control, but a high pain reaction in subjects with low perceived self-efficacy for pain control. These results raise questions for the clinical situation. When does giving control to a competent other person reduce or increase distress? In the clinic, for persons who perceive themselves as lacking control, does giving control to a healthcare provider make them feel more out of control? These questions have not yet been answered.

Matthews et al (1980) concluded that for every study that reports positive outcomes for predictability, there is a conflicting report showing no effect or a negative effect. They conclude that the only thing to be said about the effects of predictability 'is that they are unpredictable'.

Predictability is usually achieved by means of a warning signal. One issue that arises is the time gap between the warning and stimulation. In a laboratory study using electric shock (a quick, sharp, short-acting stimulus), Mittwoch et al (1990) reported that a warning signal of 5 or 30 seconds was less aversive than one of 60 or 180 seconds. With a longer-acting, repeated stimulus such as cold-pressor pain, Weisenberg et al (1996) found that the longer 180-second interval was less aversive. It seems that subjects prefer having the extra time to recover from the previous stimulus.

PREPARATION FOR TREATMENT

Many studies have been conducted that deal with the effects of preparing patients for stressful medical or dental procedures. Reviews of the literature almost uniformly point to the benefits of prior preparation (Reading 1979, Kendall & Watson 1981, Mumford et al 1982, Melamed 1984, Guggenheim 1986, Auerbach 1989). Although it is not always clear which ingredients are most important, some of the most recent studies have begun to test more specific components and their effects. Studies of repeated surgeries are also beginning to appear.

As is true with many other clinical studies, it is not always clear what is being manipulated: information, cognitive skills or other coping skills. Often a combined approach is tested. Control groups remain problematical. Many times what is compared is the 'usual' routine that remains unspecified. Process variables are still quite difficult to measure (Auerbach 1989); that is, if a specific coping skill is said to be taught, to what extent was it really taught and to what extent was it actually used?

The early work of Janis (1958) emphasized an optimal relationship between the amount of suffering expected and the amount obtained which seems conducive to inoculation and a feeling of mastery of a difficult situation and to speed of recovery. The optimal degree of worry or anxiety prior to stressful surgery is best reached when patients receive realistic information and are able to listen to and accept what is being told them. This occurs when patients experience a moderate level of anxiety. The credibility of practitioners is enhanced and patients are helped to prepare for the event. Without the 'work of worrying', there is little anticipatory fear. When the inevitable postsurgical pain is experienced, patients feel victimized.

Janis' emphasis on fear and a moderate anxiety level has not always received support (Melamed 1984). Wilson (1981) found that surgical patients who claimed that they used high levels of denial actually required less analgesia and left the hospital earlier. Cohen and Lazarus (1973) have emphasized the importance of coping strategies in dealing with the stress of surgery. When the outcome of surgery was likely to be successful, they reported the best results with an avoidance strategy.

Although the exact relationship of presurgical anxiety and outcome still remains unclear, there is enough evidence to point to the importance of considering anxiety, especially trait-anxiety status, when preparing for surgery. Thus, it would be appropriate to use any strategies that are usually successful in dealing with elevated anxiety (Johnston 1986). Jamison et al (1987) studied 50 women undergoing elective laparoscopic surgery as ambulatory patients. They found that presurgical fear and anxiety was predictive of later postoperative complications. Boeke et al (1991), in a study of 111 patients with gallstones, found that preoperative anxiety did not predict postoperative pain, but did predict length of hospitalization. Taenzer et al (1986) in a study of 40 gallbladder patients, found that trait anxiety and neuroticism were the most important factors that predicted postsurgical pain levels. Situational anxiety, measured the night before surgery, was not predictive of postsurgical pain level. Thus, it appears that although there is little support for a curvilinear relationship of anxiety and surgical outcome, there is support for the importance of presurgical anxiety in determining postsurgical outcome. It is not always clear, however, whether situational anxiety is as important as trait anxiety.

Although a period of advance notice with prior information and coping techniques does help patients, the amount of detail, the temporal spacing of information and how the personality of the subject affect the outcome are not always clear (Andrew 1970, DeLong 1970, Melamed 1984). Copers (those who attempt to deal with stress) and those called non-specific defenders (those who use both coping and avoiding strategies) seem to be able to accept more detailed information than avoiders (those who try to deny or avoid dealing with stress) (DeLong 1970). Similarly, Miller (1988) reported that gynaecological patients who are monitors (those who use an active coping style) do better with a high level of information as opposed to blunters (those who use a passive, distancing coping style) who do better with less information. Gattuso et al (1992) also reported that monitors did worst with endoscopy when provided with little information while blunters did most poorly when provided with procedural information. Scott and Clum (1984) concluded that avoiders might be better off without any information.

Faust and Melamed (1984) compared groups of children who were scheduled to have surgery the same day or the following day. Older children were able to retain more of the information provided. The preparation resulted in less physiological arousal for children who were to be operated on the next day, but greater arousal for children to be operated on the same day. Same-day patients may be better off with a distraction type of preparation (Fowler-Kerry & Lander 1987). Faust et al (1991), however, found that children (aged 4–10 years) prepared for same-day surgery showed lower arousal than the control condition. They compared participant modelling (in which a filmed model asked them to practise coping skills) with or without the presence of the mother, and a control who received the standard hospital preparation (tell – show – do in which the children could manipulate the operating room equipment). The most successful condition was the participant modelling without the presence of the mother and the least successful condition was the standard hospital preparation.

The effects of prior information, however, are not always consistent. Dworkin et al (1984) compared subjects who were provided with high or low levels of information on how nitrous oxide works to increase analgesia. Subjects were given tooth-pulp stimulation along with nitrous oxide. High- as compared to low-information subjects yielded higher sensation and pain tolerance thresholds. Wallace (1985), on the other hand, found that if the preparation leads to a greater expectation of pain, there is a more intense report of pain postsurgery. Scott et al (1983) reported that without any specific kind of preparation, higher levels of information were associated with higher levels of pain and more analgesics taken. Twardosz et al (1986) reported that when a videotape is used to prepare patients, the addition of the personal contact of a nurse increased the effectiveness of the preparation for surgery.

Information regarding sensations to be experienced seems to be more effective than information regarding the procedures to be used (Johnson 1973, Johnson & Leventhal 1974). For example, Johnson et al (1975), in a study of cast removal, found that children exposed to a brief tape-recording, which included the sound of the saw and a description of the sensations of heat and flying chalk, showed less distress and resistance to the procedure compared with a group who were only told of the procedure or not told at all. However, the results are not clear cut. Positive results were obtained for cholecystectomy but not for herniorrhaphy patients (Johnson et al 1978). The results of the intervention, therefore, remain somewhat unclear.

Litt et al (1993), in a study of oral surgery patients undergoing third molar extractions, used a dismantling design to test the relative contributions of the addition of cognitive elements to the preparation. The cognitive elements included information and cue exposure, decreased arousal, self-control attributions and enhanced self-efficacy. Four treatment groups were created into which patients were randomly assigned. Each treatment group added another of the four cognitive elements. The groups were:

1. Standard treatment (providing information, cue exposure).
2. Oral premedication (information, cue exposure, decreased arousal).
3. Relaxation only (information, cue exposure, decreased arousal, self-control attributions).
4. Relaxation plus self-efficacy (information, cue exposure, decreased arousal, self-control attributions, enhanced self-efficacy).

The information and cue exposure were given to the patient by the dentist 1–4 weeks before surgery while the other manipulations took place about 1.5 hours before surgery. The results indicated that the relaxation and the relaxation plus self-efficacy groups showed less distress than the other groups. The least distress was obtained for the relaxation plus self-efficacy group.

In a follow-up study of oral surgery, Litt et al (1995) tested the effects of self-efficacy enhancement as a function of dispositional style. Overall, a greater effect was found when more coping elements were included. However, they found that high blunters did best with the standard surgical preparation. They concluded that providing patients with a sense of control and raising their self-efficacy or confidence is effective in preparing patients for oral surgery. However, patients whose dispositional style involves distraction or ignoring of threat may benefit more from non-involving interventions.

In one of the few studies of multiple surgeries, Croog et al (1994) prepared patients for two periodontal surgeries. The positive affect enhancement (PAE) intervention was designed to stress positive feelings and benefits as an outcome of the surgery. The self-efficacy enhancement (SEE) intervention was designed to present information to promote the patient's sense of control of the sequelae of the periodontal surgery. A third group combined the two interventions (PAA–SEE). The control condition presented to patients a review of oral hygiene and dental care. The results indicated that after surgery I the SEE group tended to yield lower pain scores. The superiority of the SEE group became stronger after surgery II in comparison to the control group and even in comparison to the combined PAE–SEE group in terms of pain reduction. This result takes on added importance in that, in contrast to the laboratory studies that have shown a tendency for cognitive techniques to be less effective with repeated stimuli, the emphasis on self-efficacy and self-control in this study showed stronger results with the repeated surgery.

An added point to note before concluding this section concerns the preparation of children. Wolfer and Visitainer (1975), Melamed (1984) and Fradet et al (1990) underscore the importance of age differences among children. Children aged 3–6 compared to those aged 7–14 showed greater upset behaviour. The patient's age should also be considered in terms of the timing of the preparation. Less time in advance is desirable for younger children. Reducing parental feelings of anxiety has also been found to have a positive effect on the child patient.

PATIENT EDUCATION

An old idea has been revived and applied to pain control. Namely, it would greatly help patients cope with pain if we prepare them with educational materials. Hawley (1995) has reviewed many of these educational attempts in the treatment of rheumatoid arthritis where the majority of programmes can be found. The programmes have been classified as self-management, cognitive-behavioural or classroom educational. In the self-management there is a broadly focused approach. The patient is provided with disease-related information and assistance in learning and adapting new activities and skills. For example, patients are taught flexibility and strengthening exercise, relaxation techniques and other pain control techniques. Patients are given information while the group provides support for behavioural change. The cognitive-behavioural approach sounds like stress-inoculation training: an educational phase, a skills acquisition phase and an application to the real life setting. The educational approach uses a more traditional classroom format. The major emphasis is on information. Knowledge, however, is helpful but it is not enough to help patients cope.

The results for patients with rheumatoid arthritis indicate that patient knowledge increased. There were also some positive effects on functional ability and pain. Other positive effects were obtained for depression and in the attitudinal, self-efficacy area. With time, the effects of the programmes are weakened and require booster sessions. Hawley (1995) believes that although the effects are relatively small, they are of the same magnitude as therapy with NSAIDs but are independent of medical treatment.

The educational approach has tremendous potential in helping patients, with a minimal cost in physician time. It is starting to be applied in other pain areas as well. de Wit et al (1997) recently described a patient education programme for chronic cancer patients. Patients were taught pain management by a combination of verbal instruction, written material and an audio cassette. The goal of the programme was to instruct patients about the basic principles of pain management, on the use of a pain diary and how to communicate pain to health providers. The effectiveness of the programme appears to be strongest in increasing information. Mengshoel (1998) described a similar programme for patients with fibromyalgia. Sixteen female patients participated in a 10-week educational programme. The programme emphasized improved coping and reduction of maladaptive behaviour. At the end of the study, 12 out of the 16 patients showed a reduced visual analogue scale (VAS) and McGill Pain Questionnaire score of 35%. At 6-month follow-up the pain scores were still lower than the original baseline.

CONCLUDING COMMENT

PAIN THEORY

Conceptually, the gate-control theory (Melzack & Wall 1965, Melzack 1986) is still the most comprehensive and relevant of all pain theories for understanding the cognitive aspects of pain. There are gaps in the theory, the details of which are currently being filled in by others. According to gate-control theory, pain phenomena are viewed as consisting of sensory-discriminative, motivational-affective and cognitive-evaluative components. More than any other theoretical approach, gate-control theory emphasizes the tremendous role of psychological variables and how they affect the reaction to pain. Especially with chronic pain, successful pain control often involves changing the cognitive-motivational components while the sensory component remains intact. Hypnosis, anxiety reduction, desensitization, attention distraction and other behavioural approaches can be effective alternatives and supplements to pharmacology and surgery in the control of pain. Their effect is felt mostly on the cognitive-motivational components of pain (see Weisenberg 1977, 1980, 1983, 1987 for a more extensive review of psychological factors in pain control).

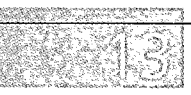

Recently, other theoretical statements have attempted to fill in the pieces of gate-control or to introduce new concepts that have not appeared in gate-control theory (cf. Algom 1992). Some of them were formulated to explain or understand the results of clinical practice (Turk & Flor 1987, Turk & Rudy 1992), while others attempted to explain the place of key concepts such as depression, emotional disturbance or other psychological phenomena of chronic pain (Rudy et al 1988, Gamsa & Vikis-Freibergs 1991).

COGNITIVE INTERVENTIONS FOR PAIN

There is little doubt that the cognitive approach has become part of the standardized approach to treating pain. The results of many studies have demonstrated that the various cognitive techniques are effective in reducing the reactions to pain. Most often, however, these techniques are applied as part of a comprehensive programme in which the cognitive approach is only one ingredient in the treatment. Such multidisciplinary programmes have been shown to be beneficial as inpatient, outpatient or as home management treatments (Cott et al 1990, Kames et al 1990, Maruta et al 1990, Peters & Large 1990, Flor et al 1992). At times the success of treatment is likely to be indirect, as a consequence of the treatment of depression or some other emotional concomitant of the pain. What appears to be quite clear is the need to consider the motivational issues as an integral part of treatment. That is, more important than the effectiveness of one technique over the other, is the perception by patients that they are capable of carrying out the tasks required of them and that this will control the pain effectively. In general, as Turk and Rudy (1990, 1991) have indicated, it is necessary to take into account motivational factors when treating pain. This is also appropriate in the use of cognitive techniques. The evidence reviewed in this chapter leaves little doubt that cognitive aspects of pain are significant in pain perception and control.

REFERENCES

Affleck G, Tennen H, Pfeiffer C, Field J 1987 Appraisals of control and predictability in adapting to a chronic disease. Journal of Personality and Social Psychology 53: 273–279

Affeck G, Urrows S, Tennen H, Higgins P 1992a Daily coping with pain from rheumatoid arthritis: patterns and correlates. Pain 51: 221–229

Affleck G, Tennen H, Urrows S, Higgins P 1992b Neuroticism and the pain–mood relation in rheumatoid arthritis: insights from a prospective study. Journal of Consulting and Clinical Psychology 60: 119–126

Algom D 1992 Psychophysical analysis of pain: a functional perspective. In: Geissler HG, Link SW, Townsend JT (eds) Cognition, information processing, and psychophysics: basic issues. Erlbaum, Hillsdale, New Jersey, p 267

Andrew JM 1970 Recovery from surgery with and without preparatory instruction for three coping styles. Journal of Personality and Social Psychology 15: 223–226

Asmundson GJG, Norton GR 1995 Anxiety sensitivity in patients with physically unexplained chronic back pain. Behaviour Research and Therapy 33: 771–777

Auerbach SM 1989 Stress management and coping research in the health care setting: an overview and methodological commentary. Journal of Consulting and Clinical Psychology 57: 388–395

Bandura A 1977 Self-efficacy: toward a unifying theory of behavioral change. Psychological Review 84: 191–215

Bandura A 1984 Recycling misconceptions of perceived self-efficacy. Cognitive Therapy and Research 8: 231–255

Bandura A 1989 Human agency in social cognitive theory. American Psychologist 44: 1175–1184

Bandura A, O'Leary A, Taylor CB, Gauthier J, Gossard D 1987 Perceived self-efficacy and pain control: opioid and nonopioid mechanisms. Journal of Personality and Social Psychology 53: 563–571

Bandura A, Cioffi D, Taylor CB, Brouillard HE 1988 Perceived self-efficacy in coping with cognitive stressors and opioid activation. Journal of Personality and Social Psychology 55: 479–488

Beck AT, Rush AJ, Shaw BF, Emory G 1979 Cognitive therapy of depression. Guilford Press, New York

Beck AT, Emory G, Greenberg RL 1985 Anxiety disorders and phobia. Basic Books, New York

Beck AT, Freeman A and Associates 1990 Cognitive therapy of personality disorders. Guilford Press, New York

Beck JS 1995 Cognitive therapy: basics and beyond. Guilford Press, New York

Berntzen D 1987 Effects of multiple cognitive coping strategies on laboratory pain. Cognitive Therapy and Research 11: 613–623

Bergdahl J, Anneroth G, Perris H 1995 Cognitive therapy in the treatment of patients with resistant burning mouth syndrome: a controlled study. Journal of Oral Pathology and Medicine 24: 213–215

Boeke S, Duivenvoorden HJ, Verhage F, Zwaveling A 1991 Prediction of postoperative pain and duration of hospitalization using two anxiety measures. Pain 45: 293–297

Chapman CR, Turner JA 1986 Psychological control of acute pain in medical settings. Journal of Pain and Symptom Management 1: 9–20

Chaves JF, Barber TX 1974 Cognitive strategies, experimenter modeling and expectation in the attenuation of pain. Journal of Abnormal Psychology 83: 356–363

Chaves JF, Brown JM 1987 Spontaneous coping strategies for pain. Journal of Behavioral Medicine 10: 263–276

Cohen F, Lazarus RS 1973 Active coping process, coping dispositions and recovery from surgery. Psychosomatic Medicine 35: 375–389

Cott A, Anchel H, Goldenberg WM, Fabich M, Parkinson W 1990 Non-institutional treatment of chronic pain by field management: an outcome study with comparison group. Pain 40: 183–194

Council JR, Ahern DK, Follick MJ, Kline CL 1988 Expectancies and functional impairment in chronic low back pain. Pain 33: 323–331

Crisson JE, Keefe FJ 1988 The relationship of locus of control to pain coping strategies and psychological distress in chronic pain patients. Pain 35: 147–154

Crombez G, Eccleston C, Baeyens F, Eelen P 1998 When somatic information threatens, catastrophic thinking enhances attentional interference. Pain 75: 187–198

Croog SH, Baume R, Nalbandian J 1994 Pain response after psychological preparation for repeated periodontal surgery. Journal of the American Dental Association 125: 1353–1359

DeLong RD 1970 Individual differences in patterns of anxiety arousal, stress-relevant information and recovery from surgery. Unpublished doctoral dissertation, University of California, Los Angeles, California

D'Eon JL, Perry CW 1984 The role of imagery and coping cognitions in response to pressure pain as moderated by choice of pain control strategy. Paper presented at the Annual Meeting of the American Psychological Association, Toronto, Canada

de Wit R, van Dam F, Zanderbelt L et al 1997 A pain education program for chronic cancer pain patients: follow-up results from a randomized control trial. Pain 73: 55–69

Dolce JJ, Doleys DM, Raczynski JM, Lossie J, Poole L, Smith M 1986a The role of self-efficacy expectancies in the prediction of pain tolerance. Pain 27: 261–272

Dolce JJ, Crocker MF, Moletteire C, Doleys DM 1986b Exercise quotas, anticipatory concern and self-efficacy expectancies in chronic pain: a preliminary report. Pain 24: 365–372

Dworkin SF, Chen ACN, Schubert MM, Clark DW 1984 Cognitive modification of pain: information in combination with NO_2. Pain 19: 339–351

Dworkin SF, von Korff MR, LeResche L 1992 Epidemiologic studies of chronic pain: a dynamic-ecologic perspective. Annals of Behavioral Medicine 14: 3–11

Eccleston C 1995 The attentional control of pain: methodological and theoretical concerns. Pain 63: 3–10

Elliott CH, Olson RA 1983 The management of children's distress in response to painful medical treatment for burn injuries. Behaviour Research and Therapy 21: 675–683

Elliott TR 1992 Problem-solving appraisal, oral contraceptive use, and menstrual pain. Journal of Applied Social Psychology 22: 286–297

Ellis A 1962 Reason and emotion in psychotherapy. Lyle Stuart, New York

Ellis JA, Spanos NP 1994 Cognitive–behavioral interventions for children's distress during bone marrow aspirations and lumbar punctures: a critical review. Journal of Pain and Symptom Management 9: 96–108

Faust J, Melamed BG 1984 Influence of arousal, previous experience, and age on surgery preparation of the same day of surgery and in-hospital pediatric patients. Journal of Consulting and Clinical Psychology 52: 359–365

Faust J, Olson R, Rodriguez H 1991 Same day surgery preparation: reduction of pediatric patient arousal and distress through participant modeling. Journal of Consulting and Clinical Psychology 59: 475–478

Fernandez E, Turk DC 1989 The utility of cognitive coping strategies for altering pain perception: a meta-analysis. Pain 38: 123–135

Flor H, Fydrich T, Turk DC 1992 Efficacy of multidisciplinary treatment centers: a meta-analytic review. Pain 49: 221–230

Folkman S, Lazarus RS, Gruen RJ, DeLongis A 1986a Appraisal, coping, health status and psychological symptoms. Journal of Personality and Social Psychology 50: 571–579

Folkman S, Lazarus RS, Dunkel-Schetter C, DeLongis A, Gruen RJ 1986b Dynamics of a stressful encounter: cognitive appraisal, coping, and encounter outcomes. Journal of Personality and Social Psychology 50: 992–1003

Forsythe CJ, Compas BE 1987 Interaction of cognitive appraisals of stressful events and coping: testing the goodness of fit hypothesis. Cognitive Therapy and Research 11: 473–485

Fowler-Kerry S, Lander JR 1987 Management of injection pain in children. Pain 30: 169–175

Fradet C, McGrath PJ, Kay J, Adams S, Luke B 1990 A prospective survey of reactions to blood tests by children and adolescents. Pain 40: 53–60

Freeman A, Pretzer J, Fleming B, Simon KM 1990 Clinical application of cognitive therapy. Plenum Press, New York

Gamsa A, Vikis-Freibergs V 1991 Psychological events are both risk factors in, and consequences of, chronic pain. Pain 44: 271–277

Gattuso SM, Litt MD, Fitzgerald TE 1992 Coping with gastrointestinal endoscopy: self-efficacy enchancement and coping style. Journal of Consulting and Clinical Psychology 60: 133–139

Guggenheim FG 1986 Psychological aspects of surgery. In: Wise TN (ed) Advances in psychosomatic medicine, vol 15. Karger, Basel

Haaga DAF (Ed.) 1997 Special section: measuring cognitive products in research and practice. Journal of Consulting and Clinical Psychology 65: 907–1000

Hackett G, Horan JJ, Buchanan J, Zumoff P 1979 Improving exposure generalization potential of stress inoculation for pain. Perceptual and Motor Skills 48: 1132–1134

Harkapaa K, Jarvikoski A, Mellin G, Hurri H, Luoma J 1991 Health locus of control beliefs and psychological distress as predictors for treatment outcome in low-back pain patients: results of a three-month follow-up of a controlled intervention study. Pain 46: 35–41

Hawley DJ 1995 Psycho-educational interventions in the treatment of arthritis. Bailliere's Clinical Rheumatology 9: 803–823

Hayes SC, Wolf MR 1984 Cues, consequences and therapeutic talk: effects of social context and coping statements on pain. Behaviour Research and Therapy 22: 385–392

Heyneman NE, Fremouw WJ, Gano D, Kirkland F, Heiden L 1990 Individual differences and the effectiveness of different coping strategies for pain. Cognitive Therapy and Research 14: 63–77

Hill A 1993 The use of pain coping strategies by patients with phantom limb pain. Pain 55: 347–353

Hill HF, Chapman CR, Kornell JA, Sullivan KM, Saeger LC, Benedetti C 1990 Self-administration of morphine in bone marrow transplant patients reduces drug requirement. Pain 40: 121–129

Hill HF, Coda BA, Mackie AM, Iverson K 1992 Patient-controlled analgesic infusions: alfentanil versus morphine. Pain 49: 301–310

Holroyd KA, Penzien DB, Hursey KG et al 1984 Change mechanism in EMG biofeedback training. Journal of Consulting and Clinical Psychology 52: 1039–1053; 59: 387–393

Horan JJ, Hacket G, Buchanan JD, Stone I, Demchik-Stone D 1977 Coping with pain: a component analysis of stress inoculation. Cognitive Therapy and Research 1: 211–221

Jamison RN, Parris WCV, Maxson WS 1987 Psychological factors influencing recovery from outpatient surgery. Behaviour Research and Therapy 25: 31–37

Janis I 1958 Psychological stress. John Wiley, New York

Jensen I, Nygren A, Gamberale F, Goldie I, Westerholm P, Jonsson E 1995 The role of the psychologist in multidisciplinary treatments for chronic neck and shoulder pain: a controlled cost-effectiveness study. Scandinavian Journal of Rehabilitation Medicine 27: 19–26

Jensen MP, Karoly P 1991 Control beliefs, coping efforts, and adjustment to chronic pain. Journal of Consulting and Clinical Psychology 59: 431–438

Jensen MP, Turner JA, Romano JM, Karoly P 1991a Coping with chronic pain: a critical review of the literature. Pain 47: 249–283

Jensen MP, Turner JA, Romano JM 1991b Self-efficacy and outcome expectancies: relationship to chronic pain coping strategies and adjustment. Pain 44: 263–269

Johnson JE 1973 Effects of accurate expectations about sensations of the sensory and distress components of pain. Journal of Personality and Social Psychology 27: 261–275

Johnson JE, Leventhal H 1974 Effects of accurate expectations and behavioral instructions on reactions during a noxious medical examination. Journal of Personality and Social Psychology 29: 710–718

Johnson JE, Kirchoff KT, Endress MP 1975 Deferring children's distress behavior during orthopaedic cast removal. Nursing Research 75: 404–410

Johnson JE, Fuller SS, Endress MP, Rice VH 1978 Altering patients' responses to surgery: an extension and replication. Research in Nursing and Health 1: 111–121

Johnston M 1986 Preoperative emotional states and postoperative recovery. Advances in Psychosomatic Medicine 15: 1–22

Kames LD, Rapkin AJ, Naliboff BD, Afifi S, Ferrer-Brechner T 1990 Effectiveness of an interdisciplinary pain management program for the treatment of chronic pelvic pain. Pain 41: 41–46

Karoly P, Lecci L 1997 Motivational correlates of self-reported persistant pain in young adults. Clinical Journal of Pain 13: 104–109

Karoly P, Ruehlman LS 1996 Motivational implications of pain: chronicity, psychological distress, and work goal construal in a national sample of adults. Health Psychology 15: 383–390

Kashikar-Zuck S, Keefe FJ, Kornguth P, Beaupre P, Holzberg A, Delong D 1997 Pain coping and the pain experience during mamography: a preliminary study. Pain 73: 165–172

Keefe FJ, Van Horn Y 1993 Cognitive-behavioral treatment of rheumatoid arthritis pain. Arthritis Care and Research 6: 213–222

Keefe FJ, Crisson J, Urban BJ, Williams DA 1990 Analyzing chronic low back pain: the relative contribution of pain coping strategies. Pain 40: 293–301

Keefe FJ, Kashikar-Zuck S, Robinson W et al 1997 Pain coping strategies that predict patients' and spouses' ratings of patients' self-efficacy. Pain 73: 191–199

Keeri-Szanto M 1979 Drugs or drums: what relieves postoperative pain? Pain 6: 217–230

Kendall PC 1985 Cognitive processes and procedures. In: Wilson GT, Franks CM, Brownell KD, Kendall PC (eds) Annual review of behavior therapy: theory and practice, vol 10. Guilford Press, New York, p 123

Kendall PC, Watson D 1981 Psychological preparation for stressful medical procedures. In: Prokop CK, Bradley LA (eds) Medical psychology: contributions to behavioral medicine. Academic Press, New York, p 197

Kendall PC, Vitousek KB, Kane M 1991 Thought and action in psychotherapy: cognitive-behavioral approaches. In: Hersen M, Kazdin AE, Bellack AS (eds) The clinical psychology handbook. Pergamon, Elmsford, p 596

Kessler R, Dane JR 1996 Psychological and hypnotic preparation for anesthesia and surgery: an individual differences perspective. International Journal of Clinical and Experimental Hypnosis XLIV: 189–207

Kirsch I 1995 Self-efficacy and outcome expectancy: a concluding comment. In: Maddux I (ed) Self-efficacy adaptation and adjustment: theory, research and application. Plenum, New York p 331

Klepac RK, Hauge G, Dowling J, McDonald M 1981 Direct and generalized effects of three components of stress inoculation for increased pain tolerance. Behavior Therapy 12: 417–424

Kores RC, Murphy WD, Rosenthal TL, Elias DB, North WC 1990 Predicting outcome of chronic pain treatment via a modified self-efficacy scale. Behaviour Research and Therapy 28: 165–169

Lawson K, Reesor KA, Keefe FJ, Turner JA 1990 Dimensions of pain-related cognitive coping: cross-validation of the factor structure of the Coping Strategy Questionnaire. Pain 43: 195–204

Lazarus RS, Folkman S 1984 Stress appraisal and coping. Springer, New York

Leventhal H 1992 I know distraction works even though it doesn't. Health Psychology 11: 208–209

Lin CC, Ward SE 1996 Perceived self-efficacy and outcome expectancies in coping with chronic low back pain. Research in Nursing and Health 19: 299–310

Litt M 1988 Self-efficacy and perceived control: cognitive mediators of pain tolerance. Journal of Personality and Social Psychology 54: 149–160

Litt MD, Nye CK, Shafer D 1993 Coping with oral surgery by self-efficacy enhancement and perceptions of control. Journal of Dental Research 72: 1237–1243

Litt M, Nye C, Shafer D 1995 Preparation for oral surgery: evaluating elements of coping. Journal of Behavioral Medicine 18: 435–459

Logan HL, Baron RS, Kohout F 1995 Sensory focus as therapeutic treatments for acute pain. Psychosomatic Medicine 57: 474–484

McArthur DL, Cohen MJ, Gottlieb HJ, Naliboff BD, Schandler SL 1987 Treating chronic low back pain. I. Admission to initial follow-up. Pain 29: 1–22

McCaul KD, Malott JM 1984 Distraction and coping with pain. Psychological Bulletin 95: 516–533

Maddux JE (ed) 1995 Self-efficacy, adaptation and adjustment: theory research and application. Plenum, New York

Malone MD, Strube MJ 1988 Meta-analysis of non-medical treatments for chronic pain. Pain 34: 231–244

Maruta T, Swanson DW, McHardy MJ 1990 Three-year follow-up of patients with chronic pain who were treated in a multidisciplinary pain management center. Pain 41: 47–53

Matthews KA, Scheier MF, Brynson BI, Carducci B 1980 Attention, unpredictability and reports of physical symptoms: eliminating the benefits of predictability. Journal of Personality and Social Psychology 38: 525–537

Meean RF, Gertman PM, Mason JH 1984 Measuring health status in arthritis: The Arthritis Impact Measurement Scales. Arthritis and Rheumatism 25: 1048–1053

Meichenbaum D 1977 Cognitive behavior modification. Plenum, New York

Meichenbaum D 1985 Stress inoculation training. Pergamon, New York

Meichenbaum D, Turk D 1976 The cognitive-behavioral management of anxiety, anger, and pain. In: Davidson PO (ed) The behavioral management of anxiety, depression and pain. Brunner/Mazel, New York, p 1

Melamed BG 1984 Health intervention: collaboration for health and science. In: Hammonds BL, Scheirer CJ (eds) Psychology and health: the master lecture series, vol 3. American Psychological Association, Washington DC

Melzack R 1986 Neurophysiological foundations of pain. In: Sternbach RA (ed) The psychology of pain. Raven, New York, p 1

Melzack R, Wall PD 1965 Pain mechanisms: a new theory. Science 150: 971–979

Mengshoel AM 1998 Pain, fatigue, and the effects of aerobic exercise and patient education programs in patients with fibromyalgia. Center for Rheumatic Diseases, The National Hospital, Oslo

Mikulincer M, 1986 Attributional processes in the learned helplessness paradigm: the behavioral effect of globality attributions. Journal of Personality and Social Psychology 51: 1248–1256

Miller ME, Bowers KS 1993 Hypnotic analgesia: dissociated experience or dissociated control? Journal of Abnormal Psychology 102: 29–38

Miller SM 1980 Why having control reduces stress: if I can stop the roller coaster, I don't want to get off. In: Garber J, Seligman MEP (eds) Human helplessness: theory and applications. Academic, New York, p 71

Miller SM 1988 The interacting effects of coping styles and situational variables in gynecologic settings: implications for research and treatment. Journal of Psychosomatic Obstetrics and Gynecology 9: 23–34

Mittwoch T, Weisenberg M, Mikulincer M 1990 The influence of warning signal timing and cognitive preparation on the aversiveness of electric shock. Pain 42: 373–381

Moses AN III, Holandsworth JG 1985 Relative effectiveness of education alone versus stress inoculation training in the treatment of dental phobia. Behavior Therapy 16: 531–537

Mumford E, Schlesinger HG, Glass GV 1982 The effects of psychological intervention on recovery from surgery and heart attacks: an analysis of the literature. American Journal of Public Health 72: 141–151

Newton CR, Barbaree HE 1987 Cognitive changes accompanying headache treatment: the use of a thought-sampling procedure. Cognitive Therapy and Research 11: 635–651

Nicholas MK, Wilson PH, Goyen J 1992 Comparison of cognitive-behavioral group treatment and an alternative non-psychological treatment for chronic low back pain. Pain 48: 339–347

O'Leary A, Brown S 1995 Self-efficacy and the physiological stress responce. In: Maddux JE (ed) Self-efficacy, adaptation, and adjustment: theory, research, and applications. Plenum, New York, pp 227–246

Patterson DR, Sharar S 1997–98 Treating patients with severe burn injuries. Advances in Medical Psychotherapy 9: 51–71

Peters JL, Large RG 1990 A randomized control trial evaluating in- and outpatient pain management programmes. Pain 41: 283–293

Pilowsky I, Spence N, Rounsefell B, Forsten C, Soda J 1995 Out-patient cognitive-behavioural therapy with amitriptyline for chronic non-malignant pain: a comparative study with 6-month follow-up. Pain 60: 49–54

Reading AE 1979 The short-term effects of psychological preparations for surgery. Social Science and Medicine 13A: 641–654

Reesor KA, Craig KD 1988 Medically incongruent chronic back-pain: physical limitations, suffering and ineffective coping. Pain 32: 35–45

Rokke PD, Al Absi M 1992 Matching pain coping strategies to the individual: a prospective validation of the cognitive coping strategy inventory. Journal of Behavioral Medicine 15: 611–625

Rosenstiel AK, Keefe FJ 1983 The use of coping strategies in chronic low back pain patients: relationship to patient characteristics and current adjustment. Pain 17: 33–44

Roskies E, Lazarus RS 1980 Coping theory and the teaching of coping skills. In: Davidson PO, Davidson SM (eds) Behavioral medicine: changing health lifestyles. Brunner/Mazel, New York, p 38

Rudy TE, Kerns RD, Turk DC 1988 Chronic pain and depression: toward a cognitive behavioral mediation model. Pain 35: 129–140

Sanders MR, Shepherd RW, Cleghorn G, Woolford H 1994 The treatment of recurrent abdominal pain in children: a controlled comparison of cognitive-behavioral family intervention and standard pediatric care. Journal of Consulting and Clinical Psychology 62: 306–314

Scott LE, Clum GA 1984 Examining the interaction effects of coping style and brief interventions in the treatment of postsurgical pain. Pain 20: 279–291

Scott LE, Clum GA, Peoples JB 1983 Preoperative predictors of postoperative pain. Pain 15: 283–293

Shilo S 1997 The influence of personal style and observing the labor pain monitor on the report of pain. Paper presented at the Annual Meeting of the Israel Pain Association, Jerusalem

Spanos NP, Radtke-Bodorik HL, Ferguson JD, Jones B 1979. The effects of hypnotic susceptibility, suggestion for analgesia and utilization of cognitive strategies on the reduction of pain. Journal of Abnormal Psychology 88: 282–292

Spence SH 1991 Cognitive-behavioural therapy in the treatment of chronic occupational pain of the upper limbs: a two-year follow-up. Behaviour Research and Therapy 29: 503–509

Spinhoven P, Linssen ACG 1991 Behavioral treatment of chronic low back pain. I. Relation of coping strategy use to outcome. Pain 45: 29–34

Stedman's Medical Dictionary 1976 23rd edn. Williams & Wilkins, Baltimore

Sternbach RA 1986 Pain and 'hassles' in the United States: findings of the Nuprin Pain Peport. Pain 27: 69–80

Sullivan MJL, D'Eon JL 1990 Relationship between catastrophizing and depression in chronic pain patients. Journal of Abnormal Psychology 99: 260–263

Sullivan MJL, Bishop SR, Pivik J 1995. The Pain Catastrophizing Scale: development and validation. Psychological Assessment 7: 524–532

Syrjala KL, Donaldson GW, Davis MW, Kippes ME, Carr JE 1995 Relaxation and imagery and cognitive-behavioral training reduce pain during cancer treatment: a controlled clinical trial. Pain 63: 180–198

Taenzer P, Melzack R, Jeans ME 1986 Influence of psychological factors on postoperative pain, mood, and analgesic requirements. Pain 24: 331–342

Ter Kuile M, Spinhoven P, Linssen ACG, Zitman FG, Van Dyck R, Rooijmans HGM 1995 Pain 58: 331–340

Thompson SC 1981 Will it hurt less if I can control it? A complex answer to a simple question. Psychological Bulletin 90: 89–101

Thorn BE, Williams GA 1989 Goal specification alters perceived pain intensity and tolerance latency. Cognitive Therapy and Research 13: 171–183

Turk DC 1978 Cognitive-behavioral techniques in the management of pain. In: Foreyt JP, Rathjen DP (eds) Cognitive behavior therapy: research and application. Plenum, New York, p 199

Turk DC, Fernandez E 1990 On the putative uniqueness of cancer pain: do psychological principles apply? Behavioural Research and Therapy 28: 1–13

Turk DC, Flor H 1987 Pain > pain behaviors: the utility and limitations of the pain behavior construct. Pain 31: 277–295

Turk DC, Rudy TE 1990 Neglected factors in chronic pain treatment outcome studies—referral patterns, failure to enter treatment, and attrition. Pain 43: 7–25

Turk DC, Rudy TE 1991 Neglected topics in the treatment of chronic pain patients – relapse, noncompliance, and adherence enhancement. Pain 44: 5–28

Turk DC, Rudy TE 1992 Cognitive factors and persistent pain: a glimpse into Pandora's Box. Cognitive Therapy and Research 16: 99–122

Turk DC, Meichenbaum D, Genest M 1983 Pain and behavioral medicine: a cognitive-behavioral perspective. Guilford Press, New York

Turner JA, Clancy S 1986 Strategies for coping with chronic low back pain: relationships to pain and disability. Pain 24: 355–364

Twardosz S, Weddle K, Borden L, Stevens E 1986 A comparison of three methods of preparing children for surgery. Behavior Therapy 17: 14–25

Tyrer SP, Capon M, Peterson DM, Charlton JE, Thompson JW 1989 The detection of psychiatric illness and psychological handicaps in a British pain clinic population. Pain 36: 63–74

Vallis TM 1984 A component analysis of stress inoculation for pain tolerance. Cognitive Therapy and Research 8: 313–329

Vallis TM, Bucher B 1986 Self-efficacy as a predictor of behavior change: interaction with type of training for pain tolerance. Cognitive Therapy and Research 10: 79–94

Wack JT, Turk DC 1984 Latent structure of strategies used to cope with nociceptive stimulation. Health Psychology 3: 27–43

Wallace LM 1985 Surgical patients' expectations of pain and discomfort: does accuracy of expectations minimize postsurgical pain and distress? Pain 22: 363–373

Weisenberg M 1977 Pain and pain control. Psychological Bulletin 84: 1008–1044

Weisenberg M 1980 Understanding pain phenomena. In: Rachman S (ed) Contributions to medical psychology, vol 2. Pergamon Press, Oxford, p 79

Weisenberg M 1983 Pain and pain control. In: Daitzman R (ed) Diagnosis and intervention in behavior therapy and behavioral medicine. Springer, New York, p 90

Weisenberg M 1984 Cognitive aspects of pain. In: Wall PD, Melzack R (eds) Textbook of pain, Ist edn. Churchill Livingstone, Edinburgh, p 162

Weisenberg M 1987 Psychological intervention for the control of pain. Behaviour Research and Therapy 25: 301–312

Weisenberg M 1989 Cognitive aspects of pain. In: Wall PD, Melzack R (eds) Textbook of pain, 2nd edn. Churchill Livingstone, Edinburgh, p 231

Weisenberg M 1994 Cognitive aspects of pain. In: Wall PD, Melzack R (eds) Textbook of pain, 3rd edn. Churchill Livingstone, Edinburgh, p 275

Weisenberg M, Wolf Y, Mittwoch T, Mikulincer M, Aviram O 1985 Subject versus experimenter control in the reaction to pain. Pain 23: 187–200

Weisenberg M, Schwarzwald J, Tepper IM 1992 The influence of warning signal timing and cognitive preparation on the aversiveness of cold-pressor pain. Pain 379–385

Weisenberg M, Schwarzwald J, Tepper I 1996 The influence of warning signal timing and cognitive preparation on the aversiveness of cold pressor pain. Pain 64: 379–385

Wells JK, Howard GS, Nowlin WF, Vargas MJ 1986 Presurgical anxiety and postsurgical pain and adjustment: effects of a stress inoculation procedure. Journal of Consulting and Clinical Psychology 54: 831–835

Wernick RL, Jaremko ME, Taylor PW 1981 Pain management in severely burned adults: a test of stress inoculation. Journal of Behavioral Medicine 4: 103–109

Wiedenfeld SA, O'Leary A, Bandura A, Brown S, Levine S, Raska K 1990 Impact of perceived self-efficacy in coping with stressors on components of the immune system. Journal of Personality and Social Psychology 59: 1082–1094

Wilhelmsen I, Haug TT, Ursin H, Berstad A 1994 Effect of short-term cognitive psychotherapy on recurrence of duodenal ulcer: a prospective study. Psychosomatic Medicine 56: 440–448

Williams DA, Thorn BE 1986 Can research methodology affect treatment outcome? A comparison of two cold pressor test paradigms. Cognitive Therapy and Research 10: 539–545

Wilson JF 1981 Behavioral preparation for surgery: benefit or harm? Journal of Behavioral Medicine 4: 79–102

Wilson L, Massoth D, Dworkin SF et al 1992 Evaluation of an early cognitive-behavioral treatment for temporomandibular disorder pain. Paper presented at the Annual Meeting of the Society of Behavioral Medicine, New York

Wolfer JA, Visitainer MA 1975 Pediatric surgical patients' and parents' stress responses and adjustments. Nursing Research 24: 244–255

Young LD, Bradley LA, Turner RA 1995 Decreases in health care resource utilization in patients with rheumatoid arthritis following a cognitive behavioral intervention. Biofeedback and Self-Regulation 20: 259–268

Zautra AJ, Manne SL 1992 Coping with rheumatoid arthritis: a review of a decade of research. Annals of Behavioral Medicine 14: 31–39

Zucker TP, Flesche CW, Germing U et al 1998 Patient controlled versus staff-controlled analgesia with pethidine after allogeneic bone marrow transplantation. Pain 75: 305–312

Assessing transient and persistent pain in animals

RONALD DUBNER & KE REN

SUMMARY

This chapter will review methods of assessing pain in animals in which the goal of the studies is to explore the phenomenon of pain itself. Most of the early studies on pain were carried out in anaesthetized animals and utilized transient stimuli to produce pain in order to avoid tissue damage. The last decade has seen the proliferation of animal models to study the effects of tissue and nerve injury on the development of persistent or chronic pain. In most of these studies the animals are awake and exposed to pain. These models attempt to mimic human clinical conditions. A major purpose of such studies is to acquire knowledge that can ultimately be applied to the management of acute and chronic pain in humans and animals. Although scientists engaged in these studies feel morally justified in conducting such experiments, there is a need to demonstrate a continuing responsibility in the proper treatment of the animals that participate in these experiments. The animals should be exposed to the minimal pain necessary to carry out the experiment (Dubner 1983). Thus, both scientific and ethical considerations require that methods of assessing pain in animals be developed.

INTRODUCTION

A committee of the International Association for the Study of Pain has defined pain in humans as an 'unpleasant sensory and emotional experience associated with actual or potential tissue damage, or described in terms of such damage' (Merskey 1979). Although animals lack the ability to verbally communicate, they exhibit the same motor behaviours and physiological responses as humans in response to pain. Such behaviours include simple withdrawal reflexes, more complex unlearned behaviours such as vocalization or escape, and learned behaviours such as pressing a bar to avoid further exposure to noxious stimulation. From these behaviours we can infer that an animal is experiencing pain. An important concept in animal studies of pain is that experimental animals should not be exposed to pain greater than humans themselves would tolerate (Bowd 1980). Another way of stating this concept is that we should apply principles used in human studies to studies of pain in animals. Human subjects are exposed only to painful stimuli that they can tolerate and they can remove a painful stimulus at any time. Thus, they establish the acceptable level of pain under which the experiment is performed.

The tolerance for pain needs to be clearly distinguished from the threshold for pain. Stimuli near threshold produce minimal aversive reactions and are well tolerated by human subjects and animals. It is only when the intensity of the stimulus approaches tolerance levels that our behaviour is dominated by attempts to avoid or escape it. Therefore, it is critical that the experimenter determine the level of pain produced by stimuli whose intensity cannot be controlled by the animal.

How does an investigator decide which is the appropriate method to minimize pain? Many experiments are performed on anaesthetized animals. There are no ethical concerns about such experiments, as long as sufficient anaesthetic is provided. This can be accomplished by the monitoring of pupillary size, stability of heart rate and blood pressure, and electroencephalographic activity. Alternatives to anaesthetic agents are surgical lesions such as those that produce a functional decerebration, thus eliminating all possibility of conscious sensation. Another approach is to study pain mechanisms in awake animals that have received analgesic agents. Experiments on pain mechanisms in animals that have been administered anaesthetics or analgesics are of limited usefulness, because the procedures used suppress the very neurobiological processes that are under study. Nevertheless, important lines of inquiry can be pursued with such methods and they can be useful in the study of neural processes that are minimally affected by such agents.

Many studies of pain today are concerned with the relationship between behaviour related to pain and neurobiological processes. Such studies require that animals be exposed to actual or potential tissue damage with electrical, thermal, mechanical or chemical stimuli. Most investigations utilize techniques in which the animal has control over the intensity and duration of the stimulus. This ensures that the animal is not exposed to intolerable levels of stimulation and can escape the stimulus. A simple example of such a method is a withdrawal reflex produced by stimulating a paw or the tail of an animal. In these experiments, animals often need to be placed under considerable restraint which may produce unwanted levels of stress which can influence the outcome of the experiment (Dubner & Bennett 1983). Such stress is minimized in animals trained to perform pain detection and discrimination tasks (Dubner 1985). These studies employ operant conditioning procedures and most closely mimic conditions under which humans participate in experimental pain studies: the animals choose to participate by initiating trials, they determine the levels of stimulation that they will accept by escaping intolerable stimuli, and they can withdraw from the experiment by ceasing to initiate new trials.

It is difficult to minimize pain in studies in which the animals cannot control the pain magnitude. In such experiments it is important that the investigator infer the level of pain by carefully monitoring the animal's general behaviour. Does the animal engage in normal activity? Does it feed properly and exhibit normal social adjustment when placed in a cage with other animals of the same species? Does it maintain its weight as compared with controls? Is its sleep–waking cycle normal? Significant changes from the normal state suggest that the magnitude of pain may be above tolerable levels. Therefore, it is necessary to determine whether the experiment can be performed with lower levels of pain.

METHODS OF ASSESSING PAIN

Animal studies on pain employ behavioural measures of two types: simple withdrawal reflexes and more complex voluntary and intentional behaviours that are unlearned or learned (Chapman et al 1985).

SIMPLE REFLEX MEASURES

These include the tail-flick test, the limb-withdrawal reflex and orofacial reflexes. In most cases latency measures are used to assess reflex responses. In the tail-flick reflex, a radiant heat stimulus is focused on the blackened area of the tail and the animal flicks its tail to escape the stimulus. The technique was introduced by D'Armour and Smith (1941) to demonstrate analgesia. The effectiveness of analgesic agents in this model is highly correlated with their effectiveness in relieving pain in humans (Grumbach 1966). It has also been used to assess nocifensive behaviour produced by brain stimulation, stress, or the microinjection of opioids or other chemical mediators (Dubner & Bennett 1983). In the limb-withdrawal test, thermal, mechanical or electrical stimuli are typically employed and the latency of a brisk motor response is used as the behavioural endpoint (Bonnett & Peterson 1975). The jaw-opening reflex (Mitchell 1964) is elicited by electrical stimulation of a tooth and electromyographic recordings from jaw muscles are used to assess the behaviour. A model involving a head-withdrawal reflex has recently been developed in which a withdrawal latency to a noxious thermal or mechanical stimulus applied to the temporomandibular joint or the perioral skin is determined in awake or lightly anaesthetized animals (Ren & Dubner 1996, Imamura et al 1997). The tail-flick reflex has the advantage that it also can be elicited under light anaesthesia (Fields et al 1983, Sandkuhler & Gebhart 1984). The tail-flick latency is faster in the lightly anaesthetized state than in the awake animal. All of these simple reflex measures permit the animal to have control over stimulus magnitude and thus ensure that the animal can control the level of pain. There are minimal ethical concerns about the use of these measures in conscious animals.

Reflex responses suffer from a number of limitations as measures of pain behaviour (Chapman et al 1985). They are a measure of reflex activity and not pain sensation. The tail-flick reflex, for example, can be elicited in spinalized animals. Although analgesia in humans and tail-flick latencies in rats are highly correlated, reflex activity in humans produced by noxious stimulation can be dissociated from pain sensation produced by the same stimulus (Willer et al 1979, McGrath et al 1981). Changes in reflex activity can result from alterations in motor as well as sensory processing. Reflex latencies also are not easily related to stimulus intensity. In fact, most investigators empirically choose a convenient endpoint and normalize distributions to avoid the problem of baseline variability in a large group of animals.

ORGANIZED UNLEARNED BEHAVIOURS

More complex organized unlearned behaviours are often used as measures of pain because they involve a voluntary purposeful act requiring supraspinal sensory processing (Chapman et al 1985). A commonly used method is the rodent hot-plate test in which a rat or mouse is placed on a plate preheated to 50–56°C. A paw-licking response, usually of the hindpaws, is measured.

Animal models of pain and hyperalgesia have been developed to study the functional changes produced by the injection of inflammatory agents into the rat or mouse hindpaw (Hargreaves et al 1988, Iadorola et al 1988a, Millan et al 1988, Qui et al 1998). The animals withdraw their limb reflexively but also exhibit more complex organized behaviours such as paw licking and guarded behaviour of the limb (Hargreaves et al 1988). A paw-withdrawal latency measure and the withdrawal duration (how long the limb remains off the glass plate) can be used to infer pain. This method appears to be particularly useful in assessing nocifensive behaviour following inflammation or partial nerve injury (Bennett & Xie 1988, Hargreaves et al 1988). Figure 14.1 shows the effect of the radiant heat stimulus used in this method on the cutaneous temperature of inflamed and saline-treated rat paws. The inflamed paws have greater initial paw temperatures than the saline-injected paws. In addition, stimulation of the inflamed paws results in shorter paw-withdrawal latencies than stimulation of the saline-treated paws, and this shorter latency corresponds to a lower threshold temperature. Withdrawal latencies using this model parallel more complex organized behaviours such as withdrawal duration and paw licking.

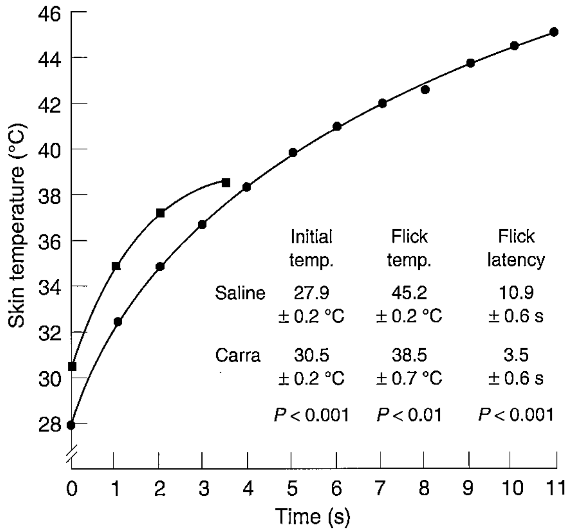

Fig. 14.1 Effect of radiant heat on cutaneous temperature of rat hindpaws after saline administration and after carrageenan (carra)-induced inflammation. Animals are unrestrained in an enclosed plastic chamber and the radiant heat stimulus was positioned under the glass floor directly beneath the hindpaw. The inset shows the mean initial temperature and the mean temperature when the rats withdrew their hindpaws (flick temperature) under both conditions. Mean withdrawal latencies are also shown. (Reproduced from Hargreaves et al 1988.)

Mechanical sensitivity after the induction of inflammation also can be quantified using paw-withdrawal latencies (Ren & Dubner 1993). Rats are placed on a meshed metal surface and a series of von Frey filaments are applied to the ventral or dorsal surface of the hindpaw. Response threshold is defined as the lowest force of two or more consecutive von Frey filaments which produces a response. Figure 14.2 shows that prior to inflammation, the median von Frey thresholds were 8.5 g for both sides. However, with this response measure, it is not clear whether the rat is withdrawing from a noxious or an innocuous stimulus. The response duration, a measure of the total time the rats withdraw and hold their hindpaw away from the mesh surface, can be quantified and used as a measure of nocifensive behaviour. The response duration is defined as the time from the start of a response to the return of the paw to the original position. A 0.2 s duration is considered a quick withdrawal, characteristic of the response to an innocuous stimulus. Figure 14.2 shows that 8.5 g forces produced average response durations that were greater than 0.2 s and likely to represent a nocifensive behaviour.

A model of visceral pain has been developed which utilizes a natural, reproducible stimulus – colorectal distension, in awake, unrestrained rats (Ness & Gebhart 1988, Ness et al 1991). Colorectal distension produces aversive behaviour measured in a passive-avoidance task. Latencies in the task vary monotonically with graded distensions above 30 mmHg (Fig. 14.3). Colorectal distension below 30 mmHg can produce non-nocifensive behaviour, because rats exhibit a visceromotor reflex consisting of contraction of the abdominal and hindlimb musculature in the innocuous and noxious range. This visceral stimulus also produces a vigorous pressor response and tachycardia that grade with increasing intensities of colorectal distension. Modulators of nociception such as morphine and capsaicin affect responses to the stimulus in a fashion consistent with the conclusion that the responses to colorectal distension are due to the noxious nature of the stimulus (Ness et al 1991). Psychophysiological studies indicate that this same stimulus is non-noxious or noxious to human subjects depending on the level of distension. Distensions below 30 mmHg are not noxious in human subjects (Ness et al 1990).

All of the above organized behaviours provide the animal with control of the intensity or duration of the stimulus because the behaviour results in removal of the aversive stimulus. By contrast, there are assessment methods in which the animal does not have control of stimulus intensity or duration. For example, the writhing response is produced in rodents by injecting pain-producing chemical substances intraperitoneally. The acute peritonitis resulting from the

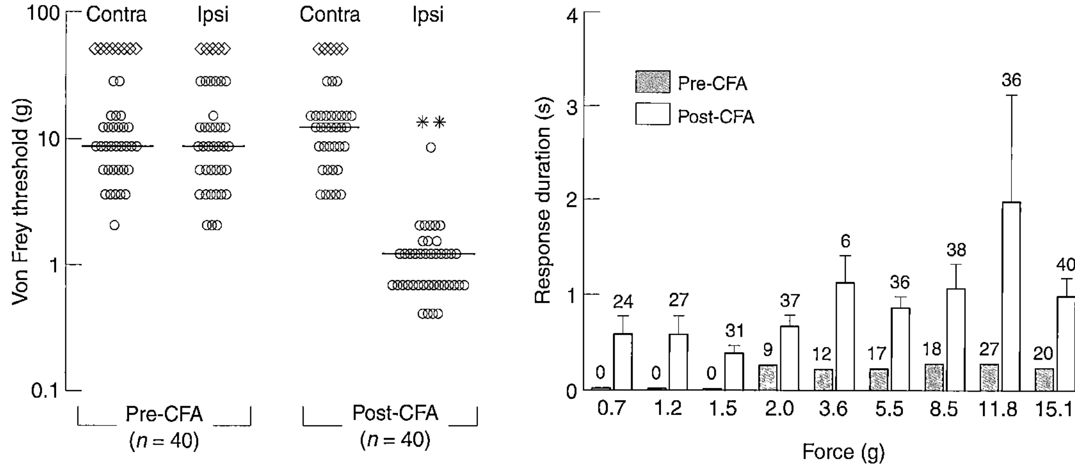

Fig. 14.2 Mechanical hyperalgesia and mechanical allodynia after CFA-induced inflammation. The mechanical thresholds of all animals (n=40) are shown as a scatter plot on the left and the medians are indicated by horizontal bars. There was a marked reduction of the mechanical threshold induced by the CFA. **Significantly different from non-injected contralateral paws, $P < 0.001$ (Mann–Whitney U). The histogram on the right shows the response duration measure of mechanical hyperalgesia and allodynia. Force is expressed in grams of each von Frey filament. The averages and SEM in each histogram are based on the responders only; the number of responders is shown above each bar (total n=40). (Adapted from Ren & Dubner 1993.)

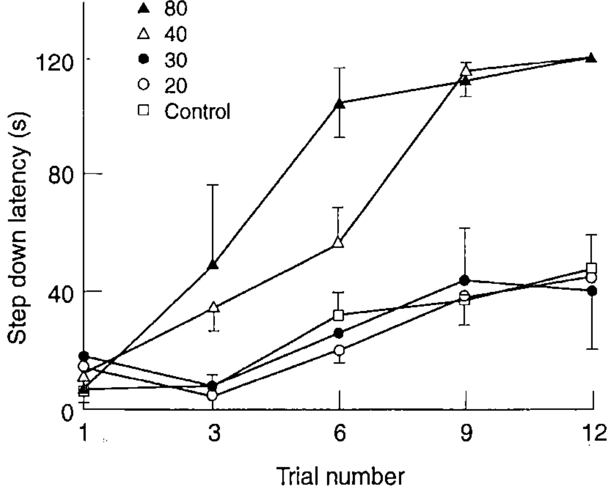

Fig. 14.3 The effect of graded colorectal distension on passive-avoidance behaviour in rats. The latency to step down from a platform was measured. When intraluminal colorectal distension pressures were either 40 or 80 mmHg, rats avoided colorectal distension by remaining on the platform. At pressures of 20 or 30 mmHg, experimental rats did not behave differently from the control rats that received no distension or distension in a different environment. Asterisks indicate significant differences between experimental and control rats at the P <0.05 level. Vertical bars indicate SEM. (Reproduced from Ness et al 1991.)

injection produces a response characterized by internal rotation of one foot, arching of the back, rolling on one side and accompanying abdominal contractions. The writhing response is considered a model of visceral pain (Vyklicky 1979). In addition to the lack of stimulus control offered the animal with this method, the experimenter cannot control the duration of the stimulus. Vocalization is another commonly used, unlearned reaction to painful stimuli (Kayser & Guilbaud 1987). The stimulus intensity necessary to elicit a vocal response from the animal is determined. The stimulus can be applied to any part of the body. The animals cannot control the intensity or duration of the stimulus.

TISSUE INJURY MODELS OF PERSISTENT PAIN

Animal models of tissue injury and inflammation have been developed which produce responses that mimic human clinical pain conditions in which the pain lasts for longer periods of time. In one test, formalin is injected beneath the footpad of a rat or cat (Dubuisson & Dennis 1977, see Abbott et al 1995 for review). The chemical produces complex response patterns that last for approximately 1 hour. The behavioural state of the animal can be graded as the effect wears off; initially the animals elevate the limb and do not place it on the cage floor, but within 15–30 min they begin to use it as a weight-bearing limb. Two phases of nocifensive behaviour are typically described: the first or acute phase lasts for about 5 min and is followed by a more long-lasting persistent phase (about 40 min) that is characterized by shaking or licking of the paw. It is generally agreed that the first phase results at least in part from direct activation of myelinated and unmyelinated fibres, both low-threshold mechanoreceptive and nociceptive types (Puig & Sorkin 1996). There has been disagreement about the underlying mechanisms of the second phase. Early studies suggested that the second phase resulted from central sensitization of dorsal horn neurons, whereas more recently it has been demonstrated that ongoing activity of primary afferents is necessary for the development of the second phase (Taylor et al 1995, Abbadie et al 1997). Many different response measures are used for assessing pain after formalin. These include single parameters such as flinching, shaking or jerking, or complex scores that are derived from several nocifensive behaviours such as licking, guarding, etc. (Clavelou et al 1995). An orofacial formalin test has been developed that uses one measure of nocifensive behaviour, the amount of time spent rubbing the injected upper lip (Clavelou et al 1989, 1995). This method has been shown to be a reliable method for assessing pain in the trigeminal region.

Models of inflammation that produce more persistent pain include the injection of carrageenan or complete Freund's adjuvant into the footpad (Hargreaves et al 1988, Iadarola et al 1988a) or into the joint of the limb (Schaible et al 1987). These models result in more persistent pain that mimics the time course of postoperative pain or other types of persistent injury. In the inflammation model elicited by injection of complete Freund's adjuvant into the footpad, the cutaneous inflammation appears within 2 hours and peaks within 6–8 hours. Hyperalgesia and oedema are present for approximately 1 week to 10 days. The physiological and biochemical effects are limited to the affected limb (Iadarola et al 1988b) and there are no signs of systemic disease. The animal cannot control the pain associated with these inflammation models. Therefore, it is important to determine that the levels of pain are below the tolerance level of the animals. Iadarola et al (1988a) observed that rats with adjuvant or carrageenan-induced inflammation exhibit minimal reductions in weight and show normal grooming behaviour. Exploratory motor behaviour is normal and no significant alterations occur in an open field locomotion test. Thus, the impact of the inflamed limb on the rat's behaviour is minimal and the rats will use the limb for support, if necessary.

The inflammation models are used to infer the presence of hyperalgesia (increased response to a noxious stimulus) or allodynia (a nocifensive behaviour in response to an innocuous stimulus). The literature on these animal models often produces the same confused use of these terms as in the clinical literature. The terms are defined based only on behaviour (Merskey 1979), although many authors attribute mechanisms to them. For example, allodynia is thought to result from either sensitization of peripheral nociceptive afferents or mediated by low-threshold mechanoreceptive afferents after increases in CNS excitability (central sensitization), or both. Hyperalgesia is thought to be due to central sensitization or to sensitization of nociceptive afferents, or both. There is thermal or mechanical allodynia and thermal or mechanical hyperalgesia. Sometimes the term hyperalgesia is used for both hyperalgesia and allodynia. For example, the paw withdrawal to a thermal stimulus after inflammation (Fig. 14.1) is thermal allodynia but it is typically described as thermal hyperalgesia (Hargreaves et al 1988). Nevertheless, a distinction can be made between these two types of behaviours in animals, and the underlying mechanisms can be investigated. Figure 14.2 shows that the injection of complete Freund's adjuvant (CFA) into the rat's paw reduced the von Frey threshold from 8.5 g to 1.2 g. This finding suggests that innocuous stimuli which are ordinarily barely perceptible are now producing paw withdrawal. However, is this hyperaesthesia or allodynia? The use of response duration as a measure (Fig. 14.2) suggests that this is mechanical allodynia. After CFA, rather than rapidly returning their paws to the mesh surface, the rats hold them off the floor for longer durations, sometimes shake them, and sometimes lick them. More intense mechanical stimuli that normally resulted in increases in response duration, now resulted in further increases, suggesting the presence of mechanical hyperalgesia (Fig. 14.2).

A model of neurogenic inflammation similar to one utilized in human subjects is the use of intradermal capsaicin to produce hyperalgesia (LaMotte et al 1991). The intradermal injection of capsaicin produces primary hyperalgesia at the site of injection and a surrounding area of secondary hyperalgesia to light touch. A flare reaction extends into the zone of secondary hyperalgesia. This model has been used in monkeys to study changes in nociceptor activity and changes in the responses of spinal dorsal horn neurons induced by the neurogenic inflammation (LaMotte et al 1991, Simone et al 1991). The model has recently been adapted to studies in the rat (Gilchrist et al 1996).

Other inflammatory agents such as mustard oil and zymosan have been used to produce behavioural and physiological changes. The effects of mustard oil are relatively short (a few minutes) when applied topically to cutaneous tissues (Ma & Woolf 1996a, Neuman et al 1996). The agent can also be injected subcutaneously or into muscle where the changes last up to 20 min (Yu et al 1994). Zymosan has been used for studies of visceral pain and results in persistent hyperalgesia (Coutinho et al 1996).

These behavioural models of hyperalgesia and allodynia have been useful in the study of peripheral and central mechanisms of hyperalgesia and allodynia. They have been correlated with neural events in primary afferent neurons and CNS neurons, particularly at the level of the medullary and spinal dorsal horns. Although correlative electrophysiological and behavioural studies have been informative (LaMotte et al 1991, Simone et al 1991, Woolf & Thompson 1991, Ren et al 1992, Ren & Dubner 1993, Yu et al 1993), only a few neurons can be studied. Recently, *Fos*, the protein product of the c-*fos* immediate early gene, has been used as a measure of neuronal activity (Hunt et al 1987, Bullitt 1990). *Fos* protein is induced by neuronal activity and appears to play a role in long-term changes in the CNS following neural activity (Goelet et al 1986). Fos expression increases in many nociceptive neurons in the dorsal horn after inflammation and these changes can be localized to specific populations of neurons using immunocytochemical methods. The findings can be correlated with behavioural hyperalgesia and allodynia after the injection of inflammatory agents such as CFA, carrageenan, mustard oil or formalin (Draisci & Iadarola 1989, Menetrey et al 1989, Presley et al 1990, Gogas et al 1991, Ma & Woolf 1996b, Ren & Ruda 1996, Wei et al 1998, 1999).

Other methods have been developed which attempt to mimic human conditions of persistent or chronic pain. Included are models of polyarthritis in which CFA is injected into the rat's tail (De Castro Costa et al 1981). The CFA results in a delayed hypersensitivity reaction, with inflammation and hyperalgesia of multiple joints occurring after 10 days to 3 weeks. Pain is inferred from scratching behaviours, reduced motor activity by the animal, weight loss, vocalization when the affected limbs are pinched, and a reduction in these behaviours following the administration of opioids. It should be noted that this is a systemic disease of the animal which includes skin lesions, destruction of bone and cartilage, impairment of liver function and a lymphadenopathy (Coderre & Wall 1987). These systemic lesions make it more difficult to associate the animal's behaviour with pain as opposed to generalized malaise and debilitation. The likely presence of central nervous system changes associated with the alterations in immune function also question the use of this model to correlate neural activity and neurochemical alterations with behaviour presumably related to pain. Other models of arthritis have been developed in which sodium urate crystals are injected into the ankle joint of rat or cat (Okuda et al 1984, Coderre & Wall 1987). The arthritis is fully developed within 24 hours. These animals reduce the weight placed on the treated hindlimb and exhibit guarded movement of the limb. In the rat, touch, pressure and thermal stimuli applied to the affected paw result in a decrease in responsiveness, presumably due to the pain associated with the movement. There are no signs of systemic disease in the urate arthritis model other than joint pathology secondary to tissue oedema and the infiltration of polymorphonuclear leucocytes (Coderre & Wall 1987). Acute arthritis can also be induced by the injection of carrageenan and kaolin into the cat or monkey knee joint just below the patella (Schaible et al 1987, Dougherty et al 1992). Changes in joint receptor and spinal dorsal horn neuronal activity begin as soon as 1–2 h following injection and build up for several hours. Behaviour studies related to this model have not been performed.

The success of many of the above models has resulted in a plethora of new inflammation models in recent years. Some examples follow. A surgical incision of the rat paw causes a reliable and quantifiable mechanical hyperalgesia (allodynia?) which can last for several days after the surgery (Brennan et al 1996). This model was developed to provide a better understanding of sensitization caused by surgery and to investigate new therapies. Bone lesions in rats produced by drilling a hole through the tibia result in secondary mechanical hyperalgesia and allodynia, and cold allodynia (Houghton et al 1997). Nocifensive behaviour is characterized by a lifting and guarding of the damaged limb. The model was developed to study mechanisms underlying bone pain. An animal model of pain has been produced by systemic administration of an immunotherapeutic antiganglioside antibody (Slart et al 1997). The antibody in rat produces mechanical allodynia and provides a model for studying the pharmacology of this allodynia which occurs in children exposed to the antibody in the treatment of neuroblastomas.

NERVE INJURY MODELS OF PERSISTENT PAIN

Approximately 2 weeks after complete sectioning of the sciatic nerve in the rat with encapsulation, the rats engage in self-mutilation of the denervated area. This begins with chewing of the toe nails and is followed by a progressive degree of amputation of the digits and the foot (Wall et al 1979). The validity of this model as a suitable model of chronic pain has been debated (Rodin & Kruger 1984, Coderre et al 1986) and redebated (Devor 1992, Kruger 1992). The critical issue is whether the self-mutilation is a response to abnormal sensations attributable to the deafferented limb, or simply a response to an insensate appendage which the animal considers a foreign body and is trying to remove. Blumenkopf and Lipman (1991) have recently provided evidence that chronic nerve block with lidocaine does not result in self-mutilation of the limb, suggesting that rats do not self-mutilate an insensate limb.

Recently developed models indicate that partial nerve injury in the rat results in signs of hyperalgesia and spontaneous pain. In one model, loose ligatures are placed around the sciatic nerve with resultant demyelination of the large fibres and destruction of some unmyelinated axons (Bennett & Xie 1988). In another model, ligation and severing of the dorsal half to one-third of the sciatic nerve produces similar behavioural changes (Seltzer et al 1990). Kim and Chung (1992) have developed a third model in which the L5 and L6 spinal nerves are tightly ligated on one side of the rat. This procedure largely reduced the variability of the extent of nerve injury because the spinal nerves are completely severed, although the surgery involved is more extensive compared with the previous two models. All three models mimic clinical conditions of painful neuropathy with evidence of persistent spontaneous pain, allodynia, hyperalgesia (Fig. 14.4) and sympathetic involvement (Kim & Chung 1991, Shir & Seltzer 1991, Desmeules et al 1995, Chung et al 1996, Ramer et al 1997). The abnormal pain sensations also appear on the uninjured side (Seltzer et al 1990, Kim & Chung 1992) and spread beyond the injured nerve territory on the ipsilateral side (Tal & Bennett 1994). It should be appreciated that although the general consequences of these nerve injury models are similar, there may be differences in underlying mechanisms. For example, the extent and modality of sympathetic involvement in these nerve injury models may be quite different (Bennett 1991, Neil et al 1991). These nerve injury models of neuropathic pain have been adapted to mice recently (Malmberg et al 1997, Ramer et al 1997), where they can be used to study pain mechanisms in transgenic animals. Patients with diabetic neuropathy often suffer from spontaneous pain and allodynia (Pfiefer et al 1993). Signs of nerve injury in diabetic rats have been reported earlier (Birchiel et al 1985). Streptozocin-induced diabetic rats provide a model that mimics chronic pain seen in diabetic neuropathy (Courteix et al 1993).

Several models of spinal injury may be used to study the mechanisms underlying central pain. Spinal injury can be induced by localized laser radiation (Hao et al 1991), weight drop (Siddall et al 1995), hemisection of the spinal cord (Christensen et al 1996) and intraspinal injection of the excitotoxic amino acid receptor agonist quisqualic acid (Yezierski et al 1998). All these manipulations produce persistent allodynia. They are particularly useful for examining CNS changes responsible for pain behaviours and the role of excitatory amino acids and neuropeptides in these effects.

All of the above nerve injury models which attempt to mimic human conditions of chronic or persistent pain produce pain that the animal cannot control. Therefore, it is important that investigators assess the level of pain in these animals and provide analgesic agents when it does not interfere with the purpose of the experiment. Pain in these studies can be inferred from on-going behavioural variables such as feeding and drinking, sleep–waking cycle, grooming and social behaviour (Sternbach 1976). Significant deviation from normal behaviour suggests that the animal is in

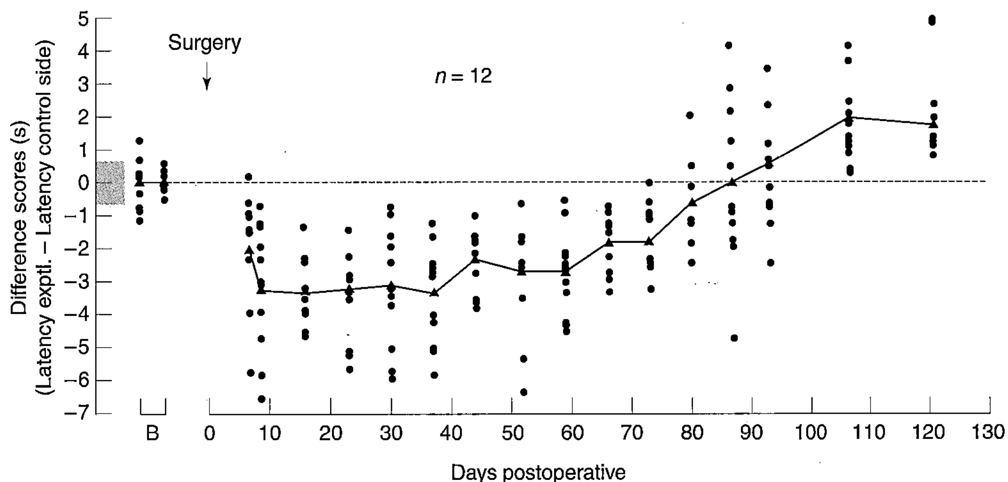

Fig. 14.4 Time course of thermal hyperalgesia produced by tying loose ligatures around the sciatic nerve of the rat. Hyperalgesia was measured using the noxious heat-evoked paw withdrawal method described in Figure 14.1. Negative difference scores indicate a lowered nociceptive threshold on the side of the sciatic nerve ligation. Filled circles indicate difference scores of individual rats and the filled triangles and solid line show the group mean difference scores. (Reproduced from Bennett & Xie 1988.)

severe and possibly intolerable pain. Additional attention should be given to those animals that may suffer from severe secondary injury. For example, autotomy behaviour has been observed in some neuropathic pain models (Bennett & Xie 1988, Xu et al 1992, DeLeo et al 1994).

ORGANIZED LEARNED BEHAVIOURS

Learned or operant responses are a separate category of behaviours from which pain has been inferred in animals. The most common and simplest method involves an animal escaping from a noxious stimulus by initiating a learned behaviour such as crossing a barrier or pressing a bar. For example, electric shock can be delivered to a grid floor in a cage and the animal can be trained to jump over a barrier partition to escape the stimulus. The latency of escape is usually measured. Another operant procedure used with electrical stimulation is the shock titration method (Weiss & Laties 1963). The animals press a bar to reduce the intensity of a continuously increasing stimulus. The animals tend to titrate the stimulus intensity at or near the noxious level. However, this method tends to assess avoidance rather than escape behaviour and it is extremely difficult to determine whether the animals are titrating the stimulus in the noxious range or below it.

Other more complex methods include reaction time experiments in which the animal detects or discriminates a noxious stimulus. In conflict paradigms (Vierck et al 1971, Dubner et al 1976), animals learn to perform a task to receive a reward, but also are exposed to noxious stimulation during the task. The animals must choose between receiving a reward or escaping the aversive stimulus on each trial. This method produces escape rather than avoidance behaviour in the animals. Reaction time tasks have been developed in which monkeys are trained to detect stimuli in the noxious heat range (Dubner 1985). This task can be designed so that the detection involves stimuli only in the noxious heat range and no cues are provided by preceding innocuous warming stimuli. Another advantage of this behavioural task is that it can be used in conjunction with the detection of innocuous stimuli. A comparison of the effects of drug manipulations on innocuous versus noxious stimuli rules out the possibility that the drug is altering attentional, motivational or motoric aspects of the animal's behaviour instead of influencing the perceived intensity of the noxious stimuli (Oliveras et al 1986). Monkeys are capable of detecting 0.10–0.20°C increases in temperature in the noxious range and wide dynamic range neurons in the medullary dorsal horn participate in the encoding process by which the monkeys perceive these sensations (Maixner et al 1986). It should be noted that operant tasks have not been developed to study mechanisms of persistent pain produced by tissue or nerve injury. There is a need for such models to study neural mechanisms of persistent pain utilizing electrophysiological approaches as well as new imaging methods.

As with unlearned behaviours related to pain, all of the above operant procedures provide only indirect measures of pain such as the latency or the probability of a motor response. However, they have the advantage over simpler, unlearned behaviours in that the magnitude of the behavioural change varies with stimulus intensity, providing more reliable evidence that the change in behaviour reflects the perception of a noxious stimulus rather than a change in motor performance. Sophisticated operant tasks in animals also allow the experimenter to rule out that changes in performance are related to attentional and motivational variables rather than changes in sensory perception. It also should be recalled that these operant procedures give the animal control over the stimulus and other parameters of the experiment to a degree comparable to that found in human studies of experimental pain.

REFERENCES

Abbadie C, Taylor KT, Peterson MA, Basbaum AI 1997 Differential contribution of the two phases of the formalin test to the pattern of c-*fos* expression in the rat spinal cord: studies with remifentanil and lidocaine. Pain 69: 101–110

Abbott FV, Franklin KBJ, Westbrook RF 1995 The formalin test: scoring properties of the first and second phases of the pain response in rats. Pain 60: 91–102

Bennett GJ 1991 The role of the sympathetic nervous system in painful peripheral neuropathy. Pain 45: 221–223

Bennett GJ, Xie Y 1988 A peripheral mono-neuropathy in rat that produces disorders of pain sensation like those seen in man. Pain 33: 87–107

Birchiel KJ, Russell LC, Lee RP, Sima AAF 1985 Spontaneous activity of primary afferent neurons in diabetic BB/wistar rats. Diabetes 34: 1210–1213

Blumenkopf B, Upman JJ 1991 Studies in autotomy: its pathophysiology and usefulness as a model of chronic pain. Pain 45: 203–209

Bonnett KA, Peterson KE 1975 A modification of the jump-flinch technique for measuring pain sensitivity in rats. Pharmacology, Biochemistry and Behaviour 3: 1–47

Bowd AD 1980 Ethics and animal experimentation. Amer Psychologist 35: 224–225

Brennan TJ, Vandermeulen EP, Gebhart GF 1996 Characterization of a rat model of incisional pain. Pain 64: 493–501

Bullitt E 1990 Expression of c-*fos*-like protein as a marker for neuronal activity following noxious stimulation in the rat. Journal of Comparative Neurology 296: 517–530

Chapman CR, Casey KL, Dubner R, Foley KM, Gracely RH, Reading AE 1985 Pain measurement: an overview. Pain 22: 1–31

Christensen MD, Everhart AW, Pickelman JT, Hulsebosch CE 1996 Mechanical and thermal allodynia in chronic central pain following spinal cord injury. Pain 68: 97–107

Chung KS, Lee BH, Yoon YW, Chung JM 1996 Sympathetic sprouting in the dorsal root ganglia of the injured peripheral nerve in a rat neuropathic pain model. Journal of Comparative Neurology 376: 241–252

Clavelou P, Dallel R, Orliaguet T, Woda A, Raboisson P 1995 The orofacial formalin test in rats: effects of different formalin concentrations. Pain 62: 295–301

Clavelou P, Pajot J, Dallel R, Raboisson P 1989 Application of the formalin test to the study of orofacial pain in the rat. Neuroscience Letters 103: 349–353

Coderre TJ, Grimes RW, Melzack R 1986 Deafferentation and chronic pain in animals: an evaluation of evidence suggesting autotomy is related to pain. Pain 26: 61–84

Coderre TJ, Wall PD 1987 Ankle joint urate arthritis (AJUA) in rats: an alternative animal model of arthritis to that produced by Freund's adjuvant. Pain 28: 379–393

Courteix C, Eschalier A, Lavarenne J 1993 Streptozocin-induced diabetic rats: behavioral evidence for a model of chronic pain. Pain 53: 81–88

Coutinho SV, Meller ST, Gebhart GF 1996 Intracolonic zymosan produces visceral hyperalgesia in the rat that is mediated by spinal NMDA and nonNMDA receptors. Brain Research 736: 7–15

D'Amour FE, Smith D 1941 A method for determining loss of pain sensation. Journal of Pharmacology and Experimental Therapeutics 72: 74–79

De Castro Costa M, De Sutter P, Gybels J, Van Hees J 1981 Adjuvant-induced arthritis in rats: a possible animal model of chronic pain. Pain 10: 173–186

DeLeo JA, Coombs DW, Willenbring S et al 1994 Characterization of a neuropathic pain model: sciatic cryoneurolysis in the rat. Pain 56: 9–16

Desmeules JA, Kayser V, Weil-Fuggaza J, Bertrand A, Guilbaud G 1995 Influence of the sympathetic nervous system in the development of abnormal pain-related behaviours in a rat model of neuropathic pain. Neuroscience 67: 941–951

Devor M 1992 Autotomy sense and nonsense. Reply to L. Kruger. Pain 49: 156

Dougherty PM, Sluka KA, Sorkin LS, Westlund KN, Willis WD 1992 Neural changes in acute arthritis in monkeys. 1. Parallel enhancement of responses of spinothalamic tract neurons to mechanical stimulation and excitatory amino acids. Brain Research Review 17: 1–13

Draisci G, Iadarola MJ 1989 Temporal analysis of increases in c-*fos*, preprodynorphin and preproenkephalin mRNAs in rat spinal cord. Molecular Brain Research 6: 31–37

Dubner R 1983 Pain research in animals. Annals of the New York Academy of Sciences 406: 128–132

Dubner R 1985 Specialization in nociceptive pathways: sensory discrimination, sensory modulation, and neural connectivity. In: Fields HL, Dubner R, Cervero F (eds) Advances in pain research and therapy, vol 9. Raven, New York, pp 111–137

Dubner R, Bennett GJ 1983 Spinal and trigeminal mechanisms of nociception. Annual Review of Neuroscience 6: 381–418

Dubner R, Beitel RE, Brown FJ 1976 A behavioral animal model for the study of pain mechanisms in primates. In: Weisenberg M, Tursky B (eds) Pain: new perspectives in therapy and research. Plenum, New York, pp 155–170

Dubuisson D, Dennis SG 1977 The formalin test: a quantitative study of the analgesic effects of morphine, meperidine, and brain-stem stimulation in rats and cats. Pain 4: 161–174

Fields H, Bry J, Hentall L, Zorman G 1983 The activity of neurons in the rostral medulla of the rat during withdrawal from noxious heat. Journal of Neuroscience 3: 545–552

Gilchrist HD, Allard BL, Simone DA 1996 Enhanced withdrawal responses to heat and mechanical stimuli following intraplantar injection of capsaicin in rats. Pain 67: 179–188

Goelet P, Castellucci VF, Schacher S, Kandel ER 1986 The long and short of long-term memory – a molecular framework. Nature 322: 419–422

Gogas KR, Presley RW, Levine JD, Basbaum AI 1991 The antinociceptive action of supraspinal opioids results from an increase in descending inhibitory control: correlation of nociceptive behavior and c-*fos* expression. Neuroscience 42: 617–628

Grumbach L 1966 The prediction of analgesic activity in man by animal testing. In: Knighton RS, Dumke PR (eds) Pain. Little Brown & Co, Boston, pp 163–182

Hao J-X, Xu X-J, Aldskogius H, Seiger A, Wesenfeld-Hallin Z 1991 Allodynia-like effects in rat after ischaemic spinal cord injury photochemically induced by laser irradiation. Pain 45: 175–186

Hargreaves K, Dubner R, Brown F, Flores C, Joris J 1988 A new and sensitive method for measuring thermal nociception in cutaneous hyperalgesia. Pain 32: 77–88

Houghton AK, Hewitt E, Westlund KN 1997 Enhanced withdrawal responses to mechanical and thermal stimuli after bone injury. Pain 73: 325–337

Hunt SP, Pini A, Even G 1987 Induction of c-*fos*-like protein in spinal cord neurons following sensory stimulation. Nature 328: 632–634

Iadarola MJ, Brady LS, Draisci G, Dubner R 1988a Enhancement of dynorphin gene expression in spinal cord following experimental inflammation: stimulus specificity, behavioral parameters and opioid receptor binding. Pain 45: 313–326

Iadarola MJ, Douglass J, Civelli O, Naranjo JR 1988b Differential activation of spinal cord dynorphin and enkephalin neurons during hyperalgesia: evidence using cDNA hybridization. Brain Research 455: 202–212

Imamura Y, Kawamoto H, Nakanishi O 1997 Characterization of heat-hyperalgesia in an experimental trigeminal neuropathy in rats. Experimental Brain Research 116: 97–103

Kayser V, Guilbaud G 1987 Local and remote modifications of nociceptive sensitivity during carrageenin-induced inflammation in the rat. Pain 28: 99–107

Kim SH, Chung JM 1991 Sympathectomy alleviates mechanical allodynia in an experimental animal model for neuropathy in the rat. Neuroscience Letters 134: 131–134

Kim SH, Chung JM 1992 An experimental model for peripheral neuropathy produced by segmental spinal nerve ligation in the rat. Pain 50: 355–363

Kruger L 1992 The non-sensory basis of autotomy in rats: a reply to the editorial by Devor and the article by Blumenkopf and Lipman. Pain 49: 153–155

LaMotte RH, Shain CN, Simone DA, Tsai E-F P 1991 Neurogenic hyperalgesia: psychophysical studies of underlying mechanisms. Journal of Neurophysiology 66: 190–211

Ma Q-P, Woolf CG 1996a Progressive tactile hypersensitivity: an inflammation-induced incremental increase in the excitability of the spinal cord, Pain 67: 97–106

Ma Q-P, Woolf CJ 1996b Basal and touch-evoked *fos*-like immunoreactivity during experimental inflammation in the rat. Pain 67: 307–316

McGrath PA, Sharav Y, Dubner R, Gracely RH 1981 Masseter inhibitory periods and sensations evoked by electrical tooth pulp stimulation. Pain 10: 1–17

Maixner W, Dubner R, Bushnell MC, Kenshalo DR Jr, Oliveras J-L 1986 Wide dynamic-range dorsal horn neurons participate in the encoding process by which monkeys perceive the intensity of noxious heat stimuli. Brain Research 374: 385–388

Malmberg AB, Chen C, Tonegawa S, Basbaum AI 1997 Preserved acute pain and reduced neuropathic pain in mice lacking PKCg. Science 278: 279–283

Menetrey D, Gannon A, Levine JD, Basbaum AI 1989 Expression of c-*fos* protein in interneurons and projection neurons of the rat spinal cord in response to noxious somatic, articular, and visceral stimulation. Journal of Comparative Neurology 285: 177–195

Merskey H (Chairman) 1979 Pain terms: a list with definitions and notes on usage. Pain 6: 249–252

Millan MJ, Czlonkowski A, Morris B et al 1988 Inflammation of the hind limb as a model of unilateral, localized pain: influence on multiple opioid systems in the spinal cord of the rat. Pain 35: 299–312

Mitchell CL 1964 A comparison of drug effects upon the jaw jerk response to electrical stimulation of the tooth pulp in dogs and cats. Journal of Pharmacology and Experimental Therapeutics 146: 1–6

Neil A, Attal N, Guilbaud G 1991 Effects of guanethidine on sensitization to natural stimuli and self-mutilating behaviour in rats with a peripheral neuropathy. Brain Research 565: 237–246

Ness TJ, Gebhart GF 1988 Colorectal distension as a noxious visceral stimulus: physiologic and pharmacologic characterization of pseudaffective reflexes in the rat. Brain Research 450: 153–169

Ness TJ, Metcalf AM, Gebhart GF 1990 A psychophysiological study in humans using phasic colonic distension as a noxious visceral stimulus. Pain 43: 377–386

Ness TJ, Randich A, Gebhart GF 1991 Further behavioral evidence that colorectal distension is a 'noxious' visceral stimulus in rats. Neuroscience Letters 131: 113–116

Neumann S, Doubell TP, Leslie T, Woolf CJ 1996 Inflammatory pain hypersensitivity mediated by phenotypic switch in myelinated primary sensory neurons. Nature 384: 360–364

Okuda K, Nakahama H, Miyakawa H, Shima K 1984 Arthritis induced in cats by sodium urate: a possible animal model for chronic pain. Pain 18: 287–297

Oliveras J-L, Maixner W, Dubner R et al 1986 The medullary dorsal horn: a target for the expression of opiate effects on the perceived intensity of noxious heat. Journal of Neuroscience 6: 3086–3093

Pfiefer MA, Ross DR, Schrager JP et al 1993 A highly successful and novel model for treatment of chronic painful diabetic peripheral neuropathy. Diabetes Care 16: 1103–1115

Presley RW, Menétrey D, Levine JD, Basbaum AI 1990 Systemic morphine suppresses noxious stimulus-evoked *Fos* protein-like immunoreactivity in the rat spinal cord. Journal of Neuroscience 10: 323–335

Puig S, Sorkin LS 1996 Formalin-evoked activity in identified primary afferent fibers: systemic lidocaine suppresses phase-2 activity. Pain 64: 345–355

Qui C, Sora I, Ren K, Uhl G, Dubner R 1998 Opioid receptor plasticity in mu opioid receptor knockout (MOR KO) mice following persistent inflammation. Society for Neuroscience Abstracts 24: 892

Ramer MS, French GD, Bisby MA 1997 Wallerian degeneration is required for both neuropathic pain and sympathetic spouting into the DRG. Pain 72: 71–78

Ren K, Dubner R 1993 NMDA receptor antagonists attenuate mechanical hyperalgesia in rats with unilateral inflammation of the hindpaw. Neuroscience Letters 163: 22–26

Ren K, Dubner R 1996 An inflammation/hyperalgesia model for the study of orofacial pain. Journal of Dental Research 75: 217

Ren K, Hylden JLK, Williams GM, Ruda MA, Dubner R 1992 The effects of an NMDA receptor antagonists, MK-801, on behavioral hyperalgesia and dorsal horn neuronal activity in rats with adjuvant-induced inflammation. Pain 50: 331–344

Ren R, Ruda MA 1996 Descending modulation of Fos expression after persistent peripheral inflammation. Neuroreport 7: 2186–2190.

Rodin BE, Kruger L 1984 Deafferentation in animals as a model for the study of pain: an alternative hypothesis. Brain Research Review 7: 213–228

Sandkuhler J, Gebhart GF 1984 Characterization of inhibition of a spinal nociceptive reflex by stimulation medially and laterally in the midbrain and medulla in the pentobarbital-anesthetized rat. Brain Research 305: 67–76

Schaible H-G, Schmidt RF, Willis WD 1987 Enhancement of the responses of ascending tract cells in the cat spinal cord by acute inflammation of the knee joint. Experimental Brain Research 66: 489–499

Seltzer Z, Dubner R, Shir Y 1990 A novel behavioral model of neuropathic pain disorders produced in rats by partial sciatic nerve injury. Pain 43: 205–218

Shir Y, Seltzer Z 1991 Effects of sympathectomy in a model of causalgiform pain produced by partial sciatic nerve injury in rats. Pain 43: 309–320

Siddall P, Xu CL, Cousins M 1995 Allodynia following traumatic spinal cord injury in the rat. Neuroreport 6: 1241–1244

Simone DA, Sorkin LS, Oh U et al 1991 Neurogenic hyperalgesia: central neural correlates in responses of spinothalamic tract neurons. Journal of Neurophysiology 66: 228–246

Slart R, Yu AL, Yaksh TL, Sorkin LS 1997 An animal model of pain produced by systemic administration of an immunotherapeutic anti-ganglioside antibody. Pain 69: 119–125

Sternbach RA 1976 The need for an animal model of chronic pain. Pain 2: 2–4

Tal M, Bennett GJ 1994 Extra-territorial pain in rats with a peripheral mononeuropathy: mechano-hyperalgesia and mechanoallodynia in the territory of an uninjured nerve. Pain 57: 375–382

Taylor BK, Peterson MA, Basbaum AI 1995 Persistent chemical nociception in the rat requires ongoing peripheral nerve input. Journal of Neuroscience 15: 7575–7584

Vierck CJ Jr, Hamilton DM, Thomby J 1 1971 Pain reactivity of monkeys after lesions to the dorsal and lateral columns of the spinal cord. Experimental Brain Research 13: 140–158

Vyklicky L 1979 Techniques for the study of pain in animals. In: Bonica JJ, Liebeskind JC, Albe-Fessard DG (eds) Advances in pain research and therapy, vol 3. Raven, New York, pp 727–745

Wall PD, Devor M, Inbal R et al 1979 Autotomy following peripheral nerve lesions: experimental anesthesia dolorosa. Pain 7: 103–113

Wei F, Ren K, Dubner R 1998 Inflammation-induced *Fos* protein expression in the rat spinal cord is enhanced following dorsolateral or ventrolateral funiculus lesions. Brain Research 782: 136–141

Wei F, Dubner R, Ren K 1999 Nucleus reticularis gigantocellularis and nucleus raphe magnus in the brain stem exert opposite effects on behavioral hyperalgesia and spinal *Fos* protein expression after peripheral inflammation. Pain 80: 127–141

Weiss B, Laties VG 1963 Characteristics of aversive thresholds measured by a titration schedule. Journal of the Experimental Analysis of Behaviour 6: 563–572

Willer JC, Boureau F, Albe-Fessard D 1979 Supraspinal influences on nociceptive flexion reflex and pain sensation in man. Brain Research 179: 61–68

Woolf CJ, Thompson SW 1991 The induction and maintenance of central sensitization is dependent on *N*-methyl-D-aspartic acid receptor activation; implications for the treatment of post-injury pain hypersensitivity states. Pain 44: 293–299

Yu X-M, Sessle BJ, Hu JW 1993 Differential effects of cutaneous and deep application of inflammatory irritant on mechanoreceptive field properties of trigeminal brain stem nociceptive neurons. Journal of Neurophysiology 70: 1704–1707

Yu X-M, Sessle BJ, Vernon H, Hu JW 1994 Administration of opiate antagonist naloxone induces recurrence of increased jaw muscle activities related to inflammatory irritant application to rat temporomandibular joint region. Journal of Neurophysiology 72: 1430–1433

Xu X-J, Hao J-X, Aldskogius H, Seiger Å, Wiesenfeld-Hallin Z 1992 Chronic pain-related syndrome in rats after ischemic spinal cord lesion: a possible animal model for pain in patients with spinal cord injury. Pain 48: 279–290

Yezierski RP, Liu S, Ruenes GL, Kajander KJ, Brewer KL 1998 Excitotoxic spinal cord injury: behavioral and morphological characteristics of a central pain model. Pain 75: 141–155

Measurement and assessment of paediatric pain

15

PATRICK J. McGRATH & ANITA M. UNRUH

SUMMARY

Appropriate management of pain in children depends on valid and reliable assessment and measurement. There have been significant improvements in pain measurement in the past decade and there are now adequate measures of short, sharp pain for all children and excellent measures of pain for children who can self report. At this time there are promising measures of longer term pain for children who cannot self report. Much remains to be done to ensure that pain is measured routinely. This chapter proposes the adoption of the WHO model of the consequences of disease for the assessment of pain. The way such a model could facilitate pain assessment is examined and existing measures in terms of the model have been recast. The review of the existing measures of pain has highlighted the significant advances that have been made in the area and has pinpointed the deficiencies that exist. Although much research remains to be done, measures are sufficiently developed and validated to call for the routine measurement of pain in all clinical situations where pain in likely to occur. Such measurement of pain is likely to improve the comfort and pain management of our young patients.

INTRODUCTION

There have been major advances in the measurement of pain in children in recent years and, generally, appropriate research attention is being paid to the reliability and validity of paediatric pain measures. However, these measures are not yet used widely enough in clinical situations.

Pain is a subjective, private event that can be measured only indirectly by one of three strategies: what children report about their experience (self-report measures), the way children react in response to pain (behavioural measures), and how children's bodies respond to pain (biological measures). Unfortunately, neonates, preverbal children and handicapped children cannot describe their experiences and thus behavioural and biological measures must be used.

Even with verbal children, measurement by self-report may be hampered by several factors. Young children have relatively limited cognitive ability to understand what is being asked of them in pain measurement, and they may have difficulty in articulating descriptions of their pain. Furthermore, our limited understanding of the developmental psychology of pain in children may prevent us from asking questions in a developmentally appropriate fashion. Finally, the preconceptions many professionals and lay persons hold about children's pain may preclude children being asked about their pain.

Behavioural and biological reactions to pain may also be considerably influenced by the age and health of the child. As young children develop, their behavioural responses to pain change. Neonates, in particular, may have substantially different biological responses than older children. In addition, seriously ill neonates and children may have substantially different behavioural and biological responses than healthy individuals of the same age.

ASSESSMENT AND MEASUREMENT

The distinction between assessment and measurement in pain research has not always been clearly drawn. Measurement refers to the application of some metric to a specific aspect, usually intensity, of pain. Measurement is like using a ruler or scale to determine the height or weight of something whereas assessment is deciding whether it is height, weight, volume, density or tensile strength that is important to measure. Assessment is a much broader endeavour which should encompass the measurement of the interplay of different factors on the total experience of pain.

While measurement of pain in children has become increasingly sophisticated, assessment has lagged behind. At least four groups have developed standardized paediatric pain assessment packages (Varni et al 1987, Savedra & Tesler 1989, Abu-Saad 1990, McGrath 1990) that are modelled on the McGill Pain Questionnaire (MPQ) (Melzack 1975). Each package measures location and intensity of pain and some factors that may be related to the pain.

The lack of a theoretical model to address the assessment of pain has left the clinician with no guide for clinical thinking and decision-making. Pain problems are more than just the physiological transmission of nociceptive impulses (even when modulated by psychological inputs). They are complex social-physiological-behavioural puzzles that require assessment on different levels. As a result, models of pain transmission alone cannot sufficiently guide the clinician in assessment and management.

THE WHO MODEL OF PAIN ASSESSMENT

The World Health Organization's (WHO) International Classification of Impairments, Disabilities and Handicaps (World Health Organization 1980) provides a model of the consequences of disease conceptualized as occurring in four planes or levels. The first plane is that of the occurrence of an abnormality (disease). The second plane (impairment) occurs when the affected individual becomes aware of the abnormality or develops a symptoms. The third plane, disability, occurs when there is a restriction or lack of ability to perform an activity in the normal way. The fourth plane, handicap, occurs when the individual's experience is socialized. Handicaps are concerned with the social disadvantages experienced by the individual as a result of impairments and disabilities. Table 15.1 illustrates the relationship between these four planes with three fictitious children who suffer from migraine.

Extensive impairment may or may not result in disability. Similarly, disability may not cause a handicap. In addition, impairment may directly result in handicap with little or no intervening disability. The causal chain may be parallel or reversed. In the parallel case, disability in one area may thwart development of new abilities or mask their expression. In the reverse situation, the effect may be from handicap to disability or impairment. That is, a handicap may cause impairment or disability. For example, a child who becomes socially isolated and bedridden (handicap) because of reflex sympathetic dystrophy may exacerbate the underlying problem by increasing muscle atrophy and bone demineralization.

When applying the model to pain (McGrath et al 1991), disease refers to the cause of the pain, such as sickle cell disease. Impairment refers to the pain itself. The WHO classification system uses pain as one example of an impairment and the detail is probably insufficient for everyday use with clinical pain problems. However, it does serve as a useful model for thinking about pain.

DISCORDANCE IN PAIN ASSESSMENT

Concordance and discordance in pain measures and assessments can occur both within and between planes or levels. Few problems are caused by concordance, so attention will be focused on discordance. Usually a discordance in which a child functions beyond the level that is expected is not only accepted, but may be seen as admirable, and the child's behaviour may be reinforced. Such discordance can be a problem, however, if a child's lack of disability or handicap and subsequent activity exacerbate damage from the disease.

Generally, the most problematical discordance occurs when the child has more disability or handicap than expected on the basis of his or her underlying disease or disorder. A common reaction to this discordance is the 'leap to the head' (Wall 1989), in which malingering or psychogenicity is assumed.

Discordance within levels may occur across behaviours, settings or time. Discordance between the child's self report

Table 15.1 The World Health Organization model of the consequences of disease as applied to migraine

	Joanna	*Bill*	*Mary*
Disease/disorder	Migraine	Migraine	Migraine
Impairment	Weekly headache	Weekly headache, nausea	Weekly headache, photophobia
Disability	Inability to concentrate	Can't play hockey	No disability
Handicap	School absence	No handicap	Social isolation

of pain and observers' evaluations of the child's pain based on his or her behaviour are not unusual. For example, children who report moderate levels of pain when asked, may be observed to be playing and seem to be unaffected. This can best be seen as a normal way for a child to cope with pain.

Discordance between levels can also be confusing to the clinician and researcher. For example, a parent or health professional may expect a low level of pain based on the amount of tissue damage suffered from an injection, but the child may exhibit and report severe pain. Conversely, a child may exhibit very little pain behaviour at the same time as reporting high levels of pain in a situation where one might expect severe pain (e.g., postoperatively; Beyer et al 1990). A clinician faced with conflicting information about the amount of pain a child is suffering may have difficulty deciding on a course of action. Should a clinician administer an analgesic when a child is not reporting pain but is behaving in a way that seems to indicate pain? Similarly, should an analgesic be given when pain report is high but pain behaviour cannot be observed? It is not unusual for clinicians to view discordance with alarm or as evidence of malingering or psychogenicity. This is unwarranted but discordant findings indicate the need for further assessment.

PSYCHOMETRICS OF PAIN MEASUREMENT

The essence of pain measurement is to assign a value to pain. The simplest level of measurement is nominal or, in the case of pain, dichotomous (Johnston 1998), that is ascertaining the presence or absence of pain. This level of measurement can be useful in screening or triage situations. The second level, ordinal, occurs when pain severity is ranked. Ordinal measures can determine if a pain is more or less severe than another pain. The third level is interval measurement in which measures have equal intervals between values. The final level is ratio in which there is a true zero point. In the case of pain measures, because a true zero point is typical (no pain), interval and ratio measures are equivalent.

Two of the most important psychometric properties of a pain measure are reliability and validity. Reliability refers to the consistency or reproducibility of the measure. In pain measurement in children the focus has been on inter-rater reliability and to some extent internal consistency. Inter-rater reliability refers to the degree of agreement if two observers use the same measure to observe the same behaviour. High inter-rater reliability is desirable. Internal reliability refers to the degree of similarity that different items in a measurement scale have. For example, if a scale uses two items measuring facial response, one measuring change in heart rate and one measuring crying to measure pain, one would hope for a moderately high degree of interrelationship or reliability among the items. Perfect reliability would suggest that fewer items would be needed and low reliability would indicate that a single concept (pain) was not being measured. Because the underlying phenomenon, pain, often varies over time there has been little interest in reliability over time.

Validity refers to how well the measure actually measures what it is supposed to measure. There are many different types of validity and the terminology in this area is often confusing. Face validity refers to how well the measure makes sense. For example, using facial response makes sense as a measure of pain and thus has high face validity. Construct validity has frequently been used in child pain measurement and refers to any evidence that adds to the believability of the measures. For example, comparing infants on a measure immediately following an invasive procedure and when they are at rest could add to the construct validity of a measure. Similarly, systematic decreases in a pain measure after the administration of an analgesic would suggest construct validity of the scale used to measure pain. Construct validity cannot be established in a single study.

It is important to determine the psychometric properties of a measure in a situation and with a sample that is similar to that being evaluated. The reader who wishes to explore issues in psychometrics of pain measures is referred to the review by Johnston (1998).

The utility of a measure refers to its usefulness. One aspect of utility is ease of use, another is versatility. A measure that requires a trained observer is less useful than an equally reliable and valid measure that can be carried out by anyone in a few seconds. Versatile measures have the advantage of being used in several different situations (e.g., across a wide age range or in both acute and chronic pain). Versatility is convenient and allows for comparisons across different situations. Whereas utility and versatility are desirable, reliability and validity are prerequisites for use. Some pain measures are used in research settings but may be too expensive or too demanding in terms of skills or time needed for clinical use. Moreover, some pain measures may not be precise enough for making specific clinical decisions but may be very useful in an epidemiological study. In addition, some clinical measures may lack the precision needed for particular research questions.

STRATEGIES OF PAIN MEASUREMENT

The three most frequently considered aspects of pain are the subjective (measured by self report), the behavioural (measured by sampling of observation and coding or rating of behaviour) and the biological (measured by sampling of physiological or electrical potentials and assaying body fluids or other biological responses). Not only are there multiple aspects, but for each there may be several different measurement strategies for each aspect.

SELF-REPORT MEASURES OF PAIN

Self-report measures depend on the child's own report of his or her subjective pain experience. This can include descriptions of pain-relevant feelings, statements and images, as well as information about the quality, intensity and temporal/spatial dimensions of the child's pain. Self-report measures, when they can be obtained, can be regarded as the 'gold standard'. Indeed, the International Association for the Study of Pain (Merskey 1986) emphasizes 'pain is always subjective'. There are two major problems with self-report measures. First of all, they require the child to have a level of cognitive and linguistic development that excludes all preverbal children and may exclude many other young children. The level of cognitive and language development depends on the type of question asked. Children at the earliest levels of language development may be able to respond to the least demanding questions, such as those about the existence of pain.

The second problem is that all self-report measures are open to bias because of the demand characteristics of the specific situation. Following surgery children may deny having pain when they are asked because they fear that if they say they have pain they will get a needle which is more feared than pain (Eland & Anderson 1977). Other contextual variables may also be important. For example, if children are asked to describe pain to their mothers they will give different answers than if they are asked to describe pain to a doctor. In addition, the type of question and the response options (e.g., open-ended versus a checklist) may also substantially alter the child's answers (Ross & Ross 1988). Clearly, demand and other contextual characteristics cannot be eliminated from the measurement of pain. We must, however, be aware that a change in context can substantially influence the measurement of pain.

The methods used to measure self-report of pain include: direct questioning, pain adjective descriptors, self-rating scales, numerical rating scales and non-verbal methods. Spontaneous reports (e.g., 'My tummy hurts') or direct questioning about pain can be useful with verbal preschoolers and school-age children. However, reliance on spontaneous reports is likely to seriously underestimate pain; some children may not spontaneously report pain because they want to be brave or because they do not know that anything can be done about it. Direct questioning may include: asking the child to make comparisons with previous pain experiences ('Is this pain like the stomach ache you had last week?'); providing the child with temporal anchors for measuring the duration of pain ('Has the pain been going on since you woke up?'); facilitating communication through the use of objects and gestures ('How much pain do you have, a little bit or a lot?').

Although direct questioning is clinically useful, several shortcomings have been observed. To a great extent, questions such as 'How is your pain today?' are more conversational gambits than pain measures. Because of their unstructured nature these methods may be particularly open to bias due to demand characteristics. As well, they lack an associated metric (i.e. there are no numbers associated with the answers) and may be biased by inaccurate memory or the recall of a previous experience. Even if specific questions are asked about pain frequency, intensity and duration, retrospective questions are likely to be inaccurate.

The typical clinical strategy is to ask the child's mother how much pain her child has been experiencing. This is similar to asking parents if they remember whether or not their child had recently appeared to have a fever. In some cases, this strategy, whether it is related to fever or pain, produces sufficient information to guide diagnosis and treatment. It is, however, likely to be insufficient in more complex situations such as those where pain is of unknown origin or where there is significant variability in the expression of pain. More precise measures of pain are likely to be obtained by the child using prospective, well-validated measures.

Pain adjective lists, such as the MPQ (Melzack 1975), have been used successfully with older adolescents to measure the sensory, affective and evaluative dimensions of pain. A major strength of this type of scale is that it is not restricted to the intensity dimension of pain but also measures affective and evaluative aspects of pain. Experience in several different laboratories has shown that children are able to select simple adjectives from word lists to describe their pain. For example, Savedra, Tesler and their colleagues have examined children's language of pain in a series of studies (e.g., Savedra et al 1990, Savedra & Tesler 1989, Wilkie et al 1990). They have developed and tested lists of words that include sensory, affective and evaluative words that can be completed by children over 8 years. A 56-item word list that measures sensory, affective and evaluative components of pain has been developed and evaluated for reliability and validity. Similar work has been undertaken in the Dutch language by Abu-Saad (1990), and by McGrath

(1990) and Varni et al (1987) in English. As yet, the meaning of different patterns of words has not been determined. Pain descriptors rely on advanced linguistic competence and are not appropriate for some children. Although these methods are appealing because the richness of the pain experience is described, the lower age limits for these methods have not yet been delineated and these methods have not been shown to be clinically superior to simpler methods that focus on the intensity of pain.

Self-rating scales of the intensity of pain vary according to the type and number of anchor points provided and may be categorized into three types: visual analogue scales, category rating scales and numerical rating scales.

Visual analogue scales (VASs) consist of either a vertical or horizontal line, usually 10 cm in length, with verbal or pictorial anchors indicating a continuum from no pain to severe pain at each end. Children are asked to indicate on the line how much pain they are experiencing. Studies have shown that for children over 5 years, VASs are reliable and valid measures of pain. Children's ratings of their pain on VASs correlate with parents', nurses' and physicians' ratings (O'Hara et al 1987, Varni et al 1987; McGrath et al 1990). Ratings on VAS also correlate with behavioural measures of pain (McGrath et al 1985, Maunuksela et al 1987). Figure 15.1 provides an example of a typical VAS.

Some authors have suggested that a vertical scale is more appropriate than a horizontal scale because children may find it easier to conceptualize the notion of greater or lesser intensity of pain with up and down rather than left or right. The VAS is versatile as it allows one to measure different dimensions such as intensity ('How bad is the pain?') and affect ('How bad do you feel about the pain?'). However, the child must have the cognitive ability necessary to translate the pain experience into an analogue format and to understand proportionality. Care must be taken when repeatedly photocopying the scale to ensure that the process does not alter the length of the line and thus confound scoring. Maunuksela et al (1987) developed and validated a variant of a VAS in the form of a 50-cm red and white wedge.

Category scales consist of a series of words along a continuum of increasing value (e.g., no pain, mild pain, medium pain, severe pain). Wilkie et al (1990) have provided data suggesting that a category scale may be valid and useful with children.

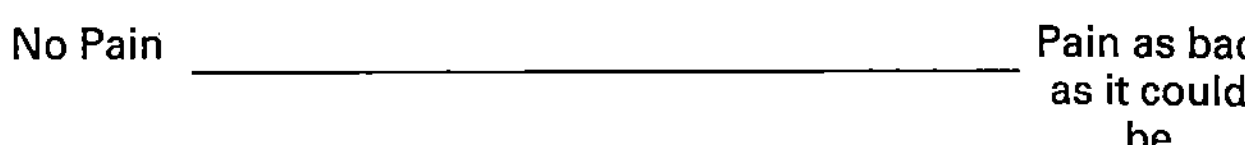

Fig. 15.1 Visual analogue scale.

The Poker Chip Tool (Hester 1979), a derivative of the category scales, is a concrete measure requiring the child to evaluate the intensity of pain by choosing one to four poker chips, representing the 'pieces of hurt' experienced. This method is reported to be appropriate for younger children between the ages of 4 and 8 years. Children's ratings correlate with overt behaviour during immunization (Hester 1979). Hester et al (1990) compared child, nurse and parental ratings of pain and demonstrated adequate convergent validity and partial support for discriminant validity of this tool.

Faces scales, another form of category scale, consist of faces expressing varying amounts of distress. Each face is assigned a numerical value reflecting its order within a series of facial expressions. Several variants of faces scales have been used to measure children's level of pain. However, if the scales do not approach being ratio scales, the numerical values assigned to each face may be deceiving unless they have been empirically tested.

The Oucher scale (Beyer 1984) is a variant of the faces scale and is designed to measure pain intensity in children aged 3–12 years. The scale is displayed in a poster format and consists of a vertical numerical scale (0–100) on the left and six photographs of children in varying degrees of pain positioned vertically to the right (Fig. 15.2).

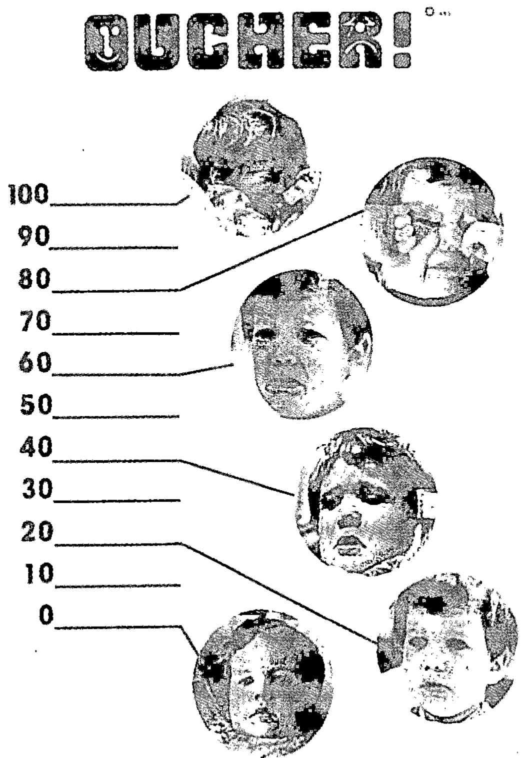

Fig. 15.2 The Oucher scale. (Reproduced from Beyer 1984 with permission.)

Validity studies indicate that children are able to classify the pictures in the correct sequence and that scores correlate highly with VASs and results from the Poker Chip measure (Beyer & Aradine 1987). Although the scale has been criticized for confounding intensity and affective measures (McGrath 1987), it correlates poorly with measures of fear (Beyer & Aradine 1987), suggesting that it does indeed tap into the pain-intensity dimension. Moreover, scores on the Oucher scale are sensitive to analgesia-caused reduction in pain. The Oucher remains one of the most thoroughly validated scales and has good psychometric properties. Variants of the Oucher have been designed and validated for African-American and Hispanic children (Beyer & Knott 1998) and a First Nations version is under development.

Bieri et al (1990) developed a faces scale to assess pain intensity in children aged 6–8 years. A unique feature of this measure is that the drawings used in the scale's development were derived from those generated by the children themselves. In addition, the faces were drawn to be reflective of the facial response to pain described by Grunau and Craig (1987). Further, strong agreement was demonstrated among children on the rank ordering of the faces according to pain severity as well as their perception of the faces as representing equal intervals. Finally, the scale demonstrated adequate test-retest reliability over a 2-week period. More recent work with this scale has affirmed the psychometric robustness of this scale (Goodenough et al 1997) and pointed out that younger children may use the extremes of scales more than older children. The scale is presented in Figure 15.3. Other faces scales have been developed (Whaley & Wong 1987, Kuttner & Lepage 1989) and there is no clear evidence that one scale is more accurate than another. In summary, faces scales are easily understood by children, are inexpensive and several have excellent psychometric characteristics.

Numerical scales use numbers (i.e. 0–5, 0–10 or 0–100) to reflect increasing degrees of pain. Children must understand number concepts in order to use this type of scale. The intervals along the scale cannot be assumed to be equal and a change between 0 and 3 is not necessarily the same as a change between 6 and 9. Although there has been no careful work on the psychometric properties of numerical rating scales, they have a place in the clinical setting. From a practical perspective, because they require no materials, are readily understood by healthcare professionals and are so easy to chart (e.g., 'James rated his pain as 7 out of 10'), numerical scales have advantages.

Pain thermometers consist of a vertical numerical rating scale ranging between 0 and 10 or 0 and 100 superimposed on a VAS. Anchors at each endpoint indicate no hurt and most hurt possible. The child is asked to point to the place on the thermometer that represents the intensity of his pain. Scores on the pain thermometer correlate with scores on other rating scales, as well as predicted changes in pain associated with burns (Szyfelbein et al 1985).

Diaries are a specific type of numerical rating scale in which repeated ratings of pain are taken. Pain diaries have been used for the measurement of headache, abdominal pain and limb pain. In a typical format, ratings range from 0 to 5 and each number corresponds to a verbal description of pain severity. The scale requires a minimum of instruction and has satisfactory inter-rater reliability when comparisons are made between parent and child ratings (Richardson et al 1983, Andrasik et al 1985). Pain diaries may be particularly useful with older children and adolescents as they encourage self-management strategies and consequently foster a sense of mastery and increased self esteem (Ross & Ross 1988). Figure 15.4 presents a diary used in our clinical and research work.

Primarily non-verbal methods have also been used to measure the self report of pain. These methods include asking children to describe the colour of their pain or to draw pictures of their pain. Children are reported typically to describe severe pain as being red or black (Eland 1974, Jeans 1983, Unruh et al 1983, Kurylyszyn et al 1987). Unfortunately, no validation of colour scales or their utility in clinical situations has been done. Red and black appear to be the preferred colours for all pain drawings, even for drawings of low intensities of pain (Kurylyszyn et al 1987). Children's pain drawings are rich in detail, are emotively powerful and provide a basis for discussion about pain. Although they can be reliably classified by raters (Unruh et al 1983) and may show developmental differences (Jeans 1983), it is not clear that drawings can tell us much about the intensity or origin of the child's pain. Kurylyszyn et al (1987) found that drawings of different intensity of headache could not be well discriminated on the basis of overall ratings of intensity or by examination of specific features of the drawings. While drawings may not have much value as measures, they may be of benefit in assessment, especially to begin discussion about pain. Drawings also provide valuable information about the location of pain.

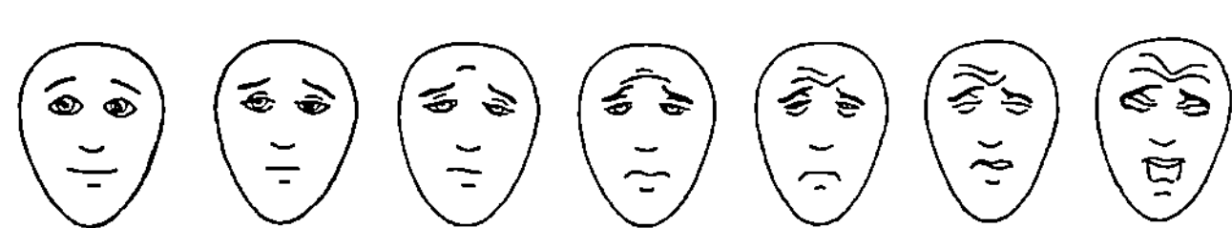

Fig. 15.3 Faces scale. (Reproduced from Bieri et al 1990 with permission.)

Introduction Week 1
Headache Diary

Fill in this form at breakfast, lunch, dinner and bedtime each day

Name: ______________________ Week beginning: ____________

Day	Time	Intensity Rating	Other Symptoms	Medication	Possible Cause
	Breakfast				
	Lunch				
	Dinner				
	Bedtime				
	Breakfast				
	Lunch				
	Dinner				
	Bedtime				
	Breakfast				
	Lunch				
	Dinner				
	Bedtime				
	Breakfast				
	Lunch				
	Dinner				
	Bedtime				
	Breakfast				
	Lunch				
	Dinner				
	Bedtime				
	Breakfast				
	Lunch				
	Dinner				
	Bedtime				
	Breakfast				
	Lunch				
	Dinner				
	Bedtime				

Intensity Ratings

0 – No headache.
1 – Headache – I am only aware of it if I pay attention to it.
2 – Headache – but I can ignore it at times.
3 – Headache – I can't ignore it but I can do my usual activities
4 – Headache – It is difficult for me to concentrate; I can only do easy activities.
5 – Headache – such that I can't do anything.

Fig. 15.4 Pain diary.

Several studies have shown that children over 6 years of age can locate their pain on a pain drawing or body outline and that these markings correspond to clinical observations and records (Varni et al 1987, Savedra & Tesler 1989).

Projective techniques have not been shown to be effective in the measurement of intensity of pain in children. For example, Eland (1974) found no relationship between responses to cartoons in which an animal was subjected to a painful experience and the child's own response. However, projective approaches may be of some use in a more broad-based assessment of children's attitudes to painful experiences, perceptions of family response to pain and coping strategies. Lollar et al (1982) developed a projective pain scale that used 24 pictures to determine how children perceive pain experienced by themselves and their parents. This scale has not been used in clinical pain measurement. The Charleston Pain Pictures (Belter et al 1988) are 17 cartoon pictures of a young child of indeterminate sex in scenes of medical, play and home situations. The scales depict situations that have been assessed by experts and by children as being no pain, low pain, moderate pain or high pain.

In summary, several self-report measures of pain that are easy to collect and use in clinical situations have been developed. However, the lower limits of these measures has not been systematically investigated, nor has it been clearly established that one measure is superior to another. Champion et al (1998) has recently reviewed self-report measures in more detail.

BEHAVIOURAL MEASURES OF PAIN

The second component of pain that can be measured is pain behaviour. Behaviours such as vocalization, facial expression and body movement are typically associated with pain. Behavioural responses are invaluable for inferring pain in children who cannot rate their pain. Anand and Craig (1996) have suggested that behaviour should be considered the equivalent of self report for preverbal children. There is, however, the ever-present challenge of distinguishing behaviour due to other forms of distress, such as hunger, thirst and anxiety, from behaviour due to pain. The best evidence for reliability and validity of behavioural measures is based on studies of short, sharp pain such as that from needle procedures, for example venepuncture, heelstick or bone marrow aspirations. Fradet et al (1990), for example, found that child self report correlated significantly with a measure of discrete pain behaviours ($r = 0.54$) and also with global estimates by nurses ($r = 0.52$) and global measures by parents ($r = 0.42$).

Some of the most interesting work on behavioural measures has been carried out with neonates. Grunau and Craig (1987) developed the Neonatal Facial Action Coding System which consists of 10 facial actions that trained coders can identify from review of videotapes. Facial movements observed in response to heel lance (the 'pain face') were: brow bulge, eye squeeze, nasolabial furrow, lip part, taut tongue, stretch mouth and chin quiver. Results indicated that facial response to heel lance was also state dependent, with increased facial responding observed in babies who were quiet and awake compared to babies who were sleeping. In a subsequent study, Grunau et al (1990) found that facial expression (especially brow bulging, eyes squeezed shut, deepening of the nasolabial furrow and open mouth) combined with a short-latency cry and long-duration first-cry cycle is the most typical (but not uniform) response to short, sharp, invasive stimuli.

Facial expressions are interesting because they are relatively free of learning biases and may represent the infant's innate response to pain. To date, the facial coding systems have been used primarily for short, sharp pain in a research context. They require video recording and time consuming scoring of responses. As a result, the full NFACS is not appropriate for routine clinical use. However, Stevens (Stevens et al 1996, Stevens 1998) has used facial actions in her Premature Infant Pain Profile. Facial action may be difficult to record in babies who have their faces obstructed due to medical interventions. Craig's recent review (Craig 1998) summarizes the recent literature in this area.

Others (Craig et al 1984, Johnston & Strada 1986, Pigeon et al 1989) have observed more gross body movements associated with pain in infants and young children. Commonly observed behaviours include: general diffuse movements in newborns, withdrawal of the affected limb in 6-month-old infants and touching the affected area in 12-month-old infants (McGraw 1945). Kicking and thrashing of limbs, tensing of limbs and a rigid, tense torso have also been observed in response to immunization (Craig et al 1984, Johnston & Strada 1986). The Infant Pain Behaviour Rating Scale (Craig et al 1984), a time-sampling scale, rates expressive body responses (rigidity, kicking) as well as vocalizations and facial expressions in infants and young children. The scale has satisfactory inter-rater reliability for most of the items, as well as validity. In a survey of neonatal nurses' perceptions of pain, similar behaviours were identified as indicative of pain in neonates but there was essentially no relationship between the various behaviours and pain intensities (Pigeon et al 1989).

The Procedural Behavioral Rating Scale (Katz et al 1980) and the Observational Scale of Behavioral Distress (Jay et al 1983) were developed to measure distress in paediatric oncology patients due to bone-marrow aspirations and lumbar punctures. Behaviours include crying, screaming, physical restraint, verbal resistance, requests for emotional support, muscular rigidity, verbal pain expression, flailing, nervous behaviour and information seeking. The scales have satisfactory inter-rater reliability, and distress behaviours on the Observational Scale of Behavioral Distress correlate with children's self report of pain and anxiety scores (Jay et al 1983).

A particular behaviour that has received considerable attention as a pain measure is crying. Investigators have attempted to differentiate the pain cry in infants in terms of its psychoacoustic properties (Johnston & Strada 1986, Grunau & Craig 1987). Johnston (1989) reported that a high-pitched, tense, non-voiced, intense cry is typical in very stressed states. Grunau and Craig (1987) found that both gender and psychological state affected crying behaviour. Specifically, in response to heel lance, boys cried sooner and had more crying cycles than girls. Also, sleeping babies cried less quickly than alert babies. Although some characteristic cry patterns have been identified during medical procedures (Johnston 1989), a cry pattern or cry template unique to painful stimuli has not been identified. Grunau et al (1990) have discussed the methodological difficulties in cry research.

Behavioural measures of longer-lasting pain are less well developed and it appears that the scales to measure short-term pain may not be valid for longer-term pain. Three scales have been developed for measuring postoperative pain in children. All have been validated in the immediate postoperative period. The Children's Hospital of Eastern Ontario Pain Scale (CHEOPS) (McGrath et al 1985) is a behavioural rating scale developed with children in the recovery room to measure postoperative pain. It consists of six behaviours (crying, facial expression, verbal expression, torso position, touch position and leg position). The scale has inter-rater reliability above 0.80 and independent pain ratings by nurses provide evidence for concurrent validity. Also, the scale is sensitive to changes in behaviour due to intravenous analgesic medication. It has excellent measurement characteristics with needle pain (Fradet et al 1990). Several variations of this scale have been developed (Splinter et al 1994, Taddio et al 1995).

Tarbell et al (1992) published a seven-item Toddler-Preschool Postoperative Pain Scale which includes items on vocal pain expression, facial pain expression and bodily pain expression. The scale has good reliability and validity data but, like the CHEOPS and the Objective Pain Scale, it has not been shown to be valid outside the immediate postoperative period. These three scales are valid for measuring pain in the recovery room but are probably not valid for measuring pain in children several hours after surgery. Beyer et al (1990) established that gross behaviours such as grimacing and body movements occur very rarely in children suffering from postoperative pain once they are out of the recovery room.

As we have noted, there is less work on longer-lasting pain. Gauvain-Piquard et al (1987) developed a 15-item behavioural rating scale for paediatric oncology patients between the ages of 2 and 6 years. The scale consists of three subscales:

1. Pain behaviours such as protective behaviours toward the affected area.
2. Psychomotor alterations such as slowing down and withdrawal.

3. Anxiety behaviours such as nervousness and irritability.

The scale appears to have adequate sensitivity between patients and satisfactory inter-rater reliability (Gauvain-Piquard et al 1987). Validity studies are ongoing and the scale is being used with other groups such as paediatric burn patients (Gauvain-Piquard & Rodary 1989).

The Postoperative Pain Measure for Parents (Chambers et al 1996) was developed from parents' reports of what behaviours they used to determine if their child was in pain (Reid et al 1995). The items of this scale are included in Table 15.2.

Initial validation has shown that the scale is highly correlated with self report and has high sensitivity and specificity in detecting clinically significant pain (Chambers et al 1996).

The Non-Communicating Children's Pain Checklist (McGrath et al in press) was developed to assist in the measurement of pain in children who cannot communicate about their pain because of physical and mental handicap. Items in the scale are presented in Table 15.3. The scale is similar to one developed by a group in France based on the observations of health professionals (Giusiano et al 1995).

In summary, there has been extensive work on measures of short, sharp pain and limited work on long-term pain. The scales range from measures of gross behaviour to measures of small changes in facial response. The behavioural measurement of long-term pain and the development of measures for special populations, such as children with disabilities, has made important strides.

Table 15.2 Postoperative pain measure for patients. (Chambers et al 1996.)

Did your child
Whine or complain more than usual?
Cry more easily than usual?
Play less than usual?
Not do the things she/he usually does?
Act more worried than usual?
Act more quietly than usual?
Have less energy than usual?
Refuse to eat?
Eat less than usual?
Hold the sore part of his/her body?
Try not to bump the sore part of his/her body?
Groan or moan more than usual?
Look more flushed than usual?
Want to be close to you more than usual?
Take medications when she/he normally refuses?

One point for each Yes answer.
Six or more points suggest clinically significant pain.

Table 15.3 The non-communicating children's pain checklist (McGrath et al 1998)

Items and areas of the checklist
Vocal
Moaning, whining, whimpering
Screaming/yelling
A specific sound or vocalization for pain, 'word', cry, type of 'laugh'
Please describe
Eating/sleeping
Eats less, not interested in food
Increase in sleep
Decrease in sleep
Social/personality
Not cooperating, cranky, irritable, unhappy
Less interaction, withdrawn
Seeks comfort or physical closeness
Difficult to distract, not able to satisfy or pacify
Facial expression of pain (cringe, grimace)
Furrowed brow
Change in eyes, including: squinching of eyes, eyes opened wide, eyes frown
Turn down of mouth, not smiling
Lips pucker up, tight, pout or quiver
Clenches, grinds teeth, chews, thrusts tongue
Activity
Not moving, less active, quiet
Jumping around, agitated, fidgety
Body and limbs
Floppy
Stiff, spastic, tense, rigid
Specify body part/limbs
Gestures to or touches part of body that hurts
Protects, favours or guards part of body that hurts
Flinch or moves body part away, sensitive to touch
Moves body in specific way to show pain (head back, arms down, curls up, etc.)
Physiological
Shivering
Change in colour, pallor
Sweating, perspiring
Tears
Sharp intake of breathe, gasping
Breath holding

BIOLOGICAL MEASURES

Biological measures of pain in children suffer from many of the same problems as behavioural measures. In particular, it is often difficult to determine if the perturbation being measured is due to causes other than pain such as hunger. Some authors (e.g. Porter 1993) have argued that the discrimination between pain and other distress may be meaningless for infants and that a search for a pain-specific measure in this age group should be abandoned in favour of a biological measure of distress. Much like behavioural measures of pain, it appears that biological indices of pain habituate in the face of longer-term pain.

There are sufficient data on heart rate, transcutaneous oxygen, sweating and the stress response to argue for their validity as measures of pain in some circumstances. There is less evidence for using endorphins, respiration and blood pressure. However, further research may elucidate their validity.

Heart rate is the most widely used biological measure of pain in infants and children. In general, heart rate increases in response to more invasive procedures. However, depending on the length of period sampled, there may be a slowing of the heart rate as the first response to pain (Johnston & Strada 1986). There appear to be major differences between healthy and ill neonates, and full-term and premature neonates, with generally weaker, more variable, disorganized responses in ill and premature babies (Field & Goldson 1984, Porter 1993). Porter (1993) has described the use of vagal tone as a direct measure of parasympathetic control and a possible index of pain and distress. However, there have been no studies to demonstrate the superiority of this measure to simple heart rate. Indeed, no studies have adequately attempted to evaluate heart rate as a measure of longer-term pain, although it is clear that heart rate is not substantially elevated by postoperative pain in older children (O'Hara et al 1987).

Transcutaneous oxygen is reduced during painful procedures such as circumcision (Rawlings et al 1980, Williamson & Williamson 1983), lumbar punctures (Porter et al 1987) and incubation (Kelly & Finer 1984), but this also occurs during non-painful handling of neonates. Transcutaneous oxygen is widely used in anaesthesia and critical care monitoring and is a frequently available measure in the intensive care unit. Transcutaneous oxygen may, however, be influenced by factors other than pain and may not be responsive in infants who have mechanically supported ventilation.

Harpin and Rutter (1983) demonstrated that, in full-term babies (but not in pre-term babies), palmar sweating, as measured by an evaporimeter, was a sensitive index of pain from heel lance. Gedaly-Duff (1989) has reviewed the use of a simpler measure, the palmar sweat index, that measures the number of active sweat glands rather than the extent of sweating. Palmar sweating has been primarily used as a measure of distress rather than pain.

Surgery or trauma triggers the release of stress hormones (corticosteroids, catecholamines, glucagon and growth hormone). This leads to a cascade of events which may have positive effects of facilitating healing but, in the sick neonate, can have disastrous results. Anand and his colleagues (Anand et al 1987a,b, Anand 1993) have detailed the stress response of premature and full-term infants to surgery. The response generally consists of marked increases in plasma catecholamines, glucagon and corticosteroids and a suppression of insulin secretion, leading to hyperglycaemia and lactic acidosis. The response in neonates is generally greater, particularly with regard to increases in plasma, adrenaline, glucagon, growth hormone, blood glucose, blood lactate and other gluconeogenic substrates. In addition, infants tend to have a uniphasic cortisol response which is smaller than the biphasic response of adults. The stress response in neonates is blunted by appropriate anaesthesia, probably by dampening input to the hypothalamus, by lessening the hypothalamic response to neural input and by altering synaptic transmission within the hypothalamus (Anand 1993). The reaction to anaesthesia indicates the validity of the measures but it is clear that the stress response is more than a measure of pain. Although useful in the research context, these measures have limited use as clinical pain measures in individual patients.

Cortisol release has been widely studied in adults and quite frequently examined in infants and children (Gunnar 1986). Cortisol release is not specific to pain and occurs with many aversive situations. Changes in cortisol level from a resting baseline are significant in response to circumcision (Gunnar et al 1981). However, sick premature babies may have very unstable levels. Thus, small perturbations from specific painful procedures may not be detectable.

Lewis and Thomas (1990), in their cross-sectional study of healthy infants who were 2, 4 and 6 months, provide insight into the complexity of the response even in healthy infants at different ages. They used the diphtheria pertussis tetanus inoculation as a standard stimulus and found that the strongest increase in cortisol levels, as measured by salivary assay, occurred with the 2-month-old children. There was little change in cortisol level in the 4-month-old children and only moderate response in the 6-month-old children. The age differences in cortisol response were eliminated if behavioural response was used as a covariate. In addition, baseline levels of cortisol were important in interpreting cortisol response to painful stimulation.

There have been recent developments in measuring CNS changes during pain (e.g., Rainville et al 1997) using advanced imaging techniques. Although these measures provide greater understanding of the central representation of pain, they do not provide clinically useful measures. Moreover, in part because many methods are invasive, none of this work has been carried out in children (Anand 1998).

Biological methods of measuring pain provide important information about the body's response to insult. These measures are particularly important to the clinician when they provide warning about responses affecting the medical stability of the child. However, biological measures are not specific to pain, often habituate and sometimes are not available in the clinical setting (Sweet & McGrath 1998).

COMPOSITE MEASURES

Because pain is a multidimensional phenomena and no one pain measure has sufficient reliability and validity, composite measures of pain have been developed (Stevens, 1998). Combining items can enhance the reliability and validity of instruments. Several scales have been developed for both neonates and for children and have been reviewed by Stevens (1998). Two of the most widely used and extensively validated scales are the Premature Infant Pain Profile (PIPP) (Stevens et al 1996) and the COMFORT Scale (Ambuel et al 1992). The PIPP consists of six items which vary in value with the gestational age at the time of the observations. The items are: behavioural state, change in heart rate, change in oxygen saturation, brow bulge, eye squeeze and nasolabial furrow. The scale has excellent psychometric properties and is now in clinical use.

The COMFORT Scale (Ambuel et al 1992) is an eight-item scale designed to measure distress (including pain) in paediatric intensive care units. The items include: alertness, calmness, respiratory response, physical movement, blood pressure, muscle tone and facial tension. The scale has excellent psychometric properties, takes only 3 minutes to administer and is used clinically.

IMPLEMENTATION OF MEASURES

The major impediment to the measurement of pain in children is the failure to implement what is already known. All children who are at risk for pain, including children who have had surgery and children who are in the active phase of potentially painful diseases or disorders such as cancer, sickle cell disease, migraine headache or juvenile arthritis, should have their pain routinely monitored. Hospitalized children's pain should be recorded on pain flow sheets on a regular basis every few hours (McGrath & Unruh 1987). Stevens (1990) has shown that pain flow sheets decrease pain by improving pain management. Pain diaries, completed by the child or by the parent, can be used with children who are at risk for significant recurrent pain. Routine measurement should be used in quality assurance programmes to ensure the adequacy of pain control in hospitals. Adequate paediatric pain measurement is an ethical imperative that all healthcare professionals are obligated to implement. There has been limited research on the implementation of pain measurement. Hester et al (1998) have outlined the process by which implementing a pain assessment strategy in a medical setting for children occurs. Attributes of innovations, such as having a standard pain measurement system in a health centre which enhances adoption include: the innovation is perceived as being better than the idea it supersedes; the innovation is compatible with existing values and practices; the innovation is simple and straightforward; the innovation can be experimented with on a limited basis and the results of the innovation are observable to others.

DISABILITY DUE TO PAIN

Disability (the restriction in ability to perform an activity) because of pain has received little systematic attention. Both Varni's pain assessment questionnaire (Thompson & Varni 1986, Varni et al 1987) and Patricia McGrath's (1990) assessment tool contain a measure of disability. However, the validity of the measures or the extent of disability in populations is unknown. Walker and Greene (1991) developed and validated the Functional Disability Inventory. The measure was carefully developed and shows excellent construct, concurrent and predictive validity. The instrument was stable over time and also sensitive to medical treatment. Instruments such as the Functional Disability Inventory will allow further investigation of disability due to various childhood pains.

HANDICAP DUE TO PAIN

The major social roles of children are as peers and as students. Consequently, handicaps include educational and social handicap. Although there are limited data on the topic, it appears that handicap due to pain is relatively rare in children. School failure is the most relevant measure of educational handicap. However, no studies have examined school failure resulting from pain. School absence could serve as a proxy measure and absence due to pain has been examined in one study. Collin et al (1985) examined the amount of school time that children between 5 and 14 years of age missed because of headache. They recorded both absence from school and attendance at sick bay. During two 12-week periods, school absence was 0.05%, which amounted to about 1% of all absences, with 85% of absences of less than 1 day. Attendance at sick bay was also low and rarely resulted in leaving school.

Pain is a frequent complaint by the child who has a phobia toward school. However, the pain symptom is usually so transparent that it is quite readily (and quite appropriately) given little attention.

The prevalence of handicap due to pain in children is clearly lower than that found in adults. However, those children who are handicapped are particularly troubling to the healthcare system and appropriate assessment may lead to more effective treatment. Little work has been done on the correlates of handicap. In a small study, we found that the mothers of adolescents who were missing school because of pain became over-involved when supervising an exercise task that might elicit pain in their adolescence (Dunn-Geier et al 1986).

REFERENCES

Abu-Saad HH 1990 Toward the development of an instrument to assess pain in children: Dutch study. In: Tyler D C, Krane E J (eds) Advances in pain research and therapy: pediatric pain. Raven Press, New York, pp 101–106

Ambuel B, Hamlett KW, Marx CM, Blumer JL 1992 Assessing distress in pediatric intensive care environments: the COMFORT scale. Journal of Pediatric Psychology 17: 95–109

Anand KJS 1998 Neurophysiological and neurobiological correlates of supraspinal pain processing: measurement techniques. In: Finley GA, McGrath PJ (eds) Measurement of pain in infants and children. Seattle: IASP Press, pp 21–46

Anand KJS 1993 The applied physiology of pain. In: Anand KJS, McGrath PJ (eds) Pain in the neonate. Elsevier, Amsterdam pp 39–66

Anand KJS, Craig KD 1996 New perspectives on the definition of pain. Pain 67: 3–6

Anand KJS, Sippell WG, Aynsley-Green A 1987a Randomized trial of fentanyl anaesthesia in preterm babies undergoing surgery: effects on the stress response. Lancet i: 243–248

Anand KJS, Sippell WG, Schofield NM et al 1987b Does halothane anaesthesia decrease the stress response of newbom infants undergoing operation? British Medical Journal 296: 668–672

Andrasik F, Burke EJ, Attanasio V et al 1985 Child, parent, and physician reports of a child's headache pain: relationships prior to and following treatment. Headache 25: 421–425

Belter RW, McIntosh JA, Finch AJ et al 1988 Preschoolers' ability to differentiate levels of pain: relative efficacy of three selfreport measures. Journal of Clinical Child Psychology 17: 329–335

Beyer JE 1984 The Oucher: a user's manual and technical report. The Hospital Play Equipment, Evanston, Illinois

Beyer JE, Aradine CR 1987 Patterns of pediatric pain intensity: a methodological investigation of a self-report scale. Clinical Journal of Pain 3: 130–141

Beyer J, Knott CB 1998 Construct validity estimation of the African-American and Hispanic versions of the Oucher Scale. Journal of Pediatric Nursing 13: 20–31

Beyer JE, McGrath PJ, Berde C 1990 Discordance between self report and behavioral pain measures in 3–7 year old children following surgery. Journal of Pain and Symptom Management 5: 350–356

Bieri D, Reeve RA, Champion GD et al 1990 The faces pain scale for the self-assessment of the severity of pain experienced by children: development, initial validation, and preliminary investigation for ratio scale properties. Pain 41: 139–150

Chambers CT, Reid GJ, McGrath PJ, Finley GA 1996 Development and preliminary validation of a postoperative pain measure for parents. Pain 68: 307–313

Champion GD, Goodenough B, von Baeyer CL, Thomas W 1998 Measurement of pain by self-report. In: Finley GA, McGrath PG (eds) Measurement of pain in infants and children. Seattle, IASP Press, pp 123–160

Collin C, Hockaday JM, Waters WE 1985 Headache and school absence. Archives of Disease in Childhood 60: 245–247

Craig KD 1998 The facial display of pain. In: Finley GA, McGrath PJ (eds) Measurement of pain in infants and children. Seattle, IASP Press, pp 103–121

Craig KD, McMahon RJ, Morison JD et al 1984 Developmental changes in infant pain expression during immunization injections. Social Science in Medicine 19: 1331–1337

Dunn-Geier BJ, McGrath PJ, Rourke BP et al 1986 Adolescent chronic pain: the ability to cope. Pain 26: 23–32

Eland IM 1974 Children's communication of pain. Master's Thesis, University of Iowa

Eland J, Anderson J 1977 The experience of pain in children. In: Jacox A (ed) A sourcebook for nurses and other health professionals. Little, Brown, Boston, pp 453–476

Field T, Goldson E 1984 Pacifying effects of nonnutritive sucking on term and preterm neonates during heelstick procedures. Pediatrics 74: 1012–1015

Fradet C, McGrath PJ, Kay S et al 1990 A prospective survey of reactions to blood tests by children and adolescents. Pain 40: 53–60

Franck LS 1986 A new method to quantitatively describe pain behavior in infants. Nursing Research 35: 28–31

Gauvain-Piquard A, Rodary C 1989 Evaluation de la douleur. In: Pichard-Leandri E, Gauvain-Piquard A (eds) La douleur chez l'enfant. Medsi/McGraw-Hill, New York, pp 38–59

Gauvain-Piquard A, Rodary C, Rezvani A et al 1987 Pain in children aged 2–6 years: a new observational rating scale elaborated in a paediatric oncology until – preliminary report. Pain 31: 177–188

Gedaly-Duff V 1989 Palmar sweat index use with children in pain research. Journal of Pediatric Nursing 4: 3–8

Giusiano B, Jimeno MT, Collignon P, Chau Y 1995 Utilization of a neural network in the elaboration of an evaluation scale for pain in cerebral palsy. Methods of Information in Medicine 34: 498–502

Goodenough B, Addicoat L, Champion GD et al 1997. Pain in 4- to 6-year-old children receiving intramuscular injections: a comparison of the Faces Pain Scale with other self-report and behavioral measures. Clinical Journal of Pain 13: 60–73

Grunau RVE, Craig KD 1987 Pain expression in neonates: facial action and cry. Pain 28: 395–410

Grunau RVE, Johnston CC, Craig KD 1990 Neonatal facial and cry responses to invasive and non-invasive procedures. Pain 42: 295–305

Gunnar ME, Fisch RO, Korsvik S et al 1981 The effects of circumcision on serum cortisol and behaviour. Psychoneuroendocrinology 6: 269–275

Gunnar MR 1986 Human developmental phoneuroendocrinology: a review of research on neuroendocrine response to challenge and threat in infancy and childhood. In: Lamb M E, Brown S L, Rogoff B (eds) Advances in developmental psychology, vol 9. Eribaum, Hillsdale, New Jersey, pp 51–103

Harpin VA, Rutter N 1983 Making heel pricks less painful. Archives of Disease in Childhood 58: 2216–2228

Hester NK 1979 The pre-operational child's reaction to immunization. Nursing Research 28: 250–255

Hester NK, Foster R, Kristensen K 1990 Measurement of pain in children: generalizability and validity of the pain ladder and the poker chip tool. In: Tyler D C, Krane E J (eds) Advances in pain research and therapy: pediatric pain. Raven Press, New York, pp 79–84

Hester NO, Foster RL, Jordan Marsh M, Ely E, Vojir CP, Miller KL 1998 Putting pain measurement into clinical practice. In: Finley GA, McGrath PJ (eds) Measurement of pain in infants and children. Seattle: IASP Press, pp 179–198

Jay SM, Ozolins M, Elliott C et al 1983 Assessment of children's distress during painful medical procedures. Journal of Health Psychology 2: 133–147

Jeans ME 1983 Pain in children: a neglected area. In: Firestone P, McGrath P J, Feldman W (eds) Advances in behavioral medicine for children and adolescents. Erlbaum, Hillsdale, New Jersey, pp 23–38

Johnston CC 1989 Pain assessment and management in infants. Pediatrician 16: 16–23

Johnston CC, Strada ME 1986 Acute pain response in infants: a multidimensional description. Pain 24: 373–382

Johnston CC 1998 Psychometric issues in the measurement of pain. In: Finley GA, McGrath PJ (eds) Measurement of pain in infants and children. Seattle, IASP Press, pp 5–20

Katz ER, Kellerman J, Seigel SE 1980 Distress behavior in children with cancer undergoing medical procedures: developmental considerations. Journal of Consulting and Clinical Psychology 48: 356–365

Kelly MA, Finer NN 1984 Nasotracheal intubation in the neonate: Physiologic responses and effects of atropine and pancuronium. Journal of Pediatrics 105: 303–309

Kurylyszyn N, McGrath PJ, Cappelli M et al 1987 Children's drawings: what can they tell us about intensity of pain? Clinical Journal of Pain 2: 155–158

Kuttner L, Lepage T 1989 Faces scales for the assessment of pediatric pain: a critical review. Canadian Journal of Behavioral Science 2 1: 198–209

Lewis M, Thomas D 1990 Cortisol release in infants in response to inoculation. Child Development 61: 50–59

Lollar DJ, Smits SJ, Patterson DL 1982 Assessment of pediatric pain:an empirical perspective. Journal of Pediatric Psychology 7: 267–277

McGrath PA 1987 An assessment of children's pain: a review of behavioral, physiological and direct scaling techniques. Pain 3 1: 147–176

McGrath PA 1990 Pain in children: nature, assessment, treatment. Guilford, New York

McGrath PJ, Unruh AM 1987 Pain in children and adolescents. Elsevier, Amsterdam

McGrath PJ, Johnson G, Goodman JT et al 1985 Tle CHEOPS: a behavioral scale to measure post operative pain in children. In: Fields H L, Dubner R, Cervero F (eds) Advances in pain research and therapy. Raven Press, New York, pp 395–402

McGrath PJ, Hsu E, Cappelli M et al 1990 Pain from pediatric cancer: a survey of an outpatient oncology clinic. Journal of Psychosocial Oncology 8: 109–124

McGrath PJ, Mathews J, Pigeon H 1991 Assessment of pain in children: a systematic psychosocial model. In: Bond MR, Charlton K E, Woolf C J (eds) Proceedings of the Vth World Congress on Pain. Pain research and clinical management, vol 5. Elsevier, Amsterdam, pp 505–521

McGrath PJ, Rosmus C, Camfield C, Campbell MA et al 1998 Behaviour caregivers use to determine pain in non-verbal, cognitively impaired individuals. Developmental Medicine and Child Neurology 40: 340–343

McGraw MB 1945 The neuromuscular maturation of the human infant. Hafner, New York

Maunuksela EL, Olkkola KT, Korpela R 1987 Measurement of pain in children with self-reporting and behavioral assessment. Clinical Pharmacology and Therapeutics 42: 137–141

Melzack R 1975 The McGill pain questionnaire: major properties and scoring methods. Pain 1: 227–299

Merskey H 1996 Classifications of chronic pain: descriptions of chronic pain syndromes and definitions of pain terms. Pain (suppl 3) 249–252

Norden J, Hannallah R, Getson P et al 1991 Concurrent validation of an objective pain scale for infants and children. Anesthesiology 75: A934

O'Hara M, McGrath PJ, D'Astous et al 1987 Oral morphine versus injected meperidine (Demerol) for pain relief in children after orthopedic surgery. Journal of Pediatric Orthopedic Surgery 7: 78–82

Pigeon H, McGrath PJ, Lawrence J et al 1989 Nurses' perceptions of pain in the neonatal intensive care unit. Journal of Pain Symptom Management 4: 179–183

Porter F 1993 Pain assessment in children: infants. In: Schechter N L, Berde C B, Yaster M (eds) Pain in infants, children and adolescents. Williams & Wilkins, Baltimore, pp 87–96

Porter F, Miller JP, Marshall RE 1987 Local anaesthesia for painful medical procedures in sick newborns. Pediatric Research 21: 374

Rainville P, Duncan GH, Price DD, Carrier B et al 1997 Pain effect encoded in human anterior cingulate but not somatosensory cortex. Science 277: 968-971

Rawlings DJ, Miller PA, Engel RR 1980 The effect of circumcision on transcutaneous Po_2 in term infants. American Journal of Diseases of Children 13: 676–678

Reid GJ, Hebb JPO, McGrath PJ, Finley GA, Forward SP 1995 Clues parents use to assess postoperative pain in their children. Clinical Journal of Pain 11: 229–235

Richardson GM, McGrath P, Cunningham SJ et al 1983 Validity of the headache diary for children. Headache 23: 184–187

Ross DM, Ross SA 1988 Childhood pain: current issues, research and management. Urban & Schwarzenberg, Baltimore

Savedra MC, Tesler MD 1989 Assessing children's and adolescents' pain. Pediatrician 16: 24–29

Savedra MC, Tesler MD, Holzemer WL, Wilkie DJ, Ward JA 1990 Testing a tool to assess postoperative pediatric and adolescent pain. In: Tyler D C, Krane E J (eds) Advances in pain research and therapy: pediatric pain. Raven, New York, pp 85–93

Splinter WM, Smallman B, Rhine EJ, Komocar L 1994 The reliability and validity of a modified CHEOPS pain score. Anesthesia and Analgesia 78: s414 [abstract]

Stevens B 1990 Development and testing of a pediatric pain management sheet. Pediatric Nursing 16: 543–548

Stevens B 1998 Composite measures of pain. In: Finley GA, McGrath PJ (eds) Measurement of pain in infants and children. Seattle, IASP Press, pp 161–178

Stevens B, Johnston CC, Petryshen P, Taddio A 1996 Premature infant pain profile: development and initial validation. Clinical Journal of Pain 12: 13–22

Sweet SD, McGrath PJ 1998 Physiological measures of pain. In: Finley GA, McGrath PJ (eds) Measurement of pain in infants and children. Seattle, IASP Press, pp 59–81

Szyfelbein SK, Osgood PF, Carr DB 1985 The assessment of pain and plasma beta-endorphin immunoactivity in bùrned children. Pain 22: 173–182

Taddio A, Nulman I, Koren BS, Stevens B, Koren G 1995 A revised measure of acute pain in infants. Journal of Pain and Symptom Management 10(6): 456–463

Tarbell SE, Cohen T, Marsh JL 1992 Tle Toddler-Preschool

Postoperative Pain Scale: an observational scale for measuring postoperative pain in children aged 1–5. Preliminary report. Pain 50: 273–280

Thompson KI, Varni JW 1986 A developmental cognitive-biobehavioral approach to pediatric pain assessment. Pain 25: 283–296

Unruh A, McGrath PJ, Cunningham SJj et al 1983 Children's drawings of their pain. Pain 17: 385–392

Varni JW, Thompson KL, Hanson V 1987 The Varni/Thompson pediatric pain questionnaire. 1. Chronic musculo-skeletal pain in juvenile rheumatoid arthritis. Pain 28: 27–38

Walker LS, Greene JW 1991 The Functional Disability Inventory: measuring a neglected dimension of child health status. Journal of Pediatric Psychology 16: 39–58

Wall PD 1989 Introduction. In: Wall P D, Melzack R (eds) Textbook of pain, 2nd edn. Churchill Livingstone, Edinburgh, p 1–18

Whaley I, Wong DL 1987 Nursing care of infants and children, 3rd edn. Mosby, St. Louis

Wilkie DJ, Holzemer WL, Tesler MD et al 1990 Measuring pain quality: validity and reliability of children's and adolescents' pain language. Pain 41: 151–159

Williamson PS, Williamson ML 1983 Physiologic stress reduction by a local anesthetic during newborn circumcision. Pediatrics 71: 36–40

World Health Organization 1980 International Classification of Impairments, Disabilities and Handicaps. World Health Organization, Geneva

Studies of pain in human subjects

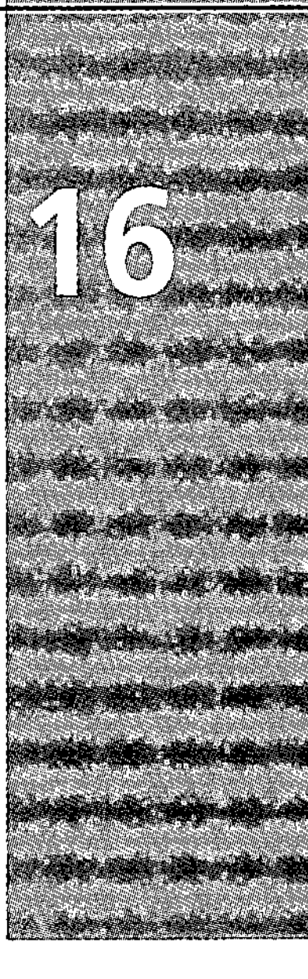

RICHARD H. GRACELY

SUMMARY

Studies of pain mechanisms in normal, pain-free individuals provide a degree of experimental control not found in studies of clinical pain, and open a window into the experience of pain that is not available in controlled studies with laboratory animals. The goals of pain studies in normal individuals can be divided into at least five overlapping categories: (1) measurement development and validation; (2) assessment of analgesic efficacy; (3) evaluation of the underlying mechanisms of pain and pain control; (4) studies of psychological variables and constructs involved in pain experience and pain report; (5) use of experimental methods as an adjunct to clinical pain assessment. This chapter will describe common methods of pain assessment in normal individuals and illustrate how these methods are used to achieve these five goals. Additional material may be found in several books, book chapters and reviews (Proacci et al 1979, Gracely 1979, 1980, 1984, 1985, 1991a,b, Melzack 1983, Bromm 1984, Chapman et al 1985, Price 1988, Chapman & Loeser 1989, Fernandes & Turk 1992, Price & Harkins 1992, Gracely & Naliboff 1996).

INTRODUCTION

METHODS OF EXPERIMENTAL PAIN STIMULATION

Studies of pain in normal man have one feature in common. An external stimulus must be applied to create the experience of pain. Once produced, this experience can be evaluated by a number of verbal, behavioural and physiological measures. Choice from the large number of combinations of stimulus and response methods ideally is based on properties of each method, and on the goals of the experiment.

The multiple properties of stimulation methods can be organized around a consideration of desirable traits. Beecher (1959) described 10 properties. An ideal pain stimulus should:

1. be applied to body parts exhibiting minimal neurohistological variation between individuals
2. provoke minimal tissue damage
3. show a relation between stimulus and pain intensity
4. provide information about discrimination between stimuli
5. result in repeatable stimulation without temporal interaction
6. be applied easily and produce a distinct pain sensation
7. allow a quantifiable determination of pain quality
8. be sensitive
9. show analgesic dose relation
10. be applicable to both man and animals.

Additional requirements have emerged as the scope of pain research broadened from the demonstration of experimental analgesia. These include:

11. rapid, controlled onset for studies in which the stimulus event must be timed precisely, such as studies using averaged measures of cortical or muscle activity
12. rapid termination is required for stimuli administered at fast rates, such as one every 1–3 seconds
13. natural stimulation that is experienced in everyday life or could be experienced by an animal in the wild
14. suppression of specific afferent activity
15. sensitisation of neurons and/or activation of processes involved with persistent pain states
16. demonstration of similar sensitivities in different individuals
17. excitation of a restricted group of primary afferents.

HEAT

Pain from radiant or contact heat is used extensively in laboratory studies. Objects heated by water baths or by contact thermodes can administer contact heat. Many modern contact thermodes use the Peltier principle in which a direct current through a semiconductor substrate results in a temperature increase on one side and a temperature decrease on the other. The magnitude and direction of stimulus change is proportional to the magnitude and polarity of the stimulating current (Kenshalo & Bergen 1975). Other contact stimulators use circulating fluid, or electrical heaters, which may be cooled by circulating fluid. A thermistor at the thermode–skin interface is used in the control circuitry to provide precise, controllable stimulation. The rate of change is relatively slow with the Peltier units and fast with electrically heated, fluid-cooled units.

Radiant heat is a classic stimulation method (Hardy et al 1952). An infrared light source is focused on a skin site usually blackened to improve absorption. Stimulus intensity is determined by lamp voltage and stimulus duration by a mechanical shutter. Modern adaptations use similar methodology (Montagne-Clavel & Oliveras 1996, Pertovaara et al 1996, Sternberg et al 1997) or employ a CO_2 or argon laser stimulus source (Meyer et al 1976, Ardent-Nielson 1990, Gibson et al 1991, Kunde & Treede 1993, Tarkka & Treede 1993, Xu et al 1995, Beydoun et al 1996, Svensson et al 1997). Measuring radiation emitted from the stimulus site can assess stimulus temperature.

COLD

Cold stimuli are administered by the contact stimulators described above, by administration of coolant sprays or by immersion in fluid. These methods can be divided into those delivering discrete stimuli and methods producing continuous stimulation. A common example of the latter is the cold pressor method in which pain is produced by immersion of a limb in very cold (0–4°C) water (Garcia de Jalon et al 1985, Casey et al 1996, Cleeland et al 1996, Sternberg et al 1997). It produces a severe pain that increases quickly and can be tolerated for only a few minutes.

ISCHAEMIA

Arresting blood flow in an arm by a tourniquet and exercising the hand produces ischaemia pain by isometric or isotonic contractions (Smith et al 1966, Fox et al 1979, Moore et al 1979, Sternbach 1983). This method produces a severe, continuous and increasing pain which can be tolerated usually for 20 minutes. It is similar to the cold pressor method and is still used extensively as a pain stimulus and as an experimental stressor.

MECHANICAL PRESSURE

Mechanical pressure is another classic method in which pain sensations are evoked by deformation of the skin by von Frey hairs and needles, by application of gross pressure to the fingers or mastoid process, by pinching (Drummond 1995a) and by distention of the oesophagus or bile duct (Beecher 1959, Sollenbohmer et al 1996). Present studies often use pressure to a finger joint (Whipple & Komisaruk 1985), muscles or deep tissue (Jensen et al 1988, 1992, Wolfe et al 1990, Lautenbacher 1994, Reid et al 1994). Distension of the oesophagus and colon are currently used in studies that include functional brain imaging. Mechanical methods produce a wide range of pain intensities and durations. However, stimulus control is difficult because tissue elasticity and stimulating area, rate and degree of compression can influence results (Wolff 1984, Jensen et al 1986, Greenspan & McGillis 1991).

ELECTRICAL

Electrical stimulation is applied to the skin (Tursky 1974, Bromm & Meier 1984), teeth (Fernandes de Lima et al 1982, Matthews et al 1974, McGrath et al 1983), muscle (Arendt-Nielsen et al 1997b) and stomach or intestine (Arendt-Nielsen et al 1997a), and directly to peripheral (Vallbo & Hagbarth 1968, Torebjork & Hallin 1970, Van Hees & Gybels 1972) and central (Davis et al 1995a, Lenz et al 1994a,b, 1995) neurons. Stimulus current is often used as the independent variable and current ranges for pulsed stimuli are usually 0–30 mA for the skin (depending on pulse density) and 0–100 μA for teeth.

CHEMICAL

Chemical stimulation has been applied to punctured or blistered skin, to the gastric mucosa or gastric ulcers, to the nasal mucosa, to teeth, to the eye or injected intramuscularly (Foster & Weston 1986, Kobal & Hummel 1990, Veerasarn & Stohler 1992, Steen and Reeh 1993, Gracely 1994, Nordin & Fagius 1995, Del Bianco et al 1996). Chemical stimuli activate unique pain processes not evoked by other methods. The degree of stimulus control is generally less, although the method developed by Kobal and his co-workers allows precise delivery of CO_2 to the nasal mucosa, resulting in orderly responses assessed by electrical brain activity (Kobal & Hummel 1990) or by psychophysical judgements (Anton et al 1992). New methods of manipulating tissue pH (Steen et al 1995, 1996) and iontophoresis of potassium (Humphries et al 1996) can also deliver controlled, repeatable chemical stimulation.

The use of topical or intradermal capsaicin, the pungent ingredient in chilli pepper, is a special case in which the primary pain of the application is of less interest than the phenomena of primary heat hyperalgesia and secondary mechanical allodynia and hyperalgesia (Simone et al 1989). The use of capsaicin and other topical agents such as mustard oil, experimental burns or freezing of the skin have been widely used to evoke a condition of central sensitization usually found only in the clinical condition of persistent pain (see Ch. 25). Capsaicin also desensitizes nociceptors, and is used both clinically and experimentally to block nociceptor activation.

PROPERTIES OF STIMULATION METHODS

The relation between research goals and types of experimental pain stimuli is shown in Table 16.1. It is apparent that specific pain-production methods satisfy some but not all criteria of an ideal pain stimulus. For example, electrical tooth pulp stimulation provides a controllable, repeatable sensation with minimal temporal effects, excites a relatively restricted group of primary afferent fibres, and exhibits a precise onset and termination. Thus, it is an ideal stimulus for many investigations. However, it is an inappropriate stimulus for studies that compare sensitivities between groups, because the range of intensities required to elicit pain sensations varies widely between individuals, probably as a consequence of individual tooth geometry. Electrical tooth pulp stimulation also bypasses receptor mechanisms to produce a synchronous barrage of afferent activity and resultant unnatural sensation. Electrical stimulation of the skin also produces unnatural sensations, but sensitivities are similar between individuals, permitting between-group comparisons. However, sensations evoked by electrical skin stimulation contain a powerful Aβ-mediated pressure-vibration component. The evoked sensation can be felt as an aversive intense stab or vibration without actually being painful. In studies of Aβ-mediated mechanical allodynia or tactile hypersensitivity, electrical stimuli can selectively activate Aβ afferents at detection-level stimulus intensities. In studies of nociceptive afferents, the contribution of Aβ stimulation may be reduced by stimulus preparation (Bromm & Meier 1984), or minimized by stimulating teeth. Although Aβ fibres have been identified in the tooth pulp, the majority of the afferent fibres are nociceptive afferents conducting in the Aδ- and C-fibre range (Dong et al 1985). The sensation evoked by electrical tooth pulp stimulation contains a measurable pre-pain component (Chatrian et al 1982, McGrath et al 1983) at near threshold levels. However, suprathreshold stimulation results in a distinct pain sensation without the significant non-pain qualities found with electrical skin stimulation.

Radiant heat stimulation produces similar sensations in different individuals, allowing comparison of pain sensitivities across groups. It excites a restricted group of primary afferents and onset is rapid. Termination is slow, however, and thus this method is less appropriate for studies in which stimulation must be repeated quickly. Contact heat stimulation has a fast termination and can be used for such studies. It excites a restricted group of primary afferent fibres but also activates slowly adapting mechanoreceptors. Laser stimulation contains all the advantages of a radiant source. The return to baseline temperature is faster due to the small area stimulated. Laser stimuli have been used to identify C-fibre-mediated brain potentials (Bromm & Treede 1987). This small area may not be adequate for studies

Table 16.1 Properties of experimental pain stimulation methods

Requirement	*Electrical*		*Thermal*		*Pressure*	*Ischaemic*	*Cold pressure*	*Chemical*
	Pulp	*Skin*	*Contact*	*Radiation*				
Fast onset	*	*	?	*	?			?
Fast offset	*	*	*					
Natural			*	*	*	*	*	*
Repeatable	*	*						?
Objective		*	*	*	?	?	?	?
Severe, constant	?	?	?	?	?	*	*	*
Few afferents	*		*	*				*

Note: Stimulation requirements are shown for electrical tooth pulp and electrical skin stimulation, thermal stimulation by contact or radiant heat, pressure stimulation, ischaemic pain produced by exercising a limb in which circulation has been occluded by a tourniquet, cold pressor stimulation achieved by immersion of a limb in cold water, and chemical stimulation of the skin, teeth or mucosa. *Indicate that the method satisfies the requirement ?Indicate that the method may satisfy the requirement under specific conditions.

of summation or warmth, which require variable or large surface stimulation. The chemical methods range from very controllable (CO_2 applied to nasal mucosa), to moderately (pH buffers) and minimally controllable (application of capsaicin or mustard oil). Stimulation is natural, and in the case of capsaicin or mustard oil is capable of mimicking many of the significant features of a clinical syndrome.

SUBJECTIVE MEASURES: PAIN PSYCHOPHYSICS

SINGLE-POINT MEASURES SUCH AS THRESHOLD AND TOLERANCE

The 'pain threshold' is an ubiquitous term in the lay person's conception of pain sensitivity. It is used to describe general pain sensitivity and its use is associated with the concept of variability between different individuals; for example, one individual may have a 'high threshold' to pain in relation to other individuals. This high threshold implies a difference in the nervous system such that it takes extra input for such a person to feel pain, and greater input to feel the same level of pain as a person with a more normal threshold. Unfortunately, the threshold is also associated with the labels chosen to describe the sensation processed by the nervous system. Minimal pain reports can represent either an insensitive nervous system or a stoical reporting style in which the label 'painful' is attached to a more intense sensation. One elusive goal in pain measurement is the assessment of pain sensitivity independent of pain labelling behaviour; that is, the assessment of subjective pain without the biases which influence verbal report.

The pain threshold is defined as the minimum amount of stimulation that reliably evokes a report of pain. Pain tolerance is similarly defined as the time that a continuous stimulus is endured, or the maximally tolerated stimulus intensity. Threshold and tolerance measures are attractive because of their simplicity for both the administrator and the subject. In addition, the response is expressed in physical units of stimulus intensity or time, avoiding the subjectivity of a psychological scale of pain. These methods are useful for many measurement situations, especially for the evaluation of sensory function in the clinic. However, these methods are problematical in a number of research scenarios. Both threshold and tolerance are single measures usually confounded with time or increasing intensity. A subject can easily be biased to respond sooner or later, or to a lower or higher intensity. Unlike determination of sensory thresholds in which a subject must choose between the presence or absence of sensation, the pain threshold in most cases is a judgement about the quality of a sensation that is always present. Pain thresholds are thus more subjective, and the judgement can be made on the basis of irrelevant stimulus features. Tolerance measures share the same problem. In addition, tolerance of a painful stimulus has been shown to be related to a separate endurance factor which is not associated with sensory intensity (Wolff 1971, Timmermans & Sternbach 1974, Cleeland et al 1996). These single-point measures are very useful, if not essential, in a number of measurement situations. However, these methods only assess the extremes of the perceptual pain range. They provide little information about levels of pain that are observed clinically and that can be produced by experimental methods.

A number of psychophysical methods can be used to assess the range of pain sensation from threshold to pain tolerance. Some consist of an ascending series and are vulnerable to the same biases which can affect ascending measures of threshold or tolerance. More sophisticated methods control many of these biases. The domain of suprathreshold pain measures can be divided into three classes:

1. Methods that treat pain as a single dimension and that assess the range from pain threshold to intense pain levels.
2. Separation of the single dimension of pain into two dimensions of sensory intensity and unpleasantness.
3. Multidimensional assessment of the many attributes of pain sensation including its intensive, qualitative and aversive aspects.

PAIN AS A SINGLE DIMENSION

Most human research studies assess 'pain', treating the experience as single dimension varying in magnitude, much like varying the sound level by turning the volume knob on a radio. Both classical threshold and suprathreshold measures treat pain as a single dimension. The following sections briefly describe these procedures.

Pain threshold

The pain threshold can be determined by the classical (Engen 1971a) Method of Limits which administers ascending and descending trials, the Method of Adjustment in which the subject adjusts stimulus intensity, and the Method of Constant Stimuli in which a set of fixed stimuli are presented several times in a random sequence (e.g., Chen et al 1996). The result of each method is a specific magnitude of stimulus intensity which is always an approximation because, as noted above, the pain threshold is not a discrete event but rather a probability function. The subjective criteria used to attach the label of 'pain' to a specific sensation varies between, and within, individuals.

There have been simple and sophisticated applications of threshold methodology to pain assessment. The simplest methods use a modification of the Method of Limits. A good example is the Marstock method described by Fruhstorfer et al (1976). A thermal stimulus slowly increases or decreases from a neutral baseline and subjects indicate either warm or cool detection threshold, or heat or cold pain threshold, by a button press which also either returns the stimulus to baseline or initiates a stimulus excursion in the opposite direction. Although this method lacks rudimentary psychophysical controls, it is very adequate for the large changes in threshold observed in many clinical conditions and, when appropriate, it efficiently describes altered thermal sensibility.

In striking contrast to the detection of large changes by the simple Marstock method, other procedures use sophisticated judgement models to evaluate pain scaling behaviour. The powerful methods of Sensory Decision Theory (SDT) have been applied both to the analysis of pain thresholds and to category responses of suprathreshold pain sensations. This method yields not one but two parameters. The beta, or response criterion, parameter is a direct measure of the subjective criteria used to attach the label of pain. For example, the criteria may be stoical, labelling only clearly painful (or greater) sensations as pain. The second SDT parameter (classically called d′) is a measure of discrimination, the ability to distinguish between two stimuli. At first glance, it seems like the application of this method could achieve the elusive goal of separating pain sensitivity from pain reporting behaviour. A number of studies investigated this goal (see Clark & Yang 1983). This research identified a number of issues and focused interest on pain measurement (Chapman 1977, Rollman 1977). One issue is the role of extraneous components of discrimination, because measures such as d′ are influenced by sensory variability and variability in choosing labels to describe sensations (Coppola & Gracely 1983). Changes in discrimination do not necessarily indicate analgesia, although unchanged discrimination is strong evidence that pain sensitivity has not changed (Clark & Clark 1980). Another issue is the interpretation of changes in response criterion. These can represent changes in labelling behaviour, or they can represent changes in other aspects of the sensation, such as unpleasantness or painfulness, that do not alter discrimination. In these situations, a change in this response parameter could represent analgesia.

The method of two alternative forced choice (2AFC) is another example of a sophisticated method that provides a measure of discrimination that is not influenced by the subject's response criterion. In this method, a stimulus is presented at one of two locations or in one of two temporal intervals during each trial, and the subject must indicate the correct location or interval. The proportion of correct responses above the 50% level that would be achieved by chance measures discrimination. This discrimination measure corresponds to the SDT parameter. However there is no corresponding SDT response criterion measure with 2AFC. The 2AFC method yields bias-free measures of discrimination but does not indicate the magnitude or direction of bias.

The precision of SDT or 2AFC is gained at the expense of extended time and increased number of stimuli. These increased requirements may be excessive due to the nature of the stimulus (very painful, prolonged) or of the subject (chronic pain patient). Other sophisticated methods have been applied to pain threshold evaluation that reduce the amount of stimulation required. The most notable are referred to as adaptive, staircase or stimulus titration procedures. Based on simple staircase rules, these methods were initially applied to the analysis of visual thresholds (Cornsweet 1962). Applications to pain expanded the response range to encompass both threshold and suprathreshold assessment, and these methods are included in the discussion of suprathreshold pain measures.

Scaling suprathreshold pain sensation: response-dependent methods

Tolerance measures and the threshold procedures described above can be considered to be 'stimulus-dependent' methods, because the dependent variable is an amount of stimulus intensity (or time) corresponding to a fixed response of pain threshold. By contrast, many of the suprathreshold scaling procedures can be classified as 'response-dependent' methods. These methods deliver a series of discrete stimuli of varying but fixed intensity in random sequence. The dependent variable is some measure of subjective response.

These response-dependent measures are more complex than methods that assess threshold or tolerance by an ascending series. However, these methods minimize the numerous biases associated with ascending methods discussed above. The presentation of randomized stimulus sequences avoids confounds associated with time or order. The difference in intensities should be small enough to create confusion between adjacent stimulus intensities, forcing choices based on judgements of sensation and not identification of specific stimulus intensities (e.g., that is the second stimulus from the bottom that I call '4'). As a further advantage, these methods deliver sensations over the entire perceptual range and do not focus only on the bottom, threshold level or the top, tolerance region.

These methods assume that subjects can meaningfully quantify the evoked sensation on a psychological scale of pain magnitude. These response-dependent methods vary both in the type of response and in analysis of these responses. Common responses include both discrete numerical (1–10) or verbal (mild, moderate, severe) categorical scales, and continuous response dimensions such as the visual analogue scale (VAS), and the psychophysical scaling techniques of magnitude estimation and cross-modality matching.

Simple category scales such as the four-point 'none, mild, moderate and severe' or the common 1–10 numerical scale can be scored in several ways. The simplest, the Method of Equal Appearing Intervals, assigns successive integers to verbal categories or uses numerical categories directly (Engen 1971b). The more complex Method of Successive Categories (Thurstone 1959) determines specific category values depending on the proportions of responses to each stimulus intensity. An additional approach (described below) determines specific numerical values for each category in a separate session. Subjects use several types of scaling methods to quantify the magnitude implied by each response category.

Category scales have been the standard in clinical trials and in many pain studies, and their reliability and validity have been demonstrated repeatedly with limited four-point scales of pain or pain relief. Issues include the resolution provided by a limited number of categories, and a number of biases associated with the limits of the available categories described below in the discussion of bounded scales. In addition, the response is easily remembered, confounding measures of repeat reliability or studies of pain memory.

The VAS consists usually of a 10-cm line labelled at the anchor points with 'no pain' and 'most intense pain imaginable' or similar descriptions. Subjects indicate their pain magnitude by marking the line at the appropriate point. The ease of administration and scoring has contributed to the widespread use of this method. The lack of a distinct response category avoids the confounds of remembering discrete responses. The validity of VASs of experimentally evoked pain sensations has been demonstrated in a number of studies (Price et al 1983, Price 1988). The reliability of the VAS has been assessed recently and found to be less than satisfactory (Yarnitsky et al 1996). However, in the absence of comparable studies with other scales, it is not possible to establish relative reliability or to distinguish whether the observed variability is due to the VAS or is a property of individuals that is accurately assessed with the VAS or other scales.

Both VAS and category scales are 'bounded', they provide a limited range of measurement confined by fixed end points. When using these scales to describe a range of painful stimuli, subjects typically spread out their responses to cover the entire range of possible responses. In the extreme case, this tendency results in the same response for any stimulus set. In most cases it makes VAS, category and other bounded scales very sensitive to stimulus range, spacing and frequency (Beck & Shaw 1965, Parducci 1974). This effect would tend to reduce the sensitivity of a scale to a pain-control intervention, because subjects would use the same responses before and after the manipulation. This tendency would be most problematical in repeated measures associated with delivering painful stimuli to normal individuals, and theoretically less of a problem in clinical assessment. This effect has been observed in pain scaling studies but not investigated in any detail (Gracely et al 1984). Despite these theoretical limitations, VASs have been used successfully for assessment of the sensory intensity and unpleasantness of experimental pain sensations, and for the evaluation of the mechanisms and efficacy of both pharmacological and non-pharmacological interventions (Price 1988, Price & Harkins 1992). Use of longer VASs (Price 1988) and specific instructions appear to avoid many of the problems of bounded scales.

Many modern psychophysical scaling methods avoid the problem of bounded scales by the use of scales with an unbounded response range. The most widely used example is the method of Magnitude Estimation (e.g., Beydoun et al 1996), in which subjects describe the magnitude of the sensation evoked by the first stimulus with a number and then assign numbers to subsequent stimuli in proportion to this judgement (Engen 1971b). If the second sensation is judged to be twice as great as the first, the number given is twice that made to the first sensation. The first stimulus may be either arbitrary or fixed (the standard), and the first response value may be either arbitrary or fixed (the modulus). These methods theoretically result in ratio scales with a true zero point that allows multiplicative statements such as 'the pain is one third of what it was before the analgesic'. Price and colleagues have provided evidence that VASs also provide ratio-level measurement (Price 1988). Although the ratio properties of these various methods have been debated in both the psychophysical and pain literature (Gracely & Dubner 1981), these methods at least provide information about the spacing between response categories not found in conventional categorical scales. They also may be less sensitive to the biases associated with the bounded response range of VAS and category scales.

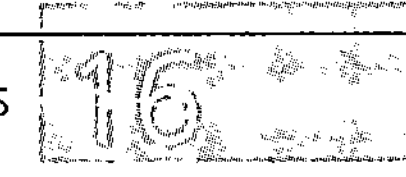

Ratio scaling methods have been used to assess pain magnitude, including variations in which the response is another adjustable stimulus modality (Tursky 1976, Gracely et al 1978a), the response is made to both painful and non-painful stimulus modalities (Duncan et al 1988), or various responses are made to the labels in a pain category scale, which determine the values used in the analysis of the scale when it is applied to pain measurement (Gracely et al 1978a,b, 1979). Quantification of category values allows random presentation of response choices, which requires a cognitive task that is uniquely different from other methods, which require matching to a response space. Randomized response lists force responses based on the meaning of the descriptor rather than its spatial location in a list. Although possibly difficult for the subject, this method may be a particularly effective means of minimizing rating biases (e.g., spreading responses over the scale) found with bounded spatial scales. Forcing choices based on meaning may facilitate the discrimination of different pain dimensions discussed below.

In addition to randomization, quantified category values permit the use of hybrid scales that combine verbal and VAS scales into graphic rating scales, which place descriptors in appropriate locations on an analogue continuum (Gracely et al 1978a, Gracely 1991a, Munakata et al 1997, Naliboff et al 1997). These and VAS scales have been incorporated into automated systems that can provide continuous measures of a pain sensation over time. Such measures can indicate pathological states, such as abnormally prolonged sensations, which are not evaluated by ordinary scaling methods (Cooper et al 1986, Gracely 1991a, Graven-Nielsen et al 1997). Additional hybrid scales include descriptors spaced appropriately over a 0–20 numerical category scale, allowing measurement without the task demands of marking a line. Such scales are useful for telephone evaluations and for studies such as brain imaging in which a motor response is difficult or undesirable (Coghill & Gracely 1996, Hostetter & Gracely 1997).

Scaling methods which require greater cognitive demands have been applied to pain assessment. Two similar methods, Functional Measurement and Conjoint Measurement, require a single response to not one stimulus, but rather to an integrated impression of two or more stimuli. These stimuli can both be painful (Jones 1980, Heft & Parker 1984) or subjects can respond to a combination of pain evoked by somatosensory stimulation and either pain implied by a verbal descriptor (Gracely & Wolskee 1983) or the discomfort of an aversive tone (Algom et al 1986). These stimulus-integration methods provide more information than that available from single-stimulus, single-response designs. They simultaneously evaluate subjective magnitude and, in addition, evaluate each subject's ability to perform the scaling task.

Scaling suprathreshold pain sensation: stimulus-dependent methods

Stimulus-dependent methods are used here to describe procedures that use a physical measure of the stimulus as a dependent measure. Staircase methods, commonly used to measure pain threshold, have been adapted to assess suprathreshold pain sensation. In these methods, an interactive computer program continuously adjusts the intensity of stimuli so that some fall within specific response categories such as 'mild' and 'moderate' or 'moderate' and 'intense'. The algorithm for this adjustment can be based on either staircase rules (Gracely 1988, Gracely et al 1988, Gracely & Gaughan 1991, Greenspan & Winfield 1992, Messinides & Naliboff 1992) or probability estimates (Duncan et al 1992). These stimulus-dependent scaling procedures may possess several advantages over commonly used response-dependent scales; they automatically equalize the psychological range of stimulus-evoked sensations, ensuring that all subjects receive a similar sensory experience. Equalization after administration of an analgesic intervention minimizes extraneous cues (e.g., reduced stimulus range) that perception has been altered. The response is expressed in units of stimulus intensity, allowing comparison of effects across different experiments.

This brief description of unidimensional pain measurement indicates how conventional measures like magnitude estimation, or procedures such as randomized verbal descriptors, magnitude-matching or stimulus-dependent scaling methods, are adapted to the measurement of suprathreshold pain magnitude. These methods may control for specific biases like those associated with spreading responses to cover the range of a scale. However, they condense the experience of pain into a single dimension of pain magnitude. They do not assess the relevant dimensions of the experience.

DUAL DIMENSIONS OF SENSORY INTENSITY AND UNPLEASANTNESS

The dual nature of pain has been recognized throughout philosophical and scientific history. Pain is both a somatic sensation and a powerful feeling state which evokes behaviours that minimize bodily harm and promote healing (Wall 1979). Single measures of pain magnitude blur this distinction and create confusion, because the underlying meaning of an expressed pain magnitude is not known.

This confusion may be minimized by scales that essentially ask, 'how intense is your sensation, and how much does it bother you?' There is a precedent for such scales, because the sensation of pain is not uniquely endowed with motivational characteristics. A sensory intensity and a feeling state also can characterize the chemical senses (taste, olfaction) and the thermal senses (warm, cool). Studies with these modalities have demonstrated different psychophysical functions for scales of sensory intensity and 'hedonic' scales of pleasantness-unpleasantness. In addition, manipulation of internal state (core temperature, hunger) has been shown to shift the hedonic responses without altering judgements of sensory intensity (Gracely et al 1978b).

The intensity and hedonic component (unpleasantness) of pain have been assessed by a number of scaling methods. In some cases, different types of scales were used to measure the two dimensions. The results of such studies must be interpreted with caution because these studies confound the different dimensions with the type of scale, thus the results could be due to method variance and not to a differential effect of pain dimension (Gracely et al 1978b).

Verbal category scales with words descriptive of each dimension have distinguished between pain intensity and unpleasantness in a number of situations (Tursky 1976, Gracely et al 1978a, Luu et al 1988, Coghill & Gracely 1996, Hostetter & Gracely 1997). The use of language specific to a dimension is assumed to facilitate the discrimination of these dimensions, although the commonly used VAS and other similar scales have also distinguished between pain intensity and unpleasantness. The results of several studies (Price 1988) suggest that the combination of instructions to the subject and the labels on a VAS ('the most intense pain sensation imaginable', 'the most unpleasant feeling imaginable') are sufficient for the discrimination of intensity and unpleasantness. These results suggest that the increased complexity of verbal methods is not needed, and problems of verbal methods, such as use with different languages, can be avoided by using VASs. On the other hand, studies which have directly compared verbal and VASs have shown greater discriminative power with the verbal methods (Gracely et al 1978b, Gracely 1979, Duncan et al 1989). The ability of subjects to describe these dimensions with each method, and the role of instructions and training, are obvious topics for future research.

The non-sensory aspect of pain experience has been termed the reaction component, the emotional component, the affective component, the evaluative component, and other terms such as discomfort, distress and suffering. The number and structure of these components has not been firmly established, although recent proposals included both an immediate unpleasantness component similar to the feelings associated with other senses, and a secondary affective component which includes emotions and feelings of distress mediated through cognitive appraisals (Wade et al 1990, Price & Harkins 1992, Gracely 1996). These types of studies, and those described in the next section, should continue to clarify the feeling and emotional components of pain sensation.

Two points are relevant in comparisons of dual scales of sensory intensity and unpleasantness to the multidimensional scales and scaling methods described below. Firstly, separate scales of sensory intensity and unpleasantness, and derivatives of such scales, assess dimensions common to all types of pain, whether chronic, acute or experimental. These scales provide a common language which is useful in describing and comparing the variety of pain experience. By contrast, multidimensional scales emphasize the differences between pain sensation, the distinguishing features which separate various pain syndromes. Secondly, sensory intensity and unpleasantness scales are a priori scales in the sense that they assume two significant dimensions of pain. By contrast, multidimensional methods empirically determine the number and character of relevant dimensions. They do not make a priori assumptions about the structure of pain experience.

MULTIPLE PAIN DIMENSIONS

Our own experience verifies the variety of pain qualities. Pain can be deep or superficial, pricking, burning, throbbing, aching or shooting. This breadth of pain experience is evaluated in normal individuals by three types of studies:

1. Multidimensional scaling of experimentally evoked pain sensation to determine scale dimensions.
2. Multidimensional scaling of verbal descriptor items to construct a scale or verify the structure of an existing scale.
3. Use of existing scales to assess experimentally evoked pain sensations.

Multidimensional scaling of sensations evoked by electrical or thermal stimulation (Clark et al 1986, Janal et al 1993) provides examples of the first type. In these studies, similarity judgements of stimulus pairs resulted in a primary dimension of sensory intensity and secondary dimensions of painfulness, or of frequency when the frequency of the stimulus was varied (Clark et al 1986, Janal et al 1991, 1993).

Examples of the second type include several studies that have examined the structure of the McGill Pain

Questionnaire (MPQ), which is the most widely-used multidimensional instrument. Melzack and Katz discuss this instrument and related studies in Chapter 17. The questionnaire was developed from a study by Melzack and Torgerson (1971) in which a large number of pain descriptors were classified into 20 categories describing sensory qualities, affective qualities and an evaluative dimension. A total of 78 descriptors appear in the present instrument, with two to six descriptors per category. Subsequent studies have replicated this method, or derived a structure by use of multidimensional scaling methods (Reading et al 1982, Kwilosz et al 1983, Boureau & Paquette 1988). Results of these experiments confirm the two main dimensions of sensory intensity and affect/unpleasantness, but have resulted in different category assignments and variations in the overall organizational scheme of hierarchical categories (Kwilosz et al 1983). The most recent and extensive of these studies has been performed by Torgerson and colleagues (1988), who have developed the Ideal Type Model which rates each descriptor on an intensity continuum and, in addition, quantifies 'quality' in terms of a number of primary ideal qualities or types. The number of primary qualities and the degree to which each of them contribute to a specific descriptor are specified, much like the primary components of a colour mixture. The MPQ, by contrast, assigns only one quality to each descriptor. A review of all of these descriptor structures reveals many commonalties. Pain sensation is described by thermal qualities, by temporal patterning, by location or changing location (superficial or deep, spreading, moving) and by a series of mechanical qualities such as punctate, traction and compression pressure. New analyses have made finer distinctions. For example, the Ideal Type Model places 'pricking' and 'stabbing' in a class separate from 'drilling' and 'boring', distinguished by the rotational character of the latter class. The most variability appears in the affective components of pain, with dimensions that describe unpleasantness, suffering, fear, autonomic reactions and fatigue. A more extensive treatment of these dimensions can be found in the references and in Chapter 17.

The third class uses multidimensional scales to assess the magnitude and quality of pain sensations produced by experimental stimulation. Few such studies have been performed because these scales are used predominantly in clinical evaluations. An early study compared the responses of both patients and normal subjects receiving painful electrical skin stimulation (Crockett et al 1977). A factor analysis identified five common factors, emphasizing the utility of assessing common dimensions of experimental and clinical pain. Another experiment by Klepac et al (1981) assessed high or low levels of either cold pressor pain or electrical tooth pulp pain in a 2 × 2 factorial design. Overall intensity scores differentiated the two types of stimulation, which also resulted in qualitatively different responses. The authors noted the problems of statistically evaluating quality differences by chi square analyses and single-item tests.

In summary, validated methods have been developed to assess one, two and more dimensions of pain experience. What should an investigator do? The answer again depends on the experimental question. Naliboff (Gracely & Naliboff 1996) identified four criteria for increasing the number of dimensions:

> *A multidimensional system may increase utility if it: 1) Leads to an increase in accuracy of pain reports. If for example a rating of intensity and affect misses or blurs critical aspects of a pain sensation then a patient or subject's pain may change due to treatment or experimental manipulation and this change could be missed. This is essentially an issue of reliability. 2) Increases greater diagnostic sensitivity. If for example the amount of prickliness of a pain is a clear marker of certain types of tissue pathology then assessment of only sensory and affective intensity (painfulness) may yield poorer diagnostic discrimination. Similarly, pain ratings with very unusual patterns of multidimensional ratings might indicate malingering or confusion. 3) Increases communication about pain, and therefore empathy with patients suffering, and 4) improves the correspondence between neurophysiological and psychological data. With the dramatic increase in sensitivity in brain imaging we might expect to see more specificity in terms of which brain areas correspond to which pain dimensions.*

Further choices between double and multiple dimensions must be made in the context of the measurement situation. As noted above, the multidimensional methods do not make assumptions about the number or kind of significant dimensions. However, the advantage of this approach over the dual dimension approach is not clear. The discussion of the above criteria also noted that the goal of multidimensional methods is to discover the salient dimensions, and that the dual dimension methods are based on the results of such discoveries (Gracely & Naliboff 1996).

NON-VERBAL MEASURES

Concerns about the reliability and validity of verbal judgements have motivated the development of physiological and behavioural 'objective measures' of pain magnitude that should be relatively insensitive to biasing factors and the psychological demands associated with requests for introspective reports (Craig & Prkachin 1983). There are also instances in which such measures are necessary, such as pain assessment in animals and in infants or in adults with poorly developed language skills.

Although arguments have been made for exclusive use of non-verbal methods, these procedures also can be influenced by extraneous factors. In addition, non-verbal methods lack the face validity of verbal report. They use similarity to verbal report to establish concurrent validity, suggesting that verbal measures are preferable if available. Generally, arguments for the superiority of one method over another often reflect the tendency of research laboratories to specialize in a single measurement method. The resulting differences have sparked lively debates, identified important measurement flaws, and generally improved the technology of pain assessment. These is a growing consensus that, in most situations, effective pain assessment may ultimately result from an approach that integrates information from these separate, complementary sources of information (Luu et al 1988, Cleeland 1989, Craig 1989, Boureau et al 1991, Gracely 1992, Kiernan et al 1995).

BEHAVIOURAL MEASURES

It is well known that pain elicits stereotypical behaviours in both man and animals. Grimace, vocalization, licking, limping and rubbing are often elicited by a painful stimulus. Both these naturally occurring reactions and trained operant behaviours (such as manipulating a bar to escape a painful stimulus) have been used to assess the magnitude of stimulus-evoked pain sensation. Many have been used more extensively for the assessment of clinical pain syndromes (Keefe & Block 1982, Craig & Prkachin 1983, Keefe & Dolan 1986, McDanial et al 1986). Recent exceptions include studies of facial expression evoked by experimental stimulation (Craig & Patrick 1985, Patrick et al 1986) or analysis of pain expressions from photographs (LeReshe 1982).

The behavioural measure of reaction time latency to pain produced by a contact thermode has been shown to be monotonically related to stimulus intensity, permitting the use of reaction time, in controlled conditions, as a measure of pain magnitude (Kenshalo et al 1989, Montagne-Clavel & Oliveras 1996, Pertovaara et al 1996).

PHYSIOLOGICAL MEASURES

The search for a physiological pain measure more objective than verbal report is not new. Previous studies have evaluated autonomic measures such as heart rate, skin conductance and temperature and correlated these measures with the magnitude of painful stimulation. Although influenced by painful stimulation, these responses habituated quickly and responded non-specifically to non-painful stressing or novel stimulation (Bromm & Scharein 1982). Recently, a number of studies have evaluated autonomic measures of vasodilatation (Drummond 1995a, Del Bianco et al 1996, Mageral & Treede 1996), vasoconstriction (Nordin & Fagius 1995) and lacrimation (Drummond 1995a). The results show evidence for both association and disassociation. In the cases of association the specificity of the response to pain is not yet known.

Progressing from the periphery to the brain, the bulk of studies of physiological consequences of pain stimulation have examined microneurographical recording of primary afferent activity, spinal reflexes, evoked cortical activity, recording and stimulation of thalamus and brain during neurosurgical procedures, and functional brain imaging.

Microneurography

Neurophysiological recording methods commonly employed in animal research have been used to investigate peripheral mechanisms in unanaesthetized normal volunteers (Vallbo & Hagbarth 1968). Human microneurography is a powerful tool which can:

1. Compare intervening primary afferent activity to both the evoking stimulus and the resulting sensation.
2. Stimulate through the recording electrode and evaluate the resulting sensation and projected sensory field (location of evoked pain sensation).

These techniques can identify all classes of primary afferent fibres, and have verified the association of specific sensations with the type of fibre stimulated (Torebjörk & Hallin 1970, Van Hees & Gybels 1972, Torebjörk et al 1992, Campero et al 1996, Marchettini et al 1996, Hallin & Wu 1998).

Reflexes

Spinal reflex measures record the electromyogram (EMG) response to a brief intense stimulus. Several measures of reflex activity, such as the H reflex, the nociceptive (RIII) reflex and the blink reflex have been investigated in human subjects. The results of several studies suggest that these reflexes can serve as a physiological correlate of subjective pain. These measures have been attenuated by TENS and by opiates such as morphine, have demonstrated stress-produced changes antagonized by naloxone, and have been correlated with other physiological parameters such as cerebral evoked potentials or concentration of administered analgesics, anaesthetics or circulating opioids (Willer 1977, Bromm & Treede 1980, Willer & Bussel 1980, Willer et al 1981, 1982, Facchinetti et al 1984, Chan & Tsang 1985, Willer 1985, McMillan & Moudy 1986, DeBroucker et al 1989, Dowman 1991, Thurauf et al 1993, Petersen-Felix et al 1995, 1996, Danziger et al 1998a,b, Piquet et al 1998). The nociceptive reflex has also been observed to be suppressed in clinical conditions such as tension headache (Langemark et al 1993) and has been used successfully as a marker of central summation in a number of studies (Andersen et al 1994, 1995a, Arendt-Nielsen et al 1994).

These reflex measures have been shown to correlate with verbal report and serve as a marker for nociceptive threshold when compared to the results of the compound action potential (Dowman 1993). However, the use of the nociceptive reflex as a surrogate for verbal pain report is challenged by a number of recent studies that have demonstrated non-linear relationships at high intensities of radiant heat stimuli (Campbell et al 1991), or dissociation of reflex and subjective measures either between patient and pain-free volunteers (Boureau et al 1991), or within subjects under conditions such as cyclic movements (Andersen et al 1995b), following cordotomy (Garcia-Larrea et al 1993) or administration of low doses of morphine (Luu et al 1988). These dissociations do not necessarily limit the utility of these measures. They suggest that these reflex measures may parallel verbal report under certain restricted conditions. In other cases, nociceptive reflexes may be complementary, providing an informative tool for the analysis of mechanisms, separating spinal from peripheral and supraspinal processes. For example, several studies have compared the relative impact of interventions on subjective report and on various physiological measures, including nociceptive reflexes and the method of cortical evoked potentials described below. Arendt-Nielsen et al (1990) found that suggestions of analgesia and hyperaesthesia produced corresponding changes in both subjective ratings and cortical evoked potentials evoked by a laser stimulus in highly susceptible subjects, indicating that hypnotic analgesia may be mediated by attenuation at the spinal level. However, Meier et al (1993) found that suggestions of either analgesia or hyperaesthesia produced expected changes in subjective ratings made to electrocutaneous stimuli in highly susceptible subjects, but no change in evoked potentials. Based on scores on the McGill Pain Questionnaire (MPQ), the authors concluded that the hypnotic effect was thus primarily on the unpleasantness component of pain assessed by these measures and not on the sensory dimension assessed either by the evoked potentials or the sensory dimensions of the MPQ. This supraspinal effect was also observed in a recent study by Kiernan et al (1995), who found independent attenuation of sensory intensity and unpleasantness over and above that indicated by the measured reduction in nociceptive reflex. These results suggest that a combination of methods can independently assess analgesic processing at spinal and supraspinal levels (Gracely 1995, Kiernan et al 1995). However, this concept is challenged by a recent study in which subjective ratings and evoked cortical potentials in individual subjects were reduced after hypnosis, while the nociceptive reflex was either strongly inhibited or facilitated (Danziger et al 1998a). This result can be interpreted in a number of ways, including the concepts that the nociceptive reflex may not always indicate the status of spinal nociceptive inhibition or that supraspinal influences can completely overwhelm the consequences of spinal modulation.

Supraspinal processing

There is an increasing growth in both the methods used to assess supraspinal processing and in the knowledge gained from these methods. As an example, the last edition of this textbook described two studies using positron emission tomography (PET), and the method of functional magnetic resonance imaging (fMRI) was in the developmental stages and had not been applied to pain. Since that time PET has become a mature technology with dozens of applications to pain, and fMRI pain studies are emerging. This section will briefly describe the methods and findings of the rapidly expanding field of physiological assessment of suprathreshold painful processing that includes these and other methods.

Cortical evoked potentials

Application of a temporally controlled stimulus can evoke a small, synchronized response in the electroencephalogram (EEG) embedded in non-synchronized (noise) EEG activity. Averaging multiple trials reduces the influence of random non-synchronized activity, revealing a waveform of about 1s duration that can be characterized by the amplitude and latency of positive and negative peaks. Early, short-latency components of the waveform have been associated with sensory components of pain input, while later components have been associated with the perceptual processing of these inputs. Measures of cortical evoked potentials have been studied extensively and under certain conditions correlate with both stimulus intensity and verbal report (Fernandes de Lima et al 1982, Chudler & Dong 1983, Hill & Chapman 1989). In the past 5 years a large number of studies have used cortical potentials evoked by electrical or laser stimulation to assess a number of research goals. Many of these have examined the waveform and topography of evoked responses to stimuli applied to various locations, including comparisons of the hand and foot (Xu et al 1995), skin and muscle (Svensson et al 1997), and anus and genitalia (Leroi et al 1997). Additional studies have assessed the topography of trigeminal stimulation (Bromm & Chen 1995) and independent stimulation of thickly (Aβ) and thinly (Aδ) myelinated fibres (Kunde & Treede 1993). Source analysis can locate areas of activation that are also found in functional imaging studies, including areas that likely correspond to primary and secondary somatosensory cortex, and anterior cingulate (Tarkka & Treede 1993). Lenz et al (1998) confirmed the presence of anterior cingulate generators by subdural recording from a grid of electrodes in a patient treated for epilepsy. Facial stimulation by a CO_2 laser evoked potentials from the contralateral anterior cingulate and supplemental motor area, with an additional weak ipsilateral response in these areas. A number of recent studies have examined the effect of visceral stimulation by balloon distention of the oesophagus (DeVault et al 1993, 1996) and electrical stimulation of the Oesophagus (Frobert et al 1995) and colon (Arendt-Nielsen et al 1997a). The successful use of balloon distention is a successful adaptation of the technique with a stimulus in which the onset is neither rapid nor precisely controlled.

Cortical evoked potentials are an effective tool in the analysis of pain processing. The amplitude of these potentials have been correlated with the magnitude of subjective pain reports and altered appropriately by experimental interventions. Evoked potential amplitudes have been modulated by pharmacological (Kochs et al 1996, Roth et al 1996) and non-pharmacological (Crawford et al 1998, Uraski et al 1998) putative analgesic treatments, and by manipulations such as noxious cooling of different extremities (Watanabe et al 1996), topical application of capsaicin (Beydoun et al 1996) and baroreceptor stimulation by lower body negative pressure (Mini et al 1995).

However, similar to reflex measures, the correspondence between cortical evoked potentials and subjective report is not preserved under all conditions. Reports of good agreement are counterbalanced by examples of disassociation in which the amplitude of evoked potentials do not covary with pain reports (Chapman et al 1981, Chudler & Dong 1983, Benedetti et al 1984, Willer et al 1987, Klement et al 1992, Meier et al 1993). A simple intervention such as passive or active movement can attenuate evoked potentials without changing verbal pain report (Kakigi et al 1993). As with reflex and other physiological measures, this dissociation does not condemn their utility for pain measurement, but rather defines the boundaries within which measurement is acceptable. Dissociation is also beneficial for the analyses of hierarchical pain processing (Gracely 1995, Kiernan et al 1995). In the case of the nociceptive reflex, a difference between this measure and verbal report can be easily interpreted as due to the influence of supraspinal processing. The same interpretation has been applied to differences between subjective report and cortical evoked potentials, with the difference attributed to the unpleasantness pain dimension (Meier et al 1993). Implicit in this interpretation is the assumption that the evoked potential is tightly coupled to the sensory intensity of pain sensation. This may be true under a restricted set of laboratory conditions, because certain manipulations may uncouple subjective pain intensity and cortical potentials independent of a change in a hierarchical pain processing stage. Like verbal report, evoked potentials may be vulnerable to certain biases (attention, movement, stimulus parameters, sedatives) which result in changes that do no reflect altered pain sensitivity.

Spontaneous EEG

Other EEG measures use clinical methods of visual inspection to identify abnormal activity that can be associated with painful conditions such as headache (Chen 1993). Spontaneous EEG has also been analysed by Fourier transformation of the signal that results in a measure of the power in specific frequency bands and in specific brain regions. Measures of the cortical power spectrum (CPS) to brief (Bromm 1984, Bromm et al 1989, Arendt-Nielsen 1990) and prolonged (Chen et al 1989, Backonja et al 1991) experimental stimulation have demonstrated increased power in specific frequency bands. Chen (1991) notes that these measures are plagued by large individual differences which may be due, in part, to haemodynamic baroreceptor-related differences. Non-contingent EEG has also been analysed to identify temporal and spatial relationships (Chen et al 1989, Veerasarn & Stohler 1992).

Magnetic methods

The electrical currents measured by the EEG can also be assessed by measuring the minute magnetic fields generated by variation in these currents. Sensitive, super-cooled detectors (superconductivity quantum induction device or SQUID) are placed near the head. An important feature is that source analysis of the magnetic signals can localize the regions responsible for evoked activity. Using this type of analysis, Hari (1983) found activity near the secondary somatosensory cortex evoked by electrical tooth pulp stimulation. Recently in a demonstration of both the spatial and temporal resolution of this technique, Howland et al (1995) administered electrical stimulation to the finger and localized the results of a source analysis to MRI anatomical scans. The results show bilateral sources in the primary sensory cortex and secondary somatosensory–insular cortex. A temporal analysis showed an initial contralateral primary sensory cortex response and subsequent intermittent bilateral primary sensory cortex and secondary somatosensory cortex–insular cortex responses.

Physiological recording and stimulation of brain structures in humans

Studies performed during stereotactic neurosurgery for pain or movement disorders have recorded from central neurons and also directly electrically stimulated these neurons. Microstimulation in areas posterior and inferior to the principle sensory nucleus of the thalamus (Vc) produces both thermal and pain sensations (Lenz et al 1994a). In some cases, stimulation evokes a previous visceral pain, such as pain from the appendix (Davis et al 1995a) or angina (Lenz et al 1994b). These evoked pain sensations do not appear to be simply an evoked, stimulus-related sensation but an entire pain memory, with attendant sensory and affective qualities (Davis et al 1995a, Lenz et al 1995). These results suggest a limbic–cortical memory system for pain similar to that for other sensory systems (Lenz et al 1997).

Brain imaging

The EEG and magnetic methods discussed above can provide spatial information by the use of numerous detectors and appropriate analysis software. The methods in this section visualize brain function in three dimensions by assessing glucose utilization or by changes in regional cerebral blood flow (rCBF). Although methods such as rCBF assessment in pain states has been performed with single-photon emission topography (SPECT) and by inhalation of tracers or NMR spectroscopy, the predominant methods are positron emission tomography (PET) and functional magnetic resonance imaging (fMRI).

PET

In this method a radioactive tracer is administered to the subject and the distribution of the tracer can be detected and imaged. Two types of studies utilize this technique. In ligand binding studies, the tracer is a labelled substance which binds at specific receptors and the distribution of these receptors and the change in this distribution can be evaluated by these techniques. In activation studies, the emitted radiation is used as a measure of glucose utilization from neural activity, or in most cases as a measure of rCBF using an O^{15} tracer. rCBF is used as an indirect measure of neural activity, an inference which depends on the localized increase in rCBF due to metabolic demands of increased neural processing.

A large number of studies have used PET to assess supraspinal responses to experimental stimuli in human subjects. Many of these evoked pain by delivering painful heat stimuli repeatedly during the 60–90 s of a PET scan (Jones et al 1991, Talbot et al 1991, Casey et al 1994, Coghill et al 1994, Craig et al 1996, Derbyshire et al 1994, 1997, Vogt et al 1996). Non-painful stimuli evoking hot, but not painful, stimuli serve as a control condition. A series of images representing the studied brain volume under these control conditions are subtracted from similar images produced during the painful conditions, resulting in a difference image that reflects regions of pain-specific pain processing. These images are smoothed, transformed into a standard space, and the results of a group of subjects are compared with standard statistics such as the *t*-test.

Brief heat stimuli consistently activate a group of brain structures in these studies. The anterior cingulate cortex is the most consistently activated, followed by the thalamus, insula, lentiform nucleus, and primary and secondary somatosensory cortex (Derbyshire et al 1997). The identification of structures activated by similar stimulus conditions can be considered a necessary first generation of studies that map general pain responses from a group of subjects receiving the same stimulation. Currently, the next generation of studies is addressing a number of issues such as the use of subjective ratings and correlational analysis to identify regions in which the amount of activation is related to stimulus intensity (Coghill et al 1997, Derbyshire et al 1997) or subjective magnitude of the evoked pain sensations (Coghill et al 1997). Additional studies have recognized the distinction between brief stimuli and clinical pain and administered tonic stimuli such as prolonged heat or cold or injection of capsaicin or ethanol, which may more closely resemble the pain of clinical conditions (Apkarian et al 1992, Di Peiro et al 1994, Casey et al 1996, Derbyshire & Jones 1998, Iadarola et al 1998, May et al 1998). These studies have demonstrated activations in many of the same regions activated by brief stimuli. This similarity may be because both brief and tonic studies deliver a painful experience that is coincident with a single scan, beginning at the start of the scan and ending or waning near the end of the scan. A study of eight subjects using a prolonged pain that persisted through three scans showed no activation in comparison to equally painful brief heat stimuli that activated primary and secondary sensory cortex, anterior cingulate and insula, suggesting that the pattern of activations observed with brief or short tonic stimuli may relate to some aspect of their episodic nature (Gracely et al 1997). Recent studies have also compared different forms of stimulation, including comparison of warmth, heat pain and cold pain (Casey et al 1996) and heat pain, ischaemic pain and re-perfusion dysaesthesias (Gracely et al 1997).

These studies could be considered as extended first, or second, generation studies that explore the effects of quantitative and qualitative stimulus parameters. With sufficient information about the sensory discriminative issues such as stimulus location, intensity, quality and duration, the stage is set for further studies of affective and cognitive processing and for studies of the modulation of supraspinal processes by pharmacological and non-pharmacological interventions. A few studies have involved these issues. The influence of nitrous oxide and fentanyl on pain evoked by tonic heat has revealed drug-related increases and decreases in rCBF. Nitrous oxide increased blood flow in the contralateral infralimbic and orbitofrontal cortices (Gyulai et al 1997), while the opioid fentanyl facilitated the activation of the contralateral supplemental motor area and ipsilateral prefrontal cortex (Adler et al 1997). Fentanyl did not attenuate any pain-evoked activation, while nitrous oxide abolished pain-evoked activation of the anterior cingulate, thalamus and supplementary motor area. A recent study by Rainville et al (1997) addressed both non-pharmacological modulation and the distinction between sensory and affective pain processing. These authors examined the influence of hypnotic induction and suggestions for reduced unpleasantness on ratings and regions of activation produced by a tonic heat stimulus. Hypnotic induction had no effect, while suggestions for increased or decreased unpleasantness resulted in corresponding increases and decreases in unpleasantness ratings and in activation of anterior cingulate cortex. This result shows a specific modulation by a non-pharmacological pain control intervention which further implicates the anterior cingulate cortex in the processing of the emotional components of pain experience.

fMRI

The use of MRI to image brain function is a recent development. These methods evaluate neural processing by detecting small changes in the magnetic environment induced by local changes in rCBF. While tracers can be used for this purpose, most studies now use the blood oxygenation level detection (BOLD) contrast method in which oxygenated and deoxygenated haemoglobin serves as an intrinsic tracer. The technical details of this method include the physics of MRI imaging and the effect of blood flow on the magnetic signal from adjacent tissue. Essentially, deoxygenated haemoglobin exhibits magnetic properties that interfere with the magnetic signal produced by surrounding tissue, suppressing the response detected by the scanner. Neural activity results in increased rCBF that overcompensates for the oxygen demand. The excess oxygenated haemoglobin, which has paramagnetic properties, produces less interference with the signal in surrounding tissue, resulting in an increased signal proportional to increased relative concentration of oxygenated haemoglobin and thus to increased neural activity. One disadvantage of fMRI in comparison to PET is that this signal is small, and numerous trials must be averaged to produce a usable measure. Slow drifts in the sensitivity of the scanner may produce equivalent changes, requiring designs that compensate for such drifts. Because of the numerous trials, head motion is a particular problem in fMRI studies. However, on the positive side, fMRI requires no ionizing radiation. A subject can be scanned repeatedly. The requirements for multiple trials are not a burden because entire volumes can be gathered quickly. Modern techniques such as echo planar imaging (EPI) can produce a functional image of the entire brain every few seconds. fMRI can trade speed for acuity, allowing functional images with a much greater spatial resolution than that obtained with PET.

Presently the status of fMRI studies of pain processing is similar to the status of PET studies at the time of the previous edition of this textbook. In each case only a small number of studies have been/were performed. fMRI has been used to localize activation of the anterior cingulate cortex produced by unilateral electrical stimulation of the median nerve. The increased spatial resolution clearly showed activation of the contralateral cingulate cortex under these conditions (Davis et al 1995b, 1997) in a region posterior and inferior to activations by an attention task (Davis et al 1997c). Electrical stimulation of the mastoid has demonstrated activations in bilateral insula and thalamus (Bucher et al 1998) and in the central sulcus (Hara et al 1997). Heat stimulation has been shown to activate many of the cortical regions observed with PET studies (Iadarola et al 1995, Ayyagari et al 1997, Becerra et al 1997). Individual analysis included a strong activation of secondary somatosensory cortex by heat (Gelnar et al 1994) which was not observed in a group analysis (Ayyagari et al 1997), suggesting a greater between-subject variability in the location of SII in comparison to SI. Painful stimulation by cold objects has been shown to activate the anterior cingulate in a relatively low-power clinical scanner (Jones et al 1998).

RELEVANCE OF EXPERIMENTAL PAIN METHODS: THE CLASSIC GOAL OF ASSESSMENT OF ANALGESIC EFFICACY

The evaluation of analgesic efficacy has been a classical goal of studies using experimental stimulation (Beecher 1959, Gracely 1991b). A validated technique promised to avoid the uncontrolled and highly variable nature of the pain 'stimulus' associated with clinical syndromes, and its report. The pioneering studies enjoyed an initial success, followed by criticism and repeated failures. Methodological improvements resulted in renewed success with the demonstration of opioid analgesia, which has been routinely observed in recent experiments (Gracely 1991b).

Many of the important features of present methods evolved from these early studies. Initially, successful methods used the pain threshold to thermal stimuli as the dependent measure in uncontrolled studies. Positive effects vanished with the introduction of double-blind placebo controls, but reappeared with the use of severe, long-lasting pain sensations produced by the continuous, increasing pain of the tourniquet ischaemia technique (Beecher 1959, Smith et al 1966) or by the use of discrete stimuli to stimulate an increasing continuous pain sensation (Parry et al 1972). The demonstration of opioid analgesia with these stimulus modalities was attributed to their severity, which was deemed enough to evoke a sufficient 'reaction component', an affective component associated with clinically significant pain but not usually found with brief discrete stimuli. Present evidence suggests that this success was not caused by the reaction component but rather by the use of suprathreshold stimulation. A wide range of discrete suprathreshold stimuli (e.g., thermal stimuli from a contact thermode or laser), double-blind placebo controls and several response methods, have repeatedly demonstrated significant effects of both pharmacological and non-pharmacological pain control interventions. Nonetheless, the reaction component has remained an influential concept in pain measurement and treatment.

Presently, experimental demonstrations of opiate analgesia are practically taken for granted. The previous version of this chapter noted 34 reports of experimental opioid analgesia, including dose–response curves (Gracely 1994). Experimental studies of the pharmacology of opioid action have found no analgesia to the morphine-6-glucuronide metabolite of morphine (Lotsch et al 1997b) but have demonstrated analgesia to a kappa agonist (Lotsch et al 1997a) in addition to the numerous demonstrations with mu agonists (Gracely 1994). Studies of experimental sensitization have demonstrated opioid attenuation of secondary hyperalgesia and the extent of mechanical allodynia following intradermal injections of capsaicin (Park et al 1995, Sethna et al 1998). The specificity of opioid effects has been evaluated by using a large battery of measures to compare opioids to local anaesthetics (Brennum et al 1993, 1994) and agents such as the sedative propofol (Petersen-Felix et al 1996). Specific patterns have been found for all three classes of drugs, with some overlap. These results suggest that either certain experimental pain measures may erroneously indicate analgesia or, in the case of propofol, that certain non-analgesics may exert analgesic properties in specific controlled situations.

The renewed interest in central sensitization has prompted a number of studies that target the putative central mechanisms responsible for secondary hyperalgesia and mechanical allodynia. In these experimental models, central sensitization is produced by experimental burns, by intradermal injection of capsaicin, or by topical application of this or other substances such as mustard oil. Davis et al (1995) showed that pretreatment of the skin by intradermal injection of a capsaicin analogue reduced the spontaneous pain of an experimental burn and eliminated evoked abnormalities of primary and secondary hyperalgesia. The NMDA receptor has been implicated in the initiation and maintenance of central sensitization, and administration of the antagonist ketamine (Park et al 1995, Andersen et al 1996, Kochs et al 1996, Sethna et al 1998) has been shown to attenuate secondary hyperalgesia and the extent of mechanical allodynia, while the antagonist dextramethorphan has been shown to reduce secondary hyperalgesia following an experimental burn (Ilkjaer et al 1997) but not after intradermal injection of capsaicin (Kinnman et al 1997a). Adrenergic influences on central sensitization have been assessed in studies administering either agonists or antagonists. Drummond (1995b) administered noradrenaline and observed increased primary heat hyperalgesia, suggesting α-adrenergic involvement in the mechanisms mediating mechanical allodynia but not mechanical punctate secondary hyperalgesia. Administration of the α-adrenergic antagonist phentolamine decreased ongoing pain and the extent of capsaicin-induced mechanical allodynia with no effect on the extent of pin-prick secondary hyperalgesia

(Liu et al 1996a, Kinnman et al 1997b). These results indicate a differential action of adrenergic mechanisms on peripheral and central hyperalgesia and provide further evidence that altered sensitivity to Aβ and to nociceptor input are mediated by independent mechanisms.

Studies of weaker analgesics have been performed less frequently, and the results are less consistent. The weak opiate codeine has demonstrated analgesia in a number of models and peripherally acting non-steroidal anti-inflammatory drugs (NSAIDs) such as aspirin or ibuprofen have significantly reduced measures of experimental pain in some studies but not in others (Gracely 1994). The topical application of agents such as acetylsalicylic acid has been shown to suppress pain evoked by tissue acidosis (Steen et al 1995) and the spontaneous pain and the area of flare, secondary hyperalgesia and mechanical allodynia produced by topical capsaicin (Schmelz & Kress 1996).

Methods using experimental pain stimulation in normal individuals have also been used to assess the effects of other drugs, including the analgesic effects observed with nitrous oxide, ketamine, tramadol, imipramine and intradermal lidocaine in combination with morphine (Gracely 1991b, Kaufman et al 1992, Thurauf et al 1993, Poulsen et al 1995, Kochs et al 1996, Atanassoff et al 1997).

The efficacy of non-pharmacological treatments has been assessed in a number of studies in normal subjects. Somatic treatments such as acupuncture or transcutaneous electrical nerve stimulation (TENS) have been investigated by several stimulation methods. Positive effects have been observed with cold pressor pain (greatest at a TENS frequency of 40 Hz) and tourniquet ischaemia, and with thermal pain thresholds but only with high TENS stimulation currents (Eriksson et al 1985, Sjölund & Eriksson 1985, Johnson et al 1989). Recent studies have examined the use of various stimulating electrodes and found that deep pain in muscle and insulated needle electrodes (Ishimaru et al 1995) was most effective for reducing pain from the periosteum. Analgesic effects of needle acupuncture have been demonstrated in several experimental studies, although the relative role of central, segmental and peripheral mechanisms has not been firmly established (Gracely 1994). At least two studies assessed the effects of low-intensity laser stimulation on experimental ischaemic pain and found no convincing evidence for any analgesic action (Mokhtar et al 1995, Lowe et al 1997).

Psychological treatments include methods such as hypnosis and meditation. A large number of studies have been performed evaluating hypnotic modification of painful stimuli, many with cold pressor pain and in some studies with thermal stimulation, electrical tooth pulp stimulation and radiofrequency heating of the chest cavity (Gracely 1994). Recent studies have examined efficacy and mechanisms by evaluating both verbal measures of pain and spinal and supraspinal physiological measures (Arendt-Nielsen et al 1990, Meier et al 1993, Kiernan et al 1995). As noted above, all studies found reductions in the verbal reports while measures of spinal nociceptive reflexes and supraspinal cortical evoked potentials produced conflicting results.

Meditation exercises, in comparison to relaxation procedures, have reduced ratings of painful cold pressor or heat stimuli when performed by either experienced (Mills & Farrow 1981) or naive subjects trained for 6 weeks (Gaughan et al 1990). Both of these studies found greater effects with scales of pain unpleasantness than with scales of pain sensory intensity.

Studies that assess analgesic efficacy by experimental methods have been criticized for being clinically irrelevant. Critics rightfully point out that laboratory administration of experimentally painful stimuli cannot duplicate the physiological features of an acute or chronic pain condition, or the accompanying psychological features such as anxiety, uncertainty, suffering and foreboding. However, this inability to exactly duplicate clinical pain syndromes only imposes modest limits on the inferential utility of these methods. The consistent results with opiates suggest that the antinociceptive efficacy of opioid agonists or antagonists can be evaluated using laboratory procedures. It is likely that any intervention which shows experimental efficacy will also show clinical efficacy. The important issues may relate to whether dose and potency relationships established experimentally predict clinical findings, and whether the models are developed sufficiently to accurately predict poor clinical analgesic action. In addition, it is increasingly clear that the pain afferent system is not a simple transmission line but a complex series of processing stages which change and increase in number as acute pain is prolonged. Specific experimental pain paradigms are able to activate specific components, such as Aδ-fibre activation, C-fibre activation, Aδ temporal summation, C-fibre 'windup', central sensitization and progressive tactile hypersensitivity (Gracely 1994, Ma & Woolf 1996, Eliav & Gracely 1998). The results of recent studies strongly suggest that the complexity of pain processing may best be assessed, and in some cases only assessed, through the administration of a battery of experimental-pain methods that target specific components of this system. In this context, the usefulness of experimental models naturally extends beyond the measurement of *if* an analgesic works to *why* it works, to the identification of mechanisms of analgesic action.

ADDITIONAL GOALS OF EXPERIMENTAL PAIN METHODS

The experimental goal of evaluating analgesic efficacy was the second goal of the five goals listed at the beginning of this chapter. The first goal of measurement development and validation is intrinsic to the methods and has been alluded to in the description of the methods. The third goal describes a major utility of experimental methods, the evaluation of mechanisms of pain and pain control. Examples of these applications are provided throughout this volume. When reviewing these, it may be helpful to divide these studies into anatomical divisions of peripheral, spinal and supraspinal mechanisms. Both psychophysical and physiological measures can assess the function of nociceptive afferents, and the recent focus on central sensitization and progressive tactile hypersensitivity has emphasized the importance of also evaluating the function of fibres which normally mediate non-painful tactile sensation. Once entering the dorsal horn, primary afferent information can be modulated by a number of mechanisms. Indeed, the attenuation of this input by either other peripheral input or by central endogenous opioid and non-opioid mechanisms has marked major milestones in pain research. In contrast to these mechanisms of attenuation, the current studies have focused on the mechanisms that exacerbate symptoms in conditions of persistent pain. Although predominantly spinal, these mechanisms are successfully investigated by all of the methods described in this chapter. Models of spinal sensitization are produced by fast trains of noxious stimuli (wind up), by application of chemicals or burns (central sensitization) and, in cases of allodynia or peripheral inflammation, use of tactile stimuli. Innocuous cold stimuli are also useful. For example, Chen et al (1996) used both an adaptive, stimulus-dependent method and the classical Method of Constant Stimuli to assess cold detection and pain thresholds and different adapting temperatures. These authors found evidence for separate afferent systems mediating the sensation of cool and of cold pain. Campero et al (1996) assessed C-polymodal nociceptors responsive to heat and mechanical stimulation and found that about 40% of these fibres were also activated by cold stimulation. These fibres may represent the afferent nociceptive channel of Chen et al (1996) and may mediate the symptom of cold hyperalgesia found in neuropathic pain syndromes (Campero et al 1996). Additional psychophysical studies and functional brain imaging studies of supraspinal processing have further identified interactions between cold and warm fibre symptoms that are responsible for the classical thermal grill illusion and likely contribute also to the symptom of cold hyperalgesia (Craig et al 1996).

The fourth goal involves the evaluation of psychological factors involved in the experience of pain and the influence of these factors in pain measurement. The controlled environment of experimental studies has demonstrated the influence of both cognitive factors such as attention, expectation, memory and suggestion, and also the influence of mood states of anxiety and depression (Gracely 1994). One important issue is the relevance of these findings for clinically significant acute and chronic pain. Like experimental measures of analgesic efficacy, these types of experiments ultimately must be cross-validated in the clinic (see Ch. 17). Many of the cited studies employed groups of patients and volunteers, or delivered experimental stimuli to pain patients. These types of studies are represented by the fifth goal, which is the use of experimental methods in the clinical situation. Methods such as experimental pain matching can be used to improve pain assessment. The growth of clinical studies employing quantitative sensory testing (see Ch. 25) is an excellent example of the successful merging of experimental procedures and clinical evaluation. New studies are now extending this concept further, exploring how clinical conditions may modulate measures of spinal and supraspinal processing. These experiments are likely to provide important parts of the puzzle of the multiple mechanisms of pain perception. They are also likely to approach one of the most elusive goals, a physiological signature associated with what is otherwise an unobservable and private event.

Acknowledgements

The author thanks Christina Bokat for her technical assistance.

REFERENCES

Adler LJ, Gyulai FE, Diehl DJ, Mintun MA, Winter PM, Firestone LL 1997 Regional brain activity changes associated with fentanyl analgesia elucidated by positron emission tomography. Anesthesia and Analgesia 84: 120–126

Algom D, Raphaeli N, Cohen-Raz L 1986 Integration of noxious stimulation across separate somatosensory communications systems: a functional theory of pain. Journal of Experimental Psychology Human Perception and Performance 12: 92–102

Andersen OK, Jensen LM, Brennum J, Arendt-Nielsen L 1994 Evidence for central summation of C and A delta nociceptive activity in man. Pain 59: 273–280

Andersen OK, Gracely RH, Arendt-Nielsen L 1995a Facilitation of human nociceptive reflex by stimulation of A beta-fibres in a secondary hyperalgesic area sustained by nociceptive input from the primary hyperalgesic area. Acta Physiologica Scandinavica 155: 87–97

Andersen OK, Jensen LM, Brennum J, Arendt-Nielsen L 1995b Modulation of the human nociceptive reflex by cyclic movements. European Journal of Applied Physiology 70: 311–321

Andersen OK, Felsby S, Nicolaisen L, Bjerring P, Jensen TS, Arendt-Nielsen L 1996 The effect of ketamine on stimulation of primary and secondary hyperalgesic areas induced by capsaicin – a double-blind, placebo-controlled, human experimental study. Pain 66: 51–62

Anton F, Euchner I, Handwerker O 1992 Psychophysical examination of pain induced by defined CO_2 pulses applied to nasal mucosa. Pain 49: 53–60

Apkarian AV, Stea RA, Manglos SH, Szeverenyi NM, King RB, Thomas FD 1992 Persistent pain inhibits contralateral somatosensory cortical activity in humans. Neuroscience Letters 140: 141–147

Arendt-Nielsen L 1990 Second pain event related potentials to argon laser stimuli: recording and quantification. Journal of Neurology, Neurosurgery and Psychiatry 53: 405–410

Arendt-Nielsen L, Zachariae R, Bjerring P 1990 Quantitative evaluation of hypnotically suggested hyperaesthesia and analgesia by painful laser stimulation. Pain 42: 243–251

Arendt-Nielsen L, Brennum J, Sindrup S, Bak P 1994 Electrophysiological and psychophysical quantification of temporal summation in the human nociceptive system. European Journal of Applied Physiology 68: 266–273

Arendt-Nielsen L, Drewes AM, Hansen JB, Tage-Jensen U 1997a Gut pain reactions in man: an experimental investigation using short and long term duration transmucosal electrical stimulation. Pain 69: 255–262

Arendt-Nielsen L, Graven-Nielsen T, Svensson P, Jensen TS 1997b Temporal summation in muscles and referred pain areas: an experimental human study. Muscle and Nerve 20: 1311–1313

Atanassoff PG, Brull SJ, Prinsev Y, Silverman DG 1997 The effect of the intradermal administration of lidocaine and morphine on the response to thermal stimulation. Anesthesia and Analgesia 84: 1340–1343

Ayyagari PV, Gelnar PA, Drauss B, Tiscione J, Szeverenvi NM, Apkarian AV 1997 Population t-maps of brain activation during painful thermal stimuli, motor and vibrotactile tasks in humans, unsin multi-slice fMRI. Society of Neuroscience Abstracts 23: 438

Backonja M, Howland EW, Wang J, Smith J, Salinsky M, Cleelend CS 1991 Tonic changes in alpha power during immersion of the hand in cold water. Electroencephalography and Clinical Neurophysiology 79: 192–203

Becerra LR, Stojanovic M, Breiter HC et al 1997 fMRI activation by noxious heat. Society of Neuroscience Abstracts 23: 439

Beck J, Shaw WA 1965 Magnitude of the standard numerical value of the standard and stimulus spacing in the estimation of loudness. Perceptual and Motor Skills 21: 151–156

Beecher HK 1959 Measurement of subjective responses. Oxford University Press, New York

Benedetti C, Colpitts Y, Kaufman E, Chapman CR 1984 Effects of methanol on evoked potentials elicited by painful dental stimuli. Pain Supplement 2: 162

Beydoun A, Dyke DB, Morrow TJ, Casey KL 1996 Topical capsaicin selectively attenuates heat pain and A delta fibermediated laser-evoked potentials. Pain 65: 189–196

Boureau F, Paquette C 1988 Translated versus reconstructed McGill Pain Questionnaires: a comparative study of two French forms. In: Dubner R, Gebhart GF, Bond MR (eds) Proceedings of the Vth World Congress on Pain. Elsevier, Amsterdam, pp 395–402

Boureau F, Luu M, Doubrère JF 1991 Study of experimental pain measures and nociceptive reflex in chronic pain patients and normal subjects. Pain 44: 131–138

Brennum J, Nielsen PT, Horn A, Arendt-Nielsen L, Secher NH, Jensen TS 1993 Quantitative sensory examination during epidural anaesthesia and analgesia in man: effects of morphine. Pain 52: 75–83

Brennum J, Nielsen PT, Horn A, Arendt-Nielsen L, Secher NH 1994 Quantitative sensory examination of epidural anaesthesia and analgesia in man: dose–response effect on bupivacaine. Pain 56: 315–326

Bromm B (ed) 1984 Neurophysiological correlates of pain. Elsevier, Amsterdam

Bromm B, Chen AC 1995 Brain electrical source analysis of laser evoked potentials in response to painful trigeminal nerve stimulation. Electroencephalography and Clinical Neurophysiology 95: 14–26

Bromm B, Meier W 1984 The intracutaneous stimulus: a new pain model for algesimetric studies. Methods and Findings in Experimental and Clinical Pharmacology 87: 431–440

Bromm B, Scharein E 1982 Response plasticity of pain evoked potentials in man. Physiology and Behavior 28: 109–116

Bromm B, Treede R-D 1980 Withdrawal reflex, skin resistance reaction and pain ratings due to electrical stimuli in man. Pain 9: 339–354

Bromm B, Treede R-D 1987 Human cerebral potentials evoked by CO_2 laser stimuli causing pain. Experimental Brain Research 67: 153–162

Bromm B, Meier W, Scharein E 1989 Pre-stimulus/post-stimulus relations in EEG spectra and their modulations by an opiodid and an antidepressant. Electroencephalography and Clinical Neurophysiology 73: 188–197

Bucher SF, Dieterich M, Wiesmann M et al 1998 Cerebral functional magnetic resonance imaging of vestibular, auditory, and nociceptive areas during galvanic stimulation. Annals of Neurology 1: 120–125

Campbell IG, Carstens E, Watkins LR 1991 Comparison of human pain sensation and flexion withdrawal evoked by noxious radiant heat. Pain 45: 259–268

Campero M, Serra J, Ochoa JL 1996 C-Polymodal nociceptors activated by noxious low temperature in human skin. Journal of Physiology 497: 565–572

Casey KL, Minoshima S, Berger KL, Koeppe RA, Morrow TJ, Frey KA 1994 Positron emission tomographic analysis of cerebral structures activated specifically by repetitive noxious heat stimuli. Journal of Neurophysiology 71: 802–807

Casey KL, Minoshima S, Morrow TJ, Koeppe RA 1996 Comparison of human cerebral activation pattern during cutaneous warmth, hot pain, and deep cold pain. Journal of Neurophysiology 76: 571–581

Chan CWY, Tsang HH 1985 A quantitative study of flexion reflex in man: relevance to pain research. In: Fields HL, Dubner R, Cervero (eds) Advances in pain research and therapy, vol 9. Raven, New York 361–370

Chapman CR 1977 Sensory decision theory methods in pain research: a reply to Rollman. Pain 3: 295–305

Chapman CR, Loeser JD (eds) 1989 Advances in pain research and therapy: issues in pain measurement, vol 12. Raven, New York 1–570

Chapman CR, Colpitts YH, Mayeno JK, Gagliardi GJ 1981 Rate of stimulus repetition changes evoked potential amplitude: dental and auditory modalities compared. Experimental Brain Research 43: 246–252

Chapman CR, Casey KL, Dubner R, Foley KM, Gracely RH, Reading AE 1985 Pain measurement an overview. Pain 22: 1–31

Chatrian GE, Fernandes de Lima VM, Lettich E, Canfield RC, Miller RC, Soso MJ 1982 Electrical stimulation of tooth pulp in humans II Qualities of sensations. Pain 14: 233–246

Chen AC 1993 Human brain measures of clinical pain: A review II Tomographic imaging. Pain 54: 133–144

Chen ACN 1991 Individual difference in human topographic EEG power: hemodynamic and psychological predictors. International Journal of Neuroscience 59: 271–280

Chen ACN, Dworkin SF, Haug J, Gehrig J 1989 Human responsivity in a tonic pain model: psychological determinants. Pain 37: 143–160

Chen ACN, Kazarians H, Scharein E, Bromm B 1993 Cerebral generators involved in pain processing: EEG response to laser stimulated trigeminal nerve. Abstract presented at the German Physiological Society Meeting, Munich

Chen CC, Rainville P, Bushnell MC 1996 Noxious and innocuous cold discrimination in humans: evidence for separate afferent channels. Pain 68: 33–43

Chudler EH, Dong WK 1983 The assessment of pain by cerebral evoked potentials. Pain 16: 221–224

Clark WC, Clark SB 1980 Pain response in Nepalese porters. Science 209: 410–411

Clark WC, Yang JC 1983 Applications of sensory decision theory to problems in laboratory and clinical pain. In: Melzack R (ed) Pain measurement and assessment. Raven, New York 15–25

Clark WC, Carroll JD, Yang JC, Janal MN 1986 Multidimensional scaling reveals two dimensions of thermal pain. Journal of Experiment Psychology (Human Perception) 12: 103–107

Cleeland CS 1989 Measurement of pain by subjective report. In: Chapman CR, Loeser JD (eds) Advances in pain research and therapy: issues in pain measurement, vol 12. Raven, New York, pp 391–403

Cleeland CS, Nakamura Y, Howland EW, Morgan NR, Edwards KR, Backonja M 1996 Effects of oral morphine on cold pressor tolerance time and neuropsychological performance. Neuropsychopharacology 15: 252–262

Coghill RC, Gracely RH 1996 Validation of combined numerical-analog descriptor scales for rating pain intensity and pain unpleasantness. American Pain Society Abstracts 15: 86

Coghill RC, Talbot JD, Evans AC et al 1994 Distributed processing of pain and vibration by the human brain. Journal of Neuroscience 14: 4095–4108

Coghill RC, Sang CN, Maisog J.Ma, Iadarola MJ 1997 Distributed representation of painful stimulus intensity in the human brain. Society of Neuroscience Abstracts 23: 439

Cooper BY, Vierck CJ Jr, Yeomans DC 1986 Selective reduction of second pain sensation by systemic morphine in humans. Pain 24: 93–116

Coppola R, Gracely RH 1983 Where is the noise in SDT pain assessment? Pain 17: 257–266

Cornsweet TN 1962 The staircase-method in psychophysics. American Journal of Psychology 75: 485–491

Craig AD, Reiman EM, Evans A, Bushnell MC 1996 Functional imaging of an illusion of pain. Nature 21: 217–218

Craig KD 1989 Clinical pain measurement from the perspective of the human laboratory. In: Chapman CR, Loeser JD (eds) Advances in pain research and therapy: issues in pain measurement, vol 12. Raven, New York 433–441

Craig KD, Patrick CJ 1985 Facial expression during induced pain. Journal of Personality and Social Psychology 48: 1080–1091

Craig KD, Prkachin KM 1983 Nonverbal measures of pain. In: Melzack R (ed) Pain measurement and assessment. Raven, New York 173–179

Crawford HJ, Knebel T, Kaplan L et al 1998 Hypnotic analgesia: 1. Somatosensory event-related potential changes to noxious stimuli and 2. Transfer learning to reduce chronic back pain. International Journal of Clinical and Experimental Hypnosis 46: 92–132

Crockett DJ, Prakchin KM, Craig KD 1977 Factors of the language of pain in patient volunteer groups. Pain 4: 175–182

Danziger N, Fournier E, Bouhassira D et al 1998a Different strategies of modulation can be operative during hypnotic analgesia: a neurophysiological study. Pain 75: 85–92

Danziger N, Rozenberg S, Bourgeois P, Charpentier G, Willer JC 1998b Depressive effects of segmental and heterotopic application of transcutaneous electrical nerve stimulatin and piezo-electric current on lower limb nociceptive flexion reflex in human subjects. Archives of Physical Medicine and Rehabilitation 79: 191–200

Davis KD, Tasker RR, Kiss ZH, Hutchison WD, Dostrovsky JO 1995a Visceral pain evoked by thalamic microstimulatin in humans. Neuroreport 6: 369–374

Davis KD, Wood ML, Crawley AP, Mikulis DJ 1995b fMRI of human somatosensory and cingulate cortex during painful electrical nerve stimulation. Neuroreport 7: 321–325

Davis KD, Meyer RA, Turnquist JL, Filloon TG, Pappagallo M, Campbell JN 1995c Cutaneous pretreatment with capsaicin analog NE-21610 prevents the pain to a burn and subsequent hyperalgesia Pain 62: 373–378

Davis KD, Taylor SJ, Crawley AP, Wook ML, Mikulis DJ 1997 Functional MRI of pain- and attention-related activations in the human cingulate cortex. American Physiological Society Journal of Neurophysiology 77: 3370–3380

Del Bianco, E, Geppetti P, Zippi P, Isolani D, Magini B, Cappugi P 1996 The effects of repeated dermal application of capsaicin to the human skin on pain and vasodilatation induced by intradermal injection of acid and hypertonic solutions. British Journal of Clinical Pharmacology 41: 1–6

DeBroucker T, Willer JC, Bergeret S 1989 The nociceptive reflex in humans: a specific and objective correlate of experimental pain. In: Chapman CR, Loeser JD (eds) Advances in pain research and therapy: issues in pain measurement, vol 12. Raven, New York, pp 337–352

Derbyshire SWG, Jones AKP 1998 Cerebral responses to a continual tonic pain stimulus measured using positron emission tomography. Pain 76: 127–135

Derbyshire SW, Jones AK, Devani P et al 1994 Cerebral responses to pain in patients with atypical facial pain measured by positron emission tomography. Journal of Neurology, Neurosurgery and Psychiatry 57: 1166–1172

Derbyshire SW, Jones AK, Gyulai F, Clark S, Townsend D, Firestone LL 1997 Pain processing during three levels of noxious stimulation produces differential patterns of central activity. Pain 73: 431–445

DeVault KR, Beacham S, Streletz LJ, Castell DO 1993 Cerebral evoked potentials. A method of quantification of central nervous system response to esophageal pain. Digestive Diseases and Science 38: 2241–2246

DeVault KR, Beacham S, Castell DO, Streletz LJ, Ditunno JF 1996 Esophageal sensation in spinal cord-injured patients: balloon distension and cerebral evoked potential recording. American Journal of Physiology 271: G937–941

Di Piero V, Ferracuti S, Sabatini U, Pantano P, Cruccu G, Lenzi GL 1994 A cerebral blood flow study on tonic pain activation in man. Pain 56: 167–173

Dong WK, Chudler EH, Martin RF 1985 Physiological properties of intradental mechanoreceptors. Brain Research 334: 389–395

Dowman R 1991 Spinal and supraspinal correlates of nociception in man. Pain 45: 269–281

Dowman R 1993 A noninvasive strategy for identifying and quantifying innocuous and nociceptive peripheral afferent activity evoked by nerve stimulation. Physiology and Behaviour 53: 1163–1169

Drummond PD 1995a Lacrimation and cutaneous vasodilatation in the face induced by painful stimulation of the nasal ala and upper lip. Journal of the Autonomic Nervous System 51: 109–116

Drummond PD 1995b Noradrenaline increases hyperalgesia to heat in skin sensitized by capsaicin. Pain 60: 311–315

Duncan GH, Miron D, Parker SR 1992 Yet another adaptive scheme for tracking threshold. Meeting of the International Society for Psychophysics, July '92 Stockholm

Duncan GH, Feine JS, Bushnell MC, Boyer M 1988 Use of magnitude matching for measuring group differences in pain perception. In: Dubner R, Gebhart GR, Bond MR (eds) Proceedings of the Vth World Congress on Pain. Elsevier, Amsterdam 383–390

Duncan GH, Bushnell MC, Lavigne GJ 1989 Comparison of verbal and visual analogue scales for measuring the intensity and unpleasantness of experimental pain. Pain 37: 295–303

Eliav E, Gracely RH 1998 Sensory changes in the territory of the lingual and inferior alveolar nerves following lower third molar extraction. Pain 77: 191–199

Engen T 1971a Psychophysics I: Discrimination and detection. In: Kling JW, Riggs LA (eds) Experimental psychology, 3rd edn. Holt, New York 11–46

Engen T 1971b Psychophysics II: Scaling methods. In: Kling JW, Riggs LA (eds) Experimental psychology, 3rd edn. Holt, New York 47–86

Eriksson MBE, Rosen I, Sjolund B 1985 Thermal sensitivity in healthy subjects is decreased by a central mechanism after TNS. Pain 22: 235–242

Facchinetti F, Sandrini G, Petraglia F, Alfonsi E, Nappi G, Genazzani AR 1984 Concomitant increase in nociceptive flexion reflex threshold and plasma opioids following transcutaneous nerve stimulation. Pain 19: 295–303

Fernandes de Lima VM, Chatrian GE, Lettich E, Canfield RC, Miller RC, Soso MJ 1982 Electrical stimulation of tooth pulp in humans. I. Relationships among physical stimulus intensities, psychological magnitude estimates, and cerebral evoked potentials. Pain 14: 207–232

Fernandez E, Turk DC 1992 Sensory and affective components of pain: separation and synthesis. Psychological Bulletin 112: 205–217

Foster RW, Weston KM 1986 Chemical irritant algesia assessed using the human blister base. Pain 25: 269–278

Fox CD, Steger HG, Jennison JH 1979 Ratio scaling of pain perception with the submaximum effort tourniquet technique. Pain 7: 21–29

Frobert O, Arendt-Nielsen L, Bak P, Funch-Jensen P, Bagger JP 1995 Oesophageal sensation assessed by electrical simuli and brain evoked potentials – a new model for visceral nociception. Gut 37: 603–609

Fruhstorfer H, Lindblom U, Schmidt WG 1976 Method for quantitative estimation of thermal thresholds in patients. Journal of Neurology, Neurosurgery and Psychiatry 39: 1071–1075

Garcia de Jalon PD, Harrison FJJ, Johnson KI, Kozma C, Schnelle K 1985 A modified cold stimulation technique for the evaluation of analgesic activity in human volunteers. Pain 22: 183–189

Garcia-Larrea L, Charles N, Sindou M, Mauguiere F 1993 Flexion reflexes following anterolateral cordotomy in man: dissociation between pain sensation and nociceptive reflex RIII. Pain 55: 139–149

Gaughan AM, Gracely RH, Friedman R 1990 Pain perception following regular practice of meditation, progressive muscle relaxation and sitting. Pain (suppl 5) 5317

Gelnar PA, Szeverenyi NM, Apkarian AV 1994 SII has the most robust response of the multiple cortical areas activated during painful thermal stimuli in humans. Society of Neuroscience Abstracts 20: 1572

Gibson SJ, La Vasseur SA, Helme RD 1991 Cerebral event-related responses induced by CO_2 laser stimulation in subjects suffering from cervico-brachial syndrome. Pain 47: 173–182

Gracely RH 1979 Psychophysical assessment of human pain. In: Bonica JJ, Liebeskind JC, Able-Fessard DG (eds) Advances in pain research and therapy, vol 3. Raven, New York 805–824

Gracely RH 1980 Pain measurement in man. In: Ng L, Bonica JJ (eds) Pain, discomfort and humanitarian care. Elsevier, New York, pp 111–137

Gracely RH 1984 Subjective quantification of pain perception. In: Bromm B (ed) Neurophysiological correlates of pain. Elsevier, Amsterdam 371–387

Gracely RH 1985 Pain psychophysics. In: Manuk S (ed) Advances in behavioral medicine, vol 1. JAI Press, New York 191–231

Gracely RH 1988 Multiple random staircase assessment of thermal pain perception. In: Dubner R, Bond M, Gebhart G (eds) Proceedings of the Fifth World Congress on Pain. Elsevier, Amsterdam, pp 391–394

Gracely RH 1991a Theoretical and practical issues in pain assessment in central pain syndromes. In: Casey KL (ed) Pain and central nervous system disease. Raven, New York, pp 85–101

Gracely RH 1991b Experimental pain models. In: Max M, Portenoy R, Laska E (eds) Advances in pain research and therapy, vol 18. The design of analgesic clinical trials. Raven, New York, pp 33–47

Gracely RH 1992 Affective dimensions of pain: How many and how measured? APS Journal 1: 243–247

Gracely RH 1994 Methods of testing pain mechanisms in normal man. In: Wall PD, Melzack R (eds) Textbook of pain, 3rd edn. Churchill Livingstone, London, pp 315–336

Gracely RH 1995 Hypnosis and hierarchical pain control systems. Pain 60: 1–2

Gracely RH 1996 Sensations, feelings and physical events. Pain Forum 5: 162–164

Gracely RH, Dubner R 1981 Pain assessment in humans: a reply to Hall. Pain 11: 109–120

Gracely RH, Gaughan AM 1991 Staircase assessment of stimulated opiate potentiation. In: Bond MR, Charlton JE, Woolf CJ (eds) Proceedings of the Sixth World Congress on Pain. Elsevier, Amsterdam, pp 547–551

Gracely RH, Dubner R, McGrath PA 1979 Narcotic analgesia: fentanyl reduces the intensity but not the unpleasantness of painful tooth pulp stimulation. Science 203: 1261–1263

Gracely RH, Wolskee PJ 1983 Semantic functional measurement of pain: integrating perception and language. Pain 15: 389–398

Gracely RH, McGrath PA, Dubner R 1978a Ratio scales of sensory and affective verbal pain descriptors. Pain 5: 5–18

Gracely RH, McGrath P, Dubner R 1978b Validity and sensitivity of ratio scales of sensory and affective verbal pain descriptors: manipulation of affect by diazepam. Pain 5: 19–29

Gracely RH, Taylor F, Schilling RM, Wolskee PJ 1984 The effect of a simulated analgesic on verbal description and category responses to thermal pain. Pain supplement. 2: 173

Gracely RH, Lota L, Walther DJ, Dubner R 1988 A multiple random staircase method of psychophysical pain assessment. Pain 32: 55–63

Gracely RH, Naliboff BD 1996 Measurement of pain sensation. In Kruger L (ed) Handbook of perception and cognition: somatosensory systems. Raven Press, New York, pp 243–313

Gracely RH, Hostetter MP, Park KM, Sang CN, Iadarola M, Coghill RC 1997 PET analysis of supraspinal processing of ischemic pain and post-ischemic dysesthesias. American Pain Society Abstracts 16: 153

Graven-Nielsen T, Arendt-Nielsen L, Svennson P, Jensen TS 1997 Stimulus–response functions in areas with experimentally induced referred muscle pain – a psychophysical study. Brain Research 744: 1221–1228

Greenspan JD, McGillis SLB 1991 Stimulus features relevant to the perception of sharpness and mechanically evoked cutaneous pain. Somatosensory Motor Research 8: 137–147

Greenspan JD, Winfield JA 1992 Reversible pain and tactile deficit associated with a cerebral tumor compressing the posterior insula and parietal operculum. Pain 50: 29–39

Gyulai FE, Firestone LL, Mintun MA, Winter PM 1997 In vivo imaging of nitrous oxide-induced changes in cerebral activation during noxious heat stimuli. Anesthesiology 86: 538–548

Hallin RG, Wu G 1998 Protocol for microneurography with concentric needle electrodes. Brain Research Brain Research Protocols. 2: 120–132

Hara K, Shimizu H, Nakasato N, Mizoi K, Yoshimoto T 1997 Evaluation of various somatosensory stimulations for function MRI. No To Skinkei 49: 65–68

Hardy JD, Wolff HG, Goodell H 1952 Pain sensation and reactions. Williams & Wilkins, Baltimore

Hari R, Kaukoranta E, Reinikainen K, Houpaniemi T, Mauno J 1983 Neuromagnetic localization of cortical activity evoked by painful dental stimulation in man. Neuroscience Letters 42: 77–82

Heft MW, Parker SR 1984 An experimental basis for revising the graphic rating scale. Pain 19: 153–161

Hill HF, Chapman CR 1989 Brain activity measures in assessment of pain and analgesia. In: Chapman CR, Loeser JD (eds) Advances in pain research and therapy: issues in pain measurement, vol 12. Raven, New York, pp 231–247

Hostetter MP, Gracely RH 1997 Disassociation of pain intensity and unpleasantness by tourniquet ischemia and modulation by PET. American Pain Society Abstracts 16: 124

Howland EW, Wakai RT, Mjaanes BA, Balog JP, Cleeland CS 1995 Whole head mapping of magnetic fields following painful electric finger shock. Brain Cognitive Brain. Research 2: 165–172

Humphries SA, Johnson MH, Long NR 1996 An investigation of the gate control theory of pain using the experimental pain stimulus of potassium iontophoresis. Perception and Psychophysics 58: 693–703

Iadarola MJ, Wen H, Coghill RC, Wolff SD, Balaban RS 1995 Spatial mapping of pain and motor activation in human cerebral cortex with fMRI at 4 Tesla. Society of Neuroscience Abstracts 20: 1387

Iadarola MJ, Berman KF, Zeffiro TA et al 1998 Neural activation during acute capsaicin-evoked pain and allodynia assessed with PET. Brain 121: 931–947

Ilkjaer S, Dirks J, Brennum J, Wernberg M, Dahl JB 1997 Effect of systemic *N*-methyl-aspartate receptor antagonist (dextromethorphan) on primary and secondary hyperalgesia in humans. British Journal of Anaesthesia 79: 600–605

Ishimaru K, Kawakita K, Sakita M 1995 Analgesic effects induced by TENS and electroacupuncture with different ytpes of stimulating electrodes on deep tissues in human subjects. Pain 63: 181–187

Janal MN, Clark WC, Carroll JD 1991 Multidimensional scaling of painful and innocuous electrocutaneous stimuli: reliability and individual differences. Perception and Psychophysics 50: 108–116

Janal MN, Clark WC, Carroll JD 1993 Multidimensional scaling of painful electrocutaneous stimulation: INDSCAL dimensions, signal detection theory indices, and the McGill Pain Questionnaire. Somatosensory and Motor Research 10: 31–39

Jensen K, Anderson HO, Olesen J, Lindblom U 1986 Pressure–pain threshold in human temporal region. Evaluation of a new pressure algometer. Pain 25: 313–323

Jensen K, Tuxen C, Olsen J 1988: Pericranial muscle tenderness and pressure-pain threshold in the temporal region during common migraine. Pain 35: 65–70

Jensen R, Rasmussen BK, Pedersen B, Lous I, Olesen J 1992 Cephalic muscle tenderness and pressure pain threshold in a general population. Pain 48: 197–203

Johnson MI, Ashton CH, Bousfield DR, Thompson JW 1989 Analgesic effects of different frequencies of transcutaneous electrical nerve stimulation on cold induced pain in normal subjects. Pain 39: 231–236

Jones AKP, Brown WD, Friston KJ, Qi LY, Frackowiak RSJ 1991 Cortical and subcortical localization of response to pain in man using positron emission tomography. Proceedings of the Royal Society of London. Series B, 244: 39–44

Jones AP, Hughes DG, Brettle DS et al 1998 Experiences with function magnetic resonance imaging at 1 tesla. British Journal of Radiology 71: 160–166

Jones B 1980 Algebraic models for integration of painful and nonpainful electric shocks. Perception and Psychophysics 28: 572–576

Kakigi R, Matsuda Y, Kuroda Y 1993 Effects of movement-related cortical activities on pain-related somatosensory evoked potentials following CO_2 laser stimulation in normal subjects. Acta Neurologica Scandinavica 88: 376–380

Kaufman E, Chastain DC, Gaughan AM, Gracely RH 1992 Staircase assessment of the magnitude and timecourse of 50% nitrous oxide analgesia. Journal of Dental Research 71: 1598–1560

Keefe FJ, Block AR 1982 Development of an observation method for assessing pain behavior in chronic low back pain patients. Behavior Therapy 13: 363–375

Keefe FJ, Dolan E 1986 Pain behavior and pain coping strategies in low back pain and myofascial pain dysfunction. Pain 24: 49–56

Kenshalo DR, Bergen DC 1975 A device to measure cutaneous sensibility in human and subhuman species. Journal of Applied Physiology 39: 1038–1040

Kenshalo DR Jr, Anton F, Dubner R 1989 The detection and perceived intensity of noxious thermal stimuli in monkey and man Journal of Neurophysiology 62: 429–436

Kiernan BD, Dane JR, Phillips LH, Price DD 1995 Hypnotic analgesia reuces R-III nociceptive reflex: further evidence concerning the multifactorial nature of hypnotic analgesia. Pain 60: 39–47

Kinnman E, Nygards EB, Hansson P 1997a Effects of dextromethorphan in clinical doses on capsaicin-induced ongoing pain and mechanical hypersensitivity. Journal of Pain Symptom Management 14: 195–201

Kinnman E, Nygards EB, Hansson P 1997b Peripheral alpha-adrenoreceptors are involved in the development of capsaicin induced ongoing and stimulus evoked pain in humans. Pain 69: 79–85

Klement W, Medert HA, Arndt JO 1992 Nalbuphine does not act analgetically in electrical tooth pulp stimulation in man. Pain 48: 269–274

Klepac RK, Dowling J, Hauge G 1981 Sensitivity of the McGill Pain Questionnaire to intensity and quality of laboratory pain. Pain 10: 199–207

Kobal G, Hummel T 1990 Brain responses to chemical stimulation of the trigeminal nerve in man. In: Green BG, Mason JR, Kare MR (eds) Chemical senses, vol 2. Irritation, Dekker, pp 123–136

Kochs E, Scharein E, Mollenberg O, Bromm B, Schulte am Esch J 1996 Analgesic efficacy of low-dose ketamine. Somatosensory-evoked responses in relation to subjective pain ratings. Anesthesiology 85: 304–314

Kunde V, Treede RD 1993 Topography of middle-latency somatosensory evoked potentials following painful laser stimuli and non-painful electrical stimuli. Electroencephalography and Clinical Neurophysiology 88: 280–289

Kwilosz DM, Green BF, Torgerson WS 1983 Qualities of hurting: the language of pain. American Pain Society Abstracts

Langemark M, Bach FW, Jensen TS, Olesen J 1993 Decreased nociceptive flexion reflex threshold in chronic tension-type headache. Archives of Neurology 50: 1061–1064

Lautenbacher S, Rollman GB, McCain GA 1994 Muli-method assessment of experimental and clinical pain in patients with fibromyalgia. Pain 59: 45–53

Lenz FA, Rios M, Chau D, Krauss GL, Zirth TA Lesser RP 1998 Painful stimuli evoke potentials recorded from the parasylvian cortex in humans. J Neurophysiol 80: 2077–2088

Lenz FA, Gracely RH, Rowland LH, Dougherty PM 1994a A population of cells in the human thalamic principal sensory nucleus respond specifically to innocuous and noxious mechanical stimuli. Neuroscience Letters 180: 46–50

Lenz FA, Gracely RH, Hope EJ et al 1994b The sensation of angina pectoris can be evoked by stimulation of the human thalamus. Pain 59: 119–125

Lenz FA, Gracely RH, Romanmoski AJ, Hope EJ, Rowland LH, Dougherty PM 1995 Stimulation in the human somatosensory thalamus can reproduce both the affective and sensory dimensions of previously experienced pain. Nature Medicine 1: 910–913

Lenz FA, Gracely RH, Zirh AT, Romanoski AJ, Doughery PM 1997 The Sensory-Limbic model of pain memory: connections from the thalamus to the limbic system mediate the learned component of the affective dimension of pain. Pain Forum 6: 22–31

LeReshe L 1982 Facial expression in pain: a study of candid photographs. Journal of Nonverbal Behavior 7: 76–186

Leroi AM, Ducrotte P, Bouaniche M, Touchais JY, Weber J, Denis P 1997 Assessment of the reliability of cerebral potentials evoked by electrical stimulation of anal canal. International Journal of Coloretral Disease 12: 335–339

Liu M, Max MB, Prada S, Rowan JS, Bennett GJ 1996a The sympathetic nervous system contributes to capsaicin-evoked mechanical allodynia but not pinprick hyperalgesia in humans. Journal of Neuroscience 16: 7331–7335

Lowe AS, McDowell BC, Walsh DM, Baxter GD, Allen JM 1997 Failure to demonstrate any hyoalgesic effect of low intensity laser irradiation (830 nm) of Erb's point upon experimental ischaemic pain in humans. Lasers in Surgery and Medicine 20: 69–76

Lotsch J, Ditterich W, Hummel T, Kobal G 1997a Antinociceptive effects of the kappa-opioid receptor agonist RP 60180 compared with pentazocine in an experimental human pain model. Clinical Neuropharmacology 20: 224–233

Lotsch J, Kobal G, Stockmann A, Brune K, Geisslinger G 1997b Lack of analgesic activity of morphine-6-glucuronide after short-term intravenous administration in healthy volunteers. Anesthesiology 87: 1348–1358

Luu M, Bonnel AM, Boureau F 1988 Multidimensional experimental pain study in normal man: combining physiological and psychological indices. In: Dubner R, Bond M, Gebhart G (eds) Proceedings of the Fifth World Congress on Pain. Elsevier, Amsterdam, pp 375–382

Ma QP, Woolf CJ 1996 Progressive tactile hypersensitivity: an inflammation-induced incremental increase in the excitability of the spinal cord. Pain 67: 97–106

Magerl W, Treede RD 1996 Heat-evoked vasodilatation in human hairy skin: axon reflexes due to low-level activity of nociceptive afferents. Journal of Physiology 497: 837–848

Marchettini P, Simone DA, Caputi G, Ochoa JL 1996 Pain from excitation of identified muscle nociceptors in humans. Brain Research 740: 109–116

Matthews B, Horiuchi H, Greenwood F 1974 The effects of stimulus polarity and electrode area on the threshold to monopolar stimulation of teeth in human subjects with some preliminary observations on the use of a bipolar pulp tester. Archives of Oral Biology 19: 35–42

May A, Kaube H, Buchel C et al 1998 Experimental cranial pain elicited by capsaicin: a PET study. Pain 74: 61–66

McDaniel LK, Anderson KO, Bradley LA et al 1986 Development of an observation method for assessing pain behavior in rheumatoid arthritis patients. Pain 24: 159–163

McGrath PA, Gracely RH, Dubner R, Heft MW 1983 Non-pain and pain sensations evoked by tooth pulp stimulation. Pain 15: 377–388

McMillan JA, Moudy AM 1986 Differences in nociception during voluntary flexion and extension. Pain 26: 329–336

Meier W, v Klucken M, Soyka D, Bromm B 1993 Hypnotic hypo- and hyperalgesia: divergent effects on pain ratings and pain-related cerebral potentials. Pain 53: 175–181

Melzack R 1983 Pain measurement and assessment. Raven, New York

Melzack R, Torgerson WS 1971 On the language of pain. Anesthesiology 34: 50–59

Messinides L, Naliboff BD 1992 The impact of depression on acute pain perception in chronic back pain patients. American Pain Society Abstracts 11: 59

Meyer RA, Walker RE, Mountcastle VB 1976 A laser stimulator for the study of cutaneous thermal pain sensation. IEEE Transactions on Biomedical Engineering 23: 54–60

Mills WM, Farrow JT 1981 The transcendental meditation technique and acute experimental pain. Psychosomatic Medicine 43: 157–164

Mini A, Rau H, Montoya P, Palomba D, Birbaumer N 1995 Baroreceptor cortical effects, emotions and pain. International Journal of Psychophysiology 19: 67–77

Mokhtar B, Baxter GD, Walsh DM, Bell AJ, Allen JM 1995 Double-blind, placebo-controlled investigation of the effect of combined phototherapy/low intensity laser therapy upon experimental ischaemic pain in humans. Lasers in Surgery and Medicine 17: 74–81

Montagne-Clavel J, Oliveras JL 1996 The 'plantar test' apparatus, a controlled infrared noxious radiant heat simulus for precise withdrawal latency measurement in the rat, as a tool for humans. Somatosensory and Motor Research 13: 215–223

Moore PA, Duncan GH, Scott DS, Gregg JM, Ghia JN 1979 The submaximal effort tourniquet test: its use in evaluating experimental and chronic pain. Pain 6: 375–382

Munakata J, Naliboff B, Harraf F et al 1997 Repetitive sigmoid stimulation induces rectal hyperalgesia in patients with irritable bowel syndrome. Gastroenterology 112: 55–63

Naliboff BD, Munakata J, Fullerton S et al 1997 Evidence for two distinct perceptual alternation in visceral perception in irritable bowel syndrome. Gut 41: 505–512

Nordin M, Fagius J 1995 Effect of noxious simulation on sympathetic vasoconstrictor outflow to human muscles. Journal of Physiology 489: 885–894

Parducci A 1974 Contextual effects: a range-frequency analysis. In: Carterette EC, Friedman MP (eds) Handbook of perception, vol 2. Academic, New York 127–141

Park KM, Max MB, Robinovitz E, Gracely RH, Bennett GJ 1995 Intradermal capsaicin as a model of chronic neuropathic pain: effects of ketamine, alfentanil, and placebo. Pain 63: 163–172

Parry WL, Smith GM, Denton JE 1972 An electric-shock method of inducing pain responsive to morphine in man. Anesthesia and Analgesia 51: 573–578

Patrick CJ, Craig KD, Prkachin KM 1986 Observer judgments of acute pain: facial action determinants. Journal of Personality and Social Psychology 50: 1292–1298

Pertovaara A, Kauppila T, Hamalainen MM 1996 Influence of skin temperature on heat pain threshold in humans. Experimental Brain Research 107: 497–503

Petersen-Felix S, Arendt-Nielson L, Bak P et al 1995 Analgesic effect in humans of subanaesthetic isoflurane concentrations evaluated by experimentally induced pain. British Journal of Anaesthesia 75: 55–60

Petersen-Felix S, Arendt-Nielson L, Bak P, Fischer M, Bjerring P, Zbinden AM 1996 The effects of isoflurane on repeated nociceptive stimuli (central temporal summation). Pain 64: 277–281

Piguet V, Desmeules J, Dayer P 1998 Lack of acetaminophen ceiling effect on R-III nociceptive flexion reflex. European Journal of Clinical Pharmacology 53: 321–324

Poulsen L, Arendt-Nielsen L, Brosen K, Nielsen KK, Gram LF, Sindrup SH 1995 The hypoalgesic effect of imipramine in different human experimental pain models. Pain 60: 287–293

Price DD 1988 Psychological and neural mechanisms of pain. Raven, New York

Price DD, Harkins SW 1992 The affective-motivational dimension of pain: a two stage model. APS Journal 1: 229–239

Price DD, McGrath PA, Rafii A, Buckingham B 1983 The validation of visual analogue scales as ratio scale measures in chronic and experimental pain. Pain 17: 45–56

Procacci P, Zoppi M, Maresca M 1979 Experimental pain in man. Pain 6: 123–140

Rainville P, Duncan GH, Price DD, Carrier B, Bushnell C 1997 Pain affect encoded in human anterior cingulate but not somatosensory cortex. Science 277: 968–971

Reading AE, Everitt BS, Sledmere 1982 The McGill Pain Questionnaire: a replication of its construction. British Journal of Clinical Psychology 21: 339–349

Reid KI, Gracely RH, Dubner R 1994 The influence of time, facial side, and location on pain pressure thresholds in chronic myogenous temporomandibular disorder. Journal of Orofacial Pain 8: 258–265

Rollman GB 1977 Signal detection theory measurement of pain: a review and critique. Pain 3: 187–211

Roth D, Petersen-Felix S, Bak P et al 1996 Analgesic effect in humans of subanaesthetic isoflurane concentrations evaluated by evoked potentials. British Journal of Anaesthesia 76: 38–42

Schmelz M, Kress M 1996 Topical acetylsalicylate attenuates capsaicin induced pain, flare and allodynia but not thermal hyperalgesia. Neuroscience Letters 214: 72–74

Sethna NF, Liu M, Gracely RH, Bennett GJ, Max MB 1998 Analgesic and cognitive effects of intravenous ketamine–alfentanil combinatios vs. either drug alone after intradermal capsaicin in normal subjects. Anesthesia and Analgesia 86: 1250–1256

Simone DA, Baumann TK, LaMotte RH 1989 Dose-dependent pain and mechanical hyperalgesia in humans after intradermal injection of capsaicin. Pain 38: 99–107

Sjölund B, Eriksson M 1985 Relief of pain by TENS. John Wiley, New York

Smith GM, Egbert LD, Markowitz RA, Mosteller F, Beecher HK 1966 An experimental pain method sensitive to morphine in man: the submaximum effort tourniquet technique. Journal of Pharmacological and Experimental Therapeutics 154: 324–332

Sollenbohmer C, Enck P, Haussinger D, Frieling T 1996 Electrically evoked cerebral potentials during esophageal distension at perception and pain threshold. American Journal of Gastroenterology 91: 970–975

Steen KH, Reeh PW 1993 Sustained graded pain and hyperalgesia from harmless experimental tissue acidosis in human skin. Neuroscience Letters 154: 113–116

Steen KH, Reeh PW, Kreysel HW 1995 Topical acetylsalicylic, salicylic acid and indomethacin suppress pain from experimental tissue acidosis in human skin. Pain 62: 339–347

Steen KH, Steen AE, Kreysel HW, Reeh PW 1996 Inflammatory mediators potentiate pain induced by experimental tissue acidosis. Pain 66: 163–170

Sternbach RA 1983 The tourniquet pain test. In: Melzack R (ed) Pain measurement and assessment. Raven, New York 27–31

Sternberg WF, Bailin D, Grant M, Gracely RH 1998 Competition alters perception of noxious heat and cold in male and female athletes. Pain 76: 231–238

Svensson P, Beydoun A, Morrow TJ, Casey KL 1997 Non-painful and painful stimulation of human skin and muscle: analysis of cerebral evoked potentials. Electroencephalography and Clinical Neurophysiology 104: 343–350

Talbot JD, Marrett S, Evans AC, Meyer E, Bushnell MC, Duncan GH 1991 Multiple representations of pain in human cerebral cortex. Science 251: 1355–1358

Tarkka IM, Treede RD 1993 Equivalent electrical source analysis of pain-related somatosensory evoked potentials elicited by a CO_2 laser. Journal of Clinical Neurophysiology 10: 513–519

Thurauf N, Hummel T, Kettenmann B, Kobal G 1993 Nociceptive and reflexive responses recorded from the human nasal mucosa. Brain Research 629: 293–299

Thurstone LI 1959 The measurement of values. University of Chicago Press, Chicago

Timmermans G, Sternbach RA 1974 Factors of human chronic pain: an analysis of personality and pain reaction variables. Science 184: 806–808

Torebjörk HE, Hallin RG 1970 C fiber units recorded from human sensory nerve fascicles in situ. Acta Societratis Medicorum Upsaliensis 75: 81–84

Torebjörk HE, Lundberg LER, LaMotte RH 1992 Central changes in processing of mechanoreceptive input in capsaicin-induced secondary hyperalgesia in humans. Journal of Physiology 448: 765–780

Torgerson WS, BenDebba M, Mason KJ 1988 Varieties of pain. In: Dubner R, Gebhart GF, Bond MR (eds) Proceedings of the Vth World Congress on Pain. Elsevier, Amsterdam, pp 368–374

Tursky B 1974 Physical, physiological and psychological factors that affect pain reaction to electric shock. Psychophysiology 11: 95–112

Tursky B 1976 The development of a pain perception profile: a psychological approach. In: Weisenberg M, Tursky B (eds) Pain: new perspectives in therapy and research. Plenum, New York 171–194

Urasaki E, Wada S, Yasukouchi H, Yokota A 1998 Effect of transcutaneous electrical nerve stimulation (TENS) on central nervous system amplification of somatosensory input. Journal of Neurology 245: 143–148

Vallbo AB, Hagbarth KE 1968 Activity from skin mechanoreceptors recorded percutaneously in awake human subjects. Experimental Neurology 21: 270–289

Van Hees J, Gybels JM 1972 Pain related to single afferent C fibres from human skin. Brain Research 48: 397–400

Veerasarn P, Stohler CS 1992 The effect of experimental muscle pain on the background electrical brain activity. Pain 49: 349–360

Vogt BA, Derbyshire S, Jones AKP 1996 Pain processing in four regions of human cingulate cortex localized with coregistered PET and MRI. European Journal of Neuroscience 8: 1461–1473

Wade JB, Price DD, Hamer RM, Schwartz SM, Hart RP 1990 An emotional component analysis of chronic pain. Pain 40: 303–310

Wall PD 1979 On the relation of injury to pain. Pain 6: 253–264

Watanabe S, Kakigi R, Hoshiyama M, Kitamura Y, Koyama S, Shimojo M 1996 Effects of noxious cooling of the skin on pain perception in man. Journal of the Neurological Sciences 135: 68–73

Whipple B, Komisaruk BR 1985 Elevation of pain threshold by vaginal stimulation in women. Pain 21: 357–367

Willer JC 1977 Comparative study of perceived pain and nociceptive flexion reflex in man. Pain 3: 69–80

Willer JC 1985 Studies on pain. Effects of morphine on a spinal nociceptive flexion reflex and related pain sensation in man. Brain Research 331: 105–114

Willer JC, Bussel V 1980 Evidence for a direct spinal mechanism in morphine induced inhibition of nociceptive reflexes in humans. Brain Research 187: 212–215

Willer JC, Dehen H, Cambier J 1981 Stress-induced analgesia in humans: endogenous opioids and naloxone reversible depression of pain reflexes. Science 212: 689–690

Willer JC, Roby A, Boulu P, Boureau F 1982 Comparative effects of electroacupuncture and transcutaneous nerve stimulation on the human blink reflex. Pain 14: 267–278

Willer JC, DeBroucker T, Barranquero A, Kahn MF 1987 Brain evoked potentials to noxious sural nerve stimulation in sciatalgic patients. Pain 30: 47–58

Wolfe F, Smythe HA, Yunus MB et al 1990 The American College of Rheumatology 1990 criteria for the classification of fibromyalgia. Report of the Multicenter Criteria Committee. Arthritis and Rheumatism 33: 160–172

Wolff BB 1971 Factor analysis of human pain responses: pain endurance as a specific pain factor. Journal of Abnormal Psychology 78: 292–298

Wolff BB 1984 Methods of testing pain mechanisms in normal man. In: Wall PD, Melzack R (eds) Textbook of pain, 1st edn. Churchill Livingstone, London

Yarnitsky D, Sprecher E, Zaslansky R, Hemli JA 1996 Multiple session experimental pain measurements. Pain 67: 327–333

Xu X, Kanda M, Shindo K et al 1995 Pain-related somatosensory evoked potentials following CO_2 laser stimulation of foot in man. Electroencephalography and Clinical Neurophysiology 96: 12–23

Pain measurement in persons in pain

17

RONALD MELZACK & JOEL KATZ

SUMMARY

Pain is a personal, subjective experience that comprises sensory-discriminative, motivational-affective and cognitive-evaluative dimensions. Approaches to the measurement of pain include verbal and numeric self-rating scales, behavioural observation scales, and physiological responses. The complex nature of the experience of pain suggests that measurements from these domains may not always show high concordance. Because pain is subjective, the patient's self report provides the most valid measure of the experience. The visual analogue scale and the McGill Pain Questionnaire are probably the most frequently used self-rating instruments for the measurement of pain in clinical and research settings. The McGill Pain Questionnaire is designed to assess the multidimensional nature of pain experience and has been demonstrated to be a reliable, valid and consistent measurement tool. A short-form McGill Pain Questionnaire is available for use in specific research settings when the time to obtain information from patients is limited and when more information than simply the intensity of pain is desired. The Descriptor Differential Scale was developed using sophisticated psychophysical techniques and is designed to measure separately the sensory and unpleasantness dimensions of pain. It has been shown to be a valid and reliable measure of pain with ratio scale properties and has recently been used in a clinical setting. Behavioural approaches to the measurement of pain also provide valuable data. Further development and refinement of pain measurement techniques will lead to increasingly accurate tools with greater predictive powers.

INTRODUCTION

People suffering acute or chronic pain provide valuable opportunities to study the mechanisms of pain and analgesia. The measurement of pain is therefore essential to determine the intensity, perceptual qualities and time course of the pain so that the differences among pain syndromes can be ascertained and investigated. Furthermore, measurement of these variables provides valuable clues which help in the differential diagnosis of the underlying causes of the pain. They also help to determine the most effective treatment, such as the types of analgesic drugs or other therapies, necessary to control the pain, and are essential in evaluating the relative effectiveness of different therapies. The measurement of pain, then, is important:

1. To determine pain intensity, quality and duration.
2. To aid in diagnosis.
3. To help decide on the choice of therapy.
4. To evaluate the relative effectiveness of different therapies.

DIMENSIONS OF PAIN EXPERIENCE

Research on pain, since the beginning of this century, has been dominated by the concept that pain is purely a sensory experience. Yet pain also has a distinctly unpleasant, affective quality. It becomes overwhelming, demands immediate attention, and disrupts ongoing behaviour and thought. It motivates or drives the organism into activity aimed at stopping the pain as quickly as possible. To consider only the sensory features of pain and ignore its motivational-affective properties is to look at only part of the problem. Even the concept of pain as a perception, with full recognition of past experience, attention and other cognitive influences, still neglects the crucial motivational dimension.

These considerations led Melzack and Casey (1968) to suggest that there are three major psychological dimensions of pain: sensory-discriminative, motivational-affective and cognitive-evaluative. They proposed, moreover, that these dimensions of pain experience are subserved by physiologically specialized systems in the brain: the sensory-discriminative dimension of pain is influenced primarily by the rapidly conducting spinal systems; the powerful motivational drive and unpleasant affect characteristic of pain are subserved by activities in reticular and limbic structures that are influenced primarily by the slowly conducting spinal systems; neocortical or higher central nervous system processes, such as evaluation of the input in terms of past experience, exert control over activity in both the discriminative and motivational systems.

It is assumed that these three categories of activity interact with one another to provide *perceptual information* on the location, magnitude and spatiotemporal properties of the noxious stimuli, *motivational tendency* toward escape or attack, and *cognitive information* based on past experience and probability of outcome of different response strategies (Melzack & Casey 1968). All three forms of activity could then influence motor mechanisms responsible for the complex pattern of overt responses that characterize pain.

THE LANGUAGE OF PAIN

Clinical investigators have long recognized the varieties of pain experience. Descriptions of the burning qualities of pain after peripheral nerve injury, or the stabbing, cramping qualities of visceral pains frequently provide the key to diagnosis and may even suggest the course of therapy. Despite the frequency of such descriptions, and the seemingly high agreement that they are valid descriptive words, studies of their use and meaning are relatively recent.

Anyone who has suffered severe pain and tried to describe the experience to a friend or to the doctor often finds himself at a loss for words. The reason for this difficulty in expressing pain experience is not because the words do not exist – as we shall soon see, there is an abundance of appropriate words. Rather, the main reason is that, fortunately, they are not words which we have occasion to use often. Another reason is that the words may seem absurd. We may use descriptors such as splitting, shooting, gnawing, wrenching or stinging as useful metaphors, but there are no external objective references for these words in relation to pain. If we talk about a blue pen or a yellow pencil we can point to an object and say 'that is what I mean by yellow' or 'this colour of the pen is blue'. But what can we point to to tell another person precisely what we mean by smarting, tingling or rasping? A person who suffers terrible pain may say that the pain is burning and add that 'it feels as if someone is shoving a red-hot poker through my toes and slowly twisting it around'. These 'as if' statements are often essential to convey the qualities of the experience.

If the study of pain in people is to have a scientific foundation, it is essential to measure it. If we want to know how effective a new drug is, we need numbers to say that the pain decreased by some amount. Yet, while overall intensity is important information, we also want to know whether the drug specifically decreased the burning quality of the pain, or if the especially miserable, tight, cramping feeling is gone.

PAIN RATING SCALES

Until recently, the methods that were used for pain measurement treated pain as though it were a single unique quality that varies only in intensity (Beecher 1959). These methods include the use of verbal rating scales (VRSs), numerical rating scales (NRSs) and visual analogue scales (VASs). These simple methods have all been used effectively in hospital clinics, and have provided valuable information about pain and analgesia. VRSs, NRSs and VASs provide simple, efficient, and minimally intrusive measures of pain intensity which have been used widely in clinical and research settings where a quick index of pain intensity is required and to which a numerical value can be assigned.

VERBAL AND NUMERICAL RATING SCALES

Verbal rating scales typically consist of a series of verbal pain descriptors ordered from least to most intense (e.g., no pain, mild, moderate, severe) (Jensen & Karoly 1992). The patient reads the list and chooses the one word that best describes the intensity of his pain at the moment. A score of zero is assigned to the descriptor with the lowest rank, a score of 1 is assigned to the descriptor with the next lowest rank, etc. Numerical rating scales typically consist of a series of numbers ranging from 0 to 10 or 0 to 100 with endpoints intended to represent the extremes of the possible pain experience and labelled 'no pain' and 'worst possible pain', respectively. The patient chooses the number that best corresponds to the intensity of his pain at the moment. Although VRSs and NRSs are simple to administer and have demonstrated reliability and validity, the advantages associated with VASs (see below) make them the measurement instrument of choice when a unidimensional measure of pain is required. However, this may not be true when assessing chronic pain in the elderly. A recent study indicates that elderly patients make fewer errors on a VRS than a VAS (Gagliese & Melzack 1997).

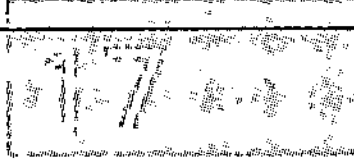

VISUAL ANALOGUE SCALES

The most common VAS consists of a 10-cm horizontal (Joyce et al 1975, Huskisson 1983) or vertical (Sriwatanakul et al 1983) line with the two endpoints labelled 'no pain' and 'worst pain ever' (or similar verbal descriptors). The patient is required to place a mark on the 10-cm line at a point which corresponds to the level of pain intensity he presently feels. The distance in centimetres from the low end of the VAS to the patient's mark is used as a numerical index of the severity of pain.

VASs for pain affect have been developed in an effort to include domains of measurable pain experience other than the sensory intensity dimension. The patient is asked to rate the unpleasantness of the pain experience (i.e., how disturbing it is). Endpoints are labelled 'not bad at all' and 'the most unpleasant feeling imaginable' (Price et al 1986, 1987).

VASs are sensitive to pharmacological and non-pharmacological procedures which alter the experience of pain (Price et al 1986, Bélanger et al 1989, Choinière et al 1990) and correlate highly with pain measured on verbal and numerical rating scales (Ohnhaus & Adler 1975, Kremer & Atkinson 1983, Ekblom & Hansson 1988). Instructions to patients to rate the amount or percentage of pain relief using a VAS (e.g., following administration of a treatment designed to reduce pain) may introduce unnecessary bias (e.g., expectancy for change and reliance on memory) which reduces the validity of the measure. It has been suggested (Carlsson 1983), therefore, that a more appropriate measure of change may be obtained by having patients rate the absolute amount of pain at different points in time such as before and after an intervention (but see Ekblom & Hansson 1988).

A major advantage of the VAS as a measure of sensory pain intensity is its ratio scale properties (Price et al 1983, Price & Harkins 1987, Price 1988). In contrast to many other pain measurement tools, equality of ratios is implied, making it appropriate to speak meaningfully about percentage differences between VAS measurements obtained either at multiple points in time, or from independent samples of subjects. Other advantages of the VAS include:

1. its ease and brevity of administration and scoring (Jensen et al 1986)
2. its minimal intrusiveness
3. its conceptual simplicity (Huskisson 1983, Chapman et al 1985)

providing that adequately clear instructions are given to the patient.

Standard VASs also have several limitations and disadvantages. These include difficulty with administration in a patient who has perceptual-motor problems, impractical scoring method in a clinical setting where immediate measurement of the patient's response may not be possible, and the occasional patient who cannot comprehend the instructions. These limitations and disadvantages of VASs have been remedied by Choinière and Amsel (1996) in their development of a visual analogue thermometer (VAT). The VAT consists of a rigid, plasticized cardboard strip of white colour with a horizontal black opening 10 cm long by 2 cm wide. The ends of the opening are labelled 'no pain' and 'unbearable pain'. A red opaque band covers the opening and slides from left to right using a tab operated from the back of the thermometer. The red strip is moved from left to right across the black opening until the patient stops at a point that corresponds to the intensity of his pain. The back of the VAT also shows a 10-cm ruler to facilitate scoring. The VAT correlates well with a standard paper-and-pencil VAS and a numerical rating scale, is sensitive to changes in pain levels and is preferred over a standard VAS by a substantial number of subjects (Choinière & Amsel 1996).

The major disadvantage of VASs is the assumption that pain is a unidimensional experience which can be measured with a single item scale (Melzack 1975). Although intensity is, without a doubt, a salient dimension of pain, it is clear that the word 'pain' refers to an endless variety of qualities which are categorized under a single linguistic label, not to a specific, single sensation which varies only in intensity or affect. The development of VASs to measure pain affect or unpleasantness has partially addressed the problem, but the same shortcoming applies within the affective domain. Each pain has unique qualities. Unpleasantness is only one such quality. The pain of a toothache is obviously different from that of a pin-prick, just as the pain of a coronary occlusion is uniquely different from the pain of a broken leg. To describe pain solely in terms of intensity or affect is like specifying the visual world only in terms of light flux without regard to pattern, colour, texture and the many other dimensions of visual experience.

THE MCGILL PAIN QUESTIONNAIRE

DEVELOPMENT AND DESCRIPTION

Melzack and Torgerson (1971) developed the procedures to specify the qualities of pain. In the first part of their study, physicians and other university graduates were asked to classify 102 words, obtained from the clinical literature, into small groups that describe distinctly different aspects of the experience of pain. On the basis of the data, the words were categorized into three major classes and 16 subclasses (Fig. 17.1). The classes are:

1. Words that describe the *sensory qualities* of the experience in terms of temporal, spatial, pressure, thermal and other properties.
2. Words that describe the *affective qualities* in terms of tension, fear and autonomic properties that are part of the pain experience.
3. *Evaluative* words that describe the subjective overall intensity of the total pain experience.

Each subclass, which was given a descriptive label, consists of a group of words that were considered by most subjects to be qualitatively similar. Some of these words are undoubtedly synonyms, others seem to be synonymous but vary in intensity, while many provide subtle differences or nuances (despite their similarities) which may be of importance to a patient who is trying desperately to communicate to a physician.

The second part of the Melzack and Torgerson (1971) study attempted to determine the pain intensities implied by the words within each subclass. Groups of physicians, patients and students were asked to assign an intensity value to each word, using a numerical scale ranging from least (or mild) pain to worst (or excruciating) pain. When this was done, it was apparent that several words within each subclass had the same relative intensity relationships in all three sets. For example, in the spatial subclass, 'shooting' was found to represent more pain than 'flashing', which in turn implied more pain than 'jumping'. Although the precise intensity scale values differed for the three groups, all three agreed on the positions of the words relative to each other. The scale values of the words for patients, based on the precise numerical values listed in Melzack and Torgerson (1971), are shown in Figure 17.1.

Because of the high degree of agreement on the intensity relationships among pain descriptors by subjects who have different cultural, socioeconomic, and educational backgrounds, a pain questionnaire (Fig. 17.2) was developed as an experimental tool for studies of the effects of various methods of pain management. In addition to the list of pain descriptors, the questionnaire contains line drawings of the body to show the spatial distribution of the pain, words that describe temporal properties of pain and descriptors of the overall present pain intensity (PPI). The PPI is recorded as a number from 1 to 5, in which each number is associated with the following words: 1, mild; 2, discomforting; 3, distressing; 4, horrible; 5, excruciating. The mean scale values of these words, which were chosen from the evaluative category, are approximately equally far apart so that they represent equal scale intervals and thereby provide 'anchors' for the specification of the overall pain intensity (Melzack & Torgerson 1971).

In a preliminary study, the pain questionnaire consisted of the 16 subclasses of descriptors shown in Figure 17.1, as well as the additional information deemed necessary for the

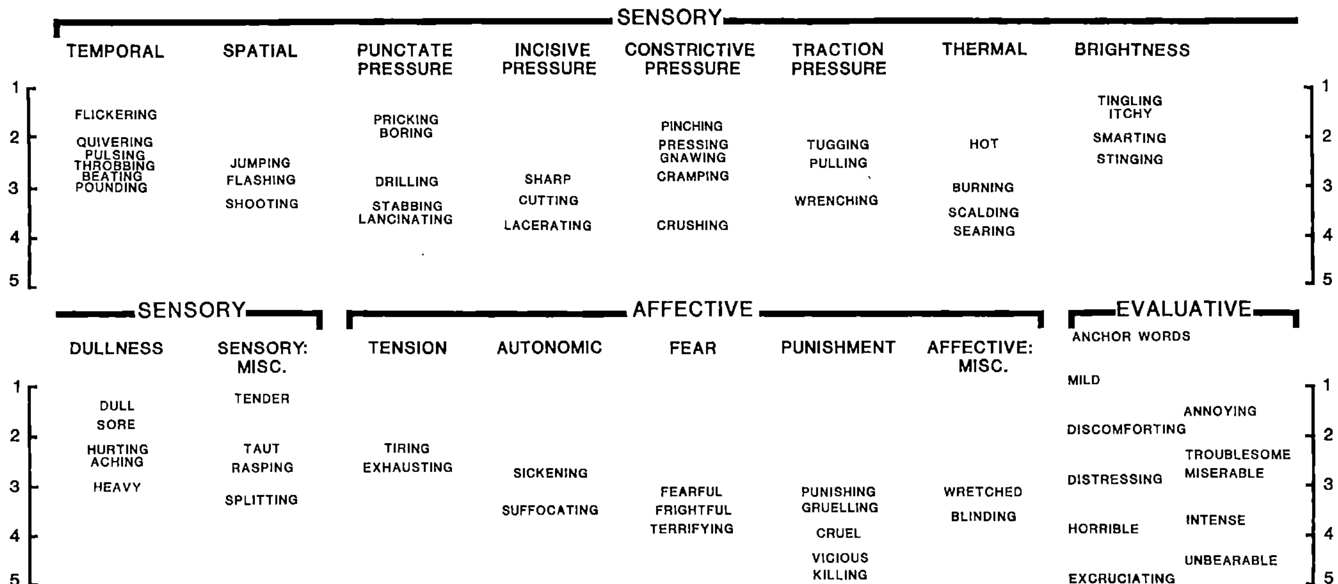

Fig. 17.1 Spatial display of pain descriptors based on intensity ratings by patients. The intensity scale values range from 1 (mild) to 5 (excruciating).

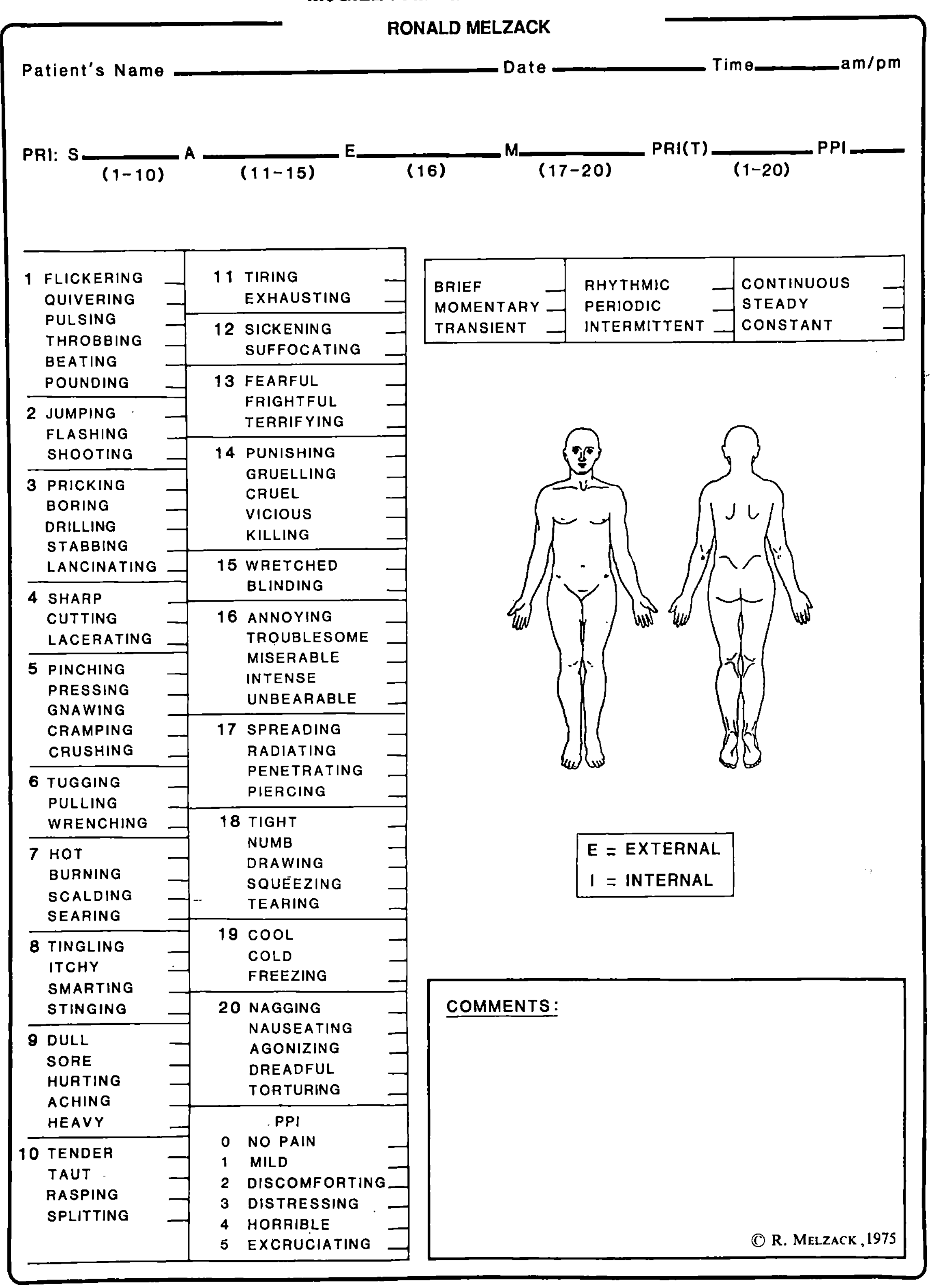

McGILL PAIN QUESTIONNAIRE

RONALD MELZACK

Patient's Name ______ Date ______ Time ______ am/pm

PRI: S ______ (1-10) A ______ (11-15) E ______ (16) M ______ (17-20) PRI(T) ______ (1-20) PPI ______

1 FLICKERING, QUIVERING, PULSING, THROBBING, BEATING, POUNDING
2 JUMPING, FLASHING, SHOOTING
3 PRICKING, BORING, DRILLING, STABBING, LANCINATING
4 SHARP, CUTTING, LACERATING
5 PINCHING, PRESSING, GNAWING, CRAMPING, CRUSHING
6 TUGGING, PULLING, WRENCHING
7 HOT, BURNING, SCALDING, SEARING
8 TINGLING, ITCHY, SMARTING, STINGING
9 DULL, SORE, HURTING, ACHING, HEAVY
10 TENDER, TAUT, RASPING, SPLITTING
11 TIRING, EXHAUSTING
12 SICKENING, SUFFOCATING
13 FEARFUL, FRIGHTFUL, TERRIFYING
14 PUNISHING, GRUELLING, CRUEL, VICIOUS, KILLING
15 WRETCHED, BLINDING
16 ANNOYING, TROUBLESOME, MISERABLE, INTENSE, UNBEARABLE
17 SPREADING, RADIATING, PENETRATING, PIERCING
18 TIGHT, NUMB, DRAWING, SQUEEZING, TEARING
19 COOL, COLD, FREEZING
20 NAGGING, NAUSEATING, AGONIZING, DREADFUL, TORTURING

PPI
0 NO PAIN
1 MILD
2 DISCOMFORTING
3 DISTRESSING
4 HORRIBLE
5 EXCRUCIATING

BRIEF	RHYTHMIC	CONTINUOUS
MOMENTARY	PERIODIC	STEADY
TRANSIENT	INTERMITTENT	CONSTANT

E = EXTERNAL
I = INTERNAL

COMMENTS:

© R. MELZACK, 1975

Fig. 17.2 McGill Pain Questionnaire. The descriptors fall into four major groups: sensory, 1–10; affective, 11–15; evaluative, 16; miscellaneous, 17–20. The rank value for each descriptor is based on its position in the word set. The sum of the rank values is the pain rating index (PRI). The present pain intensity (PPI) is based on a scale of 0–5.

evaluation of pain. It soon became clear, however, that many of the patients found certain key words to be absent. These words were then selected from the original word list used by Melzack and Torgerson (1971), were categorized appropriately and ranked according to their mean scale values. A further set of words – cool, cold, freezing – was used by patients on rare occasions but was indicated to be essential for an adequate description of some types of pain. Thus, four supplementary – or 'miscellaneous' – subclasses were added to the word lists of the questionnaire (Fig. 17.2). The final classification, then, appeared to represent the most parsimonious and meaningful set of subclasses without at the same time losing subclasses that represent important qualitative properties. The questionnaire, which is known as the McGill Pain Questionnaire (MPQ) (Melzack 1975), has become a widely used clinical and research tool (Melzack 1983, Reading 1989, Wilkie et al 1990).

MEASURES OF PAIN EXPERIENCE

The descriptor-lists of the MPQ are read to a patient with the explicit instruction that he chooses only those words which describe his feelings and sensations at that moment. Three major indices are obtained:

1. The pain rating index (PRI) based on the rank values of the words. In this scoring system, the word in each subclass implying the least pain is given a value of 1, the next word is given a value of 2, etc. The rank values of the words chosen by a patient are summed to obtain a score separately for the sensory (subclasses 1–10), affective (subclasses 11–15), evaluative (subclass 16) and miscellaneous (subclasses 17–20) words, in addition to providing a total score (subclasses 1–20). Figure 17.3 shows MPQ scores (total score from subclasses 1–20) obtained by patients with a variety of acute and chronic pains.

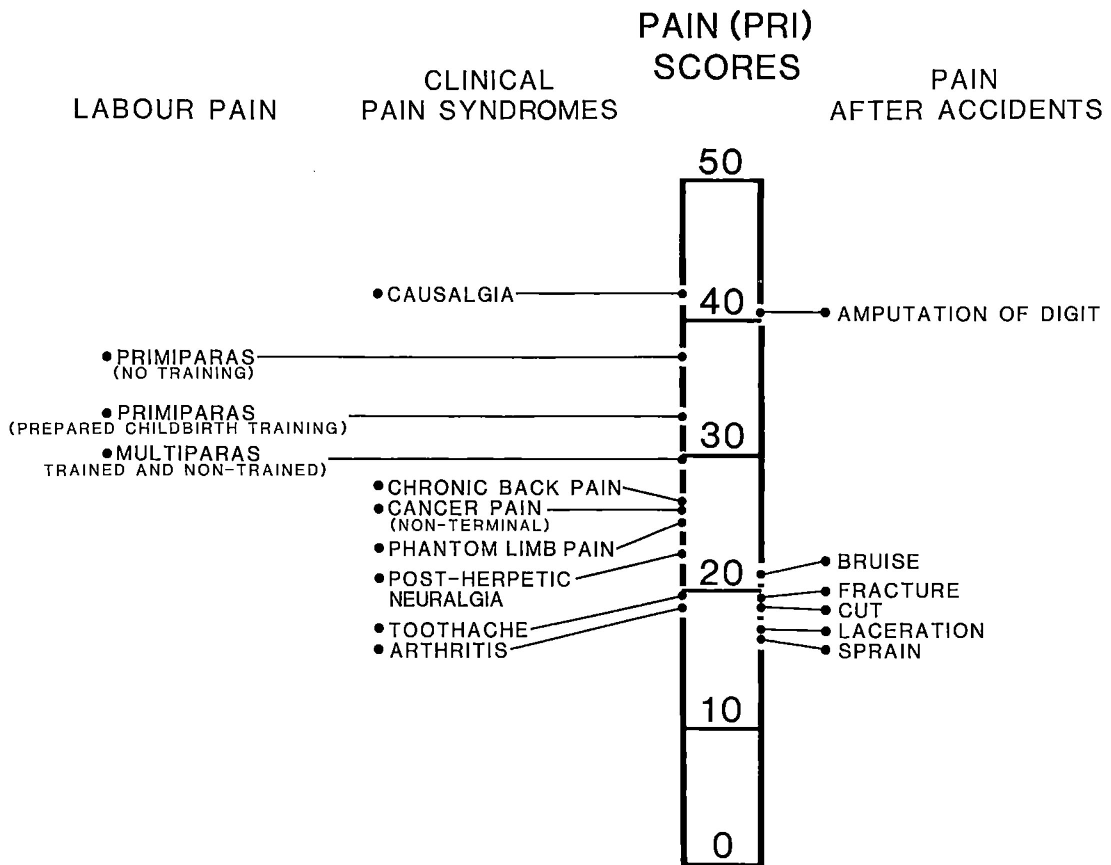

Fig. 17.3 Comparison of pain scores using the McGill Pain Questionnaire, obtained from women during labour (Melzack et al 1981), and from patients in a general hospital pain clinic (Melzack 1975) and an emergency department (Melzack et al 1982). The pain score for causalgic pain is reported by Tahmoush (1981).

 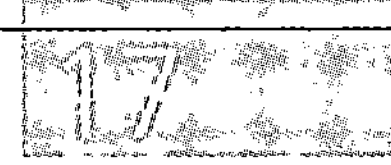

2. The number of words chosen (NWC).
3. The present pain intensity (PPI), the number–word combination chosen as the indicator of overall pain intensity at the time of administration of the questionnaire.

USEFULNESS OF THE MPQ

The most important requirement of a measure is that it be valid, reliable, consistent and above all, useful. The MPQ appears to meet all of these requirements (Melzack 1983, Chapman et al 1985, Reading 1989, Wilkie et al 1990) and provides a relatively rapid way of measuring subjective pain experience (Melzack 1975). When administered to a patient by reading each subclass, it can be completed in about 5 min. It can also be filled out by the patient in a more leisurely way as a paper-and-pencil test, although the scores are somewhat different (Klepac et al 1981).

Since its introduction in 1975, the MPQ has been used in over 350 studies of acute, chronic and laboratory-produced pains. It has been translated into several languages and has also spawned the development of similar pain questionnaires in other languages (Table 17.1).

Table 17.1 Pain questionnaires in different languages based on the McGill Pain Questionnaire

Language	*Authors*
Arabic	Harrison (1988)
Chinese	Hui & Chen (1989)
Czech (SF-MPQ)	Solcovä et al (1990)
Danish	Drewes et al (1993)
Dutch (Flemish)	Vanderiet et al (1987)
	Verkes et al (1989)
	van Lankveld et al (1992)
	van der Kloot et al (1995)
Finnish	Ketovuori & Pöntinen (1981)
French	Boureau et al (1984, 1992)
German	Kiss et al (1987)
	Radvila et al (1987)
	Stein & Mendl (1988)
Italian	De Benedittis et al (1988)
	Ferracuti et al (1990)
	Maiani & Sanavio (1985)
Japanese	Satow et al (1990)
Norwegian	Strand & Wisnes (1991)
	Kim et al (1995)
Polish	Sedlak (1990)
Portuguese	Pimenta & Teixeiro (1996)
Slovak	Bartko et al (1984)
Spanish	Laheurta et al (1982)
	Bejarano et al (1985)
	Lázaro et al (1994)
	Escalante et al (1996)
Swedish (SF-MPQ)	Burckhardt & Bjelle (1984)

Because pain is a private, personal experience, it is impossible for us to know precisely what someone else's pain feels like. No man can possibly know what it is like to have menstrual cramps or labour pain. Nor can a psychologically healthy person know what a psychotic patient is feeling when he says he has excruciating pain (Veilleux & Melzack 1976). But the MPQ provides us with an insight into the qualities that are experienced. Recent studies indicate that each kind of pain is characterized by a distinctive constellation of words. There is a remarkable consistency in the choice of words by patients suffering the same or similar pain syndromes (Van Buren & Kleinknecht 1979, Graham et al 1980, Melzack et al 1981, Grushka & Sessle 1984, Katz & Melzack 1991, Katz 1992). For example, in a study of amputees with phantom limb pain (Group PLP) or non-painful phantom limb sensations (Group PLS), every MPQ descriptor chosen by 33% or more of subjects in Group PLS was also chosen by 33% or more subjects in Group PLP, although there were other descriptors the latter group endorsed with greater frequency (Katz & Melzack 1991). These data indicated that the phantom limb experiences of the two groups have in common a paraesthetic quality (e.g., tingling, numb), although painful phantoms consist of more than this shared component.

RELIABILITY AND VALIDITY OF THE MPQ

Reading et al (1982) investigated the reliability of the groupings of adjectives in the MPQ by using different methodological and statistical approaches. Subjects sorted each of the 78 words of the MPQ into groups that described similar pain qualities. The mean number of groups was 19 (with a range of 7–31), which is remarkably close to the MPQ's 20 groups. Moreover, there were distinct subgroups for sensory and affective-evaluative words. Because the cultural backgrounds of subjects in this study and in that of Melzack and Torgerson's (1971) were different, and the methodology and data analysis were dissimilar, the degree of correspondence is impressive. More recently, Gaston-Johansson et al (1990) reported that subjects with diverse ethnic-cultural and educational backgrounds use similar MPQ adjectives to describe commonly used words such as 'pain', 'hurt' and 'ache'. Nevertheless, interesting differences between the studies were found which suggest alternative approaches for future revisions of the MPQ.

Evidence for the stability of the MPQ was provided by Love et al (1989), who administered the questionnaire to patients with chronic low back pain on two occasions (separated by several days) prior to receiving treatment. Their results show very strong test–retest reliability coefficients for the MPQ pain rating indexes as well as for some of the 20 categories. The lower coefficients for the 20 categories may be explained by the suggestion that many clinical pains show fluctuations in quality over time yet they still represent the 'same' pain to the person who experiences it.

Studies of the validity of the three-dimensional framework of the MPQ are numerous, and have been reviewed by Reading (1989). Generally, the distinction between sensory and affective dimensions has held up extremely well, but there is still considerable debate on the separation of the affective and evaluative dimensions. Nevertheless, several excellent studies (Reading 1979, Prieto et al 1980, McCreary et al 1981, Holroyd et al 1992) have reported a discrete evaluative factor. The different factor-analytic procedures that were used undoubtedly account for the reports of four factors (Reading 1979, Holroyd et al 1992), five factors (Crockett et al 1977), six factors (Burckhardt 1984) or seven factors (Leavitt et al 1978). The major source of disagreement, however, seems to be the different patient populations that are used to obtain data for factor analyses. The range includes brief laboratory pains, dysmenorrhea, back pain and cancer pain. In some studies, relatively few words are chosen, while large numbers are selected in others. It is not surprising, then, that factor-analytic studies based on such diverse populations have confused rather than clarified some of the issues.

Turk et al (1985) examined the internal structure of the MPQ by using techniques that avoided the problems of most earlier studies and confirmed the three (sensory, affective and evaluative) dimensions. Still more recently, Lowe et al (1991) again confirmed the three-factor structure of the MPQ, using elegant statistical procedures and a large number of subjects. Finally, a paper by Chen et al (1989) presents data on the remarkable consistency of the MPQ across five studies using the cold pressor task, and Pearce and Morley (1989) provided further confirmation of the construct validity of the MPQ using the Stroop color naming task with chronic pain patients.

SENSITIVITY OF THE MPQ

Recent studies show that the MPQ is sensitive to interventions designed to reduce pain (Pozehl et al 1995, Briggs 1996, Burchiel et al 1996, Eija et al 1996, Nikolajsen et al 1996, Tesfaye et al 1996). The relative sensitivity of the MPQ to change in postoperative pain following the administration of oral analgesics was evaluated by comparing it with VAS and VRS measures of pain intensity (Jenkinson et al 1995). While all three measures of pain revealed the same pattern of change over time, effect sizes for the MPQ were consistently related to self-reported directly assessed change in pain using a VRS. These findings probably underestimate the MPQ's sensitivity to change because the benchmark for change was a VRS. In support of this, the MPQ appears to provide a more sensitive measure of mild postoperative pain than does a simple VAS which assesses pain intensity only, as patients can be more precise in describing their experience by selecting appropriate descriptors (Katz et al 1994). This increased ability of the MPQ to detect differences in pain at the low end of the pain continuum most likely is a function of the multidimensional nature of the MPQ and the large number of descriptors from which to choose.

DISCRIMINATIVE CAPACITY OF THE MPQ

One of the most exciting features of the MPQ is its potential value as an aid in the differential diagnosis between various pain syndromes. The first study to demonstrate the discriminative capacity of the MPQ was carried out by Dubuisson and Melzack (1976), who administered the questionnaire to 95 patients suffering from one of eight known pain syndromes: postherpetic neuralgia, phantom limb pain, metastatic carcinoma, toothache, degenerative disc disease, rheumatoid arthritis or osteoarthritis, labour pain and menstrual pain. A multiple group discriminant analysis revealed that each type of pain is characterized by a distinctive constellation of verbal descriptors. Further, when the descriptor set for each patient was classified into one of the eight diagnostic categories, a correct classification was made in 77% of cases. Table 17.2 shows the pain descriptors that are most characteristic of the eight clinical pain syndromes in the Dubuisson and Melzack (1976) study.

Descriptor patterns can also provide the basis for discriminating between two major types of low back pain. Some patients have clear physical causes such as degenerative disc disease, while others suffer low back pain even though no physical causes can be found. Using a modified version of the MPQ, Leavitt and Garron (1980) found that patients with physical – 'organic' – causes use distinctly different patterns of words from patients whose pain has no detectable cause and is labelled as 'functional'. A concordance of 87% was found between established medical diagnosis and classification based upon the patients' choice of word patterns from the MPQ. Along similar lines, Perry et al (1988, 1991) report differences in the pattern of MPQ subscale correlations in patients with and without demonstrable organic pathology.

Further evidence of the discriminative capacity of the MPQ was furnished by Melzack et al (1986), who differentiated between the pain of trigeminal neuralgia and atypical

Table 17.2 Descriptions characteristic of clinical pain syndromes[1]

	Menstrual pain (n = 25)	*Arthritic pain (n = 16)*	*Labour pain (n = 11)*	*Disc disease pain (n = 10)*	*Toothache (n = 10)*	*Cancer pain (n = 8)*	*Phantom limb pain (n = 8)*	*Post herpetic pain (n = 6)*
Sensory	Cramping (44%) Aching (44%)	Gnawing (38%) Aching (50%)	Pounding (37%) Shooting (46%) Stabbing (37%) Sharp (64%) Cramping (82%) Aching (46%)	Throbbing (40%) Shooting (50%) Stabbing (40%) Sharp (60%) Cramping (40%) Aching (40%) Heavy (40%) Tender (50%)	Throbbing (50%) Boring (40%) Sharp (50%)	Shooting (50%) Sharp (50%) Gnawing (50%) Burning (50%) Heavy (50%)	Throbbing (38%) Stabbing (50%) Sharp (38%) Cramping (50%) Burning (50%) Aching (38%)	Sharp (84%) Pulling (67%) Aching (50%) Tender (83%)
Affective	Tiring (44%) Sickening (56%)	Exhausting (50%)	Tiring (37%) Exhausting (46%) Fearful (36%)	Tiring (46%) Exhausting (40%)	Sickening (40%)	Exhausting (50%)	Tiring (50%) Exhausting (38%) Cruel (38%)	Exhausting (50%)
Evaluative		Annoying (38%)	Intense (46%)	Unbearable (40%)	Annoying (50%)	Unbearable (50%)		
Temporal	Constant (56%)	Constant (44%) Rhythmic (56%)	Rhythmic (91%)	Constant (80%) Rhythmic (70%)	Constant (60%) Rhythmic (40%)	Constant (100%) Rhythmic (88%)	Constant (88%) Rhythmic (63%)	Constant (50%) Rhythmic (50%)

[1] Only those words chosen by more than one-third of the patients are listed, and the percentages of patients who chose each word are shown in parentheses below the word.

facial pain. Fifty-three patients were given a thorough neurological examination which led to a diagnosis of either trigeminal neuralgia or atypical facial pain. Each patient rated his or her pain using the MPQ and the scores were submitted to a discriminant analysis. Ninety-one per cent of the patients were correctly classified using seven key descriptors. To determine how well the key descriptors were able to predict either diagnosis, the discriminant function derived from the 53 patients was applied to MPQ scores obtained from a second, independent validation sample of patients with trigeminal neuralgia or atypical facial pain. The results showed a correct prediction for 90% of the patients.

Specific verbal descriptors of the MPQ have also been shown recently to discriminate between reversible and irreversible damage of the nerve fibres in a tooth (Grushka & Sessle 1984), and between leg pain caused by diabetic neuropathy and leg pain arising from other causes (Masson et al 1989). Jerome et al (1988) further showed that the MPQ discriminates between cluster headache pain and other vascular (migraine and mixed) headache pain. Cluster headache is more intense and distressing than the others and is characterized by a distinct constellation of descriptors.

It is evident, however, that the discriminative capacity of the MPQ has limits. High levels of anxiety and other psychological disturbance, which may produce high affective scores, may obscure the discriminative capacity (Kremer & Atkinson 1983). Moreover, certain key words that discriminate among specific syndromes may be absent (Reading 1982). Nevertheless, it is clear that there are appreciable and quantifiable differences in the way various types of pain are described, and that patients with the same disease or pain syndrome tend to use remarkably similar words to communicate what they feel.

MODIFICATIONS TO THE MPQ

In general, modifications to the MPQ have involved the development of alternate scoring methods (Hartman & Ainsworth 1980, Charter & Nehemkis 1983, Melzack et al 1985) and efforts to reclassify the original pain descriptors (Clark et al 1995, Fernandez & Towery 1996, Towery & Fernandez 1996). Hartman and Ainsworth (1980) have proposed transforming the MPQ data into a pain ratio or fraction: the 'pain ratio was calculated for each session by dividing the post-session rating by the sum of the pre- and post-session ratings' (p. 40). Kremer et al (1982) suggested dividing the sum of the obtained ranks within each dimension by the total possible score for a particular dimension, thus making differences between the sensory, affective, evaluative and miscellaneous dimensions more interpretable.

A final form of computation (Melzack et al 1985) may be useful because it has been argued (Charter & Nehemkis 1983) that the MPQ fails to take into account the true relative intensity of verbal descriptors as the rank-order scoring system loses the precise intensity of the scale values obtained by Melzack and Torgerson (1971). For example, Figure 17.1 shows that the affective descriptors generally have higher scale values than the sensory words. This is clear when we consider the fact that the words 'throbbing' and 'vicious' receive a rank value of 4, but have scale values of 2.68 and 4.26 respectively, indicating that the latter descriptor implies considerably more pain intensity than the former. A simple technique was developed (Melzack et al 1985) to convert rank values to weighted rank values which more closely approximate the original scaled values obtained by Melzack and Torgerson (1971). Use of this procedure may provide enhanced sensitivity in some statistical analyses (Melzack et al 1985).

Recent efforts to modify the MPQ have led to a parsimonious subset of verbal descriptors from the sensory subcategories (Fernandez & Towery 1996, Towery & Fernandez 1996). In two separate studies, university students were asked to classify the MPQ descriptors and provide an estimate of the intensity of each descriptor using a 0–10 rating scale. A three-step decision rule was applied to each descriptor to determine its inclusion or exclusion in the modified subset of words. Thirty-two out of the 84 descriptors (38%) met the criteria for inclusion. Interestingly, the intensity ratings of the modified descriptors correlated significantly ($r = 0.91$) with that of the original descriptors in the Melzack and Torgerson (1971) study, attesting to the reliability of the MPQ. Although these efforts have yielded a more parsimonious subset of adjectives, the decision to limit the descriptors to the sensory subcategories means that the resulting scale is unidimensional; the affective and evaluative dimensions of pain have been omitted. The decision to exclude important descriptors that may have diagnostic utility (e.g., numb, tingling) because they were deemed ambiguous seems excessively strict. Comparisons with the MPQ in clinical and experimental settings will determine whether there is any incremental utility associated with the modified set of descriptors over the original MPQ.

THE SHORT-FORM MCGILL PAIN QUESTIONNAIRE

The short-form McGill Pain Questionnaire (Melzack 1975) (Fig. 17.4) was developed for use in specific research settings when the time to obtain information from patients is limited and when more information is desired than that provided by intensity measures such as the VAS or PPI. The short-form McGill Pain Questionnaire (SF-MPQ) consists of 15 representative words from the sensory (n = 11) and affective (n = 4) categories of the standard, long-form (LF-MPQ). The Present Pain Intensity (PPI) and a visual analogue scale are included to provide indices of overall pain intensity. The 15 descriptors making up the SF-MPQ were selected on the basis of their frequency of endorsement by patients with a variety of acute, intermittent and chronic pains. An additional word – splitting – was added because it was reported to be a key discriminative word for dental pain (Grushka & Sessle 1984). Each descriptor is ranked by the patient on an intensity scale of 0 = none, 1 = mild, 2 = moderate, 3 = severe.

The SF-MPQ correlates very highly with the major PRI indices (sensory, affective and total) of the LF-MPQ (Melzack 1987, Dudgeon et al 1992) and is sensitive to clinical change brought about by various therapies – analgesic drugs (Melzack 1987, Harden et al 1991), epidurally or spinally administered agents (Melzack 1987, Harden et al 1991, Serrao et al 1992), TENS (Melzack 1987) and low-power light therapy (Stelian et al 1992). In addition, concurrent validity of the short form was reported in a study of patients with chronic pain due to cancer (Dudgeon et al 1992). On each of three occasions separated by at least a 3-week period, the PRI-S, PRI-A and PRI-T scores correlated highly with scores on the LF-MPQ.

Figure 17.5 shows SF-MPQ scores obtained by patients with a variety of acute and chronic pains. As can be seen, the SF-MPQ has been used in studies of chronic pain (Grönblad et al 1990, Burckhardt et al 1992, Dudgeon et al 1992, Stelian et al 1992, al Balawi et al 1996, Gagliese & Melzack 1997) and acute pain (Melzack 1987, Harden et al 1991, King 1993, McGuire et al 1993, Thomas et al 1995) of diverse aetiology and to evaluate pain and discomfort in response to medical interventions (Miller & Knox 1992, Fowlow et al 1995). Furthermore, initial data (Melzack 1987) suggest that the SF-MPQ may be capable of discriminating among different pain syndromes, which is an important property of the long-form. A Czech version (Solcovä et al 1990) and a Swedish version (Burckhardt & Bjelle 1994) of the SF-MPQ have been recently developed.

A recent study of patients with chronic arthritis suggests that the SF-MPQ may be appropriate for use with geriatric pain patients (Gagliese & Melzack 1997). In this study, the frequency of failing to complete the SF-MPQ appropriately did not differ among young, middle-aged and elderly patients. In addition, the subscales showed high intercorrelations and consistency. Although elderly patients endorsed fewer adjectives than their younger counterparts, there was a consistency among the three age groups in the most frequently chosen pain descriptors. These results suggest that pain patients across the life span approach the SF-MPQ in a similar manner. Future studies are required to demonstrate

SHORT-FORM McGILL PAIN QUESTIONNAIRE
RONALD MELZACK

PATIENT'S NAME: ____________ DATE: ________

	NONE	MILD	MODERATE	SEVERE
THROBBING	0) ____	1) ____	2) ____	3) ____
SHOOTING	0) ____	1) ____	2) ____	3) ____
STABBING	0) ____	1) ____	2) ____	3) ____
SHARP	0) ____	1) ____	2) ____	3) ____
CRAMPING	0) ____	1) ____	2) ____	3) ____
GNAWING	0) ____	1) ____	2) ____	3) ____
HOT-BURNING	0) ____	1) ____	2) ____	3) ____
ACHING	0) ____	1) ____	2) ____	3) ____
HEAVY	0) ____	1) ____	2) ____	3) ____
TENDER	0) ____	1) ____	2) ____	3) ____
SPLITTING	0) ____	1) ____	2) ____	3) ____
TIRING-EXHAUSTING	0) ____	1) ____	2) ____	3) ____
SICKENING	0) ____	1) ____	2) ____	3) ____
FEARFUL	0) ____	1) ____	2) ____	3) ____
PUNISHING-CRUEL	0) ____	1) ____	2) ____	3) ____

NO PAIN |————————————| WORST POSSIBLE PAIN

PPI

0 NO PAIN ____
1 MILD ____
2 DISCOMFORTING ____
3 DISTRESSING ____
4 HORRIBLE ____
5 EXCRUCIATING ____

© R. Melzack, 1984

Fig. 17.4 The short-form McGill Pain Questionnaire. Descriptors 1–11 represent the sensory dimension of pain experience and 12–15 represent the affective dimension. Each descriptor is ranked on an intensity scale of 0 = none, 1 = mild, 2 = moderate, 3 = severe. The Present Pain Intensity (PPI) of the standard long-form McGill Pain Questionnaire and the visual analogue scale are also included to provide overall pain intensity scores.

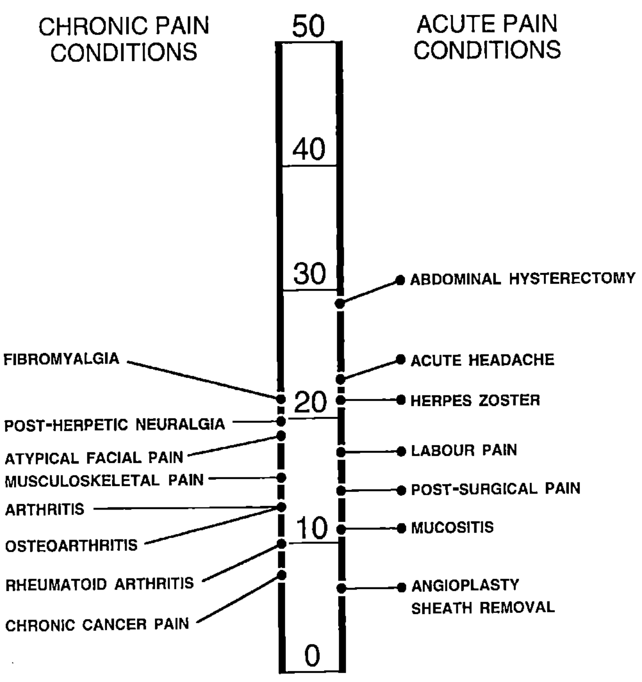

Fig. 17.5 Comparison of total pain rating index (PRI-T) scores using the short-form McGill Pain Questionnaire (SF-MPQ) for acute and chronic pain conditions. References for the various pain conditions are as follows: labour pain, musculoskeletal pain and postsurgical pain (Melzack 1987), abdominal hysterectomy (Thomas et al 1995), acute headache (Harden et al 1991), herpes zoster and postherpetic neuralgia (King 1993), mucositis (McGuire et al 1993), angioplasty sheath removal (Fowlow et al 1995), fibromyalgia and rheumatoid arthritis (Burckhardt & Bjelle 1994), atypical facial pain (al Balawi et al 1996), arthritis (Gagliese & Melzack 1997), osteoarthritis (Stelian et al 1992) and chronic cancer pain (Dudgeon et al 1992).

the reliability and validity of the SF-MPQ when used with elderly patients.

MULTIDIMENSIONAL PAIN EXPERIENCE

Turk et al (1985) and, more recently, Holroyd et al (1992) evaluated the theoretical structure of the MPQ using factor-analytical methods to analyse their data. Turk et al concluded that the three-factor structure of the MPQ – sensory, affective and evaluative – is strongly supported by the analyses; Holroyd's 'most clearly interpretable structure' was provided by a four-factor solution obtained by oblique rotation in which two sensory factors were identified in addition to an affective and an evaluative factor.

Like most others who have used the MPQ, Turk et al (1985) and Holroyd et al (1992) find high intercorrelations among the factors. However, these authors then argue that because the factors measured by the MPQ are highly intercorrelated, they are therefore not distinct. They conclude that the MPQ does not discriminate among the factors and, according to Turk et al (1985), only the PRI-T should be used. It is fallacious and potentially misleading to argue that the MPQ lacks discriminative capacity and clinical utility because factor-analytical studies reveal significant intercorrelations among the identified factors (Gracely 1992). There is, in fact, considerable evidence that the MPQ is effective in discriminating among the three factors despite the high intercorrelations.

Firstly, Gracely (1992) has convincingly argued that factor-analytical methods may be inappropriate for assessing the factor structure of the MPQ, although they provide useful information about patient characteristics. Torgerson (1988) distinguished between semantic meaning (how the MPQ descriptors are arranged) and associate meaning (how patients arrange the MPQ descriptors) to emphasize that factor analysis provides a context-dependent structure of the latter – the outcome depends on how specific patient samples make use of the MPQ descriptors. Gracely (1992) elaborates further on the difference between semantic and associative meaning and concludes that factor-analytical techniques do not 'directly evaluate the semantic structure of the questionnaire'.

Secondly, a high correlation among variables does not necessarily imply a lack of discriminant capacity. Traditional psychophysics has shown repeatedly that, in the case of vision, increasing the intensity of light produces increased capacity to discriminate colour, contours, texture and distance (Kling & Riggs 1971). Similarly, in the case of hearing, increases in volume lead to increased discrimination of timbre, pitch and spatial location (Kling & Riggs 1971). In these cases, there are clearly very high intercorrelations among the variables in each modality. But this does not mean that we should forget about the differences between colour and texture, or between timbre and pitch just because they intercorrelate highly. This approach would lead to the loss of valuable, meaningful data (Gracely 1992).

Thirdly, many papers have demonstrated the discriminant validity of the MPQ. Reading and Newton (1977) showed, in a comparison of primary dysmenorrhoea and intrauterine device (IUD) related pain, that the 'pain intensity scores were reflected in a larger sensory component with IUD users, whereas with dysmenorrhoea the affective component predominated'. In a later study, Reading (1982) compared MPQ profiles of women experiencing chronic pelvic pain and postepisiotomy pain, and showed that 'acute-pain patients displayed greater use of sensory word groups, testifying to the pronounced sensory input from the damaged perineum. Chronic pain patients used affective and reaction subgroups with greater frequency.'

In a study of hypnosis and biofeedback, Melzack and Perry (1975) found that 'there were significant decreases in both the sensory and affective dimensions, as well as the overall PRI, but that the affective dimension shows the largest decrease'. In studies on labour pain, Melzack and his colleagues (Melzack et al 1981, 1984) found that distinctly different variables correlate with the sensory, affective and evaluative dimensions. Prepared childbirth training, for example, correlates significantly with the sensory and affective dimensions but not the evaluative one. Menstrual difficulties correlate with the affective but neither the sensory nor evaluative dimension. Physical factors, such as mother's and infant's weight, also correlate selectively with one or another dimension.

Similarly, a study of acute pain in emergency ward patients (Melzack et al 1982) has 'revealed a normal distribution of sensory scores but very low affective scores compared to patients with chronic pain'. Finally, Chen et al (1989) have consistently identified a group of pain-sensitive and pain-tolerant subjects in five laboratory studies of tonic (prolonged) pain. Compared with pain-tolerant subjects, pain-sensitive subjects show significantly higher scores on all PRIs except for the sensory dimension. Atkinson et al (1982) are undoubtedly right that high affect scores tend to diminish the discriminant capacity of the MPQ, so that at high levels of anxiety and depression some discriminant capacity is lost. However, the MPQ still retains good discriminant function even at high levels of anxiety.

A recent study is of particular interest because it examines laboratory models of phasic (brief) and tonic (prolonged) pain, and compares them by using the MPQ. Chen and Treede (1985) found a very high sensory loading for phasic pain and relatively few choices of affective and evaluative words. By contrast, tonic pain was characterized by much higher scores in the affective and evaluative dimensions. Furthermore, they found that when tonic pain is used to inhibit the phasic pain, 'the sensory component is reduced by 32%, whereas the affective component vanishes almost completely'.

In summary:

1. High intercorrelations among psychological variables do not mean that they are all alike and can therefore be lumped into a single variable such as intensity; rather, certain biological and psychological variables can co-vary to a high degree yet represent distinct, discriminable entities.
2. The MPQ has been shown in many studies to be capable of discriminating among the three component factors.

THE DESCRIPTOR DIFFERENTIAL SCALE

Recently, simple but sophisticated psychophysical techniques have been applied to the development of pain measurement instruments which have been used to assess clinical and experimentally induced pain (Gracely & Dubner 1981, Hall 1981, Gracely & Kwilosz 1988 Price 1988, Gracely 1989a,b). The psychophysical approach uses cross-modality matching procedures (Gracely et al 1978a) or bimodality stimulus comparison (Doctor et al 1995) to determine the relative magnitudes of the verbal descriptors of pain.

The descriptor differential scale (Gracely & Kwilosz 1988) was developed by Gracely et al (1978a) to remedy a number of deficiencies associated with existing pain measurement instruments. The descriptor differential scale (DDS) was designed to reduce bias, assess separately the sensory intensity and 'unpleasantness' (hedonic) dimensions of pain, and provide quantification by ratio-scaling procedures (Gracely 1983). The DDS consists of two forms that measure separately the sensory intensity and unpleasantness qualities of pain. Each form consists of 12 verbal descriptors, in which each descriptor is centred over a 21-point scale with a minus sign at the low end and a plus sign at the high end. The patients rate the magnitude of the sensory intensity or unpleasantness of the pain they are experiencing. The magnitude of pain endorsed by the patient in relation to each descriptor is assigned a score of 0 (minus sign) to 20 (plus sign), where a score of 10 represents pain intensity or unpleasantness equal to the magnitude implied by the descriptor. Total mean scores may be obtained for the sensory intensity and unpleasantness dimensions by averaging the patient's scores on each 12-item form.

The DDS has been demonstrated to be differentially sensitive to pharmacological interventions that alter the sensory or unpleasantness dimensions of pain (Gracely et al 1978b, 1979, 1982). Results point to the importance of using multidimensional measures of pain with clear instructions to rate separately the sensory intensity and unpleasantness aspects of pain as opposed to the 'painfulness' of the experience (Gracely & Dubner 1987). When used in conjunction with cross-modality matching techniques, the DDS has been shown to be a reliable and valid instrument with ratio-scale properties (Gracely et al 1978a,b).

Gracely and Kwilosz (1988) assessed the psychometric properties of the DDS for use as a clinical pain measure among a sample of 91 dental patients after third molar extraction. Sensory intensity and unpleasantness DDS forms were administered to all patients 1 h and 2 h after surgery. Total scores on both forms showed high test–retest reliability coefficients as did scores derived from individual items. Correlation coefficients between individual items and the total score revealed a high degree of internal consistency for both forms of the DDS. One of the most useful features of the DDS is the potential to define a measure of scaling consistency that can be used to identify invalid patient profiles obtained by inconsistent responding. The elimination of invalid profiles improved the reliability and internal consistency of the DDS.

More recently, the intensity dimension of the DDS (DDS-I) has been found to fulfil three criteria of an ideal pain measurement tool. Doctor et al (1995) showed that the DDS-I is sensitive to small changes (1 mA) in electrical stimulation applied to the skin. Due to relatively large error variance, VAS pain intensity ratings in response to the same stimuli lacked the degree of sensitivity found for the DDS-I. The study by Doctor et al (1995) also confirmed the ratio-scale property of the DDS-I and provided evidence for its internal consistency.

BEHAVIOURAL APPROACHES TO PAIN MEASUREMENT

Recent research into the development of behavioural measures of pain has produced a wide array of sophisticated observational techniques and rating scales designed to assess objective behaviours that accompany pain experience (Keefe 1989, Turk & Melzack 1992). Techniques that have demonstrated high reliability and validity are especially useful for measuring pain in infants and preverbal children who lack language skills (McGrath & Unruh 1987, Ross & Ross 1988, McGrath 1990), adults who have a poor command of language (Reading 1989) or when mental clouding and confusion limit the patient's ability to communicate meaningfully (Cleeland 1989). Under these circumstances, behavioural measures provide important information that is otherwise unavailable from patient's self reporting. Moreover, when administered in conjunction with a subjective, patient-rated measure, behavioural measures may provide a more complete picture of the total pain experience. However, behavioural measures of pain should not replace self-rated measures if the patient is capable of rating her subjective state and such administration is feasible.

The subjective experiences of pain and pain behaviours are, presumably, reflections of the same underlying neural processes. However, the complexity of the human brain indicates that although experience and behaviour are usually highly correlated, they are far from identical. One person may be stoic so that his calm behaviour belies his true subjective feelings. Another patient may seek sympathy (or analgesic medication or some other desirable goal) and in so doing exaggerate his complaints without also eliciting the behaviours that typically accompany pain complaints of that degree. Concordance between patients' self ratings of pain and ratings of the same patients by nurses or other medically trained personnel may be modestly low (Teske et al 1983, Cleeland 1989, Loeser 1989, Van der Does 1989, Choinière et al 1990), but even in the presence of a significant correlation between physician and patient ratings of patient pain, physicians significantly underestimate the degree of pain the patients reported experiencing (Sutherland et al 1988). Moreover, when healthcare providers observe a discordance between non-verbal pain behaviour and the patient's verbal complaint of pain, the discrepancy often is resolved by disregarding the patient's self report (Craig & Prkachin 1983, Craig 1989). These studies point to the importance of obtaining multiple measures of pain and should keep us aware that because pain is a subjective experience, the patient's self report is the most valid measure of that experience.

PHYSIOLOGICAL APPROACHES TO PAIN MEASUREMENT

Profound physiological changes often accompany the experience of pain, especially if the injury or noxious stimulus is acute (Cousins 1989). Physiological correlates of pain may serve to elucidate mechanisms that underlie the experience and thus may provide clues which may lead to novel treatments (Chapman et al 1985, Price 1988). Physiological correlates of pain experience that are frequently measured include heart rate, blood pressure, electrodermal activity, electromyographic activity and cortical evoked potentials. Despite high initial correlations between pain onset and changes in these physiological responses, many habituate with time despite the persistence of pain (Gracely 1989b). In addition, these responses are not specific to the experience of pain per se, and occur under conditions of general arousal and stress. Studies that have examined the general endocrine-metabolic stress response to surgical incision indicate that under certain conditions it is possible to dissociate different aspects of the stress response and pain (Kehlet 1986, 1988). Severe injury to a denervated limb produces a significant adrenocortical response (Kehlet 1988), but the use of general anaesthesia clearly eliminates the conscious experience of pain in response to surgical incision without altering the subsequent rapid rise in plasma cortisol levels (Brandt et al 1976, Christensen et al 1982). These studies indicate that although there are many physiological and endocrine events which occur concurrently with the experience of pain, many appear to be general responses to stress and are not unique to pain.

Acknowledgements

This work was supported by a scholar award to JK from the Medical Research Council of Canada (MRC), MRC Grant MT-12052 (JK), NIH-NINDS Grant # NS35480 (JK) and Grant A7891 from the Natural Sciences and Engineering Research Council of Canada (RM).

REFERENCES

al Balawi S, Tariq M, Feinmann C 1996 A double-blind, placebo-controlled, crossover, study to evaluate the efficacy of subcutaneous sumatriptan in the treatment of atypical facial pain. International Journal of Neuroscience 86(3–4): 301–309

Atkinson JH, Kremer EF, Ignelzi RJ 1982 Diffusion of pain language with affective disturbance confounds differential diagnosis. Pain 12: 375–384

Bartko D, Kondos M, Jansco S 1984 Slovak version of the McGill–

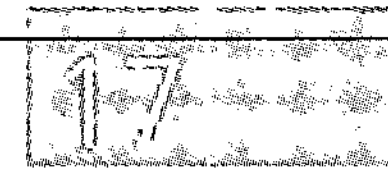

Melzack's Questionnaire on pain. Ceskoslovenska Neurologie a Neurochirurgie 47: 113–121
Beecher HK 1959 Measurement of subjective responses. Oxford University Press, New York
Bejarano PF, Noriego RD, Rodriguez ML, Berrio GM 1985 Evaluación del dolor: Adaptatión del cuestionario del McGill. [Evaluation of pain: Adaptation of the McGill Pain Questionnaire.] Revista Columbia Anesesia 13: 321–351
Bélanger E, Melzack R, Lauzon P 1989 Pain of first-trimester abortion: a study of psychosocial and medical predictors. Pain 36: 339–350
Boureau F, Luu M, Doubrère JF, Gay C 1984 Elaboration d'un questionnaire d'auto-évaluation de la douleur par liste de qualicatifs. [Development of a self-evaluation questionnaire comprising pain descriptors.] Thérapie 39: 119–129
Boureau F, Luu M, Doubrère JF 1992 Comparative study of the validity of four French McGill Pain Questionnaire (MPQ) versions. Pain 50: 59–65
Brandt MR, Kehlet H, Binder C, Hagen C, McNeilly AS 1976 Effect of epidural analgesia on the glucoregulatory endocrine response to surgery. Clinical Endocrinology 5: 107–114
Briggs M 1996 Surgical wound pain: a trial of two treatments. Journal of Wound Care 5: 456–460
Burchiel KJ, Anderson VC, Brown FD et al 1996 Prospective, multicenter study of spinal cord stimulation for relief of chronic back and extremity pain. Spine 21: 2786–2794
Burckhardt C 1984 The use of the McGill Pain Questionnaire in assessing arthritis pain. Pain 19: 305–314
Burckhardt CS, Bjelle A 1994 A Swedish version of the short-form McGill Pain Questionnaire. Scandinavian Journal of Rheumatology 23: 77–81
Burckhardt CS, Clark SR, Bennett RM 1992 A comparison of pain perceptions in women with fibromyalgia and rheumatoid arthritis: relationship to depression and pain extent. Arthritis Care and Research 5: 216–222
Carlsson AM 1983 Assessment of chronic pain. I. Aspects of the reliability and validity of the visual analogue scale. Pain 16: 87–101
Chapman CR, Casey KL, Dubner R, Foley KM, Gracely RH, Reading AE 1985 Pain measurement: an overview. Pain 22: 1–31
Charter RA, Nehemkis AM 1983 The language of pain intensity and complexity: new methods of scoring the McGill Pain Questionnaire. Perceptual and Motor Skills 56: 519–537
Chen ACN, Treede RD 1985 McGill Pain Questionnaire in assessing the differentiation of phasic and tonic pain: behavioral evaluation of the 'pain inhibiting pain' effect. Pain 22: 67–79
Chen ACN, Dworkin SF, Haug J, Gerhig J 1989 Human pain responsivity in a tonic pain model: psychological determinants. Pain 37: 143–160
Choiniere M, Amsel R 1996 A visual analogue thermometer for measuring pain intensity. Journal of Pain and Symptom Management 11: 299–311
Choinière M, Melzack R, Girard N, Rondeau J, Paquin MJ 1990 Comparisons between patients' and nurses' assessments of pain and medication efficacy in severe burn injuries. Pain 40: 143–152
Christensen P, Brandt MR, Rem J, Kehlet H 1982 Influence of extradural morphine on the adrenocortical and hyperglycaemic response to surgery. British Journal of Anaesthesia 54: 23–27
Clark WC, Fletcher JD, Janal MN, Carroll JD 1995 Hierarchical clustering of pain and emotion descriptors: toward a revision of the McGill Pain Questionnaire. In: Bromm B, Desmedt JE (eds) Advances in pain research and therapy. Raven, New York, pp 319–330
Cleeland CS 1989 Measurement of pain by subjective report. In: Chapman CR, Loeser JD (eds) Issues in pain measurement. Advances in pain research and therapy, vol 12. Raven, New York, pp 391–401
Cousins M 1989 Acute and postoperative pain. In: Wall PD, Melzack R (eds) Textbook of pain, 2nd edn. Churchill Livingstone, Edinburgh, pp 284–305
Craig KD 1989 Clinical pain measurement from the perspective of the human laboratory. In: Chapman CR, Loeser JD (eds) Issues in pain measurement. Advances in pain research and therapy, vol 12. Raven, New York, pp 433–442
Craig KD, Prkachin KM 1983 Nonverbal measures of pain. In: Melzack R (eds) Pain measurement and assessment. Raven, New York, pp 173–182
Crockett DJ, Prkachin KM, Craig KD 1977 Factors of the language of pain in patients and normal volunteer groups. Pain 4: 175–182
De Benedittis G, Massei R, Nobili R, Pieri A 1988 The Italian pain questionnaire. Pain 33: 53–62
Doctor JN, Slater MA, Atkinson JH 1995 The Descriptor Differential Scale of Pain Intensity: an evaluation of item and scale properties. Pain 61: 251–260
Drewes AM, Helweg-Larsen S, Petersen P et al 1993 McGill Pain Questionnaire translated into Danish: experimental and clinical findings. Clinical Journal of Pain 9: 80–87
Dubuisson D, Melzack R 1976 Classification of clinical pain descriptors by multiple group discriminant analysis. Experimental Neurology 51: 480–487
Dudgeon D, Ranbertas RF, Rosenthal S 1992 The Short-Form McGill Pain Questionnaire in chronic cancer pain. Journal of Pain and Symptom Management (submitted)
Eija K, Tiina T, Pertti NJ 1996 Amitriptyline effectively relieves neuropathic pain following treatment of breast cancer. Pain 64: 293–302
Ekblom A, Hansson P 1988 Pain intensity measurements in patients with acute pain receiving afferent stimulation. Journal of Neurology, Neurosurgery and Psychiatry 51: 481–486
Escalante A, Lichtenstein MJ, Rios N, Hazuda HP 1996 Measuring chronic rheumatic pain in Mexican Americans: cross-cultural adaptation of the McGill Pain Questionnaire. Journal of Clinical Epidemiology 49: 1389–1399
Fernandez E, Towery S 1996 A parsimonious set of verbal descriptors of pain sensation derived from the McGill Pain Questionnaire [published erratum appears in Pain 1996; 68: 437]. Pain 66: 31–37
Ferracuti S, Romeo G, Leardi MG, Cruccu G, Lazzari R 1990 New Italian adaptation and standardization of the McGill Pain Questionnaire. Pain (suppl 5): S300
Fowlow B, Price P, Fung T 1995 Ambulation after sheath removal: a comparison of 6 and 8 hours of bedrest after sheath removal in patients following a PTCA procedure. Heart and Lung 24: 28–37
Gagliese L, Melzack R 1997 Age differences in the quality of chronic pain: a preliminary study. Pain Research and Management 2: 157–162
Gaston-Johansson F, Albert M, Fagan E, Zimmerman L 1990 Similarities in pain descriptors of four different ethnic-culture groups. Journal of Pain and Symptom Management 5: 94–100
Gracely RH 1983 Pain language and ideal pain assessment. In: Melzack R (ed) Pain measurement and assessment. Raven, New York, pp 71–78
Gracely RH 1989a Methods of testing pain mechanisms in normal man. In: Wall PD, Melzack R (eds) Textbook of pain, 2nd edn. Churchill Livingstone, Edinburgh, pp 257–268
Gracely RH 1989b Pain psychophysics. In: Chapman CR, Loeser JD (eds) Issues in pain measurement. Advances in pain research and therapy, vol 12. Raven, New York, pp 211–229
Gracely RH 1992 Evaluation of multi-dimensional pain scales. Pain 48: 297–300
Gracely RH, Dubner R 1981 Pain assessment in humans – a reply to Hall. Pain 11: 109–120
Gracely RH, Dubner R 1987 Reliability and validity of verbal descriptor scales of painfulness. Pain 29: 175–185

Gracely RH, Kwilosz DM 1988 The Descriptor Differential Scale: applying psychophysical principles to clinical pain assessment. Pain 35: 279–288

Gracely RH, McGrath PA, Dubner R 1978a Ratio scales of sensory and affective verbal pain descriptors. Pain 5: 5–18

Gracely RH, McGrath PA, Dubner R 1978b Validity and sensitivity of ratio scales of sensory and affective verbal pain descriptors: manipulation of affect by diazepam. Pain 5: 19–29

Gracely RH, McGrath PA, Dubner R 1979 Narcotic analgesia: fentanyl reduces the intensity but not the unpleasantness of painful tooth pulp sensations. Science 203: 1361–1379

Gracely RH, Dubner R, McGrath PA 1982 Fentanyl reduces the intensity of painful tooth pulp sensations: controlling for detection of active drugs. Anesthesia and Analgesia 61: 751–755

Graham C, Bond SS, Gerkovitch MM, Cook MR 1980 Use of the McGill Pain Questionnaire in the assessment of cancer pain: replicability and consistency. Pain 8: 377–387

Grönblad M, Lukinmaa A, Konttinen YT 1990 Chronic low-back pain: intercorrelation of repeated measures for pain and disability. Scandinavian Journal of Rehabilitation Medicine 22: 73–77

Grushka M, Sessle BJ 1984 Applicability of the McGill Pain Questionnaire to the differentiation of 'toothache' pain. Pain 19: 49–57

Hall W 1981 On 'ratio scales of sensory and affective verbal pain descriptors'. Pain 11: 101–107

Harden RN, Carter TD, Gilman CS, Gross AJ, Peters JR 1991 Ketorolac in acute headache management. Headache 31: 463–464

Harrison A 1988 Arabic pain words. Pain 32: 239–250

Hartman LM, Ainsworth KD 1980 Self-regulation of chronic pain. Canadian Journal of Psychiatry 25: 38–43

Holroyd KA, Holm JE, Keefe FJ et al 1992 A multi-center evaluation of the McGill Pain Questionnaire: results from more than 1700 chronic pain patients. Pain 48: 301–311

Hui YL, Chen AC 1989 Analysis of headache in a Chinese patient population. Ma Tsui Hsueh Tsa Chi 27: 13–18

Huskisson EC 1983 Visual analogue scales. In: Melzack R (ed) Pain measurement and assessment. Raven, New York, pp 33–37

Jenkinson C, Carroll D, Egerton M, Frankland T, McQuay H, Nagle C 1995 Comparison of the sensitivity to change of long and short form pain measures. Quality of Life Research 4: 353–357

Jensen MP, Karoly P 1992 Self-report scales and procedures for assessing pain in adults. In: Turk DC, Melzack R (eds) Handbook of pain assessment. Guilford, New York, pp 135–151

Jensen MP, Karoly P, Braver S 1986 The measurement of clinical pain intensity: a comparison of six methods. Pain 27: 117–126

Jerome A, Holroyd KA, Theofanous AG, Pingel JD, Lake AE, Saper JR 1988 Cluster headache pain vs. other vascular headache pain: differences revealed with two approaches to the McGill Pain Questionnaire. Pain 34: 35–42

Joyce CRB, Zutshi DW, Hrubes V, Mason RM 1975 Comparison of fixed interval and visual analogue scales for rating chronic pain. European Journal of Clinical Pharmacology 8: 415–420

Katz J 1992 Psychophysical correlates of phantom limb experience. Journal of Neurology, Neurosurgery and Psychiatry 55: 811–821

Katz J, Melzack R 1991 Auricular TENS reduces phantom limb pain. Journal of Pain and Symptom Management 6: 73–83

Katz J, Clairoux M, Kavanagh BP et al 1994 Pre-emptive lumbar epidural anaesthesia reduces postoperative pain and patient-controlled morphine consumption after lower abdominal surgery. Pain 59: 395–403

Keefe FJ 1989 Behavioral measurement of pain. In: Chapman CR, Loeser JD (eds) Issues in pain measurement. Advances in pain research and therapy, vol 12. Raven, New York, pp 405–424

Kehlet H 1986 Pain relief and modification of the stress response. In: Cousins MJ, Phillips GD (eds) Acute pain management. Churchill Livingstone, New York, pp 49–75

Kehlet H 1988 Modification of responses to surgery by neural blockade: clinical implications. In: Cousins MJ, Bridenbaugh PO (eds) Neural blockade in clinical anesthesia and management of pain, 2nd edn. JB Lippincott, Philadelphia, pp 145–188

Ketovuori H, Pöntinen PJ 1981 A pain vocabulary in Finnish – the Finnish pain questionnaire. Pain 11: 247–253

Kim HS, Schwartz-Barcott D, Holter IM, Lorensen M 1995 Developing a translation of the McGill pain questionnaire for cross-cultural comparison: an example from Norway. Journal of Advanced Nursing 21: 421–426

King RB 1993 Topical aspirin in chloroform and the relief of pain due to herpes zoster and postherpetic neuralgia. Archives of Neurology 50: 1046–1053

Kiss I, Müller H, Abel M 1987 The McGill Pain Questionnaire – German version. A study on cancer pain. Pain 29: 195–207

Klepac RK, Dowling J, Rokke P, Dodge L, Schafer L 1981 Interview vs. paper-and-pencil administration of the McGill Pain Questionnaire. Pain 11: 241–246

Kling JW, Riggs LA 1971 Experimental psychology. Holt, Rinehart, and Winston, New York

Kremer E, Atkinson JH 1983 Pain language as a measure of effect in chronic pain patients. In: Melzack R (ed) Pain measurement and assessment. Raven, New York, pp 119–127

Kremer E, Atkinson JH, Ignelzi RJ 1982 Pain measurement: the affective dimensional measure of the McGill Pain Questionnaire with a cancer pain population. Pain 12: 153–163

Lahuerta J, Smith BA, Martinez-Lage JL 1982 An adaptation of the McGill Pain Questionnaire to the Spanish Language. Schmerz 3: 132–134

Lázaro C, Bosch F, Torrubia R, Baños JE 1994 The development of a Spanish questionnaire for assessing pain: preliminary data concerning reliability and validity. European Journal of Psychological Assessment 10: 145–151

Leavitt F, Garron DC 1980 Validity of a back pain classification scale for detecting psychological disturbance as measured by the MMPI. Journal of Clinical Psychology 36: 186–189

Leavitt F, Garron DC, Whisler WW, Sheinkop MB 1978 Affective and sensory dimensions of pain. Pain 4: 273–281

Loeser JD 1989 Pain relief and analgesia. In: Chapman CR, Loeser JD (eds) Issues in pain measurement. Advances in pain research and therapy, vol 12. Raven, New York, pp 175–182

Love A, Leboeuf DC, Crisp TC 1989 Chiropractic chronic low back pain sufferers and self-report assessment methods. Part I. A reliability study of the Visual Analogue Scale, the pain drawing and the McGill Pain Questionnaire. Journal of Manipulative and Physiological Therapeutics 12: 21–25

Lowe NK, Walker SN, McCallum RC 1991 Confirming the theoretical structure of the McGill Pain Questionnaire in acute clinical pain. Pain 46: 53–60

Maiani G, Sanavio E 1985 Semantics of pain in Italy: the Italian version of the McGill Pain Questionnaire. Pain 22: 399–405

Masson EA, Hunt L, Gem JM, Boulton AJM 1989 A novel approach to the diagnosis and assessment of symptomatic diabetic neuropathy. Pain 38: 25–28

McCreary C, Turner J, Dawson E 1981 Principal dimensions of the pain experience and psychological disturbance in chronic low back pain patients. Pain 11: 85–92

McGrath PA 1990 Pain in children: nature, assessment, and treatment. Guilford, New York

McGrath PJ, Unruh A 1987 Pain in children and adolescents. Elsevier, Amsterdam

McGuire DB, Altomonte V, Peterson DE, Wingard JR, Jones RJ, Grochow LB 1993 Patterns of mucositis and pain in patients receiving preparative chemotherapy and bone marrow transplantation. Oncology Nursing Forum 20: 1493–1502

Melzack R 1975 The McGill Pain Questionnaire: major properties and scoring methods. Pain 1: 277–299
Melzack R 1983 Pain measurement and assessment. Raven, New York
Melzack R 1987 The short-form McGill Pain Questionnaire. Pain 30: 191–197
Melzack R, Casey KL 1968 Sensory, motivational, and central control determinants of pain: a new conceptual model. In: Kenshalo D (ed) The skin senses. Thomas, Springfield, IL, pp 423–443
Melzack R, Perry C 1975 Self-regulation of pain: the use of alpha-feedback and hypnotic training for the control of chronic pain. Experimental Neurology 46: 452–469
Melzack R, Torgerson WS 1971 On the language of pain. Anesthesiology 34: 50–59
Melzack R, Taenzer P, Feldman P, Kinch RA 1981 Labour is still painful after prepared childbirth training. Canadian Medical Association Journal 125: 357–363
Melzack R, Wall PD, Ty TC 1982 Acute pain in an emergency clinic: latency of onset and description patterns related to different injuries. Pain 14: 33–43
Melzack R, Kinch R, Dobkin P, Lebrun M, Taenzer P 1984 Severity of labour pain: influence of physical as well as psychologic variables. Canadian Medical Association Journal 130: 579–584
Melzack R, Katz J, Jeans ME 1985 The role of compensation in chronic pain: analysis using a new method of scoring the McGill Pain Questionnaire. Pain 23: 101–112
Melzack R, Terrence C, Fromm G, Amsel R 1986 Trigeminal neuralgia and atypical facial pain: use of the McGill Pain Questionnaire for discrimination and diagnosis. Pain 27: 297–302
Miller RM, Knox M 1992 Patient tolerance of ioxaglate and iopamidol in internal mammary artery arteriography. Catheterization and Cardiovascular Diagnosis 25: 31–34
Nikolajsen L, Hansen CL, Nielsen J, Keller J, Arendt-Nielsen L, Jensen TS 1996 The effect of ketamine on phantom pain: a central neuropathic disorder maintained by peripheral input. Pain 67: 69–77
Ohnhaus EE, Adler R 1975 Methodological problems in the measurement of pain: a comparison between the Verbal Rating Scale and the Visual Analogue Scale. Pain 1: 374–384
Pearce J, Morley S 1989 An experimental investigation of the construct validity of the McGill Pain Questionnaire. Pain 39: 115–121
Perry F, Heller PH, Levine JD 1988 Differing correlations between pain measures in syndromes with or without explicable organic pathology. Pain 34: 185–189
Perry F, Heller PH, Levine JD 1991 A possible indicator of functional pain: poor pain scale correlation. Pain 46: 191–193
Pimenta CA, Teixeiro MJ 1996 [Proposal to adapt the McGill Pain Questionnaire into Portuguese.] Revista Da Escola de Enfermagem Da USP 30: 473–483
Pozehl B, Barnason S, Zimmerman L, Nieveen J, Crutchfield J 1995 Pain in the postoperative coronary artery bypass graft patient. Clinical Nursing Research 4: 208–222
Price DD 1988 Psychological and neural mechanisms of pain. Raven, New York
Price DD, Harkins SW 1987 Combined use of experimental pain and visual analogue scales in providing standardized measurement of clinical pain. Clinical Journal of Pain 3: 1–8
Price DD, McGrath PA, Rafii A, Buckingham B 1983 The validation of visual analogue scales as ratio scale measures for chronic and experimental pain. Pain 17: 45–56
Price DD, Harkins SW, Rafii A, Price C 1986 A simultaneous comparison of fentanyl's analgesic effects on experimental and clinical pain. Pain 24: 197–203
Price DD, Harkins SW, Baker C 1987 Sensory–affective relationships among different types of clinical and experimental pain. Pain 28: 297–307
Prieto EJ, Hopson L, Bradley LA et al 1980 The language of low back pain: factor structure of the McGill Pain Questionnaire. Pain 8: 11–19
Radvila A, Adler RH, Galeazzi RL, Vorkauf H 1987 The development of a German language (Berne) pain questionnaire and its application in a situation causing acute pain. Pain 28: 185–195
Reading AL 1982 An analysis of the language of pain in chronic and acute patient groups. Pain 13: 185–192
Reading AE 1979 The internal structure of the McGill Pain Questionnaire in dysmenorrhea patients. Pain 7: 353–358
Reading AE 1989 Testing pain mechanisms in persons in pain. In: Wall PD, Melzack R (eds) Textbook of pain, 2nd edn. Churchill Livingstone, Edinburgh, pp 269–283
Reading AE, Newton JR 1977 On a comparison of dysmenorrhea and intrauterine device related pain. Pain 3: 265–276
Reading AE, Everitt BS, Sledmere CM 1982 The McGill Pain Questionnaire: a replication of its construction. British Journal of Clinical Psychology 21: 339–349
Ross DM, Ross SA 1988 Childhood pain: current issues, research, and management. Schwartzenberg, Baltimore
Satow A, Nakatani K, Taniguchi S, Higashiyama A 1990 Perceptual characteristics of electrocutaneous pain estimated by the 30-word list and Visual Analog Scale. Japanese Psychological Review 32: 155–164
Sedlak K 1990 A Polish version of the McGill Pain Questionnaire. Pain (suppl 5): S308
Serrao JM, Marks RL, Morley SJ, Goodchild CS 1992 Intrathecal midazolam for the treatment of chronic mechanical low back pain: a controlled comparison with epidural steroid in a pilot study. Pain 48: 5–12
Solcovä I, Jacoubek B, Sÿkora J, Hnïk P 1990 Characterization of vertebrogenic pain using the short form of the McGill Pain Questionnaire. Casopis Lekaru Ceskych 129: 1611–1614
Sriwatanakul K, Kelvie W, Lasagna L, Calimlim JF, Weis OF, Mehta G 1983 Studies with different types of visual analog scales for measurement of pain. Clinical Pharmacology and Therapeutics 34: 234–239
Stein C, Mendl G 1988 The German counterpart to McGill Pain Questionnaire. Pain 32: 251–255
Stelian J, Gil I, Habot B, Rosenthal M, Abramovici I, Kutok N, Kahil A 1992 Improvement of pain and disability in elderly patients with degenerative osteoarthritis of the knee treated with narrow-band light therapy. Journal of the American Geriatrics Society 40: 23–26
Strand LI, Wisnes AR 1991 The development of a Norwegian pain questionnaire. Pain 46: 61–66
Sutherland JE, Wesley RM, Cole PM, Nesvacil LJ, Daley ML, Gepner GJ 1988 Differences and similarities between patient and physician perceptions of patient pain. Family Medicine 20: 343–346
Tahmoush AJ 1981 Causalgia: redefinition as a clinical pain syndrome. Pain 10: 187–197
Tesfaye S, Watt J, Benbow SJ, Pang KA, Miles J, MacFarlane IA 1996 Electrical spinal-cord stimulation for painful diabetic peripheral neuropathy [see comments]. Lancet 348(9043): 1698–1701
Teske K, Daut RL, Cleeland CS 1983 Relationships between Nurses' observations and patients' self-reports of pain. Pain 16: 289–296
Thomas V, Heath M, Rose D, Flory P 1995 Psychological characteristics and the effectiveness of patient-controlled analgesia. British Journal of Anaesthesia 74: 271–276
Torgerson WS 1988 Critical issues in verbal pain assessment: multidimensional and multivariate issues. American Pain Society Abstracts, Washington, DC
Towery S, Fernandez E 1996 Reclassification and rescaling of McGill Pain Questionnaire verbal descriptors of pain sensation: a replication. Clinical Journal of Pain 12: 270–276
Turk DC, Melzack R (eds) 1992 Handbook of pain assessment. Guilford, New York

Turk DC, Rudy TE, Salovey P 1985 The McGill Pain Questionnaire reconsidered: confirming the factor structures and examining appropriate uses. Pain 21: 385–397

Van Buren J, Kleinknecht R 1979 An evaluation of the McGill Pain Questionnaire for use in dental pain assessment. Pain 6: 23–33

Van der Does AJW 1989 Patients' and nurses' ratings of pain and anxiety during burn wound care. Pain 39: 95–101

van der Kloot WA, Oostendorp RA, van der Meij J, van den Heuvel J 1995 [The Dutch version of the McGill pain questionnaire: a reliable pain questionnaire.] Nederlands Tijdschrift voor Geneeskunde 139: 669–673

van Lankveld W, van't Pad Bosch P, van de Putte L, van der Staak C, Naring G 1992 [Pain in rheumatoid arthritis measured with the visual analogue scale and the Dutch version of the McGill Pain Questionnaire.] Nederlands Tijdschrift voor Geneeskunde 136: 1166–1170

Vanderiet K, Adriaensen H, Carton H, Vertommen H 1987 The McGill Pain Questionnaire constructed for the Dutch language (MPQ-DV). Preliminary data concerning reliability and validity. Pain 30: 395–408

Veilleux S, Melzack R 1976 Pain in psychotic patients. Experimental Neurology 52: 535–563

Verkes RJ, Van der Kloot WA, Van der Meij J 1989 The perceived structure of 176 pain descriptive words. Pain 38: 219–229

Wilkie DJ, Savedra MC, Holzemier WL, Tesler MD, Paul SM 1990 Use of the McGill Pain Questionnaire to measure pain: a meta-analysis. Nursing Research 39: 36–41

Measures of function and psychology

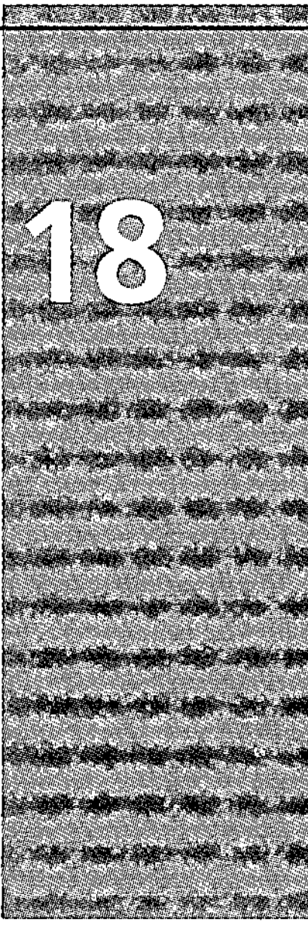

AMANDA C de C WILLIAMS

SUMMARY

This chapter is a practical guide for understanding and designing research studies concerning people in pain. Collecting and interpreting data requires a critical approach to the choice of measures, to their properties and to their claims. To that end, issues of reliability, validity and sensitivity to change are discussed, and measures in the domains of function, affect and cognition are described. The final section evaluates complex variables such as the influence of setting, treatment and interactions between patient and therapist variables on the target of study.

INTRODUCTION

In an ideal world, clinicians and researchers would have free access to a brief set of measures with good reliability and validity established in the target population, sensitive to change, acceptable to patients, easily scored, comprehensive in coverage and yielding clinically interpretable data. Such measures exist only in fantasy, but the effort required to identify 'good enough' instruments before embarking on a clinical trial, an audit or an experimental study represents an investment. Selection requires not only understanding of the science of measurement, but also resisting the temptation to underestimate human complexity and to pursue the fantasy of the perfect measure. This chapter offers ways of addressing these limitations and complications in constructive ways; for further detail, Turk and Melzack (1992), McDowell and Newell (1996), Streiner and Norman (1995), Crombie and Davies (1996) and Karoly (1985) are recommended. Factors to be considered in choosing measures include coverage of domains of interest and importance, the extent to which the measure fulfils the claim implicit in its name, and the psychometric properties upon which confident interpretation relies. Population characteristics also require attention, because heterogeneity implies large variances which may decrease confidence in between-groups differences, but narrow variance compromises generalizability of findings. Ideally, measures are obtained from multiple sources.

COVERAGE

Pain relief is rarely a necessary or sufficient condition for return to pre-pain functioning. Where targets of treatment are not covered by standardized measures used in similar studies, choices must be made among measures used in dissimilar studies within or without the pain field, direct estimation methods, or indicators within or external to the study. It is risky to use measures with unsatisfactory psychometric properties, to adapt existing measures (which changes them) or to attempt development of a new measure without adequate resources; translated scales require restandardization and revalidation (Chaturvedi 1990). Generic measures (such as the SF-36 or AIMS: Table 18.1) are an economical approach to comprehensive coverage, particularly for heterogeneous samples and multiple domains (Lambert & Hill 1994), and comparison data are usually available, but subscales often lack the reliability or validity of specific measures. However, the latter may fail to meet requirements of independence for univariate analytic methods, and multivariate analysis poses problems of interpretation in relation to the original scales.

QUALITY OF MEASURES AND PROPERTIES OF TESTS

Human experience is complex, and scales should not be confused with the hypothetical constructs they purport to measure. At worst, scores are arbitrary numbers assigned to constructs such as mood and affect; at best, they approximate phenomena rooted in current psychological, biological and/or social understanding. Generalization from findings rests on reliability and validity, not invariant properties of tests but constrained by the context of development and testing: scales standardized on young, healthy students may be inapplicable or uninterpretable for older, poorly educated people with a high prevalence of health problems. Different data are subject to different analyses: estimation methods using dichotomous data, such as odds ratios and numbers needed to treat, are the currency of evidence-based medical practice (Laupacis et al 1988, McQuay & Moore 1998). Where data are continuous, dichotomizing sacrifices efficiency, but hypothesis-testing methods may be inappropriate: an alternative is estimation of effect size (difference between means divided by standard deviation) which is clinically interpretable and permits comparison across different metrics.

RELIABILITY

Reliability refers to the consistency of a measure across conditions and occasions; its coefficient represents the ratio of true variance (i.e. due to the subject) to the sum of true variance and error variance (Rudy et al 1992, Streiner & Norman 1995). The three sources of systematic error which can be minimized are content, time and observers. Internal consistency, estimated as item intercorrelation (alpha coefficient) and/or item-total correlations, is improved by excluding items which share least variance, although this narrows meaning and applicability of the scale. Adding items tends to increase internal consistency up to about ten; beyond that, benefits are asymptotic. Test-retest reliability decreases over time, but reliability calculated over a few days may be inapplicable or inadequate over months. Intraclass correlation (McDowell & Newell 1996) with confidence intervals provides a safer estimate than simple correlation, but for some constructs, stability across time may be a chimera, given continuous reconstruction of experience. Inter-rater reliability is achieved by minimizing systematic differences between raters, for instance by clear definition of the target of observation and of rating categories, and by training and recalibrating raters, procedures which should be replicated by those using the measure. Simple correlation of raters' scores can give a misleadingly good estimate when they differ by a consistent ratio; intraclass correlation is preferable, producing a coefficient (kappa) which is a function of the base rate of the target of measurement. The non-parametric equivalent is a coefficient of concordance (Streiner & Norman 1995).

VALIDITY

Validity is commonly defined as the extent to which an instrument measures what it is intended to measure, whether an identifiable quantity or hypothetical construct. It is not inherent in a measure nor a consequence of reliability, but of its interpretation. Construct validity describes the extent to which the measurement instrument approximates a hypothetical (or hard to measure) construct beyond its bounds – such as fitness, depression or quality of life – or for which there is no agreed single indicator, such as autonomic arousal. It is established by cumulative use, and with greater difficulty than concurrent and predictive validity, both of which are aspects of it but not substitutes for it. The demonstration of concurrent validity has been compared to the convergence of torch beams in a search: they light the same area, but the construct may be elsewhere or not exist (Deary et al 1997). The issue is that naming a questionnaire 'readiness for treatment' or 'refractory personality' does not establish the hypothetical construct, which may have neither theoretical grounding nor economy in representing variables. Several statistical methods are used to investigate construct validity (Streiner & Norman 1995). Demand effects, a particular threat, are produced by contingency of financial benefits or social approval on the basis of particular responses: they may be rectified by changing questionnaire content or instructions, or estimated (Streiner & Norman 1995). Criterion validity consists of concurrent validity – coincidence with an established measure of the same latent construct – and predictive validity – coincidence with some future outcome. It is important that any instrument measures the target construct and not another; for instance, an anxiety scale should not correlate too highly with established measures of depression (although there is no consensus on the degree of independence); a measure of activity should not, as perhaps in questions about leisure activity, inadvertently measure the respondent's financial health.

SENSITIVITY TO CHANGE

If an instrument is reliable and valid, if responses are well distributed across the scale, and if conditions (such as population, training of raters, instructions) resemble those in the reliability study, it should be sensitive to change (Hays & Hadorn 1992, Streiner & Norman 1995). Ideally, this is tested against a 'gold standard' criterion, but there is no agreed coefficient (McDowell & Newell 1996).

Reference to change by units of standard deviation, as in effect sizes, can help interpretation where measurement units are arbitrary. Clinical significance cannot be extrapolated from statistical significance of a difference in scores on an instrument, which is related to the size of the standard deviation and of the sample; pretreatment and healthy population scores may be used to define clinical significance (Jacobson & Truax 1991). Cutpoints are a particular application of sensitivity and specificity and, like them, vary with the conditions under which they are estimated. Application of cutpoints to individuals rather than populations is particularly hazardous, as sensitivity varies considerably across different item sets achieving the same total (Clarke & McKenzie 1994).

DOMAINS OF MEASUREMENT

There are many ways of grouping measures into domains, given their interrelationships, so it is not possible to suggest a menu from which one measure per domain is required. As described before, it depends on the aims of the study. However, it is not unusual to draw broad conclusions from a rather narrow range of measures, as in the Quebec Task Force report (Spitzer et al 1987), which evaluated a range of pain management strategies by reference only to changes in diagnostic classifications, pain experience and work status.

MEASURES OF FUNCTION AND DISABILITY

Measures of function, disability, activity, impairment, quality of life and other overlapping constructs have arisen largely from clinical settings. While there have been attempts to use the theoretical distinctions of impairment, disability and handicap (e.g., Harper et al 1992), the model on which they draw fails to address psychosocial influences on disability. This is the more regrettable since social handicap is a neglected area of measurement. This domain includes clinical measures and instruments assessing single functions, compound and generic measures of function, and pain behaviour, the latter mainly due to the considerable overlap with behavioural measures of function.

There is no perfect solution to the conflicts of comprehensiveness versus brevity and reliability, nor that of permitting comparison across populations versus specificity and clinical meaning. Pressures to approximate diverse variables within one score cannot be avoided or ignored (Deyo 1984, Kaplan 1985, Bowling 1991), but it is difficult to conceptualize the latent variable of a measure which adds not apples and oranges, but rather apples and orangutans. For instance, one back pain rating scale combines clinical measures, patient report of pain and activity, and physician rating of dysfunction (from pain report and drug intake) in a total whose units are not specified. Subscale scores of compound measures may be more useful than the total, and many have better internal consistency and construct validity, whereas global measures may be better distributed than their component scales with superior test-retest reliability (Charlton et al 1983). Global measures are in some cases supplemented by specific scales; in other cases, subscales are omitted and the total is prorated accordingly (as in the study reported by Katz et al 1992), although this has unknown effects on psychometric qualities. Recently developed global function scales are redressing the neglect of applicability across cultural groups; it remains unaddressed in the measurement of pain behaviours, where social and cultural conditions may govern suppression and frequency of particular behaviours (Ekman 1993). A significant divergence from the earlier racial stereotyping studies, work by Bates and colleagues (Bates et al 1993) uses psychosocial variables such as degree of acculturation.

Ideally, a study concerned with function, or disability, incorporates direct or analogue measurement of relevant physical capacity or activity. However, the demands of instrument development and testing are such that progress is relatively slow, with much adaptation of existing but not entirely satisfactory instruments, and often insufficient testing of reliability, validity and sensitivity to change (Anderson et al 1993). Some instruments, such as the SF-36, have addressed this by constructing brief subscales from heavily loading items of well-established scales. Many existing tests are established for describing ill or healthy populations, but not for measuring the extent of change between states. In addition, many such measures can be criticized for taking a snapshot of capacities or performance which may poorly represent the sustained activity required by many tasks, and which is affected by unquantified psychological factors (Vasuvedan 1992).

Clinical measures

The pain field is replete with findings of supposedly pathognomic signs in symptom-free individuals (e.g., Boden et al 1990, Jensen et al 1994a), which should discourage those who would use them for patient selection or quantification of pathology. The use of biomedical diagnostic data as measurement is only appropriate within certain conditions (Keefe et al 1992a, Rudy et al 1992) and assumptions of clinical significance of test findings may generate unnecessary anxieties for the patient and unnecessary treatment; both can result in iatrogenic invalidity. Indicators of diagnostic efficiency – sensitivity, specificity, false-positive and negative rates and values derived from them – are essential data although inconsistently available. Because of dependence on base rate, the preferred index of a test's performance is the likelihood ratio: the true-positive rate (i.e. sensitivity) over the false-positive rate (Sackett et al 1991).

A number of recent studies give accounts of the generally low reliability of physical and clinical measures in common use (for instance, joint stiffness and swelling in rheumatoid arthritis), not only in outcome measurement and similar studies, but in the selection of patients for such studies. Such measures may incorporate useful data, but it is rare outside cancer populations to sample symptoms other than pain (such as numbness or weakness). Strender et al (1997) found unacceptably low inter-rater agreement for judgements such as tenderness and segmental mobility in low back pain patients. In the context of generally poor inter-rater reliability (Jensen et al 1994a) and poor specificity (Lowery et al 1992), the best available are tests described by Waddell et al (1992) and Waddell and Turk (1992). An alternative is the index of pathology (Rudy et al 1988b, Rudy et al 1990) derived from the concordance of physicians on the usefulness of various tests of adequate inter-rater reliability. However, it is not clear what we can infer from these tests, or from other functions which, while reliable when measured by automated means (e.g., Cybex: Polatin & Mayer 1992), lack demonstration of validity for the physical demands of everyday life. This was well illustrated by Dreyfuss et al (1996), who used clinical tests for sacroiliac joint pain which showed good agreement between assessors, but all of which failed to identify patients who gained at least 90% pain relief from a sacroiliac joint block with local anaesthetic.

Physiological and psychophysiological measures are relatively rarely used, not least owing to the steep requirements for specialized equipment and training, and difficulties in data reduction and interpretation. Technical details, such as electrode placement in EMG recording and practice effects, may be crucial for establishing reliability. Dynamic recording (for instance, of back muscle activity; Watson et al 1997) and changes in autonomic activity on provocation (Flor et al 1992) are superior to recording of resting EMG of muscles in the area of pain by comparison with a non-pain area, although this remains the most widely used format. The variable relationship of EMG with pain reported by the patient undermines simple interpretation. In general, EMG measures have proved more useful than measures of cardiovascular function, except where this is implicated in the pain mechanism. Blood flow, skin temperature, heart rate and blood pressure can be measured (skin temperature is commonly used in biofeedback), but reactivity rather than resting levels may be the parameter related to pain measures, and the meaning remains somewhat obscure. Recording of brain activity by EEG (Flor et al 1992, Chen 1993a) and by imaging techniques (Chen 1993b, Casey & Minoshima 1997) are technically demanding and challenging to interpret. Both are used predominantly in experimental settings and are difficult to extrapolate to clinical situations.

Unidimensional measures of function

Various self-report measures are described in the outcome literature, such as lists of activities abandoned or performed with difficulty, activities which are no longer painful after treatment and estimated hours per week of housework. Direct estimation methods – the visual analogue scale (VAS), numerical rating scale (NRS) and Likert scales – may be used for ratings such as interference of pain with activities. The important issues are the wording of questions, ideally developed using patient terminology; response categories are the second important issue response categories where seven, nine or 11 response options can usually be analysed as if they represent interval data (McCormack et al 1988, Streiner & Norman 1995), and the use of repeated measurement in diary format (Jensen & McFarland 1993) or at random or cue-determined times, possibly using pagers or electronic diaries (Stone & Shiffman 1994, Keefe et al 1997). Clinical questions, such as 'Can you sit in an ordinary chair for more than 30 minutes at a time before you need to get up and move around' (Waddell & Turk 1992) have been suggested, but cannot be assumed to be a straightforward account of everyday performance. In addition, it should be noted that patients (and doctors) can be very poor judges of distance, sometimes by a factor of ten (Sharrack & Hughes 1997). Direct measurement of the focus of the study, and of intervention, may be possible. Patient records of uptime (time out of bed) and/or downtime have been used, but are more reliably assessed mechanically (Sanders 1983) or checked against staff observation. The strength of uptime as a measure is that it is a cumulative rather than 'snapshot' measure, although without further detail on what the patient is doing, and onset/offset, interpretation is limited. It is surprising that there is not more use of cumulative measurement, such as by pedometers (Cinciripini & Floreen 1982, Bussmann et al 1998). Patients' use of orthopaedic collars and corsets, and walking and other aids, can be directly assessed by observers.

The measurement of physical performance, particularly when it is supervised during treatment, can provide face-valid data and may be useable by the patient outside the treatment setting. Recordings of speed, distance and time from treadmill or exercycle sessions, repetitions of exercises, and recordings of walk distance and stair climbing have all been used. Reliability of data collection by patients can be checked against staff counts. However, demand effects during observation may be powerful, and instructions for standardized and neutral supervision are important. Harding et al (1994) established good reliability for several measures in this category; Frost et al (1995) describe a walk test adapted from respiratory medicine. There are no comparable measures for upper limb and neck pain. In rheumatoid arthritis, measures such as grip strength, walking time and buttoning (Pincus et al 1991) appear to assess function rather than disease activity (Spiegel et al 1987).

Work status of patients is a major focus of treatment, although not routinely assessed in studies of psychological, physical, surgical or pharmacological treatment. Return to work following treatment is a contentious variable, given the many other influences on employment, such as availability of suitable work, financial contingencies and conditions imposed by third party payers. Aside from the apparently straightforward working/not working categories, work status may be assessed using hours and job demands in relation to previous performance or another criterion; it may also be assessed by using patient (and others') ratings of interference of pain with work, time taken to return to work or reasons for not returning (including entry to retraining), and termination of compensation claims and disability benefits. Some of these may be obtainable from employers or statutory records. Return to work may also be affected by local economic factors and unemployment rates (Volinn et al 1988), the type of work, and the willingness of employers to employ or re-employ a worker with significant time off work for a recurrent or chronic pain problem. Fitness for occupation is not easily measured: although many aspects of manual jobs can be measured, it is often the frequency of repetition, combinations of movements or awkward postures which mitigate against sustained work (Feuerstein & Hickey 1992); however, ergonomic measurement is beyond the scope of this chapter. Maintenance of work over the longer term is also an issue. Psychosocial factors at work may also play an important part, but there are not yet any satisfactory measures of them. The risk of developing chronic pain and work absence in workers with acute back pain can be assessed using a screening questionnaire covering pain severity, appraisal, attributions to work and current limitations (Linton & Hallden 1997).

Compensation status and work status interact: measurement of the former alone may be seriously misleading (Jamison et al 1988, Tait et al 1990, Mendelson 1992, Sanderson et al 1995). Estimation of cost savings attributable to return to work following treatment is beyond the scope of this chapter (see review by Goossens & Evers 1997). Entirely missing from pain studies is assessment of the financial impact of pain and of its treatment on the patient and his/her family, in terms of disposable income, debt and changes in socioeconomic status (Linton 1998). This is the more surprising when these financial contingencies are frequently invoked to account for disappointing treatment outcome.

Lastly, the measurement of sleep quality and quantity is often neglected, despite the prevalence of sleep problems in pain complaints, and the possibility that poor sleep adversely affects daytime function. Despite the known inaccuracy of sleepers' estimates (Lacks 1987), it appears that simple ratings of specific problems (such as difficulty falling asleep, difficulty maintaining sleep, frequent wakings, difficulty returning to sleep, and feeling poorly rested on awaking; e.g., Buysse et al 1988, Jenkins et al 1988) are adequate without concurrent polysomnographic recording, because patients' subjective sense of sleep adequacy is the more important variable.

Multidimensional measures of function

The construction of measures of function, disability or quality of life, whether de novo or using existing instruments, is fraught with problems. There are many possible domains of life or activity to be assessed, and within each an infinite number of specific activities, but the more comprehensive the questionnaire, the more liable the patient to exhaustion and error. Shorter measures may be as sensitive to change as longer ones, and far more acceptable to patients (Katz et al 1992), but the necessary exclusion of specific activities or of whole domains increases the risk of insensitivity in assessing both state and change. The question of validation is considerable, and the investment required in estimating more than concurrent validity against existing (unsatisfactory) instruments is beyond the normal scope of scale development. Choice of measure should be guided by similarity of the populations on which there are data using the measure, by validation procedures and by the purposes of assessment. Table 18.1 presents the most widely used instruments which currently have at least adequate psychometric data.

Table 18.1 Measurement of function

Measure	*Content*	*Scoring*	*Minutes for completion*	*Comments*
Short form 36 of Medical Outcomes Study SF-36	9 domains: physical, psychological, social, pain	36 items, 1–10/domain; 2–6 response categories. Rescaled 0–100. No summary score	10–15	Thorough development; widely used and translated Interpreted by reference to age and sex norms; sensitivity to change not established Possible floor effects for severely ill; report of low test-retest reliability for role limitation Supplementary questions for chronic pain treatment in development (Wagner et al 1996)
Sickness Impact Profile SIP	11 dimensions: physical, psychological, self-care, social, optional work	136 items, yes/no, weighted scores. Total score 0-10030 or calculated as %	20–45	Widely used in pain field; European translations Interview or self-administered: reliability of former better Eating, communication, work low correlation with total Sensitive to group differences; may be insensitive to change particularly improvement
Roland & Morris short SIP	Single dimension, almost entirely physical items	24 items, yes/no, unweighted, total 0–24	5	Increasingly used as brief and good psychometric properties Lacks psychosocial content
Multidimensional Pain Inventory (MPI/WHYMPI)	3 domains: pain and mood, spouse response, activity	20, 14 and 18 items/domain; totals scored as mean 0–6. Also reported as patient profile	15–20	Thorough development on chronic pain populations although predominantly male Patient profiles replicated in several US and European samples More data on group differences than on change
Oswestry Low Back Pain Disability Qu.	10 areas: physical, psychosocial, pain, sleep	1 item/area; 6 response categories. Rescaled to % for total score	5–10	Psychometric qualities need revisiting; nevertheless endorsed by medical authorities
Nottingham Health Profile NHP	6 dimensions: physical, psychological, pain, sleep	38+7 items, yes/no; 3–9 per dimension; weighted scores. No summary score	10–15	Widely used outside pain; translations not yet tested for psychometric properties Concerns about scoring system and test-retest reliability Floor effects for mild disability, limited sensitivity to small changes Authors recommend nonparametric treatment of data
Arthritis Impact Measurement Scale AIMS	9 scales: physical, psychological, social, pain	45 items, 4–7/scale. 2–6 response categories; rescaled 0–10. Total of 6 scales	15–25	Suitable for mixed or osteoarthritis or RA patients Varied findings on factor structure and sensitivity to change Dutch version, IRGL (Huiskes et al 1990), differs in content and scoring

SF-36: Ware et al 1993; see also Ware & Sherbourne 1992, Anderson et al 1993, McHorney et al 1993, McDowell & Newell 1996, Beaton et al 1997, Roberts et al 1997.
SIP: Bergner et al 1981; see also Follick et al 1985, Deyo and Centar 1986, MacKenzie et al 1986, Katz et al 1992, McDowell & Newell 1996, Beaton et al 1997.
Roland & Morris short SIP: Roland & Morris 1983, Deyo 1986, Jensen et al 1992, Stratford et al 1993
MPI (WHYMPI): Kerns et al 1985; see also Rudy 1989, De Gagne et al 1995.
Oswestry: Fairbank et al 1980; see also McDowell & Newell 1996.
NHP: Hunt et al 1985; see also Anderson et al 1993, McDowell & Newell 1996.
AIMS: Meenan et al 1982; see also Kazis et al 1983, Huiskes et al 1990, McDowell & Newell 1996.

Several questionnaires are described as instruments to assess activities of daily living, but those in common use are designed to assess the care needs of severely disabled patients, and are rarely of use. A more patient-focused measure is that of goal attainment (Kerns et al 1986), which relies heavily on the judicious choice of goals by patients, goals which are ideally independent for the purposes of analysis and are expressed in absolute rather than relative terms. These must be scored by reference to expected or ideal level of attainment, the definition of which may be influenced by a wide range of psychological variables. Not surprisingly, concurrent validity with global scales of function tends to be poor. When reported for a group of patients rather than for individuals, it effectively equates goals of different topography: for one patient the major goal may be represented by return to work, for another by being able to tie shoelaces unaided.

Quality of life measures have not been used widely in pain studies, other than in cancer. Several widely used measures arise from the intention to ration health care, and make psychologically questionable assumptions about the stability of health preferences central to their construction (Kaplan 1985, Fallowfield 1990). Two recently established instruments, the EuroQol (EuroQol Group 1990) and the WHOQoL (WHOQOL Group 1995), are undergoing extensive testing, but this is directed at describing and distinguishing populations rather than evaluating individuals or measuring change (Anderson et al 1993).

In cancer populations, none of the possible measures above has been adopted: the reader is directed to Higginson (1997) for a review and guidelines on assessment. The widely used Spitzer Quality of Life Index and the Karnofsky Performance Status (Cleeland & Syrjala 1992) are brief and focused on practical needs, making them too insensitive for many studies. The main measure with adequate psychometric data is the EORTC QLQ (European Organization for Research and Treatment of Cancer Quality of Life Questionnaire; Aaronson et al 1988), which consists of a universal core of 36 (or in the widely used short version, 30) items on physical and psychosocial function plus symptoms of cancer and adverse effects of treatment, with smaller supplementary modules specific to the site of cancer, some yet to be developed. In the diagnostic groups on which it has been tested, it appears to be sensitive to change (Anderson et al 1993).

Health-care use

Health-care use may be determined less by disease factors than by beliefs, distress and other psychosocial variables (Friedman et al 1995), a constant frustration to many clinicians. Its measurement is often unsatisfactory, not least when it stems from unarticulated models. This is clearest in the measurement of drug use, which may be classified in terminology which assumes all opioid users to be psychologically dependent. Surprisingly, there is no standard method of measuring drug intake, and so many are used, complicating comparisons between studies. Drug studies use established methods, such as dosage, assay against a drug of known efficacy, time to next analgesic and others. Classifications of drugs according to their chemical constitution is straightforward; certain properties which vary within the class, such as sedation, may also require recording. Dose data allows estimation of proportional differences across treatment or between groups, a more sensitive measure than use versus abstinence. Despite the general unreliability of self report of drug intake (Berndt et al 1993), checks for adherence to dosage are not standard. Diary recording may be the most reliable way of assessing regularity of use and whether it is contingent on time, pain or other cues.

Use of health-care facilities may be measured by frequency, type and cost. In the former categories are clinic and emergency room visits, inpatient hospital stays, outpatient treatment or diagnostic procedures, and visits to complementary health practitioners; in epidemiological studies, variables such as analgesic use and treatment access can indicate the impact of chronic pain (Purves et al 1998). Costing health care is fraught with difficulties, and the reader is referred to Friedman et al (1995) on cost offset of teaching self management; also see Caudill et al (1991) and Hill and Hardy (1996) for conservative but impressive estimates of savings within the health-care system; and Zbrozek (1994) and Linton (1998) for broader views of the issue.

Pain behaviour

Such is the overlap of concepts in the field that many of the behaviours which may be classified as pain behaviour are described elsewhere in this chapter, in particular, physical performance, uptime and use of health-care resources. As Turk and Flor (1987) pointed out in a conceptual discussion, rather than obtaining desirable outcomes or avoiding undesirable ones, pain behaviours can be strategies to reduce pain, or a consequence of a physical impairment. Patients' comments on their use of behaviours identified as pain behaviours can add novel and valuable information (Wilkie et al 1992) but are too rarely sought. Strictly, pain behaviours are identified by observation of their frequency in the context of their occurrence and of the contingencies associated with them. Self reports of pain behaviours tend to be poorly correlated with observer report of the same behaviour (Cleeland 1989), although avoidance is best sampled by self report (Waddell et al 1993). Until the important methodological development of observation and analysis of spouse–patient interaction (Romano et al 1991), assessment instruments focused on counts of frequency and testing hypotheses about associations with other variables. Major proponents of pain behaviour measurement have called for finer grained analysis and sampling of more relevant activities (Craig 1992, Keefe et al 1992a). There is also a need for the investigation of the potential application of this field to non-verbal (severely intellectually impaired) adult subjects whose pain may be overlooked, even when their distress is manifest.

The observation measure developed by Keefe and Block (1982) focuses on five observable and mutually exclusive motor patterns (rubbing, guarding, bracing, grimacing and sighing during a 10-min sequence of sitting, standing, walking and lying down), and raters require training (and recalibration) using videotaped sequences to achieve and maintain good reliability. All the behaviours distinguish chronic back pain patients from depressed and non-depressed controls and from asymptomatic subjects; all but guarding are correlated with patients' pain ratings and with naïve observers' ratings of patients' pain. A similar measure can be used with arthritis patients (McDaniel et al 1986, Keefe & Williams 1992), and in an adapted form with non-chronic back pain sufferers (Jensen et al 1989). A briefer checklist for staff use with inpatients was developed by Richards et al (1982). Ten behaviours are rated for occurrence and frequency; factor analysis suggests two main factors of facial/audible and motor behaviours; used early in low back pain absence from work, scores can predict long-term sick leave (Ohlund et al 1994). Another scale developed for nurses' use in clinical settings or for spouses at home is the Checklist for Interpersonal Pain Behavior (CHIP: Vlaeyen et al 1990b). The content is broad, including observer judgements of mood as well as mobility, verbal and non-verbal complaints, and sleep and drowsiness. The use of adults' facial expression of pain requires extensive coding of recorded samples, and is only employed in experimental studies (Craig et al 1992). Facial expression coding merits development for use in clinical settings and studies, as is occurring with the use of corrugator muscle change in the study of depression, because it appears that it is hard to suppress. The study of observer judgements of faking, exaggerating or masking pain (Poole & Craig 1992) and associated responses also offers much to clinical study, not least because facial behaviour may have primacy for observer judgements over other behaviours (Prkachin et al 1983).

Although interactions in medical settings may make a major contribution to learning and maintenance of pain and illness behaviour, there is little examination of them in this setting and no systematic measure of health professionals' behaviour. Waddell et al (1980) defined particular behaviours and responses during medical examination as non-organic signs, meaning that they were attributable to patient distress rather than to mechanical or neurological problems; inter-rater reliability is not established. However, their occurrence can be associated with biomedical as well as psychological variables (Keefe et al 1984), and the term non-organic has been widely misused as 'psychogenic'. As there are now more reliable ways to screen for psychological distress and better ways to address interaction during physical examination, this test is probably redundant.

AFFECTIVE AND COGNITIVE MEASURES

Many related constructs and measures fall into this category: the most useful are displayed in Tables 18.2 and 18.3. There is considerable overlap of constructs – for instance, mood can hardly be considered independently of its cognitive content – and it is a lively area of debate and model-building. Measures are also likely to share variance due to social desirability and cultural factors (Donaldson 1989). In contrast to measures of function, the development of many psychological measures from theoretical roots has bypassed certain clinically important areas such as social support, and produced a proliferation of measures which Lambert and Hill (1994) described as 'overwhelming if not disheartening'. Many also show shortcomings in construct definition and scope of validation.

Mood and affect

The choice of a tool to measure affect in chronic pain is fraught with difficulty. In principle, researchers and certain clinicians should be seeking not diagnoses but a broad indicator of distress which identifies individuals who require further psychological or psychiatric assessment, and which is sensitive to the effects (if any) of pain interventions. Instead, the field has been dominated by measures developed in the psychiatric diagnostic domain, some of which were designed as trait measures and therefore for stability, not sensitivity to change. In the latter category, the Minnesota Multiphasic Personality Inventory (MMPI) predominates, and remains popular despite its unsatisfactory psychometric properties and questionable applicability (Aronoff & Wagner 1987, Main et al 1991). The use of psychiatric scales flourished in pain studies on the basis of a false distinction between real/organic and functional/psychogenic pain; because pain was considered to be the product of the patient's disturbed psyche, then psychiatric measures seemed appropriate. The study of mood and mood disorder in chronic pain will benefit from setting far

Table 18.2 Measurement of mood and affect

Measure	*Content*	*Scoring*	*Purpose*	*Comments*
Beck Depression Inventory BDI	21 items; cognitive, affective, somatic	4–6 responses/item scored 0–3 for severity; total 0–63	Depression severity in psychiatric and normal patients	Psychometric data on psychiatric not pain populations Question about structure with pain patients: separate somatic factor or BDI single latent variable?
Center for Epidemiologic Studies Depression Scale CES-D	20 items; cognitive, affective, somatic	0–3 frequency rating; total 0–63	Screening of psychiatric and community samples	Psychometric data on psychiatric and community samples Question about structure with pain patients: separate somatic factor? Not very specific to depression; overlap with anxiety
General Health Questionnaire GHQ	60, 30, 28, 20 or 12 items; cognitive, affective, somatic, social	0–3 frequency compared to usual, or dichotomously; total (GHQ-28 4 subscales)	Detection of psychiatric problems in community and medical outpatients	12-item version discards items common in physically ill people GHQ-28 has 4-factor analytically derived scales Emphasis on recent change may underestimate chronic problems
Hospital Anxiety & Depression Scale HADS	14 items; 7 anxiety, 7 depression (anhedonia only)	0–3 frequency; totals 0–21 for anxiety and for depression	Detection of anxiety and depression in medical inpatients or outpatients	Depression lacks cognitive content, and may represent lack of well-being Factor structure largely upheld on testing Scores not associated with chronicity or pain rating
Modified Zung Self-Rating Depression Scale	15 items; affective and cognitive	1–4 frequency; single total	Modified for use with pain populations by removing somatic items	Psychometrics re-established on pain patients.
State Trait Anxiety Inventory STAI	20 items each state and trait anxiety	1–4 for severity; total 20–80	Severity of anxiety, normal and psychiatric populations	Lacks psychometric data on pain populations
Health Anxiety Questionnaire HAQ	21 items; health worry, fear of illness, reassurance, interference	3–8 items/cluster; 0–3 frequency	Severity of health anxiety in normal and medical populations	No pain data yet
Modified Somatic Perception Questionnaire MSPQ	13 items (of 20) All somatic	0–3 severity: total 0–39	Severity of somatic awareness/anxiety in pain patients	Part of Distress & Risk Assessment Measure (DRAM)
Pain Anxiety Symptoms Scale PASS	40 items, 4 subscales; somatic, cognitive, fear, escape and avoidance	10 items/subscale; 0–5 frequency. Subscales and total	Severity of fear of pain/pain-related fear	

BDI: Beck et al 1961; see also Wesley et al 1991, Meakin 1992, Williams & Richardson 1993, Chibnall & Tait 1994, Schuster & Smith 1994, Novy et al 1995. Cancer: Plumb & Holland 1977. Rheumatoid arthritis: Peck et al 1989.
CES-D: Radloff 1977; see also Bames & Prosen 1985, Blalock et al 1989, Snaith 1993, Turk & Okifuji 1994, McDowell & Newell 1996.
GHQ: Goldberg 1978, Goldberg & Hillier 1979; see also McDowell & Newell 1996.
HADS: Zigmond & Snaith 1983; see also Snaith 1987, Moorey et al 1991, Herrmann 1997. Cancer: Chandarana et al 1987. Rheumatoid arthritis: Clark & Steer 1994.
Modified Zung SDS: Main & Waddell 1984; see also Main et al 1991.
STAI: Spielberger 1983.
HAQ: Lucock & Morley 1996.
MSPQ: Main 1983; see also Main et al 1991, Waddell & Turk 1992.
PASS: McCracken et al 1992.

Table 18.3 Measurement of beliefs, appraisal and coping

Measure	*Items and scoring*	*Constituent scales (N of items) and item example*
Multidimensional Health Locus of Control MHLC	18 1–6 agreement	Internal locus of control (6) When I get sick, I am to blame; Powerful others locus of control (6) Health professionals keep me healthy; Chance locus of control (6) No matter what I do, I'm likely to get sick
Beliefs about Controlling Pain Questionnaire BPCQ	13 1–6 agreement	Internal control (5) I am directly responsible for my own pain; Chance (4) Being pain free is largely a matter of luck; Powerful doctors (4) I cannot get any pain relief unless I go to seek medical help
Pain Locus of Control PLC	15: 0–3 truth	Cognitive control (9) My pain will get better if I think of pleasant thoughts; Pain responsibility (6) Only I can help myself with my pain
Pain Self-Efficacy Qu. PSEQ	10: 0–6 confidence	Unidimensional, e.g., I can still accomplish most of my goals in life, despite my pain
Arthritis Self-Effecacy Scale ASE	20: 10–100 in 10s, certainty	Self-efficacy pain (5) How certain are you that you can decrease your pain quite a bit?; Self-efficacy function (9) How certain are you that you can walk 10 steps downstairs in 7 seconds?; Other Symptoms Self-Efficacy (6) How certain are you that you can control your fatigue?
Pain Beliefs and Perceptions Inventory PBPI	16: −2 to +2 (no 0) agreement	Time (9) My pain is here to stay; Mystery (4) My pain is confusing to me; Self-blame (3) I am the cause of my pain
Coping Strategies Questionnaire CSQ	42: 0–6 frequency + 2: 0–6 extent	Catastrophizing (6) I feel I can't stand it any more; Praying and hoping (6) I pray for the pain to stop; Ignoring (6) I tell myself it doesn't hurt; Reinterpreting (6) I imagine that the pain is outside my body; Increasing activity (6) I read; Diverting attention (6) I think of things I enjoy doing; Coping self-statements (6) Although it hurts, I just keep on going. Ability to decrease and to control the pain (2)
Pain Cognitions List PCL	50: 1–5 agreement	Pain impact (17) I feel less and less capable of doing something; Catastrophizing (17) The word *pain* frightens me; Outcome efficacy (7) Relaxation exercises decrease the pain; Acquiescence (4) I think the best thing to do is to wait and see what happens; Reliance on health care (5) Somebody must be able to help me
Survey of Pain Attitudes SOPA	57: 0–4 truth	Control (10) I am not in control of my pain; Disability (10) I consider myself to be disabled; Harm (8) Exercise and movement are good for my pain problem; Emotion (8) Anxiety increases the pain I feel; Medication (6) I will never take pain medications again; Solicitude (6) When I hurt I want my family to treat me better; Medical cure (9) My physical pain will never be cured
Fear Avoidance Beliefs Questionnaire FABQ	11 of 16: 0–6 agreement	Fear-avoidance beliefs about work (7) My work aggravated my pain; Fear-avoidance beliefs about physical activity (4) Physical activity makes my pain worse
Tampa Scale for Kinesiophobia TSK	17: 0–3 agreement	Unidimensional: It's really not safe for a person with a condition like mine to be physically active
Pain-Related Control Scale PRCS Pain-Related Self Statements PRSS	15 & 18: 0–5 agreement	Helplessness (7) I cannot influence my pain; Resourcefulness (8) I can do nothing about my pain; Catastrophizing (9) I have learnt to live with my pain; Coping (9) Strees aggravates my pain

MHLC: Wallston et al 1978; see also Main & Waddell 1991.
BPCQ: Skevington 1990.
PLC: Main & Waddell 1991.
PSEQ: Nicholas et al 1992; see also Coughlan et al 1995.
ASE: Lorig et al 1989; see also DeGood & Shutty 1992.
PBPI: Williams & Thom 1989; see also Herda et al 1994, Williams et al 1994.
CSQ: Rosenstiel & Keefe 1983; see also Sullivan & D'Eon 1990, Williams & Keefe 1991, Williams et al 1994, Robinson et al 1997,
Osteoarthritis: Keefe et al 1987, Main & Waddell 1991, DeGood & Shutty 1992, Swartzman et al 1994.
PCL: Vlaeyen et al 1990a.
SOPA: Jensen & Karoly 1992; see also DeGood & Shutty 1992.
FABQ: Waddell et al 1993; see also Waddell & Turk 1992.
TSK: see Vlaeyen et al 1995.
PRCS, PRSS: Flor et al 1993; see also Main & Waddell 1991.

more stringent criteria for the adoption of psychiatric measures, and turning instead to model testing using concepts from mainstream psychology such as information processing and memory. A few of the latter have emerged in pain, addressing the broad question of the relationship between pain, disability and depression (Rudy et al 1988a), or the more specific one of unidimensionality or multidimensionality of a widely used depression scale (Novy et al 1995).

A further problem of psychiatric nosology has been the rigid distinction between anxiety and depression, when the two are positively rather than negatively correlated (Lewis 1991). The doctrine of separateness dictated the exclusion of overlapping items during the development of measures (Dobson & Cheung 1990). In fact, there are reasonable arguments for making less distinction until we can better conceptualize the relationships between pain, anxiety (including both relatively specific fears associated with the impact of pain on life and somatic focus) and depression (defined more by affective and cognitive than by somatic phenomena to avoid judgements concerning origins of symptoms). Where the diagnostic systems have not been used in the construction of a measure, they are almost inevitably used in its concurrent validation, given the impossibility of specific external criteria. This remains far from ideal for measures intended for physically disabled or ill populations, given the instruction in the Diagnostic and Statistical Manual of the American Psychological Association (DSM) and International Classification of Diseases (ICD) systems to exclude symptoms due to a medical condition.

The depression questionnaires described in Table 18.2 are those with good psychometric properties and widely used in the pain field. Nevertheless, those properties were often established on populations from which those with medical conditions and symptoms have been excluded (e.g., Steer et al 1985). The import of this for use in pain populations is not fully understood, but findings of different endorsement of somatic items by pain patients and psychiatric patients, and of separate somatic factors emerging from analysis of their scores, are common within pain patients and in physically ill populations. This means that, unlike responses of psychiatric or other non-medical populations, the total scores may assess mainly somatic problems. It also means that where somatic concerns are chronic, most of the variance in change will be explained by the non-somatic symptoms, and where these are close to floor level, it renders the instrument insensitive to change.

Overall, choice of a depression measure requires careful balancing of priorities concerning content, standardization and meaning. Inspection of scores across questionnaire items can identify whether the somatic content is disproportionately represented if that is a problem for the study. Exclusion of items, however, has implications for what is measured by the resulting instrument. The Hospital Anxiety and Depression Scale (HADS), which excludes somatic items, actually arose from a model of depression as anhedonia (Snaith 1987) and measures a rather different latent construct from the Beck Depression Inventory (BDI), containing as it does questions concerning self blame, sense of failure and other cognitive concerns. In general, self-report measures of depression tend to have high sensitivity but also tend to identify more respondents as depressed than are identified by interview (Gamsa 1994); raising the cutoff point can improve specificity at a cost of sensitivity, and should in any case be established empirically.

There are fewer contenders in the measurement of anxiety, and the issue concerning the import of psychiatrically standardized instruments applies. Table 18.2 contains two relative newcomers, one specific to health-related anxieties and the other to pain-related anxieties. Given the small field of choice, reports of their use are awaited with optimism. It may be particularly appropriate in the area of specific anxieties to attempt other measurement technologies, such as recording patients' 'thinking out loud' while performing a challenging task or in an anxiogenic situation; in this case, results are subjected to qualitative rather than quantitative methods of analysis.

Controversies over the separability of anxiety and distress justify the use of a combined measure of distress, of which the General Health Questionnaire (GHQ) is by far the most widely used. Unfortunately, the SCL90-R (Derogatis 1983), which also provides a global distress score, is subject to the same preferential endorsement of somatic items by pain patients as other instruments developed in psychiatric populations, and its internal consistency, factor structure and predictive validity have been found unsatisfactory in pain studies (Buckelew et al 1986, Bradley et al 1992, Turk & Rudy 1992). The SF-36 (Table 18.1) contains a scale of general mental health and well being, whereas the Arthritis Impact Measurement Scale (AIMS) (Table 18.1) has separate depression (anhedonia) and anxiety (tension) scales. Subject to the caveats about their use, a suitably worded direct estimation method is an option, as it is for the assessment of anger, positive well being and other potentially relevant affect for which there is no clear best measure. A promising newcomer in the area is the Clinical Outcomes in Routine Evaluation system (CORE System Group 1998), a broad but brief screening instrument developed across patients of psychological treatment services, including those with physical problems.

Cognitive measures: beliefs, appraisal and coping

There are many ways of subdividing this area, but to do so assumes specificity of the latent constructs and of the measurement instruments, unattainable on the basis of the current relatively modest level of understanding in the area. Table 18.3 therefore describes measures (widely used and/or with good psychometric properties) in terms of the questions asked and response options available, to be considered in relation to the study question and the population. Choice of measure requires a balance between what is sampled by the questionnaire, whether or not it is pain-specific, and the availability of published studies describing its performance. Jensen et al (1991) tabulates a wide range of measures and findings concerning them, noting study methodology; reviews by Keefe et al (1992b) and DeGood and Shutty (1992) are also recommended.

However, readers may find themselves more confused the wider they read. The proliferation of measures is bewildering – to the extent that a leading pain researcher remarked that psychologists are more inclined to use one another's toothbrushes than questionnaires (C.J. Main) – the more so because so few offer associations of any substance. All can show correlations with other self-report measures completed concurrently and assumed to measure a variety of constructs, although glossing over the troubling issue of their interdependence. It offers more meaning when a questionnaire can predict some future outcome, preferably in a different domain such as mood, or better, observed behaviour. Few qualify in this category, although no doubt more will do so in the near future: those that do are the Coping Strategies Questionnaire (CSQ: Rosenstiel & Keefe 1983), particularly the catastrophizing subscale and the factor of pain control and rational thinking (variously shown to predict future depression and to be associated with pain-related behaviours); the Pain Beliefs and Perceptions Inventory (Williams & Thorn 1989), which predicted non-compliance with psychological and physical treatments; and the Pain Self-Efficacy Questionnaire (Nicholas et al 1992), which predicted dropout from pain management. The Survey of Pain Attitudes (Jensen & Karoly 1992) predicted self-reported health-care use, and the Arthritis Self-Efficacy Questionnaire (Lorig et al 1989) predicted depression 6 months later.

This is not to suggest that concurrent correlational findings are redundant, only that they are the first step in establishing empirical relationships with other cognitive and affective variables and with behaviour. The structure of too many questionnaires proves to be unreplicable even on apparently similar populations, and checks for contamination by social desirability and memory effects are generally lacking. The review by Clark (1988) of the psychometrics of cognitive measures is strongly recommended to anyone considering developing yet another such measure. Some measures are developed without adequate theoretical basis, making for confusion and disappointment in their use. Coping is a good example: while it appears intuitively obvious that there must be 'good' and 'bad' coping, the issue is far more complex than it appears, and a priori classification of coping strategies for checklists, without reference to intention or to outcomes, instantiates moral values or physical qualities of the strategy, both of which are somewhat remote from the assumed latent construct.

There is a general neglect of methods other than endorsement of statements according to degree of agreement, truth or falsity for the respondent, or frequency of occurrence. Recording thoughts spoken aloud during or immediately after a task, or on random or cue-dependent signals, can provide more ecologically valid data for qualitative and quantitative analysis (e.g., Heyneman et al 1990). Further, while not yet developed as measures, the use of information-processing paradigms such as task interference for attention (Crombez et al 1998) and the Stroop test for memory and cognitive bias (Pincus et al 1998) merit consideration.

Social support can be characterized by a wide range of possible variables, from marital satisfaction to size of social network (Flor et al 1987), and according to quality and quantity. Sex differences in confiding and supportive relationships may be sufficiently different that summaries across the sexes represent neither accurately. Apart from general social, familial and partner support or lack of it, measurement in this area has focused on spouse behaviour in relation to the patient and his or her pain behaviour, and until recently studies relied on associations between measures of function, mood and behaviour taken independently from spouse and patient. The development of sequential recording and analysis by Romano et al (1991) allows mapping of temporal associations between behaviours. Where the aim is to assess the pain patient's account of support, a recently developed scale (Significant Others' Scale: Power et al 1988) obtains ratings of actual and ideal emotional and practical support from standard and patient-identified important people.

PROCESS MEASURES

Properties of the setting and treatment, therapist variables and their interactions with patient variables influence the target of study, beneficially or adversely. They cannot be 'designed out', although judicious choice of control group can aid interpretation (Kazdin 1994, Schwartz et al 1997). Reviews by Roth and Fonagy (1996) and by Kazdin (1994) reveal a complex and interactive set of variables which nevertheless show certain common factors across treatments from pharmacotherapy to psychotherapy. The major contributor to outcome variance is therapeutic alliance, the patient's sense of a productive working partnership, but within that, technical skills matter: techniques without a therapeutic alliance can be harmful. The use of a manual appears to account for more variance than therapist skill, but manuals are more effective in skilled hands. To the detriment of our understanding of outcome, few of these variables are ever considered in pain treatments, and the measures require adaptation to the techniques and settings in the field.

Patient variables

The main process variables used in studies of pain populations are their participation and adherence to treatment or experimental methods, their expectations of the treatment, control or experimental condition, which constitute a measure of credibility of treatment or experimental rationale, and their satisfaction with treatment. Other than in trials of psychological treatments, patient expectations are rarely assessed, which is the more surprising when patient 'motivation' is invoked as a causative factor in outcome. Patients' expectations of benefit, or lack of them, can account for a substantial proportion of variance in change with treatment, in part by association with adherence to treatment methods (Council et al 1988). Ideally they are assessed in any outcome study, whatever the treatment: a simple scale by Borkovec and Nau (1972) is widely used. A similar measure applicable to double-blind trials, in particular of drugs, is patients' and assessors' retrospective surmise of treatment allocated to each patient. It is possible thereby to test the maintenance of blindness across the course of the trial, more often broken than triallists would like to believe (Oxtoby et al 1989). Satisfaction measurement is relatively common and can be treated as an outcome in its own right, but its reliability is generally unknown and is subject to demand effects and a tendency to positive scores (Bornstein & Rychtarik 1983). Its relationship with other outcome measures may be low and it is no substitute for them; control conditions intended to be inert and which bring about minimal measured benefits can nevertheless achieve high satisfaction ratings. Specific questions, including dissatisfactions, are likely to obtain more useful answers, but interpretation is still problematical (Chapman et al 1996).

Participation or attendance at treatment and, where relevant, completion of homework, are possible proxy measures for adherence to treatment methods, depending on the type of treatment. Arguably, attendance at outpatient treatment sessions, as in many physical and psychological therapies, is important in its own right for exposure to therapeutic methods and content. Adherence to homework and to treatment methods over follow-up periods is usually collected by self report, and its relationship with outcome is disappointingly slight (Jensen et al 1994b). The extent to which measurement techniques are responsible for this is not clear: apart from issues of reliability, frequency of use of a treatment technique is most easily collected but the relevant variables may be appropriateness of use, or independence in performance.

Treatment and therapist variables

Treatment fidelity, or validity, describes the extent to which the treatment delivered is replicable and valid in terms of its content. For instance, a programme in which staff ignore undesired behaviours but fail to attend to desired behaviours fails to qualify as operant; a placebo control condition which is not credible to patients as a treatment technique is not a true placebo control; and an epidural injection whose content does not reach the epidural space cannot contribute to understanding the effects of epidural injection. Part depends on the clear definition and specification of treatment content and methods, relevant not only to psychological treatments but to many other interventions, and including details of dose/intensity and duration of treatment, sequence of components and selection of patients (Mulrow & Pugh 1995). The usually superior methods used in research trials – such as careful verbal and written explanation, and back-up support in the case of difficulties – contribute to the generally superior results of trials over everyday clinical practice, but the gap could in principle be narrowed considerably by addressing the relevant variables. Treatment manuals, against which expert assessors may compare actual treatment, are recommended for more extensive treatments (Morley et al 1999). For complex treatments, the integration of components may be an essential aspect of treatment, although many trials treat them as additive in their analysis.

Treatment validity also includes therapist adherence to the treatment specified, and therapist competence. Adherence refers to the extent to which the therapist used the methods identified as essential components of treatment, and did not use those proscribed by the manual or equivalent (Waltz et al 1993): it can be measured in terms of occurrence/absence or in relative or absolute frequency of occurrence, and requires expert assessment of samples across treatment occasions. In principle, the concept could be applied to non-psychological treatments, such as to the appropriateness of the dose prescribed of a drug of demonstrated effectiveness, or the accuracy of targeted manipulations in physical therapy. Therapist competence refers to the skills of the therapist in applying the specified treatment, and is too rarely measured whether in trials of psychological, physical or surgical intervention. It is defined by reference to the specified treatment, rather than in universal terms of training or experience, and to its application with reference to the patient's presenting problems, the stage of treatment and other considerations specific to the therapy (Waltz et al 1993). In psychological therapies, therapist orientation or affiliation and expectations of treatment outcome may also be recorded or assessed, because they can contribute to variance in outcome measures; again, these are underused, particularly in multicentre trials where therapists' beliefs concerning trial treatments may influence their efficacy.

CONCLUSION

Measurement of human experience presents a variety of conceptual problems and technical difficulties. Nevertheless, we have some reasonable approximations, in pain itself (see Ch. 17), and in aspects of function, mood and behaviour. The gaps and shortcomings noted here not for the first time relate to subgroups of the pain population, to content (particularly the central issue of use of health care) and to the adoption of available measurement technologies to converge on specific areas of experience. Addressing those gaps from a secure theoretical standpoint, as recommended in this chapter, can improve these measures in future research.

Acknowledgements

Thanks are due to Marie Fallon, Vicki Harding and Henry McQuay for discussion of particular areas of content; to Chris Eccleston, Stephen Morley and Tony Roth for invaluable commentaries on earlier drafts; and to Gill Hancock for administrative support throughout.

REFERENCES

Aaronson NK, Bullinger M, Ahmedzai S 1988 A modular approach to quality-of-life assessment in cancer clinical trials. Recent Results in Cancer Research 111: 231–249

Anderson RT, Aaronson NK, Wilkin D 1993 Critical review of the international assessments of health-related quality of life. Quality of Life Research 2: 369–395

Aronoff GM, Wagner JM 1987 The pain center: development, structure, and dynamics. In: Burrows GD, Elton D, Stanley GV (eds) Handbook of chronic pain management. Elsevier, Amsterdam, pp 407–424

Barnes GE, Prosen H 1985 Parental death and depression. Journal of Abnormal Psychology 94: 64–69

Bates MS, Edwards WT, Anderson KO 1993 Ethnocultural influences on variation in chronic pain perception. Pain 52: 101–112

Beaton DE, Hogg-Johnson S, Bombardier C 1997 Evaluating changes in health status: reliability and responsiveness of five generic health status measures in workers with musculoskeletal disorders. Journal of Clinical Epidemiology 50: 79–93

Beck AT, Ward CH, Mendelson M, Mock N, Erbaugh J 1961 An inventory for measuring depression. Archives of General Psychiatry 4: 561–571

Bergner M, Bobbitt RA, Carter WB, Gilson BS 1981 The Sickness Impact Profile: development and final revision of a health status measure. Medical Care 19: 787–805

Berndt S, Maier C, Schutz HW 1993 Polymedication and medication compliance in patients with chronic non-malignant pain. Pain 52: 331–339

Blalock SJ, DeVellis RF, Brown GK, Wallston KA 1989 Validity of the Center for Epidemiological Studies Depression Scale in arthritis populations. Arthritis and Rheumatism 32: 991–997

Boden SD, Davis DO, Dina TS, Patronas NJ, Wiesel SW 1990 Abnormal magnetic-resonance scans of the lumbar spine in asymptomatic subjects. Journal of Bone and Joint Surgery 72A: 403–408

Borkovec TD, Nau SD 1972 Credibility of analogue therapy rationales. Journal of Behavior Therapy and Experimental Psychiatry 3: 257–260

Bornstein PH, Rychtarik RG 1983 Consumer satisfaction in adult behavior therapy: procedures, problems, and future perspectives. Behavior Therapy 14: 191–208

Bowling A 1991 Measuring health: a review of quality of life measurement scales. Open University Press, Philadelphia

Bradley LA, Haile JMcD, Jaworski TM 1992 Assessment of psychological status using interviews and self-report instruments. In: Turk DC, Melzack R (eds) Handbook of pain assessment. Guilford, New York, pp 193–213

Buckelew SP, DeGood DE, Schwartz DP, Kerler RM 1986 Cognitive and somatic item response pattern of pain patients, psychiatric patients and hospital employees. Journal of Clinical Psychology 42: 852–860

Bussmann JBJ, van de Laar YM, Neeleman MP, Stam HJ 1998 Ambulatory accelerometry to quantify motor behaviour in patients after failed back surgery: a validation study. Pain 74: 153–161

Buysse DJ, Reynolds CRF, Monk TH, Berman SR, Kupfer DJ 1988 The Pittsburgh Subjective Sleep Quality Index: a new instrument for psychiatric practice and research. Psychiatric Research 28: 193–213

Casey KL, Minoshima S 1997 Can pain be imaged? In: Jensen TS, Turner JA, Wiesenfeld-Hallin Z (eds) Proceedings of the 8th World Congress on Pain. IASP Press, Seattle, pp 855–866

Caudill M, Schnable R, Zuttermeister P, Benson H, Friedman R 1991 Decreased clinic use by chronic pain patients: response to behavioral medicine intervention. Clinical Journal of Pain 7: 305–310

Chandarana PC, Eals M, Steingart AB, Bellamy N, Allen S 1987 The detection of psychiatric morbidity and associated factors in patients with rheumatoid arthritis. Canadian Journal of Psychiatry 32: 356–361

Chapman SL, Jamison RN, Sanders SH 1996 Treatment helpfulness questionnaire: a measure of patient satisfaction with treatment modalities provided in chronic pain management programmes. Pain 68: 349–361

Charlton JRH, Patrick DL, Peach H 1983 Use of multivariate measures of disability in health surveys. Journal of Epidemiology and Community Health 37: 296–304

Chaturvedi SK 1990 Asian patients and the HAD scale [letter]. British Journal of Psychiatry 156: 133

Chen CAN 1993a Human brain measures of clinical pain: a review. Topographic mappings. Pain 54: 115–132

Chen CAN 1993b Human brain measures of clinical pain: a review II. Tomographic imagings. Pain 54: 133–144

Chibnall JT, Tait RC 1994 The short form of the Beck Depression Inventory: validity issues with chronic pain patients. Clinical Journal of Pain 10: 261–266

Cinciripini PM, Floreen A 1982 An evaluation of a behavioral program for chronic pain. Journal of Behavioral Medicine 5: 375–389

Clark DA 1988 The validity of measures of cognition: a review of the literature. Cognitive Therapy and Research 12: 1–20

Clark DM, McKenzie DP 1994 A caution on the use of cut-points applied to screening instruments or diagnostic criteria. Journal of Psychiatric Research 28: 185–188

Clark DA, Steer RA 1994 Use of nonsomatic symptoms to differentiate clinically depressed and nondepressed hospitalized patients with chronic medical illnesses. Psychological Reports 75: 1089–1090

Cleeland CS 1989 Measurement of pain by subjective report. In: Chapman CR, Loeser JD (eds) Issues in pain measurement. Raven, New York, pp 391–403

Cleeland CS, Syrjala KL 1992 How to assess cancer pain. In: Turk DC, Melzack R (eds) Handbook of pain assessment. Guilford, New York, pp 362–387

CORE System Group 1998 CORE system (information management) handbook. CORE System Group, Leeds, UK

Coughlan GM, Ridout KL, Williams ACdeC, Richardson PH 1995 Attrition from a pain management programme. British Journal of Clinical Psychology 34: 471–479

Council JR, Ahern DK, Follick MJ, Kline CL 1988 Expectancies and functional impairment in chronic low back pain. Pain 33: 323–331

Craig KD 1992 Echoes of pain. American Pain Society Journal 1: 105–108

Craig KD, Prkachin KM, Grunau RVE 1992 The facial expression of pain. In: Turk DC, Melzack R (eds) Handbook of pain assessment. Guilford, New York, pp 257–276

Crombez G, Eccleston C, Baeyens F, Eelen P 1998 When somatic information threatens, catastrophic thinking enhances attentional interference. Pain 75: 187–198

Crombie IK, Davies HTO 1996 Research in health care: design, conduct and interpretation of health services research. John Wiley, Chichester

Deary IJ, Clyde Z, Frier BM 1997 Constructs and models in health psychology: the case of personality and illness reporting in diabetes mellitus. British Journal of Health Psychology 2: 35–43

De Gagne TA, Mikail SF, D'Eon JL 1995 Confirmatory factor analysis of a 4-factor model of chronic pain evaluation. Pain 60: 195–202

DeGood DE, Shutty MS 1992 Assessment of pain beliefs, coping, and self-efficacy. In: Turk DC, Melzack R (eds) Handbook of pain assessment. Guilford, New York, pp 214–234

Derogatis L 1983 The SCL-90-R Manual II: administration, scoring and procedures. Clinical Psychometric Research, Towson, MD

Deyo RA 1984 Measuring functional outcomes in therapeutic trials for chronic disease. Controlled Clinical Trials 5: 223–240

Deyo RA 1986 Comparative validity of the Sickness Impact Profile and shorter scales for functional assessment in low-back pain. Spine 11: 951–954

Deyo RA, Centor RM 1986 Assessing the responsiveness of functional scales to clinical change an analogy to diagnostic test performance. Journal of Chronic Disease 39: 897–906

Dobson KS, Cheung E 1990 Relationship between anxiety and depression: conceptual and methodological issues. In: Maser JD, Cloninger CR (eds) Comorbidity of mood and anxiety disorders. American Psychiatric Press, Washington, pp 611–632

Donaldson GW 1989 The determining role of theory in measurement practice. In: Chapman CR, Loeser JD (eds) Issues in pain measurement. Raven, New York, pp 17–35

Dreyfuss P, Michaelsen M, Pauza K, McLarty J, Bogduk N 1996 The value of medical history and physical examination in diagnosing sacroiliac joint pain. Spine 21: 2594–2602

Ekman P 1993 Facial expression and emotion. American Psychologist 48: 384–392

EuroQol Group 1990 EuroQol: a new facility for the measurement of health-related quality of life. Health Policy 16: 199–208

Fairbank JCT, Couper J, Davies JB, O'Brien JP 1980 The Oswestry low back pain Disability Questionnaire. Physiotherapy 66: 271–273

Fallowfield L 1990 The quality of life: the missing measurement in health care. Souvenir, London

Feuerstein M, Hickey PF 1992 Ergonomic approaches in the clinical assessment of occupational musculoskeletal disorders. In: Turk DC, Melzack R (eds) Handbook of pain assessment. Guilford, New York, pp 71–99

Flor H, Behle DJ, Birbaumer N 1993 Assessment of pain-related cognitions in chronic pain patients. Behavior Research and Therapy 31: 63–73

Flor H, Miltner W, Birbaumer N 1992 Psychophysiological recording methods. In: Turk DC, Melzack R (eds) Handbook of pain assessment. Guilford, New York, pp 169–190

Flor H, Turk DC, Scholz OB 1987 Impact of chronic pain on the spouse: marital, emotional and physical consequences. Journal of Psychosomatic Research 31: 63–71

Follick MJ, Smith TW, Ahern DK 1985 The Sickness Impact Profile: a global measure of disability in chronic low back pain. Pain 21: 67–76

Friedman R, Sobel D, Myers P, Caudill M, Benson H 1995 Behavioral medicine, clinical health psychology, and cost offset. Health Psychology 14: 509–518

Frost H, Klaber Moffett JA, Moser JS, Fairbank JCT 1995 Randomised controlled trial for evaluation of fitness programme for patients with chronic low back pain. British Medical Journal 310: 151–154

Gamsa A 1994 The role of psychological factors in chronic pain. II. A critical appraisal. Pain 57: 17–29

Goldberg D 1978 Manual of the General Health Questionnaire. NFER, Windsor, UK

Goldberg DP, Hillier VF 1979 A scaled version of the General Health Questionnaire. Psychological Medicine 9: 139–145

Goossens MEJB, Evers SMAA 1997 Economic evaluation of back pain interventions. Journal of Occupational Rehabilitation 7: 15–32

Harding VR, Williams ACdeC, Richardson PH et al 1994 The development of a battery of measures for assessing physical functioning of chronic pain patients. Pain 58: 367–375

Harper AC, Harper DA, Lambert LJ et al 1992 Symptoms of impairment, disability and handicap in low back pain: a taxonomy. Pain 50: 189–195

Hays RD, Hadorn D 1992 Responsiveness to change: an aspect of validity, not a separate dimension. Quality of Life Research 1: 73–75

Herda CA, Siegeris K, Basler H-D 1994 The Pain Beliefs and Perceptions Inventory: further evidence for a 4-factor structure. Pain 57: 85–90

Herrmann C 1997 International experiences with the Hospital Anxiety and Depression Scale – a review of validation data and clinical results. Journal of Psychosomatic Research 42: 17–41

Heyneman NE, Fremouw WJ, Gano D, Kirkland F, Heiden L 1990 Individual differences and the effectiveness of different coping strategies for pain. Cognitive Therapy and Research 14: 63–77

Higginson IJ 1997 Innovations in assessment: epidemiology and assessment of pain in advanced cancer. In: Jensen TS, Turner JA, Wiesenfeld-Hallin Z (eds) Proceedings of the 8th World Congress on Pain, Progress in Pain Research and Management, vol 8. IASP Press, Seattle, pp 707–716

Hill PA, Hardy PAJ 1996 The cost-effectiveness of a multidisciplinary pain management programme in a district general hospital. Pain Clinic 9: 181–188

Huiskes CJAE, Kraaimaat FW, Bijlsma JWJ 1990 Development of a self-report questionnaire to assess the impact of rheumatic diseases on health and lifestyle. Journal of Rehabilitation Sciences 3: 65–70

Hunt SM, McEwen J, McKenna SP 1985 Measuring health status: a new tool for clinicians and epidemiologists. Journal of the Royal College of General Practice 35: 185–188

Jacobson NS, Truax P 1991 Clinical significance: a statistical approach to defining meaningful change in psychotherapy research. Journal of Consulting and Clinical Psychology 59: 12–19

Jamison RN, Mat DA, Parris WCV 1988 Effects of time-limited vs unlimited compensation on pain behavior and treatment outcome in low back pain patients. Journal of Psychosomatic Research 32: 277–283

Jenkins CD, Stantan B-A, Niemcryk SJ, Rose RM 1988 A scale for the estimation of sleep problems in clinical research. Journal of Clinical Epidemiology 41: 313–321

Jensen IB, Bradley LA, Linton SJ 1989 Validation of an observation method of pain assessment in non-chronic back pain. Pain 39: 267–274

Jensen MC, Brant-Zawadzki MN, Obuchowski N, Modic MT, Malkasian D, Ross JS 1994a Magnetic resonance imaging of the lumbar spine in people without back pain. New England Journal of Medicine 331: 69–73

Jensen MP, Karoly P 1992 Pain-specific beliefs, perceived symptom severity, and adjustment to chronic pain. Clinical Journal of Pain 8: 123–130

Jensen MP, McFarland CA 1993 Increasing the reliability and validity of pain intensity measurement in chronic pain patients. Pain 55: 195–203

Jensen MP, Strom SE, Turner JA, Romano JM 1992 Validity of the Sickness Impact Profile Roland scale as a measure of dysfunction in chronic pain patients. Pain 50: 157–162

Jensen MP, Turner JA, Romano JM 1994b Correlates of improvement in multidisciplinary treatment of chronic pain. Journal of Consulting and Clinical Psychology 62: 172–179

Jensen MP, Turner HA, Romano JM, Karoly P 1991 Coping with chronic pain: a critical review of the literature. Pain 47: 249–283

Kaplan RM 1985 Quality-of-life measurement. In: Karoly P (ed) Measurement strategies in health psychology. John Wiley, New York, pp 115–146

Karoly P (ed) 1985 Measurement strategies in health psychology. John Wiley, New York

Katz JN, Larson MG, Phillips CB, Fossel AH, Liang MH 1992 Comparative measurement sensitivity of short and longer health status instruments. Medical Care 30: 917–924

Kazdin AE 1994 Methodology, design, and evaluation in psychotherapy research. In: Bergin AE, Garfield SL (eds) Handbook of psychotherapy and behavior change, 4th edn. John Wiley, New York, pp 19–71

Kazis LE, Meenan RF, Anderson JJ 1983 Pain in the rheumatic diseases: investigations of a key health status component. Arthritis and Rheumatism 26: 1017–1022

Keefe FJ, Affleck G, Lefebvre JC, Starr K, Caldwell DS, Tennen H 1997 Pain coping strategies and coping efficacy in rheumatoid arthritis: a daily process analysis. Pain 69: 35–42

Keefe FJ, Block AR 1982 Development of an observation method for assessing pain behavior in chronic low back pain patients. Behavior Therapy 13: 363–375

Keefe FJ, Caldwell DS, Queen KT et al 1987 Pain coping strategies in osteoarthritis patients. Journal of Consulting and Clinical Psychology 55: 208–212

Keefe FJ, Dunsmore J, Burnett R 1992a Behavioral and cognitive-behavioral approaches to chronic pain: recent advances and future directions. Journal of Consulting and Clinical Psychology 60: 528–536

Keefe FJ, Salley AN, Lefebvre JC 1992b Coping with pain: conceptual concerns and future directions. Pain 51: 131–134

Keefe FJ, Williams DA 1992 Assessment of pain behavior. In: Turk DC, Melzack R (eds) Handbook of pain assessment. Guilford, New York, pp 277–292

Keefe FJ, Wilkins RH, Cook WA 1984 Direct observation of pain behavior in low back pain patients during physical examinations. Pain 20: 59–68

Kerns RD, Turk DC, Holzman AD, Rudy TE 1986 Comparison of cognitive behavioral and behavioral approaches to the outpatient treatment of chronic pain. Clinical Journal of Pain 1: 195–203

Kerns RD, Turk DC, Rudy TE 1985 The West Haven–Yale Multidimensional Pain Inventory (WHYMPI). Pain 23: 345–356

Lacks P 1987 Behavioural treatment for persistent insomnia. Pergamon, New York

Lambert MJ, Hill CE 1994 Assessing psychotherapy outcomes and processes. In: Bergin AE, Garfield SL (eds) Handbook of psychotherapy and behavior change, 4th edn. John Wiley, New York, pp 72–113

Laupacis A, Sackett DL, Roberts RS 1988 An assessment of clinically useful measures of the consequences of treatment. New England Journal of Medicine 318: 1728–1733

Lewis G 1991 Observer bias in the assessment of anxiety and depression. Social Psychiatry and Psychiatric Epidemiology 26: 265–272

Linton SJ 1998 The socioeconomic impact of chronic back pain: is anyone benefiting? Pain 75: 163–168

Linton SJ, Hallden K 1997 Risk factors and the natural course of acute and recurrent musculoskeletal pain: developing a screening instrument. In: Jensen TS, Turner JA, Wiesenfeld-Hallin Z (eds) Proceedings of the 8th World Congress on Pain. IASP Press, Seattle, pp 527–536

Lorig K, Chastain RL, Ung E, Shoor S, Holman HR 1989 Development and evaluation of a scale to measure perceived self-efficacy in people with arthritis. Arthritis and Rheumatism 32: 37–44

Lowery WD, Horn TJ, Boden SD, Wiesel SW 1992 Impairment evaluation based on spinal range of motion in normal subjects. Journal of Spinal Disorders 5: 398–402

Lucock MP, Morley S 1996 The Health Anxiety Questionnaire. British Journal of Health Psychology 1: 137–150

McCormack HM, Horne DJdeL, Sheather S 1988 Clinical applications of visual analogue scales: a critical review. Psychological Medicine 18: 1007–1019

McCracken LM, Zayfert C, Gross RT 1992 The Pain Anxiety Symptoms Scale: development and validation of a scale to measure fear of pain. Pain 50: 67–73

McDaniel LK, Anderson KO, Bradley LA et al 1986 Development of an observation method for assessing pain behavior in rheumatoid arthritis patients. Pain 24: 65–184

McDowell I, Newell C 1996 Measuring health: a guide to rating scales and questionnaires, 2nd edn. Oxford University Press, New York

McHorney CA, Ware JE, Raczek AE 1993 The MOS 36-item short-form health survey (SF-36): II. Psychometric and clinical tests of validity in measuring physical and mental health constructs. Medical Care 31: 247–263

McQuay HJ, Moore A 1998 An evidence-based resource for pain relief. Oxford University Press, Oxford

MacKenzie CR, Charlson ME, DiGioia D, Kelley K 1986 Can the

Sickness Impact Profile measure change? An example of scale assessment. Journal of Chronic Disease 39: 429–438
Main CJ 1983 The modified somatic perception questionnaire (MSPQ). Journal of Psychosomatic Research 27: 503–514
Main CJ, Waddell G 1984 The detection of psychological abnormality using four simple scales. Current Concepts in Pain 2: 10–15
Main CJ, Waddell G 1991 A comparison of cognitive measures in low back pain: statistical structure and clinical validity at initial assessment. Pain 46: 287–298
Main CJ, Wood PLR, Hollis S, Spanswick CC, Waddell G 1991 The Distress and Risk Assessment Method. Spine 17: 42–51
Meakin CJ 1992 Screening for depression in the medically ill. British Journal of Psychiatry 160: 212–216
Meenan RF, Gertman PM, Mason JH, Dunaif R 1982 The Arthritis Impact Measurement Scales: further investigation of a health status measure. Arthritis and Rheumatism 25: 1048–1053
Mendelson G 1992 Chronic pain and compensation. In: Tyrer SP (ed) Psychology, psychiatry and chronic pain. Butterworth Heinemann, Oxford, pp 68–78
Moorey S, Greer S, Watson M et al 1991 The factor structure and factor stability of the hospital anxiety and depression scale in patients with cancer. British Journal of Psychiatry 158: 255–259
Morley SJ, Eccleston C, Williams ACdeC 1999 Systematic review and meta-analysis of randomised controlled trials of cognitive behaviour therapy and behaviour therapy for chronic pain in adults, excluding headache. Pain 80: 1–13
Mulrow CD, Pugh J 1995 Making sense of complex interventions. Journal of General Internal Medicine 10: 111–112
Nicholas MK, Wilson PH, Goyen J 1992 Comparison of cognitive-behavioral group treatment and an alternative non-psychological treatment for chronic low back pain. Pain 48: 339–347
Novy DM, Nelson DV, Berry LA, Averill PM 1995 What does the Beck Depression Inventory measure in chronic pain?: a reappraisal. Pain 61: 261–270
Ohlund C, Lindstrom I, Areskoug B, Eek C, Peterson L-E, Nachemson A 1994 Pain behavior in industrial subacute low back pain. Part I. Reliability: concurrent and predictive validity of pain behavior assessments. Pain 58: 201–209
Oxtoby A, Jones A, Robinson M 1989 Is your 'double-blind' design truly double-blind? British Journal of Psychiatry 155: 700–701
Peck JR, Smith TW, Ward JR, Milano R 1989 Disability and depression in rheumatoid arthritis. Arthritis and Rheumatism 32: 1100–1106
Pincus T, Brooks RH, Callahan LF 1991 Reliability of grip strength, walking time and button test performed according to a standard protocol. Journal of Rheumatology 18: 997–1000
Pincus T, Fraser L, Pearce S 1998 Do chronic pain patients 'Stroop' on pain stimuli? British Journal of Clinical Psychology 37: 49–58
Plumb MM, Holland J 1977 Comparative studies of psychological function in patients with advanced cancer – I. Self-reported depressive symptoms. Psychosomatic Medicine 39: 264–276
Polatin PB, Mayer TG 1992 Quantification of function in chronic low back pain. In: Turk DC, Melzack R (eds) Handbook of Pain Assessment. Guilford, New York, pp 37–48
Poole GD, Craig KD 1992 Judgements of genuine, suppressed and faked facial expressions of pain. Journal of Personality and Social Psychology 63: 797–805
Power MJ, Champion LA, Aris SJ 1988 The development of a measure of social support: the Significant Others (SOS) Scale. British Journal of Clinical Psychology 27: 349–358
Prkachin KM, Currie NA, Craig KD 1983 Judging nonverbal expression of pain. Canadian Journal of Behavioral Science 15: 409–421
Purves AM, Penny KI, Munro C et al 1998 Defining chronic pain for epidemiological research – assessing a subjective definition. Pain Clinic 10: 139–147
Radloff LS 1977 The CES-D scale: a self-report depression scale for research in the general population. Applied Psychological Measurement 1: 385–401
Richards JS, Nepomuceno C, Riles M, Suer Z 1982 Assessing pain behavior: the UAB Pain Behavior Scale. Pain 14: 393–398
Roberts R, Hemingway H, Marmot M 1997 Psychometric and clinical validity of the SF-36 General Health Survey in the Whitehall II Study. British Journal of Health Psychology 2: 285–300
Robinson ME, Riley JL, Myers CD et al 1997 The Coping Strategies Questionnaire: a large sample, item level factor analysis. Clinical Journal of Pain 13: 43–49
Roland M, Morris R 1983 A study of the natural history of back pain. Part I. Development of a reliable and sensitive measure of disability in low-back pain. Spine 8: 141–144
Romano JM, Turner JA, Friedman LS, Bulcroft RA, Jensen MP, Hops H 1991 Observational assessment of chronic pain patient–spouse interactions. Behavior Therapy 22: 549–567
Rosenstiel AK, Keefe FJ 1983 The use of coping strategies in chronic low back pain patients: relationship to patient characteristics and current adjustment. Pain 17: 33–44
Roth AD, Fonagy P 1996 What works for whom? A critical review of psychotherapy research. Guilford, New York
Rudy TE 1989 Multiaxial assessment of pain: multi-dimensional Pain Inventory. Computer program, user's manual, version 2.0. Pittsburgh, University of Pittsburgh
Rudy TE, Kerns RD, Turk DC 1988a Chronic pain and depression: toward a cognitive-behavioral mediation model. Pain 35: 129–140
Rudy TE, Turk DC, Brena SF 1988b Differential utility of medical procedures in the assessment of chronic pain patients. Pain 34: 53–60
Rudy TE, Turk DC, Brena SF, Stieg RL, Brody MC 1990 Quantification of biomedical findings of chronic pain patients: development of an index of pathology. Pain 42: 167–182
Rudy TE, Turk DC, Brody MC 1992 Quantification of biomedical findings in chronic pain: problems and solutions. In: Turk DC, Melzack R (eds) Handbook of pain assessment. Oxford University Press, New York, pp 447–469
Sackett DL, Haynes RB, Guyatt GH, Tugwell P 1991 Clinical epidemiology: a basic science for clinical medicine. Little, Brown & Co, Boston
Sanders SH 1983 Automated versus self-monitoring of 'up-time' in chronic low-back pain patients: a comparative study. Pain 15: 399–405
Sanderson PL, Todd BD, Holt GR, Getty CJM 1995 Compensation, work status, and disability in low back pain patients. Spine 20: 554–556
Schuster JM, Smith SS 1994 Brief assessment of depression in chronic pain patients. American Journal of Pain Management 4: 115–117
Schwartz CE, Chesney MA, Irvine J, Keefe FJ 1997 The control group dilemma in clinical research: applications for psychosocial and behavioural medicine trials. Psychosomatic Medicine 59: 362–371
Sharrack B, Hughes RA 1997 Reliability of distance estimation by doctors and patients: cross sectional study. British Medical Journal 315: 1652–1654
Skevington SM 1990 A standardised scale to measure beliefs about controlling pain (BPCQ): a preliminary study. Psychology and Health 4: 221–232
Snaith RP 1987 Defining 'depression'. Letter American Journal of Psychiatry 144: 828–829
Snaith P 1993 What do depression rating scales measure? British Journal of Psychiatry 163: 293–298
Spiegel JS, Pulus HE, Ward NB, Spiegel TM, Leake B, Kane RL 1987 What are we measuring? An examination of walk time and grip strength. Journal of Rheumatology 14: 80–86

Spielberger CD 1983 Manual for the State-Trait Anxiety Inventory (Form 1). Consulting Psychologists Press, Palo Alto, CA

Spitzer WO et al 1987 Scientific approach to the assessment and management of activity related spinal disorders: Report of the Quebec Task Force on Spinal Disorders. Spine 12(suppl 7)

Steer RA, Beck AT, Garrison B 1985 Applications of the Beck Depression Inventory. In: Sartorius N & Ban TA (eds) Assessment of depression. Heidelberg, Springer, pp 123–142

Stone AA, Shiffman S 1994 Ecological momentary assessment (EMA) in behavioral medicine. Annals of Behavioral Medicine 16: 199–202

Stratford P, Solomon P, Binkley J, Finch E, Gill C 1993 Sensitivity of Sickness Impact Profile items to measure change over time in a low-back pain patient group. Spine 18: 1723–1727

Streiner DL, Norman GR 1995 Health measurement scales: a practical guide to their development and use, 2nd edn. Oxford University Press, Oxford

Strender L-E, Sjoblom A, Sundell K, Ludwig R, Taube A 1997 Interexaminer reliability in physical examination of patients with low back pain. Spine 22: 814–820

Sullivan MJL, D'Eon JL 1990 Relation between catastrophising and depression in chronic pain patients. Journal of Abnormal Psychology 99: 260–263

Swartzman LC, Gwadry FG, Shapiro AP, Teasell RW 1994 The factor structure of the Coping Strategies Questionnaire. Pain 57: 311–316

Tait RC, Chibnall JT, Richardson WD 1990 Litigation and employment status: effects on patients with chronic pain. Pain 43: 37–46

Turk DC, Flor H 1987 Pain > pain behaviors: the utility and limitations of the pain behavior construct. Pain 31: 277–295

Turk DC, Melzack R (eds) 1992 Handbook of pain assessment. Guilford, New York

Turk DC, Okifuji A 1994 Detecting depression in chronic pain patients: adequacy of self-reports. Behaviour Research and Therapy 32: 9–16

Turk DC, Rudy TE 1992 Classification logic and strategies in chronic pain. In: Turk DC, Melzack R (eds) Handbook of pain assessment. Guilford, New York, pp 409–428

Vasuvedan SV 1992 Impairment, disability and functional capacity assessment. In: Turk DC, Melzack R (eds) Handbook of pain assessment. Guilford, New York, pp 100–108

Vlaeyen JWS, Geurts SM, Kole-Snijders AMJ, Schuerman JA, Groenman NH, van Eek H 1990a What do chronic pain patients think of their pain? Towards a pain cognition questionnaire. British Journal of Clinical Psychology 29: 383–394

Vlaeyen JWS, Pernot DFM, Kole-Snijders AMJ, Schuerman JA, Van Eek H, Groenman NH 1990b Assessment of the components of observed chronic pain behavior: the Checklist for Interpersonal Pain Behavior (CHIP). Pain 43: 337–347

Vlaeyen JWS, Kole-Snijders AMJ, Boeren RGB, van Eek H 1995 Fear of movement (re)injury in chronic low back pain and its relation to behavioral performance. Pain 62: 363–372

Volinn E, Lai D, McKinney S, Loeser JD 1988 When back pain becomes disabling: a regional analysis. Pain 33: 33–39

Waddell G, McCullough JA, Kummel E, Venner RM 1980 Nonorganic physical signs in low back pain. Spine 5: 117–125

Waddell G, Newton M, Henderson I, Somerville D, Main CJ 1993 A Fear-Avoidance Beliefs Questionnaire (FABQ) and the role of fear-avoidance beliefs in chronic low back pain and disability. Pain 52: 157–168

Waddell G, Somerville D, Henderson I, Newton M 1992 Objective clinical evaluation of physical impairment in chronic low back pain. Spine 17: 617–628

Waddell G, Turk DC 1992 Clinical assessment of low back pain. In: Turk DC, Melzack R (eds) Handbook of pain assessment. Guilford, New York, pp 15–36

Wagner A, Sukiennik A, Kulich R et al 1996 Outcomes assessment in chronic pain treatment: the need to supplement the SF-36. Abstracts, 8th World Congress on Pain. IASP Press, Seattle, p 308

Wallston KA, Wallston BS, DeVellis R 1978 Development of the Multidimensional Health Locus of Control (MHLC) Scales. Health Education Monographs 6: 160–170

Waltz J, Addis ME, Koerner K, Jacobson NS 1993 Testing the integrity of a psychotherapy protocol: assessment of adherence and competence. Journal of Consulting and Clinical Psychology 61: 620–630

Ware JE, Sherbourne CD 1992 The MOS 36-item short-form health survey (SF-36): I. Conceptual framework and item selection. Medical Care 30: 473–483

Ware JE, Snow KK, Kosinski M, Gandek B 1993 SF-36 Health Survey: manual and interpretation guide. Health Institute, New England Medical Center, Boston

Watson PJ, Booker CK, Main CJ, Chen ACN 1997 Surface electromyography in the identification of chronic low back pain patients: the development of the flexion relaxation ratio. Clinical Biomechanics 11: 165–171

Wesley AL, Gatchel RJ, Polatin PB, Kinney RK, Mayer TG 1991 Differentiation between somatic and cognitive/affective components in commonly used measurements of depression with chronic low-back pain. Spine 16(suppl 6): S213–S215

WHOQOL Group 1995 The World Health Organization Quality of Life Assessment (WHOQOL): position paper from the World Health Organization. Social Science and Medicine 41: 1403–1409

Wilkie DJ, Keefe FJ, Dodd MJ, Copp LA 1992 Behavior of patients with lung cancer: description and associations with oncologic and pain variables. Pain 51: 231–240

Williams ACdeC, Richardson PH 1993 What does the BDI measure in chronic pain? Pain 55: 259–266

Williams DA, Keefe FJ 1991 Pain beliefs and the use of cognitive-behavioural coping strategies. Pain 46: 185–190

Williams DA, Robinson ME, Geisser ME 1994 Pain beliefs: assessment and utility. Pain 59: 71–78

Williams DA, Thorn BE 1989 An empirical assessment of pain beliefs. Pain 36: 351–358

Zbrozek AS 1994 Cost-effectiveness issues to consider in designing and interpreting pain studies. American Pain Society Bulletin Oct/Nov (5–6): 19

Zigmond AS, Snaith RP 1983 The Hospital Anxiety and Depression Scale. Acta Psychiatrica Scandinavica 67: 361–370

SECTION 2

CLINICAL STATES

- Soft tissue, joints and bones
- Deep and visceral pain
- Head
- Nerve and root damage
- Central nervous system
- Special cases

Acute and postoperative pain

MICHAEL COUSINS & IAN POWER

ISSUES IN THE MANAGEMENT OF POSTOPERATIVE AND OTHER ACUTE PAIN STATES

'It is an indictment of modern medicine that an apparently simple problem such as the reliable relief of postoperative pain remains largely unsolved' (Editorial 1978).

'Inadequate treatment of pain continues to be a problem despite more knowledge about its causes and control and despite widespread efforts of governments and multiple medical and voluntary organizations to disseminate this knowledge, particularly at the postgraduate level' (Stratton Hill 1995).

Despite substantial advances in the knowledge of acute pain mechanisms and in their treatment, acute pain is generally not effectively treated. This is partly a reflection of the emphasis in medicine on diagnosis and treatment of causative factors rather than on symptomatic treatment. In the case of acute pain, a cause is usually rapidly determined and its treatment reduces or relieves pain after a period of time. This relegates the relief of acute pain, in the minds of many doctors and nurses, to a minor level of priority. Diagnosis and treatment of the cause of acute pain resulting from trauma and acute medical and surgical conditions is the first priority. However, this should never preclude the use of appropriate effective methods of symptomatic pain relief. A well-controlled study of patients with acute abdominal pain reported that the diagnosis was not altered in a single patient by the relief of acute pain with sublingual buprenorphine, even though there were minor changes in physical signs in 12% of patients receiving pain relief compared to a control group (Zolte & Cust 1986).

The recognition of acute pain as a major problem has been unacceptably slow in view of repeated documentation of the inadequacies of its treatment. In a study of acute pain of various causes, Marks and Sacher (1973) reported that three-quarters of the patients who received narcotics for severe pain continued to experience pain. These findings have been confirmed in adults by Cohen (1980) and in children by Mather and Mackie (1983). In the USA alone 23 million patients undergo surgery every year and the majority of these experience postoperative pain (Agency for Health Care Policy and Research 1992). Trauma produced by accidents ranks third as the cause of death in industrialized societies, being surpassed only by cardiovascular disease and cancer. Trauma causes more deaths in young people between the ages of 15 and 24 years than all other causes combined. In a single year in the USA, at least 17 million civilians sustained injuries requiring hospitalization. The overall cost of all injuries in 1977 was $62 billion (Accident Facts 1978). Most of these injured patients eventually experience pain that requires management.

It is likely that all forms of acute pain are poorly managed: postoperative, post-trauma, following burns, acute medical diseases (e.g. pancreatitis, myocardial infarction), obstetric pain (Melzack et al 1981, Bonica 1985, Cousins & Phillips 1986). There are a variety of reasons for poor, ineffective, management of acute pain, as summarized in the following Box 19.1. The effective relief of labour pain with epidural block in more than 95% of patients gives hope that other types of acute pain can also be relieved (Cousins & Bridenbaugh 1988). This does not imply that neural blockade is 'the answer' to acute pain – it is one of the answers. A wide range of pharmacological, physical and psychological treatments for acute pain is now available.

Improved understanding of peripheral and central mechanisms of pain offers new treatment options. Pain treatment

BOX 19.1

Reasons for the inadequate management of acute pain. (Adapted from NHMRC 1999)

- The common idea that pain is merely a symptom and not harmful in itself
- The mistaken impression that analgesia makes accurate diagnosis difficult or impossible
- Fear of the potential for addiction to opioids
- Concerns about respiratory depression and other opioid-related side effects such as nausea and vomiting
- Lack of understanding of the pharmacokinetics of various agents
- Lack of appreciation of variability in analgesic response to opioids
- Prescriptions for opioids which include the use of inappropriate doses and/or dose intervals
- Misinterpretation of doctors' orders by nursing staff, including use of lower ranges of opioid doses and delaying opioid administration
- Thinking that patient weight is the best predictor of opioid requirement and that opioids must not be given more often than 4 hourly
- Patients' difficulties in communicating their need for analgesia

techniques depend, for their effective use, on overcoming financial, administrative and logistical hurdles (Cousins & Phillips 1986). Educational programmes need to be developed and implemented for nursing, medical and other staff. Much of this depends on a close collaboration between medical, nursing and administrative staff. The regimens chosen for each institution must be appropriate to the resources and range of expertise in that setting. A powerful aid to improving acute pain treatment would be the use of a 'pain control audit'. In some hospitals, pain is now charted, along with temperature and pulse, and orders for treatment are based on a pain score, obtained with a visual analogue scale or other techniques described in Chapter 18. Audit of the efficacy of pain control becomes feasible if a record of this type is a routine part of the medical record. Acute pain in children is a special case requiring urgent attention. This is because of the fallacious dogma that children suffer less pain than do adults. Techniques developed in adults can be applied in children; however, problems in implementation need to be overcome.

In addition to humanitarian reasons for improving acute pain treatment, there is now convincing evidence that unrelieved acute pain may result in harmful physiological and psychological effects. These adverse effects may result in significant morbidity and even mortality (Yeager et al 1987, Kehlet 1988, Scott & Kehlet 1988, Cousins 1989).

Evidence of shortened hospital stay, decreased morbidity and mortality, and increased patient satisfaction have been reported in association with the effective relief of acute pain (Modig 1976, Brandt et al 1978, Modig et al 1983, Rawal et al 1984, Cullen et al 1985, Yeager et al 1987). This has increased medical and public interest in acute pain as an important problem. In some institutions it has resulted in the setting up of 'acute pain services', sometimes in association with a comprehensive unit managing both acute and chronic pain.

The US Department of Health and Human Services recently took the unprecedented step of publishing a clinical practice guideline for acute pain management, which is based on a detailed analysis of several thousand scientific publications, examining the efficacy and safety of different methods of acute pain control. Based on this analysis, strong recommendations are made for the organization, delivery and monitoring of acute pain services (Acute Pain Management 1992).

A summary of the major elements and goals of an acute pain service is outlined in Box 19.2. The strength of the clinical trial evidence supporting the use of NSAIDs, opioids and local anaesthetics for the relief of acute postoperative pain, together with a description of the levels of clinical evidence ratings used, is presented in Table 19.1 and Box 19.3. It is apparent that a major impetus has now been provided to improve the treatment of acute pain on the basis of substantially increased scientific knowledge and by setting up 'acute pain services' (Ready et al 1988, Cousins 1989).

It is now clear that certain principles of pain management must be applied to ensure good analgesia after surgery. These include the recognition of the adverse effects of unrelieved pain, the necessity of involving the patient in the entire pain relief process, and the need for a flexible and experienced approach to the problem by the staff involved. Of course such principles can be extended to the management of all forms of acute pain, but others are more relevant for postoperative pain, such as the necessity of making clear plans for analgesia before surgery takes place. For example, this is of obvious importance in the rapidly expanding field of ambulatory surgery where the patient is discharged home soon after surgery. In all areas of acute pain management safety and efficacy can be promoted by frequent assessment of the patient, good staff and patient education, the existence of clear protocols and guidelines for staff to follow, and regular evaluation and improvement of the entire process by quality assurance programmes. These principles for the safe and effective management of acute pain are summarized in Box 19.4.

BOX 19.2

Clinical practice and acute pain: guidelines and major goals

Guidelines

- A collaborative, interdisciplinary approach to pain control, including all members of the healthcare team and input from the patient and the patient's family, when appropriate. An individualized proactive pain control plan developed preoperatively by patients and practitioners (since pain is easier to prevent than to treat)
- Assessment and frequent reassessment of the patient's pain
- Use of both drug and non-drug therapies to control and/or prevent pain
- A formal, institutional approach, with clear lines of responsibility

Major goals

- Reduce the incidence and severity of patients' postoperative or post-traumatic pain
- Educate patients about the need to communicate regarding unrelieved pain, so they can receive prompt evaluation and effective treatment
- Enhance patient comfort and satisfaction
- Contribute to fewer postoperative complications and, in some cases, shorter stays after surgical procedures

BIOLOGICAL FUNCTIONS OF ACUTE PAIN

Religious, philosophical and other connotations have been ascribed to acute pain. However, it is clear that pain usually signals impending or actual tissue damage and thus permits the individual to avoid harm. It is interesting to examine the evidence of studies in patients with congenital insensitivity to pain. Such individuals appear to have a shortened life expectancy because of unrecognized trauma and associated complications (Sternbach 1963).

Pain may also prevent harmful movement, for example, in the case of a fracture; this may be viewed as a protective role. For a finite period of time reduced mobility associated with acute pain may aid healing. However, evidence is emerging that the organism benefits only briefly from this effect and its prolongation results in an adverse outcome (Bonica 1985, Cousins & Phillips 1986, Kehlet 1988).

Pain also initiates complex neurohumoral responses (see below) that help initially to maintain homeostasis in the face of an acute disease or injury; if these changes are excessive or unduly prolonged, they may cause morbidity or mortality (Cousins & Phillips 1986, Kehlet 1988). Psychological responses to acute pain may initially be helpful in coping with the physical insult; however, if excessively severe or prolonged, they may become deleterious. In the medical context, acute pain alerts the patient to the need for medical help and helps the medical practitioner to pinpoint the

Table 19.1 Scientific evidence for pharmacological interventions to manage postoperative pain in adults. (Adapted from NHMRC 1999)

Intervention	*Level of evidence*	*Comments*
NSAIDs		
Oral (alone)	I	Effective for mild to moderate pain. Relatively contraindicated in patients with renal disease and risk of or actual coagulopathy. Risk of coagulopathy, gastrointestinal bleeding and other risk factors should be carefully sought
Oral (adjunct to opioid)	I	Potentiating effect resulting in opioid sparing. Cautions as above
Parenteral (ketorolac)	I	Effective for moderate to severe pain. Useful where opioids contraindicated or to produce 'opioid sparing', especially to minimize respiratory depression, sedation and gastrointestinal stasis. Best used as part of a multimodal analgesia regimen
Opioids		
Oral	IV	As effective as parenteral in appropriate doses. Use as soon as oral medication tolerated. Route of choice[1]
Intramuscular	I	Has been the standard parenteral route, but injections painful and absorption unreliable. Hence, avoid this route when possible[1]
Subcutaneous	I	Preferable to intramuscular because of patient comfort and a reduced risk of needlestick injury[1]
Intravenous	I	Parenteral route of choice after major surgery. Suitable for titrated bolus or continuous administration. Significant risk of respiratory depression with inappropriate dosing[1]
PCA (systemic)	I	Intravenous or subcutaneous routes recommended. Good steady level of analgesia. Popular with patients but requires special infusion pumps and staff education. See cautions about opioids above[1]
Epidural and intrathecal	I	When suitable, provides good analgesia. Risk of respiratory depression (as with opioids by other routes), but sometimes delayed in onset. Requires careful monitoring. Use of infusion pumps requires additional equipment and staff education. Expensive if infusion pumps are employed[1]

Table 19.1 (Contd.)

Intervention	*Level of evidence*	*Comments*
Local anaesthetics Epidural and intrathecal	I	Indications in particular settings. Effective regional analgesia. May blunt 'stress response' and aid recovery. Opioid sparing. Addition of opioid to local anaesthetic may improve analgesia. Risks of hypotension, weakness, numbness. Requires careful monitoring. Use of infusion pump requires additional equipment and staff education. Expensive if infusion pumps are employed[1]
Peripheral nerve block	I	Plexus block, peripheral nerve block and infitration. Effective regional analgesia. Opioid sparing

[1]The administration of opioids by any route requires monitoring.

BOX 19.3

Levels of evidence ratings. (Adapted from NHMRC 1999)

Level I
Evidence obtained from systematic review of relevant randomized controlled trials (with meta-analysis where possible)

Level II
Evidence obtained from one or more well-designed randomized controlled trials

Level III
Evidence obtained from well-designed cohort or case-control analytical studies, preferably multicentre or conducted at different times

Level IV
The opinions of respected authorities based on clinical experience, descriptive studies or reports of expert committees

location and cause of the problem. However, there is a substantial error rate in the diagnosis of some forms of acute pain. This is particularly so for acute visceral pain; for example, over 20% of diagnoses of acute appendicitis are in error. Knowledge of mechanisms of acute pain may aid clinical diagnosis and reduce this error rate, thereby supporting a more positive biological role for acute pain.

ACUTE PAIN MECHANISMS

As is the case in chronic pain, the perception of acute pain is a complex interaction that involves sensory, emotional and behavioural factors. The role of psychological factors, which

BOX 19.4

Principles of safe and effective acute pain management. (Adapted from NHMRC 1999)

- Adverse physiological and psychological effects result from unrelieved severe pain
- Proper assessment and control of pain require patient involvement
- Effective pain relief requires flexibility and tailoring of treatment to an individual rather than rigid application of formulae and prescriptions
- Pain is best treated early, because established, severe pain is more difficult to treat (Bach et al 1988, Katz et al 1996)
- While it is not possible or always desirable to completely alleviate all pain in the postoperative period, it should be possible to reduce pain to a tolerable or comfortable level
- Postoperative analgesia should be planned preoperatively, with consideration given to the type of surgery, medical condition of the patient, perioperative use of analgesics and regional anaesthetic techniques
- Ultimate responsibility for pain management should be assigned to those most experienced in its administration and not to the most junior staff members

Safe and effective analgesia also depends on:

- Frequent assessment and reassessment of pain intensity and charting of analgesia
- Adequate education of all involved in pain management, including the patient
- Formal programmes, protocols and guidelines covering acute pain management relevant to the institution
- Formal quality assurance programmes to regularly evaluate the effectiveness of pain management

include a person's emotional and behavioural responses, must always be considered to be an important component in the perception and expression of acute pain.

The biological processes involved in our perception of acute pain are no longer viewed as a simple 'hard-wired' system with a pure 'stimulus–response' relationship. The more recent conceptualization of pain seeks to take into account the changes that occur within the nervous system following any prolonged noxious stimulus. For example, trauma to any part of the body, and nerve damage in particular, can lead to changes within other regions of the nervous system, which influence subsequent responses to sensory input. There is increasing recognition that long-term changes occur within the peripheral and central nervous system following noxious input. This 'plasticity' of the nervous system then alters the body's response to further peripheral sensory input.

Recognition of these changes has fostered the concept that pain is divided into two entities: 'physiological' and 'pathophysiological' or 'clinical' (Figs 19.1, 19.2, Boxes 19.5, 19.6). It is the elucidation of these pathophysiological processes that has the most relevance for our understanding and management of acute pain in the clinical setting.

Many forms of pain arise from direct activation or sensitization of primary afferent neurons, especially C-fibre polymodal nociceptors. However the process of nociceptor activation sets in train other processes, which contribute to and modify responses to further stimuli. For example, a relatively benign noxious stimulus such as a scratch to the skin initiates an inflammatory process in the periphery, which then changes the response properties to subsequent sensory stimuli (Fig. 19.3). Under normal conditions, thermal, mechanical and chemical stimuli activate high threshold

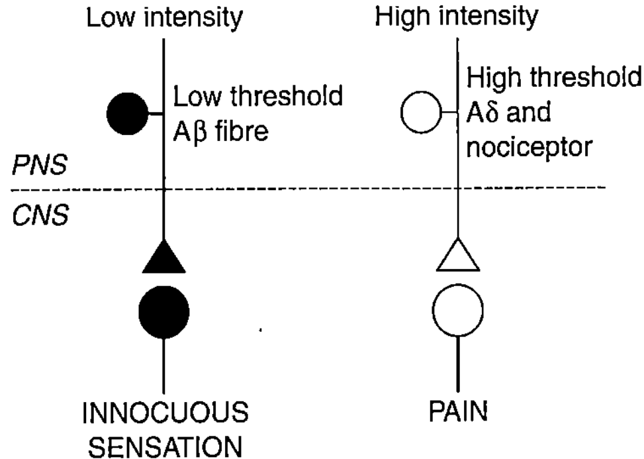

Fig. 19.1 Under 'physiological' conditions, low-intensity non-noxious stimuli activate low-threshold receptors to generate innocuous sensations, and high-intensity noxious stimuli activate high-threshold nociceptors which may lead to the sensation of pain. CNS = central nervous system; PNS = peripheral nervous system. (Reproduced from Woolf & Chong 1993.)

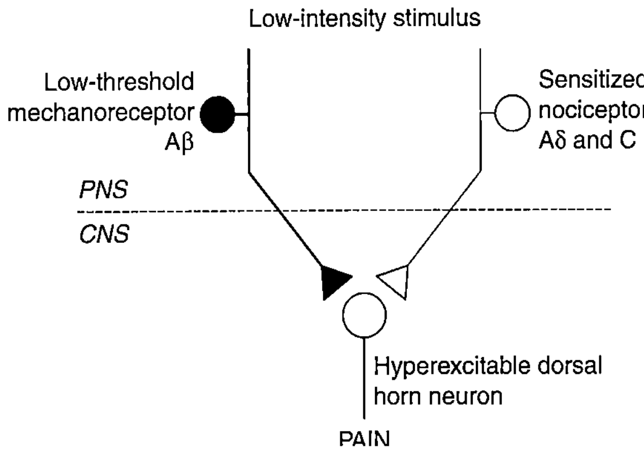

Fig. 19.2 In the clinical situation, central and peripheral changes lead to abnormal excitability in the nervous system. This means that low-intensity stimuli can produce pain. CNS = central nervous system; PNS = peripheral nervous system. (Reproduced from Woolf & Chong 1993.)

nociceptors which signal this information to the first relay in the spinal cord. However, under clinical conditions, the application of a noxious stimulus is usually prolonged, traumatic and associated with tissue damage. Tissue damage results in inflammation, which directly affects the response of the nociceptor to further stimulation.

BOX 19.5

Features of physiological pain. (Reproduced from Cousins & Bridenbaugh 1998 with permission)

- Pain (Aδ and C fibres) can be differentiated from touch (Aβ fibres)
- Pain serves a protective function
- Pain acts as a warning of *potential* damage
- Pain is transient
- Pain is well localized
- Stimulus-response pattern is the same as with other sensory modalities, e.g., touch

BOX 19.6

Features of clinical pain. (Reproduced from Cousins & Bridenbaugh 1998 with permission)

- Pain can be elicited by Aδ and C as well as Aβ fibres
- Pain is 'pathological', i.e. it is associated with inflammation, neuropathy, etc.
- Occurs in the context of peripheral sensitization
- Occurs in the context of central sensitization
- Pain outlasts the stimulus
- Pain spreads to non-damaged areas

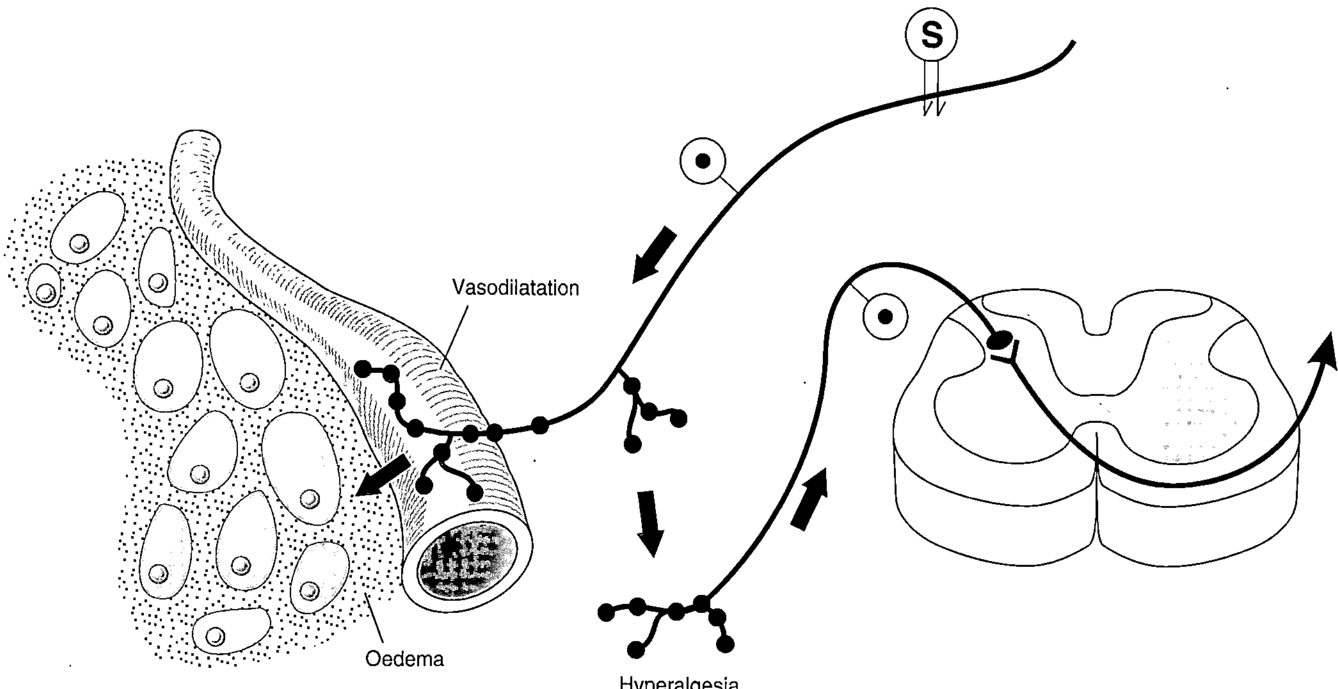

Fig. 19.3 Effect of antidromic impulses in primary afferents. Stimulation (S) of the cut end of primary afferent fibres results in the release of chemical mediators from the peripheral terminals which produce vasodilatation (flare), oedema (wheal) and hyperalgesia (triple response of Lewis). (Adapted from Fields 1987.)

Peripheral sensitization

Surgical trauma or other noxious stimuli associated with acute pain are associated with an injury response or 'inflammatory response'. Part of the inflammatory response is the release of intracellular contents from damaged cells and inflammatory cells such as macrophages, lymphocytes and mast cells. Nociceptive stimulation also results in a neurogenic inflammatory response with the release of substance P, neurokinin A and calcitonin gene-related peptide (CGRP) from the peripheral terminals of nociceptive afferent fibres (Levine et al 1993). Release of these peptides results in a changed excitability of sensory and sympathetic nerve fibres, vasodilatation, extravasation of plasma proteins as well as action on inflammatory cells to release chemical mediators. These interactions result in the release of a 'soup' of inflammatory mediators such as potassium, serotonin, bradykinin, substance P, histamine, cytokines, nitric oxide and products from the cyclooxygenase and lipoxygenase pathways of arachidonic acid. These chemicals then act to sensitize high-threshold nociceptors which results in the phenomenon of peripheral sensitization.

Following sensitization, low-intensity mechanical stimuli which would not normally cause pain are now perceived as painful. There is also an increased responsiveness to thermal stimuli at the site of injury. This zone of 'primary hyperalgesia' surrounding the site of injury is caused by peripheral changes and is a feature that is commonly observed following surgery and other forms of trauma.

NSAIDs

Non-steroidal anti-inflammatory drugs (NSAIDs) are commonly used for 'peripheral' analgesia and have as one of their actions a reduction in the inflammatory response (Walker 1995). Agents such as aspirin, paracetamol and other NSAIDs provide their anti-inflammatory action by blocking the cyclooxygenase pathway. It is now apparent that cyclooxygenase exists in two forms, COX1 and COX2. While COX1 is always present in tissues, including the gastric mucosa, COX2 is induced by inflammation (Seibert et al 1994). This presents an opportunity for the development of agents which have a selective anti-inflammatory effect without gastric side effects. COX2 inhibitor drugs are now under clinical investigation (e.g., meloxicam); initial results indicate equal efficacy to existing NSAIDs, but without toxic side effects (Laneuville et al 1994, Furst 1997, The et al 1997, Lund et al 1998). Besides the peripheral action of NSAIDs, there is increasing evidence that they exert their analgesic effect through central mechanisms (Urquhart 1993, Walker 1995).

NSAIDs are used extensively in the treatment of acute postoperative pain (Merry & Power 1995). While there has been some concern regarding the risks of NSAIDs, they continue to have a useful role as analgesics in the perioperative period. Naproxen (Comfort et al 1992), diclofenac (Laitinen & Nuutinen 1992) and ketorolac (O'Hara et al 1987) have all used either pre- or postoperatively, with a demonstrated reduction in postoperative pain and reduced opioid requirements. The different sites of action found with NSAIDs and opioids would also suggest additive, or possibly even synergistic, effects and in clinical practice they are often used in combination.

Peripheral action of opioids

Opioids have traditionally been viewed as centrally acting drugs. However, there is now evidence for the action of endogenous opioids on peripheral sites following tissue damage (Stein et al 1989, Stein 1993). Opioid receptors are manufactured in the cell body (dorsal root ganglion) and transported toward the central terminal in the dorsal horn and toward the periphery. These peripheral receptors then become active following local tissue damage. This occurs with unmasking of opioid receptors and the arrival of immunocompetent cells that possess opioid receptors and have the ability to synthesize opioid peptides. This has led to an interest in the peripheral administration of opioids, such as intra-articular administration following knee surgery or arthroscopy (Haynes et al 1994, Stein 1995) or topical administration of morphine (Tennant et al 1993). Despite initial enthusiasm with this technique, some workers have expressed doubt about the usefulness and cost-benefit of intra-articular morphine, particularly following arthroscopy or minor knee surgery (Aasbo et al 1996). However, opioids with physicochemical properties favouring peripheral action are under development and, if successful, such drugs may be useful for regional application. Medium-sized peptides are under development with a view to a localized action, thus avoiding systems uptake.

Peripheral nerve injury

Recent studies have demonstrated that section of, or damage to, a peripheral nerve results in a number of biochemical, physiological and morphological changes that act as a focus of pain in themselves (for reviews see Devor 1994, Ollat & Cesaro 1995).

Neuroplasticity changes aimed at maintaining sensory input may occur at peripheral and/or spinal levels (see Ch. 35). In the postsurgery or post-trauma patient, neuropathic pain may have an early onset within the first 24 hours; this is contrary to classic teaching. There may also be a delayed onset of the order of 10 days.

A number of agents are used with varying degrees of success in the management of peripheral neuropathic pain (Galer 1995). These include tricyclic antidepressants (Magni 1991, Max et al 1992), anticonvulsants such as carbamazepine and sodium valproate (McQuay et al 1995), clonidine (Zeigler et al 1992), opioids (Portenoy et al 1990), local anaesthetics such as lignocaine (lidocaine) (Backonja 1994) and antiarrythmic agents such as mexiletine (Chabal et al 1992). As well as these agents, which are now used extensively in the management of peripheral neuropathic pain, several new agents may be promising but as yet have not been systematically evaluated. These include new antidepressants such as venlafaxine and nefazodone, and new anticonvulsants such as gabapentin, vigabatrin and lamotrigine.

Systemic administration of local anaesthetic agents can result in a marked reduction in neuropathic pain (Backonja 1994). This effect is a result of the ability of relatively low concentrations of local anaesthetic to reduce ectopic activity in damaged nerves at levels which are below the concentration required to produce conduction block (Devor et al 1992). A puzzling feature of the response of peripheral neuropathic pain to systemic administration of local anaesthetics is the time course of pain relief. While intrathecal or peripheral nerve blockade results in temporary reduction in pain behaviour in an animal model of neuropathic pain, systemic administration of lignocaine results in a reduction in mechanical hyperalgesia that persists for 1 week (Chaplan et al 1995). This finding challenges previously accepted explanations for the mechanisms of local anaesthetics in reducing neuropathic pain, as well as suggesting possible clinical application (for discussion see Strichartz 1995).

Sympathetic nervous system

The sympathetic nervous system also has an important role in the generation and maintenance of acute pain states (McMahon 1991, Jänig & McLachlan 1994, Jänig 1996). Nerve damage and even minor trauma can lead to a disturbance in sympathetic activity (Fig. 19.4) which then leads to a sustained condition termed a 'complex regional pain syndrome', this now replaces the previously used term – 'reflex sympathetic dystrophy' (IASP Task Force on Taxonomy 1994). Complex regional pain syndromes (CRPS) are associated with features of sympathetic dysfunction including vasomotor and sudomotor changes, abnormalities of hair and nail growth and osteoporosis as well as sensory symptoms of spontaneous burning pain, hyperalgesia and allodynia, and often disturbance of motor function (Fig 19.4).

Basic studies have demonstrated that several changes involving the sympathetic nervous system may be responsible for the development of these features (Jänig & McLachlan 1994). Inflammation can result in the sensitization of primary nociceptive afferent fibres by prostanoids that are released from sympathetic fibres (Levine et al 1993). Following nerve injury, sympathetic nerve stimulation or the administration of noradrenaline can excite primary afferent fibres via an action at α-adrenoceptors; also there is innervation of the dorsal root ganglion by sympathetic terminals (McLachlan et al 1993) (see Ch. 6). This means that activity in sympathetic efferent fibres can lead to abnormal activity or responsiveness of the primary afferent fibre.

Complex regional pain syndromes may be sympathetically maintained or sympathetically independent. Pain problems that are sympathetically maintained may respond to sympathetic blockade by agents administered systemically, epidurally, regionally or around the sympathetic ganglion (Campbell et al 1994).

Following surgery or trauma, early diagnosis or CRPS is essential because early intervention is more likely to be successful than later measures. Patients with a prior history of CRPS should have preventative measures such as preoperative and peroperative regional anaesthetic techniques. Some types of surgery, such as hand surgery, pose an increased risk of CRPS.

DORSAL HORN MECHANISMS OF IMPORTANCE TO ACUTE PAIN

Termination sites of primary afferents

The dorsal horn is the site of termination of primary afferents and there is a complex interaction among afferent fibres local intrinsic spinal neurons and the endings of descending fibres from the brain. Primary afferent nociceptors terminate primarily in laminae I, II and V (Light & Perl 1979), where they connect with several classes of second order neurons in the dorsal horn of the spinal cord. Some fibres also ascend and descend several segments in Lissauer's tract before terminating on neurons that project to higher centres. This provides a mechanism for input from one spinal segment (e.g., a fractured rib) to produce reflex motor effects over as many as six segments. The end result could be muscle guarding over a sufficient area of impaired respiration. In a respiratory cripple this could precipitate respiratory failure.

Neurotransmitters

Pharmacological studies have been important in identifying the many neurotransmitters and neuromodulators that are

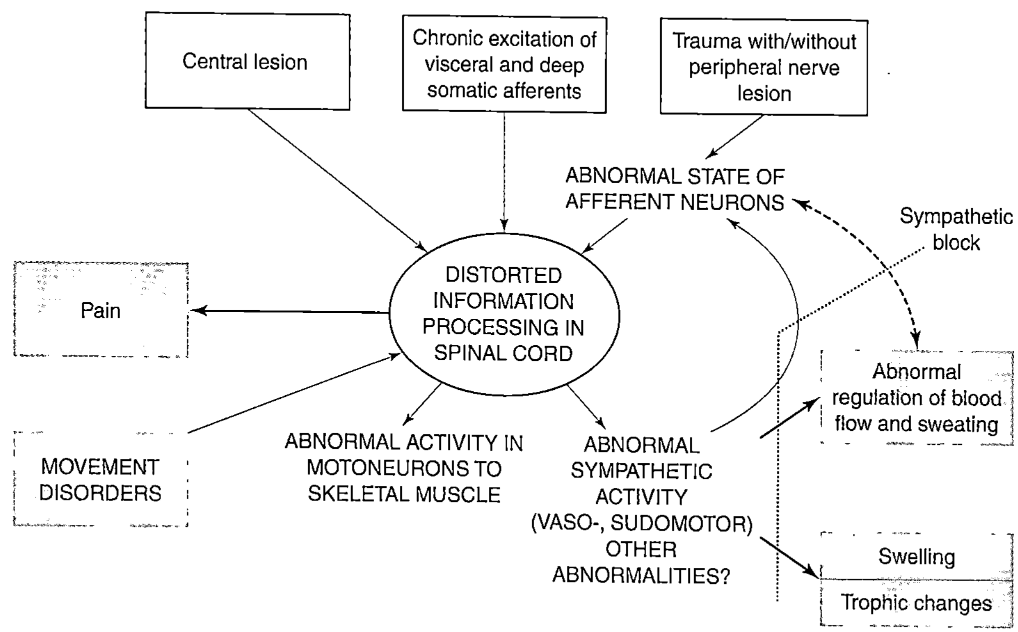

Fig. 19.4 General hypothesis about the neural mechanisms of the generation of CRPS I and II following peripheral trauma, with and without nerve lesions, chronic stimulation of visceral afferents (e.g., myocardial infarction) and deep somatic afferents and, rarely, central trauma. The clinical observations are double framed. Note the vicious circle (arrows in bold black). An important component of this circle is the excitatory influence of postganglionic sympathetic axons on primary afferent fibres in the periphery. (Reproduced from Janig 1996.)

involved in pain processes in the dorsal horn (Wilcox 1991) (see Ch. 6). The excitatory amino acids glutamate and aspartate have a major role in nociceptive transmission in the dorsal horn (Coderre 1993). The excitatory amino acids act at *N*-methyl-D-aspartate (NMDA), non-NMDA receptors such as AMPA (α-amino-3-hydroxy-5-methyl-4-isoxazolepropionic acid), kainate and metabotropic glutamate receptors (for reviews see Wilcox 1991, Price et al 1994).

There are a number of peptides released by primary afferents that have a role in acute nociception. These include substance P, neurokinin A and CGRP. Substance P and neurokinin A act on neurokinin receptors. There are a number of other receptors that are also involved in nociceptive transmission or modulation. These receptors include opioid (μ, κ and δ), α-adrenergic, γ-amino-butyric acid (GABA), serotonin (5HT) and adenosine receptors.

Traditional approaches in acute pain management have focused on classical ligand–receptor blockade as a means to reduce nociceptive or neuropathic input. The rapid progress in our understanding of the molecular and genetic mechanisms involved in nociception provides a new and potentially useful approach to acute pain management. Using this approach, it may be possible to develop drugs that regulate gene expression and selectively modify the expression of specific receptors that are involved in the transmission of nociceptive and neuropathic messages (Akopian et al 1996).

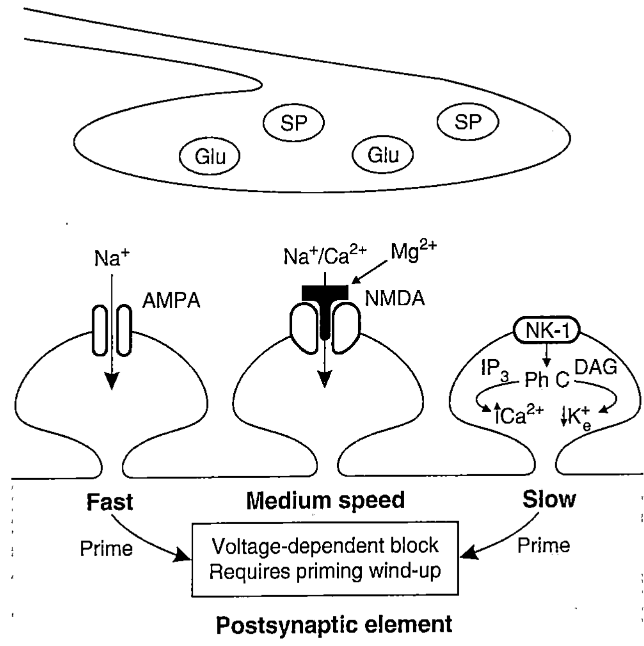

Fig. 19.5 Release of glutamate (Glu) and substance P (SP) from the terminals of nociceptive primary afferents activates AMPA and neurokinin 1 (NK-1) receptors respectively on the postsynaptic membrane. Activation of these receptors results in sodium (Na^+) influx at the AMPA receptor and activation of second messengers (IP_3, Ph C, DAG). These processes then act to prime the NMDA receptor with removal of the magnesium plug and sodium and calcium (Ca^{2+}) influx. AMPA = α-amino-3-hydroxy-5-methyl- 4-isoxazolepropionic acid; DAG = diacylglycerol; IP_3 = inositol triphosphate; NMDA = *N*-methyl-D-aspartate; Ph C = phospholipase C. (Reproduced from Cousins & Bridenbaugh 1998 with permission.)

NMDA receptors

It appears that non-NMDA receptors such as the AMPA receptor may mediate responses in the 'physiological' processing of sensory information. However, with prolonged release of glutamate or activation of neurokinin receptors, a secondary process occurs which appears to be crucial in the development of abnormal responses to further sensory stimuli. This sustained activation of non-NMDA or neurokinin receptors 'primes' the NMDA receptor, so that it is in a state ready for activation (Fig. 19.5).

There is evidence that NMDA receptors are involved in a number of phenomena that may contribute to the medium- or long-term changes that are observed in the transition from acute to chronic pain states. These phenomena include the development of 'wind-up' (Davies & Lodge 1987) facilitation, central sensitization (Woolf & Thompson 1991), changes in peripheral receptive fields, induction of oncogenes and long-term potentiation (Collingridge & Singer 1990). Long-term potentiation, in particular, refers to the changes in synaptic efficacy that occur as part of the process of memory and may play a role in the development of a cellular 'memory' for pain or enhanced responsiveness to noxious inputs. Furthermore, it appears that NMDA antagonists can attenuate these responses (Woolf & Thompson 1991), indicating a role for NMDA antagonists in the treatment of acute pain and in the prevention of chronic pain states.

While there are drugs available such as ketamine and the experimental drug MK-801 which appear to block NMDA receptor-mediated changes (Dickenson & Sullivan 1987, Trujillo & Akil 1991, Woolf & Thompson 1991), the side effects associated with their use have meant that they are limited in the clinical situation. Nevertheless, there still remains a potential for the development of clinically suitable NMDA receptor antagonists and several agents are being investigated either for analgesia or for use in other medical conditions (Lipton 1993). At present clinical options are limited to dextromethorphan, which has been demonstrated to reduce opioid requirements following oral/dental surgery and to reduce intraoperative opioid requirements in association with abdominal surgery.

Intracellular events

The activation of NMDA receptors appears to set in train a cascade of secondary events in the cell which has been activated. These events lead to changes within the cell which increase the responsiveness of the nociceptive system and lead to some of the phenomena described above (Dickenson 1996). The NMDA receptor channel in its resting state is 'blocked' by a magnesium 'plug'. Priming of the NMDA receptor by co-release of glutamate and the peptides acting on the neurokinin receptors leads to removal of the magnesium plug and subsequent calcium influx into the cell leading to secondary events such as oncogene induction (Morgan & Curran 1986), production of nitric oxide (NO), (Garthwaite et al 1988) and activation or production of a number of second messengers including phospholipases, polyphosphoinosites (IP_3, DAG), cyclic guanine monophosphate (cGMP), ecosanoids and protein kinase C. These second messengers then act directly to change the excitability of the cell or induce the production of oncogenes, which may result in long-term alterations in the responsivity of the cell. Prolonged stimulation, presumably through sustained and therefore excitotoxic release of glutamate, may result in cell death.

The exact role of NO in nociceptive processing is still unclear and it does not appear to be important in acute nociception (Malmberg & Yaksh 1993). However, the production of NO is implicated in the induction and maintenance of chronic pain states (Meller & Gebhart 1993) and may be one of the factors responsible for the cell death which has been demonstrated to occur under these conditions (Fig. 19.6). It has been suggested that NO acts as a positive feedback mechanism in the maintenance of pain. The changes in nociceptive processing, gene expression and others to be described below, form a continuum with the early effects of nociception. Thus it is no longer logical to view acute, subacute and chronic pain as being entirely separate.

The production of arachidonic acid metabolites as part of the cascade that occurs following NMDA receptor activation also raises an interesting potential avenue of intervention that is already being explored (Eisenach 1993). Although the peripheral effects of NSAIDs have been emphasized in the past, it appears that there may be a role for the spinal administration of NSAIDs. Spinal NSAIDs act either directly on receptors, such as the strychnine-insensitive glycine site of the NMDA receptor complex, or influence the production of metabolites within the cell.

Central sensitization

The changes that occur in the periphery following trauma lead to the phenomenon of 'peripheral sensitization' and primary hyperalgesia. The sensitization that occurs, however,

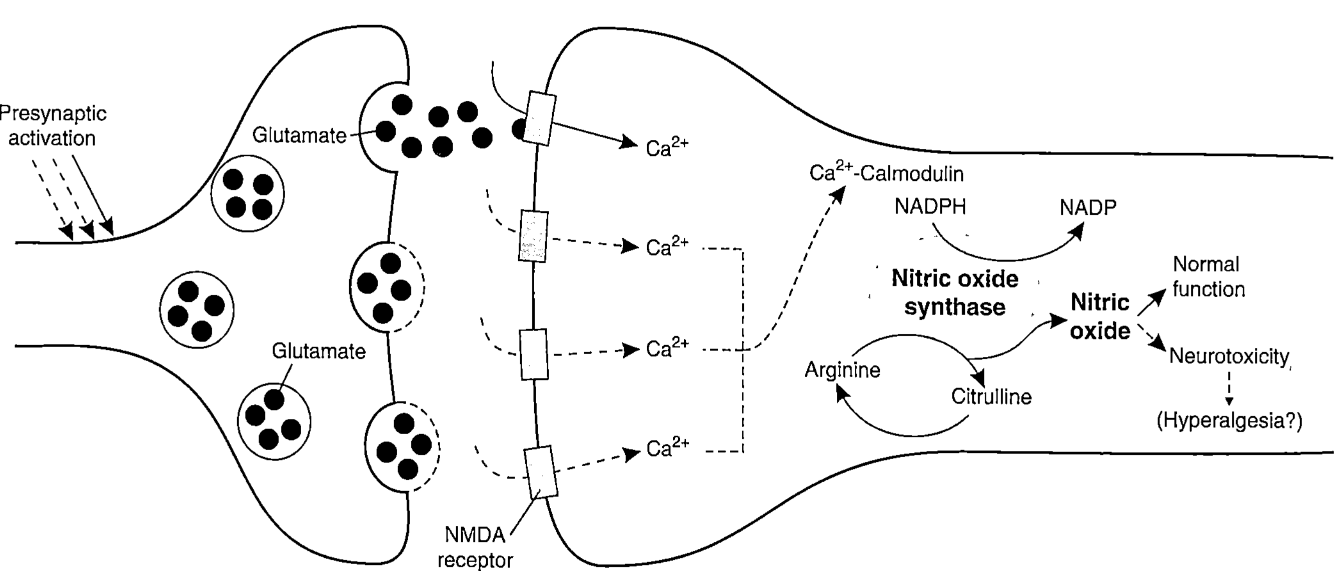

Fig. 19.6 Diagram illustrating postsynaptic events following release of glutamate from central terminals of primary afferents in the spinal cord. Following priming of the NMDA receptor complex, subsequent glutamate release results in NMDA receptor activation with subsequent calcium influx. Intracellular calcium then acts on a calmodulin-sensitive site to activate the enzyme nitric oxide synthase (NOS). In the presence of a cofactor NADPH, NOS uses arginine as a substrate to produce nitric oxide and citrulline. Nitric oxide has a role in normal cellular function, but increased production may be involved in hyperalgesia and may lead to neurotoxicity. (Reproduced from Cousins & Bridenbaugh 1998 with permission.)

can only be partly explained by the changes in the periphery. Following injury, there is an increased responsiveness to normally innocuous mechanical stimuli (allodynia) in a zone of 'secondary hyperalgesia' in uninjured tissue surrounding the site of injury. In contrast to the zone of primary hyperalgesia, there is no change in the threshold to thermal stimuli. These changes are believed to be a result of processes that occur in the dorsal horn of the spinal cord following injury (Bennett et al 1989). This is the phenomenon of central sensitization (Fig. 19.7).

These changes indicate that, in the presence of pain, the central nervous system is not 'hard-wired', but plastic, and that attempts to modify pain must take into account these changes. A barrage of nociceptive input, such as occurs with surgery, results in changes to the response properties of dorsal horn neurons (Chi et al 1993). It has been demonstrated that a painful stimulus, which is at a level sufficient to activate C fibres, not only activates dorsal horn neurons but neuronal activity also progressively increases throughout the duration of the stimulus (Mendell 1966). Therefore, with clinical pain associated with nociceptive input, there is not a simple stimulus–response relationship, but a 'wind-up' of spinal cord neuronal activity. Wind-up is dependent on activation of the NMDA receptor (Dickenson & Sullivan 1987, Woolf & Thompson 1991) and therefore has the potential to be modified by agents acting at this site. This 'wind-up' may make these neurons more sensitive to other input and is a component of central sensitisation.

Several other changes have been noted to occur in the dorsal horn with central sensitization (Dubner & Ren 1994). Firstly, there is an expansion in receptive field size so that a spinal neuron will respond to stimuli that would normally be outside the region which responds to nociceptive stimuli. Secondly, there is an increase in the magnitude and duration of the response to stimuli which are above threshold in strength. Lastly, there is a reduction in threshold so that stimuli which are not normally noxious activate neurons which normally transmit nociceptive information. These changes may be important both in acute pain states such as postoperative pain and in the development of chronic pain (Wilcox 1991).

The demonstration of the phenomenon of wind-up (Mendell 1966) has had a major impact on the current conceptualization of pain and has led to a surge of interest in approaches such as pre-emptive analgesia. Much of the philosophy and rationale behind pre-emptive analgesia lies in an attempt to reduce the development of 'sub-acute' or chronic pain by abolishing or reducing acute pain and thus preventing the changes associated with wind-up. However, the development of chronic pain may have more to do with the phenomenon of long-term potentiation (LTP) than it does with win-dup. Long-term potentiation is the strengthening of the efficacy of synaptic transmission

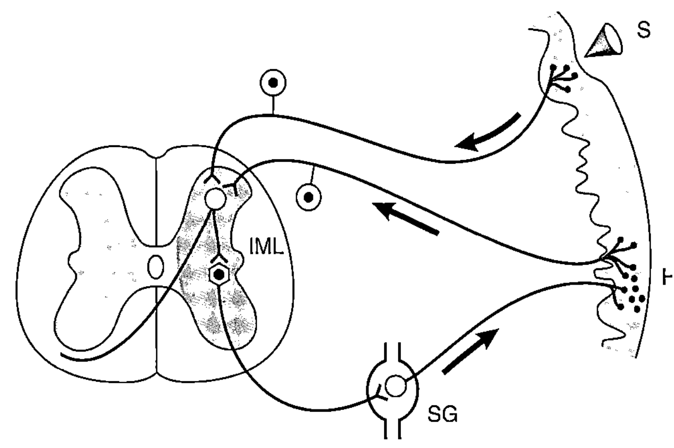

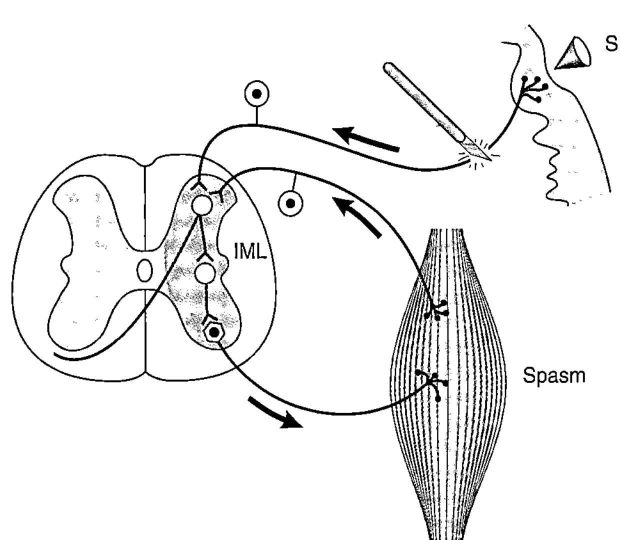

Fig. 19.7 Depiction of increased spinal neuron activity (hyperactivity) in response to various stimuli. **A** Nociceptive stimulus delivered at the skin surface (S) activates a primary afferent nociceptor that, in turn, activates the sympathetic preganglionic neuron in the interomediolateral column (IML). The preganglionic neuron activates the noradrenergic postganglionic neuron in the sympathetic ganglion (SG), which sensitizes, and can activate primary afferent nociceptors (H) that feed back to the spinal cord, maintaining the pain. Peripheral injury is associated with an increase in spinal neuron activity, so that there is an enhanced responsiveness to subsequent input. **B** Section of a peripheral nerve (e.g., following trauma) results in pronounced and long-lasting increases in spinal cord activity. Tissue injury also produces increased activity of spinal neurons causing activation of ventral horn neurons and muscle spasm. Prolonged muscle spasm activates muscle nociceptors that feed back to the spinal cord to sustain the spasm. (Modified from Fields 1987.)

that occurs following activity across that synapse and shares many of the physiological and biochemical features that are associated with the development of chronic pain. It is dependent on activation of NMDA receptors (Collingridge & Singer 1990) and LTP3 in particular, which has a longer time constant (20–30 days), is associated with the induction of immediate early genes including fos-related genes (Abraham et al 1993), which are often used as a marker in basic pain studies.

Nerve damage results in enhancement of calcium flux, nitric oxide production and protein kinase C (PKC) generation. PKC has a particularly potent effect in increasing activity at the NMDA receptor, thus causing a vicious circle. Intrathecal, or systemic, administration of morphine for neuropathic pain may also increase NMDA activity, while at the same time decreasing the efficacy of morphine at the μ-opioid receptor. Thus, unwittingly, morphine administration in neuropathic pain may progressively contribute to increasing the pain.

It has also been demonstrated that morphological changes occur within the dorsal horn following peripheral nerve injury. Peripheral nerve injury results in a redistribution of central terminals of myelinated afferents with sprouting of these terminals from lamina IV to lamina II (Woolf et al 1992, Lekan et al 1996). If functional contact is made between these terminals which normally transmit non-noxious information and neurons that normally receive nociceptive input, this may provide a framework for the pain and hypersensitivity to light touch (allodynia) that is seen following nerve injury. Such changes occur within a few days of nerve injury and thus may play a part in the development of allodynia following nerve injury as a result of surgery or trauma.

Modulation at a spinal level

Transmission of nociceptive information is subject to modulation at several levels of the neuraxis including the dorsal horn. Afferent impulses arriving in the dorsal horn initiate inhibitory mechanisms, which limit the effect of subsequent impulses. Inhibition occurs through the effect of local inhibitory interneurons and descending pathways from the brain. In the dorsal horn, incoming nociceptive messages are modulated by endogenous and exogenous agents which act on opioid, α-adreno-, GABA and glycine receptors located at pre- and postsynaptic sites (Fig. 19.8).

Opioid receptors

Opioids are widely used and generally efficacious in the management of pain. Opioid receptors are found both pre- and postsynaptically in the dorsal horn, although the majority (about 75%) are located presynaptically (Besse et al 1990). Activation of presynaptic opioid receptors results in a reduction in the release of neurotransmitters from the nociceptive primary afferent (Hori et al 1992). However the changes that occur with inflammation and neuropathy can produce significant changes in opioid sensitivity that involve a number of mechanisms. These include: an interference with opioid analgesia by cholecystokinin (CCK) (Xu et al 1993); loss of presynaptic opioid receptors (Besse et al 1990) and the formation of the morphine metabolite, morphine-3-glucuronide (Smith et al 1990), which may antagonize the analgesic action normally produced by opioid receptor activation.

It has also been demonstrated that the NMDA receptor is involved in the development of tolerance to opioids. Animal studies indicate that the administration of an NMDA antagonist reduces the development of tolerance to morphine (Wong et al 1996) and prevents the withdrawal syndrome in morphine-tolerant rats (Trujillo & Akil 1991). Therefore, agents which act as NMDA antagonists, such as dextromethorphan, have the potential to interfere with the development of pain states, potentiate the action of opioids (Advokat & Rhein 1995) and prevent the development of opioid tolerance.

α adrenoceptors

Activation of α adrenoceptors in the spinal cord has an analgesic effect either by endogenous release of noradrenaline by descending pathways from the brainstem, or by exogenous spinal administration of agents such as clonidine (Yaksh & Reddy 1981). Furthermore, α-adrenoceptor agonists appear to have a synergistic effect with opioid agonists (Meert & De Kock 1994). There are a number of α-adrenoceptor subtypes and the development of selective α-adrenoceptor subtype agonists has the potential to provide effective new analgesic agents with reduced side effects.

GABA and glycine

Both GABA and glycine are involved in tonic inhibition of nociceptive input and loss of their inhibitory action can result in features of neuropathic pain such as allodynia (Sivilotti & Woolf 1994). Although both $GABA_A$ and $GABA_B$ receptors have been implicated at both pre- and postsynaptic sites, it has been demonstrated that $GABA_A$-receptor-mediated inhibition occurs through largely postsynaptic mechanisms (Lin et al 1996). By contrast, $GABA_B$ mechanisms may be preferentially involved in presynaptic inhibition through suppression of excitatory amino acid release from primary afferent terminals. This finding may help to understand the disparity between laboratory findings which demonstrate that $GABA_B$ receptor agonists such as baclofen have an antinociceptive action (Wilson & Yaksh 1995) and clinical experience which has found that

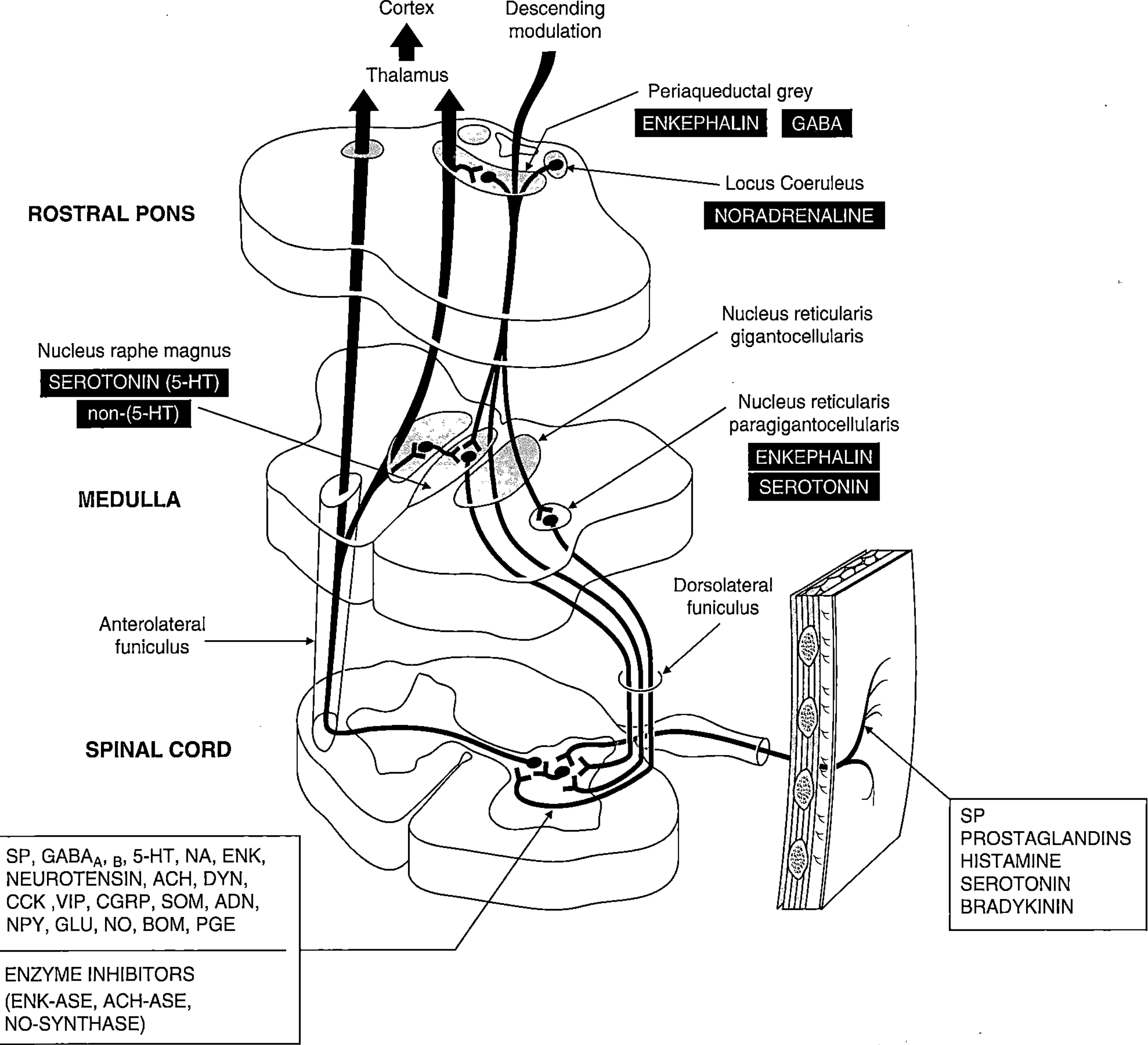

Fig. 19.8 Simplified diagram of afferent sensory pathways (left) and descending modulatory pathways (right). Stimulation of nociceptors in the skin surface leads to impulse generation in the primary afferent. Concomitant with this impulse generation, increased levels of various endogenous algesic agents (substance P, prostaglandins, histamine, serotonin, bradykinin) are detected near the area of stimulation in the periphery. Primary afferent nociceptors relay to projection neurons in the dorsal horn, which ascend in the anterolateral funiculus to terminate in the thalamus. En route, collaterals of the projection neurons activate multiple higher centres, including the nucleus reticularis gigantocellularis (NRG). Neurons from the NRG project to the thalamus and also activate the nucleus raphe magnus (NRM) and periaqueductal grey (PAG) of the midbrain. Descending fibres from the PAG project to the NRM and reticular formation adjacent to the NRM. These neurons activate descending inhibitory neurons which are located in these regions and travel via the dorsolateral funiculus to terminate in the dorsal horn of the spinal cord. Descending projections also arise from a number of brainstem sites including the locus coeruleus (LC). A number of neurotransmitters are released by afferent fibres, descending terminations, or local interneurons in the dorsal horn and modulate peripheral nociceptive input. These include substance P (SP), γ-aminobutyric acid (GABA), serotonin (5-HT), noradrenaline (NA), enkephalin (ENK), neurotensin, acetylcholine (ACH), dynorphin (DYN), cholecystokinin (CCK), vasoactive intestinal peptide (VIP), calcitonin gene-related peptide (CGRP), somatostatin (SOM), adenosine (ADN), neuropeptide Y (NPY), glutamate (GLU), nitric oxide (NO), bombesin (BOM) and prostaglandins (PGE). Inhibitors of enzymes such as enkephalinase (ENK-ASE), acetylcholinesterase (ACH-ASE) and nitric oxide synthase (NO-SYNTHASE) may act to modify the action of these neurotransmitters. (Reproduced from Cousins & Bridenbaugh 1998 with permission.)

intrathecal baclofen is of limited use in the management of chronic pain (Fromm 1994). Particularly in neuropathic pain, where there is increased excitability of second-order neurons with no direct relationship to the amount of excitatory amino acids (EAAs) released by primary afferents, intrathecal administration of $GABA_A$ agonists may be more effective. There is recent evidence that $GABA_A$ active drugs may also have analgesic effects via the δ opioid receptor.

DESCENDING INHIBITION

Descending inhibition (see Ch. 51) involves the action of endogenous opioid peptides as well as other neurotransmitters, including serotonin and noradrenaline and GABA (for review see Fields & Basbaum 1994). Many of the traditional strategies available in acute pain management such as the use of opioids act via these inhibitory mechanisms. The elucidation of inhibitory mechanisms has resulted in the use of new techniques which aim to stimulate these inhibitory pathways. It has also provided a clearer rationale for techniques already in use and used empirically. These include the use of techniques such as transcutaneous electrical nerve stimulation, acupuncture and epidural/ intrathecal opioid and non-opioid drug administration.

AETIOLOGY AND FEATURES OF ACUTE PAIN

Acute pain may arise from cutaneous, deep somatic or visceral structures. Careful mapping of the principal superficial dermatomes is important for the effective use of neural blockade techniques. Visceral pain is much more vaguely localized than somatic pain and has other unique features (Table 19.2). The convergence of visceral and somatic afferents has been proven and this helps to explain referred pain. Also important viscerosomatic reflexes have been identified (Fig. 19.9).

The relief of visceral pain requires blockade of visceral nociceptive fibres that travel to the spinal cord by way of the sympathetic chain. The viscera and the spinal cord segments associated with their visceral nociceptor afferents are shown in Table 19.3. Visceral pain is 'referred' to the body surface areas, as shown in Figure 19.10. It should be noted that there is considerable overlap for the various organs. Thus it is not surprising that there is a substantial error rate in the diagnosis of visceral pain. Also, there are important viscerosomatic and somaticovisceral reflexes that may make diagnosis and treatment difficult (Fig. 19.9).

The temporary relief of visceral pain by blockade of the somatic referred area poses potential problems of interpretation of 'diagnostic' local anaesthetic nerve blocks. It appears that the processes of peripheral and central sensitization which have been described previously in this chapter may be shared by somatic as well as visceral structures. This may account for the heightened response of visceral structures to a relatively benign stimulus following inflammation or tissue damage ('visceral hyperalgesia').

FEATURES OF ACUTE PAIN

There are important differences between most types of acute pain and chronic pain. In acute pain the nervous system is usually intact; the pain is caused by trauma, surgery, acute 'medical' conditions or a physiological process (e.g., labour). Facial grimaces and signs of increased autonomic activity and other potentially harmful effects may be evident: for example, hypertension, tachycardia, vasoconstriction, sweating, increased rate and decreased depth of respiration, skeletal muscle spasm, increased gastrointestinal secretions, decreased intestinal motility and increased sphincter tone, urinary retention, venous stasis and potential for thrombosis, and possible pulmonary embolism; anx-

Table 19.2 Visceral pain compared with somatic pain. (Reproduced from Cousins & Bridenbaugh 1998 with permission)

Factors	*Somatic: well localized*	*Visceral: poorly localized*
Radiation	May follow distribution of somatic nerve	Diffuse
Character	Sharp and definite	Dull and vague (may be colicky, cramping, squeezing, etc.)
Relation to stimulus	Hurts where the stimulus is; associated with external factors	May be 'referred' to another area; associated with internal factors
Time relations	Often constant (sometimes periodic)	Often periodic and builds to peaks (sometimes constant)
Associated symptoms	Nausea usually only with deep somatic pain owing to bone involvement	Often nausea, vomiting, sickening feeling

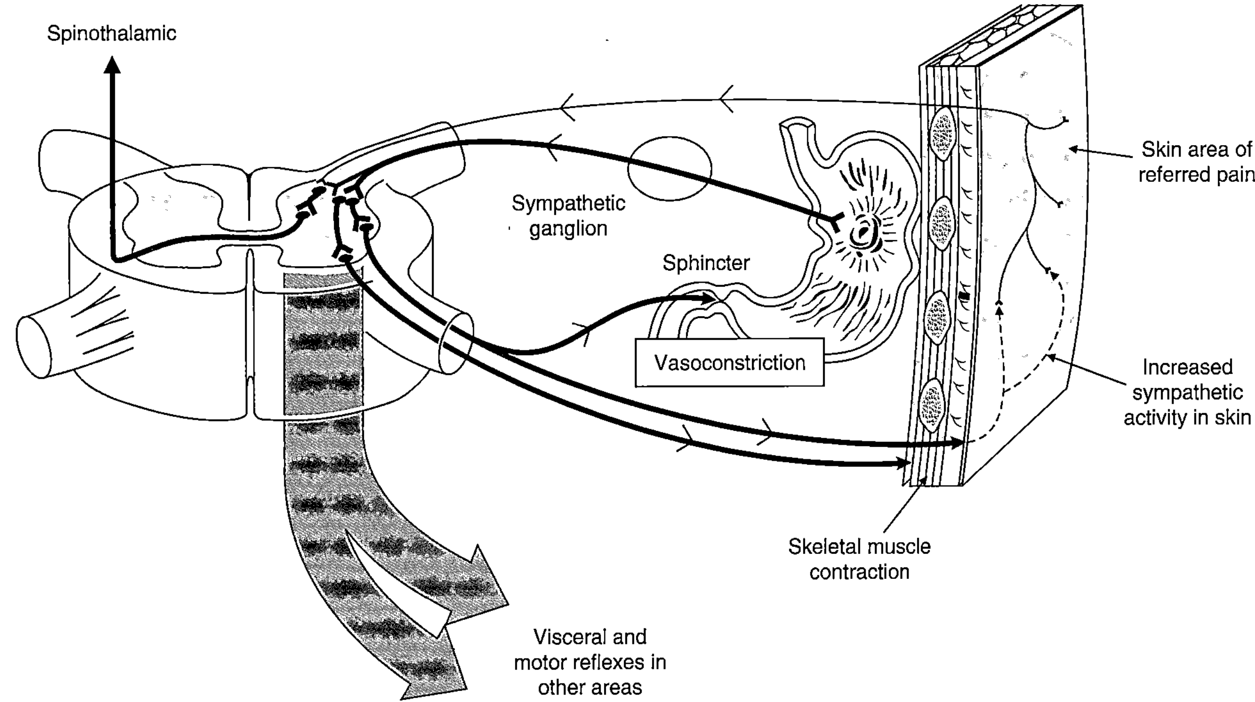

Fig. 19.9 Visceral pain: convergence of visceral and somatic nociceptive afferents. Visceral nociceptive afferents converge on the same dorsal horn neuron as do somatic nociceptive afferents. Viceral noxious stimuli are then conveyed, together with somatic noxious stimuli, by means of the spinothalamic pathways to the brain. Notes: (1) Referred pain is felt in the cutaneous area corresponding to the dorsal horn neuron upon which visceral afferents converge. This is accompanied by allodynia and hyperalgesia in this skin area. (2) Reflex somatic motor activity results in muscle spasm, which may stimulate parietal peritoneum and initiate somatic noxious input to dorsal horn. (3) Reflex sympathetic efferent activity may result in spasm of sphincters of viscera over a wide area, causing pain remote from the original stimulus. (4) Reflex sympathetic efferent activity may result in visceral ischaemia and further noxious stimulation. Also, visceral nociceptors may be sensitized by noradrenaline release and microcirculatory changes. (5) Increased sympathetic activity may influence cutaneous nociceptors, which may be at least partly responsible for referred pain. (6) Peripheral visceral afferents branch considerably, causing much overlap in the territory of individual dorsal roots. Only a small number of visceral afferent fibres converge on dorsal horn neurons compared with somatic nociceptor fibres. Also, visceral afferents converge on the dorsal horn over a wide number of segments. Thus dull, vague visceral pain is very poorly localized. This is often called deep visceral pain. (Reproduced from Cousins & Bridenbaugh 1998 with permission.)

iety, confusion and delirium. Also, the pain usually ceases when the wound heals or the medical condition improves. Patients are usually aware that the pain will improve as they recover, and thus an end is in sight. This may not be so if patients are ill prepared and poorly informed.

Some severe and prolonged acute pain may progressively become more like chronic pain (see below). Some patients with chronic pain may have superimposed acute pain (e.g., when they require further surgery or develop a bone fracture owing to metastatic cancer) (Foley 1985). Such patients may not have an intact nervous system and may have marked pre-existing psychological problems, opioid tolerance and other problems.

Extensive somatic and sympathetic blockade may be required to relieve acute pain associated with some types of major surgery. For example, the following may be required for pain after thoracoabdominal oesophagogastrectomy with cervical anastomosis: C3–C4 and T2–T12 sensory nerves (somatic structures in neck, thorax and abdomen); cervicothoracic sympathetic chain and coeliac plexus (intrathoracic and abdominal viscera); C3, C4 phrenic nerve sensory afferents (pain from incision in central diaphragm referred to shoulder tip).

Segmental and suprasegmental reflex responses to acute pain result in muscle spasm, immobility, vasospasm and other adverse effects, as described above. This may intensify the pain by way of various vicious cycles (Fig. 19.9), which include increased sensitivity of peripheral nociceptors. Acute pain that is unrelieved results in anxiety and sleeplessness, which in turn increase pain. Also anxiety and a feeling of helplessness, before as well as after surgery, increase pain. Their prevention and relief are valuable adjuncts to other treatments. Psychological journals contain much of relevance to acute pain. After major surgery, or severe trauma, or painful medical conditions (e.g., pancreatitis), acute pain may persist for more than 10 days (Bonica 1985). In such

Table 19.3 Viscera and their segmental nociceptive nerve supply. (Reproduced from Cousins & Bridenbaugh 1998 with permission)

Viscus	Spinal segments of visceral nociceptive afferents[1]
Heart	T1–T5
Lungs	T2–T4
Oesophagus	T5–T6
Stomach	T6–T10
Liver and gallbladder	T6–T10
Pancreas and spleen	T6–T10
Small intestine	T9–T10
Large intestine	T11–T12
Kidney and ureter	T10–L2
Adrenal glands	T8–L1
Testis, ovary	T10–T11
Urinary bladder	T11–L2
Prostate gland	T11–L1
Uterus	T10–L1

[1]These travel with sympathetic fibres and pass by way of sympathetic ganglia to the spinal cord. However, they are *not* sympathetic (efferent) fibres. They are best referred to as visceral nociceptive afferents. *Note*: Parasympathetic afferent fibres may be important in upper abdominal pain (vagal fibres, coeliac plexus).

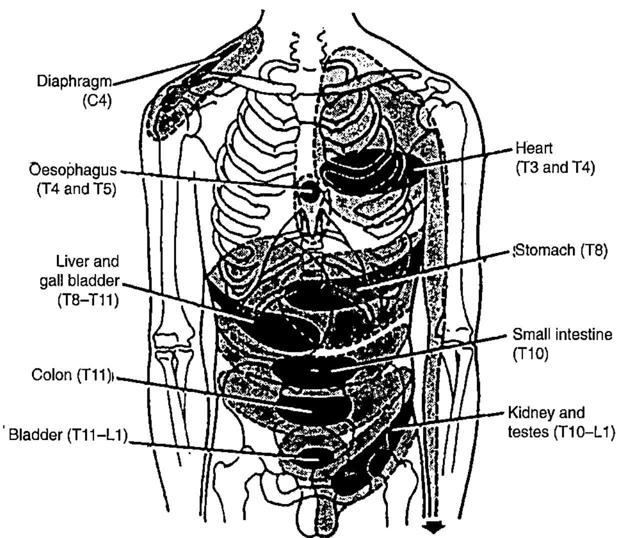

Fig. 19.10 Viscerotomes. Approximate superficial areas to which visceral pain is referred, with related dermatomes in brackets. The dark areas are those most commonly associated with pain in each viscus. The grey areas indicate approximately the larger area that may be associated with pain in that viscus. (Reproduced from Cousins 1987.)

situations the pain and its sequelae become similar to chronic pain. It is not uncommon for such patients to show anger, depression and other characteristics of chronic pain (Bonica 1985, Cousins & Phillips 1986). Thus one should be wary of drawing too sharp a distinction between acute and chronic pain: as acute pain persists, more emphasis may need to be placed on psychological in addition to physical and pharmacological approaches to treatment. An increasingly important role of acute pain services is to identify patients with emerging chronic pain problems. In many situations such patients can be identified by 2–3 weeks post surgery or trauma. However, a clear diagnosis may require assessment of the relative roles of physical, psychological and environmental factors.

PAIN MANAGEMENT: CLINICAL ISSUES

SPINAL ADMINISTRATION OF AGENTS

The elucidation of the types of receptors present pre- and postsynaptically around nociceptive transmission neurons in the dorsal horn has led to the use of spinal drug administration as a pain management technique. The application of relatively low doses of agents acting at specific receptor types within the spinal cord with the relative avoidance of side effects has been a major advance in the management of some pain problems.

Although their use is largely experimental at this stage, the availability of spinal drug administration has led to interest in the use of agents which are not traditionally considered for use by the spinal route. NSAIDs have an action at the glycine receptor of the NMDA receptor complex and tricyclic antidepressants also have an action at a receptor within the NMDA complex. Both types of agents have been administered by the spinal route with some success.

PRE-EMPTIVE ANALGESIA

The discovery of the changes associated with the phenomenon of central sensitization has led to attempts to prevent these changes occurring. It has been demonstrated that early postoperative pain is a significant predictor of long-term pain (Katz et al 1996). It was hoped that steps which would reduce or abolish noxious input to the spinal cord during a painful event such as surgery would reduce or minimize spinal cord changes and thereby lead to reduced pain postoperatively and in the long term. However, it is still not known what duration or degree of noxious input is required before these long-term changes occur.

It is also not known how much these long-term changes are dependent on the afferent barrage during surgery and how much they are dependent on continuing inputs from the wound after surgery. At both stages there will be sustained noxious input and therefore both stages have the capacity to produce central sensitization. However, it would be expected that intervention which pre-empts central sensitization and seeks to prevent it occurring, rather than attempts to treat it after it has occurred, would be more successful.

This concept has led to an increasing interest in the use of pre-emptive analgesia. Local anaesthetics, opioids and NSAIDs have been used alone or in combination and have been administered locally, epidurally, intrathecally or systemically. They have also been administered pre-, intra- and postoperatively. There have been many trials that have purported to show that pre-emptive analgesia results in reduced pain, decreased analgesic requirements, improved morbidity and decreased hospital stay (for reviews see Dahl & Kehlet 1993, Woolf & Chong 1993). However the variability in agent, and timing and method of administration, as well as differences in the type of surgery and anaesthetic procedures, has made it difficult to compare trials which examine the effectiveness of pre-emptive analgesia. There have also been several problems with the design of these studies that has made it difficult to draw definite conclusions concerning outcomes. Therefore despite studies which appear to indicate the advantages of pre-emptive analgesia, the logical appeal of this approach and its ready application to the clinical arena, two recent reviews (Dahl & Kehlet 1993, Woolf & Chong 1993) both conclude that further trials are necessary before a definitive statement can be made regarding its benefits and advantages.

Most studies have focused on the effect of pre-emptive analgesia in reducing pain in the early postoperative period. However pre-emptive analgesia may also be important in reducing the incidence of chronic pain. One study which has generated interest was the finding by Bach and colleagues (1988) that preoperative epidural blockade of patients undergoing lower limb amputation resulted in a lower incidence of phantom limb pain at 6 and 12 months following surgery when compared to the control group which had intraoperative block alone. Although it has been pointed out that there are several inadequacies in the design of this study (Dahl & Kehlet 1993), it does demonstrate that pre-emptive analgesia may have the potential to prevent the development of chronic pain states and further studies should be carried out to address this important question. A second study reports that the degree of pain after thoracic surgery predicts long-term post-thoracotomy pain (Katz et al 1996).

CONCLUSION

There has been substantial progress in our understanding of pain mechanisms in recent years. Our understanding of the pharmacology and physiology of nociceptive processes and the identification of neurotransmitters and pathways involved in nociceptive transmission has led to the development of new agents and more effective use of agents that were previously available. The recognition and characterization of nervous system changes that occur with pain has also had a profound influence on our conceptualization of pain and indicates the potential that exists to modify or prevent the development of chronic pain states, by managing acute pain more effectively and in different ways.

ACUTE PAIN AND MULTIMODAL ANALGESIA

There is now good evidence that patients benefit from the use of multimodal, or balanced, analgesia after surgery. NSAIDs, paracetamol, local anaesthetics, other non-opioid analgesics and opioids are employed in combination to improve pain relief (Kehlet & Dahl 1993a, b). Multimodal analgesia employs a variety of drugs, given perhaps by different routes, to achieve analgesia, with a reduction in the incidence and severity of side effects (Kehlet 1989, 1997). For example, the addition of regular postoperative injections of the NSAID ketorolac to a regimen previously based on intercostal nerve blocks and patient controlled (PCA) morphine significantly improved analgesia after thoracotomy (Power et al 1994). Non-opioid analgesics contribute significantly to multimodal analgesia and postoperative recovery of the patient by minimizing opioid side effects including the inevitable opioid-induced gastrointestinal stasis that delays the resumption of normal enteral nutrition after surgery. After bowel surgery multimodal analgesia comprising epidural analgesia using a mixture of local anaesthetics and low-dose opioid provides excellent analgesia and hastens the rate of recovery of gastrointestinal function after surgery of the colon, especially if systemic NSAIDs are used to avoid the need for opioid administration after the epidural has been ceased (Liu et al 1995a).

It is possible to eliminate pain after surgery using multimodal analgesia with a significant reduction in total opioid consumption (Schulze et al 1988, Dahl et al 1990). However the effect on morbidity and mortality has been disappointing in some studies (Moiniche et al 1994a), demonstrating that very good pain control is not automatically associated with an improvement in outcome. Recent research has suggested, however, that the use of multimodal analgesia after major surgery may improve recovery and thus reduce costs (Brodner et al 1998). Kehlet has proposed that the 'pain free state' should be employed as a fundamental component of an aggressive regimen of postoperative mobilization and early oral feeding in a process of acute rehabilitation after surgery (Kehlet & Dahl 1993a). Clearly, multimodal analgesia employing non-opioids to minimize opioid requirements has the particular advantage over unimodal systemic opioid administration of providing excellent pain relief upon movement allowing early mobilization. In addition, by using non-opioids as part of a balanced analgesic plan, the patient can return to normal enteral nutrition much more quickly by avoiding the undesirable opioid problems of gastrointestinal stasis and nausea and vomiting (Moiniche et al 1994a, b, Bardram et al 1995).

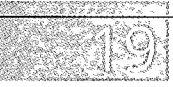

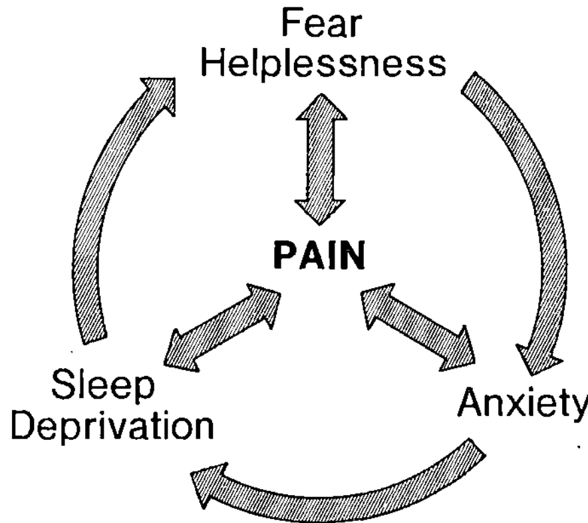

Fig. 19.11 Vicious circle of pain, anxiety, fear, helplessness, sleep deprivation. If pain persists unrelieved for several days, anger and depression also begin to contribute to the vicious circle as patients become demoralized and lose confidence in the ability (and motivation) of their medical attendants to relieve their pain. Sleeplessness compounds the problem.

PSYCHOLOGICAL FACTORS AND ACUTE PAIN

PSYCHOLOGICAL RESPONSE

Severe pain can cause a number of changes in an individual's behaviour, including increased self absorption and concern, withdrawal from interpersonal contact, and an increased sensitivity to external stimuli such as light and sound. Fear and anxiety are the major emotional concomitants of acute pain and are especially pronounced when associated with fear of death. When pain is prolonged and unrelieved, the sufferer may express a range of emotions including anger and resentment, especially if it is believed that pain relief is being withheld. It is important to recognize that severe acute pain which remains unrelieved for days on end may lead to depression and helplessness as a result of patients experiencing a loss of control over their environment (Fig. 19.11). It is now generally agreed that unrelieved severe acute pain exacerbates premorbid tendencies for anxiety, hostility, depression or preoccupation with health. In a few cases, the inability to cope with pain may create an acute psychotic reaction (Peck 1986). Acute pain is one of the important factors contributing to the development of delirium in the intensive care unit. Intensive care units and surgical high-dependency wards can introduce a number of factors which may increase patients' susceptibility to acute pain (Cousins & Phillips 1986): sleep deprivation and abnormal sleep patterns; excessive noise (peak levels approximating those of heavy traffic); disturbing sounds; unguarded conversations; lack of communication; preoccupation of staff with equipment; lack of windows and associated deprivation of day–night cycles; deprivation of information on seasonal and weather conditions; disturbances of visual and auditory vigilance; inability to concentrate; increased boredom, and depression. Reporting a case of postoperative psychosis following massive facial surgery, Cranin and Sher (1979) observed: 'when one is undiverted pain hurts more, fear becomes more intense, the usual conscious control mechanisms fall away'.

It should be acknowledged that much of the literature on the psychological response to acute pain has been gained from the experimental laboratory using various types of experimental pain. An important challenge remains for more clinical psychologists to come into the clinical setting where various types of acute pain are experienced by patients.

PSYCHOLOGICAL FACTORS AFFECTING THE ACUTE PAIN RESPONSE

In both the clinical setting and the laboratory, large individual differences in responsiveness to noxious stimuli are well documented. Psychological factors affecting the pain response are summarized in Box 19.7. The clinical observations by Beecher (1946) of wounded soldiers were the first clear description of individual differences in pain response to acute injury. He reported that 65% of soldiers who were severely wounded in battle felt little or no pain. He attributed this to the positive meaning of the situation, because being wounded meant that the individual was still alive and would be taken back to the safety of a hospital and then possibly sent home. The meaning of the situation may also be important in civilian surgery. For example, civilian surgical teams visiting developing countries comment on the lack of requirement for postoperative pain medication in many patients who are treated by these teams. Presumably this is because the opportunity to have corrective surgery is viewed by the patients in a very positive sense. However, in developed parts of the world it has also been documented that approximately 20% of civilians who undergo major surgery feel very little pain after the operation (quoted in Peck 1986). In a study of patients in an emergency unit, 30% did not feel pain at the time of injury and some experienced delays of up to 9 hours before the onset of pain. Melzack et al (1982) concluded: 'Clearly the link between injury and pain is highly variable: injury may occur without pain and pain without injury'. There is now considerable evidence that a substantial proportion of the variance in pain response is due to psychological factors. As indicated in Box 19.7, many factors have some effect on the experience of acute pain, such as the anxiety state of the patient, which seems to be particularly important in patients who were inadequately prepared psychologically and who experience a great deal of uncertainty and fear (Averill 1973). Unfortunately, the majority of studies have investigated the effect of differences in patients' characteristics on acute pain response. The effects of situational or environmental variables have been shown to be important, as exemplified by the powerful effect of anxiety and perceived control over the situation (Peck 1986). Another important area of investigation has been the interaction between individual and situational variables, such as the interaction between coping style and the control the patient has over the situation (Andrew 1970).

A detailed analysis of the psychological factors affecting the acute pain response (Box 19.7) has been made by Peck (1986). She observes that anxiety is the psychological variable which is most reliably related to high levels of pain. Fear of death and general anxiety about bodily well-being are probably the most pervasive and intense emotions known to mankind. Circumstances associated with acute postoperative pain, trauma pain and other situations of acute pain are probably some of the most potent in aggravating such fears. Fear of the unknown is also a major component of the general anxiety which patients experience. The routine of a postoperative ward or intensive therapy unit will continue to be stressful to patients (Cousins & Phillips 1986). Hospitalization itself produces many threats, including possible disability, loss of life, coping with a new situation, loss of normal freedom and separation from one's family and normal routine (Johnson 1980).

BOX 19.7

Psychological factors affecting pain response

- Cultural differences
- Observational learning (modelling)
- Cognitive appraisal (meaning of pain)
- Fear and anxiety
- Neuroticism and extroversion
- Perceived control of events
- Coping style
- Attention/distraction

Some patients may interpret the use of sophisticated monitoring equipment as implying that their situation is one of imminent disaster (Cousins 1970). The anxiety experienced by family members is often transferred directly to the patient and serves to reinforce or reactivate his or her own fears.

Some important implications for treatment have arisen from knowledge of the psychological factors affecting the acute pain response:

1. Measures to reduce anxiety levels have an important bearing on the acute pain experienced by patients and their need for pain treatment (Egbert et al 1964, Fortin & Kirovac 1976, Chapman & Cox 1977, Peck 1986).
2. Approaches which give patients more control are likely to be successful in reducing anxiety and decreasing the requirement for pain and medication. Patient-controlled analgesia (PCA) is a highly successful example.
3. The relief of acute pain is likely to reduce the risks of unwanted psychological sequelae, such as depression, poor motivation to return to normal activities, antipathy towards further surgical procedures and, in some situations, psychotic reactions.

Psychological methods for reducing pain have been discussed by Peck (1986) and Melzack (1988). Some of these methods are summarized in Box 19.8. It is worth emphasizing that placebo and expectation effects can sometimes play a very powerful role. One aspect of these effects is the patient's confidence and belief that the healthcare professional will be able to provide pain relief, and clearly such a placebo response is augmented by a positive doctor–patient or nurse–patient relationship (Dimatteo & DiNicola 1982). Studies suggest that the initial relief experienced in a new situation may be an important determinant of future relief, because the patient's expectations may be conditioned at that time. On the other hand, inadequate relief may condition a negative expectation which could adversely affect

BOX 19.8

Psychological methods for reducing pain

- Placebo and expectation
- Psychological support
- Procedural and instructional information
- Sensory information
- Filmed modelling
- Relaxation training
- Cognitive coping strategies
- Stress inoculation

later pain control. This indicates the importance of providing adequate pain control as quickly as possible and conveying the expectation that the pain control procedures will continue to provide effective pain relief (Voudoris & Peck 1985).

PATHOPHYSIOLOGY AND COMPLICATIONS OF UNRELIEVED ACUTE PAIN

In general, severe acute pain results in abnormally enhanced versions of the physiological and psychological responses described above. Such responses set up pronounced reflex changes which result in so-called vicious circles with progressively increasing pathophysiology. If this situation is allowed to continue, it may result in significant dysfunction in a substantial number of organ systems which may progress to organ damage and even failure. We must also now include pathophysiology in the nervous system itself leading to severe persistent pain (Fig. 19.7). Thus it is possible for acute severe unrelieved pain to result in significant morbidity and even mortality.

Treatment should be instituted before or during the period of functional impairment resulting from the pathophysiology of acute severe pain. Clearly, there is a critical time interval before morbidity such as atelectasis or pneumonia ensues (see below). Most of the information concerning the pathophysiology of acute pain has been obtained in patients following surgery. However, the information is also applicable to patients who have been injured in motor vehicle accidents and other situations of acute trauma.

RESPIRATORY SYSTEM

After surgery or trauma to the chest or abdominal region, respiratory dysfunction is the most common and most important result of the pain that is associated with such situations. Involuntary spinal reflex responses to the noxious input from the injured area result in reflex muscle spasm in the immediate region of the tissue injury, as well as in muscle groups cephalad and caudad to the injury site. This is not surprising when one considers that nociceptive afferents commonly travel two to three segments above or below their site of entry into the tract of Lissauer before synapsing in the dorsal horn. The patient's appreciation of pain may also result in voluntary reduction of muscle movement in the thorax and abdominal area. The end result is often described in the clinical setting as 'muscle splinting', which means muscle contraction on either side of the injured area in an attempt to 'splint' the area to prevent movement, comparable to the way one would apply an external splint to a fractured bone (Fig. 19.12). This splinting is often associated with partial closure of the glottis, which produces a 'grunting' sound during breathing. The glottic closure is probably part of a primitive response which permits an increase in intra-abdominal and intrathoracic pressure, associated with muscle spasm, to brace the individual against an impending injury.

Such a response becomes totally inappropriate in a patient who has received corrective surgery, or whose trauma has been effectively treated. The pattern of ventilation is illustrated in Figure 19.13, where the small tidal volume and high inspiratory and expiratory pressures are seen in association with acute pain. In addition to decreased tidal volume, there are decreases in vital capacity, functional residual capacity (FRC) and alveolar ventilation. FRC may become less than the volume at which small airway closure occurs. The potential for this problem is exaggerated in elderly patients, smokers and those with respiratory disease. This situation progresses to regional lung collapse (atelectasis), associated with considerable impairment of pulmonary gas exchange as a result of alteration of the relationship between ventilation and perfusion of the lung (V/Q inequality) leading to hypoxaemia. The low volume of ventilation also causes hypercarbia and contributes to the hypoxaemia. As a result of the muscle splinting, the patient is unable to cough and clear secretions, and this contributes to lobular or lobar collapse (Craig 1981). Infection often follows this situation, leading to pneumonia. Inability to cooperate with chest physiotherapy further complicates treatment and greatly prolongs the course of pulmonary complications and in turn prolongs hospital stay.

It is not commonly recognized that elderly patients and those in poor general condition may suffer pulmonary complications following lower abdominal and peripheral limb surgery, as a result of unrelieved severe pain which causes them to become immobile, resulting in a hypostatic pneumo-

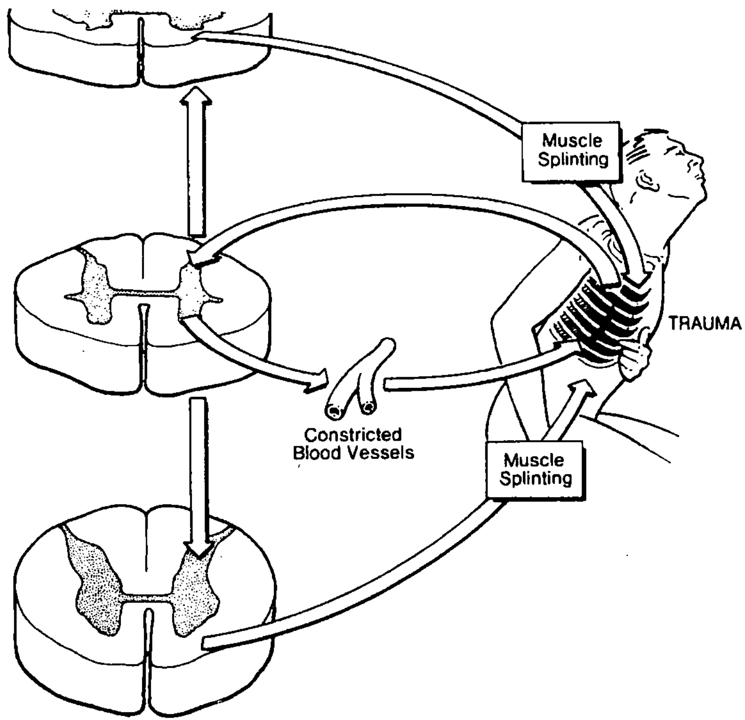

Fig. 19.12 Some effects of postoperative pain. Surgery or trauma may result in a vicious circle of pain–muscle spasm–increased sympathetic activity and other reflex changes. Note that interneuronal activity increases several segments above and below pain stimulus. This may result in widespread increase in motor and sympathetic activity. Increased motor activity results in muscle spasm, causing further stimulus at the site of pain stimulus and more pain. Increased sympathetic activity releases noradrenaline, which sensitizes pain receptors. Local microcirculatory vasospasm results in changes in local pH and release of algogenic substances, further increasing pain. These vicious circles can be broken by peripheral (intercostal) or epidural neural blockade. (Reproduced from Cousins & Phillips 1986 with permission.)

nia, initially at the base of the lung. This was demonstrated by Modig (1976), who reported on a group of elderly patients following total hip replacement. Those patients who were managed with routine intramuscular opioids had low tidal volumes and high respiratory rates associated with hypoxaemia. It seemed likely that the hypoxaemia was due to immobility and other adverse reflexes resulting from pain, because patients who were managed with epidural analgesia, and were completely pain free, did not show these abnormalities in pulmonary function (Fig. 19.13).

Recent basic and clinical studies have demonstrated a 'viscerosomatic' reflex involving the diaphragm, with changes in amplitude and pattern of diaphragm activity in response to noxious visceral stimuli. This can be blocked by epidural bupivacaine (Mankikian et al 1988).

The classic clinical picture of the patient with unrelieved severe pain and impending respiratory failure is as follows: obvious splinting of abdominal and thoracic muscles; grunting on expiration, and small tidal volume and very rapid respiratory rate. Unfortunately, this is a very inefficient and energy-consuming method of respiration and may result in a high oxygen consumption which is not matched by an increase in cardiac output. This may cause excessive desaturation of mixed venous blood which will contribute to hypoxaemia (Bowler et al 1986). Impressive correction of the majority of these abnormalities in pulmonary function can be obtained with effective pain relief associated with epidural block (Bowler et al 1986, Scott 1988). The cumulative evidence of many clinical trials, when subjected to meta-analysis, has confirmed the superiority of epidural over systemic opioid administration in minimizing postoperative pulmonary morbidity (Fig. 19.14).

CARDIOVASCULAR SYSTEM

It is generally agreed that severe acute pain results in sympathetic overactivity with increases in heart rate, peripheral resistance, blood pressure and cardiac output. The end result is an increase in cardiac work and myocardial oxygen consumption. Because heart rate is greatly increased, diastolic filling time is decreased and this may result in reduced oxygen delivery to the myocardium. Thus an imbalance results between myocardial oxygen demand and oxygen

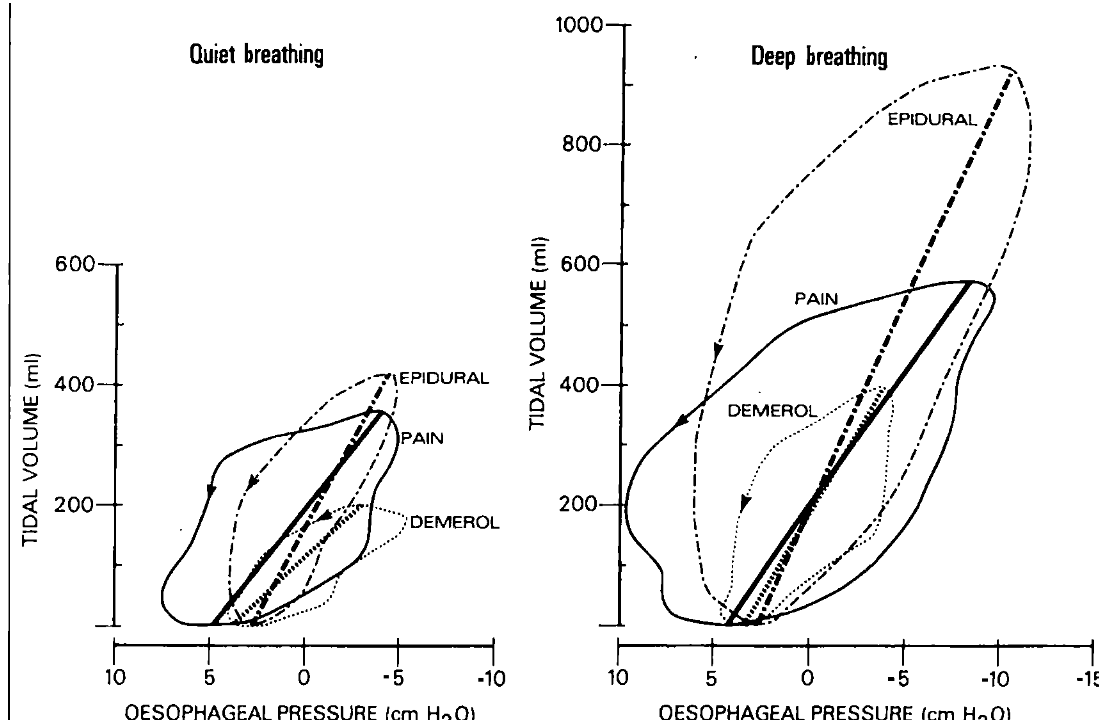

Fig. 19.13 Effect of pain and analgesia on thoracic pressure–volume relationships. Pressure–volume loops are shown 2–6 h after cholecystectomy during quiet breathing and deep breathing. Pain is associated with decreased tidal volume, which is marked when deep breathing is attempted. During expiration there is high positive pressure, particularly during deep breathing. Such high pressure would be associated with glottic closure, abdominal splinting and grunting type of respiration. Demerol decreases tidal volume but also decreases the high pressure during expiration, thus grunting diminishes, an apparent and deceptive improvement. Epidural blockade increases tidal volume, particularly during deep breathing. This is achieved with much lower positive pressure during expiration, and would be accompanied by elimination of grunting and abdominal splinting. A tidal volume of close to 1000 ml would be associated with effective coughing. (Reproduced from Bromage 1978 with permission.)

supply, with a resultant risk of hypoxaemia. Also, it is now known that α receptors in the coronary vasculature may respond to intense sympathetic stimulation by producing coronary vasoconstriction. The end result of this pathophysiology may be myocardial ischaemia associated with anginal pain and even myocardial infarction. The potential for this situation is increased in patients with pre-existing coronary artery disease (Bowler et al 1986, Scott 1988). Anginal pain is associated with increased anxiety, further increases in circulating catecholamines and further potential for coronary artery constriction.

The effects of postoperative pain on cardiovascular variables have been demonstrated by Sjögren and Wright (1972) and are summarized in Figure 19.15. That the cardiovascular changes were predominantly due to noxious stimuli is illustrated by the effect of epidural analgesia in preventing and reversing these abnormalities (Sjögren & Wright 1972, Hoar & Hickey 1976, Kumar & Hibbert 1984). There is impressive evidence from animal studies that noxious stimulation results in coronary artery vasoconstriction and potential for myocardial ischaemia.

Prevention of these noxious stimuli with thoracic epidural analgesia greatly improves the oxygen supply to the myocardium and reduces the myocardial ischaemic insult (Vik-Mo et al 1978, Klassen et al 1980). These findings have recently been supported by evidence in man of a lesser incidence of myocardial ischaemic episodes intraoperatively when noxious stimuli are impeded by epidural blockade (Reiz et al 1982). There is a decreased incidence of postoperative cardiovascular complications when effective pain relief is provided by epidural block (Yeager et al 1987). In this study by Yeager et al there was an overall decrease in mortality associated with effective pain relief produced by epidural blockade compared with conventional and less effective methods of pain relief. A recent study has shown that there is an increase in myocardial ischaemia upon cessation of epidural analgesia in patients who have had aortic surgery (Garnett et al 1996). Acute anginal pain in non-surgical patients can be relieved with thoracic epidural block and, at the same time, blood flow in 'at risk' myocardium is improved by increasing the diameter of stenosed coronary artery segments (Blomberg et al 1990).

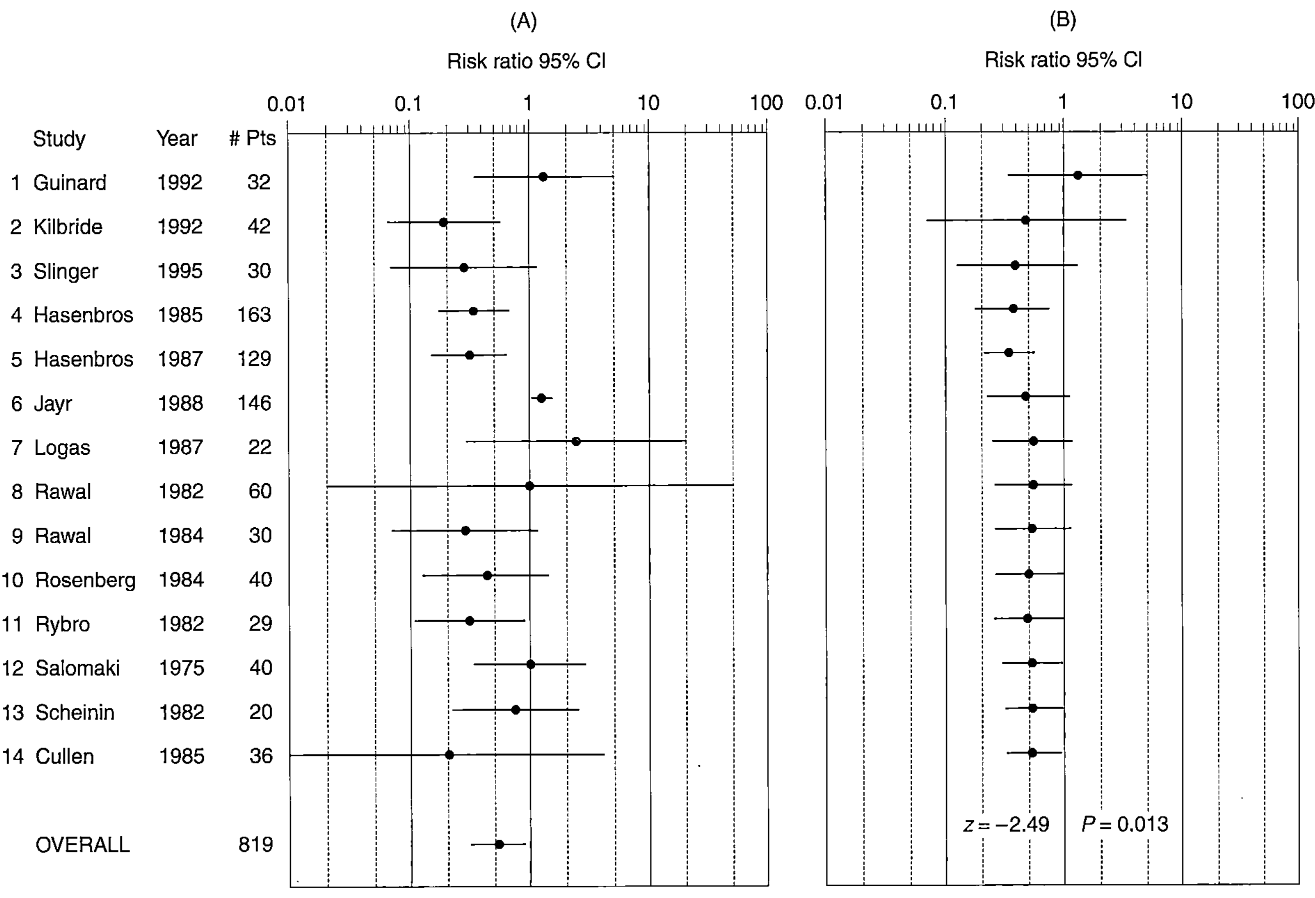

Fig. 19.14 Risk ratios and confidence intervals (CI) for postoperative pulmonary dysfunction in randomized controlled trials of epidural opioid versus intramuscular as-needed opioid, intravenous opioid by continuous infusion or patient-controlled intravenous opioid bolus doses. **A** Results from individual trials. **B** Estimates obtained by stepwise accumulation of results from successive trials. (Reproduced from Ballantyne et al 1997.)

It is important to realize that there is evidence that other analgesics can reduce the incidence of myocardial ischaemia after surgery. In a recent study of patients having elective hip or knee arthroplasty, Beattie et al found that the addition of a continuous infusion of ketorolac (5 mg/hour for 24 hours) to a PCA morphine regimen reduced pain scores and arterial blood pressure, heart rate and the duration of myocardial ischaemia (Beattie et al 1997). It is not clear whether this is a benefit of improved analgesia per se, a consequence of NSAID inhibition of thromboxane production, or an intrinsic effect on the heart.

In the peripheral circulation, acute pain is associated with decreased limb blood flow and this can be particularly serious in patients undergoing vascular grafting procedures. Relief of pain with epidural blockade results in a reversal of reductions in blood flow associated with surgical trauma and acute pain (Cousins & Wright 1971), and in an improved outcome (Tuman et al 1991). Severe postoperative pain and high levels of sympathetic activity may be associated with reduced arterial inflow and decreased venous emptying (Modig et al 1980). In association with changes in blood coagulability and immobility of patients, this may lead to venous thrombosis and pulmonary embolism (Modig et al 1983). Although increased sympathetic activity due to pain would be expected to reduce renal blood flow and also hepatic blood flow, data documenting such changes in patients with pain have not been obtained.

MUSCULOSKELETAL SYSTEM

As noted above, segmental and suprasegmental motor activity in response to pain results in muscle spasm which may further increase pain, thus setting up a vicious circle. This vicious circle may also activate marked increases in sympathetic activity, which further increases the sensitivity

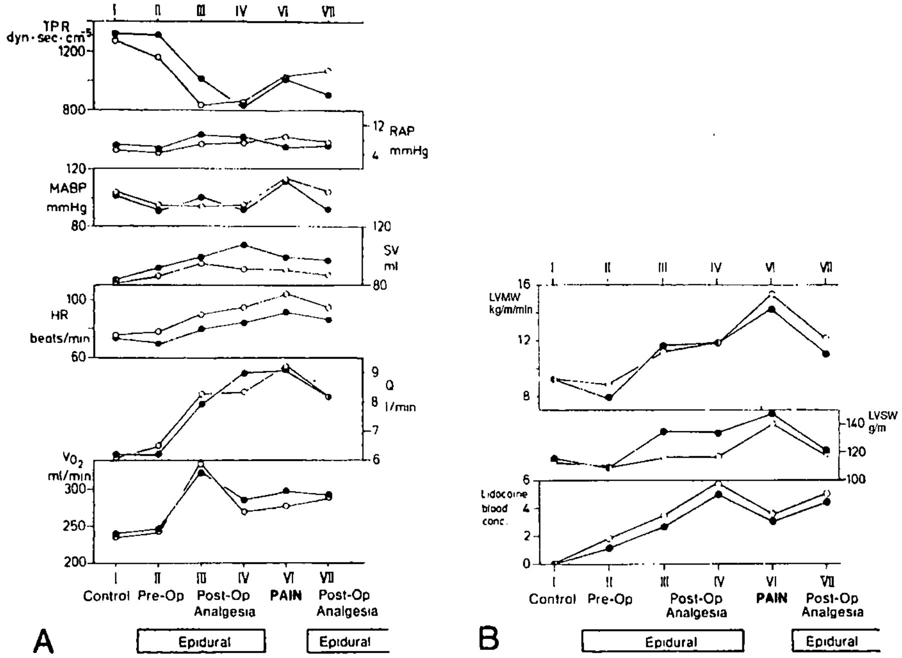

Fig. 19.15 Effect of epidural block on cardiovascular sequelae of severe pain. 1 = Period of control cardiovascular measurements; II = 30 min after epidural injection of 2% lidocaine either in the lumbar region (15 ml) (open circles) or thoracic region (8 ml) (closed circles); III = 1 h after cholecystectomy, analgesia maintained with 0.4% lidocaine drip; IV = on the morning after surgery, after 17 h of continuous pain relief by epidural; V (not shown) = pain returning, when epidural drip ceased for 30–60 min; VI = 60–90 min after epidural drip ceased, severe pain present; VII = 90 min after pain relief re-established by epidural drip. In both A and B: open circles = lumbar epidural, closed circles = thoracic epidural. **A** Changes in total peripheral resistance (TPR); right atrial pressure (RAP); mean arterial blood pressure (MABP); stroke volume (SV); heart rate (HR); cardiac output (Q); oxygen uptake (Vo_2). **B** Changes in left ventricular minute work (LVMW); left ventricular stroke work (LVSW); and lidocaine venous blood concentrations. Note: in A and B, pain is associated with increased TPR, MABP, HR and Q. As well as increased LVMW and LVSW. Pain relief by the thoracic epidural route restored all these variables to levels close to those prior to the emergence of pain. (Reproduced from Sjögren & Wright 1972 with permission.)

of peripheral nociceptors. This situation can result in widespread disturbances, even in patients with relatively localized nociceptive foci in the long bones or other areas of the bony skeleton. Recent data indicate that persistent postoperative pain and limitation of movement may be associated with marked impairment of muscle metabolism, muscle atrophy and significantly delayed normal muscle function. These changes appear to be due to pain and reflex vasoconstriction, and possibly reflex responses which can be at least partly reversed by the relief of pain with epidural analgesia. Patients managed in this manner appear to have a much quicker return to normal function (Bonica 1985).

GASTROINTESTINAL AND GENITOURINARY SYSTEMS

Increased sympathetic activity increases intestinal secretions and smooth muscle sphincter tone, whereas it decreases intestinal motility. Gastric stasis and even paralytic ileus may occur. These changes are at least partly related to severe pain and a resultant increase in sympathetic activity. However, recent data indicate that the administration of opioid analgesic drugs may also make a significant contribution to delayed gastric emptying (Nimmo 1984). There is some evidence that pain relief with neural blockade may reduce the transit time of X-ray contrast media through the gut, from up to 150 hours in a control group to 35 hours in a group receiving epidural analgesia (Ahn et al 1988).

There is also evidence that the pain-related impairment of intestinal motility may be relieved by epidural local anaesthetic but not by epidural opioid (Scheinin et al 1987, Thoren et al 1989, Wattwil et al 1989, Thorn et al 1992, Liu et al 1995a, b).

Interestingly, there is good evidence that the systemic, intravenous, administration of lignocaine speeds the return of bowel function after radical prostatectomy, as well as reducing pain and shortening hospital stay (Groudine et al 1998).

Increased sympathetic activity also results in increased urinary sphincter activity which may result in urinary retention. Once again the precise role of pain in this situation is difficult to assess, because the administration of opioid analgesic drugs may result in a significant incidence of urinary retention.

GENERAL STRESS RESPONSE TO ACUTE INJURY

Surgery and other forms of trauma generate a catabolic state by changes in endocrine hormonal control with increased secretion of catabolic hormones and decreased secretion or action of anabolic hormones. The results for the patient include: pain; nausea, vomiting and intestinal stasis; alterations in blood flow, coagulation and fibrinolysis; alterations in substrate metabolism; alterations in water and electrolyte handling by the body; increased demands on the cardiovascular and respiratory systems. This stress response to surgery and trauma, together with the modifying effects of analgesics, has been discussed recently by Kehlet (1996, 1998) and Liu et al (1995b).

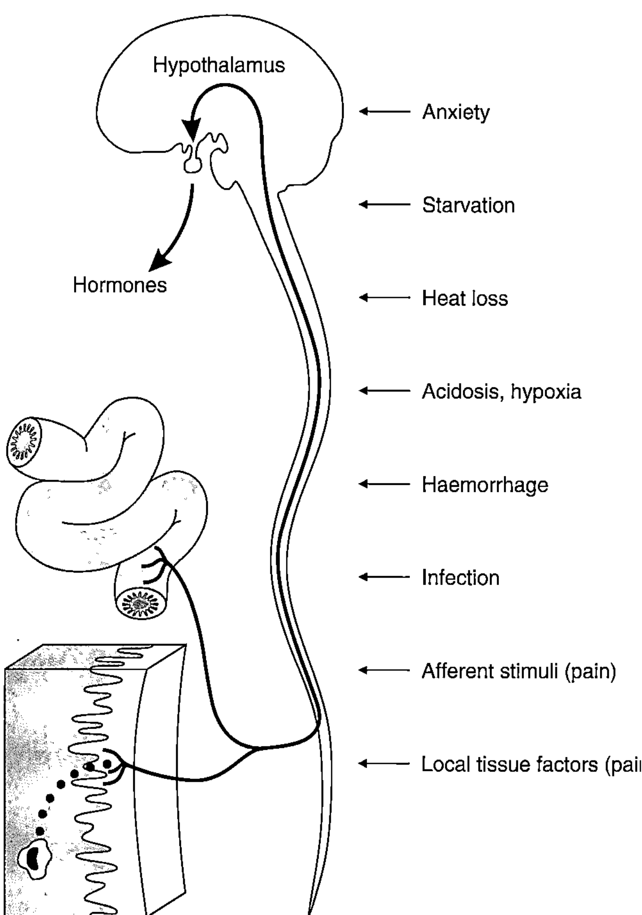

Fig. 19.16 Release mechanisms of the endocrine metabolic response to surgery. The principal mechanisms are afferent neural stimuli (arrows on right) due to noxious surgical/trauma stimuli and local tissue factors released at the trauma site; both of these categories of stimuli may be associated with pain. Interleukin 1 black dots is released from circulating macrophages and forms part of the 'inflammatory soup' that sensitizes nociceptors. Secondary amplifiers of the response are psychological factors (e.g., anxiety), starvation, heat loss, acidosis, hypoxia, haemorrhage and infection. Noxious stimuli from viscera (e.g. gut) travel via visceral nociceptive afferents (via sympathetic ganglia) and contribute to the trauma stimuli, and local tissue factors are also involved. Central responses to afferent stimuli involve hypothalamus and other CNS areas mediating the efferent humoral and neural components of the endocrine-metabolic response. (Reproduced from Cousins & Bridenbaugh 1998 with permission.)

The responses to surgical and other trauma may be divided into two phases. The initial acute 'ebb' or 'shock phase' is characterized by a hypodynamic state, a reduction in metabolic rate and depression of most physiological processes. With surgical trauma this phase is either absent or very transient during the operative period.

The second phase is the hyperdynamic or 'flow phase', which may last for a few days or weeks depending on the magnitude of the surgical or traumatic insult or on the occurrence of complications. Characteristically in this phase, metabolic rate and cardiac output are elevated (Kehlet 1998). There is some evidence that nociceptive impulses play an important part in the ebb phase and in the early part of the flow phase. However, there are a substantial number of other factors which contribute to initiation of the stress response (Fig. 19.16), and it seems likely that these play an increasingly important part in the flow phase. This is an important area for investigation, because clinical experience indicates that the major benefits from the relief of severe postoperative pain with potent techniques may be obtained in the first 48 h following surgery (Cousins & Phillips 1986).

A summary of the endocrine and metabolic changes which are elicited by surgical trauma is given in Box 19.9. It should be emphasized that it is assumed that nociceptive stimuli originating from the surgically traumatized area are partly responsible for these responses. However, it is almost certain that other factors, such as those presented in Figure 19.16, contribute. Although the precise contribution of pain has not been defined, it is clear that the changes in energy metabolism and substrate flow are predominantly determined by the injury response. The intensity of the stress response to surgery is in general related to the degree to tissue trauma (but see above). Thus procedures of short duration on the body surface and other minor procedures evoke a slight and transient response, whereas procedures involving the thorax and abdominal cavity elicit a more pronounced response in which the flow phase may last up to several days or weeks if there are complications. A detailed description of the endocrine metabolic response to surgery and trauma has been provided by Kehlet (1998) and Wilmore (1983). The role of different factors in modifying the stress response is also reviewed by Kehlet (1996, 1998) and Liu et al (1995b).

The specific role of nociceptive stimuli in initiating the injury response was first raised by the hypothesis of anoci-association, which suggested that disruption of nociceptive stimuli by neural blockade might favourably affect post-traumatic outcome (Crile 1910). In contrast to this proposal was the demonstration by Cannon (1939) of the importance of the sympathetic nervous system in maintaining homeostasis in response to a variety of stresses such as fluid deprivation, haemorrhage and cold. The theory of anoci-association was supported by experimental studies, which demonstrated that spinal anaesthesia given before injury reduced the mortality due to blunt hind limb trauma (O'Shaughnessey & Slome 1934). This was supported by classic studies by Hume and Egdahl (1959), demonstrating the importance of the peripheral as well as the central nervous system in mediating the adrenocortical responses to trauma.

More recently a large amount of data has indicated that blockade of noxious impulses by local anaesthetic and opioid neural blockade may produce a powerful modification of the responses to surgical injury (Kehlet 1989, 1996, 1998). Neural blockade with local anaesthetics may diminish a predominant part of the physiological response to surgical procedures in the lower abdomen and to procedures on the lower extremities (Table 19.4). This usually occurs in situations where postoperative pain is completely alleviated. The inhibitory effect is much less pronounced during and following major abdominal and thoracic procedures, possibly because of the difficulty in obtaining sufficient afferent neural blockade by the currently available techniques. In order to obtain a pronounced reduction of the surgical stress response, it is necessary to maintain pain relief with continuous epidural analgesia for at least 48–72 hours postoperatively (Kehlet 1989, 1996, 1998, Liu et al 1995b).

Current data indicate that pain relief by epidural or intrathecal administration of opioids is less efficient in reducing the stress response (Liu et al 1995b) (Fig. 19.17). However, studies of mixtures of local anaesthetics and opioids indicate that this combination may be capable of a more potent modification of the stress response. A convincing demonstration of the efficacy of pain relief with epidural blockade in modifying the stress response is the significant improvement in cumulative nitrogen balance that is obtained when pain relief is provided both intra- and postoperatively with continuous epidural neural blockade (Brandt et al 1978) (Fig. 19.18).

Changes in coagulation and fibrinolysis associated with major surgery may be partly modified by pain relief with neural blockade (Jorgensen et al 1991). However, interpretation of these results is complex, because factors other than pain may be involved. Also the absorption of local anaesthetics associated with neural blockade may result in an antithrombotic effect (Kehlet 1998). Encouragingly, a clin-

BOX 19.9

Neuroendocrine and metabolic responses to surgery

Endocrine

Catabolic

Due to increase in: ACTH, cortisol, ADH, GH, catecholamines, renin, angiotensin II, aldosterone, glucagon, interleukin-1

Anabolic

Due to decrease in: insulin, testosterone

Metabolic

Carbohydrate – hyperglycaemia, glucose intolerance, insulin resistance

Due to increase in: hepatic glycogenolysis (epinephrine, glucagon) – gluconeogenesis (cortisol, glucagon, growth hormone, epinephrine, free fatty acids)

Due to decrease in: insulin secretion/action

Protein – muscle protein catabolism, increased synthesis of acute-phase proteins

Due to increase in: cortisol, epinephrine, glucagon, interleukin-1

Fat – increased lipolysis and oxidation

Due to increase in: catecholamines, cortisol, glucagon, growth hormone

Water and electrolyte flux – retention of H_2O and Na^+, increased excretion of K^+, decreased functional extracellular fluid with shifts to intracellular compartments

Due to increase in: catecholamines, aldosterone, ADH, cortisol, angiotensin II, prostaglandins and other factors

Table 19.4 Influence of regional (spinal/epidural) anaesthesia on the endocrine response to lower abdominal (gynaecological) surgery or procedures on the lower extremities.[1] (Data from Kehlet 1982, 1984)

	Intraoperative response	*Postoperative response*
Prolactin	↓	↓
Growth hormone	↓	↓
ACTH	↓	↓
ADH	↓	↓
TSH	?	?
FSH	→	↘
LH	→	↘
Beta-endorphin	↓	?
Cortisol	↓	↓
Aldosterone	↓	↓
Renin	↓	↓
Adrenalin	↓	↓
Norepinephrine	↓	↓
Insulin	↘	↘
C-peptide	↘	↘
Glucagon	?	?
T_3	→	→
T_4	→	→
Testosterone	?	?
Oestradiol	?	?
Glucose	↓	↓
Glucose tolerance	↑	→
Free fatty acids	↓	?
Sodium balance		→
Potassium balance		↑
Water balance		→
Nitrogen balance		↑
Creatinine phosphokinase		↓
Acute phase proteins		→
Oxygen consumption		↓

[1]Continuous epidural analgesia only.
? = No data; ↑ = improvement or normalization (nitrogen balance, glucose tolerance); ↘ = slight inhibition; ↓ = inhibition of response; → = no effect on response; ACTH = adrenocorticotropic hormone; ADH = antidiuretic hormone; TSH = thyroid-stimulating hormone; FSH = follicle-stimulating hormone; LH = luteinizing hormone; T_3 = triiodothyronine; T_4 = tetraiodothyronine.

ical study comparing the effects of epidural and general anaesthesia in peripheral vascular surgery has found that the epidural group needed fivefold fewer repeat operations for graft failure within 1 month (Christopherson et al 1993). Changes in immunocompetence and acute-phase proteins are well documented in association with surgical trauma. Pain relief with neural blockade has a mild influence on various aspects of the surgically induced impairment of immunocompetence. The mechanism has not been completely elucidated, but may be partly explained by the concomitant inhibition of various endocrine metabolic responses. It is currently not clear if the mechanism of this

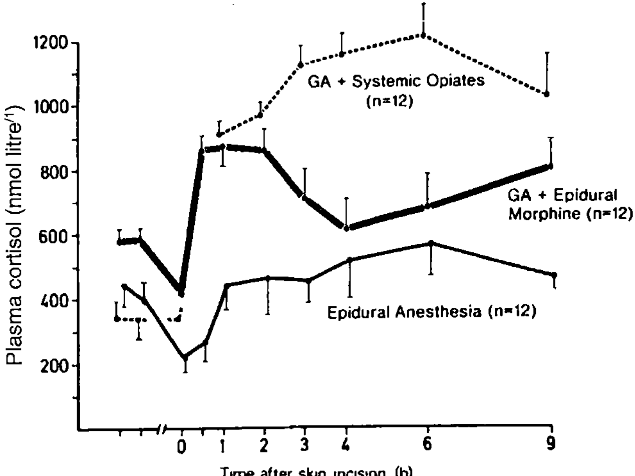

Fig. 19.17 Plasma cortisol: comparison of systemic opiates with epidural local anaesthesia or morphine. In patients receiving general anaesthesia followed by systemic opiates: during surgery (0–2 h), there is a large increase in plasma cortisol which continues into the postoperative period (2–9 h). In patients receiving general anaesthesia followed by epidural morphine: during surgery there is only slight modification of cortisol response; postoperatively cortisol response is modified but not to normal levels. In patients receiving epidural local anaesthesia intra- and postoperatively: plasma cortisol remains unchanged. (Reproduced from Christensen et al 1982 with permission.)

effect is predominantly a result of blockade of nociception. Elucidation of this mechanism is important because post-traumatic immunodepression has been impossible to modulate by other therapeutic measures (Kehlet 1998).

Adverse effects of unrelieved pain are likely to manifest themselves in failure in more than one system, particularly in high-risk surgical patients. This question was examined by Yeager et al (1987) in a controlled study of high-risk patients undergoing major surgery. Patients were randomly assigned to receive general anaesthesia and epidural local anaesthetic during surgery followed by epidural opioid after surgery, or general anaesthesia alone during surgery followed by parenteral opioid postoperatively. The results of the study showed a striking difference in morbidity in several systems and in mortality between the two groups. Although the number of patients studied was rather small, the results are so consistently in favour of the group receiving epidural analgesia that it is unlikely that a Type I error resulted, particularly in view of the powerful randomized, controlled design. Of further interest was the substantial reduction in cost of treatment for the group receiving epidural analgesia. The precise role of pain relief in producing these more favourable results with epidural analgesia is not certain from the results of the study. Intraoperatively, epidural local anaesthesia permitted a reduction in doses of anaesthetic agents and resulted in efferent sympathetic

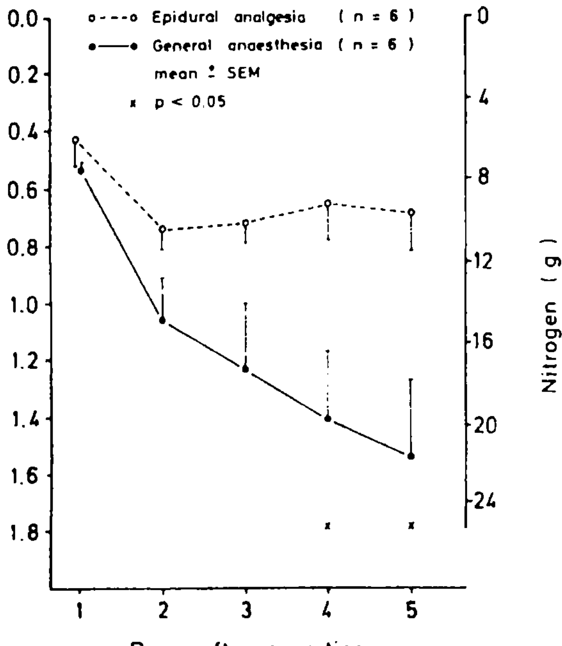

Fig. 19.18 Nitrogen balance: comparison of urinary nitrogen excretion during the initial 5 days after abdominal hysterectomy in patients under general anaesthesia with halothane, or continuous epidural analgesia for 24 h with intermittent injections of plain bupivacaine 0.5%. Sensory level of analgesia was held from T4 to S5. During the 5-day postoperative period, both groups received a hypocaloric oral intake amounting to 20 g of nitrogen and about 2900 calories. Patients receiving epidural analgesia had no intraoperative and postoperative increase in plasma cortisol and glucose, and concomitantly, urinary nitrogen excretion was significantly reduced. (Reproduced from Brandt et al 1978 with permission.)

blockade, in addition to blockade of nociceptive afferents. Postoperatively, however, it is likely that the effects of epidural opioids were predominantly due to pain relief. Unfortunately, corroborative evidence of reduced morbidity and mortality following potent methods of pain relief is hard to find (Scott & Kehlet 1988, Liu et al 1995b).

OTHER FORMS OF ACUTE PAIN

Tissue trauma usually, but not always, results in immediate sharp pain, probably associated with the rapidly conducting Aδ fibres. 'Second' pain then follows, partly due to more slowly arriving impulses in C fibres, but also due to the complex neurochemical events associated with the inflammatory response (Fig. 19.19). In the case of musculoskeletal pain, mechanical factors such as physical distension of joints or fascial compartments may contribute, as may ischaemia. In acute visceral trauma, distension, obstruction, ischaemia, chemical irritation from rupture of viscera into the peritoneal cavity, infection and other factors may also play a part.

Patients with multiple trauma often need assessment and treatment by a number of different specialities because they have pain and injury in different systems. However, their resuscitation, pain relief and overall care is frequently coordinated by specialists in emergency medicine or intensive care; indeed it is often most appropriate for such specialists to maintain knowledge and expertise in pain relief for critically ill patients. There have been major developments in pain management in these settings which have been reviewed by Cousins and Phillips (1986). Algorithms have been developed to help staff in emergency and intensive care departments assess and treat pain in patients who may have multiple acute life-threatening conditions (Fig. 19.20).

Patients with more localized and minor trauma were studied by Melzack et al (1982). The patients presented to an emergency department with simple fractures, dislocations, strains, sprains, lacerations and bruises. Of the 138 patients studied, 37% did not feel pain at the time of injury; of 46 patients with injuries limited to the skin, 53% had a pain-free period, whereas of 86 patients with deep tissue injuries (e.g., fractures, sprains, amputation, bruises, stabs and crushes) only 28% had a pain-free period. Delay periods varied from a few minutes up to several hours (Melzack et al 1982).

Using the McGill Pain Questionnaire, it was found that the sensory scores were similar to those of patients with chronic pain, but the affective scores were lower. The descriptions used were very similar for the types of injury: 'hot' or 'burning' characterized fractures, cuts and bruises; cuts and lacerations had a 'throbbing' or 'beating' quality; sprains or fractures and bruises had a 'sharp' quality (Melzack et al 1982).

In the case of pain following major trauma, it is likely that the injury and pathophysiological response is almost identical to that of postoperative pain. However, there has been only a moderate degree of investigation of this important area. Because of the lack of preparation, suddenness of the injury and associated severe psychological responses, anxiety levels are usually very high; segmental, suprasegmental and cortical responses are extreme and initiate pronounced versions of the changes in various body systems that have been described above (Hume & Egdahl 1959, Wilmore et al 1976, Wilmore 1983). It has been claimed that excessive vasoconstriction may result in splanchnic ischaemia with hypoxic damage, particularly to the gut region; continued pain may result in further vasoconstrictor activity and further initiation of nociceptive impulses. It is

 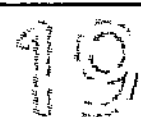

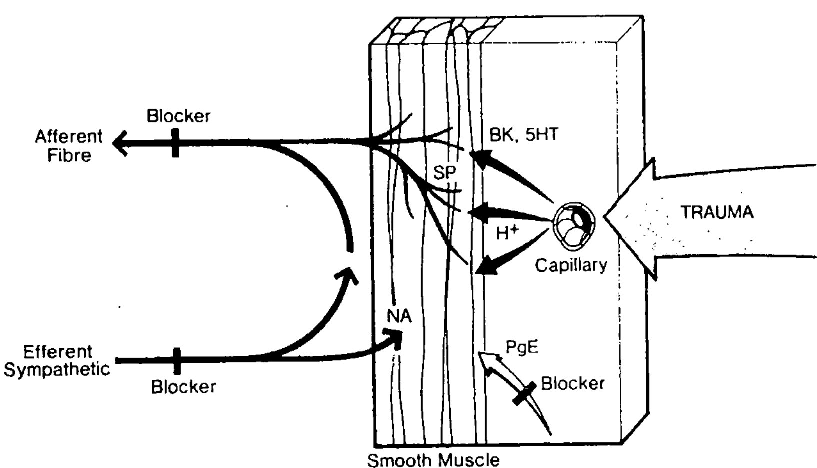

Fig. 19.19 Acute trauma and pain: simplified schema of some proposed mechanisms. Tissue trauma evokes nociceptive afferent activity which travels back to spinal cord. Action potentials also travel antidromatically, by axon collaterals into the surrounding vascular bed to release substance P (SP) which is proposed to cause vasodilatation and increased vascular permeability. The latter results in local oedema and also permits the release of potentially algogenic agents from the circulation, e.g. bradykinin (BK). Some algogenic agents may be derived from traumatized tissue, e.g. potassium (see text). The algogenic agents sensitize sensory afferent terminals, producing a state of hyperalgesia. Prostaglandins (PgE) have a facilitating effect on the algogenic agents. Note also that noradrenaline (NA) release may increase nociceptor sensitivity, further increasing afferent input to spinal cord and initiating reflex increases in sympathetic activity. A vicious circle is signified by the circular arrow from efferent to afferent fibre (this is not a direct neural connection). Increased sympathetic activity may cause vasoconstriction, local tissue ischaemia, increased hydrogen ion (H^+) concentration and further increases in nociceptor sensitivity. Some possible sites of modification of peripheral nociception are depicted by the notation 'Blocker': e.g. afferent fibre blockade by local anaesthetics or modification of local nociceptive activity by depletion of substance P and diverse other options (see text); PgE synthesis blockade by aspirin-like drugs, and efferent sympathetic blockade at the level of sympathetic fibre by local anaesthetics, or at sympathetic terminals by depletion of NA (e.g., guanethidine). (Reproduced from Cousins & Phillips 1986 with permission.)

hypothesized that toxic peptides with vasoactive properties may be released from the gut region and may be responsible for cardiovascular depression. The role of severe unrelieved pain in initiating these postulated events is currently unproven (Bonica 1985).

Acute pancreatitis is an example of an acute medical condition which may be accompanied by severe pain and pronounced abnormal reflex responses. The abdominal pain is usually accompanied by severe abdominal muscle spasm, with a resultant decrease in diaphragmatic movement, and progressive hypoventilation with a potential for hypoxaemia and hypercarbia. The release of pancreatic enzymes and other substances into the peritoneal cavity is associated with severe pain. It is also possible that depressant toxic substances are released which may result in cardiovascular depression and shock. Once again, the precise role of pain in contributing to these events is unclear. There are clinical reports of the relief of pain of acute pancreatitis with epidural local anaesthetics or opioids and an associated improvement in the overall condition of the patient (Cousins & Phillips 1986).

Myocardial infarction produces a disruption of the usual reciprocal relationship between sympathetic and parasympathetic control of cardiac function, frequently with overactivity of both systems. It is likely that these changes are substantially induced by haemodynamic alterations associated with myocardial infarction. However, it is possible that pain and associated increases in sympathetic activity, as well as increases in vagal activity, may contribute to the problem. Sudden changes in vagal activity may result in severe bradycardia, atrioventricular block, peripheral vasodilatation (faint response) and severe hypotension that may progress to cardiogenic shock. As indicated above, experimental evidence in animals (Vik-Mo et al 1978, Klassen et al 1980) and in man (Reiz et al 1982, Yeager et al 1987, Blomberg et al 1990) indicate that epidural neural blockade may substantially modify these adverse effects. It is not known how much of this effect is due to blockade of efferent sympathetic activity and how much is due to blockade of afferent nociceptive impulses from the myocardium. It has recently been reported that the pain of myocardial infarction can be relieved by spinal administration of opioids (Pasqualucci et al 1980), thus it should be possible to dissect out the relative role of pain relief and efferent sympathetic blockade (see also Blomberg et al 1990).

The relief of pain in emergency departments need not be delayed by undue concerns that important symptoms may be masked as a consequence. Indeed the early administra-

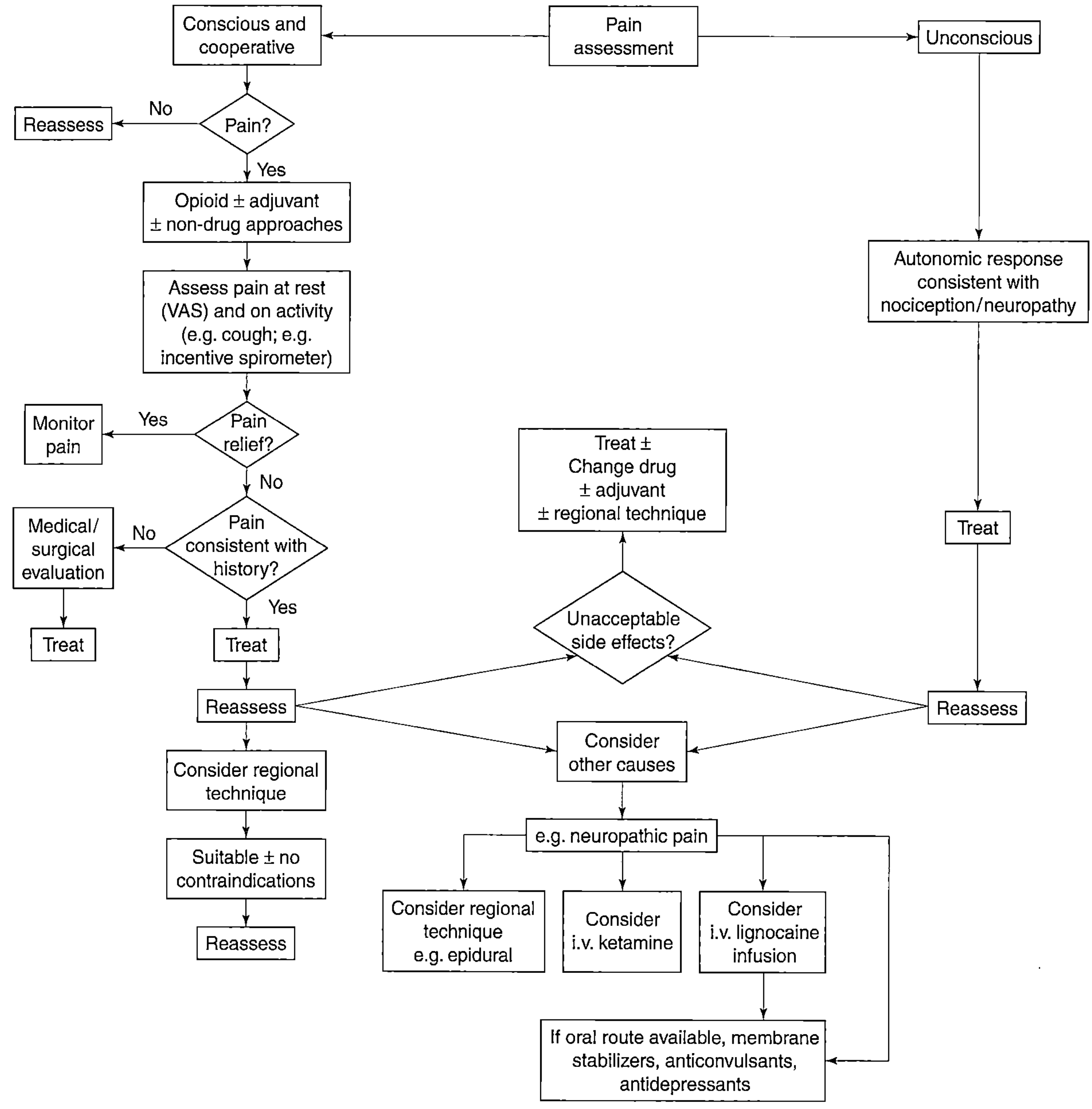

Fig. 19.20 Pain assessment in the intensive care environment. VAS = visual analogue scale. (Adapted from Molloy & Cousins 1998.)

tion of opioids in patients with an 'acute abdomen' does not impair the diagnosis of serious pathology, but may facilitate it. Therefore, appropriate analgesia must not be withheld from such patients (Attard et al 1992, Zolte & Cust 1986).

Recent advances in the pharmacology of analgesic agents are now having important consequences in emergency departments and intensive care units. In the emergency department an example of this is the recognition that the common and severe pain of renal colic responds better to NSAIDs than to opioids (Hetherington & Philp 1986). In the intensive care unit the introduction of new concepts of the use of shorter-acting opioids (e.g., alfentanil, remifentanil) over long periods of time will shift the rational for the choice of opioids for use in intensive care towards consideration of the biophase (i.e. effect site) and the 'context-sensitive half-time' (i.e., the time taken for the effect site drug concentration to decrease by 50%) rather than on the length of the elimination half-life (Shafer & Varvel 1991).

CLINICAL SYNDROMES OF ACUTE PAIN: IMPLICATIONS FOR DIAGNOSIS AND TREATMENT

As indicated above there is a wide variety of situations that may produce acute pain. These include: pain following surgery; post-traumatic pain; burns and various acute medical and surgical emergencies, such as myocardial infarction, acute pancreatitis and renal and biliary colic. It should also be recognized that a number of conditions, which are usually regarded as being chronic in nature, may have acute exacerbations that are associated with acute pain. Prominent in this respect is the patient with cancer who is subject to acute episodes of pain as a result of pathological fractures of long bones, acute intestinal obstructions and other problems. It would be quite wrong to regard this type of pain in the same category as other forms of chronic cancer pain. Patients with chronic occlusive vascular disease may also suffer acute episodes of pain during an exacerbation of their condition in winter months. Another chronic condition that may present with acute episodes of pain is the acquired immune deficiency syndrome (AIDS). The special problems of pain associated with labour and acute pain in children are discussed in Chapters 29 and 42.

Acute pain may arise from cutaneous, deep somatic or visceral structures. Careful mapping of the precise area of the pain is important. In the case of pain arising entirely from cutaneous structures, it is helpful to determine which dermatomes or superficial nerves are involved in the pain. In the case of deep somatic or visceral pain, some guidance as to the source of pain can be obtained by reference to classic viscerotome regions and also to superficial areas to which visceral pain is referred (Fig. 19.10). There is considerable overlap in the viscerotomes for various body organs, which undoubtedly results in a high error rate in the diagnosis of acute visceral pain. It is important to be aware of the spinal cord segments which are associated with nociceptive input from the various viscera (Table 19.3).

There are a number of general differences between visceral and somatic pain and these are summarized in Table 19.2. Further complicating the differentiation of somatic and visceral pain are viscerosomatic and somatovisceral reflexes (Fig. 19.21). A classic example of various neural pathways associated with acute pain is acute appendicitis. During the early phases of inflammation of the appendix, pain is conveyed by visceral nociceptive afferents arising from the appendix and conveyed to segment T10 of the spinal cord. As indicated in Figure 19.10, this viscerotome is represented centrally around the umbilical area. The inflammation associated with the appendicitis spreads to the parietal peritoneum in the region of the right iliac fossa and pain becomes localized in this region, as somatic nociceptive afferents in the T10 and L1 region become involved. However there may be wide variations in this pattern as the result of anatomical placement of the appendix, the initiation of viscerovisceral and viscerosomatic reflexes and other factors (Fig. 19.21).

Clear delineation of the neural pathways involved in acute pain may be important for treatment, particularly if neural blockade techniques are contemplated. Extensive somatic and visceral nociceptive afferent blockade may be required to relieve acute pain associated with some types of major surgery. For example, the following pathways may need to be blocked for pain associated with thoracoabdominal oesophagectomy with anastomosis of the oesophagus and bowel in the cervical region: C3–C4 and T2–T12 sensory nerves (somatic structures in neck, thorax and abdomen); C8–T4 cervicothoracic sympathetic chain and coeliac plexus (intrathoracic and abdominal viscera), and C3, C4 phrenic nerve sensory afferents (pain from incision in central diaphragm referred to shoulder tip). Also neural pathways associated with acute gynaecological pain have generally not been well understood (Cousins 1987).

In the diagnosis and treatment of acute pain associated with medical emergencies or acute trauma, a clear definition of the involvement of visceral and/or somatic structures may play an important part in deciding upon the treatment of the underlying cause of the pain. Quite clearly, diagnosis and treatment of the causes of the pain must take precedence over the symptomatic relief of pain. However, the availability of a wide range of clinical diagnostic techniques can now supplement the clinical history and physical examination, in which the patient's report of pain and response to examination is an important part. The availability of opioid drugs with rapid onset and offset of action when given intravenously makes it possible to provide periods of pain relief for the patient, while still permitting reassessment at a later time. The use of intravenous boluses or controlled intravenous infusions of rapidly acting drugs such as fentanyl and alfentanil permits a more humanitarian approach to the early relief of acute pain.

In differentiating between the various causes of acute pain, the following are of particular importance: onset, time relations after onset, characteristics and intensity of pain, site and radiation, and symptoms associated with the pain. Usually, but not always, it is possible to determine whether the pain has a somatic or visceral origin by reference to the factors outlined in Table 19.2. In the case of visceral pain, a rapid onset suggests mechanisms such as rupture of an organ or arterial occlusion due to embolus. More gradual onset is

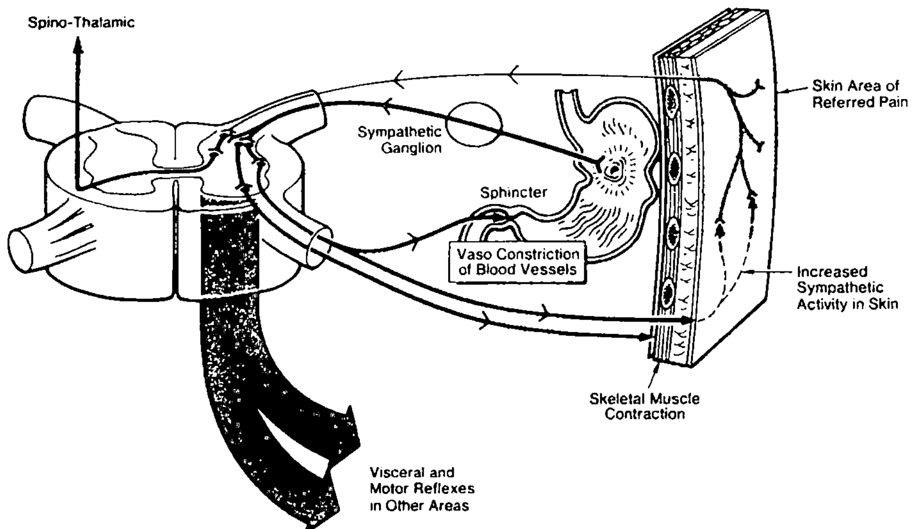

Fig. 19.21 Visceral pain: convergence of visceral and somatic nociceptive afferents. Visceral sympathetic afferents converge on the same dorsal horn neuron as do somatic nociceptive afferents. It is possible that visceral afferents activate interneurons that synapse at a deeper level than for somatic afferents. Visceral noxious stimuli are then conveyed, together with somatic noxious stimuli, by means of the spinothalamic pathway to the brain. Notes: (1) Referred pain is felt in the cutaneous area corresponding to the dorsal horn neuron upon which afferents converge. This is accompanied by allodynia and hyperalgesia in this skin area. (2) Reflex somatic motor activity results in muscle spasm, which may stimulate parietal peritoneum and initiate somatic input to dorsal horn. (3) Reflex sympathetic efferent activity may result in spasm of sphincters of viscera over a wide area, causing pain remote from the original stimulus. (4) Reflex sympathetic efferent activity may result in visceral ischaemia and further noxious stimulation. Also, visceral nociceptors may be sensitized by noradrenaline release and microcirculatory changes (see Fig. 19.4). (5) Increased sympathetic activity may influence cutaneous nociceptors (see Fig. 19.7), which may be at least partly responsible for referred pain. (6) Peripheral visceral afferents branch considerably, causing much overlap in the territory of individual dorsal roots. Only a small number of visceral afferent fibres converge on dorsal horn neurons compared with somatic nociceptor fibres. Also, visceral afferents converge on the dorsal horn over a wide number of segments. Thus dull vague visceral pain is very poorly localized. This is often called 'deep visceral pain'. (Reproduced from Cousins & Phillips 1986 with permission.)

suggestive of inflammation or infection. Constant pain may be associated with ischaemia or inflammation, whereas intermittent pain may be associated with periodically increased pressure in hollow organs due to obstruction.

An important example of referred pain is provided by the life-threatening situation of a torn spleen, with bleeding under the diaphragm which results in stimulation of phrenic afferent fibres (C3 and C4) and thus referral of pain to the shoulder tip region. In the thoracic region, pain due to acute trauma in the apical region of the lung may activate somatic afferents in the brachial plexus (C5–T1), resulting in pain on the outer aspect of the arm and shoulder and radiation into other regions of the arm. Pain emanating from trauma to the mediastinum may be diffusely located over the retrosternal area but may also radiate into the neck and abdomen. Because of the involvement of sympathetic afferent fibres which may involve segments from at least C8–T5, it is possible for pain to be referred into one or other arm. The pain of acute gallbladder and bile duct disease is usually located either diffusely in the upper abdomen or the right upper quadrant and may radiate to the back near the right scapula. This is often a colicky pain which is related to eating and may be relieved by vomiting. Acute pain involving the liver is also located diffusely in epigastrium and right upper quadrant. It may be a constant dull pain and have a sickening component. Acute pancreatitis pain is usually located high in the upper abdomen or left upper quadrant and radiates directly through to the back in the region of the first lumbar vertebra to the left of this area or to the interscapular region. The pain is usually described as being very severe, constant and dull.

Pain from the kidney usually radiates from the region of the loin to the groin and sometimes to the penis if the ureter is also involved, for example due to a stone in the ureter (renal colic). It seems likely that reflex increase in sympathetic activity associated with renal colic may intensify the pain and set up a vicious circle, which prevents the passage of the stone due to intense spasms of the ureter. Relief of such pain with continuous epidural block will sometimes not only result in highly effective pain relief, but also the passage of the stone (Scott 1988). The irritant presence of a stone in the ureter sets up a painful cycle of uncoordinated ureteric muscle contraction by stimulating local prostaglandin release and hence smooth muscle spasm. By inhibition of prostaglandin production, NSAID are more

 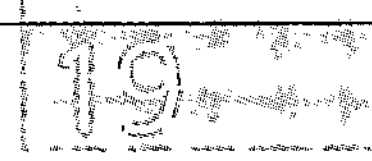

effective than opioids in relieving the pain of renal colic (Hetherington & Philp 1986).

Following surgery, the treatment of acute pain cannot be carried out without reference to the cause of the pain. This is so because of different requirements for drug treatment of somatic and visceral pain; also, as indicated above, the use of neural blockade techniques may be greatly influenced by neural pathways involved in the pain. 'Incident pain' is pain occurring other than at rest, such as during deep breathing and coughing or during ambulation. This pain usually, not unexpectedly, has a higher requirement for analgesia. Another cause of apparently increased levels of pain is opioid tolerance in patients treated with opioids for 7–10 days or more before surgery. Of particular importance, pain of certain patterns may be indicative of the development of postoperative complications which require surgical correction rather than pressing on blindly with the treatment of pain. A sudden increase in the requirements for intravenous opioid infusion, epidural administration of opioids or local anaesthetics should be carefully examined, bearing in mind the possibility that a new event has occurred (Fig. 19.22). A similar situation exists in patients treated in a critical care unit following trauma and who have been stabilized initially on an analgesic regimen. In the experience of this author, the development of an important complication is frequently associated with pain which will break through an analgesic regimen which was previously successful (Cousins & Phillips 1986).

The possibility of the development of neuropathic pain should be borne in mind after surgery as it is often missed in patients with acute pain, and may require specific therapy (Hayes & Molloy 1997). A useful definition is pain associated with injury, disease or surgical section of the peripheral or central nervous system. One diagnostic clue after surgery or trauma is an unexpected increase in opioid consumption, as neuropathic pain often responds poorly to opioids. Features that suggest the development of neuropathic pain are summarized in Box 19.10.

LONG-TERM EFFECTS OF SURGICAL INCISION AND ACUTE TISSUE TRAUMA

It might be assumed that surgical incision would be followed by a rather orderly healing process with minimal residual potential for continuing pain. However, surgical incision is inevitably complicated by the division of small peripheral nerves and sometimes larger nerves, in addition to a variable amount of tissue trauma, retraction and compression of tissues, and other factors. Interestingly, there is no convincing evidence that pain problems are less frequent after elective surgical incision and associated tissue trauma compared to traumatic injuries.

The subject of continuing pain following traumatic injury is very large and is considered in many other chapters in this book. Important examples are the following: stump pain, phantom limb pain, complex regional pain syndrome (CRPS types I and II), trigeminal neuralgia secondary to trauma, occipital neuralgia due to trauma, cervical sprain or whiplash syndrome, acute postmastectomy pain, post-thoracotomy pain, abdominal cutaneous nerve entrapment syndrome, and a large variety of postoperative neuralgias involving peripheral nerves such as the iliohypogastric, ilioinguinal, genitofemoral, lateral femoral cutaneous, obturator, femoral, sciatic and ulnar nerves. The specific features, associated symptoms and diagnostic criteria for all of these syndromes will not be repeated here, because they have been described well in published classifications of chronic pain (Merskey 1986, IASP Task Force on Taxonomy 1994). Rather, the reader is directed to some important chapters in the basic section of this text which explain the underlying mechanisms of these disorders and to chapters in the clinical section and treatment section which discuss diagnosis and management.

EFFECTS OF INJURY TO NERVES

As pointed out by Wall in the Introduction to this volume, there are inevitable primary, secondary and tertiary effects of injury to nerve terminals. Although the immediate effects in generating impulses in Aδ and C fibres are generally understood, it is often forgotten that powerful secondary changes occur due to the release of chemicals from nerves, from damaged cells and as a result of the release of enzyme products. Even more neglected is an appreciation of the tertiary phase with invasion of the injured area by phagocytes and fibroblasts. It is of great significance that damaged nerve endings and capillaries 'sprout' and infiltrate into the area. The sprouting nerves include sensory, sympathetic and motor fibres. The C fibres are involved in detecting or 'tasting' the altered chemical environment and perhaps transporting abnormal chemicals to the area. Clinically, this tertiary phase probably coincides with the beginning of formation of reparative scar tissue. It is a critical time for close observation of the patient, because early detection of continuing pain at this stage is a signal for early intervention to prevent the development of some of the very difficult postincisional and post-traumatic pain syndromes (Cousins 1989, 1991).

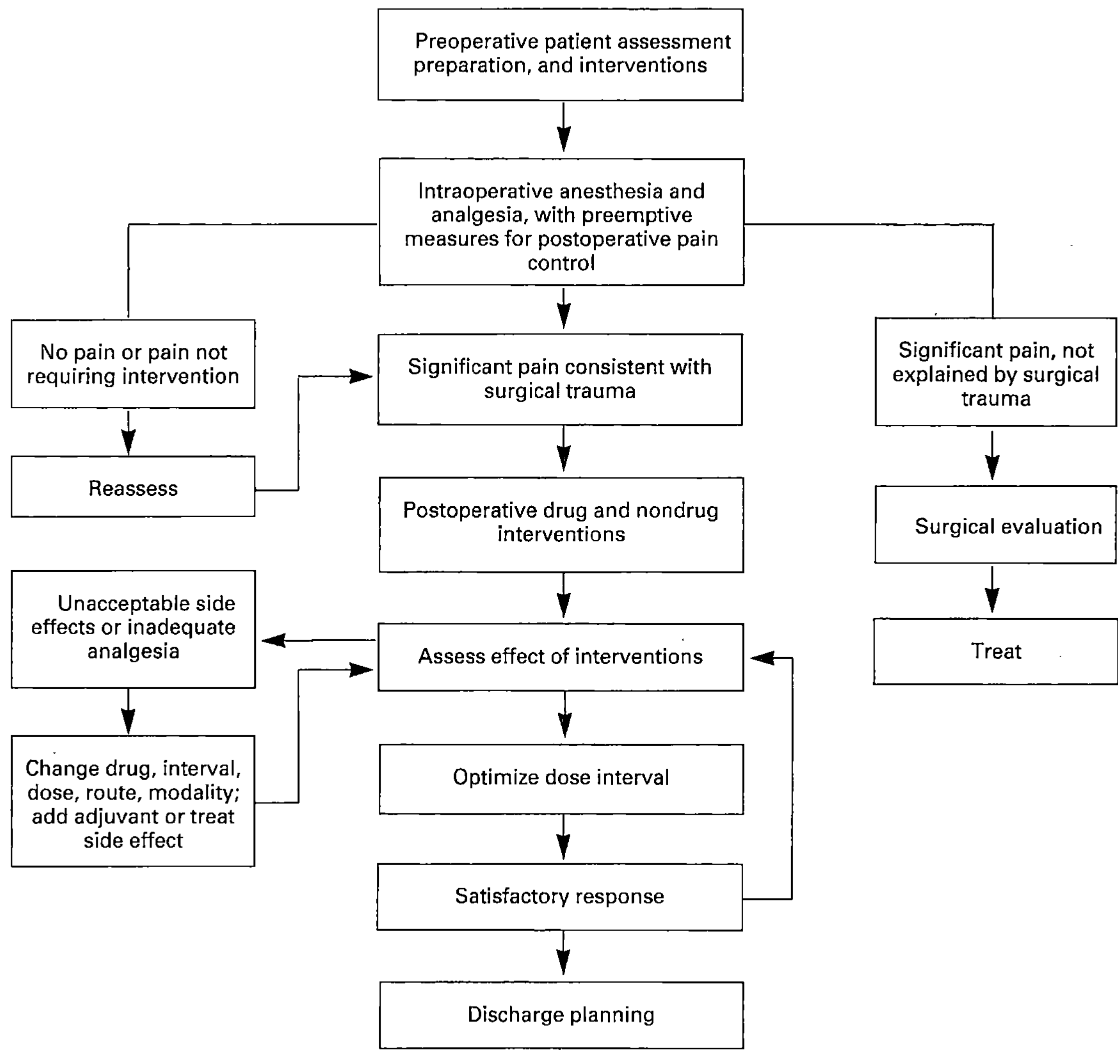

Fig. 19.22 Postoperative pain management: a brief flow chart.

The majority of long-term effects of incision and trauma appear to begin with damage to axon terminals, axon sheaths or dorsal root ganglia. This has been covered extensively in this book (see Ch. 4) by Devor, who proposes that there is normal and pathological pain. Normal pain results from activity in nociceptive afferents aroused by intense stimuli. Pain produced in any other way is said to be pathological. There is a considerable number of possibilities for the development of pathological pain (Wall & Devor 1978). Briefly, abnormalities may occur at the periphery, due to sensitization of nociceptors or damaged axons, permitting abnormal (ectopic) locations for excitation, or from abnormal activity originating within the central nervous system itself (Lindblom 1979, Tasker et al 1983). As discussed in the section below on clinical syndromes, neuroma formation may sometimes be the dominant mechanism of the pain, reflex increases in sympathetic activity may be prominent at other times and, more rarely, loss of sensory input from a substantial area (deafferentation) may be the basis of the problem.

An important aspect of understanding persistent pain following surgical incision and trauma is the process of wallerian degeneration and regeneration of nerves. The process is summarized in Figure 19.23. It is not commonly recognized that the formation of a neuroma is inevitable whenever peripheral nerves are cut. These are the fibres that failed to reach end organs. Substantial nerve-end neuromas always form after limb amputation. Axons trapped in suture lines will form tangled sprouts which result in a neuroma in continuity along the course of the nerve. After partial injury, regions of external regeneration may be arrested, forming microneuromas.

BOX 19.10

Features that suggest neuropathic pain. (Adapted from NHMRC 1999)

- Pain in the absence of ongoing tissue damage
- Pain in an area of sensory loss
- Paroxysmal or spontaneous pain
- Allodynia (pain in response to non-painful stimuli)
- Hyperalgesia (increased pain in response to painful stimuli)
- Dysaesthesias (unpleasant abnormal sensations)
- Characteristic of pain different from nociception: burning, pulsing, stabbing pain
- Sometimes a delay in onset of pain after nerve injury (*note*: some neuropathic pain has immediate onset)
- Hyperpathia: increasing pain with repetitive stimulation; 'after response' (continued exacerbation of pain after stimulation); radiation of pain to adjacent areas after stimulation
- Tapping of neuromas (spontaneously firing growth buds from damaged peripheral nerves) produces a radiating electric shock sensation in the distribution of the nerve (Tinel's sign)
- Poor response (not unresponsiveness) to opioids
- Presence of a major neurological deficit (e.g. brachial plexus avulsion, spinal injury, etc.)

Neuromas, whether at a cut nerve ending or along the course of an axon, are capable of spontaneous discharge, have greatly enhanced and prolonged discharges in response to stimuli and show minimal accommodation to stimuli. In animal experiments, and also in the clinical setting, the sensitivity of neuromas appears to be related to the time since nerve injury. It seems to be most intense within the first 2 weeks of neuroma development, but then continues at a lesser but sustained level. Clinically, this situation is recognized by the production of intense radiating pain in response to tapping on the neuroma (Tinel's sign) and in extreme tenderness to palpation of the neuroma region. This situation may be accompanied by allodynia (pain due to a stimulus which does not normally provoke pain) and hyperalgesia (an increased response to a stimulus which would normally only provoke minimal pain). Of clinical importance in the treatment of neuroma pain is the finding that neuroma activity is enhanced by a number of chemical mediators, including noradrenaline, and thus can be decreased by noradrenaline depletion with agents such as guanethidine or bretylium. It should also be recognized that damage to axon sheaths may produce demyelination, resulting in an area which is capable of generating abnormal nerve impulses. This state of hyperexcitability results in paroxysms of pain and the afferent activity may initiate reflex motor activity causing muscle spasm.

Although it has not been possible to confirm that events occurring in damaged axons in animals are directly applicable to man, evidence is accumulating and this may be the case. In keeping with animal studies, Nystrom and Hagbarth (1981) found that spontaneous discharge and phantom pain associated with stump neuromas could not be blocked with local anaesthetic injection of stump neuromas. This implies a central as well as peripheral abnormality. Thus, although there may be initially an abnormality which is predominantly of a peripheral nature, this rapidly involves more central portions of axons, dorsal root ganglia and cells in dorsal horn. Increased sympathetic activity enhances peripheral nociception, and ephaptic 'cross-talk' between high- and low-threshold sensory channels may contribute to the problem. The underlying problem in all situations appears to be increased nerve excitability. Considerable recent progress in treatment has resulted from the early use of sympathetic nerve blocks, if sympathetic hyperactivity is a predominant part of the problem.

Even more promising has been recent evidence that the systemic administration of drugs acting on the sodium channel may switch off excitable cells and attack the problem at all of the major sites of abnormality. The prototype drugs in this treatment are the local anaesthetic drugs (Boas et al 1982), such as lidocaine and its longer-acting congeners, tocainide, mexiletine and flecainide, and the antiepileptics such as sodium valproate and carbamazepine. There is evidence that systemic administration of the local anaesthetics produces a rather selective depression of C-afferent fibre-evoked activity in the spinal cord (Woolf & Wiesenfield-Hallin 1985). This opens the way for the development of drugs which have a very selective and safe effect in reducing the abnormal neuronal excitability associated with nerve damage following surgical incision and traumatic injury. Another finding of possible significance to the treatment of pain associated with neuromas is the report that corticosteroids suppress ectopic neural discharge originating in experimental neuromas (Devor et al 1985). Pathophysiology at a spinal level undoubtedly plays a part in the genesis of pain following nerve injury (Woolf 1983, 1989, Woolf et al 1992).

CLINICAL PAIN SYNDROMES FOLLOWING INCISION

The precise incidence of persistent pain following surgical incision and trauma is difficult to determine. However, in this author's experience, it is seen in at least 10% of surgical

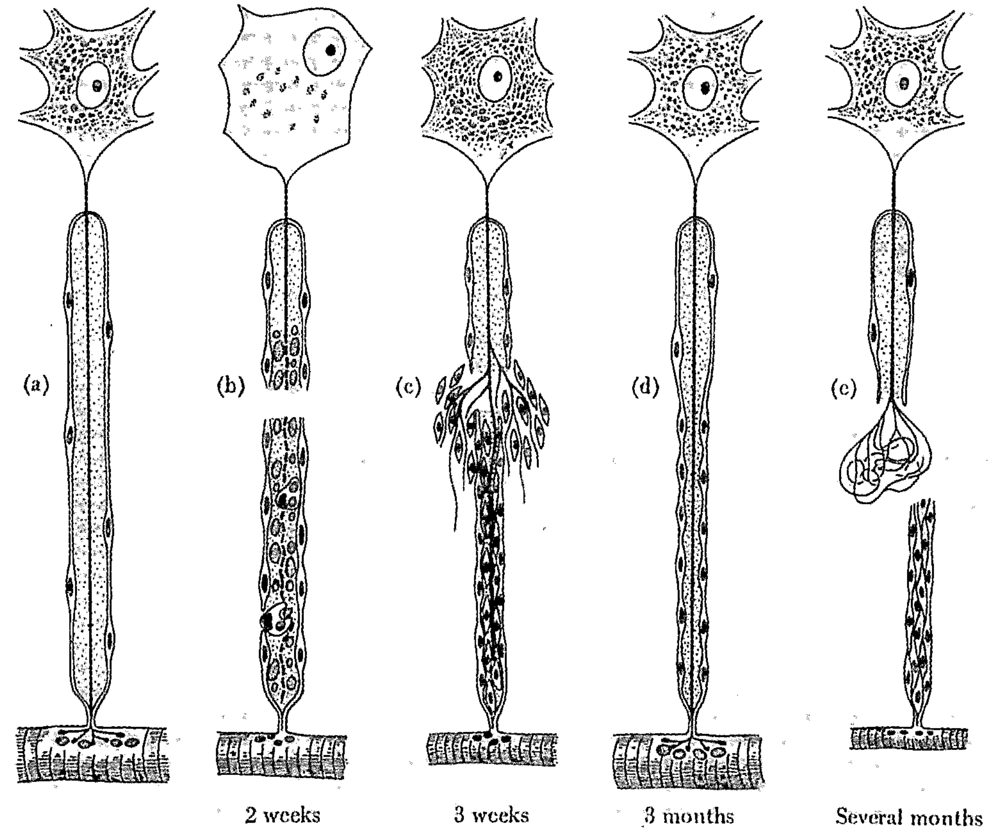

Fig. 19.23 Major changes associated with nerve fibre regeneration. (a) Normal nerve fibre with its perikaryon and its effector cell (striated skeletal muscle). The axon is surrounded by myelin generated by Schwann cells. (b) When the fibre is injured, the neuronal nucleus moves to the periphery and Nissel bodies in the perikaryon become greatly reduced in number. The nerve fibre distal to the injury degenerates along with its myelin sheath–wallerian degeneration. The blood–nerve barrier is damaged, and debris is phagocytosed by macrophages. (c) By 3 weeks the muscle fibre shows a pronounced disuse atrophy. Schwann cells proliferate, forming a compact cord through which an axon may grow. The axon grows at a rate of 1 mm/day. (d) In this example, the nerve fibre has regenerated successfully 3 months after injury. (e) In other cases, however, the axon may not successfully find its original and organ if growth is impeded by mechanical obstacles or is unorganized for other reasons. It is almost invariably the case that some axons form neuromas, which then gradually recede. However if a number of axons have their path obstructed, a large tangled mass of neuroma may form. (Reproduced from Ross & Reigh 1985 with permission.)

operations. There is strong evidence from animal studies that there is a genetic predisposition to the development of spontaneous activity in neuromas. This evidence is supported by observations that patients who develop neuromas and incisional pain frequently have similar problems if an attempt is made to remove the neuroma tissue surgically. Such patients tend to have similar problems when operations on other parts of the body are carried out. Thus, the preceding history of the patient is important and may point to the need for careful surveillance and the early use of appropriate treatment measures.

Surgical textbooks discuss factors in wound healing such as gentleness of handling tissues, different methods of suturing, use of appropriate suture material, avoidance of haematoma and infection and other factors (Sabiston 1982). However, there appears to have been only limited investigation of factors that have a significant influence on the development of various pain syndromes following surgical incision. It is generally held that incisions which cut across muscle fibres cause more postoperative pain than those that separate fibres. One of the few studies to test this hypothesis compared a dorsal approach to the kidney (muscle-separating) with the classic flank approach (muscle-cutting). The former was associated with a lesser requirement for postoperative analgesia and shorter hospital stay (Freiha & Zeineh 1983). Unfortunately patients were not followed up to determine the comparative incidence of postincisional pain.

Clinical observation suggests that the following operations are particularly prone to be associated with long-term pain in or near the surgical incision: lateral thoracotomy; cholecystectomy; nephrectomy (flank incision); radical mastectomy; vein-stripping (especially long saphenous because of proximity to saphenous nerve); inguinal herniorrhaphy; episiotomy; various operations on the arm and hand; facial surgery (Litwin 1962, White & Sweet 1962, Applegate 1972, Lindblom 1979, Tasker et al 1983, Kitzinger 1984). However, there are few data to indicate which surgical factors are important in the genesis of postincisional pain. Patient factors such as genetic makeup (Inbal et al 1980), middle to old age (Tasker et al 1983) and the presence of unrelieved pain prior to surgery may be important (Melzack 1971). The latter is supported in animal studies, where injury prior to denervation of a limb by neurectomy resulted in increased self mutilation (autotomy) compared to animals who were not injured prior to neurectomy (Coderre et al 1986). The study suggests that tissue damage and unrelieved pain prior to surgery may predispose to persistent pain problems following surgery. This is supported by the clinical observation that patients with pain due to occlusive vascular disease have a lower incidence of postamputation pain if their pain is relieved by neurolytic sympathectomy (Cousins et al 1979) or by epidural block (Bach et al 1988) prior to amputation.

The long-term effects of surgical incision can be considered in three broad categories: the postoperative neuralgias, complex regional pain syndromes (types I and II) and deafferentation syndromes.

Postoperative neuralgias

The postoperative neuralgias may involve numerous peripheral nerves, as indicated above. A classic example is post-thoracotomy neuralgia which presents as pain that either recurs or persists along a thoracotomy scar, characterized by a change from the usual aching sensation to a burning, dysaesthetic component. The skin may sometimes but not always show hyperaesthesia. In this situation it is most likely that neuroma formation has occurred, but it is also possible for the syndrome to follow stretching or scarring of intercostal nerves, following either incisional trauma or infection.

If treated early, this condition may sometimes respond to transcutaneous electrical nerve stimulation, but may require a number of other modalities, including nerve blocks of both distal and proximal tissues with local anaesthetic, sympathetic blocks, intravenous local anaesthetic infusion, oral membrane stabilizing drugs, and the use of centrally acting drugs such as the tricyclic antidepressant drugs, anticonvulsants and phenothiazines.

Complex regional pain syndromes

It is very important to recognize the development of complex regional pain syndromes (CRPS) after surgery or trauma. As noted earlier, CRPS type I was previously known as 'reflex sympathetic dystrophy' and CRPS type II as 'causalgia' (IASP Task Force on Taxonomy 1994). CRPS type I is defined as a syndrome that usually develops after an initial noxious event, is not limited to the distribution of a single peripheral nerve, and is disproportionate to the inciting event. It is associated with various combinations of oedema, changes in skin blood flow, abnormal sudomotor activity in the region of the pain, allodynia, hyperalgesia and disordered motor function. CRPS type II is a syndrome of burning pain, allodynia and hyperpathia usually in the hand or foot after injury of a nerve.

With CRPS the pain tends to be a burning sensation with hyperalgesia, allodynia, excessive sweating and vasomotor changes producing redness to a blue blotchy appearance. Many of these features are associated with sympathetic hyperactivity, thus the use of the term 'sympathetically maintained pain' (SMP). However, SMP is not always a feature of CRPS and the term 'sympathetically independent pain' (SIP) has been introduced. This may be the reason why some patients with CRPS respond to sympathetic blocking drugs (SMP) and others do not (SIP).

The many factors involved in the genesis of CRPS have been extensively reviewed (Sunderland 1978, Bonica 1979, Roberts 1986, Schott 1986). The nerves most commonly involved are the median, the sciatic and its two main branches, and the brachial plexus. Sunderland proposes that these nerves are most at risk because they carry the bulk of the sensory fibres and postganglionic supply to the hand and foot respectively (Sunderland 1978). However, CRPS can involve other nerves. There seems to be a particular risk of CRPS type I following surgery of the hand.

It is also important to recognize that in some cases early forms of CRPS type I may present with an appearance of sympathetic hypoactivity, increase in skin temperature, congestion and swelling of the extremity. The pain is diffuse but localized to the hand or other region and the skin is usually warm, dry and pink. This picture often changes with time and manifests the features of sympathetic overactivity with cold, sweaty, cyanosed skin. Trophic changes then follow in the skin and nails.

The critical aspect of the treatment of CRPS is early recognition and the use of sympathetic blocking techniques with local anaesthetics, intravenous sympathetic techniques (e.g., guanethidine) or systemic-acting sympathetic drugs in combination with vigorous physical therapy and rehabilitation (Sunderland 1978, Bonica 1979, Bonelli et al 1983,

Hannington-Kiff 1984, Holder & Mackinnon 1984, Horowitz 1984).

Deafferentation syndromes

The third major category, the deafferentation syndromes (Lindblom 1979, Tasker et al 1983), are less common and usually only occur after major surgery, such as extensive back surgery. These syndromes usually present clinically with a substantial area of sensory loss. However, sometimes there is a less noticeable area of sensory loss, for example following thoracotomy, where only one intercostal nerve was cut or traumatized (Tasker et al 1983). The pathophysiology is complex, but is at least partly due to loss of normal sensory input and consequent reduction in normal modulatory mechanisms (Wall 1983, Woolf et al 1992). Treatments such as transcutaneous and dorsal column stimulation are based on this concept. However, as the syndrome progresses clinically, more complex mechanisms seem to operate and treatment often involves the use of centrally acting drugs such as the tricyclic antidepressants and phenothiazines. Severe forms of this problem, such as brachial plexus avulsion, are usually the result of trauma.

There is some evidence that an important part of the pathophysiology in this situation is in disturbed activity in the region of the dorsal horn. The treatment of a dorsal root entry zone (DREZ) lesion is based on this assumption and initial results have shown considerable promise.

The unfortunate consequence of some extensive and repeated back surgeries has been the development of large areas of sensory denervation. It is important to document this area of sensory loss, because it is often a vital guide to treatment. In general such problems are not responsive to treatment with the usual analgesic drugs such as NSAIDs and opioids.

Evidence of pathophysiology and neuroanatomical reorganisation in the dorsal horn of the spinal cord, following nerve trauma, has raised the possibility of treatment aimed at the NMDA receptor, or associated receptors. Thus there are some anecdotal reports now appearing of patients with severe neuropathic pain which has persisted following surgery and which has been responsive to the epidural or intrathecal administration of opioids, with or without the addition of drugs such as clonidine. At this early stage, there is no indication of how effective such treatment will prove to be in the long term, nor is it clear how long such treatment would be required before it could be discontinued without reappearance of the pain.

THE ORGANIZATION OF ACUTE PAIN SERVICES

Much of the responsibility for supervising the provision of relief of acute pain in hospitals has been allocated to formal acute pain services, often staffed by anaesthetists and nurses. In an elegant and well-designed study performed in Cardiff, Gould found that the introduction of an acute pain service to the general surgical wards in his hospital led to considerable improvement in the level of postoperative pain as assessed by visual analogue scores (Gould et al 1992). Such a formal service offers: continuing education of staff about pain; standardization of orders of analgesic prescription and monitoring of patients; the introduction of new methods of pain relief; the employment of specialized or invasive analgesic techniques; daily review and supervision of patients referred to the service; audit and clinical research of acute pain managements. Acute pain services are therefore a valuable clinical, educational and organizational resource within any hospital. The roles and the organization of acute pain services have been described by Ready et al (1995) (Box 19.11).

One purpose of an acute pain service is to construct algorithms that other less experienced members of staff can follow to provide safe and effective pain relief for their patients, as commended by the work of Gould et al (1992). The figure shown below is an algorithm used in the Royal North Shore Hospital, Sydney, for subcutaneous morphine administration after surgery, designed by members of the acute pain service. An important aspect of such algorithms is the frequent assessment of the patient to ensure safety and efficacy of the treatment. Clinical assessments include pain and sedation scores, respiratory rate and arterial blood pressure. The algorithm should include a clear description of recommended doses and instructions on how to treat recognized side-effects as respiratory depression (Fig. 19.24)

In the future the various roles of the members of acute pain services will be integrated much more closely with those of surgical and other staff, to provide a complete perioperative care service for the patient. This is consistent with recent suggestions that multimodal analgesia, nutrition and mobilization must be approached and addressed in a unifying manner to facilitate rapid functional recovery, or acute rehabilitation, after surgery (Kehlet 1994, 1997, Brodner et al 1998) (Fig. 19.25).

CONCLUSION

Acute pain has emerged as an important issue because of humanitarian aspects, associated morbidity and mortality,

BOX 19.11

Organizational aspects of an anaesthesiology- based postoperative pain programme. (Reproduced from Ready et al 1995)

1. **Education (initial, updates):**
   Anaesthetists
   Surgeons
   Nurses
   Pharmacists
   Patients and families
   Hospital administrators
   Health insurance carriers
2. **Areas of regular administrative activity:**
   Maintenance of clear lines of communication
   Manpower – 24-hour availability of pain service personnel
   Evaluation (including safety) of equipment (e.g. pumps)
   Secretarial support
   Economic issues
   Continuous quality improvement
   Resident medical teaching (if applicable)
   Pain management-related research
3. **Collaboration with nursing services:**
   Job description of pain service nurse (if applicable)
   Nursing policies and procedures
   Nurses in-service and continuing education
   Definition of roles in patient care
   Institutional administrative activities
   Continuous quality improvement
   Research activities (if applicable)
4. **Elements of documentation:**
   Preprinted orders
   Procedures
   Protocols
   Bedside pain management flow sheets
   Daily consultation notes
   Educational packages

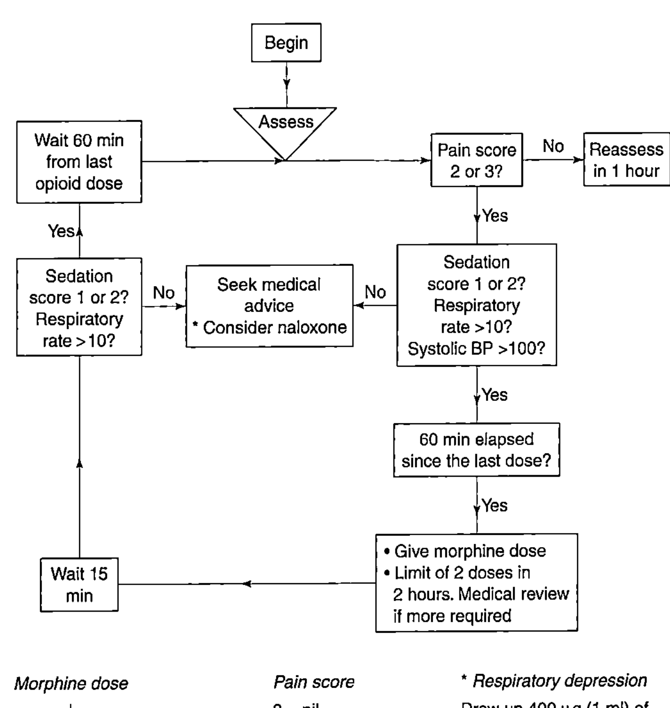

Age (yrs)	Dose (mg)
<55	7.5–10
56–70	5.0–7.5
>70	2.5–5.0

Fig. 19.24 Subcutaneous morphine treatment of acute postoperative or acute severe pain.

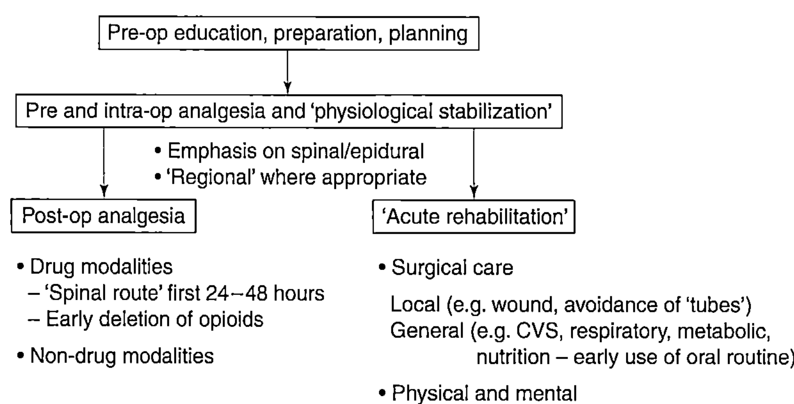

Fig. 19.25 The concept of acute pain treatment and acute rehabilitation. The diagram emphasizes the need for an integrated approach to pain relief and acute rehabilitation, in order to return patients to normal activity as soon as possible.

and important financial consequences. Substantial progress in understanding peripheral, spinal cord and brain mechanisms involved in acute pain continues to be made with important consequences for treatment. The diagnosis and treatment of the cause of acute pain must always have high priority. However, new methods of pain relief have sufficient flexibility to provide early pain relief while still permitting reassessment of patients. Acute pain management now focuses on important issues as preventive measures, multimodal analgesia, mobilization, nutrition, acute rehabilitation, careful surveillance to identify important acute pain syndromes that may lead to persisting pain, the application of greatly improved methods of treatment, and, above all, the eventual outcome for the patient. The introduction of acute pain services has been shown to improve postoperative pain relief, but it is foreseeable that their role should expand and integrate into general perioperative care. The challenge is to approach and employ multimodal and pre-emptive analgesia, early nutrition and rapid mobilization after surgery and trauma in a unifying manner to aid acute rehabilitation to the benefit of the patient. The aim should be that the majority of patients have good relief of acute pain together with rapid functional recovery. To achieve this result requires a substantial educational and organizational effort to apply the knowledge and methodology that is now available, with close cooperation between anaesthetic, surgical and nursing staff. If this is achieved, we will truly be able to enter a new era of acute pain management.

REFERENCES

Aasbo V, Raeder JC, Grogaard B, Roise O 1996 No additional analgesic effect of intra-articular morphine or bupivacaine compared with placebo after elective knee arthroscopy. Acta Anaesthesiologica Scandinavica 40: 585–588

Abraham WC, Mason SE, Demmer J et al 1993 Correlations between immediate early gene induction and the persistence of long-term potentiation. Neuroscience 56: 717–727

Accident Facts 1978 National Safety Council, Chicago

Advokat C, Rhein FQ 1995 Potentiation of morphine-induced antinociception in acute spinal rats by the NMDA antagonist dextrorphan. Brain Research 699: 157–160

Agency for Health Care and Policy Research 1992 Acute pain management: operative or medical procedures and trauma. Clinical practice guidelines. AHCPR pub no 92-0032. Agency for Health Care Policy and Research, Public Health Service, US Department of Health and Human Services, Rockville, MD

Ahn H, Andaker L, Bronge A et al 1988 Effect of continuous epidural analgesia on gastro-intestinal motility. British Journal of Surgery 75: 1176–1178

Akopian AN, Abson NC, Wood JN 1996 Molecular genetic approaches to nociceptor development and function. Trends in Neurosciences 19: 240–246

Andrew J 1970 Recovery from surgery with and without preparation instruction, for three coping styles. Journal of Personality and Social Psychology 17: 233

Applegate W V 1972 Abdominal cutaneous nerve entrapment syndrome. Surgery 71: 118

Attard AR, Corlett MJ, Kidner NJ et al 1992 Safety of early pain relief for acute abdominal pain. British Medical Journal 305: 554–556

Averill J R 1973 Personal control over aversive stimuli and its relationship to stress. Psychological Bulletin 80: 286

Bach S, Noreng M F, Tjellden N U 1988 Phantom limb pain in amputees during the first 12 months following limb amputation, after preoperative lumbar epidural blockade. Pain 33: 297–301

Backonja MM 1994 Local anesthetics as adjuvant analgesics. Journal of Pain and Symptom Management 9: 491–499

Ballantyne JC, Carr DB, Chalmers TC et al 1998 Comparative effects of postoperative analgesic therapies upon respiratory function: meta-analysis of initial randomized control trials. Anesthesia and Analgesia 86(3): 598–612

Bardram L, Funch-Jensen P, Jensen P, Crawford ME, Kehlet H 1995 Recovery after laparoscopic colonic surgery with epidural analgesia, and early oral nutrition and mobilisation. Lancet 345: 763–764

Beattie WS, Warriner CB, Etches R et al 1997 The addition of continuous intravenous infusion of ketorolac to a patient-controlled analgetic morphine regime reduced postoperative myocardial ischemia in patients undergoing elective total hip or knee arthroplasty. Anesthesia and Analgesia 84: 715–722

Beecher H K 1946 Pain in men wounded in battle. Annals of Surgery 123: 96

Bennett GJ, Kajander KC, Sahara Y, Iadarola MJ, Sugimoto T 1989 Neurochemical and anatomical changes in the dorsal horn of rats with an experimental painful peripheral neuropathy. In: Cervero F, Bennett GJ, Headley PM (eds) Processing of sensory information in the superficial dorsal horn of the spinal cord. Plenum, Amsterdam, pp 463–471

Besse D, Lombard MC, Zakac JM, Roques BP, Besson J-M 1990 Pre- and postsynaptic distribution of mu, delta and kappa opioid receptors in the superficial layers of the cervical dorsal horn of the rat spinal cord. Brain Research 521: 15–22

Blomberg S, Emanuelsson H, Kuist H, Lamm C et al 1990 Effects of thoracic epidural anaesthesia on coronary arteries and arterioles in patients with coronary artery disease. Anesthesiology 73(5): 840–847

Boas R A, Covino B G, Shahwarian A 1982 Analgesic response to iv lidocaine. British Journal of Anaesthesia 54: 501

Bonelli S, Conoscente F, Movilia P G et al 1983 Regional intravenous guanethidine vs stellate ganglion block in reflex sympathetic dystrophies: a randomized trial. Pain 16: 297–307

Bonica J J 1979 Causalgia and other reflex sympathetic dystrophies. In: Bonica J J, Liebeskind J C, Albe-Fessard D (eds) Advances in pain research and therapy, vol 3. Raven, New York, pp 141–166

Bonica J J 1985 Biology, pathophysiology and treatment of acute pain. In: Lipton S, Miles J (eds) Persistent pain. Grune & Stratton, Orlando, pp 1–32

Bowler G, Wildsmith J, Scott D B 1986 Epidural administration of local anaesthetics. In: Cousins M J, Phillips G D (eds) Acute pain management. Churchill Livingstone, New York, pp 187–236

Brandt M R, Fernandes A, Mordhorst R, Kehlet H 1978 Epidural analgesia improves postoperative nitrogen balance. British Medical Journal 1: 1106–1108

Brodner G, Pogatzki E, Van Aken H, Buerkle H, Goeters C, Schulzki C, Nottberg H, Mertes N 1998 A multimodal approach to control postoperative pathophysiology and rehabilitation in patients undergoing abdominothoracic esophagectomy. Anesthesia and Analgesia 86: 228–234

Cannon W B 1939 The wisdom of the body. Norton, New York

Campbell JN, Raja SN, Selig DK, Belzberg AJ, Meyer RA 1994 Diagnosis and management of sympathetically maintained pain. In: Fields HL, Liebeskind JC (eds) Progress in pain research and management. IASP Press, Seattle, pp 85–100

Chabal C, Jacobson L, Mariano A, Chaney E, Britell CW 1992 The use of oral mexiletine for the treatment of pain after peripheral nerve injury. Anesthesiology 76: 513

Chaplan SR, Bach FW, Shafer SL, Yaksh TL 1995 Prolonged alleviation of tactile allodynia by intravenous lidocaine in neuropathic rats. Anesthesiology 83: 775–785

Chapman C R, Cox G B 1977 Anxiety, pain and depression surrounding elective surgery: a multivariate comparison of abdominal surgery patients with kidney donors and recipients. Journal of Pyschosomatic Research 21: 7

Chi S-I, Levine JD, Basbaum AI 1993 Effects of injury discharge on the persistent expression of spinal cord fos-like immunoreactivity produced by sciatic nerve transection in the rat. Brain Research 617: 220–224

Christopherson R, Beattie C, Frank SM et al 1993 The perioperative ischemia randomized anesthesia trial study group: perioperative morbidity in patients randomized to epidural or general anesthesia for lower-extremity vascular surgery. Anesthesiology 79: 422–434

Clark WC, Clark SB 1980 Pain responses in Nepalese porters. Science 209: 410

Coderre TJ 1993 The role of excitatory amino acid receptors and intracellular messengers in persistent nociception after tissue injury in rats. Molecular Neurobiology 7: 229

Coderre T, Grimes RW, Melzack R 1986 Autonomy after nerve section in the rat is influenced by tonic descending inhibition from locus coeruleus. Neuroscience Letters 67: 81–86

Cohen FL 1980 Postsurgical pain relief: patients' status and nurses' medication choice. Pain 9: 265

Collingridge G, Singer W 1990 Excitatory amino acid receptors and synaptic plasticity, Trends in Pharmacological Science 11: 290–296

Comfort VK, Code WE, Rooney ME, Yip RW 1992 Naproxen premedication reduces postoperative tubal ligation pain. Canadian Journal of Anaesthesia 39: 349–352

Cousins MJ 1987 Visceral pain. In: Andersson S, Bond M, Mehta M, Swerdlow M (eds) Chronic non-cancer pain: assessment and practical management. MTP Press, Lancaster 119–132

Cousins MJ 1989 Acute pain and the injury response: immediate and prolonged effects. Regional Anaesthesia 14: 162–178

Cousins MJ 1991 Prevention of postoperative pain. In: Bond MR, Charlton JE, Woolf CJ (eds) Proceedings of the VIth World Congress on Pain. Elsevier, Amsterdam, pp 41–52

Cousins MJ, Bridenbaugh PO (eds) 1988 Neural blockade in clinical anaesthesia and management of pain, 2nd edn. JB Lippincott, Philadelphia

Cousins MJ, Bridenbaugh PO (eds) 1998 Neural blockade in clinical anaesthesia and management of pain, 3rd edn. Lippincott-Raven, Philadelphia

Cousins MJ, Phillips GD (eds) (1986) Acute pain management. Clinics in critical care medicine. Churchill Livingstone, Edinburgh

Cousins MJ, Wright CJ 1971 Graft, muscle and skin blood flow after epidural block in vascular surgical procedures. Surgery, Gynecology and Obstetrics 133: 59

Cousins MJ, Reeve TS, Glynn CJ, Walsh JA, Cherry DA 1979 Neurolytic lumbar sympathetic blockade: duration of denervation and relief of rest pain. Anaesthesia and Intensive Care 7: 121–135

Cousins N 1970 Anatomy of an illness as perceived by the patient. Norton, New York

Craig DB 1981 Postoperative recovery of pulmonary function. Anesthesia and Analgesia 60: 46

Cranin AN, Sher J 1979 Sensory deprivation. Oral Surgery 47: 416

Crile GW 1910 Phylogenetic association in relation to certain medical problems. Boston Medical and Surgical Journal 103: 893

Cullen ML, Staren ED, el Ganzouri A, Logas WG, Ivankovitch AD, Economov SG 1985 Continuous epidural infusion for analgesia after major abdominal operations; a randomized, prospective double blind study. Surgery 98: 718

Dahl JB, Kehlet H 1993 The value of pre-emptive analgesia in the treatment of postoperative pain. British Journal of Anaesthesia 70: 434

Dahl JB, Rosenberg J, Dirkes WE, Morgensen T, Kehlet H 1990 Prevention of postoperative pain by balanced analgesia. British Journal of Anaesthesia 64:518–520

Davies SN, Lodge D 1987 Evidence for involvement of *N*-methylaspartate receptors in 'wind-up' of class 2 neurons in the dorsal horn of the rat. Brain Research 424: 402–406

Devor M 1994 The pathophysiology of damaged peripheral nerves. In: Wall PD, Melzack R (eds) Textbook of pain, 3rd ed. Churchill Livingstone, London, pp 79–100

Devor M, Govrin-Lippmann R, Raber P 1985 Corticosteroids suppress ectopic neural discharge originating in experimental neuromas. Pain 22: 127

Devor M, Wall PD, Catalan N 1992 Systemic lidocaine silences ectopic neuroma and DRG discharge without blocking nerve conduction. Pain 48: 261

Dickenson AH 1996 NMDA receptor antagonists as analgesics. In: Fields HL, Liebeskind JC (eds) Pharmacological approaches to the treatment of chronic pain: Concepts and critical issues. Progress in pain research and management, vol 1. Seattle, IASP Press, pp 173–187

Dickenson AH, Sullivan AF 1987 Evidence for a role of the NMDA receptor in the frequency dependent potentiation of deep rat dorsal horn nociceptive neurons following C fiber stimulation. Neuropharmacology 26: 1235–1238

Dimatteo MR, Di Nicola DD 1982 Achieving patient compliance: the psychology of the medical practitioner's role. Pergamon Press, New York

Dubner R, Ren K 1994 Central mechanisms of thermal and mechanical hyperalgesia following tissue inflammation. In: Boivie J, Hansson P, Lindblom U (eds) Touch, temperature, and pain in health and disease: mechanisms and assessments. IASP Press, Seattle, pp 267–277

Editorial 1978 Post-operative pain. British Medical Journal 2: 517

Egbert LD, Battit GE, Welch CE et al 1964 Reduction of postoperative pain by encouragement and instruction of patients. New England Journal of Medicine 270: 825

Eisenach JC 1993 Aspirin, the miracle drug – spinally, too? Anesthesiology, 79: 211–213

Fields HL 1987 Pain. McGraw-Hill, New York

Fields HL, Basbaum AI 1994 Central nervous system mechanisms of pain modulation. In: Wall PD, Melzack R (eds) Textbook of pain, vol 3. Churchill Livingstone, Edinburgh, pp 243–257

Foley KM 1985 The treatment of cancer pain. New England Journal of Medicine 313: 84

Fortin F, Kirovac S 1976 A randomized controlled trial of pre-operative patient education. Educational Journal of Nursing Studies 13: 11

Freiha F, Zeineh S 1983 Dorsal approach to upper urinary tract. Urology 21: 15–16

Fromm GH 1994 Baclofen as an adjuvant analgesic [Review]. Journal of Pain and Symptom Management 9: 500–509

Furst DE 1997 Meloxicam – selective cox-2 inhibition in clinical practice [Review]. Seminars in Arthritis & Rheumatism 26: 21–27

Galer BS 1995 Neuropathic pain of peripheral origin – advances in pharmacologic treatment. Neurology 45: S17–S25

Garnett RL, MacIntyre A, Lindsay P 1996 Perioperative ischemia in aortic surgery: combined epidural/general anesthesia and epidural analgesia vs general anesthesia and IV analgesia. Canadian Journal of Anaesthesia 43: 769–778

Garthwaite J, Charles SL, Chess-Williams R 1988 Endothelium-derived relaxing factor release on activation of NMDA receptors suggests role as intercellular messenger in the brain. Nature 336: 385–388

Gould TH, Crosby DL, Harmer M et al 1992 Policy for controlling pain after surgery: effect of sequential changes in management. British Medical Journal 305: 1187–1193

Groudine SB, Fisher HAG, Kaufman RP et al 1998 Anesthesia and Analgesia 86: 235–239

Hannington-Kiff JG 1984 Pharmacologic target blocks in hand surgery and rehabilitation. Journal of Hand Surgery 9: 29–36

Haynes TK, Appadurai IR, Power I, Rosen M, Grant A 1994 Intra-articular morphine and bupivacaine analgesia after arthroscopic knee surgery. Anaesthesia 49: 54–56

Hayes C, Molloy AR 1997 Neuropathic pain in the perioperative period. In: Molloy AR, Power I (eds) International anesthesiology clinics. Acute and chronic pain. Lippincott–Raven, Philadelphia, pp 67–81

Hetherington JW, Philp NH 1986 Diclofenac sodium versus pethidine in acute renal colic. British Medical Journal 292: 237–338

Hoar PF, Hickey RF 1976 Systemic hypertension following myocardial revascularization: a method of treatment using epidural anesthesia. Journal of Thoracic and Cardiovascular Surgery 71: 859

Holder LE, Mackinnon SE 1984 Reflex sympathetic dystrophy in the hands: clinical and scintigraphic criteria. Radiology 152: 517–522

Horowitz SH 1984 Iatrogenic causalgia: clarification, clinical findings and legal ramifications. Archives of Neurology 41: 819–824

Hori Y, Endo K, Takahashi T 1992 Presynaptic inhibitory action of enkephalin on excitatory transmission in superficial dorsal horn of rat spinal cord. Journal of Physiology 450: 673–685

Hume DM, Egdahl RH 1959 The importance of the brain in the endocrine response to injury. Annals of Surgery 150: 697

IASP Task Force on Taxonomy 1994 Classification of chronic pain. IASP Press, Seattle

Inbal R, Devor M, Tuchendler O, Lieblich L 1980 Autonomy following nerve injury: genetic factors in the development of chronic pain. Pain 9: 327–337

Jänig W 1996 The puzzle of 'reflex sympathetic dystrophy': mechanisms, hypotheses, open questions. In: Janig W, Stanton-Hicks M (eds) Reflex sympathetic dystrophy: a reappraisal. IASP Press, Seattle, pp 1–24

Jänig W, McLachlan EM 1994 The role of modifications in noradrenergic peripheral pathways after nerve lesions in the generation of pain. In: Fields HL, Liebeskind JC (eds) Progress in pain research and management. IASP Press, Seattle, pp 101–128

Johnson M 1980 Anxiety in surgical patients. Psychological Medicine 10: 145

Jorgensen L, Rasmussen L, Nielsen A, Leffers A, Albrecht-Beste E 1991 Antithrombotic efficacy of continuous extradural analgesia after knee replacement. British Journal of Anaesthesia 66: 8–12

Katz J, Jackson M, Kavanagh BP, Sandler AN 1996 Acute pain after thoracic surgery predicts long-term post-thoracotomy pain. Clinical Journal of Pain 12: 50–55

Kehlet H 1982 The modifying effect of general and regional anesthesia on the endocrine-metabolic response to surgery. Regional Anesthesia 7: 538

Kehlet H 1984 The stress response to anaesthesia and surgery: release mechanisms and modifying factors. Clinical Anaesthesiology 2: 315

Kehlet H 1988 Modification of responses to surgery by neural blockade: clinical implications. In: Cousins MJ, Bridenbaugh PO (eds) Neural blockade in clinical anesthesia and management of pain, 2nd edn. JB Lippincott, Philadelphia, pp 145–188

Kehlet H 1989 Surgical stress: the role of pain and analgesia. British Journal of Anaesthesia 63: 189–195

Kehlet H 1994 Postoperative pain relief – what is the issue? British Journal of Anaesthesia 72: 375–378

Kehlet H 1996 Effect of pain relief on the surgical stress response. Regional Anesthesia 21(6S): 35–37

Kehlet H 1997 Multimodal approach to control postoperative pathophysiology and rehabilitation. British Journal of Anaesthesia 78: 606–617

Kehlet H 1998 Modification of responses to surgery by neural blockade: clinical implications. In: Cousins MJ, Bridenbaugh PO (eds) Neural blockade in clinical anesthesia and management of pain, 3rd edn Lippencott-Raven Philadelphia, pp 129–178

Kehlet H, Dahl JB 1993a The value of 'multimodal' or 'balanced analgesia' in postoperative pain treatment. Anesthesia and Analgesia 77: 1048–1056

Kehlet H, Dahl JB 1993b Postoperative pain [Review]. World Journal of Surgery 17: 215–219

Kitzinger S 1984 Episiotomy pain. In: Wall PD, Melzack R (eds) Textbook of pain, 1st edn. Churchill Livingstone, Edinburgh, pp 293–303

Klassen GA, Bramwell PR, Bromage RS, Zborawska-Sluis DT 1980 Effect of acute sympathectomy by epidural anesthesia on the canine coronary circulation. Anesthesiology 52: 8–15

Kumar B, Hibbert GR 1984 Control of hypertension during aortic surgery using lumbar extradural blockade. British Journal of Anesthesia 56: 797

Laitinen J, Nuutinen L 1992 Intravenous diclofenac coupled with PCA fentanyl for pain relief after total hip replacement. Anesthesiology 76: 194–198

Laneuville O, Breuer DK, Dewitt DL, Hla T, Funk CD, Smith WL 1994 Differential inhibition of human endoperoxide H synthases-1 and -2 by non-steroidal anti-inflammatory drugs. Journal of Pharmacology and Experimental Therapeutics 271: 927–934

Lekan HA, Carlton SM, Coggeshall RE 1996 Sprouting of A-beta fibers into lamina II of the rat dorsal horn in peripheral neuropathy. Neuroscience Letters 208: 147–150

Levine JD, Fields HL, Basbaum AI 1993 Peptides and the primary afferent nociceptor. Journal of Neurosciences 13: 2273–2286

Light AR, Perl ER 1979 Spinal termination of functionally identified primary afferent neurons with slowly conducting myelinated fibers. Journal of Comparative Neurology 186: 133–150

Lin Q, Peng YB, Willis WD 1996 Role of GABA receptor subtypes in inhibition of primate spinothalamic tract neurons – difference between spinal and periaqueductal gray inhibition. Journal of Neurophysiology 75: 109–123

Lindblom U 1979 Sensory abnormalities in neuralgia. In: Bonica JJ, Liebeskind JC, Albe-Fessard DL (eds) Advances in pain research and therapy, vol 3. Raven Press, New York, pp 111–120

Lipton SA 1993 Prospects for clinically tolerated NMDA antagonists: open-channel blockers and alternative redox states of nitric oxide. Trends in Neurosciences 16: 527–532

Litwin MS 1962 Postsympathectomy neuralgia. Archives of Surgery 84: 591–595

Liu SS, Carpenter RL, Mackey DC et al 1995a Effects of perioperative analgesic technique on rate of recovery after colon surgery. Anesthesiology 83: 757–765

Liu SS, Carpenter RL, Neal JM 1995b Epidural anesthesia and analgesia. Their role in postoperative outcome. Anesthesiology 82: 1474–1506

Lund B, Distel M, Bluhmki E 1998 A double-blind, randomized, placebo-controlled study of efficacy and tolerance of meloxicam treatment in patients with osteoarthritis of the knee. Scandinavian Journal of Rheumatology 27: 32–37

McLachlan EM, Jänig W, Devor M, Michaelis M 1993 Peripheral nerve injury triggers noradrenergic sprouting within dorsal root ganglia. Nature 363: 543–546

McMahon SB 1991 Mechanisms of sympathetic pain. British Medical Bulletin 47: 584–600

McQuay HJ, Carroll D, Jadad AR, Wiffen PJ, Moore A 1995 Anticonvulsants drugs for management of pain: a systematic review. British Medical Journal 311: 1047–1052

Magni G 1991 The use of antidepressants in the treatment of chronic pain: a review of the current evidence. Drugs 42: 730–748

Malmberg AB, Yaksh TL 1993 Spinal nitric oxide synthesis inhibition blocks NMDA-induced thermal hyperalgesia and produces antinociception in the formalin test in rats. Pain 54: 291–300

Mankikian B Cantineau JP, Bertrand M et al 1988 Improvement of diaphragmatic dysfunction by extradural block after upper abdominal surgery. Anesthesiology 68: 379–386

Marks RM, Sacher EJ 1973 Undertreatment of medical patients with narcotic analgesics. Annals of Internal Medicine 78: 173

Mather LE, Mackie J 1983 The incidence of postoperative pain in children. Pain 15: 271

Max MB, Lynch SA, Muir J, Shoaf SE, Smoller B, Dubner R 1992 Effects of desipramine, amitriptyline, and fluoxetine on pain in diabetic neuropathy. New England Journal of Medicine 326: 1250–1256

Meert TF, De Kock M 1994 Potentiation of the analgesic properties of fentanyl-like opioids with α_2-adrenoceptor agonists in rats. Anesthesiology 81: 677–688

Meller ST, Gebhart GF 1993 Nitric oxide (NO) and nociceptive processing in the spinal cord. Pain 52: 127–136

Melzack R 1971 Phantom limb pain. Anesthesiology 35: 409

Melzack R 1988 Psychological aspects of pain, implications for neural blockade. In: Cousins MJ, Bridenbaugh PO (eds) Neural blockade in clinical anesthesia and management of pain, 2nd edn. JB Lippincott, Philadelphia, pp 845–860

Melzack T, Taenzer P, Feldman P, Kinch RA 1981 Labour is still painful after prepared childbirth training. Canadian Medical Association Journal 125: 357

Melzack R, Wall PD, Ty TC 1982 Acute pain in an emergency clinic: latency of onset and description patterns. Pain 14: 33

Mendell LM 1966 Physiological properties of unmyelinated fiber projection to the spinal cord. Experimental Neurology 16: 316–332

Merry A, Power I 1995 Perioperative NSAIDs: towards greater safety. Pain Reviews 2: 268–291

Merskey H 1986 Classification of chronic pain. Descriptions of chronic pain syndromes and definition of pain terms. Pain 3(suppl): S1–S225

Modig J 1976 Respiration and circulation after total hip replacement surgery: a comparison between parenteral analgesics and continuous lumbar epidural block. Acta Anaesthesiologica Scandinavica 20: 225–236

Modig J, Malmberg P, Karlstom G 1980 Effect of epidural versus general anesthesia on calf blood flow. Acta Anaesthesiologica Scandinavica 24: 305

Modig J, Borg T, Karlstom G, Maripuu E, Sahlstedt B 1983 Thromboembolism after hip replacement: role of epidural and general anesthesia. Anesthesia and Analgesia 62: 174–180

Moiniche S, Hjortso NC, Hansen BL et al 1994a The effect of balanced analgesia on early convalescence after major orthopaedic surgery. Acta Anaesthesiologica Scandinavica 38: 328–335

Moiniche S, Dahl JB, Rosenberg J, Kehlet H 1994b Colonic resection with early discharge after combined subarachnoid-epidural analgesia, preoperative glucocorticoids, and early postoperative mobilization and feeding in a pulmonary high-risk patient. Regional Anesthesia 19: 352–356

Molloy AR, Cousins MJ 1999 Pain management. In: Webb AR, Shapiro MJ, Singer M, Suter PM (eds) Oxford Textbook of Critical Care. Oxford University Press. pp 544–547

Morgan JI, Curran T 1986 Role of ion flux in the control of *c-fos* expression. Nature 322: 552–555

NHMRC 1999 Acute pain management: Scientific evidence of Australia. National Health and Medical Research Council of Australia, Canberra

Nimmo WS 1984 Effect of anaesthesia on gastric motility and emptying. British Journal of Anaesthesia 56: 29–37

Nystrom B, Hagbarth KE 1981 Microelectrode recordings from transected nerves in amputees with phantom limb pain. Neuroscience Letters 27: 211–216

O'Hara DA, Fragen RJ, Kinzer M, Pemberton D 1987 Ketorolac tromethamine as compared with morphine sulfate for the treatment of postoperative pain. Clinical Pharmacology and Therapeutics 41: 556–561

Ollat H, Cesaro P 1995 Pharmacology of neuropathic pain. Clinical Neuropharmacology 18: 391–404

O'Shaughnessey L, Slome D 1934 Aetiology of traumatic shock. British Journal of Surgery 22: 589

Pasqualucci V, Moricca G, Solinas P 1980 Intrathecal morphine for the control of the pain of myocardial infarction. Anaesthesia 35: 68

Peck C 1986 Psychological factors in acute pain management. In: Cousins M J, Phillips G D (eds) Acute pain management. Churchill Livingstone, Edinburgh, pp 251–274

Portenoy RK, Foley KM, Inturrisi CE 1990 The nature of opioid responsiveness and its implications for neuropathic pain: new hypotheses derived from studies of opioid infusions. Pain 43: 273–286

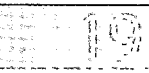

Power I, Bowler GMR, Pugh GC, Chambers WA 1994 Ketorolac as a component of balanced analgesia after thoracotomy. British Journal of Anaesthesia 72: 224–226

Price DD, Mao JR, Mayer DJ (1994) Central neural mechanisms of normal and abnormal pain states. In: Fields HL, Liebeskind JC (eds) Progress in pain research and management. IASP Press, Seattle, pp 61–84

Rawal N, Sjostrand U, Christoffersson E, Dahlstrom B, Avril A, Raymond H 1984 Comparisons of intramuscular and epidural morphine for postoperative analgesia in the grossly obese: influence on postoperative ambulation and pulmonary function. Anesthesia and Analgesia 63: 583–592

Ready LB, Oden R, Chadwick HS et al 1988 Development of an anesthesiology-based postoperative pain service. Anesthesiology 68: 100–106

Ready LB, Ashburn M, Caplan RA et al 1995 Practice guidelines for acute pain management in the peri-operative setting – a report of the American Society of Anesthesiologists task force on pain management. Anesthesiology 82: 1071–1081

Reiz S, Balfors E, Sorensen MR et al 1982 Coronary hemodynamic effects of general anesthesia and surgery. Regional Anesthesia 7(suppl): S8–S18

Roberts WJ 1986 An hypothesis on the physiological basis for causalgia and related pains. Pain 24: 297–311

Sabiston DC 1982 Davis Christopher textbook of surgery: the biological basis of modern surgical practice, 2nd edn. W B Saunders, Philadelphia, pp 265–286

Scheinin B et al 1987 The effect of bupivacaine and morphine on pain and bowel function after colonic surgery. Acta Anaesthesiologica Scandinavica 31: 161–164

Schott GD 1986 Mechanisms of causalgia and related clinical conditions: the role of the central and of the sympathetic nervous systems. Brain 109: 717–738

Schulze S, Roikjaer O, Hasseistrom L, Jensen NH, Kehlet H 1988 Epidural bupivacaine and morphine plus systemic indomethacin eliminates pain but not systemic response and convalescence after cholecystectomy. Surgery 103: 321–327

Scott DB 1988 Acute pain management. In: Cousins MJ, Bridenbaugh PO (eds) Neural blockade in clinical anesthesia and management of pain, 2nd edn. JB Lippincott, Philadelphia, pp 861–864

Scott N, Kehlet H 1988 Regional anaesthesia and surgical morbidity. British Journal of Surgery 75: 199–204

Seibert K, Zhang Y, Leahy K 1994 Pharmacological and biochemical demonstration of the role of cyclooxygenase 2 in inflammation and pain. Proceedings of the National Academy of Science of USA 91: 12013–12017

Shafer S, Varvel JR 1991 Pharmacokinetics, pharmacodynamics and rational opioid selection. Anesthesiology 74: 54–63

Sivilotti L, Woolf CJ 1994 The contribution of $GABA_A$ and glycine receptors to central sensitization: disinhibition and touch-evoked allodynia in the spinal cord. Journal of Neurophysiology 72: 169–179

Sjogren S, Wright B 1972 Circulatory changes during continuous epidural blockade. Acta Anaesthesiologica Scandinavica 46(suppl): 5

Smith MT, Watt JA, Cramond T 1990 Morphine-3-glucuronide: a potent antagonist of morphine analgesia. Life Sciences 47: 579–585

Stein C 1993 Peripheral mechanisms of opioid analgesia. Anesthesia and Analgesia 76: 182–191

Stein C 1995 Morphine – a local 'analgesic'. Pain: Clinical Updates 3: 1–4

Stein C, Millan MJ, Shippenberg TS 1989 Peripheral opioid receptors mediating antinociception in inflammation: evidence for involvement of mu, delta, and kappa receptors. Journal of Pharmacology and Experimental Therapeutics 248: 1269–1275

Sternbach RA 1963 Congenital insensitivity to pain: a critique. Physiological Bulletin 60: 252–264

Stratton Hill C 1995 When will adequate pain treatment be the norm? [Editorial.] Journal of the American Medical Association 274(23): 1881–1882.

Strichartz G 1995 Protracted relief of experimental neuropathic pain by systemic local anesthetics – how, where, and when. Anesthesiology 83: 654–655

Sugimoto T, Takemura M, Sakai A, Ishimaru M 1987 Rapid transneuronal destruction following peripheral nerve transection. Pain 30: 385–394

Sunderland S 1978 Neroes and nerve injuries, 2nd edn. Churchill Livingstone, Edinburgh

Tasker RR, Tsuda T, Hawrylyshyn P 1983 Clinical neurophysiological investigation of deafferentation pain. In: Bonica JJ, Lindblom U, Iggo A (eds) Advances in pain research and therapy, vol 5. Raven, New York, pp 713–738

Tennant F, Moll D, Depaulo V 1993 Topical morphine for peripheral pain. Lancet 342: 1047–1048

The HSG, Lund B, Distel MR, Bluhmki E 1997 A double-blind, randomized trial to compare meloxicam 15 mg with diclofenac 100 mg in the treatment of osteoarthritis of the knee. Osteoarthritis & Cartilage 5: 283–288

Thoren T, Sundberg A, Wattwil M, Garvill JE et al 1989 Effects of epidural bupivacaine and epidural morphine on bowel function and pain after hysterectomy. Acta Anaesthesiologica Scandinavica 33: 181–195

Thorn SE, Wattwil M, Naslund I et al 1992 Post-operative epidural morphine but not epidural bupivacaine, delays gastric emptying on the first day after cholecystectomy. Regional Anesthesia 17 (2) 91–94

Trujillo KA, Akil H 1991 Inhibition of morphine tolerance and dependence by the NMDA receptor antagonist MK-801. Science 251: 85–87

Tuman KJ, McCarthy RJ, March RJ et al 1991 Effects of epidural anesthesia and analgesia on coagulation and outcome after major vascular surgery. Anesthesia and Analgesia 73: 696–704

Urquhart E 1993 Central analgesic activity of nonsteroidal antiinflammatory drugs in animal and human pain models. Seminars in Arthritis and Rheumatism 23: 198–205

Vik-Mo H, Ottsen S, Renck H 1978 Cardiac effects of thoracic epidural analgesia before and during acute coronary artery occlusion in openchest dogs. Scandinavian Journal of Clinical and Laboratory Investigation 38: 737–746

Voudoris N, Peck C 1985 Conditional placebo responses. Journal of Personality and Social Psychology 48: 47

Walker JS 1995 NSAID: an update on their analgesic effects. Clinical and Experimental Pharmacology and Physiology 22: 855–860

Wall PD 1983 Alterations in the central nervous system after deafferentation. In: Bonica JJ, Lindblom U, Iggo A (eds) Advances in pain research and therapy, vol 5. Raven, New York, pp 677–689

Wall PD, Devor M 1978 Physiology of sensation after peripheral nerve injury, regeneration and neuroma formation. In: Waxman SG (ed) Physiology and pathobiology of axons. Raven, New York

Wattwil M, Thoren T, Hennerdal S, Garvill JE et al 1989 Epidural analgesia with bupivacaine reduces postoperative paralytic ileus after hysterectomy. Anesthesia and Analgesia 68: 353–358

White JC, Sweet WH 1962 Pain and the neurosurgeon. CC Thomas, Springfield, Illinois, pp 11–49

Wilcox GL 1991 Excitatory neurotransmitters and pain. In: Bond MR, Charlton JE, Woolf CJ (eds) Proceedings of the VIth World Congress on Pain. Elsevier, Amsterdam, pp 97–117

Wilmore DW 1983 Alterations in protein, carbohydrate and fat metabolism in injured and septic patients. Journal of the American College of Nutrition 2: 3

Wilmore DW, Long JM, Mason AD, Pruitt BA 1976 Stress in surgical patients as a neurophysiologic reflex response. Surgery, Gynecology and Obstetrics 142: 257

Wilson PR, Yaksh TL 1995 Baclofen is antinociceptive in the spinal intrathecal space of animals. European Journal of Pharmacology 51: 323–330

Wong CS, Cherng CH, Luk HN, Ho ST, Tung CS 1996 Effects of NMDA receptor antagonists on inhibition of morphine tolerance in rats – binding at mu-opioid receptors. European Journal of Pharmacology 297: 27–33

Woolf CJ 1983 Evidence for a central component of post injury pain hypersensitivity. Nature 306: 686–688

Woolf CJ 1989 Recent advances in the pathophysiology of acute pain. British Journal of Anaesthesia 63: 139–146

Woolf C, Shortland P, Coggeshall RE 1992 Peripheral nerve injury triggers central sprouting of myelinated afferents. Nature 355: 75–78

Woolf CJ, Chong MS 1993 Preemptive analgesia – treating postoperative pain by preventing the establishment of central sensitization. Anesthesia and Analgesia 77: 362–379

Woolf CJ, Thompson SWN 1991 The induction and maintenance of central sensitization is dependent on *N*-methyl-*D*-aspartic acid receptor activation; implications for the treatment of post-injury pain hypersensitivity states. Pain 44: 293–299

Woolf CJ, Wiesenfield-Hallin Z 1985 The systemic administration of local anaesthetics produces a selective depression of c-afferent fiber evoked activity in the spinal cord. Pain 23: 361–374

Woolf CJ, Shortland P, Coggeshall RE 1992 Peripheral nerve injury triggers central sprouting of myelinated afferents. Nature 355: 75–78

Xu X-J, Puke MJC, Verge VMK, Wiesenfeld-Hallin Z, Hughes J, Hokfelt T 1993 Up-regulation of cholecystokinin in primary sensory neurons is associated with morphine insensitivity in experimental neuropathic pain in the rat. Neuroscience Letters 152: 129–132

Yaksh TL, Reddy SVR 1981 Studies in the primate on the analgetic effects associated with intrathecal actions of opiates, alpha-adrenergic agonists and baclofen. Anesthesiology 54: 451–467

Yeager MP, Glass DD, Neff RK, Brinck-Johnson T 1987 Epidural anesthesia and analgesia in high risk surgical patients. Anesthesiology 66: 729–736

Zeigler D, Lynch SA, Muir J, Benjamin J, Max MB 1992 Transdermal clonidine versus placebo in painful diabetic neuropathy. Pain 48: 403–408

Zolte N, Cust MD 1986 Analgesia in the acute abdomen. Annals of the Royal College of Surgeons of England 68: 209–210

Osteoarthritis

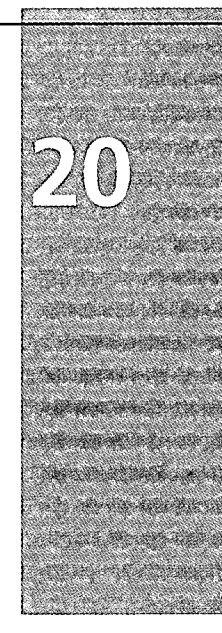

PAUL CREAMER

SUMMARY

Osteoarthritis (OA) is the most common form of arthritis, and is a major cause of morbidity, limitation of activity and health-care utilization (Van Saase et al 1989, Lawrence et al 1990). Pain is the major symptom of OA and the main reason why affected individuals elect to seek medical care. Pain is also a major determinant of functional loss. Despite its importance, there is much about OA pain that remains unclear including, for example, the anatomical cause of pain and the reason for the poor correlation between pain and radiographic change.

This chapter will provide a brief overview of OA before a more detailed description of the nature, causes and treatment of pain. Back pain is dealt with elsewhere: this chapter will concentrate on peripheral joint OA with particular emphasis on the knee.

AETIOPATHOGENESIS OF OSTEOARTHRITIS

Osteoarthritis is a disorder of synovial joints characterized by destruction of articular cartilage and remodelling of subchondral bone. Cartilage loss is mediated by a range of degradative enzymes, notably the matrix metalloproteinases, which are capable of breaking down both proteoglycan and type II collagen. Cartilage breakdown is accompanied by an increase in the number and activity of chondrocytes representing an attempt at tissue repair. OA is thus far from a passive, 'degenerative' process but may be viewed as a failure of the normal balance which exists between cartilage formation and catabolism. Thickening of subchondral bone, detectable by an increase in activity on bone scan, is also an early feature and may predict the future development of OA in otherwise asymptomatic joints in both the hand (Fig. 20.1) (Hutton et al 1986) and the knee (Dieppe et al 1993). It is unclear whether bone or cartilage represent the primary lesion in OA but clearly both are potential areas for therapeutic intervention.

Macroscopically, these changes result in focal cartilage fibrillation and thinning, sclerosis and cyst formation in the underlying bone, and formation of bony spurs (osteophytes) at the joint margins. Some of these features correspond to radiographic changes on which the diagnosis of

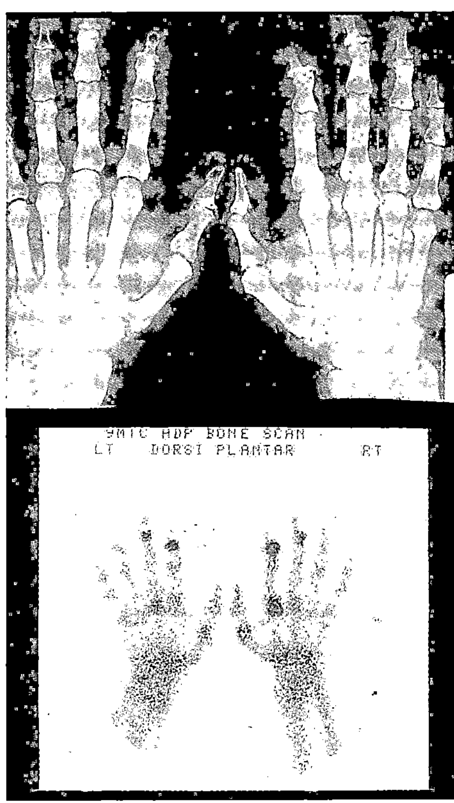

Fig. 20.1 Plain radiograph (top) and Tc^{99} scintigraphy (bottom) of a patient with hand OA. Note the 'hot' joints on scan, corresponding to sites of radiographic change.

OA is usually made (Fig. 20.2, Table 20.1). It is, however, increasingly clear that OA is not a single disorder but rather a group of overlapping distinct diseases: risk factors, clinical features, radiographic features and outcomes may vary from site to site. The term 'osteoarthritic disorders' has been suggested as a more appropriate descriptor. Radiographically, for example, some patients develop an erosive form of OA, particularly at the hand; another variant is 'atrophic' OA, seen mostly at the hip (Fig. 20.3) in which bony response in terms of osteophyte is minimal.

There are a number of predisposing factors for OA, including genetic factors, age, gender, obesity and race. However, local biomechanical factors including joint shape, usage and trauma probably determine which joints get OA in a susceptible individual. Thus, removal of a meniscus greatly increases the risk of subsequent OA at the knee. Although OA is found in other animals, humans appear to be at greater risk: perhaps because they live longer or because their joints are relatively maladapted in an evolutionary sense to, for example, the stresses of bipedal locomotion.

CLINICAL FEATURES OF OSTEOARTHRITIS

The main joints to be affected by OA include the interphalangeal joints of the hand (Fig. 20.4), the thumb base, the knees, hips and facet joints of the cervical and lumbar spine. Much OA appears to be asymptomatic: when it does cause clinical problems these include pain, stiffness after inactivity, deformity, swelling and loss of function.

The diagnosis of OA still relies on radiographic features, although it is clear that considerable pathological change may occur before radiographs become abnormal (Fife et al 1991).

The interpretation of radiographs usually refers to a standard atlas of composite features, such as the Kellgren and Lawrence grading system (Kellgren & Lawrence 1963) which ranges from grade 0 (normal) to grade 4 (severe advanced OA). There is some evidence that the relationship between radiographs and pain is better for osteophytes than for other features, at least at the knee (Spector et al 1993, Lethbridge-Cejku et al 1995, Cicuttini et al 1996). Arthroscopy allows direct visualization of cartilage (but not underlying bone) and scoring systems are now available to standardize recording of cartilage damage (Ayral et al 1996). Magnetic resonance imaging (MRI) (Fig. 20.5) has the advantage of being non-invasive and allowing assessment of non-bony structures: however, the cost and expertise required for interpretation make it impractical for routine use.

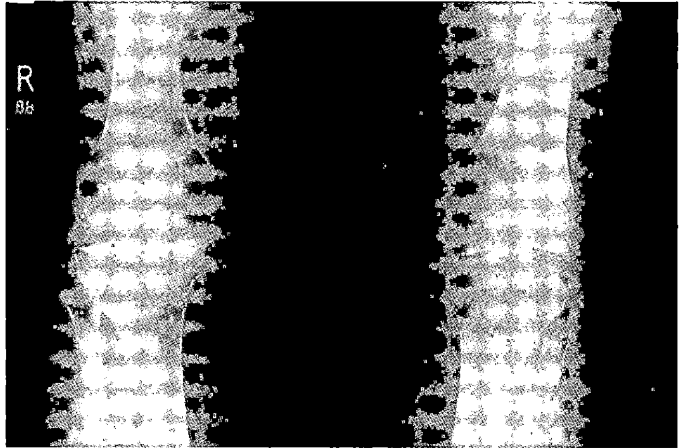

Fig. 20.2 Radiograph of tibiofemoral OA, showing joint space narrowing, sclerosis and osteophyte formation.

PATHOPHYSIOLOGY OF JOINT PAIN

Detailed descriptions of the pathophysiology of joint pain are beyond the scope of this chapter and have been recently reviewed elsewhere (Kontinnen et al 1994, Kidd 1996). Most afferent fibres in articular nerves are unmyelinated, comprising C (group IV) fibres and postganglionic sympathetic fibres. Heavily myelinated Aβ (group II) fibres and thinly myelinated Aδ (group III) fibres comprise about 20% of the total fibres. There is rich innervation to articular

Table 20.1 Relationship between pathological and radiographic features of osteoarthritis

Pathological features	*Radiographic features*
Focal areas of loss of articular cartilage	Asymmetric loss of interbone distance ('joint space narrowing')
Marginal lipping and overgrowth	Osteophytosis of bone
Remodelling of subchondral bone	Sclerosis and cysts in subchondral bone, altered bony contour
Capsular thickening and mild chronic synovitis	

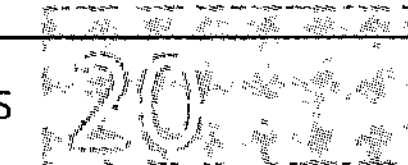

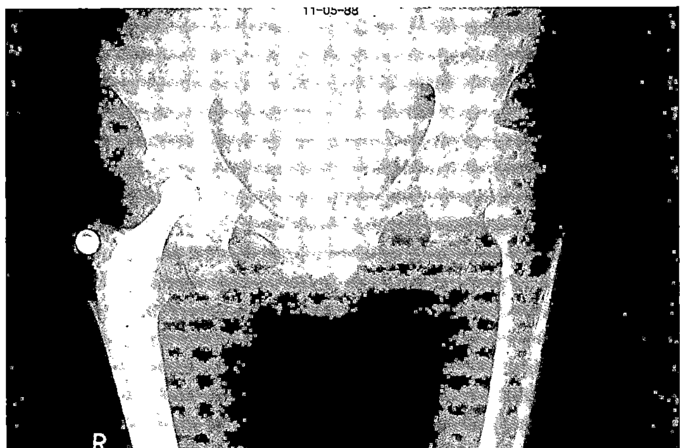

Fig. 20.3 Atrophic OA of the hip.

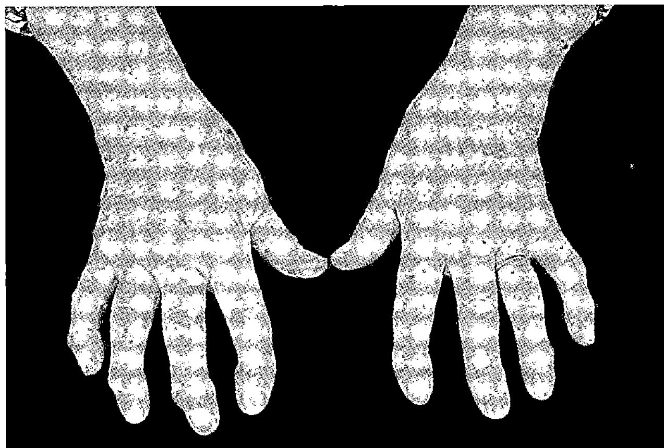

Fig. 20.4 Interphalangeal OA.

capsule, tendons, ligaments synovium and periosteum via a mixture of free nerve endings and receptors. These sensory nerves respond to mechanical stimuli such as stretching of the joint capsule but also to chemical mediators such as lactic acid, histamine, kinins and substance P. Such inflammatory mediators may stimulate pain fibres directly but may also sensitize fibres to mechanical stimuli. Many fibres, for example, are non-responsive under normal conditions but react after inflammation. There is therefore potential for acute injury or inflammation to sensitize nerves such that they respond even when the original stimuli is removed. This 'neurogenic plasticity' may operate at both peripheral and spinal levels and is likely to be mediated by upregulation of specific receptors such as those for *N*-methyl-D aspartate (NMDA). Clearly these represent potential targets for therapeutic intervention. Although there is evidence for a central role for pain production in some patients, peripheral mechanisms are probably more important; for example, intra-articular local anaesthetic effectively abolishes pain

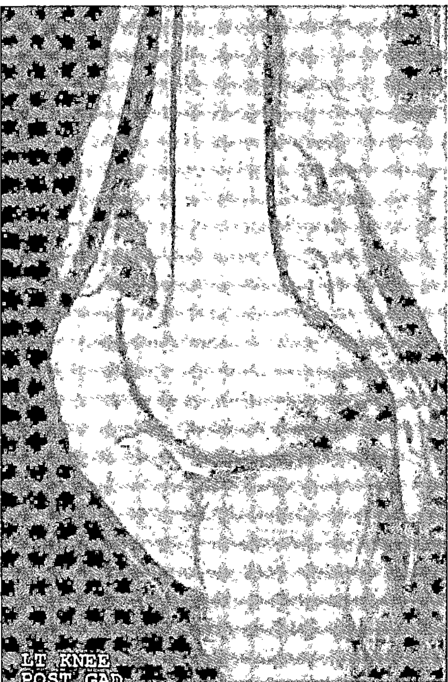

Fig. 20.5 MRI of knee, showing extensive patellofemoral OA.

temporarily in many patients with knee OA (Creamer et al 1996).

MEASUREMENT OF PAIN IN OSTEOARTHRITIS

In epidemiological studies, the presence of knee pain is usually ascertained by a simple question such as the NHANES-I question: 'Have you ever had pain in or around the knee on most days for at least a month?' (Lawrence et al 1990). Subjects responding positively are said to have 'ever' knee pain. Subjects reporting pain within the last year have 'current' pain. This question has been criticized as being too specific, and may fail to capture subjects with intermittent or mild pain. It is clear that small alterations in the exact wording may result in large differences in the prevalence of reported pain (O'Reilly et al 1996).

Severity is a separate aspect of the pain experience; the risk factors for presence of pain may differ from those for severity. Subjective pain intensity may be graded using a simple Likert scale (none, mild, moderate, severe, very severe) or a visual analogue scale. The stem question may be a simple 'how bad is your (knee, hip, hand) pain?', but additional valuable information can be obtained by asking about pain with different activities: stairs, walking, rest and so on. Such information is obtained in at least three questionnaires specifically designed to assess lower limb OA: the WOMAC (Bellamy et al 1988) and Lequesne (1991) indices and the Knee Pain Scale (Rejeski et al 1995).

An attempt is sometimes made to assess the quality of pain in OA, using the McGill Pain Questionnaire (MPQ; Melzack 1975). This instrument allows subjects to select words (total = 76) which describe their pain. The MPQ was not specifically designed for arthritis pain and some of the descriptors used may reflect mood disturbance rather than pure pain.

Finally, attempts have been made to examine the effect of pain on observed behaviour in OA (Keefe et al 1987a), usually by videotaping patients while they undergo a standard programme of activities. Five components are identified: guarding, active rubbing, unloading the joint, rigidity and joint flexing. Pain behaviour correlates only modestly with reported pain severity (r=0.46), suggesting that they identify different facets of the pain experience. A number of factors have been shown to correlate with pain behaviour in knee OA: these include coping strategies, age (older patients showing more pain behaviour), obesity and disability support status. These were predictive of pain behaviour even after controlling for gender, obesity and radiographic disease severity.

EPIDEMIOLOGY OF OSTEOARTHRITIC PAIN

Most studies of pain in OA have looked at the knee. The prevalence of knee pain (as a dichotomous variable – present or absent) in relation to radiographic OA has been reported in several community studies. Using the question 'have you had pain within the last year in and around the knee that occurred on most days for at least a month?', a recent postal survey (O'Reilly et al 1996) of 40–79-year-old community dwellers in the UK found a positive response in 25.3%. Radiographic knee OA was reported in 76%. Other examples are given in Table 20.2. Less data is available on other joints. Using a definition of 'mild to severe pain during the last month', Carman (1989) reported a prevalence of hand pain of 37% in 50–74 year olds, of whom 45% had definite OA.

A consistent finding is that, although the chances of reporting pain increase with increasing radiographic severity, a significant number of people in the community report knee pain despite normal knee radiographs. At the other end of the spectrum many individuals with unequivocal knee OA apparently deny having pain. Further evidence of discrepency between radiographic change and symptoms comes from studies examining pain severity rather than presence/absence. Individuals with severe OA do not necessarily report higher levels of pain than those with mild OA. Finally, longitudinal studies (Ledingham et al 1995, Dieppe et al 1997) show that radiographic change and symptoms do not always progress in parallel.

How do we account for this lack of association between pain and structural damage? One explanation may be the relative lack of sensitivity of radiographs: structures responsible for pain (e.g. ligaments or menisci) may not show up on a plain X-ray. Some studies rely on inadequate views of the joint: for example, at the knee, plain anteroposterior views fail to visualize the patellofemoral joint which is a frequent site of OA (Fig. 20.6).

Our attempts to link radiographic changes to pain reporting stem from the belief that the cause of knee pain is visible on an X-ray. This may not be so. Non-pharmacological

Table 20.2 Prevalence of knee pain by radiographic severity (Kellgren and Lawrence/KL grade) in selected community studies. In all studies, prevalence figures given indicate a positive response to the question: 'Have you ever had pain in and around your knee on most days for at least 1 month':* = pain occurring within last 1 year. ** = pain occurring within last 2 years. No asterisk = pain occurring at any time in the past ("ever pain").

	Felson et al 1987	*Hochberg et al 1989*	*Carman et al 1989*	*Davis et al 1992*		*Lethbridge-Cejku et al 1995*	
Age range (yr)	63–94	25–74	50–74	45–74		19–92	
Gender	M/F**	M/F	M/F	M	F	M/F*	M/F*
KL grade (%)							
0	7.6	—	22	7.6	8.4	14.4	9.4
1	10.8	—	34	11.0	21.4	21.9	11.8
2	19.2	39	58	42.5	31.6	29.9	20.4
3/4	40.0	61	80	76.0	51.9	65.8	56.1

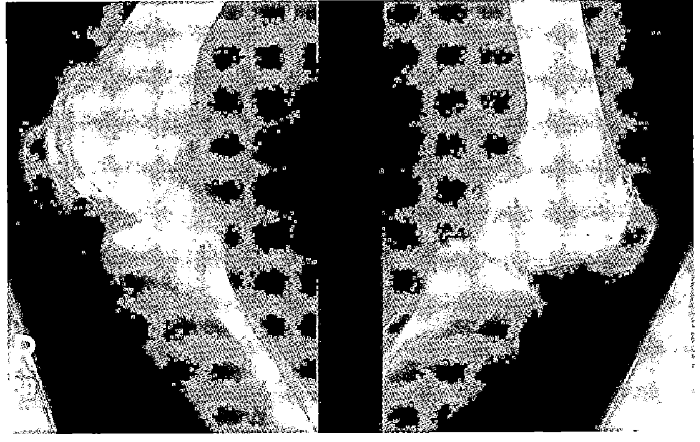

Fig. 20.6 Lateral view of knee, showing patellofemoral OA. The anteroposterior views of this patient appeared normal.

interventions such as simply talking to patients by telephone, use of acupuncture or weight loss and aerobic exercise programmes can have significant effects on pain severity. Interventions on one knee may have a profound effect on pain perception in the other (Creamer et al 1996). Pain severity is reported by some patients as greater at weekends and less on weekdays (Bellamy et al 1990). It is therefore likely that pain in OA is not simply the result of structural changes but, rather, the outcome of a complex interplay between structural change, peripheral and central pain processing mechanisms and subjective differences in what constitutes pain, in turn influenced by cultural, gender and psychosocial factors. It is perhaps more helpful to regard knee pain and radiographic knee OA as separate problems: certainly they appear to differ in their risk factors (Davis 1992).

Subjects with clinical features such as crepitus and morning stiffness are more likely to report pain. For a given degree of radiographic severity, women tend to report pain more often than men. Age does not appear to be related to pain reporting. Increasing body mass index has been found to be a risk factor for pain in knee OA in some studies. Quadriceps weakness is a major risk factor for knee pain and subsequent disability (McAlindan et al 1993).

ANATOMICAL CAUSES OF PAIN IN OSTEOARTHRITIS

The anatomical cause of pain in OA remains unclear. Any theory must take account of the fact that the principal structure involved (articular cartilage) possesses few pain-sensitive fibres: pain must therefore be arising from other tissues.

BONE PAIN

Bony changes at the joint margin and beneath focal areas of damaged cartilage are probably major sources of pain in OA. As chondrophytes and osteophytes grow they result in elevation and stretching of the richly innervated periosteum (Kellgren 1983). Many subjects with knee OA report well-localized pain and tenderness at the inferomedial part of the joint which may represent osteophyte growth. It is possible that osteophytes may only be painful at certain phases in their development.

Raised intraosseous pressure can be demonstrated in OA and there is much evidence to link this with pain, particularly at rest (Arnoldi et al 1980). Osteotomy provides rapid relief from pain in OA (Insall et al 1974); the fact that even simple drilling to reduce pressure has a similar benefit suggests that this is not only operating by altering bony mechanics (Astrom 1975).

INFLAMMATION

Although traditionally OA has been regarded as a non-inflammatory disease, there is accumulating evidence that an inflammatory component may be present in some patients at some phases of the disease. For example, synovial histology may show marked focal synovial hyperplasia and a dense mononuclear cell infiltrate, indistinguishable from that seen in rheumatoid arthritis (RA) (Revell et al 1988, Haraoui et al 1991). Recently, expression of oncoproteins (Roivainen et al 1996) and NF-kB (Marok et al 1996), an essential transcription factor for expression of a variety of proinflammatory genes, has also been demonstrated in OA synovium. Finally, systemic markers of inflammation such as C-reactive protein (CRP) and serum hyaluronic acid (HA) are elevated in many patients and may predict progression (Sharif et al 1995, Spector et al 1997).

The cause of inflammation in OA remains unclear: the role of cartilage-derived macromolecules and calcium-containing crystals is controversial (Schumacher 1995). Once initiated, the release of wear particles may contribute to a cycle of inflammation resulting in further activation of synovium and release of cytokines (Evans & Mears 1981). Inflammation may play an important role in the symptoms of OA; most notably by modulating pain perception (Kontinnen et al 1994). Some products of inflammation such as bradykinin or histamine are capable of directly stimulating primary afferent nociceptive (PAN) fibres, while others (prostaglandins, leukotrienes and interleukins 1 and 6) may sensitize PANs to mechanical or other stimuli. Corticosteroids, by inhibiting phospholipase A2, reduce the production of these mediators and hence reduce inflammatory pain.

SOFT-TISSUE PAIN

The joint capsule contains many pain fibres. Capsular changes are found in OA; it is possible that stretching the capsule is one cause of pain. Ligaments are similar pain-sensitive structures. Periarticular pain is common in OA and may arise from a number of structures (Lynn & Kellgren 1986). These include bursae (particularly around the knee joint, the anserine bursa), tendons and their insertions (entheses). In addition, there may be referred tender spots (Lynn & Kellgren 1986): that is, areas of local tenderness away from the joint.

PSYCHOSOCIAL FACTORS

Depression is a feature of most chronic painful conditions. A 25.9% prevalence of 'possible' depression was found in a survey of elderly community-based subjects with OA hip or knee (Dexter & Brandt 1994). Depression scores were positively associated with black race, living in subsidized housing and perceiving the problem as severe and negatively associated with older age and higher education. Subjects with knee OA who attend hospital have higher rates of depression: 33% of hospital outpatients with hip/knee OA had 'possible' depression (Hawley & Wolfe 1993), contrasting with a population prevalence using the same criteria of 19%. While differences between hospital and community subjects may reflect severity of disease, it is also possible that depression may play a role in the decision by patients to seek medical care.

Are subjects with or without radiographic evidence of OA more likely to report knee pain if they are depressed or anxious? In summary, community surveys in which pain is treated as a dichotomous variable (present or absent) suggest that psychological factors are associated with reporting of knee pain. Although some early studies (Lawrence et al 1966) found no relationship between 'psychological factors' (using a fairly crude four-point scale of neurosis) and knee pain, data from the New Haven Survey of Joint Disease (Acheson & Ginsburg 1973), the NHANES-I cohort (Carman 1989, Hochberg et al 1989) and the Baltimore Longitudinal Study of Aging (Creamer et al 1998) all suggest a link between psychological factors and knee pain, independent of radiographic changes.

In patients who have symptomatic knee OA, to what extent do depression and anxiety influence pain intensity scores? A study (Summers et al 1988) of hospital outpatients with hip or knee OA found that both depression and anxiety correlated with pain severity as measured by the MPQ. Also using the MPQ in a study of hospital outpatients with knee OA, Salaffi et al (1991) found significant correlations between all facets of the MPQ and anxiety and depression, using the Zung inventories. The strongest correlations were with 'affective' pain: for anxiety r=0.56; for depression r=0.62. These reports from hospital outpatients have recently been supported by a community survey of elderly subjects reporting sporadic, episodic or chronic knee pain (Hopman-Rock et al 1996). Chronicity and severity of pain were associated with higher psychosocial disability when compared with age-matched pain-free controls from the same community.

In addition to depression and anxiety, personality traits such as hypochondriasis have been shown to be associated with greater pain severity in OA of the hip (Lunghi et al 1978) and knee (Lichtenberg et al 1984, 1986). 'Life stress' may also be a risk factor for pain reporting (Lichtenberg et al 1984), although there is some evidence that 'daily hassles' (repetitive, chronic irritations such as troubles with family life or work, excessive noise, frustrations with living conditions) are equally important (Lichtenberg et al 1986). Lower formal education level has been reported to be a risk factor for both radiographic and symptomatic knee OA (Hannan et al 1992).

The mechanisms by which psychosocial factors are related to knee pain are unclear and cross-sectional studies do not allow us to make inferences about cause and effect. Chronic pain may result in a range of psychological reactions, including uncertainty, anxiety, depression and anger. Conversely, psychological processes themselves may be responsible for pain or pain amplification. Pathophysiological effects of anxiety or depression include increased muscle tension which may be painful. Anxiety, manifested by persistent attempts to avoid knee pain, may lead to loss of muscle bulk and generalized deconditioning and loss of confidence. Quadriceps strength is an important determinant of knee pain and function (McAlindon et al 1993) and it is possible that overavoidance of movement in knee pain leads to a chronic cycle of inactivity, muscle wasting and weakness and further pain and inactivity (Dekker et al 1993). Depression may also result in maladapted 'coping strategies' or affect the patient's belief about their ability to cope with pain, which in itself results in higher reported pain severity (Keefe et al 1987b).

It should be noted that these two explanations are not mutually exclusive, indeed, it is likely that a chronic cycle exists in which pain results in psychological distress, which in turn results in pain amplification. Psychological factors may also be important in predicting response to therapies and determining patients' adherence to treatment. In a study of exercise for patients with knee arthritis, for example, the most powerful predictors of maintaining exercise at 3 months were baseline anxiety and depression (Minor & Brown 1993).

THE NATURE OF OSTEOARTHRITIC PAIN

Pain due to OA is generally insidious in onset, localized and not associated with any systemic disturbance. The severity of OA pain is comparable to that of RA (Huskisson et al 1979). However, the words used to describe pain may be different: OA tends to be a persistent ache, interspersed with episodes of stabbing pain provoked by movement of the affected joint, whereas in RA the pain is said to be more 'hot' or 'burning' (Wagstaff et al 1985). Using the MPQ, the most frequent words selected by subjects with knee OA to describe their pain were 'aching', 'throbbing' and 'sharp'.

Characteristically, pain is worse on use of the affected joint (e.g. going up or down stairs for knee OA), worse in the evenings and eased by rest. A significant proportion of subjects, however, do complain of pain at night: such patients have generally had symptoms for longer than those without night pain and may have more severe disease. In addition to diurnal variation, some patients show a day-to-day variation, with symptoms being worse at the weekends (Bellamy et al 1990).

The location of pain in OA generally corresponds to the affected joint but referred pain may be seen: for example, pain from hip OA may be felt in the knee and pain from spinal OA may be felt in the hip or buttock. At the knee, most pain is either diffusely felt anteriorly over the surface of the patella or is more localized to the inferomedial aspect of the joint: these differences are not simply explained by the location of radiographic change. A number of structures may cause inferomedial knee pain including the medial collateral ligament, the anserine bursa and osteophytes at the medial tibial plateau. Tender spots are also common around the knee, the most frequent being the insertion and origin of the medial collateral ligament and the medial and lateral joint lines. Even more frequently tenderness is found at a point about 5 cm below the medial joint line: this does not correspond to any clear structure and may represent a referred tender spot.

MANAGEMENT OF PAIN IN OSTEOARTHRITIS

Pain is the most frequent symptom of OA and, in the absence of therapies which may modify the underlying disease process, treatments for OA are primarily assessed by their ability to reduce pain. Ideally, treatments would be based on knowledge of pathogenesis: however, because we do not know the cause of pain in OA, treatment is to some extent empirical. Nevertheless, four areas may be identified: correction of abnormal mechanical stress; control of disease processes driving OA; modulation of central perception of pain and, finally, surgery.

CORRECTION OF ABNORMAL BIOMECHANICS

Load reduction may be achieved at the hip or knee by the use of a walking stick, which can reduce load bearing in the affected joint by 20–30% with a consequent reduction in symptoms. The adaption of footwear, for example by use of shock-absorbing insoles or lateral heel wedges (Keating et al 1993), can also reduce pain. Other orthotic devices, such as splints, braces and neck collars, aim to correct deformity and instability: at the knee, for example, braces may correct lateral thrust. Patients with knee OA who have patellofemoral joint disease have been shown to benefit from medial taping of the patella (Cushnaghan et al 1994).

Many cross-sectional studies have shown a strong association between overweight and OA, particularly at the knee and particularly in women (Felson et al 1988, Schouten et al 1992). Weight loss is associated with a lower chance of developing symptomatic OA and incident radiographic OA (Felson et al 1997). Despite the obvious importance of obesity as a potentially modifiable risk factor for knee OA, there are few studies showing that weight reduction reduces symptoms. In a study of overweight postmenopausal women with symptomatic knee OA (Martin et al 1996), weight loss during a 6-month programme of dietary counselling and exercise was associated with a reduction in both pain and impaired function as measured by the WOMAC Osteoarthritis Index. The paucity of other data may reflect that losing weight by diet alone is clearly not easy, particularly in the elderly who may be relatively immobile.

Quadriceps weakness may be a risk factor for radiographic OA (Slemenda et al 1997) and is clearly an important determinant of function and pain (Dekker et al 1993, McAlindon et al 1993). Several studies, of 3–6 months in duration, have documented that quadriceps strengthening exercises are effective in reducing pain and improving function in patients with knee OA (Chamberlain et al 1982, Fisher et al 1993). Quadriceps strengthening can be accomplished by both isometric and isotonic, resistive exercise. The preferred technique for patients with knee OA is currently unclear.

Aerobic conditioning exercise, either supervised fitness walking or aquatics, has been shown to be well tolerated and more effective than conventional physical therapy or standard medical care in patients with OA of the hip and/or knee. Home exercises are as effective as outpatient hydrotherapy in hip OA. A recent multicentre study (Ettinger et al 1997) on community-dwelling adults with knee OA and self-reported physical disability aged 60 and above demonstrated that participation in either aerobic or resistive exercise was superior to patient education alone.

CONTROL OF DISEASE PROCESS DRIVING OSTEOARTHRITIS

Anti-inflammatories

Non-steroidal anti-inflammatory drugs are widely prescribed in OA, although evidence for the superiority of non-steroidal anti-inflammatory drugs (NSAIDs) over paracetamol is largely lacking and, at least under trial conditions, many patients on chronic NSAID therapy for knee OA can cease this medication without apparent deterioration in symptoms. A small proportion of patients with OA do seem to derive sustained benefit from NSAIDs: it is tempting to suggest that these patients have a more 'inflammatory' type of OA, but it is not possible from clinical examination to predict those patients who will respond (Bradley et al 1992). The use of NSAIDs is associated with appreciable morbidity, particularly in the elderly (the group most likely to have OA). Intra-articular (IA) steroids are also widely used. Controlled trials, confined to the knee, provide some evidence supporting their efficacy, but only for up to 4 weeks (Creamer 1997). This contrasts with clinical practice which suggests that some patients have a sustained response lasting up to 6 months. Efforts to identify predictors of response have proved largely unsuccessful, although some studies have reported that the presence of effusion (Gaffney et al 1995) or local tenderness (Jones & Doherty 1996) may be associated with a better response. There is much less data on steroid injection in joints other than the knee. A recent report (Griffith et al 1997) found significant improvement in pain, stiffness and range of movement after steroid or anaesthetic injection at the hip but both injections were equally effective. Anecdotally, injection of the carpometacarpal joint can be very helpful in thumb-base OA.

Intra-articular hyaluronic acid

Hyaluronic acid forms the backbone of the proteoglycan molecule and is the major constituent of synovial fluid. In addition to its mechanical role as a lubricant, shock absorber and buffer between articular cartilage surfaces, it also may have a role in binding inflammatory mediators and neuropeptides associated with pain production. Preparations of HA are available for use by intra-articular injection in knee OA. Several studies suggest a modest benefit when compared to placebo injections (Dougados et al 1993, Puhl et al 1993, Lohmander et al 1996) or intra-articular steroids (Jones et al 1995). Given the reluctance to use NSAIDs in the elderly, there may be a role for intra-articular hyaluronic acid in the treatment of selected elderly patients with knee OA: for example, in those in whom surgery is contraindicated and whose pain is not controlled by simple oral and/or topical analgesics.

Nutritional supplements

Glucosamine is an amino-monosaccaride which is essential for the formation of the glycosaminoglycans in articular cartilage. Several studies (Noack et al 1994) of 3–8 weeks in duration suggest that glucosamine sulfate at doses of 500 mg three times a day produces significantly greater improvement in pain than placebo and is as effective as ibuprofen 1200 mg daily (Muller-Fassbender et al 1994) with fewer gastrointestinal adverse reactions.

CENTRAL PAIN MODIFICATION

Simple analgesics such as paracetamol, codeine and tramadol are all effective in OA and should form the first line of drug therapy. Low doses of tricyclics given at night can also help. Other, non-pharmacological interventions have also been shown to reduce pain. For example, several randomized controlled trials (Weinberger et al 1989, Maisiak et al 1996) have shown that the provision of social support through routine telephone contact can improve functional status and pain in patients with OA. Patients who received monthly telephone calls by trained non-medical personnel to discuss issues such as presence and amount of joint pain, compliance with medications and other treatments, drug side effects and potential problems with keeping appointments, had a greater improvement in joint pain and function without significantly higher medical costs (Weinberger et al 1993). The content of the telephone calls seems to be important: symptom monitoring is not as effective as specific advice and counselling (Maisiak et al 1996).

Cognitive behavioural approaches, designed to teach patients ways of coping with their pain, are also beneficial. These interventions emphasize the control of pain by understanding the interaction of emotions and cognition with the physical and behavioural aspects of pain. In one study (Keefe et al 1996), patients with knee OA who participated in a programme that involved their spouse had greater improvement in pain, psychological disability, self efficacy and pain behaviours, as well as better marital adjustment and coping skills, compared to patients who participated in a traditional programme without their spouse.

Finally, patient education is an effective treatment. The Arthritis Self-Help Course has been shown to be effective. This course consists of six weekly education sessions focusing on exercise, relaxation techniques, joint protection techniques and a description of the various medications used in treating patients with arthritis. Studies by Lorig and colleagues (Lorig & Holman 1993) have shown that patients with OA who participate in this programme have significant improvement in knowledge, pain and quality of life, and a decreased frequency of physician visits and lower health-care costs.

SURGICAL PROCEDURES

Tidal lavage (the instillation and drainage of 500 ml–2 L of saline) is effective in some patients with knee OA that has not responded to standard medical therapy, and is particularly useful in those for whom surgery is contraindicated or refused (Ike et al 1992). Traditionally, lavage has been performed at the same time as arthroscopy but can also be achieved using a 'needle' arthroscope or even a sterile disposable 14-gauge cannula, thereby avoiding the need for an operating room and anaesthesia. The mechanism of action of lavage is unknown: reduction of secondary synovitis induced by crystals or joint debris, removal of inflammatory mediators and stretching of joint capsule have all been suggested. An improvement in quadriceps muscle function after lavage has been demonstrated (Gibson et al 1992).

Finally, total joint replacement (TJR) (Buckwalter & Lohmander 1994) is an excellent treatment for OA and has been responsible for a dramatic improvement in the quality of life of individuals with severe symptomatic lower limb OA who have failed to respond to medical management. Highly significant changes in pain, mobility, social function and global health status are detectable at 3 months; improvement may continue for up to a year (Liang et al 1990).

FUTURE DEVELOPMENTS IN OSTEOARTHRITIS

OA is a difficult disease to study for several reasons. Its onset is in middle to late life and it has a very slow progression, making intervention studies difficult. It is clearly a heterogeneous disease and what works for OA at one site may not work at another. There may even be differences within the same joint: for example, at the knee the risk factors and progression of patellofemoral OA may differ from those for tibiofemoral OA (Cooper et al 1994). There is no clear agreement of what constitutes OA and no easy way of diagnosing early disease. However, advances in imaging techniques such as MRI have great potential not only in diagnosis but also in assessing interventions, for example in allowing quantitation of cartilage volume. Biochemical markers of cartilage and bone metabolism are now available with the potential to detect early disease and even predict progression (Sharif et al 1995). Genetic studies have clearly shown that isolated gene mutations can cause OA, although the extent to which these cause the majority of 'typical' OA remains uncertain. There are also likely to be developments in the treatment of OA and its pain. The development of selective COX-2 inhibitors may provide safer NSAIDs, which will improve the management of symptoms in patients with OA (Spangler 1996). Studies of a number of novel agents, including chemically modified tetracyclines and other metalloproteinase inhibitors (Brand 1995, Ryan et al 1996) and interleukin-1 receptor antagonist (Caron et al 1996), with the potential to reverse the structural or biochemical abnormalities of OA, are currently being investigated. In addition, autologous cartilage transplantation may be useful in patients with early disease and focal cartilage defects (Brittberg et al 1994). Hopefully, these advances will alter the prognosis and improve the quality of life for patients with OA in the next century.

REFERENCES

Acheson RM, Ginsburg GN 1973 New Haven survey of joint diseases. XVI. Impairment, disability, and arthritis. British Journal of Preventive and Social Medicine 27: 168–176

Arnoldi CC, Djurhuus JC, Heerfordt J, Karte A 1980 Intraosseous phlebography, intraosseous pressure measurements and 99mTc polyphosphate scintigraphy in patients with painful conditions in the hip and knee. Acta Orthopaedica Scandinavica 51: 19–28

Astrom J 1975 Preoperative effect of fenestration upon intraosseous pressure in patients with osteoarthritis of the hip. Acta Orthopaedica Scandinavica 46: 963–967

Ayral X, Dougados M, Listrat V et al 1996 Arthroscopic evaluation of chondropathy in osteoarthritis of the knee. Journal of Rheumatology 23: 698–706

Bellamy N, Buchanan WW, Goldsmith CH et al 1988 Validation study of

WOMAC: a health status instrument for measuring clinically important patient relevant outcomes to antirheumatic drug therapy in patients with osteoarthritis of the hip or knee. Journal of Rheumatology 15: 1833–1840

Bellamy N, Sothern R, Campbell J 1990 Rhythmic variations in pain perception in osteoarthritis of the knee. Journal of Rheumatology 17: 364–372

Bradley JD, Brandt KD, Katz BP et al 1992 Treatment of knee osteoarthritis: relationship of clinical features of joint inflammation to the response to a nonsteroidal antiinflammatory drug or pure analgesic. Journal of Rheumatology 19: 1950–1954

Brandt KD 1995 Modification by oral doxycycline administration of articular cartilage breakdown in osteoarthritis. Journal of Rheumatology 22 (suppl 43): 149–151

Brittberg M, Lindahl A, Nilsson A et al 1994 Treatment of deep cartilage defects in the knee with autologous chondrocyte transplantation. New England Journal of Medicine 331: 889–895

Buckwalter JA, Lohmander S 1994 Operative treatment of osteoarthrosis: current practice and future development. Journal of Bone and Joint Surgery 76A: 1405–1418

Carman WJ 1989 Factors associated with pain and osteoarthritis in the Tecumseh Community Health Study. Seminars in Arthritis and Rheumatism 18: 10–13

Caron JP, Fernandes JC, Martel-Pelletier J et al 1996 Chondroprotective effect of intraarticular injections of interleukin-1 receptor antagonist in experimental osteoarthritis. Suppression of collagenase-1 expression. Arthritis and Rheumatism 39: 1535–1544

Chamberlain MA, Care G, Harfield B 1982 Physiotherapy in osteoarthrosis of the knees. A controlled trial of hospital versus home exercises. International Rehabilitation Medicine 4: 101–106

Cicuttini FM, Baker J, Hart D, Spector TD 1996 Association of pain with radiological changes in different compartments and views of the knee joint. Osteoarthritis and Cartilage 4: 143–147

Cooper C, McAlindon T, Snow S et al 1994 Mechanical and constitutional risk factors for symptomatic knee osteoarthritis: differences between medial tibiofemoral and patellofemoral disease. Journal of Rheumatology 21: 307–313

Creamer P 1997 Intra-articular steroid injections in osteoarthritis: do they work and if so how? (Editorial). Annals of the Rheumatic Diseases 56: 634–635

Creamer P, Hunt M, Dieppe PA 1996 Pain mechanisms in osteoarthritis of the knee: effect of intraarticular anesthetic. Journal of Rheumatology 23: 1031–1036

Creamer P, Lethbridge-Cejku M, Costa P et al 1999 The relationship of anxiety and depression with self reported knee pain in the community. Data from the Baltimore Longitudinal Study of Aging (BLSA). Arthritis Care Research 12(2)

Cushnaghan J, McCarthy C, Dieppe P 1994 Taping the patella medially: a new treatment for osteoarthritis of the knee joint? British Medical Journal 308: 753–755

Davis M, Ettinger W, Neuhaus J et al 1992 Correlates of knee pain among US adults with and without radiographic knee osteoarthritis. Journal of Rheumatology 19: 1943–1949

Dekker J, Tola P, Aufdemkampe G, Winckers M 1993 Negative affect, pain and disability in osteoarthritis patients: the mediating role of muscle weakness. Behaviour Research and Therapy 31: 203–206

Dexter P, Brandt K 1994 Distribution and predictors of depressive symptoms in osteoarthritis. Journal of Rheumatology 21: 279–286

Dieppe PA, Cushnaghan J, Young P, Kirwan J 1993 Prediction of the progression of joint space narrowing in osteoarthritis of the knee by scintigraphy. Annals of the Rheumatic Diseases 52: 557–563

Dieppe PA, Cushnaghan J, Shepstone L 1997 The Bristol 'OA500' study: progression of osteoarthritis (OA) over 3 years and the relationship between clinical and radiographic features at the knee joint. Osteoarthritis and Cartilage 5: 87–97

Dougados M, Nguyen M, Listrat V, Amor B 1993 High molecular weight sodium hyaluronate (hyalectin) in osteoarthritis of the knee: a 1 year placebo-controlled trial. Osteoarthritis and Cartilage 1: 97–103

Ettinger WH, Burns R, Messier SP et al 1997 A randomized trial comparing aerobic exercise and resistance exercise with a health education program in older adults with knee osteoarthritis. Journal of the American Medical Association 277: 25–31

Evans CH, Mears DC 1981 Release of neutral proteinases from mononuclear phagocytes and synovial cells in response to cartilaginous wear particles in vitro. Biochemica et Biophysica Acta 677: 287–294

Felson DT, Naimark A, Anderson J et al 1987 The prevalence of knee osteoarthritis in the elderly: The Framingham Osteoarthritis Study. Arthritis and Rheumatism 30: 914–918

Felson DT, Anderson J, Naimark A et al 1988 Obesity and knee osteoarthritis. Annals of Internal Medicine 109: 18–24

Felson DT, Zhang Y, Hannan MT et al 1997 Risk factors for incident radiographic knee osteoarthritis in the elderly. Arthritis and Rheumatism 40: 728–733

Fife RS, Brandt K, Braunstein E et al 1991 Relationship between arthroscopic evidence of cartilage damage and radiographic evidence of joint space narrowing in early osteoarthritis of the knee. Arthritis and Rheumatism 34: 377–382

Fisher NM, Gresham GE, Abrams M et al 1993 Quantitative effects of physical therapy on muscular and functional performance in subjects with osteoarthritis of the knees. Archives of Physical Medicine and Rehabilitation 74: 840–847

Gaffney K, Ledingham J, Perry JD 1995 Intra-articular triamcinolone hexacetonide in knee osteoarthritis: factors influencing the clinical response. Annals of the Rheumatic Diseases 54: 379–381

Gibson JN, White MD, Chapman VM, Strachan RK 1992 Arthroscopic lavage and debridement for osteoarthritis of the knee. Journal of Bone and Joint Surgery 74B: 534–537

Griffith SM, Dziedzic K, Cheung NT et al 1997 Clinical outcomes: a double blind randomised controlled trial to compare the effect of intra-articular local anaesthetic and local anaesthetic plus steroid in hip arthritis. British Journal of Rheumatology 36(suppl 2): 21

Hannan MT, Anderson JJ, Pincus T, Felson DT 1992 Educational attainment and osteoarthritis: differential associations with radiographic changes and symptom reporting. Journal of Clinical Epidemiology 45: 139–147

Haraoui B, Pelletier JP, Cloutier JM et al 1991 Synovial membrane histology and immunopathology in rheumatoid arthritis and osteoarthritis. Arthritis and Rheumatism 34: 153–163

Hawley DJ, Wolfe F 1993 Depression is not more common in RA: a 10 year longitudinal study of 6153 patients with rheumatic disease. Journal of Rheumatology 20: 2025–2031

Hochberg MC, Lawrence RC, Everett DF, Cornoni-Huntley J 1989 Epidemiological associations of pain in osteoarthritis of the knee. Seminars in Arthritis and Rheumatism 18 (suppl 2): 4–9

Hopman-Rock M, Odding E, Hofman A et al 1996 Physical and psychosocial disability in elderly subjects in relation to pain in the hip and/or knee. Journal of Rheumatology 23: 1037–1044

Huskisson EC, Dieppe PA, Tucker AK, Cannell LB 1979 Another look at osteoarthritis. Annals of the Rheumatic Diseases 38: 423–428

Hutton CW, Higgs ER, Jackson PC et al 1986 99mTc HMDP bone scanning in generalised nodal osteoarthritis. II The four hour bone scan predicts radiographic change. Annals of the Rheumatic Diseases 45: 622–626

Ike RW, Arnold WJ, Rothschild EW, Shaw HL 1992 Tidal irrigation versus conservative medical management in patients with osteoarthritis of the knee: a prospective randomized study. Journal of Rheumatology 19: 772–779

Insall J, Shoji H, Mayer V 1974 High tibial osteotomy. A 5-year evaluation. Journal of Bone and Joint Surgery 56A: 1397–1405

Jones A, Doherty M 1996 Intra-articular corticosteroids are effective in osteoarthritis but there are no clinical predictors of response. Annals of the Rheumatic Diseases 55: 829–832

Jones AC, Pattrick M, Doherty S, Doherty M 1995 Intra-articular hyaluronic acid compared to intra-articular triamcinolone hexacetonide in inflammatory knee osteoarthritis. Osteoarthritis and Cartilage 3: 269–273

Keating EM, Faris PM, Ritter MA, Kane J 1993 Use of lateral heel and sole wedges in the treatment of medial osteoarthritis of the knee. Orthop Review 22: 921–924

Keefe FJ, Caldwell DS, Queen K et al 1987a Osteoarthritis knee pain: a behavioral analysis. Pain 28: 309–321

Keefe FJ, Caldwell DS, Queen KT et al 1987b Pain coping strategies in osteoarthritis patients. Journal of Consulting and Clinical Psychology 55: 208–212

Keefe FJ, Caldwell DS, Baucom D et al 1996 Spouse-assisted coping skills training in the management of osteoarthritic knee pain. Arthritis Care and Research 9: 279–291

Kellgren JH 1983 Pain in osteoarthritis. Journal of Rheumatology 10(suppl 9): 108–109

Kellgren JH, Lawrence JS 1963 The epidemiology of chronic rheumatism: atlas of standard radiographs, vol 2. Blackwell Scientific, Oxford

Kidd B 1996 Problems with pain – is the messenger to blame? Annals of the Rheumatic Diseases 55: 276–283

Kontinnen YT, Kemppinen P, Segerberg M et al 1994 Peripheral and spinal neural mechanisms in arthritis with particular reference to treatment of inflammation and pain. Arthritis and Rheumatism 37: 965–982

Lawrence RC, Everett DF, Hochberg MC 1990 Arthritis. In: Huntley R, Cornoni-Huntley J (eds) Health status and well being of the elderly: National Health and Nutrition Examination I epidemiologic follow-up study. Oxford University Press, New York, pp 133–151

Lawrence JS, Bremner JB, Bier F 1966 Osteoarthritis: prevalence in the population and relationship between symptoms and X-ray changes. Annals of the Rheumatic Diseases 25: 1–24

Ledingham J, Regan M, Jones A, Doherty M 1995 Factors affecting radiographic progression of knee osteoarthritis. Annals of the Rheumatic Diseases 54: 53–58

Lethbridge-Cejku M, Scott WW Jr, Reichle R et al 1995 Association of radiographic features of osteoarthritis of the knee with knee pain: data from the Baltimore Longitudinal Study of Aging. Arthritis Care and Research 8: 182–188

Lequesne M 1991 Indices of severity and disease activity for osteoarthritis. Seminars in Arthritis and Rheumatism 20(suppl 2): 48–54

Liang M, Fossel A, Larson M 1990 Comparison of five health status instruments for orthopaedic evaluation. Medical Care 28: 632–642

Lichtenberg PA, Skehan MW, Swensen CH 1984 The role of personality, recent life stress and arthritic severity in predicting pain. Journal of Psychosomatic Research 28: 231–236

Lichtenberg PA. Swensen CH. Skehan MW 1986 Further investigation of the role of personality, lifestyle and arthritic severity in predicting pain. Journal of Psychosomatic Research 30: 327–337

Lohmander LS, Dalen N, Englund G et al 1996 Intra-articular hyaluronan injections in the treatment of osteoarthritis of the knee: a randomized, double blind, placebo controlled trial. Annals of the Rheumatic Diseases 55: 424–431

Lorig KR, Holman HR 1993 Arthritis self management studies: a 12 year review. Health Education Quarterly 20: 17–28

Lunghi M, Miller P, McQuillan W 1978 Psychosocial factors in osteoarthritis of the hip. Journal of Psychosomatic Research 22: 57–63

Lynn B, Kellgren JH 1986 Pain. In: Scott JT (ed) Copeman's textbook of the rheumatic diseases, 6th edn. Churchill Livingstone, Edinburgh, pp 143–160

McAlindon T, Cooper C, Kirwan JR, Dieppe PA 1993 Determinants of disability in osteoarthritis of the knee. Annals of the Rheumatic Diseases 52: 258–262

Maisiak R, Austin J, Heck L 1996 Health outcomes of two telephone interventions for patients with rheumatoid arthritis or osteoarthritis. Arthritis and Rheumatism 39: 1391–1399

Marok R, Winyard PG, Coumbe A et al 1996 Activation of the transcription factor nuclear factor-kappaB in human inflamed synovial tissue. Arthritis and Rheumatism 39: 583–591

Martin K, Nicklas BJ, Bunyard LB et al 1996 Weight loss and walking improve symptoms of knee osteoarthritis. Arthritis and Rheumatism 39(suppl): S225

Melzack R 1975 The McGill pain questionnaire: major properties and scoring methods. Pain 1: 277–299

Minor MA, Brown JD 1993 Exercise maintenance of persons with arthritis after participation in a class experience. Health Education Quarterly 20: 83–95

Muller-Fassbender H, Bach GL, Haase W et al 1994 Glucosamine sulfate compared to ibuprofen in osteoarthritis of the knee. Osteoarthritis and Cartilage 2: 61–69

Noack W, Fischer M, Foster KK, Rovati LC, Setnikar I 1994 Glucosamine sulfate in osteoarthritis of the knee. Osteoarthritis and Cartilage 2: 51–59

O'Reilly S, Muir KR, Doherty M 1996 Screening for pain in knee osteoarthritis: which question? Annals of the Rheumatic Diseases 55: 931–933

Puhl W, Bernau A, Greiling H et al 1993 Intra-articular sodium hyaluronate in osteoarthritis of the knee: a multicenter, double-blind study. Osteoarthritis and Cartilage 1: 233–241

Rejeski WJ, Ettinger WH, Shumaker S et al 1995 The evaluation of pain in patients with knee osteoarthritis: the knee pain scale. Journal of Rheumatology 22: 1124–1129

Revell PA, Mayston V, Lalor P, Mapp P 1988 The synovial membrane in OA: a histological study including the characterisation of the cellular infiltrate present in inflammatory OA using monoclonal antibodies. Annals of the Rheumatic Diseases 47: 300–307

Roivainen A, Soderstrom KO, Pirila L et al 1996 Oncoprotein expression in human synovial tissue: an immunohistochemical study of different types of arthritis. British Journal of Rheumatology 35: 933–942

Ryan ME, Greenwald RA, Golub LM 1996 Potential of tetracyclines to modify cartilage breakdown in osteoarthritis. Current Opinions in Rheumatology 8: 238–247

Salaffi F, Cavalieri F, Nolli M, Ferraccioli G 1991 Analysis of disability in knee osteoarthritis. Relationship with age and psychological variables but not with radiographic score. Journal of Rheumatology 18: 1581–1586

Schouten JS, van den Ouweland, Valkengurg HA 1992 A 12 year follow up study in the general population on prognostic factors of cartilage loss in OA of the knee. Annals of the Rheumatic Diseases 51: 932–937

Schumacher HR Jr 1995 Synovial inflammation, crystals, and osteoarthritis. Journal of Rheumatology Supplement 43: 101–103

Sharif M, George E, Shepstone L et al 1995 Serum hyaluronic acid level as a predictor of disease progression in osteoarthritis of the knee. Arthritis and Rheumatism 38: 760–767

Slemenda C, Brandt KD, Heilman DK et al 1997 Quadriceps weakness and osteoarthritis of the knee. Annals of Internal Medicine 127: 97–104

Spangler RS 1996 Cyclooxygenase 1 and 2 in rheumatic disease: implications for nonsteroidal anti-inflammatory drug therapy. Seminars in Arthritis and Rheumatism 26: 435–446

Spector TD, Hart DJ, Byrne J et al 1993 Definition of osteoarthritis for epidemiological studies. Annals of the Rheumatic Diseases 52: 70–74

Spector TD, Hart DJ, Nandra D et al 1997 Low level increases in serum

C-reactive protein are present in early osteoarthritis of the knee and predict progressive disease. Arthritis and Rheumatism 40: 723–727

Summers MN, Haley WE, Reveille JO, Alarcon GS 1988 Radiographic assessment and psychological variables as predictors of pain and functional impairment in osteoarthritis of the knee or hip. Arthritis and Rheumatism 31: 204–209

Van Saase JLCM, Van Romunde LKJ, Cats A et al 1989 Epidemiology of osteoarthritis: the Zoetermeer survey. Annals of the Rheumatic Diseases 48: 271–280

Wagstaff S, Smith OV, Wood PHN 1985 Verbal pain descriptors used by patients with arthritis. Annals of the Rheumatic Diseases 44: 262–265

Weinberger M, Tierney WM, Booher P, Katz BP 1989 Can the provision of information to patients with osteoarthritis improve functional status? A randomized, controlled trial. Arthritis and Rheumatism 32: 1577–1583

Weinberger M, Tierney WM, Cowper PA et al 1993 Cost-effectiveness of increased telephone contact for patients with osteoarthritis. A randomized, controlled trial. Arthritis and Rheumatism 36: 243–246

Rheumatoid arthritis

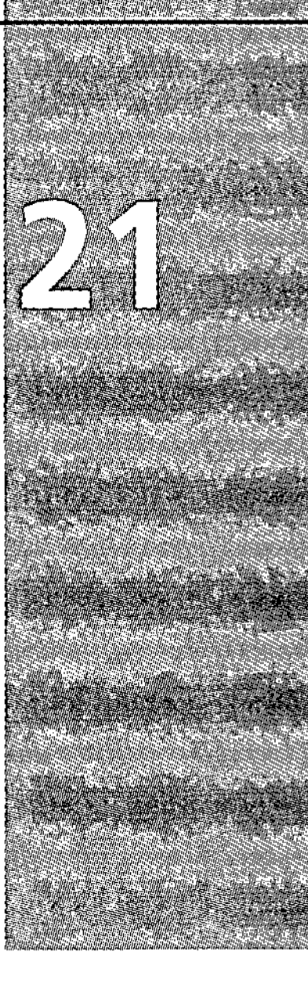

MALCOLM I. V. JAYSON

INTRODUCTION

Rheumatoid arthritis (RA) is a multicomplex system inflammatory disorder in which the principle problems affect the synovial linings of the joints and tendons. In acute disease many patients develop generalized malaise and weight loss and specific complications may affect other organ systems. Occasionally these features predominate.

The cause of RA is unknown but the prevailing view is that both inherited and environmental factors are important, with systemic autoimmune reactions precipitating a cascade of inflammatory changes.

There is an increased familial aggregation of the disease and, in particular, greater concordance in monozygotic than dizygotic twins. The best documented genetic marker for RA is the class II major histocompatibility complex (MHC) antigen HLA DR4. The presence of this inherited HLA marker conveys a sixfold increase in the relative risk of developing this disease. Some 50% of patients with RA carry the DR4 antigen. In particular it is associated with more severe disease and systemic complications (Westedt et al 1986). The presence of this tissue type acts as a susceptibility factor for autoimmune events but the mechanism for this remains to be determined.

Against this background environmental factors are believed to precipitate the development of this problem. Much effort has gone into identifying a possible infective basis for the development of RA in genetically predisposed individuals. A wide variety of organisms have been implicated, but in contrast to reactive arthritis and other forms of chronic inflammatory disease, no definitive evidence of a specific causative microorganism has been identified.

Many patients blame the onset of RA on a stressful event. The evidence for this is weak but undoubtedly psychological distress exacerbates patients' perception of severity of the disease.

Despite many claims, diet plays little role in RA. Some patients have individual allergies and may develop acute synovitis on exposure to specific types of food but this is very different from the rheumatoid process. Numerous studies have been undertaken on the effects of diet on arthritis but with little positive results. A very high intake of fish oil may lead to a decrease in the ability to generate certain inflammatory cytokines and have a limited anti-inflammatory effect.

The prevalence of the disease varies considerably between different populations. In part this is due to different genetic make-ups but environmental factors also play their part. For example, in Africa there is a considerably lower prevalence in rural black groups than urbanized populations (Beighton et al 1975).

PATHOLOGY

The normal synovial lining of diarthrodial joints is a delicate tissue layer up to three cells thick and a loosely arranged stroma with connective tissue, microvasculature and lymphatics. In early active disease the synovium becomes swollen, hypertrophic and inflamed. Microscopically the stroma is invaded by lymphocytes and plasma cells. Fibrin deposition may occur on the surface of the hypertrophic synovium. The synovial stroma is replaced by proliferation of local connective tissue cells by the process of mesenchymoid transformation. Excess production of synovial fluid leads to joint swelling and clinically detectable effusions.

The cellular content of rheumatoid synovial fluid consists principally of polymorphonuclear leucocytes. The destructive phase of the disease is associated with the production of chronic granulation tissue or pannus, which spreads over the articular cartilage surface. Cartilage destruction appears on the deep surface of the pannus and is seen as loss of joint space on X-ray. Bone erosions usually appear first at the joint margins at the point of normal synovial reflection and where bone is relatively unprotected by cartilage. Neutral proteolytic enzymes (Barrett & Saklatvala 1981) secreted by macrophages in the pannus, and acidic lysosomal enzymes secreted by polymorphonuclear leucocytes in the synovial fluid, both play a part in bone and cartilage destruction. In severe forms of the disease continued bone and cartilage destruction are associated with irreversible deformity and, particularly in weight-bearing joints, secondary osteoarthritis may occur.

CLINICAL FEATURES

RA occurs in both sexes but is two or three times more common in females than males. It may start at any age but with an increasing incidence in older people. The overall prevalence is about 1% of the population. In recent years the incidence of the disease appears to be decreasing and its effects less severe.

RA is a generalized disease with the most obvious problems affecting the joints. Severe forms of the disease may be associated with both articular and extra-articular features and the symptoms and signs of a systemic disease process. These include general malaise and lassitude, weight loss and low-grade pyrexia. The disease onset is insidious in up to 70% of patients but may be acute and associated with systemic upset and fever.

ARTICULAR CLINICAL FEATURES

Established rheumatoid disease is typically a symmetrical peripheral inflammatory polyarthritis which most often involves the small joints of the hands and feet, the wrists, ankles, knees and cervical spine. The shoulders and elbows may be involved and the hips and lumbar spine less frequently. In severe forms of the disease any synovial joint may be affected.

In early active rheumatoid disease there is pain, soft-tissue swelling and stiffness. The pain and stiffness of active inflammation are typically worse in the early morning and improve with activity during the day, although many patients develop further symptoms when they become tired in the early evening. Gelling or stiffening of the joints with rest or inactivity are also typical of inflammatory disease. On examination the soft-tissue joint swelling of active RA is due to synovial hypertrophy and effusion and is warm and tender. Muscle wasting appears rapidly around painful swollen joints and there is sometimes periarticular inflammatory oedema.

In late-stage destructive RA problems of deformity and loss of function predominate with relatively little active inflammation.

HANDS

Early active disease typically is associated with involvement of the proximal interphalangeal joints producing spindling of the fingers and synovitis of the metacarpophalangeal joints (Fig. 21.1). Synovial hypertrophy may also involve the flexor tendon sheaths of the fingers, producing diffuse swelling of the palmar aspects of the fingers and contributing to impaired finger movement and poor grip. Synovitis of the wrists may lead to compression of the median nerve beneath the flexor retinaculum and produce features of the carpal tunnel syndrome. These include paraesthesiae and numbness of the fingers, which are worse at night. Sometimes this is a presenting feature of the disease. Severe forms of carpal tunnel syndrome are associated with wasting of the thenar eminence and sensory loss in a median nerve distribution. Such wasting should be distinguished from generalized muscle wasting because of disuse with active joint disease. Synovitis of the extensor aspect of the wrist may rupture the extensor tendons, particularly the extensor pollicis longus, leading to loss of ability to extend the thumb.

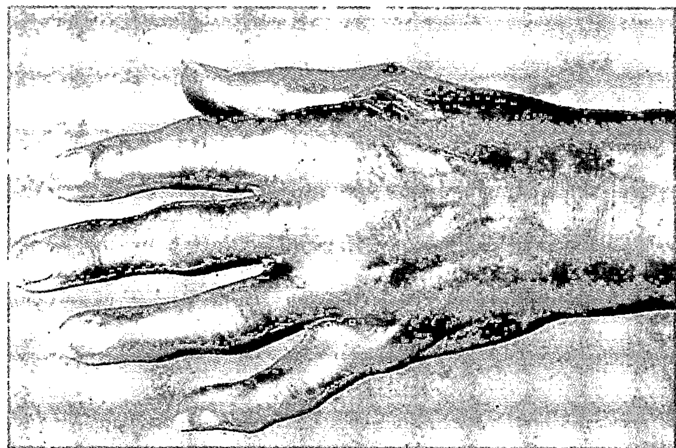

Fig. 21.1 Early rheumatoid inflammation of the proximal interphalangeal and metacarpophalangeal joints of the hand.

The deformities of chronic RA in the hands are produced by chronic synovial inflammation and swelling, giving rise to stretching and rupture of capsules surrounding ligaments and tendons (Wyn Parry 1984). They include the following:

1. Swan-neck deformity of the fingers with hyperextension of the proximal interphalangeal joints and flexion at the distal interphalangeal joints.
2. The boutonnière or buttonhole deformity (Fig. 21.2), which is associated with hyperflexion at the proximal interphalangeal joint, stretching or rupture of the central slip of the extensor and buttonholing of the joint between the lateral extensor tendon slips.
3. Continued inflammation at the metacarpophalangeal joints, which produces flexion deformity and ulnar deviation (Fig. 21.3).
4. The more frequent deformity of the thumb is the Z associated with continued inflammation at the first metacarpophalangeal joint. This deformity consists of flexion at the metacarpophalangeal joint produced by volar displacement of the long extensor and hyperextension at the distal joints. Other thumb deformities may result from chronic inflammation at the first metacarpal joint, resulting in abduction of the thumb and hyperextension of either the distal or proximal phalanx.
5. Dorsal subluxation of the ulnar head at the wrist ('caput ulnae') is associated with a high risk of rupture of fourth and fifth extensor tendons and 'dropped fingers' (Fig. 21.4). Prophylactic surgical resection of the ulnar head with synovectomy usually prevents this complication.

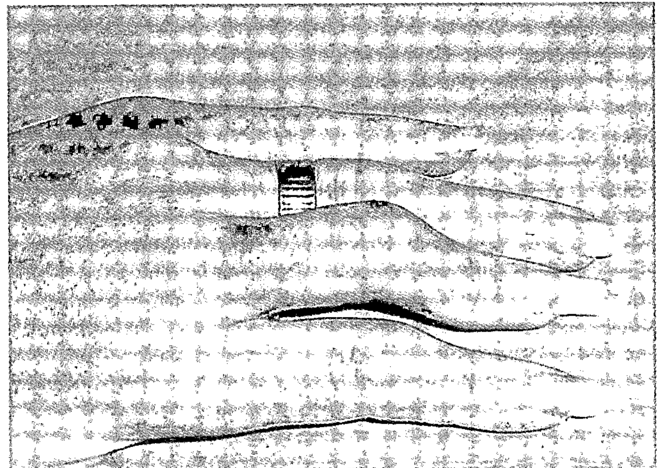

Fig. 21.2 The boutonnière, or buttonhole, deformity of the middle finger.

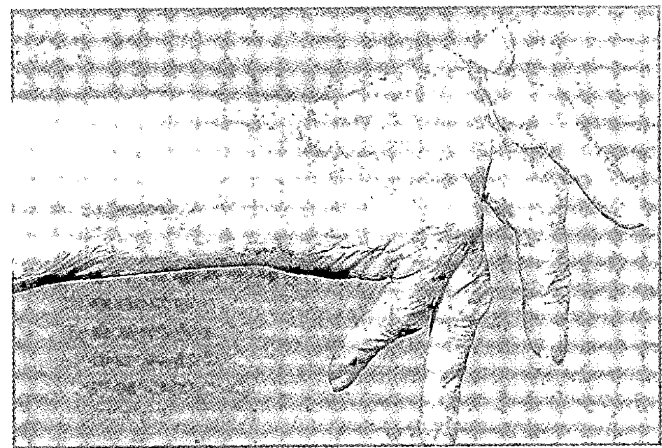

Fig. 21.3 Ulnar deviation of the fingers.

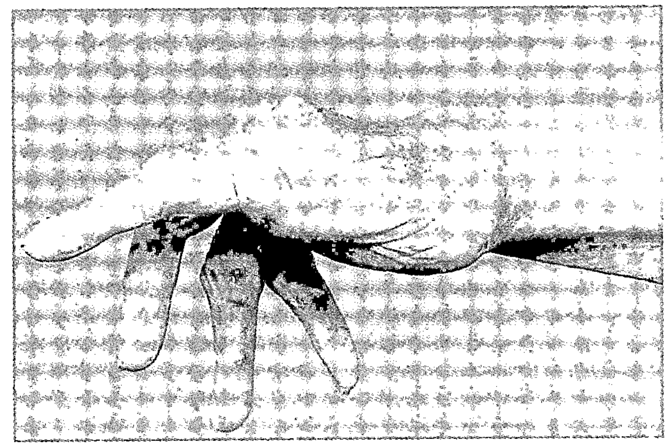

Fig. 21.4 Rupture of extensor tendons with 'dropped fingers'.

FEET AND ANKLES

Foot involvement is an important but often neglected aspect of the disease (Jayson & Smidt 1987). Both active synovitis and radiological changes are most frequent at the metatarsophalangeal joints and may be detected by the presence of swelling and tenderness around the joints. Erosions of the metatarsophalangeal joints are common even in the absence of symptoms and may be found in over 80% of rheumatoid patients admitted to hospital. Active synovitis may also produce symptoms in ankles, subtalar and midtarsal joints. Synovial hypertrophy may produce symptoms laterally as a result of peroneal tendon sheath involvement and medially as a result of flexor tendon sheath involvement.

The most frequent rheumatoid foot deformity is associated with subluxation at the metatarsophalangeal joints and displacement of the normally weight-bearing fat pad distally. The subluxated metatarsal heads may be felt in the sole and are often associated with callosities. Patients with this deformity often complain of a feeling like 'walking on stones'. Other toe deformities found in RA include hallux valgus and cock-up toes.

Chronic synovitis in the midtarsal and subtalar regions may cause destruction of the ligaments supporting the longitudinal and transverse arches of the feet. This results in broadening and flattening of the foot and production of the characteristic pronated foot deformity. Uncommonly, a pes varus deformity may be produced, but it has been suggested that such patients have a pre-existing pes cavus.

Other foot symptoms may result from rheumatoid nodules in weight-bearing regions. Rheumatoid disease may also cause symptoms in the region of the plantar fascia and Achilles tendon insertion with the calcaneus, although these features are more typical of ankylosing spondylitis and other seronegative arthritides.

KNEES

Active synovitis in the knees is associated with soft-tissue swelling and effusions, which are often visible around the knee itself and in the suprapatellar pouch. Quadriceps muscle wasting commonly accompanies inflammation of the joint.

Effusions of the joint may be associated with a gastrocnemius–semimembranous bursa or Baker's cyst in the popliteal fossa, which may be uncomfortable. Sometimes this cyst extends down the calf to produce swelling and discomfort, and this joint or the cyst may rupture to give acute pain, swelling and tenderness. The signs and symptoms of rupture may exactly mimic and be misdiagnosed as deep venous thrombosis. The correct diagnosis can often be made on clinical grounds. Patients with a ruptured cyst may previously have noted pain and swelling in the knee and popliteal fossa, which decreases in size immediately the pain in the calf begins. Cyst rupture is often associated with physical activity, while deep vein thrombosis is more likely to occur after rest or immobilization of the leg. The diagnosis of a ruptured cyst may be confirmed by an arthrogram, ultrasound or MRI scan when free fluid is seen extravasating into the calf. Treatment of a ruptured cyst is by rest and local injection of steroid into the knee. Rarely, ruptured cysts and deep vein thrombosis occur together. In general, anticoagulants should be given to rheumatoid patients with calf pain only if thrombosis has been proven by venography.

Chronic synovitis of the knee may produce instability of the joint by destruction of cruciate or medial and lateral ligaments.

ELBOWS

Synovial effusions in the elbows may produce limitation of extension of the joint and be detected clinically as a bulge felt on either side of the olecranon as the joint is extended. Pronation and supination may be affected if the superior radioulnar joint is involved.

CERVICAL SPINE

Pain on movement of the neck is a common feature of active RA. However, radiological abnormalities of the cervical spine are often asymptomatic, and may be found in up to 80% of patients (Bland et al 1963, Conlon et al 1966). They include osteoporosis, apophyseal joint erosions, erosions of the vertebral endplates, loss of disc space without osteoporosis, atlantoaxial and subaxial subluxations and erosions of the odontoid peg.

Both anterior atlantoaxial and subaxial subluxations may be associated with neurological complications. Subluxations at the atlantoaxial region occur in about 25% of rheumatoid patients seen in hospital (Conlon et al 1966, Mathews 1974), although only a minority have features of neurological involvement. This deformity is caused by destruction within the network of ligaments, which normally maintains the odontoid peg in apposition to the posterior aspect of the anterior arch of the atlas during movements of the head and neck. This ligamentous framework includes the transverse ligament, which forms part of the cruciate ligament, the apical ligament of the odontoid peg, the alar ligaments and posterior longitudinal ligament. Anterior atlantoaxial subluxation is demonstrated by lateral X-ray of the cervical spine with the neck in flexion, when the gap between the odontoid peg and the anterior arch of the atlas should not become greater than 3 mm. Vertical subluxation of the odontoid peg may also occur and is diagnosed when the tip of the odontoid peg is seen more than 3 mm above McGregor's line, drawn from the posterior edge of the hard palate to the margin of the occipital curve. Less common forms of atlantoaxial subluxation include lateral and posterior subluxations (Brunton et al 1978).

The presence of gross forms of atlantoaxial subluxation may be suspected because of a peculiar posture of the head and neck. Typical symptoms include upper cervical pain which may radiate to the occiput or retro-orbital areas. Cervical cord compression may result from both atlantoaxial and subaxial subluxation. Clinical features of neurological involvement include weakness in arms and legs which is out of proportion to the degree of articular involvement, bladder or bowel symptoms, shooting pains in the arms and sometimes symptoms suggestive of a peripheral neuropathy. There is a risk that a subsequent fall or accident may convert a minor neurological deficit into complete quadriplegia. Uncommonly, sudden death has occurred after vertical subluxation of the odontoid peg into the foramen magnum.

Pain or minor neurological symptoms resulting from cervical spine involvement may respond to immobilization of the neck in a Plastazote fitted collar. Severe pain or neurological features that fail to respond to conservative measures may require fusion of the cervical spine by surgery.

OTHER

Any synovial joint may become involved by the more severe forms of RA. Pain in the shoulder may be due to periarticular involvement and synovitis of the glenohumeral or acromioclavicular joints. A minority of patients are seen who develop severe destructive changes of the glenohumeral joint and if such patients also have elbow disease they may have severe functional difficulties. Hip joint involvement may occur occasionally. Both bilateral and unilateral forms of temporomandibular involvement may occur and affect chewing and mouth opening. The lumbar spine may be affected by synovitis of apophyseal joints. They develop a scoliosis which can be very gross, causing pain and neurological damage. Occasionally more unusual joints are affected, such as the cricoarytenoid, which produces difficulty on swallowing, and the joints of the middle ear leading to hearing difficulties.

EXTRA-ARTICULAR CLINICAL FEATURES

Extra-articular features are found particularly in patients with the most severe forms of articular disease.

The pathogenesis of many of the systemic features, such as vasculitis and nodules, are thought to be related to the local deposition of circulating immune complexes containing IgM and possibly IgG rheumatoid factors.

NODULES

Rheumatoid nodules are found most frequently in subcutaneous regions subject to recurrent mechanical stress. Common sites include the subcutaneous borders of the forearms, the olecranon, often in association with an olecranon bursa, and also over sites such as the tips of the fingers and sacrum. Rheumatoid nodules in these sites are firm, non-tender and larger and less transient than the small nodules of rheumatic fever. In certain areas, such as over the sacrum, nodules may ulcerate and become infected bedsores. They can form a potential focus for systemic infections. Although most frequently found in the subcutaneous regions, these nodules may also occur as intracutaneous nodules and within other tissues such as the sclera, lung, pleura and myocardium.

The histology of the rheumatoid nodule is almost specific for RA and consists of a central area of fibrinoid necrosis surrounded by a palisade layer of histiocytes and peripherally by a zone of loose connective tissue (Gardner 1992). The presence of rheumatoid nodules may be helpful for clinical diagnosis and their presence indicates an adverse prognosis.

VASCULITIS

This is an uncommon but potentially fatal complication found in the most severe forms of the disease. All sizes of blood vessels may become affected. Cutaneous vasculitis is most often seen as nailfold haemorrhages in the fingers. Patients with these lesions do not always develop the more serious forms of vasculitis although they are at increased risk of doing so. More serious forms of cutaneous vasculitis may be associated with persistent cutaneous ulceration which often appears in the lower leg and may prove resistant to treatment. Medium or large blood vessels may become involved and present clinically with gangrene of the fingers, small bowel infarction or perforation and pulmonary hypertension. Small-vessel vasculitis is thought to underline many of the other extra-articular disease features such as peripheral neuropathy and probably nodule formation.

The histological changes found in rheumatoid vasculitis range from intimal hyperplasia to an inflammatory reaction affecting all layers of the vessel wall and are sometimes associated with necrosis (Fassbender 1975). Immunological tests often show high titres of circulating IgM rheumatoid factors, antinuclear antibodies and evidence of circulating immune complex activity, such as reduced serum complement levels and sometimes circulating cryoglobulins (Ansell & Loewi 1977).

Patients with severe forms of vasculitis are medical emergencies and often require aggressive treatment with corticosteroids and immunosuppressive drugs.

HAEMATOLOGY

The anaemia of RA is similar to that found in other chronic disorders such as malignancy, chronic infections and uraemia. This anaemia is usually normocytic normochromic, but may be hypochromic and, less commonly, macrocytic (Bennett 1977). The degree of anaemia in rheumatoid disease roughly correlates with the erythrocyte sedimentation rate (ESR). Typically the serum iron and total iron binding capacity are reduced and serum ferritin is elevated. The anaemia is associated with an increased affinity of the reticuloendothelial system for iron and bone marrow iron stores are plentiful. The anaemia of rheumatoid disease is to be distinguished from that of iron deficiency; the latter commonly results from gastrointestinal blood loss, which is frequently a side effect of non-steroidal anti-inflammatory drug (NSAID) therapy. In an iron deficiency anaemia serum iron is low but the total iron binding capacity is elevated and the bone marrow iron stores are reduced. Two types of anaemia may coexist and factors which might suggest that iron deficiency is contributing to anaemia include a history of melaena or recent dyspepsia, a sudden drop in haemoglobin or a haemoglobin value much lower than 9 g/dl. Unless there is coincidental iron deficiency, oral iron therapy does not improve the anaemia of RA. Parenteral iron is occasionally used, but the main treatment of this anaemia consists of measures directed at suppressing the underlying disease process.

The main reason for the development of anaemia in rheumatoid arthritis (Vreugdenhil & Swaak 1990) is the high affinity of the reticuloendothelial system for iron which is then sequestered in a non-utilizable form. Other factors which may contribute include ineffective erythropoiesis and haemolysis and possibly inadequate erythropoietin production. Serum folate levels may be low as a non-specific feature of inflammation but folate therapy is usually unhelpful.

Felty's syndrome is the association of RA with splenomegaly and leucopenia. Other features of the syndrome may include normocytic normochromic anaemia, thrombocytopenia, lymphadenopathy, cutaneous ulceration and pigmentation. The major hazard of the condition is recurrent major or minor infection. Patients with Felty's syndrome tend to have more severe forms of articular disease and on serological testing usually have high titres of IgM rheumatoid factor and antinuclear factors.

The leucopenia of Felty's syndrome usually lies between 800 and 2500 cells per mm^3 and is associated with a fall in granulocyte number. Occasionally a leucopenia of less than 800 per mm^3 is seen. The most frequent bone marrow abnormality found is granulocyte maturation arrest. The pathogenesis of Felty's syndrome is multifactorial and includes both an increased peripheral destruction partly attributable to circulating immune complexes as well as depression of granulopoiesis by a splenic humoral factor. Excessive margination of leucocytes in the peripheral circulation may account for some of the apparent fall in circulating cell counts.

The treatment of Felty's syndrome is only indicated if the leucopenia is associated with significant recurrent infection. Although corticosteroid therapy may increase the peripheral white cell count, it also increases the susceptibility to infection and is of uncertain value in the treatment of Felty's syndrome. Gold or penicillamine therapy can be very effective but these drugs must be used carefully because of their potential toxic effects on the bone marrow. A proportion of patients with this condition respond to splenectomy, although the operation itself is associated with significant postoperative mortality. Rarely, despite a rise in the peripheral white cell count after splenectomy, susceptibility to infection does not improve and patients die of fulminating septicaemia. The removal of splenic factors normally helpful in the defence against infection may be responsible. Immunization against disease and prompt aggressive treatment of any infections becomes essential.

Thrombocytosis or an increase in the circulating platelet count may be seen in active rheumatoid disease and probably represents a non-specific effect of inflammation. This thrombocytosis is not usually clinically significant.

SJÖGREN'S SYNDROME

Sjögren's syndrome is the association of keratoconjunctivitis sicca (KCS) and/or xerostomia with RA or other connective tissue disorders. Dysfunction of lacrimal and salivary glands is associated with lymphocytic infiltration, which may progress to fibrosis and complete loss of acinar tissue. This is distinguished from the gland dysfunction due to simple atrophy in old age. Estimates of the prevalence of Sjögren's syndrome vary between 13 and 58% of rheumatoid patients (Benedek 1993).

The symptoms of KCS are a gritty feeling or irritation of the eyes. This is often worse first thing in the morning when patients find it difficult to open their eyes. The lysozyme content of tears is reduced and the eyes may be subject to recurrent infection. The diagnosis of KCS is best confirmed with a slit lamp, when absence of the normal tear film will be noted. In addition, thick strands of mucus may be seen sticking to the conjunctiva and cornea. Two drops of 1% rose bengal instilled into the eye can be used to show up the mucus strands and abnormal epithelium of the dry conjunctiva. In the absence of a slit lamp the reduction in tear secretion may be demonstrated by the Schirmer tear test. A strip of filter paper is hooked over the lower lid at the junction of the middle and outer thirds and wetting of less

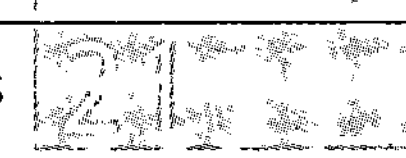

than 10 mm of the paper over a 5-min period is considered abnormal. The symptoms of KCS are usually relieved by the regular instillation of artificial tear drops into the affected eyes. Occasionally, tarsorrhaphy or lacrimal canal ablation is indicated.

The xerostomia may be associated with recurrent salivary gland swelling. A clinical diagnosis of xerostomia may be made if the patient complains of a dry mouth and on examination there is no salivary pool in the floor of the mouth. Again it is advisable to consider other non-specific factors such as drug therapy and anxiety before attributing all complaints of mouth dryness to this condition. Biopsy of minor salivary glands from the lip may be used to confirm the diagnosis. Other investigations that have been used in the formal assessment of xerostomia include measurement of salivary flow rate following cannulation of the parotid duct, sialography and radioisotope imaging of the salivary glands. Treatment of the xerostomia of Sjögren's syndrome is unsatisfactory.

Artificial saliva is available and may prove helpful. Dental hygiene is important, as patients with the condition are susceptible to dental caries. Local radiotherapy to the involved glands is not helpful and increase the risk of these patients developing lymphoma to which they already have an increased susceptibility.

Secretions from other endothelial surfaces may also be affected, so that other features of the condition may include dysphagia, dyspareunia and dryness of the skin. Sjögren's syndrome may be associated with a number of immunological symptoms, including renal tubular acidosis and autoimmune thyroid disease.

OPHTHALMIC

Keratoconjunctivitis sicca is the most frequent eye feature of rheumatoid disease. Scleritis (Jayson & Jones 1971) is less common but is potentially more serious. It may occur in diffuse or nodular forms. Rarely, a severe necrotizing form of scleritis is seen. The complications of untreated scleritis include perforation of the sclera, glaucoma and cataract. Systemic steroids in dosages of around 60 mg daily, local steroid drops, and sometimes immunosuppressive drugs, may be required for the treatment to this condition. Milder attacks may respond to NSAIDS.

RESPIRATORY

Pleurisy and pleural effusions are the most common forms of pulmonary involvement by the disease. Rheumatoid pleural effusions show lymphocytosis and reduced glucose content in the absence of infection. Sometimes macrophages containing IgM inclusions (ragocytes) are present and immunological tests for antinuclear antibodies and IgM rheumatoid factor may be positive. The histology of the underlying pleura often shows non-specific changes of chronic inflammation, but occasionally rheumatoid nodule formation is seen.

Interstitial fibrosis (fibrosing alveolitis) may occur uncommonly as the cause of progressive breathlessness in seropositive, nodular rheumatoid disease, particularly in smokers (Hyland et al 1983). The associated features found in the idiopathic condition are also found in the form associated with rheumatoid disease and include finger clubbing, coarse pleural crepitations and widespread pulmonary shadows on chest X-ray. Treatment with corticosteroid drugs is usually disappointing but occasionally immunosuppressive drugs appear to help. Asymptomatic impairment of carbon monoxide diffusion capacity in the absence of radiological change is common in rheumatoid disease, as in other forms of connective tissue disease, and usually does not progress to symptomatic interstitial fibrosis.

Rheumatoid nodules may appear in the lungs as nodules of varying size and need to be differentiated from other causes of pulmonary shadowing such as neoplasms and tuberculosis.

Seropositive rheumatoid arthritics who are coal miners or are exposed to industrial dusts may develop gross forms of pulmonary fibrosis and nodules. Caplan (1953) originally described such lesions in coal miners.

Destructive airways disease has been shown to be more frequent in RA patients than in controls matched for smoking habits. A rare and progressively fatal form of obstructive bronchiolitis has also been described in a group of rheumatoid patients.

CARDIOVASCULAR

Pericardial effusions may be detected by echocardiography. They are frequently asymptomatic. Rarely, cardiac tamponade may result from massive effusions (Hara et al 1990).

Clinical forms of rheumatoid disease affecting the myocardium or cardiac valve structures are rare. However, postmortem studies have shown non-specific valvulitis in up to 30% of rheumatoid patients. Rheumatoid granulomas of the myocardium have also been noted in postmortem studies. Rheumatoid disease is an uncommon cause of chronic valve malfunction, but granulomas have been frequently noted in the aortic and mitral valves in patients receiving cardiac valve surgery.

NEUROLOGICAL

Peripheral nerve symptoms in rheumatoid patients may arise from entrapment neuropathies and cervical myelopathy. Symptoms of entrapment neuropathy can usually be relieved by appropriate decompression. The sites of entrapment include compression of the median nerve at the wrist (carpal tunnel syndrome), compression of the posterior tibial nerve at the ankle (tarsal tunnel syndrome) and ulnar nerve compression at the elbow (ulnar neuritis).

Rheumatoid peripheral neuropathies fall into two pain groups – severe sensorimotor neuropathy and milder sensory neuropathy (Chamberlain & Bruckner 1970). The former is associated with a sudden loss of motor and sensory function and often picks out isolated nerves in a mononeuritis multiplex pattern. It is associated with the more severe forms of seropositive nodular disease and there is often evidence of vasculitis elsewhere. Nerve conduction tests usually show features of muscle denervation and the condition is thought to be produced by vasculitis of the vasa nervorum. The sensory type of neuropathy usually occurs as a glove-and-stocking pattern of sensory loss, and if motor signs occur they are usually minor. Nerve conduction tests may be normal or may show slowing of motor and sensory conduction.

Cervical myelopathy from atlantoaxial or subaxial subluxation of the cervical spine can be confused with a peripheral neuropathy and has been discussed earlier.

RENAL

Slight impairment of renal function is common in rheumatoid patients (Wish & Kammer 1993). The most frequent histological abnormalities found on biopsy are interstitial nephritis and amyloidosis. Interstitial nephritis may result from chronic bacterial infection or anti-inflammatory analgesic drug therapy. Renal papillary necrosis is a less common renal side effect of drugs, but in man probably only results from chronic ingestion of compound analgesics containing both phenacetin and aspirin. More frequent causes of drug-induced renal disease are gold and penicillamine therapy, both of which may induce an immune complex-associated vasculitis. Occasionally, in vasculitic forms of rheumatoid disease, a mild form of disease-associated glomerulonephritis may occur.

HEPATIC

Liver enlargement is found clinically in about 11% of rheumatoid patients (Whaley & Webb 1977). Liver biopsies in these patients are often normal but otherwise show non-specific fatty change or mild lymphocytic infiltration of portal tracts. Asymptomatic increases in serum alkaline phosphatase are also common in rheumatoid patients and sometimes reflect hepatotoxicity from salicylates and other anti-inflammatory drugs.

SEPTIC ARTHRITIS

This severe and potentially fatal complication is found particularly in patients with the most severe forms of rheumatoid disease. Presentation may be acute, with one disproportionately painful and inflamed joint and pyrexia. At other times septic arthritis may present in a more obscure fashion such as feeling unwell or even with an apparent flare of the disease. Fever and leucocytosis may be absent in elderly debilitated and steroid-treated patients most prone to develop this condition (Ostensson & Geborek 1991). *Staphylococcus aureus* is the organism most frequently isolated. Prompt diagnosis and treatment are essential in order to minimize joint damage and to preserve life.

LABORATORY FINDINGS

The diagnosis of RA is made mainly on clinical grounds but laboratory investigations may help. They provide objective measurements of disease activity and sometimes have prognostic value. The anaemia of rheumatoid disease has been discussed. In active disease the ESR, plasma viscosity and acute-phase reactants such as C-reactive protein are elevated and provide a rough guide to disease activity. As a non-specific feature of chronic inflammation, serum albumin may be reduced and alpha and gamma globulin elevated on protein electrophoresis. All the immunoglobulin components (IgG, IgA and IgM) may be elevated or sometimes just IgG is increased.

The serological tests for IgM rheumatoid factor become positive in 75% of patients with RA. However, the higher the titre of rheumatoid factor and the earlier in the disease course that the test becomes positive, the worse the prognosis tends to be. Antinuclear antibodies are also found in a proportion of patients and again tend to be associated with extra-articular disease. None of these autoantibodies are specific for RA and they may be found in association with other autoimmune diseases. They may be of some help in diagnosis. Significant titres of rheumatoid factor would be in keeping with a diagnosis of RA, while high titres of antinuclear antibodies in association with low or absent titres of IgM rheumatoid factor suggest systemic lupus erythematosus.

PROGNOSIS

The natural history of RA is variable. A high proportion of patients with the disease have a mild illness with a good prognosis. In a 10-year follow-up of a group of rheumatoid patients who were treated fairly conservatively by present-day practices, Duthie and colleagues found that over 50% had an eventual satisfactory outcome while only 11% became completely disabled (Duthie et al 1955). The following are adverse prognostic factors: development of erosions within 1 year of onset, poor functional capacity early in the disease course, the presence of extra-articular disease features, a persistently high ESR and failure to respond to NSAIDs. Some studies also suggest that the histocompatibility antigen DR4 may be associated with severe disease (Westedt et al 1986).

THERAPY

Decisions on effective treatment depend on the stage and activity of the disease. When there is early active inflammation the emphasis is on suppression of inflammation by general measures and antirheumatic drugs. In the late stages when destructive disease and secondary osteoarthritis predominate, the emphasis of management shifts towards relief of pain by provision of simple analgesics, improving joint function and reconstructive surgery. The prognosis in the majority of patients is reasonable and the aim of treatment is to suppress the disease process to prevent and limit the onset of erosions and the development of deformities and disabilities.

GENERAL MEASURES

The long-term management of patients with RA is undertaken by a management team which includes not only rheumatologists but also orthopaedic surgeons, physiotherapists, occupational therapists, chiropodists/podiatrists, social workers, disablement resettlement officers and nurses. The programme includes advice and education about the nature of the disease and the aims and limitations of treatment. During phases of active disease many patients require an extra rest period during the day. Physiotherapists and occupational therapists help by prescribing exercises designed to maintain and restore muscle function and ranges of joint movements, providing splints to prevent or reduce deformities and providing aids to improve function. During major disease exacerbations short periods in bed, together with splinting of particularly inflamed joints, are helpful. Individual inflamed joints may be controlled by aspirating synovial effusions and injection of slow-release corticosteroids under strict aseptic conditions.

DRUG THERAPY

The drugs used in the treatment of RA can be considered under the following headings:

1. simple analgesics
2. NSAIDs
3. second-line antirheumatic drugs
4. immunosuppressives and corticosteroids.

Simple analgesics

These include paracetamol, often in mixtures with codeine, dextropopoxyphene and others, which act on the central nervous system. They are not very effective in relieving the pain of acute inflammation and are of more use for the pain of secondary osteoarthritis and for a top-up effect in patients in whom the NSAIDs prove inadequate. These drugs do not have the gastrointestinal effects of the non-steroidal anti-inflammatory agents which are discussed in detail in Chapter 49. Narcotic analgesics are virtually never required for RA.

Non-steroidal anti-inflammatory drugs

Drugs in this group provide symptomatic relief of pain and stiffness. However, they do not alter the natural history of the disease and on their own do not prevent the development of progressive joint damage. These agents may be adequate for many rheumatoid patients but now we believe that second-line antirheumatic agents should be the initial treatment at an early stage.

Soluble aspirin was the prototype of this type of drug but is now largely replaced by newer agents such as the propionic acid derivatives. These are better tolerated but are not significantly more effective.

There is some evidence from studies of osteoarthritis that some anti-inflammatory drugs such as indomethacin may actually exacerbate damage to articular cartilage. All these drugs may cause gastrointestinal ulceration and bleeding in susceptible patients. If a patient suffers from dyspepsia it may be possible to administer the drug successfully as a suppository, as it is then absorbed more slowly and lower peak levels occur in the peripheral blood. Other alternatives include the prophylactic use of antiulcer drugs or the use of prodrugs, such as benoxaprofen, in which the agent is taken in an inactive form and only activated after absorption through the intestinal muscosa. Both the anti-inflammatory properties and the gastrointestinal adverse toxicity of these agents are in part due to their abilities to inhibit the cyclooxygenase enzymes involved in prostaglandin synthesis.

Second-line antirheumatic drugs

Active RA is now treated aggressively in most units and the second-line antirheumatic drugs are instituted rapidly if there is evidence of active inflammation. These drugs are given on a long-term basis and all have a delay from the start of treatment until the onset of action of commonly 2 or 3 months.

Sulphasalazine

This agent is effective in causing remission of RA. The usual regimen is to start with 0.5–1.0 g of the enteric-coated form daily and increase by weekly increments to a maximum of 1 g three times per day. Gastrointestinal side effects such as nausea may occur but more serious problems such as blood dyscrasias are rare. Sulphasalazine may uncommonly cause hepatotoxicity and in males a fall in sperm count. Regular monitoring of the blood count, urea, creatinine and liver function is required.

Antimalarials

Chloroquine and hydroxychloroquine have definite disease-suppressing properties. There is a small risk of producing retinopathy and visual impairment but this is minimized if the daily dosage is kept as low as possible and the eyes are monitored by an ophthalmologist. Gastrointestinal problems are uncommon and these agents lack the haematological and renal side effects which are found in many more potent antirheumatic drugs.

Gold therapy

Gold salts have been used in the treatment of RA since the 1930s. Intramuscular sodium aurothiomalate (Myocrisin) is the gold salt most commonly used in the UK, although an oral preparation has also been introduced. In a commonly used regimen, after incremental test doses, the drug is given as 50 mg weekly by intramuscular injections to a maximum of 1 g or until there is disease remission or toxicity. Once remission has occurred and maximum benefit appears to have been achieved, it is usual to lengthen the intervals between injections and reduce the dose to a monthly maintenance regimen. If there has been no response to the gold after a cumulative dose of 1 g has been given, most physicians withdraw the drug, but it is possible to try increasing the weekly injection dose (Rothermick et al 1976).

Possible side effects of gold therapy include minor skin rashes, itching, exfoliative dermatitis, stomatitis, renal problems, blood dyscrasias, hepatotoxicity and penumonitis. All patients receiving gold therapy will require regular monitoring of the skin, blood and urine.

D-Penicillamine

This drug was initially used as a chelating agent in the treatment of Wilson's disease. It is given orally but otherwise has indications and side effects similar to gold salts. The usual starting dose is 125 mg or 250 mg daily and it is important to take this drug well away from food as it can combine with food nutrients. Some patients respond to doses as low as this but if there is no improvement the dosage is slowly increased by similar amounts, at intervals, to a maximum of 750 mg daily. Most commonly the final dose is around 375 mg per day. Adverse effects include skin rashes, blood dyscrasias and renal problems. Rare side effects include immunological syndromes such as myasthenia gravis and drug-induced systemic lupus erythematosus. Regular monitoring of the skin, blood and urine for toxicity is essential.

Immunosuppressives and corticosteroids

Immunosuppressive agents, and in particular methotrexate, are frequently used for patients with severe persistent disease not controlled by more conservative measures. Methotrexate is a folic acid antagonist with immunosuppressive properties. It is given in a weekly dose, starting at 5 mg, and then increasing usually to a maximum of 15 mg per week but occasionally more. It appears much more effective than the second-line antirheumatic agents (Ward 1985). The onset of benefit commonly does not start for at least a month after initiating treatment. Adverse effects are uncommon but may affect blood, liver and lungs and the drug is contraindicated in patients with a high alcohol intake. Careful monitoring of the blood and liver function is essential. Co-prescription of folic acid, usually on the third day after the methotrexate, may reduce the risk of gastrointestinal problems.

Alternative immunosuppressive agents such as cyclophosphamide are used for very severe individual cases and are sometimes given as bolus infusions. They are usually reserved for patients with complications such as severe forms of vasculitis and for patients who have failed to respond to more conservative therapy.

Cyclosportin is an immunosuppressive agent used following transplantation surgery. It is effective in severe and resistant forms of RA. Common problems of treatment include some impairment of renal function and the development of hypertension. Careful monitoring is essential.

Oral corticosteroids such as prednisolone have dramatic effects in relieving symptoms. Unfortunately, once patients have started on steroids it is commonly very difficult, if not impossible, to withdraw them. Patients receiving steroid therapy over a number of years frequently develop severe adverse effects such as osteoporosis, hypertension, dermal atrophy, etc., and in the long run these may outweigh the benefits in relieving the arthritis symptoms. The decision to start corticosteroids is a major one and should only be taken after careful consideration. The bone mineral density should be checked in patients maintained on steroids. If necessary, bone strengthening measures such as calcium and vitamin D, oestrogens or biophosphates are added.

Local steroid injections are helpful when one or two joints or tendon sheaths show continued inflammation. If there is any suspicion of infection, the synovial fluid should be aspirated and cultured and the steroid injection given later. Slow-acting steroid preparations are usually used. Fluorinated steroids should be avoided for very superficial injections, as they are more likely to cause dermal atrophy than other steroid preparations.

SURGERY

Surgery is indicated for the relief of pain and prevention of loss of function when medical measures prove inadequate. The programme is best planned in a combined clinic held jointly by the rheumatologist and the orthopaedic surgeon.

In early disease synovectomy may be helpful symptomatically when synovial swelling is localized to one or two joints and significant erosions have not appeared. Tenosynovectomy may help when synovial hypertrophy has involved tendon sheaths and is affecting hand function or threatening tendon rupture. Decompression may be required for the relief of nerve entrapment syndromes.

In advanced cases, joint replacements are now available for a variety of joints and are continually being improved. Hip and knee replacements are commonplace and are the most successful. Replacements are available for the shoulder, and elbow and ankle.

Other surgical procedures sometimes used include excision arthroplasty, fusion and repair of ruptured tendons.

REFERENCES

Ansell BM, Loewi G 1977 Rheumatoid arthritis – general I'catures. Clinics in Rheumatic Diseases 3: 385–401

Barrett AJ, Saklatvala H 1981 Proteinases in joint disease. In: Kelley WN, Harris ED, Ruddy SF, Sledge CB (eds) Textbook of rheumatology. WB Saunders, Philadelphia, pp 195–209

Beighton P, Soloman L, Valkenburgh HA 1975 Rheumatoid arthritis in a rural South African population. Annals of Rheumatic Disease 34: 136–141

Benedek TG 1993 Association between rheumatic diseases and neoplasia. In: Maddison PH et al (eds) Oxford textbook of rheumatology. Oxford University Press, Oxford, pp 1070–1082

Bennett RM 1977 Haematological changes in rheumatoid disease. Clinics in Rheumatic Diseases 3: 433–465

Bland JH, David PH, London MG, Van Buskirk FW, Duarte EG 1963 Rheumatoid arthritis of cervical spine. Archives of Internal Medicine 122: 892–898

Brunton RW, Grennan DM, Palmer DG, de Silva RTA 1978 Lateral subluxation of the atlas in rheumatoid arthritis. British Journal of Radiology 51: 963–967

Caplan A 1953 Certain unusual radiological appearances in the chest of coalminers suffering from rheumatoid arthritis. Thorax 8: 29–37

Chamberlain MA, Bruckner FE 1970 Rheumatoid neuropathy. Clinical and electrophysiological features. Annals of the Rheumatic Diseases 29: 609–616

Conlon PW, Isdale IC, Rose BS 1966 Rheumatoid arthritis of the cervical spine. Annals of the Rheumatic Diseases 25: 120–126

Duthie JR, Thompson M, Wier MM, Fletcher WB 1955 Medical and social aspects of the treatment of rheumatoid arthritis with special reference to factors affecting prognosis. Annals of the Rheumatic Diseases 14: 133–149

Fassbender HG 1975 Rheumatoid arthritis in pathology of rheumatic diseases. Springer Verlag, Berlin, pp 70–210

Gardner DL 1992 Pathological basis of the connective tissue disease. Edward Arnold, London, pp 485–487

Hara KS et al 1990 Rheumatoid pericarditis: clinical features and survival. Medicine 69: 81–91

Hyland RH, Gordon DA, Broder I, Davies GM et al 1983 A systemic controlled study of pulmonary abnormalities in rheumatoid arthritis. Journal of Rheumatology 10: 395–405

Jayson MIV, Jones DEP 1971 Scleritis and rheumatoid arthritis. Annals of the Rheumatic Diseases 30: 343–347

Jayson MIV, Smidt LA 1987 The foot in arthritis. In: Baillière's Clinical Rheumatology 1: 2

Lawrence JS 1970 Rheumatoid arthritis – nature or nurture. Annals of the Rheumatic Diseases 29: 357–379

Mathews JA 1974 Atlanto-axial subluxation in rheumatoid arthritis – a 5 year follow-up. Annals of the Rheumatic Diseases 33: 526–531

Ostensson A, Geborek P 1991 Septic arthritis as a non-surgical complication in rheumatoid arthritis and relation to disease severity and therapy. British Journal of Rheumatology 30: 35–38

Rothermick NO, Philips VK, Bergen W, Rhomas MH 1976 Chrysotherapy. A prospective study. Arthritis and Rheumatism 19: 1321–1327

Vreugdenhil G, Swaak AJG 1990 Anaemia in rheumatoid arthritis:

pathogenesis, diagnosis and treatment. Rheumatology International 9: 243–257
Ward T 1985 Historical perspective on the use of methotrexate for the treatment of rheumatoid arthritis. Journal of Rheumatology (suppl i): 3–6
Westedt ML, Breedveld FC, Schrevder GM Th, d'Amato J, Cats N, de Vries RRP 1986 Immunogenetic heterogeneity of rheumatoid arthritis. Annals of the Rheumatic Diseases 45: 534–538
Whaley K, Webb J 1977 Liver and kidney disease in rheumatoid arthritis. Clinics in Rheumatic Diseases 3: 527–547
Wish JB, Kammer GM 1993 Nephrological aspects of management in the rheumatic diseases. In: Maddison PH et al (eds) Oxford text book of rheumatology. Oxford University Press, Oxford, pp 179–187
Wyn Parry CB 1994 The hand. In: Clinics in Rheumatic Disease. WB Saunders, London 10: 3

Muscles, tendons and ligaments

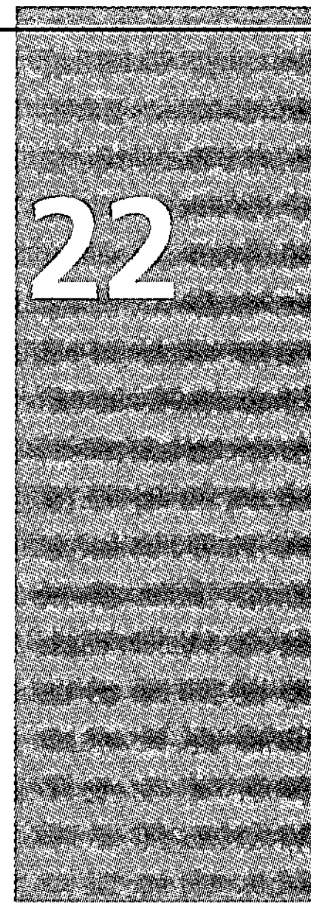

DIANNE J. NEWHAM & KERRY R. MILLS

Musculoskeletal soft tissue is composed of muscle, tendon and ligament and it is often difficult for the patient and clinician to distinguish which of these tissues are the source of pain. Due to their physical and functional proximity more than one is likely to be affected at the same time. The cardinal signs of damage to the non-contractile soft tissues are pain, tenderness, swelling and loss of function.

Most individuals will have experienced musculoskeletal pain, particularly that of muscular origin. Usually it is clearly associated with trauma or exercise and is of a temporary nature. There are, however, a considerable number of people who experience this type of pain which, because of its severity or chronicity, causes them to seek advice. A wide variety of pathological conditions may give rise to myalgia. Diseases of collagen and connective tissue are relatively rare but often have a devastating effect (Pope 1998).

This chapter commences by considering the structures responsible for the perception of pain from these tissues.

NOCICEPTORS

At the turn of the century Sherrington (1900) thought that specific afferent nerve fibres did not exist for the transmission of noxious stimuli from skeletal muscle and that 'adequate' stimulation of muscle spindles and tendon organs would elicit pain. Later workers have shown that, as in the skin, the thin myelinated (Group III or Aδ) and unmyelinated (Group IV or C) fibres are responsible for transmitting nociceptive impulses from muscle (Knighton & Dumke 1966), tendons and ligaments. Group I and II fibres from muscle spindles and tendon organs do not transmit noxious information from skeletal muscle. Electrical stimulation of Group I fibres (which elicit the H reflex) is not at all painful and known algesic agents such as bradykinin do not excite Group I or II muscle afferent units (Mense 1977).

The unencapsulated, freely branching endings of these afferents are found throughout soft musculoskeletal tissues with particularly dense projections in the region of tendons, fascia, capsules and aponeuroses (Stacey 1969, Schiable & Grubb 1993, Schmidt et al 1994). Experimental access to these endings is complicated by their intimate connections with surrounding tissue, but despite technical difficulties the receptors of muscular Group III (Paintal 1960, Bessou & Laporte 1961) and IV (Iggo 1961) fibres have been shown to be activated by a variety of noxious stimuli. Physiological mechanisms of pain in the musculoskeletal system have been reviewed by Zimmermann (1988).

The receptive properties of the chemo- and mechano-nociceptors indicate that they are a heterogeneous group; some may respond to a single chemical substance while others are polymodal and respond to a variety of chemical, mechanical and thermal stimuli (Kumazawa & Mizumura 1977, Mense & Schmidt 1977).

The most effective substances for activation of these receptors are bradykinin, 5-hydroxytryptamine (serotonin), histamine, potassium and hydrogen ions. Aspirin has been shown to reduce the increased activity in Group III and IV muscle afferents which is induced by bradykinin, but not by 5-hydroxytryptamine (Mense 1982).

In addition to transmitting nociceptive information, muscle afferents play a role in the cardiovascular and respiratory adjustments occurring during exercise. Electrical stimulation produces changes similar to those during exercise (Coote & Perez-Gonzales 1971). Nerve-blocking techniques established that the reflex responses to exercise are mediated by muscle Group III and IV afferents (Kalia et al 1972, McCloskey & Mitchell 1972). Afferent units fulfilling this function have been termed 'ergoreceptors', but they are not a distinct population, as many afferents have both nociceptive and ergoreceptive properties (Kniffki et al 1978).

Recent evidence indicates that thick myelinated afferents may transmit information which is perceived as pain in some circumstances. Thus the conventional classification of nociceptors and nociception may be misleading (McMahon & Koltzenburg 1990).

The density of nociceptors in ligaments is relatively low in comparison to muscle and joint capsules (McLain & Weinstein 1994). Four basic types of afferent nerve endings have been described in articular tissues. In addition to the nociceptive role of the Group IV fibres, the endings of Groups I–III are capable of responding to excessive joint movement with noxious stimuli and are thought to be effective in reflex control mechanisms that maintain joint stability (Freeman & Wyke 1967, Barrack & Skinner 1990).

Nociceptors in tendons appear to be located primarily close to the muscle attachment. Total tendon ruptures often do not cause pain and may often be missed, because loss of strength and function can often be largely compensated for by other intact tissues.

MUSCLE PAIN

ASSOCIATION WITH EXERCISE

In normal healthy subjects there is usually a clear association between muscle pain and exercise but two very different time courses may occur. In one case, pain occurs during the exercise and rapidly increases in intensity until the contractions stop and blood flow is restored, whereupon the pain disappears very rapidly, within seconds or a few minutes. This is termed ischaemic muscle pain. Alternatively, the pain may occur with a delayed onset of some hours after exercise and may persist for days.

Ischaemic muscle pain

Intermittent claudication and angina pectoris are two well-known clinical presentations of this type of pain. It occurs in muscles whose blood supply is compromised: a situation that occurs in normal muscle as the result of the increase in intramuscular pressure during muscular activity. In normal subjects it disappears within seconds of the contractions stopping and the circulation being restored, leaving no residual effects.

Hypoxia was thought to cause this type of pain but a preliminary period of hypoxia does not reduce the time for which ischaemic contractions can be performed (Park & Rodbard 1962). It is now accepted that accumulation of metabolites is, at least in part, responsible for ischaemic pain, although the metabolic stimulus, or combination of stimuli, is not clear. Lactic acid was thought by many to be the prime algesic substance, but it has been eliminated from this role by the finding that patients with myophosphorylase deficiency (McArdle's syndrome) experience particularly severe ischaemic muscle pain during exercise, despite an inability to produce lactic acid (Schmid & Hammaker 1961, Cady et al 1989). Data, acquired by magnetic resonance spectroscopy, have shown that clearance of intramuscular lactic acid at the end of exercise or vascular occlusion is slower than the disappearance of pain. Possible agents, acting alone or in combination, are currently thought to include histamine, acetylcholine, serotonin and bradykinin. Potassium (Lendinger & Sjogaard 1991) and adenosine (Sylven et al 1988) are currently receiving considerable attention in this respect.

Ischaemic muscle pain also has mechanical determinants and the effects of contraction force and frequency have been investigated by many workers. The repetition rate of intermittent contractions has a marked effect, the onset and severity of pain increasing with increasing contraction frequency (Park & Rodbard 1962, Rodbard & Pragay 1968, Mills et al 1982a).

Delayed-onset muscle pain

Heavy or unaccustomed exercise has long been associated with muscle pain which has a delayed onset of about 8 h and persists for days. Asmussen (1956) was the first to establish that it is particularly associated with unaccustomed eccentric contractions – those in which the active muscle is lengthened by external forces. This observation has since been confirmed by many workers (Newham et al 1983c, 1988, Stauber 1989). Eccentric contractions generate a higher force per active fibre (Katz 1939, Abbott et al 1952) and have a lower metabolic cost per unit force than other types of muscle activity (Curtin & Davies 1973, Menard et al 1991). Thus delayed-onset muscle pain is likely to be caused by mechanical, rather than metabolic, factors and differs from ischaemic pain in time course as well as underlying mechanisms.

Delayed onset pain is associated with considerable muscle damage, as shown by structural (Newham et al 1983b, Friden 1984, Jones et al 1986, Newham 1988), biochemical (Newham 1983a, 1986a,b, Stauber 1989) and radioisotopic changes (reviewed by Clarkson & Newham 1995). The damage is presumably initiated by the high forces generated in active fibres during eccentric contractions, but none of these damage markers follow the same time course as the pain (Jones et al 1986, Newham et al 1986b), the cause of which remains unknown. Recent evidence increasingly indicates connective tissue damage (Brown et al 1997) which may cause pain, along with the inflammatory process. The affected muscles are tender and often feel swollen. Increased intramuscular pressures have been reported in muscles in non-compliant compartments (Friden et al 1986), but not in others (Newham & Jones 1985), and the increased pressure precedes pain.

There is conflicting evidence about the effect of steroidal and non-steroidal anti-inflammatory agents on delayed-onset pain (Janssen et al 1983, Kuipers et al 1983, Headley et al 1986).

CLINICAL MYALGIA

Signs and symptoms

The vocabulary of patients presenting with myalgia is relatively restricted. Common terms for the symptom are stiffness, soreness, aching, spasms or cramps. Tenderness is a common self-reported sign. The symptom of stiffness usually means discomfort on muscle movement, rather than a change of compliance.

Muscle pain is most often reported as having a dull, aching quality. Sharp, lancinating pain is relatively rare, although acute tenderness from a 'trigger point' (Travell & Simons 1998) may occur. Even severe cramps have a relatively dull quality. Muscle pain is usually exacerbated by voluntary contraction, although rarely the opposite may be the case.

The terms cramp, contracture, spasm and tetanus or tetany have precise definitions but are often used inaccurately (Simons & Mense 1998). Cramps are strong, involuntary contractions of rapid onset which are extremely painful and are associated with electromyographic signals similar to those of a normal voluntary contraction (Mills et al 1982b). A contracture is an extremely rare form of involuntary contraction due to depletion of muscle adenosine triphosphate (ATP) and is electrically silent. It is a sign of rare metabolic disorders (e.g., myophosphorylase deficiency) and only occurs in healthy individuals after death as rigor mortis because force fatigue prevents ATP depletion. Spasm usually implies a reflex contraction of the muscles surrounding an injured or inflamed structure and is seen in the abdominal muscles during visceral inflammation or obstruction. Tetany is an involuntary contraction, often in carpopedal muscles, and is usually associated with hypocalcaemia or hypocapnia (Layzer & Rowland 1971).

Less common are myotonia and dystonia. The former is a prolongation of muscle contraction and delayed relaxation; it is most often associated with dystrophia myotonica. Dystonia is an involuntary contraction of muscles acting over the same joint, but which have opposing actions and may be described as either spasm or cramp.

Associated signs and symptoms

Patients with myalgia often complain of weakness, fatigability or exercise intolerance (discussed under 'Investigation of muscle pain' below). Swelling of painful muscles is often reported, but rarely substantiated. If it is, it almost always implies serious underlying pathology and occurs in polymyositis, dermatomyositis, myophosphorylase and phosphofructokinase deficiencies and acute alcoholic myopathy.

Enquiry should be made about alcohol, diet and fasting. A drinking bout in an alcoholic may precipitate acute alcoholic myopathy and even myoglobinuria. A diet deficient in vitamin D is associated with osteomalacia, causing bone and muscle pain (Smith & Stern 1967). Attacks of pain and weakness occur in carnitine palmityltransferase deficiency, particularly during prolonged exercise after fasting or after a high-fat, low-carbohydrate diet or meal (Di Mauro & Di Mauro 1973, Bank et al 1975). Fasting may be used as a provocative test for this condition (Carroll et al 1979).

Both muscle pain and dyskinesia are associated with poor sleep patterns, although it is not known which is the primary event (Lavigne et al 1991).

Differentiation of muscle pain from pain in other tissues

Pain localization is poor in skeletal muscle and patients may also be unable to differentiate it from pain arising from tendons, ligaments and bones, as well as from joints and their capsules. Several conditions (e.g., systemic lupus erythematosus) involve both muscles and joints. It is obviously important to identify the painful tissue but this may be very difficult due to poor localization and referred pain; pain from an arthritic hip may be referred to the thigh muscles or knee joint, from a carpal tunnel syndrome to the forearm muscles or from cervical spondylosis to the arm muscles.

Pain from joints and their capsules tends to be more localized than myalgia and arthralgia is often worsened by passive joint movement. Capsular pain may be present only in specific joint positions (e.g., painful arc syndrome in the shoulder). Bone pain also tends to be poorly localized but, unlike myalgia, usually has a deep, boring quality. It is usually worse at night and tends to be unaffected by either movement or muscle activity.

Myalgia, exercise and rest

Many patients presenting with myalgia describe a relationship between exercise and muscle pain that has one of the two time courses found in normal subjects. Others find no relationship or even that their pain is relieved by moderate exercise.

The paradigm of exercise-related muscle pain is intermittent claudication, in which pain occurs in the calf muscles during exercise then disappears after a period of rest. This is a pathological form of ischaemic muscle pain caused by stenosis of the feeding artery and is experienced distal to the stenosis. Thus thrombosis of the terminal aorta leads to pain in the buttocks (Leriche's syndrome), narrowing of the axillary artery by a cervical rib gives rise to forearm pain and arteritis of cranial arteries may result in pain in the muscles of mastication during chewing. Reduced blood supply can also occur due to increased blood viscosity (e.g., Waldenström's macroglobulinaemia). Ischaemia can also arise with a normal blood flow if the oxygen-carrying capacity of blood is reduced, as in anaemia.

Other conditions in which myalgia is clearly related to exercise involve an impaired energy supply to a contracting muscle; the mechanism is presumably the same as ischaemic muscle pain. Myophosphorylase deficiency (Schmid & Mahler 1959), glycolytic disorders of muscle (McArdle 1951) and phosphofructokinase deficiency (Tarui et al 1965) all present as exercise-related myalgia with cramps and contracture. Contracture is a potentially serious event, because it leads to irreversible muscle breakdown and the release of large amounts of myoglobin may lead to renal cast formation and failure. A clear association between exercise and myalgia is also found in several of the mitochondrial myopathies (Land & Clark 1979) and in carnitine palmityltransferase deficiency (Bank et al 1975).

In those individuals where failure of energy or blood supply has been eliminated, the relationship of pain to exercise or rest appears to have no diagnostic or prognostic value (Mills & Edwards 1983).

AETIOLOGY (TABLE 22.1)

Primary infective myositis

Direct infection of muscle with bacteria is uncommon. Tropical myositis (Taylor et al 1976) is an infection with *Staphylococcus aureus*, probably secondary to a viral myositis. It affects children and young adults in the tropics and is characterized by fever, muscle pains (often severe and localized to a single limb) and deep intramuscular abscesses. It usually responds to antibiotics and surgical drainage.

Parasitic infections of muscle that cause muscle pain and tenderness include trichinosis (Gould 1970), sparganonosis (Wirth & Farrow 1961), sarcosporidosis (Jeffrey 1974) and cysticercosis. Infection with *Trichinella spiralis*, usually by eating undercooked pork, is common in many parts of the world, especially the USA, but many cases are asymptomatic. The disease is ushered in with fever and periorbital oedema. Later myalgia and muscle weakness develop to reach a peak at 3 weeks. The prognosis depends on the heaviness of the infection; 2–10% of cases are fatal. Treatment with thiabendazole and steroids has been successful.

Table 22.1 Principal medical conditions associated with myalgia

Trauma and sports injuries
Primary infective myositis
Inflammatory myopathies
Polymyositis
Dermatomyositis
Polymyositis or dermatomyositis in association with connective tissue disease
Viral myositis
Polymyalgia rheumatica
Myalgia of neurogenic origin
Muscle cramp
Impaired muscle energy metabolism
Cytosolic enzyme defects
Lipid storage myopathies
Mitochondrial myopathies
Drug-induced myalgia
Myalgic encephalomyelitis
Muscle pain of uncertain cause

Inflammatory myopathies

Polymyositis and dermatomyositis
(Pachman 1998, Targoff 1998)

The idiopathic inflammatory myopathies, polymyositis and dermatomyositis, classified by Bohan and Peter (1975a,b) and Carpenter and Karpati (1981), have been reviewed extensively (Currie 1981, Mastaglia 1988, Dalakas 1988, Pachman 1998, Targoff 1998). In a few cases muscle pain may be a prominent feature but usually the presentation is of muscle weakness. It was originally thought that the two diseases represented part of the same spectrum, with skin lesions being present only in dermatomyositis. This view has now been challenged and there are both clinical and pathological distinctions between them. Dermatomyositis presents more commonly in the female with acute or subacute onset of limb girdle weakness, dysphagia, muscle tenderness and skin involvement. There is often involvement of other systems, such as the lungs and heart, and in 20% of cases there may be an associated carcinoma. Pathologically in dermatomyositis, there is evidence of a microangiopathy with immunoglobulin deposits on vessel walls which lead to microinfarcts. On muscle biopsy there may be striking perivascular atrophy. Polymyositis on the other hand presents equally in males and females, has a chronic course, respiratory muscle involvement is unusual and muscle tenderness infrequent. There is no skin involvement or involvement of other systems. Pathologically, muscle biopsy shows endomysial lymphocyte infiltration and cytotoxic T cells predominate.

Diagnosis rests on the findings of:

1. A muscle biopsy showing muscle cell necrosis, lymphocyte infiltration, phagocytosis, variation in size of both fibre types and basophilic fibres reflecting regeneration.
2. EMG showing brief, small-amplitude polyphasic potentials and fibrillations (Marinacci 1965).
3. Plasma creatine kinase (CK) which is raised in the acute phase but may be normal in 30% of cases.
4. A raised erythrocyte sedimentation rate in 60% of cases.

The treatment remains controversial. Despite widespread clinical use of high-dose corticosteroids, no well-controlled trial has been performed. Nevertheless, the clinical usefulness of steroid therapy is a widely held view and the complications of long-term steroid therapy are said to be uncommon (Riddoch & Morgan-Hughes 1975, Bunch et al 1980, Currie 1981), although they must always be borne in mind (Carpenter et al 1977, Edwards et al 1981). Other immunosuppressive drugs such as azathioprine, cyclophosphamide, methotrexate and cyclosporin, immunoglobulin infusions, whole-body irradiation and plasmapheresis have all been tried but the results and the benefits are not clear cut. Estimates of prognosis and mortality in polymyositis vary; in the 20 cases studied by Riddoch & Morgan-Hughes over a 5-year period, eight patients died and only four improved. De Vere & Bradley (1975) reported a 25–30% mortality over 5 years. The prognosis of dermatomyositis is rather better, with many patients showing full recovery of muscle function; although the disease will eventually burn itself out, this may take several years.

Muscle pain is not a feature of inclusion body myositis (Lotz et al 1989).

Polymyositis in association with connective tissue disease

Polymyositis may be seen in association with systemic lupus erythematosus (Tsokos et al 1991), progressive systemic sclerosis, mixed connective tissue disease, rheumatoid disease (Haslock et al 1970), Sjögrens syndrome, polyarteritis nodosa and, occasionally, myasthenia gravis. In polyarteritis nodosa muscle changes are probably due to infarction, but in the other conditions findings are similar to those in idiopathic polymyositis, although the changes of steroid myopathy are often superimposed.

Viral polymyositis

Myalgia is a feature of several acute viral infections; in the vast majority of cases, influenza virus A or B or coxsackie virus A or B are the agents involved. Coxsackie B virus is the agent responsible for epidemic myalgia (Bornholm disease) in which there is fever, headache and muscle pain in the chest and abdomen. The disease is rapidly self limiting, as is benign acute childhood myositis which can follow influenza A or B virus infection. In these conditions, the CK may be raised and in the few patients who have been tested, electromyography (EMG) may show myopathic features. A syndrome of muscle cramps, aching and fatigability following an influenza-like illness, has been described and designated 'benign post-infectious polymyositis' (Schwartz et al 1978). The symptoms may persist for 2 years after the initial febrile episode. Occasionally, a viral infection is thought to precipitate idiopathic polymyositis or dermatomyositis, and it has recently been suggested that inclusion body myositis may be a slow mumps virus infection (Chou 1988).

Polymyalgia rheumatica

This condition affects patients over the age of 55 and is characterized by pain and stiffness of the proximal muscles especially the shoulder girdle (Hamrin 1972). There may be mild anaemia, weight loss and malaise. The erythrocyte sedimentation rate is typically over 50 mm in the first hour, but Creatinine Kinase (CK), muscle biopsy and EMG are normal. Occasional cases show arthritic change within muscle and there appears to be a close relationship between this condition and temporal, cranial or giant cell arteritis. The response to steroids is usually immediate and dramatic (Bird et al 1979), most authorities advising a high initial dose of 40–60 mg per day.

Myalgia of neurogenic origin

Pain which appears to be localized to muscle may be a predominant feature in a number of neurogenic diseases.

Cervical radiculopathy with pain radiating into the myotomal distribution of the roots, or nerve compression (e.g., carpel tunnel syndrome), may produce pain radiating into the forearm or upper arm muscles. Peripheral neuropathies may produce pain especially when they affect small fibres, but this is usually distinguishable on its peripheral and superficial characteristics. Spasticity of any origin can give rise to flexor 'spasms' which can be very distressing. Treatment is difficult but diazepam and baclofen can be tried.

Muscle cramps

Apart from the benign 'ordinary' muscle cramps experienced by most individuals, cramps are also seen in glycolytic disorders (see below), in dehydration, in uraemia, with certain drugs such as salbutamol, phenothiazine, vincristine, lithium, cimetidine and bumetanide (Lane & Mastaglia 1978), after haemodialysis and in tetanus (Layzer 1994).

The 'stiff man' syndrome, first described by Moersch and Woltman (1956) and reviewed by Gordon et al (1967) and Layzer (1994), is characterized by continuous board-like stiffness of muscles, paroxymsms of intense cramp, abolition of muscle stiffness during sleep and a normal motor and sensory examination. Stiffness treatment with diazepam, often in very large doses, has been reported.

Neuromyotonia (Isaacs' syndrome) features widespread fasciculation, generalized stiffness, excessive sweating and continuous motor unit activity, which persist during sleep and anaesthesia (Isaacs 1961, Newsom-Davis & Mills 1992). A family with cramps in the distal muscles with fasciculation (Lazaro et al 1981), and a muscular pain and fasciculation syndrome (Hudson et al 1978), have also been reported. In all the above conditions the defect is thought to be in the spinal cord or motor axons.

Impaired muscle energy metabolism

Cytosolic enzyme defects

Myophosphorylase deficiency (McArdle's disease) In 1951 McArdle first described a patient with exercise-induced muscle pain and contractures, and postulated a defect in muscle glycolysis. Myophosphorylase deficiency was demonstrated by Mommaerts et al (1959) and Schmid and Mahler (1959) in further cases. The symptoms usually begin in early adolescence with painful muscle stiffness, cramps, contractures and muscle weakness induced by vigorous exercise. The symptoms disappear after a period of rest but contractures may persist for several hours. Moderate exercise may be performed for long periods without symptoms developing, but if they do, further exercise may result in resolution of the pain. This is the 'second wind' phenomenon (Pernow et al 1967), thought to be due to a combination of increased muscle blood flow and the mobilization of free fatty acids and glucose from the liver. The condition has a relatively benign course, symptoms becoming less troublesome after the age of 40 years. Patients often have no physical signs at rest, although quadriceps weakness may be demonstrated by quantitative testing. CK is elevated at rest and reaches very high values as contractures resolve. EMG may be normal or show myopathic changes, but the definitive investigation is muscle biopsy showing excessive glycogen deposition and a reduction or absence of myophosphorylase. Biopsy in an acute attack may, in addition, show muscle cell necrosis.

Phosphofructokinase deficiency This condition was described initially by Tarui et al (1965). The symptoms are very similar to those of McArdle's disease but may begin early in childhood and contractures are less frequent. The second wind phenomenon has also been reported (Layzer et al 1967). Diagnosis is achieved by the demonstration of the absence of phosphofructokinase (PFK) activity and of glycogen accumulation in muscle. CK is elevated between attacks of pain and, as in McArdle's disease, there is no rise in venous lactate on the ischaemic exercise test. PFK is also present as an isoenzyme in erythrocytes and patients with the deficiency have mild haemolysis with a raised reticulocyte count.

Other cytosolic enzyme defects A number of other enzyme deficiencies have been reported which cause exercise intolerance, exercise-induced muscle pains and muscle fatigue. Phosphoglycerate kinase deficiency (type 9 glycogenesis) (Di Mauro et al 1983), phosphoglycerate mutase deficiency (type 10 glycogenesis) (Di Mauro et al 1982) and lactate dehydrogenase deficiency (Kanno et al 1980) have been reported in only a few cases.

Lipid storage myopathies

Transport of long-chain fatty acids to the interior of the mitochondrion depends on the enzyme carnitine palmityltransferase (CPT) located on the inner membrane and the carrier molecule carnitine. Deficiency of either would be expected to lead to a block in energy supply once intramuscular glycogen stores were depleted. Syndromes due to carnitine palmityltransferase deficiency, to carnitine deficiency and to both have been described.

Systemic carnitine deficiency, in which both muscle and plasma carnitine are low, presents in childhood with episodes of nausea, vomiting, encephalopathy and muscle weakness (Karpati et al 1975). Muscle carnitine deficiency (Willner et al 1979), in which plasma carnitine is normal, presents in young adults with proximal muscle weakness and pain. CK is usually raised and the EMG myopathic. Muscle biopsy shows lipid accumulation beneath the plasma membrane and between myofibrils, and low levels of carnitine. Response to treatment with carnitine (Angelini et al 1976, Carroll et al 1980) has been variable, possibly indicating heterogeneity in the disease.

CPT deficiency usually presents in adolescence with attacks of muscle pain, weakness and myoglobinuria precipitated by prolonged exercise, especially after fasting or after a low-carbohydrate, high-fat diet (Bertorini et al 1980). CK is usually normal between attacks but rises markedly during and after attacks of pain. Muscle biopsy at the height of an attack may show lipid accumulation and/or muscle cell necrosis and assay for CPT shows very low levels. Management with a high-carbohydrate, low-fat diet has achieved some increase in exercise tolerance. Ionasescu et al (1980) have described a mother and son who had attacks of muscle cramp and myoglobinuria and whose muscle biopsies showed deficiencies of both carnitine and CPT.

Mitochondrial myopathies

This is a heterogeneous group of conditions, often presenting with muscle weakness and/or exercise-induced pain, and distinguished by the finding, usually on electron microscopy, of mitochondria of abnormal size, shape or numbers, often with crystalline inclusions. Many patients may have 'ragged red fibres' on the modified Gomori trichrome stain. With increasingly sophisticated biochemical investigations, metabolic abnormalities isolated to particular segments of the cytochrome chain can now be distinguished (Petty et al 1986, Morgan-Hughes et al 1987, Holt et al 1989). For example, patients have been described with cytochrome B deficiency (Morgan-Hughes et al 1979), with NADH cytochrome B reductase deficiency (Land & Clark 1979) and cytochrome B deficiency (complex 3) (Hayes et al 1984). Several other mitochondrial cytopathies have been associated with a bewildering number of other abnormalities: deafness, myoclonus, encephalopathy, ophthalmoplegia, growth retardation and retinitis pigmentosa (Kearns–Sayre syndrome), as reviewed by Petty et al (1986).

Drug-induced myalgia

A large number of agents have now been catalogued as the cause of muscle pain (Lane & Mastaglia 1978). A polymyositis can be produced by d-penicillamine, with myopathic features on EMG, muscle cell necrosis and an inflammatory infiltrate on muscle biopsy samples. A severe acute rhabdomyolysis with myoglobinuria and the threat of renal failure can be induced by diamorphine, amphetamine, phencyclidine and alcohol.

Myalgic encephalomyelitis/ chronic fatigue syndrome

The well-publicized syndrome of myalgic encephalomyelitis (ME) commonly presents with diffuse muscle pain, which is exacerbated by muscle activity, marked exercise intolerance, weakness and fatigability. Other symptoms include loss of concentration and sleep disturbance. A proportion of cases relate the onset of symptoms to a viral illness, giving rise to the term postviral (fatigue) syndrome. The multiplicity of possible symptoms often makes diagnosis difficult and a consensus has recently been agreed on diagnostic criteria (Dawson 1990). It may occur sporadically or in epidemics and is most common in young and middle-aged women (Behan & Bakheit 1991). Currently there is much debate about whether the aetiology is physical or psychological (Wessely 1990). Irrespective of the underlying mechanisms, the symptoms affect a large number of individuals, some of whom will recover over a few months or years, while others are transformed into chronic invalids (Wessely & Newham 1993). A recent publication presents a series of expert reviews on the diagnosis, aetiology, clinical findings and management of the syndrome (Behan et al 1991).

There is a lack of agreement about whether the patients show immunological indications of chronic viral infections. Hyperventilation is reported as being a common finding, which when treated brings symptomatic improvement. There is neurophysiological evidence of attentional deficits and slowed information processing (Prasher et al 1990). There appears to be an increased incidence of psychiatric disorder in these patients, compared to normal individuals and those with muscle disease (Wessley & Powell 1989, Wood et al 1991).

On objective muscle testing there is no evidence of muscle wasting, weakness or abnormal fatigability, due to either central or peripheral mechanisms (Stokes et al 1988, Edwards et al 1991, Lloyd et al 1991, Rutherford & White 1991). Neither are there consistent histochemical or metabolic changes, other than the non-specific changes associated with immobility. Blood levels of skeletal muscle cytoplasmic enzymes (e.g., CK), usually raised with muscle damage, are normal.

Muscle pain of uncertain cause

Vague muscle aches and pains commonly form part of the symptomatology in depressive illness and in individuals with a neurotic or obsessive personality disorder. However, care must be taken not to dismiss these symptoms; the depression may be secondary to an organic muscle abnormality.

In large studies a group of patients always appears who complain of muscle pain, in whom no abnormality can be found despite exhaustive investigation (Serratrice et al 1980, Mills & Edwards 1983, Simons & Mense 1998). Rational criteria to filter out those patients with organic abnormalities appear to be the measurement of ESR and CK. If either of these is abnormal, then muscle biopsy, EMG, exercise and strength testing should be performed. However, there exists a considerable group of patients with muscle pain in whom no definite muscle abnormality can be found. Undoubtedly, a number of specific muscle abnormalities remain to be characterized.

The term 'repetitive strain injury' has recently gained popularity as a catch-all term for pain developing as the consequence of some repetitive occupation. Although changes in muscle biopsy specimens have been reported (Fry 1986), there has been no firm confirmation of any neurological or rheumatological abnormality (Barton et al 1992).

Primary fibromyalgia (Bengtsson 1986) or 'fibrositis' (Bennett 1981) is a disorder in which histological abnormalities have been detected (Bartels & Danneskiold-Samsoe 1986, Bengtsson et al 1986a), as have reduced high-energy phosphate levels (Bengtsson et al 1986b), although the clear definition of the syndrome remains controversial (Hazleman 1998).

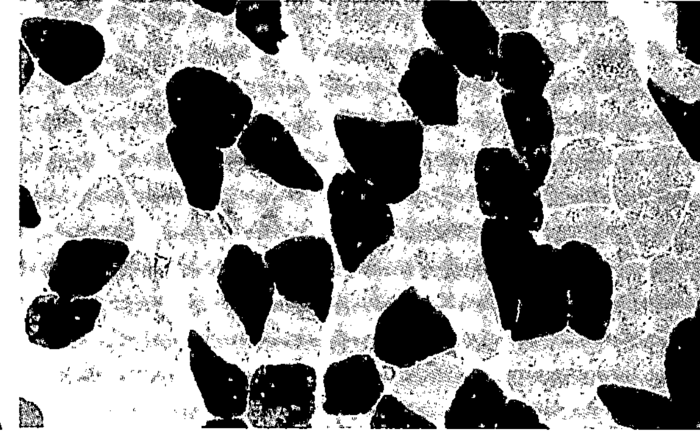

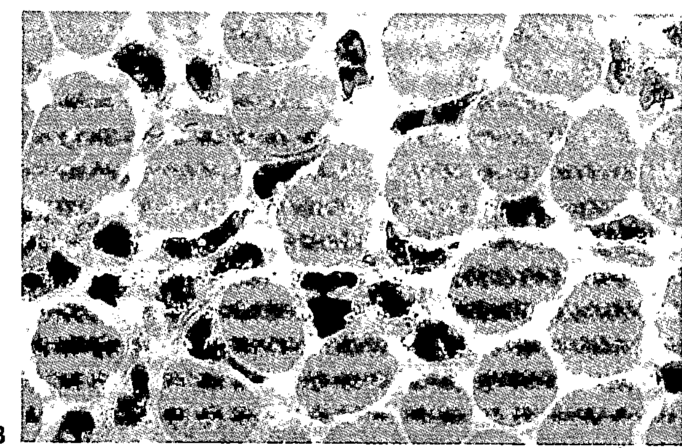

Fig. 22.1 Needle biopsy from a human gastrocnemius muscle, with Type II, fast twitch fibres staining dark. **A** No histochemical abnormalities. **B** Inflammatory changes (rounded fibres with increased extracellular fluid and infiltration of white cells) typical of an inflammatory myopathy and also Type II fibre degeneration. The samples were taken from the same normal individual 4 (A) and 12 (B) days after eccentric exercise. On day 4 they had severe delayed-onset muscle pain which disappeared by day 12. ATPase stain at pH 9.4. Original magnification ×100.

INVESTIGATION OF MUSCLE PAIN

Muscle biopsy

This is often the definitive investigation in the management of a patient with myalgia. Percutaneous muscle biopsy is suitable for histological, histochemical, electron microscopic and metabolic characterization (Fig. 22.1). With needle biopsies (Edwards et al 1980) all these procedures may be performed, despite the fact that only a small quantity (100–300 mg) of tissue is obtained. The conchotome technique allows the percutaneous removal of larger tissue samples (Dietrichson et al 1987). These procedures are relatively atraumatic and can be used serially for following progress.

Muscle biopsy can be useful in the diagnosis of inflammatory myopathies with demonstration of muscle cell necrosis and inflammatory cell infiltrate. There is, however, a poor correlation between muscle morphology and myalgia. Where the pain is of neurogenic origin, fibre-type grouping may be found. In the case of metabolic disorders, histochemical staining techniques reveal the absence or reduction of enzymes such as myophosphorylase. Direct measurement can be made of enzymes such as carnitine palmityltransferase and mitochondrial activity.

Muscle biopsy is essential in the analysis of mitochondrial myopathies in which there is a defect in either mitochondrial substrate transport or in electron transport. The defective components of the electron transport chain can be identified on relatively small biopsy samples obtained by needle biopsy (Gohil et al 1981).

Open biopsy is still practised and may have advantages in 'patchy' diseases such as focal polymyositis or in arthritic diseases (e.g., polyarteritis nodosa). In the majority of primary investigations of myalgia we consider it unnecessary and unethical.

Biochemical markers of muscle damage

Myoglobinuria and myoglobinaemia

Myoglobinuria is an important sign of muscle disease and has many causes (Rowland et al 1964). It may be the presenting complaint in a number of conditions with exercise-induced muscle pain or may be a concomitant of severe polymyositis, viral myositis or alcoholic myopathy.

Myoglobin is a muscle protein involved in oxygen storage and transport; when muscle fibres degenerate, myoglobin leaks out into the plasma and is a sufficiently small molecule (molecular weight 17 500) to pass into the urine. This is important to recognize because of the potentially fatal complication of oliguric renal failure due to acute tubular necrosis (Paster et al 1975). Myoglobinuria can also occur in normal individuals after prolonged strenuous exercise, especially when performed at high ambient temperatures (Demos et al 1974). Although patients may report 'muddy' coloured urine after exercise, the pigment may only be detectable by appropriate testing of the urine. Myoglobinaemia may be seen in up to 74% of patients with myositis and may precede the elevation of CK in relapses.

Creatine kinase

CK is the enzyme responsible for catalysing the breakdown and synthesis of phosphoryl creatine and plays a central role in the metabolism of muscle contraction. It is present as three isoenzymes, MM, MB and BB; the MB and BB isoenzymes are not generally found much in normal skeletal muscle. Probably because of the regeneration of immature muscle fibres in various myopathies, all three isoenzymes may occasionally be seen. However, in most muscle diseases the MM isoenzyme, which comprises 95–99% in muscle, is predominantly elevated. It has been suggested that the MB fraction which emanates from heart muscle can be used as an indicator of cardiac involvement in polymyositis. However, this enzyme can be elevated in as many as 28% of patients with polymyositis uncomplicated by cardiac disease.

Leakage of the enzyme into plasma is usually taken as evidence of muscle damage, but this must be seen in perspective because it is known that moderate exercise in normal individuals will cause a rise in CK (Thomson et al 1975, Brooke et al 1979) and that CK is higher in outpatients with a higher level of habitual activity than inpatients (Griffiths 1966). Intramuscular injection and electromyographic investigation are also known to cause a rise in CK.

CK is many times higher than normal in the muscular dystrophies, especially Duchenne dystrophy, and may be elevated in spinal muscular atrophy, motor neurone disease, postpoliomyelitis muscular atrophy, hypothyroidism and toxic muscle damage. In acute rhabdomyolysis, CK can reach very high values and is then associated with myoglobinuria. CK can nevertheless be used as a screening test in painful myopathies of less dramatic onset, because it may be elevated in asymptomatic periods between attacks. In McArdle's disease, for example, CK is usually 5–15 times the upper limit of normal with habitual daily activity, but may rise to 100 times this level during and after a painful cramp or contracture. CK is said to be elevated in myoadenylate deaminase deficiency (Fishbein et al 1978), but is normal between attacks of muscle pain in carnitine palmityltransferase deficiency (Morgan-Hughes 1982). In polymyositis and dermatomyositis CK is usually elevated, but even in acute myositis it may be normal. Only in 3% of patients does the CK remain persistently normal throughout the entire clinical course of polymyositis. It has been reported to be of use in following the course of polymyositis (Bohan & Peter 1975b), rising 5–6 weeks before a relapse and decreasing 3–4 weeks before an improvement in muscle strength. CK is usually normal in polymyalgia rheumatica.

3-Methylhistidine

Myofibrillar protein contains the amino acid 3-methylhistidine; when protein is broken down, this amino acid is not reutilized but is excreted in the urine unchanged and may therefore, if related to the total excretion of creatinine (generally taken as an index of total muscle mass), be used as an indicator of muscle breakdown (McKeran et al 1977). However, although muscle contains the largest amount of 3-methylhistidine, other actin-containing tissues such as skin and gut may turn over 3-methylhistidine much faster and thus there are uncertainties in using 3-methylhistidine excretion as an indicator of muscle breakdown.

Erythrocyte sedimentation rate

Inflammatory myopathies, particularly polymyalgia rheumatica (Panayi 1998), cause a rise in the erythrocyte sedimentation rate (ESR). This simple investigation is useful as a screening test for active disease and in following the progress of treatment.

Magnetic resonance techniques

Spectroscopy

Phosphorus magnetic resonance spectroscopy (MRS) of skeletal muscle enables muscle metabolism to be monitored by the determination of the amount of the phosphocreatine (PCr), inorganic phosphate (Pi) and ATP. Intramuscular pH can also be calculated. It is assumed that the volume sampled equates to the muscle of interest, but this may not be the case where relatively large coils are used over small muscles, as in the forearm, and this is particularly important in exercise studies (Fleckenstein et al 1989a).

Patients with the metabolic disorders of myophosphorylase deficiency (Ross et al 1981, Radda et al 1984) and phosphofructokinase deficiency (Chance et al 1982, Edwards et al 1982a, Cady et al 1985, 1989) usually have normal spectra at rest, as do patients with an alcoholic myopathy (Bollaert et al 1989). Exercise causes unusually large metabolic changes, with the exception of the internal pH in myophosphorylase deficiency which shows no or little change.

Mitochondrial myopathies are associated with excessive changes in pH, Pi and PCr during exercise. Abnormal amounts of these metabolic markers may also be found in unexercised, resting muscle (Gadian et al 1981, Narayana et al 1989, Matthews et al 1991a,b). Similar findings occur in numerous neuromuscular diseases (Barany et al 1989). Patients with peripheral vascular disease (PVD) often show signs of excessive metabolism at rest (Hands et al 1986), as do those with hypothyroidism (Kaminsky et al 1992). In PVD patients the metabolic abnormalities are greater in those with rest pain (Hands et al 1990). Vascular surgery eliminates symptoms and abolishes the metabolic abnormalities (Hands et al 1986).

MRS has failed to detect metabolic abnormality in the tender points of patients with fibromyalgia (De Blecourt et al 1991).

Normal individuals with delayed-onset muscle pain have an unusually high Pi concentration in resting muscle (Aldridge et al 1986, McCully et al 1988). However, this metabolic abnormality precedes the onset of pain. It is also found in some patients with primary muscle diseases (Barany et al 1989) which are not usually painful. This may be a non-specific finding which has no direct relationship with myalgia (Newham & Cady 1990).

Imaging

Magnetic resonance imaging (MRI) techniques have the advantage of allowing tissue visualization which is precise enough for differentiating one tissue from another. Individual muscle groups and also their relative composition of fat and water can be seen, enabling sensitive monitoring of therapies (Fleckenstein et al 1991b). In patients presenting with muscle pain, intramuscular masses (Turner et al 1991), abscesses (Stephenson et al 1991) and anomalous muscles (Paul et al 1991, Sanger et al 1991) have been identified.

Valuable information can be obtained for differential diagnosis and also in cases of referred pain (Chevalier et al 1991, Halpern et al 1997, Stollen 1997). MRI can determine the aetiology of shoulder (Fritz et al 1992) and foot pain (Kier et al 1991) with greater accuracy than either computerized tomographic (CT) arthrography or ultrasonography (Nelson et al 1991) and conventional radiographs (Kier et al 1991). Myositis ossificans circumspecta (pseudomalignant osseous soft-tissue tumour) may be differentiated from malignant neoplasms (Ehara et al 1991). Imaging techniques may be combined with spectroscopy to study tumour site, size and metabolic characteristics (Zlatkin et al 1990).

In patients with an existing diagnosis of primary skeletal muscle disease, the distribution and severity of individual muscle involvement can be determined (Lamminen 1990, Fleckenstein et al 1991b). Exercise testing may reveal further abnormalities (Amendola et al 1990, Fleckenstein et al 1991a).

Traumatic and sports injuries are readily visualized (Fig. 22.2) (Fleckenstein et al 1989b, Greco et al 1991, Farley et al 1992), although the actual level and extent of damage is not always clear. They may be accompanied by haemorrhage (De Smet et al 1990).

As with other investigations, the technique to be used should be chosen with care (Erlemann et al 1990, Greco et al 1991), and both the operator and obesity of the subject may affect accuracy (Nelson et al 1991).

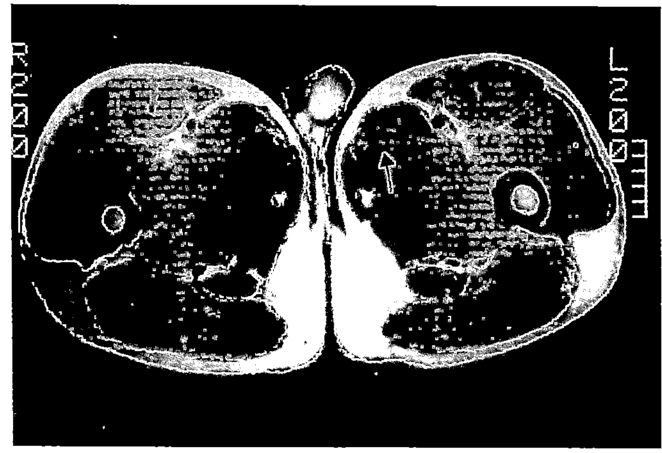

Fig. 22.2 Magnetic resonance image (T2 weighted) from a footballer presenting with pain in the left groin. The image shows a tear with resolving haematoma in the belly of the left adductor longus muscle. (Courtesy of Professor Graham Whitehouse, University Department of Radiodiagnosis and Magnetic Resonance Research Centre, University of Liverpool.)

Radioisotope scanning

This technique also allows the identification of individual muscles, showing abnormal isotopic uptake and the extent and distribution of abnormality in affected muscles (Fig. 22.3). An excessive uptake of radioisotope-labelled complexes into muscle has been shown in a variety of muscle diseases, the majority of which are pain free (Bellina et al 1978, Giraldi et al 1979). It has been suggested that the extent of uptake in patients with polymyositis and dermatomyositis has prognostic value (Buchpiguel et al 1991).

These techniques allow the affected bone and soft tissues to be identified in cases of trauma and sports injuries (Elgazzar et al 1989, Rockett & Freeman 1990, Halpern et al 1997). Muscular involvement may be identified in cases of ischaemic damage (Yip et al 1990, Rivera-Luna & Spiegler 1991) and peripheral vascular disease (Sayman & Urgancioglu 1991).

Increased muscle uptake of isotope has been observed after exercise in normal, pain-free individuals (Matin et al 1983, Valk 1984). When the pectoral muscles are involved there is the possibility of a false diagnosis of exercise-induced left ventricular dysfunction (Campeau et al 1990). Similar findings occur in those with delayed-onset muscle pain (Jones et al 1986, Newham et al 1986b). Serial studies show that the time course of changes in muscle uptake parallel the changes in blood levels of CK (Jones et al 1986, Newham et al 1986b) and both presumably reflect changes in the integrity of the sarcolemma. The mechanism of increased isotope uptake is unclear (for a review see Brill 1981) and it appears that different mechanisms may be involved in different situations.

Exercise testing

The energy supply for muscle contraction is held in essentially three pools:

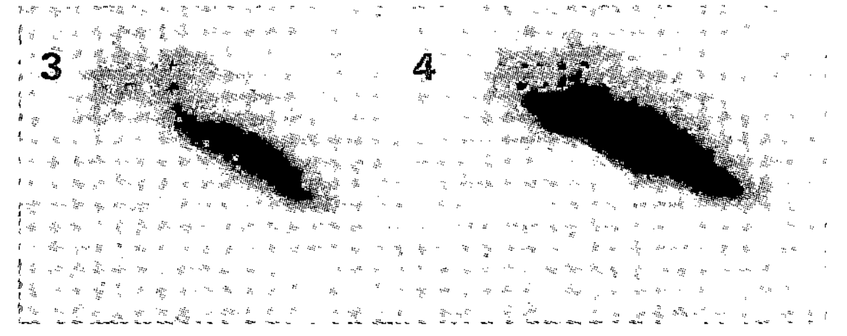

Fig. 22.3 Lateral views of the lower limb showing an abnormal increase of radioisotope (technetium-99m pyrophosphate) uptake in the calf muscles. The scans were taken 3 and 4 days after eccentric exercise by a normal individual, when the muscles were painful. Note greater area of increased uptake on day 4. The biopsy sample taken from the gastrocnemius muscle on day 4 is shown in Figure 22.1A.

1. Creatine phosphate interacts with ADP to reform ATP, which forms an instantly available energy buffer but which can sustain energy supply for only a very short time.
2. Glycogen stores within muscle provide an intermediate energy supply system. Glycogen is a large glucose polymer linked by means of α_{1-4} linkages with α_{1-6} linkages at each branch point. Myophosphorylase cleaves glucose molecules from glycogen which is then degraded to provide ATP, with lactate produced as a by-product. Phosphofructokinase is the controlling enzyme in this metabolic sequence.
3. Long-term energy supply to muscle is provided by carbohydrate and fat. This energy supply is used in long-term, endurance-type exercise. The degree to which carbohydrate oxidation and fat oxidation are used to provide energy depends on the duration of the exercise and the availability of oxygen.

It can be seen that the energy supply to muscle is complex and exercise testing needs to be tailored to test specific aspects of the system.

There is a large literature on the response to exercise of normal individuals and in many disease categories exercise testing may be revealing (Jones et al 1975). The performance of whole-body exercise, such as cycle ergonometry, stresses not only the neuromuscular system but also the cardiovascular and respiratory systems and is of course dependent on the motivation of the subjects. The technique may be useful not only for assessing the overall work fitness of an individual, but it can also provoke symptoms in patients with muscle pain which can then be analysed further. Exercise testing can also be useful in the management of patients, in that they can be reassured that they can perform adequately without producing excessive pain.

Many protocols for progressive exercise tests on a cycle ergometer are available (Jones et al 1975, McArdle et al 1991). The aim is to assess the cardiovascular, respiratory and metabolic responses to exercise; blood pressure, heart rate, ventilation and blood lactate and pyruvate may be measured during and after the exercise. Submaximal exercise tests are usually performed at a work rate that is a fixed proportion of the previously determined maximal rate and continue for a fixed time with regular and frequent monitoring. Exercise testing is useful in patients with muscle pain when a metabolic muscle disease is suspected. In many mitochondrial myopathies (see below) there is a raised resting lactate which rises markedly after moderate exercise.

The prolonged exercise test (Brooke et al 1979) attempts to measure the individual's ability to switch to fatty acid oxidation once glycogen in muscle has been depleted.

Ischaemic forearm exercise tests (McArdle 1951, Munsat 1970, Sinkeler et al 1986) are designed to test the phosphorylase system in muscle. Essentially, a catheter is placed in a superficial vein and, with the arm rendered ischaemic by a cuff, the patient performs hand grips once a second for 1 min. A workload of between 4 and 7 kg is required and blood is sampled at intervals for lactate. In normal subjects, lactate rises to between three and five times the resting level at 3 min. In McArdle's disease and phosphofructokinase deficiency, there is no rise in lactate. The tests should be performed with care because they are invasive and can also produce contractures in myophosphorylase-deficient patients.

Electromyography

Electrical activity can be recorded from muscles, either with surface electrodes or with intramuscular recording needles. With the former, activity from a large volume of tissue can be recorded and this can be useful in the study of abnormalities in the gross pattern of muscle activation (e.g., kinaesiological studies) and in the study of fatigue. The electrical properties of the skin, however, effectively filter out diagnostic information from the muscle signal. For diagnostic purposes, needle electromyography (EMG) is required (Hayward & Willison 1973, Dause 1983, Desmedt 1983). Conventional concentric EMG needles record from a tissue volume of 1 mm radius and therefore sample from a large number of fibres, but only from a small proportion of the fibres belonging to one motor unit. EMG is useful in distinguishing primary muscle diseases from those conditions associated with abnormalities of the anterior horn cell or motor axons. In primary muscle disease, motor unit potentials recorded with a conventional concentric needle electrode consist of brief, small-amplitude potentials. These summate to form a crowded recruitment pattern when the muscle is moderately activated. By contrast, in muscle which has undergone denervation followed by reinnervation, motor unit potentials of high amplitude and broad simple waveform are seen and, even when the muscle is producing its maximal force, they occur as discrete potentials repeating at high rates. In primary muscle disease, motor unit potentials may have maximal amplitude of 0.5–1 mV, whereas in chronic reinnervation due to a neurogenic process, motor unit potentials may be up to 20 mV in amplitude (Mills & Wilson 1987).

Healthy muscle at rest is electrically silent. Spontaneous muscle fibre potentials (fibrillations) are most characteristically seen in acute denervating processes, but may also be seen in muscular dystrophies and inflammatory muscle diseases.

Apart from this major function in distinguishing primary muscle and neurogenic diseases, EMG may also be useful in the investigation of muscle pain in other situations. It can detect myotonia when clinical myotonia is absent, and can distinguish the electrically silent contracture of McArdle's disease from the excessive motor unit activity of a muscle cramp. Combined with nerve conduction studies, EMG can be used to assess the distribution of muscles affected by denervation, and may help to provide information about which nerve or nerve roots are involved. EMG may also be useful in deciding which muscle is active in focal dystonia prior to botulinum toxin injection and can be helpful in selecting the appropriate muscle for biopsy, although clearly the site of needle entry should be avoided.

Measurements of muscle force

The two most common force-related symptoms are weakness and excessive fatigability. The two should be differentiated; weakness is a failure to achieve the expected force, while fatigue is an excessive loss of force generation during or after activity.

Measurements of maximal voluntary force generation, using either strain-gauge systems or dynamometers ranging from simple hand-held devices to expensive dynamic systems, provide information about the presence and distribution of weakness, as well as about longitudinal changes in strength (Edwards 1982, Edwards et al 1980, 1983). Percutaneous electrical stimulation, either through the motor nerve or its intramuscular nerves, can provide useful information about abnormalities in muscle contractile properties, i.e. force : frequency characteristics, relaxation rate and fatigability (Edwards et al 1977).

Patients with both myalgia and weakness are likely to have a specific muscle problem. The distribution may be informative, for example, pain and weakness in the forearm and fingers may simply be a nerve entrapment syndrome, whereas weakness of proximal muscles is often associated with primary muscle disease.

Muscle weakness and wasting are associated with, and may be the main presenting symptom of, both neuropathic and myopathic conditions, the former usually being pain free. Electromyographic studies and clinical examination enable the two to be distinguished. Myopathies are subdivided into the atrophic and destructive forms. Atrophic myopathies may cause muscle pain (hypothyroid, osteomalacia) but others do not (steroid, Cushing's). The destructive myopathies are further subdivided into those of a destructive nature (the muscular dystrophies) and inflammatory (polymyositis and dermatomyositis). In both categories the relationship with pain is very variable and does not appear to correlate well with any findings. When muscular discomfort is reported it is usually described as aching, especially on activity but sometimes at rest, and also as muscle tenderness. Muscle weakness and pain are reported by some, but not all, former victims of poliomyelitis. The underlying mechanism is unclear (Agre et al 1991).

In unilateral conditions the extent of weakness may be estimated by comparison of the muscle strength on the affected and unaffected sides. There is also a substantial body of literature on the strength of a number of muscle groups in healthy individuals in a wide age range.

With measurements of voluntary force there is always the possibility that poor motivation or central fatigue is preventing the generation of the maximal force of the muscle. The superimposition of electrical or magnetic stimulation on a voluntary contraction determines if it is maximal or not (Fig. 22.4) (Belanger & McComas 1981, Rutherford et al 1986, Gandevia et al 1995), because additional force is generated only if the voluntary contraction is submaximal. Furthermore, the true strength of the muscle can be estimated when the voluntary contraction is not maximal (Bigland-Ritchie et al 1986). Interestingly, patients with primary myopathy and myalgia rarely show central fatigue (Rutherford et al 1986). By contrast, mechanical joint damage, which may be completely pain free, is strongly associated with a failure of voluntary activation (Newham et al 1989).

Peripheral fatigue is a failure of force generation despite the muscle being fully activated by either a voluntary or externally stimulated contraction. Undue fatigability of this type is seen without pain in myasthenia gravis and myotonic disorders (Wiles & Edwards 1977, Ricker et al 1978). Fatigability and pain are found in mitochondrial myopathies (De Jesus 1974, Edwards et al 1982b).

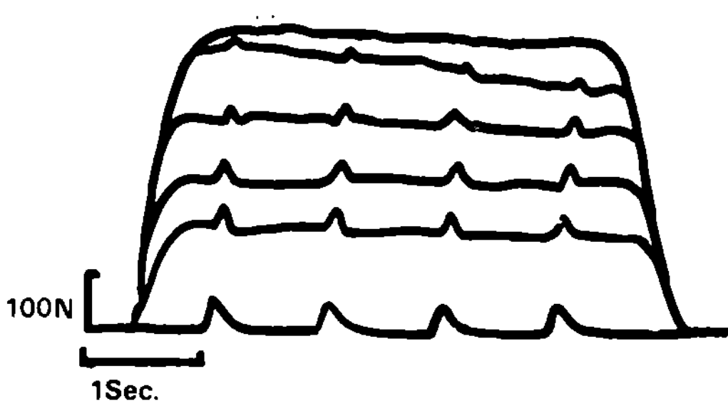

Fig. 22.4 Force traces from human muscle stimulated electrically with single impulses at 1 Hz. The muscle was stimulated at rest and during a series of voluntary contractions at varying forces up to maximum (top trace). Additional force is generated by electrical stimulation only when the voluntary contraction is submaximal and increases in amplitude as the level of voluntary activation decreases.

Using motor nerve stimulation, simultaneous measurements of force and the compound muscle action potential allow the investigation of excitation and activation. These techniques have revealed that the excessive peripheral fatigue in myophosphorylase deficiency is mainly due to a failure of muscle membrane excitation (Wiles et al 1981, Linssen et al 1990).

TREATMENT

Specific drug therapy for a specific disease is rarely attainable and even when the diagnosis is clear, treatment may be either unknown or controversial. In polymyositis, for example, steroid therapy may contribute to the pathological changes by superimposing a steroid myopathy (Edwards et al 1980).

A number of drugs are available for myalgia. Aspirin and many other steroidal and non-steroidal anti-inflammatory drugs (e.g., ibuprofen, flurbiprofen, naproxen, indomethacin) may be used, but no single preparation has been shown to be superior. Diazepam and other benzodiazepines may be effective for muscle 'spasm', as may baclofen or dantrolene sodium, although the latter may impair force generation.

Quinine sulphate has long been used to treat night cramps and those associated with haemodialysis. In the latter case the drug appears to reduce the frequency but not the severity (Kaji et al 1976). Verapamil has helped some patients with exertional muscle pain (Lane et al 1986). A wide range of physical therapies is used, particularly in the case of trauma and sport and traumatic injuries. The repertoire includes ice, transcutaneous nerve stimulation and a variety of electrical treatments. Despite the high incidence of these conditions, the effectiveness of these therapies in any particular situation has rarely been compared (Renstrom 1991). Both immobilization and mobilization are considered important at different stages (Lehto & Jarvinen 1991, Renstrom 1991). Immobilization results in marked muscle atrophy which, although reversible, may delay full rehabilitation (Appell 1990).

Surgical intervention is indicated in cases of severe or complete muscle tears, severe haematomas and compartment syndromes.

Patients with myalgia of unknown aetiology may be offered a variety of treatments as part of behavioural therapy. The elimination of serious underlying pathology may be of reassurance. Those with diffuse myalgia may be profoundly unfit as a result of inactivity and some may have a degree of postural hypotension (Newham & Edwards

1979). A logical approach is to provide a well-supervised exercise programme (Edwards 1986), although the individual response to this is very variable. Most patients with ME report their symptoms to be increased by excessive exercise, although a carefully graded programme may be beneficial.

Dietary supplementation of essential fatty acids in ME (Behan et al 1990) and protein in McArdle's syndrome (Jensen et al 1990) has been reported to improve symptoms.

Occasionally, patients with mitochondrial cytopathies have been reported to respond to vitamins. The best-documented example (Eleff et al 1984) is a patient with complex III deficiency in whom vitamins K3 and C (which might be expected to bypass the metabolic defect) resulted in rapid clinical improvement.

TRAUMA AND SPORTS INJURIES

Direct trauma from many causes ranging from intramuscular injections to sports and severe crush injuries, is an obvious cause of muscle pain. If sufficient muscle tissue is damaged, life is threatened by hypercalcaemia and acute renal failure from myoglobinuria. Sports injuries, from minor muscle sprains to complete rupture (e.g., hamstring rupture), may include direct trauma. They are increasingly common in exercise-conscious cultures (Renstrom 1991, Harries et al 1994, de Lee & Prez 1994).

MUSCLE

Traumatic muscular damage is invariably associated with pain, which may have a gradual or immediate onset. It may also be detected by imaging techniques, blood biochemistry and the immunohistochemical (Fechner et al 1991) and routine histochemical examination of tissue samples as described in this chapter. The combination of damage and immobilization (Appell 1990) results in considerable weakness and wasting, which may only be reversed by relatively long periods of rehabilitation.

In many cases the cause of injury is obvious and associated with a forced lengthening of an active muscle, but spontaneous ruptures of many muscle groups, particularly the hamstrings and pectoralis major (Kretzler & Richardson 1989), occur frequently. Muscle ruptures and tears of limb muscle may mimic a compartment syndrome, while those of the abdominal musculature may cause groin pain. They are commonly associated with muscle spasms, which in turn give rise to additional muscle pain. Myositis ossificans is a potentially disabling complication of muscle trauma which may be confused with a sarcoma (Booth & Westers 1989).

Activity-related compartment syndromes occur in muscle groups within a relatively inextensible fascial sheath, such as the anterior tibial muscles (Vincent 1994). Pain occurs during exercise and increases in intensity as the blood supply to the active tissue is inadequate. Symptoms include pain and cramp-like sensations, very similar to the symptoms of intermittent claudication. They usually disappear at rest but tenderness may persist. Weakness, paralysis and numbness may occur in acute cases, which tend to result in continued symptoms and raised intramuscular pressures at rest (Martens & Moeyersoons 1990).

LIGAMENTS AND TENDONS

There are only subtle morphological differences between these two structures (Oakes 1994). Mature adult ligaments and collagen are composed of large-diameter type I collagen fibrils tightly packed together with smaller type III collagen. These are dispersed in an aqueous gell which contains small amounts of proteoglycans and elastic fibres.

Tendons require greater flexibility and the ability to resist high forces. Ligaments are passive structures which are superior to tendons in their ability to sustain constant tension. Healthy structures are extremely strong, their strength being related to cross-sectional area. Forces of >2000 N are required to disrupt the healthy anterior cruciate ligament of the human knee. However forces of up to 4000 N have been recorded in the Achilles tendon (Komi 1992) and so it is not surprising that injury occurs. Injuries are thought to be caused by both overt trauma and also to repeated, cumulative micro-trauma associated with intense functional use, particularly in structures with a small cross-sectional area. Conversely, immobilization also weakens ligamentous collagen (Amiel et al 1983) as well as bone.

Injuries range in severity from microscopic damage through partial tears to complete ruptures. In addition to soft-tissue injuries, the high forces involved may detach some bone which remains attached to the tendon or ligament. Muscles acting over two joints, such as the hamstrings and rectus femoris, appear to be particularly susceptible. This may be due to the complex neuromuscular control needed for co-contraction and relaxation in muscle groups with opposing actions. The intrinsic cause of these injuries is largely unknown.

Clinically it is extremely difficult to determine the exact location and extent of damage. Pain and tenderness usually accompany such lesions, but localization can be difficult. Palpation always involves the tendon as well as its sheath and muscle contraction will apply force to both. Imaging techniques tend to overestimate the size of a lesion. Depending on the extent of damage, pain may be absent, may occur only on activity or be constant and severe.

Tendon injuries

Many sporting activities stress tendons to a high proportion of their theoretical maximum (Alexander & Vernon 1975). The incidence of tendinitis and rupture tends to increase with changes in the nature or intensity of activity, but often there is no recognizable change in activity.

The musculo-tendinous junction is a common site of failure (Curwin 1994). The last sarcomere of a muscle fibre shows increased folds which are thought to increase surface area and reduce stress at the junction (Oakes 1994). These are probably not reproduced during repair and might explain the frequent occurrence of repeat injuries. Intrinsic causes of the injury remain unknown, but are thought to include inadequate muscle/tendon length (e.g., tight hamstrings), muscle weakness and fatigue.

Repetitive use, combined with overuse and micro-trauma, may cause a progressive attrition of tendon. Spontaneous tendon rupture is uncommon in young people. It usually occurs in association with the age-related degeneration. It is also rare under normal loading in the absence of previous injury or disease (Barfred 1971).

Compressive forces, such as those from the individual's own anatomy or tight shoes, etc, may be an external cause of tendon damage.

Ligament injuries

These have a high incidence, particularly in association with sporting injuries. Sprains of the ankle ligaments, possibly with bone avulsion, are the single most common specific injury (McBride 1994). They may be acute or have a gradual onset. Mechanical joint damage, including ligament injury, appears to be associated with voluntary activation failure (Hurley et al 1994).

Acute knee injuries are one of the most common career-ending events for competitive sports men and women (Johnson 1994) and may involve one or more of the ligaments and menisci. Meniscal damage inevitably results in pain and functional impairment, but a damaged anterior cruciate ligament may mean either normal function or significant symptoms and substantial functional disability.

Injuries to the rotator cuff occurs particularly in those active in sports such as swimming, tennis and baseball (Bowen & Warren 1994). Involved structures could involve the supra- and infra-spinati, teres major and subscapularis muscles and their tendons and joint capsule as well as ligaments (Itio & Tabata 1992). The supraspinatus appears to be highly susceptible to injury, perhaps due to a relatively poor vasculature near the tendon. There is frequently some degree of glenohumeral instability. Pain is poorly localized and may radiate down the affected arm. Night pain is common.

The prognosis for function is poor unless effective treatment is instigated early

Treatment

Ligaments and tendons are poorly vascularized and so tend to heal slowly. Soft-tissue injuries present a challenge for treatment due to the conflicting demands of maintaining or increasing mobility and the requirement of injured tissues for low stress for healing (Curwin 1994). However effective treatment is essential because many injuries will fail to heal spontaneously and chronic conditions tend to develop.

Remodelling and mobilization of connective tissue takes place and can continue for up to a year (Oakes 1994). Scar collagen and adjacent normal collagen matrices may shorten the affected region and small-diameter collagen fibrils are retained instead of the original larger ones. The area is weaker than before and susceptible to repeated injury.

Reduced activity leads to atrophy in collagen as well as muscle tissue, however regenerating fibres cannot tolerate high forces. Once fibrils are strong enough, application of load causes the fibrils to become larger and stronger or to change their material properties to increase strength per unit area (Butler et al 1978). Muscle hypertrophy probably also involves connective tissue.

Trauma frequently results in bleeding into the extravascular space and often needs to be removed. Extravascular blood in itself may increase tissue pressure to the point where increased pressure causes pain and also acts as an irritant, leading to further pressure increases and possibly tissue necrosis.

The basic issue for treatment is whether initially it is to be conservative or surgical. Improved imaging techniques have increased the ability to determine the location and extent of injury (Stoller 1997, Halpern et al 1997). The criteria are usually on symptoms and functional loss. Ruptures involving more than a small proportion of the structure are unlikely to spontaneously reunite with any degree of functional improvement and often lead to chronic conditions.

In general, the approach for the first few days after surgery or injury is with ice, rest and anti-inflammatory agents.

Applied forces are kept to a minimum to avoid further collagen, including that of regenerating fibrils. From about 5 days to 3 weeks gentle movement and stress is introduced to increase collagen regeneration, fibril size and cross-sectional area and prevent the adverse consequences of immobilization and disuse atrophy. From 3 weeks onwards progressive stresses are placed on the tissue to increase cross-linking, size and strength. Physical therapy is widely and intensively used and is thought to be essential for optimal healing and rehabilitation outcome (De Lee & Prez 1994, Harries et al 1994, Sallis & Massimo 1997). A prime goal is to prevent repeated injury, so attention must be paid to possible internal and external contributing factors to the initial injury.

OVERUSE

Great emphasis has been placed on the ability of training to protect against injury in sports (Safran et al 1989). Nevertheless, it is currently accepted that for many athletes overtraining in itself can produce a wide variety of symptoms, both physical and psychological (Fry et al 1991), which are generally poorly understood. Depression of the immune system is associated with overuse in athletes (Shepherd 1998).

There seems to be considerable individual variation in the susceptibility to sports-related injuries, which is little understood and may be caused by a combination of physical and psychological factors (Taimela et al 1990). The syndrome also involves tendons and ligaments (Renstrom 1994). This syndrome affects a wide range of people ranging from elite athletes to sedentary individuals involved in low-intensity, highly repetitive occupations (Simons & Mense 1998). Predisposing factors are thought to be classified as external (intensity, repetition, duration, environmental, clothing, footware, etc.) and internal (anatomical or postural abnormalities, muscle weakness, decreased flexibility and previous disorders). As is usually the case in syndromes which are poorly understood, there is multiple nomenclature, mostly involving words such as repetitive, strain or overuse.

In the last decade there has been a virtual epidemic of these syndromes but optimal treatment or prevention regimens remain unclear. However these are important issues due to the high incidence and the fact that acute pain that persists tends to become chronic and processed differently in the brain (Hsieh et al 1995).

REFERENCES

Abbott BC, Bigland B, Ritchie JM 1952 The physiological cost of negative work. Journal of Physiology 117: 380–390

Agre JC, Rodriquez AA, Tafel JA 1991 Late effects of polio: a critical review of the literature on neuromuscular function. Archives of Physical Medicine and Rehabilitation 72: 923–931

Alexander DS, Vernon P 1975 The dimensions of knee and ankle muscles and the force they exert. Journal of Human Movement Studies 41: 115–123

Aldridge R, Cady EB, Jones DA, Obletter G 1986 Muscle pain after exercise is linked with an inorganic phosphate increase as shown by ^{31}P NMR. Bioscience Reports 6: 663–667

Amendola A, Rorabeck CH, Vellett D, Vezina W, Rutt B, Nott L 1990 The use of magnetic resonance imaging in extertional compartment syndromes. American Journal of Sports Medicine 18: 29–34

Amiel D, Akesan WH, Harwood FL, Frank CB 1983 Stress deprivation effect on metabolic turnover of medial collateral ligament collagen; a comparison between 9 and 12 week immobilisation. Clinical Orthopaedics and Related Research 172: 265–270

Angelini C, Luke S, Cantarutti F 1976 Carnitine deficiency of skeletal muscle: report of a treated case. Neurology 26: 633–637

Appell HJ 1990 Muscular atrophy following immobilisation. A review. Sports Medicine 10: 42–58

Asmussen E 1956 Observations on experimental muscular soreness. Acta Rheumatologica Scandinavica 2: 109–116

Bank WJ, Di Mauro S, Bonilla E, Capuzzi DM, Rowland LP 1975 A disorder of muscle lipid metabolism and myoglobinuria. Absence of carnitine palmityl transferase. New England Journal of Medicine 292: 443–449

Barany M, Siegel IM, Venkatasubrananian PN, Mok E, Wilbur AC 1989 Human leg neuromuscular diseases: P-31 MR spectroscopy. Radiology 172: 503–508

Barfred T 1971 Experimental rupture of Achilles tendon: comparison of various types of experimental rupture in rats. Acta Orthopaedica Scandinavica 42: 528–543

Barrack RL, Skinner HB 1990 Senesory function of knee ligaments. In: Daniel P, Akeson W, O'Connor J (eds) Knee ligaments: sensory function in injury and repair. Raven Press, New York, pp 95–114

Bartels EM, Danneskiold-Samsoe B 1986 Histological abnormalities in muscle from patients with certain types of fibrositis. Lancet 7: 755–757

Barton NJ, Hooper G, Noble J, Steel WM 1992 Occupational causes of disorders in the upper limb. British Medical Journal 304: 309–311

Behan PO, Bakheit AMO 1991 Clinical spectrum of postviral fatigue syndrome. In: Behan PO, Goldberg DP, Mowbray JF (eds) Postviral fatigue syndrome. British Medical Bulletin 47: 793–809

Behan PO, Behan WM, Horrobin D 1990 Effects of high doses of essential fatty acids on the postviral fatigue syndrome. Acta Neurologica Scandinavica 82: 209–216

Behan PO, Goldberg DP, Mowbray JF (eds) 1991 Postviral fatigue syndrome. British Medical Bulletin 47

Belanger AY, McComas AJ 1981 Extent of voluntary unit activation during effort. Journal of Applied Physiology 51: 1131–1135

Bellina CR, Biachi R, Bombardini S et al 1978 Quantitative evaluation of ^{99m}Tc pyrophosphate muscle uptake in patients with inflammatory and non-inflammatory muscle diseases. Journal of Nuclear Medicine 22: 89–96

Bengtsson A 1986 Primary fibromyalgia. A clinical and laboratory study. Linkoping University, dissertation no. 224

Bengtsson A, Henriksson K-G, Jarson J 1986a Muscle biopsy in primary fibromyalgia. Light microscopical and histochemical findings. Scandinavian Journal of Rheumatology 15: 1–6

Bengtsson A, Henriksson K-G, Jarson J 1986b Reduced high energy phosphate levels in painful muscle in patients with primary fibromyalgia. Arthritis and Rheumatism 29: 817–821

Bennett RM 1981 Fibrositis: misnomer for a common rheumatic disorder. Western Journal of Medicine 134: 405–413

Bertorini T, Yeh YY, Trevisan C, Standlan E, Sabesin S, Di Mauro S 1980 Carnitine plamityltransferase deficiency: myoglobinuria and respiratory failure. Neurology 30: 263–271

Bessou P, Laporte Y 1961 Some observations on receptors of the soleus muscle innervated by group III afferent fibers. Journal of Physiology 155: 19P

Bigland-Ritchie B, Jones DA, Hosking GP, Edwards RHT 1978 Central and peripheral fatigue in sustained maximum voluntary contractions of human quadriceps muscle. Clinical Science and Molecular Medicine 54: 609–614

Bigland-Ritchie B, Furbush F, Woods JJ 1986 Neuromuscular transmission and muscular activation in human post-fatigue ischaemia. Journal of Physiology 337: 76P

Bird HA, Esselinck W, Dixon A St J, Mowat AG, Wood PHN 1979 An evaluation of the criteria for polymyalgia rheumatica. Annals of the Rheumatic Diseases 38: 424–439

Bohan A, Peter JB 1975a Polymyositis and dermatomyositis: part 1. New England Journal of Medicine 292: 344–347

Bohan A, Peter JB 1975b Polymyositis and dermatomyositis: part 2. New England Journal of Medicine 292: 402–407

Bollaert PE, Robin-Lherbier B, Escanye JM, et al 1989 Phosphorus nuclear magnetic resonance evidence of abnormal skeletal muscle metabolism in chronic alcoholics. Neurology 39: 821–824

Booth DW, Westers BM 1989 The management of athletes with myositis ossificans traumatica. Canadian Journal of Sport Science 14: 10–16

Bowen MK, Warren RF 1994 Injuries of the rotator cuff. In: Harries M, Williams C, Stanish WD, Micheli LJ (eds) Oxford textbook of sports medicine. Oxford Medical Press, Oxford, pp 442–452

Brill DR 1981 Radionuclide imaging of non-neoplastic soft tissue disorders. Seminars in Nuclear Medicine 11: 277–288

Brooke MH 1986 A clinician's view of neuromuscular diseases, 2nd edn. Williams & Wilkins, Baltimore

Brooke MH, Carroll JE, Hagberg JM 1979 The prolonged exercise test. Neurology 29: 636–643

Brown SJ, Child RB, Day SH, Donnelly A 1997 Indices of skeletal muscle damage and connective tissue breakdown following eccentric muscle contractions. European Journal of Applied Physiology 75: 369–374

Buchpiguel CA, Roizenblatt S, Lucena-Fernandes MF et al 1991 Radioisotopic assessment of peripheral and cardiac muscle involvement and dysfunction in polymyositis/dermatomyositis. Journal of Rheumatology 18: 1359–1363

Bunch TW, Worthington JW, Combs JJ, Ilstrup DM, Engel AG 1980 Azathioprine with prednisone for polymyositis. Annals of Internal Medicine 92: 365–369

Butler DL, Grood ES, Noyes FR, Zernicke RG 1978 Biomechanics of ligaments and tendons. Exercise and Sports Science Reviews 6: 125–182

Cady EB, Griffiths RD, Edwards RHT 1985 The clinical use of nuclear magnetic resonance spectroscopy for studying human muscle metabolism. International Journal of Technological Assessment in Health Care 1: 631–645

Cady EB, Jones DA, Lynn J, Newham DJ 1989 Changes in force and intracellular metabolites during fatigue of human skeletal muscle. Journal of Physiology 418: 311–325

Campeau RJ, Garcia OM, Correa OA, Mace JE 1990 Pectoralis muscle uptake of thallium-201 after arm exercise ergometry. Possible confusion with lung thallium-201 activity. Clinical Nuclear Medicine 15: 303–306

Carpenter S, Karpati G 1981 The major inflammatory myopathies of unknown cause. Pathological Annual 16: 205–237

Carpenter JR, Bunch TW, Angel AG, O'Brien PC 1977 Survival in polymyositis: corticosteroids and risk factors. Journal of Rheumatology 4: 207–214

Carroll JE, De Vivo DC, Brooke MH, Planner GJ, Hagberg JH 1979 Fasting as a provocative test in neuromuscular diseases. Metabolism 28: 683–687

Carroll JE, Brooke MH, De Vivo DC et al 1980 Carnitine 'deficiency': lack of response to carnitine therapy. Neurology 30: 618–626

Chance B, Eleff S, Bank W, Leigh JR, Warnell R 1982 ^{31}P NMR studies of control of mitochondrial function in phosphofructokinase deficient human skeletal muscle. Proceedings of the National Academy of Sciences USA 79: 7714–7718

Chevalier X, Wrona N, Avouac B, Larget B 1991 Thigh pain and multiple osteonecrosis: value of magnetic resonance imaging. Journal of Rheumatology 18: 1627–1630

Chou SM 1988 Viral myositis. In: Mastaglia FL (ed) Inflammatory diseases of muscle, 1st edn. Blackwell, Oxford, pp 125–153

Clarkson PM, Newham DJ 1995 Associations between muscle soreness, damage and fatigue. In: Gandevia SC et al (eds) Fatigue: neural and muscular mechanisms. Advances in Experimental medicine and biology, vol 384. Plenum Press, New York, pp 457–470

Coote JH, Perez-Gonzales JF 1971 The reflex nature of the pressure response to muscular exercise. Journal of Physiology 215: 789–804

Currie S 1981 Inflammatory mypathies. Polymyositis and related disorders. In: Walton JN (ed) Disorders of voluntary muscle, 4th edn. Churchill Livingstone, Edinburgh, pp 525–568

Curtin NA, Davies RE 1973 Chemical and mechanical changes during stretching of activated frog muscle. Cold Spring Harbor Symposia on Quantitative Biology 37: 619–626

Curwin SL 1994 The aetiology and treatment of tendinitis. In: Harries M, Williams C, Stanish W D, Micheli LJ (eds) Oxford textbook of sports medicine. Oxford Medical Press, Oxford, pp 512–528

Dalakas MC (ed) 1988 Polyositis and dermatomyositis, 1st edn. Butterworths, Boston

Daube JR 1983 Disorders of neuromuscular transmission: a review. Archives of Physical Medicine and Rehabilitation 64: 195–200

Dawson J 1990 Consensus on research into fatigue syndrome. British Medical Journal 300: 832

De Blecourt AC, Wolf RF, van Rijswijk MH et al 1991 In vivo ^{31}P magnetic resonance spectroscopy (MRS) of tender points in patients with primary fibromyalgia syndrome. Rheumatology International 1: 51–54

De Jesus PV 1974 Neuromuscular physiology in Luft's syndrome. Electroencephalography and Clinical Neurophysiology 14: 17–27

de Lee JC, Prez D 1994 Orthopaedic sports medicine, vol 11. WB Saunders, Philadelphia

Demos MA, Gitlin EL, Kagen L 1974 Exercise myoglobinuria and acute exertional rhabdomyolysis. Archives of Internal Medicine 134: 669–673

De Smet AA, Fischer DR, Heiner JP, Keene JS 1990 Magnetic resonance imaging of muscle tears. Skeletal Radiology 19: 283–286

Desmedt JE (ed) 1983 Computer aided electromyography. Progress in clinical neurophysiology, vol 10. Karger, Basle

De Vere R, Bradley WG 1975 Polymyositis: its presentation, morbidity and mortality. Brain 98: 637–666

Dietrichson P, Oakley J, Smith PEM, Griffiths RD, Helliwell TR, Edwards RHT 1987 Conchotome and needle percutaneous biopsy of skeletal muscle. Journal of Neurology, Neurosurgery and Psychiatry 50: 1461–1476

Di Mauro S, Di Mauro PM 1973 Muscle carnitine palmityltransferase deficiency and myoglobinuria. Science 182: 929–931

Di Mauro S, Miranda AF, Olarte M, Friedman R, Hays AP 1982 Muscle phosphoglycerate mutase (GAM) deficiency: a new metabolic myopathy. Neurology 32: 584–591

Di Mauro S, Dalakas M, Miranda AF 1983 Phosphoglycerate kinase

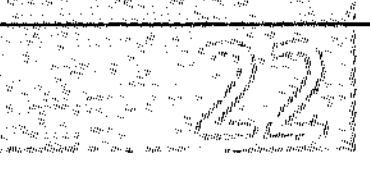

deficiency: another cause of recurrent myoglobinuria. Annals of Neurology 13: 11–19
Douglas JG, Ford MJ, Innes JA, Munro JF 1979 Polymyalgia arteritica: a clinical review. European Journal of Clinical Investigation 9: 137–140
Edwards RHT 1982 Weakness and fatigue of skeletal muscles. In: Sarner M (ed) Advanced medicine 18. Pitman Medical, London, pp 100–119
Edwards RHT 1986 Muscle fatigue and pain. Acta Medica Scandinavica (suppl) 711: 179–188
Edwards RHT, Young A, Hosking GP, Jones DA 1977 Human skeletal muscle function: description of tests and normal values. Clinical Science and Molecular Medicine 52: 283–290
Edwards RHT, Young A, Wiles CM 1980 Needle biopsy of skeletal muscle in diagnosis of myopathy and the clinical study of muscle function and repair. New England Journal of Medicine 302: 261–271
Edwards RHT, Isenberg DA, Wiles CM, Young A, Snaith ML 1981 The investigation of inflammatory myopathy. Journal of the Royal College of Physicians 15: 19–24
Edwards RHT, Dawson MJ, Wilkie DR, Gordon RE, Shaw D 1982a Clinical use of nuclear magnetic resonance in the investigation of myopathy. Lancet i: 725–731
Edwards RHT, Wiles CM, Gohil K, Krywawych S, Jones DA 1982b Energy metabolism in human myopathy. In: Schotland DC (ed) Disorders of the motor unti. Wiley, London, pp 715–728
Edwards RHT, Wiles CM, Mills KR 1983 Quantitation of human muscle function. In: Dyck P, Thomas PK, Lambert EH (eds) Peripheral neuropathy. WB Saunders, Philadelphia, pp 1093–1102
Edwards RHT, Newham DJ, Peters TJ 1991 Muscle biochemistry and pathophysiology in postiviral fatigue syndrome. In: Behan PO, Goldberg DP, Mowbray JF (eds) Postviral fatigue syndrome. British Medical Bulletin 47: 826–837
Ehara S, Nakasato T, Tamakawa Y et al 1991 MRI of myositis ossificans circumscripta. Clinical Imaging 15: 130–134
Eleff S, Kennaway NG, Buist NRM et al 1984 ^{31}P-NMR studies of improvement of oxidative phosphorylation by vitamins K3 and C in a patient with a defect in electron transport and complex III in skeletal muscle. Proceedings of the National Academy of Sciences USA 81: 3529–3533
Elgazzar AH, Malki AA, Abdel-Dayem HM et al 1989 Indium-111 monoclonal anti-myosin antibody in assessing skeletal muscle damage in trauma. Nuclear Medicine Communications 10: 661–667
Engel AG, Sieckert RG 1972 Lipid storage myopathy responsive to prednisone. Archives of Neurology 27: 174–181
Erlemann R, Vassallo P, Bongartz G et al 1990 Musculoskeletal neoplasm: fast low-angle shot MR imaging with and without Gd-DTPA. Radiology 176: 489–495
Farley TE, Neumann CH, Steinbach LS, Jahnke AJ, Petersen SS 1992 Full-thickness tears of the rotator cuff of the shoulder: diagnosis with MR imaging. American Journal of Roentgenology 158: 347–351
Fechner G, Hauser R, Sepulchre MA, Brinkman B 1991 Immunohistochemical investigations to demonstrate vital direct damage of skeletal muscle. International Journal of Legal Medicine 104: 215–219
Fishbein WN, Armbrustmacher KW, Griffin JL 1978 Myoadenylate deaminase deficiency: a new disease of muscle. Science 200: 545–548
Fleckenstein JL, Bertocci LA, Nunnally RL, Parkey RW, Peshock RM 1989a Exercise-enhanced MR imaging of variations in forearm muscle anatomy and use; importance in MR spectroscopy. American Journal of Roentgenology 153: 693–698
Fleckenstein JL, Weatherall PT, Parkey RW, Payne JA, Peshock RM 1989b Sports-related muscle injuries: evaluation with MR imaging. Radiology 172: 793–798
Fleckenstein JL, Haller RG, Lewis SF et al 1991a Absence of exercise-induced MRI enhancement of skeletal muscle in McArdle's disease. Journal of Applied Physiology 71: 961–969
Fleckenstein JL, Weatherall PT, Bertocci LA et al 1991b Locomotor system assessment by muscle magnetic resonance imaging. Magnetic Resonance Quarterly 7: 79–103
Freeman MAR, Wyke BD 1967 The innervation of the knee joint. An anatomical and histological study in the cat. Journal of Anatomy 101: 505–532
Friden J 1984 Muscle soreness after exercise: implications of morphological changes. International Journal of Sports Medicine 5: 57–66
Friden J, Sfakianos PN, Hargens AR 1986 Delayed muscle soreness and intramuscular fluid pressure: comparison between eccentric and concentric load. Journal of Applied Physiology 61: 2175–2179
Fritz RC, Helms CA, Steinbach LS, Genant KK 1992 Suprascapular nerve entrapment: evaluation with MR imaging. Radiology 182: 437–444
Fry HJH 1986 Overuse syndrome of the upper limb in musicians. Medical Journal of Australia 144: 182–185
Fry RW, Morton AR, Keast D 1991 Overtraining in athletes. An update. Sports Medicine 12: 32–65
Gadian DG, Radda GK, Ross BD et al 1981 Examinations of a myopathy by phosphorus nuclear magnetic resonance. Lancet ii: 774–775
Gandevia SC, Allen GM, McKenzie DK 1995 Central fatigue: critical issues, quantification and practical issues. In: Gandevia SC et al (eds) Fatigue: neural and muscular mechanisms. Advances in experimental medicine and biology, vol 384. Plenum Press, New York, pp 281–294
Giraldi C, Marciani G, Molla N, Rossi B 1979 ^{99m}Tc-pyrophosphate muscle uptake in four subjects with Becker's disease. Journal of Nuclear Medicine 23: 45–47
Gohil K, Jones DA, Edwards RHT 1981 Analysis of muscle mitochondrial function with techniques applicable to needle biopsy samples. Clinical Physiology 1: 195–207
Gordon EE, Januszko DM, Kaufman L 1967 A critical survey of stiff-man syndrome. American Journal of Medicine 42: 582–599
Gould SE (ed) 1970 Trichinosis in man and animals. CC Thomas, Springfield, Illinois, pp 147–189
Greco A, McNamara MT, Escher RM, Trifilio G, Parienti J 1991 Spin-echo and STIR imaging of sports related injuries at 1.5 T. Journal of Computer Assisted Tomography 15: 994–999
Griffiths PD 1966 Serum levels of ATP and creatine phosphotranferase (creatine kinase). The normal range and effect of muscular activity. Clinica Chimica Acta 13: 413–420
Halpern B, Herring SA, Altchelk D, Herzog R (eds) 1997 Imaging in muscle and sports medicine. Blackwell Science, Malden, MA
Hamrin B 1972 Polymyalgia rheumatica. Acta Medica Scandinavica (suppl) 553: 1–131
Hands CJ, Bone PJ, Galloway G, Morris PJ, Radda GK 1986 Muscle metabolism in patients with peripheral vascular disease investigated by ^{31}P nuclear magnetic resonance spectroscopy. Clinical Science 71: 283–290
Hands LJ, Sharif MH, Payne GS, Morris PJ, Radda GK 1990 Muscle ischaemia in peripheral vascular disease studied by ^{31}P-magnetic resonance spectroscopy. European Journal of Vascular Surgery 4: 637–642
Harries M, Williams C, Stanish WD, Micheli LJ (eds) 1994 Oxford textbook of sports medicine. Oxford Medical Press, Oxford
Haslock DI, Wright V, Harriman DGF 1970 Neuromuscular disorders in rheumatoid arthritis. A motor-point muscle biopsy study. Quarterly Journal of Medicine 39: 335–358
Hayes DJ, Lecky BRF, Landon DN, Morgan-Hughes JA, Clark JB 1984 A new mitochondrial myopathy: biochemical studies revealing a deficiency in the cytochrome b–c1 complex (complex III) of the respiratory chain. Brain 107: 1165–1177

Hayward M, Willison RG 1973 The recognition of myogenic and neurogenic lesions by quantitative EMG. In: Desmedt JE (ed) New developments in electromyography and clinical neurophysiology, vol 2. Karger, Basle, pp 448–453

Hazelman B 1998 Soft tissue rheumatology. In: Maddison PJ, Isenberg DA, Woo P, Glass D (eds) The Oxford textbook of rheumatology, 2nd edn. Oxford Medical Press, Oxford, pp 1489–1514

Headley SA, Newham DJ, Jones DA 1986 The effect of prednisolone on exercise induced muscle pain and damage. Clinical Science 70: 85P

Hsieh JC, Beifrage M, Stone-Elander P, Hansson P, Ingvar M 1995 Central representation of chronic ongoing neuropathic pain studied by positron emission tomography. Pain 63: 224–236

Holt IJ, Harding AE, Cooper JM et al 1989 Mitochrondrial myopathies: clinical and biochemical features of 30 patients with major deletions of muscle mitochondrial DNA. Annals of Neurology 29: 600–608

Hudson J, Brown WF, Gilbert JJ 1978 The muscular pain–fasciculation syndrome. Neurology 28: 1105–1109

Hurley MV, Jones DW, Newham DJ 1994 Arthrogenic quadriceps inhibition and rehabilitation of patients with traumatic knee injury. Clinical Science 86: 305–310

Iggo A 1961 Non-myelinated afferent fibers from mammalian skeletal muscle. Journal of Physiology 155: 52–53P

Ionasescu V, Hug G, Hoppel C 1980 Combined partial deficiency of muscle carnitine palmityltransferase and carnitine with autosomal dominant inheritance. Journal of Neurology, Neurosurgery and Psychiatry 43: 679–682

Isaacs H 1961 A syndrome of continuous muscle fibre activity. Journal of Neurology, Neurosurgery and Psychiatry 24: 319–325

Itoi E, Tabata S 1992 Conservative treatment of rotator cuff tears. Clinical Orthopaedics 275: 165–173

Janssen E, Kuipers H, Venstrappen FTJ, Costill DL 1983 Influence of an anti-inflammatory drug on muscle soreness. Medicine and Science in Sports and Exercise 15: 165

Jeffrey HC 1974 Sarcosporidosis in man. Transactions of the Royal Society of Tropical Medicine and Hygiene 68: 17–29

Jensen KE, Jakobsen J, Thomsen C, Henriksen O 1990 Improved energy kinetics following high protien diet in McArdle's syndrome. A ^{31}P magnetic resonance spectroscopy study. Acta Neurologica Scandinavica 81: 499–503

Johnson RL 1994 Acute knee injuries. In: Harries M, Williams C, Stanish WD, Micheli LJ (eds) Oxford textbook of sports medicine. Oxford Medical Press, Oxford, pp 350–363

Jones DA, Newham DJ, Round JM, Tolfree SEJ 1986 Experimental human muscle damage: morphological changes in relation to other indices of damage. Journal of Physiology 375: 435–448

Jones NL, Campbell EJM, Edwards RHT, Robertson DG 1975 Clinical exercise testing. WB Saunders, Philadelphia

Kaji DM, Ackad A, Nottage WG, Stein RM 1976 Prevention of muscle cramps on haemodialysis patients by quinine sulphate. Lancet ii: 66–67

Kalia M, Serapati BP, Panda A 1972 Reflex increase in ventilation by muscle receptors with non-modulated fibers (C-fibers). Journal of Applied Physiology 32: 189–193

Kaminsky P, Robin Lherbier B, Brunotte F, Escanye JM, Walker P 1992 Energetic metabolism in hypothyroid skeletal muscle, as studied by phosphorus magnetic resonance spectroscopy. Journal of Clinical Endocrinology and Metabolism 74: 124–129

Kanno T, Sudo K, Takeuchi I et al 1980 Hereditary deficiency of lactate dehydrogenase M subunit. Clinica Chimica Acta 108: 267–276

Karpati G, Carpenter S, Engel A et al 1975 The syndrome of systemic carnitine deficiency. Neurology 25: 16–24

Katz B 1939 The relation between force and speed in muscular contraction. Journal of Physiology 96: 46–64

Kier R, McCarthy S, Dietz MJ, Rudicel S 1991 MR appearance of painful conditions of the ankle. Radiographics 11: 401–414

Kniffki KD, Mense S, Schmidt RF 1978 Response of group IV afferent units from skeletal muscle to stretch, contraction and chemical stimulation. Experimental Brain Research 31: 511–522

Knighton RS, Dumke PR 1966 Pain. Little Brown, Boston

Komi PV 1992 Strength-shortening cycle. In: Komi PV (ed) Strength and power in sport. Blackwell Scientific, Oxford, pp 169–179

Kretzler HH Jr, Richardson AB 1989 Rupture of the pectoralis major muscle. American Journal of Sports Medicine 17: 453–458

Kuipers H, Kieren HA, Venstrappen FTJ, Costill DL 1983 Influence of a prostaglandin inhibiting drug on muscle soreness after eccentric work. Journal of Sports Medicine 6: 336–339

Kumazawa T, Mizumura K 1977 Thin fibre receptors responding to mechanical, chemical and thermal stimulation in the skeletal muscle of the dog. Journal of Physiology 273: 179–194

Lamminen AE 1990 Magnetic resonance imaging of primary skeletal diseases: patterns of distribution and severity of involvement. British Journal of Radiology 63: 946–950

Land JM, Clark JB 1979 Mitochondrial myopathies. Biochemical Society Transactions 7: 231–245

Lane RJM, Mastaglia FL 1978 Drug-induced myopathies in man. Lancet ii: 562–566

Lane RJM, Turnbull DM, Welch JL, Walton J 1986 A double blind placebo controlled cross-over study of verapamil on exertional muscle pain. Muscle and Nerve 9: 635–641

Layzer RB 1986 Muscle pain, cramps and fatigue. In: Engel AG (ed) Myology, 1st edn. McGraw-Hill, New York, pp 1907–1922

Layzer RB 1994 Muscle pain, cramps and fatigue. In: Engel AG, Franzini-Armstrong C (eds) Myology, vol 2, 2nd edn. McGraw-Hill, New York, pp 1754–1768

Layzer RB, Rowland LP 1971 Cramps. New England Journal of Medicine 285: 31–40

Layzer RB, Rowland LP, Ranney HM 1967 Muscle phosphofructokinase activity. Archives of Neurology 17: 512–523

Lavigne GJ, Velly-Miguel AM, Montplaisir J 1991 Muscle pain, dyskinesia and sleep. Canadian Journal of Physiology and Pharmacology 69: 678–682

Lazaro RP, Rollinson RD, Fenichez GM 1981 Familial cramps and muscle pain. Archives of Neurology 38: 22–24

Lehto MU, Jarvinen MJ 1991 Muscle injuries, their healing processes and treatment. Annales Chirurgiae et Gynaecologiae 80: 102–108

Lendinger MI, Sjogaard G 1991 Potassium regulation during exercise and recovery. Sports Medicine 11: 382–401

Linssen WH, Jacobs M, Stegman DF, Joosten EM, Moleman J 1990 Muscle fatigue in McArdle's disease. Muscle fibre conduction velocity and surface EMG frequency spectrum during ischaemic exercise. Brain 113: 1779–1793

Lloyd AR, Gandevia SC, Hales JP 1991 Muscle performance, voluntary activation, twitch properties and perceived effort in normal subjects and patients with the chronic fatigue syndrome. Brain 114: 85–98

Lotz BP, Enger AG, Nishino H, St Evens JC, Litchy WJ 1989 Inclusion body myositis. Observations on 40 cases. Brain 122: 727–747

McArdle B 1951 Myopathy due to a defect in muscle glycogen breakdown. Clinical Science 10: 13–33

McArdle WD, Katch FI, Katch VL 1991 Exercise physiology: Energy, nutrition and human performance. Lea and Febiger, Philadelphia

McBride AM 1994 The acute ankle sprain. In: Harries M, Williams C, Stanish WD, Micheli LJ (eds) Oxford textbook of sports medicine. Oxford Medical Press, Oxford, pp 471–482

McCloskey DI, Mitchell JH 1972 Reflex cardiovascular and respiratory responses originating in exercising muscle. Journal of Physiology 224: 173–186

McCully KK, Argov Z, Boden BA, Brown RL, Blank WJ, Chance B 1988 Detection of muscle injury in humans with ^{31}P magnetic resonance spectroscopy. Muscle and Nerve 11: 212–216

McKeran RO, Halliday D, Purkiss D 1977 Increased myofibrillar protein catabolism in Duchenne muscular dystrophy measured by 3-methylhistidine excretion in the urine. Journal of Neurology, Neurosurgery and Psychiatry 40: 979–981

McLain RF, Weinstein JN 1994 Orthopaedic surgery. In: Wall PD, Melzack R (eds) Textbook of pain, 3rd edn. Churchill Livingstone, Edinburgh, pp 1095–1112

McMahon S, Koltzenburg M 1990 The changing role of afferent neurones in pain. Pain 43: 269–272

Martens MA, Moeyerssoons JP 1990 Acute and recurrent effort-related compartment syndrome in sports. Sports Medicine 9: 62–68

Mastaglia FL (ed) 1988 Inflammatory diseases of muscle, 1st edn. Blackwell, Oxford

Matthews PM, Allaire C, Shoubridge EA, Karpati G, Carpenter S, Arnold DL 1991a In vivo muscle magnetic resonance spectroscopy in the clinical investigation of mitochondrial disease. Neurology 41: 114–120

Matthews PM, Berkovic SF, Shoubridge EA, et al 1991b In vivo magnetic resonance spectroscopy of brain and muscle in a type of mitochondrial encephalomyopathy (MERRF). Annals of Neurology 29: 435–438

Marinacci AA 1965 Electromyography in the diagnosis of polymyositis. Electromyography 5: 255–268

Matin P, Lang G, Ganetta R, Simon G 1983 Scintiographic evaluation of muscle damage following extreme exercise. Journal of Nuclear Medicine 24: 308–311

Menard MR, Penn AM, Lee JE, Dusik LA, Hall LD 1991 Relative metabolic efficiency of concentric and eccentric exercise determined by 31P magnetic resonance spectroscopy. Archives of Physical Medicine and Rehabilitation 72: 976–983

Mense S 1977 Nervous outflow from skeletal muscle during chemical noxious stimulation. Journal of Physiology 267: 75–88

Mense S 1982 Reduction of the bradykinin induced activation of feline group III and IV muscle receptors by acetylsalicylic acid. Journal of Physiology 376: 269–283

Mense S, Schmidt RF 1977 Muscle pain: which receptors are responsible for the transmission of noxious stimuli? In: Clifford Rose F (ed) Physiological aspects of clinical neurology. Blackwell, Oxford, pp 265–278

Middleton PJ, Alexander RM, Szymanski MT 1970 Severe myositis during recovery from influenza. Lancet ii: 532

Mills KR, Edwards RHT 1983 Investigative strategies for muscle pain. Journal of the Neurological Sciences 58: 73–88

Mills KR, Willison RG 1987 Quantification of EMG on volition. In: The London Symposia (electroencephalography and clinical neurophysiology, suppl 39). Elsevier, Amsterdam, pp 27–32

Mills KR, Newham DJ, Edwards RHT 1982a Force, contraction frequency and energy metabolism as interactive determinants of ischaemic muscle pain. Pain 14: 149–154

Mills KR, Newham DJ, Edwards RHT 1982b Severe muscle cramps relieved by transcutaneous nerve stimulation. Journal of Neurology, Neurosurgery and Psychiatry 45: 539–542

Millward DJ, Bates PC, Grimble GK, Brown JG, Nathan M, Rennie MJ 1980 Quantitative importance of non-skeletal muscle sources of NT methylhistidine in urine. Biochemical Journal 190: 225–228

Moersch FP, Woltman HW 1956 Progressive fluctuating muscular rigidity and spasm ('stiff man' syndrome): report of a case and some observations in 13 other cases. Proceedings of the Staff Meetings of the Mayo Clinic 31: 421–427

Mommaerts WFHM, Illingworth B, Pearson CM, Guillory RJ, Seraydarian K 1959 A functional disorder of phosphorylase. Proceedings of the National Academy of Sciences USA 45: 791–797

Morgan-Hughes JA 1982 Defects of the energy pathways of skeletal muscle. In: Matthews WB, Glaser GH (eds) Recent advances in clinical neurology 3. Churchill Livingstone, Edinburgh, pp 1–46

Morgan-Hughes JA, Darveniza P, Landon DN, Land JM, Clark JD 1979 A mitochondrial myopathy characterised by a deficiency of reducible cytochrome B. Brain 100: 617–640

Morgan-Hughes JM, Cooper JM, Schapira AHV, Hayes DJ, Clark JB 1987 The mitochondrial myopathies. Defects of the mitochondrial respiratory chain and oxidative phosphorylation system. In: Ellingson JR, Murray NMF, Halliday AM (eds) The London Symposia (electroencephalography and clinical neurophysiology, suppl 39). Elsevier, Amsterdam, pp 103–114

Munsat TL 1970 A standardised forearm ischaemic test. Neurology 20: 1171–1178

Narayana PA, Slopis JM, Jackson EF, Jazle JD, Kulkarni MV, Butler IJ 1989 In vivo muscle magnetic resonance spectroscopy in a family with mitochondrial cytopathy. A defect in fat metabolism. Magnetic Resonance Imaging 7: 33–39

Nelson MC, Leather GP, Nirschl RP, Pettrone FA, Freedman MT 1991 Evaluation of the painful shoulder. A prospective comparison of magnetic resonance imaging, computerized tomographic arthrography, ultrasonography and operative findings. Journal of Bone and Joint Surgery 73A: 707–716

Newham DJ 1988 The consequences of eccentric contractions and their relation to delayed onset muscle pain. European Journal of Applied Physiology 57: 353–359

Newham DJ, Cady EB 1990 A ^{31}P study of fatigue and metabolism in human skeletal muscle with voluntary, intermittent contractions at different forces. NMR in Biomedicine 3: 211–219

Newham DJ, Edwards RHT 1979 Effort syndromes. Physiotherapy 65: 52–56

Newham DJ, Jones DA 1985 Intramuscular pressure in the painful human biceps. Clinical Science 69: 27P

Newham DJ, Jones DA, Edwards RHT 1983a Large and delayed plasma creatine kinase changes after stepping exercise. Muscle and Nerve 6: 36–41

Newham DJ, McPhail G, Mills KR, Edwards RHT 1983b Ultrastructural changes after concentric and eccentric contractions. Journal of Neurological Science 61: 109–122

Newham DJ, Mills KR, Quigley BM, Edwards RHT 1983c Pain and fatigue after eccentric contractions. Clinical Science 64: 55–62

Newham DJ, Jones DA, Edwards 1986a Plasma creatine changes after eccentric and concentric contractions. Muscle and Nerve 9: 59–63

Newham DJ, Jones DA, Tolfree SEJ, Edwards RHT 1986b Skeletal muscle damage: a study of isotope uptake enzyme efflux and pain after stepping exercise. European Journal of Applied Physiology 55: 106–112

Newham DJ, Hurley MV, Jones DW 1989 Ligamentous knee injuries and muscle inhibition. Journal of Orthopaedic Rheumatology 2: 163–173

Newsom-Davies JM, Mills KR 1992 Immunological associations in acquired neuromyotonia (Isaacs' syndrome): report of 5 cases and literature review. Brain 116: 453–469

Oakes B 1994 Tendons and ligaments – basic science. In: Harries M, Williams C, Stanish WD, Micheli LJ (eds) Oxford textbook of sports medicine. Oxford Medical Press, Oxford, pp 493–511

Pachman LM 1998 Polymyositis and dermatomyositis in children. In: Maddison PJ, Isenberg DA, Woo P, Glass D (eds) The Oxford textbook of rheumatology, 2nd edn. Oxford Medical Press, Oxford, pp 1287–1300

Paintal AS 1960 Functional analysis of group III and IV afferent fibers of mammalian muscle. Journal of Physiology 152: 250–270

Panayi GS 1998 Polymyalgia rheumatica. In: Maddison PJ, Isenberg DA, Woo P, Glass D (eds) The Oxford textbook of rheumatology, 2nd edn. Oxford Medical Press, Oxford, pp 1373–1381

Park SR, Rodbard S 1962 Effects of load and duration of tension on pain induced by muscular tension. American Journal of Physiology 203: 735–738

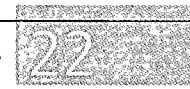

Paster SB, Adams DI, Hollenberg NK 1975 Acute renal failure in McArdle's disease and myoglobinuric states. Radiology 114: 567–570

Paul MA, Imanse J, Golding RP, Koomen AR, Meijer S 1991 Accessory soleus muscle mimicking a soft tissue tumour. Acta Orthopaedica Scandinavica 62: 609–611

Pearson CM, Bohan A 1977 The spectrum of polymyositis and dermatomyositis. Medical Clinics of North America 61: 349–357

Perkoff GT, Hardy P, Velez-Garcia E 1966 Reversible acute muscular syndrome in chronic alcoholism. New England Journal of Medicine 274: 1277–1285

Pernow BB, Havel RJ, Jennings DB 1967 The second wind phenomenon in McArdle's syndrome. Acta Medica Scandinavica (suppl) 472: 294–307

Petty RKH, Harding AE, Morgan-Hughes JA 1986 The clinical features of mitochondrial myopathy. Brain 109: 915–938

Pope FM 1998 Molecular abnormalities of collagen and connective tissue. In: Maddison PJ, Isenberg DA, Woo P, Glass D (eds) The Oxford textbook of rheumatology, 2nd edn. Oxford Medical Press, Oxford, pp 353–404

Prasher D, Smith A, Findley L 1990 Sensory and cognitive event-related potentials in myalgic encephalomyelitis. Journal of Neurology, Neurosurgery and Psychiatry 53: 247–253

Radda GK, Bone PJ, Rajagoplan B 1984 Clinical aspects of 31P NMR spectroscopy. British Medical Bulletin 40: 155–159

Renstrom P 1991 Sports traumatology today. A review of common sports injury problems. Annales Chirugiae et Gynaecologiae 80: 81–93

Renstrom PAFH 1994 Introduction to chronic overuse injuries. In: Harries M, Williams C, Stanish WD, Micheli LJ (eds) Oxford textbook of sports medicine. Oxford Medical Press, Oxford, pp 531–545

Ricker K, Haass A, Hertel G, Mertens HG 1978 Transient muscular weakness in severe recessive myotonia congenita. Journal of Neurology 218: 253–262

Riddoch J, Morgan-Hughes JA 1975 Prognosis in adult polymyositis. Journal of the Neurological Sciences 26: 71–80

Rivera-Luna H, Spiegler EJ 1991 Incidental rectus abdominis muscle visualization during bone scanning. Clinical Nuclear Medicine 16: 523–527

Rockett JF, Freeman BL 1990 3D scintigraphic demonstration of pectineus muscle avulsion injury. Clinical Nuclear Medicine 15: 800–803

Rodbard S, Pragay EB 1968 Contraction frequency, blood supply and muscle pain. Journal of Applied Physiology 24: 142–145

Ross BD, Radda GK, Gadian DG, Rolker G, Esiri M, Falloner-Smith J 1981 Examination of a case of suspected McArdle's syndrome with ^{31}P nuclear magnetic resonance. New England Journal of Medicine 304: 1338–1342

Rowland LP, Tahn S, Hirschberg E, Harter DH 1964 Myoglobinuria. Archives of Neurology 10: 537–562

Rutherford OM, White J 1991 Human quadriceps strength and fatigability in patients with post-viral syndrome. Journal of Neurology, Neurosurgery and Psychiatry 54: 961–964

Rutherford OM, Jones DA, Newham DJ 1986 Clinical and experimental application of the switch superimposition technique for the study of human muscle activation. Journal of Neurology, Neurosurgery and Psychiatry 49: 1288–1291

Safran MR, Seaber AV, Garrett WE Jr 1989 Warm-up and muscular injury prevention. An update. Sports Medicine 8: 239–249

Sallis RE, Massimo F (eds) 1997 ACSM's essentials of sports medicine. Mosby, London

Sanger JR, Krasniak CL, Matloub HS, Yousif NJ, Kneeland JB 1991 Diagnosis of an anomalous superficialis muscle in the palm by magnetic resonance imaging. Journal of Hand Surgery (America) 16: 98–101

Sayman HB, Urgancioglu I 1991 Muscle perfusion with technetium-MIBI in lower extremity peripheral arterial diseases. Journal of Nuclear Medicine 32: 1700–1703

Schiable HG, Grubb BD 1993 Afferent and spinal mechanisms of joint pain. Pain 55: 5–54

Schmid R, Mahler R 1959 Chronic progressive myopathy with myoglobinuria: demonstration of a glycogenolytic defect in muscle. Journal of Clinical Investigation 38: 2044–2058

Schmid R, Hammaker L, 1961 Hereditary absence of muscle phosphorylase (McArdle's syndrome). New England Journal of Medicine 264: 223–225

Schmidt RF, Schiable HG, Melinger K, Heeppelmann B, Hanesch U, Pawlak M 1994 Silent and active nociceptors: structure, function and clinical implications. In: Gebhart GF, Hammond DL, Jensen TS (eds) Proceedings of the 7th World Congress of Pain. Progress in pain research and management, Vol 2. IASP, Seattle, pp 213–250

Schwartz MS, Swash M, Gross M 1978 Benign post-infection polymyositis. British Medical Journal 2: 1256–1257

Serratrice G, Gastaut JL, Schiand A, Pellissier JF, Carrelet P 1980 A propos de 210 cas de myalgies diffuses. Semaine des Hopitaux de Paris 56: 1241–1244

Shepherd JRL 1998 Acute and chronic over exercise: do depressed immune responses provide useful markers? Internation Journal of Sports Medicine 19: 59–171

Sherrington CS 1900 Cutaneous sensations. In: Schäfer's textbook of physiology, vol 2. YJ Pentland, London, pp 920–1001

Shumate JB, Katnik R, Ruiz M et al 1979 Myoadenylate deaminase deficiency. Muscle and Nerve 2: 213–216

Simons DG, Mense S 1998 Understanding of muscle tone as related to clinical muscle pain. Pain 75: 1–17

Sinkeler SP, Wevers RA, Joosten EM et al 1986 Improvement of screening of exertional myalgia with a standardised ischaemic forearm test. Muscle and Nerve 9: 731–737

Smith R, Stern G 1967 Myopathy, osteomalacia and hyperparathyroidism. Brain 90: 593–602

Stacey MJ 1969 Free nerve endings in skeletal muscle of the cat. Journal of Anatomy 105: 231–254

Stälberg E 1980 Macro EMG, a new recording technique. Journal of Neurology, Neurosurgery and Psychiatry 43: 475–482

Stauber W 1989 Eccentric action of muscles: physiology, injury and adaptation. In: Pandolf KB (ed) Exercise and sports sciences reviews, vol 17. Williams & Wilkins, Baltimore, pp 157–186

Stephenson CA, Seibert JJ, Golladay ES et al 1991 Abscess of the iliopsoas muscle diagnosed by magnetic resonance imaging and ultrasonography. Southern Medical Journal 84: 509–511

Stokes M, Cooper R, Edwards RHT 1988 Normal strength and fatigability in patients with effort syndrome. British Medical Journal 297: 1014–1018

Stollen DW 1997 Magnetic resonance in orthopaedic and sports medicine. Lippincott, Philadelphia

Stout AP 1946 Rhabdomyosarcoma of the skeletal muscles. Annals of Surgery 123: 447–472

Sylven C, Jonzon B, Fredholm BB, Kaijser L 1988 Adenosine injection into the brachial artery produces ischaemia-like pain or discomfort in the forearm. Cardiovascular Research 22: 674–678

Taimela S, Kujala UM, Osterman K 1990 Intrinsic risk factors and athletic injuries. Sports Medicine 9: 205–215

Targoff IN 1998 Polymyositis and dermatomyositis in adults. In: Maddison PJ, Isenberg DA, Woo P, Glass D (eds) The Oxford textbook of rheumatology, 2nd edn. Oxford Medical Press, Oxford, pp 1249–1286

Tarui S, Okuno G, Ikura Y, Tanaka T, Suda M, Nishikawa M 1965 Phosphofructokinase deficiency in skeletal muscle: a new type of glycogenosis. Biochemical and Biophysical Research Communications 19: 517–523

Taylor JF, Fluck D, Fluck D 1976 Tropical myositis: ultrastructural studies. Journal of Clinical Pathology 29: 1081–1084

Thomson WHS, Sweetin JC, Hamilton IJD 1975 ATP and muscle enzyme efflux after physical exertion. Clinica Chimica Acta 59: 241–245

Travell JG, Simons DG 1998 Myofascial pain and dysfunction. The Trigger Point Manual, 2nd edn. Williams & Wilkins, Baltimore, MD

Tsokos GC, Moutsopoulos HM, Steinberg AD 1981 Muscle involvement in systemic lupus erythematosus. Journal of the American Medical Association 246: 766–768

Turner RM, Peck WW, Prietto C 1991 MR of soft tissue chloroma in a patient presenting with left pubic and hip pain. Journal of Computer Assisted Tomography 15: 700–702

Valk P 1984 Muscle localisation of Tc 99m MDP after exertion. Clinics in Nuclear Medicine 9: 492–494

Vincent NE 1994 Compartment syndromes. In: Harries M, Williams C, Stanish WD, Micheli LJ (eds) Oxford textbook of sports medicine. Oxford Medical Press, Oxford, pp 564–568

Wessley S 1990 Old wine in new bottles: neurasthenia and ME. Psychological Medicine 20: 35–53

Wessely S, Newham DJ 1993 Virus syndromes and chronic fatigue. In: Vaeroy H, Merskey H (eds) Pain research and clinical management, vol 6. Progress in fibromyalgia and myofascial pain. Elsevier, Amsterdam, pp 349–360

Wessley S, Powell R 1989 Fatigue syndromes: a comparison of postviral fatigue with neuromuscular and affective disorders. Journal of Neurology, Neurosurgery and Psychiatry 52: 940–948

Wiles CM, Edwards RHT 1977 Weakness in myotonic syndromes. Lancet ii: 598–601

Wiles CM, Jones DA, Edwards RHT 1981 Fatigue in human metabolic myopathy. In: Porter R, Whelan J (eds) Human muscle fatigue: physiological mechanisms. Ciba Foundation Symposium 82. Pitman, London, pp 264–282

Willison RG 1971 Quantitative electromyography. In: Licht S (ed) Electrodiagnosis and electromyography, 3rd edn. Elizabeth Licht, New Haven, CN, pp 390–411

Willner J, Di Mauro S, Eastwood A, Hays A, Roohi R, Lovelace R 1979 Muscle carnitine deficiency: genetic heterogeneity. Journal of the Neurological Sciences 41: 235–246

Wirth WA, Farrow CC 1961 Human sparganosis. Case report and review of the subject. Journal of the American Medical Association 177: 6–9

Wood GC, Bentall RP, Gopfert M, Edwards RHT 1991 A comparative psychiatric assessment of patients with chronic fatigue syndrome and muscle disease. Psychological Medicine 21: 619–628

Yip TC, Houle S, Hayes G, Forrest I, Nelson L, Walker PM 1990 Quantitation of skeletal muscle necrosis using ^{99}Tc pyrophosphate with SPECT in a canine model. Nuclear Medicine Communications 11: 143–149

Zimmermann M 1988 Physiological mechanisms of pain in the musculoskeletal system. In: Emre M, Mathies H (eds) Muscle spasms and pain. Parthenon Publishing, Carnforth, pp 7–17

Zlatkin MB, Leninski RE, Shinkwin M et al 1990 Combined MR imaging and spectroscopy of bone and soft tissue tumours. Journal of Computer Assisted Tomography 14: 1–10

Chronic back pain

23

DONLIN M. LONG

INTRODUCTION

Chronic back pain, often with associated leg pain, is the most common medical complaint in developed countries (Bigos et al 1994). Headache is its only peer (Lawrence 1977). Costs associated with back pain are enormous (Kelsey 1982). While it is doubtful that any of the cost estimates currently available are entirely accurate, they all emphasize that direct and indirect costs of this disabling complaint are huge (Frymoyer & Cats-Baril 1991). A complaint of back pain is the most common reason for early social security disability in the USA. The disability issues are so important that several countries and many organizations have convened to examine the problem (Damkot et al 1984, Anderson 1996, Riihimaki 1985). Back pain is one of the most common reasons why patients see physicians, one of the most common reasons for secondary referral, and both operative and non-operative treatment of back pain ranks high in terms of total expenditures of healthcare dollars in the USA (Moeri et al 1899, Bush et al 1992, Davis 1994).

In spite of the obvious importance of back pain as a complaint, the problem is poorly understood and few treatments have been validated (Bigos et al 1994). One of the major issues is the lack of an appropriate classification system. Back pain is simply a complaint which originates in a large heterogeneous spectrum of diseases. Another major issue is that the actual pathophysiological causes of complaints are unknown (Kuslich et al 1991). Even when the complaints can be associated with definable diseases, what is causing the back pain is unclear (Boden et al 1990a, Jonsson & Stromqvist 1993). There is reasonable evidence that overt instability causes pain and elimination of that instability will reduce pain (Cholewicki & McGill 1996). The strongest evidence is that root compression is associated with pain and neurological deficit (Saal & Saal 1989, Saal et al 1990, Weber 1994). Decompression is a satisfactory treatment for a majority of patients (Bohannon & Gajdosik 1987). However, these two conditions are relatively rare in the spectrum of patients with back and/or leg pain complaints, and for the majority the association of complaints with demonstrated structural abnormalities is tenuous at best (Saal & Saal 1989, Weber 1994).

It is not surprising that therapies are problematical in a condition without known causes of pain (Bell & Rothman 1984, Basmajian 1989). Much research will be required to examine the unanswered questions in low back pain in a rational way. Until there is a better scientific basis for understanding back pain and its treatment, we must use what is known to decide upon the best current therapy for these patients. All too often speciality bias is substituted for rational treatment (Evans 1930, Brown 1960, Goebert et al 1960, Harley 1967, Kim & Sadove 1975, Heyse-Moore 1978, Berman et al 1984, Postacchini et al 1988, Hsieh et al 1992, Koes et al 1992a,b, Shekelle et al 1992, Bowman et al 1993, Pope et al 1994, Weber 1994, Meade et al 1995, Triano et al 1995).

In order to reach supportable decisions concerning the evaluation and treatment of these patients, the physician involved in their care must have an organized classification framework in which to work (Box 23.1). Knowing what the various diagnostic tests available can be expected to demonstrate is important. A rigorous evaluation of claims of therapeutic efficacy for all modalities of treatment is required. It is also important to have an equally rigorous understanding of outcomes measurement to assess these claims (Wiesel et al 1980).

BOX 23.1

Temporal classification of low back pain with or without sciatica

Transient
Self-limited; duration is hours to days; comes to medical attention when episodic

Acute
Self limited, but protracted; duration is days to weeks; often seen by physicians; treatment is symptomatic; most recover spontaneously; evaluation and treatment required for severe symptoms

Persistent
Lasts more than 3–6 months; does not relent with time; high correlation with spondylotic disease; no psychological co-morbidities; surgical intervention occurs mostly in this group

Chronic (pain syndrome)
Lasts more than 6 months; worsens with time; associated with major co-morbidities, especially psychological. Multidisciplinary therapy is commonly required

The goal of this chapter is to provide the framework for the evaluation, diagnosis, treatment, choice and assessment of treatment outcome for patients complaining of chronic low back pain with or without sciatica.

CLASSIFICATION OF THE COMPLAINT OF LOW BACK PAIN

The most practical classification yet devised describes low back pain in terms of temporal characteristics. While incomplete, this classification is useful because so much of low back pain is still idiopathic (Bigos et al 1994). *Transient* low back pain typically lasts for a very short period of time and does not come to medical attention, except by history later. Treatment is usually symptomatic and instituted by the patient. The causes are virtually never known and the problem does not have great significance for practice or disability.

Acute low back pain is generally defined as pain which lasts from a few days to a few months. Back pain with or without leg radiation is common. Experience and some evidence says that the majority of these problems are self limited and resolve spontaneously. Standard treatments have little influence upon the natural history. Typical treatment algorithims include short periods of bedrest, adequate analgesia, local physical measures and watchful waiting. Some patients, particularly those with acute disc herniation, have intractable pain which cannot be allowed to resolve spontaneously because of its severity. Rarely, a significant neurological deficit may accompany pain. Both situations usually lead to prompt surgical intervention (Bigos et al 1994).

PERSISTENT LOW BACK PAIN

Most commonly it is assumed that pain which persists for 6 months progressively leads to the chronic state, defined by preoccupation with pain, depression, anxiety and disability. In the recent past, a large group of patients has been identified in whom pain persists for more than 6 months without any concomitants of the chronic pain syndrome. Ninety-five per cent of patients seen demonstrated complaints of pain and dysfunction which reduced, but did not seriously affect, all activities otherwise. Psychological testing in these patients revealed patterns similar to those expected in any ill normal population. There was a 5% incidence of psychological dysfunction in the overall group. We have termed this constellation the *persistent pain syndrome* to differentiate it from the implications of the word chronic in the pain field. The majority of these patients suffered from spondylotic disease. There was no significant worsening or improvement with longitudinal evaluation and these patients did not respond to typical modalities of therapy employed for them.

THE CHRONIC PAIN SYNDROME

For the past 20 years, there has been general agreement about the symptoms and signs which define a group of patients who chronically complain of pain (Waddell et al 1980). Virtually irrespective of the cause of the pain, these patients present with similar complaints and findings. They are preoccupied with pain and pain is the cause of their impairment. A very high percentage are depressed and anxious. There is an unusually high incidence of psychiatric diagnoses among them. An even larger number have features consistent with personality disorder. Drug misuse is common, although addictive behaviour is relatively rare. These patients use medical resources heavily and are consistently disabled from pain. Specialized treatment facilities have been developed throughout the world to deal with them. Patients with low back pain and leg pain complaints who fall into this category do not seem to have different anatomical diagnoses than those patients in the persistent pain syndrome who do not exhibit the co-morbidities of the chronic pain patient.

EVALUATION OF BACK AND LEG PAIN

The evaluation should begin with a careful history which describes the pain severity, location and influences (Deyo et al 1992). Back pain only is unlikely to be associated with root compression (Hakelius & Hindmarsh 1972a). When only radicular pain is present, instability will not be a problem. Physical examination is unlikely to be diagnostic but will assess neurological and musculoskeletal abnormalities. Posture and range of motion are helpful (Heliovaara 1987). Routine neurological examination is needed as a baseline at least. Vascular examination is important (Hurme et al 1983).

During these examinations, listen for the danger signals such as night pain (intraspinal tumour), constant pain (cancer or infection), systemic symptoms (cancer or infection) and symptoms of other organ or systemic disease.

Also, observe the patient's behaviour during the examination. Is there much pain behaviour? Are actions consistent with complaints? Is motor examination reliable (Hurme et al 1987, McCombe et al 1989)?

Unlike the acute pain problems, imaging is important in the chronic patients. Plain films with flexion/extension are important. Magnetic resonance imaging (MRI) is best for most screening. Computed tomography (CT) can be used if bony pathology is suspected: with 2–3D reconstructions fixator artefacts can be reduced. CT myelogram is needed rarely, most commonly in patients with previous surgery (Hakelius & Hindmarsh 1972b, Wiesel et al 1984, Boden et al 1990b, Deyo et al 1994).

There is no need for psychological testing unless symptoms suggestive of psychiatric disturbance are present. If concerned, carry out a thorough evaluation of the DSM-designated factors rather than relying on screening tests (Waddell et al 1980).

CAUSES OF CHRONIC BACK AND LEG PAIN (BOX 23.2)

Another way to categorize patients with chronic back and leg pain is to list the causes. The prevalence is hard to determine for any of these conditions because reported series are always biased by referral patterns and adequate population studies have not been done. However, most experts agree that the preponderance of these patients have spondylotic disease which is at least associated with the pain problem, if not proven to be causative yet (Spangfort 1972, Weber 1983, Waddell 1987a).

BOX 23.2

Causes of chronic back and leg pain

1. As a symptom of intercurrent disease
Bony tumour or spinal cord tumour
Lumbar metastases
Lumbar spinal infection
Retroperitoneal inflammation
Renal disease
Aortic aneurysm
Endometriosis
Abdominal or pelvic cancer

2. Osteoporosis
Secondary to compression fracture
Osseous pain (?)

3. Spondylitis
Rheumatoid arthritis
Ankylosis spondylitis
Psoriatic arthritis
Acromegalic spondylitis

4. Myofascial-ligamentous pain
Myofascial-pain syndrome
Associated with HIV/AIDS

5. Pain as a symptom of psychiatric disease
Depression
Somatiform disorder
Schizophrenia
Personality disorder
State-anxiety
Early dementia

6. Hip disease

7. Peripheral nerve entrapment
Pyriformis syndrome
Pudenal syndrome
Meralgia paraesthetica

8. Congenital spinal anomalies
Transverse facets
Spondylolysis
Myelomeningocele – forme frustes
Sacral cysts – usually with Marfan's syndrome or Ehlers–Danlos syndrome

9. Sacral abnormalities
Tumour (chordoma)
Fracture (osteoporosis)
Sacroiliac joint disease

BACK AND LEG PAIN AS A MANIFESTATION OF UNEXPECTED OR INTERCURRENT DISEASE

In our own series of patients, an unexpected systemic disease was found in only 3% of patients. All had symptoms or signs which suggested something other than common spondylotic disease. Osseous metastases are the most common. Retroperitoneal inflammatory processes, sometimes associated with chronic gastrointestinal disease, pancreatitis, chronic and acute renal disease all may cause back pain rarely. The clues that these do not represent spondylotic disease are usually obvious, although differentiation may occasionally be obscure. The pain from any of these processes is usually local. Leg radiation may occur secondary to lumbosacral plexus involvement, but is rarely typically sciatic. These pains are constant, tend not to be exacerbated by activity or relieved by rest, and are often associated with other signs or symptoms of systemic disease. Leg pain is non-radicular, as are the physical findings associated with infiltration of the plexus. Signs and symptoms which suggest intercurrent disease are intractable pain, unremitting pain, neurological deficit suggestive of lumbosacral plexus involvement, a history of cancer or inflammatory disease, a history of any disease likely to be complicated by infection and a history of significant trauma.

Evaluation of patients with any of these should include plain spine films and MRI for diagnosis. Treatment will depend upon the cause of the presenting symptoms.

Osteoporosis

There is still an argument about whether osteoporosis alone can cause back pain (Bigos et al 1994). Many experts in spinal pain believe it can. However, the most common cause of intractable pain with osteoporosis is compression fracture. Pain with compression fracture is local and extremely severe. If the collapse is great enough, then individual nerve root compression signs and symptoms may occur. However, typically the pain does not radiate, it is focal in the back, and can be localized with great accuracy over the collapsed segment. Those at risk include postmenopausal women, and anyone with other disorders of calcium and oestrogen metabolism, heavy smokers, prolonged steroid users and any patient with prolonged immunosuppression. The diagnosis is made by plain X-ray. Treatment usually consists of rest, external support, limitation of activity and time with therapy for the underlying problem. The pain often persists for 6 months or more following compression fracture.

Recently, vertebroplasty has been introduced (Fig. 23.1). In this procedure, the acutely compressed segment is visualized with fluoroscopy. A needle is placed through the pedicle into the vertebral body and methyl methacrylate is injected to reinforce the collapse. Pain relief is usually immediate and may be very gratifying. The procedure is much more effective when applied early, rather than in the chronic phase of pain.

Spondylitis

The most common inflammatory condition to be associated with chronic back pain is *rheumatoid arthritis* (Lawrence 1977). Back pain is usually not an early characteristic of the disease, so the diagnosis is known when back pain occurs. If systemic manifestations are not prominent, it can be difficult to be certain about the diagnosis on clinical grounds. Plain films, CT, and MRI all suggest inflammatory spondylotic disease. The diagnosis is confirmed by serological testing. Treatment consists of three phases. The first is treatment of the underlying disease. The second is an exercise programme for lifelong maintenance of axial muscle strength. The third is surgical therapy for spinal instability or root compression syndromes. The majority of rheumatoid spinal problems requiring surgery are cervical, but spinal stenosis in the lumbar region does occur. The syndrome is typical neurogenic claudication. Surgery requires decompression and frequently fusion.

The second common problem is *ankylosing spondylitis* (Lawrence 1977). This is a disease of males predominantly. Symptoms usually begin with back pain early in life and a progressive history of constant back pain is typical. Radicular or cord compression symptoms are uncommon. The diagnosis is made by the typical 'bamboo spine' appearance on plain X-ray or MRI. Treatment is typically symptomatic. As spontaneous fusion progresses up the spine, pain relents in the lumbar region, only to reappear at higher levels progressively.

Psoriatic arthritis is a rare similar disease (Lawrence 1977). The problem is more facet arthropathy with synovial proliferation (Liu et al 1990, Xu et al 1990). Thus in psoriatic arthritis, root compression syndromes are common and spinal stenosis is typical. Back pain alone is best treated symptomatically. Surgical decompression and occasional stabilization is required for root compression syndromes.

Acromegalic spondylitis is common in untreated patients. Fortunately, with the quality of therapy now available for these pituitary tumours, this problem has become very rare. The syndrome is similar to ankylosing spondylitis, with progressive pain usually beginning in the lumbar region and which ceases with spontaneous fusion. Treatment is symptomatic.

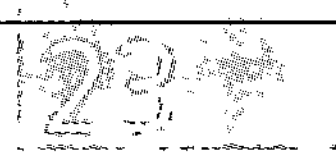

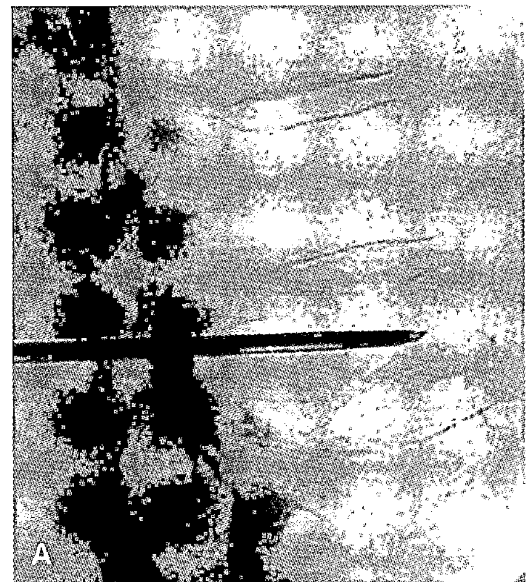

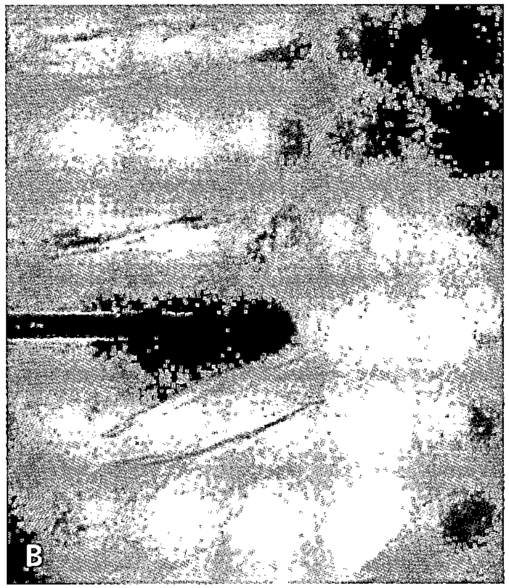

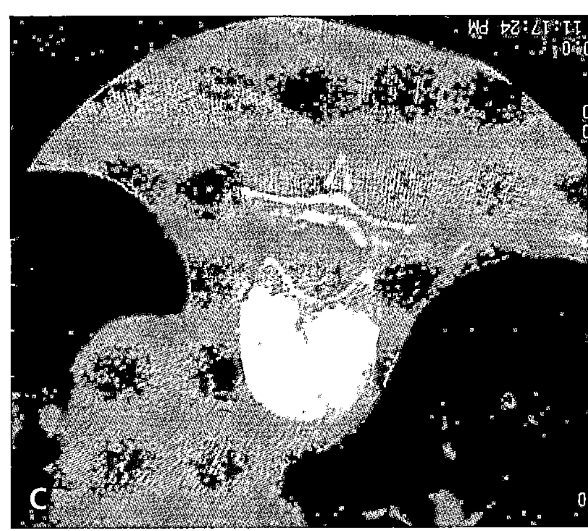

Fig. 23.1 Vertebroplasty. **A** The thoracic compression fracture with a transpedicular needle in the vertebro body. **B** The injection of methacrylate into the body as seen under fluoroscopy. **C** The finished product after bilateral transpedicular injection. The body is now filled with methacrylate and strength is restored. Pain relief was immediate.

MUSCULOSKELETAL PAIN SYNDROMES

There are a group of people with idiopathic back and leg pain for whom no correlated underlying abnormality can be found (Lawrence 1977). Most complain of muscular tenderness and pain (Kalimo et al 1989). Most have associated spasm and focal tenderness, with loss of range of motion. There are no associated neurological signs. The back pain is typically local, but radiates diffusely upward and diffusely into the hips and upper thighs (Macintosh & Bogduk 1987). The problem may be isolated to the lumbar spine or be a part of the larger syndrome called **'myofascial pain'** (Mense 1991). Diagnosis is made by history and through the non-specific physical findings which typically are loss of range of motion, local pain and tenderness in muscles or at muscular insertions and the presence of focal areas of myositis (Panjabi et al 1982). Imaging studies typically are normal or have non-diagnostic spondylotic abnormalities. Treatment consists of anti-inflammatories, local passive therapy measures for focal areas of abnormality, and a long-term exercise programme (Bell & Rothman 1984, Basmajian 1989, Bigos et al 1994).

There is much debate concerning the basis for these symptoms. Some experts believe that this is an inflammatory disease and eventually will become as well defined as rheumatoid arthritis. Others believe that these symptoms are non-specific and have no underlying unifying diagnosis. Still others suggest that these symptoms are largely psychosomatic and frequently are a part of somatization. Currently available data do not allow a precise definition of this symptom complex. Symptomatic therapy is all that is available now. It does appear that the co-morbidities associated with the chronic pain syndrome appear with uncommon frequency in patients with these diffuse myofascial complaints. As in all such patients, these co-morbidities should be defined carefully and treated individually (Waddell et al 1980, 1987a).

The myofascial pain syndrome generates one of the controversial treatment programmes in the chronic back pain field. These are patients who undergo prolonged courses of multiple injections of the so-called trigger points. Sometimes these trigger points are not treated by direct injection, but acupuncture and various forms of other local direct treatments are employed repetitively as the areas of tenderness in muscle are identified. As yet, there are no controlled studies demonstrating the value of local measures for these specific areas of tenderness. Most clinicians expert in the management of back pain recognize that the occasional local treatment of these foci of pain and tenderness is beneficial. The controversial issue occurs when these treatments are both multiple and prolonged. As an adjunct to a vigorous general rehabilitation programme, many of these local measures appear to have value. There is little or no convincing evidence that they are useful as independent prolonged treatment plans.

ABDOMINAL AND PELVIC DISEASE CAUSING LOW BACK PAIN

It is rare for abdominal, pelvic or hip disease to mimic spondylotic or idiopathic low back pain, but a few specific diseases are important. The most common is likely to be metastatic disease to the lumbar spine which can be diagnosed with appropriate imaging. Retroperitoneal inflammatory disease or cancer are other definable causes. Chronic pelvic inflammatory disease and endometriosis both produce low back pain and leg pain. Aortic aneurysm may produce chronic back pain associated with vascular claudication, although dissection is usually an acutely painful event. Intra-abdominal disease of other organs is so rarely confused with idiopathic chronic back pain that any are unlikely to be important in diagnosis. Renal, gallbladder and bowel disease are so commonly associated with other symptoms that confusion in diagnosis is unlikely to occur.

BACK PAIN AS A MANIFESTATION OF PSYCHIATRIC DISEASE

There is a strong tendency among physicians and many others involved in the treatment of chronic pain to assume that all pain for which no diagnosable cause can be found is psychosomatic. Nowhere where is this more true than with chronic back pain. The National Low Back Pain Study data indicates that the incidence of psychopathology is no greater in back pain patients than would be expected in any ill population. Three per cent of patients in that study had a psychiatric diagnosis which was thought by the examiners to be the primary cause of the complaint. However, in a population of more than 2000 patients admitted to a pain treatment programme for manifestations of the chronic pain syndrome, the incidence of psychopathology was much higher. Between 15 and 20% of these patients had a primary psychiatric diagnosis which was thought to be the origin of the pain complaint or at least an important mediator. Endogenous depression was the most common diagnosis. The psychiatrists involved with these patients separated this diagnosis from the reactive depression seen much more commonly. Somatiform disorder was the next most common diagnosis made, followed by schizophrenia. There is an important difference of opinion among pain specialists about what is the most common diagnosis in some experiences, personality disorder. Some experts find an increased incidence of diagnosable personality disorder among patients with chronic pain syndrome. Others note the increased frequency of symptoms suggestive of personality disorder without a truly diagnosable syndrome by DSM criteria. Often, there is imprecise separation of psychosocial symptoms which follow an acute pain event and those which are present antecedent to the noxious event. Then, there is the added factor that the presence of a psychiatric diagnosis or these personality traits does not eliminate the possibility of a bona fide painful problem with the back. This chapter is not the place for an exhaustive review of these psychological factors. In this context, it is only important to emphasize that psychiatric disease may have pain as an important symptom. The presence of psychiatric disease does not eliminate the probability that the patient has a diagnosable separate cause. The presence of traits suggestive of personality disorder cannot be construed as causative of the complaint of back pain. However, the increased incidence of co-morbidities which will be discussed under the heading of chronic pain syndrome in patients with these traits is important therapy (Waddell et al 1980).

It is much more likely that symptoms in patients with idiopathic low back pain are ascribed to psychosomatic causes than for patients with symptoms secondary to psychiatric disease to be misdiagnosed as organic problems. In typical patients with chronic back pain, psychological issues are uncommon. Even in the so-called chronic pain syndrome, overt psychiatric disease is unusual. The psychosomatic side of disability compensation is poorly defined at present, but may be more important than in the general population. The chicken–egg issue of psychiatric symptoms in chronic pain syndrome is not yet settled and deserves further investigation.

SPONDYLOTIC LOW BACK PAIN (IDIOPATHIC) (FIG. 23.2, BOX 23.3)

The majority of patients who present complaining of low back pain with or without leg pain, have associated spondylotic spinal disease. These spondylotic changes may be defined as the primary loss of hydration of lumbar discs with subsequent change in signal characteristics and associated ligament thickening, chronic inflammatory changes in ligaments and adjacent endplates, loss of disc height, facet arthropathy and hypertophy with or without associated canal and foraminal stenosis, or evidence of instability. The presence of spondylosis and the complaints are at least correlated, but the correlation is far from certain (Boden et al 1990a, Weber 1994). Even if the relationship is causative, the mechanisms by which the pain is produced are largely unknown. The diagnostic problem is that a substantial number of patients have spondylotic changes without any apparent related symptoms. Most of the studies that document this observation are limited in scope and only indicate that the patient is not having problems at that time or that back problems are not the predominant issue at the time. Careful population studies with detailed histories outlining past and present history for these patients have not been done. Nevertheless, virtually every physician has had the experience of seeing a patient with profound spondylotic changes who has no complaints currently and has never had complaints. These observations make the correlation of back pain with spondylotic changes difficult and more evidence is needed than the simple occurrence of spondylosis to prove causation. Nevertheless, in a sizeable majority of patients with chronic back pain complaints, spondylotic changes are present and are the only abnormalities which seem to explain the pain. The history of the problem is the most important diagnostic tool. Patients with pain of apparent spondylitic origin characteristically have more pain when standing or load bearing. The symptoms are improved by rest in most. A minority are worsened by reclining, although this is usually limited to reclining in extension. Non-steroidal analgesics are of limited use and pain is temporarily relieved by simple local modalities such as heat and massage. The pain is local in the lumbar region and the patient often can precisely identify an origin with a fingertip. Severe back pain is often associated with non-radicular leg pain, usually diffuse and aching in the anterior or posterior thighs. Associated true radicular pain is common, as is neurogenic claudication. Nearly all patients have pain worsened by activity and improved by rest. The pain is usually best in the morning and worsens with activity in contradistinction to osteoarthritis and the other spondylitic problems.

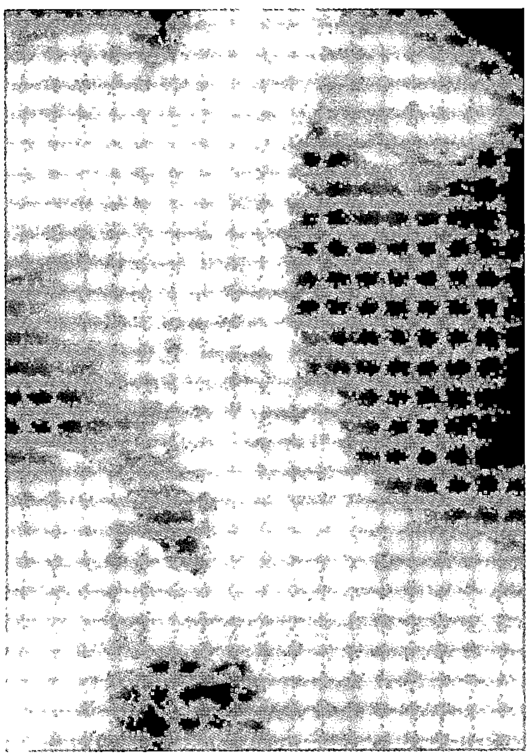

Fig. 23.2 Anteroposterior plain radiograph of lumbar spine demonstrating dramatic kyphoscoliosis involving lumbar vertebrae 1–4 and the lower thoracic spine. These structural deformities are often associated with severe pain and respond well to surgical correction.

BOX 23.3

Back pain syndromes commonly associated with spondylosis

1. Diffuse spondylotic disc degeneration
2. Focal spondylotic disc degeneration
3. Facet arthropathy
4. Facet arthropathy with synovial root compression
5. Canal stenosis (lateral recess)
6. Foraminal stenosis
7. Degenerative spondylolisthesis
8. Compression fractures
9. Loss of lordotic curve (flat back Syndrome)
10. Progressive deformity of spine:
    - Scoliosis
    - Kyphosis
    - Rotoscoliosis
    - Angular deformity

Diagnosis

Diagnosis is made with plain X-ray (Fig. 23.3), CT or MRI, all of which demonstrate different characteristics of the disease (Hakelius & Hindmarsh 1972a). The earliest changes are dissication of the disc. The nucleus loses its definitive character and the disc narrows, becomes irregular and loses water. First acute and then chronic inflammatory changes occur in the surrounding bone of the endplate and beyond. Discs erode the endplates and interosseous herniation occurs. There is associated ligamentous thickening, anterior and posterior disc bulges occur, and traction spurs appear anteriorly or posteriorly. The canal may narrow and degenerative changes in facets are typical. Canal narrowing is a combination of facet overgrowth, synovial hypertrophy, ligamentous thickening and bony enlargement (Annertz et al 1990).

Treatment

Surgical procedures are of value only for the relief of demonstrated nerve root compression, the correction of a fixed deformity or stabilizing an unstable segment (Spangfort 1972, Weber 1983, Hurme & Alaranta 1987). Patients who do not demonstrate any of these abnormalities are not likely to be benefited by surgical procedures. Pain-associated spondylosis alone does not constitute a reason for surgery. The selection of patients for surgery will be discussed in greater detail under the specific headings for which surgery is a reasonable choice. For the majority of patients, no direct intervention is likely to be of value. Therapy is symptomatic (Bell & Rothman 1984). For patients whose symptoms have been present for 6 months or longer, there is strong new evidence that spontaneous improvement will not occur. The evidence is equally good that the usual conservative measures, as they are applied in a typical practice, are not useful and cannot be differentiated from no treatment. Our studies have examined many forms of standard physical therapy, manipulation therapy and a wide variety of other treatments, including acupuncture, back schools, nutritional therapies, pain treatment centres and cognitive therapies. We were unable to determine any effect of any of these treatments as currently applied in practice. Therefore, it will not suffice to simply refer patients for any of these treatments. A programme based on the best available data should be individualized for each patient (Waddell 1987a).

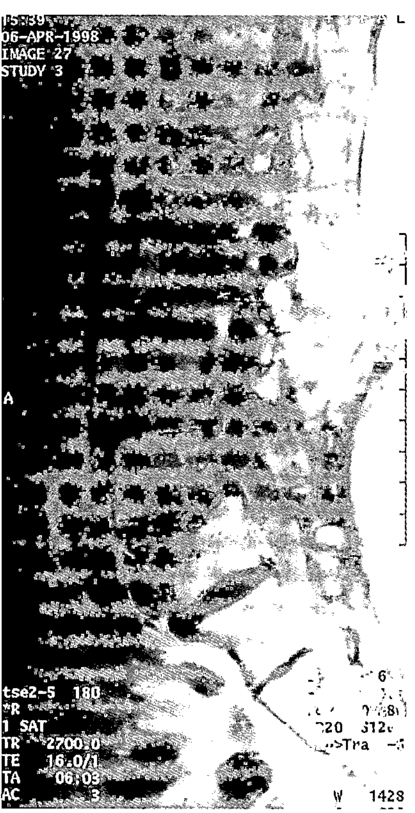

Fig. 23.3 Sagittal MRI demonstrating spondylitic degeneration of all lumbar discs. L3–4 and L4–5 are particularly degenerated with loss of disc height and substance with a change in water signal as well. There is a grade 1 spondylolisthesis. Correlation of these changes with specific pain syndromes is difficult.

Adequate analgesia is a first choice. Non-steroidal anti-inflammatory analgesics are standard (Basmajian 1989). Some investigators are examining the use of long-acting narcotics for the relief of pain of benign origin. It has been our experience that very few patients with spondylotic disease will tolerate the side effects of narcotics and refuse to use them. Some patients will be benefitted by short-term bracing, especially when active; so, a trial lumbosacral support is worthwhile. There is reasonable evidence that an individualized exercise programme to strengthen the paravertebral and abdominal muscles, combined with local measures to restore painless range of motion, will benefit many patients. These programmes are typically not available from the usual physical medicine sources, but if such a programme can be obtained, many patients will benefit. Elderly patients are particularly helped by a general physical conditioning programme as well, but any deconditioned patient can be helped. Weight loss has not been proven to be beneficial, but reduction in weight makes intuitive sense and is included in most vigorous rehabilitation efforts. Patients must be convinced that the exercise programme is worth doing and told that it will require 1–2 years to see maximum improvement. These vigorous physical therapy programmes require real commitment from patient and physician if they are to be successful. Serious osteoporosis should be treated as well (Koes et al 1992b).

THE FACET SYNDROME

A small subset of patients have pain which apparently is generated from lumbar zygapophyseal joints. Typically, these patients complain of local pain and often can point to the involved joint. Movement is painful. Rest is helpful and axial loading particularly produces pain (Schwarzer et al 1994b).

Imaging studies demonstrate arthropathy. Joints are hypertrophied. Synovial cysts are common. The cartilage endplates are eroded and both acute and chronic inflammatory changes occur around the articular surfaces. Subluxations are common.

A diagnosis is validated when injection of local anaesthetic into the joint or its innervation produces pain relief. The so-called 'facet block' has all of the negatives of any diagnostic block, but if expertly done and interpreted, it does define a group of patients whose pain is partly or largely from arthritic joints. Radiofrequency destruction of the innervation has proven to be useful, providing lasting relief for the majority of patients who fit the diagnostic criteria. In our experience, this is a very small percentage, being no more than 1–2% of patients presenting with back pain (Schwarzer et al 1994a, 1995c).

There is still considerable controversy over the reality of the diagnosis. It is odd that pain from arthritic joints should be so easily accepted in every other part of the body and yet denied by some in the spine.

Patients who are identified with apparent pain generators in zygapophyseal joints may be treated by radiofrequency destruction of the innervation of the symptomatic joints. Several papers, indicating that steroid injection in and around the joints are ineffective, have been published. Radiofrequency thermal destruction has been recommended for years, the assumed thermal lesion has been thought to disrupt the nerve anatomy and thus extinguish function. As yet, there are no well-controlled studies of the beneficial effect of denervation, but the personal experience of a number of spinal experts suggests that destruction of the innervation of symptomatic zygapophyseal joints will relieve pain often for long periods of time. There is some question about whether the lesion created is thermal, but the efficacy of the technique in a limited number of patients is recognized by many experts in the field.

SPINAL STENOSIS

The syndrome of spinal stenosis is signified by back pain and leg pain with claudication. Patients typically present first with simple gait disturbance. That is, they have trouble walking well after ambulating for more than a short time. Then pain occurs and the hallmark of the diagnosis is painful weakness in both legs brought on by walking. Typically, these patients are relieved immediately upon cessation of walking and often assume a flexed position to speed resolution of symptoms. These features differentiate it from vascular claudication whose symptoms take longer to resolve after cessation of activity. Sensory complaints are usually stocking-like and suggestive of metabolic peripheral neuropathy with which the problem is often confused. The neurological examination may be entirely normal at rest, but both motor and sensory loss can appear after activity.

The diagnosis is made with imaging studies. Plain X-rays are misleading, but either MR (Fig. 23.4) or CT will make the diagnosis.

The treatment for spinal stenosis when symptoms are severe is surgical decompression. The outcomes are excellent. The issue is when are symptoms serious enough to warrant operation. The majority of patients have mild to moderate incapacity and do not necessarily require surgery. When symptoms become significantly incapacitating or when progressive important neurological deficits occur, then surgery is indicated. Prior to that time, symptomatic treatment is warranted. The symptomatic therapies include modification of lifestyle, adequate analgesia, and an exercise activity programme designed to maximize function and minimize symptoms.

The surgical treatment consists of decompressive laminectomy with foraminotomies and stabilization, if

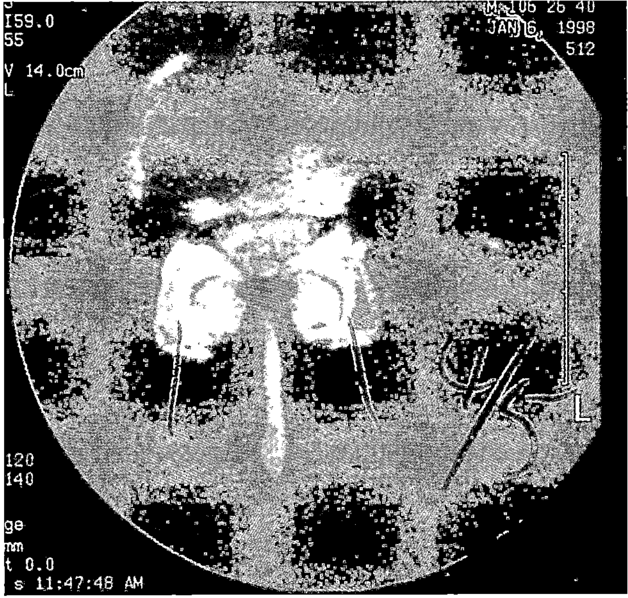

Fig. 23.4 Axial MRI at L4–5 demonstrating moderate canal stenosis with a trefoil appearance. There is significant foraminal stenosis and dramatic facet arthropathy. These are the typical changes of spinal stenosis.

necessary. When severe back pain is an important part of the syndrome, it is probable that fusion will be required. When the syndrome is claudication, then decompression alone will be adequate. It is our experience that over 90% of patients will achieve satisfactory relief of claudication symptoms, while back pain as a complaint is more likely to persist. Even with fusion, it is our experience that no more than 60–70% of these patients achieve satisfactory relief of back pain.

FORAMINAL ROOT COMPRESSION SYNDROME

A variation of the spinal stenosis problem occurs when there is compression of an isolated root in a spondylotic foramen. Patients present much with similar complaints as in acute disc herniation, but the time course is protracted and the onset has usually been gradual. Patients complain of sciatica or femoral pain in the accepted distribution of a single root. Sometimes root involvement is bilateral and occasionally more than one root on one side is affected. However, the syndrome is not of claudication but of ongoing root compression. That is, the pain tends to be constant, although it is often exacerbated by activity, being upright and axial loading. The associated reflex, motor and sensory changes relate to the individual root. A positive straight-leg raising is unusual, which is different, than the tension sign of the acute disc herniation. Diagnosis is made by MRI (Fig. 23.5) and CT, which visualize the neural foramina and the compression of the nerve root.

There is little evidence that any conservative measures will benefit such patients, but if the pain is tolerable and there is no major neurological deficit, then a thorough trial of an individualized exercise activity programme is indicated. If the rehabilitation programme is not effective and pain is intractable, or if there are associated neurological deficits, then surgery should proceed. The operation consists of decompression through adequate foraminotomy. The outcome of surgery should be as good as that enjoyed for acute disc herniation.

SPINAL INSTABILITY AND PROGRESSIVE DEFORMITY SYNDROMES

A significant number of patients with spondylotic disease will develop progressive spinal deformities. These are degenerative in nature for the majority, although congenital and traumatic instability certainly can occur and will be similar in presentation. Fortunately, the treatment is very much the same, so the aetiology makes very little difference (Panjabi et al 1984, Olerud et al 1986, Dvorak et al 1991).

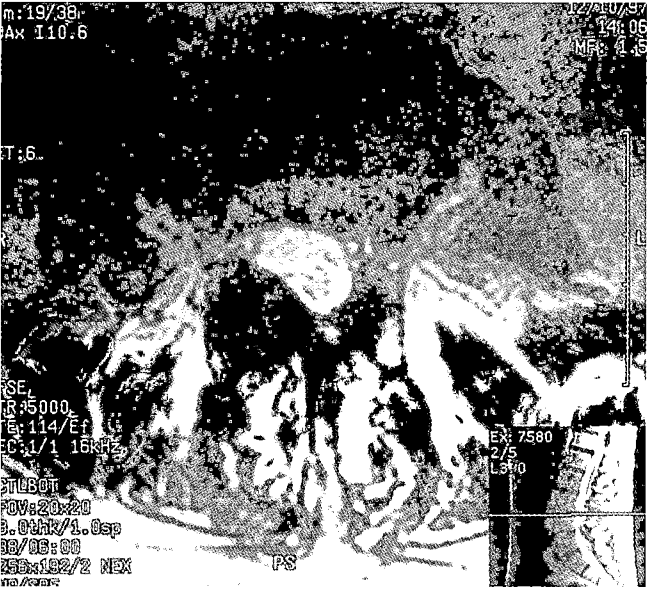

Fig. 23.5 Axial view MRI demonstrating unilateral facet hypertrophy with encroachment upon the spinal canal and foraminal stenosis. The change is at L3–4 and the patient's symptoms were right-sided anterior thigh pain.

Degenerative spondylolisthesis

This is the most common of the apparent instability syndromes encountered (Annertz et al 1990). However, the apparent movement expected because of the malalignment of adjacent vertebral bodies may not be seen on flexion-extension films. It may be slowly progressive and occasionally may be fixed. Patients typically complain of back pain in the lumbar area with or without associated root signs. Diagnosis is made by plain X-rays, which should include dynamic films to be certain whether the spine is moving actively.

Treatment should be symptomatic, unless pain is intractable or significant nerve root compression with neurological deficit is occurring. Symptomatic therapies include bracing, modification of lifestyle, and individualized active exercise for axial muscle strengthening, range of motion, and leg strength. Surgery should be considered when axial back pain, radicular pain, or both, are severe and disabling. Most patients with progressive listhesis or slowly progressive scoliotic deformities of any kind will require fixator use for stabilization and fusion. It is best to proceed when it is apparent that symptoms are serious enough to warrant surgery, but before extremely severe deformities occur. The surgeon should be experienced in the use of fixators and in this complex reconstructive spinal surgery. The goal of surgery is to restore or maintain lumbar lordosis in association with the decompression of individual lumbar roots and

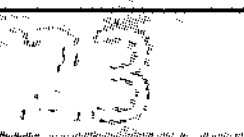

the stabilization of all required segments (Turner et al 1992, Zdeblick 1993, Temple et al 1994).

THE FAILED BACK SYNDROME

The failed back syndrome is an imprecise term usually used to categorize a large group of patients who have undergone one or more operations on the lumbar spine without benefit. It serves no useful purpose and should be abandoned. The patient who has not been benefited from one or more operations needs an evaluation which, if anything, is more complex than the patient who has not undergone surgery (Fig. 23.6) (Cherkin et al 1994). It may be possible to make a specific diagnosis about the cause of pain with greater frequency than in most idiopathic spondylitic back pain problems. The goal of the evaluation should be the most precise definition of abnormalities possible, so that an individualized treatment plan can be prescribed (La Rocca 1990). Patients fall into broad categories within this heterogeneous group that are useful in order to guide the evaluation and the therapeutic plans. The first of these broad categories is a group of patients for whom *surgery was probably not indicated in the first place* (Cherkin et al 1994). The second group of patients is those with clear indications for surgery, but in whom *surgery did not correct the original abnormality.* A third category of patients is those in whom some *significant complication of surgery* occurred and is now the pain generator (Fager & Freidberg 1980). There is another very small group of patients in whom an *intercurrent diagnosis has been missed.* A typical example is the patient with chronic back pain who harbours a tumour, usually a schwannoma or ependymoma, of the cauda equina.

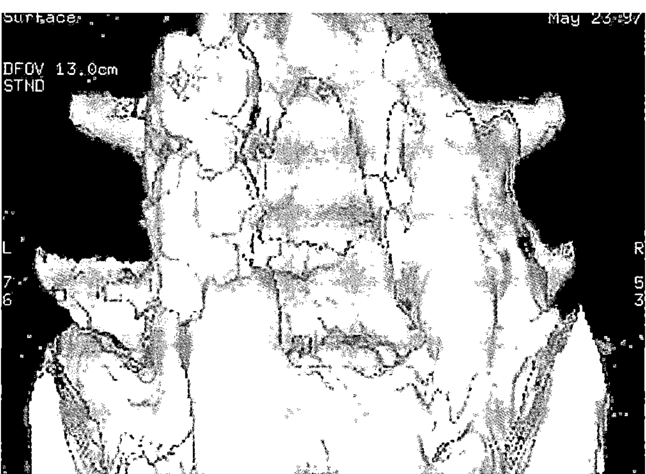

Fig. 23.6 Three dimensional reconstruction demonstrating the previous laminectomy and fusion. These are most useful in reconstructing the postsurgical changes and in assessing fusion stability; remember the averaging techniques used will always overstate the solidity of fusion.

Whatever the proposed treatment plan, precise definition of the abnormalities which are likely to be generating the pain and which must be treated, is imperative. Specifically, if any reoperative surgery is to be done, it should be planned for abnormalities which are as well defined as for first surgery. It is still true in these patients that surgery will only benefit individuals who have nerve root compression or clearly demonstrable instability. Utility of surgery for removal of scar, which is not compressive, removal of tissues which potentially generate noxious substances in the inflammatory chain or the correction of micromovement in painful segments has not been proven and we do not use any of these concepts to justify reoperation.

In an extensive review of a small group of patients for whom all preoperative studies were available and complete records detailed status before failed lumbar surgery, we determined that the majority did not meet commonly accepted criteria for lumbar operation. Therefore, it is not surprising that surgery failed to relieve them. In a recent multicentre nationwide prospective study of the outcome of first-time-back surgery, we determined that over 90% of patients were improved when chosen for surgery by expert spinal surgeons. By contrast, in a small group of patients rejected for surgery by these same experts, only 10% were improved by operation carried out outside our study and worsening of symptoms following surgery was the rule. In examining patients who have failed lumbar surgery, it is important to determine the original indications for the procedure if possible. Of course, it is still quite possible for such patients to have had a surgical complication which now requires correction. Even though patients have not had appropriate indications for original surgery, they still require evaluation to determine the current cause of the problem. If symptoms remain the same and no new abnormalities are found, it is unlikely that any surgical procedure will be beneficial. However, the original surgeons may have failed to correct an abnormality or some complication may have occurred which will influence a decision about additional surgery. Therefore, whatever the original indications, complete evaluation of patients is required (La Rocca 1990).

The first questions relate to the pain. Is it the same or has something new occurred? Does the pain suggest a mechanical back problem only or is there a radicular component? Does the radicular pain sound neuropathic, suggesting nerve root injury?

Physical examination is unlikely to be helpful in the diagnosis, but will record the patient's current physical state.

Imaging studies begin with plain films with flexion-extension. These should include obliques to evaluate the zygapophyseal joints. CT imaging, particularly with multi-dimensional reconstructions, will demonstrate bony detail, the effects of previous surgery, the status of zygapophyseal joints, the size of neural foramina and such common complications as pars fracture. MRI is more useful for the examination of discs, nerve root relations in the neural foramina, the size of the spinal canal and inflammation (Ross et al 1987, Hochhauser et al 1988, Hueftle et al 1988, Cavanagh et al 1993). If fixators are in place, 3D reconstruction will eliminate the metallic artefact and provide a view of the placement of the fixator as well (Firooznia et al 1987). CT myelography is sometimes required, particularly when fixators are in place (Hashimoto et al 1990).

COMMON POSTOPERATIVE PAIN SYNDROMES

INAPPROPRIATE PATIENT SELECTION

Analysis of patients who present with failure of pain relief after first-time lumbar surgery often suggests that the majority have not met accepted criteria before operation and were lacking symptoms, signs and imaging demonstration of either root compression or instability syndromes (Spengler & Freeman 1979, Bigos et al 1991, Cherkin et al 1994). When previous studies and records are available, they will validate or refute the original indications for surgery (Cauchoix et al 1978). Remember that the imaging studies are not entirely accurate and that some patients will harbour correctable problems in spite of negative imaging. However, the fact that the original surgery was not obviously indicated does not imply that the patient does not now have a correctable problem. Re-evaluation is warranted (Hochhauser et al 1988, Hueftle et al 1988, Montaldi et al 1988). It is important to remember that failure of first surgery with residual pain is not an indication for a second surgery. There is a tendency for some surgeons to first carry out a decompressive procedure with or without discectomy and then to follow that with fusion when the first procedure fails to relieve the patient. The problem is frequently that the first surgery was ill chosen. Therefore, there is no indication that a second procedure with fusion will be beneficial. The indications for surgery in reoperation should be as stringent as those applied for first surgery. Stereotyped addition of fusion because of a failed first procedure is unwarranted (Waddell 1987b).

FAILURE TO CORRECT THE INITIAL PATHOLOGY

Another common problem is that the original surgeon simply did not perform an operation designed to completely correct the original disease (O'Connell 1951). Common examples are failure to decompress a nerve root or roots through foraminotomy, failure to decompress the spinal canal, wrong level, failure to remove a disc entirely and failure to recognize and stabilize unstable segments (Adkins 1955). Repeat of the imaging studies will usually demonstrate the residual abnormality. When these abnormalities are concordant with the patient's complaints, surgical repair is virtually as successful as first-time operation (Finnegan et al 1979, Dawson et al 1981, Zdeblick 1993).

SURGICAL COMPLICATIONS

A large number of complications can occur. These include nerve root injury, pseudomeningocele, surgically induced instability, infection and excessive scar formation (Frymoyer et al 1978, Hanley & Shapiro 1989, Wetzel & LaRocca 1991).

Fixators have their own set of problems. Fusions may fail (pseudarthrosis). Hardware may loosen and even extrude. Sometimes hardward is inappropriately placed. It is important to examine all patients who have undergone fusion to assess the competency of bony fusion, the location of fixators and their stability, and the appropriateness of fixator placement (Raugstad et al 1982, Kozak & O'Brien 1990, Steinmann & Herkowitz 1992, Yuan et al 1994).

There are other problems related to surgery which are not direct or even immediate complications. The fixation of one or more spinal segments may lead to degeneration of the segment above. Sometimes this is acute, but more typically it is a chronic problem. The symptoms are those of instability and stenosis above the fusion (Dawson et al 1981, Lin et al 1983, O'Brien et al 1986, Srdjan 1994).

A large number of patients have obviously thick scar which may deform the thecal sac following surgery. The significance of these scars is uncertain. There is no evidence that operating upon those that are not compressive will benefit the patient (Braun et al 1985, Bundschuh et al 1988, Bandschuh et al 1990).

DONOR-SITE PAIN

A commonly over-looked problem is pain in the donor site over the hip where bone graft was harvested (Spangfort 1972). Many patients complain of seriously disabling pain in the donor site. The cause is unknown and the problem is extremely difficult to treat. The diagnosis is usually made by point tenderness over the donor site, although it may spread to hip and thigh. Local injection virtually always relieves the pain. No consistently effective treatments have been described. The problem does seem to ameliorate with time.

ARACHNOIDITIS

This is an unusual problem if viewed as a clinical syndrome not a radiological finding (Fitt & Stevens 1995). Many patients who have undergone spinal surgery with or without myelography demonstrate root adhesions and adherence of nerve roots to the dural sac (Fig. 23.7). Most of these findings have no obvious clinical significance, but some do seem to be associated with symptoms. However, chronic adhesive arachnoiditis is rarely progressive and needs to be considered with some patients. Symptoms of this rare syndrome are diffuse lower extremity pain, often burning in character, with slowly progressive loss of function. MRI may suggest arachnoiditis, but myelography is required to really be certain of the degree of arachnoiditis, particularly when spinal stenosis is present (Fitt & Stevens 1995). Arachnoiditis was most commonly associated with infection when first described and then was described as a complication of myelography and surgery. Arachnoiditis is now seen in patients who have not had myelography, as a complication of surgery alone. When the rare progressive problem is present, there is little question of the relationship between the myelographic findings of arachnoiditis and the symptomatology. However, for the majority of patients, the relationship between arachnoiditis and symptoms is still uncertain. Simply finding arachnoiditis does not imply that this pathological process is the cause of the patient's complaints.

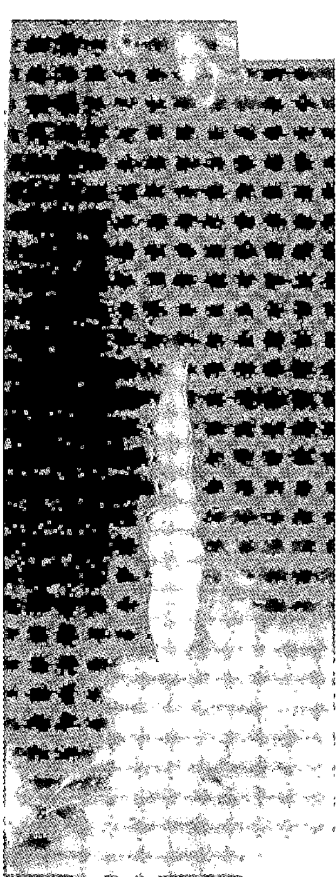

Fig. 23.7 Anteroposterior view of a myelogram carried out with water-based agent demonstrating the typical changes of epidural fibrosis and arachnoiditis. The thecal sac is deformed laterally from epidural scar, from L3 to L5. No root sheaths are seen; roots are adherent to the dura and no internal structures within the thecal sac are seen. This is a typical form of arachnoiditis. The patient's complaints were of migratory pains involving different nerve roots at different times. She was treated first with narcotics to which the pains were unresponsive and then to a series of novel drugs for neuropathic pain.

EVALUATION AND TREATMENT OF POSTOPERATIVE COMPLICATIONS

A careful history is the most important part of the initial evaluation. It is important to determine whether the problem being described is the same one for which the patient was operated upon or something that has developed following surgery. The character of the pain and its spatial and temporal characteristics are no different than what will be described in patients who have not had surgery. Pain which is predominantly in the back is suggestive of a local mechanical problem (Hanley & Shapiro 1989). Non-radicular leg pain has no localizing significance. Radicular leg pain should conform to accepted dermatomes. Patients are routinely worsened by activity and improved by rest, axial loading and repetitive bending are common activities which increase complaints. Constant pain is more suggestive of infection if in the back, and nerve root injury if radicular in character.

The major problem in evaluating patients with postoperative pain is that, with our current diagnostic techniques, no obvious cause can be found in the majority. It is our experience that significantly less than half of these patients have a defined correctable anatomical problem (Waddell 1987b). In the majority, a number of abnormalities are found. Diffuse epidural scarring is one such process, but it has never been demonstrated that the scar in patients complaining of pain is different from the scar present in all patients (Sotiropoulos et al 1989, Tullberg et al 1994). All surgeons have observed that some patients have much more postoperative scarring than others, when reoperation is required. Whether this is an individual patient reaction to surgery or a product of surgical technique is uncertain. Moreover, the relationship to pain is unproven. Sunderland (personal communication) suggested traction scar as a source of pain. He postulated that irritation of the root occurred because it was fixed and did not move with changes in the spine. This mechanism has never been substantiated. Many patients with fusion, solid or with pseudarthrosis, are symptom free (Hanley et al 1991). Others have chronic back pain and many of these can be relieved by local anaesthetic infusion on the fusion mass. This suggests that the scar attaching muscle to fusion bone or the surface of the fusion itself is a pain generator, but the real origins of pain in these patients is unproven. Some patients with pseudarthrosis are relieved by injection in and around the pseudarthrosis. In others, the pain is unaffected. Provocative disc injection demonstrates that many patients complaining with pain after surgery have reproduction of that pain by injection into one or more lumbar discs. The predictive power of these concordant blocks for relief of pain by surgery is as yet unproven. All of these observations identify painful segments in the lumbar spine, but as yet have not elucidated the origins of the pain. For the majority of patients with postoperative complaints, there are no consistent explanations for the origins of pain.

BOX 23.4

Theoretical cause of back and leg pain syndromes

1. Micromovement
It is postulated that imperceptible movements occur at endplates and facets to produce pain. Simple loading may be enough stimulus

2. Noxious chemical release
Some products of disc degeneration are known to produce pain when applied in epidural space. Role in humans is uncertain

3. Painful scar with microneuroma
Formation: blockade of these scars sometimes produces pain relief

4. Traction scar
Local tethering excites nociceptors due to mechanical traction on root during movement

5. Central excitation
Local factors excite field changes in cord or higher now susceptible to non-painful stimuli

THEORETICAL CAUSES OF LOW BACK PAIN (BOX 23.4)

Because back and leg pain often are unaccompanied by obvious diagnosable instability or clearly defined nerve root compression, there have been extensive investigations into possible causes of the pain. In some patients, it appears that the pain arises mostly from ligaments and muscles. At least, no other causes have been defined (Mense 1991). Three other lines of investigation are being followed. The first of these suggests that the pain may be neuropathic in type and may originate from minor degrees of demyelinization and sensitization, probably accompanied by central receptor changes (Wall & Gutnick 1974, Seltzer & Devor 1979, Calvin et al 1982, Sugimoto et al 1990, Basbaum et al 1991, Devor et al 1991, 1994, Gracely et al 1992, McLachlan et al 1993, Wagner et al 1993, Woolf et al 1994, Kinnman & Levine 1995). A variety of factors and possible mechanisms are being examined. None of these are clearly applicable to typical patients with chronic back and leg pain, as yet.

A second important line of inquiry suggests that the nerve activation and sensitization is secondary to the release of inflammatory products secondary to degeneration, spondylotic changes and/or surgical trauma (Rothwell & Relton 1993, Gronblad et al 1994).

A third general category is termed by its originators' micromovement. In this concept, the noxious stimuli come from small but abnormal degrees of movement in zygapophyseal joints and in and around the disc. These movements presumably would activate nocioceptors in ligaments, periosteum and muscles (Bogduk 1991). None of these are proven to be important in patients as yet, and investigations are ongoing. All have clinical implications. The concept that the pain is neuropathic has led to trials of drugs that are known to effect neuropathic pain. The concept of micromovement has led to fusion, mainly of the interbody type. The theory of release of noxious products of the inflammatory cascade has led some to postulate total disc removal to eliminate the inflammatory process and stabilize the spine.

FURTHER EVALUATION OF THE PATIENT WITHOUT AN APPARENT CAUSE OF PAIN

After all these specific abnormalities have been diagnosed or excluded there remains a majority of patients for whom no currently definable cause of pain has been found. Some of them respond well to non-specific conservative measures, but many do not. Many spinal experts have continued to examine these patients with physiological techniques to try to add information to the anatomical data available from imaging studies.

The hypothesis that underlies the use of *temporary diagnostic blockade* to augment clinical decision making is straightforward; that is, anaesthetization of a pain generator should produce relief of the pain being produced (April 1992). Additions include production of pain by mechanical irritation of the generator and control by placebo injections.

There is probably no current area in the field of spinal disease more misunderstood than the use of diagnostic blocks to aid the clinician in identifying painful segments or structures in the lumbar spine (Bogduk et al 1995b). A few principles must be understood if blocks are to be applied appropriately. Current evidence indicates that these blocks are effective in identifying painful segments, but are not necessarily specific for individual structures blocked, because there appears to be much overlap in multiple blocks of different types in the same segment. Placebo-controlled blocks are more accurate than others. Blocks without a negative control are suspect (Bogduk 1994b). The problem of placebo can be partially overcome by the use of anaesthetic agents of varying durations of action and by carefully constructed block protocols in which the patient does not know specifically what structure is blocked and evaluation of outcome of the block is carried out by someone other than the treating physician. It is also important to recognize that interpretation of what patients say about block results requires understanding of blocks and their uses. The unwary can be misled either positively or negatively by the way questions to patients are constructed. It is also important to remember that anaesthetization of a site to which pain is referred will often block the pain of which the patients complain. This non-specific effect can be erroneously interpreted as identification of a pain generator. It is important to recognize that diagnostic blocks have no truth in themselves and must be used as adjuncts in a comprehensive patient evaluation.

With these caveats, it does appear that the blocks are useful adjuncts in the diagnosis of some patients with spinal disease. There is not enough evidence yet available to suggest they can be more than aids to the expert clinician.

Another cause of confusion is the widespread use of therapeutic blocks such as epidural steroid injection (Goebert et al 1960, Harley 1967, Heyse-Moore 1978). While time honoured in practice, there is not much evidence to support their use in chronic back pain. The blocks described here are not therapeutic, but used only for diagnosis.

Blocks in current use include blockade of zygapophyseal joints, individual root blocks, block of donor site and pseudarthroses, and provocative disc blockade (Bogduk 1994a).

Zygapophyseal joint blocks can be carried out by blocking the innervation of the joints in question, or direct injection of small amounts of anaesthetic into them. Relief of pain suggests that the joints blocked play a role in the painful process.

Individual root blockade is used to be certain about the root which is injured or compressed when clinical and radiological differentiation is not clear.

Provocative disc blockade is probably the most controversial of these blocks currently (Bogduk et al 1995a). Part of this is because of the use of the name discography which confuses the current procedures with the radiological studies proposed in the 1950s for the identification of degenerated discs (Holt 1968, Simmons et al 1988). At that time, the hypothesis was that the simple identification of a degenerated disc should lead to reparative surgery. That hypothesis has long been rejected. Current blocks should provoke pain by injection and pain should be relieved when local anaesthetic is used. While many people carry out an injection with radiopaque contrast material and describe anatomical abnormalities, none of these have been correlated with specific syndromes, as yet. Their meaning is uncertain (Bogduk 1991, Schwarzer et al 1995b).

Bogduk and associates have also demonstrated that placebo-controlled positive block, that is one provoking and relieving pain, has a chance of being accurate of greater than 90%, while negative blocks are no more than 50% accurate.

The current use of these blocks is to support a clinical impression of the origin of the complaint of pain (Moran et al 1988, Schwarzer et al 1995a). As yet, the next major step has not been taken. That is, there is no study available that clearly demonstrates the predictive power of any of these blocks to estimate the chance of a good result from a rationally chosen interventional procedure (Knox & Chapman 1993). Nevertheless, they are useful in the hands of an expert clinician who performs them well and interprets them without bias.

So-called facet blocks may lead to denervation of facets or fusion (Bogduk et al 1987, Schwarzer et al 1995d). Positive root blocks can lead to exploration and decompression (Bogduk et al 1995b). Discogenic pain has been treated with interbody fusion. In the hands of experts, fully informed patients may benefit (Bogduk 1991).

ALTERNATIVES FOR CARE OF CHRONIC LOW BACK PAIN (BOX 23.5)

It is not surprising that a clinical problem as poorly understood as low back pain should generate a huge number of therapies which are devised to be helpful. Most are as yet unproven, although many are supported by long-standing practice (Bigos et al 1994).

The first general category comprises all those adjuncts which claim to make people more comfortable. The list is long: adjustable beds, firm mattresses, chairs, pillows, supports and whirlpools to name a few. Patients may try the ones that seem attractive to them, and use those that are comfortable. I tend to discourage use of those that are excessively expensive and will not prescribe any.

Many patients are in long-term programmes of passive therapy measures such as heat, massage, electrical stimulation, or active programmes of massage, electrical stimulation, or active programmes of massage plus manipulation. The value of any of these is not supported by strong evidence in chronic back pain. I tell patients to continue if they are convinced they are symptomatically better (Wiesel et al 1980, Bell & Rothman 1984, Heliovaara 1987).

Patients also seek accupuncture, and a variety of related and unrelated therapies such as are available from mail-order catalogues. None are supported by scientific data on chronic back pain, and I do not recommend any. This is also true of the many herbal remedies patients bring.

A large number of books, tapes and videos are available on the topic of back pain. Most are helpful; a few could be dangerous. It is best to find some you like and recommend them, rather than allowing the patient to choose indiscriminantly.

Many minimally invasive techniques have and are appearing which promise patients no risk relief. Some of the most popular were and are chymopapain intradiscal injection, steroid in epidural or intradiscal spaces, percutaneous discectomy, endoscopic laser discectomy, endoscopic discectomy, endoscopic fusion and microdiscectomy. All are techniques for experts. Some have come and gone. Some are being evaluated. None are clearly established to have an important role in chronic low back and leg pain (Martins et al 1978, Choy et al 1987, Kambin 1988, 1991a,b, Kahanovitz et al 1990, Onik et al 1990, Nordby et al 1993, Revel et al 1993, Regan et al 1995).

BOX 23.5

Non-surgical management of chronic back/leg pain

1. Adequate analgesia: the role of long-acting narcotics is still controversial
2. Weight loss: unproven but intuitively a good idea
3. Passive measures to correct *specific* areas of myofascial tenderness and pain
4. Restore flexibility
5. Restore strength: paraspinal and abdominal muscles first
6. Restore general conditioning
7. Teach posture and body mechanics
8. Teach how to do things without injury
9. Maximize function and return to activity
10. Educate to prevent recurrence

CONCLUSION

Low back and *leg pain* are ubiquitous complaints found throughout the world. Although there is a strong correlation with spondylosis, the causes of pain remain unknown in most patients. In the acute phase, the prudent physician excludes serious illness and waits. Most patients resolve spontaneously.

In the persistent pain problems another search for intercurrent disease is warranted, although one will be found rarely. No certain diagnosis may be possible. A small number of patients will have spinal root compression or instability. Surgery will predictably relieve both. For the majority this will not be true.

When no correctable cause is found, an individualized programme of weight control, conditioning, modification of activity, prevention of recurrence and education/understanding can provide satisfactory relief.

One of our great research goals must be to find out why the spine hurts so that better more specific therapies can be devised (Box 23.6).

BOX 23.6

Causes of the failed back syndrome

1. Initial surgery was not indicated:
physical and imaging criteria not met
co-morbidities very important

2. Intercurrent diagnosis missed at initial surgery:
intraspinal tumour at higher level
cervical stenosis
thoracic disc herniation

3. Initial surgery failed to correct spinal abnormality:
wrong level operated upon
disc missed
stenosis not relieved
unstable spine not fused

4. Complication of initial surgery:
recurrent disc
excessive compressing scar
collapse of foramen (may be opposite side)
spondylolisthesis
disciitis
non-disc infection
arachnoiditis
pseudomeningocoele
radiculopathy – traumatic
pseudoarthrosis
loosen or broken fixators
misplaced fixators
donor site pain (fracture)

5. Late complications of surgery:
stenosis above a fusion (transition syndrome)
instability above a fusion
root compression above or below a scoliotic curve

REFERENCES

Adkins EWO 1955 Lumbo-sacral arthrodesis after laminectomy. Journal of Bone and Joint Surgery 37B: 208–223

Anderson GBJ 1996 The epidemiology of spinal disorders. In: Frymoyer JW (ed) The adult spine, principles and practice, 2nd edn. Philadelphia, PA, JB Lippincott, pp 277–288

Annertz M, Holtas S, Cronqvist S et al 1990 Isthmic lumbar spondylolisthesis with sciatica: MR imaging vs myelography. Acta Radiologica 31: 449–453

Aprill CN 1992 The role of anatomically specific injections into the sacroiliac joint. In: Vleeming A, Mooney V, Snijders C et al (eds) First Interdisciplinary World Conference on Low Back Pain and its Relation to the Sacroiliac Joint. San Diego, CA, University of California, pp 373–380

Basbaum AI, Gautron M, Jazat F et al 1991 The spectrum of fiber loss in a model of neuropathic pain in the rat: an electron microscopic study. Pain 47: 359–367

Basmajian JV 1989 Acute back pain and spasm: a controlled multicenter trial of combined analgesic and antispasm agents. Spine 14: 438–439

Bell GR, Rothman RH 1984 The conservative treatment of sciatica. Spine 9: 54–56

Berman AT, Garbarino JL Jr, Fisher SM et al 1984 The effects of epidural injection of local anesthetics and corticosteroids on patients with lumbosciatic pain. Clinical Orthopedics 188: 144–151

Bigos SJ, Battie MC, Spengler DM et al 1991 A prospective study of work perceptions and psychosocial factors affecting the report of back injury. Spine 16: 1–6

Bigos SJ, Bowyer O, Braen G et al 1994 Acute low back problems in adults. In: Clinical Practice Guideline No 14 (AHCPR Publication

No 95-0642). US Department of Health and Human Services, Rockville, MD

Boden SD, Davis DO, Dina TS et al 1990a Abnormal magnetic-resonance scans of the lumbar spine in asymptomatic subjects: a prospective investigation. Journal of Bone and Joint Surgery 72A: 403–408

Boden SD, Davis DO, Dina TS et al 1990b Abnormal magnetic-resonance scans of the lumbar spine in asymptomatic subjects: a prospective investigation. Journal of Bone and Joint Surgery 72A: 403–408

Bogduk N 1991 The lumbar disc and low back pain. Neurosurgery Clinics of North America 2: 791–806

Bogduk N 1994a Diskography. American Pain Society Journal 3: 149–154

Bogduk B 1994b Proposed discography standards. In: ISIS Newsletter, vol 2. International Spinal Injection Society, Daly City, CA, pp 10–13

Bogduk N, Macintosh J, Marsland A 1987 Technical limitations to the efficacy of radiofrequency neurotomy for spinal pain. Neurosurgery 20: 529–535

Bogduk N, Aprill C, Derby R 1995a Discography. In: White AH (ed) Spine care: diagnosis and conservative treatment. CV Mosby, St Louis, MO, pp 219–238

Bogduk N, Aprill C, Derby R 1995b Selective nerve root blocks. In: Wilson DJ (ed) Interventional radiology of the musculoskeletal system. Edward Arnold, London, pp 121–132

Bohannon RW, Gajdosik RL 1987 Spinal nerve root compression: some clinical implications. A review of the literature. Physical Therapy 67: 376–382

Bowman SJ, Wedderburn L, Whaley A et al 1993 Outcome assessment after epidural corticosteroid injection for low back pain and sciatica. Spine 18: 1345–1350

Braun IF, Hoffman JC Jr, Davis PC et al 1985 Contrast enhancement in CT differentiation between recurrent disk herniation and postoperative scar: Prospective study. American Journal of Neuroradiology 6: 607–612

Brown JH 1960 Pressure caudal anesthesia and back manipulation: conservative method for treatment of sciatica. Northwestern Medicine 59: 905–909

Bundschuh CV, Modic MT, Ross JS et al 1988 Epidural fibrosis and recurrent disk herniation in the lumbar spine: MR imaging assessment. American Journal of Roentgenology 150: 923–932

Bundschuh CV, Stein L, Slusser JH et al 1990 Distinguishing between scar and recurrent herniated disk in postoperative patients: value of contrast-enhanced and MR imaging. American Journal of Neuroradiology 11: 949–958

Bush K, Cowan N, Katz DE et al 1992 The natural history of sciatica associated with disc pathology: a prospective study with clinical and independent radiologic follow-up. Spine 17: 1205–1212

Calvin WH, Devor M, Howe JF 1982 Can neuralgias arise from minor demyelination? Spontaneous firing, mechanosensitivity and after-discharge from conducting axons. Experimental Neurology 75: 755–763

Cauchoix J, Ficat C, Girard B 1978 Repeat surgery after disc excision. Spine 3: 256–259

Cavanagh S, Stevens J, Johnson JR 1993 High-resolution MRI in the investigationof recurrent pain after lumbar discectomy. Journal of Bone and Joint Surgery 75B: 524–528

Cherkin DC, Deyo RA, Loeser JD et al 1994 An international comparison of back surgery rates. Spine 19: 1201–1206

Cholewicki J, McGill SM 1996 Mechanical stability of the in vivo lumbar spine: implications for injury and chronic low back pain. Clinical Biomechanics 11: 1–15

Choy DS, Case RB, Field W et al 1987 Letter: percutaneous laser nucleolysis of lumbar disks. New England Journal of Medicine 317: 771–772

Damkot DK, Pope MH, Lord J et al 1984 The relationship between work history, work environment and low-back pain in men. Spine 9: 395–399

Davis H 1994 Increasing rates of cervical and lumbar spine surgery in the United States, 1979–1990. Spine 19: 1117–1124

Dawson EG, Lotysch M III, Urist MR 1981 Intertransverse process lumbar arthrodesis with autogenous bone graft. Clinical Orthopedics 154: 90–96

Devor M, Basbaum AI, Bennett GJ et al 1991 Mechanisms of neuropathic pain following peripheral injury. In: Basbaum AI, Besson JMR (eds) Towards a new pharmacotherapy of pain. John Wiley, Chichester, pp 417–440

Devor M, Lomazov P, Matzner O 1994 Na^+ channel accumulation in injured axons as a substrate for neuropathic pain. In: Boivie J, Hansson P, Lindblom U (eds) Touch, temperature and pain in health and disease: mechanisms and assessments. IASP, Seattle, WA, pp 207–230

Deyo RA, Rainville J, Kent DL 1992 What can the history and physical examination tell us about low back pain? Journal of the American Medical Association 268: 760–765

Deyo RA, Haselkorn J, Hoffman R et al 1994 Designing studies of diagnostic tests for low back pain or radiculopathy. Spine 19(suppl 18): 2057S–2065S

Dvorak J, Panjabi MM, Novotny JE et al 1991 Clinical validation of functional flexion-extension roentgenograms of the lumbar spine. Spine 16: 943–950

Evans W 1930 Intrasacral epidural injection in the treatment of sciatica. Lancet ii: 1225–1229

Fager CA, Freidberg SR 1980 Analysis of failures and poor results of lumbar spine surgery. Spine 5: 87–94

Finnegan WJ, Fenlin JM, Marvel JP et al 1979 Results of surgical intervention in the symptomatic multiply-operated back patient: analysis of sixty-seven cases followed for three to seven years. Journal of Bone and Joint Surgery 61A: 1077–1082

Firooznia H, Kricheff II, Rafii M et al 1987 Lumbar spine after surgery: examination with intravenous contrast-enhanced CT. Radiology 163: 221–226

Fitt GJ, Stevens JM 1995 Postoperative arachnoiditis diagnosed by high resolution fast spin-echo MRI of the lumbar spine. Neuroradiology 37: 139–145

Frymoyer JW, Cats-Baril WL 1991 An overview of the incidences and costs of low back pain. Orthopedic Clinics of North America 22: 263–271

Frymoyer JW, Matteri RE, Hanley EN et al 1978 Failed lumbar disc surgery requiring second operation: a long-term follow-up study. Spine 3: 7–11

Goebert HW Jr, Jallo SJ, Gardner WJ et al 1960 Sciatica: treatment with epidural injections of procaine and hydrocortisone. Cleveland Clinic Quarterly 27: 191–197

Gracely RH, Lynch SA, Bennett GJ 1992 Painful neuropathy: altered central processing maintained dynamically by peripheral input. Pain 51: 175–194

Gronblad M, Virri J, Tolonen J et al 1994 A controlled immunohistochemical study of inflammatory cells in disc herniation tissue. Spine 19: 2744–2751

Hakelius A, Hindmarsh J 1972a The significance of neurological signs and myelographic findings in the diagnosis of lumbar root compression. Acta Orthopaedica Scandinavica 43: 239–246

Hakelius A, Hindmarsh J 1972b The comparative reliability of preoperative diagnostic methods in lumbar disc surgery. Acta Orthopaedica Scandinavica 43: 234–238

Hanley EN Jr, Shapiro DE 1989 The development of low-back pain after excision of a lumbar disc. Journal of Bone and Joint Surgery 71A: 719–721

Hanley EN Jr, Phillips ED, Kostuik JP 1991 Who should be fused? In:

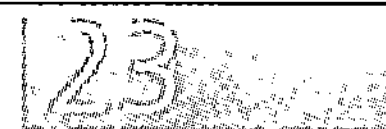

Frymoyer JW, Ducker TB, Hadler NM et al (eds) The adult spine: principles and practice, vol 2. Raven, New York, pp 1893–1917

Harley C 1967 Extradural corticosteroid infiltration: a follow-up study of 50 cases. Annals of Physical Medicine 9: 22–28

Hashimoto K, Akahori O, Kitano K et al 1990 Magnetic resonance imaging of lumbar disc herniation: comparison with myelography. Spine 15: 1166–1169

Heliovaara M 1987 Body height, obesity, and risk of herniated lumbar intervertebral disc. Spine 12: 469–472

Heyse-Moore GH 1978 A rational approach to the use of epidural medication in the treatment of sciatic pain. Acta Orthopaedica Scandinavica 49: 366–370

Hochhauser L, Kieffer SA, Cacayorin ED et al 1988 Recurrent postdiskectomy low back pain: MR-surgical correlation. American Journal of Roentgenology 151: 755–760

Holt EP Jr 1968 The question of lumbar discography. Journal of Bone and Joint Surgery 50A: 720–726

Hsieh CY, Phillips RB, Adams AH et al 1992 Functional outcomes of low back pain: comparison of four treatment groups in a randomized controlled trial. Journal of Manipulative Physiological Therapeutics 15: 4–9

Hueftle MG, Modic MT, Ross JS et al 1988 Lumbar spine: postoperative MR imaging with Gd-DTPA. Radiology 167: 817–824

Hurme M, Alaranta H 1987 Factors predicting the result of surgery for lumbar intervertebral disc herniation. Spine 12: 933–938

Hurme M, Alaranta H, Torma T et al 1983 Operated lumbar disc herniation: epidemiological aspects. Annales de Chirurgie et Gynaecologiae 72: 33–36

Jonsson B, Stromqvist B 1993 Symptoms and signs in degeneration of the lumbar spine: a prospective, consecutive study of 300 operated patients. Journal of Bone and Joint Surgery 75B: 381–385

Kahanovitz N, Viola K, Goldstein T et al 1990 A multicenter analysis of percutaneous discectomy. Spine 15: 713–715

Kalimo H, Rantanen J, Viljanen T et al 1989 Lumbar muscles: structure and function. Annals of Medicine 21: 353–359

Kambin P 1988 Percutaneous lumbar discectomy: current practice. Surg Rounds Orthop 2: 31–35

Kambin P 1991a Arthroscopic microdiskectomy. Seminars in Orthopaedics 6: 97–108

Kambin P 1991b Arthroscopic microdiscectomy laser nucleolysis. Philadelphia Med 87: 548–549

Kelsey JL 1975 An epidemiological study of acute herniated lumbar intervertebral discs. Rheumatological Rehabilitation 14: 144–159

Kelsey JL 1982 Idiopathic low back pain: magnitude of the problem. In: White AA III, Gordon SL (eds) American Academy of Orthopaedic Surgeons Symposium on Idiopathic Low Back Pain. CV Mosby, St Louis, MO, pp 5–8

Kieffer SA, Witwer GA, Cacayorin ED et al 1986 Recurrent post-discectomy pain: CT surgical correlation. Acta Radiologica 369(suppl): 719–722

Kim SI, Sadove MS 1975 Caudal-epidural corticosteroids in post-laminectomy syndrome: Treatment for low-back pain. Comprehensive Therapy 1: 57–60

Kinnman E, Levine JD 1995 Sensory and sympathetic contributions of nerve injury-induced sensory abnormalities in the rat. Neuroscience 64: 751–767

Koes BW, Bouter LM, van Vameren H et al 1992a A blinded randomized clinical trial of manual therapy and physiotherapy for chronic back and neck complaints: physical outcome measures. Journal of Manipulative and Physiological Therapy 15: 16–23

Koes BW, Bouter LM, van Mameren H et al 1992b The effectiveness of manual therapy, physiotherapy, and treatment by the general practitioner for nonspecific back and neck complaints: a randomized clinical trial. Spine 17: 28–35

Kozak JA, O'Brien JP 1990 Simultaneous combined anterior and posterior fusion: an independent analysis of a treatment for the disabled low-back pain patient. Spine 15: 322–328

Knox BD, Chapman TM 1993 Anterior lumbar interbody fusion for discogram concordant pain. Journal of Spinal Discordance 6: 242–244

Kuslich SD, Ulstrom CL, Michael CJ 1991 The tissue origin of low back pain and sciatica: a report of pain response to tissue stimulation during operations on the lumbar spine using local anesthesia. Orthopedic Clinics of North America 22: 181–187

La Rocca H 1990 Failed lumbar surgery: principles of management. In: Weinstein JN, Wiesel SW (eds) The lumbar spine. WB Saunders, Philadelphia, PA, pp 872–881

Lawrence JS (ed) 1977 Rheumatism in populations. London, Heinemann Medical, 1977

Lin PM, Cautilli RA, Joyce MF 1983 Posterior lumbar interbody fusion. Clinical Orthopedics 180: 154–168

Liu SS, Williams KD, Drayer BP et al 1990 Synovial cysts of the lumbosacral spine: diagnosis by MR imaging. American Journal of Roentgenology 154: 163–166

McCombe PF, Fairbank JC, Cockersole BC et al 1989 Reproducibility of physical signs in low-back pain. Spine 14: 908–918

Macintosh JE, Bogduk N 1987 The morphology of the lumbar erector spinae. Spine 12: 658–668

McLachlan EM, Janig W, Devor M et al 1993 Peripheral nerve injury triggers noradrenergic sprouting within dorsal root ganglia. Nature 363: 543–546

Martins AN, Ramirez A, Johnston J et al 1978 Double-blind evaluation of chemonucleolysis for herniated lumbar discs: late results. Journal of Neurosurgery 49: 816–827

Meade TW, Dyer S, Browne W et al 1995 Randomised comparison of chiropractic and hospital outpatient management for low back pain: results from extended follow up. British Medical Journal 311: 349–351

Mense S 1991 Considerations concerning the neurobiological basis of muscle pain. Canadian Journal of Physiology and Pharmacology 69: 610–616

Moeri R, Balague F., Carron R et al 1991 Chronic backache and occupational rehabilitation: prognostic factors. Schweizerische Medizinische Wochenschrift 121: 1897–1899

Montaldi S, Fankhauser H, Schnyder P et al 1988 Computer tomography of the postoperative intervertebral disk and lumbar spinal canal: investigation of twenty-five patients after successful operation for lumbar disk herniation. Neurosurgery 22: 1014–1022

Moran R, O'Connell D, Walsh MG 1988 The diagnostic value of facet joint injections. Spine 13: 1407–1410

Nelson DA 1993 Intraspinal therapy using methylprednisolone acetate: twenty-three years of clinical controversy. Spine 18: 278–286

Nordby EJ, Wright PH, Schofield SR 1993 Safety of chemonucleolysis: adverse effects reported in the United States, 1982–1991. Clinical Orthopedics 293: 122–134

O'Brien JP, Dawson MH, Heard CW et al 1986 Simultaneous combined anterior and posterior fusion: a surgical solution for failed spinal surgery with a brief review of the first 150 patients. Clinical Orthopedics 203: 191–195

O'Connell JEA 1951 Protrusions of the lumbar intervertebral discs: a clinical review based on five hundred cases treated by excision of the protrusion. Journal of Bone and Joint Surgery 33B: 8–30

Olerud S, Sjostrom L, Karlstrom G et al 1986 Spontaneous effect of increased stability of the lower lumbar spine in cases of severe chronic back pain: the answer to an external transpeduncular fixation test. Clinical Orthopedics 203: 67–74

Onik G, Mooney V, Maroon JC et al 1990 Automated percutaneous discectomy: a prospective multi-institutional study. Neurosurgery 26: 228–233

Panjabi MM, Goel VK, Takata K 1982 Physiologic strains in lumbar spinal ligaments: an in vitro biomechanical study. Spine 7: 192–203

Panjabi MM, Krag MH, Chung TQ 1984 Effects of disc injury on mechanical behavior of the human spine. Spine 9: 707–713

Pope MH, Phillips RB, Haugh LD et al 1994 A prospective randomized three-week trial of spinal manipulation, transcutaneous muscle stimulation, massage and corset in the treatment of subacute low back pain. Spine 19: 2571–2577

Postacchini F, Facchini M, Palieri P 1988 Efficacy of various forms of conservative treatment in low back pain: a comparative study. Neuro-orthopedics 6: 28–35

Raugstad TS, Harbo K, Oogberg A et al 1982 Anterior interbody fusion of the lumbar spine. Acta Orthopaedica Scandinavica 53: 561–565

Regan JJ, Guyer RD, McAfee P et al 1995 Early clinical results of laparoscopic fusion of the L-5 S-1 disc space. Orthop Trans 19: 776–777

Revel M, Payan C, Vallee C et al 1993 Automated percutaneous lumbar discectomy versus chemonucleolysis in the treatment of sciatica: a randomized multicenter trial. Spine 18: 1–7

Riihimaki H 1985 Back pain and heavy physical work: a comparative study of concrete reinforcement workers and maintenance housepainters. British Journal of Industrial Medicine 42: 226–232

Ross JS, Masaryk TJ, Modic MT et al 1987 Lumbar spine: postoperative assessment with surface-coil MR imaging. Radiology 164: 851–860

Rothwell NJ, Relton JK 1993 Involvement of cytokines in acute neurodegeneration in the CNS. Neuroscience Biobehavioural Review 17: 217–227

Saal JA, Saal JS 1989 Nonoperative treatment of herniated lumbar intervertebral disc with radiculopathy: an outcome study. Spine 14: 431–437

Saal JA, Saal JS, Herzog RJ 1990 The natural history of lumbar intervertebral disc extrusions treated nonoperatively. Spine 15: 683–686

Schwarzer AC, Derby R, Aprill, CN et al 1994a The value of the provocation response in lumbar zygapophyseal joint injections. Clinical Journal of Pain 10: 309–313

Schwarzer AC, Aprill CN, Derby R et al 1994b Clinical features of patients with pain stemming from the lumbar zygapophysial joints: is the lumbar facet syndrome a clinical entity? Spine 19: 1132–1137

Schwarzer AC, Aprill CN, Bogduk N 1995a The sacroiliac joint in chronic low back pain. Spine 20: 31–37

Schwarzer AC, Aprill CN, Derby R et al 1995b The prevalence and clinical features of internal disc disruption in patients with chronic low back pain. Spine 20: 1878–1883

Schwarzer ZC, Wang SC, Bogduk N et al 1995c Prevalence and clinical features of lumbar zygapophysial joint pain: a study in an Australian population with chronic low back pain. Annals of Rheumatic Disorders 54: 100–106

Schwarzer AC, Wang SC, O'Driscoll D et al 1995d The ability of computed tomography to identify a painful zygapophysial joint in patients with chronic low back pain. Spine 20: 907–912

Seltzer Z, Devor M 1979 Ephaptic transmission in chronically damaged peripheral nerves. Neurology 29: 1061–1064

Shekelle PG, Adams AH, Chassin MR et al 1992 Spinal manipulation for low-back pain. Annals of Internal Medicine 117: 590–598

Simmons JW, Aprill CN, Dwyer AP et al 1988 A reassessment of Holt's data on 'the question of lumbar discography'. Clinical Orthopedics 237: 120–124

Sotiropoulos S, Chafetz NI, Lang P et al 1989 Differentiation between postoperative scar and recurrent disk herniation: prospective comparison of MR, CT, and contrast-enhanced CT. American Journal of Neuroradiology 10: 639–643

Spangfort EV 1972 The lumbar disc herniation: a computer-aided analysis of 2,504 operations. Acta Orthopaedica Scandinavica 142(suppl): 1–95

Spengler DM, Freeman CW 1979 Patient selection for lumbar discectomy: an objective approach. Spine 4: 129–134

Srdjan M 1994 The role of surgery for nonradicular low-back pain. Current Opinions in Orthopedics 5: 37–42

Steinmann JC, Herkowitz HN 1992 Pseudarthrosis of the spine. Clinical Orthopedics 284: 80–90

Sugimoto T, Bennett GJ, Kajander KC 1990 Transsynaptic degeneration in the superficial dorsal horn after sciatic nerve injury: effects of a chronic constriction injury, transection, and strychnine. Pain 42: 205–213

Temple HT, Kruse RW, van Dam BE 1994 Lumbar and lumbosacral fusion using Steffee instrumentation. Spine 19: 537–541

Triano JJ, McGregor M, Hondras MA et al 1995 Manipulative therapy versus education programs in chronic low back pain. Spine 20: 948–955

Tullberg T, Grane P, Rydberg J et al 1994 Comparison of contrast-enhanced computer tomography and gadolinium-enhanced magnetic resonance imaging one year after lumbar diskectomy. Spine 19: 183–188

Turner JA, Ersek M, Herron L et al 1992 Patient outcomes after lumbar spinal fusions. Journal of the American Medical Association 268: 907–911

Waddell G 1987a A new clinical model for the treatment of low-back pain. Spine 12: 632–644

Waddell G 1987b Failures of disc surgery and repeat surgery. Acta Orthopaedica Belgica 53: 300–302

Waddell G, McCulloch JA, Kummel E et al 1980 Nonorganic physical signs in low back pain. Spine 5: 117–125

Wagner R, DeLeo JA, Coombs DW et al 1993 Spinal dynorphin immunoreactivity increases bilaterally in a neuropathic pain model. Brain Research 629: 323–326

Wall PD, Gutnick M 1974 Ongoing activity in peripheral nerves: the physiology and pharmacology of impulses originating from a neuroma. Experimental Neurology 43: 580–593

Weber H 1983 Lumbar disc herniation: a controlled, prospective study with ten years of observation. Spine 8: 131–140

Weber H 1994 The natural history of disc herniation and the influence of intervention. Spine 19: 2234–2238

Wetzel FT, LaRocca H 1991 The failed posterior lumbar interbody fusion. Spine 167: 839–845

Wiesel SW, Cuckler JM, Deluca F et al 1980 Acute low-back pain: an objective analysis of conservative therapy. Spine 5: 324–330

Wiesel SW, Tsourmas N, Feffer HL et al 1984 A study of computer-assisted tomography: I. The incidence of positive CAT scans in an asymptomatic group of patients. Spine 9: 549–551

Woolf CJ, Safieh-Garabedian B, Ma QP et al 1994 Nerve growth factor contributes to the generation of inflammatory sensory hypersensitivity. Neuroscience 62: 327–331

Xu GL, Haughton VM, Carrera GF 1990 Lumbar facet joint capsule: appearance at MR imaging and CT. Radiology 177: 415–420

Yuan HA, Garfin SR, Dickman CA et al 1994 A historical cohort stud of pedicle screw fixation in thoracic, lumbar, and sacral spinal fusions. Spine 19(suppl 20): 2279S–2296S

Zdeblick TA 1993 A prospective, randomized study of lumbar fusion: preliminary results. Spine 18: 983–991

Upper extremity pain

ANDERS E. SOLA

INTRODUCTION

Upper extremity pain may be related to many different conditions: degeneration of cervical spine processes, degeneration of the affected joint, trauma to the cervical spine or affected joint, vascular compromise, nerve impingement, thoracic or abdominal pathology or any combination of these elements. Further, pain which emanates from a joint area may involve muscle, ligaments, tendons or the capsule. This chapter describes procedures for determining the aetiology of the pain and the clinical management of the various forms of upper extremity pain. Cervical sprain or 'whiplash' injury is also discussed in terms of mechanisms and management.

Upper extremity pain can be an enigma to physicians because it may be related to many different conditions: degeneration of cervical spine processes, degeneration of the affected joint, trauma to the cervical spine or affected joint, vascular compromise, nerve impingement, thoracic or abdominal pathology or any combination of these elements. Further, pain which emanates from a joint area may involve muscle, ligaments, tendons or the capsule. Therefore unless the aetiology of pain is obvious, the clinical management of upper extremity pain begins with a determination, through history and examination, of whether the pain is intrinsic to the shoulder area, extrinsic or of combined aetiologies (Table 24.1) (DePalma 1973, Bateman 1978, Calliet 1981).

Table 24.1 Causes of shoulder pain (adapted from Gerhart et al 1985)

Intrinsic causes
The joint
Acromioclavicular separation
Acute with instability
Chronic with degenerative joint disease
Adhesive capsulitis (idiopathic, secondary)
Glenohumeral instability (capsular laxity, labrum tear)
Periarticular
Myofascial syndromes
Bursitis, tendinitis (supraspinatus, infraspinatus, bicipital)
Impingement (subacromial)
Rotator cuff tear
Other
Fracture (proximal humerus, scapula, clavicle)
Myofascial trigger points in interscapular, periscapular muscles
Tumour (metastatic, primary)
Extrinsic causes of shoulder pain
Elbow or wrist pathology (carpal tunnel syndrome)
Cervical or thoracic nerve root irritation; spondylosis; herniated disc
Injuries to the brachial plexus
Myofascial trigger points in the trapezii, levator scapulae, scalenae, pectoralis muscles
Thoracic outlet syndrome (cervical rib, scalenus anticus)
Somatic disorders (free air under diaphragm)
Visceral disorders (gallstones, cholecystitis, hepatitis, myocardial infarction, pneumonitis or tumours of lung/spinal cord)

INTRINSIC SHOULDER PAIN

Intrinsic pain is most often caused by acute trauma, minor chronic trauma (overuse or strain), arthritides (osteoarthritis is fairly common, rheumatoid arthritis less so), local infection or tumour, infectious arthritis and capsulitis in association with any condition that causes splinting. When the supraspinatus tendon, acromioclavicular joint, sternoclavicular joint or anterior subacromial area is implicated as the source of pain, the specific structure will be exquisitely sensitive to touch (Steindler 1959, DePalma 1973).

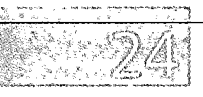

Examination for trigger points requires more diligence and pressure to identify the cause of pain referral (Travell & Simons 1983).

EXTRINSIC SHOULDER PAIN

Cervical radiculopathy affecting the C5–T1 roots is a common neurological cause of shoulder pain; however, cervical lesions may cause multilevel nerve root irritation without radiculitis (Bateman 1978). Other neurological disorders affecting the shoulder are pathology in the cervical roots, the brachial plexus and the axillary, suprascapular or other peripheral nerves (Gerhart et al 1985).

Additional causes of extrinsic pain are myofascial trigger points in the muscles of the neck and shoulder, severe temporomandibular joint disease, cervicodorsal ligamental sprains, thoracic outlet syndromes, injuries to the brachial plexus and referred pain from visceral disorders, such as gallstones, cholecystitis, hepatitis, myocardial infarction, pneumonitis or tumours of the lung or spinal cord (Bonica 1990). When pain is referred to the shoulder, a common site of pain is the anterior-superior portion of the shoulder. Three clues suggest exclusively extrinsic causes:

1. virtual absence of objective findings in the shoulder joint
2. normal active and passive range of movement (ROM) without pain
3. absence of point tenderness with direct pressure on the bicipital tendon, supraspinatus tendon and the clavicular joints.

Pain referred from the shoulder is rarely felt beyond the insertion of the deltoid; therefore a primary or secondary extrinsic cause is suggested when the extremities are affected. Pain of combined intrinsic and extrinsic aetiology increases with ageing, i.e. in older patients shoulder pain is more likely to be complicated by spondylosis or multiple involvement of nerve root and degeneration of the joint, particularly of muscles of the rotator cuff. Myofascial disorders are often present as a secondary disorder in conjunction with acute or nonacute trauma and degenerative conditions.

Finally, there are a number of factors that may contribute to the aetiology and intensity of a painful event. These include stressors, either physical or psychological, latent trigger points from previous injuries and the patient's physical and psychological 'interpretation' of the pain and its importance.

IMPORTANT ELEMENTS OF THE HISTORY

The first purpose of the history is to determine whether the pain experienced in the upper extremity actually originates in the structures of the neck, shoulder, forearm or wrist. Observation of the total patient is important. Does the patient appear ill? Is he or she feverish or reporting recent illness? What is the patient's age and general health status? Does the patient appear tense or report unusual stresses?

Pertinent data can usually be elicited by asking what the patient thinks the problem is. If it is necessary to lead the patient, the examiner should ask what has happened recently, if the patient has been involved in a motor vehicle accident in the past or whether there has been any change in work or recreational activities.

Always using the vocabulary of the patient, the history taker should question him or her closely about the chronological development of the symptoms and the onset and nature of the pain. Where is it felt? Does it feel superficial or deep, such as bone pain? What does it feel like? 'Pins and needles', 'burning sensations' and 'shooting pains' are terms easily understood. Does the patient experience a 'grating feeling' when turning the head or neck? Does he or she experience electric-like pain on flexion or extension of the neck? Has the patient experienced any arthritis/gout/rheumatic problems? Does the patient have other aches and pains? Difficulty in swallowing? Does the patient have unusual sensations into the hand or fingers? Has the patient had the same problem before? If so, what was the diagnosis and treatment?

It is wise also to question the effects of the pain. Is there anything the patient normally does that he or she cannot do because of pain? Does riding in a car aggravate the condition? Does pain result in limitation of movements or weakness? Is it worse at night? Does it interfere with sleep or result in the patient's assuming different sleeping positions?

The history should also include recent medical care and medication or drug use. Has the patient been treated recently by another physician? Were any X-rays taken? Has the patient been hospitalized, particularly because of injury to the back or upper extremity? Is the patient taking any drugs, antibiotics? Heavy alcohol consumption may be a significant clue and exposure to industrial chemicals may play a part in upper extremity pain. (See also Ch. 35 for a discussion of peripheral neuropathies caused by diabetes or thyroid disease, nutritional deficiencies, metabolic disorders, infections and other entities.)

EXAMINATION

Head, neck, and cervical spine

A thorough screening to determine the probable aetiology of upper extremity pain usually begins with at least a routine evaluation of head, neck and cervical spine. The few procedures outlined below are adequate to eliminate these structures as the probable source of pain in the initial assessment.

1. Visual inspection, looking for deformities, atrophy, loss of normal contour
2. Palpation of spinous and transverse processes, thyroid gland and carotid pulse
3. Range of movement of head and neck, with rotation right to left, flexion/extension and lateral bending
4. Distraction or evaluation of the effect of cervical traction by placing hands on occiput and under chin
5. Compression: if neural foramina are compromised, this may produce or intensify pain
6. Valsalva manoeuvre to determine if straining with breath holding reproduces pain
7. Lhermitte's sign: flexion or extension of the head and neck causes lancinating or 'electric' shock radiating from neck into hands (Brody & Wilkins 1969)
8. Adson's test: in the modified Adson's test, the patient's arm is abducted to 90° and externally rotated with the elbow flexed. The patient turns the head toward the abducted arm, takes a deep breath and coughs. The test is positive if the radial pulse is reduced or absent. This may indicate compression of the subclavian artery (Adson 1951).

Testing for radiculitis is based on radiation of symptoms such as sensory changes, weakness and loss of reflexes. If the symptoms are aggravated by cervical tests that stretch the nerve roots, increase intraspinal pressure (Valsalva manoeuvre) or decrease the spinal formina (head compression), the diagnosis is implied.

Cervical spondylosis, which results in gradually increasing clinical signs, may present multiple levels of nerve root irritation and contribute to confusion of diagnosis, particularly in patients over 55 years of age. In younger age groups, single nerve root involvement due to cervical herniation is more common (see Chs 37 and 54).

A summary of neurological levels relating to the upper extremity is shown in Table 24.2. Weakness in any of these extremity structures calls for further evaluation of the cervical spine in addition to assessment of the extremity itself.

Local structures

The shoulder joint has the most complex motions of the body (Saha 1961, Post 1987). They are possible because the shoulder girdle is composed of three joints (the sternoclavicular, acromioclavicular and glenohumeral) which work with the scapulothoracic articulation in a synchronized pattern to provide extension, flexion, abduction, adduction, internal and external rotation. ROM in any of the three joints may be inhibited because of pain, neurological deficit or skeletal or soft tissue pathology. Both extremities should be tested for active and passive ROM to characterize the pain pattern and compared. ROM should also be tested against resistance. If any weakness is noted, a thorough muscle test and grading should be done.

Table 24.2 Summary of neurological levels relating to upper extremity pain and/or dysfunction

	Motor	*Sensory*	*Reflex*
C5	Shoulder abduction, deltoids, biceps	Lateral aspect, arm (C5 axillary nerve)	Biceps
C6	Wrist extension	Lateral forearm, musculocutaneous	Brachioradialis
C7	Wrist flexion Finger extension	Middle finger	Triceps
C8	Finger flexion	Medial forearm	Finger flexion Hand intrinsics
T1	Finger abduction	Medial arm	Hand intrinsics

Pain upon abduction between 60–120° suggests supraspinatus tendinitis; pain with forward flexion up to 90° with internal rotation suggests rotator cuff involvement due to impingement; pain at 140–180° of abduction suggests acromioclavicular joint pain. In testing ROM, the first 30–40° involve only glenohumeral motion and patients may compensate for restriction in this area with scapulothoracic motion.

Observations of joint noises, crepitation or loss of normal gliding motion suggest that degenerative changes and intrinsic injury must be ruled out. A not uncommon condition is friction rub secondary to exostoses either on the scapula or rib, causing pain, although ROM may be normal. When this is suspected, special thoracic and scapular X-ray views are required.

Point tenderness examination of the two clavicular joints, supraspinatus tendon, bicipital tendon and anterior subacromial region (for impingement syndrome) will usually be sufficient to identify local pathology. Figure 24.1 provides a review of shoulder structures with common points of tenderness. Palpation must be done gently, as excessive pressure will be painful and may irritate sensitive tissues. To palpate the bicipital groove, the arm is rotated externally (Yergason's test). The groove lies between the medial lesser tuberosity and the more lateral greater tuberosity. Passive extension of the shoulder will allow examination of the bursa and the cuff as it moves these

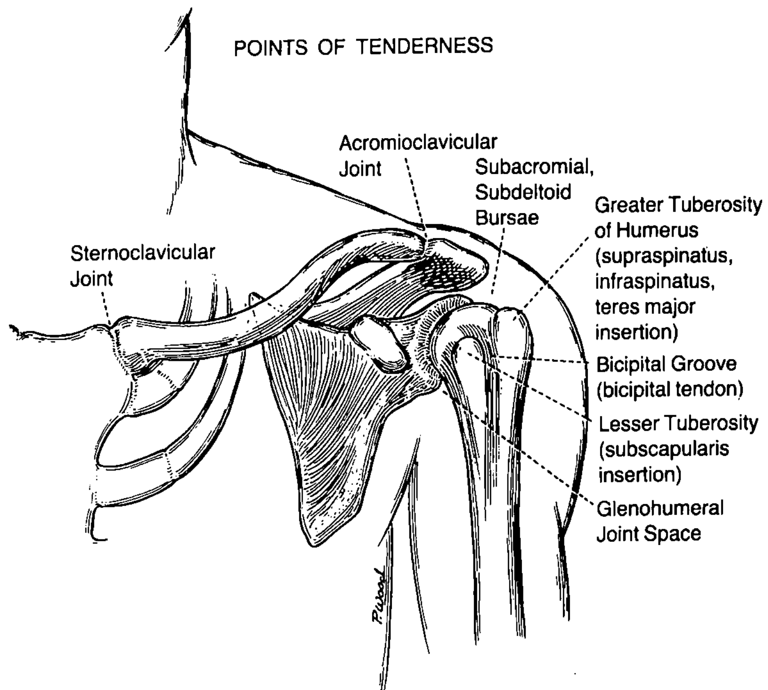

Fig. 24.1 Shoulder joint pain can arise from the greater tuberosity, the lesser tuberosity, the subacromial bursa, the subdeltoid bursa, bicipital groove and the long head of the biceps, the glenohumeral joint and the acromioclavicular joint. When degenerative changes interact with clinical findings, severe pain, dysfunction or loss of range of movement may result. Poor muscle tone, often associated with ageing, tends to exacerbate shoulder lesions.

structures forward; the insertion of the subscapularis is not palpable. Swelling and unusual warmth should be noted. Careful examination may reveal abnormal masses or thickening. Fluid can never be palpated in a normal synovial joint and its presence is a sign of joint pathology. If a ligament is tender or painful on palpation, the ligament has been injured or there is pathology at the joint. Palpation of muscle will identify sensitive trigger points that may be the primary or secondary cause of pain.

SUPPORTING DIAGNOSTIC PROCEDURES

Often careful history taking, palpation and range of motion will establish a clear aetiology for upper extremity pain on the initial visit. However, with more complex problems or combined aetiologies, two or three evaluation visits may be necessary and it may be helpful to utilize supporting diagnostic procedures such as special roentgenographs or electromyograms (EMG) with peripheral nerve conduction studies.

Diagnostic radiographic studies

Radiographic studies are done on joints as indicated by the initial work-up. In any situation where diagnosis is difficult, these studies should include anterior/posterior and lateral views of the neck in extended, neutral and flexed positions and also oblique views to visualize the neuroforamina. Routine shoulder films include anterior and posterior views and abduction, axillary and bicipital groove views. Note that negative findings do not rule out pathology. Even positive findings do not necessarily explain the cause of pain or other symptoms.

High-resolution ultrasonography is particularly helpful as a non-invasive procedure to rule out rotator cuff tears. If there is any question or a tear is suspected, it is most easily confirmed by arthrography and magnetic resonance imaging (MRI). MRI holds great promise for evaluation and diagnosis of soft tissue injuries. MRI technology is particularly valuable in diagnosing damage to tendons, ligaments and fibrocartilage and tears in the rotator cuff or glenoid labrum.

EMG and peripheral nerve conduction studies

EMG is particularly valuable for identifying peripheral neuropathies and for eliminating cervical lesions, discogenic disease and nerve root entrapment as probable contributors to pain and dysfunction in the upper extremity. It is the only reliable tool for identifying peripheral neurocervical radiculitis.

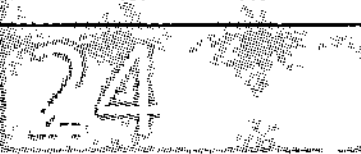

ROTATOR CUFF INJURIES

TENDINITIS

Tendinitis is generally a non-traumatic lesion which occurs as the result of gradual degenerative changes in the rotator cuff. These changes may or may not be accompanied by calcium deposits in the tendon. A mild ache or discomfort may be present for months. In calcific tendinitis the ache may suddenly develop into an intolerable, unremitting pain, usually referred to the top or lateral aspect of the shoulder. The patient will usually hold the arm immobile against the body. Deep breathing may increase the pain. This acute episode may be associated with acute bursitis as a result of calcium, which may form in the tendon in response to injury, penetrating into the bursal sac. Since the condition is related to degenerative changes, it is more common after the fifth decade of life (Calliet 1981).

Signs and symptoms

It is usually possible to arrive at a working diagnosis of shoulder tendinitis through physical examination, including resisted range of motion. With involvement of the supraspinatus tendon, pain is often localized at the greater tuberosity of the humerus. The patient may be unable or unwilling to move the arm but full passive range of motion is possible. Pain upon resisted abduction is an indication of supraspinatus tendinitis. Infraspinatus involvement is also associated with pain localized at the greater tuberosity, but it is resisted external rotation which exacerbates the pain. Tendinitis of teres minor results in pain at the greater tuberosity which is aggravated by resisted external rotation. Pain experienced locally at the lesser tuberosity may be tendinitis of the subscapularis. This will be further confirmed if the pain is associated with resisted medial rotation. Bicipital tendinitis most frequently involves the long head of the biceps muscle. Pain is experienced locally in the bicipital groove and at its attachment at the superior rim of the glenoid fossa.

Treatment course and prognosis

Calcific tendinitis in the acute stage may require immobilization of the arm in a sling, the use of cold packs, medication with oral anti-inflammatory and non-steroidal anti-inflammatory products, local anaesthetic and steroid injections. Some patients may require the use of a narcotic for several days. If this treatment course is not successful, some physicians prefer to aspirate the joint. Milder cases usually respond to conservative treatment. The most important aspect of treatment is early mobilization of the shoulder starting with passive pendular exercises. These are followed by active pendular exercises as soon as tolerated.

BURSITIS

Unfortunately, the term 'bursitis' is often used inappropriately for any painful shoulder. Specifically, bursitis is an acute inflammatory response usually associated with the deposition of calcific material. The bursa swells and impinges upon surrounding structures, causing excruciating pain. Primary bursitis is an uncommon entity, but it does occur. Inflammation of the bursa is more likely to occur secondarily to a tear or inflammation of adjacent tendon or muscle or to direct trauma. It is essentially a disease of middle age, being associated with degenerative changes of tendon, muscle or the rotator cuff, although it is occasionally seen in a young patient.

Signs and symptoms

Subdeltoid bursitis is characterized by painful passive arc. Passive abduction is limited by pain at approximately 70° through 110–115°, after which point the pain disappears. The pain is usually sharp and localized. Abduction and external rotation increase the pain dramatically, although any motion can cause pain. Pain seems to be aggravated at night. Roentgenograms may confirm the presence of calcific deposits. It is important to note, however, that only 35% of patients with X-ray evidence of calcium develop symptoms. Symptoms usually accompany calcium deposits greater than 1.5 cm.

Treatment course and prognosis

Treatment for bursitis is much the same as for calcific tendinitis. An unfortunate sequela of bursitis is adhesive capsulitis, particularly without proper treatment to ensure range of motion.

BICIPITAL TENDINITIS

The long head of the big tendon passes through the bicipital groove across the shoulder joint and is attached to the superior rim of the glenoid cavity. As a result of degenerative changes, chronic irritation may occur over the anterior aspect of the shoulder. This is often related to repetitious movement. This condition is frequently misdiagnosed as bursitis because of the similarity of location of pain.

Signs and symptoms

Bicipital tendinitis should be suspected if there is pain and tenderness to pressure over the bicipital groove. Yergason's sign (increased pain on resistance to supination) is a positive indicator, as is a palpable, swollen tendon. The pain of bicipital tendinitis may occur after heavy lifting and is associated with unusual athletic activity in young adults.

Treatment course and prognosis

Most of these patients respond to conservative treatment of resting the arm in a sling and providing analgesics for pain. Some clinicians advise local injections of steroids, but this writer has seen several cases in which this treatment has resulted in rupture of the tendon. Range of motion must be maintained during treatment to prevent 'frozen shoulder' or adhesive capsulitis. This is usually done passively until pain is adequately controlled, at which time active exercises are introduced.

ROTATOR CUFF TEARS

The rotator cuff is a band of tendinous-fibrous tissue composed of the tendons of the subscapularis, supraspinatus, infraspinatus and teres minor muscles, which fuse around the anatomic neck of the humerus where it inserts with the joint capsule. This part of the cuff is characterized by a marginal blood supply, which contributes to early degeneration, which in turn is associated with minor tears from normal activities.

Tears of the rotator cuff should be considered in conjunction with injuries sustained while working with arms overhead, with falls involving striking the shoulder or breaking the force of the fall with an outstretched hand and with fractures or dislocations of the shoulder and greater tuberosity of the humerus. Residual pain subsequent to an earlier injury with loss of range of motion should also suggest rotator cuff tear. Degenerative cervical disease is a predisposing factor. Small tears may not require treatment. It has been reported that 30% of cadavers have rotator cuff tears.

Signs and symptoms

Rotator cuff tears are associated with pain at the anterolateral margin of the acromion. They are rare in patients under 40 years with the exception of those using the joint heavily. The patient, most often a labourer between the ages of 40 and 65, reports feeling a tear or snap in the shoulder, followed by severe pain if the tear is extensive. With less severe tears, the pain may increase in intensity, reaching a peak after 48 hours and remaining in an acute stage for several days. Shoulder motion increases the pain, which is usually felt first in the shoulder joint but may spread to the posterior scapular area and to the deltoid and forearm. Frequently the pain is described as a deep, throbbing sensation and it may interfere with sleep.

Physical findings may include exquisite tenderness on pressure over the greater tuberosity, reduced abduction or pain on resisted abduction and weakness on forward flexion or pain on internal rotation. Scapulohumeral dysrhythm may be present. The patient may be unable to control lowering of the arm to his side and it may drop freely. This is a useful guide for rotator cuff tears, but it should be noted that injuries to the suprascapular and axillary nerves, as well as fifth cervical root lesions, produce the same clinical sign. Atrophy of the rotator cuff suggests an injury several weeks old which involves the supraspinatus or infraspinatus muscles.

To rule out a diagnosis of rotator cuff impingement, 5 ml of local anaesthetic is injected laterally into the subacromial bursa just underneath the acromial arch. Relief of pain and improved strength around the shoulder joint following injection confirm rotator cuff impingement syndrome.

Treatment course and prognosis

Suspected lesions must be confirmed by contrast radiography, ultrasonography or MRI. Minor tears respond to nonsurgical treatment and usually heal within 2 months. Since tears are often associated with some degree of degenerative process, they tend to be a chronic problem. Severe tears should be evaluated by an orthopaedic surgeon for possible repair (Neviaser 1975, Post 1987) (Table 24.3).

ADHESIVE CAPSULITIS

Adhesive capsulitis affects the glenohumeral joint. Adhesions form as a result of an inflammatory response which produces saturation with a serofibrinous exudate. It is a common finding secondary to heavy use, immobilization, injury, tendonitis, fractures about the shoulder, infections, neoplasms, general surgery and heart attacks. Bicipital tenosynovitis is also reported as a frequent cause. McLaughlin (1961) maintains that a shoulder which is put through the full range of movement a few times daily will not develop adhesive capsulitis, indicating that prolonged dependency is the initiating factor. The condition is unusual in patients under 40 years of age.

Table 24.3 Shoulder pain: clinical findings and treatment (adapted from Lippert & Teitz 1987)

Differential diagnosis	*Key findings*	*Key tests*	*Treatment*
Imingement syndrome	Acromial pain on lumeral forward flexion beyond 90°, tenderness on anterior insertion supraspinatus tendon	Reduced pain with subacromial lidocaine	NSAID; subacromial steroid injection (× 3 max); cuff-strengthening exercises; acromioplasty
Rotator cuff tears	Weak external rotation; supraspinatus atrophy; painful arc 60–120°; difficulty initiating abduction; usually more painful at night; uncommon in patients under 40 years	Drop-arm test positive; subacromial dye extravasation on arthrogram	Cuff-strengthening exercises for small tears; surgery large tears
Supaspinatus tendinitis	Pain tenderness; pain with external rotation	Calcification on X-ray	NSAID; acromioplasty
Biceps tendinitis	Positive Yergason's test; tender bicipital groove; anterior shoulder pain	None	NSAID; restricted-activity; surgery
Frozen shoulder	Diffuse pain and tenderness; decreased passive glenohumeral motion	Reduced capsular space on arthrogram	Range of movement exercises
Glenohumeral arthritis	Increased pain with activity; barometric sensitivity	X-rays	NSAID; arthroplasty
AC joint arthritis	AC; joint tenderness and pain with adduction 140–180°	X-ray, injections of lidocaine into AC joint decreases pain	NSAID; AC joint steroid injection (×3 max); distal clavicle resection

AC = acromioclavicular; NSAID = nonsteroidal antiinflammatory drug.

Signs and symptoms

The patient may report pain with a gradual onset without any known injury. It is often seen in sedentary persons who have recently begun to participate in an activity involving the upper extremities, such as golf, tennis or bowling (Neer & Welsh 1977). The patient will have difficulty putting on a shirt, combing hair or placing the hand in a back pocket. There may be little pain on palpation, but it will be aggravated by both external and internal rotation. Pain may seem to localize in the deltoid, particularly at its insertion, and frequently causes suffering at night.

A tentative diagnosis of adhesive capsulitis must be confirmed with arthrography to differentiate a simple stiff shoulder from the inflammatory condition. Neviaser (1975) classifies patients according to how much of the injected dye is accepted into the capsule and what the patient's range of passive abduction indicates. Abduction to more than 90° and dye acceptance of more than 10 ml indicates a mild form. Moderate involvement includes patients who cannot abduct over 90° and whose capsular joint space measures from 5 to 10 ml. A third classification is severe capsulitis, which is usually seen only after proximal humerus fracture in patients with osteoporosis or following severe shoulder dislocation.

Treatment course and prognosis

The best treatment for adhesive capsulitis is prevention with regular, daily range of movement exercises. Fortunately, many cases respond to a conservative treatment programme consisting mainly of steroid therapy and pain management in conjuction with an aggressive physical therapy programme carried out by a qualified physical therapist. The judicious use of steroids injected into the rotator cuff and intra-articular space may be helpful when applied in combination with intensive physical therapy (Sheon et al 1987).

Local anaesthetics may be adequate to facilitate therapy but local nerve block, particularly of the suprascapular nerve, may be indicated. Muscle relaxants are sometimes helpful. Trigger points can be injected with either lidocaine or procaine to reduce the possibility of a pain cycle. Manipulation is frequently used. When the degree of involvement is greater, manipulation may require anaesthesia. The arm may be positioned in 90° abduction during a period of 2 weeks bedrest, followed by a 3–6-month therapy programme usually leading to full recovery. The use of narcotics is not recommended over an extended period of time. Depression is not uncommon in these patients and it should be recognized and treated as necessary.

BICIPITAL LESIONS

BICIPITAL SUBLUXATION

The same type of degenerative process that precipitates tendonitis can predispose older patients toward subluxation of the tendon. In younger individuals this condition may be associated with sports activities.

Signs and symptoms

When the transverse ligament is torn, local tenderness is normally experienced. The clinician may be able to feel the muscle 'snap' in and out of the groove upon passive rotation of the arm in the abducted position.

Treatment course and prognosis

When subluxation occurs in a young active person, surgery is indicated. Bicipital subluxation can lead to chronic tenosynovitis. In the older individual, restriction of activity may be the preferable course unless the patient is experiencing severe pain.

BICIPITAL RUPTURE

Bicipital rupture is another condition which is usually related to degenerative changes in the biceps tendon or muscle. It may be a painless condition in which the biceps has completely separated between the muscle belly and the tendon or away from the supraglenoid fossa.

Signs and symptoms

Complete separation can usually be visualized. The flaccid biceps muscle bulges.

Treatment course and prognosis

In younger patients surgical repair is indicated. In older patients, if decrease of upper extremity strength would not impair lifestyle, no treatment is required although it may be desirable for cosmetic reasons.

ACROMIOCLAVICULAR JOINT LESIONS

Lesions of the acromioclavicular joint are one of the most overlooked causes of shoulder and arm pain. The joint is subject to arthritic involvement, to various injuries including sprains, contusions and separations, and to tumours, although these are rare (DePalma 1957).

Signs and symptoms

Pain associated with the acromioclavicular joint is usually local without referral. It is aggravated by shrugging the shoulder and by full passive adduction of the arm across the chest. X-rays are not particularly useful for diagnostic purposes if the aetiology is an arthritic process, but they will rule out separation of the joint. Separation usually involves pain over the entire shoulder, often accompanied by weakness of all shoulder movements and loss of function. Palpation of the clavicular attachment may reveal subluxation, in which the clavicle usually displaces upward.

The symptoms of degenerative arthritis include tenderness, swelling and/or warmth over the joint.

Treatment course and prognosis

In the case of mild injury of the joint, a shoulder elbow strap is used for immobilization for 1–2 weeks as needed. If the injury is more severe (subluxation) the strap is worn for up to 5–6 weeks. Surgery may be necessary if immobilization is not successful. The shoulder joint must be passively put through the range of movement as tolerated by pain. In addition, appropriate measures to prevent disabilities to the hand, wrist and elbow must be taken.

ARTHRITIS

The shoulder joint has only minimal susceptibility to arthritis, probably because it is not a weight-bearing joint and only under certain conditions is it a power-bearing joint. To a great extent it escapes the destructive degenerative changes of repeated pressure and trauma. The major exception to this is athletes, particularly those who load the joint in 'bursts'. Osteoarthritis is moderately common among persons who play baseball and overhead racquet sports, skiers and musicians, being activity related rather than disease related. However, osteoarthritis and traumatic arthritis do occur in other patients and symptoms of painful, swollen, warm joints should suggest a systematic work-up for arthritic involvement. Other arthritides, including rheumatoid arthritis, are discussed elsewhere in this book.

HEMIPLEGIA

Shoulder pain is a common complaint of people with hemiplegia. It can be so severe that it interferes with the rehabilitation programme that is so crucial immediately after 'stroke'. Appropriate splinting to prevent capsular stretching and resultant subluxation of the glenohumeral joint is necessary early in therapy and should help to prevent the complication of pain.

Treatment of the pain is comparable to that used in other painful shoulder conditions: injections of steroids, local anaesthetics, suprascapular nerve block and oral medications consistent with the medical status of the patient. These patients should be managed by medical personnel trained in rehabilitation or by a healthcare team which includes a physical therapist.

PAIN OF COMBINED AETIOLOGIES

MYOFASCIAL DISORDERS

An understanding of myofascial disorders, their pain patterns, incidence, origins and proper treatment is absolutely essential in treatment of upper extremity pain (Travell & Rinzler 1952, Sola & Kuitert 1955, Sola et al 1955, Sola & Williams 1956, Kraft et al 1968, Kraus 1970, Simons 1975, 1976, Travell 1976, Melzack et al 1977, Sola 1981, Sola 1984, Bonica 1990, Roberts & Hedges 1991, Travell & Simons 1998).

Like the lower back, the shoulder and neck region are commonly the 'storehouse' of numerous latent points that, when challenged by physical (and, to some degree, emotional) stressors, can cause pain. The mechanism of pain can be described as follows: from an initiating stimulus such as trauma, fatigue or stress, a physiological response is generated and a particular trigger point begins to send distress signals to the central nervous system. Muscles associated with the trigger point become tense and soon muscle fatigue is experienced. Local ischaemia occurs, leading to change in the extracellular environment of the affected cells, including release of algesic agents. These feed into a cycle of increasing motor and sympathetic activity and other trigger points 'flare up', contributing to the cycle (Zimmerman 1980). Thus a painful event may be magnified far out of proportion to its precipitating challenge (Fig. 24.2). Furthermore, once established as a cycle, a painful event may sustain itself in spite of control of the stimulus which originally initiated the cycle. Thus, proper

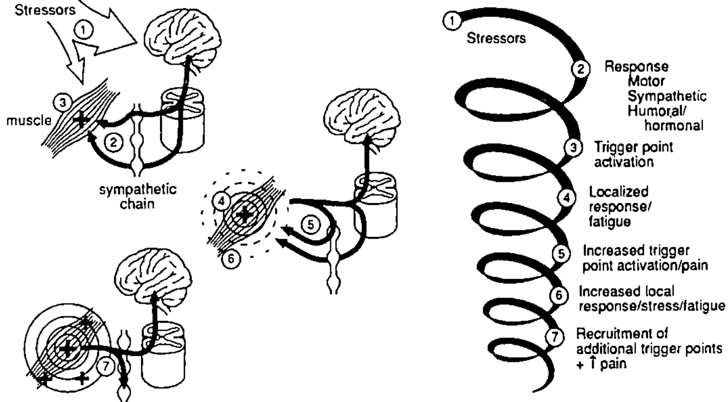

Fig. 24.2 The pain cycle. The individual, subjected to the physical and emotional stresses of daily living (1), responds with defence mechanisms (2) that include various physiological changes, such as splinting and bracing of muscles, vasomotor changes, increased sympathetic discharge and hormonal and other humoral changes in the plasma and extracellular fluids. A particular point in a braced, stressed muscle or fascia that is more sensitive than the surrounding tissue, perhaps due to previous injury or genetic mandate, fatigues and begins to signal its distress to the central nervous system (3). A number of responses may result. The most readily understood involves the motor reflexes. Various muscles associated with the trigger point become more tense and begin to fatigue. Sympathetic responses lead to vasomotor changes within and around the trigger point. Local ischaemia after vasoconstriction or increased vascular permeability after vasodilatation may lead to changes in the extracellular environment of the affected cells, release of algesic agents (bradykinins, prostaglandins), osmotic changes and pH changes, all of which may increase the sensitivity or activity of nociceptors in the area. Sympathetic activity may cause smooth muscle contraction in the vicinity of nociceptors, increasing their activity (4), which contributes to the cycle by increasing motor and sympathetic activity. This in turn leads to increased pain (5). The pain is shadowed by growing fatigue, adding an overall mood of distress to the patient's situation and feeding back to the cycle (6). As tense muscles in the affected area begin to fatigue in an environment of sympathetic stimulation and local biochemical change, latent trigger points within these muscles may also begin to fire, adding to the positive feedback cycle and spreading the pain to these adjacent muscle groups. The stress of pain and fatigue, coupled with both increased muscle tension and sympathetic tone through the body (conceivably with ipsilateral emphasis through the sympathetic change), may lead to flare-ups or trigger points in other muscles remote from the initial area of pain (7).

and adequate treatment of a local injury may not provide alleviation of pain.

Trigger-point syndromes affect virtually everyone, either in a primary role of translating stress responses into pain or in a secondary role in which activation intensifies or prolongs pain from another stimulus. Trigger-point pain varies from slight discomfort to severe unrelenting pain and is described as either sharp or dull. It can also simulate the pain of visceral disorders which are referred to the shoulder area.

THE 'INJURY POOL' CONCEPT

Trigger points (TPs) seem to be involved in a phenomenon by which the body 'remembers' previous injury. Tissues that were affected by an earlier injury become prone to react to a new challenge. Each new insult may provide additional TPs that become part of an 'injury pool'. These 'pooled' TPs may in turn be recruited into the pain cycle in response to a later injury (Fig. 24.3). Thus a painful stimulus in a young person may be painful in direct proportion to the damage with little or no myofascial involvement in the pain process. However, in an individual with an established 'pool' of repeated injuries (generally an older individual), an injury may well be accompanied by myofascial pain and muscle involvement out of proportion to the insult (Sola 1984).

Many physicians are only now becoming aware of TPs and their significance. Most of the scapular muscles can cause shoulder pain, including the cuff muscles (infraspinati, supraspinati, subscapularis, teres minor), pectoralis major and minor, teres major and trapezii (Fig. 24.4). The erector spinii are often overlooked as a frequent source of TPs. Posterior and anterior strap muscles can also refer pain to the shoulder and TPs present in the lumbar-gluteal region can activate TPs in the shoulder girdle.

It is important to note that although trigger-point pain can affect both sides of the body, it is commonly confined to one side and is often associated with ipsilateral hypersensitivity in muscles seemingly quite removed from the reported problem. For example, pain in the neck and shoulder is commonly associated with gluteal TPs that are exquisitely sensitive to pressure even though the patient may not report overt pain in these muscles. In such cases treatment must involve the remote ipsilateral TPs as well as those in the painful area (see Fig. 24.5).

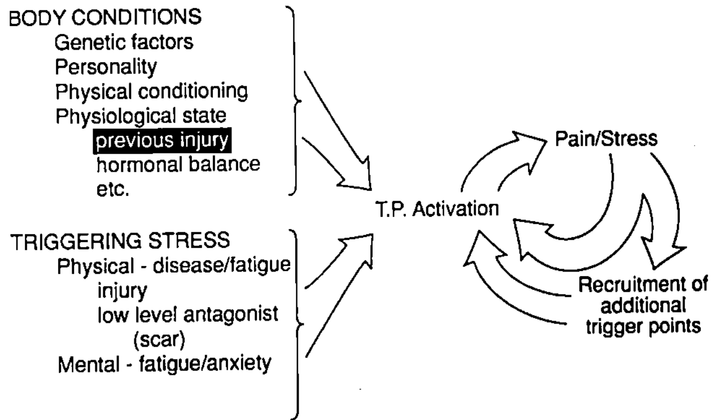

Fig. 24.3 Injury pool. A variety of stress-inducing stimuli may be implicated in the onset of myofascial pain. The power of these stimuli to induce pain is moderated by the genetics, personality, conditioning and physiological state of a particular individual. Once established, however, a painful event may sustain itself despite control or elimination of the initiating stimuli.

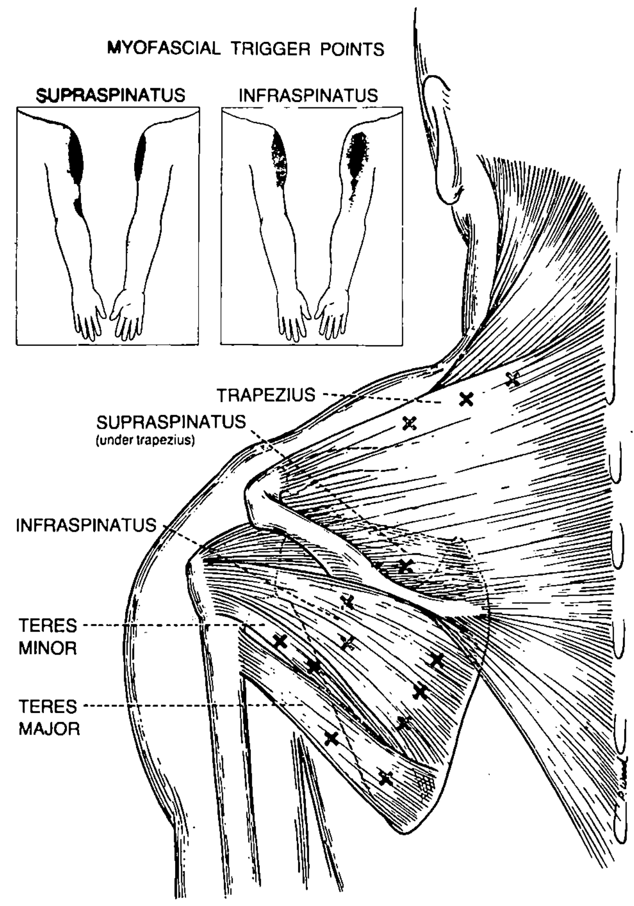

Fig. 24.4 Trigger points tend to concentrate in groups of muscles, such as the shoulder. When activated, adjacent muscle groups may become involved. The scapular muscles refer pain to the posterior or lateral surface of the shoulder girdle. The trapezius usually has local pain at the trigger points and refers to the posterior scalp and neck. Myofascial pain from the shoulder area can be reflected to the proximal arm, wrist or hand and symptoms may include weakness of grip, paraesthesia and hyperhydrosis.

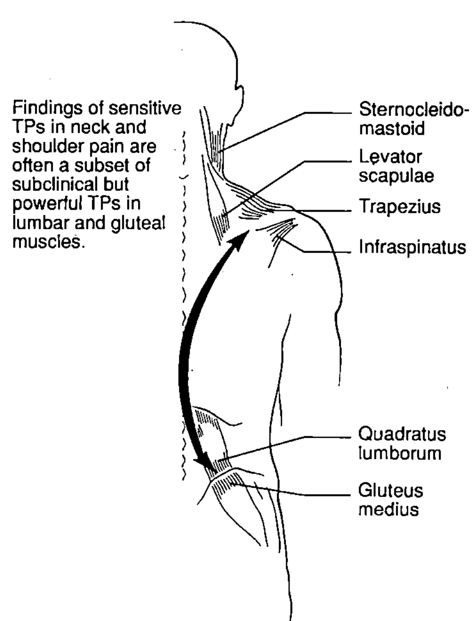

Fig. 24.5 Ipsilateral pain, a diagnostic key to treatment of refractory local pain. An ipsilateral pattern of pain is very common, with simultaneously active painful trigger points in the neck and shoulder, quadratus lumborum and gluteal muscles. The patient may not be aware of pain in the lumbar gluteal region but may confirm aching or stiffness in the hip area, sciatica-like pain or fatigue in the lower back and extremities. Hyperactive trigger points (TPs) in the lumbar gluteal muscles must be treated before positive results can be expected from treatment of TPs in head, neck or extremities.

Treatment course and prognosis

An injection of local anaesthetic or physiological saline into the TPs is often adequate to break the pain cycle (Bray & Sigmond 1941, Frost et al 1980, Tfelt-Hansen et al 1980). The use of vasocoolants, such as fluoromethane spray, has been shown to be a helpful technique by Travell & Daitz (1990). The insertion of thin solid needles alone (dry needling as described by Gunn 1996) has often been found to be as effective as injection without subjecting the patient to the added tissue disruption caused by edged hypodermic needles. When dry needling, local anaesthetic or saline injection prove inadequate, injection of a weak solution of dexamethasone (1 cc diluted in 100 cc of normal saline) is a useful procedure (Edagawa 1994). This treatment presumes that there are no contraindications to steroid use such as diabetes or clotting disorders. When the pain is secondary to another stimulus, particularly nerve root lesions or nerve compression, the treatment is never more than moderately successful in relieving pain. Therefore this procedure is useful as a differential diagnostic tool, as it interrupts the pain cycle and allows exposure of the underlying disorder. Other treatments are being explored. Periosteal stimulation reportedly enhances the effectiveness of TP injection, reducing myofascial pain (Lawrence 1978). There is also new work in the use of laser therapy and interesting work in progress on electromagnetic fields to relieve pain.

REFLEX DYSTROPHY-LIKE SYNDROMES

Reflex dystrophies are part of the group of sympathetic disorders whose features may include throbbing, burning or aching pain, hyperaesthesia, hyperalgesia and oedema and/or erythema. These are serious, painful and disabling disorders. Onset may be triggered by coronary ischaemia, hemiplegia, adhesive capsulitis, bicipital tendinitis, trauma or even simple bruises or sprains. In a study of 140 patients with reflex dystrophy, 40% of the cases occurred following soft tissue injury, 25% following fractures, 20% were post-operative, 12% followed myocardial infarction and 3% followed CVA. It was also noted that 37% of these patients had significant emotional disturbances at the time of onset. Thus elements of the process include CNS involvement and the entire myofascial pain cycle of stressors, trigger-point activation, pain and sympathetic involvement (Fig. 24.2) (Pak et al 1970). Treatment must be instituted immediately and includes injection of the affected trigger points with an anaesthetic–corticosteroid mixture by a specialist and physical therapy. If this provides no relief, one must resort to sympathetic blocks, oral corticosteroids and, finally, sympathectomy. Early treatment of the affected TPs has shown great promise in breaking this cycle.

SHOULDER–HAND SYNDROME

Signs and symptoms

The disease has several stages. Onset is usually insidious. The patient may present with a burning pain involving the shoulder and vasomotor changes in the hand and fingers. This phase may last several months. After this initial phase, shoulder pain may ease but trophic changes appear: atrophy of the muscles in the affected extremity, thickening of palmar fascia, demineralization and atrophy of the nails. By the time these trophic changes have occurred, it is extremely difficult to reverse the disease process despite aggressive treatment and the end result is flexion deformities of the fingers. At this stage vasomotor changes are absent.

Treatment course and prognosis

This condition requires aggressive treatment. Residual damage is usually irreversible; surgery has not proven successful in restoring function. The pain associated with shoulder–hand syndrome can be excruciating and the patient will normally require narcotics for pain management. Phenobarbital should not be given but other sedatives may be used. Sympathetic blocks done early in the course of the disease may be helpful, as well as corticosteroid therapy. Injection of local anaesthetics into hypersensitive areas of the shoulder or the suprascapular nerve may also be helpful. From the outset, treatment must be accompanied by an intensive physical therapy programme to maintain function.

OVERUSE SYNDROMES

Although a given action or set of actions may be well within the body's capabilities, excessive repetition may, through interference with circulation, repeated microinjury, build-up of waste products or any of these and other factors, stress a tissue beyond its anatomical or physiological limits. The stressor may be either dynamic, as in the case of repetitive movement, or static, as in the case of prolonged bracing or maintenance of a particular posture. In 1990 the US Bureau of Statistics reported that more than 180 000 workers suffered overuse injuries. Workers who performed more than 2000 manipulations per hour were particularly vulnerable. Those performing highly repetitive, forceful jobs were most at risk (LaDou 1990).

One should suspect an overuse syndrome when a patient reports that he or she:

1. performs a repetitive task
2. maintains a fixed posture for long periods of time
3. lifts above or below a mechanically strainful height
4. performs a tedious or monotonous task.

Furthermore, it should be suspected when numerous other workers or participants have been disabled performing the same tasks. Such a finding would suggest that an evaluation of the ergonomics of the workplace would be in order (Sheon et al 1987, Khalil et al 1994).

The repeated movements of certain sports such as tennis, swimming and baseball and extended periods of wrist pressure involved in cycling are well-documented sources of overuse injury. So too are certain occupations. For example, musicians are particularly vulnerable to a variety of overuse phenomena. Pianists, clarinettists and oboists may suffer carpal tunnel syndrome or De Quervain's tenosynovitis (both dynamic stressor related), while string and wind players frequently have shoulder problems (static stressor related), especially impingement syndrome, subdeltoid and subacromial bursitis and bicipital tendinitis, and may also demonstrate dynamic problems in the hand or wrist such as carpal tunnel syndrome. Inflammation is rarely apparent on physical examination in patients with overuse syndrome and it is often not clear if the injured structure is tendon, muscle, ligament, joint capsule or a combination of these (Sataloff et al 1990).

CARPAL TUNNEL SYNDROME

Carpal tunnel syndrome is the second most common industrial injury in the United States, surpassed only by low back pain. Workers in occupations which require heavy wrist activity, such as data entry operators, grocery checkers, pipefitters, tool workers, carpenters, secretaries and pianists, are considered most at risk for this syndrome. Recent findings suggest that the condition is exacerbated by psychological stressors such as boredom, insecurity or the stress of other painful processes. Furthermore, recent studies of the wrist using computed tomography suggest that workers with carpal tunnel syndrome tend to have carpal bones of a smaller cross-sectional area (Bleecker 1987). This suggests a potential for screening for those most at risk.

Carpal tunnel syndrome is caused by pressure on the median nerve; this may be due to increased synovial hypertrophy, as it occurs in rheumatoid arthritis, gout, hypothyroidism, diabetes, ganglion tumours or lipomas, pregnancy and trauma. Biomechanical studies have shown that intracarpal pressure is particularly increased with flexon and ulnar deviation. Rosenbaum and Ochoa (1993) suggest that Phalen's wrist flexion test is more reliable than Tinel's nerve stimulation of the median nerve at the wrist in diagnosis of carpal tunnel syndrome.

Signs and symptoms

This syndrome causes paraesthesias and dysthaesias along the median nerve into the hand and wrist. The pain may be localized at the wrist, but may also show retrograde spread to the elbow or shoulder. Shaking or moving the hand may relieve symptoms, suggesting a pressure gradient involving the lymphatic or circulatory system. However, if such shaking causes increased pain, cervical radiculitis should be suspected. Thenar atrophy may be present.

Treatment course and prognosis

Conservative treatment measures include splinting, cortisone injections, rest and/or change in activities. Treatment of trigger points in the forearm, shoulder, neck and, often, gluteal region may help relieve both the pain and dystrophy-like syndromes. In difficult cumulative disorders the patient should ideally begin a 'work-hardening' programme under the supervision of trained hand, occupational or physical therapists to develop strength and endurance. Ergonomic improvements in the workplace may also be required. When other treatments are not effective, surgical release is recommended. Although Silverstein et al (1987) have reported that 58% of surgically treated patients return to their former job, none of these returned to jobs that required forceful repetitive motion.

OTHER PERIPHERAL ENTRAPMENT SYNDROMES

Among the most puzzling pains of the extremity are the peripheral neuropathies (Fig. 24.6). The causes are obscure and differential diagnosis is not easy, especially since cervical nerve root irritation must be considered (Kopell & Thompson 1973, Dyck et al 1976). There is evidence that radiculitis increases the susceptibility to nerve entrapment (Upton & McComas 1973, Bland 1987). Table 24.4 gives some guidelines to differentiate between entrapment and peripheral radiculopathy (Dawson et al 1983, 1990). Peripheral radiculopathy must also be differentiated from cervical spondylosis and other less common entities that

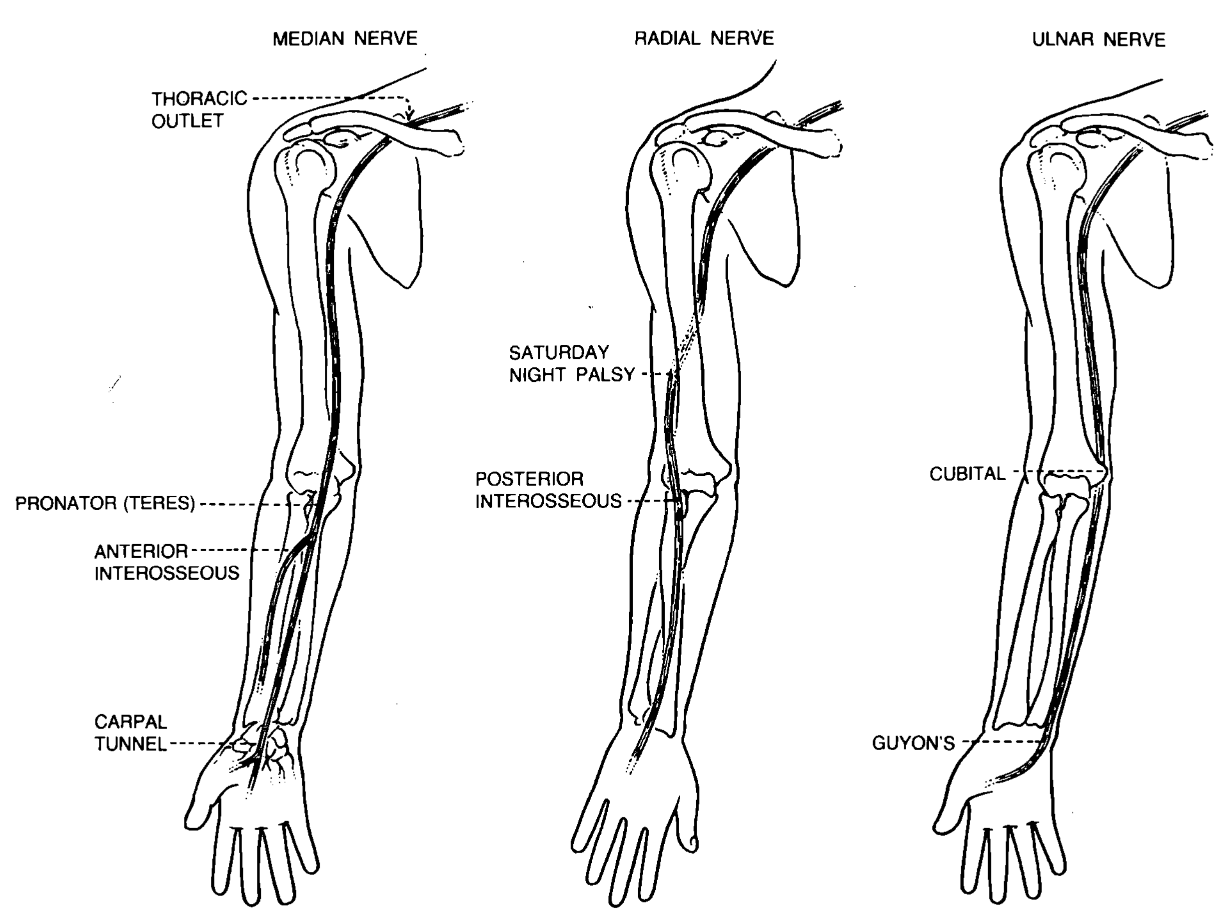

Fig. 24.6 Common neurovascular and peripheral entrapment syndromes. There are four thoracic outlet syndromes: scalenus anticus, costoclavicular syndrome, cervical rib syndrome and hyperabduction syndrome. Peripheral entrapment syndromes affect the radial, ulnar or median nerves and can cause pain at the area of entrapment and in muscles distal to the entrapment. These are often inconsistent or intermittent pains.

Table 24.4 Differentiating between radiculopathy and entrapment syndromes

Radiculopathy	*Entrapment*
Involves posterior division of cervical root; radiation along medial border of scapula	Signs uncommon with entrapment
Pain with coughing, sneezing, Valsalva manoeuvre, highly specific for radiculopathy when present	Signs not associated with entrapment
Pain increases with use of hand	Carpal tunnel syndrome pain is relieved by massage, shaking hand, immersion of hand in water, changing positions
Muscle weakness rarely severe. Most easily identified; deltoid, infraspinatus (C5); biceps, wrist extensors (C6); triceps, long finger flexors, finger extensors (C7); intrinsic muscles of hand and wrist flexors (C8); arm and when testing muscle	Not a diagnostic feature
Electrophysiological studies Nerve conduction studies almost always normal with uncomplicated radiculopathy. EMGs done on a number of arm muscles may show changes in a radicular pattern. Paraspinus muscles may be denervated, confirming nerve root damage. Myelography/computerized tomography delineates lateral disc protrusion	*Electrophysiological studies* local changes may be present
Treatment Successful response to several weeks of conservative treatment (traction, cervical collar, local massage and analgesics) confirms diagnosis	*Treatment* In early stages is likely to respond to conservative treatment; splinting, cortisone, rest. More advanced may require surgical release

cause cervical root irritation, such as tumours, infection, osteophytes, prolapsed disc, fractures and epidural abscess, all of which are considered in Chapter 37 in this book. Note that patients can usually distinguish between pain that radiates from the hand to the shoulder and pain that originates in the neck or shoulder and spreads to the hand. The only definitive way to diagnose peripheral neuropathy is by electromyography and nerve conduction studies in addition to routine radiological studies.

Any one of the entrapment syndromes can cause hand, forearm and shoulder pain which is not consistent in character. Generally, there is some local pain at the area of entrapment, but muscles distal to the entrapment may or may not have pain involvement. Frequently the pain experienced is intermittent, low grade and worse at night. Scapulocostal irritation and myofascial disturbances tend to distort the pain patterns to peripheral nerve compression. Carpal tunnel syndrome is the most common of the nerve compression syndromes affecting the median nerve. Two other conditions related primarily to median nerve compression are pronator teres syndrome and anterior interosseous nerve syndrome. Conditions affecting the radial nerve are radial palsy and posterior interosseous syndrome. Ulnar nerve compression is associated with cubital tunnel syndrome and Guyon's canal compression. In addition to the conditions described below, compression of the suprascapular nerve can cause dull, deep pain in the rhomboid area and dorsal scapular nerve syndrome can cause pain particularly in the posterolateral aspect of the shoulder.

Treatment course and prognosis

Treatment for these syndromes follows much the same pattern as treatment for carpal tunnel syndrome and includes splinting, cortisone injections, rest and/or change in activities, as well as treatment of trigger points in the affected and related areas to help relieve both the pain and dystrophy-like syndromes.

PRONATOR TERES SYNDROME

This syndrome occurs when the median nerve is trapped as the nerve passes below the two heads of the muscle. Pain and paraesthesias occur in flexor muscles of the forearm and in the thenar muscles. There is associated weakness in the muscles.

ANTERIOR INTEROSSEOUS NERVE SYNDROME

This nerve supplies the flexor pollicis longus, the flexor digitorus profundus and the pronator quadratus muscle. Pressure causes weakness or paralysis in the index and middle fingers. When the elbow is flexed, the pronator teres will be weak; the pronator quadratus will be weak in pronation.

RADIAL PALSY

Radial palsy occurs because of excessive pressure over the spiral groove. This affects all muscles of the forearm supplied by the radial nerve. This condition is usually painless, but frequently hyperparaesthesia is present.

POSTERIOR INTEROSSEOUS SYNDROME

Posterior interosseous nerve syndrome describes compression of the radial nerve, where the nerve penetrates the supinator. The patient is able to extend the wrist but unable to extend metacarpophalangeal joints of the fingers, unable to abduct the thumb and unable to extend the distal joint of the thumb.

CUBITAL TUNNEL SYNDROME

Cubital tunnel syndrome describes a condition of pressure on the ulnar nerve as it passes under the medial epicondyle. The patient may experience pain along the ulnar border of the forearm, weakness of intrinsic muscles of the hand and hyperaesthesias.

GUYON'S CANAL COMPRESSION

Guyon's canal compression is impingement on the ulnar nerve where it enters the hand through the canal of Guyon, between the piriform and hamate bones. The condition is associated with fractures or aneurysm of the small artery. The patient may experience local pain and numbness in the ulnar distribution of the fourth and fifth fingers.

TENNIS ELBOW OR EPICONDYLITIS

Signs and symptoms

The patient complains of severe pain in the elbow, frequently radiating to wrist or shoulder. Any grasping movements are painful and the patient may drop things from the hand. The pain is usually described as 'deep'. Pressure applied over the lateral condyles causes extreme pain. Dorsiflexion of the wrist may be painful. This clinical picture of pain is usually accompanied by a history of overuse of the extensors and supinators of the wrist in sports such as tennis and golf and in occupations requiring similar motions such as hammering. It can also be associated with excessive hand shaking. In older patients, this lesion is more likely to be a chronic condition unrelated to a specific activity and much less amenable to treatment. Chronic inflammation of periosteal nerves and blood vessels may contribute to the pain.

Treatment course and prognosis

When a clear association with activity is not present from the history, X-rays may be indicated to eliminate the possibility of fracture or pathological bone formations. Treatment depends on the structures involved. Common extensor and flexor tendons will usually respond to steroids and local anaesthetic. When the extensor carpi radialis tendon is involved, the pain may originate with muscle rather than on the epicondyle and a local anaesthetic may be indicated. Muscle involvement is uncommon at the supracondylar ridge. Joint dysfunction at any of the three elbow joints can cause pain simulating tennis elbow. These are treated by manipulation. Refractory cases of tennis elbow are frequently treated by surgery. Trigger points may occur in any of the muscles around the elbow joint and these frequently respond to injection therapy. Trigger points in the scalenus anticus muscle can frequently refer pain to this area (Zohn & Mennell 1976).

OLECRANON BURSA

Signs and symptoms

The olecranon bursa, which lies over the bony olecranon process, is frequently injured by constant mechanical pressure. Clinically, the bursa sac area becomes red and swollen, warm to the touch and tender on palpation. Occasionally it may become infected. Patients who have gout and rheumatoid arthritis are prone to this disorder.

Treatment course and prognosis

Pain and swelling usually subside if a cushioning ring is used around the area of irritation to prevent further mechanical pressure. If pain persists, fluid can be aspirated from the bursal sac and examined for evidence of infection and/or to differentiate between aetiologies. If the condition is persistent or recurrent, surgical excision may be the treatment of choice.

LIGAMENTAL INJURIES

Ligamental injuries are common at the wrist. Diagnosis is made on the basis of local pain and tenderness. The most frequent of these injuries is sprain of the ulnar collateral ligament, which is characterized by pain on radial deviation. When the radial ligament is sprained or torn, pain is present on ulnar deviation. The ulnar-capitate sprain is also quite common. With flexion of the wrist, pain is felt at the dorsal aspect.

Treatment course and prognosis

Local management with steroid injection treatment is usually effective for ligamental injuries. Ruptures may require surgical intervention.

GANGLION CYST

Signs and symptoms

Ganglia are the most common tumours of the hand and wrist. They are most frequently found on the dorsal aspect of the wrist joint and occasionally on the volar aspect of the wrist. The cystic swelling is found near, and often attached to, a tendon sheath and it is believed that the cyst may be derived from these structures. Ganglia are often painless; however, they can be locally tender and painful.

Treatment course and prognosis

Ganglia are known to disappear spontaneously. However, the usual treatment is puncture of the cyst and aspiration of its contents. Some clinicians inject a corticosteroid into the cyst after aspiration.

DE QUERVAIN'S DISEASE (CONSTRICTIVE TENOSYNOVITIS)

Signs and symptoms

De Quervain's disease may have slow or acute onset precipitated by an injury to the wrist which causes swelling in tendons thickened by the disease process. The patient will present with pain in the wrist and thumb area and weakness of grip. In the acute state, there may be local swelling with symptoms similar to wrist sprain. Examination will reveal marked tenderness to pressure over the styloid process and over the tendons, abductor pollicis longus and extensor pollicis brevis.

The pain is related to thickening and stenosis of the sheath surrounding the tendons. It is most commonly seen in female workers doing heavy hard work, such as cooks and dressmakers who lift heavy material. Diagnosis of De Quervain's disease is affirmed by holding the patient's thumb in flexion and abducting the wrist. This will elicit a pain response.

Treatment course and prognosis

Immobilization is recommended and the area is injected with long-acting anaesthetic. Injectable steroid therapy is also appropriate. In one study, symptoms of infectious arthritis were present in one-quarter of the patients with this condition.

TRIGGER FINGER

As result of injury, small tears in the flexor tendon curl into a ball and form a nodule, usually at the proximal end of the tendon sheath. This nodule interferes with normal gliding motion and abnormal tension is required to force it through the tendon sheath, causing the finger to snap in extension. Palpation of the tendon sheath will usually be painful.

Treatment is the same as for De Quervain's disease: immobilization, steroid injection and surgical release if necessary.

IMPINGEMENT SYNDROMES

Diagnosis of shoulder pain is facilitated by an understanding of impingement syndromes, which are common in athletes and persons doing heavy physical labour. Impingement is diagnosed by point tenderness over the anterior insertion of the supraspinatus tendon and positive findings on forward flexion with internal rotation. The critical test is relief of symptoms with use of local anaesthetic injected into the anterior acromial process (coracoid acromial ligament).

Tendinitis, rotator cuff tears and adhesive capsulitis may all be components of a degenerative process beginning with impingement. When impingement syndromes are present in young persons, they are almost always associated with racquet sports, swimming, baseball, football and repetitive overhead motions (Moseley 1969, Post 1987, Nichols & Hershman 1990).

Neer and Welsh (1977) have suggested three stages.

- Stage I is characterized by oedema and/or inflammation and usually occurs in patients between the ages of 15 and 30 years. Treatment at this stage is conservative; restriction of shoulder movement, anti-inflammatory medications and ice packs. Occasionally steroid injections are given if these measures do not provide relief.

- Stage II is characterized by fibrosis and thickening of the rotator cuff which further compromises subacromial mechanisms. If the patient does not respond to conservative treatment and cuff tear has been ruled out, a partial anterior acromioplasty and sectioning of the coracoid acromial ligament may be necessary.
- Stage III is usually associated with patients over the age of 40 years, when further degeneration has taken place, and it may include partial tears of the rotator cuff and bony changes. Surgery may be necessary to correct the condition, particularly if tears are involved (Post 1987). The diagnosis can be confirmed by an arthrogram (see Table 24.3).

THORACIC OUTLET SYNDROME

Thoracic outlet syndrome (TOS) involves discomfort caused by compression or irritation of the neurovascular bundle by the scalene muscles, rib, clavicle or pectoralis minor muscle. Most commonly, it is the inferior portion of the brachial plexus which is involved, affecting the ulnar and, sometimes, the medial nerves. In a small percentage of cases the subclavian vein may also be compressed.

Signs and symptoms

In this condition, there is a gradual increase in discomfort until the patient experiences pain involving the upper extremity, lower neck region, shoulder and arm. The pain tends to be intermittent and is associated with movement, particularly with lifting objects overhead. The patient may describe a 'pins and needles' sensation in the forearm and wrist and may experience weakness or numbness in the fourth or fifth finger. Symptoms are usually worse in the morning than later in the day. The condition is seen most often in young adult patients with poor posture and is reported more frequently in women.

Palpation or percussion during examination may indicate tenderness of the brachial plexus. A confirming test for TOS is to have the patient assume the 'hold up' position for 3 minutes while slowly opening and closing the hands. If radial pulses remain strong but the patient experiences the usual symptoms, the test is positive for TOS. (The 'hold up' position consists of sitting with both arms elevated to 90° abduction with external rotation. The elbows are maintained somewhat behind the frontal plane.)

Treatment course and prognosis

Insofar as TOS may be related to poor posture, a conservative approach is to recommend posture-related therapy and mild exercise to strengthen shoulder muscles. If the problem can be associated with a particular type of activity or position during sleeping, these should be modified. Medication for muscle relaxation may be indicated. However, all these measures are limited if the condition has progressed to the extent that only surgical procedures can provide decompression. Surgery will establish the presence of congenital fibromuscular bands which could not be identified by X-ray. When these bands are present, they usually affect both sides of the body.

CERVICAL SPRAIN

Cervical sprain or 'whiplash' injury is associated with the rapid acceleration of the neck into hyperextension and/or flexion with subsequent rebound and reflex splinting. Although 'whiplash' can cause cord damage it is most commonly associated with some trauma to the supporting muscles, tendons and ligaments (see Fig. 24.7). It may also be associated with damage or functional compromise of the cervical nerve roots either directly or through the pressures of subsequent muscle spasm (Bland 1987, Bonica 1990, Johnson 1996). Common causes of such injury include automobile or other transportation accidents, falls or high-velocity sports injuries. People also become more vulnerable to these injuries as they age.

The short-term signs of cervical sprain include stiffness and pain in the neck and shoulder girdle, hoarseness or dysphagia (in anterior damage), headache and various sympathetic dystrophy-like symptoms. A normal neurological examination with no swelling or apparent trauma to the neck may be taken as a good indication that there is no spinal or cord damage. Even if the injury appears minimal, the patient must be carefully followed for several days following the incident (Borchgrevink et al 1998). Muscles and ligaments heal within 4–6 weeks, whereas intervertebral discs heal slowly because they have no blood supply. If there is any suspicion of damage to the cervical spine or cord, one must obtain a transtable lateral view of the entire cervical spine.

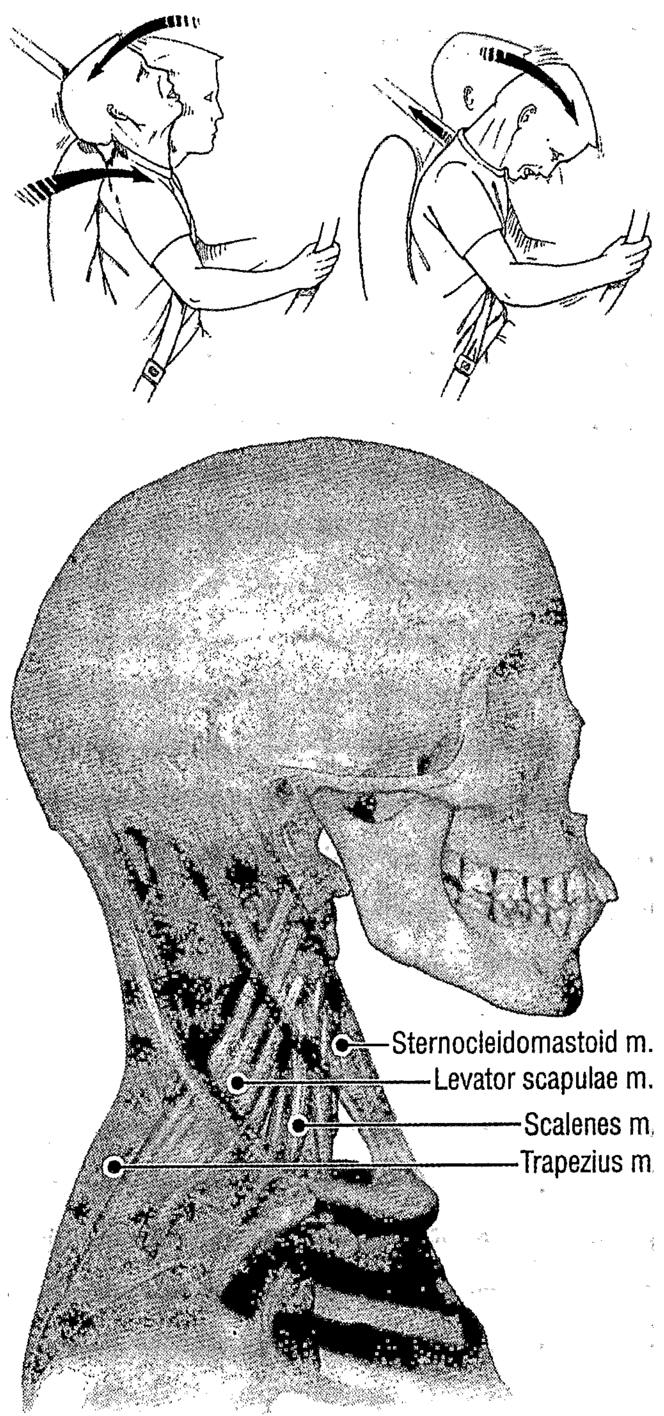

Fig. 24.7 Cervical sprain or 'whiplash' injury from rapid hyperextension and/or flexion and subsequent rebound. 'Whiplash' commonly causes some trauma to the supporting muscles, tendons and ligaments. The scalene, levator scapulae, sternocleidomastoid and posterior cervical muscles are most commonly involved. (Derived from Graney et al, with permission.)

If spinal injury has been ruled out, immediate treatment includes applying mild cervical traction and physical therapy and administration of non-steroidal anti-inflammatory medications. A soft cervical collar may be indicated for a short time although these have not generally been found to be effective. Injury may well involve the scalene, levator scapulae, sternocleidomastoid and posterior cervical muscles. Spasm and TPs in these muscles may affect nerve roots as low as T7 (see Fig. 24.8). Related pain in the muscles of the lower back, becoming apparent at some time after the injury, is also quite common. Thus one must examine the lower torso for painful foci and trigger points with particular attention to the paraspinal muscles and the gluteal muscle group. Trigger points in these areas are often deep and easily overlooked yet they are important. They are not only sources of localized pain but, since they also can exacerbate problems in the neck and shoulders, they may make treatment in those areas less effective if left untreated (see Fig. 24.5).

The application of vasocoolant sprays, injection or dry needling of trigger points in the neck, shoulder girdle and lower back may help to relieve muscle spasm and interrupt the potential for the establishment of a long-term pain cycle precipitated by the injury (see Fig. 24.2). The sternocleidomastoid in particular is a source of such long-term, low intensity TPs.

Usually 85% of those injured have returned to their jobs at the end of 3 months. About 75% of accident cases do not

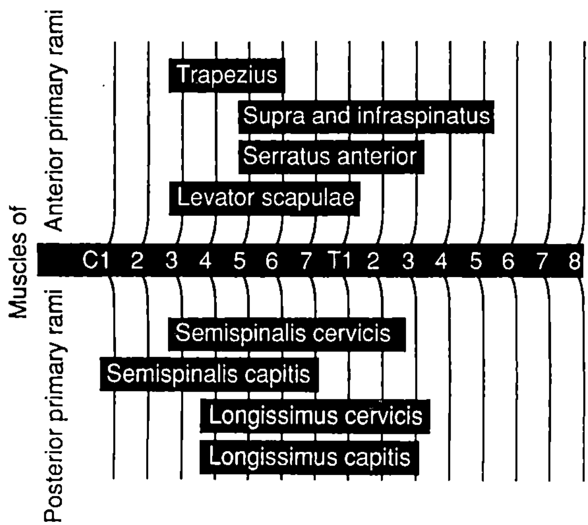

Fig. 24.8 This schematic illustration gives examples of upper extremity muscles supplied by the anterior primary rami of the cervical spine. Note the length of the muscles supplied by the posterior rami shown for the same cervical region. Activation of trigger points (TPs) that exist along the entire length of a muscle can cause or intensify pain felt in muscles supplied by any common nerve segment. Therefore, pain experienced along a muscle such as the semispinalis capitis can contribute to shoulder pain. Injection treatment of posterior primary rami muscles beginning at T6 is indicated if hypersensitive TPs are found in the muscles.

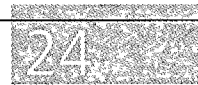

involve litigation. When pain persists beyond 6 months, these cases are labelled as chronic. Post-traumatic syndromes are common with whiplash injuries. This may include balance problems, narrowing of visual fields, insomnia, confusion, memory loss and anxiety. Post-traumatic syndromes are frequent with those patients who have, in addition, residual injuries, socioeconomic stresses, depression, anger and the complicating problem of litigation (Bland 1987). These are often relieved by treatment of the specific cervical lesions and the contributing lower back TPs. Acupuncture may also be helpful in relieving these symptoms.

MULTIPLE UPPER EXTREMITY LESIONS

One of the problems in managing upper extremity pain is that several lesions may be contributing to it. This is particularly true in the case of a middle-aged or older patient who sustains an injury as result of a fall in which the first contact was made by his or her outstretched hand, an elbow or shoulder (Fig. 24.9). The initial contact injury may be a fracture, contusion, ligamental sprain or muscle/soft tissue injury. After successful treatment, the patient experiences residual pain, dysfunction or limitation of movement.

When this is the history, the first accessory injury site to be considered is the cervical region, especially if cervical spondylosis is present. Slight injuries can occur at the nerve roots, involving nerve fibres in the root sleeves. When these are injured, they set up a radiculitis which continues to feed impulses to the original injury site (Gunn & Milbrandt 1978, Sola 1984). Unrelieved or persistent pain following seemingly satisfactory healing of the point of injury should always suggest further evaluation for potential cervical problems. In treating cervical radiculitis, it is important to remember that it takes several months of treatment with traction and supportive physical therapy for recovery of damaged nerves.

Further assessment should also include examination of the shoulder for hypersensitive TPs which, as stated before, may be perpetuating a pain cycle even though the initial stimulus has been negated. The elbow should be examined to rule out joint dysfunction and painful hypersensitive TPs.

If cervical and myofascial pain sources have been eliminated, further evaluation of tendons, bursae, rotator cuff and joint capsule should be carried out to eliminate the possibility of undiagnosed injuries along the path of shock absorption. Any injury site has the potential for setting up a dystrophy-like syndrome, a possibility which must be recognized and prevented. An extremity which has residual sequelae from a previous injury is much more vulnerable to pain and dysfunction following another injury to the same extremity. It is unfortunate for the patient if the clinician overlooks these sequelae, since they can usually be treated effectively and the pain eliminated.

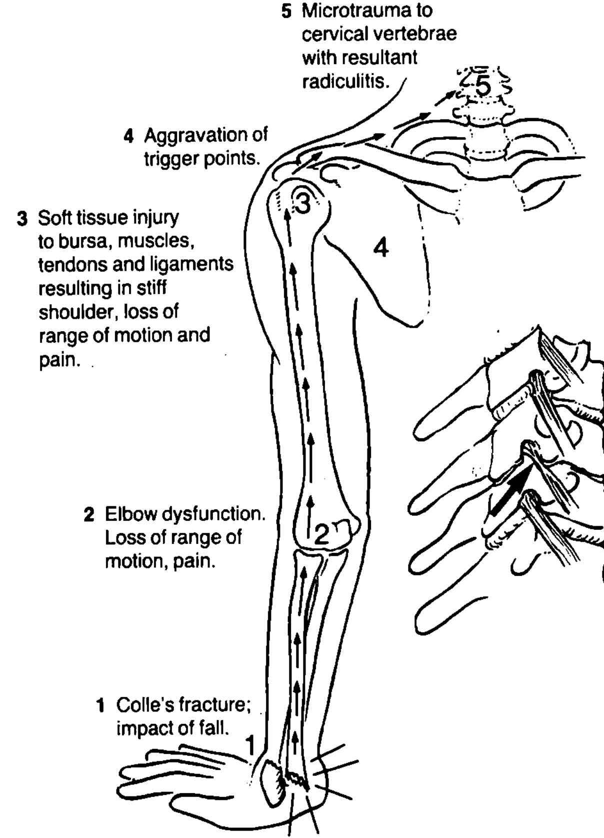

5 Microtrauma to cervical vertebrae with resultant radiculitis.

2 Elbow dysfunction. Loss of range of motion, pain.
1 Colle's fracture; impact of fall.

Fig. 24.9 Even a relatively minor force applied to a distal extremity can cause injury at any of these points on the shock pathway or can cause flare-up of residual sequelae which were not identified at the time of an earlier injury. Minimal changes of EMG can reflect presence of radiculitis (Gunn 1980).

REFERENCES

Adson AW 1951 Cervical ribs: symptoms, differential diagnosis and indications for section of the insertion of the scalenus anticus muscle. Journal of the International College of Surgeons 16: 546

Bateman JE 1978 The shoulder and neck, 2nd edn. WB Saunders, Philadelphia

Bland JH 1987 Disorders of the cervical spine: diagnosis and medical management. WB Saunders, Philadelphia, chs 13, 20

Bleecker ML 1987 Medical surveillance for carpal tunnel syndrome and workers. Journal of Hand Surgery 12A: 845

Bonica JJ 1990 The management of pain, 2nd edn. Lea & Febiger, Philadelphia, chs 21, 40, 47, 52

Borchgrevink GE, Kaasa A, McDonagh D, Stiles TC, Haraldseth O, Lereim I 1998 Acute treatment of whiplash neck sprain injuries. A randomized trial of treatment during the first 14 days after a car accident. Spine: 23(1): 25–31

Bray EA, Sigmond H 1941 The local and regional injection treatment of low back pain and sciatica. Annals of Internal Medicine 15: 840–852

Brody IA, Wilkins RH 1969 Lhermitte's sign. Archives of Neurology 21: 338

Calliet R 1981 Shoulder pain, 2nd edn. FA Davis, Philadelphia

Dawson DM, Hallet M, Millender LH 1983 Entrapment neuropathies. Little, Brown, Boston

Dawson DM, Hallet ML, Millender LH 1990 Entrapment neuropathies, 2nd edn. Little, Brown, Boston

DePalma AF 1957 Degenerative changes in sternoclavicular and acromioclavicular joints in various decades. CC Thomas, Springfield

DePalma AF 1973 Surgery of the shoulder, 2nd edn. JB Lippincott, Philadelphia

Dyck PJ, Lambert EH, O'Brien PC 1976 Pain in peripheral neuropathy related to rate and kind of nerve fiber degeneration. Neurology 26: 466–477

Edagawa N 1994 Body wall medicine. W4 Group, Mississauga, Ontario

Frost FA, Jeason B, Siggaard-Anderson JA 1980 A controlled, double-blind comparison of mepivacaine injection versus saline injection for myofascial pain. Lancet 1: 499–501

Gerhart TN, Dohlman LE, Warfield CA 1985 Clinical diagnosis of shoulder pain. Hospital Practice 20(9) 134–141

Gunn CC 1980 'Prespondylosis' and some pain syndromes following denervation supersensitivity. Spine 5: 185–192

Gunn CC 1989 Treating myofascial pain: intramuscular stimulation (IMS) for myofascial pain syndromes of neuropathic origin. Health Sciences Center for Educational Resources, University of Washington, Seattle

Gunn CC, Milbrandt WE 1978 Tennis elbow and the cervical spine. Canadian Medical Association Journal 114: 803–809

Johnson G 1996 Hyperextension soft tissue injuries of the cervical spine – a review. Journal of Accident and Emergency Medicine 13(1): 3–8

Khalil T, Abdel-Moty E, Steele-Rosomoff R, Rosomoff H 1994 The role of ergonomics in the prevention and treatment of myofascial pain. In: Rachlin ES (ed) Myofascial pain and fibromyalgia. Mosby, St Louis

Kopell HP, Thompson W 1973 Peripheral entrapment neuropathies. Williams & Wilkins, Baltimore

Kraft GH, Johnson EW, LaBan MM 1968 The fibrositis syndrome. Archives of Physiological Medicine and Rehabilitation 49: 155–162

Kraus H 1970 Clinical treatment of back and neck pain. McGraw-Hill, New York

LaDou J 1990 Occupational medicine. Appleton & Lange, Hoaglund, Maryland

Lawrence RM 1978 New approach to the treatment of chronic pain: combination therapy. American Journal of Acupuncture 6: 59–62

Lippert FG III, Teitz CC 1987 Diagnosing musculoskeletal problems – a practical guide. Williams & Wilkins, Baltimore

McLaughlin HL 1961 The 'frozen shoulder'. Clinical Orthopedics 20: 126–131

Melzack R, Stillwell DM, Fox EJ 1977 Trigger points and acupuncture points for pain: correlations and implications. Pain 3: 3

Moseley HF 1969 Shoulder lesions, 3rd edn. E & S Livingstone, Edinburgh, pp 75–81, 243–292

Neer CS II, Welsh RP 1977 The shoulder in sports. Orthopedic Clinics of North America 8: 583–591

Neviaser JS 1975 Arthrography of the shoulder: the diagnosis and management of the lesions visualized. CC Thomas, Springfield

Nichols JA, Hershman EB 1990 The upper extremity in sports medicine. CV Mosby, St Louis

Pak TJ, Martin GM, Magnes JL, Kavanaugh GJ 1970 Reflex sympathetic dystrophy. Minnesota Medicine 53: 507–512

Post M 1987 Physical examination of the musculoskeletal system. Year Book Medical Publishers, Chicago

Roberts JR, Hedges JR 1991 Clinical procedures in emergency medicine, 2nd ed. WB Saunders, Philadelphia, ch 64

Rosenbaum RB, Ochoa JL 1993 Carpal tunnel syndrome and other disorders of the median nerve. Butterworth-Heinemann, New York

Saha AK 1961 Theory of shoulder mechanism. CC Thomas, Springfield

Sataloff RT, Brandfonbrenner AG, Lederman RJ 1990 Textbook of performing arts medicine. Raven Press, New York

Sheon RP, Moskowitz RW, Goldberg VM 1987 Soft tissue rheumatic pain, 2nd edn. Lea & Febiger, Philadelphia

Silverstein B, Fine L, Stetson D 1987 Hand-wrist disorders among investment casting plant workers. Journal of Hand Surgery 12A: 838

Simons DG 1975 Muscle pain syndromes. Part I. American Journal of Physical Medicine 54: 289–311

Simons DG 1976 Muscle pain syndromes. Part II. American Journal of Physical Medicine 55: 15–42

Sola AE 1981 Myofascial trigger point therapy. Resident Staff Physicians 27: 38–48

Sola AE 1984 Treatment of myofascial pain syndromes. In: Benedetti C et al (eds) Advances in pain research and therapy. Raven Press, New York, p 13

Sola AE, Kuitert JH 1955 Myofascial trigger point pain in the neck and shoulder girdle: 100 cases treated by normal saline. Northwest Medicine 54: 980–984

Sola AE, Williams RL 1956 Myofascial pain syndromes. Neurology 6: 91–95

Sola AE, Rodenberg ML, Getty BB 1955 Incidence of hypersensitive areas in posterior shoulder muscles. American Journal of Physical Medicine 34: 585–590

Steindler A 1959 Lectures on the interpretation of pain in orthopedic practice. CC Thomas, Springfield

Tfelt-Hansen P, Olesen J, Lous I et al 1980 Lignocaine versus saline in migraine pain. Lancet 1: 1140

Travell J 1976 Myofascial trigger points. In: Bonica JJ (ed) Advances in pain research and therapy. Raven Press, New York

Travell J, Daitz B 1990 Myofascial pain syndromes: the Travell trigger point tapes. Williams & Wilkins Electronic Media, Baltimore

Travell J, Rinzler SH 1952 The myofascial genesis of pain. Postgraduate Medicine 11: 425–434

Travell J, Simons DG 1983 Myofascial pain and dysfunction: the trigger point manual. Williams & Wilkins, Baltimore

Upton ARM, McComas AJ 1973 The double crush syndrome in nerve entrapment syndromes. Lancet 2: 359

Zimmermann M 1979 Peripheral and central nervous mechanisms of nociception, pain and Pain therapy: facts and hypotheses. P.3 In Bonica JJ, Liebeskind JC, Albe-Fessard DG (eds) Advances in Pain Research and Therapy. Vol. 3 Lippincott. Raven. Philadelphia

Zohn DA, Mennell JM 1976 Musculoskeletal pain: diagnosis and physical treatment. Little, Brown, Boston

Fibromyalgia

ROBERT M. BENNETT

INTRODUCTION

Fibromyalgia is a common syndrome that is characterized by chronic, widespread pain. The diagnosis of fibromyalgia is currently based on the American College of Rheumatology 1990 classification criteria. These require a history of widespread pain and 11 or more tender points out of 18 defined locations. Its pathogenesis is currently thought to involve both abnormal sensory processing (central sensitization) and peripheral pain generators. There is no tissue-specific pathology and pain generators include painful joints, muscle injuries, inflammation and visceral pain. The course of fibromyalgia is prolonged and most patients seen in tertiary referral centres have lifelong symptoms which negatively affect quality of life and employability. Current management is palliative and aims to modulate pain, improve sleep, maintain function, treat psychological distress and diminish the impact of associated syndromes.

Fibromyalgia is a syndrome of chronic, widespread pain that has been largely defined by rheumatologists (Smythe & Moldofsky 1977, Bennett 1981, Yunus et al 1981, Goldenberg 1987, Wolfe et al 1990). This group of patients accounts for a large proportion of patients who consult rheumatologists in North America (Marder et al 1991, White et al 1995b). Not all rheumatologists are comfortable with this situation (Carette 1995, Solomon & Liang 1997, Winfield 1997, Wolfe 1997), since contemporary fibromyalgia research points towards a neuropathological rather than a rheumatological basis for the symptomatology. However, some neurologists have been the most vocal critics of the fibromyalgia concept (Bohr 1995, 1996). The evolution of the fibromyalgia concept has a long, contentious history.

HISTORICAL PERSPECTIVE

In the 19th century Balfour (1816) noted an association of muscular rheumatism and tender points and a similar connection was later made by Helleday (1876). The first use of the word 'fibrositis' is attributed to Sir William Gowers in a lecture on the subject of lumbago published in the *British Medical Journal* in 1904 (Gowers 1904). He wrote: 'I think we need a designation for inflammation of the fibrous tissue – we may conveniently follow the analogy of "cellulitis" and term it "fibrositis"'. Ralph Stockman, a Glasgow pathologist, described foci of inflammation in the interstitium of muscle bundles, the so-called 'myalgic nodules', that same year (Stockman 1904).

The first half of the 20th century was characterized by fibrositis speculation and controversy. Most of the reports during this period did not differentiate between focal fibrositis and generalized fibrositis (presumably akin to the current concept of fibromyalgia). More recently, research was focused on finding a local pathology in muscle to account for the indurated tender point. For instance, Brendstrup et al (1957) performed a carefully controlled study on the paraspinal muscles of patients operated on for disc herniation. In 12 patients, biopsies were made of indurated areas of muscles that were palpated under general anaesthesia. In all 12 'fibrositic nodules' there was an accumulation of acid mucopolysaccharides in the interstitial tissues. Awad (1973) reported similar findings, but his study was not controlled. Miehlke et al (1960) analysed 77 trapezius biopsies in patients with varying degrees of trapezius myalgia and found that patients with widespread pain had no muscle abnormalities, but patients with focal pain and associated hardening of muscle exhibited variations in the width of individual fibres, had increased numbers of sarcolemmal nuclei and often displayed degeneration of myofibres in association with a sparse infiltration of lymphocytes and histiocytes.

Subsequently, Fassbender (1975) reported that there were no distinctive light microscopic features in trapezius muscle biopsies from 11 patients with 'muscular rheumatism,' but electron microscopy showed a moth-eaten appearance of myofibrils and swelling of mitochondria. In more severe lesions, there was a disruption of sarcomere structure with destruction of myofilaments in the area of the I band. In some patients, there were areas of focal contraction of sarcomeric units. In six of the 11 cases the endothelial cells were swollen to the extent of almost obliterating the capillary lumen. Fassbender interpreted the capillary changes as being due to ischaemia – a result of focal muscle contraction.

The modern era of fibrositis research can be traced to the 1970s and the recognition by Smythe and Moldofsky (1977) that a history of widespread pain, sleep disturbance and the presence of multiple tender points was useful in defining patients with diffuse non-articular rheumatism. At about the same time they described α rhythm intrusion into sleep stages 3 and 4 of non-REM sleep as being a common occurrence in these patients (Moldofsky et al 1975) and that experimental disruption of non-REM induced a 'fibrositis-like' pain syndrome (Moldofsky & Scarisbrick 1976). A few years later Yunus et al (1981) made a detailed study of 50 fibrositis patients compared to healthy controls, confirming the usefulness of the tender point exam in diagnosis and describing the common co-morbidities such as irritable bowel syndrome and restless legs. Bennett (1981) described fibrositis as a misnomer for a common rheumatic disease and, with his colleagues (Campbell et al 1983), showed that quantitative dolorimetry could distinguish between subjects with widespread pain and healthy controls and also between tender points and control points (non-tender areas). After a flurry of interest by North American rheumatologists (Wolfe & Cathey 1983, 1985, Wallace 1984, Yunus 1984, Clark et al 1985b, Felson & Goldenberg 1986, Russell et al 1986, Simms et al 1988, Bennett 1989a,b, Yunus et al 1989b) and then Scandinavian rheumatologists (Henriksson et al 1982, Danneskiold-Samsoe et al 1983, Bengtsson et al 1986a,b, 1989, Lund et al 1986, Jacobsen & Danneskiold-Samsoe 1987, Vaeroy et al 1988), the American College of Rheumatology (ACR) commissioned a multicentre study to provide diagnostic guidelines. The results of this study were published in 1990 (Wolfe et al 1990) and are generally referred to as the 1990 ACR guidelines. They adopted the name of fibromyalgia; Kahler Hench had originally suggested this name in 1976, as the preferred name for a syndrome of widespread pain and tender points (Hench PK 1976). The old name of 'fibrositis' was considered to represent a pathological notion that was now discredited.

DIAGNOSIS OF FIBROMYALGIA

The 1990 ACR guidelines for making a diagnosis of fibromyalgia are the most widely used criteria (Wolfe et al 1990). They comprise one historical feature and one physical finding. The historical feature is widespread pain of 3 months or more. Widespread is defined as pain in an axial distribution plus pain of both left and right sides of the body and pain above and below the waist. Thus, a patient with axial pain plus pain in three body segments would qualify. The physical finding is a requisite number of tender points. The diagnosis requires the patient to experience pain in 11 or more out of 18 specified tender point sites on digital palpation with an approximate force of 4 kg (the amount of pressure required to blanch a thumbnail). The locations of the 18 tender points are shown in Figure 25.1. Symptoms and signs such as sleep disturbance, fatigue, stiffness, skinfold tenderness and cold intolerance are common in FM patients, but their inclusion did not improve diagnostic accuracy. The 1990 criteria suggested abolishing the distinction between primary and secondary FM. This concept is important as some FM patients get extensive work-ups to exclude another diagnosis. The number of tender points out of 11 or more was originally derived from a receiver-operating curve and relates to the number giving the best sensitivity and specificity. In clinical practice, the diagnosis of FM can be entertained when less than 11 tender points are present.

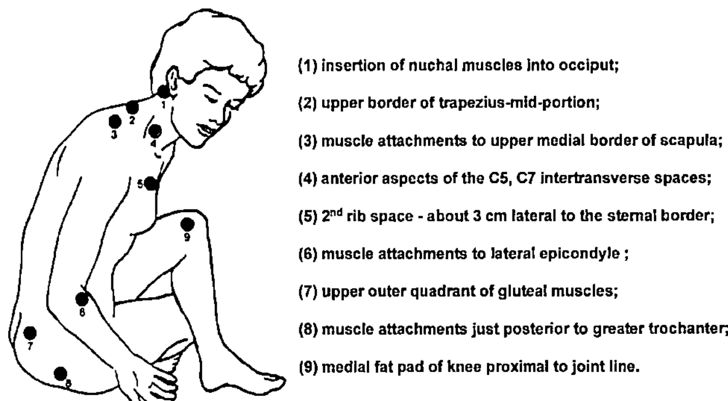

Fig. 25.1 The diagnosis of fibromyalgia requires a history of axial pain plus pain in at least three of the four segments of the body and the finding of at least 11 tender points on digital palpation of 18 designated tender points. (Adapted from Wolfe et al 1990.)

When examining a tender point area, the patient usually has a reflex response to pain, such as an involuntary exclamation or a flinch. These reflex actions are difficult to fake (Smythe et al 1997). In patients with widespread pain and other features typical of FM who have less than 11 out of 18 tender points it is useful to palpate other locations that are commonly tender; these include the infraspinatus, the quadratus lumborum, the upper portion of the sternocleidomastoid, the mandibular insertion of the masseter, the upper portion of the latissimus dorsi, the scapular insertion of the levator scapulae, the humeral insertion of the deltoid, the interossei muscles in the first webspace of the hand, the junction of the tensor fascia lata and the iliotibial tract, the junction of the soleus and Achilles' tendon and the origin of the foot flexor muscles from the medial aspect of the calcaneum. In general, designated tender points are more tender than control areas (distal dorsal third of forearm, thumbnail and mid-foot of the midpoint of the dorsal third metatarsal); however, it is now appreciated that such a differentiation cannot be used to exclude FM or indicate malingering (Wolfe 1998).

It is appreciated that the 1990 ACR guidelines are a compromise, but they have been invaluable in the research setting to standardize communication between investigators. Problems with these criteria include:

1. there is no gold standard pathology or other test to make a diagnosis of fibromyalgia.
2. they are too restrictive, as epidemiological studies have reported that a history of widespread pain is several times more common than ACR-defined fibromyalgia.
3. the number of tender points tested is only 18, which represents only about 3% of the potential tender point locations.
4. the criteria do not reflect the current concept of fibromyalgia being a disorder of sensory processing.

EPIDEMIOLOGY

Chronic musculoskeletal pain is commonly encountered in the general population (Skootsky et al 1984, Jacobsson et al 1989, Makela & Heliovaara 1991, Harvey 1993, Prescott et al 1993, Borenstein 1995, Mikkelsson et al 1997). Patients with rheumatic symptoms often have areas of hyperalgesia in muscles and nearby structures – so-called 'tender points'. Croft et al (1993) reported prevalence rates of 11.2% for chronic widespread pain, 43% for regional pain and 44% for no pain. When subjects with widespread pain were examined, 21.5% had 11 or more tender points, 63.8% had between one and 10 tender points and 14.7% had no tender points (Croft et al 1994). In general, there was a positive correlation between the finding of a tender point and a history of pain in that location. The tender point count did not correlate with widespread pain, but it did correlate with depression, fatigue and poor sleep, independently of pain status. Wolfe et al (1995) conducted a similar study in Wichita, Kansas, and found that the prevalence of chronic widespread musculoskeletal pain was more common in women and increased progressively from ages 18 to 70, with a 23% prevalence in the seventh decade. Chronic regional pain had a similar prevalence in men and women, approaching 30% by the eighth decade (Fig. 25.2). When Wolfe examined patients with a history of widespread pain, 25.2% of women and 6.8% of men had 11 or more tender points. The overall (M+F) prevalence of fibromyalgia in the Wichita population was 2%, with a prevalence of 3.4% in women and 0.5% in men. There was an almost linear increase in the prevalence of fibromyalgia, reaching nearly 8% of females in their eighth decade.

The results of both Croft's and Wolfe's studies suggest that a history of chronic widespread pain is more prevalent than the ACR-defined diagnosis of fibromyalgia. It is now conceptualized that fibromyalgia is at one end of a continuous spectrum of chronic pain.

CLINICAL FEATURES

PAIN

The core symptom of the FM syndrome is chronic widespread pain (Wolfe et al 1990). The pain is usually perceived as arising from muscle, but many fibromyalgia patients also report joint pain (Reilly & Littlejohn 1992). Stiffness,

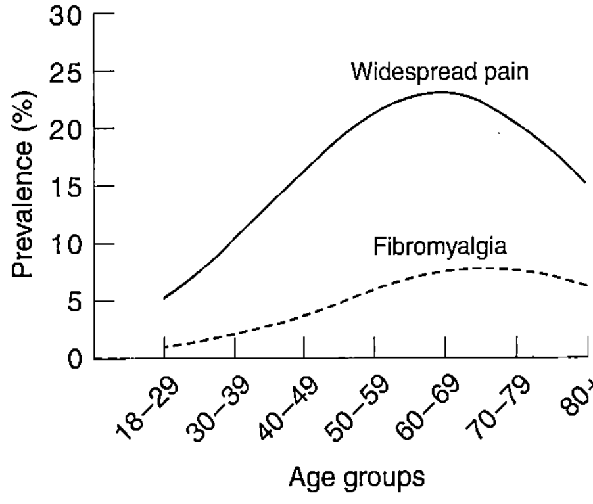

Fig. 25.2 Chronic widespread pain is several-fold more common than fibromyalgia defined according to the 1990 American College of Rheumatology diagnostic guidelines. (Adapted from Wolfe et al 1995.)

worse in the early morning, is a prominent symptom of most FM patients; along with the perception of articular pain, this may reinforce the impression of an arthritic condition. Fibromyalgia pain and stiffness typically have a diurnal variation, with a nadir during the hours of about 11.00 am to 3.00 pm (Moldofsky 1994). Symptoms also wax and wane in intensity over days and weeks, with flares occurring with increased exertion, systemic infections, soft tissue injuries, lack of sleep, cold exposure and psychological stressors. Many FM patients describe increased pain with cold damp weather, in particular low pressure fronts (Quick 1997); however, these claims have not been objectively verified (Guedj & Weinberger 1990, De Blecourt et al 1993, Hagglund et al 1994). Although most patients have widespread body pain, there are typically one or two locations that are the major foci. These pain centres often shift to other locations, often in response to new biomechanical stressess or trauma. Hyperalgesia is a *sine qua non* for diagnosis; some patients exhibit widespread allodynia and have been labelled as having 'touch-me-not' syndrome.

FATIGUE

Easy fatiguability from physical exertion, mental exertion and psychological stressors are typical of fibromyalgia (Yunus et al 1981, Bengtsson et al 1986a, Bennett 1989a, Wolfe et al 1990). The aetiology of fatigue in fibromyalgia is multifaceted and is thought to include non-restorative sleep, deconditioning, depression, poor coping mechanisms and secondary endocrine dysfunction involving the hypothalamic-pituitary-adrenal axis and growth hormone deficiency (Crofford et al 1994, Bennett et al 1997, Pillemer et al 1997, Kurtze et al 1998). Patients with chronic fatigue syndrome (CFS) have many similarities with FM patients (Komaroff & Buchwald 1991). Characteristically, patients with CFS have an acute onset of symptoms after an infectious type of illness, with subsequent persistence of debilitating fatigue and postexertional malaise (Komaroff & Buchwald 1991). Other prominent symptoms include myalgias, sleep disturbances, cognitive impairment and features suggestive of infections such as low-grade fevers, pharyngitis and adenopathy. Despite the attribution of a viral aetiology, an infectious cause has never been convincingly demonstrated. About 75% of patients who meet the diagnostic criteria of CFS also meet the criteria for diagnosis of FM (Goldenberg et al 1990).

DISORDERED SLEEP

Fibromyalgia patients invariably report disturbed sleep (Moldofsky et al 1975, Campbell et al 1983, Bengtsson et al 1986a, Wolfe et al 1990). Even if they report 8–10 hours of continuous sleep, they wake up feeling tired. This is referred to as non-restorative sleep. Most relate to being light sleepers, being easily aroused by low-level noises or intrusive thoughts. Many exhibit an α-δ EEG pattern, which diminishes the restorative stages 3 and 4 of non-REM sleep (Moldofsky 1989, Drewes et al 1995). α activity during sleep in fibromyalgia patients has been associated with the perception of shallow sleep and an increased tendency to awaken in relation to auditory stimuli (Perlis et al 1997). However, an α intrusion rhythm in δ sleep is not invariable in fibromyalgia and nor is it specific (Hauri & Hawkins 1973, Donald et al 1996, Shaver et al 1997). The experimental induction of α-δ sleep in healthy individuals has been reported to induce musculoskeletal aching and/or stiffness as well as increased muscle tenderness (Moldofsky & Scarisbrick 1976). Similarly, a poor night's sleep is often followed by a worsening of fibromyalgia symptoms the next day (Affleck et al 1996). There is probably a partial correlation between cognitive dysfunction, psychological distress and disturbed sleep in fibromyalgia patients (Jennum et al 1993, Perlis et al 1997, Shaver et al 1997).

ASSOCIATED DISORDERS

It is not unusual for fibromyalgia patients to have an array of somatic complaints other than musculoskeletal pain (Bennett 1989a, Clauw 1995). It is now thought that these symptoms are in part a result of abnormal sensory processing.

Restless leg syndrome

This strictly refers to daytime (usually maximal in the evening) symptoms of (1) unusual sensations in the lower limbs (but can occur in arms or even scalp) that are often described as paraesthesias (numbness, tingling, itching, muscle crawling) and (2) a restlessness, in that stretching or walking eases the sensory symptoms. This daytime symptomatology is nearly always accompanied by a sleep disorder – now referred to as periodic limb movement disorder (formerly nocturnal myoclonus) (Moldofsky et al 1986, Krueger 1990, MacFarlane et al 1996b). Restless leg syndrome has been reported in 31% of fibromyalgia patients compared to 2% of controls (Yunus & Aldag 1996).

Irritable bowel syndrome

This common syndrome of GI distress that occurs in about 20% of the general population is found in about 60% of fibromyalgia patients (Veale et al 1991, Sivri et al 1996).

The symptoms are those of abdominal pain and distension with an altered bowel habit (constipation, diarrhoea or an alternating disturbance). Typically, the abdominal discomfort is improved by bowel evacuation.

Irritable bladder syndrome

This is found in 40–60% of fibromyalgia patients (Wallace 1990, Paira 1994, Alagiri et al 1997, Clauw et al 1997). The initial incorrect diagnoses are usually recurrent urinary tract infections, interstitial cystitis or a gynaecological condition. Once these possibilities have been ruled out a diagnosis of irritable bladder syndrome (also called female urethal syndrome) should be considered. The typical symptoms are those of suprapubic discomfort with an urgency to void, often accompanied by frequency and dysuria.

Cognitive dysfunction

This is a common problem for many fibromyalgia patients (Wolfe et al 1990, Henriksson 1994, Landro et al 1997). It adversely affects employment and may cause concern about the early presentation of a neurodegenerative disease. In practice, this concern has never been a documented problem and patients can be reassured. The cause of poor memory and problems with concentration is, in most patients, related to the distracting effects of chronic pain, mental fatigue and psychological distress (Sletvold et al 1995, Kurtze et al 1998).

Cold intolerance

About 30% of fibromyalgia patients complain of cold intolerance (Bengtsson et al 1986a, Wolfe et al 1990). In most cases this amounts to needing warmer clothing or turning up the heat in their homes. Some patients develop a true primary Raynaud's phenomenon, which may mislead an unknowing physician to consider diagnoses such as lupus (SLE) or scleroderma (Dinerman et al 1986, Bennett et al 1991). Many fibromyalgia patients have cold hands and feet and some have cutis marmorata (a lace-like pattern of violaceous discoloration of their extremities on cold exposure) (Caro 1984).

Multiple sensitivities

One result of disordered sensory processing is that many sensations are amplified in fibromyalgia patients. Thus patients with fibromyalgia are more likely to receive other diagnoses such as multiple chemical sensitivity (MCS), sick building syndrome and drug intolerance. One report cites an MCS prevalence of 52% in fibromyalgia (Slotkoff et al 1997). Buchwald found a large overlap between fibromyalgia, chronic fatigue syndrome and MCS (Buchwald & Garrity 1994). In general fibromyalgia patients are less tolerant of adverse weather, medications, loud noises, bright lights and other sensory overloads.

Dizziness

This is a common complaint of fibromyalgia patients (Wolfe et al 1990). Before this symptom is attributed to fibromyalgia, a thorough search for other causes should be pursued (e.g. postural vertigo, vestibular disorders, eighth nerve tumours, demyelinating disorders, brainstem ischaemia and cervical myelopathy). In many cases no obvious cause is found, despite sophisticated testing. Treatable causes related to fibromyalgia include: proprioceptive dysfunction secondary to muscle deconditioning, proprioceptive dysfunction secondary to myofascial trigger points in the sternocleidomastoids and other neck muscles, neurally mediated hypotension and medication side effects.

Neurally mediated hypotension (NLM)

This syndrome is a lesser variant of 'neurocardiogenic syncope'. Its prevalence in one report was 60% (Bou-Holaigah et al 1997). Similar results have been noted in patients with chronic fatigue syndrome (Freeman & Komaroff 1997). NLM results from a paradoxical reflex when venous pooling reduces filling of the heart (right ventricle). In predisposed patients, this causes an inappropriately high secretion of catecholamines. This in turn leads to a vigorous contraction of the volume-depleted ventricle and an overstimulation of ventricular mechanoreceptors which signal the midbrain to reduce sympathetic tone and increase vagal tone, with resulting syncope or presyncope. In fibromyalgia patients this may be manifest by severe fatigue after exercise, on prolonged standing or in response to stressful situations. Although many fibromyalgia patients have a low BP with postural changes, orthostasis is not a prerequisite for diagnosis. A tilt-table test is the most reliable way to confirm NLM (Wilke et al 1998).

PSYCHOLOGICAL DISTRESS

As in many chronic pain syndromes, there is an increased prevalence of psychological diagnoses in fibromyalgia patients (Table 25.1). Several studies have noted elevations of certain scales on the Minnesota Multiphasic Personality

Table 25.1 Psychiatric testing in fibromyalgia patients

Diagnosis	*Prevalence*
Current major depression	21.4%
Lifetime major depression	42.8%
Current generalized anxiety disorder	6.1%
Lifetime generalized anxiety disorder	19.1%
Somatization disorder	13.7%
Pain profile on MMPI	50%
MMPI > 3 elevated T scores	27%

These results are based on a computerized assessment of DSM-III-R diagnoses and MMPI results in 131 fibromyalgia patients (from Bennett et al 1996)

Inventory (MMPI), especially the hypochondriasis, hysteria and depression scales (Payne et al 1982, Ahles et al 1984, Hawley et al 1988). Using criteria proposed by Bradley et al (1978) to delineate subgroups based on MMPI testing, about one-third of fibromyalgia patients can be categorized as being psychologically disturbed while the remainder have a normal or chronic pain profile. Using contemporary MMPI norms, Ahles et al (1986) found that only 18% of fibromyalgia patients could be classified as being psychologically disturbed. Smythe (1984) contended that any chronic pain patient would give positive answers on the MMPI to questions relating to pain and somatic symptoms; he concluded that there was a 40% bias of labelling a chronic pain patient as being 'neurotic'. In a subanalysis of the 117 statements relating to depression, hypochondriasis and hysteria, Leavitt and Katz (1989) noted that 18 MMPI statements were able to differentiate fibromyalgia from rheumatoid arthritis, with inappropriate health concerns and non-somatic symptoms being more prevalent in fibromyalgia patients.

Depression is more common in fibromyalgia patients than in healthy controls (Burckhardt et al 1994, Yunus 1994, Katz & Kravitz 1996). In four studies it was more common in fibromyalgia than rheumatoid arthritis (Hudson et al 1985, Uveges et al 1990, Hawley & Wolfe 1993, Alfici et al 1998) and in another three studies there was no difference (Kirmayer et al 1988, Dailey et al 1990, Ahles et al 1991). Importantly, fibromyalgia is not common in patients with major depression; even those depressed individuals who complained of pain did not have multiple tender points (Fassbender et al 1997).

Psychological distress in fibromyalgia may in part determine who becomes a patient. Clark et al (1985a) found no differences in three tests (SCL-90R, Spielberger State and Trait Anxiety, and Beck Depression Inventory) in subjects attending a general medical clinic who did not have fibromyalgia and subjects meeting criteria for fibromyalgia who were not seeking treatment for their pain (i.e. fibromyalgia non-patients). A similar study supported the notion that psychological distress in part determines who becomes a patient with fibromyalgia (Aaron et al 1996). Although psychiatric disorders are more prevalent in fibromyalgia patients than fibromyalgia non-patients, they do not seem to be intrinsically related to the pathophysiology of the fibromyalgia syndrome, but rather appear to be a result of symptom severity (Yunus 1994, Aaron et al 1996).

There are several reports of emotional and physical abuse in fibromyalgia patients (Goldberg 1994, Boisset-Pioro et al 1995, Taylor et al 1995, Toomey et al 1995, Walker et al 1997). The current consensus is that these childhood experiences do not cause fibromyalgia, but adversely affect coping mechanisms (Hudson & Pope 1995, Aaron et al 1997).

The psychiatric diagnoses that are often considered in the differential diagnosis of fibromyalgia are the somatoform disorders, especially somatization disorder and pain disorder as defined in the current *Diagnostic and statistical manual of mental disorders* (DSM-IV) (Hales & Clonginger 1994). *Somatization* is the communication of psychological and interpersonal distress in terms of somatic symptoms that suggest an organic disease. Formal studies of fibromyalgia patients have reported a diagnosis of somatization disorder in 14–23% patients (Aaron et al 1996, Bennett et al 1996d). Thus the concept of somatization may apply to a subset of fibromyalgia patients, but obviously this cannot explain the symptoms in the majority of patients. If somatization was the major aetiological factor in the generation of fibromyalgia symptomatology, the diagnosis would be found in the preponderance of patients. There are two subgroups of *pain disorder*.

1. Pain associated with psychological factorss (307.80). In this subgroup psychological factors are judged to have the major role in the onset, severity, exacerbation or maintenance of the pain.
2. Pain associated with both psychological factors and a general medical condition (307.89). In this subgroup both psychological factors and a general medical condition are judged to have the major role in the onset, severity, exacerbation or maintenance of the pain.

Another diagnostic category is also described: pain disorder associated with a general medical condition. It implies that the pain results from a general medical condition and psychological factors are judged to play either no role or a minimal role in the onset or maintenance of pain. This is not considered a mental disorder and is coded on Axis III (general medical disorders) rather than Axis I (mental disorders). Many fibromyalgia patients would fit into this latter category, and some patients with high levels of psychological distress could be classified under DSM-IV 307.89. One can of course debate whether a general medical condition characterized by dysfunction of sensory processing (i.e. fibromyalgia) should ever be classified in terms of a somatoform disorder! For instance, a psychiatric diagnosis that depends on 'the presence of physical symptoms that suggest a general medical condition and are not explained by a general medical condition' will become a non-psychiatric diagnosis once the general medical condition adequately explains the symptoms (McWhinney et al 1997).

INITIATION AND MAINTENANCE OF FIBROMYALGIA

Fibromyalgia seldom emerges out of the blue. Most patients relate an acute injury, repetitive work-related pain, athletic injuries or another pain state. Others attribute its onset to stress, infections and toxins. Fibromyalgia is commonly found as an accompaniment of rheumatoid arthritis (Wolfe et al 1984, Urrows et al 1994), low back pain (Borenstein 1995, Lapossy et al 1995) and osteoarthritis. A recent study documented a 22% prevalence of fibromyalgia 1 year after automobile accidents causing whiplash; this compares to a 1% prevalence after accidents involving leg fractures (Buskila et al 1997). This would suggest that nociceptive afferent input from neck muscles is a potent inducer of central sensitization. However, most injured subjects do not develop fibromyalgia and only 20–35% of patients with rheumatoid arthritis or lupus (SLE) have a concomitant fibromyalgia syndrome.

A striking familial prevalence of fibromyalgia has been reported by Buskila (Buskila et al 1996, Buskila & Neumann 1997) (Fig. 25.3). This suggests that subjects destined to develop fibromyalgia are either genetically predisposed (nature) or have past life events or experiences that favour its later development (nurture). Interestingly, fibromyalgia patients have an increased prevalence of other pain/dysthetic disorders, such as irritable bowel, female urethral syndrome and restless legs syndrome (Wallace 1990, Veale et al 1991, Yunus & Aldag 1996). It is possible that abnormal processing of normally non-nociceptive afferent impulses permits the expression of these commonly associated syndromes. It is also germane to speculate as to the relative importance of the nociceptive input from such associated conditions in maintaining central sensitization. This could occur through the extensive convergence of visceral and muscle afferents onto second-order wide-dynamic neurons in the dorsal horn (Kramis et al 1996).

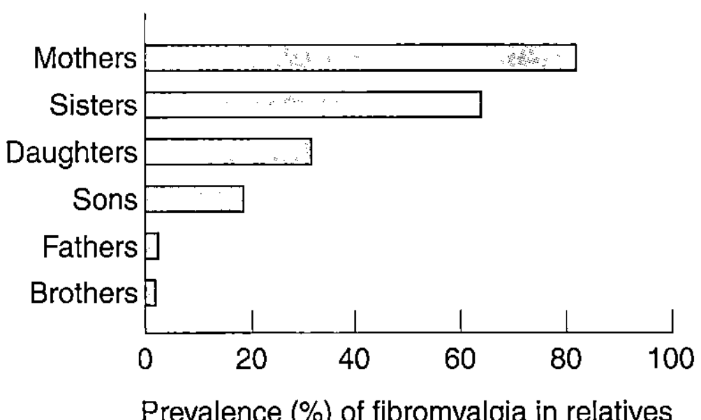

Fig. 25.3 A study of the familial clustering of fibromyalgia in Israelis showed a striking aggregation of cases in female family members. (Adapted from Buskila et al 1997.)

Chronic pain states may also develop during or after some infections (Dinerman & Steere 1990, Simms et al 1990, Leventhal et al 1991, Barkhuizen et al 1996, Rivera et al 1997) or in association with ongoing inflammatory diseases such as SLE and Sjogren's (Vitali et al 1989, Middleton et al 1994, Morand et al 1994, Bonafede et al 1995, Wallace et al 1995, Bennett 1997). In SLE there is a growing awareness that associated fibromyalgia is a major cause of morbidity in terms of pain, fatigue and a reduced quality of life (Wysenbeek et al 1992, Calvo-Alen et al 1995, Gladman et al 1997, Wang et al 1998). A series of elegant experiments in rats has described a complex neural pathway whereby proinflammatory cytokines can cause a hyperalgesic state (Maier et al 1993, Watkins et al 1994, 1995a,b,c,d, 1994a,b, Wiertelak et al 1997). This pathway involves proinflammatory cytokines (IL-1, IL-6, TNF) that activate cytokine-binding sites on vagal paraganglia with afferent impulses travelling to the nucleus of the tractus solitarus. Subsequent cross-stimulation of the nucleus raphe magnus activates descending spinal tracts which sensitize second-order dorsal horn neurons via an NMDA/substance P/nitrous oxide cascade. Thus, one can hypothesize that several discrete stimuli may initiate fibromyalgia via a common final pathway that involves the generation of a central pain state through the sensitization of second-order spinal neurons. The machinery whereby this may occur in relation to focal pain states as well as infection/inflammation is now much clearer thanks to the efforts of basic researchers.

PROGNOSIS AND IMPACT

Several long-term follow-up studies of FM patients have indicated that fibromyalgia symptomatology persists over many years (Felson & Goldenberg 1986, Ledingham et al 1993, Bengtsson et al 1994). Kennedy and Felson (1996) reported on follow-up of 39 patients, mean age 55, who had experienced fibromyalgia symptoms for 15 years. All of them still had fibromyalgia. Moderate to severe pain or stiffness was present in 55% of patients; significant sleep difficulties were reported in 48%; and notable levels of fatigue were present in 59%. Despite continuing symptoms, 66% of patients reported that FMS symptoms were somewhat improved compared to when first diagnosed. Chronic musculoskeletal pain often has a severe impact on a patient's quality of life (Burckhardt et al 1993). Wolfe et al (1997c) analysed 1604 fibromyalgia patients followed for 7 years in academic rheumatology centres. Symptoms of pain, fatigue, sleep disturbance, functional status, anxiety, depression and health status were abnormal at initiation and were the same after 7 years of follow-up. Fifty-nine per cent of the patients rated their health as only fair or poor.

There is some evidence that fibromyalgia patients seen in the community, rather than tertiary care centres, have a better prognosis. Granges et al (1994) reported a 24% remission rate after 2 years in patients seen in an ambulatory care setting. This is similar to the remission rate of chronic widespread pain in the community reported by Macfarlane. He found that 15% of patients with chronic widespread pain were pain free after 27 months, whereas 35% continued to have widespread pain and 50% had reverted to regional pain (MacFarlane et al 1996a). Siegel has reported a better prognosis for children and adolescents with fibromyalgia, seen at the University of Rochester, than adults seen in tertiary referral centres (Siegel et al 1998).

The consequences of pain and fatiguability influence motor performance. Henriksson (1994) has noted that everyday activities take longer in fibromyalgia patients, they need more time to get started in the morning and often require extra rest periods during the day. They have difficulty with repetitive sustained motor tasks, unless frequent rests are taken. Tasks may be well tolerated for short periods of time but when carried out for prolonged periods become aggravating factors (Waylonis et al 1994). Prolonged muscular activity, especially under stress or in uncomfortable climatic conditions, was reported to aggravate the symptoms of fibromyalgia (Waylonis et al 1994). The adaptations that fibromyalgia patients have to make in order to minimize their pain experience have a negative impact on both vocational and avocational activities.

DISABILITY

Despite the superficial appearance of normality, many fibromyalgia patients have difficulty remaining competitive in the workforce (Bennett 1996a). Most FM patients report that chronic pain and fatigue adversely affect the quality of their life and negatively impact their ability to be competitively employed (Hawley & Wolfe 1991, Henriksson et al 1992, Henriksson 1995). The extent of reported disability in FM varies greatly from country to country (Bengtsson et al 1986a, Bruusgaard et al 1993, Ledingham et al 1993), probably reflecting differences in political philosophies and socioeconomic realities. A survey of fibromyalgia patients seen in six US centres reported that 42% were employed and 28% were homemakers. Seventy per cent perceived themselves as being disabled. Twenty-six per cent were receiving at least one form of disability payment (Wolfe et al 1997c). Sixteen per cent were receiving Social Security benefits; this compares to 2.2% of the US population.

A similar high rate of disability was found in Canada. Bombardier evaluated 402 patients from a university-based chronic fatigue/fibromyalgia clinic (Bombardier & Buchwald 1996). Unemployment was 26% in chronic fatigue syndrome and 51% in patients with both chronic fatigue and fibromyalgia. Using the Stanford Health Assessment Questionnaire (HAQ), Wolfe compared 1522 patients with rheumatoid arthritis, fibromyalgia, hand osteoarthritis, neck pain and low back pain (Hawley & Wolfe 1991). Dysfunction in activities of daily living were comparable in patients with rheumatoid arthritis and fibromyalgia and higher than in the other conditions. Rheumatoid arthritis patients and healthy controls were directly compared to fibromyalgia patients using a 'work simulator' (Cathey et al 1988). Fibromyalgia patients performed 59% and rheumatoid arthritis patients performed 62% of the workload achieved by the healthy controls. The HAQ disability index best predicted the extent of objective functional disability; other correlates were pain severity and psychological status.

Disability in fibromyalgia and its assessment is a controversial topic for which there is currently no consensus (McCain et al 1989, Wolfe 1993, White et al 1995a, Wolfe & Potter 1996, Gjesdal & Kristiansen 1997, Mannerkorpi & Ekdahl 1997, Cohen & Quintner 1998). The problems encountered in assessing disability in fibromyalgia patients are related to four issues:

1. pain is a purely subjective sensation which is usually interpreted in an emotional context.
2. chronic pain cannot be fully understood in terms of the classic model of disease that equates pathogenesis with tissue damage or dysfunction.
3. many 'non-sick' people have persistent pain but are not disabled.
4. disability due to pain results from a complex interplay between past experiences, education, income level, work-related self-esteem, motivation, psychological distress, fatigue, personal value systems, ethnocultural

background and the availability of financial compensation.

It is increasingly evident that dysfunction in chronic pain states is poorly correlated with the severity of pain (Tait et al 1988, Loeser 1991). Disabled pain patients usually link impaired functioning to having persistent pain and cannot conceive of living a normal life as long as they are in pain (Reesor & Craig 1988, Talo et al 1989). They pursue a fruitless search for a cure which is never realized, thus rationalizing their continued disability. In the process they not only remain dysfunctional, but also overutilize medical care and develop increasing personal distress. Interestingly, it is the *belief* that pain is the major cause of disability that seems to determine the actual degree of dysfunction, rather than the absolute level of pain (Riley et al 1988). These psychosocial and behavioural issues are clearly relevant to some fibromyalgia patients seeking disability, but should not be generalized. Each patient has to be thoughtfully evaluated according to his or her unique set of circumstances. There is an extensive literature on the nature of disability in chronic pain patients which is presumably relevant to the problem in fibromyalgia (Gerdle & Elert 1995, Teasell & Merskey 1997, Estlander et al 1998, Leserman et al 1998, Li & Moore 1998).

PATHOGENESIS

There is still considerable debate as to whether fibromyalgia is a 'distinct entity', whether the symptoms emanate from the 'body or the mind' and whether the fibromyalgia concept is useful or detrimental to patient management. Most serious students of the fibromyalgia concept reject the notion that fibromyalgia is a discrete entity based on a distinctive pathology. The current paradigm is that of a complex hyperalgesic pain syndrome, in which abnormalities of central sensory processing interact with peripheral pain generators and psychoneuroendocrine dysfunction to generate a wide spectrum of patient symptomatology and distress. Some of the experimental underpinnings that have influenced this paradigm shift are now presented.

PERIPHERAL PAIN MECHANISMS

For most of the 20th century fibrositis/fibromyalgia was considered to be a muscle disease. It is now appreciated that there are no distinctive muscle changes that can define fibromyalgia in terms of a specific tissue pathology. It is now thought that both peripheral and central factors contribute in varying degrees to the expression of symptoms labelled as fibromyalgia.

Muscle biopsy studies

Bengtsson et al (1986b) reported on one of the first controlled muscle biopsy studies in FM patients. Biochemical analysis demonstrated a significant decrease in high-energy phosphate levels (ATP and PCr) in the areas of trigger points in the trapezius muscle compared to the trapezius muscle in healthy controls and the anterior tibial muscles from the same fibromyalgia patient. It was hypothesized that these changes represented areas of focal muscle ischaemia. Yunus et al (1989b) reported on a carefully controlled and blinded study of electron microscopic findings in the trapezius muscle in fibromyalgia. They found several abnormalities (papillary projections, myotubular lysis, sarcolemmal glycogen deposition and interstitial lipid deposition) to be common in both fibromyalgia patients and the healthy controls. It was concluded that microscopic abnormalities in the trapezius muscle are a frequent *normal* finding that probably results from the persistent chronic biomechanical stresses that act on this muscle.

The most rigorous study of the trapezius muscle to date is that of Lindman et al (1991a,b). They compared subjects with fibromyalgia or trapezius myalgia with healthy individuals and postmortem muscle biopsies from healthy young females who had suffered accidental death. Muscle fibre size in female patients was almost half that in the males and the degree of capillarization and mean volume density of mitochondria in female trapezii were lower than that in other muscles. In the patients with focal myalgia, type 1 fibres were significantly larger in biopsies of myalgic areas and the number of capillaries per cross-sectional area (both type 1 and type 2A fibres) was lower than in healthy controls. Levels of both ATP and PCr were also lower in these same fibres. In the fibromyalgia group, capillary endothelial cells were often swollen and deranged. The total capillary area and the thickness of the endothelial cells were larger in the fibromyalgia patients than in healthy controls or in patients with focal myalgia. Some of Lindman's results are in accord with the earlier findings of Fassbender (i.e. capillary abnormalities) and the findings of Bengtsson et al (low levels of ATP and PCr).

Magnetic resonance spectroscopy

There have been eight studies of NMR spectroscopy in fibromyalgia patients, both in resting muscle and in muscle that has been exercised (Mathur & Gatter 1988, De

Blecourt et al 1991, Jacobsen et al 1992, Roy 1993, Jacobsen et al 1994, Jubrias et al 1994, Simms et al 1994, Park et al 1998). Most studies failed to show any global defect in muscle metabolism in fibromyalgia. The exception was a study by Park et al (1998) that reported significantly lower than normal PCr and ATP levels ($P < 0.004$) and PCr: Pi ratios ($P < 0.04$). This study also showed a trend to an increased prevalence of phosphodiester peaks in fibromyalgia patients compared to controls, supporting an earlier report by Jubrias et al (1994). Phosphodiester peaks occur in musculodystrophies (Younkin et al 1987) and also with increasing age (Satrustegui et al 1988). They are thought to result from the lipid peroxidation of sarcolemmal membrane proteins. This process occurs in calcium-activated muscle damage (muscle microtrauma) (Armstrong et al 1991) – the cause of muscle pain on overexertion. Muscle microtrauma, a normal occurrence in healthy individuals, has been postulated to be one cause of peripheral nociceptive input in fibromyalgia patients (Bennett 1993).

Respiratory gas exchange

Respiratory gas exchange studies in fibromyalgia patients have shown that most patients have a low VO_2 max for their age (i.e. they are aerobically unfit) (Bennett et al 1989, Mengshoel et al 1990, Sietsem et al 1993). However, most attained an anaerobic threshold at a reasonable workload. These findings suggest that global muscle metabolism is normal in fibromyalgia patients. Interestingly, the majority of fibromyalgia patients perceive the level of their exertion correctly. A subset (about 20%) who never reached an anaerobic threshold over-reported their level of exertion in one study (Clark et al 1993).

Muscle blood flow

It has been hypothesized that focal changes in muscle blood flow may be important in the pathophysiology of fibromyalgia and myofascial pain syndromes (Henriksson 1994). Some support for this notion comes from the muscle biopsy findings showing swollen capillary endothelial cells (Fassbender 1975, Lindman et al 1992). Lund et al (1986) applied an oxygen-sensitive electrode directly to surgically exposed fibromyalgia tender point areas in the trapezius muscle. They reported an abnormal distribution of oxygenation compared to controls; it was hypothesized that the abnormal distribution was a result of focal areas of ischaemia. Klemp et al (1982), using a ^{33}Xenon clearance technique in focal trapezius myalgia, found no difference in resting blood flow between patients and controls. Bennett et al (1989), using a ^{33}Xenon clearance method in peroneal muscles, found that the exercising muscle blood flow in fibromyalgia patients was significantly lower than that in controls matched for age, sex, weight and aerobic capacity.

Muscle strength

Studies of both isometric and isokinetic muscle strength in fibromyalgia patients have reported values approximately 50% of those found in healthy individuals (Jacobsen & Danneskiold-Samsoe 1987, Mengshoel et al 1990, Elert et al 1992, Nordenskiöld & Grimby 1993, Lindh et al 1994). Muscular endurance is also reduced in FM patients compared to controls (Jacobsen & Danneskiold-Samsë 1992, Elert et al 1995). Jacobsen et al (1991) found a negative correlation between the number of fibromyalgia tender points and isokinetic muscle strength. It was hypothesized that this reduction in strength is partly related to central inhibition mechanisms due to pain. Backman et al (1988) reported that the handgrip strength of fibromyalgia patients was 64% that of controls, but after electrical stimulation of the adductor pollicis (via the ulnar nerve) they had a normal grip strength. In a similar study, additional twitches delivered to the quadriceps femoris by transcutaneous electrical nerve stimulation during voluntary maximal voluntary contraction (the 'twitch interpolation' technique) showed that 65% of fibromyalgia patients submaximally activated their muscles compared to 15% of controls (Jacobsen et al 1991). In a similar study, superimposed electrical stimulation of the quadriceps induced an increased torque output in 79% of FM patients compared to 10% of controls (Lindh et al 1994). These results are most consistent with the notion that muscle contraction in fibromyalgia patients causes pain that reflexly inhibits maximal voluntary muscle contraction. The source of the muscle pain is most likely to be focal in origin.

Experimentally induced muscle pain

Focal loci of muscle pain are referred to clinically as myofascial trigger points. These are hyperalgesic zones in muscle that often feel indurated on palpation. Prolonged pressure over these areas may cause a pattern of pain that is referred distally – hence the label 'trigger points' (Travell & Rinzler 1952, Travell & Simons 1983, 1992). Kellgren (1938, 1939) pioneered studies using hypertonic saline to evaluate the correlates of painful foci within muscle.

Recently Graven-Nielsen (1997) has refined this technique in a series of elegant studies. In particular he found that hypertonic saline-induced muscle pain demonstrates temporal and spatial summation that are influenced by central facilitatory and inhibitory mechanisms (Basbaum & Fields 1984, Fields et al 1994). This observation is in keeping with the findings of Wall and Woolf (1984) regarding the propensity of nociceptive input from muscle to induce a state of central sensitization. In these experiments a decerebrate rat model was used to explore the effects on reflex withdrawal of the hind limb of a noxious stimulus. The pain stimulus was applied both before and after stimulating either the sural nerve (a purely cutaneous nerve) or the gastrocnemius-soleus nerve (a predominantly muscle afferent) at 1 Hz for 20 seconds. Stimulation of the sural nerve induced an increased excitability of the withdrawal reflex that lasted for only about 10 minutes. Stimulation of the gastrocnemius-soleus nerve produced a prolonged increase in reflex activity that lasted up to 90 minutes. Importantly, these results were also seen in the contralateral limb. It was surmised that intraspinal changes evoked by stimulation of muscle C afferent fibres induced long-lasting spinal changes. These experiments highlight the importance of focal muscle pain in inducing a state of central sensitization and are postulated to be relevant to abnormal sensory processing in fibromyalgia patients (Henriksson 1994, Bennett 1996c).

CENTRAL PAIN MECHANISMS

There are several lines of evidence to suggest that the pain experience of fibromyalgia patients is in part the result of disordered sensory processing at a central level.

Qualitative differences in pain

An objective measure of applied force to a tender point can be obtained by dolorimetry (Campbell et al 1983). A study using an electronic dolorimeter recorded the subject's assessment of pain intensity on a 0–10 cm visual analogue scale (VAS) at varying levels of applied force (Bendtsen et al 1997). Distinctly different response curves were obtained for controls and fibromyalgia patients. It was found that in pain-free controls there is a threshold at about 160 dolorimeter units beyond which there was an almost linear increase in pain intensity. In comparison fibromyalgia subjects exhibited a linear increase in pain from the baseline dolorimeter force of 80 units. This is a demonstration of qualitatively altered nociception in fibromyalgia and suggests that fibromyalgia patients differ from pain-free subjects in their processing of sensory information. Similar abnormalities of pain processing in fibromyalgia patients have also been reported for heat and cold (Kosek et al 1996b). When a muscle is isometrically contracted there is normally an increase in the pain threshold to palpation (Pertovaara 1992). In fibromyalgia patients there is a decrease in the pain threshold (Kosek et al 1996a). It has been hypothesized that this is a result of either sensitization of mechanoreceptors in fibromyalgia or dysfunction of afferent inhibition activated by muscle contraction (Kosek et al 1996a). Whatever the mechanism, it provides a partial explanation for the increased pain experienced by fibromyalgia patients on exertion.

Deficient pain modulation in response to repeated thermal stimuli

Diffuse noxious inhibitory control (DNIC) was investigated in 25 female patients with fibromyalgia and 26 age-matched healthy women (Lautenbacher & Rollman 1997). Tonic thermal stimuli at painful and non-painful intensities were used to induce pain inhibition. The patients with fibromyalgia had significantly lower heat pain thresholds than the healthy subjects, but similar electrical detection and pain thresholds. Concurrent tonic thermal stimuli, at both painful and non-painful levels, significantly increased the electrical pain threshold in the healthy subjects but not in the fibromyalgia patients. It was concluded that DNIC was deficient in fibromyalgia patients, suggesting that they either had deficient pain modulation or were unable to tolerate a tonic stimulus that was of sufficient intensity to stimulate an inhibitory effect.

Hyper-responsive somatosensory induced potentials

Somatosensory induced potentials recorded by skull electrodes in response to peripheral sensory stimulation have been studied in FM patients. Gibson et al (1994) reported that an increased late nociceptive (CO_2-laser stimulation of skin) evoked somatosensory response in 10 FM patients compared to 10 matched controls. Lorenz et al (1996) have recently reported increased amplitude of the N170 and P390 brain somatosensory potentials in fibromyalgia compared to controls evoked by laser stimulation of the skin (Fig. 25.4). Furthermore, they observed a response in both hemispheres, while in controls the somatosensory potential was strictly localized to one side of the brain. They controlled for increased hypervigilance (a psychological concept related to a conditioned expectation response) by using interspersed auditory stimuli; the somatosensory potentials to these stimuli were no different in fibromyalgia patients than controls. These two studies provide objective

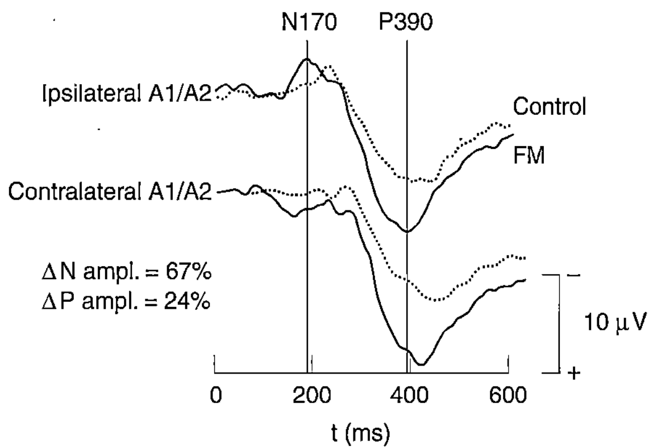

Fig. 25.4 Laser-induced skin pain results in significantly increased EEG potentials at the 170 and 390 msec peaks in fibromyalgia patients compared to controls. (Adapted from Lorenz et al 1996.)

evidence that fibromyalgia patients have an altered processing of nociceptive stimuli in comparison to pain-free controls.

Secondary hyperalgesia on electrocutaneous stimulation

Primary hyperalgesia is the normal perception of pain from nociceptor stimulation in an injured tissue. Secondary hyperalgesia refers to pain elicited from uninjured tissues (Magerl et al 1998). Torebjork et al (1992) have convincingly demonstrated this phenomenon in humans. Synergism between substance P and NMDA (N-methyl D-aspartate) receptors play an important role in the perpetuation of secondary hyperalgesia (Dickenson & Sullivan 1991, Dougherty & Willis 1992). Arroyo and Cohen (1993), while attempting to treat fibromyalgia patients with electrical nerve stimulation that would elicit only non-painful sensations in normal individuals, noted that the pain was made worse and often caused dysthetic sensations. Compared to controls, fibromyalgia patients had a reduced pain tolerance and two unexpected phenomena: (i) a spread of dysthesia (mainly tingling and burning) that was felt both distally and proximally to the stimulator, and (ii) a persistence of dysthesia around the stimulated locus that lasted for 12–20 minutes after the stimulation was terminated. Thus electrical stimulation of the skin in fibromyalgia patients results in phenomena that are characteristic of secondary hyperalgesia. This experiment provides further evidence of altered non-nociceptive processing in fibromyalgia patients.

Abnormalities on SPECT imaging

It is now evident that pain-related functional CNS changes can be demonstrated by imaging techniques. For instance, positron emission tomography (PET) studies have shown increased activity in the anterior cingulate gyrus in response to painful stimuli (Hsieh et al 1995). Mountz et al (1995) reported that fibromyalgia patients, characterized by low pain thresholds, had a decreased regional blood flow compared to healthy controls on SPECT (single photon emission computed tomography) imaging. The decreased perfusion was particularly prominent in the thalamic and caudate nuclei (structures involved in the processing of nociceptive stimuli). A similar finding has been reported in patients with unilateral chronic neuropathic pain, using O-15 PET (Iadarola et al 1995). It is interesting that chronic pain states have been associated with reduced thalamic blood flow, whereas acute pain increases thalamic blood flow. The reason for this difference is postulated to be a disinhibition of the medial thalamus which results in activation of a limbic network (Craig 1998). Thus functional imaging studies are supportive of an altered processing of sensory input in fibromyalgia patients.

Elevated levels of substance P in the CSF

Substance P is an important nociceptive neurotransmitter. It lowers the threshold of synaptic excitability, permitting the unmasking of normally silent interspinal synapses and the sensitization of second-order spinal neurons (Sastry 1979, Arnetz & Fjellner 1986, Coderre et al 1993). Activation of NMDA receptors has a permissive effect on substance P release in the dorsal horn (Liu et al 1997). Furthermore, substance P can diffuse widely in the spinal cord and sensitize dorsal horn neurons at some distance from the initial input locus. This results in an expansion of receptive fields and the activation of WDR neurons by non-nociceptive afferent impulses. An increased production of neurotransmitters within the spinal cord may be detected as increased levels in CSF (Tsigos et al 1993). There are two definitive studies that have shown a three-fold increase of substance P in the CSF of fibromyalgia patients compared to controls (Vaeroy et al 1988, Russell et al 1994). Animal models of hyperalgesia and hypoalgesia have implicated substance P as a major aetiological factor in central sensitization (Dougherty & Willis 1992, Abbadie et al 1996, Mantyh et al 1997, De Felipe et al 1998) and have highlighted the relevance of substance P in human pain states (Abbadie et al 1996). Thus the finding of elevated levels of substance P in patients is in accord with the notion that central sensitization is germane to the pathogenesis of fibromyalgia.

Beneficial response to an NMDA receptor antagonist

The excitatory amino acid glutamine reacting with NMDA receptors plays a central role in the generation of non-nociceptive pain. If this were relevant to pain in fibromyalgia, one would expect NMDA receptor antagonists to have a beneficial therapeutic effect. Two recent studies from Sweden reported that intravenous ketamine (an NMDA receptor antagonist) attenuates pain and increases pain threshold, as well as improving muscle endurance in FM patients (Sorensen et al 1995, 1997). In some patients a single intravenous infusion over a course of 10 minutes (0.3 mg/kg) resulted in a significant reduction in pain that persisted for up to 7 days. Ketamine, at this subanaesthetic dose, was more potent than intravenous morphine (10 gm) and intravenous lidocaine (5 mg/kg). This is a therapeutic demonstration that helps to elucidate the molecular basis for altered pain processing in fibromyalgia patients.

Experimentally induced central hyperexcitability

Sorensen et al (1998) injected hypertonic saline (2 ml of 5.7% saline over 8 minutes) into the anterior tibial muscle of fibromyalgia patients and healthy controls. Importantly, this muscle was not a site of spontaneous pain in any of the subjects. Pain intensity was assessed continually by an electronic visual analogue scale and the area of both local and referred pain was charted on a drawing. Compared to controls, fibromyalgia patients experienced a longer duration of pain and a larger area of referral. The same subjects were also compared as to pressure pain threshold over the anterior tibial muscle and pain threshold to both single and repetitive electrical stimulation of the overlying skin and electrical intramuscular stimulation. Pressure pain threshold was significantly lower in the fibromyalgia group. No differences were found between the two groups in cutaneous pain threshold or cutaneous summation pain threshold, nor in the intramuscular pain threshold to single stimulation. However, the intramuscular summation pain threshold was significantly lower in fibromyalgia patients. These results were interpreted as being due to a state of central hyperexcitability in fibromyalgia that could be revealed by stimulation of muscle nociceptors in a muscle exhibiting no spontaneous pain.

MANAGEMENT

The management of fibromyalgia patients is an exercise in symptom palliation and maintenance of physical and emotional functionality. A follow-up of 530 fibromyalgia patients from six US tertiary referral centres over 7 years highlighted the refractoriness of fibromyalgia symptoms (Wolfe et al 1997b). Basically there was no significant improvement in pain, functional disability, fatigue, sleep disturbance and psychological status over the course of 7 years. Half the patients were dissatisfied with their health and 59% rated their health as fair or poor. These results were achieved in the setting of a high use of medical resources (Wolfe et al 1997a). Fibromyalgia patients averaged almost 10 outpatient medical visits per year and were hospitalized at a rate of one hospitalization every 3 years (50% for fibromyalgia-associated problems). Fibromyalgia patients used an average of 2.7 fibromyalgia-related drugs in every 6-month period. The mean yearly per-patient cost in 1996 dollars was $2274.

Despite this gloomy picture there is some evidence that fibromyalgia patients can be helped, but not cured, by a multidisciplinary approach that emphasizes education, cognitive-behavioural therapy, therapeutic treatment of pain, participation in a stretching and aerobic exercise programme and prompt treatment of psychological problems such as depression (Clark 1994, Goldenberg et al 1994, 1996, Masi 1994, Bennett et al 1996d, Martin et al 1996, Wigers et al 1996, Dwight et al 1998).

Education and support

Patients need to understand that fibromyalgia does not cause crippling or reduced life expectancy and that the treating physician is prepared to provide empathic and continuing support. As in any chronic incurable condition, education is an important resource (Gonzalez et al 1990, Burckhardt & Bjelle 1994). Patients also need to realize that their symptoms cannot be eradicated in toto and that the aim of treatment is to make them more functional and not to eliminate all pain (Rosen 1994).

Psyche

Patients with poor coping strategies often tend to catastrophize adverse life events, which they perceive themselves as being helpless to influence. Psychological intervention in terms of improving the internal locus of control and more effective problem solving is important in such patients. Techniques of cognitive-behavioural therapy seem particularly well suited to effect these changes and may be enhanced when done as a part of group therapy (Nielson et al 1992, Goldenberg et al 1994). Specific psychological problems such as depression, anxiety states, alcoholism and childhood abuse need to be recognized early on and appropriately treated (Goldberg 1994, Boisset-Pioro et al 1995, Taylor et al 1995, Linton et al 1996, Walker et al 1997).

Sleep

Non-restorative sleep is a problem for most fibromyalgia patients and contributes to their feelings of fatigue and seems to intensify their experience of pain (Affleck et al 1996). Effective management involves:

1. ensuring an adherence to the basic rules of sleep hygiene
2. regular low-grade exercise
3. adequate treatment of associated psychological problems (depression, anxiety, etc.)
4. the prescription of low-dose tricyclic antidepressants (amitryptiline, trazadone, doxepin, imipramine, etc.) (Bennett et al 1988, Goldenberg 1989, Carette et al 1994).

Some fibromyalgia patients cannot tolerate TCAs due to unacceptable levels of daytime drowsiness or weight gain. In these patients benzodiazopine-like medications such as aprazolam (Russell et al 1991), zolpidem (Moldofsky et al 1996) and zopiclone (Drewes et al 1991) may be used. Some fibromyalgia patients suffer from a primary sleep disorder, which requires specialized management. About 25% of male and 15% of female fibromyalgia patients have sleep apnoea. Unless specific questions about this possibility are asked, sleep apnoea will often be missed. Patients with sleep apnoea usually require treatment with positive airway pressure (CPAP) or surgery. By far the commonest sleep disorder in fibromyalgia patients is restless leg syndrome. This can be effectively treated with L-dopa/carbidopa (Sinemet 10/100 mg at suppertime) or clonazepam (Klonipin 0.5 or 1.0 mg at bedtime) (Montplaisir et al 1992).

Pain

Attempts to break the pain cycle, to enable patients to be more functional, are especially important. In general, most FM patients do not derive a great deal of benefit from NSAID preparations or acetaminophen. Prednisone has been shown to be ineffective (Clark et al 1985b). Tramadol (Ultram) has recently been shown to be a moderately effective analgesic in fibromyalgia patients (Russell et al 1997, Biasi et al 1998). Currently opiates are the most effective medications for managing most chronic pain states (Friedman 1990, Portenoy 1996). Their use is often condemned out of ignorance regarding their propensity to cause addiction, physical dependence and tolerance (Melzack 1990, Portenoy et al 1997, Wall 1997). While physical dependence (defined as a withdrawal syndrome on abrupt discontinuation) is inevitable, this should not be equated with addiction (Portenoy 1996). Addiction is a dysfunctional state occurring as a result of the unrestrained use of a drug for its mind-altering properties; manipulation of the medical system and the acquisition of narcotics from non-medical sources are common accompaniments. Addiction should not be confused with 'pseudo-addiction'. This is a drug-seeking behaviour generated by attempts to obtain appropriate pain relief in the face of undertreatment of pain (Weissman 1989). Opiates should not be the first choice of analgesia in fibromyalgia, but they should not be withheld if less powerful analgesics have failed. A study of their utility in fibromyalgia is needed.

Physical modalities such as heat, massage, acupuncture and passive stretching often provide some palliative relief. When the patient has a major focus of regional pain, it is worthwhile trying a course of trigger point injections, using 1% procaine or lidocaine (Travell & Simons 1983). The technique of fluorimethane spray and stretch can be taught to family members and can minimize repetitive office visits for pain management (Travell & Simons 1983).

Exercise

FM patients cannot afford *not* to exercise, as deconditioned muscles are more prone to microtrauma and inactivity begets dysfunctional behavioural traits (McCain et al 1988, Bennett et al 1989). However, musculoskeletal pain and severe fatigue are powerful conditioners for inactivity. All FM patients need to have a home programme with muscle stretching, gentle strengthening and aerobic conditioning. There are several points that need to be stressed about exercise in FM patients (Clark 1994).

1. Exercise is health training, not sports training.
2. Exercise should be non-impact loading.
3. Aerobic exercise should be done for 30 minutes each day. This may be broken down into three 10-minute periods or other combinations, such as two 15-minute periods, to give a cumulative total of 30 minutes. This should be the aim – it may take 6–12 months to achieve this level.
4. Strength training should emphasize concentric work and avoid eccentric muscle contractions.
5. Regular exercise needs to become part of the usual lifestyle; it is not merely a 3–6 month programme to restore them to health.

Suitable aerobic exercise includes: regular walking, the use of a stationary exercycle or Nordic track (initially not using the arm component). Patients who are very deconditioned or incapacitated should be started with water therapy using a buoyancy belt (Aqua-jogger). Fibromyalgia patients have to be seen regularly and encouraged to continue with their exercise programme.

Endocrine replacement therapy

There is no good evidence that fibromyalgia is primarily due to endocrine dysfunction. However, common problems such as hypothyroidism and menopausal symptoms will often aggravate pain and fatigue and appropriate replacement therapy is usually indicated. There has been much interest in abnormalities of the hypothalamic-pituitary-adrenal (HPA) axis in fibromyalgia patients (Crofford et al 1994, Pillemer et al 1997). The general impression is that fibromyalgia patients have a somewhat reduced HPA responsiveness. However, replacement therapy with prednisone 15 mg/day was not shown to be therapeutically useful (Clark et al 1985b). Bennett et al (1992, 1997) have reported that about one-third of fibromyalgia patients are growth hormone deficient and that replacement therapy is of benefit to many of these (Bennett et al 1998). However, growth hormone is very expensive and it is difficult to justify its use in fibromyalgia at the present time.

Fibromyalgia-associated problems

Recognition and treatment of problems that are commonly associated with fibromyalgia are important in the overall management scheme.

Chronic fatigue

The common treatable causes of chronic fatigue in fibromyalgia patients are:

1. inappropriate dosing of medications (TCAs, drugs with antihistamine actions, benzodiazapines, etc.)
2. depression
3. aerobic deconditioning
3. a primary sleep disorder (e.g. sleep apnoea)
4. non-restorative sleep
5. neurally mediated hypotension
6. growth hormone deficiency (Bennett et al 1992, 1997, 1998).

Restless leg syndrome

Treatment is simple and very effective – L-dopa (Sinemet) in an *early* evening dose of 10/100 mg (a minority require a higher dose or use of the long-acting preparations). Some patients respond to gabapentin. Recalcitrant cases are often helped by low-dose opioid therapy.

Irritable bowel syndrome

Treatment involves:

1. elimination of foods that aggravate symptoms
2. minimizing psychological distress
3. adhering to basic rules for maintaining a regular bowel habit
4. prescribing medications for specific symptoms: constipation (stool softener, fibre supplementation and gentle laxatives such as bisacodyl), diarrhoea (loperamide or diphenoxylate) and antispasmodics (dicyclomine or anticholinergic/sedative preparations such as Donnatal).

Irritable bladder syndrome

Treatment involves:

1. increasing intake of water
2. avoiding bladder irritants such as fruit juices (especially cranberry)
3. pelvic floor exercises (e.g. Kagel exercises)
4. the prescription of antispasmodic medications (e.g. oxybutinin, flavoxate, hyoscamine).

Cognitive dysfunction

This is a common problem for many fibromyalgia patients. It adversely affects employment and may cause concern about an early dementing type of neurodegenerative disease. In practice, the latter concern has never been a problem and patients can be reassured. The cause of poor memory and problems with concentration is, in most patients, related to the distracting effects of chronic pain and mental fatigue. Thus the effective treatment of cognitive dysfunction in fibromyalgia is dependent on the successful management of the other symptoms.

Cold intolerance

Treatment involves:

1. keeping warm
2. low-grade aerobic exercise (which improves peripheral circulation)
3. treatment of neurally mediated hypotension (see below)
4. the prescription of vasodilators such as the calcium

channel blockers (but these may aggravate the problem in patients with hypotension).

Multiple sensitivities

Treatment involves being aware that this is a fibromyalgia-related problem, so that medications often need to be started at half the usual doses.

Dizziness

Treatable causes related to fibromyalgia include:

1. proprioceptive dysfunction secondary to muscle deconditioning
2. proprioceptive dysfunction secondary to myofascial trigger points in the sternocleidomastoids and other neck muscles
3. neurally mediated hypotension (see below)
4. medication side effects.

Treatment is dependent on making an accurate diagnosis.

Neurally mediated hypotension

Treatment involves:

1. education as to the triggering factors and their avoidance
2. increasing plasma volume (increased salt intake, prescription of florinef)
3. avoidance of drugs that aggravate hypotension (e.g. TCAs, antihypertensives)
4. preventing reflex (β-adrenergic antagonists or disopyramide)
5. minimizing the efferent limb of the reflex (α-adrenergic agonists or anticholinergic agents).

MULTIDISCIPLINARY TEAM THERAPY

Most of the recommendations for management given so far have been directed at the one-on-one doctor–patient encounter. In the current era of cost-effective medicine it is often difficult to accommodate the demands of these patients. However, most of these same recommendations can be incorporated into a multidisciplinary treatment programme. The fibromyalgia treatment group at Oregon Health Sciences University has pioneered this concept using a team of interested health professionals (nurse practitioners, clinical psychologists, exercise physiologists, mental healthcare workers and social workers) (Bennett 1996b, Bennett et al 1996). In this way groups of 10–30 patients can be seen in designated sessions several times a month. Patients usually appreciate meeting others who share similar problems and the dynamics of group therapy is often a powerful aid to cognitive-behavioural modifications. Such groups can be encouraged to develop a sense of camaraderie in solving mutual problems. This form of therapy has proved beneficial in one 6-month programme, with continuing improvement out to 2 years after leaving the programme (Bennett et al 1996) (Fig. 25.5).

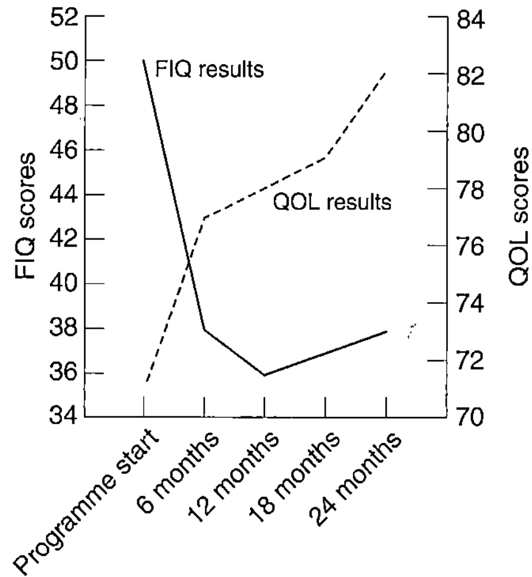

Fig. 25.5 A 6-month multidisciplinary fibromyalgia treatment programme resulted in worthwhile improvements in the Fibromyalgia Impact Questionnaire (FIQ) and the Quality of Life Questionnaire. These improvements persisted for up to 24 months after patients left the programme. (From Bennett et al 1996.)

REFERENCES

Aaron LA, Bradley LA, Alarcon GS et al 1996 Psychiatric diagnoses in patients with fibromyalgia are related to health care-seeking behavior rather than to illness. Arthritis and Rheumatism 39: 436–445

Aaron LA, Bradley LA, Alarcon GS et al 1997 Perceived physical and emotional trauma as precipitating events in fibromyalgia. Associations with health care seeking and disability status but not pain severity. Arthritis and Rheumatism 40: 453–460

Abbadie C, Brown JL, Mantyh PW, Basbaum AI 1996 Spinal cord substance P receptor immunoreactivity increases in both inflammatory and nerve injury models of persistent pain. Neuroscience 70: 201–209

Affleck G, Urrows S, Tennen H, Higgins P, Abeles M 1996 Sequential daily relations of sleep, pain intensity, and attention to pain among women with fibromyalgia. Pain 68: 363–368

Ahles TA, Yunus MB, Riley SD, Bradley JM, Masi AT 1984 Psychological factors associated with primary fibromyalgia syndrome. Arthritis and Rheumatism 27: 1101–1106

Ahles TA, Yunus MB, Gaulier B, Riley SD, Masi AT 1986 The use of contemporary MMPI norms in the study of chronic pain patients. Pain 24: 159–163

Ahles TA, Khan SA, Yunus MB, Spiegel DA, Masi AT 1991 Psychiatric status of patients with primary fibromyalgia, patients with rheumatoid arthritis, and subjects without pain: a blind comparison of DSM-III diagnoses. American Journal of Psychiatry 148: 1721–1726

Alagiri M, Chottiner S, Ratner V, Slade D, Hanno PM 1997 Interstitial cystitis: unexplained associations with other chronic disease and pain syndromes. Urology 49: 52–57

Alfici S, Sigal M, Landau M 1998 Primary fibromyalgia – a variant of depressive disorder? Psychotherapy and Psychosomatics 51: 156–161

Armstrong RB, Warren GL, Warren JA 1991 Mechanisms of exercise-induced muscle fibre injury. Sports Medicine 12: 184–207

Arnetz BB, Fjellner B 1986 Psychological predictors of neuroendocrine responses to mental stress. Journal of Psychosomatic Research 30: 297–305

Arroyo JF, Cohen ML 1993 Abnormal responses to electrocutaneous stimulation in fibromyalgia. Journal of Rheumatology 20: 1925–1931

Awad EA 1973 Interstitial myofibrositis: hypothesis of the mechanism. Archives of Physical Medicine 54: 449–452

Backman E, Bengtsson A, Bengtsson M, Lennmarken C, Henriksson KG 1988 Skeletal muscle function in primary fibromyalgia. Effect of regional sympathetic blockade with guanethidine. Acta Neurologica Scandinavica 77: 187–191

Balfour W 1816 Observations, with cases illustrative of a new, simple and expeditious mode of curing rheumatism and sprains. J & C Muirhead, Edinburgh, p 110

Barkhuizen A, Schoeplin GS, Bennett RM 1996 Fibromyalgia: a prominent feature in patients with musculoskeletal problems in chronic hepatitis C: a report of 12 patients. Journal of Clinical Rheumatology 2: 180–184

Basbaum AI, Fields HL 1984 Endogenous pain control systems: brainstem spinal pathways and endorphin circuitry. Annual Review of Neuroscience 7: 309–338

Bendtsen L, Norregaard J, Jensen R, Olesen J 1997 Evidence of qualitatively altered nociception in patients with fibromyalgia. Arthritis and Rheumatism 40: 98–102

Bengtsson A, Henriksson KG, Jorfeldt L et al 1986a Primary fibromyalgia. A clinical and laboratory study of 55 patients. Scandinavian Journal of Rheumatology 15: 340–347

Bengtsson A, Henriksson KG, Larsson J 1986b Reduced high-energy phosphate levels in the painful muscles of patients with primary fibromyalgia. Arthritis and Rheumatism 29: 817–821

Bengtsson A, Backman E, Lindblom B, Skogh T 1994 Long term follow-up of fibromyalgia patients: clinical symptoms, muscular function, laboratory tests – an eight year comparison study. Journal of Musculoskeletal Pain 2: 67–80

Bengtsson M, Bengtsson A, Jorfeldt L 1989 Diagnostic epidural opioid blockade in primary fibromyalgia at rest and during exercise. Pain 39: 171–180

Bennett RM 1981 Fibrositis: misnomer for a common rheumatic disorder. Western Journal of Medicine 134: 405–413

Bennett RM 1989a Confounding features of the fibromyalgia syndrome: a current perspective of differential diagnosis. Journal of Rheumatology 16 (suppl 19): 58–61

Bennett RM 1989b Physical fitness and muscle metabolism in the fibromyalgia syndrome: an overview. Journal of Rheumatology 16 (suppl 19): 28–29

Bennett RM 1993 The origin of myopain: an integrated hypothesis of focal muscle changes and sleep disturbance in patients with the fibromyalgia syndrome. Journal of Musculoskeletal Pain 1: 95–112

Bennett RM 1996a Fibromyalgia and the disability dilemma. A new era in understanding a complex, multidimensional pain syndrome. Arthritis and Rheumatism 39: 1627–1634

Bennett RM 1996b Multidisciplinary group programs to treat fibromyalgia patients. Rheumatic Diseases Clinics of North America 22: 351–367

Bennett RM 1996c The contribution of muscle to the generation of fibromyalgia symptomatology. Journal of Musculoskeletal Pain 4: 35–59

Bennett RM 1997 The concurrence of lupus and fibromyalgia: implications for diagnosis and management. Lupus 6: 494–499

Bennett RM, Gatter RA, Campbell SM et al 1988 A comparison of cyclobenzaprine and placebo in the management of fibrositis. A double-blind controlled study. Arthritis and Rheumatism 31: 1535–1542

Bennett RM, Clark SR, Goldberg L et al 1989 Aerobic fitness in patients with fibrositis. A controlled study of respiratory gas exchange and ^{133}xenon clearance from exercising muscle. Arthritis and Rheumatism 32: 454–460

Bennett RM, Clark SR, Campbell SM et al 1991 Symptoms of Raynaud's syndrome in patients with fibromyalgia. A study utilizing the Nielsen test, digital photoplethysmography, and measurements of platelet alpha 2-adrenergic receptors. Arthritis and Rheumatism 34: 264–269

Bennett RM, Clark SR, Campbell SM, Burckhardt CS 1992 Low levels of somatomedin C in patients with the fibromyalgia syndrome. A possible link between sleep and muscle pain. Arthritis and Rheumatism 35: 1113–1116

Bennett RM, Burckhardt CS, Clark SR, O'Reilly CA, Wiens AN et al 1996 Group treatment of fibromyalgia: a 6 month outpatient program. Journal of Rheumatology 23: 521–528

Bennett RM, Cook DM, Clark SR, Burckhardt CS, Campbell SM 1997 Hypothalamic-pituitary-insulin-like growth factor-I axis dysfunction in patients with fibromyalgia. Journal of Rheumatology 24: 1384–1389

Bennett RM, Clark SC, Walczyk J 1998 A randomized, double-blind, placebo-controlled study of growth hormone in the treatment of fibromyalgia. American Journal of Medicine 104: 227–231

Biasi G, Manca S, Manganelli S, Marcolongo R 1998 Tramadol in the fibromyalgia syndrome: a controlled clinical trial versus placebo. International Journal of Clinical Pharmacology Research 18: 13–19

Bohr TW 1995 Fibromyalgia syndrome and myofascial pain syndrome. Do they exist? Neurologic Clinics 13: 365–384

Bohr TW 1996 Problems with myofascial pain syndrome and fibromyalgia syndrome. Neurology 46: 593–597

Boisset-Pioro MH, Esdaile JM, Fitzcharles MA 1995 Sexual and physical abuse in women with fibromyalgia syndrome. Arthritis and Rheumatism 38: 235–241

Bombardier CH, Buchwald D 1996 Chronic fatigue, chronic fatigue syndrome, and fibromyalgia. Disability and health-care use. Medical Care 34: 924–930

Bonafede RP, Downey DC, Bennett RM 1995 An association of fibromyalgia with primary Sjogren's syndrome: a prospective study of 72 patients. Journal of Rheumatology 22: 133–136

Borenstein D 1995 Prevalence and treatment outcome of primary and secondary fibromyalgia in patients with spinal pain. Spine 20: 796–800

Bou-Holaigah I, Calkins H, Flynn JA et al 1997 Provocation of hypotension and pain during upright tilt table testing in adults with fibromyalgia. Clinical and Experimental Rheumatology 15: 239–246

Bradley LA, Prokop CK, Margolis R, Gentry WD 1978 Multivariate analysis of MMPI profiles of low back pain patients. Journal of Behavioral Medicine 1: 253–272

Brendstrup P, Jespersen K, Asboe-Hansen 1957 Morphological and chemical connective tissue changes in fibrositis muscles. Annals of Rheumatic Diseases 16: 438–440

Bruusgaard D, Evensen AR, Bjerkedal T 1993 Fibromyalgia – a new cause for disability pension. Scandinavian Journal of Social Medicine 21: 116–119

Buchwald D, Garrity D 1994 Comparison of patients with chronic fatigue syndrome, fibromyalgia, and multiple chemical sensitivities. Archives of Internal Medicine 154: 2049–2053

Burckhardt CS, Bjelle A 1994 Education programmes for fibromyalgia patients: description and evaluation. Baillière's Clinical Rheumatology 8: 935–955

Burckhardt CS, Clark SR, Bennett RM 1993 Fibromyalgia and quality of life: a comparative analysis. Journal of Rheumatology 20: 475–479

Burckhardt CS, O'Reilly CA, Wiens AN et al 1994 Assessing depression in fibromyalgia patients. Arthritis Care Research 7: 35–39

Buskila D, Neumann L 1997 Fibromyalgia syndrome (FM) and nonarticular tenderness in relatives of patients with FM. Journal of Rheumatology 24: 941–944

Buskila D, Neumann L, Hazanov I, Carmi R 1996 Familial aggregation in the fibromyalgia syndrome. Seminars in Arthritis and Rheumatism 26: 605–611

Buskila D, Neumann L, Vaisberg G, Alkalay D, Wolfe F 1997 Increased rates of fibromyalgia following cervical spine injury. A controlled study of 161 cases of traumatic injury. Arthritis and Rheumatism 40: 446–452

Calvo-Alen J, Bastian HM, Straaton KV et al 1995 Identification of patient subsets among those presumptively diagnosed with, referred, and/or followed up for systemic lupus erythematosus at a large tertiary care center. Arthritis and Rheumatism 38: 1475–1484

Campbell SM, Clark S, Tindall EA, Forehand ME, Bennett RM 1983 Clinical characteristics of fibrositis. I.A 'blinded' controlled study of symptoms and tender points. Arthritis and Rheumatism 26: 817–824

Carette S 1995 Fibromyalgia 20 years later: what have we really accomplished? Journal of Rheumatology 22: 590–594

Carette S, Bell MJ, Reynolds WJ et al 1994 Comparison of amitriptyline, cyclobenzaprine, and placebo in the treatment of fibromyalgia. Arthritis and Rheumatism 37: 32–40

Caro XJ 1984 Immunofluorescent detection of IgG at the dermal-epidermal junction in patients with apparent primary fibrositis syndrome. Arthritis and Rheumatism 27: 1174–1179

Cathey MA, Wolfe F, Kleinheksel SM et al 1988 Functional ability and work status in patients with fibromyalgia. Arthritis Care Research 1: 85–98

Clark S, Campbell SM, Forehand ME, Tindall EA, Bennett RM 1985a Clinical characteristics of fibrositis. II. A 'blinded,' controlled study using standard psychological tests. Arthritis and Rheumatism 28: 132–137

Clark S, Tindall E, Bennett RM 1985b A double blind crossover trial of prednisone versus placebo in the treatment of fibrositis. Journal of Rheumatology 12: 980–983

Clark SR 1994 Prescribing exercise for fibromyalgia patients. Arthritis Care Research 7: 221–225

Clark SR, Burckhardt CS, Campbell S, O'Reilly C, Bennett RM 1993 Fitness characteristics and perceived exertion in women with fibromyalgia. Journal of Musculoskeletal Pain 1: 191–197

Clauw DJ 1995 Fibromyalgia: more than just a musculoskeletal disease. American Family Physician 52: 843–851, 853–854

Clauw DJ, Schmidt M, Radulovic D et al 1997 The relationship between fibromyalgia and interstitial cystitis. Journal of Psychiatric Research 31: 125–131

Coderre TJ, Katz J, Vaccarino AL, Melzack R 1993 Contribution of central neuroplasticity to pathological pain: review of clinical and experimental evidence. Pain 52: 259–285

Cohen ML, Quintner JL 1998 Fibromyalgia syndrome and disability: a failed construct fails those in pain. Medical Journal of Australia 168: 402–404

Craig AD 1998 A new version of the thalamic disinhibition hypothesis of central pain. Pain Forum 7: 1–14

Crofford LJ, Pillemer SR, Kalogeras KT et al 1994 Hypothalamic-pituitary-adrenal axis perturbations in patients with fibromyalgia. Arthritis and Rheumatism 37: 1583–1592

Croft P, Rigby AS, Boswell R, Schollum J, Silman A 1993 The prevalence of chronic widespread pain in the general population. Journal of Rheumatology 20: 710–713

Croft P, Schollum J, Silman A 1994 Population study of tender point counts and pain as evidence of fibromyalgia. British Medical Journal 309: 696–699

Dailey PA, Bishop GD, Russell IJ, Fletcher EM 1990 Psychological stress and the fibrositis/fibromyalgia syndrome. Journal of Rheumatology 17: 1380–1385

Danneskiold-Samsoe B, Christiansen E, Lund B, Anderson RB 1983 Regional muscle tension and pain ('fibrositis'): effect of massage on myoglobin in plasma. Scandinavian Journal of Rehabilitation Medicine 15: 17–20

De Blecourt AC, Wolf RF, van Rijswijk MH et al 1991 In vivo 31P magnetic resonance spectroscopy (MRS) of tender points in patients with primary fibromyalgia syndrome. Rheumatology International 11: 51–54

De Blecourt AC, Knipping AA, De Voogd N, Van Rijswijk MH 1993 Weather conditions and complaints in fibromyalgia. Journal of Rheumatology 20: 1932–1934

De Felipe C, Herrero JF, O'Brien JA et al 1998 Altered nociception, analgesia and aggression in mice lacking the receptor for substance P. Nature 392: 394–397

Dickenson AH, Sullivan AF 1991 NMDA receptors and central hyperalgesic states. Pain 46: 344–345

Dinerman H, Steere AC 1990 Fibromyalgia following Lyme disease: association with neurologic involvement and lack of response to antibiotic therapy. Arthritis and Rheumatism 33: 136

Dinerman H, Goldenberg DL, Felson DT 1986 A prospective evaluation of 118 patients with the fibromyalgia syndrome: prevalence of Raynaud's phenomenon, sicca symptoms, ANA, low complement, and Ig deposition at the dermal-epidermal junction. Journal of Rheumatology 13: 368–373

Donald F, Esdaile JM, Kimoff JR, Fitzcharles MA 1996 Musculoskeletal complaints and fibromyalgia in patients attending a respiratory sleep disorders clinic. Journal of Rheumatology 23: 1612–1616

Dougherty PM, Willis WD 1992 Enhancement of spinothalamic neuron responses to chemical and mechanical stimuli following combined micro-iontophoretic application of N-methyl-D-aspartic acid and substance P. Pain 47: 85–93

Drewes AM, Andreasen A, Jennum P, Nielsen KD 1991 Zopiclone in the treatment of sleep abnormalities in fibromyalgia. Scandinavian Journal of Rheumatology 20: 288–293

Drewes AM, Gade K, Nielsen KD et al 1995 Clustering of sleep electroencephalographic patterns in patients with the fibromyalgia syndrome. British Journal of Rheumatology 34: 1151–1156

Dwight MM, Arnold LM, O'Brien H et al 1998 An open clinical trial of venlafaxine treatment of fibromyalgia. Psychosomatics 39: 14–17

Elert JE, Rantapäa-Dahlqvist SB, Henriksson-Larsën K, Lorentzon R, Gerdlë BU 1992 Muscle performance, electromyography and fibre type composition in fibromyalgia and work-related myalgia. Scandinavian Journal of Rheumatology 21: 28–34

Elert JE, Dahlqvist SR, Almay B, Eismann M 1995 Muscle endurance, muscle tension, and personality traits in patients with muscle or joint pain – a pilot study. Journal of Rheumatology 20: 1550–1556

Estlander AM, Takala EP, Viikari-Juntura E 1998 Do psychological factors predict changes in musculoskeletal pain? A prospective, two-year follow-up study of a working population. Journal of Occupational and Environmental Medicine 40: 445–453

Fassbender HG 1975 Pathology of rheumatic disease. Springer Verlag, New York, pp 304–307

Fassbender K, Samborsky W, Kellner M, Muller W, Lautenbacher S 1997

Tender points, depressive and functional symptoms: comparison between fibromyalgia and major depression. Clinical Rheumatology 16: 76–79

Felson DT, Goldenberg DL 1986 The natural history of fibromyalgia. Arthritis and Rheumatism 29: 1522–1526

Fields HL, Basbaum AI, Wall PD, Melzack R 1994 Central nervous system mechanisms of pain modulation. In: Melzack R, Wall PD (eds) Textbook of pain. Churchill Livingstone, Edinburgh, pp 243–257

Freeman R, Komaroff AL 1997 Does the chronic fatigue syndrome involve the autonomic nervous system? American Journal of Medicine 102: 357–364

Friedman OP 1990 Perspectives on the medical use of drugs of abuse. Journal of Pain and Symptom Management 5: S2–S5

Gerdle B, Elert J 1995 Disability and impairment in fibromyalgia syndrome: possible pathogenesis and etiology. Critical Reviews in Physical and Rehabilitative Medicine 7: 189–232

Gibson SJ, Littlejohn GO, Gorman MM, Helme RD, Granges G 1994 Altered heat pain thresholds and cerebral event-related potentials following painful CO2 laser stimulation in subjects with fibromyalgia syndrome. Pain 58: 185–193

Gjesdal S, Kristiansen AM 1997 Norwegian fibromyalgia epidemic – its rise or possible decline. What is the trend based on disability statistics? Tidsskrift for den Norske Laegforening 117: 2449–2453

Gladman DD, Urowitz MB, Gough J, MacKinnon A 1997 Fibromyalgia is a major contributor to quality of life in lupus. Journal of Rheumatology 24: 2145–2148

Goldberg RT 1994 Childhood abuse, depression, and chronic pain. Clinical Journal of Pain 10: 277–281

Goldenberg DL 1987 Fibromyalgia syndrome. An emerging but controversial condition. Journal of the American Medical Association 257: 2782–2787

Goldenberg DL 1989 A review of the role of tricyclic medications in the treatment of fibromyalgia syndrome. Journal of Rheumatology 19 (suppl): 137–139

Goldenberg DL, Simms RW, Geiger A, Komaroff AL 1990 High frequency of fibromyalgia in patients with chronic fatigue seen in a primary care practice. Arthritis and Rheumatism 33: 381–387

Goldenberg DL, Kaplan KH, Nadeau MG et al 1994 A controlled study of a stress-reduction, cognitive-behavioral treatment program in fibromyalgia. Journal of Musculoskeletal Pain 2: 53–66

Goldenberg DL, Mayskiy M, Mossey C, Ruthazer R, Schmid C 1996 A randomized, double-blind crossover trial of fluoxetine and amitriptyline in the treatment of fibromyalgia. Arthritis and Rheumatism 39: 1852–1859

Gonzalez VM, Goeppinger J, Lorig K 1990 Four psychosocial theories and their application to patient education and clinical practice. Arthritis Care Research 3: 132–143

Gowers WR 1904 Lumbago: its lessons and analogues. BMJ 1: 117–121

Granges G, Zilko P, Littlejohn GO 1994 Fibromyalgia syndrome: assessment of the severity of the condition 2 years after diagnosis. Journal of Rheumatology 21: 523–529

Graven-Nielsen T 1997 Sensory manifestations and sensory-motor interactions during experimental muscle pain in man. PhD thesis, Aalborg University

Guedj D, Weinberger A 1990 Effect of weather conditions on rheumatic patients. Annals of Rheumatic Diseases 49: 158–159

Hagglund KJ, Deuser WE, Buckelew SP, Hewett J, Kay DR 1994 Weather, beliefs about weather, and disease severity among patients with fibromyalgia. Arthritis Care Research 7: 130–135

Hales RE, Clonginger CRBJF 1994 Somatoform disorders. In: Diagnostic and statistical manual of mental disorders (DSM-IV). American Psychiatric Association, Washington DC, pp 445–469

Harvey CK 1993 Fibromyalgia. Part II. Prevalence in the podiatric patient population. Journal of the American Podiatric Medical Association 83: 416–417

Hauri P, Hawkins DR 1973 Alpha-delta sleep. Electroencephalography and Clinical Neurophysiology 34: 233–237

Hawley DJ, Wolfe F 1991 Pain, disability, and pain/disability relationships in seven rheumatic disorders: a study of 1,522 patients. Journal of Rheumatology 18: 1552–1557

Hawley DJ, Wolfe F 1993 Depression is not more common in rheumatoid arthritis: a 10-year longitudinal study of 6,153 patients with rheumatic disease. Journal of Rheumatology 20: 2025–2031

Hawley DJ, Wolfe F, Cathey MA 1988 Pain, functional disability, and psychological status: a 12-month study of severity in fibromyalgia. Journal of Rheumatology 15: 1551–1556

Helleday U 1976 Om myitis chronica (rheumatica). Ett bidrag till dess diagnostik och behandling. Nord Med Ark 8: 1–17

Hench PK 1976 Nonarticular rheumatism. Rheumatism Reviews 22: 1081–1088

Henriksson CM 1994 Longterm effects of fibromyalgia on everyday life. A study of 56 patients. Scandinavian Journal of Rheumatology 23: 36–41

Henriksson CM 1995 Living with continuous muscular pain–patient perspectives. Part I: Encounters and consequences. Scandinavian Journal of the Caring Sciences 9: 67–76

Henriksson CM, Gundmark I, Bengtsson A, Ek AC 1992 Living with fibromyalgia. Consequences for everyday life. Clinical Journal of Pain 8: 138–144

Henriksson KG 1994 Chronic muscular pain: aetiology and pathogenesis. Baillière's Clinical Rheumatology 8: 703–719

Henriksson KG, Bengtsson A, Larsson J, Lindstrom F, Thornell LE 1982 Muscle biopsy findings of possible diagnostic importance in primary fibromyalgia (fibrositis, myofascial syndrome). Lancet 2: 1395

Hsieh JC, Belfrage M, Stone-Elander S, Hansson P, Ingvar M 1995 Central representation of chronic ongoing neuropathic pain studied by positron emission tomography. Pain 63: 225–236

Hudson JI, Pope HG Jr 1995 Does childhood sexual abuse cause fibromyalgia? Arthritis and Rheumatism 38: 161–163

Hudson JI, Hudson MS, Pliner LF, Goldenberg DL, Pope HG Jr 1985 Fibromyalgia and major affective disorder: a controlled phenomenology and family history study. American Journal of Psychiatry 142: 441–446

Iadarola MJ, Max MB, Berman KF 1995 Unilateral decrease in thalamic activity observed in positron emission tomography in patients with chronic neuropathic pain. Pain 63: 55–64

Jacobsen S, Danneskiold-Samsoe B 1987 Isometric and isokinetic muscle strength in patients with fibrositis syndrome. New characteristics for a difficult definable category of patients. Scandinavian Journal of Rheumatology 16: 61–65

Jacobsen S, Danneskiold-Samsoe B 1992 Dynamic muscular endurance in primary fibromyalgia compared with chronic myofascial pain syndrome. Arch. Phys. Med. Rehabil. 73: 170–173

Jacobsen S, Wildschiodtz G, Danneskiold-Samsoe B 1991 Isokinetic and isometric muscle strength combined with transcutaneous electrical muscle stimulation in primary fibromyalgia syndrome. Journal of Rheumatology 18: 1390–1393

Jacobsen S, Jensen KE, Thomsen C, Danneskiold-Samsoe B, Henriksen O 1992 31P magnetic resonance spectroscopy of skeletal muscle in patients with fibromyalgia. Journal of Rheumatology 19: 1600–1603

Jacobsen S, Jensen KE, Thomsen C, Danneskiold-Samsoe B, Henriksen O 1994 [Magnetic resonance spectroscopy in fibromyalgia. A study of phosphate-31 spectra from skeletal muscles during rest and after exercise]. Ugeskrift for Laeger 156: 6841–6844

Jacobsson L, Lindgärde F, Manthorpe R 1989 The commonest rheumatic complaints of over six weeks' duration in a twelve-month period in a defined Swedish population. Prevalences and relationships. Scandinavian Journal of Rheumatology 18: 353–360

Jennum P, Drewes AM, Andreasen A, Nielsen KD 1993 Sleep and other symptoms in primary fibromyalgia and in healthy controls. Journal of Rheumatology 20: 1756–1759

Jubrias SA, Bennett RM, Klug GA 1994 Increased incidence of a resonance in the phosphodiester region of 31P nuclear magnetic resonance spectra in the skeletal muscle of fibromyalgia patients. Arthritis and Rheumatism 37: 801–807

Katz RS, Kravitz HM 1996 Fibromyalgia, depression, and alcoholism: a family history study. Journal of Rheumatology 23: 149–154

Kennedy M, Felson DT 1996 A prospective long-term study of fibromyalgia syndrome. Arthritis and Rheumatism 39: 682–685

Kellgren JH 1938 Observations on referred pain arising from muscle. Clinical Science 3: 175–190

Kellgren JH 1939 On the distribution of pain arising from deep somatic structures with charts of segmental pain areas. Clinical Science 4: 35–46

Kirmayer LJ, Robbins JM, Kapusta MA 1988 Somatization and depression in fibromyalgia syndrome. American Journal of Psychiatry 145: 950–954

Klemp P, Nielsen HV, Korsgard J et al 1982 Blood flow in fibromyotic muscles. Scandinavian Journal of Rehabilitation Medicine 14: 81–86

Komaroff AL, Buchwald D 1991 Symptoms and signs of chronic fatigue syndrome. Reviews of Infectious Diseases 13: S8–S11

Kosek E, Ekholm J, Hansson P 1996a Modulation of pressure pain thresholds during and following isometric contraction in patients with fibromyalgia and in healthy controls. Pain 64: 415–423

Kosek E, Ekholm J, Hansson P 1996b Sensory dysfunction in fibromyalgia patients with implications for pathogenic mechanisms. Pain 68: 375–383

Kramis RC, Roberts WJ, Gillette RG 1996 Non-nociceptive aspects of persistent musculoskeletal pain. Journal of Orthopaedic and Sports Physical Therapy 24: 255–267

Krueger BR 1990 Restless legs syndrome and periodic movements of sleep. Mayo Clinic Proceedings 65: 999–1006

Kurtze N, Gundersen KT, Svebak S 1998 The role of anxiety and depression in fatigue and patterns of pain among subgroups of fibromyalgia patients. British Journal of Medical Psychology 71: 185–194

Landro NI, Stiles TC, Sletvold H 1997 Memory functioning in patients with primary fibromyalgia and major depression and healthy controls. Journal of Psychosomatic Research 42: 297–306

Lapossy E, Maleitzke R, Hrycaj P, Mennet W, Muller W 1995 The frequency of transition of chronic low back pain to fibromyalgia. Scandinavian Journal of Rheumatology 24: 29–33

Lautenbacher S, Rollman GB 1997 Possible deficiencies of pain modulation in fibromyalgia. Clinical Journal of Pain 13: 189–196

Leavitt F, Katz RS 1989 Is the MMPI invalid for assessing psychological disturbance in pain related organic conditions? Journal of Rheumatology 16: 521–526

Ledingham J, Doherty S, Doherty M 1993 Primary fibromyalgia syndrome–an outcome study. British Journal of Rheumatology 32: 139–142

Leserman J, Li Z, Hu YJ, Drossman DA 1998 How multiple types of stressors impact on health. Psychosomatic Medicine 60: 175–181

Leventhal LJ, Naides SJ, Freundlich B 1991 Fibromyalgia and parvovirus infection. Arthritis and Rheumatism 34: 1319–1324

Li L, Moore D 1998 Acceptance of disability and its correlates. Journal of Social Psychology 138: 13–25

Lindh MH, Johansson LG, Hedberg M, Grimby GL 1994 Studies on maximal voluntary muscle contraction in patients with fibromyalgia. Arch. Phys. Med. Rehabil. 75: 1217–1222

Lindman R, Eriksson A, Thornell LE 1991a Fiber type composition of the human female trapezius muscle: enzyme-histochemical characteristics. American Journal of Anatomy 190: 385–392

Lindman R, Hagberg M, Angqvist KA et al 1991b Changes in muscle morphology in chronic trapezius myalgia. Scandinavian Journal of Work and Environmental Health 17: 347–355

Lindman R, Hagberg M, Bengtsson A, Henriksson KG, Thornell LE 1992 Capillary structure and mitochondrial volume density in the normal trapezius muscle and in chronic trapezius myalgia and in fibromyalgia. In: Chronic Trapezius Myalgia – a morphological study. PhD Thesis University of Umea, Sweden

Linton SJ, Larden M, Gillow AM 1996 Sexual abuse and chronic musculoskeletal pain: prevalence and psychological factors. Clinical Journal of Pain 12: 215–221

Liu H, Mantyh CR, Basbaum AI 1997 NMDA-receptor regulation of substance-P release from promary afferent nociceptors. Nature 386: 721–724

Loeser JD 1991 What is chronic pain? Theoretical Medicine 12: 213–225

Lorenz J, Grasedyck K, Bromm B 1996 Middle and long latency somatosensory evoked potentials after painful laser stimulation in patients with fibromyalgia syndrome. Electroencephalogr. Clinical Neurophysiology 100: 165–168

Lund N, Bengtsson A, Thorborg P 1986 Muscle tissue oxygen pressure in primary fibromyalgia. Scandinavian Journal of Rheumatology 15: 165–173

MacFarlane GJ, Thomas E, Papageorgiou AC et al 1996a The natural history of chronic pain in the community: a better prognosis than in the clinic? Journal of Rheumatology 23: 1617–1620

MacFarlane JG, Shahal B, Mously C, Moldofsky H 1996b Periodic K-alpha sleep EEG activity and periodic limb movements during sleep: comparisons of clinical features and sleep parameters. Sleep 19: 200–204

Magerl W, Wilk SH, Treede RD 1998 Secondary hyperalgesia and perceptual wind-up following intradermal injection of capsaicin in humans. Pain 74: 257–268

Maier SF, Wiertelak EP, Martin D, Watkins LR 1993 Interleukin-1 mediates the behavioral hyperalgesia produced by lithium chloride and endotoxin. Brain Research 623: 321–324

Makela M, Heliovaara M 1991 Prevalence of primary fibromyalgia in the Finnish population. British Medical Journal 303: 216–219

Mannerkorpi K, Ekdahl C 1997 Assessment of functional limitation and disability in patients with fibromyalgia. Scandinavian Journal of Rheumatology 26: 4–13

Mantyh PW, Rogers SD, Honore P et al 1997 Inhibition of hyperalgesia by ablation of lamina I spinal neurons expressing the substance P receptor. Science 278: 275–279

Marder WD, Meenan RF, Felson DT et al 1991 Editorial: the present and future adequacy of rheumatology manpower: a study of health care needs and physician supply. Arthritis and Rheumatism 34: 1209–1217

Martin L, Nutting A, MacIntosh BR et al 1996 An exercise program in the treatment of fibromyalgia. Journal of Rheumatology 23: 1050–1053

Masi AT 1994 An intuitive person-centred perspective on fibromyalgia syndrome and its management. Baillière's Clinical Rheumatology 8: 957–993

Mathur AK, Gatter RA 1988 Abnormal 31P-NMR spectroscopy of painful muscles of patients with fibromyalgia. Arthritis and Rheumatism 31: S23

McCain GA, Bell DA, Mai FM, Halliday PD 1988 A controlled study of the effects of a supervised cardiovascular fitness training program on the manifestations of primary fibromyalgia. Arthritis and Rheumatism 31: 1135–1141

McCain GA, Cameron R, Kennedy JC 1989 The problem of longterm disability payments and litigation in primary fibromyalgia: the Canadian perspective. Journal of Rheumatology 19(suppl): 174–176

McWhinney IR, Epstein RM, Freeman TR 1997 Rethinking somatization. Annals of Internal Medicine 126: 747–750

Melzack R 1990 The tragedy of needless pain. Scientific American 262: 27–33

Mengshoel AM, F??rre O, Komnaes HB 1990 Muscle strength and aerobic capacity in primary fibromyalgia. Clinical and Experimental Rheumatology 8: 475–479
Middleton GD, McFarlin JE, Lipsky PE 1994 The prevalence and clinical impact of fibromyalgia in systemic lupus erythematosus. Arthritis and Rheumatism 37: 1181–1188
Miehlke K, Schulze G, Eger W 1960 Klinische and experimentelle untersuchungen zum fibrositis syndrom. Zeitschrift fur Rheumaforschung 19: 310–330
Mikkelsson M, Salminen JJ, Kautiainen H 1997 Non-specific musculoskeletal pain in preadolescents. Prevalence and 1-year persistence. Pain 73: 29–35
Moldofsky H 1989 Sleep and fibrositis syndrome. Rheumatic Diseases Clinics of North America 15: 91–103
Moldofsky H 1994 Chronobiological influences on fibromyalgia syndrome: theoretical and therapeutic implications. Baillière's Clinical Rheumatology 8: 801–810
Moldofsky H, Scarisbrick P 1976 Induction of neurasthenic musculoskeletal pain syndrome by selective sleep stage deprivation. Psychosomatic Medicine 38: 35–44
Moldofsky H, Scarisbrick P, England R, Smythe H 1975 Musculoskeletal symptoms and non-REM sleep disturbance in patients with "fibrositis syndrome" and healthy subjects. Psychosomatic Medicine 37: 341–351
Moldofsky H, Tullis C, Lue FA 1986 Sleep related myoclonus in rheumatic pain modulation disorder (fibrositis syndrome). Journal of Rheumatology 13: 614–617
Moldofsky H, Lue FA, Mously C, Roth-Schechter B, Reynolds WJ 1996 The effect of zolpidem in patients with fibromyalgia: a dose ranging, double blind, placebo controlled, modified crossover study. Journal of Rheumatology 23: 529–533
Montplaisir J, Lapierre O, Warnes H, Pelletier G 1992 The treatment of the restless leg syndrome with or without periodic leg movements in sleep. Sleep 15: 391–395
Morand EF, Miller MH, Whittingham S, Littlejohn GO 1994 Fibromyalgia syndrome and disease activity in systemic lupus erythematosus. Lupus 3: 187–191
Mountz JM, Bradley LA, Modell JG et al 1995 Fibromyalgia in women. Abnormalities of regional cerebral blood flow in the thalamus and the caudate nucleus are associated with low pain threshold levels. Arthritis and Rheumatism 38: 926–938
Nielson WR, Walker C, McCain GA 1992 Cognitive behavioral treatment of fibromyalgia syndrome: preliminary findings. Journal of Rheumatology 19: 98–103
Nordenskiöld UM, Grimby G 1993 Grip force in patients with rheumatoid arthritis and fibromyalgia and in healthy subjects. A study with the Grippit instrument. Scandinavian Journal of Rheumatology 22: 14–19
Paira SO 1994 Fibromyalgia associated with female urethral syndrome. Clinical Rheumatology 13: 88–89
Park JH, Phothimat P, Oates CT, Hernanz-Schulman M, Olsen NJ 1998 Use of P-31 magnetic resonance spectroscopy to detect metabolic abnormalities in muscles of patients with fibromyalgia. Arthritis and Rheumatism 41: 406–413
Payne TC, Leavitt F, Garron DC et al 1982 Fibrositis and psychologic disturbance. Arthritis and Rheumatism 25: 213–217
Perlis ML, Giles DE, Bootzin RR et al 1997 Alpha sleep and information processing, perception of sleep, pain, and arousability in fibromyalgia. International Journal of Neuroscience 89: 265–280
Pertovaara AKP 1992 Lowered cutaneous sensitivity to nonpainful electrical stimulation during isometric exercise in humans. Experimental Brain Research 89: 447–452
Pillemer SR, Bradley LA, Crofford LJ, Moldofsky H, Chrousos GP 1997 The neuroscience and endocrinology of fibromyalgia. Arthritis and Rheumatism 40: 1928–1939
Portenoy RK 1996 Opioid therapy for chronic nonmalignant pain: a review of the critical issues. Journal of Pain and Symptom Management 11: 203–217
Portenoy RK, Dole V, Joseph H et al 1997 Pain management and chemical dependency. Evolving perspectives. Journal of the American Medical Association 278: 592–593
Prescott E, Kjeller M, Jacobsen S et al 1993 Fibromyalgia in the adult Danish population: I. A prevalence study. Scandinavian Journal of Rheumatology 22: 233–237
Quick DC 1997 Joint pain and weather. A critical review of the literature. Minnesota Medicine 80: 25–29
Reesor KA, Craig KD 1988 Medically incongruent chronic back pain: physical limitations, suffering, and ineffective coping. Pain 32: 35–45
Reilly PA, Littlejohn GO 1992 Peripheral arthralgic presentation of fibrositis/fibromyalgia syndrome. Journal of Rheumatology 19: 281–283
Riley JF, Ahern DK, Follick MJ 1988 Chronic pain and functional impairment: assessing beliefs about their relationship. Arch Phys Med Rehabil 69: 579–582
Rivera J, Diego A, Monforte GA 1997 Fibromyalgia-associated hepatitis C virus infection. British Journal of Rheumatology 36: 981–985
Rosen NB 1994 Physical medicine and rehabilitation approaches to the management of myofascial pain and fibromyalgia syndromes. Baillière's Clinical Rheumatology 8: 881–916
Roy SH 1993 Combined use of surface electromyography and 31P-NMR spectroscopy for the study of muscle disorders. Physical Therapy 73: 892–901
Russell IJ, Vipraio GA, Morgan WW, Bowden CL 1986 Is there a metabolic basis for the fibrositis syndrome? American Journal of Medicine 81: 50–54
Russell IJ, Fletcher EM, Michalek JE, McBroom PC, Hester GG 1991 Treatment of primary fibrositis/fibromyalgia syndrome with ibuprofen and alprazolam: A double-blind, placebo-controlled study. Arthritis and Rheumatism 34: 552–560
Russell IJ, Orr MD, Littman B et al 1994 Elevated cerebrospinla fluid levels of substance P in patients with the fibromyalgia syndrome. Arthritis and Rheumatism 37: 1593–1601
Russell IJ, Kamin M, Sager D et al 1997 Efficacy of Ultram™ [Tramadol HCL] treatment of fibromyalgia syndrome: preliminary analysis of a multi-center, randomized, placebo-controlled study. Arthritis and Rheumatism 40: S214
Sastry BR 1979 Substance P effects on spinal nociceptive neurones. Life Sciences 24: 2178
Satrustegui J, Berkowitz H, Boden B et al 1988 An in vivo phosphorus nuclear magnetic resonance study of the variations with age in the phosphodiers content of human muscle. Mechanisms of Aging and Development 42: 105–114
Shaver JL, Lentz M, Landis CA et al 1997 Sleep, psychological distress, and stress arousal in women with fibromyalgia. Research in Nursing and Health 20: 247–257
Siegel DM, Janeway D, Baum J 1998 Fibromyalgia syndrome in children and adolescents: clinical features at presentation and status at follow-up. Pediatrics 101: 377–382
Sietsema KE, Cooper DM, Caro X, Leibling MR, Louie JS 1993 Oxygen uptake during exercise in patients with primary fibromyalgia syndrome. Journal of Rheumatology 20: 860–865
Simms RW, Goldenberg DL, Felson DT, Mason JH 1988 Tenderness in 75 anatomic sites. Distingushing fibromyalgia patients from controls. Arthritis and Rheumatism 31: 182–187
Simms RW, Ferrante N, Craven DE 1990 High prevalence of fibromyalgia syndrome (FMS) in human immunodeficiency virus type 1 (HIV) infected patients with polyarthralgia. Arthritis and Rheumatism 33(9): S135–S136
Simms RW, Roy SH, Hrovat M et al 1994 Lack of association between

fibromyalgia syndrome and abnormalities in muscle energy metabolism. Arthritis and Rheumatism 37: 794–800
Sivri A, Cindas A, Dincer F, Sivri B 1996 Bowel dysfunction and irritable bowel syndrome in fibromyalgia patients. Clinial Rheumatology 15: 283–286
Skootsky SA, Jaeger B, Dye RK 1984 Prevalence of myofascial pain in general internal medicine practice. Western Journal of Medicine 151: 157–160
Sletvold H, Stiles TC, Landro NI 1995 Information processing in primary fibromyalgia, major depression and healthy controls. Journal of Rheumatology 22: 137–142
Slotkoff AT, Radulovic DA, Clauw DJ 1997 The relationship between fibromyalgia and the multiple chemical sensitivity syndrome. Scandinavian Journal of Rheumatology 26: 364–367
Smythe HA 1984 Problems with the MMPI. Journal of Rheumatology 11: 417–418
Smythe HA, Moldofsky H 1977 Two contributions to understanding of the 'fibrositis' syndrome. Bulletin on the Rheumatic Diseases 28: 928–931
Smythe HA, Gladman A, Mader R, Peloso P, Abu-Shakra M 1997 Strategies for assessing pain and pain exaggeration: controlled studies. Journal of Rheumatology 24: 1622–1629
Solomon DH, Liang MH 1997 Fibromyalgia: scourge of humankind or bane of a rheumatologist's existence? Arthritis and Rheumatism 40: 1553–1555
Sorensen J, Bengtsson A, Backman E, Henriksson KG, Bengtsson M 1995 Pain analysis in patients with fibromyalgia: effects of intravenous morphine, lidocaine and ketamine. Scandinavian Journal of Rheumatology 24: 360–365
Sorensen J, Bengtsson A, Ahlner J et al 1997 Fibromyalgia – are there different mechanisms in the processing of pain? A double blind crossover comparison of analgesic drugs. Journal of Rheumatology 24: 1615–1621
Sorensen J, Graven-Nielsen T, Henriksson KG, Bengtsson M, Arendt-Nielsen L 1998 Hyperexcitability in fibromyalgia. Journal of Rheumatology 25: 152–155
Stockman R 1904 The causes, pathology and treatment of chronic rheumatism. Edinburgh Medical Journal 15: 107–116
Tait RC, Margolis RB, Krause SJ, Liebowitz E 1988 Compensation status and symptoms reported by patients with chronic pain. Arch. Phys. Med. Rehabil. 69: 1027–1029
Talo S, Hendler N, Brodie J 1989 Effects of active and completed litigation on treatment results: workers' compensation patients compared with other litigation patients. Journal of Occupational Medicine 31: 265–269
Taylor ML, Trotter DR, Csuka ME 1995 The prevalence of sexual abuse in women with fibromyalgia. Arthritis and Rheumatism 38: 229–234
Teasell RW, Merskey H 1997 Chronic pain disability in the workplace. Pain Forum 6: 228–238
Toomey TC, Seville JL, Mann JD, Abashian SW, Grant JR 1995 Relationship of sexual and physical abuse to pain description, coping, psychological distress, and health-care utilization in a chronic pain sample. Clinical Journal of Pain 11: 307–315
Torebjork HE, Lundberg LER, Lamotte RH 1992 Central changes in processing of mechanoreceptive input in capsaicin-induced secondary hyperalgesia in humans. Journal of Physiology 448: 765–780
Travell J, Rinzler SH 1952 The myofascial genesis of pain. Postgraduate Medicine 11: 425–434
Travell JG, Simons DG 1983 Myofascial pain and dysfunction: the trigger point manual. Williams, Wilkins & Baltimore
Travell J, Simons D 1992 Myofascial pain and dysfunction: the trigger point manual, volume 2. Williams & Wilkins, Baltimore
Tsigos C, Diemel LT, White A, Tomlinson DR, Young RJ 1993 Cerebrospinal fluid levels of substance P and calcitonin-gene-related peptide: correlation with sural nerve levels and neuropathic signs in sensory diabetic polyneuropathy. Clinical Science 84: 305–311
Urrows S, Affleck G, Tennen H, Higgins P 1994 Unique clinical and psychological correlates of fibromyalgia tender points and joint tenderness in rheumatoid arthritis. Arthritis and Rheumatism 37: 1513–1520
Uveges JM, Parker JC, Smarr KL 1990 Psychological symptoms in primary fibromyalgia syndrome: relationship to pain, life stress and sleep disturbance. Arthritis and Rheumatism 33: 1279–1283
Vaeroy H, Helle R, Forre O, Kass E, Terenius L 1988 Elevated CSF levels of substance P and high incidence of Raynaud phenomenon in patients with fibromyalgia: new features for diagnosis. Pain 32: 21–26
Veale D, Kavanagh G, Fielding JF, Fitzgerald O 1991 Primary fibromyalgia and the irritable bowel syndrome: different expressions of a common pathogenetic process. British Journal of Rheumatology 30: 220–222
Vitali C, Tavoni A, Neri R et al 1989 Fibromyalgia features in patients with primary Sjögren's syndrome. Evidence of a relationship with psychological depression. Scandinavian Journal of Rheumatology 18: 21–27
Walker EA, Keegan D, Gardner G et al 1997 Psychosocial factors in fibromyalgia compared with rheumatoid arthritis: II. Sexual, physical, and emotional abuse and neglect. Psychosomatic Medicine 59: 572–577
Wall PD 1997 The generation of yet another myth on the use of narcotics. Pain 73: 121–122
Wall PD, Woolf CJ 1984 Muscle but not cutaneous C-afferent input produces prolonged increases in the excitability of the flexion reflex in the rat. Journal of Physiology 356: 443–458
Wallace DJ 1984 Fibromyalgia: unusual historical aspects and new pathogenic insights. Mt Sinai Journal of Medicine NY 51: 124–131
Wallace DJ 1990 Genitourinary manifestations of fibrositis: an increased association with the female urethral syndrome. Journal of Rheumatology 17: 238–239
Wallace DJ, Schwartz E, Chi-Lin H, Peter JB 1995 The 'rule out lupus' rheumatology consultation: clinical outcomes and perspectives. Journal of Clinical Rheumatology 1: 158–164
Wang B, Gladman DD, Urowitz MB 1998 Fatigue in lupus is not correlated with disease activity. Journal of Rheumatology 25: 892–895
Watkins LR, Wiertelak EP, Furness LE, Maier SF 1994 Illness-induced hyperalgesia is mediated by spinal neuropeptides and excitatory amino acids. Brain Research Bulletin 664: 17–24
Watkins LR, Goehler LE, Relton J, Brewer MT, Maier SF 1995a Mechanisms of tumor necrosis factor-alpha (TNF-alpha) hyperalgesia. Brain Research 692: 244–250
Watkins LR, Maier SF, Goehler LE 1995b Cytokine-to-brain communication: a review and analysis of alternative mechanisms. Life Sciences 57: 1011–1026
Watkins LR, Maier SF, Goehler LE 1995c Immune activation: the role of pro-inflammatory cytokines in inflammation, illness responses and pathological pain states. Pain 63: 289–302
Watkins LR, Maier SF, Goehler LE 1995d Immune activation: the role of pro-inflammatory cytokines in inflammation, illness responses and pathological pain states. Pain 63: 289–302
Watkins LR, Wiertelak EP, Goehler LE et al 1994a Neurocircuitry of illness-induced hyperalgesia. Brain Research 639: 283–299
Watkins LR, Wiertelak EP, Goehler LE et al 1994b Characterization of cytokine-induced hyperalagesia. Brain Research 654: 15–26
Waylonis GW, Ronan PG, Gordon C 1994 A profile of fibromyalgia in occupational environments. Am. J. Phys. Med. Rehabil. 73: 112–115
Weissman DE HJ 1989 Opioid pseudo-addiction: an iatrogenic syndrome. Pain 36: 363–364

White KP, Harth M, Teasell RW 1995a Work disability evaluation and the fibromyalgia syndrome. Semin. Arthritis and Rheumatism 24: 371–381

White KP, Speechley M, Harth M, Ostbye T 1995b Fibromyalgia in rheumatology practice: a survey of Canadian rheumatologists. Journal of Rheumatology 22: 722–726

Wiertelak EP, Roemer B, Maier SF, Watkins LR 1997 Comparison of the effects of nucleus tractus solitarius and ventral medial medulla lesions on illness-induced and subcutaneous formalin-induced hyperalgesias. Brain Research 748: 143–150

Wigers SH, Stiles TC, Vogel PA 1996 Effects of aerobic exercise versus stress management treatment in fibromyalgia. A 4.5 year prospective study. Scandinavian Journal of Rheumatology 25: 77–86

Wilke WS, Fouad-Tarazi FM, Cash JM, Calabrese LH 1998 The connection between chronic fatigue syndrome and neurally mediated hypotension. Cleveland Clinical Journal of Medicine 65: 261–266

Winfield JB 1997 Fibromyalgia: what's next? Arthritis Care Research 10: 219–221

Wolfe F 1993 Disability and the dimensions of distress in fibromyalgia. Journal of Musculoskeletal Pain 1: 65–87

Wolfe F 1997 The fibromyalgia problem. Journal of Rheumatology 24: 1247–1249

Wolfe F 1998 What use are fibromyalgia control points? Journal of Rheumatology 25: 546–550

Wolfe F, Cathey MA 1983 Prevalence of primary and secondary fibrositis. Journal of Rheumatology 10: 965–968

Wolfe F, Cathey MA 1985 The epidemiology of tender points: a prospective study of 1520 patients. Journal of Rheumatology 12: 1164–1168

Wolfe F, Potter J 1996 Fibromyalgia and work disability: is fibromyalgia a disabling disorder? Rheumatic Diseases Clinics North America 22: 369–391

Wolfe F, Cathey MA, Kleinheksel SM 1984 Fibrositis (Fibromyalgia) in rheumatoid arthritis. Journal of Rheumatology 11: 814–818

Wolfe F, Smythe HA, Yunus MB et al 1990 The American College of Rheumatology 1990 criteria for the classification of fibromyalgia: report of the Multicenter Criteria Committee. Arthritis and Rheumatism 33: 160–172

Wolfe F, Ross K, Anderson J, Russell IJ, Hebert L 1995 The prevalence and characteristics of fibromyalgia in the general population. Arthritis and Rheumatism 38: 19–28

Wolfe F, Anderson J, Harkness D et al 1997a A prospective, longitudinal, multicenter study of service utilization and costs in fibromyalgia. Arthritis and Rheumatism 40: 1560–1570

Wolfe F, Anderson J, Harkness D et al 1997b Health status and disease severity in fibromyalgia: results of a six-center longitudinal study. Arthritis and Rheumatism 40: 1571–1579

Wolfe F, Anderson J, Harkness D et al 1997c Work and disability status of persons with fibromyalgia. Journal of Rheumatology 24: 1171–1178

Wysenbeek AJ, Leibovici L, Amit M, Weinberger A 1992 Disease patterns of patients with systemic lupus erythematosus as shown by application of factor analysis. Journal of Rheumatology 19: 1096–1099

Younkin DP, Berman P, Sladky J et al 1987 31P NMR studies in Duchenne muscular dystrophy: age-related metabolic changes. Neurology 37: 165–169

Yunus MB 1984 Primary fibromyalgia syndrome: current concepts. Comprehensive Therapy 10: 21–28

Yunus MB 1994 Psychological aspects of fibromyalgia syndrome: a component of the dysfunctional spectrum syndrome. Baillière's Clinical Rheumatology 8: 811–837

Yunus MB, Aldag JC 1996 Restless legs syndrome and leg cramps in fibromyalgia syndrome: a controlled study. British Medical Journal 312: 1339

Yunus MB, Masi AT, Calabro JJ, Miller KA, Feigenbaum SL 1981 Primary fibromyalgia (fibrositis): clinical study of 50 patients with matched normal controls. Semin. Arthritis and Rheumatism 11: 151–171

Yunus MB, Masi AT, Aldag JC 1989a A controlled study of primary fibromyalgia syndrome: clinical features and association with other functional syndromes. Journal of Rheumatology 19(suppl): 62–71

Yunus MD, Kalyan-Raman UP, Masi AT, Aldag JC 1989b Electromicroscopic studies of muscle biopsy in primary fibromyalgia syndrome: a controlled and blinded study. Journal of Rheumatology 16: 97–101

Abdominal pain

26

LAURENCE M. BLENDIS

The symptom of pain in the abdomen is one of the most common presenting complaints in family practice, from childhood through to the elderly. Yet, in the vast majority of patients, no physical cause is apparent and in most of these, the symptoms are short-lived. In the minority, the pain persists or recurs and yet usually, even after investigation, no cause is found, suggesting that the pain is psychogenic in origin. With many causes of pain there are both organic and non-organic elements, with one or other factor dominating. Thus, although we classify abdominal pain as organic or non-organic, this only refers to the precipitating cause. The fact that a pathological process causes pain may depend on psychological factors, whereas even non-organic pain can often be shown to have a clearcut physical mechanism.

THE ACUTE ABDOMEN

Sudden onset of abdominal pain is a very common and important surgical diagnostic problem, since the surgeon must often decide relatively quickly whether or not the patient requires an operation. Less than 5% of young people presenting with this symptom are admitted to hospital for observation and even fewer undergo surgery (Stevenson 1985). One helpful approach to diagnosis is to divide the abdomen into four quadrants and the central abdomen and to discuss the differential diagnosis for each quadrant.

RIGHT LOWER QUADRANT PAIN

Acute appendicitis

Pain in the right lower quadrant is common and the main differential diagnosis is that of acute appendicitis. The pain, associated with anorexia, nausea and vomiting, often starts in the periumbilical area and moves to the right lower quadrant after some hours, often associated with a slight temperature of up to 38°C with or without frequency of bowel action or micturition. It is important to enquire about previous similar attacks since up to 10% may be suffering from recurrent appendicitis (Barber et al 1997). The patient is usually exquisitely tender in the right lower quadrant, except for patients with retrocaecal appendix, and there may be a sensation of a mass. The patient is also tender in the right side on rectal examination. Abdominal X-rays are unlikely to show any diagnostic features other than a faecolith in 25% of cases in young children. Blood tests usually reveal a polymorphonuclear leucocytosis and urinalysis shows increased white cells. In one study the 10–40% incidence of negative surgical explorations was more than halved in uncertain cases by a simple 24-hour observation period, during which more than 60% were found to have an infection not requiring surgery (Wenham 1982).

The clinical challenge is, first, to make the correct diagnosis of appendicitis and, second, early enough to prevent complications, such as perforation, which increase morbidity (Malt 1986). To this end, additional technologies have been incorporated into the diagnostic work-up, such as appendiceal ultrasonography, with the abdomen compressed. With this technique, no patients were operated upon unnecessarily for a normal appendix (100% specificity) but the sensitivity was only 75% (Puylaert et al 1987). Since in women the differential diagnosis is longer, laparoscopy has been added. This reduced unnecessary appendicectomy from 37% to 7% (Olsen et al 1993).

More recently, computed tomography (CT) of the appendix has been shown to be more accurate. One hundred consecutive patients in the emergency room were to be hospitalized for suspected acute appendicitis. Appendiceal CT was performed routinely and was 98% accurate, changing the proposed management in 59 patients (Rao et al 1998). This included unnecessary surgery or admission for 24-hour observation. The overall savings were $447 per patient. Nonetheless, CT involves more irradiation and expense than ultrasound. Therefore expertise in appendiceal ultrasound should be encouraged (Balthazar et al 1994), as well as maintenance of clinical skills (McColl 1998).

Mesenteric lymphadenitis

This differential diagnosis is a large one and is among the more common disorders shown in Box 26.1. In children and young adolescents, who are at the commonest age of presentation of acute appendicitis, mesenteric lymphadenitis is a likely alternative. This usually occurs in a setting of an 'epidemic' or contact history of virus infections, usually of the upper respiratory tract. Symptomatically, the patients closely resemble those with acute appendicitis. One helpful differentiating point is that in mesenteric lymphadenitis, the white blood count is usually normal with a relative lymphocytosis, although it may be surprisingly high. Abdominal imaging should reveal a lymphadenopathy and normal appendix, hopefully reducing the number of young people with this condition having a normal appendix removed.

Acute distal ileitis

Patients with distal ileitis due to Yersinia very often give a history of swimming in a lake or drinking possibly contaminated water. Serial serological studies for Yersinia should be performed (Attwood et al 1987).

Crohn's disease

In contrast, patients with Crohn's disease usually, but not always, give a past history of abdominal symptoms such as intermittent discomfort with distension and alteration in bowel habit and weight loss, with or without other systemic manifestations. On examination, the most important differential diagnostic sign is that of a mass in the right lower quadrant. Barium radiographs are diagnostic in patients with Crohn's disease, but they are inadvisable in a patient with acute appendicitis who is about to undergo surgery. Instead, non-invasive techniques such as an abdominal flat plate, ultrasonography and CT scan may provide further diagnostic support (Weill 1982).

BOX 26.1

Some common causes of acute abdomen: differential diagnosis

Right lower quadrant
- Acute appendicitis
- Mesenteric lymphadenitis
- Infective distal ileitis
- Crohn's disease
- In females, tubo-ovarian disorders, e.g.:
  - Ectopic pregnancy
  - Rupture of ovarian cyst
  - Acute salpingitis
- renal disorders, e.g.:
  - Right ureteric calculus
  - Acute pyelonephritis
  - Acute cholecystitis
  - Acute rheumatic fever
  - Pyogenic sacroiliitis

Right upper quadrant
- Acute cholecystitis
- Biliary colic
- Acute hepatic distension or inflammation
- Perforated duodenal ulcer

Central abdominal pain
- Gastroenteritis
- Small intestinal colic
- Acute pancreatitis

Left upper quadrant
- Perisplenitis
- Splenic infarct
- Disorders of splenic flexure

Left lower quadrant
- Acute diverticulitis
- Pyogenic sacroiliitis

Ovarian tubular disorders

In young women in the third and fourth decades, ovario-tubal disorders become more important. Thus, it is extremely important to obtain a complete menstrual history. A period of amenorrhoea suggests the possibility of an ectopic pregnancy, whereas a history of promiscuity would suggest the possibility of acute salpingitis. However, this is usually bilateral. These conditions usually give rise to tenderness on vaginal examination.

Renal ureteric pain

Renal pain is usually due to acute renal colic caused by a ureteric calculus. In this condition, the calculus passes from the renal pelvis into the ureter where it causes obstruction and the pain results from increasing peristaltic contractions as the calculus is forced distally toward the bladder. Colicky pain characteristically comes in waves which gradually build up in intensity, causing the patient to sweat and to feel nauseated. As the wave of pain recedes, the patient feels considerable relief, although he may feel a residual soreness until the next wave. The symptoms are similar, regardless of the source of colicky pain, but the sites are different. Thus, with renal colic, the pain starts in either flank and radiates around and down into the groin. The patient will often be tender in the loin or flank of the painful side.

Pyogenic sacroiliitis

Pyogenic sacroiliitis commonly presents in the second and third decades with a history of about 1 week of gluteal pain on walking. There is then acute onset of right or left lower quadrant pain and fever and pain also when the patient is examined with the leg extended or flexed and externally rotated or abducted at the hip. The commonest predisposing factors are intravenous drug abuse, trauma and skin injections. The diagnosis is made by the aspiration of sacroiliac joint fluid (Cohn & Schoetz 1986).

RIGHT UPPER QUADRANT PAIN

Biliary colic and acute cholecystitis

Biliary colic usually starts in the right upper quadrant and radiates around to the back with or without referred pain to the right shoulder tip. Such patients are often tender in the right upper quadrant, particularly on deep inspiration. In contrast, in acute inflammation of the gallbladder or cholecystitis without the passage of a gallstone, the pain is constant and the patient is exquisitely tender in the right upper quadrant. At least two other conditions have to be considered in acute right upper quadrant pain: acute duodenal ulcer perforation and acute hepatic congestion.

Acute duodenal ulcer perforation

Acute perforation of a duodenal ulcer produces pain. Acute ulcers are often precipitated by stress. The sudden onset of severe pain in the region is followed by symptoms and signs of peritonism with 'boardlike' rigidity of the anterior abdominal wall and 'guarding'. A straight abdominal radiograph may show a telltale gas shadow outside the duodenal lumen under the right diaphragm.

Acute hepatic congestion (enlargement)

The major organ in the right upper quadrant, the liver, occasionally causes acute pain which is usually associated with acute enlargement and stretching of the hepatic capsule, due either to inflammation, as in acute viral hepatitis, or to acute congestion secondary to acute heart failure or hepatic vein obstruction (the Budd–Chiari syndrome). All conditions result in a variable degree of jaundice and an acute release into the bloodstream of hepatic enzymes, especially the transaminases with levels rising from less than 50 to greater than 1000 iu/l. Clinical examination should reveal the presence of heart failure.

If acute Budd–Chiari syndrome is suspected, a liver–spleen radionuclide scan may show the characteristic pattern of hepatic 'wipe-out' with sparing of the caudate lobe due to its drainage directly into the inferior vena cava. The diagnosis must be confirmed by Doppler ultrasound and hepatic venography to demonstrate the blockage.

CENTRAL ABDOMEN

Colic of the small intestine

The third type of colic is intestinal and is most commonly due to acute inflammation of the bowel, such as acute gastroenteritis, in which the patient suffers from acute nausea, with or without vomiting, and crampy or colicky abdominal pain, repeatedly relieved by defaecation of loose or watery stools. The infection is either viral, usually by contact during an epidemic, or bacterial from contaminated food. In contrast, intestinal colic may be secondary to intestinal obstruction, the cause of which will depend on the site and on the age of the patient. Table 26.1 shows some of the conditions that can cause gastrointestinal colic. In contrast to infection, this is associated with partial or complete constipation and abdominal distension. Vomiting occurs in relation to the site of the obstruction; the more proximal the lesion, the more likely the associated vomiting.

Non-invasive techniques are most useful in the diagnosis of colicky conditions. A flat plate of the abdomen may reveal a calcified stone in the ureter, gallbladder or bile duct, whereas a non-calcified stone may be seen on ultrasonography (Weill 1982). With intestinal obstruction, a supine and erect film will show distension of the bowel proximal to the obstruction whilst the erect film will show multiple air–fluid levels.

Acute pancreatitis

One of the few pains to begin in the centre of the abdomen is pancreatic. Acute pancreatitis is one of the severest of all

Table 26.1. Some common causes of intestinal obstruction

Age group	*Stomach*	*Small intestine*	*Large intestine*
Neonates	Pyloric stenosis	Congenital lesions Cystic fibrosis	Imperforate anus
Infants		Intussusception	
Young adults	Duodenal ulcer	Crohn's disease Coeliac syndrome Pseudo-obstruction	Crohn's disease
Middle-aged adults and elderly		Crohn's disease	Carcinoma of colon Diverticular disease Faecal impaction

pains and has a number of causes (Box 26.2). This central pain is constant in nature and commonly bores through to the back so that relief may be attained by the patient sitting forward hugging his knees. If the diagnosis is considered from a suggestive history, it cannot be made by examination but by estimation of the pancreatic enzymes, serum amylase or lipase which are greatly elevated, the amylase rising from less than 200 to over 1000 iu. This test has a 75% sensitivity and 90% specificity. More recently, a urinary trypsinogen 2 dipstick test was shown to have 95% sensitivity and specificity and 99% negative predictive value (Kemppainen et al 1997). This should make the diagnosis simpler and cheaper.

Abdominal angina

Central abdominal pain associated with large as opposed to small meals may be due to intestinal ischaemia. The diagnosis can only be made by angiographic demonstration of narrowed coeliac or superior mesenteric vessels and confirmed by the demonstration of a pressure difference across the stricture.

LEFT UPPER QUADRANT

Splenic pain

The left side of the abdomen is an uncommon site of acute abdominal pain. The left upper quadrant is occupied by the spleen, which rarely causes pain except following a splenic infarct or when involved in a serositis, as in familial Mediterranean fever. Much more commonly, the spleen causes discomfort or a dragging sensation when it becomes enlarged due to any cause.

BOX 26.2

Some common causes of acute pancreatitis

Alcohol
Gallstones
Drugs, e.g. thiazides, frusemide, the pill
Metabolic: parathyroidism, hyperlipidaemia
Local inflammation: gastric or duodenal ulcer
Postoperative

Splenic flexure of colon

The splenic flexure of the colon may cause pain if distended acutely, for example in patients with toxic megacolon secondary to ulcerative colitis, although this usually occurs in the transverse or descending colon. It is a common site of involvement in elderly patients with ischaemic colitis and secondary stricture formation may occur in the area.

Miscellaneous

Pain originating from the stomach due to distension or ulceration, or from the tail of an inflamed pancreas, may radiate to this area.

LEFT LOWER QUADRANT

Acute diverticulitis

The left lower quadrant is the classic site of pain in elderly patients with acute diverticulitis. Characteristically, they suffer from fever, pain and either bloody stools or constipation. On examination, they will have a painful, sometimes 'hot' mass in this area and a polymorphonuclear leucocytosis on the blood film.

Non-specific ulcerative colitis

The commonest site of pain in patients with ulcerative colitis is the left lower quadrant, since the commonest site of involvement is the distal colon. The patient is often tender over the descending colon. The diagnosis is made by observing the classic characteristics of the colonic and rectal muscosa on sigmoidoscopy. However, this condition, by spreading proximally, can involve any amount of the colon and thus cause pain and tenderness over the surface markings of the colon, especially in patients with toxic megacolon.

Peritonitis

This can present either as acute or chronic abdominal pain. Acute peritonitis usually occurs secondarily to perforation of a viscus or from direct involvement with an inflamed organ, such as the pancreas (Box 26.3). The pain is usually generalized, although it may start in the area of the perforated organ. The patient learns to lie very still, since any movement of the abdomen increases the pain. Thus, on examination, the abdomen is still and the anterior abdominal wall is not involved in respiration. It feels 'boardlike' on palpation as the anterior abdominal wall muscles 'guard' the inflamed mucosa underneath. The secondary effect of peritonitis is a loss of bowel sounds as the bowel becomes paralysed by contact with the inflammation and an ileus develops. Abdominal radiographs show large dilated loops of both large and small bowel.

From the clinical viewpoint, the physician has to make the following decisions. Is the cause surgical (e.g. perforation) or medical, infectious or just inflammatory? Then, clearly, the cause will determine the management.

ACUTE ABDOMINAL PAIN IN GENERAL MEDICAL CONDITIONS

All physicians must be aware of the possibility of a generalized medical condition presenting as acute abdominal pain.

AIDS

Patients with AIDS can suffer from a variety of infections with gastrointestinal manifestations but most commonly diarrhoea and abdominal pain. One of the most common is cytomegalovirus (CMV), which can involve any part of the GI tract (Goodgame 1993). Other important causes are tuberculosis, the common GI pathogens, salmonella and shigella, cryptospiridia and *Clostridium difficile* as well as neutropenic enterocolitis.

BOX 26.3

Some common causes of peritonitis

Acute

Infectious
- Appendicitis
- Diverticulitis
- Toxic megacolon in inflammatory bowel disease
- Perforated duodenal ulcer
- Postoperative
- Spontaneous peritonitis in cirrhosis

Non-infectious
- Familial Mediterranean fever
- Biliary: perforated gallbladder
- Pancreatic: acute haemorrhagic pancreatitis

Chronic

Tuberculosis

Chemotherapeutic enterocolitis (neutropenic enteropathy)

This condition occurs in patients with AIDS and cancer patients on chemotherapy. It presents with acute abdominal pain and neutropenia, fever greater than 37.8°C, with or without diarrhoea or melaena and diffuse or localized tenderness. The symptoms usually resolve with antibiotic therapy (Starnes et al 1986).

Collagen vascular disorders (mesenteric arteritis)

Abdominal pain is a feature of juvenile rheumatoid arthritis or Still's disease. However, it does not lead to complications or major problems in management. In contrast, acute abdominal pain may be the presenting feature in patients with polyarteritis nodosa and polyangiitis (Jennette & Falk 1997). The pain may be due to intestinal perforation or infarction resulting in significantly higher mortality rates (Jacobsen et al 1985). The pain may also be associated with a purpuric rash, arthralgia and nephritis or Henoch–Schönlein purpura (Martinez-Frontanilla et al 1984).

Familial Mediterranean fever

This is an autosomal recessive disorder characterized by recurrent acute attacks of fever and serositis, including peritonitis, giving rise to abdominal pain. It affects certain ethnic groups, i.e. Sephardic Jews, Armenians, Turks and Arabs. Recently, the FMF gene has been cloned on the short arm of chromosome 16. The treatment of choice is colchicine.

Diabetes mellitus

These patients, usually young, can present with acute abdominal pain. Commonly, the diabetes is poorly controlled, with ketoacidosis. The pain may be associated with hyperamylasaemia, but in the majority of cases they do not have acute pancreatitis. Alternatively, it may be associated with an autonomic neuropathy.

Tabes dorsalis

One of the symptoms of this condition is acute abdominal pain known as a tabetic crisis. This should rarely be confused with an acute surgical abdomen.

Sickle cell anaemia

The onset of acute abdominal pain in a black person should always make the clinician think of sickle cell anaemia. Undergoing a sickle cell crisis (sickling of red cells in small blood vessels) is thought to be the cause of this, precipitated by dehydration, hypoxia, infection, etc. The diagnosis is made by observing sickling on blood smear slides.

Acute intermittent porphyria (Kauppinen & Mustajorkil 1992)

Colicky acute abdominal pain is a cardinal presenting symptom of this inherited disorder of haem synthesis. The pain may be extremely severe, colicky and either localized to the epigastrium or right lower quadrant or generalized and associated with mild tenderness, vomiting and constipation. It may be associated with an autonomic neuropathy and a cutaneous photodermatitis and precipitated by drugs metabolized by microsomal cytochrome P_{450} enzymes, such as phenobarbitone, anticonvulsants and alcohol. The diagnosis is made by detecting urinary porphyrins.

Opiate withdrawal

Opiate withdrawal can give rise to severe abdominal pains.

Lead poisoning

Lead poisoning most commonly occurs in children as the result of sucking lead-painted toys or other objects. The diagnosis, if considered, can be confirmed by detecting a black 'lead line' on the gingival margins, basophilic stippling of erythrocytes and elevated blood lead levels.

Acute rheumatic fever

Epigastric or right lower quadrant pain with anorexia, nausea and vomiting may be an early presentation. However, 50% have a history of sore throat and associated symptoms include fever, migratory arthritis, erythema marginatum, heart murmur and an inappropriate tachycardia for the height of the fever.

Jogger's pain

With the recent popularity of physical exercise, it has become apparent that intense physical exertion, even in extremely fit individuals, can result in acute severe abdominal pain and vomiting, possibly due to acute splanchnic ischaemia. The relationship of the pain to exercise should suggest the diagnosis.

Abdominal migraine

This is characterized by episodic attacks of abdominal pain and vomiting, often in the absence of headaches (Lundberg 1975). It is commoner in male children and the symptoms often respond to antimigraine therapy, usually giving way to the more typical headaches as the individual grows older (Kunkel 1986).

DIAGNOSIS OF DIFFICULT CASES OF ACUTE ABDOMINAL PAIN

When the diagnosis of acute abdominal pain is in doubt and laparotomy is being considered, there are a number of diagnostic prelaparotomy tests that can be used to help with the decision. These include simple paracentesis (Baker et al 1967), peritoneal lavage (Evans et al 1975) and peritoneoscopy (Sugarbaker et al 1975). More recently, a new method of fine catheter aspiration cytology was described by (Stewart et al 1986). Cytological specimens were prepared by the cytosieve technique and the number of neutrophils per 500 cells counted. Of 27 patients, 25 had a successful test. Prelaparotomy diagnosis was correct in 14 patients before the test, compared to 20 after the test.

CHRONIC ABDOMINAL PAIN

CHRONIC ABDOMINAL WALL PAIN

Before discussing the causes of chronic visceral pain, it is important to exclude the above condition. This is done first and foremost by considering this diagnosis and then looking for the characteristic findings on examination of this pain, namely, superficial tenderness which persists when the patient tenses the anterior abdominal wall. The pain and tenderness should disappear following injection of local anaesthetic directly into the tender area. The most likely explanation for this pain is entrapment and stretching of the anterior cutaneous branch of the thoracoabdominal nerve and the treatment is by local anaesthetic injection. However, the presence of a small ventral hernia must be excluded.

ORGANIC CAUSES OF CHRONIC ABDOMINAL PAIN

Atypical gastro-oesophageal reflux disorders (GERD)

Although the vast majority of patients suffering from GERD present with heartburn and other thoracic symp-

 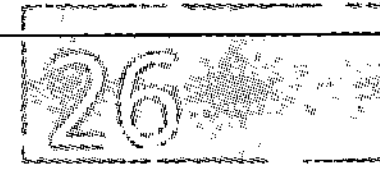

toms, a minority present with epigastric pain. A careful history is essential to raise suspicions of the diagnosis. When suspected, the diagnosis will require some or all of the following tests: barium swallow with video, manometry with 24-hour monitoring for acid reflux, radionuclide technetium swallows for reflux, endoscopy with biopsy, especially looking for the presence of *Helicobacter pylori* infection, and serological tests for *H. pylori*. If present, then eradication of the infection with triple therapy, including a proton pump inhibitor, should bring relief. However, since the majority of the population can be demonstrated to have reflux during a 24-hour period, psychological factors may sensitize certain patients to perceive heartburn (Johnstone et al 1995). For example, in 60% of patients a stress factor can be identified (Bradley et al 1993) and such patients can be helped with relaxation therapy (McDonald et al 1994).

Gastric ulcer

Patients with gastric ulcer complain of periodic upper abdominal pain over a fairly large area, that is frequently related to meals and occurs soon after the patient starts eating. The pain may radiate in any direction and is usually relieved to some extent by antacid medication. Other gastric symptoms such as nausea and vomiting are uncommon. Gastric ulcer patients may lose a little weight in association with decreased food intake. It is now clear that the major factor in the aetiology of peptic ulcer disease is infection with *H. pylori*, cagA genotype. This organism infects the mucosal environment and results in inflammation and ulceration. Probably most individuals are infected in childhood. The treatment is one of a number of 1-week courses of triple therapy with two antibiotics and antacid therapy, such as a proton pump inhibitor.

Gastric malignancy

The major differential diagnosis of a gastric ulcer is whether it is benign or malignant. Malignant ulcers are usually associated with atypical, constant pain, unrelated to meals. They are often associated with anorexia and considerable weight loss. Associated symptoms will be caused by variation in the site of the cancer. Fundic cancer causes dysphagia and regurgitation whereas prepyloric lesions will cause gastric outlet obstruction with vomiting. The malignant ulcers differ in their appearance. Carcinomatous ulcers classically have heaped-up edges and nodular involvement of the gastric wall and should be diagnosed by biopsy or brush cytology.

Primary low-grade lymphoma of the mucosa-associated lymphoid tissue (MALT) of the stomach is relatively rare, accounting for up to 10% of gastric malignancies. It is now clear that *H. pylori* infection is involved in the pathogenesis and that eradication of the infection may lead to disappearance of the lymphoma (Sackman 1997).

Duodenal ulcer

In contrast to gastric ulcer, patients with duodenal ulcer are often able to localize their periodic epigastric pain with one finger, most commonly to the right of the midline or very high up in the midline, with or without radiation through to the back. The pain is also characteristically associated with the fasting state, often waking the patient in the early hours of the morning, and is then relieved by eating or drinking or antacid medication.

Nausea, abdominal distension and vomiting are these days uncommon symptoms. These patients do not usually lose weight and may actually gain weight due to eating frequently to relieve the pain.

The mechanism of pain in peptic ulcer disease remains controversial; suggestions include smooth muscle spasm and low intraluminal pH. Recently, intravenous boluses of adenosine produced typical epigastric pain in duodenal ulcer patients (Watt et al 1987), possibly through both mechanisms.

Diagnosis

The diagnosis of peptic ulcer disease can now be made with confidence by upper gastrointestinal endoscopy, which is the investigation of choice. At the same time biopsies should be taken for the diagnosis of *H. pylori*, either by a rapid urease activity test or by histology.

Treatment

Once the diagnosis has been made, the aim of therapy is eradication of *H. pylori* infection, with one of the triple therapy combinations. These generally include two antibiotics such as clarithromycin, amoxicillin, tetracycline, with or without metronidazole, in addition to antacid therapy with a proton pump inhibitor, H2-receptor antagonist or bismuth compound (Maastricht Consensus Report 1997).

Gastroparesis

There is little doubt that gastric distension can cause pain. Some of the best evidence comes from patients with gastroparesis, most of whom are diabetic. At one time this was thought to be only poorly manageable with prokinetic agents. Recently, gastric pacing with cardiac pacing wires implanted on the serosal surface has been used. Pacing entrained the gastric slow wave and converted tachygastria into regular 3-cpm slow waves with an improvement in both gastric emptying and symptoms, including pain (McCallum et al 1998).

Chronic intestinal pseudo-obstruction (Colemont & Camilleri 1989)

Disorders of the myenteric plexus and smooth muscle result in loss of peristaltic control and the migrating motor complex and intestinal distension. The patient's symptoms mimic chronic intestinal obstruction with abdominal distension and pain, with or without vomiting, and diarrhoea associated with bacterial overgrowth and malabsorption. Or there may be involvement of the oesophageus, stomach, with gastroparesis, or colon, with constipation. There may be a family history or a history of drug ingestion. The numerous causes can be classified in various ways as for example in Box 26.4.

Therefore the diagnosis will involve clinical history, examination, radiology, endoscopy and finally surgery with full-thickness biopsy of the intestinal wall. The treatment will depend on the diagnosis.

Chronic pancreatitis and carcinoma of the pancreas

Chronic pancreatitis develops in less than 10% of patients following an attack of acute pancreatitis. The majority of these patients suffer from chronic relapsing pancreatitis with recurrent bouts of pain similar to the acute attacks and associated with elevation of pancreatic enzymes. In less than 20% the pain is chronically persistent. There are two theories for this pain. The first is that there is involvement of the pancreatic nerves by inflammatory or scar tissue and therefore the treatment is by medical nerve block. The second is that the pain is due to pancreatic ductular hypertension secondary to stricture formation. The medical treatment for this is to reduce pancreatic secretion. However, in a double-blind crossover study subcutaneous octreotide was not more effective than saline in relieving pain (Malfertheimer et al 1995).

The pain of carcinoma of the pancreas is usually central abdominal, deep and radiating through to the back. Unrelated to meals, it is characteristically severe and requires powerful analgesics. Once the diagnosis is suspected, abdominal CT is the test of choice, showing pancreatic enlargement. This can be confirmed by endoscopic retrograde cholangiopancreatography (ERCP) examination. Unfortunately, only a small percentage of such cancers are operable.

BOX 26.4

The causes of chronic intestinal pseudo-obstruction

1. Disorders of the Myenteric Plexus
   a. Developmental disorders
   b. Familial visceral disorders
   c. Sporadic visceral disorders
   d. Diffuse small intestinal diverticulosis
   e. Amyloidosis
   f. Toxic damage e.g. laxatives, anticholinergics etc.
2. Disorders of smooth muscle
   a. Primary (familial) visceral myopathies
   b. Secondary myopathies e.g. systemicsclerosis

BOX 26.5

The Rome Criteria for IBS

Continuous or recurrent symptoms for at least 3 months of:

1. Abdominal pain or discomfort, relieved by defaecation or associated with a change in frequency or consistency of stool, associated with:

2. Irregular bowel habit at least 25% of the time with three or more of the following:
   altered stool frequency
   altered stool consistency
   altered stool passage (straining, urgency, etc.)
   passage of mucus per rectum
   abdominal bloating or distension

Gastrointestinal food hypersensitivity

In 1949 Ingelfinger et al stated that 'Gastrointestinal allergy is a diagnosis frequently entertained, occasionally evaluated, but rarely established'. Today, in the era of naturopaths and allergists, it may be even more so. Nevertheless, particularly in atopic individuals, it is a true entity, most frequently involving cow's milk, wheat, eggs, fish and nuts. There is a clear symptom complex with bloating, abdominal pain and diarrhoea. Whatever the mechanism, recognition of the possibility and withdrawal of the offending food can result in the disappearance of symptoms (Crowe & Perdue 1992).

Leishmaniasis (Post Desert Storm Syndrome) (Magill et al 1993)

Some veterans of Operation Desert Storm complained of unexplained fever, chronic fatigue and malaise, intermittent abdominal pain, or diarrhoea for several months. The diagnosis of Leishmania tropica infection was made from isolates of bone marrow aspirates of lymph node biopsy. Following treatment with sodium stibogluconate the symptoms including the abdominal pain improved.

Mesenteric panniculitis (sclerosing mesocolitis, Weber–Christian disease)

This is characterized by recurrent episodes of moderate to severe, generalized or focal abdominal pain, associated with intermittent nausea, vomiting, malaise, low-grade fever and occasionally weight loss. On examination, a tender, central abdominal mass is commonly found, with or without chylous ascites. Barium small bowel radiographs show irregularity, nodularity, thickening and strictures. The principal differential diagnosis is malignant disease, particularly abdominal lymphoma, the diagnosis being made by laparotomy and biopsy (Steely & Gooden 1986). The final diagnosis may be of retractile mesenteritis with or without retroperitoneal fibrosis (Tedeschi & Botta 1962).

Grumbling appendicitis

One to two per cent of patients with appendicular inflammation suffer from chronic right lower quadrant pain (Mattei et al 1994). The differential diagnosis in long and abdominal imaging usually fails to provide a diagnosis. However, colonoscopy can be diagnostic with the appearance of inflammation localized to the root of the appendix in the caecal region (Johnson & De Cosse 1998).

Carbohydrate maldigestion and malabsorption

Five grams of indigestible carbodydrate can produce 1000 ml carbon dioxide, 400 ml methane (in methane producers) and 200 ml hydrogen via colonic bacterial fermentation (Hightower 1977). However, it has recently been shown that it is important to distinguish excess gas formation, as in hypolactasia, from a sensation of bloating, as in irritable bowel syndrome with normal gas production (Levitt et al 1996).

Hypolactasia

However, patients with certain carbohydrate maldigestion or malabsorption syndromes will still produce excessive amounts of gas even with low-residue carbohydrates such as disaccharides. The best example of this is patients with disaccharidase deficiency, the commonest form of which is hypolactasia. Lactases are situated at the tips of the jejunal villi. Caucasians in Europe and the United States, unlike most of the rest of the world, retain lactase activity throughout life. However, diseases of the jejunum, resulting in atrophy of the villi, will result in loss of lactase activity, for example, coeliac syndrome, tropical sprue and postgastroenteritis enteropathy. The result is that on drinking milk or eating certain dairy foods, lactose malabsorption occurs, leading to colonic gaseous fermentation. The patient will then complain of crampy abdominal pain over the colon and diarrhoea and excessive flatus. The diagnosis can frequently be made from the history and confirmed by the lactose hydrogen breath test (Metz et al 1975). Management consists of treating any underlying pathology such as coeliac syndrome, in this case with a gluten-free diet, and then putting the patient on a lactose-free diet. Alternatively, if the patient needs or likes milk and dairy foods, these can be given together with synthetic lactases.

Lactose maldigestion was detected in 24% of 137 children with recurrent abdominal pain, which improved with a lactose free diet (Webster et al 1995).

Hyposucrasia and multiple sugar malabsorptions

Because of their position further down the villi and their greater number and quantity, other disaccharidase deficiencies are either extremely rare or never occur. For example, there are only a few case reports of sucrase deficiency. The patients present in the same way after eating foods containing sucrose, are diagnosed by the sucrose hydrogen breath test (Metz et al 1976a) and are treated by the elimination of sucrose from the diet. However, if symptoms do not improve other sugars may be involved, such as fructose and sorbitol (Mishkin et al 1997).

Stagnant loop syndrome

Carbohydrate maldigestion may also occur in patients who have bacterial colonization of the small intestine. Normally, the upper small intestine is only significantly colonized after meals and the bacteria are 'swept downstream' with the food. In patients with certain pathologies of the small intestine, luminar contents stagnate and become colonized, resulting in malabsorption. Examples of this are jejunal diverticulosis; systemic sclerosis of the duodenum and jejunum; fistulae producing a blind loop, such as Crohn's disease, and incomplete obstruction, such as radiation enteropathy (Newman et al 1973). These conditions are grouped under the heading of 'stagnant loop syndrome' and if the abnormality is proximal enough, monosaccharide fermentation may even occur, leading to increased hydrogen production from glucose (Metz et al 1976b). The symptomatology is similar but the site of the crampy pain is central or periumbilical over the area of the small intestine. The diagnosis can be suspected by evidence of bile acid or vitamin B12 malabsorption and confirmed by anatomical demonstration of the lesion by radiology.

Colonic maldigestion

Colonic 'maldigestion' of carbohydrate occurs normally if the diet contains large amounts of indigestible carbohydrate (Hickey et al 1972). These can be classified as cereal fibres such as wheat bran, gums from certain beans, such as guar, and pectins from citrus fruits. It has already been noted that 5 g of such carbohydrate can produce more than 1500 ml of gas. Providing the individual has a regular bowel action, as a result of adequate amounts of cereal fibre in the diet, the gas will either be absorbed or passed as flatus.

Constipation

In constipated individuals, increasing amounts of faecal material and gas build up in the colon, causing crampy pain. This may occur in the absence of any colonic pathology or, commonly, in association with diverticular disease of the colon in the elderly. This diagnosis is made by barium enema examination and treatment consists of normalizing the bowel action with a combination of diet and laxatives. Constipation is also a particularly common cause of abdominal pain in children, but a long list of causes have to be excluded first (Seth & Heyman 1994).

NON-ORGANIC OR PSYCHOGENIC PAIN

The criteria for psychogenic abdominal pain were reviewed by Glaser and Engel (1977).

1. The location, distribution, timing, quality and intensity of the pain do not relate to established pathophysiological patterns.
2. There is often a marked discrepancy between the severity of the pain and the patient's behaviour.
3. The patient usually has or has had multiple pains in many other parts of the body which may have been fully investigated without any obvious abnormality being discovered. In other words, the patient is 'pain prone'.
4. The onset of pain may bear an obvious temporal relationship to stress. This is particularly the case with bereavement, where the onset may coincide with the death of a close relative or friend in whom abdominal pain may have been a major symptom.

The abdomen is the third commonest site of pain in psychiatric patients (Spear 1967), whereas in patients suffering from chronic pain the abdomen is the second commonest site (Merskey 1965). Of a large unselected series of children, 15% complained of chronic or recurrent abdominal pain (Apley & Naish 1958). In the majority of older children and adolescents chronic abdominal pain is functional (Daum 1997). High incidences of parents with abdominal pain, large sibships and bereavement have all been described in association with non-organic abdominal pain (Hill & Blendis 1967) and the relationship of pain to the emotions has been previously reviewed (Blendis et al 1978). Extensive research into brain–gut relationships should lead to further elucidation of this problem and advances in therapy (Aziz & Thompson 1998). Non-organic abdominal pain has classically been divided into different symptom complexes. However, it has been suggested that they are all regional manifestations of visceral hypersensitivity with increased excitability of spinal neurons (Mayer & Gebhart 1994) and that multiple events result in short-term or long-term sensitization of these pathways.

GASEOUS DISTENSION

The major stimulus of normal gut is stretch and tension receptors have been demonstrated electrically in series with muscle cells. Gas is a normal constituent of the gastrointestinal tract. However, no obvious function has as yet been ascribed to it. The main sources of gas are swallowed air (oxygen and nitrogen), endogenous production of carbon dioxide from gastrointestinal secretions and bacterial fermentation of non-absorbable carbohydrates and proteins (carbon dioxide, hydrogen and methane) (Calloway 1966, Levitt & Bond 1970). Certain foods, such as broad beans, produce more gas than others, related to the oligosaccharides, stachyose and raffinose (Steggerda 1968).

Surprisingly, some individuals appear to be unable to produce hydrogen and this may vary from 2% to 20% (Gilat et al 1978). Hydrogen will readily diffuse across the colonic mucosa into the portal bloodstream and luminal hydrogen production can readily be measured by gas chromatography from samples of expired air (Levitt 1969). In contrast, methane is produced by only about one-third of the population (Levitt & Bond 1970) who have methane bacteria in their colon. Methane production was found to be commoner in white females than in males and commoner in

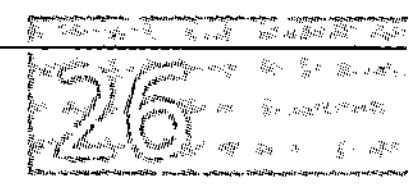

Orientals and Indians (Pitt et al 1980). As with hydrogen production, methane production will vary from day to day and may increase with ingestion of unabsorbed carbohyrate (Pitt et al 1980).

GASEOUS DISTENSION SYNDROMES

Aerophagy

Aerophagy or excessive air swallowing is due to both organic and non-organic causes. Organic conditions are those that cause pain or discomfort of the pharynx and oesophagus and include acute pharyngitis and peptic oesophagitis. The patient experiences relief of discomfort momentarily by swallowing air since, presumably, this results in a 'cushion' of air separating the inflamed surfaces.

The non-organic and far more common causes of aerophagy include anxiety and depression (Song et al 1993). Anxious people tend to swallow more air and tend to eat more quickly and take in excessive amounts of air whilst swallowing food. Gradually the air builds up in the fundus of the stomach until it starts to produce discomfort and eventually pain throughout the gastrointestinal tract by stimulation of stretch receptors in the wall of the viscera. The patient will then gain temporary relief by belching the air out and the process is repeated.

The amount of air required to produce symptoms in the stomach is unknown, although insufflation of approximately 200 ml of air via a gastroscope reproduced symptoms in patients presenting with non-organic upper abdominal pain (Hill & Blendis 1967). Normally, there is up to 150 ml of gas in the entire gastrointestinal tract at any one time, although ten times this amount may pass through in 24 hours (Danhot 1978).

The pain in such patients was constant, non-radiating and associated with abdominal distension, poorly localized and never woke the patients at night. It was variably related to meals associated with nausea (but rarely vomiting), flatulence and borborygmi as the air passed down the bowel. It was unrelieved by antacids. Most patients were tender in the upper abdomen. By definition, all investigations were negative. Most of the patients had suffered for years. There was a high incidence of bereavement and of a family history of the symptoms or of a close friend who had died with abdominal pain. In a small group of these patients, the pain responded to antidepressant therapy (Hill & Blendis 1967).

Non-ulcer dyspepsia

Up to 60% of patients complaining of non-specific upper abdominal discomfort, one of the commonest symptoms causing patients to visit physicians, have no obvious pathology. However, it appears that on investigation 30–60% of these will be found to be infected with *H. pylori* with or without gastritis. It is still unclear whether this infection is the cause of the symptoms, although in a percentage of patients the symptoms will disappear with triple therapy (Talley et al 1998). If symptoms persist following successful eradication then an alternative cause is likely. For example, delayed gastric emptying with gastric distension has been detected in up to 35% of dyspeptic patients in a referral centre (Stanghellini et al 1996). This syndrome was associated with female sex, postprandial fullness and vomiting and tended to respond to prokinetic agents. Although anecdote and clinical suspicion strongly favour a psychological cause for non-ulcer dyspepsia, due to stress and life events, etc., the cause and effects remain unproven (Thompson 1997).

IRRITABLE BOWEL SYNDROME (LYNN & FRIEDMAN 1993, DROSSMAN ET AL 1997)

Definition

As indicated at the beginning of the chapter, most people at some time or other suffer from a bout of non-organic abdominal pain associated with stress or after a bout of gastroenteritis. However, in the majority, the symptoms gradually disappear. Therefore, in children, irritable bowel syndrome (IBS) has been classified as symptoms lasting for longer than 3 months (Apley & Naish 1958) and a similar period seems reasonable for adults. Thus, IBS may be defined as symptoms of abdominal pain and disturbance of bowel action of more than 3 months' duration without any organic cause. However, separating patients into diagnoses of non-ulcer dyspepsia and IBS may be artificial since 50% of patients may change their symptoms from one category to the other over a 1-year period (Agreus et al 1995).

Incidence

A recent study in the United States indicates that about 20% of the population suffer from IBS symptoms. IBS affects females more commonly than males, with ratios in published series varying from 1.5:1 (Waller & Misiewicz 1969) to 5.2:1 (Keeling & Fielding 1975). A recent study found that in up to 44% of women presenting with IBS, there is a history of sexual and physical abuse (Drossman et al 1990). The peak age of onset is in the third decade, although it also affects children (Bonamico et al 1995) and old people (Hislop 1971). However, up to 70% of persons with identical IBS symptoms do not seek medical attention (Hahn et al 1997).

Clinical features

Abdominal pain is predominantly periumbilical in children (Stone & Barbero 1970) whereas in adults it tends to occur over the surface markings of the colon with the commonest site in the left lower quadrant (Waller & Misiewicz 1969). Occasionally, it may be in either the right or left upper quadrant over the hepatic or splenic flexures. The pain varies from a dull ache to attacks of excruciating severity requiring powerful analgesic injections. It may last from minutes to several hours. Often the pain lasts all day, but it rarely prevents the patient from sleeping through the night. 'Meteorism' is due to 'air trapping' in which segmental accumulation of gas occurs.

Alterations of bowel habit occur in up to 90% of the patients and vary from diarrhoea to constipation or both. A classic history is that on waking, the patient immediately has a loose bowel action and then three or four more watery bowel actions during the morning. After midday, the patient may not have any further bowel actions or may have a normally formed stool later in the day. In the constipated patient, the patient passes 'rabbity' small, hard stools irregularly. In about half the patients pain is aggravated by eating and relieved by defaecation. However, the patient's appetite is rarely affected and therefore a history of significant weight loss (i.e. more than 3.5 kg) is unusual and should raise suspicions of an alternative diagnosis.

As in patients with non-organic upper abdominal pain, IBS pain is associated with nausea without vomiting, dyspepsia, urinary symptoms, especially dysuria, gynaecological symptoms, especially dysmenorrhoea, and headache. There may be a clearcut history of IBS symptoms beginning after an attack of gastroenteritis (Gwee et al 1996). Approximately 60% of women attending gynaecological clinics with pelvic pain had symptoms suggestive of IBS (Crowell et al 1994) and 40% having elective hysterectomy, compared to 32% of age-matched controls (Longstreth et al 1990). Thus, these patients fit another of the criteria of non-organic pain by being multisymptomatic and prone to pain. They frequently have a past history of appendicectomy for 'chronic appendicits' and dilatation and curettage for dysmenorrhoea (Waller & Misiewicz 1969). Cancer phobia is another frequent observation in these patients.

Several authors have attempted to identify symptom complexes that will reliably distinguish IBS patients. Manning et al (1978) identified four such symptoms: pain onset with loose bowel movement; pain relieved by bowel movement; increased bowel movements with pain, and bloating. More recently, Talley and co-workers (1989) described the following cluster of symptoms: more than one episode of pain per week; of greater than 2 hours' duration; diffuse localization; associated with eating; and bowel disturbance. Finally, Whitehead et al (1990), in a factor analysis of 23 symptoms, found a cluster of four: relief of pain with defaecation; looser stools with pain onset; more frequent stools with pain; and symptoms with eating, thus verifying at least three of Manning's four. These criteria have been used to identify an unexpectedly high prevalence of IBS in Africans (Olubuyide et al 1995). Although control patients and individuals identified as having abdominal pain but not having sought medical advice have similar symptoms, in patients with IBS, abdominal pain occurred six times more frequently (Heaton et al 1991). Finally, at a conference in Rome on IBS, the Rome Criteria were born (Box 26.4).

The Rome Criteria are excellent for standardization of therapeutic trials and the discipline that they brought to the field but their very rigidity brings artificial constraints which have to be reconsidered in the future (Camilleri 1998).

Psyche

Historical evidence of an affective disorder is common. Continuous fatigue is almost universal, some patients waking up tired after a full night's sleep, although insomnia may also be a problem. Alternatively, they may feel depressed and frequently close to tears (Hislop 1971). Occasionally, the patient may be suicidal. On formal testing, patients scored higher for anxiety, neuroticism and introversion than normal controls or than patients with ulcerative colitis (Esler & Goulston 1973). Their neurosis score may lie midway between normal and frank neurosis (Palmer et al 1974), even in those patients with acute gastroenteritis before they have developed IBS (Gwee et al 1996). Women with IBS and a history of sexual abuse have altered pain perception and typical psychosocial features (Scarinci et al 1994). However, more recent studies suggest that the psychological abnormalities undoubtedly found in IBS are secondary to their patient status and not primary factors causing IBS (Drossman et al 1988, Kumar et al 1990, Talley et al 1990). Indeed, as with organic disease, they were the determinants of health-care seeking (Smith et al 1990).

Examination

On examination, there is usually a disparity between the severity of the patient's symptoms and his or her physical condition. Far from looking ill, they look well, often slightly or moderately overweight. The main finding is in the abdomen where the patient will be tender over an area of the colon, most commonly the descending colon, which is also palpable, and less commonly over the transverse colon or the entire colon. Some patients are exquisitely tender on rectal examination. Sigmoidoscopic examination is usually normal but it is extremely difficult to proceed beyond the rectosigmoid junction with a rigid scope because of spasm and pain. The patients may also have mucosal hyperalgesia to light touch via the sigmoidoscope. Routine blood tests, including sedimentation rate, should be normal.

Investigations

Any evidence of anaemia, leucocytosis, etc. should be further investigated to exclude other disease such as inflammatory bowel disease. Although it is important psychologically not to overinvestigate these patients, most of them eventually have a barium enema or colonoscopy, which is normal apart from a variable amount of spasm, usually in the descending or sigmoid colon, which should be relieved by intravenous antispasmodics. Up to 25% of patients with IBS may have lactose intolerance (Vernia et al 1995, Bohmer & Tuynman 1996) or some other form of food intolerance (Nanda et al 1989). Furthermore, removal of the offending food may lead to a marked improvement in symptoms.

Motility studies

Intestinal motility has frequently been shown to be abnormal in IBS patients. Initially, all the studies were on the colon, hence the name 'spastic colon'. More recent studies on the upper gastrointestinal tract, including the oesophagus, have shown abnormalities, associated with hypersensitivity of lumbar splanchnic afferents (Lembo et al 1994, Accarino et al 1995). Hence 'irritable gut' or 'gastrointestinal tract syndrome' would be a more appropriate name. Using balloons and open-ended tubes, distension of the appropriate area of intestine reproduced the pain (Swarbrick et al 1980), particularly with distension of the rectum and sigmoid colon (Kendall 1985). In 1973 Ritchie showed that the pain threshold in IBS patients from distension of the sigmoid colon was much lower than that of normal volunteers. This was the first description of what has now come to be recognized as the hypersensitivity phenomenon (Mayer & Gebhart 1994). Furthermore, pain did not originate from hypercontractions (Trotman & Misiewicz 1988).

Other manometric studies have shown a variety of other motility abnormalities; for example, patients have been separated into the diarrhoeal types, in which colonic motor activity was increased and disordered, and the constipation type, in which it was significantly reduced. It has now been shown that the diarrhoeal subgroup have an adrenergic abnormality, while the constipated subgroup is associated with a cholinergic disorder (Aggarwal et al 1994). Another characteristic finding is that of decreased resting activity in the fasting state with an exaggeration of the colonic motor response to eating and other stimuli (Connell et al 1965).

Recent motility studies have confirmed that the whole gut is affected in IBS (Moriarty & Dawson 1982, Kumar & Wingate 1985); that decreased lower oesophageal sphincter pressure and disordered oesophageal motility (Whorwell et al 1981) lead to gastro-oesophageal reflux with oesophagitis (Smart et al 1986); and that superficial gastritis is a frequent finding (Fielding & Doyle 1982). In addition, it has been found that there is disordered small bowel motility associated with mechanoreceptor-related hypersensitivity (Evans et al 1996). Clusters of jejunal pressure activity and ileal propulsive waves (Kellow & Phillips 1987) and excessive responses to infusions of cholecystokinin (Kellow et al 1988) have been reported, leading to slowing of transit (Cann et al 1983), particularly in the constipation group (Nielsen et al 1986). Technetium brain scans have shown that the ileocaecal valve clearance is slower (Trotman & Price 1986), but not especially in patients with bloating (Hutchinson et al 1995).

Gastrointestinal hormones

One explanation for these later findings could be abnormalities in gastrointestinal hormones. Both gastrin and cholecystokinin (Harvey & Read 1973) increase colonic and small intestinal motor activity and some IBS patients have an exaggerated response to these hormones. It is conceivable, therefore, that IBS patients could have either abnormalities of excretion of these or other gastrointestinal hormones, or increased sensitivity to them, as previously shown for neostigmine.

Treatment (Drossman et al 1997)

The essence of treatment of IBS is a sympathetic physician who is prepared to spend time discussing the patient's symptoms and the pathogenesis of IBS as far as it is known, and who is willing to try various therapeutic regimes without growing impatient. A high-fibre diet using cereal fibre such as natural bran has been proposed as the basis of therapy but is not universally accepted. Fibre appears to normalize abnormal transit time, whether too rapid or too slow (Harvey et al 1973). As in normal subjects, abdominal symptoms occur frequently in IBS patients following the ingestion of lactose, fructose and sorbitol due to malabsorption (Rumessen & Gudmand-

Hoyer 1988, Nelis et al 1990). Therefore, it may be worth attempting to exclude these carbohydrates, in the form of confectionery and soft drinks, from the diet. In addition, stool-softening agents such as diocyte sodium 100 mg twice daily can be given. Antispasmodic agents with or without sedatives have been tried with some success for patients with bloating and cramps. Tricyclic antidepressants and serotonin reuptake antagonists have been advocated for patients with frequent severe pain, since their neuromodulatory and analgesic properties function at lower doses (Clouse 1994).

Many controlled trials have shown variable efficacy despite a placebo response of greater than 50% (Drossman et al 1997). Controlled trials of various forms of psychotherapy, cognitive-behavioural therapy, hypnotherapy and relaxation have shown a significant symptomatic improvement over standard medical therapy maintained with up to 18 months follow-up (Whorwell et al 1984, Guthrie et al 1991). However, in an extensive review, Klein (1988) remained sceptical about any form of therapy.

Prognosis

Irritable bowel syndrome is considered a chronic pain condition lasting for many years. However, in a report of the aggressive use of high-fibre diets and bulking agents, nearly 70% of patients were reported to be pain free at 5 years (Harvey et al 1987).

Postsurgical pain

In a significant number of patients pain may recur following a surgical operation. This may follow the removal of a normal organ or one showing mild chronic inflammation only, as with an appendix or gallbladder. Other pains may result from a complication of surgery such as ulcer surgery. Some patients complain of obscure abdominal pain following surgery, such as hysterectomy or trauma. Balloon insufflation of the rectum or sigmoid colon may reproduce their pain (Kendall 1985).

Postcholecystectomy syndrome (Spangou et al 1995)

This is a fairly well-defined entity of right upper quadrant pain which occurs usually after a 3–6-month latent period. The pain often resembles the patient's preoperative pain although it is frequently more severe and persistent. The patient is often tender in the right upper quadrant but all routine investigations may be normal and an ERCP examination must be performed to exclude retained stones in the bile duct or a stricture. However, if normal, a characteristic finding is reproduction of the pain on ERCP examination when contrast material is injected under pressure. This is an important observation since it enables the physician to discuss the mechanism of the pain with the patient even though medical therapy is disappointing. Recently anecdotal information suggests that ursodeoxycholic acid may be helpful symptomatically in such patients.

Postgastrectomy pain

Postgastrectomy pain, when associated with rapid satiety on eating and a feeling of distension, is usually due to 'small stomach syndrome' and is managed by small frequent meals.

A more severe pain with easily localized tenderness may indicate a stomal ulcer and requires maximum antiulcer therapy with either cimetidine or sucralfate.

Thus, there are many causes of abdominal pain which present the physician with one of the commonest and most difficult diagnostic problems. Management of abdominal pain is one of the best examples of the importance of a full, carefully taken history as well as clinical examination. The inter-relationships of the physical and the psychological have been probed but a great deal more investigation is required to understand the mechanisms of abdominal pain.

REFERENCES

Accarino AM, Azpiroz F, Malagelada J-R 1995 Selective dysfunction of mechanosensitive intestinal afferents in irritable bowel syndrome. Gastroenterology 108: 636–643

Aggarwal A, Cutts TF, Abell TL, Cardoso S, Familoni B et al 1994 Predominant symptoms in irritable bowel syndrome correlate with specific autonomic nervous system abnormalities. Gastroenterology 106: 945–950

Agreus L, Svardsudd K, Nyren O, Tibblin G 1995 Irritable bowel syndrome and dyspepsia in the general population: overlap and lack of stability. Gastroenterology 109: 671–680

Apley J, Naish N 1958 Recurrent abdominal pains; a field survey of 1000 school children. Archives of Diseases in Childhood 33: 165–167

Attwood SEA, Mealy K, Cafferkey MT et al 1987 *Yersinia* infection and acute abdominal pain. Lancet 1: 529–533

Aziz Q, Thompson DG 1998 Brain-gut axis in health and disease. Gastroenterology 114: 559–578

Baker WNW, Mackie DR, Newcombe JF 1967 Diagnostic paracentesis in the acute abdomen. British Medical Journal 3: 393–398

Balthazar EJ, Megibow AJ, Siegel SE, Birnbaum BA 1994 Acute appendicitis. Radiology 190: 31–35

Barber MD, McLaren J, Rainey JB 1997 Recurrent appendicitis. British Journal of Surgery 84: 110–112
Blendis LM, Hill OW, Merskey H 1978 Abdominal pain and the emotions. Pain 5: 179–191
Bohmer CJM, Tuynman HARE 1996 The clinical relevance of lactose malabsorption in irritable bowel syndrome. European Journal of Gastroenterology and Hepatology 8: 1013–1016
Bonamico M, Culasso F, Colombo C, Giunta AM 1995 Irritable bowel syndrome in children: an Italian multicentre study. Italian Journal of Gastroenterology 27: 13–20
Bradley LA, Richter JE, Pulliam TJ, Haile S, Scarinci IC, Schan CA 1993 The relationship between stress and symptoms of gastroesophageal reflux. American Journal of Gastroenterology 88: 11–19
Calloway DH 1966 Respiratory hydrogen and methane as affected by consumption of gas-forming foods. Gastroenterology 51: 383–389
Camilleri M 1998 What's in a name? Roll on Rome II. Gastroenterology 114: 237
Cann PA, Read NW, Brown C, Hobson N, Holdsworth CD 1983 Irritable bowel syndrome; relationship of disorders in the transit of a single solid meal to symptom patterns. Gut 24: 405–411
Clouse RE 1994 Antidepressants for functional gastrointestinal syndromes. Digestive Diseases and Sciences 39: 2352–2363
Cohn SM, Schoetz DJ 1986 Pyogenic sacroiliitis: another imitator of the acute abdomen. Surgery 100: 95–98
Colemont IJ, Camilleri M 1989 Chronic intestinal pseudo-obstruction: diagnosis and treatment. Mayo Clinic Proceedings 64: 60–70
Connell AM, Jones FA, Rowlands EN 1965 Motility of the pelvic colon. Part IV. Abdominal pain associated with colonic hypermotility after meals. Gut 6: 105–112
Crowe SE, Perdue MH 1992 Gastrointestinal food hypersensitivity: basic mechanisms of pathophysiology. Gastroenterology 103: 1075–1095
Crowell MD, Dubin NH, Robinson JC et al 1994 Functional bowel disorders in women with dysmenorrhea. American Journal of Gastroenterology 89: 1973–1977
Danhot I 1978 The clinical gas syndromes, a pathophysiologic approach. Annals of the New York Academy of Science 150: 127–130
Daum F 1997 Functional abdominal pain in older children and adolescents. Gastrointestinal Diseases Today 6: 7–12
Drossman DA, McKee DC, Sandler RS et al 1988 Psychosocial factors in the irritable bowel syndrome. Gastroenterology 95: 701–708
Drossman DA, Leserman J, Nachman G et al 1990 Sexual and physical abuse in women with functional gastrointestinal disorders. Annals of Internal Medicine 113: 808–833
Drossman DA, Whitehead WE, Camilleri M 1997 Irritable bowel syndrome. Gastroenterology 112: 2118–2137
Esler MD, Goulston KJ 1973 Levels of anxiety in colonic disorders. New England Journal of Medicine 288: 16–20
Evans C, Rashid A, Rosenberg IL, Pollock AV 1975 An appraisal of peritoneal lavage in the acute abdomen. 62: 119–120
Evans PR, Bennett EJ, Bak Y-T, Tennant CC, Kellow JE 1996 Jejunal sensorimotor dysfunction in irritable bowel syndrome: clinical and psychosocial features. Gastroenterology 110: 393–404
Evans PR, Bak Y-T, Shutter B, Hoschl R, Kellow JE 1997 Gastroparesis and small bowel dysmotility in irritable bowel syndrome. Digestive Diseases and Sciences 42: 2087–2093
Fielding JF, Doyle GD 1982 The prevalence and significance of gastritis in patients with lower intestinal irritable bowel (irritable colon) syndrome. Journal of Clinical Gastroenterology 4: 507–510
Gilat T, Ben-Hur H, Gelman-Malachi E, Terdiman R, Peled Y 1978 Alterations of the colonic flora and their effect on the hydrogen breath test. Gut 19: 602–605
Glaser JP, Engel GL 1977 Psychodynamics, psychophysiology and gastrointestinal symptomatology. Clinics in Gastroenterology 6: 507–531
Goodgame RW 1993 Gastrointestinal cytomegalovirus disease. Annals of Internal Medicine 119: 924–925
Guthrie E, Creed F, Dawson D, Tomenson B 1991 A controlled trial of psychological treatment for the irritable bowel syndrome. Gastroenterology 100: 450–457
Gwee KA, Graham JC, McKendrick MW, Collins SM, Walters SJ, Read NW 1996 Psychometric scores and persistence of irritable bowel after infectious diarrhoea. Lancet 347: 150–153
Hahn BA, Saunders WB, Maier WC 1997 Differences between individuals with self-reportable irritable bowel syndrome (IBS) and IBS-like symptoms. Digestive Diseases and Sciences 42: 2585–2590
Harvey RF, Read AE 1973 Effect of cholecystokinin on colonic motility and symptoms in patients with irritable bowel syndrome. Lancet 1: 1–3
Harvey RF, Pomare EW, Heaton KW 1973 Effects of increased dietary fiber on intestinal transit. Lancet 1: 1278–1280
Harvey RF, Mauad EC, Brown AM, 1987 Prognosis in the irritable bowel syndrome: a 5-year prospective study. Lancet 1: 963–965
Heaton KW, Ghosh S, Braddon FEM 1991 How bad are the symptoms of patients with irritable bowel syndrome? Gut 32: 73–79
Hickey CA, Calloway DH, Murphy E 1972 Intestinal gas production following ingestion of fruits and fruit juices. American Journal of Digestive Diseases 17: 383–387
Hightower NC 1977 Intestinal gas and gaseousness. Clinical Gastroenterology 6: 597–606
Hill OW, Blendis LM 1967 Physical and psychological evaluation of non-organic abdominal pain. Gut 8: 221–229
Hislop IG 1971 Psychological significance of the irritable colon syndrome. Gut 12: 452–455
Hutchinson R, Notghi A, Smith NB, Harding LK, Kumar D 1995 Scintigraphic measurement of ileocaecal transit in irritable bowel syndrome and chronic constipation. Gut 36: 585–589
Ingelfinger FJ, Lowell FC, Franklin W 1949 Gastrointestinal allergy. New England Journal of Medicine 241: 303–340
Jacobsen SEH, Petersen P, Jenson P 1985 Acute abdomen in rheumatoid arthritis due to mesenteric arteritis. Danish Medical Bulletin 32: 191–193
Jennette JC, Falk RJ 1997 Small-vessel vasculitis. New England Journal of Medicine 337: 1512–1523
Johnson TR, De Cosse JJ 1998 Colonoscopic diagnosis of grumbling appendicitis. Lancet 351: 495
Johnstone BT, Lewis SA, Love AHG 1995 Psychological factors in gastro-oesophageal reflux disease. Gut 36: 481–482
Kauppinen R, Mustajorki P 1992 Prognosis of acute porphyria. Medicine 71: 1–12
Keeling PWN, Fielding JF 1975 The irritable bowel syndrome. A review of 50 consecutive cases. Journal of the Irish College of Physicians and Surgeons 4: 91–94
Kellow JE, Phillips SF 1987 Altered small bowel motility in irritable bowel syndrome is correlated with symptoms. Gastroenterology 92: 1885–1893
Kellow JE, Phillips SF, Muler LJ, Zinsmeister AR 1988 Dysmotili of the small intestine in irritable bowel syndrome. Gut 29: 1236–1243
Kemppainen EA, Hedstrom JI, Puolakkainen PA et al 1997 Rapid measurement of urinary trypsinogen-2 as a screening test for cute pancreatitis. New England Journal of Medicine 336: 1788–1793
Kendall GPN 1985 Visceral pain. British Journal of Surgery 72 (suppl): 64–65
Klein KB 1998 Controlled treatment trials in the irritable bowel syndrome. A critique. Gastroenterology 95: 232–241
Kumar D, Wingate DL 1985 The irritable bowel syndrome, a paroxysmal bowel disorder. Lancet 2: 973–977
Kumar D, Pfeffer J, Wingate DL 1990 Role of psychological factors in the irritable bowel syndrome. Digestion 45: 80–85

Kunkel RS 1986 Acephalgic migraine. Headache 26: 198–201
Lembo T, Munakata J, Mertz H et al 1994 Evidence for the hypersensitivity of lumbar splanchnic afferents in irritable bowel syndrome. Gastroenterology 107: 1686–1696
Levitt MD 1969 Production and excretion of hydrogen gas in man. New England Journal of Medicine 281: 122–127
Levitt MD, Bond JH Jr 1970 Volume composition and source of intestinal gas. Gastroenterology 59: 921–929
Levitt MD, Furne J, Olsson S 1996 The relation of passage of gas and abdominal bloating to colonic gas production. Annals of Internal Medicine 124: 422–424
Longstreth GF, Preskill DB, Youkeles L 1990 Irritable bowel syndrome in women having diagnostic laparoscopy of hysterectomy. Digestive Diseases and Sciences 35: 1285–1290
Lundberg PW 1975 Abdominal migraine–diagnosis and therapy. Headache 15: 122–128
Lynn RB, Friedman LS 1993 The irritable bowel syndrome. New England Journal of Medicine 329: 1940–1945
Maastricht Consensus Report 1997 The management of H. pylori infection. Gut 41: 8–13
Magill AJ, Grogi M, Gasser RA, Sun W, Oster CN 1993 Visceral infection caused by leishmania tropica in veterans of Operation Desert Storm. New England Journal of Medicine 328: 1383–1387
Malfertheimer P, Mayer D, Buchler M, Dominguez-Monoz JE, Schiefer B, Ditschuneit H 1995 Treatment of pain in chronic pancreatitis by inhibition of pancreatic secretion with octreotide. Gut 36: 450–454
Malt RA 1986 Editorial: the perforated appendix. New England Journal of Medicine 315: 1546–1547
Manning AP, Thompson WE, Heaton KW, Morris AF 1978 Towards positive diagnosis of the irritable bowel. British Medical Journal 3: 762–763
Martinez-Frontanilla LA, Haase GM, Ernster JA 1984 Surgical complications of Henoch–Schonlein purpura. Journal of Pediatric Surgery 19: 434–436
Mattei P, Sola JE, Yeo CH 1994 Chronic and recurrent appendicitis are uncommon entities often misdiagnosed. Journal of the American College of Surgeons 178: 385–389
Mayer EA, Gebhart GF 1994 Basic and clinical aspects of visceral hyperalgesia. Gastroenterology 107: 271–293
McCallum RW, Chen J de Z, Lin Z, Schirmer BD, Williams RD, Ross RA 1998 Gastric pacing improves emptying and symptoms in patient with gastroparesis. Gastroenterology 114: 456–461
McColl I 1998 More precision in diagnosing appendicitis. New England Journal of Medicine 338: 190–191
McDonald HJ, Bradley LA, Bailey MA, Schan CA, Richter JE 1994 Relaxation training reduces symptom reports and acid exposure in gastroesophageal reflux disease (GERD) patients. Gastroenterology 107: 61–69
Merskey H 1965 Psychiatric patients with persistent pain. Journal of Psychosomatic Research 9: 299–309
Metz G, Jenkins DJA, Peters TJ, Newman A, Blendis LM 1975 Breath hydrogen as a diagnostic method for hypolactasia. Lancet 1: 1155–57
Metz G, Jenkins DJA, Newman A, Blendis LM 1976a Breath hydrogen in hyposucrasia. Lancet 1: 119–120
Metz G, Gassull, MA, Draser BS, Jenkin DJA, Blendis LM 1976b Breath hydrogen test for small intestinal bacterial colonization. Lancet 1: 668–669
Mishkin D, Sablauskas L, Yalosky M, Mishkin S 1997 Fructose and sorbitol malabsorption in ambulatory patients with functional dyspepsia. Digestive Diseases and Sciences 42: 2591–2598
Moriarty KH, Dawson AM 1982 Functional abdominal pain: further evidence that the whole gut is affected. British Medical Journal 284: 1670–1677
Nanda R, James R, Smith H, Dudley CR, Jewell DP 1989 Food intolerance and the irritable bowel syndrome. Gut 30: 1099–1104
Nelis GF, Vermeeren MAP, Jansen W 1990 Role of fructose sorbitol malabsorption in the irritable bowel syndrome. Gastroenterology 99: 1016–1020
Newman A, Katsaris J, Blendis LM, Charlesworth M, Walter LH 1973 Small intestinal injury in women who received pelvis radiotherapy. Lancet 2: 1471–1473
Nielsen OH, Gjoru PT, Christensen FN 1986 Gastric emptying rate and small bowel transit time in patients with irritable bowel syndrome. Digestive Diseases and Sciences 31: 1287–1292
Olubuyide IO, Olawuyi F, Fasanmade AA 1995 A study of irritable bowel syndrome diagnosed by Manning criteria in an African population. Digestive Diseases and Sciences 40: 983–985
Olsen JB, Myren CI, Haahr PE 1993 Randomised study of the value of laparoscopy before appendectomy. British Journal of Surgery 80: 922–923
Palmer RL, Stonehill E, Crisp AH, Waller SL, Misiewicz JJ 1974 Psychological characteristics of patients with the irritable bowel syndrome. Postgraduate Medical Journal 50: 416–419
Pitt P, Bruijn KM, Beeching M, Goldberg E, Blendis LM 1980 Studies on breath methane: the effect of ethnic origins and lactulose. Gut 21: 951–954
Puylaert JB, Rutgers PH, Lalisang RI et al 1987 A prospective study of ultrasonography in the diagnosis of appendicitis. New England Journal of Medicine 317: 666
Rao PM, Rhea JT, Novelline RA, Mostafavi AA, McCabe CJ 1998 Effect of computerised tomography of the appendix on treatment of patients and use of hospital resources. New England Journal of Medicine 338: 141–146
Ritchie JA 1973 Pain from distension of the pelvic colon by inflating a balloon in the irritable colon syndrome. Gut 14: 125–132
Rumessen JJ, Gudmand-Hoyer E 1988 Functional bowel disease. Gastroenterology 95: 694–700
Sackman M, Morgner A, Rudolph B et al 1997 Regression of gastric MAL lymphoma after eradication of H. pylori is predicted by endosonographic staging. Gastroenterology 113: 1087–1090
Scarinci IC, McDonald-Haile JM, Bradley LA, Richter JE 1994 Altered pain perception and psychological features among women with gastrointestinal disorders and history of abuse: a preliminary model. American Journal of Medicine 97: 108–118
Seth R, Heyman MB 1994 Management of constipation and encopresis in infants and children. Gastroenterology Clinics of North America 23: 621–636
Smart HL, Nicholson DA, Atkinson M 1986 Gastroesophageal reflux in the irritable bowel syndrome. Gut 27: 1127–1131
Smith RC, Greenbaum DS, Vancouver JB et al 1990 Psychosocial factors are associated with health care seeking rather than diagnosis in irritable bowel syndrome. Gastroenterology 98: 293–301
Song JY, Merskey H, Sullivan S, Noh S 1993 Anxiety and depression in patients with abdominal bloating. Canadian Journal of Psychiatry 38: 475–479
Spear FG 1967 Pain in psychiatric patients. Journal of Psychosomatic Research 11: 187–193
Stanghellini V, Tosetti C, Paternico A et al 1996 Risk indicators of delayed gastric emptying of solids in patients with functional dyspepsia. Gastroenterology 110: 1036–1042
Stangou AJ, Devlin E, Howard E, Williams R 1995 Is common bile duct dysmotility a common cause of post-cholecystectomy biliary pain? Gut 36: 9
Starnes HF, Moore FD, Mentzer S, Osteen RT, Steele GD, Wilson RE 1986 Abdominal pain in neutropenic cancer patients. Cancer 57: 616–619
Steely WM, Gooden SM 1986 Sclerosing mesocolitis. Diseases of the Colon and Rectum 29: 266–268
Steggerda FR 1968 Gastrointestinal gas following food consumption. Annals of the New York Academy of Science 150: 57–66

Stevenson RJ 1985 Abdominal pain unrelated to trauma. Surgical Clinics of North America 65: 1181–1215

Stewart RJ, Gupta RK, Purdie GL, Isbister WH 1986 Fine catheter aspiration cytology of peritoneal cavity in difficult cases of acute abdominal pain. Lancet 2: 1414–1415

Stone RT, Barbero GJ 1970 Recurrent abdominal pain in childhood. Pediatrics 45: 732–738

Sugarbaker PK, Bloom BS, Sanders JH, Wilson RE 1975 Preoperative laparoscopy in diagnosis of acute abdominal pain. Lancet 1: 442–445

Swarbrick ET, Hegarty JE, Bat L, Williams CB, Dawson AM 1980 Site of pain from the irritable bowel. Lancet 2: 443–446

Talley NJ, Phillips SF, Melton J, Wiltgen C, Zinsmeister AR 1989 A patient questionnaire to identify bowel disease. Annals of Internal Medicine 111: 671–674

Talley NJ, Phillips SF, Bruce B et al 1990 Relation among personality and symptoms in non-ulcer dyspepsia and the irritable bowel syndrome. Gastroenterology 99: 327–333

Talley NJ, Silverstein MD, Agreus L, Nyren O, Sonnenberg A, Holtmann G 1998 AGA technical review: evaluation of dyspepsia. Gastroenterology 114: 579–592

Tedeschi CG, Bota GC 1962 Retractile mesenteritis. New England Journal of Medicine 266: 1035–1040

Thompson WB 1997 Dyspepsia world-wide and the role of stress. European Journal of Gastroenterology and Hepatology 9: 7–8

Trotman IF, Misiewicz JJ 1988 Sigmoid motility in diverticular disease and the irritable bowel syndrome. Gut 29: 218–222

Trotman IF, Price CC 1986 Bloated irritable bowel syndrome defined by dynamic 99mTC brain scan. Lancet 2: 364–366

Vernia P, Ricciardi R, Frandina C, Bilotta T, Friere G 1995 Lactose malabsorption and irritable bowel syndrome. Italian Journal of Gastroenterology 27: 117–121

Waller SL, Misiewicz JJ 1969 Prognosis in the irritable bowel syndrome. Lancet 2: 753–756

Watt AH, Lewis DJM, Horne JJ, Smith PH 1987 Reproduction of epigastric pain of duodenal ulceration by adenosine. British Medical Journal 294: 10–12

Webster RB, Di Palma JA, Gremse DA 1995 Lactose maldigestion and recurrent abdominal pain in children. Digestive Diseases and Sciences 40: 1506–1510

Weill FS 1982 Ultrasonography of digestive disease, 2nd edn. CV Mosby, St Louis

Wenham PW 1982 Viral and bacterial associations of acute abdominal pain in children. British Journal of Clinical Practice 36: 321–326

Whitehead WE, Crowell MD, Bosmajian L et al 1990 Existence of irritable bowel syndrome supported by factor analysis of symptoms in two community samples. Gastroenterology 98: 336–340

Whorwell PJ, Clouter C, Smith CL 1981 Oesophageal motility in the irritable bowel syndrome. British Medical Journal 282: 1101–1103

Whorwell PH, Prior A, Faragher EB 1984 Controlled trial of hypnotherapy in the treatment of severe refractory irritable bowel syndrome. Lancet 2: 1232–1233

Heart, vascular and haemopathic pain

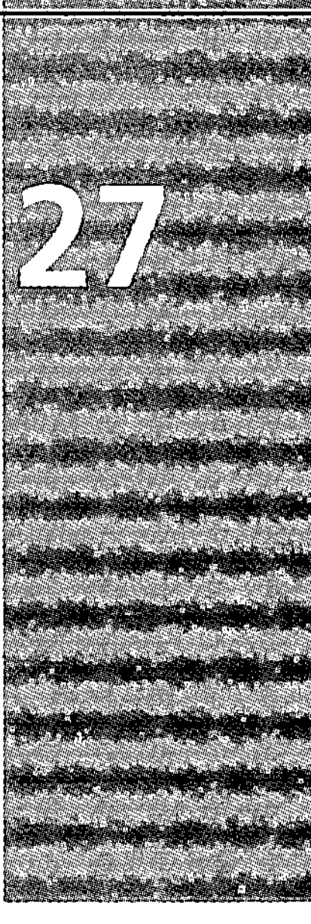

PAOLO PROCACCI, MASSIMO ZOPPI & MARCO MARESCA

INTRODUCTION

This chapter will attempt a study of the clinical aspects of:

1. heart pain
2. vascular pain
3. pain in haemopathies.

The reader is referred to specific textbooks for laboratory and instrumental investigations.

HEART PAIN

The main diagnostic problem for a clinician who sees a patient suffering from chest pain is whether he is affected by heart disease. Particular attention is focused on exploring for possible cardiac ischaemia. We have, however, to remember that many diseases cause chest pain. Apart from angina pectoris and myocardial infarction, pain can be present in some valvular heart diseases and in pericarditis. Many thoracic diseases may cause chest pain that often resembles pain from the heart, including:

1. some diseases of the aorta, such as dissection and atherosclerotic aneurysms
2. some diseases of the lungs, such as pulmonary embolism, infarction, pneumonia, cancer
3. pleuritis
4. diseases of the oesophagus, such as alterations of motility and inflammation.

Chest wall pain may also accompany or follow herpes zoster, chest injury or Tietze's syndrome (i.e. discomfort localized in swelling of the costochondral and costosternal joints, which are painful to palpation).

Differential diagnosis between chest pain from visceral organs and that from somatic diseases, such as cervicodorsal osteoarthritis and myofascial pain of the thoracic muscles, may be difficult. The diagnosis is even more complex when there are intricate problems, i.e. algogenic summation and/or interaction from different structures, such as those observed in cholecystocardiac syndromes, in vertebrocoronary syndromes and in the association of hiatus hernia or peptic ulcer with ischaemic cardiopathies (see Complex problems, below). Lastly, great care should be taken not to make a diagnosis of functional painful disease when organic alterations are not clearly evident.

A careful investigation of the characteristics of pain, of other sensory disturbances and of accompanying symptoms should not be neglected because, together with laboratory and instrumental examinations, they are of fundamental importance for a correct diagnosis.

HISTORICAL NOTES ON CARDIAC PAIN

In a historical review on heart pain (Procacci & Maresca 1985a) the first term found for cardiac pain is *passio cardiaca propria* used by Caelius Aurelianus, a fifth-century Roman physician (published 1722). The phrase was translated from the Greek physician Soranus of Ephesus who lived in the second century. After the Middle Ages, many scientists, such as Castelli (1598), Lieutaud (1759), Morgagni (1765) and Van Swieten (1768), mentioned pain in the chest referred to the heart. The term angina pectoris was introduced by Heberden in 1768 in a lecture to the Royal College of Physicians of London (published in 1772) to designate a very distinctive 'disorder of the breast' attended with 'a sense of strangling and anxiety'. Heberden probably read this term in Celsus' works and adopted it because of the similarity of the symptoms to those of the inflammatory diseases of the throat, accompanied by a feeling of choking and strangling, for which ancient Greek and Latin writers such as Celsus and Aretaeus used the term angina. The word derives from the Indo-European root *agh* and, nasalized, *angh*, which means 'to choke, to oppress, to suffer'. In English, from the same root we have *ake* (Middle English), *ache*, *anguish*, *anger* and *anxious* (Skeat 1882, Procacci & Maresca 1985b).

Heberden (1772) observed the typical relationship between effort and the onset of pain. He wrote that patients suffering from angina pectoris:

> *... are seized, while they are walking, and more particularly when they walk soon after eating, with a painful and most disagreeable sensation in the breast which seems as if it would take their life away if it were to increase or to continue: the moment they stand still, all this uneasiness vanishes...*

In the *Commentarii*, translated into English from the original Latin and published by Heberden's son in 1802, the localization of pain is carefully described:

> *...the pain is sometimes situated in the upper part, sometimes in the middle, sometimes at the bottom of the os sterni, and often more inclined to the left than to the right side. It likewise very frequently extends from the breast to the middle of the left arm.*

Heberden differentiated between angina pectoris and other forms of chest pain which were assembled under the heading of dolor pectoris. He observed that angina pectoris was often accompanied by anguish of the mind (*angor animi*).

A few years after Heberden's description, Fothergill (1776), Jenner (mentioned by Parry 1799), Parry (1799), Burns (1809) and Testa (1810) discovered that the severity of angina, often leading to sudden death, was due to a severe sclerosis (ossification) of the coronaries.

Good descriptions of anginal pain were given by Laënnec (1826) and by Trousseau (1861), who observed the radiation of pain to the thoracic muscles, clearly indicating the deep parietal component of pain, and the radiation to the internal surface of the arm.

Other important contributions in this field were: the discovery by Brunton (1867) that inhaled amyl nitrite relieved the anginal pain; the clear separation of myocardial infarction from angina pectoris by Obrastzow and Straschesko (1910) and Herrick (1912); and the description of electrocardiographic changes during attacks of angina pectoris by Bousfield (1918) and Fiel and Siegel (1928).

GENERAL CONSIDERATIONS ON PAIN FROM ISCHAEMIC HEART DISEASE

Pain from ischaemic heart disease is a symptom well known to every physician, for it is frequently observed. However, descriptions in textbooks and everyday experience give the impression of a wide variety of symptoms because of different areas of reference, different kinds of pain in the same area and involvement of areas far away from the heart. This pain, therefore, seems not to follow any rules. We believe that for this reason the attention of the physician is given less to an exact observation of the pain and more to laboratory and instrumental investigations.

The absence of rules for cardiac pain is only apparent if we examine in detail the various types of pain perceived by the patient. Indeed, it is not enough to investigate where pain is felt, but it is also necessary to distinguish between true visceral pain and referred pain and to determine whether pain is referred in deep or superficial parietal structures. Only an adequate and careful investigation of the patient can give us such information. Consequently, the description of cardiac pain should be preceded by a few clinical concepts on the characteristics of visceral pain.

The subsequent discussion on pain from the heart and from other chest organs is mainly based on observations made in the Medical School of Florence over the last 50 years (Teodori & Galletti 1962, Procacci 1969, Procacci et al 1986, Procacci & Maresca 1987a).

CLINICAL CHARACTERISTICS OF VISCERAL PAIN

The qualities of true visceral pain are clearly different from those of deep pain or cutaneous pain. Visceral pain is dull, aching or boring; it is not well localized and is described differently by the patient. It is always accompanied by a sense of malaise and of being ill. It is associated with strong autonomic reflexes, such as diffuse sweating, vasomotor responses, changes of arterial pressure and heart rate, and with an intense alarm reaction. This deep pain was defined as splanchnic pain by Ross (1887) and as direct pain of viscera (*direkter Schmerz der Eingeweide*) by Hansen and Schliack (1962).

When an algogenic process affecting a viscus recurs frequently or becomes more intense and prolonged, the location is more exact and pain is gradually felt in more superficial structures, even, sometimes, far from the site of origin. This phenomenon is usually called referred pain in

English, whereas German authors use the less common but, in our opinion, more appropriate term transferred pain (*übertragener Schmerz*).

Referred pain can be divided into:

1. deep referred pain – this pain shows a segmental pattern. It is felt in bones (sclerotomes) and muscles (myotomes)
2. superficial referred pain – this pain is felt in the skin within the dermatomes related to the affected viscus.

Both deep and superficial referred pain may be accompanied by autonomic reflexes. Cutaneous hyperalgesia and zones of muscular tenderness are often present.

With unpleasant visceral feelings, the patient often declines to apply the word pain, selecting words such as discomfort, pressure, tightness or squeezing. Between the lack of sensory symptoms and the true pain we have a continuum of intensity and unpleasantness. For these intermediate sensations, which are unpleasant but not painful, we can use the term proposed by Keele and Armstrong (1964): metaesthesia. These sensations should be carefully investigated before defining a visceral disease as 'silent'.

PAIN IN MYOCARDIAL INFARCTION

This pain arises with various modalities: suddenly during more or less stressful activities, after a large meal or during rest or sleep. Occasionally, it is preceded by a feeling of chest discomfort or slight dyspnoea or unpleasant gastric sensations described as fullness of the stomach or indigestion. The patient has often experienced previous paroxysms of angina pectoris. The early pain is deep, central, anterior and sometimes also posterior; it lasts from a few minutes to a few hours, showing the characteristics of true visceral pain. It is defined by most patients as pressing, constricting or squeezing or with phrases such as 'a band across the chest'. This kind of pain is central, often behind the lower sternum, less frequently on the epigastrium or in both these sites. Anterior pain may be concomitant with central back pain; in some patients pain is only posterior (Fig. 27.1). Pain is often accompanied by nausea and vomiting and by diffuse sweating. This pain is very intense and often accompanied by a strong alarm reaction, sometimes with a feeling of impending death.

In a following phase, after a period which varies from 10 minutes to a few hours, the pain reaches the parietal structures, assuming the characteristics of deep referred pain. It may be the first perceived pain. This pain is often defined as pressing or constricting and tends to radiate. The spatial localization is more exact than for visceral pain; it is often accompanied by sweating and rarely by nausea and vomiting. This pain is often referred beneath the sternum or in the precordial area, sometimes spreading to both sides of the anterior chest or, in a few cases, only to the right. The radiation is accompanied by feelings such as numbness, cramp or squeezing of the elbow or wrist. Frequently the pain radiates to the whole left arm or to both arms or involves the left forearm and hand; in a few cases it radiates only to the right arm. Another uncommon radiation is to the neck, jaw and temporomandibular joint on both sides simultaneously. In rare cases a posterior pain is felt in the interscapulovertebral region and may radiate to the ulnar aspect of the left arm. In patients not treated with drugs, the duration of this parietal pain varies from half an hour to 12 or more hours. It always lasts longer than true visceral pain.

Muscular tenderness follows the onset of this pain after a delay that varies from a few hours to half a day. It mainly involves the pectoralis major, the deep muscles of the interscapular region, the muscles of the forearm and, less frequently, the trapezius and deltoid muscles (Fig. 27.2).

In some patients a superficial referred pain arises, localized within the dermatomes C8–T1, that is, on the ulnar side of the arm and forearm (Fig. 27.3). This pain is rarely the only starting symptom. It lasts from half an hour to 6 hours and is intense, stabbing or lancinating. In the areas of reference cutaneous hyperalgesia is often found. There are no clear correlations between the type of infarction (inferior, anterior, transmural, non-transmural) and the pattern of pain.

PAIN IN ANGINA PECTORIS

The pain is generally deep, more rarely superficial, with the same qualities and radiations as those described in myocardial infarction, but the intensity and duration are less. Pain is not accompanied by a feeling of impending death and seldom by nausea and vomiting. The alarm reaction with the accompanying symptoms is less intense than in myocardial infarction. In these patients deep muscular tenderness is found in the same areas as in infarction and is constant and independent of pain attacks.

The deep referred pain with muscular tenderness in many cases does not replace but only inhibits the perception of true visceral pain. In patients suffering from angina of effort, Procacci and Zoppi (1983) observed that pain

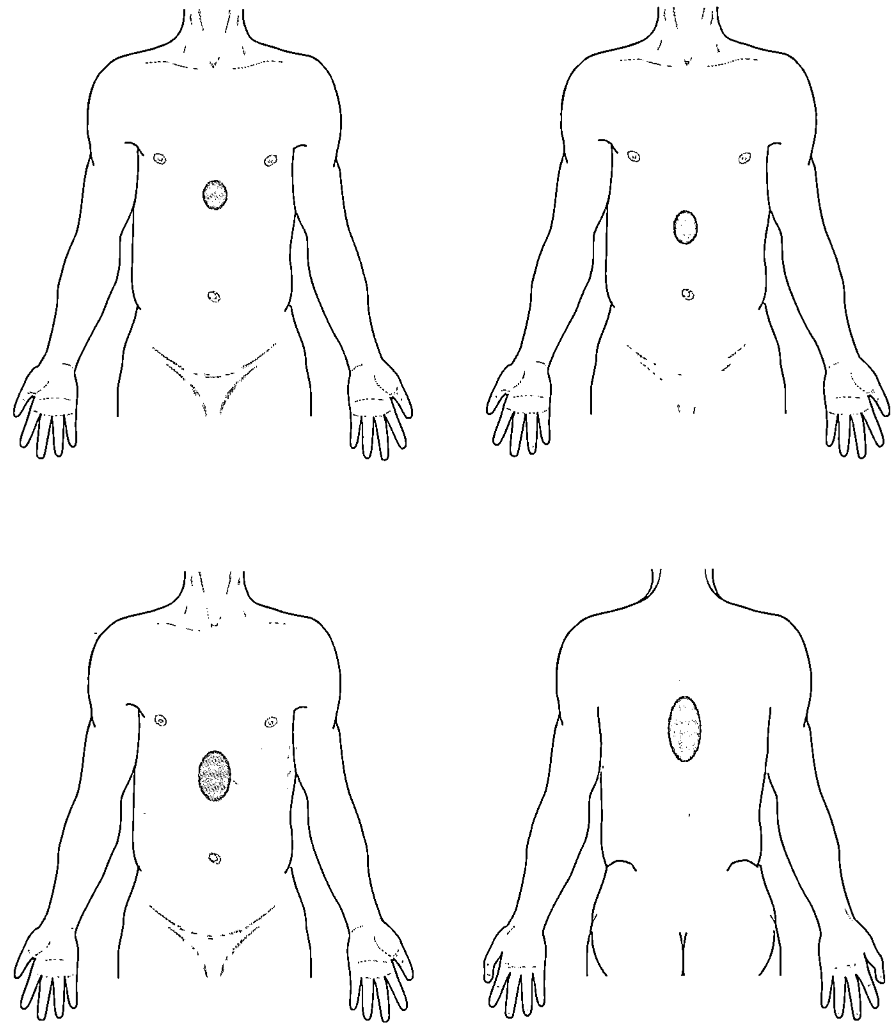

Fig. 27.1 Areas of deep visceral pain in myocardial infarction and in angina. (From Teodori & Galletti 1962 with permission.)

during stress testing was referred anteriorly on the chest wall. These patients had areas of deep tenderness on the chest wall which were blocked with a local anaesthetic. After the block, during stress testing and at S-T segment displacement in the electrocardiogram, the patients experienced a new type of pain or a general discomfort which had never been felt before. The new pain was substernal or epigastric, with the characteristics of true visceral pain.

In recent classifications of angina pectoris, the following anginal syndromes are distinguished: stable angina, unstable angina and variant (Prinzmetal's) angina (Rogers 1996, Gersh et al 1997).

STABLE ANGINA

Patients with stable angina usually have angina with effort or exercise or during other conditions in which myocardial oxygen demand is increased. The quality of sensation is sometimes vague and may be described as a mild pressure-like discomfort or an uncomfortable numb sensation. Anginal 'equivalents' (i.e. symptoms of myocardial ischaemia other than angina) such as breathlessness, faintness, fatigue and belching have also been reported (Gersh et al 1997). A classic feature of stable angina is the disappearance of pain after the use of nitroglycerine or the inhalation of amyl nitrite.

UNSTABLE ANGINA

The term unstable angina, previously also known as preinfarction angina, acute coronary insufficiency and intermediate coronary syndrome, indicates angina pectoris characterized by one or more of the following features:

1. crescendo angina (more severe, prolonged or frequent) superimposed on a pre-existing pattern of relatively stable, exertion-related angina pectoris

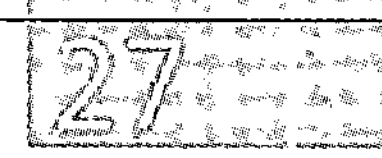

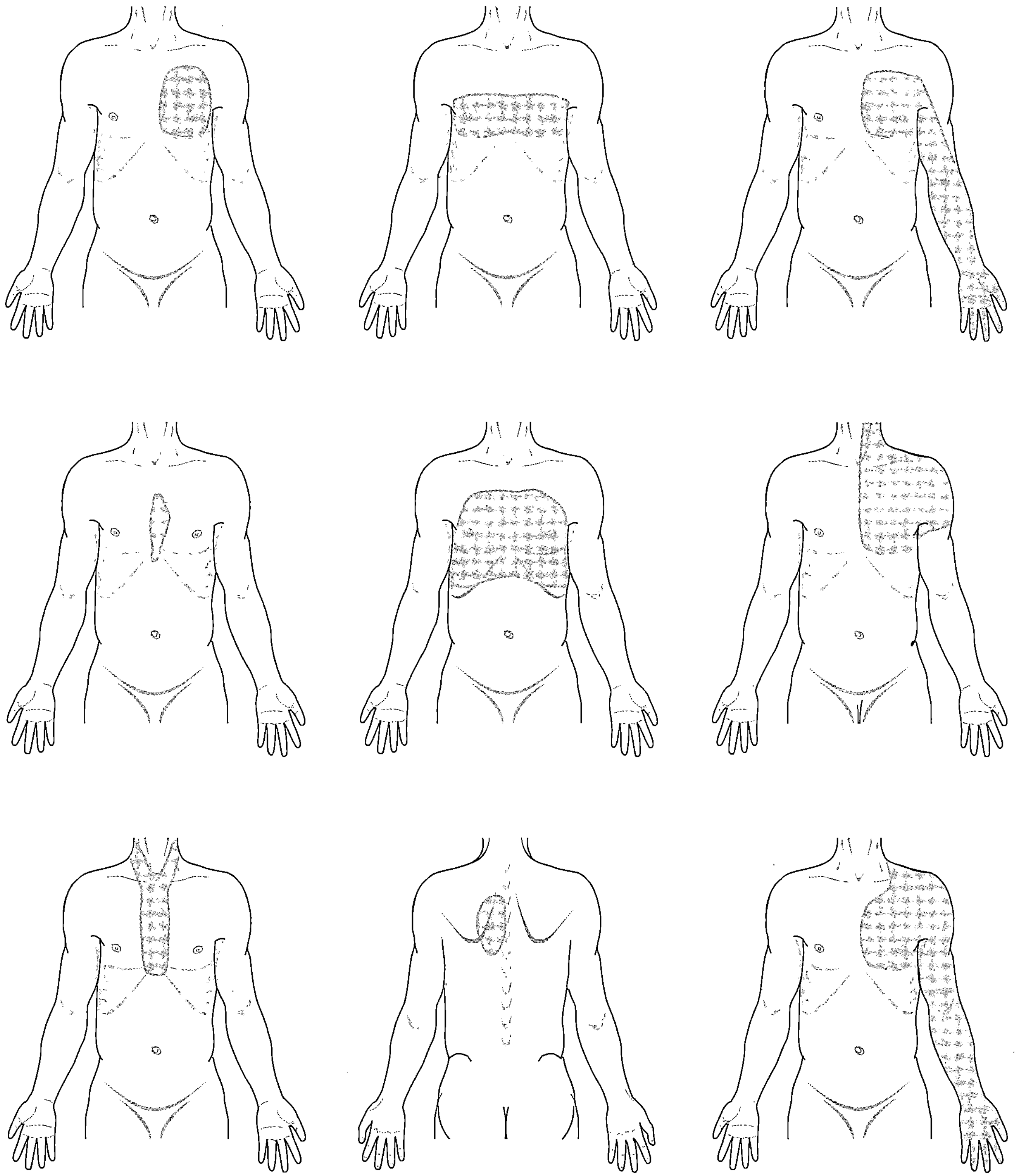

Fig. 27.2 Areas of deep referred pain in myocardial infarction and in angina. (From Teodori & Galletti 1962 with permission.)

2. angina pectoris at rest as well as with minimal exertion
3. angina pectoris of new onset (usually within 1 month), which is brought on by minimal exertion (Gersh et al 1997).

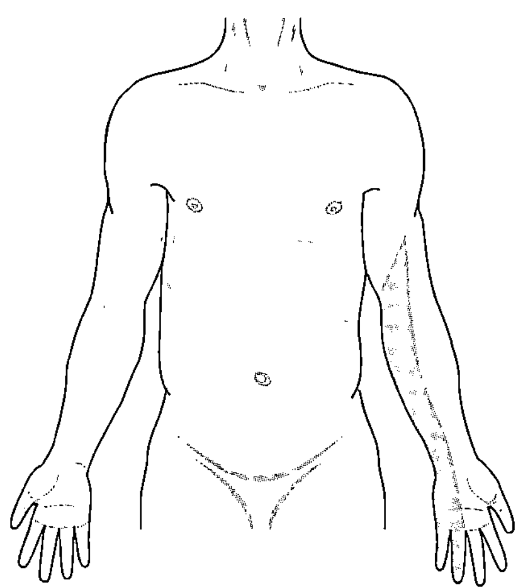

Fig. 27.3 Superficial referred pain in myocardial infarction and in angina. (From Teodori & Galletti 1962 with permission.)

In unstable angina the chest discomfort is similar in quality to that of chronic stable angina, although it is usually more intense, is usually described as pain, may persist for as long as 30 minutes and occasionally awakens the patient from sleep. When it lasts more than 30 minutes, an infarction should be suspected. One of the characteristics of this pain is that its intensity varies greatly, from very slight to (more frequently) intermediate, sometimes reaching maximal intensity, like that described in infarction.

Several clues should alert the physician to a changing anginal pattern. These include an abrupt reduction in the threshold of physical activity which provokes angina; an increase in the frequency, severity and duration of angina; radiation of the discomfort to a new site; onset of new features associated with the pain, such as nausea and decreased relief of pain afforded by nitroglycerine. Some authors observed that the natural history of stable angina and that of unstable angina are in many cases different except that in some patients stable angina evolves into unstable angina, whereas unstable angina almost never evolves into stable angina (Poggesi et al 1992). Moreover, recent studies suggest that lymphocyte activation in patients with active, unstable angina indicate that the outbursts of unstable angina appear to be an acute, transient inflammatory phase, repeatedly occurring only in a subgroup of the patients with coronary atherosclerotic disease (Neri Serneri et al 1997).

VARIANT ANGINA

Variant (Prinzmetal's) angina is an unusual syndrome of cardiac pain that occurs almost exclusively at rest, usually is not precipitated by physical exertion or emotional stress and is associated with S-T segment elevations on the electrocardiogram (Prinzmetal et al 1959). This syndrome has been demonstrated convincingly to be due to coronary artery spasm. However, in arteriographic studies Maseri et al (1978) observed that in many patients the coronary vasospasm occurring during an anginal attack was associated with S-T segment elevation or depression, blurring the distinction between variant (Prinzmetal's) angina and unstable angina. Selwyn and Braunwald (1998) consider variant angina as a peculiar form of unstable angina.

SYNDROME X

Under the broad definition of syndrome X (Kemp 1973), some studies have included a variety of patients with chest pain with a pattern of chronic stable angina and angiographically normal coronary arteries. Some patients, however, may have had a non-cardiac origin of symptoms (Maseri 1995). In some of the subjects ischaemic-appearing S-T segment responses are evident with exercise test, while in some ischaemia is undetectable by currently available techniques (Maseri 1995). It was proposed that patients with cardiac syndrome X have an exaggerated response of small coronary vessels to vasoconstrictor stimuli (Gersh et al 1997).

The absence of definitive evidence of ischaemia in some patients with syndrome X has focused attention upon other causes of chest pain, e.g. upon pain originating from oesophagus. An increased sensitivity to, and decreased tolerance of, forearm tourniquet and electrical skin stimulation were observed in women with typical angina and normal coronary arteries compared with patients with coronary artery obstructions; an exaggerated sensitivity to cardiac, potentially painful stimuli, but also an overlap between increased sensitivity to cardiac and oesophageal pain were also reported (Maseri 1995). Thus, a generalized increase in somatic and visceral pain sensitivity seems to be a common feature in patients with syndrome X. Whether this phenomenon represents an abnormal activation of somatic and visceral receptors or an abnormal processing of afferent neural impulses is unknown.

THE PROBLEM OF PAINLESS CORONARY HEART DISEASES

It is well known that myocardial infarction has been found in electrocardiographic studies or at postmortem examinations in patients in whom there was no history of a well-defined episode of chest pain. The occurrence of painless infarctions has not been correlated with the location, size or age of the infarction, nor with the age of the patients (Rinzler 1951, Friedberg 1956, Teodori & Galletti 1962, Stern 1998). During long-term follow-up in the Framingham Study, one-quarter of patients had 'unrecognized' myocardial infarction, detected only on routine 2-yearly electrocardiogram, and of these approximately half of the episodes were truly silent (Kannel & Abbott 1984). Other population studies suggest that between 20% and 60% of non-fatal myocardial infarctions are unrecognized by the patient and are discovered only on subsequent routine electrocardiographic or postmortem examination (Antman & Braunwald 1997). These differences are partly due to the use of different methods of investigating and understanding the symptoms. If, indeed, we assemble an accurate history of patients in whom a diagnosis of asymptomatic previous myocardial infarction is suspected in the course of routine examination, we may find a transient episode of chest discomfort or sudden and unusual thoracic paraesthesias (tingling, pricking, numbness) radiating to the left arm or a slight pain which was judged unimportant by the patient or an episode of nausea and vomiting interpreted as due to gastric fullness or indigestion (Procacci et al 1976). The history should be very accurate, since often these episodes are underestimated and have been forgotten by patients. Taking these factors into account, the frequency of asymptomatic myocardial infarction is reduced.

Recently the term and concept of silent myocardial ischaemia have been introduced to indicate all forms of painless myocardial ischaemia. The frequency of silent myocardial ischaemia is higher in patients with diabetes, probably because of neuropathy involving the visceral afferent fibres.

Two forms of silent myocardial ischaemia are recognized (Gersh et al 1997). The first and less common form, designated type I silent ischaemia, occurs in patients with obstructive coronary artery disease, sometimes severe, who do not experience angina at any time; some type I patients do not even experience pain in the course of myocardial infarction. These patients may be considered to have a decreased cardiac sensitivity, a condition opposed to that of syndrome X. The second and more frequent form, designated type II silent ischaemia, occurs in patients with the usual forms of chronic stable angina, unstable angina and variant angina. When monitored with a dynamic ECG, these patients exhibit some episodes of ischaemia that are associated with chest discomfort and other episodes that are not, i.e. episodes of silent (asymptomatic) ischaemia.

Some interesting investigations have been carried out to explain the mechanisms of silent myocardial ischaemia. According to Neri Serneri et al (1993), silent ischaemia in unstable angina is related to a disorder in cardiac norepinephrine handling, i.e. increased selective cardiac spillover and reduced cardiac norepinephrine extraction. Malliani (1995) observed that the temporal sequence of ischaemic episodes, sometimes more than one per hour, about 70% of which are unaccompanied by pain, seems to furnish a most intriguing clinical puzzle. In our opinion, different modalities of activation of peripheral sensory terminals and different modalities of central processing of potentially painful stimuli are likely to play a major role in determining the presence or absence of cardiac pain.

PAINFUL COMPLICATIONS OF MYOCARDIAL INFARCTION

Angina may evolve into myocardial infarction. After myocardial infarction, stable or unstable angina may develop.

Persistent pain after myocardial infarction, especially transmural, may be due to pericarditis. It is important to diagnose the chest pain of pericarditis accurately, since failure to appreciate it may lead to the erroneous diagnosis of recurrent ischaemic pain and/or extension of the infarction and to the inappropriate use of anticoagulants, nitrates, β-adrenergic blocking agents or narcotics. The pain can often be distinguished from that of an extending infarction by its characteristic pericardial pattern: the pain is relieved by leaning forward and exacerbated by deep breathing.

Pleuropericardial chest pain with fever may begin in a few cases 1–6 weeks after myocardial infarction. This post-myocardial infarction syndrome (or Dressler's syndrome) is thought to be caused by a pericarditis and pleuritis, possibly due to an autoimmune mechanism (Dressler 1956, Lorell 1997). The syndrome usually benefits from treatment with aspirin-like agents or corticosteroids. Since effusions associated with Dressler's syndrome may be haemorrhagic, anticoagulants should be discontinued if they are being administered.

Left scapulohumeral periarthritis, giving a picture of frozen shoulder, with pain, stiffness and marked limitation of motion of the shoulder joint, may complicate some cases of long-lasting angina and 5% of cases of myocardial infarction. In some cases, 3–6 weeks after myocardial infarction, a progressive reflex dystrophy of the left arm begins. It mainly involves the shoulder, the wrist and the hand (shoulder–hand syndrome). The evolution may be very severe and includes advanced stages of osteoporosis, muscular and cutaneous atrophy, glossy skin, loss of hair and vasomotor changes, etc. As in other reflex dystrophies, it often improves with blocks of the stellate ganglion.

FUNCTIONAL OR PSYCHOGENIC CHEST PAIN

Patients with chest pain and without instrumental signs of ischaemic heart disease are frequently observed. A precordial pain, often radiating with characteristics that resemble those of angina, worries many anxious patients, often with a depressive trait. They frequently undergo medical visits and examinations, the normality of which reassures them for only a short while.

Pain is variously described as stabbing, piercing, burning, dull, squeezing, annoying, slight, intense, variable and synchronous with the cardiac beats, etc. First of all, the physician must consider other causes of chest pain.

Some characteristics of this pain distinguish it from true angina: the duration varies from a few moments to some days; it is often not related to effort; patients are restless and nervous, while during an attack of angina they remain relatively immobile. The behaviour of patients often differs when they are asked where they feel pain: the patient with angina puts an open hand on the sternum, the anxious patient touches, with his index finger, the left submammary region or often zones of the precordial area.

In spite of these differences, great caution should be exercised in diagnosing functional or psychogenic chest pain, because differentiation between a true angina and an anxious depressive syndrome is often difficult. Tiresome patients, dismissed too soon and labelled as anxious or depressed, may develop an acute myocardial infarction. A careful instrumental study of these patients is important. We must remember that an anxious reaction is typical of long-lasting visceral pain.

DIAGNOSIS OF ISCHAEMIC HEART PAIN

We shall limit the description to the criteria based on the characteristics of the pain. The duration of pain is usually from a few seconds to a few minutes in stable angina, variable but not exceeding 30 minutes in unstable angina and longer in infarction; the pain of myocardial infarction is often accompanied by a feeling of impending death. Other symptoms, such as nausea and vomiting, are often present in infarction but rarely in angina. The importance of other characteristics of pain and their limits for diagnosis have been previously explained.

Some acute diseases of abdominal organs, such as peptic ulcer, acute cholecystitis and pancreatitis, may simulate heart pain, just as heart pain may simulate those diseases. Sometimes a multifactorial pain is present (see Complex problems, below).

OTHER CAUSES OF HEART PAIN

AORTIC STENOSIS

Angina pectoris has been noted in about two-thirds of cases of symptomatic aortic stenosis. Angina pectoris occurs more frequently in aortic stenosis than in other valvular lesions. The pain is usually a typical angina of effort. Patients with severe chronic aortic stenosis tend to be free of cardiovascular symptoms until relatively late in the course of the disease. Once patients become symptomatic the average survival is 2–5 years (Braunwald 1997). Obviously the course of this disease changes after cardiac surgery or angioplasty. The pain is generally related to a coronary narrowing or to myocardial hypertrophy with increased oxygen demand.

AORTIC INSUFFICIENCY

It is well known that angina pectoris has long been regarded as a symptom of aortic insufficiency. According to Friedberg (1956), angina pectoris is uncommon in uncomplicated aortic insufficiency, but it may occur because of coronary atherosclerosis or because superimposed calcification of the aortic valve leads to stenosis of the coronary arteries.

MITRAL STENOSIS

In the course of mitral stenosis the patient may have a posterosuperior pain on the left side of the chest, which is sometimes deep and sometimes superficial. Hope (1832) wrote that pain in the course of mitral stenosis is a rather frequent event. Vaquez (1922) identified a myalgic spot on the left interscapulovertebral region which is particularly evident in the phase of mitral stenosis that precedes heart failure. More recently, it has been pointed out that about 15% of patients suffering from mitral stenosis have a pain with the same characteristics as that of angina pectoris (Braunwald 1997). The observation of pain in mitral stenosis is now rare, following the development of cardiac surgery.

MITRAL VALVE PROLAPSE

Mitral valve prolapse is an anatomical and clinical entity, characterized by systolic bowing in the left atrium of one or both mitral leaflets and by typical auscultatory findings (midsystolic clicks and late systolic murmurs) (Barlow et al 1963, Braunwald 1997). Chest pain is sometimes reported. In some cases, in which mitral valve prolapse is associated with coronary heart disease, a typical anginal pain is present. Maresca et al (1989) carefully examined a group of patients with mitral valve prolapse in whom association with any other valvular or heart disease had been ruled out. A characteristic which did emerge was that most of them suffered a typical myofascial pain of the muscles of the chest.

INFLAMMATORY DISEASES OF THE HEART

Pain can occur in all inflammatory diseases of the heart, i.e. pericarditis, myocarditis and endocarditis. Pain is, however, much more frequent in pericarditis than in myocarditis or endocarditis; consequently we shall describe only the pain from pericarditis.

Pain in pericarditis is less frequent than in pleurisy, so when pain is present, pleural involvement should be suspected. For these reasons the pericardium is considered to be less sensitive to pain than the pleura (Teodori & Galletti 1962).

In acute pericarditis the onset of pain often coincides with fever or it may follow a shivering chill. Pain is often deep and substernal, usually involving the upper two-thirds of the sternum, less commonly precordial; it is continuous and lasts from a few hours to 3 days. It may appear repeatedly, always for brief periods. It is aggravated by deep inspiration, cough and lateral movements of the chest. Pain is reduced by sitting up and leaning forward.

In about half the cases, together with this deep pain, there is a superficial referred pain. The pain may radiate to the left shoulder, scapula and arm, to the neck and the epigastrium. It may appear during exertion, resembling angina. Pain is often accompanied by tenderness of the subclavicular fossa, of the superior ridge of the trapezius muscle and of the coracoid process and, more rarely, of the left chest base. (As regards pericarditis after myocardial infarction, see Painful complications of myocardial infarction, p 627.)

Chronic pericarditis is often painless, but on careful questioning the patient may report a deep, dull, slight pain or sensation of heaviness or fullness in the chest.

COR PULMONALE

In many cases of acute cor pulmonale (pulmonary embolism) a true visceral pain is observed that has the same qualities and radiation as myocardial infarction, including a strong alarm reaction.

Some patients suffering from chronic cor pulmonale have pain that shows great similarities with that of angina. The pain may be present in all diseases in which pulmonary hypertension is present: chronic cor pulmonale, mitral stenosis, some congenital heart diseases and idiopathic pulmonary hypertension. Anginal pain in patients with pulmonary hypertension is similar to that of angina pectoris: both types of pain have the same location, radiation, quality and intensity. A careful analysis, however, will show that during spontaneous or exertional pain in pulmonary hypertension, the severity of cyanosis increases (*angor coeruleus*), whereas in coronary angina the patient is pale (*angor pallidus*). The duration of pain in pulmonary hypertension is often longer than in heart angina; it may last some hours and afterwards gradually disappears. In some cases the pain worsens during inspiration and this does not happen in heart angina. This phenomenon is probably due to an increase in pulmonary pressure during this phase of breathing.

CAUSES OF CHEST PAIN (FROM ORGANS OTHER THAN THE HEART)

DISEASES OF THE AORTA

Aneurysms

The aneurysms that give rise to chest pain are those of the thoracic aorta, while aneurysms of the abdominal aorta are often asymptomatic but are sometimes accompanied by abdominal and low back pain (Isselbacher et al 1997).

Pain in thoracic aortic aneurysms is probably due to the excitation of aortic end organs and to compression and erosion of adjacent musculoskeletal structures. It is usually steady and boring and occasionally may be pulsating.

Congenital coarctation of the aorta is painless. Acquired coarctation of the aorta, which is generally due to extensive atherosclerosis with or without thrombosis, may produce symptoms of arterial insufficiency, such as intermittent claudication or coldness of the lower extremities.

Aortic dissection

According to Isselbacher et al (1997), by far the commonest presenting symptom of aortic dissection is severe pain, which is found in 74–90% of cases. The pain of dissection is often unbearable, forcing the patient to writhe in agony or pace restlessly in an attempt to gain some measure of relief.

Pain resembles that of myocardial infarction but several features of the pain may arouse suspicion of aortic dissection. The quality of the pain as described by the patient is often remarkably appropriate to the actual event. Adjectives such as 'tearing', 'ripping' and 'stabbing' are frequently used. Another characteristic of the pain of aortic dissection is its tendency to migrate from the point of its origin to other sites, following the path of the dissecting haematoma as it extends through the aorta. Pain felt maximally in the anterior thorax is more frequent with proximal dissection, whereas pain that is most severe in the interscapular area is much more common with the involvement of a distal site. Nausea and vomiting, diffuse sweating, fainting and hiccup, resistant to drugs and to manoeuvres which would ordinarily stop it, can frequently accompany the pain.

Syphilitic aortitis

Syphilitic aortitis is generally an asymptomatic lesion. The symptoms attributed to it are probably due to its complications: coronary ostial stenosis, aortic insufficiency or aneurysm.

DISEASES OF THE LUNGS

Thoracic or thoracobrachial pain is present in many patients with lung diseases, always in pulmonary infarction and sometimes in pneumonia. Pain is usually due to the involvement of the pleura. However, in patients with early cancer of the lungs not involving the pleura, Marino et al (1986) observed that pain was present in 40% of cases. Pain was always deep, referred on the chest anteriorly or posteriorly, with a good correlation between its location and the site of pulmonary lesion (Procacci 1969).

PLEURISY

Chest pain is frequently observed in the course of pleurisy because the pain sensitivity of the pleura is very high.

We shall first consider which kind of stimulus determines the pain in pleuritis. Two components are present: a mechanical component, due both to the friction between the two adjacent pleural surfaces (particularly when they are covered with fibrinous exudate) and to the stretching of the parietal pleura during inspiration; a chemical component, due to the high algogenic power of the pleural liquid, rich in pain-producing substances (Procacci 1969).

The pain shows a more exact spatial localization than in diseases of the lung. Its onset is more frequently sudden than progressive, often preceding other symptoms such as fever, dyspnoea and cough, and lasts a few days.

The location of pain varies according to the location and extent of the inflammation (Teodori & Galletti 1962).

1. In effusive pleurisy, it is felt in a region corresponding to the site of inflammation and frequently referred to the submammary area.
2. In diaphragmatic pleurisy, pain is often felt on the trapezius ridge and on the base of the affected side of the chest.
3. In apical pleurisy, pain is in the interscapulovertebral region.

Almost always, in effusive pleurisies, pain is steady, aggravated by deep inspiration, cough, movements of the chest and lying on the affected side. Shoulder pain with diaphragmatic pleurisy and interscapulovertebral pain with apical pleurisy are less localized, constrictive and not aggravated by movement, cough or deep inspiration. Pain is very intense in effusive pleurisy, especially when it is located in the submammary area, in empyema, in pleurisy that follows a pulmonary or subdiaphragmatic abscess and in pleurisy that complicates pneumonia or cancer of the lung. Pain is often associated with superficial and/or deep hyperalgesia and with slight contraction of the hyperalgesic muscles.

DISEASES OF THE OESOPHAGUS

Experimental and spontaneous oesophageal pain shows the typical characteristics of visceral pain: it is poorly localized, accompanied by autonomic reflexes and by emotions and becomes referred.

The fundamental algogenic stimuli for the oesophagus are:

1. strong mechanical stimulation from oesophageal stenosis and motor disorders, such as cancer, achalasia, diffuse oesophageal spasm, nutcracker oesophagus (symptomatic peristalsis) and aspecific motor disorders (Goyal 1998)
2. gastro-oesophageal reflux and inflammation. In patients with gastro-oesophageal reflux, the most common symptom is heartburn. The term 'burning' rather than 'pain' is usually used, although heartburn can increase in intensity until it is perceived as pain. Pain can be long-lasting or present during swallowing (odynophagia).

In patients with oesophagitis, pain was experimentally induced with the introduction of liquids at 5°C and 30°C (Teodori & Galletti 1962). These individuals felt a very unpleasant, deep, burning pain behind the sternum, mainly at the level of the xyphoid process. Oesophageal pain may be induced in routine exams by oesophageal infusion of 0.1 N hydrochloric acid (Bernstein test) or by inflating a balloon.

The areas of reference of oesophageal pain are the higher sternum for diseases of the proximal third of the oesophagus and lower sternum for diseases of the distal third. Diseases of the intermediate third give rise to pain referred to one or other area. The zones to which pain radiates are many and may be the same for diseases of the upper and lower oesophagus. The more frequently observed are the interscapular and central dorsal areas at the level of the sixth and seventh thoracic vertebrae, the neck, the ear, the jaw, the precordium, the shoulders, the upper limbs and the epigastrium (Teodori & Galletti 1962).

Oesophageal pain can mimic that of myocardial ischaemia. Discomfort is often relieved by nitroglycerine, sometimes by calcium antagonists and also, unlike angina, by milk or antacids.

COMPLEX PROBLEMS

Frequently heart pain is mingled with pain arising from other structures (*angors coronariens intriqués*) (Froment & Gonin 1956). For instance, a myocardial ischaemia may be accompanied by cervicothoracic osteoarthritis (vertebrocoronary syndrome), by chest fibromyalgias or by many diseases of the gastrointestinal tract, such as diseases of the oesophagus, hiatus hernia, gastroduodenitis, peptic ulcer, calculous and non-calculous cholecystitis (cholecystocoronary syndrome). It is difficult to ascertain whether these intricate conditions are due to a simple addition of impulses from different sources in the central nervous system or to somatovisceral and viscerosomatic reflexes which may induce a classic 'vicious circle' between different structures (Procacci et al 1986). Pain may vary from typical angina pectoris to chest pain with different patterns.

MECHANISMS OF CARDIAC PAIN

The mechanisms of cardiac pain seem to be partly similar to those of visceral and partly similar to those of skeletal muscles. For instance, a solution of NaCl 5%, a well-known algogenic stimulus for the skeletal muscles, injected in the left ventricular wall of the cat induces a powerful discharge of A-δ afferent fibres from the heart (Brown 1967). The problem of spasm of the coronaries during painful attacks is much debated. The coronary artery spasm is typical of variant angina and can be observed in both stable and unstable angina. Constriction of a small coronary vessel is supposed to be the cause of some cases of syndrome X (Maseri 1995).

According to Aviado and Schmidt (1955), the necessary stimuli in the heart for the onset of pain and of reflex phenomena were the following:

1. reduced coronary arterial pressure distal to an occlusion, acting on coronary arterial pressoreceptors
2. ischaemia, stimulating the myocardial pressoreceptors and chemoreceptors
3. release of pain-producing substances formed by tissue breakdown or platelet disintegration.

To these mechanisms, Teodori and Galletti (1962) added distension of the cardiac chambers and possibly of the large vessels. This mechanism probably prevails for posterior chest pain in early phases of mitral stenosis and may be important for pain in the course of other clinical conditions accompanied by enlargement of cardiac ventricles (cor pulmonale, aortic valve diseases, etc.).

The first mechanism, a localized hypotension, finds experimental support in Brown's experiments on the cat (1967): the pseudoaffective reaction, an indirect sign of pain, begins in fact only 1 second after experimental coronary occlusion, too short a time for the release and/or activation of pain-producing substances (Iggo 1974). This mechanism could therefore be prevalent in early phases of cardiac pain. These findings were supported by research in the cat which showed an increased discharge of the afferent C-fibres from the left ventricle following mechanical and biochemical stimuli.

The problem of the presence of true cardiac nociceptors is still debated (Cervero 1994, 1995). Malliani and his school (Malliani & Lombardi 1982, Malliani 1995) observed in animals an increased discharge of cardiac afferent C-fibres after powerful stimuli, such as the intracoronary injection of bradykinin, but never observed that coronary occlusion or bradykinin administration induced a recruitment of silent afferents. Malliani (1995) concluded that the 'intensity mechanism' was the most likely candidate to account for the properties of the neural substrate subserving cardiac nociception.

Together with mechanical factors, the biochemical component of cardiac pain in ischaemic heart disease is relevant. This component is multifactorial; increase of lactic acid, release of potassium ions and production of kinins and of other pain-producing substances must be considered.

In recent years, attention has focused on adenosine as a potential biochemical mediator of anginal pain (Cannon 1995). Malliani (1995) found that adenosine can potentiate the excitation induced by myocardial ischaemia on the impulse activity of ventricular afferent fibres. It is probable that a group of pain-producing substances act in concert. Whatever the pain-producing substances could be, the metabolic disturbance during angina pectoris induces changes in the peripheral microenvironment and is responsible for pain which shows similarities to pain from skeletal muscles. Keele and Armstrong (1964) suggested a parallel between the biochemical and algogenic phenomena of myocardial infarction and those of myonecrosis of skeletal muscles, as observed in idiopathic myoglobinuria, Haff disease and sea-snake poisoning. In both infarction and myonecrosis, the release of pain-producing substances from the necrotic tissue could be the fundamental stimulus for the severe, long-lasting pain characteristic of these afflictions.

We believe that another important mechanism is the development of an ischaemic neuropathy of heart nerves. Such a neuropathy is present in atherosclerotic arterial disease of the legs with intermittent claudication (*claudicatio intermittens*) in which, according to Lewis (1942), pain resembles that of effort angina (*claudicatio cordis*).

The various mechanisms for cardiac pain intermingle, one or other being prevalent in different conditions and in different patients (Procacci et al 1986, Maseri 1995). We can endorse the opinion of Malliani (1986) and Cervero (1994) that the link between myocardial ischaemia and cardiac pain is neither strong nor unequivocal, for cardiac pain can occur in the absence of ischaemia and, conversely, episodes of myocardial ischaemia can be painless.

MNEMONIC TRACES

Every level of the central nervous system can hold learned experiences and replay when necessary. It has been demonstrated that the mnemonic process is facilitated if the experience to be retained is repeated many times or is accompanied by pleasant or unpleasant emotions. Like other sensory modalities, pain is, at least in part, a learned experience (Melzack 1973). The processes of retained painful experience were termed memory-like processes by Melzack (1973). Nathan (1962) observed that in some subjects different kinds of stimuli could call to mind forgotten pain experiences.

We performed experiments in patients with previous myocardial infarction but with normal sensibility as judged by accurate examination. Ischaemia of the upper limbs was provoked with two pneumatic cuffs according to the technique of our school (Procacci et al 1986). In most patients ischaemia caused pain with characteristics similar to those of the pain felt during the episode of infarction. Some patients felt common sensations accompanied by alarm reaction with sweating, nausea, tachycardia and tachypnoea. No ECG changes were observed. The test was promptly interrupted at the onset of these symptoms. We also examined patients with previous painless myocardial infarction. Some of these patients remembered an episode variously defined as fullness of the stomach, nausea or indigestion, whereas in other patients the history was completely silent. In most of the patients, the ischaemia of the upper limbs provoked the onset of diffuse unpleasant common sensations, often accompanied by autonomic and emotional reactions (Procacci et al 1976).

Ischaemia of the upper limbs was also induced in patients suffering from angina pectoris. Most patients whose anginal pain radiated to the left arm reported pain in the same limb and with the same radiation as their spontaneous pain. Most patients whose anginal pain was felt only in the chest or radiated to both upper limbs reported pain in both limbs (Procacci et al 1986).

These results suggest that ischaemic pain induced in the limbs can evoke mnemonic traces left by heart pain.

THERAPY

Pain in angina pectoris is relieved by a group of drugs which are ineffective in other types of pain. The first drugs used were amyl nitrite (Brunton 1867) and, a few years later, nitroglycerine. The relief of pain with nitrates is often dramatic. Other drugs are used to prevent ischaemic attacks, such as β-blocking agents, long-lasting organic nitrates and calcium antagonists. The mechanism of these drugs is as controversial as the mechanism of pain.

We should also mention the useful association of antianginal drugs with aspirin which presumably has a direct action on cardiac pain and contributes to the elimination of the algogenic summation from myalgic spots, often present in patients with angina. This latent afferent input may assume an important role in reflexes which facilitate the attacks of angina. Aspirin is also useful for its antithrombotic effect, due to inhibition of platelet aggregation. Intravenous heparin has been used in the control of myocardial ischaemia in patients with unstable angina (Neri Serneri et al 1995).

The drug of choice in myocardial infarction is morphine, which generally induces relief of pain and good sedation. Morphine in myocardial infarction not only relieves pain but also centrally interrupts reflexes that may worsen the cardiovascular state or induce life-threatening arrhythmias.

In myocardial infarction intracoronary thrombolysis with streptokinase, urokinase and other drugs is useful in the first hours after the onset of symptoms. When intracoronary thrombolysis cannot be performed, intravenous thrombolysis is used.

As far back as 1955, White and Sweet gave a detailed description of the method of injecting the four upper thoracic sympathetic ganglia with procaine and alcohol for relief of persistent pain in angina pectoris.

Epidural blockade of the upper thoracic sympathetic segments has been shown to offer good pain relief in patients with severe unstable angina or acute myocardial infarction (Blomberg et al 1990, Kirnö et al 1994, Olausson et al 1997). The mechanism of action of this therapy is surely multifactorial, as both visceral afferent fibres and sympathetic efferent fibres are blocked.

In cardiac surgery, it is well known that most patients with angina have good relief of pain after coronary angioplasty or aortocoronary bypass. The disappearance of pain is generally related to an improvement of coronary flow. It should, however, be considered that during the operation of coronary bypass some of the cardiac afferent fibres running in sympathetic nerves are cut. This denervation may be relevant to the relief of heart pain.

The treatment of ischaemic heart disease with drugs, peripheral nerve blocks or surgery is rapidly developing and the interested reader is referred to specialized journals and textbooks.

VASCULAR PAIN

Vascular pain is a complex area. It may be divided into three sections: arterial pain; pain due to lesion or dysfunction of the microvessels (arterioles, capillaries, small venules); and venous pain.

Obviously many traumas, frequent in daily life, can damage the vascular tree with different consequences.

Vascular pain due to haemorrhage in the brain is described in Chapter 33.

ARTERIAL PAIN

Pain originating in coronary vessels and in the aorta has been covered in previous sections of this chapter.

Arterial pain may be due to different diseases such as: atherosclerosis and/or thrombosis of the arterial bed; arteritis or arteriolitis; and dysfunction of the arterioles.

Atherosclerosis and/or thrombosis of arterial bed

Atherosclerosis and/or thrombosis in the coronary vessels give rise to the pain of angina pectoris and of myocardial infarction. In arterial occlusive diseases of the limbs, it gives rise to intermittent claudication or to rest pain. Intermittent claudication is defined as a pain, ache, cramp, numbness in the muscles; it occurs during exercise and is relieved by rest. As in angina pectoris, in intermittent claudication of lower limbs the onset of pain after a given effort is an important clue to judge the severity of the syndrome. If the free interval before the onset of pain is constant, the condition is stable, as in stable angina pectoris; if the free interval shortens, the condition is similar to unstable angina. This clinical observation is obviously important for medical or surgical therapy.

Leriche's syndrome is due to isolated aortoiliac occlusive arterial disease, which produces a characteristic clinical picture: intermittent claudication of the low back, buttocks and thigh or calf muscles, impotence, atrophy of the limbs and pallor of the skin of the feet and legs. In rare cases, when atherosclerotic processes involve abdominal vessels, the patient suffers from angina abdominis. As in angina pectoris, the pain of chronic mesenteric insufficiency occurs under conditions of increased demand for splanchnic blood flow. There is usually intermittent dull or cramping midabdominal pain, characteristically beginning 15–30 minutes after eating and lasting for 1–2 hours. The arteriographic studies of angina abdominis demonstrate occlusion or high-grade stenosis of the superior or inferior mesenteric artery or the coeliac axis.

Arteritis or arteriolitis

Some diseases, such as thromboangiitis obliterans, Takayasu's syndrome and systemic giant cell arteritis, are well known (Rosenwasser 1996, Fauci 1998).

Thromboangiitis obliterans (Bürger's disease) is an obstructive arterial disease caused by segmental inflammatory and proliferative lesions of the medium and small arteries and veins of the limbs (Kontos 1996). The symptoms result mainly from impairment of arterial blood supply to the tissues and to some extent from local venous insufficiency. The symptoms are: intermittent claudication; rest pain when severe ischaemia of tissues has developed; pain from ulcerations and gangrene; and pain from ischaemic neuropathy, which must be considered an important component. Raynaud's phenomenon and migratory superficial thrombophlebitis are common.

Takayasu's syndrome (aortic arc syndrome) is due to arteritis and arteriolitis of the vessels of the upper part of the body as far as the arterioles of the eye. It is prevalent in adolescent girls and young women. In a prodromic phase about two-thirds of the patients complain of malaise, fever, limb-girdle stiffness and arthralgia; this prodromic phase is similar to that seen in giant cell arteritis, rheumatic diseases and systemic lupus erythematosus. In many instances this is soon followed by local pain over the affected arteries, erythema nodosum and erythema induratum. In some cases the disease evolves in angina pectoris or myocardial infarction.

Giant cell arteritis (temporal arteritis) is an inflammation of medium and large arteries. It characteristically involves one or more branches of the carotid artery, particularly the temporal artery, hence the name cranial or temporal arteritis. It occurs almost exclusively in individuals older than 55 years and is more common in women than in men. Headaches are often intense and almost unbearable. Headache typically occurs over involved arteries, usually the temporal arteries, but occasionally in the occipital region. A typical tenderness and induration along the vessels is observed. The area around arteries is exquisitely sensitive to pressure. Claudication in the jaw muscles while chewing occurs in up to two-thirds of patients.

Giant cell arteritis is considered a systemic disease and can involve arteries in multiple locations (Fauci 1998). The patient often describes an illness that begins like a 'flu syndrome', with severe malaise, slight fever and myalgia. The muscle pain progresses and may become severe, involving mainly the neck, shoulder girdle and pelvic girdle and also the trunk and the distal limbs to a lesser degree; the involvement is bilateral but not necessarily equal in severity. Intermittent claudication, myocardial infarctions and infarctions of visceral organs have been reported. This syndrome is considered strictly related to polymyalgia rheumatica and consequently it is classified with rheumatic diseases.

The borderline between Takayasu's syndrome and giant cell arteritis is often not clear. Today they are both considered connective tissue diseases. Rosenwasser (1996) classifies cranial or temporal arteritis and Takayasu's arteritis as subgroups of giant cell arteritides.

Dysfunction of arterioles

Raynaud's phenomenon is characterized by episodes of intense pallor of the fingers and toes (ischaemic phase), generally followed by rubor and cyanosis. The phenomenon is due to a sudden arteriolar constriction, followed by a paralytic phase. The patients usually feel an intense burning or throbbing pain during the ischaemic phase and a less intense pain together with paraesthesias during the cyanotic phase. This condition may be classified as primary or idiopathic Raynaud's phenomenon (Raynaud's disease) and as Raynaud's phenomenon secondary to other diseases, trauma or drugs. In Raynaud's disease, different alterations of the arterioles, characteristic of different kinds of arteriolitis, have been described. Calcium antagonists, adrenergic-blocking drugs and other sympathicolytic agents are considered the specific therapy for Raynaud's phenomenon (Creager & Dzau 1998).

Erythromelalgia (erythermalgia) is a syndrome characterized by the following symptoms in the extremities: red discoloration and increased temperature of the skin; deep and superficial burning pain, often accompanied by tingling and pricking; and in many cases oedema. The symptoms simultaneously involve the distal part of the lower limbs and, less frequently, of the upper limbs as well. The attacks of erythromelalgia are induced by increased temperature, either in the environment or locally, and are aggravated by a dependent position. The duration of attacks varies from a few minutes to hours. Erythromelalgia may be primary or secondary and is sometimes familial. The most common recognized cause of secondary erythromelalgia is thrombocytosis due to essential thrombocythaemia or to other myeloproliferative disorders (see Pain in haemopathies, below) (Ball 1996). Other reported associations with erythromelalgia include diabetes mellitus. Arteriolar inflammation and thrombotic occlusions were found on skin punch biopsy samples. Erythromelalgia due to thrombocytosis disappears for 3 or 4 days after a single dose of aspirin which is the duration of its inhibition of platelet aggregation. It is pertinent to ask whether primary erythromelalgia could be classified with reflex sympathetic dystrophies. As a matter of fact, excellent results, with complete disappearance of the symptoms, were observed with local anaesthetic blocks of the sympathetic chain (Zoppi et al 1985).

Mechanisms of arterial pain

The mechanisms of pain in arterial diseases are many and often intermingle.

1. Ischaemia per se. The most evident examples of diseases due to this mechanism are: angina at rest, pain occurring in arterial embolism and Raynaud's phenomenon. Ischaemia can give rise to a continuous pain in the limb when:

   a. the ischaemia is very severe
   b. myalgic spots with the characteristics of trigger points are present in the limbs (Dorigo et al 1979)
   c. a reflex sympathetic dystrophy arises which contributes to pain and dystrophy through different mechanisms: vasomotor changes; fast and slow changes in permeability of microvessels and tissue imbibition; release of active substances; direct control of some enzymatic reactions; and direct modulation of sensory receptors (Procacci 1969, Maresca et al 1984, Geppetti & Holzer 1996, Jänig 1996).
2. Ischaemia occurring during muscular exercise because of a discrepancy between the supply and demand of oxygen carried to muscles. This mechanism, according to Lewis (1942), is typical of effort angina pectoris (stable chronic angina) and intermittent claudication of the limbs. Typical myalgic spots are found in many patients with intermittent claudication and are a component of pain (Procacci 1969, Dorigo et al 1979, Maresca et al 1984).
3. Ischaemia plus inflammation and/or metabolic disorders, typical of thromboangiitis obliterans, inflammatory arteriolitis and diabetic arteriolitis.

The process of vascular thrombosis is generally considered a common arrival point of different pathways. However, in many vascular diseases the two mechanisms, thrombosis and inflammation, are in part overlapping, as is clear from clinical observations, e.g. in thromboangiitis obliterans or in angina or infarction that sometimes occur in giant cell arteritis and in thrombophlebitis.

PAIN DUE TO DYSFUNCTION OF MICROVESSELS

Pain originating from microvessels must be distinguished from classic arterial and venous pain for pathophysiological and clinical reasons.

Firstly, both arterial and venous vessels are involved in some classic syndromes, such as Raynaud's phenomenon, pernio (chilblains) and erythromelalgia (erythermalgia) (Kontos 1996, Creager & Dzau 1998). Obviously, in these cases an alteration of capillary filtration is also present, with changes in the microenvironment important for the onset of pain, as stated by Zimmermann (1979) and Jänig (1996). Many substances may be active in inducing pain. Only some of these have been identified: histamine, 5-hydroxytriptamine, kinins and substance P. The temporal relationships involved in the release of active substances in different cases are unknown. Neurogenic inflammation, i.e. the antidromic release from afferent C-fibres of substance P, calcitonin gene-related peptide (CGRP), neurokin-A and possibly other substances (Geppetti & Holzer 1996), probably plays a role in many diseases of microvessels; certainly neurogenic phenomena are important in Raynaud's phenomenon and erythromelalgia. It must be noted that Raynaud's phenomenon is often induced by cold, applied not on the hands but on the face; a disorder of the hypothalamic centres of thermoregulation may be considered probable.

VENOUS PAIN

A typical venous pain is observed in thrombophlebitis. In superficial thrombophlebitis the vein may be apparent as a red, tender cord. Pain at rest is often observed. In deep vein thrombophlebitis about half of the patients may be asymptomatic. Tenderness to palpation and pain on the voluntary dorsiflexion of the foot can be observed (Kontos 1996, Creager & Dzau 1998). Many factors are active in inducing pain: biochemical factors and mechanical factors, especially venous stasis. Much more than in arterial pain, in venous pain perivascular tissues, muscles and tendons are involved in inflammation and hence are painful. The importance of these additional factors is demonstrated by the fact that, when thrombophlebitis is resolved, a postphlebitis pain often remains in the limbs. We have observed that in many cases pain originates not only from the vein which remains painful, but also from myalgic spots, often accompanied by skin hyperalgesia. In conclusion, a postphlebitic myofascial pain syndrome is observed, which sometimes responds to aspirin-like drugs.

In every vascular disease, as well as in myocardial infarction, a reflex sympathetic dystrophy can arise. In this case skin dystrophy (glossy skin), muscle atrophy, osteoporosis and clear vasomotor and sudomotor phenomena are observed in the limbs. The classic treatment of reflex sympathetic dystrophies with sympathetic blocks can be opportune (Procacci & Maresca 1987b, Bonica 1990).

PAIN IN HAEMOPATHIES

In many haemopathies pain, due to different mechanisms, can be observed. In multiple myeloma a typical bone pain can be present. In rare cases of chronic leukaemia, a neuropathic pain is observed with different clinical manifestations. In paroxysmal nocturnal haemoglobinuria, paroxysmal cold haemoglobinuria and other acute haemolytic crises, frequent clinical complaints include abdominal, back and musculoskeletal pain. Such pain may be associated with intravascular haemolysis and haemoglobinuria or it may be ischaemic, secondary to the complication of thrombosis of major or minor vessels (Schreiber 1996). In many haemopathies a vascular pain can be observed, due to alterations of microvessels and haemostasis. However, pain is not a frequent symptom.

In four haemopathies, pain is a fundamental symptom: sickle cell disease, in which strong pain crises in trunks and limbs are frequent; essential thrombocythaemia, in which an erythromelalgic syndrome is frequently observed; haemophilic disorders; multiple myeloma, in which bone pain can be observed. We shall describe these four syndromes in detail.

PAIN IN SICKLE CELL DISEASE

Sickle cell disease is a genetic disorder, inherited with an autosomal recessive pattern which is more frequent in certain African populations, in which the sickle cell gene conferred a selective advantage, i.e. resistance to infection with malaria. The disease is present in black populations of African ancestry in America and in other parts of the world in which the presence of African groups is relevant, i.e. in the United Kingdom.

Sickle cell disease is characterized by the presence of haemoglobin S, which differs from normal haemoglobin by a single amino acid substitution in the β-globin chain (Beutler 1998). The decreased solubility of the deoxygenated form of haemoglobin S provokes the formation of haemoglobin polymers, with a typical change in red cell shape, which becomes similar to a sickle. Sickle red cells are rigid and traverse small vessels with great difficulty: vaso-occlusion may occur, with distal areas of ischaemia or infarction. The change in shape (sickling) of red cells containing haemoglobin S depends upon the degree of oxygenation of haemoglobin, the concentration of haemoglobin S in the cell, the pH and the temperature (Beutler 1998).

The main clinical manifestations of sickle cell disease include haemolytic anaemia and different complications related to the rheologic abnormalities: haematuria due to renal papillary necrosis, stroke due to cerebral infarction, painful crises due to infarctions of different organs. Acute pain is often the first symptom of disease and is the most frequent complication after the newborn period. The frequency of pain is highest in the third and fourth decades and after the second decade frequent pain is associated with increased mortality rates (Embury 1996). Painful crises may be induced by precipitating factors, such as cold, infection, fever, dehydration, menses, alcohol consumption and exposure to low oxygen tension. However, the majority of painful episodes have no clear precipitant. Apart from these factors, the frequency of painful crises varies greatly from patient to patient.

Pain may be localized in different parts of the body. An acute chest syndrome is described, characterized by fever, chest pain, dyspnoea, leucocytosis and pulmonary infiltrates on radiography (Embury 1996). The syndrome is usually due to vaso-occlusion and infection. The back, extremities and abdomen are also commonly affected in painful episodes. In the abdominal crises, pain simulates intra-abdominal disorders; consequently it is difficult to distinguish between painful episodes of sickle cell disease and other acute processes as appendicitis, biliary colic and perforated viscus. The clue to the differential diagnosis is the presence of increased sickling of red cells on peripheral blood smears and evidence of haemolysis. The episodes last from hours to weeks, followed by a return to baseline. Onset and resolution can be sudden or gradual. Some patients may experience chronic, persistent pain. Severe skeletal pain is related to bone infarctions. Periarticular infarctions may provoke arthritic pain, swelling and effusion. Frequent pain may cause despair, depression and apathy, with consequent psychosocial problems such as poor family relationships and social isolation. Shapiro et al (1995) observed that the impact of pain on psychosocial function can also affect school attendance of children and adolescents with sickle cell disease.

The treatment of painful episodes of sickle cell disease is mainly based on the administration of steroidal and non-steroidal anti-inflammatory drugs, associated with mild or strong opioids in more severe crises. Antibiotic therapy is also necessary in acute chest syndrome and other cases in which infection is present. Therapy with hydroxyurea, which induces an improvement of other clinical manifestations of sickle cell disease, may also decrease the incidence of painful episodes. The mechanism of action of hydroxyurea is mainly related to interference with normal erythropoiesis with increased production of γ-globin chains and hence of fetal haemoglobin. The increased levels of fetal haemoglobin interfere with the sickling process. Hydroxyurea also improves rheologic properties of sickle cells independently of its effect on the production of fetal haemoglobin. A comprehensive approach to the problem of pain in sickle cell disease includes the administration of antidepressive drugs and psychosocial support.

PAIN IN ESSENTIAL THROMBOCYTHAEMIA

The predominant disease expression in essential thrombocythaemia is thrombocytosis, a condition also observed in other acute or chronic myeloproliferative disorders such as granulocytic leukaemia and polycythaemia vera (Tefferi & Silverstein 1996). By far the most frequent painful disorder is erythromelalgia but headache, angina and myocardial infarction can be observed. In the cases we observed, some had a true erythromelalgia while others had attacks of acute pain in the inferior limbs without any cutaneous manifestation. In all cases the symptomatology disappeared with the administration of aspirin.

PAIN IN HAEMOPHILIC DISORDERS

Haemophilia is a group of disorders of blood coagulation due to a functional deficiency of a specific plasma-clotting factor. Classic haemophilia (haemophilia A) and Christmas disease (haemophilia B) are deficiencies of factor VIII and IX respectively. Approximately 80% of haemophiliac patients have haemophilia A. Both haemophilia A and B are X-linked recessive diseases and are associated with recurrent spontaneous and traumatic haemarthroses. The frequency and severity of the bleeding complications of haemophilia are related to the level of deficiency of the coagulation factor.

Pain may complicate haemophiliac arthropathy in different ways.

1. Haemarthroses characterized by load pain and joint swelling: the most involved joints are the knees, ankles, elbows and shoulders
2. Septic arthritis: this complication is not rare and is accompanied by fever and allodynia in the affected joints (Rasner & Bhogal 1991, Gilliland 1998)
3. Subacute or chronic arthritis with intra-articular effusion and synovitis whose typical symptom is morning stiffness and pain on awakening in the morning, lasting up to 2–3 hours
4. Endstage haemophiliac arthritis: pain in this case is continuous and exacerbated by little movements of the joints; the joint appears enlarged and 'knobby' owing to osteophytic bony overgrowth. Pain is due to severe restriction of motion, fibrous ankylosis, subluxation, joint laxity and malalignment. The joint changes stimulated by repeated intra-articular bleeding resemble those of rheumatoid arthritis (Gilliland 1998)
5. Muscle and soft tissue haemorrhage; bleeding into muscles and soft tissues is common and provokes spontaneous pain which worsens on moving the affected muscle. The most frequently involved muscle is the iliopsoas; iliopsoas haemorrhage produces acute groin pain mainly on hip extension and flexion accompanied by muscle contractures (Upchurch & Brettler 1997, Gilliland 1998). Another quite common compartment syndrome involves volar forearm muscles: if the pressure remains elevated for several hours cramplike pain worsens and the normal function of muscles and nerves is compromised and, over time, muscle infarction and nerve injury lead to Volkman's ischaemic contracture accompanied by a continuous very intense pain on the volar surface of the hand which interferes with sleep (Heck 1997).

The best therapy is infusion of recombinant factor VIII to stop bleeding. Non-steroidal anti-inflammatory drugs are contraindicated as they may worsen bleeding (York 1998).

PAIN IN MULTIPLE MYELOMA

Multiple myeloma is a malignant proliferation of plasma cells derived from a single clone. The tumour, its products and the host response to it result in a number of organ dysfunctions and symptoms. Bone pain, due to bone destruction, is the most common symptom, affecting nearly 70% of patients. The pain usually involves the back and ribs and, unlike the pain of metastatic carcinoma which is often worse at night, the pain of myeloma is precipitated by movement. Persistent localized pain in a patient with myeloma usually signifies a pathologic fracture (Longo 1998). Bony damage and collapse may lead to cord compression, radicular pain and loss of bowel and bladder control. Infiltration of peripheral nerves by amyloid can be a cause of carpal tunnel syndrome and other sensorimotor mono- and polyneuropathies.

REFERENCES

Antman EM, Braunwald E 1997 Acute myocardial infarction. In: Braunwald E (ed) Heart disease, 5th edn. WB Saunders, Philadelphia, pp 1184–1288

Aviado DM, Schmidt CF 1955 Reflexes from stretch receptors in blood vessels, heart and lungs. Physiological Reviews 35: 247–300

Ball EV 1996 Erythromelalgia. In: Bennett JC, Plum F (eds) Cecil textbook of medicine, 20th edn. WB Saunders, Philadelphia, p 1528

Barlow JB, Pocock WA, Marchand P, Denny M 1963 The significance of late systolic murmurs. American Heart Journal 66: 443–452

Beutler E 1998 Disorders of hemoglobin. In: Fauci AS, Braunwald E, Isselbacher KJ et al (eds) Harrison's principles of internal medicine, 14th edn. McGraw-Hill, New York, p 645–652

Blomberg S, Emanuelsson H, Kvist H et al 1990 Effects of thoracic epidural anesthesia on coronary arteries and arterioles in patients with coronary artery disease. Anesthesiology 75: 840–847

Bonica JJ 1990 Causalgia and other reflex sympathetic dystrophies. In: Bonica JJ (ed) The management of pain, 2nd edn. Lea & Febiger, Philadelphia, pp 220–243

Bousfield G 1918 Angina pectoris: changes in the electrocardiogram during paroxysm. Lancet 2: 457

Braunwald E 1997 Valvular heart disease. In: Braunwald E (ed) Heart disease. WB Saunders, Philadelphia, pp 1007–1076

Brown AM 1967 Excitation of afferent cardiac sympathetic nerve fibers during myocardial ischaemia. Journal of Physiology 190: 35–53

Brunton TL 1867 On the use of nitrite of amyl in angina pectoris. Lancet 2: 97

Burns A 1809 Observations on diseases of the heart. Murray & Callow, London

Caelius Aurelianus 1722 De morbis acutis et chronicis. Wetseniana, Amsterdam

Cannon RO 1995 Cardiac pain. In: Gebhart GF (ed) Visceral pain. IASP Press, Seattle, pp 373–389

Castelli B 1598 Lexicon medicum graeco-latinum ex Ippocrate et Galeno desumptum. Breae, Messanae

Cervero F 1994 Sensory innervation of the viscera: peripheral basis of visceral pain. Physiological Reviews 74: 95–137

Cervero F 1995 Mechanisms of visceral pain: past and present. In: Gebhart GF (ed) Visceral pain. IASP Press, Seattle, pp 25–40

Creager MA, Dzau VJ 1998 Vascular diseases of the extremities. In: Fauci AS, Braunwald E, Isselbacher KJ et al (eds) Harrison's principles of internal medicine, 14th edn. McGraw-Hill, New York, pp 1398–1406

Dorigo B, Bartoli V, Grisillo D, Beconi D 1979 Fibrositic myofascial pain in intermittent claudication. Effect of anesthetic block of trigger points on exercise tolerance. Pain 6: 183–190

Dressler W 1956 Post-myocardial infarction syndrome; preliminary report of a complication resembling idiopathic, recurrent, benign pericarditis. Journal of the American Medical Association 160: 1379–1383

Embury SH 1996 Sickle cell anemia and associated hemoglobinopathies. In: Bennett JC, Plum F (eds) Cecil textbook of medicine, 20th edn. WB Saunders, Philadelphia, pp 882–893

Fauci AS 1998 The vasculitis syndromes. In: Fauci AS, Braunwald E, Isselbacher KJ et al (eds) Harrison's principles of internal medicine. McGraw-Hill, New York, pp 1910–1922

Fiel H, Siegel ML 1928 Electrocardiographic changes during attacks of angina pectoris. American Journal of Medical Sciences 175: 255–259

Fothergill J 1776 Further account of the angina pectoris. Medical Observer and Inquiry 5: 252–281

Friedberg CK 1956 Disease of the heart, 2nd edn. WB Saunders, Philadelphia

Froment R, Gonin A 1956 Les angors coronariens intriqués. Expansion Scientifique Française, Paris

Geppetti P, Holzer P (eds) 1996 Neurogenic inflammation. CRC Press, Boca Raton

Gersh BJ, Braunwald E, Rutherford JD 1997 Chronic coronary artery disease. In: Braunwald E (ed) Heart disease, 5th edn. WB Saunders, Philadelphia, pp 1289–1365

Gilliland BC 1998 Relapsing polychondritis and other arthritides. In: Fauci AS, Braunwald E, Isselbacher KJ et al (eds) Harrison's principles of internal medicine, 14th edn. McGraw-Hill, New York, pp 1951–1963

Goyal RK 1998 Diseases of the esophagus. In: Fauci AS, Braunwald E, Isselbacher KJ et al (eds) Harrison's principles of internal medicine, 14th edn. McGraw-Hill, New York, pp 1588–1596

Hansen K, Schliack H 1962 Segmentale Innervation. Thieme, Stuttgart

Heberden W 1772 Some account of a disorder of the breast. Medical Transactions of the Royal College of Physicians of London 2: 59–67

Heberden W 1802 Commentarii de morborum historia et curatione. Payne, London

Heck LV Jr 1997 Arthritis associated with hematologic disorders, storage diseases, disorders of lipid metabolism and dysproteinemias. In: Koopman WJ (ed) Arthritis and allied conditions, 13th edn. Williams & Wilkins, Baltimore, pp 1697–1717

Herrick JB 1912 Clinical features of sudden obstruction of the coronary arteries. Journal of the American Medical Association 72: 2015–2021

Hope J 1832 A treatise on the diseases of the heart. Kidd, London

Iggo A 1974 Pain receptors. In: Bonica JJ, Procacci P, Pagni CA (eds) Recent advances on pain. CC Thomas, Springfield, pp 3–35

Isselbacher EM, Eagle KA, Desanctis RW 1997 Diseases of the aorta. In: Braunwald E (ed) Heart disease, 5th edn. WB Saunders, Philadelphia, pp 1546–1581

Jänig W 1996 The puzzle of 'reflex sympathetic dystrophy': mechanisms, hypotheses, open questions. In: Jänig W, Stanton-Hicks M (eds) Reflex sympathetic dystrophy: a reappraisal. IASP Press, Seattle, pp 1–24

Kannel WB, Abbott RD 1984 Incidence and prognosis of unrecognized myocardial infarction. New England Journal of Medicine 311: 1144–1147

Keele CA, Armstrong D 1964 Substances producing pain and itch. Arnold, London

Kemp HG 1973 Left ventricular function in patients with the anginal syndrome and normal coronary arteriograms. American Journal of Cardiology 32: 375–376

Kirnö K, Friberg P, Grzegorczyk A et al 1994 Thoracic epidural anesthesia during coronary artery bypass surgery: effects on cardiac sympathetic activity, myocardial blood flow and metabolism, and central hemodynamics. Anesthesia and Analgesia 79: 1075–1081

Kontos HA, 1996 Vascular diseases of the limbs. In: Bennett JC Plum F (eds) Cecil textbook of medicine, 20th edn. WB Saunders, Philadelphia, pp 346–357

Laënnec RTH 1826 Traité de l'auscultation médiate, 2nd edn. Broffon & Chaude, Paris

Lewis T 1942 Pain. Macmillan, New York

Lieutaud J 1759 Précis de médecine pratique. Vincent, Paris

Longo DL 1998 Plasma cell disorders. In: Fauci AS, Braunwald E, Isselbacher KJ et al (eds) Harrison's principles of internal medicine, 14th edn. McGraw-Hill, New York, pp 712–718

Lorell BH 1997 Pericardial diseases. In: Braunwald E (ed) Heart disease, 5th edn. WB Saunders, Philadelphia, pp 1478–1534

Malliani A 1986 The elusive link between transient myocardial ischaemia and pain. Circulation 73: 201–204

Malliani A 1995 The conceptualization of cardiac pain as a nonspecific and unreliable alarm system. In: Gebhart GF (ed) Visceral pain. IASP Press, Seattle, pp 63–74

Malliani A, Lombardi F 1982 Considerations of fundamental mechanisms eliciting cardiac pain. American Heart Journal 103: 575–578

Maresca M, Nuzzaci G, Zoppi M 1984 Muscular pain in chronic occlusive arterial diseases of the limbs. In: Benedetti C, Chapman CR, Moricca G (eds) Recent advances in the management of pain. Raven Press, New York, pp 521–527

Maresca M, Galanti G, Castellani S, Procacci P 1989 Pain in mitral valve prolapse. Pain 36: 89–92

Marino C, Zoppi M, Morelli F et al 1986 Pain in early cancer of the lungs. Pain 27: 51–55

Maseri A 1995 Ischemic heart disease. Churchill Livingstone, New York

Maseri A, Severi S, Nes MD et al 1978 'Variant' angina: one aspect of a continuous spectrum of vasospastic myocardial ischemia. Pathogenetic mechanisms, estimated incidence and clinical and arteriographic findings in 138 patients. American Journal of Cardiology 42: 1019–1035

Melzack R 1973 The puzzle of pain. Penguin, Harmondsworth

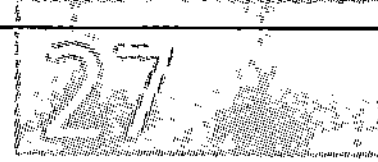

Morgagni JB 1765 De sedibus et causis morborum per anatomen indagatis. Remondini, Padua
Nathan PW 1962 Pain traces left in the central nervous system. In: Keele CA, Smith R (eds) The assessment of pain in man and animals. Livingstone, Edinburgh, pp 129–134
Neri Serneri GG, Boddi M, Arata L et al 1993 Silent ischemia in unstable angina is related to an altered cardiac norepinephrine handling. Circulation 87: 1928–1937
Neri Serneri GG, Modesti PA, Gensini GF et al 1995 Randomised comparison of subcutaneous heparin, intravenous heparin, and aspirin in unstable angina. Lancet 345: 1201–1204
Neri Serneri GG, Prisco D, Martini F et al 1997 Acute T-cell activation is detectable in unstable angina. Circulation 95: 1806–1812
Obrastzow WP, Straschesko ND 1910 Zur Kenntnis der Thrombose der Koronararterien des Herzens. Zeitschrift für Klinische Medizin 71: 116–132
Olausson K, Magnusdottir H, Lurje L et al 1997 Anti-ischemic and anti-anginal effects of thoracic epidural anesthesia versus those of conventional medical therapy in the treatment of severe refractory unstable angina pectoris. Circulation 96: 2178–2182
Parry CH 1799 An inquiry into the symptoms and causes of the syncope anginosa, commonly called angina pectoris. Murray & Callow, London
Poggesi L, Balli E, Comeglio M et al 1992 Comparative natural history of unstable and effort angina. Thrombosis Research 65 (suppl 1): S71
Prinzmetal M, Kennamer R, Merliss R et al 1959 A variant form of angina pectoris. American Journal of Medicine 27: 375–388
Procacci P 1969 A survey of modern concepts of pain. In: Vinken PJ, Bruyn GW (eds) Handbook of clinical neurology, vol 1. North-Holland, Amsterdam, pp 114–146
Procacci P, Maresca M 1985a Historical consideration of cardiac pain. Pain 22: 325–335
Procacci P, Maresca M 1985b A philological study on some words concerning pain. Pain 22: 201–203
Procacci P, Maresca M 1987a Clinical aspects of heart pain. In: Tiengo M, Eccles J, Cuello AC, Ottoson D (eds) Advances in pain research and therapy, vol 10: Pain and mobility. Raven Press, New York, pp 127–133
Procacci P, Maresca M 1987b Reflex sympathetic dystrophies and algodystrophies: historical and pathogenic considerations. Pain 31: 137–146
Procacci P, Zoppi M 1983 Pathophysiology and clinical aspects of visceral and referred pain. In: Bonica JJ, Lindblom U, Iggo A (eds) Advances in pain research and therapy, vol 5: proceedings of the Third World Congress on Pain. Raven Press, New York, pp 643–658
Procacci P, Zoppi M, Padeletti L, Maresca M 1976 Myocardial infarction without pain. A study of the sensory function of the upper limbs. Pain 2: 309–313
Procacci P, Zoppi M, Maresca M 1986 Clinical approach to visceral sensation. In: Cervero F, Morrison JFB (eds) Visceral sensation. Elsevier, Amsterdam, pp 21–28
Rasner SM, Bhogal RS 1991 Infectious arthritis in a hemophiliac. Journal of Rheumatology 8: 519–523
Rinzler SH 1951 Cardiac pain. CC Thomas, Springfield
Rogers WJ 1996 Angina pectoris. In: Bennett JC, Plum F (eds) Cecil textbook of medicine, 20th edn. WB Saunders, Philadelphia, pp 296–301
Rosenwasser LJ 1996 The vasculitic syndromes. In: Bennett JC, Plum F (eds) Cecil textbook of medicine, 20th edn. WB Saunders, Philadelphia, pp 1490–1495
Ross J 1887 On the segmental distribution of sensory disorders. Brain 10: 333–361
Schreiber AD 1996 Autoimmune hemolytic anemia. In: Bennett JC, Plum F (eds) Cecil textbook of medicine, 20th edn. WB Saunders, Philadelphia, pp 859–868
Selwyin AP, Braunwald E 1998 Ischemic heart disease. In: Fauci AS, Braunwald E, Isselbacher KJ et al (eds) Harrison's principles of internal medicine, 14th edn. McGraw-Hill, New York, pp 1365–1375
Shapiro BS, Dinges DF, Orne EC et al 1995 Home management of sickle cell-related pain in children and adolescents: natural history and impact on school attendance. Pain 61: 139–144
Skeat WW 1882 Etymological dictionary of the English language. Clarendon Press, Oxford
Stern S 1998 Silent myocardial ischemia. Martin Dunitz, London
Tefferi A, Silverstein MN 1996 Chronic myeloproliferative diseases. In: Bennett JC, Plum F (eds) Cecil textbook of medicine, 20th edn. WB Saunders, Philadelphia, pp 922–925
Teodori U, Galletti R 1962 Il dolore nelle affezioni degli organi interni del torace. Pozzi, Roma
Testa AG 1810 Delle malattie di cuore. Loro cagioni, specie, segni e cure. Lucchesini, Bologna
Trousseau A 1861 Clinique médicale de l'Hotel-Dieu de Paris. Baillière, Paris
Upchurch KS, Brettler DB 1997 Arthritis as a manifestation of other systemic diseases. In: Kelley WN, Harris ED, Ruddy S, Sledge CB (eds) Textbook of rheumatology, 5th edn. WB Saunders, Philadelphia, pp 1485–1492
Van Swieten GB 1768 Commentaria in omnes aphorismos Hermani Boerhaave, de cognoscendis et curandis morbis. Remondini, Venice
Vaquez H 1922 Malattie del cuore. UTET, Torino
White JC, Sweet WH 1955 Pain. Its mechanisms and neurosurgical control. CC Thomas, Springfield
York JR 1998 Endocrine and hemoglobin-related arthropathies and storage diseases. In: Klippel JH, Dieppe PA (eds) Rheumatology, 2nd edn. CV Mosby, London, pp 8–24
Zimmermann M 1979 Peripheral and central nervous mechanisms of nociception, pain and pain therapy: facts and hypotheses. In: Bonica JJ, Liebeskind JC, Albe-Fessard D (eds) Proceedings of the Second World Congress on Pain. Raven Press, New York, pp 3–32
Zoppi M, Zamponi A, Pagni E, Buoncristiano U 1985 A way to understand erythromelalgia. Journal of the Autonomic Nervous System 13: 85–89

Chronic pelvic pain

ANDREA J. RAPKIN

INTRODUCTION

Chronic pelvic pain (CPP) is defined as pain which persists for more than 6 months. It is one of the most common but taxing problems for women's health providers and represents an increasing proportion of visits to specialized pain clinics. Even after a thorough evaluation, the aetiology of the pain may remain obscure and the relationship between certain types of pathology such as adhesions, endometriosis, pelvic congestion and the pain response can be inconsistent. In the patient who has no obvious pathology, it may be tempting to remove pelvic structures for their physiologic variations. The exact prevalence of chronic pelvic pain is unknown, but one study sited a prevalence of 12% and a lifetime occurrence rate of 33% (Walker et al 1991). Approximately 10% of referrals to gynaecologists are for CPP and 44% of laparoscopies are performed to evaluate CPP (Howard 1993). Whereas 12% of hysterectomies are performed for the treatment of pelvic pain, 30% of women who present to pain clinics have already undergone a hysterectomy (Reiter 1990a, Howard 1993). The purpose of this chapter is to outline the relevant pelvic anatomy and to review the differential diagnosis and management of chronic pelvic pain.

NEUROANATOMY

The afferent innervation of the pelvic viscera is dependent on their embryologic origin (Kumazawa 1986). The reproductive organs are innervated by the sympathetic and parasympathetic autonomic nervous systems with contributions from the somatic sensory nervous system (Cervero & Tattersall 1986, Kumazawa 1986, Wesselmann & Lai 1997). The major afferent pathways for nociception from the female pelvic organs travel with the sympathetic nerve bundles and have cell bodies in a thoracolumbar distribution (T10–L3). Sensory afferents which travel with the parasympathetic (sacral) fibres may also be important for pain transmission from the pelvic organs. These latter nerves have their cell bodies in the sacral dorsal root ganglia (Kumazawa 1986). The terms 'sympathetic' and 'parasympathetic' are currently used to describe only efferent innervation (Cervero 1994). The afferents are, therefore, described by their anatomic pathway of projection, i.e. thoracolumbar or hypogastric and sacral or pelvic afferents. The innervation of the female pelvic viscera and somatic structures is depicted in Figures 28.1 and 28.2.

The genital tract afferent innervation travels through the vaginal, cervical and uterine plexes to the hypogastric plexus (paracervical ganglia) to the hypogastric nerve, through the superior hypogastric plexus and to the lower thoracic and lumbar sympathetic chain (Kumazawa 1986). The afferents then pass through the dorsal roots of T10, T11, T12 and L1 and enter the spinal cord at this level. There is some duplication of afferent fibres in the thoracolumbar and sacral regions and there are probably some pain impulses from the upper vagina, cervix and lower uterine segment which travel in the pelvic nerve (nerve erigentes) via pelvic parasympathetics (sacral autotomics) to S2–4 (Kumazawa 1986). Both the thoracolumbar and sacral innervation of the pelvic viscera pass through the inferior hypogastric plexus. Multiple pelvic organs including the upper vagina, cervix, uterine corpus, inner one-third of the fallopian tube, broad ligament, upper bladder, proximal urethra, distal ureter, terminal ilium and terminal large bowel are innervated via the inferior hypogastric plexus. Urogenital sinus structures including the lower vagina,

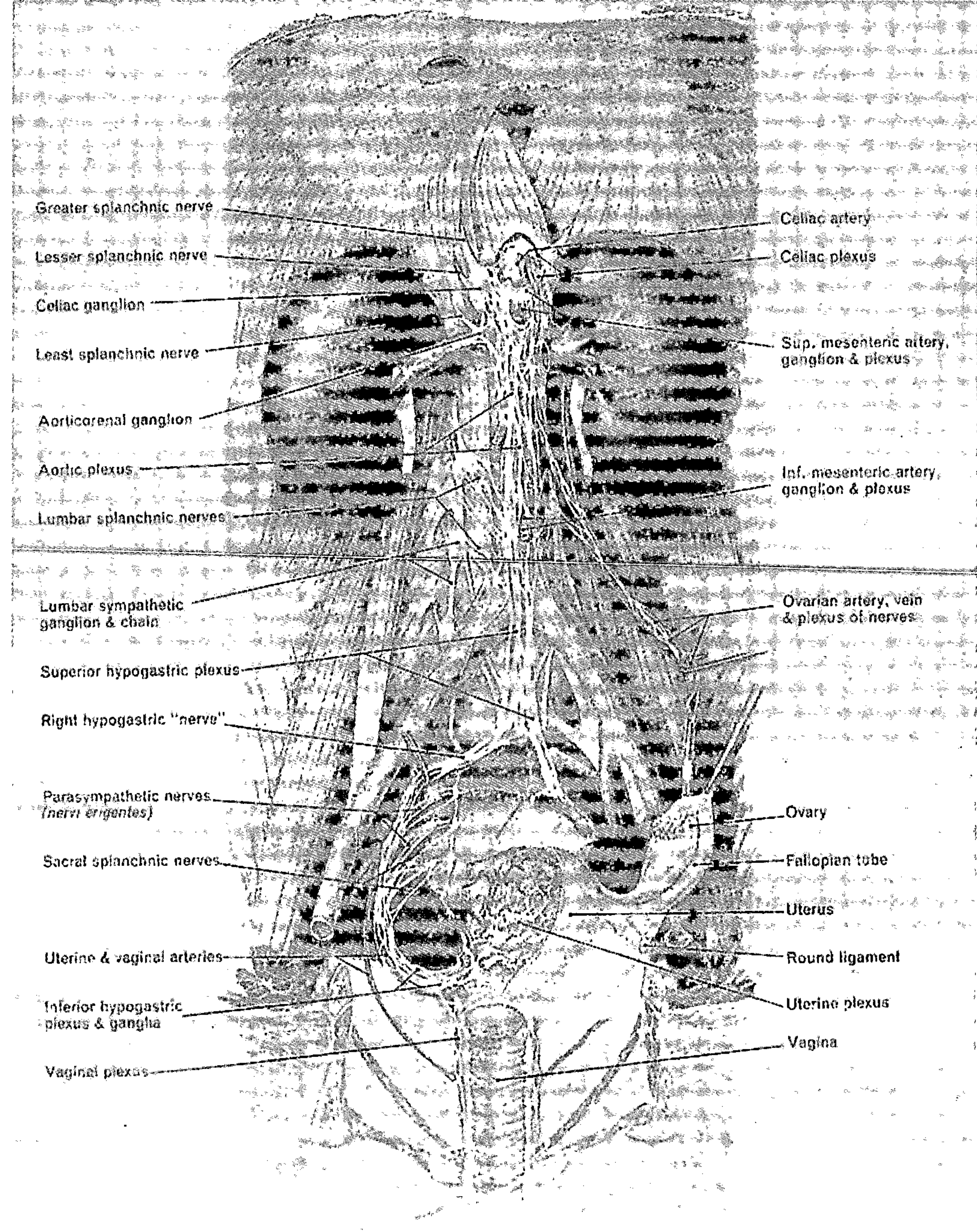

Fig. 28.1 Nerve supply of the internal genitalia (from Bonica JJ 1960 What's new. Abbott Laboratories, Chicago, p 20).

rectum and lower bladder are innervated by both thoracolumbar and sacral afferents (Kumazawa 1986).

Afferents from the ovary, outer fallopian tube and upper ureter travel with the ovarian artery, entering the sympathetic nerve chain at lumbar spinal segment 4 (L4) ascending with the sympathetic chain to penetrate the spinal cord at T9 and T10 (Kumazawa 1986). The superior hypogastric plexus carries no afferents from the ovary. In summary, the transmission of painful stimuli from the pelvic organs relies on an intact sympathetic nervous system (Cervero & Tattersall 1986). However, the parasympathetic (sacral) system is crucial for sensation and motor control of urination, defaecation and reflex regulation of the reproductive organs (Kumazawa 1986). The role of the sacral autonomics in the genesis of pelvic pain remains to be delineated.

The lower abdominal wall and anterior vulva, urethra and

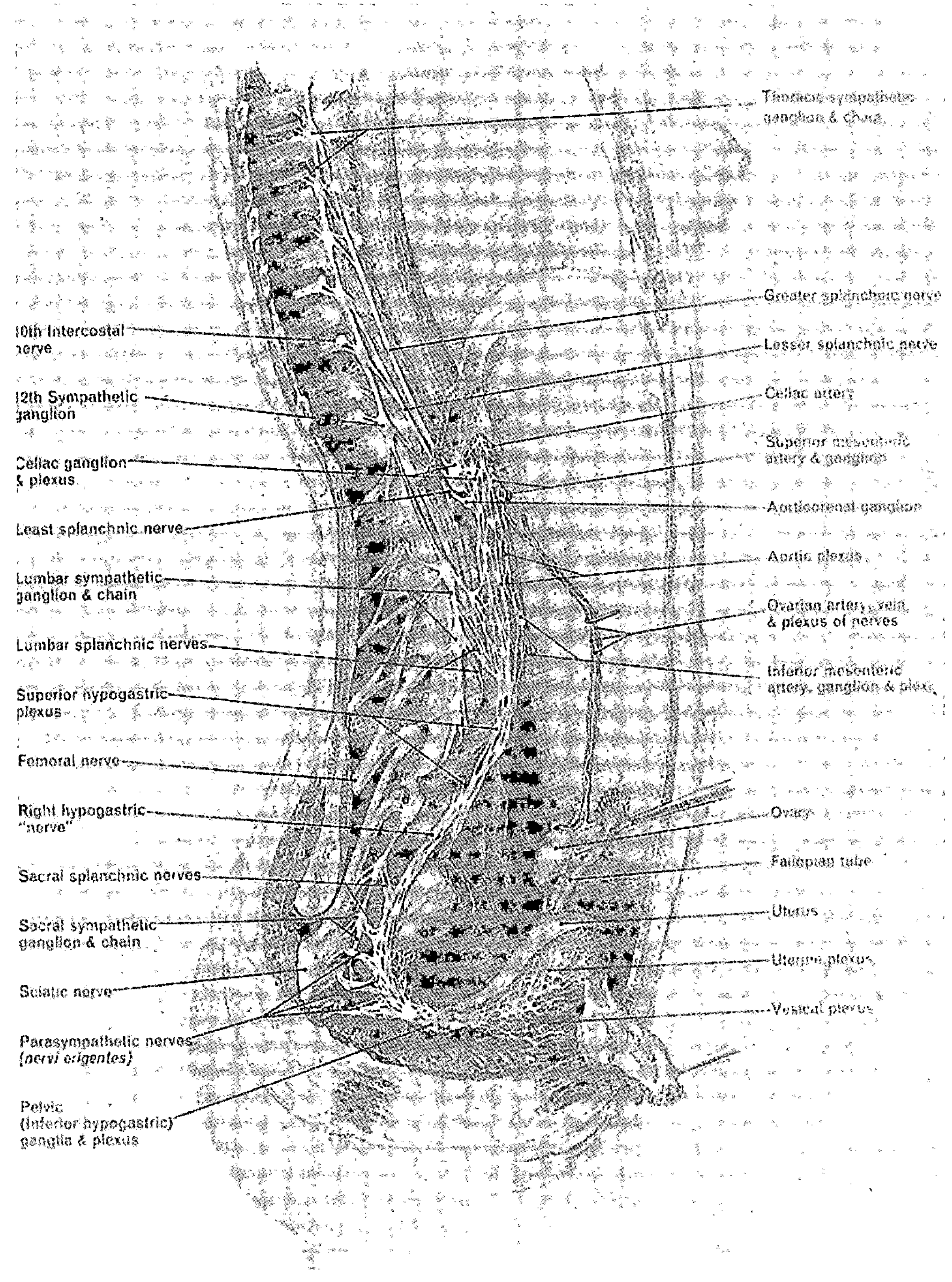

Fig. 28.2 Sagittal view of the nerve supply of the internal genitalia (from Bonica JJ 1960 What's new. Abbott Laboratories, Chicago, p 21).

clitoris are innervated by mixed (motor and sensory) somatic nerves deriving from L1 and L2: iliohypogastric, ilioinguinal, genitofemoral nerves (Hughes 1990). The dorsal rami derived from L1 and L2 innervate the lower back, often a region of referred pelvic pain. The anal canal (external and internal sphincter and puborectalis muscle), urethra, perineum and lower vagina and clitoris are innervated by somatic branches of the pudendal nerve, which is derived from S2–4.

The cell bodies of the afferent axons from the pelvic organs are located in the dorsal (sensory) ganglia of the spinal nerves (Fields 1987). Before entering the spinal grey matter of the dorsal horn, branches of these afferent axons may extend for two or more segments beyond the level at which the original axons entered the cord.

The dorsal horn is an important site of modulation of afferent input (Cervero & Tattersall 1986). Recent animal studies continue to expand the knowledge of the interactions of spinal and supraspinal centres in the transmission, modulation and perception of sensory information from the pelvic viscera (De Groat 1994, Berkley & Hubscher 1995). Clearly, the perception of pain ultimately depends on the complex central processing of peripheral neuronal activity (Cervero 1994).

GENERAL CONSIDERATIONS OF VISCERAL PAIN

The neurophysiology of pain transmission from the viscera (internal organs such as bowel, bladder, rectum, uterus, ovaries and fallopian tubes) differs from that of somatic structures (cutaneous elements, fascia, muscles, parietal peritoneum, mesentery, external genitalia, anus, urethra). Visceral pain, in contrast to somatic pain, is usually deep and difficult to localize and is frequently associated with various autonomic reflexes such as restlessness, nausea, vomiting and diaphoresis (Procacci et al 1986). However, these reflex responses are characteristic of acute not chronic visceral pain.

Viscerosomatic convergence characterizes the visceral input to the dorsal horn. The second-order neurons in the dorsal horn receive either somatic or visceral and somatic input. There are no second-order neurons receiving only visceral input. Additionally, there are also many more somatic second-order neurons than there are viscerosomatic neurons (Cervero & Tattersall 1986). Both of these facts may account for the poorly localizable quality of visceral pelvic pain. Whereas somatic structures manifest specific receptors called nociceptors which are exquisitely sensitive to tissue-damaging stimuli, the sensitivity of the viscera to different types of stimulation varies greatly. This difference between somatic and visceral pain is a subject of current debate concerning the existence of specific visceral nociceptors, similar to those found in somatic structures such as skin.

Pain from the pelvic reproductive organs seems to result from high-intensity or noxious activity in non-specific wide dynamic range receptors, not nociceptors (Berkley 1994, Cervero 1994). Cutting, crushing or burning the bowel, for example, evokes no pain, whereas significant distension of muscular organs or hollow viscera, stretching of the capsule of solid organs, hypoxia or necrosis of viscera, production of algesic (pain producing) substances, rapid compression of ligaments or vessels and inflammation may cause severe acute pain. In contrast, cutting or crushing a somatic structure produces exquisite pain which is well localized (Procacci et al 1986).

Chronic pelvic pain is generally not attributable to these classes of noxious stimuli but acutely painful gynaecologic conditions, frequently seen in the emergency room rather than the surgery, tend to result from these noxious stimuli. For example, muscular contraction of a hollow viscous is exemplified by the uterine contractions associated with labour, spontaneous abortion or transcervical passage of a submucosal myoma; sudden stretching of the capsule of a solid organ is associated with a haemorrhagic ectopic pregnancy or corpus luteum cyst; hypoxia of viscera produces the pain associated with adnexal torsion; exposure of the peritoneum to algesic substances occurs with haemoperitoneum, ruptured cystic teratoma or endometrioma or inflammation secondary to pelvic inflammatory disease. Increasingly intense or repetitive visceral stimuli or inflammation result in increased pain sensitivity, characterized by central changes in processing of sensory information by the spinal cord (Cervero 1994). Enhanced excitability of visceral sensory receptors has also been reported. For example, the repeated distension of the rat uterine horn or application of algesic agents has been shown to produce increased responsiveness of hypogastric afferent fibres (Berkley et al 1988). Oestrus also sensitizes hypogastric afferents (Robbins et al 1992).

Visceral pain is also characterized by referred pain. This referred pain is superficial, well localized and perceived to arise in the same dermatome or spinal cord segment receiving the visceral stimulus. Various acute and chronic gynaecologic pain conditions are characterized by referred pain to the dermatomes associated with pelvic organ innervation, i.e. T10–L2 (anterior abdominal wall and anterior thighs) and dorsal rami of L1–2 (lower back) (Slocumb 1984, Giamberardino et al 1995. Wesselmann & Lai (1997) developed a model of inflammatory uterine pain in the rat to investigate these mechanisms of referred pain. In this model, experimentally induced uterine inflammation led to neurogenic plasma extravasation in the regions of referred uterine pain: the skin over the abdomen, groin, lower back and perineal area. The neuronal pathways mediating the dye extravasation in the skin are the subject of future investigation which will further the understanding of visceral pain from the reproductive organs.

PERIPHERAL CAUSES OF CHRONIC PELVIC PAIN

ADHESIONS

The differential diagnosis of the peripheral component of pelvic pain is listed in Box 28.1. Laparoscopic studies for the evaluation of chronic pelvic pain would suggest that

BOX 28.1

Peripheral causes of chronic pelvic pain

1. Gynaecologic

Non-cyclic
- Adhesions
- Endometriosis
- Salpingo-oophoritis
- Ovarian remnant syndrome
- Pelvic congestion syndrome (varicosities)
- Ovarian neoplasms
- Pelvic relaxation

Cyclic
- Primary dysmenorrhoea
- Secondary dysmenorrhoea
  - a. Imperforate hymen or transverse vaginal septum
  - b. Cervical stenosis
  - c. Uterine anomalies (congenital malformation, bicornuate uterus, blind uterine horn)
  - d. Intrauterine synechiae (Asherman's syndrome)
  - e. Endometrial polyps
  - f. Uterine leiomyoma
  - g. Adenomyosis
  - h. Pelvic congestion syndrome (varicosities)
  - i. Endometriosis
- Atypical cyclic
  - a. Endometriosis
  - b. Adenomyosis
  - c. Ovarian remnant syndrome
  - d. Chronic functional ovarian cyst formation

II. Gastrointestinal

Irritable bowel syndrome
Ulcerative colitis
Granulomatous colitis (Crohn's disease)
Carcinoma
Infectious diarrhoea
Recurrent partial small bowel obstruction
Diverticulitis
Hernia
Abdominal angina
Recurrent appendiceal colic

III. Genitourinary

Recurrent or relapsing cystourethritis
Urethral syndrome
Interstitial cystitis
Ureteral diverticuli or polyps
Carcinoma of the bladder
Ureteral obstruction
Pelvic kidney

IV. Neurologic

Nerve entrapment syndrome
Neuroma
Trigger points

V. Musculoskeletal

Low back pain syndrome
- Congenital anomalies
- Scoliosis and kyphosis
- Spondylolysis
- Spondylolisthesis
- Spinal injuries
- Inflammation
- Tumours
- Osteoporosis
- Degenerative changes
- Coccydynia

Myofascial syndrome
Fibromyalgia
Pelvic floor muscle tension/spasm or trigger points

VI. Systemic

Acute intermittent porphyria
Abdominal migraine
Systemic lupus erythematosus
Lymphoma
Neurofibromatosis

adhesions play a prominent role. However, when these laparoscopic studies were performed, non-obvious or 'occult' sources of pelvic pain such as abdominal wall or pelvic floor muscle pain, pelvic congestion, irritable bowel syndrome and interstitial cystitis were generally not excluded prior to laparoscopy. Adhesions were found in 16–44% of the patients undergoing laparoscopy for chronic pelvic pain (Liston et al 1972, Lundberg et al 1973, Kresch et al 1984, Rapkin 1986, Hughes 1990).

The role of pelvic adhesions in the genesis of pelvic pain has been debated from various perspectives. One approach has been to compare the prevalence of adhesions in women with CPP and asymptomatic controls. Adhesions are more prevalent in women with CPP than asymptomatic controls but the prevalence of adhesions in the control group depends on the comparison group selected (i.e. sterilization or infertility). Kresch et al (1984) noted adhesions in 51% of CPP patients and 14% of women undergoing sterilization and the adhesions in the CPP group more often involved bowel. Rapkin (1986) reported adhesions in 26% of CPP patients and 39% of asymptomatic infertility patients. There were no differences in the location or density of adhesions between the two groups. The latter findings were confirmed by Koninckx et al (1991) who laparoscoped 227 patients and again noted a similar prevalence and distribution of adhesions between CPP patients and asymptomatic infertility patients. Some 'adhesions' may be physiologic, such as the tethering of the ileum and ascending colon to right sidewall and sigmoid colon to left sidewall.

In summary, although women with CPP have a higher prevalence of adhesions than women undergoing sterilization, one cannot conclude that these findings are causal or even highly associated. If adhesions cause pain, adhesiolysis should relieve it. There is only one randomized controlled trial of lysis of adhesions in women with CPP (Peters et al 1992). Patients with CPP and laparoscopic diagnosis of stage III–IV adhesions proceeded to surgical adhesiolysis via laparotomy or expectant management. Follow-up assessment of pain was performed 16 months postoperatively. Three scoring systems were used to evaluate pain response. Adhesiolysis was of no more benefit than expectant management. Only those patients with severe vascularized adhesions involving the serosa of the small bowel and to a lesser extent the colon benefited and improvement was only noted on two of the three assessment scales. These patients tended to have symptoms and physical findings consistent with intermittent partial small bowel obstruction.

A prospective non-randomized study of adhesiolysis also did not note improvement in pain at the time of the 8-month follow-up (Steege & Scott 1991). There was, however, significant relief of pain after adhesiolysis in the subgroup of women without 'CPP syndrome'. CPP syndrome was defined as manifesting four or more of the following:

1. pain duration >6 months
2. incomplete relief by previous treatments
3. impaired physical functioning secondary to pain
4. vegetative signs of depression
5. altered family roles.

In this study, the location of the pain overlapped with location of adhesion in 90% of patients and large bowel adhesions were prevalent (70–80%). The intensity of pain did not correlate with amount of disease. Steege and Scott (1991) concluded that lysis of adhesions may be a useful procedure in many circumstances but women with 'CPP syndrome' were unlikely to benefit from adhesiolysis. Other retrospective non-controlled studies of adhesiolysis demonstrated relief of pain in 50–80% of patients (Chan & Wood 1985, Daniell 1989, Fayez & Clark 1994, Saravelos et al 1995). There was no difference in outcome if adhesiolysis was performed via laparoscopy or laparotomy. In addition to 'CPP syndrome', women who have had a prior hysterectomy or laparotomy are less likely to benefit from lysis of adhesions (Saravelos et al 1995).

Future studies of laparoscopy under local anesthesia may allow 'pain mapping' to determine the sensitivity of peritoneal surfaces and adhesions in women with and without pain. 'Pain mapping' is a new and untested procedure. It is unclear whether it will be specific for intraperitoneal 'pathology' or if any tissue manipulation in the dermatomal distribution of pain will be perceived as painful.

ENDOMETRIOSIS

Another 'peripheral' cause of chronic pelvic pain is endometriosis. The incidence of endometriosis has been estimated to be 1–2% in the general female population, although in infertile women the incidence is 15–25%. There has been an apparent increase in incidence of endometriosis over the last 10 years which may be a reflection of the more liberal use of laparoscopy combined with the recent recognition of atypical forms of endometriosis. Endometriosis is found in approximately 28–74% of the patients undergoing laparoscopy for chronic pelvic pain (Liston et al 1972, Lundberg et al 1973, Kresch et al 1984, Rapkin 1986, Reese et al 1996). The diagnosis of endometriosis is usually made in the third or fourth decade but it has been noted to be a prominent diagnosis in adolescents and women in their 20s who are evaluated for chronic pelvic pain (Chatman & Ward 1982).

Endometriosis is defined as the presence of endometrial glands and stroma located outside the uterine cavity, most commonly in the cul-de-sac, ovaries and pelvic visceral and parietal peritoneum. The favoured theory of aetiology is retrograde menses with implantation of endometrium in susceptible women and probably involves a local disorder of immune modulation (D'Hooghe et al 1996).

The most common symptoms of endometriosis are dysmenorrhoea, dyspareunia, infertility and abnormal uterine bleeding, usually from a secretory endometrium. Pelvic pain in women with endometriosis may occur at any time in the menstrual cycle, though dysmenorrhoea is the most classic symptom. Dysmenorrhoea may begin 7–10 days before the onset of the menstrual period and persist after the bleeding has ceased. The patient often describes pressure-like or sharp pain in the lower abdomen, back and rectum with radiation to the vagina, thighs or perineum. Dyspareunia or dyschezia (pain with bowel movements) is common when the disease involves the cul-de-sac (pouch of Douglas), uterosacral ligaments or rectovaginal septum. Although the serosa of the intestine is involved in many patients, only rarely is the mucosa affected, leading to cyclic haematochezia. Urinary urgency, frequency, bladder pain and, rarely, haematuria can also be associated with urinary tract involvement. Rarely, patients may develop bowel or ureteral obstruction. Postmenopausal women on oestrogen replacement can continue to experience symptomatic endometriosis. However, without oestrogen replacement the diagnosis is highly debatable.

Examination of patients with endometriosis often reveals focal tenderness and nodularity on the rectovaginal examination of the uterosacral or broad ligaments and posterior cul-de-sac (D'Hooghe et al 1996). Progressive disease will result in obliteration and fibrosis of the cul-de-sac and fixed retroversion of the uterus. Enlarged ovaries filled with 'chocolate cysts' (endometriomas) with decreased mobility are often noted on examination or ultrasound of the pelvis.

Laparoscopy is necessary for definitive diagnosis of endometriosis though the diagnosis may be suggested by history and pelvic examination. Clinical diagnosis is accurate only 50% of the time (Martin et al 1989) and the histologic confirmation laparoscopic diagnosis is approximately 60% (Cornillie et al 1990). Ultrasound is not diagnostic as small implants are not detectable and an endometrioma can resemble a cystic ovarian neoplasm. CA 125 and erythrocyte sedimentation rate (ESR) can be elevated in women with endometriosis, but are not specific enough to aid in diagnosis.

Endometriosis is usually progressive and, untreated, approximately 50% of women will have worsening of the disease over a 2-year period. Endometriosis can be treated hormonally using androgenic hormones (Danocrine®), high doses of progestins or gonadotrophin-releasing hormone analogues to lower oestrogen levels and create pseudomenopause, thereby leading to atrophy of implants (D'Hooghe et al 1996). Laparoscopic electrodessication resection or laser vaporization or laparotomy with resection of disease is usually recommended and is necessary for the treatment of severe endometriosis or endometriomas. Patients who do not desire fertility may opt for radical surgery, consisting of a total abdominal hysterectomy with bilateral salpingo-oophorectomy and appendectomy as well as removal of any residual GI, GU or peritoneal disease. Those who are less symptomatic often benefit from continuous or cyclic oral contraceptive pills. Additional benefit can be derived from adjunctive acupuncture or multidisciplinary pain management (Rapkin & Kames 1987).

Endometriosis is a common finding in women of reproductive age, but it is clear that in many women with chronic pelvic pain and endometriosis the latter may not be the cause of the pain or may only represent a contributing factor. At least 30% of patients with recurrent pain after treatment of endometriosis do not have residual disease at the time of repeat laparoscopy. There is no significant correlation between the amount of disease and pain severity although higher stage disease tends to be associated with a greater prevalence and increased intensity of pain. Additionally, there is no correlation between location of pain and site of endometriotic lesions (Fukaya et al) and as many as 30–50% of patients regardless of stage have no pain. However, deeply infiltrating lesions, particularly of the uterosacral ligaments, are strongly associated with pain (Cornillie et al 1990).

Clinically it is possible to determine if there is a relationship between pain and endometriosis in a specific patient because of the hormonal sensitivity of the disease and the potential to excise disease surgically. Pain that does not respond to adequate surgical and medical management of endometriosis should be re-evaluated for another source of pain or other contributing factors.

TUMOURS AND CYSTS OF THE REPRODUCTIVE ORGANS

Most tumours and cysts of the reproductive organs can cause acute pain from adnexal torsion or degeneration or torsion of leiomyomata. Outside the settings of an acute event, however, vague lower abdominal discomfort and fullness may be related to pelvic tumours such as leiomyomata or ovarian neoplasms, both benign and malignant. Ultrasound is diagnostic.

Uterine leiomyomata are the most common pelvic neoplasms. They undergo malignant transformation in approximately 2–3/100 000 of women and growth is usually slow. Pelvic discomfort from myomata is present when the neoplasms encroach on adjacent bladder or rectum. This pain is not usually severe. Surgery, myomectomy or hysterectomy, is warranted for abnormal bleeding or discomfort due to uterine size (usually greater than 14 cm). If the diagnosis is uncertain, a laparoscopy may be necessary.

PELVIC CONGESTION

For the last 40 years, there has been interest in the role of 'pelvic congestion' or uterine and ovarian vein varicosities in the genesis of chronic pelvic pain. Taylor (1954) proposed the concept that emotional stress could lead to autonomic nervous system dysfunction manifested by smooth muscle spasm and congestion of the ovarian and uterine veins. Recently, substance P binding sites were localized to the endothelium of pelvic veins and may have a role in controlling vascular tone and pain (Stones et al 1995). Clinically, the syndrome includes abdominal and low back pain, dysmenorrhoea, dyspareunia and menorrhagia. The pain is usually bilateral, lower pelvic in distribution and exacerbated by the menstrual period. Anxiety, chronic fatigue, breast tenderness, symptoms of irritable bowel, as well as premenstrual syndrome are associated complaints. On examination, there is tenderness over the uterus, parametria and especially the uterosacral ligaments and polycystic ovaries are often noted (Taylor 1954, Beard et al 1988).

Beard performed a blinded study of venograms in patients with chronic pelvic pain and controls noted larger mean ovarian vein diameters, delayed disappearance of contrast medium and ovarian plexus congestion in a significantly greater proportion of women with chronic pelvic pain without pathology than those with pathology or controls (Beard et al 1984, 1988).

Until recently, the diagnosis of pelvic congestion was a clinical diagnosis. Clearly, the symptoms overlap with irritable bowel, myofascial pain and secondary dysmenorrhoea. Beard and colleagues (1988) have published studies in which the diagnosis was made via transuterine venogram. However, this test was technically not feasible or unreadable in 21% of Beard's sample. Additionally, the diameter of the veins and time for disappearance of contrast material from the uterine and ovarian veins must be compared with standard pain-free controls. There are a few small studies concerning the utility of pelvic ultrasound with Doppler or MRI for the diagnosis of pelvic congestion (Stones et al 1990).

Since many patients were noted to have polycystic ovaries and all were of reproductive age, hormonal suppression providing a hypo-oestrogenic environment has been used to treat pelvic congestion. Medroxyprogesterone acetate (MPA) 30 mg was administered daily for 3 months in a randomized, placebo-controlled treatment trial (Farquhar et al 1989). Patients given MPA reported a 50% reduction in pain score compared with a 33% reduction in pain after receiving placebo. However, after discontinuation of treatment, the pain returned in the MPA group but did not return in the placebo group. Psychotherapy did not reduce pain in the short term, but there was a positive interaction between MPA and psychotherapy 9 months after the treatment was concluded. Contrary to expectation, one study failed to show improvement after gonadotrophin-releasing hormone suppression with low-dose oestrogen and progestin hormone addback (Gangar et al 1993). Total abdominal hysterectomy with bilateral salpingo-oophorectomy eliminated pain in 33 of 36 patients followed for 1 year (Beard et al 1991). Transcatheter embolization of pelvic veins has been performed in a limited number of subjects with promising outcome but the long-term risks and benefits remain unknown (Sichlau et al 1994).

SALPINGO-OOPHORITIS

Salpingo-oophoritis can cause chronic pelvic pain, though patients usually present with symptoms and signs of acute or subacute infection before the pain becomes chronic. In the past, frequent recurrent acute infections were typical but with the advent of potent broad-spectrum aerobic and anaerobic antibiotic regimens, this problem is less common.

Sweet and Gibbs (1985) proposed criteria for making the diagnosis of acute salpingitis on clinical grounds. Two of the three must be present: lower abdominal pain as well as lower abdominal tenderness (with or without rebound), cervical motion tenderness and adnexal tenderness. In addition, one of the following minor criteria must be present: temperature greater than 38°C, leucocytosis (more than 10 500 white blood cells per mm^3), culdocentesis fluid containing white cells and bacteria and Gram stain, presence of an inflammatory mass, elevated ESR, a Gram stain from the endocervix revealing Gram-negative intracellular diplococci or a monoclonal smear from the endocervical secretions revealing chlamydia or gonorrhoea.

Patients may complain of having had numerous episodes of pain associated with fever and may have been given the diagnosis of pelvic inflammatory disease. However, the patient may not have salpingitis at all. Clinical diagnosis leads to error in 50% of cases (Sweet & Gibbs 1985). Laparoscopy with visualization of pelvic organs and peritoneal fluid cultures is diagnostic. Intravenous aerobic and anaerobic antibiotic therapy is the standard treatment for salpingo-oophoritis. Only rarely is hysterectomy and salpingo-oophorectomy required, generally for tubo-ovarian abscesses.

OVARIAN REMNANT SYNDROME

A hysterectomy and bilateral salpingo-oophorectomy performed in the setting of severe anatomic distortion, such as with severe endometriosis or pelvic inflammatory disease, may result in the ovarian remnant syndrome, in which residual ovarian cortical tissue is left in situ (Steege 1987, Siddall-Allum et al 1994). The incidence of ovarian remnants in this setting is unknown but is probably high. Pain associated with an ovarian remnant is, however, a rare event.

The diagnosis is suspected on the basis of history, physical examination and hormonal evaluation (Steege 1987, Price et al 1990). Pelvic pain, usually arising 2–5 years after surgery, is often cyclic, accompanied by flank pain and, on occasion, urinary tract infection and intermittent, partial bowel obstruction. Pelvic examination may reveal a tender mass in the lateral region of the pelvis. Ultrasound following ovarian stimulation with clomiphene usually confirms a mass with the sonographic characteristics of ovarian tissue. In a patient who has had bilateral salpingo-oophorectomy and is not on hormonal replacement, oestradiol and follicle-stimulating hormone (FSH) levels reveal a characteristic premenopausal picture, though on occasion the remaining ovarian tissue may not be active enough to suppress FSH levels. Laparotomy and removal of residual ovarian tissue is necessary for treatment (Pettit & Lee 1988). Surgical management via laparoscopy is not advisable. Complications including haemorrhage, ureteral, bladder and bowel injury and postoperative ileus are common. Recurrent remnants occur in 15% of cases. Treatment with GnRH agonists and oestrogen and progestin addback therapy may be an appropriate alternative (Steege 1987, Carey & Slack 1996).

CYCLIC PELVIC PAIN

Cyclic pelvic pain implies pain occurring with a specific relationship to the menstrual cycle. It consists of primary and secondary dysmenorrhoea but also includes atypical cyclic pain, such as pain beginning 2 weeks prior to menses. Atypical cyclic pain is a variant of secondary dysmenorrhoea. The diagnosis of cyclic pain often depends on the review of a daily pain and menstrual diary.

Dysmenorrhoea or 'painful monthly flow' is a common gynaecologic disorder affecting up to 50% of menstruating women (ACOG 1983). Primary dysmenorrhoea refers to pain with menses when there is no pelvic pathology, whereas secondary dysmenorrhoea is painful menses with underlying pelvic pathology. Primary dysmenorrhoea usually appears 1–2 years after menarche, with the establishment of ovulatory cycles, but may persist into the 40s. The pain consists of suprapubic cramping radiating down the anterior thighs and to the lumbosacral region often accompanied by nausea, vomiting and diarrhoea. The pain occurs prior to or just after the onset of menses and lasts for 48–72 hours.

The pain of dysmenorrhoea derives from activation of primarily thoracolumbar and pelvic afferent innervation. The effective stimulus causing this activation is unclear but the following factors are clearly relevant:

1. myometrial contractions leading to intense intrauterine pressure and uterine hypoxia
2. hyperproduction of leukotrienes and other hormonal factors effectively increasing afferent terminal excitability
3. altered CNS processing of the afferent barrage possibly mediated by opioid or GABAergic mediations
4. environmental and behavioural factors (Rapkin et al 1997).

Secondary dysmenorrhoea, on the other hand usually, though not always, occurs years after menarche and may occur with anovulatory cycles. The most common causes of secondary dysmenorrhoea are endometriosis and adenomyosis, a condition in which the endometrial glands penetrate the myometrium. Other common causes are listed in Box 28.1 and include vaginal, cervical, uterine, fallopian tube, adnexal and peritoneal pathology (Rapkin & Reading 1991). The differential diagnosis of secondary dysmenorrhoea includes primary dysmenorrhoea and non-cyclic pelvic pain and entails ruling out primary dysmenorrhoea and confirming the cyclic nature of the pain. The distinction between primary and secondary dysmenorrhoea requires a thorough history as to the timing and duration of the pain, a pain diary and a careful pelvic examination, with focus on the size, contour, mobility and tenderness of the uterus, adnexal structures, nodularity of the uterosacral ligaments and rectovaginal septum. Genital studies for gonorrhoea and chlamydia and a complete blood count with ESR and possibly a transvaginal ultrasound are warranted. If no abnormalities are found, a tentative diagnosis of primary dysmenorrhoea can be made.

Prostaglandin synthetase inhibitors are effective for the treatment of primary dysmenorrhoea in up to 80% of cases (Medical Letter 1979). For the patient with primary dysmenorrhoea who has no contraindications to oral contraceptive agents, the birth control pill is the second agent of choice (Chan & Dawood 1980). More than 90% of women with primary dysmenorrhoea have relief with oral contraceptive control pills (Chan & Dawood 1980). Narcotic analgesics can be administered for pain control. Prior to the addition of narcotic medication, organic pathology should be ruled out, generally via laparoscopy and, if indicated, hysteroscopy. Other modes of hormonal menstrual suppression include high-dose progestins (oral or depot intramuscular injection), continuous oral contraceptive pill administration or gonadotrophin-releasing hormone agonists with continous low (menopausal) dosage hormone addback. Breakthrough bleeding with associated pain are potential problems with these regimens. Acupuncture or transcutaneous electrical nerve stimulation may be successful (Mannhemier & Whaler 1985, Helms 1987).

If treatment fails, laparoscopy is warranted to rule out secondary dysmenorrhoea, in particular endometriosis. A strong family history of endometriosis, infertility or any clinical signs of endometriosis on examination may suggest that laparoscopy be performed sooner. With the availability of non-steroidal anti-inflammatory agents and compounds which alter the female sex steroids, such as oral contraceptive pills, progestins (oral or depot injectable) or gonadotrophin-releasing hormone (GnRH) agonists, cyclic pelvic pain has become significantly more manageable (Smith 1993).

Surgical approaches to dysmenorrhoea include laparoscopic uterosacral ligament ablation, presacral neurectomy and, in selected cases of secondary dysmenorrhoea, hysterectomy (Malinak 1980). The uterosacral ligaments carry the main afferent supply from the uterus and, if complete, the uterosacral ablation should be as effective as the presacral neurectomy, though Doyle (1955) described a 70% success rate. Long-term or controlled studies of the neurectomy procedures are lacking (see Management of chronic pelvic pain, p. 654). The treatment of secondary dysmenorrhoea depends on the nature of the underlying pathology.

GASTROENTEROLOGIC CAUSES OF CHRONIC PELVIC PAIN

Many patients referred to gynaecologists with chronic pelvic pain actually have gastroenterologic (GI) pathology (Reiter 1990b, Walker et al 1996). Since the cervix, uterus, adnexa, lower ileum, sigmoid colon and rectum share the same visceral innervation, with pain signals travelling via the sympathetic nerves to spinal cord segments T10–L1, it is often difficult to determine if lower abdominal pain is of gynaecologic or enterocolic origin (Rapkin & Mayer 1993). In addition, as is true with other types of visceral pain, pain sensation from the GI tract is often diffuse and poorly localized (Mayer & Gebhart 1993). Skilful medical history and examination are usually necessary to make the diagnosis.

Irritable bowel syndrome (IBS) is one of the more common causes of lower abdominal pain and may account for as many as 7–60% of referrals to a gynaecologist for chronic pelvic pain (Reiter 1990b). The predominant symptom of irritable bowel syndrome is abdominal pain, usually intermittent, crampy and predominantly left lower quadrant in location (Rapkin & Mayer 1993). Other symptoms include excessive flatulence, bloating and alternating diarrhoea and constipation. Pain is often improved after a bowel movement and worse prior to a bowel movement. The pain may last for only a few minutes, but 50% of patients may have pain for hours to days and 20% of patients may complain of pain for weeks or longer. Symptoms are usually worse after eating, during periods of stress, tension, anxiety, or depression and with the premenstrual and menstrual phases of the cycle (Rapkin & Mayer 1993).

The diagnosis of the irritable bowel syndrome is usually made on the basis of the history but cannot be made without first excluding other conditions. Red flags such as blood in stool, recent antibiotic usage, nocturnal awakening, family history of colon cancer, weight loss and abnormal pelvic or abdominal exam do not support a diagnosis of IBS and colonoscopy or barium enema is often necessary to rule out pathology.

Irritable bowel syndrome is a waxing and waning disorder and treatment consists of dietary alterations, bulk-forming agents and high-fibre diet, reassurance, education, stress reduction and anxiolytic, anticholinergic or other antispasmodic pharmaceutical agents. Low-dose tricyclic antidepressants are also useful (Drossman & Thompson 1992).

Though appendicitis is a common cause of abdominal pain, the abdominal pain of appendicitis is usually severe and accompanied by anorexia, nausea or fever, localized right lower quadrant tenderness and peritoneal signs on examination. Occasionally, a patient under care for chronic pelvic pain will develop acute appendicitis or other acute pelvic condition such as ectopic pregnancy, pelvic inflammatory disease or a ruptured cyst. Chronic appendicitis is a controversial entity; it probably does exist and responds to appendectomy (Lee et al 1985).

Another cause of chronic enterocolic pain is diverticular disease of the colon (Drossman & Thompson 1992). Five to 40% of individuals over the age of 40 have diverticulosis, although most patients never develop diverticulitis. Though diverticulosis is usually asymptomatic, diverticulitis results in severe, acute left lower quadrant pain associated with fever, a tender mass and leucocytosis.

Inflammatory bowel disease such as ulcerative colitis or granulomatous disease (Crohn's disease) similarly do not usually present as chronic pelvic pain because their presentation is usually more acute, with diarrhoea, fever, vomiting and anorexia. A colonoscopy or barium study is diagnostic.

Tumours of the GI tract can cause chronic lower abdominal pain in women. The most frequent and early symptoms of bowel carcinomas are change in bowel habits (74% of patients) and abdominal pain (65% of patients). Rectal bleeding and weight loss may be signs of advanced disease. Most rectal tumours can be palpated on rectal examination. Sigmoidoscopy or barium enema is diagnostic.

HERNIA

Hernia is included in the differential diagnosis of lower abdominal pain. There is a relatively low incidence of inguinal hernia in females (Hightower & Roberts 1981). Anterior and posterior perineal hernias are usually limited to cystocoele, rectocoele or enterocoele and may cause lower pressure-like abdominal/perineal pain in women. This type of pain will usually respond to a pessary followed by surgical management. Another cause of abdominal pain in women is Spigelian hernias. These hernias produce lower abdominal pain located between the semilunar line (transition between the muscle and the aponeurosis of the transversalis muscle) and the lateral border of the rectus muscle. This hernia is a weakness in the transversalis fascia (Spangen 1984). Increased pain with Valsalva, clinical examination and ultrasound are helpful for diagnosis. The management is surgical repair.

UROLOGIC CAUSES OF CHRONIC PELVIC PAIN

Chronic pain of urologic origin may present as pelvic pain due to the close developmental and anatomic relationship of the urinary and genital tracts. The urethra, bladder, vagina and vestibule are all derived from the embryologic urogenital sinus. Recurrent cystoureteritis, urethral syndrome, urethral diverticulae, urgency, frequency syndrome, interstitial cystitis, infiltrating bladder tumours, ectopic pelvic kidney and various ureteral causes of pelvic pain such as urolithiasis, ureteral obstructions or endometriosis can present as pelvic pain in approximately 5% of women with chronic pelvic pain (Reiter 1990b, Summit 1993). The medical history should query symptoms such as urgency, frequency, hesitancy, incontinence, nocturia, dyspareunia and past history of treatment of urinary tract problems.

The patient with infectious cystitis presents with complaints of suprapubic pain, dysuria, frequency and urgency and has pyuria and a positive urine culture. The symptoms usually respond to adequate antibiotic therapy. Relapses and reinfection can be diagnosed with the aid of history, urinalysis and culture. The antibiotic and duration of therapy may have to be adjusted and on occasion, if the patient has recurrent cystourethritis, antibiotics may have to be administered postcoitally or for a prolonged period of time. Chlamydial infection is responsible for about 25% of cases of pyuria and urethritis in women (Summit 1993).

The urethral syndrome may present as chronic pelvic pain or irritative lower urinary tract symptoms such as dysuria, urinary frequency and dyspareunia (Bergman et al 1989, Summit 1993). The diagnosis is one of exclusion. At negative urinalysis, negative or a low colony count (e.g. $< 10^4$ col/ml) on urine culture, negative chlamydia study and evaluation for vulvovaginitis will increase the suspicion for the diagnosis of urethral syndrome. The aetiology of the syndrome is unknown: chronic inflammation of the periurethral glands or urethral spasticity with periurethral muscle fatigue have been suggested. Treatment consists of re-education of voiding habits through pelvic floor muscle biofeedback (Summit 1993), chronic suppression with 3–6-month low-dose course of broad-spectrum antibiotics or tetracycline for 2–3 weeks if chlamydia is suspected. Urethral dilatation has also been utilized. Vaginal oestrogen for peri- and postmenopausal women is important (Bergman et al 1989). Consideration should be given to pelvic floor muscle biofeedback, muscle relaxants and psychotherapy.

Symptoms of urinary frequency, urgency, nocturia and suprapubic pain with negative laboratory studies are consistent with both interstitial cystitis (IC) or urgency/frequency syndrome (Karram 1993). The consensus criteria for the diagnosis of IC include at least two of the following: pain on bladder filling relieved by emptying, pain in suprapubic, pelvic, urethral, vaginal or perineal region, glomerulations on endoscopy or decreased compliance on cystometrogram (Gillenwater & Wein 1988). Symptoms that do not meet IC criteria can be termed urgency/frequency syndrome. Interstitial cystitis is an inflammatory condition of uncertain aetiology although autoimmune disease, defect of the glycosaminoglycan layer of the bladder mucosa, and activated bladder sensory neuropeptides have been proposed (Gillenwater & Wein 1988). The evaluation of patients with the above symptoms should include cystoscopy under anaesthesia with hydrodistension and possible biopsy. Therapy consists of bladder diet (Box 28.2), intravesical hydrodistension, instillation of dimethylsulphoxide or analogues of glycosaminoglycan, transcutaneous electrical nerve stimulation (TENS), physical therapy, biofeedback to the pelvic floor muscles or repeated anaesthetic blocks (hypogastric plexus). The treatment of the condition remains empiric and less than optimal. Oral pharmacologic agents such as anticholinergic, antispasmodic, NSAIDs, tricyclic antidepressants and narcotics have all been utilized with some success.

Very severe chronic suprapubic pain may be caused by infiltrating carcinomas of the bladder, cervix, uterus or rectum. These conditions should be apparent after performing the history, pelvic examination, urine analysis and cystoscopy, though intravenous pyelogram (IVP) or CT urogram may be necessary.

BOX 28.2

LIST B: Foods to Substitute for List A Foods	LIST A: Foods to AVOID
Alcohol or wines for flavouring	All alcoholic beverages
Almonds	Apples
Apple, small	Apple juice
Blueberries	Avocados
Carob	Bananas
Coffee, no acid (Kava)	Beer
Extracts, brandy, rum, etc.	Brewer's yeast
French Sauternes	Cantaloupe
Imitation Sour Cream	Champagne
Onions, cooked	Cheese
Orange juice, reduced acid	Chicken livers
Peanuts	Chilies/spicy foods
Pears	Chocolate
Pine nuts	Citrus fruits
Processed cheeses, not aged	Coffee
Spring water	Corned beef
Strawberries, 1/2 cup	Cranberries
Sun tea	Fava beans
Tomatoes, low acid	Grapes
White chocolate	Guava
Wines, late harvest	Lemon juice
Zest of orange or limes	Lentils
Shallots, green onions	Lima beans
All other foods not on List A	Mayonnaise
	NutraSweet
	Nuts
	Onions
	Peaches
	Pickled herring
	Pineapple
	Plums
	Prunes
	Raisins
	Rye bread
	Saccharine
	Sour cream
	Soy sauce
	Strawberries
	Tea
	Tomatoes
	Vinegar
	Vitamins buffered w/aspartate
	Yogurt

NERVE ENTRAPMENT OR INJURY

Abdominal cutaneous nerve entrapment or injury should be considered in the differential diagnosis of chronic lower abdominal pain, especially if no visceral aetiology is apparent. The syndrome most commonly occurs months to years after Pfannenstiel skin or other lower abdominal and even laparoscopic incisions (Sippo et al 1987) but can also follow trauma, automobile accidents or exercise. Commonly involved nerves include ilioinguinal (T_{12}, L_1), iliohypogastric (T_{12}, L_1) and genitofemoral (L_1, L_2).

Symptoms of nerve entrapment include pain, typically elicited by exercise and relieved by bedrest (Hammeroff et al 1981, Suppo et al 1987). The pain is described as stabbing and colicky, located along the lateral edge of the rectus margin, often associated with a burning or aching pain radiating to the hip or sacroiliac region. Nausea, bloating, menstruation and a full bladder or bowel exacerbate the pain.

On examination, the pain can be localized with the fingertip (MacDonald 1993). The maximal point of tenderness is the neuromuscular foramen at the rectus margin medial and inferior to the anterior iliac spine or, in the case of spontaneous nerve entrapment, at the site of exit from the aponeurosis of the other thoracic/abdominal cutaneous nerves. A manoeüvre which helps to make the diagnosis is to ask the patient to tense the abdominal wall by raising the shoulders or raising and extending the lower limbs in a straight leg-raising movement. The outer side of the rectal muscle is then pressed with a single finger. The pain will be exacerbated if abdominal wall pain is present (Thompson & Francis 1977). In a series of 46 women with a clinical diagnosis of ilioinguinal nerve entrapment, 88% had hyperasthesia and 53% dysasthesia. The tentative diagnosis is confirmed with a diagnostic nerve block consisting of injection of 2–3 ml of 0.25% bupivacaine (Hahn 1989). Immediate relief is usually reported and many patients require up to five biweekly injections. Cryoneurolysis may lead to a longer pain-free interval. Only as a last resort should consideration be given to surgical removal of the involved nerves. Deafferentation pain is a possible sequel of this surgery. One non-controlled study noted a 'good to excellent' response rate of 76% at the time of 1-year follow-up in 39 operative nerve transections for ilioinguinal nerve entrapment (Hahn 1989). Medications such as low-dose tricyclic antidepressants, anticonvulsants and acupuncture are also useful for pain control. Physical therapy or lifestyle change may be necessary to strengthen other muscles and avoid reinjury.

MUSCULOSKELETAL CAUSES OF CHRONIC PELVIC PAIN

Women complaining of lower back pain without complaints of pelvic pain rarely have gynaecologic pathology as the cause of their pain, but low back pain may accompany pelvic pathology. Back pain may be caused by gynaecologic, vascular, neurologic, psychogenic or spondylogenic (related to the axial skeleton and its structures) pathology (Morscher 1981, Baker 1993). Musculoskeletal abnormalities commonly contribute to the symptoms of chronic pelvic pain (Baker 1993). A physical therapist who can evaluate posture, muscle length and strength and joint range of motion should improve the efficacy of treatment (Baker 1993).

MYOFASCIAL PAIN

Reports of the prevalence of myofascial pain as a cause of pelvic pain vary. Reiter and Gambone found myofascial syndrome in 15% of their patients with somatic pathology (Reiter 1990b). (Patients with somatic pathology represented 47% of all patients referred to their pelvic pain clinic (Reiter et al 1991)). Slocumb (1984, 1990), in comparison, noted 'trigger points' in 89% of women presenting with chronic pelvic pain irrespective of underlying pelvic pathology. The painful tissue, according to Slocumb, was Camper's fascia. Whether pain is primarily myofascial or is a manifestation of referred pain is not known.

Clinically, musculoskeletal pain, similar to visceral pain, is dull, aching and poorly localized and may be altered by the phases of the menstrual cycle. Any structure or muscle innervated via T12–L4 can refer pain to the lower abdomen (i.e. vertebrae, joint capsule, ligaments, discs, muscles such as the rectus, iliopsoas, quadratus lumbarum, piriformis and obturators). Similarly, due to T10–S4 innervation, the reproductive organs refer pain to the abdominal wall, low back, thighs and pelvic floor (Baker 1993). Myofascial pain is exacerbated by activity within the affected part and by activity in deeper visceral structures which share the same dermatomal innervation (Slocumb 1984, 1990, Travell 1976) (bladder or colon activity or pathology, menses, cervical motion and intercourse). On digital examination of dermatomes of the abdomen, back or vagina, pressure on the trigger point evokes local and referred pain. Pain is exacerbated by the straight leg-raising manoeuvre described above.

Treatment of myofascial trigger points includes injecting the trigger points with local anaesthetic as well as physical therapy and treatment of associated psychological factors such as depression, anxiety and learned behaviour patterns which may accompany and exacerbate the condition (Travell 1976, Slocumb 1984). Medications such as tricyclic antidepressants and anticonvulsants may also be useful.

PSYCHOLOGICAL FACTORS IN CHRONIC PELVIC PAIN

From a psychological perspective, there are various factors which may promote the chronicity of pain. Studies of women with chronic pelvic pain have documented a high level of psychological disturbance. The MMPI conversion 'V' profile was described (Castelnuova-Tedesco & Krout 1970) in a survey of 40 women with pelvic pain. Gross et al (1980) reported high levels of psychopathology in women with pelvic pain, as well as a past exposure to childhood sexual abuse in 90% of their sample. Studies using the MMPI have failed to find a correspondence between psychological and physical findings. MMPI profiles of women with chronic pain without obvious pathology were compared with those of women with pain arising from endometriosis and a control group (Renaer et al 1979). The two pain groups differed from controls but not from each other.

Other studies have focused on the specific diagnosis of depression and pain (Magni et al 1984, Walker et al 1988). Higher depression scores and family histories of affective disorder were described in women with chronic pelvic pain without pathology compared to women with chronic pelvic pain and pathology as established by laparoscopy (Magni et al 1984). A comparison of women with pelvic pain of unknown aetiology, IBS and a pain-free control group revealed the pelvic pain group had significantly higher prevalence of major depression, dysthymic disorder, panic disorders, somatization disorder and sexual abuse. Often, the depression preceded the onset of the pain, but no prospective studies have been performed (Magni et al 1984, Walker et al 1988, Mayer & Gebhart 1993).

Studies have also examined the role of sexual abuse as a specific risk factor for chronic pelvic pain. Gross et al (1980) reported a high prevalence (90%) of sexual abuse. Harrop-Griffiths et al (1988) compared a group of women with pelvic pain to a control group of pain-free gynaecological patients and found a higher prevalence of prior substance abuse, dyspareunia, inhibited sexual desire, higher scores on the SCL-90 and a greater prevalence of sexual abuse. A history of childhood sexual abuse and a past history of depression were strongly related to the subsequent persistence of pelvic pain.

Rapkin et al (1990), in a study designed to assess whether sexual or physical abuse was more prevalent, noted the prevalence of childhood sexual abuse did not differ significantly between the three groups: 19% of women with pelvic pain, 16% of women with 'other' pain locations and

12% of control women. There was, however, a significant difference in the prevalence of physical abuse: pelvic pain patients (39%), other pain patients (18%) and controls (9%). This study suggested that abuse of any kind is associated with chronic pain. Abuse may predispose to chronicity of pain because it increases the vulnerability to depression and helplessness in the face of adversity (Abramson et al 1978). Toomey et al (1993) reaffirmed the importance of obtaining sexual and physical abuse histories in chronic pelvic pain patients.

Renaer (1980) has suggested the diagnosis 'chronic pelvic pain without obvious pathology' for patients who lack somatic pathology. Often, these patients have been considered to have psychogenic pain. As noted in the previous discussion, the majority of patients with chronic pain have abnormal psychogenic profiles. Patients without pathology do not appear to be psychologically different from those with 'organic' disease. The role of as yet unknown neurophysiologic mechanisms within the brain and spinal cord in the maintenance of chronic pain cannot be overestimated (Rapkin 1995). Trigger points, nerve entrapment, pelvic congestion syndrome, pelvic pain without pathology or with pathology such as endometriosis or adhesions which fail to respond to exterpative therapy, irritable bowel syndrome and interstitial cystitis represent the most common sources of chronic pelvic pain, all of which probably entail alterations of central processing. The stimulus for these alterations and mechanisms, underlying maintenance of changes in central processing without an inflammatory stimulus or nerve damage, is unknown. Wall (1988) has suggested that it is 'necessary to consider the lability of central transmission pathways as well as seeking peripheral pathology in all painful conditions'. It is reasonable, therefore, to suggest that chronic pelvic pain without, or even with, 'pathology' is likely to involve all levels of the neuroaxis and to direct management approaches accordingly.

DIAGNOSIS AND MANAGEMENT OF CHRONIC PELVIC PAIN

Successful diagnosis and management of patients with chronic pelvic pain, as with other chronic pain conditions, requires a meticulous yet compassionate, multidisciplinary approach. A thorough history should be obtained. The nature of the pain, location and radiation, aggravating and alleviating factors, timing, effect of menses, exercise, work, stress, intercourse and orgasm should be queried. Ascertain the context in which the pain arose and is maintained, including previous episodes of pain, inability to perform family role or occupation, litigation or worker's compensation. Other somatic symptoms should be noted: genital tract (abnormal vaginal bleeding, discharge, Mittelschmerz, dysmenorrhoea, dyspareunia, infertility), enterocolic (constipation, diarrhoea, flatulence, tenesmus, blood, changes in colour or calibre of stool), musculoskeletal (predominant low back distribution, pain radiation, association with injury, fatigue, postural changes), urologic (dysuria, urgency, frequency, suprapelvic pain). Historical questions specific to all the peripheral pathologies noted in Box 28.1 should be queried. Past history including medical, surgical, gynaecologic, obstetric, medication intake and prior evaluations for the pain should be documented. Operative and pathology reports are important if the patient has had surgery.

Current and past psychological history, including psychosocial factors, history of past (or current) physical, sexual and/or emotional abuse, history of hospitalization, suicide attempts and chemical (drug or alcohol) dependency, should be elicited. The attitude of the patient and her family toward the pain, resultant behaviour of the patient's family with respect to the pain and current upheavals in the patient's life should be discussed. The part of the history addressing sensitive issues may have to be reobtained after establishing rapport with the patient.

Symptoms of an acute process such as fever, anorexia, nausea, emesis, significant diarrhoea or recurrent constipation, ascites, uterine bleeding, pregnancy or recent abortion should alert one to the possibility of an acute condition requiring immediate medical or surgical intervention, especially if accompanied by orthostasis, peritoneal signs, pelvic or abdominal mass, abnormal CBC, positive genital or urinary tract cultures or a positive pregnancy test.

One should perform a complete physical examination, with particular attention to the abdominal, back, vaginal, urethrovesicle, bimanual, rectovaginal and pelvic floor muscle examination. The exam should include evaluation of the abdomen with the straight leg-raising manoeuvre to discern abdominal wall sources of pain. Abdominal wall pain is augmented and visceral pain is diminished with the above manoeuvres (Slocumb 1984, 1990). The patient should be examined while standing for hernias, abdominal (inguinal, femoral and Spigelian) and pelvic (cystocoele, rectocele, enterocoele). An attempt should be made to reproduce the patient's pain by fingertip palpation of the tissues (abdominal, pelvic, external genital and lower back). The appearance, support and tenderness of the bladder, urethra and rectum should be determined. A neurologic examination of the lower extrem-

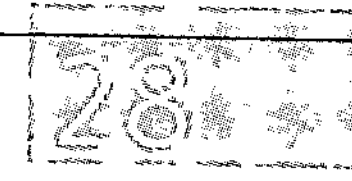

ities and perineum can aid the assessment of S3–5 and L2–4 nerve roots. Vaginal oestrogenization should also be determined when visualizing the vaginal epithelium. The patient should be evaluated by, or in concert with, a gynaecologist.

Laboratory studies, if not already performed, include CBC, ESR, urinalysis and culture, cervical and urethral cultures (gonorrhoea and chlamydia), wet mount of vaginal secretions, Pap smear, stool guaiac and, if diarrhoea is present, stool culture. If the pelvic or abdominal examination is inadequate or suggestive of a mass, ultrasound or MRI evaluation is indicated. If symptoms and signs are suggestive of other system involvement, fibreoptic or other appropriate imaging studies of other organ systems should be considered.

A daily pain diary to note the occurrence and intensity of pain and mood should be undertaken. Medication intake, menses, aggravating and alleviating factors should be noted in the diary. A simple diary utilizes a visual analogue scale from 1 (no pain) to 10 (most severe pain ever). The diary should be maintained for at least 2 months.

The patient should be evaluated by a psychologist familiar with the management of chronic pain. The psychologist should preferably be located within the same clinic suite. Psychological referral accomplishes evaluation and also provides the opportunity for introducing stress reduction, relaxation and behavioural therapies. The assessment should be designed to evaluate the pain complaint, its impact on life circumstances, controlling factors and coping mechanisms. Assessment in the context of chronic pain involves a broad range of measures, reflecting biological, social and psychological influences and sequelae.

Pelvic pain is likely to affect sexual functioning, which may have additional repercussions in terms of mood and quality of relationships and self-esteem. A careful history is needed to establish whether the sexual problems existed before the pain or developed subsequently. Previous or current physical abuse, sexual abuse or trauma should be evaluated. The impact of the pain on day-to-day functioning should be determined. Standardized psychological testing is helpful to determine if affective disturbance is present, as well as to establish a baseline against which to measure treatment response and guide treatment approaches.

If specific pathology is confirmed, management should proceed (see Box 28.1). Patients with cyclic or atypical cyclic pain based on evaluation of the pain diary should be evaluated and treated for primary or secondary dysmenorrhoea. Consultation with a urologist, gastroenterologist, orthopaedist or neurologist should be requested if indicated.

Evaluation of pelvic pain, especially cyclic pain, may require a diagnostic laparoscopy. Pelvic ultrasound, MRI or transuterine venography, if available, may be indicated if pelvic congestion is suspected but treatment can proceed on the basis of clinical suspicion. If trigger points were injected and pain has persisted, injection should be repeated weekly or biweekly for up to five injections and consideration should be given to a physical therapy consultation, especially if activity increases the pain or if low back pain is prominent. Pharmacologic management of CPP mirrors that of chronic pain in general (see Chs. 48–53). Tricyclic antidepressants and anticonvulsants have been used successfully in pelvic pain patients although controlled studies are lacking. Narcotics administered appropriately and with a narcotic contract are useful in the control of pelvic pain. Depression is treated with selective serotonin reuptake inhibitors. The patient should continue to have scheduled visits with the gynaecologist on a regular basis.

SURGICAL MANAGEMENT OF CHRONIC PELVIC PAIN

Only rarely is the surgical management of CPP studied in a randomized controlled trial. Postoperative follow-up is often less than 6 months and pain measurement scales are generally not adequate.

DIAGNOSTIC LAPAROSCOPY

Diagnostic laparoscopy has become a standard procedure in the evaluation of patients with chronic pelvic pain. Although exceedingly useful in the diagnosis and management of acute pelvic pain, the role of the laparoscope in the management of chronic pelvic pain has been controversial. Fourteen to 77% of patients have no obvious pathology and two-thirds of patients have findings of adhesions which may or not play a role in their pain (Stout et al 1991, Reese et al 1996). Furthermore, non-surgical management of chronic pelvic pain is successful in 65–90% of patients regardless of presence of 'pathology' (Slocumb 1984, Rapkin & Kames 1987, Peters et al 1991, Reiter et al 1991). Peters et al (1991) randomized women with chronic pelvic pain to two different management approaches: a standard approach group in which laparoscopy was routinely performed and results guided by findings (n = 49) and an integrated approach group with attention to somatic, psychological, dietary and physiotherapeutic factors, laparoscopy not routinely performed (n = 57). Of the 49 patients in the standard group, 65% had no abnormality, 5% had endometriosis, 18% had adhesions and the remainder myomata, ovarian cysts or pelvic varices. The integrated approach was significantly more effective in the reduction of pelvic pain (75% vs 41%; $P < 0.01$).

Laparoscopy is helpful to provide reassurance and in the surgical management of adhesions and endometriosis but should probably be reserved for patients in whom other non-gynaecologic pathology has been ruled out or those with signs and/or symptoms of endometriosis, cyclic pelvic pain or infertility (Baker & Symonds 1992, Reese et al 1996). Additional randomized controlled trials are needed.

HYSTERECTOMY

Nineteen per cent of hysterectomies are performed for the sole indication of chronic pelvic pain (Howard 1993). However, 30% of patients presenting to pelvic pain clinics have already undergone hysterectomy without experiencing relief of pain (Reiter 1990a). Reiter et al (1991) noted a decline in the incidence of hysterectomy for the indication of chronic pelvic pain from 16.3% to 5.8% after the initiation of a multidisciplinary approach to the diagnosis and treatment of chronic pelvic pain. Patients with cyclic pain or dysfunctional uterine bleeding are excellent candidates for hysterectomy, especially if they have relief of pain with hormonal suppression. A prospective cohort study, the Maine Women's Health Study, revealed that 18% of women had undergone hysterectomy for the indication of chronic pelvic pain. Significant improvement in pain and associated symptoms was noted in 95% of the women. The underlying diagnoses, and whether pain was cyclic, were not described (Carlson et al 1994a,b). In a retrospective study of 99 women with CPP felt to be of 'uterine' origin (i.e. associated with uterine tenderness), 77% had relief but 25% experienced persistent or worsening pain at the time of the 1-year follow-up (Storall èt al 1990). Hillis et al (1995) similarly noted a 74% response rate for hysterectomy. Persistent pain was associated with multiparity, prior history of PID, lack of pathology and Medicare payer status. Hysterectomy remains an option for appropriately selected patients with pain of 'uterine' origin (Hillis et al 1995).

PRESACRAL NEURECTOMY

Presacral neurectomy or sympathectomy (PSN) was first described for the indication of dysmenorrhoea (Cotte 1937). The presacral nerve, which is actually the superior hypogastric plexus, receives the major afferent supply from the cervix, uterus and proximal fallopian tubes. Afferents travelling with the sympathetic nerve supply from the bladder and rectum also pass through the superior hypogastric plexus but normal micturition and defaecation are dependent on an intact sacral autonomic nerve supply and are relatively unaffected by resection of the superior hypogastric plexus. Afferents from the adnexal structures travel with sympathetic fibres accompanying the spinal cord at T9–10 and therefore, lateralizing pain of visceral origin will not be relieved by PSN.

PSN has not been studied in a controlled fashion, but has been described for the management of central pelvic pain in the setting of both cyclic (dysmenorrhoea) and non-cyclic pain (Ingersoll & Meigs 1948, Polan & DeCherney 1980, Vercellini et al 1991, Candiani et al 1992). In one study, only 26% of women experienced relief of pain with resection of endometriosis alone as compared with 75% of patients who also underwent PSN (Polan & DeCherney 1980). The surgery is technically difficult to perform via laparoscopy (Chen & Soong 1997). Complications of haemorrhage and ureteral injury are not uncommon, even during laparotomy. The LUNA procedure or laparoscopic transection of the uterosacral ligaments, and thus uterine afferents, has been subjected to only one randomized controlled trial (Lichten & Bombard 1987). Eighty-one per cent had relief with LUNA but the improvement at the 1-year follow-up was only significant in 45% of the 10 subjects. None of the controls improved, however (Lichten & Bombard 1987).

MULTIDISCIPLINARY PAIN MANAGEMENT

Multidisciplinary pain management is an excellent approach to chronic pelvic pain. The team usually includes a gynaecologist or internist as pain manager, psychologist and often a physical therapist, anaesthesiologist and dietitian. Non-steroidal anti-inflammatory medications, narcotics, tricyclic antidepressants, gabaergics and trigger point injections and nerve blocks (i.e. pudendal, ilioinguinal, iliohypogastric, genitofemoral and occasionally hypogastric) are utilized.

One programme utilizing cognitive-behavioural therapy, acupuncture and tricyclic antidepressants was successful in reducing pain by at least 50% in 85% of the subjects (Rapkin & Kames 1987, Kames et al 1990). Other studies have suggested that similar results may be obtained with a multidisciplinary team (Gambone & Reiter 1990, Wood et al 1990, Peters et al 1991, Reiter et al 1991, Milburn et al 1993). In a prospective randomized, controlled study, the multidisciplinary approach combining traditional gynaecologic treatment, psychological, dietary and physical therapy input was found to be more effective than traditional gynaecologic (medical and surgical) management or cure (Peters et al 1991).

REFERENCES

Abramson LY, Seligman MEP, Teasdale JD 1978 Learned helplessness in humans: critique and reformation. Abnormal Psychology 87: 49–74

American College of Obstetricians and Gynecologists 1983 Dysmenorrhea. ACOG, Washington DC Technical Bulletin 68

Baker PK 1993 Musculoskeletal origins of chronic pelvic pain. In: Ling FW (ed) Obstetrics and gynecology clinics of North America: contemporary management of chronic pain. WB Saunders, Philadelphia, pp 719–742

Baker PN, Symonds MD 1992 The resolution of chronic pelvic pain after normal laparoscopy findings. American Journal of Obstetrics and Gynecology 166: 835–836

Beard RW, Highman JH, Pearce S, Reginald PW 1984 Diagnosis of pelvic varicosities in women with chronic pelvic pain. Lancet 2: 946–949

Beard RW, Kennedy RG, Gangar KF et al 1991 Bilateral oophorectomy and hysterectomy in the treatment of intractable pelvic pain associated with pelvic congestion. British Journal of Obstetrics and Gynaecology 98: 988–992

Beard RW, Reginald PW, Wadsworth J 1988 Clinical features of women with chronic lower abdominal pain and pelvic congestion. British Journal of Obstetrics and Gynaecology 95: 153–161

Bergman A, Karram M, Bhatia NN 1989 Urethral syndrome: a comparison of different treatment modalities. Journal of Reproductive Medicine 34: 157–160

Berkley KJ 1994 Communications from the uterus (and other tissues). In: Besson JM (ed) Pharmacological aspects of peripheral neurons involved in nociception, pain research and clinical management. Elsevier, Amsterdam, pp 39–47

Berkley KJ, Hubscher CH 1995 Visceral and somatic sensory tracks through the neuraxis and their relation to pain: lessons from the rat female reproductive system. In: Gebhart GF (ed) Visceral pain: progress in pain research and management, vol. 5. IASP Press, Seattle, pp 195–216

Berkley KJ, Robbins A, Sato Y 1988 Afferent fibers supplying the uterus in the rat. Journal of Neurophysiology 59: 142–163

Candiani GB, Fedele L, Vercellini P, Bianchi S, Di Nola G 1992 Presacral neurectomy for the treatment of pelvic pain associated with endometriosis: a controlled study. American Journal of Obstetrics and Gynecology 167: 100–103

Carey MP, Slack MC 1996 GnRH analogue in assessing chronic pelvic pain in women with residual ovaries. British Journal of Obstetrics and Gynaecology 103: 150–153

Carlson KJ, Miller BA, Fowler FJ Jr 1994a The Maine women's health study: I. outcomes of hysterectomy. Obstetrics and Gynecology 83: 557–565

Carlson KJ, Miller BA, Fowler FJ Jr 1994b The Maine women's health study: II. outcomes of nonsurgical management of leiomyomas, abnormal bleeding, and chronic pelvic pain. Obstetrics and Gynecology 83: 566–572

Castelnuova-Tedesco P, Krout BM 1970 Psychosomatic aspects of chronic pelvic pain. Psychiatric Medicine 1: 109–126

Cervero F 1994 Sensory innervation of the viscera: peripheral basis of visceral pain. Physiological Reviews 74: 95–138

Cervero F, Tattersall JEH 1986 Somatic and visceral sensory integration in the thoracic spinal cord. In: Cervero F, Morrison J (eds) Visceral sensation. Elsevier, New York, pp 189–205

Chan CLK, Wood C 1985 Pelvic adhesiolysis: the assessment of symptom relief by 100 patients. Australian and New Zealand Journal of Obstetrics and Gynaecology 25: 295–298

Chan WY, Dawood MY 1980 Prostaglandin levels in menstrual fluid of non-dysmenorrheic and of dysmenorrheic subjects with and without oral contraceptive or ibuprofen therapy. Advances in Prostaglandin, Thromboxane and Leukotriene Research 8: 1443–1447

Chatman DL, Ward AB 1982 Endometriosis in adolescents. Obstetrics and Gynecology 27: 186–190

Chen F-P, Soong Y-K 1997 The efficacy and complications of laparoscopic presacral neurectomy in pelvic pain. Obstetrics and Gynecology 90: 974–977

Cornillie FJ, Oosterlynck D, Lauweryns JM et al 1990 Deeply infiltrating pelvic endometriosis: histology and clinical significance. Fertility and Sterility 53: 978–983

Cotte G 1937 Resection of the presacral nerves in the treatment of obstinate dysmenorrhea. American Journal of Obstetrics and Gynaecology 33: 1034–1040

D'Hooghe TM, Hill JA 1996 Endometriosis. In: Berek JS, Adashi EY, Hillard PA (eds) Novak's gynecology, 12th edn. Williams & Wilkins, Baltimore, pp 887–914

Daniell JP 1989 Laparoscopic enterolysis for chronic abdominal pain. Journal of Gynecological Surgery 5: 61–66

De Groat WC 1994 Neurophysiology of the pelvic organs. In: Rushton DN (ed) Handbook of neuro-urology. Marcel Dekker, New York, pp 55–93

Doyle IB 1955 Paracervical uterine denervation by transection of the cervical plexus for the relief of dysmenorrhea. American Journal of Obstetrics and Gynecology 70: 1–16

Drossman DA, Thompson WG 1992 The irritable bowel syndrome: review and a graduated multicomponent treatment approach. Annals of Internal Medicine 116: 1009–1016

Farquhar CM, Rogers V, Franks S, Pearce S, Wadsworth J, Bland RW 1989 A randomized controlled trial of medroxyprogesterone acetate and psychotherapy for the treatment of pelvic congestion. British Journal of Obstetrics and Gynaecology 96: 1153–1162

Fayez JA, Clark RR 1994 Operative laparoscopy for the treatment of localized chronic pelvic-abdominal pain caused by postoperative adhesions. Journal of Gynecological Surgery 10: 79–83

Fields H 1987 Pain. McGraw-Hill, New York, p 41

Fukaya T, Hoshiai H, Yajima A 1993 Is pelvic endometriosis always associated with chronic pain? A retrospective study of 618 cases diagnosed by laparoscopy. American Journal of Obstetrics and Gynecology 169: 719–722

Gambone JC, Reiter RC 1990 Nonsurgical management of chronic pelvic pain: a multidisciplinary approach. Clinical Obstetrics and Gynecology 33: 205–211

Gangar KV, Stones RW, Saunders D et al 1993 An alternative to hysterectomy? GnRH analogue combined with hormone replacement therapy. British Journal of Obstetrics and Gynaecology 100: 360–364

Giamberardino MA, Berkley KJ, Iezzi S, di Bigotina P, Vecchiet L 1997 Pain threshold variations in somatic wall tissues as a function of menstrual cycle. Segmented site and tissue depth in non-dysmenorrheic women, dysmenorrheic women and men. Pain 71: 187–197

Gillenwater JY, Wein AJ 1988 Summary of the National Institute of Arthritis, Diabetes, Digestive and Kidney Diseases Workshop on interstitial cystitis. National Institutes of Health, Bethesda, MD, August 28–29. Journal of Urology 140: 203–206

Gross RJ, Doerr H, Caldirola D, Guzinski G, Ripley H 1980 Borderline syndrome and incest in chronic pelvic pain patients. International Journal of Psychiatric Medicine 10: 79–96

Hahn L 1989 Clinical findings and results of operative treatment in ilioinguinal nerve entrapment syndrome. British Journal of Obstetrics and Gynaecology 96: 1080–1083

Hammeroff SR, Carlson GL, Brown BR 1981 Ilioinguinal pain syndrome. Pain 10: 253–257

Harrop-Griffiths J, Katon W, Walker E, Helm L, Russo J, Hickok C 1988 The association between chronic pelvic pain, psychiatric diagnoses and childhood sexual abuse. Obstetrics and Gynecology 71: 589–594

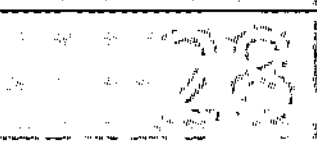

Helms JM 1987 Acupuncture for the management of primary dysmenorrhea. Obstetrics and Gynecology 69: 51–56

Hightower NC, Roberts JW 1981 Acute and chronic lower abdominal pain of enterologic origin in chronic pelvic pain. In: Renaer MR (ed) Chronic pelvic pain in women. Springer-Verlag, New York, pp 110–137

Hillis SD, Marchbanks PA, Peterson HB 1995 The effectiveness of hysterectomy for chronic pelvic pain. Obstetrics and Gynecology 86: 941–945

Howard FM 1993 The role of laparoscopy in chronic pelvic pain: promise and pitfalls. Obstetrical and Gynecological Survey 48(6): 357–387

Hughes JM 1990 Psychological aspects of pelvic pain. In: Rocker I (ed) Pelvic pain in women. Diagnosis and management. Springer-Verlag, London, pp 13–20

Ingersoll FM, Meigs JV 1948 Presacral neurectomy for dysmenorrhea. New England Journal of Medicine 238: 357–360

Kames LD, Rapkin AJ, Naliboff BD, Afifi S, Ferrer-Brechner T 1990 Effectiveness of an interdisciplinary pain management program for the treatment of chronic pelvic pain. Pain 41: 41–46

Karram MM 1993 Frequency, urgency, and painful bladder syndrome. In: Walters MD, Karram MM (eds) Clinical Urogynecology. CV Mosby, St Louis, pp 285–298

Koninckx PR, Meuleman C, Demeyere S, Lesaffre E, Cornillie FJ 1991 Suggestive evidence that pelvic endometriosis is a progressive disease, whereas deeply infiltrating endometriosis is associated with pelvic pain. Fertility and Sterility 55: 759–770

Kresch AJ, Seifer DB, Sachs LB, Barrese I 1984 Laparoscopy in 100 women with chronic pelvic pain. Obstetrics and Gynecology 64: 672–674

Kumazawa T 1986 Sensory innervation of reproductive organs. In: Cervero F, Morrison J (eds) Visceral sensation. Elsevier, New York, pp 115–131

Lee AW, Bell RM, Griffen WO Jr, Hagihara P 1985 Recurrent appendiceal colic. Surgery Gynecology and Obstetrics 161: 21–24

Lichten EM, Bombard J 1987 Surgical treatment of primary dysmenorrhea with laparoscopic uterine nerve ablation. Journal of Reproductive Medicine 32: 37–41

Liston WA, Bradford WP, Downie J, Kerr MG 1972 Laparoscopy in a general gynecologic unit. American Journal of Obstetrics and Gynecology 113: 672–677

Lundberg WI, Wall JE, Mathers JE 1973 Laparoscopy in the evaluation of pelvic pain. Obstetrics and Gynecology 42: 872–876

MacDonald JS 1993 Management of chronic pain. In: Ling FW (ed) Obstetrics and gynecology clinics of North America: contemporary management of chronic pain. WB Saunders, Philadelphia, pp 817–839

Magni G, Salmi A, deLeo D, Ceola A 1984 Chronic pelvic pain and depression. Psychopathology 17: 132–136

Malinak LR 1980 Operative management of pelvic pain. Clinical Obstetrics and Gynecology 23: 191–199

Mannheimer JS, Whaler EC 1985 The efficacy of transcutaneous electrical nerve stimulation in dysmenorrhea. Clinical Journal of Pain 1: 75–83

Martin DC, Hubert GD, VanderZwaag R 1989 Laparoscopic appearances of peritoneal endometriosis. Fertility and Sterility 51: 63

Mayer EA, Gebhart GF 1993 Functional bowel disorders and the visceral hyperalgesia hypothesis. In: Mayer EA, Raybould HE (eds) Pain research and clinical management, vol 9. Elsevier, Amsterdam, pp 3–28

Medical Letter 1979 Drugs for dysmenorrhea. Medical Letter on Drugs and Therapeutics 21: 81–84

Milburn A, Reiter RC, Rhomberg AT 1993 Multidisciplinary approach to chronic pelvic pain. In: Ling FW (ed) Obstetrics and gynecology clinics of North America: contemporary management of chronic pelvic pain. WB Saunders, Philadelphia, pp 643–661

Morscher E. 1981 Low back pain in women. In: Renaer MR (ed) Chronic pelvic pain in women. Springer-Verlag, New York, pp 137–154

Peters AA, Van Dorst E, Jellis B, Van Zuuren E, Hermans J, Trimbos JB 1991 A randomized clinical trial to compare two different approaches in women with chronic pelvic pain. Obstetrics and Gynecology 77: 740–744

Peters AAW, Trimbos-Kemper GCM, Admiraal C, Trimbos JB 1992 A randomized clinical trial on the benefit of adhesiolysis in patients with intraperitoneal adhesions and chronic pelvic pain. British Journal of Obstetrics and Gynaecology 99: 59–62

Pettit PD, Lee RA 1988 Ovarian remnant syndrome: diagnostic dilemma and surgical challenge. Obstetrics and Gynecology 71: 580–583

Polan ML, DeCherney A 1980 Presacral neurectomy for pelvic pain in infertility. Fertility and Sterility 34: 557–560

Price FV, Edwards R, Buchsbaum HJ 1990 Ovarian remnant syndrome: difficulties in diagnosis and management. Obstetrical and Gynecological Surgery 45: 151–156

Procacci P, Zoppi M, Maresen M 1986 Clinical approach to visceral sensation. In: Cervero F, Morrison J (eds) Visceral sensation. Elsevier, New York, pp 21–36

Rapkin AJ 1986 Adhesions and pelvic pain: a retrospective study. Obstetrics and Gynecology 68: 13–15

Rapkin AJ 1995 Gynecological pain in the clinic: is there a link with the basic research? In: Gebhart GF (ed) Visceral pain: progress in pain research and management. IASP Press, Seattle, pp 469–488

Rapkin AJ Kames LD 1987 The pain management approach to chronic pelvic pain. Journal of Reproductive Medicine 32: 323–327

Rapkin AJ, Kames LD, Darke LL 1990 History of physical and sexual abuse in women with chronic pelvic pain. Obstetrics and Gynecology 76: 90–96

Rapkin AJ, Mayer EA 1993 Gastroenterologic causes of chronic pelvic pain. In: Ling FW (ed) Obstetrics and gynecology clinics of North America: contemporary management of chronic pain. WB Saunders, Philadelphia, pp 663–684

Rapkin AJ, Rasgon NL, Berkley KJ 1997 Dysmenorrhea. In: Yaksh TL et al (eds) Anesthesia: biologic foundations. Lippincott-Raven, Philadelphia, pp 785–793

Rapkin AJ, Reading AE 1991 Chronic pelvic pain. Current Problems in Obstetrics, Gynecology and Fertility XIV: 102–137

Reese KA, Reddy S, Rock JA 1996 Endometriosis in an adolescent population: the Emory experience. Journal of Pediatric and Adolescent Gynecology 9: 125–128

Reiter RC 1990a A profile of women with chronic pelvic pain. Clinical Obstetrics and Gynecology 33: 130–136

Reiter RC 1990b Occult somatic pathology in women with chronic pelvic pain. Clinical Obstetrics and Gynecology 33: 154–160

Reiter RC, Gambone JC, Johnson SR 1991 Availability of a multidisciplinary pelvic pain clinic and frequency of hysterectomy for pelvic pain. Journal of Psychosomatic Obstetrics and Gynaecology 12(suppl): 109

Renaer M 1980 Chronic pelvic pain without obvious pathology in women: personal observation and a review of the problem. European Journal of Obstetrics and Gynecology 10: 415–463

Renaer M, Vertommen H, Nijs P, Wagemans M, Van Hemelrijk T 1979 Psychosocial aspects of chronic pelvic pain in women. American Journal of Obstetrics and Gynecology 134: 75–80

Robbins A, Berkley KJ, Sato Y 1992 Estrous cycle variation of afferent fibers supplying reproductive organs in the female rat. Brain Research 596: 353–356

Saravelos HG, Li T-C, Cooke ID 1995 An analysis of the outcome of microsurgical and laparoscopic adhesiolysis for chronic pelvic pain. Human Reproduction 10: 2895–2901

Sichlau MJ, Yao JST, Vogelzang RL 1994 Transcatheter embolotherapy for the treatment of pelvic congestion syndrome. Obstetrics and Gynecology 83: 892–896

Siddall-Allum J, Rae T, Rogers V, Witherow R, Flanagan A, Beard RW

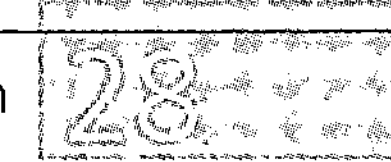

1994 Chronic pain caused by residual ovaries and ovarian remnants. British Journal of Obstetrics and Gynaecology 101: 979–985

Sippo WC, Burghardt A, Gomez AC 1987 Nerve entrapment after pfannensteil incision. American Journal of Obstetrics and Gynecology 157: 420–421

Slocumb JC 1984 Neurological factors in chronic pelvic pain: trigger points and the abdominal pelvic pain syndrome. American Journal of Obstetrics and Gynecology 149: 536–543

Slocumb JC 1990 Chronic somatic myofascial and neurogenic abdominal pelvic pain. In: Porreco RP, Reiter RC (eds) Clinical obstetrics and gynecology. JB Lippincott, Philadelphia, pp 145–153

Smith RP 1993 Cyclic pelvic pain and dysmenorrhea. In: Ling FW (ed) Obstetrics and gynecology clinics of North America: contemporary management of chronic pain. WB Saunders, Philadelphia, pp 753–764

Spangen L 1984 Spigelian hernia. Surgical Clinics of North America 64: 351–366

Steege JF 1987 Ovarian remnant syndrome. Obstetrics and Gynecology 70: 64–67

Steege JF, Scott AL 1991 Resolution of chronic pelvic pain after laparoscopic lysis of adhesions. American Journal of Obstetrics and Gynecology 165: 278–283

Stones RW, Loesch A, Beard RW, Burnstock G 1995 Substance P: endothelial localization and pharmacology in the human ovarian vein. Obstetrics and Gynecology 85: 273–278

Stones RW, Rae T, Rogers V, Fry R, Beard RW 1990 Pelvic congestion in women: evaluation with transvaginal ultrasound and observation of venous pharmacology. British Journal of Radiology 63: 710–711

Stout AL, Steege JF, Dodson WC, Hughes CL 1991 Relationship of laparoscopic findings to self-report of pelvic pain. American Journal of Obstetrics and Gynecology 164: 73–79

Stovall TG, Ling FW, Crawford DA 1990 Hysterectomy for chronic pelvic pain of presumed uterine etiology. Obstetrics and Gynecology 75: 676–679

Summit RL 1993 Urogynecologic causes of chronic pelvic pain. In: Ling FW (ed) Obstetrics and gynecology clinics of North America: contemporary management of chronic pain. WB Saunders, Philadelphia, pp 685–698

Sweet RL, Gibbs RS 1985 Pelvic inflammatory disease. In: Infectious diseases of the female genital tract. Williams & Wilkins, Baltimore, pp 53–77

Taylor HC Jr 1954 Pelvic pain based on a vascular and autonomic nervous system disorder. American Journal of Obstetrics and Gynecology 67: 1177–1196

Thomson H, Francis DMA 1977 Abdominal-wall tenderness: a useful sign in the acute abdomen. Lancet Volume 2 pp1053–1055

Toomey TC, Hernandez JT, Gittelman DF, Hulka JF 1993 Relationship of sexual and physical abuse to pain and psychological assessment variables in chronic pelvic pain patients. Pain 53: 105–109

Travell J 1976 Myofascial trigger points: clinical view. Advances in Pain Research and Therapy 1: 919–926

Vercellini P, Fedele L, Bianchi S, Candiani GB 1991 Pelvic denervation for chronic pain associated with endometriosis: fact or fancy? American Journal of Obstetrics and Gynecology 165(3): 745–749

Walker EA, Katon WJ, Harrop-Griffiths J 1988 Relationship of chronic pelvic pain of psychiatric diagnoses and childhood sexual abuse. American Journal of Psychology 145: 75–80

Walker EA, Gelfand AN, Gelfand MD, Green C, Katon WJ 1996 Chronic pelvic pain and gynecological symptoms in women with irritable bowel syndrome. Journal of Psychosomatic Obstetrics and Gynecology 17(1): 39–46

Walker EA, Katon WJ, Alfrey H, Bowers M, Stenchever MA et al 1991 The prevalence of chronic pain and irritable bowel syndrome in two university clinics. Journal of Psychosomatic Obstetrics and Gynaecology 12(suppl): 66–69

Wall PD 1988 The John J Bonica distinguished lecture. Stability and instability of central pain mechanisms. In: Dubner R (ed) Proceedings of the Fifth World Congress on Pain. Elsevier, Amsterdam, pp 13–24

Wesselmann U, Lai J 1997 Mechanisms of referred visceral pain: uterine inflammation in the adult virgin rat results in neurogenic plasma extravasation in the skin. Pain 73: 209–317

Wood DP, Weisner MG, Reiter RC 1990 Psychogenic chronic pelvic pain. Clinical Obstetrics and Gynecology 33: 179–195

Obstetric pain

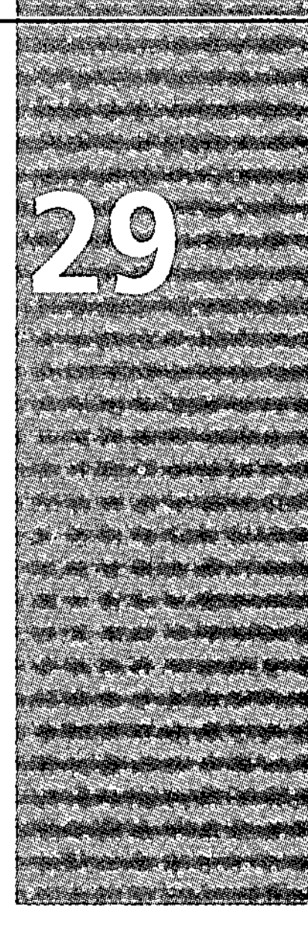

JOHN S. McDONALD

The purpose of this chapter is to give an overview of the nature of pain of childbirth, and its impact on the mother, the fetus and newborn. The chapter is organized under the following headings:

- Introduction.
- Mechanisms and pathways of the pain of childbirth.
- Physiological and psychological effects of labour pain.
- Current methods to relieve childbirth pain.

INTRODUCTION

Fortunately, for both the mother and her baby, effective control of the pain of childbirth continues to be forged today even at the close of the twentieth century (Crawford 1984, Albright et al 1986, Shnider & Levinson 1986, Chestnut 1994, Bonica & McDonald 1995). In past editions of this book, it was pointed out that proponents of natural childbirth believed that labour pain had an important biological function and, therefore, should not be relieved. In addition, others thought that the heavily directed pharmacological methods of pain relief had deleterious effects on the mother and fetus and should be avoided (Dick-Read 1933, 1953, Lamaze 1956). This is mentioned to put into perspective that in the past obstetrics was largely clinically driven by the basics of history, physical and pelvic examination. Now, almost 30 years later, obstetrics has matured considerably and is technology driven with surveillance by both fetal electronic and ultrasonographic methods. In addition, constant improvement of obstetric anaesthesia has occurred over the last 30 years by those fully dedicated to this new discipline.

During the past two decades, there has been a surge of interest in obstetric pain among all those involved in labour and delivery management. These include anaesthetists, obstetricians, paediatricians, neonatologists, labour nurses and the even the lay public. Such widespread interest has promoted an impressive growth in basic and clinical research in perinatology. This has brought forth huge interest and understanding of the physiology and pathophysiology of the mother, fetus and newborn. This research advance has been paralleled by a similar clinical advance with an ever-increasing number of anaesthetists entering the specialty of obstetric anaesthesia. Additionally, two solid interest groups of world-wide stature, the Society of Obstetric Anesthesia and Perinatology (SOAP) in the United States and Canada, and the Obstetric Anaesthesia Association (OAA) in the United Kingdom, have captured the imagination of health care-givers and stirred interest in this challenging subspecialty. As evidence of these solid and separate interests in obstetric anaesthesiology, an impressive number of textbooks, monographs, articles, major journals and other types of communication have been generated nationally and internationally. Labour and delivery is said all over the world to be the most beautiful time in a couple's life, and certainly the more we can do to make this process enjoyable and safe, the more we do to further the science of medicine. The overall protection of the mother and baby must be kept in mind regardless of the method of analgesia chosen. The modern mother wants to have pain relief and wants to be in touch with herself, her environment and, most of all, her baby. In addition and paramount above all, she wants to be in control while assuring safety is maintained for her unborn baby.

Pain is the single most predominant sentinel of the beginning of labour. It is well appreciated that the maturation of the cervix by effacement and dilatation prior to the onset of labour is painless and very effective as a physiological process to set the stage for the eventual onset of labour (Huszar et al 1986). The modern theory of pain management in labour and delivery points out that pain should and must be relieved effectively, as persistent severe pain and its stress generate harmful effects for the mother and, possibly, the fetus. Many notable anaesthetists have paved the way for a better understanding and designed the concept of regional pain relief to offer the parturient a pleasant and respectable labour and delivery. A few of the early giants would include Cleland, Hingson and Bonica, who all pushed hard for cross education of the obstetrician and anaesthetist by a thorough understanding by both groups of the many complex issues of childbirth pain. Even though today it is acknowledged that improperly administered analgesia can result in serious complications and even maternal and perinatal morbidity and mortality, there is impressive clinical evidence that *properly* administered analgesia actually reduces maternal and perinatal mortality and morbidity (Crawford 1984, Albright et al 1986, Shnider & Levinson 1986, Gabbe & Steven 1991, Bonica & McDonald 1995).

There have been many inaccurate and confusing notions about the nature of the pain of parturition over the centuries. Most of these have been perpetrated by those who have no concept of the pain endured. As early as 1844 Lee noted that labour was a 'painless process' (Lee 1844). Even in the early 1900s, Behan stated clearly in his classic book of that time that childbirth should be a painless process just like menstruation. Further, with the advancement of human cultures there has been development pain in labour because in primitive women labour pain is non-existent (Behan 1914). By around the 1930s a similar voice was heard in support of this same erroneous thesis by Dick-Read (1953). It is important to recall that this individual was an evangelist who spent much of his time condemning pharmacological pain relief methods and supported only 'natural childbirth'. The modern psychoprophylactic method now popular in some parts of the USA really grew from a modification of the natural childbirth method of Dick-Read. Psychoprophylaxis, popular in the then USSR, was spread throughout Europe in the name of its French hero who locally modified the harsh natural childbirth method and coined his own name 'Lamaze' (1956). The claim of painless childbirth is now said to be a well-accepted myth because of several studies that dispute its existence (Freedman & Ferguson 1950, Ford).

Present-day obstetricians have adopted a much more conservative attitude regarding maternal medication. There is an acute awareness of the fact that drugs administered to mothers can have fetal and neonatal depressant effects. Furthermore, mothers are by far more appreciative of a lucid, coherent participation in their childbirth experience (Lamaze & Vellay 1952, Atlee 1956). Modifications and improvements in analgesic techniques have been substantial, and communication and coordination between the specialities have been gratifying. Today, the obstetric scenario is highly stable and effective, and in which patients receive not only antepartum evaluation and consultation, but also careful consideration and management augmented by monitoring during the intrapartum period. The most sensitive index of the proficiency of such a system of care is the perinatal mortality rate, which is now at its lowest level in the history of the USA. The early pioneering work of Dr John Bonica boasted records on some 2700 parturients, which confirmed 65% had moderate to severe pain in labour (Scott-Palmer & Skevington 1981). Much of that work came from personal observation or interviews and was not standardized. However, subsequent systematic epidemiological work using the McGill Pain Questionnaire essentially confirmed Dr Bonica's work. Melzack determined about 65–68% of primiparas and multiparas rated their labour pain as severe or very severe in nature; moreover, 23% of primiparas and 11% of multiparas rated their pain as 'horrible' (Melzack 1984). Finally, highly developed countries now cognizant of the benefits of modern analgesia because of physician lectures, the news media and other sources, fully expect effective pain relief throughout their labour and delivery.

MECHANISMS AND PATHWAYS OF THE PAIN OF CHILDBIRTH

The mechanisms and pathways of the pain of childbirth are outlined here to provide an understanding and foundation upon which to build the logical application of pain relief in labour. The innervation of the reproductive organs can be divided into five general sections: (i) uterus; (ii) lower uterine segment; (iii) cervix; (iv) vagina, and (v) perineum.

The uterus and lower uterine segment is innervated by afferents with cell bodies in the dorsal root ganglia of the T10–T12 and L1 segments. Afferent pathways course alongside the sympathetic nerves that make up the pelvic plexus and cervical plexus. Eventually these afferents from the four aforementioned segments move through the three hypogastric pelvic plexi (inferior, medial and superior). Lastly, they make the transition up the lumbar sympathetic chain, and finally to the thoracic sympathetic chain where they eventually exit by the individual rami communicants of

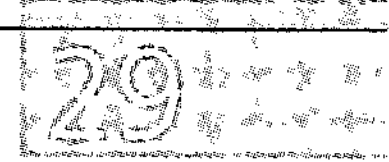

the lower thoracic and upper lumbar roots. Refer to Figure 29.1 for an appreciation of the complexity of the transitional and eventual CNS linkage of the nociceptive process of labour.

The Aδ and C primary afferent nerves that supply the uterus and cervix accompany the sympathetic nerves in the following sequence: the uterine and cervical plexus, the pelvic (inferior hypogastric plexus, the middle hypogastric plexus or nerve, and the superior hypogastric) and aortic plexuses. The nociceptive afferents then pass to the lumbar sympathetic chain and course cephalad through the lower thoracic sympathetic chain, which they leave by way of the rami communicants associated with the T10, T11, T12 and L1 spinal nerves. Finally they pass through the posterior roots of these nerves to make synaptic contact with interneurons in the dorsal horn. Typical of pain arising from the viscera, the pain caused by uterine contractions is referred to the dermatomes supplied by the same spinal cord segments which receive input from the uterus and cervix (Fig. 29.2).

The lower uterine segments and the cervix are innervated by afferents that traverse though the sympathetic plexi just noted above. The initial classical report was by Head in 1893. Cleland supported this original work by his innovative research in 1949. The problem is Cleland argued that the cervix and lower uterine segments were innervated by pelvic nerve afferents (nervi erigentes). However, studies by Bonica utilizing human regional nerve blocks substantiated that cervical innervation travels the T10–T12 pathways with the innervation of the uterus and not via the sacral plexus, S2–S4 (Bonica 1969).

Innervation of the perineum, however, is in another separate location. For this innervation pathway we must proceed on to the sacral nerve roots and then on directly to the

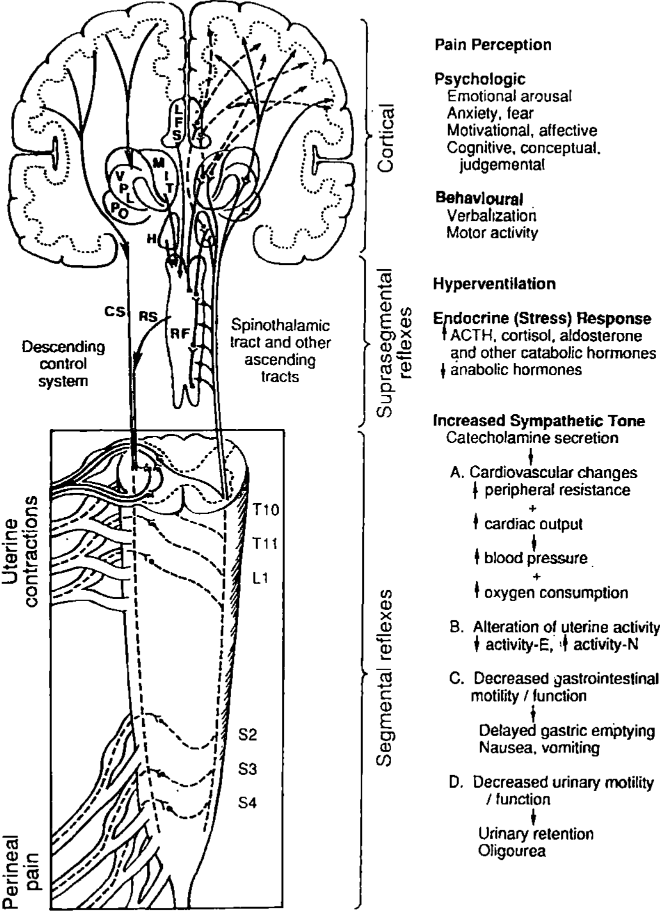

Fig. 29.1 Schematic depiction of the nociceptive input to the spinal cord, provoked by uterine contractions throughout labour and stimulation of the perineum during the second and third stages of labour. The spinothalamic tract and other ascending tracts in the neuraxis are primarily involved in central transmission of nociceptive information to the anterior and anterolateral horn cells of the spinal cord, which provoke segmental reflex responses and impulses that reach the brainstem provoking the suprasegmental responses listed on the right. The nociceptive impulses that reach the brain provoke the cortical responses that include perception of pain, initiation of psychological mechanisms and behavioural responses. On the left is a simple schematic illustration of descending pathways that convey modulating influence from the brain to the spinal cord. RF = reticular formation; RS = reticulospinal; CS = corticospinal; H = hypothalamus; PO = posterior thalamus; VPL = ventral posterolateral thalamus; MIT = medial and intralaminar thalamic nuclei; LFS = limbic forebrain structures. (Modified from Bonica 1990.)

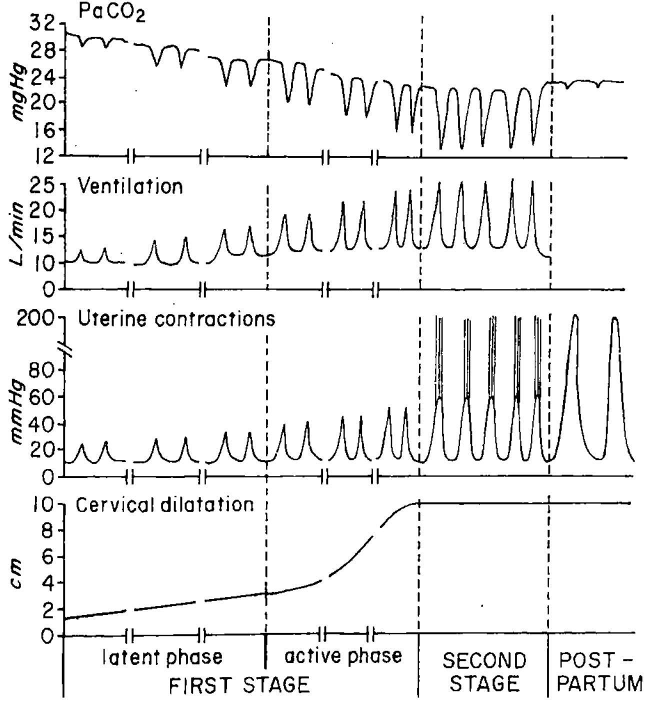

Fig. 29.2 The intensity and distribution of parturition pain during the various phase of labour and delivery. **A** anterior view; **B** lateral view; **C** posterior view. (Reproduced from Bonica 1980.)

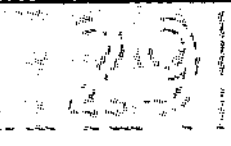

spinal dorsal horn via the pudendal nerves. There are some mixed areas of overlap in the vagina with over 70% of the afferents from the uterine-cervical area linking up with the inferior hypogastric plexus of nerves on each side of the cervix, while the remainder of the afferents from the vagina and lower genital tract link up to the pudendal nerve. Innervation of the uterine horns is also separate, via the sympathetic nerves (Kawatani & de Groat 1991). The fibre types of the reproductive tract are consistent with other visceral organ innervation. Thus, the principle fibre types of the uterus and cervix are Aa (small myelinated) and C (unmyelinated) fibres.

Thus, the vagina and the perineum are innervated by the same neural pathways as the second and third stages of labour. These involve the pudendal nerve and other smaller nerves which are derived from S2, S3 and S4. However, the peculiar pain caused by pressure on the intrapelvic structures, and which is felt in the thigh and upper legs, usually involves fibres as high as the L2 nerves and as low as the S3 spinal segments.

PAIN OF THE FIRST STAGE OF LABOUR

The first stage of labour pain is caused by uterine contractions and stretching of the cervix. This continues throughout the first stage until complete dilatation is achieved. For nearly a century, based on the results published by Head (1893) and subsequently by Cleland (1949), the Aδ and C primary afferent fibres that supply the uterus and cervix accompany the sympathetic nerves as follows; first, the uterine and cervical plexus; second, the pelvic (inferior hypogastric) plexus; third, the middle hypogastric plexus or nerve, and fourth, the superior hypogastric and aortic plexuses (Head 1893, Cleland 1949). The nociceptive afferents then pass to the lumbar sympathetic chain and onward cephalad through the lower thoracic sympathetic chain. As is often the case, pain from the viscera, such as the pain caused by uterine contractions, is directly referred to dermatomes supplied by the same spinal cord segments that receive input from the uterus and cervix.

This work was recently confirmed in animal experiments (Kawatani et al 1986, Peters et al 1987, Berkley et al 1988, 1993a,b, Berkley & Wood 1989, Berkley 1990). Some of these investigators, such as Berkeley and her associates, have carried out a systematic and comprehensive series of experiments, using in vitro and in vivo electrophysiological and behavioural studies of the nerve supply of the uterus and other pelvic organs. These findings concluded that afferent fibres in the hypogastric and sympathetic nerves are the transmission linkage of nociceptive information. These uterine pelvic nerve afferents are able to transmit less stressful information, like more physiologically structured data.

PAIN OF THE SECOND AND THIRD STAGES OF LABOUR

When complete dilatation of the cervix occurs there is a notable reduction of nociceptive signals, but uterine contractions persist even against impressive forces of resistance. The pain that develops in the second stage emanates from continued distention of the entire vaginal canal as the fetus descends toward the vaginal outlet. Some of the painful signalling comes from muscular tension and tearing during this final descent and dilatation of the birth canal. Continued distension causes intense stretching and actual fascia tearing. Duration of the second stage of labour may be as short as less than 1 hour. Yet a duration of 1, 2 or even 3 hours can occur. During this interval there is descent of the fetus until the fetal head begins to negotiate the mid-pelvis at the anatomical level of the ischeal spines. The eventual passage of the fetal head through the mid-pelvis results in distension and stretching of the tissues of the mid and lower vagina, distention of the outlet and eventual dilatation to make way for the passage of the largest portion of the fetus – the fetal head. As will be considered below, these latter anatomical changes are accomplished with maximum stimulation via the nociceptive pathways by way of the pudendal nerves to dorsal root ganglia located at the S2–4 levels. There is also a significant sensory spillover to other adjacent pathways via the lower sacrum, perianal and even upper thigh regions. Just like the pain caused by stimulation of superficial somatic structures, the perineal pain is sharp and well localized. This pain can be eliminated by blockade of the aforementioned nerves (Klink 1953, Bonica 1967).

As complete dilatation occurs, the pain may be overwhelming and too much to push against the strong tension of the perineal muscles until analgesia is accomplished. This can be accomplished in the form of an epidural with sacral distribution or a caudal regional analgesic method. In the late part of the first stage and during the second stage, a number of parturients develop aching, burning or cramping discomfort in the thigh and less frequently in the legs. This can be the result of the stimulation of pain-sensitive structures in the pelvic cavity that include traction on the pelvic peritoneum, stretching and tension of the bladder, urethra and rectum, stretching and tension of ligaments, fascia and muscles of the pelvic cavity and abnormal pressure on roots of the lumbosacral plexus. As noted earlier, the neural pathways for the second and third stages of labour involve the pudendal nerve and other smaller branches, which are derived from S2, S3, and S4.

PHYSIOLOGICAL AND PSYCHOLOGICAL EFFECTS OF LABOUR PAIN

CHANGES IN VENTILATION

Because of the significant maternal, anatomical and physiological changes that involve the respiratory system during pregnancy, there are changes in the airways, changes in lung volumes, changes in dynamics of breathing and, therefore, substantial changes in ventilation (Bonica 1973). By the third month of gestation, there is an increase in respiratory rate and tidal volume resulting in a 50% increase in minute volume. Because the dead space remains normal, alveolar ventilation increases by 70%. The decrease in lung volumes and the increase in ventilation effect a reduction of arterial and alveolar carbon dioxide tension to around 32 mmHg, and a consequential increase in oxygen tension to about 105 mmHg (Prowse & Gaensler 1965) (Figs 29.3–29.5). The pain experienced at the time of labour and delivery serves as a powerful respiratory stimulus. This results in a further marked increase in tidal volume and minute ventilation, and an even greater increase in alveolar ventilation. This physiological change causes a further reduction of $Paco_2$ from the pregnancy level of 32 mmHg to a value of as low as 16–20 mmHg, or occasionally even as low as 10–15 mmHg (Fig. 29.6). This causes a reflex increase in pH to 7.5–7.6 (Cole & Nainby-Luxmoore 1962, Fisher & Prys-Roberts 1968, Bonica 1973, Huch et al 1977, Peabody 1979). This respiratory alkalosis, which occurs at the peak of each uterine contraction, results in decreases in cerebral and uterine blood flow and a shift to the left of the maternal oxygen dissociation curve. With the onset of the relaxation phase, pain no longer stimulates respiration so that the hypocapnia causes a transient period of hypoventilation that decreases the maternal $Paco_2$ by 10–50% with a mean value of 25–30% (Huch et al 1977, Peabody 1979). Mothers who have received an opioid for pain relief have the depressant effect of the respiratory alkalosis then enhanced by the action of the opioids. When the maternal $Paco_2$ falls below 70 mmHg, it has a significant effect on the fetus, namely a decrease in fetal $Paco_2$ and late decelerations (Myers 1975) (Fig. 29.6). For a summary of the various ventilatory changes associated with pregnancy refer to Table 29.1.

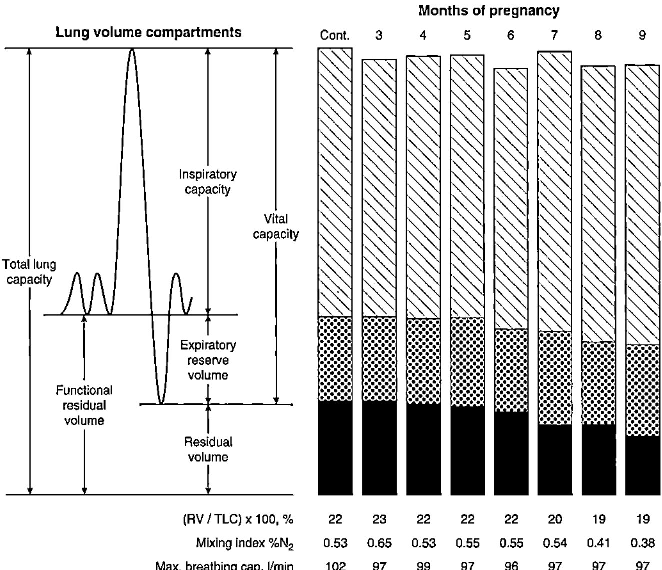

Fig. 29.3 Serial measurements of lung volume compartments during pregnancy. The control values were computed from the same woman at 4–9 months postpartum. (Reproduced from Bonica & McDonald 1995 with permission.)

NEUROENDOCRINE EFFECTS

Some of the previously described changes that have been discussed, such as reduced carbon dioxide and increases in catecholamine levels (20–40%) caused by noxious stimulation, produce a net reduction in uterine blood flow in the animal model (Jouppila 1977, Morishima et al 1978, Shnider & Levinson 1987, Berkley & Wood 1989).

The chief increase in catecholamine levels is caused by elevations of noradrenaline, the latter has the most impressive effect upon placental vasculature with a low of 35%, and a high of 70% decrease in uterine blood flow (Fig. 29.7). On the human studies side, data has shown that severe pain and anxiety during active labour can cause a 300–600% increase in the adrenaline (A) level, a 200–400% increase in the noradrenaline (NA) level; a 200–300% increase in the cortisol level and significant increases in corticosteroid and ACTH levels during labour. These all reach peak values at or just after delivery (Lederman et al 1977, 1982, Ohno et al 1986). Lederman's work revealed A-level increases by nearly 300%, NA levels by 150% and the cortisol levels by 200%. Of great interest was the fact that increased A and cortisol levels correlated with anxiety and pain. More recent research in a comprehensive study of catecholamines and cyclic nucleotides during labour and following delivery noted a nearly twofold increase in the dopamine levels, a threefold increase in the A level and a twofold increase in the NA level, as well as a small increase

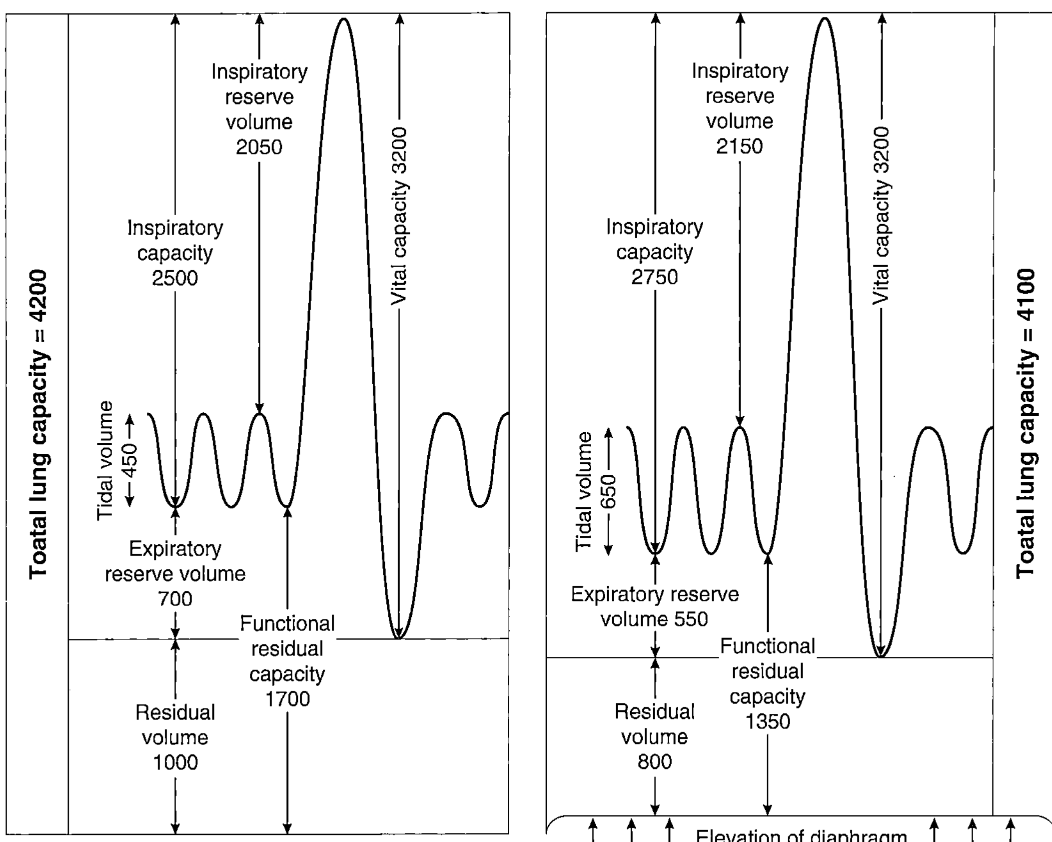

Fig. 29.4 Pulmonary volumes and capacitances in the non-pregnant and term gravida. This demonstrates the effect of elevation of the diaphragm. (Reproduced from Bonica & McDonald 1995 with permission.)

in the cyclic adenosine monophosphate (cAMP) level. They also noted a positive correlation between the A level and heart rate and systolic blood pressure, along with a correlation between NA and cAMP levels during labour (Ohno et al 1986).

CARDIOVASCULAR CHANGES

Ueland and Hansen are given credit for unravelling the mystery of why pregnant patients were thought not to have increased cardiac outputs after the second trimester of pregnancy. Until the late 1960s all studies on cardiac output were carried out with patients in the supine position. Ueland and Hansen measured cardiac outputs in the lateral decubitus position and showed increased outputs throughout pregnancy for the first time. It was already common knowledge that around 6–8 weeks of pregnancy, the total blood, plasma and red cell volumes progressively increased, and topped out at 28–32 weeks (Adams & Alexander 1958, Hansen & Ueland 1966, Lees 1970) This elevated blood volume was accompanied by a similar increase in cardiac output from increased stroke volume and heart rate. In labour, cardiac output increased further above prelabour levels. The percentage increase in cardiac output was higher when the parturient was in the supine position than when she was in the lateral position. With the parturient in the supine position, between contractions cardiac output during the early first stage was about 15% above that of prelabour, during the late first stage it was about 30%, during the second stage about 45% and immediately after delivery 65–80% above prelabour (Hendricks & Quilligan 1956, Adams & Alexander 1958, Hansen & Ueland 1966). During painful uterine contractions, there was even a further increase of 15–20% in cardiac output (Fig. 29.8).

It is believed that nearly 50% of the increase during contractions is caused by the extrusion of 250–300 ml of blood from the uterus and by increased venous return from the pelvis and lower limbs into the maternal circulation. The remainder is caused by an increase in sympathetic activity provoked by pain, anxiety, apprehension and the physical effort of labour, which contribute to the progressive rise in cardiac output as labour advances. Uterine contractions in the absence of analgesia also cause increases of 20–30 mmHg in the systolic and diastolic blood pressures

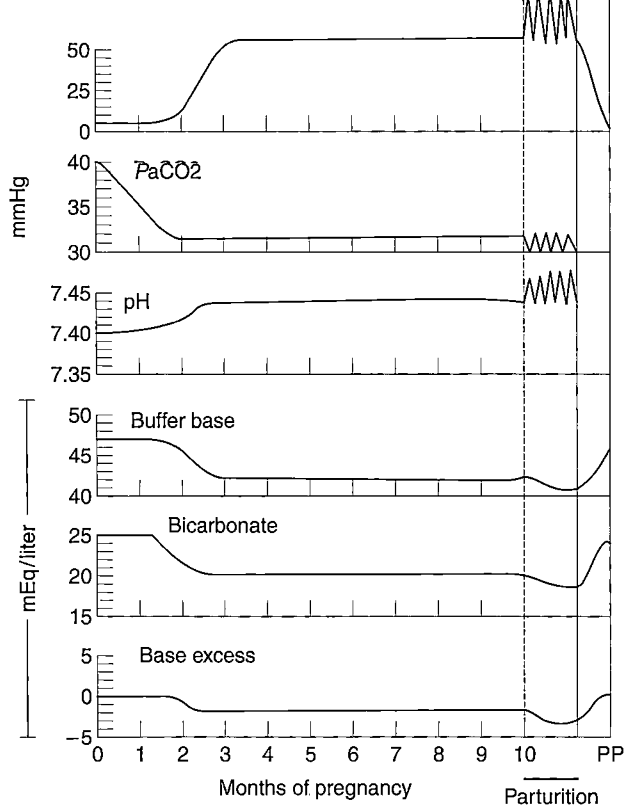

Fig. 29.5 Changes in alveolar ventilation, arterial CO2, pH and acid–base changes during pregnancy phases and through the postpartum period. (Reproduced from Bonica & McDonald 1995 with permission.)

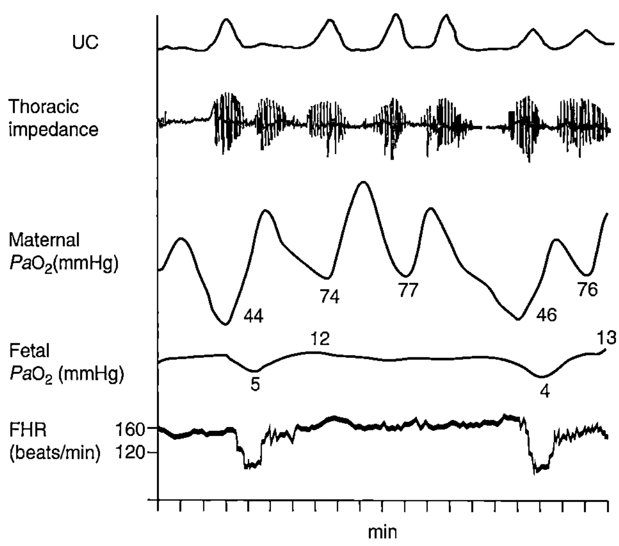

Fig. 29.6 Continuous recording of uterine contractions (UC), maternal thoracic impedance, maternal transcutaneous oxygen tension, fetal oxygen tension and fetal heart rate (FHR) in a primipara 120 min before spontaneous delivery of an infant with an Apgar score of 7. Marked hyperventilation during uterine contractions was followed by hypoventilation or apnoea in between contractions. With the parturient breathing air during and after the first and fourth periods of hyperventilation, the maternal Pao_2 fell to 44 and 46 mmHg with a consequent fall of fetal Pao_2 and variable decelerations which reflected fetal hypoxia. (Modified from Huch et al 1977.)

(Fig. 29.9). The increase in cardiac output and systolic blood pressure leads to a significant increase in left ventricular work. This is tolerated by healthy parturients, but it can prove deleterious if the parturients have heart disease, pre-eclampsia, essential hypertension or pulmonary hypertension (Hendricks & Quilligan 1956, Hansen & Ueland 1966, Robson et al 1987).

METABOLIC EFFECTS

It would be expected during pregnancy that the basal metabolic rate and oxygen consumption progressively increase; and, at term, their values rise to an imposing 20% above normal (Bonica 1967, 1969, 1980, Bonica & McDonald 1995). During parturition, the metabolism and oxygen consumption increase further (Bonica & McDonald 1990). It is believed that in labour, free fatty acids and lactate levels increase significantly as a result of pain-induced catecholamine release and the resultant sympathetic-induced lipolytic metabolism (Bonica & McDonald 1990). This is based on the fact that, with complete blockade of nociceptive afferent and efferent pathways with epidural analgesia, only small increases in maternal free fatty acid, lactate levels and acidosis are observed (Mary & Greene 1964). With poor analgesia during the second stage of labour, maternal acidosis can occur. This is caused by maternal pain and physical exertion inherent in the repetitive active bearing-down efforts (Fig. 29.10). The increased sympathetic activity elicited by labour pain and anxiety also increase metabolism and oxygen consumption, as mentioned above. The increased oxygen consumption inherent in the work of labour, together with the loss of bicarbonate from the kidney as compensation for the pain-induced respiratory alkalosis, produce a progressive maternal metabolic acidosis that is transferred to the fetus (Marx & Greene 1964, Buchan 1980, Bonica & McDonald 1990). The maternal pyruvate level increases, alongside a greater increase in the lactate level; soon a progressive accumulation of excess lactate occurs which is reflected by a progressive offset increase in base excess (Marx & Greene 1964, Buchan 1980, Bonica & McDonald 1990).

GASTROINTESTINAL AND URINARY FUNCTION

Once again the pain of labour and the consequent increase in sympathetic activity has another effect, this time on the

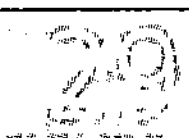

Table 29.1 Ventilatory changes during pregnancy. (Reproduced from Bonica & McDonald 1995 with permission)

Parameters	*Normal non-pregnant female*	*Gravida at term*	*Change*[1]
Tidal volume (ml)	450	650	+ 45%
Respiratory rate per min	15	16	+ 10%
Minute ventilation (litres)	6.5	10	+ 55%
Inspiratory capacity (IC) (litres)	2.5	2.75	+ 10%
Expiratory reserve volume (ERV) (litres)	0.7	0.55	− 20%
Residual volume (RV) (litres)	1.0	0.8	− 20%
Functional residual capacity (FRC) (litres)	1.7	1.35	− 20%
Vital capacity (VC) (litres)	3.2	3.2	None
Timed vital capacity			
1 s	82%	80%	Insignificant
2 s	93%	94%	Insignificant
3 s	98%	98%	None
Maximum breathing capacity (MBC) (litres)	102	97	− 5%
Total lung volume (litres)	4.2	4.1	− 5%
Maximum air flows (litres/min)			
Inspiratory	150	135	− 13%
Expiratory	100	98	− 2%
Airway resistance in cmH_2O/litres	2.5	2.5	None
Walking ventilation (litre/min)	15	19	+ 30%
Walking dyspnoea index (%)	15	21	+ 40%

[1]Calculated in round figures. Based on data of Cugell 1953.

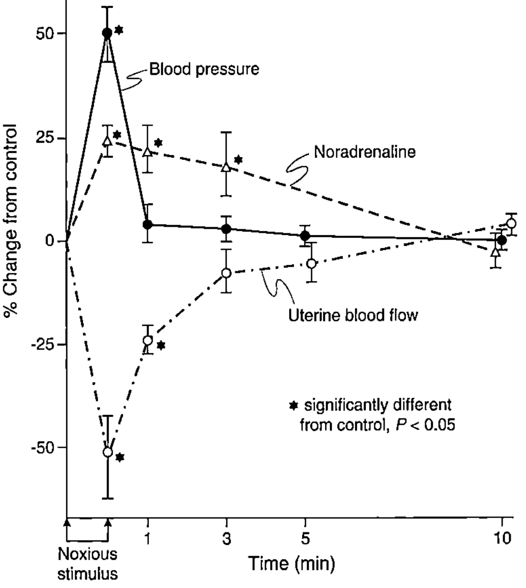

Fig. 29.7 The effects of a noxious stimulus on maternal arterial blood pressure, noradrenaline blood level and uterine blood flow. The stress was induced by application of an electric current on the skin of a ewe at term. Note that the increase in arterial pressure is very transient but the decay in noradrenaline level is more protracted and is reflected by a mirror-image decrease in uterine blood flow. (Reproduced from Shnider et al 1979 with permission.)

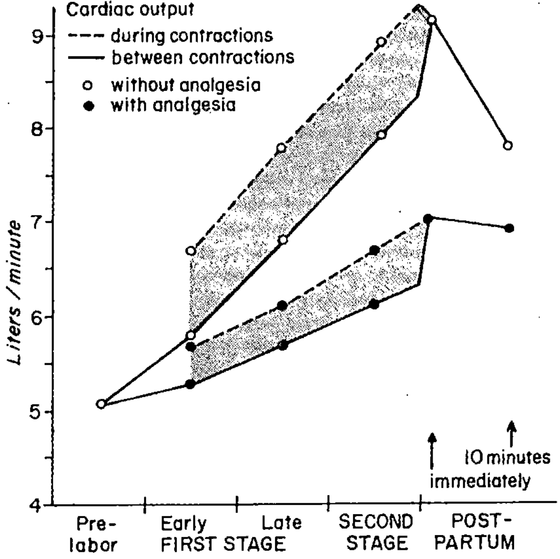

Fig. 29.8 Cardiac output during various phases of labour between contractions and during contractions. In a group of patients labouring without analgesia, the progressive increase between contractions and the further increase during each contraction were much greater than the changes in the group of patients who received continuous epidural analgesia. (Developed from data of Hendricks & Quilligan 1956, Ueland & Hansen 1969.)

function of the gastrointestinal and urinary tracts. Pain during labour stimulates gastrin release and results in increased gastric acid secretion (Marx & Greene 1964). Additionally, pain, anxiety and emotional stress create segmental and suprasegmental reflex inhibition of gastrointestinal and urinary motility with delays in gastric and urinary bladder

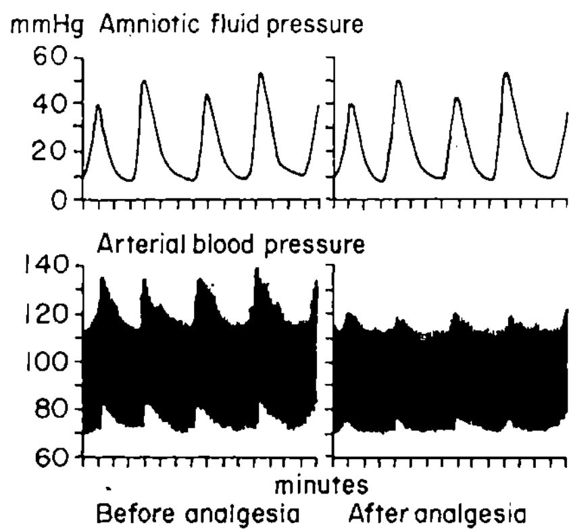

Fig. 29.9 The fluctuation in blood pressure produced by uterine contractions before and after induction of continuous epidural analgesia. Like the cardiac output changes, complete relief of pain resulted in decreasing the contraction-induced fluctuations to nearly half of the values measured before analgesia.

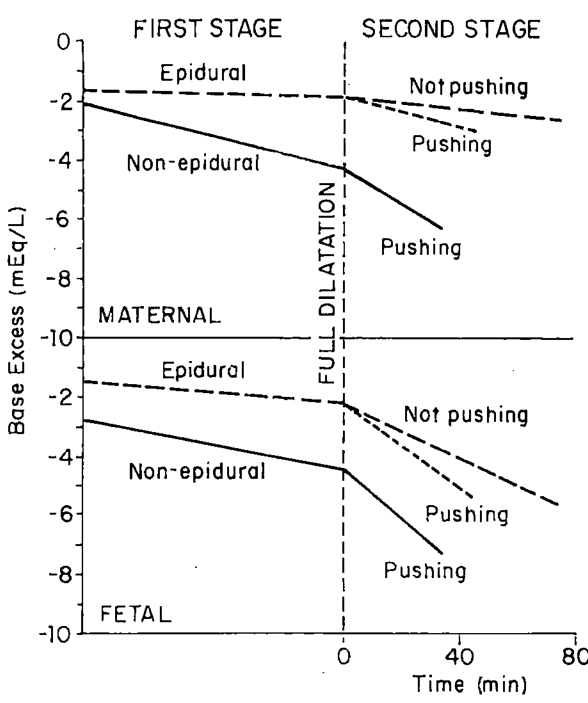

Fig. 29.10 Mean changes in extent of maternal (above) and fetal (below) metabolic acidosis, during the first and second stages of labour, in a group of parturients managed without lumbar epidural analgesia and in two similar groups managed with epidural analgesia, one of which retained the bearing down reflex while the other did not. The parturients were delivered by outlet forceps. Significant metabolic acidosis was experienced by those in the nonepidural group of parturients, whereas those given epidural analgesia experienced little or no change in their acid–base status. Fetuses born of mothers managed without epidural also developed significant metabolic acidosis during the first stage and to an even greater degree during the second stage. In contrast, fetuses of mothers given epidural analgesia had no change in acid–base status during the first stage but showed a time-dependent increase in metabolic acidosis during the second stage, due to the process of birth (see text). (Reproduced from Bonica 1980, based on data from Pearson & Davies 1974.)

function. Such reflex effects of nociception are aggravated by recumbent positions, opioids and depressant medications (Marx & Greene 1964, Pearson & Davies 1973a, 1974, Buchan 1980). The combined effects of pain and depressant drugs can thus cause food and fluids other than water to be retained for as long as 36 hours or more. During this period, swallowed air and gastric juices accumulate progressively, with gradual gastric pH decline below the critical value of pH 2.5. Therefore, delayed gastric emptying of the acidic gastric contents increases the risk of regurgitation and pulmonary aspiration, especially during the induction of general anaesthesia. This hazard has long been, and still today remains, one of the most common causes of maternal mortality and morbidity due to general anaesthesia (Hayes et al 1972).

EFFECTS ON UTERINE ACTIVITY AND LABOUR

The same increased secretion of catecholamines and cortisol caused by pain and emotional stress can either increase or decrease uterine contractility, which, of course, influences the duration of labour. Noradrenaline increases uterine activity, whereas it is decreased by adrenaline and cortisol (Nimmo et al 1975). An early animal study revealed nociceptive stimulation increased uterine activity by about 60% that was associated with a decrease in fetal oxygen tension and fetal heart rate characterized by ominous signs of late decelerations (Holdsworth 1978). Lederman and associates (Lederman et al 1977, 1978) noted that in some parturients severe pain and anxiety caused such an increase in adrenaline and cortisol levels such that uterine activity was decreased and labour was prolonged. In a small percentage of parturients, pain and anxiety even produced 'incoordinate uterine contractions' manifested by a decrease in intensity and an increase in frequency and uterine tone with ineffectual labour patterns (Moir & Willocks 1967, Holdsworth 1978, Tomkinson et al 1982).

PSYCHOLOGICAL EFFECTS

There is no question that psychological factors do affect the incidence and intensity of parturition pain and impact the mental attitude and mood of the patient during labour. Fear, apprehension and anxiety further enhance pain perception and pain behaviour (Deutsch 1955, Zuckerman et al 1963, Moir & Willocks 1967, Bonica & Hunter 1969, Brown et al 1972, Morishima et al 1980, Tomkinson et al

1982). Ignorance or misinformation is the classic generator of fear and anxiety for the parturient. An uninformed patient, especially a primipara, can be disturbed by fear of the unknown, suffering, complications and even the possibility of death. In addition, she may also be concerned that her fetus may be damaged (Myers 1975, Tomkinson et al 1982, Reading & Cox 1985). Studies have demonstrated patients who have an unplanned or illegitimate pregnancy or have an ambivalent or negative reaction to gestation report more pain during labour and delivery (Reading & Cox 1985).

The relationship between the parturient and her spouse also plays an important role in the degree of pain she experiences. Melzack reported in 1984 that the effective pain scores were higher when the husband was in the labour room than when he was absent. He suggested that this may reflect genuinely higher effective pain scores or may be due to a deliberate choice of descriptors in the attempt to impress the husband or express anger at him, but in any case, the finding was not spurious. Wallach found a similar effect in an independent study in 1982. By contrast, Nettelbladt and associates (1976), Norr et al (1977) and Fridh et al (1988) found that positive feelings of the expectant father toward the pregnancy seemed to be an important factor in decreasing the mother's feelings of apprehension during pregnancy. When expectant fathers were very supportive of their mates during pregnancy and labour, the women experienced less pain during parturition.

Other emotional factors, such as intensive motivation and cultural influences, can affect modulation of sensory transmissions and certainly can influence the effective and behavioural dimensions of pain. Cognitive intervention, such as giving the parturient preparatory information about labour, reduces uncertainty, while producing distraction and dissociation from pain reduces pain behaviour. In a study of 134 low-risk parturients at term, Lowe found in 1989 that confidence in ability to handle labour was the most significant predictor of all components of pain during active labour. The greater the confidence the parturient had, the less the pain she experienced and vice versa (Lowe 1989).

Severe labour pain can produce serious long-term emotional disturbances that might impair the parturient's mental health, negatively influence her relationship with her baby during the first few crucial days and cause a fear of future pregnancies that could affect her sexual relationship with her husband (Marx & Greene 1964). Melzack and associates (1981), Gaston-Johansson and associates (1988) and Stewart (1982) all reported that a significant number of women who had participated in natural childbirth developed or had aggravation of prelabour depression, or had other deleterious emotional reactions in the postpartum period, consequent to the pain experienced during their childbirth without analgesia. Melzack also noted that some women experienced an added burden of guilt, anger and failure when they anticipated 'a natural painless childbirth', but had to convert to the use of analgesia when confronted with severe pain. Stewart reported that such patients became miserable, depressed and even suicidal and lost interest in sex. In some cases, the husbands of women who anticipated 'natural' childbirth had to undergo psychotherapy for serious reactions after seeing their wives experience such severe pain as they themselves developed feelings of guilt and subsequent impotence and phobias.

CURRENT METHODS TO RELIEVE CHILDBIRTH PAIN

In centres where anaesthesia coverage is available, regional analgesia is preferred by far to any other technique offered today. In the past two decades there were questions about what was the safest technique for pain relief for the first stage of labour. Throughout the last 20 years, regional analgesia by lumbar epidural (LE) method was scrutinized by every possible investigative modality. The LE method has withstood the test of time and is clearly the favourite of the mother, the nurse, the anesthetist and, finally, the obstetrician. Of course, there is no one standard of anaesthesia available in all countries and thus we will also discuss other methods that are more common in countries where full-time anaesthesia coverage is not available. Currently, many drugs and techniques are available to provide for the relief of childbirth pain. All of these can be arbitrarily classified into four categories:

1. psychological analgesia
2. simple methods of pharmacological analgesia
3. inhalation analgesia/anaesthesia
4. regional analgesia/anaesthesia.

During the past two decades, but especially since the previous editions of this book appeared, there have been significant changes in the methods used for the relief of pain of childbirth. This is suggested by four major surveys of the practice of obstetric analgesia/anaesthesia carried out in the USA during the past three decades, and two surveys which included current practice in the UK, Scandinavian countries and a number of other countries throughout the world (Marx & Green 1964, Bonica & McDonald 1995). These

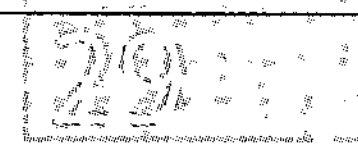

surveys indicate that in major hospitals where obstetric services are well organized and an obstetric anaesthesia service is available, there has been a trend of increasing use of continuous lumbar epidural block with a dilute solution of local anaesthetics and opioids and a decrease in the use of regional analgesia and inhalation analgesia.

In the USA, about 20–30% of parturients select psychological analgesia, but eventually two-thirds of them receive lumbar epidural or other forms of regional analgesia. There has also been a general trend not to use inhalation anaesthesia for labour and vaginal delivery. However, in the UK and in Scandinavian countries, inhalation analgesia is still being used, alone or together with the systemic opioids, in 20–50% of parturients. In the UK, nevertheless, there has been a steady increase in the use of continuous lumbar epidural blocks as opposed to the use of inhalation analgesia for the first stage of labour.

In developing countries there are, as anticipated, still many problems because of the limited availability of regional anaesthesia experts and because of deficient equipment and support systems. Most parturients receive either no analgesia or simple methods of inhalation and local anaesthesia (Marx & Green 1964, Bonica & McDonald 1995). On the basis of these data, psychological analgesia and simple techniques of inhalation and regional anaesthesia are briefly commented upon below and adequate emphasis is given to the use of continuous lumbar epidural analgesia/anaesthesia (Brownridge 1991).

PSYCHOLOGICAL ANALGESIA

Three of the most well known methods of psychological analgesia will be discussed in the following paragraphs. These methods have been used for many years with varying degrees of success.

Natural childbirth

Natural childbirth has been used with great success for some relief of labour pain, which has really never been well understood and even today is the brunt of many misconceptions. Confusion about the exact nature of labour pain and its specific treatment are often caused by frank ignorance. In some instances, poor understanding of the effects of the emotional and psychological aspects of labour and delivery has blocked the use of this method of pain relief by obstetricians. On the other hand, overzealous insistence on the tenet that pain could be entirely eradicated by natural childbirth has also blocked the ancillary use of other methods of pain relief, such as regional analgesic methods combined in late labour for beneficial effect.

Dick-Read popularized natural childbirth at a time when little else could be offered for pain relief, and for that contribution he should be appreciated. His original emphasis was centred upon the mother entirely (Dick-Read 1953). It was paramount she be in excellent physical condition so that she could endure the challenge of labour. Therefore, conditioning became very important in the early phases of the development of the technique and later on the psychological aspects were added, but this was not a sole emphasis made by Dick-Read himself, who did stress the need for patient control over the process of labour. This method was enhanced greatly by the cooperation of a friendly and helpful nurse who would act as a coach and facilitator for the patient during stressful times.

Psychoprophylactic method

The psychoprophylactic method of analgesia modified the Dick-Read method with another method of analgesia that was popularized in Russia. These techniques were used for many years and soon were accepted elsewhere in Europe with success. By the middle of the century, the psychological methods were known by many different names, but the most popular names were 'psychoprophylaxis' and 'childbirth without pain', as Dick-Read originally described it. The method was popularized by Lamaze (1954) of France, who successfully introduced it to the USA around the same time that regional anaesthesia was being reintroduced, thanks to pioneers such as Bonica (1967), Cleland (1949) and Edwards and Hingson (1942). At this time, various exercises in ventilation were added and it was understood that control of this aspect of breathing could have a salutary effect on the pain experience. This occurred in the mid 1970s, when there were still not many physicians involved in obstetric anaesthesia. All of these methods demanded the close communication and coordination of the teachers, the nurses, the patient and the obstetrician. The healthcare team helped to foster confidence and optimism in the parturient, which was very important in developing a pleasing, fulfilling experience at childbirth.

Hypnotic method

The hypnotic method demands complete cooperation between the obstetric patient and the obstetrician. Often the obstetrician may act as the teacher for the hypnosis sessions. This author had the distinct pleasure to observe sessions of learning by patients during intense hypnotic lessons with their obstetrician a few years ago, and was impressed by the patients who were so genuinely enthusiastic about the method. The relationship between the patient and her obstetrician is usually very strong and very positive, which of course makes learning hypnosis from the physician quite effective. Continued enthusiasm for this method demands time, concentration, dedication to learning a new technique and a belief in the patient's own inner self and strength.

In all of the above methods, the role of the nurse in the success of the patient is vital. It cannot be emphasized too much that the patients need, seek and appreciate understanding and kindness during such a first encounter with the labour process. Here is a wonderful example of an area where there is still much to be done in the area of cooperation and coordination of these patients and the fulfilment of the goals set forth by the obstetrician early in the pregnancy. It really emphasizes the importance of the fact that obstetrics is really a team effort among many individuals, including the patient, the nurse, the obstetrician, the anaesthetist and the paediatrician. It is only with close adherence to cooperation, communication, coordination and mutual respect and admiration for each other, that success and enjoyment of the entire process can be assured.

Bonica summarized his evaluation of the above methods in relieving pain during labour and made the following three conclusions:

1. 5–10% experience little or no pain and will require no analgesia/anaesthesia during the entire process.
2. In an additional 15–20%, the pain is decreased to a moderate degree, and the parturient will require less pharmacological analgesia/anaesthesia
3. In the remainder, the pain is not influenced but fear and anxiety will be less and the patients will manifest less pain behaviour (Bonica 1967, 1980).

It would seem that those who are so vocal in recruiting patients to the psychological methods are often quite biased in their evaluations of its efficacy. Some reports indicate that prepared childbirth patients have a shorter labour, fewer operative deliveries, fewer intrapartum and postpartum complications, less blood loss and better and happier babies than patients given drug-induced analgesia/anaesthesia (Davenport-Slack & Boylan 1974), while other reports indicate no significant differences regarding these variables between prepared and unprepared anaesthesia groups (Scott & Rose 1976, Melzack et al 1981, Gerdin et al 1990). The personal observations by Bonica in the former Soviet Union and in Western European and American hospitals suggested that the discrepancies are due to:

1. Differences in motivation, attitude and personality of the parturient and her instructor.
2. The practices of the obstetrician.
3. Most importantly, the skill with which pharmacological analgesia/anaesthesia was used.

On the basis of his observations and from long personal experience with regional analgesia, Bonica agreed with Melzack et al (1981) in recommending that prepared childbirth training should be combined with regional analgesia in order to achieve the best results for the mother and her infant.

SIMPLE TECHNIQUES OF PHARMACOLOGICAL ANALGESIA

Simple techniques in many parts of the world, where anaesthetists are not available, are the mainstay of pain relief for labour. Many times there just is no analgesia available and birth occurs without any pain relief period. In some instances, mothers in labour must rely on the use of prepared childbirth and drug analgesia only. Sometimes early first-stage pain can be relieved by using just suggestion and mild sedatives and tranquillizers. When this is not effective, various opioid drugs may be used with success.

Now for a brief discussion of sedatives for anxiety in patients in early labour or with Braxton Hicks type contractions. Popular sedatives include the hypnotic barbiturate class with secobarbital and pentobarbital most often chosen. Next in line are the phenothiazine sedatives like hydroxyzine hydrochloride and promethazine hydrochloride. These were used as potentiating drugs and primary sedatives. Benzodiazepine drugs are used commonly with diazepam being a favourite.

Barbituates include the mainstays of obstetrics such as phenobarbital or nemutal and secobarbital or seconal. One must recall that the primary effect of these drugs is sedation. As such, they are very effective in early labour situations where some anxiety is prominent and disruptive to sleep patterns. Especially in false labour situations, these drugs can relax the mother, help her to develop a calm, collected mental state and perhaps enable her to get good restorative sleep the night before that will prepare here for a full day of labour when she does go into labour for real.

Anticholinergics such as scopolamine have been used successfully in obstetrics to obtain a tranquil state or even an amnestic state in certain unpleasant situations. When administered with an opioid such as morphine, a special state referred to as 'twilight sleep' occurs. In such cases, often mother did not even remember they had had a delivery once they emerged from the sedative effects of the drugs. Its popularity has dropped substantially in the USA, but again, it is a good drug with which to be familiar in third world countries.

Hyroxyzine or vistaril is a potent sedative that is really an antihistaminic agent. It is very effective in providing sedation early in labour. When given with opioids, it potentiates their effect, with the result being better sedation and better analgesia. It can be given via the intramuscular route with good results.

Promethazine or phenergan is a popular phenothiazine. It produces sedation also and seems to have a potent effect with very mild respiratory depressant effects. It can be given separately in small IV doses of 25 mg or it can be given via the intramuscular route (Table 29.2).

Systemic analgesics

Narcotics, or more correct opioids, are the primary agents used for pain relief in labour not managed by regional analgesic methods. These agents are simple to use with intramuscular delivery by a labour nurse who really serves as the primary healthcare person responsible for decision-making in regard to comfort of the patient. Thus the nurse would establish contact with the patient during regular rounds and contact the patient's physician only when necessary. Often an initial order was given for meperidine (Demerol) after good active labour was established. Additional narcotic drugs, such as morphine, alphaprodine, nalbuphine and

Table 29.2 Sedatives, hypnotics, ataractics. (Reproduced from Bonica & McDonald 1995 with permission)

			Therapeutic effect[1]					
Drug	*Synonym*	*Dose (mg)*	*Sedation*	*Sleep*	*Tranquillizer*	*Antiemetic*	*Antihistaminic*	*Analgesia*
A. Barbiturates								
1. Secobarbital	Seconal	50–200	4	4	2	2	0	–
2. Pentobarbital	Nembutal	50–200						
3. Cyclobarbital	Phanodorn	100–300						
4. Vinbarbital	Delvinal	50–200						
B. Ataractics								
1. Phenothiazines								
a. Chlorpromazine	Thorazine Largactil	25	3	1	4	3	1	1
b. Promethazine	Phenergan	25–50	3	1	4	3	4	–
c. Promazine	Sparine	25–50	3	1	3	1	1	1
d. Perphenazine	Trilafon Fentazin	10	2	1	3	4	1	–
e. Prochlorperazine	Compazine Stemetil	15	3	1	4	4	1	–
f. Triflupromazine	Vesprin Vespral	50	3	1	4	3	1	–
g. Mepazine	Pacatal Pecazine	50	2	1	3	0	0	–
2. Propanediols								
a. Meprobamate	Equanil Miltown	500	3	3	2	0	0	0
3. Diphenylmethanes								
a. Hydroxyzine	Atarax Vistaril	100	3	1	4	0	0	1
C. Non-barbiturate sedative-hypnotics								
1. Ethinamate	Valmid	500–1000	3	3	1	0	0	0
2. Glutethimide	Doriden	250–500	3	3	1	0	0	0
3. Ethchlorvynol	Placidyl	250–500	3	3	1	0	0	0
4. Methyprylon	Noludar	200–400	3	3	1	0	0	0
5. Chloral hydrate		1–2 g	4	3	1	0	0	0
6. Scopolamine	Hyoscine	0.3 mg (gr. 1/200)	2	1	2	0	0	0

[1] 0 = no effect; 1 = minimum effect; 2 = moderate effect; 3 = good effect; 4 = maximum effect; – = analgesic effect.

fentanyl, were used. Although these narcotics were initially used via the intramuscular route in earlier years, they are now given in small intravenous doses to decrease the total amount needed for labour pain and thus decrease the amount available for effect upon the fetus.

Morphine was perhaps the oldest and the most long-standing opioid of choice for many obstetricians for many years. When combined with scopolamine to provide twilight sleep, it had a dramatic analgesic effect. This effect was impressive, but so was the depressant effect upon the mother and the neonate (Table 29.3). In an attempt to decrease the depressant effect, intravenous boluses of small amounts of morphine were tried. When administered just before uterine contractions, there may have been some fetal protective effect (Gerdin et al 1990).

Meperidine or demoral was the most popular opioid for

Table 29.3 Opioid analgesics used in labour. (Reproduced from Bonica & McDonald 1995 with permission)

Class generic name; proprietary names	*Routes*	*Equianalgesic dose (mg)*[1]	*Peak (h)*[2]	*Duration (h)*[3]	*Half-life (h)*	*Comments*	*Precautions*
Agonists							
Naturally occurring opium derivatives							
Morphine	IM[3]	10–15	0.5–1	3–5'[4]	2–3.5	Standard of comparison for opioid-type analgesics	Impaired ventilation; bronchial asthma; increased intracranial pressure; liver failure; renal failure
	PO[3]	30–60[1]	1.5–2	4			
Codeine	IM	120	0.5–1	4–6	3	Less potent than morphine; excellent oral potency	Like morphine
	PO	30–200		3–4			
Partially synthetic derivatives of morphine							
Hydromorphone (Dilaudid)	IM	1–2	0.5–1	3–4	2–3	Slightly shorter acting than morphine, possibly less sedation, N/V	Like morphine
	PO	2–4	1.5–2	4–6			
Oxymorphone (Numorphan)	IM	1–1.5	0.5–1	3–5	NA	Like morphine	Like morphine
Heroin	IM	4	0.5–1	3–4	2–3	Slightly shorter acting	Like morphine
	PO	4–8	1.5–2	3–4			
Oxycodone	PO	30	1	4–6	NA	Available only (5-mg doses) in combination with acetaminophen (Percocet) or aspirin (Percodan), which limits dose escalation	Like morphine
Synthetic compounds							
Morphonans							
Levorphanol (Levo-Dromoran)	IM	2	0.5–1	5–8	12–16	Like methadone	Like methadone
	PO	4	1.5–2				
Phenylheptylamines							
Methadone (Dolophine)	IM	8–10	0.5–1	4–8	15–30	Good oral potency; long plasma half-life	Like morphine, accumulative with repeated doses
	PO	10	1.5–2	4–12			
Propoxyphene HCl (Darvon)	PO	32–65		4–6	3.5	'Weak' opioid, often used in combination with non-opioid analgesics	Accumulative with repeated doses, convulsions with overdose
Phenylpiperidines							
Meperidine (Demerol)	IM	75–100	0.5–1	2–3		Shorter acting and about 10% as potent as morphine; has mild atrophine-like anti spasmatic effects	Normeperidine accumulates with repetitive dosing, causing CNS excitation; not for patients with impaired renal function or for those receiving monoamine oxidase inhibitors
	PO	200–300	1–2	2–3			

Table 29.3 (Contd.)

Class generic name; proprietary names	*Routes*	*Equianalgesic dose (mg)*[1]	*Peak (h)*[2]	*Duration (h)*[3]	*Half-life (h)*	*Comments*	*Precautions*
Alphaprodine (Nisentil)	IM	40		1.5–2		Similar to meperidine but shorter acting, low placental transfer – not available in USA	Like meperidine
Fentanyl	IV	50–100 µg		0.75–1		Short-acting potent opioid, mostly used in anaesthesia or continuous infusion	More severe side effects than morphine
Sufentanil	IV	5–10 µg					
Diffentanil	IV	500–1000 µg		0.25–0.4			
Agonist–Antagonists							
Buprenorphine (Temgesic)	IM	0.3–0.6	0.5–1	6–8	NA	Partial agonist of the morphine type, less abuse liability than morphine	Can precipitate withdrawal in narcotic-dependent patients
	SL	0.4–0.8	2–3	6–8			
Butorphanol (Stadol)	IM	2	0.5–1	4	2.3–3.5	Like nalbuphine	Like pentazocine
Pentazocine (Talwin)	IM	40–60	0.5–1	3–4	2–3	Mixed agonist-antagonist; less abuse liability than morphine; included in Schedule IV of Controlled Substances Act	Can cause psychotomimetic effects; might precipitate withdrawal in narcotic-dependent patients, not for those with myocardial infarction
	PO	50–200	1.5–2	3–4			
Nalbuphine (Nubain)	IM	10–20	0.5–1	4–6	5	Like pentazocine but not scheduled	Incidence of psychotomimetic effects lower than with pentazocine

[1]These doses are recommended starting doses from which the optimal dose for each patient is determined by titration and the maximal dose is limited by adverse effects.
[2]Peak time and duration of analgesia are based on mean values and refer to the stated equianalgesic doses.
[3]For a single oral dose the ratio of IM/oral is 1 : 6; for repeated doses the ratio is closer to 1 : 3.
[4]Plasma half-life at least for morphine is age-dependent; it increases with age.
IM = intramuscular; PO = oral; SL = sublingual; NA = not available; IV = intravenous.

many years in the USA and worldwide. It is a synthetic opioid with an intermediate half-life of about 3 hours. For some time there was confusion about its efficacy because of its active metabolite normeperidine. The latter is a potent respiratory depressant and the serious impact to consider is its long half-life of over 48 hours in the neonate (Caldwell et al 1978).

Alphaprodine or nisentil was popular in the 1950s, 1960s and 1970s. Its use was based upon its rapid analgesic effect within 3–5 minutes after intramuscular or subcutaneous administration. Its popularity for some 30 years was overshadowed by its propensity to cause a fetal heart sinusoidal pattern and its powerful respiratory depressant effect upon the neonate. It has not been used in obstetrics since the late 1980s.

Nalbuphine or nubain is both an agonist and antagonist-type opioid. Its respiratory depressant effect is similar to morphine. The advantage of nalbuphine is that its depressant characteristic has a ceiling effect. In other words, a dosage that gives maximum depression can be increased without further evidence of increased depression upon the neonate. This opioid is 80% as potent as morphine. See Table 29.4 for relative comparisons. The onset of 2–3 minutes after intravenous injection was appealing for the management of labour pain.

Fentanyl is a highly lipid soluble synthetic opioid that is 100 times more potent than morphine. It was used primarily for its quick analgesic effect, but its other advantage was that it did produce active metabolites that could act as respiratory depressants. Small doses of 50 µg IV were used

Table 29.4 Equivalent analgesic narcotic doses. (Reproduced from Bonica & McDonald 1995 with permission)

Drug	*Oral dose (mg)*	*Intramuscular dose (mg)*
Alphaprodine (Nisentil)	–	45.0
Anileridine (Leritine)	–	35.0
Codeine	200.0	130.0
Diacetylmorphine (heroin)	–	3.0
Fentanyl (Sublimaze)	–	0.1
Hydromorphone (Dilaudid)	7.5	1.5
Meperidine (Demerol)	400.0	100.0
Methadone	10.0	8.0
Morphine	30.0	10.0
Oxycodone (Percodan)	30.0	15.0
Oxymorphone (Numorphan)	–	1.5
Pentazocine (Talwin)	180.0	6.0

with success in the first stage of labour, but there was little if any advantage noted over morphine and the latter had a much longer analgesic effect. Because of its high lipid solubility, it also crossed the placenta and appeared rapidly in the fetal circulation (Rosaeg et al 1992).

Once the first stage of labour is managed, it is time to consider a good second-stage technique that will be reliable and offer full pain relief. With the onset of the moderate pain of the second stage, opioids are required. Narcotics produce adequate relief of moderate pain in 70–80% and relief of severe pain in about 35–60% of parturients (Bonica 1967, 1969). Small doses do not produce significant maternal respiratory depression, but can produce some neonatal depression. For delivery, inhalation analgesia with nitrous oxide can be used with intermittent or continuous administration via a mask connected to an anaesthesia machine. This technique can be useful right at delivery, with the crowning of the fetal head causing maximum dilatation of the perineum (Marx & Katsnelson 1992). An alternative analgesic technique is bilateral pudendal nerve block or infiltration of the perineum for similar pain relief during the delivery of the fetus.

Labour pain is not well appreciated still in many parts of the world and is a major problem today in regard to pain control. There is such a wide variance in care given from modern centres with 90% benefiting from regional analgesic methods to third world countries where no pain relief exists whatsoever. In modern centres, there are even classes to allay the patient's fears and reassure them that they will be cared for with the utmost consideration for their comfort and the baby's safety. Discussions like this emphasize the importance of the nurse who helps both the obstetrician and the anaesthetist by offering support to the patient in a time of need.

INHALATIONAL ANALGESIA/ANAESTHESIA

The next logical step up from systemic analgesia is inhalation analgesia. Today it is still a popular method of relieving labour pain because it rapidly produces moderately effective pain relief at a time when it is sorely needed without causing loss of consciousness or significant maternal/neonatal depression. Commonly agents such as these are 40–50% nitrous oxide in oxygen, or sevoflurane or desflurane in oxygen can be used (Swart et al 1991). Nitrous oxide can be administered intermittently during uterine contractions by the assistant to the anaesthetist or the anaesthetist (Carstoniu et al 1994). Premixed cylinders of 50% nitrous oxide and 50% oxygen are used in some parts of the world just for this purpose, but most of the time it is administered by an anaesthetic machine in the operating room or delivery room setting for safety purposes. Safety and optimal analgesia principles dictate that the inhalation of the drug should be given administered by someone in the specialty of anaesthesia. Inhalation should be given some 10–15 seconds before the painful period of each contraction. Properly used, inhalational analgesia produces good analgesia in one-third and partial relief in another one-third of parturients (Norman et al 1992).

Inhalational anaesthesia for very brief time periods and for actual delivery is still employed, because it can be rapidly induced and affords maximum control of depth and duration of action and is rapidly eliminated at the end of the procedure. On the other hand, general anaesthesia is very dangerous and carries the risk of maternal mortality caused by difficult endotracheal intubation with consequent asphyxia (Glassenberg 1991). This, and regurgitation and pulmonary aspiration, are the two leading causes of anaesthesia-related maternal mortality in Britain and the USA. For this reason, general anaesthesia should be avoided but, if necessary, should be given only by a properly trained anaesthetist who has secured the airway by endotracheal intubation prior to the induction of anaesthesia. Refer to Figure 29.11 for proper protection against regurgitation with the use of the cricoid pressure manoeuvre. Some have advocated the use of the laryngeal mask airway to administer anaesthesia in cases where intubation by the normal means is difficult or impossible (Fig. 29.12). This is a controversial issue at this time as there is not enough experience with the use of the laryngeal mask airway in obstetrics to make claims for the safety of the mother. Furthermore, this is one of the most difficult areas of obstetric anaesthesia. Until more experience is gained with this technique, it should be reserved for those expert in its application and then only under special indications.

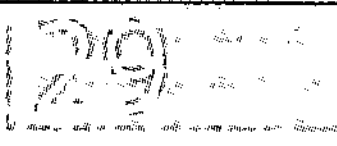

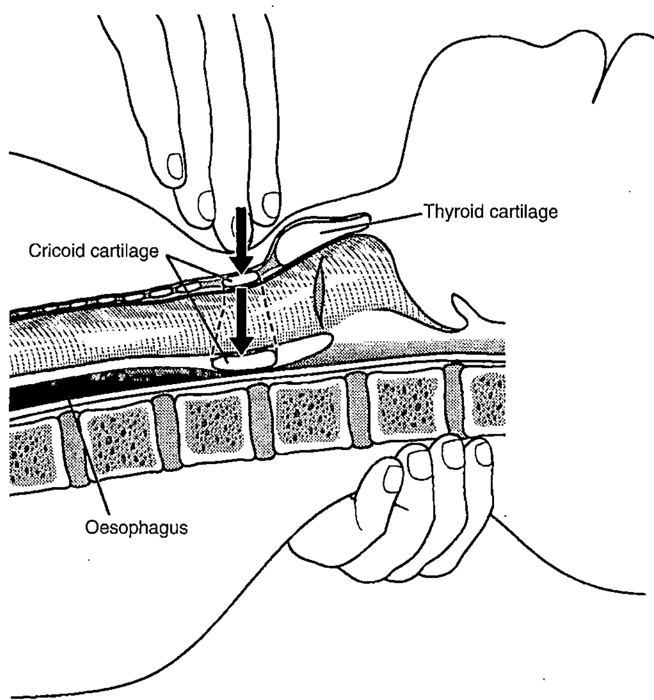

Fig. 29.11 The use of the cricoid pressure manoeuvre.

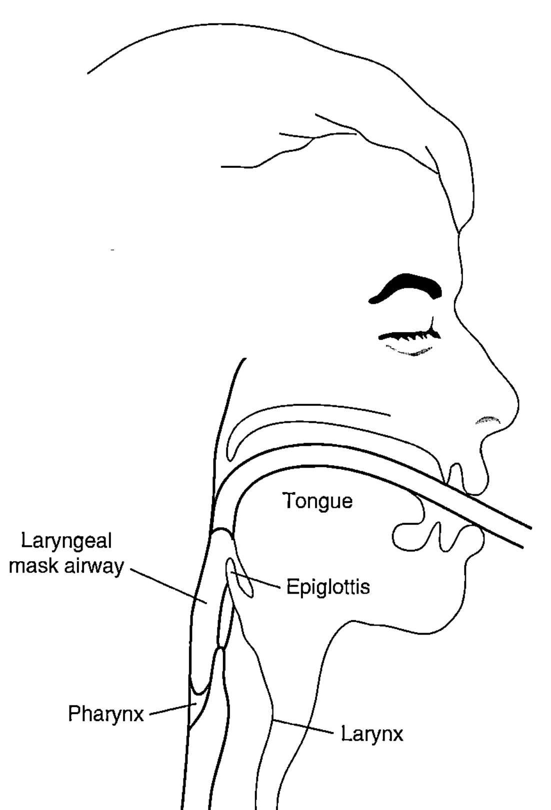

Fig. 29.12 The laryngeal mask airway in situ.

The estimation of the difficulty of intubation is still problematical; refer to Figure 29.13 for the different classes of airways. Every centre should establish their own method for evaluation of the difficult airway patient. Figure 29.14 shows both a preoperative and operative evaluation that can be used for such purposes. The use of inhalational analgesia is by definition the administration of dilute amounts of anaesthetic such that the patient has control of her airway. Its purpose is to smooth out some of the pain experienced just at the end of delivery. It is not under any circumstances to hazard the mother's safety. The use of inhalational anaesthesia is reserved for general anaesthesia techniques associated with caesarean section delivery. Again, if the anaesthetist deems that the patient presents as a very difficult intubation, then a discussion with the obstetrician needs to follow with the options mentioned. Some of these options might include local anaesthesia for caesarean section with oxygen administration via mask and some IV sedation. The latter may sound confrontational, but the

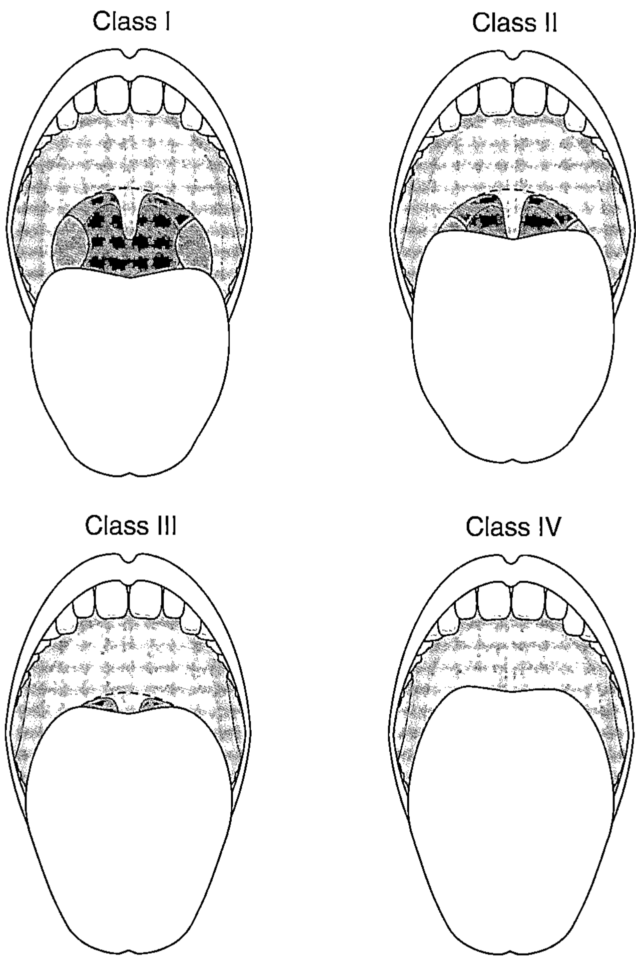

Fig. 29.13 Different classes of airways.

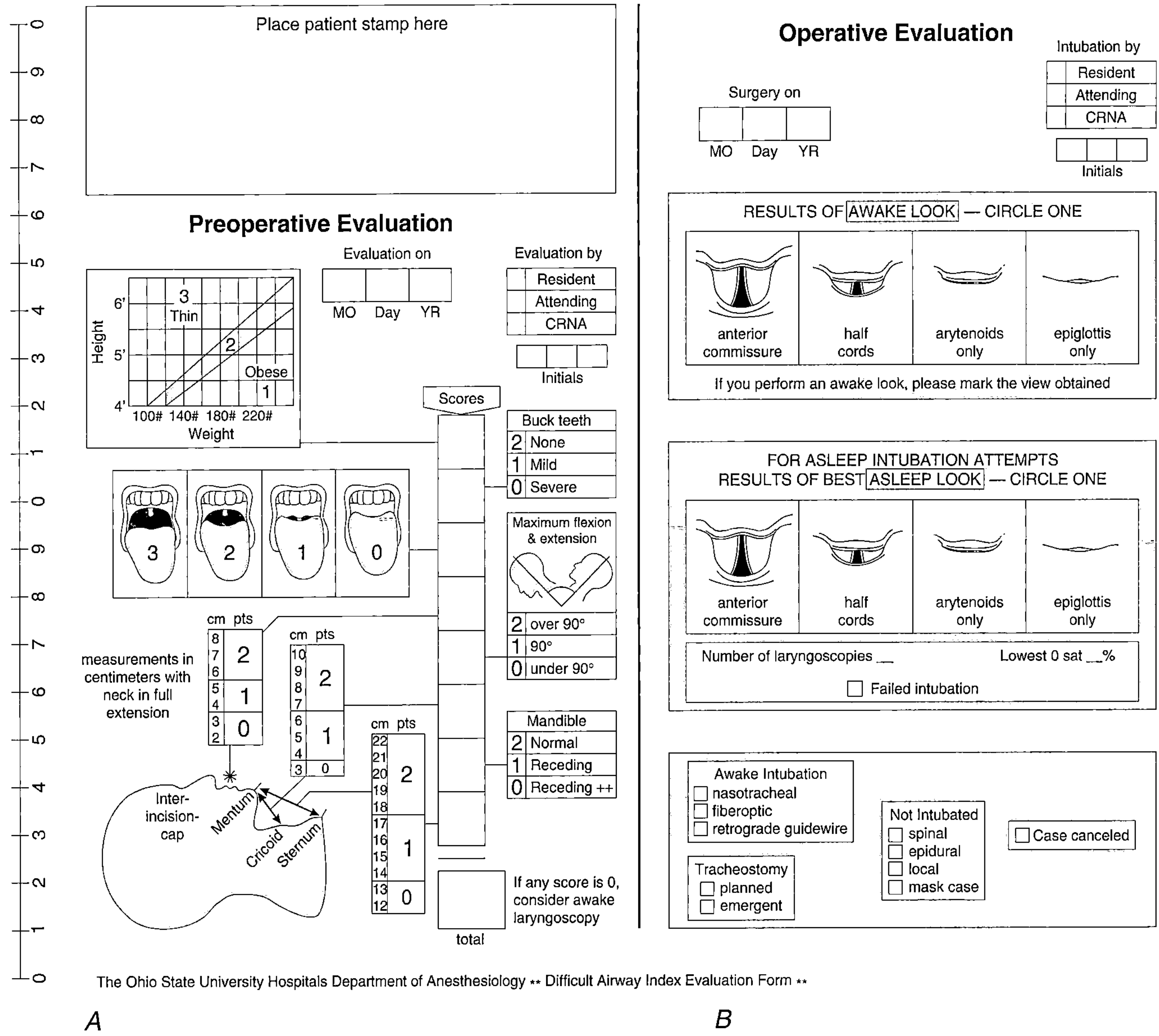

Fig. 29.14 The components of a preoperative evaluation carried out in 1992. **A** The eight scores compiled as a result of the evaluation. **B** The eventual awake or asleep look and the results of the intubation. (Reproduced from Bonica & McDonald 1995 with permission.)

anaesthetist must remember that the prime regard must be patient protection. This includes a professional opinion of the hazard of a 'crash' induction that may lead to failed intubation, hypoxia, cardiac embarrassment, cardiac arrest or even eventual brain damage or death. The anaesthetist must remain the final protector of the health and well-being of the primary patient in the obstetric equation – the mother. Our professional opinion cannot be second-guessed by the obstetrician who may be stressed because of fetal jeopardy that is threatening the life of the baby. At best, such situations are very very difficult, but must be managed with a cool head, logic and a collegial effort directed at what is best for the family at risk. The two prime healthcare givers must work out a strategic scenario that will accomplish the aforementioned goal. It must be done with mutual respect, one for the other. Both physicians must try to see the other's viewpoint, but in the end must compromise and present a unified decision-making plan to the mother and to the father or other loved one personally involved. These difficult intubation scenarios have various solutions that are noted in Figure 29.15. However, of these, at least nine are untenable in emergency crises such as those outlined here. The only logical solutions for such a serious challenge as proposed above with failed intubation

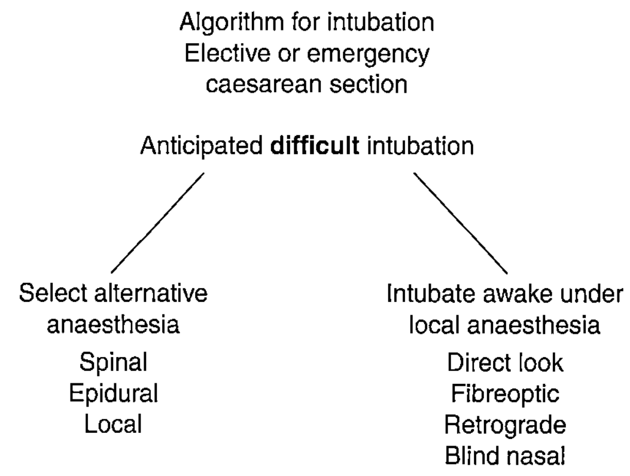

Fig. 29.15 Algorithm for intubation. Elective or emergency caesarean section. Anticipated difficult intubation. (Reproduced from Bonica & McDonald 1995 with permission. Redrawn from The Ohio State University Hospitals, Department of Anesthesiology.)

and an impossible intubation are direct fibreoptic laryngoscopy via the oral airway device, cricothyroidotomy, tracheostomy or mask ventilation with continuous cricoid pressure (and even this is highly controversial). The best solution of all may be to obviate the entire worry about using inhalation anaesthesia and place a continuous spinal catheter in such high-risk patients and thus allow rapid analgesia to be obtained for a 'stat' caesarean section, when and if indicated.

REGIONAL ANALGESIA/ANAESTHESIA

The popularity and use of regional analgesia in the form of epidurals for labour and delivery has increased incredibly since the 1970s. The most common techniques are:

- Continuous lumbar epidural.
- Subarachnoid block.
- Bilateral paracervical block.
- Double catheter-combined epidural/low caudal.

Over the years, many have extolled the virtues of regional analgesia, primarily because it offered excellent pain relief without any central nervous system depression. In other words, the mother can enjoy the beauty of the experience of her lifetime in complete control and with all her faculties intact. With the current methods of delivery and selection of local anaesthetics, there are few if any complications for either the mother or the fetus, and there is little if any deleterious effect upon the pattern or length of labour. By selecting regional techniques, the use of depressant medications during labour that adversely affect the mother and baby, along with the use of general anaesthesia for operative delivery with the complications of aspiration, are avoided.

At the same time the disadvantages of regional analgesia must be kept in mind also, because one thing that must be remembered is that the mother at all costs does not want anything to adversely affect the outcome of her baby regardless of how much pain she suffers. For example, the complications of hypotension, toxic systemic reactions and unexpected high spinal with potential cardiac arrest must always be guarded against.

Maternal hypotension is reduced by infusing fluids before inducing spinal, epidural or caudal block to compensate for the increased vascular capacitance experienced after sympathetic block; the parturient is also placed in the lateral decubitus position during labour to avoid the aortocaval compression inherent in the supine position. Systemic toxic reactions may be prevented by avoiding excessive doses or accidental intravenous injection of therapeutic doses and by the administration of local anaesthetic doses in small quantities with repeated injections over several small intervals of time. In addition, the use of small quantities of adrenaline was found to reduce the maternal and fetal exposure to the local anaesthetic agent used for the epidural (McLintic et al 1991). Sometimes this complication can be picked up by use of the test dose and careful monitoring of the maternal heart rate from injection until a 3-minute period. The adrenaline in the test dose will cause an acute increase in the heart rate for a transient period of time.

Very high or total spinal anaesthesia may result from accidental subarachnoid injection of a local anaesthetic dose intended for extradural block. Because the dosage of local anaesthetic is huge compared to what would be administered in the subarachnoid space, the effect upon the sympathetic system that is responsible for the maintenance of tone in the capacitance vessels is profound, and results in a progressive reduction in blood pressure with eventual shock if not diagnosed and treated in a timely fashion.

The latter two complications can be virtually obviated by attempting to aspirate blood or cerebrospinal fluid and injecting a test dose of 2–3 ml of solution containing 5–7.5 mg bupivacaine and 15 mg adrenaline. If the injection is accidentally subarachnoid, the parturient will develop a low (T10–S5) spinal anaesthesia. As mentioned above, if the injection is intravenous the adrenaline will produce moderate tachycardia and hypertension within 20–30 seconds of the injection and this will last for 30–60 seconds (Moore & Batra 1981). Only when neither occurs should large therapeutic doses be injected.

Paracervical and pudendal block

Techniques of paracervical block combined with pudendal block (Fig. 29.16) offer excellent first-stage and second-

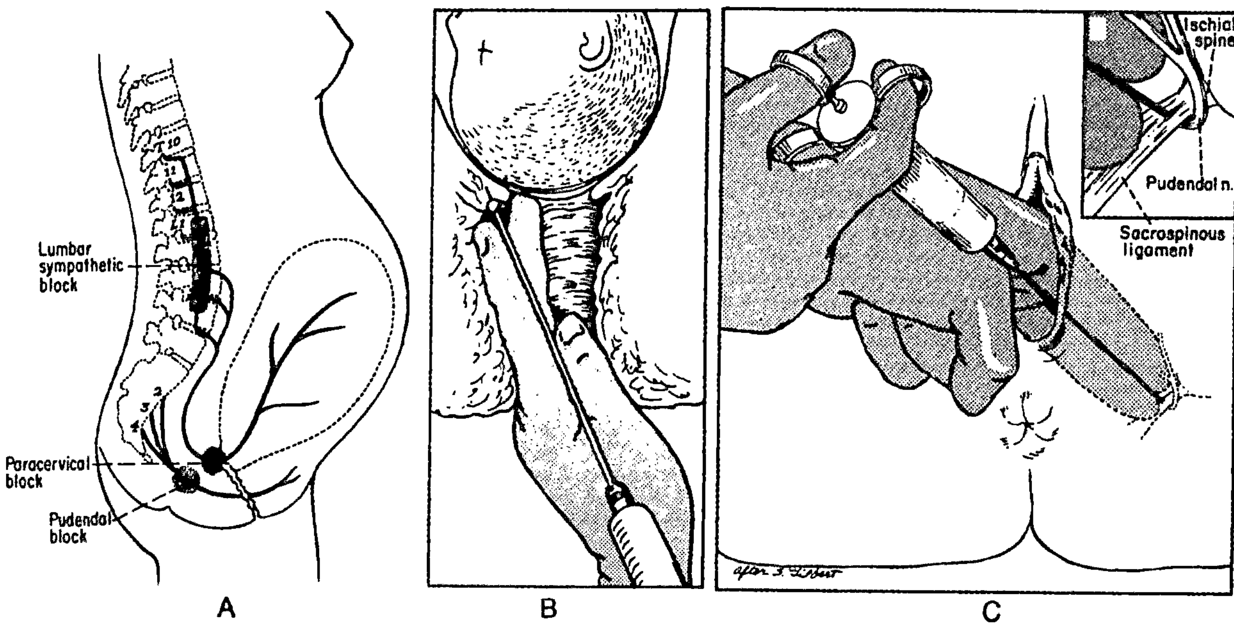

Fig. 29.16 **A** Sites of three regional techniques for obstetric analgesia. Lumbar sympathetic block is rarely used but is highly effective in relieving pain of the first stage and may be preferable to paracervical block, especially in high-risk pregnancies. **B** Schematic coronal section of vagina and lower part of the uterus containing the fetal head, showing the techniques of paracervical block. The 22-gauge. needle is within a guide, with its point protruding only 5–7 mm beyond the end of the guide. This prevents insertion of the needle more than 5–7 mm beyond the surface of the mucosa. After negative aspiration, an injection of 8–10 ml of 0.25% bupivacaine at 4 and 8 o'clock of the cervical fornix will produce relief of uterine pain for several hours. **C** Transvaginal technique of blocking the pudendal nerve. The two fingers of the left hand are inserted into the vagina to guide the needle point into the sacrospinous ligament. As long as the bevel of the needle is in the ligament, there is some resistance to the injection of local anaesthetic, but as soon as the bevel passes through the ligament, there is sudden lack of resistance, indicating that the needle point is next to the nerve. (Modified from Bonica 1967.)

stage analgesia if performed by an expert who is skilled in the anatomy of those specific nerve areas. The paracervical block (Fig 29.17) is used in some centres now in dilute local anaesthetic concentrations only. However, in many parts of the country, this excellent regional block has been abandoned because of the problems of bradycardia in the fetus after administration of the drug to the mother. It was a very popular method of pain relief and was extremely effective for many years. The reasons are that it could be given by the obstetrician, took effect immediately and gave really excellent analgesia for much of the painful period of labour. However, unless the technique can be rejuvenated with the discovery of agents that do not stimulate fetal bradycardia, it will probably not be used with much frequency as a first-stage analgesic method. On the other hand, bilateral pudendal block is still being used by obstetricians in those institutions where obstetric anaesthesia services are unavailable.

Epidural analgesia

Over the past several decades epidural analgesia for labour and vaginal delivery and for caesarean section has become increasingly popularized (Shnider et al 1993). The technique has undergone a number of modifications since the 1960s. Initially, the method entailed the intermittent injection of 12–15 ml of 1–1.5% lidocaine or equianaesthetic concentrations of another local anaesthetic that usually produced analgesia from T9–10 to S5 (Fig. 29.18A). While usually effective in providing pain relief throughout labour and delivery, the use of such a relatively high dose of local anaesthetic increased the risk of systemic toxic reactions from accidental intravenous injection or total spinal anaesthesia from accidental subarachnoid injection. In many parturients each injection of local anaesthetic produced a transitory decrease in uterine activity and weakness or even paralysis of the lower limbs and perineal muscles. With loss of control of the lower limbs, this caused discomfort and inconvenience to the patient. Perineal muscle weakness or paralysis diminished resistant forces essential for internal rotation of the presenting part. Sacral anaesthesia also eliminated the afferent limb of the reflex urge to bear down. All of these effects combined to result in prolongation of the second stage and often the need for instrumental delivery (Bonica 1967, 1969, 1980, 1990, Bonica & McDonald 1995).

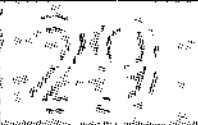

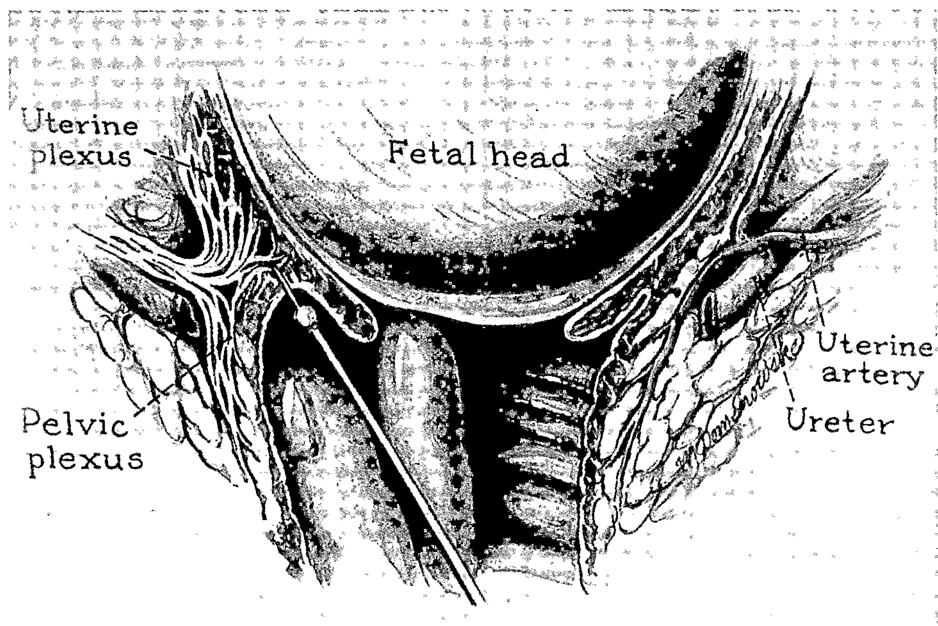

Fig. 29.17 Technique for the paracervical block. (Reproduced from Bonica & McDonald 1995 with permission.)

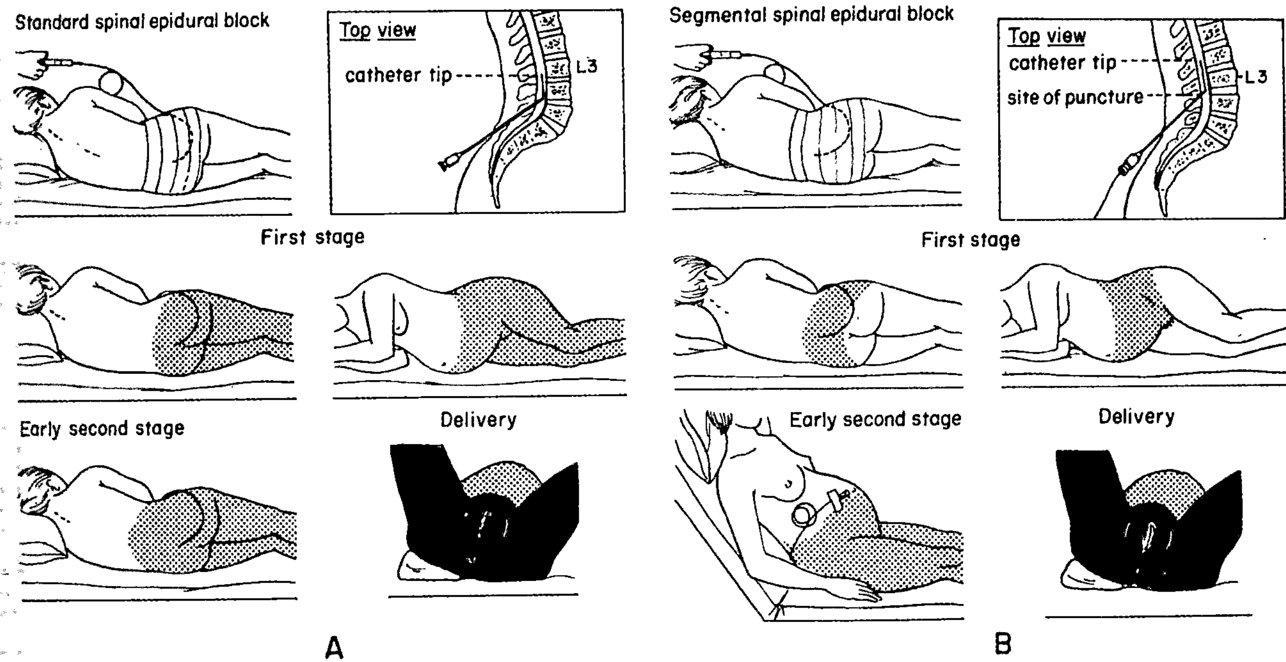

Fig. 29.18 Techniques of lumbar epidural block for labour and vaginal delivery. **A** The standard continuous technique, which is carried out as follows: after starting a preload infusion of fluid, a continuous catheter is inserted through a needle placed in the L4 interspace and advanced until its tip is at the L3 vertebra. With the onset of moderate pain, a test dose is injected and, if negative, 10–12 ml of a local anaesthetic (e.g. 0.25% bupivacaine) is injected to produce analgesia extending from T10–S5. The patient is then made to lie on her side, is given oxygen and frequently monitored, and 'top-up' analgesic doses are injected as soon as pain returns, to produce continuous analgesia. After flexion and internal rotation have occurred, a high concentration of local anaesthetic is injected with the patient in the semirecumbent position to produce perineal relaxation and anaesthesia as depicted (black) in the lower right figure. For the delivery, a wedge is placed under the right buttock to displace the uterus towards the left away from the inferior vena cava and aorta. **B** The technique of segmental epidural analgesia differs slightly from the standard technique in that the catheter is placed higher (L2) and for the first stage the dose is limited to 5–6 ml of local analgesic solution. At the onset of perineal pain, analgesia is extended to the lower lumbar and sacral segments by injecting 10–12 ml of local analgesic solution with the patient in Fowler's position.

These and other concerns led to a series of modifications (Bonica 1995). The first was limiting analgesia to T10–11 during the first stage and then extended to the sacral segments (Fig. 29.18B). As previously mentioned, the continuous epidural block provides an excellent form of obstetric analgesia and anaesthesia (Cleland 1949, Eddleston et al 1992). The advantage of this technique is that less medication is required than with other epidural block techniques mentioned above. It causes no premature numbness or weakness of the lower limbs and no premature weakness of the perineal muscles. So, consequently, there is no interference with flexion or internal rotation. It or its discontinuous counterpart, i.e. patient-controlled epidural infusion, is now used routinely for parturients who request this option. In the 1980s, at obstetric centres where the anaesthetists have had extensive experience with caudal blocks as well as lumbar epidural blocks, the double catheter technique was also used in some of the parturients who required analgesia (Bonica & McDonald 1995). Over several years, the practices have become more widespread of adding opioids to the infusion solution, to enhance the analgesic efficacy of the local anaesthetics and of using infusion pumps that permit more precise administration of the analgesic solution. This last technique has become very popular. In many institutions where anaesthetists provide an obstetric anaesthesia service, it has replaced all other regional techniques for labour and vaginal delivery because it has been shown to:

1. Produce more stable levels of analgesia.
2. Lead to a smaller incidence of maternal hypotension.
3. Decrease the risk of systemic toxic reaction or accidental total spinal anaesthesia.
4. Decrease and, in some instances, eliminate the incidence of motor block, thus obviating the problems mentioned above (Bonica & McDonald 1995).

The lumbar epidural block really became popular only in the late 1960s and early 1970s, although it was a method used by pioneers in the field of anaesthesia for many years prior to this. In the late 1950s, medical papers began to identify the fact that babies born of mothers who received regional anaesthesia were more active and vigorous at delivery than babies born of mothers who received general anaesthesia. In those days, general anaesthesia often meant deep anaesthesia, which meant significant placental transfer and depression of the fetus caused by agents like cyclopropane and ether. Soon afterwards the use of epidural analgesia rather than narcotics and other systemic drugs was found to decrease maternal work, oxygen consumption and maternal and fetal metabolic acidosis (Thalme et al 1974, Zador & Nilsson 1974a, Zador et al 1974b, Sangoul et al 1975, Coalson & Glosten 1991). Another advantage soon discovered was the continuous technique, which meant the mother could benefit from uninterrupted pain relief throughout the entire first stage of labour, and enjoy the benefits of continued pain relief during the second and third stages (Ramanathan 1988).

In the early 1970s, the use of modified techniques came into vogue to try to decrease the amount of drug the fetus would be exposed to. Early attempts included the use of smaller volumes of 8–10 ml of local anaesthetic to get only a T10–12 block for early labour and to increase it slightly to a T10 to L2 block for later labour. This method worked nicely and started the trend in the use of various dosages and agents which has continued. Today the patient gets a very small injection of 8–10 ml of 0.25% bupivacaine followed by a continuous dosage throughout the rest of her labour. The continuous infusion dosage includes a dilute local anaesthetic (0.625% bupivacaine and adrenaline), and a dilute concentration of sufentanil (Bonica & McDonald 1995). The combination is pumped via a pump throughout labour until the patient is ready for delivery. For those who wish to read a more detailed account of the various aspects of this method please refer to the following excellent articles on lumbar epidural for obstetrics: Bonica 1969, Albright et al 1986, Shnider et al 1987, Crosby 1990, Meiklejohn 1990, Gaylard et al 1990, Candido & Winnie 1992, Zarzur & Ganzalves 1992.

The caudal epidural block was popularized before lumbar epidural block as a method of pain relief for labour. It was championed by Cleland and Hingson, who were strong advocates of regional methods of pain relief for mothers as early as the late 1930s and early 1940s. In fact a tremendous popularity was generated around that time and it would have undoubtedly provided for a much earlier acceptance of regional analgesia for labour and delivery had not neurological complications occurred which were secondary to resterilization of equipment and contamination with cleansing solutions. These caused many spinal complications to be recorded in the literature around the mid to late 1940s and early 1950s, so that it retarded the popularity and spread of regional analgesia significantly. Today with our readily disposable needles and catheters the problem is non-existent, except for situations of poor preparation or less than optimum sterile precautions before and during the block. The caudal block, while being ideal for second-stage analgesia, is not perfectly suited for first-stage pain relief because of the fact that a generous amount of local anaesthetic must be used to obtain analgesia at the T10 level from where the catheter tip resides at S4 or S2. In some instances as much as a 20–25 ml volume has been used to effect first-stage pain relief. Of course, all the intermediary segments are also blocked so that the patient does have a resultant large degree sympathetic block with all the attendant complications therein. Nevertheless, it is mentioned because it is such an effective method of pain relief for labour and was the mainstay for so many years earlier in the history of obstetric anaesthesia. More detailed information on performing caudal analgesia can be found in numerous texts (Bonica 1973, Albright et al 1986, Shnider et al 1987, Meiklejohn 1990).

Technique of continuous epidural infusion

A detailed description of the technique of achieving lumbar epidural analgesia is beyond the scope of this chapter. Most clinicians use a single catheter placed with its tip in the upper lumbar epidural space (Gieraerts et al 1992). To introduce the catheter, I prefer the use of a Touhy needle via the paramedian technique (Bonica 1980). Once the catheter is fixed in place and all the monitoring and resuscitation equipment is available for immediate use, anaesthetic consisting of 3 ml 0.25% bupivacaine and 1 : 200 000 adrenaline is injected. Alternatively, 10 ml of bupivacaine 0.125% with 12.5 μg of adrenaline can be used (Williams et al 1990). If no signs of intravenous or subarachnoid injection develop within 5 minutes, a single bolus of 5 ml of 0.25% bupivacaine is injected as a priming dose. This usually produces analgesia extending from T9–T10 to L1–L2 (Fig. 29.19). As soon as this is achieved, a continuous infusion of a solution containing 0.0625% bupivacaine and 0.002% fentanyl (2 μg/ml) is initiated at a rate of 10–12 ml/h, and this is subsequently increased or decreased to maintain analgesia with the upper level at T10. Usually a total of 120 ml of solution is prepared. Some clinicians use a mixture of 30 ml of 0.25% bupivacaine, 60 μg of sufentanyl and 200 μg of adrenaline in a 120 ml volume (McIntosh & Rayburn 1991). It is easy to deliver precisely the needed amounts of drugs and the unit is small and portable so that ambulation during the early part of labour is feasible. Some obstetricians prefer this in the early first stage because they believe it enhances labour. A unique advantage related to portability is that it has a self-contained medication cassette with a capacity of 100 ml of solution and thus obviates the need to have a separate medication bottle that requires a pole for its suspension. There are many infusion pumps now available that subserve the needs of the labouring patient.

Throughout labour and until delivery, if the patient prefers to lie in bed, she is placed in the left or right lateral position with the upper part of the body raised about 15–20°. With each subsequent hour, the extent of cephalad level of analgesia remains fairly constant at T10, but the caudal level tends to extend. After about the third or fourth hour, analgesia usually involves all of the lumbar and sacral segments (Fig. 29.19E). In about 50–60% of the parturients, the sacral analgesia is sufficient for perineal analgesia. The patient is examined prior to delivery, and if sacral analgesia is incomplete 10 ml of 1% lidocaine or 2% chloroprocaine are given with the patient in the sitting position. This usually produces sufficient analgesia and perineal relaxation for the actual delivery.

The extension of the continuous epidural infusion is the patient controlled epidural analgesic delivery system. The studies that have compared these two techniques reveal similar advantages for the patients and no real differences in patient preferences of one over the other (Bonica 1980, Gambling et al 1990, Ferrante et al 1991).

Technique of spinal–epidural

One last technique must be mentioned that has gained momentum recently, the spinal–epidural combination technique where a 27-gauge spinal needle is passed via the standard 18-gauge thin-walled epidural needle for delivery of a small amount of subarachnoid opioid. First the lumbar epidural needle is placed and the usual entry into the epidural space is assured. Next the small-gauge spinal needle is passed through the epidural needle until the dura is contacted. After the spinal needle contacts the dura a puncture is made and a small amount of opioid is injected for the purpose of providing analgesia without significant sympathetic blockade and without significant motor paralysis of the lower extremities. Some refer to this method as the 'walking epidural', because the patient is able to control her legs and has good first-stage pain relief due to the opioid in the subarachnoid space, but has no motor loss of any note (Norris et al 1998). The last advantage mentioned is especially important during the second stage; the incidence of lack of rotation of the presenting part is decreased and the mother can voluntarily mobilize her expulsive forces to augment those of labour to achieve spontaneous delivery. In centres with obstetric anaesthesia services, standard continuous epidural block or continuous segmental block (Fig. 29.18) were the procedures of choice for most parturients up to a decade ago. Continuous caudal block was formerly used widely, but, as mentioned, the increasing use of continuous lumbar epidural block has replaced it almost entirely in most centres. It is still being used infrequently in a few academic centres as part of the double catheter epidural technique. Unfortunately, in the USA, the UK and other countries, there is now little training in the caudal block technique.

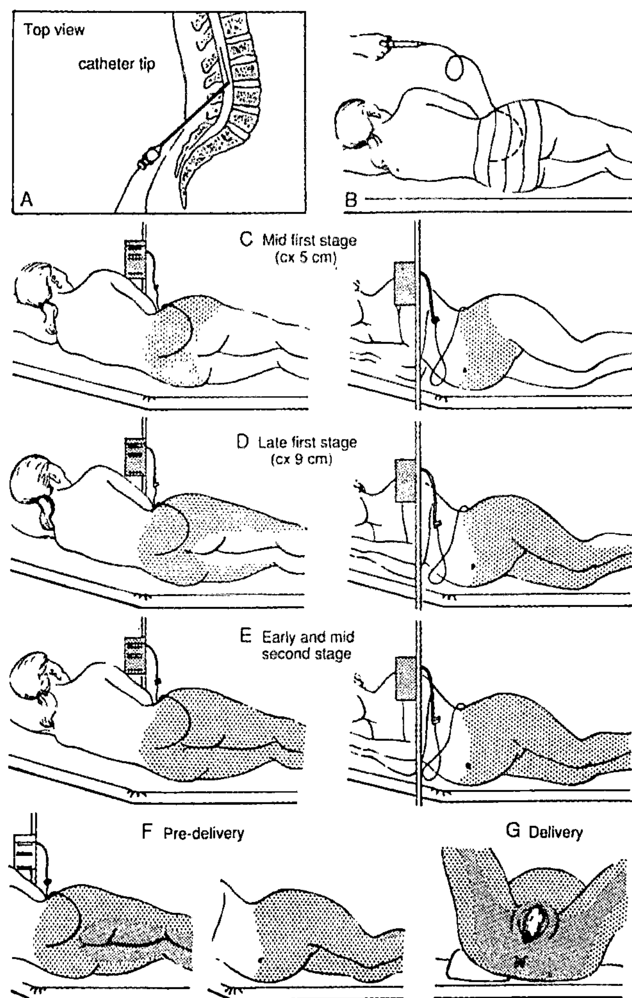

Fig. 29.19 Schematic illustration showing technique of continuous epidural analgesia and the extent and intensity of analgesia during the first and second stages of labour and for delivery. **A** The epidural needle and catheter in place. After removing the needle, the catheter is taped to the patient's back and a test dose of local anaesthetic given. **B** If after 5 min there is no sign of accidental intravenous or subarachnoid injection, a bolus of 5 ml of local anaesthetic is injected while the patient is in the lateral position. **C** After signs of epidural analgesia of T9–10 to 1–2 are noted, the catheter is connected to the continuous infusion system and the solution is administered at a rate of 10–12 ml/h with the patient in a 15–20° head-up position, lying on her side. **D** Extent of analgesia after 1.5–2 h of infusion. **E** Extent of analgesia in the early and mid-second stage. **F** After internal rotation has occurred, injection of a bolus of 10 ml of local anaesthetic solution (e.g. 1% lidocaine) produces an increase in the intensity of analgesia indicated by the more heavily shaded area involving the lower sacral segments. **G** The patient is ready for delivery. Note the wedge under the right hip and lower region to help displace the uterus to the left. (See text for details.)

Technique of continuous epidural infusion

A detailed descriptive of the actual technique of performing and achieving lumbar epidural analgesia will not be found in this chapter. However for the purpose of general description it can be said that: most clinicians use a single catheter with its tip near T10–T11 from needle entry at the second or third lumbar epidural space. Most clinicians prefer to use a Touhy needle via the midline or the paramedian technique (Bonica & McDonald 1995). A catheter is fixed in place and all monitoring and resuscitation equipment is checked, a test dose of 3 ml of 0.25% bupivacaine and 1 : 200 000 adrenaline is injected. Signs of intravenous or subarachnoid injection are carefully watched for within the next 5 minutes. A single bolus of 5 ml of 0.25% bupivacaine is injected as a priming dose. This usually produces analgesia extending from T9–10 to L1–2 (Fig. 34.18C). As soon as this is achieved, a continuous infusion of a solution containing 0.0625% bupivacaine and 0.0002% fentanyl (2 mg/ml) is administered at a rate of 10 ml/h and this is subsequently increased or decreased to maintain analgesia with the upper level at T10. Usually a total of 120 ml of solution is prepared. Some clinicians use a mixture of 30 ml of 0.25% bupivacaine, 60 μg of sufentanil and 200 μg of epinephrine in a 120 ml volume.

This method makes it easy to deliver precisely the needed amounts of medication; the pump unit is small and portable so that ambulation during the early part of labour is feasible. Some obstetricians prefer this method of delivery in early first stage because they believe it enhances labour. A unique advantage related to portability is that it has a self-contained medication cassette with a capacity of 100 ml of solution and thus obviates the need to have a separate medication bottle that requires a pole for its suspension. There are many infusion pumps now available that subserve the needs of the labouring patient.

During all of labour and until delivery, if the patient prefers to lie in bed, she can be put in the left or right lateral decubitus position with the upper part of the body raised just slightly. Throughout labour hour after hour, the cephalad level of analgesia stays constant at T10, but an interesting phenomena occurs at the caudal level because it tends to extend downward. By the third or fourth hour, analgesia usually involves all of the lumbar and sacral segments (Fig. 29.19E). We found that in 50–60% of the parturients, the sacral analgesia is sufficient for perineal analgesia. The patient is examined prior to delivery and if sacral analgesia is incomplete, 10 ml of 1% lidocaine or 2% chloroprocaine is injected in the epidural catheter with the patient in the sitting position; if analgesia is still unacceptable a bilateral pudendal block is given. This usually produces sufficient analgesia and perineal relaxation for the actual delivery.

REFERENCES

Adams JQ, Alexander Jr AM 1958 Alterations in cardiovascular physiology during labour. Obstetrics and Gynecology 12: 542–549

Albright GA, Ferguson JE, Joyce TH, Stephenson DK 1986 Anaesthesia in obstetrics: maternal, fetal and neonatal aspects, 2nd edn. Butterworths, London

Atlee HB 1956 Natural childbirth. Springfield, Charles C Thomas

Behan RJ 1914 Pain. Appleton, New York

Berkley KJ 1990 The role of various peripheral afferent fibers in pain sensation produced by distension of the vaginal canal in rats. Pain (suppl 5): S239

Berkley KJ, Wood E 1989 Responses to varying intensities of vaginal distension in the awake rat. Society of Neuroscience Abstracts 15: 979

Berkley KJ, Robbins A, Sato Y 1988 Afferent fibres supplying the uterus in the rat. Journal of Neurophysiology 59: 142–163

Berkley KJ, Robbins A, Sato Y 1993a Functional differences between afferent fibres in hypogastric and pelvic nerves innervating the female reproductive organs in the rat. Journal of Neurophysiology 69: 533–544

Berkley KJ, Hubscher CH, Wall PD 1993b Neuronal responses to stimulation of the cervix, uterus, colon and skin in the rat spinal cord. Pain 69: 545–556

Bonica JJ 1967 Principles and practice of obstetric analgesia and anesthesia, vol 1. FA Davis, Philadelphia

Bonica JJ 1969 Principles and practice of obstetric analgesia and anesthesia, vols 1, 2. Philadelphia, FA Davis

Bonica JJ 1973 Matérnal respiratory changes during pregnancy and parturition. In: Marx GF (ed) Parturition and perinatology. FA Davis, Philadelphia

Bonica JJ 1980 Obstetric analgesia and anaesthesia, 2nd edn. World Federation of Societies of Anaesthesiologists, Amsterdam/University of Washington Press, Seattle

Bonica JJ, Hunter Jr CA 1969 Management in dysfunction of the forces of labor. In: Bonica JJ (ed) Principles and practice of obstetric analgesia and anesthesia, vol 2. FA Davis, Philadelphia

Bonica JJ, McDonald JS 1990 The pain of childbirth. In: Bonica JJ (ed) The management of pain, 2nd edn. Lea & Febiger, Malvern, Pennsylvania, pp 1313–1343

Bonica JJ, McDonald JS (eds) Principles and practice of obstetric analgesia and anesthesia, 2nd edn. Lea & Febiger, Malvern, Pennsylvania, p 1

Bonica JJ, McDonald JS 1995 Principles and practice of obstetric analgesia and anesthesia, 2nd edn. Williams & Wilkins, Baltimore

Brown WA, Manning T, Grodin J 1972 The relationship of antenatal and perinatal variables to the use of drugs in labor. Psychosomatic Medicine 34: 119–127

Brownridge P 1991 Treatment options for the relief of pain during childbirth. Drugs 41: 69–80

Buchan PC 1980 Emotional stress in childbirth and its modification by variations in obstetric management – epidural analgesia and stress in labor. Acta Obstetricia et Gynecologica Scandinavica 59: 319–321

Caldwell J, Wakile LA, Notarianni LJ et al 1978 Maternal and neonatal disposition of pethidine in childbirth – a study using quantitative gas chromotography – mass spectometry. Life Sciences 22: 589–596

Candido KD, Winnie AP 1992 A dual-chambered syringe that allows identification of the epidural space using the loss of resistance technique with air and with saline. Regional Anesthesia 17: 163–165

Carstoniu J, Levytam S, Norman P et al 1994 Nitrous oxide in labour: safety and efficacy assessed by a double-blind placebo controlled study. Anesthesiology 80: 30–35

Chestnut DH 1994 Obstetric anesthesia principles and practice.

Cleland JGP 1949 Continuous peridural and caudal analgesia in obstetrics. Current Research in Anesthesia and Analgesia 28: 61

Coalson DW, Glosten B 1991 Alternatives to epidural analgesia. Seminars in Perinatology 15: 375–385

Cole PV, Nainby-Luxmoore RC 1962 Respiratory volumes in labour. British Medical Journal 1: 1118

Crawford JS 1984 Principles and practice of obstetric analgesia and anaesthesia, 5th edn. Blackwell, Oxford

Crosby ET 1990 Epidural catheter migration during labour and hypothesis for inadequate analgesia. Canadian Journal of Anesthesia 37: 789–793

Cugell DW et al 1953 Pulmonary function in pregnancy; serial observations in normal women. American Review of Tuberculosis 67: 568

Davenport-Slack B, Boylan CH 1974 Psychological correlates of childbirth pain. Psychosomatic Medicine 36: 215–223

Deutsch H 1955 Psychology of pregnancy, labour and puerperium. In: Greenhill JP (ed) Obstetrics, 11th edn. WB Saunders, Philadelphia, pp 349–360

Dick-Read G 1933 Natural childbirth. Heinemann, London

Dick-Read G 1953 Childbirth without fear. Harper, New York

Eddleston JM, Maresh M, Horsman EL, Young H 1992 Comparison of maternal and fetal effects associated with intermittent or continuous infusion or extradural analgesia. British Journal of Anaesthesia 69: 154–158

Ferrante FM, Lu L, Jamison SB, Datta S 1991 Patient-controlled epidural analgesia: demand dosing. Anesthesia and Analgesia 73: 547–552

Fisher A, Prys-Roberts C 1968 Maternal pulmonary gas exchange: a study during normal labour and external blockade. Anaesthesia 23: 350–355

Ford CS A comparative study of human reproduction. Yale University Press, New Haven, Connecticut

Freedman LZ, Ferguson VS 1950 The question of 'painless childbirth' in primitive cultures. American Journal of Orthopsychiatry 20: 363–379

Fridh G, Kopare T, Gaston-Johansson F, Norvell KT 1988 Factors associated with more intense labor pain. Research in Nursing and Health 11: 117–124

Gabbe, Steven G 1991 Obstetrics – normal and problem pregnancies, 2nd edn. Churchill Livingstone, Edinburgh

Gambling DR, McMorland GH, Yu P, Laszlo C 1990 Comparison of patient-controlled epidural analgesia and conventional intermittent 'top-up' injections during labor. Anesthesia and Analgesia 70: 256–261

Gaston-Johansson F, Fridh G, Turner-Norvell K 1988 Progression of labor pain in primiparas and multiparas. Nursing Research 37: 86–90

Gaylard D 1990 Epidural analgesia by continuous infusion. In: Reynolds F (ed) Epidural and spinal blockade in obstetrics. Baillière Tindall, London, pp 49–58

Gerdin A, Salmonson T, Lindberg B, Rane A 1990 Maternal kinetics of morphine during labor. Journal of Perinatal Medicine 18: 479–487

Gieraerts R, Van Zundert A, De Wolf A, Vaes L 1992 Ten ml bupivacaine 0.125% with 12.5 μ epinephrine is a reliable epidural test dose to detect inadvertent intravascular injection in obstetric patients. A double-blind study. Acta Anaesthesiologica Scandinavica 36: 656–659

Glassenberg R 1991 General anesthesia and maternal mortality. Seminars in Perinatology 15: 386–396

Hansen JM, Ueland K 1966 The influence of caudal analgesia on cardiovascular dynamics during normal labour and delivery. Acta Anaesthesiologica Scandinavica 23 (suppl 10): 449–452

Hayes JR, Ardill J, Kennedy TL, Shanks RG, Buchanan KD 1972 Stimulation of gastrin release by catecholamines. Lancet i: 819–821

Head H 1893 On disturbances of sensation with special reference to the pain of visceral disease. Brain 16: 1

Hendricks CH, Quilligan EJ 1956 Cardiac output during labor. American Journal of Obstetrics and Gynecology 71: 953–972

Holdsworth JD 1978 Relationships between stomach contents and analgesia in labour. British Journal of Anaesthesia 50: 1145–1148

Huch A, Huch R, Schneider H, Rooth G 1977 Continuous transcutaneous monitoring of foetal oxygen tension during labour. British Journal of Obstetrics and Gynaecology 84 (suppl 1): 1–39

Hughey MJ, McElin TW, Young T 1978 Maternal and fetal outcome of Lamaze-prepared patients. Obstetrics and Gynecology 51: 643–647

Huszar G, Cabrol D, Naftolin F 1986 The relationship between myometrial contractility and cervical maturation. In: Huszar G (ed) The physiology and biochemistry of the uterus in pregnancy and labor. CRC Press, Baca Raton, FL

Jouppila R 1977 The effect of segmental epidural analgesia on hormonal and metabolic changes during labour. Acta Universitatis Ouluensis, Series D, Medica No 16, Anaesthesiologica No 2

Jouppilla R, Hollmen A 1976 The effect of segmental epidural analgesia on maternal and foetal acid-base balance, lactate, serum potassium and creatine phosphokinase during labour. Acta Anaesthesiologica Scandinavica 20: 259–268

Kawatani M, de Groat WC 1991 A large proportion of afferent neurons innervating the uterine cervix of the cat contain VIP and other neuropeptides. Cell and Tissue Research 266: 191–196

Kawatani M, Takeshige C, Narasimhan S, De Groat WC 1986 An analysis of the afferent and efferent pathways to the uterus of the cat using axonal tracing techniques. Society of Neuroscience Abstracts 12: 1055

Klink EW 1953 Perineal nerve block: an anatomic and clinical study in the female. Obstetrics and Gynecology 1: 137–146

Lamaze F 1956 Qu'est-ce que l'accouchement sans douleur par la méthode psychoprophylactique? Ses principles, sa réalization, ses résultants. Savoir et Connâitre, Paris

Lamaze F, Vellay P 1952 L'accouchement sans douleur par la methode psycholophysique: premiers resultats portant sur 500 cas. Gaz Med Fr 59: 1445

Lederman RP, McCann DS, Work B, Huber MJ 1977 Endogenous plasma epinephrine and norepinephrine in last-trimester pregnancy and labour. American Journal of Obstetrics and Gynecology 129: 5–8

Lederman RP, Lederman E, Work BA Jr, McCann DS 1978 The relationship of maternal anxiety, plasma catecholamines, and plasma cortisol to progress in labor. American Journal of Obstetrics and Gynecology 132: 495–500

Lee R 1844 Lectures on the theory and practice of midwifery. Barrington and Hoswell, Philadelphia

Lees MM, Scott DB, Kerr MG 1970 Haemodynamic changes associated with labour. Journal of Obstetrics and Gynaecology of the British Commonwealth 77: 29–36

Lowe NK 1989 Explaining the pain of active labor: the importance in maternal confidence. Research in Nursing and Health 12: 237–245

McIntosh DG, Rayburn WF 1991 Patient-controlled analgesia in obstetrics and gynecology. Obstetrics and Gynecology 70: 202–204

McLintic AJ, Danskin SH, Reid JA, Thorburn J 1991 Effects of adrenaline on extradural anesthesia, plasma lignocaine concentrations and feto-placental unit during elective cesarean section. British Journal of Anaesthesia 67: 683–689

Marx GF, Greene NM 1964 Maternal lactate, pyruvate and excess lactate production during labor and delivery. American Journal of Obstetrics and Gynecology 90: 786–793

Marx GF, Katsnelson T 1992 The introduction of nitrous oxide into obstetrics. Obstetrics and Gynecology 80: 715–718

Meiklejohn BH 1990 Distance from the skin to the lumbar epidural space in an obstetric population. Regional Anesthesia 3: 134–136

Melzack R 1984 The myth of painless childbirth. The John J. Bonica Lecture. Pain 19: 321

Melzack R, Taenzer P, Feldman P, Kinch RA 1981 Labour is still painful after prepared childbirth training. Canadian Medical Association Journal 125: 357–363

Moir DD, Willocks J 1967 Management of incoordinate uterine action under continuous epidural analgesia. British Medical Journal 3: 396–400

Moore DC, Batra MS 1981 The components of an effective test dose prior to epidural block. Anesthesiology 55: 693–696

Morishima HO, Pedersen H, Finster M 1978 The influence of maternal psychological stress on the fetus. American Journal of Obstetrics and Gynecology 131: 286–290

Morishima HO, Pedersen H, Finster M 1980 Effects of pain on mother, labour and fetus. In: Marx GF, Bassel GM (eds) Obstetric analgesia and anaesthesia. Elsevier/North Holland, Amsterdam, pp 197–210

Myers RE 1975 Maternal psychological stress and fetal asphyxia: a study in the monkey. American Journal of Obstetrics and Gynecology 122: 47–59

Nettelbladt P, Fagerstrom CF, Uddenberg N 1976 The significance of reported childbirth pain. Journal of Psychosomatic Research 20: 215–221

Nimmo WS, Wilson J, Prescott LF 1975 Narcotic analgesics and delayed gastric emptying during labour. Lancet i: 890

Norman PH, Kavanagh B, Daley MD et al 1992 Nitrous oxide analgesia in labour (abstract). Anesthesia and Analgesia 74: S222

Norr KL, Block CR, Charles A, Meyering S, Meyers E 1977 Explaining pain and enjoyment in childbirth. Journal of Health and Social Behavior 18: 260–275

Norris MC, Fogel ST, Holtmann B 1998 Intrathecal sufentantil (5 vs. 10 microg) for labor analgesia: efficacy and side effects. Regional Anesthesia and Pain in Medicine 23: 252–257

Ohno H, Yamashita K, Yahata et al 1986 Maternal plasma concentrations of catecholamines and cyclic nucleotides during labor and following delivery. Research Communications in Chemical Pathology and Pharmacology 51: 183–194

Peabody JL 1979 Transcutaneous oxygen measurement to evaluate drug effect. Clinical Perinatology 6: 109–121

Pearson JF, Davies P 1973 The effect of continuous epidural analgesia on the acid-base status of maternal arterial blood during the first state of labour. Journal of Obstetrics and Gynaecology of the British Commonwealth 80: 218–224

Pearson JF, Davies P 1974 The effect of continuous lumbar epidural analgesia on the acid-base status of maternal arterial blood during the first state of labour. Journal of Obstetrics and Gynaecology of the British Commonwealth 81: 975–979

Peters LC, Kristal MB, Komisaruk BR 1987 Sensory innervation of the external and internal genitalia of the female rat. Brain Research 402: 199–204

Prowse CM, Gaensler EA 1965 Respiratory and acid-base changes during pregnancy. Anesthesiology 26: 381–392

Ramanathan S 1988 Obstetric anesthesia. Lea & Febiger, Philadelphia

Reading AE, Cox DN 1985 Psychosocial predictors of labor pain. Pain 22: 309–315

Robson SC, Dunlop W, Boys RJ, Hunter S 1987 Cardiac output during labor. British Medical Journal 295: 1169–1172

Rosaeg OP, Kitts JB, Koren G, Byford LL 1992 Maternal and fetal effects of intravenous patient-controlled fentanyl analgesia during labour in a thrombocytopenic parturient. Canadian Journal of Anesthesia 39: 277–281

Sangoul F, Fox GS, Houle GL 1975 Effect of regional analgesia on maternal oxygen consumption during the first stage of labor. American Journal of Obstetrics and Gynecology 121: 1080

Scott JR, Rose NB 1976 Effect of psychoprophylaxis on labor and delivery in primiparas. New England Journal of Medicine 294: 1205–1207

Scott-Palmer J, Skevington SM 1981 Pain during childbirth and menstruation: a study of locus of control. Journal of Psychosomatic Research 25: 151

Shnider SM, Levinson G 1986 Anesthesia for obstetrics, 2nd edn. Williams & Wilkins, Baltimore

Shnider SM, Levinson G 1987 Anesthesia for obstetrics, 3rd edn. Williams & Wilkins, Philadelphia

Shnider SM, Levinson G, Ralston DH 1993 Regional anesthesia in labor and vaginal delivery. In: Shnider SM, Levinson G (eds) Anesthesia for obstetrics, 3rd edn. Williams & Wilkins, Baltimore, pp 135–153

Stewart DE 1982 Psychiatric symptoms following attempted natural childbirth. Canadian Medical Association Journal 127: 713–716

Swart F, Abboud TK, Zhu J et al 1991 Desflurance analgesia in obstetrics: maternal and neonatal effects (abstract). Anesthesiology 75: A844

Thalme B, Belfrage P, Raabe N 1974 Lumbar epidural analgesia in labour. Acta Obstetricia et Gynaecologica Scandinavica 53: 27–35, 113–119

Tomkinson J et al 1982 Report on confidential inquiries into maternal death in England and Wales 1976–1978. Report on Health and Social Subjects No 16. HMSO, London

Williams B, Kwan K, Chen B, Wu Y 1990 Comparison of 0.0312% bupivacaine plus sufental and 0.0625% bupivacaine plus sufental for epidural anesthesia during labor and delivery. Anesthesiology 73: A950

Zador G, Nilsson BA 1974a Low-dose intermittent epidural anesthesia with lidocaine for vaginal delivery. II. Influence of labour and foetal acid-base status. Acta Obstetricia et Gynaecologica Scandinavica Supplementum 34: 17

Zador G, Englesson S, Nilsson BA 1974b Low dose intermittent epidural anaesthesia with lidocaine for vaginal delivery

Zarzur E, Gonzalves JJ 1992 The resistance of the human dura mater to needle penetration. Regional Anesthesia 17: 216–218

Zuckerman M, Nurnberger JI, Gardiner SH, Vandiveer JM, Barrett BH, den Breeijen A 1963 Psychological correlates of somatic complaints in pregnancy and difficulty in childbirth. Journal of Consulting and Clinical Psychology 27: 324–329

Genitourinary pain

URSULA WESSELMANN & ARTHUR L. BURNETT

INTRODUCTION

Chronic non-malignant pain syndromes (longer than 6 months' duration) of the genitourinary tract are well described but poorly understood, and often very frustrating for the patients and their physicians. Pain in these areas of the body is usually very embarrassing for the male and female patient, who may be afraid to discuss his/her symptoms with family members, friends and healthcare providers. Except in those cases in which a specific secondary cause can be identified, the aetiology of the chronic genitourinary pain syndromes often remains unknown. The controversy that surrounds these pain syndromes ranges from questioning their existence to dismissing them as purely psychosomatic. This is counterbalanced by an extensive literature attesting to their organicity. Patients with these pain syndromes often suffer for many years, have seen numerous physicians in numerous subspecialties, and are frustrated, embarrassed and frequently depressed. Despite the challenge inherent in the management of chronic genitourinary pain, many patients can be treated successfully. Effective treatment modalities, although often empirical only, are available to lessen the impact of pain and offer reasonable expectations of an improved functional status. The focus of this chapter is on chronic non-malignant genitourinary pain syndromes. Another very important issue is the management of pain syndromes associated with cancer of the genitourinary tract (see Ch. 45 for a discussion of cancer pain). The present chapter first reviews the current knowledge of the neurobiology of the genitourinary tract, which is a prerequisite for trying to understand the chronic pain syndromes in this area. We will then discuss, the clinical presentation, aetiology and differential diagnosis of chronic genitourinary pain and review treatment options are discussed.

NEUROBIOLOGY OF THE GENITOURINARY TRACT

The foundation for understanding the neurobiology of the genitourinary tract relates to a proper familiarity with the neuroanatomical and neurochemical principles that characterize the neuroregulation and sensory processing of genitourinary organs. This section is organized with the purpose of presenting initially a generalized overview of the peripheral neuronal supply of the genitourinary tract and then including a more detailed discussion of the precise innervation and neurochemical basis required for functional aspects of various regions of the genitourinary tract. The description of the neuroanatomy adheres to the anatomical nomenclature (Nomina Anatomica 1977), with terms often applied in clinical usage indicated in brackets (Baljet & Drukker 1980). While this summary attempts to derive as much information as possible from studies involving humans, some generalizations had to be taken necessarily from animal studies, where human data were not available.

The innervation of the genitourinary tract is commonly appreciated to be served by both divisions of the autonomic nervous system, the sympathetic and parasympathetic divisions, as well as the somatic and sensory nervous systems (Morrison 1987, de Groat et al 1993, de Groat 1994). Autonomic pathways are represented by dual projections from the thoracolumbar and sacral segments of the spinal cord that converge primarily into discrete neuronal plexuses which then provide nerve fibres extending throughout the retroperitoneum and pelvis (Figs 30.1, 30.2). Visceral afferents travel with the sympathetic and parasympathetic divisions and are sometimes labelled sympathetic and parasympathetic afferents. This nomenclature, however, has

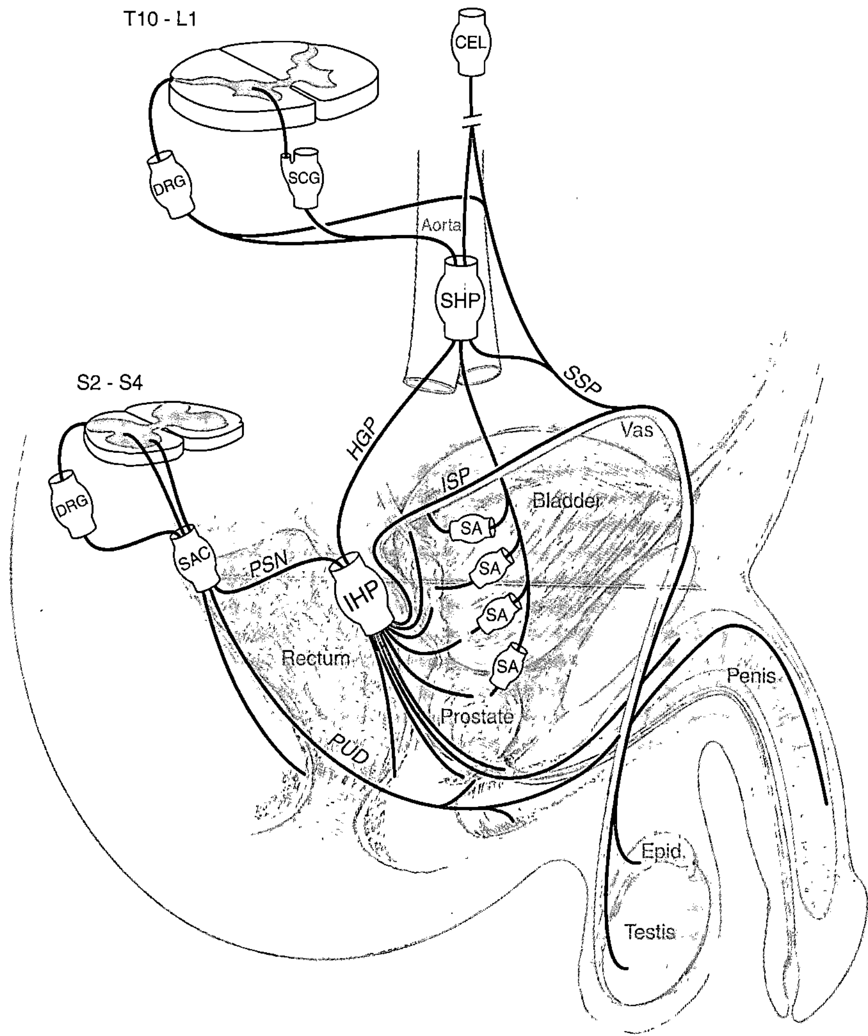

Fig. 30.1 The innervation of the urogenital and rectal area in *males*. Although this diagram attempts to show the innervation in humans, much of the anatomical information is derived from animal data (see text). CEL = coeliac plexus; DRG = dorsal root ganglion; Epid. = epididymis; HGP = hypogastric plexus; IHP = inferior hypogastric plexus; ISP = inferior spermatic plexus; PSN = pelvic splanchnic nerve; PUD = pudendal nerve; SA = short adrenergic projections; SAC = sacral plexus; SCG = sympathetic chain ganglion; SHP = superior hypogastric plexus; SSP = superior spermatic plexus. (Reproduced from Wesselmann et al 1997 with permission.)

been criticized, because of the lack of an unequivocal correlation between pathway of projection and functional role (Cervero 1994), and it has been suggested that visceral afferents should be described by their anatomical, rather than their functional pathway of projection. In reference to origins at the spinal cord level, autonomic preganglionic efferents arise for the most part in the intermediolateral cell column, referred to as the sacral parasympathetic nucleus at sacral levels, whereas cell bodies of corresponding afferents are contained within dorsal root ganglia. The sympathetic thoracolumbar outflow of particular relevance to the genitourinary tract involves preganglionic projections to the coeliac plexus and to the superior hypogastric plexus [presacral nerve] (Ferguson & Bell 1993, Lincoln & Burnstock 1993). The coeliac plexus, which lies on the anterior aorta surrounding the coeliac arterial trunk and connects with paired coeliac ganglia laterally, provides the majority of the autonomic innervation to the adrenal, kidney, renal pelvis and ureter, as well as some sympathetic input to the testes along the course of the internal spermatic vessels. The superior hypogastric plexus (presacral nerve), situated at the lower extent of the abdominal aorta at its bifurcation, represents the majority of the sympathetic input to the pelvic urinary organs and genital tract. In addition to this route in supplying pelvic structures, thoracolumbar preganglionic nerves also synapse on postganglionic nerves in sympathetic chain ganglia that commingle with autonomic sacral nerve projections as well

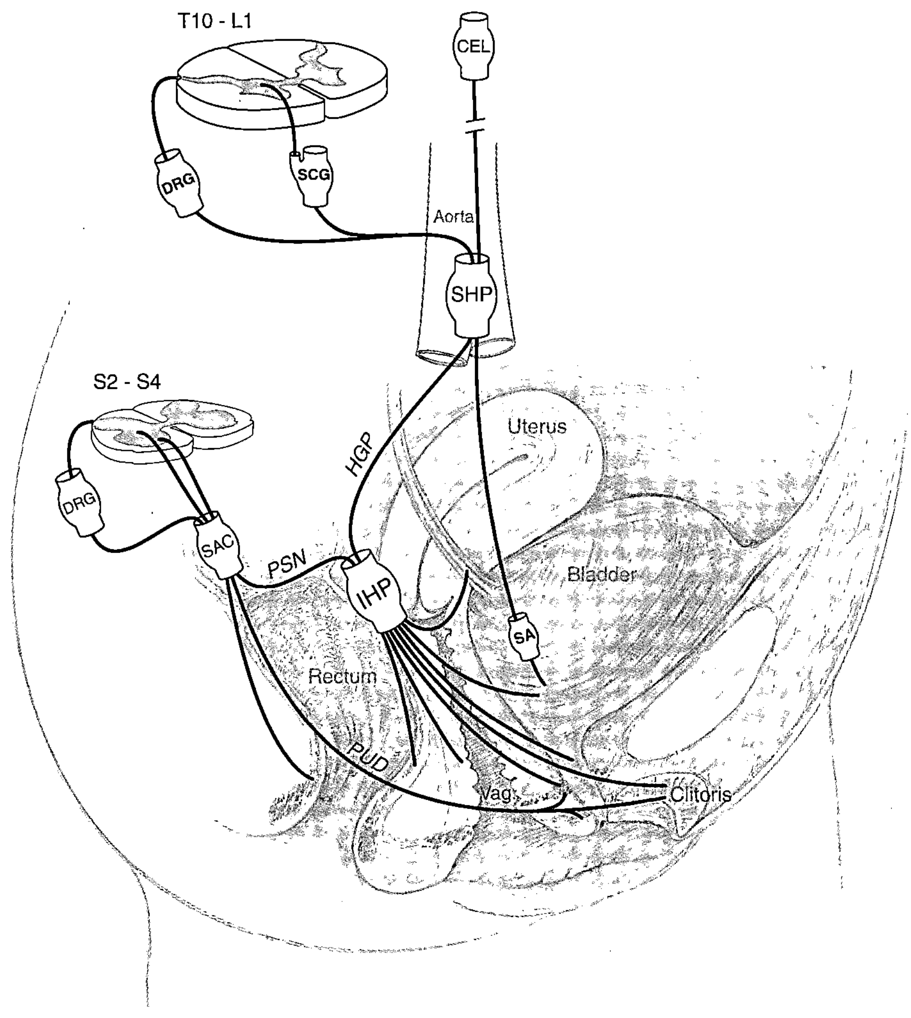

Fig. 30.2 The innervation of the urogenital and rectal area in *females*. Although this diagram attempts to show the innervation in humans, much of the anatomical information is derived from animal data (see text). CEL = coeliac plexus; DRG = dorsal root ganglion; HGP = hypogastric plexus; IHP = inferior hypogastric plexus; PSN = pelvic splanchnic nerve; PUD = pudendal nerve; SA = short adrenergic projections; SAC = sacral plexus; SCG = sympathetic chain ganglion; SHP = superior hypogastric plexus; Vag. = Vagina. (Reproduced from Wesselmann et al 1997 with permission.)

as with pelvic somatic neuronal pathways (McKenna & Nadelhaft 1986). Parasympathetic sacral outflow (S2–S4) consists of preganglionic nerves that are referred to as the pelvic splanchnic nerves (pelvic nerve). Within the pelvis, the inferior hypogastric plexus (pelvic plexus) is the major autonomic neuronal relay centre that supplies visceral structures of the pelvis (Lincoln & Burnstock 1993). It receives sympathetic input from the superior hypogastric plexus (presacral nerve) and its caudal extension, the hypogastric plexus (hypogastric nerve), as well as a component from the sympathetic chain ganglia, and parasympathetic input from the pelvic splanchnic nerve (pelvic nerve) (de Groat 1994). Both efferent and afferent fibres are understood to course in these sympathetic and parasympathetic projections (Jänig & Koltzenburg 1993).

Somatic neuronal outflow to the pelvis also originates from sacral spinal cord levels (S2–S4), represented by efferents originating within Onuf's nucleus in the ventral horn and afferents having cell bodies contained within dorsal root ganglia at these levels (Lincoln & Burnstock 1993). The central level overlapping of somatic afferents with pelvic nerve afferents theoretically affords coordination of somatic and visceral motor activity (McKenna & Nadelhaft 1986). Sacral nerve roots emerge from the spinal cord to form the sacral plexus, from which arises the pudendal nerve as the primary efferent and afferent somatic distribution with various branches involving pelvic viscera and the pelvic floor musculature (Elbadawi 1996). The pudendal nerve also receives terminations of postganglionic axons arising from the caudal sympathetic chain ganglia (de Groat 1994).

UPPER URINARY TRACT NEUROBIOLOGY

The autonomic innervation of the kidney is served by the renal plexus, which is situated behind the ostium of each renal artery (Ferguson & Bell 1993, Kabalin 1998). The plexus represents a confluence of thoracolumbar sympathetic neuronal projections from the coeliac ganglion, aorticorenal ganglion, the aortic plexus, the lowest thoracic nerves and the first lumbar splanchnic nerve, as well as parasympathetic input from the vagus nerve. Using the main renal artery as a scaffold, postganglionic efferents course into the kidney hilum supplying the substance of the kidney. Small renal ganglia may also exist within the renal plexus with distributions along the renal artery. Within the kidney, efferent nerve endings are primarily vasomotor with terminations in proximity to renal vessels, glomeruli and tubules. Afferent fibres originating in the region of the renal capsule and cortex follow the course of the renal artery as well before forming neuronal pathways primarily entering the spinal cord at T11–L2 segmental levels. Some afferent fibres otherwise merge with the vagus nerve. The sympathetic nerves supplying the kidney contain noradrenaline, dopamine, an assortment of neuropeptides, and possibly purinergic substances with a distribution suggesting roles in renal blood flow, renin release and tubular function (Ferguson & Bell 1993). Substance P and calcitonin gene-related peptide have been localized in renal sensory nerves, suggesting their roles in mechanoreceptive, chemoreceptive and nociceptive activities (Ferguson & Bell 1993).

The autonomic innervation of the ureter derives from separate neuronal sources in association with three divisions (Kabalin 1998). The upper third of the ureter is supplied by branches of the renal and aortic plexuses, the middle third by projections from the superior hypogastric plexus (presacral plexus), and the lower third by the hypogastric plexus (hypogastric nerve) and inferior hypogastric plexuses (pelvic plexuses). Noradrenergic, cholinergic and peptidergic nerve fibres have been identified in the ureter, with possible roles in the regulation of motility, epithelial transport and ureterovesical sphincteric activity (Ferguson & Bell 1993).

LOWER URINARY TRACT NEUROBIOLOGY

The direct autonomic nerve supply to the lower urinary tract including the urinary bladder, proximal urethra and lower ureter derives principally from the inferior hypogastric plexus (pelvic plexus) (Lincoln & Burnstock 1993). Postganglionic efferent projections commonly originate within this ganglion, although vesical or intramural ganglia that do not relay in the pelvic plexus also serve as origins for postganglionic axons. While the autonomic innervation from the pelvic plexus supplies the smooth muscle components of the lower urinary tract, it may also contribute to the innervation of the striated musculature of the distal intrinsic urethral sphincter (rhabdosphincter) (Donker 1986, Kumagai et al 1987). The rhabdosphincter is also supplied by somatic innervation consisting of an intrapelvic projection from the pudendal nerve that merges with the pelvic splanchnic nerve (pelvic nerve) and separate pudendal nerve perineal branches (Tanagho et al 1982, Juenemann et al 1988, Zvara et al 1994). Given the extensive appearance of cholinergic terminals within the detrusor smooth muscle, the contractile function of the bladder is generally perceived to be cholinergically mediated (Elbadawi 1996), although other 'transmitter-like substances' such as adenosine 5′-triphosphate are contended to exert a contributory effect in this response (Bo & Burnstock 1995). α_1-adrenergic influences produce smooth muscle contraction at the level of the bladder neck and proximal urethra, with a role in maintaining outlet closure for urinary continence (Krane & Olsson 1973). Non-adrenergic, non-cholinergic influences, most appreciably nitric oxide, may exert effects on proximal urethral smooth muscle relaxation as part of normal micturition (Vizzard et al 1994, Burnett et al 1997). Sensory nerve terminals have been identified throughout the lower urinary tract, with higher concentrations in the bladder neck region and within subepithelial layers of the bladder and urethra (Lincoln & Burnstock 1993). The content of these nerves probably includes neuropeptides, most notably substance P and calcitonin gene-related peptide (De Groat 1987, Maggi & Meli 1988).

MALE REPRODUCTIVE TRACT NEUROBIOLOGY

The autonomic nerve supply to the male internal reproductive tract structures including the prostate, seminal vesicles and the prostatic end of the vas deferens derives mostly from the hypogastric ganglion, the terminal portion of the hypogastric plexus (hypogastric nerve) that also forms the anterior part of the inferior hypogastric plexus (pelvic plexus) (Lincoln & Burnstock 1993). Sympathetic preganglionic efferents typically course through this ganglion and synapse on short adrenergic neurons, termed for postganglionic projections that originate close to and sometimes within the intramural portions of these organs (Dail 1993). Afferent fibre distributions for these organs also include the inferior hypogastric plexus (pelvic plexus) and the hypogastric plexus (hypogastric nerve) (Jänig & Koltzenburg 1993).

The autonomic nerve supply to the male external reproductive tract structures, which refers to the epididymal end of the vas deferens, epididymis and testis, consists of the inferior and superior spermatic plexuses (Hodson 1970, Dail 1993). The inferior spermatic plexus derives from the inferior hypogastric plexus (pelvic plexus) and provides local distributions in following the course of the vas deferens to the caudal epididymis. The superior spermatic plexus accompanies the internal spermatic vessels as a primary neuronal source to the testis and caput and corpus portions of the epididymis, although contributions to these structures include neuronal projections from the inferior spermatic plexus, superior hypogastric plexus (presacral plexus), and other sympathetic chain ganglia. While the superior spermatic plexus is perceived to provide afferent input for the testis and epididymis, the inferior hypogastric plexus (pelvic plexus) may also provide an afferent source with relays through the inferior spermatic plexus (Zorn et al 1994). Afferent innervation involving the parietal and visceral layers of the tunica vaginalis and cremaster is carried by the genital branch of the genitofemoral nerve originating in L1–L2 segments (Peterson & Brown 1973).

The adrenergic effector, noradrenaline, primarily influences contractile properties of male reproductive tract structures, whereas cholinergic mechanisms primarily influence their secretory aspects (McConnell et al 1982). Some evidence exists for the possible roles of purines, neuropeptides and possibly nitric oxide in seminal fluid processing and propulsion (Dail 1993). Adrenergic and cholinergic mechanisms are believed to account for vasomotor responses in the testis (Dail 1993).

MALE AND FEMALE GENITAL ORGAN NEUROBIOLOGY

The innervation of the male and female genitalia combines autonomic and somatic components. In the male, the autonomic component consists of the cavernous nerve, a projection of nerve fibres that derives from the inferior hypogastric plexus (pelvic plexus) and courses distally between the rectum and dorsolateral aspect of the prostate bilaterally within the lateral pelvic fascia (Walsh & Donker 1982, Lue et al 1984, Lepor et al 1985). After penetrating the urogenital diaphragm in proximity to the muscular wall of the urethra at the prostatic apex, it distributes some local terminations within these structures with additional further terminations involving proximal regions of the corpora cavernosa and corpus spongiosum (Paick et al 1993, Burnett & Mostwin 1998). The somatic component consists of the dorsal nerve of the penis which represents an initial branch of the pudendal nerve that terminates with dorsal branches supplying the glans penis and lateral branches supplying lateral and ventral aspects of the penile shaft and distal regions of the corpus spongiosum (Yang & Bradley 1998). Multiple communications appear to exist between the cavernous nerve and dorsal nerve of the penis at the penile hilum, suggesting that the dorsal nerve may serve as an autonomic carrier to the distal portions of the penis or itself contain autonomic nerve fibres (Paick et al 1993). Sensory influences in the penis involve afferent fibres carried in the dorsal nerve projections and possibly also in the cavernous nerve.

In the female, the autonomic component consists of nerve trunks that mostly derive from the paracervical ganglia part of the inferior hypogastric plexus and course in the adventitia of the vagina parallel to its long axis, before distributing anterior branches to the clitoris and periurethral tissues and local branches to the vaginal smooth muscle (Baljet & Drukker 1980, Donker 1986, Hilliges et al 1995, Ball et al 1997). As in the male, the somatic component is served by the dorsal nerve branch of the pudendal nerve (Goss 1973). Nerve density is observed to be greater in the distal part of the vagina compared with proximal regions (Hilliges et al 1995).

Genital organ blood engorgement which commonly occurs with both penile erection in men and clitoral swelling with vaginal fluid transudation in women has been associated with parasympathetic vasodilator mechanisms, with evidence for nitric oxide, acetylcholine and vasoactive intestinal peptide as principal co-mediators of these responses (De Groat & Booth 1993a,b, Burnett 1997). The unstimulated, flaccid genital organ state evidently is governed by adrenergic and possibly peptidergic sympathetic mechanisms (De Groat & Booth 1993a). Sensory experiences in the genital region including the skin, prepuce, glans and connective tissue septa of the corpora cavernosa are received by significantly dense afferent receptors and conveyed by pudendal nerve pathways (De Groat & Booth 1993a,b). The content of afferent nerve terminals in the dermis of the penis, testis and male reproductive tract includes calcitonin gene-related peptide and substance P (Dail 1993). These neuropeptides are also prominently contained in the afferent nerve distributions within the vascular and non-vascular smooth muscle of the vagina (Papka & Traurig 1993).

PERINEAL NEUROBIOLOGY

In addition to providing nerve branches to the penis (or clitoris), anal canal and urethral sphincter, the pudendal nerve distributes nerve branches to the anterior perineal musculature (bulbospongiosus and ischiocavernosus muscles) (Donker 1986). Nerve branches arising from sacral nerve root S4 generally supply the posterior perineal musculature (pubococcygeus and iliococcygeus muscles). Nerve branches of sacral nerve roots S4–S5 form the coccygeal plexus with nerve fibre extensions to perineal, perianal and scrotal (or labial) skin (Matzel et al 1990). Cholinergic nerve release likely governs the somatic mechanisms of the perineal musculature (Vodusek & Light 1983). Neuropeptide release appears to account for perineal sensations (Jänig & Koltzenburg 1993).

CHRONIC PAIN SYNDROMES OF THE GENITOURINARY TRACT: CLINICAL PRESENTATION. AETIOLOGY. DIFFERENTIAL DIAGNOSIS AND TREATMENT STRATEGIES

KIDNEY AND URETER PAIN

There are few chronic non-malignant pain syndromes of the upper urinary tract. Most pain syndromes of the kidney and ureter are acute, colicky in character and caused by acute distension due to an obstructing lesion or by infection. With improved diagnostic techniques cases of idiopathic nephralgia, as they were frequently diagnosed earlier this century (Harris & Harris 1930), have become extremely rare. As in other visceral disease, patients with diseases of the kidney and/or ureter present with true visceral pain and referred visceral pain to somatic structures (Head 1893). The distribution of the referred pain pattern from the kidney and the ureter has been studied since the beginning of this century (Lennandier 1906, McLellan & Goodell 1942). The referred pain is typically radiating from the costovertebral angle laterally around to the lower quadrant and into the testicle or labia. In patients suffering from colics due to renal or ureteral calculosis pain thresholds in the referred zone are still lower 8 months after lithotripsy as compared to controls (Giamberardino et al 1994), suggesting that the referred hyperalgesia is only in part linked to the continuing presence of the stone in the urinary tract. This might explain why some patients with a history of renal/ureteral calculosis complain about persistent chronic flank pain long after the stones that originally caused the acute renal/ureteral colic have either been removed or passed spontaneously. Thus, the referred hyperalgesia becomes independent of the primary focus, probably as a result of plastic neuronal changes in the central nervous system, which are initially triggered by afferent visceral inputs, but are maintained even after their removal. This persistent pain in the referred zone is often reported as a dull, continuous pain, mild to moderate in intensity, in contrast to the intermittent and colicky, often excruciating pain described by patients with renal/ureteral colic.

Loin pain/haematuria syndrome is a descriptive diagnosis given to patients with recurrent attacks of unilateral or bilateral loin pain accompanied by microscopic or macroscopic haematuria in whom no cause can be identified (Little et al 1967, Editorial 1992). The syndrome is more frequent in women than men (Little et al 1967, Bultitude et al 1998). No consistent histological changes have been described in renal specimen (Editorial 1992, Weisberg et al 1993). The diagnosis is made by exclusion, and because no aetiological treatment is possible to this date, treatment is symptomatic to relieve pain. Sometimes the syndrome resolves spontaneously. Most patients require large doses of analgesics, usually opioids, for pain control (Bultitude 1995). Transcutaneous electrical nerve stimulation (TENS) has been reported to result in partial pain relief, some women have benefited from stopping birth control pills and anticoagulation has been beneficial in several patients (Burden et al 1975, Aber & Higgins 1982). Surgical approaches have included renal denervation and even nephrectomy or autotransplantation (with the aim of achieving complete denervation while preserving kidney function). However, after nephrectomy or autotransplantation the pain often returns on the contralateral side (Editorial 1992). Bultitude et al (1998) recently reported symptomatic pain relief in 65% of patients with loin pain/haematuria syndrome after local irrigation of the renal pelvis and ureter with capsaicin solution, which lasted for several months. This treatment results in degeneration of afferent fibres of the ureter and renal pelvis (Allan et al 1997).

INTERSTITIAL CYSTITIS

Interstitial cystitis (IC) is a chronic, painful and often debilitating disease (Ratliff et al 1994, Slade et al 1997), whose aetiology and pathophysiology is largely unknown (Ruggieri et al 1994, Toozs-Hobson et al 1996, Elbadawi 1997). It is characterized by pelvic and suprapubic pain, urinary symptoms such as frequency and urgency, and in females often by dyspareunia that may be relieved by voiding. IC subdivides into an ulcerative and non-ulcerative type, as determined by cystoscopic findings of either Hunner's ulcer or glomerulations without ulcer on the bladder wall (Johansson & Fall 1994, Elbadawi 1997, Messing et al 1997, Nigro et al 1997). While prevalence estimates vary widely, it has been suggested that somewhere between 450 000 (Slade et al 1997) and 1 million people (Jones & Nyberg 1997) in the USA suffer from IC or IC-like conditions. Based on the National Household Interview Survey (Jones & Nyberg 1997), it was estimated that among IC patients the mean age is 49 years and the female to male ratio is 9 : 1.

Aetiologies that have been considered include infection (Ratliff et al 1994, Warren 1994, Ducan & Schaeffer 1997), lymphatic or vascular obstruction (Ratliff et al 1994), immunological deficiencies (Ratliff et al 1994), glycosaminoglycan layer deficiency (Ratliff et al 1994, Mobley & Baum 1996, Parsons 1997), presence of toxic urogenous substance (Ratliff et al 1994), neural factors and primary mast cell disorders (Sant & Theoharides 1994, Elbadawi 1997, Hofmeister et al 1997). It has also been considered that the cause leading to the onset of IC has resolved, leaving in its wake a chronic visceral pain syndrome, such as occurs with chronic chest pain (Cannon 1995) and chronic pelvic pain (Wesselmann 1998). This is consistent with the report of Baskin and Tanagho (1992), where several cases of removal of the bladder in IC patients did not lead to a resolution of pain. Rare cases of the coexistence of vulvodynia and IC have been reported and it has been proposed that these syndromes represent a generalized disorder of urogenital sinus-derived epithelium (Fitzpatrick et al 1993). In 60% of men with prostate pain without bacteriuria there might be an association with IC or a related condition (Miller et al 1995, Berger et al 1998).

An assortment of oral, intravesical, surgical, local and behaviourally based treatments have been suggested for the management of IC. Surgical approaches include removal or modification of the bladder (Irwin & Galloway 1994, Peeker et al 1998). Local treatments include laser therapy (Malloy & Shanberg 1994), hydrodistension (Irwin & Galloway 1994, Sant & LaRock 1994, Zimmern 1995) and urethral dilatation (Irwin & Galloway 1994), infusions of various materials into the bladder such as dimethyl sulfoxide (DMSO) (Fowler 1981, Barker et al 1987, Childs 1994, Sant & LaRock 1994, Parkin et al 1997), silver nitrate (Sant & LaRock 1994), heparin (Sant & LaRock 1994), chlorpactin (Sant & LaRock 1994) and hyaluronic acid (Morales et al 1997). Oral medications range from those used for other chronic pain syndromes such as amitriptyline (Hanno 1994, Pontari et al 1997, Pranikoff & Constantino 1998) and calcium channel blockers (Fleischmann 1994), to medications acting against a possible allergic mechanism such as hydroxyzine and other antihistamines (Simmons & Bunce 1958, Theoharides & Sant 1997). Pentosanpolysulphate sodium, a mild anticoagulant with properties of sulphated glycosaminoglycans and an affinity for mucosal membranes, has been used for the treatment of IC based on the hypothesis that a defect in the glycosaminoglycan layer contributes to the pathogenesis (Fritjofsson et al 1987, Hanno 1997, Jepsen et al 1998). Non-medical treatment strategies such as TENS (Fall & Lindstrom 1994), acupuncture (Geirsson et al 1993), behavioural interventions (including the keeping of voiding diaries, pelvic floor muscle training) and acid-lowering diets have been advocated (Chaiken et al 1993, Whitmore 1994). Most reports of treatment of IC so far have suffered from lack of agreement about what constitutes a case and the lack of agreeable, valid outcome data. The National Institutes of Health in the USA has established research diagnostic criteria for IC (Gillenwater & Wein 1988), and the development of IC symptom and pain indices has recently been reported (Keller et al 1994, O'Leary et al 1997). Several multicentre controlled trials are currently underway comparing different treatment strategies for the management of IC, and it is to be hoped that this clinical research will result in improved – logical and systematic – treatment approaches in the near future.

URETHRAL SYNDROME

Many women present to the urologist, gynaecologist or family physician with painful micturition but no evidence of organic disease and the urine culture is negative by standard techniques. To describe this problem the term 'urethral syndrome' was coined by Gallagher et al in 1965. He reported that 41% of women seen in general practice with symptoms of a urinary tract infection had in fact sterile urine. The urethral syndrome is defined as an entity characterized by urinary urgency, frequency, dysuria and, at times, by suprapubic and back pain and urinary hesitancy in the absence of objective urological findings. Few epidemiological data for the urethral syndrome have been reported. The urethral syndrome typically occurs in women during their reproductive years (Carson et al 1979, Smith 1979, Kaplan et al 1980, Mabry et al 1981), but it has also been reported in children (Kaplan et al 1980) and in men (Barbalias 1990).

The aetiology of the urethral syndrome is not clear. Several theories have been proposed, however, with little supporting evidence. One popular theory is that symptoms are caused by urethral obstruction and are thus surgically treatable (Davis 1955, Bergman et al 1989, Sand et al 1989). Although surgical procedures aimed at relieving a urethral obstruction claim excellent results, it has to be cautioned that diagnostic criteria were unfortunately poorly documented (Splatt & Weedon 1981). Most importantly, there is rarely evidence to support an anatomically obstructive aetiology (Mabry et al 1981). These procedures involve some risk of incontinence and are of uncertain and usually temporary efficacy (Mabry et al 1981, Schmidt & Tanagho 1981). Many studies have investigated the role of infection in the urethral syndrome, but there is little evidence supporting the concept of an inflammatory or infectious aetiology for the urethral syndrome (reviewed in Messinger 1992). Urinary hesitance, which is often reported by patients with urethral syndrome, might be due to spasms of the external urethral sphincter. Several studies reported a staccato or prolonged flow phase during uroflowmetry and increased external sphincter tone detected on urethral pressure profilometry in patients with urethral syndrome (Raz & Smith 1976, Kaplan et al 1980, Schmidt & Tanagho 1981). However, these urodynamic findings are difficult to interpret in support of a neurogenic aetiology of the urethral syndrome, because they may also be produced voluntarily in a neurologically intact person (Messinger 1992). In contrast to other chronic non-malignant pain genitourinary pain syndromes, the rates of spontaneous remission are very high in this patient population (85% in Carson et al 1980 and 100% in Zufall 1978).

A thorough diagnostic evaluation is crucial. The urethral syndrome is a diagnosis of exclusion, its symptoms are indistinguishable from those caused by urinary infections, tumours, stones, interstitial cystitis and many other entities and these conditions have to be ruled out. The first diagnostic step is a thorough urological examination including urine analysis, culture and cytology. In selected patients further radiographic studies, urodynamic studies and cystoscopy are necessary (Messinger 1992). In females a gynaecological problem needs to be ruled out. The symptoms of the urethral syndrome can be part of the symptoms of systemic diseases affecting the innervation of the urogenital area, including multiple sclerosis, collagen diseases and diabetes mellitus. A psychological evaluation should be part of the multidisciplinary evaluation to rule out a psychogenic aetiology and to assess for symptoms of depression associated with the chronic pain syndrome.

Various invasive and medical treatment options have been suggested for patients with the urethral syndrome (reviewed in Messinger 1992). Endoscopic and open surgical procedures have been reported with the aim of eliminating a presumed urethral stenosis. Fulguration, scarification, resection or cryosurgery have been advocated to obliterate cystoscopically apparent urethritis. Bladder instillations with a variety of anti-inflammatory or cauterizing agents and systemic therapy with anticholinergics, α-adrenergic blockers and muscle relaxants have been considered. Electrical stimulation and biofeedback have been advocated to correct neurogenic causes. High rates of success were found with skeletal muscle relaxants or electrostimulation combined with biofeedback techniques (Kaplan et al 1980, Schmidt & Tanagho 1981). While exercising caution toward invasive and irreversible therapeutic procedures, a conservative approach is recommended because this is usually as effective as surgery, less expensive and, most importantly, less subject to risk (Carson et al 1980, Bodner 1988).

VULVODYNIA

Interestingly, hyperaesthesia of the vulva was a well-described entity in American (Thomas 1880) and European (Pozzi 1897) gynaecological textbooks in the last century. Thomas (1880) wrote in his textbook *Practical Treatise of the Disease of Women*:

> *The disease which I proceed to describe under this name, although to all appearances one of trivial character, really constitutes, on account of its excessive obstinacy and the great influence which it obtains over the mind of the patient, a malady of a great deal of importance. ... This disorder, although fortunately not very frequent, is by no means very rare. So commonly it is met with at least, that it becomes a matter of surprise that it has not been more generally and fully described. ... It is not a true neuralgia, but an abnormal sensitiveness; 'a plus state of excitability' in the diseased nerves.*

Surprisingly, despite early detailed reports, there was little interest in chronic vulvar pain until the early 1980s. The International Society for the Study of Vulvar Disease Task Force (1984) defined vulvodynia as chronic vulvar discomfort (McKay 1984), characterized by the patient's complaint of a burning and sometimes stinging sensation in the vulvar area. The term vulvodynia includes several disorders, all of which result in chronic vulvar pain: vulvar dermatosis, cyclic vulvovaginitis, vulvar vestibulitis, vulvar papillomatosis and essential vulvodynia (McKay 1989). It is important to recognize the different subsets of vulvodynia, because treatment options differ. These subsets may occur alone, simultaneously or sequentially, and treatment of one condition may affect the onset of another (McKay 1988, 1989). The recognition of multiple factors in the

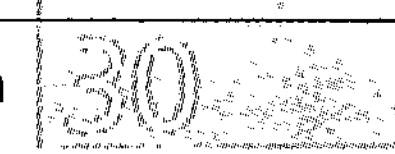

aetiology of vulvodynia is the key to appropriate evaluation and treatment.

The incidence or prevalence of vulvodynia is not known, but, as was already pointed out by Thomas (1880), this pain syndrome is probably more common than generally thought. It is estimated that at least 200 000 women in the USA suffer from significant vulvar discomfort that greatly reduces their quality of life (Jones & Lehr 1994). Unlike some other chronic pain syndromes that have a low incidence in the population, there appears to be a sufficient number of women with vulvodynia (Goetsch 1991) to perform controlled studies. The age distribution ranges from the twenties to late sixties (Lynch 1986, Paavonen 1995a,b). Goetsch (1991) reported that 15% of all patients seen in her general gynaecological private practice fulfilled the definition of vulvar vestibulitis. The subjects included in this study had not come for a gynaecological evaluation because of vulvar pain. Fifty per cent of these patients had always experienced entry dyspareunia and pain with inserting tampons, most since their teenage years. They had often wondered whether they were unique or had a hidden emotional aversion to sex.

The aetiology of vulvodynia remains unclear. Although many aetiological hypotheses have been proposed, our current understanding of vulvodynia is limited because most of the proposed causal explanations are derived from clinical case reports. Twenty-five to thirty-two per cent of women with vulvodynia know of a female relative with dyspareunia or tampon intolerance, raising the question of a genetic predisposition (Goetsch 1991, Bergeron et al 1997). Chronic vulvodynia often has an acute onset, but sometimes no associated event can be recalled by the patient. In many cases the onset can be linked to episodes of a vaginal infection, local treatments of the vulvar or vaginal area (application of steroid or antimicrobial cream, cryo- or laser surgery), or changes in the pattern of sexual activity. The pain is typically described at the vaginal introitus, the vestibule, which is the only genital tissue derived from endoderm and may have unique developmental features. The vestibule is the inner portion of the vulva, which extends from the so-called Hart's line (mucocutaneous line) on the labia minora to the hymenal ring, which marks the beginning of the vaginal mucous membrane. Anteriorly the vestibule extends to the area just beneath the clitoris and posteriorly to the fourchette (Friedrich 1983, Woodruff & Foster 1991). There are very few studies on the innervation of the vagina in humans. The first survey of the innervation pattern in the human vagina using a marker claimed to detect all nerves was published in 1995 (Hilliges et al 1995). Free intraepithelial nerve endings were only detected in the introitus vaginae region. These very superficial free nerve endings are generally considered to be nociceptive or thermoceptive (Iggo & Andres 1982). Further, nerve fibres containing nitric oxide synthase, neuropeptide Y, vasoactive intestinal peptide, calcitonin gene-related peptide and substance P closely associated with capillary loops in the epithelial papillae of the human vagina have been reported (Hoyle et al 1996). It has been suggested that these neurotransmitters are responsible for controlling blood flow and capillary permeability in the human vagina; further studies are necessary to evaluate whether they play a role in vaginal nociception as well.

On physical examination patients with vulvodynia usually present with no abnormalities. In patients with vulvar vestibulitis pain can easily be elicited or exacerbated by a simple 'Swabtest' (Goetsch 1991, Paavonen 1995a,b): touching the vulvar vestibule with a moist cotton swab results in sharp, burning pain.

Vulvar dermatoses are a frequent cause of chronic vulvar pain. A recent prospective study (Fischer et al 1995) of 144 patients presenting with vulvar pain showed that the majority of patients had a corticosteroid-responsive dermatosis. In contrast to most other subsets of vulvodynia, vulvar dermatoses are associated with physical signs: redness, blisters and erosions that can be recognized during a careful physical examination (Paavonen 1995a,b). The differential diagnosis of these physical signs is complex and may include inflammatory dermatoses, chronic contact dermatitis, lichen planus, lichen sclerosus, lichen simplex chronicus, seborrheic dermatitis, psoriasis, herpetic infections and systemic autoimmune diseases such as Behçet's disease and systemic lupus erythematosus (McKay 1988, 1992, Perniciaro et al 1993). The diagnosis usually needs to be confirmed by vulvar biopsy, vulvar neoplasia needs to be excluded.

Cyclic vulvovaginitis is characterized by episodic 'flares' of vulvar pain, often after sexual intercourse (pain is typically worst the next day) or during the luteal phase of the menstrual cycle (McKay 1988). Cyclic symptoms have been reported after hormonal changes, such as starting or discontinuing birth control pills, or during pregnancy. Hypersensitivity to the candida antigen (Ashman & Ott 1989), IgA deficiency (Scrimin et al 1991) and cyclic changes in the vaginal environment (McKay 1988) have been suggested as factors contributing to the aetiology. Prolonged maintenance therapy with antimycotics, topically or systemically, is usually effective if cultures show candida (Paavonen 1995a,b).

Women with vulvar vestibulitis describe entry dyspareunia, pain at the introitus of the vagina when inserting a tampon, and painful sensations when wearing pants, or with bicycle and horseback riding. Approximately one-half of the patients eventually experience spontaneous remission (Peckham et al 1986). On gynaecological examination there is vestibular erythema, touch of the vestibule is very painful (Friedrich 1987, Marinoff & Turner 1991). The clinical observation of vestibular erythema associated with dyspareunia was described in 1928 by Kelly:

> *'Exquisitely sensitive deep-red spots in the mucosa of the hymenal ring are a fruitful source of dyspareunia – tender enough at times to make a vaginal examination impossible. Inflamed caruncles with or without these spots often stand guard at the introitus labeled "noli me tangere".'*

Earlier studies implicated that chronic vulvar vestibulitis is the result of persistent infection and inflammation, but histological studies have not supported this (McKay 1988, Pyka et al 1988, Bazin et al 1994). Vestibular biopsies show mild to moderate inflammation in the epithelial stroma (Pyka et al 1988). A recent study reported vestibular neural hyperplasia (Westrom & Willen 1998) which might provide a morphological explanation of the pain in vulvar vestibulitis syndrome; however, functional studies are necessary to test this hypothesis. Early reports suggested that human papilloma virus (HPV) plays a major role in the pathogenesis of vulvar vestibulitis (Di Paola & Ruedo 1986, Reid et al 1988, Turner & Marinoff 1988). However, this could not be confirmed by studies using molecular techniques (Wilkinson et al 1993, De Deus et al 1995, Bernstein et al 1996). In women undergoing surgical therapy for vulvar vestibulitis no difference was found between women with HPV-associated vestibulitis and HPV-negative disease in the clinical presentation or response to surgical therapy (Bornstein et al 1997). Interestingly, while common HPV lesions such as condyloma acuminatum do not cause pain (Bornstein et al 1996), another viral vulvar lesion – herpes genitalis (infection with herpes simplex virus) – can be extremely painful. However, there is no evidence of herpes simplex virus infection in patients with vulvar vestibulitis (Bornstein et al 1996).

Medical and surgical treatment strategies have been suggested for vulvar vestibulitis. In mild cases of vulvar vestibulitis topical applied lidocaine cream is often sufficient to decrease dyspareunia markedly (Goetsch 1996). Oestrogen cream applied to the vaginal introitus has been reported to relieve pain in 20% of patients in an uncontrolled study (Yount et al 1997). One case report associated vulvar vestibulitis with oxalate crystalluria (Solomons et al 1991) – the patient experienced pain relief with calcium citrate and a low-oxalate diet. However, a subsequent larger study with 130 patients with vulvar pain and 23 volunteers without symptoms showed that urinary oxalates may be non-specific irritants that aggravate vulvodynia, but that the role of oxalates as instigators is doubtful (Baggish et al 1997). Intralesional alpha interferon injections have been suggested as a treatment modality, with about 50% of patients reporting substantial or partial improvement (Mann et al 1992, Marinoff et al 1993). Isoprenosine, another agent reported to enhance immune function, was found to improve pain in six of ten patients (Petersen & Weismann 1996). It is of concern that no long-term follow-up was reported in any of these patients. Surgical approaches have been suggested with the aim of removing the painful skin area. The most common procedure is perineoplasty (Woodruff & Foster 1991): the vulvar vestibule (the hyperalgesic area) is excised and the vaginal mucosa is then advanced to cover the defect. Cure rates are reported as follows: Woodruff & Friedrich 1985 – 36/44; Peckham et al 1986 – 7/8; Friedrich 1987 – 23/38; Mann et al 1992 – 41/56; Marinoff et al 1993 – 18/19; Bornstein et al 1995 – 9/11; Chaim et al 1996 – 15/16. Unfortunately these conclusions are hampered by multiple methodological flaws: therapeutic success is seldom clearly defined, control groups are missing in most of the studies, pain measurement is rudimentary or not specified at all, and there is lack of long-term follow-up data. Risks include general anaesthesia, prolonged healing period, intraoperative bleeding and postoperative disfigurement (Goetsch 1996). A simplified surgical revision under local anaesthesia has recently been suggested by Goetsch (1996), resulting in complete resolution of vulvar vestibulitis in 10 of 12 patients. Biofeedback of the pelvic floor musculature has been reported to result in pain improvement in 83% of 33 patients suffering from vulvar vestibulitis (Glazer et al 1995). Before considering any more invasive treatment strategies, a trial of biofeedback is warranted, given that this treatment modality is not associated with any side effects and given the high response rate reported in the literature.

In vulvar papillomatosis small papillae are seen around the vulvar vestibule. While in some cases this is a normal variant, in others these papillae are seen in conjunction with lichen simplex chronicus, or with subclinical infection with HPV. Colposcopy and biopsy are important to rule out an infection with HPV. Treatment of the papillomatosis is usually unnecessary (Paavonen 1995a,b). If pain persists, symptomatic treatment of the vulvar pain is indicated.

When no secondary cause of vulvodynia can be identified, chronic vulvar pain is referred to as essential vulvodynia, also known as dysaesthetic vulvodynia (McKay 1988). This subtype of vulvodynia is more common in perimenopausal or postmenopausal women. Essential vulvody-

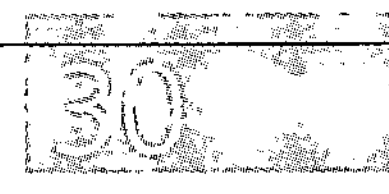

nia is characterized by constant hyperalgesia in the vulvar area, often extending to the urethral and rectal area. Using quantitative sensory testing of the vulvar area with topically applied acetic acid solutions, Sonni et al (1995) demonstrated that in essential vulvodynia the pain threshold for acid solutions is decreased. In contrast to patients with vulvar vestibulitis, patients with essential vulvodynia have less focal tenderness by the swab test and complain less about dyspareunia. It has been hypothesized that the vulvar hyperalgesia is due to altered cutaneous perception, such as in other neuropathic pain syndromes, and that pudendal neuralgia should be considered if the hyperaesthesia extends from the mons pubis to the upper inner thighs and posteriorly across the ischial tuberosities (McKay 1988, 1992). Many patients can be helped with medications recommended for other neuropathic pain syndromes (Watson et al 1982, Max et al 1992). A retrospective study by McKay (1993) demonstrated that low-dose amitriptyline was effective in women over 40 years old, but rarely in younger patients with essential vulvodynia.

Lastly iatrogenic causes have to be considered when evaluating a patient with vulvodynia. Local agents applied to the vulvar region such as topical steroids can cause irritant reactions. Vulvodynia has been recognized as a complication of CO_2 laser therapy to the vulva (McKay 1992). Few studies have examined the long-term effects of vaginal and perineal trauma as occurs with episiotomy or spontaneous perineal tears associated with delivery on vaginal and perineal pain perception. This literature might be sparse, either because long-term pain is not a significant problem in this patient population, or because women are reluctant to discuss pain associated with delivery, especially if the pain persists after the postpartum period. In a retrospective study (Rageth et al 1989), 16–47% of the women interviewed still reported dyspareunia 1–5 years after episiotomy.

CLITORAL PAIN

In contrast to the emerging literature about chronic pain syndromes of the vulva/vagina, very few reports exist on clitoral pain. Occasionally clitoral pain is seen as part of the essential vulvodynia pain syndrome complex in clinical practice. The patients report a burning stinging sensation that is exacerbated by touch (U. Wesselmann, unpublished data). Chronic pain is reported as one of the complications of female circumcision which involves excision of the clitoris and the labia minora and is still performed on young females in many parts of the world, where it is favoured as an instrument to control female sexuality and maintain cultural pride (Dirie & Lindmark 1992, Hanly & Ojeda 1995, Briggs 1998). With increasing mobility some of these women have moved to western countries. It is estimated that 2000 young women living in the UK undergo this ritual every year (Hanly & Ojeda 1995). However, the incidence of pain in these women is not known, because few of them seek medical attention.

TESTICULAR PAIN

Chronic testicular pain (orchialgia) can be one of the most vexing pain problems for men and their treating physician. Because pain syndromes in the genital region are often considered taboo in our society, men with testicular pain are usually embarrassed to talk about it, similar to women who suffer from vulvodynia. The incidence and prevalence is not known. Patients from adolescence to old age have been described who suffered from chronic testicular pain (Zvieli et al 1989, Davis et al 1990, Costabile et al 1991): the majority are in their mid to late thirties (Davis et al 1990, Costabile et al 1991). Many patients cannot recall any precipitating event that led to the onset of the chronic pain syndrome (Costabile et al 1991, Wesselmann & Burnett 1996). Chronic testicular pain can be unilateral or bilateral and may be confined to the scrotal contents or can radiate to the groin, penis, perineum, abdomen, legs and back. Some patients have constant pain, in others the pain is intermittent – either spontaneously or precipitated by certain movements or pressure on the testis. There is usually no sexual dysfunction associated with chronic orchialgia (Davis et al 1990, U. Wesselmann & A.L. Burnett, unpublished observation).

A careful history, physical examination, urological evaluation and selected imaging studies will uncover most secondary causes of chronic testicular pain. For the physician evaluating a patient with chronic testicular pain it is important to understand the nerve supply of the testis, so that the diagnostic evaluation can be guided by the functional neuroanatomy including the referred pain pattern (see Fig. 30.1). However, in many cases the patients present with a completely normal physical examination of the scrotum, testis, epididymis and spermatic cord. The pain remains unexplained despite a very thorough diagnostic work-up (Davis et al 1990). Secondary causes of chronic orchialgia include infection, tumour, testicular torsion, varicocele, hydrocele, spermatocele, trauma (such as a bicycle accident) and previous surgical interventions (Davis et al 1990, Costabile et al 1991). Testicular pain can be a sign of referred pain from the ureter or hip (Goldberg & Witchell 1988, Holland et al 1994) or from entrapment neuropathies of the ilioinguinal or genitofemoral nerve (Yeates 1985, Bennini 1992). There have been case reports about referred testicular pain from aneurysms of the common iliac artery or aorta due to pressure on the genitofemoral nerve (Ali 1983, McGee 1993), however, usually this pain is acute rather than chronic. Testicular pain can be due to intervertebral disc protrusion (White & Leslie 1986). Neuropathic testicular pain has been described in men with diabetic neuropathy (Hagen 1993). Vasectomy can result in chronic orchialgia and is probably far more common than realized (Selikowitz & Schned 1985, McCormack 1988, McMahon et al 1992, Hayden 1993). It has been hypothesized that this postvasectomy pain syndrome is due to impairment of the genital branch of the genitofemoral nerve by sperm granuloma (Yeates 1985), but others have questioned this theory (Silber 1981, McCormack 1988). Chronic testicular pain can be one of the symptoms of retroperitoneal fibrosis, usually associated with abdominal pain and low back pain (Mitchinson 1972, Baker et al 1987). Rare cases of orchialgia due to periarteritis nodosa have been reported (Lee et al 1983, McLean & Burnett 1983, Rosenthal et al 1987). There are two case reports in the neurological literature describing episodic testicular pain as a manifestation of epilepsy (York et al 1979, Bhaskar 1987). Schneiderman and Voytovich (1988) reported a patient who was overly concerned about developing testicular cancer and palpated his testis numerous times per day, resulting in 'self-palpation orchitis'.

The diagnostic work-up should include a thorough urological evaluation. If the urological evaluation is unrevealing further gastroenterological evaluations may be necessary to rule out referred pain from the lower pelvic organs and evaluation for hernia. Ekberg et al (1988) suggested herniography to evaluate for an occult hernia in patients who present with testicular pain. A neurological evaluation is directed toward the lumbosacral roots, the ilioinguinal, genitofemoral, pelvic and pudendal nerves. Placebo-controlled nerve blocks with local anaesthetic may help to differentiate which nerves are mediating the chronic pain problem. A discogram might be helpful to assess whether a protruding disc is the cause of the pain problem. A psychological evaluation should be included in a multidisciplinary comprehensive work-up to assess for depression or other psychological issues. It is important to be aware that in nearly 25% of patients, despite thorough evaluations, no aetiology of the pain can be found (Davis et al 1990).

The treatment of chronic testicular pain is directed towards the underlying aetiology, if one can be found. We agree with Holland et al (1994) that hydrocele, varicocele or spermatocele usually are not the cause of chronic testicular pain, but a coincidental finding. We have seen many patients with chronic testicular pain (U. Wesselmann & A. L. Burnett, unpublished observation) who had previously undergone testicular surgery for these conditions without any pain relief. It is important that the physician is not impelled by the lack of findings to institute more invasive procedures in an effort to find a non-existent pathological condition (Costabile et al 1991). Drastic surgical procedures have been recommended for the treatment of chronic orchialgia, including epididymectomy (Davis et al 1990, Chen & Ball 1991) and orchiectomy (Davis et al 1990). Several studies recently suggested microsurgical denervation of the spermatic cord as an alternative to orchiectomy for chronic testicular pain (Choa & Swami 1992, Levine et al 1996). However, before any invasive and irreversible measures are considered for pain relief, medical pain management should be attempted. Traditionally, urologists prescribed only a trial of antibiotics and NSAIDs for men presenting with chronic testicular pain, with the aim of treating a possible occult inflammatory process (Davis et al 1990). Recent research has demonstrated that medications used for other chronic pain syndromes (Galer 1995), such as low-dose antidepressants, anticonvulsants, membrane-stabilizing agents and opiates, often result in excellent pain relief in patients with chronic testicular pain (Costabile et al 1991, Hagen 1993, Hayden 1993, Wesselmann et al 1996). TENS might be helpful (Hayden 1993, Holland et al 1994). The testes receive a rich sympathetic innervation and sympatholytic procedures such as a lumbar sympathetic block with local anaesthetic or phentolamine infusions have resulted in marked pain relief in a subgroup of men with chronic testicular pain (Wesselmann et al 1995, Wesselmann & Burnett 1996).

PROSTATODYNIA

Prostatodynia is defined as persistent complaints of urinary urgency, dysuria, poor urinary flow and perineal discomfort, without evidence of bacteria or purulence in the prostatic fluid (Drach et al 1978). Patients report pain in the perineum, lower back, suprapubic area and groin, as well as pain on ejaculation. They typically range from 20 to 60 years of age (Moul 1993). Often the term 'prostatitis' is used to describe any unexplained symptom or condition that might possibly originate from the prostate gland (Nickel 1998). In the USA approximately 25% of all office visits of male patients for genitourinary tract problems are diagnosed with prostatitis (Lipsky 1989, Meares 1992). Drach et al (1978) defined four categories of prostatitis:

1. acute bacterial prostatitis
2. chronic bacterial prostatitis
3. non-bacterial prostatitis (including non-bacterial infections, allergic and autoimmune prostatitis)
4. prostatodynia.

Prostatodynia accounts for approximately 30% of patients presenting with prostatitis (Brunner et al 1983).

On physical examination the prostate is typically normal with no sign of tenderness on palpation (Orland et al 1985). A thorough urological evaluation should include urinalysis, urine culture, urine cytology and urethral cultures (de la Rosette et al 1992). In selected patients urodynamic evaluation should be performed, because several studies have demonstrated detrusor striated sphincter dyssynergy, abnormalities in urethral closing pressure and urethral narrowing in patients with prostatodynia (Segura et al 1979, Barbalias et al 1983, Barbalias 1990). Prostatodynia is a diagnosis of exclusion, where it is assumed that the chronic pain syndrome is related to the prostate, but no inflammatory prostatic process can be identified. It is important to consider in the differential diagnosis other diseases which can mimic prostatodynia. A gastroenterological examination is indicated if referred pain from the colon or rectum is suspected. The neurological examination is directed towards the nerve supply of the prostate (Fig. 30.1). Osteitis pubis, a well-recognized disease in active participants in strenuous sports and exercises, can mimic prostatodynia. Pelvic X-ray and bone scan confirm the diagnosis of osteitis pubis (Buck et al 1982). In some patients prostatodynia is one of the presenting symptoms of interstitial cystitis (see above).

Various medical and invasive treatment options have been suggested for patients with prostatodynia, most of which are anecdotal reports. Despite the fact that in patients with prostatodynia no infection can be demonstrated (Brunner et al 1983), the most frequently advocated treatment is antibiotics, probably based on the assumption that there might be an infection that is undiagnosed. De la Rosette et al (1992) reviewed the diagnostic and therapeutic results of 409 patients diagnosed with pain from the prostate: antibiotic treatment resulted in the relief of complaints in 36% of the patients and cure in 24%. Interestingly, however, similar results were found, even if no antibiotic was administered: 32% of the patients reported relief and 30% reported cure. As the urodynamic abnormalities observed in some patients with prostatodynia suggest increased sympathetic activity (Barbalias et al 1983), treatment with oral α-adrenergic blockers has been proposed to improve the voiding abnormalities as well as the pain. Prazosin, terazosin and doxazosin are the most frequently used agents (Orland et al 1985, Moul 1993, Barbalias et al 1998), but their use is often limited by side effects, most frequently hypotension.

In cases where a functional urinary outlet obstruction can be documented on urodynamic testing, retrograde transurethral balloon dilatation of the prostate has been suggested. This resulted in marked improvement of the voiding symptomatology but no results were given regarding the effect on the pain scores (Lopatin et al 1990). Transurethral microwave hyperthermia has been suggested for non-bacterial prostatitis and prostatodynia (Montorsi et al 1993, Nickel & Sorenson 1994). Pain relief has been reported with pelvic floor relaxation techniques (Segura et al 1979) and muscle-relaxing medications (Moul 1993).

PENILE PAIN

In contrast to other chronic pain syndromes of the genitourinary tract, chronic penile pain seems to be extremely rare. If a patient presents with persistent penile pain, the pain can usually be treated by treating the underlying disease (paraphimosis, priapism, Peyronie's disease, herpes genitalis – see Gee et al 1990). One of the most frequently reported acute penile pain events is the intracavernous injection of drugs for the treatment of erectile dysfunction (Godschalk et al 1996). Acute penile pain has been examined with regards to penile prosthesis (Althof et al 1987, Pedersen et al 1988, Tiefer et al 1988). Patients undergoing penile prostheses surgery report that postoperative pain is one of the most negative sequelae of surgery (Tiefer et al 1988). However, there are no reports indicating that a chronic pain syndrome develops after these acute noxious events. Also, surgical trauma to the penis such as occurs during routine circumcision does not seem to result in a chronic penile pain syndrome. A case report in the British literature described a man with recurrent penile pain attacks (Corder 1989). Physical examination revealed an inguinal hernia, which was surgically repaired. No recurrence of his episodic penile pain attacks was reported, and it was hypothesized that the penile pain in this case was due to irritation of the ilioinguinal nerve in the inguinal canal, which supplies the ventral base of the penis. Men who seek urological consultation for sexual impotence do not seem to suffer from penile (or testicular – see above) pain. Pudendal nerve injury in men results in sensory loss over the shaft and bulb of the penis and difficulty with erection, but persistent pain associated with the nerve injury has not been reported (Goodson 1981, Hofmann et al 1982).

PERINEAL PAIN

Perineal pain can be part of one of the more specific genitourinary pain syndromes discussed here such as interstitial cystitis, urethral syndrome, clitoral pain, vulvodynia, testicular pain or prostatodynia, all of which might present with pain radiating into the perineal region. However, often chronic perineal pain is an entity of its own, although poorly defined. The differential diagnosis of chronic perineal pain is extensive: gastroenterological, proctological, urological, gynaecological and neurological pathology needs to be excluded. Systemic diseases associated with painful peripheral neuropathies such as diabetes mellitus or AIDS can present with perineal pain. Several French studies report pudendal nerve entrapment in up to 91% of patients with perineal pain referred to a pain clinic (Bensignor et al 1996). Surgical neurolysis-transposition resulted in pain improvement in 67% of the patients (Robert et al 1993). The best results were seen in patients where the pudendal nerve entrapment was diagnosed early. Local anaesthetic blocks of the pudendal nerve and electromyography and nerve conduction studies of the pelvic floor might be helpful to confirm the diagnosis (Beck et al 1994). Imaging studies of the thoracolumbosacral spine can be considered if there is suspicion of rare cases of meningeal cysts (Van De Kleft & Van Vyve 1993) or meningiomas (Pagni & Canavero 1993) resulting in perineal pain. Surgical resection of sacral meningeal cysts has been reported to result in complete resolution of symptoms in 10/12 patients with perineal pain (Van de Kleft & Van Vyve 1993). Rare cases of perineal pain caused by plexiform neurofibromas involving the nerves of the perineum have been reported (Batta et al 1989). Ford et al (1994, 1996) recently reported perineal pain as a symptom of movement disorders:

1. Painful tardive perineal pain syndromes occurred as a complication of neuroleptic drug exposure (Ford et al 1994). Catecholamine depletors resulted in resolution of the painful sensations.
2. Perineal pain was reported as a rare – but in those rare cases very prominent feature – of Parkinson's disease (Ford et al 1996), responding to medications regularly used for the treatment of Parkinson's disease.

PSYCHOLOGICAL ASPECTS OF CHRONIC GENITOURINARY PAIN

As with other chronic pain syndromes in the absence of obvious organic pathology, many theories regarding a psychogenic origin of chronic non-malignant genitourinary pain have been entertained (see Wesselmann et al 1997 for review). The location of pain may be a significant predictor for appraisals of pain, affective response and disclosure of pain complaints. This is likely to play an important role in pain syndromes of the genitourinary region, an area often considered taboo. It is not surprising that subjects asked to imagine pain in their genitals reported that they would be least likely to disclose genital pain and would be more worried, depressed and embarrassed by pain in the genitals than in all other areas. They appraised themselves more ill than if they were asked to imagine chest, stomach, head or mouth pain (Klonoff et al 1993). Preliminary psychological research has been published on most of the genitourinary pain syndromes, however most studies have suffered from lack of adequate control groups, retrospective design, lack of standardized measures, small sample size and samples with significant self-selection factors. Of major concern is that most studies have neglected to assess whether the psychological findings in patients with genitourinary pain were likely to be pre-existing or reactive (see Wesselmann et al 1997 for review). Genitourinary pain affects many aspects of the quality of life of women and men, and it would not be surprising or necessarily indicative of psychiatric disease if a patient with chronic genitourinary pain was emotionally distressed or had an impaired sexual life. The questions to be asked and answered are:

1. Did these psychological symptoms occur before or after the chronic pain syndrome developed?
2. Did mood and sexual life return to normal after successful treatment of the chronic pain syndrome?

Further, a history of sexual and physical abuse has been associated with a variety of pain syndromes (Kinzl et al 1995) and that association appears to be especially strong with chronic gynaecological pain (Walker & Stenchever 1993). However, these studies may wrongly assume cause and effect between abuse history and the development of chronic gynaecological pain. Often sexual and physical abuse are symptoms of multiproblem families, characterized by chaos, alcohol and substance abuse and general neglect which results in children not being adequately protected. A completely unexplored question is whether physical injury to the genitourinary tract, as occurs during sexual abuse, can make the victim more prone to develop chronic genitourinary pain.

CONCLUSION

Chronic genitourinary pain syndromes are well described but poorly understood. Patients with chronic genitourinary pain have often suffered for many years and have frequently seen multiple physicians and undergone endless tests without finding a cure or even a diagnosis. A specific secondary cause can only be identified in the minority of patients. For the physician who is consulted by a patient with genitourinary pain, it is important to be familiar with these pain syndromes of body areas that are often considered taboo. The approach to the patient begins with acknowledging that the genitourinary pain syndromes are well described, searching for a secondary cause, and performing a careful psychological evaluation. It is usually very reassuring for the patient to learn that he/she is suffering from a well-described pain syndrome and is not the only case with this syndrome. Some patients present with more than one genitourinary pain syndrome (e.g., interstitial cystitis and vulvodynia). It has been suggested that this might be due to a generalized disorder of urogenital sinus derived epithelium (Fitzpatrick et al 1993). Realizing the extensive convergence of visceral afferent input on the spinal cord level and in the neuronal plexuses in the pelvis demonstrated in animal studies (Wesselmann 1987, Jänig et al 1991, Cervero 1994, Wesselmann & Lai 1997), it would not be surprising if a chronic pain syndrome in one area of the genitourinary tract could trigger the development of chronic pain and dysfunction in another area of the genitourinary system (Fig. 30.3). Although complete cures are uncommon, some pain relief can be provided to almost all patients using a multidisciplinary approach including pain medications, local treatment regimens, local anaesthetic techniques, physical therapy and psychological approaches, all the while exercising caution toward invasive and irreversible therapeutic procedures.

The aetiology of most genitourinary pain syndromes is not known and further research is desperately needed. These areas of the body, which are often considered taboo in our society, have been largely neglected in neuroanatomical, neurophysiological and neuropharmacological research. Current treatment approaches are empirical only. Better knowledge of the underlying pathophysiological mechanisms of chronic genitourinary pain will allow the development of treatment strategies specifically targeted against the pathophysiological mechanisms.

Acknowledgements

Ursula Wesselmann is supported by the Blaustein Pain Research Foundation, the Reflex Sympathetic Dystrophy Syndrome Association of America and USPHS-grant DA10802 and NS 36553.

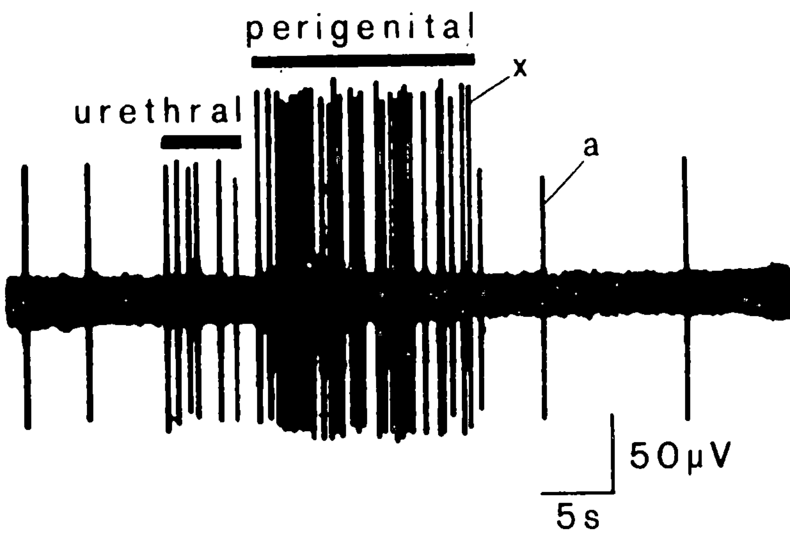

Fig. 30.3 Recordings from sympathetic neurons projecting in the hypogastric nerves in cats. Neuron a: Postganglionic neuron with ongoing activity, which was excited on mechanical stimulation of the urethra (by slight distoproximal movements of the urethral catheter) and inhibited by mechanical stimulation of the perigenital skin. Neuron x: Postganglionic neuron with no on-going activity, which was activated by mechanical stimulation of the perigenital skin. (Modified from Wesselmann 1987.)

REFERENCES

Aber GM, Higgins PM 1982 The natural history and management of the loin pain/haematuria syndrome. British Journal of Urology 54: 613–615

Ali MS 1983 Testicular pain in a patient with aneurysm of the common iliac artery. British Journal of Urology 55: 447–448

Allan JDD, Bultitude MI, Bultitude MF, Wall PD, McMahon SB 1997 The effect of capsaicin on renal pain signaling systems in humans and Wistar rats. Journal of Physiology 505: 39P

Althof SE, Turner LA, Levine SB et al 1987 Intracavernosal injection in the treatment of impotence: a prospective study of sexual, psychological, and marital functioning. Journal of Sex and Marital Therapy 13: 155–167

Ashman RB, Ott AK 1989 Autoimmunity as a factor in recurrent vaginal candidosis and the minor vestibular gland syndrome. Journal of Reproductive Medicine 4: 264–266

Baggish MS, Sze EHM, Johnson R 1997 Urinary oxalate excretion and its role in vulvar pain syndrome. American Journal of Obstetrics and Gynecology 177: 507–511

Baker LR, Mallinson WJ, Gregory MC et al 1987 Idiopathic retroperitoneal fibrosis. A retrospective analysis of 60 cases. British Journal of Urology 60: 497–503

Baljet B, Drukker J 1980 The extrinsic innervation of the pelvic organs in the female rat. Acta Anatomica 107: 241–267

Ball TP, Teichman JMH, Sharkey FE, Rogenes VJ, Adrian EK 1997 Terminal nerve distribution to the urethra and bladder neck: considerations in the management of stress urinary incontinence. Journal of Urology 158: 827–829

Barbalias GA 1990 Prostatodynia or painful male urethral syndrome? Urology 36: 146–153

Barbalias GA, Meares EM Jr, Sant GR 1983 Prostatodynia: clinical and urodynamic characteristics. Journal of Urology 130: 514–517

Barbalias GA, Nikiforidis G, Liatsikos EN 1998 Alpha-blockers for the treatment of chronic prostatitis in combination with antibiotics. Journal of Urology 159: 883–887

Barker SB, Matthews PN, Philip PF, Williams G 1987 Prospective study of intravesical dimethyl sulphoxide in the treatment of chronic inflammatory bladder disease. British Journal of Urology 59: 142–144

Baskin LS, Tanagho EA 1992 Pain without pelvic organs. Journal of Urology 147: 683–686

Batta AG, Gundian JC, Myers RP 1989 Neurofibromatosis presenting as perineal pain and urethral burning. Urology 33: 138–140

Bazin S, Bouchard C, Brisson J, Morin C, Meisels A, Fortier M 1994 Vulvar vestibulitis syndrome: an exploratory case-control study. Obstetrics and Gynecology 83: 47–50

Beck R, Fowler CJ, Mathias CJ 1994 Genitourinary dysfunction in disorders of the autonomic nervous system. In: Rushton DN (ed) Handbook of neuro-urology. Marcel Dekker, New York, pp 281–301

Bennini A 1992 Die Ilioinguinalis- und Genitofemoralisneuralgie. Schweizerische Rundschau der Medizin 81: 1114–1120

Bensignor MF, Labat JJ, Robert R, Ducrot P 1996 Diagnostic and therapeutic pudendal nerve blocks for patients with perineal non-malignant pain. Abstract, 8th World Congress on Pain, p 56

Berger RE, Miller JE, Rothman I, Krieger JN, Muller CH 1998 Bladder petechiae after cystoscopy and hydrodistension in men diagnosed with prostate pain. Journal of Urology 159: 83–85

Bergeron S, Bouchard C, Fortier M, Binik YM, Khalife S 1997 The surgical treatment of vulvar vestibulitis syndrome: a follow-up study. Journal of Sex and Marital Therapy 23: 317–325

Bergman A, Karram M, Bhatia NN 1989 Urethral syndrome: a comparison of different treatment modalities. Journal of Reproductive Medicine 34: 157–160

Bhaskar PA 1987 Scrotal pain with testicular jerking: an unusual manifestation of epilepsy. Journal of Neurology, Neurosurgery and Psychiatry 50: 1233–1234

Bo X, Burnstock G 1995 Characterization and autoradiographic localization of [^{3}H], alpha-beta-methylene adenosine 5′-triphosphate binding sites in human urinary bladder. British Journal of Urology 76: 297–302

Bodner DR 1988 The urethral syndrome. Urologic Clinics of North America 15: 699–704

Bornstein J, Zarfati D, Goldik Z, Abramovici H 1995 Perineoplasty compared with vestibuloplasty for severe vulvar vestibulitis. British Journal of Obstetrics and Gynaecology 102: 652–655

Bornstein J, Shapiro S, Rahat M et al 1996 Polymerase chain reaction search for viral etiology of vulvar vestibulitis syndrome. American Journal of Obstetrics and Gynecology 175: 139–144

Bornstein J, Shapiro S, Goldshmid N, Goldik Z, Lahat N, Abramovici H 1997 Severe vulvar vestibulitis, relation to HPV infection. Journal of Reproductive Medicine 42: 514–518

Briggs LA 1998 Female circumcision in Nigeria – is it not time for government intervention. Health Care Analysis 6: 14–23

Brunner H, Weidner W, Schiefer HC 1983 Studies on the role of *Ureaplasma urealyticum* and *Mycoplasma hominis* in prostatitis. Journal of Infectious Diseases 126: 807–813

Buck AC, Crean M, Jenkins IL 1982 Osteitis pubis as a mimic of prostatic pain. British Journal of Urology 54: 741–744

Bultitude M, Young J, Bultitude M, Allan J 1998 Loin pain haematuria syndrome: distress resolved by pain relief. Pain 76: 209–213

Bultitude MI 1995 Capsaicin in treatment of loin pain/haematuria syndrome. Lancet 345: 921–922

Burden RP, Booth LJ, Ockenden BG, Boyd WN, Higgins P McR, Aber GM 1975 Intrarenal vascular changes in adult patients with recurrent haematuria and loin pain: a clinical, histological and angiographic study. Quarterly Journal of Medicine 175: 433–447

Burnett AL 1997 Nitric oxide in the penis: physiology and pathology. Journal of Urology 157: 320–324

Burnett AL, Calvin DC, Chamness SL et al 1997 Urinary bladder-urethral sphincter dysfunction in mice with targeted disruption of neuronal nitric oxide synthase models idiopathic voiding disorders in humans. Nature Medicine 3: 571–574

Burnett AL, Mostwin JL 1998 In situ anatomical study of the male urethral sphincteric complex: relevance to urinary continence preservation following major pelvic surgery. Journal of Urology 160: 1301–1306

Cannon RO 3rd 1995 The sensitive heart. A syndrome of abnormal cardiac pain perception (Clinical Conference). Journal of The American Medical Association 273: 883–887

Carson CC, Osborne D, Segura JW 1979 Psychological characteristics of patients with female urethral syndrome. Journal of Clinical Psychology 35: 312–315

Carson CC, Segura JW, Osborne DM 1980 Evaluation and treatment of the female urethral syndrome. Journal of Urology 124: 609–610

Cervero F 1994 Sensory innervation of the viscera: peripheral basis of visceral pain. Physiological Reviews 74: 95–138

Chaiken DC, Blaivas JG, Blaivas ST 1993 Behavioral therapy for the treatment of refractory interstitial cystitis. Journal of Urology 149: 1445–1448

Chaim W, Meriwether C, Gonik B, Qureshi F, Sobel JD 1996 Vulvar vestibulitis subjects undergoing surgical intervention: a descriptive analysis and histopathological correlates. European Journal of Obstetrics and Gynecology and Reproductive Biology 68: 165–168

Chen TF, Ball RY 1991 Epididymectomy for post-vasectomy pain: histological review. British Journal of Urology 68: 407–413

Childs SJ 1994 Dimethyl Sulfone in the treatment of interstitial cystitis. Urologic Clinics of North America 21: 85–88

Choa RG, Swami KS 1992 Testicular denervation: a new surgical procedure for intractable testicular pain. British Journal of Urology 70: 417–419

Corder AP 1989 Penile pain and direct inguinal hernia. British Journal of Hospital Medicine 42: 238

Costabile RA, Hahn M, McLeod DG 1991 Chronic orchialgia in the pain prone patient: the clinical perspective. Journal of Urology 146: 1571–1574

Dail WG 1993 Autonomic innervation of male reproductive genitalia. In: Maggi CA (ed) Nervous control of the urogenital system. Harwood Academic, Chur, Switzerland, pp 69–101

Davis BE, Noble MJ, Weigel JW, Foret J, Mebust WK 1990 Analysis and management of chronic testicular pain. Journal of Urology 143: 936–939

Davis DM 1955 Vesicle orifice obstruction in women and its treatment by transurethral resection. Journal of Urology 73: 112–117

De Deus JM, Focchi J, Stavale JN, De Lima GR 1995 Histologic and biomolecular aspects of papillomatosis of the vulvar vestibule in relation to human papillomavirus. Obstetrics and Gynecology 86: 758–763

De Groat WC 1994 Neurophysiology of the pelvic organs. In: Rushton DN (ed) Handbook of neuro-urology. Marcel Dekker, New York, pp 55–93

De Groat WC 1987 Neuropeptides in pelvic afferent pathways. Experientia 43: 801–812

De Groat WC, Booth AM 1993a Neural control of penile erection. In: Maggi CA (ed) Nervous control of the urogenital system. Harwood Academic, Chur, Switzerland, pp 467–524

De Groat WC, Booth AM 1993b Synaptic transmission in pelvic ganglia. In: Maggi CA (ed) Nervous control of the urogenital system. Harwood Academic, Chur, Switzerland, pp 291–347

De Groat WC, Booth AM, Yoshimura N 1993 Neurophysiology of micturition and its modification in animal models of human disease. In: Maggi CA (ed) Nervous control of the urogenital system. Harwood Academic, Chur, Switzerland, pp 227–290

De la Rosette JJMCH, Hubregtse MR, Karhaus HFM, Debruyne FMJ 1992 Results of a questionnaire among Dutch urologists and general practitioners concerning diagnostics and treatment of patients with prostatitis syndrome. European Journal of Urology 22: 14–19

di Paola GR, Ruedo NG 1986 Deceptive vulvar papillomavirus infection. A possible explanation for certain cases of vulvodynia. Journal of Reproductive Medicine 31: 966–970

Dirie MA, Lindmark G 1992 The risk of medical complications after female circumcision. East African Medical Journal 69: 479–482

Donker PJ 1986 A study of the myelinated fibres in the branches of the pelvic plexus. Neurourology and Urodynamics 5: 185–202

Drach GW, Fair WR, Meares EM, Stamey TA 1978 Classification of benign diseases associated with prostatic pain: prostatitis or prostatodynia? Journal of Urology 120: 266

Duncan JL, Schaeffer AJ 1997 Do infectious agents cause interstitial cystitis? Urology 49: 48–51

Editorial 1992 Loin pain/haematuria syndrome. Lancet 340: 701–702

Ekberg O, Abrahamsson P-A, Kesek P 1988 Inguinal hernia in urological patients: the value of herniography. Journal of Urology 139: 1253–1255

Elbadawi A 1996 Functional anatomy of the organs of micturition. Urologic Clinics of North America 23: 177–210

Elbadawi A 1997 Interstitial cystitis: a critique of current concepts with a new proposal for pathologic diagnosis and pathogenesis. Urology 49: 14–40

Fall M, Lindstrom S 1994 Transcutaneous electrical nerve stimulation in classic and nonulcer interstitial cystitis. Urologic Clinics of North America 21: 131–139

Ferguson M, Bell C 1993 Autonomic innervation of the kidney and ureter. In: Maggi C A (ed) Nervous control of the urogenital system. Harwood Academic, Chur, Switzerland, pp 1–31

Fischer G, Spurrett B, Fisher A 1995 The chronically symptomatic vulva: aetiology and management, British Journal of Obstetrics and Gynaecology 102: 773–779

Fitzpatrick CC, Delancey JOL, Elkins TE, McGuire EJ 1993 Vulvar vestibulitis and interstitial cystitis: a disorder of urogenital sinus-derived epithelium? Obstetrics and Gynaecology 81: 860–862

Fleischmann J 1994 Calcium channel antagonists in the treatment of interstitial cystitis. Urologic Clinics of North America 21: 107–112

Ford B, Greene P, Fahn S 1994 Oral and genital tardive pain syndromes. Neurology 44: 2115–2119

Ford B, Louis ED, Greene P, Fahn S 1996 Oral and genital pain syndromes in Parkinson's disease. Movement Disorders 11: 421–426

Fowler JE 1981 Prospective study of intravesical dimethyl sulphoxide in treatment of suspected early interstitial cystitis. Urology 18: 21–26

Friedrich EG 1983 The vulvar vestibule. Journal of Reproductive Medicine 28: 773–777

Friedrich EG 1987 Vulvar vestibulitis syndrome. Journal of Reproductive Medicine 32: 110–114

Fritjofsson A, Fall M, Juhlin R, Persson E, Ruutu M 1987 Treatment of ulcer and nonulcer interstitial cystitis with sodium pentosanpolyphosphate: a multicenter trial. Journal of Urology 138: 508–512

Galer BS 1995 Neuropathic pain of peripheral origin: advances in pharmacologic treatment. Neurology 45: S17–S25

Gallagher DJA, Montgomerie JZ, North JDK 1965 Acute infections of the urinary tract and the urethral syndrome in general practice. British Medical Journal 1: 622–626

Gee WF, Ansell JS, Bonica JJ 1990 Pelvic and perineal pain of urologic origin. In: Bonica JJ (ed) The management of pain, vol 2. Lea & Febiger, Philadelphia, pp 1368–1394

Geirsson G, Wang YG, Lindstrom S, Fall M 1993 Traditional acupuncture and electrical stimulation of the posterior tibial nerve. A trial in chronic interstitial cystitis. Scandinavian Journal of Urology and Nephrology 27: 67–70

Giamberardino MA, de Bigontina P, Martegiani C, Vecchiet L 1994 Effects of extracorporeal shock-wave lithotripsy on referred hyperalgesia from renal/ureteral calculosis. Pain 56: 77–83

Gillenwater JY, Wein AJ 1988 Summary of the National Institute of Arthritis, Diabetes, Digestive and Kidney Diseases Workshop on Interstitial Cystitis, National Institutes of Health, Bethesda, Maryland, August 28–29, 1987. Journal of Urology 140: 203–206

Glazer HI, Rodke G, Swencionis C, Hertz R, Young A W 1995 Treatment of vulvar vestibulitis syndrome with electromyographic biofeedback of pelvic floor musculature. Journal of Reproductive Medicine 40: 283–290

Godschalk M, Gheorghiu D, Katz PG, Mulligan T 1996 Alkalization does not alleviate penile pain induced by intracavernous injection of prostaglandin E1. Journal of Urology 156: 999–1000

Goetsch MF 1991 Vulvar vestibulitis: prevalence and historic features in a general gynecologic practice population. American Journal of Obstetrics and Gynecology 164: 1609–1616

Goetsch MF 1996 Simplified surgical revision of the vulvar vestibule for vulvar vestibulitis. American Journal of Obstetrics and Gynecology 174: 1701–1707

Goldberg SD, Witchell SJ 1988 Right testicular pain: unusual presentation of obstruction of the ureteropelvic junction. Canadian Journal of Surgery 31: 246–247

Goodson JD 1981 Pudendal neuritis from biking. New England Journal of Medicine 304: 365

Goss CM 1973 The external genital organs. In: Gray's anatomy of the human body, 29th edn. Lea & Febiger, Philadelphia, p 1331

Hagen NA 1993 Sharp, shooting neuropathic pain in the rectum or genitals: pudendal neuralgia. Journal of Pain and Symptom Management 8: 496–501

Hanly MG, Ojeda VJ 1995 Epidermic inclusion cysts of the clitoris as a complication of female circumcision and pharaonic infibulation. Central African Journal of Medicine 41: 22–24

Hanno PM 1994 Diagnosis of interstitial cystitis. Urologic Clinics of North America 21: 63–66

Hanno PM 1997 Analysis of long-term elmiron therapy for interstitial cystitis. Urology 49: 93–99

Harris SH, Harris RGS 1930 Sympathicotonus, renal pain and renal sympathectomy. British Journal of Urology 2: 367–374

Hayden LJ 1993 Chronic testicular pain. Australian Family Physician 22: 1357–1365

Head H 1893 On disturbances of sensation with special reference to the pain of visceral disease. Brain 16: 1–113

Hilliges M, Falconer C, Ekman-Ordeberg G, Johansson O 1995 Innervation of the human vaginal mucosa as revealed by PGP 9.5 immunohistochemistry. Acta Anatomica 153: 119–126

Hodson N 1970 The nerves of the testis, epididymis, and scrotum. In: Johnson AD, Gomes WR, Vandemark NL (eds) The testis. Academic, New York, pp 47–99

Hofmann A, Jones RE, Schoenvogel R 1982 Pudendal nerve neurapraxia as a result of traction on the fracture table. Journal of Bone and Joint Surgery 64: 136–138

Hofmeister M, He F, Ratliff TL, Mahoney T, Becich MJ 1997 Mast cell and nerve fibers in interstitial cystitis: an algorithm for histological diagnosis via quantitative image analysis and morphometry. Urology 49: 41–47

Holland JM, Feldman JL, Gilbert HC 1994 Phantom orchalgia. Journal of Urology 152: 2291–2293

Hoyle CHV, Stones W, Robson T, Whitely K, Burnstock G 1996 Innervation of vasculature and microvasculature of the human vagina by NOS and neuropeptide-containing nerves. Journal of Anatomy 188: 633–644

Iggo A, Andres KH 1982 Morphology of cutaneous receptors. Annual Revues of Neuroscience 5: 1–31

Irwin PP, Galloway NTM 1994 Surgical management of interstitial cystitis. Urologic Clinics of North America 21: 145–152

Jänig W, Koltzenburg M 1993 Pain arising from the urogenital tract. In: Maggi CA (ed) Nervous control of the urogenital system. Harwood Academic, Chur, Switzerland, pp 525–578

Jänig W, Schmidt M, Schnitzler A, Wesselmann U 1991 Differentiation of sympathetic neurones projecting in the hypogastric nerve in terms of their discharge patterns in cats. Journal of Physiology (London) 437: 157–179

Jepsen JV, Sall M, Rhodes PR, Schmid D, Messing E, Bruskewitz RC 1998 Long-term experience with pentosanpolysulfate in interstitial cystitis. Urology 51: 381–387

Johansson SL, Fall M 1994 Pathology of interstitial cystitis. Urologic Clinics of North America 21: 55–62

Jones CA, Nyberg LM 1997 Epidemiology of interstitial cystitis. Urology 49: 2–9

Jones KD, Lehr ST 1994 Vulvodynia: diagnostic techniques and treatment modalities. Nurse Practitioner 19: 34–46

Juenemann KP, Lue TF, Schmidt RA, Tanagho EA 1988 Clinical significance of sacral and pudendal nerve anatomy. Journal of Urology 139: 74–80

Kabalin JN 1998 Surgical anatomy of the retroperitoneum, kidneys, and ureters. In: Walsh PC, Retik AB, Vaughan ED, Wein AJ (eds) Campbell's urology, vol 1, 7th edn. WB Saunders, Philadelphia, pp 49–88

Kaplan WE, Firlit CF, Schoenberg HW 1980 The female urethral syndrome: external sphincter spasm as etiology. Journal of Urology 124: 48–49

Keller ML, McCarthy DO, Neider RS 1994 Measurement of symptoms of interstitial cystitis: a pilot study. Urologic Clinics of North America 21: 67–72

Kelly HA (ed) 1928 Gynecology. Appelton and Company, New York, p 236

Kinzl JF, Traweger C, Biebl W 1995 Family background and sexual abuse associated with somatization. Psychotherapy and Psychosomatics 64: 82–87

Klonoff EA, Landrine H, Brown M 1993 Appraisal and response to pain may be a function of its bodily location. Journal of Psychosomatic Research 37: 661–670

Krane RJ, Olsson CA 1973 Phenoxybenzamine in neurogenic bladder dysfunction. I. A theory of micturition. Journal of Urology 110: 650–652

Kumagai A, Koyanagi T, Takahashi Y 1987 The innervation of the external urethral sphincter; an ultrastructural study in male human subjects. Urological Research 15: 39–43

Lee LM, Moloney PJ, Wong HCG, Magil AB, McLoughlin MG 1983 Testicular pain: an unusual presentation of polyarteritis nodosa. Journal of Urology 129: 1243–1244

Lennandier KG 1906 Über lokale Anaesthesie und über Sensibilität in Organ und Gewebe. Weitere Beobachtungen. Mitteilungen aus den Grenzgebieten der Medizin und Chirurgie 15: 465–494

Lepor H, Gregerman M, Crosby R, Mostofi FK, Walsh PC 1985 Precise localization of the autonomic nerves from the pelvic plexus to the corpora cavernosa: a detailed anatomical study of the adult male pelvis. Journal of Urology 133: 207–212

Levine LA, Matkov TG, Lubenow TR 1996 Microsurgical denervation of the spermatic cord: a surgical alternative in the treatment of chronic orchialgia. Journal of Urology 155: 1005–1007

Lincoln J, Burnstock G 1993 Autonomic innervation of the urinary bladder and urethra. In: Maggi CA (ed) Nervous control of the urogenital system. Harwood Academic, Chur, Switzerland, pp 33–68

Lipsky BA 1989 Urinary tract infections in men. Annals of Internal Medicine 110: 138

Little PJ, Sloper JS, de Wardener HE 1967 A syndrome of loin pain and haematuria associated with disease of peripheral renal arteries. Quarterly Journal of Medicine 36: 253–259

Lopatin WB, Martynik M, Hickey DP, Vivas C, Hakala TR 1990 Retrograde transurethral balloon dilation of prostate: innovative management of abacterial chronic prostatitis and prostadynia. Urology 36: 508–510

Lue TF, Zeineh SJ, Schmidt RA, Tanagho EA 1984 Neuroanatomy of penile erection: its relevance to iatrogenic impotence. Journal of Urology 131: 273–280

Lynch PJ 1986 Vulvodynia: a syndrome of unexplained vulvar pain, psychologic disability and sexual dysfunction. Journal of Reproductive Medicine 31: 773–780

Mabry EW, Carson CC, Older RA 1981 Evaluation of women with chronic voiding discomfort. Urology 18: 244–246

Maggi CA, Meli A 1988 The sensory-efferent function of capsaicin-sensitive neurons. General Pharmacology 19: 1–43

Malloy TR, Shanberg AM 1994 Laser therapy for interstitial cystitis. Urologic Clinics of North America 21: 141–144

Mann MS, Kaufman R, Brown D, Adam E 1992 Vulvar vestibulitis: significant clinical variables and treatment outcome. Obstetrics and Gynecology 79: 122–125

Marinoff SC, Turner MLC 1991 Vulvar vestibulitis syndrome: an overview. American Journal of Obstetrics and Gynecology 165: 1228–1233

Marinoff SC, Turner ML, Hirsch RP, Richard G 1993 Intralesional alpha interferon cost effective therapy for vulvar vestibulitis syndrome. Journal of Reproductive Medicine 38: 19–24

Matzel KE, Schmidt RA, Tanagho EA 1990 Neuroanatomy of the striated muscular anal continence mechanism: implications for the use of neurostimulation. Diseases of the Colon and Rectum 33: 666–673

Max MB, Lynch SA, Muir J, Shoaf SE, Smoller B, Dubner R 1992 Effects of desipramine, amitriptyline, and fluoxetine on pain in diabetic neuropathy. New England Journal of Medicine 326: 1250–1256

McConnell J, Benson GS, Wood JG 1982 Autonomic innervation of the urogenital system: adrenergic and cholinergic elements. Brain Research Bulletin 9: 679–694

McCormack M 1988 Physiologic consequences and complications of vasectomy. Canadian Medical Association Journal 138: 223–225

McGee SR 1993 Referred scrotal pain: case reports and review. Journal of General Internal Medicine 8: 694–701

McKay M 1984 Burning vulva syndrome. Journal of Reproductive Medicine 29: 457

McKay M 1988 Subsets of vulvodynia. Journal of Reproductive Medicine 33: 695–698

McKay M 1989 Vulvodynia. A multifactorial problem. Archives of Dermatology 125: 256–262

McKay M 1992 Vulvodynia: diagnostic patterns. Dermatologic Clinics 10: 423–433

McKay M 1993 Dysesthetic ('essential') vulvodynia, treatment with amitriptyline. Journal of Reproductive Medicine 38: 9–13

McKenna KD, Nadelhaft I 1986 The organization of the pudendal nerve in the male and female cat. Journal of Comparative Neurology 248: 532–549

McLean NR, Burnett RA 1983 Polyarteritis nodosa of epididymis. Urology 21: 70–71

McLellan AN, Goodell H 1943 Pain from the bladder, the ureter and kidney pelvis. Research Publications – Association for Research in Nervous and Mental Disease 23: 252–262

McMahon AJ, Buckley J, Taylor A, LLoyd SN, Deane RF, Kirk D 1992 Chronic testicular pain following vasectomy. British Journal of Urology 69: 188–191

Meares EMJ 1992 Prostatitis and related disorders. In: Walsh PC, Retik AB, Stanley TA, Vaughan EDJ (eds) Campbell's urology, 6th edn. WB Saunders, Philadelphia, pp 807–822

Messing E, Pauk D, Schaeffer A et al 1997 Associations among cystoscopic findings and symptoms and physical examination findings in women enrolled in the interstitial cystitis data base study. Urology 49: 81–85

Messinger EM 1992 Urethral syndrome. In: Walsh PC, Retik AB, Stanley TA, Vaughan EDJ (eds) Campbell's urology, 6th edn. WB Saunders, Philadelphia, pp 997–1005

Miller JL, Rothman I, Bavendam TG, Berger RE 1995 Prostatodynia and interstitial cystitis: one and the same? Urology 45: 587–589

Mitchinson MJ 1972 Some clinical aspects of idiopathic retroperitoneal fibrosis. British Journal of Surgery 59: 58–60

Mobley DF, Baum N 1996 Interstitial cystitis: when urgency and frequency mean more than routine inflammation. Postgraduate Medicine 99: 201–208

Montorsi F, Guazzoni G, Bergamaschi F et al 1993 Is there a role for transrectal microwave hyperthermia of the prostate in the treatment of abacterial prostatitis and prostatodynia. Prostate 22: 139–146

Moralès A, Emerson L, Nickel JC 1997 Intravesical hyaluronic acid in the treatment of refractory interstitial cystitis. Urology 49: 111–113

Morrison JFB 1987 Role of higher levels of the central nervous system. In: Torrens M, Morrison JFB (eds) The physiology of the lower urinary tract. Springer-Verlag, London, pp 237–274

Moul JW 1993 Prostatitis: sorting out the different causes. Postgraduate Medicine 94: 191–194

Nickel JC 1998 Prostatitis – myths and realities. Urology 51: 363–366

Nickel JC, Sorenson R 1994 Transurethral microwave thermotherapy of nonbacterial prostatitis and prostatodynia: initial experience. Urology 44: 458–460

Nigro DA, Wein AJ, Foy M et al 1997 Associations among cystoscopic and urodynamic findings for women enrolled in the interstitial cystitis data base study. Urology 49: 86–92

Nomina Anatomica, 4th edn 1977 Excerpta Medica, Amsterdam

O'Leary MP, Sant GR, Fowler FJ, Whitmore KE, Spolarich-Kroll J 1997 The interstitial cystitis symptom index and problem index. Urology 49: 58–63

Orland SM, Hanno PM, Wein AJ 1985 Prostatitis, prostatosis, and prostatodynia. Urology 25: 439–459

Paavonen J 1995a Diagnosis and treatment of vulvodynia. Annals of Medicine 27: 175–181

Paavonen J 1995b Vulvodynia – a complex syndrome of vulvar pain. Acta Obstetricia et Gynecologica Scandinavica 74: 243–247

Pagni CA, Canavero S 1993 Paroxysmal perineal pain resembling tic douloureux, only symptom of a dorsal meningioma. Italian Journal of Neurological Sciences 14: 323–324

Paick JS, Donatucci CF, Lue TF 1993 Anatomy of cavernous nerves distal to prostate: microdissection study in adult male cadavers. Urology 42: 145–149

Papka RE, Traurig HH 1993 Autonomic efferent and visceral sensory innervation of the female reproductive system: special reference to neurochemical markers in nerves and ganglionic connections. In: Maggi CA (ed) Nervous control of the urogenital system. Harwood Academic, Chur, Switzerland, pp 423–466

Parkin J, Shea C, Sant GR 1997 Intravesical dimethyl sulfoxide for interstitial cystitis – a practical approach. Urology 49: 105–107

Parsons CL 1997 Epithelial coating techniques in the treatment of interstitial cystitis. Urology 49: 100–104

Peckham BM, Maki DG, Patterson JJ, Hafez GR 1986 Focal vulvitis: a characteristic syndrome and cause of dyspareunia. American Journal of Obstetrics and Gynecology 154: 855–864

Pedersen B, Tiefer L, Ruiz M, Melman A 1988 Evaluation of patients and partners 1 to 4 years after penile prosthesis surgery. Journal of Urology 139: 956–958

Peeker R, Aldenborg F, Fall M 1998 The treatment of interstitial cystitis with supratrigonal cystectomy and ileocystoplasty – difference in outcome between classic and nonulcer disease. Journal of Urology 159: 1479–1482

Periciaro C, Bustamante Jr AS, Gutierrez MM 1993 Two cases of vulvodynia with unusual causes. Acta Dermato-Venereologica (Stockholm) 73: 227–228

Petersen CS, Weismann K 1996 Isoprenosine improves symptoms in young females with chronic vulvodynia. Acta Dermato-Venereologica (Stockholm) 76: 404

Peterson DF, Brown AM 1973 Functional afferent innervation of testis. Journal of Neurophysiology 36: 425–433

Pontari MA, Hanno PM, Wein AJ 1997 Logical and systematic approach to the evaluation and management of patients suspected of having interstitial cystitis. Urology 49: 114

Pozzi SJ 1897 Traite de gynecologie clinique et operatoire, Masson, Paris

Pranikoff K, Constantino G 1998 The use of amitriptyline in patients with urinary frequency and pain. Urology 51(suppl 5A): 179–181

Pyka RE, Wilkinson EJ, Friedrich EG, Croker BP 1988 The histopathology of vulvar vestibulitis syndrome. International Journal of Gynecological Pathology 7: 249–257

Rageth JC, Buerklen A, Hirsch HA 1989 Spätkomplikationen nach Episiotomie. Zeitschrift für Geburtshilfe und Perinatologie 193: 233–237

Ratliff TL, Klutke CG, McDougall EM 1994 The etiology of interstitial cystitis. Urologic Clinics of North America 21: 21–30

Raz S, Smith RB 1976 External sphincter spasticity syndrome in female patients. Journal of Urology 115: 443–446

Reid R, Greenberg MD, Daoud Y, Husain M, Selvaggi S, Wilkinson E 1988 Colposcopic findings in women with vulvar pain syndromes. Journal of Reproductive Medicine 33: 523–532

Robert R, Brunet C, Faure A et al 1993 La chirurgie du nerf pudental lors de certaines algies perineales: evolution et resultats. Chirurgie 119: 535–539

Rosenthal S, Kim YD, Wise GJ 1987 Neuropathy and orchialgia in a 40-year old man. Journal of Urology 138: 114–115

Ruggieri MR, Chelsky MJ, Rosen SI, Shickley TJ, Hanno PM 1994 Current findings and future research avenues in the study of interstitial cystitis. Urologic Clinics of North America 21: 163–176

Sand PK, Bowen LW, Ostergard DR, Bent A, Panganibaum R 1989 Cryosurgery versus dilation and massage for treatment of recurrent urethral syndrome. Journal of Reproductive Medicine 34: 499–504

Sant GR, LaRock DR 1994 Standard intravesical therapies for interstitial cystitis. Urologic Clinics of North America 21: 73–84

Sant GR, Theoharides TC 1994 The role of mast cell in interstitial cystitis. Urologic Clinics of North America 21: 41–54

Schmidt RA, Tanagho EA 1981 Urethral syndrome or urinary tract infection? Urology 18: 424–427

Schneiderman H, Voytovich A 1988 Self-palpation orchitis. Journal of General Internal Medicine 3: 97

Scrimin F, Volpe C, Tracanzan G, Toffoletti FG, Barciulli F 1991 Vulvodynia and selective IgA deficiency. Case reports. British Journal of Obstetrics and Gynecology 98: 592–593

Segura JW, Opitz JL, Greene LF 1979 Prostatosis, prostatitis or pelvic floor tension myalgia? Journal of Urology 122: 168–169

Selikowitz SM, Schned AR 1985 A late post-vasectomy syndrome. Journal of Urology 134: 494–497

Silber SJ 1981 Reversal of vasectomy and the treatment of male infertility: role of microsurgery, vasoepididymostomy, and pressure-induced changes of vasectomy. Urologic Clinics of North America 8: 53–62

Simmons JL, Bunce PL 1958 On the use of antihistamine in the treatment of interstitial cystitis. American Journal of Surgery 24: 664–667

Slade D, Ratner V, Chalker R 1997 A collaborative approach to managing interstitial cystitis. Urology 49: 10–13

Smith PJB 1979 The management of the urethral syndrome. British Journal of Hospital Medicine 22: 578–587

Solomons CC, Melmed MH, Heitler SM 1991 Calcium citrate for vulvar vestibulitis. Journal of Reproductive Medicine 36: 879–882

Sonni L, Cattaneo A, De Marco A, De Magnis C, Carli P, Marabini S 1995 Idiopathic vulvodynia clinical evaluation of the pain threshold with acetic acid solutions. Journal of Reproductive Medicine 40: 337–341

Splatt AJ, Weedon D 1981 The urethral syndrome: morphological studies. British Journal of Urology 53: 263–265

Tanagho EA, Schmidt RA, De Araujo CG 1982 Urinary striated sphincter: what is its nerve supply? Urology 20: 415–417

Theoharides TC, Sant GR 1997 Hydroxyzine therapy for interstitial cystitis. Urology 49: 108–110

Thomas TG (ed) 1980 Practical treatise on the diseases of woman, Henry C Lea's Son, Philadelphia, pp 145–147

Tiefer L, Pederson B, Melman A 1988 Psychosocial follow-up of penile prosthesis implant patients and partners. Journal of Sex and Marital Therapy 14: 184–201

Toozs-Hobson P, Gleeson C, Cardozo L 1996 Interstitial cystitis – still an enigma after 80 years. British Journal of Obstetrics and Gynaecology 103: 621–624

Turner ML, Marinoff SC 1988 Association of human papillomavirus with vulvodynia and the vulvar vestibulitis syndrome. Journal of Reproductive Medicine 33: 533–537

Van de Kleft E, Van Vyve M 1993 Sacral meningeal cysts and perineal pain. Lancet 341: 500–501

Vizzard MA, Erdman SL, Forstermann U, De Groat WC 1994 Differential distribution of nitric oxide synthase in neural pathways to the urogenital organs (urethra, penis, urinary bladder) of the rat. Brain Research 646: 279–291

Vodusek DB, Light JK 1983 The motor nerve supply of the external sphincter muscles: an electrophysiological study. Neurourology and Urodynamics 293: 193–200

Walker EA, Stenchever MA 1993 Sexual victimization and chronic pelvic pain. Obstetrics and Gynecology Clinics of North America 20: 795–807

Walsh PC, Donker PJ 1982 Impotence following radical prostatectomy: insight into etiology and prevention. Journal of Urology 128: 492–497

Warren JW 1994 Interstitial cystitis as an infectious disease. Urologic Clinics of North America 21: 31–40

Watson CP, Evans RJ, Reed K, Merskey H, Goldsmith L, Warsh J 1982 Amitriptyline versus placebo in postherpetic neuralgia. Neurology 32: 671–673

Weisberg LS, Bloom PB, Simmons RL, Viner ED 1993 Loin pain haematuria syndrome. American Journal of Nephrology 13: 229–237

Wesselmann U 1987 Untersuchungen der Impulsübertragung im Ganglion Mesentericum Inferius. Dissertation, Medizinische Fakultät der Christian-Albrechts-Universität zu Kiel, Germany, pp 1–244

Wesselmann U 1998 Management of chronic pelvic pain. In: Aronoff GM (ed) Evaluation and treatment of chronic pain, 3rd edn. Williams and Wilkins, Baltimore 19: 269–279

Wesselmann U, Burnett AL 1996 Treatment of neuropathic testicular pain. Neurology 46 (suppl): 206

Wesselmann U, Lai J 1997 Mechanisms of referred visceral pain: uterine inflammation in the adult virgin rat results in neurogenic plasma extravasation in the skin. Pain 73: 309–317

Wesselmann U, Burnett AL, Campbell JN 1995 The role of the sympathetic nervous system in chronic visceral pain. Society for Neuroscience (Abstracts) 21: 1157

Wesselmann U, Burnett AL, Heinberg LJ 1996 Chronic testicular pain – a neuropathic pain syndrome: diagnosis and treatment. Abstract, 8th World Congress on Pain, p 256

Wesselmann U, Burnett AL, Heinberg LJ 1997 The urogenital and rectal pain syndromes. Pain 73: 269–294

Westrom LV, Willen R 1998 Vestibular nerve fiber proliferation in vulvar vestibulitis syndrome. Obstetrics and Gynecology 91: 572–576

White SH, Leslie IJ 1986 Pain in scrotum due to intervertebral disc protrusion. Lancet i: 504

Whitmore KE 1994 Self-care regimens for patients with interstitial cystitis. Urologic Clinics of North America 21: 121–130

Wilkinson EJ, Guerrero E, Daniel R et al 1993 Vulvar vestibulitis is rarely associated with human papillomavirus infection types 6, 11, 16, or 18. International Journal of Gynecological Pathology 12: 344–349

Woodruff JD, Foster DC 1991 The vulvar vestibule. Postgraduate Obstetrics and Gynecology 11: 1–5

Woodruff JD, Friedrich EG Jr 1985 The vestibule. Clinical Obstetrics and Gynecology 28: 134–141

Yang CC, Bradley WE 1998 Peripheral distribution of the human dorsal nerve of the penis. Journal of Urology 159: 1912–1917

Yeates WK 1985 Pain in the scrotum. British Journal of Hospital Medicine 33: 101–104

York GK, Gabor AJ, Dreyfus PM 1979 Paroxysmal genital pain: an unusual manifestation of epilepsy. Neurology 29: 516–519

Yount JJ, Solomons CC, Willems JJ, Amand RP St 1997 Effective nonsurgical treatments for vulvar pain. Women's Health Digest 3: 88–93

Zimmern PE 1995 Hydrodistension in suspected interstitial cystitis patients: diagnosis and therapeutic benefits. Urology 153: 290A

Zorn BH, Watson LR, Steers WD 1994 Nerves from pelvic plexus contribute to chronic orchialgia. Lancet 343: 1161

Zufall R 1978 Ineffectiveness of treatment of urethral syndrome in women. Urology 12: 337–339

Zvara P, Carrier S, Kour NW, Tanagho EA 1994 The detailed neuroanatomy of the human striated urethral sphincter. British Journal of Urology 74: 182–187

Zvieli S, Vinter L, Herman J 1989 Nonacute scrotal pain in adolescents. Journal of Family Practice 28: 226–228

Orofacial pain

YAIR SHARAV

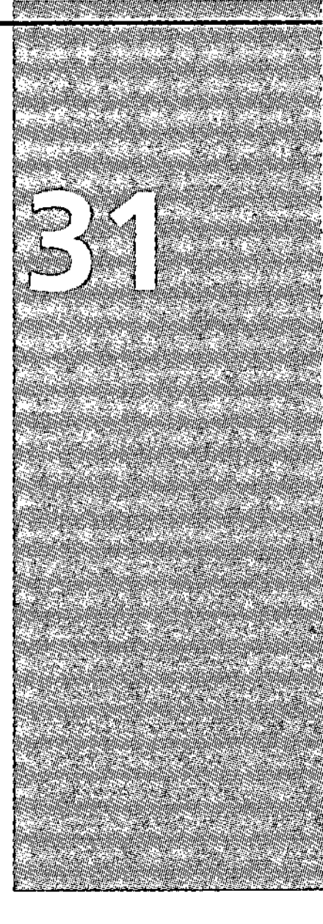

INTRODUCTION

Diagnosis and treatment of orofacial pain are complicated by the density of anatomical structures in the area, mechanisms of referred pain and the important psychological meaning attributed to the face and the oral cavity.

The most prevalent pain in the orofacial region originates from the teeth and their surrounding structures. This is dealt with in detail in the section on oral pain, subdivided into dental, periodontal, gingival and mucosal pain, and is summarized in Table 31.1. Temporomandibular disorders (TMD) is another prevalent entity of orofacial pain. Its controversial aetiology, diagnosis and treatment are thoroughly

Table 31.1 Differential diagnosis of oral pain

	History				*Physical examination*		*Radiography*	
Source of pain	*Ability to locate*	*Character of pain*	*Pain intensified by*	*Pain intensity*	*Associated signs*	*Pain duplicated by*	*Bite-wing*	*Periapical*
Dental								
Dentinal	Poor	Evoked, does not outlast stimulus	Hot, cold, sweet, sour	Mild to moderate	Caries, defective restorations exposed dentine	Hot or cold application, scratching dentine	Interproximal carries, defective restorations	NA
Pulpal	Very poor	Spontaneous, explosive, intermittent	Hot, cold, sometimes chewing	Usually severe	Deep caries, extensive restoration	Hot or cold, caries probing sometimes percussion	Deep caries and deep restoration with no secondary dentine	Limited use, sometimes periapical change
Periodontal								
Periapical	Good	For hours on same level, deep, boring	Chewing	Moderate to severe	Periapical swelling and redness, tooth mobility	Percussion, palpation of periapial area	Limited use, deep caries and deep restorations	Sometimes periapical changes
Lateral	Good	For hours on same level, boring	Chewing	Moderate to serve	Periodontal swelling, deep pockets with pus exudating, tooth mobility	Percussion, palpation of periodontal area	Sometimes alveolar bone resorpion	Very useful when X-rayed with probe inserted into pocket

Table 31.1 Differential diagnosis of oral pain (Contd.)

	History				*Physical examination*		*Radiography*	
Source of pain	*Ability to locate*	*Character of pain*	*Pain intensified by*	*Pain intensity*	*Associated signs*	*Pain duplicated by*	*Bite-wing*	*Periapical*
Periodontal (Contd.)								
Gingival	Good	Pressing, annoying	Food impaction, tooth-brushing	Mild to serve	Acute gingival inflammation	Touch, percussion	NA	NA
Mucosal	Usually good	Burning, sharp	Sour, sharp and hot food	Mild to moderate	Erosive or ulcerative lesions, redness	Palpation of lesion	N/A	N/A

NA = not applicable.

discussed in two distinct entities: temporomandibular myofascial pain (TMP) and internal derangement of the temporomandibular joint. Modern concepts associated with possible relationships between TMP, headache mechanisms and fibromyalgia are examined. Next is a new section on primary vascular-type craniofacial pain, summarized in Table 31.2; typical vascular-type facial pains such as cluster headache and paroxysmal hemicrania are described and a new diagnostic entity, vascular orofacial pain, is proposed and discussed in detail. Ill-defined *atypical oral and facial pain* is discussed next, possible mechanisms are reviewed and suggested therapies are indicated. The 'burning mouth' syndrome (BMS) is considered in detail.

To conclude, the differential diagnosis of orofacial pain is discussed. It is subclassified into pain associated with defined local injury and pain not related to defined injury and is summarized in Table 31.3.

ORAL PAIN

Oral pain is primarily associated with the teeth and their supporting structures, i.e. the periodontium. Most frequently, dental pain is a sequela of dental caries. Initially, when the carious lesion is confined to the dentine, the tooth is sensitive both to changes in temperature and to sweet substances, but pain is not spontaneous. As the lesion penetrates deeper into the tooth, the pain produced by these stimuli becomes stronger and lasts longer. Eventually, when the carious lesion invades the tooth pulp, an inflammatory process develops (pulpitis) associated with acute, intermittent spontaneous pain. If micro-organisms and products of tissue disintegration invade the area around the root apex (periapical periodontitis), the tooth becomes very sensitive to chewing, touch and percussion. At that stage the explosive, intermittent pain acquires a continuous boring nature and the tooth is no longer sensitive to changes in temperature. In clinical practice the demarcation between these various stages is sometimes indistinct; for example, the tooth may be sensitive simultaneously to temperature changes and to chewing. Other sources of oral pain are associated with direct insult to the tissues surrounding the teeth, resulting in lateral periodontal or gingival pain. Pain arising from the oral mucosa can be localized and associated with a detectable erosive or ulcerative lesion or be of a diffuse nature resulting from widespread irritation of the oral mucosa. It is important to realize that there is no correlation between the amount of tissue damage to dental or other oral tissues and reported presence or absence of pain. Pain alone is an insufficient diagnostic tool for oral disease and must be validated by other diagnostic procedures for each individual case.

DENTAL PAIN

Dentinal pain

The pain originating in dentine is described as a sharp, deep sensation that is usually evoked by an external stimulus and subsides within a few seconds. Natural external stimuli are normally produced by food and drinks when hot, cold, sweet, sour and sometimes salty changes are produced. Although extreme changes in temperature (e.g. hot soup followed by ice cream) may cause pain in intact, non-affected teeth, in most cases pain evoked by natural stimuli indicates a hyperalgesic state of the tooth. The pain is poorly localized, often only to an approximate area within two or three teeth adjacent to the affected tooth. Frequently, the patient is unable to distinguish whether the pain originates from the lower or the upper jaw. However, patients rarely make localization errors across the midline and posterior teeth are more difficult to localize than anterior ones (Friend & Glenwright 1968). A wide two-point discrimination threshold is believed to exist when teeth are electrically stimulated (Van Hassel & Harrington 1969).

Duplication of pain produced by controlled application of cold or hot stimuli to various teeth in the suspected area can aid in identifying the affected, hyperalgesic tooth. Most frequently, this hyperalgesic state is associated with dental caries, which can be found by means of direct observation and probing with a sharp dental explorer. The 'bite-wing' intraoral dental radiograph (Fig. 31.1) is a very useful diagnostic aid in these cases. Defective restorations and any other cavity, e.g. abrasion and erosion of the enamel or roots exposed due to gingival recession, are other causes for pain. In these instances, scratching the exposed dentine with a sharp probe can evoke pain and aid in locating its source.

In addition to these symptoms, the patient may also complain of a sharp pain, elicited by biting, that ceases immediately when pressure is removed from the teeth. Localization of the source of pain is not precise, although the affected area can often be limited to two or three adjacent teeth. The patient complains of pain and discomfort associated with cold and hot stimuli in the area. These complaints indicate that there may be a crack in the dentine, the so-called 'cracked tooth syndrome' (Cameron 1976, Goose 1981). Although the diagnosis is frequently difficult because the affected tooth is not readily localized and radiographs are unhelpful, diagnosis and localization of the affected tooth can be achieved by the following:

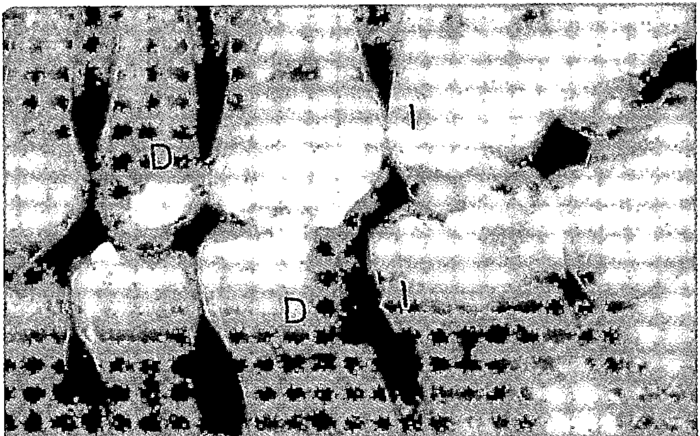

Fig. 31.1 Bite-wing radiograph demonstrating the coronal parts of the posterior teeth on the left. I=initial caries associated with dentinal pain; D= deep caries associated with pulpal pain.

1. percussing the cusps of the suspected teeth at different angles
2. asking the patient to bite on individual cusps using a fine wooden stick
3. probing firmly around margins of fillings and in suspected fissures
4. applying cold stimuli to various areas of the suspected tooth.

Other possible additional diagnoses include occlusal abrasion with exposed dentine or a cracked filling. However, these can be detected visually with the aid of a sharp explorer.

Treatment

Dentinal pain due to caries is best treated by removal of the carious lesion and restoring the tooth by a filling. Sensitivity usually disappears within a day. Treatment of the 'cracked tooth' consists of covering the crown of the tooth with a crown. Treatment of exposed, hypersensitive dentine is somewhat controversial (Seltzer 1978). It has been the author's experience that good oral hygiene is essential in reducing the sensitivity of dentine exposed at the root surface and that acidic foods and beverages will enhance dentinal sensitivity.

Pulpal pain

Pain associated with pulp disease is spontaneous, strong and often throbbing and is exacerbated by temperature change, sweet foods and pressure on the carious lesion. When pain is evoked it outlasts the stimulus (unlike stimulus-induced dentinal pain) and can be excruciating for many minutes. Similarly to dentinal pain, localization is poor and seems to be even poorer when pain becomes more intense. Pain tends to radiate or refer to the ear, temple and cheek but does not cross the midline (Fig. 31.2). Pain may be described by patients in different ways and a continuous dull ache can be periodically exacerbated (by stimulation or spontaneously) for short (minutes) or long (hours) periods (Cohen 1996). Pain may increase and throb when the patient lies down and in many instances wakes the patient from sleep (Sharav et al 1984). The pain of pulpitis is frequently not continuous and abates spontaneously; the precise explanation for such abatement is not clear (Seltzer 1978).

This interrupted, sharp, paroxysmal, non localized pain may lead to the misdiagnosis of other conditions that may mimic pain of pulpal origin (e.g. trigeminal neuralgia). The initial aim of the diagnostic process is to identify the

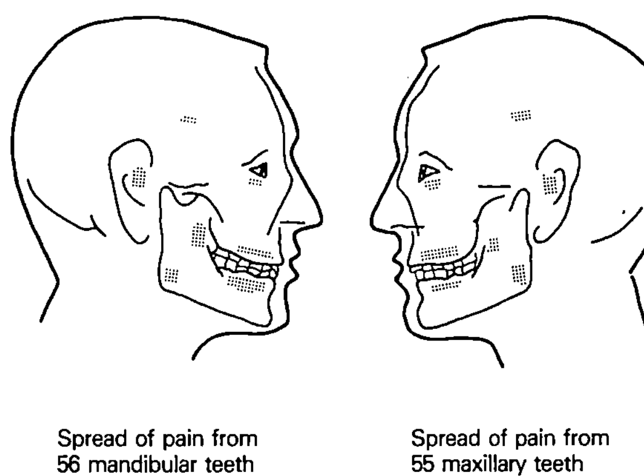

Fig. 31.2 The distribution of pain in the face from dental and periodontal sources. Each dot represents a painful area pointed to by the patient. There is a considerable overlap in pain reference locations for maxillary and mandibular sources.

affected tooth and then to assess the state of the tooth pulp in order to determine treatment. Localization of the affected tooth is achieved through the same methods detailed in the previous section on dentinal pain. The application of heat and cold to the teeth should be done very carefully because these can cause excruciating pain. Percussion aids in localizing the affected tooth. The state of the pulp cannot be judged from one single symptom and should be based on the combination of several signs and symptoms (Seltzer & Bender 1975, Cohen 1996). Although pain is the most common symptom of a diseased pulp, no correlation exists between specific pain characteristics and the histopathological status of the pulp (Seltzer et al 1963, Tyldesley & Mumford 1970).

Treatment

Depending on the prognosis of the pulp, treatment may aim at conserving the pulp, extirpating it or extracting the tooth. Pulpal pain normally disappears immediately after treatment.

MECHANISMS OF DENTAL SENSITIVITY AND PAIN

Recently erupted human teeth with uncompleted roots are often insensitive to tooth pulp stimulation (Tal & Sharav 1985). This cannot be explained by the absence of innervation, as nerve fibres are already present at the time of eruption (Avery 1971). Tal and Sharav (1985) demonstrated that masseteric reflex activity could be evoked in the absence of sensation when teeth were electrically stimulated in children. They proposed that segmental reflex connections appear to be established before the cortical sensory projections are functional.

It is agreed that under certain conditions of tooth pulp stimulation sensations other than pain can be evoked (Sessle 1979). Recent studies address the question of whether non-pain and pain sensations are mediated by two distinct populations of afferents (McGrath et al 1983, Brown et al 1985, Virtanen et al 1987). When temporal summation stimuli were employed it was suggested by McGrath et al (1983) that non-pain sensations are mediated by a distinct population of afferents. Brown et al (1985), utilizing spatial summation techniques, favoured the hypothesis of a single modality innervation for both non-pain and pain sensations. Based upon their temporal summation experiments, Virtanen et al (1987) concluded that 'prepain' and painful sensations from electrical tooth pulp stimulation are both evoked by the same A-fibre populations.

The mechanisms of dentinal sensitivity and pain have been extensively reviewed and deal with the problems of pain conduction in a non-innervated, yet very sensitive, dentine (Anderson et al 1970, Dubner et al 1978, Seltzer 1978, Brannstrom 1979, Närhi 1985, Olgart 1985). Morphologically, nerve fibres may penetrate into the dentine as far as 150–200 mm only (Byers & Kish 1976). Furthermore, the concept that the odontoblast has a role as a sensory receptor of the dentine has not been substantiated (Byers et al 1982).

Experimentally induced pain was produced by applying various stimuli to exposed dentine, i.e. drying by application of absorbent paper or a blow of air, mechanical stimulation (e.g. cutting, scratching, probing) and changes in osmotic pressure, pH or temperature. However, the application of various pain-inducing substances, such as potassium chloride, acetylcholine, 5-hydroxytryptamine (5 HT), bradykinin and histamine to exposed dentine does not evoke pain (Anderson & Naylor 1962, Brannstrom 1962). All these substances can produce pain when placed on a blister base on the skin (Armstrong et al 1953). The limited distribution of nerve fibres in dentine and the fact that neuroactive chemical agents fail to stimulate or anaesthetize dentine led to the proposal of the hydrodynamic mechanism by Brannstrom (1963). The movement of the extracellular fluid that fills the dentinal tubules will, according to Brannstrom's hypothesis, distort the pain-sensitive nervous structure in the pulp and predentinal area and activate mechanoreceptors to produce pain (Brannstrom 1979). Mumford and Newton (1969) and Horiuchi and Matthews (1973), however, could detect an electrical potential across the dentine of extracted teeth to which hydrostatic pressure was applied. It is not clear whether these currents would be

 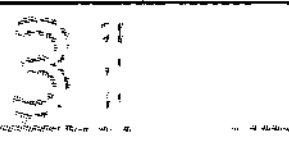

sufficient to excite nerves in the pulp (Greenwood et al 1972).

Many possible pain mechanisms have been suggested for pulpal pain. These have been summarized by Seltzer (1978), Mumford (1982) and Olgart (1985), are related to pulp inflammation and include a host of mediators found in the pulp, such as cholinergic and adrenergic neurotransmitters (probably the most important among these is 5HT), prostaglandins and cyclic adenosine monophosphate (cAMP). Most of these are hypothetical mechanisms, suggested only because such agents produce pain in other parts of the body (Keele & Armstrong 1968). Recent studies do confirm, however, the effect of some substances, such as prostaglandins (probably PGE_2), serotonin and bradykinin (Inoki et al 1993) on tooth pulp nerve excitability. It is suspected that, unlike pulpal C-fibres, A-fibres are relatively insensitive to inflammatory mediators (Olgart 1985). It has recently been found, however, that leukotriene B_4 can sensitize pulpal A-δ fibres (Madison et al 1992). Other factors to be considered are lowered oxygen tension and impaired microcirculation associated with increased intrapulpal pressure. The latter should be considered, taking into account the unique features of the pulp that is rigidly encased within dentin (Trowbridge & Kim 1996).

DIFFERENTIAL DIAGNOSIS OF ODONTALGIA

Diagnosis of toothache is challenging because teeth often refer pain to other teeth as well as to other craniofacial locations (Sharav et al 1984) and other craniofacial pain disorders (Benoliel et al 1997) or pain from more remote structures (Tzukert et al 1981) may refer to teeth. The latter may mimic the symptoms of a toothache. In this respect vascular orofacial pain, to be discussed later, is of great diagnostic importance. Conditions mimicking odontalgia are listed below and should be considered in the differential diagnosis of intraoral pain disorders, especially when toothache is atypical.

Conditions mimicking odontalgia

Musculoskeletal
Arthralgia
Myalgia
Neuropathic
Trigeminal neuralgia
Postherpetic neuralgia
Phantom (deafferentation) toothache
Vascular
Vascular orofacial pain
Cluster headache
Paroxysmal hemicrania
Inflammatory
Papillitis/food impaction
Acute otitis media
Acute maxillary sinusitis
Obstructive sialoadenitis
Herpes zoster infection
Neoplastic
Local/metastatic tumours
CNS lesions
Referred pain not from head and neck
Cardiogenic

PERIODONTAL PAIN

Pain originating in the structures surrounding the teeth is readily localized; the affected teeth are very tender to pressure. Periodontal pain usually results from an acute inflammatory process of the gingiva, the periodontal ligament and alveolar bone due to bacterial infection. Aetiologically, two modes of affection are possible:

1. a sequela of pulp infection and pulp necrosis which results in periapical inflammation
2. gingival and periodontal infection and pocket formation that result in a lateral periodontal involvement.

Although pain characteristics, ability to localize and pain-producing situations are similar in both cases (see Table 31.1), treatment differs for aetiological reasons and these categories are therefore discussed separately.

Acute periapical periodontitis

Pain associated with acute periapical inflammation is spontaneous and moderate to severe in intensity for long periods of time (hours). Pain is exacerbated by biting on the tooth and, in more advanced cases, even by closing the mouth and bringing the affected tooth into contact with the opposing teeth. In these cases, the tooth feels highly extruded and is very sensitive to touch. Frequently the patient reports that pulpal pain preceded the pain originating from the periapical area. The latter, although of a more continuous nature, is usually better tolerated than the paroxysmal and excruciating pulpal pain. Localization of pain originating from the periapical area is usually precise and the patient is able to indicate the affected tooth. In this respect periodontal pain differs from the poorly localized dentinal and pulpal pain. The improved ability to localize the source of pain may be attributed to the proprioceptive and mechanoreceptive sensibility of the periodontium (Harris 1974, Van Steenberghe 1979) that is lacking in the pulp. However, although localization of the affected tooth is usually precise, in approximately half the cases the pain is diffuse and spreads into the jaw on the affected side of the face (Sharav et al 1984).

During examination the affected tooth is readily located by means of tooth percussion. The periapical vestibular area is usually tender to palpation. The pulp of the affected tooth is non-vital, i.e. it does not respond to thermal changes or to electrical pulp stimulation. However, as mentioned above, in clinical practice pulpitis may not be sharply distinguished from acute periapical periodontitis and pulpal as well as periapical involvement could occur at the same time. In these cases, although the periapical area has been invaded by endogenous pain-producing substances due to pulp tissue damage (e.g. 5HT, histamine, bradykinin) and exogenous pain-producing substances (e.g. bacterial toxins) the pulp has not yet completely degenerated and can still react to stimuli such as temperature changes. These instances are fairly common (Okeson 1995). In more severe, purulent cases, swelling of the face associated with cellulitis is sometimes present and can be associated with fever and malaise. The affected tooth may be extruded and mobile. Usually, when swelling of the face occurs, pain diminishes in intensity due to rupture of the periostium of the bone around the affected tooth and the decrease in pus pressure.

The radiographic picture is of limited use in the diagnosis of acute periapical periodontitis as no periapical radiographic changes are detected in the early stages. If a radiographic periapical rarefying osteitis is noticed in a tooth that is sensitive to touch and percussion, the condition is then classified as reacutization of chronic periapical periodontitis. Often, however, such a rarefying osteitis lesion is present in an otherwise symptomless situation. This lack of correlation between pain and the radiographic picture is also true for pain and the type of periapical inflammation and infection present (Block et al 1976, Langeland et al 1977).

Treatment

While the pain originates from the periodontal periapical tissues, the source of insult and infection usually lies within the pulp chamber and the root canal. The primary aim of treatment is to eliminate the source of irritation. The pulp chamber is opened and the root canal cleansed. Grinding the tooth to prevent contact with the opposing teeth also relieves pain. If cellulitis, fever and malaise are present, systemic administration of antibiotics is recommended. Incision and drainage are very effective when a fluctuating abscess is present. Pain usually subsides within 24–48 hours.

Lateral periodontal abscess

Pain characteristics of the lateral periodontal abscess are very similar to those of acute periapical periodontitis. The pain is continuous, moderate to severe in intensity and is exacerbated by biting on the affected tooth. The pain is well localized. During examination swelling and redness of the gingiva may be noticed, usually located more gingivally than in the case of the acute periapical lesion. The affected tooth is sensitive to percussion and is often mobile and slightly extruded. In more severe cases, cellulitis, fever and malaise may occur. A deep periodontal pocket is usually located around the tooth; once probed, there is pus exudation and subsequent relief from pain. The tooth pulp is usually vital, i.e. it reacts normally to temperature changes and electrical stimulation. The pulp may occasionally be slightly hyperalgesic in these cases and sometimes pulpitis and pulpal pain may develop due to retrograde infection (Fig. 31.3). Abscess formation usually results from a blockage of drainage from a periodontal pocket and is frequently associated with a deep infrabony pocket and teeth with root furcation involvement (Fig. 31.3).

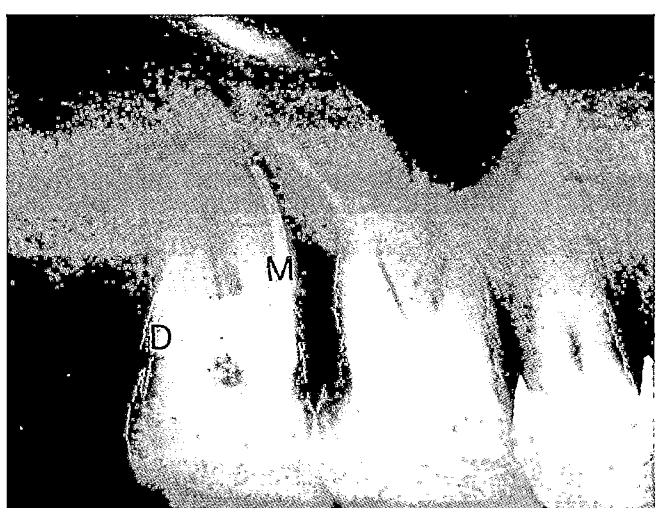

Fig. 31.3 Periapical radiograph of the molar area in the right maxillary region. Radiopaque probes were inserted into mesial (M) and distal (D) periodontal pockets of the second molar to demonstrate the depth of these pockets. Lateral periodontal and pulpal pain were both present. Pulpal pain in this case was not associated with caries but with 'retrograde' infection of the pulp through the deep mesial pocket.

Treatment

Gentle irrigation and curettage of the pocket should be performed. The tooth is ground in order to avoid contact with the opposing teeth. When cellulitis, fever and malaise are present, systemic antibiotic administration is recommended. Direct incision and drainage are recommended when the abscess cannot be approached through the pocket and it is ripe for incision.

Pain usually subsides within 24 hours of treatment.

GINGIVAL PAIN

Gingival pain may occur as a result of mechanical irritation, due to acute inflammation associated with a gingival pocket or as a result of infection when specific underlying factors prevail.

Food impaction

The patient complains of localized pain that develops between two teeth after meals, especially when food is fibrous (e.g. meat, celery). The pain is associated with a feeling of pressure and discomfort that is very annoying. The patient reports that the pain may gradually disappear until evoked again at the next meal or the pain may be relieved immediately by removing the food impacted between the teeth. Upon examination, a faulty contact between two adjacent teeth is noticed so that food is usually trapped between these teeth; the gingival papilla is tender to touch and bleeds easily. The two adjacent teeth are usually sensitive to percussion. The cause of the faulty contact between the teeth is often a carious lesion and restoring the tooth will eliminate pain.

Pericoronitis

Pain, which may be severe, is usually located at the distal end of the arch of teeth in the lower jaw. Pain is spontaneous and may be exacerbated by closing the mouth. In more severe cases, pain is aggravated by swallowing and trismus may occur. Acute pericoronal infections are common in teeth that are incompletely erupted and are partially covered by flaps of gingival tissue.

Upon examination, the flap of gingiva is acutely inflamed, red and oedematous. Frequently, an indentation of the opposing tooth can be seen imprinted on the oedematous gingival flap. Occasionally, fever and malaise are associated with this infection.

Treatment includes irrigation of debris between the flap and the affected tooth and eliminating trauma by the opposing tooth (by grinding or extraction). Systemic antibiotic administration is commonly recommended, especially when trismus occurs.

Acute necrotizing ulcerative gingivitis

Soreness and pain are felt at the margin of the gums. Pain is intensified by eating and brushing the teeth; these activities are usually accompanied by gingival bleeding. In the early stages some patients may complain of a feeling of tightness around the teeth. Metallic taste is sometimes experienced and usually there is a foetid smell from the mouth. Pain is fairly well localized to the affected areas, but in cases when lesions are spread all over the gums pain is experienced all over the mouth. Fever and malaise are sometimes present. Upon examination necrosis and ulceration are noticed on the marginal gingiva with different degrees of gingival papillary destruction. An adherent greyish slough represents the so-called pseudomembrane that is present in the acute stage of the disease. Swabbing this slough is associated with pain and bleeding. Although basically a bacterial disease that responds dramatically to antibiotics, it is not clear whether the bacteria actually initiate the disease or are merely secondary to some underlying factors. Local as well as systemic factors are suggested as possible underlying factors. These include, locally, gross neglect of oral hygiene, heavy smoking and mouth breathing. Systemically, any underlying debilitating factors are suggested, but there is no doubt that these are secondary to the more important local factors (Burket & Greenberg 1977).

Treatment includes swabbing and gentle irrigation of the ulcerative lesions, preferably with an oxidizing agent (hydrogen peroxide), and scaling and cleaning the teeth. Systemic antibiotics are recommended when fever and malaise are present.

INTENSITY AND LOCATION OF ACUTE ORAL PAIN

Acute dental and periodontal pain is frequently rated as moderate to severe in intensity or from 60–100 on a 100 mm visual analogue scale (Sharav et al 1984). Pain is conceived of as deep and unpleasant. In about 60% of cases pain is not localized only at the affected site but spreads into remote areas in the head and face (Fig. 31.2). There is a considerable overlap in pain reference locations for maxillary and mandibular sources (Fig. 31.2). Pain spread is correlated positively with pain intensity and unpleasantness (Fig. 31.4). Two factors which may be important for this

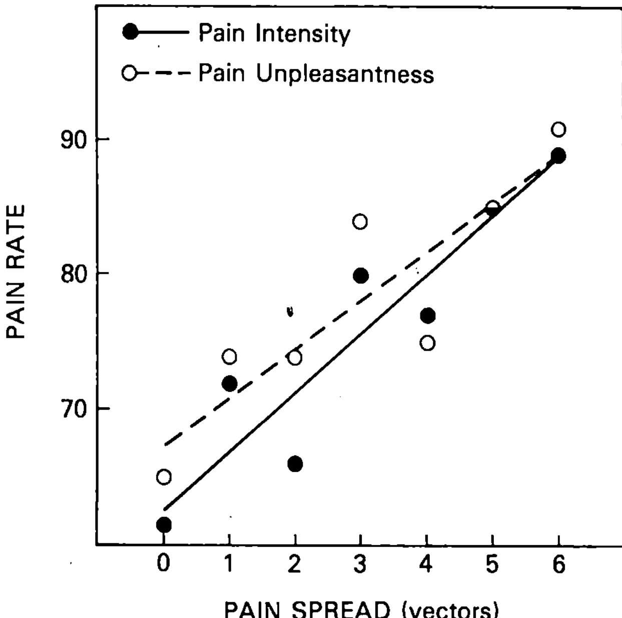

Fig. 31.4 Pain spread in the face, from dental and periodontal sources, as a function of pain intensity and pain unpleasantness ratings. Pain spread is rated as the number of pain reference locations (vectors). Pain intensity and pain unpleasantness are visual analogue scale ratings.

pain spread are the large receptive fields of wide dynamic-range neurons with extensive gradient sensitivity and the somatotopic organization (Sharav et al 1984).

MUCOSAL PAIN

Pain originating from the oral mucosa can be either localized or of a more generalized diffuse nature. The localized pain is usually associated with a detectable erosive or ulcerative lesion; the diffuse pain may be associated with a widespread infection, a systemic underlying deficiency disease or other unknown factors.

The localized pain that is associated with a detectable lesion results from physical, chemical or thermal trauma, viral infection or lesions of unknown origin. Pain is usually mild to moderate but may become quite severe when there is irritation, mechanically or by sour, spicy or hot foods. This exacerbation of pain may last for some minutes. Detailed descriptions of the various lesions of the oral mucosa are beyond the scope of this chapter and only the most common lesion (recurrent aphthous stomatitis) will be described briefly.

Presumably of autoimmune nature and aggravated by stress, recurrent aphthous stomatitis is characterized by a prodromal burning sensation from 2 to 48 hours before an ulcer appears. Although small in diameter (0.3–1.0 cm) this lesion may be quite painful (Greenberg 1977). In the mild form, healing occurs within 10 days and pain is usually mild to moderate in severity. In the more severe forms (major aphthous ulcers), deep ulcers occur which may be confluent, are extremely painful and interfere with speech and eating. Such lesions may last for months, heal slowly and leave scars. Treatment is mostly symptomatic, including the application of a topical protective emollient for the mild form and the use of topical corticosteroids and tetracycline to decrease healing time for the severe form.

When a generalized diffuse pain occurs in the oral mucosa, it usually has a burning nature and may be accompanied by a change in taste, predominantly of a bitter metallic quality. This pain may result from a direct insult to the tissues due to bacterial, viral or fungal infection, which can be identified by the characteristic appearance of the oral mucosa. Diagnosis is aided by microbiological laboratory examinations. In cases of chronic fungal infection (candidiasis), possible underlying aetiological factors such as prolonged broad-spectrum antibiotic therapy, immunodeficiencies and other debilitating factors should be investigated. Radiation therapy to the head and neck region may result in acute mucositis with severe generalized mucosal pain (Kolbinson et al 1988). Decreased salivary flow is a later sequela that may result in chronic pain and discomfort of the oral mucosa.

Burning sensation of the oral mucosa, particularly the tongue, may result from systemic deficiency disease, such as chronic iron deficiency anaemia. This is usually associated with observable atrophic changes, in particular that of the filiform and fungiform papillae of the tongue. However, there is a large proportion of patients, mostly women between the ages of 50 and 70 years, who complain of a burning sensation in the mouth and the tongue, with no observable changes in the oral mucosa and with no detectable underlying systemic changes. This group of patients is discussed further in the section on the burning mouth syndrome.

TEMPOROMANDIBULAR DISORDERS

This prevalent entity of orofacial pain and mandibular dysfunction (Helkimo 1979, Dworkin et al 1990a) has acquired more than a dozen names (De Boever 1979, McNeill 1997) since it was first described by Costen in 1934. In addition to a variety of names, a variety of different criteria have been used for defining this disorder (Rugh & Solberg 1979). Indeed, the criteria for the syndrome were such that they encompassed disorders which under today's concepts would be diagnosed differently (Eversole & Machado 1985, McNeill 1997, Okeson 1997). By the 1950s it was becoming obvious that many of these patients suffered from a masticatory muscle disorder apparently unrelated to the temporomandibular joint (TMJ). However, it was only during the last decade that, with the aid of modern TMJ imaging techniques (Dolwick et al 1983), we began to understand that there was also a temporomandibular disorder of the joint proper that justified separate classification. The definition of internal derangements (ID) of the TMJ finally dissociated the temporomandibular joint from this 'syndrome' and the justification for a separate entity of temporomandibular myofascial pain (unrelated to TMJ pathology), as opposed to the 'general' myofascial pain dysfunction (MPD) syndrome, was further questioned. Indeed, the 1986 International Association for the Study of Pain (IASP) classification combines temporomandibular pain and dysfunction and tension headache under the same category of 'craniofacial pain of musculoskeletal origin'. The justification for segregation of temporomandibular myofascial pain and dysfunction from other myofascial pain disorders of a more generalized type, such as primary fibromyalgia, has more recently been questioned by others (Widmer 1991). The question of whether temporomandibular pain is a localized symptom of a more generalized condition or a discrete entity will be addressed in more detail later.

Recently, the American Academy of Orofacial Pain recommended that orofacial pain and mandibular dysfunction be termed temporomandibular disorders (TMD) (Okeson 1996). TMD are defined as a collective term embracing a number of clinical problems that involve the masticatory musculature, the temporomandibular joint and associated structures or both. These are characterized by pain that is usually aggravated by manipulation or function, limited range of motion, asymmetric mandibular movement and/or locking and joint sounds. It is felt, however, that such 'an all-embracing collective term' is too wide to be usefully discussed. I have chosen therefore to approach TMD as two distinct entities: one associated primarily with pain and dysfunction of myofascial origin, that will be referred to as temporomandibular myofascial pain (TMP); the other associated primarily with intra-articular disorders and referred to as internal derangement (ID) of the TMJ.

TEMPOROMANDIBULAR MYOFASCIAL PAIN

Patients usually describe a poorly localized, dull, continuous ache, typically around the ear, the angle of the mandible and the temporal area. However, pain has also been described in the jaws, teeth and diffusely throughout one side of the face (Okeson 1995). Pain may also occur bilaterally; there is some evidence that bilateral pain is more commonly associated with underlying psychogenic factors (Gerschman et al 1990). The temporal pain pattern varies considerably, with some patients experiencing the most intense pain in the morning or late afternoon and others having no fixed pattern (Laskin 1969). Duration can be from weeks to several years, but fortunately the pain rarely wakes the patient from sleep. Pain may be aggravated during function with transient spikes of pain occurring spontaneously or induced by jaw movements (Okeson 1995).

In addition to pain, there may be deviation of the mandible on opening, fullness of the ear, dizziness and soreness of the neck (Schwarz 1959, Molin 1973, Gelb & Tarte 1975, Block 1976, Sharav et al 1978, Blasberg & Chalmers 1989). Dizziness has been associated with pain in the sternomastoid muscle (Sharav et al 1978) and ear stuffiness with spasm of the medial pterygoid (Block 1976).

Examination may reveal limited mouth opening (less than 40 mm, interincisal). Masticatory and neck muscles are tender to palpation (Butler et al 1975, Gelb & Tarte 1975, Sharav et al 1978) and pain often refers (Travell 1960, Okeson 1995). Trigger points in the muscles may also be detected (Travell & Simons 1983). Diagnosis is usually based on the history and clinical examination of the patient. However, clinical signs are difficult to measure with consistency (Kopp & Wenneberg 1983, Carlsson et al 1980); moreover, inter-rater reliability for some signs of TMD is not good (Dworkin et al 1990b).

Neurophysiological studies

Numerous physiological investigations have been performed in temporomandibular pain patterns (Dubner et al 1978, Yemm 1979, Lund et al 1991). It has been shown that these patients have a substantially reduced biting force compared to controls, which has been attributed to muscle pain and tenderness (Molin 1972). In 1971, Bessette et al reported that the interruption of sustained electromyographic (EMG) activity of the masseter by a tap to the chin (the so-called 'silent period'), was longer in patients than in controls. This was later confirmed by some (Wildmalm 1976, Baily et al 1977), but not by others (Zulqarnain et al 1989). Subject selection and experimental methodological variations could account for some of these differences. Sharav et al (1982) found that masseteric inhibitory periods were shorter in patients than in controls when evoked by electrical tooth pulp stimulation. Shorter inhibitory periods were also described in patients in response to tooth tapping (De Laat et al 1985, Zulqarnain et al 1989). Sharav et al (1982) suggested that there was an increase in excitability of the central motor neuron pool in these patients and muscle hyperactivity was suggested by De Laat et al (1985). A further demonstration of an association between hyperactivity of masticatory muscles and temporomandibular disorders is that EMG inhibitory responses following initial tooth contact are either absent or reduced and that EMG activity, not normally detected when the mouth is open, is found in 50% of temporomandibular patients (Munro 1975). Several other studies report that patients with TMP have higher resting masseter and temporalis EMG activity than non-patients (Glaros et al 1989). No difference was found in the duration of the masseteric inhibitory period between the painful and the non-painful sides (Sharav et al 1982). Comparison of the bilateral activity in the anterior temporalis and the masseter muscles during clenching showed, however, that patients with muscle pain demonstrate asymmetrical recruitment of these muscles in contrast to the more symmetrical recruitment seen in normal individuals (Nielsen et al 1990).

Epidemiology

Temporomandibular pain and dysfunction disorders are recognized as the most common chronic orofacial pain condition (Dworkin et al 1990a). However, information on the prevalence of TMD signs and symptoms was based mainly on studies of patients seeking treatment (Greene & Marbach 1982). A further major problem is the definition of inclusion and exclusion criteria (Rugh & Solberg 1979). Moreover, given poor inter-rater reliability, comparing data seems perilous. The advent of the diagnosis of ID of the TMJ certainly questions the validity of much of the epidemiological research done before this diagnostic entity was defined. In the available epidemiological studies of the general population, TMD signs and symptoms appear to be equally distributed between the sexes (Helkimo 1979, Christensen 1981) or the differences are minor (Locker & Slade 1988). In Agerberg and Carlsson's classic cross-sectional study (1972), about half of the 15–44-year-old population had at least one symptom of dysfunction and one-third had two or more symptoms. Reporting symptoms in a population over 18 years old, Locker and Slade (1988) describe a prevalence of 48.8% while the percentage of those needing treatment was estimated at 3.5–9.7%. Of much interest in this respect is the study of Wanman and Agerberg (1986a) who reported a prevalence of 20% in a study group of 17-year-olds. They followed up this group for 2 years and found that although the incidence was 8% there was no general increase in the severity or number of symptoms in this study period; the explanation offered was that new symptoms appear as often as old ones disappear (Wanman & Agerberg 1986b). Thus, spontaneous remission seems to be quite prevalent in this disorder.

While signs and symptoms of TMD are equally distributed between the sexes in the general population, the majority of patients who seek treatment (up to 80%) are females (Butler et al 1975, Sharav et al 1978, Helkimo 1979, Rugh & Solberg 1985). Signs and symptoms of mandibular dysfunction have been found in all age groups (Helkimo 1979, Nielsen et al 1990), with a tendency to increase with age (Rugh & Solberg 1985, Torvonen & Knuuttila 1988). Dworkin et al (1990a,b) report that TMJ pain, however, is less common among the elderly. Signs of mandibular dysfunction have been described in children and adolescents with a higher prevalence than was previously suspected (Perry 1973, Nielsen et al 1990). The syndrome occurs also in edentulous patients (Carlsson 1976, Agerberg 1988).

Aetiological factors

Bruxism and occlusal derangement

The association between TMP, the teeth and dental occlusion stems back to Costen (1934), who believed that overclosure of the mandible due to loss of teeth was responsible for TMJ pain. More recent theories consider occlusal disturbances a prerequisite for the development of dysfunction and pain. Whilst the extent of the occlusal 'interference' may be minute, the important fact is that such interference can upset proprioceptive feedback and thus cause bruxism and spasm of masticatory muscles (Krogh-Poulsen & Olsson 1968). These assumptions were recently refuted by Rugh et al (1984) who demonstrated that occlusal discrepancies, produced experimentally, tend to reduce bruxism rather than enhance it. Furthermore, data by Thomson (1971), Solberg et al (1972), Clarke (1982) and presented in Greene and Marbach's review (1982) indicate that there are no significant differences between the occlusal relationship in patients and in asymptomatic controls. Finally, in a recent paper, Clark et al (1997) state that the relationship made between occlusion and TMD is not convincing, powerful or practical enough to make any recommendations about a causal association.

Bruxism is no longer perceived as related to occlusal 'disharmonies' but rather as a physiological behaviour that may sometimes be associated with TMP (Rugh & Harlan

1988). Clark et al (1980) suggest that bruxism is stress related. They demonstrated a positive relationship between increased urinary epinephrine and high levels of nocturnal masseter muscle activity. The forces exerted during nocturnal tooth grinding are quite high and were found to exceed maximal conscious clenches (Clarke et al 1984). However, the association between bruxism and TMP is not entirely clear. Bruxism is viewed as an arousal phenomenon (Satoh & Harada 1973) or as a sleep parasomnia (American Sleep Disorder Association 1990). Some preliminary results suggest that a majority of patients with bruxism have pain levels and sleep quality comparable with TMP patients (Lavigne et al 1991). On the other hand, patients having bruxism without muscle pain did not show differences in any of the sleep variables compared to matched controls (Velly-Miguel et al 1991).

A specific relationship between bruxism and TMP is based on the vicious cycle theory where an occlusal interference or a painful lesion of a muscle is supposed to induce a spasm in the affected muscle, which in turn leads to ischaemia because of the compression of blood vessels. Ischaemic contractions are painful and activate muscle nociceptors; by this mechanism the vicious cycle is closed. However, this concept is not supported by experimental data (Mense 1991). If muscle hyperactivity, presumably associated with stress and bruxism, is not the cause of pain but is rather a 'pain adaptation' response (Lund et al 1991) then bruxism can no longer be considered as a specific aetiological mechanism of pain in TMP.

Psychosocial correlates

Early studies emphasize the contribution of psychological factors to TMP (Schwarz 1959). Lascelles (1966) described a background of depressive illness in the majority of his 93 facial pain patients and a significantly larger number of Fine's (1971) TMP patients were depressed compared to controls. However, on the basis of an extensive literature review, Rugh and Solberg (1979) concluded that there was little evidence suggesting that TMP is related to any specific personality trait. Thus, Marbach et al (1978) found no significant difference in either state anxiety or trait anxiety between patients with intractable facial pain and groups of general dental and general medical patients. In a later study Marbach and Lund (1981) found no difference in depression and anhedonia between TMP patients and a normal, non-patient group. Salter et al (1983) challenge the idea that TMP patients represent a population whose pain results from their emotional state. They found that the comparison of TMP patients and patients with facial pain and lesions or pathophysiological disorders showed little evidence of neuroticism in either group. Furthermore, examining the premorbid characteristics of TMP patients did not reveal abnormal parental bonding attitudes in this group (Salter et al 1983) nor did they show any other measures of previous premorbid personality traits (Merskey et al 1987). Sharav et al (1987) found that only two out of 32 patients with chronic facial pain were cortisol non-suppressors on the dexamethasone suppression test (DST). In a recent study Schnurr et al (1990) classified their TMD patients according to the diagnostic criteria of Eversole and Machado (1985), enabling a separate comparison of myogenic (TMP) and of TMJ facial pain to non-facial injury 'pain controls' and healthy controls. The results of Schnurr et al (1990) suggested that TMP and TMJ pain patients do not appear to be significantly different from other pain patients or healthy controls in personality type, response to illness, attitudes toward healthcare or ways of coping with stress.

While psychological factors seem to play a minor role in the aetiology of TMP, research supports the appropriateness of a dual diagnostic approach for TMD based on physical and psychological axes, that allows for treatment customized to address the physical as well as the psychological characteristics of the patient (Turk 1997).

Vascular mechanisms and headache

Muscle tenderness is a frequent finding in headache patients (Raskin & Appenzeller 1980) and the distribution may be distinctly similar to that in TMP patients (Butler et al 1975, Sharav et al 1978, Tafelt-Hansen et al 1981, Clark et al 1987). Patients with signs of TMP report a significantly higher incidence of tension headache than controls (Magnusson & Carlsson 1978, Watts et al 1986); indeed, epidemiological data suggest great similarity and possible overlap between patients suffering from headache and TMP (Magnusson & Carlsson 1978). The sex ratio is similar – about 75% females in both groups; age distribution and contributing psychophysiological mechanisms are also shared (Rugh & Solberg 1979, Raskin & Appenzeller 1980). It seems, therefore, that two of the fundamental symptoms of TMP, i.e. pain of daily occurrence and tenderness of muscles to palpation, fail to properly differentiate between tension-type headache and TMP patients. As previously mentioned, the 1986 IASP classification combines these two under 'craniofacial pain of musculoskeletal origin'. However, most TMP patients have pain and muscle tenderness on palpation unilaterally (Butler et al 1975, Sharav et al 1978) while tension-type headache causes pain bilaterally.

The association between migraine and temporomandibular dysfunction was studied by Watts et al (1986). A total of 50 patients with mixed headache syndromes were compared to 50 TMP patients. The authors stated that the rate of migraine in the TMP group did not differ from that in the general population and concluded that TMP and migraine patients are two segregated groups. That TMP and vascular headache are two distinct entities can also be inferred from studies of sleep physiology. Bruxism, associated with TMP (Lavigne et al 1991), occurred mostly in non-rapid eye movement (N-REM) stages of sleep (Satoh & Harada 1973, Wieselmann et al 1986, Rugh & Harlan 1988), while vascular headache is REM 'locked' (Dexter & Weizman 1970). Recently, however, a severe tooth-destructive form of bruxism has been found in REM sleep (Ware & Rugh 1988), which may suggest that in some cases vascular mechanisms could be associated with TMP.

Fibromyalgia

Much controversy exists in the medical literature concerning muscle tenderness and its diagnosis in specific cases. The boundaries between fibromyalgia (FM) and myofascial pain dysfunction (MPD) are at times poorly demarcated although specific criteria have been established (Scudds et al 1989). In the light of the possibility that on the one hand FM may begin as a localized pain disorder and later become widespread, and on the other hand that persistent MPD may involve multiple sites and cause systemic symptoms (Bennet 1986, Wolfe 1988), some authors believe that all local 'syndromes' of myofascial pain should be conflated to form one entity. Thus, it is claimed by Widmer (1991) that when the symptoms of FM patients are compared with those of patients with temporomandibular disorders without joint pathology, no symptoms are specific to TMP. TMP seems to be a localized condition but the evidence needs to be examined carefully. Blasberg and Chalmers (1989) retrospectively reviewed a series of TMP patients for evidence of generalized musculoskeletal pain. They conclude that there are great similarities between these and primary fibromyalgia (PFM) patients. Eriksson et al (1988) studied eight patients with PFM and found that six had severe signs of mandibular dysfunction using the Helkimo Anamnestic Dysfunction Index, thus promoting the hypothesis that a connection may exist between these entities.

These conclusions should be viewed very carefully; PFM, by definition, is characterized by a widespread pain on both sides of the body and in both the upper and the lower parts of the body in 97.6% of PFM patients (Henriksson & Bengtsson 1991), whereas TMP is mostly a local, unilateral, pain syndrome (Sharav et al 1978, Okeson 1995).

TMJ damage

Theoretically, trauma or noxious stimulation of TMJ tissues can produce a sustained excitation of masticatory muscles that may serve to protect the masticatory system from potentially damaging movements and stimuli (Sessle & Hu 1991). However, injection into the TMJ of algesic chemicals resulted in sustained reflex increase in EMG activity of jaw-opening muscles; excitatory effects were also seen in jaw-closing muscles but were generally weaker (Broton & Sessle 1988). While such effects might be related to clinically based concepts of myofascial dysfunction (e.g. splinting, myospastic activity and trigger points), the weak effects in muscles that are invoked clinically to show such dysfunction (jaw closing) and the stronger effects in antagonist muscles (jaw opening) suggest associations more in keeping with protective, withdrawal-type reflexes (Sessle & Hu 1991). Based upon the available data, it seems that pain originating in the TMJ contributes minimally to the development of TMP.

Conclusions

Bruxism and TMJ derangements do not seem to be primary aetiological factors of TMP. The role that vascular mechanisms, related to other craniofacial pains (e.g. migraine, cluster headache, paroxysmal hemicrania), play in TMP is not entirely clear. Whilst the importance of vascular mechanisms may not yet be fully appreciated, one should not dismiss their contribution to TMP. Some data (Ware & Rugh 1988) point to a REM-locked destructive form of bruxism that may link certain forms of TMP with vascular mechanisms. Recent findings strongly suggest that neurogenic inflammation may play the major role in vascular headache (Moskowitz et al 1989). In view of the cardinal role of the trigeminal system in conveying vascular headache (Dostrovsky et al 1991), the possibility of interrelated central mechanisms of headache and facial pain cannot be discounted. Research in the area of TMP should concentrate more on central generators of pain mechanisms rather than peripheral inputs such as occlusal interferences and 'muscle hyperactivity' (Lund et al 1991). One attractive way to understand TMP better is to study the role of trigeminal neurogenic inflammation and the contribution of the sympathetic nervous system (Basbaum & Levine 1991) regarding the pain mechanisms of TMP.

Differential diagnosis

TMP should be differentiated from pain due to TMJ derangement and other specific TMJ disease (e.g. psoriasis, rheumatoid arthritis). Of particular importance are instances where TMP can mask underlying malignancies such as nasopharyngeal carcinoma (Sharav & Feinsod 1977, Roistacher & Tanenbaum 1986).

Treatment

Like other chronic pain syndromes, TMP is a complex entity associated with behavioural changes, secondary psychological gains, changes in mood and attitudes to life and drug abuse. While alleviation of pain and dysfunction remain the primary goals of therapy, restoring the patient's attitudes by modelling behavioural changes and controlling drug abuse should also be achieved. Often reassurance of the patient, combined with simple muscle exercises for masticatory and neck muscles, will result in pain alleviation and restored mandibular function (Schwarz 1959, Selby 1985). Muscle tenderness may be treated with vapocoolant sprays and injections of local anaesthetics into identified trigger points (Travell & Simons 1983). Diazepam is significantly more effective than placebo in the relief of pain, while ibuprofen has had minimal therapeutic benefit in TMP patients (Singer et al 1987). Sharav et al (1987) demonstrated the beneficial effect of low doses of amitriptyline (less than 30 mg/day) in patients with chronic facial pain of myofascial origin. The efficacy of amitriptyline in relieving chronic facial pain, such as TMP, is through a direct analgesic effect not associated with the antidepressive effect of the drug (Sharav et al 1987). Occlusal splint therapy is a widely used mode of treatment (Clarke et al 1984), and may be associated with the reduction of nocturnal bruxism (Clark et al 1979). Some investigators found occlusal splint therapy to be superior to relaxation procedures (Okeson et al 1983).

It is widely believed that chronic pain patients lack psychological insight and therefore do not respond to psychodynamic interpretation (Sternbach 1978). Consequently other psychological interventions such as relaxation training, biofeedback and cognitive behaviour approaches (Carlsson & Gale 1976, Stem et al 1979) would be more appropriate for these patients.

Prognosis in the majority of patients is good and remission of pain and dysfunction is readily achieved for long periods.

INTERNAL DERANGEMENT OF THE TEMPOROMANDIBULAR JOINT

Internal derangement (ID) of the TMJ is defined as an abnormal relationship of the articular disc to the mandibular condyle, fossa and articular eminence. Usually the disc is displaced in an anteromedial direction (Dolwick & Riggs 1983). In addition to pain, limited mouth opening, or deviation of mouth opening, patients complain of clicking in the TMJ. Clicking refers to a distinct cracking, snapping sound associated with opening and closing of the mouth. Farrar (1971) introduced the term 'reciprocal clicking' to describe patients with opening and closing clicks. Reciprocal click is considered pathognomonic to internal derangement. Patients may report an increase in the intensity of the pain prior to the click with relief after the click occurs. Pain is usually limited to the TMJ area. The TMJ will generally be tender to palpation and the muscles of mastication may sometimes be tender. Crepitus and multiple scraping sounds are best detected with the aid of a stethoscope placed over the TMJ while the patient opens and closes the mouth. Crepitus frequently indicates a disruption of the disc or its posterior attachment and heralds more advanced disease.

The final, definitive diagnosis of ID is made by arthrography of the TMJ using radiopaque contrast material injected into the joint space, usually the lower one (Katzberg et al 1979). While the diagnostic 'gold standard' has been arthrography, MRI is now the imaging technique of choice for the TMJ IDs (Rao 1995) and CT for hard tissue imaging (Larheim 1995). However, these seem justified only in appropriately selected cases (doubtful or suspicion of tumour) or candidates for surgery. In combination with SPECT, MRIs demonstrate a sensitivity of 0.96 for IDs. The invasive nature of arthrography and the high cost involved in MRIs that would otherwise need to be performed routinely support a conservative approach.

On the basis of clinical signs and arthrographic findings, ID of the TMJ has been further classified (Dolwick & Riggs 1983, Eversole & Machado 1985, Roberts et al 1985). This classification includes:

1. disc displacement with reduction
2. disc displacement with intermittent locking
3. disc displacement without reduction
4. disc displacement with perforation.

Clinical signs and arthrographic findings are usually in good agreement (Roberts et al 1985).

Anatomical studies on nerve fibre distribution in the joint disclose the fact that the adult joint possesses no nerve endings within the disc. Specialized and free nerve endings are located in the retrodiscal tissues (Griffin & Harris 1975). Unlike rheumatoid arthritis, ID of the TMJ is not associated with an inflammatory cell reaction in the joint capsule. However, deposits of extravasated erythrocytes and altered composition of the connective tissue are present. The presence of these pain-initiating breakdown products and that of nerve fibres trapped in the posterior disc attachment, which become compressed during movement, may be responsible for TMJ arthralgia (Isacsson et al 1986). There are no proven aetiological factors for IDs of the TMJ. Proposed aetiological factors include jaw trauma, muscle hyperactivity and hyperextension of the mandible.

Recent findings may challenge the relationship between TMJ pain dysfunction and the concept of disc displacement (Westesson et al 1989, Nitzan et al 1991). Westesson et al (1989) demonstrated that 15% of healthy asymptomatic volunteers were radiographically abnormal with displacement of the disc; Nitzan and Dolwick (1991) showed that more than 50% of patients in a most advanced stage of ID (closed-locked) had normally shaped discs. Although in both studies there may be a sample selection bias, they still indicate that factors other than disc position may be considered, at least in some patients, for the genesis of pain and dysfunction associated with the TMJ. These may include decreased volume of synovial fluid with high viscosity or a 'vacuum effect' (Nitzan et al 1991, 1992).

Treatment

Conservative treatment modalities recommended for TMP are utilized for ID of the TMJ. Unfortunately, as has long been known, the elimination of joint sounds is the single most resistant feature in most studies dealing with these patients (Eversole & Machado 1985). Interocclusal anterior repositioning splints are of value in eliminating clicks, but are of short-term benefit with no known long-term effect (Lundh et al 1985). In more advanced cases which do not respond to non-surgical treatment, surgery is recommended (Dolwick & Riggs 1983). However, long-term evaluation of non-surgical treatment of advanced cases demonstrated favourable results (Yoshimura et al 1982) and it seems that most individuals with internal derangement do not deteriorate and, indeed, demonstrate remarkable adaptive potential (Okeson 1995). In selected cases, arthrographic surgery or rinsing and lavage seems to be the treatment of choice (Nitzan et al 1991). On the basis of current data, one is unable to conclusively recommend any specific treatment modality.

PRIMARY VASCULAR-TYPE CRANIOFACIAL PAIN

The differential diagnosis of primary vascular-type craniofacial pain includes migraine-type headaches, cluster headaches, paroxysmal hemicranias, SUNCT, cold stimulus ('ice cream') headache and a recently proposed (Sharav et al 1996) vascular orofacial pain (Table 31.2). Each diagnostic entity has specific criteria for diagnosis (Headache Classification Committee 1988 & Mersky, Bogduk 1994) but in general craniofacial vascular pains have some common signs and symptoms:

Pain is:	*Accompanied by:*
a. Periodic	a. Ocular: tearing, redness
b. Severe	b. Nasal: rhinorrhoea, congestion
c. Unilateral	c. Local swelling and redness
d. Pulsatile	d. Nausea, vomiting
e. Wakes from sleep	e. Photo/phonophobia

MIGRAINE

Migraine with or without aura is a periodic, unilateral headache mostly in the forehead and temple areas. Pain may persist from a couple of hours to 2 days. Pain intensity is moderate to severe, usually throbs and may be accompanied by photo- and phonophobia and is associated with nausea and occasional vomiting (Table 31.2).

As migraine headache is discussed in detail in Chapter 33, it will not be further discussed here.

CLUSTER HEADACHE

Cluster headache (CH) was first recognized in the 1950s. Episodic CH refers to a temporal pattern consisting of a series of pain attacks, or 'active' episodes, occurring in succession over a period of 4–12 weeks with 'inactive' periods that last from 6 to 18 months. In the active period pain occurs daily or almost daily. Patients with continuous cluster headache, or constantly 'active', were also recognized and are termed 'chronic CH' (Nappi & Russell 1993).

Pain pattern

Pain is unilateral, occurs in the ocular, frontal and temporal areas, is excruciatingly severe, paroxysmal and may last from 15 to 120 minutes. Nocturnal attacks are typical.

Accompanying phenomena

Pain attacks are accompanied by ipsilateral cojunctival injection, lacrimation, stuffiness of the nose and/or rhinorrhoea. Ipsilateral ptosis and miosis may be associated with some attacks; occasionally they persist after attacks and may remain permanently (Mersky & Bogduk 1994). Onset is at 30–40 years, with predominantly a male population. Alcohol precipitates attacks in the active period (Table 31.2).

Table 31.2 Differential diagnosis of primary vascular-type craniofacial pain

	Migraine headache	*Cluster headache*	*Paroxysmal hemicrania*	*Vascular orofacial pain*
Onset (age)	20–40	30–40	30–40	40–50
M:F	1:2	5:1	1:2	1:2.5
Location (mostly unilateral)	Forehead, temple	Orbital and periorbital	Temporal and periauricular	Intraoral/lower face
Duration	Hours to days	15–120 min	Minutes	Mins to hours
Time course	Periodic	Periodic/chronic	Chronic	Periodic/chronic
Character of pain	Throbbing, deep, continuous	Paroxysmal, boring In clusters	Paroxysmal, lancinating	Throbbing, may be paroxysmal
Pain intensity	Moderate to severe	Severe	Severe	Moderate to severe
Precipitating factors	Stress, hunger, menstrual period, etc.	Alcohol	Movement of head	Sometimes cold foods
Associated signs	Nausea, photophobia, visual aura	Lacrimation, rhinorrhoea, ptosis, miosis	Lacrimation, rhinorrhoea, eye redness	Cheek swelling and redness, tearing
Treatment: *abortive*	NSAID, ergot, sumatriptan	Oxygen, ergot, sumatriptan	Indomethacin	NSAID
Treatment: *prophylactic*	Amitriptyline, β-blockers, valproates	Ergot, methysergide, lithium carbonate	Indomethacin	Amitriptyline, β-blockers

Treatment

Treatment consists of abortive and prophylactic approaches. Most effective abortive treatment is the administration of 100% oxygen at a rate of 7–8 l/min for 15 minutes during an attack (Nappi & Russell 1993). Ergot preparations and sumatriptan (s.c.) have a beneficial effect. Prophylactic treatment is administered during the active period. Ergot preparations should not exceed 10 mg per week. Methysergide can be administered for short (weeks) periods. Lithium carbonate is utilized for the chronic-type cluster headache.

PAROXYSMAL HEMICRANIA

Paroxysmal hemicrania (PH) was first described by Sjaastad and Dale in 1974 and was thought initially to be a rare variant of cluster headache. As new cases appear and the clinical features of this syndrome (Table 31.2) are further defined, it is doubtful that subclassifying PH under CH will be justified (Benoliel & Sharav 1998b). The International Association for the Study of Pain (IASP), in their most recent classification (Mersky & Bogduk 1994), thus defined a separate category for PH. This seems justified, based on a number of features that distinguish PH from CH (Table 31.2).

Temporal pattern

The attacks in PH are short (10–25 minutes), sharp and excruciating; hence the term 'paroxysmal' (Antonaci & Sjaastad 1989). Frequency is higher than that usually seen in cluster headaches; about eight attacks per 24 hours in PH, but with as many as 30 (Haggag & Russell 1993). The first reported cases of PH were of a continuous nature and were categorized as chronic paroxysmal hemicrania (CPH). In contrast to CH, only a scant number of PHs behaved episodically (EPH) and many of these eventually developed into a chronic form (CPH:EPH = 4:1) (Antonaci & Sjaastad 1989). A high number of patients report nocturnal attacks of PH that wake the patient from sleep (Antonaci & Sjaastad 1989). However, the same nocturnal tendency as in CH is not apparent. Like most vascular-type craniofacial pain, PH is considered to be REM sleep related (Sahota & Dexter 1990).

Location

Pain occurs typically in the temporal, periauricular and periorbital areas, hence the term hemicrania. Referral to the shoulder, neck and arm has been reported. Unlike CH that may change sides, the vast majority of PH cases do not. Most cases in PH are unilateral and do not become bilateral but strong pain may cross the midline.

Accompanying Phenomena

As in other primary vascular-type headaches, PH is accompanied by a number of usually ipsilateral autonomic phenomena. These may occur bilaterally but the symptomatic side is more pronounced. The most commonly seen are lacrimation (62%), nasal congestion (42%), conjunctival injection and rhinorrhoea (36% each) (Benoliel & Sharav 1998b).

Treatment

The response to indomethacin in PH is usually absolute and clearly distinguishes it from CH, which is non-responsive. Recently, however, the inclusion of an absolute indomethacin response as part of PH's criteria has been questioned.

SUNCT

Short-lasting, Unilateral, Neuralgiform, headache attacks with Conjunctival injection and Tearing (SUNCT) syndrome was introduced by Sjaastad (Sjaastad et al 1989). It is a unilateral headache/facial pain characterized by brief, triggered, paroxysmal pain accompanied by ipsilateral local autonomic signs, usually conjunctival injection and lacrimation (Benoliel & Sharav 1998a). Multiple attacks occur usually during daytime, with less than 2% occurring at night. Each attack lasts from 15 to 120 seconds (Pareja et al 1996a).

Triggering

SUNCT may be triggered by light mechanical stimuli in the areas innervated by the trigeminal nerve, in a way similar to trigeminal neuralgia. Neck movements have also been shown to trigger attacks (Mersky & Bogduk 1994).

Pain typically appears in the ocular and periocular regions, corresponding to the area innervated by the first branch (ophthalmic) of the trigeminal nerve. However, pain may be felt in the temporal and auricular regions.

Accompanying phenomena

By definition, SUNCT is accompanied by marked ipsilateral conjunctival injection and lacrimation, but these can also be seen in trigeminal neuralgia (Benoliel & Sharav 1998c). Nasal stuffiness, rhinorrhoea and sweating may also accompany attacks, but are rarer and may be subclinical.

Treatment

A further distinct factor in SUNCT is its absolute resistance to both antineuralgic and antivascular drug therapy.

COLD STIMULUS ('ICE CREAM') HEADACHE

Application of ice to the palate or to the posterior pharyngeal mucosa produces facial pain in the midfrontal region or around the ears, referred probably by the trigeminal and glossopharyngeal nerves respectively (Lance 1993). Pain follows the passage of cold material over the palate and posterior pharyngeal wall and does not originate in the teeth. It is postulated that incoming impulses due to cold cause disinhibition of central pain pathways. Cold stimulus headache or 'ice cream' headache occurs particularly in individuals with a history of migraine and is not associated with dental pathology.

Treatment

No treatment is needed other than sensible caution in ingestion of cold substances.

VASCULAR OROFACIAL PAIN

Recently, Sharav et al (1996) proposed a new diagnostic entity: vascular orofacial pain (VOP), that was detailed in a later publication (Benoliel et al 1997). The rationale for introducing such a separated diagnostic entity is based on the specific features of VOP, that segregate it from other primary vascular-type craniofacial pain and justify a unique diagnosis (Table 31.2). Furthermore, orofacial pain of vascular origin is of great diagnostic and therapeutic importance. The similarities between dental pulpitis and VOP, especially when it affects only the oral structures, have obviously caused diagnostic difficulties (Brooke 1978, Rees & Harris 1979, and see Benoliel et al 1997).

As can be seen from Table 31.2, vascular orofacial pain (VOP) is characterized by strong, episodic, unilateral, intraoral pain. In about half of cases the pain throbs and wakes the patient from sleep. Pain may last from minutes to hours

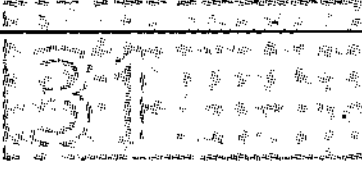

(70% of cases) or can go on for days (30% of cases). Pain can be accompanied by various local autonomic signs, such as tearing or nasal congestion, or by other phenomenon such as photo- or phonophobia and nausea (Benoliel et al 1997). The onset of VOP is around 40–50 years of age and it affects females at a rate of 2.5 times more than males.

Mechanisms of VOP

The trigeminovascular system

There is unequivocal evidence for the existence of sensory axons innervating cephalic blood vessels. Together they have been termed the trigeminovascular system (Moskowitz 1993). These trigeminal axons relay nociceptive information to the central nervous system and, when stimulated antidromically, promote a neurogenic inflammation. Because the neurogenic inflammation takes place within the restricted space of the cranium, the pain may be more severe than if it occurred in a more flexible space. Such pain mechanisms are possible in other craniofacial structures within confined spaces. Thus, the pain in cluster headache may be associated with a perivascular inflammatory process of the carotid artery in its bony canal or, as supported by findings of increased intraocular pressure, within the confines of the eye (Pareja et al 1996b). It is not surprising, then, that such a neurogenic inflammatory process, when confined to another limited space, i.e. the tooth pulp chamber or inferior alveolar canal, may cause strong intraoral pain that mimic pulpitis.

Neurogenic inflammation in oral tissues and the dental pulp

Nerve fibres entering the dental pulp have been identified as unmyelinated nerve fibres that are C-fibres and autonomic nerves (Trowbridge & Kim 1996). Additionally, myelinated A-δ fibres and A-β fibres have also been demonstrated (Byers 1984). Nerve fibres exhibiting SP and CGRP positive immunoreactivity have been demonstrated in the dental pulp and oral mucosa in several species including humans (Wakisaka 1990, Gyorfi et al 1992). Following antidromic electrical nerve stimulation, neurogenic inflammation has been demonstrated in the dental pulp of dogs (Inoki et al 1973) and in the dental pulp and lower lip of rats (Ohkubo et al 1993). Since the role of neurogenic inflammation in the trigeminovascular system seems to play a central role in the genesis of vascular-type headaches, the same mechanism could function in the oral mucosa and teeth.

It is tempting to further extrapolate the model and compare the trigeminovascular system causing its effects within the space limited by the skull to the neurovascular system in the dental pulp similarly confined by the dental hard tissues. It is possible that pressure build-up plays a role in intrapulpal pain sensation. A-δ fibres have been shown to be sensitive to the increased intrapulpal pressure following extravasation (Wallin 1976).

Differential diagnosis of VOP

Dental pain

The extensive involvement of the teeth and oral structures accompanied by common dental symptomatology (e.g. thermal hypersensitivity) in VOP often leads to confusion with pulpitis.

Primary vascular-type headaches

Although exhibiting some similarities to other primary vascular headaches, there may be enough differentiating factors to define VOP separately (Table 31.2). If VOP were simply a migraine variant one would expect to see the majority of patients with long pain attacks (hours–days) and no local autonomic signs. Cluster headache is often misdiagnosed as pain of dental origin, but is usually located primarily periocularly (Nappi & Russell 1993). The similarities to the cluster headache group are limited by the fact that systemic symptoms (such as nausea and photo/phonophobia) are often present in VOP, with an overwhelming female preponderance, and that treatment response is not similar.

Neuropathic-type pains

Trigeminal neuralgia is a short-lasting pain with a particular triggering pattern not usually accompanied by frank autonomic signs, making it clinically distinct from VOP.

Treatment

Successful abortive treatment in VOP has been attained with non-steroidal anti-inflammatory drugs. No particularly preferential response to indomethacin (see paroxysmal hemicrania) has been noted and sodium naproxen (275–550 mg stat) has proved effective abortive therapy. Prophylactic treatment using amitriptyline at doses up to 50 mg and the use of β-adrenergic blocking agents (in antihypertensive dosage) are effective.

ATYPICAL ORAL AND FACIAL PAIN

This ill-defined category includes a variety of pain descriptions such as phantom tooth pain (Marbach 1978), atypical odontalgia (Rees & Harris 1979, Brooke 1980) and atypical facial neuralgia (Marbach et al 1982). Chronic pain, usually at a constant intensity, is a common feature of all the above. The pain has a burning quality which occasionally intensifies to produce a throbbing sensation. The pain is not triggered by remote stimuli, but may be intensified by stimulation of the painful area itself. Autonomic phenomena are usually not seen. Grushka et al (1987a) demonstrated that pain in the burning mouth syndrome was comparable in intensity to toothache and was more severe than has previously been suggested. The pain does not usually wake the patient from sleep. The location is ill defined. Although the pain usually starts in one quadrant of the mouth, it often spreads across the midline to the opposite side. Frequently, the pain changes location, which may result in extensive dental work, alcohol nerve blocks and surgery; this does not usually alleviate the pain. Unfortunately, it has been the author's experience and that of others (Marbach et al 1982) to see patients who have had more than 70(!) operations performed in their mouth (e.g. pulp extirpation, apicoectomy, tooth extraction) for the relief of this type of pain.

Typically in most of these patients there is a lack of objective signs and all other tests are negative. The age range is wide (20–82 years), but the mean age of patients with atypical odontalgia is around 45–50 years (Marbach 1978, Rees & Harris 1979, Brooke 1980, Vickers et al 1998), and of patients with sore mouth and other oral complaints (e.g. burning sensation) around 55 years (Grushka et al 1987a). All reports indicate an overwhelming majority of females (82–100%) in the series of atypical oral and facial pain studied.

There is no identified uniform aetiology of atypical oral and facial pain (Loeser 1985). Several underlying mechanisms have been proposed. A number of reports have suggested that atypical facial pain is a psychiatric disorder (Engel 1951, Lascelles 1966, Feinmann et al 1984, Remick & Blasberg 1985). Depression is considered the most likely diagnosis and is explained on the basis of the catecholamine hypothesis of affective disorders (Rees & Harris 1979). However, Sharav et al (1987) showed that only two of their 28 patients were cortisol non-suppressors on the dexamethasone suppression test and that half the patients were not depressed at all. Grushka et al (1987a) conclude that the personality characteristics of patients with burning mouth syndrome are similar to those seen in other chronic pain patients and that these personality disturbances tend to increase with increased pain. Marbach (1978) postulates that phantom tooth pain associated with previous trauma such as tooth extraction and tooth pulp extirpation interferes with central nervous system pain modulatory mechanisms. This idea is supported by the observation that experimental tooth extraction produces lesions in the trigeminal nucleus caudalis (Westrum et al 1976, Gobel & Binck 1977). It was also found that more extensive tooth pulp injury is associated with greater excitatory changes of central trigeminal neurons (Hu et al 1990). Although far from proven, a deafferentation associated with peripheral nerve injury may be responsible for some types of atypical facial pain. Recently, Jaaskelainen et al (1998) studied the eye blink reflex (BR) in 17 patients with atypical facial pain. Twelve demonstrated electrophysiological signs of hyperexcitability such as lack of habituation of the BR. These were explained as correlates of allodynia, because the stimulus intensities used in the study were not noxious (Jaaskelainen et al 1998). Furthermore, the atypical facial pain group demonstrated higher stimulus thresholds for the R1 component of the BR, indicating altered tactile sensory function (Jaaskelainen et al 1998). It is too early to say, however, whether the BR can be considered a diagnostic tool that specifically identifies patient with atypical facial pain.

Vascular changes are other possible underlying mechanisms for atypical facial pain (Reik 1985). Rees and Harris (1979) and Brooke (1980) found a history of migraine in about a third of their patients (and see previous section on vascular orofacial pain).

Atypical facial pain should be differentiated from pains associated with a causative lesion. Chronic atypical facial pain can be a presenting symptom of a slow-growing cerebellopontine angle tumour (Nguyen et al 1986).

While various treatment modalities are used for atypical oral and facial pain, the predominant trends are clear. All authors firmly recommend against any surgical or dental interventions for the relief of pain (Loeser 1985). Since such interventions usually exacerbate the condition, reassurance, psychological counselling and the use of antidepressants, particularly from the tricyclic group, have been found to be a very promising mode of therapy. Two double-blind controlled studies demonstrated that tricyclic antidepressive drugs were superior to placebo in reducing chronic facial pain (Feinmann et al 1984, Sharav et al 1987). Furthermore, Sharav et al (1987) showed that amitriptyline was effective in a daily dose of 30 mg or less and that the relief of pain was independent of the antidepressive activity. In a recent paper, Vickers et al (1998) analyse the effects of various modes of therapy on 50 cases with 'atypical odontalgia'; the application of a topical anaesthetic (ELMA) results in 60% reduction of pain, while phentolamine infusion reduces pain by 31% and topical application of capsaicine results in 58% pain reduction. It is hard to conclude from their results what the underlying mechanism is. Vickers et al (1998) suggest a possible neuropathic pain mechanism, but point out that it cannot explain all cases. One should also note that 10 out of their 50 cases have periodic, rather than constant pain, which could indicate a vascular type orofacial pain (and see section on vascular orofacial pain). Finally, Vickers et al (1998) suggest that some of their cases may fit the diagnosis of complex regional pain syndrome (Mersky & Bogduk 1994).

THE BURNING MOUTH SYNDROME

The burning mouth syndrome (BMS) is an intraoral pain disorder that is unaccompanied by clinical signs. Its vague definition and unknown aetiology warrant its inclusion under atypical oral and facial pain. Inclusion criteria of patients with BMS may differ in different studies, e.g. the presence of systemic disorders may or may not be an exclusion criterion (Grushka 1987, Van der Ploeg et al 1987). Numerous names have been given to this disorder, such as: glossodynia, glossopyrosis, oral dysaesthesia, oral galvanism or the more widely accepted name burning mouth syndrome (Hampf et al 1987, Zilli et al 1989, Cekic-Arambasin et al 1990, Grushka & Sessle 1991).

The prevalence of BMS is in the range of 1.5–2.5% of the general population but may be as high as 15% in women over 40 years of age (Grushka & Sessle 1991).

Clinical features

Burning pain often occurs at more than one oral site, with the anterior two-thirds of the tongue, the anterior hard palate and the mucosal aspect of the lower lip most frequently affected (Main & Basker 1983, Grushka et al 1987a). The pain is intense and quantitatively similar to toothache pain but differs from toothache in quality. While toothache was mostly described as annoying and sharp, BMS pain was most commonly described as burning (Grushka et al 1987a). Burning pain is constant throughout the day or begins by mid-morning and reaches maximum intensity by early evening, but is not usually present at night and does not disturb sleep (Gorsky et al 1987, Grushka 1987). Many studies indicate, however, that BMS patients have difficulty falling asleep (Grushka 1987, Lamey & Lamb 1988, Zilli et al 1989). Grushka (1987) reported no significant difference between BMS and controls in any clinical oral features including number of teeth, oral mucosal conditions, presence of Candida and parafunctional habits.

Psychophysical assessment

There is evidence for taste dysfunction in BMS, especially in those individuals with self-reported dysgeusia (Grushka et al 1987c). Sweet thresholds were significantly higher for BMS than control subjects. At suprathreshold concentrations, perception intensity was significantly higher for the BMS cases than for controls for sweet tastes and for sour at some of the lower suprathreshold concentrations (Grushka & Sessle 1991). No differences were found between BMS and control subjects in somatosensory modalities such as two-point discrimination, temperature perception and stereognostic ability at any of eight intraoral and facial sites tested (Grushka et al 1987b). Grushka et al (1987b) did, however, find that heat pain tolerance was significantly reduced at the tongue tip of BMS subjects and suggested as an explanation the possibility that hyperalgesia in these patients may depend on prolonged temporal or spatial central summation.

Recently, Jaaskelainen et al (1997) studied the BR in 11 patients with BMS. As a group, the BMS patients demonstrated higher stimulus thresholds for the R1 component of the BR, indicating altered tactile sensory function (Jaaskelainen et al 1997). In 50% of the BMS subjects, R3 components of the BR were present at non-painful stimulus intensities. Four of the patients demonstrated electrophysiological signs of hyperexcitability such as lack of habituation of the BR. These findings were explained as correlates of allodynia, because the stimulus intensities used in the study were not noxious (Jaaskelainen et al 1997). BMS patients thus demonstrated changes on the BR similar to other atypical facial pain subjects (Jaaskelainen et al 1998).

Aetiology

Many possible aetiologies have been suggested and include local, intraoral factors as well as general, systemic ones.

Local factors

These include galvanic currents, denture allergy and mechanical irritation and decreased salivary secretion or change in saliva composition. No difference was found in electric currents, potential or energy capacity in the dental metallic restorations between BMS patients and controls

(Hampf et al 1987). Most studies have not supported an allergic or mechanical irritation cause for BMS (Grushka & Sessle 1991). Most salivary flow rate studies have not demonstrated a significant decrease in salivary output, stimulated or unstimulated (Glick et al 1976, Syrjanen et al 1984, Lamey & Lamb 1988). On the other hand, some studies found significant alterations in salivary components such as proteins, immunoglobulins and phosphates as well as differences in saliva pH buffering capacity (Glick et al 1976, Syrjanen et al 1984, Hampf et al 1987, Grushka & Sessle 1991). Whether these alterations in salivary composition are a causal or a coincidental event in BMS is unknown (Grushka & Sessle 1991).

Systemic factors

Among these are menopause and hormonal imbalance, nutritional deficiencies and psychogenic factors.

A wide range of prevalence rates (18–80%) was given to BMS during menopause or after oophorectomy (Storer 1965, Ferguson et al 1981, Wardrop et al 1989), pointing to different definition criteria and possibly to various sampling methods. In a recent study Wardrop et al (1989) found significantly more oral discomfort in menopausal women. The oral discomfort was not associated with any of the vasomotor symptoms of menopause nor did it show any relationship to mucosal health. The presence of oral discomfort bore no relationship to follicle-stimulating hormone (FSH) or oestradiol levels measured in menopausal women, but hormone replacement therapy was accompanied with a significant reduction in oral discomfort (Wardrop et al 1989). However, as no control group was utilized it was difficult to assess how much of this reduction was due to a placebo effect. In spite of the conflicting data on the effect of menopause and oestrogen replacement therapy on oral discomfort, the high frequency of oral complaints in menopausal women clearly indicates a significant, although poorly understood, association between menopause and BMS (Grushka & Sessle 1991).

Iron serum deficiency was observed in 40% of patients with BMS (Brooke & Seganski 1977) but no control group was used. Lamey et al (1986) did not find any deficiency in A, C, D or E vitamins but did observe deficiency of vitamins B1, B2 and B6. With appropriate replacement therapy, Lamey et al (1986) produced clinical resolution of symptoms in most cases but no lasting effect in non-vitamin deficient BMS subjects. It is difficult to draw conclusions from this study since a double-blind crossover design was not used and a double-blind placebo-controlled study (Hugoson & Thorstensson 1991) could not demonstrate any effect of B1, B2 and B6 vitamin replacement therapy in vitamin-deficient BMS patients. Recently serum zinc levels were found to be significantly lower in BMS patients than in matched controls (Maragou & Ivanyi 1991). However, only nine out of 30 BMS patients demonstrated zinc levels less than the minimum normal levels. There is certainly a need for more controlled studies in order to determine the role of these nutrient elements in BMS.

Numerous studies have used psychological questionnaires and psychiatric interviews to demonstrate psychological disturbances such as depression, anxiety and irritability in patients with BMS (Grushka et al 1987a, Van der Ploeg et al 1987, Hammaren & Hugoson 1989, Zilli et al 1989). BMS patients showed elevation in certain personality characteristics which were similar to those seen in other chronic pain patients (Grushka et al 1987a). Zilli et al (1989) indicate that psychiatric illness, especially depression, may play an important role in BMS. However, most investigators cannot say whether depression and other personality characteristics are causative or the result of the pain (Grushka et al 1987a, Van der Ploeg et al 1987, Zilli et al 1989, Grushka & Sessle 1991).

In conclusion, no clear aetiology is available today and it is possible that a further subclassification of this 'syndrome' is needed. A more rigorous definition of inclusion and exclusion criteria may help in future studies of aetiology and possible therapy.

Treatment

Before treatment is instigated, local and systemic underlying factors should be ruled out and treated. Thus, faulty irritating prosthetic devices should be corrected and underlying diseases, such as diabetes or anaemia, should be treated. Unfortunately, as noted above, in many instances these corrections may not improve the burning sensation and oral discomfort. Symptomatic treatment with psychotropic drugs, such as amitriptyline or clonazepam, may be of some benefit, but no good controlled studies are available to demonstrate a real effect of these drugs. The local application of various medications was recently examined. Interestingly, burning sensation increased after local application of topical anaesthesia, while dysgeusia symptoms were more likely to decrease (Ship et al 1995). Ship et al (1995) suggested a centrally based neuropathic condition for the burning sensation and that the topical anaesthesia may be releasing peripheral inhibition of central sensory pathways. However, the application of capsaicin to oral mucosa in patients with intraoral neuropathic pain was beneficial in about 50% of patients (Epstein & Marcoe 1994).

The potential importance of a placebo effect cannot be ruled out in this open study (Epstein & Marcoe 1994) and double-blind controlled studies are warranted before this treatment can be recommended for BMS.

DIFFERENTIAL DIAGNOSIS OF OROFACIAL PAIN

PAIN AND DEFINED LOCAL INJURY

Diagnosis of pain in the orofacial region is complicated by the density of anatomical structures, rich innervation, high vascularity of the area and the important psychological meaning that is attributed to the face and the oral cavity. Most prevalent is pain in the area that results from local injury to fairly well-defined anatomical structures. Injury can result from trauma, infection and neoplasia. Pain in these cases can be defined and described in terms of anatomical structures and thus originates from the oral cavity, the jaws, salivary glands, paranasal sinuses or the TMJ. Oral pain has been extensively reviewed above and can be divided into dental, periodontal and mucosal pain. These have been summarized in Table 31.1.

Pain from the jaws can be associated with acute infection, malignancies and direct trauma. Unless infected, cysts, retained roots or impacted teeth are usually not responsible for pain in the jaws. Radiation therapy to this area may result in severe pain due to infection and osteomyelitis associated with osteoradionecrosis. Odontogenic and other benign tumours of the bone do not normally produce pain in the jaws except for the osteoid osteoma, which is known to be associated with severe pain. However, this tumour is extremely rare in the jaws (Shafer et al 1974). Malignant tumours, both primary and those metastasized to the jaws, usually produce deep, boring pain, associated with paraesthesia (Massey et al 1981). Pain from salivary glands is localized to the affected gland, may be quite severe and, when associated with a blocked salivary duct, is intensified by increased saliva production, such as that occurring before meals. The salivary gland is swollen and extremely sensitive to palpation. Salivary flow from the affected gland is usually reduced and sometimes abolished completely. Pain may be associated with fever and malaise. In children, the most common causes are acute recurrent parotitis and mumps. In adults, pain from salivary glands usually results from blockage of a salivary duct by calculus or mucin plug formation. Pain results from salivary retention, resulting in pressure and sometimes ascending infection. In acute parotitis, mouth opening exerts pressure on the gland by the posterior border of the mandible, resulting in severe pain (see Table 31.3).

Pain from the maxillary sinus is deep and boring and may become quite severe. Usually the maxillary posterior teeth on the affected side are tender to pressure and percussion. Pain is commonly felt all over the maxillary sinus. In some cases, the infraorbital nerve on the affected side is very sensitive to pressure and there is hyperaesthesia in the area supplied by this nerve. Pain is intensified by either moving the head rapidly or by lowering the head. Pain may be associated with fever and malaise (Table 31.3).

Pain from the TMJ is usually intensified by movement of the mandible; the joint is tender when palpated via the external auditory meatus. Pain may result from acute infection, trauma, rheumatoid arthritis, psoriasis and primary or secondary malignant tumours. When acutely inflamed the joint may be swollen and warm to touch. A splinting protective mechanism by the masticatory muscles may result in muscle spasm, producing secondary pain.

PAIN NOT RELATED TO DEFINED INJURY

Pain in the orofacial area can result from mechanisms other than local injury described above. These are usually associated with chronic orofacial pain and can be generated by musculoskeletal, vascular, neuropathic, referred and psychogenic mechanisms (Okeson 1995). Trauma to the head and neck, especially high-velocity trauma, may be associated with a combination of mechanisms (Benoliel et al 1994).

Musculoskeletal pain is related to TMP and was discussed extensively above.

Vascular pain was discussed under the section on primary vascular-type craniofacial pain. In addition, pain in the facial area may also be associated with occlusive vascular disease, such as temporal arteritis (Paine 1977). External carotid occlusive disease has been described as a cause of facial pain (Herishanu et al 1974) and carotid system arteritis is an important entity in the differential diagnosis of facial pain (Troiano & Gaston 1975). Neuropathic pain is primarily expressed in the facial area as idiopathic trigeminal neuralgia, also known as tic douloureux. Classic features are: paroxysmal pain which lasts only seconds; pain produced by non-noxious stimuli applied to a trigger zone; pain confined to the trigeminal nerve and unilateral in any one paroxysm; the patient is pain free between attacks and there is no accompanying sensory loss. (Dubner et al 1987). A rare form of facial neuralgic pain, associated with sweet food intake, was recently described (Sharav et al 1991, Helcer et al 1998). Neuralgic pain of a completely different type may be associated with herpes zoster, which is a bor-

Table 31.3 Differential diagnosis of orofacial (excluding primary vascular-type) pain

	Dental	*TMP*	*TMJ (ID)*	*Sinusitis (maxillary)*	*Salivary glands*	*Trigeminal neuralgia*	*Atypical deaferrent*
Location	Mouth, ear, jaws, cheek	Angle of mandible, temple, jaws	TMJ, ear	Cheek, zygomatic area	Area of gland	Nerve distribution	Diffuse, may cross midline
Localization	Poor, radiating, does not cross midline	Diffuse but usually unilateral	Localized, usually good	Usually localized, may radiate	Usually good	Good, in the trigeminal distribution	Poor, may change location
Duration	Minutes to hours	Weeks to years	Weeks to years	Days to weeks	Hours to days	Seconds	Weeks to years
Character of pain	Intermittent, sharp, paroxysmal	Dull, continuous, annoying	Deep, boring	Dull, boring, pressing	Drawing, pulling	Lancinating, paroxysmal	Dull, boring, continuous
Pain intensity	Mild to severe	Mild to moderate	Mild to moderate	Mild to severe	Moderate to severe	Severe	Mild to severe
Precipitating factors	Hot and cold foods	yawning, chewing	yawning, chewing	Bending, head movement	Eating, especially sour food	Touch, vibration, cold wind	Stress, fatigue
Associated signs	Caries	Limited mouth opening	Click in TMJ, deviation of mouth opening	Cheek oedema, infraorbital nerve hypoaesthesia	Blockage of salivary flow, salivary gland swelling	Facial tic	Sometimes scarring
Pain duplication	Cold/hot application	Masticatory muscle palpation	TMJ palpation	Pressure on sinus wall, head bending	Pressure to gland, citric acid to tongue	Touch of trigger point	Rubbing of scar if present
Sleep association	May disturb	Does not disturb	May disturb	May disturb	May disturb	Does not disturb	Does not disturb
Treatment	Endodontic, tooth restoration	Physiotherapy Behavioural TCA	Bitegaurd, NSAID, TCA	Antibiotic decongestants	Antibiotics, blockage removal	Carbamazepine baclofen, nerve block, neurosurgery	TCA, clonazepam behavioural

TMP = temporomandibular pain; ID = internal derangement; TMJ = temporomandibular joint; NSAID = non-steroidal anti-inflammatory drugs; TCA = tricyclic antidepressant drugs

ing, burning pain of long duration and high intensity. Postherpetic neuralgia may develop in some of these cases.

Referred pain is a frequent feature in the facial area: pain may refer from teeth to remote areas in the head and face (Sharav et al 1984) and muscle pain from both neck and masticatory muscle is referred to the oral and facial areas (Travell 1960). Pain in the teeth may also be referred from the ear (Silverglade 1980). Of special interest is pain due to cardiac ischaemia that is referred to the orofacial area (Tzukert et al 1981). Facial pain can also be an expression of a central nervous system lesion (Bullitt et al 1986).

Psychogenic pain in the orofacial area is associated with many emotional disorders; however, depression is apparently the most frequent (Lascelles 1966, Harris 1974, Remick & Blasberg 1985). Psychogenic pain overlaps many of the features of atypical oral and facial pain that have been described previously. It is possible that apparent atypical oral and facial pain is often psychogenic in nature.

REFERENCES

Agerberg G 1988 Mandibular function and dysfunction in complete denture wearers – a literature review. Journal of Oral Rehabilitation 15: 237–249

Agerberg G, Carlsson GE 1972 Functional disorders of the masticatory system. Distribution of symptoms accordings to age and sex as judged from investigation by questionnaire. Acta Odontologica Scandinavica 30: 597–613

American Sleep Disorder Association 1990 International classification of sleep disorders: diagnosis and coding manual. American Sleep Disorder Association, Rochester, Minnesota, pp 181–185

Anderson DJ, Naylor MN 1962 Chemical excitants of pain in human dentine and dental pulp. Archives of Oral Biology 7: 413

Anderson DJ, Hannam AG, Matthews B 1970 Sensory mechanisms in mammalian teeth and their supporting structures. Physiological Review 50: 171

Antonaci F, Sjaastad O 1989 Chronic paroxysmal hemicrania (CPH): a review of the clinical manifestations. Headache 29: 648–656

Armstrong D, Dry RML, Keele CA, Harkham JN 1953 Observations of chemical excitants of cutaneous pain in man. Journal of Physiology 120: 326

Avery JK 1971 Structural elements of the young normal human pulp. Oral Surgery 32: 113

Baily JO, McCall WD, Ash MM Jr 1977 Electromyographic silent periods and jaw motion parameters; quantitative measures of temporomandibular joint dysfunction. Journal of Dental Research 56: 249

Basbaum AI, Levine JD 1991 The contribution of the nervous system to inflammation and inflammatory disease. Canadian Journal of Physiology and Pharmacology 69: 647–651

Bennet RM 1986 Current issues concerning management of the fibrositis/fibromyalgia syndrome. American Journal of Medicine (suppl 3A): 1–115

Benoliel B, Sharav Y 1998a SUNCT syndrome: case report and literature review. Oral Surgery, Oral Medicine, Oral Pathology, Oral Radiology and Endodontics 85: 158–61.

Benoliel R. Sharav Y 1998b Paroxysmal hemicrania: case studies and review of the literature. Oral Surgery, Oral Medicine, Oral Pathology, Oral Radiology and Endodontics 85: 285–292

Benoliel R, Sharav Y 1998c Trigeminal neuralgia with lacrimation or SUNCT syndrome? Cephalalgia 18: 85–90

Benoliel R, Eliav E, Elishoov H, Sharav Y 1994 The diagnosis and treatment of persistant pain following trauma to the head and neck. Journal of Oral and Maxillofacial Surgery 52: 1138–47

Benoliel R, Elishoov H, Sharav Y 1997 Orofacial pain with vascular-type features. Oral Surgery, Oral Medicine, Oral Pathology, Oral Radiology and Endodontics 84: 506–512

Bessette RW, Bishop B, Mohl N 1971 Duration of masseteric silent period in patient with TMJ syndrome. Journal of Applied Physiology 30: 864

Blasberg B, Chalmers A 1989 Temporomandibular pain and dysfunction syndrome associated with generalized musculoskeletal pain: a retrospective study. Journal of Rheumatology (suppl 19): 87–90

Block SL 1976 Possible etiology of ear stuffiness (barohypoacusis) in MPD syndrome. Journal of Dental Research 55: B250 abstract 752

Brannstrom M 1962 The elicitation of pain in human dentine and pulp by chemical stimuli. Archives of Oral Biology 7: 59

Brannstrom M 1963 Dentine sensitivity and aspiration of odontoblasts. Journal of the American Dental Association 66: 366

Brannstrom M 1979 The transmission and control of dentinal pain. In: Crossman LI (ed) Mechanism and control of pain. Masson, New York, p 15

Brooke RI 1978 Periodic migrainous neuralgia: a cause of dental pain. Oral Surgery 46: 511

Brooke RI 1980 Atypical odontalgia. Oral Surgery 49: 196

Brooke RI, Seganski DP 1977 Aetiology and investigation of the sore mouth. Journal of the Canadian Dental Association. 10: 504

Broton JG, Sessle BJ 1988 Reflex excitation of masticatory muscles induced by algesic chemicals applied to the temporomandibular joint of the cat. Archives of Oral Biology 33: 741–747

Brown AC, Beeler WJ, Kloka AC, Fields EW 1985 Spatial summation of pre-pain and pain in human teeth. Pain 21: 1

Bullitt E, Tew J, Boyd J 1986 Intracranial tumors in patients with facial pain. Journal of Neurosurgery 64: 865–871

Burket LW, Greenberg MS 1977 Disease primarily affecting the gingiva. In: Lynch MA (ed) Burket's oral medicine, 7th edn. JB Lippincott, Philadelphia, p 175

Butler JH, Folke LE, Brandt CL 1975 A descriptive survey of signs and symptoms associated with the myofascial pain-dysfunction syndrome. Oral Surgery 90: 635

Byers MR 1984 Dental sensory receptors. International Review of Neurobiology 25: 39–94

Byers MR, Neuhaus SJ, Gehirg JD 1982 Dental sensory receptor structure in human teeth. Pain 13: 221

Byers MR, Kish SJ 1976 Delineation of somatic nerve endings in rat teeth by radioautography of axon-transported protein. Journal of Dental Research 55: 419

Cameron CE 1976 The cracked tooth syndrome: additional findings. Journal of the American Dental Association 93: 971

Carlsson GE, 1976 Symptoms of mandibular dysfunction in complete denture wearer. Journal of Dentistry 4: 265

Carlsson GE, Gale EN 1976 Biofeedback treatment for muscle pain associated with the temporomandibular joint. Journal of Behavioural, Therapeutic and Experimental Psychiatry 7: 383

Carlsson GE, Egermark-Eriksson I, Magnusson T 1980 Intra- and inter-observer variation in functional examination of the masticatory system. Swedish Dental Journal 4: 187–194

Cekic-Arambasin A, Vidas I, Stipetic-Mravak M 1990 Clinical oral test for the assessment of oral symptoms of glossodynia and glossopyrosis. Journal of Oral Rehabilitation 17: 495–502

Christensen LV 1981 Facial pains and the jaw muscles: a review. Journal of Oral Rehabilitation 8: 193

Clark GT, Beemsterboer PL, Solberg WK, Rugh JD 1979 Nocturnal electromyographic evaluation of myofascial pain dysfunction in patients undergoing occlusal splint therapy. Journal of the American Dental Association 99: 607–611

Clark GT, Rugh JD, Handelman SL 1980 Nocturnal masseter muscle activity and urinary acid catecholamine levels in bruxers. Journal of Dental Research 59: 1571–1576

Clark GT, Green EM, Dornan MR, Flack VF 1987 Craniocervical dysfunction levels in a patient sample from a temporomandibular joint clinic. Journal of the American Dental Association 115: 251–256

Clark GT, Tsukiyama Y, Baba K, Simmons M 1997 The validity and utility of disease detection methods and of occlusal therapy for temporomandibular disorders. Oral Surgery, Oral Medicine, Oral Pathology, Oral Radiology and Endodontics 83: 101–116

Clarke NG 1982 Occlusion and myofascial pain dysfunction: is there a relationship? Journal of the American Dental Association 85: 892

Clarke NG, Townsend GC, Carey SE 1984 Bruxing patterns in man during sleep. Journal of Oral Rehabilitation 11: 123–127

Cohen S 1996 Endodontic diagnosis. In Cohen S, Burns RC (eds) Pathways of the pulp, 7th edn. CV Mosby, St Louis

Costen JB 1934 Syndrome of ear and sinus symptoms dependent upon disturbed function of the temporomandibular joint. Annals of Otorhinolaryngology 43: 1

De Boever JA 1979 Functional disturbances of the temporomandibular

joint. In: Zarb GA, Carlsson GE (eds) Temporomandibular joint. Munksgaard, Copenhagen, p 193
De Laat A, Van der Glas HW, Weytjens JLF, Van Steenberghe D 1985 The masseteric post-stimulus electromyographic-complex in people with dysfunction of the mandibular joint. Archives of Oral Biology 30: 177
Dexter JD, Weizman ED 1970 The relationship of nocturnal headaches to sleep stage patterns. Neurology 20: 513–518
Dolwick MD, Riggs RR 1983 Diagnosis and treatment of internal derangements of the temporomandibular joint. Dental Clinics of North America 27: 561
Dolwick MF, Katzberg RW, Helms CA 1983 Internal derangements of the temporomandibular joint: fact or fiction? Journal of Prosthetic Dentistry 49: 415
Dostrovsky JO, Davis KD, Kawakita K 1991 Central mechanisms of vascular headaches. Canadian Journal of Physiology and Pharmacology 69: 652–658
Dubner R, Sessle BJ, Storey AT 1978 The neural basis of oral and facial function. Plenum, New York
Dubner R, Sharav Y, Gracely RH, Price DD 1987 Idiopathic trigeminal neuralgia: sensory features and pain mechanisms. Pain 31: 23–33
Dworkin SF, Huggins KH, LeResche L et al 1990a Epidemiology of signs and symptoms in temporomandibular disorders: clinical signs in cases and controls. Journal of the American Dental Association 120: 273–281
Dworkin SF, LeResche L, DeRouen T, Von-Kroff M 1990b Assessing clinical signs of temporomandibular disorders: reliability of clinical examiners. Journal of Prosthetic Dentistry 63: 574–579
Engel GL 1951 Primary atypical facial neuralgia. An hysterical conversion symptom. Psychosomatic Medicine 13: 375
Epstein JB, Marcoe JH 1994 Topical application of capsaicin for treatment of oral neuropatic pain and trigeminal neuralgia. Oral Surgery, Oral Medicine and Oral Pathology 77: 135–140
Eriksson PO, Lindmen R, Stal P, Bengtsson A 1988 Symptoms and signs of mandibular dysfunction in primary fibromyalgia syndrome (PSF) patients. Swedish Dental Journal 12: 141
Eversole LR, Machado L 1985 Temporomandibular joint internal derangements and associated neuromuscular disorders. Journal of the American Dental Association 110: 69
Farrar W 1971 Diagnosis and treatment of anterior dislocation of the articular disc. New York Journal of Dentistry 41: 348
Feinmann C, Harris M, Cawley R 1984 Psychogenic facial pain: presentation and treatment. British Medical Journal 288: 436
Ferguson MM, Carter J, Boyle P et al 1981 Oral complaints related to climacteric symptoms in oophorectomized women. Journal of the Royal Society of Medicine 74: 492
Fine EW 1971 Psychological factors associated with non-organic temporomandibular joint pain dysfunction syndrome. British Dental Journal 131: 402
Friend LA, Glenwright HD 1968 An experimental investigation into the localisation of pain from the dental pulp. Oral Surgery 25: 765
Gelb H, Tarte J 1975 A two-year dental clinical evaluation of 200 cases of chronic headache: craniocervical-mandibular syndrome. Journal of the American Dental Association 91: 1230
Gerschman JA, Reade PC, Hall W, Wright J, Holwill B 1990 Lateralization of facial pain, emotionality and affective disturbance. Pain 5 (suppl): S42
Glaros AG, McGlynn FD, Kapel L 1989 Sensitivity, specificity and the predictive value of facial electromyographic data in diagnosing myofascial pain-dysfunction. Cranio 7: 189–193
Glick D, Ben Aryeh H, Gutman D et al 1976 Relation between idiopathic glossodynia and salivary flow rate and content. International Journal of Oral Surgery 5: 161
Gobel S, Binck JM 1977 Degenerative changes in primary trigeminal axons and in neurons in nucleus caudalis following tooth pulp extirpations in the cat. Brain Research 132: 347
Goose DH 1981 Cracked tooth syndrome. British Dental Journal 2: 224
Gorsky M, Silverman S Jr, Chinn H 1987 Burning mouth syndrome: a review of 98 cases. Journal of Oral Medicine 42: 7
Greenberg MS 1977 Ulcerative, vesicular and bullous lesions. In: Lynch MA (ed) Burket's oral medicine, diagnosis and treatment, 7th edn. JB Lippincott, Philadelphia, p 33
Greene CS, Marbach JJ 1982 Epidemiologic studies of mandibular dysfunction: a critical review. Journal of Prosthetic Dentistry 48: 184–190
Greenwood F, Horiuchi H, Matthews B 1972 Electrophysiological evidence on the types of nerve fibres excited by electrical stimulation of teeth with a pulp tester. Archives of Oral Biology 17: 701
Griffin CJ, Harris E 1975 Innervation of the temporomandibular joint. Australian Dental Journal 20: 78
Grushka M 1987 Clinical features of burning mouth syndrome. Oral Surgery 63: 30
Grushka M, Sessle BJ 1991 Burning mouth syndrome. Dental Clinics of North America 35: 171
Grushka M, Sessle BJ, Miller R 1987a Pain and personality profiles in burning mouth syndrome. Pain 28: 155
Grushka M, Sessle BJ, Howley TP 1987b Psychophysical assessment of tactile pain and thermal sensory functions in burning mouth syndrome. Pain 28: 169
Grushka M, Sessle BJ, Howley TP 1987c Taste dysfunction in burning mouth syndrome (BMS). Annals of the New York Academy of Sciences 510: 321
Gyorfi A, Fazekas A, Rosivall L 1992 Neurogenic inflammation and the oral mucosa. Journal of Clinical Periodontology 19: 731–736
Haggag KJ, Russell D 1993 Chronic paroxysmal hemicrania. In: Olesen J, Tafelt-Hansen P, Welch K M A (eds) The headaches. Raven Press, New York, pp 601–608
Hammaren M, Hugoson A 1989 Clinical psychiatric assessment of patients with burning mouth syndrome resisting oral treatment. Swedish Dental Journal 13: 77–88
Hampf G, Ekholm A, Salo T et al 1987 Pain in oral galvanism. Pain 29: 301
Harris SM 1974 Psychogenic aspects of facial pain. British Dental Journal 136: 199
Headache Classification Committee of the International Headache Society 1988 Classification and diagnostic criteria for headache disorders, cranial neuralgias and facial Pain. cephalalgia 8(suppl 7): 19–41
Helcer M, Schnarch A, Benoliel R, Sharav Y 1998 Trigeminal neuralgic-type pain and vascular-type headache due to gustatory stimulus. Headache 38: 129–131
Helkimo M 1979 Epidemiological surveys of dysfunction of the masticatory system. In: Zarb GA, Carlsson GE (eds) Temporomandibular joint. Munksgaard, Copenhagen, p 175
Henriksson KG, Bengtsson A 1991 Fibromyalgia – a clinical entity? Canadian Journal of Physiology and Pharmacology 69: 672–677
Herishanu Y, Bendheim P, Dolberg M 1974 External carotid occlusive disease as a cause of facial pain. Journal of Neurology, Neurosurgery and Psychiatry 8: 963
Horiuchi H, Matthews B 1973 In-vitro observations on fluid flow through human dentine caused by pain-producing stimuli. Archives of Oral Biology 18: 275
Hu JW, Sharav Y, Sessle BJ 1990 Effect of one- or two-stage deafferentation of mandibular and maxillary tooth pulps on the functional properties of trigeminal brainstem neurons. Brain Research 516: 271–279
Hugoson A, Thorstensson B 1991 Vitamin B status and response to replacement therapy in patients with burning mouth syndrome. Acta Odontologica Scandinavica 49: 367–375

Inoki R, Toyoda Y, Yamamoto I 1993 Elaboration of a bradykinin-like substance in dog's canine pulp during electrical stimulation and its inhibition by narcotic and non-narcotic analgesics. Nyunyn-Schemiedeberg's Archives of Pharmacology 279: 387–398

Isacsson G, Isberg A, Johansson A-S, Larson D 1986 Internal derangement of the temporomandibular joint: radiographic and histologic changes associated with severe pain. Journal of Maxillofacial Surgery 44: 771

Jaaskelainen SK, Forsssell H, Tenovuo O 1997 Abnormalities of the blink reflex in burning mouth syndrome. Pain 73: 455–460

Jaaskelainen SK, Forsssell H, Tenovuo O 1998 Electrophysiological testing of the trigeminofacial system: aid in the diagnosis of atypical facial pain. Pain (in press)

Katzberg RW, Dolwick MF, Bles DJ, Helms CA 1979 Arthrography of the temporomandibular joint: new technique and preliminary observations. American Journal of Roentgenology 132: 949

Keele CA, Armstrong D 1968 Mediators of pain. In: Lim RDS, Armstrong D, Pardo EG (eds) Pharmacology of pain. Pergamon, Oxford, pp 3–24

Kolbinson DA, Schubert MM, Flournoy N, Truelove EL 1988 Early oral changes following bone marrow transplantation. Oral Surgery, Oral Medicine and Oral Pathology 66: 130–138

Kopp S, Wenneberg B 1983 Intra- and interobserver variability in the assessment of signs of disorder in the stomatognathic system. Swedish Dental Journal 7: 239–246

Krogh-Polsen WG, Olsson A 1968 Management of the occlusion of the teeth, Part 1: Background, definitions, rationale. In: Schwartz L and Chayes CM (Eds). Facial pain and mandibular dysfunction. Saunders, Philadelphia pp 239–249

Lamey PJ, Lamb AB 1988 Prospective study of aetiological factors in burning mouth syndrome. British Medical Journal 296: 1243

Lamey PJ, Hammond A, Allam BF, McIntosh WB 1986 Vitamin status of patients with burning mouth syndrome and the response to replacement therapy. British Dental Journal 160: 81

Lance JW 1993 Miscellaneous headaches unassociated with a structural lesion. In: Olesen J, Tafelt-Hansen P, Welch KMA (eds) The headaches. Raven Press, New York, pp 609–617

Langeland K, Block RM, Grossman LI 1977 A histopathologic and histobacteriologic study of 35 periapical endodontic surgical specimens. Journal of Endodontics 3: 8

Larheim TA 1995 Current trends in temporomandibular joint imaging. Oral Surgery, Oral Medicine, Oral Pathology, Oral Radiology and Endodontics 80: 555–576

Lascelles RG 1966 Atypical facial pain and psychiatry. British Journal of Psychiatry 112: 654

Laskin DM 1969 Etiology of the pain dysfunction syndrome. Journal of the American Dental Association 79: 147

Lavigne GJ, Velly-Miguel AM, Montplaisir J 1991 Muscle pain, dyskinesia, and sleep. Canadian Journal of Physiology and Pharmacology 69: 678–682

Locker D, Slade G 1988 Prevalence of symptoms associated with temporomandibular disorders in a Canadian population. Community Dental and Oral Epidemiology 16: 310–313

Loeser JD 1985 Tic douloureux and atypical facial pain. Journal of the Canadian Dental Association 12: 917

Lund JP, Donga R, Widmer CG, Stohler CS 1991 The pain adaptation model: a discussion of the relationship between chronic musculoskeletal pain and motor activity. Canadian Journal of Physiology and Pharmacology 69: 683–694

Lundh H, Westesson P-L, Kopp S, Tillström B 1985 Anterior repositioning splint in the treatment of temporomandibular joints with reciprocal clicking: comparison with a flat occlusal splint and untreated control group. Oral Surgery 60: 131

Madison S, Whitsel EA, Suarez-Roca H, Maixner W 1992 Sensitizing effects of leukotriene B_4 on intradental primary afferents. Pain 49: 99

Magnusson T, Carlsson GE 1978 Comparison between two groups of patients in respect of headache and mandibular dysfunction. Swedish Dental Journal 2: 85–92

Main DMG, Basker RM 1983 Patients complaining of a burning mouth. British Dental Journal 154: 206

Maragou P, Ivanyi L 1991 Serum zinc levels in patients with burning mouth syndrome. Oral Surgery, Oral Medicine and Oral Pathology 71: 447–450

Marbach JJ 1978 Phantom tooth pain. Journal of Endodontics 4: 362

Marbach JJ, Lund P 1981 Depression, anhedonia and anxiety in temporomandibular joint and other facial pain syndromes. Pain 11: 73–84

Marbach JJ, Lipton J, Lund P et al 1978 Facial pains and anxiety levels: considerations for treatment. Journal of Prosthetic Dentistry 40: 434–437

Marbach JJ, Hulbrock J, Hohn C, Segal AG 1982 Incidence of phantom tooth pain: a typical facial neuralgia. Oral Surgery 53: 190

Massey EW, Moore J, Schold SC 1981 Dental neuropathy from systemic cancer. Neurology 31: 1227

McGrath PA, Gracely RH, Dubner R, Heft M 1983 Non-pain and pain sensations evoked by tooth pulp stimulation. Pain 15: 377

McNeill C 1997 History and evolution of TMD concepts. Oral Surgery, Oral Medicine, Oral Pathology, Oral Radiology and Endodontics 83: 51–60

Mense S 1991 Considerations concerning the neurobiological basis of muscle pain. Canadian Journal of Physiology and Pharmacology 69: 610–616

Merskey H, Bogduk N (eds) 1994 International Association for the Study of Pain. Classification of chronic pain: descriptions of chronic pain syndromes and definition of pain terms, 2nd edn. IASP Press, Seattle, pp 68–71

Merskey H, Lau CL, Russel ES et al 1987 Screening for psychiatric morbidity. The pattern of psychological illness and premorbid characteristics in four chronic pain populations. Pain 30: 141–157

Molin C 1972 Vertical isometric muscle forces of the mandible. A comparative study of subjects with and without manifest mandibular pain dysfunction syndrome. Acta Odontologica Scandinavica 30: 485

Molin C 1973 Studies in mandibular pain dysfunction syndrome. Swedish Dental Journal 66 (suppl 4): 1

Moskowitz MA 1993 The trigeminovascular system. In: Olesen J, Tafelt-Hansen Welch KMA (eds) The headaches. Raven Press, New York, pp 97–104

Moskowitz MA, Buzzi MG, Sakas DE, Linik MD 1989 Pain mechanisms underlying vascular headaches. Revue Neurologique (Paris) 145: 181–193

Mumford JM 1982 Orofacial pain, 3rd edn. Churchill Livingstone, Edinburgh

Mumford JM, Newton AV 1969 Transduction of hydrostatic pressure to electric potential in human dentine. Journal of Dental Research 48: 226

Munro R 1975 Electromyography of the masseter and anterior temporalis muscles in the open-close-clench cycle in temporomandibular joint dysfunction. In: Griffin CJ, Harris R (eds) The temporomandibular joint syndrome. Monographs in oral sciences. Karger, Basel, p 117

Nappi G, Russell D 1993 Cluster headache clinical features. In: Olesen J, Tafelt-Hansen P, Welch KMA (eds) The headaches. Raven Press, New York, pp 577–584

Närhi MVO 1985 The characteristic of intradental sensory units andtheir responses to stimulation. Journal of Dental Research 64: 564

Nguyen M, Maciewicz R, Bouckoms A, Poletti C, Ojemann R 1986 Facial pain symptoms in patients with cerebellopontine angle tumors: a report of 44 cases of cerebellopontine angle meningioma and review of the literature. Clinical Journal of Pain 2: 3

Nielsen LL, McNeil C, Danzig W, Goldman S, Levy J, Miller AJ 1990

Adaptation of craniofacial muscles in subjects with craniomandibular disorders. American Journal of Orthodontics and Dentofacial Orthopedics 97: 20–34

Nitzan DW, Dolwick MF 1991 An alternative explanation for the genesis of closed-lock symptoms in the internal derangement process. Journal of Oral and Maxillofacial Surgery 49: 810–815

Nitzan DW, Dolwick MF, Martinez GA (1991) Temporomandibular joint arthrocentesis: a simplified treatment for severe, limited mouth opening. Journal of Oral and Maxillofacial Surgery 49: 1163–1167

Nitzan DW, Mahler Y, Simkin A 1992 Intra-articular pressure measurements in patients with suddenly developing severely limited mouth opening. Journal of Maxillofacial Surgery 50: 1038

Ohkubo T, Shibata M, Yamada Y, Kaya H, Takahashi H 1993 Role of substance P in neurogenic inflammation in the rat incisor pulp and the lower lip. Archives of Oral Biology 38: 151–158

Okeson JP 1995 Bell's orofacial pains, 5th edn. Quintessence, Chicago, pp 135–184

Okeson JP (ed) 1996 Orofacial pain: guidelines for assessment, diagnosis and management. Quintessence, Chicago

Okeson JP 1997 Current terminology and diagnostic classification schemes. Oral Surgery, Oral Medicine Oral, Pathology, Oral Radiology and Endodontics 83: 61–64

Okeson JP, Moody PM, Kemper JT, Haley JV 1983 Evaluation of occlusal splint therapy and relaxation procedures in patients with temporomandibular disorders. Journal of the American Dental Association 107: 420

Olgart LM 1985 The role of local factors in dentine and pulp in intradental pain mechanisms. Journal of Dental Research 64: 572

Paine R 1977 Vascular facial pain. In: Alling CC III, Mahan PE (eds) Facial pain, 2nd edn. Lea & Febiger, Philadelphia, p 57

Pareja JA, Shen JM, Kruszewski P, Caballero V, Pamo M, Sjaastad O 1996a SUNCT syndrome: duration, frequency, and temporal distribution of attacks. Headache 36: 161–165

Pareja JA, White LR, Sjaastad O 1996b Pathophysiology of headaches with a prominent vascular component. Pain Research and Management 1(2): 93–108

Perry HT 1973 Adolescent temporomandibular dysfunction. American Journal of Orthodontics 63: 517

Rao VM 1995 Imaging of the temporomandibular joint. Seminars in Ultrasound, CT and MRI 16: 513–526

Raskin NH, Appenzeller O (1980) Headache. WB Saunders, Philadelphia, pp 132–136

Rees RT, Harris M 1979 Atypical odontalgia. British Journal of Oral Surgery 16: 212

Reik L 1985 Atypical facial pain: a reappraisal. Headache 25: 30

Remick RA, Blasberg B 1985 Psychiatric aspects of atypical facial pain. Journal of the Canadian Dental Association 12: 913

Roberts CA, Tallents RH, Espeland MA, Handelman SL, Katzberg RW 1985 Mandibular range of motion versus arthrographic diagnosis of the temporomandibular joint. Oral Surgery 60: 244

Roistacher SL, Tanenbaum D 1986 Myofascial pain associated with oropharyngeal cancer. Oral Surgery 61: 459

Rugh JD, Harlan J 1988 Nocturnal bruxism and temporomandibular disorders. Advances in Neurology 49: 329–341

Rugh JD, Solberg WK 1979 Psychological implications in temporomandibular pain and dysfunction. In: Zarb GA, Carlsson GE (eds) Temporomandibular joint. Munksgaard, Copenhagen, p 239

Rugh JD, Solberg WK 1985 Oral health status in the United States: temporomandibular disorders. Journal of Dental Education 49: 398–405

Rugh JD, Barghi N, Drago CJ 1984 Experimental occlusal discrepancies and nocturnal bruxism. Journal of Prosthetic Dentistry 51: 548

Sahota PK, Dexter JD 1990 Sleep and headache syndromes: a clinical review. Headache 30: 80–84

Salter M, Brooke RL, Merskey H et al 1983 Is the temporomandibular pain and dysfunction syndrome a disorder of the mind? Pain 17: 151–166

Satoh T, Harada Y 1973 Electrophysiological study on tooth grinding during sleep. Electroencephalography and Clinical Neurophysiology 35: 267–275

Schnurr RF, Brooke RI, Rollman GB 1990 Psychosocial correlates of temporomandibular joint pain and dysfunction. Pain 42: 153–165

Schwarz C 1959 Disorders of the temporomandibular joint. WB Saunders, Philadelphia

Scudds RA, Trachsel LC, Luckhurst BJ, Percy JS 1989 A comparative study of pain, sleep quality and pain responsiveness in fibrositis and myofascial pain syndrome. Journal of Rheumatology 19 (suppl): 120–126

Selby A 1985 Physiotherapy in the management of temporomandibular disorders. Australian Dental Journal 30: 273–280

Seltzer S 1978 Pain control in dentistry–diagnosis and management. JB Lippincott, Philadelphia

Seltzer S, Bender IB 1975 The dental pulp, 2nd edn. JB Lippincott, Philadelphia, p 203

Seltzer S, Bender IB, Ziontz M 1963 The dynamics of pulp inflammation: correlation between diagnostic data and actual histologic findings in the pulp. Oral Surgery 16: 846

Sessle B 1979 Is the tooth pulp a 'pure' source of noxious input? Advances in Pain Research and Therapy 3: 245

Sessle BJ, Hu JW 1991 Mechanisms of pain arising from articular tissues. Canadian Journal of Physiology and Pharmacology 69: 617–626

Shafer WG, Hine MK, Levy BM 1974 A textbook of oral pathology, 3rd edn. WB Saunders, Philadelphia, p 152

Sharav Y, Benoliel R, Elishoov H 1996 Vascular orofacial pain: diagnostic features. 8th World Congress on Pain, Vancouver. IASP Press, Seattle, p 155

Sharav Y, Feinsod M 1977 Nasopharyngeal tumor manifested as myofascial pain dysfunction syndrome. Oral Surgery 44: 54

Sharav Y, Tzukert A, Refaeli B 1978 Muscle pain index in relation to pain dysfunction and dizziness associated with myofascial pain-dysfunction syndrome. Oral Surgery 46: 742

Sharav Y, McGrath PA, Dubner R, Brown F 1982 Masseteric inhibitory periods and sensations evoked by electric tooth-pulp stimulation in patients with oral-facial pain and mandibular dysfunction. Archives of Oral Biology 27: 305

Sharav Y, Leviner E, Tzukert A, McGrath PA 1984 The spatial distribution, intensity and unpleasantness of acute dental pain. Pain 20: 363

Sharav Y, Singer E, Schmidt E, Dionne RA, Dubner R 1987 The analgesic effect of amitriptyline on chronic facial pain. Pain 31: 199

Sharav Y, Benoliel R, Schnarch A, Greenberg L 1991 Idiopathic trigeminal pain associated with gustatory stimuli. Pain 44: 171–174

Ship J, Grushka M, Lipton J, Mott AE, Sessle BJ, Dionne RA 1995 Burning mouth syndrome: an update. Journal of the American Dental Association 126: 842–853

Silverglade D 1980 Dental pain without dental etiology: a manifestation of referred pain from otitis media. Journal of Dentistry for Children 47: 358

Singer EJ, Sharav Y, Dubner R, Dionne RA 1987 The efficacy of diazepam and ibuprofen in the treatment of the chronic myofascial orofacial pain. Pain 4 (suppl): 583

Sjaastad O, Dale I 1974 Evidence for a new (?) treatable headache entity. Headache 14: 105–108

Sjaastad O, Saunte C, Salvesen R, Fredrikson TA, Seim A, Roe OD et al 1989 Short-lasting unilateral neuralgiform headahce attacks with conjunctival injection, tearing, sweating and rhinorrhea. Chaphalalgia 9: 1947–1956

Solberg WK, Flint RT, Brantner JP 1972 Temporomandibular joint pain and dysfunction: a clinical study of emotional and occlusal components. Journal of Prosthetic Dentistry 28: 412

Stem PG, Mothersill KJ, Brooke RI 1979 Biofeedback and a cognitive behavioral approach to treatment of myofascial pain dysfunction syndrome. Behavioural Therapy 10: 29

Sternbach RA 1978 Clinical aspects of pain. In: Sternbach RS (ed) The psychology of pain. Raven Press, New York, p 241

Storer R 1965 The effects of the climacteric and of aging on prosthetic diagnosis and treatment planning. British Dental Journal 119: 340–354

Syrjanen S, Piironen P, Yli-Urpo A 1984 Salivary content of patients with subjective symptoms resembling galvanic pain. Oral Surgery 58: 387

Tafelt-Hansen P, Lous I, Olesen J 1981 Prevalence and significance of muscle tenderness during common migraine attacks. Headache 21: 49–54

Tal M, Sharav Y 1985 Development of sensory and reflex responses to tooth-pulp stimulation in children. Archives of Oral Biology 30: 467

Torvonen T, Knuuttila M 1988 Prevalance of signs and symptoms of mandibular dysfunction among adults aged 25, 35, 50 and 60 years in Osthrobotnia, Finland. Journal of Oral Rehabilitation 15: 455–463

Thomson H 1971 Mandibular dysfunction syndrome. British Dental Journal 130: 187

Travell J 1960 Temporomandibular joint pain referred from muscles of head and neck. Journal of Prosthetic Dentistry 10: 475

Travell J, Simons D 1983 Myofascial pain and dysfunction: the trigger point manual. Williams & Wilkins, Baltimore, pp 165–182

Troiano MF, Gaston GW 1975 Carotid system arteritis: an overlooked and misdiagnosed syndrome. Journal of the American Dental Association 91: 589

Trowbridge H, Kim S 1996 Pulp development structure and function. In: Cohen S, Burns RC (eds) Pathways of the pulp, 7th edn. CV Mosby, St Louis, 296–336

Turk DC 1997 Psychosocial and behavioral assessment of patients with temporomandibular disorders: diagnostic and treatment implications. Oral Surgery, Oral Medicine, Oral Pathology, Oral Radiology and Endodontics 83: 65–71

Tyldesley WR, Mumford JM 1970 Dental pain and the histological condition of the pulp. Dental Practice and Dental Research 20: 333

Tzukert A, Hasin Y, Sharav Y 1981 Orofacial pain of cardiac origin. Oral Surgery 51: 484

Van der Ploeg HM, Van der Wal N, Ejkman MAJ et al 1987 Psychological aspects of patients with burning mouth syndrome. Oral Surgery 63: 664

Van Hassel HJ, Harrington GW 1969 Localization of pulpal sensation. Oral Surgery 28: 753

Van Steenberghe D 1979 The structure and function of periodontal innervation. Journal of Periodontal Research 14: 185

Velly-Miguel A, Montplaisir J, Lavigne G 1991 Nocturnal bruxism, jaw movements and sleep parameters: a controlled pilot study. Journal of Dental Research 70 (abstract): 1970

Vickers ER, Cousins MJ, Walker S, Chisholm K 1998 Analysis of 50 patients with atypical odontalgia. Oral Surgery, Oral Medicine, Oral Pathology, Oral Radiology and Endodontics 85: 24–32

Virtanen ASJ, Huopaniemi T, Nahri MVO, Perovaara A, Wallgren K 1987 The effect of temporal parameters on subjective sensations evoked by electrical tooth stimulation. Pain 30: 361

Wakisaka S 1990 Neuropeptides in the dental pulp: distribution, origins, and correlation. Journal of Endodontics 16: 67–69

Wallin G, Torbjork E, Hallin R 1976 Preliminary observations of the pathophysiology of hyperalgesia in the causalgic pain syndrome. in: Zotterman Y (Ed) Sensory functions of the skin in primates. Pergammon Press, Oxford 489–499

Wanman A, Agerberg G 1986a Mandibular dysfunction in adolescents. I. Prevalence of symptoms. Acta Odontologica Scandinavica 44: 47–54

Wanman A, Agerberg G 1986b Two year longitudinal study of symptoms of mandibular dysfunction in adolescents. Acta Odontologica Scandinavica 44: 321–331

Wardrop RW, Hailes J, Burger H et al 1989 Oral discomfort at menopause. Oral Surgery 67: 535

Ware JC, Rugh JD (1988) Destructive bruxism: sleep state relationship. Sleep 11: 172–181

Watts PG, Peet KM, Juniper RP 1986 Migraine and the temporomandibular joint: the final answer? British Dental Journal 161: 170–173

Westesson PL, Eriksson L, Kurita K 1989 Reliability of negative clinical temporomandibular joint examination: prevalence of disc displacement in asymptomatic temporomandibular joints. Oral Surgery, Oral Medicine and Oral Pathology 68: 551–554

Westrum LE, Canfield RC, Black RG 1976 Transganglionic degeneration in the spinal trigeminal nucleus following removal of tooth pulps in adult cats. Brain Research 101: 137

Widmer CG 1991 Introduction III. Chronic muscle pain syndromes: an overview. Canadian Journal of Physiology and Pharmacology 69: 659–661

Wieselmann G, Permann R, Korner E 1986 Distribution of muscle activity during sleep in bruxism. European Neurology 25 (suppl 2): 111–116

Wildmalm SE 1976 The silent period in the masseter muscle of patients with TMJ dysfunction. Acta Odontologica Scandinavica 34: 43–52

Wolfe F 1988 Fibrositis, fibromyalgia, and musculoskeletal disease: the current status of the fibrositis syndrome. Archives of Physical Medicine and Rehabilitation 69: 527–531

Yemm R 1979 Neurophysiologic studies of temporomandibular joint dysfunction. In: Zarb GA, Carlsson GE (eds) Temporomandibular joint. Munksgaard, Copenhagen, p 215

Yoshimura Y, Yoshida Y, Oka M, Miyoshi M, Uemura S 1982 Long-term evaluation of non-surgical treatment of osteoarthrosis of temporomandibular joint. International Journal of Oral Surgery 11: 7

Zilli C, Brooke RI, Lau CL et al 1989 Screening for psychiatric illness in patients with oral dysaesthesia by means of the General Health Questionnaire – twenty-eight item version (GHQ-28) and the Irritability, Depression and Anxiety Scale (IDA). Oral Surgery 67: 384

Zulqarnain BJ, Furuya R, Hedegard B, Magnusson T 1989 The silent period in the masseter and the anterior temporalis muscles in adult patients with mild or moderate mandibular dysfunction symptoms. Journal of Oral Rehabilitation 16: 127–137

Trigeminal, eye and ear pain

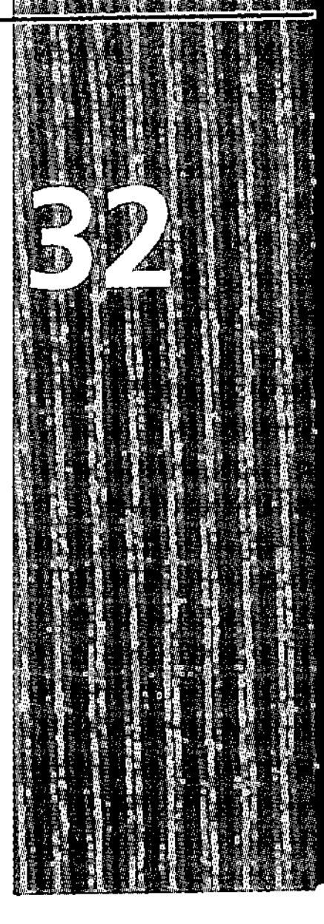

JOANNA M. ZAKRZEWSKA

INTRODUCTION, AIMS AND OBJECTIVES

This chapter covers pain that can occur in the area of the face bounded by the distribution of the trigeminal nerve. It includes pain in and around the eyes and ears but excludes pain in the oral cavity or associated with the temporomandibular joint. Although mention will be made of acute pain presenting in this region, this is often relatively easy for primary healthcare workers to diagnose and manage. Chronic pain, defined here as pain persisting beyond 3 months, is more difficult to diagnose and treat and often falls to the remit of pain clinics or specialists.

It is hoped that this chapter will enable a clinician to adopt an evidence-based approach to the management of facial pain. It aims to combine clinical expertise with the best clinical evidence. The latter is based on clinically relevant, high-quality research. Wherever possible, evidence from systematic reviews or randomized controlled trials will be used as it is now well recognized that experts are highly biased in their views. Systematic reviews, abstracts of reviews of effectiveness and registers of controlled trials can be found in the Cochrane Library which is updated quarterly. The diagnostic criteria proposed by the International Association for the Study of Pain (IASP) (Anonymous 1994) or the International Headache Society (IHS) (Anonymous 1988) will be used throughout this chapter.

Trigeminal neuralgia, glossopharyngeal neuralgia, acute herpes zoster, postherpetic neuralgia, sinusitis, optic neuritis and phantom eye pain will be reviewed under the following headings: definition, epidemiology, aetiology/pathophysiology, clinical features, investigations, management; and wherever possible some guidelines for management will be proposed. Other rare causes of facial pain and common ear and eye diseases will only be summarized in tables with appropriate references to randomized controlled trials. Table 32.1 provides a differential diagnosis and gives the IASP and IHS code classification.

TRIGEMINAL NEURALGIA

DEFINITION

The IASP definition of trigeminal neuralgia is 'sudden, usually unilateral, severe, brief, stabbing, recurrent pains in the distribution of one or more branches of the fifth cranial nerve'. Secondary or symptomatic trigeminal neuralgia is caused by a demonstrable, structural lesion such as a tumour, aneurysm or multiple sclerosis.

EPIDEMIOLOGY

The diagnostic criteria for trigeminal neuralgia are complex and do not lend themselves to epidemiological surveys carried out through mailed questionnaires. In order to achieve sufficient accuracy, interviews and examinations by trained staff are required. In a French village where they were assessing prevalence of neurological disease, Munoz et al (1988) found that 2.7% reported facial and head pain. Of this group, 0.1% (one male patient) had trigeminal neuralgia. Incidence data have been collected since 1945 in Rochester (USA) (Katusic et al 1990). The annual incidence, when age adjusted, was 5.9 per 100 000 in women and 3.4 per 100 000 in men. The average annual incidence increased with age and was highest over 80 years of age. The disease most frequently linked with trigeminal neuralgia is multiple sclerosis and Katusic et al (1990) estimated that

Table 32.1 Differential diagnosis of facial pain by location or type

	Condition	*Prevelance incidence*	*ISAP*	*IHS*
Eye	Corneal abrasions	Relatively common		
	Iritis, ant. uveitis	Relatively rare		
	Optic neuritis	Relatively rare		12.1.2
	Acute angle closure glaucoma	Relatively common		11.3.1
	Tolosa–Hunt	Rare	002.X3a, 11–14	12.1.5
	Ophthalmoplegic migraine	Extremely rare		1.3
	Raeder's syndrome	Rare	002.x8	
Otolaryngological	Sinusitis	Common	031.X2a	11.5
	Otitis externa	Relatively common		11.4
	Otitis media	Relatively common		11.4
Orodental	Salivary gland	Rare		11.6
	TMJ	Common	034.X8a	11.7
	Dental disease	Very common	034–031	11.6
Neuralgias	Trigeminal	Relatively rare	006.X8a, 11–1	12.2
	Glossopharyngeal	very rare	006.x8b, 11–8	12.3
	Postherpetic	Relatively rare	003.X2b, 11–5	12.1.4
	Pretrigeminal	Rare		
	SUNCT	Rare	006.X8j	
	Cluster headaches	Relatively rare	004.X8a	3.1–3.3
	Geniculate neuralgia (Ramsay Hunt)	Relatively rare	006.X2	
Psychogenic/somatizers	Atypical facial pain	Infrequent		12.8
Vascular	Migraine	Common	004.x7	1.1–1.2
	Giant cell arteritis	Relatively rare	023.X3, V–12	6.5
	Aneurysym	Rare		
Neoplasia	Sinus, posterior fossa, ear	Rare		
Referred	From other organs			

the relative risk was 20 (95% confidence interval, 4.1–58.6). Rothman and Monson (1973) assessed risk factors using a case control group and found that relative to controls, trigeminal neuralgia patients smoked less, consumed less alcohol, had fewer tonsillectomies and were less likely to be Jewish or immigrants. More population-based studies are required to estimate the prevalence of this condition and its impact on quality of life and economic cost.

AETIOLOGY AND PATHOPHYSIOLOGY

Research on the aetiology and the pathophysiology of trigeminal neuralgia is hampered by the lack of a good animal model. Considerable advances have been made in our understanding of the mechanisms of damage to peripheral nerves, which can be applied to the trigeminal nerve. These aspects are discussed in greater detail in Section 1.

Several theories have been proposed for the mechanism of trigeminal neuralgia but, to date, none explains all the clinical features of this condition. One of the diagnostic criteria for trigeminal neuralgia, that of short-lasting but severe paroxysmal pain, has continued to puzzle basic neuroscientists. The uniqueness of the pain, its mainly unilateral distribution with occasional radiation beyond the trigeminal nerve distribution, its triggering by non-noxious stimuli and the presence of specific trigger points are factors that need to be explained and recent neurophysiological research has begun to address some of these questions.

Based on clinical observation, it has been postulated that trigeminal neuralgia is caused by compression of the trigeminal nerve by either vessels or tumours. This compression occurs at what is termed the root entry zone. This is defined as an area at which the trigeminal nerve enters the brainstem in the pontine area and is a point at which there is transition between peripheral and central myelin. A mismatch may occur here or this point may be more susceptible to damage by outside pressure. As a result of pressure on the nerve at this point, myelin is lost and this leads to abnormal depolarization and reverberations resulting in ectopic impulses which manifest themselves in the form of pain. Support for this theory is gained from neurosurgical observations of compression of the nerve at this point and the association of multiple sclerosis with trigeminal neuralgia.

Surgeons and neuroscientists are not unanimous in their support of this theory as some argue that the root entry zone is a very small, microscopic area whereas compression and distortion of the trigeminal nerve is gross. Mere contact of vessels or tumours with the trigeminal nerve does not cause trigeminal neuralgia. Some surgeons will argue that if surgery is delayed then nerve dysfunction becomes irreversible and that this results in recurrence of pain.

Most experimental models suggest that peripheral nerve damage results in central changes. These mechanisms are discussed in greater depth by Devor in Chapter 5.

CLINICAL FEATURES

At present the diagnosis of trigeminal neuralgia is made principally on the history. There has not been a single report of a case control series to either ascertain the key features of trigeminal neuralgia or assess the validity of the IHS and IASP criteria for the diagnosis of trigeminal neuralgia in clinical practice. The major diagnostic features of trigeminal neuralgia are summarized in Table 32.2.

As the history plays such a crucial role in the diagnosis of trigeminal neuralgia, it is essential that it is taken with utmost care and that non-verbal behaviour is also recorded. Patients should be encouraged to 'tell their own story' as the words used to describe the character of the pain, such as shock-like, lightning, shooting, an electric current, its severity and periodicity are often pathognomonic of the condition.

Table 32.2 Trigeminal Neuralgia: Diagnostic Clinical Criteria

1. *Character	Shooting, electric shock, sharp, superficial
2. *Severity	Moderate to most severe
3. Duration	Each episode of pain lasts no more than 2 minutes, numerous episodes during the day
4. *Periodicity	Periods of weeks, months when no pain; also, pain-free periods between attacks
5. *Site	Distribution of the trigeminal nerve area, mostly unilateral
6. Radiation	Within trigeminal nerve area or beyond
7. *Provoking features	Light touch such as eating, talking, washing
8. Relieving features	Often sleep, anticonvulsant drugs
9. Associated features	Trigger areas, weight loss, poor quality of life, depression

**The IHS classification suggests that at least four of these must be present to make the diagnosis.*

Pain measurement in trigeminal neuralgia has largely been limited to single-dimensional rating scales, such as a verbal rating scale using 4–5 words. Yet, the McGill Pain Questionnaire has been shown to be an extremely useful tool for discriminating between trigeminal neuralgia and atypical facial pain (Melzack et al 1986). Not only does the McGill Pain Questionnaire provide details of the characteristics of the pain but it also gives an indication of its severity. The most frequently used words are sharp, shooting, unbearable, stabbing, exhausting, tender, vicious, terrifying and torturing. The McGill Pain Questionnaire has also shown that some patients additionally have a dull, aching, continuous component to their pain (Zakrzewska et al 1999). Neurosurgeons have noted that patients who have this latter type of pain do less well after surgery but this has not been measured (Szapiro et al 1985).

The severity of trigeminal neuralgia varies from moderate to most severe. It is generally accepted that pain severity increases with time but there have been no formal studies to validate this. During an attack of severe pain the face may be distorted or 'freeze' and hands may be put in front of the face as if to protect it without touching it. Patients may also cry out with pain. These non-verbal behaviours are useful clues as to the severity of the pain.

Another important characteristic is the siting of the pain, unilaterally distributed along the trigeminal nerve. Around 4% of patients will have bilateral pain but it rarely occurs simultaneously. There is a slight right-sided predominance, around 60%, but there seems to be no relationship to handedness (Rothman & Wepsic 1974). All three divisions may be affected and the most commonly affected divisions are the second and third, together. The rarest division is that of the ophthalmic branch. An epidemiological review showed that pain in the mandibular division occurred in patients with an earlier onset of disease and that more right-sided cases were associated with upper face involvement (Rothman & Beckman 1974).

The timing of the pain attacks is highly significant. Each burst of severe pain usually lasts for a maximum of 2 minutes but several of these may follow in quick succession before the nerve becomes refractory. After such attacks patients often report residual, dull ache or burning sensations. These attacks of pain diminish at night (Rasmussen 1991). Rasmussen (1990) found in his 109 trigeminal neuralgia patients that patients could be free of pain for years (6%), months (36%), weeks (16%) or only days (16%). Diurnal constant pain was present in 4% of patients and 23%

had no recordable pain-free intervals. Katusic et al (1990), in their epidemiological survey of 75 patients, found that the median length of an episode of pain was 49 days and the mean was 116 days with a range of 1–462 days. Using Kaplan–Meier life table methodology, they estimated that 65% of patients would have a second episode of pain within 5 years and 77% within 10 years. The proportion of people having recurrences after a second or third episode was similar to that after a first episode. Age did not appear to correlate with the timing of the next episode. Kurland (1958), in his epidemiological survey, reported that up to 58% of patients have long, spontaneous remission periods and that these tended to occur early in the disease process.

Pain is characteristically triggered by light touch and Rasmussen (1991), in his series of 229 patients, reported that only 4% had no precipitating factors. The major precipitating factors he identified were chewing and talking (76%), touching (65%) and cold (48%). He also found that a trigger zone could be identified in 50% of these patients. Apart from avoiding touching and moving their faces, patients can do little to gain relief without recourse to drug therapy.

It is important to enquire how patients cope with the pain and what strategies they adopt to deal with it. Many patients will avoid precipitating factors and so will lose weight, avoid cleaning their teeth on the affected side and will reduce their socializing, especially if it involves eating and talking. An assessment of the psychological and emotional factors that affect the pain needs to be made. Patients with trigeminal neuralgia, especially when going through a bout of severe pain, will suffer from anhedonia and even depression (Zakrzewska & Thomas 1993, Zakrzewska 1999). These factors, however, have only been measured in a handful of studies and need to be addressed further.

Using a variety of measures, including the Spielberger State-Trait Anxiety Inventory, Marbach and Lund (1981) failed to differentiate between different facial pain syndromes. On the Illness Behaviour Questionnaire patients with trigeminal neuralgia scored higher on denial and low on effective inhibition when compared to other facial pain patients. They had normal scores on hypochondriasis and irritability but were convinced that there was a physical cause for their disease (Gordon & Hitchcock 1983). Patients with trigeminal neuralgia also score lower on neuroticism when tested on the Eysenck Personality Inventory (Gordon & Hitchcock 1983). No other psychological or quality of life assessments have been reported. To date, no attempts have been made to measure the consequences of trigeminal neuralgia in terms of economic costs or cost to the patient in terms of disability, handicap or psychological problems or to compare these to other pain patients or before and after different forms of treatment.

EXAMINATION

Gross neurological examination rarely shows up any abnormalities in idiopathic trigeminal neuralgia. However, instrumental examination shows that over 50% of patients may have at least one abnormal measure of sensation, not only in the trigger zone division but also in the adjacent division (Nurmikko 1991). There is currently no evidence to suggest that these subtle findings reflect severity of disease or predict the presence of compression. Patients with gross neurological abnormalities or progressive intractable pain often have secondary trigeminal neuralgia.

INVESTIGATIONS

There is, as yet, no highly specific or sensitive test to confirm the diagnosis of trigeminal neuralgia. Several investigations have been advocated but few of them have undergone rigorous evaluation and specificity, sensitivity and predictive value are rarely quoted. Magnetic resonance imaging (MRI) has been used to identify patients with multiple sclerosis or tumours and to assess possible compression of the trigeminal nerve. Yang et al (1996) showed that the pattern of pain did not correlate with MRI findings and concluded that the sensitivity and specificity of MRI are still low. Magnetic resonance tomographic angiography (MRTA) has been put forward as the definitive investigation but there are insufficient controlled randomized trials to assess its sensitivity and specificity (Meaney et al 1995). Electronic facial thermography has been evaluated in a wide variety of patients with oral, facial and dental pains but although matched controls were used, there was no attempt at randomization or blinding. The technique was not sensitive enough to distinguish between different forms of pain (Graff-Radford et al 1995, Gratt et al 1996).

MANAGEMENT

The wide range of treatments currently in use for trigeminal neuralgia are ample evidence that there is no simple answer to how trigeminal neuralgia should be managed. A survey among 159 British consultants with an interest in neurogenic pain showed that the treatment with greatest consensus was carbamazepine, with 99 consultants using it as their treatment of choice (Davies et al 1993). There are remarkably few randomized controlled trials and no reports of large, multinational trials.

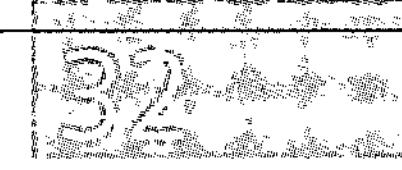

Trials in patient with trigeminal neuralgia are difficult to conduct for a number of reasons: its relative rarity, its unknown aetiology, its natural history of spontaneous remissions, its varying severity and lack of an objective diagnostic test. These, however, are also strong arguments in favour of randomized controlled trials. Many new drugs and operations have been introduced over the years and each time, the opportunity to do a randomized controlled trial was not taken up at the time of introduction of the new treatment.

Currently, there are no agreed guidelines on the conduct of trials such as have been prepared in other disciplines, e.g. cluster headaches (Lipton et al 1995). There is no consensus on what outcome parameters should be used and how they should be measured. No surveys have been done to ascertain what outcomes the patients themselves would expect given that a complete cure is rarely achieved and most treatments have side effects.

Anticonvulsant drugs, especially initially, are the treatment of choice but the timing of surgery is controversial. Most physicians and patients opt for surgery when medical management either fails to give pain relief or results in unacceptable side effects. However, some surgeons argue that surgery reduces damage to the trigeminal nerve and results in fewer recurrences if done early and that fewer postoperative complications occur, as patients are younger and medically fitter.

A systematic review of the use of anticonvulsants in the management of acute and chronic neuropathic pain, which includes trigeminal neuralgia, has recently been completed (McQuay et al 1995) and is kept updated on the Cochrane database. This review identified three placebo-controlled, randomized controlled trials and three active treatment-controlled, randomized controlled trials using carbamazepine for the controlled arm, which are listed in Table 32.3.

The three placebo-controlled trials all used carbamazepine and involved 151 patients in total. Carbamazepine was used in dosages up to 1 g and follow-up was for up to 46 months. The number needed to treat for effective control was 2.6, that is, around 70% of patients will gain a response from using carbamazepine. The number needed to obtain an adverse effect was 3.4, that is, 3.4 patients needed to be treated before one adverse reaction occurred. The number needed to treat for severe side effects resulting in withdrawal from the study was 24. The incidence of side effects is often higher in the elderly and those in whom the drug and dose escalations are introduced rapidly. Haematological adverse reactions include a lowering of the white cell count and megaloblastic anaemia associated with folic acid deficiency. Carbamazepine hypersensitivity in the form of an allergic rash may occur in up to 10% of patients. At high concentrations, fluid retention can occur in patients with cardiac problems and the risk of hyponatraemia increases with age, higher carbamazepine serum concentrations and the use of diuretics. As carbamazepine is a potent hepatic enzyme inducer, it results in numerous drug interactions which can result in variable side effects..

Three other randomized controlled trials were analysed in McQuay et al's systematic review (McQuay et al 1995). When carbamazepine was compared with tizanidine (Vilming et al 1986), carbamazepine was found to be superior whereas when compared with tocainide (Lindstrom &

Table 32.3 Drugs used in the management of trigeminal neuralgia which have been evaluated in randomized controlled trials or controlled trials

Report	*Drug*	*Type of study*	*No. of patients*
Campbell et al 1998	Carbamazepine	Randomized controlled trial	77
Killian & Fromm 1968	Carbamazepine	Randomized controlled trial	30
Nicol 1969	Carbamazepine	Randomized controlled trial	54
Vilming et al 1986	Tizanidine/carbamazepine	Randomized controlled trial	12
Fromm et al 1993	Tizanidine/carbamazepine	Controlled trial, double blind	11
Lindstrom & Lindblom 1987	Tocainide/carbamazepine	Randomized controlled trial	12
Lechin et al 1989	Pimozide/carbamazepine	Randomized controlled trial	68
Zakrzewska et al 1997	Lamotrigine	Randomized controlled trial	13
Fromm et al 1984	Baclofen/carbamazepine	Not randomized double-blind trial	10
Fromm & Terrence 1987	Racemic baclofen/L-baclofen	Not randomized, double-blind trial	15
Kondziolka et al 1994	Proparcaine eyedrops	Randomized controlled trial	25

Lindblom 1987), both were equally effective. Pimozide produced better results than carbamazepine but 40 out of 48 patients reported adverse reactions which limited its use (Lechin et al 1989).

Lamotrigine 400 mg daily has recently been evaluated in a placebo-controlled, randomized controlled trial which used it as an add-on medication to suboptimal doses of carbamazepine or phenytoin (Zakrzewska et al 1997). In 13 patients the number needed to treat was found to be 7. There were no adverse reactions and side effects such as dizziness, constipation, nausea, tiredness were reported but these could have been due to concomitant anticonvulsant therapy. The commonest side effect with lamotrigine, a skin rash, was not encountered in this study, probably due to the short-term use of the drug (2 weeks).

Kondziolka et al (1994) reported a randomized controlled trial on a single application of proparacaine (local anaesthetic) in 25 patients with ophthalmic trigeminal neuralgia. The trial showed that topical anaesthetics do not have a role to play in the control of trigeminal neuralgia pain.

Baclofen, an antispasmodic drug, has been compared to carbamazepine in trials that were double blind but not randomized (Fromm et al 1980, 1984, Fromm & Terrence 1987). They suggest that baclofen may be useful but that it is not as effective as carbamazepine.

Numerous other drugs that have never been evaluated in any form of trial are still being used. Some of these are listed in Table 32.4, with proposed maximum dosages.

Hundreds of reports have been published on the surgical management of trigeminal neuralgia but only two randomized controlled trials have been located, both of which used peripherally injected streptomycin. There are no well-designed cohort studies done prospectively with concurrent or even historical controls. Most of the cohort studies are retrospective and have no controls. There is only one prospective, longitudinal study and a few prospective ones. Available data are mostly descriptive studies and few have used independent observers to assess outcome. Very few studies give full details of diagnostic criteria, including inclusion and exclusion criteria. Rarely are the criteria for classification of recurrences given and few authors provide definitions of the terminology used, e.g. anaesthesia dolorosa, dysaesthesia, hyperaesthesia. An outcome measure is rarely defined and in the vast majority pain is measured solely on a verbal rating scale using an ordinal scale of 1–3. Only a handful of papers give measurements of preoperative pain. Length of follow-up is extremely variable, some series do not even provide details and others exclude patients lost to follow-up. Timings of the assessments are extremely variable as most studies are conducted at a particular time point and so the patients are at different stages of follow-up. Data analysis is very variable and it is only possible to compare those series that have used analysis such as the Kaplan–Meier probability methodology. No studies have assessed outcome in terms of quality of life or ability to carry out daily activities. No economic evaluations are available for a single surgical procedure.

The ideal procedure should fulfil the following criteria: be easy to perform, require no sophisticated equipment, be repeatable if necessary, give immediate pain relief, have no or low recurrence rates, be free of risks and side effects, provide excellent quality of life and be low cost. The following account of surgical management at three different levels, peripheral, Gasserian ganglion and posterior fossa, is, unfortunately, biased due to lack of evidence. The major procedures will be described and they are compared in Table 32.5.

Table 32.4 Recommended daily dosages of drugs used in trigeminal neuralgia. Many of these have not been evaluated in trials and dosages are based on case series

Drug	*Daily dose*
Baclofen	50–80 mg*
Carbamazepine	300–1000 mg
Clonazepam	4–8 mg
Gabapentin	1800–3600 mg
Lamotrigine	200–400 mg*
Oxcarbazepine	300–1200 mg
Phenytoin	200–300 mg
Tizanidine	6–18 mg
Valproic acid	600–1200 mg

**Slow dose escalation is recommended*

Peripheral surgery

Peripheral surgery was the first surgery used for the management of trigeminal neuralgia and relies on the location of a specific trigger point that relates to a terminal nerve branch that can be isolated and, therefore, treated. Two randomized controlled trials have been done to assess the value of injections of streptomycin with lignocaine as compared to lignocaine on its own (Stajcic et al 1990, Bittar & Graff-Radford 1993). Both studies showed that lignocaine on its own was as effective as streptomycin. Table 32.6 lists, in general, the advantages and disadvantages of peripheral treatments which vary depending on whether the nerve is visualized, as in cryotherapy or neurectomy, or whether the procedures are done using a blind technique, e.g. alcohol,

Table 32.5 Comparison of different surgical techniques used for the management of trigeminal neuralgia at the level of the Gasserian ganglion or posterior fossa (Zakrzewska 1995, Burchiel 1996, Kondziolka et al 1997)

	Radiofrequency thermocoagulation	*Glycerol*	*Microcompression*	*Gamma lesion*	*MVD*
Age of patient	Any age	Any age	Any age	Any age	Preferably under 65 years
Medical fitness of patient	Care needed if bleeding problems	Care needed if bleeding problems	Care needed with cardiac patients	Any patient	Medically fit only
Ease of technique	Need to wake patient during procedure +	No need to wake patient ++	Need a larger bore needle so may be more difficult to cannulate +	++	Needs considerable skill
Specialized equipment	Need lesioning machine	None needed	None needed	Specialized equipment needed	Operating microscope
Type of anaesthesia	Short-acting GA, sedation	Light GA, sedation, no need to wake patient	Light GA, sedation, no need to wake patient	Local anaesthesia with sedation	Full general anaesthesia
Peroperative complications	Haemorrhage	Bradycardia, hypotension	Bradycardia, hypertension	None reported	All the usual reported with neurosurgical procedures
Repeatability	Easy	Easy	Easy	Probably can be repeated	Rarely repeated
Length of stay in hospital	Day stay	Day stay	Day stay	24 hours	One week
Expertise of surgeon	+++	++	+	Needs a team	++++
Specificity of area lesioned	Difficult to be specific	Can vary area of treatment	Difficult to be specific	Difficult to be specific	Highly specific
Immediacy of pain relief	Immediate	Can be delayed for days	Immediate	Median time 4 weeks	May be delayed
Recurrence rates	Mean 3–5 years	Mean 2–3 years	Mean 4.5–6.5 months	33% recurrence at 18 months	Low, 2 years 72% pain free, 2% recur per year
Morbidity	Low outside trigeminal nerve	Low outside trigeminal nerve	Low outside trigeminal nerve	Low outside trigeminal nerve	Transient cranial nerve, may be up to 10%
Mortality	Very low	None reported	None reported	None reported	Up to 1%
Sensory loss	+++, related to temperature used	+	V3 often affected	10% partial loss	None
Anaesthesia dolorosa	0.3–4%	None reported	None reported	None reported	None reported
Eye complications	Keratitis, 0.5–3%	None reported	Very rare	None reported	Diplopia rare
Hearing complications	1%	None reported	None reported	None reported	23% may have hearing loss
Masticatory complications	10%	None reported	Common, 100% for 3 months, permanent 3%	None reported	May occur
Numbers of treatments reported	++++	+++	++	+	+++

++++most difficult, + easiest

streptomycin injections, peripheral radiofrequency thermocoagulation.

Most of these procedures can be done under local anaesthesia with sedation although in some it is technically easier to use a general anaesthetic. The various techniques used for each of the individual procedures are described in greater detail in the chapter on peripheral surgery in *Trigeminal neuralgia* (Zakrzewska 1995).

Surgery at the level of the Gasserian ganglion

Surgery at this level relies on the principle that a needle is guided through the foramen ovale into the Gasserian

Table 32.6 Advantages and disadvantages of peripheral treatments

Advantages	*Disadvantages*
Most do not require general anaesthesia	Short-term relief – months
Can be done at any age	Often need adjuvant therapy
Patients do not need to be medically fit	Repeat procedures common
Relatively easy to perform	Sensory loss can occur
Most reversible	Only possible if there is a discrete trigger point
Can be repeated	
Minor side effects	
No mortality	
Immediate treatment in the case of injections	

ganglion or the surrounding trigeminal cistern. This is done utilizing fluoroscopic techniques and then other instruments or substances can be passed through this wide-bore needle. These techniques are mostly done under sedation or a brief general anaesthetic which rarely requires endotracheal intubation. Patients, therefore, can have these procedures done as day cases or, at the most, a 1–2-day inpatient stay. Each of the techniques will be described in general and the reader is referred to more surgical details in textbooks on trigeminal neuralgia (Anonymous 1987, Anonymous 1990) or to Burchiel (1996). Mortalities with these techniques are very rare and morbidity is mainly in relation to more extensive damage to the trigeminal nerve, the major complication being sensory loss. Recurrence rates are between 3–5 years. The expertise of the neurosurgeon contributes considerably to the success or otherwise of these techniques.

Radiofrequency thermocoagulation

The principle of this technique is to use a precisely controlled heat source to differentially destroy pain fibres, A-δ and C, while preserving light-touch A-fibres. Once the needle is in place and its position confirmed on fluoroscopy, the stilette is removed and a radiofrequency electrode thermistor, of varying length depending on the number of divisions to be treated, is inserted. The patient is woken while small pulses are passed so that details can be obtained as to the stimulation of the trigger zone and the potential area of anaesthesia to be achieved. The patient is then anaesthetized more fully and the lesions are made at temperatures varying from 69° to 90° for periods varying from 30 to 300 seconds.

Percutaneous retro-Gasserian glycerol injection

Glycerol is a chemoneurotoxic substance which preferentially destroys small, myelinated or unmyelinated fibres and large, damaged myelinated fibres as it diffuses slowly out of the cistern.

Once the needle is introduced into the cistern, this is visualized by the injection of radiocontrast medium. The radiocontrast medium is then drained out and glycerol slowly injected by the same amount as previously estimated on cisternography. By the use of careful positioning and injection, the ophthalmic branch may be spared.

Microcompression of the Gasserian ganglion

This technique relies on compression of the trigeminal nerve with a small balloon. This induces ischaemic and mechanical damage to the rootlets and ganglion cells.

Once entry has been gained into the Gasserian ganglion, a Fogarty embolectomy catheter is inserted through the needle and inflated with non-ionic water-soluble radiocontrast until it assumes a pear shape. The length of time for inflation varies from 0.5 to 1 minute.

Posterior fossa surgery

Apart from the use of the gamma knife, surgery at the level of the posterior fossa is major surgery which, inevitably, carries with it a risk of mortality, may be up to 1% in some centres, and a morbidity of around 10%.

Microvascular decompression

Microvascular decompression entails entry into the posterior fossa and visualization of the trigeminal nerve at its junction with the pons. Using microscopic techniques, blood vessels and lesions are identified and removed from direct contact with the trigeminal nerve. This surgical procedure purports to address the aetiological basis of trigeminal neuralgia in that it decompresses the trigeminal nerve from blood vessels or tumours which have resulted in demyelination of the nerve.

If no compression of the nerve is identified, some neurosurgeons will proceed to partial sensory rhizotomy. This involves the division of the sensory root of the trigeminal nerve. It will, inevitably, result in sensory loss.

Gamma knife irradiation

Radiation energy has been shown to affect ephaptic transmission but not normal axonal conduction. For trigeminal neuralgia, the irradiation is aimed at the proximal nerve and root entry zone in the pons as it is hypothesized that the change in myelin from central to peripheral type may be most affected by radiobiological effects. Magnetic resonance has allowed identification of this part of the nerve and, hence, delivery of the radiation to a highly specific area.

The procedure is carried out under local anaesthesia with light sedation and patients can be discharged within 24 hours. MRI sequencing is performed in order to identify the trigeminal nerve in its course from the pons into the Gasserian ganglion. Radiosurgical doses of between 70–90 Gy are normally used although the best dosage to get maximum pain relief with minimal complications is still being evaluated. The radiosurgery planning and dose selection are performed by a combination of neurosurgeons, radiation oncologists and medical physicists. The morbidity from gamma knife irradiation is much smaller given that this is a non-invasive procedure.

Additional management

It is inevitable that severe and intractable chronic pain leads to psychological and behavioural disturbances. Little attention has been paid to this aspect of management when describing medical or surgical procedures. Referral to a psychiatrist or clinical psychologist may, in some patients, be of more importance than other forms of treatment, especially in those patients who do not present with classic features.

Allaying fear and anxiety and reducing depression, if present, can have considerable effect on reducing pain. Patients should be taught how to develop coping strategies and pain diaries are extremely useful in monitoring response to drugs. Patients in control of their management are likely to do better. Support or self-help groups fulfil an important role as they allow consumers to have a greater say in the direction of research. In the USA there is a National Trigeminal Neuralgia Association which is now attempting to set up a branch in the UK.

All patients should be given adequate information, both verbally and in writing. Physicians and surgeons must avoid bias and be prepared to explain all forms of treatment even if they do not do the full range, as only then will patients be able to give fully informed consent.

GUIDELINES FOR MANAGEMENT

1. Detailed history and examination.
2. MRI on patients with rapidly progressing, severe trigeminal neuralgia, marked sensory loss or other symptoms in relation to possible lesion or multiple sclerosis. Very young patients.
3. Medical management initially with carbamazepine up to 1 g daily. There is less evidence for the possible addition of baclofen up to 80 mg or lamotrigine up to 400 mg daily.
4. Surgical management is proposed if drug therapy becomes ineffective or quality of life is adversely affected by side effects. Elderly and medically unfit patients should be offered peripheral surgery if the pain is very localized or surgery at the level of the Gasserian ganglion. In deciding which surgery to choose, the recurrence rate and sensory loss, with its effect on quality of life, need to be taken into account. Surgery at the posterior fossa level is only advocated for the medically fit patient and, in some centres, those under 65 years. Patients need to be aware of the risks and balance these against a high chance of long-term but not permanent relief of pain.
5. Psychological support, treatment of anxiety and depression is important. Contact with a support group can be extremely helpful.

Trigeminal neuralgia remains an enigma and its management remains controversial, not least because of the lack of multicentre, randomized controlled trials.

GLOSSOPHARYNGEAL NEURALGIA

DEFINITION

Sudden, severe, brief, stabbing, recurrent pains in the distribution of the glossopharyngeal nerve is the definition provided by the IASP.

EPIDEMIOLOGY

This is a rare condition and there are no data on its prevalence. Its incidence has been assessed in Rochester, USA, to be 0.7 per 100 000 (Katusic et al 1991a). The peak age was found to be between 70 and 79 years with a slight male predominance. A review of all the published case series, however, reported a lower peak age of around 50 years for both sexes and no difference in sex distribution (Bruyn 1983).

AETIOLOGY AND PATHOPHYSIOLOGY

This is unknown for glossopharyngeal neuralgia but it is assumed that the mechanism may be similar to that of trigeminal neuralgia with compression of appropriate nerve roots. Patients have been reported who have both trigeminal neuralgia and glossopharyngeal neuralgia (Rushton et al 1981).

CLINICAL FEATURES

The pain is unilateral, distributed within the posterior part of the tongue, tonsillar fossa and pharynx or beneath the angle of the jaw or even the ear and, depending on which predominates, it can be termed either pharyngeal or otalgic type. Radiation to the mandibular area, eye, nose and maxilla has also been reported. The left side appears to predominate in all reports (Katusic et al 1991b). Although the pain is described as being of a sharp, shooting quality, a dull, aching, burning pain is often present in the background (Rushton et al 1981, King 1987). Although the pain can be extremely severe, it tends to be less severe than trigeminal neuralgia (Katusic et al 1991b). The pain is episodic and in the series described by Katusic et al (1991a) the time interval between episodes was 0.5–9 years. There appear to be fewer recurrences than in patients with trigeminal neuralgia (Katusic et al 1991b).

Provoking factors are not only swallowing but also contact with fluids, especially cold ones. Yawning, talking and moving the head can all precipitate the pain. The most immediate relieving factor is the application of a 10% solution of cocaine to the trigger zone (Rushton et al 1981). Anticonvulsant drugs relieve the pain. Attacks of pain may be associated with syncope and cardiac arrhythmias (Rushton et al 1981). Examination shows no neurological deficits.

INVESTIGATION

MRI of the posterior fossa or vertebral angiograms have been used but there have been no studies specifically to investigate glossopharyngeal neuralgia and assess their specificity and sensitivity.

MANAGEMENT

Not a single randomized controlled trial has been carried out in this group of patients. Treatment, therefore, is based on case series and relies on comparison with trigeminal neuralgia. Ceylan et al (1997) reported on six cases, four of which responded to antineuralgic therapy and two of which required surgical management. Drugs used are the same as for trigeminal neuralgia while surgery has included radiofrequency thermocoagulation and microvascular decompression. Only 77 cases have been reported in the literature. Side effects of surgery include hoarseness, dysphagia, inability to speak loudly and persistent coughing. There have been reports of two deaths and three patients who sustained permanent ninth nerve palsies (Resnick et al 1995).

GUIDELINES FOR MANAGEMENT

The very few case reports suggest that most cases can be managed with an anticonvulsant such as carbamazepine in doses similar to trigeminal neuralgia. Intracranial section or microvascular decompression should be reserved for those patients who cannot be managed medically.

ACUTE HERPES ZOSTER TRIGEMINAL

DEFINITION

Pain in the distribution of the trigeminal nerve associated with acute herpes zoster. The IASP classification uses this definition to describe pain associated with the eruption of vesicles, before, during or after. The IHS definition includes pain prior to vesicle eruption and one that subsides within 6 months of the rash. Both classifications have separate definitions for postherpetic neuralgia. In clinical studies, however, the definition varies considerably. This is probably because most patients feel their pain as a continuum although the quality and pathophysiology of acute pain of herpes zoster are different from that of postherpetic neuralgia.

EPIDEMIOLOGY

Herpes zoster is a fairly common condition and can occur in up to 20% of the population. In this group, up to 20% of patients may have trigeminal herpes zoster and out of this group, 50% will have involvement of the eye itself. There appears to be no predilection for either sex but the elderly are most at risk. The ophthalmic form of herpes zoster causes the most serious side effects and can threaten sight. Acute and long-term complications are common, especially in the elderly.

AETIOLOGY AND PATHOPHYSIOLOGY

The respiratory system is the route of entry of the varicella virus and provides for the initial replication of the virus in the reticuloendothelial system. A viraemia occurs and then the virus seeds target organs which include the skin and lungs. The virus tracks along sensory, peripheral nerves and becomes latent in the satellite cells of the dorsal root ganglion. The initial pain is caused by the acute neuritis, which occurs both peripherally and in the dorsal root ganglion. Histological changes show classic features of acute inflammation with destruction of myelin and axonal degeneration extending along the sensory nerve.

It appears that reduced cell-mediated immunity leads to increased susceptibility to herpes zoster as it is commoner in the elderly and patients who are immunosuppressed and those susceptible to haematological and lymphoreticular carcinomas.

CLINICAL FEATURES

The pain can be in any of the divisions of the trigeminal nerve and there may be some radiation. The mouth will be involved in maxillary and mandibular cases whereas the nasolabial area is often involved in ophthalmic division pain. The pain is extremely severe and is described as being burning and tingling with sharp, shooting exacerbation. The continuous pain may occur at any time, either before the eruption of the vesicles, during the eruption or after. It can last from one to several weeks but can gradually merge into postherpetic neuralgia pain. There appear to be no provoking factors and only drug therapy will provide relief of symptoms. Associated with the pain is a generalized fever, headaches and malaise.

Vasculitis also occurs within the ophthalmic division. Any structure within or surrounding the orbit may be involved, leading to any of the following: eyelid scarring, keratitis and scleritis, iritis, glaucoma and retinal necrosis. Ulceration and chronic scarring of the cornea can result in future blindness. Involvement of extraocular muscles occurs if optic neuritis develops.

The condition is nearly always unilateral. The eye may initially be red prior to the eruption of the vesicles. The small cluster of vesicles in the distribution of the affected nerve slowly enlarge, become pustular and later haemorrhagic. The lesions take 1–2 weeks to crust over. The lymph nodes draining the area may become tender and enlarged. Immunocompromised patients are at risk of more systemic complications such as pneumonia, encephalitis, polyneuritis and motor neuropathies.

INVESTIGATION

In most patients laboratory confirmation is not necessary although immunocompromised patients and those who have an unusual form or progression may need further investigations which would include polymerase chain reactions on vesicle scrapings, CSF or vitreous aspirates.

MANAGEMENT

The aim of treatment is to reduce the duration and spread of the rash. It is also important to attempt to reduce the frequency and severity of complications, including those of postherpetic neuralgia. Lancaster et al (1995) carried out a systematic review of primary care management of acute herpes zoster from randomized controlled trials up until 1993. Since then, the British Society for the Study of Infection has also produced guidelines for the management of shingles (Anonymous 1995). The guidelines given below are made on the basis of these reports.

If there is involvement of the eye, then oral antiviral drug therapy is recommended whatever the age of the patient and within 72 hours of appearance of the lesions. There is currently insufficient evidence to say that systemic or topical antiviral drugs will prevent ophthalmic complications but it is suggested that early use of these agents may reduce the incidence of complications. Since the systematic review, valaciclovir and famciclovir have been introduced but, as yet, there is insufficient evidence to suggest their routine use. It is extremely important, however, to ensure that any patient who has a red eye or other ocular involvement is referred within 3 days for a specialist ophthalmological opinion and for possible treatment with topical steroids.

Oral aciclovir is used in dosages of 800 mg five times daily for 7 days. The newer antiviral agents can be used on three times dosage scales due to their improved bioavailability: valaciclovir 100 mg tds and famciclovir 500 mg tds (Tyring et al 1995, Beutner et al 1995). In those patients with no ocular involvement, antiviral therapy is only required in patients over the age of 60 years presenting within 72 hours of rash appearance or those who have very severe, acute pain within 72 hours of the rash who are below 60 years of age. Highly immunocompromised patients should receive aciclovir intravenously and oral therapy should be substituted later. Steroids have been suggested but the evidence is inconclusive. Amitryptiline, to reduce incidence of postherpetic neuralgia, may be of value only in those over 60 years of age (Bowsher 1997). Nerve blocks have been used but there is no evidence to suggest that they are effective. There is also no evidence to suggest that nerve blockade can be used as part of a pre-emptive measure for the treatment of postherpetic neuralgia.

GUIDELINES FOR MANAGEMENT

1. Oral antiviral agent, e.g. aciclovir 800 mg tds or valaciclovir 100 mg tds or famciclovir 500 mg tds within 72 hours of onset, continued for 7 days.
2. Ophthalmological opinion within 72 hours.
3. Topical steroids – only under the guidance of an ophthalmologist.

POSTHERPETIC NEURALGIA

DEFINITION

The IHS classification defines this as facial pain developing during the acute phase of herpes zoster and persisting for more than 6 months thereafter. The IASP classification defines it as chronic pain with skin changes in the distribution of one or more roots of the fifth cranial nerve subsequent to acute herpes zoster. It remains difficult to establish when the pain of acute herpes zoster changes to postherpetic neuralgia as improvements can occur for up to 3 years.

EPIDEMIOLOGY

There is conflicting evidence on the incidence of postherpetic neuralgia although it is known to be strongly age related. It is considered that a significant proportion of patients over 60 years will suffer from postherpetic neuralgia and that it is uncommon in those below 50 years. Numerous studies have been carried out to see whether it is possible to predict patients who are likely to suffer from postherpetic neuralgia. These studies have identified three predictors but firm evidence is still lacking. They include severe or prolonged prodromal pain, zoster affecting the trigeminal nerve and a history of anxiety or depression prior to illness or excessive anxiety and depression or increased illness behaviour during acute zoster (Dworkin et al 1992).

AETIOLOGY AND PATHOPHYSIOLOGY

The pathophysiology needs to explain the allodynia and sensory deficits but also the origin of the pain. The initial acute herpes zoster results in the loss of many large fibres in the affected sensory nerve. Chronic inflammatory changes probably also result in the loss of axons and myelin in the sensory nerve route fibres leading to deafferentation of nociceptive fibres which then result in new synaptic connections being made (Morris et al 1995). Immunological mechanisms may also play a role as in the elderly the response to the herpes zoster antigen and hence the cytotoxic efficacy could be altered.

CLINICAL FEATURES

Patients present with three different types of pain, all in the distribution of the affected cranial nerve or division. The pain does not radiate extensively, may be described as aching, burning or lancinating and is usually of moderate severity although it can become intolerable. The pain can last from months to years. The allodynia is often triggered by light touch such as clothing or washing the face. It can be cold induced. Associated with the pain is a sensory deficit in all modalities including perception of warmth, cold, heat, pain, touch, pinprick, vibration and two-point discrimination. Patients will often be anxious and depressed. Cutaneous scarring and pigmentary changes may be seen. Abnormal responses are noted on sensory testing.

MANAGEMENT

A systematic review of randomized controlled trials on the treatment of postherpetic neuralgia was carried out by Volminck et al (1996), using trials up to December 1993. The British Society for the Study of Infections has also published guidelines for the management of postherpetic neuralgia (Anonymous 1995). Treatment remains difficult and there is no ideal method. Application of cold packs and occlusive dressings with local anaesthetic are often inappropriate for facial application. Vibrators and TENS (transcutaneous electrical nerve stimulation) may be useful in some patients. Antidepressants, amitryptiline and desipramine, are effective whereas clomipramine and lorazepam are ineffective. Topical capsaicin and topical 5% lignocaine gel may be beneficial but more randomized controlled trials using less heterogeneous groups are needed to prove their efficacy. Anticonvulsants are not useful in this condition and surgical therapy is contraindicated.

GUIDELINES FOR MANAGEMENT

1. Amitryptiline 75 mg daily.
2. Desipramine 167 mg daily.
3. Topical capsaicin 0.075%.
4. Topical lignocaine gel 5%.

It must be remembered that postherpetic neuralgia continues to be a very difficult condition to treat and only modest results can be expected.

SINUSITIS

DEFINITION

Inflammation of any sinus leading to a constant burning pain over the site of the sinus with a nasal discharge. Patients may have disease in only one sinus, bilaterally or in several. The signs and symptoms are very similar in each case and the discussion will be based mainly on maxillary sinusitis which is the commonest form. Both the IASP and IHS classifications consider chronic forms to be incomplete resolutions of acute sinusitis and not a separate entity.

EPIDEMIOLOGY

Sinusitis, especially maxillary sinusitis, is extremely common and it is estimated that 0.5–5% of upper respiratory tract infections are complicated by sinusitis. It occurs equally in both sexes and in all age groups.

AETIOLOGY AND PATHOPHYSIOLOGY

Retention of secretions in the paranasal sinuses for any reason – change in secretion, viscosity or overproduction, obstruction of ostia, changes in the number or impairment in the function of cilia – results in sinusitis. The infection in most cases is due to bacterial causes and the common organisms are *Haemophilus influenzae* and *Streptococcus pneumoniae*. Infections occur either from an upper respiratory tract infection or for odontological reasons such as dental extraction or penetration of instruments and materials into the maxillary sinus.

CLINICAL FEATURES

The pain overlies the involved sinus or sinuses and, therefore, may be unilateral or bilateral. Radiation often occurs to surrounding structures. Frontal sinusitis will radiate to the vertex and behind the eyes while maxillary sinusitis will radiate to the upper teeth or to the forehead. Ethmoiditis is located between and behind the eyes and may radiate to the temporal area and sphenoiditis is located in the occipital area of the vertex, the frontal region or behind the eyes. Sinusitis is a dull, burning, aching, continuous pain of mild to moderate severity. It occurs just as patients are recovering from an upper respiratory tract infection and lasts for a few days. Touching the affected area and, in a case of maxillary sinusitis, bending or biting on the affected side will increase the pain. Drainage of the sinus provides the best form of relief. Associated with the pain is a purulent nasal discharge.

INVESTIGATIONS

It can sometimes be difficult to differentiate between upper respiratory tract infection and maxillary sinusitis and yet the correct diagnosis is important, as there is evidence of overdiagnosis and subsequent overuse of antibiotics. With this in mind, a protocol has been registered with the Cochrane Collaboration which is going to do a systematic review of 'ultrasonography, radiography and clinical examination in the diagnosis of acute maxillary sinusitis in primary health care' (Varonen & Makela 1998). A study by Lindboek et al (1996b) assessed the use of symptoms, signs and blood tests in the diagnosis of acute sinus infections in primary care. They assessed 27 signs and symptoms, blood tests and sinus radiography and sinus CT. They found that only four were significantly associated with the presence of infection and they were purulent rhinorrhoea by history, double sickening (an upper respiratory infection that initially improved and then worsened), purulent secretions in the nasal cavity and an ESR >10 mm per hour. If a patient has the four relevant signs and symptoms the probability of a correct diagnosis increases to 95% while with three of the four it is around 80%. If none of these is present there is only a 15% chance that the patient may have sinusitis. Radiographic investigations, either as plain radiography or CT scanning, will show opacities in the sinusitis, air–fluid levels and mucosal thickening.

MANAGEMENT

Acute sinusitis is a self-limiting illness for most patients and over 50% will respond well to decongestants alone. The other 50% may benefit from the use of antibiotics but this must be weighed against the increased risk of side effects, especially gastrointestinal. As yet, there are no published placebo-controlled trials to evaluate therapies such as topical and oral decongestants, antihistamines, systemic glucocorticoids and irrigation of the nasal cavity. A systematic review of the role of antibiotics has not yet been done. Low et al (1997) attempted a review of the literature and found that a 10-day course of amoxycillin should be the first line of therapy. However, a randomized controlled trial (Van Buchem et al 1997) suggested that amoxycillin did not improve the course of maxillary sinusitis in primary care, in contrast to Lindboek et al (1996a) who showed that both penicillin V and amoxycillin improved health status in adults with confirmed sinusitis. A small randomized controlled trial also showed that 3 days of trimethoprim-sulphamethoxazole treatment was as effective as 10 days and should therefore be used in otherwise healthy patients in conjunction with a nasal decongestant (Williams et al 1995). Further randomized controlled trials on management of acute sinusitis can be found in the Cochrane database of trials which is updated quarterly.

GUIDELINES FOR MANAGEMENT

1. Careful assessment of symptoms and signs.
2. Sinus radiography, either plain or CT.
3. ESR.
4. Nasal decongestants.
5. Antibiotics in those patients with bacterial maxillary sinusitis: penicillin V, amoxycillin are most commonly used for 7–10 days; consider using 3 days of trimethoprim-sulphamethoxazole. Other newer antibiotics are under review.

RARE PAINS OF THE FACE

Table 32.7 lists the principal features of some rare pains of the face that need to be considered if other common causes are excluded. The data for all these conditions is based on case series and there is very little evidence at present on how these conditions should be managed.

EYE PAIN

Eye pain may be from eye disease itself or from other extraocular structures or may be referred to the region of the eye. The majority of ocular diseases are not painful and referred pain may be from structures as distant as the neck, jaws, sinuses or teeth (see Table 32.1). Most eye pain needs to be evaluated by an ophthalmologist because of the specialized nature of the disease and the equipment required to evaluate the problem.

Eye pain can originate from the surface or from the deeper structures of the globe. Superficial pain originating from structures like the cornea typically results in acute, sharp pain which is easily relieved by local anaesthetic solutions. Diseases within the globe cause a dull, aching, deep type of pain which results in tenderness of the globe on palpation. Iritis and keratitis can cause reflex spasm of the ciliary muscles and the iris sphincter and this can lead to pain over the brow area and painful light sensitivity. These deeper pains are more difficult to treat.

Refractory errors due to hypermetropia, astigmatism or presbyopia or the wearing of incorrect glasses can result in pain either in the eyes or referred to the frontal region. These are relatively mild headaches which develop throughout the day as more prolonged visual tasks are undertaken. Typically, the patient has no pain on wakening. Uncorrected squints can also lead to mild to moderate headaches in the frontal region and can also be associated with intermittent blurred vision or diplopia and difficulty in adjusting focus from near to distant objects. Closing an eye often relieves the symptoms. These conditions can easily be rectified by an ophthalmologist.

Conditions that most often cause eye pain are summarized in Table 32.8. The general principles of management are given but the reader is referred to randomized controlled trials for more evidence-based treatments.

OPTIC NEURITIS

This is a broad term denoting inflammation or demyelination of the optic nerve. One form of optic neuritis is retrobulbar neuritis which is often diagnosed late, as the optic disc is involved deeply and so signs are not seen on ophthalmological examination.

Epidemiology

The optic neuritis treatment trial (ONTT) conducted between 1988 and 1993 recruited 457 patients. In this group 77% of patients were women and the mean age was 32 years (Beck et al 1992). Rodriguez et al (1995) determined the incidence and prevalence of optic neuritis in a population-based study. The median age of onset was 31 years and the age- and sex-adjusted prevalence rate was 115.3 per 100 000 (95% CI, 95.2–135.4/100 000). Optic neuritis is most closely linked with multiple sclerosis and progression increases with length of follow-up, that is,

Table 32.7 Rare conditions that cause pain in the trigeminal, ear and eye regions

	Tolosa–Hunt syndrome	*SUNCT**	*Geniculate neuralgia (Ramsay Hunt)*	*Raeder's syndrome (paratrigeminal)*	*Pretrigeminal neuralgia*
Defintion	Episodic unilateral orbital pain associated with ophthalmoplegia	Repetitive paroxysms of short-lasting pain associated with eye and nasal symptoms	Severe pain in external auditory meatus following herpes zoster	Painful type of Horner's syndrome	Prodromal pain prior to trigeminal neuralgia
Epidemiology	Rare, mean age of onset 40 yrs, M=F	Very rare, middle age M:F, 4:0.25	Rare, incidence 5/100 000 per year	Rare, mainly males, middle age	Rare, 52 cases reported, age late 50s
Aetiology	Fibrous tissue formation in the cavernous sinus and surrounding area, venous vasculitis	Unknown, may be abnormal cerebral circulation	Related to herpes zoster infection	Tumour, trauma for type 1, unknown for type 2	As for trigeminal neuralgia
Site	Eye, unilateral	Ocular, periocular, unilateral	Deep in external auditory meatus	Unilateral	Unilateral, trigeminal distribution
Radiation	Periorbital, behind the eye	Frontotemporal, upper jaw, palate	Postauricular	Upper part of face, forehead	Other divisions, teeth
Character	Ache	Burning, electrical, stabbing	Sharp, lancinating	Aching, non-pulsatile	Dull, aching, toothache-like
Severity	Moderate to severe	Moderate to severe	Severe	Mild to severe, fluctuates	Moderate
Duration	Average 8 weeks	5–250 sec, mean 61 sec	Several days to weeks	Long-lasting pain which gradually builds up & then diminishes	Up to several hours
Periodicity	Average 1 year, not all recur	Several attacks a day, mean 28, periods of weeks to months and then remissions	Continuous, a week or so after eruption	Weeks to months, rarely recurs	3 months to 10 yrs before trigeminal neuralgia develops
Provoking factors	May be stress	Mechanical, neck movements		Strenuous exercise, cardiovascular factors	Movement, temperature but not always
Relieving factors	Drugs	Drugs slightly	Drugs	Analgesia	Carbamazepine
Associated factors	Back pain, cold feet, arthralgia, gut problems, may get other facial pain in between without ophthalmoplegia, nasal, hearing deficit may also occur	Conjunctival injection, lacrimation, nasal stuffiness, rhinorrhoea	These may also be present: hearing loss, tinnitus, hyperacusis, vertigo, Bell's palsy, dysgeusia, epiphora	Ptosis, miosis, hypohidrosis in type 1, also involvement of any of the following cranial nerves II, III, IV, V, VI	Often thought to have dental problems
Clinical signs	Paralysis of one or more nerves 3rd, 4th 6th occurs either at time of pain or later	Conjunctival injection, forehead sweating unilateral	Nil	Cranial nerve abnormalities, most commonly discrete involvement of V	Nil
Investigations	Orbital phlebography shows venous, collateral venous flow and obstruction of cavernous sinus, ESR, serum inflammatory changes may be raised, MRI	Orbital phlebography shows venous vasculitis, MRI	MRI shows enhancement of geniculate ganglion & facial nerve, auditory tests to assess hearing loss	Type 1 numerous to find underlying pathology, MRI	Nil
Medical treatment	Steroids during an episode, rapid response, resistant cases azothioprine	Poor response, cortisone may help, does not respond to carbamazepine, indomethacin or anaesthetic blockades	Aciclovir-prednisolone (not RCT)	Analgesia for type 2	Carbamazepine, baclofen

Table 32.7 (Contd.) Rare conditions that cause pain in the trigeminal, ear and eye regions

	Tolosa–Hunt syndrome	*SUNCT**	*Geniculate neuralgia (Ramsay Hunt)*	*Raeder's syndrome (paratrigeminal)*	*Pretrigeminal neuralgia*
References	Anon (1994), Anon (1988), Hannerz (1992), Yousem et al (1990), Odabasi et al (1997)	Anon (1994), Pareja et al (1995, 1997), Pareja & Sjaastad (1997), Goadsby & Lipton (1997), Benoliel & Sharav (1998)	Anon (1994), Wayman et al (1990), Murakami et al (1997)	Anon (1994), Grimson & Thompson (1980)	Mitchell (1980) Fromm et al (1990)

**SUNCT = short-lasting, unilateral neuralgiform pain with conjunctival injection and tearing. Other conditions that need to be considered in the differential diagnosis, such as cluster headaches, paroxysmal hemicrania and cluster tic syndrome, are discussed in the chapter on headaches. Atypical facial pain and TMJ pain are covered in the chapter on orofacial pain.*

Table 32.8 Causes, presentation and management of eye pain

Location	*Cause*	*Signs & symptoms*	*Principles of management*	*References RCTs*
Corneal abrasion	Foreign body, metallic fragments, scratch, contact lens	Sharp stabbing, severe pain, worse on blinking, often acute, blepharospasm, photophobia, red eye, lacrimation	Local anaesthesia may aid removal of foreign body, topical antibiotic, mydriatic, may patch the eye if no overt infection	Kaiser (1995), Patterson et al (1996), Brahma et al (1996) Haynes et al 1996), Jayamanne et al (1997)
Corneal infection, keratitis, peripheral corneal ulcers	Viral, e.g. herpes simplex, bacterial, chronic use of eye medication	Dull, throbbing, persistent severe pain, worse on moving eyelid, photophobia, tearing, ulceration	Antibiotics, antiviral	Kosrirukvongs (1997)
Episcleritis, scleritis	Often associated with rheumatoid arthritis, herpes zoster	Ocular discomfort, dull, throbbing photophobia, lacrimation, vision normal or reduced, cornea clear, pupil normal or miosed	Nil to topical steroids of varying strength and frequency, non-steroidal anti-inflammatories, cycloplegic agents	Watson et al (1973)
Iritis, anterior uveitis, granulomatous or non-granulomatous	Granulomatous caused by infective agents, non-granulomatous due to hypersensitivity reaction	Pain most marked in non-granulomatous , red eye, photophobia, blurred vision, often reduced vision, pupil miosed, fixed	Steroids of varying strengths, frequency, systemic analgesics	
Acute angle closure glaucoma	Elevated intraocular pressure due to impaired access of aqueous to the drainage system	Sudden onset, pain: throbbing, dull, very severe at times; vomiting, dehydrated, blurring, halos, red eye, raised intraocular pressure, oedematous cornea, mid dilated oval fixed pupil, with pupillary block, reduced vision, cornea cloudy, tender to touch, swollen	Emergency, carbonic anhydrase inhibitors, hyperosmotics, topical β-blockers, miotic drops, topical steroids, may need surgery	Rossetti et al (1993)
Optic neuritis	Associated with multiple sclerosis	Pain with eye movements, tenderness of the globe	High-dose steroids	Beck et al (1992, 1993), Rodriguez et al (1995)

RCT = randomized controlled trials

progression to multiple sclerosis was 39% at 10 years but 60% at 40 years. The only factors that were linked with the development of multiple sclerosis were the presence of perivenous sheathing and recurrent optic neuritis.

Aetiology

Optic neuritis is regarded as an immune-mediated inflammatory disorder, which may affect any part of the optic nerve.

Clinical features

Typically, in over 90% of patients, pain is a prominent feature, often beginning before loss of visual function. The pain is deep-seated, of a dull, throbbing character and, in 50% of patients, is made worse with specific eye movements. The pain usually resolves prior to visual improvement and occurs within the first 2 weeks. Other symptoms include loss of vision, which can vary and last for 2–6 weeks; central scotomas are the most common visual field defects although any unilateral field change may occur. The pupillary light reflex is sluggish and there may also be impairment of colour vision. In the ONTT survey the optic disc was initially normal in 65% of patients. Hyperaemia of the optic disc with distension of large veins is common but other changes may be seen on ophthalmological examination although these are relatively rare.

Differential diagnosis

The main differential diagnosis is that of papilloedema. Although multiple sclerosis is the most likely disease, lupus erythematosus or optic neuropathy due to other demyelinating diseases such as diabetes or B12 deficiency may also occur. Optic neuritis may also be drug induced or related to syphilis, sarcoidosis and vascular disorders.

Investigations

Abnormal visual evoked potentials are noted.

Management

Treatment of acute optic neuritis with intravenous methylprednisolone improves short-term (6 months) visual outcome but this tends not to influence the final disability or rate of further relapse (ONTT) (Beck et al 1992). Oral steroid therapy, however, resulted in a high incidence of recurrent optic neuritis when compared with either intravenous steroids or placebo (Beck et al 1993).

Guidelines for management

Intravenous methylprednisolone (1 g/day).

PHANTOM EYE PAIN

Definition

Phantom eye pain occurs following ocular bulb amputation, most commonly for orbital cancer.

Epidemiology

As orbital cancer is a rare condition, phantom eye pain is rare and there are no epidemiological data. The largest reported series is by Nicolodi et al (1997), who reported 53 subjects collected over a period of 8 years.

Aetiology

This is presumed to be the same as after amputation of other bodily parts. In the series of Nicolodi et al (1997), 62% of patients complained of non-painful phantom sensations, 43% had photopsia (appearance of sparks or flashes within the eye) and 28% complained of phantom pain. They also found that these patients were more likely to suffer from headaches than those who were non-headache sufferers prior to surgery.

Treatment

None has been described but it would be expected that these patients would respond to neuropathic-type drugs.

EAR PAIN

Otalgia can be due to primary causes or may be referred pain (see Table 32.1). The primary causes of otalgia are summarized in Table 32.9. Only the general features and treatment are given, as most patients will need to be seen by an ear, nose and throat specialist for specific management.

CONCLUSION

Pain in the trigeminal, ear and eye regions is extremely complex and may be due to a wide variety of causes. Diagnosis may be difficult but in most cases is based on a careful history. Treatments involve a wide range of specialists and currently, in some conditions, there are very few randomized controlled trials to help a-clinician in managing the condition.

Table 32.9 Causes, presentation and management of primary otalgia

Location	*Condition*	*Clinical features*	*General principles of management*	*References to RCTs on management*
Pinna	Haematoma	Blow to ear results in haematoma, ballooned blue pinna	Aspiration of clot and compression	
Pinna	Perichondritis	Pain on moving pinna or tragus	Antibiotic, incision	
Pinna	Acute dermatitis	Oedematous, red auricle, serous fluid, painful when pinna moved	Debridement, topical steroids	
	Frostbite or burn to pinna	Itchiness		
External auditory meatus	Foreign body	History of insertion often by children	Removal of foreign body by otologist	
	Wax impaction	Deafness, itchiness	Soften wax, remove	
	Otitis externa	Bacterial or fungal, pain moderate to severe, increased by jaw movement, irritation, scanty discharge, deafness, tender on compression of tragus, red desquamated meatal skin	Swab for culture and sensitivity, aural toilet, appropriate topical therapy	
	Furunculosis	Infection of hair follicle in meatus, severe pain worse with jaw movement and movement of pinna, deafness, tenderness on compression of tragus, boils seen in meatus on examination	Analgesics, aural dressing, only in severe cases systemic antibiotic	
	Malignant disease	Pain becomes intractable and very severe, bloodstained discharge from the ear, presents as ulcer or friable mass	Radiotherapy and/or surgery	
	Acute otitis media	Earache is severe, throbbing, not exacerbated by movement of pinna or tragus, child will cry and scream, deafness, pyrexia, tenderness, depending on stage of disease tympanic membrane may be bulging or perforated	If bacterial antibiotics, myringotomy, aural toilet if discharge, follow-up, xylitol chewing gum	Rosenfeld et al (1994), Kozyrskyj et al (1998), Glasziou et al (1998), Uhari et al (1996)
	Chronic otitis media		Topical antibiotics, in children adenoidectomy	
	Acute mastoiditis	Persistent throbbing pain with tenderness over the mastoid antrum, creamy discharge, increasing deafness, pyrexial, malaise, swelling over mastoid	Antibiotics, cortical mastoidectomy if indicated	
	Petrositis (Gradenigo's syndrome)	Pain in trigeminal area, diplopia, headache, signs of middle ear infection	Antibiotics and mastoidectomy	
	Secretory otitis media (glue ear)	Deafness, stuffy feeling in the ear, transient pain, fluid in the middle ear, common in children	Systemic steroids combined with antibiotics, myringotomy, grommets, adenoidectomy	Rosenfeld & Post (1992), Acuin et al (1998)

RCT = randomized controlled trials

REFERENCES

Anonymous 1987 The medical and surgical management of trigeminal neuralgia. In: Fromm GH (ed) Part 11B Relatively localised symptoms of the Head and Neck pp 59–99 Futura, New York

Anonymous 1988 Classification and diagnostic criteria for headache disorders, cranial neuralgias and facial pain. Headache Classification Committee of the International Headache Society. Cephalalgia 8 (suppl 7): 1–96

Anonymous 1990 Trigeminal neuralgia. In: Rovit RL, Murali R, Jannetta PJ (eds) Part 11B Relatively localised symptoms of the Head and Neck pp 59–99 Williams and Wilkins, Baltimore

Anonymous 1994 In: Merskey H, Bogduk N (eds) Classification of chronic pain. Descriptors of chronic pain syndromes and definitions of pain terms. IASP Press, Seattle

Anonymous 1995 Guidelines for the management of shingles. Report of a working group of the British Society for the Study of Infection (BSSI). Journal of Infection 30(3): 193–200

Acuin J, Smith A, Mackenzie I 1998 Treatment of chronic suppurative otitis media (protocol). Issue 2, Update Software. Cochrane Library, Oxford

Beck RW, Cleary PA, Anderson MM Jr et al 1992 A randomized, controlled trial of corticosteroids in the treatment of acute optic neuritis. The Optic Neuritis Study Group [see comments]. New England Journal of Medicine 326(9): 581–588

Beck RW, Cleary PA, Trobe JD et al 1993 The effect of corticosteroids for acute optic neuritis on the subsequent development of multiple sclerosis. The Optic Neuritis Study Group. New England Journal of Medicine 329(24): 1764–1769

Benoliel R, Sharav Y 1998 SUNCT syndrome: case report and literature review. Oral Surgery, Oral Medicine, Oral Pathology, Oral Radiology and Endodontics 85(2): 158–161

Beutner KR, Friedman DJ, Forszpaniak C, Andersen PL, Wood MJ 1995 Valaciclovir compared with acyclovir for improved therapy for herpes zoster in immunocompetent adults. Antimicrobial Agents and Chemotherapy 39(7): 1546–1553

Bittar GT, Graff-Radford SB 1993 The effects of streptomycin/lidocaine block on trigeminal neuralgia: a double blind crossover placebo controlled study. Headache 33(3): 155–160

Bowsher D 1997 The effects of pre-emptive treatment of postherpetic neuralgia with amitriptyline: a randomized, double-blind, placebocontrolled trial. Journal of Pain and Symptom Management 13(6): 327–331

Brahma AK, Shah S, Hillier VF et al 1996 Topical analgesia for superficial corneal injuries. Journal of Accident and Emergency Medicine 13(3): 186–188

Bruyn GW 1983 Glossopharyngeal neuralgia. Cephalalgia 3(3): 143–157

Burchiel KJ 1996 Pain in neurology and neurosurgery: tic douloureux (trigeminal neuralgia). In: Campbell JN (ed) Pain 1996 – an updated review. IASP Press, Seattle, pp 41–60

Campbell FG, Graham JG, Zilkha KJ 1998 Clinical trial of carbamazepine (Tegretol) in trigeminal neuralgia. Journal of Neurology, Neurosurgery and Psychiatry 29: 265–267

Ceylan S, Karakus A, Duru S, Baykal S, Koca O 1997 Glossopharyngeal neuralgia: a study of 6 cases. Neurosurgical Review 20(3): 196–200

Davies HT, Crombie IK, Macrae WA 1993 Polarised views on treating neurogenic pain. Pain 54(3): 341–346

Dworkin RH, Hartstein G, Rosner HL, Walther RR, Sweeney EW, Brand L 1992 A high-risk method for studying psychosocial antecedents of chronic pain: the prospective investigation of herpes zoster. Journal of Abnormal Psychology 101(1): 200–205

Fromm GH, Terrence CF 1987 Comparison of L-baclofen and racemic baclofen in trigeminal neuralgia. Neurology 37(11): 1725–1728

Fromm GH, Terrence CF, Chattha AS, Glass JD 1980 Baclofen in trigeminal neuralgia: its effect on the spinal trigeminal nucleus: a pilot study. Archives of Neurology 37(12): 768–771

Fromm GH, Terrence CF, Chattha AS 1984 Baclofen in the treatment of trigeminal neuralgia: double-blind study and long-term follow-up. Annals of Neurology 15(3): 240–244

Fromm GH, Graff-Radford SB, Terrence CF, Sweet WH 1990 Pre-trigeminal neuralgia. Neurology 40(10): 1493–1495

Fromm GH, Aumentado D, Terrence CF 1993 A clinical and experimental investigation of the effects of tizanidine in trigeminal neuralgia. Pain 53(3): 265–271

Glasziou PP, Hayem M Del Mar CB 1998 Antibiotic versus placebo for acute otitis media in children. Issue 2, Update Software. Cochrane Library, Oxford

Goadsby PJ, Lipton RB 1997 A review of paroxysmal hemicranias, SUNCT syndrome and other short-lasting headaches with autonomic features, including new cases. Brain 120(Pt 1): 193–209

Gordon A, Hitchcock ER 1983 Illness behaviour and personality in intractable facial pain syndromes. Pain 17(3): 267–276

Graff-Radford SB, Ketelaer MC, Gratt BM, Solberg WK 1995 Thermographic assessment of neuropathic facial pain. Journal of Orofacial Pain 9(2): 138–146

Gratt BM, Graff-Radford SB, Shetty V, Solberg WK, Sickles EA 1996 A 6-year clinical assessment of electronic facial thermography. Dentomaxillofacial Radiology 25(5): 247–255

Grimson BS, Thompson HS 1980 Raeder's syndrome. A clinical review. Survey of Ophthalmology 24(4): 199–210

Hannerz J 1992 Recurrent Tolosa–Hunt syndrome. Cephalalgia 12(1): 45–51

Haynes RJ, Walker S, Kirkpatrick JN 1996 Topical diclofenac relieves pain from corneal rust ring. Eye 10(Pt 4): 443–446

Jayamanne DG, Fitt AW, Dayan M, Andrews RM, Mitchell KW, Griffiths PG 1997 The effectiveness of topical diclofenac in relieving discomfort following traumatic corneal abrasions. Eye 11(Pt 1): 79–83

Kaiser PK 1995 A comparison of pressure patching versus no patching for corneal abrasions due to trauma or foreign body removal. Corneal Abrasion Patching Study Group [see comments]. Ophthalmology 102(12): 1936–1942

Katusic S, Beard CM, Bergstralh E, Kurland LT 1990 Incidence and clinical features of trigeminal neuralgia, Rochester, Minnesota, 1945–1984. Annals of Neurology 27(1): 89–95

Katusic S, Williams DB, Beard CM, Bergstralh EJ, Kurland LT 1991a Incidence and clinical features of glossopharyngeal neuralgia, Rochester, Minnesota, 1945–1984. Neuroepidemiology 10(5–6): 266–275

Katusic S, Williams DB, Beard CM, Bergstralh EJ, Kurland LT 1991b Epidemiology and clinical features of idiopathic trigeminal neuralgia and glossopharyngeal neuralgia: similarities and differences, Rochester, Minnesota, 1945–1984. Neuroepidemiology 10(5–6): 276–281

Killian JM, Fromm GH 1968 Carbamazepine in the treatment of neuralgia. Use of side effects. Archives of Neurology 19(2): 129–136

King J 1987 Glossopharyngeal neuralgia. Clinical and Experimental Neurology 24: 113–121

Kondziolka D, Lemley T, Kestle JR, Lunsford LD, Fromm GH, Jannetta PJ 1994 The effect of single-application topical ophthalmic anesthesia in patients with trigeminal neuralgia. A randomized double-blind placebo-controlled trial. Journal of Neurosurgery 80(6): 993–997

Kondziolka D, Lunsford LD, Habeck M, Flickinger JC 1997 Gamma knife radiosurgery for trigeminal neuralgia. Neurosurgical Clinics of North America 8(1): 79–85

Kosrirukvongs P 1997 Topical piroxicam and conjunctivitis. Journal of the Medical Association of Thailand 80(5): 287–292

Kozyrskyj AL, Hildes-Ripstein GE, Longstaffe SEA, Wincott JL, Sitar DS, Klassen TP 1998 Antibiotics for acute otitis media: short vs 7–10 day course (protocol). Issue 2, Update Software. Cochrane Library, Oxford

Kurland LT 1958 Descriptive epidemiology of selected neurological and myopathic disorders with particular reference to a survey in Rochester, Minnesota. Journal of Chronic Diseases 8: 378–418

Lancaster T, Silagy C, Gray S 1995 Primary care management of acute herpes zoster: systematic review of evidence from randomized controlled trials. British Journal of General Practice 45(390): 39–45

Lechin F, Van der Dijs B, Lechin ME et al 1989 Pimozide therapy for trigeminal neuralgia. Archives of Neurology 46: 960–963

Lindbock M, Hjortdahl P, Johnsen UL 1996a Randomised, double blind, placebo controlled trial of penicillin V and amoxycillin in treatment of acute sinus infections in adults. British Medical Journal 313(7053): 325–329

Lindbock M, Hjortdahl P, Johnsen UL 1996b Use of symptoms, signs, and blood tests to diagnose acute sinus infections in primary care: comparison with computed tomography. Family Medicine 28(3): 183–188

Lindstrom P, Lindblom V 1987 The analgesic effect of tocainide in trigeminal neuralgia. Pain 28: 45–50

Lipton RB, Micieli G, Russell D, Solomon S, Tafelt-Hansen P, Waldenlind E 1995 Guidelines for controlled trials of drugs in cluster headache. Cephalalgia 15(6): 452–462

Low DE, Desrosiers M, McSherry J et al 1997 A practical guide for the diagnosis and treatment of acute sinusitis [see comments]. Canadian Medical Association Journal 156 (suppl 6): S1–14

Marbach JJ, Lund P 1981 Depression, anhedonia and anxiety in temporomandibular joint and other facial pain syndromes. Pain (11): 73–84

McQuay H, Carroll D, Jadad AR, Wiffen P, Moore A 1995 Anticonvulsant drugs for management of pain: a systematic review. British Medical Journal 311(7012): 1047–1052

Meaney JF, Eldridge PR, Dunn LT, Nixon TE, Whitehouse GH, Miles JB 1995 Demonstration of neurovascular compression in trigeminal neuralgia with magnetic resonance imaging. Comparison with surgical findings in 52 consecutive operative cases. Journal of Neurosurgery 83(5): 799–805

Melzack R, Terrence C, Fromm G, Amsel R 1986 Trigeminal neuralgia and atypical facial pain: use of the McGill Pain Questionnaire for discrimination and diagnosis. Pain 27(3): 297–302

Mitchell RG 1980 Pre-trigeminal neuralgia. British Dental Journal 149(6): 167–170

Morris GC, Gibson SJ, Helme RD 1995. Capsaicin-induced flare and vasodilation in patients with postherpetic neuralgia. Pain 63: 93–101

Munoz M, Dumas M, Boutros-Toni F et al 1988 [A neuro-epidemiologic survey in a Limousin town] [French]. Revue Neurologique (Paris) 144(4): 266–271

Murakami S, Hato N, Horiuchi J, Honda N, Gyo K, Yanagihara N 1997 Treatment of Ramsay Hunt syndrome with acyclovir-prednisone: significance of early diagnosis and treatment. Annals of Neurology 41(3): 353–357

Nicol CF 1969 A four year double-blind study of tegretol in facial pain. Headache 9(1): 54–57

Nicolodi M, Frezzotti R, Diadori A, Nuti A, Sicuteri F 1997 Phantom eye: features and prevalence. The predisposing role of headache. Cephalalgia 17(4): 501–504

Nurmikko TJ 1991 Altered cutaneous sensation in trigeminal neuralgia. Archives of Neurology 48(5): 523–527

Odabasi Z, Gokcil Z, Atilla S, Pabuscu Y, Vural O, Yardim M 1997 The value of MRI in a case of Tolosa–Hunt syndrome. Clinical Neurology and Neurosurgery 99(2): 151–154

Pareja JA, Sjaastad O 1997 SUNCT syndrome. A clinical review. Headache 37(4): 195–202

Pareja JA, Kruszewski P, Sjaastad O 1995 SUNCT syndrome: trials of drugs and anesthetic blockades. Headache 35(3): 138–142

Pareja JA, Kruszewski P, Sjaastad O 1997 SUNCT syndrome. Diagnosis morbi. Shortlasting Unilateral Neuralgiform headache attacks, with Conjunctival injection, Tearing and rhinorrhoea. Neurologia 12 (suppl 5): 66–72

Patterson J, Fetzer D, Krall J, Wright E, Heller M 1996 Eye patch treatment for the pain of corneal abrasion. Southern Medical Journal 89(2): 227–229

Rasmussen P 1990 Facial pain. II. A prospective survey of 1052 patients with a view of: character of the attacks, onset, course, and character of pain. Acta Neurochirurgica (Wien) 107(3–4): 121–128

Rasmussen P 1991 Facial pain. IV. A prospective study of 1052 patients with a view of: precipitating factors, associated symptoms, objective psychiatric and neurological symptoms. Acta Neurochirurgica (Wien) 108(3–4): 100–109

Resnick DK, Jannetta PJ, Bissonnette D, Jho HD, Lanzino G 1995 Microvascular decompression for glossopharyngeal neuralgia. Neurosurgery 36(1): 64–68; discussion 68–69

Rodriguez M, Siva A, Cross SA, O'Brien PC, Kurland LT 1995 Optic neuritis: a population-based study in Olmsted County, Minnesota [see comments]. Neurology 45(2): 244–250

Rosenfeld RM, Post JC 1992 Meta-analysis of antibiotics for the treatment of otitis media with effusion. Otolaryngology–Head and Neck Surgery 106(4): 378–386

Rosenfeld RM, Vertrees JE, Carr J et al 1994 Clinical efficacy of antimicrobial drugs for acute otitis media: metaanalysis of 5400 children from thirty-three randomized trials [see comments]. Journal of Pediatrics 124(3): 355–367

Rossetti L, Marchetti I, Orzalesi N, Scorpiglione N, Torri V, Liberati A 1993 Randomized clinical trials on medical treatment of glaucoma. Are they appropriate to guide clinical practice? [see comments]. Archives of Ophthalmology 111(1): 96–103

Rothman KJ, Beckman TM 1974 Epidemiological evidence for two types of trigeminal neuralgia. Lancet 1(845): 7–9

Rothman KJ, Monson RR 1973 Epidemiology of trigeminal neuralgia. Journal of Chronic Diseases 26(1): 3–12

Rothman KJ, Wepsic JG 1974 Site of facial pain in trigeminal neuralgia. Journal of Neurosurgery 40(4): 514–523

Rushton JG, Stevens JC, Miller RH 1981 Glossopharyngeal (vagoglossopharyngeal) neuralgia: a study of 217 cases. Archives of Neurology 38(4): 201–205

Stajcic Z, Juniper RP, Todorovic L 1990 Peripheral streptomycin/lidocaine injections versus lidocaine alone in the treatment of idiopathic trigeminal neuralgia. A double blind controlled trial. Journal of Craniomaxillofacial Surgery 18(6): 243–246

Szapiro J Jr, Sindou M, Szapiro J 1985 Prognostic factors in microvascular decompression for trigeminal neuralgia. Neurosurgery 17(6): 920–929

Tyring S, Barbarash RA, Nahlik JE et al 1995 Famciclovir for the treatment of acute herpes zoster: effects on acute disease and postherpetic neuralgia. A randomized, double-blind, placebo-controlled trial. Collaborative Famciclovir Herpes Zoster Study Group [see comments]. Annals of Internal Medicine 123(2): 89–96

Uhari M, Kontiokari T, Koskela M, Niemela M 1996 Xylitol chewing gum in prevention of acute otitis media: double blind randomised trial. British Medical Journal 313(7066): 1180–1184

Van Buchem FL, Knottnerus JA, Schrijnemaekers VJ, Peeters MF 1997 Primary-care-based randomised placebo-controlled trial of antibiotic treatment in acute maxillary sinusitis. Lancet 349(9053): 683–687

Varonen H, Makela M 1998 Ultasonography, radiography and clinical examination in the diagnosis of acute maxillary sinusitis in primary health care. Update Software. Cochrane Library, Oxford

Vilming ST, Lyberg T, Latase X 1986 Tizanidine in the management of trigeminal neuralgia. Cephalalgia 6: 181–182

Volminck J, Lancaster T, Gray S, Silagy C 1996 Treatments for postherpetic neuralgia–a systematic review of randomized controlled trials. Family Practice 13(1): 84–91

Watson PG, McKay DA, Clemett RS, Wilkinson P 1973 Treatment of episcleritis. A double-blind trial comparing betamethasone 0.1 per cent, oxyphenbutazone 10 per cent, and placebo eye ointments. British Journal of Ophthalmology 57(11): 866–870

Wayman DM, Pham HN, Byl FM, Adour KK 1990 Audiological manifestations of Ramsay Hunt syndrome. Journal of Laryngology and Otology 104(2): 104–108

Williams JW Jr, Holleman DR Jr, Samsa GP, Simel DL 1995 Randomized controlled trial of 3 vs 10 days of trimethoprim/sulfamethoxazole for acute maxillary sinusitis [see comments]. Journal of the American Medical Association 273(13): 1015–1021

Yang J, Simonson TM, Ruprecht A, Meng D, Vincent SD, Yuh WT 1996 Magnetic resonance imaging used to assess patients with trigeminal neuralgia. Oral Surgery, Oral Medicine, Oral Pathology, Oral Radiology, Endodopathy 81(3): 343–350

Yousem DM, Atlas SW, Grossman RI, Sergott RC, Savino PJ, Bosley TM 1990 MR imaging of Tolosa-Hunt syndrome. American Journal of Roentgenology 154(1): 167–170

Zakrzewska JM 1995 Trigeminal neuralgia. WB Saunders, London

Zakrzewska JM, Thomas DG 1993 Patient's assessment of outcome after three surgical procedures for the management of trigeminal neuralgia. Acta Neurochirurgica (Wien) 122(3–4): 225–230

Zakrzewska JM, Chaudhry Z, Nurmikko TJ, Patton DW, Mullens EL 1997 Lamotrigine (Lamicatal) in refractory trigeminal neuralgia: results from a double blind placebo controlled crossover trial. Pain 73: 223–230

Zakrzewska JM, Sawsan J, Bulman JS (1999). A prospective, longitudinal study on patients with trigeminal neuralgia who underwent radiofrequency thermocoagulation of the Gasserian ganglion Pain 79: 51–58

Headache

JEAN SCHOENEN & PETER S. SÁNDOR

INTRODUCTION

Headache is the most common pain syndrome. It is also the most frequent symptom in neurology where it may be a disease in itself or indicate an underlying local or systemic disease. Many excellent textbooks on headache have been published in recent years (see bibliography). We felt therefore that a comprehensive synthesis would be more useful to the reader than detailed descriptions of the various headache types. We decided to follow the headache classification of the International Headache Society (IHS 1988) although it is about to be revised. This classification system has indeed been validated in many countries and it has proven useful for clinical and research purposes. It has been taken over by the International Classification of Diseases, 10th revision (ICD-10-Neurological Adaptation; Cephalalgia 1997, 17: Suppl.19) and the new version will probably not contain fundamental changes. For each of the most common types of headache, this chapter will summarize present knowledge on diagnosis, epidemiology, pathogenesis and therapy.

Most of the brain parenchyma itself is insensitive to pain. Nociceptive input can be generated from cranial sinuses and veins, proximal parts of cerebral arteries, dura mater mainly in the vicinity of the large vessels, cranial nerves and upper cervical roots, as well as from extracranial structures. Headache must be due to excessive nociceptive input from these intra- or extracranial sites, a disturbed central control of these inputs or a combination of both. If one applies to the brain and its envelopes the scenario for pain generators as proposed for other viscera (Cervero & Jänig 1992), peripheral and central sensitization including activation of 'silent nociceptors' would allow small-calibre trigeminovascular afferents, some of which play a role in physiological vasoregulation, to produce long-lasting, so-called vascular headaches. Activation of high-threshold mechanoceptors would be responsible for brief, stabbing headaches (Fig. 33.1).

Many classifications of headache have been proposed. One can schematically distinguish primary and secondary headaches. Primary (or idiopathic) headaches are autonomous diseases or syndromes, in which there is a transient or permanent functional disorder without a structural lesion. These are by far the most frequent headache types, comprising migraine, tension headache and cluster headache. Secondary (or symptomatic) headaches are due to a local organic lesion or to a systemic disease. In several headache types, however, such a simplistic distinction is not applicable.

The IHS headache classification is hierarchically constructed and based on operational diagnostic criteria for all headache disorders. The hierarchical system coding with up to four digits makes it possible to use the classification at different levels of sophistication. Table 33.1 represents the headings of the various headache groups and subgroups. Codes 1–4 comprise most of the so-called primary headaches. Although this classification grades headaches and not patients, it represents a major advance in headache research because it offers a common denominator, allowing for better comparison of clinical data between centres. Because of space limitations, we will cover only the primary and the most frequent secondary headaches, leaving aside some very common but generally obvious causes of pain in head or face, such as systemic infections (code 9), metabolic disorders (code 10), eye disorders (code 11.3) or nose and sinus diseases (code 11.5).

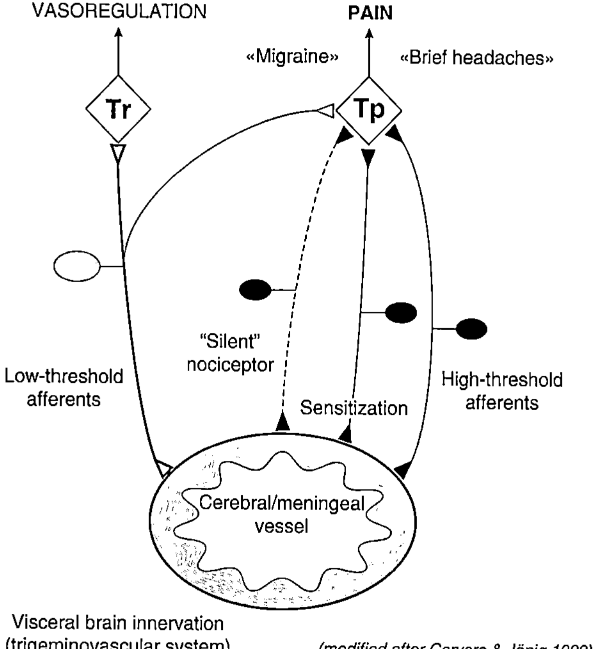

Fig. 33.1 Cervero and Jänig's (1992) proposal of functional roles for the different types of visceral sensory receptors applied to the 'trigeminovascular' system of the brain. The brain's trigeminal visceral afferents are supposed to activate two central neuronal systems, one (Tr) responsible for regulatory vasomotor reflexes via low-threshold afferents and the other (Tp) for the triggering of brief pain via high-threshold afferents and of prolonged pain such as migraine via the latter and 'silent' nociceptors. High-threshold receptors probably dominate in the brain as, like the biliary system or the ureter, it has no visceral sensory experience but pain. They may be activated by transient high-intensity stimuli, which may lead to acute, brief pain such as 'idiopathic stabbing headache', cough, exertional or ice cream headache. More prolonged forms of visceral stimulations, including those leading to hypoxia and inflammation of the tissue, result in the sensitization of high-threshold receptors and the bringing into play of previously unresponsive 'silent' nociceptors, which evokes more persistent pain, such as the migraine headache. Tr = central trigeminal neurons responsible for vasoregulation; Tp = central trigeminal nociceptor responsible for pain transmission.

1. MIGRAINE

DIAGNOSIS AND CLINICAL FEATURES

Migraine is a multifaceted disorder, of which the head pain is only one component. It is an autonomous disease, but in some instances it may occur for the first time in close temporal relation to one of the disorders listed in groups 5–11 of Table 33.1, e.g. to head trauma (Weiss et al 1991, Solomon & Newman 1998). Migraine is a paroxysmal disorder characterized by attacks which are separated by symptom-free intervals. As with epilepsy, it is the repetition of attacks that characterizes the disorder and not a single attack which may occur in many individuals under certain circumstances.

Table 33.1 Classification and Diagnostic Criteria for Headache Disorders, Cranial Neuralgias and Facial Pain (Cephalalgia 1988) (*& ICD-10 codes*)

1. Migraine *(G43)*
- 1.1 Migraine without aura (*G43.0*)
- 1.2 Migraine with aura (*G43.1*)
  - 1.2.1 Migraine with typical aura (*G43.10*)
  - 1.2.2 Migraine with prolonged aura (*G43.11*)
  - 1.2.3 Familial hemiplegic migraine *(G43.1x5)*
  - 1.2.4 Basilar migraine *(G43.1x3)*
  - 1.2.5 Migraine aura without headache *(G43.1x4)*
  - 1.2.6 Migraine with acute onset aura *(G43.12)*
- 1.3 Ophthalmoplegic migraine *(G43.80)*
- 1.4 Retinal migraine *(G43.81)*
- 1.5 Childhood periodic syndromes that may be precursors to or associated with migraine *(G43.82)*
  - 1.5.1 Benign paroxysmal vertigo of childhood *(G43.821)*
  - 1.5.2 Alternating hemiplegia of childhood *(G43.822)*
- 1.6 Complications of migraine
  - 1.6.1 Status migrainosus *(G43.2)*
  - 1.6.2 Migrainous infarction *(G43.3)*
- 1.7 Migrainous disorder not fulfilling above criteria *(G43.83)*

2. Tension-type headache *(G44.2)*
- 2.1 Episodic tension-type headache
  - 2.1.1 Episodic tension-type headache associated with disorder of pericranial muscles *(G44.20)*
  - 2.1.2 Episodic tension-type headache unassociated with disorder of pericranial muscles *(G44.21)*
- 2.2 Chronic tension-type headache
  - 2.2.1 Chronic tension-type headache associated with disorder of pericranial muscles *(G44.22)*
  - 2.2.2 Chronic tension-type headache unassociated with disorder of pericranial muscles *(G44.23)*
- 2.3 Headache of the tension-type not fulfilling above criteria *(G44.28)*

3. Cluster headache and chronic paroxysmal hemicrania
- 3.1 Cluster headache *(G44.0)*
  - 3.1.1 Cluster headache periodicity undetermined *(G44.00)*
  - 3.1.2 Episodic cluster headache *(G44.01)*
  - 3.1.3 Chronic cluster headache *(G44.02)*
    - 3.1.3.1 Unremitting from onset *(G44.020)*
    - 3.1.3.2 Evolved from episodic *(G44.021)*
- 3.2 Chronic paroxysmal hemicrania *(G44.03)*
- 3.3 Cluster headache-like disorder not fulfilling above criteria *(G44.08)*

4. Miscellaneous headaches unassociated with structural lesion *(G44.8)*
- 4.1 Idiopathic stabbing headache *(G44.800)*
- 4.2 External compression headache *(G44.801)*
- 4.3 Cold stimulus headache *(G44.802)*
  - 4.3.1 External application of a cold stimulus *(G44.8020)*
  - 4.3.2 ngestion of a cold stimulus *(G44.8021)*
- 4.4 Benign cough headache *(G44.803)*
- 4.5 Benign exertional headache *(G44.804)*
- 4.6 Headache associated with sexual activity *(G44.805)*
  - 4.6.1 Dull type *(G44.8050)*
  - 4.6.2 Explosive type *(G44.8051)*
  - 4.6.3 Postural type *(G44.8052)*

Table 33.1 (Contd.)

5. Headache associated with head trauma
- 5.1 Acute post-traumatic headache *(G44.880)*
  - 5.1.1 With significant head trauma and/or confirmatory signs *(S06)*
  - 5.1.2 With minor head trauma and no confirmatory signs *(S09.9)*
- 5.2 Chronic post-traumatic headache (G44.3)
  - 5.2.1 With significant head trauma and/or confirmatory signs *(G44.30)*
  - 5.2.2 With minor head trauma and no confirmatory signs *(G44.31)*

6. Headache associated with vascular disorders *(G44.81)*
- 6.1 Acute ischaemic cerebrovascular disease
  - 6.1.1 Transient ischaemic attack (TIA)
  - 6.1.2 Thromboembolic stroke
- 6.2 Intracranial haematoma
  - 6.2.1 Intracerebral haematoma
  - 6.2.2 Subdural haematoma
  - 6.2.3 Epidural haematoma
- 6.3 Subarachnoid haemorrhage
- 6.4 Unruptured vascular malformation
  - 6.4.1 Arteriovenous malformation
  - 6.4.2 Saccular aneurysm
- 6.5 Arteritis
  - 6.5.1 Giant cell arteritis
  - 6.5.2 Other systemic arteritides
  - 6.5.3 Primary intracranial arteritis
- 6.6 Carotid or vertebral artery pain
  - 6.6.1 Carotid or vertebral dissection
  - 6.6.2 Carotidynia (idiopathic)
  - 6.6.3 Postendarterectomy headache
- 6.7 Venous thrombosis
- 6.8 Arterial hypertension
  - 6.8.1 Acute pressor response to exogenous agent
  - 6.8.2 Phaeochromocytoma
  - 6.8.3 Malignant (accelerated) hypertension
  - 6.8.4 Pre-eclampsia and eclampsia
- 6.9 Headache associated with other vascular disorder

7. Headache associated with non-vascular intracranial disorder *(G44.82)*
- 7.1 High cerebrospinal fluid pressure
  - 7.1.1 Benign intracranial hypertension
  - 7.1.2 High pressure hydrocephalus
- 7.2 Low cerebrospinal fluid pressure
  - 7.2.1 Postlumbar puncture headache
  - 7.2.2 Cerebrospinal fluid fistula headache
- 7.3 Intracranial infection
- 7.4 Intracranial sarcoidosis and other non-infectious inflammatory diseases
- 7.5 Headache related to intrathecal injections
  - 7.5.1 Direct effect
  - 7.5.2 Due to chemical meningitis
- 7.6 Intracranial neoplasm
- 7.7 Headache associated with other intracranial disorder

8. Headache associated with substances or their withdrawal *(G44.4)*
- 8.1 Headache induced by acute substance use or exposure *(G44.40)*
  - 8.1.1 Nitrate/nitrite-induced headache

Table 33.1 (Contd.)

8. Headache associated with substances or their withdrawal *(G44.4)* (Contd.)
  - 8.1.2 Monosodium glutamate-induced headache
  - 8.1.3 Carbon monoxide-induced headache
  - 8.1.4 Alcohol-induced headache
  - 8.1.5 Other substances
- 8.2 Headache induced by chronic substance use or exposure *(G44.41)*
  - 8.2.1 Ergotamine-induced headache
  - 8.2.2 Analgesics abuse headache
  - 8.2.3 Other substances
- 8.3 Headache from substance withdrawal (acute use)
  - 8.3.1 Alcohol withdrawal headache (hangover)
  - 8.3.2 Other substances
- 8.4 Headache from substance withdrawal (chronic use)
  - 8.4.1 Ergotamine withdrawal headache
  - 8.4.2 Caffeine withdrawal headache
  - 8.4.3 Narcotics abstinence headache
  - 8.4.4 Other substances
- 8.5 Headache associated with substances but with uncertain mechanism
  - 8.5.1 Birth control pills or oestrogens
  - 8.5.2 Other substances

9. Headache associated with non-cephalic infection *(G44.881)*
- 9.1 Viral infection
  - 9.1.1 Focal non-cephalic
  - 9.1.2 Systemic
- 9.2 Bacterial infection
  - 9.2.1 Focal non-cephalic
  - 9.2.2 Systemic (septicaemia)
- 9.3 Headache related to other infection

10. Headache associated with metabolic disorder *(G44.882)*
- 10.1 Hypoxia
  - 10.1.1 High-altitude headache
  - 10.1.2 Hypoxic headache
  - 10.1.3 Sleep apnoea headache
- 10.2 Hypercapnia
- 10.3 Mixed hypoxia and hypercapnia
- 10.4 Hypoglycaemia
- 10.5 Dialysis
- 10.6 Headache related to other metabolic abnormality

11. Headache or facial pain associated with disorder of cranium, neck, eyes, ears, nose, sinuses, teeth, mouth or other facial or cranial structures *(G44.84)*
- 11.1 Cranial bone *(G44.840)*
- 11.2 Neck
  - 11.2.1 Cervical spine *(G44.841)*
  - 11.2.2 Retropharyngeal tendinitis *(G44.842)*
- 11.3 Eyes *(G44.843)*
  - 11.3.1 Acute glaucoma
  - 11.3.2 Refractive errors
  - 11.3.3 Heterophoria or heterotropia
- 11.4 Ears *(G44.844)*
- 11.5 Nose and sinuses *(G44.845)*
  - 11.5.1 Acute sinus headache
  - 11.5.2 Other diseases of nose or sinuses
- 11.6 Teeth, jaws and related structures *(G44.846)*

Table 33.1 (Contd.)

11. Headache or facial pain associated with disorder of cranium, neck, eyes, ears, nose, sinuses, teeth, mouth or other facial or cranial structures *(G44.84) (Contd.)*

- 11.7 Temporomandibular joint disease

12. Cranial neuralgias, nerve trunk pain and deafferentation pain

- 12.1 Persistent (in contrast to tic-like) pain of cranial nerve origin *(G44.848)*
  - 12.1.1 Compression or distortion of cranial nerves and second or third cervical roots
  - 12.1.2 Demyelinization of cranial nerves
    - 12.1.2.1 Optic neuritis (retrobulbar neuritis)
  - 12.1.3 Infarction of cranial nerves
    - 12.1.3.1 Diabetic neuritis
  - 12.1.4 Inflammation of cranial nerves
    - 12.1.4.1 Herpes zoster
    - 12.1.4.2 Chronic postherpetic neuralgia *(G53.00)*
  - 12.1.5 Tolosa–Hunt syndrome *(G44.850)*
  - 12.1.6 Neck–tongue syndrome
  - 12.1.7 Other causes of pesistent pain of cranial nerve origin
- 12.2. Trigeminal neuralgia *(G50.0)*
  - 12.2.1 Idiopathic trigeminal neuralgia *(G50.00)*
  - 12.2.2 Symptomatic trigeminal neuralgia *(G50.09)*
    - 12.2.2.1 Compression of trigeminal root or ganglion
    - 12.2.2.2 Central lesions
- 12.3 Glossopharyngeal neuralgia *(G52.1)*
  - 12.3.1 Idiopathic glossopharyngeal neuralgia
  - 12.3.2 Symptomatic glossopharyngeal neuralgia
- 12.4 Nervus intermedius neuralgia *(G51.80)*
- 12.5 Superior laryngeal neuralgia *(G52.20)*
- 12.6 Occipital neuralgia *(G52.80)*
- 12.7 Central causes of head and facial pain other than tic douloureux
  - 12.7.1 Anaesthesia dolorosa *(G97.8)*
  - 12.7.2 Thalamic pain *(G46.21)*
- 12.8 Facial pain not fulfilling criteria in groups 11 or 12

13. Headache non-classifiable

In 10–15% of patients, premonitory symptoms (or prodromes) may precede the migraine attack by hours or by a day or two (Blau 1980). These consist of symptoms which are unspecific but often reproducible in a given patient, such as sudden mood changes, repetitive yawning or craving for special foods. At the other end of the spectrum, the migraine attack can be followed by so-called 'postsyndromes', such as fatigue. The clinical diagnosis of migraine is based on the repetition and characteristics of the attack.

The diagnostic criteria for *migraine without aura* (code 1.1) (formerly common migraine) are illustrated in Table 33.2. In *migraine with aura* (code 1.2), the headache phase is immediately preceded by focal neurological symptoms (Table 33.3). Visual disturbances are the most common aura symptoms, occurring in 90% of patients. Aura symptoms of sensory, motor or speech disturbances seldom occur without pre-existing visual symptoms (Rasmussen & Olesen 1992).

Table 33.2 Migraine without aura (MO) (Code 1.1): diagnostic criteria

A) n ≥ 5

B) 4 - 72 h

C) 2/4
1. /
2.
3. ++ / +++
4.

D) 1/2
1. +
2. /

E) normal

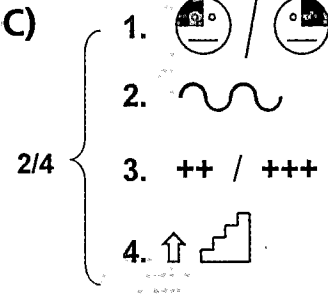

- A – at least 5 attacks fulfilling B–D
- B – headache attacks lasting 4–72h (untreated or unsuccessfully treated)
- C – headache has at least 2 of the 4 following characteristics:
  1. unilateral location
  2. pulsating quality
  3. moderate or severe intensity (inhibits or prohibits daily activities
  4. aggravated by walking stairs or similar routine physical activity
- D – during headache at least 1 of the 2 following symptoms occur:
  1. phonophobia and photophobia
  2. nausea and/or vomiting
- E – at least 1 of the following 3 characteristics is present:
  1. history and physical and neurological examinations do not suggest 1 of the disorders listed in groups 5–11 (please see table 33.1)
  2. history and/or physical and/or neurological examinations do suggest such a disorder, but it is ruled out by appropriate investigations
  3. such a disorder is present, but migraine attacks do not occur for the first time in close temporal relation to the disorder

Table 33.3. Migrane with aura (MA) (Code 1.2): diagnostic criteria

A) $n \geq 2$

B) 3/4

1. / +

2. 4 min /

3. 60 min

4. 60 min

C) normal

A. at least 2 attacks fulfilling B
B. headache has at least three of the following four characteristics:
 1. one or more fully reversible aura symptoms indicating focal cerebral cortical and/or brain stem functions.
 2. at least one aura symptom develops gradually over more than 4 min, or two or more symptoms occur in succession.
 3. no aura symptom lasts more than 60 min; if more than one aura symptom is present, accepted duration is proportionally increased.
 4. headache follows aura with free interval of <60 min (it may also simultaneously begin with the aura.
C. at least one of the following three characteristics is present:
 1. history, physical and neurological examinations do not suggest one of the disorders listed in groups 5–11 (please see IHS classification and diagnostic criteria)
 2. history and/or physical and/or neurological examinations do suggest such a disorder, but it is ruled out by appropriate investigations.
 3. such a disorder is present, but migrane attacks do not occur for the first time in close temporal relation to the disorder.

Migrainous aura symptoms can be distinguished from those produced by a seizure or by a transient ischaemic attack (TIA) by their progressive onset, march over time and quality (Table 33.4).

In *migraine with prolonged aura* (code 1.2.2), all the criteria for migraine with typical aura (code 1.2.1) are fulfilled but at least one symptom lasts more than 60 minutes and less than a week. Compared to migraine without aura, migraine with aura is characterized on average by headache of lower intensity and shorter duration. The headache may even be completely absent (code 1.2.5). Many patients have attacks of both migraine with and migraine without aura. In so-called 'early morning' migraine, it is impossible to ascertain whether the attack was preceded by an aura or not.

Table 33.4 Differential diagnosis of focal paroxysmal neurological symptoms

	TIA	*Epilepsy*	*Migraine*
Onset	Sudden	Sudden	Progressive
Progression rate	None	Fast	Slow
Different symptoms	Simultaneous	In succession	In succession
Type of symptoms if visual	Negative	Positive coloured	Negative/ positive b&w, grey
Territory	Vascular	Cortical	Cortical
Duration	Short (10–15 min)	Short (min)	Longer (1/2–1 h)

In *basilar migraine* (code 1.2.4) two or more aura symptoms are of the following types: visual symptoms in both the temporal and nasal fields of both eyes, dysarthria, vertigo, tinnitus, decreased hearing, double vision, ataxia, bilateral paraesthesias, bilateral pareses, decreased level of consciousness. The differential diagnosis between *migraine with acute onset aura* (code 1.2.6) and thromboembolic transient ischaemic attacks may be difficult.

Familial hemiplegic migraine (FHM) is a rare subtype of migraine characterized by the occurrence during the aura phase of hemiparesis/-plegia with a varying duration from minutes to days, by an autosomal dominant transmission and onset before age 20. In some families the migraine may be associated with cerebellar ataxia. FHM has attracted much interest in recent years because of the finding of a mutation in a chromosome 19 gene coding for the $\alpha 1$ subunit of a voltage dependent P/Q calcium channel (see Pathophysiology) in some families.

In children below the age of 12 years, migraine attacks often last less than 4 hours and the duration criterion of Table 33.2 does not apply. Associated symptoms may be unremarkable in certain children affected with migraine in which case the differential diagnosis with tension-type headache may be difficult. Sometimes GI symptoms are at the forefront of the attack symptomatology. It is possible that *childhood periodic syndromes* (code 1.5), such as cyclical vomiting, abdominal pains or benign vertigo, are precursors of adult migraine and of similar pathophysiology. It has been reported in some studies that childhood somnambulism is frequently found in the history of adult migraineurs (Pradalier et al 1987).

The two major complications of migraine are *status migrainosus* (code 1.6.1) and *migrainous infarction* (code 1.6.2). In the former the headache lasts more than 72 hours without interruption, despite treatment, or headache-free intervals do not exceed 4 hours. To qualify for migrainous infarction, a neurological deficit has to occur during a migraine attack that is typical of those previously experienced by a patient, to last more than 7 days and/or to be associated with ischaemic infarction in the relevant area on neuroimaging techniques. Most importantly, other causes of infarction have to be ruled out by appropriate investigations (Welch & Levine 1990).

EPIDEMIOLOGY

The results of epidemiological studies performed in various countries are remarkably consistent. The prevalence of migraine is around 15% whatever the study design: 15% in a cross-sectional epidemiological survey of the Danish population aged between 25 and 64 years and diagnosed following a structured interview as well as a neurological examination (Rasmussen et al 1991); 12% in a nationwide survey performed by mailed questionnaire in a representative sample of French residents aged 15 years or older (Henry et al 1992); and 23.3% in a study using a self-administered questionnaire sent to a sample of 15 000 US households (Stewart et al 1992). In Third World countries, prevalence of migraine is similar to that found in Western Europe and North America. Migraine therefore presents with a uniform worldwide distribution. Up to now, the only exception to this seems to be China where a lower prevalence of 8% was reported (Wang et al 1997).

Migraine without aura is almost twice as frequent as migraine with aura in population-based studies. In many patients both types of attack may coexist. Female preponderance is a characteristic feature of migraine, but also of other primary headaches. Male: female ratios vary between studies. Boys and girls are affected in the same proportions (Bille 1962, Chu & Shinnar 1991), while from age 16, migraine is 2–3 times more frequent in females than in males, suggesting that migraine attacks may disappear in boys after puberty. Females around age 40 have the highest prevalence (±25%). Onset of migraine is nearly always below age 50 with peak incidences at age 10–12 for males and at age 14–16 for females (Abu-Arefeh et al 1994, Stewart et al 1994b).

About 50% of migraineurs have less than two attacks per month, the median attack frequency being 1.5 per month. At least 10% of patients have weekly attacks (Stewart et al 1994a); 5% of the general population have at least 18 migraine days per year and 1% at least one day per week (Ferrari 1998). The annual cost of migraine-related productivity loss is therefore enormous (Lipton et al 1994).

The most common precipitating (or trigger) factors of attacks are mental stress, menstruation and alcohol (Amery and Vandenbergh 1987). It remains controversial whether other dietary factors can consistently precipitate attacks in certain patients. The majority of female migraineurs report occurrence of attacks in the perimenstrual period. In less than 10%, however, attacks occur exclusively at this stage of the ovarian cycle and this corresponds to 'menstrual migraine' (MacGregor et al 1990).

Comorbidity of migraine was shown with psychiatric disorders such as anxiety and panic disorders, depression and bipolar disorder (Breslau et al 1996). The comorbidity of migraine and epilepsy is weak and controversial (Ottman & Lipton 1994). In young females only, migraine is a risk factor for ischaemic stroke (Tzourio et al 1995).

PATHOPHYSIOLOGY

In recent years the general consensus has emerged that in migraine both neuronal and vascular components are relevant and most probably inter-related (Lance et al 1983, Welch 1987, Olesen 1991, Ferrari 1991).

Migraine aura

Wolff's theory that the aura is caused by vasoconstriction and the headache by vasodilatation has not been confirmed by modern blood flow studies during migraine attacks. In the early phase of the attack a focal hypoperfusion can indeed be recorded over the cortical area which is responsible for the aura symptoms, but it may precede and outlast the latter and it spreads from posterior to more anterior parts of the hemisphere, halted by anatomical rather than vascular boundaries. In the later stages of the attack, cerebral hyperperfusion may appear but this is not chronologically related to the headache (Olesen et al 1990, Olesen 1992).

There is indirect evidence that the migraine aura is the clinical manifestation of cortical spreading depression rather than of ischaemia (Lauritzen 1992). The clinical aura symptoms progress at a pace (Lashley 1941, Milner 1958) similar to that of the wave of cortical spreading depression in the animal brain (Leão 1944, Leão & Morrison 1945) and of the spreading oligaemia observed during migraine with aura (Olesen et al 1981). A recent study using functional perfusion-weighted magnetic resonance imaging during the aura also favours a depression of neuronal activity with secondary flow changes rather than ischaemia (Cutrer et al 1998). Spreading depression, however, although easily elicited in animals, has been recorded only in the hippocampus and caudate nucleus of man (Bures et al 1974). It remains to be demonstrated whether the DC shifts and activity reductions observed with magneto-electroencephalography (Barkley et al 1990) may be related to the phenomenon of cortical spreading depression.

In migraine without aura normal cerebral blood flow was reported by some investigators (Olesen 1992), diffuse or focal hyperperfusion not related to headache intensity or localization by others (Bès & Fabre 1992). Unilateral reductions of EEG activity, however, have been reported with quantified methods during attacks of migraine without aura (Schoenen et al 1987a) and more recently anteroposterior spreading oligaemia was found during a positron emission tomography (PET) study with visual activation in a patient who developed an attack of migraine apparently without aura (Woods et al 1994).

Spreading depression is not specific to migraine. In animals it can be triggered by ionic shifts (high K^+), ischaemia or mechanical stimuli. As brain K^+ is buffered by glial cells, the visual cortex may be prone to spreading depression because of its low ratio of glial to neuronal cells.

The trigeminovascular system

Experimental studies in animals suggest that the trigeminovascular system is the final common pathway where the migraine headache is generated (Moskowitz 1984). Activation of trigeminal afferent fibres arising from the ophthalmic division and surrounding the proximal parts of large cerebral vessels, pial vessels, large venous sinuses and dura mater produces local release of neuropeptides, leading to plasma extravasation (substance P, neurokinin A) and vasodilatation (CGRP). The latter are accompanied by platelet as well as mast cell activation and may favour sensitization of high-threshold afferents (Strassman et al 1996) (see Fig. 33.1) and produce a visceral nociceptive input which is relayed in the nucleus trigeminus caudalis and reaches the thalamus via the quintothalamic tract. Pain, though of visceral origin and therefore not strictly localized, is referred to the somatic territory of the first division of the trigeminal nerve and the superior cervical roots because of convergence of visceral and somatic afferents in the brainstem. The elevation of neuropeptides such as calcitonin gene-related peptide (CGRP) in the external jugular vein blood during migraine attacks (Goadsby et al 1989), which is also found in cluster headache, could support the trigeminovascular theory. Via the superior salivary nucleus, the greater superficial petrosal nerve and the pterygopalatine ganglion trigeminal afferents can activate parasympathetic fibres which participate in the innervation of cerebral and dural vessels and corelease acetylcholine and VIP (Goadsby 1997) (Fig. 33.2).

Drugs that are highly effective in treating migraine (and cluster headache) attacks, such as ergot alkaloids or selective $5HT_{1B/1D}$ agonists ('triptans'), can block the dural neurogenic plasma extravasation produced in the rat by electrical stimulation of the trigeminal ganglion, but this effect does not necessarily predict antimigraine efficacy (Goadsby 1997). These drugs may exert their therapeutic action at at least three sites: at $5HT_{1D}$ receptors, located presynaptically on perivascular trigeminal fibres and inhibiting peptide release, as suggested by animal experiments (Moskowitz 1991, Buzzi & Moskowitz 1992) and some clinical data (Goadsby et al 1990); at $5HT_{1D}$ receptors located centrally in the trigeminocervical system and inhibiting glutamate release (Goadsby & Hoskin 1996, Longmore et al 1997); or at vascular $5HT_{1B}$ receptors constricting cerebral/dural vessels, as suggested by pharmacology (Humphrey 1991) and some human studies using transcranial Doppler (Friberg et al 1991, Caekebeke et al 1992). Their precise mechanism of action remains to be determined, including whether their effect on other receptor subtypes such as $5HT_{1F}$ is relevant in migraine.

It must be pointed out that the trigeminovascular system is the major pain-signalling system of the visceral organ brain and the final common pathway for disorders other than migraine, such as the headaches of meningitis, vasculitis, arteriovenous malformation, ischaemic cerebrovascular disease, subarachnoid haemorrhage and post-traumatic vascular headaches. Experimental cortical spreading depression is able to activate the trigeminovascular system (Moskowitz & MacFarlane 1993).

Role of NO and 5HT

Nitric oxide (NO) may play a pivotal role in activation of the trigeminovascular system and hence in the migraine headache. Nitroglycerine, an NO donor, is a well-known trigger of migraine attacks and compared with healthy controls, migraineurs who received placebo-controlled intravenous infusions of nitroglycerine showed greater dilatation of the middle cerebral artery and were more likely to develop migraine-like headaches (without aura) (Olesen et al 1993). The migraine attack only appeared an average of 6 hours after the infusion, suggesting that an intermediate pathway has to be activated first. Activation of $5HT_{2B}$ receptors located on the endothelium of cerebral and

The trigeminovascular system and possible sites of action of antimigraine drugs

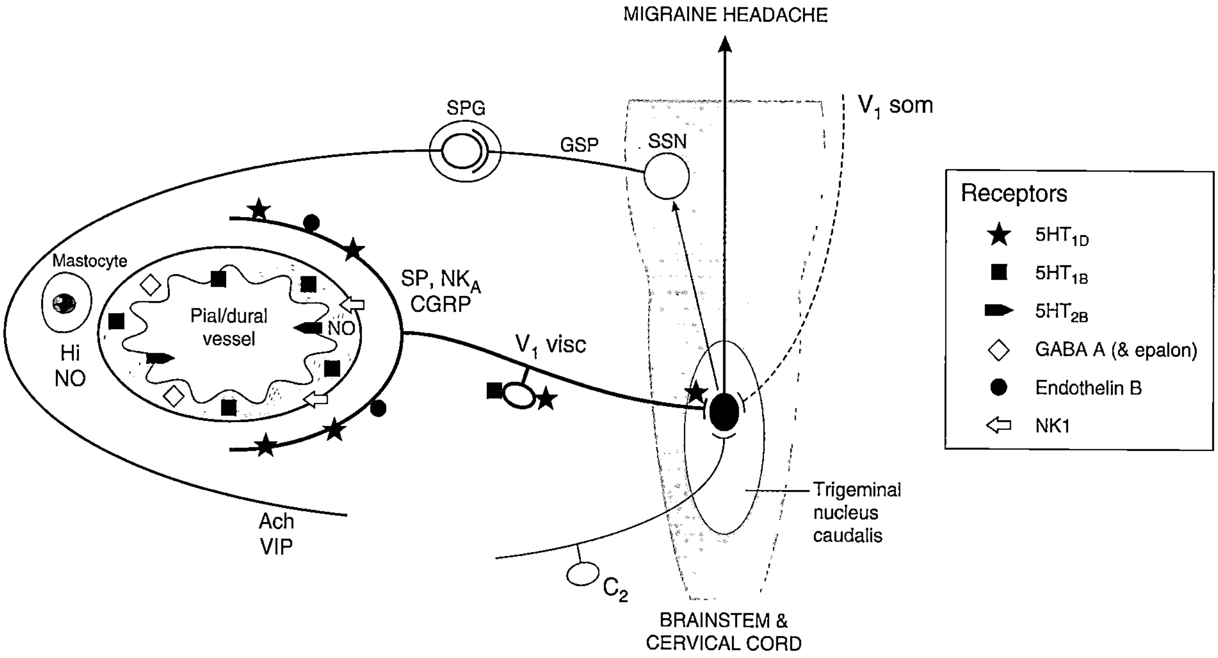

Fig. 33.2 Schematic view of the visceral arm of the trigeminovascular system showing the localization of various neurotransmitters and receptors supposedly acting in the generation of migraine headache and targeted by currently available acute antimigraine drugs. Note the connexion with the parasympathetic system and with the C2 upper cervical root. SSN = Superior solitary nucleus: GSP = Greater superficial Petrosol nerve; SPG = Sphenopalatine ganglion.

meningeal vessels (see Fig. 33.2) is able to promote NO release and vasodilatation. Whether this plays a role in migraine remains to be determined.

Various modifications of neurotransmitters (Ferrari 1992) or platelets (Ollat & Gurruchaga 1992) in the peripheral blood have been described in migraine between and during attacks. It is still not clear whether these peripheral changes contribute to the pathophysiology of migraine or are just an epiphenomenon of the central migrainous process. Migraine patients have a low systemic turnover of 5HT between attacks and an ictal 5HT release from platelets with rise of plasma levels, the latter probably presenting a self-defence mechanism (Ferrari 1992). Earlier anecdotal reports that parenteral administrations of 5HT were able to abort migraine attacks at the expense of severe side effects inspired the development of a selective $5HT_1$ agonist to treat acute migraine more safely (Humphrey & Feniuk 1991).

Role of the brainstem

Besides the above-mentioned $5HT_{1D}$ receptors in the nucleus trigeminus caudalis able to decrease activation of second-order nociceptors, the brainstem has recently received attention in migraine for another reason. During attacks, PET has identified an area of increased blood flow in the dorsolateral part of the brainstem opposite to the hemicrania (Weiller et al 1995). Since this persisted after pain relief with sumatriptan, while activation of cortical areas associated with pain perception had disappeared, it was hypothesized that a 'migraine generator' could exist in the region of the dorsal raphe nucleus, locus coeruleus and periaqueductal grey which would not be influenced by symptomatic acute antimigraine drugs (Ferrari 1998). With present neuroanatomical knowledge, however, it is difficult to conceive how a contralateral 'generator' would be able to activate the trigeminovascular system on the side of the headache, although it may modulate pain transmission upstream. The brainstem area may thus more likely be a 'migraine modulator or reliever', i.e. a neuronal population instrumental in terminating the attack during its natural course. The fact that the same brainstem areas play a role in central pain modulation as well as in sleep, which is the most efficient natural reliever of a migraine attack, is of relevance to such an interpretation.

Interictal abnormalities of the migrainous brain

During the headache-free interval, an abnormal functioning of the migrainous brain can be demonstrated by neurophysiological and metabolic studies. Neurophysiological methods show that cortical information processing in migraineurs is characterized by a deficient habituation during repetition of the stimulation (Schoenen 1998b). This has been demonstrated for event-related (Maertens de Noordout et al 1986, Kropp & Gerber 1993, Wang & Schoenen 1998) and visual evoked potentials (Schoenen et al 1995, Afra et al 1998a) (Fig. 33.3).

Moreover, intensity dependence of auditory evoked cortical potentials is increased in migraine with or without aura patients compared with normal controls (Wang et al 1996). The cortical abnormality is likely to be due to dysfunctioning monoaminergic subcorticocortical pathways which are known to 'set the tone' for sensory cortices. For instance, low activity in the raphe-cortical serotonergic pathway would reduce cortical preactivation levels, increasing activation thresholds but allowing a wider range for suprathreshold cortical activation and thus enhancing intensity dependence (Hegerl & Juckel 1993). In concordance with this hypothesis, increased thresholds for electromagnetic activation of visual and motor cortices were found interictally in migraine with aura (Afra et al 1998a). During and up to 24 hours before an attack, there is a dramatic change in cortical excitability with quasi-normalization of event-related (Kropp & Gerber 1995) and evoked potentials (Afra et al 1998b).

Metabolic studies using nuclear magnetic resonance spectroscopy have suggested reduction of magnesium (Ramadan et al 1989) and a low phosphorylation potential (Welch et al 1989, Barbiroli et al 1992, Montagna et al 1994) in the brain of migraineurs. Low magnesium, which might be related to the decrease of magnesium in erythrocytes (Schoenen et al 1991c), could increase the excitability of N-methyl-D-aspartate (NMDA) receptors. The mitochondrial dysfunction could impair the brain's ability to handle energy demands under conditions of repeated and prolonged stimulations (Montagna et al 1989). Since one function of habituation is to protect the cortex against over-

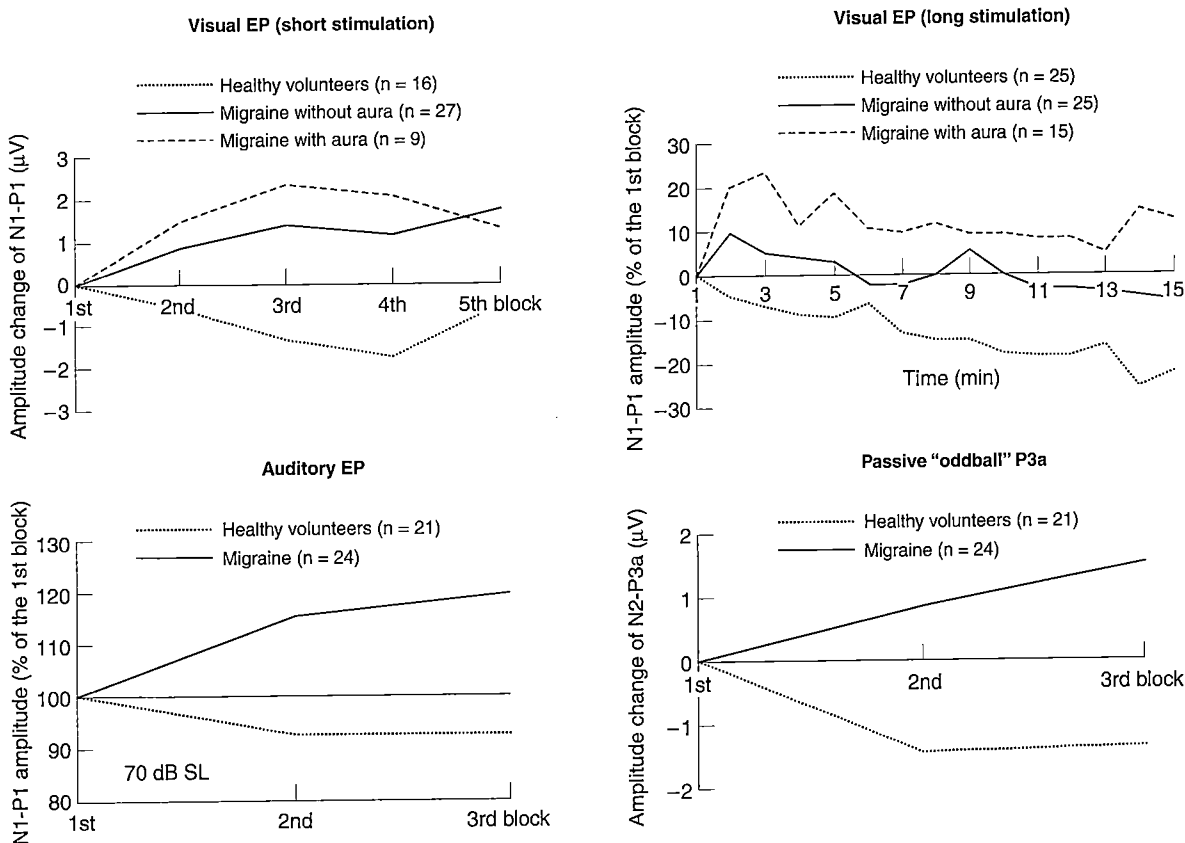

Fig. 33.3 Composite graph showing habituation, i.e. decrease of amplitude, in healthy volunteers, but lack of habituation or potentiation, i.e. increase of amplitude, in MO and MA for visual evoked potentials during 2 min (short) and 16 min (long) of continuous stimulation, for auditory evoked cortical responses at a repeated 70dB stimulation and for the auditory event-related potential P3a.

stimulation and lactate accumulation (Sappey-Marinier et al 1992), the interictal cortical dysfunction found in migraineurs might favour biochemical shifts leading to spreading depression, trigeminovascular activation and thus to a migraine attack which would restore a metabolic equilibrium (Schoenen 1994).

Migraine genes

The familial character of migraine has been known for many years and has been confirmed by recent studies of genetic epidemiology (Russell & Olesen 1995). The weight of genetic factors seems to be greater in migraine with than in migraine without aura. These common forms of migraine are likely to be polygenic, but new insight into their genetic basis has been gained from the discovery of a gene for the rare subtype of migraine, familial hemiplegic migraine (FHM), which is an autosomal dominant monogenic disorder with incomplete penetrance (Joutel et al 1993). The gene (CACNA1A) located on chromosome 19 codes for the α-1 subunit, i.e. the ionophore, of a neuronal P/Q calcium channel which controls neurotransmitter, e.g. 5HT, release (Ophoff et al 1996). Missense mutations are found in half of families with FHM while truncating mutations cause episodic ataxia type 2 and CAG repeat at the 3′ end spinocerebellar ataxia type 6. Depending on the missense mutation of the chromosome 19 gene, there may be a gain or a loss of function in the voltage-dependent calcium channel (Kraus et al 1998). Some FHM families are linked to another, yet to be identified, locus on chromosome 1 (Ducros et al 1997, Gardner & Hofman 1997). In about one-third of families, the genetic locus has not yet been determined. It is likely that the chromosome 19 gene is also involved in the commoner forms of migraine (Terwindt et al 1997).

Other genetic factors determining migraine susceptibility may be related to the dopamine D2 receptor gene (Peroutka et al 1997), the serotonin transporter gene (Ogilvie et al 1998) or a locus on chromosome X (Nyholt et al 1998).

For the time being, migraine can thus be regarded as a genetically determined CNS channelopathy which lowers the threshold for an internally or externally triggered brain and/or brainstem dysfunction leading to activation of the trigeminovascular system. The pathogenetic concept proposed by Liveing a century ago is thus far from being outdated:

> …the fundamental cause … is to be found … in a primary and often hereditary vice or morbid disposition of the nervous system itself…
>
> …the immediate antecedent of an attack is a condition of unstable equilibrium and gradually accumulating tension in … the nervous system… while the paroxysm itself may be likened to a storm, by which this condition is dispersed and the equilibrium for the time restored. Liveing, 1873, *On megrim*)

TREATMENT

Any therapeutic regimen in migraine has to be tailored to the individual patient, taking into account his demands, disability, previous medical history and psychosocial profile. Some general therapeutic rules can nonetheless be defined. Therapy can be divided into acute treatment of the attack and prophylactic treatment. Figures 33.4 and 33.5 are tentative algorithms which may guide the decision process in treating migraine patients.

Whenever possible, precipitating factors should be avoided or treated. Strategies for coping with stress, or dietary measures, can be advised. Attacks occurring during the perimenstrual period can sometimes be prevented by treatment with transdermal oestradiol and/or a non-steroidal anti-inflammatory drug (NSAID) such as naproxen.

Acute treatment

All the acute treatments of migraine are more effective if combined with a short resting period or a nap.

Many migraine attacks can be effectively treated with high doses of aspirin, paracetamol or NSAIDs. Because of the gastrointestinal symptoms that accompany the attack, all these drugs are more effective when administered by the rectal or parenteral route and usually need to be associated with an antiemetic such as metoclopramide or domperidone (Tfelt-Hansen et al 1995).

At present, the most effective drugs for interrupting a migraine attack are the $5HT_{1B/1D}$ agonists, the so-called triptans (Schoenen 1997, Goadsby 1998). Subcutaneous sumatriptan (6 mg) has the highest efficacy rate and the quickest onset of action, but is bedevilled by unpleasant side effects. Intranasal and oral sumatriptan have a lower and slower efficacy. After oral administration some of the newer triptans (zolmi-, riza-, ele-, almo-, frovatriptan) may be slightly more efficacious than sumatriptan. The principal explanation for this is their superior lipophilicity which allows a better bioavailability and brain penetration (Proietti Cecchini et al 1997a). Unfortunately, the latter may also be responsible for increased CNS side effects like somnolence (Fig. 33.6).

Because of their vasoconstrictor action, the triptans are contraindicated in the presence of cardio- or cerebrovascular disorders. Selective agonists of the $5HT_{1F}$ receptor, which is also activated by the triptans, are new promising com-

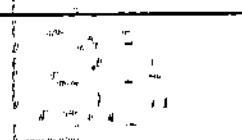

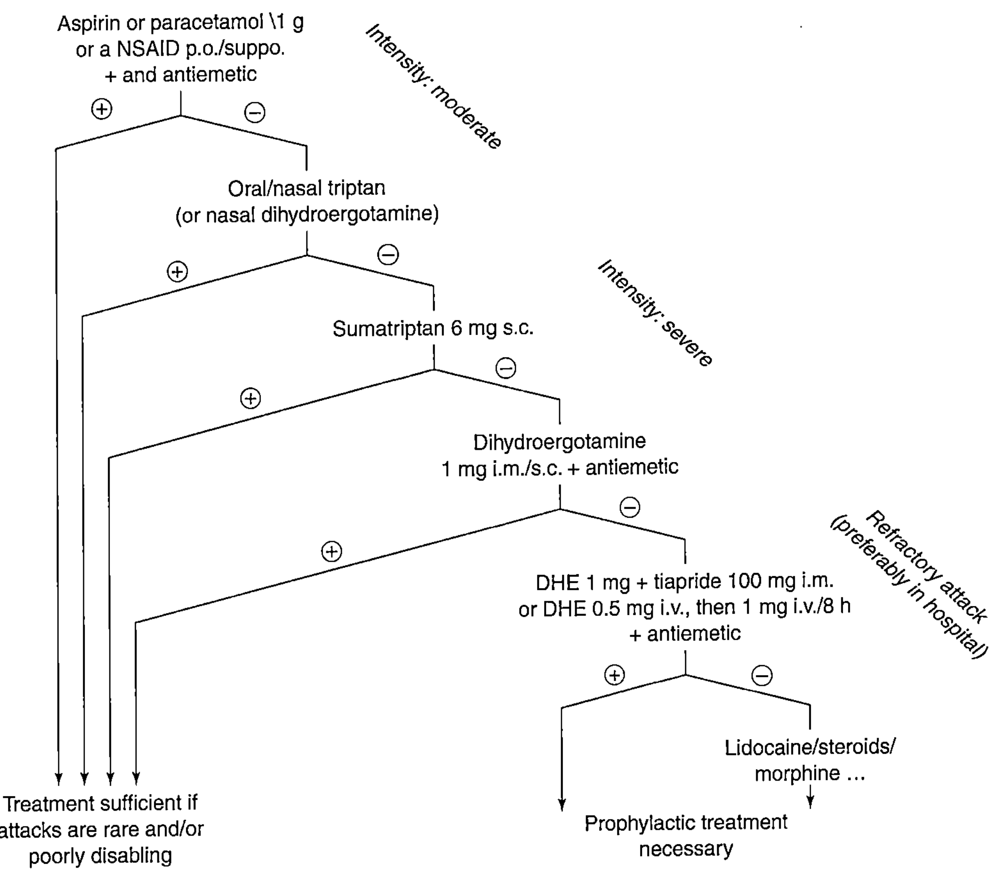

Fig. 33.4 An algorithm for acute migraine treatment. Circles with plus sign = disappearance of migraine within 2 h and absence of unpleasant side effects.

pounds devoid of a coronary vasoconstrictor action but not of central side effects. At present, the major reason for not considering the triptans as first-choice treatments, however, is their high cost. Despite their high efficacy score, they are nonetheless far from having solved all migraineurs' problems (Fig. 33.7).

Other options for routine acute treatment are intranasal dihydroergotamine or lidocaine. Contrary to previous habits, there is nowadays little, if any, place for ergotamine in migraine management because of its unselective receptor profile, unreliable bioavailability and unfavourable efficacy: side effect ratio as well as its propensity to induce overuse and headache chronification.

Prophylactic treatment

Prophylactic antimigraine treatment should be considered when attacks are frequent and/or disabling. On average, the long-term efficacy of prophylactic treatments does not exceed 50–60%. Drugs effective for preventing migraine attacks include: β blockers devoid of intrinsic sympathomimetic activity (Massiou & Bousser 1992); sodium valproate (Hering & Kuritzky 1992, Jensen et al 1994, Mathew et al 1995); serotonin antagonists such as methysergide or pizotifen (Ollat 1992); and calcium channel blockers, especially verapamil and flunarizine. In some patients tricyclics may be useful as an adjuvant therapy. A major drawback of most prophylactic agents are side effects. Other better tolerated, but less effective options are high-dose magnesium (Peikert et al 1996) or cyclandelate (Diener et al 1996).

A novel preventive treatment for migraine is high-dose (400 mg) riboflavin which has an excellent efficacy: side effect ratio (Schoenen et al 1998) (Fig. 33.8). Riboflavin may improve the reduced mitochondrial phosphorylation potential (see Pathophysiology) while the other antimigraine prophylactics are chiefly acting on neurotransmission.

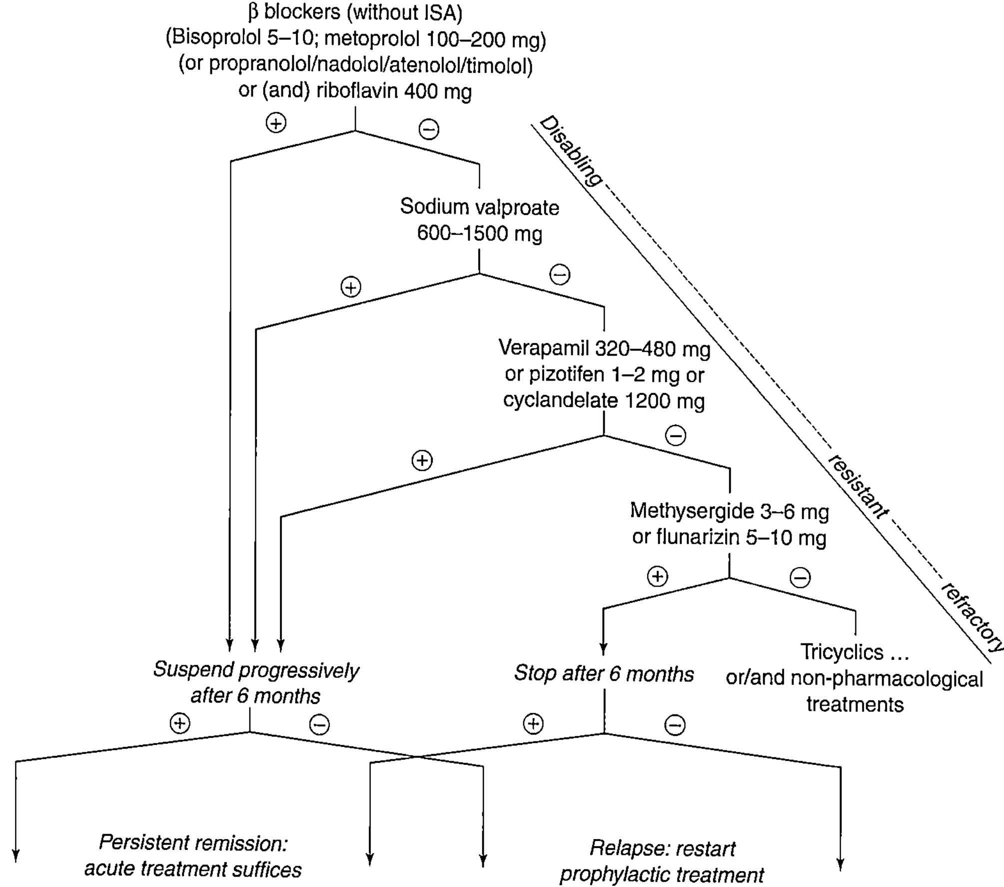

Fig. 33.5 An algorithm for prophylactic migraine treatment. Circles with plus sign = reduction by at least 50% of attack frequency and intensity and absence of unpleasant side effects.

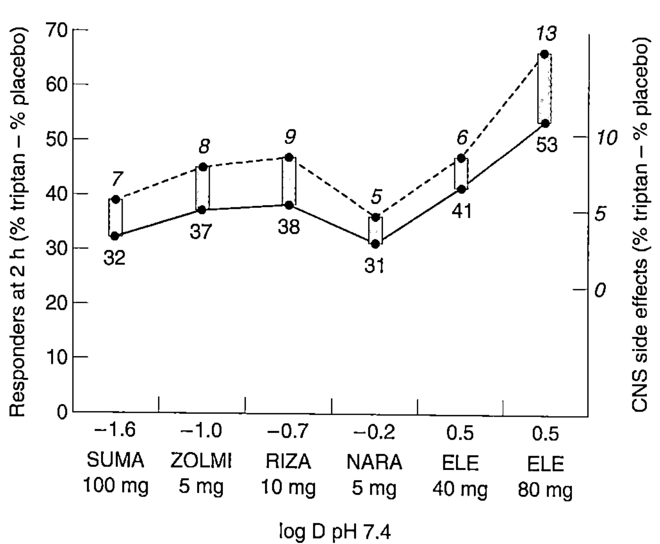

Fig. 33.6 Therapeutic 'gain' (left ordinate) and therapeutic 'harm' (for CNS side effects) over placebo of triptans with increasing lipophilicity as assessed by their logD pH 7.4 value.

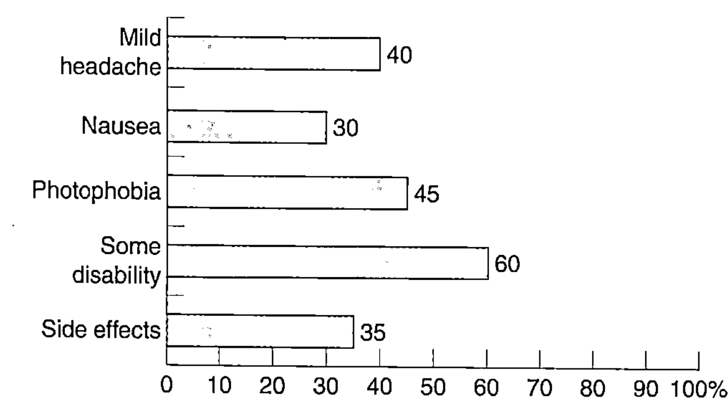

Fig. 33.7 Survival of symptoms and incidence of side effects 2 h after successful treatment of a migraine attack with an oral triptan. Treatment success is defined in most trials as a reduction of headache intensity from severe or moderate to mild or nil. Average percentages from recent trials with zolmitriptan and rizatriptan are shown. Average responder rate in these studies is 65%.

Among the non-pharmacological treatments of migraine, behavioural therapies, such as relaxation and

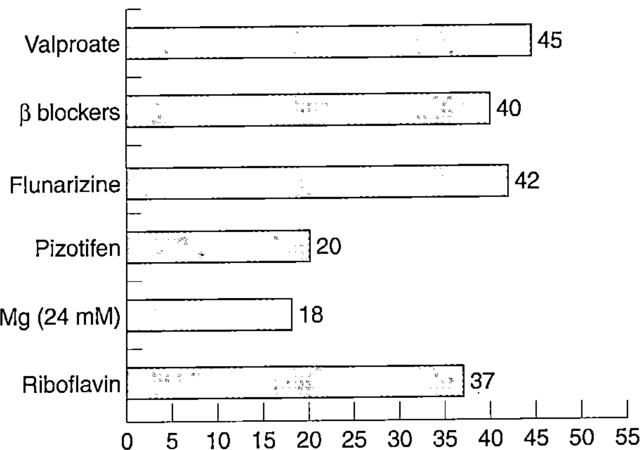

Fig. 33.8 Therapeutic gain over placebo for responder rates of various prophylactic drugs studied with double-blind randomized controlled trials in migraine. 'Responders' have at least a 50% reduction of monthly attack frequency after 3–4 months of treatment. Average values from several trials are shown for valproate, β blockers, flunarizine and pizotifen.

biofeedback, have shown some efficacy in many studies (Holroyd et al 1984) and acupuncture has been found effective in a few reports. Homeopathy, on the other hand, seems to be of no utility (Wallach et al 1997, Whitmarsh et al 1997).

2. TENSION-TYPE HEADACHE

DIAGNOSIS AND CLINICAL FEATURES

The headaches formerly described as 'muscle contraction', 'psychogenic', 'stress' or 'essential' are classified in this group. It is thus a heterogeneous group which can appear controversial and may undergo modifications in the future. The term 'tension-type' has been chosen in order to offer a new heading, underlining the uncertainties about the precise pathogenesis, but indicating nevertheless that some kind of mental or muscular tension may play a causative role.

The diagnostic criteria of *episodic tension-type headache* (code 2.1) (ETH) are illustrated as visual symbols in Table 33.5.

In *chronic tension-type headache* (code 2.2) (CTH), the average headache frequency is equal to or greater than 15 days per month or 180 days per year. The characteristics of the headache are similar to those of episodic tension-type headache except that nausea can be accepted as an isolated associated symptom.

Table 33.5 tension-type headache (TH) (code 2.1): diagnostic criteria

A) n ≥ 10

B) 30 min - 7 days

C) 2/4
1.
2. (no)
3. + / ++
4. no

D) 2/2
1. no (/)
2. no (/)

E) normal

A. at least 10 previous headache episodes fulfilling criteria B–D listed below. Number of days with such headache ,180/year (<15/month).
B. headache lasting from 30 min to 7 days
C. at least 2 of the followig pain characteristics:
   1. pressing/tightening (non-pulsating) quality
   2. mild or moderate intensity (may inhibit, but does not prohibit activities)
   3. bilateral location
   4, no aggravation by walking up/downstairs or similar routine physical activity
D. both of the following:
   1. no nausea or vomiting (anorexia may occur)
   2. photophobia and phonophobia are absent, or one but not both is present
E. at least one of the following:
   1. history, physical- and neurological examinations do not suggest one of the disorders listed in groups 5–11 (please see table 33.1)
   2. history and/or physical- and/or neurological examinations do suggest such disorder, but it is ruled out by appropriate investigations
   3. such disorder is present, but tension-type headache does not occur for the first time in close temporal relation to the disorder

The third digit code number reflects the existence of two kinds of tension-type headache: associated (codes 2.1.1 and

2.2.1) or unassociated (2.1.2 and 2.2.2) with disorder of the pericranial muscles. Such a disorder is supposed to be present when pericranial muscles are excessively tender by manual palpation or pressure algometer measurements or when increased electromyographic (EMG) levels can be recorded in pericranial muscles at rest or during physiological tests. Although pericranial tenderness and pericranial muscle activity vary greatly between patients, there is at present no conclusive evidence that patients with higher levels of these differ from those with normal findings in clinical presentation, pathogenesis of pain or response to therapy (Schoenen et al 1991b).

The single episode of tension-type headache is the least distinct of all headache types since clinical diagnosis is chiefly based on negative features, e.g. the absence of symptoms that characterize other idiopathic or symptomatic headache. These include the absence of unilaterality, pulsatility, aggravation by physical activity and associated symptoms. Moreover, as demonstrated in population-based studies (Rasmussen et al 1991), a substantial proportion of patients may present with atypical symptoms such as unilateral pain (10%), aggravation by routine activity (27.7%), anorexia (18.2%), photophobia (10.6%) or nausea (4.2%). Episodic tension-type headache can therefore be difficult to distinguish from migraine without aura (code 1.1) or from organic brain disease (see below). The diagnosis of chronic tension-type headache is straightforward in most cases with a long enough clinical course. The late exteroceptive suppression period of temporalis muscle may be abolished in patients with daily tension-type headache (Schoenen et al 1987b).

Chronic daily headache may affect up to 4% of the general population (Solomon et al 1992). It comprises patients with chronified migraine or tension-type headache due to analgesic and/or ergotamine overuse, with chronic tension-type headache and a puzzling minority of patients having new chronic daily headache.

The fourth digit code number for tension-type headache gives an indication of the most probable causative or precipitating factors. In many patients several of these factors may be associated, as described in the pathophysiology section.

EPIDEMIOLOGY

In many epidemiological studies the prevalence of muscle contraction headache or psychogenic headache has been found to be equal to or greater than that of migraine. In the Danish population-based study (Rasmussen et al 1991) the lifetime prevalence of tension-type headache was 79%; 59% of Danish subjects had tension-type headache 1 day per month or less and, at the other extreme, 3% more than 15 days per month, i.e. CTH. The 1-year prevalence of frequent tension-type headache (more than one per month) is estimated at 20–30%. Tension headache seems to be more prevalent in women than in men and in both sexes the prevalence tends to decline with age.

Since most patients with ETH do not consult a doctor, the proportion of patients with chronic tension-type headache is much higher in specialized headache or pain centres than in the general population. In this selected patient population, coexistence of migraine and tension-type headache is also frequently found, which may give the impression that both headache types have a common pathophysiological denominator (Olesen 1991) and that they are at the opposite ends of a disease spectrum. On the contrary, however, recent population-based epidemiological studies demonstrate that tension-type headache is not significantly more prevalent in migraineurs than in non-migraineurs (Rasmussen et al 1992), supporting the contention that these types of headache are distinct entities.

PATHOPHYSIOLOGY

From the clinical heterogeneity of TH, one may infer that pathophysiological mechanisms are multiple. Traditionally, muscular factors have been thought to play an important role as illustrated by the previously used term muscle contraction headache. Another previously used denomination, psychogenic headache or 'stress headache', suggests that 'psychological factors' play a dominant role. The controversy between peripheral and central pathogenic aspects is still ongoing. It may be a false debate since both peripheral and central factors could be at work, interacting and varying in importance between patients and TH subtypes or even during the course of the disorder. The following is a synthesis of available data arguing in favour of one or the other pathophysiological mechanism (Schoenen et al 1997).

Peripheral aspects

Experimental ischaemic exercise of temporal muscle may cause pain. Blood flood studies, however, have ruled out the possibility that TH is caused by ischaemia of the temporal muscles (Langemark et al 1990b). Cerebral blood flow is normal in TH but in transcranial Doppler studies, increased flow velocities have been reported in ETH compared to CTH or controls (Reinecke et al 1991, Wallasch 1992, 1993).

The results of biochemical studies performed in TH have been synthesized by Ferrari. Results are in part contradictory because of varying methodologies. Several recent biochemical studies tend to indicate nonetheless that serotonin (D'Andrea et al 1993, Jensen & Hindberg 1994) and met-enkephalin (Ferrarri et al 1990, Longemark et al 1990a) turnover may be high in TH, which contrasts with migraine.

Evidence both for and against a myofascial origin of pain has accumulated over recent years. EMG levels in pericranial muscles may be on average increased in TH, but there is no correlation between EMG activity and headache severity. Lower pressure pain thresholds (PPTs) are found on average at pericranial sites in CTH patients and in population-based studies (Jensen et al 1993a); palpation tenderness is increased in patients, more so during an actual headache. In ETH, however, cephalic PPTs are usually normal (Drumoand 1987, Bovim 1992, Göbel et al 1992, Jensen et al 1993a, Bendtsen et al 1996b). Compared with normal controls a qualitative difference of pericranial myofascial tenderness with a linear stimulus-response function was found in CTH over the temple, suggesting sensitization of nociceptors (Bendtsen et al 1996b). Studies of extracephalic pain thresholds are scarce. In one study (Drummond 1987), a more rapid increase of pain in fingers was found in ETH; in another study (Schoenen et al 1991a), PPTs were decreased over the Achilles tendon in CTH. During isometric contraction, PPTs tend to decrease over the temporal muscle in TH patients while they increase in healthy controls (Proietti Cecchini et al 1997). After tooth clenching, pericranial palpation tenderness increases in subjects who develop an episode of TH (Jensen & Olesen 1996). In addition to sensitization of peripheral nociceptors, central disnociception may therefore play a role in the increased pericranial tenderness of TH patients.

Central nervous system aspects

EEG and evoked potentials are normal in TH (see Schoenen (1992) for a review). Contingent negative variation, an event-related potential, was normal in most studies, but a reduced amplitude was found in one study (Wallasch et al 1993).

Many psychological abnormalities have been associated with TH. It remains to be determined whether these are related to TH aetiology or are just consequences of the headache (see Andrasik & Passchier (1993) for a review).

In recent years, much attention has been paid to an inhibitory reflex of jaw-closing muscles, called exteroceptive suppression or silent period. The second exteroceptive suppression of temporalis muscle (ES2) may be shortened or abolished in CTH patients. Although not confirmed in two recent studies differing in methodology and patient selection (Bendtsen et al 1996b, Lipchick et al 1996), this observation is of potential pathophysiological interest. ES2 duration does reflect excitability of inhibitory brainstem interneurons, which receive afferent inputs from several brainstem centres and limbic structures, in particular from serotonergic raphe nuclei. The following data suggest that the descending control, and not the inhibitory interneurons themselves, is abnormal in TH: inhibition of ES2 by a preceding peripheral stimulus is greatly enhanced; habituation of ES2 at high-frequency stimulation is normal in chronic but increased in episodic tension-type headache; direct suppression of temporalis activity by exteroceptive stimuli at the upper limbs is normal (Wang & Schoenen 1994 a,b, 1996).

A model for TH pathogenesis

Considering the heterogeneous pathophysiological abnormalities found in TH, a comprehensive model was recently proposed as a working hypothesis (Olesen & Schoenen 1993). According to this concept, TH may be the result of an interaction between changes of the descending control of nociceptive brainstem neurons and inter-related peripheral changes, such as myofascial pain sensitivity and strain in pericranial muscles (Fig. 33.9).

An acute episode of ETH may occur in most individuals otherwise perfectly normal. It can be brought on by physical stress usually combined with psychological stress or non-physiological working positions. In such cases, increased nociception from strained muscles may be the primary cause of the attack, possibly favoured by a central temporary change in pain control due to stress. Emotional mecha-

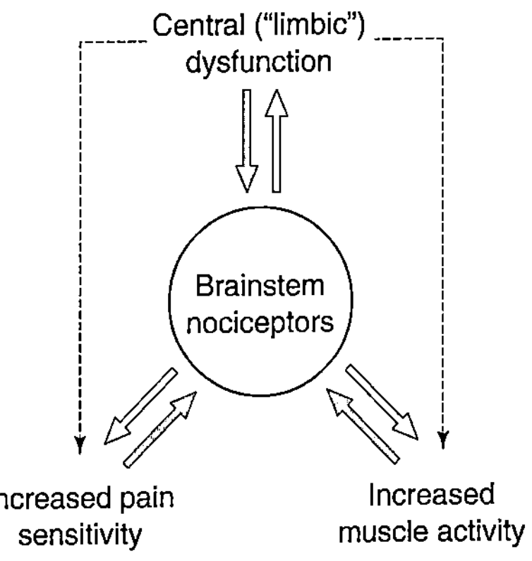

Fig. 33.9 Tension-type headache: model of potential mechanisms.

nisms may indeed increase muscle tension via the limbic system of muscle control and at the same time reduce tone in the endogenous antinociceptive system. With more frequent episodes of headache, central changes may become increasingly more important. Long-term potentiation/sensitization of nociceptive neurons and decreased activity in the antinociceptive system could cause CTH. This is probably the most important mechanism in frequent ETH and in CTH.

The relative importance of peripheral and central factors, however, may vary between patients and over time in the same patient. The complex inter-relation between various pathophysiological aspects in TH may explain why this disorder is so difficult to treat. It certainly suggests that various therapeutic approaches should be used in sequence or in combination and that in the future determining the relative importance of peripheral and central mechanisms might be of some utility in deciding on a therapeutic strategy. Management of TH should strive to prevent chronification.

TREATMENT

Various treatment modalities are used in TH (Schoenen & Wang 1997). Only some of them have been proved effective in good quality controlled clinical trials. Guideliness for clinical drug trials in TH have been proposed by the International Headache Society (1995); they can be recommended to the reader as a standard against which to compare the scientific value of treatment trials published in the literature. As in the case of migraine, therapies for TH can be schematically subdivided into short-term, abortive (mainly pharmacologic) treatments of the individual headache attack and long-term, prophylactic (pharmacologic or non-pharmacologic) treatments that may prevent headache.

Acute pharmacotherapy

Many controlled studies of simple analgesics and NSAIDs have been performed in TH, using the headache attack as a model for acute pain. From these studies (see Mathew (1993) for a review), one may conclude that NSAIDs are the drugs of first choice (Fig. 33.10).

Ibuprofen 400 or 800 mg is significantly more effective than placebo or aspirin (Schachtel et al 1996). Other NSAIDs such as naproxen, ketoprofen (Dahlöf & Jacobs 1996), ketoralac or indomethacin are also effective, but less well studied. Because of the overall lower prevalence of gastrointestinal side effects (Ryan 1977), ibuprofen (800 mg) is probably the first choice, followed by naproxen sodium (825 mg).

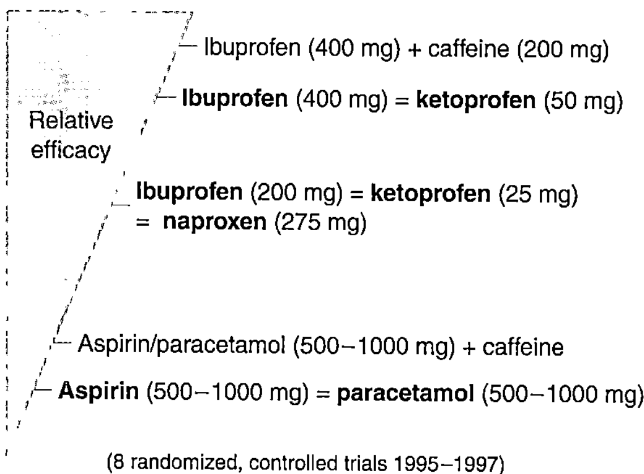

Fig. 33.10 Hierarchy of NSAIDs according to their relative efficiency in aborting tension-type headache episodes. Summary of eight comparative, randomized controlled trials performed between 1995 and 1997.

In some patients, combination of analgesics with caffeine, sedatives or tranquillizers may be more effective than simple analgesics or NSAIDs, but in many cases this impression comes from too low a dosage of the latter. Whenever possible, combination analgesics for TH should be avoided because of the risk of dependency, abuse and chronification of the headache. There is at present no scientific basis for the use of muscle relaxants, such as the mephenesin-like compounds, baclofen, diazepam, tizanidine, cyclobenzaprine or dantrolene sodium, in the treatment of TH.

Prophylactic pharmacotherapy

The tricyclic antidepressants are the most widely used first-line therapeutic agents for CTH. Surprisingly, few controlled studies have been performed and not all of them have found an efficacy superior to placebo (Table 33.6).

One major problem that arises with trials showing statistical superiority of tricyclics over placebo is to evaluate whether the observed effect is clinically relevant. Nonetheless, in clinical practice the tricyclic antidepressants remain useful prophylactic drugs for CTH or frequent ETH. Amitriptyline is the most frequently used; clomipramine may be slightly superior, but has more side effects. Other antidepressants, such as doxepin, maprotiline or mianserin, can be used as a second choice. The average dose of amitriptyline in CTH is 75–100 mg per day (Couch & Micieli 1993), but many patients will be satisfied with a lower dose. If the headache is improved by at least 80% after 4 months, it is reasonable to attempt discontinuation of the medication. Decreasing the daily dose by 20–25% every

Table 33.6 Global efficacy of pharmacotherapies in TH. (Reproduced from Schoenen & Wang 1997)

Drugs	*Amitryptiline (several studies)*	*Maprotiline (1 study)*	*Doxepine (1 study)*	*Citalopram (1 study)*	*Mianserine (1 study)*
Therapeutic 'gain' vs placebo	10–46%	32%	15%	12%	5%

2–3 days may avoid rebound headache. Selective 5HT reuptake inhibitors have little usefulness (Bendtsen et al 1996a).

The mechanism of action of antidepressants in CTH remains to be determined. Their effect on the headache may be partly independent from their antidepresssant effect. Tricyclics have a variety of pharmacological activities. Serotonin increase by inhibition of its reuptake, endorphin release or inhibition of NMDA receptors that play a role in pain transmission may all be relevant for the pathophysiology of TH.

Non-pharmacological treatments

Psychological and behavioural techniques

There is solid scientific support for the usefulness of relaxation and EMG biofeedback therapies in the management of TH (Diamond 1984, Blanchard et al 1987, Schoenen et al 1998). Across studies, relaxation training, EMG biofeedback training and their combination have all yielded a near 50% reduction in headache activity. Improvements are similar for each treatment modality, but significantly greater than those observed in untreated patients or patients with false or non-contingent biofeedback (Table 33.7) (Holroyd & Penzien 1986). Nonetheless, these treatments do not seem to be interchangeable since some patients who fail to respond to relaxation training may benefit from subsequent EMG biofeedback training.

Cognitive-behavioural interventions, such as stress management programmes, alone can effectively reduce TH activity, but they seem to be most useful when added to biofeedback or relaxation therapies in patients with higher levels of daily hassles. Limited contact treatment based on the patient's guidance at home by audiotapes and written materials with only three or four monthly clinical sessions may be a cost-effective alternative to fully therapist-administered treatment in many patients (Haddock et al 1997). Despite this alternative, behavioural therapies are time consuming for patients and therapists.

Although there is no infallible means of predicting treatment outcome, a number of factors have been identified that may have some predictive value. In one study, relaxation producing at least 50% reduction of EMG activity at the fourth session was predictive of an excellent outcome. Excessive analgesic or ergotamine use limits the therapeutic benefits. Short duration of headache complaints and young age improve treatment outcome (Bogaards & ter Kuile 1994). Patients with continuous headache are less responsive to relaxation or biofeedback therapies and those with elevated scores on psychological tests that assess depression or psychiatric disturbance have done poorly with behavioural treatment in some studies (Holroyd 1993).

Other non-pharmacologic treatments

Physical therapy techniques are employed in the treatment of TH and include positioning, ergonomic instruction, massage, transcutaneous electrical nerve stimulation, heat or cold application and manipulations. None of these techniques has been proven to be effective in the long term. Physical treatment such as massage may be useful for acute episodes of TH.

Oromandibular treatment may be helpful in selected TH patients. Unfortunately, most studies claiming efficacy of treatments such as occlusal splints, therapeutic exercises for masticatory muscles or occlusal adjustment are uncontrolled. In one single trial comparing occlusal equilibration

Table 33.7 Global efficacy of behavioural therapies in TH (data summarized from Holroyd 1993)

Techniques	*EMG biofeedback*	*Relaxation*	*Relaxation & biofeedback*	*Non-contingent biofeedback*	*Controls (monitoring)*
Improvement range (%)	13–87	17–94	29–88	–14–40	–28–12

or a placebo equilibration in 56 TH patients, headache frequency was reduced in 80% and intensity in 47% of patients in the active group compared to 50% and 16% in the placebo group (Forsell et al 1985). In another study (Schokker et al 1990) headache frequency decreased in 56% of patients treated with occlusal stabilization splints compared to 32% in patients receiving neurologic treatments. Considering the large number of headache-free subjects who display signs and symptoms of oromandibular dysfunction (Jensen et al 1993b), caution should be taken not to advocate irreversible dental treatments in TH. A minority of selected patients may, however, benefit from oromandibular treatment.

To conclude, there is little scientific evidence to guide the selection of treatment modalities in TH. The best treatment is often found by trial and error. Because the success rates with the different therapeutic strategies, both pharmacologic and non-pharmacologic, appear very similar, it is not surprising that the likelihood of dental treatment is much higher if the patient sees a dentist, that of behaviour therapy if he sees a psychologist and that of pharmacological treatment if he consults a neurologist. This situation is unfortunate because the multifactorial aetiopathogenesis of TH suggests that therapy should be tailored individually to each patient and that a combination of different therapeutic methods, such as the combination of pharmacologic and non-pharmacologic treatments, may yield better results than either treatment by itself. To prove this superior efficacy of combination therapies, multidisciplinary collaborations and large-scale comparative trials will be required.

3. CLUSTER HEADACHE

Cluster headache and chronic paroxysmal hemicrania share common features such as location of pain and associated autonomic symptoms, but differ by sex preponderance, frequency and duration of attacks and drug effects.

DIAGNOSIS AND CLINICAL FEATURES

The diagnostic criteria of cluster headache are listed in Table 33.8. A most typical feature of cluster headache is, as suggested by the term itself, the temporal clustering of attacks during periods usually lasting between 2 weeks and 3 months, separated by remissions of at least 14 days, but usually of several months. This is the temporal profile of *episodic cluster headache* (code 3.1.2). When onset of the disease is too recent to determine periodicity, the headache is coded 3.1.1. *Chronic cluster headache* (code 3.1.3) is characterized by absence of remissions of at least 14 days for more than 1 year. This may be the case from onset (primary chronic, code 3.1.3.1) or an evolution over time from the episodic form (code 3.1.3.2).

Table 33.8 Cluster headache (code 3.1): diagnostic criteria

A. At least five attacks fulfilling B–D

B. Severe unilateral orbital, supraorbital and/or temporal pain lasting 15–180 minutes untreated

C. Headache is associated with at least one of the following signs which have to be present on the pain side.
1. Conjunctival injection
2. Lacrimation
3. Nasal congestion
4. Rhinorrhoea
5. Forehead and facial sweating
6. Miosis
7. Ptosis
8. Eyelid oedema

D. Frequency of attacks: from one every other day to eight per day

Although pain is maximal periorbitally, it may spread in some patients to other regions of the face or the cranium on the same side (Fig. 33.11).

Attacks recur on the same side of the head during a cluster period. In some patients, pain may shift sides from one cluster to another or, rarely, in the midst of a cluster period. Cluster headache causes the most intense and excruciating pain among the primary non-symptomatic headaches. Patients tend to be agitated and to pace the floor which is clearly different from migraine where patients seek rest. Other features distinguishing the cluster headache attack from the migraine attack are shorter duration, presence of autonomic symptoms and absence of gastrointestinal disturbances. During a cluster period attacks can be provoked by alcohol (or histamine or nitroglycerine) and tend to occur in the evening or during sleep. In the general population and among general practitioners, cluster headache is often confused with trigeminal neuralgia (see p. 791) from which it is clearly different by duration of attacks, associated symptoms and temporal profile (Table 33.9).

Cluster migraine is a variant of migraine not sufficiently validated, but characterized by unilateral autonomic features, such as conjunctival injection or tearing, accompanying an otherwise typical migraine attack. A very rare syndrome is the so-called cluster-tic syndrome where periods of cluster headache attacks can alternate with episodes of trigeminal neuralgia. There are a few reports in the literature linking cluster headache attacks to an organic

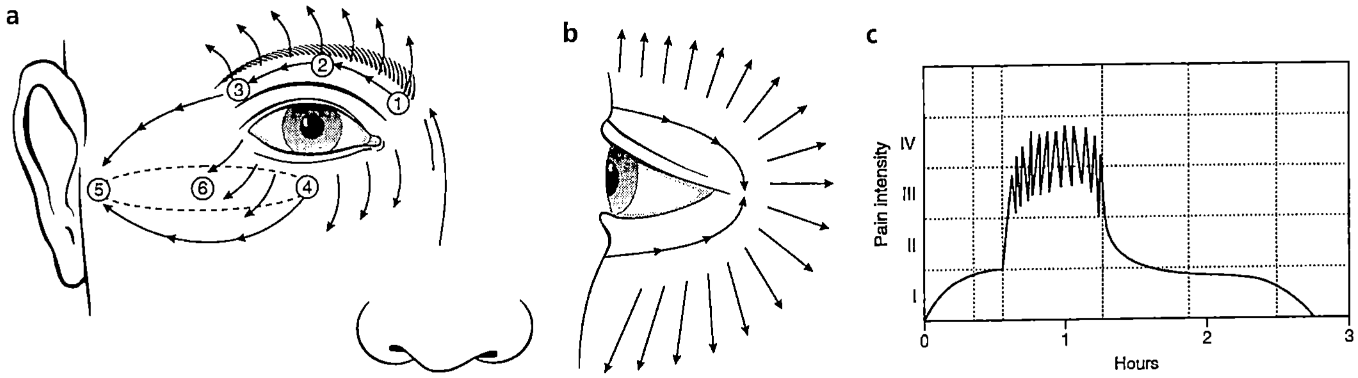

Fig. 33.11 A patient's drawing of the topographic and temporal patterns of an attack of cluster headache. Comments given by the patient: (a,b) 1 starting pain and 2–6 successive spread of pain; the most intense pain is located within the 1–3–4 triangle; slight pain in areas 4, 5 and 6 may outlast the attack. (c) Grading of pain intensity: I slight; II moderate; III violent; IV excruciating pain.

Table 33.9 Differential diagnosis

Characteristics	*Cluster headache*	*Trigeminal neuralgia*	*Migraine*
Sex	m > f	m = f	f > m
Localization	Unilateral, periorbital	Unilateral V_2 / V_3	Uni-/bilateral
Pain quality	Continuous, severe	Paroxysmal, 'electric discharge'	+/– pulsating
Duration, time and frequency of attacks	15–180 min, in the morning, during the night, 1 or more/24 h	(Milli)seconds, during the day, during meals, several / 24 h	4–72 h, time and frequency variable
Associated symptoms	Ipsilateral autonomic signs, agitation	Trigger zones, grimacing	Nausea, vomiting, photo- & phonophobia, prostration
Neurologic examination	Normal	Normal	Normal
Course of disease	'Clusters' of headache with free intervals or chronic form	Periods of exacerbations	Changes of attack frequency over time

lesion, e.g. pituitary adenoma, upper cervical meningioma or cerebral arteriovenous malformations (Sjaastad 1992). In 16% of patients, the onset of cluster headache can be preceded by (even minor) head trauma (Turkewitz et al 1992).

EPIDEMIOLOGY

Epidemiological surveys of cluster headache are rare and/or controversial. Comparing various studies, the overall prevalence is around 0.04–0.09% (Sjaastad 1986). The relative incidence of the chronic form (code 3.1.3) in various published series of cluster headache patients is, on average, 10% (Ekbom 1986). There is a clear preponderance of the male sex in all large series with an average male: female ratio of 5:1. Cluster headache may begin at any age but most often the first attack occurs between 20 and 40 years. It is associated with cigarette smoking, head trauma and a positive family history for headache (Italian Cooperative Study Group).

Some familial cases with an autosomal dominant pattern of inheritance have been described (Russell & Olesen

1995), but genetic influences seem to be less pronounced than in migraine.

PATHOPHYSIOLOGY

There is at present no pathogenetic theory of cluster headache that accounts for all aspects of this disorder, i.e. the pain location and characteristics, autonomic features, temporal profile of attacks and clusters and the male preponderance. Several pathophysiological abnormalities have been demonstrated both during and between attacks (Table 33.10). They point on the one hand towards the cavernous sinus as a potential crossroad where nociceptive peptidergic afferents of the ophthalmic nerve, preganglionic parasympathetic fibres running in the greater superficial petrosal nerve and postganglionic sympathetic fibres of the pericarotid plexus can be impaired and give rise to both the pain and the autonomic symptoms of the cluster headache attack (Hardebo & Moskowitz 1993). On the other hand, a central hypothalamic dysfunction is suggested by the circadian and circannual pattern of attacks, the dysruption of neuroendocrine tests and neurophysiological data. With positron emission tomography an area of increased blood flow was recently found in the ventromedial hypothalamus ipsilateral to nitroglycerine-provoked attacks (May et al 1998). The activated area most probably comprises the suprachiasmatic nucleus where biological rhythms are generated and its ictal activation suggests that, like migraine, cluster headache is a neurovascular disorder with a primary underlying CNS dysfunction (Fig. 33.12).

The significance of reduced choline levels and G-protein subunits in peripheral blood cells (Gardiner et al 1998) is not clear. It is noteworthy, however, that although the signalling pathways in the suprachiasmatic nucleus change with the time domain in the circadian rhythm, the critical gating takes place at a molecular level downstream from the second messengers. One may hypothesize that these gating mechanisms are malfunctioning in cluster headache and that this is related to the abnormal membrane-dependent transduction mechanisms reported by De Belleroche et al in blood cells and possibly to the therapeutic effect of lithium which is able to modulate G-proteins and the phosphatidylinositol signalling pathway (Schoenen 1998a).

TREATMENT

Acute treatment

To abate the single attack, inhalation of 100% oxygen (7–10 l/min) using a facemask is effective within 10–15 minutes in 60–70% of cases. Because of its delayed effectiveness, orally or rectally administered ergotamine tartrate is rarely useful, unless attacks are of long duration. In contrast, intranasal application of dihydroergotamine is effective in about 50% of patients.

At present, subcutaneous injection of sumatriptan, a $5HT_{1B/1D}$ agonist also effective in migraine, is the most efficient treatment of cluster headache attacks. At a dose of 6 mg, it alleviates the attack within 15 minutes in more than 80% of patients without tachyphylaxis in the long term (Wilkinson et al 1995). Sumatriptan was not able to prevent attacks when given on a daily prophylactic basis (Monstad et al 1995).

Prophylactic treatment

There is no general agreement on a standard prophylactic therapy for cluster headache (Ekbom 1995).

Table 33.10 Putative causal factors in cluster headache

Peripheral (trigeminovascular)	*Central (hypothalamic)*
• Trigeminovascular activation and sensitization (Goadsbye, Edvinsson 1994, Fanciullacci et al 1995, Lozza et al 1997)	• Phase shifts of circadian rhythm (Nappi et al 1981)
• High efficacy of sumatriptan (SCHSG 1991)	• Blunted circadian and circannual melatonin / cortisol level (Waldenlind et al 1994, Leone et al 1994 Strittmatter et al 1996
• Parasympathetic activation (Goadsbye, Edvinsson 1994, Sjaastad 1992)	• Increased ictal vasopressin levels (Franceschini et al 1995)
• Sympathetic hypofunction (Fanciullacci et al 1995)	
• Cavernous sinus as pathophysiological focus (Hardebo & Moskowitz 1993, Afra et al 1998c)	• Increased blood flow in ipsilateral anteroventral hypothalamus during nitroglycerin-provoked attacks (May et al 1998)

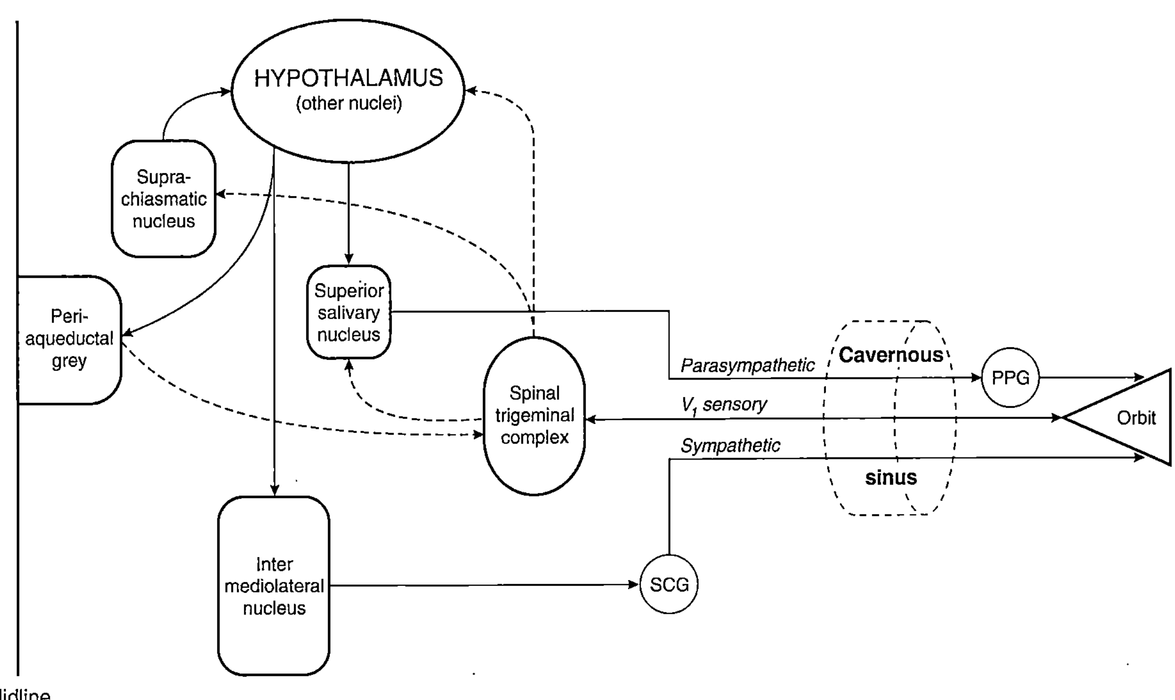

Fig. 33.12 Putative neurovascular mechanisms in cluster headache (CH) in the light of the recent PET findings by May et al (1998). In the hypothesis of a primary central cause, hypothalamic activation, as found during an attack, could induce vascular changes in the cavernous sinus loggia with subsequent irritation of the local plexus of nerve fibres via autonomic preganglionic neurons in the superior salivary and cervicothoracic intermediolateral nuclei. The hypothalamus might also modulate the control of trigeminal pain through its projections to the periaqueductal grey and other pain-controlling nuclei in the brainstem. Phase shifting in the suprachiasmatic nuclei may be relevant for the circadian and circannual rhythmicity of CH attacks; it could be related to abnormal membrane-dependent transduction mechanisms or signalling pathways. Alternatively, thinking of a peripheral origin of symptoms in the cavernous sinus, one has to keep in mind that strong somatosensory input from the trigeminal complex during the attack is able to influence the functioning of hypothalamic structures (for details see text). SCG = superior cervical ganglion; PPG = pterygopalatine ganglion.

Verapamil is probably the most effective preventive treatment (Lewis & Solomon 1996). The average dose is 240 mg bid, but daily doses up to 960 mg or more if tolerated, may be necessary in some patients. The most common adverse effects are constipation, fatigue and hypotension.

Lithium carbonate is an effective treatment at doses inducing plasma levels between 0.7 and 1 mmol/1. The effectiveness of lithium may decrease during successive clusters. Lithium may be more effective in the chronic form.

Methysergide has been used with success in cluster headache for many years. Daily dosage should be as low as possible, preferably 3–4 mg. Methysergide has to be interrupted every 5–6 months for 1 month to avoid retroperitoneal fibrosis.

Ergotamine tartrate given orally at bedtime may be useful to prevent nocturnal attacks.

Corticosteroids at high doses are able to interrupt a cluster in many patients. However, their use should be restricted to incapacitated and resistant patients with the episodic form. Tapering or interruption of cortisone treatment is indeed frequently followed by recurrence of attacks. Suboccipital injection of corticosteroids, associated or not with a local anaesthetic, is used as an adjuvant therapy in some centres. By itself, this may interrupt a cluster in a few patients, but whether this is due to a systemic or to a local effect of the drug remains to be determined.

In some patients, it can be helpful to combine two of the above-mentioned substances. Other drugs like pizotifen, indomethacin or sodium valproate may have an effect in selected patients.

Various invasive treatments have been tried in cluster headache: alcoholization or radiofrequency lesions (Sanders & Zuurmond 1997), cryosurgery or resection of the pterygopalatine ganglion; radiofrequency lesions or glycerol injections of the Gasserian ganglion; gamma knife radiosurgery of the trigeminal nerve root entry zone (Ford et al 1998). None of these procedures gives consistent long-lasting relief and some of them are not yet sufficiently validated. They should therefore be considered only in the minority (+/–1%) of patients who resist a full trial of medical therapy.

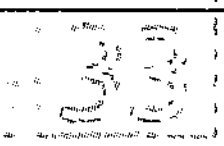

PAIN SYNDROMES RELATED TO CLUSTER HEADACHE

Chronic paroxysmal hemicrania (CPH) is a rare disorder first described by Sjaastad and Dale (1974), affecting adult females almost exclusively and noteworthy because of its absolute responsiveness to indomethacin. Attacks resemble those of cluster headache, but they last for a shorter time (mean duration 15 minutes), are more frequent (more than five a day for more than half of the time; mean of about 12 per day) and have no nocturnal preponderance. The chronic stage, which characterizes most reported cases, may be preceded by an episodic, 'pre-CPH' stage.

The exact pathogenesis of CPH is not known. Various abnormalities (e.g. corneal indentation or temperature changes, intraocular pressure changes) are similar to those reported in cluster headache (Sjaastad 1992). Several symptomatic cases occurring with sellar or parasellar neoplasms have been reported.

The absolute responsiveness of CPH to indomethacin is part of the diagnostic criteria. As a diagnostic test, 50 mg of indomethacin injected intramuscularly is able to increase significantly the time to the next attack. The effective oral dosage for continuous treatment varies between patients (up to 150 mg or more). On discontinuation of the drug, attacks frequently reappear but long-lasting remissions have been observed in some patients. Recently, other NSAIDs, such as ketoprofen, have been found effective in a few patients.

Short-lasting, unilateral, neuralgiform orbital pain attacks with conjunctival injection, tearing, sweating and rhinorrhoea, the so-called SUNCT syndrome, may be a new entity which has similarities to CPH and trigeminal neuralgia (Sjaastad et al 1989). SUNCT is characterized by a multiplicity of short (usually less than 120 s) paroxysms of moderate to severe intensity with massive autonomic symptoms in the eye. Only a few cases have been described in the literature up to now; most of them are males.

4. MISCELLANEOUS HEADACHES UNASSOCIATED WITH STRUCTURAL LESION

This section comprises several rather characteristic headaches which are benign in nature. Pathophysiologically, they are triggered by stimulation of the trigeminal nerve territory or changes in intracranial pressure. Some of them have been more frequently reported in migraineurs.

Idiopathic stabbing headache (code 4.1), previously called ice-pick pains or 'jabs and jolts', is characterized by short-lasting pains in the distribution of the first division of the trigeminal nerve, occurring at irregular intervals. It was found in 2% of the general population (Rasmussen et al 1992) and is significantly more prevalent in migraineurs. If treatment is necessary, indomethacin or other NSAIDs are usually effective.

External compression headache (code 4.2), also called 'swim-goggle headache', is a dull constant pain felt in an area of the scalp subjected to prolonged pressure. Up to 4% of the population may present with such a headache (Rasmussen et al 1992), preferentially individuals suffering also from migraine.

Cold stimulus headache (code 4.3) includes headaches developing during external exposure to cold (sub-zero weather, cold water) or during ingestion of a cold food or drink (previously called 'ice cream headache'). This type of headache seems to be frequent in the general population, affecting 15% of individuals in the Danish study; it is also more frequent in migraineurs.

Benign cough headache (code 4.4) and *benign exertional headache* (code 4.5) are rare (1% of the population) and not associated with migraine or tension-type headache (Rasmussen et al 1992). Note that cough headache is benign in only about 50% of cases, with a male preponderance and an onset after 45 years of age. For the other 50%, cough headache is most often due to Chiari type I malformation, equally distributed in both sexes and beginning under age 50 (Pascual et al 1996). Benign exertional headache has an earlier onset than benign cough headache and it is frequently related to benign sexual headache. It can be prevented in some patients by taking indomethacin before exercise. Ergotamine tartrate, methysergide and propranolol have also been used. When it is symptomatic, exertional headache is often due to subarachnoid haemorrhage.

Headache associated with sexual activity (code 4.6) may present in three different forms: a dull pain in the head and neck that intensifies as sexual excitement increases (code 4.6.1); a sudden severe, explosive, headache occurring at orgasm (code 4.6.2) or a postural headache resembling that of low cerebrospinal fluid pressure developing after coitus (code 4.6.3). Sexual headaches are reported by only 1% of subjects in the general population (Rasmussen et al 1992).

When a sudden severe headache occurs for the first time during sexual activity or exertion, an intracranial aneurysm has to be excluded (see p. 785).

5. HEADACHE ASSOCIATED WITH HEAD TRAUMA

DIAGNOSIS AND CLINICAL FEATURES

The diagnostic criteria for *acute post-traumatic headache* (code 5.1) are listed in Table 33.11. In the *chronic form* (code 5.2) the headache continues for more than 8 weeks after regaining consciousness or after trauma, if there has been no loss of consciousness. Acute post-traumatic headache is often moderate to severe, throbbing in quality, with accompanying nausea, vomiting, photo- and phonophobia, memory impairment, irritability or drowsiness, or vertigo. It is usually exacerbated by physical exercise, described as incapacitating by the patient, and bears many similarities to migraine, except the attack pattern.

Although the quality of chronic post-traumatic headache is not characteristic, it is usually a generalized headache, almost permanent like chronic tension-type headache, but aggravated by physical effort and mental strain. The pain may be focused on the area that the patient believes to have been damaged and which tends to be tender. Migrainous features, such as a pulsating quality or nausea, may occur.

Many patients with chronic post-traumatic headache fulfil DSMIII-R criteria for post-traumatic stress disorder (Hickling et al 1992). Depressive features are common and decreased amplitude of contingent negative variation has been reported (Schoenen & Timsit-Berthier 1993).

Table 33.11 Acute post-traumatic headache (code 5.1): diagnostic criteria

5.1.1 *With significant head trauma and/or confirmatory signs*

A. Significance of head trauma documented by at least one of the following:
   1. Loss of consciousness
   2. Post-traumatic amnesia lasting more than 10 minutes
   3. At least two of the following exhibit relevant abnormality: clinical neurological examination, X-ray of skull, neuroimaging, evoked potentials, spinal fluid examination, vestibular function test, neuropsychological testing

B. Headache occurs less than 14 days after regaining consciousness (or after trauma, if there has been no loss of consciousness)

C. Headache disappears within 8 weeks after regaining consciousness (or after trauma, if there has been no loss of consciousness)

5.1.2 *With minor head trauma and no confirmatory signs*

A. Head trauma that does not satisfy 5.1.1. A

B. Headache occurs less than 14 days after injury

C. Headache disappears within 8 weeks after injury

As mentioned elsewhere, migraine or cluster headache may appear de novo after a head trauma. The incidence of post-traumatic migraine was as high as 3% in one study (Kelly 1986). Worsening of pre-existing headache is coded according to pre-existing headache form.

EPIDEMIOLOGY AND PATHOPHYSIOLOGY

Headache is a major factor in the symptomatology of head trauma. It is obvious, however, that the severity of trauma has little relationship to the intensity or duration of the headache. There is even some evidence that the incidence of post-traumatic headache is inversely related to the severity of head injury (Kay et al 1971). In a recent study severe post-traumatic headache was found in 72% of mildly injured and 33% of severely injured patients, despite the fact that cervical X-ray and CT scan abnormalities were more frequent in the latter group (Yamaguchi 1992).

Acute post-traumatic headache is very common. The incidence of chronic post-traumatic headache varies between studies from 15% to 40% (Jensen & Nielsen 1990). Patients suffering from headache before the trauma are no more at risk of having traumatic headache than patients who did not suffer from headache before the trauma. For an unexplained reason, post-traumatic headache is, like many other headaches, reported by more women than men (Jensen & Nielsen 1990).

Russell (1932) and Cook (1972) observed that persistence of post-traumatic symptoms and duration of absence from work were longer in patients claiming financial compensation from the employer or insurance company. In Lithuania where litigation is not possible, a recent survey found no increased prevalence of headache in a cohort of subjects who had experienced a rear-end car collision 1–3 years before (Schrader et al 1996). In a long-term follow-up of over 800 patients with the chronic post-traumatic syndrome, Kelly (1986) found that only 0.06% of patients had not already returned to work before settlement of their claim for litigation and that for this subgroup of patients it was unusual to return to work after the case had come to settlement irrespective of whether the latter was favourable or not.

TREATMENT

Treatment of acute post-traumatic headache is part of the general management of the cerebral concussion syndrome: physical and mental rest in a supine position and simple analgesics or anti-inflammatory drugs. After the immediate acute stage, the practitioner frequently has to deal with the other symptoms of the postconcussion syndrome such as memory impairment, mood and personality changes and social dysfunctioning.

Treatment of chronic post-traumatic headache is difficult because of the complex inter-relation between organic and psychosocial factors. Daily consumption of analgesics are a well-established but often neglected chronifying factor (Warner & Fenichel 1996) (see p. 789). Moreover, there is often an outstanding claim for compensation from the employer (when trauma occurred at work) or from insurance companies (for traffic accidents) and, until this claim is settled, a complete failure of any proposed treatment may be observed. The first and possibly major step is to recognize that the condition does exist and is not always a 'figment of the patient's cupidity' (Kelly 1986). Once this is accepted, therapeutic strategy has to be planned for each patient individually. In patients who have migrainous features, prophylactic antimigraine drugs can be useful (see above). Behavioural treatments, such as biofeedback, have provided persistent relief in some patients. In many of them antidepressants, tricyclics or MAO inhibitors, are necessary. In all cases of resistant post-traumatic headache, psychosocial guidance is the cornerstone of management with the objective of helping the patient to recover progressively his social and professional status.

Unfavourable prognostic factors in chronic post-traumatic headache are age higher than 40, low intellectual, educational and socioeconomic level, previous head trauma and a history of alcohol abuse. Initial severe headache, extensive mobility decrease of the cervical spine, depressive mood and vegetative symptoms are additional factors which tend to prolong headache after whiplash injury (Keidel & Diener 1997).

6. HEADACHE ASSOCIATED WITH VASCULAR DISORDER

All headaches coded to this group fulfil the following criteria: symptoms and/or signs of vascular disorder; appropriate investigations demonstrate the vascular disorder; headache as a new symptom or of a new type occurring in close temporal relation to onset of vascular disorder.

As previously, worsening of pre-existing headache is coded according to pre-existing headache form.

ACUTE ISCHAEMIC CEREBROVASCULAR DISEASE (CODE 6.1)

Although it has been repeatedly emphasized for many years, the importance of headache as a symptom of occlusive cerebrovascular disease is still neglected by many physicians. Comprehensive reviews have been undertaken by Edmeads (1986) and Mitsias and Ramadan (1992). Their major conclusions can be summarized as follows.

1. The incidence of headache accompanying transient ischaemic attacks (TIAs) or strokes varies from 15% to 65% between studies, with an average incidence of 30%. The literature suggests that headache is more likely to occur in patients with posterior circulation ischaemia, independent of mechanism.
2. The headache can precede the ischaemic event in about 10% of patients ('sentinel headache').
3. The headache is usually on the side of the affected artery when the carotid circulation or the posterior cerebral artery is involved and in most cases its location is frontal. In basilar artery or vertebral occlusion or stenosis the headache is most often occipital and non-lateralized; sometimes it is occipitofrontal and lateralized.
4. The quality of headache in ischaemic cerebrovascular disease varies widely among patients. The headache may be continuous or throbbing. It is usually of moderate intensity.
5. Headache at the onset of the ischaemic stroke does not help to distinguish embolic from atherothrombotic stroke. Headache may be less frequent in lacunar infarcts.

Whether or not migraine is an independent risk factor for ischaemic stroke is still debated. Recent surveys suggest that it is so only in young females (Tzourio et al 1995).

INTRACRANIAL HAEMATOMA (CODE 6.2)

The overall incidence of headache as a major symptom in various series of *intracerebral haemorrhages* (code 6.2.1) ranges from 36% to 66% (Edmeads 1986). Impaired consciousness or aphasia can prevent patients from complaining of headache. In all the published series there is nevertheless a proportion of non-comatose, non-aphasic patients, ranging from 10% in putaminothalamic to 30% in lobar haemorrhages, who do not have headaches. The occurrence, acuity and severity of headache will depend largely on the location, rate of evolution and size of the haemorrhage.

Headache is a useful and common indicator of the late development of an acute *epidural* (code 6.2.3) or *subdural* (code 6.2.2) haematoma in patients who have recovered consciousness and subsequently appear to deteriorate. It may be similar to that due to raised intracranial pressure (see p. 786). Subdural haematomata can sometimes produce a characteristic paroxysmal headache that returns on and off irregularly throughout the day, lasts only minutes and is accompanied by generalized sweating and an increase in pulse rate (Kelly 1986). The headache is usually frontal, but when the subdural haematoma is in the posterior fossa, it is likely to be occipital. Occipital headache associated with neck stiffness may indicate the onset of cerebellar pressure coning from the presence of an unrelieved supratentorial bilateral subdural haematoma.

SUBARACHNOID HAEMORRHAGE (CODE 6.3)

The headache of subarachnoid haemorrhage is typically abrupt in onset and incapacitating in severity. Time from onset to maximal pain intensity is less than 60 minutes in the case of ruptured aneurysm and less than 12 hours if it is an arteriovenous malformation. The headache is diffuse, often posterior and radiating into the neck. It can be accompanied by blunting of consciousness, vomiting, stiff neck and sometimes subhyaloid haemorrhages. The diagnosis is confirmed by CT scan, which may be normal in 10% of cases, and CSF examination.

UNRUPTURED VASCULAR MALFORMATION (CODE 6.4)

About one-quarter of patients with an intracranial aneurysm present prerupture manifestations. The most frequent of these is the so-called 'sentinel headache' (or 'premonitory headache', 'minibleeds' or 'warning leaks'), suggesting that an aneurysm might leak intermittently into the subarachnoid space (Edmeads 1986). Fortunately, not every severe global headache of abrupt onset, the so-called 'thunderclap' headache, is the first symptom of an *intracranial aneurysm* (code 6.4.1). Two recent studies have shown that patients struck by 'thunderclap' headache who have normal CT scan and lumbar puncture results do not subsequently develop subarachnoid haemorrhage (Wijdicks et al 1988, Markus 1991). Consequently, the following guidelines may be helpful in patients with an abrupt 'worst headache of my life' thunderclap and a normal neurological examination: perform CT scan; if normal, perform lumbar puncture; if normal, the patient can be reassured and the headache considered to be benign (but it may recur in some patients). If any aspect of the CT scan or lumbar puncture is abnormal, an angiography is required.

Arteriovenous malformations (code 6.4.1), which account for 6% of all subarachnoid haemorrhages (Edmeads 1986), often cause focal seizures or neurological deficits. Although the relationship of migraine and other headaches to unruptured arteriovenous malformation (AVM) is poorly substantiated, there are several case reports in the literature of AVMs mimicking attacks of migraine with aura. Possible diagnostic clues are symptom localization being always on the same side; absent family history for migraine; absence of visual aura symptoms and atypical auras.

ARTERITIS (CODE 6.5)

Giant cell arteritis (code 6.5.1)

Diagnosis and clinical features

In the IHS classification, the diagnostic criteria for giant cell arteritis (temporal arteritis or Horton's disease) are the presence of typical histopathological features on temporal artery biopsy and one or more of the following: swollen and tender scalp artery; elevated erythrocyte sedimentation rate and disappearance of headache within 48 hours of steroid therapy.

Other clinical characteristics, however, may be helpful for the diagnosis at an earlier stage. For instance, giant cell arteritis is a disease of the elderly. Its prevalence increases after the age of 50 years and was found to be 78.1 per 100 000 in the ninth decade in some studies (Ross Russell 1986). In two recent series the mean age was over 65 years and women predominated by 2:1 (Berlit 1992, Chmelewski et al 1992). The headache is usually temporal, of variable severity, of a constant boring quality and temporarily relieved by analgesics such as aspirin. Pulsation in branches of the superficial temporal artery or the facial artery may be absent. Symmetrical arthralgia-myalgia in pectoral or pelvic girdle areas ('polymyalgia rheumatica') frequently accompanies this systemic disease as well as general malaise, anorexia or mild fever. Early morning large joint stiffness may be the only manifestation of polymyalgia rheumatica. Typical complications are claudication of jaw muscles and visual loss due to ischaemia of the optic nerve and retina. The frequency of visual loss has been variously reported to be between 7% and 60% (Ross Russell 1986). Visual disturbances require immediate and energetic treatment, because the prognosis for recovery of vision lost for more than a few hours' duration is poor. Stroke due to involvement of cerebral arteries may occur in exceptional cases.

Pathology

Temporal artery biopsy confirms the diagnosis of a granulomatous arteritis, but it may be normal in a minority of patients. Treatment should nevertheless be undertaken if the clinical and biological picture of the disease is suggestive

(Berlit 1992). Although reported otherwise in some series, bilateral temporal artery biopsy does not increase the incidence of positive results (Chmelewski et al 1992).

Treatment

The treatment of choice of giant cell arteritis is corticosteroids. Initial steroid dosage ranges from 40 to 90 mg/d prednisone. The clinical response to treatment is rapid and severe headache disappears within 48 hours. Whenever necessary, corticosteroid treatment can be initiated before temporal artery biopsy is performed since this does not appear immediately to suppress diagnostic histopathologic abnormalities.

Once symptoms are controlled, doses of steroids should gradually be reduced over a period of weeks to months. The erythrocyte sedimentation rate is a helpful guide at this stage for determining the lowest effective dose. With doses of steroids below 20 mg of prednisone, as many as 30% of patients may have a relapse. Unfortunately, in these elderly patients the long-term side effects of prednisone are manifold and troublesome. It is therefore recommended that the prednisone dosage should be brought down to 10–15 mg/d by the third month, while monitoring the erythrocyte sedimentation rate value as the first, early indication of potential relapse. If side effects of corticosteroids are severe, it may be possible to control the arteritis with immunosuppressive drugs such as azathioprine.

CAROTID OR VERTEBRAL ARTERY PAIN (CODE 6.6)

Ipsilateral headache and/or cervical pain may be the only manifestation of *carotid or vertebral dissection* (code 6.6.1) or may accompany the neurological symptoms (Biousse et al 1992). *Carotidynia* (code 6.6.2) is a controversial entity. It is doubtful whether an idiopathic form of carotidynia exists, but there is clear evidence that a number of diseases of the carotid artery or of the neck are able to produce symptoms suggestive of carotidynia, such as tenderness, swelling and increased pulsation of the carotid artery.

Postendarterectomy headache (code 6.6.3) is defined as an ipsilateral headache beginning within 2 days of carotid endarterectomy, in the absence of carotid occlusion or dissection. Recent studies suggest that these criteria are not satisfactory and that endarterectomy headache may be multifactorial. In a prospective study of 50 patients, 62% reported headache, which occurred in the first 5 days after surgery in 87% of cases. The headache was mostly bilateral (74%), mild or moderate (78%) and requiring no treatment (77%). In this series only five patients met the IHS criteria for postendarterectomy headache (Tehindrazanarivelo et al 1992).

VENOUS THROMBOSIS (CODE 6.7)

Headache is the most frequent symptom in cerebral venous thrombosis and most often the first one. It is more frequently diffuse than localized and more often subacute than acute. Its intensity is highly variable. Associated neurological signs (focal deficit or seizures) and/or raised intracranial pressure causing papilloedema are present in the majority of cases. Headache can, however, occasionally be the only symptom of cerebral venous thrombosis. This is thus another reason why recent, persisting headache should prompt appropriate investigations including CT scan, magnetic resonance imaging and, if necessary, angiography.

ARTERIAL HYPERTENSION (CODE 6.8)

There is convincing evidence from several epidemiological studies that chronic hypertension of mild or moderate degree does not cause headache. Arterial hypertension is considered to be the cause of headache in four conditions which are not usually difficult to diagnose: acute pressor response to exogenous agent (code 6.8.1); phaeochromocytoma (code 6.8.2); malignant hypertension and hypertensive encephalopathy (code 6.8.3) and pre-eclampsia and eclampsia (code 6.8.4).

7. HEADACHE ASSOCIATED WITH NON-VASCULAR INTRACRANIAL DISORDER

In the IHS classification this category comprises mainly headaches associated with changes in intracranial pressure. Some of the disorders, such as intracranial infections, need no further comment, as their diagnosis is usually straightforward. Others have to be considered in more detail, because they are frequent and/or because their diagnosis is difficult at a stage when headache is the only symptom. This is the case for benign intracranial hypertension, postlumbar puncture headache and headache associated with brain tumour.

HIGH CEREBROSPINAL FLUID PRESSURE (CODE 7.1)

Benign intracranial hypertension (code 7.1.1)

Diagnosis and clinical features

The diagnostic criteria for benign intracranial hypertension, also called pseudotumour cerebri or idiopathic intracranial hypertension, are listed in Table 33.12.

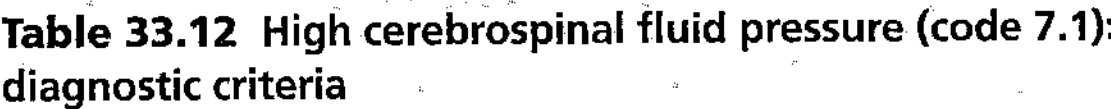

Table 33.12 High cerebrospinal fluid pressure (code 7.1): diagnostic criteria

A. Patient suffers from benign intracranial hypertension fulfilling the following criteria:
   1. Increased intracranial pressure (>200 mm H_2O) measured by epidural or intraventricular pressure monitoring or by lumbar puncture
   2. Normal neurological examination except for papilloedema and possible VI nerve palsy
   3. No mass lesion and no ventricular enlargement on neuroimaging
   4. Normal or low protein concentration and normal white cell count in CSF
   5. No clinical or neuroimaging suspicion of venous sinus thrombosis

B. Headache intensity and frequency related to variations of intracranial pressure with a time lag of less than 24 hours

The headache accompanying this condition may mimic that of chronic tension-type headache: it is generalized, non-throbbing and of low or moderate intensity. It is usually increased, however, on suddenly jolting or rotating the head. In the study by Wall (1990) the following features were found to be characteristic for the diagnosis: predominant occurrence in young obese women (93%); the most severe headache ever experienced by the patient (93%); pulsatile character (83%); nausea (57%); vomiting (30%); orbital pain (43%); transient visual obscuration (71%); diplopia (38%) and visual loss (31%). Papilloedema, without neuroradiological abnormalities (except for a possible 'empty sella'), is pathognomonic for this condition, but may be lacking in a small subgroup of patients (Marcelis & Silberstein 1991). The resting spinal pressure varies from 220 to 600 mmH_2O. CSF cytology is normal, but protein content may be low. Computed axial tomography may show narrow, 'slit-like' ventricles.

Pathogenesis

Pathogenetic factors which may be associated with benign intracranial hypertension include, in addition to intracranial venous occlusion, menstrual dysfunction, deficiency of the adrenals, corticosteroid therapy, hypoparathyroidism, vitamin A intoxication, insecticides (e.g. kepone) and administration of tetracycline in infants (Dalessio 1989). In many cases no precise cause is found.

Treatment

The treatment of elevated intracranial pressure syndromes depends on the underlying cause. If the diagnosis is benign intracranial hypertension, secondary causes should be sought and if possible eliminated. The headache has been reported to respond to standard headache treatment, including β-adrenergic blockers, calcium channel antagonists, antidepressants, MAO inhibitors, anticonvulsants, analgesics and ergotamine preparations. If such therapy is unsuccessful, then a 4–6-week trial of furosemide or a potent carbonic anhydrase inhibitor (acetazolamide) should be given. The use of high-dose corticosteroid is controversial, but may be effective in benign intracranial hypertension. Lumbar puncture typically relieves headache, but the long-term usefulness of repeated lumbar puncture is uncertain.

Careful ophthalmological follow-up is necessary in all patients. Surgical treatment has been directed toward preventing visual loss secondary to papilloedema. Optic nerve sheath fenestration can produce improvement of headache as a felicitous side effect. Ventriculoperitoneal shunts can be performed successfully in selected patients.

High-pressure hydrocephalus (code 7.1.2)

High-pressure hydrocephalus may not cause headache when it develops progressively. The acute increase in intracranial pressure which occurs, for example, with ventricular obstruction or shunt malfunction in a treated hydrocephalic usually causes severe headache followed by visual disturbance.

LOW CEREBROSPINAL FLUID PRESSURE (CODE 7.2)

Diagnosis and clinical features

The clinical hallmark of low CSF pressure headache is that the pain is aggravated by upright position and relieved with recumbency ('orthostatic headache'). The headache may be frontal, occipital or diffuse. The pain is severe, dull or throbbing in nature and not usually relieved with analgesics. Other symptoms include anorexia, nausea, vomiting, vertigo and tinnitus. The pain is aggravated by head shaking and jugular compression. Physical examination may show mild neck stiffness and a slow pulse rate, but is most often normal. Spinal fluid pressure usually ranges from 0 to 30 mmH_2o in the lateral supine position.

Aetiology

The most frequent cause of low CSF pressure is lumbar puncture. Theories concerning pathogenesis of *postlumbar puncture headache* (code 7.2.1) have nonetheless been contradictory. Although the weight of the evidence supports the view that it is related to a loss of CSF secondary to leakage through the dural hole, other factors may favour the syndrome: for instance, postlumbar puncture headache, the prevalence of which may be as high as 40–50% in some studies, is more frequent in young, healthy, female patients with low body mass and in subjects who have a history of previous headaches (Göbel & Schenkl 1989, Kuntz et al 1992).

There are many other causes of low-pressure headache syndrome including post-traumatic, postoperative or idiopathic *cerebrospinal fluid leak* (code 7.2.2) or systemic illnesses such as dehydration, diabetic coma, hyperpnoea or uraemia. Moreover, a syndrome of spontaneous intracranial hypotension has been described (Rando & Fishman 1992). Leptomeningeal enhancement on magnetic resonance imaging is a hallmark of intracranial hypotension.

Treatment

The incidence of postlumbar puncture headache may be lower when small-diameter (20 or 22 G) or 'atraumatic' needles are used, but this lacks definitive proof (Kuntz et al 1992, Lenaerts et al 1993). Contrary to previous belief, recommendation of a resting period in the supine position after the procedure makes no difference to the incidence (Vilming et al 1988).

Treatment of postlumbar puncture headache and spontaneous intracranial hypotension is similar. It begins with non-invasive therapeutic modalities of bedrest and, eventually, an abdominal binder. If there is no improvement, intravenous or oral caffeine may produce significant relief, possibly associated with the use of corticosteroids for a short period if necessary. If the patient continues to be symptomatic after a non-invasive medical approach for 2 weeks, an epidural blood patch is indicated. If the headache of intracranial hypotension recurs, an epidural blood patch can be repeated or a continuous intrathecal saline infusion may be attempted (Silberstein & Marcelis 1992).

INTRACRANIAL NEOPLASM (CODE 7.6)

Headache occurs at presentation in 36–50% of adult patients with brain tumours and develops in the course of the disease in 60% (Silberstein & Marcelis 1992). The headache is usually generalized, of the dull, deep, aching type. It is usually intermittent and relieved by simple analgesics. If there is any variation in intensity during the 24-hour cycle, it is worse in the early morning and it may be ameliorated by breakfast. Elevation of intracranial pressure is not necessary for its production. It is said to be more prominent with rapidly growing tumours than with those of slower growth, but this has been challenged in some studies. Headache is a rare initial symptom in patients with pituitary tumours, craniopharyngiomas or cerebellopontine angle tumours.

In 30–80% of patients the headache overlies the tumour. Some general rules concerning headache as an aid to localization in patients with brain tumour have been proposed by Dalessio (1989).

1. Although the headache of brain tumour may be referred from a distant source it approximately overlies the tumour in about one-third of all patients.
2. If the tumour is above the tentorium, the pain is frequently at the vertex or in the frontal region.
3. If the tumour is below the tentorium, the pain is occipital and cervical muscle spasms may be present.
4. Headache is always present with posterior fossa tumour.
5. If the tumour is midline, it may be increased with cough or strain or sudden head movement.
6. If the tumour is hemispheric, the pain is usually felt on the same side of the head.
7. If the tumour is chiasmal, at the sella, the pain may be referred to the vertex.

Headache may be a more common symptom of brain tumour in children (over 90%). The following characteristics were found to occur frequently in children with brain tumour headache: headache awakening the child from sleep or present on arising; increased severity or frequency of headache; and increased frequency of vomiting. The majority of children presenting with headache because of a brain tumour have abnormal signs on neurological examination.

In specialized headache or pain clinics, brain tumours account for less than 1% of cases. There is significant overlap between the headache of brain tumour and migraine and tension-type headache. The following clues indicate that a thorough neuroradiological examination is recommended: any headache of recent onset; a headache that has changed in character; a focalized headache not resembling one of the vascular headaches; and morning or nocturnal headache, associated with vomiting, in a non-migraineur.

8. HEADACHE ASSOCIATED WITH SUBSTANCES OR THEIR WITHDRAWAL

A new headache including migraine, tension-type headache or cluster headache in close temporal relation to substance use or withdrawal is coded to this group. As usual, type of headache may be specified with the fourth digit. As stated in the IHS classification, effective doses and temporal relationships have not yet been determined for most substances. Although headache may be caused by a number of different substances, the most significant and intriguing headaches in clinical practice are those which are induced by misuse of antiheadache medications, i.e. ergotamine and analgesic compounds.

HEADACHE INDUCED BY ACUTE SUBSTANCE USE OR EXPOSURE (CODE 8.1)

General surveys suggest that a vast number of drugs can cause headaches (Askmark et al 1989). To establish that any substance really induces headache, double-blind, placebo-controlled experiments are necessary.

There is evidence that headache can be produced by nitrates/nitrites ('hot dog headache') (code 8.1.1), monosodium glutamate ('Chinese restaurant syndrome') (code 8.1.2), carbon monoxide (code 8.1.3) or alcohol (code 8.1.4).

HEADACHE INDUCED BY CHRONIC SUBSTANCE USE OR EXPOSURE (CODE 8.2)

Diagnosis and clinical features (Table 33.13)

It can be estimated that around 10% of the patients attending a specialized headache clinic, of whom only half originally had migraine, suffer this condition (Steiner et al 1992, Olesen 1995). Drug-induced headache is a chronic, usually daily headache involving the whole skull, often described as a pressing helmet over the head (Henry 1992). Pain is exacerbated by physical exercise and intellectual effort and is often accompanied by asthenia, irritability, sleep and memory disturbances. The characteristics of chronic drug-induced headache are very similar to those of tension-type headache, except that nausea, photo- and phonophobia are much more frequent in drug-induced headache. These patients use analgesics for even the mildest headaches or even before pain appears and have a long-lasting history of abortive drug intake, with escalation over months or years of the doses needed to provide some relief. Concomitant depression or anxiety is common, as is the tendency towards tranquillizer abuse. Ergotamine, usually associated with caffeine, and combination analgesics containing codeine and/or caffeine are most often responsible for the syndrome, but more recently abuse of the selective antimigraine drugs, the triptans, was also reported in migraineurs who had a previous history of ergotamine/analgesic misuse.

Table 33.13 Headache induced by chronic substance use or exposure (code 8.2): diagnostic criteria

A. Occurs after daily doses of a substance for >3 months
B. A certain minimum dose should be indicated
C. Headache is chronic (15 days or more a month)
D. Headache disappears within 1 month after withdrawal of the substance

8.2.1 *Ergotamine-induced headache*
A. Is preceded by daily ergotamine intake (oral >2 mg, rectal >1 mg)
B. Is diffuse, pulsating and distinguished from migraine by absent attack pattern and/or absent associated symptoms

8.2.2 *Analgesic abuse headache*
One or more of the following:
1. >50 g of aspirin a month or equivalent of other analgesics
2. >100 tablets a month of analgesics combined with barbiturates or other non-narcotic compounds
3. One or more narcotic analgesics

Pathophysiology

So far, headache induced by chronic use of ergotamine and analgesics has only been described when the drugs were taken for headaches and not when they were taken for other disorders such as chronic low back pain. It remains to be determined whether pain syndromes such as the latter might also be rendered chronic by analgesic abuse. Although some side effects of ergotamine and analgesics are well known, many physicians still ignore the fact that use of these drugs in large amounts can induce chronic headaches. Moreover, analgesic abuse seems to nullify the effects of prophylactic drugs given for the original headache condition (Mathew et al 1990).

In the criteria of the IHS classification, the cumulative doses of ergotamine or analgesics capable of inducing chronic headaches are obviously overestimated. Individual susceptibility must play a role and like others, we have seen many otherwise typical cases of chronic drug-induced headache whose consumption was far less than reported in the classification (Schoenen et al 1989). The repetition of intake rather than the total dose of medication seems to be a crucial factor. The mechanisms of drug abuse headache are still poorly understood. A familial predisposition is possible. A similar clinical pattern is encountered in patients using such different drugs as analgesics, ergotamine, barbiturates or opiates. Analgesics and ergotamine might modify central neurotransmitter systems (e.g. norepinephrine, serotonin and endorphins) playing a role in the control of nociception and mood (Mathew 1987, Saper 1987). Considering the role of dopamine in central reward systems and substance abuse, the hypersensitivity of dopamine receptors (Mascia et al 1998) and DRD2 gene polymorphism (Peroutka et al 1997) found in certain migraineurs is of potential interest.

Treatment

The only treatment of drug misuse headache is complete withdrawal of the substance(s) involved (Kudrow 1982, Dichgans et al 1984). This can be done on an ambulatory basis, but management of withdrawal reactions may require a short hospitalization in some patients. These reactions include nervousness, restlessness, increased headaches, nausea, vomiting, insomnia, diarrhoea, tremor, autonomic dysfunction and even seizures in the case of barbiturate or benzodiazepine abuse (Saper 1987, Mathew et al 1990). They can be alleviated by temporary prescription of neuroleptics or tranquillizers, e.g. tiapride (75–100 mg/d) or acamprosate (1332 mg/d). We use infusions (100 mg/d for 8 days) or oral administration (75 mg/d) of clomipramine, followed by decreasing oral dosage for 2–3 months in association with prophylactic antimigraine drugs like valproate. Results of withdrawal in 121 patients were excellent in the short term (73% at 10 days, 65% at 90 days), but there was a recurrence in about 20% of patients at 6 months (Schoenen et al 1989). Kudrow (1982) suggests use of amitryptiline with the same beneficial effect; over two-thirds of patients were headache free when discharged.

Long-term prognosis primarily depends on the ability of the patient to remain free of the drug, the physician's skill in prescribing efficient prophylaxis for the original headache condition and providing appropriate psychological support (Henry et al 1985).

Education of patients and their physicians is obviously important in the prevention of this syndrome. Important steps include: limiting the prescription of ergotamine/analgesics; avoiding treatment with combined drugs including psychotropics; preferentially using single NSAID, aspirin or paracetamol compounds and triptans for the acute headache treatment; and considering prophylactic therapy whenever headache is frequent and/or incapacitating (Schoenen et al 1989).

11. HEADACHE OR FACIAL PAIN ASSOCIATED WITH DISORDER OF CRANIUM. NECK. EYES. EARS. NOSE. SINUSES. TEETH. MOUTH OR OTHER FACIAL OR CRANIAL STRUCTURES

CERVICAL SPINE (CODE 11.2.1)

Diagnosis and clinical features

Cervicogenic headache is not well defined by the criteria shown in Table 33.14. Edmeads (1988) underlines the similarities between diagnostic criteria of migraine without aura and cervicogenic headache, an opinion partly challenged by Sjaastad et al (1990). They describe cervicogenic headache as a unilateral headache, without sideshift (unlike migraine), affecting mostly women. It can be provoked by passive movements of the neck or pressure over the ipsilateral neck region. Pain can extend to ipsilateral neck, shoulder and arm, without radicular distribution. It is usually of moderate intensity, non-throbbing, starting in the neck and eventually spreading to anterior areas. Pain episodes vary in duration without clustering or there is fluctuating, almost continuous pain. If present, photophobia or blurred vision of the ipsilateral eye is mild to moderate. There is often a history of whiplash, but in Sjaastad's description, no overt reference is made to X-ray abnormalities described in the IHS diagnostic criteria (point D in Table 33.14).

Table 33.14 Cervical spine (code 11.2.1): diagnostic criteria

A. Pain localized to neck and occipital region. May project to forehead, orbital region, temple, vertex or ears

B. Pain is precipitated or aggravated by special neck movements or sustained neck posture

C. At least one of the following:
  1. Resistance to or limitation of passive neck movements
  2. Changes in neck muscle contour, texture, tone or response to active and passive stretching and contraction
  3. Abnormal tenderness of neck muscles

D. Radiological examination reveals at least one of the following:
  1. Movement abnormalities in flexion/extension
  2. Abnormal posture
  3. Fractures, congenital abnormalities, bone tumours, rheumatoid arthritis or other distinct pathology (not spondylosis or osteochondrosis)

Pathophysiology

In many cases, pain is transiently relieved by anaesthetic blockade of the greater occipital nerve (GON) not only posteriorly but also in the supraorbital area (Bovim & Sand 1992). The latter suggests that the GON might play a role in the pathophysiology of cervicogenic headache and that pain in the area of the ophthalmic division of the trigeminal nerve might indeed be due in this condition to the projection of upper cervical root (C2–C3) fibres to the spinal trigeminal complex (Kerr 1961). However, other possibly damaged structures located in the neck area (bones, muscles and arteries) can induce pain. The actual origin of the pain remains unknown and, like tension-type headache, cervicogenic headache (although triggered initially by peripheral mechanisms) might be caused in its chronic form by dysfunction of central rather than peripheral structures.

Treatment

Pharmacological treatment of cervicogenic headache is often disappointing. Analgesics and NSAIDs can provide temporary relief, but side effects of such drugs often preclude long-term treatment. Tricyclic antidepressants can also produce some benefit. As with tension-type headaches, physical therapy, relaxation and biofeedback can provide some relief (Graff-Radford et al 1987, Jaeger 1989). Besides anaesthesia of the GON, neurolysis of this nerve or of C2 roots has been performed, but results were short-lasting (Bovim et al 1992). Radiofrequency electrocoagulation has also been proposed (Blume et al 1982).

TEMPOROMANDIBULAR JOINT DISEASE (CODE 11.7)

Diagnosis and clinical features

Temporomandibular joint disease is a pain in the jaw, located to the temporomandibular joint and/or radiating from there, usually of mild to moderate intensity. It is often precipitated by movement and/or clenching the teeth. Range of movement of the joint is reduced, with tenderness of the capsule and noise ('click') during joint movements. Plain X-rays and/or scintigraphy of the temporomandibular joint are abnormal.

Pathophysiology

Pain from temporomandibular joints is common, but is rarely due to definable organic disease. By far the most frequent cause of temporomandibular pain is a myofascial one, due to oromandibular dysfunction and related to tension-type headache (see code 2). Patients with rheumatoid arthritis or generalized osteoarthrosis often show X-ray involvement of the temporomandibular joints but do not experience significantly more pain in that area than the normal population (Chalmers & Blair 1973, 1974). The so-called Costen's syndrome includes impaired hearing, tinnitus, pain in the region of the ear and vertical or occipital headache, attributed by Costen (1934) to retroposition of the head of the mandibular condyle, causing irritation of the auriculotemporal or chorda tympani nerves. Treatment of this condition would rest on the fitting of dental prostheses, stabilization splint or physical therapy (Schokker 1989).

However, 60 years after Costen's original description, pathological proof of the existence of this syndrome is still missing. Moreover, there is strong evidence that many patients with temporomandibular pain syndrome suffer from concomitant anxiety or depression and should be treated accordingly (Feinmann et al 1984).

12. CRANIAL NEURALGIA, NERVE TRUNK PAIN AND DEAFFERENTATION PAIN

HERPES ZOSTER (CODE 12.1.4.1) AND CHRONIC POSTHERPETIC NEURALGIA (CODE 12.1.4.2)

Herpes zoster affects the trigeminal ganglions in 10–15% of patients, with particular affinity for the ophthalmic division (80% of cases). Third, fourth or sixth cranial nerve palsies are sometimes observed. Herpes zoster may also involve the geniculate ganglion, with an eruption in the external auditory meatus often associated with facial nerve palsy or acoustic symptoms.

Postherpetic neuralgia (code 12.1.4.2) is a chronic pain developing during the acute phase of infection and persisting more than 6 months after the eruption. It is a frequent sequela of herpes zoster infection, affecting up to 50% of patients, particularly those of older age (Watson & Evans 1988). Its incidence is reduced by acyclovir treatment at the acute phase. Pain is felt in the area formerly involved by the infection. It is constant, moderate to severe, often described as burning. Paraesthesia or hypoaesthesia is frequent. Treatment of postherpetic neuralgia rests on tricyclic antidepressants (amitryptiline) (Max et al 1988, Watson & Evans 1988) or, when side effects are unbearable, other classes of antidepressants such as maprotiline (Watson et al 1992). Such treatments improve symptoms in about half of the patients (Watson et al 1991). Better outcome seems to be related to early treatment. Topical administration of capsaicin or analgesics can be tried in refractory cases and recently lamotrigine was found most promising.

TRIGEMINAL NEURALGIA (TIC DOULOUREUX) (CODE 12.2)

Idiopathic trigeminal neuralgia (code 12.2.1)

Diagnosis and clinical features

Trigeminal neuralgia or tic douloureux is described in detail in Chapter 32. In summary, it is characterized by very short-lasting (a few seconds to 2 minutes) attacks of intense, electric shock-like pain limited to the distribution of one or more divisions of the trigeminal nerve (see Table 33.9). Idiopathic trigeminal neuralgia more often affects women than men (ratio 3:2) and usually starts after 50 years of age. Pain can often be triggered by trivial stimuli such as washing, shaving, chewing, brushing the teeth or speaking. It may also occur spontaneously. Painful episodes start and end abruptly, may recur dozens of times in a single day but interfere little with sleep. Remissions of variable duration are described. In most cases, pain is restricted to the second or third divisions of the trigeminal nerve. It never crosses the midline, but a few patients (less than 5%) have bilateral attacks. The pain often induces reflex spasms of facial muscles on the affected side, hence the name 'tic douloureux'.

Pathophysiology

It is currently believed that in many cases, so-called idiopathic trigeminal neuralgia might result from local demyelination of the trigeminal root entry zone due to compressions in the posterior fossa, usually by small tortuous arteries or veins (Jannetta 1970). Favouring this hypothesis, it has been shown that surgical decompression of the trigeminal root can induce prolonged remissions (Taarnhoj 1982). Thus, many cases of idiopathic trigeminal neuralgia should in fact be considered symptomatic. The painful episodes are thought to result from repetitive and aberrant electric discharges (ephaptic transmission) originating in the axons of the demyelinated segment (Loeser et al 1977).

Treatment

More than two-thirds of patients with idiopathic trigeminal neuralgia respond favourably to drug treatment with carbamazepine (200–400 mg tid) or in refractory cases, carbamazepine plus baclofen (25 mg tid) or plus clonazepam (2 mg tid) or phenytoin (200–300 mg/d) or lomotrigine (200–400 mg/d). For refractory cases, thermocoagulation of the Gasserian ganglion can be proposed or microsurgical decompression of the trigeminal root in the posterior fossa (Jannetta 1970). Radiofrequency thermocoagulation of the Gasserian ganglion is safe and can be performed even in very old patients. The relapse rate is variable (21–85%), depending on the duration of follow-up and the depth of anaesthesia produced. Side effects include anaesthesia dolorosa (2–3%), numbness and paraesthesia (15–50%) and corneal anaesthesia (1–8%). Posterior fossa decompression is a more serious procedure, although the reported perioperative mortality is low (1–2%) (Jannetta 1981, Apfelbaum 1982). Long-term complete relief is achieved in about 70–75% of cases, but some patients still need some drugs and a minority (4–6%) develop permanent cranial nerve palsies (usually of the eighth, but sometimes of the fourth or seventh nerves).

Symptomatic trigeminal neuralgia (code 12.2.2)

Besides microvascular compressions, several diseases can produce trigeminal neuralgia, such as acoustic neurinomas, brainstem infarcts and, chiefly, multiple sclerosis. The main differences from the idiopathic form are a younger age at onset, persistence of aching between paroxysms and signs of sensory impairment in the distribution of the corresponding trigeminal division.

GLOSSOPHARYNGEAL (CODE 12.3) AND NERVUS INTERMEDIUS (CODE 12.4) NEURALGIAS

These forms of neuralgia are uncommon and their pathophysiology and treatment are similar to those of trigeminal neuralgia. The attack pattern is also similar, with very short paroxysms. Glossopharyngeal neuralgia is characterized by unilateral attacks of transient stabbing pain in the ear, base of tongue, tonsillar fossa or beneath the angle of the jaw. It is provoked by swallowing, talking and coughing. Neuralgia of the nervus intermedius is felt deeply in the ear, lasting for seconds or minutes, with a trigger zone in the posterior wall of the auditory canal.

FACIAL PAIN NOT FULFILLING CRITERIA IN GROUPS 11 AND 12 (CODE 12.8)

Many patients, usually middle-aged women, complain of facial pain which cannot be put into one of the previous categories (atypical facial pain). Pain is described as burning or aching, is present daily and persists for most of the day. At onset, it is confined to a limited area on one side of the face but later it may spread to the upper and lower jaws or a wider area of the face and neck. It is poorly localized and does not fit with the sensory distribution of a trigeminal branch. Clinical examination and paraclinical investigations are fully normal. Pain is often triggered by operations or injuries to the face or dental problems, but becomes chronic without any demonstrable lesion. Such patients often exhibit depressive traits (Lascelles 1966). Tricyclic antidepressants may provide some relief.

Exceptionally, unilateral facial pain mimicking atypical facial pain is due to lung cancer compressing the vagus nerve (Schoenen et al 1992).

 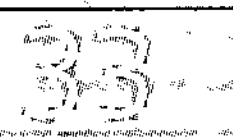

CONCLUSION

The operational diagnostic criteria of the IHS headache classification allow a more uniform grouping of headache types for research purposes. Their usefulness in routine clinical practice is limited. When confronted with a headache patient, the practitioner first has to decide whether the headache is symptomatic of an underlying disease or whether it is a 'primary' headache.

With few exceptions, any headache of recent onset should, as a rule, be considered to be symptomatic. Recognizing the cause needs, above all, clinical skill and an adequate choice of paraclinical investigations.

Most chronic headaches correspond to one of the primary headache types. Many, if not all, are probably biobehavioural disorders, resulting from a complex, variable interplay between neurobiological (in part genetically determined) mechanisms and behavioural processes influenced by environmental factors. Treatment of these patients, besides alleviating the symptom 'head pain', has to be directed towards both body and mind.

REFERENCES

Abu-Arefeh I, Russell G 1994 Prevalence of headache and migraine in schoolchildren. British Medical Journal 309: 765–769

Afra J, Mascia D, Gèrard P et al 1998a Interictal cortical excitability in migraine: a study using transcranial magnetic stimulation of motor and visual cortices. Annals of Neurology, 44: 209–215

Afra J, Proietti Cecchin A, De Pasqua V et al 1998b Visual evoked potentials during long-lasting pattern-reversal stimulations in migraine. Brain 121: 233–241

Afra J, Proietti Cecchini A, Schoenen J 1998c Craniometric measures in cluster headache patients. Cephalalgia 18: 143–145

Amery WK, Vandenbergh V 1987 What can precipitating factors teach us about the pathogenesis of migraine? Headache 27: 146–150

Andrasik F, Passchier J 1993 Tension-type headache, cluster headache, and miscellaneous headaches: psychological aspects. In: Olesen J, Tfelt-Hansen P, Welch KMA (eds) The headaches. Raven Press, New York, pp 489–492

Apfelbaum RI 1982 Microvascular decompression for tic douloureux. In: Brackman DE (ed) Neurological surgery of the ear and skull base. Raven Press, New York, pp 175–180

Askmark H, Lundberg O, Olsson S 1989 Drug related headache. Headache 29: 441–444

Barbiroli B, Montagna P, Cortelli P et al 1992 Abnormal brain and muscle energy metabolism shown by 31P magnetic resonance spectroscopy in patients affected by migraine with aura. Neurology 42: 1209–1214

Barkley GL, Tepley N, Simkins RT et al 1990 Neuromagnetic findings in migraine. Preliminary findings. Cephalalgia 10: 171–176

Bendtsen L, Jensen R, Olesen J 1996a A non-selective (amitriptyline), but not a selective (citalopram), serotonin reuptake inhibitor is effective in the prophylactic treatment of chronic tension-type headache. Journal of Neurology, Neurosurgery and Psychiatry 61: 285–290

Bendtsen L, Jensen R, Olesen J 1996b Qualitatively altered nociception in chronic myofascial pain. Pain 65: 259–264

Berlit P 1992 Clinical and laboratory findings with giant cell arteritis. Journal of the Neurological Sciences 111: 1–12

Bès A, Fabre N 1992 Débit sanguin cérébral et migraine sans aura. Pathologie et Biologie 40: 325–331

Bille B 1962 Migraine in school children. Acta Paediatrica 51, (suppl. 136): 3–151

Biousse V, Woimant F, Amarenco P et al 1992 Pain as the only manifestation of internal carotid artery dissection. Cephalalgia 12: 314–317

Blanchard EB, Appelbaum KA, Guarnieri P et al 1987 Five year follow-up on the treatment of chronic headache with biofeedback and/or relaxation. Headache 27: 580–583

Blau JN 1980 Migraine prodromes separated from the aura: complete migraine. British Medical Journal 281: 658–660

Blume H, Kakolewski R, Richardson R 1982 Radiofrequency denaturation in occipital pain: results in 450 cases. Applied Neurophysiology 45: 543–548

Bogaards MC, ter Kuile MM 1994 Treatment of recurrent tension headache: a meta-analytic review. Clinical Journal of Pain 10: 174–190

Bovim G 1992 Cervicogenic headache, migraine and tension-type headache. Pressure pain thresholds measurements. Pain 51: 169–173

Bovim G, Sand T 1992 Cervicogenic headache, migraine without aura and tension-type headache. Diagnostic blockade of greater occipital and supraorbital nerves. Pain 51: 43–48

Bovim G, Fredriksen TA, Stolt-Nielsen A, Sjaastad O 1992 Neurolysis of the greater occipital nerve in cervicogenic headache. A follow-up study. Headache 32: 175–179

Breslau N, Merikangas K, Bowden CL 1996 Comorbidity of migraine and major affective disorders. Neurology 44, (suppl. 7): S56–62

Bures J, Buresova O, Krivanek J 1974 The mechanism and applications of Leão's spreading depression on electroencephalographic activity. Academic Press, New York

Buzzi G, Moskowitz MA 1992 The trigeminovascular system and migraine. Pathologie et biologie 40: 313–317

Caekebeke JFV, Ferrari MD, Zwetsloot CP et al 1992 Antimigraine drug sumatriptan increases blood flow velocity in large cerebral arteries during migraine attacks. Neurology 42: 1522–1526

Cervero F, Jänig W 1992 Visceral nociceptors: a new world order? Trends in Neuroscience 15: 374–378

Chalmers IM, Blair GS 1973 Rheumatoid arthritis of the temporomandibular joint. Quarterly Journal of Medicine 42: 369–386

Chalmers IM, Blair GS 1974 Is the temporomandibular joint involved in primary osteoarthrosis? Oral Surgery, Oral Medicine, Oral Pathology 38: 74–79

Chmelewski WL, McKnight KM, Agudelo CA, Wise CM 1992 Presenting features and outcomes in patients undergoing temporal artery biopsy: a review of 98 patients. Archives of Internal Medicine 152: 1690–1695

Chu ML, Shinnar S 1991 Headaches in children younger than 7 years of age. Archives of Neurology 49: 79–82

Cook JB 1972 The postconcussional syndrome and factors influencing after minor head injury admitted to hospital. Scandinavian Journal of Rehabilitation Medicine 4: 27–30

Costen JB 1934 A syndrome of ear and sinus symptoms dependent upon disturbed function of the temporomandibular joint. Annals of Otology, Rhinology and Laryngology 43: 1–15

Couch JR, Micieli G 1993 Tension-type headache, cluster headache, and miscellaneous headaches: prophylactic pharmacotherapy. In: Olesen J, Tfelt-Hansen P, Welch KMA (eds): The headaches. Raven Press, New York, pp537–542

Cutrer FM, Sorensen AG, Weisskoff RM et al 1998 Perfusion-weighted imaging defects during spontaneous migrainous aura. Annals of Neurology 43: 25–31

D'Andrea G, Hasselmark L, Alecci M et al 1993 Increased platelet serotonin content and hypersecretion from dense and α-granules in vitro in tension-type headache. Cephalalgia 13: 349–353

Dahlöf CGH, Jacobs LD 1996 Ketoprofen paracetamol and placebo in the treatment of episodic tension-type headache. Cephalalagia 16: 117–123

Dalessio DJ 1989 Headache. In: Wall PD, Melzack R (eds) Textbook of pain 2nd edn. Churchill Livingstone, Edinburgh, pp386–401

Diamond S 1984 The value of biofeedback in the treatment of chronic headache: a four-year retrospective study. Headache 25: 5–18

Dichgans J, Diener HC, Gerber WD et al 1984 Analgetikainduzierter Dauerkopfsschmerz. Deutsche Medizinische Wochenschrift 109: 369–373

Diener HC, Föh M, Iaccarino C et al on behalf of the Study Group 1996: Cyclandelate in the prophylaxis of migraine: a randomized, parallel, double-blind study in comparison with placebo and propranolol. Cephalalgia 16: 441–447

Drummond PD 1987 Scalp tenderness and sensitivity to pain in migraine and tension-type headache. Headache 27: 45

Ducros A, Juotel A, Vahedi K et al 1997 Mapping of a second locus for familial hemiplegic migraine to 1q21–23 and evidence of further genetic heterogeneity. Annals of Neurology 45: 885–890

Edmeads J: Headache in cerebrovascular disease 1986 In: Viken PJ, Bruyn GW, Klawans HL (eds) Handbook of clinical neurology, vol 4 (48), Elsevier, Amsterdam, pp 273–290

Edmeads J 1988 The cervical spine and headache. Neurology 38: 1874–1878

Ekbom K 1986 Chronic migrainous neuralgia. In: Vinken PJ, Bruyn GW, Klawans HL (eds) Handbook of clinical neurology, vol 4(48), Elsevier, Amsterdam pp 247–255

Ekbom K 1995 Treatment of cluster headache: clinical trials, design and results. Cephalalgia, 15: 33–36

Fanciullacci M, Alessandri M, Figini M et al 1995 Increase in plasma calcitonin gene-related peptide from the extracerebral circulation during nitroglycerin-induced cluster headache attack. Pain 60: 119–123

Feinmann C, Harris M, Cawley R 1984 Psychogenic facial pain: presentation and treatment. British Medical Journal 88: 436–438

Ferrari MD 1992 Biochemistry of migraine. Pathologie et Biologie 40: 287–292

Ferrari MD 1998 Migraine. The Lancet 351: 1043–1051

Ferrari MD, Odink J, Frölich M et al 1990 Methionine-Enkephalin in migraine and tension headache. Differences between classic migraine, common migraine and tension headache, and changes during attacks. Headache 30: 160–164

Ford ERG, Ford KT, Swaid S et al 1998 Gamma knife treatment of refractory cluster headache. Headache 38: 3–9

Forsell H, Kirveskari P, Kangasniemi P 1985 Changes in headache after treatment of mandibular dysfunction. Cephalalgia 5: 229–236

Franceschini R, Leandri M, Cataldi A et al 1995 Raised plasma arginine vasopressin concentrations during cluster headache attacks. Journal of Neurology, Neurosurgery and Psychiatry 59: 381–383

Friberg L, Olesen J, Iversen HK et al 1991 Migraine pain associated with middle cerebral artery dilatation: reversal by sumatriptan. Lancet 338: 13–17

Gardiner IM, Ahmed F, Steiner TJ et al 1998 A study of adaptive responses in cell signaling in migraine and cluster headache: correlations between headache type and changes in gene expression. Cephalalgia 18: 192–196

Gardner K, Hofman EP 1997 Current status of genetic discoveries in migraine: familial hemiplegic migraine and beyond. Current Opinion in Neurology 11: 211–216

Goadsby PJ 1997 Pathophysiology of migraine: a disease of the brain In: Headache. Blue books of practical neurology. vol 14. Butterworth-Heinemann, Newton, pp 5–24

Goadsby PJ 1998 A triptan too far. Journal of Neurology, Neurosurgery and Psychiatry 64: 143–147

Goadsby PJ, Hoskin KJ 1996 Inhibition of trigeminal neurons by intravenous administration of the serotonin (5-HT) 1B/D receptor agonist zolmitriptan (311C90): are brain stem sites therapeutic target in migraine? Pain 67: 355–359

Goadsby PJ, Edvinsson L, Ekman R 1989 Extracerebral levels of circulating vasoactive peptides during migraine headache. Cephalalgia 9 (suppl. 10): 292–293

Goadsby PJ, Edvinsson L 1994 Human in vivo evidence for trigeminovascular activation in cluster headache. Neuropeptide changes and effects of acute attacks therapies. Brain 117: 427–434

Goadsby PJ, Edvinsson L, Ekman R 1990 Vasoactive peptide release in the extracerebral circulation of humans during migraine headache. Annals of Neurology 28: 183–187

Goadsby PJ, Edvinsson 1994 Human in vivo evidence for trigeminovascular activation in cluster headache. Neuropeptide changes and effects of acute attacks therapies. Brain 117: 427–434

Graff-Radford SB, Reeves JL, Jaeger B 1987 Management of chronic head and neck pain: effectiveness of altering factors perpetuating myofascial pain. Headache 27: 180–185

Göbel H, Schenkl S 1989 Post-lumbar puncture headache: the relation between experimental suprathreshold pain sensitivity and a quasi-experimental clinical pain syndrome. Pain 40: 267–278

Göbel H, Weigle L, Kropp P et al 1992 Pain sensitivity and pain reactivity of pericranial muscles in migraine and tension-type headache. Cephalalgia 12: 142–151

Haddock CK, Rowan AB, Andrasik F et al 1997 Home-based behavioral treatments for chronic benign headache: a meta-analysis of controlled trials. Cephalalgia 17: 113–118

Hardebo JE, Moskowitz MA 1993 Synthesis of cluster headache pathophysiology. In: Olesen J, Tfelt-Hansen P, Welch KMA (eds) The headaches. Raven Press, New York, pp 576–596

Hegerl U, Juckel G 1993 Intensity dependence of auditory evoked potentials as an indicator of central serotonergic neurotransmission: a new hypothesis. Biological Psychiatry 33: 173–187

Henry P 1992 Drug abuse in headache. Functional Neurology 6 (suppl. 7) 5–6

Henry P, Dartigues JF, Benetier MP et al 1985 Ergotamine and analgesic induced headache. Controlled study of the use of electrical stimulation by high frequency current. In: Clifford-Rose F (ed) Migraine: clinical and research advances. Karger, Basle, pp 195–207

Henry P, Michel P, Brochet B et al 1992 A nationwide survey of migraine in France: prevalence and clinical features in adults. Cephalalgia 12: 229–237

Hering R, Kuritzky A 1992 Sodium valproate in the prophylactic treatment of migraine: a double-blind study versus placebo. Cephalalgia 12: 81–84

Hickling EJ, Blanchard EB, Silverman DJ et al 1992 Motor vehicle accidents, headaches and post-traumatic stress disorder: assessment findings in a consecutive series. Headache 32: 147–151

Holroyd KA 1993 Tension-type headache, cluster headache, and miscellaneous headaches: Psychological and behavioral techniques. In: Olesen J, Tfelt-Hansen P, Welch KMA (eds) The headaches. Raven Press, New York, pp 515–520

Holroyd KA, Penzien DB 1986 Client variables and behavioral treatment of recurrent tension headaches: a meta-analytic review. Journal of Behavioural Medicine 9: 515–536

Holroyd KA, Penzien DB, Holm JE et al 1984 Behavioural treatment of tension and migraine headache: what does the literature say? Headache 24: 167–168

Humphrey PPA 1991 5-hydroxytryptamine and the pathophysiology of migraine. Journal of Neurology 238: S38–44

Humphrey PPA, Feniuk W 1991 Mode of action of the anti-migraine drug sumatriptan. Trends in Pharmacology 12: 444–446

International Headache Society 1998 Classification and diagnostic criteria for headache disorders, cranial neuralgias and facial pain. Cephalalgia 8 (suppl. 7) 1–96

International Headache Society Committee on Clinical Trials 1995 Guidelines for trials of drug treatments in tension-type headache. Cephalalgia 15: 165–179

Italian Cooperative Study Group on the Epidemiology of Cluster Headache (ICECH) 1995 Case-control study on the epidemiology of cluster headache. I: Etiological factors and associated conditions. Neuroepidemiology 14: 123–127

Jaeger B 1989 Are (cervicogenic) headaches due to myofascial pain and cervical spine dysfunction? Cephalalgia 9: 157–164

Jannetta PJ 1970 Observations on the etiology of trigeminal neuralgia, hemifacial spasm, acoustic nerve dysfunction and glossopharyngeal neuralgia: definitive microsurgical treatment and results in 117 cases. Neurochirurgia 20: 145–154

Jannetta PJ 1981 Vascular decompression in trigeminal neuralgia. In: Samii M, Jannetta PJ (eds): The cranial nerves. Springer, Berlin, pp 331–340

Jensen OK, Nielsen FF 1990 The influence of sex and pre-traumatic headache on the incidence and severity of headache after head injury. Cephalalgia 1: 285–294

Jensen R, Hindberg I 1994 Plasma serotonin increase during episodes of tension-type headache. Cephalalgia 14: 219–222

Jensen R, Olesen J 1996 Initiating mechanisms of experimentally induced tension-type headache. Cephalalgia 16: 175

Jensen R, Rasmussen BK, Pedersen B et al 1993a Cephalic muscle tenderness and pressure pain threshold in headache. Pain 52: 193–199

Jensen R, Rasmussen BK, Pedersen B et al 1993b Oromandibular disorders in a general population. Journal of Craniomandibular Disorders, Facial and Oral Pain 7: 175–182

Jensen R, Brinck T, Olesen J 1994 Sodium valproate has a prophylactic effect in migraine without aura: a triple-blind, placebo-controlled crossover study. Neurology 44: 647–651

Joutel A, Bousser MG, Biousse V et al 1993 A gene for familial hemiplegic migraine maps to chromosone 19. Nature Genetics 5: 40–45

Kay DWK, Kerr TA, Lassman LP 1971 Brain trauma and the postconcussional syndrome. Lancet 2: 1052–1055

Keidel M, Diener HC 1997 Post-traumatic headache. Nervenarzt 68: 769–777

Kelly RE 1986 Post-traumatic headache. In: Vinken PJ, Bruyn GW, Klawans HL (eds) Handbook of clinical neurology, vol 4(48) Elsevier, Amsterdam, pp 383–390

Kerr FWL 1961 Structural relation of the trigeminal spinal tract to upper cervical roots and the solitary nucleus in cat. Experimental Neurology 4: 134–148

Kraus RL, Sinnegger MJ, Glossmann H et al 1998 Familial hemiplegic migraine mutations change (1A Ca2+ channel kinetics. Journal of Biological Chemistry 273: 5586–5590

Kropp P, Gerber WD 1993 Is increased amplitude of contingent negative variation in migraine due to cortical hyperativity or to reduced habituation? Cephalalgia 13: 37–41

Kropp P, Gerber WD 1995 Contingent negative variation during migraine attack and interval: evidence for normalization of slow cortical potentials during the attack. Cephalalgia 15: 123–128

Kudrow L 1982 Paradoxical effects of frequent analgesic use. Advances in Neurology 3: 335–341

Kuntz KM, Kohmen E, Stevens JC et al 1992 Post-lumbar puncture headaches: experience in 501 consecutive procedures. Neurology 42: 1884–1887

Lance JW, Lambert GA, Goadsby PJ et al 1983 Brain-stem influences on the cephalic circulation: experimental data from cat and monkey of relevance to mechanisms of migraine. Headache 23: 258–265

Langemark M, Bach FW, Ekman R, Olesen J 1990a Increased CSF levels of met-enkephalin in chronic tension-type headache. Pain, suppl 5: S43

Langemark M, Jensen K, Olesen J 1990b Temporal muscle blood flow in chronic tension-type headache. Archives of Neurology 47: 654–658

Lascelles RG 1966 Atypical facial pain and depression. British Journal of Psychiatry 112: 651–659

Lashley KS 1941 Patterns of cerebral integration indicated by the scotomas of migraine. Archives of Neurology and Psychiatry 46: 331–339

Lauritzen M 1992 Spreading depression and migraine. Pathology et Biologie 40: 332–337

Leão AA 1944 Spreading depression of activity in cerebral cortex. Journal of Neurophysiology 7: 359–390

Leão AA, Morrison RS 1945 Propagation of spreading cortical depression. Journal of Neurophysiology 8: 33–35

Lenaerts M, Pepin J-L, Tombu S, Schoenen J 1993 No significant effect of an 'atraumatic' needle on incidence of post-lumbar puncture headache or traumatic tap. Cephalalgia 13: 296–297

Leone M, Maltempo C, Gritti A, Bussone G 1994 The insulin tolerance test and ovine corticotrophin-releasing-hormone test in episodic cluster headache. II: comparison with low back pain patients. Cephalalgia 14: 357–364

Lewis TA, Solomon GD 1996 Advances in cluster headache management. Cleveland Clinic Journal of Medicine 63: 237–244

Lipchick GL, Holroyd KA, France CR et al 1996 Central and peripheral mechanisms in chronic tension-type headache. Pain 64: 467–475

Lipton RB, Stewart WF, Von Korff M 1994 The burden of migraine: a review of cost to society. Pharmacoeconomics 6: 215–221

Loeser JD, Calvin WH, Howe JF 1977 Pathophysiology of trigeminal neuralgia. Clinical Neurosurgery 24: 527–537.

Longmore J, Shaw D, Hopkins R et al 1997 Differential distribution of 5HT1D- and 5HT1B-immunoreactivity within the human trigemino-cerebrovascular system: implications for the discovery of new antimigraine drugs. Cephalalgia 17: 833–842

Lozza A, Schoenen J, Delwaide PJ 1997 Inhibition of the blink reflex R2 component after supraorbital and index finger stimulations is reduced in cluster headache: an indication for both segmental and suprasegmental dysfunction? Pain 7: 81–88

MacGregor EA, Chia H, Vohrah RC et al 1990 Migraine and menstruation: a pilot study. Cephalalgia 10: 305–310

Maertens de Noordhout A, Timsit-Berthier M, Schoenen J 1986 Contingent negative variation in headache. Annals of Neurology 1: 78–80

Marcelis J, Silberstein SD 1991 Idiopathic intracranial hypertension without papilloedoma. Archives of Neurology 48: 392–399

Markus HS 1991 A prospective follow-up thunderclap headache mimicking subarachnoid haemorrhage. Journal Neuro Neurosurgery Psychiatry 54: 1117–1118

Mascia A, Áfra J, Schoenen J 1998 Dopamine and migraine: a review of pharmacological, biochemical, neurophysiological, and therapeutic data. Cephalalgia 18: 174–182

Massiou H, Bousser MJ 1992 Bêta-bloquants et migraine. Pathologie et Biologie 40: 373–380

Mathew NT 1987 Transformed or evolutive migraine. In: Clifford-Rose F (ed) Advances in headache research. John Libbey, London, pp 241–247

Mathew NT 1993 Tension-type headache, cluster headache, and miscellaneous headaches: Acute pharmacotherapy. In: Olesen J, Tfelt-Hansen P, Welch KMA (eds) The headaches. Raven Press, New York, pp.531–536

Mathew NT, Kurman R, Perez F 1990 Drug induced refractory headache. Headache 30: 634–638
Mathew NT, Saper JR, Silberstein SD et al 1995 Migraine Prophylaxis with Divalproex. Archives of Neurology 52: 2481–286
Max B, Schafer SC, Culnane M et al 1988 Amitriptyline, but not lorazepam, relieves post-herpetic neuralgia. Neurology 38: 1427–1432
May A, Bahra A, Büchel C et al 1998 First direct evidence for hypothalamic activation in cluster headache attacks. Lancet 352: 275–278
Milner PM 1958 Note on a possible correspondence between the scotomas of migraine and spreading depression of Leão. EEG and Clinical Neurophysiology 10: 705
Mitsias P, Ramadan NM 1992 Headache in cerebrovascular disease. Part I: Clinical features. Cephalalgia 12: 269–274
Monstad I, Krabbe A, Micieli G et al 1995 Preemptive oral treatment with sumatriptan during a cluster period. Headache 35: 607–613
Montagna P, Sayuegna T, Cortelli P et al 1989 Migraine as a defect of brain oxidative metabolism: a hypothesis. Journal of Neurology 236: 124–125
Montagna P, Cortelli P, Monari L et al 1994 31P-Magnetic resonance spectroscopy in migraine without aura. Neurology 44: 666–668
Moskowitz MA 1984 Neurobiology of vascular head pain. Annals of Neurology 6: 157–168
Moskowitz MA 1991 The visceral organ brain: implications for the pathophysiology of vascular head pain. Neurology 41: 182–186
Moskowitz MA, MacFarlane R 1993 Neurovascular and molecular mechanisms in migraine headaches. Cerebrovascular Brain Metabolism Review 5: 159–177
Nappi G, Ferrari E, Polleri A et al 1981 Chronobiological study in cluster headache. Chronobiologia 2: 140
Nyholt DR, Dawkins JL, Brimage PJ et al 1998 Evidence for an X-linked genetic component in familial typical migraine. Human Molecular Genetics 7: 459–463
Ogilvie AD, Russell MB, Dhall P et al 1998 Altered allelic distributions of the serotonin transporter gene in migraine without aura and migraine with aura. Cephalalgia 18: 23–26
Olesen J 1991 Clinical and pathophysiological observations in migraine and tension-type headache explained by integration of vascular, supraspinal and myofascial inputs. Pain 46: 125–132
Olesen J 1992 Cerebral blood flow in migraine with aura. Pathologie et Biologie 40: 318–324
Olesen J, Analpesic headache. British Medical Journal 370: 479–480.
Olesen J, Schoenen J 1993 Tension-type headache, cluster headache, and miscellaneous headaches: synthesis. In: Olesen J, Tfelt-Hansen P, Welch KMA (eds) The headaches. Raven Press, New York pp 493–496
Olesen J, Larsen B, Lauritzen M 1981 Focal hyperemia followed by spreading oligemia and impaired activation of rCBF in classic migraine. Annals of Neurology 9: 344–352
Olesen J, Friberg L, Olsen TS et al 1990 Timing and topography of cerebral blood flow, aura, and headache during migraine attacks. Annals of Neurology 28: 791–798
Olesen J, Iversen HK, Thomsen LL 1993 Nitric oxide supersensitivity. A possible molecular mechanism of migraine pain. Neuroreport 4: 1027–1030
Ollat H 1992 Agonistes et antagonistes de la sèrotonine et migraine. Pathologie et Biologie 40: 389–396
Ollat H, Gurruchaga JM 1992 Plaquettes et migraine. Pathologie et Biologie 40: 305–312
Ophoff RA, Terwindt GM, Vergouwe MN et al 1996 Familial hemiplegic migraine and episodic ataxia type-2 are caused by mutations in the Ca2+ channel gene CACNL1A4. Cell 87: 543–552
Ottman R, Lipton RB 1994 Comorbidity of migraine and epilepsy. Neurology 44: 2105–2110
Pascual J, Iglesias F, Oterino A et al 1996 Cough, exertional, and sexual headaches: an analysis of 72 benign and symptomatic cases. Neurology 46: 1520–1524
Peikert A, Wilimzig C, Köfhne-Volland R 1996 Prophylaxis of migraine with oral magnesium: results from a prospective, multi-center, placebo-controlled and double-blind randomized study. Cephalalgia 16: 257–263
Peroutka SJ, Wilhoit T, Jones K 1997 Clinical susceptibility to migraine with aura is modified by dopamine D2 receptor (DRD2) NcoI alleles. Neurology 49: 201–206
Pradalier A, Giroud M, Dry J 1987 Somnambulism, migraine and propranolol. Headache 27: 143–145
Proietti Cecchini A, Afra J, Schoenen J 1997a Intensity dependence of the cortical auditory evoked potentials as a surrogate marker of CNS serotonin transmission in man: demonstration of a central effect for the 5-HT 1B/1D agonist zolmitriptan (311C90, Zomig().Cephalalgia 17: 849–854
Proietti Cecchini A, Afra J, Maertens de Noordhout A et al 1997b Modulation of pressure pain thresholds during isometric contraction in patients with chronic tension-type headache and/or generalized myofascial pain compared to healthy volunteers. Neurology 48: A258, PO4.118
Ramadan NM, Halvorsen H, Vande-Linde A et al 1989 Low brain magnesium in migraine. Headache 29: 590–593
Rando TA, Fishman RA 1992 Spontaneous intracranial hypotension. Neurology 42: 481–487
Rasmussen BK, Olesen J 1992 Migraine with aura and migraine without aura: an epidemiological study. Cephalalgia 12: 221–228
Rasmussen BK, Jensen R, Schroll M et al 1991 Epidemiology of headache in a general population – a prevalence study. Journal of Clinical Epidemiology 44: 1147–1157
Rasmussen BK, Jensen R, Schroll M, Olesen J 1992 Interrelations between migraine and tension-type headache in the general population. Archives of Neurology 49: 914–918
Reinecke M, Konen T, Langohr HD 1991 Autonomic cerebrovascular reactivity and exteroceptive suppression of temporalis muscle activity in migraine and tension-type headaches. In: Clifford Rose F (ed). New advances in headache research. Smith-Gordon,
Ross Russell RW 1986 Giant cell (cranial) arteritis. In: Vinken PJ, Bruyn GW, Klawans HL (eds) Handbook of clinical neurology, vol. 4(48) Elsevier, Amsterdam, pp 309–328
Russell MB, Olesen J 1995 Increased familial risk and evidence in genetic factor in migraine. British Medical Journal 311: 541–544
Russell WR 1932 Cerebral involvement in head injury; a study based on the examination of 200 cases. Brain 55: 549–570
Ryan RE 1977 Motrin – a new agent for symptomatic treatment of muscle contraction headache. Headache 16: 280–283
Sanders M, Zuurmond WW 1997 Efficacy of sphenophalatine ganglion blockade in 66 patients suffering from cluster headache: a 12- to 70-month follow-up evaluation. Journal of Neurosurgery 87: 876–880
Saper JR 1987 Ergotamine dependency. A review. Headache 27: 435–438
Sappey-Marinier D, Galabrese G, Fein G et al 1992 Effect of photic stimulation on human visual cortex lactate and phosphates using 1H and 31P magnetic resonance spectroscopy. Journal of Cerebral Blood Flow and Metabolism 12: 584–592
Schachtel BP, Furey SA, Thoden WR 1996 Nonprescription ibuprofen and acetaminophen in the treatment of tension-type headache. Journal of Clinical Pharmacology 36: 1120–1125
Schoenen J 1992 Clinical neurophysiology studies in headache: a review of data and pathophysiological hints. Functional Neurology 7: 191–204
Schoenen J 1994 Pathogenesis of migraine: the biobehavioural and hypoxia theories reconciled. Acta Neurologica Belgica 94: 79–86

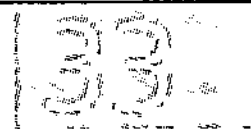

Schoenen J 1997 Acute migraine therapy: the newer drugs. Current Opinion in Neurology 10: 237–243

Schoenen J 1998a Cluster headache – Central or peripheral in origin. Lancet 352: 253–255

Schoenen J 1998b Cortical electrophysiology in migraine and possible pathogenetic implications. Clinical Neuroscience 5: 10–17

Schoenen J, Timsit-Berthier M 1993 Contingent negative variation: methods and potential interest in headache. Cephalalgia 13: 28–32

Schoenen J, Wang W 1997 Tension-type headache. In : Goadsby PJ, Silberstein SJ (eds): Headache Butterworth-Heinemann, Boston, pp 177–200

Schoenen J, Jamart B, Delwaide PJ 1987a Topographic EEG mapping in common and classic migraine during and between attacks. In: Clifford Rose F (ed) Advances in headache research. Smith Gordon, London, pp 25–33

Schoenen J, Jamart B, Gèrard P et al 1987b Exteroceptive suppression of temporalis muscle activity in chronic headache. Neurology 37: 1834–1836

Schoenen J, Lenarduzzi P, Sianard-Gainko J 1989 Chronic headaches associated with analgesics and/or ergotamine abuse: a clinical survey of 434 consecutive out patients. In: Clifford Rose F (ed) New advances in headache research. Smith Gordon, London, pp 255–259

Schoenen J, Bottin D, Hardy F, Gèrard P 1991a Cephalic and extracephalic pressure pain thresholds in chronic tension-type headache. Pain 47: 145–149

Schoenen J, Gèrard P, De Pasqua V, Sianard-Gainko J 1991b Multiple clinical and paraclinical analyses of chronic tension-type headache associated or unassociated with disorder of pericranial muscles. Cephalalgia 11: 135–139

Schoenen J, Sianard-Gainko J, Lenaerts M 1991c Blood magnesium levels in migraine. Cephalalgia 11: 97–99

Schoenen J, Broux R, Moonen G 1992 Unilateral facial pain as the first symptom of lung cancer: are there diagnostic clues? Cephalalgia 12: 178–179

Schoenen J, Wang W, Albert A, Delwaide PJ 1995 Potentiation instead of habituation characterizes visual evoked potentials in migraine patients between attacks. European Journal of Neurology 2: 115–122

Schoenen J, Jacquy J, Lenaerts M 1998 Effectiveness of high-dose riboflavin in migraine prophylaxis: a randomized controlled trial. Neurology 50: 466–470

Schokker P 1989 Craniomandibular disorders in headache patients. Thesis. University of Amsterdam

Schokker RP, Hansson TL, Ansink BJ 1990 The results of treatment of the masticatory system of chronic headache patients J Craniomandib Disord Facial Oral Pain 4: 126–130

Schrader H, Obelieniene D, Bovim G et al 1996 Natural evolution of late whiplash syndrome outside the medicolegal context. Lancet 347 (9010): 1207–1211

Silberstein SD, Marcelis J 1992 Headache associated with changes in intracranial pressure. Headache 32: 84–94

Sjaastad O 1986 Cluster headache. In: Vinken PJ, Bruyn GW, Klawans HL (eds) Handbook of clinical neurology, vol. 4(48). Elsevier, Amsterdam, pp 217–246

Sjaastad O 1992 Cluster headache syndrome. In: Major problems in neurology vol 23. WB Saunders, London

Sjaastad O, Dale I 1974 Evidence for a new (?) treatable headache entity. Headache 14: 105–108

Sjaastad O, Saunte C, Salvesen R et al 1989 Shortlasting, unilateral, neuralgiform headache attacks with conjunctival injection, tearing, sweating, and rhinorrhea. Cephalalgia 9: 147–156

Sjaastad O, Fredriksen TA, Pfaffenrath V 1990 Cervicogenic headache diagnostic criteria. Headache 30: 25–26

Solomon S, Newman LC 1998 Classification of post-traumatic migraine. Neurology 48: PO4.128

Solomon S, Lipton RB, Newman LO 1992 Evaluation of chronic daily headache – comparison to criteria for chronic tension-type headache. Cephalalgia 12: 365–368

Steiner TJ, Couturier EGM, Catarci T, Hering R 1992 Social aspects of drug abuse in headache. Functional Neurology 6 (suppl).: 11–14

Stewart WF, Lipton RB, Celentano DD et al 1992 Prevalence of migraine headache in the United States. Journal of the American Medical Association 267: 64–69

Stewart WF, Schechter A, Lipton RB 1994a Migraine heterogeneity: disability, pain intensity, and attack frequency and duration. Neurology 44, (suppl) 4: S24–39

Stewart WF, Schechter A, Rasmussen BK 1994b Migraine prevalence: a review of population-based studies. Neurology 44 (suppl) 4: S17–23

Strassman AM, Raymond SA, Burstein R 1996 Sensitization of meningeal sensory neurons and the origin of headaches. Nature 384: 560–564

Strittmatter M, Hamann GF, Grauer M et al 1996 Altered activity of the sympathetic nervous system and changes in the balance of hypophyseal, pituitary and adrenal hormones in patients with cluster headache. Neuroreport 17: 1229–1234

Sumatriptan Cluster Headache Study Group 1991 Treatment of acute cluster headache with sumatriptan. New England Journal of Medicine 325: 322–326

Taarnhoj P 1982: Decompression of the posterior trigeminal root in trigeminal neuralgia: a 30 year follow-up review. Journal of Neurosurgery 57: 14–17

Tehindrazanarivelo AD, Lutz G, Petitjean C, Bousser M-G 1992 Headache following carotid endarterectomy: a prospective study. Cephalalgia 12: 380–382

Terwindt GM, Ophoff RA, Sandkuijl LA et al for the DMGRG 1997 Involvement of the familial hemiplegic migraine gene on 19p13 in migraine with and without aura. Cephalalgia 17: 332

Tfelt-Hansen P, Henry P, Mulder LJ et al 1995 The effectiveness of combined oral lysine acetylsalicylate and metoclopramide compared with oral sumatriptan for migraine. Lancet 346: 923–926

Turkewitz JL, Wirth O, Dawson GA, Casaly JS 1992 Cluster headache following head injury: a case report and review of the literature. Headache 32: 504–506

Tzourio C, Tehindrazanarivelo A, Iglèsias S et al 1995 Case-control study of migraine and risk of ischaemic stroke in young women. British Medical Journal 310: 830–833

Vilming ST, Schrader H, Monstad I 1988 Post-lumbar puncture headache: the significance of body posture. A controlled study of 300 patients. Cephalalgia 8: 75–78

Waldenlind E, Ekbom K, Wetterberg L et al 1994 Lowered circannual urinary melatonin concentrations in episodic cluster headache. Cephalalgia 14: 199–204

Wall M 1990 The headache profile of idiopathic intracranial hypertension. Cephalalgia 10: 331–335

Wallach H, Haeusler W, Lowes T et al 1997 Classical homeopathic treatment of chronic headaches. Cephalalgia 17: 119–126

Wallasch TM 1992 Transcranial doppler ultrasonic features in episodic tension-type headache. Cephalalgia 12: 293–296

Wallasch TM 1993 Transcranial doppler ultrasonic findings in episodic and chronic tension-type headache. In: Olesen J, Schoenen J (eds) Tension-type headache: classification, mechanisms, and treatment. Raven Press, New York, pp 127–130

Wallasch TM, Kropp P, Weinschütz T et al 1993 Contingent negative variation in tension-type headache. In: Olesen J, Schoenen J (eds) Tension-type headache: classification, mechanisms, and treatment. Raven Press, New York, pp 173–175

Wang SJ, Liu HC, Fuh JL et al 1997 Prevalence of headaches in a Chinese elderly population in Kinmen: age and gender effect and cross-cultural comparisons. Neurology 49: 195–200

Wang W, Schoenen J 1994a Habituation of temporalis ES2 in healthy volunteers, migraine and tension-type headache patients.

Proceedings of the EHF 2nd International Conference, Liège, Belgium

Wang W, Schoenen J 1994b Reduction of temporalis ES2 by peripheral electrical stimulation in migraine and tension-type headaches. Pain 59: 327–334

Wang W, Schoenen J 1996 Suppression of temporalis EMG by upper limb stimulations: results in healthy volunteers, migraine and tension-type headache patients. Functional Neurology 11: 307–315

Wang W, Schoenen J 1998 Interictal potentiation of passive 'oddball' auditory event-related potentials in migraine. Cephalalgia 18: 261–265

Wang W, Timsit-Berthier M, Schoenen J 1996 Intensity dependence of auditory evoked potentials is pronounced in migraine: an indication of cortical potentiation and low serotonergic neurotransmission? Neurology 46: 1404–1409

Warner JP, Fenichel GB 1996 Chronic posttraumatic headache often a myth? Neurology 46: 915–916

Watson CPN, Evans RJ 1988 Post-herpetic neuralgia: 208 cases. Pain 35: 289–297

Watson CPN, Watt VR, Chipman M, Birkett N, Evans RJ 1991 The prognosis with post-herpetic neuralgia. Pain 46: 195–199

Watson CPN, Chipman M, Reed K et al 1992 Amitriptyline versus maprotiline in post-herpetic neuralgia: a randomized, double blind, cross-over trial. Pain 8: 29–36

Weiller C, May A, Limmroth V et al 1995 Brain stem activation in spontaneous human migraine attacks. Nature Medicine 1: 658–660

Weiss HD, Stern BJ, Goldberg J 1991 Post-traumatic migraine: chronic migraine precipitated by minor head or neck trauma. Headache 31: 451–456

Welch KMA 1987 Migraine, a biobehavioural disorder. Archives of Neurology 44: 323–327

Welch KMA, Levine SR 1990 Migraine-related stroke in the context of the International Headache Society Classification of head pain. Archives of Neurology 47: 458–462

Welch KMA, Levine SR, D'Andrea G et al 1989 Preliminary observations on brain energy metabolism in migraine studied by in vivo 31-phosphorus NMR spectroscopy. Neurology 39: 538–541

Whitmarsh TE, Coleston-Shields DM, Steiner TJ 1997 Double-blind randomized placebo-controlled study of homoeopathic prophylaxis of migraine. Cephalalgia 17: 600–604

Wijdicks EF, Kerkhoff H, van Gijn J 1988 Long-term follow-up of 71 patients with thunderclap headache mimicking subarachnoid haemorrhage. Lancet 2: 68–70

Wilkinson M, Pfaffenrath V, Schoenen J et al 1995 Migraine and cluster headache. Their management with sumatriptan: a critical review of the current clinical experience. Cephalalgia 15: 337–357

Woods RP, Iacoboni M, Mazziotta JC 1994 Brief report: bilateral spreading cerebral hypoperfusion during spontaneous migraine headache. New England Journal of Medicine 331: 1689–1692

Yamaguchi M 1992 Incidence of headache and severity of head injury. Headache 32: 427–431

Phantom pain and other phenomena after amputation

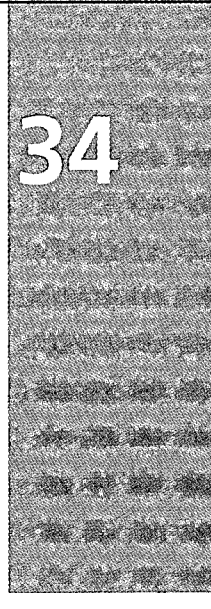

TROELS STAEHELIN JENSEN & LONE NIKOLAJSEN

INTRODUCTION

Sensations referred to a lost body part have been a mystery to laymen and scientists for a long time. Yet the literature on the subject dates back only to the end of the last century. Before that, phantom phenomena were sporadically described by authors as Ambroise Paré (16th century), René Descartes (17th century), Albrecht von Haller (18th century), and Charles Bell (19th century). Ambroise Paré noticed that amputees could complain of pain in the missing limb a long time after amputation. In the medical profession phantom pain was considered to represent a mere psychological phenomenon and interest was therefore limited. The first studies came from Gueniot (1861), Mitchell (1872) and Pitres (1897), to mention some of the most important authors. In this century, World War II, Vietnam, Israeli and former Jugoslavia wars have provided many cases of amputations and phantom phenomena have eventually become accepted in the medical sphere.

Today phantom limb is a natural and expected consequence of amputation and it does not necessarily present any therapeutic problems. However, in some amputees the phantom or the amputation stump itself becomes the site of severe and excruciating pain, presenting a major obstacle to successful rehabilitation.

This chapter will describe the clinical characteristics of postamputation phenomena. This is followed by a review of the possible mechanisms underlying pain in amputees and finally, the question whether phantom pain can be prevented will be discussed.

Definition and classification

Although a painless and a painful part of the missing limb may be at either end of the same clinical spectrum, it is useful to distinguish between:

- *phantom pain*: painful sensations referred to the missing limb
- *stump pain*: pain referred to the stump
- *phantom sensation*: any sensation of the missing limb except pain.

CLINICAL CHARACTERISTICS

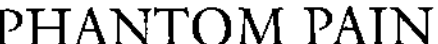

PHANTOM PAIN

Incidence of phantom pain

The incidence of phantom pain shows great discrepancy in the literature. Some figures are in the range of 2–4% (Ewalt et al 1947, Henderson & Smyth 1948, Abramson & Feibel 1981), whereas most recent studies report an incidence of 60–80% (Parkes 1973, Carlen et al 1978, Sherman & Sherman 1983, Jensen et al 1983, Houghton et al 1994, Nikolajsen et al 1997a) (Table 34.1). This variation may be due to several factors, including methods of estimating pain. Studies based on analgesic requirements must be interpreted with particular care. Sherman and Sherman (1983) found that although 61% of amputees with phantom pain had discussed the problem with their doctors, only 17% were offered treatment.

The incidence of phantom pain does not seem to be influenced by age, gender, side or level of amputation (Jensen et al 1983) or cause (civilian versus traumatic) of amputation (Sherman & Sherman 1985, Houghton et al 1994). Phantom pain is less frequent in young children (Riese & Bruck 1950, Simmel 1962) and in congenital amputees (Weinstein & Sersen 1961, Flor et al 1998). Gradual loss of a limb does not prevent the occurrence of

Table 34.1 Incidence of phantom pain as reported in previous studies

Authors	*Year*	*No. of amputees*	*% with phantom pain*
Riddoch	1941	?	50
Ewalt et al	1947	2284	2
Henderson and Smyth	1948	300	4
Cronholm	1951	122	35
Appenzeller and Bicknell	1969	34	56
James	1973	38	62
Parkes	1973	46	61
Carlen et al	1978	73	67
Finch et al	1980	133	54
Abramson and Feibel	1981	2000	2
Jensen et al	1983	58	72
Sherman and Sherman	1983	764	85
Krebs et al	1985	86	52
Wall et al	1985	25	88
Pohjolainen	1991	124	59
Dillingham and Braverman	1994	14	64
Houghton et al	1994	176	78
Krane and Heller	1995	24	83
Warten et al	1997	526	55
Montoya et al	1997	32	50
Nikolajsen et al	1997	56	75

phantom pain as phantom phenomena are reported to occur among patients with limb shortening due to leprosy (Price 1976).

Time course of phantom pain

The onset of phantom pain is usually in the first week (Lunn 1948, Parkes 1973, Carlen et al 1978, Jensen et al 1983, Krane & Heller 1995, Nikolajsen et al 1997a). In a prospective study 48% developed their pain within the first 24 hours and 83% within 4 days. In less than 10% was phantom pain delayed for more than 1 week (Jensen et al 1983). This is confirmed by another prospective study in which 56 patients scheduled for amputation of the lower limb were interviewed about pain before the amputation and after 1 week, 3 and 6 months. Only two patients developed significant phantom pain (i.e. >20 on a VAS 0–100) after 1 week (Nikolajsen et al 1997a). However, case reports suggest that the onset of phantom pain may be delayed for several years after amputation (Nathan 1962).

It is generally believed that phantom pain gradually diminishes with time and eventually fades away. In a retrospective study by Houghton et al (1994), 176 amputees were asked to assess phantom pain severity at different times after the amputation as they remembered it. On a scale from 0 to 10, phantom pain score decreased from four immediately after the amputation to one 5 years postoperatively. In the prospective study by Nikolajsen et al (1997a) the incidence of phantom pain was 67%, 68% and 75% after 1 week, 3 and 6 months, respectively. Although the incidence did not decline with time, duration of pain attacks decreased significantly.

Frequency, character and location of phantom pain

Phantom pain is usually intermittent; only few patients are in constant pain. Episodes of pain are reported to occur daily or at daily or weekly intervals with only a few reporting monthly, yearly or rarer episodes. Duration of individual pain attacks is seconds, minutes and hours, but rarely days or longer (Parkes 1973, Finch 1980, Jensen et al 1983, 1985, Sherman & Sherman 1983, 1985, Montoya et al 1997).

Phantom pain is described as shooting, stabbing, pricking, boring, squeezing, throbbing and burning (Parkes 1973, Carlen et al 1978, Jensen et al 1983, 1985, Sherman & Sherman 1983, 1985, Krane & Heller 1995). Shooting, pricking and boring are the words most often used to describe it (Nikolajsen et al 1997a).

Phantom pain is mainly localized distally in the phantom limb (Lunn 1948, Sliosberg 1948, Carlen et al 1978, Jensen et al 1983, 1985, Sherman & Sherman 1983, 1985, Katz & Melzack 1990, Nikolajsen et al 1997a) (Fig. 34.1). Thus, among 64 above-knee amputees with phantom pain in Lunn's series (Lunn 1948), 66% had pain in the foot or the toes, 39% also in the calves and only 6% had additional pain in the thigh.

Preamputation pain and phantom pain

Some previous studies (Riddoch 1941, Appenzeller & Bicknell 1969, Parkes 1973), but not all (Henderson & Smyth 1948), have reported that preamputation pain increased the risk of phantom pain. A few more recent studies have examined the relation between preamputation pain and phantom pain. Wall et al (1985) failed to find such a relation in 25 patients who had amputation because of cancer: in 16 patients with preamputation pain, 14 had phantom pain and in nine patients without preamputation pain, eight had phantom pain. Krane and Heller (1995) interviewed 24 children and adolescents with limb amputations because of cancer, trauma, infection or congenital anomaly. Twenty of the patients had phantom pain and only 13 of these had experienced pain preoperatively. Houghton et al

(1994) studied 176 amputees: in vascular amputees there was a significant relation between preamputation pain and phantom pain immediately after the amputation and after 6 months, 1 and 2 years. In traumatic amputees phantom pain was only related to preamputation pain immediately after the amputation.

Jensen et al (1983, 1985) prospectively followed 58 amputees who had amputation mainly because of vascular disease. Phantom pain was significantly more frequent after 8 days and 6 months but not after 2 years in patients who had pain in the limb before the amputation than in those who were free of pain. Nikolajsen et al (1997a) found that phantom pain was more frequent after 1 week (Fig. 34.2a) and 3 months (Fig. 34.2b), but not after 6 months, in patients who had moderate or severe preamputation pain compared to patients with less preamputation pain.

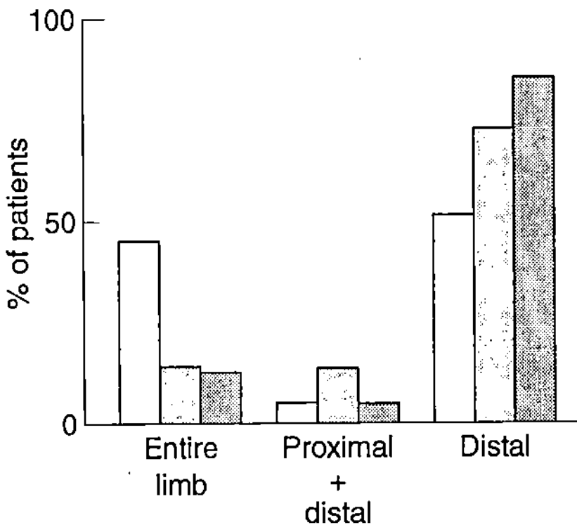

Fig. 34.1 Percentage of amputees with phantom pain localization 8 days (open bars, n=42), 6 months (pale bars, n=33) and 2 years (dark bars, n=20) after amputation. (From Jensen et al 1985 with permission.)

Similarity between preamputation pain and phantom pain

The literature contains numerous case reports of the continuation of preamputation pain in the phantom. Bailey and Moersch (1941) described an amputee who had his arm amputated following an accident. A week before the accident he had had a sliver under the nail of his finger. The feeling of the sliver was present until 2 years after the amputation. Hill et al (1996) described a woman who had recurrent infections of a leg wound. The most distressing preamputation pain consisted of cleaning and packing the wound twice daily. After the amputation the patient reported phantom pain localized to the open drainage site of the wound which was no longer there. Pain was described as a tearing sensation which felt like the dried wick being pulled out of the wound and a deep pressing pain which resembled the wound being repacked.

Other descriptions include the reactivation of pain experienced before the amputation, but which was not present at the time of the amputation. Nathan (1962) described an

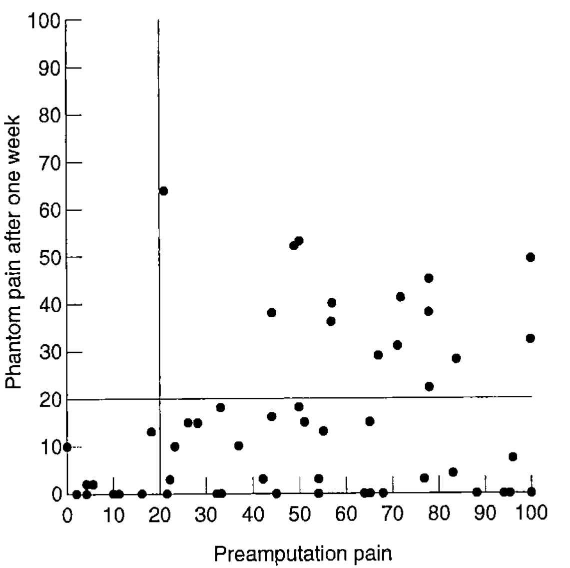

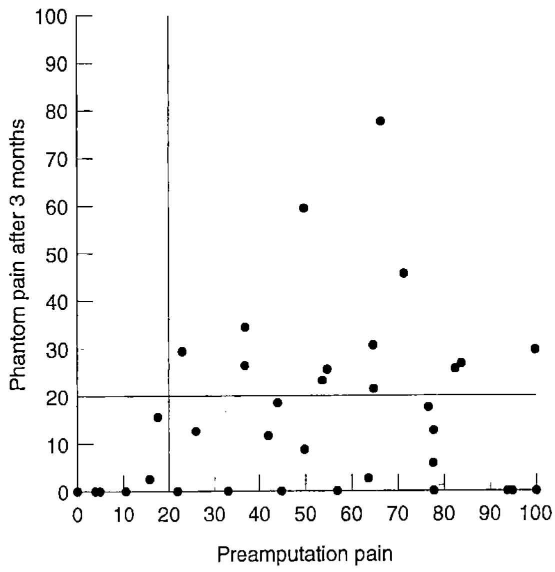

Fig. 34.2 (a) Preamputation pain ≥20 increases the risk of phantom pain ≥20 after 1 week (VAS 0–100 mm). P = 0.04, Fischer's exact test. Each dot represents one patient, n = 54. (From Nikolajsen et al 1997a with permission.) (b) Preamputation pain ≥20 increases the risk of phantom pain ≥20 after 3 months (VAS 0–100 mm). P = 0.03, Fischer's exact test. Each dot represents one patient, n = 37. (From Nikolajsen et al 1997a with permission.)

amputee who, following a noxious stimulus to the stump, re-experienced pain from a skating injury which he had sustained 5 years earlier.

Only a few studies have examined the incidence with which preamputation pain persists as phantom pain. The incidence has been reported as being from 12.5% to nearly 80% (Appenzeller & Bicknell 1969, Parkes 1973, Wall et al 1985, Jensen et al 1985, Katz & Melzack 1990). In a prospective study of 58 amputees, Jensen et al (1985) found a similarity between preamputation pain and phantom pain regarding both character and location in 36% of patients after 8 days, but only in 10% of patients after 6 months and 2 years. Katz and Melzack (1990) interviewed 68 amputees about phantom pain from 20 days to 46 years after the amputation. If phantom pain was present the amputees were asked whether the pain was similar to any pain they had ever had in the limb before the amputation. Fifty-seven per cent of those who reported having had preamputation pain claimed that their phantom pain resembled the pain they had at the time of the amputation. Fourteen per cent found that their phantom pain resembled a pain they had experienced previously but which was not present at the time of the amputation. Nikolajsen et al (1997a) recorded location and character of pain (pain was described using the patients' own words, different word descriptors and the McGill Pain Questionnaire) before the amputation and after 1 week, 3 and 6 months. Although 42% of patients claimed that their phantom pain resembled the pain they had experienced before the amputation, there was no relation between the patient's own opinion about similarity and the actual similarity found when comparing pre- and postoperative recordings of pain. It is possible that some patients with phantom pain would try to explain their pain by comparing it to pain experienced previously, thus giving a false estimate of the number of patients with identical preamputation pain and phantom pain.

Modulating factors

Phantom pain may be modulated by several internal and external factors. Attention, anxiety and autonomic reflexes such as coughing and urination may increase pain, whereas rest and distraction ameliorate pain. Phantom pain may be provoked by changes in the weather, cooling and pressure at the stump (Krebs et al 1985) (Table 34.2).

Other factors

Feinstein et al (1954) showed and Nordenbos (1959) confirmed that counterirritation with hypertonic saline injected in the L4–L5 interspinous tissue first exacerbated phantom limb pain and then produced transient awareness of the whole phantom followed by a long-lasting, sometimes permanent, phantom pain relief. Spinal anaesthesia in amputees may cause appearance of phantom pain in otherwise pain-free subjects (Mackenzie 1983). However, in a prospective study of 23 spinal anaesthetics in 17 amputees, only one developed transient phantom pain (Tessler & Kleiman 1994).

Table 34.2 Modulating factors

Aggravating factors	*Relieving factors*
Attention	Distraction
Emotional distress	Rest
Weather change	Cold or heat
Stump touch or pressure	Massage of stump
Autonomic reflexes	Stump movement
Pain of other origin	
Wearing a prosthesis	

An existing phantom limb experience, whether painful or not, may be altered by spinal cord or brain lesions. A focal brain infarct in the posterior internal capsule made a former phantom limb disappear (Yarnitsky et al 1988).

An unsolved question is whether phantom pain has a heritable component. In an animal model of neuropathic pain, Devor and Raber (1990) showed that autotomy (a self-mutilating behaviour of the animal to the denervated limb) was likely to be inherited as an autosomal recessive trait. On the other hand, Schott (1986) described a family in which five members sustained traumatic amputations of their limbs. The development of phantom phenomena, including pain, was unpredictable, despite their being first-degree relatives.

Psychological factors

Losing a limb is a traumatic experience and amputees often exhibit a range of psychological symptoms such as depression, anxiety and isolation.

Henderson and Smyth (1948) suggested that the emotional importance of preamputation pain may play a role in its persistence as phantom pain. They described a soldier who sprained his ankle when jumping from a truck and therefore could not keep up with his companions. A few minutes later he was wounded in the same leg and the pain of the sprain was replaced by a different pain in the wound. The leg was amputated a few days later but he continued to experience the pain only from the ankle sprain. The soldier remarked that he would have succeeded in escaping had it not been for the sprained ankle.

Parkes (1973) proposed that complaints of persisting pain were related to patients with a rigid, self-reliant personality and to unemployment or retirement. However, there is no evidence that phantom pain represents a psychological disturbance. On the basis of a literature survey, Sherman et al (1987) were unable to find a relation between phantom pain and any psychological variables. Katz and Melzack (1990) studied 60 amputees and found no difference between amputees with and amputees without phantom pain when comparing scores obtained from different personality, depression and anxiety questionnaires.

STUMP PAIN

Incidence and time course of stump pain

Virtually all amputees experience stump pain immediately after the amputation. This is expected and is a normal result of major surgery. If the pain does not decrease substantially within the first few days or if it subsides and then worsens, there is usually a problem with the amputation. In some patients, however, stump pain persists despite proper healing of the stump. Persistent stump pain is reported to occur in 5–21% of patients (Finch et al 1980, Abramson & Feibel 1981, Jensen et al 1983, 1985, Pohjolainen 1991). In the 1985 study by Jensen et al, 57% of the patients experienced stump pain immediately after the amputation. After 6 months and 2 years, stump pain was reported by 22% and 21% respectively. Nikolajsen et al (1997a) prospectively recorded incidence and intensity of postamputation stump pain in 56 amputees. All patients had some stump pain during the first week after amputation, but in most patients pain subsided. However, in two patients stump pain worsened. The severity of persistent stump pain may be illustrated by the following case history (Nikolajsen et al 1997b).

A 61-year-old man presented with severe pain in both stumps following amputation at knee level bilaterally 5 months previously. The patient never experienced phantom pain and stump pain only presented minor discomfort. However, after 3 months he suddenly developed severe stump pain after a ride on a gravel walk in his wheelchair. Pain was described as shooting, cutting, burning, killing, unbearable and torturing and the intensity of pain was 100 on VAS 0–100. Stump pain was present constantly and interfered with his sleep. Examination revealed allodynia bilaterally but no palpable neuromas. As no pain relief was obtained by slow-release morphine, tricylic antidepressants or paracetamol and the patient was considered to be suicidal, treatment was started with ketamine, an anaesthetic agent with N-methyl-D-aspartate receptor-blocking properties. Oral ketamine produced almost complete pain relief for 3 months. After that time the patient was admitted to hospital because of bedsores and treatment with ketamine was stopped. Stump pain recurred but treatment with ketamine was never started again as the patient died of sepsis before discharge from hospital.

Character of stump pain

In the study by Jensen et al (1985), stump pain was described as either pressing, throbbing, burning or squeezing. Other descriptions include a stabbing sensation or an electric current, which is strictly localized to the stump and often to its posterior aspect close to the scar (Browder & Gallagher 1948). These pains can easily be triggered by stimulating the stump with pinpricks or pressing tender neuromas. A variant of this type is what Sunderland (1978) termed 'nerve storms', with painful attacks of up to 2 days' duration. Several amputees complain of spontaneous movements, also known as chorea of the stump, tic douloureux, *épilepsie du moignon* or jactitation. These movements range from painful, hardly visible, myoclonic jerks to severe clonic contractions of the stump. Although rarely reported, Sliosberg (1948) observed it in nearly 50% of amputees and considered it to be even more common.

Stump and phantom pain are inter-related phenomena

Parkes (1973) studied 46 amputees and found that stump pain within the first 3 weeks after amputation was significantly associated to phantom pain 1 year later. In a survey of 648 amputees, Sherman and Sherman (1983) found that stump pain was present in 61% of amputees with phantom pain but only in 39% of those without phantom pain. Carlen et al (1978) noted that phantom pain was decreased by the resolution of stump-end pathology. Jensen et al (1985) found that 2 years after amputation phantom pain was significantly more frequent in patients with stump pain than in patients without stump pain: seven of 20 patients with phantom pain had stump pain, none of 14 patients without phantom pain had stump pain. Nikolajsen et al (1997a) found that stump and phantom pain were significantly related 1 week after amputation.

The association between stump and phantom pain is consistent with experimental studies in amputees. Nystrøm and Hagbarth (1981) observed abnormal activity in peroneal and median nerve fibres of two amputees with ongoing pain in their phantom foot and hand, respectively.

Percussion of neuromas in these two patients produced increased nerve fibre discharges and an augmentation of their phantom pain. Other studies have shown that temperature and muscle activity at the stump are related to phantom pain. Sherman and Glenda (1987) examined 30 amputees and found a consistent inverse relationship between temperature at the stump and burning, throbbing and tingling phantom pain. A direct relationship was found between the intensity of pain and changes in EMG in eight patients with cramping phantom pain (Sherman et al 1992). Katz (1992) found a significantly lower temperature at the stump than at the control side in a group of 20 amputees with phantom pain and sensation but no difference of temperature was seen in a group of eight patients with no phantom pain or sensation.

Stump pathology associated with pain

Examinations of stumps often disclose definite pathological findings which may account for the pain in the stump and/or the phantom:

- skin pathology
- circulatory disturbances
- infection of the skin or underlying tissue or bone
- bone spurs
- neuromas.

Although stump and phantom pain is significantly more frequent in patients with obvious stump pathology than in those without pathological findings, pain may occur in perfectly healed stumps. In preliminary work careful examination of stump sensibility has revealed areas of altered sensitivity (e.g. hypoalgesia, hyperalgesia, hyperpathia or allodynia) in almost all amputees (Jensen et al, unpublished data). The incidence of hyperalgesia, allodynia and wind-up pain (pain evoked by repetitive stimulation of the skin) was examined in a prospective study of 43 amputees. After 6 months allodynia was found in 58% of amputees and wind-up pain could be elicited in 32%. One week after amputation mechanical thresholds (pressure algometry and von Frey hairs) at the stump were related to ongoing stump and phantom pain and after 6 months wind-up pain was related to ongoing pain (Nikolajsen et al, submitted).

PHANTOM LIMB

Phantom limb sensation

Non-painful phantom sensations rarely pose a clinical problem and will only be discussed briefly. Phantom pain and phantom sensation often coexist but phantom sensations are more frequent than phantom pain. Previous reports indicate that 80–100% of all amputees will experience phantom sensations following amputation (Lunn 1948, Carlen et al 1978, Jensen et al 1983, Krane & Heller 1995). The onset is usually within the first days after amputation (Henderson & Smyth 1948, Lunn 1948, Carlen et al 1978, Jensen et al 1983, 1984) (Fig. 34.3). The amputee often wakes up from the anaesthesia with a feeling that the amputated limb is still there. This feeling may be so real that the amputee tumbles when trying to get out of bed. In some cases phantom sensations may be very vivid and include feelings of movement and posture (Riddoch 1941, Henderson & Smyth 1948, Lunn 1948, Cronholm 1951); in other cases only suggestions of the phantom are felt.

In a prospective study of 58 amputees, the incidence of phantom limb sensation was 84%, 90% and 71% 8 days, 6 months, and 2 years after amputation, respectively. While the incidence of phantom sensation did not decrease during follow-up, both duration and frequency of phantom phenomena declined significantly. Approximately three-quarters of patients had kinaesthetic sensations in the limb during the first 6 months after amputation (i.e. feeling of length, volume or other spatial sensation) but less than half of patients had this later in the course (Jensen et al 1984).

A 62-year-old patient who had undergone below-knee amputation 3 months previously still had a vivid feeling of the missing limb. He reported that the phantom was in a strange position, angled to the stump and moving freely around in the air (Fig. 34.5a). When he put on his prosthesis in the morning the phantom limb slipped back to a normal position inside the prosthesis. The phantom sensation faded away and was not present after 1 year.

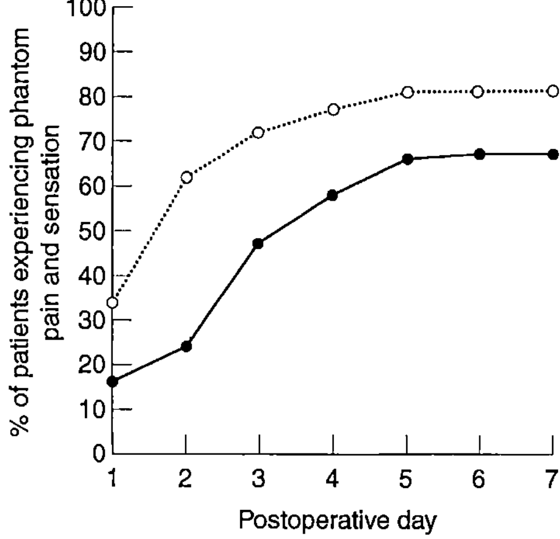

Fig. 34.3 Cumulative incidence of patients who have experienced phantom pain (●) and phantom sensation (O) in the first week after amputation.

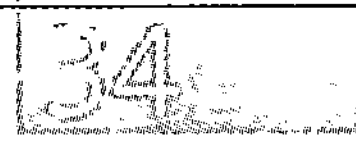

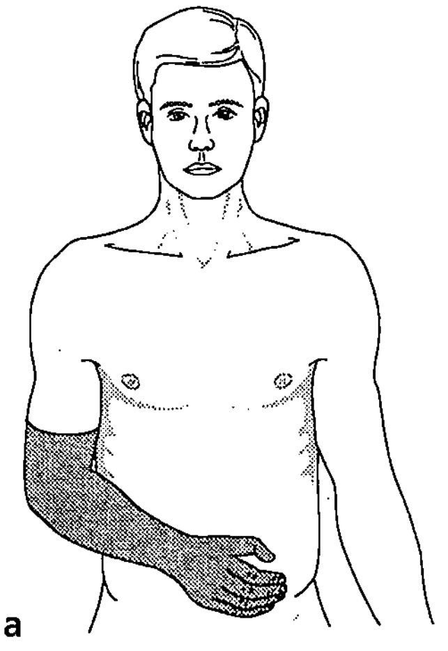

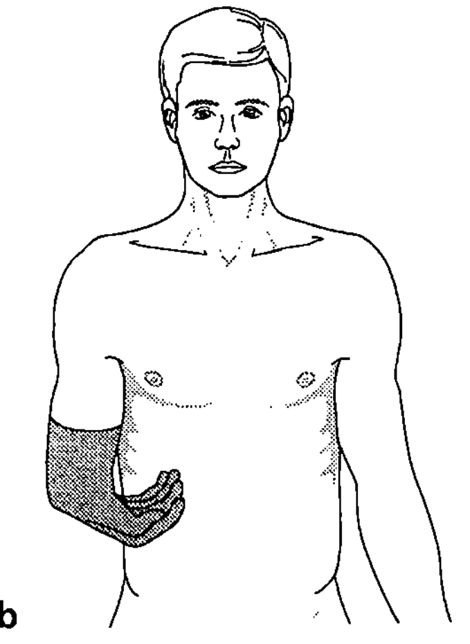

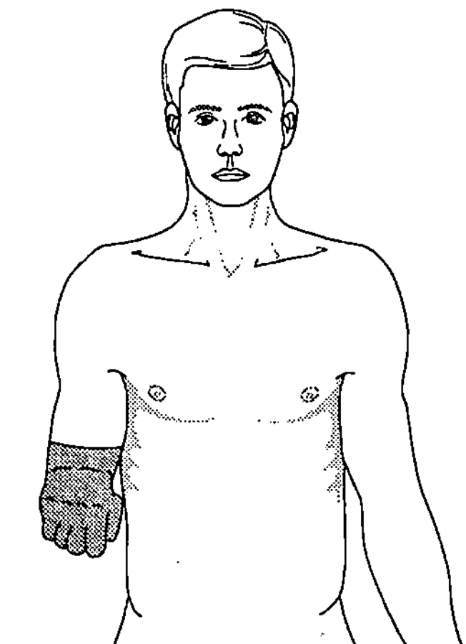

Fig. 34.4 (a–c) Telescoping

Another patient had his arm amputated following an accident. The phantom arm was stuck in a position in front of the chest and in addition to the feeling that he could still move his phantom fingers, the fingers also had involuntary movements (Fig. 34.5b).

Another phenomenon is telescoping, which refers to shrinkage of the phantom (Fig 34.4). Telescoping is reported to occur in about half of patients. It has been postulated that phantom pain prevents or retards shrinkage of the phantom but Montoya et al (1997) failed to find such a relation: 12 of 16 patients with phantom pain and five of 10 patients without pain reported telescoping.

A 39-year-old woman who had her leg amputated at thigh level felt that her foot gradually approached the stump and eventually became located inside the stump (Fig. 34.5c). Her only complaint was that the prosthesis squeezed her phantom foot.

AETIOLOGY AND PATHOPHYSIOLOGICAL MECHANISMS

The mechanisms underlying pain in amputees are not known exactly, despite great efforts to explain them

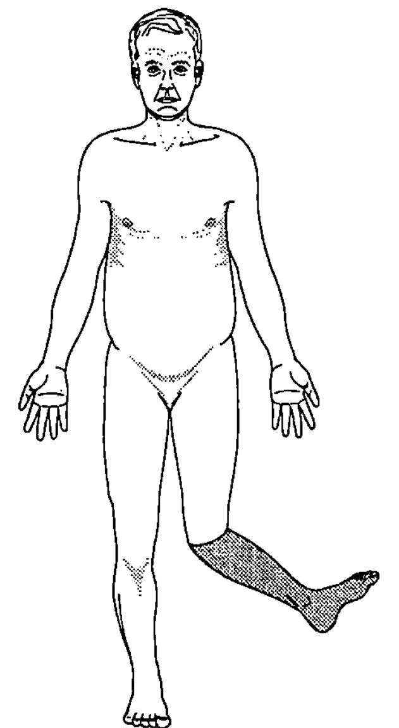

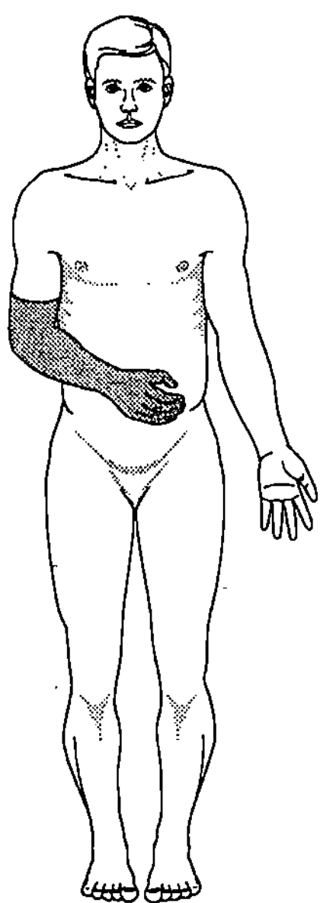

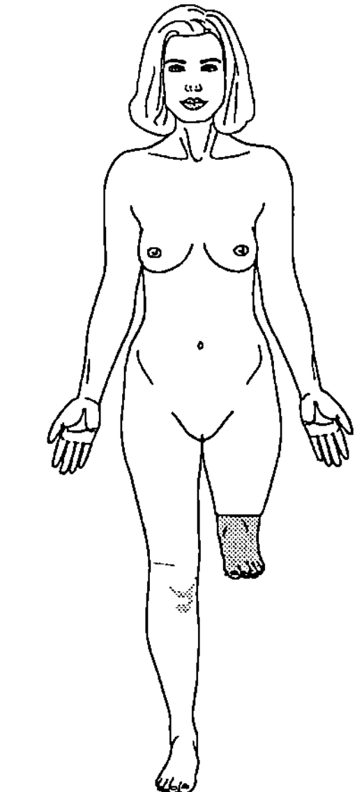

Fig. 34.5 (a,b) Unusual kinaesthetic sensations. (c) Telescoping.

(Frederiks 1963, Van Wirdum 1965, Melzack 1971, Melzack & Loeser 1978, Sunderland 1978, Lawrence 1980, Wall 1981, Sherman 1989, Coderre & Katz 1997). Amputation is the most radical form of nerve injury. An extensive experimental and clinical literature documents that following nerve injury a number of morphological, physiological and chemical events take place both in the peripheral and central nervous system (see Chs 5 & 6). These changes may lead to chronic neuropathic pain. It is well established that neuropathic pains, irrespective of underlying cause and site of lesion, are characterized by a series of clinical events:

- ongoing and evoked pain in the region of nerve injury
- no signs of tissue injury
- paroxysms of pain
- coexistent sensory loss, hyperalgesic phenomena, summation and aftersensations following repetitive stimuli.

Many of these features, but not necessarily all, are seen in amputees with phantom pain. While much of the pathology related to amputation occurs at the level of the primary afferent neuron and in the spinal cord (see below), it is also obvious that the phantom limb image with its complex, perceptual, emotional and cognitive qualities involves interaction of some cerebral structure(s). The starting point in understanding phantom limb phenomena, painful or not, must be that amputation of a limb causes a sudden cessation of a normal patterned afferent input. This normal input is substituted by an as yet unknown, but certainly different, new input which may furnish the spinal cord and the brain with the necessary information to create a phantom.

A comparison of the clinical aspects of phantom pain, its related phenomena and the effects of experimental nerve sections may give clues about possible pathophysiological mechanisms involved in generating phantom limb phenomena.

PERIPHERAL MECHANISMS

Several clinical observations suggest that mechanisms in the periphery (i.e. in the stump or in central parts of sectioned primary afferents) may play a role in the phantom limb percept:

- phantom limb sensations can be modulated by various stump manipulations
- phantom limb sensations are temporarily abolished after local stump anaesthesia
- stump revisions and removal of tender neuromas often reduce pain transiently
- phantom pain is significantly more frequent in those amputees with long-term stump pain than in those without persistent pain
- although obvious stump pathology is rare, altered cutaneous sensibility in the stump is a common if not universal feature
- finally, changes in stump blood flow alter the phantom limb perception.

Experimental studies have shown that nerve injury induces several changes in the peripheral nervous system. Sprouts emerge from near the cut and if regeneration is prevented, as in limb amputation, nerve-end neuromas are created. These neuromas acquire the capability of spontaneous activity and an increased sensitivity to mechanical stimuli and various neurochemicals, e.g. noradrenaline (norepinephrine) (Wall & Gutnick 1974, Devor & Rappaport 1990; see also Ch. 5). The increased sensitivity of sprouts and neuromas to noradrenaline may in part explain the exacerbation of phantom pain by stress and other emotional states associated with increased catecholamine release from sympathetic efferent terminals which are in close proximity to afferent sensory nerves and sprouts.

Nyström and Hagbarth (1981), in microelectrode recordings from transected nerves in two amputees, found that tapping of neuromas induced activity in afferent fibres (some probably of C-fibre type) and that such activity was associated with increased phantom limb pain. Chabal et al (1989) studied the effect of a potassium channel blocker, gallamine, injected into neuromas of human amputees suffering from phantom pain. It was found that gallamine increased pain, whereas saline had no effect. This suggests that ion channel permeability in neuromas does play a role in phantom pain. The chaotic reinnervation of stumps with formation of ectopic excitation sites and ephaptic synapses may contribute to the changed sensitivity of stumps and to alterations in evoked sensations (e.g. allodynia) (Devor & Rappaport 1990).

In addition to abnormal activity from nerve-end neuromas, cell bodies in the dorsal root ganglion show similar abnormal spontaneous activity and increased sensitivity to mechanical and neurochemical stimulation (Kajander et al 1992). Thus, abnormal activity from at least two sources – neuromas and dorsal root ganglion cell bodies – may contribute to the phantom limb percept, including pain.

SPINAL CORD MECHANISMS

Spinal cord lesions and root avulsions from the plexus brachialis are sometimes associated with pain of the same character and localization as seen in amputees with phantom pain (Bors 1951, Melzack & Loeser 1978, Wynn Parry 1980). Case reports support the notion that spinal mechanisms may play a role in the phantom limb pain. Brihaye (1958) described a patient with a right lower limb phantom which disappeared after herniation of a cervical disc causing myelopathy. After removal of the herniated disc and upon recovery from myelopathy, the phantom limb percept reappeared. Catchlove (1983) reported a case in which a paraplegic patient with a full sensory loss below Th11 had phantom limb pain after amputation of one leg. Mackenzie (1983) described the appearance of phantom limb pain during spinal anaesthesia in two amputees who formerly had not experienced phantom pains. Similar induction or reduction of phantom limb pain following spinal anaesthesia has been noted by others (Carrie & Glynn 1986, Jacobsen et al 1989). While these findings suggest that spinal cord mechanisms modulate the phantom limb percept, including pain, it is noteworthy that extramedullary processes, such as herniated discs, neurinomas, meningiomas and malignant tumours, are only rarely associated with phantom-like pain.

More than 30 years ago, Nordenbos (1959) suggested that disinhibition of dorsal horn neurons which have lost their neuronal afferent input may play a role in triggering phantom limb phenomena. Recent studies support this idea. Experimental nerve injury produced by tight or loose ligation of the sciatic nerve results in a behavioural syndrome characterized by guarding of the affected limb and hyperalgesia and allodynia in and surrounding the territory innervated by the ligated nerve (Bennett & Xie 1988, Kim & Chung 1992). This behavioural syndrome mimicks the symptoms of nerve injury pain in humans, including phantom pain. Following nerve constriction, a cascade of morphological, physiological and neurochemical changes are seen in the dorsal horn, including spontaneous neuronal activity, induction of immediate early genes, increase in spinal cord metabolic activity (Price et al 1997) and expansion of receptive fields (Cook et al 1987) with the result that dorsal horn neurons that have lost their normal afferent input begin to respond to nearby intact afferent nerves (see Ch. 6). The clinical significance of these experimental findings is at present incompletely understood. However, it is of interest to note that phantom limb phenomena, whether painful or not, are most vivid in the distal parts of a limb and that these sensations can be induced by stimulating the stump. One possible explanation could be that medial dorsal horn neurons in the spinal cord, with skin receptive fields located in distal parts of a limb, show spontaneous activity and expansion of receptive fields after limb amputation with the result that these cells can be driven from areas located more proximally (e.g. stump).

The pharmacology of spinal sensitization involves an increased activity in N-methyl-D-aspartate (NMDA) receptor-operated systems and many aspects of the central sensitization can be reduced by NMDA receptor antagonists (see Ch. 10). In human amputees one aspect of such central sensitization, the evoked stump or phantom pain produced by repetitive stimulation of the stump by non-noxious pinprick, can be reduced by the NMDA receptor antagonist ketamine (Nikolajsen et al 1996).

SUPRASPINAL MECHANISMS

The phantom limb percept, with its complex perceptual qualities and its modification by a variety of internal stimuli (e.g. attention, distraction or stress), clearly indicates that the phantom image is ultimately integrated in the brain. Some case reports suggest that cortical and thalamic structures modulate phantom limb and phantom pain. Head and Holmes (1915) noted the disappearance of a left leg phantom after a cerebral lesion in the right hemisphere. Others (Appenzeller & Bicknell 1969, Yarnitsky et al 1988) have suggested that cortical or subcortical lesions may erase a contralateral phantom limb experience. Finally, electrical stimulation of the parvocellular part of the nucleus ventralis posterolateralis in the thalamus is reported to reduce phantom limb and phantom pain (Merienne & Mazars 1981). Davis et al (1998) have shown in a small series of amputees that thalamic stimulation results in phantom sensation and pain. Normally such stimulation does not evoke pain. This suggests that plastic changes in the thalamus are involved in generation of chronic pain.

Recent electrophysiological studies have documented the existence of nociceptive specific neurons and wide dynamic-range neurons in the cerebral cortex (see Ch. 7). In view of the plasticity in nociceptive and antinociceptive systems, it is reasonable to assume that amputation not only produces a cascade of events in the periphery and in the spinal cord, but that these changes eventually sweep more centrally and alter neuronal activity in cortical and subcortical structures.

Studies in humans have documented a cortical reorganization after amputation. In a series of studies Flor and colleagues (1995, 1998) have shown a correlation between phantom pain and the amount of reorganization in the somatosensory cortex. They therefore suggested that phantom limb pain may be a result of plastic changes in the somatosensory cortex.

THERAPY

GENERAL

Treatment of chronic pain following amputation is difficult and has not been successful. In a survey of 764 amputees, Sherman and Sherman (1983) found that 44% of those who discussed their phantom pain with the physician were told that they were mentally disturbed. Only 17% were offered treatment.

Various treatments have been and are currently in use for chronic pain after amputation. In another survey, Sherman and Sherman (1980) identified 68 different treatment methods, of which 50 were in current use. Only a few were described as being effective and today the majority of these treatments have probably been abandoned. Examples of treatment are presented in Table 34.3.

Most studies dealing with pain treatment in amputees suffer from severe methodological errors:

- samples are small, heterogeneous and non-randomized
- studies are open
- controls are often lacking
- follow-up periods are short.

A success rate of any previous reported treatment rarely exceeds a placebo response of 30%. With a pathophysiology that is still unclear, it is not possible to give precise directions for pain treatment in amputees. In general, treatment should be based on non-invasive techniques. Educational programmes for amputees, their relatives and those health professionals dealing with amputees may perhaps contribute to a reduction of chronic pain after amputation. Surgery on the peripheral or the central nervous system in cases of deafferentation pain always implicates further deafferentation and thereby an increased risk of persistent pain. However, for historical reasons some invasive treatment methods will be mentioned briefly.

Table 34.3 Examples of treatments used for phantom pain

Medical	*Surgical*	*Other*
Conventional analgesics	Neurectomy	TENS
Tricyclic antidepressants	Stump revision	Acupuncture
Neuroleptics	Rhizotomy	Biofeedback
Anticonvulsants	Sympathectomy	Hypnotherapy
β blockade	Cordotomy	Massage
Calcitonin	Tractotomy	Ultrasound
Ketamine	Lobectomy	
Epidural treatment	Dorsal column stimulation	
Nerve blocks	Brain stimulation	
Sympathetic blocks		

NON-INVASIVE TECHNIQUES

Non-medical

Transcutaneous electrical nerve stimulation (TENS), acupuncture, relaxation training, ultrasound and hypnosis may in some cases have a beneficial effect on stump and phantom pain. Physical therapy involving massage, manipulation and passive movements may prevent trophic changes and vascular congestion in the stump. Induction of sensory input from the stump area by physical therapy could play a role in the ameliorating effect of such types of treatment.

TENS either on the stump or on the contralateral extremity has been used with some success in the treatment of phantom pain (Thoden et al 1979, Sherman et al 1980, Carabelli & Kellerman 1985, Lundeberg 1985, Katz & Melzack 1991). Thus Lundeberg (1985) found that in 24 patients with phantom pain given either peripheral vibratory stimulation or placebo, 75% reported pain reduction during stimulation, while 44% noted pain reduction during placebo. The advantage of peripheral nerve stimulation is the absence of side effects and complications and the fact that the treatment can be easily repeated.

Medical

No drug treatment is specifically effective and persistent long-term phantom pain may be resistant to any treatment. In some cases carbamazepine has a splendid effect and can relieve the patient from pain if the membrane-stabilizing drug is administered in ordinary neuralgic doses (Elliott et al 1976, Patterson 1988). Certain antidepressants (e.g. clomipramine) may also have a beneficial effect in some patients. Used in the treatment of pain, antidepressants may be effective at doses lower than those corresponding to their antidepressant effect. In single cases the antidepressant doxepin has been reported to be effective (Iacono et al 1987). Others have found β blockers to be of value (Marsland et al 1982). Permanent phantom pain should not be accepted until opioids have been tried. It is our experience (as well as that of others; Urban et al 1986) that

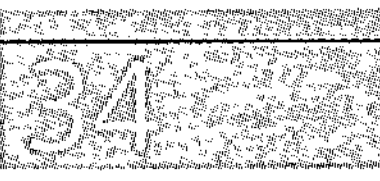

opioids can be used safely for years with a limited risk of drug dependence. In a double-blind, crossover study Jaeger and Maier (1992) recently reported a beneficial effect of intravenous calcitonin on phantom limb pain. Jacobsen et al (1990) found that intrathecal fentanyl abolished pain in eight patients with established stump pain. Others have found that stump and phantom pain was reduced by ketamine, a NMDA receptor antagonist (Stannard & Porter 1993, Nikolajsen et al 1996). However, well-controlled studies with a sufficient number of patients are lacking.

INVASIVE TECHNIQUES

Stump revision

Surgery on amputation neuromas and more extensive amputation have played important roles in the treatment of stump and phantom pain. By surgical stump revision, Baumgartner and Riniker (1981) achieved considerable relief of both stump and phantom pain in 87 out of 100 patients. In order to avoid the development of traumatic neuromas in amputees, others have performed encapsulation with Millipore, fascicle ligation (Battista 1979) and centrocentral anastomosis (Samii 1981). Formation of neuromas is a universal phenomenon after peripheral nerve cut. Excision of tender neuromas may relieve pain transiently but usually leads to the formation of new bulbs which are as painful as the first. Stump revision should probably be limited to those few amputees with obvious stump pathology. Embedding tender neuromas deep into tissue and thereby protecting them from mechanical compression may in some cases eliminate symptoms of increased mechanosensitivity (Herndon et al 1976). In properly healed stumps there is almost never any indication for proximal extension of the amputation because of pain.

Neurectomy/rhizotomy and sympathectomy

Denervation between the amputation stump and the spinal nerve roots was previously used in the treatment of amputation pains, but because of the poor results it has now been almost entirely abandoned.

While both clinical and experimental findings support the notion that sympathetic activity influences phantom and/or stump pain (see above), sympathectomy has only a limited effect on stump and phantom pain. The role of chemical sympathectomy after guanethidine (see Ch. 36) in phantom pain is not clear.

Dorsal root entry zone lesions

This treatment, primarily introduced for the treatment of painful brachial plexus avulsions, has also been used in the treatment of phantom pain (Nashold & Ostdahl 1979, Samii & Moringlane 1984, Saris et al 1985, 1988, Wiegand & Winkelmüller 1985). It is generally believed that dorsal root entry zone lesions have a limited effect on phantom pain. Saris et al (1985) studied 22 patients with postamputation stump and/or phantom pain. All underwent dorsal root entry zone lesions and were followed for 6 months to 4 years after surgery. Only 36% of the patients obtained pain relief from the operation. However, in patients suffering from phantom pain alone, a good result was obtained in six patients (Saris et al 1985).

Spinal cord stimulation

Spinal cord stimulation has been widely used in the treatment of amputation pain. Krainick et al (1980) stimulated 64 patients with postamputation pain and obtained a 50–100% pain reduction in 45% of patients and a 25–50% pain reduction in 11%. At a follow-up examination 5 years later, 23% still had 50–100% pain relief. Siegfried and Cetinalp (1981) analysed the material of nine authors and found that among 148 patients, 51% obtained 50–100% pain relief, while 18% obtained 25–50% pain reduction.

Brain stimulation

Mundinger and Salomáo (1980) treated 32 patients with thalamic pains, persisting zoster pains, anesthesia dolorosa and phantom pains and achieved more than 50% pain relief in 53% of the patients. Out of 14 amputees, 13 (93%) treated with a combination of deep brain stimulation and transcutaneous stimulation had a pain reduction of more than 50% (Mundinger & Neumüller 1981).

Cordotomy

This operation was used for many years in the treatment of phantom pain (Doupe et al 1944, De Gutierrez-Mahoney 1948). In a survey, Siegfried and Cetinalp (1981) summarized the results of five small studies comprising 52 patients in whom cordotomy had been performed: 38% had a 50–100% reduction of pain, 44% had a 25–50% reduction. This treatment has been almost abandoned today.

PREVENTION

Some previous studies found that patients who had severe pain before the amputation had a higher risk of developing phantom pain than patients who had less or no pain before the amputation (Riddoch 1941, Appenzeller & Bicknell 1969, Parkes 1973, Jensen et al 1983, 1985). Also, several case reports suggested that pain experienced before the amputation (i.e. a painful ulcer) might continue to be present in the phantom (Bailey & Moersch 1941, Nathan 1962).

These observations prompted Bach et al (1988) to carry out a controlled study in which patients scheduled for amputation of the lower limb were randomized to receive either epidural pain treatment for 3 days before the amputation or conventional pain treatment. They found that the incidence of phantom pain was significantly lower after 6 months among 11 patients who received epidural pain treatment than among 14 patients who received conventional pain treatment. Subsequent clinical trials have confirmed their findings (Jahangiri et al 1994, Shug et al 1995, Katsuly-Liapis et al 1996). Jahangiri et al (1994) examined the effect of perioperative epidural infusion of diamorphine, bupivacaine and clonidine on postamputation stump and phantom pain. Thirteen patients received the epidural treatment 24–48 hours preoperatively and for at least 3 days postoperatively. A control group of 11 patients received opioid analgesia on demand. All patients had general anaesthesia for the amputation. The incidence of severe phantom pain was lower in the epidural group 7 days, 6 months and 1 year after amputation. No effect was seen on stump pain. In another prospective study by Shug et al (1995), 23 patients had either epidural analgesia before, during and after the amputation (n=8), intra- and postoperative epidural analgesia (n=7) or general anaesthesia plus systemic analgesia (n=8). After 1 year the incidence of phantom pain was significantly lower among the patients who received pre-, intra- and postoperative epidural analgesia relative to patients who received general anaesthesia plus systemic analgesia. Katsuly-Liapis et al (1996) presented in abstract form a study in which 45 patients were allocated to one of three groups: group A (n=15) received epidural bupivacaine and morphine for 3 days prior to amputation and the infusion was maintained for 72 hours postoperatively; group B (n=12) received conventional analgesics before the amputation and epidural pain treatment after the amputation; group C (n=18) had conventional analgesics both before and after the amputation. After 6 months the incidence of phantom pain was significantly lower in group A compared to groups B and C.

Others have examined the effect of peri- or intraneural blockade on phantom pain. Fischer and Meller (1991) introduced a catheter into the transsected nerve sheath at the time of amputation and infused bupivacaine for 72 hours in 11 patients. None developed phantom pain during a 12-month follow-up. In a retrospective study Elizaga et al (1994) found no effect of such a treatment. Pinzur et al (1996) prospectively randomized 21 patients to continuous postoperative infusion of either bupivacaine or saline, but failed to find any difference between the two groups with regard to the incidence of phantom pain after 3 and 6 months.

However, a number of methodological problems, such as small sample sizes, no or insufficient randomization and non-blinded assessment of pain, limit the validity of all these studies. Nevertheless, the impact of the Bach et al (1988) study is immense and in many anaesthesiological departments procedures have been changed so that patients undergoing amputation are offered an epidural catheter before amputation in order to prevent phantom pain. Starting an epidural treatment before rather than at the time of the amputation is associated with extra hospital costs so simply from a cost–benefit point of view, it is important to know whether patients should be taken into the anaesthesiological department for epidural pain treatment before the amputation.

We therefore carried out a randomized, double-blind and placebo-controlled study to clarify whether postoperative stump and phantom pain is reduced by preoperative pain treatment with epidural bupivacaine and morphine (Nikolajsen et al 1997c). Sixty patients scheduled for lower limb amputation were randomly assigned into one of two groups:

1. a blockade group that received epidural bupivacaine and morphine before the amputation and during the operation (29 patients)
2. a control group that received epidural saline and oral/intramuscular morphine (31 patients).

Both groups had general anesthesia for the amputation and all patients received epidural analgesics for postoperative pain management. Patients were interviewed about preamputation pain on the day before the amputation and about stump and phantom pain after 1 week, 3, 6 and 12 months. Median duration of preoperative epidural blockade (blockade group) was 18 hours. After 1 week the percentage of patients with phantom pain was 51.9 in the blockade group and 55.6 in the control group. Subsequently the figures were (blockade/control): at 3 months, 82.4/50; at 6 months, 81.3/55; and at

12 months, 75/68.8. Intensity of stump and phantom pain and consumption of opioids were also similar in the two groups at all four postoperative interviews. Thus, we were not able to confirm the findings by others that perioperative epidural blockade prevents phantom pain. The above-mentioned studies are listed in Table 34.4.

CONCLUSION

Phantom pain is a common consequence of limb amputation and has also been reported following visceral removal. Approximately two-thirds of patients complain of phantom pain following limb removal, but in less than 10% of amputees does pain represent a severe incapacitating condition. The incidence of severe phantom pain is therefore similar to other chronic neuropathic pain states. Experimental studies within the last two decades have shown that a nerve cut gives rise to a series of morphological, physiological and biochemical changes which result in a hyperexcitability in the nervous system. Spontaneous pain and abnormally evoked pain from the stump of amputees reflect this hyperexcitability, which is amenable for modulation and treatment by the same remedies used for neuropathic pain in general. Although it was thought that

Table 34.4 Summary of studies on the prevention of phantom pain

Authors	*Randomization*	*Blinding*	*No. of patients*	*Treatment*	*Effect*
Bach et al 1988	+	?	25	A (n=11): epidural bupivacaine and morphine for 72 h before amputation B (n=14): systemic analgesia	+
Fischer and Meller 1991	–	–	11	A (n=11): nerve sheath block with bupivacaine for 72 h after amputation	+
Elizaga et al 1994	–	–	21	A (n=9): nerve sheath block with bupivacaine for at least 72 h after amputation B (n=12): systemic analgesia	–
Jahangiri et al 1994	–	–	24	A (n=13): epidural bupivacaine, clonidine and diamorphine for 24–48 h before amputation and continued 72 h after amputation B (n=11): systemic analgesia	+
Shug et al 1995	–	–	23	A (n=8): epidural bupivacaine and morphine for 24 h before, during and after amputation B: (n=7): epidural bupivacaine and morphine during and after amputation C (n=8): systemic analgesia	+
Katsuly Liapis et al 1996	+	?	45	A (n=15): epidural bupivacaine and morphine for 72 h before, during and after amputation B: (n=12): epidural bupivacaine and morphine after amputation C (n=18): systemic analgesia	+
Pinzur et al 1996	+	?	21	A (n=11): nerve sheath block with bupivacaine for 72 h after amputation B (n=10): nerve sheath block with saline for 72 h after amputation	–
Nikolajsen et al 1997c	+	+	60	A (n=29): epidural bupivacaine and morphine 18 h before, during and after amputation B (n=31): systemic analgesia before amputation, epidural bupivacaine and morphine after amputation	–

phantom pain could be prevented by pre-emptive types of treatments, e.g. epidurally administered local anaesthetics and opioids before amputation, recent data suggest that a short-lasting blockade of afferent input before amputation is not sufficient to prevent the development of central sensitization, hyperalgesia and pain. Further studies are needed to determine the role of peripheral and central mechanisms in phantom limb phenomena, including phantom pain, in order to find better types of treatments.

REFERENCES

Abramson AS, Feibel A 1981 The phantom phenomenon; its use and disuse. Bulletin of the New York Academy of Medicine 57: 99–122

Appenzeller O, Bicknell JM 1969 Effects of nervous system lesions on phantom experience in amputees. Neurology 19: 141–146

Bach S, Noreng MF, Tjéllden NU 1988 Phantom limb pain in amputees during the first 12 months following limb amputation after preoperative lumbar epidural blockade. Pain 33: 297–301

Bailey AA, Moersch FP 1941 Phantom limb. Canadian Medical Association Journal 45: 37–42

Battista AF 1979 Pain of peripheral nerve origin: fascicle ligation for prevention of painful neuroma. In: Bonica JJ, Liebeskind JC, Albe-Fessard DG (eds) Advances in pain research and therapy 3. Raven Press, New York

Baumgartner R, Riniker C 1981 Surgical stump revision as a treatment of stump and phantom pains. Results of 100 cases. In: Siegfried S, Zimmermann M (eds) Phantom and stump pain. Springer Verlag, Berlin, pp 118–122

Bell C 1830 The nervous system of the human body. Longman, London

Bennett GJ, Xie Y-K 1988 A peripheral mononeuropathy in rat that produces disorders of pain sensation like those seen in man. Pain 33: 87–107

Bors E 1951 Phantom limbs of patients with spinal cord injury. Archives of Neurology and Psychiatry 66: 610–631

Brihaye J 1958 Extinction of phantom limb in leg amputated during medullary compression by cervical discal hernia: revival of phantom after surgical removal of hernia. Acta Neurologica et Psychiatrica Belgica 58: 536

Browder J, Gallagher JP 1948 Dorsal cordotomy for pain phantom limbs. Annals of Surgery 128: 456–469

Carabelli RA, Kellerman WC 1985 Phantom limb pain: relief by application of TENS to contralateral extremity. Archives of Physical Medicine and Rehabilitation 66: 466–477

Carlen PL, Wall PD, Nadvorna H, Steinbach T 1978 Phantom limbs and related phenomena in recent traumatic amputations. Neurology 28: 211–217

Carrie LES, Glynn CJ 1986 Phantom limb pain and epidural anesthesia for cesarean section. Anesthesiology 65: 220–221

Catchlove RF 1983 Phantom pain following limb amputation in a paraplegic. A case report. Psychotherapy and Psychosomatics 39: 89–93

Chabal C, Jacobsen L, Russell LC, Burchiel KJ 1989 Pain responses to perineuromal injection of normal saline, gallamine and lidocaine in humans. Pain 36: 321–325

Coderre TJ, Katz J 1997 Peripheral and central hyperexcitability: differential signs and symptoms in persistent pain. Behavioural and Brain Sciences 20: 404–419

Cook AJ, Woolf CJ, Wall PD, McMahon SB 1987 Dynamic receptive field plasticity in rat spinal cord dorsal horn following C-primary afferent input. Nature 325: 151–153

Cronholm B 1951 Phantom limb in amputees. Acta Psychiatrica et Neurologica Scandinavica 72 (suppl): 1–310

Davis KD, Kiss ZH, Luo L 1998 Phantom sensations generated by thalamic microstimulation. Nature 391 (6665): 385–387

De Gutierrez-Mahoney CG 1948 The treatment of painful phantom limb. A follow-up study. Surgical Clinics of North America 28: 481–483

Devor M, Raber P 1990 Heritability of symptoms in an experimental model of neuropathic pain. Pain 42: 51–67

Devor M, Rappaport ZH 1990 Pain and the pathophysiology of damaged nerve. In: Fields HL (ed) Pain syndromes in neurology. Butterworths, London, pp 47–83

Dillingham TR, Braverman SE 1994 Persian Gulf War amputees: Injuries and rehabilitative needs. 159: 635–639

Doupe J, Cullen CH, Chance GQ 1944 Post-traumatic pain and the causalgic syndrome. Journal of Neurology, Neurosurgery and Psychiatry 7: 33–48

Elizaga AM, Smith DG, Sharar SR, Edwards T, Hansen ST 1994 Continuous regional analgesia by intraneural block: effect on postoperative opioid requirements and phantom limb pain following amputation. Journal of Rehabilitation Research and Development 31: 179–187

Elliott F, Little A, Milbrandt W 1976 Carbamazepine for phantom limb phenomena. New England Journal of Medicine 295: 678

Ewalt JR, Randall GC, Morris H 1947 The phantom limb. Psychosomatic Medicine 9: 118–123

Feinstein B, Luce JC, Langton JNK 1954 The influence of phantom limbs. In: Klopsteg P, Wilson P (eds) Human limbs and their substitutes. McGraw-Hill, New York, pp 19–138

Finch DRA, MacDougal M, Tibbs DJ, Morris PJ 1980 Amputation for vascular disease: the experience of a peripheral vascular unit. British Journal of Surgery 67: 233–237

Fischer A, Meller Y 1991 Continuous postoperative regional analgesia by nerve sheath block for amputation surgery – a pilot study. Anesthesia and Analgesia 72: 300–303

Flor H, Elbert T, Knecht S 1995 Phantom limb pain as a perceptual correlate of cortical reorganization following arm amputation. Nature 375: 482–484

Flor H, Elbert T, Mühlnickel W 1998 Cortical reorganization and phantom phenomena in congenital and traumatic upper-extremity amputees. Experimental Brain Research 119: 205–212

Frederiks JAM 1963 Occurrence and nature of phantom limb phenomena following amputation of body parts and following lesions of the central and peripheral nervous system. Psychiatria Neurologica et Neurochirurgica 66: 73–97

Guéniot M 1861 D'une hallucination du toucher (ou hétérotopie subjective des extrémités) particulière a certains amputés. Journal de la Physiologie de l'Homme et des Animaux 4: 416

Head H, Holmes G 1915 Sensory disturbances from cerebral lesions. Brain 34: 102–254

Henderson WR, Smyth GE 1948 Phantom limbs. Journal of Neurology, Neurosurgery and Psychiatry 11: 88–112

Herndon JH, Eaton RG, Little JW 1976 Management of painful neuromas in the hand. Journal of Bone and Joint Surgery 58: 369–373

Hill A, Niven CA, Knussen C 1996 Pain memories in phantom limbs: a case story. Pain 66: 381–384

Houghton AD, Nicholls G, Houghton AL, Saadah E, McColl L 1994 Phantom pain: natural history and association with rehabilitation. Annals of the Royal College of Surgeons of England 76: 22–25

Iacono RP, Sandyk R, Baumford CR, Awerbuch G, Malone JM 1987 Post-amputation phantom pain and autonomous stump movements responsive to doxepin. Functional Neurology 2: 343–348

Jacobsen L, Chabal C, Brody MC 1989 Relief of persistent postamputation stump and phantom limb pain with intrathecal fentanyl. Pain 37: 317–322

Jacobsen L, Chabal C, Brody MC 1990. A comparison of the effects of intrathecal fentanyl and lidocaine on established postamputation stump pain. Pain 40: 137–141

Jaeger H, Maier C 1992 Calcitonin in phantom limb pain: a double-blind study. Pain 48: 21–27

Jahangiri M, Jayatunga AP, Bradley JWP, Dark CH 1994 Prevention of phantom pain after major lower limb amputation by epidural infusion of diamorphine, clonidine and bupivacaine. Annals of the Royal College of Surgeons of England 76: 324–326

James U 1973 Unilateral above-knee amputees. A clinico-orthopedic evaluation of healthy active men, fitted with a prosthesis. Scandinavian Journal of Rehabilitative Medicine 5: 23–34

Jensen TS, Krebs B, Nielsen J, Rasmussen P 1983 Phantom limb, phantom pain and stump pain in amputees during the first 6 months following limb amputation. Pain 17: 243–256

Jensen TS, Krebs B, Nielsen J, Rasmussen P 1984 Non-painful phantom limb phenomena in amputees: incidence, clinical characteristics and temporal course. Acta Neurologica Scandinavica 70: 407–414

Jensen TS, Krebs B, Nielsen J, Ramussen P 1985 Immediate and long-term phantom limb pain in amputees: incidence, clinical characteristics and relationship to preamputation limb pain. Pain 21: 267–278

Kajander KC, Wakisaka S, Bennett GJ 1992 Spontaneous discharge originates in the dorsal root ganglion at the onset of a painful peripheral neuropathy in the rat. Neuroscience Letters 138: 225–228

Katsuly Liapis I, Georgakis P, Tierry C 1996 Preemptive extradural analgesia reduces the incidence of phantom pain in lower limb amputees. British Journal of Anaesthesia 76: 125

Katz J 1992 Psychophysical correlates of phantom limb experience. Journal of Neurology, Neurosurgery and Psychiatry 50: 811–821

Katz J, Melzack R 1990 Pain 'memories' in phantom limbs: review and clinical observations. Pain 43: 319–336

Katz J, Melzack R 1991 Auricular transcutaneous electrical nerve stimulation (TENS) reduces phantom limb pain. Journal of Pain and Symptom Management 6 (2): 73–83

Keil G 1990 Sogenannte erstbeschreibung des phantomschmerzes von Ambroise Paré. Fortschritte der Medicine 108: 58–66

Kim SH, Chung JM 1992 An experimental model for peripheral neuropathy produced by segmental spinal nerve ligation in the rat. Pain 50: 335–363

Krainick J-U, Thoden U, Riechert T 1980 Pain reduction in amputees by long-term spinal cord stimulation. Journal of Neurosurgery 52: 346–350

Krane EJ, Heller LB 1995 The prevalence of phantom sensation and pain in pediatric amputees. Journal of Pain and Symptom Management 10: 21–29

Krebs B, Jensen TS, Krøner K, Nielsen J, Jørgensen HS 1985 Phantom limb phenomena in amputees 7 years after limb amputation. In: Fields HL, Dubner R, Cervero F (eds) Advances in pain research and therapy 9. Raven Press, New York, pp 425–429

Lawrence RM 1980 Phantom pain: a new hypothesis. Medical Hypotheses 6: 245–248

Lundeberg T 1985 Relief of pain from nine phantom limbs by peripheral stimulation. Journal of Neurology 232: 79–82

Lunn V 1948 Om legemsbevidstheden. Munksgaard, Copenhagen

Mackenzie N 1983 Phantom limb pain during spinal anaesthesia. Anaesthesia 38: 886–887

Marsland AR, Weekes JWN, Atkinson RL, Leong MG 1982 Phantom limb pain: a case for beta blockers? Pain 12: 295–297

Melzack R 1971 Phantom limb pain: implications of treatment of pathological pain. Anesthesiology 35: 409–419

Melzack R, Loeser JD 1978 Phantom body pain in paraplegics: evidence for a central 'pattern generating mechanism' for pain. Pain 4: 195–210

Merienne L, Mazars G 1981 Transformation of body scheme caused by thalamic stimulation. Thalamic stimulation for painful phantom limb. Neurochirurgie 27: 121–123

Mitchell SW 1872 Injuries of nerves and their consequences. JB Lippincott, Philadelphia

Montoya P, Larbig W, Grulke N 1997 Relationship of phantom limb pain to other phantom limb phenomena in upper extremity amputees. Pain 72: 87–93

Mundinger F, Neumüller H 1981 Programmed transcutaneous (TNS) and central (DBS) stimulation for control of phantom limb pain and causalgia: a new method for treatment. In: Siegfried J, Zimmermann M (eds) Phantom and stump pain. Springer Verlag, Berlin, pp 167–178

Mundinger F, Salomáo JF 1980 Deep brain stimulation in mesencephalic lemniscus medialis for chronic pain. Acta Neurochirurgica 30: 245–258

Nashold BS, Ostdahl RH 1979 Dorsal root entry zone lesions for pain relief. Journal of Neurosurgery 51: 59–69

Nathan PW 1962 Pain traces left in the central nervous system. In: Keele CA, Smith R (eds) The assessment of pain in man and animals. E & S Livingstone, Edinburgh, pp 129–134

Nikolajsen L, Hansen CL, Nielsen J, Keller J, Arendt-Nielsen L, Jensen TS 1996 The effect of ketamine on phantom pain: a central neuropathic disorder maintained by peripheral input. Pain 67: 69–77

Nikolajsen L, Ilkjær S, Krøner K, Christensen JH, Jensen TS 1997a The influence of preamputation pain on postamputation stump and phantom pain. Pain 72: 393–405

Nikolajsen L, Hansen PO, Jensen TS 1997b Oral ketamine therapy in the treatment of postamputation stump pain. Acta Anaesthesiologica Scandinavica 41: 427–429

Nikolajsen L, Ilkjær S, Krøner K, Christensen JH, Jensen TS 1997c Randomised trial of epidural bupivacaine and morphine in prevention of stump and phantom pain in lower-limb amputation. Lancet 350: 1353–1357

Nordenbos W 1959 Pain. Elsevier, Amsterdam

Nyström B, Hagbarth KE 1981 Microelectrode recordings from transected nerves in amputees with phantom limb pain. Neuroscience Letters 27: 211–216

Parkes CM 1973 Factors determining the persistence of phantom pain in the amputee. Journal of Psychosomatic Research 17: 97–108

Patterson JF 1988 Carbamazepine in the treatment of phantom limb pain. Southern Medical Journal 81: 1100–1102

Pinzur MS, Garla PGN, Pluth T, Vrbos L 1996 Continuous postoperative infusion of a regional anaesthetic after an amputation of the lower extremity. Journal of Bone and Joint Surgery 78: 1501–1505

Pitres A 1897 Étude sur les sensations illusoires des amputés. Annales Medico-psychologiques 55: 177–192

Pohjolainen T 1991 A clinical evaluation of stumps in lower limb amputees. Prosthetics and Orthotics International 15: 178–184

Price DB 1976 Phantom limb phenomena in patients with leprosy. Journal of Nervous and Mental Disease 163: 108–116

Price DD, Mao J, Mayer DJ 1997 Central consequences of persistent pain states. In: Jensen TS, Turner JM, Wiesenfeld-Hallin Z (eds) Proceedings of the 8th World Congress on Pain, Progress in Pain Research and Management, vol. 8. IASP Press, Seattle, pp 155–184

Riddoch G 1941 Phantom limbs and body shape. Brain 64: 197–222

Riese W, Bruck G 1950 Le membre fantôme chez l'enfant. Revue Neurologique 83: 221–222
Samii M 1981 Centrocentral anastomosis of peripheral nerves: a neurosurgical treatment of amputation neuromas. In: Siegfried J, Zimmermann M (eds) Phantom and stump pain. Springer Verlag, Berlin, pp 123–125
Samii M, Moringlane JR 1984 Thermocoagulation of the dorsal root entry zone for the treatment of intractable pain. Neurosurgery 15: 953–955
Saris SC, Iacono RP, Nashold BS Jr 1985 Dorsal root entry zone lesions for post-amputation pain. Journal of Neurosurgery 62: 72–76
Saris SC, Iacono RP, Nashold BS Jr 1988 Successful treatment of phantom pain with dorsal root entry zone coagulation. Applied Neurophysiology 51: 188–187
Schott GD 1986 Pain and its absence in an unfortunate family of amputees. Pain 25: 229–231
Sherman RA 1989 Stump and phantom limb pain. Neurologic Clinics 7: 249–264
Sherman RA, Glenda GM 1987 Concurrent variation of burning phantom limb and stump pain with near surface blood flow in the stump. Orthopedics 10: 1395–1402
Sherman R, Sherman C 1983 Prevalence and characteristics of chronic phantom limb pain among American veterans: results of a trial survey. American Journal of Physical Medicine 62: 227–238
Sherman RA, Sherman CJ 1985 A comparison of phantom sensations among amputees whose amputations were of civilian and military origins. Pain 21: 91–97
Sherman RA, Sherman CJ, Gall NG 1980 A survey of current phantom limb pain treatment in the United States. Pain 8: 85–99
Sherman RA, Sherman CJ, Bruno GM 1987 Psychological factors influencing chronic phantom limb pain: an analysis of the literature. Pain 28: 285–295
Sherman RA, Vernice GD, Evans CB 1992. Temporal relationship between changes in phantom limb pain intensity and changes in surface electromyogram of the residual limb. International Journal of Psychophysiology 13: 71–77
Shug SA, Burell R, Payne J, Tester P 1995 Preemptive epidural anaesthesia may prevent phantom limb pain. Regional Anesthesia 20: 256
Siegfried J, Cetinalp E 1981 Neurosurgical treatment of phantom limb pain: a survey of methods. In: Siegfried J, Zimmermann M (eds) Phantom and stump pain. Springer Verlag, Berlin, pp 148–155
Simmel ML 1962 Phantom experiences following amputation in childhood. Journal of Neurology, Neurosurgery and Psychiatry 25: 69–78
Sliosberg A 1948 Les algies des amputés. Masson, Paris
Stannard CF, Porter GE 1993 Ketamine hydrochloride in the treatment of phantom limb pain. Pain 54: 227–230
Sunderland S 1978 Nerves and nerve injuries. Williams & Wilkins, Baltimore
Tessler MJ, Kleiman SJ 1994 Spinal anaesthesia for patients with previous lower limb amputations. Anaesthesia 49: 439–441
Thoden U, Gruber RP, Krainick J-U, Huber-Mück L 1979 Langzeitergebnisse transkutaner Nervenstimulation bei chronisch neurogenen Schmerzzuständen. Nervenarzt 50: 179–184
Urban BJ, France RD, Steinberger EK, Scoot DL, Maltbie AA 1986 Long-term use of narcotic/antidepressant medication in the management of phantom limb. Pain 24: 191–196
Van Wirdum P 1965 A new explanation of phantom symptoms. Psychiatrica Neurologica et Neurochirurgica 68: 306–313
Wall PD 1981 On the origin of pain associated with amputation. In: Siegfried J, Zimmermann M (eds) Phantom and stump pain. Springer Verlag, Berlin, pp 2–14
Wall PD, Gutnick M 1974 Ongoing activity in peripheral nerves: the physiology and pharmacology of impulses originating from a neuroma. Experimental Neurology 43: 580–593
Wall R, Novotny-Joseph P, Macnamara TE 1985 Does preamputation pain influence phantom limb pain in cancer patients? Southern Medical Journal 78: 34–36
Warten SW, Hamann W, Wedley JR, McColl I 1997 Phantom pain and sensation among British veteran amputees. British Journal of Anaesthesia 78: 652–659
Weinstein S, Sersen EA 1961 Phantoms in cases of congenital absence of limbs. Neurology 11: 905–911
Wiegand H, Winkelmüller W 1985 Treatment of deafferentation pain by high-frequency intervention of the dorsal root entry zone. Deutsche Medizinische Wochenschrift 100: 216–220
Wynn Parry CB 1980 Pain in avulsion lesions of the brachial plexus. Pain 9: 40–53
Yarnitsky D, Barron SA, Bental E 1988 Disappearance of phantom pain after focal brain infarction. Pain: 32: 285–287

Peripheral neuropathies

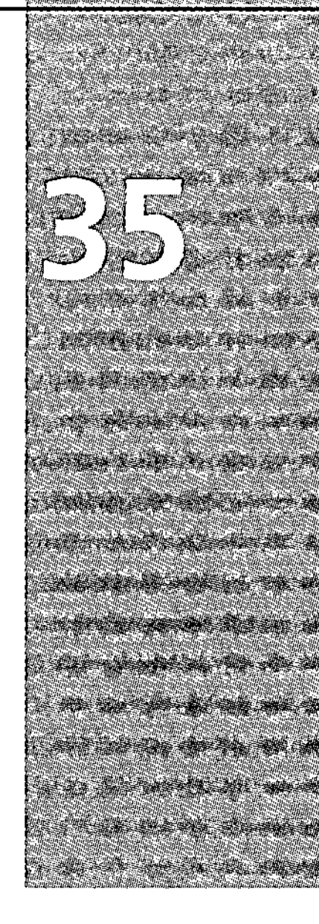

J. W. SCADDING

The primary sensory nerve may be affected in a number of different ways by a great variety of diseases. Motor or sensory fibres may be preferentially affected, but in most neuropathies both are involved, leading to various patterns of sensorimotor deficit. Sensory neuropathies are frequently accompanied by positive sensory symptoms, which usually take the form of paraesthesiae which are not troublesome and which are overshadowed by the symptoms of sensory or motor deficits. However, there are neuropathies in which pain and severe paraesthesiae are typical and troublesome features. In these neuropathies, the dysaesthesiae may be the presenting and most severe continuing symptoms. This chapter is concerned with these neuropathies, which include many polyneuropathies and mononeuropathies. Experimental animal studies, trigeminal neuropathies, amputation and phantom pain, complex regional pain syndrome (causalgia and reflex sympathetic dystrophy) and the treatment of pain due to peripheral neuropathies are topics considered in other chapters in this volume.

The relationship of painful symptoms to morphological and electrophysiological changes in peripheral nerves has been a subject of interest for many years, particularly since the introduction of nerve biopsy (see Thomas 1970, Dyck et al 1993) and the development of clinical electrophysiological techniques (Kimuna 1993, Lambert & Dyck 1993). Since it was established that the transmission of impulses in different classes of peripheral nerve fibre depended on the type of peripheral stimulus in animals and man (Adrian 1931, Lewis et al 1931, Clark et al 1935, Collins et al 1960), the early observations have been greatly expanded by single-fibre recordings in animals and man (Burgess & Perl 1973, Iggo 1977, Valbo et al 1979, Yaksh & Hammond 1982). Wortis et al (1942) noted the similarity of the burning pain in patients with alcoholic neuropathy to the sensations that were obtained by peripheral stimulation after prolonged anoxia of a limb in normal subjects and, in the light of the observations of Gasser's group (Clark et al 1935), suggested that the burning pain in alcoholic neuropathy might be due to a predominantly C-fibre input, with loss of the normal large-fibre input.

Subsequently, Weddell et al (1948) examined nerve fibres in biopsies of hyperpathic skin, finding a decreased number of fibres in small dermal nerves with a reduced fibre density in the hyperpathic skin, and postulated that the presumed decreased afferent barrage from these areas was responsible for hyperpathia. Lourie and King (1966) also reported a decreased fibre density in hyperpathic skin and noted a preponderance of small-diameter fibres. In particular, they found that hyperpathic hairs arose from follicles innervated predominantly by small fibres. In a study of herpes zoster neuropathy, Noordenbos (1959) found a predominant loss of larger myelinated fibres in affected nerves.

These observations seemed to suggest that in situations where there was either preferential regeneration of small fibres or selective loss of large fibres, dysaesthesiae might result. This idea and the formation of the gate control theory (Melzack & Wall 1965) stimulated interest in the further investigation of peripheral neuropathy in man.

TYPE OF PAIN IN PERIPHERAL NEUROPATHY

Many terms may be used by patients with neuropathies to describe their painful sensations. The symptoms may be divided into those which are unprovoked (spontaneous) and those which are provoked by manoeuvres such as skin stimulation, pressure over affected nerves, changes in temperature or emotional factors. The most commonly described spontaneous symptoms are a deep aching in the extremities and a superficial burning, stinging or prickling pain. Some patients also report paroxysmal, shock-like lancinating pains, sometimes radiating through a whole limb (Dyck et al 1976, Thomas 1979, Thomas & Ochoa 1993).

Allodynia may be particularly incapacitating in some neuropathies and accompanying hyperpathia is not uncommon (Lindblom 1979, Noordenbos 1979). In the following descriptions of the different neuropathies, the major painful complaints typical of each condition are given, but it should be emphasized that, within a single aetiological or pathological diagnostic category, considerable symptom variation occurs in different individuals. The clinical features of neuropathic pain are summarized in Table 35.1 and the neuropathies which are commonly associated with pain are listed in Table 35.2.

INVESTIGATION OF PERIPHERAL NEUROPATHIES

The cause of some neuropathies may become apparent after a few simple tests and there is no need for specialized investigation. Nevertheless, as pointed out by Thomas and Ochea (1993), even after extensive investigation the cause of a substantial minority of neuropathies remains uncertain. Detailed discussion of basic clinical diagnostic aspects of peripheral neuropathies and of specialized investigative techniques is beyond the scope of this chapter, but some aspects of the morphological techniques are considered, with regard particularly to their limitations. Full accounts of these topics are to be found in reviews by Thomas (1970), Kimuna (1993), Lambert and Dyck (1993) and Dyck et al (1993).

Table 35.1 Clinical features of neuropathic pain

Abnormal quality: raw, burning, gnawing
Paroxysmal pains
Sensory impairment
Associated allodynia, hyperalgesia, hyperpathia
Evidence of abnormal sympathetic function
Sometimes associated with changes of complex regional pain syndrome
Immediate or delayed onset of pain following injury in mononeuropathy
Intensity of pain markedly altered by emotion and fatigue

NERVE BIOPSY

A major problem of structure–function correlation in peripheral neuropathies is the sampling error inherent in relating sensory abnormalities and whole-nerve electrophysiology to the morphology of a small fascicular nerve biopsy. To overcome this, Dyck and co-workers (Dyck et al 1971b, Lambert & Dyck 1993) took long multifascicular biopsies of sural nerve and investigated these electrophysiologically in vitro, by measurement of compound action potentials, and morphologically, the main emphasis being fibre populations and teased fibre studies. Biopsies from normal volunteers were compared with biopsies from patients with Friedreich's ataxia, dominantly inherited amyloidosis, hereditary motor and sensory and sensory neuropathies and chronic relapsing inflammatory polyneuropathy. In Friedreich's ataxia, a substantial reduction of the A α potential with preservation of A δ and C potentials correlated well with the decrease in the large myelinated fibre population and with the sensory deficit of touch-pressure and two-point discrimination with preservation of pain and temperature sensation. In dominantly inherited amyloidosis, the absent C-fibre potentials, greatly reduced A δ potential and only moderately reduced A α potential correlated well both with a near absence of C fibres and reduced small myelinated fibre population and with the injured pain and temperature sensation and autonomic function in this patient. Similar good correlations were found in the two types of hereditary sensory neuropathy and in uraemic neuropathy, but not in chronic relapsing inflammatory neuropathy. This was thought to be due to extensive segmental demyelination and remyelination, leading to dispersion of large-fibre action potentials, some of which were considered to have contributed to the C-fibre potential.

These observations established that a selective loss of small myelinated and unmyelinated fibres leads to impaired pain sensation in man and indicated that reasonable predictions about fibre population could be made from physiological observations, except where segmental demyelination was a prominent feature. It should be emphasized, however, that such extensive nerve biopsy and in vitro electrophysiology remain research investigations.

Some problems of standard nerve biopsy morphological observations require mention here. Examination of transverse sections by light microscopy will fail to recognize segmentally demyelinated axons and will thus underestimate the myelinated fibre population. An increase in the density of small fibres does not necessarily imply a selective loss of

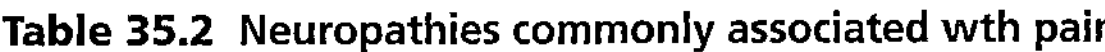

Table 35.2 Neuropathies commonly associated wth pain

Traumatic mononeuropathies		
Entrapment neuropathies		Painful scars
Transection (partial or complete)		Post-thoracotomy
Causalgia		Stump pain
Other mononeuropathies and multiple mononeuropathies		
Diabetic mononeuropathy		Neuralgic amyotrophy
Diabetic amyotrophy		Malignant nerve/plexus invasion
Postherpetic neuralgia		Radiation plexopathy
Trigeminal neuralgia		Connective tissue disease
Glossopharyngeal neuralgia		
Polyneuropathies		
Metabolic/nutritional:	Diabetic	Strachan's (Jamaican neuropathy)
	Alcoholic	Cuban neuropathy
	Pellagra	Tanzanian neuropathy
	Amyloid	Burning feet syndrome
	Beriberi	
Drugs:	Isoniazid	Nitrofurantoin
	Cisplatin	Disulfiram
	Vincristine	
Toxic:	Thallium	
	Arsenic	
	Clioquinol	
Hereditary:	Fabry's disease	
	Dominantly inherited sensory neuropathy	
Malignant:	Myeloma	
	Carcinomatous	
Others:	Acute idiopathic polyneuropathy (Guillain–Barré)	
	Idiopathic	

large fibres, since regeneration will increase the population of small fibres. By relating axonal diameter to myelin sheath thickness by electron microscopic examination and using certain criteria for differentiating the sprouts of myelinated and unmyelinated fibres, this problem can be overcome to some extent (Ochoa 1970, Morris et al 1972, Dyck et al 1993).

The two major pathological processes in peripheral neuropathy are axonal degeneration and segmental demyelination. The division of polyneuropathies into either of these pathological categories is somewhat artificial, since both processes are usually present, albeit in varying proportions (Thomas 1971). This has been evidence since the introduction of routine examination of teased fibres (Dyck et al 1968, Thomas 1970) which permits easier recognition of demyelination, remyelination and degenerative changes, which may be graded according to severity (Dyck et al 1971b). Since teased fibres may also subsequently be examined by electron microscopy (Dyck & Lais 1970, Spencer & Thomas 1970, Dyck et al 1993).

The various patterns of axonal degeneration, affecting distal parts of the axon or the cell body or both, and details of segmental demyelination, remyelination and onion bulb formation and of pathological reactions of unmyelinated fibres are reviewed by Dyck et al (1993) and Ochoa (1978).

POLYNEUROPATHIES

From the point of view of understanding mechanisms of pain in human neuropathies, information is limited. Standard neurophysiological tests are essentially diagnostic, but tell us little about the properties which may be responsible for pain. Single-fibre microneurographic recordings up to the present time have been performed almost exclusively on normal subjects and there is little direct information in human polyneuropathies concerning the presence of the abnormal properties of ectopic impulse generation, catecholamine sensitivity and interactions between fibres, which have been so extensively studied in experimental animals (see Ch. 14). As a result of the technical limitations of neurophysiological investigation in man, the morphological changes in nerve biopsies and their correlation with nerve conduction studies have provided the only basis on which to consider mechanisms underlying the development of pain in neuropathy.

Following the earlier indications that an imbalance between large and small-fibre input might be of particular importance, fibre size distribution in different neuropathies became a particular focus of attention. In the account of the polyneuropathies, it is convenient to follow the subdivision of the neuropathies on this basis, both to trace the development of ideas about mechanisms of pain in neuropathy and also as a means of showing that fibre size distribution per se is unlikely to be an important factor leading to pain. Table 35.3 lists some neuropathies important to the present discussion, divided on the basis of painfulness and fibre size distribution.

POLYNEUROPATHIES WITH SELECTIVE LOSS OF PAIN SENSATION

These comprise a rare, poorly defined group of inherited disorders in which, from an early age, an insensitivity to pain is evident. It is important to distinguish those disorders in which the peripheral and central nervous systems are intact, where the problem appears to be a lack of recognition of pain, an indifference or asymbolia, from insensitivity (Schilder et al 1931), which can be explained on the basis of observed structural abnormalities. In the former group, patients are able to identify noxious stimuli and sensory thresholds are normal but they do not react behaviourally or physiologically in the expected way (Ogden et al 1959, Winkelmann et al 1962). Peripheral nerves, spinal cord and thalamus are all normal in these patients (Feindel 1953, Baxter & Olszewski 1960). Asymbolia for pain may also be acquired, recent evidence suggesting a crucial role for the insular cortex, damage to which may lead to disconnection between sensory cortex and the limbic system (Berthier et al 1988).

Table 35.3 Painful and painless polyneuropathies

Polyneuropathies with selective loss of pain sensation
Congenital analgesia with anhidrosis
Congenital analgesia with other sensory impairment
Tangier disease (familial α-lipoprotein deficiency)
Painful polyneuropathies with selective large-fibre loss
Isoniazid neuropathy
Pellagra neuropathy
Painless polyneuropathies with selective large-fibre loss
Friedreich's ataxia
Chronic renal failure
Painful polyneuropathies with selective small-fibre loss
Diabetic neuropathy
Amyloid neuropathy
Fabry's disease
Dominantly inherited sensory neuropathy
Painful polyneuropathies with non-selective fibre loss
Alcoholic neuropathy
Myeloma neuropathy
Miscellaneous painful polyneuropathies
Acute inflammatory polyneuropathy
Nutritional neuropathies
Beriberi
Strachan's syndrome
Burning feet syndrome
Arsenic neuropathy
Subacute myelo-optic neuropathy

Leaving such cases aside, two major subgroups may be recognized. In congenital analgesia with anhidrosis (Swanson 1963), impairment of pain sensation predisposes to tissue-damaging injury, leading on occasion to loss of fingers (Mazar et al 1976) or severe mutilation of the tongue (Pinsky & DiGeorge 1966). Sweet (1981) reviewed reports of 15 such patients. Typically, pain and, to a lesser extent, thermal sensation are severely defective, while other sensory modalities remain intact. The associated anhidrosis may lead to episodes of hyperpyrexia. Of the 15 patients, only four were of normal intelligence and these children mutilated themselves less severely. Pathologically, a case coming to autopsy showed evidence of a severe sensory neuropathy with a total absence of small dorsal root ganglion cells, of small fibres in dorsal roots and of Lissauer's tract, together with a reduction in size of the spinal tract of the trigeminal nerve (Swanson et al 1965).

In the second group, an insensitivity to pain is evident in childhood, accompanied by symptoms and signs of a sensory polyneuropathy, but the impairments of pain sensation is out of proportion to impairment of other modalities; 21 such cases were reviewed by Sweet (1981), in which the degree of selectivity of pain sensation impairment was variable. The case reports of a brother and sister aged 6 and $2\frac{1}{2}$ years by Haddow et al (1970) exemplify the most extreme form. Both siblings had extensive mutilating lesions of the fingers and in the 6-year-old a pin was not painful anywhere, while there was a much milder distal loss to other modalities. The pathological peripheral nerve changes in this group range from a complete absence of myelinated fibres to a marked non-selective reduction, with normal unmyelinated fibres (Sweet 1981). It seems likely that some of these cases were examples of dominantly inherited sensory neuropathy, considered below.

Tangier disease

Tangier disease, familial α-lipoprotein deficiency, is an extremely rare lipid disorder in which a neuropathy occurs in at least half those affected (Yao & Herbert 1993). The complex biochemistry of this disorder is reviewed by Yao and Herbert (1993). Two patients with a remarkable

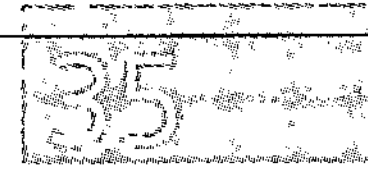

dissociated sensory loss of pain and temperature sensation over most of the body have been reported (Kocen et al 1967, Fredrickson et al 1972). Kocen et al (1973) reported the radial nerve biopsy features in one of these. Small myelinated fibres were selectively lost and unmyelinated fibres were virtually absent.

PAINFUL POLYNEUROPATHIES WITH SELECTIVE LOSS OF LARGE FIBRES

Isoniazid neuropathy

Pain as a feature of polyneuropathies in which a selective large-fibre loss occurs would accord with the predications of the gate control theory. An example is isoniazid neuropathy, which was first recognized by Pegum (1952); clinical features were described by Gammon et al (1953). Initial symptoms of distal numbness and tingling paraesthesiae are later accompanied by pain, which may be felt as a deep ache or burning. The calf muscles are often painful and tender and the exacerbation of symptoms produced by walking may prevent the patient from walking. Spontaneous pain and paraesthesiae may be particularly troublesome at night. Examination shows signs of a sensorimotor neuropathy, often confined to the legs. Cutaneous hyperaesthesia is a frequent finding. Ochoa (1970) examined sural nerve biopsies from nine patients, reporting a primary axonal degeneration in myelinated fibres with evidence of degeneration in unmyelinated fibres and regeneration in both types, together with degeneration of regenerated myelinated fibres. Using several ultrastructural criteria, Ochoa (1970) was able to distinguish as yet unmyelinated sprouts of myelinated fibres from unmyelinated fibres and was also able to make an accurate assessment of differential myelinated fibre damage, finding that large fibres were preferentially lost. The relative resistance of unmyelinated fibres to isoniazid was shown by Hopkins and Lambert (1972), who reported preservation of the C-fibre compound action potential in severe experimental isoniazid neuropathy. Prevention and treatment with pyridoxine was described by Biehl and Wilter (1954); the biochemical pathogenesis is discussed by Windebank (1993).

Pellagra neuropathy

Peripheral neuropathy is one of the many neurological manifestations of pellagra, due to niacin deficiency (Spillane 1947). A predominant feature of the sensorimotor neuropathy is spontaneous pain in the feet and lower legs, with tenderness of the calf muscles and cutaneous hyperaesthesia of the feet (Lewy et al 1940). There are no recent pathological studies of this neuropathy and no ultrastructural study. Wilson (1913–1914) reported changes suggesting a predominant axonal degeneration and, in a later investigation, Aring et al (1941) observed a decreased density of myelinated fibres, with a preferential loss of larger fibres. In spinal cord, extensive degeneration was found in the dorsal and lateral tracts by Anderson and Spiller (1940) in two patients at autopsy, while others, for example Greenfield and Holmes (1939), observed degeneration mainly in the posterior columns, with less marked changes in the pyramidal tracts. Pellagra neuropathy would thus appear to be a further example of a painful neuropathy in which large fibres are selectively lost. The possibility that regenerated myelinated fibres biased the fibre population studies of Aring et al (1941) is made less likely, but is not excluded, by the overall decrease in fibre density. The spinal cord changes suggest that this is an example of a central–peripheral distal axonopathy.

Hypothyroid neuropathy

Pollard et al (1982) reported the pathological changes in sural nerve biopsies from two patients with untreated hypothyroidism. One presented with a long history of pain in the feet and progressive difficulty in walking, the other with pain and paraesthesiae in the hands. In both there were signs of a sensorimotor neuropathy. The biopsies showed a mainly axonal degeneration with occasional segmental demyelination. In both patients, myelinated fibre densities were decreased with a relative loss of large fibres, but there were regenerating myelinated fibres which may have contributed to the small-fibre bias, though probably not to a significant extent. Unmyelinated fibre densities were increased, due to small-diameter regenerating axons. Dyck and Lambert (1970) also found reduced myelinated fibre densities in two hypothyroid patients, associated with reduced A α and δ potentials in vitro, with normal C-fibre potentials. Teased fibres showed more marked segmental demyelination and remyelination with less axonal degeneration than in the patients of Pollard et al (1982).

PAINLESS POLYNEUROPATHIES WITH SELECTIVE LARGE-FIBRE LOSS

In contrast to the polyneuropathies described above, there are two conditions associated with neuropathies in which a selective loss of large fibres is not generally associated with painful symptoms. These are Friedreich's ataxia and chronic renal failure.

Friedreich's ataxia

The physiological and pathological characteristics of the neuropathy of Friedreich's ataxia were referred to earlier (Dyck et al 1971b). Pain is an unusual complaint in this condition and is only occasionally severe. Friedreich himself mentioned it, though others with a large experience of the condition do not report pain as an important feature (Thomas 1974, 1979, Dyck 1993). It is worth emphasizing that the selective loss of myelinated fibres occurs only in the earlier stages of the disorder and eventually loss of all fibre sizes occurs (Dyck 1993). The pathology is an axonal degeneration with secondary segmental demyelination (Dyck & Lais 1973). Pain might be expected as a regular feature in the earlier stages of Friedreich's ataxia, during the period of selective fibre loss, but this is not the case (Dyck 1993).

Chronic renal failure

Chronic renal failure due to any cause may be associated with a neuropathy in which a selective loss of large fibres occurs, but which is rarely painful. A complaint of restless legs is an early symptom, followed by distal numbness and paraesthesiae, with distal weakness usually confined to the legs. The rate of progression and eventual extent of the disability are extremely variable (Asbury et al 1963, Asbury 1993). Thomas et al (1971) noted that painful symptoms were uncommon, though Asbury (1993) reported burning on the soles of the feet in some patients. Extensive pathological studies have been performed in patients coming to autopsy (Marin & Tyler 1961, Asbury et al 1963, Forno & Alston 1967) and showed axonal degeneration in distal parts of the lower limb nerves, with chromatolysis of anterior horn cells and, in one case of Asbury et al (1963) with a neuropathy of long duration, there were myelin degenerative changes in the cervical dorsal columns, suggesting that this may be a central–peripheral distal axonopathy. Demyelination and remyelination in teased fibres have caused some to take the view that pathology is primarily a segmental demyelination (Dayan et al 1970, Dinn & Crane 1970) but the extensive studies of Thomas et al (1971) and Dyck et al (1971a) leave little doubt that it is a primary axonal degeneration.

Thomas et al (1971) observed a reduced myelinated fibre density in five of six biopsies, with selective loss of larger fibres, without significant numbers of regenerating fibres in teased fibres. This was also found in Dyck et al (1971a), who noted a non-random distribution of demyelination of fibres about to degenerate as a result of primary axonal pathology. None of the eight patients in the two investigations had experienced major painful symptoms. Improvement in chronic renal failure neuropathy may occur with dialysis (Thomas et al 1971) and after renal transplantation (Dyck 1982).

PAINFUL POLYNEUROPATHIES WITH SELECTIVE SMALL-FIBRE LOSS

It is perhaps surprising that small-fibre neuropathies should be painful, but there are several examples, including some patients with diabetic polyneuropathy, amyloid, Fabry's disease and some hereditary neuropathies.

Diabetes

Diabetes is associated with several types of polyneuropathy of which the commonest is a symmetrical sensory polyneuropathy (Thomas 1973). Numbness and paraesthesiae are common presenting complaints, the paraesthesiae sometimes having a burning quality. In addition, some patients complain of a spontaneous deep, aching pain and lightning pain may be reported. The prevalence of these severe dysaesthetic symptoms is not known but in the experience of Thomas and Tomlinson (1993), pain is frequently troublesome, even when sensory and motor deficits are mild. Severe sensory neuropathy in diabetes may lead to painless perforating foot ulcers and in such patients the upper limbs may also be involved and there may be an associated autonomic neuropathy. The pathology and biochemical factors in the sensory neuropathy due to diabetes are complex controversial topics (Thomas & Tomlinson 1993). As with other neuropathies, uncertainty as to whether the pathology is primarily an axonal degeneration of Schwann cell dysfunction leading to demyelination has been the major issue. Segmental demyelination and remyelination, sometimes leading to onion bulb formation, has been reported (Thomas & Lascelles 1966, Ballin & Thomas 1968) but axonal loss has also been observed (Greenbaum et al 1964, Thomas & Lascelles 1966). In addition, dorsal root ganglion cell degeneration occurs (Olsson et al 1968) and loss of anterior horn cells has been reported (Greenbaum et al 1964). The characteristic marked slowing of conduction velocity in most cases of diabetic neuropathy (Gilliatt 1965) suggests that demyelination is the usual primary pathology, but it is not recognized that at times extensive demyelination may occur as a result of pathological processes primarily affecting axons (Thomas 1971). Overall, the evidence indicates that demyelination is the predominant pathology in the majority of patients and axonal degeneration in a minority. Earlier suggestions that the neuropathy might

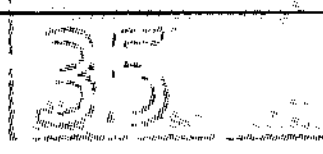

result from a diabetic microangiopathy have not been supported by more recent observations (Thomas & Tomlinson 1993), though a vascular pathology in diabetic mononeuropathy is likely.

Brown et al (1976) reported clinical and pathological findings in three patients with severe pain due to diabetic polyneuropathy. Two of the patients had shooting pains in the legs. In all three there was a distal sensory impairment, but tendon reflexes were preserved. Nerve biopsies suggested a predominant axonal degeneration affecting mainly small myelinated and unmyelinated fibres. There were also myelinated fibre sprouts and their presence in appreciable numbers led Brown et al (1976) to suggest that the pain in these patients might have been due to abnormal impulse generation, as in sprouts forming experimental neuromas (Wall & Gutnick 1974).

They also reviewed patients with diabetic polyneuropathy with attention to painfulness in relation to physical signs. Patients without pain tended to have areflexia with distal sensory loss particularly involving joint position sense, while patients with severe burning pain and hyperaesthesia tended to have sensory loss with a relative preservation of position sense and intact reflexes and more often had evidence of an accompanying autonomic neuropathy.

Said et al (1983) reported three patients similar to those of Brown et al (1976), with a striking selective loss of pain and temperature sensation, producing a pseudosyringomyelic picture. However, some of the patients with chronic sensorimotor neuropathy reported by Behse et al (1977) had pain. Nerve biopsies showed a non-selective fibre loss. A similar non-selective fibre loss, but accompanied by evidence of regeneration, characterized the nerve biopsies of the patients with the acute painful neuropathy reported by Archer et al (1983).

Britland et al (1992) report a morphometric study of sural nerve biopsies from six diabetics, four with active acute painful neuropathy and two with recent remission from this type of neuropathy. Myelinated and unmyelinated fibre degeneration and regeneration were present in all of the nerves, the only discernible differences between the nerves from patients with and without pain being that those with remission from the pain had a less abnormal axon: Schwann cell calibre ratio, more successful myelinated fibre regeneration and less active myelinated fibre regeneration. However, these were all differences in the severity and the authors emphasize the similarity of the pathological changes in the two groups.

In a cross-sectional study, Guy et al (1985) found that loss of thermal sensation occurred in isolation or in combination with loss of vibration sensation but the reverse pattern, selective loss of vibration sensation, did not occur. These observations indicate that small fibres are affected early and large fibres later in diabetic polyneuropathy. However, no longitudinal studies have been reported.

Over and above the structural and physiological alterations common to many types of peripheral nerve damage which may lead to pain, two other factors may be of importance in diabetic neuropathy. Hyperglycaemia in diabetics may itself lower pain threshold and tolerance, compared with non-diabetic controls (Morley et al 1984). Further, it has been found in animal experiments that hyperglycaemia reduces the antinociceptive effect of morphine (Simon & Dewey 1981), indicating a possible effect of glucose on opiate receptors. This raises the further possibility that hyperglycaemia might modulate the abnormal properties such as ectopic impulse generation, which develop in damaged nerve.

The other factor is blood flow. Autonomic involvement in diabetic neuropathy increases peripheral blood flow. Archer et al (1984) compared peripheral blood flow and its response to sympathetic stimulation in diabetics with severe non-painful sensory polyneuropathy and diabetics with acute severe painful neuropathies of the type described by Archer et al (1983). High flow was present in both groups, but was reduced by sympathetic stimulation in the group with painful neuropathy and this reduction was accompanied by an improvement in pain. The explanation of this effect is uncertain; a decrease in temperature may be important. The observations seem to conflict with the experimental observation of an increase in ectopic impulse generation in neuromas produced by sympathetic stimulation (Devor & Janig 1981).

The primary prevention and treatment of diabetic neuropathy is good control of the diabetes (Thomas & Tomlinson 1993), though neuropathies have occasionally developed soon after initiation of treatment either with insulin or oral hypoglycaemic drugs (Ellenberg 1958).

Amyloid neuropathy

A second example of a painful small-fibre neuropathy is that caused by amyloid, both the inherited and sporadic varieties (Dyck & Lambert 1969, Dyck et al 1971b, Thomas & King 1974). Patients typically present with a distal sensory loss which initially affects pain and thermal sensations, often with autonomic involvement. As the neuropathy progresses, all modalities are affected, reflexes are lost and there is motor involvement. The physiological and morphological findings of Dyck and Lambert (1969) and Dyck et al (1971b), referred to earlier, showed that small myelinated and unmyelinated fibres are selectively lost and this was confirmed by Thomas and King (1974). It is thus a surprising but common experience that this type of polyneuropathy is often very painful, the pain usually having a deep aching quality, sometimes with superimposed shooting pains.

Fabry's disease

Fabry's disease, angiokeratoma corpus diffusum, is a rare lipid storage disorder in which a painful peripheral neuropathy is the usual presenting feature. The dermatological manifestation is telangiectasia with proliferation of keratin and epidermal cells (Wise et al 1962) and most tissues, including heart, kidneys and lungs, may be involved (Brady 1993). There is a deficiency of ceramide trihexosidase in this sex-linked recessive disease, leading to accumulation of ceramide trihexoside in the tissues (Brady et al 1967). Typically, boys or young men present with tenderness of the feet and spontaneous burning pain in the legs, which may be extremely severe (Wise et al 1962), occasionally leading to suicide (Thomas 1974). The accompanying sensorimotor deficit is often mild. A rash is usually present early on and this should always suggest the diagnosis of Fabry's disease in a young man. Heterozygous carrier females occasionally develop symptoms later in life (Brady 1993). The central nervous system is relatively spared, though patients with mental retardation have been reported (Rahman & Lindenberg 1963). Dorsal root ganglion cells are variably affected, but in peripheral nerves there is a selective loss of small myelinated fibres and a decrease in unmyelinated axons, particularly those of larger diameter (Kocen & Thomas 1970, Ohnishi & Dyck 1974). On electron microscopy the accumulated lipid appears as lamellated, often concentric inclusions known as zebra bodies.

Hereditary sensory neuropathy

The last example of a painful small-fibre neuropathy is dominantly inherited sensory neuropathy, in which symptoms develop slowly from the second decade onwards, mainly in the feet. Distal sensory impairment, particularly affecting pain and temperature sensation in the early stages, with little motor involvement and distal autonomic involvement are the major clinical features. The selective loss of pain sensation may lead to painless penetrating foot ulcers and eventually loss of large parts of the feet (Dyck 1993). Severe lancinating pains are well recognized in this condition and are not related to the severity or the rate of progression of the disease. In their combined electrophysiological and morphological study, Dyck et al (1971b) found a preferential reduction in Aδ and C-fibre potentials associated with a selective loss of unmyelinated and small myelinated fibres, though there was also a considerable reduction of larger myelinated fibres. It is interesting to compare this neuropathy with recessively inherited sensory neuropathy, in which touch-pressure sensation is initially preferentially impaired, though in which a painless mutilating acropathy may eventually occur. Pain is not a feature. Recordings in vitro showed absent myelinated fibre potentials with reduced C-fibre potentials, associated with a histological absence of myelinated fibres and reduced numbers of unmyelinated axons (Ohta et al 1973).

PAINFUL POLYNEUROPATHIES WITH NON-SELECTIVE FIBRE LOSS

Two commonly painful polyneuropathies are associated with a non-selective fibre loss. These are alcoholic and myeloma neuropathies. They are discussed separately from the miscellaneous group of painful neuropathies that follow, since they have been extensively studied pathologically, particularly with regard to the question of differential fibre involvement.

Alcoholic neuropathy

The incidence of neuropathy in chronic alcoholism is in the region of 9% (Victor & Adams 1953), including asymptomatic patients. Of the symptomatic patients, approximately one-quarter complain of pain or paraesthesiae as the first symptom (Windebank 1993). Burning pain and tenderness of the feet and legs are the characteristic complaints, the upper limbs being only rarely involved. Examination reveals a sensorimotor neuropathy and the occurrence of painful symptoms is not related to the severity of the deficit. In a pathological study, Walsh and McLeod (1970) examined sural nerve biopsies from 11 patients who were divided into those with acute and those with chronic neuropathies and, in addition, their diet was assessed. Myelinated fibre densities were decreased in all the biopsies. Fibre-size histograms in five biopsies showed reduction of all fibre sizes in three, but in two there was a relative excess of small-diameter fibres. Teased-fibre preparations showed that these were regenerating sprouts. Patients presenting with an acute neuropathy and a poor diet had active axonal degeneration, whereas those with chronic neuropathies and a better diet had less degeneration and regeneration was present. However, Walsh and McLeod (1970) did not relate this to painfulness in their patients.

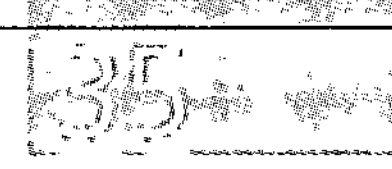

In the early stages of alcoholic neuropathy in some patients, clinical evidence of large sensory fibre involvement is slight or even absent and abnormal thermal thresholds indicate a preferential affectation of unmyelinated afferent fibres. This is thus another example of a painful neuropathy with selective small-fibre involvement.

Treatment of alcoholic neuropathy consists of stopping drinking and ensuring an adequate diet. Poor diet is a major contributory factor to the development of the neuropathy and there are obvious clinical similarities to the neuropathies caused by specific vitamin deficiencies; pellagra has already been discussed and some further examples are considered below. The therapeutic effect of thiamine in alcoholic peripheral neuropathy was demonstrated by Victor and Adams (1961). Victor (1975) drew attention to the causalgic nature of the pain in alcoholic neuropathy and reported good temporary pain relief with sympathetic blockade.

Myeloma

Both multiple and solitary myeloma may be associated with a peripheral sensorimotor neuropathy (Walsh 1971, Davis & Drachman 1972, Kyle & Dyck 1993). The neuropathy is extremely variable in severity and rate of progression, ranging from mild, predominantly sensory neuropathy to a complete tetraplegia. Bone pain is of course a common symptom but, in addition, pain attribution to the associated neuropathy occurs. In reviewing reported patients, Davis and Drachman (1972) calculated an incidence of painful symptoms of 59% in patients with neuropathy. In five sural nerve biopsies from patients with neuropathies but without painful symptoms, Walsh (1971) found a loss of myelinated fibres of all sizes and in teased fibres the appearances suggested a primary axonal degeneration. Unmyelinated axon counts in two patients showed a substantial decrease in numbers, without regeneration. Amyloid has only occasionally been found in nerves of patients with myeloma neuropathy and is not the cause of the neuropathy (Davies-Jones & Esiri 1971). The neuropathy responds well to myeloma chemotherapy or radiotherapy for solitary myeloma and this includes resolution of the painful symptoms.

MISCELLANEOUS PAINFUL NEUROPATHIES

Some further polyneuropathies not included in the above categories and which may be painful are considered here. They have been excluded from the foregoing sections either because of inadequate pathological studies or because the primary demyelinating pathology precludes an accurate assessment of differential fibre loss.

Acute inflammatory polyneuropathy (AIP)

In AIP of the Guillain–Barré type, pain is a common early symptom, often preceding sensory impairment or weakness. It may present in a distal distraction, as generalized muscular pain or as root pain, which sometimes leads to diagnostic difficulties. It has been suggested by Thomas (1979) that such pain may be due to local inflammation in roots, mediated by the nervi nervorum, rather than neuropathic pain due to the pathological processes involving the root fibres themselves. Pain in AIP may be severe but is usually transient. Persisting pain is more often in a distal distribution. In patients with chronic relapsing and chronic progressive inflammatory polyneuropathy, pain is not usually a prominent symptom. The pathology of AIP is demyelination, usually predominantly affecting the roots, and in the great majority of patients full recovery occurs.

Nutritional neuropathies

In addition to niacin deficiency neuropathy and nutritional factors in the pathogenesis of alcoholic neuropathy already discussed, several other painful neuropathies attributed to specific nutritional deficiencies have been described (reviewed by Windebank 1993). Many accounts in the literature provide descriptions of clinical features but lack biochemical or neuropathological investigation. Other problems of aetiological differentiation are that nutritional deficiency of a single vitamin seldom occurs and that in some cases, for example alcoholic neuropathy, a known neurotoxin is also involved. Three painful polyneuropathies of probable or possible nutritional origin are relevant here: beriberi, Strachan's syndrome (Jamaican neuropathy) and the burning feet syndrome.

Beriberi neuropathy

In beriberi, a painful sensorimotor polyneuropathy is very common. There is spontaneous pain in the feet and sometimes the hands, often with a burning character. The calf muscles may be particularly painful and although sensory thresholds are raised, skin stimulation may produce extremely unpleasant paraesthesiae. It is likely, though not completely proven, that thiamine deficiency is the cause of this neuropathy and the associated cardiac disorder and improvement with thiamine is well recorded (Victor 1975). In experimental studies, Swank (1940) showed peripheral nerve degeneration in thiamine-deficient pigeons and North and Sinclair (1956) and Prineas (1970) in rats. In Swank's (1940) investigation, the large myelinated fibres degenerated before the smaller fibres and the longest fibres were preferentially affected. In man, the reported pathological studies are all in the older literature. In an extensive post-mortem study, Peklharing and Winkler (1889; quoted by Victor 1975) described degenerative changes which were most marked in the distal part of peripheral nerves and in the posterior columns and their nuclei. Wright (1901) observed degeneration of dorsal root ganglion cells and anterior horn cells. The animal and human pathology suggest that beriberi neuropathy is primary axonal degeneration of the central peripheral distal type. Reversal of the experimental neuropathy with thiamine was shown by Swank and Prados (1942).

Strachan's syndrome (Jamaican neuropathy)

In 1897, Strachan described 510 cases of a neuropathy observed in Jamaica. Patients presented with pain, paraesthesiae and sensory impairment in the feet and hands, together with pains proximally around the shoulder and hip girdles, visual impairment, deafness and orogenital dermatitis, in some cases resembling the lesions of pellagra. Many of the patients were ataxic, though whether this was peripheral or central in origin is not clear. More recent studies have shown that the neuropathy of Jamaican neuropathy is accompanied by features of spinal cord disease (Montgomery et al 1964) and that a pure peripheral disorder of the type described by Strachan (1897) is not now seen.

There is no evidence that the patients described by Strachan (1897) had a specific nutritional deficiency, though nutritional or toxic factors may have been important in some patients included in this clinically heterogeneous group. Those patients with spinal cord disturbances almost certainly included what is now recognized as tropical spastic paraparesis, due to HTLV1 infection (Gessain & Gout 1992).

Burning feet syndrome

This syndrome was seen in many prisoners of war during the Second World War (Cruickshank 1946, Simpson 1946, Smith & Woodruff 1951). The symptoms were severe aching or causalgic-like burning pains with unpleasant paraesthesiae, starting on the soles of the feet and sometimes spreading up the legs. The symptoms were often worse at night and were relieved by cold. Objective signs of neuropathy were not always present in these patients, some of whom also had amblyopia and orogenital dermatitis (Simpson 1946). Hyperhidrosis of the feet was sometimes a prominent feature. A single nutritional deficiency was not identified in this condition and most patients responded to an improvement in general diet and vitamin B-rich foods.

Cuban neuropathy

A very large epidemic of painful sensory neuropathy and bilateral optic atrophy occurred in western Cuba between 1991 and 1993, with more than 45 000 people reported to have been affected. Clinical features in 25 patients are reported by Thomas et al (1995) and include bilateral optic neuropathy with centrocaecal scotomas or a predominantly sensory polyneuropathy, sometimes associated with deafness, or a combination of optic and peripheral neuropathies. There are clearly similarities between the Cuban disease and Strachan's syndrome. In a further study the Cuban Neuropathy Field Investigation Team (1995) examined 123 patients and assessed dietary factors and exposure to potential toxins. It was found that smoking, particularly cigars, was associated with an increased risk of optic neuropathy and the risk was lower amongst patients with higher dietary intakes of methionine, vitamin B12, riboflavin and niacin and higher serum concentrations of antioxidant carotenoids. In support of a nutritional basis for Cuban neuropathy is the fact that the numbers of new cases began to decrease after vitamin supplementation was initiated in the population.

Tanzanian neuropathy

A syndrome similar to Strachan's syndrome and Cuban neuropathy has also been observed in coastal Tanzania since 1988. The clinical features in 38 affected patients have been described by Plant et al (1997). An optic neuropathy, with primary retinal involvement in some patients, was associated with a dysaesthetic peripheral neuropathy. It was suspected, but not proven, that the condition had a nutritional basis.

Arsenic neuropathy

The polyneuropathy caused by arsenic may be painful, though it is as often painless. It is the commonest of the heavy metal neuropathies and presents as a pure sensory or mixed sensorimotor neuropathy (Goldstein et al 1975). Patients may complain of intense pain or painful paraesthesiae of the extremities (the feet more than the hands) with

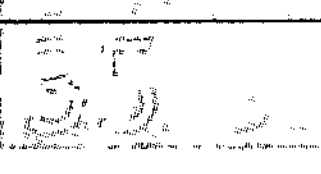

tenderness. Nerve biopsies show axonal degeneration involving fibres of all classes (Goldstein et al 1975).

CENTRAL–PERIPHERAL DISTAL AXONOPATHIES

An advance in the understanding of diseases affecting the primary sensory neuron was the recognition that some pathological processes may have differential effects on the peripheral and central axons. Several references have already been made to the process of dying back or distal axonopathy and it seems likely that this is a common pattern in peripheral neuropathies in which axonal degeneration is the primary pathology. The process of distal axonopathy is now well established in a number of experimental neuropathies, for example those caused by triorthocresyl phosphate (Cavanagh 1954) and acrylamide (Fullerton & Barnes 1966, Prineas 1969), and the underlying cellular processes involved have been the subject of several investigations (Spencer & Schaumburg 1976, Schoental & Cavanagh 1977). In man, anatomical information concerning the central processes of primary sensory neurons is rather more difficult to obtain than the peripheral processes, but there is now physiological evidence that central processes may be selectively involved in some diseases, for example in subacute myelo-optic neuropathy (SMON) due to clioquinol poisoning in Japan and in pure hereditary spastic paraplegia (Thomas 1982). A more common pattern in distal axonopathies is probably affectation of both central and distal axons but, as pointed out by Thomas (1982), differential recovery of function in peripheral and central axons may occur, as is probably the case in SMON, where there is poor resolution of the painful symptoms after removal of the toxin, and in a patient with vitamin E deficiency, in whom differential electrophysiological recovery was documented by Harding et al (1982). The implications of differential vulnerability and recovery in relation to pain in neuropathies other than SMON are at present not clear.

MONONEUROPATHIES AND MULTIPLE MONONEUROPATHIES

Clinical and pathological observations on mononeuropathies have drawn attention to several potentially important mechanisms underlying the production of painful symptoms, which may also be relevant to pain production in some polyneuropathies. Nerve transection with neuroma formation and other types of nerve trauma are discussed in other chapters, but brief reference is made to entrapment neuropathies. The other mononeuropathies considered here include postherpetic neuralgia, diabetic mononeuropathies, ischaemic neuropathy, neuralgic amyotrophy and carcinomatous neuropathies.

POSTHERPETIC NEURALGIA

Definition and description

Postherpetic neuralgia (PHN) is one of the commonest intractable conditions seen in pain clinics. There is no generally agreed definition of PHN. Pain persisting past the stage of healing of the rash, at 1 month after the onset, is the time chosen by many investigators (e.g. Hope-Simpson 1965). However, as PHN tends to diminish in severity with time and may cease to be troublesome many months or even years later (see below), most now accept the longer interval of 3 months after the onset of the acute eruption (Watson et al 1988).

It is unusual for shingles to be entirely painless in middle-aged or older people. Pre-eruptive pain for up to 3 weeks is well described (Juel-Jenson & MacCallum 1972), though pain for more than 2 days before the rash is uncommon. Acute herpetic neuralgia is often severe. There are no features of the pain unique to the acute neuralgia and it merges into PHN. The pain is most often of two types: an ongoing pain described as burning, raw, severe aching or tearing, and superimposed paroxysmal pains, stabbing or electric shock-like. Both the ongoing and paroxysmal pains may be present throughout the whole of the affected dermatome, but commonly become concentrated in one part of the dermatome, particularly after a period of more than 6 months.

The pain is frequently accompanied by a very unpleasant sensitivity of the skin, which again is often most severe in part of the dermatome. The scars themselves tend to be hypoaesthetic, but elsewhere there is hyperaesthesia, allodynia and sometimes hyperpathia (Watson et al 1988). Allodynia may take the form of an exacerbation of the underlying ongoing pain or the evoked dysaesthesiae may be different, often a severe itching sensation. These evoked sensations constitute the most unbearable part of PHN for many patients, usually produced by clothes contact and skin stretching with movement. The patient's emotional state (there is often associated depression), environmental temperature and fatigue may profoundly affect the severity of the ongoing and evoked pains.

Incidence of PHN

PHN, defined as pain persisting at 1 month, has an incidence of between 9% (Ragozzino et al 1982) and 14.3% (Hope-Simpson 1975). Of these patients, the number with pain at 3 months is between 35% and 55% and at 1 year is between 22% and 33% (Demoragas & Kierland 1957, Raggozzino et al 1982). Watson et al (1988) draw attention to an incidence at 1 year of only 3% and in a further study of 91 patients with PHN defined as pain persisting at more than 3 months (Watson et al 1988), found that at a median of 3 years follow-up (range 3 months to 12 years), 52 patients (56%) either had no pain or pain which had decreased to a level of no longer being troublesome. More than half of these 52 patients had had PHN for longer than 1 year at the time of first being seen.

This study underlines the tendency of PHN to gradually improve in many patients even after long periods, an important fact which has often been overlooked in studies of treatment for PHN. It is also of interest that Watson et al (1988) found that a good or bad outcome did not depend on age, sex or affected dermatome. In a further study of prognosis of PHN, Watson et al (1991a) in general confirmed these findings, but found that those patients with longer duration PHN at the time of presentation tended to do worse and some patients were identified whose pain appeared to gradually worsen, despite all attempts at pain relief.

The commonest sites for PHN are the mid-thoracic dermatomes and the ophthalmic division of the trigeminal nerve, but may occur in any dermatome. Women are more often affected than men, in a ratio of approximately 3:2 (Hope-Simpson 1975, Watson et al 1988).

Pathology and pathogenesis of pain

There have been few pathological studies in PHN. Head and Campbell (1900) were the first to document the changes in the DRG and sensory roots but of 21 patients only one was reported to have PHN. Lhermitte and Nicholas (1924) studied a patient with acute zoster myelitis, who had acute haemorrhagic inflammatory in DRG, posterior roots and peripheral nerve, with demyelination and axonal degeneration. Denny-Brown et al (1944) observed similar changes in three patients, with marked lymphocytic infiltration at the sites of inflammation. Noordenbos (1959) found a reduction in the large myelinated fibre population in intercostal nerves. In peripheral nerves of patients biopsied early and late after the acute eruption, Zachs et al (1964) found Wallerian degeneration, followed by marked fibrotic change, leading to severe myelinated fibre depletion with preservation of small myelinated fibres only in some patients. Esiri and Tomlinson (1972) described a patient with myeloma who died in the acute phase of ophthalmic zoster. Skin, nerve and DRG all contained virus particles and the nerve showed severe degenerative changes which were unevenly distributed in nerve fascicles.

In an autopsy study of a 67-year-old man with PHN for 5 years before death in a right T7–8 dermatome, Watson et al (1988) found atrophy of the dorsal horn on the right from T4 to T8 with loss of myelin and axons. Only the T8 DRG and dorsal root were affected by fibrosis and cell loss. Markers of unmyelinated fibres (substance P levels), substantia gelatinosa neurons (opiate receptors), glial cells (glial fibrillary acidic protein) and monoaminergic descending spinal projections (dopamine β-hydroxylase and serotinin levels) were all normal.

In a further autopsy study, Watson et al (1991b) examined spinal cords, DRG, dorsal roots and peripheral nerves from five patients, three of whom had had severe persistent PHN and two of whom had had no pain. Dorsal horn atrophy was only found in those patients with PHN. Axonal and myelin loss and fibrosis were found in one DRG from all the patients without pain. In all patients the peripheral nerve showed severe loss of myelin and axons. In these nerves, there was a relative loss of larger myelinated fibres. The dorsal roots in all patients with PHN and in one patient without pain showed loss of myelin and axons but in the other pain-free patient the dorsal root was normal. Substance P and CGRP levels were measured in two patients with PHN. Staining was absent in the affected DRG but apparently normal in the dorsal horn. Quantitative study of the unmyelinated fibres was not performed in either study, so the degree to which unmyelinated afferents were affected in patients with PHN remains uncertain. An additional finding of interest in one patient who had had PHN for 22 months prior to death was marked inflammatory change with lymphocytic infiltration bilaterally in the DRG of four adjacent segments and in the respective peripheral nerves, suggesting that an ongoing inflammatory process may result following acute zoster in some patients.

Clearly, further studies of this type are needed in a larger number of patients, before the interpretation of the findings of Watson et al (1988a, 1991a, 1991b) in relation to pain pathogenesis. As yet, the pathological studies have not revealed a specific change present in patients with PHN and absent in patients without pain, which might offer a clue as to the mechanism of pain. Preferential loss of larger

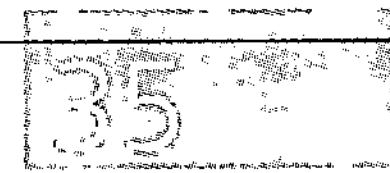

myelinated fibres appears to be a feature common to both patients with and without PHN. Watson et al (1991a) speculate whether the persistent inflammation found in one patient at a longer interval after acute zoster might indicate continuing low-grade infection and might be a feature of those patients whose pain gradually worsens.

Prevention

Treatment options for PHN are discussed by Fields (Ch. 67). The important issue of prevention of PHN has received considerable attention. There are obvious difficulties in conducting an adequate trial of any treatment to answer this question, given the low and decreasing incidence of PHN at intervals between 3 and 12 months after the acute eruption. In a trial of 40% idoxuridine in DMSO in a fairly small group of patients, Juel-Jenson et al (1970) showed a reduction in incidence of PHN. However, subsequent widespread use of this treatment has been disappointing. Systemic corticosteroids may be effective, as suggested in two controlled trials (Eaglstein et al 1970, Keczkes & Basheer 1980) and in other studies (Appleman 1955, Elliott 1964). There is a danger of dissemination (Merselis et al 1964), though this may be confined to those patients with underlying malignancy or other serious disease leading to immune suppression. Acyclovir has been advocated as an effective preventive drug but controlled studies have not confirmed earlier hopes that it would substantially reduce the incidence of PHN, though some studies have shown shorter periods of acute zoster neuralgia and faster healing of the rash (Esman et al 1982, Bean et al 1982, Balfour et al 1983). Colding (1969) reported that PHN could be reduced by sympathetic blockade, but this was not a controlled study and the finding has not been confirmed by others.

DIABETIC MONONEUROPATHY AND AMYOTROPHY

Mononeuropathies occur more frequently in diabetes than in the normal population, affecting particularly the motor nerves to the extraocular muscles but also single peripheral nerves including median, ulnar, peroneal, femoral and lateral cutaneous nerve of the thigh. It is particularly interesting that approximately half the patients with acute lesions of the third, fourth and sixth cranial nerves have pain, which may precede the ocular palsy by a few days (Zorilla & Kozak 1967). Third nerve palsy is the most common and is usually pupil staring. Pain is felt around or behind the eye and may be severe. Since there are no somatosensory fibres in these nerves, where is the pain arising? Two suggestions have been put forward: the first is that the lesions involve the nervi nervorum, producing pain (Thomas 1974), and the second is that there may be concurrent lesions of the branches of the trigeminal nerve in the cavernous sinus, in support of which Zorilla and Kozak (1967) reported discrete facial sensory impairment in some of their patients. With regard to the acute peripheral nerve lesions, pain is a common symptom, though usually transient. Thomas (1979) reported a diabetic patient with an acute radial nerve palsy which was heralded by severe pain in the upper arm, but there was no pain distally. A fascicular biopsy of the nerve in the upper arm showed only small-diameter regenerating myelinated fibres and the endoneurial vessels showed the changes of diabetic microangiopathy. This case is again suggestive of pain arising as a result of activity in nervi nervorum, also termed nerve trunk pain (Asbury & Fields 1984).

Postmortem studies of the pathology of diabetic mononeuropathy include a patient reported by Dreyfus et al (1957), who died 5 weeks after developing a unilateral third cranial nerve palsy. The nerve was swollen retro-orbitally, with degenerative changes in the central parts of nerve and Wallerian degeneration distally. This lesion was considered to have a vascular cause, on the basis of arteriolar changes observed, though no vessel occlusion was seen. Raff et al (1968) reported the presence of punctate lesions in the nerve of a diabetic patient who had developed mononeuritis multiplex in the legs 6 weeks before death, which also suggested a vascular pathology. A particularly interesting patient who died a month after the onset of a third nerve palsy and who had had a contralateral transient third nerve palsy 3 years earlier was studied by Asbury et al (1970). As in the patient of Dreyfus et al (1957), the changes in the acutely affected nerve were maximal in the central parts of the nerve, though they were less severe, consisting mainly of demyelination. The contralateral previously affected nerve was structurally normal.

Diabetic amyotrophy, also now known as painful proximal diabetic neuropathy (PDN), is an asymmetrical predominantly motor neuropathy, sometimes related to poor diabetic control, found in middle-aged and elderly diabetics (Thomas & Tomlinson 1993). In a clinical and pathological study of PDN, Said et al (1997) examined nerve biopsies of the intermediate cutaneous nerve of the thigh. Inflammatory changes and ischaemic lesions associated with vasculitis of epineurial and perineurial vessels were found. There was an associated mixed axonal and demyelinating neuropathy, with degeneration of unmyelinated axons, together with evidence of regeneration. Endoneurial and perineurial inflammatory infiltrates were common. The findings were considered by Said et al (1997) to be in keeping with an ischaemic mechanism secondary to occlusion of blood vessels. In view of the marked inflammatory component of PDN, it is likely that the pain may in part be another example of pain mediated by nervi nervorum, nerve trunk pain (Thomas 1979).

ENTRAPMENT NEUROPATHIES

Entrapment neuropathies or sensory or mixed nerves, such as carpal tunnel syndrome, are usually characterized in the early stages by paraesthesiae and pain. Morphologically, entrapment lesions cause damage to myelinated fibres in the first instance (Thomas & Fullerton 1963, Neary et al 1975, Ochoa & Noordenbos 1979), with a near absence of myelinated fibres only in severe lesion, in which there is preservation only of C fibres. Local pain and tenderness at the site of nerve entrapment in many patients is likely to be nerve trunk pain, mediated by nervi nervorum, as discussed in relation to diabetic mononeuropathy. Paraesthesiae of non-painful type with entrapment neuropathies presumably reflect activity in damaged myelinated fibres, as demonstrated microneurographically in experimental nerve ischaemia in man by Ochoa and Torebjork (1980).

The explanation of pain in entrapment neuropathies (other than nerve trunk pain) is more difficult. Severe pain, sometimes with a burning quality, is frequently a symptom, albeit often in short-lived episodes in electrophysiologically mild carpal tunnel syndrome, in which myelinated fibre conduction is relatively mildly affected and thus it is difficult to imagine that C fibres are damaged. Whether pain is due to activity in myelinated afferents alone in this situation remains uncertain.

Morton's neuralgia is an example of a frequently histologically severe entrapment neuropathy in which a plantar digital nerve becomes compressed in the region of the metatarsal heads in the foot. In badly affected nerves, many myelinated fibres may be disrupted within the region of compression, producing a nerve which is populated almost exclusively by C fibres. However, explanations of pain pathogenesis based on these findings have to take account of the fact that similar changes are often found in control nerves from subjects who never suffered this type of neuralgia (Scadding & Klenerman 1987).

ISCHAEMIC NEUROPATHY

Polyarteritis nodosa, rheumatoid arthritis and systemic lupus erythematosus may all be associated with painful peripheral mononeuropathies, which probably have a microangiopathic basis (Dyck et al 1972, Chalk et al 1993). In a study of nerves involved in rheumatoid arthritis, Dyck et al (1972) found degenerative changes in the central parts of fascicles in nerves from the upper arm and thigh and postulated that these represented watershed areas in these nerves. The probable ischaemic basis for these changes is supported by the experimental ischaemic peripheral nerve lesions produced by injection of arachidonic acid in rats (Parry & Brown 1982), which produced similar central fascicular degenerative changes, in which small myelinated fibres and unmyelinated fibres were affected to a greater extent than large myelinated fibres. Lacomis et al (1997) reported two patients with small-fibre neuropathies, found on biopsy to be due to vasculitis. One patient had systemic lupus erythematosus. It was proposed that the mechanism of the pain might be preferential affection of small fibres by ischaemia.

The effects of whole-limb ischaemia on peripheral nerves were shown by Eames and Lange (1967), who found clinical signs of sensory neuropathy in 87.5% of patients undergoing amputation for major vessel atheromatous disease and observed loss of myelinated fibres with segmental demyelination, remyelination and Wallerian degeneration in nerves from these patients. Ischaemia to the nerves of a limb may, of course, be associated with ischaemia to non-neural structures, which may be the source of pain rather than the neuropathic changes.

There is good evidence that ischaemia may precipitate or potentiate painful symptoms in nerves already damaged by other factors. Gilliatt and Wilson (1954) demonstrated an abnormally rapid onset of paraesthesiae with cuff ischaemia in patients with carpal tunnel syndrome and Harding and Le Fanu (1977) reported precipitation of symptoms of carpal tunnel syndrome in patients during haemodialysis with antebrachial arteriovenous fistulae.

NEURALGIC AMYOTROPHY

Neuralgic amyotrophy, or cryptogenic brachial plexus neuropathy, is a condition characterized by acute onset of severe pain around the shoulder girdle or in the arms, often in a root distribution, which is followed within 2 weeks by weakness in the limb. This is most frequently distributed around the shoulder girdle and upper limb but may involve distal muscle groups. A minority of patients report a minor, possibly viral, preceding illness (Tsairis et al 1972). The ensuing paralysis is extremely variable in severity and duration, but good recovery is usual within 2 years. Little is known about the pathology of the condition or even

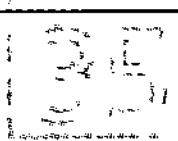

whether the site of the initial lesion is in the roots or more distally in the brachial plexus, though the patchy distribution favours involvement of the plexus and its branches rather than the roots in the majority of patients. The time course of milder lesions suggests demyelination without axonal disruption, whereas that of severe lesions indicates that axonal degeneration probably occurs. There are similarities between neuralgic amyotrophy and the brachial neuritis which occurs in serum sickness. In the latter condition, severe lancinating pain around the shoulder girdle and in the arms is a leading symptom, tending to be more common on the side of handedness, though it may be bilateral (Doyle 1933). Pathological studies are few, but marked swelling of roots has been observed (Roger et al 1934) and it has been suggested that in some patients the swollen roots may become entrapped in the cervical exit foraminae and that this is the cause of the radicular pain. Neuralgic amyotrophy is reviewed by Wilbourn (1993).

CARCINOMATOUS NEUROPATHIES

Neuropathies of various types are well documented as non-metastatic complications of malignant disease, the commonest being a progressive sensory neuropathy which is only occasionally painful (Croft & Wilkinson 1969). However, it was subsequently reported that causalgia may occur as a result of direct invasion of peripheral nerves by carcinoma, responding to sympathectomy (Hupert 1978).

HUMAN MICRONEUROGRAPHY

Single-fibre recordings made by microneurography in nerve damage are still few in number but have confirmed some of the abnormal properties found in animal experiments. Ochoa et al (1982) recorded mechanical sensitivity in fibres proximal to a peroneal nerve lesion. Similarly, Nordin et al (1984) found ectopic impulse generation provoked by light mechanical stimulation over an ulnar nerve entrapment at the elbow. Perhaps the most interesting observation to date is the ongoing activity and mechanical sensitivity recorded by Nystrom and Hagbarth (1981) proximal to a median nerve neuroma in an amputee with phantom limb pain. Following local anaesthetic blockade of the nerve distal to the recording site, impulses evoked by mechanical stimulation of the neuroma were abolished, but ongoing activity at the recording site continued. It is likely that this residual activity arose from the DRG, as observed experimentally by Wall and Devor (1983). One further microneurographic observation of interest is that neuropathic pain of peripheral nerve origin can be reproduced by intraneural microstimulation of single afferent fibres (Ochoa et al 1985).

SUMMARY OF HUMAN EVIDENCE

As stated earlier, the emphasis of most investigations of human neuropathy has been on morphological correlation of fibre size distribution with nerve conduction and painfulness, but a review of the data shows that there are too many exceptions to a general hypothesis of fibre size imbalance as a cause of pain for it to be tenable. This has been recognized for some time (Thomas 1974, 1979). Dyck et al (1976) reviewed 72 patients who had had nerve biopsies, looking at the type and rate of myelinated fibre degeneration and correlating this with painfulness. There was inevitably bias in the diseases represented in this study, but it was concluded that pain was a feature of those neuropathies in which there was acute axonal degeneration and this bore no relationship to fibre size distribution. It is interesting to note here that a recent morphological study of an animal model of hyperalgesia due to nerve injury produced by loose ligatures (Bennett & Xie 1988) has revealed very acute degenerative changes in both myelinated and unmyelinated fibres (Basbaum et al 1991).

Overall, the human evidence may be summarized as follows:

1. Pain is not related to fibre size distribution alone, if at all.
2. Those neuropathies in which there is rapid degenerative change are more likely to be painful.
3. Neuropathies involving small fibres, with or without large-fibre involvement, are often painful.
4. The coexistence of degenerative and regenerative changes appears to be an important factor (e.g. in some diabetic neuropathies).
5. Some pain may be sympathetic dependent. This evidence derives from studies in traumatic mononeuropathies in man, particularly causalgia (see Ch. 36). The extent to which this is important in polyneuropathies remains uncertain.
6. Ischaemia in nerves may exacerbate paraesthesiae and pain due to peripheral damage and, in certain circumstances, severe ischaemia is the cause of neuropathies which may be very painful.
7. Nerve trunk pain is a feature of mononeuropathies and this mechanism may also be important in certain polyneuropathies.

EVIDENCE FROM ANIMAL EXPERIMENTS

The above conclusions leave us far short of an adequate explanation for pain in peripheral neuropathy and we must turn to animal experiments to provide clues about other mechanisms. This evidence is discussed in detail by Devor (Ch. 5). Following a brief injury discharge in damaged nerve fibres, a chronic afferent barrage of impulses develops. There are sites of ectopic impulse generation both at the point of injury, with or without axonal disruption (demyelination is sufficient to produce this), and proximal to the injury, at the DRG. In addition, an abnormal mechanical sensitivity and noradrenaline sensitivity develop in damaged axons, both of these properties increasing the magnitude of the afferent impulse discharge. Warming tends to increase the A-fibre discharge, while cooling increases the C-fibre discharge. Ephaptic impulse transmission, from motor to sensory axons, develops in a small proportion of fibres and another type of interaction, crossed after discharge, also develops. The ongoing activity in damaged peripheral nerve (experimental neuromas) is reduced by phenytoin and carbamazepine and by locally applied corticosteroid and glycerol.

Other than in the special case of trigeminal neuralgia in which systemic carbamazepine and local glycerol are often highly effective, the therapeutic actions of the drugs mentioned are usually disappointing in peripheral neuropathic pain, but the experimental observations do provide some evidence for a peripheral action for these agents.

Central factors are also likely to be of great importance. These include reduced inhibitions and altered sensitivities of dorsal horn cells and more rostral changes, all of which may occur following peripheral nerve damage (see Ch. 6). The identification of these peripheral and central abnormal physiological and pharmacological properties following peripheral nerve damage has opened up a new range of possible explanations of the mechanisms of peripheral neuropathic pain. However, to what extent each of the experimentally observed properties exists in different neuropathies in man remains uncertain, as do the balance and interactions of the various peripheral and central factors. This continues to be a considerable and crucial gap in our understanding of mechanisms of pain in neuropathy. However, the experimental observations provide a powerful stimulus to the further investigation of human neuropathies. This is a prerequisite for the establishment of rational and specific treatment. Clinicians who regularly deal with patients suffering from pain resulting from peripheral neuropathies are the first to admit the inadequacies and unpredictability of the present range of treatments which can be offered to this unfortunate group of patients.

REFERENCES

Adrian ED 1931 The messages in sensory nerve fibres and their interpretation. Proceedings of the Royal Society of London Series B 109: 1–18

Anderson PV, Spiller WG 1940 Pellagra, with a report of two cases with necropsy. American Journal of the Medical Sciences 141: 307–312

Appleman DH 1955 Treatment of herpes zoster with ACTH. New England Journal of Medicine 253: 693–695

Archer AG, Watkins PJ, Thomas PK, Sharma AK, Payan J 1983 The natural history of acute painful neuropathy in diabetes mellitus. Journal of Neurology, Neurosurgery and Psychiatry 46: 491–499

Archer AG, Roberts VC, Watkins PJ 1984 Blood flow patterns in painful diabetic neuropathy. Diabetologia 27: 563–567

Aring CD, Bean WB, Roseman E, Rosenbaum M, Spies TD 1941 Peripheral nerves in cases of nutritional deficiency. Archives of Neurology and Psychiatry 45: 772–787

Asbury AK 1993 Neuropathies with renal failure, hepatic disorders, chronic respiratory insufficiency, and critical illness. In: Dyck PJ, Thomas PK, Griffin JW, Low PA, Poduslo JF (eds) Peripheral neuropathy, 3rd edn. WB Saunders, Philadelphia, pp 1251–1265

Asbury AK, Fields HL 1984 Pain due to peripheral nerve damage: an hypothesis. Neurology 34: 1587–1590

Asbury AK, Victor M, Adams RD 1963 Uremic polyneuropathy. Archives of Neurology 8: 413–428

Asbury AK, Aldredge H, Hershberg R, Fisher CM 1970 Oculomotor palsy in diabetes mellitus: a clinico-pathology study. Brain 93: 555–556

Balfour H, Bean B, Laskin OL et al 1983 Acyclovir halts progression of herpes zoster in immunocompromised patients. New England Journal of Medicine 308: 1453

Ballin RHM, Thomas PK 1968 Hypertropic changes in diabetic neuropathy. Acta Neuropathologica 11: 93–102

Basbaum AI, Gautrum M, Jazat F, Mayes M, Guilbaud G 1991 The spectrum of fibre loss in a model of neuropathic pain in the rat: an electron microscopic study. Pain 47: 357–367

Baxter DW, Olszewski J 1960 Congenital universal insensitivity to pain. Brain 83: 381–393

Bean B, Braun C, Balfour HH 1982 Acyclovir therapy for acute herpes zoster. Lancet ii: 118–121

Behse F, Buchthal F, Carlsen F 1977 Nerve biopsy and conduction studies in diabetic neuropathy. Journal of Neurology and Psychiatry 40: 1072–1082

Bennett GJ, Xie Y-K 1988 A peripheral mononeuropathy in rat that produces disorders of pain like those seen in man. Pain 33: 87–108

Berthier M, Starkstein S, Leignarda R 1988 Asymbolia for pain: a sensory-limbic disconnection syndrome. Annals of Neurology 24: 41–49

Biehl JP, Wilter RW 1954 The effect of isoniazid on vitamin B6 metabolism, and its possible significance in producing isoniazid neuritis. Proceedings of the Society for Experimental Biology and Medicine 85: 389–392

Brady RO 1993 Fabry disease. In: Dyck PJ, Thomas PK, Griffin JW, Low PA, Poduslo JF (eds) Peripheral neuropathy, 3rd edn. WB Saunders, Philadelphia, pp 1169–1178

Brady RO, Gal AE, Bradley RM, Martensson E, Warshaw AL, Laster L

1967 Enzymatic defect in Fabry's disease: ceramidetrihexosidase deficiency. New England Journal of Medicine 276: 1163–1167
Britland ST, Young RJ, Sharma AK, Clarke BF 1992 Acute and remitting painful diabetic polyneuropathy: a comparison of peripheral nerve fibre pathology. Pain 48: 361–370
Brown MJ, Martin JR, Asbury AK 1976 Painful diabetic neuropathy. A morphometric study. Archives of Neurology 33: 164–171
Burgess PR, Perl ER 1973 Cutaneous mechanoreceptors and nociceptors. In: Iggo A (ed) Handbook of sensory physiology, vol 2. Springer Verlag, Berlin, pp 29–78
Cavanagh JB 1954 The toxic effects of tri-ortho-cresyl phosphate on the nervous system. Journal of Neurology, Neurosurgery and Psychiatry 17: 163–172
Chalk CH, Dyck PJ, Conn DL 1993 Vasculitic neuropathy. In: Dyck PJ, Thomas PK, Griffin JW, Low PA, Poduslo JF (eds) Peripheral neuropathy, 3rd edn. WB Saunders, Philadelphia, pp 1424–1436
Clark D, Hughes J, Gasser HS 1935 Afferent function in the group of nerve fibres of the slowest conduction velocity. American Journal of Physiology 114: 69–76
Colding A 1969 The effect of sympathetic blocks on herpes zoster. Acta Anaesthesiologica Scandinavica 13: 113–141
Collins WF, Nulsen FE, Randt CT 1960 Relation of peripheral nerve fibre size and sensation in man. Archives of Neurology 3: 381–397
Croft PB, Wilkinson M 1969 The course and prognosis in some types of carcinomatous neuromyopathy. Brain 92: 1–8
Cruickshank EK 1946 Painful feet in prisoners of war in the Far East. Lancet ii: 369–381
Cuban Neuropathy Field Investigation Team 1995 Epidemic optic neuropathy in Cuba – clinical characterization and risk factors. New England Journal of Medicine 333: 1176–1182
Davies-Jones GAB, Esiri MM 1971 Neuropathy due to amyloid in myelomatosis. British Medical Journal 2: 444
Davis LE, Drachman DB 1972 Myeloma neuropathy: successful treatment of two patients and a review of cases. Archives of Neurology 27: 507–511
Dayan AD, Gardner-Thorpe C, Down PF, Gleadle RI 1970 Peripheral neuropathy in uremia. Neurology (Minneapolis) 20: 649–658
Demoragas JM, Kierland RR 1957 The outcome of patients with herpes zoster. Archives of Dermatology 75: 193–196
Denny-Brown D, Adams RD, Fitzgerald PJ 1944 Pathologic features of herpes zoster: a note on 'geniculate herpes'. Archives of Neurology and Psychiatry 77: 337–349
Devor M, Janig W 1981 Activation of myelinated afferents ending in a neuroma by stimulation of the sympathetic supply in the rat. Neuroscience Letters 24: 43–47
Dinn JJ, Crane DL 1970 Schwann cell dysfunction in uremia. Journal of Neurology, Neurosurgery and Psychiatry 33: 605–608
Doyle JB 1933 Neurological complications of serum sickness. American Journal of the Medical Sciences 185: 484–492
Dreyfus PM, Hakim S, Adams RD 1957 Diabetic ophthalmoplegia. Archives of Neurology and Psychiatry 77: 337–347
Dyck PJ 1982 Current concepts in neurology: the causes, classification and treatment of peripheral neuropathy. New England Journal of Medicine 307: 283–285
Dyck PJ 1993 Neuronal atrophy and degeneration predominantly affecting peripheral sensory and autonomic neurons. In: Dyck PJ, Thomas PK, Griffin JW, Low PA, Poduslo JF (eds) Peripheral neuropathy, 3rd edn. WB Saunders, Philadelphia, pp 1065–1093
Dyck PJ, Lais AC 1970 Electron microscopy of teased nerve fibres: method permitting examination of repeating structures of same fibre. Brain Research 23: 418–424
Dyck PJ, Lais AC 1973 Evidence for segmental demyelination secondary to axonal degeneration in Friedreich's ataxia. In: Kakulas BA (ed) Clinical studies of myology. Excerpta Medica, Amsterdam, pp 253–263
Dyck PJ, Lambert EH 1969 Dissociated sensation in amyloidosis. Archives of Neurology 20: 490–507
Dyck PJ, Lambert EH 1970 Polyneuropathy associated with hypothyroidism. Journal of Neuropathology and Experimental Neurology 29: 631–658
Dyck PJ, Gutrecht JA, Bastron JA, Karnes WE, Dale AJD 1968 Histologic and teased-fibre measurement of sural nerve in disorders of lower motor and primary sensory neurons. Mayo Clinic Proceedings 43: 81–114
Dyck PJ, Johnson WJ, Lambert EH, O'Brien PC 1971a Segmental demyelination secondary to axonal degeneration in uremic neuropathy. Mayo Clinic Proceedings 46: 400–431
Dyck PJ, Lambert EH, Nichols PC 1971b Quantitative measurement of sensation related to compound action potentials and number and sizes of myelinated and unmyelinated fibres of sural nerve in health, Friedreich's ataxia, hereditary sensory neuropathy and tabes dorsalis. In: Remond A (ed) Handbook of electroencephalography and clinical neurophysiology, vol 9. Elsevier, Amsterdam, pp 83–118
Dyck PJ, Conn DL, Okazaki H 1972 Necrotizing angiopathic neuropathy: three-dimensional morphology of fibre degeneration related to sites of occluded vessels. Mayo Clinic Proceedings 47: 461
Dyck PJ, Lambert EH, O'Brien PC 1976 Pain in peripheral neuropathy related to rate and kind of fibre degeneration. Neurology 28: 466–471
Dyck PJ, Giannini C, Lais A 1993 Pathologic alteration of nerves. In: Dyck PJ, Thomas PK, Griffin JW, Low PA, Poduslo JF (eds) Peripheral neuropathy, 3rd edn. WB Saunders, Philadelphia, pp 515–595
Eaglstein WH, Katz R, Brown JA 1970 The effects of early corticosteroid therapy on the skin eruption and pain of herpes zoster. Journal of the American Medical Association 211: 1681–1683
Eames RA, Lange LS 1967 Clinical and pathological study of ischaemic neuropathy. Journal of Neurology, Neurosurgery and Psychiatry 30: 215–226
Ellenberg M 1958 Diabetic neuropathy precipitating after institution of diabetic control. American Journal of the Medical Sciences 238: 418
Elliott FA 1964 Treatment of herpes zoster with high doses of prednisolone. Lancet ii: 610–611
Esiri MM, Tomlinson AH 1972 Herpes zoster. Demonstration of virus in trigeminal neuralgia and ganglion by immunofluorescence and electron microscopy. Journal of the Neurological Sciences 15: 35–48
Esman V, Ipsen J, Peterslund NA et al 1982 Therapy of acute herpes zoster with acyclovir in the non-immunocompromised host. American Journal of Medicine 73: 320–325
Feindel W 1953 Note on nerve endings in a subject with arthropathy and congenital absence of pain. Journal of Bone and Joint Surgery 35B: 402–407
Forno L, Alston W 1967 Uremic polyneuropathy. Acta Neurologica Scandinavica 43: 640–654
Frederickson DS, Gotto AM, Levy RI 1972 Familial lipoprotein deficiency (abetalipoproteinemia, hypobetalipoproteinemia and Tangier disease). In: Stanbury JB, Wyngaarden JB, Fredrickson DS (eds) The metabolic basis of inherited disease. McGraw-Hill, New York, pp 493–530
Fullerton PM, Barnes JM 1966 Peripheral neuropathy in rats produced by acrylamide. British Journal of Industrial Medicine 25: 210–221
Gammon GD, Burge FW, King G 1953 Neural toxicity in tuberculous patients treated with isoniazid (isonicotinic acid hydrazide). Archives of Neurology and Psychiatry 70: 64–69
Gessain A, Gout O 1992 Chronic myelopathy associated with human T-lymphotropic virus type I (HTLV-1). Annals of Internal Medicine 117: 933–946
Gilliatt RW 1965 Clinical aspects of diabetes. In: Cummings JN, Kremer M (eds) Biochemical aspects of neurological disorders, 2nd series. Blackwell, Oxford, pp 117–142

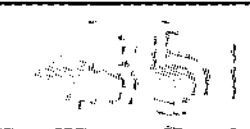

Gilliatt RW, Wilson TG 1954 Ischaemic sensory loss in patients with peripheral nerve lesions. Journal of Neurology, Neurosurgery and Psychiatry 17: 104–123

Goldstein NP, McCall JT, Dyck PJ 1975 Metal neuropathy. In: Dyck PJ, Thomas PK, Lambert EH (eds) Peripheral neuropathy, 2nd edn. WB Saunders, Philadelphia, pp 1227–1262

Greenbaum D, Richardson PC, Salmon MV, Urich H 1964 Pathological observation on six cases of diabetic neuropathy. Brain 87: 201–214

Greenfield JG, Holmes JM 1939 A case of pellagra: the pathological changes in the spinal cord. British Medical Journal 815–819

Guy RJC, Clark CA, Malcolm PN, Watkins PJ 1985 Evaluation of thermal and vibration sensation in diabetic neuropathy. Diabetologia 28: 131–137

Haddow JE, Shapiro SR, Gall DG 1970 Congenital sensory neuropathy in siblings. Paediatrics 45: 651–655

Harding AE, Le Fanu J 1977 Carpal tunnel syndrome related to antebrachial Cimmino-Brescia fistula. Journal of Neurology, Neurosurgery and Psychiatry 40: 511–513

Harding AE, Muller DPR, Thomas PK, Willison HJ 1982 Spinocerebellar degeneration secondary to chronic intestinal malabsorption: a vitamin E deficiency syndrome. Annals of Neurology 12: 419–424

Head H, Campbell AW 1900 The pathology of herpes zoster and its bearing on sensory localisation. Brain 23: 353–523

Hope-Simpson RE 1965 The nature of herpes zoster: a long term study and a new hypothesis. Proceedings of the Royal Society of Medicine 58: 9–20

Hope-Simpson RE 1975 Post-herpetic neuralgia. Journal of the Royal College of General Practitioners 25: 571–575

Hopkins AP, Lambert EH 1972 Conduction in unmyelinated fibres in experimental neuropathy. Journal of Neurology, Neurosurgery and Psychiatry 35: 63–69

Hupert C 1978 Recognition and treatment of causalgic pain occurring in cancer patients. Pain Abstracts 1: 47

Iggo A 1977 Cutaneous and subcutaneous sense organs. British Medical Bulletin 33: 97–102

Juel-Jenson BE, MacCallum of 1972 Herpes simplex varicella and zoster. JB Lippincott, Philadelphia

Juel-Jenson BE, MacCallum FO, MacKenzie AMR, Pike MC 1970 Treatment of zoster with idoxuridine in dimethyl sulphoxide. Results of two double blind controlled trials. British Medical Journal iv: 776–780

Keczkes K, Basheer AM 1980 Do corticosteroids prevent post-herpetic neuralgia? British Journal of Dermatology 102: 551–555

Kimuna J 1993 Nerve conduction studies and electromyography. In: Dyck PJ, Thomas PK, Griffin JW, Low PA, Poduslo JF (eds) Peripheral neuropathy, 3rd edn. WB Saunders, Philadelphia, pp 598–644

Kocen RS, Thomas PK 1970 Peripheral nerve involvement in Fabry's disease. Archives of Neurology 22: 81–87

Kocen RS, Lloyd JJ, Lascelles PT, Fosbrooke AS, Williams D 1967 Familial alpha-lipoprotein deficiency (Tangier disease) with neurological abnormalities. Lancet I: 1341–1345

Kocen RS, King RHM, Thomas PK, Haas LF 1973 Nerve biopsy findings in two cases of Tangier disease. Acta Neuropathologica 26: 317–327

Kyle RA, Dyck PJ 1993 Neuropathy associated with the monoclonal gammopathies. In: Dyck PJ, Thomas PK, Griffin JW, Low PA, Poduslo JF (eds) Peripheral neuropathy, 3rd edn. WB Saunders, Philadelphia, pp 1275–1287

Lacomis D, Giuliani MJ, Steen V, Powell HC 1997 Small fibre neuropathy and fasculitis. Arthritis and Rheumatism 40: 1173–1177

Lambert EH, Dyck PJ 1993 Compound action potentials of sural nerve in vitro in peripheral neuropathy. In: Dyck PJ, Thomas PK, Griffin JW, Low PA, Poduslo JF (eds) Peripheral neuropathy, 3rd edn. WB Saunders, Philadelphia, pp 672–684

Lewis T, Pickering GW, Rothschild P 1931 Centripetal paralysis arising out of arrest block flow to the limb, including notes on a form of tingling. Heart 16: 1–32

Lewy FH, Spies TD, Aring CD 1940 Incidence of neuropathy in pellagra; effect of carboxylase upon its neurologic signs. American Journal of the Neurological Sciences 199: 840–849

Lhermitte J, Nicholas M 1924 Les lesions spinales du zona. La myelite zosterienne. Revue Neurologique 1: 361–364

Lindblom U 1979 Sensory abnormalities in neuralgia. In: Bonica JJ, Liebeskind JC, Albe-Fessard DG (eds) Advances in pain research and therapy 3. Raven Press, New York, pp 11–120

Lourie H, King RB 1966 Sensory and neurohistological correlates of cutaneous hyperpathia. Archives of Neurology 14: 313–320

Marin OSM, Tyler HR 1961 Hereditary interstitial nephritis associated with polyneuropathy. Neurology 111: 999–1005

Mazar A, Herold HZ, Vardy PA 1976 Congenital sensory neuropathy with anhidrosis. Orthopaedic complications and management. Clinical Orthopaedics 118: 184–187

Melzack R, Wall PD 1965 Pain mechanisms: a new theory. Science 150: 971–979

Merselis JG, Kaye D, Hook EW 1964 Disseminated herpes zoster. Archives of Internal Medicine 113: 679–686

Montgomery RD, Cruickshank EK, Robertson WB, McMenemey WH 1964 Clinical and pathological observations on Jamaican neuropathy – a report on 206 cases. Brain 87: 425–462

Morley GK, Mooradian AD, Levine AL, Morley LE 1984 Mechanisms of pain in diabetic peripheral neuropathy: effect of glucose on pain perception in humans. American Journal of Medicine 77: 79

Morris JH, Hudson AR, Weddell G 1972 A study of degeneration and regeneration in the divided rat sciatic nerve based on electron microscopy. Zeitschrift fur Zellforeschung und Mikroskopische Anatomie 124: 76–203

Neary D, Ochoa J, Gilliatt RW 1975 Sub-clinical entrapment neuropathy in man. Journal of the Neurological Sciences 24: 283–298

Noordenbos W 1959 Pain. Elsevier, Amsterdam

Noordenbos W 1979 Sensory findings in painful traumatic nerve lesions. In: Bonica JJ, Liebeskind JC, Albe-Fessard DG (eds) Advances in pain research and therapy 3. Raven Press, New York, pp 91–102

Nordin M, Nystrom B, Wallin U et al 1984 Ectopic sensory discharges and paraesthesiae in patients with disorders of peripheral nerves, dorsal roots and dorsal columns. Pain 20: 231–245

North JDK, Sinclair HM 1956 Nutritional neuropathy: chronic thiamine deficiency in the rat. Archives of Pathology 62: 341–353

Nystrom B, Hagbarth K-E 1981 Microelectrode recordings from transected nerves in amputees with phantom limb pain. Neuroscience Letters 27: 211–216

Ochoa J 1970 Isoniazid neuropathy in man. Brain 93: 831–850

Ochoa J 1978 Recognition of unmyelinated fibre disease: morphologic criteria. Muscle and Nerve 1: 375–387

Ochoa J, Noordenbos W 1979 Pathology and disordered sensation in local nerve lesions: an attempt at correlation. In: Bonica J et al (eds) Advances in pain research and therapy, vol 3. Raven Press, New York

Ochoa J, Torebjork HE 1980 Paraesthesiae from ectopic impulse generation in human sensory nerves. Brain 103: 835

Ochoa JL, Torebjork HE, Culp WL et al 1982 Abnormal spontaneous activity in single sensory nerve fibres in humans. Muscle and Nerve 5: 574–577

Ochoa JL, Torebjork HE, Marchettini P et al 1985 Mechanisms of neuropathic pain: cumulative observations, new experiments and further speculation. In: Fields HL, Dubner R, Cervero F (eds) Advances in pain research and therapy, vol 9. Proceedings of the Fourth World Congress on Pain. Raven Press, New York, pp 431–450

Ogden TE, Robert F, Carmichael EA 1959 Some sensory syndromes in children: indifference to pain and sensory neuropathy. Journal of Neurology, Neurosurgery and Psychiatry 22: 267–276
Ohnishi A, Dyck PJ 1974 Loss of small peripheral sensory neurons in Fabry's disease. Archives of Neurology 31: 120–127
Ohta M, Ellefson RD, Lambert EH, Dyck PJ 1973 Hereditary sensory neuropathy type II: clinical, electrophysiologic, histologic and biochemical studies in a Quebec kinship. Archives of Neurology 29: 23–37
Olsson Y, Save-Soderbergh J, Sourander P, Angervaall L 1968 A pathoanatomical study of the central and peripheral nervous system in diabetes of early onset and long duration. Pathologia Europaea 3: 62–79
Parry GJ, Brown MJ 1982 Selective fibre vulnerability in acute ischaemic neuropathy. Annals of Neurology 11: 147–154
Pegum JS 1952 Nicotinic acid and burning feet. Lancet ii: 536
Pinsky L, Di George AM 1966 Congenital familial sensory neuropathy with anhidrosis. Journal of Paediatrics 68: 1–13
Plant GT, Mtanda AT, Arden GB, Johnson GJ 1997 An epidemic of optic neuropathy in Tanzania: characterisation of the visual disorder and associated peripheral neuropathy. Journal of Neurological Sciences 145: 127–140
Pollard JD, McLeod JG, Honnibal TGA, Verheijden MA 1982 Hypothyroid polyneuropathy. Clinical, electrophysiological and nerve biopsy findings in two cases. Journal of Neurological Sciences 53: 461–471
Prineas J 1969 The pathogenesis study of experimental triortho-cresyl phosphate intoxification in the cat. Journal of Neuropathology and Experimental Neurology 28: 571–597
Prineas J 1970 Peripheral nerve changes in thiamine-deficient rats. Archives of Neurology 23: 541–548
Raff MC, Sangaland V, Asbury AK 1968 Ischaemic mononeuropathy multiplex associated with diabetes mellitus. Archives of Neurology 18: 487
Ragozzino MW, Melton LJ, Kurland LT et al 1982 Population based study of herpes zoster and its sequelae. Medicine 21: 310–316
Rahman AN, Lindenberg R 1963 Neuropathy of hereditary dystrophic lipidosis. Archives of Neurology 9: 373–385
Roger H, Poursines Y, Recordier M 1934 Polynevrite apres serotherapie antitetanique curative, avec participation due nevraxe et des meninges (observation automoclinique). Revue Neurologique 1: 1078–1088
Said G, Slama G, Selva J 1983 Progressive centripetal degeneration of axons in small fibre diabetic polyneuropathy. A clinical and pathological study. Brain 106: 791–807
Said G, Elgrably F, Lacroix C 1997 Painful proximal diabetic neuropathy: inflammatory nerve lesions and spontaneous favourable outcome. Annals of Neurology 41: 762–770
Scadding JW, Klenerman LE 1987 Light and electron microscopic observations in Morton's neuralgia. Pain (suppl 4) 5: 246
Schilder P, Schmidt BJ, Leon L 1931 Asymbolia for pain. Archives of Neurology and Psychiatry 25: 598–600
Schoetnal R, Cavanagh JB 1977 Mechanisms involved in the dying-back process – an hypothesis implicating coenzymes. Neuropathology and Applied Neurobiology 3: 145–158
Simon GS, Dewey WL 1981 Narcotics and diabetes. The effect of streptozoticin-induced diabetes on the antinociceptive potency of morphine. Journal of Pharmacology and Experimental Therapeutics 218: 318–323
Simpson J 1946 'Burning feet' in British prisoners of war in the Far East. Lancet I: 959–961
Smith DA, Woodruff MF 1951 Deficiency diseases in Japanese prison camps. Medical Research Council, Special Report Series 274. HMSO, London
Spencer PS, Schaumburg HH 1976 Central peripheral distal axonopathy – the pathology of dying back polyneuropathies. Progress in Neuropathology 3: 253–295
Spencer PS, Thomas PK 1970 The examination of isolated nerve fibres by light and electron microscopy with observations on demyelination proximal to neuromas. Acta Neuropathologica 16: 177–186
Spillane JD 1947 Nutritional disorders of the nervous system. Williams & Wilkins, Baltimore
Strachan H 1897 On a form of multiple neuritis prevalent in the West Indies. Practitioner 59: 477–484
Swank RL 1940 Avian thiamine deficiency. Journal of Experimental Medicine 71: 683–702
Swank RK, Prados M 1942 Avian thiamine deficiency. II. Pathologic changes in the brain and cranial nerves (especially vestibular) and their relation to the clinical behaviour. Archives of Neurology and Psychiatry 47: 97–131
Swanson AG 1963 Congenital insensitivity to pain with anhidrosis. Archives of Neurology 8: 299–306
Swanson AG, Buchan GC, Alvord EC 1965 Anatomic changes in congenital insensitivity to pain. Archives of Neurology 12: 12–18
Sweet WH 1981 Animal models of chronic pain: their possible validation from human experience with posterior rhizotomy and congenital analgesia. Pain 10: 275–295
Thomas PK 1970 The quantitation of nerve biopsy findings. Journal of the Neurological Sciences 11: 285–295
Thomas PK 1971 Morphological basis for alterations in nerve conduction in peripheral neuropathy. Proceedings of the Royal Society of Medicine 64: 295–298
Thomas PK 1973 Metabolic neuropathy. Journal of the Royal College of Physicians of London 7: 154–160
Thomas PK 1974 The anatomical substratum of pain. Canadian Journal of Neurological Science 1: 92
Thomas PK 1979 Painful neuropathies. In: Bonica J, Liebeskind JC, Albe-Fessard DG (eds) Advances in pain research and therapy 3. Raven Press, New York, pp 103–110
Thomas PK 1982 The selective vulnerability of the centrifugal and centripetal axons of primary sensory neurons. Muscle and Nerve 5: S 117–121
Thomas PK, Fullerton PM 1963 Nerve fibre size in the carpal tunnel syndrome. Journal of Neurology, Neurosurgery and Psychiatry 26: 520–527
Thomas PK, King RHM 1974 Peripheral nerve changes in amyloid neuropathy. Brain 97: 395–406
Thomas PK, Lascelles RG 1966 The pathology of diabetic neuropathy. Quarterly Journal of Medicine 35: 489–509
Thomas PK, Ochoa J 1993 Clinical features and differential diagnosis. In: Dyck PJ, Thomas P K, Griffin JW, Low PA, Poduslo JF (eds) Peripheral neuropathy, 3rd edn. WB Saunders, Philadelphia, pp 749–774
Thomas PK, Tomlinson DR 1993 Diabetic and hypoglycaemic neuropathy. In: Dyck PJ, Thomas PK, Griffin JW, Low PA, Poduslo JF (eds) Peripheral neuropathy, 3rd edn. WB Saunders, Philadelphia, pp 1219–1250
Thomas PK, Hollinrake K, Lascelles RG et al 1971 The polyneuropathy of chronic renal failure. Brain 94: 761–780
Thomas PK, Plant GT, Baxter P, Bates C, Santiago Luis R 1995 An epidemic of optic atrophy and painful sensory neuropathy in Cuba: clinical aspects. Journal of Neurology 242: 629–638
Tsairis P, Dyck PJ, Mulder DW 1972 Natural history of brachial plexus neuropathy: report on 99 patients. Archives of Neurology 27: 109–117
Valbo AB, Hagbarth KE, Torebjork HE, Wallin BG 1979 Somatosensory, proprioceptive and sympathetic activity in human peripheral nerves. Physiological Reviews 59: 919–957
Victor M 1975 Polyneuropathy due to nutritional deficiency and alcoholism In: Dyck PJ, Thomas PK, Lambert EH (eds) Peripheral neuropathy, 2nd edn. WB Saunders, Philadelphia, pp 1030–1066

Victor M, Adams RD 1953 The effect of alcohol on the nervous system. Research Publications – Association for Research in Nervous and Mental Disease 32: 526–573
Victor M, Adams RD 1961 On the aetiology of the alcoholic neurologic diseases. With special reference to the role of nutrition. American Journal of Clinical Nutrition 9: 379–397
Wall PD, Devor M 1983 Sensory afferent impulses originate from dorsal root ganglia as well as from the periphery in normal and nerve injured rats. Pain 17: 321–339
Wall PD, Gutnick M 1974 Ongoing activity in peripheral nerves: the physiology and pharmacology or impulses originating from a neuroma. Experimental Neurology 43: 580–593
Walsh JC 1971 The neuropathy of multiple myeloma. Archives of Neurology 25: 404–414
Walsh JC, McLeod JG 1970 Alcoholic neuropathy. An electrophysiological and histological study. Journal of the Neurological Sciences 10: 457–469
Watson CPN, Morshead C, Van der Koog D, Deck JH, Evans RJ 1988 Post-herpetic neuralgia: post mortem analysis of a case. Pain 34: 129–138
Watson CPN, Watt VR, Chipman M, Birkett N, Evans R 1991a The prognosis with post-herpetic neuralgia. Pain 46: 195–199
Watson CPN, Deck JH, Morshead C, Van der Koog D, Evans RJ 1991b Post-herpetic neuralgia: further post mortem studies of cases with and without pain. Pain 44: 105–117
Weddell G, Sinclair DC, Feindel WH 1948 An anatomical basis for alterations in quality of pain sensibility. Journal of Neurophysiology 11: 99–109
Wilbourn AJ 1993 Brachial plexus disorders. In: Dyck PJ, Thomas PK, Griffin JW, Low PA, Poduslo JF (eds) Peripheral neuropathy, 3rd edn. WB Saunders, Philadelphia, pp 911–950
Wilson SAK 1913–1914 The pathology pellagra. Proceedings of the Royal Society of Medicine 7: 31–41
Windebank AJ 1993 Polyneuropathy due to nutritional deficiency and alcoholism. In: Dyck PJ, Thomas PK, Griffin JW, Low PA, Poduslo JF (eds) Peripheral neuropathy, 3rd edn. WB Saunders, Philadelphia, pp 1310–1321
Winkelmann RK, Lambert EH, Hayes AB 1962 Congenital absence of pain. Archives of Dermatology 85: 325–339
Wise D, Wallace HJ, Jellinek EH 1962 Angiokeratoma corporis diffusum. Quarterly Journal of Medicine 31: 177–206
Wortis H, Stein MH, Jolliffe M 1942 Fibre dissociation in peripheral neuropathy. Archives of Internal Medicine 69: 222–237
Wright H 1901 Changes in the neuronal centres in beri-beri neuritis. British Medical Journal i: 1610–1616
Yaksh TL, Hammond DL 1982 Peripheral and central substrates involved in the rostrad transmission of nociceptive information. Pain 13: 1–86
Yao JK, Herbert PN 1993 Lipoprotein deficiency and neuromuscular manifestations. In: Dyck PJ, Thomas PK, Griffin JW, Low PA, Poduslo JF (eds) Peripheral neuropathy, 3rd edn. WB Saunders, Philadelphia, pp 1179–1193
Zachs SI, Langfit TW, Elliot FA 1964 Herpetic neuritis: a light and electron microscopic study. Neurology 14: 644–750
Zorilla E, Kozak GP 1967 Ophthalmoplegia in diabetes mellitus. Annals of Internal Medicine 67: 968–976

Complex regional pain syndrome

J. W. SCADDING

INTRODUCTION

Complex regional pain syndrome (CRPS) is the name now given to a group of conditions previously described as reflex sympathetic dystrophy (RSD), causalgia, algodystrophy, Sudeck's atrophy and a variety of other diagnoses (Box 36.1 and see Rizzi et al 1984). These conditions share a number of clinical features including pain with associated allodynia and hyperalgesia, autonomic changes, trophic changes, oedema and loss of function. The term causalgia was retrospectively applied by Mitchell to describe a syndrome of burning pain, hyperaesthesia, glossy skin and colour changes in the limbs of soldiers sustaining major nerve injuries from gunshot wounds, seen during the American Civil War (Mitchell et al 1864, Richards 1967a,b). It was later recognized that a very similar clinical picture could be produced by a variety of other illnesses and injuries which did not include major limb nerve injury, and the term RSD has, for many years, been used to embrace these conditions (Evans 1946, Bonica 1953, 1979).

BOX 36.1

Conditions comprising complex regional pain syndrome

- Reflex sympathetic dystrophy
- Post-traumatic sympathetic dystrophy
- Algodystrophy
- Algoneurodystrophy
- Causalgia (major, minor)
- Sudeck's atrophy
- Post-traumatic painful osteoporosis
- Transient osteoporosis
- Acute bone atrophy
- Migratory osteolysis
- Post-traumatic vasomotor syndrome
- Shoulder-hand syndrome

INVOLVEMENT OF THE SYMPATHETIC NERVOUS SYSTEM IN CAUSALGIA AND REFLEX SYMPATHETIC DYSTROPHY: HISTORICAL ASPECTS

It is worthwhile re-examining the early observations that led to a widespread acceptance that the sympathetic nervous system is crucially involved in the pathogenesis and maintenance of these syndromes. This has influenced subsequent thinking to the extent that some have even proposed response of the conditions to sympathetic blockade or sympathectomy as diagnostic criteria. However, this illogical and scientifically unjustified approach to conditions of uncertain, and quite possibly heterogeneous, pathogenesis has now been abandoned.

Leriche (1916) described the relief of causalgia in a patient with a brachial plexus injury and thrombosis of the brachial artery by surgical sympathectomy, resecting the adventitia of a length of the brachial artery. In this and subsequent patients, pain relief combined with an improvement in discolouration and sweating changes led Leriche to conclude that the sympathetic nervous system was involved in the pathogenesis of causalgia (Leriche 1939). As described by Schott (1995), peri-arterial sympathectomy was replaced by preganglionic sympathectomy and became standard treatment for painful nerve injuries sustained during the two World Wars, although without further critical evaluation of effectiveness.

For the conditions without major nerve or blood vessel injury, later described by the term RSD, in which very similar clinical features to causalgia are present, attempts to relieve pain and restore function by sympathectomy or repeated sympathetic blockade have, for many years, been standard treatment. Evidence of efficacy is examined later but it is recognized by those regularly treating these patients that while temporary pain relief may occur, long-term results are poor. It is probable that sympathetic block has only survived as standard treatment because of the lack of more effective therapy.

CAUSES OF COMPLEX REGIONAL PAIN SYNDROME

According to the previous IASP definitions of causalgia and RSD, causalgia referred to the syndrome associated with nerve injury, while RSD included patients whose pain and associated features followed a variety of insults, most commonly relatively minor, and normally fully recoverable injuries. These are listed in Box 36.2 (Richards 1967a, Schwartzman & McLellan 1987).

BOX 36.2

Causes of complex regional pain syndrome

- Peripheral tissues
  - Fractures and dislocations
  - Soft-tissue injury
  - Fasciitis, tendonitis, bursitis, ligamentous strain
  - Arthritis
  - Mastectomy
  - Deep vein thrombosis
  - Immobilization
- Peripheral nerve and dorsal root
  - Peripheral nerve trauma
  - Brachial plexus lesions
  - Post-herpetic neuralgia
  - Root lesions
- Central nervous system
  - Spinal cord lesions, particularly trauma
  - Head injury
  - Cerebral infarction
  - Cerebral tumour
- Viscera
  - Abdominal disease
  - Myocardial infarction
- Idiopathic

DEFINITION AND TAXONOMY OF COMPLEX REGIONAL PAIN SYNDROME

The need for a new classification and terminology stems from a poor understanding of the clinical limits of the conditions concerned, the underlying pathophysiology and how variable this may be, and the unsatisfactory existing terminology and particularly RSD with its clear pathogenic implication. The term 'sympathetically maintained pain' (SMP) introduced in recent years is also redefined within the context of CRPS and is discussed later in this chapter.

The new definition results from an IASP consensus conference (Stanton-Hicks et al 1995) and is summarized in Box 36.3, reproduced from Boas (1996). The first criterion for CRPS is that there is an initiating noxious event. However, there are a few patients otherwise fulfilling the diagnostic criteria for CRPS in whom there is no history of any such initiating event (Veldman et al 1993, Veldman & Goris 1996).

CLINICAL FEATURES OF COMPLEX REGIONAL PAIN SYNDROME

It can be seen from Box 36.3 that CRPS II is in all respects similar to CRPS I, except that included in the definition is the additional condition that it follows a nerve injury and thus corresponds to the condition previously known as causalgia.

Some of the clinical features merit further comment. The symptoms and signs of CRPS are found in a regional distribution, often widely in a limb and in both types of CRPS the symptoms and signs often spread well beyond the limits of the causative injured territory.

PAIN

Spontaneous and evoked pain (allodynia and hyperalgesia) coexist in the great majority of patients and are essential features of the conditions. Pain is disproportionate to the initiating cause in distribution, severity and duration, and may have various qualities. Commonly patients describe burning, aching or throbbing pain and in the case of CRPS II, superimposed paroxysmal pains are common. Allodynia, hyperalgesia and hyperpathia are often severe so that any contact with the affected part and active or passive movement may be extremely painful, leading to protection of the limb and frequently severe loss of function. This in turn

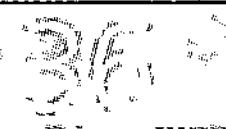

BOX 36.3

Diagnostic criteria for complex regional pain syndrome. (Reproduced from Boas 1996)

CRPS describes a variety of painful conditions that usually follow injury, occur regionally, have a distal predominance of abnormal findings, exceed in both magnitude and duration the expected clinical course of the inciting event, often result in significant impairment of motor function, and show variable progression over time

CRPS Type I (RSD)

1. Follows an initiating noxious event
2. Spontaneous pain and/or allodynia and hyperalgesia occur beyond the territory of a single peripheral nerve(s), and is disproportionate to the inciting event
3. There is or has been evidence of oedema, skin blood flow abnormality, or abnormal sudomotor activity, in the region of the pain since the inciting event
4. The diagnosis is excluded by the existence of conditions that would otherwise account for the degree of pain and dysfunction.

CRPS II (Causalgia)

This syndrome follows nerve injury. It is similar in all other respects to CRPS type I

1. Is a more regionally confined presentation about a joint or area, associated with a noxious event
2. Spontaneous pain and/or allodynia and hyperalgesia are usually limited to the area involved, but may spread variably distal or proximal to the area, not in the territory of a dermatomal or peripheral nerve distribution
3. Intermittent and variable oedema, skin blood flow change, temperature change, abnormal sudomotor activity, and motor dysfunction, disproportionate to the inciting event, are present about the area involved

may lead to secondary effects of prolonged immobilization, including muscle wasting and joint stiffness sometimes with contracture, and these are frequent compounding factors in CRPS.

Occasional patients who otherwise fulfill the diagnostic criteria for CRPS do not complain of spontaneous pain. Of the 829 patients studied by Veldman et al (1993), 7% did not have spontaneous pain at the time they were evaluated, although they may have had pain at some time during the illness and it is not clear how many of these patients had allodynia or hyperalgesia. This raises a problem of classification and nomenclature for patients with features of CRPS who have had pain at some stage which has spontaneously resolved leaving other persistent symptoms and signs of the condition. It is possible that there may be some patients who otherwise satisfy the diagnostic criteria for CRPS, who never experience pain which is disproportionate to the initiating event. This question will only be answered by careful prospective study.

AUTONOMIC SIGNS

The definition of CRPS is careful to state that autonomic signs are or have at some time been present, but are not necessarily constant features in a particular patient. Abnormalities of temperature and colour are common and there are frequently descriptions of marked variation in these signs and of sweating. Oedema is often present as an early sign (Blumberg & Janig 1994b), which later resolved in about half of patients. These autonomic changes could, in part, be secondary to immobilization.

MOTOR SIGNS

Objective motor signs are variable but loss of function of the affected part is almost universal. Wasting and weakness are common and tremor and dystonia are observed in a small proportion of patients.

DYSTROPHIC CHANGES

Some of these outlined below may simply result from prolonged disuse. Skin changes include thinning, sometimes with a shiny appearance, but other patients develop flaky, thickened skin. Hair may be lost or become abnormally coarse and the nails may become thickened. Osteoporosis, again explicable on the basis of disuse, is a frequent finding in many patients but occasionally a more profound loss of bone mineral content occurs (Sudeck's atrophy).

PREDISPOSITION TO CRPS

It has been postulated that certain individuals might be predisposed to the development of CRPS but there is no conclusive evidence in favour of this (Covington 1996) and individual patients with two similar injuries, one leading to CRPS and the other not, argue against any such tendency.

PSYCHOLOGICAL FACTORS

The absence of a clear pathogenesis and pathophysiological basis for CRPS, and the disproportionate pain and loss of function, have understandably led to examination of potential psychological aetiology, including secondary gains from injury. The evaluation of papers on this aspect of CRPS emphasizes the difficulties and importance of accurate diagnosis. Patients with conversion disorder and factitious illnesses may present with symptoms that can closely resemble CRPS and indeed because diagnosis of CRPS is based on assessment of symptoms and signs, not all of which are necessarily present at the time of diagnosis, it is not surprising that some patients with primary psychiatric morbidity are erroneously diagnosed as having CRPS. A diagnosis of CRPS as distinct from conversion disorder may only emerge in some patients after a period of time and a series of diagnostic assessments. These are likely to include careful clinical examination on more than one occasion, investigation for a possible ongoing cryptic cause for pain and loss of function and psychiatric examinations.

The severe pain of CRPS with loss of function and lack of a clear diagnosis produces anxiety, fear and depression in many patients. Whether or not such secondary psychological features developing early following an injury might then predispose to the development of CRPS remains controversial. This and other psychological aspects of CRPS are reviewed by Covington (1996).

Some of the patients reported by Ochoa and Verdugo (1995) with so-called pseudoneuropathy mimicking CRPS type I undoubtedly had primarily psychiatric illnesses, again emphasizing the need for careful and often repeated clinical assessment over a period of time.

RELATIVE FREQUENCY OF CLINICAL FEATURES IN CRPS

Case ascertainment is clearly a difficulty in CRPS and all the large series reported in the literature suffer from referral bias to some extent. Prospective studies examining patients after a particular known cause, for example Colles fracture (Bickerstaff & Kanis 1994), avoid such bias but only provide a single cause perspective of the condition. A report from a centre known to have an interest in CRPS, and thus attracting referrals from many other hospitals in the Netherlands, inevitably suffered from referral bias to some extent, but analysis of 829 patients with CRPS from all causes provides a fairly reliable insight into the relative frequency of the various symptoms and signs comprising CRPS (Veldman et al 1993). These were categorized by Veldman et al (1993) as inflammatory, neurological, dystrophic and sympathetic and were evaluated with respect to duration of CRPS. Table 36.1 presents data from Veldman et al (1993).

Table 36.1. Symptoms and signs of complex regional pain syndrome. (Data adapted from Veldman et al 1993)

Symptom/sign	*Duration of CRPS*	
	2–6 months (%)	*> 12 months (%)*
Inflammatory		
Pain	88	97
Colour difference	96	84
Temperature difference	91	91
Limited movement	90	83
Exacerbation with exercise	95	97
Oedema	80	55
Neurological		
Hyperaesthesia	75	85
Hyperpathia	79	81
Incoordination	47	61
Tremor	44	50
Involuntary spasms	24	47
Muscle spasm	13	42
Paresis	93	97
Pseudoparalysis	7	26
Dystrophy		
Skin	37	44
Nails	23	36
Muscle	50	67
Bone	41	52
Sympathetic		
Hyperhidrosis	56	40
Changed hair growth	71	35
Changed nail growth	60	52

STAGING OF CLINICAL FEATURES IN CRPS

Earlier studies of RSD suggested that three stages could be recognized: an acute warm phase in which pain and oedema predominated, a dystrophic phase categorized by muscle wasting and vasomotor instability with pale cyanotic skin, and a later cold, atrophic stage categorized particularly by bone and skin changes (Stenbrocker 1947, Blumberg & Janig 1994b). The value of staging has been questioned as patients do not all follow the same course, the duration of the recognizable phases is variable and not all patients progress to the third stage (Walker & Cousins 1997). Veldman et al (1993) found that in 95% of their patients the acute phase was categorized by pain, oedema, vasomotor changes, changes in temperature and loss of function, all of which were intensified by exercise of the affected limb, signs which they interpreted as characteristic of inflammation. With regard to temperature, patients with longer duration symptoms were more likely to have a cold limb. Of those patients seen from the onset of the illness, 13% had primarily cold limbs without any initial warm phase. More

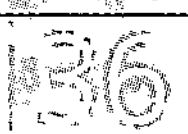

than half their patients did not develop signs of tissue dystrophy or atrophy in the later stages.

LESS COMMON CLINICAL FEATURES OF CRPS

Very infrequently, CRPS may be migratory, relapsing or occur in two or more extremities (Johnson 1943, Bentley & Hameroff 1980, Veldman et al 1993). In 53% of the patients with relapsing or multiple RSD described by Velman et al (1993), no initiating injury or illness could be identified, raising the possibility that very rarely a predisposition to develop CRPS may exist in certain subjects. Other less common features of CRPS include intractable or relapsing skin infections (associated with chronic oedema), spontaneous haematomas, increased skin pigmentation, nodular fasciitis of palmar or plantar skin and clubbing of the nails (Veldman et al 1993).

CRPS IN CHILDREN

It is only relatively recently that the occurrence of CRPS in children has been recognized (Bernstein et al 1978, Olsson et al 1990, Wilder et al 1992, Wilder 1996, Fermaglich 1997). Certain differences between CRPS in children and adults are apparent. Delay in diagnosis due to lack of awareness of the condition amongst paediatricians is still more likely in children. The lower limb is much more frequently affected than the upper limb (ratio about 5 : 1), whereas the opposite is true in adults. Most studies of CRPS in adults show a female preponderance, but this is more marked in children (ratio about 4 : 1). Although young children with CRPS have been reported, sufferers are typically pubertal adolescent girls. Approximately half the children affected will get better with complete resolution of symptoms and signs and only a relatively small proportion continue to experience severe pain. There are indications that recovery is helped by physiotherapy, transcutaneous electrical stimulation and cognitive and behavioural pain management techniques. Many children with CRPS participate in competitive sports and other physical activities, putting them at greater risk of musculoskeletal injury.

Interest has focused on the role of psychological factors with the suggestion that injury and persistent pain provide a means of escape from stressful competition and the parental expectations associated with this (Sherry & Weisman 1998). Sympatholytic treatment is as unpredictable in its efficacy as in adults and long-term results are disappointing, although comparisons are not easy due to the higher rate of spontaneous resolution or cure in children than in adults.

DIAGNOSTIC TESTS: SYMPATHETICALLY MAINTAINED PAIN AND SYMPATHETICALLY INDEPENDENT PAIN

There are no diagnostic tests for CRPS, the diagnostic criteria at present being clinical. Three-phase isotope bone scans are frequently abnormal (Goldsmith et al 1989, Barrera et al 1992), but a normal bone scan does not exclude the diagnosis. Although the existence of a sympathetic influence on pain in CRPS and other pain states has been questioned (Ochoa et al 1994, Schott 1995), there is substantial experimental and clinical evidence in favour of such an influence (see Ch. 5 and see later discussion Loh & Nathan 1978, Loh et al 1980, Torebjork et al 1995). Sympathetically maintained pain (SMP) is the component of a patient's pain which is maintained by efferent noradrenergic sympathetic activity and circulating catecholamines, whereas sympathetically independent pain (SIP) is the component which is not (Roberts 1986). A variety of neurogenic pains, including some central pains as well as peripheral neuropathic pains, may be partly, if only temporarily, responsive to sympathetic blockade (Loh et al 1980, Bonica 1990, Arner 1991, Raja et al 1991, Wahren et al 1991). A conceptual framework for the relationship between SMP and some painful conditions is shown in Figure 36.1 from Boas (1996). SMP as assessed clinically by the affect of sympathetic blockade is a very variable component of pain in CRPS I and II, not only between different individuals but also in the same individual at different times. SMP is correctly not included in the diagnostic criteria for either type of CRPS. A useful algorithm for the diagnosis of CRPS arose from the IASP consensus meeting shown in Box 36.4.

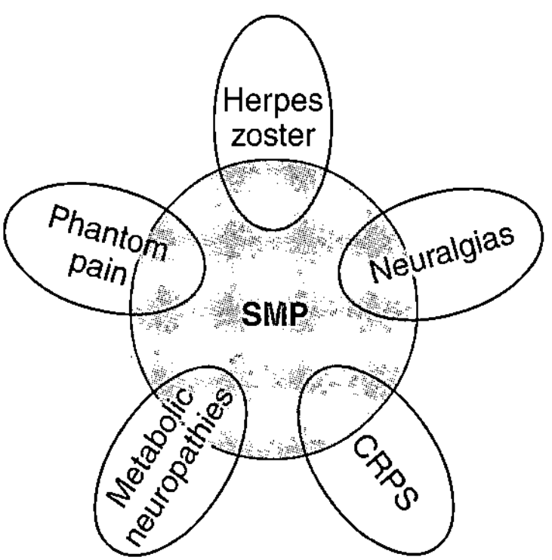

Fig. 36.1 Diagrammatic representation of the relationship of sympathetically maintained pain (SMP) and some painful conditions, demonstrating the existence of SMP in these conditions. (Reproduced from Boas 1996 with permission.)

INCIDENCE AND NATURAL HISTORY OF COMPLEX REGIONAL PAIN SYNDROME

One of the problems with the current defining diagnostic criteria for CRPS of both types is establishing the limits of the diagnosis. When is pain judged to be disproportionate in severity, distribution and duration to the initiating event? Furthermore, some degree of oedema or vasomotor or sudomotor change following many injuries is extremely common. At what stage can these changes be said to be excessive and indicative of the development of CRPS? These uncertainties, together with the fact that there are very few prospective studies, currently permit limited conclusions about incidence and natural history.

The development of CRPS I following fractures is well recognized. In a prospective study of 274 patients with Colles fractures of varying severity, Bickerstaff and Kanis (1994) measured tenderness of the fingers, hand swelling and grip strength, together with symptomatic assessment of pain, vasomotor symptoms and finger stiffness at intervals up to 1 year following the fracture. At 2 weeks following removal of the plaster cast, 54% had one of the measured features, swelling being the most common (45%). However, only 28% had all four features (bone tenderness, vasomotor symptoms, swelling and stiffness). These patients were more likely to complain of pain in the hand or shoulder and had a more markedly impaired grip strength. At 1 year 18%, 14% and 12% still had finger tenderness, pain and swelling respectively and these features were usually found in the same patients. Some 50% of patients still had finger stiffness. These authors' conclusion that each of these symptoms indicated the presence of algodystrophy is at variance with the new diagnostic criteria for CRPS (Stanton-Hicks et al 1995), and it would not be accepted that about 20% of their patients had developed CRPS at 1 year. However, the study of Bickerstaff and Kanis (1994) does indicate that careful prospective study following a common fracture usually considered to be associated with excellent recovery, presents a truer picture and draws attention to the underestimation of continuing painful symptoms. Prospective study has yielded similar results in other conditions potentially giving rise to chronic painful symptoms, for example amputation (Carlen et al 1978).

Other estimates for the incidence of CRPS, though not from prospective studies, include 1–2% after fractures (Bohm 1985), 1–5% after peripheral nerve injury (Omer & Thomas 1971, Veldman et al 1993) and the shoulder–hand syndrome in 5% of patients with myocardial infarction (Rosen & Graham 1957).

PATHOPHYSIOLOGY OF COMPLEX REGIONAL PAIN SYNDROME

Animal and human investigations into the underlying mechanisms of CRPS have focused on three areas. Firstly, evidence of abnormal coupling between the efferent sympathetic nervous system and sensory afferents; secondly, the nature and importance of inflammatory processes in peripheral tissues, both with and without nerve injury, and, thirdly, the development of secondary central changes explaining the wide radiation of the clinical features of CRPS and the maintenance of the syndrome long after the initiating cause has healed or been removed. While it is not yet possible to build a complete picture of pathophysiology and still less possible to translate this into effective treatment, several lines of investigations have provided important insights.

THE SYMPATHETIC NERVOUS SYSTEM AND PAIN: NERVE DAMAGE

Three sites of sympathetic sensory interaction after nerve injury have been identified; the region of the nerve damage itself, undamaged fibres distal to the nerve lesion and the dorsal root ganglion.

Following severe injury, for example nerve section with neuroma formation, somatosensory fibres develop an abnormal sensitivity to catecholamines, an effect mediated by α receptors. Both circulating catecholamines and endogenously released transmitter following sympathetic trunk stimulation can be shown to stimulate damaged sprouting sensory fibres. The effect is maximal within the first few weeks in all the species studied but is present to some extent as a long-term property in the region of nerve damage and it also occurs when continuity of the nerve is restored by resuture following nerve section. All classes of afferent fibre are affected, both from skin and deep tissue, including C fibres (Wall & Gutnick 1974, Govrin-Lippmann & Devor 1978, Devor & Janig 1981, Korenman & Devor 1981, Scadding 1981, Blumberg & Janig 1984a, Burchiel 1984, Habler et al 1987, Janig 1996; and see Ch. 5). Following partial nerve lesions of different types, the development of catecholamine sensitivity in intact or partly damaged afferents also occurs. Shyu et al (1990) found an increase in the amplitude of the C-fibre compound action potential after sympathetic stimulation with a compressive lesion of rat peroneal nerve. In a single fibre study, Sato and Perl (1991) showed that after a partial lesion of the auricular nerve in the rabbit, a proportion of C fibres which were undamaged by the lesion could be activated by sympathetic

BOX 36.4

Algorithm for the diagnosis of complex regional pain syndrome. (Reproduced from Wilson et al 1996)

Pain

The diagnosis of CRPS cannot be made in the absence of pain; it is a pain syndrome. However, the characteristics of the pain may vary with the initiating event and other factors. The pain is often described as burning, and might be spontaneous or evoked in the context of hyperalgesia or allodynia. Both spontaneous and evoked pain may occur together

History

- Develops after an initiating noxious event or immobilization
- Unilateral extremity onset (rarely may spread to another extremity)
- Symptom onset usually within a month

Exclusion criteria:

- Identifiable major nerve lesion (CRPS II)
- Existence of anatomical, physiological, or psychological conditions that would otherwise account for the degree of pain and dysfunction

Symptoms (patient report)

A. Pain (spontaneous or evoked)
   Burning
   Aching, throbbing
B. Hyperalgesia or allodynia (at some time in the disease course) to mechanical stimuli (light touch or deep pressure), to thermal stimulation or to joint motion
C. Associated symptoms (minor)
   Swelling
   Temperature or colour: asymmetry and instability
   Sweating: asymmetry and instability
   Trophic changes: hair, nails, skin

Signs (observed)

Hyperalgesia or allodynia (light touch, deep pressure, joint movement, cold)
Oedema (if unilateral and other causes excluded)
Vasomotor changes: colour, temperature instability, asymmetry
Sudomotor changes
Trophic changes in skin, joint, nail, hair
Impaired motor function (may include components of dystonia and tremor)

Criteria required for diagnosis of CRPS I

History of pain:

- Plus allodynia, hyperalgesia, or hyperaesthesia
- Plus two other signs from the above list

Characteristics of spontaneous pain:
Sympathetically maintained pain (SMP)
Sympathetically independent pain (SIP)
Combined SMP + SIP

stimulation. Shir and Seltzer (1991) demonstrated that systemic guanethidine reduced heat and mechanical hyperalgesia after a partial nerve lesion in the rat, and similar observations were reported by Kim et al (1993) using surgical sympathectomy or systemic phentolamine. It has been suggested that these findings are consistent with an upregulation of α receptors in the membrane of intact nociceptive fibres (Bossut et al 1996).

The normal spontaneous discharge of dorsal root ganglion neurons is greatly enhanced by peripheral nerve injury (Kirk 1974, Wall & Devor 1993), and this may be further increased by sympathetic stimulation (Devor et al 1994). However, subsequent studies have indicated that this sympathetic sensory coupling occurs mainly in non-nociceptive afferents and is present only transiently following nerve injury. Furthermore, at later intervals, sympathetic stimulation may exert an inhibitory effect on dorsal root ganglion neuron activity (Devor et al 1994, Chen et al 1996, Michaelis et al 1996).

There are limited but important human investigations which indicate a sympathetic influence on pain following peripheral nerve injury. Fifty years ago Walker and Nulsen (1948) showed that intraoperative sympathetic chain stimulation exacerbated pain in patients with causalgia. In patients with successfully treated causalgia, Wallin et al (1976) found that the patient's original pain could be rekindled by cutaneous application of noradrenaline. Injection of noradrenaline around amputation stump neuromas may cause severe pain (Chabal et al 1992). The study of Torebjork et al extended the earlier observations of Wallin et al (1976). Two findings are of particular interest. In patients with nerve injury and pain responsive to sympathetic blockade (SMP), only 28% experienced an increase in pain when noradrenaline was injected into the sensitive skin. Because the pain in all these patients had been shown to be reduced by sympathectomy, one might expect all these patients to have experienced exacerbation of their pain with noradrenaline injected into the skin. Torebjork et al (1995) and Wall (1995) suggest three possible reasons for these observations. Firstly, that all the α receptors on the abnormal nerve fibres are occupied by circulating or endogenously released noradrenaline. It is not known if injected noradrenaline in unsympathectomized patients fails to increase pain, as would be expected if this were the case. Secondly, that noradrenaline-sensitive fibres are present also in deep tissues and thus unaffected by cutaneous injection of noradrenaline. Thirdly that, as shown by Wall and Devor (1983), a second source of ectopic impulse generation after nerve injury of dorsal root ganglion neurons, which are also sensitive to the alpha effect of noradrenaline, are unaffected by cutaneous injection. Wall (1995) further suggests that there might then be patients who fail to respond to a peripheral sympathetic block with regional guanethidine but do respond to a sympathetic ganglion block, which eliminates both sources of adrenergic stimulation. Systematic study has not yet addressed this important question.

The second finding of interest in the investigation of Torebjork et al (1995) is that some of the patients examined in the earlier study of Wallin et al (1976), and who at that time had SMP, were found at the later examination to have pain that did not respond to sympathetic blockade. In line with this, most of those subjects in the earlier study whose pain was rekindled or exacerbated with injected noradrenaline had pain at the later time which did not respond in this way. This indicates changing pathophysiology in CRPS over long periods of pain, presenting further difficulties in targeting treatments.

In a clinical condition which may be likened to experimental situations in which partly damaged regenerated or undamaged afferents in partial nerve injury become sensitive to catecholamines, Choi and Rowbotham (1997) showed that intracutaneous injections of noradrenaline or adrenaline in an area affected by postherpetic neuralgia, increased both spontaneous pain and allodynia.

THE SYMPATHETIC NERVOUS SYSTEM AND PAIN: WITHOUT NERVE DAMAGE

Investigation of possible sympathetic influences on painful sensation without nerve injury, in other words, in conditions which are more representative of the clinical situations in which CRPS type I may develop, has been more recent than the studies of nerve injury. The complex mechanisms underlying the development of spontaneous pain, hyperalgesia and allodynia to various types of stimulation following experimental heat and chemically induced cutaneous inflammation using irritants such as mustard oil and capsaicin, are summarized by Koltzenburg (1996). Both peripheral and central factors are involved. Some components of experimental cutaneous inflammation have been shown to be influenced by noradrenergic α-receptor agonists or antagonists. This was first demonstrated by Drummond (1995) who reported an increase in heat-induced hyperalgesia in skin inflamed by topical capsaicin after iontophoresis of noradrenaline. In inflammation produced by intradermal capsaicin, Kinman et al (1997) showed that spontaneous pain could be reduced by locally injected phentolamine, although the evoked pain in capsaicin-induced inflammation was not influenced by intravenous phentolamine in the experiments of Liu et al (1996).

It might be argued that the demonstrated sympathetic influence occurred as a secondary effect of altered local blood supply in the area of inflammation. However, in a microneurographic study, Elam et al (1996) found that the discharge from axons sensitized by cutaneous application of mustard oil was not influenced by physiological reflex alterations of sympathetic vasoconstrictor neurons. In addition,

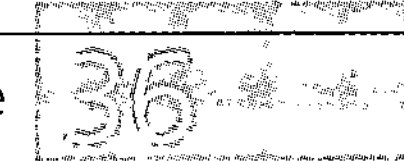

Baron et al (1998) have reported that cutaneous sympathetic vasoconstrictor activity does not alter the intensity of ongoing pain induced by capsaicin inflammation.

In addition to the alteration of heat hyperalgesia reported by Drummond (1995), other components of secondary hyperalgesia may also be under sympathetic influence. Kinman et al (1997) showed that mechanical hyperalgesia to strong stimulation, mediated by Aδ and C fibres in topically induced capsaicin inflammation, could be reduced by locally injected phentolamine. Again, using capsaicin inflammation, dynamic mechanical allodynia mediated by Aβ fibres was reduced by systemic phentolamine (Liu et al 1996).

The sensitization of somatosensory afferents may be caused by direct stimulation by noradrenaline or indirectly through release of inflammatory substances, particularly prostaglandins. Levine and others have shown that in certain experimental situations, noradrenaline released from sympathetic postganglionic neurons causes release of prostaglandins (Levine et al 1986, Gold et al 1994). In an experimental sciatic neuropathy in rats, Tracey et al (1995) found hyperalgesia which was enhanced by local injection of noradrenaline and decreased by injection of indomethacin, strongly suggesting mediation of the hyperalgesia by prostaglandins and perhaps other inflammatory substances. It was further shown that the observed sympathetic enhancement of hyperalgesia was an α_2-receptor effect, as both phentolamine and yohimbine (a selective α_2-adrenergic receptor blocker) relieved the hyperalgesia but prazosin (an α_1-receptor blocker) was ineffective.

Finally, returning to inflammation in the absence of nerve injury, Sanjue and Juu (1989) demonstrated that the degree of nociceptor sensitivity to noradrenaline varies with the pre-existing activity of the nociceptor. In the absence of injury with nociceptors in a non-sensitized state, the action of noradrenaline was weak in contrast to marked enhancement of activity in a nociceptor sensitized by a cocktail of inflammatory substances.

PAIN IN CRPS RELATED TO INFLAMMATION AND INDEPENDENT OF THE SYMPATHETIC NERVOUS SYSTEM

The experimental animal and human evidence outlined above would appear to indicate an important adrenergic sympathetic postganglionic influence in the processes which may lead to pain, both with and without nerve injury. The singular lack of long-term effectiveness of sympathetic blockade and sympathectomy in clinical practice in CRPS, both type I and type II in the majority of patients, has led some to question the existence of any significant sympathetic involvement in CRPS or indeed any type of pain syndrome. Arguments are based on the poor quality of clinical investigations, including lack of proper controls and the questionable relevance of animal models to the human situation, together with possible underestimation of psychological factors (Ochoa 1994, Ochoa et al 1994, Ochoa & Verdugo 1995, Schott 1995, 1997). Schott (1995, 1997) proposes a mechanism for the analgesic effect of sympathetic blockade that does not depend on a reduction of peripheral noradrenergic activity. He suggests that pain relief after sympathectomy may be explained by a reduction of activity of visceral afferent fibres which travel in sympathetic nerves (Cervero 1994, Schott 1994), rather than any peripheral effect on efferent noradrenergic function.

Schott (1995) proposes inflammatory mechanisms that are independent of noradrenergic efferent function as the cause of pain in CRPS (Dray 1996). In a subsequent paper Schott (1997) draws attention to the evidence indicating an inflammatory basis for the bone atrophy that occurs in CRPS, leading in its extreme form to Sudeck's atrophy. This evidence is reviewed by Kozin (1992) and Oyen et al (1993). Treatments, including calcitonin to reverse the marked osteopenia which may occur in CRPS, have been advocated in the past but without adequate controlled trials. Interest recently has focused on the biphosphonates, which prevent bone resorption by inhibiting osteoclast activity and dissolution of calcium apatite crystals. However, this property of biphosphonates is unlikely to explain the very rapid relief of bone pain that has been observed in bone pain due to cancer, and it is possible that additional effects of biphosphonates on prostaglandin E_2 and other inflammatory mediators may be responsible for analgesia (Strang 1996). Further investigation may clarify the mechanisms of bone atrophy in CRPS and possibly atrophic changes in other tissues, which are frequent features of CRPS.

Relevant to the issue of visceral and somatic afferents in sympathetic nerves, Kramis et al (1996) review a curious but well-recognized consequence of sympathetic chain interruption, the development of a new pain which occurs days to weeks after sympathectomy, and propose mechanisms for such pain. This so-called sympathalgia, or post-sympathectomy pain, tends to be distributed in the proximal parts of the sympathectomized limb and extends onto the trunk. Distally in the limb there is usually evidence of sympathetic denervation but proximally there may be excessive sweating and other features include deep muscular tenderness and proximal cutaneous allodynia and hyperalgesia (Tracy & Crockett 1957, Raskin et al 1974).

The incidence of postsympathectomy pain following sympathetic trunk lesioning, but not after local anaesthetic block or more distal sympathetic nerve blockade either with local anaesthetic or guanethidine, is estimated to occur in 30–50% of patients, although it is not usually severe. Kramis et al (1996) propose that postsympathectomy pain develops as a result of transection of paraspinal somatic and visceral afferents travelling within the sympathetic trunk, and that this in turn leads to cell death of many of the axotomized neurons, causing central deafferentation. Pain related to the deafferentation may be worse as a result of prior sensitization of dorsal horn cells produced by the painful state for which the sympathectomy was performed.

CENTRAL NERVOUS SYSTEM CHANGES

Central nervous system physiological and pharmacological changes secondary to prolonged nociceptive inputs, with and without nerve injury, are reviewed in Chs 6 and 10. A detailed description is beyond the scope of this chapter. The acute response to a noxious input is to induce a suppressed state in which the inhibitory mechanisms are activated which influence the forward transmission of the nociceptive input. These inhibitions are mediated at segmental level in the spinal cord and via descending mechanisms from the brainstem. Prolonged or abnormal noxious inputs from tissue or nerve injury may lead to a sensitized state in which wide dynamic range (WDR) neurons show increasing responses to C-fibre inputs (wind up). This change is mediated by NMDA and neurokinin receptors. Further biochemical changes may ensue, leading to prostaglandin and nitric oxide synthesis, both of which lower the threshold of WDR, which may then respond to normally non-noxious inputs. Under circumstances that are poorly understood, if the state of hyperexcitability of WDR becomes excessive, further changes may occur which may lead to degenerative and thus permanent effect. Following peripheral nerve injury there is withdrawal of terminals of primary afferents from lamina II, degeneration of primary afferent terminals and variable dorsal root ganglion cell death. There are associated chemical changes, including upregulation of some substances and downregulation of other transmitters, with resultant altered signalling at the first synapse.

A prolonged C-fibre input can lead to excitotoxicity, resulting in degenerative changes. Experimentally observed trans-synaptic changes include upregulation of some postsynaptic receptors, denervation hypersensitivity and reduced segmental inhibition. Later, regeneration may occur in the central terminals of primary afferent fibres through expression of growth-associated proteins. One potentially important observation is that Aβ-fibre terminals may grow into lamina II of the dorsal horn. If functional synapses form, this new and inappropriate connectivity could lead to pain, with impulse activity in low-threshold fibres now leading to activity in second-order neurons, which was previously exclusively activated by high-threshold C fibres. It is likely that such a re-organized state of the dorsal horn could be permanent.

Changes of the sort briefly outlined above may clearly be important in relation to the pain of CRPS.

SUMMARY OF MECHANISMS IN CRPS

The pathophysiology of pain and other clinical features in CRPS remain poorly understood and although experimental studies outlined here represent a considerable advance in knowledge, we are still some way from a clear understanding of these conditions. The diagrammatic representation in Figure 36.2 sets out some components of CRPS which are currently thought to be of importance in pathogenesis. The basic concept of a vicious circle, first proposed by Livingston (1943), remains evident. The importance of the sympathetic nervous system may be overrated, and that of chronic inflammatory changes in deeper tissues underestimated, in the scheme presented. The potential for some central changes to become permanent, and thus possibly limit the effectiveness of any treatment directed towards the initiating peripheral event, is not shown in Figure 36.2. These factors, together with further knowledge of the somatic and visceral sensory sympathetic coupling in peripheral tissues, require elucidation through further research.

TREATMENT OF COMPLEX REGIONAL PAIN SYNDROME

Few conditions can match CRPS types I and II for the variety of treatment modalities and drugs suggested – a sure indication that no single treatment is superior to others and that nothing is consistently successful. Controlled trials have been few and comparisons of treatments in different reports are made difficult by patient populations which are heterogeneous in causation, clinical features and severity. This is not surprising in a condition which has proved so difficult to define and whose limits, even with the now generally accepted definition provided by the IASP consensus conference, are uncertain. The older term, RSD, has focused undue attention upon sympatholytic procedures to the exclusion of consideration of other treatments,

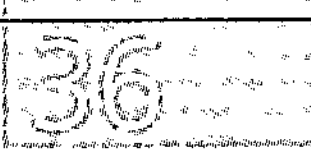

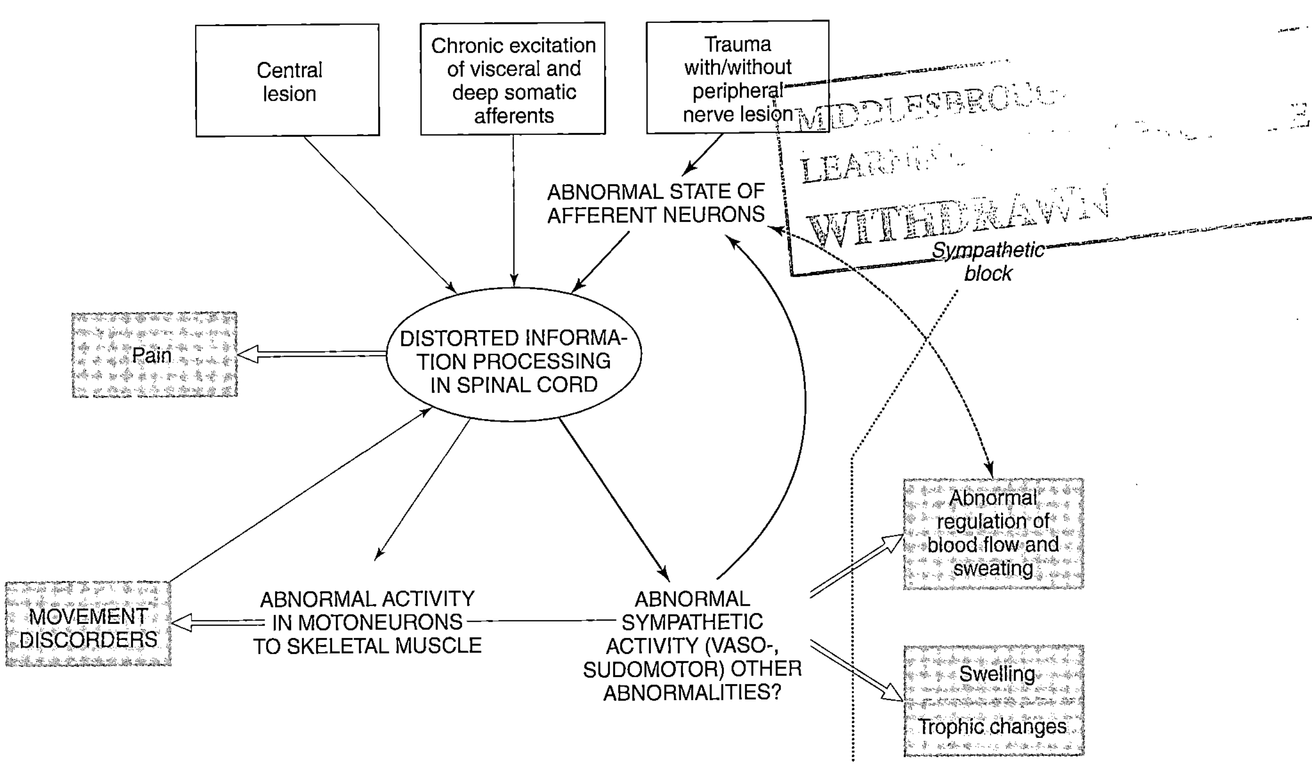

Fig. 36.2 Relationship of various peripheral and central factors important in the mechanisms of pain and other clinical features of CRPS types I and II. See text for further explanation. (Reproduced from Janig 1996 with permission.)

although this is now changing. The research on mechanisms of CRPS types I and II is recent, particularly for type I, and many treatments suggested have previously been based on ideas and speculation rather than fact. This state of affairs is now set to change.

DOES EARLY TREATMENT IMPROVE OUTCOME?

It has long been accepted that early recognition and institution of active treatment improves the outcome in CRPS. While this seems intuitively correct, it has never been subjected to systematic study. Clearly, the management of injuries and diseases known to have the potential of leading to the development of CRPS should be optimally managed in the acute stages, but again there is no evidence that it is only badly managed patients who are prone to develop CRPS. However, immobilization and disuse are undoubtedly factors which contribute to the development of CRPS, and it makes sense to minimize these factors by instituting physiotherapy at an early stage after injury.

This raises an important point about the aims of treatment in established cases of CRPS. It is always gratifying, both to patient and clinician, to obtain analgesia by whatever means, but pain relief alone is insufficient. A hallmark of CRPS is loss of function of the affected part and every period of even partial analgesia should be utilized to begin mobilization and rehabilitation. This emphasizes the importance of a multidisciplinary approach to treatment.

SYMPATHOLYTIC PROCEDURES

Intravenous regional guanethidine blocks

Guanethidine reduces noradrenaline concentrations in adrenergic neurons and blocks reuptake. The technique of intravenous regional guanethidine block (IVRGB) described by Hannington-Kiff (1974) quickly became established as a simple and reliable method of peripheral sympathetic blockade and is now widely used. The treatment has, however, only been subject to controlled study in recent years. In open studies it has been common experience that some patients respond, usually transiently, for hours or days but many patients do not and some patients report a transient increase in pain following IVRGB. Multiple blocks over a period of time have been advocated in the hope of producing a cumulative effect (Girgis & Wynn Parry 1989).

Two recent studies of IVRGB have been helpful in evaluating the treatment in patients with CRPS. Many other studies have used patients with a number of painful conditions and the results are difficult to assess. Jadad et al (1995) reviewed seven randomized controlled trials from the literature. In most of these guanethidine was used, but reserpine, bretylium, droperidol and ketanserin were used in some as alternatives. In the four guanethidine studies, none demonstrated a difference in analgesia between guanethidine and control and none of the studies was designed to determine a dose–response effect. Jadad et al (1995) criticized the methodology of these investigations, with problems identified including poor defined diagnostic criteria, inadequate wash-out periods, an incomplete crossover, open administration of some treatments and a high proportion of withdrawals. In a subsequent controlled trial, Jadad et al (1995) recruited patients with CRPS who had reported analgesia following an open trial of IVRGB. Nine patients completed the trial and no significant difference was shown between guanethidine and saline control (lignocaine was not used in this study).

Ramamurthy and Hoffman (1995) randomized 60 patients to receive up to four IVRGBs with lignocaine, control injections being lignocaine and saline. Although there was no difference between guanethidine and control treated patients, patients in all treatment groups showed a decrease in oedema and pseudomotor, trophic and vasomotor changes. All patients had at least one IVRGB and those receiving up to four blocks gained no greater degree of pain relief. Campbell et al (1988) investigated the effects of a tourniquet inflated to suprasystolic pressure as used in IVRGB. Hyperalgesia was relieved but temperature sensation was not affected. It was suggested that hyperalgesia was mediated via Aβ-mechanoreceptor fibres, these being most susceptible to pressure block.

Sympathetic ganglion block

Local anaesthetic stellate ganglion or lumbar chain blocks have been much used in the treatment of CRPS but no adequately controlled study has been done, and indeed would be difficult to do. Aggressive early treatment has often been suggested (Wang et al 1985, Bonica 1990) but without clear supporting evidence. Kozin (1992) analysed reports in seven studies of sympathetic blocks in more than 500 patients and concluded that 46% of patients had significant prolonged analgesia. Again, these were uncontrolled observations. Wang et al (1985) compared 71 patients with CRPS treated over a 3-year period. Twenty-seven patients did not receive sympathetic blocks and 43 patients did. At 3 years 41% and 65% respectively had improved, suggesting some effect from the treatment.

In patients with early CRPS associated with severe limb swelling, sympathetic blocks may dramatically reduce swelling and produce pain relief. It is suggested that this is due to interruption of vasoconstrictor activity with opening of venules (Blumberg and Janig, 1994).

The intravenous phentolamine test has been advocated as a test to assess the likely efficacy of subsequent sympathetic blocks (Arner 1991). Patients who may obtain pain relief with IVRGB or sympathetic ganglion block may not respond to phentolamine due to the less complete α-noradrenergic receptor blockade achievable with systemic rather than local administration. The phentolamine test is widely used in many centres to identify those likely to respond to more prolonged local sympathetic blockade.

Sympathectomy

Surgical, chemical or radiofrequency sympathectomy may produce good short-term results but long-term pain relief is poor (Tasker 1990, Rocco 1995), leading most to abandon these procedures. The problems of sympathalgia following sympathectomy have already been referred to.

Other drugs used in regional blocks

Ketanserin, a selective serotonin type II receptor blocker, and bretylium, which reduces release of noradrenaline, have both been given by the Biers block technique and in controlled trials have been found to be analgesic in CRPS (Ford et al 1988, Hanna & Peat 1989). Clonidine was not effective by the same root (Glynn & Jones 1990). The nonsteroidal anti-inflammatory drug ketorolac, which reduces prostaglandin release, has been reported to be effective in a small group of patients with CRPS, of interest in relation to pathophysiology (Vanos et al 1992).

EPIDURAL AND INTRATHECAL DRUGS

The role of long-term administration of drugs by the epidural or intrathecal root is uncertain. When CRPS involves the lower limb opiate, with or without local anaesthetic, will produce partial analgesia, although often at the cost of imparied bladder and bowel sphincter function and some degree of weakness. In patients with severe allodynia and hyperalgesia, short-term percutaneous infusions for 1–2 weeks may help by allowing weight bearing on a previously useless leg and the start of rehabilitation. Long-term intrathecal morphine has been reported to produce useful analgesia in CRPS (Becker et al 1995).

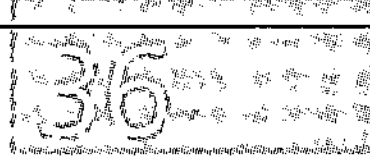

Clonidine, an alpha 2 receptor agonist given epidurally has been reported to relieve pain in CRPS affecting both upper and lower limbs over long periods (Rauck et al 1993, Walker & Cousins 1997). Given orally, clonidine is limited by adverse effects and does not produce analgesia in CRPS (Walker & Cousins 1997).

ORAL DRUGS

Numerous drugs have been tried in CRPS by the oral route. Many patients report analgesic effects from simple analgesics, codeine and non-steroidal anti-inflammatory drugs, and continue to take these drugs in the absence of more effective treatment. No controlled trials substantiate the effectiveness of these drugs in CRPS. Of the anticonvulsant drugs, recent interest has focused on gabapentin which is reported to help in CRPS, but again controlled trials are awaited (Mellick & Mellick 1997). Other reports of benefit in uncontrolled studies include phenoxybenzamine (Ghostine et al 1984, Muizelaar et al 1997), tricyclic antidepressants (Wilder et al 1992), phenytoin (Chaturvedi 1989) and nifedipine (Prough et al 1985, Muizelaar et al 1997). Biphosphonates via the intravenous route have been reported to relieve pain in CRPS in open label studies (Adami et al 1997, Cortet et al 1997). Trials with oral biphosphonates are awaited.

TRANSCUTANEOUS AND DORSAL COLUMN STIMULATION

Transcutaneous electrical nerve stimulation has been reported to be beneficial in children with CRPS (Wilder et al 1992) but not in adults. Dorsal column stimulation may be helpful (Law 1993).

PSYCHOLOGICAL MEASURES AND REHABILITATION

As in all chronic pain syndromes, psychological interventions may have a vital part to play in treatment. Fear, anxiety, depression, loss of function, job and income, and domestic and marital stresses may all take their toll in CRPS. Many patients find psychological management extremely helpful, particularly when, as is often the case, physical treatments fail. Efforts to rehabilitate the patient as far as is possible should be initiated at an early stage and pursued with vigour. The role of straightforward support for these unfortunate patients cannot be overemphasized. Patients with established CRPS should always be referred to a centre where a multidisciplinary programme of pain management is available.

REFERENCES

Adami S, Fossaluzza V, Gatti D, Fracassi E, Braga V 1997 Biphosphonate therapy of reflex sympathetic dystrophy syndrome. Annals of the Rheumatic Disease 56: 201–204

Arner S 1991 Intravenous phentolamine test: diagnostic and prognostic use in reflex sympathetic dystrophy. Pain 46: 17–22

Baron R, Wasner GL, Borgstedt R 1998 Interaction of sympathetic nerve activity and capsaicin evoked spontaneous pain and vasodilatation in humans. Neurology 50: 45

Barrera P, Van Riel PLCM, De Jong AJL 1992 Recurrent and migratory reflex sympathetic dystrophy syndrome. Clinical Rheumatology 11: 416–421

Becker WJ, Ablett DP, Harris CJ, Dold ON 1995 Long term treatment of intractable reflex sympathetic dystrophy with intrathecal morphine. Canadian. Journal of Neurological Sciences 22: 153–159

Bentley JB, Hameroff SR 1980 Diffuse reflex sympathetic dystrophy. Anaesthesiology 53: 256–257

Bernstein BH, Singsen BH, Kent JT et al 1978 Reflex neurovascular dystrophy in children. Journal of Pediatrics 93: 211–215

Bickerstaff DR, Kanis JA 1994 Algodystrophy: an under-recognised complication of minor trauma. British Journal of Rheumatology 33: 240–248

Blumberg H, Janig W 1994 Discharge pattern of afferent fibres from a neuroma. Pain 20: 335–353

Blumberg H, Janig W 1994 Clinical manifestation of reflex sympathetic dystrophy and sympathetically maintained pain. In: Wall PD, Melzack R (eds) Textbook of pain, 3rd edn. Churchill Livingstone, Edinburgh, pp 685–698

Boas RA 1996 Complex regional pain syndromes: symptomas, signs, and differential diagnosis. In: Janig W, Stanton-Hicks M (eds) Reflex sympathetic dystrophy: a reappraisal. Progress in pain research and management, vol 6. IASP, Seattle, pp 79–92

Bohm E 1985 Das Sudecksche Syndrom. Hefte zur Unfallheilkunde 174: 241–250

Bonica JJ 1953 The management of pain. Kimpton, London

Bonica JJ 1979 Causalgia and other reflex sympathetic dystrophies. In: Bonica JJ, Liebeskind JC, Albe-Fessard DG (eds) Proceedings of the Second World Congress on Pain. Advances in pain research and therapy, vol 3. Raven, New York, pp 141–166

Bonica JJ 1990 Causalgia and other reflex sympathetic dystrophies. In: Bonica JJ (ed) The management of pain, 2nd edn. Lea and Febriger, Philadelphia, pp 230–243

Bossut DF, Shea VK, Perl ER 1996 Sympathectomy induces adrenergic excitability of cutaneous C-fiber nociceptors. Journal of Neurophysiology 75: 514–517

Burchiel KJ 1984 Spontaneous impulse generation in normal and denervated dorsal root ganglia: sensitivity to alpha-adrenergic stimulation and hypoxia. Experimental Neurology 85: 257–272

Campbell JN, Raja SN, Meyer RA, Mackinnon SE 1988 Myelinated afferents signal the hyperalgesia associated with nerve injury. Pain 32: 89–94

Carlen PL, Wall PD, Nadvorna H, Steinbach T 1978 Phantom limbs and related phenomena in recent traumatic amputations. Neurology 28: 211–217

Cervero F 1994 Sensory innervation of the viscera: peripheral basis of visceral pain. Physiological Reviews 74: 95–138

Chabal C, Jacobson L, Russell LC, Burchiel KJ 1992 Pain response to perineuronal injection of normal saline, epinephrine, and lidocaine in humans. Pain 49: 9–12

Chaturvedi SK 1989 Phenytoin in reflex sympathetic dystrophy. Pain 36: 379–380

Chen Y, Michaelis M, Janig W, Devor M 1996 Adrenoreceptor subtype mediating sympathetic-sensory coupling in injured sensory neurons. Journal of Neurophysiology 76: 3721–3730

Choi B, Rowbotham MC 1997 Effects of adrenergic receptor activation on post-herpetic neuralgia pain and sensory disturbances. Pain 69: 55–63

Cortet B, Flipo R-M, Coquerelle P, Duquesnoy B, Delcambre B 1997 Treatment of severe, recalcitrant reflex sympathetic dystrophy: assessment of efficacy and safety of the second generation biphosphonate pamidronate. Clinical Rheumatology 16: 51–56

Covington EC 1996 Psychological issues in reflex sympathetic dystrophy. In: Janig W, Stanton-Hicks M (eds) Reflex sympathetic dystrophy: a reappraisal. Progress in pain research and management, vol 6. IASP, Seattle, pp 191–216

Devor M, Janig W 1981 Activation of myelinated afferents ending in a neuroma by stimulation of the sympathetic supply in the rat. Neuroscience Letters 24: 43–47

Devor M, Janig W, Michaelis M 1994 Modulation of activity in dorsal root ganglion neurons by sympathetic activation in nerve-injured rats. Journal of Neurophysiology 71: 38–47

Dray A 1996 Neurogenic mechanisms and neuropeptides in chronic pain. Progress in Brain Research 110: 85–94

Drummond PD 1995 Noradrenaline increases hyperalgesia to heat in skin sensitised by capsaicin. Pain 60: 311–315

Elam M, Skarphedinsson JO, Olhausson B, Wallin BG 1996 No apparent modulation of single C-fiber afferent transmission in human volunteers. In: Abstract of the 8th World Congress on Pain. IASP, Seattle, p 398

Evans JA 1946 Reflex sympathetic dystrophy. Surgery, Gynecology and Obstetrics 82: 36–43

Fermaglich DR 1977 Reflex sympathetic dystrophy in children. Pediatrics 60: 881–883

Ford SR, Forrest WH, Eltherington L 1988 The treatment of reflex sympathetic dystrophy with intravenous regional bretylium. Anesthesiology 68: 137–140

Ghostine SY, Comair YG, Turner DM, Kassell NF, Azar CG 1984 Phenoxybenzamine in the treatment of causalgia. Journal of Neurosurgery 60: 1263–1268

Girgis FL, Wynn Parry CB 1989 Management of causalgia after peripheral nerve injury. International Disability Studies 11: 15–20

Glynn CJ, Jones PC 1990 An investigation of the role of clonidine in the treatment of reflex sympathetic dystrophy. In: Stanton-Hicks, M, Janig W, Boas RA (eds) Reflex sympathetic dystrophy. Kluwer Academic, Massachusetts, pp 187–196

Gold MS, White DM, Ahlgeru SC, Guo M, Levine JD 1994 Catecholamine-induced mechanical sensitisation of cutaneous nociceptors in the rat. Neuroscience Letters 175: 166–170

Goldsmith DP, Vivino FB, Eichenfield AH, Athreya BH, Heyman S 1989 Nuclear imaging and clinical features of childhood reflex neurovascular dystrophy: comparison with adults. Arthritis and Rheumatism 32: 480–485

Govrin-Lippmann R, Devor M 1978 Ongoing activity in severed nerves. Source and variation with time. Brain Research 159: 406–410

Habler HJ, Janig W, Koltzenburg M 1987 Activation of unmyelinated afferents in chronically lesioned nerves by adrenaline and excitation of sympathetic efferents in the cat. Neuroscience Letters 82: 35–40

Hanna MH, Peat SJ 1989 Ketanserin in reflex sympathetic dystrophy. A double blind placebo controlled cross-over trial. Pain 38: 145–150

Hannington-Kiff JG 1974 Intravenous regional sympathetic block with guanethidine. Lancet i 1019–1020

Jadad AR, Carroll D, Glynn CJ, McQuay HJ 1995 Intraevous regional sympathetic blockade for pain relief in reflex sympathetic dystrophy: a systematic review and a randomised, double-blind crossover study. Journal of Pain and Symptom Management 10: 13–20

Janig W 1996 The puzzle of 'Reflex Sympathetic Dystrophy' mechanisms, hypotheses, open questions. In: Janig W, Stanton-Hicks M (eds) Reflex sympathetic dystrophy: a reappraisal. Progress in Pain Research and Management, vol 6. IASP, Seattle, pp 1–24

Johnson AC 1943 Disabling changes in the hands resembling sclerodactylia following myocardial infarctions. Annals of Internal Medicine 19: 433–456

Kim SH, Na HS, Sheen K, Chung JM 1993 Effects of sympathectomy on a rat model of peripheral neuropathy. Pain 55: 85–92

Kinman E, Nygards EB, Hausson P 1997 Peripheral alpha-adrenoreceptors are involved in the development of capsaicin induced ongoing and stimulus evoked pain in humans. Pain 69: 79–85

Kirk EJ 1974 Impulses in dorsal spinal nerve rootlets in cats and rabbits arising from dorsal root ganglia isolated from the periphery. Journal of Comparative Neurology 155: 165–176

Koltzenburg M 1996 Afferent mechanisms mediating pain and hyperalgesias in neuralgia. In: Janig W, Stanton-Hicks M (eds) Reflex sympathetic dystrophy: a reappraisal. Progress in pain research and management, vol 6. IASP, Seattle, pp 123–150

Korenman EM, Devor M 1981 Ectopic adrenergic sensitivity in damaged axons. Experimental Neurology 72: 63–81

Kozin F 1992 Reflex sympathetic dystrophy: a review. Clinical and Experimental Rheumatology 10: 401–409

Kramis RC, Roberts WJ, Gillette RG 1996 Post-sympathectomy neuralgia: hypotheses on peripheral and central neuronal mechanisms. Pain 64: 1–9

Law JD 1993 Spinal cord stimulation for intractable pain due to reflex sympathetic dystrophy. CNI Review 17–22

Leriche R 1916 De la causalgie envisagee comme au nevrite de sympathique et de son traitement par la denudation et l'excision des plexus nerveax peri-arteriels. Presse Medicin 24: 177–180

Leriche R 1939 The surgery of pain. (Translated by A Young.) Baillière, Tindall and Cox, London

Levine JD, Taiwo YO, Collins SD, Tam JK 1986 Noradrenaline hyperalgesia is mediated through interaction with sympathetic postganglionic neurone terminals rather than activation of primary afferent nociceptors. Nature 323: 158–160

Liu M, Max MB, Parada S, Rowan JS, Bennett GJ 1996 The sympathetic nervous system contributes to capsaicin-evoked mechanical allodynia but not pinprick hyperalgesia in humans. Journal of Neuroscience 16: 7331–7335

Livingston WK 1943 Pain mechanisms: a physiological interpretation of causalgia and its related symptoms. Macmillan, London

Loh L, Nathan PW 1978 Painful peripheral states and sympathetic blocks. Journal of Neururology, Neurosurgery and Psychiatry 41: 664–671

Loh L, Nathan PW, Schott GD, Wilson PG 1980 Effects of regional guanethidine infusion in certain pain states. Journal of Neurology Neurosurgery and Psychiatry 43: 446–451

Mellick GA, Mellick LB 1997 Reflex sympathetic dystrophy treated with gabapentin. Archives of Physical Medicine and Rehabilitation 78: 98–105

Michaelis M, Devor M, Janig W 1996 Sympathetic modulation of activity in dorsal root ganglion neurons changes over time following peripheral nerve injury. Journal of Neurophysiology 76: 753–763

Mitchell SW, Morehouse GR, Keen WW 1864 Gunshot wounds and other injuries of nerves. Lippincott, Philadelphia.

Muizelaar JP, Kleyer M, Hertogs IAM, De Lange DC 1997 Complex regional pain syndrome (reflex sympathetic dystrophy and causalgia): management with the calcium channel blocker nifedipine and/or the alpha-sympathetic blocker phenoxybenzamine in 59 patients. Clinical Neuorology and Neurosurgery 99: 26–30

Ochoa JL 1994 Pain mechanisms in neuropathy. Current Opinions in Neurology 7: 407–414

Ochoa JL, Verdugo RJ 1995 Reflex sympathetic dystrophy. A common clinical avenue for somatoform expression. Neurologic Clinics 13: 351–363

Ochoa JL, Verdugo RJ, Campero M 1994 Pathophysiological spectrum of organic and psychogenic disorders in neuropathic pain patients fitting the description of causalgia or reflex sympathetic dystrophy. In: Proceedings of the 7th World Congress on Pain. Progress in pain research and management, vol 2. IASP, Seattle, pp 483–494

Olsson GL, Arner S, Hirsch G 1990 Reflex sympathetic dystrophy in children. In: Tyler DC, Krane KJ (eds) Pediatric pain, vol 15. Raven, New York, pp 323–331

Omer GC, Thomas MS 1971 Treatment of causalgia. Texas Medicine 67: 93–96

Oyen WJM, Arntz IE, Claessens RAMJ, Van der Meer JWM, Corstens FHM, Goris RJA 1993 Reflex sympathetic dystrophy of the hand: an excessive inflammatory response? Pain 55: 151–157

Prough DS, McLeskey CH, Poehling GG et al 1985. Efficacy of oral nifedipine in the treatment of reflex sympathetic dystrophy. Anesthesiology 62: 796–799

Raja SN, Treede RD, Davis KD, Campbell JN 1991 Systemic alpha-adrenergic blockade with phentolamine: a diagnostic test for sympathetically maintained pain. Anesthesiology 74: 691–698

Ramamurthy S, Hoffman J 1995 Intravenous regional guanethidine in the treatment of reflex sympathetic dystrophy/causalgia: a randomised, double-blind study. Anaesthesia and Analgesia 81: 718–723

Raskin NH, Levinson SA, Hoffman PM, Pickett JBE, Fields HL 1974 Post-sympathectomy neuralgia. American Journal of Surgery 128: 75–78

Rauck RL, Eisenach JC, Jackson K, Young LD, Southern J 1993 Epidural clonidine treatment for refractory reflex sympathetic dystrophy. Anesthesiology 79: 1163–1169

Richards RL 1967a Causalgia: a centennial review. Archives of Neurology 16: 339–350

Richards RL 1967b The term 'causalgia'. Medical History 11: 97–99

Rizzi R, Visentin M, Mazzetti G 1984 Reflex sympathetic dystrophy. In: Benedetti C, Chapman CR, Moricca G (eds) Recent advances in the management of pain. Advances in pain research and therapy, vol 7. Raven, New York, pp 451–465

Roberts WJ 1986 A hypothesis on the physiological basis for causalgia and related pains. Pain 24: 297–311

Rocco AG 1995 Radiofrequency lumbar sympatholysis. The evolution of a technique for managing sympathetically maintained pain. Regional Anaesthesie 20: 3–12

Rosen PS, Graham W 1957 The shoulder–hand syndrome: historical review with observations on 73 patients. Canadian Medical Association Journal 77: 86–91

Sanjue H, Juu Z 1989 Sympathetic facilitation of sustained discharges of polymodal nociceptors. Pain 38: 85–90

Sato J, Perl ER 1991 Adrenergic excitation of cutaneous pain receptors induced by peripheral nerve injury. Science 251: 1608–1610

Scadding JW 1981 Development of ongoing activity, mechanosensitivity and adrenaline sensitivity in severed peripheral nerve axons. Experimental Neurology 73: 345–364

Schott GD 1994 Visceral afferents: their contribution to 'sympathetic dependent pain'. Brain 117: 397–413

Schott GD 1995 An unsympathetic view of pain. Lancet 345: 634–636

Schott GD 1997 Biphosphonates for pain relief in reflex sympathetic dystrophy. Lancet 350: 1117

Schwartzman RJ, McLellan TL 1987 Reflex sympathetic dystrophy: a review. Archives of Neurology 44: 555–561

Sherry DD, Weisman R 1988 Psychologic aspects of childhood reflex neurovascular dystrophy. Pediatrics 81: 572–578

Shir Y, Seltzer Z 1991 Effects of sympathectomy in a model of causalgiform pain produced by partial sciatic nerve injury in rats. Pain 45: 309–320

Shyu BC, Danielsen N, Andersson SA, Dahlin LB 1990 Effects of sympathetic stimulation on C-fibre response after peripheral nerve compression: an experimental study in the rabbit common personeal nerve. Acta Physiologica Scandinavica 140: 237–243

Stanton-Hicks M, Janig W, Hassenbusch S, Haddox JD, Boas R, Wilson P 1995 Reflex sympathetic dystrophy: changing concepts and taxonomy. Pain 63: 127–133

Steinbrocker O 1947 The shoulder–hand syndrome: associated pain homolateral disability of the shoulder and hand with swelling and atrophy of the hand. American Journal of Medicine 3: 402–407

Strang P 1996 Analgesic effect of biphosphonates on bone pain in breast cancer patients. Acta Oncologica 35 (Suppl): 50–54

Tasker RR 1990 Reflex sympathetic dystrophy – neurosurgical approaches. In: Stanton-Hicks M, Janig W, Boas RA (eds) Reflex sympathetic dystrophy. Kluwer Academic, Massachusetts, pp 125–134

Torebjork HE, Wahren LK, Wallin BG, Hallin RG, Koltzenburg M 1995 Noradrenaline-evoked pain in neuralgia. Pain 63: 11–20

Tracey DJ, Cunningham JE, Romm MA 1995 Peripheral hyperalgiesia in experimental neuropathy: mediation by alpha-2 adreno-receptors on post-ganglionic sympathetic terminals. Pain 60: 317–327

Tracy GD, Cockett FB 1957 Pain in the lower limb after sympathectomy. Lancet i 12–14

Vanos DN, Ramamurthy S, Hoffman J 1992 Intravenous regional block using ketorolac: preliminary results in the treatment of reflex sympathetic dystrophy. Anesthesia and Analgesia 74: 139–141

Veldman PJHM, Goris JA 1996 Multiple reflex sympathetic dystrophy. Which patients are at risk for developing a recurrence of reflex sympathetic dystrophy in the same or another limb? Pain 64: 463–466

Veldman PJHM, Reynen HM, Arntz IE, Goris JA 1993 Signs and symptoms of reflex sympathetic dystrophy: prospective study of 829 patients. Lancet 342: 1012–1016

Wahren LK, Torebjork HE, Nystrom B 1991 Quantitative sensory testing before and after regional guanethidine block in patients with neuralgia in the hand. Pain 46: 23–30

Walker AE, Nulsen F 1948 Electrical stimulation of the upper thoracic portion of the sympathetic chain in man. Archives of Neurology and Psychiatry 59: 559–560

Walker SM, Cousins MJ 1997 Complex regional pain syndromes: including 'reflex sympathetic dystrophy' and 'causalgia'. Anaesthesia and Intensive Care 25: 113–125

Wall PD 1995 Noradrenaline-evoked pain in neuralgia. Pain 63: 1–2

Wall PD, Devor M 1983 Sensory afferent impulses from dorsal root ganglia. Pain 17: 321–339

Wall PD, Gutnick M 1974 Ongoing activity in peripheral nerves. The physiology and pharmacology of impulses originating in a neuroma. Experimental Neurology 43: 580–593

Wallin BG, Torebjork HE, Hallin RG 1976 Preliminary observations on the pathophysiology of hyperalgesia in the causalgic pain symdrome. In: Zolterman Y (ed) Sensory functions of the skin in primates. Pergamon, Oxford, pp 489–499

Wang JK, Johnson KA, Ilstrap DM 1985 Sympathetic blocks for reflex sympathetic dystrophy. Pain 23: 13–17

Wilder RT 1996 Reflex sympathetic dystrophy in children and adolescents: differences from adults. In: Janig W, Stanton-Hicks M (eds) Reflex sympathetic dystrophy: A reappraisal. Progress in pain research and management, vol 6. IASP, Seattle, pp 67–77

Wilder RT, Berde CB, Wolohan M, Vieyra MA, Masele BJ, Michell LJ 1992 Reflex sympathetic dystrophy in children. Clinical characteristics and follow-up of seventy patients. Journal of Bone and Joint Surgery 74(A): 910–919

Wilson PR, Low PA, Bedder MD, Covington EC, Rauck RL 1996 Diagnostic algorithm for complex regional pain syndromes. In: Janig W, Stanton-Hicks M (eds) Reflex sympathetic dystrophy: a reappraisal. Progress in pain research and management, vol 6. IASP, Seattle, pp 93–106

Nerve root disorders and arachnoiditis

37

DAVID DUBUISSON

It is appealing to be able to diagnose one or more sites of nerve root compression as the cause of a patient's chronic pain. The great majority of patients with root compression will be relieved of their symptoms eventually, either by simple conservative measures and passage of time or by a decompressive operation. A large population of chronic pain sufferers fall into the category of failed back or neck surgery and many of them may, on reinvestigation, turn out to have problems amenable to treatment. Close attention to the history, details of the neurological examination and radiological findings will suffice in most cases to determine whether the spaces around spinal roots have been made as anatomically correct as possible. It often happens that efforts directed at a single root have led the physician to ignore relevant problems at other neighbouring levels of the spine. It is also frequent to find pain patients and their referring physicians who are too quickly convinced that something is bothering a nerve root and if only a surgical exploration were done, everything would be solved. It is important for clinicians with special interest in chronic pain to be wary of the abuse of surgery in such patients, but at the same time to be willing to seek objective evidence of root compression. Again, the clinical history, examination and radiology will point the way to proper care for the patient, often avoiding needless additional tests or surgery. The first half of this chapter gives most of the salient details needed to investigate or reinvestigate possible nerve root problems.

An unfortunate and more difficult problem of pain management is the patient whose underlying condition and failed surgery have resulted in a chronic, intractable state of nerve root damage. In some instances, the condition known as arachnoiditis is present. Chronic root damage and arachnoiditis are among the most frequent, and difficult to treat, causes of severe chronic pain.

Often, pain is not the only issue at stake in cases of root damage and arachnoiditis. Muscle weakness, loss of sensation, gait disorder or loss of bowel and bladder control may supervene and, in some instances, direct the further approach to management. The neurological examination should be carefully and repeatedly documented in these patients. Progression of neurological damage might require surgery even at a time when pain is resolving.

In the assessment, careful thought must be given to the number and location of roots involved. A common but unreliable approach is to investigate and treat as if the patient's pain were due entirely to damage of a single nerve root. In the author's practice, few patients complaining of pain in the back, neck or extremities will ultimately be shown to have an isolated root lesion as the cause of their symptoms. Clinics that treat intractable pain may see even fewer patients whose complaints result from damage of only one root. The underlying disease processes causing root compression tend, especially in the older population, to occur at multiple levels of the spine. Sometimes, previous surgery or other invasive treatment measures have increased the extent of the problem. One lesson that we are learning especially well in the era of computerized imaging is that spondylosis is often far more extensive than we anticipate on first meeting a new patient with root problems.

SIGNS AND SYMPTOMS

The essential quality of pain associated with root damage is referral along the peripheral distribution of fibres in the root. In many cases but not in all, this follows one of the dermatomes down the arm or leg or around the trunk. When a patient describes pain radiating down an extremity or in a segment of the chest or abdomen, it is important to record the exact distribution of pain on several occasions when it is actually present. It is useful to do this on diagrams which do not depict peripheral nerve territories or dermatomes. Plain diagrams counteract the clinician's urge to make the findings fit neatly into his own concept of what is happening. Comparison with standard charts can be made later if necessary.

The cutaneous afferent distributions of the spinal nerves are not yet adequately defined in humans. The dermatomes are certainly not constant from individual to individual (see Foerster 1933) and no two dermatomal charts agree in all details. There is particular confusion about the cervical thoracic and lumbosacral junctions. Not all authors agree, for instance, that the second and third thoracic dermatomes involve the arm or that the fourth lumbar and second sacral dermatomes extend to the toes. Some charts show the fourth and fifth lumbar dermatomes spiralling across the anterior thigh; others place the second lumbar dermatome there (see Fig. 37.1). These issues have not been resolved.

Lack of agreement of dermatomal charts, frustrating for the clinician, is due to the various methods used to define the dermatomes. Head and Campbell (1900) devised a dermatomal chart based on cutaneous eruptions in herpes zoster. It was assumed that the lesions were confined to single dorsal root ganglia, although it is known that the lesions of herpes zoster may also involve the spinal cord (Adams 1976). Head and Campbell showed dermatomes with contiguous borders but Sherrington's (1898) studies in monkeys made it clear that extensive overlap was present. Subsequently, Foerster (1933) revised the dermatomes in accordance with his examination of a series of patients in whom he had sectioned several adjacent dorsal roots, leaving a zone of remaining skin sensation. In addition, Foerster used electrical stimulation of the distal end of divided dorsal roots to produce cutaneous vasodilatation which approximated the dermatome. Like Sherrington, he found large overlapping dermatomes (Figs 37.1, 37.2). In zones of remaining sensation, the borders for complete anaesthesia were smaller than those for analgesia with some preservation of touch sensation. Individual variations in the size and shape of isolated dermatomes were frequent. Some 60 years later, Foerster's diagrams still provide some of our best information about the extent and variability of the dermatomes in man. As pointed out by White and Sweet (1969), these experiments are not likely to be repeated by any modern surgeon because it is now appreciated that extensive deafferentation of a limb makes it useless and may add to the patient's pain.

In some instances, root compression by herniated intervertebral discs may produce distinct areas of sensory loss. On this basis, Keegan and Garrett (1948) constructed a

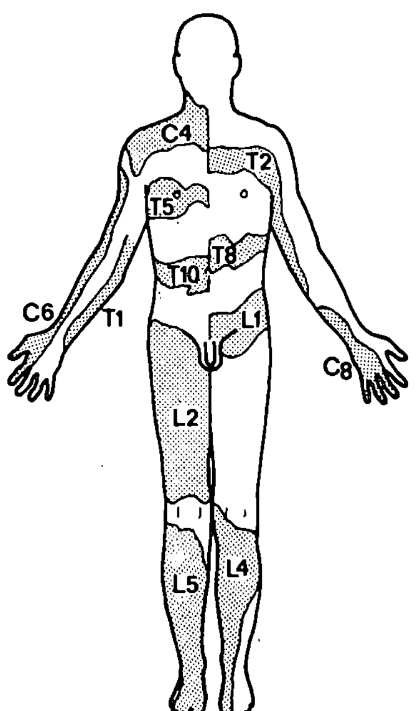

Fig. 37.1 Examples of dermatomes isolated by multiple root section: anterior aspect (after Foerster 1933).

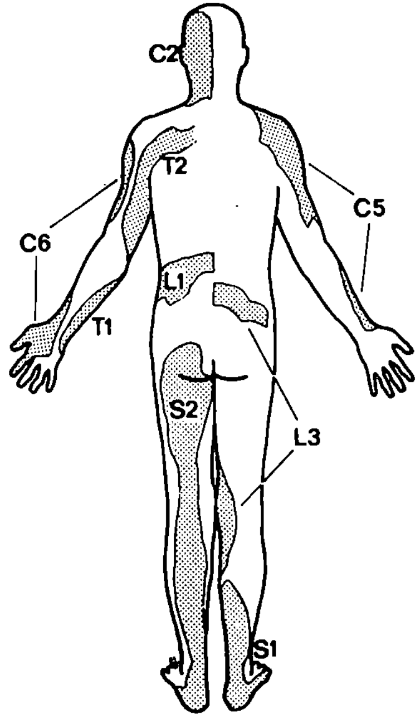

Fig. 37.2 Further examples of dermatomes isolated by multiple root section: posterior aspect (after Foerster 1933).

map of the dermatomes which depicted them as sharply demarcated bands extending to the middle in front and back. In some areas, the zones of hyposensitivity to pinscratch extended much farther proximally than Foerster's maps had indicated. The precise organization of dermatomes shown by Keegan and Garrett has received little experimental confirmation. Instead, physiological studies in monkeys (Dykes & Terzis 1981) suggests that the cutaneous region served by each spinal nerve root is even wider and more variable in location than that envisaged by Sherrington or Foerster. The apparent size of an isolated dermatome also depends on the integrity of distant roots and of the Lissauer tract (Kirk & Denny-Brown 1970, Denny-Brown et al 1973).

The segmental distributions in muscle, fascia and joints are less well known. It is known that a radicular pattern of pain may result from ideas of a spinal apophyseal (facet) joint. The pattern of pain may be difficult to interpret, since each facet joint is innervated by branches of two nerve roots. Certainly the pattern of innervation in muscles and other deep structures does not conform strictly to the overlying dermatomes. Kellgren (1939) injected hypertonic saline into the paraspinous muscles and ligaments to produce pain which was referred in segmental patterns. His map of deep segmental sensory innervations suggested that some myotomes and sclerotomes in the vicinity of the cervicothoracic and lumbosacral junctions were confined to the trunk while the corresponding dermatomes extended down the leg or arm. A clinical situation which illustrates this principle is pain referred to the anterior chest in compression of lower cervical roots (Davis 1957). The serious anterior and pectoral muscles are innervated by these roots while the corresponding dermatomes are restricted to the arm and hand. Charts of myotomes and sclerotomes are available (Inman & Saunders 1944) but perhaps not widely used, due to difficulty in applying stimuli accurately to deep structures. In a clinical setting, involvement of muscle is usually detected as weakness, decreased bulk, visible fasciculation or an electromyographic change. A detailed compilation of segmental muscle innervations is given by Kendall et al (1971) in their excellent monograph on muscle function and testing.

SPECIFIC ROOT LESIONS

SEVENTH CRANIAL NERVE (NERVUS INTERMEDIUS COMPONENT)

The nervus intermedius, a component of the seventh cranial nerve, is known to contain sensory afferents whose cell bodies are located in the geniculate ganglion in the roof of the temporal bone. These axons supply part of the external auditory canal and tympanic membrane, the skin in the angle between ear and mastoid process, the tonsillar region and some other deep structures of the head and neck. The nervus intermedius may be involved in attacks of pain referred to the ear. Recurrent stabbing or shooting pain of a paroxysmal nature felt deep in the ear and sometimes in the ipsilateral face, neck or occiput suggests the possibility of geniculate neuralgia. The condition is not likely to be encountered in most clinical practices because of its rarity. Stimulating or cutting the nervus intermedius distinguishes the condition from glossopharyngeal neuralgia.

Patients with geniculate neuralgia are typically young or middle-aged adults. In most cases, a vesicular rash in the external ear and mastoid, typical of herpes zoster, precedes the onset of pain by several days. This has been called the Ramsay Hunt syndrome when it is accompanied by ipsilateral facial paralysis. Attacks of pain lasting seconds, minutes or sometimes hours may be entirely spontaneous. Less commonly, they can be triggered by touching the external ear canal. Dull background pain may persist between attacks. Other possible symptoms include tenderness in or near the external ear, salivation, nasal discharge, tinnitus, vertigo or a bitter taste during attacks. Further details of several cases are summarized in the volume by White and Sweet (1969).

NINTH AND 10TH CRANIAL NERVES

Pain in the afferent distribution of the glossopharyngeal and vagus nerves may be felt in the larynx, base of the tongue, tonsillar region, ear and occasionally ipsilateral face, neck or scalp. Paroxysms of pain of unknown aetiology occurring in this distribution may be due to glossopharyngeal neuralgia, also known as vagoglossopharyngeal neuralgia in recognition of the role of the upper vagal rootlets (Robson & Bonica 1950, White & Sweet 1969). The uncommon variant known as neuralgia of the superior laryngeal nerve (vagus nerve neuralgia) is a syndrome of pain around the thyroid cartilage and pyriform sinus. Pure glossopharyngeal neuralgia is more likely to be felt in the tonsillar region. The attacks are usually described as stabbing, sharp, 'like a knife', 'like an electric shock', and sometimes hot or burning. Their intensity ranges from mild to severe. The attacks are probably less intense than typical bouts of trigeminal neuralgia, which is 70–100 times as common (Rushton et al 1981). Patients with glossopharyngeal neuralgia are almost always above the age of 20. Men and women are about equally affected. There is a slight predominance of left-sided cases in most large series. Attacks are bilateral in less than 2% of cases. Individual attacks commonly last seconds or minutes and rarely occur at night (Deparis 1968). Constant dull aching, burning or pressure may persist between attacks (Rushton et al 1981). It is characteristic of glossopharyngeal neuralgia that the pain is triggered by such innocuous stimuli as swallowing, yawning, coughing and chewing. Other reported triggers are laughing, touching the throat, ear or neck, turning the head or moving the arm. In unusual cases, particular tastes may trigger attacks (White & Sweet 1969).

A variety of cardiovascular and other symptoms may accompany the attacks. They include cardiac arrhythmias or cardiac arrest, hiccups, spells of intractable coughing, inspiratory stridor, excessive salivation and seizures. These accompanying symptoms can be especially troublesome during and after surgical manipulation of the 10th nerve in the posterior fossa (White & Sweet 1969, Nagashima et al 1976).

UPPER CERVICAL ROOTS

Pain in the territory of the C1–4 roots may involve the posterior scalp; the periorbital, temporal and mandibular regions; the external ear and mastoid region; and the neck and shoulder. The border zone of innervation by the upper cervical nerve roots and innervation by the cranial nerves was determined by Foerster (1933) who cut all the cervical roots on one side in 12 of his patients. With more selective root sections, Foerster demonstrated a region innervated by the C2 and C3 posterior roots (Fig. 37.3). Posterior roots are absent in the human C1 cord segment in 50–70% of cases (Rhoton & Oliveira 1990, Dubuisson 1995). The C2 and C3 dermatomes have been mapped more specifically

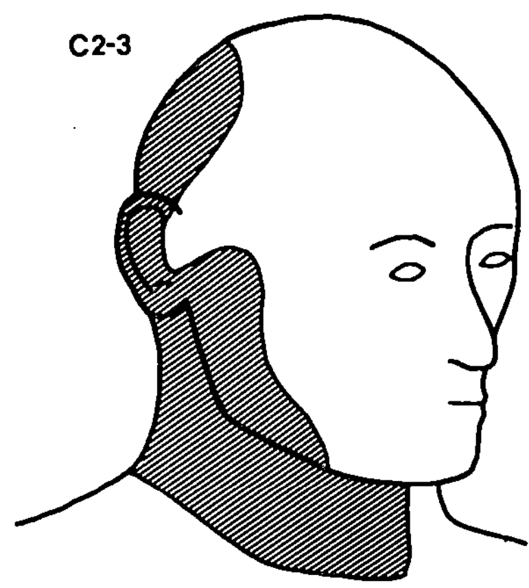

Fig. 37.3 The cutaneous field of the upper cervical roots (after Foerster 1933).

(Bogduk 1980, 1982, Poletti 1991). The C2 dermatome mainly involves the territory of the greater occipital nerve, which is a direct extension of the C2 root. This includes the occipital region from foramen magnum to skull vertex, and from the midline to the mastoid. The C3 dermatome involves mainly the territory of the lesser occipital nerve, which also receives a C2 contribution. This includes the ear, mastoid, and angle of the jaw, and side of the head. Poletti (1996) describes a clinical syndrome associated with compression of the C3 nerve root or ganglion consisting of radiating pain, dysaesthesias, numbness, and sensory deficit in the C3 territory. C4 radicular pain involves mainly the neck and upper shoulder. In the author's experience, it is often associated with chronic headache and may include a subtle sensory deficit in the side of the neck.

Pain at the craniocervical junction is frequently associated with trauma or structural abnormalities of the upper cervical spine and is not infrequently bilateral. Unilateral symptoms are often caused by traumatic rotational injuries (Hunter & Mayfield 1949). Occipital neuralgia is a syndrome of recurrent attacks of pain in the C2 and C3 territory. Patients may report frontal, periorbital or retro-orbital radiation of pain that is sometimes relieved by partial posterior rhizotomy at C1–3 (Dubuisson 1995). Attacks of occipital neuralgia may be paroxysmal and lancinating in some cases or prolonged for hours in others. Discrete trigger zones are seldom found, but pain can often be reproduced by pressure over the greater occipital nerve. In some cases, pain may be triggered by pressure over the site of an old craniectomy or depressed skull fracture. Pain may often be aggravated or reproduced by mechanical factors such as neck movements, pressure on the C2 spinous process, or downward pressure on the head (Dugan et al 1962). Tingling paraesthesias may be felt in the scalp or ear and blunting of sharp point sensation is commonly found in the scalp if the patient is examined carefully.

The motor supply to neck muscles is derived from multiple spinal and cranial nerves. Because of this overlap, weakness and atrophy are not frequently detected in cases of upper cervical radiculopathy. Patients whose upper cervical roots are stretched by downward displacement of the cerebellar tonsils, as is seen in Chiari malformation and cerebellar tumours, often complain of bilateral radiating occipital pain with sneezing, coughing or neck movements. An unusual syndrome of pain in the neck or suboccipital region with simulataneous paraesthesias of the ipsilateral half of the tongue is known as 'neck–tongue syndrome' (Lance & Anthony 1980) and is thought to be due to the presence of afferents to C2–3 through the ansa hypoglossi.

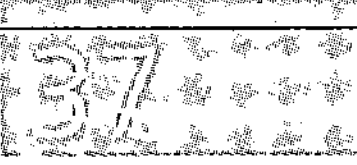

LOWER CERVICAL ROOTS

In nerve root lesions associated with protruded cervical intervertebral discs, certain patterns of pain are fairly constant (Murphey et al 1973). Some typical neurological signs which accompany lower cervical root pain are listed in Table 37.1. Compression of the C5 root may produce pain in the neck, shoulder, anterior chest, medial scapular region and lateral aspect of the arm. Lesions affecting the C6 or C7 root are often associated with pain in the neck, shoulder, anterior chest, scapular region, lateral aspect of the arm and dorsum of the forearm. Compression of C8 is suggested by pain in the neck, medial scapular region, sometimes in anterior chest and usually along the medial aspect of the arm and forearm. A similar pattern may be seen in damage of the first thoracic root. It is somewhat unusual to find a patient with pain in the hand due to cervical root compression (Murphey et al 1973) even though the dermatomes of C6, C7 and C8 clearly include the fingers (see Figs 37.1, 37.2). Numbness and tingling paraesthesias ('pins and needles') are often described in a wider zone than the painful one. These innocuous but annoying sensations frequently radiate into the fingers while the pain does not. They therefore provide important clues to the level of involvement (Table 37.1).

Table 37.1 Typical findings in cervical root compression (after Murphey et al 1973)

C5 root compression (C4–5 disc)
Pain – neck, shoulder, medial scapula, anterior chest, lateral aspect of upper arm
Numbness – sometimes lateral upper arm or area over deltoid
Weakness – deltoid, supraspinatus, infraspinatus, biceps, brachioradialis
Hyporeflexia – biceps, brachioradialis reflexes

C6 root compression (C5–6 disc)
Pain – neck, shoulder, medial scapula, anterior chest, lateral aspect of upper arm, dorsal aspect of forearm
Numbness – thumb and index finger (sometimes absent)
Weakness – biceps (mild to moderate), extensor carpi radialis
Hyporeflexia – biceps reflex

C7 root compression (C6–7 disc)
Pain – same as in C6 root compression
Numbness – index and middle fingers (sometimes absent)
Weakness – triceps
Hyporeflexia – triceps reflex

C8 root compression (C7–T1 disc)
Pain – neck, medial scapula, anterior chest, medial aspect of arm and forearm
Numbness – fourth and fifth fingers, occasionally middle finger
Weakness – triceps, all extensors of wrist and fingers except extensor carpi radialis; all flexors of wrist and fingers except flexor carpi radialis and palmaris longus; all intrinsic hand muscles
Hyporeflexia – triceps reflex

T1 root compression (T1–2 disc)
Pain – same as in C8 root compression
Numbness – ulnar aspect of forearm (usually subjective)
Weakness – only intrinsic muscles of hand
Hyporeflexia – none
Miscellaneous – Horner's syndrome

As noted above, chest pain may be of lower cervical root origin. When it is severe, it may imitate the pain of angina or myocardial infarction. Davis (1957) presented convincing histories of patients whose attacks of substernal and praecordial pain closely resembled the events of coronary insufficiency. It was shown that all the symptoms could be reproduced by manipulation of the neck. Firm pressure over the lower cervical or uppermost thoracic vertebrae caused excruciating pain in the chest. Spine films confirmed the existence of spondylosis which was thought to be the cause of root compression.

Pain associated with cervical disc protrusions is usually constant with daily exacerbations related to activity, especially movements of the neck. Coughing, sneezing, pushing and any type of straining may severely aggravate the pain and reproduce the paraesthesias. In some cases, a Valsalva manoeuvre or bilateral jugular compression for 5–10 seconds will reproduce the pain or the paraesthesias. When the intervertebral foramina are narrowed by protruding discs and by spondylotic changes of the vertebral bodies ('osteophytes') and articulator facets, the contained roots may be subject to marked compression during extension of the neck or tilting of the head to the involved side.

Chronic compression of an individual cervical root produces a continuous aching pain with sharp, shooting sensations superimposed during movements. Murphey (1968, Murphey et al 1973) performed a large number of cervical discectomies under local anaesthetic. Touching the damaged root produced severe pain in the arm, whereas touching normal cervical roots produced only electric sensations. When an involved root was blocked with local anaesthetic and retracted, it was sometimes possible to reproduce pain in the neck, shoulder, chest or scapular region by pressing on the posterior longitudinal ligament and torn annulus fibrosus. It was postulated that these stimuli activated in the sinuvertebral nerves which enter the spinal canal as recurrent branches of the roots (Petersen et al 1956).

A special type of pain seen in cases of traumatic avulsion of cervical nerve roots was described by Wynn Parry (1980) who found that of 108 cases of brachial plexus avulsion injury, 98 patients suffered significant pain. Pain was not a problem in 167 additional patients whose brachial plexus lesions were distal to the dorsal root ganglia. A remarkably consistent description of the pain was given which differed substantially from that of cervical disc protrusions. Pain was almost invariably felt in the hand and forearm after C6, C7, C8 or T1 root avulsions, conforming fairly well to the dermotome of the avulsed root. Some patients with avulsed C5 root felt pain in the shoulder. Almost all the patents used the term 'hot' or 'burning' to describe the pain; many had a feeling that the hand was on fire or that boiling water was being poured over it. Some had a sensation of severe pressure, of pounding or of 'electric shock'. This formed a constant background of severe pain in which, in 87 cases, additional sudden paroxysms occurred. These lasted usually for a few seconds, came without warning and were sometimes of unbearable intensity. They radiated from the fingers to the shoulder and were described as sharp, shooting, cutting or 'like lightning'. The paroxysms came unpredictably at intervals of 10 minutes to 1 week. Typically the patient would stop what he was doing and grip the arm or cry out. Paraesthesias were also common and almost all the patients complained of tingling, 'pins and needles' or feelings of electricity. Nearly all were aware of a phantom limb with sensations of movement when effort was made to use paralysed muscles. The pain of root avulsion was aggravated by worry and emotional stress and relieved by relaxation and by distraction. Some patients reported less pain when gripping, striking or massaging the painful limb. Others had moderate relief when moving the neck or the paralysed arm. In this series, all the patients were young men between the ages of 18 and 30 and nearly all sustained their injuries in motorcycle accidents.

THORACIC ROOTS

Root lesions from T2 to L1 mainly involve the trunk. Radicular pain at truncal levels often appears as a discrete band around the chest or abdomen. When due to a spinal tumour, it may be constant, becoming worse at night when the patient is recumbent for hours. It may involve a single root initially and later more than one adjacent root or the contralateral root at the same level. Radicular pain of thoracic spinal tumours or disc protrusions is typically aggravated by coughing, sneezing and straining. It often has an aching, constrictive quality. When due to herpes zoster, it is apt to be described as sharp, tender, tugging or pulling (Dubuisson & Melzack 1976). The skin may be exquisitely sensitive in the involved dermatome. Characteristic vesicles usually appear as viral particles are distributed along peripheral branches of the spinal nerve. Subjective numbness, tingling and other paraesthesias are common but objective loss of sensation is unusual in solitary thoracic root lesions. When present, it suggests either involvement of several adjacent roots or an intramedullary lesion of the spinal cord at the equivalent level.

Weakness of the trunk muscles is not typical of solitary thoracic root lesions or, at least, not clinically detectable. If several adjacent roots are damaged, weakness of the abdominal wall may give rise to visible bulging of the abdomen (Boulton et al 1984). Autonomic signs are rare. Marked tenderness over the spine at a corresponding level may signal infectious or tumorous destruction of bone. Metastatic lesions of vertebrae may announce their presence with a sudden collapse, occasionally audible to the patient, followed by abrupt radicular pain. Root pain accompanied by fever, spinal ache with local tenderness, nuchal rigidity or paraparesis is a warning of spinal epidural abscess which is most common in the thoracic region (Baker et al 1975).

LUMBOSACRAL ROOTS

This group includes two broad categories: involvement of individual roots and involvement of the cauda equina as a bundle of roots. Individual root lesions will be considered here. As with cervical root lesions, patterns of pain, numbness, weakness and loss of reflexes are fairly consistent in the lumbosacral region (Keegan & Garrett 1948, Bertrand 1975, Davis 1982). Pain associated with L3 root compression is usually felt in the lower back, anteromedial thigh and knee. Numbness may be reported in the anterior thigh and knee. Pain in the lower back, with radiation down the anterolateral thigh to the front of the knee or shin, suggests L4 root involvement. Sometimes numbness can be detected around the medial aspect of the lower leg. An L5 root lesion characteristically produces pain in the lower back, posterolateral thigh, lateral aspect of the lower leg and sometimes lateral malleolus of the ankle or dorsum of the foot. Accompanying numbness or paraesthesias may be present in the dorsum of the foot, great toe and second or third toe. Pain of S1 lesions usually radiates from the lower back and buttock down the posterior thigh to the calf and sometimes to the heel, with tingling or numbness in the sole of the foot, lateral border of the foot, little toe and sometimes fourth toes. Continuous pain in the foot itself is not typical of lumbosacral disc protrusions (Davis 1982) and suggests instead some local problem of the foot. Numbness is of good localizing value since it frequently extends distally in the dermatome when the pain does not. Foerster (1933) argued that the dorsal aspect of the foot was predominantly supplied by L5 while the entire plantar surface was supplied by S1. Nevertheless, the medial-lateral distinction seems more useful in distinguishing L5 from S1 root compression. Numbness along the lateral border of the foot is most consistent with an S1 lesion. These features are summarized in Table 37.2.

Paraesthesias consisting of subjective numbness, tingling, 'pins and needles' or a wooden sensation are often more widespread than the pain. Due to the overlap of dermatomes, zones of objective sensory loss defined by touch and pinprick are usually small or absent. Some patients show hypoaesthesia over a large part of a dermatome (Keegan & Garrett 1948).

Radicular pain associated with ordinary lumbosacral disc protrusions is described as sharp, tender and shooting by a majority of patients given a verbal questionnaire. Other descriptive terms commonly chosen are cramping, throbbing, aching, heavy and stabbing. Bertrand (1975) described a group of patients suffering from 'battered root', a permanent radiculopathy with severe pain and paraesthesias in the lower extremity following unsuccessful lumbar disc surgery. Pain from the 'battered root' was constant, not intermittent as with most ordinary disc protrusions. It was described as burning or 'ice cold' by many patients and was often superimposed on a zone of residual numbness. Similar pain was sometimes reported following rhizotomy or ganglionectomy. Despite the patient's description of thermal qualities, autonomic signs were subtle or absent. This type of pain is distinct from the discomfort of ordinary root compression in its severity and in the terms used by the patient to describe it. It is typically more distressing to the patient than the original pain of disc protrusion.

Table 37.2 Typical findings in lumbosacral root compression

L3 root compression (L2–3 disc)
Pain – low back, anterior or anteromedial thigh, anterior knee
Numbness – anterior thigh, knee (sometimes absent)
Weakness – quadriceps, iliopsoas
Hyporeflexia – knee jerk (may be normal)
Miscellaneous – positive reversed-leg raising test

L4 root compression (usually L3–4 disc)
Pain – low back, anterior thigh, sometimes medial aspect of lower leg
Numbness – medial aspect of lower leg (may be absent)
Weakness – quadriceps, sometimes tibialis anterior
Hyporeflexia – knee jerk
Miscellaneous – positive straight-leg raising and reversed-leg raising test

L5 root compression (usually L4–5 disc)
Pain – low back, buttock, posterolateral thigh, lateral aspect of lower leg, lateral malleolus, sometimes dorsum of foot
Numbness – dorsum of foot, big toe, occasionally second toe or lateral aspect of lower leg
Weakness – tibialis anterior, extensor hallucis longus, extensor digitorum brevis, sometimes gluteals
Hyporeflexia – occasionally biceps femoris reflex
Miscellaneous – positive straight-leg raising test

S1 root compression (usually L5–S1 disc)
Pain – low back, buttock, posterior thigh, calf, heel
Numbness – lateral border of foot, sole, heel, sometimes fourth and fifth toes
Weakness – gastrocnemius/soleus, gluteals, occasionally hamstrings
Hyporeflexia – ankle jerk
Miscellaneous – positive straight-leg raising test

Bending at the waist is usually restricted in painful lumbosacral radiopathies of any cause. If the patient is able to touch his toes comfortably from a standing position or, lying supine, to hold both heels off the examining table for some time, a mechanical lesion of the lumbosacral roots is unlikely. Passive straight-leg raising in the supine position is almost always painful in the presence of mechanical L4–L5–S1 root lesions. This manoeuvre, which stretches the sciatic nerve and its tributaries, causes pain to radiate into the appropriate dermatome or muscles. In the apprehensive patient and in the malingerer, the same postural manipulation can often be produced without the patient's knowledge by passively extending his knee while he is seated. Passive reverse-leg raising with the knee flexed stretches the femoral nerve and is often painful when the L3 or L4 root is involved (Deyck 1976).

LOWER SACRAL AND COCCYGEAL ROOTS

The sacrococcygeal dermatomes are known mainly from stimulation of the roots at the time of rhizotomy for painful sacral and pelvic disorders. Stimulation of S2 produces pain in the buttock, groin, posterior thigh and genitalia. Foerster (1933) mapped portions of an isolated S2 dermatome on the sole of the foot (see Fig. 37.2). During stimulation of S3, pain is felt in the perianal region, rectum and genitalia. Stimulation of S4 may evoke pain in the vagina. Pain in the anus and around the coccyx is felt with stimulation of S4, S5 and coccygeal roots (Bohm & Franksson 1959, White & Sweet 1969).

Severe burning pain around the coccyx in the absence of tumour or other disease is termed coccygodynia. The pain can be unilateral or bilateral and usually occurs in middle-aged or elderly women. The S4, S5 and coccygeal roots are involved in some cases (White & Sweet 1969). In others, the pain may be referred from L4, L5 or S1 (Long 1982). Sensory deficits are not typical, nor are signs of bowel and bladder involvement, despite the known innervation of the bladder and anal sphincter by the S2–4 roots. Objective loss of sensation, diminished bladder tone and loss of the bulbocavernosus reflex suggest destruction of the roots.

A particularly intractable type of pain can occur in the sacral dermatomes in association with the finding of sacral cysts. These cysts are in fact abnormal dilatations of the meninges around the sacral nerve roots, filled with cerebrospinal fluid, expanding the sacral neural canal and foramina. On surgical exploration, which the author rarely advises, the sacral roots are found to be embedded in the meningeal wall of the cyst, stretched and thinned from growth of the fluid-filled compartment. There may or may not be a visible spinal fluid communication with the rest of the subarachnoid space. Terminology used to describe this condition includes 'sacral arachnoid cyst', 'sacral meningocoele' and 'sacral root sleeve diverticula'. The anatomy of the meningeal cystic anomaly varies from case to case, but the symptomatology seems to have in common some unusual and relentless, painful sensations and dysaesthesias around the saddle region, rectum or vagina. The symptoms may be positional, with bizarre-sounding descriptions of pulsation or formication in the region. The usual pertinent neurological findings can often be brought out by a thorough examination. Consultation with a urologist and, for women, a gynaecologist is usually appropriate to complete the assessment of these patients.

MULTISEGMENTAL ROOT SYNDROMES

CERVICAL SPONDYLOSIS

Cervical spondylosis sometimes declares its presence by pain in the distribution of one root, but more often the picture is multisegmental, diffuse and bilateral. A clinical hallmark of cervical spondylosis is restriction of neck motion with discomfort on attempting a complete range of movement. Multiple root constriction in the intervertebral foramina leads to symptoms of numbness in the hands and forearms, in a pattern not conforming to that of any peripheral nerve territory. Weakness and diminished reflexes point to loss of innervation of muscles. Weakness of the wrist extensors, triceps and shoulder girdle is detectable in a typical case. Long tract signs such as upgoing plantar reflexes, difficulty maintaining balance on attempting to walk a straight line in heel-to-toe fashion and clumsy fine movements of the toes and fingers may indicate cord compression in the spondylotic canal. In the author's practice, it has been common to find concomitant lumbar spondylosis of a degree resembling that found in the neck, so that reflex changes in the legs are unpredictable. In cases with both cervical and lumbar spondylosis, there may be loss of tendon reflexes in the lower limbs, instead of the expected hyperreflexia due to cervical cord compression. It is also undoubtedly true that in patients with documented lumbar spondylosis, studies of the cervical spine will usually reveal cervical spondylosis. Occasionally, paraesthesias such as tingling or electrical sensations can occur in the trunk and legs with cervical spondylosis, particularly during neck extension. Frank pain in the legs is rarely if ever due to cervical spondylosis; at least, this author has never seen a believable example of it. Occipital pain due to bony encroachment on the upper cervical roots may add to the confusing picture of a patient with pain and paraesthesias all over the body! The character of pain in cervical spondylosis resembles that of chronic compression of individual roots and the same aggravating factors may be present (Wilkinson 1971). In general, patients with single lateral cervical disc protrusions of soft nucleus pulposus tend to form a younger group than patients with multiple degenerated cervical discs and extensive bony spurs and ridges.

LUMBAR SPONDYLOSIS

Pain distributed in several dermatomes of the lower extremities, often bilateral and otherwise resembling the pain of a solitary lumbar disc protrusion, may be due to widespread spondylotic changes of the lumbar spine. Regardless of whether disc protrusions are present, back pain and leg pain are prominent complaints. Weinstein et al (1977) found that 66% of patients with narrowed lumbar canals due to spondylosis suffered from back pain; 36% had unilateral leg pain and 36% had bilateral leg pain. Painful muscle spasms and cramps in the back and legs were frequent but the localization of pain was not consistent or helpful in diagnosis. Of 227 cases, pain was felt in the buttock or hip in 25, in the thigh in 23 and in the groin or genitalia in nine. In many cases, the pain was aggravated by extension of the lumbar spine. Twenty cases were classified as 'neurogenic claudication', which is discussed below. Objective sensory abnormalities were present in only half of the cases and often did not follow a discrete dermatomal pattern. In a few cases, perianal or 'saddle' hypoaesthesia was noted. Muscle weakness was observed in 64% and was often most marked in the extensor hallucis longus and tibialis anterior, suggesting predominant L5 root involvement. Tendon stretch reflexes in the ankles or knees were decreased or absent in 70% of cases. In about 10% there was additional evidence of cauda equina involvement consisting of bowel or bladder incontinence, urinary retention or impotence. A positive response to straight-leg raising was found in only 30% of the 227 cases, a useful point in distinguishing the pain of lumbar spondylosis and canal stenosis from that of simple disc protrusion.

Neurogenic claudication

A prominent caudal radiculopathy caused by lumbar spondylosis or by congenital lumbar spinal stenosis has come to be known as neurogenic claudication. This syndrome of the narrow spinal canal was described by Verbiest (1954). Typically there is a distinctly unpleasant sensation in the legs which can be frankly painful in some cases. It is variably described as numb, cold, burning or cramping (Weinstein et al 1977). This sensation characteristically appears after assumption of an upright posture or during prolonged extension of the lumbar spine. The symptoms may begin in the feet and spread proximally or vice versa. Paraesthesias often appear even when the patient is standing still, but they are typically brought on by walking. These points help to distinguish the syndrome from peripheral vascular claudication, in which cramps affect the leg muscles after exercise regardless of posture. A useful rule of thumb is that the patient whose intermittent claudication is due to arterial insufficiency would rather walk downhill than uphill. The reverse is true of the patient with a narrow spinal canal since the back is slightly flexed in climbing. Descending places the spine in lordosis with further constriction of the cauda equina. Objective sensory deficits are usually slight or absent in cases of neurogenic claudication and straight-leg raising does not usually cause pain.

ARACHNOIDITIS

There is often diffuse involvement of nerve roots in chronic spinal arachnoiditis. In recent decades, reported cases have been predominately lumbosacral (Shaw et al 1978) but any part of the spine may be affected. Almost always, pain is the first symptom. The pain of arachnoiditis may obey a radicular pattern but more often it involves portions of two or more root distributions. In some cases, widely separated zones are involved in an irregular distribution (Whisler 1978). In others, the painful region is large with poorly demarcated borders. Pain tends to be bilateral (Elkington 1951). The low back is often a focal point from which pain seems to be distributed to both legs. The locations of painful zones in the extremities may shift over days or weeks and so may be patient's description of his symptoms. The sensory quality of the pain is described as stinging, burning, aching or gnawing (Elkington 1951). It is continuous but worsened by movement. Jarring, straining, coughing or sneezing may aggravate the pain (Fedar & Smith 1962). It may be particularly severe in the morning or after prolonged bedrest (Christensen 1942). Cramping sensations and painful muscle spasms suggest ventral root involvement later confirmed by atrophy and fasciculation. Painful spasms of the extremities may also indicate spinal cord involvement at a higher level.

With lumbosacral arachnoiditis, the straight-leg raising test is positive on one or both sides in the vast majority of cases (French 1946). There is typically stiffness and tenderness of the paravertebral muscles and marked limitation of the lumbar spine flexion. Pain in the lower extremities may be aggravated by flexing the neck. Numbness and paraesthesias are common. They are often widespread, poorly localized and inconstant from day to day. The paraesthesias may be described as dull, tingling, hot, burning, cold, constricting or 'like pins and needles' (Rocovich 1947). Occasional patients complain of an inexorable feeling of fullness in the rectum. Tingling in the extremities can often be reproduced by flexing the neck. Objective sensory examination by touch and pinprick may be vague or entirely normal despite bizarre subjective complaints. Autonomic signs and trophic changes are not commonly found.

Like lumbosacral disc disease, to which it is related, arachnoiditis affects men more often than women in a ratio of almost 2:1. The typical age of onset is between 25 and 65 (French 1946). When extensive spondylosis or multiple disc protrusions are present it will be difficult to blame arachnoiditis for the patient's symptoms even when the myelogram shows diagnostic signs. Only the history, extent and variability of symptoms and occasional involvement of the spinal cord distinguish arachnoiditis clinically from disc protrusions and entrapment of nerve roots.

MENINGEAL CARCINOMATOSIS

Multiple nerve roots may be involved at different levels by leptomeningeal metastases from solid tumours. The subject of nerve and root pain in cancer is reviewed elsewhere in this volume and will be mentioned only briefly here. The typical clinical syndrome of meningeal carcinomatosis consists of neurological dysfunction at several levels of the neuraxis without radiological evidence of brain metastasis or of epidural spinal metastasis. About two-thirds of the patients in one reported series were women (Wasserstrom et al 1982). Patients ranged in age from 30 to 74 years in this series. Breast cancer was the commonest primary source, followed by lung cancer and malignant melanoma. Spinal root infiltrates are also a common problem in leukaemic patients, who are frequently children (Neiri et al 1968).

Root symptoms, including radicular pain, may be the first sign of meningeal carcinomatosis. Olson et al (1974) found that 25% of patients whose leptomeninges were infiltrated by metastatic cancer had only root symptoms initially. Another 15% had spinal root symptoms plus symptoms of other sites of neurological damage. In a series of 90 patients with known carcinomatous invasion of the meninges, Wasserstrom et al (1982) reported that 74 had spinal symptoms and signs. Pain in a radicular pattern was a prominent feature in 19, while back pain or neck pain was present in 23. Other frequent complaints were of weakness, usually of the legs, paraesthesias in the extremities and bowel or bladder dysfunction. Seven patients had nuchal rigidity and 11 had back pain on straight-leg raising; 30 patients had signs of cauda equina involvement. The tendency for lumbosacral root involvement has also been noted in leukaemic patients (Neiri et al 1968). It is thought to be due to the gravitation of malignant cells in the cerebrospinal fluid as well as the relatively long course of the lumbosacral roots within the subarachnoid space (Little et al 1974). Headaches are a frequent accompanying complaint. Some patients experience pain when the neck is manipulated, others show tenderness to percussion over the spine. Absence of one or more of the tendon stretch reflexes is typical, as is muscle wasting and fasciculation. Additional signs and symptoms due to systemic cancer may complicate the picture.

PSEUDORADICULAR SYNDROMES

MULTIPLE SCLEROSIS

Limb pain and paroxysmal pain are not uncommon in patients with multiple sclerosis (Clifford & Trotter 1984, Moulin et al 1988). In some cases, this takes the form of a radicular syndrome mimicking the pain of nerve root compression and prompting a diagnostic search for disc protrusion or other spine disease. Ramirez-Lassepas et al (1992) described 11 patients presenting with acute radicular pain, in whom root compression was ruled out by careful imaging studies. Multiple sclerosis was eventually determined to be the cause of the pseudoradicular pain, which was lumbosacral in six cases, cervical in three and thoracic in two. In about half the cases, acute radicular symptoms appeared in association with trauma. These patients represented only 4% of newly diagnosed cases of MS in the authors' practices over a 15-year interval. Uldry and Regli (1992) reported four additional cases of pseudoradicular pain associated with demyelinating plaques in the cervical spinal cord diagnosed with MRI. It is important not to ignore the fact that disc protrusions and spondylosis are still the most common causes of radicular pain in the MS population and the diagnosis of demyelinating disease does not necessarily preclude surgical treatment. The diagnosis of pseudoradicular pain due to MS is best established by MRI, which is quite sensitive to the presence of demyelinating plaques in the spinal cord (Gebarski et al 1985, Paty et al 1988). The author has seen one instance in which a tiny demyelinating plaque in the high cervical cord of a patient with MS was associated with pain otherwise indistinguishable from occipital neuralgia.

NEUROSYPHILIS AND DIABETES

In tabetic neurosyphilis (tabes dorsalis), degeneration of dorsal roots and dorsal columns is associated with a clinical syndrome of lancinating pains and visceral crises. Patients are typically 40–60 years of age because the symptoms rarely appear less than 10–20 years after the disease begins (Storm-Mathisen 1978). The most frequent complaint is of 'lightning pains': sudden intense, fleeting pains in the legs, less often in the back and arms. They are described as cramping, crushing, burning, lancinating or 'like an electric shock'. They tend to occur in clusters and may shift unpredictably in location. Occipital neuralgia has been reported as an unusual presenting feature of neurosyphilis (Smith et al 1987). Numbness or tingling and aching paraesthesias are common in the trunk and soles of the feet. Hyperaesthesia to touch may occur. Objective sensory loss is said to appear in characteristic patterns: the middle of the face, ulnar forearm, nipple area, and perianal region (Storm-Mathisen 1978). Additional signs of neurosyphilis may include Charcot joints, absent joint position sense in the legs, ataxia and Argyll Robertson pupil.

Diabetic pseudotabes is a pseudoradicular pain syndrome seen in diabetes mellitus. Brief, shooting pains may be restricted to a single dermatome. Paraesthesias and other signs of dorsal column dysfunction may be found. The presence of an irregular pupil that accommodates but reacts poorly to light may sometimes further confuse the clinical picture (Gilroy & Meyer 1975).

PELVIC LESIONS

Pelvic tumours and inflammatory diseases affecting the lumbosacral plexus may closely mimic lumbosacral radicular syndromes. When adequate CT or MRI studies of the lumbosacral spine fail to show a cause for sciatica, it is probably wise to proceed to imaging of the pelvic region. In patients with advanced vascular disease, atherosclerotic aneurysms of the hypogastric or common iliac arteries may produce sciatica, sometimes with abrupt onset (Chapman et al 1964).

REFERRED PAIN FROM ZYGOPOPHYSEAL JOINTS

Because the spinal zygopophyseal (facet) joints are innervated by medial branches of the posterior primary rami of nerve roots, there is an anatomical substrate for referred pain to the limb from abnormalities of these joints. Injections into the facet joints may produce apparent radicular pain, as may injections into a variety of ligamentous, fascial and other soft tissue structures in and around the spine (North et al 1994). Diagnosis of chronic referred pain is somewhat complicated and depends upon a process of elimination. Imaging of the discs and intervertebral foramina should fail to demonstrate direct root compression and objective radicular neurological deficits should not be found. It may be possible to elicit tenderness to palpation over the involved facet joints. Pain may be provoked by injection into the joint and should be consistently relieved by repeated, selective local anaesthetic blocks directed at the nerve branches innervating the joints (Bogduk & Long 1979, Barnsley et al 1993).

PERIPHERAL NERVE ENTRAPMENT

Peripheral nerve entrapment syndromes may produce symptomatology closely resembling limb pain of nerve root compression. Saal et al (1988) identified 45 patients with peripheral nerve entrapments as the primary cause of pseudoradicular leg pain, out of a population of approximately 4000 patients evaluated for sciatica. Sites of nerve entrapment included the femoral nerve proximal to the inguinal ligament in nine cases; the saphenous nerve around the knee in seven; the common peroneal nerve at or above the popliteal space in 20; and the tibial nerve within the popliteal space in nine. Diagnosis was established by electromyography and nerve conduction studies and by selective spinal and peripheral nerve blocks. Back pain was noted in 49% of these patients and 44% showed a positive straight-leg raising sign.

Piriformis syndrome is a form of entrapment of the sciatic nerve at the greater sciatic notch due to an abnormality of the piriformis muscle that can sometimes be identified by MRI. Pain is usually located in the buttock and upper thigh but may radiate distally to resemble radicular pain. Pain is said to be aggravated by prolonged hip flexion, adduction and internal rotation and there is typically tenderness around the buttock and sciatic notch (Barton 1991).

TIME COURSE AND PROGNOSIS

Few generalities apply to pain of root damage. Lesions of single roots are usually of recent onset in young individuals, while multiradicular syndromes are apt to be of chronic duration in an older age group. Pain of individual root origin is often due to benign mechanical lesions which compress or distort. Pain of multiradicular origin suggests a diffuse degenerative, neoplastic or inflammatory cause, frequently intradural. In general, pain due to mechanical distortion of a single root is more amenable to surgery than is pain of multiple root damage.

Possibly the great majority of root compressions due to disc protrusion are asymptomatic. In a series of 300 patients having no symptoms referrable to cervical or lumbar roots, myelography showed root-sleeve deformities and other abnormalities characteristic of disc protrusion in 110 (37%). Multiple defects were shown in 18% (Hitselberger & Witten 1968). In a similar study using computed tomography of the lumbar spine in asymptomatic individuals, there was a 35% incidence of abnormalities. In the group under 40 years of age, there were changes typical of disc protrusion in every case. In the over-40 age group, there was a 50% incidence of abnormalities, including disc protrusion, facet joint degeneration and spinal stenosis (Wiesel et al 1984). It is likely that many instances of root compression by bulging discs are transient and that healing of the torn annulus takes place (Davis 1982). In a study of 47 patients followed prospectively for symptomatic disc herniations, without significant joint disease or stenosis, 42 patients tolerated conservative management without surgery until signs of radiculopathy subsided (Maigne et al 1992). Serial CT scans documented shrinkage of the disc herniations over periods of 1–40 months, with the largest herniations tending to decrease the most. A majority of patients who experience an episode of low back pain can be expected to be asymptomatic within a month with no treatment (Nachemson 1977). When radicular pain is also present, the percentage is less but many patients will still recover with rest. In most instances of cervical radiculopathy due to spondylosis, the symptoms will resolve over about 6 weeks (Wilkinson 1971).

The typical patient with radicular pain due to cervical or lumbosacral disc protrusion has a history of one or more previous episodes of neck or back pain which cleared with rest. These episodes took place during preceding months or years and usually lasted several days or weeks at a time. The onset of new, severe symptoms then commenced with neck or back pain, often brought on by exercise or by some twisting movement. This improved somewhat over days or weeks but was replaced by radicular pain. In some cases, the radicular pain then spread distally in a saltatory fashion.

A few patients do not fit this pattern but instead develop sudden severe radiating pain as the initial symptom. After a radicular pattern is established, some patients with disc protrusion still obtain relief by resting in bed but they are very susceptible to future attacks of a similar nature. More commonly, the pain persists with fluctuations which are closely related to physical activity. Sudden disappearance of radicular pain is cause for concern since this might indicate destruction of the root. Increasing numbness and weakness or further diminution of tendon reflexes signal worsening of the root lesion even when the pain is improving (Murphey 1968).

In many cases, particularly when the patient is unable to function at work, the sequence of events will be interrupted by disc surgery. Spangfort (1972) concluded that complete relief of both back pain and leg pain occurs in 60% of patients undergoing discectomy on the basis of clearcut mechanical and neurological findings supported by indisputable abnormalities. Many neurosurgeons would find this figure to be an underestimate of the success rate of disc surgery today. Even before the advent of microsurgical techniques, a 96% success rate in 779 patients undergoing 'radical' lumbar disc operations was reported. There is a good correlation between the degree of pain relief and the degree of disc herniation which indicates the severity of root compression prior to surgery. It is among the unfortunate minority of patients failing surgery that we find cases of chronic pain associated with root damage and arachnoiditis.

Some patients who are not relieved by operation may continue to experience pain because of surgical trauma to the root. In this group of patients who have prolonged pain and paraesthesias, the chronology is often difficult to follow because the patient, unhappy with his treatment, migrates from place to place seeking relief. It can become almost impossible to reconstruct the course of events, but this is what is needed in such cases. If the previous records and X-ray films are gathered and studied, one of three chronological patterns may emerge (Bertrand 1975). The sequence: *radicular pain → operation → relief for weeks or months → return of pain in the same or in a different distribution* does not usually indicate permanent root damage but rather suggests that recurrent root compression at the same level or at a different level is present. The sequence: *radicular pain → operation → no change* suggests that the cause of pain was not identified at surgery. A disc fragment may have migrated out of reach or the root may have been trapped in a hidden zone. The sequence: *radicular pain → operation → relief of pain but severe numbness* suggests surgical trauma to the root or its vascular supply. A fourth pattern might be added: *radicular pain → operation → increased radicular pain and severe bilateral leg cramps → temporary improvement → chronic bilateral pain* suggests the development of arachnoiditis (Auld 1978). In this syndrome, severe cramps and spasms in both legs, sometimes accompanied by fever and chills, begin on the first, second or third postoperative day and last for 4–20 days. There is usually some improvement but signs of chronic arachnoiditis develop over the following months or years with new neurological deficits and relentless bilateral back and leg pain.

The long-range prognosis of arachnoiditis is poor in that the neurological deficits tend to persist permanently. Late onset of urinary frequency, urgency or frank incontinence was noted in 23% of a group of arachnoiditis patients followed over 10–21 years (Guyer et al 1989). Of the patients in that study, 90% had undergone Pantopaque myelography and disc surgery prior to developing arachnoiditis. Progression of neurological disability did not appear to be the typical natural course of the disease. When increased neurological deficits were seen, they were most often due to surgical intervention. A majority of the patients depended on daily narcotic analgesics; alcohol abuse, depression and two deaths by suicide were also noted.

The time course of pain due to various other forms of root damage depends on the aetiology. The pain of paroxysmal cranial neuralgias usually appears suddenly and unexpectedly in previously healthy adults and recurs at irregular but increasingly frequent intervals of months, weeks, days or hours. Attacks may appear in clusters with pain-free periods lasting less than an hour. Spontaneous remissions lasting as long as 20 years were described in 161 of 217 cases of glossopharyngeal neuralgia (Rushton et al 1981). Neuralgias associated with upper cervical root lesions can also be expected to persist with repeated aggravations for months or years in the absence of treatment.

The course of radiculopathies due to fractures and other mechanical disorders is similar to that described above for disc protrusions in that there is a tendency for pain to persist as long as the root is distorted or compressed. Exacerbations are closely related to physical activity and the patient is understandably reluctant to return to work. Pain associated with cervical or lumbar spondylosis, including the syndrome of neurogenic claudication, can be considered permanent in the absence of treatment. The neurological symptoms tend to be slowly progressive over years. Generous laminectomy and decompression of the involved roots at the intervertebral foramina usually arrest the process.

Pain of spinal tumours tends to be overshadowed by signs of spinal cord or cauda equina compression during succeeding weeks or months depending on the histological nature of the tumour. Relief can be expected following surgical excision of benign masses, particularly if only a single root is involved, if a rhizotomy is done and if neighbouring roots are not traumatized.

There is a disturbing tendency for lumbosacral arachnoiditis to ascend, causing cord compression by tense, fluid-filled loculations. In a few unfortunate cases, adhesions reform at accelerating intervals despite repeated surgical lysis until the patient is paraplegic and incontinent. However, this is by no means the typical expected course of arachnoiditis. In mild cases relief is imminent for many patients within a year or two. It has not been possible to predict which patients will improve and which will deteriorate. The number of roots involved gives some indication of the severity of the process.

Diabetic root pain may also improve spontaneously in some cases and this does not necessarily depend on rigorous control of blood sugar levels. In most cases of herpes zoster, segmental pain may precede the appearance of cutaneous vesicles by 3–4 days. Healing of the skin lesions takes place over 2–3 weeks. Pain lasts an additional week or two in young patients and usually disappears, leaving hypo- or hyperaesthesia. Pain persists for over 2 months in 70% of patients over 60 years of age, even though the skin lesions heal normally (Ray 1980). Intractable postherpetic neuralgia occurs mainly in elderly patients. When it has been present for 6 months or more, the prognosis for recovery is very poor (Lipton 1979).

The prognosis of meningeal carcinomatosis depends on the response to intrathecal chemotherapy and radiation as well as the tumour histology and extent of disease. The pain of root destruction by trauma, scarring, avulsion, very severe herpetic or syphilitic lesions, or advanced arachnoiditis, is usually a protracted affair with a component of deafferentation in many cases. Pain continues for years or for the rest of the patient's life unless effective treatment can be found.

AETIOLOGY AND DIAGNOSTIC STUDIES

Some common conditions associated with radicular pain are listed in Table 37.3. Most of these have already been

Table 37.3 Some common aetiologies of radicular pain

Lower cranial roots
Glossopharyngeal neuralgia
  idiopathic
  associated with vascular anomaly
Cerebellopontine angle tumour
Skull base tumour
Geniculate neuralgia

Upper cervical roots
Occipital neuralgia
  idiopathic
  associated with C1–2 arthrosis
  associated with rheumatoid arthritis
  post-traumatic
Postherpetic neuralgia
Metastatic spine tumour
Chiari malformation

Lower cervical roots
Cervical disc protrusion
Cervical spondylosis
Metastatic spine tumour
Brachial plexus avulsion injury
Cervical spine fracture or dislocation
Intradural tumour

Thoracic roots
Postherpetic neuralgia
Intercostal neuralgia
  idiopathic
  following thoracotomy
  associated with systemic malignancy
Thoracic disc protrusion
Metastatic spine tumour
Intradural tumour
Meningeal carcinomatosis, lymphoma, leukaemia
Spinal epidural abscess
Diabetic neuropathy
Thoracic spine fracture or dislocation
Tabes dorsalis

Lumbar and first sacral roots
Lumbar disc protrusion
Lumbar spondylosis
  spinal stenosis
  superior facet syndrome
Postsurgical epidural scarring
Arachnoiditis
Spondylolisthesis
Occult postoperative facet fracture
Metastatic spine tumour
Intradural tumour
Meningeal carcinomatosis, lymphoma, leukaemia
Spinal epidural abscess
Lumbar spine fracture or dislocation
Perineurial or leptomeningeal cyst
Tabes dorsalis

Sacrococcygeal roots
Coccygodynia
Metastatic sacral tumour
Meningeal carcinomatosis, lymphoma, leukaemia
Perineurial cyst

mentioned in the preceding discussion of symptoms, time course and prognosis. Here we are concerned with the pathophysiology of radicular pain, which may vary greatly depending on the segmental level involved. The related topic of trigeminal neuralgia is reviewed in Chapter 32.

Pain in the sensory distribution of the lower cranial nerves may be due to orofacial cancers and metastatic tumours of the skull base or it may be secondary to nerve compression by intracranial tumours of the posterior fossa, usually benign, or vascular malformations in this region. In other cases, the pain is idiopathic, although some of these cases may be due to compression of the nerves by vessels or arachnoidal adhesions near the brainstem. Geniculate neuralgia may be entirely idiopathic or it may appear subsequent to an attack of herpes zoster involving the external auditory canal (Hunt 1915). The exact mechanism of the virus in causing pain is not known, but the syndrome might be considered a variant of postherpetic neuralgia. At spinal levels, inflammation and necrosis of dorsal root ganglia have been well documented in pathological reports of herpes zoster (Adams 1976). The middle ear cavity is innervated in part by the tympanic branch of the glossopharyngeal nerve and some cases of paroxysmal otalgia are a variant of vagoglossopharyngeal neuralgia, in which case the herpetic prodrome is not seen. Both types of neuralgia may be associated with vascular compression and some surgeons advise exploration with the aim of microvascular decompression of the fifth, ninth and 10th cranial nerves as well as section of the nervus intermedius in the management of primary otalgia (Rupa et al 1991, Lovely & Jannetta 1997).

In more typical cases of vagoglossopharyngeal neuralgia, neurovascular compression (Laha & Jannetta 1977) is now known to be frequent and may be a causative factor since microvascular decompression can provide long-term pain relief in 89–95% of cases (Resnick et al 1995, Kondo 1998). The vessels most likely to compress the ninth and 10th cranial nerves are the posterior inferior cerebellar artery, the vertebral artery and, less often, the anterior inferior cerebellar artery. Microvascular decompression and rhizotomy of the lower cranial nerves are discussed in more detail in Chapter 51. Neurovascular compression is not found in all cases. In many, no definite aetiology is found. In others, trauma, local infection, an elongated styloid process or a calcified stylohyoid ligament is responsible. Similar abnormalities have been found in the vagal variant, in which pain is restricted to the larynx. Partial demyelination of the glossopharyngeal nerve has been shown postmortem in some cases of vagoglossopharyngeal neuralgia, but the syndrome is rarely associated with multiple sclerosis (Rushton et al 1981).

Diagnosis of vagoglossopharyngeal neuralgia is most easily distinguished from third division trigeminal neuralgia by the location of pain trigger zones. While trigeminal neuralgia is sometimes triggered from the oral mucosa and teeth, vagoglossopharyngeal neuralgia is more typically triggered from the tonsillar region. Attacks may sometimes be aborted by spraying the tonsil with a topical anaesthetic (Rushton et al 1981). Pain due to vagal involvement tends to be deeper in the throat and may be inactivated by superior laryngeal nerve block. Non-paroxysmal pain in the throat and deep in the ear is suggestive of tumour involvement. All cranial neuralgias should be investigated with plain and contrast-enhanced MRI of the posterior fossa and skull base region. Unexplained ear and throat pain warrants consultation with an otolaryngologist.

As noted earlier, pain in the territory of the upper cervical nerve roots may be due to occipital neuralgia, but this diagnosis includes many possible aetiologies. Many cases are post-traumatic or associated with arthritis, fractures or arthrosis of the upper cervical facet joints (Ehni & Benner 1984). In some instances, trauma to the scalp or skull, or cranial surgery, directly injures branches of the greater and lesser occipital nerves with persistent neuropathic pain. The author has encountered cases of occipital neuralgia, often bilateral, following laminectomies to treat cervical spondylosis, presumably because the surgical incision and retraction traumatize the origins of the greater occipital nerves. Following trauma, occipital pain is probably most often due to stretch injury and subsequent swelling and spasm of the posterior cervical muscles, some of which attach on the occipital bone in the territory of the C2 and C3 roots. The occipital nerves themselves may be stretched or constricted by fibrotic bands in the surrounding muscles and ligaments. Occasionally, pain in the occipital region will lead to a diagnosis of Chiari malformation, spinal cord or nerve root tumour or metastases in the occipital bone. Adequate investigation of 'occipital neuralgia' should include a set of cervical spine films with oblique, flexion-extension and open-mouth odontoid views and imaging by plain and contrast-enhanced CT or MRI. Diagnostic blocks of the greater and lesser occipital nerves in the scalp may be helpful and, if combined with small amounts of depository steroids, may be therapeutic.

Radiation of pain to the frontal and orbital region in occipital neuralgia patients is probably due to overlap of synaptic inputs from trigeminal and upper cervical afferents to neurons in the trigeminal nucleus caudalis, which extends into the upper cervical spinal cord and blends with the cervical dorsal horn. Kerr (1961) demonstrated in awake patients that pain radiated to the frontal and periorbital region during electrical stimulation of identified C1 dorsal rootlets but not C2 rootlets. This might imply a C1 contribution in cases of occipital neuralgia with periorbital radiation, but Dubuisson (1995) noted periorbital pain in four patients in whom no C1 dorsal rootlets could be found; relief of periorbital pain in two patients following partial posterior rhizotomy at C2–3; and failure to relieve pain in one patient when identified C1 rootlets were completely divided.

At lower cervical, thoracic and lumbar levels, spinal nerve roots may be compressed and distorted in a variety of ways (Figs 37.4, 37.5). An enlarged facet joint and thickened ligamentum flavum may compress the root posteriorly. Free fragments of herniated disc material may be trapped within the spinal canal or in an intervertebral foramen. In the lumbar spine, spondylotic changes of the facet joints may entrap roots passing caudally in the lateral recess of the spinal canal, producing lateral recess stenosis, also known as 'superior facet syndrome' (Epstein et al 1972), with symptoms indistinguishable from those of disc herniation (Figs 37.5, 37.6). Compression of roots within the foramina may be produced, or aggravated, by spinal instability, due to disc and joint degeneration (degenerative spondylolisthesis) or to a congenital lytic defect of the pars interarticularis of a vertebra (congenital spondylolisthesis with spondylolysis). The portion of the defective arch still attached to the upper vertebra may be dragged forward against the root in the foramen (Fig. 37.4, lower right). Further root entrapment can result from chronic fibrosis around the root near the site of the bony defect. A less frequently diagnosed cause of radicular pain following surgery

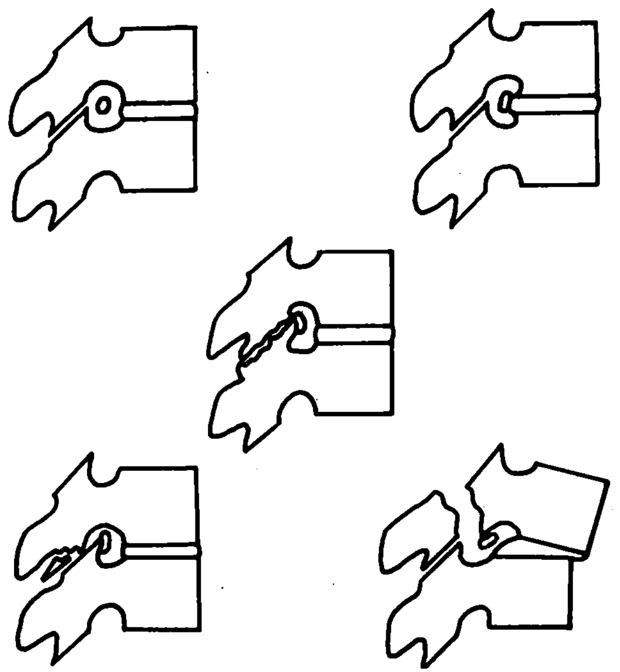

Fig. 37.4 Mechanical root lesions (lateral view). **Upper left** Normal relationship of nerve root to disc and vertebrae. **Upper right** Disc protrusion and osteophytes. **Centre** Facet joint degeneration. **Lower left** Fracture of inferior articular process. **Lower right** Spondylolysis with spondylolisthesis.

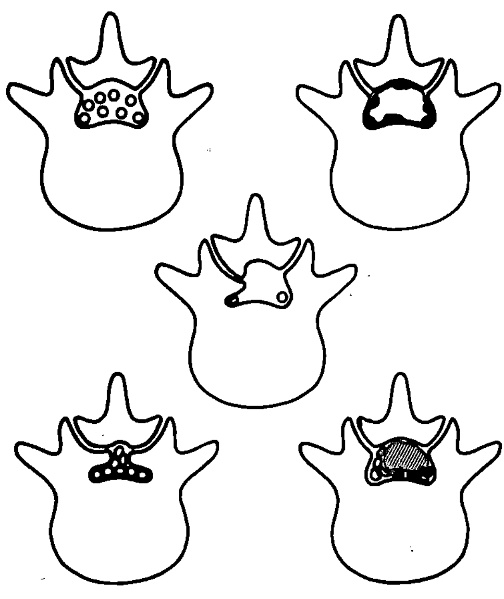

Fig. 37.5 Lumbosacral root lesions (horizontal view). **Upper left** Normal configuration of the spinal canal and cauda equina. **Upper right** Chronic adhesive arachnoiditis and atrophic roots. **Centre** Entrapment of a root descending in narrow lateral recess ('superior facet syndrome'). **Lower left** Lumbar spinal stenosis due to spondylosis. **Lower right** Intradural tumour compressing the cauda equina.

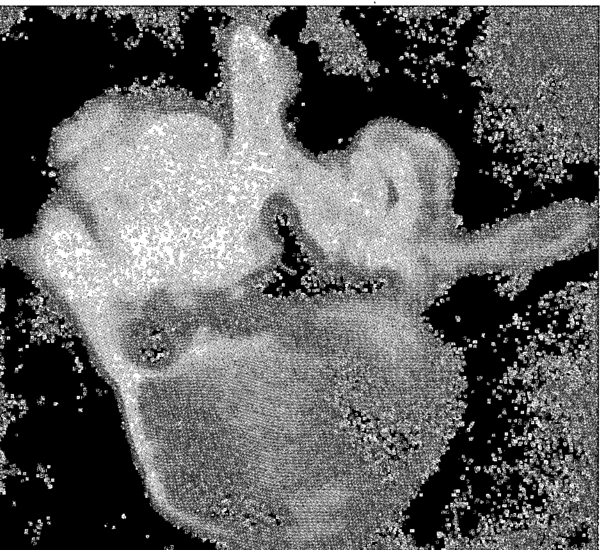

Fig. 37.6 Computed tomographic (CT) scan in horizontal plane showing severely degenerated, hypertrophic facet joint at the L4–5 level (left side of photograph; compare this with Fig. 37.5, centre).

is an occult fracture of the inferior articular process of a vertebra. This typically follows overly aggressive bone removal around the medial aspect of the facet joint (medial facetectomy) at the time of disc removal or laminectomies for spinal stenosis and may not develop until the patient resumes activities in an upright posture. The unopposed superior articular process of the vertebra below may encroach into the foramen to pinch an existing root (Fig. 37.4, lower left). Occult facet fractures were found on routine postoperative CT scans in 6% of patients undergoing lumbar spine surgery (Rothman et al 1985). This type of occult facet fracture is not easily identified on axial images and is best seen on sagittally reformatted CT or MRI.

Postoperative epidural fibrosis is a common finding after laminectomies and disc surgery. It is widely believed that epidural fibrosis may lead to adhesions around nerve roots, with compression or tethering of the roots, which may in turn lead to recurrent radicular pain and physical impairment. Cervellini et al (1988) used CT to study 20 asymptomatic operated patients and 20 patients with recurrent radicular pain after disc surgery, none with stenosis, recurrent disc herniation or other non-fibrosis causes. They found the degree and type of fibrosis to be unrelated to recurrent symptoms. However, more recently the correlation of recurrent radicular pain with amount of lumbar epidural fibrosis was studied in a randomized, double-blind, controlled multicentre clinical trial using gadolinium-enhanced MRI (Ross et al 1996). Patients were studied at 1 and 6 months after first-time, single-level discectomies. At 6 months, the results showed that patients having extensive epidural scar were 3.2 times more likely to experience recurrent radicular pain. Descriptions of pain 'on average' and 'when most severe' were analysed and only pain when most severe showed a significant correlation with amount of scar tissue.

Epidural fibrosis has also been reported as a complication of implanted epidural catheters, appearing 21–320 days after implantation and manifested by pain or resistance to flow on injection of the catheter (Aldrete 1995). This appears to be a type of foreign body reaction due to the presence of the catheter in the epidural space and may limit the permanency of the catheter.

Epidural fibrosis in the lumbosacral region binds nerve roots and dural tube to surrounding structures such as the disc annulus and posterior longitudinal ligament and probably prevents normal elastic stretch and sliding motion of the root sleeves during spine motion and leg elevation.

Reasons for scar formation following spinal surgery are beginning to be understood and may include inflammatory reaction to foreign matter. Traces of surgical swab debris retained in the epidural space after spinal surgery were identified histologically within dense fibrous connective tissue in 55% of cases submitted to biopsy (Hoyland et al 1988). Moreover, herniated discs are a potent source of phospholipase A_2, an enzymatic marker of inflammation. According to Saal et al (1990), human lumbar disc phospholipase A_2 activity is from 20- to 100 000-fold more active than any previously described source. Because the enzyme is responsible for liberation of arachnoidonic acid from cell membranes, phospholipase A_2 represents the rate-limiting step in the production of prostaglandins and leukotrienes, some of which may in turn affect adjacent nerve roots so as to cause root inflammation, venous congestion and oedema (Lundborg 1988, Vishnawath et al 1988) and hyperalgesia (Levine et al 1984).

Other mechanical causes of root distortion include primary and metastatic tumours of the vertebrae, which encroach upon the intervertebral foramen as the pedicle is destroyed. Spinal intradural tumours may grow directly from the root (e.g. schwannoma, neurofibroma) or so close to it that compression in inevitable (e.g. meningioma, ependymoma). Vertebral metastases may occur at all levels. Meningiomas and schwannomas are commonly thoracic, while ependymomas are more likely to develop in the lumbar region. Tumours of the lumbar canal and cauda equina may produce crowding of the lumbosacral roots similar to that found in lumbar spinal stenosis (see Fig. 37.5).

Focal deposits of leukaemic cells, lymphoma or metastatic carcinoma within the cerebrospinal fluid pathways cause radicular pain. Some types of carcinoma actually infiltrate the dorsal roots, spinal nerve trunks and dorsal root ganglia (Barron et al 1960). In addition, a syndrome of slowly progressive sensory neuropathy, which may be painful, has been described as a remote effect of carcinoma. In three autopsied cases, this syndrome was associated with inflammation and degeneration of the dorsal root ganglia and dorsal roots (Horwich et al 1977).

The pathophysiology of root dysfunction causing pain and claudication in lumbar stenosis is not known with certainty. When narrow spinal canal is present, compression of the cauda equina when the lumbar spine is in extension may cause mechanical distortion of the roots, venous stasis and swelling of the roots and relative ischaemia and hypoxia of the roots in the face of an increased neuronal oxygen demand during exercise (Weinstein et al 1977).

Coccygodynia is a loosely defined syndrome which undoubtedly has more than one possible aetiology. Fibrosis, inflammation and demyelination of sacral roots have been reported in some cases of coccygodynia (Bohm & Franksson 1959). In other cases, sacral root cysts or arachnoiditis have been found. Some instances of coccygodynia are thought to be referred pain from degenerative disease of the lumbosacral facet joints.

ARACHNOIDITIS

Arachnoiditis is a chronic condition of inflammation and sometimes atrophy of neural structures within the subarachnoid space. Multiple predisposing factors have been identified (Table 37.4). While arachnoiditis is usually an aseptic process seen in patients who have undergone multiple spine surgery, some cases are associated with active or healed infectious diseases such as tuberculosis. The older literature on arachnoiditis is based largely on myelographic descriptions of filling defects in the subarachnoid space, absence of root sleeves, an irregular contrast pattern resembling 'candle drippings', arachnoid cysts and sometimes complete blockage of flow (Seaman et al 1953, Smith & Loeser 1972). In older patients who in past years may have had myelography with oil-based contrast agents such as iophendylate (Myodil, Pantopaque), it is not unusual to find droplets and sometimes larger collections of residual contrast material permanently lodged within arachnoid adhesions and loculations. The severe adhesive arachnoiditis associated with these agents is rarely seen today, partly because newer water-soluble contrast agents were developed and partly because myelography has given way to CT and MRI. Although iophendylate is frequently incriminated in lumbar arachnoiditis, two retrospective follow-up studies of large numbers of patients who underwent ventriculography with this contrast agent showed no cases of chronic lumbar arachnoiditis and no increased incidence of back pain (Hughes & Isherwood 1992, Hill et al 1992).

Table 37.4 Some factors predisposing to arachnoiditis

Chronic lumbosacral root compression
Disc protrusion
Spinal stenosis
Spine surgery
Infection
Bacterial meningitis, including tuberculous
Fungal meningitis
Cryptococcal meningitis
Viral meningitis
Syphilis
Haemorrhage
From spinal vascular malformation
Following trauma
Following lumbar puncture
Following surgery
Implanted epidural catheters
Irritant chemicals
Myelographic contrast agents
iophendylate
meglumine iocarmate
methiodal
? metrizamide
Anaesthetic agents
Amphotericin B
Methotrexate
? Steroids
Polyethylene glycol
2-Chloroprocaine

The process of laminectomy and discectomy may itself contribute to the development of arachnoiditis. Serial MRI examinations of 10 patients following lumbar surgery for stenosis or disc herniation revealed cauda equina adhesions that were most severe at the level of laminectomy (Matsui et al 1995). Transient focal shrinkage of the dural tube and subarachnoid space were also noted over a 3-week interval following surgery, with eventual re-expansion in all cases.

Metrizamide can produce signs of meningeal irritation, including fever, nuchal rigidity and the appearance of inflammatory cells in the cerebrospinal fluid (Junck & Marshall 1983). Methiodal myelography was shown to cause the known radiographic changes of arachnoiditis in 29% of non-operated cases and 48% of those who had subsequent spinal surgery (Skalpe 1976). Typical adhesive arachnoiditis has been demonstrated after administration of either meglumine iocarmate or metrizamide in monkeys (Haughton et al 1977). Even though blood is known to increase the chance of arachnoiditis after myelography with iophendylate, the addition of blood to cerebrospinal fluid along with aqueous contrast agents failed to increase the incidence of experimental arachnoiditis in monkeys (Haughton & Ho 1982). Adhesive arachnoiditis was described in 15 patients who underwent lumbar radiculography with a combination of meglumine iocarmate and depository steroids. This complication may have been due partly to steroids, since patients studied with melumine iocarmate alone did not show arachnoiditis (Dullerud & Morland 1976).

Chronically compressed lumbar nerve roots and dorsal root ganglia may develop swelling and histological signs of an inflammatory reaction inside the root sleeve (Lindahl & Rexed 1951). In chronic arachnoiditis, some or all of the lumbosacral roots may be encased by dense leptomeningeal adhesions within the dura. The final stage of this process is a lumbar canal in which the roots are bound circumferentially to the dura (see Fig. 37.5). Burton (1978) suggested the following sequence of events:

1. The pia of individual roots is inflamed, with root swelling and hyperaemia (radiculitis).
2. The roots adhere to each other and to the surrounding arachnoid trabeculae and fibroblasts proliferate.
3. There is atrophy of the roots, which are displaced circumferentially and encased in collagen deposits.

The changes characteristic of arachnoiditis can often be demonstrated by MRI or CT. The lumbar nerve roots can sometimes be shown to cluster together and to adhere to the surrounding meninges, leaving the centre of the spinal canal void. With many long-standing cases of arachnoiditis, one sees trapped radiographic contrast material of high density which may produce scattering artefacts on CT images. This is more of a problem with older CT scanners than with the current generation. Magnetic resonance imaging does accurately diagnose arachnoiditis, comparing favourably with CT myelography and plain film myelography for that purpose (Delamarter et al 1990). However, use of gadolinium during MR imaging does not reveal significant additional information about the condition (Johnson & Sze 1990).

Arachnoiditis is usually worst in the lumbosacral subarachnoid space, although it can involve any level of the spinal canal or even the intracranial cisterns. In many cases, arachnoiditis seems to result from an initial focus of inflammation such as nerve root compressed by lumbar stenosis or disc protrusion. The presence of blood in the cerebrospinal fluid after lumbar puncture, myelography or surgery aggravates this. The additional presence of an irritating foreign substance such as iophendylate greatly augments the effect of blood in the subarachnoid space. Intrathecal drugs and infection of the meninges may also contribute. Drugs with known risk of arachnoiditis include the antifungal agent amphotericin B, methotrexate, 2-chloroprocaine and methylprednisolone acetate (for references, see Esses & Morley 1983). Wilkinson (1992) reviewed the literature on intrathecal methylprednisolone and concluded that most of the evidence implicating the drug in arachnoiditis was circumstantial; also, most of the complications of intrathecal steroids appeared to be related to frequent injections and large doses. All types of infectious meningitis, including viral, parasitic, cryptococcal, tuberculous and ordinary bacterial, may be followed by arachnoiditis.

The exact cause of root dysfunction in arachnoiditis is not known, but direct compression by scar encasement, arachnoid cysts and tense fluid loculations must certainly contribute. Caplan et al (1990) postulated that central spinal cord ischaemia and altered cerebrospinal fluid flow patterns associated with chronic arachnoiditis may lead to formation of cystic regions of myelomalacia in the cord or even frank syrinx formation. Possibly the encasement of roots by collagen deposits leads to atrophy on an ischaemic basis. It is also reasonable to think that roots which are tethered by scarred meninges are no longer free to slide during flexion/extension motions of the spine and legs, so that recurring stretch injury to individual nerve fibres would be likely. In some cases, the arachnoid is known to contain chronic inflammatory cells as well as collagen deposits and hyaline material (Quiles et al 1978). Macrophages may also be found (Dujovny et al 1978).

INVESTIGATIONS

For diagnosis of spinal disorders, conventional X-ray films and myelography have been almost entirely replaced by CT and MRI. Either modality can demonstrate disc protrusions, spondylosis, fractures, spinal tumours and cysts at any level of the spine. Use of CT with intravenous contrast has an accuracy of 67–100% in distinguishing epidural fibrosis from disc material (Teplick & Haskin 1984, Braun et al 1985). MRI has the advantage of multiplanar imaging and avoids loading the patient with radiographic contrast. Gadolinium-enhanced MRI with pre- and postcontrast images distinguishes scar from disc with 96% accuracy (Hueftle et al 1988, Ross et al 1989). In an animal model of postoperative epidural scarring, it was shown that gadolinium enhancement of epidural scar was heightened by increasing the dose of contrast from 0.1 to 0.3 mmol/kg and obtaining MR images within 15 minutes of injection.

High-resolution CT can be very helpful in demonstrating osteophytes and other bone pathology (see Fig. 37.6). MRI is clearly superior for demonstrating syringomyelic cavities, demyelinating plaques and other abnormalities within the spinal cord. Patients with implanted programmable cardiac pacemakers, spinal cord stimulation pulse generators and drug infusion pumps and those with spine instrumentation made of ferromagnetic materials may not be able to undergo MRI safely. CT with or without intravenous or intrathecal contrast may be substituted. Plain films of the spine are useful mainly to assess stability by means of dynamic range-of-motion views and sometimes to look for osteophytes encroaching into foramina on oblique cervical views. These views can provide a quick and inexpensive way to screen for spondylolisthesis or foraminal constriction within the time constraints of an initial clinic visit and may provide justification for the patient to return for a scheduled MRI at a later date. In the author's clinical practice, conventional myelography, epidurography and discography have not been found to be necessary or helpful in the investigation of nerve root disorders and arachnoiditis. Selective nerve root blocks with local anaesthetic are not used for diagnostic purposes, but are sometimes used for prognostic purposes when planning treatment. The method of puncturing an individual nerve root sleeve for injection of contrast or local anaesthetic (MacNab 1971, Schutz et al 1973) is very painful and risks further injury to a root which may already be damaged. Lumbar puncture for CSF evaluation is occasionally needed to rule out tuberculous meningitis or to aid in the diagnosis of demyelinating disease.

Various electromyographic techniques are useful to identify sites of nerve root damage (Stewart 1987). In radicular pain of recent onset, signs of active denervation appear in muscles innervated by the damaged root and not in other muscles. These signs of active denervation include fibrillation potentials and positive sharp waves. In chronic lesions, active denervation is no longer seen. Instead, an increased number of polyphasic potentials may be the only evidence of root damage. Electromyogram (EMG) abnormalities tend to appear sooner in the deep paraspinous muscles than in limb muscles. Changes in the paraspinous muscle EMG may persist for 2 years after spinal surgery (See & Kraft 1975). In patients who have undergone previous root decompressions, the most valuable finding would therefore be a normal EMG (Eisen 1981).

Recordings of selective somatosensory-evoked potentials have been shown to be helpful in determining the sites of cervical and lumbosacral root lesions (Eisen & Elleker 1980, Aminoff et al 1985). Recordings of peripheral nerve and muscle responses to stimulation may serve to distinguish central damage (cord, roots or ganglia) from peripheral nerve injury. If there is a history of trauma and a paralysed, anaesthetic arm, the finding of normal sensory nerve action potentials and absence of muscle action potentials on nerve stimulation suggests that nerve roots of the brachial plexus have been avulsed from the cord (Warren et al 1969). Similar findings could occur in syringomyelia (Fincham & Cape 1968) which might also develop after spine trauma and which may mimic the segmental anaesthesia and severe pain of root avulsion.

PHYSIOLOGICAL CORRELATES OF RADICULAR PAIN

The physiological events which cause root pain are controversial. Some authors (e.g. Kelly 1956) maintain that nerve compression per se is not painful. This may be so in many cases of asymptomatic disc protrusion, as noted earlier (Hitselberger & Witten 1968). Acute mechanical injuries of nerve roots in laboratory animals cause only short (1–50 s) trains of repetitive firing in sensory axons (Wall et al 1974). Clearly, this brief injury discharge is not the physiological correlate of chronic sciatica in humans.

Some of the pain associated with root compression is referred from regions of distortion of neighbouring muscle insertions, joint capsules and ligaments. Truncal pain can be produced during surgery under local anaesthesia by direct pressure on these structures, whereas pain radiating to the extremity is best reproduced by stimulation of the root itself (Frykholm 1951, Murphey 1968). Even gentle mechanical stimuli to dorsal roots, such as stroking with a probe or slight stretching, can elicit segmental pain in humans (Smyth & Wright 1958).

It is unlikely that axons in chronically compressed, ischaemic, inflamed or otherwise damaged roots would behave in normal fashion. Many of the physical events which damaged nerve roots lead to either focal loss of myelin or loss of axons. This is most likely to occur at sites between the dorsal root ganglia and the dorsal root entry zone. Ectopic impulse generation is known to occur in fibres of chronically injured nerves and in compressed dorsal root ganglia (Howe et al 1977). At least in myelinated axons, long periods (5–15 min) of repetitive firing may result. The dorsal root ganglion itself is subject to compression in some cases of disc disease (Lindblom & Rexed 1948). The ganglion is undoubtedly affected in some cases of perineural cysts and arachnoiditis as well. Slight root movements may serve as mechanical triggers of abnormal impulse generation in mechanosensitive chronically injured roots and ganglia when they are tethered by adhesions or compressed by disc, bone or tumour. Dorsal root ganglion cells can also be a source of ectopic afferent impulses in sensory fibres after peripheral nerve damage (Wall & Devor 1983). This latter finding may be relevant to cases of so-called 'double-crush' syndrome (Upton & McComas 1973), in which peripheral nerve entrapment and nerve root entrapment coexist. Nordin et al (1984) demonstrated ectopic neuronal activity in human dorsal root afferents by means of microneurography and correlated this activity with subjective dysaesthesias referred to the foot during a straight-leg raising manoeuvre.

In a case of L5 radiculopathy, in which transcutaneous electrical stimulation of the sciatic nerve reproduced the patient's pain, after local anaesthetic block at the ankle, pain from stimulation was felt only in the thigh and calf but not in the foot (Xavier et al 1990). It was suggested that the stimulation was sending antidromic impulses distally and directly exciting nociceptors in the foot and that this mechanism was prevented by the block.

An explanation of the paroxysmal pain which occurs in cranial neuralgia might include ectopic impulse generation at sites of nerve compression where there is focal demyelination, reflection of impulses at these sites and others to produce reverberation in the nerve and recruitment of small afferent fibres by means of strong presynaptic depolarization of their terminals (Calvin et al 1977). Another possible mechanism for recruitment of thinly myelinated and unmyelinated fibres might be hepatic impulse transmission at sites lacking myelin, similar to that which is thought to occur in ventral roots of dystrophic mice (Rasminsky 1980).

In cases of chronic root avulsion, transection or destruction, the chronic deafferentation of spinal sensory transmission neurons might cause paroxysmal pain. Deafferented cord neurons are thought to discharge in an uncontrolled fashion (Loeser et al 1968). It follows that lesions of the dorsal horn might stop the abnormal discharge, a theory which helps to explain the success of dorsal root entry zone lesions for controlling root avulsion pain (Nashold et al 1983). Traumatic, syphilitic and herpetic lesions of the dorsal roots can sometimes involve portions of the Lissauer tract and substantia gelatinosa which are thought to be involved in the physiological mechanisms of pain suppression (Wall 1980). This suggests that some types of deafferentation pain may be due to an indirect rather than a direct disinhibition of dorsal horn transmission cells.

The quality of pain and the size of the painful region must depend on:

1. the population of fibres which are destroyed
2. the population of normally functioning afferents
3. the number and types of fibres which are discharging excessively, and
4. the interaction of impulses in the cord.

In laboratory animals, the receptive fields of individual dorsal horn neurons show marked long-term plasticity after chronic root section (Wall 1977). Pain is sometimes abolished temporarily by root blocks distal to the site of root damage (Kibler & Nathan 1960), so that some 'normal' afferent impulses must play a facilitating role. Local anaesthetic block of neighbouring roots might have a similar effect, reducing the total afferent input to cord transmission neurons. Therefore the results of diagnostic nerve root blocks must be interpreted with caution. When pain is referred to the distal portion of the dermatome from a source located proximally, local anaesthetic blockade of branches to that proximal source may alleviate the referred pain. Thus, in some cases of severe lumbar facet joint degeneration, injection into the facet joint itself (facet block) may rid the patient of pain radiating down the leg. Similar phenomena undoubtedly occur when local anaesthetic is injected into trigger points in the back muscles and ligaments.

The role of the ventral rootlets in radicular pain is speculative. Ectopic efferent activity in ventral root fibres could lead to muscle spasm, which might in turn generate painful afferent activity in the associated myotome (Frykholm 1951). However, the territory of pain radiation to muscles correlates poorly with electromyographic evidence of damage to the ventral roots (Fisher et al 1978).

TREATMENT

The emphasis in this section is on management of chronic radicular pain disorders that are refractory to conservative management. However, some advice will also be offered regarding the treatment of acute nerve root pain in some common conditions. It is assumed that a careful clinical evaluation has first been performed to document the history, neurological deficits and mechanical signs.

Pain of neuralgias of the lower cranial nerves is usually managed initially with carbamazepine or other medications of the anticonvulsant type. Drugs such as baclofen or amitriptyline may also be helpful in some cases. Refractory cases should be considered for surgery, as discussed in Chapter 51. It is prudent to pursue a conservative course of treatment initially because spontaneous remissions can occur and all the available surgical procedures carry significant risks. For vagoglossopharyngeal neuralgia, the choice of surgery may include percutaneous radiofrequency rhizotomy at the jugular foramen or open exploration by posterior fossa craniectomy. When neurovascular compression is identified, microvascular decompression (MVD) may be feasible although it carries risks similar to those of root section. Some of the most impressive results in the current neurosurgical literature on vagoglossopharyngeal neuralgia are those of MVD, which in the hands of experienced neurosurgeons is reported to have an initial success rate of 85–90% and little likelihood of recurrence in the long term (Resnick et al 1995, Kondo 1998). Equally impressive results were reported by Taha and Tew (1995) who described good or excellent relief of pain with no mortality and minimal morbidity in all 12 of their patients after intracranial section of the ninth nerve and some upper rootlets of the 10th. Taha and Tew recommend that percutaneous RF lesions of the ninth nerve should be limited to use in cancer cases because of the high incidence of hoarseness, vocal cord paralysis and dysphagia after the RF technique. For cases of geniculate neuralgia, surgical treatment is somewhat controversial, but would in any case include either excision of the geniculate ganglion or intracranial section of the nervus intermedius component of the seventh cranial nerve. Bearing in mind that otalgia may result from processes affecting several different cranial nerves, some authors now add exploration and MVD of cranial nerves 5, 9 and 10 if neurovascular compression is found (Rupa et al 1991, Lovely & Jannetta 1997).

Most cases of occipital neuralgia can be managed conservatively with non-steroidal anti-inflammatory drugs, amitriptyline and periodic injection of local anaesthetic and steroids around the greater or lesser occipital nerves in the scalp. Several effective surgical options for treating refractory occipital neuralgia are discussed in Chapter 51. They include decompression of constricted upper cervical nerve roots (Poletti 1983, 1996), C2 ganglionectomy (Lozano et al 1998) and partial posterior rhizotomy at C1–3 (Dubuisson 1995). Some cases involving structural upper cervical spine disease or instability may require surgical stabilization. A technique of electrical spinal cord stimulation for chronic pain in the cervical and occipital regions has also been reported (Barolat 1998) and the long-term effectiveness of this remains to be determined. The choice of surgical procedure can be decided according to results of preliminary radiological investigations and local anaesthetic blocks and the experience of the treating neurosurgeon.

Pain and dysaesthesias associated with avulsion injuries of the brachial or lumbosacral plexus are usually unresponsive to medications. This syndrome is usually best managed by a programme of behavioural pain management and vocational rehabilitation (Wynn Parry 1980). For severe and intractable cases, dorsal root entry zone (DREZ) lesions of the relevant segments of the spinal cord have now been shown to be effective in many surgical series, with long-term pain relief reported in 37–100% of cases (Iskandar & Nashold 1998). A majority of authors report success rates above 65%.

Postherpetic neuralgia, meaning persistent radicular pain 3 or more months after an acute attack of herpes zoster, can be prevented in about 50% of cases by pre-emptive use of amitriptyline or nortriptyline at time of diagnosis of shingles, according to Bowsher (1997). Treatment with oral acyclovir within 72 hours of the appearance of a zoster rash reduces the incidence of residual neuralgic pain at 6 months by 46% (Jackson et al 1997). In a randomized, double-blind, placebo-controlled trial (Tyring et al 1995), famciclovir prescribed for acute herpes zoster led to approximately two times faster resolution of postherpetic neuralgia and decreased the median duration of pain by about 2 months. In established postherpetic neuralgia, chronic radicular pain may still sometimes respond to amitriptyline or topical lidocaine gel (Rowbotham et al 1995). High doses of the putative NMDA receptor blocker dextromethorphan are not more effective than placebo (Nelson et al 1997). Some cases benefit from transcutaneous electrical nerve stimulation (Nathan & Wall 1974) or epidural steroid injections (Forrest 1980). In 3960 patients with postherpetic neuralgia, dermatomal subcutaneous infiltrations with a combination of local anaesthetics and dexamethasone were said to give relief in 28%; another 57% had relief after two injections and 11% after three injections, while 4% had no response (Bhargava et al 1998). Ablative surgical procedures have not been conspicuously successful in treating postherpetic neuralgia. Dorsal rhizotomy carries about a 29% long-term success rate (see Table 51.1), similar to the long-term outcome after DREZ lesions (Iskandar & Nashold 1998). Somewhat better results have been reported for electrical spinal cord stimulation. In a review of literature on treatment of postherpetic neuralgia with cord stimulation through 1991, it was noted that 19 out of 21 reported cases responded well to this modality beyond the first 3 months (Spiegelmann & Friedman 1991).

Most patients with nerve root compression by a disc protrusion will need a temporary period of oral analgesics and reduced physical activity while the diagnostic tests are completed. Some patients with acute cervical disc protrusions may benefit from use of a soft cervical collar, especially during sleep when the patient may be totally unaware of his neck position. In cases of new lumbar radicular pain associated with disc protrusions or facet hypertrophy, a short period of bedrest can be helpful. A randomized clinical trial (Deyo et al 1986) showed that a 2-day period of bedrest was as effective as longer periods, even when minor motor and sensory deficits were present. Most cases of mild radicular pain will settle down over a few weeks. In this author's practice, for mild radiculopathies it has been helpful to prescribe a combination of acetaminophen plus a non-steroidal anti-inflammatory drug every 4–6 hours on a daily basis, remaining within the range of recommended safe dosages. Usually an opiate analgesic is added, the choice of which depends on the severity of pain. Use of cyclobenzaprine, doxepin, amitriptyline or nortriptyline at night can ensure adequate sleep, if the patient is able to tolerate the prolonged sedative effects of these medications. When muscle cramping and spasm are a part of the picture, use of heat or ice, massage, very gentle stretching exercises and muscle relaxants can be helpful.

For more persistent radicular pain, many patients will

experience at least transient relief from a short course of oral steroids in tapering dose. In one series of 100 patients with signs of acute lumbosacral radiculopathy, conservative management and occasional short-term use of oral corticosteroids produced satisfactory relief in 95% (Johnson & Fletcher 1981). Another series of 100 patients with radicular pain due to herniated lumbar discs were treated with an initially high but tapering dose of intramuscular dexamethasone for 7 days. All had relief of pain in 24–48 hours and only nine subsequently required surgery (Green 1975). Oral steroids do have potentially serious adverse effects, most of which can be prevented by brief duration of use and by precautions to reduce gastric acidity.

Epidural steroid injection is sometimes advocated for pain associated with nerve root compression due to disc protrusions and spondylosis. Unfortunately, most of the available literature suffers from poor methodological design, usually with inadequate radiological documentation of the sites of root compression. As noted earlier, the presence of inflammatory mediators associated with herniated disc material suggests a role for early use of anti-inflammatory drugs including corticosteroids in these cases. However, it appears that when frank root damage is already present, the chances of benefit from epidural steroids are greatly diminished. Following mild disc protrusions prior to surgery, reported success rates range from 0% to 70% using rather lenient criteria for success (Dilke et al 1973, Brevik et al 1976, Snoek et al 1977, Cuckler et al 1985). In patients with cervical radicular pain persisting more than 12 months but not considered candidates for disc surgery, a randomized comparison of epidural lidocaine and triamcinolone versus the same combination plus epidural morphine showed no significant difference in outcome (Castagnera et al 1994). Patients with chronic sciatica do not fare too well with epidural steroids and those with previous surgery, entrapment of nerve roots by bone or scar tissue or demonstrable behavioural disturbances are even less likely to respond (White et al 1980). In successful cases, as many as three injections may be needed and the beneficial effects are often delayed for 2–6 days (Green et al 1980). There is some evidence that intrathecal steroids can lead to arachnoiditis, probably due to the vehicle propylene glycol (Nelson et al 1973). Intrathecal steroid injection may aggravate radicular pain acutely and administration by this route is inadvisable (Johnson et al 1991). In a review of literature on this topic, Wilkinson (1992) found most of the evidence for harmful effects of intrathecal methylprednisolone to be circumstantial and most complications followed multiple, large-dose or frequent injections. Epidural injections of the steroid triamcinolone in cats failed to produce any histological signs of damage in lumbar nerve roots (Delaney et al 1980). Steroids given in this way are absorbed systemically and can suppress adrenal function for 3 weeks (Gorski et al 1982).

If pain and deficits do not improve or if the radicular pain is severe, it is the author's practice to proceed with MRI or CT and to formulate a surgical treatment plan. If the diagnosis remains in doubt, electromyography, imaging of the lumbar or brachial plexus or other tests may be needed. Surgical decompression of compromised nerve roots is warranted by progression of neurological deficits or by intractable pain. In the cervical region, pain of solitary root compression can be relieved in most cases by discectomy and foraminotomy or by foraminotomy alone. When pain of cervical disc protrusion has been present for 3 months or more, it has been suggested that physical therapy or use of a cervical collar may be as effective as surgery (Persson et al 1997). In the thoracic region, disc protrusions may be removed by posterolateral, extracavitary approach, by transthoracic approach or thoracoscopically in some centres. Lumbar discectomy is usually performed today with microsurgical techniques, although not all surgeons attempt to work through a tiny incision. Adequate root decompression may require removal of not only the protruding portion of a disc but also osteophytes, portions of enlarged facet joints and thickened ligament. Several series of lumbar microdiscectomies, using minimal incisions, have been reported in which over 90% of patients were relieved of their symptoms and returned to their previous activities (Wilson & Kenning 1979, Goald 1980, Williams 1983, Maroon & Abla 1986). Wilson and Harbaugh (1981) reported a 50% earlier return to work with microdiscectomy than with standard laminectomy, but Kahanovitz et al (1989) found that the main advantage of microdiscectomy was that the patients left the hospital earlier. Bertrand (1975) and Fager (1986) criticized the use of microdiscectomy on the grounds that bony and ligamentous pathology may not be fully accessible through a tiny incision. Moreover, limited exposure during discectomy may require greater retraction on an exposed nerve root, causing root damage. The topic of nerve root decompression is discussed further in Chapter 51 and disc surgery is discussed in Chapter 52.

Postoperative epidural fibrosis, thought to be a frequent cause for failure of disc surgery, may be demonstrated radiologically by gadolinium-enhanced MRI or CT with intravenous contrast, as discussed earlier (see Investigations). Epidural scar tends to develop over 5–6 weeks and its appearance stabilizes by 3–6 months after surgery (Boden & Wiesel 1992, Van Goethem et al 1996). The clinical course of discectomy patients also appears to reach a plateau around this time, so that the outcome 3–6 months after surgery predicts long-term outcome (Abramovitz & Neff 1991). Numerous methods have been advocated to reduce the likelihood of postoperative scarring after spinal surgery, most with little or no proven value. Epidural fat grafts do not consistently prevent fibrosis and may sometimes become a part of the scarring process (Martin-Ferrer 1989). A prospective, randomized multicentre clinical trial of a resorbable anti-adhesion gel, ADCON-L, was conducted in 298 patients undergoing first-time lumbar discectomy (De Tribolet et al 1998). This study showed significant inhibition of epidural scar formation, with significantly better clinical outcomes in treatment patients compared to controls.

Patients with significant degrees of lumbar or cervical spinal stenosis, multilevel foraminal root compression or structural lesions such as tumours or cysts within the spinal canal may require more extensive operations designed to relieve cord and root compression. These operations carry risks of epidural fibrosis that are at least as great as those of disc surgery. In cases of chronic radicular pain after failed back surgery, factors other than scarring may be identified on postoperative studies. If persistent root distortion by osteophytes, thick ligaments or residual disc material is found, reoperation and completion of the root decompression should be considered. However, pain of chronically damaged roots seldom responds to these measures. Repeated exploration and decompression of traumatized roots is usually futile and may further increase the patient's pain. In a study of 34 patients with failed back surgery syndrome, some with MRI-documented epidural fibrosis, trials of epidurography and attempted lysis of adhesions by fluid injection produced some improvement of contrast spread without any lasting improvement of pain (Devulder et al 1995). Rhizotomy at the time of re-exploration is not apt to be beneficial (Bertrand 1975) and may lead to a very unpleasant deafferentation syndrome. Approximately 2–3% of patients with chronic low back pain and sciatica due to failed back surgery syndrome may be relieved temporarily by local anaesthetic block of one or two lumbosacral roots (Taub et al 1995). Dorsal root ganglionectomy in these cases was said to relieve sciatica, but not back pain, in 59% of cases. However, there was a high incidence of dysaesthesias often requiring additional treatment measures afterward. Other authors have found ganglionectomy ineffective for chronic sciatica in failed back surgery syndrome (Gybels & Sweet 1989, North et al 1991a). Electrical spinal cord stimulation is a safer and less destructive means of treating this condition and should be considered the current surgical procedure of choice, as discussed below.

The management of pain in chronic arachnoiditis continues to be a discouraging problem. Initially, cultures of cerebrospinal fluid should be done to eliminate the possibility of a chronic low-grade infection. The presence of fibrosis in the spinal canal may make it dangerous to attempt administration of epidural drugs for pain management in these cases (O'Connor et al 1990). Steroids have been advocated; there is no objective proof of their effectiveness and, as noted above, their use intrathecally may even contribute to arachnoiditis. The rationale of steroid therapy has its basis in animal studies showing diminution of the aseptic maningeal inflammatory reaction to blood and radiographic contrast agents (Howland & Curry 1966). This may not be analogous to the severe chronic adhesive process seen in humans. Lumbar air insufflation and radiation therapy have not been shown to have any value in this condition (Whisler 1978). In occasional cases, the inflammatory process is focal enough that dorsal rhizotomies or dorsal root ganglionectomies help (Jain 1974), but the risks of postoperative dysaesthesias and deafferentation pain are unattractive ones. Lysis of intradural adhesions by tedious microsurgery has its proponents, but the results are equivocal. Microscopic lysis in 28 patients did not produce better results than conservative treatment, according to Johnston and Matheny (1978). Myelography showed reaccumulation of arachnoid loculations in all cases examined. Wilkinson and Schuman (1979) reported initial pain relief in 76% of cases after extensive dissection of adhesions under the operating microscope and 50% were still relieved after 1 year. Gourie-Devi and Satish (1984) described intrathecal use of the proteolytic enzyme hyaluronidase in chronic spinal arachnoiditis. Early improvement of neurological status was seen in 11 of 15 patients, with no serious toxic effects. Of 66 patients with spinal arachnoiditis secondary to tuberculous meningitis, 39 were given intrathecal hyaluronidase in addition to the usual antituberculous drugs. These patients appeared to have reduced mortality and improved functional deficit scores in comparison with the group not receiving hyaluronidase (Gourie-Devi & Satishchandra 1991). Hyaluronidase therapy has not received widespread usage outside India so far and its potential role in the treatment of arachnoiditis after failed back surgery remains to be determined.

In a randomized, double-blind 6-month crossover trial of d-penicillamine versus placebo to treat chronic arachnoiditis, 13 of 17 patients reported no clear preference and one actually preferred the placebo, while the remaining three strongly preferred d-penicillamine (Grahame et al 1991). Although no statistically significant effect of d-penicillamine could be demonstrated, the authors felt that there might be a small subgroup of patients with arachnoiditis who could benefit from the drug.

Currently the most promising treatment for chronic radicular pain associated with epidural fibrosis or arachnoiditis is electrical spinal cord stimulation (SCS). Technological advances in stimulation equipment have made this procedure increasingly attractive for large numbers of patients. In particular, bilateral electrode arrays and multichannel stimulator systems make it feasible to treat bilateral sciatica and even low back pain in cases of failed back surgery syndrome. Although SCS has a long-term success rate equal to or better than that of reoperation (North et al 1991b), SCS is clearly less risky. Although patients strongly habituated to narcotics and those with prominent behaviour disorders or long-standing unresolved compensation claims may be poor candidates, SCS is still applicable to a much larger proportion of the population of patients with failed back surgery syndrome than is ablative nerve root surgery. Moreover, implantation of a spinal cord stimulator is a reversible procedure that is very unlikely to leave permanent dysaesthesias or other neurological complications. Electrode placements for lumbar radiculopathy are typically between T8 and T12. Therefore, patients wary of further spinal surgery are usually relieved to learn that a trial of cord stimulation will not require surgical reopening of the laminectomy site.

In the literature review by North (1998), a majority of authors reporting long-term results of SCS specifically for failed back surgery syndrome saw good or excellent results in more than 60% of their cases. However, this excludes cases subjected to preliminary trials of SCS without permanent implantation. SCS is somewhat more effective for unilateral than for bilateral sciatica (Meilman et al 1989, Kumar et al 1991). When arachnoiditis is present, the outcome of SCS appears to be primarily related to the number of roots involved (Meilman et al 1989). As might be expected, patients with injury to a single root respond more favourably than do patients with multiple root damage. Technical difficulties such as hardware infection, electrode migration and difficulty finding or maintaining an effective target in the cord may impede the success of SCS. Nevertheless, when SCS is effective, it can provide a welcome respite for these patients.

REFERENCES

Abramovitz JN, Neff SR 1991 Lumbar disc surgery: results of the prospective lumbar discectomy study of the Joint Section on Disorders of the Spine and Peripheral Nerves of the American Association of Neurological Surgeons and the Congress of Neurological Surgeons. Neurosurgery 29: 301–308

Adams JH 1976 Virus diseases of the nervous system. In: Blackwood W, Corsellis JAN (eds) Greenfield's neuropathology. Edward Arnold, London, pp 292–326

Aldrete JA 1995 Epidural fibrosis after permanent catheter insertion and infusion. Journal of Pain Symptom Management 10: 624–631

Aminoff MJ, Goodin DS, Barbaro NM, Weinstein PR, Rosenblum ML 1985 Dermatomal somatosensory evoked potentials in unilateral lumbosacral radiculopathy. Annals of Neurology 17: 171–176

Auld AW 1978 Chronic spinal arachnioditis. A postoperative syndrome that may signal its onset. Spine 3: 88–91

Baker AS, Ojemann RG, Swartz MN, Richardson EP 1975 Spinal epidural abscess. New England Journal of Medicine 293: 463–468

Barnsley L, Lord SM, Bogduk N 1993 Comparative local anaesthetic blocks in the diagnosis of cervical zygapophyseal joint pain. Pain 55: 99–106

Barolat G 1998 Spinal cord stimulation for persistent pain management. In: Gildenberg PL, Tasker R R (eds) Textbook of sterotactic and functional neurosurgery. McGraw-Hill, New York, pp 1519–1537

Barron KD, Rowland LP, Zimmerman HM 1960 Neuropathy with malignant tumour metastases. Journal of Nervous and Mental Diseases 131: 10–31

Barton PM 1991 Piriformis syndrome: a rational approach to management. Pain 47: 345–352

Bertrand G 1975 The 'battered' root problem. Orthopedic Clinics of North America 6: 305–309

Bhargava R, Bhargava S, Haldia KN, Bhargava P 1998 Jaipur block in postherpetic neuralgia. International Journal of Dermatology 37: 465–468

Boden SC, Wiesel S W 1992 The multiply operated low back patient. In: Rothman RH, Simeone FA (eds) The spine, 3rd edn. W B Saunders, Philadelphia, pp 1899–1906

Bogduk N 1980 The anatomy of occipital neuralgia. Clinical and Experimental Neurology 17: 167–184

Bogduk N 1982 The clinical anatomy of the cervical dorsal rami. Spine 7: 319–330

Bogduk N, Long DM 1979 The anatomy of the so-called 'articular nerves' and their relationship to facet denervation in the treatment of low back pain. Journal of Neurosurgery 51: 172–177

Bohm E, Franksson C 1959 Coccygodynia and sacral rhizotomy. Acta Chirurgica Scandinavica 116: 268–274

Boulton AMJ, Angus E, Ayyar DR, Weiss R 1984 Diabetic thoracic polyradiculopathy presenting as abdominal swelling. British Medical Journal 289: 798–799

Bowsher D 1997 The management of postherpetic neuralgia. Postgraduate Medical Journal 73: 623–629

Braun IF, Hoffman JC, David PC, Landman JA, Tindall GT 1985 Contrast enhancement in CT differentiation between recurrent disc herniation and postoperative scar: prospective study. American Journal of Radiology 145: 785–790

Brevik H, Hesla PE, Molnar I, Lind B 1976 Treatment of chronic low back pain and sciatica: comparison of caudal epidural steroid injections of bupivacaine and methylprednisolone with bupivacaine followed by saline. In: Bonica J J, Albe-Fessard D (eds) Advances in pain research and therapy, vol 1. Raven Press, New York, pp 927–932

Burton CV 1978 Lumbosacral arachnoiditis. Spine 3: 24–30

Calvin WH, Loeser JD, Howe JF 1977 A neurophysiological theory for the pain mechanism of tic douloureux. Pain 3: 147–154

 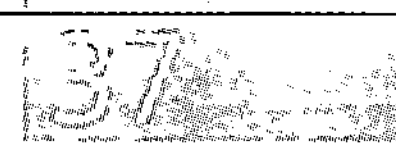

Caplan LR, Norohna AB, Amico LL 1990 Syringomyelia and arachnioditis. Journal of Neurology, Neurosurgery and Psychiatry 53: 106–113

Castagnera L, Maurett P, Pointilart V, Vital JM, Erny P, Senegas J 1994 Long-term results of cervical epidural steroid injection with and without morphine in chronic cervical radicular pain. Pain 58: 239–243

Cervellini P, Curri D, Volpin L, Bernardi L, Pinna V, Benedetti A 1988 Computed tomography of epidural fibrosis after discectomy: a comparison between symptomatic and asymptomatic patients. Neurosurgery 23: 710–713

Chapman EM, Shaw RS, Kubik CS 1964 Sciatic pain from arteriosclerotic aneurysm of pelvic arteries. New England Journal of Medicine 271: 1410–1411

Christensen E 1942 Chronic adhesive spinal arachnoiditis. Acta Psychiatrica Scandinavica 17: 23–38

Clifford DB, Trotter JL 1984 Pain in multiple sclerosis. Archives of Neurology 41: 1270–1272

Cuckler JM, Bernini PA, Wiesel SW, Booth RE, Rothman RH, Pickens GT 1985 The use of epidural steroids in the treatment of lumbar radicular pain: a prospective, randomized, double-blind study. Journal of Bone and Joint Surgery 67A: 63–66

Davis CH 1982 Extradural spinal cord and nerve root compression from benign lesions of the lumbar area. In: Youmans J R (ed) Neurological surgery. W B Saunders, Philadelphia, pp 2535–2561

Davis D 1957 Radicular syndromes. Year Book, Chicago

Delamarter RB, Ross JS, Masaryk TJ, Modic MT, Bohlman H H 1990 Diagnosis of lumbar arachnoiditis by magnetic resonance imaging. Spine 15: 304–310

Delaney TJ, Rowlingson JC, Carron HC, Butler A 1980 Epidural steroid effects on nerves and meninges. Anesthesia and Analgesia 59: 610–614

Denny-Brown D, Kirk EJ, Yanagisawa N 1973 The tract of Lissauer in relation to sensory transmission in the dorsal horn of the spinal cord in the macaque monkey. Journal of Comparative Neurology 151: 175–200

Deparis M 1968 Glossopharyngeal neuralgia. In: Vinken P J, Bruyn G W (eds) Handbook of clinical neurology, vol 5. Headaches and cranial neuralgias. North-Holland, Amsterdam, pp 350–361

De Tribolet N, Porchet F, Lutz TW et al 1998 Clinical assessment of a novel antiadhesion barrier gel: prospective, randomized, multicenter, clinical trial of ADCON-L to inhibit postoperative peridural fibrosis and related symptoms after lumbar discectomy. American Journal of Orthopedics 27: 111–120

Devulder J, Bogaert L, Castille F, Moerman A, Rolly G 1995 Relevance of epidurography and epidural adhesiolysis in chronic failed back surgery patients. Clinical Journal of Pain 11: 147–150

Deyck P 1976 The femoral nerve traction test with lumbar disc protrusions. Surgical Neurology 6: 163–166

Deyo RA, Diehl AK, Rosenthal M 1986 How many days of bed rest for acute low back pain? A randomized clinical trial. New England Journal of Medicine 315: 1064–1070

Dilke TFW, Burry HC, Grahame R 1973 Extradural corticosteroid injection in management of lumbar nerve root compression. British Medical Journal 2: 635–637

Dubuisson D 1995 Treatment of occipital neuralgia by partial posterior rhizotomy at C1–3. Journal of Neurosurgery 82: 581–586

Dubuisson D, Melzack 1976 Classification of clinical pain descriptions by multiple group discriminant analysis. Experimental Neurology 51: 480–487

Dugan MC, Locke S, Gallagher JR 1962 Occipital neuralgia in adolescents and young adults. New England Journal of Medicine 267: 1166–1172

Dujovny M, Barrionuevo PJ, Kossovsky N, Laha RK, Rosenbaum AE 1978 Effects of contrast media on the canine subarachnoid space. Spine 3: 31–35

Dullerud R, Morland TJ 1976 Adhesive arachnoiditis after lumbar radiculography with Dimer-X and Depo-Medrol. Radiology 119: 153–155

Dykes RW, Terzis JK 1981 Spinal nerve distributions in the upper limb: the organization of the dermatome and afferent myotome. Philosophical Transactions of the Royal Society of London (Biology) 293: 509–554

Ehni G, Benner B 1984 Occipital neuralgia and the C1–2 arthrosis syndrome. Journal of Neurosurgery 61: 961–965

Eisen A 1981 Identifying a spinal nerve lesion. American Academy of Neurology, Special Courses 22: 81–92

Eisen A, Elleker G 1980 Sensory nerve stimulation and evoked cerebral potentials. Neurology 30: 1097–1105

Elkington J St C 1951 Arachnoiditis. In: Feiling A (ed) Modern trends in neurology. Hoeber, New York, pp 149–161

Epstein JA, Epstein BS, Rosenthal AD, Carras R, Lavine LS 1972 Sciatica caused by nerve root entrapment in the lateral recess: the superior facet syndrome. Journal of Neurosurgery 36: 584–589

Esses SI, Morley TP 1983 Spinal arachnoiditis. Canadian Journal of Neurological Sciences 10: 2–10

Fager CA 1986 Lumbar microdiscectomy: a contrary opinion. Clinical Neurosurgery 33: 419–456

Fedar BH, Smith JL 1962 Roentgen therapy in chronic spinal arachnoiditis. Radiology 78: 192–198

Fincham RW, Cape CA 1968 Sensory nerve conduction in syringomyelia. Neurology 18: 200–201

Fisher MA, Shivde AJ, Texera C, Grainer LS 1978 Clinical and electrophysiological appraisal of the significance of radicular injury in back pain. Journal of Neurology, Neurosurgery and Psychiatry 41: 303–306

Foerster O 1933 The dermatomes in man. Brain 56: 1–39

Forrest JR 1980 The response to epidural steroid injections in chronic dorsal root pain. Canadian Anesthetists Society Journal 27: 40–46

French JD 1946 Clinical manifestations of lumbar spinal arachnoiditis. Surgery 20: 718–729

Frykholm R 1951 Cervical root compression resulting from disc degeneration and root sleeve fibrosis. Acta Chirurgica Scandinavica 160 (suppl): 1–149

Gebarski SS, Gabrielsen TO, Gilman S, Knake JE, Latack JT, Aisen AM 1985 The initial diagnosis of multiple sclerosis: clinical impact of magnetic resonance imaging. Annals of Neurology 17: 469–474

Gilroy J, Meyer JS 1975 Medical neurology, Macmillan, New York

Goald H 1980 Microlumbar discectomy: follow-up of 477 patients. Journal of Microsurgery 2: 95–100

Gorski DW, Rao TLK, Glisson SN, Chintagada M, El-Etr A 1982 Epidural triamcinolone and adrenal response to hypoglycemic stress in dogs. Anesthesiology 57: 364–366

Gourie-Devi M, Satish P 1984 Intrathecal hyaluronidase treatment of chronic spinal arachnoiditis of noninfective etiology. Surgical Neurology 22: 231–234

Gourie-Devi M, Satishchandra P 1991 Hyaluronidase as an adjuvant in the management of tuberculous spinal arachnoiditis. Journal of the Neurological Sciences 102: 105–111

Grahame R, Clark B, Watson M, Polkey C 1991 Toward a rational therapeutic strategy for arachnoiditis. A possible role for d-penicillamine. Spine 16: 172–175

Green LN 1975 Dexamethasone in the management of symptoms due to herniated lumbar disc. Journal of Neurology, Neurosurgery and Psychiatry 38: 1211–1217

Green PWB, Burke AJ, Weiss CA, Langan P 1980 The role of epidural cortisone injection in the treatment of discogenic low back pain. Clinical Orthopedics 153: 121–125

Guyer DW, Wiltse LL, Eskay ML , Guyer BH 1989 The long-range prognosis of arachnoiditis. Spine 14: 1332–1341
Gybels JM, Sweet WH 1989 Neurosurgical treatment of persistent pain. Physiological and pathological mechanisms of human pain. Karger, New York
Haughton VM, Ho KC 1982 Effect of blood on arachnoiditis from aqueous myelographic contrast media. American Journal of Roentgenology 139: 569–570
Haughton VM, Ho KC, Larson SJ, Unger GF, Correa-Paz F 1977 Experimental production of arachnoiditis with water-soluble myelographic media. Radiology 123: 681–685
Head H, Campbell AW 1900 The pathology of herpes zoster and its bearing on sensory localization. Brain 23: 353–523
Hill CA, Hunter JV, Moseley IF, Kendall BE 1992 Does Myodil introduced for ventriculography lead to symptomatic lumbar arachnoiditis? British Journal of Radiology 65: 1105–1107
Hitselberger WE, Witten RM 1968 Abnormal myelograms in asymptomatic patients. Journal of Neurosurgery 28: 204–206
Horwich MS, Cho L, Porro RS, Posner JB 1977 Subacute sensory neuropathy: a remote effect of carcinoma. Annals of Neurology 2: 7–19
Hosobuchi Y 1980 The majority of unmyelinated afferent axons in human ventral roots probably conduct pain. Pain 8: 167–180
Howe JF, Loeser JD, Calvin WH 1977 Mechanosensitivity of dorsal root ganglia and chronically injured axons: a physiological basis for the radicular pain of nerve root compression. Pain 3: 25–41
Howland WJ, Curry JL 1966 Pantopaque arachnoiditis. Experimental study of blood as a potentiating agent and corticosteroids as an ameliorating agent. Acta Radiological 5: 1032–1041
Hoyland JA, Freemont AJ, Denton J, Thomas AM, McMillan JJ, Jayson MI 1988 Retained surgical swab debris in post-laminectomy arachnoiditis and peridural fibrosis. Journal of Bone and Joint Surgery 70: 659–662
Hueftle MG, Modic MT, Ross JS et al 1988 Lumbar spine: postoperative MR imaging with Gd-DPTA. Radiology 167: 817–824
Hughes DG, Isherwood I 1992 How frequent is chronic lumbar arachnoiditis following intrathecal Myodil? British Journal of Radiology 65: 758–760
Hunt JR 1915 The sensory field of the facial nerve: a further contribution to the symptomatology of the geniculate ganglion. Brain 38: 418–446
Hunter CR, Mayfield FH 1949 Role of the upper cervical roots in the production of pain in the head. American Journal of Surgery 78: 743–751
Inman VT, Saunders JB, De CM 1944 Referred pain from skeletal structures. Journal of Nervous and Mental Diseases 99: 660–667
Iskandar BJ, Nashold BS 1988 Spinal and trigeminal DREZ lesions. In: Gildenberg PL, Tasker R R (eds) Textbook of stereotactic and functional neurosurgery. McGraw-Hill, New York, pp 1573–1583
Jackson JL, Gibbons R, Meyer G, Inouye L 1997 The effect of treating herpes zoster with oral acyclovir in preventing postherpetic neuralgia. Archives of Internal Medicine 157: 909–912
Jain KK 1974 Nerve root scarring and arachnoiditis as a complication of lumbar intervertebral disc surgery. Surgical treatment. Neurochirurgia 17: 185–192
Johnson A, Ryan MD, Roche J 1991 Depo-Medrol and myelographic arachnoiditis. Medical Journal of Australia 155: 18–20
Johnson CE, Sze G 1990 Benign lumbar arachnoiditis: MR imaging with gadopentetate dimeglumine. American Journal of Neuroradiology 11: 763–770
Johnson EW, Fletcher ER 1981 Lumbosacral radiculopathy: review of 100 consecutive cases. Archives of Physical Medicine and Rehabilitation 62: 321–323
Johnston JDH, Matheny JB 1978 Microscopic lysis of lumbar adhesive arachnoiditis. Spine 3: 36–39
Junck L, Marshall WH 1983 Neurotoxicity of radiological contrast agents. Annals of Neurology 13: 469–484
Kahanovitz N, Viola K, McCulloch J 1989 Limited surgical discectomy and microdiscectomy. A clinical comparison. Spine 14: 79–81
Keegan JJ, Garrett FD 1948 The segmental distribution of the cutaneous nerves in the limbs of man. Anatomical Record 102: 409–437
Kellgren JH 1939 On the distribution of pain arising from deep somatic structures with charts of segmental pain areas. Clinical Science 4: 35–46
Kelly M 1956 Is pain due to pressure on nerves? Neurology 6: 32–36
Kendall HO, Kendall FP, Wadsworth GE 1971 Muscles: testing and function. Williams & Wilkins, Baltimore
Kerr FWL 1961 A mechanism to account for frontal headache in cases of posterior fossa tumors. Journal of Neurosurgery 18: 605–609
Kibler RF, Nathan PW 1960 Relief of pain and paresthesiae by nerve block distal to the lesion. Journal of Neurology, Neurosurgery and Psychiatry 23: 91–98
Kirk EJ, Denny-Brown D 1970 Functional variation in dermatomes in the macaque monkey following dorsal root lesions. Journal of Comparative Neurology 139: 307–320
Kondo A 1998 Follow-up results of using microvascular decompression for treatment of glossopharyngeal neuralgia. Journal of Neurosurgery 88: 221–225
Kumar K, Nath R, Wyant GM 1991 Treatment of chronic pain by epidural spinal cord stimulation: a 10 year experience. Journal of Neurosurgery 75: 402–407
Laha RK, Jannetta PJ 1977 Glossopharyngeal neuralgia. Journal of Neurosurgery 47: 316–320
Lance JW, Anthony M 1980 Neck-tongue syndrome on sudden turning of the head. Journal of Neurology, Neurosurgery and Psychiatry 43: 97–101
Levine JD, Lau W, Kwiat G, Goetzl EJ 1984 Leukotriene B4 produces hyperalgesia that is dependent on polymorphonuclear leukocytes. Science 225: 743–745
Lindahl O, Rexed B 1951 Histologic changes in spinal nerve roots of operated cases of sciatica. Acta Orthopaedica Scandinavica 20: 215–225
Lindblom K, Rexed B 1948 Spinal nerve injury in dorsalateral protrusions of lumbar discs. Journal of Neurosurgery 5: 413–432
Lipton S 1979 Relief of pain in clinical practice. Blackwell, Oxford, pp 231–248
Little JR, Dale AJD, Okazaki H 1974 Meningeal carcinomatosis: clinical manifestations. Archives of Neurology 30: 138–143
Loeser JD, Ward AA, White LE 1968 Chronic deafferentation of human spinal cord neurons. Journal of Neurosurgery 29: 48–50
Long DM 1982 Pain of spinal origin. In: Youmans J R (ed) Neurological surgery. W B Saunders, Philadelphia, pp 3613–3626
Lovely TJ, Jannetta PJ 1997 Surgical management of geniculate neuralgia. American Journal of Otolaryngology 18: 512–517
Lozano AM, Vanderlinden G, Bachoo R, Rothbart P 1998 Microsurgical C2 ganglionectomy for chronic intractable occipital pain. Journal of Neurosurgery 89: 359–365
Lundborg G 1988 Intraneural microcirculation. Orthopedic Clinics of North America 19: 1–12
MacNab I 1971 Negative disc exploration. An analysis of the causes of nerve root involvement in 68 patients. Journal of Bone and Joint Surgery 53A: 891–903
Maigne J-Y, Rime B, Deligne B 1992 Computed tomographic follow-up study of forty-eight cases of nonoperatively treated lumbar intervertebral disc herniation. Spine 17: 1071–1074
Maroon JC, Abla AA 1986 Microlumbar discectomy. Clinical Neurosurgery 33: 407–417
Martin-Ferrer S 1989 Failure of autologous fat grafts to prevent postoperative epidural fibrosis in surgery of the lumbar spine. Neurosurgery 24: 718–721

Matsui H, Tsuji J, Kanamori M, Kawaguchi Y, Yudoh K, Futatsuya R 1995 Laminectomy-induced arachnoradiculitis: a postoperative serial MRI study. Neuroradiology 37: 660–666

Meilman PW, Leibrock LG, Leong FT 1989 Outcome of implanted spinal cord stimulation in the treatment of chronic pain: arachnoiditis versus single nerve root injury and mononeuropathy. Clinical Journal of Pain 5: 189–193

Moulin DE, Foley KM, Ebers GC 1988 Pain syndromes in multiple sclerosis. Neurology 38: 1830–1834

Murphey F 1968 Sources and patterns of pain in disc disease. Clinical Neurosurgery 15: 343–350

Murphey F, Simmons JCH, Brunson B 1973 Ruptured cervical discs, 1939 to 1972. Clinical Neurosurgery 20: 9–17

Nachemson AL 1977 Pathophysiology and treatment of back pain: a critical look at the different types of treatment. In: Buerger A A, Tobis J S (ed) Approaches to the validation of manipulation therapy. Charles C Thomas, Springfield, Illinois, pp 769–779

Nagashima C, Sakaguchi A, Kamisasa A, Kawanuma S 1976 Cardiovascular complications on upper vagal rootlet section for glossopharyngeal neuralgia. Journal of Neurosurgery 44: 248–253

Nathan P, Wall PD 1974 Treatment of postherpetic neuralgia by prolonged electric stimulation. British Medical Journal 14: 645–647

Neiri RL, Burgert EO, Groover RV 1968 Central nervous system leukemia: a review. Mayo Clinic Proceedings 43: 70–79

Nelson DA, Vates TS, Thomas RB 1973 Complications from intrathecal steroid therapy in patients with multiple sclerosis. Acta Neurologica Scandinavica 49: 176–188

Nelson KA, Park KM, Robinovitz E, Tsigos C, Max MB 1997 High-dose oral dextromethorphan versus placebo in painful diabetic neuropathy and postherpetic neuralgia. Neurology 48: 1212–1218

Nordin M, Nystrom B, Wallin U, Hagbarth K-E 1984 Ectopic sensory discharges and paresthesiae in patients with disorders of peripheral nerves, dorsal roots and dorsal columns. Pain 20: 231–245

North RB 1998 Spinal cord stimulation for the failed back surgery syndrome. In: Gildenberg PL, Tasker RR (eds) Textbook of functional and stereotactic neurosurgery. McGraw-Hill, New York, pp 1611–1620

North RB, Campbell JN, James CS et al 1991b Failed back surgery syndrome: five year follow-up in 102 patients undergoing repeated operation. Neurosurgery 28: 685–691

North RB, Han M, Zahurak M, Kidd D H 1994 Radiofrequency lumbar facet denervation: analysis of prognostic factors. Pain 57: 77–83

North RB, Kidd DH, Campbell JN, Long DM 1991a Dorsal root ganglionectomy for failed back surgery syndrome: a 5-year follow-up study. Journal of Neurosurgery 74: 236–242

O'Connor M, Brighouse D, Glynn CJ 1990 Unusual complications in the treatment of chronic spinal arachnoiditis. Clinical Journal of Pain 6: 240–242

Olson ME, Chernik NL, Posner JB 1974 Infiltration of the leptomeninges by systemic cancer. A clinical and pathologic study. Archives of Neurology 30: 122–137

Paty DW, Oger JJF, Kastrukoff LF et al 1988 MRI in the diagnosis of MS: a prospective study with comparison of clinical evaluation, evoked potentials, oligoclonal banding, and CT. Neurology 38: 180–185

Pedersen HE, Blunck CFJ, Gardner E 1956 The anatomy of the lumbosacral posterior rami and meningeal branches of spinal nerves (sinu-vertebral nerves), with an experimental study of their functions. Journal of Bone and Joint Surgery 38A: 377–391

Persson LC, Carlsson CA, Carlsson JY 1997 Long-lasting cervical radicular pain managed with surgery, physiotherapy, or a cervical collar. A prospective, randomized study. Spine 22: 751–758

Poletti CE 1983 Proposed operation for occipital neuralgia: C2 and C3 root decompression. Neurosurgery 12: 221–224

Poletti CE 1991 C2 and C3 pain dermatomes in man. Cephalalgia 11: 155–159

Poletti CE 1996 Third cervical nerve root and ganglion compression: clinical syndrome, surgical anatomy, and pathological findings. Neurosurgery 39: 941–949

Quiles M, Marchisello PJ, Tsairis P 1978 Lumbar adhesive arachnoiditis. Etiologic and pathologic aspects. Spine 3: 45–50

Ramirez-Lassepas M, Tulloch JW, Quinones MR, Snyder BD 1992 Acute radicular pain as a presenting symptom in multiple sclerosis. Archives of Neurology 49: 255–258

Rasminsky M 1980 Ephaptic transmission between single nerve fibres in the spinal nerve roots of dystrophic mice. Journal of Physiology 305: 151–169

Ray CG 1980 Chickenpox (varicella) and herpes zoster. In: Isselbacher K J et al (eds) Harrison's principles of internal medicine. McGraw-Hill, New York, pp 801–804

Resnick DK, Jannetta PJ, Bisonette D, Jho H-D, Lanzino G 1995 Microvascular decompression for glossopharyngeal neuralgia. Neurosurgery 36: 64–69

Rhoton AL Jr, Oliveira E 1990 Microsurgical anatomy of the region of the foramen magnum. In: Wilkins RH, Rengachary SS (eds) Neurosurgery update I. McGraw-Hill, New York, pp 434–460

Robson JT, Bonica JJ 1950 The vagus nerve in surgical consideration of glossopharyngeal neuralgia. Journal of Neurosurgery 7: 482–484

Rocovich PM 1947 Adhesive spinal arachnoiditis. Bulletin of the Los Angeles Neurological Society 12: 69–77

Ross JS, Delamarter R, Hueftle MG et al 1989 Gadolinium-DPTA-enhanced MR imaging of the postoperative lumbar spine. American Journal of Neuroradiology 10: 37–46

Ross JS, Robertson JT, Frederickson RCA et al 1996 Association between peridural scar and recurrent radicular pain after lumbar discectomy: magnetic resonance evaluation. Neurosurgery 38: 855–863

Rothman SLG, Glenn WV, Kerber CW 1985 Postoperative fractures of lumbar articular facets: occult cause of radiculopathy. American Journal of Neuroradiology 145: 779–784

Rowbotham MC, Davies PS, Fields HL 1995 Topical lidocaine gel relieves postherpetic neuralgia. Annals of Neurology 37: 246–253

Rupa V, Saunders RL, Weider DJ 1991 Geniculate neuralgia: the surgical management of primary otalgia. Journal of Neurosurgery 75: 505–511

Rushton JG, Stevens JC, Miller RH 1981 Glossopharyngeal (vagoglossopharyngeal) neuralgia. Archives of Neurology 38: 201–205

Saal JA, Dillingham MF, Gamburd RS, Fanton GS 1988 The pseudoradicular syndrome. Lower extremity peripheral nerve entrapment masquerading as lumbar radiculopathy. Spine 13: 926–930

Saal JS, Franson RC, Dobrow R, Saal JA, White AH, Goldthwaite N 1990 High levels of inflammatory phospholipase A2 activity in lumbar disc herniations. Spine 15: 674–678

Schutz H, Lougheed WM, Wortzman G, Awerbuck BG 1973 Intervertebral nerve root in the investigation of chronic lumbar disc disease. Canadian Journal of Surgery 16: 217–221

Seaman WB, Marder SN, Rosenbaum HE 1953 The myelographic appearance of adhesive spinal arachnoiditis. Journal of Neurosurgery 10: 145–153

See DH, Kraft GH 1975 Electromyography in paraspinal muscles following surgery for root compression. Archives of Physical Medicine and Rehabilitation 56: 80–83

Shaw MDM, Russell JA, Grossart KW 1978 The changing pattern of spinal arachnoiditis. Journal of Neurology, Neurosurgery and Psychiatry 41: 97–107

Sherrington CS 1898 Experiments in the examination of the peripheral distribution of the fibres of the posterior roots of some spinal nerves. Part II. Philosophical Transactions B 190: 45–186

Skalpe IO 1976 Adhesive arachnoiditis following lumbar radiculography with water-soluble agents. A clinical report with special reference to metrizamide. Radiology 121: 647–651

Smith DL, Lucas LM, Kumar KL 1987 Greater occipital neuralgia: an unusual presenting feature of neurosyphilis. Headache 27: 552–554

Smith RW, Loeser JD 1972 A myelographic variant in lumbar arachnoiditis. Journal of Neurosurgery 36: 441–446

Smyth MJ, Wright V 1958 Sciatica and the intervertebral disc. Journal of Bone and Joint Surgery 40A: 1401–1418

Snoek W, Weber H, Jorgensen B 1977 Double blind evaluation of extradural methylprednisolone for herniated lumbar disc. Acta Orthopaedica Scandinavica 48: 635–641

Spangfort EV 1972 The lumbar disc herniation. Acta Orthopaedica Scandinavica 142 (suppl): 1–95

Spiegelmann R, Friedman W A 1991 Spinal cord stimulation: a contemporary series. Neurosurgery 28: 65–71

Stewart JD 1987 Focal peripheral neuropathies. Elsevier, New York

Storm-Mathisen A 1978 Syphilis. In: Vinken PJ, Bruyn G W (eds) Handbook of clinical neurology. North-Holland, Amsterdam, pp 337–394

Taha JM, Tew JM Jr 1995 Long-term results of surgical treatment of idiopathic neuralgias of the glossopharyngeal and vagal nerves. Neurosurgery 36: 926–929

Taub A, Robinson F, Taub E 1995 Dorsal root ganglionectomy for intractable monoradicular sciatica. In: Schmidek HH, Sweet WH (eds) Operative neurosurgical techniques, 3rd edn. W B Saunders, Philadelphia, pp 1585–1593

Teplick JG, Haskin ME 1984 Intravenous contrast-enhanced CT of the postoperative lumbar spine: improved identification of recurrent disk herniation, scar, arachnoiditis, and diskitis. American Journal of Roentgenology 143: 845–855

Tyring S, Barbarash RA, Nahlik JE et al 1995 Famciclovir for the treatment of acute herpes zoster: effects on acute disease and postherpetic neuralgia. A randomized, double-blind, placebo-controlled trial. Collaborative Famciclovir Herpes Zoster Study Group. Annals of Internal Medicine 123: 89–96

Uldry PA, Regli F 1992 Pseudoradicular syndrome in multiple sclerosis. Four cases diagnosed by magnetic resonance imaging. Revue Neurologique 148: 692–695

Upton ARM, McComas AJ 1973 The double crush in nerve entrapment syndromes. Lancet 2: 359–360

Van Goethem JW, Van de Kleft E, Biltjes IG et al 1996 MRI after successful lumbar discectomy. Neuroradiology 38 (suppl 1): S90–S96

Verbiest H 1954 A radicular syndrome from developmental narrowing of the lumbar vertebral canal. Journal of Bone and Joint Surgery 36B: 230–237

Vishnawath B, Fawzy A, Franson R 1988 Edema inducing activity of phospholipase A2 purified from human synovial fluid and inhibition by aristolochic acid. Inflammation 12: 549

Wall PD 1977 The presence of ineffective synapses and the circumstances which unmask them. Philosophical Transactions of the Royal Society of London 278: 361–372

Wall PD 1980 The role of substantia gelatinosa as a gate control. In: Bonica J J (ed) Pain. Raven Press, New York, pp 205–231

Wall PD, Devor M 1983 Sensory afferent impulses originate from dorsal root ganglia as well as from the periphery in normal and nerve-injured rats. Pain 17: 321–339

Wall PD, Waxman S, Basbaum AI 1974 Ongoing activity in peripheral nerve: injury discharge. Experimental Neurology 45: 576–589

Warren J, Guttman L, Figueroa AP, Bloor BM 1969 Electromyographic changes of brachial plexus root avulsions. Journal of Neurosurgery 31: 137–140

Wasserstrom WR, Glass JP, Posner JB 1982 Diagnosis and treatment of leptomeningeal metastases from solid tumours. Cancer 49: 759–772

Weinstein PR, Ehni G, Wilsou CB 1977 Lumbar spondylosis. Year Book, Chicago

Whisler WW 1978 Chronic spinal arachnoiditis. In: Vinken PJ, Bruyn GW (eds) Handbook of clinical neurology, vol 33. North-Holland, New York, pp 263–274

White AA, Derby R, Wynne G 1980 Epidural injections for the diagnosis and treatment of low back pain. Spine 5: 78–86

White JC, Sweet WH 1969 Pain and the neurosurgeon. Charles C Thomas, Springfield, Illinois

Wiesel SW, Tsoumas N, Feffer HL, Citrin CM, Patronas N 1984 A study of computer-assisted tomography. The incidence of positive CAT scans in an asymptomatic group of patients. Spine 9: 549–551

Wilkinson HA 1992 Intrathecal Depo-Medrol: a literature review. Clinical Journal of Pain 8: 49–52

Wilkinson HA, Schuman N 1979 Results of surgical lysis of lumbar adhesive arachnoiditis. Neurosurgery 4: 401–409

Wilkinson M 1971 Cervical spondylosis. Heinemann, London

Williams RW 1983 Microsurgical discectomy: a surgical alternative for initial disc herniation. In: Cauthen J (ed) Lumbar spine surgery. Williams & Wilkins, Baltimore, pp 85–98

Wilson DH, Harbaugh R 1981 Microsurgical and standard removal of the protruded lumbar disc: a comparative study. Neurosurgery 8: 422–425

Wilson DH, Kenning J 1979 Microsurgery lumbar discectomy: preliminary report of 83 corrective cases. Neurosurgery 4: 137–140

Wynn Parry CB 1980 Pain in avulsion lesions of the brachial plexus. Pain 9: 41–53

Xavier AV, Farrell CE, McDanal J, Kissin I 1990 Does antidromic activation of nociceptors play a role in sciatic radicular pain? Pain 40: 77–79

Central pain

JÖRGEN BOIVIE

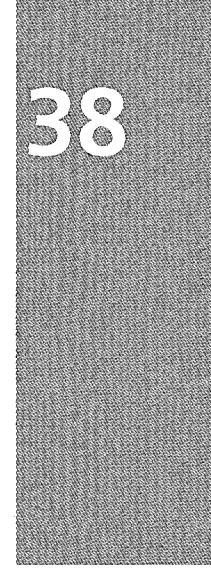

SUMMARY

The International Assocation for the Study of Pain (IASP) has defined central pain as pain caused by a lesion or dysfunction in the central nervous system (CNS) (Merskey & Bogduk 1994). Note that the cause is a primary process in the CNS. Thus peripherally induced pain with central mechanisms is not central pain, even if the central mechanisms are prominent. As with all definitions, there are conditions which may or may not be included. In the present context pain due to brachial plexus avulsion and phantom pain are such examples. They will not be discussed in this chapter. Painful epileptic seizures are evoked by primary processes in the CNS and may thus be considered central pain.

The term 'thalamic pain' is often used in a general sense for all central pain and the expression 'pseudothalamic pain' is sometimes used for central pain caused by extrathalamic lesions. The term 'dysaesthetic pain' is also sometimes used for central pain in general, probably due to the belief that all or almost all central pain has a predominantly dysaesthetic character, which is incorrect. Dysaesthetic pain can have either central or peripheral causes. It is recommended that the general term central pain be used in most instances, and that only central pain caused by lesions in the thalamus should be labelled thalamic pain.

The term 'anaesthesia dolorosa' has chiefly been used for head and face pain, and in particular for the neurogenic pain that sometimes develops after neurosurgical lesions of the trigeminal nerve or ganglion, or after destructive nerve blocks carried out to treat trigeminal neuralgia. It has also been used for central pain in an anaesthetic region caused by neurosurgical brain lesions created in the treatment of severe pain.

The term 'deafferentation pain' is used for similar conditions, but it is more commonly used in patients with lesions of spinal nerves.

INTRODUCTION AND HISTORICAL PERSPECTIVE

Central pain is commonly thought of as being excruciating pain with bizarre character, and covering large areas of the body. This is only part of the truth, however, because central pain can appear in many guises. It can have a trivial character and be restricted to a relatively small area, such as distal pain in one arm, or in the face. It is true, though, that central pain is mostly severe in the sense that it causes the patient much suffering, even though its intensity may be relatively low. This is because central pain is commonly very irritating and is largely constant.

Central pain has often been overlooked as a possibility in patients with CNS diseases, because of poor knowledge of its characteristics. This may cause puzzling symptoms when several coexisting pains of unusual nature exist. Not infrequently central pain has been thought to be of psychogenic origin. One reason for the lack of knowledge concerning central pain is the fact that relatively little systematic research has been carried out on the clinical aspects of central pain. Publications in the literature largely consist of case reports, reviews and studies on particular aspects, rather than more general studies characterizing central pain occurring after various kinds of lesions and diseases in the CNS. The lack of experimental models for central pain until recently has also contributed to the situation, because this has hampered research into its mechanisms.

Historically central pain appears to have first been knowingly described as early as 1883 by Greiff in a patient who, following cerebrovascular lesions, developed lasting pain ('reissende Schmetzen' – tearing pain) (Greiff 1883). The lesion included the thalamus. Eight years later Edinger (1891) presented arguments for the existence of central pain. By then it was known that sensory pathways project to the thalamus, which was therefore at an early stage thought to play a crucial role in central pain. Throughout the years thalamic pain, i.e. pain caused by thalamic lesions, has remained the best-known form of central pain. For this reason all kinds of central pain are often called thalamic pain, although only a minority is related to thalamic lesions.

The most cited early description of central pain is Dejerine and Roussy's classic report (Dejerine & Roussy 1906). They studied six patients with thalamic syndromes including central pain. According to them the syndrome is characterized by:

1. slight hemiplegia
2. disturbances of superficial and deep sensibility
3. hemiataxia and hemiastereognosia
4. intolerable, persistent and paroxysmal pain
5. choreoathetoid movements.

The cause of the syndrome is usually a thalamic infarction or haemorrhage (Garcin 1968). However, in the three patients in which Dejerine and Roussy carried out post-mortem microscopy, the lesions extended lateral to the thalamus to include the posterior part of the internal capsule where the thalamocortical fibres from the ventroposterior thalamic region pass to the cerebral cortex. This has been a common feature in other patients with thalamic lesions reported in the literature. Few patients have had complete thalamic syndromes, which are evidently very rare, but thalamic pain, i.e. pain caused by a thalamic lesion, is less rare (Riddoch 1938, Schott et al 1986, Bogousslavsky et al 1988, Leijon et al 1989, Bowsher 1996, Bowsher et al 1998).

Although interest in central pain was mainly focused on thalamic pain for many years, Edinger had already in 1891 introduced the idea that cortical lesions might also cause pain (Edinger 1891). He further mentioned that the aura of epileptic seizures can include the experience of pain, which has since been reported by several authors. It has now also been demonstrated beyond doubt that lesions above the thalamus can cause central pain (e.g., Davidson & Schick 1935, Schuster 1936 (cases 29 and 32), Ajuraguerra 1937, Biemond 1956, Garcin 1968, Fields & Adams 1974, Leijon et al 1989, Michel et al 1990, Schmahmann & Leifer 1992, Bowsher et al 1998, Pagni 1998), but it is still uncertain whether a lesion strictly limited to the cortex can lead to central pain, because in all cases published, the lesions have also included some subcortical white matter (Breuer et al 1981, Sandyk 1985, Michel et al 1990).

Evidence showing that lesions in the brainstem can evoke central pain has also been accumulating (Riddoch 1938, Garcin 1968, Cassinari & Pagni 1969, Tasker 1990, Bowsher et al 1998, Pagni 1998). The most common site of these lesions has been the medulla oblongata, whereas few cases of pontine and midbrain lesions with central pain have been reported. Only rare cases of midbrain lesions are known, mainly after mesencephalic tractotomies (Drake & Mckenzie 1953). Pontobulbar lesions have been dominated by infarctions in the territory of the posterior inferior cerebellar artery (PICA), but also syringobulbia, multiple sclerosis and tumours can give rise to central pain.

An early description of central pain after traumatic spinal cord injuries (SCI) was published by Holmes, who had noticed this form of pain in soldiers injured in the First World War (Holmes 1919). In the report he did not use the term central pain, but remarked that the pain and hypersensitivity resembled that found in thalamic syndromes. This pain started shortly after the injury and subsided spontaneously after about 1 month. It has since been shown that long-lasting central pain is common after SCI, and is actually one of the major problems in patients with traumatic SCI. Central pain is also common in several other forms of myelopathy, for instance in multiple sclerosis, syringomyelia and vascular malformations.

Many descriptions of central pain syndrome were published during the first three decades of the twentieth century, showing that the character of this pain can vary considerably from patient to patient and that central pain can be excruciating. Because these case reports vividly illustrate this kind of pain, some of the descriptions given by Head and Holmes will be cited: 'crushed feeling, scalding sensation, as if boiling water was being poured down the arm, cramping, aching, soreness, as if the leg was bursting, something crawling under the skin, pain pumping up and down the side, as if the painful region was covered with ulcers, as if pulling a dressing from a wound, as if a log of wood was hanging down from the shoulder, as if little pins were sticking into the fingers, like a wheel running over the arm, cold stinging feeling' (Head & Holmes 1911); 'as if knives heated in Hell's hottest corner were tearing me to pieces' (Holmes 1919). In a more recent report of a patient with central poststroke pain with unknown location, the following pain components were described: 'boiling hot, deep as though in the bones, showers of pain like electric shocks or red-hot needles evoked by touch, as though the arm and leg were being twisted, continuous sensation of pins and needles, a strange sensation of the limbs being abnormally full' (Loh et al 1981).

AETIOLOGY AND EPIDEMIOLOGY

LESIONS CAUSING CENTRAL PAIN

Structure and location of the lesion

It appears that all kinds of lesion in the brain and spinal cord can cause central pain (Box 38.1). These lesions and

BOX 38.1

Causes of central pain

Vascular lesions in the brain and spinal cord
- infarct
- haemorrhage
- vascular malformation

Multiple sclerosis
Traumatic spinal cord injury
- cordotomy

Traumatic brain injury
Syringomyelia and syringobulbia
Tumours
Abscesses
Inflammatory diseases other than MS; myelitis caused by viruses, syphilis
Epilepsy
Parkinson's disease

dysfunctions are caused by many different disease processes. The macrostructure of the lesion is probably less important than its location as regards the probability that it will induce central pain. This does not mean that the structure of the lesion has no significance, because it is conceivable that the microstructure of the lesion in some instances is critical, but there is to date no information from research on this matter.

Pain in Parkinson's disease has previously not been considered central pain. Recent surveys show that pain is common in this disease, but it is at present not clear to what extent this pain is caused directly by the brain pathology. It is possible though that much of the pain is of central origin and thus is central pain.

The lesions that lead to central pain include rapidly and slowly developing lesions. There appears to be no difference in the tendency to cause central pain between rapidly developing haemorrhages, infarcts (Leijon et al 1989, Pagni 1998, Bowsher et al 1998), and traumatic spinal cord lesions, and slowly developing demyelination or arteriovenous malformations. Syringomyelia very often leads to central pain, but it is unlikely that this has anything to do with the fact that the lesion develops extremely slowly. As the prevalence of central pain is very low in patients with intracranial tumours and spinal tumours, it is difficult to know whether or not they differ in this respect, and if there is any difference between intra- and extraparenchymal tumours. Besides the common kind of constant central pain, tumours may also cause painful epileptic seizures.

It is now clear that lesions at any level along the neuraxis can cause central pain. Thus lesions at the first synapse in the dorsal horn of the spinal cord or trigeminal nuclei, along the ascending pathways through the spinal cord and brainstem, in the thalamus, in the subcortical white matter and probably in the cerebral cortex have all been reported to cause central pain (Riddoch 1938, Garcin 1968, Cassinari & Pagni 1969, Leijon et al 1989, Tasker 1990, Bowsher 1996, Bowsher et al 1998, Pagni 1998). The highest prevalences have been noticed after lesions in the spinal cord, lower brainstem and ventroposterior part of the thalamus (Tasker 1990, Bonica 1991, Boivie 1992).

The location of lesions that produce central pain has been best studied in central poststroke pain (CPSP). The role of thalamic lesions is one of the recurrent questions in this context. In one study it was found that nine of 27 patients had lesions involving the thalamus (33%), but the lesions were restricted to the thalamus in only two of these (Leijon et al 1989). These results were based on X-ray CT scans. In their prospective study, Andersen et al had 25% thalamic involvement among the CPSP patients (by CT scans), but in a recently published study of 70 patients using magnetic resonance imaging (MRI) it was found that about 60% had lesions engaging the thalamus (Bowsher et al 1998).

The importance of the location of the thalamic lesion within the thalamus was elucidated in a study of the clinical consequencies of thalamic infarcts. The results showed that only patients with lesions including the ventroposterior thalamic region developed central pain (Bogousslavsky et al 1988). Three of 18 patients with such infarcts had central pain at follow-up, whereas none of the 22 patients with other locations, including a medially located one, had central pain. In studies carried out by Bowsher et al (1998) and Leijon et al (1989) all thalamic lesions included part of the ventroposterior thalamic region. This is in accordance with Hassler's idea that the posterior inferior part of the ventroposterior region, i.e. his V.c.p.c or VPI in recent terminology, is the crucial location for thalamic lesions causing central pain (Hassler 1960). This region receives a particularly dense spinothalamic projection in primates (Boivie 1979).

It was recognized at an early stage that subcortical lesions can induce central pain, but there has been continuing argument whether superficial lesions in the cerebral cortex can also have that effect. This question can still not be given a definite answer, because lesions restricted to the cortex are rare. Usually the lesions damage more or less of the subcortical white matter too. Several central pain patients with such combined lesions and lesions located just deep to the cortex have been published, particularly with lesions in the insular region, i.e. in the second somatosensory region (Michelson 1943, Biemond 1956, Bender &

Jaffe 1958, Michel et al 1990, McNamara et al 1991, Schmahmann & Leifer 1992, Pagni 1998). These lesions have included infarcts, haematomas, meningiomas and traumatic lesions. Some of the patients with superficial lesions have had painful partial epileptic seizures. This is a strong argument for the idea that cortical lesions can lead to central pain, because epileptic seizures are cortical phenomena.

Lesions affect somatic sensibility

The first requisite for a disease process to produce central pain seems to be that it affects structures involved in somatic sensibility, which is not surprising, because pain is part of somaesthesia. This notion is based on previous reviews, case reports and recent studies in patients with central pain caused by stroke, multiple sclerosis and syringomyelia, which indicate that central pain is independent of non-sensory symptoms and signs (Leijon et al 1989, Tasker 1990, Andersen et al 1995, Bowsher 1996, Bowsher et al 1998, Pagni 1998; J Boivie and U Rollsjö, unpublished observations). This excludes many lesion sites as possible causes of central pain. Fortunately, however, only a minority of the patients with lesions that carry a risk will develop central pain. The risk differs very much between diseases and locations of the lesion (see below).

Most patients with central pain reported in the literature have had sensory abnormalities, and the dominating features have been abnormal sensibility to temperature and pain, and hyperaesthesia (Riddoch 1938, Tasker 1990, Pagni 1998). Depending on the location of the lesion, the sensibility profiles differ, often in a predictable way. For instance, after ventroposterior thalamic lesions there is usually a general profound loss of all modalities. After low brainstem infarcts of the Wallenberg type there is a crossed dissociated sensory loss, and after complete spinal cord injuries all sensibility is lost. However if one looks for a common denominator among these patients, abnormal pain and temperature sensibility, together with hyperaesthesia, stand out.

These observations, and results from studies on patients with central pain as a result of cerebrovascular lesions, multiple sclerosis, traumatic spinal cord injuries and syringomyelia employing quantitative methods to assess the sensory abnormalities, form the basis for the hypothesis that central pain only occurs after lesions that affect the spinothalamic pathways, i.e. the pathways that are most important for temperature and pain sensibility (Berić et al 1988, Boivie et al 1989, Boivie 1992, Vestergaard et al 1995, Bowsher et al 1998, Pagni 1998). If this hypothesis turns out to be correct it means that lesions of the dorsal column-medial lemniscal pathways are not a requisite for the occurrence of central pain. Such lesions were for many years thought to be essential in the mechanism of central pain (see below). This hypothesis states that central pain is the result of lesions of the lemniscal system, which remove the inhibition normally exerted on the spinothalamic projections. Undoubtedly the lemniscal projections are affected in many central pain patients, but the question is whether or not this part of the lesion is of importance for the pain. It certainly affects sensibility. No patients with central pain and lesions unequivocally restricted to the lemniscal pathways appear to have been published, whereas many cases of lesions strictly limited to the spinothalamic pathways have been reported, for instance in the Wallenberg syndrome and after cordotomy.

EPIDEMIOLOGY

There are large differences in the prevalence of central pain among the disorders that may lead to such pain (Table 38.1; Bonica 1991). To some extent the figures are estimates, because few epidemiological studies have been carried out. Such estimates are difficult to make, because it is sometimes difficult to distinguish central pain from other possible causes of the pain. This, for instance, is the case in many patients with pain after spinal injury and multiple sclerosis. Nevertheless the figures given in Table 38.1 are probably in the right range, which means that even if pain in epilepsy and Parkinson's disease are excluded, about 278 000 Americans have central pain, i.e. a prevalence of about 115 per 100 000 individuals.

The only prospective epidemiological study that has been carried out concerns central poststroke pain (Andersen et al 1995). In this study 191 patients were followed for 12 months after stroke onset with regard to sensory abnormalities and the development of spontaneous and evoked central pain. Sixteen of these developed central

Table 38.1 Estimated prevalences of major disorders with central pain in the USA 1989 (population around 250 million). (From Bonica 1991 and Österberg & Boivie, in preparation)

Disease	*Total patients (no.)*	*Patients with CP (no.)*	*Patients with CP (%)*
Spinal cord injury	225 000	68 000	30
Multiple sclerosis	150 000	42 000	28
Stroke	2000 000	168 000	8.4
Epilepsy	1600 000	44 800	2.8
Parkinson's disease	500 000	50 000	10

pain, i.e. 8.4%, which is a much higher incidence than had previously been predicted or suspected. Among patients with somatosensory deficits (42% of all stroke patients), the incidence of central pain was 18%. The corresponding figure in a mainly retrospective study of central pain in 63 patients with brainstem infarcts was 44% (MacGowan et al 1997). In this study the overall incidence for CPSP was 25%.

A recent study of the prevalence of central pain in 371 patients with multiple sclerosis has found that 28% of MS patients experience, or have experienced, central pain (A Österberg and J Boivie, in preparation; see below).

The highest prevalences are found with traumatic spinal cord injuries, multiple sclerosis and syringomyelia. The latter is a rare disease with a very high incidence of central pain, probably the highest of any disease. In a recent survey of 22 patients it was found that most had central pain at some stage of the disease (J Boivie and U Rollsjö, unpublished observations).

PATHOPHYSIOLOGY

HYPOTHESES CONCERNING THE MECHANISMS INVOLVED

The lesions that cause central pain vary enormously in location, size and structure. There is no study indicating that a small lesion in the dorsal horn of the spinal cord carries less risk for central pain than a huge infarct involving much of the thalamus and large parts of the white matter lateral and superior to the thalamus. This raises the question whether or not the same pathophysiology underlies all central pain. The fact that the character of the pain also differs widely between patients with the same kind of lesion, and between groups, points in the same direction. However, this does not exclude the possibility that some common pathophysiological factors may be involved in central pain.

For many reasons knowledge about the pathophysiology of central pain is incomplete. This has stimulated several investigators to propose hypotheses concerning the mechanisms involved. The most important will be briefly summarized.

Irritable focus

One of the first hypotheses was that the pain is the result of activity produced by an irritable focus created at the site of injury. This was Dejerine and Roussy's (1906) explanation for thalamic pain.

Disinhibition by lesions in the medial lemniscal pathways

The notion that central pain is caused by lesions in the dorsal column–medial lemniscal pathway has been one of the most favoured hypotheses. The crucial physiological consequence of the lesions is thought to be a disinhibition of neurons in the pain-signalling system, i.e. in the spinothalamic pathways (when this term is used in this chapter it also includes the thalamocortical projections activated via the spinothalamic and spinoreticulothalamic pathways, and the cortical projections via the spinomesencephalic tract). Head and Holmes (1911) were among the first to embrace this notion. They mainly discussed it with regard to corticothalamic connections. Later Foerster (1927) formulated the hypothesis slightly differently when he argued that the epicritic sensibility normally exerts control over the protopathic sensibility. The term epicritic sensibility includes the sensory modalities thought to depend on activity through the lemniscal pathways, i.e. touch, pressure, vibration and kinaesthesia, whereas protopathic sensibility includes pain and temperature. According to this hypothesis central pain can only occur when there is a loss of epicritic sensibility, i.e. a lesion in the lemniscal system.

Lesions in the spinothalamic pathway

In recent years most investigators have found indications that the spinothalamic system is affected in the majority of central pain patients (Beric et al 1988, Boivie et al 1989, Tasker 1990, Bowsher 1995, Vestergaard et al 1995, Bowsher et al 1998, Pagni 1998). These indications include, for instance, the finding that central pain patients have abnormal temperature and pain sensibility, but they may have normal threshold to touch, vibration and joint movements (Beric et al 1988, Boivie et al 1989, Vestergaard et al 1995, Bowsher et al 1998), and that low brainstem infarcts (=Wallenberg syndrome) and cordotomies, in which the spinothalamic but not the lemniscal pathways are injured, cause central pain. This is the basis for the hypothesis that central pain only occurs after lesions affecting the spinothalamic system (Boivie et al 1989, Bowsher 1995, Bowsher et al 1998, Pagni 1998). In many patients the lemniscal pathways are also affected by the lesion, but this does not appear to be necessary for the occurrence of central pain. It even appears possible that the involvement of the lemniscal pathway in no way affects the character of the pain, but it does of course affect the character of the sensory abnormalities. Further elaboration has been made on this hypothesis and it has been proposed that the crucial lesion is one that affects the neospinothalamic projections, by which is meant the projections to the ventroposterior thalamic region (Garcin 1968, Bowsher 1995, Pagni 1998). This kind of lesion is thought to leave the more medially and inferiorly terminating paleospinothalamic projections anatomically intact. This idea is somewhat related to the hypothesis proposing that a lemniscal lesion is crucial, because it is based on the idea that the neospinothalamic projections carry the sensory-discriminative aspects of pain and temperature sensibility (location, intensity, sensory character). There is some support in the literature for this notion, but it cannot be considered proven.

Disinhibition by removal of cold activated spinothalamic projections

Based on results from experimental studies in cats, monkeys and humans, Craig has put forward a new hypothesis about the mechanisms of central pain. The hypothesis states that 'central pain is due to the disruption of thermosensory integration and the loss of cold inhibition of burning pain' (Craig 1998). This disruption is, according to the hypothesis, caused by a lesion somewhere along the spinothalamic projections to the thalamus (to the ventroposterior, posterior and mediodorsal nuclear regions; nuclei VPI, VMpo, MDvc). These projections are thought to tonically inhibit nociceptive thalamocortical neurons, which by the lesion increase their firing, and produce pain. The pathway is activated by cold receptors in the periphery, which in turn activate cold-specific and polymodal lamina I cells in the grey matter of the spinal cord. The supporting results from humans includes psychophysical and PET studies with the thermal grill, by which the skin can be simultaneously stimulated with both cold and warm bars in an interlaced way. By some combinations of inoccuous stimuli, burning painful sensations are evoked without using temperatures that normally evoke pain. Like several other hypotheses, this one might be applicable in some patients, but not in others, because of the location of the lesions and the character of the pain (only about 40–60% of all central pain has a burning character).

Removal of inhibition exerted by the reticular thalamic nucleus

This hypothesis focuses on the role of the reticular thalamic nucleus, and the medial and intralaminar thalamic regions receiving spinothalamic projections. According to this hypothesis the lesion removes the suppressing activity exerted by the reticular thalamic nucleus on medial and intralaminar thalamic nuclei, thereby releasing abnormal activity in this region, which in turn leads to pain and hypersensitivity (Schott et al 1986, Mauguiere & Desmedt 1988, Cesaro et al 1991). Experimental studies have shown that the reticular thalamic nucleus receives collateral input from the thalamocortical projections, and that it in turn projects to the medially located spinothalamic projection zones. In an investigation aimed at showing if there was neuronal hyperactivity in the brain of four patients with central pain caused by cerebrovascular lesions in the thalamus (one patient) and in the thalamocortical projection path (three patients), using the SPECT technique (= single photon emission computerized tomography), Cesaro et al (1991) found signs of hyperactivity in the thalamus, possibly in its medial part, in two patients with hyperpathia, but not in the other two patients without hyperpathia. It is interesting to note that in one of the patients hyperactivity was not found during successful treatment with amitriptyline, but reappeared when the treatment had to be stopped and the pain had returned. The technique, however, has a poor spatial resolution, so it could not be determined in which part of the thalamus the hyperactivity was located. In accordance with this hypothesis it appears from the literature that most thalamic lesions that cause central pain might involve part of the reticular nucleus, as well as parts of the ventroposterior nuclei (Edgar et al 1993).

Cellular pain

A theory of 'cellular pain' was proposed 60 years ago (Foix et al 1922). The hypothesis proposes that central pain is the result of 'disorganization of integration at the level of cellular relays' (cited from Garcin 1968). This is a modern idea that fits well with current knowledge about the neurophysiological correlates of pain (see below).

Sympathetic mechanisms

Sympathetic dysfunction has long been suspected of playing a role in central pain, because signs of abnormal sympathetic activity have been observed in many patients, including oedema, decreased sweating, lowered skin temperature, change in skin colour and trophic skin changes (Riddoch 1938, Bowsher 1996). It is difficult to evaluate the significance of these abnormalities, however, because they may be secondary to the change in mobility. Many patients with central pain avoid using the painful arm or foot because of the hypersensitivity to skin contact and the aggravating effect of movements, or because of paresis. This total or

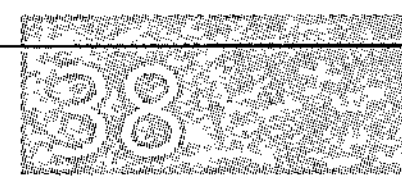

partial immobilization could, itself, lead to changes in the sympathetic outflow and in the microcirculation of the region. Attempts have been made to study these relationships, but it has been difficult to determine if the abnormalities are causal or coincidental with regard to central pain, or caused by the central pain. The results of sympathetic blockade might give some clue about these relationships, but the case reports show contradictory results with only some patients reporting pain relief (Loh et al 1981; G Leijon, J Boivie, J Sörensen, unpublished observations).

THALAMIC AND CELLULAR MECHANISMS

In most hypotheses the thalamus is believed to play a major role in the mechanism of central pain. Three of its regions are in focus, namely the ventroposterior part including also the posteriorly and inferiorly located nuclei bordering on this region, the medial-intralaminar region and the reticular nucleus (see above). All three regions receive spinothalamic projections, directly or indirectly. The role of the ventroposterior region in central pain was analysed in a series of articles in the 'APS Journal' (Boivie 1992, Jones 1992, Lenz 1992, Salt 1992). Lenz proposed that the ventroposterior thalamic region is heavily involved in the mechanism of central pain, and summarized data showing that in primates large parts of the ventroposterior nuclei (VP) receive nociceptive inputs, although these may be concentrated to the so-called shell zones in the outer part of the complex. Many of these thalamic neurons appear to be wide dynamic range neurons, receiving inputs via the lemniscal pathways as well, but there are also nociceptive-specific neurons in the nuclei.

Neurophysiological studies in the human ventroposterior thalamus

Burst activity and neurochemistry of sensory projections

Recordings from the thalamus in patients with central pain following spinal cord injuries have demonstrated increased spontaneous activity characterized by bursts of action potentials in the portions of the ventroposterior nuclei representing the anaesthetic or painful area of the body. This activity has similarities to calcium spikes shown in animal studies, i.e. activity related to the function of calcium channels, and it has been proposed that excitatory amino acids acting through NMDA receptors are involved (Lenz 1992). In this context it is of interest to note that such receptors are crucial in the relaying of inputs from nociceptors in the thalamus (Eaton & Salt 1990) and that the spinothalamic and lemniscal systems differ neurochemically, for instance with regard to the calcium-binding proteins. Thus parvalbumin immunoreactivity has been found in the lemniscal projections, whereas calbindin is present in the spinothalamic system. Jones (1992) concluded that current evidence suggests that the calbindin cells in the posterior, anterior pulvinar, caudal intralaminar, ventral posterior inferior, ventroposterior lateral (VPL), ventroposterior medial (VPM), and parts of the ventral lateral and ventral medial nuclei form a small-celled spinothalmic- and caudal trigeminothalamic-recipient matrix that projects diffusely to widespread areas of the cerebral cortex. In monkeys with long-term deafferentation after cervical rhizotomy there was an increase in calbindin in this small-celled matrix (Rausell et al 1991). It was speculated that this might underlie the signs of deafferentation pain that were observed.

Pain memory – possible long-term potentiation

Lenz, Tasker, Dostrovsky and collaborators showed that electrical stimulation in a ventroposterior zone deprived of its peripheral input due to a spinal cord lesion or amputation might evoke pain in the deafferented, but painful, region (Lenz et al 1988). Stimulation at these thalamic sites in patients without pain did not evoke pain. The fact that the stimulation evoked pain in deafferented regions indicates that there remains a representation in the CNS of the somatic sensibility for the deafferented region, a kind of long-term memory, which need not necessarily be located in the thalamus. Hypothetically it is possible that such a memory could be activated long after the lesion appeared, which may explain the long delay in the onset of central pain in some patients. Long-term potentiation is thought to be an important aspect in the memory processes. It seems probable that some kind of long-term potentiation is involed in chronic central pain, which is really a long-term process. NMDA receptors and associated calcium conduction have been implicated in long-term potentiation, thus representing another possible connection with excitatory amino acids (Bear & Molinka 1994).

Lesions in the ventroposterior thalamus and central pain

An important question regarding Lenz's hypothesis is whether the observed abnormal activity observed in the ventroposterior thalamus is the primary event, or if it is mainly a reflection of primary events occurring somewhere else in the CNS, for instance in the spinal cord, the brainstem, some other part of the thalamus or in the cerebral cortex. This question can not be answered at present.

The observations reviewed above have been made in patients with spinal cord injuries. It is reasonable to suspect some common mechanisms in all central pain conditions, but it is also conceivable that there are differences depending on where the primary lesion is located. It would thus be surprising if the physiological abnormalities are identical in a patient with a large supratentorial cerebrovascular lesion affecting much of the thalamus, including the ventroposterior region, and one with a small spinal cord lesion mainly affecting the dorsal horn. As regards the hypothesis postulating a crucial role for abnormal neuronal activity in the ventroposterior thalamic region in central pain, the mere location of the lesion sometimes makes this impossible, because in some patients with central pain this region is completely silent, namely in many patients with central pain as a result of thalamic infarct or haemorrhage. In fact, it appears that this is where the thalamic lesions that cause central pain have to be located (see 'Lesions in the spinothalamic pathway' above).

In a study of the clinical consequences of thalamic infarct it was found that only patients with thalamic lesions, including the ventroposterior thalamic region, developed central pain (Bogousslavsky et al 1988). Three of 18 patients with such infarcts had central pain at follow-up, whereas none of the 22 patients with other locations had central pain. In our own material with CPSP, all nine thalamic lesions included part of the ventroposterior thalamic region (Leijon et al 1989a). The same was found by Bowsher et al (1998). This is in accordance with Hassler's idea that the posterior inferior part of the ventroposterior region, i.e. his V.c.p.c or ventroposterior inferior nucleus (VPI) in recent terminology, is the crucial target for thalamic lesions causing central pain (Hassler 1960).

Mediodorsal nucleus (MDvc)

This medially located thalamic nucleus, which corresponds to the submedius nucleus (Sm) of the cat, has been proposed to play a role in the pathophysiology of central pain (Craig 1991, 1998). Nociceptive projections from lamina I cells of the spinal cord have been shown to the MDvc, which projects to the ventral lateral orbital cortex (VLO). This cortical zone is reciprocally connected with area 3a, the caudal aspect of the second somatosensory region (SII), area 5a and the anterior cingulate region. It has descending projections to the ventrolateral PAG. These connections support a sensory role of the submedius nucleus, possibly in affect aspects of pain. 'A lesion of lateral spinothalamic terminations in the ventral caudal part of the VP nuclei that produced a contralateral hypalgesia could result in release of corticocortical control by the ventral VP projection areas on the Sm projection area in VLO' (Craig 1991). This would lead to 'dysfunctional activity' in the Sm and VLO, which could possibly be part of the mechanism causing central pain.

A POSSIBLE EXPERIMENTAL MODEL FOR CENTRAL PAIN

Experience from many fields of medical research has shown that experimental models are most valuable in the search for mechanisms and treatments. Experience from techniques to produce experimental lesions in the spinal cord gives hope that the use of the model will lead to new insights into central pain. In one model ischaemic lesions are produced by a photochemical process involving the injection of Erythrosin B parenterally, followed by irradiation with an argon laser (Watson et al 1986). The size of the lesions depends on the energy transferred to the spinal cord by the laser, but it has so far not been possible to predetermine the exact location and size of the lesions. In a series of studies Wiesenfeld-Hallin and collaborators have tested the model on rats and reported interesting results (for references see Wiesenfeld-Hallin et al 1997). It has been shown for instance that the lesion strikes both white and grey matter, that the rats almost immediately after induction of the lesion develop tactile allodynia which is morphine resistant but responds to the GABA-B agonist baclofen given systemically, that the allodynia is prevented by pretreatment with the NMDA-antagonist MK-801 in rats with short irradiation times, that pretreatment with guanethidine or the opioid antagonist naltrexone does not prevent the development of allodynia, and that the sensitivity of wide dynamic range neurons in Rexed's lamina I–V to mechanical pressure is greatly increased with lowered threshold and more vigorous response. Intrathecally administered clonidine and morphine reduced the allodynic reaction. Injections of an antagonist of the B-receptor for cholecystokinin (CCK-B) also reduced the allodynic reaction, which the investigators propose is caused by the removal of a normally active tonic inhibition by the CCK-B system on endogenic opioid systems, thereby increasing the activity of this system (Xu et al 1994).

In the other model the lesions are produced by injecting cytotoxic substances such as quisqualic acid and AMPA, which results in cavities. About 10–21 days postinjection the animals start to develop pain-like behaviours. Electrophysiological studies with this model have obtained results that are similar to those with the ischaemic model (Yezierski 1996).

The models are no doubt promising experimental models of central pain, but further studies are needed to establish their similarity to chronic central pain in humans.

SUMMARY OF PATHOPHYSIOLOGY

1. The disease process, here called the lesion, involves the spinothalamic pathways, including the indirect spino-reticulo-thalamic and spino-mesencephalic projections, as indicated by abnormalities in the sensibility to pain and temperature.
2. The lesion probably does not have to involve the dorsal column–medial lemniscal pathways to invoke central pain.
3. The lesion can be located at any level of the neuraxis, from the dorsal horn to the cerebral cortex.
4. It is probable that all kinds of disease processes may cause central pain, but the probability of central pain occurring varies greatly between these diseases, from being rare to occurring in the majority of patients.
5. As yet no single region has been shown to be crucial in the processes underlying central pain, but three thalamic regions have been focused upon, namely the ventroposterior, reticular and medial/intralaminar regions. The role of the cerebral cortex in central pain is unclear, but this issue has not been specifically studied.
6. The pain and hypersensitivity experienced by central pain patients are compatible with the increased burst activity that has been found in the ventroposterior thalamic region in spinal cord injury patients with central pain. It is conceivable that this kind of cellular activity is also present at other levels of the sensory pathways, including the cerebral cortex.
7. The cellular processes underlying central pain are still unknown, but processes involving excitatory amino acids, and particularly glutaminergic NMDA-receptors, have been implicated.

CLINICAL CHARACTERISTICS

DIAGNOSIS OF A CNS PROCESS

The definition of central pain states that it is caused by a lesion or dysfunction in the CNS. The first step in the diagnostic procedure is therefore to ensure that the patient has a CNS disorder. This is often obvious, as in many patients with stroke or multiple sclerosis (MS), but it is sometimes not clear that there is a CNS lesion, as in some patients with moderate spinal trauma or suspected minor stroke. A detailed history of the neurological symptoms and a neurological examination are important parts of the diagnostic procedure, but laboratory examinations are often necessary. These include computerized tomography with X-ray or magnetic resonance, i.e. a CT scan or MRI, assays of the cerebrospinal fluid (CSF), neurophysiological examinations and other tests.

In addition to confirming the presence of a CNS process, one must also consider whether or not the patient has pain as a result of peripheral neuropathy. Polyneuropathy is not uncommon in, for instance, stroke patients, a group with a high incidence of diabetes. Neurography and electromyography are therefore indicated in some patients. Quantitative sensory tests are also valuable in the diagnosis of neuropathy. They include examination of sensibility to temperature and pain, as well as to vibration and touch (Lindblom 1994). Whereas neurography can only demonstrate abnormalties in large fibres, these tests can show dysfunction in both large and small sensory fibres.

DIFFERENTIAL DIAGNOSIS OF CENTRAL VERSUS NOCICEPTIVE AND PSYCHOGENIC PAIN

Central pain can usually be distinguished from other forms of pain provided that one is familiar with the characteristics of central pain, but in some patients it is difficult to determine whether the pain is central, peripheral neurogenic, nociceptive or psychogenic. Some patients have more than one kind of pain. A hemiplegic stroke patient, for instance, can have a nociceptive shoulder pain in addition to central pain. The examination of patients suspected of having central pain has to be individually tailored in order to identify possible non-central causes of the pain. Diagnostic problems are particularly difficult in some patients with MS and spinal cord injury (SCI), because of the complex clinical picture, with a mixture of motor and sensory symptoms and pain. Paresis and dyscoordination may lead to abnormal strain in musculoskeletal structures and development of nociceptive pain. The diagnostic procedure often calls for consultations by specialists, particularly in orthopaedics.

Psychogenic factors are important in central pain, as in all pain, but with increasing knowledge of the characteristics of central pain it rarely turns out that pain suspected of being central is truly psychogenic. Psychiatric and psychological consultations may be indicated in some patients, even if there is certain central pain, because the patient may also be depressed, although patients with central pain do not appear to be more depressed than other pain patients.

PAIN CHARACTERISTICS

The next step is to analyse the chacteristics of the pain, i.e. its location, quality, intensity, onset and development after onset, variation with time, and influence by external and internal events.

Pain location

It is usually stated with considerable emphasis that central pain is diffusely located. This notion appears to be largely derived from the fact that central pain often extends over large areas of the body, for instance the whole right or left side, or the lower half of the body. However, central pain can also involve one hand only, or just the ulnar or radial side of the hand, or one side of the face. Even patients with extensive central pain find it relatively easy to describe the extent of the painful regions, as shown in studies of patients with central pain after stroke and MS (Leijon et al 1989, A Österberg & J Boivie, unpublished observations from MS-patients). It is therefore more correct to state that most central pain is extensive than to describe it as diffuse.

The location of the lesion determines the location of the pain (Box 38.2). Thus large lesions in the ventroposterior thalamic region or the posterior limb of the internal capsule tend to cause hemibody pain, whereas large spinal cord lesions cause bilateral pain involving the body regions innervated by the segments caudal to the lesion. Even lesions that cause extensive loss of somatic sensibility may lead to central pain restricted to a small portion of the deafferented region. Examples of central pain engaging small regions were shown in patients with superficial cortical/subcortical vascular lesions by Michel et al (1990).

Cerebrovascular lesions in the medulla oblongata, i.e. mainly lesions caused by thrombosis in the posterior inferior cerebellar artery leading to Wallenberg syndromes, can induce central pain on both sides, the face and head being involved on the lesion side, and the rest of the body on the contralateral side (Riddoch 1938, Leijon et al 1989, Bowsher et al 1998). This pattern is caused by injury to the ipsilateral spinal trigeminal nucleus and the crossed spinothalamic tract. Lesions affecting the spinothalamic tract in the spinal cord will lead to pain on the contralateral side, after cordotomy for example. In syringomyelia central pain may be restricted to part of one side of the thorax, but it may also be more extensive, including the arm too, and even the lower body regions.

Central pain is experienced as superficial or deep pain, or with both superficial and deep components, but the high incidence of cutaneous hyperaesthesias contribute to the impression that superficial pain dominates, although deep pain is common too. Among 27 central poststroke (CPSP) patients, eight described the pain as superficial, eight as deep and the remaining 11 as both superficial and deep (Leijon & Boivie 1989c).

Quality of pain

No pain quality is pathognomonic for central pain. Central pain is thus not always burning or 'dysaesthetic', as one might believe from reading some of the literature on the subject. In fact central pain can have any quality, and the variation between patients is great, although some qualities are more common than others (Box 38.3).

Another basic feature is the presence of more than one pain quality in many patients. The different pains can coexist in a body region, or may be present in different parts of the body. A patient with CPSP, for instance, may have burning and aching pain in the leg and arm, and burning and stinging pain in the face. Other patients have a less complex

BOX 38.2

Common locations of central pain

Stroke
All of one side
All of one side except the face
Arm and/or leg on one side
Face on one side, extremities on the other side
The face

Multiple sclerosis
Lower half of the body
One or both legs
Arm and leg on one side
Trigeminal neuralgia

Spinal cord injury
Whole body below the neck
Lower half of the body
One leg

Syringomyelia
Arm and thorax on one side
One arm
Thorax on one side
One leg in addition to one of the above

BOX 38.3

Qualities of pain reported by patients with central pain:* indicates the most common qualities

*Burning	Shooting	Stabbing
*Aching	Squeezing	Cramping
*Lancinating	Throbbing	Smarting
*Pricking	Cutting	Pulling
*Lacerating	Crushing	Sore
*Pressing	Splitting	Icy feeling
	Stinging	

pain condition, with aching pain in the arm or leg. Some patients have pain with bizarre character, as was illustrated by citations from the early literature in the 'Introduction'.

One would expect the location of the lesion to be a deciding factor regarding the quality of pain. This appears to be partly true, but it is also apparent that similar lesions can lead to different pain qualities, as illustrated by central pain caused by cerebrovascular lesions in the thalamus. Nine patients with such pain reported more than eight types of pain, and none of these qualities was experienced by all patients (Leijon et al 1989). All of the lesions involved the ventroposterior thalamic region, but in seven of the patients the lesions extended lateral to the thalamus. It was not possible to correlate a particular pain character to the site of the lesion.

The description of the various central pain conditions given later in this chapter shows that, just as with central pain in general, no pathognomonic pain character has been found in any of these conditions. Perhaps the most homogeneous group consists of patients with central pain after spinal cordotomy, in whom the pain has mostly been described as dysaesthetic (see below), but the incidence is low, so only small numbers of patients have been reported from each centre (Cassinari & Pagni 1969, White & Sweet 1969, Tasker 1990). When comparing central pain conditions one gets the impression that the variation in pain qualities may be largest among stroke patients (Table 38.3). This is not surprising, because the variation in the structure and location of the lesion is largest in this group.

The most common central pain quality is probably burning pain, which has been found to be frequent in most central pain conditions (Cassinari & Pagni 1969, Schott et al 1986, Berić et al 1988, Moulin et al 1988, Leijon et al 1989, Tasker 1990, Boivie 1995, Bowsher 1996a, Bowsher et al 1998, Pagni 1998). However, it was reported that burning pain is rare in patients with cortical/subcortical lesions (Michel et al 1990). As mentioned above, dysaesthetic pain has been reported to be common in some conditions, for instance in MS and incomplete SCI, and after cordotomy, which also is a form of incomplete SCI. However, the term has not been well defined and evidently it has often been used to indicate a combination of dysaesthesias and spontaneous pain of differing qualities. This is indicated by Davidoff & Roth (1991) results in 19 SCI patients with 'dysaesthetic pain syndrome'. They experienced the following pain qualities: cutting (63%), burning (58%), piercing (47%), radiating (47%), tight (37%). The descriptions 'cruel' and 'nagging' were each used by 37%. Since dysaesthesias are common in most central pain conditions, this results in high figures for 'dysaesthetic' pain. It would seem logical to reserve this term for painful dysaesthesias, which occur spontaneously or are evoked by cutaneous stimuli, and also to specify any other forms of pain that the patient experiences.

Central pain caused by spinal cord processes commonly include a pressing belt-like pain (= a girdle pain) at the level of the upper border of the lesion, in addition to other pains. This pain occurs in patients with MS and traumatic SCI, and is similar to pain caused by lesions or inflammation affecting the spinal dorsal roots, which may present a diagnostic problem in SCI patients. For instance, an MS patient with a complete transverse lesion at T9 experienced a girdle pain with the character of tight armour at the level of the umbilicus, in addition to a constant burning pain in both legs and feet (A Österberg & J Boivie, in preparation).

Intensity of pain

From much of the early literature one gets the impression that central pain is always excruciating. This is incorrect, because the intensity of central pain ranges from low to extremely high. However, even if the pain is of low or moderate intensity the patients assess the pain as severe because it causes much suffering due to its irritating character and constant presence. Thus a patient may indicate a pain intensity of 28 on a visual analogue scale (VAS 0–100), and yet explain that the pain is a great burden making life very miserable. Interviews with patients show that many patients with central pain and severe motor handicap following strokes, MS or SCI often rate the pain as their worst handicap (Britell & Mariano 1991; G Leijon, J Boivie and A Österberg, unpublished observations). SCI patients with minor motor handicap have stated that they would prefer to trade their pain for a severe paresis if it was possible (Nepomuceno et al 1979). The results of such surveys differ, though, as shown by Davidoff et al (1987b), who reported that many SCI patients did not consider their pain to be a great problem.

In a study of patients with central poststroke pain with different lesion sites, it was found that the pain intensity was highest in the groups with lesions in the thalamus and low brainstem lesions, with mean VAS values of 79 and 61, respectively, compared to patients with suprathalamic lesion, who scored 50 (Table 38.2; Leijon et al 1989). The ranges were large and the number of patients in each group was small, so no definite conclusions can be drawn from these data, but a picture emerges that the pain intensity is higher with some lesion sites than with others. Thalamic lesions probably tend to cause more intense pain than non-thalamic lesions, because all patients with such lesions scored high.

Central pain may have a constant intensity or the intensity may vary. These variations seem to occur spontaneously or under the influence of external somatic or psychological stimuli, or as a result of internal events. In patients with more than one central pain quality, the variation in intensity may differ between pain forms.

Onset and other temporal aspects

Central pain may start almost immediately after occurrence of the lesion, or it may be delayed for up to several years. Delays are well known in poststroke central pain. This delay may be as long as 2–3 years, but in most patients the pain starts within a couple of weeks of the stroke (Fig. 38.1; Mauguiere & Desmedt 1988, Michel et al 1990, Leijon & Boivie 1991, Andersen et al 1995, Bowsher 1996). In some patients the pain starts immediately after the stroke. Andersen et al noticed that 63% had pain onset within 1 month post stroke (Andersen et al 1995). When the onset is delayed it frequently coincides with changes in the subjective sensory abnormalities. For example, a patient with dense sensory loss may start to experience paraesthesias or dysaesthesias, and soon afterwards the pain starts. With successively developing lesions such as the lesions of patients with spinal vascular malformations, MS and syringomyelia, it is difficult to know the temporal relationship between the lesion and onset of pain. In such diseases the pain can be the first symptom, or start later at any stage of the disease. In MS the prevalence of central pain is higher after the fifth year than earlier in the disease (Moulin et al 1988). The situation is complex in SCI because these patients frequently have multiple injuries with a mixture of different kinds of pain during the initial period following injury, which makes it more difficult to distinguish central pain in the early stages.

Table 38.2 Pain intensity in patients with central poststroke pain. Assessment with VAS 0–100. (Reproduced from Leijon et al 1989)

Lesion site	*No.*	*Mean*	*Range*
Brainstem	8	61	39–94
Thalamus	9	79	68–98
Extrathalamic	6	50	30–91

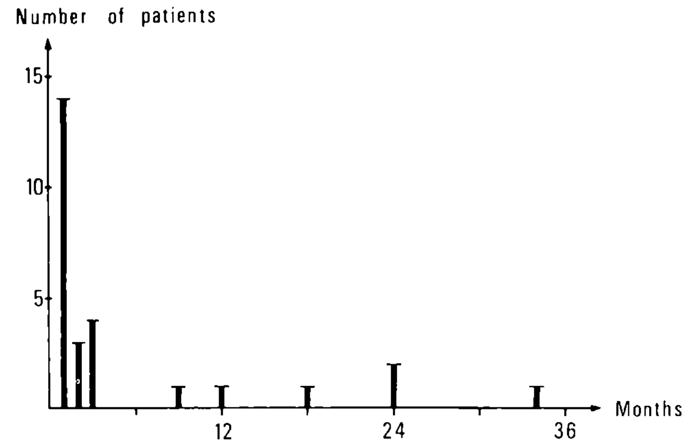

Fig. 38.1 Interval between onset of stroke and onset of central poststroke pain in 27 patients. (Reproduced from Boivie & Leijon 1991.)

Most spontaneous central pain is constantly present, with no pain-free intervals. In central poststroke pain 23 of 27 patients reported constant pain, whereas the other four patients had some pain-free intervals lasting at most a few hours each day (Leijon & Boivie 1989b). In addition to the spontaneous pain, many patients experience intermittent pain evoked by external and internal stimuli. Intermittent pain is well known in MS as part of tonic painful seizures and as trigeminal neuralgia. MS patients may also develop intermittent aching pain during physical activity, for instance during walking.

Unfortunately central pain is commonly permanent, but it may remit completely. This occurs spontaneously, or as a result of new lesions or other changes in the underlying disease. Some CPSPs successively cease completely, but most CPSP continues throughout life (Leijon & Boivie 1996). A few cases have been reported in which a new supratentorial stroke abolished the pain (Soria & Fine 1991). In SCI the central pain can be temporary lasting a few months only, but more commonly it is permanent (Berić et al 1988, Britell & Mariano 1991), which is similar to central pain in MS. A few patients with syringomyelia have described temporary pain with features characteristic of central pain during the early phase of the disease, but no central pain later (J Boivie and U Rollsjö, unpublished observations).

Stimuli affecting central pain

Many internal and external events influence central pain, such as cutaneous stimuli, body movements, visceral stimuli, emotions and changes in mood. Allodynia, i.e. pain evoked by a stimulus that is normally not painful, for example touch, light pressure or moderate heat or cold, is common in patients with central pain (Riddoch 1938, Berić et al 1988, Boivie et al 1989, Pagni 1989, Tasker 1990, Boivie 1992, Hansson & Lindblom 1992, Bowsher 1996). Such stimuli often give prolonged aftereffects, and they may increase ongoing pain. Patients with central pain frequently experience an increase in pain associated with body movement, such as changes in body posture, non-strenuous walking or movement of the extremities (Leijon & Boivie 1989c; A Österberg & J Boivie, unpublished observations in MS). Visceral stimuli, particularly from a full bladder or rectum, have long been thought to influence central pain (Riddoch 1938). Several case reports in the early literature and current experience from SCI patients support this notion.

It is also common that patients with central pain experience an immediate increase in pain after sudden fear, joy, loud noise or bright light (Riddoch 1938, Leijon & Boivie 1989b, Tasker 1990, Bowsher 1996). Experience from clinical practice indicates that central pain is as affected by psychological factors as other pain conditions, i.e. anxiety and depression aggravate central pain. This has not been well documented, however, although studies from SCI patients point in this direction (Britell & Mariano 1991). On the other hand, there is no reason to believe that psychological factors per se are important in the development of central pain, which is clearly somatic organic pain caused by lesions in the CNS. This concept is supported by studies of 22 CPSP patients, none of whom had major depression or other psychiatric disease (G Leijon & J Boivie, unpublished observations).

NEUROLOGICAL SYMPTOMS AND SIGNS

Because central pain is a neurological symptom emanating from processes in the CNS, it is of interest to know if central pain is accompanied by any other particular neurological symptoms and signs, which should then be included in the criteria for diagnosis. All investigators agree that central pain is caused by perturbations of the somatosensory systems, usually a lesion. It is thus a somatosensory symptom and it is therefore natural that abnormalities in somatic sensibility are the only symptoms and signs besides pain that are present in all patients with central pain. Several studies have shown that central pain is independent of abnormalities in muscle function, coordination, vision, hearing, vestibular functions and higher cortical functions (Riddoch 1938, Berić et al 1988, Leijon et al 1989, Pagni 1989, Tasker 1990, Bowsher 1996). In a study on CPSP all 27 patients had sensory abnormalities, whereas only 48% had paresis and 58% ataxia (see Table 38.5; Leijon et al 1989). Other neurological symptoms were present in a few patients. Similar results have been obtained in MS patients with central pain (see Table 38.5).

This statement is not contradicted by the fact that symptoms of the aforementioned kind are common in patients with central pain, because these non-sensory symptoms are a natural consequence of the lesion, which is seldom restricted to somatosensory structures. The important point is that the non-sensory symptoms are not necessary for the development of central pain. This is supported by the fact that many patients with central pain lack non-sensory symptoms. This has been shown in CPSP (Riddoch 1938, Leijon et al 1989, Bowsher 1996), MS (A Österberg & J Boivie, unpublished observations) and syringomyelia (J Boivie and U Rollsjö, unpublished observations).

SOMATOSENSORY ABNORMALITIES

Abnormalities in somatic sensibility are important in patients with central pain, both as criteria for diagnosis and as symptoms contributing to the patient's handicap. All central pain is probably accompanied by such symptoms and signs, although they may be subtle and may elude detection with clinical test methods which only provide a rough qualitative estimate. To be able to demonstrate small changes in sensibility one needs to use quantitative sensory tests (QSTs). Devices for such tests are now available for clinical use. They include calibrated vibrameters, and sets of von Frey filaments for the analysis of touch, devices for quantitative testing of temperature and temperature pain sensibility with Peltier element stimulators, and devices for measuring mechanical pain (Boivie et al 1989, Lindblom 1994, Yarnitsky & Sprecher 1994). It is postulated that central pain is always accompanied by sensory abnormalities, but we have examined a few patients in whom the clinical criteria have strongly indicated central pain and yet not even quantitative tests have shown abnormal sensibility (J Boivie, G Leijon, A Österberg, unpublished observations).

There is a large variation in the spectrum of sensory abnormalities among patients with central pain. It ranges from a slightly raised threshold for one of the submodalities, to complete loss of all somatic sensibility in the painful region. Hyperaesthesia also occurs often, as well as abnormal sensations. The most important sensory abnormalities are listed in Box 38.4. They include changes in detection thresholds and in stimulus–response function, spontaneous or evoked abnormal sensations, radiation of sensations from the stimulus site, prolonged response latency, and spatial and temporal summation. They represent both quantitative and qualitative abnormalities. The occurrence of these abnormalities in patients with central pain will be briefly summarized.

Hypoaesthesia

This term is usually used to denote a raised threshold, but it can also mean that the sensation evoked by a stimulus is weaker than normal. Raised thresholds or total loss of sensibility is common in central pain. It can affect some or all submodalities. In a study of CPSP, it was found that all patients had hypoaesthesia to temperature, whereas only about half of the patients had hypoaesthesia to touch, vibration and kinaesthesia (Boivie et al 1989). Similar results, but less pronounced, were found in other CPSP materials (Vestergaard et al 1995, Bowsher & Nurmikko 1996b, Bowsher et al 1998). Hypoaesthesia to noxious thermal and mechanical stimuli (heat, cold, pinprick or pinching), i.e. hypoalgesia, was also found. In other studies using quantitative sensory tests (QST), similar observations were made in patients with MS (Österberg et al 1994, Boivie 1995) and SCI with central pain (Berić et al 1988), and in syringomyelia (J Boivie and U Rollsjö, unpublished observations). This is the basis for the hypothesis that central pain only occurs in patients who have dysfunctions in the spinothalamic systems, i.e. in the pathways that are most important for temperature and pain sensibility (Boivie et al 1989, Bowsher 1995).

Hyperaesthesia

This denotes increased sensation to a stimulus, i.e. a steeper than normal stimulus–response curve. If this hypersensitivity occurs to noxious stimuli it is termed 'hyperalgesia'. 'Allodynia' is the name for pain evoked by stimuli that under normal conditions do not evoke pain, for example touch, vibration, moderate joint movements or moderate heat or cold. It often occurs as touch-evoked painful dysaesthesia. Hyperaesthesia to touch, moderate cold and heat, allodynia to touch and cold, and hyperalgesia to cold, heat or pin-prick are common in many central pain conditions (Riddoch 1938, Garcin 1968, Boivie et al 1989, Pagni 1989, Tasker 1990, Hansson & Lindblom 1992, Bowsher 1996). Combinations of hypoaesthesia and allodynia to touch or cold are not uncommon. For instance, some CPSP patients with severely decreased touch sensibility, even with total loss, have allodynia to touch (Boivie et al 1989). Head and Holmes as early as 1911 claimed that overreaction to somatic stimuli was the most typical sign of central pain.

BOX 38.4

Somatosensory abnormalities

Threshold (detection)	Numbness
hypo-, hyper-	Allodynia
Intensity functions	Radiation of sensation
hypo-, hyper-	Prolonged response latency
Abnormal sensations	Prolonged aftersensations
paraesthesias	Spatial and temporal summation
dysaesthesias	Hyperpathia

Paraesthesias and dysaesthesias

These are common in central pain (Riddoch 1938, Garcin 1968, Pagni 1989, Tasker 1990). In a study of CPSP 85% and 41% of the patients reported spontaneous and evoked dysaesthesia respectively, whereas 41% experienced paraesthesia (Boivie et al 1989). Dysaesthesia is often evoked by touch and cold and is sometimes painful. It is possible that painless dysaesthesia together with non-dysaesthetic central pain may result in the pain being classified as dysaesthetic (see 'Quality of pain' above). This could partly explain the claim expressed in some articles that dysaesthetic pain dominates in central pain, because dysaesthesia is one of the most frequent symptoms in central pain patients. This kind of pain has been reported to be common in MS (Moulin et al 1988) and after incomplete SCI (Davidoff et al 1987b, Berić et al 1988).

Numbness

Many central pain patients experience numbness, but it is not clear what underlies the perception of numbness. Is it primarily related to loss of tactile sensibility? Undoubtedly total sensory loss leads to numbness, but evidently it can also occur with normal threshold to touch, as shown in CPSP (Boivie et al 1989). Patients will sometimes use the term numbness when they experience paraesthesias or dysaesthesias.

Radiation, prolonged response latency, aftersensations, summation

These features are indicative of neurogenic pain and seem to be more common in central pain than in peripheral

 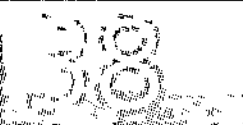

neurogenic pain. The term radiation means that the sensation spreads outside the site of stimulation, such as when touch with cotton wool or pin-prick on the dorsum of the foot evokes a sensation in both the leg and foot. Radiation was demonstrated in 12 of 24 patients with CPSP (Boivie et al 1989), and is also found in other central pain conditions (Riddoch 1938, Garcin 1968, Tasker et al 1991).

Prolonged latency between the stimulus and perception of the sensation can in some patients be demonstrated with tactile and pin-prick stimulation. This appears to occur only when there is a hyperaesthetic/hyperalgesic response, which includes spatial and temporal summation. It is then that the delay in sensation is mostly prolonged, and it may also be of an explosive hyperpathic kind. Hyperalgesia is found in many, but not all central pain patients.

Neurophysiological examinations

The central somatosensory pathways can be examined with neurophysiological techniques, which offer objective information regarding the function of the pathways. The most commonly employed method is to study somatosensory evoked postentials (SEP) evoked by electrical stimulation of the median and tibial/sural nerves. This method tests the function of the dorsal column–medial lemniscal pathways, because the stimulation activates large primary afferent fibres innervating low-threshold mechanoreceptors. Studies have shown that abnormalities in SEP evoked with this technique correlate well with abnormalities in the sensibility to touch and vibration (Schott et al 1986, Mauguiere & Desmedt 1988, Holmgren et al 1990).

As the sensory disturbances in central pain indicate that the lesions affect the spinothalamic pathways, it is of interest to study SEP evoked by peripheral stimulation of afferents that activate the spinothalamic pathways. This can be done by using lasers to stimulate cutaneous heat receptors (Bromm & Treede 1987, Pertovaara et al 1988, Treede et al 1988). A study with this technique on patients with CPSP showed that abnormalities in the laser-evoked cortical potentials, which have a long latency, correlate well with abnormalities in the sensibility to temperature and pain, but not to touch and vibration (Casey et al 1996).

Willer and collaborators have extensively studied the flexion reflex in patients with central pain and found that the latency of this reflex is prolonged in these patients. This reflex, the R III reflex, is dependent on activation of nociceptor afferents. Lesions in the CNS leading to decreased pain sensibility have been found to result in a delay of this reflex following electrical stimulation of the sural nerve (Dehen et al 1983).

PSYCHOLOGICAL FACTORS

Central pain patients have CNS disease that is mostly chronic and, in many cases, causes severe handicap. It is therefore natural that these diseases per se can lead to depression, for example poststroke depression, and depression in MS and SCI patients. Because many investigations have shown that there are mutual correlations between pain and depression (see chapter on psychiatric aspects of pain), one would expect to find a high incidence of depression in central pain patients. This has not been well studied and available data are incomplete and somewhat conflicting. In a group of SCI patients depression, anxiety, loneliness and several other psychosocial factors correlated significantly with the degree of pain, but this study also included nociceptive pain (Umlauf et al 1992), whereas studies of 24 and 16 CPSP patients could not identify any signs of depression (G Leijon & J Boivie, unpublished observations; Andersen et al 1995). Nor were these CPSP patients different from a control group with regard to social situation or major life events.

There has previously been a tendency among those not familiar with central pain to consider it as psychogenic pain. It is now absolutely clear that central pain is somatic organic pain and that it is not caused by psychologic factors, but like all other pains the experience of central pain is influenced by such factors and may of course also affect the afflicted both psychologically and socially.

TREATMENT

GENERAL ASPECTS

Treating central pain is no easy task, because there is no universally effective treatment. This means that one often has to try various treatment modalities to get the best results, which sometimes are achieved with combinations of treatments (Box 38.5). With each treatment it is important that the patient is well informed about possible adverse side effects, and how these should be regarded and when they should contact the doctor responsible. Treatment usually reduces the pain, rather than giving complete relief, and patients should be aware of this, so that they have realistic expectations. In this context it is interesting to note that relatively small decreases in pain intensity are often highly valued by the patients, with the result that they want to continue treatment even if the clinician responsible is doubtful about doing so.

Most treatment regimens for central pain are empirical and based on clinical experience. Many treatments have

BOX 38.5

Treatment modalities for central pain, including methods with unproven effect

Pharmacological
Antidepressant drugs (AD)
Antiepileptic drugs (AED)
Antiarrhythmic drugs, local anaesthetics
Analgesics
Other drugs
- adrenergic drugs
- cholinergic drugs
- GABA-ergic drugs
- glutaminergic drugs
- naloxone
- neuroleptic drugs

Sensory stimulation
Transcutaneous electrical stimulation (TENS)
Dorsal column stimulation (DCS)
Deep brain stimulation (DBS)

Neurosurgery
Cordotomy
Dorsal root entry zone (DREZ) lesions
Cordectomy
Mesencephalic tractotomy
Thalamotomy
Cortical and subcortical ablation

Sympathetic blockade

been claimed to be effective in the literature, mostly based on experience with small groups of patients. Few treatments have been tested in well-designed clinical trials. There is thus a great need for such trials on homogeneous patient groups. Furthermore, because it is conceivable that treatment affects some aspects of central pain but not others, it would be desirable to assess the effect of treatment on each pain modality separately. The practical problems in performing such studies are obvious. One has therefore to compromise, which often results in a global assessment of the effect on the spontaneous pain, whereas the effect on the painful hyperaesthesia is not assessed.

An important but still largely unanswered question concerning treatment is whether or not the different central pain conditions respond differently to one particular treatment. This has not been systematically studied, but such differences appear to exist. From a study of the literature and from clinical experience one gets the impression that CPSP responds better to antidepressants than the central pain in SCI and MS. Conversely paroxysmal pain in MS seems to respond much better to antiepileptic drugs than the other kinds of central pain.

One of the similarities between central pain and peripheral neurogenic pain is treatment. In both pain categories antidepressants and antiepileptic drugs are the most frequently used drugs. These are also the ones with the best documented effects, and virtually the only ones tested in well-conducted clinical trials. They are the first-line treatments, together with transcutaneous electrical nerve stimulation (TENS), which can only have a chance of giving relief, however, if the dorsal column–medial lemniscal pathways are not totally damaged. The other treatments listed in Box 38.4 have more of an experimental character, although some of them are used quite frequently by some pain specialists.

The ideal would be to use only treatments with well-documented effects, and this is the goal for the future. This goal can only be reached through carefully planned and well-designed evaluation of the results of treatment. This can be included in everyday practice, by choosing methods that are manageable in clinical practice. Scientific studies require more rigid and elaborate regimens. Treatments may affect spontaneous and/or painful hyperaesthesia, or both. It is desirable that both effects are evaluated. It has also been strongly recommended that the effects are analysed separately with regard to pain intensity (sensory aspect) and unpleasantness (affective aspect) of the pain (Gracely 1991; see Ch. 16). Further features to consider are the effects on anxiety, depression and other psychological factors. There is thus a risk for overload in evaluation, and this should be taken into account when studies are planned.

ANTIDEPRESSANTS

Documentation of effects, clinical aspects

Box 38.6 presents the first-line drugs for central pain. Controlled trials have been done only on CPSP and the central pain in SCI, with conflicting results. The CPSP study was a crossover study on 15 patients (mean age 66 years) in which the effects of amitriptyline (25 plus 50 mg), carbamazepine (400 mg b.i.d.) and placebo, given in randomized order, were assessed during three treatment periods, each 4 weeks long (Fig. 38.2; Leijon & Boivie 1989a). Assessment was done by daily ratings of pain intensity with a 10-step verbal scale (morning and evening), post-treatment global ratings of pain relief and depression scores (Comprehensive Psychopathological Rating Scale = CPRS) on days 0 and 28. The cut-off for responders was 20% pain

BOX 38.6

Antidepressant drugs used in central pain

Relatively unselective with regard to 5HT and NA
Amitriptyline
Doxepine
Nortriptyline

Some selectivity for 5HT
Clomipramine
Imipramine

High selectivity for 5HT
Citalopram
Fluoxetin
Fluvoxamine
Paroxetine
Trazodone

Some selectivity for NA
Desipramine
Maprotiline
Mianserine

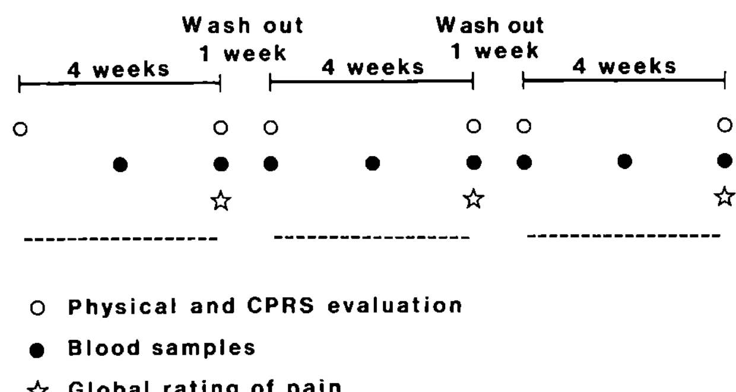

Fig. 38.2 Design of a study of the treatment with amitriptyline, carbamazepine and placebo in patients with central poststroke pain (CPSP). CPRS=comprehensive psychopathological rating scale. (Reproduced from Leijon & Boivie 1989c.)

reduction, as compared to the placebo period. Ten of the 15 patients were responders to amitriptyline with both assessment modes, and there was a statistically significant reduction in pain as compared to placebo. No difference was noted between patients with thalamic (five patients) and non-thalamic lesions, but the groups were small. The order in which the drugs were given did not affect the outcome. There appeared to be a correlation between pain relief and the plasma concentrations of amitriptyline and its active metabolite nortriptyline (Fig. 38.3), the responders having a mean concentration of 497 nmol/l, whereas the corresponding value was 247 mmol/l for the non-responders. Other studies of treatment with tricyclics have not supported these results (Rascol et al 1987). The results have also indicated that the pain-relieving effect could not depend on an improvement of depression because none of the patients were depressed according to assessment and their depression scores did not decrease during treatment.

These results contrast with those from a controlled study of the effect of trazodone, a tricyclic antidepressant (AD) with specific action on serotonin reuptake, on central pain in 18 patients with SCI (Davidoff et al 1987a). No significant effects were found compared to placebo. The trial was done with parallel groups, so only nine patients tried each treatment, but there was not even a tendency towards an effect of the active drug.

One possible explanation for the differences in effect on the two pain conditions is a difference in pharmacodynamics, i.e. specific serotonin reuptake inhibitors may be less effective than drugs also acting on the noradrenergic systems (see below). Another possible explanation is differences in susceptibility to treatment with AD in the two central pain conditions. The idea that central pain conditions may respond differently to AD therapy is supported by clinical experience from the use of AD in an open way. However, such conclusions may be affected by strong bias.

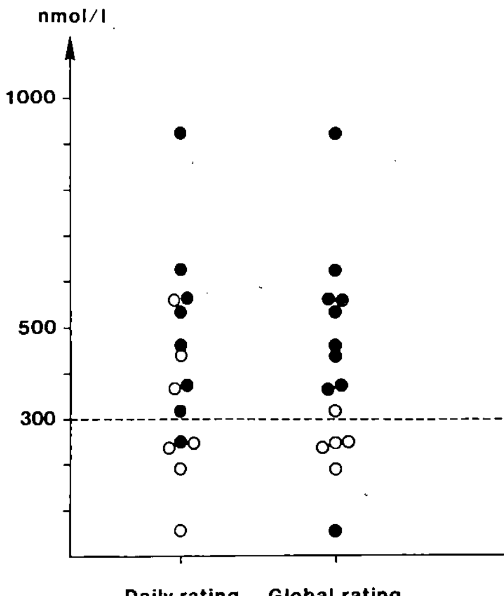

Fig. 38.3 The relationship between plasma concentration of amitriptyline and nortriptyline, and response in 15 patients with central poststroke pain (CPSP). ● = responder (median 497); ○ = non-responder (median 247). (Reproduced from Leijon & Boivie 1989.)

It is our impression that CPSP may be more amenable to relief by AD than the central pain in MS and SCI (J Boivie & G Leijon, unpublished observations). The favourable responsiveness in CPSP has also been found by Bowsher and collaborators (Bowsher & Nurmikko 1996b), and by Tourian (1987) in 10 patients treated with a combination of doxepin and propranolol. About 50% of these patients had long-lasting pain relief with AD.

Mechanisms of action, adverse side effects

The mechanisms underlying the pain-relieving effect of AD are unclear. For a long time it has been believed that it depends on inhibition of the reuptake of serotonin, but this idea has been contested. Instead it has been argued that it depends on their effects on the noradrenergic systems (Lenz 1992). This conclusion is based on observations that AD, having major effects on noradrenaline function and minor or no effects on serotonin (e.g., desipramin, maprotilin, mianserin), appear to be more effective in relieving neurogenic pain than the specific serotonin uptake inhibitors (=SSRIs; including among others citalopram, fluoxetin, fluvoxamin, paroxetin, trazodone, zimelidin; Watson & Evans 1985). However, this issue has not been finally clarified yet, because results have been obtained indicating a weak effect of SSRIs on peripheral neurogenic pain (Sindrup et al 1990, Max et al 1992). No controlled studies have been carried out using these drugs on central pain.

Amitriptyline, clomipramine and doxepin have effects on both noradrenergic and serotonergic systems, in addition to rather strong anticholinergic, and even some dopaminergic effects. It appears probable that it is an advantage to use drugs with mixed effects, because several of the transmitter systems that they affect are involved in pain and pain inhibition. However, there are undoubtedly problems in managing treatment with the first-generation tricyclics because of their side effects, mainly the anticholinergic ones. Thorough pretreatment information, slow dose increases, the whole dose at bedtime, and close monitoring with frequent contacts are important steps to minimize the problems of treatment. In this way most patients can tolerate the drugs and test the effect. The SSRIs also have adverse effects that prevent their use in some patients, which is not surprising considering that they are very potent drugs. It is too early to recommend general use of the new ADs in the treatment of central pain, because there are still uncertainties regarding their effects in clinical use.

The new antidepressants with mixed serotinergic and noradrenergic effects have not yet been studied systematically with respect to their possible effects on central pain or other neuropathic pains.

Several studies on AD and neurogenic pain have shown that their pain-relieving effect is independent of their effect on depression (see Ch. 50). In addition to relieving the pain, the ADs may thus decrease depression and may also allow the patient to sleep better. The temporal relationship between the onset and full development of the analgesic and antidepressive effects is unclear, as with many other questions regarding the place of the AD in the treatment of central pain. One such aspect is the dose–response relationship.

Dose–response relationships

In the CPSP study of amitriptyline the results indicated a correlation between the plasma concentration and the degree of pain relief (Leijon & Boivie 1989a, 1991); some other studies have yielded similar results (Watson et al 1982, Max et al 1988, Sindrup et al 1990), but results to the contrary have also been obtained (Boivie & Leijon 1996). Usually doses of 50–100 mg/day are used, but it has also been claimed that small doses in the order of 10–20 mg of tricyclics are sufficient for some patients. No controlled studies have provided support for this. In one of the studies on postherpetic neuralgia the results indicated that there might be a therapeutic window for the tricyclics (Watson et al 1982), but the study on CPSP was not in accordance with that idea, because good responses were only found in some patients with high plasma concentrations.

The large interindividual differences in plasma concentration between patients on the same dose probably results, to a large extent, from genetically determined differences in the rate of drug metabolism (Gram 1990). A fixed dose regimen will thus lead to underdosage in some patients and toxic levels in others. This is well illustrated by investigations on imipramine showing that to obtain similar plasma concentrations the dose may vary between 25 and 350 mg/day. It is therefore recommended that the dose be titrated individually. If insufficient effect is obtained with doses of 50–100 mg/day, one should either check the plasma concentration or try a higher dose, provided that side effects do not prevent dose increase.

ANTIEPILEPTIC DRUGS

Documentation of effects, clinical aspects

These drugs are widely used for central and peripheral neurogenic pain. However, an effect has not been demon-

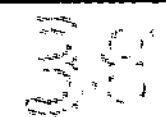

strated in well-designed clinical trials, except in idiopathic tic douloureux (Tomson 1980). In the only two controlled studies on the effect of an antiepileptic drug (AED) (carbamazepine) on central pain, an effect significantly better than placebo could not be demonstrated in one (Leijon & Boivie 1989a), and in the other only three MS patients were studied, all of whom obtained good pain relief (Espir & Millac 1970). Their use in central pain is thus largely based on tradition rather than on results from systematic research. This does not mean that they have no effect on central pain. Clinical experience speaks strongly in favour of an effect on tic douloureux and painful tonic seizures in MS (Osterman & Westerberg 1975). Based on experience it has been suggested that AED can only be expected to relieve paroxysmal central pain. Although this may be the most suitable condition to treat with AED, it is conceivable that other kinds of central pain may also respond. This conclusion is supported by the results from the CPSP study mentioned above, in which the responders did not have paroxysmal pain (Leijon & Boivie 1989a). It is recommended that an AED is included in the list of treatments for central pain.

In the study on the effect of carbamazepine on CPSP, 800 mg/day for 4 weeks was compared with amitriptyline and placebo in 14 patients (Leijon & Boivie 1989a). Five patients responded, but the effect did not reach statistical significance. In the other study all three MS patients with pain responded to carbamazepine (Espir & Millac 1970). From two open-label studies on paroxysmal central pain it was reported that all six MS patients and all seven patients with tabetic lightning pain had excellent results with carbamazepine (Ekbom 1966, Shibasaki & Kuroiwa 1974). A few cases have also been reported in which phenytoin was found to be beneficial in CPSP and MS (for references see Leijon & Boivie 1991). Clonazepam was likewise reported to be better than other AEDs in seven out of nine central pain patients (Swerdlow 1986).

A controlled trial with sodium valporate for the treatment of central pain following spinal cord injury showed no analgesic effect by the drug.

In recent years gabapentin has been widely recommended in the treatment of neuropathic pain, and two studies have shown a positive effect on postherpetic neuralgia and polyneuropathy pain (Attal et al 1997, Backonja et al 1997), but so far no studies on central pain have been published. In clinical practice the results with gabapentine have differed from good to poor. It should be noticed that the currently recommended daily doses are in the range of 2000–3600 mg.

Mechanism of action

The commonly used AEDs are listed in Box 38.7. Carbamazepine is probably the most widely used drug, but clonazepam has gained popularity (Swerdlow 1986). The rationale underlying the use of AEDs for central pain is their ability to suppress discharge in pathologically altered neurons, an effect that is also the basis for their use in epilepsy. Carbamazepine and phenytoin probably exert their effect by the inactivation of sodium channels (McLean & Macdonald 1986). Clonazepam, like other benzodiazepines, binds to a receptor associated with the GABA–chloride iontophoric complex, thus facilitating GABA-mediated inhibition, which is also thought to be the mechanism for sodium valproate (Budd 1989).

Dose–response relationships, adverse side effects

In trigeminal neuralgia it is clear that the pain-relieving effect of carbamazepine is strongly correlated with the plasma concentration, as in epilepsy (Tomson 1980), but it is not known whether or not this is also the case with AEDs in central pain. No such correlation was found in the study on CPSP (Leijon & Boivie 1989a).

Like the antidepressants the AEDs have a tendency to cause troublesome side effects, and must therefore be managed with caution. It is possible that some groups of central pain patients are more amenable to the side effects than other patients with neurological diseases, because many neurologists have the impression that carbamazepine, and possibly also other AEDs, cause more problems in MS patients than in patients with idiopathic trigeminal neuralgia or epilepsy. This could be explained by the fact that carbamazepine has effects on cerebellar centres for the coordination of movements which are frequently affected by the disease process in MS.

BOX 38.7

Antiepileptic drugs used in central pain

Carbamazepine
Phenytoin
Barbiturates
Clonazepam
Sodium valproate
Gabapentin
Vigabatrin
Topiramate

LOCAL ANAESTHETICS, ANTIARRHYTHMIC DRUGS

These substances have structural similarities and are thought to act on the same kind of pathophysiology as the antiepileptic drugs, i.e. to reduce pathological neuronal activity to a more normal level, mainly by acting on ion channels in the peripheral and central nervous systems Wiesenfeld-Hallin & Lindblom 1985, Woolf & Wiesenfeld-Hallin 1985, Chabal et al 1989). In controlled clinical trials, intravenous lidocaine (= lignocaine) and oral mexiletine have been shown to have a pain-relieving effect in painful diabetic neuropathy (Dejgard et al 1988, Kastrup et al 1987), and oral tocainide in trigeminal neuralgia (Lindström & Lindblom 1987). The duration of effect of an intravenous infusion of lidocaine is short, lasting 3–21 days in diabetics (Kastrup et al 1987). Tocainide was probably about as effective as carbamazepine in trigeminal neuralgia, but it had to be withdrawn from the market because of serious adverse effects.

No controlled clinical trials have been published on the use of these substances in central pain, but according to results from a placebo-controlled study of intravenous lidocaine in 10 CPSP patients, four of the patients responded with short-term relief, two on placebo and two on lidocaine (A Coe, G Leijon, J Dean, F McGlone, P McCarthy, unpublished observations). A few patients with central pain have responded well in open-label treatment studies using lidocaine (Boas et al 1982, Edwards et al 1985). Similar experiences were made with oral mexiletine in seven CPSP patients, of whom five responded well (Awerbuch 1990). Controlled clinical trials are evidently needed to establish the role of these substances in the treatment of central pain.

ANALGESICS

The question whether or not neurogenic pain responds to analgesics is controversial. Some claim that their material indicates that neuropathic pain in general responds poorly or not at all. Others report experience to the contrary. Apparently most clinicians agree that neurogenic pain in general responds less well to analgesics than does most nociceptive pain, and that many patients do not respond at all to opioids. Portenoy, Foley and collaborators reason that neurogenic pain may respond to some but not to all opioids, in other words, that differences in pharmacological properties may be important, and that it is partly a matter of dosage (Portenoy & Foley 1986, Portenoy et al 1990). There may also be differences between different neurogenic pains in this respect, presumably because of differences in the pathophysiology involved. The positive effects of morphine on postherpetic neuralgia shown in a well-designed trial might be an illustration of this (Rowbotham et al 1991).

Most of the patients referred to specialists because of central pain have tried analgesics, often in relatively high doses, without experiencing relief, but a few have obtained some pain reduction, mostly with weak opioids such as codeine and dextropropoxyphene. The results from acute, single-blind tests of opioids on central pain also provide strong evidence for a low sensitivity to opioids (Arnér & Meyerson 1991, Kupers et al 1991, Kalman et al 1993). We tried doses in the order of 30–50 mg morphine over 2 hours, i.e. close to doses causing the patient to sleep or develop confusion, and found analgesic effects only in a few patients with CPSP (unpublished observations) and central pain in MS (Kalman et al 1993). It is also common that patients with central pain who undergo operations and receive opioids postoperatively report that they have a good effect on the pain related to the operation, but no effect on the central pain. Portenoy et al, however, have reported good effects of long-term treatment with moderate doses of opioids in central pain (Portenoy & Foley 1986, Portenoy et al 1990).

A reasonable conclusion from the evidence available seems to be that a few central pain patients may benefit from analgesics, and that it is important to evaluate these effects carefully in each individual before prescribing them for long-term use. If the patient reports that the opioid clearly reduced the pain, and thereby the suffering significantly, then she should not be denied this relief.

ADRENERGIC, CHOLINERGIC, GABA-ERGIC AND GLUTAMINERGIC DRUGS, NALOXONE

Adrenergic synapses play a role in the mechanisms of pain. It has therefore been postulated that adrenergic drugs may contribute to pain relief (Scadding et al 1982, Glynn et al 1986). For some years the interest focused on the α_2-agonist clonidine, which has been shown to block the release of transmitters and peptides in primary afferent terminals by presynaptic action. In a double-blind study, patients with pain induced by arachnoiditis responded equally well to 150 μg clonidine as to morphine, both given epidurally (Glynn et al 1988), as well as in an open trial in patients with MS/SCI and painful spasms (Glynn et al 1986). Clonidine gave fewer side effects and longer lasting relief. Agents acting on β-adrenergic receptors have also been tried in neurogenic pain.

The β_2-antagonist propranolol was found to relieve trigeminal neuralgia, phantom pain and diabetic neuropathy pain, but none of eight patients with post-traumatic neuralgia responded to 240 mg/day (Scadding et al 1982). Tourian (1987) reported that propranolol enhances the effectiveness of doxepin, a tricyclic antidepressant, in open-label treatment of CPSP.

Cholinergic systems are involved in pain and analgesia (Hartvig et al 1989). Acetylcholinesterase inhibitors and muscarinic receptor agonists increase pain thresholds after both systemic and spinal administration. In an open study two out of five patients reported long-term relief of CPSP during treatment with physostigmine and pyridostigmine (Schott & Loh 1984). One group has extensively tried the combination of distigmine and tricyclic antidepressants in an open-label trial and found this to be beneficial in CPSP patients, but it is unclear if this is obtained by suppression of the anticholinergic side effects of the tricyclic or by more effective analgesia, or both (Hampf & Bowsher 1989). However, data from well-designed clinical trials are needed before this combination can be recommended for general use.

In experimental and clinical spinal cord injury pain the $GABA_B$ agonist baclofen has been shown to reduce tactile allodynia and clinical pain, respectively, but only when given intrathecally (Hao et al 1992, Herman et al 1992, Taira et al 1994). Clinically oral baclofen is used to reduce spasticity, but in severely affected patients the intrathecal route has been found to be more effective.

When administered intravenously ketamine, an NMDA-antagonist, has been found to reduce allodynia and painful dysaesthesia in patients with central pain (Backonja et al 1994, Wood & Sloan 1997), but presently available NMDA-antagonists have serious psychotropic effects that prevent their use in clinical practice.

The μ-receptor opioid antagonist naloxone has been given to CPSP patients in high doses to alleviate the pain, but the results are conflicting (Budd 1985, Bainton et al 1992). Budd, who introduced the therapy, claims that one injection of huge doses of about 20–50 mg gives good long-lasting relief in many patients, whereas Bowsher found in a controlled study that 10 mg did not differ from placebo. Budd reported that X-ray CT scans showed signs of increased blood flow in the thalamus on the injured side after naloxone injections, but the methods employed did not have sufficiently high sensitivity to show this.

NEUROLEPTIC DRUGS

There is a long clinical tradition for the use of phenothiazines and other neuroleptic drugs in pain treatment. They are believed to increase the effect of analgesics and to have analgesic properties of their own. In neurogenic pain they are particularly used for dysaesthesia and hyperaesthesia. However, such effects have not been shown in controlled studies on any pain condition, or in any form of convincing study. Their potentially severe and partially irreversible adverse effects and the lack of documented effects are strong enough reasons to caution against the use of these drugs in the treatment of central pain. This is particularly so as many of these patients have brain lesions which increase the risk for the occurrence of irreversible tardive dyskinesia, which is the most serious side effect of neuroleptics.

SENSORY STIMULATION

Transcutaneous nerve stimulation

This form of treatment provides relief for some central pains and has the advantage of few and mild adverse side effects, apart from possible effects on cardiac pacemakers (Sjölund 1991). It is applied in one of two modes: high-frequency stimulation (80–100 Hz; called conventional transcutaneous nerve stimulation (TENS) by Sjölund), aiming at activation of myelinated cutaneous sensory fibres, or low-frequency stimulation (short trains of impulses with 1–4 Hz repetition rate; called acupunture-like TENS), aiming at activation of muscle efferents or muscle cells, thereby evoking muscle afferent inputs to the CNS. The mechanisms are believed to be mainly segmental, but suprasegmental mechanisms exist too (see Ch. 57). It is unclear how the effect of TENS in central pain is explained, but it appears that TENS can only reduce central pain if the dorsal column–medial lemniscal pathways are uninjured or only mildly injured.

This hypothesis is based on a study of TENS in CPSP. Three of 15 CPSP patients obtained long-term relief (Leijon & Boivie 1989c). All three had normal or almost normal thresholds to touch and vibration, indicating good function in the lemniscal pathways. Two of the three suffered from brainstem infarction, but in the third the location of the lesion could not be identified. One of the Wallenberg patients had facial pain on one side and extremity pain on the other. He used high-frequency TENS for the facial pain, but this had no effect on the arm or leg. High- and low-frequency stimulation had approximatly equal effect in the other two. Our continued use of TENS in CPSP follows these results, but a better yield had been reported in an earlier study (Eriksson et al 1979). In this study good results were also reported in SCI patients, with seven of 11 patients responding well to TENS. These patients probably had incomplete lesions, because it would be surprising if one could obtain relief with stimulation that cannot affect the structures located rostral to the lesion, which would be the case with a complete SCI.

Spinal cord and deep brain stimulation

From a review of the literature and of his own patients Tasker and colleagues (Tasker 1990, Tasker et al 1991) concluded that spinal cord stimulation is not effective enough in central pain to be recommended, a view shared by Gybels and Sweet (1989), Nashold and Bullitt (1981) and Pagni (1998), although he and others have had patients with successful results from spinal cord stimulation in central pain due to SCI. Instead he favours deep brain stimulation (DBS). Richardsson et al observed good results at 1-year follow-up in six of 19 paraplegics, and Siegfried reported good to excellent relief at 1- to 4-year follow-up in about 70% of 84 patients with 'deafferentation' pain caused by various central and peripheral lesions (Richardsson et al 1980 Siegfried 1983).

DBS is an exclusive mode of treatment that should be reserved for particularly severe and treatment-resistant pain conditions. The exquisite pain suffered by many central pain patients fulfils these criteria. The periaqueductal and periventricular grey regions (PAG, PVG) are the primary targets for stimulation in the treatment of nociceptive pain, whereas stimulation for neurogenic pain is usually carried out along the lemniscal pathways in the ventroposterior thalamic region or the posterior limb of the internal capsule. Tasker et al (1991) reported successful results in five out of 12 patients following thalamic stimulation, similar to the results of Siegfried and Demierre (1984), whereas only three out of 19 gained relief from stimulation of the PVG (Siegfried & Demierre 1984, Tasker et al 1991). Excellent results were reported following surface stimulation of the motor cortex in central pain (Peyron et al 1995, Tsubokawa 1995, Yamamoto et al 1997).

NEUROSURGICAL ABLATIVE PROCEDURES

Many different surgical lesions have been tried to find relief for central pain, but no particular lesion has been found that reliably results in successful outcome (Tasker 1990, Sjölund 1991, Tasker et al 1991, Pagni 1998). Lesions have been made at almost all levels of the neuraxis from the spinal cord to the cerebral cortex. Even lesions of peripheral nerves, mainly rhizotomy, have been tried. It is interesting to note that such lesions have not had an effect on steady ongoing pain, but in some cases there has been improvement of hyperaesthesia (Tasker 1990). According to Tasker et al (1991), ablative procedures in the spinal cord and the brain have also given better results with the intermittent and evoked components of central pain.

Three main kinds of spinal cord lesion have been performed for the treatment of central pain, namely anterolateral cordotomy, dorsal root entry zone (DREZ) lesion and cordectomy. The underlying lesion has usually been a traumatic cord lesion. A fair proportion of patients with sacrococcygeal lesions have been found to obtain relief from cordotomy, but there has been a tendency for the pain to recur, as after cordotomy for nociceptive pain (Tasker 1990). The more rostral the lesion, the lesser the chance that cordotomy will do anything for the patient.

DREZ lesions have gained interest over recent years for the treatment of central SCI pain (Nashold & Bullitt 1981, Edgar et al 1993). The procedure aims at destroying the Lissauer tract and the superficial part of the dorsal horn. One would thus expect the DREZ lesion to affect pain emanating from the segment where the original lesion is located, i.e. in the transitional zone of partially injured cord tissue. So far results have not been consistent, but some centres have reported a success rate of about 50% (Nashold & Bullitt 1981, Gybels & Sweet 1989, Tasker 1990, Sjölund 1991, Edgar et al 1993). Cordectomy is a more robust method to achieve a similar goal as the DREZ lesion, namely to interfere with the local pain-generating process. As with cordotomy, and probably also DREZ lesions, it appears that cordectomy rarely affects steady ongoing pain, but rather intermittent pain and hyperaesthesia, but has a low success-rate (Gybels & Sweet 1989, Tasker 1990).

Among the many intracranial ablative procedures that have been tried for central pain are mesencephalic tractotomy, medial and lateral thalamotomies, cingulotomy and cortical ablation. None of these have turned out to produce successful long-term outcomes. Some operations have resulted in postoperative pain relief in some patients, but the overall results have not been good, because of unacceptably high complication rates or return to preoperative pain levels after some time. From a review of the literature and of his own material, Tasker concluded that the only procedures that can be recommended in selected cases are stereotactic mesencephalic tractotomy and/or medial thalamotomy (Tasker 1990). Of his own nine patients with central pain caused by brain lesions in whom such operations were performed, only three had 'modest' relief of steady pain, and another four had some effect on intermittent pain. Three had transient complications. It has been suggested that the pain-relieving effect of the mesencephalic lesion is obtained by interfering with the spino-reticulo-thalamic projections. Medial thalamotomy appears to affect the spinal and trigeminal projections to the intralaminar-submedius region. This kind of thalamotomy has been strongly advocated by Jeanmonod and collaborators (Jeanmonod et al 1996), but many neurosurgeons are sceptical about these lesions in the treatment of pain.

SYMPATHETIC BLOCKADE

In the section on pathophysiology the idea that sympathetic dysfunction may be part of the mechanism underlying central pain was discussed. Oedema, decreased sweating, lowered skin temperature, change in skin colour and trophic skin changes occur in regions affected by central pain (Bowsher 1996). Based on these observations sympathetic blockade has been tried in the treatment of central pain. Loh et al (1981) gave a detailed report of the results of sympathetic blockade in three patients with CPSP, one with a traumatic brainstem lesion, two with MS, one with a spinal cord tumour and one with traumatic SCI. The short-term effects were remarkable. All patients experienced at least 50% reduction in pain and disappearance or improvement of hyperaesthesia, but the effects usually lasted only 1–24 hours, apart from the patient with a traumatic brainstem lesion who experienced long-term relief. In some cases symptom reduction was noticed outside the region involved by the sympathetic block, for instance in the leg after a stellate ganglion block. These results are interesting and raise important questions that ought to be explored further. Firstly, these clinical effects need to be studied in larger patient groups because experience with sympathetic blockade in clinical practice has shown this procedure does not give consistent results. Secondly, what can be the explanation for the dramatic effects of a distal regional block in the arm on symptoms caused by a lesion in the brain? Could this indicate that there is a peripheral component affecting the central pain generator, or that the spinal grey matter also plays a role in the central pain caused by brain lesions and that altered peripheral input affects this mechanism? And furthermore, can similar effects be obtained by the blockade of somatic nerves?

INDIVIDUAL CENTRAL PAIN CONDITIONS

Some features of particular interest regarding individual central pain conditions will be summarized in this section. Many of the features of individual central pain conditions have been discussed above. Much of this information will not be repeated in this section. For a more detailed presentation on central pain following SCI the reader is referred to Chapter 39.

CENTRAL POSTSTROKE PAIN

The lesions

All kinds of cerebrovascular lesion (CVL) can cause central poststroke pain (CPSP). There appears to be no difference between haemorrhages and infarcts as regards the tendency to induce central pain (Leijon et al 1989, Bowsher 1996, Bowsher et al 1998). The consequence of this is that there are many more patients with CPSP caused by infarct than haemorrhages, because approximately 85% of all strokes are caused by infarct.

Different principles can be used to classify CVL. One principle is according to the artery involved, giving two major groups, namely carotid and vertebrobasilar strokes. About 80% of all infarcts occur in the carotid territories. Infarcts in the territories of the thalamostriate and the posterior inferior cerebellar arteries (PICA) are particularly interesting, because they engage the ventroposterior part of the thalamus and the lower brainstem, respectively. These infarcts are probably among the most frequent causes of central pain.

Haemorrhages can only induce central pain when they damage the brain parenchyma. It is thus unusual that subarachnoid haemorrhage causes central pain, but it occurs when severe vasospasm develops and leads to an infarct and when the bleeding causes direct tissue injury (Bowsher et al 1989).

As regards central pain caused by vascular malformation, this mainly concerns arteriovenous malformations (AVM) and the result is similar to CVL. They can cause central pain in two ways, namely through rupture and haemorrhage, or if they increase in size and cause parenchymal damage. Patients with CPSP due to both these forms of lesion have been reported. The lesions were located cortically and subcortically in the parietal region and in the thalamus (Silver 1957, Waltz & Ehni 1966).

The location of the CVL, and not its size, is crucial as regards the probability that it will produce central pain (see 'Pathophysiology' above). The following major locations have been shown to be associated with central pain: lateral medulla oblongata (PICA), thalamus, posterior limb of the internal capsule, subcortical and cortical zones in the post-central gyrus (i.e., in the regions of the first somatosensory area, SI), and the insular regions (second somatosensory area, SII). A crude picture of the relative prevalence of

CPSP according to the different lesion locations was obtained in a study of 27 patients, of whom eight had low brainstem lesions, nine had thalamic lesions, and six had supratentorial, extrathalamic lesions (Leijon et al 1989). Only two of the thalamic lesions were restricted to the thalamus, the other seven extended laterally and superior to the thalamus; the location could not be determined in the four remaining patients.

A recent prospective study of 191 stroke patients followed for 12 months showed that the incidence of CPSP is 8% (Andersen et al 1995). The exact figures at 1, 6 and 12 months follow-up were: 4.8%, 6.5% and 8.4%. It appears that CVL in the lower brainstem and thalamus more often result in central pain than CVL in other locations, because these are not the most frequent locations of CVL and yet these locations are common in CPSP materials (Riddoch 1938, Garcin 1968, Leijon et al 1989, Andersen et al 1995, Bowsher et al 1998). The incidence of central pain after lateral medullary infarcts may be as high as 25% (MacGowan et al 1997). In studies carried out by Leijon et al (1989) and by Andersen et al (1995), 33% and 25%, respectively, of the patients with CPSP had CVL involving the thalamus. These conclusions were based on X-ray CT scans. A later study using MRI indicated that about 60% of all CPSP patients have lesions engaging the thalamus (Bowsher et al 1998). It appears probable that about half of all CPSP patients have lesions that involve the thalamus.

CPSP associated with thalamic lesions has attracted much attention over the years, probably because Dejerine and Roussy's early description of cases of thalamic pain provided the archetypal characteristics of central pain (Dejerine & Roussy 1906). The reader is referred to the section on 'Pathophysiology' above for a discussion of the role of thalamic lesions in central pain. In brief, recent and old data indicate that lesions in the ventroposterior thalamic region relatively often cause central pain. In one study three of 18 patients with such lesions developed central pain (Bogousslavsky et al 1988). It has also been shown that a small but strategically located thalamic lesion may result in central pain.

Pain characteristics

The major problem in the diagnosis of CPSP is to distinguish central pain from nociceptive pains of various kinds, particularly hemiplegic shoulder pain, which is common in hemiplegic stroke patients. The development of shoulder pain can to a large extent be prevented by physiotherapy and information to everyone involved in the care of the patient.

The onset of CPSP is delayed in many patients. In one study, about half of the patients noticed the pain within a few days or during the first month, but in half of the patients the onset was delayed by more than 1 month (Fig. 38.1; Leijon et al 1989). The longest delay was 34 months. In the Danish prospective study 63% had onset of pain within 1 month (Andersen et al 1995) and after brainstem infarcts the figure was 56% (MacGowan et al 1997).

CPSP is commonly experienced in a large part of the right or left side. This was the case in 20 of 27 patients in our study, but the face was involved in only six of them (Leijon et al 1989). However, some patients only have pain in a small region, such as the distal part of the arm and hand, or in the face. Two of the eight patients with brainstem infarcts had pain in the face on one side and in the rest of the body on the other side. The most common pain location after lateral medullary infarcts appears to be ipsilaterally around the eye (MacGowan et al 1997).

In our study two-thirds of the patients had left-sided pain, which was in accord with the material of Schott et al (1986) and a summary of published patients with thalamic stroke (Nasreddine & Saver 1997), but dominance of one side did not appear in a large study from one centre (Bowsher et al 1998).

Patients with CPSP report a large variety of pain qualities. Most patients experience two to four qualities. A burning sensation is the most frequent quality reported by about 60% of patients, with aching, pricking and lacerating sensations being next in frequency (Table 38.3). In another study 32 patients described the pain as principally burning and 30 patients described it as principally non-burning (Bowsher et al 1998). Bizarre pain qualities do occur, as mentioned in the first part of this chapter, but they are the exception rather than the rule.

Table 38.3 Quality of central poststroke pain: proportion of patients (%). (Reproduced from Leijon et al 1989)

	BS (n = *8)*	*TH* (n = *9)*	*SE* (n = *6)*	*UI* (n = *4)*	*All* (n = *27)*
Burning	75	22	83	75	59
Aching	38	22	33	25	30
Pricking	25	22	33	50	30
Lacerating	0	44	33	25	26
Shooting	13	22	0	0	11
Squeezing	13	22	0	0	11
Throbbing	0	22	17	0	11
Other	13	22	17	25	19

BS = CVL in brainstem; TH = CVL involving thalamus; SE = supratentorial, extrathalamic CVL; UI = location of CVL not identified.

Assessment of the intensity of CPSP reveals large individual variations (Table 38.4). In a global sense most patients consider the pain to be severe, although some of them rate the pain intensity rather low on scales such as the VAS, but a few patients have a mild form of CPSP. There are also patients in whom it is difficult to determine whether the sensation experienced should be classified as pain or not. This for instance is true for some dysaesthesias, because there is no sharp transition from non-painful to painful dysaesthesias.

In many patients the pain is affected by internal and external stimuli. Such stimuli usually increase the pain (Leijon et al 1989). Table 38.4 provides some information on this (see also Bowsher 1996). Many patients report that body movement increases the pain. CPSP patients are also sensitive to cold (see also Michel et al 1990). In the cited study relatively few patients had observed that strong emotions affected the pain, but this has been common in previous case reports.

Neurological symptoms and signs

Because pain is a somatosensory symptom it is not surprising that somatosensory symptoms and signs regularly accompany CPSP, whereas other symptoms may or may not be present in patients with CPSP (Table 38.5). Among 27 CPSP patients more than half had no paresis (Leijon et al 1989), and other non-sensory symptoms were much more uncommon. In a subgroup of nine patients with thalamic lesions only one had choreoathetosis, a symptom that others have found to be more common.

Some of the sensory abnormalities are subtle, and are not noticed by the patients or revealed in the clinical sensory examination, but can be demonstrated by quantitative sensory testing (QST). However, we and others have had a few patients with CPSP, and other forms of central pain, in whom it has not been possible even with quantitative methods to show any sensory disturbances.

Table 38.4 Factors increasing central poststroke pain: proportion of patients (%). (Reproduced from Leijon et al 1989)

	BS (n = 8)	*TH* (n = 9)	*SE* (n = 6)	*UI* (n = 4)	*All* (n = 27)
Movements	38	89	83	75	70
Cold	63	33	33	75	48
Warmth	20	11	33	35	22
Touch	63	4	17	50	44
Emotions	25	33	0	0	19

For definition of abbreviations, see Table 38.3.

Table 38.5 Neurological signs in 27 patients with central poststroke pain and multiple sclerosis: proportion of patients (%). (From Leijon et al 1989 and Österberg & Boivie, in preparation)

	CPSP	*MS*
Sensory abnormality	100	97
Paresis (moderate/severe)	37/11	48/11
Ataxia	62	29
Choreoatetosis	4	0
Agnosia	17	
Apraxia	17	
Dysphasia (light)	7	
Hemianopia	22	0

Some of the sensory abnormalities are of a quantitative nature, others are more qualitative (Box 38.4). The spectrum of quantitative and qualitative abnormalities are shown in Tables 38.6 and 38.7 for CPSP patients with different lesion locations (results from Boivie et al 1989). The dominating features are abnormal temperature and pain sensibility, which was found in all of the patients examined, and hyperaesthesias and dysaesthesias, which were found in about 85% of the patients. The abnormalities in temperature sensibility were pronounced. Eighty-one per cent could not identify temperatures between zero and 50°C. About half of these patients had normal thresholds to touch and vibration. These results indicate that all CPSP patients have lesions affecting the spinothalamic pathways, which are those most important for the sensibility of temperature and pain, whereas only some of the patients have lesions that affect the dorsal column–medial lemniscal pathways. A similar, but less pronounced tendency has been found in larger studies (Bowsher 1996, Bowsher et al 1998). These results are the basis for the hypothesis that CPSP only occurs in patients who have lesions affecting the spinothalamic pathways (see above).

Treatment

The reader is referred to the general section on treatment of central pain for details. In this section only a few comments will be made. It is recommended that transcutaneous electrical stimulation (TENS) is tried as the primary treatment in patients who have not lost touch and vibration sensibility in the painful region, because this relatively inexpensive treatment with almost no adverse side effects will give some patients long-lasting relief.

Antidepressants have undoubtely been the most useful of the drugs. About 50–70% of CPSP patients have been found to benefit from these drugs. Next in order are

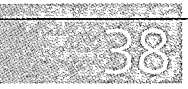

Table 38.6 Sensory abnormalities in 27 patients with central poststroke pain as revealed with quantiative (Q) and clinical (CL) tests: proportion of patients (%). (From Boivie et al 1989)

	BS (n = 8)	*TH* (n = 9)	*SE* (n = 6)	*UI* (n = 4)	*All* (n = 27)
Vibration (Q)					
Moderate	0	22	0	0	7
Severe	12	56	50	0	33
Touch (Q)					
Moderate	0	22	33	50	23
Severe	25	67	0	0	29
Innocuous temperature (Q)					
Moderate	25	11	17	25	19
Severe	75	89	83	75	81
Temperature pain (Q)					
Moderate	12	0	33	25	15
Severe	75	100	50	75	78
Touch (CL)					
Hypo	50	33	50	75	48
Hyper	38	56	33	0	37
Pinprick (CL)					
Hypo	63	11	33	50	37
Hyper	38	89	50	50	59
Kinaesthesia (CL)					
Hypo	0	78	25	33	37

For definition of abbreviations, see Table 38.3.

Table 38.7 Quantitative sensory abnormalities in 27 patients with central poststroke pain (CPSP): proportion of patients (%). (Reproduced from Boivie et al 1989)

	BS	*TH*	*SE*	*UI*	*All*
Numbness	3/8	5/9	6/8	4/4	18/22(67%)
Paraesthesia	3/8	1/9	5/6	2/4	11/27(41%)
Dysaesthesia	7/8	7/9	5/6	4/4	23/27(85%)
Hyperaesthesia	7/7	8/9	3/5	4/4	22/25(88%)
Allodynia	2/7	3/8	0/4	0/3	5/22(23%)
Radiation	2/7	4/8	3/4	3/3	12/22(55%)
Aftersensations	4/7	4/8	2/4	0/3	10/22(45%)

For definition of abbreviations, see Table 38.3.

antiepileptic drugs, which should not be restricted to patients with tic-like pain. Other drugs are not well documented, but may nevertheless be tried. The same is true for sympathetic blockade.

MULTIPLE SCLEROSIS

Epidemiology and pain characteristics

Multiple sclerosis (MS) is a severe chronic neurological disease that in many patients causes serious handicap and suffering. The disease process is of a neuroinflammatory nature and results in destruction of myelin, and eventually of the axons and cell bodies, in the CNS. The characteristic lesion is the plaque, which is a zone of demyelination. Such plaques may occur anywhere in the CNS, and in the optic nerves, but are most frequently found in the spinal cord, particularly in the dorsal columns, in the brainstem, and periventricularly in the forebrain. The two major clinical forms are the slowly progressive and remitting-relapsing forms. The cause of the inflammatory process is as yet unknown, but much is known about the various stages in the process in which different lymphatic T-cell populations play a crucial role.

In a fairly comprehensive monograph on MS it was stated that pain is uncommon in MS (Tourtellotte & Baumhefner 1983). This reflects a common view of MS, which is believed to be dominated by problems concerning mobility, incoordination of movements, balance control and vision, when in fact pain is a major problem for many MS patients. Ironically trigeminal neuralgia, which is one of the most infrequent pain types associated with MS, has been the MS-related pain usually quoted.

As soon as investigations were made on the prevalence of pain in MS it became evident that the majority of MS patients experience pain. Four studies obtained prevalence figures indicating that 42–65% of all MS patients have clinically significant pain (Table 38.8). These results were based on interviews and examination of 723 patients. The figures include almost all forms of pain except headache. In one of the studies it was found that 45% had pain at the time of the investigation, and that 32% considered the pain to be one of their worst symptoms (Stenager et al 1991).

Not all MS pain is central. It is to be expected that MS patients with paresis, spasticity and incoordination of movements will develop nociceptive musculoskeletal pain, and this is indeed the case. Vermote et al (1986) found that about 20% had such pain, including back pain, which is comparable to the 14% with back pain reported by Moulin et al (1988). It is also conceivable that peripheral neurogenic pain will be found in some MS patients. Primary psychogenic pain, i.e. pain as part of a major psychiatric disease, appears to be rare in MS. Vermote et al (1986) found only two such cases in their material of 83 patients.

It is important to carefully analyse the characteristics of the various pains experienced by MS patients to form a basis for the optimal management of the pain. According to the prevalence studies cited in Table 38.8, such an analysis will show that the majority of MS patients with pain have central pain caused by the disease itself. The figures for central pain in Table 38.8 are estimates made from the descriptions of the pain, and were not made by the authors themselves. They are thus somewhat uncertain and may be an overestimation. The figures include both paroxysmal/acute and chronic pain. Box 38.8 lists most of the pain types classified as central pain, and gives the prevalences found by Moulin et al (1988). These relative prevalences of the various forms of central pains are in accordance with most other studies.

Idiopathic trigeminal neuralgia is usually considered to be peripherally induced, but it appears likely that in MS this pain is caused by demyelination in the brainstem, and it is therefore classified as central pain in this context. Its prevalence has now been shown to be 5%, which is higher than the previous estimates (A Österberg and J Boivie, in preparation).

In a retrospective study it was concluded that pain increases with age in MS (Clifford & Trotter 1984). A similar trend was found by Moulin et al (1988). No such trend was found regarding the age at onset of MS or disease duration, apart from the fact that pain was less common during the first 5 years of the disease than later (Clifford & Trotter 1984, Moulin et al 1988, Stenager et al 1991). These relationships were not analysed specifically for central pain, however.

Pain characteristics and neurological symptoms

The characteristics of trigeminal neuralgia is described in Chapter 32. Its character is similar in MS and idiopathic tic douloureux.

The Lhermitte sign is classical of MS. It consists of rapidly spreading paraesthesias or dysaesthesias, sometimes like an electric current, down the back and radiating to the

BOX 38.8

Location of central pain in 86 patients with multiple sclerosis (A Österberg and J Boivie, in preparation)

Lower extremities	90%
Trunk	22%
Upper extremities	36%
Unilaterally	24%
Bilaterally	76%

Table 38.8 Results from prevalence studies of pain in multiple sclerosis

Study	*Clifford-Trotter 1984*	*Vermote et al 1986*	*Moulin et al 1988*	*Stenager et al 1991*	*Österberg-Boivie 1998*
Patients (no.)	317	83	159	117	364
Patients with pain (%)	29	54	55	65	65
Patients with central pain(%)	17	31	34	52	28
Trigeminal neuralgia (%)	1.6	4	4.4	1	4.9
Paroxysmal pain (%)	6	4	5	6	2
Pain quality/no. of patients	Burning/18 Toothache/15	Burning/12 Pricking/10 Stabbing/9 Dull/5	Burning/46		Burning/34 Aching/34 Pricking/21 Stabbing/13 Squeez/8

extremities. It is mostly bilateral and sometimes painful. It is usually evoked by bending the head forward and it has been proposed that it is produced when the cervical part of the inflamed dorsal columns are stretched.

Painful tonic seizures constitute another kind of paroxysmal pain in MS. A detailed description of these attacks is found in Shibasaki and Kuroiwa's (1974) report. They found 11 such cases among 64 patients with MS, which is higher than in our large material in which only 2% of the patients with central pain has this component. The attacks consist of spreading paraesthesias, pain and muscle spasm in the spinal segments involved. They are evoked by light touch or movement. No correlation was found between the pain and the degree of paresis or spasticity, but with sensory signs. The attacks usually occurred during exacerbation of spinal cord symptoms, i.e. during bouts of increased myelopathy. Painful paroxysms without muscle engagement also occur, but very infrequently (Osterman & Westerberg 1975).

The most common form of central pain in MS is non-paroxysmal extremity pain, usually termed dysaesthetic pain. The quality of this pain shows a large interindividual variation and most patients experience more than one pain quality. Burning and aching pain are most frequent, occurring in about 40%, with pricking, stabbing and squeezing being next in frequency (Table 38.8). In Box 38.8 percentage figures for the location of central pain in MS are listed, showing that there is a large dominance for pain in the lower extremities.

The combination of different pain locations and qualities can be illustrated by one of our patients. He is a 53-year-old clerk with central pain of 4 years' duration. The pain started about 2 months after he rapidly developed signs of a transverse myelitis at T9, with total loss of voluntary motor and bladder control, and total sensory loss below the waist. He now has steady pain of three distinctly different kinds. The first is a burning pain from the waist down. The second is a tight belt-like pressing pain just above the waist; it feels like tight armour. The third pain is described as if he is sitting heavily on a tennis ball. It is interesting to know that the first symptom this patient noticed was hyperaesthesia to heat, i.e. an indication of dysfunction in the spinothalamic pathways.

Most investigators have found that MS patients with non-paroxysmal central pain have disturbed somatic sensibility. It has usually been found that the patients have sensory abnormalities indicating posterior column involvement, whereas not all patients have shown signs of dysfunction in the spinothalamic pathways (Moulin et al 1988). These results have been based on clinical examinations of sensibility. In our study of 63 patients using both clinical and quantitative sensory tests, only two patients were found to have completely normal sensibility (A Österberg & J Boivie, in preparation). The abnormalities found were dominated by abnormal temperature and pain sensibility, only two patients having normal pain and temperature sensibility, whereas more than one-third of the patients had normal threshold to touch. The vibration sense was also severely affected, but not to the same degree as temperature and pain. These results have similarities with the results from patients with central poststroke pain (see above).

As regards non-sensory symptoms and signs it appears that, at most, half of MS patients with non-paroxysmal central pain have paresis, ataxia or bladder dysfunction (A Österberg & J Boivie, in preparation). Only 11 of 99 patients had severe paresis, whereas 29% had ataxia. This conforms with the results of other studies failing to find any covariation between central pain and disability (Vermote et al 1986, Moulin et al 1988, Stenager et al 1991). This also seems to be true for central pain and depression in MS (Stenager et al 1991, Österberg et al 1993). Stenager et al (1991) found no differences between MS patients with and without pain with respect to depressive symptoms.

Treatment

Antiepileptic drugs (AED) are the treatment of choice for trigeminal neuralgia and other paroxysmal pains in MS (Shibasaki & Kuroiwa 1974). These treatments are generally very successful. Carbamazepine is the first-line drug, but most other AED have a good effect too (see section on 'Antiepileptic drugs' above). The effects of treatment are dependent on the plasma concentration. It appears that many MS patients have difficulty in tolerating sufficiently high doses of carbamazepine, probably more so than other patient groups. One possible way around such problems is to try a combination of baclofen and an AED.

The AED have generally not been found effective against steady extremity pain (Clifford & Trotter 1984, Moulin et al 1988). In a controlled trial investigating the pain-relieving effects of carbamazepine and amitriptyline in 21 MS patients, it was found that carbamazepine did not have a significant effect, whereas amitriptyline had a weak effect on the spontaneous constant pain (A Österberg and J Boivie, in preparation). In this study it was noticed that MS patients do indeed have more problems with side effects than what has previously been found in patients with poststroke pain. The outcome of treatment with antidepressants has varied. Thus Clifford and Trotter (1984) reported excellent results, while Moulin et al (1988) had a poor

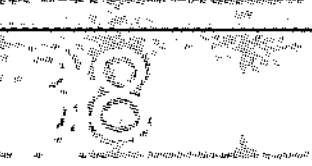

outcome with only nine of 46 patients responding well to amitriptyline and imipramine.

TENS can be tried in patients with at least some preservation of dorsal column function. Electrical stimulation of the spinal cord (DCS) has been tried quite extensively, but the outcome has been poor (Rosen & Barsoum 1979, Young & Goodman 1979, Tasker 1990) and the method is not recommended. Intrathecal baclofen has been used successfully to treat severe spasticity, but the experience of its possible effect on central pain in MS is poorly known, although some centres have reported promising results (Herman et al 1992).

SPINAL CORD INJURY

The reader is referred to Chapter 39 for more detailed information about pain following spinal cord injury (SCI).

Differential diagnosis of pain categories and epidemiology

Five studies from the last 13 years show that many SCI patients have chronic pain, with a moderate to severe pain prevalence of 42–77% of all SCI patients (from Britell & Mariano 1991). Bonica estimated that about 30% of these patients have central pain (Bonica 1991). This calculation is difficult because many of the patients have more than one kind of neurogenic pain, for instance pain due to lesions of the nerve roots and peripheral nerves. Some of the pain emanating from all three kinds of lesion has been described as dysaesthetic, although most of the dysaesthetic pain after SCI is considered to be central. Dysaesthetic pain is said to be more common after high spinal lesions than after low lesions, which on the other hand often result in lesions of the cauda equina, i.e. root lesions, and such lesions are known to cause severe pain. Many SCI patients suffer from visceral pain. Some of this pain may be central.

The lesions are classified as complete or incomplete, depending on whether they result in total loss of voluntary motor control, i.e. complete paralysis, and total loss of sensibility below the lesion, or in partial loss of these functions, which reflects the extent of the damage to the white and grey matter in the cord. A rare cause of spinal injury pain is cordotomies performed to relieve intractable pain. It has been estimated that about 3–5% of cordotomies induce central pain (Tasker 1990).

Characteristics of central pain in SCI

Currently available information about the characteristics of central pain in SCI patients is incomplete. It is thus uncertain whether or not the character of central pain is different in patients with complete and incomplete lesions. In studies over recent years, the term 'dysaesthetic' has been used for all SCI pain (Davidoff et al 1987a, Berić et al 1988, Britell & Mariano 1991), although one might get the impression from one of the studies that dysaesthetic pain occurs mainly after incomplete lesions (Berić et al 1988). By analysing pain in 19 patients, Davidoff et al (1987a) showed that the term dysaesthetic pain corresponds to many pain qualities. When these SCI patients described their central pain according to the McGill Pain Questionnaire (MPQ), it was found that 58% experienced cutting pain 47% burning pain, 47% radiating pain and 37% tight pain. Thirty-seven per cent chose the word 'cruel' and 37% the word 'nagging'. In most of the patients the pain was deep (83%), whereas it was both deep and superficial in the others. All of the 13 patients reported by Lenz et al (1988) had burning pain. Most patients have constant pain, but paroxysmal pain is not uncommon. The onset of central pain in SCI is sometimes immediate; in other patients there is a considerable delay (Berić et al 1988).

The profile of the sensory abnormalities was investigated by quantitative sensory testing (QST) in 13 patients with 'dysaesthetic' burning central pain following SCI (Berić et al 1988). All but one had incomplete lesions. The sensibility to temperature and pain were more severely affected than vibration and touch. These results are in accordance with the results from patients with CPSP, i.e. they may indicate that spinothalamic tract lesions are more important for central pain than lesions in the dorsal column–medial lemniscal pathways.

Painful hyperaesthesias, for instance touch and cold allodynia, occur in some SCI patients. Their spontaneous central pain is sometimes also influenced by body movement, external stimuli and emotions.

SYRINGOMYELIA AND SYRINGOBULBIA

Syringomyelia (in the spinal cord) and syringobulbia (in the lower brainstem) are rare diseases with a very high incidence of central pain. From a scientific point of view they are of particular interest for the understanding of the mechanisms that underlie central pain and sensory disturbances, because they illustrate the possible consequences of internal lesions in the spinal cord and brainstem. The lesion is a cystic cavity filled with a fluid that is similar to normal CSF. The size and extension of the cavity, i.e. the syrinx (from the greek word for flute), varies enormously between patients, from a small lesion in the dorsal part of the spinal cord over a couple of segments to huge cavities extending from the most caudal part of the cord into the medulla oblongata, as illustrated by findings at autopsy, and in recent years by examination with MRI (Foster & Hudgson 1973, Schliep 1978, Milhorat et al 1996). The largest cavities leave only a thin layer of spinal cord tissue undamaged at the maximally cavitated regions.

Much is still unknown about how the cavities develop, and particularly about the cause of the disease. According to the most embraced theory hydromechanical forces are important for the expansion of the cavity. This theory states that the cavity develops as an enlargement of the central canal. Waves of increased pressure are thought to descend from the fourth ventricle in moments of increased intracranial pressure. Incomplete closure of the upper part of the central canal may enhance such a process. This means that the cavity starts in the centre of the spinal cord, which is where the spinothalamic fibres cross the midline to reach their position in the ventrolaterally located spinothalamic tract. A lesion with this location will affect the sensibility to temperature and pain, i.e. a dissociated sensory loss will appear. Studies have shown that this in fact happens, because this sensory abnormality was found in 248 of 250 patients with syringomyelia and syringobulbia (Foster & Hudgson 1973, Schliep 1978). Syringomyelia can also be post-traumatic and be caused by spinal cord haematomas.

Pain is common in syringomyelia (when this term is used in this chapter it also includes syringobulbia). In a recent survey of 22 patients it was found that all had pain, and that 16 (73%) had central pain (J Boivie and U Rollsjö, unpublished results). This pain was in most patients located in one of the upper extremities, seldom in both. The thorax was another rather common location, and a few had pain in the lower extremities. Burning, aching and pressing were the most common pain qualities. Pain, often central pain, was a frequent initial symptom in this disease which usually progresses slowly over decades.

The results from our study cast doubt on the notion that the somatosensory symptoms of syringomyelia, including central pain, are mainly caused by damage to the spinothalamic fibres as they cross the midline, because it has been found that the symptoms and signs are strictly unilateral in several patients who are probably in an early stage of the disease. Thus some patients have central pain and dissociated sensory loss in one arm and hand. This could be explained by either a lesion affecting the dorsal horn or one affecting the spinothalamic fibres on that side, before they cross. Unfortunately no MRI verification is available for these patients. It can be speculated that the syrinx expands from the central canal into the dorsal horn grey matter, because the mechanical resistance is lower there than in the white matter. This would fit with the clinical features. However, there is as yet no support for this idea from MRI or postmortem examinations, which usually show that the cavities are very extensive both longitudinally and across the cord. The results from MRI or postmortem examinations do not contradict this idea.

Quantitative sensory tests show that all patients with syringomyelia have abnormal temperature and pain sensibility (Boivie 1984) (J Boivie and U Rollsjö, unpublished results). These abnormalities are mostly pronounced with total loss of temperature sensibility. Patients in advanced stages of the disease have abnormal touch, vibration and kinesthaesia too, indicating that either the dosal root fibres or the dorsal columns are affected by the syrinx. Some, but not all patients with central pain have hyperaesthesias of the hyperpathic kind or allodynia.

The treatment of central pain in syringomyelia is similar to that of central pain after traumatic spinal cord injuries. In our clinical experience tricyclic antidepressants have been moderately successful.

PARKINSON'S DISEASE

Parkinson's disease (PD) is rightfully considered to be a movement disorder. The dominating symtoms are rigidity, bradykinesia, tremor and defective postural control. However, it is becoming increasingly clear that many patients with PD have pain and sensory symptoms (Snider et al 1976, Koller 1984, Goetz et al 1985, Schott 1985, Quinn et al 1986). In some patients these symptoms precede the onset of the motor symptoms. The mechanisms behind these symptoms are unknown. It is thus unclear to what extent the pain in PD should be classified as central pain, but it appears likely that at least part of it is of primarily central origin, i.e. central pain. A brief summary of published reports on this pain will be made.

In an investigation of 105 ambulatory PD patients it was found that 43% had sensory symptoms (pain, tingling, numbness; Snider et al 1976). Pain was the most common complaint, reported by 29%: 'It was usually described as an intermittent, poorly localized, cramp-like or aching sensation, not associated with increased muscle contraction and not affected by movement or pressure. It was often proximal and in the limb of greatest motor deficit.' Eleven per cent had burning sensations and 12% had painful muscle spasm or cramps. In 7% the pain preceded the motor symptoms. In a similar study of 94 patients, 46% were found to have pain (Goetz et al 1985). The major pains were 'muscle cramps or tightness' (34% of all patients) and painful dystonias (13% of all patients).

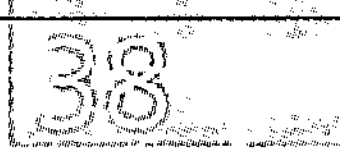

A classification for the pain directly related to PD was proposed by Quinn et al (1986):

A. Pain preceding the diagnosis of PD.
B. Off-period pain (without dystonia) in patients with fluctuating response to levodopa (four subgroups).
C. Painful dystonic spasms (four subgroups).
D. Peak-dose pain.

Quinn et al (1986) did not give any prevalence figures for the four groups. They concluded that most of the pain is related to fluctuations in motor symptoms, which in turn are related to the response to the drug treatment. This idea was supported by observations in two patients in which the fluctuations in motor symptoms and pain were recorded (Nutt & Carter 1984). These observations are compatible with a modulatory influence of the basal ganglia on somatic sensibility, including pain. In all of the studies cited no significant abnormalities in the sensibility to cutaneous stimuli were found.

From the case reports of Quinn et al (1986), it appears that much of the pain in PD can be relieved by careful adjustment of the anti-parkinson medication, but they also show that this is sometimes a difficult task.

EPILEPSY, BRAIN TUMOURS AND ABSCESSES

Central pain in these disease states will be briefly discussed. In a survey of 858 patients with epilepsy it was found that 2.8% had pain as part of epileptic seizures (Young & Blume 1983). In several of the patients the cause of the epilepsy was unknown. Many were children. No patients with cerebrovascular lesions were included. The pain was either a symptom during the major part of the seizure, or part of the aura.

Three groups were recognized:

1. Unilateral pain in the face, arm, leg or trunk (10 patients). Various pain qualities were experienced, including, for instance, burning, tingling, cramp-like, aching, throbbing, stinging, like a sharp knife or like an electric shock. These seizures were thought to emanate from activity in the first somatosensory cortical region in the postcentral gyrus.
2. Head pain, mainly headache (11 patients). These attacks included pain described as throbbing, pricking or diffuse headache. The cortical focus of these attacks could not be determined.
3. Abdominal pain (three patients). These attacks were different from the epigastic rising sensations that are sometimes part of the aura of temporal lobe seizures, but the attacks were still considered to be a feature of temporal lobe epilepsy.

Since then the same investigations have described a patient with bilateral extremity pain during epileptic seizures, which they proposed to originate in the second somatosensory cortical region (Young et al 1988).

Patients with cerebrovascular lesions that engage the cerebral cortex may develop epilepsy. Fine (1967) reported five such patients with epileptic seizures that included severe pain. This pain had qualities similar to CPSP, but it occurred spontaneously in short attacks, and disappeared completely when antiepileptic drugs were given.

In general brain tumours rarely induce central pain, but several patients with meningiomas and central pain have been reported (Bender & Jaffe 1958). Surprisingly not even thalamic tumours have a tendency to cause central pain. In a retrospective study only one of 49 patients with thalamic tumours had central pain (Tovi et al 1961).

Finally a late twentieth century illustration of the fact that all kinds of lesion can result in central pain – two patients with brain abscesses in the thalamus and internal capsule and central pain were reported (Gonzales et al 1992). The cause of the abscesses was toxoplasma infection – the patients had AIDS!

CONCLUDING COMMENTS

For the patient it is important to identify central pain when present because this is the basis for its rational management. An ad hoc committee in the Special Interest Group on Central Pain of the International Association for the Study of Pain (IASP) has worked out an examination protocol for the diagnosis of central pain. This protocol can be recommended for clinical use. It has the following components:

Historical information:

1. Is pain the major or primary complaint? If not, indicate the alternative.
2. Nature of primary neurological disability:
   a. primary diagnosis (e.g., stroke, tumour, etc.)
   b. location of disability (e.g., left hemiparesis).
3. Date of onset of neurological signs/symptoms.
4. Date of onset of pain.

5. Description of pain:
   a. location:
      body area – preferably use pain drawing
      superficial (skin) and/or deep (muscle, viscera)
      radiation or referral.
   b. intensity (1–10 or VAS or categorical scaling):
      most common intensity; at maximum; at minimum
   c. temporal features:
      steady, unchanging; intermittent
      fluctuates over minutes, hours, days, weeks
      paroxysmal features (shooting pain, tic-like).
   d. quality:
      thermal (burning, freezing, etc.)
      mechanical (pressure, cramping, etc.)
      chemical (stinging, etc.)
      other (aching, etc.).
   e. factors increasing the pain (cold, emotions, etc.).
   f. factors decreasing the pain (rest, drugs, etc.).
6. Neurological symptoms besides pain:
   a. motor (paresis, ataxia, involuntary movements)
   b. sensory (hypo-, hyperaesthesia, paraesthesia, dysaesthesia, numbness, overreaction)
   c. others (speech, visual, cognitive, mood, etc.).

Examination:

1. Neurological disease – results of CT, MRI, SPECT, PET, CSF assays, neurophysiological examinations, etc.
2. Major neurological findings (e.g., spastic paraparesis).
3. Sensory examination – preferably use sensory chart with the dermatomes. Indicate if modalities listed have normal, increased or decreased threshold, and paraesthesias or dysaesthesias are evoked.
   a. vibratory sense (tuning fork, Biothesiometer or Vibrameter)
   b. tactile (cotton wool, hair movement)
   c. skin direction sense, graphaesthesis
   d. kinaesthesia
   e. temperature (specify how tested; cold and warm, noxious and innocuous)
   f. pinprick
   g. deep pain (specify how tested)
   h. allodynia to mechanical stimuli, cold, heat
   i. hyperpathia (specify how tested)
   j. other abnormalities like radiation, summation, prolonged aftersensation.

CRITERIA FOR THE DIAGNOSIS OF CENTRAL PAIN

The examination protocol will in most patients lead to information that will enable the examiner to determine if central pain is at hand. For this decision the following criteria for central pain may be used:

1. The presence of CNS disease. The lesion/dysfunction can be located at any level of the neuraxis from the dorsal horn grey matter of the spinal cord, and the trigeminal spinal nucleus, to the cerebral cortex, i.e. either engaging the ascending pathways and/or their brainstem or cortical relays.
2. Pain that started after the onset of this disease. The pain can be steady, intermittent or paroxysmal, or be present in the form of painful hyperaesthesias such as allodynia or hyperpathia. Its onset can be immediate, or delayed up to several years.
3. The pain can have virtually any quality, including trivial aching pain. More than one pain quality is often experienced, in the same region or in different regions.
4. The pain can engage large parts of the body (hemipain, one-quarter, lower body half, etc.) or be restricted to a small region such as one arm or the face.
5. The pain can be of high or low intensity. It is often increased, or evoked, by various internal or external stimuli, such as touch, cold and sudden emotions.
6. The presence of abnormalities in somatic sensibility. The abnormalities can be subtle and in some patients it takes quantitative sensory tests to demonstrate their presence. However, in rare cases not even the quantitative methods can show such abnormalities. They are dominated by abnormal sensibility to temperature and pain, indicating involvement of the spinothalamic pathways. Abnormalities are common in touch, vibration and kinaesthesia too, but their presence is not mandatory in central pain, and many patients with central pain have normal thresholds for these submodalities. Hyperaesthesias such as allodynia, hyperalgesia and hyperpathia are common, but not demonstrable in all patients with central pain. Most patients with central pain experience paresthaesias or dysaesthesias that are sometimes painful, and thus themselves are a kind of central pain.
7. Non-sensory neurological symptoms and signs may or may not be present. There is thus no correlation between central pain and motor disturbances.
8. Psychological or psychiatric disturbances may or may not be present. A large majority of central pain patients are normal in these respects.
9. The pain should not appear to be of psychic origin.
10. The diagnosis of certain central pain should be ascertained on clinical grounds/criteria or with the help of laboratory examinations that show that the pain is not of nociceptive or peripheral neurogenic origin.

TREATMENT

Because no universally effective treatment is available for central pain it is important to try available modalities in a systematic way to find the best treatment for the individual patient. Therefore it is important to keep the patient well informed and to monitor treatment closely because of potential side effects. When drugs are used increases in dosage should be gradual. It is also wise to inform the patient that the treatment may not relieve the pain completely, which it seldom does.

Central pain is truly chronic pain, often lasting for the rest of patient's lives, and it mostly causes patients much suffering. It is therefore important that patients have a reliable long-lasting relationship with their physicians so that they know whom to contact when the pain brings them into despair when support by a psychotherapist may be indicated. Furthermore there is reason to include physiotherapy in the treatment programme, aiming at increased activity and rehabilitation.

The first-line specific treatments are TENS, antidepressants and antiepileptic drugs. The reader is referred to the sections on these treatments or on the individual pain conditions for detailed information. In some patients the treatment of the central pain needs to be combined with other forms of treatment, because other pains may also be present.

REFERENCES

Ajuraguerra dJ 1937 La douleur dans les affections du système nerveux central. Doin, Paris

Andersen G, Vestergaard K, Ingeman-Nielsen M, Jensen TS 1995 Incidence of central post-stroke pain. Pain 61: 187–193

Arnér S, Meyerson BA 1991 Genuine resistance to opioids – fact or fiction? Pain 47: 116–118

Attal N, Parker F, Brasseur L, Chauvin M, Bouhassira D 1997 Efficacy of gabapentin on neuropathic pain: a pilot study. In: Abstracts of the American Pain Society Meetings, p 108

Awerbuch 1990 Treatment of thalamic pain syndrome with Mexiletone. Annals of Neurology 28: 233

Backonja M, Arndt G, Gombar KA, Check B, Zimmermann M 1994 Response of chronic neuropathic pain syndromes to ketamine: a preliminary study. Pain 56: 51–57

Backonja M, Hes MS, LaMoreaux LK, Garafolo EA, Koto EM 1997 Gabapentin reduces pain in diabetics with painful peripheral neuropathy: results of a double blind, placebo-controlled clinical trial. In: Abstracts of the American Pain Society Meetings, p 108

Bainton T, Fox M, Bowsher D, Wells C 1992 A double-blind trial of naloxone in central post-stroke pain. Pain 48: 159–162

Bear MS, Molinka RC 1994 Synaptic plasticity: LTP and LTD. Current Opinions in Neurobiology 4: 389–399

Bender MB, Jaffe R 1958 Pain of central origin. Medical Clinics of North America 49: 691–700

Berić A, Dimitrijević MR, Lindblom U 1988 Central dysesthesia syndrome in spinal cord injury patients. Pain 34: 109–116

Biemond A 1956 The conduction of pain above the level of the thalamus opticus. Archives of Neurology and Psychiatry 75: 231–244

Boas RA, Covino BG, Shahnarian A 1982 Analgesic responses to i.v. lignocaine. British Journal of Anaesthesia 54: 501–505

Bogousslavsky J, Regli F, Uske A 1988 Thalamic infarcts: clinical syndromes, etiology, and prognosis. Neurology 38: 837–848

Boivie J 1979 An anatomic reinvestigation of the termination of the spinothalamic tract in the monkey. Journal of Comparative Neurology 168: 343–370

Boivie J 1984 Disturbances in cutaneous sensibility in patients with central pain caused by the spinal cord lesions of syringomyelia. Pain. Supplement 2: S 82

Boivie J 1992 Hyperalgesia and allodynia in patients with CNS lesions. In: Willis WDJ (ed) Hyperalgesia and allodynia. Raven, New York, pp 363–373

Boivie J 1995 Pain syndromes in patients with CNS lesions and a comparison with nociceptive pain. In: Bromm B, Desmeth JE (ed) Advances in pain research and therapy. Raven, New York, pp 367–375

Boivie J, Leijon G 1991 Clinical findings in patients with central post-stroke pain. In: Casey KL (ed) Pain and central nervous system disease: the central pain syndromes. Raven, New York, pp 65–75

Boivie J, Leijon G 1996 Central post-stroke pain (CPSP)-longterm effects of amitryptiline. In: Abstracts 8th World Congress on Pain. IASP Press, Seattle, p 380

Boivie J, Leijon G, Johansson I 1989 Central post-stroke pain – a study of the mechanisms trough analyses of the sensory abnormalities. Pain 37: 173–185

Bonica JJ 1991 Introduction: semantic, epidemiologic, and educational issues. In: Casey KL (ed) Pain and central nervous system disease: the central pain syndromes. Raven, New York, pp 13–29

Bowsher D 1995 Central pain. Pain Reviews 2: 175–186

Bowsher D 1996 Central pain: clinical and physiological characteristics. Journal of Neurology, Neurosurgery and Psychiatry 61: 62–69

Bowsher D, Nurmikko T 1996a Central post-stroke Pain drug treatment options. Disease Management 5: 160–165

Bowsher D, Nurmikko T 1996b Central post-stroke pain. Drug Treatment Options. CNS Drugs 5: 160–165

Bowsher D, Foy PM, Shaw MDM 1989 Central pain complicating infarction following subarachnoid haemorrhage. British Journal of Neurosurgery 3: 435–442

Bowsher D, Leijon G, Thuomas K-Å 1998 Central post-stroke pain: correlation of magnetic resonance imaging with clinical pain characteristics and sensory abnormalities. Neurology 51: 1352–1358

Breuer AC, Cuervo H, Selkoe DJ 1981 Hyperpathia and sensory level due to parietal lobe arteriovenous malformation. Archives of Neurology 38: 722–724

Britell CW, Mariano AJ 1991 Chronic pain in spinal cord injury. Physical Medicine and Rehabilitation: State of Art Reviews 5: 71–82

Bromm B, Treede RD 1987 Human cerebral potentials evoked by CO_2 laser stimuli causing pain. Experimental Brain Research 67: 153–162

Budd K 1985 The use of the opiate antagonist naloxone in the treatment of inreactable pain. Neuropeptides 5: 419–422

Budd K 1989 Sodium valproate in the treatment of pain. In: Chadwick D (ed) Fourth international symposium on sodium valproate and epilepsy. Royal Society of Medicine, London, pp 213–216

Casey KL, Beydoun A, Boivie J et al 1996 Laser-evoked cerebral potentials and sensory function in patients with central pain. Pain 64: 485–491

Cassinari V, Pagni CA 1969 Central pain. A neurosurgical survey. Harvard University Press, Cambridge, Massachusetts, pp 1–192

Cesaro P, Mann MW, Moretti JL et al 1991 Central pain and thalamic hyperactivity: a single photon emission computerized tomographic study. Pain 47: 329–336

Chabal C, Russel LC, Burchiel KJ 1989 The effect of intravenous lidicaine, tocainide, and mexiletine on spontaneous active fibers originating in rat sciatic neuromas. Pain 38: 333–338

Clifford DB, Trotter JL 1984 Pain in multiple sclerosis. Archives of Neurology 41: 1270–1272

Craig AD 1991 Supraspinal pathways and mechanisms relevant to central pain. In: Casey KL (ed) Pain and central nervous disease: the central pain syndromes. Raven, New York, pp 157–170

Craig AD 1998 A new version of the thalamic disinhibition hypothesis of central pain. Pain Forum 7: 1–14

Davidoff G, Guarrachini M, Roth E, Sliwa J, Yarkony G 1987a Trazodone hydrochloride in the treatment of dysesthetic pain in traumatic myelopathy: a randomized, double-blind, placebo-controlled study. Pain 29: 151–161

Davidoff G, Roth EJ, Guarracini M, Sliwa J, Yarkony G 1987b Function-limiting dysesthetic pain syndrome among traumatic spinal cord injury patients: a cross-sectional study. Pain 29: 39–48

Davidoff G, Roth EJ 1991 Clinical characteristics of central (dysesthetic) pain in spinal cord injury patients. In: Casey KL (ed) pain and central nervous disease: the central pain syndromes. Raven Press, New York, pp 77–83

Davidson C, Schick W 1935 Spontaneous pain and other subjective sensory disturbances: a clinicopathological study. Neurology 34: 1204–1237

Dehen H, Willer JC, Cambier J 1983 Pain in thalamic syndrome: electrophysiological findings in man. Advances in Pain Research and Therapy 5: 936–940

Dejerine J, Roussy G 1906 La syndrome thalamique. Revue Neurologique (Paris) 14: 521–532

Dejgard A, Pewtersen P, Kastrup J 1988 Mexiletine for treatment of chronic painful diabetic neuropathy. Lancet i: 9–11

Drake CG, Mckenzie KG 1953 Mesencephalic tractotomy for pain. Journal of Neurosurgery 10: 457–462

Eaton SA, Salt TE 1990 Thalamic NMDA receptors and nociceptive sensory synaptic transmission. Neuroscience Letters 110: 297–302

Edgar RE, Best LG, Quail PA, Obert AD 1993 Computer-assisted DREZ microcoagulation: posttraumatic spinal deafferentation pain. Journal of Spinal Disease 6: 48–56

Edinger L 1891 Giebt es central antstehender Schmerzen. Deutche Zeitschrift fur Nervenheilkunde 1: 262–282

Edwards WT, Habib F, Burney RG, Begin G 1985 Intravenous lidocaine in the management of various chronic pain states. Regional Anaesthesia 10: 1–6

Ekbom K 1966 Tegretol, a new therapy of thabetic lightning pains. Acta Medica Scandinavica 179: 251–252

Eriksson MBE, Sjölund BH, Nielzén S 1979 Long term results of pheripheral conditioning stimulation as an analgesic measure in chronic pain. Pain 6: 335–347

Espir MLE, Millac P 1970 Treatment of paroxysmal disorders in multiple sclerosis with carbamazepine (Tegretol). Journal of Neurology, Neurosurgery and Psychiatry 33: 528–531

Fields HL, Adams JE 1974 Pain after cortical injury relieved by electrical stimulation of the internal capsule. Brain 97: 169–178

Fine W 1967 Post-hemiplegic epilepsy in the elderly. British Medical Journal 1: 199–201

Foerster O 1927 Die Lactungsbahnen des Schmerzgefuhls und die chirurgische Behandlung der Schmerzzustande. Urban & Schwarzenberg, Berlin, pp 77–80

Foix C, Thévenard A, Nicolesco 1922 Algie faciale dórigine bulbo-trigéminale au cours de la Syringomyélie.-Troubles sympathiques concomitants. -Douleur á type cellulaire. Revue Neurologique 29: 990–999

Foster JB, Hudgson P 1973 Clinical features of syringomyelia. In: Barnett HJ, Foster JB, Hudgson P (eds) Syringomyelia. Saunders, London, pp 1–123

Garcin R 1968 Thalamic syndrome and pain central origin. In: Soulairac A, Cahn J, Charpentier J (eds) Pain. Academic, London, pp 521–541

Glynn CJ, Jamous MA, Teddy PJ, Moorem RA, Lloyd JW 1986 Role of spinal noradrenergic system in transmission of pain in patients with spinal cord injury. Lancet ii: 1249–1250

Glynn C, Dawson D, Sanders RA 1988 A double-blind comparison between epidural morphine and epidural clonidine in patients with chronic non-cancer pain. Pain 34: 123–128

Goetz CG, Tanner CM, Levy M, Wilson RS, Garron DG 1985 Pain in idiopathic Parkinson's disease. Neurology 35: 200

Gonzales GR, Herskovitz S, Rosenblum M et al 1992 Central pain from cerebral abscess: thalamic syndrome in AIDS patients with toxoplasmosis. Neurology 42: 1107–1109

Gracely RH 1991 Theoretical and practical issues in pain assessment in central pain syndromes. In: Casey KL (ed) Pain and central nervous system disease: the central pain syndromes. Raven, New York, pp 85–101

Gram L 1990 Inadequate dosing and pharmacokinetic variability as confounding factors in assessment of efficacy of antidepressants. Clinical Neuropharmacology 13 (suppl 1): 35–44

Greiff 1883 Zur Localisation der Hemichorea, Archiv fur der Psychologie und Nervenkrankheiten 14: 598

Gybels JM, Sweet WH 1989 Neurosurgical treatment of persistant pain. Karger, Basel

Hampf G, Bowsher D 1989 Distigmine and amitriptyline in the treatment of chronic pain. Anesthesia Progress 36: 58–62

Hansson P, Lindblom U 1992 Hyperalgesia assessed with quantitative sensory testing in patients with neurogenic pain. In: Willis WDJ (ed) Hyperalgesia and allodynia. Raven, New York, pp 335–343

Hao JX, Xu XJ, Yu YX, Sieger Å, Wiesenfeldt-Hallin Z 1992 Baclofen reverses the hypersensitivity of dorsal horn wide dynamic range neurons to mechanical stimulation after transient spinal cord ischemia – implications for a tonic GABA-ergic inhibitory control of myelinated fiber input. Journal of Neurophysiology 68: 392–396

Hartvig P, Gillberg PG, Gordh T, Post C 1989 Cholinergic mechanisms in pain and analgesia. TIPS (suppl Dec 89): 75–79

Hassler R 1960 Die zentrale Systeme des Schmerzes. Acta Neurochirurgica 8: 353–423

Head H, Holmes G 1911 Sensory disturbances from cerebral lesions. Brain 34: 102–254

Herman RM, Luzansky SCD, Ippolito R 1992 Intrathecal baclofen supresses central pain in patients with spinal lesions. Clinical Journal of Pain 8: 338–345

Holmes G 1919 Pain of central origin. In: Osler W (ed) Contributions to medical and biological research. Paul B Hoeber, New York, pp 235–246

Holmgren H, Leijon G, Boivie J, Johansson I, Ilievska L 1990 Central post-stroke pain – somatosensory evoked potentials in relation to location of the lesion and sensory signs. Pain 40: 43–52

Jeanmonod D, Magnin M, Morel A 1996 Low-threshold calcium spike bursts in the human thalamus. Common physiopathology for sensory, motor and limbic positive symptoms. Brain 119: 363–375

Jones EG 1992 Thalamus and pain. APS Journal 1: 58–61

Kalman S, Sörensen J, Österberg A, Boivie J, Bertler Å 1993 Is central pain in multiple sclerosis opioid sensitive? In: Abstracts 7th World Congress on Pain. IASP Press, p 407

Kastrup J, Petersen P, Dejgård A, Angelo HR, Hilsted J 1987 Intravenous lidocaine infusion- a new treatment of chronic painful diabetic neuropathy? Pain 28: 69–75

Koller WC 1984 Sensory symptoms in Parkinson's disease. Neurology 34: 957–959

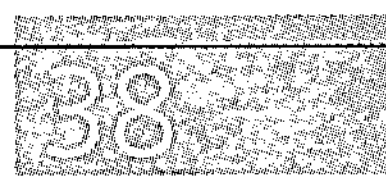

Kupers RC, Konings H, Adriasen H, Gybels JM 1991 Morphine differentially affects the sensory and affective ratings in neurogenic and ideopathic forms of pain. Pain 47: 5–12

Leijon G, Boivie J 1989a Central post-stroke pain – a controlled trial of amitriptyline and carbamazepine. Pain 36: 27–36

Leijon G, Boivie J 1989b Treatment of neurogenic pain with antidepressants. Nordisk Psykiatrisk Tidsskrift 43 (suppl 20): 83–87

Leijon G, Boivie J 1989c Central post-stroke pain – the effect of high and low frequency TENS. Pain 38: 187–191

Leijon G, Boivie J 1991 Pharmacological treatment of central pain. In: Casey KL (ed) Pain and central nervous system disease: the central pain syndromes. Raven, New York, pp 257–266

Leijon G, Boivie J 1996 Central post-stroke pain (CPSP) – A longterm follow up. In: Abstracts 8th World Congress on Pain. IASP Press, Seattle, p 380

Leijon G, Boivie J, Johansson I 1989 Central post-stroke pain – neurological symptoms and pain characteristics. Pain 36: 13–25

Lenz FA 1992 Ascending modulation of thalamic function and pain; experimental and clinical data. In: Sicuteri F (ed) Advances in pain research and therapy. Raven, New York, pp 177–196

Lenz AF, Tasker RR, Dostrovsky JO et al 1988 Abnormal single-unit activity and response to stimulation in the presumed ventrocandal nucleus of patients with central pain. In: Dubner R, Gebhart GF, Bond MR (ed) Pain research and clinical management. Elsevier, Amsterdam, pp 157–164

Lindblom U 1994 Analysis of abnormal touch, pain, and temperature sensation in patients. In: Boivie J, Hansson U, Lindblom U (ed) Touch, temperature, and pain in health and disease. IASP Press, Seattle, pp 63–84

Lindström P, Lindblom U 1987 The analgesic effect of tocainide in trigeminal neuralgia. Pain 28: 45–50

Loh L, Nathan PW, Schott GD 1981 Pain due to lesions of central nervous system removed by sympathetic block. British Medical Journal 282: 1026–1028

MacGowan DJL, Janal MN, Clark WC et al 1997 Central post-stroke pain and Wallenberg's lateral medullary infarction: frequency, character, and determinants in 63 patients. Neurology 49: 120–125

McLean MJ, Macdonald RL 1986 Carbamazepine and 10,11-epoxycarbamazepine produce use- and voltage-dependent limitation of rapidly firing action potentials of mouse central neurons in cell culture. Journal of Pharmacology and Experimental Therapeutics 238: 727–738

McNamara PJ, Tanaka Y, Miyazaki M, Albert ML 1991 Pain associated with cerebral lesions. Pain (suppl 5): 434

Mauguiere F, Desmedt JE 1988 Thalamic pain syndrome of Dejérine–Roussy. Differentation of four subtypes assisted by somatosensory evoked potentials data. Archives of Neurology 45: 1312–1320

Max MB, Schafer SC, Culnane M, Smoller B, Dubner R, Gracely RH 1988 Amitriptyline, but not lorazepam, relieves postherpetic neuralgi. Neurology 38: 1427–1432

Max MB, Lynch SA, Muir J, Shoaf SE, Smoller B, Dubner R 1992 Effects of desipramine, amitriptyline, and flouxetine on pain in diabetic neuropathy. New England Journal of Medicine 326: 1250–1256

Mersky H, Bogduk N 1994 Classification of chronic pain. IASP Press, Seattle, pp 1–222

Michel D, Laurent B, Convers P et al 1990 Douleurs corticales. Étude clinique, électrophysiologique et topographie de 12 cas. Revue Neurologique (Paris) 146: 405–414

Michelson JJ 1943 Subjective disturbances of the sense of pain from lesions of the cerebral cortex. Research Publications – Association for Research in Nervous and Mental Disease 23: 86–99

Milhorat TH, Kotzen RM, Mu HTM, Copocelli AL, Milhorat RH 1996 Dysesthetic pain in patients with syringomyelia. Neurosurgery 38: 940–947

Moulin DE, Foley KM, Ebers GC 1988 Pain syndromes in multiple sclerosis. Neurology 38: 1830–1834

Nashold BS, Bullitt E 1981 Dorsal root entry zone lesions to control central pain in paraplegics. Journal of Neurosurgery 55: 414–419

Nasreddine ZS, Saver JL 1997 Pain after thalamic stroke: right dienchephalic predominance and clinical features in 180 patients. Neurology 48: 1196–1199

Nepomuceno C, Fine PR, Richards S et al 1979 Pain in patients with spinal cord injury. Archives of Physical Medicine and Rehabilitation 60: 605–609

Nutt JG, Carter JH 1984 Sensory symptoms in parkinsonism related to central dopaminergic function. Lancet 2: 456–457

Österberg A, Boivie J, Henriksson A, Holmgren H, Johansson I 1993 Central pain in multiple sclerosis. In: Abstracts 7th World Congress on Pain, p 407

Österberg A, Boivie J, Holmgren H, Thomas K-Å, Johansson I 1994 The clinical characteristics and sensory abnormalities of patients with central pain caused by multiple sclerosis. In: Gebhart GF, Hammond DL, Jensen TS (eds) Progress in pain research and management. IASP Press, Seattle, pp 789–796

Osterman PO, Westerberg C-E 1975 Paroxysmal attacks in multiple sclerosis. Brain 98: 189–202

Pagni CA 1989 Central pain due to spinal cord and brainstem damage. In: Wall PD, Malzack R (eds) Textbook of pain. Churchill Livingstone, Edinburgh, pp 634–655

Pagni C 1998 Central pain. A neurosurgical challenge. Edizioni Minerva Medica, Turin, p 211

Pertovaara A, Morrow TJ, Casey KL 1988 Cutaneous pain and detection thresholds to short CO_2 laser pulses in humans: evidence on afferent mechanisms and the influence of varying stimulus conditions. Pain 34: 261–269

Peyron R, Garcia-Larrea L, Deiber MP et al 1995 Electrical stimulation of precentral cortical area in the treatment of central pain: electrophysiological and PET study. Pain 62: 275–286

Portenoy RK, Foley KM 1986 Chronic use of opioid analgesics in non-malignant pain: report of 38 cases. Pain 25: 171–186

Portenoy RK, Foley KM, Inturrisi CE 1990 The nature of opioid responsiveness and its implications for neuropathic pain: new hypothesis derived from studies of opioid infusions. Pain 43: 273–286

Quinn NP, Koller WC, Lang AE, Marsden CD 1986 Painful Parkinson's disease. Lancet 1: 1366–1369

Rascol O, Tran M-A, Bonnevialle P et al 1987 Lack of correlation between plasma levels of amitryptiline (and nortriptyline) and clinical improvement of chronic pain of peripheral neurologic origin. Clinical Neuropharmacology 10: 560–564

Rausell E, Cusick CG, Taub E, Jones EG 1991 Chronic deafferentation in monkeys differentially affects nociceptive and non-nociceptive pathways distinguished by specific calcium binding proteins and down regulates GABA-A receptors at thalamic levels. Proceedings of the National Academy of Sciences USA 89: 2571–2575

Richardsson RR, Meyer PR, Cerullo L 1980 Neurostimulation in the modulation of intractable paraplegic and traumatic neuroma pains. Pain 8: 75–84

Riddoch G 1938 The clinical features of central pain. Lancet 234: 1093–1098, 1150–1156, 1205–1209

Rosen JA, Barsoum AH 1979 Failure of chronic dorsal column stimulation in multiple sclerosis. Annals of Neurology 6: 66–67

Rowbotham MC, Reisner-Keller LA, Fields HL 1991 Both intravenous lidocaine and morphine reduce the pain of postherpetic neuralgia. Neurology 41: 1024–1028

Salt TE 1992 The possible involvement of exitatory amino acids and NMDA receptors in thalamic pain mechanisms and central pain syndromes. ASP Journal 1: 52–54

Sandyk R 1985 Spontaneous pain, hyperpathia and wastings of the hand due to parietal lobe haemorrhage. European Neurology 24: 1–3
Scadding JW, Wall PD, Parry CBW, Brooks DM 1982 Clinical trial of propranolol in post-traumatic neuralgia. Pain 14: 283–292
Schliep G 1978 Syringomyelia and syringobulbia. In: Vinken G, Bruyn G (eds) Handbook of neurology. North-Holland Publishing Company, Amsterdam, pp 255–327
Schmahmann JD, Leifer D 1992 Parietal pseudothalamic pain syndrome. Clinical features and anatomic correlates. Archives of Neurology 49: 1032–1037
Schott B, Laurent B, Mauguière F 1986 Les douleurs thalamiques: étude critique de 43 cas. Revue Neurologique (Paris) 142: 308–315
Schott GD 1985 Pain in Parkinson's disease. Pain 22: 407–411
Schott GD, Loh L 1984 Anticholinesterase drugs in the treatment of chronic pain. Pain 20: 201–206
Schuster P 1936 Beiträge zur patologie des Thalamus opticus. Archiv fur Psychiatrie und Nervkrankheiten 105: 550–622
Shibasaki H, Kuroiwa Y 1974 Painful tonic seizure in multiple sclerosis. Archives of Neurology 30: 47–51
Siegfried J 1983 Long term results of electrical stimulation in the treatment of pain by means of implanted electrodes. In: Rizzi C, Visentin TA (eds) Pain therapy. Elsevier, Amsterdam, pp 463–475
Siegfried J, Demierre B 1984 Thalamic electrostimulation in the treatment of thalamic pain syndrome. Pain (suppl 2): 116
Silver ML 1957 'Central pain' from cerebral arteriovenous aneurysm. Journal of Neurosurgery 14: 92–97
Sindrup SH, Gram LF, Brosen K, Eshöj O, Mogensen EF 1990 The selective serotonin reuptake inhibitor paroxetine is effective in the treatment of diabetic neuropathy symptoms. Pain 42: 135–144
Sjölund BH 1991 Role of transcutaneous electrical nerve stimulation, central nervous system stimulation, and ablative procedures in central pain syndromes. In: Casey KL (ed) Pain and central nervous disease: the central pain syndromes. Raven, New York, pp 267–274
Snider SR, Fahn S, Isgreen WP, Cote LJ 1976 Primary sensory symptoms in parkinsonism. Neurology 26: 423–429
Soria ED, Fine EJ 1991 Disappearance of thalamic pain after parietal subcortical stroke. Pain 44: 285–288
Stenager E, Knudsen L, Jensen K 1991 Acute and chronic pain syndromes in multiple sclerosis. Acta Neurologica Scandinavica 84: 197–200
Swerdlow M 1986 Anticonvulsants in the therapy of neuralgig pain. The Pain Clinic 1: 9–19
Taira T, Tanikawa T, Kawamura H, Iseki H, Takamura K 1994 Spinal intrathecal baclofen suppresses central pain after stroke. Journal of Neurology, Neurosurgery and Psychiatry 57: 381–382
Tasker R 1990 Pain resulting from central nervous system pathology (central pain). In: Bonica JJ (ed) The management of pain. Lea and Febiger, Philadelphia, pp 264–280
Tasker RR, de Carvalho G, Dostrovsky JO 1991 The history of central pain syndromes, with observations concerning pathophysiology and treatment. In: Casey KL (ed) Pain and central nervous disease: the central pain syndromes. Raven, New York, pp 31–58
Tomson T 1980 Carbamazepine therapy in trigeminal neuralgia. Archives of Neurology 37: 699–703
Tourtellotte WW, Baumhefner WW 1983 Comprehensive management of multiple sclerosis. In: Hallpike JF, Adams CWM, Tourtellotte WW (eds) Multiple sclerosis. Williams & Wilkins, Baltimore, pp 513–578
Tourian AY 1987 Narcotic responsive 'thalamic' pain treatment with propranolol and tricyclic antidepressants. Pain (suppl 4): 411
Tovi D, Schisano G, Liljequist B 1961 Primary tumours of the region of the thalamus. Journal of Neurosurgery 18: 730–740
Treede RD, Kief S, Hölzer T, Bromm B 1988 Late somatosensory evoked cerebral potentials in response to cutaneous heat stimuli. Electroencephalography and Clinical Neurophysiology 70: 429–441
Tsubokawa T 1995 Motor cortex stimulation for deafferentation pain relief in various clinical syndromes and its possible mechanisms. In: Besson JM, Guildbaud G, Ollat H (eds) Forebrain areas involved in pain processing. John Libby Eurotext, Paris, pp 261–276
Umlauf RL, Moore JE, Britell CW 1992 Relevance and nature of the pain experience in spinal cord injured. Journal of Behavioural Medicine 37: 254–261
Vermote R, Ketelaer P, Carton H 1986 Pain in multiple sclerosis patients. Clinical Neurology and Neurosurgery 88: 87–93
Vestergaard K, Nielsen J, Andersen G, Ingeman-Nielsen M, Arendt-Nielsen L, Jensen TS 1995 Sensory abnormalities in consecutive, unselected patients with central post-stroke pain. Pain 61: 177–186
Waltz TA, Ehni G 1966 The thalamic syndrome and its mechanism. Journal of Neurosurgery 24: 735–742
Watson BD, Prado R, Diedrich WD 1986 Photochemically induced spinal cord injury in the rat. Brain Research 367: 296–300
Watson C, Evans RJ 1985 A comparative trial of amitryptiline and zimilidine in post-herpetic neuralgia. Pain 23: 387–394
Watson CP, Evans RJ, Reed K, Merskey H, Goldsmith L, Warsh J 1982 Amytriptyline versus placebo in postherpetic neuralgia. Neurology 32: 671–673
White JC, Sweet WH 1969 Pain and the neurosurgeon. A forty-year experience. Charles C Thomas, Springfield
Wiesenfeld-Hallin Z, Lindblom U 1985 The effect of systemic tocaimide, lidocaine and bupivacaine on nociception in the rat. Pain 23: 357–360
Wiesenfeld-Hallin Z, Hao J-X, Xu X-J 1997 Mechanisms of central pain. In: Jensen TS, Turner JA, Wiesenfeld-Hallin Z (eds) Progress in pain research and management. IASP Press, Seattle, pp 575–588
Wood T, Sloan R 1997 Successful use of ketemine for central pain. Palliative Medicine 11: 57–58
Woolf CJ, Wiesenfeld-Hallin Z 1985 The systematic administration of local anesthetics produces a selective depression of C-afferent fibre evoked activity in the spinal cord. Pain 23: 361–374
Xu X-J, Hao JX, Seiger Å 1994 Chronic pain-related behaviors in spinally injured rats: evidence for functional alterations of the endogenous cholecystokinin and opioid systems. Pain 56: 271–277
Yamamoto T, Latayama Y, Hirayama T, Tsubokawa T 1997 Pharmacological classification of central post-stroke pain: comparison with the results of chronic motor cortex stimulation therapy. Pain 72: 5–12
Yarnitsky D, Sprecher E 1994 Different algorithms for thermal threshold measurement. In: Boivie J, Hansson P, Lindblom U (eds) Touch, temperature, and pain in health and disease: mechanisms and assessments. IASP Press, Seattle, pp 105–112
Yezierski RP 1996 Pain following spinal cord injury: the clinical problem and experimental studies. Pain 68: 185–194
Young BG, Blume WT 1983 Painful epileptic seizures. Brain 106: 537–554
Young GB, Barr HWK, Blume WT 1988 Painful epileptic seizures involving the second sensory area. Neurology 19: 412
Young RF, Goodman SJ 1979 Dorsal spinal cord stimulation in the treatment of multiple sclerosis. Neurosurg 5: 225–230

Spinal cord damage: injury

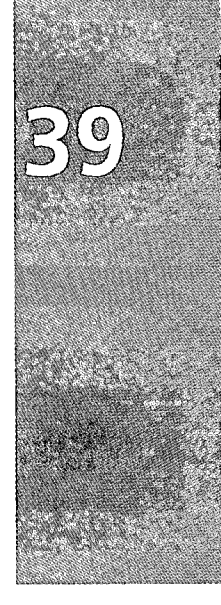

ALEKSANDAR BERIĆ

SUMMARY

Spinal cord injury pain encompasses a number of different pain syndromes. The spectrum includes transitional zone pain, cauda equina pain, central dysaesthesia syndrome, double lesion syndrome, anterior spinal artery syndrome, syringomyelia, musculoskeletal pains, and other pains and borderline syndromes, such as autonomic dysreflexia. The characteristics of chronic pains are presented together with their diagnosis and management. Two more contemporary classifications are presented and discussed together with a putative aetiology of spinal cord injury pains.

INTRODUCTION

Spinal cord injury (SCI) usually results from severe spinal column damage. Frequently, there is a concomitant ligamentous, joint, disc and soft-tissue injury. That contributes to an acute phase of pain (Berić 1997a). To a large extent, this pain usually subsides with general pain treatment and the management of acute SCI (Cairns et al 1996, Sved et al 1997). Although the acute phase is physically and psychologically the most traumatic, pain may become a significant problem only later (Tasker et al 1991, Berić 1997a, Kennedy et al 1997, Johnson et al 1998). Usually SCI pains appear after a few months and not infrequently after several years, sometimes changing their characteristics as they appear or disappear. It is actually the chronic pain that may be so devastating that it may override any other motor, bladder and bowel, and functional disabilities in the postacute phase (Nepomuceno et al 1979). Fortunately, only a fraction of SCI patients suffer from such severe pain (Bonica 1991).

In this brief introduction, it is already obvious that SCI is a very dynamic process. This is fortunate for mildly injured people because as a result of reorganization of the spinal cord and brain and collateral reinnervation, there may not be any permanent clinical deficits or pain after a few months. However, in more severe SCI patients, the nervous system attempts to reorganize and regenerate, which leads to an incomplete recovery plagued with weakness, spasticity, bladder problems and, frequently, pain. With good rehabilitative and urological measures, the majority of SCI-related problems can be minimized (Levi et al 1995a), while some of the pains remain uncontrollable (Berić 1997b).

The use of the term 'pains' is deliberate to emphasize the existence of a multitude of pains. There are different pains present in different patients and also different pains present in the same patient at different times or simultaneously. This leads us to an even more complex and unrewarding issue – SCI pain classification. Almost every paper dealing with pain in SCI has suggested some classification; however, there is no consensus regarding even a simple approach (Riddoch 1938, Davis & Martin 1947, Freeman & Heimburger 1947, Kaplan et al 1962, Burke 1973, Burke & Woodward 1976, Maury 1977–78, Donovan et al 1982, Waisbrod et al 1984, Tunks 1986, Davidoff et al 1987, Berić et al 1988, Bonica 1991, Mariano 1992, Bowsher 1996, Loubser & Akman 1996, New et al 1997, Ragnarsson 1997, Demirel et al 1998). The International Association for Study of Pain (IASP) has avoided SCI pain classification for years. Only recently have some more extensive attempts been made to classify SCI pains (Berić 1997a,b, Siddall et al 1997). Very recently, a task group on SCI pain has been proposed and organized to try to move this field forward (Yezierski 1996).

The treatment of SCI is a very difficult task and should be addressed together with classification. There are no SCI pain-specific medications, reflecting our poor understanding of underlying pain mechanisms. Due to a variety of pain disorders, a practical classification would help in developing clinical therapeutic guidelines. However, this is only a part of the solution, as there is still no optimal therapy for some of the pains, for example central pains. Another complicating factor is the fragility of the SCI patient's medical condition regarding pain medication. Spasticity, bladder and bowel function, blood pressure regulation, etc., are all by different degrees influenced by our current pain medications and control measures.

The term 'pain' is used generically throughout this chapter, although it sometimes denotes more than one type of pain. Referrals to pain generally include dysaesthesia because it is difficult to distinguish between these conditions before considering a detailed description of the patient's complaint, including its distribution as well as neurological findings.

PAIN INCIDENCE IN SPINAL CORD INJURY

Pain is usually present in acute SCI and can take different courses. It may subside with or without treatment when early musculoskeletal abnormalities slowly subside. If it is caused by root injury or SCI, it may also subside if the injury is mild and does not trigger persistent central changes or may persist into the chronic stage. As previously mentioned, pains sometimes appear weeks or months later in the course of SCI. Therefore, it is not easy to estimate the incidence of pain. On the other hand, once the spinal cord dysfunction becomes stable, usually 6–12 months after more severe injury, SCI patients after rehabilitation do not visit SCI clinics often. Furthermore, sometimes after poor pain control, persons with SCI seek other help and alternative approaches and are not readily available for pain assessments and interviews. Incidence statistics are, therefore, variable and, depending on the methodology, range from 10% to 90% (Lamid et al 1985, Rose et al 1988, Berić 1990, Levi et al 1995b, Stormer et al 1997). Recently, both inpatient and outpatient reports and telephone interviews estimate a 50% incidence of pain in the SCI population. Intractable pain is present in about one-third of these patients. If SCI patients are asked historically if they have ever experienced pain, the numbers rise to 90% and even higher (New et al 1997).

The problem with these reports, however, is that the numbers do not reflect the variety of pains in the SCI population. Some pains are spasticity related while others are due to muscle overuse problems. There are yet others that are genuine neurogenic SCI pains, which are the most difficult to manage. Sometimes the cauda equina (CE) injuries are included because there are many overlapping features between CE injuries and SCI. Different types of injuries lead to different spinal cord syndromes with a wide range of pain intensities (Richards et al 1990). There are some specific features of injuries at different spinal levels, i.e., cervical, thoracic, etc. Most studies use a presumed mechanism of pain to report its incidence. The lack of consensus in pain classification as previously mentioned leads to more confusion when comparing different studies (Richards 1992).

It would be advantageous to report the severity, distribution, quality, onset and course of pain, together with the neurological condition of the patient, according to the American Spinal Injury Association (ASIA) criteria (Maynard et al 1997). Another parameter would be previous pain treatments, especially if destructive. As some treatments change the characteristics of pain, it would be useful to state these changes in relation to treatment.

RECOGNIZED PAIN CONDITIONS IN SPINAL CORD INJURY

TRANSITIONAL ZONE PAIN

The cause of some pains in post-SCI is intuitively obvious based on the site and distribution of pain and its relationship to the primary injury. Among these types of pains are root pains, also called transitional zone segmental pains, which occur at the level of the SCI (Davis 1975, Burke & Woodward 1976). Among the 88 patients who complained of dysaesthesias and pain in our study, approximately one-third had a primary transitional zone-root pain associated with all levels of injury (Berić 1990). However, there was a disproportionately higher incidence of pain among patients with thoracic injuries compared with patients with cervical injuries. As expected, chronic transitional pain was present more often in patients with clinically complete sensory and motor dysfunction based on the severity of impact that is generally necessary to result in thoracic injury. The distribution was most often within a few contiguous segments and asymmetrical. Descriptions of pain sensation included aching, burning and stinging. In general, pain descriptions resembled those for pain that patients have experienced in the past unrelated to SCI. Frequently, there is an early allodynia to touch and hyperalgesia similar to reflex sympathetic dystrophy (RSD) or poststroke central pain that generally improves spontaneously. However, if severe,

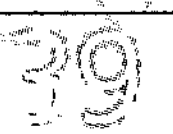

resolution of this pain may require a series of blocks or even DREZ surgery (Nashold & Bullitt 1981, Moossy & Nashold 1988, Edgar et al 1993, Sampson et al 1995, Sindou 1995).

Transitional zone segmental pains may last for some time. However, they are frequently managed by pharmacological and local block treatments. Therefore, their natural course is usually modified in the relatively early stages due to a range of reasonably effective treatment modalities.

CAUDA EQUINA PAIN

When the spinal column lesion involves levels below L1, the CE is usually injured. The pain associated with this injury may involve the legs, feet, perineum, genitals and rectum. The mechanism is similar to that of transitional zone pain in SCI. CE pain is considered a root neurogenic type of pain. In severe complete lesions of the lumbosacral segments, the upper- and mid-lumbar segments are partially injured and those dermatomes (anterior thigh) demonstrate hyperalgesia, allodynia to touch and spontaneous pain. If the injury is lower at the L4 and L5 levels, hyperalgesia and pain affect the feet or perineum and rectum. The pain usually has a burning, causalgic quality. These pains are among the most severe in spinal injuries.

CENTRAL DYSAESTHESIA SYNDROME

One of the most frequently described pain states in SCI is the diffuse burning sensation below the level of the lesion. Many terms have been used to describe this pain syndrome: burning dysaesthetic pain, function-limiting dysaesthesias, central pain, phantom pain and, more recently, central dysaesthesia syndrome (CDS) (Davis & Martin 1947, Pollock et al 1951, Davis 1975, Davidoff et al 1987, Berić et al 1988, Woodward & Vulpe 1991). The intriguing feature of this syndrome, almost invariably seen in these patients, is the relative dissociation between the anterolateral spinothalamic and dorsal column systems. Temperature, pinprick and pain perception is severely impaired in these patients. However, in most cases light-touch sensitivity and discriminatory and vibratory senses are relatively spared, with some preserved motor function below the level of the lesion that is sufficient even to allow ambulation. The CDS represents a genuine central pain syndrome (CPS) (Berić 1998).

In our series, CDS was the second most frequent pain syndrome, which occurred in 29.4% of patients (Berić 1990). The pain was relatively symmetrical, with uniform diffuse burning below the level of the lesion. It was almost equally distributed between the lower cervical and thoracic segments of the primary SCI, with a slightly higher relative incidence in the upper cervical segments. The majority of patients had dissociated sensory loss with spinothalamic deafferentation. Clinically, only 6 of 26 patients had complete absence of motor and sensory functions below the level of the lesion, including 2 patients who had undergone prior multilevel phenol rhizotomies.

There are two caveats to this general description:

1. There was some asymmetry in pain distribution.
2. There was the possibility of fluctuation in symptom intensity and, therefore, in symptom distribution in patients who had longer-term follow-ups.

Overall, total diffuseness and uniformity of pain were not present at all points of assessment (Berić 1990).

CDS is a rare entity in the general population, as it is present only in severe spinal cord pathology, usually in patients with incomplete SCI. Compared with poststroke pain, the evoked dysaesthesia component is less frequent; however, that does not mean that it is not the most prominent feature in some patients. It is usually not difficult to recognize a sensory deficit; nevertheless, it is a challenge to quantify it because there is a disproportionately greater involvement of the anterolateral modalities compared with dorsal column modalities (Berić et al 1988). In addition, it is easier to diagnose in cervical SCI patients as some diffuseness of pain below the level of the lesion is always present. It can be confused with double lesion syndrome (DLS) as DLS pain is usually sacral and lumbosacral and can be a real challenge in thoracic SCI, especially if transitional zone pain is also present. Under those circumstances, the pain can mimic CDS as it appears to cover the entire area below the level of the lesion.

Similar to poststroke pain, CDS usually appears with some functional recovery in more severe cases and can appear months after the injury. This dysaesthesia usually increases slowly in intensity and can follow three possible courses. The first and most frequent is a stable course that can linger for an indefinite number of years, with some fluctuations in symptom intensity as seen in our patient population. The second more unusual possible course of pain is continuous escalation, requiring more aggressive treatment involving possibly a destructive procedure such as cordectomy. This type of procedure may change the underlying neurological substrate but may not influence the intensity of pain significantly. The third and certainly the best possible course is the slow decrease in pain intensity within a few years. At that point, while the pain may still be present, it does not affect the patient or limit his or her functional activities. There have been a few reports from patients of a CDS type of pain that appears for the first time or is exacerbated following implantation of intrathecal baclofen administered for reduction of spasticity (Loubser & Akman 1996). It is more difficult to treat CDS in SCI than post-stroke pain because some of the relatively minor nuisances of treatment can be disastrous in SCI. Dryness of mouth, for example, in quadriplegic patients is of different significance than in hemiparetic patients. Furthermore, constipation and bladder retention in quadriplegic or paraplegic patients can have dire consequences, including a major increase in intensity of their baseline pain.

DOUBLE LESION SYNDROME

DLS represents dysfunction of the sacral and lumbosacral segments that are distant from the primary SCI, most frequently at the cervical or upper thoracic levels. In thoracic and cervical SCI patients, DLS consists of sacral dysfunction with amyotrophy and CE progressive degeneration, which is usually asymmetrical, along with bladder and sphincteric abnormalities (Berić et al 1987). DLS may be followed by a specific pain syndrome (Beric et al 1992). In the majority of patients who developed distant asymmetrical and localized lumbosacral and sacral pain, a double lesion was demonstrated neurophysiologically and, in a few cases, morphologically. Approximately 25% had some clinically preserved sensation below the level of the lesion, whereas the other 75% were described as clinically complete. However, in almost all the clinically complete cases, there was evidence of some degree of both motor and sensory incompleteness.

Patients describe DLS pain as a constant aching and burning that generally occurs in the rectal area, perineum or feet (Berić et al 1992). If it is felt in the legs, it is more often asymmetrical than symmetrical. Frequently, it is observed in patients with so-called complete SCI who do not have any detectable movement or sensation below the level of the lesion based on routine clinical examinations. This pain as well as CDS and CE pain have been referred to as phantom pains in SCI. They are considered similar to the phantom pain experienced by amputees. Supposedly, there is no communication above and below the level of the spinal cord lesion. Therefore, any sensation including pain that is referred to the body part below the level of the lesion is presumed to be brain generated and thus a phantom pain. The concept, however, that the lesion is complete if the patient cannot move parts of the body or feel a light touch or movement of an object over an area below the level of the lesion has been successfully challenged. Firstly, some communication above and below the level of the lesion has been documented in the motor system, although not necessarily for voluntary movement. However, the recognized communication has been significant enough to prove that lesions determined to be clinically complete may not be morphologically, functionally and/or neurophysiologically complete (Berić 1997a).

There is a small but significant group of patients who may appear clinically complete on a routine sensory examination, who nevertheless may perceive some sensations upon prolonged, repeated or continuous application of different stimuli. These patients may be able to transmit some afferent information from below the level of the lesion to the brain consciousness. There is another subgroup of patients in whom different sensory modalities including transcutaneous nerve stimulation, dorsal column stimulation and application of blocks below the level of the lesion may alter their stable pain in a repeated and predictable fashion. This indicates that pain manipulation below the level of the lesion in clinically complete patients may either decrease or increase their pain, suggesting the existence of communication between the nervous system structures below the level of the lesion and the brain (Berić et al 1992).

In our series, 20% of patients complained of pain similar to that related to DLS (Berić 1990). The most frequent characteristic of pain was sharp pricking and electric shock sensations, with occasional burning, as well as aching and dull pain. The distribution was for the most part asymmetrical and localized to the leg, groin, thigh or foot with frequent inclusion of the perineum, rectum and genitals. These patients usually had progressive neurological syndrome with progressive muscle atrophy and conversion of the upper motor neuron (UMN) bladder to the lower motor neuron (LMN) bladder. Therefore, the diagnosis of this syndrome was based not only on the pain characteristics but also on the presence of neurological, neurophysiological and urodynamic evidence of dysfunction of the lumbosacral segment along with cauda equina progressive dysfunction.

Patients with DLS pain tend to develop pain within a year after the time of injury. However, it is not uncommon for patients to develop pain later, along with a deterioration of function in the sacral and lumbosacral segments. In these patients, there is generally a conversion of the UMN bladder to the LMN bladder, which may sometimes be a positive development. In other situations, however, in which urological procedures were already employed, this LMN development would result in added morbidity. Their pain condition often stabilizes within several months or several

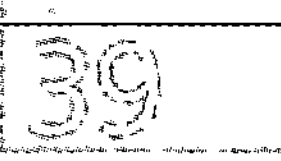

years but remains constant, with minimal fluctuation. Most patients eventually adapt to their pain over time.

ANTERIOR SPINAL ARTERY SYNDROME

Anterior spinal artery syndrome (ASAS) can be considered a subsyndrome in SCI because it can be traumatic, although the pure syndrome is generally a vascular event and is also described as iatrogenic (Triggs & Berič 1992). It is the exaggeration of the CDS in SCI. There is profound anterolateral sensory system involvement, usually a complete absence of temperature and thermal pain perception, with a variable degree of motor paralysis and excellent preservation of the dorsal column modalities. It resembles a bilateral, deep and extremely well-done surgical anterolateral cordotomy (Nathan & Smith 1979) with some additional complication (motor deficit).

SYRINGOMYELIA

Syringomyelia is classified as a complication of SCI that generally appears much later in the post-SCI period (Williams et al 1981). Therefore, late appearance of pain in some SCI patients, for example, 5–10 years after the initial SCI, should alert us to the possibility of syringomyelia. It should not, however, be used to suggest that the onset of CPS in SCI can be delayed as long as 10 years because this is not the case. The time from onset of progressive syringomyelia to onset of pain is certainly less than that, probably weeks to months as in other CPSs. Its hallmark is the development of an expanding post-traumatic cyst with ascension of the motor and sensory levels, increasing motor disability, and development of new pain (Vernon et al 1982, Dworkin & Staas 1985, Rossier et al 1985). Once the motor and sensory abnormalities are recognized and appropriate imaging studies obtained, it is not difficult to determine the cause of the new pain. However, if pain is one of the first symptoms of syringomyelia and superimposed on other post-SCI pain states, it becomes extremely difficult to diagnose initially. Patients with syringomyelia usually complain of an aching and burning pain at the level of the lesion, sometimes extending above and below the level of the lesion. The ascending cyst may increase the level of disability and even convert low cervical SCI, which is functionally considered as paraplegia, to quadriplegia. In some patients, it has led to the development of neuropathic joints (Griffiths & McCormick 1981). Rigorous and expedient assessment of sensory and motor functions coupled with magnetic resonance imaging (MRI) help determine the diagnosis (Wang et al 1996). If MRI is not possible due to prior surgical intervention–spinal stabilization, delayed computer tomography (CT) myelogram should be performed and intervention instituted as soon as possible.

There is another similar condition that can be sometimes differentiated from syringomyelia by MRI – progressive post-traumatic myelomalacic myelopathy. This subentity may lead to transitional zone pain and may be treated surgically by attempting to untether the abnormal spinal cord (Ragnarsson et al 1986, Lee et al 1997).

Continuous escalation in pain is the natural course of pain associated with syringomyelia. Appropriate diagnosis and intervention, however, are usually initiated before the pain becomes unmanageable. Unfortunately, once the pain appears, surgical intervention including shunting of the cyst may not bring the pain under control or completely abolish it. In a significant percentage of cases, it improves but does not necessarily disappear completely (Dworkin & Staas 1985, Milhorat et al 1996, Kramer & Levine 1997).

OTHER PAINS

Musculoskeletal pain most commonly occurs in patients with thoracic spine injuries. The pain is frequently localized around the level of the injury or just above the injury, due to stretching of the long muscles of the trunk. Shoulder pain in quadriplegics is an example of musculoskeletal pain (Silfverskiold & Waters 1991, Waring & Maynard 1991, Campbell & Koris 1996). It is most frequently triggered by a change in physical activity and aggravated by increased muscle activity and movement. A subgroup of these patients have reflex sympathetic dystrophy (RSD) of the hand that is infrequently seen in patients with cervical SCI (Wainapel 1984, Wainapel & Freed 1984, Davidoff & Roth 1991, Aisen & Aisen 1994). The pain, however, can also be present below the level of the lesion (Gallien et al 1995). Muscle, ligament and joint pains in the lower extremities of patients with incomplete SCI are also musculoskeletal pains, including pains due to heterotopic ossification with muscle and soft-tissue calcification. These patients have ambulatory potential and asymmetrical corticospinal left/right leg deficits and asymmetrical spasticity, with more involvement in some muscle groups than in others.

Patients with absent voluntary activity below the level of the lesion can also have pain due to uncontrollable spasms. These pains are generally of the crescendo type, paralleling an increase in the intensity and spread of the spasm.

Musculoskeletal pain tends to appear when the patient becomes more active, with transfers, wheelchair activities or ambulation in the case of incomplete SCI. The pain is usually proportional to the amount of offending activity.

Rest alleviates or at least decreases pain. As treatment is instituted early, the pain generally subsides. In thoracic SCIs, however, sometimes sitting and abnormal positioning in the wheelchair cannot be easily modified. The long thoracic muscles can be stretched for an extended time, resulting in intractable pains that can resemble transitional zone or even CDS pain.

Carpal tunnel syndrome in paraplegics deserves a special consideration as it is a neurogenic pain syndrome triggered usually by overuse of hands, especially by propelling wheelchairs (Davidoff & Roth 1991, Sie et al 1992).

Visceral pain is deep abdominal pain usually related to urological procedures and concomitant bladder infections that are aggravated by bowel and bladder activity. The debate is far from resolved regarding the question of whether or not visceral pain warrants a separate classification. Should it perhaps be classified as central pain, with symptoms expressed mainly within visceral organs and less in the somatosensory system? To further complicate the matter, a recent series of reports from the Galveston group suggest that posterior funiculi may signal visceral pain and that dorsal myelotomy may be beneficial for visceral pain relief (Hirshberg et al 1996, Nauta et al 1997).

In SCI patients, special consideration should be given to non-SCI-related pains including those due to urinary tract infections, bowel dysfunction with impaction, or abdominal infections such as acute abdomen due to appendicitis or cholecystitis. Typical physical signs of these conditions, such as localized muscle spasms, localized pain sensitivity, or even fever, are absent. Often changes in bowel and bladder patterns and sometimes an increase or decrease in spasticity are the only indicators of infection. Such changes should alert physicians to perform a more complete clinical examination, especially in the event of new pain, for example visceral or abdominal pain. Unfortunately, due to the primary spinal cord dysfunction, there is poor localization of muscle spasms in acute abdomen, which therefore represents a rare but life-threatening condition. Due to SCI, the presentation of pains associated with bladder infection, bowel infection or other abdominal causes is not typical of these conditions and may mimic genuine SCI pains. Therefore, with the appearance of new pain or exacerbation of otherwise stable pain in patients with SCI, evaluation of blood pressure, pulse, temperature, rectal examination, urinary analysis and white blood cell count is necessary. On the other hand, even the presence of a relatively simple condition such as sciatica in incomplete cervical SCI patients can be difficult to diagnose. In incomplete and especially ambulatory SCI patients, it is important to be aware of the possible appearance of other neurological conditions with manifestations that may be modified by the primary spinal cord lesion.

A separate condition in upper thoracic and cervical SCI is autonomic dysreflexia (Clinchot & Colachis 1996, Curt et al 1997). This can be brought on by a number of triggers: bladder distention, sphincter dyssynergia (concomitant contraction of the bladder and sphincter, with increasing pressure inside the bladder), bowel movements and impaction, and dysfunction due to severe spasms. This can be a life-threatening situation, causing an increase in blood pressure, the presence of headache, a possible increase in intracranial pressure, and the occurrence of a fatal intracranial haemorrhage. This is not a simple pain syndrome. The presence of discomfort, headache and unpleasant internal sensations should be recognized. The cause of these symptoms should be determined and the condition treated appropriately. These episodes tend to be repetitive, short term and acute.

SPECIAL CONSIDERATIONS

PHANTOM SENSATIONS VERSUS PHANTOM PAINS

Phantom sensations should be distinguished from so-called phantom pains as described by Pollock et al (1957). In general, phantom sensations appear early, almost immediately after SCI, and vanish within hours or days of SCI. Rarely do they persist for months or longer. Furthermore, the quality and intensity of these sensations rarely interfere with activities of daily living. They are not painful or functionally limiting, although they are frequently bizarre in nature (Sweet 1975). On the other hand, pain in the paralysed and insensitive segment below the level of the lesion generally appears later in the post-SCI period, when phantom sensations fade.

CAUDA EQUINA VERSUS CONUS MEDULLARIS

Close proximity of CE to conus medullaris blurs the distinction between the lesion of purely nerve roots as in CE and the lesion of the spinal cord as in conus medullaris. Both types of lesions are frequently seen with SCI at T12 and L1 vertebral levels. It is, however, important to describe the extent of the root lesion versus the extent of the spinal cord lesion. There are some tools that can help assess the difference, such as videourodynamics and lumbosacral somatosensory evoked potentials (LSEPs). These procedures can show the difference in degree of involvement between the spinal cord and CE lesions.

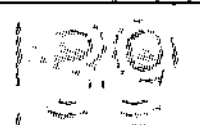

ROLE OF PRIOR TREATMENT IN CHRONIC SCI PAIN

Failure to consider past treatments when assessing the current SCI condition and deciding on appropriate treatment has led to a number of misconceptions about its associated pain states. It is an especially important consideration when previous treatment includes destructive procedures that would alter residual functions of the nervous system. For example, a group of patients developed lower extremity and perianal pains after low thoracic and lumbar injuries. They received a series of phenol injections, chemical or surgical rhizotomies, and ultimately even cordotomies or cordectomies after variable time from pain onset. After these procedures, there was still no pain relief and destruction of the spinal cord was surgically documented. Such examples have been used to further support the concept of phantom pain in SCI (Melzack & Loeser 1978). However, these findings reveal only that deafferentation after the pain had already developed did not reduce or abolish pain. In other words, the pain, having been present for an extended period of time, does not require continuous ongoing afferent input from the pain site for it to continue. This, however, does not exclude the possibility that other afferent inputs maintain that pain from different systems, including non-nociceptive inputs. The failure of anterolateral cordotomy to relieve pain in central pain syndromes is not surprising, as there is already significant anterolateral system deafferentation present. Therefore, further deafferentation appears useless and invalidates any conclusion pertaining to the pathogenesis of pain with regard to a lack of response to surgical intervention.

CLINICAL CLASSIFICATION

Classifications are plagued with uncertainty of either the aetiology of SCI pain or even which system is involved. There are some new classifications that try to use the advantage of the tri-axial system to better delineate different SCI pains (Siddall et al 1997). However, only the site of the pain is non-disputable. The system, for example musculoskeletal, visceral or neuropathic, is very much questionable in a large proportion of SCI pains, as it requires more than just a location and quality to be defined, contrary to the suggestion by Frisbie and Aguilera (1990). The third axis, which is presumably a source of pain, is highly debatable as the aetiology remains in question. I have used a combined presumed aetiological and syndromatological classification for quite some time with some success (Berić et al 1988, 1992, Berić 1990). It does presume the aetiology, which is speculative. However, it does require a number of other parameters to be assessed, increasing the probability of this presumed aetiology. The combination of these two classifications might be a next intermediate step before we succeed in better defining all SCI pains. Therefore, modified versions of the two most recent classification efforts are presented (Table 39.1, Box 39.1) (Berić 1997a, Siddall et al 1997).

DIAGNOSTIC APPROACH

CLINICAL INTERVIEW

Work-up of every SCI patient with pain should include a detailed history of pain in relation to SCI pain onset. An inventory of pain characteristics should be obtained: course;

Table 39.1 Spinal cord injury pain classification. (Modified from Siddall et al 1997 with permission.)

Axis 1 (system)	*Axis 2 (site)*	*Axis 3 (source)*
Musculoskeletal		
Visceral		
Neuropathic	at level	radicular central
Other	below level	

BOX 39.1

Chronic post-spinal cord injury pain states. (Modified from Beric 1997a with permission.)

Nociceptive
Musculoskeletal
Spasm
Other

Neurogenic
Peripheral
- Transitional zone
- Double lesion syndrome
- Cauda equina
- Visceral

Central
- Central dysaesthesia syndrome
- Syringomyelia
- Anterior spinal artery syndrome
- Visceral

quality; distribution; factors affecting pain, especially spasms; transfers; and impact of physical therapy (PT). The relationship of pain onset to recovery or deterioration of sensory and motor function and overall functional status should also be determined. In addition, history of intercurrent episodes of infection, surgeries, new injuries and pain treatments, followed by changes in pain character, are also important to the work-up for post-SCI pain. A standardized Pain Questionnaire (PQ) is usually useful as it can be used in follow-up studies. The PQ should include the visual analogue scale, pain drawing, and the standard or modified McGill PQ.

CLINICAL EXAMINATION

Neurological examination is mandatory and should include sensory, motor and functional assessments and scales as recommended by the ASIA (Maynard et al 1997). The pain is localized within a region of a large sensory deficit. The presence of allodynia and hyperalgesia is helpful, if there are no local causes of irritation. Although the light touch allodynia or proprioceptive allodynia can have bizarre clinical manifestations, intolerance of the skin to warm or cool is also frequently present as a more conventional continuous dull or burning pain. Overall, allodynia and hyperalgesia are less frequently present in SCI than in stroke and other CPSs. A finding of dissociated sensory loss on clinical grounds is also helpful for the diagnosis of CDS, but is not required.

LABORATORY AND ELECTRODIAGNOSTIC TESTS

Laboratory tests are not useful in the diagnosis and classification of pain. However, they are extremely important in excluding urinary tract infections and other non-SCI pain-related conditions. Complete gastrointestinal and urological work-ups are recommended for visceral pains. Neurophysiological testing is useful for root and cauda equina as well as for conus medullaris lesion and is mandatory in DLS. Neurophysiological tests used in DLS pain include LSEPs and nerve conduction study and electromyography.

IMAGING

MRI is invaluable for syringomyelia diagnosis. Sometimes, in addition to allowing observation of the level of the lesion, MRI can provide useful information regarding the cord below the level of the lesion. For example, it can provide evidence of suspected vascular extension of the lesion, i.e., an extended downward infarct with cord atrophy – spinal amyotrophy. MRI is not very useful, however, for the assessment of completeness of the lesion, except if the cord is totally separated at the injury level, which is rare.

URODYNAMIC TESTING

Urodynamic evaluation is important for differentiation of upper motor neuron (UMN) from lower motor neuron (LMN) bladder. Sometimes if pain and/or dysaesthesias are diffuse and located in lumbar and sacral segments, CDS and DLS can be differentiated based on the presence of UMN bladder in CDS and LMN bladder in DLS. Urodynamic testing with pressure-flow studies is mandatory for bladder neck and sphincter function assessment.

QUANTITATIVE SENSORY TESTING AND OTHER ANCILLARY PROCEDURES

In CDS, quantitative sensory testing (QST) at the lesion level and at standard sites below the level of the lesion is necessary to document incompleteness as well as different degrees of dissociated sensory loss. In syringomyelia, QST may be used for follow-ups for assessment of progression. QST is useful for overall sensory function and especially in follow-ups, as it is non-invasive for the determination of ascension of sensory level and documentation of dissociated sensory loss.

Some pain syndromes can be better recognized by additional testing, while others are determined only through treatment trials and modification of PT and overall activity. In nociceptive musculoskeletal pains, PT and rehabilitation programme modifications are used as assessment tools in addition to their possible therapeutic effects. Psychological tests with a multiaxial approach have been recommended (Wegener & Elliott 1992). The Hamilton Depression Scale and Beck Inventory are useful, including both self-inventory and interview approaches, for the assessment of depression. When the question of lesion completeness is raised, at least several of the following different tests and modalities should be employed: central EMG, TENS, spinal cord stimulation, epidural and intrathecal blocks, vibration and repetitive brushing. Furthermore, other modalities appropriate for the situation should be tested.

NERVE AND SPINAL BLOCKS

In transitional zone pain, anaesthetic blocks are employed diagnostically and repeatedly as a therapeutic option. Spinal blocks have been employed for all SCI pains and usually provide, as expected, temporary and frequently only a partial relief of pain (Loubser & Donovan 1991, Loubser & Clearman 1993). Intrathecal baclofen is very useful in alleviating spasms. However, it has only at best a mixed effect on pain. Diagnostic anaesthetic blocks are of no prognostic value as further deafferentation is not a desired goal. Although there has been much debate regarding sympathetic system dysfunction or its preservation as a pain ascending system, this has never been proven and sympathetic blocks are not routinely required. Nevertheless, some patients receive a significant temporary decrease of evoked pains with local, regional and sympathetic blocks.

MANAGEMENT OF SPINAL CORD INJURY PAINS

There is no single treatment modality that can manage all the different post-SCI pain states. Some syndromes are easier to treat, while some are notorious for their intractability. The problem in assessing the value of any particular treatment for any of these syndromes is how precisely and thoroughly patients were described in accordance with the criteria for the particular pain syndrome, for example CDS. This is certainly more difficult in DLS and visceral pain. In these patients, an adequate description can only be achieved through longer-term follow-ups that help to provide a perspective on the natural progression of the pain, which can be evaluated by the use of a variety of radiological, neurophysiological and urological techniques. This is certainly not standardized and, therefore, the efficacy of treatment in these syndromes is unknown.

GENERAL GUIDELINES

The treatment of CPS follows the general rules of a stepwise conservative approach (Fenollosa et al 1993, Gonzales 1994). Antidepressants with antinoradrenergic properties are first-line therapy, usually followed by membrane-stabilizing drugs and anticonvulsants. Narcotics should be used as adjuvants, especially at the peaks of pain or periods of increased intensity of pain. Stimulation techniques may follow, from simple non-invasive ones, such as TENS, to trials with spinal cord stimulation and possibly deep brain stimulation in very selected cases. Experimental drugs and experimental drug deliveries may follow, and finally surgical destructive modalities may be contemplated.

ANTIDEPRESSANTS

Antidepressants with noradrenergic properties are first-line therapy for most SCI pains. Tricyclic antidepressant effectiveness has been shown in both non-controlled clinical trials and double-blind studies in CPS (Leijon & Boivie 1989, Sanford et al 1992). Amitriptyline appears to be most effective, but it also has the most side effects, which are mainly anticholinergic, including urinary retention, mouth dryness, drowsiness and provoking glaucoma. Effective pain doses are below antidepressant doses. Due to frequent side effects, however, a very low starting dose is suggested based on the patient's weight and age, with no more than 10 mg at bedtime. Increments should be gradual, sometimes no more than 10 mg a week. If there is no response at approximately 2 weeks with an average daily dose of 75 mg, at least two different antidepressants from the same noradrenergic group should be tried.

ANTIEPILEPTICS AND MEMBRANE STABILIZERS

Second-line therapy includes antiepileptics and membrane-stabilizing drugs. Carbamazepine is probably most effective (Sanford et al 1992). The dosage is often above antiseizure recommendations. The blood level is irrelevant, unless there is an issue of non-compliance. Side effects are dose limiting and blood work-up is standard. Recently, a negative study on the effect of valproate on SCI pain was reported (Drewes et al 1994). There are a number of relatively new medications that have not undergone either rigorous double-blind studies or simply a test of time, such as gabapentine and lamotrigine. Because of relatively low side-effect profile, however, and some promising trials in neurogenic pains, they may be tried possibly in conjunction with other drugs. Mexiletine was tried in CPS (Edmondson et al 1993); however, it was not beneficial in SCI (Chiou-Tan et al 1996). The key to mexiletine therapy is a very low starting dose with minimal increments as there can be associated gastric irritation, which is a major problem.

NARCOTICS

Low-dose narcotics are useful in SCI as they are effective in nociceptive pains. They are, however, not effective in neurogenic pains (Arner & Meyerson 1988), especially CDS. High doses are limited because of side effects (Portenoy et al 1990). Narcotics should be used as adjuvants, especially at the peaks of pain or periods of increased intensity of pain, in addition to antidepressants and antiepileptics. Combinations with NSAIDs are useful for short courses, but the long-term use of NSAIDs may cause gastric disturbances or be renally toxic and therefore should be avoided. Sometimes intrathecal opioids can be a viable option (Winkelmuller & Winkelmuller 1996).

GABA AGONISTS

GABA-A agonists have been used for a long time. Valium has both antispastic and analgesic effects; however, it is a non-specific sedative that impairs cognitive function and tolerance usually develops. GABA-B agonists, such as baclofen, in oral preparations are not effective for pain relief. Intrathecally administered in SCI patients, GABA-B agonists may occasionally have an analgesic effect (Herman et al 1992, Mertens et al 1995, Loubser & Akman 1996). It is, however, unclear if they affect CPS or other neurogenic, spastic and musculoskeletal pains in these patients, as they all can coexist.

OTHER MEDICATIONS

There is a potential beneficial effect of *N*-methyl-D-aspartate (NMDA) antagonists, although ketamine is limited by its adverse effects and only used for research trials (Eide et al 1995). Clonidine, neuroleptics and even naloxone are sometimes tried (Middleton et al 1996). All other medications are investigational. Their efficacy is yet unproven and, therefore, they have not been approved.

STIMULATION TECHNIQUES

In some cases, stimulation techniques may also be useful such as low- and high-frequency TENS, and spinal cord and deep brain stimulation (Davis & Lentini 1975, Richardson et al 1980, Richardson 1995). Because I am not a proponent of destructive surgical procedures, I will not review their indications and results and only refer to excellent extensive newer and older texts (Maspes & Pagni 1974, Pagni 1974, 1976, 1979).

PAIN SYNDROME-SPECIFIC TREATMENTS

Opiates alone or in combination with other analgesics and antidepressants are helpful in most of the transitional zone pains, with adjunctive use of intercostal and peripheral blocks. For conus medullaris and CE injuries, in addition to previously mentioned measures for transitional zone pain, DREZ surgery may be effective. It may, however, move the neurological levels for a few segments proximally with a consequent increase in disability.

CDS is unfortunately very difficult to treat and trials with antidepressants, anticonvulsants and oral congeners of local anaesthetics are always warranted, probably in that order. There are anecdotal reports of the usefulness of intravenous lidocaine, deep brain stimulation or even deafferentation. Syringomyelia pain resembles pain of CDS, therefore treatment should be similar to that for both CDS and CPS. However, surgical intervention is almost always necessary, including drainage and shunting of the cyst (Vernon et al 1983). A new approach was recently reported, with use of a human embryonic spinal cord graft for cyst obliteration (Falci et al 1997).

In some DLS patients, our own anecdotal reports demonstrate the efficacy of spinal cord stimulation below the level of the lesion, as well as TENS or a combination of spinal blocks and analgesics (Berić 1990, Berić et al 1992).

Musculoskeletal pain syndromes usually respond well to analgesics, local blocks and trigger injections. The most effective treatment includes adjustment of activity level and use of certain muscle groups, as well as appropriate PT. Pain caused by spasms responds excellently to muscle relaxants, baclofen in particular, especially to intrathecal baclofen infusion (Loubser & Akman 1996).

Psychological interventions should also be employed (Umlauf 1992), as there are substantial psychosocial implications of pain and disability in SCI patients (Richards et al 1980, Lundquist et al 1991, Summers et al 1991, Mariano 1992, Stormer et al 1997). In general, destructive chemical and surgical procedures should be avoided as they further alter pre-existing abnormal function of the nervous system and broaden the gap between normal and abnormal nervous system function. Although some of these procedures may temporarily alleviate pain, in the long term they are detrimental. Furthermore, they may create conditions in these patients that disqualify them for procedures developed in the future.

Acknowledgements

Portions of the text were taken with permission from: Beric A 1997 Post-spinal cord injury pain states. Anesthesiology Clinics of North America 15:445–463; Berić A 1998 Central pain and dysesthesia syndromes. Neurology Clinics of North America 16: 899–918.

REFERENCES

Aisen PS, Aisen ML 1994 Shoulder-hand syndrome in cervical spinal cord injury. Paraplegia 32: 588–592

Arner S, Meyerson BA 1988 Lack of analgesic effect of opioids on neuropathic and idiopathic forms of pain. Pain 33: 11–23

Berić A 1990 Altered sensation and pain in spinal cord injury. In: Dimitrijevic MR, Wall PD, Lindblom U (eds) Recent achievements in restorative neurology 3: altered sensation and pain. Karger, Basel, pp 27–36

Berić A 1997a Post-spinal cord injury pain states. Anesthesiology Clinics of North America 15: 445–463

Berić A 1997b Post-spinal cord injury pain states. Pain 72: 295–298

Berić A 1998 Central pain and dysesthesia syndrome. Neurology Clinics of North America 16: 899–918

Berić A, Dimitrijevic MR, Light JK 1987 A clinical syndrome of rostral and caudal spinal injury: neurologic, neurophysiologic and urodynamic evidence for occult sacral lesion. Journal of Neurology, Neurosurgery and Psychiatry 50: 600–606

Berić A, Dimitrijevic MR, Lindblom U 1988 Central dysesthesia syndrome in spinal cord injury patients. Pain 34: 109–116

Berić A, Dimitrijevic MR, Light JK 1992 Pain in spinal cord injury with occult caudal lesions. European Journal of Pain 13: 1–7

Bonica JJ 1991 Introduction: sematic, epidemiologic, and educational issues. In: Casey KL (ed) Pain and central nervous system disease: the central pain syndromes. Raven, New York, pp 13–29

Bowsher D 1996 Central pain of spinal origin. Spinal Cord 34: 707–710

Burke DC 1973 Pain in paraplegia. Paraplegia 10: 297–313

Burke DC, Woodward JM 1976 Pain and phantom sensation in spinal paralysis. In: Vinken PJ, Bruyn GW (eds) Handbook of clinical neurology, vol 26, injuries of the spine and spinal cord, part II. North-Holland Publishing, Amsterdam, pp 489–499

Cairns DM, Adkins RH, Scott MD 1996 Pain and depression in acute traumatic spinal cord injury: origins of chronic problematic pain? Archives of Physical Medicine and Rehabilitation 77: 329–335

Campbell CC, Koris MJ 1996 Etiologies of shoulder pain in cervical spinal cord injury. Clinical Orthopedics and Related Research 322: 140–145

Chiou-Tan FY, Tuel SM, Johnson JC, Priebe MM et al 1996 Effect of mexiletine on spinal cord injury dysesthetic pain. American Journal of Physical Medicine and Rehabilitation 75: 84–87

Clinchot DM, Colachis SC 1996 Autonomic hyperreflexia associated with exacerbation of reflex sympathetic dystrophy. Journal of Spinal Cord Medicine 19: 225–257

Curt A, Nitsche B, Rodic B, Schurch B, Dietz V 1997 Assessment of autonomic dysreflexia in patients with spinal cord injury. Journal of Neurology, Neurosurgery and Psychiatry 62: 473–477

Davidoff G, Roth EJ 1991 Clinical characteristics of central (dysesthetic) pain in spinal cord injury patients. In: Casey KL (ed) Pain and central nervous system disease: the central pain syndromes. Raven, New York, pp 77–83

Davidoff G, Roth E, Guarracini M et al 1987 Function-limiting dysesthetic pain syndrome among traumatic spinal cord injury patients: a cross-sectional study. Pain 29: 39–48

Davis R 1975 Pain and suffering following spinal cord injury. Clinical Orthopedics 112: 76–80

Davis R, Lentini R 1975 Transcutaneous nerve stimulation for treatment of pain in patients with spinal cord injury. Surgical Neurology 4: 100–101

Davis L, Martin J 1947 Studies upon spinal cord injuries II. The nature and treatment of pain. Journal of Neurosurgery 4: 483–491

Demirel G, Yllmaz H, Gencosmanoglu B, Kesiktas N 1998 Pain following spinal cord injury. Spinal Cord 36: 25–28

Donovan WH, Dimitrijevic MR, Dahm L et al 1982 Neurophysiological approaches to chronic pain following spinal cord injury. Paraplegia 20: 135–146

Drewes AM, Andreasen A, Poulsen LH 1994 Valproate for treatment of chronic pain after spinal cord injury. A double-blind cross-over study. Paraplegia 32: 565–569

Dworkin GE, Staas WE 1985 Posttraumatic syringomyelia. Archives of Physical Medicine and Rehabilitation 66: 329–331

Edgar RE, Best LG, Quail PA, Obert AD 1993 Computer-assisted DREZ microcoagulation: posttraumatic spinal deafferentation pain. Journal of Spinal Disorders 6: 48–56

Edmondson EA, Simpson RK, Stubler DK et al 1993 Systemic lidocaine therapy for poststroke pain. Southern Medical Journal 86: 1093–1096

Eide PK, Stubhaug A, Stenehjem AE 1995 Central dysesthesia pain after traumatic spinal cord injury is dependent on *N*-methyl-D-aspartate receptor activation. Neurosurgery 37: 1080–1087

Falci S, Holtz A, Akesson E et al 1997 Obliteration of posttraumatic spinal cord cyst with solid human embryonic spinal cord grafts: first clinical attempt. Journal of Neurotrauma 14: 875–884

Fenollosa P, Pallares J, Cervera J et al 1993 Chronic pain in the spinal cord injured: statistical approach and pharmacological treatment. Paraplegia 31: 722–729

Freeman LW, Heimburger RF 1947 Surgical relief of pain in paraplegic patients. Archives of Surgery 55: 433–440

Frisbie JH, Aguilera EJ 1990 Chronic pain after spinal cord injury: an expedient diagnostic approach. Paraplegia 28: 460–465

Gallien P, Nicolas B, Robineau S et al 1995 The reflex sympathetic dystrophy syndrome in patients who have had a spinal cord injury. Paraplegia 33: 715–720

Gonzales GR 1994 Central pain. Seminars in Neurology 14: 255–262

Griffiths ER, McCormick CC 1981 Post-traumatic syringomyelia (cystic myelopathy). Paraplegia 19: 81–88

Herman RM, D'Luzansky SC, Ippolitio R 1992 Intrathecal baclofen suppresses central pain in patients with spinal lesions. Clinical Journal of Pain 8: 338–345

Hirshberg RM, Al-Chaer ED, Lawand NB, Westlund KN, Willis WD 1996 Is there a pathway in the posterior funiculus that signals visceral pain? Pain 67: 291–305

Johnson RL, Gerhart KA, McCray J, Menconi JC, Whiteneck GG 1998 Secondary conditions following spinal cord injury in a population-based sample. Spinal Cord 36: 45–50

Kaplan LI, Grynbaum BB, Lloyd E et al 1962 Pain and spasticity in patients with spinal cord dysfunction. Journal of the American Medical Association 182: 918–925

Kennedy P, Frankel H, Gardner B, Nuseibeh I 1997 Factors associated with acute and chronic pain following traumatic spinal cord injuries. Spinal Cord 35: 814–817

Kramer KM, Levine AM 1997 Posttraumatic syringomyelia. Clinical Orthopedics and Related Research 334: 190–199

Lamid S, Chia JK, Kohli A, Cid E 1985 Chronic pain in spinal cord injury: comparison between inpatients and outpatients. Archives of Physical Medicine and Rehabilitation 66: 777–778

Lee TT, Arias JM, Andrus HL, Quencer RM, Falcone SF, Green BA 1997 Progressive posttraumatic myelomalacic myelopathy: treatment with untethering and expansive duraplasty. Journal of Neurosurgery 86: 624–628

Leijon G, Boivie J 1989 Central post-stroke pain – a controlled trial of amitriptyline and carbamazepine. Pain 36: 27–36

Levi R, Hultling C, Nash MS, Sieger A 1995a The Stockholm spinal cord injury study: 1. medical problems in a regional SCI population. Paraplegia 33: 308–315

Levi R, Hultling C, Seiger A 1995b The Stockholm spinal cord injury study: 2. Associations between clinical patient characteristics and post-acute medical problems. Paraplegia 33: 585–594

Loubser PG, Akman NM 1996 Effects of intrathecal baclofen on chronic spinal cord injury pain. Journal of Pain and Symptom Management 12: 241–247

Loubser PG, Clearman RR 1993 Evaluation of central spinal cord injury pain with diagnostic spinal anesthesia. A case report. Anesthesiology 79: 376–378

Loubser PG, Donovan WH 1991 Diagnostic spinal anaesthesia in chronic spinal cord injury pain. Paraplegia 29: 25–36

Lundqvist C, Siosteen A, Blomstrand C, Lind B, Sullivan M 1991 Spinal cord injuries: clinical, functional and emotional status. Spine 16: 78–83

Mariano AJ 1992 Chronic pain and spinal cord injury. Clinical Journal of Pain 8: 87–92

Maspes PE, Pagni CA 1974 A critical appraisal of pain surgery and suggestions for improving treatment. In: Bonica JJ, Procacci P, Pagni CA (eds) Recent advances in pain. Charles C Thomas, Springfield, pp 201–255

Maury M 1977–78 About pain and its treatment in paraplegics. Paraplegia 15: 349–352

Maynard FM, Bracken MB, Creasey G et al 1997 International standards for neurological and functional classification of spinal cord injury. Spinal Cord 35: 266–274

Melzack R, Loeser JD 1978 Phantom body pain in paraplegics: evidence for a central 'pattern generating mechanism' for pain. Pain 4: 195–210

Mertens P, Parise M, Garcia-Larrea L et al 1995 Long-term clinical, electrophysiological and urodynamic effects of chronic intrathecal baclofen infusion for treatment of spinal spasticity. Acta Neurochirurgica. Supplementum 64: 17–25

Middleton JW, Siddall PJ, Walker S, Molloy AR, Rutkowski SB 1996 Intrathecal clonidine and baclofen in the management of spasticity and neuropathic pain following spinal cord injury: a case study. Archives of Physical Medicine and Rehabilitation 77: 824–826

Milhorat TH, Kotzen RM, Mu HTM, Capocelli AL, Milhorat RH 1996 Dysesthetic pain in patients with syringomyelia. Neurosurgery 38: 940–947

Moossy JJ, Nashold BS 1988 Dorsal root entry zone lesions for conus medullaris root avulsions. Applied Neurophysiology 51: 198–205

Nashold BS, Bullitt E 1981 Dorsal root entry zone lesions to control central pain in paraplegics. Journal of Neurosurgery 55: 414–419

Nathan PW, Smith MC 1979 Clinico-anatomical correlation in anterolateral cordotomy. In: Bonica JJ et al (eds) Advances in pain research and therapy, vol 3. Raven, New York, pp 921–926

Nauta HJW, Hewitt E, Westlund KN, Willis WD 1997 Surgical interruption of a midline dorsal column visceral pain pathway. Journal of Neurosurgery 86: 538–542

Nepomuceno C, Fine PR, Richards JS et al 1979 Pain in patients with spinal cord injury. Archives of Physical Medicine and Rehabilitation 60: 605–609

New PW, Lim TC, Hill ST, Brown DJ 1997 A survey of pain during rehabilitation after acute spinal cord injury. Spinal Cord 35: 658–663

Pagni CA 1974 Pain due to central nervous system lesions: physiopathological considerations and therapeutical implications. Advances in Neurology 4: 339–350

Pagni CA 1976 Central pain and painful anesthesia. Progress in Neurological Surgery 8: 132–257

Pagni CA 1979 General comments on ablative neurosurgical procedures. In: Bonica JJ, Ventafrida V (eds) Advances in pain research and therapy, vol 2. Raven, New York, pp 405–423

Pollock LJ, Brown M, Boshes B et al 1951 Pain below the level of injury of the spinal cord. Archives of Neurology and Psychiatry 65: 319–322

Pollock LJ, Boshes B, Arieff AJ et al 1957 Phantom limb in patients with injuries to the spinal cord and cauda equina. Surgery, Gynecology and Obstetrics 104: 407

Portenoy RK, Foley KM, Inturrisi CE 1990 The nature of opioid responsiveness and its implications for neuropathic pain: new hypotheses derived from studies of opioid infusions. Pain 43: 273–286

Ragnarsson KT 1997 Management of pain in persons with spinal cord injury. Journal of Spinal Cord Medicine 20: 186–199

Ragnarsson TS, Durward QJ, Nordgren RE 1986 Spinal cord tethering after traumatic paraplegia with late neurological deterioration. Journal of Neurosurgery 64: 397–401

Richards JS 1992 Chronic pain and spinal cord injury: review and comment. Clinical Journal of Pain 8: 119–122

Richards JS, Meredith RL, Nepomuceno C et al 1980 Psycho-social aspects of chronic pain in spinal cord injury. Pain 8: 355–366

Richards JS, Stover SL, Jaworski T 1990 Effect of bullet removal on subsequent pain in persons with spinal cord injury secondary to gunshot wound. Journal of Neurosurgery 73: 401–404

Richardson DE 1995 Deep brain stimulation for the relief of chronic pain. Neurosurgery Clinics 6: 135–143

Richardson RR, Meyer PR, Cerullo LJ 1980 Neurostimulation in the modulation of intractable paraplegic and traumatic neuroma pains. Pain 8: 75–84

Riddoch G 1938 The clinical features of central pain. Lancet 1150–1156

Rose M, Robinson JE, Ells P et al 1988 Pain following spinal cord injury: results from a postal survey. Pain 34: 101–102

Rossier AB, Foo D, Shillito J et al 1985 Posttraumatic cervical syringomyelia. Incidence, clinical presentation, electrophysiological studies, syrinx protein and results of conservative and operative treatment. Brain 108: 439–461

Sampson JH, Cashman RE, Nashold BS, Friedman AH 1995 Dorsal root entry zone lesions for intractable pain after trauma to the conus medullaris and cauda equina. Journal of Neurosurgery 82: 28–34

Sanford PR, Lindblom LB, Haddox JD 1992 Amitriptyline and carbamazepine in the treatment of dysesthesia pain in spinal cord injury. Archives of Physical Medicine and Rehabilitation 73: 300–301

Siddall PJ, Taylor DA, Cousins MJ 1997 Classification of pain following spinal cord injury. Spinal Cord 35: 69–75

Sie IH, Waters RL, Adkins RH et al 1992 Upper extremity pain in the postrehabilitation spinal cord injured patient. Archives of Physical Medicine and Rehabilitation 73: 44–48

Silfverskiold J, Waters RL 1991 Shoulder pain and functional disability in spinal cord injury patients. Clinical Orthopedics and Related Research 272: 141–145

Sindou M 1995 Microsurgical dreztomy (MDT) for pain, spasticity and hyperactive bladder: a 20-year experience. Acta Neurochirurgica 137: 1–5

Stormer S, Gerner HJ, Gruninger W et al 1997 Chronic pain/dysaesthesiae in spinal cord injury patients: results of a multicentre study. Spinal Cord 35: 446–455

Summers JD, Rapoff MA, Varghese G et al 1991 Psychosocial factors in chronic spinal cord injury pain. Pain 47: 183–189

Sved P, Siddall PJ, McClelland J, Cousins MJ 1997 Relationship between surgery and pain following spinal cord injury. Spinal Cord 35: 526–530

Sweet WH 1975 Phantom sensations following intraspinal injury. Neurochirurgia 18: 139–154

Tasker RR, de Carvalho G, Dostrovsky JO 1991 The history of central pain syndromes, with observations concerning pathophysiology and treatment. In: Casey KL (ed) Pain and central nervous system disease: the central pain syndromes. Raven, New York, pp 31–58

Triggs W, Beric A 1992 Sensory abnormalities and dysaesthesia in the anterior spinal artery syndrome. Brain 115: 189–198

Tunks E 1986 Pain in spinal cord injured patients. In: Block RF, Basbaum M (eds) Management of spinal cord injuries. Williams and Wilkins, Baltimore, pp 180–211

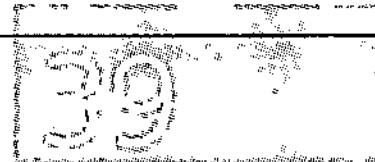

Umlauf RL 1992 Psychological interventions for chronic pain following spinal cord injury. Clinical Journal of Pain 8: 111–118

Vernon JD, Silver JR, Ohry A 1982 Post-traumatic syringomyelia. Paraplegia 20: 339–364

Vernon JD, Chir B, Silver JR et al 1983 Post-traumatic syringomyelia: the results of surgery. Paraplegia 21: 37–46

Wainapel SF 1984 Reflex sympathetic dystrophy following traumatic myelopathy. Pain 18: 345–349

Wainapel SF, Freed MM 1984 Reflex sympathetic dystrophy in quadriplegia: case report. Archives of Physical Medicine and Rehabilitation 65: 35–36

Waisbrod H, Hansen D, Gerbershagen HU 1984 Chronic pain in paraplegics. Neurosurgery 15: 933–934

Wang D, Bodley R, Sett P, Gardner B, Frankel H 1996 A clinical magnetic resonance imaging study of the traumatised spinal cord more than 20 years following injury. Paraplegia 34: 65–81

Waring WP, Maynard FM 1991 Shoulder pain in acute traumatic quadriplegia. Paraplegia 29: 37–42

Wegener ST, Elliott TR 1992 Pain assessment in spinal cord injury. Clinical Journal of Pain 8: 93–101

Williams B, Terry AF, Jones F et al 1981 Syringomyelia as a sequel to traumatic paraplegia. Paraplegia 19: 67–80

Winkelmuller M, Winkelmuller W 1996 Long-term effects of continuous intrathecal opioid treatment in chronic pain of nonmalignant etiology. Journal of Neurosurgery 85: 458–467

Woodward KG, Vulpe M 1991 The proximal tap or 'central Tinel' sign in central dysesthetic syndrome after spinal cord injury. Journal of the American Paraplegia Society 14: 136–138

Yezierski RP 1996 Pain following spinal cord injury: the clinical problem and experimental studies. Pain 68: 185–194

Pain and psychological medicine

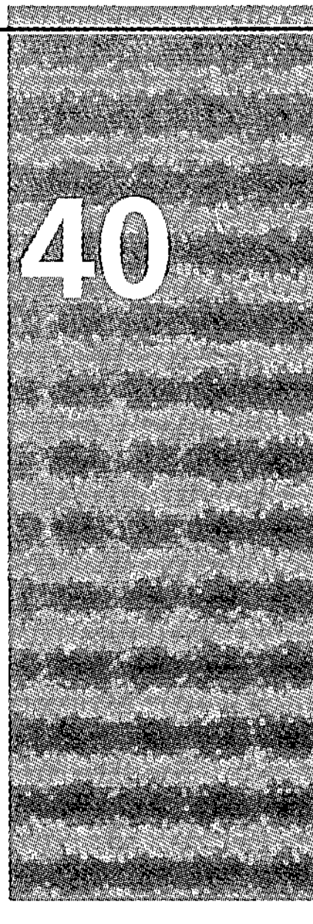

HAROLD MERSKEY

SUMMARY

Psychological illness may promote pain in several ways. Headache is common as a consequence of depression. Pain anywhere else in the body may be produced as a result of depression or anxiety or other psychological mechanisms but is less frequent. The mechanisms responsible have not been fully determined. Hysterical conversion or hypochondriacal mechanisms (somatoform conditions) are often invoked but much less often proven. Probably more often than any of the above mechanisms, depression or anxiety may make pain worse.

Psychological changes are common in patients seen in pain clinics. Selection factors are unquestionably important in this respect. Pain is also highly liable to cause depression. Population studies have shown that patients with mild or more severe chronic pain have approximately twice the normal rate for depression. There is a modest amount of prospective follow-up evidence that shows that those with pain develop depression in the long term somewhat more often than those with depression who later develop pain. Clinical studies have demonstrated striking relief of depression, anxiety and associated psychological symptoms following the successful relief of pain.

A psychological cause for pain is frequently misdiagnosed on the basis of types of physical sign which are said to indicate psychological illness. Plasticity of the nervous system however may well be responsible for regional changes, and behavioural signs of the presence of pain are primarily signs of an organic disorder. Disability assessments based upon pain behaviour theories are frequently suspect of being ethically questionable.

Psychiatric treatment in the pain clinic is appropriate for patients with independent psychological problems and may be useful in relieving the distress of those with physical causes of pain.

INTRODUCTION

Psychological medicine means psychiatry but also conveys an emphasis on topics which involve bodily function. When bodily complaints occur, the psychological aspect may be related to the contribution of emotion to them, or to the often considerable effects of somatic illness upon the psyche. Both phenomena may occur independently or together and they involve a much broader field than illness alone, as can be seen in Chapters 12 and 13 on the emotional and cognitive aspects of pain as well as elsewhere in this book. Various aspects of psychological medicine are also often covered by the terms general hospital psychiatry and consultation liaison psychiatry.

This chapter describes, firstly, the ways in which psychological illness is believed to be responsible for pain, and secondly, the ways in which sustained noxious input which is experienced as moderately severe or severe pain may itself affect the emotional state. Common features of the pain in psychiatric patients and in pain-clinic patients with psychiatric problems will then be described. This approach reverses the order of proceeding from symptom and pattern of illness to aetiology and treatment. It does so mainly because the patterns of pain in psychological illness are not so distinct that they form neat and convenient groupings for diagnostic purposes. It is true that they have some idiosyncrasies and special features which enable them to be distinguished at times, but these are less important than the general understanding of the relationship between emotion and pain.

PSYCHOLOGICAL CAUSES OF PAIN

Pain is frequent in psychiatric patients. Klee et al (1959) found it occurred in 61% of a Veterans Administration outpatient population. Spear (1967) found it in 65.6% of psychiatric inpatients and outpatients. It was a spontaneous complaint in more than 50% of them. Delaplaine et al

(1978) examined patients in a psychiatric hospital on admission and found the lowest rate, namely 38%, with 22% of the patients having no physical cause to account for their symptoms. It was anticipated that these figures would be relatively low in a psychiatric hospital, because the association of pain with lesser degrees of anxiety and depression is much more prominent than that of pain with psychosis or many types of personality disorder (Merskey 1965a). In any case, the view generally goes without challenge that there is an important minority of psychiatric patients in whom pain results from their mental state. In many instances the pain is not a major complaint; it is incidental and is mentioned only after rather full enquiries have been made. Even so, severe or moderately severe pain affects a minimum of 25% of psychiatric patients (Delaplaine et al 1978). In other settings (e.g., clinics for headache and low-back pain and in pain clinics generally) the importance of emotional disorders as a cause of pain, or as an agent in increasing it, is usually taken to be a matter of course.

The sample of patients which is seen by any practitioner – whether family practitioner, psychiatrist, neurologist, neurosurgeon or anaesthetist or any other clinician – is almost always influenced by psychological and social selection factors. People who are concerned about their bodies, hypochondriacal or tenacious, will seek medical help more often than those who do not have these characteristics. It is easy to see this, for example, with migraine. Studies which rely on clinic patients find them to have marked psychological disturbance (Klee 1968). When migraine-clinic patients were compared with migraine patients who did not attend a special clinic, the former were the more emotionally disturbed (Henryk-Gutt & Rees 1973). When a more complete epidemiological study was carried out (Crisp et al 1977), it was found that there was a little excess anxiety in patients with migraine but that overall they much resembled the general population, as might be expected. There is probably a relationship between episodes of depression and an increased frequency of migraine, as any clinician will observe. However, the overall link between migraine and the emotional state is less strong than is sometimes suggested (Merskey 1982).

Hospital clinics inevitably acquire some patients who do not rest content when symptoms have not been completely removed by their doctors. However, even general practitioners only see a selected sample of the illnesses or symptoms in a population. In one study, patients were asked to keep a sickness diary of the number of episodes of illness which they underwent (Banks et al 1975). Only 3% of such complaints as headache, vomiting, diarrhoea, etc. were reported to the general practitioners. The scope for self-selection in this context is enormous. A general practitioner can expect to see patients more often whose personal and psychological characteristics differ from those of the general population. Accordingly, no medical practitioner can expect to find that the patients whom he sees with chronic pain will be free from a relative excess of emotional disorder. In fact, the more specialized and highly regarded his practice, the more this will happen. Thus it must always be recognized that the clinical material on which we form our opinion about pain is biased by these selection problems. General conclusions about the psychology of pain which would apply to all groups with pain must be made very cautiously. On the other hand, the role of psychiatry in accounting for pain in psychiatric patients is quite well developed, because psychiatric patients with pain have been studied by a number of authors. It is merely necessary to recognize that the psychiatry of patients with pain, seen by a psychiatrist, or seen in pain clinics, only allows qualified generalizations about pain overall.

DEFINITION OF PAIN

Before proceeding to discuss the psychiatry of pain it is important to emphasize that the pain which psychiatric patients have, often without lesions, is as 'real' as that of those people whose pain is due to lesions or pathophysiological states. This observation is embodied in the definition of the International Association for the Study of Pain (IASP), which is: 'an unpleasant sensory and emotional experience associated with actual or potential tissue damage or described in terms of such damage' (International Association for the Study of Pain 1979).

PAIN IN PSYCHIATRIC PATIENTS

Walters (1961) was the first to describe a large series of psychiatric patients with pain and demonstrate their main diagnostic and personal characteristics. In 430 patients whom he had seen in consultation concerning pain, 185 had a pain in the head and neck, 133 in the chest and upper limbs, 112 in the low back and the lower limbs, 61 in the trunk and back, 50 in the genitals or pelvis and seven had pain all over. Others had pain in the abdomen, all four limbs or both limbs on one side. Sometimes, but not invariably, the pain was described dramatically. Only 26 patients had conversion hysteria and only 68 had psychoses (including 45 with depression). The majority (336) had 'other neuroses and situational states'. Walters emphasized, besides, that many patients had minor physical lesions which gave rise to much more pain in the presence of emotional disturbance than would otherwise have been expected. Merskey and Spear (1967) found, like Walters, that pain was more often located in the head than in any other region of the body in psychiatric patients. Apart from psychiatric practice the low back is ordinarily the commonest site of chronic pain. Merskey (1965a), examining a group of psychiatric patients with pain as a major complaint and with no physical lesions, found that compared with a control group of psychiatric patients who did not have pain, the proportions with anxiety, depression, hysterical (conversion) and hypochondriacal complaints were very much higher and the proportions with severe depression of an endogenous type, schizophrenia and other diagnoses were lower.

The frequency of the diagnosis of hysteria either on the basis of a history of conversion symptoms or personality disorder was relatively high. Spear (1967), whose patients were less chronic, found lower percentages of hysteria but still showed the same predominance of anxiety, depressive or hysterical conditions relating to psychiatric illness in those who had pain compared with those who did not have pain. The above work was some of the earliest to provide controlled comparisons of psychiatric patients with pain and without pain, but the diagnosis of hysterical complaints today requires much stricter criteria than were acceptable at that time and comes under different headings such as conversion or somatoform disorders. Large (1980), examining patients referred to a psychiatrist in a pain clinic, found that those patients who had pain with psychological illness appeared to be suffering for the most part from anxiety or depressive disorders.

Pilowsky and Spence (1976) used an illness behaviour questionnaire (IBQ) to characterize pain-clinic patients and observed six taxonomic clusters which have much in common with the traditional findings described above. Psychological test studies yield comparable results. Pilling et al (1967) showed the occurrence of the conversion V triad pattern in the Minnesota Multiphasic Personality Inventory (MMPI) in patients who had pain as a presenting symptom with psychological illness. In this pattern, the scale for hypochondriasis is elevated, that for depression is elevated but less than that for hypochondriasis, and the scale for hysteria is also elevated more than for depression. These findings were attributed early on to low-back pain (Hanvik 1956) and have been found in a wide range of studies of patients with chronic pain (Merskey 1980). It is noteworthy however that, as Fordyce (1976) recognizes, this pattern is common to pain patients whether or not they have physical lesions. Watson (1982) showed that chronic pain patients obtained elevated hysteria and hypochondriasis scores on the MMPI because they endorsed items that were relevant to their problem and not because they were hypochondriacal. Smythe (1985) and Merskey et al (1985) have emphasized that the use of these scales in the MMPI can be seriously misleading. They rely to a considerable extent upon symptoms like pain in different locations, fatigue, other bodily complaints and insomnia as evidence for hypochondriasis, depression (Hs,D) and hysteria (Hy). In the presence of physical illness this will often be invalid. Love and Peck (1987) reviewed 56 studies and concluded that the MMPI should not be used in the attempt to distinguish psychological causes of pain. Some use remains for the MMPI as a measure of severity or for the analysis of different profiles (Bradley et al 1978).

Sternbach (1974), who demonstrated the conversion V pattern in many pain clinic patients, also showed that it was especially associated with chronicity and could improve with treatment (Sternbach et al 1973). Naliboff et al (1988) confirmed that reductions appear in MMPI scores with successful treatment. This may be as much because physical symptoms abate as because psychological improvement occurs.

It is worth mentioning that the term 'hysterical pain', which the writer sometimes considers to be justified, is usually best avoided. There are a number of practical reasons for this, especially the difficulty in conveying the concept directly to patients. Another term used for patients who seem to have pain for psychological reasons is 'operant pain'. The writer has reservations about this term, about its applications to the theory of pain and psychological illness, and about the validity of many of the claims which have been made for treatments based upon the notion of operant pain. Those grouped under it probably include patients whose pain is related to anxiety, depression and many psychiatric characteristics. The same is true for patients who are said to have 'somatoform' complaints. These include a mixture of individuals with anxiety and depression, and sometimes widespread physically unexplained symptoms (Kirmayer & Robbins 1991). It is important to distinguish these phenomena in order to apply appropriate treatment, whether antidepressants, psychotherapy or rehabilitative measures.

The literature on pain patients has frequently commented upon a number of characteristics which are said to be typical of them (Hart 1947, Engel 1959). In fact, more than 30 authors who mention such characteristics have been listed (Merskey & Spear 1967). The traits noted particularly include guilt, resentment, hostility, multiple somatic complaints, excessive consultations and numerous operations. Most of these features have been confirmed and reconfirmed in subsequent literature. Many of the reports are anecdotal but the systematic ones have shown an increased frequency of operations (Spear 1967) in psychiatric patients with pain and an increased frequency of resentment in the same group compared with those without pain (Merskey 1965b). The marital relationships of the patients have been noted to be disturbed (Merskey 1965b, Mohamed et al 1978, Rowat & Knafl 1985, Payne & Norfleet 1986). Several investigators, including Rowat and Knafl (1985), have found the spouses of patients with pain suffer in addition (Flor et al 1987, 1989, Romano et al 1989, Watt Watson et al 1988, Thomas & Roy 1989). On the whole, among these reports the tendency is greater for the wives of male patients to be affected by their partner's pain rather than for the husbands to be affected by their wives' pain. However, Dura and Beck (1988) did show that a wife's chronic pain also had an effect on the husband. Labbe (1988) concluded that the literature suggests that about two-thirds of all back pain patients report sexual problems after the onset of pain, the frequency and quality of activity both being affected. Also, there are now many reports of sexual abuse in childhood among patients with chronic pain, but the material is not yet sufficient to evaluate satisfactorily. The problems of sampling and comparisons with the base rate for sexual abuse in the population have yet to be dealt with adequately, as well as the effects of concomitant emotional and physical deprivation in childhood.

PSYCHOLOGICAL ILLNESS IN PAIN CLINICS

Engel (1959) advanced the view, which has been supported also by Blumer (1975), that many patients could adapt themselves to life only by reason of having a traumatic social or personal relationship, such as a bad marriage in which they played a masochistic role, or by suffering from chronic pain.

Engel's hypothesis has been quite influential but only partly confirmed. It suffers from a lack of controlled evidence and the possibility that the cases reported were very highly selected. Merskey (1965b) did find that psychiatric patients with chronic pain were more resentful than psychiatric patients without pain, and irritability in pain patients is a common observation which probably has a biological basis. If pain reflects damage to the body which can, on occasion, result from the actions of an aggressor, it may be expected that it will not only promote rest or retreat, but also a more active defence by aggression. However while resentment was shown to be a feature of some chronic pain, Spear (1967) was quite unable to demonstrate that psychiatric patients with pain were more hostile either covertly or overtly than those without. Adler et al (1989) in a small-scale but intensive controlled study found that female pain patients experienced more brutality, sexual abuse, punishment and guilt feelings in childhood than three other types of patient. They saw more illness and pain in their parents as well. This evidence is not strong, and could be related to social class differences and differences in employment. However, it matches a popular view in support of Violon-Jurfest (1980) who argued that, because of their past experiences, patients could only relate to other individuals through the experience of pain and could not have an affectionate or loving relationship except if they suffered in that way. In other words, one would suppose that although they did not necessarily seek masochistic patterns of relationship, pain offered the same function for them, enabling them to feel that they could be loved. These views are speculative and are not well supported by controlled evidence, but they might apply to some patients whether or not they have lesions to promote their pain.

Several reports from pain clinics have been discussed already. They represent only some samples from the earlier papers in the very large literature on the psychological aspects of patients in pain clinics. In particular, the number of reports of MMPI findings and of other psychological test results is very great. Perhaps the most important observation in regard to all these reports is that they inevitably reflect the variety of types of clinics, the pattern of selection (also called referral bias) and the different tests employed. Many of the findings include reports on the frequency of depression which will be considered further below. They also provide information on the diagnosis of conditions such as anxiety or hysteria, or characteristics which are held to be typical of anxiety or hysterical personality patterns.

Except where the results are defined by sets of criteria on psychological test scores, these findings may be hard to replicate and criteria are not uniform. However, even where the criteria are uniform, it is not clear that they are reliable or always meaningful. For example, criteria for hypochondriasis which are invariably linked with the MMPI depend on the proof of the absence of physical illness, which is almost never provided in these populations. The problems of relying upon such test data have been considered by a number of authors.

Where psychiatric techniques are used for the diagnosis

of anxiety, depression, conversion and hypochondriacal disorders, the criteria are often somewhat variable and it is only lately that the same criteria have been used, even in a semistandardized form, by different investigators. The principal agent for this purpose has been the Diagnostic and Statistical Manual of the American Psychiatric Association in its third and fourth editions (DSM-III 1980, DSM-III[R] 1987 and DSM-IV 1994). After working steadily through these editions the current version (DSM-IV) describes a category of 'Pain Disorder' which has dropped previous appellations of Psychogenic Pain Disorder and Somatoform Pain Disorders, although it is still found, like hypochondriasis, in the section dealing with Somatoform Disorders. This category of Pain Disorder is not to be diagnosed if the pain is better accounted for by 'a Mood, Anxiety, or Psychotic Disorder' or if it meets criteria for Dyspareunia. It is thus restricted to circumstances where it is possible to show that a psychological factor, other than those just mentioned, can account for the 'onset, severity, exacerbation or maintenance of the pain'.

The International Classification of Diseases, 10th revision (ICD-10 1992) has a similar category of persistent somatoform pain disorder about which it says that the pain occurs in association with emotional conflict or psychosocial problems that are sufficient to allow the conclusion that they are the main causative influences. It is important only to make such a diagnosis on the basis of substantial psychological evidence. The exclusion of organic disorders is certainly not sufficient on its own to warrant such a diagnosis. There must be positive evidence and, in practice, if the criteria are followed carefully, this diagnosis will rarely be made.

Weighty evidence on this topic exists from another direction. In a series of studies Bogduk and his colleagues (Wallis et al 1997) have provided double-blind controlled prospective evidence that psychological changes associated with the cervical sprain syndrome (whiplash) diminish substantially when the pain of the disorder is relieved.

As one might expect, psychiatric illness is most often found in those patients where no lesion is evident and it is found less often in patients who do have a lesion. Chaturvedi et al (1984) made a psychiatric diagnosis in only 50% of patients who had lesions with chronic pain, and in 86% of patients who had no lesions. Magni and Merskey (1987) recorded psychiatric diagnoses in 61% of patients with lesions and in 97% of patients without lesions.

Another approach to the examination of psychiatric illness in pain clinics is to undertake screening tests, not measuring the severity of psychiatric illness but its frequency. This does not necessarily give a diagnostic breakdown but it will indicate the extent to which a population is thought to suffer from psychiatric illness. A survey by Merskey et al (1987) used the General Health Questionnaire 28-item version (GHQ-28). This questionnaire has some advantages over the usual psychiatric questionnaires when employed in non-psychiatric populations, because it tends to be based on items concerning physical function in the first instance, and then only secondarily does it ask about psychological status. One disadvantage is that it requires adjustment for the presence of physical illness, but this can be made. It has been standardized in numerous studies in the past. When several different types of clinic were compared it was found that in an anaesthetist's pain clinic serving a mixed urban and rural population, 37% of patients were positive for psychiatric illness. In an oral medicine facial pain clinic the figures were 30% positive for psychiatric illness and in a rural hospital pain clinic 37% positive for psychiatric illness. In the writer's own personal series of patients, using the same test, 51% were positive for psychiatric illness. This demonstrates the effects of selection on the psychiatric characteristics of different pain populations. However it should be noted that current psychiatric illness was only present in approximately half of the population. This is a much lower rate than that found either by Reich et al (1983) or by Fishbain et al (1986). It is certainly possible that some of the difference relates to a lack of sensitivity on the part of the screening test, although this seems somewhat unlikely considering that it is usually more than 80% sensitive and specific in comparison with psychiatric interview. Some part of the difference between the screening test paper by Merskey et al and these two papers may be due to a superior technique of case finding in the other papers.

Retrospective examination of the writer's own practice by chart review showed that a much higher proportion of the patients than 50% had a psychological problem *at some time*. Some 47% were positive for definite psychiatric illness by DSM-III criteria and a further 37% had atypical or minor forms of psychological disturbance, making 84% affected altogether. Perhaps the most important observation here is that psychological illness in the presence of chronic pain with lesions tends to fluctuate and that it will be present at one time and not at another. This may well depend on the severity of the pain and the process through which the patient is going. For example, after injury many patients suffer difficulties in employment and marital relationships, as well as continuing insomnia from pain, and become depressed. After a while treatment may take the edge off the worst of their pain, and some of their social difficulties may be resolved, so that although the pain persists, depression and other psychological problems subside. This observation would indicate that much of the depression found with chronic pain with lesions is secondary rather than primary in causing the pain.

Fibromyalgia provides another group of patients in whom psychological changes are evident without accounting for all the cases. It appears from a review of several sources that between 35% and 72% of patients with fibromyalgia have current or past psychiatric disturbance (Merskey 1989). Such a finding leads to the conclusion that while psychiatric factors might promote some cases of fibromyalgia, they are very unlikely to be a principal cause of the illness and the same conclusion probably applies to most cases with chronic pain in medical practice.

Overall, there is no doubt that there is an increased frequency of psychological illness in pain-clinic patients, although it does not necessarily rise to 100%. The most characteristic findings in the psychiatric population within a pain clinic are that depression is found in a significant minority of the patients as well as other anxiety symptoms and social dysfunction; irritability is also a marked feature of the depression seen in pain clinics, especially in comparison with depression seen in other settings. Epidemiological evidence supports this position. Crook et al (1984), in a community survey, found chronic pain in 11% of the adult population and acute pain in a further 5%. Crook et al (1989) have since shown that, compared with the community sample, patients in a pain clinic were more likely to have been injured, reported a greater intensity and constancy of pain and had more difficulties with the activities of daily living. They were more depressed and withdrawn socially and showed more long-term consequences as a result of unemployment, litigation and alcohol and drug abuse.

Magni et al (1990) reported the relationship between pain and depression in a very carefully chosen epidemiological sample. Data was obtained from the United States National Center for Health Statistics based on a survey of a stratified sample of 3023 subjects, aged 25–74 years, 1319 males and 1704 females. Of these, 416 (14.4%) definitely suffered from pain in the musculoskeletal system which had been present on most days for at least 1 month in the 12 months preceding the interview. A total of 219 patients (7.4%) were 'uncertain' cases in the sense that they had some pain, but it was not possible to determine that the duration of their symptoms was at least 1 month, or that they had been present during the previous 12 months. The remaining 2388 (78.1%) had no chronic pain. All these subjects were also given the Depression Scale of the Center for Epidemiologic Studies (CES-D). The chronic pain subjects scored significantly higher than normals, and those with pain of uncertain duration scored similar to the definite chronic pain population. Using a conservative (i.e. high) cut-off score for depression, 18% of the population with chronic pain were found to have depression compared with 8% of the population who did not have chronic pain. To date, these are the most definitive data we have on the relationship in the population between chronic pain and depression, indicating that depression occurs twice as frequently in those with chronic pain as in a control sample. There are two questions in the CES-D which relate to somatic items that could be due to physical effects (e.g. insomnia), but the use of the high cut-off score effectively cancels their possible influence. In the pain group there were also significantly more females and older people and people with a lower income.

Incidentally, it is worth noting that Merskey et al (1987) obtained a measure of the personality features of the pain population with the hysteroid-obsessoid questionnaire of Caine and Hope (1967), and the mean score for the pain population was slightly towards the obsessional side of the hysteroid-obsessoid continuum. A significant difference was found by clinic, with the psychiatric clinic population being somewhat more obsessoid than the populations of the other three clinics. Premorbid personality did not appear to contribute to the pain complaints themselves nor to social dysfunction. Tauschke et al (1990) also obtained evidence that adult defence mechanisms in patients with pain were related to the presence or absence of psychiatric illness and immature defence mechanisms were greater in patients who had psychiatric illness with or without pain than in those who did not have psychological illness.

A number of the studies in pain clinics have reported on the frequency of depression in the patients there. Studies of pain in psychiatric patients have also produced data about the frequency of depression. This is an important topic which has been much discussed lately. Before considering it, it is desirable to examine the accepted mechanisms by which psychological illness may produce pain, and also the question of hysteria or 'somatoform' conditions.

STRESS FACTORS AND CHRONIC PAIN

The influence of psychological factors in causing pain is often thought to be mediated through stress. Vulnerable individuals faced with difficult circumstances may develop pain in response. Three principal phenomena should be associated with this hypothesis. Firstly, there should be evidence of stress sufficient to cause emotional change.

 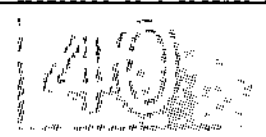

Secondly, there should be evidence of emotional change. Thirdly, the people affected should be at greater risk than average.

Although it is often recognized that stress occurs in conjunction with chronic pain, particularly the sort of chronic pain for which patients are referred to hospital, there has been little satisfactory evidence on the topic until lately. Good evidence is hard to obtain because the task is very time consuming. The popular checklists for stress are not efficient or satisfactory and an adequate measure usually requires a lengthy interview to determine prior life events. The methodology is difficult (Brown et al 1973). Jensen (1988) compared patients with low-back pain, with and without nerve-root compression, and two groups of headache patients. Comparison of the frequency of single life events within the previous 12 months revealed no statistically significant differences among the diagnostic groups. The same applied to the total number of life events and the number of life events with transient distress or enduring distress. A number of life events with transient distress were found to show a significant negative association with the persistence of pain in patients with headache but not in other groups. However, even this finding does not appear to be significant after correction for multiple tests.

Atkinson et al (1988) hypothesized that low-back pain patients with depressed mood would report significantly more untoward life events and ongoing life difficulties than chronic low-back pain patients without depressed mood and controls. Their prediction was confirmed. However, the increased stress reported by the depressed group appeared to be a direct consequence of life events related to back pain rather than from other life problems. This supports a model of pain causing disability or disadvantage rather than the latter causing the pain. Kukull et al (1986) showed similarly that, among outpatients in a general medical clinic, depression appeared to result most often from physical illness. Those who were not depressed initially but became depressed also had more new physical illness.

Marbach et al (1988) undertook a thorough study of life events in patients with temporomandibular pain and dysfunction syndrome. They found no preponderance of life events in the patients with facial pain compared with controls except after the onset of the symptom. The occurrence of other physical illness was more common in these patients. This may suggest an association of types of musculoskeletal change but it does not suggest an effect of stress in producing the illnesses originally. Speculand et al (1984) found some evidence with a similar syndrome which they felt favoured the occurrence of life events as a precipitating factor.

In none of this work does it appear that life events reflect even a large subordinate portion of the variance in explaining the appearance of pain. By contrast, the NUPRIN Study (Sternbach 1986) showed that individuals approached by telephone in the community reported a strong association between stress and pain, in that minor ongoing stresses and strains of daily living – 'hassles' – were related to pain in different locations, including headache and backache. It would fly in the face of ordinary experience to suggest that stress does not cause chronic pain but it seems equally clear that the contribution is not large. Most studies have not shown that stressful life events will precipitate or increase headache or low-back pain, and life events have not been used for predicting the results of treatment (Jensen 1988).

Another perspective is suggested by the Boeing study in Seattle, Washington (Bigos et al 1991). This study has been widely taken as indicating that one of the most important factors in back pain is the satisfaction of the employee with his or her job. This was a prospective study of workers in an aircraft factory of whom 279 out of 3020 reported back problems when followed longitudinally. The subjects who stated they 'hardly ever' enjoyed their job tasks were 2.5 times more likely to report a back injury ($P = 0.0001$) than subjects who 'almost always' enjoyed their job tasks. There are some limitations to this study. Only 75% of those who were solicited to take part in the study actually participated, and only 54% of these respondents, i.e. only 40.5% of the total, were studied. Some 279 out of 1569 reported back pain but only 89 of them (32%) actually did not enjoy their job. After deducting from this figure the 40% who presumably had other reasons for sickness, although they were also discontented, we are left with 53 workers (19%) who are likely to have been off work because they were discontented. In any case, this is a short-term study, dealing with relatively acute pain and does not demonstrate the factors involved in chronic pain. There is reason to believe that many people who dislike work, and have an adequate income when they are not working, will take extra time off, or take some time off, when they have a modest illness, but not that they will prolong this into chronic pain which requires much more substantial treatment and is much more disruptive to the working life.

In a substantial study of large numbers of patients with chronic pain in different centres, Gamsa (1990) provided evidence that psychological changes were more related to the occurrence of pain than to premorbid characteristics. The same implication appears from several studies in which we have undertaken screening procedures for psychological illness in relation to chronic pain (Salter et al 1983, Merskey et al 1985, 1987, Zilli et al 1989). As we have already noticed, less than 50% of patients receiving treatment for chronic pain show significant evidence of psychiatric illness. This means that even if all such cases had pain because of their emotional state, the hypothesis of psychogenesis of pain could fit only a minority. There is also only a small relationship at most between previous personality and current symptoms of anxiety and depression in patients with pain (Merskey et al 1987). The foregoing indicates that although there may be a relationship between stress and the production of pain, the relationship is not a strong one and in the absence of psychological illness has not been shown to account for pain syndromes which appear to have a pathophysiological or organic basis.

MECHANISMS OF PAIN

There are five ways in which psychological illness may be causally related to the appearance or increase of pain. The first is perhaps one of the most common and has to do with the increase of pain which occurs when patients who have a lesion are worried about it. The precise psychological mechanism of this effect is unknown. Nevertheless, patients in a state of anxiety frequently experience much greater pain from lesions than would otherwise be expected. A reduction of their anxiety leads to a reduction in their pain. Perhaps this is the situation in which gate-theory-type explanations are most relevant to pain due to psychological causes. It is plausible to suppose that pain which is related to some existing activity in peripheral nerve pathways may be greatly increased as a result of heightened arousal in the patient, so that an effect is transmitted through descending pathways to the spinal cord, thus increasing the abnormal activity which itself is ultimately the basis for the experience of pain in consciousness. This explanation remains speculative, but acute or subacute pain in clinical practice is frequently much relieved by measures which reduce the patient's anxiety about the provocative lesion.

Pain may also at times, but very rarely, be due to psychotic hallucinations. The most clear cut and most rare example of this is in schizophrenia. Typical schizophrenic hallucinations are almost never concerned with pain. Schizophrenic patients do have some pains, for example dull headache, which may be hallucinatory but which are not readily recognizable as such. They have frequent bodily experiences of other people doing things to them, such as hypnotizing them, influencing them with rays and so forth, but it is astonishing how rarely they indicate that these bodily changes are painful. In a series of 78 patients with schizophrenia only one was found whose pain might be attributed to her delusion (Watson et al 1981) and, as it happens, that patient was suffering from an atypical or schizoaffective illness. Perhaps slightly more often, depressive patients may have delusions which appear to give rise to hallucinations – for example, a patient who felt that she was being punished and who was experiencing stabbing pains in her buttocks and genitals. Usually it is reasonable to suppose that the pain associated with depression is like that found with anxiety or with hysterical conditions, which is to be discussed below.

The third mechanism of the production of pain which may be considered is the well-known tension pain mechanism. There is no doubt that if muscles are exercised in the absence of adequate circulation, they will give rise to discomfort and even very severe pain. This was demonstrated well over 60 years ago (Lewis et al 1931). The common hypothesis holds that inadequate removal of waste products from the tissues provides noxious stimulation.

Unaccustomed exercise of almost any bodily part, especially under conditions of emotional tension, may hence give rise to pain which is attributable to muscle contraction. The very term 'muscle contraction headache', which is a popular diagnostic category, implies this aetiological theory. Anyone who has driven a new car (or one with which he or she was not very familiar) in difficult driving conditions over long distances may have experienced comparable aching and discomfort in muscles which were used in an unaccustomed fashion. Thus the notion of muscle tension pain is easily understood and widely popular. It is a perfectly acceptable explanation for many cases in ordinary life and also for many people who have anxiety and who have increased muscle tension. The limitation to this theory is that it is probably excessively applied to all types of pain from psychological causes. Thus there are many patients who have chronic pain who do not show the increase in muscular tension which might be expected (Sainsbury & Gibson 1954). This has been particularly well known in studies where patients with so-called muscle contraction headache had less frontal muscle tension than patients with migraine (Pozniak-Patewicz 1976, Bakal & Kaganov 1977). Muscle tension in patients with chronic headache only accounts for a very small proportion of the pain, as little as 5% of the variance (Epstein et al 1978, Martin & Mathews 1978). The pain is more related to personality disorder and measures thereof (Harper & Steger 1978).

Lund and his colleagues (1993) have reviewed the literature that describes motor function in fibromyalgia and several other muscle pain conditions such as tension-type headache, temporomandibular disorders, chronic lower back pain and postexercise muscle soreness and are satisfied that muscular hyperactivity is not associated with those conditions. On the other hand, they find that there is a lot of evidence that these chronic pain patients have a reduced level of maximum voluntary contraction in agonist muscles and an increase of co-contraction in antagonist muscles in a body part that is painful. These changes are probably protective. Moreover, traditional methods of relieving anxiety and muscle tension (relaxation, psychotherapy, anxiolytic-medication) are largely ineffective in these chronic cases. It is therefore felt that there is a group of patients for whom another explanation must be provided.

The fourth explanation, and one which presumably applies to many of the patients with chronic headache and other chronic pains without clear evidence of physical illness, is the production of pain by hysterical (conversion) mechanisms. The idea that pain can be a hysterical symptom has been recognized since antiquity and has been popular since the Middle Ages at least. Perhaps it has been too popular and some pains which were not due to hysteria were too readily explained in that way. One of the main problems is that 'hysteria' has meant different things at various times in medical history. Thus, 19th century hysteria often included anxiety and depression (Merskey 1995) with different implications from modern conversion, hysteria or pain disorder. However, there are several anecdotal and observational instances which give an indication of how such a pain might appear. The best example of pain due to the patient's thoughts or due to a hysterical process may be that of the couvade syndrome where husbands have the pains which their wives would normally experience in labour. This has been well studied by Reik (1914), Bardhan (1965a, b), Curtis (1965), Trethowan and Conlon (1965) and Trethowan (1968).

Another striking example of pain due to hysterical mechanisms is probably to be found in the report by Rawnsley and Loudon (1964), who were able to show that many patients in a group whom they studied and who had a history of headache had a previous history of gross hysterical fits. Anecdotal instances which have some theoretical significance have been described in several places by the present writer. The most relevant type of pain to 'hysteria' today would come under the category of somatoform disorder, including somatization disorder. Purported hysterical conversion mechanisms may also be included under pain disorder (as described above).

Fifth, while this may not be a mechanism of pain in exactly the same way as the other factors just discussed, hypochondriasis is liable to promote pain and may transform a minor physical complaint into a substantial psychological and medical problem. Occasionally too, the hypochondriacal nature of the pain symptom is more marked than any other pattern and represents the principal diagnosis and explanation. Mild hypochondriasis amounts to excessive concern with bodily symptoms and is often dispelled by reassurance when that can be given appropriately. It is then a form of expression of anxiety, very well considered by Kellner (1986) and Barsky and Klerman (1983). Barsky and Wyshak (1990) provided evidence of a tendency of hypochondriacal patients to amplify bodily sensations in response to a questionnaire. This extends the earlier fundamental work of Pilowsky (1967), in which it was well demonstrated that the other principal phenomena of hypochondriasis are fear of disease combined with a conviction that disease is present, as well as bodily preoccupation. Such tendencies are common among patients who have chronic pain, but the recognition should not, as with hypochondriasis in general, overshadow the need to appreciate the existence of a physical mechanism in many instances.

PROBLEMS OF HYSTERIA OR SOMATOFORM ILLNESS

Some comments have already been made on hysteria. However, no discussion of hysteria as a cause of pain is sufficient without a warning. The mere absence of physical evidence for a cause of pain does not justify a diagnosis of hysteria. This diagnosis must always be made on positive evidence. In cases of paralysis and some other types of loss of function, it can be shown by neurological examination that there is positive evidence that the patient is able to do things which he or she thinks are not feasible. In the case of pain itself, that opportunity does not exist. On the contrary, there are probably certain signs which are traditionally taken to be evidence of hysteria but which are misleading in patients with pain.

The first of these signs is the so-called 'give-way' weakness. Many patients in a state of pain who frankly are able to use their limbs in different ways will refuse to do so, knowing that to comply with the examiner's request would hurt them. Either consciously or unconsciously they are affected by 'pain inhibition'. That should not be taken to suggest that they have hysteria or even that they are 'hysterical'.

Further, the occurrence of non-anatomical sensory loss is not necessarily hysterical either. Wall (1984) summarized evidence which has consistently increased over the 15 years since then and which indicates that at least some cells in the dorsal horn may have receptive fields from the whole of a limb. Thus, as Fishbain et al (1986) point out, the issue of non-dermatomal sensory abnormalities and their significance may need more research. These findings are extremely frequent and may well reflect an aspect of pain physiology which has not been properly understood.

In view of the findings by Wall and his colleagues that receptive fields of cells in the spinal cord can change enormously in response to pain in a limb, it becomes evident that regional non-dermatomal changes cannot be relied upon as signs of hysteria. This view is reinforced from another direction by the work of Gould et al (1986), who examined 30 patients with acute organic disease of the nervous system and demonstrated that they showed a high frequency of signs which are supposed to be characteristic of hysteria. Seven traditional signs were examined; namely, a history suggestive of hypochondriasis, potential secondary gain, belle indifference, non-anatomical or patchy sensory loss, changing boundaries of hypalgesia, sensory loss (to pinprick or vibratory stimulation) that splits at the midline and give-way weakness. All the patients demonstrated at least one of the above. Of these 30 patients, 29 showed at least one feature of a supposedly non-physiological sensory examination. The mean number of these items per patient was 3.4. The authors infer that hysteria is easily misdiagnosed if the above signs or items of history are accepted as pathognomonic, and many tests which are said to provide good evidence of hysteria lack validity.

There are several conditions which are basically physical and have been mistaken for hysteria or even for malingering. The writer has known some of them to be diagnosed as psychiatric, for example pain from ectopia cerebelli, facial pain with dyskinetic movements, and even the thoracic outlet syndrome in the presence of physical signs. In recent years the FM syndrome (IASP category 1.9, code X33.X8a) has been well characterized as a physical disorder (Smythe 1985, Wolfe et al 1990, Vaeroy 1996). Localized myofascial syndromes have also been increasingly recognized (Littlejohn 1986, International Association for the Study of Pain 1994). Such relatively subtle syndromes which depend for their recognition on advances or improvement in clinical method may have often been misdiagnosed as hysteria in the past and the possibility still exists of such a misdiagnosis.

If the diagnosis of hysteria is to be made on psychiatric grounds, there must be evidence for this from psychological examination, to an extent which shows that psychological problems and causes are present in proportion to the symptom. Ideally, they should be accepted by the patient as the principal causes of her complaint. This situation is rarely achieved.

It is relevant at this point to comment on the relationship between psychiatry and pain in routine practice. Most psychiatric patients are seen in outpatient departments, and pain is only a major problem in a minority. Even when they do present with pain, particularly headache, which is the commonest type of pain in psychiatric patients (Merskey 1965b, Spear 1967), the pain is frequently relegated to a secondary place while the psychiatrist concentrates on the psychiatric disorders and causes of illness which he is able to find. More often, patients who have pain about which they are particularly concerned tend to appear in headache clinics or in pain clinics, and the psychiatrist there has the extra task of adding his advice on the care of individuals who are generally disinclined to think of their illness in psychological terms and are more prone to think of it in physical terms. This is perhaps even more often a problem for non-psychiatrists who seek to refer the patient to the psychiatrist. The management of this objection is difficult for all physicians and surgeons, and it is normally handled in several different ways depending on the individual case. Some patients who are able to accept the advice that they need psychological help – or who even volunteer for it themselves – are readily referred. Others are persuaded to see psychiatrists because they are told that the individual doctor has experience or an interest in the treatment of pain which goes beyond his particular specialty, and this is a justifiable approach. Still others are seen in psychiatric practice because the patients are told that everybody entering a pain clinic or centre is assessed automatically in both physical and psychological respects. This is perhaps one of the easiest and most effective ways of providing a psychological assessment and is one of the particular advantages of pain clinics.

PHYSICAL SIGNS AND PSYCHOLOGICAL ILLNESS

The detection of psychological illness, or a psychological problem, by means of supposedly 'non-organic' physical signs has long been popular, and it was noted above that this can be a useful method for demonstrating the presence of psychological problems. Difficulties were recognized in applying some of these approaches to patients with pain. Nevertheless, an impressive sustained effort has been made to do this, particularly by Waddell and his colleagues (1980, 1984a & 1984b, 1989, Waddell 1987). The fundamental initial study in this series demonstrated the use of five types of physical sign to indicate the occurrence of psychological problems. They were tenderness (superficial or non-anatomic), simulated physical stresses leading to a report of pain (either from axial loading or rotation), distraction (in straight-leg raising), regional alterations (weakness or sensory change) and overreaction. Patients without back pain had none of these. British patients with previously untreated back pain referred to a routine hospital orthopaedic clinic had one or more of these signs in about 10% of cases. This figure compares with one-third of cases in both Canadian and British patients with more persistent problems (failed surgery, chronic disability, etc.). These signs had a strong relationship to the judgement by a surgeon that the condition was 'non-organic' or that the patient was unsuitable for surgery. They also had a strong relationship to general somatic and neurotic symptoms, so-called disability behaviour and 'inappropriate symptoms'. There was a low but consistent correlation in one study in which the neurotic triad of scores of the MMPI was used but no relationship with the Eysenck Personality Questionnaire (EPQ) in British patients.

Subsequent work demonstrated consistency and reliability in the measurements of these signs (Waddell & Main 1984) and that both objective physical impairment and psychological distress accounted for significant proportions of the disability observed. Thus, physical impairment was thought to account for about 40% of the disability observed, depression and increased bodily awareness for 22.5% between them and 'magnified illness behaviour' for 8.4% of the variance (Waddell et al 1984b). Four patients with partial cord lesions, three with cauda equina lesions and two with lumbosacral injuries did not show these signs. The authors concluded that 'Disability in low back pain can be understood in terms of physical impairment, psychological distress and illness behaviour, each of which can be defined, observed and measured'. Those patients who had more evidence of inappropriate illness behaviour received more treatment (Waddell et al 1984a). The implications of these findings and further studies were explored by Waddell et al (1989) with the use of the Illness Behaviour Questionnaire of Pilowsky and Spence (1976). Disease affirmation or disease conviction were observed to be prominent in patients with chronic low-back pain.

This series of studies is unmatched in methodology, numbers and attention to detail. The result might be thought to imply that much disability from back pain is due to the mental state of the patients rather than the physical illness. The authors themselves are cautious about such a conclusion. They suggested that these signs should not be thought to indicate psychological problems in patients who are over the age of 55–69 or who have acute causes of pain. Waddell et al (1980) also point out that it is wise to assume that there is a physical basis in most cases of back pain. Further, the figures quoted show that 40% of the variance with disability is related to demonstrable physical illness and 31% to the psychological state. The contributions of the two types of factor appear to be fairly similar.

Two more qualifications should be expressed concerning this phenomenon. The first qualification is that some of the so-called non-organic physical signs are less non-organic than was thought. The difficulty of proving that signs of 'hysteria' were free from organic influence as shown by Gould et al (1986) was discussed earlier. It is true that the work of Waddell does not utilize the same signs as that of Gould, except for give-way weakness which only appeared in one of Gould's cases. Nevertheless as with regional weakness it is not accurate to interpret superficial tenderness or regional pain syndromes as due to psychological factors. Among the other signs on which reliance has been placed, simulation and overreaction place a burden (which may be legitimate) on the judgement of the examiner. One also has to note that in the instructions connected with the measurement of responses to simulated stresses, the stress of pressure on the neck giving rise to pain is found to be common and should be discounted, whereas the same effect lower down the vertebral column is not common and is taken into account as psychological. Further, if the more severe cases of pain have more of these findings is it because they are a non-specific accompaniment of the more intense physical disorder or because they are due primarily to a psychological cause? This is a substantial problem which has not been resolved and indeed if non-specific – but organic – disorder is the explanation of these signs then they would not be 'non-organic', but instead the pathophysiological outcome of myofascial pain or 'mechanical back pain'.

In order to show that the 'non-organic' signs are attributable to something other than the severity of the painful disorder, and are due to an independent variable, such as a wish for compensation or a state of depression due to bereavement and not connected with the physical disorder, it is necessary to establish the occurrence of stressful events or other psychological causes more often in those individuals who show significant amounts of 'non-organic' signs compared with those who have a comparable physical state but do not show those signs. This does not appear to have been done. As noted above it is not an easy task. However, in so far as investigations of stress factors in relation to chronic pain have been successful they have mostly shown that the worst stresses appear to arise in relation to consequences of pain and the disability associated with it.

Some other correlates of the 'non-organic' signs are also misleading. A modest relationship with the MMPI is not meaningful in terms of a psychological aetiology because, as mentioned earlier, that test merely counts symptoms, many of which on the most relevant scales relate to complaints about the physical state of the body.

Lastly, and most importantly, even if pain is due to a physical cause it will in that case, as in any other case, be experienced as a subjective condition. This is inherent in all accepted definitions of pain. The final statement about pain is subjective. The associated experience of the patient is subjective. Subjective psychological measures, whether they reflect independent psychological causes, or the mental state of an individual suffering from significant physical problems, will always show the closest relationships between pain and subjective measures. Pain cannot be better expressed than through reports of distress and subjective experience. Measures of distress will always be powerfully influenced by it. It follows that the patient's subjective awareness may well give a better estimate of the actual physical state than the physician's external measurements.

BEHAVIOURAL THEORIES OF PAIN – BEHAVIOURAL MEASURES

Fordyce et al (1981) have shown systematically that exercise helps to reduce pain or the behaviour related to it. It has long been recognized that exercise can be beneficial in some cases of pain. Stiffness produced by overactivity may be abated by further activity (a day or two later). In clinical practice, however, it remains very difficult at times to know which patients will benefit from exercise and which will be made worse. Hilton (1863) argued that rest is also beneficial for pain and despite some qualifications this remains true for many cases. Pain which is related to disuse and inactivity of muscles may be the sort which will respond best to behavioural measures. Pain which is related to current tenderness and spasm is much less likely to benefit. Hence exercise programmes which are increasingly common in North America appear to have great success with relatively easy cases but give rise to a good deal of discontent on the part of patients when the effort is made to apply exercise in the more protracted cases. This is most notable when there are continuing indications of some sort of musculoskeletal dysfunction, and no improvement after continuing effort.

The question of exercise is a subordinate topic within the larger issue of behavioural treatment of patients with chronic pain. Indeed, it can be separated from it because it also has a physiological rationale. Efforts to treat patients by behavioural means which discourage so-called 'pain behaviour' and encourage activity have continued through the 1980s. Current books or articles on pain frequently indicate a behavioural element in programmes for the treatment of pain (Sternbach 1987, Aronoff 1988, Loeser & Egan 1989, Bonica 1990). The theory of this treatment has been advanced (Fordyce et al 1985, 1988, Rachlin 1985) and criticized (Atkinson & Kremer 1985, Merskey 1985, Schmidt 1987, 1988). Critics of the theoretical position of the operant school of treatment are extremely wary of Fordyce's view that '... *behavioural methods* in pain treatment programs *are intended to treat excess disability and expressions of suffering*'. They wonder if the clinician is going to be as skilful as is necessary in defining 'excess disability and expressions of suffering'. Anyone who gets this wrong is going to be pushing patients repeatedly to do things which are increasingly difficult and painful for them. We have seen this often and it is not a pretty matter. This is a lesser point, though a grievous one in practice, than the fundamental issue which Fordyce (1976) previously stated, namely, that the subjective state of the patient is not a matter of concern to him, provided behaviour can change. Rachlin (1985) complained that Fordyce makes it harder to defend his valid position by this particular notion. Schmidt (1988), however, demonstrated that the operant approach by Fordyce and colleagues has confused pain, ratings of pain by the sufferer and pain behaviours, although Fordyce (1990) disputes this.

The culmination of the behavioural approach appears in 'Back pain in the workplace' (Fordyce 1995), a monograph written on behalf of a Task Force of the IASP which recommends that, after 6 weeks of treatment by conservative measures, patients with so-called non-specific back pain and without any surgically correctible lesion, are to be treated as suffering from 'activity intolerance' and denied benefits. Waddell is also one of the members of this Task Force, and like Rachlin noted earlier with respect to the denial of pain, has shown ambivalence about the approach in the Report, saying that it was meant to stimulate debate but that '... it is not the answer' (Waddell 1996). No matter how much argument there is around this topic, it seems that the notion of treating pain behaviour involves some denial of the patient's experience.

Although I have not seen this discussed there is a significant potential problem of conflict of interest in programmes that aim to treat patients behaviourally. Of course all practitioners who follow such a policy are likely to establish a contract with the patient and obtain the patient's agreement and informed consent. In many countries such as the UK or Canada the problem of conflict of interest in this connection will not often arise because doctors are mostly overworked and medical care is often wholly funded from public sources or directly by the patient. A different situation obtains in the USA, where a considerable proportion of the patients in pain clinics, if not all of them, have their treatment funded by insurance carriers. The best interests of an insurance company lie in getting the insured person back to health and strength, and in establishing that the insured person will receive treatment directed to her employability. That, too, is in the interest of the insured. Nevertheless, patients are more interested than insurance companies in relieving pain, but in order to satisfy the companies, clinics have to provide programmes which offer to remove *disability* rather than necessarily remove *pain*. In fact one aim is often sacrificed for the sake of another. The considerable popularity of behavioural programmes in the USA may have something to do with the need to talk to insurance companies in terms which encourage them to provide funds for treatment of the affected individuals. The style of treatment adopted in consequence is not necessarily one which would otherwise be favoured.

As an alternative, many psychologists have adopted cognitive approaches which are dealt with elsewhere in this volume. It is worthwhile pointing out here that Flor and Turk (1989) have shown that cognitive variables in rheumatoid arthritis explain between 32% and 60% of the variance in pain and disability and did so more effectively than physical measures. There is increasing recognition that the patient's awareness of disability and distress predicts outcome better than the physician's estimate of the physical status in a number of instances. Perhaps this is because the patient's awareness effectively takes into account both her physical state and her feelings.

Anderson et al (1988) showed that psychological variables did not independently predict pain behaviour in rheumatoid arthritis. Their study was accompanied by a thorough rating of pain behaviours such as guarding, bracing, grimacing, sighing, rigidity, passive rubbing and active rubbing. One of the most striking findings was that pain behaviour was most closely related to physical illness. This ought to be in accordance with expectation, because the model of pain behaviour was developed out of the model of physical disease. Pain behaviour is thought to be anomalous only when it is not matched by physical disease to a considerable extent. Thoughts on this have been confused at times by the fact that some physical measures are not very satisfactory, for example X-ray measurements are a poor organic index for the pain of patients with osteoarthritis. Anderson et al, like Keefe et al (1990), demonstrate effectively that the strongest relationship of pain behaviour is found to be with physical illness. As Anderson et al state: 'in our prior investigations ... rigidity and guarding were the behaviours that were the most highly associated with disease activity variables and self report of functional disability ... the results of multiple studies support the validity of guarding and rigidity as measures of RA pain...'.

Meanwhile, the studies of Keefe and his colleagues do identify a subgroup of patients with low-back pain who have some evidence of pain behaviour and only moderate complaints of pain. This group remains a focus of attention and amounted to 19% of the sample of Keefe et al taken from patients referred to a pain management programme who were participating in structured inpatient treatment. Whether or not this group had its pain from mainly psychological or behavioural reasons is not clear. The findings are somewhat reminiscent of the conclusions of Leavitt et al (1982) on another occasion that perhaps 10% of patients with chronic back pain are not adequately diagnosed psychiatrically or physically. Keefe's subgroup may also only have had less severe pain than others. In summary, the work of this group suggests that pain behaviour can be measured quite effectively but that it should not be misinterpreted as merely a sign of operant pain. This type of pain behaviour is more marked with movement and cannot easily be measured without inducing movement.

Psychological studies of coping and behaviour bear obvious links with other issues that we have been considering. Thus, the way in which individuals cope may be influenced by or may influence the relationships within the family, the frequency of pain or its severity and the extent of the emergence of depression. Watt-Watson et al (1988) have demonstrated relationships between depression and coping responses, pain intensity and family function. Coping responses also had a significant relationship with pain intensity and family functioning. This is but one of numerous papers which indicate the importance of a comprehensive appraisal of the situation of individuals with chronic pain.

DEPRESSION IN PATIENTS WITH PAIN

In the discussion of psychiatric illness in patients with pain and also in examining the frequency of psychiatric illness in patients attending pain clinics, it was observed that depression is often found in both such populations. Some workers have reported that a particularly high proportion of pain-clinic patients have depression. For example, Lindsay and Wyckoff (1981), from the University of Washington Pain Clinic in Seattle, indicated that, out of 150 consecutive referrals to the clinic of patients with non-malignant pain, at least 85% had depression according to the research diagnostic criteria of Feighner et al (1972). Perhaps those criteria were easier to satisfy than some others. By contrast, Large (1980) found 46 diagnoses of one type of depression or another among 172 pain-clinic patients. Using quite stringent psychological screening tests, Pilowsky et al (1977) demonstrated that depression affected only 10% of their series of patients. Pelz and Merskey (1982) observed that 83 pain-clinic patients, all with lesions, had a mean score on the Levine–Pilowsky depression questionnaire of 7.13, which placed them in the 'non-depressed group'. Even 12 patients who were receiving tricyclic antidepressants were also in this category. Although occasional cases of depressive illness were recognized in pain-clinic patients, they were only a minority. On the other hand, a far larger number of patients may express some complaint of dysphoric mood or depression as a symptom, such as 'feeling blue'. Thus, 26.5% of patients confessed to feeling blue compared with the very small number who admitted to depression in that study.

A specific study by Kramlinger et al (1983), using Research Diagnostic Criteria (Spitzer et al 1978), found that 25 were definitely depressed, 39 were probably depressed and 36 were not depressed. In the author's own chart review of patients seen in psychiatric consultation for painful conditions, at some time nine out of 32 patients had major affective disorder and 12 had atypical affective disorder (Merskey et al 1987). Thus, the proportion with a well-defined affective illness was limited to 28%. Only with the inclusion of atypical affective disorder does the figure for depression reach 66%. The latter diagnosis, incidentally, was dropped from DSM-III(R) and DSM-IV in which the equivalent would be depressive disorder not otherwise specified. This longitudinal evaluation fits with clinical experience. Patients with chronic pain from injuries are not depressed initially. They often become depressed as the pain persists, and improve somewhat in their depression as they adjust to their altered circumstances. The importance to be given to depression when it is found frequently in pain-clinic patients may thus be very much diminished if the finding of high frequency is based on a very mild state.

The numerous reports of pain in relation to depression have been reviewed by Roy et al (1984), Romano and Turner (1985) and Gupta (1986). All these reviews point to the inconsistency of the data available in the literature and the limitations of the different studies and their methodological differences. There are few controlled studies and the diagnostic criteria in relation to both depression and pain are often not rigorous enough. The populations are extremely heterogeneous, different instruments are used, some patients come from one source and some from another, as already considered, and some have organic lesions and some not. Overall, while there is probably an increased frequency of depression in pain-clinic patients and of pain in patients with depression, the frequency will vary with the sample and with the method used for measuring depression, and the writer estimates that in most pain-clinic populations, other than specialized centres, the frequency of sustained depression will be of the order of about 10–30%. The frequency of depression in patients with chronic musculoskeletal pain is 18% compared with a population incidence of depression of 8% (Magni et al 1990). However, we cannot tell from that finding alone whether the pain causes depression or the depression is due to pain.

Other data which suggest that the depression is often due to pain were discussed above, particularly the appearance of depression in patients whose burdens from pain become sufficiently high, and whose depression declines when the severity of the pain and its burden decrease. Some direct, albeit retrospective evidence, comes from the work of Atkinson et al (1991) who showed that patients with chronic pain from industrial injuries had depression twice as often after their injury as prior to it. The same patients also showed more evidence of alcoholism prior to their injuries compared with controls, which tends to suggest that the recording of illness before and after the injury was objective.

Another condition which provides increasing evidence to suggest organic effects in causing depression or psychological change is the cervical sprain ('whiplash') syndrome. Macnab (1964) has long established that this is a condition with an important physical basis in terms of torn muscles, ligaments and even disks. Taylor (1991) has shown from postmortem examinations that many patients with relatively 'minor' cervical injury suffer splitting of their cervical disks. Radanov et al (1991) found that the only variable which they could discover to predict cognitive function at 6 months was the severity of the pain at the time of the initial injury. Patients with this problem frequently become depressed in the course of the illness when they were not depressed previously. Bogduk and his colleagues, discussed above, have provided impeccable studies implicating the facet joints as the cause of much whiplash pain (Lord et al 1996).

One aspect of the relationship between pain and depression which has often been considered deserves further comment. There are some patients who appear to have no explanation for their pain physically and who also do not seem to be depressed. Moreover, no other psychiatric diagnosis seems to be feasible. No doubt in some of these cases further inquiry and time will reveal an unknown physical cause or a psychiatric one. Magni et al (1987a) collected a group of patients who had such a pattern of pain and examined them systematically for phenomena associated with depression, such as a family history of depressive disorders and related phenomena. They found that this group of patients had an increased family history of so-called 'depressive spectrum disorders' compared with a normal group. Further they found that imipramine binding was reduced in patients with this pattern of illness in the same direction as patients with depression but not to the same extent. These authors then went on to show (Magni et al 1987b) that the pain responded to antidepressant treatment, particularly in those patients who had a reduced number of imipramine binding sites and also a family history of depression. This leads to the conclusion that there are sometimes patients whose cerebral pathophysiology is such that they will respond to antidepressants in the same way as patients with depression, but who lack the evidence of a depressed mood.

Patients who have this condition, or this state, have previously been diagnosed as having 'depressive equivalents'. Such a diagnosis, however, lacks clinical criteria and ought to be avoided. The best term for those patients for whom no physical or organic cause can be shown is probably 'indeterminate pain'. Magni (1987) has reviewed the evidence for the explanation of indeterminate pain as being related to depression at times.

PAIN PROMOTING PSYCHOLOGICAL ILLNESS

Most authors who have worked with patients with chronic pain due to lesions have come to the conclusion that changes are liable to occur in the emotional state of people who are otherwise normal as a result of their experience of prolonged pain. Weir Mitchell (1872) observed the condition of a man with causalgia who, from being 'one of gay and kindly temper', became morose and apparently furious. Patients with pain, and especially with chronic pain from physical lesions, may be expected to be worn down and generally made miserable by their experience. Taub (A Taub, personal communication) observed that patients in a neurological clinic with such conditions tended to present a picture initially of anxiety and depression. This contrasts with the expectation that patients with pain of psychological origin will have slightly more hypochondriacal or hysterical aspects to their emotional disorder. Comparing patients with physical lesions and those without, Woodforde and Merskey (1972) found that those who had their pain from lesions actually became more anxious, more depressed and more subject to signs of neuroticism than patients whose pain had no physical cause and who were known to have psychiatric illness. Patients with physical causes for their pain did, however, tend to see themselves as being persons who in the past were well adjusted, stable, successful and well controlled. This gave them high scores on the L-scale of the Eysenck Personality Inventory. That scale was at first thought to indicate a tendency to falsify the account of the individual's previous personality by 'faking good'. Evidence from other studies such as Morgenstern (1967) and Bond (1971) indicates that higher scores are also associated with physical disability, and it appears that, in patients with pain of organic origin, high L scores accompanied by raised neuroticism scores may have the following explanation (Woodforde & Merskey 1972); they represent the response of individuals struggling to keep themselves stable in the face of damage done to their personalities who nevertheless feel that they were once fit, well and effective people. Despite increasing anxiety and depression, the patient looks back to a time when perhaps, in fact, he was free from those psychological troubles because he was not beset by intractable pain.

Evidence from another direction supports this, in that Sternbach et al (1973) showed that chronic-pain patients had increased hysteria, depression and hypochondriasis scores on the MMPI compared with patients with acute back pain, while Sternbach and Timmermans (1975) showed a reduction of 'neuroticism' in patients whose pain was relieved by back surgery. Crown and Crown (1973) showed that patients with late rheumatoid arthritis had more personality change than those with early arthritis (who resembled normals). In the case of animals, experimental pain gives rise to aggressive responses – biting the bars of the cage or the neighbour (O'Kelly & Steckley 1939). Aggression in response to pain is presumably part of the fight or flight mechanism, the alternative being retreat. Thus it seems that we should also expect emotional change to appear quite consistently in patients who have chronic lesions.

Studies which enable us to discriminate between patients with lesions and those without lesions on the basis of MMPI scores or other psychological techniques are rather few or slight. Other studies using the MMPI have, however, been used to predict successfully which patients would respond to organic treatment (chemonucleolysis), to surgery (Wiltse & Rocchio 1975, Smith & Duerksen 1980, Oostdam et al 1981) or to conservative treatment (McCreary et al 1979). Not all studies have agreed that it is possible to discriminate in this way (Waring et al 1976). Another approach to the separation of patients by psychological techniques on the basis of their psychiatric characteristics has been made by Bradley et al (1978) who have tried to discern MMPI groupings which would signify different types of pain patients. Sternbach did so earlier (1974) and the effort should be continued. Meanwhile, one approach which has helped in the discrimination, by psychological means, of groups of patients with lesions and without lesions is the use of the McGill Pain Questionnaire (MPQ). Although it has been argued by the present writer that in general the descriptions of pain by patients with lesions and without lesions are remarkably similar (Devine & Merskey 1965), it appears that there are times and occasions when a distinction can be made between the two groups of patients on the basis of their response to the adjectival checklists of the MPQ. Leavitt and Garron (1979a,b) reported substantial success in this respect. They were also able to show that patients who did not have a detectable lesion, but who did not have psychiatric illness either, used language which suggested that they fell in the group of patients with organic lesions which had not yet been discovered.

PAIN AND DISABILITY

As mentioned above the culmination of the behavioural approach resulted in a report which rejected medical care and disability payments for individuals after 6 weeks' treatment of non-specific back pain. The bases for this report were held to be, firstly, a lack of proven organic lesions, secondly, a large rise in disability claims and payments in many countries and, thirdly, evidence that this rise was influenced by psychosocial factors. There is, in fact, a great deal of evidence that regional pain – of which non-specific low back pain is one form – has important physical and physiological causes (Merskey 1988) and should not be confused with hysteria (somatoform illness). The physiological sections of this book give pause to anyone who doubts this view. Likewise the work of Bogduk and his colleagues (Lord et al 1996) has shown that percutaneous radiofrequency coagulation of the terminal nerve supply to the cervical zygapophyseal joints in patients with the cervical sprain syndrome, undertaken in a controlled double-blind fashion, produces prolonged relief of pain in those patients who had the active treatment with concomitant relief of psychiatric symptoms. This gives very strong support to the idea that psychological changes may not only be primary factors in causing pain and disability, but also – and probably more often – are no more than consequences or secondary modifiers of pain and disability. In addition to the evidence already cited on this matter, an extensive study by Gatchel et al (1995) on a cohort of 421 patients within 6 weeks of the onset of acute back pain and 12 months after onset, found that:

> *Major pathophysiology, such as depression and substance abuse, was not found to be a precursor or predictive of chronic disability. Such data are important in indicating that the high rates of psychopathology seen in chronic pain disability conditions develop as a result of the chronicity and do not cause it.*

Those authors did find that self-reported pain and disability scores on scale three of the Minnesota Multiphasic Personality Inventory (MMPI), Workers' Compensation Board and Personal Injury Insurance Status, and female sex work correlated with chronicity. However it could be argued that much of the effect can also be accounted for by the severity of pain; the MMPI is known to be an indicator of somatic pain severity, and the presence of compensation may have been associated with more severe injuries.

The most detailed critique to date of Back Pain in the Workplace has been undertaken by Teasell and Merskey (1997). These authors concluded that in addition to some of the observations mentioned here already, the approach of the report runs the risk of hurting those patients who can least afford it – individuals who perform jobs with heavy or physical demands, are less well educated, lack transferable skills, and are older and in a lower socioeconomic class.

PATTERNS OF ILLNESS

Overall, the patterns of psychological illness which are associated with pain are essentially those of the particular psychological conditions with which the pain is occurring. Pain does not differ significantly in patients according to psychiatric diagnosis. Nevertheless, there are some patterns of pain which may be recognized in patients whose pain is primarily of psychological origin. The pain may be expected to occur more often in women than in men, but if it occurs in men it will be more often in association with a disability that has occurred at work and provides some compensatory

 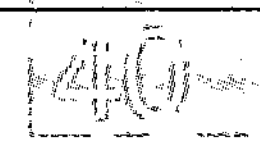

benefits, at least financially. In chronic pain of psychological origin, the pain is usually severe. The commonest site in the USA and the UK is the head. The genitals may be affected in as many as 10% of patients, but special enquiry may be needed to show this. Frequently the patient has pain in more than one part of the body and unless an organic diagnosis is evident, pain in more than two sites of the body is suggestive of pain of psychological origin. The pain is bilateral or symmetrical in approximately half the patients and there is a tendency in some studies for it to be commoner on the left side (Merskey & Watson 1979). It has been disputed whether this is true for all pain, and it has been suggested that it applied only to pain of psychological origin and especially to pain where there are hysterical features (Hall et al 1981). The only safe conclusion on this point is that pain on the left side has only been shown to be commoner in patients where there is evidence of hysterical patterns. Pain of psychological origin usually appears with the illness and is coexistent with it. If pain has been present before the onset of the psychological illness, it may be presumed to be due to another cause. It will usually become worse with the illness and improve afterwards.

Pain from psychological illness is usually continuously present with rather irregular fluctuations. It rarely, if ever, keeps the patient awake at night and it rarely, if ever, wakens the patient from sleep. If pain actually wakes the individual (and he is not merely conscious of pain after waking for some other reason) it gives very strong reason to think that the diagnosis is not wholly psychiatric. In studies of the actual words used by patients to describe their pains, it has been found that approximately 50% do not use unusual descriptions (Gittleson 1961, Devine & Merskey 1965). Physical factors sometimes relieve pain even though it is of psychological origin – mild analgesics, heat or cold may help. The response never appears to be great, at least not for long. Many patients with pain of psychological origin may recognize the relationship between it and worry or emotional difficulties.

The psychiatric conditions associated with pain of psychological origin are primarily those of anxiety, depression and somatoform complaints, as already indicated. No description will be given of these in general, because one chapter cannot be a textbook on psychiatry. It is worth emphasizing that the common associations of hysterical patterns, anxiety and situational or reactive depression, in that order, will be found more often in patients with chronic pain, whereas with acute pain anxiety may well be the most frequent phenomenon. The endogenous type of depressive illness represents a small but significant group which, if recognized, responds very well to treatment. Schizophrenia is a very rare cause indeed of chronic pain.

The primary treatment of these pain problems is that of the underlying psychiatric condition. Perhaps the most important distinction from ordinary psychiatric work is a careful study of the pain. This itself is therapeutic for those patients in whom it is a very prominent and troublesome aspect of their symptoms. So many of them feel that physicians and others have neglected to consider their pain while diagnosing them as having something wrong with their minds. Thus the practice of taking a careful direct history from the patient about this pain, before even beginning to look at psychological aspects, is frequently helpful in forming a relationship with the patient. One does not have to accept that pain has an organic basis when it is largely of psychological origin. One must accept the need to take seriously the patient's description of his symptoms and to treat this as a priority at the initial part of the relationship. Once that is done, it is usually possible to take an ordinary or conventional psychiatric history and establish at least some information about the psychological disorder which may be promoting the illness. In patients with chronic pain and psychiatric illness, and where the clinician is not initially acquainted with the individual, the interview normally takes more than 1 hour. If only 1 hour has been booked, it is best to say that more time is needed and allow for a second hour before coming to a moderately definitive opinion. This works well enough with many patients who have had the experience of seeing other doctors either for short periods which proved unsatisfactory or for longer periods which were demonstrably necessary in order to review the total history of the individual's experience.

If a diagnosis has been made and the clinician is satisfied that she has appropriate guidelines for treatment of the individual, psychiatric treatment may then proceed in conventional fashion whether by marital guidance, psychotherapy, drug treatment or whatever is most appropriate. Many of these different forms of treatment are considered in other chapters and so their special application to pain will not be described here. It should be noted, however, that it is occasionally worth giving minor analgesics if only to establish that they do not work. Patients for whom other forms of treatment are more appropriate will perhaps accept them somewhat more readily if it has been shown that the physician has a sincere interest in attempting to use the sort of medication and the sort of approach which, on commonsense grounds, the patient favours. A 1-week trial of a non-narcotic anti-inflammatory drug, whether it is acetylsalicylic acid or indomethacin or nabumetone, is frequently useful in demonstrating the open-mindedness of the clinician and the effectiveness, or lack of effectiveness, of the medication.

REFERENCES

Adler RH, Zlot S, Hüray C, Minder C 1989 Engel's psychogenic pain and the pain-prone patient. A retrospective controlled study. Psychosomatic Medicine 51: 87–101

Anderson KO, Keefe FR, Bradley LA et al 1988 Prediction of pain behavior and functional status of rheumatoid arthritis patients using medical status and psychological variables. Pain 3: 25–32

Aronoff GM 1988 Pain centers: a revolution in health care. Raven, New York.

Atkinson JH, Kremer EF 1985 Behavioral definition of pain: necessary but not sufficient. Behavioral and Brain Sciences 8: 54–55

Atkinson JH, Slater MA, Grant I, Patterson TL, Garfn SR 1988 Depressed mood in chronic low back pain: relationship with stressful life events. Pain 35: 47–55

Atkinson JH, Slater MA, Patterson TL, Grant I, Garfn SR 1991 Prevalence, onset, and risk of psychiatric disorders in men with chronic low back pain: a controlled study. Pain 45: 111–121

Bakal DA, Kaganov JA 1977 Muscle contraction and migraine headache: psychophysiological comparison. Headache 17: 208–215

Banks MH, Beresford SHA, Morrell DC, Waller JJ, Watkins CJ 1975 Factors infuencing demand for primary medical care in women aged 20–40 years; a preliminary report. International Journal of Epidemiology 4: 189–255.

Bardhan PN 1965a The fathering syndrome. US Armed Forces Medical Journal 20: 200–208

Bardhan PN 1965b The couvade syndrome. British Journal of Psychiatry 111: 908–909

Barsky AJ, Klerman GL 1983 Overview: hypochondriasis, bodily complaints, and somatic styles. American Journal of Psychiatry 140: 273–283

Barsky AJ, Wyshak G 1990 Hypochondriasis and somatosensory amplification. British Journal of Psychiatry 157: 404–409

Bigos SJ, Battie MC, Spengler DM et al 1991 A prospective study of work perceptions and psychosocial factors affecting the report of back injury. Spine 16: 1–6

Blumer D 1975 Psychiatric considerations in pain. In: Rothman RH, Simeone FA (eds) The spine. Vol II WB Saunders, Philadelphia pp 871–906

Bond MR 1971 The relation of pain to the Eysenck Personality Inventory, Cornell Medical Index and Whiteley Index of Hypochondriasis. British Journal of Psychiatry 119: 671–678

Bonica JJ 1990 The management of pain, 2nd edn. Lea & Febiger, Philadelphia

Bradley LA, Prokop CK, Margolis R, Gentry WD 1978 Multivariate analysis of the MMPI profiles of low back pain patients. Journal of Behavioral Medicine 1: 253–272

Brown GW, Sklair F, Harris TO, Birley JLT 1973 Life events and psychiatric disorders. Part I: Some methodological issues. Psychological Medicine 3: 74–87

Caine TH, Hope K 1967 Manual of the hysteroid-obsessed questionnaire. University of London Press, London

Chaturvedi SK, Varma VK, Malhotra A 1984 Non-organic intractable pain: a comparative study. Pain 19: 87–94

Crisp AH, Kalucy RS, McGuinness B, Ralph PC, Harris G 1977 Some clinical, social and psychological characteristics of migraine subjects in the general population. Postgraduate Medical Journal 53: 691–697

Crook J, Rideout E, Browne G 1984 The prevalence of pain complaints in a general population. Pain 18: 299–314

Crook J, Weir R, Tunks E 1989 An epidemiological follow-up survey of persistent pain sufferers in a group family practice and specialty pain clinic. Pain 36: 49–61

Crown S, Crown JM 1973 Personality in early rheumatic disease. Journal of Psychosomatic Research 17: 189–196

Curtis JL 1965 A psychiatric study of 55 expectant fathers. US Armed Forces Medical Journal 6: 937–950

Delaplaine R, Ifabumuyi OI, Merskey H, Zarfas J 1978 Significance of pain in psychiatric hospital patients. Pain 4: 361–366

Demjen S, Bakal DA 1981 Illness behavior and chronic headache. Pain 10: 221–229

Devine R, Merskey H 1965 The description of pain in psychiatric and general medical patients. Journal of Psychosomatic Research 9: 311–316

Dura JR, Beck SJ 1988 A comparison of family functioning when mothers have chronic pain. Pain 35: 79–89

Engel GL 1959 'Psychogenic' pain and the pain prone patient. American Journal of Medicine 26: 899–918

Epstein LH, Abel GG, Collin F, Parker L, Cinciripini PM 1978 The relationship between frontalis muscle activity and self-reports of headache pain. Behaviour Research and Therapy 16: 153–160

Feighner P, Robins E, Guze SB et al 1972 Diagnostic criteria for use in psychiatric research. Archives of General Psychiatry 26: 56–63

Fishbain DA, Goldberg M, Meagher BR et al 1986 Male and female chronic pain patients categorized by DSM-III psychiatric diagnostic criteria. Pain 26: 181–197

Flor H, Kerns RD, Turk DC 1987 The role of the spouse in the maintenance of chronic pain. Journal of Psychosomatic Research 31: 251–260

Flor H, Turk DC 1988 Chronic back pain and rheumatoid arthritis: predicting pain and disability from cognitive variables. Journal of Behavioral Medicine 11: 231–265

Flor H, Turk DC, Rudy TE 1989 Relationship of pain impact and significant other reinforcement of pain behaviors: the mediating role of gender, marital status and marital satisfaction. Pain 38: 45–50

Fordyce WE 1976 Behavioural methods in chronic pain and illness. CV Mosby, St Louis, p 236

Fordyce WE 1990 A response to Schmidt et al (1989 Pain 38: 137–140). Pain 43: 133–134

Fordyce WE 1995 Back pain in the workplace: management of disability in non-specific conditions. Task Force on Pain in the Workplace. International Association for the Study of Pain. IASP, Seattle

Fordyce WE, McMahon R, Rainwater G et al 1981 Pain complaint–exercise performance relationship in chronic pain. Pain 10: 311–321

Fordyce WE, Roberts AH, Sternbach RA 1985 The behavioral management of chronic pain: a response to critics. Pain 22: 113–125

Fordyce WE, Roberts AH, Sternbach RA 1988 The behavioral management of pain: a critique of a critique (letter to the editor). Pain 33: 385–387

Gamsa A 1990 Is emotional status a precipitator or a consequence of pain? Pain 42: 183–195

Gatchel RJ, Polatin PB, Mayer TG 1995 The dominant role of psychosocial risk factors in the development of chronic low back pain disability. Spine 20: 270–279

Gittleson NL 1961 Psychiatric headache: a clinical study. Journal of Mental Science 107: 403–416

Gould R, Miller BL, Goldberg MA, Benson DF 1986 The validity of hysterical signs and symptoms. Journal of Nervous and Mental Diseases 174: 593–598

Gupta MA 1986 Is chronic pain a variant of depressive illness? A critical review. Canadian Journal of Psychiatry 31: 241–248

Hall W, Hayward L, Chapman CR 1981 On 'the lateralization of pain'. Pain 10: 337–351

Hanvik LH 1956 MMPI profiles in patients with low-back pain. Journal of Consulting and Clinical Psychology 15: 350–353

Harper RC, Steger JC 1978 Psychological correlates of frontalis EMG and pain in tension headache. Headache 18: 215–218
Hart H 1947 Displacement, guilt and pain. Psychoanalysis Review 34: 259–273
Henryk-Gutt R, Rees WL 1973 Psychological aspects of migraine. Journal of Psychosomatic Research 17: 141–153
Hilton J 1863 Rest and pain. London
International Association for the Study of Pain (Subcommittee on Taxonomy) 1979 Pain terms: a list with definitions and notes on usage. Pain 6: 249–252
International Association for the Study of Pain (Subcommittee on Taxonomy) 1986 Classification of chronic pain: descriptions of chronic pain syndromes and definitions of pain terms. Pain (suppl 3). Elsevier, Amsterdam
Jensen J 1988 Life events in neurological patients with headache and low back pain (in relation to diagnosis and persistence of pain). Pain 27: 203–210
Keefe FJ, Bradley LA, Crisson JE 1990 Behavioral assessment of low back pain: identification of pain behavior subgroups. Pain 40: 153–160
Kellner R 1986 Somatization and hypochondriasis. Prager, New York
Kirmayer LJ, Robbins JM 1991 Three forms of somatization in primary care: prevalence, co-occurence and sociodemographic characteristics. Journal of Nervous and Mental Disease 179: 647–655
Klee A 1968 A clinical study of migraine with particular reference to the most severe cases. Munksgaard, Copenhagen
Klee GD, Ozelis S, Greenberg I, Gallant LJ 1959 Pain and other somatic complaints in a psychiatric clinic. Maryland State Medical Journal 8: 188–191
Kramlinger KG, Swanson DW, Maruta T 1983 Are patients with chronic pain depressed? American Journal of Psychiatry 140: 6
Kukull WA, Koepsell TD, Inui TS et al 1986 Depression and physical illness among elderly general medical clinic patients. Journal of Affective Disorders 10: 153–162
Labbe EE 1988 Sexual dysfunction in chronic back pain patients. Clinical Journal of Pain 4: 143–149
Large RG 1980 The psychiatrist and the chronic pain patient: 172 anecdotes. Pain 9: 253–263
Leavitt F, Garron DC 1979a Validity of a back pain classification scale among patients with low back pain not associated with demonstrable organic disease. Journal of Psychosomatic Research 23: 301–306
Leavitt F, Garron DC 1979b Psychological disturbance and pain report differences in both organic and non-organic low back pain patients. Pain 7: 187–195
Leavitt F, Garron DC, McNeill TW et al 1982 Organic status, psychological disturbance, and pain report characteristics in low-back pain patients on compensation. Spine 7: 398–402
Lewis T, Pickering GW, Rothschild P 1931 Observations upon muscular pain in intermittent claudication. Heart 15: 359–383
Lindsay PG, Wyckoff M 1981 The depression-pain syndrome and its response to antidepressants. Psychosomatics 22: 571–577
Littlejohn GO 1986 Repetitive strain syndrome: an Australian experience (editorial). Journal of Rheumatology 13: 1004–1006
Locser J, Egan KJ 1989 Managing the chronic pain patient. Raven, New York
Lord SM, Barnsley L, Wallis BJ, Bogduk N 1996 A randomised double-blind controlled trial of percutaneous radiofrequency neurotomy for the treatment of chronic cervical zygapophysial joint pain. New England Journal of Medicine 335: 1721–1726
Love AW, Peck DL 1987 The MMPI and psychological factors in chronic low back pain: a review. Pain 28: 1–12
Lund JP, Stohler CS, Widmer CG 1993 The relationship between pain and muscle activity in fibromyalgia and similar conditions. In: Vaeroy H, Merskey H (eds) Progress in fibromyalgia and myofascial pain. Elsevier Science, Amsterdam, pp 311–327
McCreary RP, Turner J, Dawson E 1979 The MMPI as a predictor of response to conservative treatment for low back pain. Journal of Clinical Psychology 35: 278–284
Macnab I 1964 Acceleration injuries of the cervical spine. Journal of Bone and Joint Surgery 46A: 1797–1799
Magni G 1987 On the relationship between chronic pain and depression when there is no organic lesion. Pain 31: 1–21
Magni G, Merskey H 1987 A simple examination of the relationships between pain, organic lesions and psychiatric illness. Pain 29: 295–300
Magni G, Andreoli F, Arduino C et al 1987a ^{3}H imipramine binding sites are decreased in platelets of chronic pain patients. Acta Psychiatrica Scandinavica 75: 108–110
Magni G, Andreoli F, Arduino C et al 1987b Modifications of ^{3}H-imipramine binding sites in platelets of chronic pain patients treated with mianserin. Pain 30: 311–320
Magni G, Caldieron C, Rigatti-Luchini S, Merskey H 1990 Chronic musculoskeletal pain and depressive symptoms in the general population. An analysis of the 1st National Health and Nutrition Examination survey data. Pain 43: 299–307
Marbach JJ, Lennon MC, Dohrenwend BP 1988 Candidate risk factors for temporomandibular pain and dysfunction syndrome: psychosocial, health behaviour, physical illness and injury. Pain 34: 139–151
Martin PR, Mathews AM 1978 Tension headaches: psychophysiological investigation and treatment. Journal of Psychosomatic Research 22: 389–399
Merskey H 1965a The characteristics of persistent pain in psychological illness. Journal of Psychosomatic Research 9: 291–298
Merskey H 1965b Psychiatric patients with persistent pain. Journal of Psychosomatic Research 9: 299–309
Merskey H 1980 The role of psychiatrist in the investigation and treatment of pain. In: Bonica JJ (ed) Pain. Raven, New York, pp 249–260
Merskey H 1982 Pain and emotion: their correlation in headache. In: Critchley M et al (eds) Advances in neurology, 3rd edn. Raven, New York, pp 135–143
Merskey H 1985 A mentalistic view of 'Pain and behaviour'. Commentary on Rachlin. Behavioral and Brain Sciences 8: 68
Merskey H 1988 Regional pain is rarely hysterical. Archives of Neurology 45: 915–918
Merskey H 1995 The analysis of hysteria: understanding dissociation and conversion, 2nd edn. Gaskell, London
Merskey H, Spear FG 1967 Pain: psychological and psychiatric aspects. Baillière, Tindall & Cassell, London
Merskey H, Watson GD 1979 The lateralization of pain. Pain 7: 271–280
Merskey H, Brown A, Brown J, Malhotra L, Morrison D, Ripley C 1985 Psychological normality and abnormality in persistent headache patients. Pain 23: 35–47
Merskey H, Lau CL, Russell ES et al 1987 Screening for psychiatric morbidity: the pattern of psychological illness and premorbid characteristics in four chronic pain populations. Pain 30: 141–147
Merskey H 1989 Physical and psychological considerations in the classification of fibromyalgia. Journal of Rhematology (suppl 19) 16: 72–79
Mitchell SW 1872 Injuries of nerves and their consequences. Reprinted 1965 Dover Publications, New York
Mohamed SN, Weisz GM, Waring EM 1978 The relationship of chronic pain to depression, marital adjustment and family dynamics. Pain 5: 285–292
Morgenstern FS 1967 Chronic pain. DM Thesis, Oxford
Naliboff BD, McCreary CP, McArthur DL, Cohen MJ, Gottlieb HJ 1988 MMPI changes following behavioral treatment of chronic low back pain. Pain 35: 271–277
O'Kelly LE, Steckley LC 1939 A note on long enduring emotional

responses in the rat. Journal of Psychology 8: 125. (Cited by Ulrich RE, Hutchinson PR, Azrin NH 1965 Pain-elicited aggression. Psychological Research 15: 11)

Oostdam EMM, Duivenvoorden HJ, Pondaag W 1981 Predictive value of some psychological tests on the outcome of surgical intervention in low back pain patients. Journal of Psychosomatic Research 3: 227–235

Payne B, Norfleet MA 1986 Chronic pain and the family: a review. Pain 26: 1–22

Pelz M, Merskey H 1982 A description of the psychological effects of chronic painful lesions. Pain 14: 293–301

Pilling LF, Brannick TL, Swenson WM 1967 Psychological characteristics of patients having pain as a presenting symptom. Canadian Medical Association Journal 97: 387–394

Pilowsky I 1967 Dimensions of hypochondriasis. British Journal of Psychiatry 113: 89

Pilowsky I, Spence DN 1976 Pain and illness behaviour: a comparative study. Journal of Psychosomatic Research 20: 131–134

Pilowsky I, Chapman CR, Bonica JJ 1977 Pain, depression and illness behaviour in a pain clinic population. Pain 4: 183–192

Pozniak-Patewicz E 1976 'Cephalgic' spasm of head and neck muscles. Headache 15: 261–266

Rachlin H 1985 Pain and behavior. Behavioral and Brain Sciences 8: 43–83

Radanov BP, Stefano GD, Schnidrig A, Ballinari P 1991 Role of psychosocial stress in recovery from common whiplash. Lancet 338: 712–715

Rawnsley K, Loudon JB 1964 Epidemiology of mental disorders in a closed community. British Journal of Psychiatry 110: 830–839

Reich J, Tupin JP, Abramowitz SI 1983 Psychiatric diagnosis of chronic pain patients. American Journal of Psychiatry 140: 1495–1498

Reik T 1914 Ritual: psychoanalytical studies. Hogarth, London

Romano JM, Turner JA 1985 Chronic pain and depression: does the evidence support a relationship? Psychological Bulletin 97: 18–34

Romano JM, Turner JA, Clancy SL 1989 Sex differences in the relationship of pain patient dysfunction to spouse adjustment. Pain 39: 289–295

Rowat KM, Knaf KA 1985 Living with chronic pain: the spouse's perspective. Pain 23: 259–271

Roy R, Thomas M, Matas M 1984 Chronic pain and depression. Comprehensive Psychiatry 25: 96–105

Sainsbury P, Gibson JG 1954 Symptoms of anxiety and tension and the accompanying physiological changes in the muscular system. Psychosomatic Medicine 17: 216–224

Salter M, Brooke RI, Merskey H, Fichter GF, Kapusianyk DH 1983 Is the temporomandibular pain and dysfunction syndrome a disorder of the mind? Pain 17: 151–166

Schmidt AJM 1987 The behavioral management of pain: a criticism of a response. Pain 30: 285–291

Schmidt AJM 1988 Reply to letter from Fordyce, Roberts and Sternbach (letter to the editor). Pain 33: 388–389

Smith WL, Duerksen DL 1980 Personality in the relief of chronic pain: predicting surgical outcome. In: Smith WL, Merskey H, Gross SC (eds) Pain: meaning and management. pp 119–126 Spectrum, New York

Smythe HA 1985 Fibrositis and other diffuse musculoskeletal syndromes. In: Kelley WN, Harris ED Jr, Ruddy S et al (eds) Textbook of rheumatology. WB Saunders, Philadelphia, pp 481–489

Spear FG 1967 Pain in psychiatric patients. Journal of Psychosomatic Research 11: 187–193

Spitzer RL, Endicott Robins E 1978 Research diagnostic criteria: rationale and reliability. Archives of General Psychiatry 35: 773–782

Sternbach RA 1974 Pain patients. Traits and treatment. Academic, New York

Sternbach RA 1986 Survey of pain in the United States: the NUPRIN Pain Report. Clinical Journal of Pain 2: 49–53

Sternbach RA 1987 Mastering pain. GP Putnam's Sons, New York

Sternbach RA, Timmermans G 1975 Personality changes associated with reduction of pain. Pain 1: 177–181

Sternbach RA, Wolf SR, Murphy RW, Akeson WH 1973 Traits of pain patients: the low-back 'loser'. Psychosomatics 14: 226–229

Tauschke E, Merskey H, Helmes E 1990 A systematic inquiry into recollections of childhood experience and their relationship to adult defence mechanisms. British Journal of Psychiatry 157: 392–398

Taylor JR, Kakulas BA 1991 Neck injuries. Lancet 338, 1343

Teasell RW, Merskey H 1997 Chronic pain disability in the workplace. Pain Research and Management 2: 197–205

Thomas M, Roy R 1989 Pain patients and marital relations. Clinical Journal of Pain 5: 255–259

Trethowan WH 1968 The couvade syndrome – some further observations. Journal of Psychosomatic Research 12: 107–115

Trethowan WH, Conlon MF 1965 The couvade syndrome. British Journal of Psychiatry 3: 57–76

Vaeroy H 1996 Contribution to the understanding of pain in fibromyalgia based on cerebro-spinal fluid investigations. Pain Research and Management 1: 45–49

Violon-Jurfest A 1980 The onset of facial pain: a psychological study. Psychotherapy and Psychosomatics 34: 11–16

Waddell G 1987 A new clinical model for the treatment of low-back pain. Spine 12: 632–644

Waddell G 1996 Back pain in the workplace. Pain 65: 114

Waddell G, Main CJ 1984 Assessment of severity in low-back disorders. Spine 9: 204–208

Waddell G, McCulloch JA, Kummel EG, Venner RM 1980 Non-organic physical signs in low back pain. Spine 5: 117–125

Waddell G, Gircher M, Finlayson D, Main CJ 1984a Contemporary themes: symptoms and signs: physical disease or illness behaviour? British Medical Journal 289: 739–741

Waddell G, Main CJ, Morris EW, Di Paola M, Gray ICM 1984b Chronic low-back pain, psychologic distress, and illness behaviour. Spine 9: 209–213

Waddell G, Pilowsky I, Bond MR 1989 Clinical assessment and interpretation of abnormal illness behaviour in low back pain. Pain 39: 41–53

Wall PD 1984 Introduction In: Wall & Melzack (eds) Textbook of Pain 3E Churchill Livingstone, Edinburgh pp 1–7

Wallis BJ, Lord SM, Bogduk N 1997 Resolution of psychological distress of whiplash patients following treatment by radiofrequency neurotomy: a randomised double-blind placebo controlled trial. Pain 73: 15–22

Walters A 1961 Psychogenic regional pain alias hysterical pain. Brain 84: 1–18

Waring EM, Weisz GM, Bailey SI 1976 Predictive factors in the treatment of low back pain by surgical intervention. In: Bonica JJ, Albe-Fessard D (eds) Advances in pain research and therapy. Raven, New York, pp 939–942

Watson D 1982 Neurotic tendencies among chronic pain patients: an MMPI item analysis. Pain 14: 365–385

Watson GD, Chandarana PC, Merskey H 1981 Relationships between pain and schizophrenia. British Journal of Psychiatry 138: 33–36

Watt-Watson JH, Evans RJ, Watson CPN 1988 Relationships among coping responses and perceptions of pain intensity, depression, and family functioning. Clinical Journal of Pain 4: 101–106

Wiltse LL, Rocchio PD 1975 Preoperative psychological tests as predictors of success of chemonucleolysis in the treatment of low-back syndrome. Journal of Bone and Joint Surgery 57AI: 478–483

Wolfe F, Smythe HA, Yunus MB et al 1990 The American College of Rheumatology 1990 criteria for the classification of fibromyalgia. Report of the Multicenter Criteria Committee. Arthritis and Rheumatism 33: 160–172

Woodforde JM, Merskey H 1972 Personality traits of patients with chronic pain. Journal of Psychosomatic Research 16: 167–172

Zilli C, Brooke RI, Merskey H, Lau CL 1989 Screening for psychiatric illness in patients with oral dysaesthesia using the GHQ-28 and the IDA. Oral Surgery, Oral Medicine, Oral Pathology 67: 384–389

Sex and gender differences in pain

KAREN J. BERKLEY & ANITA HOLDCROFT

SUMMARY

Epidemiological and psychophysical studies, together with disease-prevalence estimates, consistently reveal that the burden of pain is greater, more varied and more variable for women than for men. With encouragement during the past decade from some governmental legislative and funding agencies for basic and clinical researchers in many fields to address the issue of sexual difference, evidence is rapidly accumulating demonstrating that sex differences in pain are brought about by a confluence of genetic, physiological, anatomical, neural, hormonal, lifestyle and cultural factors. These factors in turn provide women with a wider array than men of both sex-linked biological and gender-related sociocultural mechanisms that can act to reduce pain. Thus, while women generally are more vulnerable to pain than men, they have more ways to deal with it. The clinical applicability of these findings, now under intense scrutiny, appear significant for both sexes, with considerable implications for health economics. Indeed, a few recommendations for research and healthcare have already emerged from these ongoing basic and clinical studies that can be implemented immediately to improve not only diagnosis but also treatment with a full range of drugs, somatic and situational therapies for both male and female individuals.

INTRODUCTION

Sexual difference is probably the issue in our time which could be our 'salvation' if we thought it through.

So announced Louise Irigeray, at the beginning of a series of lectures she delivered in 1982 at Erasmus University in Rotterdam (Irigeray 1993, p 5). Although this philosophical statement may sound overly dramatic here, increasing societal respect for sex and gender differences in the past decade has influenced basic and clinical research, as well as public policy on drug development, resulting in an expanding literature that addresses the issue in many arenas from molecular-genetic to sociocultural[1]. Pain is clearly one of these arenas, evidenced by six recent comprehensive reviews (Fillingim & Maixner, 1995, Jensvold et al 1996, Unruh 1996, Berkley 1997a, Ciccone & Holdcroft 1998, Riley et al 1998). Importantly, as implied by Irigeray's statement, what is also becoming apparent is that a continuing analysis and synthesis of the developing evidence is likely to lead to significant advances in our understanding of pain modulation from fetus to old age, with concomitant development of new therapeutic strategies for the care of individuals of either sex in pain. In this chapter these reviews and more recent publications containing useful literature syntheses are used to summarize the evidence for sex differences in pain and the mechanisms that might underlie them. We then consider the clinical relevance of this information and discuss future directions.

WHAT ARE THE DIFFERENCES?

As shown in Figure 41.1, evidence for sex differences in human pain derives from four main lines of research.

EPIDEMIOLOGY AND SEX PREVALENCE IN DISEASE

Community epidemiological studies consistently reveal that women report more severe levels of pain, more frequent pain, pain in more areas of the body, and pain of longer duration then men (Unruh 1996, Berkley 1997a). In addition, as shown in Table 41.1, there are many more painful

[1]Gender is defined as the sex with which an individual identifies.

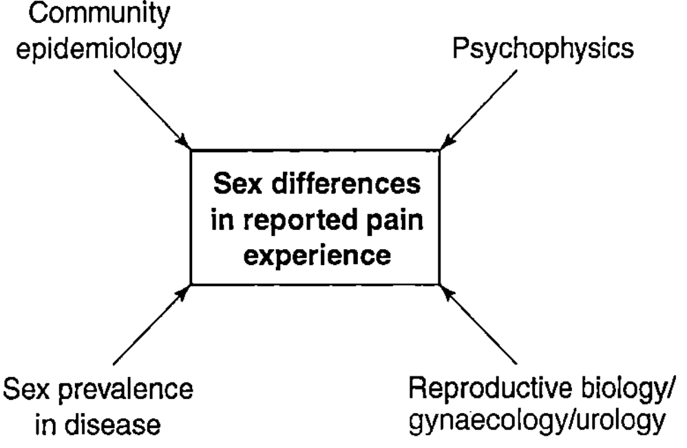

Fig. 41.1 Sources of evidence for sex differences in human pain.

diseases that have a documented female prevalence than have a male prevalence, particularly those of the head and neck, of musculoskeletal or visceral origin and of autoimmune aetiology. Some authors have attributed this apparent female vulnerability to an increased willingness for women to report pain and seek healthcare. While that may be a factor, it is only one of many. Thus, much of the female prevalence can be accounted for by parturition or gynaecological problems. In addition, overall prevalence patterns in both sexes for many types of pain (such as those of temporomandibular disorder, fibromyalgia, migraine, chest, abdomen and joint) change across the lifespan

Table 41.1 Sex prevalence of some common painful syndromes and potential contributing causes[1]

	Female prevalence	*Male prevalence*
Head and neck	Migraine headache with aura Chronic tension headache Postdural puncture headache Cervicogenic headache Tic douloureux Temporomandibular disorder Occipital neuralgia Atypical odontalgia Burning tongue Carotidynia Temporal arteritis Chronic paroxysmal hemicrania	Migraine without aura Cluster headache Post-traumatic headache Paratrigeminal syndrome[2]
Limbs	Carpal tunnel syndrome Raynaud's disease Chilblains Reflex sympathetic dystrophy Chronic venous insufficiency Piriformis syndrome Peroneal muscular atrophy[4]*	Thromboangiitis obliterans[3] Haemophilic arthropathy* Brachial plexus neuropathy
Internal organs	Oesophagitis Gallbladder disease† Irritable bowel syndrome Interstitial cystitis Proctalgia fugax Chronic constipation	Pancoast tumour[5]† Pancreatic disease Duodenal ulcer
General	Fibromyalgia syndrome Multiple sclerosis‡ Rheumatoid arthritis‡ Acute intermittent porphyria* Lupus erythematosis‡	Postherpetic neuralgia

[1]Sex prevalences were taken mainly from Merskey and Bogduk (1994) and cross-checked using Medline and other search sources.
[2]Raeder's syndrome.
[3]Buerger's disease.
[4]Charcot–Marie–Tooth disease.
[5]Bronchogenic carcinoma.
Potential contributory causes: *sex-linked inheritance; †lifestyle; ‡autoimmune.

(LeResche & Von Korff 1998, Von Korff et al 1998). Thus, the sex prevalence of some painful disorders can diminish or reverse with age. Further complicating the issue is that in some disorders, such as irritable bowel syndrome, acute appendicitis, migraine headaches, rheumatoid arthritis and coronary heart disease, the clinical signs differ between the sexes (Berkley 1997a, b, Weyand et al 1998). And finally, in the context of major disease or illness, sex differences in pain reports disappear (Turk & Okifuji 1998). Thus, while overall women are more vulnerable than men to acute, intermittent and chronic pain, the pertinant individual circumstances vary and there are many exceptions (Unruh 1996).

Importantly, these overall sex differences are accompanied by differences in the strategies used by women and men to alleviate their pains. Women not only report using more medications and are more willing to seek out and combine different types of therapeutic approaches (Jensvold et al 1996), but also they appear able to derive more benefit from some of them, for example cognitive therapies (Fig. 41.2). Therefore, ironically, women may have developed a better array of strategies than men for coping with different types of pain (see Ch. 64; Unruh 1996, Berkley 1997b).

PSYCHOPHYSICAL STUDIES

A recent meta-analysis of experimental psychophysical studies of healthy individuals on sex differences in the attribution of somatic stimulation as painful showed that women have lower pain thresholds, higher ratings and less tolerance than men (Riley et al 1998). Thus, similar to the epidemiological/clinical findings, even in safe experimental settings where the subject knows that the pains she or he will experience will be brief and are not signs of a disease condition, it appears that females generally report more pain than men.

As in the epidemiological/clinical findings, some authors attribute nearly all of the higher female pain sensitivity observed in psychophysical studies to response bias or 'somatosensory amplification' (Berkley 1997b). However, here again, the existence and even the direction of the sex differences are affected by numerous factors. One group of factors is the *stimulus* – its type and manner of presentation. Thus, both pressure and electrical stimuli consistently produce large sex differences, whereas results from studies using themal or ischaemic stimuli are inconsistent (Riley et al 1998). However, greater female sensitivity to thermal stimuli does indeed become evident when the stimuli are delivered repeatedly (Fillingim et al 1998). The *testing paradigm* also affects sex differences; for example, effect size depends on whether thresholds or tolerance are being measured (Riley et al 1998). The *stimulus location* is important; for example, in a reversal of the usual difference, males show greater sensitivity than females when the stimuli are applied to the lower abdominal region (near the genitalia) rather than to the limbs (Giamberardino et al 1997). Other significant factors include *situational variables*, such as the sex and attractiveness of the experimenter or the setting in which the experiment is carried out (e.g. clinic versus science laboratory), and *psychological variables*, such as anxiety, or efficacy and control beliefs. Physiological factors are also important. Examples are:

1. *Blood pressure* is inversely related to pain sensitivity, even for normotensive subjects (Fillingim & Maixner 1996).
2. The presence of *stress* induces analgesia, the effects being different in the two sexes (Sternberg & Liebeskind 1995).
3. *Nutrition* (sugar and fat intake) and the presence of certain *disease* conditions can significantly increase or decrease pain sensitivity (Berkley 1997a).

REPRODUCTIVE BIOLOGY/GYNAECOLOGY/UROLOGY

Reproductive organs differ between the sexes, thereby affecting the relative arrangements of other pelvic organs. For example, female urethras are shorter and less tortuous than those of males. These differences create sex-specific pains of pelvic origin, reviewed by Wesselmann in Chapter 30. Another significant difference concerns the relative proportions and lifetime fluctuations from embryo through senescence of sex hormones. Recently, new data are emerging that pain symptomatology of many diseases/illnesses sometimes varies with reproductive status, especially at puberty, across the menstrual cycle, during pregnancy, immediately postpartum, and during and after the menopause and the longer course of andropause (Murray & Holdcroft 1989, Marcus 1995, Unruh 1996, Berkley 1997a, b, Jones 1997, LeResche & Von Korff 1998). Similarly, experimental pain sensitivity in both humans and animals has been shown to change at puberty and vary with the menstrual cycle, during pregnancy and lactation, as well as with the use of exogenous hormones (Fillingim & Maixner 1995, Berkley 1997a, Fillingim et al 1998). Again, however, the reported effects vary. One result of this situation, rarely addressed in most human experimental and clinical studies, is that whether or not a sex difference is found for a given type of pain or even the direction of the difference may depend on the reproductive or hormonal status of the comparison groups. Overall, however, an important consequence of the impact of reproductive status is that there is more variability in women's pains than in men.

HOW MIGHT THESE DIFFERENCES OCCUR?

The varied and sometimes contradictory findings of the many studies of sex differences in both experimentally induced and endogenous pain, together with fluctuations associated with reproductive and hormonal status, make application of the information to specific clinical circumstances difficult. Of value for the developing translation process are considerations of potential mechanisms of sex differences in pain, derived from widespread areas of research on animals and humans (Fig. 41.2).

GENETICS

John Liebeskind presented to the National Academy of Sciences the challenge that 'the study of the genetic differences in pain-related traits has been largely neglected' (Mogil et al 1996, p 3048). There are at least four means by which these traits could manifest themselves in sex-specific ways. First are *sex-linked genetic diseases* that underly some of the pain syndromes listed in Table 41.1, such as haemophilia, porphyria and the X-linked recessive type of peroneal muscular atrophy (Charcot–Marie–Tooth). Second are some sex-related genetic variations of *metabolizing enzyme systems* that could underly differences in both pain mechanisms and response to therapies. An example includes the cytochrome P450 (CYP) enzyme families in which genetic variations in the CYP2 family manifest themselves differently in females and males (Jensvold et al 1996, Ciccone & Holdcroft 1998). Third are sex-linked genetic differences in both *nociception and responses to manipulations of exogenous and endogenous analgesics* recently discovered by several investigators in mice and rats. Using quantitative trait locus (QTL) mapping techniques, Mogil et al (1997a) localized a male-specific QTL on chromosome 4 that appears to account for variability between two strains of mice in δ-opioid associated nociception as assessed by the hot-plate assay method. This same group also localized, on chromosome 8, a female-specific QTL that accounts for variability in stress-induced analgesia (SIA; Mogil et al 1997b). They concluded that it may be part of the basis for a female-specific SIA mechanism in rats that is ontogenetically organized, non-opioid, varies with reproductive status and is oestrogen-dependent. Fourth are sex differences that may be associated with oestrogen regulation of *gene expression*, recently discovered in rats for neurofilament proteins, nerve growth factor and substance P (Sohrabji et al 1994, Scoville et al 1997, Villablanca & Hanley 1997).

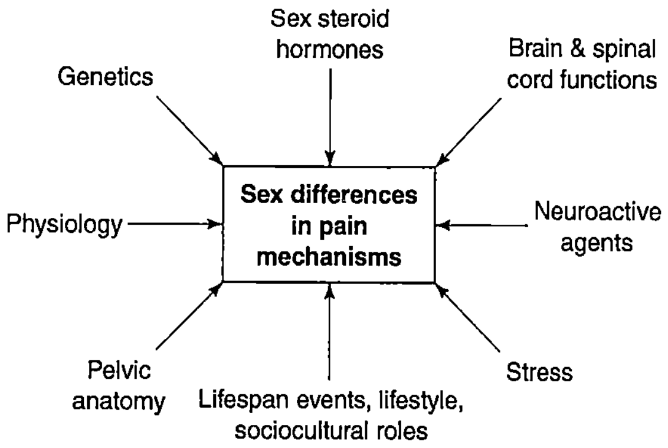

Fig. 41.2 Potential mechanisms of sex differences in pain.

PHYSIOLOGY, BODY COMPOSITION

Women, on average, relative to men, have a higher percentage of body fat, smaller muscle mass, lower blood pressure, and fluctuations associated with reproductive condition in gastrointestinal transit time, urinary creatinine clearance, metabolism and thermoregulation. These differences have implications not only for sex prevalence differences in various pain conditions (e.g. musculoskeletal), but also for both the pharmacodynamics and pharmacokinetics of analgesics, anaesthetics and adjuvants used for pain management (Jensvold et al 1996, Ciccone & Holdcroft 1998). Furthermore, pain estimates are inversely proportional to resting blood pressure, a situation that, due to higher blood pressure in males, may be one of the contributors to male hypoalgesia relative to females for pain induced by thermal and ischaemic stimuli (Fillingim & Maixner 1995).

PELVIC ANATOMY

Differences in pelvic organ structures and arrangements create large sex differences in pain (see Ch. 30). In addition, as argued by Berkley (1997a), sex differences in the reproductive tract create in females a greater vulnerability to both local and remote central sensitization. This situation could partly explain the greater vulnerability in women for multiple referred pains, particularly in muscles and the head/neck, as evidenced in Table 41.1. It might also be part of the underlying basis for sex differences in clinical signs of some diseases, for example the more widespread neck and shoulder pains in women with coronary heart disease (Douglas & Ginsberg 1996, described below). Support for this argument lies in considering six pieces of information, as follows:

1. Afferent innervation of internal pelvic organs is extensive and mainly by C fibres.
2. Dorsal root axons of C fibres diverge as they enter the spinal cord, giving rise to long-ranging axonal branches that synapse with dorsal horn neurons along many remote segments above and below their level of entry, including a large component at upper cervical levels.
3. C fibres are activated and sensitized by trauma, injury or disease. This peripheral sensitization can persist long after the organ damage abates, thereby helping to maintain central sensitization of dorsal horn neurons and consequent referred hyperalgesia.
4. A greater proportion of the reproductive tract is internal in females than in males (e.g. vaginal canal and cervix versus penis).
5. Internal female reproductive organs are more frequently subject to trauma, injury and disease than those in men (e.g. vagina – tampons, intercourse, examination, parturition; uterus – periodic strong contractions, pregnancy, parturition).
6. Uterine disorders give rise to widespread hyperalgesia much greater in muscles than in skin (Giamberardino et al 1997).

STRESS

There are enormous sex differences in responses to and the effects of stress in every realm of biology (i.e. genetic through sociocultural), and much research is underway in this arena forming a major component of a new discipline called psychoneuroimmunology. Studies in progress relevant to sex difference in pain include those on:

1. The hypothalamic–pituitary axis, which, while most well known for the integration of sexual and reproductive functions, is differentially affected by stress in males and females (Aloisi et al 1996, Aloisi 1997).
2. Exercise-induced cardiovascular, respiratory and pain responses, studied mainly in the context of angina, that differ in males and females (Forslund et al 1998).
3. Mechanisms of stress-induced analgesia that exhibit sex differences in opiate/non-opiate involvement (Sternberg et al 1995, Sternberg & Liebeskind 1995).

Also of relevance here is that major life events, which are stressful, are accompanied by changes in sex steroid hormones (puberty, pregnancy, parturition, menopause, andropause; Jones 1997).

SEX STEROID HORMONES

The influence of gonadal hormones has been described as having 'organizing' or 'activating' effects. Organizing effects occur during embryonic development to set up sex differences in the adult that are either independent of or activated by contemporary hormonal conditions. For hormone-dependent situations, three aspects are relevant. The first involves two mechanisms by which hormones affect cellular function. One, genomic, acts via intracellular messengers to effect gene transcription; the other, non-genomic, acts directly on cell membrane receptors. The second aspect includes overall sex differences in the relative amounts of oestrogens, progestins, androgens and other sex hormones. The third involves lifetime temporal features of those differences, including effects on the embryo, at puberty, during fertile adulthood (menstrual cyclicity, pregnancy and labour) and changes at senescence (menopause, andropause).

Sex steroid organizing and activating effects on cellular function are pervasive, modifying the functioning of virtually every bodily organ including the CNS in complex ways, still little understood. With respect to pain, five examples of some of the many potentially important hormonal influences include those on:

1. Metabolism (with implications for drug action, discussed later).
2. The immune system (with implications for painful autoimmune diseases, up to nine times more common in women, see Table 41.1 and Fox 1995).
3. Trauma-induced inflammation (modulated by sex hormones, e.g. Ashcroft et al 1997, Roof et al 1997).
4. The hypothalamic–pituitary axis (with implications for the interactions between stress and pain and cardiovascular variables; see Fillingim & Maixner 1995, Aloisi 1997, Forslund et al 1998).
5. Neuroactive agents (discussed below).

Little is yet known about the impact on pain experience of either *naturally occurring* sex differences in the relative amounts of sex steroid hormones or the effects of *supplemental hormones* (e.g. birth control drugs, peri- and postmenopausal hormone replacement, hormonal treatment of cancer in women and men). Part of the reason for this ignorance is the failure until recently of most studies on pain, whether animal or human, experimental or clinical, to take these factors into account. Another reason is the difficulty in measuring hormones due to the lack of rapid, easy assay techniques, although solutions for some of the problems are now actively being sought (Stern & McClintock 1996).

Because some pain conditions such as migraine resolve during pregnancy or are reduced during the midluteal phase of the menstrual cycle, and other pains are reduced in animals during lactation (when progesterone levels are high), and some anaesthetics are progesterone based (e.g. alphaxolone), and progesterone can protect against the effects of trauma, progesterone has been associated with analgesia and anaesthesia. Similarly, because some pain conditions increase after the menopause when oestrogen decreases (e.g., joint pain, vaginal pain) and some are alleviated by oestrogen (e.g. vaginal pain) and oestrogen can accelerate wound healing (Ashcroft et al 1997), oestrogen has also been associated with analgesia. So has testosterone, because of the consistent increase in older men (when testosterone concentrations decline) of some painful conditions, such as angina pain. However, for each of these examples, either no effects or opposite examples can be found, such as the emergence in men at puberty (when testosterone increases) of cluster headaches, the decrease in older men and postmenopausal women (when testosterone, oestrogen and progesterone levels decline) of abdominal pain (including irritable bowel disease), migraine and tension headaches, and new evidence in women demonstrating that supplemental hormones increase the risk for temporomandibular pain (LeResche et al 1997). Of great significance here is that the effects just described (reviewed in Unruh 1996, Berkley 1997a, LeResche & Von Korff 1998) likely depend not solely on the current concentration of one hormone, but on the duration or previous fluctuations of that hormone and its concentration relative to the others (Marcus 1995, Majewska 1996), together with neural and, more importantly, lifestyle factors (both discussed below). As more information accumulates, however, it is apparent that hormone therapy is likely to become a useful adjuvant for the treatment of certain painful conditions.

CNS FUNCTION AND NEUROACTIVE AGENTS

Currently, few would disagree with the general statement that there are sex differences in the brain and spinal cord. Regarding specifics, while there are unpleasant arguments on the validity of the evidence for and functional significance of sex differences in the *sizes* of various structures (e.g., Bishop & Wahlsten 1997), constructive progress is occurring in research concerning the organizing and activating, genomic and non-genomic effects of sex steroid hormones on the CNS (Jensvold et al 1996, Majewska 1996). Unfortunately, how the influences of sex steroid hormones on cells and systems in the CNS relate to sex differences in central pain mechanisms is at present largely unknown, partly because the relevance and importance of these influences is only now just beginning to be appreciated by pain researchers (Ruda 1998). It is likely that the relationship will prove to be wide ranging and complex.

Part of the reason for this complexity relates to observations emerging from brain imaging studies that used SPECT, PET or fMRI to study activations associated with reports of pain produced by the delivery of noxious stimuli (see Ch. 8). Although the results of these studies are creating some controversy, they are consistent in two ways. Firstly, they show surprising activations of rather widespread regions of the brain, including many not traditionally associated with pain. Secondly, they show large intersubject variations in activation patterns. Thus, there are multiple CNS 'targets' within which the organizational and activating effects of sex steroid hormones, together with sociocultural and lifespan factors (see below), can act in individuals to effect a myriad of sex differences in pain (Derbyshire 1997).

Two recent studies support this conclusion. The first (Silverman et al 1997) used PET to compare brain activation patterns produced by distention of the distal intestine in men and women suffering from irritable bowel syndrome (IBS) with normal subjects. There were no sex differences in the activation pattern of normal men and women, and this pattern differed from that of males and females with IBS in whom there was an additional activation of the left prefrontal cortex and an absence of perigenual anterior cingulate cortex activation. Importantly, however, among the IBS patients, significant activation was observed in right premotor cortex and left anterior insula only in the men. The second study (Becerra et al 1998) used fMRI to compare brain activation patterns induced by noxious thermal stimulation in men and women in two stages of their menstrual cycle (midfollicular stage – low progesterone/oestradiol, high testosterone, and midluteal stage – high progesterone/oestradiol, low testosterone). Their results showed similar patterns of activation of multiple regions in men and women in their midfollicular stage, but significant reduction of activity in the anterior cingulate, insula and frontal lobes in women during their midluteal phase, despite identical pain ratings in the two phases. These exciting data suggest that if we are to understand sex differences and other individual variations in pain mechanisms, it is imperative to adopt some form of an 'ensemble' (or 'distributed') conceptualization of neural mechanisms for pain which accommodates more easily than does our traditional 'fascicular' conceptualization of the multiple means by which the nervous system can create pain in both sexes (Melzack 1989, Berkley & Hubscher 1995).

In addition to sex differences that are organizationally established during development, sex steroids exert sex-specific effects within the CNS by their genomic and non-genomic neuromodulatory actions on neurons, either directly or via modification of the actions of other neuroactive agents (McEwen 1991a, b). It is not surprising that these effects occur in CNS regions associated with reproductive function. Interestingly, however, for neuroactive agents such as preproenkephalin, enkephalins, dopamine, serotonin, galanin, *N*-methyl-D-aspartate (NMDA), γ-aminobutyric acid (GABA), glutamate, cholecystokinin, bombesin, substance P, neurokinin A, nitric oxide, cytokines and growth factors, located variously in the 'non-reproductive' areas such as the neocortex, hippocampus, basal forebrain, striatum, central grey, cerebellum, inferior olive, dorsal column and trigeminal nuclei and spinal cord, there is substantive evidence, mainly from animal research, about each of them for one or more of the following:

1. Quantitative sex differences in their distribution.
2. Quantititive variations in immunoreactivity, receptors or function with reproductive status.
3. Colocalization with sex steroid hormones or their receptors.
4. Modulation by hormones of their gene expression.

Herewith is a sample of 17 recent relevant research reports that support this conclusion and are also important for the reviews they contain: Micevych et al 1988, Woolley & McEwen 1993, Abbud et al 1994, Sohrabji et al 1994, McCarthy 1995, Al-Dahan & Thalmann 1996, Duval et al 1996, Majewska 1996, Newton & Hamill 1996, Scoville et al 1997, Smith 1997, Turcotte & Blaustein 1997, VanderHorst & Holstege 1997, Villablanca & Hanley 1997, Weaver et al 1997, Weiner et al 1997, Xiao & Becker 1997).

Although research is just beginning on how these complex factors yield sex, age and other chronobiological variations in pain mechanisms, pain experience and pain treatment efficacy, some promising directions are evident. Six of many examples are given below:

1. If one compiles lists of the most popular CNS areas studied by researchers interested in sex differences in reproductive behaviour and those interested in pain, it is evident there has been much territorial but not communicative overlap. Recently, however, researchers studying animals are beginning to recognize that sex steroid interactions with other neuroactive substances in the regulation of reproductive behaviours has relevance to pain behaviours. One example is a group of studies on GABA–hormone interaction in the spinal cord studied in the context of lordosis behaviours (McCarthy 1995). A second example concerns descending regulation from the brainstem of input and output associated with the hindlimbs and pelvic reproductive organs (Hubscher & Johnson 1996, 1998). A third example relates to studies on the hypothalamic–pituitary axis and stress (Aloisi 1997).
2. The now-popular concept of central sensitization is an important component of putative neural mechanisms underlying hyperalgesia and persistent pain, and involves changes in gene expression related to NMDA, cytokines, growth factors, excitatory amino acids (e.g. glutamate), and peptides such as substance P and CGRP (see Ch. 14). As discussed above, all of these agents are potently affected by sex steroids and some show sex differences, suggesting that reproductive and/or hormonal status at the time of trauma may be important for the subsequent development of chronic pains.
3. There appear to be organizationally determined sex differences in CNS sensitivity to morphine, a μ-opioid, with male rats being more sensitive than females (Cicero et al 1996). This difference intersects with studies showing that female rats have their own non-opioid, but oestrogen-dependent SIA (see above). Furthermore, in humans, studies on acute postoperative pain (after molar tooth extraction) indicate that κ opioids may produce greater analgesia in females than males (Gear et al 1996), an observation that likely relates to the finding that analgesia during pregnancy in rats involves a κ-opioid mechanism (Dawson-Basoa & Gintzler 1996). These data may prove to be one of the contributory components for females seemingly having a wider range of mechanisms than men for alleviating pain.
4. Sex differences in the organization of the sympathetic nervous system and neuromodulatory action of its adrenergic and other agents (e.g. nitric oxide and purinergic) may increase female vulnerability to neuropathic and 'sympathetically mediated' pain conditions. (Coyle et al 1995, Newton & Hamill 1996, Berkley 1997a).
5. One of the interesting outcomes of imaging studies of pain is the inclusion in the activated regions of areas normally thought of as 'motor' (see Ch. 8), which fits with the view that pain is a context-dependent experience created by the nervous system as a means to motivate the individual to plan her/his own care (Wall 1994). As discussed above, some of these regions, for example, cerebellum, striatum, inferior olive, show

potent sex differences in steroidal influences on their somatosensory functions.

6. As more is learned about sex differences in the effectiveness of cognitive therapies (see Ch. 64), it may become increasingly important to integrate knowledge of the potent effects that sex hormones have on neuroplasticity within the hippocampus, now being extensively studied in the context of Alzheimer's disease (Yaffe et al 1998).

LIFESPAN EVENTS, LIFESTYLE AND SOCIOCULTURAL ROLES

Individual differences in pain are clearly influenced across the lifespan by major events (both individually unique and universally associated with reproductive status and ageing), by personal characteristics that can be loosely termed 'lifestyle', and by changing sociocultural roles. Despite their obvious importance, these factors have been only loosely integrated into our conceptualizations of pain mechanisms and individualized treatment strategies. However, as society moves away from disease models of illness towards holistic ones, and as can be seen here in several chapters (e.g. Chs 11, 15, 17, 40, 43, 63, 64, 68), this situation is changing. Although it remains difficult to assess precisely how the factors might participate in generating sex differences, there are some emerging constructive directions that should help. One useful perspective is to consider how the changing characteristics during each stage of human development – fetus, childhood, puberty/adolescence, fertile adulthood, menopause, senescence – accumulate their potential influences on sex differences across the lifespan.

Fetus, childhood, puberty

Major sex differences in future bodily structure, physiology and brain function (including some aspects of nociceptive sensitivity and stress modulation) are established during fetal life, gradually manifesting themselves as childhood progresses. These factors, together with family lifestyle and schooling, all influenced by sociocultural sex roles, operate uniquely on each child, gradually producing overall sex-specific patterns of reported pain sensitivity and other behaviours (see Ch. 15). During puberty and adolescence, dramatic alterations in hormonal status (Jones 1997) exert their activating effects within the nervous system and other bodily organs, rapidly producing enormous sex differences in body structure, physiology, and behaviour that add to the childhood lifestyle influences to bring about lifelong sex-specific traits. It is at this time that some pain-relevant, sex-different lifestyle patterns begin to be established, all influenced by the cultural milieu, such as tendency towards risk-taking behaviours (smoking, dangerous activities, violent behaviours), occupational goals, social roles and attitudes towards injury and disease both in oneself and others. Sex differences in some painful disorders also emerge at this time (e.g. cluster headaches in males, dysmenorrhoea in females).

Fertile adulthood

It is during the long period of fertile adulthood that an individual's occupation, social roles and lifestyle, while slowly changing, become entrenched. Although societal attitudes are rapidly occurring in many cultures, it remains the case to varying degrees in most of them that women still predominate as caregivers and organizers with wide-ranging obligations and duties spanning family and workplace realms, while men still predominate in aggressive and focused, physically demanding occupational and leisure activities with a relatively narrower range than women of social obligations and duties. Such differences have enormous implications for sex differences in the following: vulnerability to different types of injury (work- or sport-related for men; assault/rape for women); greater female duty, obligations and willingness to seek healthcare; higher female sensitivity towards the recognition of conditions as being 'painful' (i.e. those that demand tending) both in others and in themselves; greater female freedom to access healthcare; and, finally, sex-specific attitudes of healthcare givers towards the significance of pain in their patients.

Some of the lifestyle differences evidence themselves specifically in sex prevalence of some diseases. One example relates to injury-induced conditions, such as brachial plexus neuropathy, more common in men (e.g. motor bike crashes), and pelvic pains, more common in women (physical assault; see Ch. 28). A second includes smoking- and alcohol-associated disorders, more common in men, such as thromboangiitis obliterans (Buerger's disease), which, interestingly, is increasing in women because more are smoking. A third includes gallbladder disorders, more common in women, in which sex differences in lifestyle are but part of a complex multifactorial aetiology that can be traced to a combination of nutritional, metabolic pathways and hormone effects.

Sex differences in lifestyle are also one of the big components underlying the overall female vulnerability to pain, with its companion strategy of marshalling multiple approaches to deal with it. These sex differences are exaggerated by the repetitive pain cycles of dysmenorrhoea, as well as by pregnancy and parturition. As discussed above, the severe dysmenorrhoea suffered by a substantial proportion of women induces a constant and generalized muscle hyperalgesia (Giamberardino et al 1997). During pregnancy and premenstrually, fluid retention can increase tissue pressure around nerves, thereby precipitating or exacerbating painful neuropathies such as carpel tunnel syndrome and lateral femoral cutaneous nerve pain (Zager et al 1998). The trauma associated with parturition clearly generates its own extremely severe pain (Melzack 1993), and can increase the severity of postpartum pain after subsequent deliveries (Murray & Holdcroft 1989) as well as sensitivity to noxious stimulation in a manner similar to that in men resulting from comparable experiences, such as severe injury sustained during war, sport, a phenomenon that appears to be associated with long-term changes in gene expression induced by injury in animals (see Ch. 14).

Menopause, andropause and scenescence

Following the fertile years, there is at first, for women, a 5–10-year period of menopausal alterations in hormone patterns terminating in their sharp decline, while in men more complex changes in hormone metabolism occur over a longer period between the ages of about 48 and 70 (Jones 1997). Accompanying this are changes in general metabolism, physiology and structure. Lifestyle changes also occur relatively rapidly during this period, as children leave home and both occupational duties and leisure activities are altered. These changes together give rise to an increasing disease burden for both sexes, alterations of drug metabolism that while most dramatic for women also occur in men, and modified attitudes towards and access of healthcare. While the net result is a decrease in many sex differences in pain, especially as chronic disease burden becomes significant in both sexes (Turk & Okifuju 1998), sex differences in strategic therapeutic approaches by individuals persist (see Ch. 64).

WHAT ARE THE CLINICAL IMPLICATIONS?

Clearly, it will always remain the case that diagnostic and treatment strategies are best carried out by focusing on the individual, regardless of sex. However, as more information accumulates and is codified (Fig. 41.2), sex differences in reported pain experience and pain mechanisms will have increasingly potent and useful implications for both diagnosis and treatment as well as for health economics.

DIAGNOSIS

The first component of the diagnostic process involves gathering evidence of the patient's symptoms, signs and drug usage. It is during these first steps that knowledge about sex differences will lead informed clinicians towards establishing a partnership with the patient, to ease the process of obtaining patient details they might not otherwise have collected to improve their differential diagnoses and treatment decisions. Some of these details include:

1. Signs and symptoms that are distant as well as focused on the presenting illness.
2. The timing characteristics of those symptoms (both by memory and, if possible, some form of diary).
3. Family history of painful disease and how it was dealt with.
4. History of major life events in the patient's life.
5. Detailed characteristics of the individual's lifestyle (including such things as risk-taking behaviours, smoking, occupational goals, leisure activities, attitudes towards healthcare).
6. Reproductive status.

Of obvious significance for women is gaining complete knowledge of her parosity, menstrual history or menopausal status (along with, when it becomes easy/inexpensive to assay, hormone levels; see below), and for both sexes usage of supplemental hormones. Other important details for both sexes include knowledge of any history of abuse or other trauma, and assessment of tenderness or pain symptoms throughout the body, including 'minor' ones the patient might discount or fail to report.

To examine how this strategy could improve diagnosis, let us consider coronary heart disease as an example. When a patient presents with chest pain, it is often difficult to assess the likelihood that coronary artery disease is present, with its attendant need for further invasive and expensive testing. Recently, Douglas and Ginsberg (1996) reviewed the literature to arrive at a clear set of sex differential features. Three are described below. Regarding pain distribution, they state: 'Ischemia produces a slightly different pattern of pain in women with known coronary heart disease [than in men]; chest pain while at rest or the presence of other symptoms beyond typical angina during exertion [such as neck and shoulder pain] does not decrease the likelihood of coronary heart disease in women, as it does in men.' Regarding associated medical conditions such as diabetes and hypertension, they state: 'The presence of diabetes mellitus is a more powerful predictor of coronary heart disease and its prognosis in women than in men,' and

'Among the elderly, hypertension is a stronger predictor of coronary heart disease in women than in men.' The importance of these three statements for the practising cardiologist or general practitioner seems obvious. When a patient presents with 'atypical' chest pain, it might not in the past have been considered relevant to ask about other pains. However, by including as diagnostic a detailed history of pain complaints and their distribution, as well as, particularly for the postmenopausal woman, observing that she is diabetic and hypertensive, could be lifesaving.

THERAPY

As shown in Figure 41.2, there are three broad categories of pain therapies – drugs, somatic manipulations and situational adjustments. While it is now usually the case, especially for acute pain conditions, that only one is selected by the clinician (primarily drugs), strategies are slowly changing towards suitable combinations chosen in partnership with the patient. Here we consider for each category how knowledge of sex differences might in the future be applied towards developing strategies that include considerations of the patient's sex and reproductive condition.

Drugs

Potential sources of sex differences in drug action

As reviewed in Ciccone and Holdcroft (1998) and Jensvold et al (1996), there are clear body composition and sex hormone-related differences between women and men that can modify drug pharmacokinetics and pharmacodynamics. Potential sources of sex differences in *pharmacokinetics* include drug absorption, protein binding, volume of distribution, renal excretion, total drug clearance and metabolism (Gleiter & Gunder-Remy 1996).

Regarding absorption, women are affected by changes in gastric function during the menstrual cycle, leading to decreased absorption during the periovulatory stage (midcycle) of some drugs such as aspirin (and alcohol). Intestinal transit times are longer for women in the late luteal phase, as well as during pregnancy and hormone supplementation. Regarding protein binding, levels of α_1-acid glycoprotein are slightly lower in women than in men and change with birth control medication and pregnancy, so that free lidocaine is increased if used in nerve blocks.

Body compositional differences would seem relevant to the volume of distribution, but they appear not to be, even if the drug is highly lipophilic. They do, however, alter renal excretion. Creatinine clearance is higher in men than women, because of a larger muscle mass and the fact that glomerular filtration is proportional to body weight (lower on average in women). However, glomerular filtration is increased in pregnancy so that antiepileptic drugs require increased dosage. When total drug clearance is considered, measurements are limited because they do not differentiate between the various excretory processes. Age is an important factor in this process and clear sex differences in clearance with age have been demonstrated for the short-acting opioid drug alfentanil (Lemmens et al 1990). Thus, in females and males of similar weight, total median alfentanil clearance was highest in women less than 50 years of age, decreasing thereafter to rates similar to men at any age.

Regarding drug metabolism, there are well-known sex-specific effects in hepatic metabolism of drugs. Firstly, some components of the CYP2 enzyme family display genetic polymorphism, and some of the CYP3 family (that metabolize drugs such as lidocaine and midazolam) are regulated by androgens. Secondly, exogenous sex steroid hormones can have facilitatory or inhibitory activity on drug-metabolizing enzyme systems, for example the half-life of prednisolone used as an adjunct in pain medication increases when birth control medication is prescribed. Thirdly, not only are there quantitative differences in enzyme activity but there are also qualitative effects. Thus, the metabolic fate of some chiral drugs such as mephobarbital, an anticonvulsant, is sex specific, with its clearance greater and elimination half-life shorter in young men than in women or older men (Hooper & Qing 1990). It may therefore be important to consider that as chiral drugs are introduced to reduce the side effects of racemic mixtures or to enhance potency, some may be metabolized in a sex-specific manner.

In the developing area of human sex differences in *pharmacodynamics*, the analgesic effectivess of partial κ opioids such as nalbuphine, buprenophine and pentazocine for postoperative pain relief, compared with morphine, was significantly better in young nulliparous females than in young males (Gear et al 1996). Because, as described above, sex hormones have been shown in animals to affect the function of many neuroactive agents associated with pain, it is likely that new drugs targeted on these agents will also exhibit sex differences in their pharmacodynamics.

Adverse drug events

At least two aspects of drug usage lead to sex differences in adverse effects. Firstly, the prevalence of such effects is twice as much for women than men (Haddi et al 1990), probably not a result of differences in body composition (e.g. weight), but of drug sensitivity and interactions produced by a greater overall use by women of all medications as well as supplemental hormones (25% of childbearing women, Jensvold et al 1996). Contributing to this polypharmacy are women's use of medications such as iron and anti-inflammatory agents for the anaemia and pain associated with menstruation and the fact that some painful infections are more common in women (e.g. urinary tract infections), necessitating greater use of antibiotics. Secondly, new evidence is emerging for sex differences in the side effects of individual drugs. For example, morphine reduces the slope of the ventilatory response to carbon dioxide more in young adult women than in men (Dahan et al 1998).

Implications for drugs currently in use for pain

Figure 41.2 summarizes some of the rapidly emerging evidence on sex differences in the efficacy and safety of pain therapies, along with implications for their clinical usage. When the information on drugs in this figure is considered together with the above review, several generalities and specific recommendations emerge:

- The efficacy of some classes of drugs such as opioids could be improved by considering the use of different specific agonists for women and men or by titrating dosage in women to account for variations with age (e.g. alfentanil), with care taken to monitor respiratory depression. As more data on humans become available, adjustments of dosage by sex, reproductive status and supplemental hormone use are likely to improve efficacy not only for opiate drugs but also for other classes of analgesics and adjuvants.
- While a cyclical history of pain may or may not be diagnostic of any particular pain condition, its impact could be used to advantage in treatment. It would not be unreasonable to consider increasing drug dose just before pain is expected to increase and reducing it when pain decreases. Such strategies could also be coordinated with other therapies, such as exercise titrated to cyclical conditions. For example, in women with rheumatoid arthritis who exhibit exacerbations of their pain and mobility perimenstrually, doses of their non-steroidal anti-inflammatory drugs (NSAIDs) might be increased perimenstrually and plans for activities requiring dexterity scheduled during other menstrual stages (Wetherby 1995).
- Because of relatively common drug interactions, it is indeed important to collect information *routinely* about the patient's supplemental sex hormone usage (as well as other medications) and to adjust drug choice and dose appropriately. Safety could be further improved for some drugs by using dosing schedules related to body weight.
- Adjuvant hormones or similar agents are likely to prove useful as important components of pain prevention and management.
- The speed with which new clinically applicable information is being published on sex differences and hormonal influences on the efficacy and safety of all drugs (including those used for pain management) warrants continuous attention by clinicians.

Future drug development and clinical trials

Sex differences and hormone interactions in the specificity of pharmacological action and half-life or clearance are likely for some new drugs, particularly chiral forms. If such factors were considered initially at the outset of drug development, enzyme specificity would then be determined before clinical trials, and would therefore help to avoid needless potential adverse drug effects or discovering after the fact (as in κ opioids) that there are differences in effectiveness. This same logic applies to phase one (toxicity) trials, which in the USA, but not Europe, are now being carried out routinely in both sexes. During all clinical trials, much is to be gained from analyses stratified by sex, age, menstrual stage, menopausal status, andropause status and supplemental hormone use.

Somatic (physical) interventions

Little is known about sex differences in the effectiveness of some of the simpler forms of somatic therapies (Fig. 41.2), but, for some effective forms such as relaxation, heat or cold application, massage and vibration, women are generally more willing to use them, suggesting that men might benefit from further encouragement and education on their value. In addition, psychophysical studies in healthy women show that their sensitivity to some forms of somatic stimuli (pressure, thermal) can change with menstrual status (see above), which could affect efficacy when heat, cold, vibration or massage is used for pain alleviation by women. Regarding exercise and physical therapy, sports medicine studies report greater risks of injury in women than men (Jones et al 1993), and more problems for women perimenstrually. In addition, the differences in exercise-induced cardiovascular responses in males and females may affect pain either by way of the relationship between blood pressure and pain discussed above or by other mechanisms (Fillingim & Maixner 1996, Forslund et al 1998). For

Table 41.2 A growing list of therapies for pain and possible sex differences in their effects with implications for usage.

Drugs

Drug	*Sex-related effects*	*Considerations in use*
PRIMARY ANALGESICS		
NSAIDS (e.g. aspirin) AND ACETAMINOPHEN	PK: faster conjugation in ♂ than ♀, and ♀-oc	Duration: poss longer in ♀ than ♂ ↑ dose for ♀-oc
OPIOIDS (e.g. morphine)	PD: μ agonists: ♂ > ♀ κ agonist: ♀ > ♂ response to CO_2: ♀ < ♂	For ♀, ↑ titrate with age or change to κ agonist Care: respir depression may be ♀ > ♂
LOCAL ANAESTHETICS (e.g. lidocaine)	PK: CYP3A activity: ♀ > ♂ $\alpha_1$acidGP (see text)	Care toxicity: free lidocaine: ♀ (esp preg) > ♂
OTHER ANALGESICS		
ANTICONVULSANTS (e.g. phenytoin)	PK: ↓ plasma conc. in ♀-oc and ♀-preg	Monitor plasma concentration to maintain therapeutic levels
ANTIDEPRESSANTS	PK: oc alters met	oc have variable effects, monitor closely
CORTICOSTEROIDS	PK: ↓ met if using supplemental hormones	Care toxicity in ♀-oc and ♀-HRT
α_2 AGONISTS (e.g. clonidine) β ADRENERGIC ANTAGONISTS (e.g., propranolol)	ADR: ↓ libido	Check compliance (esp ♂)
Ca^{2+} CHANNEL BLOCKERS (e.g. amlodipine)	ADR: oedema ♀ > ♂	Awareness
CANNABINOIDS	PD: efficacy varies with oestrous stage[1]	Efficacy: poss-MC
ADJUVANTS SEX HORMONES	PK, PD – multiple	See text[2]

Somatic manipulations

Manipulation	*Sex-related effects*	*Considerations in use*
RELAXATION	♀ willing to use > ♂	Encourage, educate ♂
HEAT OR COLD APPLICATION	♀ willing to use > ♂	Encourage, educate > ♂
VIBRATION	poss-MC	Uncertain
MASSAGE	♀ willing to use > ♂ skin blood flow is improved ♀ > ♂ poss-MC	Encourage, educate ♂ Uncertain Uncertain
TENS	♂ may respond > ♀ (in some conditions)	Uncertain
EXERCISE AND PHYSICAL THERAPY	Training injuries: ♀ > ♂ Pain may ↑ in ♀ perimenstrually CVS: ♀ differ from ♂ SIA ♀ differ from ♂	Awareness Adjust levels if necessary Uncertain Uncertain
REGIONAL NERVE BLOCKS (EPIDURAL/SPINAL)	Efficacy ♀ > ♂	Improve pt selection and therapies for ♂
SYMPATHETIC BLOCKS	AD: libido ↓ ♂ > ♀	Inform ♂ (and ♀) and spouses preintervention
SURGICAL PROCEDURES	ADP: ♀ > ♂ MC: ADP and efficacy	Awareness

Situational adjustments

Adjustment	*Sex-related effects*	*Considerations in use*
CLINICIAN (EDUCATION/ATTITUDE)	Beliefs about ♀ vs ♂	Recognition and modification
CLINICAL SETTING AND ARRANGEMENT	Could → different stress responses in ♀ & ♂ ♀ verbal skills > ♂	Adjust examination and treatment environment
SELF-EDUCATION	♀ willing to use > ♂ ♀ verbal skills > ♂	Encourage, educate ♂
DIET AROMATHERAPY ART MUSIC POETRY PERFORMING ARTS SPORTS GARDENING RELIGION HYPNOSIS BIOFEEDBACK SUPPORT GROUPS, ADVOCACY GROUPS, NETWORKING SELF-HELP GROUPS	♀ willing to use > ♂	Encourage, educate ♂
GROUP THERAPY FAMILY COUNSELLING JOB COUNSELLING COGNITIVE THERAPY BEHAVIOURAL THERAPY PSYCHOTHERAPY MULTIDISCIPLINARY CLINIC	♀ hierarchy may reduce effectiveness in structured settings ♂ may benefit more from some of them	Recognize sex differences in group activities

Information provided only on specific therapies for which evidence currently exists for potential sex and gender differences. Supporting references are discussed and cited throughout the text. The table's format was adapted from Table 1 in Berkley (1997c), to which the reader is referred for a fuller list of therapies.[1] Data available only from animal research.[2] Sex hormone therapy is already used prophylactically to prevent painful conditions such as osteoporosis in ♀ as well as for treatment of painful malignancies.

Abbreviations: ♀ = women; ♀-oc = women using oc; ♂ = men; AD = adverse effects; ADP = adverse postoperative effects; ADR = adverse drug reactions; CVS = cardiovascular (see text); GP = glycoprotein; HRT = hormone replacement therapy; met = metabolism; oc = oral contraceptives; PD = pharmacodynamics; PK = pharmacokinetics; poss-MC = possible menstrual cycle variations; preg = pregnant; pt K = patient; SIA = stress-induced analgesia; TENS = transcutaneous electrical nerve stimulation.

surgical interventions, emerging evidence suggests that hormonal or menstrual status may in some cases affect surgical outcome. This evidence is currently most compelling for mastectomy (Hrushesky 1996), but may soon extend to other surgeries including those for painful conditions, as information about the effects of hormones on trauma-induced inflammation (discussed above) accumulates. Although sex differences in acute postoperative pains have in the past not been well studied, a recent prospective study of 4173 patients (45% female) showed that women have more 'minor' postoperative pains of sore throat, headache and backache than men (Myles et al 1997). This difference may relate to drugs used in women during anaesthesia (such as succinylcholine, known to produce more muscle pain in women than men), or to the choice of postoperative analgesics, or to reporting bias. Attempts to assess such sex differences by analysing postoperative drug usage with patient-controlled analgesic machines have been inconclusive (Lehmann 1993).

Situational manipulations

When pain is chronic, situational changes in the patient's environment and social interactions may not eliminate the pain, but there is much evidence that they reduce it by changing expectations, enhancing productive activity and improving quality of life. Several studies of relevance here indicate not only that women are more likely than men to make use of many of these forms of therapy, but also that they may derive more benefit from some of them, particularly cognitive ones (see Ch. 64). Part of the basis for this difference may lie in women's greater verbal abilities (reviewed in Harasty et al 1997) and their lifestyles and occupations, but whatever the cause(s), it seems clear that it is important for the clinician to consider that male more than female patients might need education and encouragement to consider situational adjustments, including not only changes in their personal environment (music, diet, meditation, etc.), but also in their use of various interactive services (Fig. 41.2). Of obvious relevance here is recognition by the clinician that her/his attitudes are an important aspect of the situation. These attitudes, warranting continual reassessment, include the clinician's general beliefs about the differences between women and men in the validity of their pain reports or responses to treatment, and about the value of various situational manipulations (Unruh 1996, Berkley 1997a).

Deliberate combinations of therapies

It should be evident from these discussions that the best clinical treatment for the patient in pain is the design for that patient of a flexible ***combination of drugs***, ***somatic therapies*** and ***situational manipulations***. How to apply what we are learning about sex differences in pain to this process can be illustrated by considering labour pain as an example. The acute pain of labour is severe in 60% of primiparous women (Melzack 1993). In expectation of this suffering, pre-emptive situational therapy can be applied which begins before childbirth. Women are educated on how their body functions, how to relax, how to use coping strategies and somatic manipulations (massage, body position), and how to choose or combine various drugs to maintain control during painful contractions. Despite wide variations in age, socioeconomic status, previous dysmenorrhoea, body size, maternal body mass, time of day and multiparity, such combined therapies can be considerably successful for the woman during her labour and delivery, not only in reducing her pre- and postpartum pain and other morbidity, but also in reducing her need for analgesics. However, what is not usually considered is the effect on the woman's male partner. If the initial training ignores her male partner, he could suffer considerably, experiencing feelings of helplessness and guilt with long-lasting consequences. On the other hand, if the training includes the male partner, not only could his morbidity be reduced during the labour and delivery events, but, if the training were to be carried out with this goal in mind, it could affect his approach towards his own painful conditions later on.

HEALTH ECONOMICS

All of the issues discussed above have implications for health economics. Here are four reasons:

1. Diagnosis would be improved by strategies that include awareness of potential sex and gender differences in signs and symptoms, along with their temporal variations. Such improvement would lead to the choice of more effective, more efficient and safer treatments, thus lessening costs.
2. Increasing awareness by healthcare insurers/servicers, clinicians and patients, particularly men, of the effectiveness of simpler forms of situational and somatic therapies, especially when they are combined with more expensive and invasive procedures, could obviously greatly reduce costs.
3. As new drugs are developed, attention during the very first stages of research and clinical trials to possible sex, gender and hormonal differences in pharmacokinetics and pharmacodynamics could improve their eventual safety and effectiveness when they are put into use for individuals in the general population. Part of what will

help this process is the development, now underway, of simple, fast and inexpensive hormone assay techniques for both sexes (Jensvold et al 1996).

4. Estimations of quality assurance figures associated with particular types of surgical procedures or other interventions currently in use would be improved if the results were stratified by sex- and hormone-related factors (menstrual cycle, reproductive status, supplemental hormone use).

REFERENCES

Abbud R, Hoffman GE, Smith MS 1994 Lactation-induced deficits in NMDA receptor-mediated cortical and hippocampal activation: changes in NMDA receptor gene expression and brainstem activation. Molecular Brain Research 25: 323–332

Al-Dahan MI, Thalmann RH 1996 Progesterone regulates gamma-aminobutyric acid B (GABAB) receptors in the neocortex of female rats. Brain Research 727: 40–48

Aloisi, AM 1997 Sex differences in pain-induced effects on the septo-hippocampal system. Brain Research Reviews 25: 397–406

Aloisi AM, Albonetti ME, Carli G 1996 Formalin-induced changes in adrenocorticotropic hormone and corticosterone plasma levels and hippocampal choline acetyltransferase activity in male and female rats. Neuroscience 74: 1019–1024

Ashcroft GS, Dodsworth J, van Boxtel E et al 1997 Estrogen accelerates cutaneous wound healing associated with an increase in TGF-betal levels. Nature Medicine 3: 1209–1215

Becerra L, Comite A, Breiter H, Gonzalez RG, Borsook D 1998 Differential CNS activation following a noxious thermal stimulus in men and women: and fMRI study. Society for Neuroscience Abstracts 24: (in press)

Berkley KJ 1997a Sex differences in pain. Behavioral and Brain Sciences 20: 371–380

Berkley KJ 1997b Female vulnerability to pain and the strength to deal with it. Behavioral and Brain Sciences 20: 473–479

Berkley KJ 1997c On the dorsal columns: translating basic research hypotheses to the clinic. Pain 70: 103–107

Berkley KJ, Hubscher CH 1995 Are there separate central nervous pathways for touch and pain? Nature Medicine 1: 766–773

Bishop KM, Wahlsten D 1997 Sex differences in the human corpus callosum: myth or reality? Neuroscience and Biobehavioral Reviews 21: 581–601

Ciccone G, Holdcroft A 1998 Drugs and sex differences: a review of drugs relating to anaesthesia. British Journal of Anaesthesia (in press)

Cicero TJ, Nock B, Meyer ER 1996 Gender-related differences in the antinociceptive properties of morphine. Journal of Pharmacology and Experimental Therapeutics 279: 767–773

Coyle DE, Sehlhorst CS, Mascari C 1995 Female rats are more susceptible to the development of neuropathic pain using the partial sciatic nerve ligation (PSNL) model. Neuroscience Letters 186: 135–138

Dahan A, Sarton E, Teppema L, Olievier C 1988 Sex-related differences in the influence of morphine on ventilatory control in humans. Anesthesiology 88: 903–913

Dawson-Basoa ME, Gintzler AR 1996 Estrogen and progesterone activate spinal kappa-opiate receptor analgesic mechanisms. Pain 64: 608–615

Derbyshire SWG 1997 Sources of variation in assessing male and female responses to pain. New Ideas in Psychology 15: 83–95

Douglas PS, Ginsberg GS 1996 The evaluation of chest pain in women. New England Journal of Medicine 334: 1311–1315

Duval P, Lenoir V, Moussaoui S, Garret C, Kerdelhue B 1996 Substance P and neurokinin A variations throughout the rat estrous cycle; comparison with ovariectomized and male rats: II. Trigeminal nucleus and cervical spinal cord. Journal of Neuroscience Research 45: 610–616

Fillingim RB, Maixner W 1995 Gender differences in the responses to noxious stimuli. Pain Forum 4: 209–221

Fillingim RB, Maixner W 1996 The influence of resting blood pressure and gender on pain responses. Psychosomatic Medicine 58: 326–332

Fillingim RB, Maixner W, Kincaid S, Silva S 1998 Sex differences in temporal summation but not sensory-discriminative processing of thermal pain. Pain 75: 121–127

Forslund L, Hjemdahl P, Held C, Bjorkander I, Eriksson SV, Rehnqvist N 1998 Ischaemia during exercise and ambulatory monitoring in patients with stable angina pectoris and healthy controls. Gender differences and relationships to catecholamines. European Heart Journal 19: 578–587

Fox HS 1995 Sex steroids and the immune system. In: Bock GR, Goode JA (eds) Non-reproductive actions of sex steroids. John Wiley, Chichester, pp 203–217

Gear RW, Miaskowski C, Gordon NC, Paul SM, Heller PH, Levine JD 1996 Kappa-opioids produce significantly greater analgesia in women than in men. Nature Medicine 2: 1248–1250

Giamberardino MA, Berkley KJ, Iezzi S, de Bigontina P, Vecchiet L 1997 Pain threshold variations in somatic wall tissues as a function of menstrual cycle, segmental site and tissue depth in non-dysmenorrheic women, dysmenorrheic women and men. Pain 71: 187–197

Gleiter CH, Gundert-Remy U 1996 Gender differences in pharmacokinetics. European Journal of Drug Metabolism and Pharmacokinetics 21: 123–128

Haddi E, Sharpin D, Tafforeau M 1990 Atopy and systemic reactions to drugs. Allergy 45: 1–4

Harasty J, Double KL, Halliday GM, Kril JJ, McRitchie DA 1997 Language-associated cortical regions are proportionally larger in the female brain. Archives of Neurology 54: 171–176

Hooper WD, Qing MS 1990 The influence of age and gender on the stereoselective metabolism and pharmacokinetics of mephobarbital in humans. Clinical Pharmacology and Therapeutics 48: 633–640

Hrushesky WJM 1996 Breast cancer, timing of surgery, and the menstrual cycle: call for prospective trial. Journal of Women's Health 5: 555–566

Hubscher CH, Johnson RD 1996 Responses of medullary reticular formation neurons to input from the male genitalia. Journal of Neurophysiology 76: 2474–2482

Irigeray L 1993 An ethics of sexual difference. Athlone Press, London

Jensvold MF, Halbreich U, Hamilton JA (eds) 1996 Psychopharmacology and women. Sex Gender and Hormones, American Psychiatric Press, Washington, DC

Johnson RD, Hubscher CH 1998 Brainstem microstimulation differentially inhibits pudendal motoneuron reflex inputs. Neuroreport 9: 341–345

Jones BH, Bovee MW, Harris JM 3rd, Cowan DN 1993 Intrinsic risk factors for exercise-related injuries among male and female army trainees. American Journal of Sports Medicine 21: 705–710

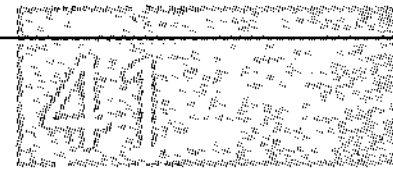

Jones, RE 1997 Human reproductive biology, 2nd edn. Academic Press, San Diego

Lehmann KA 1993 Intravenous patient-controlled analgesia: postoperative pain management and research. In: Chrubasik J, Cousins M, Martin E (eds) Advances in pain therapy II. Springer-Verlag, Berlin, pp 65–93

Lemmens HJM, Burm AGL, Hennis PJ, Gladines MPPR, Bovill JG 1990 Influence of age on the pharmacokinetics of alfentanil: gender dependence. Clinical Pharmacokinetics 19: 416–422

LeResche L, Von Korff M 1998 Epidemiology of chronic pain. In: Block AR, Kremer EF, Fernandez E (eds) Handbook of pain syndromes: biopsychosocial perspectives. Lawrence Erlbaum, Mahwah, NJ (in press)

LeResche L, Saunders K, Von Korff MR, Barlow W, Dworkin SF 1997 Use of exogenous hormones and risk of temporomandibular disorder pain. Pain 69: 153–160

McCarthy MM 1995 Functional significance of steroid modulation of GABAergic neurotransmission: analysis at the behavioral, cellular, and molecular levels. Hormones and Behavior 29: 131–140

McEwen BW 1991a Non-genomic and genomic effects of steroids on neural activity. Trends in Pharmacological Sciences 12: 141–147

McEwen BW 1991b Steroid hormones are multifunctional messengers to the brain. Trends in Endocrinology and Metabolism 2: 62–67

Marcus DA 1995 Interrelationships of neurochemicals, estrogen, and recurring headache. Pain 62: 129–141

Majewska MD 1996 Sex differences in brain morphology and pharmacodynamics. In: Jensvold MF, Halbreich U, Hamilton JA (eds) Psychopharmacology and women. Sex gender and hormones. American Psychiatric Press, Washington, DC, pp 73–83

Melzack R 1989 Phantom limbs, the self and the brain (the D.O. Hebb memorial lecture). Canadian Psychology 30(1989): 1–16

Melzack R 1993 Labor pain as a model of acute pain. Pain 53: 117–120

Merskey H, Bogduk N (eds) 1994 Classification of chronic pain: descriptions of chronic pain syndromes and definitions of pain terms, 2nd edn. IASP Press, Seattle

Micevych PE, Matt DW, Go VLW 1988 Concentrations of cholecystokinin, Substance P, and bombesin in discrete regions of male and female rat brain: sex differences and estrogen effects. Experimental Neurology 100: 416–425

Mogil JS, Sternberg WF, Marek P, Sadowski B, Belknap JK, Liebeskind JC 1996 The genetics of pain and pain inhibition. Proceedings of the National Academy of Sciences USA 93: 3048–3055

Mogil JS, Richards SP, O'Toole LA et al 1997a Identification of a sex-specific quantitative trait locus mediating nonopioid stress-induced analgesia in female mice. Journal of Neuroscience 17: 7995–8002

Mogil JS, Richards SP, O'Toole LA, Helms ML, Mitchell SR, Belknap JK 1997b Genetic sensitivity to hot-plate nociception in DBA/2J and C57BL/6J inbred mouse strains: possible sex-specific mediation by delta2-opioid receptors. Pain 70: 267–277

Murray A, Holdcroft A 1989 Incidence and intensity of postpartum lower abdominal pain. British Medical Journal 298: 1619

Myles PS, Hunt JO, Moloney JT 1997 Postoperative 'minor' complications: comparison between men and women. Anaesthesia 52: 300–306

Newton BW, Hammill RW 1996 Sexual differentiation of the autonomic nervous system. In: Unsicker K (ed) Autonomic–endocrine interactions. Harwood Academic, Amsterdam, pp 425–463

Riley III JL, Robinson ME, Wise EA, Myers CD, Fillingim RB 1998 Sex differences in the perception of noxious experimental stimuli: a meta-analysis. Pain 74: 181–187

Roof RL, Hoffman SW, Stein DG 1997 Progesterone protects against lipid peroxidation following traumatic brain injury in rats. Molecular and Chemical Neuropathology 31: 1–11

Ruda MA 1998 Gender and pain: a focus on how pain impacts women differently than men. Conference sponsored by National Institutes of Health Pain Research Consortium, Bethesda

Scoville SA, Bufton SM, Liuzzi FJ 1997 Estrogen regulated neurofilament gene expression in adult female rat dorsal root ganglion neurons. Experimental Neurology 146: 596–599

Silverman DHS, Munakata J, Hoh C, Mandelkern E, Mayer EA 1997 Gender differences in regional cerebral activity associated with visceral stimuli. Abstracts of the Society for Neuroscience 23: 1955

Smith SS 1997 Estrous hormones enhance coupled, rhythmic olivary discharge in correlation with facilitated limb stepping. Neuroscience 82: 83–95

Sohrabji F, Miranda RC, Toran-Allerand DC 1994 Estrogen differentially regulates estrogen and nerve growth factor receptor mRNAs in adult sensory neurons. Journal of Neuroscience 14: 459–471

Stern KN, McClintock MM 1996 Individual variation in biological rhythms: accurate measurement of preovulatory LH surge and menstrual cycle phase. In: Jensvold MF, Halbreich U, Hamilton JA (eds) Psychopharmacology and women. Sex gender and hormones. American Psychiatric Press, Washington, DC, pp 393–413

Sternberg WF, Liebeskind JC 1995 The analgesic response to stress: genetic and gender considerations. European Journal of Anaesthesiology 10: 14–17

Sternberg WF, Mogil JS, Kest B et al 1995 Neonatal testosterone exposure influences neurochemistry of non-opioid swim stress-induced analgesia in adulthood. Pain 63: 321–326

Turcotte JC, Blaustein JD 1997 Convergence of substance P and estrogen receptor immunoreactivity in the midbrain central gray of female guinea pigs. Reproductive Neuroendocrinology 66: 28–37

Turk DC, Okifuji A 1998 Chronic pain and pain associated with cancer: do men and women respond differently? (under review)

Unruh AM 1996 Gender variations in clinical pain experience. Pain 65: 123–167

VanderHorst VGJM, Holstege G 1997 Estrogen induces axonal outgrowth in the nucleus retroambiguus-lumbosacral motoneuronal pathway in the adult female cat. Journal of Neuroscience 17: 1122–1136

Villablanca AC, Hanley MR 1997 17beta-estradiol stimulates substance P receptor gene expression. Molecular and Cellular Endocrinology 135: 109–117

Von Korff M, Dworkin SF, Le Resche L, Kruger A 1988 An epidemiologic comparison of pain complaints. Pain 32: 173–183

Wall PD 1994 Introduction to the edition after this one. In: Wall PD, Melzack R (eds) Textbook of pain, 3rd edn. Churchill Livingstone, Edinburgh, pp 1–7

Weaver Jr CE, Park-Chung M, Gibbs TT, Farb DH 1997 17β-Estradiol protects against NMDA-induced excitotoxicity by direct inhibition of NMDA receptors. Brain Research 761: 338–341

Weiner CP, Lizasoain I, Baylis SA, Knowles RG, Charles IG, Moncada S 1994 Induction of calcium-dependent nitric oxide synthases by sex hormones. Proceedings of the National Academy of Sciences USA 91: 5212–5216

Wetherby MMC 1995 Fluctuations of pain and the menstrual cycle in rheumatoid arthritis. Thesis, Florida State University

Weyand CM, Schmidt D, Wagner U, Goronzy JJ 1998 The influence of sex on the phenotype of rheumatoid arthritis. Arthritis and Rheumatism 41: 817–822

Woolley CS, McEwen BS 1993 Roles of estradiol and progesterone in regulation of hippocampal dendritic spine density during the estrous cycle in the rat. Journal of Comparative Neurology 336: 293–306

Xiao L, Becker JB 1997 Hormonal activation of the striatum and the nucleus accumbens modulates paced mating behavior in the female rat. Hormones and Behavior 32: 114–124

Yaffe K, Sawaya G, Lieberburg I, Grady D 1998 Estrogen therapy in postmenopausal women: effects on cognitive function and dementia. Journal of the American Medical Society 279: 688–695

Zager EL, Pfeifer SM, Brown MJ, Torosian MH, Hackney DB 1998 Catamenial mononeuropathy and radiculopathy: a treatable neuropathic disorder. Journal of Neurosurgery 88: 827–830

Cancer pain and palliative care in children

42

CHARLES B. BERDE & JOHN J. COLLINS

SUMMARY

Most of us expect that we and our children will live a full lifespan, and will die only after growing old. The prospect of life-threatening or terminal illness in a child strikes us as especially cruel, undeserved and unnatural. This chapter outlines approaches to pain management, symptom management, supportive care and palliative care for children with life-threatening illnesses. Much of the literature on palliative care in adults and children concerns cancer, and this chapter will focus in large measure on cancer. Some similar considerations and supportive/palliative care approaches apply to children and young adults with a range of other life-threatening conditions, including neurodegenerative disorders, AIDS and more rapidly progressive cases of cystic fibrosis. Each of the latter conditions differs from cancer in its natural history, clinical course, patterns of symptoms and prognosis; these differences are important to individualized approaches to palliative care. A traditional view creates a strong dichotomy between curative treatment and palliative treatment. There are many reasons for this distinction to be blurred, and for curative, supportive and palliative care to be regarded as a continuum. Aspects of a supportive care approach should be incorporated in the care of all children with life-threatening illnesses, even while curative or life-prolonging therapies continue.

CANCER IN CHILDREN: EPIDEMIOLOGY AND PROGNOSIS

For several of the most common adult cancers, including cancers of the lung, stomach and pancreas, gains in long-term survival have been only incremental over the past 40 years. By contrast, the treatment of childhood cancer has in many cases seen much more dramatic improvements in survival. Over half of children diagnosed with malignancy in developed countries, who have access to state-of-the-art treatment, will have long-term disease-free survival. Acute lymphoblastic leukaemia, the most common form of childhood cancer, was uniformly fatal in the early 1950s; now disease-free long-term survival rates exceed 70%. Prognosis is much less optimistic with some of the primary CNS neoplasms, although recent advances have improved survival.

Compared with adults, multimodal treatment with chemotherapy, radiation therapy and surgery is performed more commonly with curative intent. Although more frequently successful, curative cancer therapy in children can be arduous, requiring a year or longer of repetitive cycles of chemotherapy, frequent diagnostic and therapeutic procedures, with associated medical complications, pain, nausea and other symptoms.

Many children with widely advanced cancer participate in experimental protocols of chemotherapeutic agents and other novel treatment approaches. They and their families are often willing to undertake treatments with low a priori probability of cure.

The gains in survival in childhood cancer are not shared worldwide. Many developing countries lack the economic resources to provide the costly medications, blood products, radiation therapy, surgical expertise and intensive medical support required to deliver curative therapy. Recognition of these economic realities prompted the WHO Cancer Unit to emphasize straightforward, cost-effective, non-technological methods of palliative care. Regulatory barriers continue to limit patients' access to effective analgesics (Joranson & Gilson 1998).

PAIN AND DISTRESS AT THE TIME OF INITIAL DIAGNOSIS OF CANCER

At initial diagnosis, many children report tumour-related pain (Miser et al 1987a). Miser surveyed children at initial presentation and found that 62% of the children reported pain with their first physician visit prior to diagnosis, and in the majority, pain had been present for over 2 months.

Tumour-related pain at presentation commonly involves bone, viscera, soft tissues and nerves. Bone pain may be caused by periosteal stretch, as with bone sarcomas. Leukaemias and other malignancies that proliferate in the bone marrow can cause pain due as a result of filling and compression of bone marrow spaces. Leukaemias, lymphomas, neuroblastoma and hepatoblastoma proliferate in abdominal viscera, especially in liver and spleen, and cause pain predominantly due to capsular stretch. Nephroblastoma (Wilm's tumour) may cause marked renal enlargement and flank pain, although commonly it is recognized in younger children by an asymptomatic abdominal mass or haematuria. Headache is quite common among children presenting with brain tumours, although others present first with neurological deficits. The majority of children with spinal cord tumours have back or neck pain at the time of diagnosis (Hahn & McLone 1984). Metastatic spinal cord compression is unusual at diagnosis and is more likely to occur later in the child's illness (Lewis et al 1986). Back pain, as a sign of spinal cord compression in children, usually occurs before abnormal neurological signs or symptoms at presentation (Lewis et al 1986).

Analgesics are often required for short periods of time following the initial diagnosis of cancer. The initiation of cancer therapy brings relief of pain in the great majority of cases, typically within 2 weeks. Resolution of bone marrow and visceral pain is particularly rapid for haematological malignancies, but resolution of pain may be somewhat slower for children with solid tumours of bone and soft tissues. Headache from brain tumours may improve with the initiation of corticosteroid therapy, or with the relief of increased intracranial pressure, either from surgical resection or from shunting of cerebrospinal fluid (CSF).

Children and their families are 'shell-shocked' at the time of diagnosis. An atmosphere of fear, anxiety, anger, denial and panic is common. It is essential that all clinicians caring for these children and families recognize the acute trauma of the situation. Explanations should be simple, forthright and calmly stated. Because of the overwhelming amount of information presented, patients and parents may not process or remember instructions or descriptions.

Psychological support should be provided and individualized with consideration of the child's development and coping style, and the family's cultural and spiritual values. For many children and families, support by clergy provides great comfort. A range of interventions for emotional and spiritual support should be available. Many children best express their fears and emotions through play, art or music. Child life programmes have taken a lead in advocating for the emotional support of children and families facing illness (Brazelton & Thompson 1988, Anonymous 1993, Ruffin et al 1997) (Box 42.1).

PAIN AS A RESULT OF CANCER TREATMENT

As the treatment progresses, treatment-related rather than tumour-related causes of pain predominate (Miser et al 1987a,b). Possible causes of treatment-related pain include postoperative and procedure-related pain (e.g. needle puncture, bone marrow aspiration, lumbar puncture, removal of central venous line, mucositis, phantom limb pain, infection antineoplastic therapy-related pain).

BOX 42.1

Reasons to view palliative care as a continuum rather than an abrupt transition of care

1. Patients at all stages of care, not just end-of-life, benefit from psychosocial support and broad-based symptom management. Kindness should not be restricted only to the dying patient
2. Issues of quality of life and goals of care should be raised at all stages of treatment, not just when treatments appear futile
3. Prediction of longevity is a very inexact science
4. Patients, parents and health providers often differ among themselves in their views of chances of cure and futility
5. A child who is terrorized and isolated during the initial phase of curative treatment will more likely feel fearful and isolated during late-stage care. In many cases, inadequate treatment of symptoms and inadequate support during treatment has led to adolescents refusing further treatment with a high likelihood of cure
6. Conversely, if the child feels safe and cared for during curative treatment, they may better face subsequent curative treatments, as well as coping better during end-of-life care
7. An abrupt shift in the goals of care and therapeutic approach may make the patient and family feel abandoned. Physicians, nurses, psychologists, and child life specialists who have cared for the child during their long illness have formed a unique connection to the child that can continue in palliative care

PAINFUL DIAGNOSTIC AND THERAPEUTIC PROCEDURES

Needle procedures are a major source of distress for children with cancer; many long-term cancer survivors recall needles as the worst part of their experience of cancer therapy (Zeltzer et al 1989). Common procedures include venepuncture, venous cannulation, lumbar puncture, bone marrow aspirate and biopsy, and removal of central venous lines. Other procedures, including radiation therapy, are not painful per se, but they are distressing, and often require sedation or general anaesthesia to facilitate cooperation and immobility.

For many previously well children, initial diagnostic and therapeutic needle procedures may be their first experience of intensive medical intervention. It is crucial to treat the pain and distress of initial diagnostic procedures very effectively. Children need adequate preparation before needle procedures to minimize their fear and anxiety. This preparation includes involving the child's parents, to obtain an insight into their child's coping style, to explain to them the nature of the procedure and to enlist their support. An age-appropriate explanation to the child should follow with consideration of a particular child's previous experience and coping style (Zeltzer et al 1989).

Effective treatment will set a pattern of trust and confidence for patients and families. Conversely, if a first bone marrow aspirate or lumbar puncture is a horrific experience, there will be a carry-over effect of persistent fear and distress into future procedures. A follow-up study of children in a clinical trial supports this belief. A randomized controlled trial compared a method of rapid opioid delivery, oral transmucosal fentanyl citrate (OTFC), versus placebo for the pain of lumbar puncture and bone marrow aspirate (Schechter et al 1995). (Regulatory agencies insisted on a placebo group, despite the objections of some of the investigators.) The investigators were permitted to give OTFC unblinded to all patients for subsequent procedures. The group who had received the active agent for the first procedure showed less distress and pain for the group of subsequent procedures, implying a persistent carry-over effect of inadequately treated pain (Weisman et al 1998).

The management of painful and distressing procedures is best carried out by a combination of non-pharmacological and pharmacological approaches, which are individualized to the particular child's developmental level, coping style, medical and psychological condition, and type of procedure (Berde 1995). Some aspects of the non-pharmacological approach are commonsense, as outlined in Box 42.2.

BOX 42.2

Commonsense, but frequently forgotten, aspects of paediatric procedures

1. Minimize unnecessary procedures, especially repeated venipuncture
2. Use age-appropriate explanations
3. Involve the parents to support the child and be allies, not to assist or restrain the child
4. In most cases, use a treatment room rather than the patient's room, so that their own room remains a 'safe' place
5. Skilled and expeditious, but not rushed, performance shortens the period of distress. Get all supplies and equipment prepared beforehand, so that the procedure goes as quickly as possible
6. Assign practitioners' pagers ('beepers') to other clinicians during the procedure whenever feasible, to minimize interruptions
7. Where feasible, trainees should learn first by watching, by in vitro models, and in some cases by supervised performance of procedures on anaesthetized patients

In addition to these commonsense measures, there are a number of specific psychological techniques for managing the pain and distress of procedures, including hypnosis, relaxation training and guided imagery (Katz et al 1987, Kuttner et al 1988, 1989, Steggles et al 1997). Other cognitive-behavioural interventions include preparatory information, positive coping statements, modelling and/or behavioural rehearsal. There are many variations of these methods, and the optimal techniques depend on the experience of the practitioners and the developmental level and personal style of the child. Training programmes are provided by many organizations; the Society for Behavioral Pediatrics has taken a lead in this regard in North America.

There is an extensive literature supporting the efficacy of psychological techniques for managing painful procedures in children with cancer (Jay et al 1987, 1995). In our opinion, these should be taught to children with cancer whenever possible. They have several advantages. They are exceedingly safe, and the child can develop a sense of mastery and confidence. Children can generalize the use of these techniques to new situations. Although it would be an ideal to prevent all painful situations (Schechter et al 1997), it is unlikely that this can ever be accomplished. Hypnosis is a skill that, once learned, travels anywhere. However, hypnosis should not be used as an excuse for withholding adequate analgesics for moderate to severe pain. Some children may be too traumatized to use these techniques, or may have developmental or cognitive limitations that prevent their use.

Cutaneous analgesia can be provided by several local anaesthetic formulations and delivery systems, including a eutectic mixture of the local anaesthetics lidocaine and prilocaine (EMLA), tetracaine gel (amethocaine) and iontophoresis of lidocaine. EMLA has been used widely (Maunuksela & Korpela 1986, Halperin et al 1989, Miser et al 1994). It is available either as a patch or as a cream, which is applied under an occlusive dressing. While the standard recommendation is to apply EMLA for 60 minutes, the depth and reliability of analgesia increases with longer application times, for example 90–120 minutes (Bjerring & Arendt-Nielsen 1993). EMLA has been proven to be safe, with low plasma local anaesthetic concentrations and a negligible risk of methaemoglobinaemia. EMLA provides no analgesia for structures deep to the dermis, but it can make subsequent deeper infiltration with local anaesthetic less noxious. Tetracaine gel (amethocaine, Ametop) appears to be as effective as EMLA, and may have more rapid onset (Doyle et al 1993). Tetracaine gel is available in much of Europe and Canada, but is not available commercially in the USA at present. Some hospital pharmacies make their own preparations. Further study is needed of the preparative issues with 'home-made' formulations, particularly regarding pH and stability issues that may alter efficacy. Topical cooling using ice or fluorocarbon coolant sprays has been used with some success (Abbott & Fowler-Kerry 1995). Both skin cooling and EMLA may produce vasoconstriction, which may make venous cannulation more difficult in some patients. Iontophoresis is a method that employs electric current to accelerate drug penetration through skin. A packaged formulation of lidocaine is marketed as 'Numby-Stuff'. Iontophoresis can produce skin analgesia very rapidly and with a good depth of penetration (Zeltzer et al 1991). Several series have reported very good efficacy and safety, although we continue to hear anecdotal reports of occasional cases of skin burns.

Topical skin analgesia with local anaesthetics is extremely useful, and should be widely available in paediatric centres. It is not a panacea, however. For a child who has experienced repeated distressing procedures, they will likely remain anxious despite the use of EMLA, because of their fear and lack of trust. Consider a situation in which a child is promised a pain-free venous cannulation: EMLA is applied to one or two sites, but these sites are not feasible, and it becomes necessary to stick a third site; then the procedure will be painful, and the child will lose trust.

Local anaesthetic infiltration can reduce pain from deeper needle procedures. Prior use of topical anaesthesia, such as EMLA or amethocaine, can reduce the discomfort of the infiltrating needle. Lidocaine and other local anaesthetics are dispensed as acid solutions, because this increases their stability and shelf life. Neutralizing the local anaesthetic solutions with sodium bicarbonate reduces the pain of infiltration. For lidocaine 1% solution, a common recommendation is to combine 9 ml of the commercial lidocaine solution with 1 ml of sodium bicarbonate, which is generally available as a 0.88 mEq/ml solution. The solubility of bupivacaine at neutral pH is much lower, and 1 ml of sodium bicarbonate should be mixed with at least 25 ml of bupivacaine 0.25% solution; even at these ratios, bupivacaine 0.25% and 0.5% solutions will precipitate with time at neutral pH (Peterfreund et al 1989).

'Conscious' sedation and general anaesthesia (Box 42.3)

For more painful or extensive procedures, or for children who have a limited ability to cope or cooperate, conscious sedation or general anaesthesia should be readily available.

BOX 42.3

Recommendations for conscious sedation in children

1. Establish protocols, education programmes, and an assessment programme to track efficacy and complications. Efficacy should be judged by patients as well as practitioners
2. Standardize the choice of drugs and doses for the majority of procedures, so that practitioners are comfortable with a consistent approach
3. Reduce doses in patients with risk factors for hypoventilation
4. Observe fasting guidelines for solids and clear liquids to reduce the risk of aspiration
5. Employ an observer whose only job is to assess level of consciousness and adequacy of respiration
6. Use pulse oximetry to assess oxygenation
7. Keep available an oxygen delivery source, suction, a bag and mask, and an airway management cart with a proper range of equipment
8. Keep available reversal agents, especially naloxone and flumazenil
9. Recognize that conscious sedation is a continuum, and in some patients, standard doses may produce deep sedation
10. Recognize that conscious sedation does not permit complete lack of responses to events; it is not general anaesthesia
11. Refer higher risk patients and more extensive procedures for management by paediatric anaesthetists or similar specialists

In many paediatric centres, both approaches are used. Conscious sedation refers to the administration of anxiolytics and analgesics to render the child sedated and comfortable, but able to respond to stimuli and able to maintain airway reflexes and ventilation. For both conscious sedation and general anaesthesia, safe practice necessitates administration by practitioners with expertise in airway management and with knowledge of the relevant pharmacology and medical issues. Protocols for monitoring and drug dosing can help reduce the risk. Monitoring with oximetry is widely recommended.

Some procedures, such as radiation therapy, are not painful, but require sedation to permit immobility. In these circumstances, pure sedatives, such as pentobarbital, chloral hydrate and midazolam, are widely used. Where procedures involve significant pain that cannot be relieved by local anaesthesia, such as a bone marrow aspirate, it is generally preferable to combe a sedative-anxiolytic, such as midazolam (Sievers et al 1991), with an analgesic, either an opioid or ketamine. The combination of midazolam with either fentanyl or low-dose ketamine has been shown to be safe and effective in several studies (Marx et al 1997, Parker et al 1997). The intravenous route is useful because of rapid onset, complete bioavailability, and the ability to titrate incremental doses to effect.

Ketamine has received widespread use because it produces excellent analgesia, dissociation and stable respiration in most children. While ketamine is extremely useful, it should not be regarded as risk-free or devoid of adverse reactions. Occasional children have very prolonged sedation or confusion. Although respiration is generally well maintained, perhaps better than with opioids dosed to comparable effect, ketamine has the disadvantage of no pharmacological reversal agent. Severe respiratory sequelae in children have been reported (Mitchell et al 1996, Litman 1997, Green & Rothrock 1997, Roelofse & Roelofse 1997). In our view, ketamine should be used primarily in a setting where personnel with advanced airway skills are readily available. The incidence of dysphoria or bad dreams remains in some dispute. While several series report bad dreams and dysphoria to be insignificant problems, others disagree (Valentin & Bech 1996). The co-administration of ketamine with benzodiazepines appears to diminish this risk.

Although many children with cancer have indwelling central venous lines or easy peripheral venous access, others do not. For these children, needle-free routes of administration are helpful. Oral benzodiazepine-opioid or benzodiazepine-ketamine mixtures can be effective, although there is considerable variation in absorption, and the oral/parenteral ratios are only rough approximations (Hollman & Perloff 1995, Qureshi et al 1995). If oral sedation is used, sufficient time should elapse to give peak drug effect. Because of the variability in onset and offset, children need to be observed for the development of deep sedation or respiratory depression. Some children will become restless or will try to get up and walk, and may injure themselves if unattended. An oral-transmucosal preparation of fentanyl has rapid absorption and intense analgesia. Studies by Weisman, Schechter and their colleagues have shown very good efficacy for bone marrow aspiration and lumbar puncture.

Nitrous oxide can be used for conscious sedation (Miser et al 1988, Gamis et al 1989, Bouffet et al 1996). Advantages include very rapid onset and offset, no requirement for intravenous access and good analgesia. Nitrous oxide in concentrations of 30–50% in oxygen has a generally good safety record. Some children will resist the mask, will report bothersome dreams (particularly with concentrations in excess of 50%), or will find nitrous oxide inadequate for portions of more painful procedures. The combination of nitrous oxide with other sedatives or analgesics requires some experience, because there is considerable variability in the responses (Litman et al 1996, 1997). Scavenging of exhaled gas and high flow turnover of room air is recommended to reduce environmental exposure for health personnel.

The development of shorter duration general anaesthetic agents has greatly facilitated providing general anaesthesia for these procedures, either in or near operating room areas, or in remote locations and clinics. If intravenous access is available, propofol is widely favoured because of its rapid onset, rapid, pleasant emergence and antiemetic effects (Van Gerven et al 1992, Frankville et al 1993). If inhalation anaesthesia is required, the newer potent vapour anaesthetic sevoflurane has become popular because of its sweet smell and extremely rapid onset and offset. Some children may fear the mask or dislike the pungent aroma of volatile anaesthetics, especially halothane and isoflurane (Jay et al 1995).

There is considerable controversy regarding the relative risks and benefits of brief deep sedation or general anaesthesia provided by anaesthetists (Maunuksela et al 1986), versus conscious sedation provided by non-specialists (Cote 1994, Maxwell & Yaster 1996). Many paediatric centres employ a two-tiered approach, with conscious sedation for certain procedures by oncologists and other non-anaesthetists according to protocol guidelines, and with a 'sedation service' staffed by paediatric anaesthetists for higher risk patients, for more extensive or demanding procedures, or in cases of failed sedation by non-anaesthetists. It is essential that there be close communication and collaboration between paediatricians and anaesthetists, and recognition of each others' practice constraints. It is important that paediatric residents receive sufficient experience and training in the use of conscious sedation in preparation for a wide range of subsequent practice settings.

Lumbar puncture

A significant portion of the pain of lumbar puncture is caused by skin puncture by the spinal needle, though if the interspace is difficult to locate, there may be significant pain as a result of needle contact with bony spinous processes or laminae. Topical anaesthesia can facilitate deeper infiltration (Kapelushnik et al 1990). The distress of lumbar puncture for children with cancer is related in part to the required body position and the necessity to remain still. The distress of lumbar puncture in many cases will benefit from cognitive and behavioural techniques, conscious sedation or, in some cases, general anaesthesia.

Lumbar puncture may produce a sustained CSF fluid leak, leading to low intracranial pressure. The epidemiology of postdural puncture headache in children with cancer is not known. The risk of dural-puncture headache can be reduced by the use of smaller gauge needles with noncutting points (Lambert et al 1997). The treatment of this headache, should it occur, is generally by simple analgesics, adequate hydration and supine position. In adults, caffeine (Camann et al 1990) and sumatriptan have both been reported to provide relief in some cases (Carp et al 1994, Choi et al 1996), but not others (de las Heras-Rosas et al 1997). In refractory cases an epidural blood patch (i.e. the injection of autologous blood in the epidural space) may be required to alleviate this symptom (Carrie 1993).

Bone marrow aspiration

Bone marrow aspiration produces pain both with passage of a large needle through the periosteum, but also with application of suction to the marrow space. The former pain is only partially relieved by local anaesthetic infiltration near the periosteum, the latter pain is unrelieved by local anaesthetic. Bone marrow aspiration is a source of severe distress in children (Katz et al 1980, Jay et al 1983). Guided imagery, relaxation, hypnosis, conscious sedation and general anaesthesia have been shown to be effective modalities for reducing distress in this setting (Jay et al 1987, 1995).

Removal of central venous lines

Tunnelled central venous lines require removal, either electively when treatment courses are completed or, more urgently, in cases of infection or occlusion. Brief general anaesthesia and conscious sedation are widely used for these procedures.

As noted above, choice among treatments depends on the child's age, temperament, preferences, previous experience with procedures and on the local availability of services. For example, a 12 year old who is an excellent hypnotic subject and who experiences severe nausea or dysphoria with sedation or general anaesthesia may prefer hypnosis to pharmacological measures. Conversely, a 3 year old who has had severely traumatic experiences with previous procedures may do better with a brief general anaesthetic. Ideally, options should be tailored to individual needs (Berde 1995). Pharmacological and psychological approaches should be seen as complementary, not mutually exclusive (Jay et al 1995). Many children will benefit from combining cognitive-behavioural techniques with analgesics.

MUCOSITIS

Cancer chemotherapy and radiation therapy attack the rapidly dividing cells of the epithelial lining of the oral cavity and gastrointestinal tract. Mucosal injury and cell death impair barrier function, and produces pain and inflammation known as mucositis. The extent and severity of this condition is variable.

A number of topical therapies have been used, including diphenhydramine, kaolin suspensions, sodium bicarbonate, hydrogen peroxide, sucralfate, clotrimazole, nystatin, viscous lidocaine and diclonine. There is little uniformity in the use of these drugs, and data regarding efficacy are limited for children. The excessive use of topical local anaesthetics can occasionally block protective airway reflexes, resulting in aspiration, or can cause systemic accumulation, with a risk of seizures. When pain persists despite topical therapies, opioids should be used.

The mucositis following conditioning for bone marrow transplantation is more intense and prolonged than that associated with routine chemotherapy. Mucositis in transplant patients has a continuous component, with sharp exacerbation during mouth care and swallowing. Preventive strategies may reduce the incidence and severity of mucositis (Symonds et al 1996, Larson et al 1998). Opioids are generally partially effective, but for some patients the pain can preclude talking, eating and, on occasions, swallowing. Continuous opioid infusions, patient-controlled analgesia (PCA) and nurse-controlled analgesia via a PCA pump are widely used (Hill et al 1991). PCA appears safe and effective for mucositis pain following bone marrow transplantation in children (Mackie et al 1991, Collins et al 1996a). In one comparison, the PCA group required less morphine, had less sedation and less difficulty concentrating, but equivalent analgesia to the group receiving staff-controlled morphine continuous infusion; in other comparisons, PCA groups have lower opioid use and side effects, as well as lower pain scores (Zucker et al 1998). For some children, the pain remains severe despite very high doses of opioids. There is a need for further study of optimal methods of management.

GRAFT VERSUS HOST DISEASE

Donor-derived immune cells attack host tissues following bone marrow transplantation to create a multiorgan inflammatory process known as graft versus host disease. Abdominal pains and limb pains are common. Abdominal pain may arise from both hepatic and intestinal inflammation and veno-occlusion. Despite pre-emptive anti-T-cell therapies in bone marrow transplant protocols, this problem remains quite common, and is a frequent source of pain, which is usually treated with opioids.

INFECTION

Immunocompromised children are susceptible to painful bacterial, viral, fungal and protozoal infections in a range of sites. These infections include mouth sores, perirectal abscesses and skin infection, especially at sites of intravenous access. Analgesics may be required until antimicrobial therapies reduce inflammation.

Acute herpes zoster in children with cancer and AIDS can be quite painful, and merits use of opioids as needed. Overall, zoster infection in children is less likely to produce prolonged postherpetic neuralgia than in adults, although there is a small subgroup of children with postherpetic severe burning pain, episodic shooting pain, itching and skin hypersensitivity that persists for years. Early antiviral therapy should be encouraged (Wood et al 1996, Grant et al 1997). Therapies for postherpetic neuralgia are adapted from those used in adults (Watson 1995), including tricyclic antidepressants (Bowsher 1997), anticonvulsants, topical (Rowbotham et al 1996), regional and systemic local anaesthetics, and opioids (Watson & Babul 1998).

ACUTE ABDOMINAL EMERGENCIES

Oncology patients may have any of the causes of an acute abdomen that afflict other patients, such as appendicitis, a perforated ulcer or a bowel obstruction.

Neutropenic patients with cancer may present with acute abdominal pain as a result of bowel inflammation; this is known as tiflitis. Although they show the signs of an acute surgical abdomen, this condition is usually treated conservatively, and surgical exploration is usually restricted to cases of overt bowel perforation or severe bleeding. Many of these patients are quite ill and require opioids despite their effects on bowel motility.

Pre-emptive treatment of constipation is important in all cancer patients taking opioids, but it is especially important in sick neutropenic patients. The delayed administration of oral laxatives for routine mild ileus and mild constipation can lead to a difficult situation in which a patient has severe abdominal distension, is suspected of developing tiflitis, is vomiting and may appear toxic. In this setting, treatment options become limited, because they can no longer receive oral cathartics, and cannot receive enemas or rectal medications because of their risks of producing bacteraemia.

POSTOPERATIVE PAIN AND PERIOPERATIVE CARE

Postoperative pain management in general is discussed in detail in Chapter 19. In approaching perioperative care for children with cancer, it is to be expected that there will be considerable anxiety and fear for the patient and parents. Heavy premedication may be required, and early anticipation of the need for larger-than-average doses for premedication may prevent unpleasant scenes and distress in the preoperative waiting area.

Children who have become opioid tolerant may have a higher risk of intraoperative awareness during anaesthesia, particularly if a nitrous oxide–opioid-relaxant-based anaesthetic technique is used without adjustment for these increased opioid requirements. Unless there is severe haemodynamic instability, the incorporation of either volatile anaesthetic agents or adequate doses of hypnotics (e.g. propofol infusions) is recommended to ensure unconsciousness.

Postoperatively, patients who have been receiving preoperative opioids should have their daily dose of opioids calculated, and this dose used as a baseline to which additional opioids are added for the purposes of postoperative pain control. It is our experience that this principle is commonly ignored in postoperative care, leading to dramatic undermedication of oncology patients. Cancer resection can be especially painful postoperatively because of the need to cut across tissues, rather than dividing in natural tissue planes, in order to obtain clear margins.

Epidural analgesia can be used with very good effect for cancer surgery in children (Tobias et al 1992). As with systemic opioids, it is our experience that initial dosing of epidural infusions in children with cancer is often too conservative. Rapid and aggressive bedside titration should be used to relieve their pain. Maximum weight-based local anaesthetic dosing is limited by strict guidelines, as outlined in Chapter 52, while dosing of epidural opioids should be titrated upwards to clinical effect. If limiting doses of amino amide local anaesthetics are inadequate, the amino-ester local anaesthetic 2-chlororprocaine can be used because of its rapid plasma clearance and high margin of safety. Whenever feasible, placement of the epidural catheter tip at the level of the dermatomes innervating the surgical field permits the optimal use of local anaesthetic–opioid synergism. If epidural catheter tips are below the level of surgical dermatomes, or if there is inadequate analgesia with combinations of local anaesthetics with lipid-soluble opioids (e.g. fentanyl), clinicians should not hesitate to switch the opioid component of the epidural mixture to a water-soluble drug such as morphine and hydromorphone to achieve adequate neuraxial spread.

Postsurgical neuropathic pains

Damage to peripheral nerves is unavoidable in many types of tumour resection, particularly with limb sarcomas, and nerve injury may sometimes produce prolonged neuropathic pain. Human studies of pre-emptive analgesia with local anaesthetic blockade in preventing neuropathic pain are limited, but in view of the difficulties in treating neuropathic pain once established, we favour the use of perioperative pre-emptive blockade whenever feasible for limb sarcoma resections. If a child shows signs and symptoms of neuropathic pain following cancer surgery, early use should be made of tricyclic antidepressants and anticonvulsants. In many cases they appear beneficial, and are required for several weeks to months. For a tricyclic, a typical regimen is to begin with nortriptyline in doses of 0.1–0.2 mg/kg at night-time and increase dosing every few days until there is relief, or there are side effects, or full antidepressant levels are achieved, often with the addition of a smaller morning dose.

Recently, gabapentin has become extremely popular for the treatment of neuropathic pains. At this time, randomized controlled trials are limited for adults, and are nonexistent for children. Our experience with its use in children with cancer has been very favourable, both because of its efficacy and its apparent safety. Some children experience headaches, sedation, abdominal upset and behavioural disturbances.

Pain due to antineoplastic therapy

Several chemotherapy drugs can produce local necrosis or irritation when a peripheral vein infiltrates. Some forms of chemotherapy are painful when injected via peripheral veins, even when no extravasation occurs. Intrathecal chemotherapy can produce backache, headache, and signs of arachnoiditis or meningeal irritation.

Vincristine commonly produces peripheral nerve dysfunction, with hyporeflexia, sensory abnormalities, paraesthesias and gastrointestinal hypomotility as common sequelae. Although in many cases these impairments are not painful, a small subgroup of children report burning or shooting pains and paraesthesias. These cases are often treated with opioids, tricyclic antidepressants and anticonvulsants. There are insufficient paediatric data to support a best drug class for treatment. In the majority of patients in our experience, these symptoms improve over several months, but are likely to recur with repeated cycles of chemotherapy.

Granulocyte colony stimulating factor (GCSF) accelerates neutrophil production and shortens the duration of neutropenic episodes. It may produce bone marrow pain.

Some experimental anticancer therapies have produced new and unanticipated sources of pain. For example, a monoclonal antibody therapy for advanced neuroblastoma was shown to produce an acute peripheral sensory neuropathy with severe pain. Gabapentin appears promising for the relief of this pain, based both on human experience and animal model studies (Gillin & Sorkin 1998).

CHRONIC PAINS IN LONG-TERM SURVIVORS OF CHILDHOOD CANCER

In our clinics in Boston and Sydney, a number of children and adolescents have been followed who are long-term survivors of childhood cancer who have chronic pain despite apparent cure of their tumour. Neuropathic pains most commonly seen include causalgia of the lower extremity, phantom limb pain, postherpetic neuralgia and central pain after spinal cord tumour resection. Several patients have chronic lower extremity pain as a result of a mechanical problem with an internal prosthesis, failure of bony union or avascular necrosis of multiple joints. Several have longstanding myofascial pains and chronic abdominal pain of uncertain aetiology. A number of patients treated with shunts for brain tumours have recurrent headaches that appear to be unrelated to intracranial pressure or changes in shunt functioning.

Phantom sensations and phantom limb pain are common among children following amputation for cancer in an extremity (Dangel 1998). Unlike adults, the experience in children tends to decrease with time. There is evidence that preoperative pain in the diseased extremity may be a predictor for subsequent phantom pain and in adults preoperative regional anaesthesia may be effective in preventing phantom pain. Krane and Heller suggested that phantom pain was quite common in children following cancer resection, and was often under-recognized by physicians (Krane et al 1991). Melzack and co-workers reported that phantom sensation and pain can occur in children with congenital absence of limbs, although the prevalence of pain is less than among children who received amputations (Melzack et al 1997).

Survivors of childhood cancer and their families have the ever-present worry that pains and other symptoms may imply relapse or a second treatment-induced malignancy. It can be a difficult issue to determine what degree of investigation is appropriate in surveillance for recurrent tumour. Approaches to the care of these children and young adults should be multidisciplinary and should include psychological interventions, physical therapy and efforts to help these children and young adults return to school and work.

A small percentage of long-term survivors take oral opioid analgesics on a daily basis for long-term treatment of pain as part of a multidisciplinary programme.

PAIN AS A RESULT OF TUMOUR PROGRESSION

When tumours progress, they can produce pain by infiltration in or pressure on bone, viscera, soft tissues or nerves.

Even in cases of widespread disease where there is no longer a curative intent, chemotherapy and radiation therapy may be used to help relieve pain by shrinking the tumour. Several excellent recent reviews of symptom management and palliative care in children with advanced cancer are available (Stevens et al 1994, Frager 1996, Goldman 1996, 1998, Liben 1996, Dangel 1998).

Chapter 42 describes the general difficulties with pain assessment in preverbal children. Several points are worth reiterating here. Behavioural signs of persistent pain may differ from those in the setting of acute medical procedures. Behavioural distress scales that were developed for acute procedures often under-rate pain in this setting.

Gauvain-Piquard et al (1984, 1987) designed a behavioural observation scale to be used in the assessment of tumour-related pain in children aged 2–6 years. The 17 items in the scale assessed pain, depression and anxiety. There are some practical implementation issues with the use of this scale in clinical practice. This scale is attractive conceptually because it assesses both affective and sensory dimensions of pain, as well as the impact of pain on daily functioning.

Many children with pain as a result of widespread cancer will lie still, close their eyes and inhibit body movements. While sometimes this response is caused by oversedation, in other cases a withdrawal from their surroundings is a response to undertreated pain. When in doubt, a trial of opioid titration may be diagnostic. If the child becomes more interactive and moves around more freely after opioid dosing, then it is likely that they were previously undermedicated, not oversedated.

Trends in physiological signs, including heart rate and blood pressure, can provide some information about pain intensity, but should not be used as isolated measures of pain. Many processes unrelated to pain can alter heart rate and blood pressure. Autonomic signs may habituate with persistent pain.

ANALGESICS FOR PAIN CAUSED BY ADVANCED CANCER

The WHO analgesic ladder approach outlined for adults with cancer is in many respects applicable for children as well. General aspects of paediatric analgesic pharmacology are reviewed in Chapter 65. Dosing guidelines for non-opioid and opioid analgesics are summarized in Tables 42.1 and 42.2 and Box 42.4, respectively.

Acetaminophen

Acetaminophen is the most commonly used non-opioid analgesic in children with cancer, particularly because it lacks the antiplatelet and gastric effects of NSAIDs and aspirin. Oral dosing of 10–15 mg/kg every 4 hours is recommended, with a daily maximum dose of 90 mg/kg/day in children and 60 mg/kg/day in infants. An intravenous prodrug, propacetamol, is available in Europe, but not the USA. It may be useful in selected circumstances for fever control and for analgesia in children unable to take oral medications.

Table 42.1 Dosing recommendations for non-opioid analgesics for children

Drug	*Recommended dosing*	*comments*
Acetaminophen (paracetamol)	Single doses of 15–20 mg/kg Repeated doses of 10–15 mg/kg every 4 h orally, up to 90 mg/kg/day in children and 60 mg/kg/day in infants	Generally safe. Does not cause gastric irritation or bleeding
Choline-magnesium salicylate	10–15 mg/kg every 8–12 h orally	Lower gastric and bleeding risk than most NSAIDs
Ibuprofen	8–10 mg/kg every 6–8 h orally	Largest paediatric experience among NSAIDs. Potential for bleeding and gastritis limits use in children with cancer
Naproxen	5–7 mg/kg every 8–12 h orally	Risks similar to ibuprofen. Longer duration permits less frequent dosing
Amitriptyline or nortriptyline	Begin at 0.1–0.2 mg/kg at bedtime, increase incrementally as limited by side effects and as needed for efficacy up to 2 mg/kg day	Clearance is variable, so that some patients will benefit from a small morning dose in addition. Plasma concentrations may be a helpful guide at higher dose ranges
Gabapentin	Begin at 100 mg orally at bedtime, or with 50 mg (1/2 of the smallest capsule's contents) in younger children. If tolerated, advance to twice daily then three times daily over several days. If tolerated, escalate as needed and tolerated up to 60 mg/kg/day, divided in three times daily dosing	These recommendations are provisional, because current experience is limited

Aspirin and NSAIDs

Aspirin and NSAIDs are frequently contraindicated in paediatric oncology patients because of bleeding concerns. In selected children with adequate platelet number and function, NSAIDs may be very useful, both alone and in combination with opioids. The effectiveness of NSAIDs in cancer is not limited to bone pains (Eisenberg et al 1994).

Choline magnesium salicylate (Trilisate) and related non-acetylated salicylates appear in adult studies to produce less gastric irritation and antiplatelet effects than most NSAIDs. Data are too limited to warrant extrapolating these conclusions to patients with severe thrombocytopenia.

The newer cyclooxygenase-2 (COX-2) inhibitors are likely to be enormously beneficial for pain management for children with cancer. If initial studies in adults are replicated, then they should be very safe and effective in many situations, both alone and in combination with opioids.

Weak opioids: codeine and low-dose oxycodone

The WHO ladder distinguishes between weak opioids and strong opioids, although this is a function of dose as well as drug. For children, codeine is widely used. Dosing of codeine is rarely escalated beyond 2 mg/kg because of an impression that this produces more side effects than comparable doses of other opioids. Recommended paediatric oral dosing is 0.5–1 mg/kg every 4 hours. Oxycodone can be regarded as either a 'weak' or a 'strong' opioid depending on the dose used. Dosing of oxycodone can be escalated as long as it is not given in a fixed preparation with acetaminophen (e.g. Percocet) in doses that would risk acetaminophen toxicity.

The practical advantage of the so-called weak opioids is that they can be prescribed in some locations by telephone more easily than many other opioids. In many parts of the USA, there is greater acceptance of telephone prescribing of combinations of acetaminophen with either codeine (e.g. Tylenol #3 or #4) or hydrocodone (e.g. Vicodin).

Most available evidence recommends the use of standard μ-opioid agonists for cancer pain in preference to mixed agonist–antagonist opioids or opioids acting primarily at κ receptors. Somnolence and dysphoria are common with the latter drugs, and they may cause withdrawal symptoms in patients receiving μ opioids. The κ agonist buprenorphine

BOX 42.4

General guidelines for opioid use for cancer pain in children

1. Use sufficient doses to keep the patient comfortable and dose frequently enough to prevent most recurrences of pain
2. Use the oral route first in most circumstances
3. Use appropriate oral : parenteral conversion ratios
4. The 'right' dose is whatever it takes to relieve the pain
5. Treat opioid side effects promptly
6. Treat constipation pre-emptively
7. If side effects are bothersome with one opioid, consider opioid switching

is widely used for children in countries with limited availability of morphine. It is more properly regarded as a strong opioid, and it can have very prolonged duration of action.

Strong opioids: morphine, hydromorphone, fentanyl, meperidine, methadone

For moderate to severe pain, μ-opioid agonists are the cornerstone of treatment. Initial dose recommendations for opioid prescribing for children with cancer are outlined in Table 42.2.

Morphine is the most widely used strong opioid, and is a proper first choice in most circumstances. Age-related differences in morphine conjugation and excretion are summarized in Chapter 42. A typical starting dose for immediate-release oral morphine in opioid-naive subjects is 0.3 mg/kg every 4 hours.

Sustained-release preparations of morphine and oxycodone are widely available, and a sustained release preparation of hydromorphone is under development. They permit oral dosing at intervals of either twice or three times daily. Crushing these tablets produces immediate release of morphine, which limits their use for children unable to swallow pills. Sustained-release oral suspensions of morphine are under investigation. Hunt, Goldman and their co-workers (personal communication) recently examined the pharmacokinetics of immediate- and sustained-release oral morphine (MST) in children with cancer. Based on the peak-to-valley fluctuations in plasma concentrations, they concluded that sustained-release oral morphine should probably be given three times daily in children to achieve a constant effect.

Hydromorphone is an opioid that is roughly five to eight times as potent as morphine. It is otherwise similar in many respects to morphine in its actions, but it may be used in settings where there are dose-limiting side effects from morphine. A double-blinded, randomized cross-over comparison of morphine to hydromorphone using PCA in children and adolescents with mucositis following bone marrow transplantation showed that hydromorphone was well tolerated, and had an approximate potency ratio of 6:1 relative to morphine in this setting (Collins et al 1996a). Because of its high potency and high aqueous solubility, hydromorphone is convenient for high-dose subcutaneous infusion. It is commercially available in 10 mg/ml solutions, and can be prepared in concentrations up to 50 mg/ml if needed. Little is known about pharmacokinetics in infants or biological actions of metabolites.

Fentanyl is about 50–100 times as potent as morphine, depending on whether infusion or intravenous single dose comparisons are used. It has a rapid onset and offset following intravenous administration, which is convenient for brief painful procedures. With infusions, the clinical duration of action becomes much more prolonged (Ginsberg et

Table 42.2 Starting doses of commonly used opioids in paediatrics. (Adapted from Collins & Berde 1997)

Drug	*Usual IV starting dose (<50 kg)*	*Usual IV starting dose (>50 kg)*	*Usual PO starting dose (<50 kg)*	*Usual PO starting dose (>50 kg)*
Morphine	0.1 mg/kg q3–4 h	5–10 mg q3–4 h	0.3 mg/kg q3–4 h	30 mg q3–4 h
Hydromorphone	0.015 mg/kg q3–4 h	1–1.5 mg q3–4 h	0.06 mg/kg q3–4 h	6 mg q3–4 h
Oxycodone	N/A	N/A	0.3 mg/kg q3–4 h[1]	10 mg q3–4 h
Meperidine[2]	0.75 mg/kg q2–3 h	75–100 mg q3 h	N/R	N/R
Fentanyl	0.5–1.5 μg/kg q1–2 h	25–75 μg/kg q1–2 h	N/A	N/A

[1]Smallest tablet size is 5 mg.
[2]Meperidine is not recommended for chronic use because of the accumulation of the toxic metabolite normeperidine.
N/A = not available; N/R = not recommended.

al 1996, Scholz et al 1996). Fentanyl is commonly used for patients who have excessive pruritus from morphine.

Meperidine should be avoided for ongoing use if other opioids are available, because its major metabolite normeperidine can cause dysphoria, excitation and convulsions, particularly in patients with impaired renal function. Meperidine can be used for brief painful procedures, and it has a specific indication in low doses (0.25–0.5 mg/kg IV) for the treatment of severe shivering or rigors following the infusion of amphotericin and blood components.

Methadone is long acting due to its slow hepatic metabolism. In single parenteral doses, it is equipotent to morphine. Oral absorption is efficient, with an oral : parenteral ratio of approximately 1.5–2:1. Elixir preparations are convenient for prolonged duration in children who are unable to swallow sustained-release morphine tablets. Episodic intravenous dosing may be convenient for patients with intravenous access, to maintain sustained analgesia without the requirement for an infusion pump (Berde et al 1991).

Methadone is somewhat more tricky to titrate than several of the other commonly used opioids. There is considerable variation in its duration of action (Plummer et al 1988), and careful assessment is required. Accumulation can produce delayed sedation and hypoventilation several days after a dosing change. Once comfort is achieved, it is often necessary to lower the dose or extend the interval to avoid subsequent oversedation. Some have advocated p.r.n. dosing as a method of initial dose titration. Methadone sometimes carries an unfortunate stigma because of its use in opioid addiction programmes.

From all of the above discussion, it should be apparent that opioids are more similar than different, and no single opioid is right for all patients in all situations.

Choice among routes of opioid administration

The oral route of opioid administration is convenient, inexpensive and non-technological, and therefore to be favoured whenever feasible. A number of strategies have been described for helping children take oral medications (McGrath et al 1994). Some children with advanced cancer either refuse to take oral medications, or cannot take them because of nausea, ileus, painful swallowing or obtundation.

Intravenous administration permits rapid dosing and titration with complete bioavailability. Where available, indwelling central venous lines obviate the need for repeated intravenous cannulation. Small portable infusion pumps are widely available in many countries, permitting consistent plasma concentrations (Miser et al 1980).

Continuous subcutaneous infusions are a useful intermediate technology for parenteral opioid administration for children with poor intravenous access (Miser et al 1983) (Grimshaw et al 1995). A small catheter or butterfly needle may be placed under the skin of the thorax, abdomen or thigh, with sites changed every 3–7 days as needed. Solutions are generally concentrated so that infusion rates do not exceed 1–3 ml/h, although higher rates have been used (Bruera et al 1994). Morphine and hydromorphone are commonly used, and are well tolerated; methadone should be avoided because it can produce local irritation and skin necrosis. Needle placement can be made less noxious by the prior use of topical local anaesthetic preparations as described above. Pain at the injection site can be diminished by mixing small amounts of lidocaine in the infusion, as long as cumulative lidocaine dosing does not exceed 1.5 mg/kg/h. Intravenous and subcutaneous infusions can be made more convenient for the home by the use of small portable infusion pumps.

Many of the home infusion pumps are equipped with a PCA bolus option as well as a continuous infusion mode. In most locations in the USA, there is no greater operating cost in adding a PCA option. Most children with cancer have fluctuations in pain intensity and in opioid requirements. A PCA option is a straightforward method to permit rescue medication via either intravenous or subcutaneous routes (Bruera et al 1988). In general, it is simpler and more convenient for patients or parents to push a button than it is to open vials, draw medication into a syringe and inject medication into the infusion line. General discussion of PCA use in children is given in Chapter 42. In palliative care, pushing the PCA button is often not limited to patients, and parents and nurses frequently participate in dosing.

Transdermal administration of fentanyl via a patch is a convenient method to provide sustained analgesia without the need for intravenous access or infusion pumps (Payne 1992, Patt et al 1993). Paediatric studies are in progress, but preliminary analyses suggest good efficacy and safety in a small population of paediatric oncology patients. These formulations should be used with caution in opioid-naïve patients or in patients with rapidly changing analgesic requirements. The lowest delivery rate currently available in the USA is 25 μg/h, which may be excessive for some children. There is a considerable delay in obtaining steady-state concentrations, and initial titration to comfort by other routes is required (Zech et al 1992). Absorption may be impaired by severe oedema or impaired circulation, which can be a factor in end-of-life care. For patients with fluctuating pain intensity, another method of opioid administration is required for rescue dosing. These considerations are especially important in the treatment of terminal symptoms, such as air hunger.

Oral transmucosal fentanyl produces a rapid onset of effect and bypasses first-pass hepatic clearance. As noted above, OTFC is effective for painful procedures, but it has also been used successfully for adults for breakthrough pain due to tumour (Fine et al 1991). Data on OTFC for tumour-related pain in children are limited.

Management of opioid side effects

As with adults, the key to the successful use of opioids lies in individualized dosing and the treatment of side effects (Table 42.3). Constipation should be prevented and treated with laxatives. Several classes of antiemetics, including $5HT_3$ antagonists, phenothiazines, butyrophenones, antihistamines and cannabinoids, have been used effectively for opioid-induced nausea in children. The largest studies of nausea in children have either been for postoperative nausea

Table 42.3 Management of opioid side effects. (Adapted from Collins & Berde 1997)

Side effect	*Treatment*
Constipation	1. Regular use of stimulant and stool softener laxatives (fibre, fruit juices are often insufficient) 2. Ensure adequate water intake
Sedation	1. If analgesia is adequate, try dose reduction 2. Unless contraindicated, add non-sedating analgesics, such as acetaminophen or NSAIDs, and reduce opioid dosing as tolerated 3. If sedation persists, try methylphenidate or dextroamphetamine 0.05–0.2 mg/kg PO b.i.d. in early a.m. and midday 4. Consider an opioid switch
Nausea	1. Exclude disease processes (e.g. bowel obstruction, increased intracranial pressure) 2. Antiemetics (phenothiazines, ondansetron, hydroxyzine) 3. Consider an opioid switch
Urinary retention	1. Exclude disease processes (e.g. bladder neck obstruction by tumour, impending cord compression, hypovolaemia, renal failure, etc.) 2. Avoid other drugs with anticholinergic effects (e.g. tricyclics, antihistamines) 3. Consider short-term use of bethanechol or Crede manoeuvre 4. Consider short-term catheterization 5. Consider opioid dose reduction if analgesia adequate or an opioid switch if analgesia inadequate
Pruritus	1. Exclude other causes (e.g. drug allergy, cholestasis) 2. Antihistamines (e.g. diphenhydramine hydroxyzine) 3. Consider an opioid dose reduction if analgesia adequate, or an opioid switch. Fentanyl causes less histamine release
Respiratory depression Mild–Moderate	1. Awaken, encourage to breathe 2. Apply oxygen 3. Withhold opioid dosing until breathing improves, reduce subsequent dosing by at least 25%
Severe	1. Awaken if possible, apply oxygen, assist respiration by bag and mask as needed 2. Titrate small doses of naloxone (0.02 mg/kg increments as needed) stop when respiratory rate increases to 8–10/min in older children or 12–16/min in infants, do not try to awaken fully with naloxone DO NOT GIVE A BOLUS DOSE OF NALOXONE AS SEVERE PAIN AND SYMPTOMS OF OPIOID WITHDRAWAL MAY ENSUE 3. Consider a low-dose naloxone infusion or repeated incremental dosing 4. Consider short-term intubation in occasional cases where risk of aspiration is high
Dysphoria/confusion/ hallucinations	1. Exclude other pathology as a cause for these symptoms before attributing them to opioids 2. When other causes excluded, change to another opioid 3. Consider adding a neuroleptic such as haloperidol (0.01–0.1 mg/kg PO/IV every 8 h to a maximum dose of 30 mg/day)
Myoclonus	1. Usually seen in the setting of high-dose opioids, or alternatively, rapid dose escalation 2. No treatment may be warranted, if this is infrequent and not distressing to the child 3. Consider an opioid switch or treat with clonezepam (0.01 mg/kg PO every 12 h to a maximum dose of 0.5 mg/dose) or a parenteral benzodiazepine (e.g. diazepam) if the oral route is not tolerated

or chemotherapy-induced nausea, rather than in palliative care, but similar dosing is generally used.

Opioid dose escalation

Opioid dose requirements for children with widespread cancer vary greatly. Opioids are likely to be similar in their population prevalence of side effects, but there may be marked individual variability in these effects. Recently, Galer et al (1992) described a series of cases which showed incomplete cross-tolerance when switching from one opioid to another, and markedly different efficacy or ratio of analgesia to side effects with different opioids. Incomplete cross-tolerance between opioids is especially pronounced when switching from morphine or hydromorphone to methadone. This appears to be a consequence of the NMDA receptor blocking activity of the d-isomer of methadone in the racemic commercial preparations (Elliott et al 1995, Bilsky et al 1996, Gorman et al 1997).

If intolerable side effects are found with dose escalation with one opioid, a trial of a second opioid should be considered, beginning at perhaps 25–50% of the equianalgesic dose in the case of most opioids, or 15–25% of the equianalgesic dose if methadone is chosen. Tolerance to sedation, nausea and vomiting, pruritus often develop within the first week of commencing opioids.

Patients and parents are often reluctant to increase dosing because of a fear that tolerance will make opioids ineffective at a later date. They should be reassured that tolerance usually can be managed by simple dose escalation, the use of adjunctive medications or opioid switching. There is no justification for withholding opioids to save them for a later time of need. Fears of drug addiction can also be a barrier to opioid use.

Among adults with cancer, rapid opioid dose escalation is most commonly a result of tumour spread, rather than rapidly progressive tolerance (Collin et al 1993). We reported on patterns of opioid administration among 199 children who died of malignancy at Boston Children's Hospital and the Dana-Farber Cancer Institute from 1989 to 1993, a time during which the WHO programme was more consistently applied (Collins et al 1995a). Over 90% remained comfortable during their terminal course with standard opioid dose escalation and side-effect management.

Two subgroups required more intensive management. One group of six patients had intolerable side effects before reaching dose escalation more than 100-fold above standard starting rates (i.e. above 3 mg/kg/h IV morphine equivalents). All of these patients could be made comfortable by regional anaesthetic approaches (see below). A second group of 12 patients (6% of the overall group) escalated their systemic dosing to greater than 3 mg/kg/h intravenous morphine equivalent. Rapid dose escalation was most common in the final weeks of life. Eleven out of 12 of these patients had solid tumours metastatic to the spine, central nervous system or major nerve plexus. Maximum opioid dosing ranged from 3.8 to 518 mg/kg/h IV morphine equivalent. Among these 12 patients, four were comfortable primarily with opioid escalation, but the rest required either regional anaesthesia or continuous sedation.

Adjunctive medications

Tricyclic antidepressants are widely used for neuropathic pain, as well as to facilitate sleep. Paediatric use of tricyclics for pain is largely extrapolated from adult trials. Reviews of antidepressants in children are given elsewhere (Steingard et al 1995, Birmaher 1998). Commence with a single night-time dosing of tricyclics in most patients. If dose escalation is tolerated without sedation, a smaller morning dose can be added. Plasma levels can be useful to guide titration. Electrocardiograms are recommended for screening for rhythm disturbances and to follow changes on therapy, but little is known about their predictive value for risk of severe arrhythmias or cardiac events due to tricyclics. Additional caution should be exercised with patients who have signs of cardiac dysfunction or ectopy due to anthracyclines. In selected cases where the oral route is not feasible, an injectable preparation of amitriptyline can be used intravenously with very slow infusion and monitoring of dose titration (Collins et al 1995b).

For children with limiting sedation from opioids, some success has been found with the use of stimulants, especially methylphenidate and dextroamphetamine (Bruera et al 1989, Yee & Berde 1994). Overall, the lack of serious adverse reactions, and the improvement in alertness in many cases, have been impressive. Typically, methylphenidate is started with morning and noontime dosing of 0.1 mg/kg, with dose escalation as necessary up to roughly 0.6 mg/kg/day.

Benzodiazepines are useful for sedation for noxious procedures. They are often overused for persistent anxiety. The prolonged use of benzodiazepines for sleep disturbance is discouraged, because with chronic use they disrupt sleep cycles, produce tolerance and dependence, and can exacerbate daytime somnolence and confusion.

Corticosteroids are used in adults in a range of settings for cancer pain, including headache as a result of brain tumours, for nerve compression, for epidural spinal cord compression and for metastatic bone disease (Watanabe & Bruera 1994). They can be useful for shorter-term pain relief in children as well, although a number of sequelae can arise from prolonged use, including mood disturbances, a cushingoid body habitus, cataracts, immunosuppression and fractures.

Anticonvulsants

Anticonvulsants should be considered for pain of neuropathic origin. It has been taught that anticonvulsants are more effective for lancinating pains and paroxysmal pains rather than burning pains, but this has been questioned. Lancinating neuropathic pain and other episodic neuropathic pains characterized by a paroxysmal onset are considered to be an indication for a trial of anticonvulsants. Carbamazepine, phenytoin, clonezepam, gabapentin and valproate have all been used, but the evidence is not clear on the relative risks and benefits among these agents in children. Sedation, ataxia and dysphoria are common symptoms.

Neuroleptics

Phenothiazines and butyrophenones can be used as antiemetics. Their use as 'chemical straightjackets' for patients with pain should be discouraged. In general, they are not analgesic, but may reduce the reporting of pain. Methotrimeprazine is used in some centres more specifically as an adjuvant analgesic (Beaver et al 1966), although published experience in children is limited. Methotrimeprazine is highly sedating, and may diminish acute agitation in some patients.

INTERVENTIONAL APPROACHES TO PAIN MANAGEMENT FOR CHILDREN WITH CANCER

Epidural and spinal analgesic infusions

A percentage of adults with widespread cancer and difficult to control pain can be made comfortable by the use of spinal analgesic infusions (Plummer et al 1991, Eisenach et al 1995) and neurodestructive procedures (Brown et al 1987, Plancarte et al 1990). Experience with these approaches in children is more limited (Patt et al 1995, Staats & Kost-Byerly 1995, Collins et al 1996b), and we approach them with considerable caution.

In considering such an approach it is essential first to optimize pharmacological and non-pharmacological approaches. It is crucial to consider the wishes of the child and her parents in the context of a realistic appraisal of her disease and its likely progression.

Our recommendations for the use of regional anaesthetic approaches for the management of pain caused by advanced cancer in children is outlined in Box 42.5.

It is important to emphasize that spinal infusions can be excellent for relieving pain in refractory cases, but they

BOX 42.5

Recommendations for use of epidural and spinal infusions for the management of pain due to widespread cancer in children

1. Optimize use of non-pharmacological approaches, opioids and adjuvants first
2. Do not promise perfect pain relief
3. Be clear with patients and their parents regarding the potential for adverse events and side effects. Where local anaesthetics are used, warn them about the potential for degrees of motor and sensory blockade and impairment of bowel or bladder function
4. Place catheters under general anaesthesia or deep sedation, not awake
5. Use fluoroscopic guidance whenever available to ensure proper localization while the child is asleep
6. It is preferable to tunnel catheters with initial placement for improved skin care
7. The key to success is precise dermatomal application of local anaesthetics; opioids alone are rarely sufficient to achieve an improved therapeutic index. Combine opioids with local anaesthetics, and occasionally add other drugs, such as clonidine
8. For pain below the umbilicus, lumbar subarachnoid catheters are preferred; for pain in higher dermatomes, thoracic epidural placement with the catheter tip in the middle of the most important dermatomes innervating the painful area is preferred. The subarachnoid route gives the greatest flexibility in escalating local anaesthetic dosing to achieve de-afferentation with a margin of safety. With prolonged epidural infusions, local anaesthetic dosing is restricted by concerns for systemic toxicity
9. Epidural tumour may impede placement, or prevent drug spread to intended sites. Radiographic confirmation of spread of contrast helps ensure a likelihood of access of drug to intended target sites
10. The optimal combination of drugs must be individualized based on both previous analgesic use, the nature and location of the pain, and the patient's individual preferences in balancing analgesia with side effects. Dose escalation is often needed

require a great deal of individualized attention, and should not be undertaken by inexperienced practitioners without guidance. Dose requirements vary dramatically, and the process of converting from a systemic to a spinal drug is often quite unpredictable, with the potential for either oversedation or withdrawal symptoms. If children with spinal infusions are to be managed at home, it is essential to have resources available to manage new symptoms, such as terminal dyspnoea and air hunger.

Neurodestructive procedures

As with adults (Mercadante 1993), coeliac plexus blockade can provide excellent pain relief for children with severe pain due to massively enlarged upper abdominal viscera caused by tumour (Berde et al 1990, Staats & Kost-Byerly 1995). Many children and parents are reluctant to consider procedures with the potential for irreversible loss of somatic function. A discussion of considerations for neurosurgical approaches to pain in childen has been summarized elsewhere (Rossitch & Madsen 1993). Cordotomy was successfully applied in an era when opioid use in children was less refined (Matson 1969). Decompressive operations on the spine can in some cases produce dramatic relief of pain (Rossitch & Madsen 1993). Treatment algorithms for epidural spinal cord compression depend on a number of issues, and may also involve the use of high-dose steroids, chemotherapy and radiation therapy (Greenberg et al 1980).

SEDATION IN END-OF-LIFE CARE

Opioids generally relieve pain with a partial preservation of clarity of sensorium, although many patients require doses of opioids that make them sedated when undisturbed, but rousable when spoken to (Coyle et al 1990). Patients and their families can be told that comfort can be achieved with opioids in most situations (Foley 1997). Providers need to reassure parents that by treating pain with opioids they are not causing their child's death; that the child's disease is the cause of death.

There remains a very small subgroup of patients who have intolerable side effects and/or inadequate analgesia despite the extremely aggressive use of analgesics as outlined above. While regional anaesthetic approaches may be chosen by some patients and families, others will chose continuous sedation as a means of relieving suffering.

The choice of sedation as a method of relief of suffering generally assumes there is no feasible or acceptable means for providing analgesia with preservation of alertness. If sedation is chosen, we favour continuing high-dose opioid infusions to reduce the possibility that a patient might experience unrelieved pain but be too sedated to report on it. The ethical and practical issues around providing sedation in the terminally ill have been discussed (Truog et al 1992, Foley 1997). Sedation for terminally ill patients is widely regarded as providing comfort, not euthanasia, according to the principle of double-effect (Foley 1997), although others describe some difficult logical consequences in the use of this ethical justification (Quill et al 1997). Many clinicians and ethicists with a range of views regarding assisted suicide and euthanasia agree on the following position: no child or parent should choose death because of our profession's inadequate efforts to relieve pain and suffering, to ameliorate depression, fear and isolation, or to provide spiritual and emotional support.

HUMAN IMMUNODEFICIENCY VIRUS AND THE ACQUIRED IMMUNE DEFICIENCY SYNDROME

Infants now acquire the human immunodeficiency virus (HIV) predominantly through transplacental infection from their mothers (Grossman 1988). Transfusion-acquired HIV is declining in prevalence in developed countries, although new cases of transfusion-acquired disease continue in some developing countries. Adolescents become infected through sexual contact and infected needles.

In developed countries, the prognosis for congenitally acquired HIV infection has improved dramatically in recent years as a result of multidrug therapies. Access to these treatments is severely limited in developing countries, and the majority of infants with the acquired immune deficiency syndrome (AIDS) in Africa continue to suffer cachexia, neurological devastation and early death.

Children with HIV infection with access to sophisticated medical treatment undergo an enormous number of invasive diagnostic and therapeutic procedures which produce pain and distress (Hirschfeld et al 1996). Many of the principles outlined above for the treatment of oncological procedures apply for children with HIV.

In developing countries and in infants in developed countries with less access to care, HIV-induced neurological degeneration can produce severe irritability and the appearance of poorly localized pain. Experience by M. Strafford and co-workers (personal communication) found that, in many cases, opioids diminished these distress behaviours better than sedative-hypnotics. This experience differs somewhat from the general impression of treatment of infants with some other neurodegenerative disorders, as outlined below.

Many infants and children with HIV are orphaned or in foster care. Many are cared for by grandparents or other relatives, but some remain in hospital or hospice care during palliative care because they have no other place to go. In major cities, infants and children with HIV represent a growing population for whom hospice, as opposed to home palliative care, may be a reasonable option. Because some of their parents were infected through needles in illicit drug use, there may be considerable resistance by relatives to administering opioids to these infants.

CYSTIC FIBROSIS

Cystic fibrosis is the most common life-shortening genetic disorder in Caucasian populations. It is a multisystem disorder that arises in different families from one of a series of similar autosomal recessive mutations in a gene encoding a chloride channel. Cystic fibrosis affects a range of organs, including pancreas, intestines, liver, paranasal sinuses and sweat glands, but the predominant cause of morbidity, mortality and suffering is chronic obstructive lung disease. The ion channel abnormality leads to viscous pulmonary secretions, bronchiectasis, and a particular susceptibility to airways colonization or infection with mucoid strains of *Pseudomonas aeruginosa*.

Longevity among patients with cystic fibrosis has improved dramatically over the past 30 years. The median age at death was less than age 20 in the 1960s. In many centres today, the median survival is approaching age 40. There remains a smaller subgroup of patients with rapidly progressive lung disease who are in respiratory failure during their teenage years.

Improved survival has been ascribed to better antibiotics, better nutritional support or the use of chest physiotherapy, although there is little consensus on the relative importance of each of these therapies. Newer approaches include the use of inhaled antibiotics, and inhaled deoxyribonuclease enzyme (to reduce sputum viscosity).

Patients with advanced lung disease suffer several types of distressing symptoms. There can be severe near-constant dyspnoea and air hunger. There is a constant need to cough in an attempt to clear their airways of tenacious sputum, and often the coughing is extremely intense. The high airways resistance and high ratio of alveolar dead space to tidal volume leads to dramatically increased work of breathing and fatigue.

Sleep is often disturbed, and many people with cystic fibrosis develop a fear that they will suffocate during sleep. This may lead them to stay up much of the night and sleep in the daytime. Small evening doses of antidepressants may improve sleep. Some tolerate tricyclics, such as nortriptyline. Others are bothered by the peripheral anticholinergic actions in drying their secretions, and instead prefer the tetracyclic, trazodone.

Ravilly and co-workers (1996) in our group documented a high prevalence of chronic daily headache and chest pain in patients with advanced cystic fibrosis. Headache appears multifactorial, and is usually poorly characterized. Although in many cases hypoxaemia and hypercapnia are present and appear to worsen headache, others experience daily headache before blood-gas abnormalities can be demonstrated. Constant violent coughing may contribute to the headache, both by associated muscle contraction of the scalp and neck muscles, and possibly because of frequent and profound fluctuations in intracranial pressure. Nasal polyposis and sinusitis is ubiquitous, and often contributes to headache.

Chest pain in cystic fibrosis is also multifactorial. Chronic daily chest pain may be caused, in part, by intercostal muscle fatigue and overuse, both due to the work of breathing, and due to coughing. Acute episodes of chest pain with localized rib tenderness may indicate a rib fracture. In many cases of acute rib pain with normal radiographs, there is a periosteal tear of the intercostal muscle attachments, or a stress fracture. This view is supported by the finding that many of these patients with normal radiographs have a 'hot spot' on a bone scan at the site of their acute pain. Acute-onset chest pain with dyspnoea may also herald a pneumothorax.

The prevalence of headache and chest pain increases dramatically in the final year of life, and the majority of patients in their final 6 months of life have chronic daily headache and chest pain.

With a genetic disorder such as cystic fibrosis, the psychological implications for end-of-life and palliative care are different from those for patients with cancer. Most of these patients are aware of their shortened lifespan from an early age. Conversely, as the natural history of the disease has changed, patients' concepts of their illness have changed. Many adults with cystic fibrosis currently in the age range 35–45 years were told during childhood not to expect to live beyond age 20.

Patients with cystic fibrosis die predominantly as a result of respiratory failure, with progressive hypoxaemia and hypercapnia. Prominent symptoms at the end of life are fatigue, dyspnoea, severe coughing, air hunger and headache. Opioids can provide some relief of these symptoms. In some cases, opioids may exacerbate headache by worsening hypercapnia. Benzodiazepines are often administered as well for the relief of agitation and anxiety associated with terminal dyspnoea.

Patients' concepts of their illness have also been dramatically altered by the development of lung transplantation and heart–lung transplantation. While in the past cystic fibrosis was regarded as a disorder with no definitive treatment, lung transplantation offers the hope to many of an end to their dyspnoea and coughing. Lung transplantation at present is severely limited by several factors:

1. A severe shortage of organ donors.
2. A significant early mortality because of acute rejection, infection and perioperative complications.
3. Late mortality as a result of progressive pulmonary deterioration known as bronchiolitis obliterans, which may a form of chronic rejection.

A few centres are attempting to circumvent the shortage of cadaveric organ donors by having living related donation of lung segments from two family members. Many patients who have received lung transplantation in general report improved quality of life, despite their need for intensive medical support.

Even though lung transplantation is currently available for only a small percentage of people with cystic fibrosis, its availability has altered views of the illness and end-of-life care. Robinson and co-workers (1997) in our group documented a dramatic increase in the use of intensive care units for end-of-life care since the beginning of a lung transplant programme at our hospital. Before this, the vast majority of patients with cystic fibrosis in our centre died on the adolescent-young adult unit, not in the intensive care unit. In the current era, the great majority of patients with advanced disease in our centre now die on a waiting list for transplantation, and a higher percentage are in an intensive care unit. Non-invasive assisted ventilation is frequently tried, but is of limited effectiveness in this disorder in its advanced stages. Home care for end-of-life care is rarely chosen by our patients with cystic fibrosis. Many of our patients report fear of suffocation, and say that they prefer to be in hospital for end-of-life care, to ensure that they will receive adequate opioids and sedatives to relieve air hunger. This preference for hospital care is also shared by the subgroup of patients who have made longstanding decisions in favour of do-not-resuscitate and do-not-intubate orders. This pattern of preference for in-hospital care is not universal; in other centres, a greater proportion of patients with cystic fibrosis die at home (Westwood 1998).

NEURODEGENERATIVE DISORDERS

There is a wide range of neurological or neuromuscular disorders among infants and children that may be associated with suffering (Hunt & Burne 1995) and/or a shortened lifespan. Although any one of these conditions is relatively rare, taken together they affect considerable numbers of children who may require symptom management, palliative care or end-of-life care. These disorders vary greatly in their effects on longevity and quality of life, and on their spectrum of cognitive versus motor impairments. Some disorders, such as Tay–Sachs disease, may cause profound cognitive and motor devastation and death in the first years of life. Conversely, patients with spinal muscular atrophy have intact intelligence, and a range of motor impairments according to subtype. At another other end of the spectrum, Duchenne's muscular dystrophy leaves cognition intact and produces slowly progressive weakness, cardiomyopathy and restrictive lung disease. Depending on its course and on the use of mechanical ventilation, many people with Duchenne's muscular dystrophy are now living well into their twenties.

Decision making in these disorders is complicated by several factors. Making a specific diagnosis in some cases is difficult or delayed. Even when a diagnosis is made, the prognosis can be extremely variable, with the same condition having either a rapidly progressive or slow clinical course (Davies 1996).

Many neurological and neuromuscular disorders impair cognition and communication abilities. These factors may make it extremely difficult to determine whether the child is experiencing pain and, if so, to determine what is causing the pain.

Some children with neurodegenerative disorders may have persistent screaming or agitation with no apparent cause after extensive medical evaluation to exclude the common treatable cause, such as gastro-oesophageal reflux, hip dislocation or otitis media. These children can be extraordinarily distressing to their parents, who want physicians to find out what is causing pain and fix it. A limited experience with drug trials suggests that many of these children continue to be agitated despite intravenous opioid titration to near-apnoea. Even when an opioid trial is ineffective for relieving pain, it may be a comfort to the parents that an attempt was made to relieve distress. By contrast, some of these children with distress of unknown origin have reduced distress with anticonvulsants, even when there are no clinical or electroencephalographic signs of seizures. In other cases, the GABA agonist baclofen has appeared effective. There is a need for more systematic study of the roles and risk benefit ratios of anticonvulsants and sedatives in children with unremitting agitation.

Mechanical ventilation is traditionally regarded as an invasive, painful, extreme or extraordinary measure for many illnesses. Increasingly, many children with myopathies and other disorders characterized predominantly by motor weakness, are now receiving mechanical ventilation both to prolong survival and to improve quality of life. Improvements in nasal or face-mask non-invasive positive-pressure devices have made it possible in many cases to support the work of breathing and maintain lung volumes without the need for tracheotomy. Many children use these devices at night-time only, with sustained improvement in their sleep quality and daytime functioning. Non-invasive assisted ventilation may be insufficient for more severely affected children, particularly for those who can no longer control bulbar musculature.

HOME, HOSPICE OR HOSPITAL CARE

There is no single 'correct' location for end-of-life care. Children and their families should feel free to choose home, a free-standing hospice, a community hospital or a paediatric tertiary care hospital for end-of-life care (Stevens et al 1994, Frager 1996, Liben 1996, Goldman 1996, Goldman 1998, Dangel 1998).

Home has the advantage of a 'natural' and 'safe' environment where the child may feel loved, more in control of her surroundings, and less susceptible to the torments of medical intervention. World-wide experience from well-organized paediatric palliative care teams shows that they are able to provide services effectively, and most children and parents appear to feel safe and well cared for at home (Goldman 1996, Kopecky et al 1997). Families should not be 'pushed out the door' against their wishes because of a belief by the medical and nursing staff that 'home is best'.

Optimum home care requires planning for contingencies that account for issues related to making things work in the child's community. Support from the local community including clergy can be extremely beneficial. Home care requires local solutions to a range of practical problems, including availability of supplies (e.g. medications, oxygen, special beds). For children with severe pain, the importance of anticipatory planning for adequate opioid availability cannot be emphasized enough. Children in remote areas may use up all their opioid on a weekend day, and be left in pain for extended periods of time. Direct contact with home-care pharmacies and nurses can anticipate or fix these problems in many cases. Some pharmacies will accept faxed prescriptions in these situations.

For some children and families, there is a safety and security in continued care by the physicians, nurses, psychologists, child life specialists and other caregivers who have guided them through curative therapy. There is a strong connection with their nurses and their specialist physicians in oncology, infectious diseases, pulmonology or neurology who have guided them through diagnosis and treatment for cancer, AIDS, cystic fibrosis or spinal muscular atrophy.

Because of the strong connection between families and their caregivers in paediatric tertiary centres, in many parts of the world a predominant model involves home care with ongoing connection to tertiary hospital specialist physicians and nurses who had previously been involved in curative care (Sirkia et al 1997). Another model involves home care with transfer of care to specific palliative care physicians and nurses (Goldman 1996, 1998). There are few data to recommend one model over another. In great measure, the success or failure of one or another approach will depend both on organizational factors that facilitate delivery of care, as well as on the personal style, expertise, commitment and manner of the caregivers.

Free-standing hospices have been established in many parts of the world, both as a place for children to come to for end-of-life care and as a site for coordinating home care (Eng 1995, Davies 1996, Aquino & Perszyk 1997, Faulkner 1997, Deeley et al 1998, Thompson 1998). Paediatric free-standing hospices face formidable challenges related to size of appropriate populations, staffing, finances and patterns of relationship to paediatric medical centres.

One approach to facilitate staffing and coverage is to have these centres provide two distinct services: (i) hospice/end-of-life care and (ii) respite care for children with profound disabilities. Caring for a child with serious illness or major disabilities is physically and emotionally exhausting for parents. Respite care for as brief a time as 2–5 days can help the parents and siblings get a break from this work.

Discussions regarding do-not-resuscitate and do-not-intubate orders and no heroic measures must be tailored to the child's particular prognosis, to the child's and parents' views of illness and cure, and to their coping and cognitive styles. Caregivers must be aware of ethnic, cultural and sociological differences in how families will respond to these discussions. The truth can be told in many ways (De Trill & Kovalcik 1997).

DEATHS IN INTENSIVE CARE UNITS AND IN THE OPERATING ROOM

Many neonates, infants and children die in intensive care units. In some cases, critical illness and death have no warning, as in infants with sudden infant death syndrome or children following motor vehicle accidents. In other cases, death follows prenatal diagnosis (Pearson 1997), long-standing critical illness or planned surgery with known risks, such as cardiac operations. Efforts can be made even in these technologically oriented settings to relieve suffering, preserve dignity and permit parents' closeness to their child (Burns J, Truog R, Geller M, manuscript submitted). The removal of mechanical ventilation need not produce air hunger and distress; terminal sedation and analgesia should be provided as a comfort measure (Truog 1993). Many parents later report how important it was that they were permitted to hold their dying infant or child.

Bereavement programmes should be encouraged to provide ongoing support and connection (Carroll & Griffin 1997). Parents may respond very differently to the loss of a child, and these differences in their patterns of expressing grief can further strain their relationship (Vance et al 1995).

Siblings of children with terminal illness must confront a range of emotions, including sadness and grief over the loss of their sibling, jealousy and loneliness during the course of treatment because of parents directing more attention towards their sibling's needs, guilt because of a mistaken fantasy that something they did may have caused their sibling's illness and fear that a similar fate could befall them (Lehna 1995, Mahon & Page 1995, Gillance et al 1997).

CONCLUSIONS

Children with life-threatening illnesses should receive symptom management, emotional support and spiritual support that is adapted to their needs continuously from the time of diagnosis to end-of-life care. These approaches should be family centred and should consider developmental and cultural factors. More research is needed on assessing outcomes of different models of delivery of services. There is a need for more attention to supportive care for illnesses other than cancer, particularly neurodegenerative disorders.

REFERENCES

Abbott K, Fowler-Kerry S 1995 The use of a topical refrigerant anesthetic to reduce injection pain in children. Journal of Pain and Symptom Management 584

Anonymous 1993 American Academy of Pediatrics Committee on Hospital Care: child life programs. Pediatrics 91: 671–673

Aquino JY, Perszyk S 1997 Hospice Northeast and Nemours Children's Clinic, Jacksonville, Florida. American Journal of Hospice & Palliative Care 14: 248–250

Beaver WT, Wallenstein S, Houde RW, Rogers A 1966 A comparison of the analgesic effects of methotrimeprazine and morphine in patients with cancer. Clinical Pharmacology and Therapeutics 7: 436–446

Berde C 1995 Pediatric oncology procedures: to sleep or perchance to dream? Pain 62: 1–2

Berde CB, Sethna NF, Fisher DE, Kahn CH, Chandler P, Grier HE 1990 Celiac plexus blockade for a 3-year-old boy with hepatoblastoma and refractory pain Pediatrics 86: 779–781

Berde CB, Beyer JE, Bournaki MC, Levin CR, Sethna NF 1991 Comparison of morphine and methadone for prevention of postoperative pain in 3- to 7-year-old children. Journal of Pediatrics 136–141

Bilsky EJ, Inturrisi CF, Sadee W, Hruby VJ, Porreca F 1996 Competitive and non-competitive NMDA antagonists block the development of antinociceptive tolerance to morphine, but not to selective mu or delta opioid agonists in mice. Pain 68: 229–237

Birmaher B 1998 Should we use antidepressant medications for children and adolescents with depressive disorders? Psychopharmacology Bulletin 34: 35–39

Bjerring P, Arendt-Nielsen L 1993 Depth and duration of skin analgesia to needle insertion after topical application of EMLA cream. British Journal of Anaesthesia 64: 173–177

Bouffet E, Douard MC, Annequin D, Castaing MC, Pichard-Leandri E 1996 Pain in lumbar puncture. Results of a 2-year discussion at the French Society of Pediatric Oncology [in French]. Archives de Pediatrie 3: 22–27

Bowsher D 1997 The effects of pre-emptive treatment of postherpetic neuralgia with amitriptyline: a randomized, double-blind, placebo-controlled trial. Journal of Pain and Symptom Management 13: 327–331

Brazelton TB, Thompson RH 1988 Child life Pediatrics 81: 725–726

Brown DL, Bulley CK, Quiel EC 1987 Neurolytic celiac plexus block for pancreatic cancer pain. Anesthesia and Analgesia 66: 869–873

Bruera E, Brenneis C, Michaud M, MacMillan K, Hanson J, MacDonald RN 1988 Patient-controlled subcutaneous hydromorphone versus continuous subcutaneous infusion for the treatment of cancer pain. Journal of the National Cancer Institute 80: 1152–1154

Bruera E, Brenneis C, Paterson A, MacDonald R 1989 Use of methyphenidate as an adjuvant to narcotic analgetics in patients with advanced cancer. Journal of Pain and Symptom Management 4: 3–6

Bruera E, Brenneis C, Perry B, MacDonald RN 1994 Continuous subcutaneous administration of narcotics for the treatment of cancer pain. Knoll Pharmaceuticals, Edmonton

Camann WR, Murray RS, Mushlin PS, Lambert DH 1990 Effects of oral caffeine on postdural puncture headache. A double-blind, placebo-controlled trial. Anesthesia and Analgesia 70: 181–184

Carp H, Singh PJ, Vadhera R, Jayaram A 1994 Effects of the serotonin-receptor agonist sumatriptan on postdural puncture headache: report of six cases. Anesthesia and Analgesia 79: 180–182

Carrie LE 1993 Postdural puncture headache and extradural blood patch. British Journal of Anaesthesia 71: 179–181
Carroll ML, Griffin R 1997 Reframing life's puzzle: support for bereaved children. American Journal of Hospice and Palliative Care 14: 231–235
Choi A, Laurito CE, Cunningham FE 1996 Pharmacologic management of postdural puncture headache [Review]. Annals of Pharmacotherapy 30: 831–839
Collins JJ, Berde CB 1997 Pain management. In: Pizzo PA, Poplack DG (eds) Principles and practice of pediatric oncology. Philadelphia: Lippincott–Raven, pp 1183–1199
Collin E, Poulain P, Gauvain-Piquard A, Petit G, Pichard-Leandri E 1993 Is disease progression the major factor in morphine 'tolerance' in cancer pain treatment? Pain 55: 319–326
Collins JJ, Kerner J, Sentivany S, Berde CB 1995a Intravenous amitriptyline in pediatrics. Journal of Pain and Symptom Management 10: 471–475
Collins JJ, Grier HE, Kinney HC, Berde CB 1995b Control of severe pain in children with terminal malignancy [see comments]. Journal of Pediatrics 126: 653–657
Collins JJ, Geake J, Grier HE et al 1996a Patient-controlled analgesia for mucositis pain in children: a three-period crossover study comparing morphine and hydromorphone. Journal of Pediatrics 129: 722–728
Collins JJ, Grier HE, Sethna NF, Wilder RT, Berde CB 1996b Regional anesthesia for pain associated with terminal pediatric malignancy. Pain 65: 63–69
Cote CJ 1994 Sedation for the pediatric patient. A review. Pediatric Clinics of North America 41: 31–58
Coyle N, Adelhardt J, Foley KM, Portenoy RK 1990 Character of terminal illness in the advanced cancer patient: pain and other symptoms during the last four weeks of life [see comments]. Journal of Pain and Symptom Management 5: 83–93
Dangel T 1998 Chronic pain management in children. Part I: Cancer and phantom pain. Paediatric Anaesthesia 8: 5–10
Davies H 1996 Living with dying: families coping with a child who has a neurodegenerative genetic disorder. Axone 18: 38–44
de las Heras-Rosas MA, Rodriguez-Perez A, Ojeda-Betancor N, Boralla-Rivera G, Gallego-Alonso JI 1997 [Failure of sumatriptan in post-dural puncture headache (letter)] [Spanish]. Revista Espanola de Anestesiologia y Reanimacion 44: 378–379
De Trill M, Kovalcik R 1997 The child with cancer. Influence of culture on truth-telling and patient care. Annals of the New York Academy of Sciences 809: 197–210
Deeley L, Stallard P, Lewis M, Lenton S 1998 Palliative care services for children must adopt a family centred approach [letter]. British Medical Journal 317: 284
Doyle E, Freeman J, Im NT, Morton NS 1993 An evaluation of a new self-adhesive patch preparation of amethocaine for topical anaesthesia prior to venous cannulation in children. Anaesthesia 48: 1050–1052
Eisenach JC, DuPen S, Dubois M, Miguel R, Allin D 1995 Epidural clonidine analgesia for intractable cancer pain. The Epidural Clonidine Study Group. Pain 61: 391–399
Eisenberg E, Berkey CS, Carr DB et al 1994 Efficacy and safety of nonsteroidal antiinflammatory drugs for cancer pain: a meta-analysis. Journal of Clinical Oncology 12: 2756–2765
Elliott K, Kest B, Man A, Kao B, Inturrisi CE 1995 *N*-methyl-D-aspartate (NMDA) receptors, mu and kappa opioid tolerance, and perspectives on new analgesic drug development [Review]. Neuropsychopharmacology 13: 347–356
Faulkner KW 1997 Pediatric hospice reference library. American Journal of Hospice and Palliative Care 14: 228–230
Fine P, Marcus M, De Boer A, Van der Oord B 1991 An open label study of oral transmucosal fentanyl citrate (OTFC) for the treatment of breakthrough cancer pain. Pain 45: 149–153
Foley KM 1997 Competent care for the dying instead of physician-assisted suicide. New England Journal of Medicine 336: 54–58
Frager G 1996 Pediatric palliative care: building the model, bridging the gaps [Review]. Journal of Palliative Care 12: 9–12
Frankville DD, Spear RM, Dyck JB 1993 The dose of propofol required to prevent children from moving during magnetic resonance imaging. Anesthesiology 79: 953–958
Galer BS, Coyle N, Pasternak GW, Portenoy RK 1992 Individual variability in the response to different opioids: report of five cases. Pain 49: 87–91
Gamis AS, Knapp JF, Glenski JA 1989 Nitrous oxide analgesia in a pediatric emergency department. Annals of Emergency Medicine 18: 177–181
Gauvain-Piquard A, Rodary C, Rezvani A, Lemerle J 1984 Development of a new rating scale for the evaluation of pain in young children (2–6 years) with cancer. In: Rizzi R, Viscentin M (eds) Pain. Piccin/Butterworths, Padua, Italy, pp 383–390
Gauvain-Piquard A, Rodary C, Rezvani A, Lemerle J 1987 Pain in children aged 2–6 years: a new observational rating scale elaborated in a pediatric oncology unit – preliminary report. Pain 31: 177–188
Gillance H, Tucker A, Aldridge J, Wright JB 1997 Bereavement: providing support for siblings. Paediatric Nursing 9: 22–24
Gillin S, Sorkin LS 1998 Gabapentin reverses the allodynia produced by the administration of anti-GD2 ganglioside, an immunotherapeutic drug. Anesthesia and Analgesia 86: 111–116
Ginsberg B, Howell S, Glass PS et al 1996 Pharmacokinetic model-driven infusion of fentanyl in children. Anesthesiology 85: 1268–1275
Goldman A 1996 Home care of the dying child. Journal of Palliative Care 12: 16–19
Goldman A 1998 ABC of palliative care. Special problems of children [Review]. British Medical Journal 316: 49–52
Gorman AL, Elliott KJ, Inturrisi CE 1997 The d- and l-isomers of methadone bind to the non-competitive site on the *N*-methyl-D-aspartate (NMDA) receptor in rat forebrain and spinal cord. Neuroscience Letters 223: 5–8
Grant DM, Mauskopf JA, Bell L, Austin R 1997 Comparison of valaciclovir and acyclovir for the treatment of herpes zoster in immunocompetent patients over 50 years of age: a cost-consequence model. Pharmacotherapy 17: 333–341
Green SM, Rothrock SG 1997 Transient apnea with intramuscular ketamine [letter; comment]. American Journal of Emergency Medicine 15: 440–441
Greenberg HS, Kim J, Posner JB 1980 Epidural spinal cord compression from metastatic tumor: results with a new treatment protocol. Annals of Neurology 8: 361–366
Grimshaw D, Holroyd E, Anthony D, Hall DM 1995 Subcutaneous midazolam, diamorphine and hyoscine infusion in palliative care of a child with neurodegenerative disease. Child: Care, Health and Development, 21: 377–381
Grossman M 1988 Children with AIDS. Infectious Disease Clinics of North America 2: 533–541
Hahn YS, McLone DG 1984 Pain in children with spinal cord tumors. Child's Brain 11: 36–46
Halperin DL, Koren G, Attias D, Pellegrini E, Greenberg ML, Wyss M 1989 Topical skin anesthesia for venous, subcutaneous drug reservoir and lumbar punctures in children. Pediatrics 84: 281–284
Hill HF, Mackie AM, Coda BA, Iverson K, Chapman CR 1991 Patient-controlled analgesic administration. A comparison of steady-state morphine infusions with bolus doses. Cancer 67: 873–882
Hirschfeld S, Moss H, Dragisic K, Smith W, Pizzo PA 1996 Pain in pediatric human immunodeficiency virus infection: incidence and characteristics in a single-institution pilot study [see comments]. Pediatrics 98: 449–452
Hollman GA, Perloff WH 1995 Efficacy of oral ketamine for providing

sedation and analgesia to children requiring laceration repair [letter]. Pediatric Emergency Care 11: 399

Hunt A, Burne R 1995 Medical and nursing problems of children with neurodegenerative disease. Palliative Medicine 9: 19–26

Jay S, Elliot C, Katz E, Siegal S 1987 Cognitive-behavioral and pharmacologic interventions for children's distress during painful medical procedures. Journal of Consulting and Clinical Psychology 55: 860–865

Jay S, Elliott CH, Fitzgibbons I, Woody P, Siegel S 1995 A comparative study of cognitive behavior therapy versus general anesthesia for painful medical procedures in children [see comments]. Pain 62: 3–9

Jay SM, Ozolins M, Elliot C, Caldwell S 1983 Assessment of children's distress during painful medical procedures. Journal of Health Psychology 2: 133–147

Joranson DE, Gilson AM 1998 Regulatory barriers to pain management. Seminars in Oncology Nursing 14: 158–163

Kapelushnik V, Koren G, Solh H, Greenberg M, DeVeber L 1990 Evaluating the efficacy of EMLA in alleviating pain associated with lumbar puncture: comparison of open and double-blinded protocols in children. Pain 42: 31–34

Katz ER, Kellerman J, Siegel SE 1980 Behavioral distress in children with cancer undergoing medical procedures: developmental considerations. Journal of Consulting Care 48: 356–365

Katz E, Kellerman J, Ellenberg L 1987 Hypnosis in the reduction of acute pain and distress in children with cancer. Journal of Pediatric Psychology 12: 379–394

Kopecky EA, Jacobson S, Joshi P, Martin M, Koren G 1997 Review of a home-based palliative care program for children with malignant and non-malignant diseases. Journal of Palliative Care 13: 28–33

Krane EJ, Heller LB, Pomietto ML 1991 Incidence of phantom sensation and pain in pediatric amputees. Anesthesiology 75: A691

Kuttner L 1989 Management of young children's acute pain and anxiety during invasive medical procedures. Pediatrician 16: 39–44

Kuttner L, Bowman M, Teasdale M 1988 Psychological treatment of distress, pain and anxiety for young children with cancer. Developmental and Behavioral Pediatrics 9: 374–381

Lambert DH, Hurley RJ, Hertwig L, Datta S 1997 Role of needle gauge and tip configuration in the production of lumbar puncture headache. Regional Anesthesia 22: 66–72

Larson PJ, Miaskowski C, MacPhail L et al 1998 The PRO-SELF Mouth Aware program: an effective approach for reducing chemotherapy-induced mucositis. Cancer Nursing 21: 263–268

Lehna CR 1995 Children's descriptions of their feelings and what they found helpful during bereavement. American Journal of Hospice and Palliative Care 12: 24–30

Lewis DW, Packer RJ, Raney B, Rak IW, Belasco J, Lange B 1986 Incidence, presentation, and outcome of spinal cord disease in children with systematic cancer. Pediatrics 78: 438–443

Liben S 1996 Pediatric palliative medicine: obstacles to overcome. Journal of Palliative Care 12: 24–28

Litman RS 1997 Apnea and oxyhemoglobin desaturation after intramuscular ketamine administration in a 2-year-old child [letter; comment]. American Journal of Emergency Medicine 15: 547–548

Litman RS, Berkowitz RJ, Ward DS 1996 Levels of consciousness and ventilatory parameters in young children during sedation with oral midazolam and nitrous oxide [see comments]. Archives of Pediatrics and Adolescent Medicine 150: 671–675

Litman RS, Kottra JA, Berkowitz RJ, Ward DS 1997 Breathing patterns and levels of consciousness in children during administration of nitrous oxide after oral midazolam premedication. Journal of Oral and Maxillofacial Surgery 55: 1372–1379

McGrath PJ, Finley GA, Ritchie J 1994 Pain, Pain, Go Away. Association for the care of Children's Health, Bethesda, MD.

Mackie AM, Coda BC, Hill HF 1991 Adolescents use patient-controlled analgesia effectively for relief from prolonged oropharyngeal mucositis pain. Pain 46: 265–269

Mahon MM, Page ML 1995 Childhood bereavement after the death of a sibling. Holistic Nursing Practice 9: 15–26

Marx CM, Stein J, Tyler MK, Nieder ML, Shurin SB, Blumer JL 1997 Ketamine-midazolam versus meperidine-midazolam for painful procedures in pediatric oncology patients. Journal of Clinical Oncology 15: 94–102

Matson DD 1969 Neurosurgery of infancy and childhood, 2nd edn. Charles C. Thomas, Springfield IL, pp 847–851

Maunuksela EL, Rajantie J, Siimes MA 1986 Flunitrazepam-fentanyl-induced sedation and analgesia for bone marrow aspiration and needle biopsy in children. Acta Anaesthesiologica Scandinavica 30: 409–411

Maxwell LG, Yaster M 1996 The myth of conscious sedation [editorial; comment]. Archives of Pediatrics and Adolescent Medicine 150: 665–667

Melzack R, Israel R, Lacroix R, Schultz G 1997 Phantom limbs in people with congenital limb deficiency or amputation in early childhood. Brain 120: 1603–1620

Mercadante S 1993 Celiac plexus block versus analgesics in pancreatic cancer pain. Pain 52: 187–192

Miser AW, Miser JS, Clark BS 1980 Continous intravenous infusion of morphine sulfate for control of severe pain in children with terminal malignancy. Journal of Pediatrics 96: 930–932

Miser AW, Davis DM, Hughes CS, Mulne AF, Miser JS 1983 Continuous subcutaneous infusion of morphine in children with cancer. American Journal of Diseases of Children 137: 383–385

Miser AW, Dothage JA, Wesley M, Miser JS 1987a The prevalence of pain in a pediatric and young adult cancer population. Pain 29: 73–83

Miser AW, McCalla J, Dothage JA, Wesley M, Miser JS 1987b Pain as a presenting symptom in children and young adults with newly diagnosed malignancy. Pain 29: 85–90

Miser AW, Ayash D, Broda E et al 1988 Use of a patient controlled device for nitrous oxide administration to control procedure related pain in children and young adults with cancer. Clinical Journal of Pain 4: 5–10

Miser AW, Goh TS, Dose AM et al 1994 Trial of a topically administered local anesthetic (EMLA cream) for pain relief during central venous port accesses in children with cancer. Journal of Pain and Symptom Management 9: 259–264

Mitchell RK, Koury SI, Stone CK 1996 Respiratory arrest after intramuscular ketamine in a 2-year-old child [see comments]. American Journal of Emergency Medicine 14: 580–581

Parker RI, Mahan RA, Giugliano D, Parker MM 1997 Efficacy and safety of intravenous midazolam and ketamine as sedation for therapeutic and diagnostic procedures in children [see comments]. Pediatrics 99: 427–431

Patt R, Lustik S, Litman R 1993 The use of transdermal fentanyl in a six-year-old patient with neuroblastoma and diffuse abdominal pain. Journal of Pain and Symptom Management 8: 317–319

Patt R, Payne R, Farhat G, Reddy S 1995 Subarachnoid neurolytic block under general anesthesia in a 3-year-old with neuroblastoma. Clinical Journal of Pain 11: 143–146

Payne R 1992 Transdermal fentanyl: suggested recommendations for clinical use. Journal of Pain and Symptom Management 7: S40–44

Pearson L 1997 Family-centered care and the anticipated death of a newborn. Pediatric Nursing 23: 178–182

Peterfreund RA, Datta S, Ostheimer GW 1989 pH adjustment of local anesthetic solutions with sodium bicarbonate: laboratory evaluation of alkalinization and precipitation. Regional Anesthesia 14: 265–270

Plancarte R, Amescua C, Patt RB, Aldrete JA 1990 Superior hypogastric plexus block for pelvic cancer pain. Anesthesiology 73: 236–239

Plummer JL, Gourlay GK, Cherry DA, Cousins MJ 1988 Estimation of methadone clearance: application in the management of cancer pain. Pain 33: 313–322

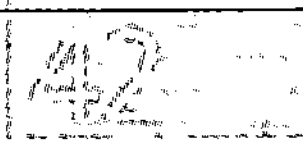

Plummer JL, Cherry DA, Cousins MJ, Gourlay GK, Onley MM, Evans KH 1991 Long-term spinal administration of morphine in cancer and non-cancer pain: a retrospective study. Pain 44: 215–220

Quill TE, Dresser R, Brock DW 1997 The rule of double effect – a critique of its role in end-of-life decision making [see comments]. New England Journal of Medicine 337: 1768–1771

Qureshi FA, Mellis PT, McFadden MA 1995 Efficacy of oral ketamine for providing sedation and analgesia to children requiring laceration repair. Pediatric Emergency Care 11: 93–97

Ravilly S, Robinson W, Suresh S, Wohl ME, Berde CB 1996 Chronic pain in cystic fibrosis. Pediatrics 98: 741–747

Robinson WM, Ravilly S, Berde C, Wohl ME 1997 End-of-life care in cystic fibrosis. Pediatrics 100: 205–209

Roelofse JA, Roelofse PG 1997 Oxygen desaturation in a child receiving a combination of ketamine and midazolam for dental extractions [Review]. Anesthesia Progress 44: 68–70

Rossitch E, Madsen JR 1993 Neurosurgical procedures for relief of pain in children and adolescents. In: Schechter NI, Berde CB, Yaster M (eds) Pain in infants, children and adolescents. Williams and Wilkins, Baltimore, pp 237–243

Rowbotham MC, Davies PS, Verkempinck C, Galer BS 1996 Lidocaine patch: double-blind controlled study of a new treatment method for post-herpetic neuralgia. Pain 65: 39–44

Ruffin JE, Creed JM, Jarvis C 1997 A retreat for families of children recently diagnosed with cancer [Review]. Cancer Practice 5: 99–104

Schechter N, Weisman S, Rosenblum M, Bernstein B, Conard P 1995 The use of oral transmucosal fentanyl citrate for painful procedures in children. Pediatrics 95: 335–339

Schechter NL, Blankson V, Pachter LM, Sullivan CM, Costa L 1997 The ouchless place: no pain, children's gain. Pediatrics 99: 890–894

Scholz J, Steinfath M, Schulz M 1996 Clinical pharmacokinetics of alfentanil, fentanyl and sufentanil. An update [Review]. Clinical Pharmacokinetics 31: 275–292

Sievers TD, Yee JD, Foley ME, Blanding PJ, Berde CB 1991 Midazolam for conscious sedation during pediatric oncology procedures: safety and recovery parameters. Pediatrics 88: 1172–1179

Sirkia K, Saarinen UM, Ahlgren B, Hovi L 1997 Terminal care of the child with cancer at home. Acta Paediatrica 86: 1125–1130

Staats PS, Kost-Byerly S 1995 Celiac plexus blockade in a 7-year-old child with neuroblastoma. Journal of Pain and Symptom Management 10: 321–324

Steggles S, Damore-Petingola S, Maxwell J, Lightfool N 1997 Hypnosis for children and adolescents with cancer: an annotated bibliography, 1985–1995. Journal of Pediatric Oncology Nursing 14: 27–32

Steingard RJ, DeMaso DR, Goldman SJ, Shorrock KL, Bucci JP 1995 Current perspectives on the pharmacotherapy of depressive disorders in children and adolescents [Review]. Harvard Review of Psychiatry 2: 313–326

Stevens M, Dalla Pozza L, Cavalletto B, Cooper M, Kilham H 1994 Pain and symptom control in paediatric palliative care [Review]. Cancer Surveys 21: 211–231

Symonds RP, McIlroy P, Khorrami J et al 1996. The reduction of radiation mucositis by selective decontamination antibiotic pastilles: a placebo-controlled double-blind trial. British Journal of Cancer 74: 312–317

Thompson M 1998 Children's hospices: 15 years on. Paediatric Nursing 10: 24

Tobias JD, Oakes L, Rao B 1992 Continuous epidural anesthesia for postoperative analgesia in the pediatric oncology patient. American Journal of Pediatric Hematology and Oncology 14: 216–221

Truog R, Brennan T 1993 Participation of physicians in capital punishment (see comments). New England Journal of Medicine 329: 1346–1350

Truog RD, Berde CB 1993 Pain, euthanasia, and anesthesiologists [see comments]. Anesthesiology 78: 353–360

Truog RD, Berde CB, Mitchell C, Grier HE 1992 Barbiturates in the care of the terminally ill. New England Journal of Medicine 327: 1678–1682

Valentin N, Bech B 1996 Ketamine anaesthesia for electrocochleography in children. Are psychic side effects really rare? Scandinavian Audiology 25: 39–43

Van Gerven M, Van Hemelrijck J, Wouters P, Vandermeersch E, Van Aken H 1992 Light anaesthesia with propofol for paediatric MRI. Anaesthesia 47: 706–707

Vance JC, Boyle FM, Najman JM, Thearle MJ 1995 Gender differences in parental psychological distress following perinatal death of sudden infant death syndrome. British Journal of Psychiatry 167: 806–811

Watanabe S, Bruera E 1994 Corticosteroids as adjuvant analgesics [Review]. Journal of Pain and Symptom Management 9: 442–445

Watson CP, Babul N 1998 Efficacy of oxycodone in neuropathic pain: a randomized trial in postherpetic neuralgia. Neurology 50: 1837–1841

Westwood AT, 1998 Terminal care in cystic fibrosis: hospital versus home? [letter]. Pediatrics 102: 436–437

Wood MJ, Kay R, Dworkin RH, Soong SJ and Whitley RJ 1996 Oral acyclovir therapy accelerates pain resolution in patients with herpes zoster: a meta-analysis of placebo-controlled trials. Clinical Infectious Diseases 22: 341–347

Yee JD, Berde CB 1994 Dextroamphetamine or methylphenidate as adjuvants to opioid analgesia for adolescents with cancer. Journal of Pain and Symptom Management 9: 122–125

Zech D, Ground S, Lynch J, Dauer H, Stollenwerk B, Lehmann K 1992 Transdermal fentanyl and initial dose-finding with patient-controlled analgesia in cancer pain. A pilot study with 20 terminally ill cancer patients. Pain 50: 293–301

Zeltzer L, Jay S, Fisher D 1989 The management of pain associated with pediatric procedures. Pediatric Clinics of North America 36: 941–964

Zeltzer L, Regalado M, Nichter LS, Barton D, Jennings S, Pitt L 1991 Iontophoresis versus subcutaneous injection: a comparison of two methods of local anesthesia delivery in children. Pain 44: 73–87

Zucker TP, Flesche CW, Germing U et al 1998 Patient-controlled versus staff-controlled analgesia with pethidine after allogeneic bone marrow transplantation. Pain 75: 305–312

Pain in the elderly

LUCIA GAGLIESE, JOEL KATZ & RONALD MELZACK

SUMMARY

Despite growing empirical attention, much remains to be learned about the effects of ageing on pain. There appear to be age differences in experimental, acute and chronic pain. Increasing age is associated with higher pain threshold, lower tolerance and impaired ability to discriminate between suprathreshold levels of noxious stimuli. Clinically, the elderly are less likely than younger patients to report pain associated with acute pathology, and they may report lower levels of postoperative pain. The prevalence of chronic pain appears to peak at mid-life and decrease thereafter. Nonetheless, many elderly people report pain. Among chronic pain patients, there may be a change in the quality but not the intensity of chronic pain with age. The affective and cognitive components of pain do not appear to be age related. Each of these conclusions, however, is limited by the pain scales employed in the studies. These measures have only begun to be validated for use with the elderly. These data suggest that verbal descriptor scales of pain intensity as well as the McGill Pain Questionnaire are appropriate across the adult lifespan, but this may not be true of visual analogue scales. Chronic pain in the elderly is often undertreated. This may be due, in part, to the increased risks associated with pharmacotherapy in this group. However, the elderly benefit substantially from psychological and physical treatment methods. Multidisciplinary approaches may be the treatment of choice for the elderly patient. Misconceptions regarding the relationship between pain and ageing and the willingness of the elderly to participate in non-pharmacological treatments may hamper appropriate care in this group. However, intense pain which interferes with functioning is not a normal part of ageing and should never be accepted as such.

INTRODUCTION

Despite growing empirical attention to the problems of pain assessment and management in the elderly, much remains to be learned about the effects of ageing on pain. The elderly, especially those over 80 years of age, are the fastest growing segment of the population (US Department of Commerce 1991). This trend, known as the 'graying of the population', has been documented throughout the world (Ferrell 1996) and has important implications for the study of pain. With increasing numbers of elderly people, it becomes ever more urgent that age-related changes in the experience and management of pain be understood so that appropriate steps can be taken to diminish needless suffering among this especially vulnerable age group (Melzack 1988).

Unfortunately, the research in this area is replete with studies which report radically different effects of ageing on pain. The inconsistencies in this literature have been so great, in fact, that various reviewers have drawn contradictory conclusions from the same data. This may be due to several factors, including methodological weaknesses and variability across studies, and the use of measures which have not been validated for the elderly.

This chapter describes the validity and reliability of popular pain scales in the elderly. While some of the most commonly used scales have been shown to be appropriate for this age group, the validity of the visual analogue scale may be compromised by low completion rates and lack of agreement with other measures. The data regarding age differences in the experience of experimental, acute and chronic pain will then be critically reviewed. These different types of pain each have their own function, emotional meanings and perceived consequences, which may make generalizations across them questionable (Melzack & Wall 1988). For instance, an increase in the experimental pain threshold in the elderly does not imply that comparable differences will be seen in the clinical setting. Finally, pain management strategies for the elderly will be discussed for this group. Although there are few rigorous well-controlled studies, those available suggest that the elderly may obtain substantial relief from various treatment modalities including pharmacological, psychological and physical treatments. Although it is far too early to draw definitive conclusions, we will attempt to present a balanced portrayal of the disparate findings, to offer potential explanations for some of the inconsistencies, and to make useful suggestions for urgently needed research into pain and ageing.

PSYCHOMETRIC TOOLS

MEASURES OF PAIN INTENSITY

Most pain assessment instruments were designed for use with younger adults. Preliminary data regarding the psychometric properties of these instruments for elderly samples have become available only recently. These studies have assessed the elderly's ability to complete the scales, their preferences among them, and the consistency of intensity estimates obtained from different measures.

The most commonly used measures of pain intensity are visual analogue scales (VAS) (Huskisson 1974), verbal descriptor scales (VDS) and numerical rating scales (NRS) (see Jensen & Karoly 1992 for a review). The elderly may have deficits in abstract reasoning which make use of the VAS difficult (Kremer et al 1981). In fact, increasing age has been associated with a higher frequency of incomplete or unscorable responses on the VAS (Kremer et al 1981, Jensen et al 1986, Gagliese & Melzack 1997a) but not on the VDS (Jensen et al 1986, Gagliese & Melzack 1997a), the behavioural rating scale (BRS) (Jensen et al 1986, Gagliese & Melzack 1997a) or the NRS (Jensen et al 1986). Consistent with this, the elderly report that the VAS is more difficult to complete and is a poorer description of pain than scales made up of verbal descriptors (Herr & Mobily 1993, Benesh et al 1997). However, the sample sizes in the studies of subject preferences were small and age differences were not assessed.

Another potential difficulty with the VAS is a lack of agreement with other measures in estimates of pain intensity levels. Specifically, in elderly samples, VAS scores may be significantly different from other intensity measures, including the VDS and BRS (Herr & Mobily 1993, Gagliese & Melzack 1997a) which do not differ from each other. This pattern was not found in young and middle-aged chronic pain patients (Gagliese & Melzack 1997a).

Although the data are preliminary, taken together, they raise important problems for the use of the VAS with the elderly. As many as 30% of cognitively intact elderly may be unable to complete this scale (Gagliese & Melzack 1997a). Furthermore, among those who can complete the scale, intensity estimates may be significantly different from those obtained using verbal descriptor or numerical rating scales. Reasons for this and strategies to improve the validity and reliability of this scale in the elderly require further study.

THE MCGILL PAIN QUESTIONNAIRE

The McGill Pain Questionnaire (MPQ) (Melzack 1975), the most widely used multidimensional pain inventory (Wilke et al 1990), measures the sensory, affective, evaluative, and miscellaneous components of pain. There is much evidence for the validity, reliability and discriminative abilities of the MPQ when used with younger adults (Melzack & Katz 1992). Although Herr and Mobily (1991) have suggested that this scale may not be appropriate for the elderly, they do not present data to support this claim. Instead, recent evidence suggests that the psychometric properties of the MPQ may not be age related. Specifically, Gagliese (1998) has found that the latent structure, internal consistency and pattern of subscale correlations of the MPQ are very similar in young and elderly chronic pain patients who have been matched for pain diagnosis, location and duration, and for gender. Although further studies are needed, these results suggest that the MPQ is indeed appropriate for use with older patients. It appears to measure the same constructs in the same way across the adult lifespan.

The short form of the MPQ (SF-MPQ) (Melzack 1987), which measures the sensory and affective dimensions of pain, also may be appropriate for use with the elderly (Gagliese & Melzack 1997a). In a sample of adults with chronic arthritis pain, there were no age differences in error rates on this scale (Gagliese & Melzack 1997a). Consistent with a previous report (Helme et al 1989), SF-MPQ subscale scores were highly correlated and gave comparable estimates of pain levels (Gagliese & Melzack 1997a). Although the elderly endorsed fewer words than younger subjects, the same adjectives were chosen to describe arthritis pain with the greatest frequency regardless of age (Gagliese & Melzack 1997a). Although these findings are promising, they must be replicated in larger samples with more detailed psychometric analyses before final conclusions can be drawn.

In summary, the assessment of pain in the elderly should include a verbal descriptor scale measure of pain intensity and either the MPQ or SF-MPQ. This combination of scales also would be the most appropriate for the assessment of age differences in pain. Larger studies are needed to more adequately assess the psychometric properties of these scales across the adult lifespan. Future work should examine the factors that hinder appropriate use of the VAS by the elderly, the age-related sensitivity of these scales to experimental or therapeutic manipulations, and their appropriateness in the assessment of acute pain in the elderly. These scales have been used extensively, even though data on their psychometric properties in elderly samples are limited. As a result, the validity of this research remains unclear until it is shown that these tools are appropriate for use in the elderly.

AGE DIFFERENCES IN EXPERIMENTAL PAIN

PAIN DETECTION THRESHOLD

Much of the literature on age differences in pain has focused on pain in the laboratory. There are 23 studies of age differences in pain threshold, 'the lowest value at which the person reports that the stimulation feels painful' (Melzack and Wall 1988, p 17). The results of these studies have been inconsistent with reports that pain threshold increases, decreases or does not change with increasing age (Table 43.1). These disparate findings may be the result, in part, of methodological weaknesses and diversity of the studies. For example, studies show considerable variability in the mean age of the groups being compared, the pain induction methods employed, and the psychophysical endpoints measured (Harkins et al 1994). Subject inclusion/exclusion criteria and sufficient statistical data to allow comparison across studies are rarely provided. In addition, several studies do not include adequate numbers of elderly subjects, further limiting interpretation of the data. Keeping in mind these limitations, the majority of the studies nonetheless suggest that there is an increase in pain threshold with age, especially for cutaneous thermal pain (Table 43.1). More rigorous, systematic studies which adequately sample across the lifespan are required before firm conclusions can be drawn. The cross-sectional design of these studies also limits conclusions. Data from longitudinal studies would allow for an examination of age-related changes in the response to experimental pain independent of cohort effects.

PAIN TOLERANCE THRESHOLD

Much less attention has been paid to the effect of age on pain tolerance, the 'lowest stimulation level at which the subject withdraws or asks to have the stimulation stopped' (Melzack & Wall 1988, p 17). Decreased pain tolerance with age has been found using several different pain induction methods, including mechanical pressure applied at the Achilles tendon (Woodrow et al 1972), cold pressor pain (Walsh et al 1989) and cutaneous electric current (Collins & Stone 1966) (but see Neri & Agazzani 1984 for an exception). A possible interaction between sex and age on pain tolerance has been investigated but remains unclear (Collins & Stone 1966, Woodrow et al 1972). Although research with more directly comparable methodologies is needed, the conclusion, at this time, is that pain tolerance decreases with age.

SIGNAL DETECTION THEORY

It is not clear whether a sensory deficit, a reluctance to report painful stimuli, or an interaction of both factors underlie age differences in experimentally induced pain (Harkins & Chapman 1976). Signal detection theory (Green & Swets 1966) has been used to separate these factors (Clark & Mehl 1971, Harkins & Chapman 1976, 1977). These studies have found only subtle age differences in sensitivity. As well, the elderly adopt a more conservative response bias than younger subjects when labelling noxious stimuli. Specifically, they are more reluctant to label weak vaguely noxious stimuli as painful; however, at higher intensities, they are more likely to do so than younger groups. Furthermore, elderly subjects may have greater difficulty than young subjects in discriminating between different stimulus intensities.

These results suggest that reported age differences in pain threshold may be a result of the elderly's conservative response bias. Their reluctance to label weak stimuli as painful may artificially inflate threshold scores relative to younger subjects. However, the use of signal detection methodology in pain studies has been criticized, and the interpretation of the results has been questioned (Rollman 1977, Coppola & Gracely 1983). Nonetheless, the conclusions of these studies are widely accepted and have had important implications for the assessment of pain in the clinical setting. It has been assumed that the elderly adopt a more conservative attitude than younger patients towards reporting painful symptoms (Tremblay 1994).

RATINGS OF SUPRATHRESHOLD NOXIOUS STIMULI

Age differences in the perception of suprathreshold painful stimuli have been assessed using direct psychophysical scaling and cross-modality matching. Despite one failed replication (Heft et al 1996), the elderly have been found to rate suprathreshold thermal stimuli as less intense and unpleasant than do younger subjects (Gibson et al 1991, Tremblay

Table 43.1 Studies of age differences in pain threshold

Noxious stimulus	*Reference*	*Subjects (age range and no. of subjects)*	*Site of stimulation*	*Results*
Thermal stimuli				
Radiant heat	Chapman & Jones 1944	10–85 years *n*=60	Mid-forehead	Threshold increases with age
	Hall & Stride 1954	18–70 years *n*=256	Mid-forehead	Threshold increases with age
	Sherman & Robillard 1960	20–97 years *n*=200	Mid-forehead	Threshold increases with age
	Schluderman & Zubek 1962	12–83 years *n*=171	Mid-forehead, arms and legs	Threshold increases with age
	Procacci et al 1970	18–70+ years *n* = 525	Forearm	Threshold increases with age
	Schumacher et al 1940	No age range reported *n*=150	Mid-forehead	No age differences
	Hardy et al 1943	10–80 years *n*=200	Mid-forehead	No age differences
	Birren et al 1950	19–82 years *n*=16	Mid-forehead	No age differences
	Clark & Mehl 1971	18–67 years *n* = 64	Forearm	No age differences
Contact heat	Gibson et al 1991	20–99 years *n* = 66	Hand	Threshold increases with age
	Lautenbacher & Strian 1991	17–63 years *n* = 64	Foot Hand	Threshold increases with age No age differences
	Heft et al 1996	20–89 years *n* = 189	Upper lip and chin	Threshold increases with age
	Chakour et al 1996	20–65+ *n* = 30	Hand	Threshold increases with age
	Kenshalo 1986	19–84 years *n* = 47	Hand and foot	No age differences
Electric current				
Cutaneous	Tucker et al 1989	5–105 years *n* = 520	Upperarm	Threshold increases with age
	Neri & Agazzani 1984	20–82 years *n* = 100	Forearm	Threshold increases with age
	Collins & Stone 1966	18–53 years *n* = 56	Fingers	Threshold decreases with age
Tooth pulp	Mumford 1963	10–73 years *n* not reported	Variety of healthy teeth	No age differences
	Mumford 1968	18–63 years *n* = 111	Healthy unfilled incisor	No age differences
	Harkins & Chapman 1976	21–85 years *n* = 20	Healthy unfilled incisor	No age differences
	Harkins & Chapman 1977	20–81 years *n* = 20	Healthy unfilled incisor	No age differences
Pin prick				
	Horch et al 1992	9–83 years *n* = 130	Fingers	No age differences
Visceral pain				
	Lasch et al 1997	18–87 years *n* = 27	Intraoesophageal balloon distension	Threshold increases with age

1994, Chakour et al 1996). However, at higher intensities, the elderly rate the stimulus as more intense and unpleasant than do younger subjects (Harkins et al 1986). This pattern is consistent with increased threshold but decreased tolerance with age, and suggests that differences are apparent in both the affective and sensory dimensions of pain.

PROPOSED MECHANISMS

Mechanisms for the age differences in reactivity to experimental pain have been proposed at both the peripheral and central levels of the nervous system. In the periphery, age-related changes in the characteristics of the skin and of nociceptors have been put forward as possible mechanisms (Procacci et al 1970). However, age-related histological changes in the skin have not been reported consistently (Kenshalo 1986), and there is no direct evidence for changes in free-nerve receptor function, morphology or density with age (Harkins et al 1984). Age-related changes in peripheral nerves have also been implicated, and there is evidence that C- (Helme & McKernan 1985, Parkhouse & Le Quesne 1988, Harkins et al 1996) and Aδ- (Chakour et al 1996, Harkins et al 1996) fibre function decrease with age. The implications and clinical relevance of these changes remain to be clarified.

Explanations involving central neural mechanisms, namely age-related decreases in the capacity or speed of processing of nociceptive stimuli (Harkins et al 1984), have also been proposed to account for the age differences in sensitivity. There is some evidence to support this view. An age-related decrease in EEG amplitude and an increase in response latency to painful stimuli have been reported (Gibson et al 1991). In response to painful thermal stimuli, both young and older adults show activation of midline and central cortical regions, but older adults also show activation in more frontal and lateral sites, implying wider recruitment of neurons and slower cognitive processing in response to painful stimuli in the elderly (Gibson et al 1994).

The mechanisms responsible for the age-related differences in experimental pain require further elucidation. Undoubtedly, there is an interaction of both peripheral and central changes, including changes in emotional and cognitive factors. However, the implications of these changes for clinical painful states remain to be determined (Procacci et al 1979). Experimental pain paradigms provide an oversimplified approximation to both the acute and chronic pain experience. The important role that psychological and emotional factors play in pathological pain states can not be modelled in the experimental setting (Procacci et al 1979). The relevance of peripheral and central mechanisms which contribute to differences in experimental pain reactivity must be evaluated in the clinical setting.

CLINICAL PAIN

EPIDEMIOLOGICAL STUDIES

Most of the epidemiological studies conducted in community settings have found that the prevalence of pain complaints (Andersson et al 1993), of headache (Lipton et al 1993, Schwartz et al 1998), migraine (Cook et al 1989) and low back pain (Wright et al 1995, de Zwart et al 1997) peaks in middle age and decreases thereafter. An age-related decrease in the prevalence of pain problems for all sites other than the joints has also been reported (Sternbach 1986). By contrast, there have been several reports of an age-related increase in the prevalence of persistent (Crook et al 1984) and recurrent (Brattberg et al 1997) pain, musculoskeletal pain (Badley & Tennant 1992, de Zwart et al 1997) and fibromyalgia (Wolfe et al 1995). At present, strong conclusions regarding the pattern of age differences in pain prevalence cannot be drawn.

There may be several reasons for these inconsistent results. Firstly, in community samples, decreases in pain prevalence with age may be an artifact of higher rates of mortality or institutionalization among the elderly with chronic pain (Harkins & Price 1992). Secondly, there may be age differences in the willingness to report painful symptoms (Prohaska et al 1987). Thirdly, different definitions of chronic and/or acute pain have been employed, making comparison of the results difficult.

Nonetheless, these studies indicate that a considerable proportion of elderly people experience pain. Approximately 2–27% of the elderly report migraine or tension headache (Lipton et al 1993), 14–49% report low back pain (Sternbach 1986, Valkenburg 1988) and 24–71% report joint pain (Sternbach 1986, Valkenburg 1988). Higher prevalence estimates are obtained from institutionalized samples of elderly people. In this setting, 71–83% of patients report at least one current pain problem (Roy & Thomas 1986, Ferrell et al 1990).

The characteristics and impact of these pain complaints have not been clarified. The majority of elderly people report mild to moderate, intermittent pain (Lavsky-Shulan et al 1985, Roy & Thomas 1986, Ferrell et al 1990, Cook & Thomas 1994). Although the pain may interfere with activities (Ferrell et al 1990), others have reported that activity restriction due to pain in the elderly is as great as that reported by middle-aged people (Brattberg et al 1989). Surprisingly, activity levels and use of healthcare services among elderly people with and without chronic pain do not differ (Roy & Thomas 1987, Cook & Thomas 1994). In summary, a large proportion of elderly individuals reports pain complaints. It is not clear from the available data what the significance of these complaints may be. Future studies should focus on documenting the frequency, duration, intensity, qualities and impact of pain throughout the adult lifespan.

ACUTE PAIN

The most striking and consistently reported age differences are in the experience of acute pain. Acute pain, in this context, refers to pain related to specific, brief pathological insults such as tissue damage or infectious processes (Cousins 1994). In general, the elderly present with few of the symptoms typically associated with acute clinical syndromes, including pain. When pain is reported, it is likely to be referred from the site of origin in an atypical manner. In fact, pathological conditions that are painful to young adults may, in the elderly, produce only behavioural changes such as confusion, restlessness, aggression, anorexia and fatigue (Butler & Gastel 1980). These differences may contribute to delayed seeking of treatment, misdiagnosis and increased mortality in the elderly (Albano et al 1975). For example, a dramatic increase with age in the incidence and prevalence of asymptomatic and atypical myocardial infarction has been reported (Bayer et al 1986, Sigurdsson et al 1995). Although relatively uncommon in younger patients, up to 30% of elderly survivors of myocardial infarction did not report any acute symptoms, while another 30% had an atypical presentation (see review by Ambepitiya et al 1993). Similar age differences have been documented in the presentation of duodenal ulcer (Scapa et al 1989), acute intra-abdominal infection (Cooper et al 1994), appendicitis (Albano et al 1975) and pancreatitis (Gullo et al 1994).

Although there is considerable evidence that the prevalence of acute pain decreases with age, only one study has assessed age differences in the intensity of the acute pain. Among patients diagnosed with duodenal ulcer or acute myocardial infarction, the elderly were more likely than younger patients to report mild pain (Scapa et al 1992). Although more research is needed, it appears that the elderly are less likely to report pain associated with acute pathology and, when pain is reported, it tends to be less intense than that experienced by younger subjects. Mechanisms to account for the differences in the reporting of acute pain with age are poorly understood (Ambepitiya et al 1993).

POSTOPERATIVE PAIN

Postoperative pain in the elderly has only recently begun to receive empirical attention, although this age group has the highest rate of surgical procedures (Politser & Schneidman 1990). Proper assessment and management of acute postoperative pain is critical, as postoperative confusion (Cousins 1994, Lynch et al 1998), suppression of the immune and respiratory systems and high rates of mortality (Ergina et al 1993) have been associated with inadequate pain control. Age differences reported in postoperative pain levels have been inconsistent. Several studies have suggested that elderly patients report lower pain intensity than younger patients (Bellville et al 1971, Oberle et al 1990), while others have found that age is not related to levels of postoperative pain intensity (Giuffre et al 1991, Duggleby & Lander 1994). Nonetheless, age-related increases in the analgesic efficacy of opioids have been consistently reported (Kaiko 1980, Moore et al 1990). Elderly patients obtain greater analgesia than younger patients in response to a fixed dose of opioids (Bellville et al 1971, Kaiko 1980). Compared with younger patients, the elderly self-administer significantly less drug when using patient-controlled analgesia (PCA) (Burns et al 1989, Giuffre et al 1991, Macintyre & Jarvis 1995). The increased analgesic efficacy of opioids may be due to age differences in the pharmacokinetics and pharmacodynamics of these agents (Popp & Portenoy 1996).

The management of postoperative pain in the elderly continues to be inadequate, even though many of the standard treatment strategies, especially the use of opioids and NSAIDs, are effective (Pasero & McCaffery 1996). The elderly are more vulnerable to the adverse effects of these drugs, and it has been recommended that initial doses be reduced to 25–50% of those given to younger patients (Pasero & McCaffery 1996). PCA may provide adequate analgesia in elderly patients (Egbert et al 1990, Macintyre & Jarvis 1995, Badaoui et al 1996) and has been associated with fewer pulmonary and cognitive complications than intramuscular injection of opioids (Egbert et al 1990). However, barriers to the effective use of PCA by the elderly include difficulty in learning to use the equipment (Monk et al 1990, Badaoui et al 1996) and fear of opioid addiction (Hofland 1992). It should be noted that age differences in these barriers have not been studied. Other strategies to control postoperative pain, such as the use of pre-emptive analgesia (Katz et al 1992), have been advocated for the elderly (Pasero & McCaffery 1996), although the efficacy of this intervention has not been tested in this age group. Studies are needed to document age differences in the efficacy of these pain management strategies, in patient satisfaction and learning needs, as well as possible modifications which may enhance pain control across the lifespan.

CHRONIC PAIN

Chronic pain 'persists after all possible healing has occurred or, at least, long after pain can serve any useful function' (Melzack & Wall 1988, p 36). The evidence for age differences in the experience of chronic pain remains controversial. Although several studies have found no age differences in pain intensity measured with the VAS (Harkins 1988, Middaugh et al 1988, Benbow et al 1995, Harkins et al 1995) or NRS (Sorkin et al 1990, McCracken et al 1993), there have also been occasional reports that pain intensity, measured with the NRS (Turk et al 1995) and VAS (Parker et al 1988), decreases with age, and still other reports that elderly patients rate their pain as more intense than younger patients on both the VDS (Puder 1988) and VAS (Wilkieson et al 1993). Comparisons between age groups using the MPQ have also been inconsistent. Of the six studies using this measure, two found no age differences (Lichtenberg et al 1986, Corran et al 1993), while four reported that advancing age was associated with lower MPQ scores (Lichtenberg et al 1984, McCracken et al 1993, Benbow et al 1996, Corran et al 1997).

These disparate findings are difficult to reconcile. It appears that the observed age differences may be dependent on the scale used to measure pain. However, because of the large cross-study variability in age range, pain tools, sample size and characteristics, it is difficult to draw firm conclusions. More instructive is the interesting pattern of results found in studies that employ multiple measures of pain in the same sample. Gagliese and Melzack (1997a) found no age differences in the intensity of pain as measured by several unidimensional scales, including the VAS, VDS and BRS. However, on the SF-MPQ, the elderly obtained significantly lower sensory and affective scores and endorsed fewer words than younger groups. Similar results were reported by McCracken et al (1993).

There are several possible explanations for the dissociation between scale scores. One may be that there are age-related changes in the quality but not the intensity of chronic pain. On the other hand, the dissociation may reflect the elderly's reluctance to endorse the 'most intense' words on the MPQ (Oberle et al 1990). If so, however, this should also lead the elderly to endorse lower levels of pain on the intensity measures, which the data show is not the case. Thirdly, there may be other words of equal or greater intensity, not included on the MPQ, which would more accurately capture the experience of pain in this group. The elderly may not group or rank the adjectives in the same ways as did subjects in the original validation studies (Melzack 1975), or they may simply fail to comprehend the demands of either or both types of tools (Herr & Mobily 1991). Our interpretation of this dissociation must await further data on the validity and reliability of these pain measures in the geriatric population.

The cognitive dimension of chronic pain

The cognitive dimension of pain refers to the appraisal of and attempts to cope with painful symptoms (Weisenberg 1994). The appraisals and coping strategies employed by chronic pain patients have been consistently associated with levels of pain intensity, disability and emotional distress. Specifically, increased emotional distress, impairment and pain intensity have been associated with increased use of maladaptive coping strategies (see review by Katz et al 1996).

Pain beliefs

Pain beliefs represent an important component in the process of appraising potential stressors. Pain beliefs are personally formed or culturally shared cognitive configurations about the causes, meanings, consequences and effective treatments of pain (De Good & Shutty 1992). These beliefs may influence symptom reporting, treatment seeking, compliance and outcome (De Good & Shutty 1992). It has been proposed that the elderly have the belief that pain is a normal part of the ageing process and, therefore, they do not appraise such symptoms as threats to their health. Instead, painful sensations are expected, tolerated and not considered worthy of medical treatment (Hofland 1992). In addition, the elderly may be more reluctant than other age groups to acknowledge the contribution of psychological factors to the pain experience (Blazer & Houpt 1979).

There is little empirical evidence to support these widely held views. In fact, one study found that only 2% of the elderly attributed their chronic health conditions to ageing and that health beliefs in general were not strongly associated with age (Segall & Chappell 1991). Another study found that a significant proportion of the elderly did not agree with items reflecting beliefs that pain is a normal part of ageing (Brockopp et al 1996). In addition, Gagliese and Melzack (1997b) recently found no age differences in pain beliefs in both pain-free adults and in those with arthritis pain. The elderly were not more likely than the younger groups to believe that pain was normal at their age, nor were they more likely to associate pain with the normal ageing process than with organic factors such as tissue damage. Furthermore, they did not deny the importance of psychological factors to the pain experience.

Locus of control

The locus of control for health-related outcomes is important in the determination of strategies employed to cope with pain. Health-related locus of control can be internally or externally situated. External locus of control can be further subdivided into beliefs about the control of powerful others and beliefs about fate/luck (Wallston et al 1978). In a recent review, Melding (1997) concluded that health locus of control becomes more external with advancing age. The elderly are more likely than younger patients to relinquish control of their health to powerful others. Although this has been associated with poorer outcomes and increased use of maladaptive coping strategies in younger patients (Gold et al 1991), in the elderly it may actually be predictive of increased treatment compliance (Nagy & Wolfe 1984). However, in both young and older groups, an external fate/luck locus of control has been associated with increased depression, pain and impairment (Crisson & Keefe 1988), while a strong internal locus of control is related to decreased pain and emotional distress (Rudy et al 1988). Age differences in locus of control are very subtle, and their implications for treatment have not been fully explored.

Coping

The elderly are more likely than younger patients to employ externally mediated passive coping strategies such as praying and hoping (Keefe & Williams 1990, Sorkin et al 1990, Corran et al 1993, McCracken et al 1993). These differences, however, are not large, and their clinical significance is not clear. A lack of significant age differences in perceived effectiveness of coping strategies and in perceived ability to control pain has been consistently reported (Harkins 1988, Keefe & Williams 1990, Corran et al 1993, Gagliese & Melzack 1997b). This pattern of results implies that the elderly with chronic pain may be more amenable to psychological pain management strategies than has previously been assumed, because many of these treatments are designed to modify this dimension of the pain experience (Turk & Meichenbaum 1994).

The affective dimension of chronic pain

Pain and anxiety

The affective consequences of chronic pain are most often conceptualized in terms of depression and/or anxiety. Age differences in anxiety have received far less empirical attention than depression. It appears that elderly chronic pain patients report lower anxiety levels than younger patients (Corran et al 1993, McCracken et al 1993; but see Middaugh et al 1988). Nonetheless, anxious elderly individuals report more pain complaints and pain of greater intensity than those with lower levels of anxiety (Parmelee et al 1991). This relationship may be independent of concurrent depressive symptomatology (Parmelee et al 1991). These data suggest that, in elderly chronic pain patients, anxiety may be a significant problem that requires assessment and treatment.

Pain and depression

It has been well documented that the majority of chronic pain patients have significant depressive symptoms and that depressed individuals are more likely to report painful symptoms than non-depressed individuals (Fishbain et al 1997). Although it has been suggested that this relationship may be enhanced in the elderly (Kwentus et al 1985, Harkins & Price 1992), there is convincing evidence that there are no age differences in the severity (Sorkin et al 1990, McCracken et al 1993, Turk et al 1995, Gagliese & Melzack 1997b) or prevalence (Corran et al 1993, Turk et al 1995) of depressive symptoms experienced by chronic pain patients.

Recently, Turk et al (1995) reported that the relationship between pain intensity and depression may differ in young and elderly chronic pain patients. Although the relationship between these variables is mediated by perceived life control and the extent to which pain interferes with functioning in both age groups, it is only in elderly patients that the direct relationship between depression and pain intensity may be significant. As such, in elderly, but not younger, patients changes in pain intensity may directly influence levels of depression and vice versa, independent of other factors. Consistent with this possibility, depressed elderly people report more intense pain and more pain complaints than do the non-depressed elderly (Parmelee et al 1991, Casten et al 1995). In addition, elderly people with chronic pain obtain higher scores on depression scales than

 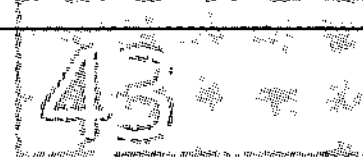

those who are pain free (Roy & Thomas 1986, Williamson & Schulz 1992, Black et al 1998, Werner et al 1998) (but see Ferrell et al 1990 and Harkins & Price 1992). Further work is needed to clarify the pathway between pain and depression across the adult lifespan.

There is significant co-morbidity of pain and depression in the elderly. Differentiation of these states may be difficult as the symptoms are often similar (see Herr & Mobily 1991 for guidelines). In fact, some elderly people use pain complaints to explain symptoms of depression (Kwentus et al 1985). However, the elderly are also more likely to present with atypical pain (see above), so that the suspicion of depression does not reduce the importance of a comprehensive pain assessment. Pain assessments should routinely include an evaluation of the patient's psychological well-being.

There are several well-validated instruments for the assessment of depression in the elderly (Brink et al 1982). Users of these instruments should be aware of potential problems with these scales for the elderly in pain. Many of the items assess the vegetative or somatic symptoms of depression, which may also be part of the pain problem. This would inflate the depression scores obtained on these scales by chronic pain patients (Bourque et al 1992). Clinicians are advised to use only scales validated for the elderly and, whenever feasible, more than one scale should be used (Gibson et al 1994).

CHRONIC PAIN AND IMPAIRMENT

Both chronic pain (Brattberg et al 1989) and increasing age (Forbes et al 1991) have been associated with impairment in functional abilities and the performance of activities of daily living (ADLs). In fact, it has been proposed that high rates of co-morbidity, deconditioning, polypharmacy and social isolation make the elderly more susceptible than younger groups to impairments associated with pain (Kwentus et al 1985). Consistent with this, some studies have found that elderly chronic pain patients report more disability and impairment in the performance of ADLs than pain-free elderly (March et al 1998, Scudds & Robertson 1998). However, several others have not found this relationship (Roy & Thomas 1987, Ross & Crook 1998, Werner et al 1998). Therefore, it is not yet clear whether pain increases the disability associated with ageing.

Furthermore, it is not clear whether the impact of pain is different in younger and older chronic pain patients. Although the elderly may have greater physical pathology, they report similar levels of interference of pain in their lives, relationships and performance of daily activities as do younger chronic pain patients (Brattberg et al 1989, Sorkin et al 1990, Corran et al 1997). In fact, impairment due to pain is reported to be more emotionally distressing for younger than older individuals (Williamson & Schulz 1995). A recent study (Corran et al 1997) classified chronic pain patients on the basis of pain, depression and pain impact measures and found that comparable proportions of young and elderly patients had made a positive adaptation to pain, or had achieved good pain control. However, in each age group, a unique subgroup was identified. Among younger patients, this subgroup was characterized by high levels of pain, depression and functional impact, while among the elderly, the subgroup was characterized by low levels of pain but high levels of depression and functional impact. The authors suggest that the high impact may be an artifact of co-morbidity within this group (Corran et al 1997). Interestingly, the results of this study suggest that the relationship between pain and functional impairment may change with age. Further studies are required to document the age-related differences in the impact of chronic pain on functioning and quality of life.

PAIN AND DEMENTIA

Differential diagnosis between pain and dementia is often necessary in the elderly patient. Pain complaints may be the first signs of dementia (Kisely et al 1992), or may be used to explain or hide mild cognitive impairment (Harkins et al 1984). Also, acute pathologies, which often are associated with pain in younger patients, may manifest only as confusion in the elderly (see above).

The assessment of pain in the demented elderly has recently begun to receive empirical attention. Experimental pain threshold does not differ between the cognitively impaired and intact elderly (Cornu 1975, Jonsson et al 1977). In the clinical setting, the prevalence (Takeshima et al 1990, Marzinski 1991, Parmelee et al 1993) and intensity of painful conditions (Cohen-Mansfield & Marx 1993, Parmelee et al 1993) may decrease as dementia progresses. However, these results must be interpreted with great caution. Memory and language impairments may confound reports of pain, especially if patients are asked, for instance, to recall pain in the previous 2 weeks (Farrell et al 1996). Furthermore, studies based on self-report do not provide evidence that the cognitively impaired subjects understood the demands of the task. Specifically, it is not clear that the protocols assessed each subject's understanding of the concept of pain or of the method used to quantify intensity. None of the studies included modified pain assessment tools which accommodate for the cognitive limitations of the respondents. For instance, scales designed for children may be more appropriate for this population (Harkins & Price 1992). A recent study (Herr et al 1998) has suggested that the Faces Pain Scale (Bieri et al 1990) may be valid for the intact elderly, but the feasibility of using this scale with the demented elderly has not been assessed.

It has been suggested that modifications to existing pain assessment tools are not necessary because mild to moderate cognitive impairment does not affect the successful completion of standard pain instruments (Ferrell et al 1995). However, Ferrell et al studied cognitively impaired patients who were able to verbally report pain, of whom 17% were unable to complete any of the five intensity scales presented. Unfortunately, the relationship between degree of cognitive impairment and the ability to complete the scales was not explored. Further research into the relationship between pain and dementia is required. The initial challenge is the development of a reliable, quantitative pain assessment instrument for use with this population.

As dementia progresses, patient self-report of pain may become invalid. At this point, valuable information may be obtained from significant others (Werner et al 1998) or through direct observation of behaviour (Weiner et al 1996), especially abrupt changes in behaviour or disruption in usual functioning (Marzinski 1991). Hurley and colleagues (1992) have developed a scale to measure possible behavioural indicators of discomfort in non-communicative patients with advanced Alzheimer's disease. This appears to be a promising start. However, it is not clear whether consistent pain behaviours are displayed by the elderly and how these might change as a result of dementia (Marzinski 1991, Parke 1992).

Facial expressions have been shown to provide reliable indicators of painful states among non-verbal populations (Craig et al 1992). However, there is little information regarding the facial expression of pain among the demented elderly. In two small studies, an increase in the number of facial movements during exposure to noxious stimuli was found, but the responses were highly variable (Asplund et al 1991, Porter et al 1996). Specific facial movements associated with pain could not be identified, and complex facial expressions, which are indicators of emotion (Collier 1985), were not seen (Asplund et al 1991, Porter et al 1996). Much more work is needed in order to develop systematic guidelines for the assessment of pain in the non-verbal demented elderly.

MANAGEMENT OF PAIN IN THE ELDERLY

A significant proportion of elderly people do not receive adequate pain treatment. Approximately 47–80% of community-dwelling (Roy & Thomas 1987, Woo et al 1994) and 16–27% of institutionalized individuals do not receive any treatment for their pain (Roy & Thomas 1986, Lichtenberg & McGrogan 1987). Among the demented elderly, an even greater proportion of those with potentially painful diagnoses may not receive any analgesic medication (Marzinski 1991). Although inadequate pain management is not limited to the elderly, several unique factors may contribute to the poor treatment of pain in this group. These include, but are not limited to, increased risks of pharmacotherapy, misconceptions regarding the efficacy of non-pharmacological pain management strategies, as well as ageist attitudes that may contribute to a reluctance to offer multidisciplinary treatments to the elderly.

PHARMACOLOGICAL THERAPY

Analgesics are the most frequently used method of pain control, and it has been shown that this modality, including the use of opioids, is safe for the elderly when used with appropriate medical supervision (Portenoy & Farkash 1988). Nonetheless, it is well documented that the elderly are more likely than younger patients to develop adverse reactions to opioids at much lower dosages (Portenoy & Farkash 1988). This may be due to age-associated changes in the metabolism and clearance rates of drugs which lead to altered pharmacokinetics and pharmacodynamics (McCaffery & Beebe 1989, Popp & Portenoy 1996). The AGS (American Geriatrics Society) Panel on Chronic Pain in Older Persons (1998) has recently developed detailed clinical practice guidelines, which are applicable to all classes of analgesic medication. Because pharmacotherapy requires special attention in this group, it is important to recognize that there are alternative potentially safer modalities of therapy commonly available in the management of chronic pain. These include both physical and psychological treatments.

PSYCHOLOGICAL TREATMENT

The efficacy of psychological interventions for the management of chronic pain has been well established for younger patients (Melzack & Wall 1988). Comparable data from elderly samples are limited yet promising (Gagliese & Melzack 1997c). Most of the available studies are retrospective, uncontrolled and lack appropriate comparison groups. Nonetheless, the elderly have been shown to benefit from cognitive-behavioural therapy (Puder 1988), relaxation and biofeedback training (Nicholson & Blanchard 1993), and behaviour therapy (Miller & LeLieuvre 1982).

In some of these studies, the elderly made treatment gains comparable to those of younger patients (Middaugh et al 1988, Puder 1988), although modifications to the interventions may be required to maximize compliance and treatment benefits (Arena et al 1988, 1991). These modifications have not been tested with younger patients and may prove to be of equal benefit across the adult lifespan (Gagliese & Melzack 1997c). Overall, although more systematic, large-scale studies are needed, it appears that elderly chronic pain patients may benefit substantially from psychological interventions.

PHYSICAL THERAPIES

Elderly patients have been shown to benefit from physical interventions such as transcutaneous electrical nerve stimulation (Thorsteinsson 1987), massage (Eisenberg et al 1993) and the application of heat and cold (Eisenberg et al 1993). In addition to these more passive strategies, there is considerable evidence that elderly chronic pain patients, especially those with musculoskeletal pain, may derive substantial benefit from regular exercise (Ferrell et al 1997). An additional advantage to these treatment modalities is that they involve little risk of adverse events when carried out under appropriate medical supervision (AGS Panel on Chronic Pain in Older Persons 1998).

MULTIDISCIPLINARY TREATMENT

Multidisciplinary treatment has been recognized as essential to the effective management of chronic pain in younger individuals (Flor et al 1992). However, the data concerning the elderly are scant and often contradictory. It has been suggested that the elderly may not have access to such treatment (Harkins & Price 1992, Kee et al 1998). The age distribution of patients referred to pain clinics peaks in mid-life and decreases thereafter, with 7–20% of patients over the age of 65 (Harkins & Price 1992, Gagliese & Melzack 1997d). This pattern is consistent with both the age distribution of the prevalence of many common pain disorders and the proportion of elderly in the general population (Gagliese & Melzack 1997d). Therefore, it is not clear that the elderly are underrepresented in these clinics.

Nonetheless, some clinics do set an upper age limit on the patients they will treat (Sorkin & Turk 1995). This is most likely related to a 'return to work' outcome objective (Kee et al 1998), but may also be the result of the myth that chronic pain is a normal consequence of ageing and is not amenable to treatment (Harkins & Price 1992, Kee et al 1998). This belief may contribute to a referral bias on the part of healthcare workers (Harkins & Price 1992). Another factor which may hinder referral of elderly patients is the misconception that they are less willing to participate in multidisciplinary treatment (Sorkin & Turk 1995, Kee et al 1998). However, studies have not found age-related differences in treatment expectations (Harkins & Price 1992), acceptance, compliance or drop-out rates (Sorkin et al 1990).

Although there have been reports that increasing age is a predictor of poor outcome following multidisciplinary pain management (Aronoff & Evans 1982, Guck et al 1986, Graff-Radford & Naliboff 1988), there is also evidence that the elderly may derive substantial benefit (Hallett & Pilowsky 1982, Moore et al 1984, Ysla et al 1986, Sandin 1993, Cutler et al 1994) comparable to that seen with younger patients (Middaugh et al 1988). More systematic work is needed to clarify the relationship between age and treatment outcome. To date, there is no compelling evidence to suggest that elderly patients should be denied such treatment. In fact, the potential adverse effects of untreated pain and/or polypharmacy suggest that multidisciplinary treatment should be considered for all geriatric patients with significant pain complaints.

CONCLUSIONS

Despite the abundance of inconsistent results and the need for more systematic research, several tentative conclusions can be drawn. There appear to be age differences in experimental, acute and chronic pain. The most consistent findings in the experimental setting are that increasing age is associated with higher pain threshold, lower tolerance, and reduced ability to discriminate between suprathreshold levels of noxious stimuli. Clinically, the elderly are less likely than younger patients to report pain associated with acute pathology, such as intra-abdominal infection, and they may report lower levels of postoperative pain. The prevalence of chronic pain appears to peak at mid-life and decrease thereafter. Nonetheless, many elderly people report some type of pain. Among chronic pain patients, there may be a change in the quality but not the intensity of chronic pain with age. The affective and cognitive components of pain do not appear to be age related. The similarities within the cognitive domain suggest that the elderly may be as amenable to psychological treatments as younger patients. The evidence that the emotional distress, especially depression, experienced by chronic pain patients is of comparable intensity throughout the adult lifespan suggests that the need for these treatments does not decrease with age. Each of these conclusions, however, is limited by the pain scales employed in the studies. These measures have only begun to be validated for use with the elderly. These data suggest that verbal descriptor scales of pain intensity as well as the MPQ may be appropriate across the adult lifespan; however, this may not be true of VASs. Future work must continue to explore the psychometric properties of different pain scales in the elderly in order to provide adequate assessment to this group and to elucidate the age differences described above.

Chronic pain in the elderly is often undertreated. This may be due, in part, to the increased risks associated with pharmacotherapy in this group. However, the elderly benefit substantially from psychological and physical treatment methods. Multidisciplinary approaches remain the treatment of choice for younger patients and this may also be true of the elderly patient. It may be that the elderly benefit more from brief exposure to multiple treatments, including pharmacotherapy, than from a prolonged trial of any one treatment. Misconceptions regarding the relationship between pain and ageing and the willingness of the elderly to participate in non-pharmacological treatments may also hamper appropriate care in this group. Intense pain which interferes with functioning is not a normal part of ageing and should never be accepted as such. Fortunately, there has recently been an increase in the empirical attention devoted to pain in the elderly. It is hoped that the results of more rigorous studies will soon resolve some of the inconsistencies highlighted throughout this chapter. This knowledge will be invaluable to the growing numbers of elderly people and to those committed to their care.

Acknowledgements

This work was supported by a scholar award to J.K. from the Medical Research Council of Canada (MRC), MRC Grant MT-12052 (J.K.), NIH-NINDS Grant No. NS35480 (J.K.) and Grant A7891 from the Natural Sciences and Engineering Research Council of Canada (R.M.).

REFERENCES

AGS Panel on Chronic Pain in Older Persons 1998 The management of chronic pain in older persons. Journal of the American Geriatrics Society 46: 635–651

Albano WA, Zielinski CM, Organ CH 1975 Is appendicitis in the aged really different? Geriatrics 30: 81–88

Ambepitiya GB, Iyengar EN, Roberts ME 1993 Review: silent exertional myocardial ischaemia and perception of angina in elderly people. Age and Ageing 22: 302–307

Andersson HI, Ejilertsson G, Leden I, Rosenberg C 1993 Chronic pain in a geographically defined population: studies of differences in age, gender, social class and pain localization. Clinical Journal of Pain 9: 174–182

Arena JG, Hightower NE, Chong GC 1988 Relaxation therapy for tension headache in the elderly: a prospective study. Psychology, Aging 3: 96–98

Arena JG, Hannah SL, Bruno GM, Meador KJ 1991 Electromyographic biofeedback training for tension headache in the elderly: a prospective study. Biofeedback, Self-Regulation 16: 379–390

Aronoff GM, Evans WO 1982 The prediction of treatment outcome at a multidisciplinary pain center. Pain 14: 67–73

Asplund K, Norberg A, Adolfsson R, Waxman HM 1991 Facial expressions in severely demented patients: a stimulus-response study of four patients with dementia of the Alzheimer type. International Journal of Geriatric Psychiatry 6: 599–606

Badaoui R, Riboulot M, Ernst C, Ossart M 1996 L'analgésie postopératoire autocontrolée par le patient agé. Cahiers d'Anesthésiologie 44: 519–522

Badley EM, Tennant A 1992 Changing profile of joint disorders with age: findings from a postal survey of the population of Calderdale, West Yorkshire, United Kingdom. Annals of Rheumatic Disease 51: 366–371

Bayer AJ, Chadha JS, Pathy J 1986 Changing presentation of myocardial infarction with increasing old age. Journal of the American Geriatrics Society 34: 263–266

Bellville JW, Forrest WH, Miller E, Brown BW 1971 Influence of age on pain relief from analgesics. Journal of the American Medical Association 217: 1835–1841

Benbow SJ, Cossins L, Bowsher D 1995 A comparison of young and elderly patients attending a regional pain centre. Pain Clinic 8: 323–332

Benbow SJ, Cossins L, Wiles JR 1996 A comparative study of disability, depression and pain severity in young and chronic pain patients. VIIIth World Congress on Pain, Vancouver

Benesh LR, Szigeti E, Ferraro FR, Gullicks JN 1997 Tools for assessing chronic pain in rural elderly women. Home Healthcare Nurse 15: 207–211

Bieri D, Reeve R, Champion G 1990 The Faces Pain Scale for the self-assessment of the severity of pain experienced by children: development, initial validation, and preliminary investigation for ration scale properties. Pain 41: 139–150

Birren JE, Schapiro HB, Miller JH 1950 The effect of salicylate upon pain sensitivity. Journal of Pharmacological and Experimental Therapy 100: 67–71

Black SA, Goodwin JS, Markides KS 1998 The association between chronic diseases and depressive symptomatology in older Mexican Americans. Journal of Gerontology: Medical Sciences 53A: M188–M194

Blazer DG, Houpt JL 1979 Perception of poor health in the healthy older adult. Journal of the American Geriatrics Society 27: 330–334

Bourque P, Blanchard L, Saulnier J 1992 L'impact des symptômes somatiques dans l'evaluation de la dépression chez une population gériatrique. Revue Canadienne des Sciences du Comportement 24: 118–128

Brattberg G, Thorslund M, Wikman A 1989 The prevalence of pain in a general population. The results of a postal survey in a county of Sweden. Pain 37: 215–222

Brattberg G, Parker MG, Thorslund M 1997 A longitudinal study of pain: reported pain from middle age to old age. Clinical Journal of Pain 13: 144–149

Brink TL, Yesavage JA, Lum O, Heersema PH, Adey M, Rose TL 1982 Screening tests for geriatric depression. Clinical Gerontologist 1: 37–43

Brockopp D, Warden S, Colclough G, Brockopp G 1996 Elderly people's knowledge of and attitudes to pain management. British Journal of Nursing 5: 556–562

Burns JW, Hodsman NBA, McLintock TTC, Gillies GWA, Kenny GNC, McArdle CS 1989 The influence of patient characteristics on the requirements for postoperative analgesia. Anaesthesia 44: 2–6

Butler RN, Gastel B 1980 Care of the aged: perspectives on pain and discomfort. In: Ng LK, Bonica J (eds) Pain, discomfort and humanitarian care. Elsevier North Holland, New York, pp 297–311

Casten RJ, Parmelee PA, Kleban MH, Lawton MP, Katz IR 1995 The relationships among anxiety, depression, and pain in a geriatric institutionalized sample. Pain 61: 271–276

Chakour MC, Gibson SJ, Bradbeer M, Helme RD 1996 The effect of age on A delta and C-fibre thermal pain perception. Pain 64: 143–152

Chapman WP, Jones CM 1944 Variations in cutaneous and visceral pain sensitivity in normal subjects. Journal of Clinical Investigation 23: 81–91

Clark CWM, Mehl L 1971 Thermal pain: a sensory decision theory analysis of the effect of age and sex on the various response criteria and 50% pain threshold. Journal of Abnormal Psychology 78: 201–212

Cohen-Mansfield J, Marx MS 1993 Pain and depression in the nursing home: corroborating results. Journal of Gerontology: Psychological Sciences 48: 96–97

Collier G 1985 Emotional expression. Erlbaum, Hillsdale, NJ

Collins LG, Stone LA 1966 Pain sensitivity, age and activity level in chronic schizophrenics and in normals. British Journal of Psychiatry 112: 33–35

Cook AJ, Thomas MR 1994 Pain and the use of health services among the elderly. Journal of Aging and Health 6: 155–172

Cook NR, Evans DA, Funkenstein HH et al 1989 Correlates of headache in a population-based cohort of elderly. Archives of Neurology 46: 1338–1344

Cooper GS, Shlaes DM, Salata RA 1994 Intraabdominal infection: differences in presentation and outcome between younger patients and the elderly. Clinical Infectious Diseases 19: 146–148

Coppola R, Gracely RH 1983 Where is the noise in SDT pain assessment? Pain 17: 257–266

Cornu FR 1975 Disturbances of the perception of pain among persons with degenerative dementia. Journal de Psychologie Normale et Pathologique 72: 461–464

Corran TM, Helme RD, Gibson SJ 1993 Comparison of chronic pain experience in young and elderly patients. Paper presented at the VIIth World Congress on Pain, Paris, France

Corran TM, Farrell MJ, Helme RD, Gibson SJ 1997 The classification of patients with chronic pain: age as a contributing factor. Clinical Journal of Pain 13: 207–214

Cousins M 1994 Acute and postoperative pain. In: Wall PD, Melzack R (eds) Textbook of pain, 3rd edn. Churchill Livingstone, UK, pp 357–386

Craig KD, Prkachin KM, Grunau RVE 1992 The facial expression of pain. In: Turk DC, Melzack R (eds) Handbook of pain assessment. Guilford, New York, pp 257–274

Crisson JE, Keefe FJ 1988 The relationship of locus of control to pain coping strategies and psychological distress in chronic pain patients. Pain 35: 147–154

Crook J, Rideout E, Browne G 1984 The prevalence of pain complaints in a general population. Pain 18: 299–314

Cutler RB, Fishbain DA, Rosomoff RS, Rosomoff HL 1994 Outcomes in treatment of pain in geriatric and younger age groups. Archives of Physical Medicine and Rehabilitation 75: 457–464

De Good DE, Shutty MS 1992 Assessment of pain beliefs, coping and self-efficacy. In: Turk DC, Melzack R (eds) Handbook of pain assessment. Guilford, New York, pp 214–234

de Zwart BCH, Broersen JPJ, Frings-Dresen MHW, van Dijk FJH 1997 Musculoskeletal complaints in the Netherlands in relation to age, gender and physically demanding work. International Archives of Occupational and Environmental Health 70: 352–360

Duggleby W, Lander J 1994 Cognitive status and postoperative pain: older adults. Journal of Pain and Symptom Management 9: 19–27

Egbert AM, Parks LH, Short LM, Burnett ML 1990 Randomized trial of postoperative patient-controlled analgesia vs intramuscular narcotics in frail elderly men. Archives of Internal Medicine 150: 1897–1903

Eisenberg DM, Kessler RC, Foster C 1993 Unconventional medicine in the United States: prevalence, costs and patterns of use. New England Journal of Medicine 328: 246–252

Ergina PL, Gold SL, Meakins JL 1993 Perioperative care of the elderly patient. World Journal of Surgery 17: 192–198

Farrell MJ, Katz B, Helme RD 1996 The impact of dementia on the pain experience. Pain 67: 7–15

Ferrell BA 1996 Overview of aging and pain. In: Ferrell BR, Ferrell BA (eds) Pain in the elderly. IASP, Seattle, pp 1–10

Ferrell BA, Ferrell BR, Osterweil D 1990 Pain in the nursing home. Journal of the American Geriatrics Society 38: 409–414

Ferrell BA, Ferrell BR, Rivera L 1995 Pain in cognitively impaired nursing home residents. Journal of Pain and Symptom Management 10: 591–598

Ferrell BA, Josephson KR, Pollan AM, Loy S, Ferrell BR 1997 A randomized trial of walking versus physical methods for chronic pain management. Aging: Clinical and Experimental Research 9: 99–105

Fishbain DA, Cutler RB, Rosomoff HL, Rosomoff RS 1997 Chronic pain-associated depression: antecedent or consequence of chronic pain? A review. Clinical Journal of Pain 13: 116–137

Flor H, Fydrich T, Turk DC 1992 Efficacy of multidisciplinary pain treatment centers: a meta-analytic review. Pain 49: 221–230

Forbes WF, Hatward LM, Agwani N 1991 Factors associated with the prevalence of various self-reported impairments among older people residing in the community. Canadian Journal of Public Health 82: 240–244

Gagliese L 1998 Age differences in the experience of pain in humans and animals. Unpublished doctoral thesis, McGill University, Montreal, Canada

Gagliese L, Melzack R 1997a Age differences in the quality of chronic pain: a preliminary study. Pain Research and Management 2: 157–162

Gagliese L, Melzack R 1997b Lack of evidence for age differences in pain beliefs. Pain Research and Management 2: 19–28

Gagliese L, Melzack R 1997c Chronic pain in elderly people. Pain 70: 3–14

Gagliese L, Melzack R 1997d The assessment of pain in the elderly. In: Lomranz J, Mostofsky DI (eds) Handbook of pain and aging. Plenum, New York, pp 69–96

Gibson SJ, Gorman MM, Helme RD 1991 Assessment of pain in the elderly using event-related cerebral potentials. In: Bond MR, Charlton JE, Woolf CJ (eds) Proceedings of the VIth World Congress on Pain. Elsevier, New York, pp 527–533

Gibson SJ, Katz B, Corran TM, Farrell MJ, Helme RD 1994 Pain in older persons. Disability and Rehabilitation 16: 127–139

Giuffre M, Asci J, Arnstein P, Wilkinson C 1991 Postoperative joint replacement pain: description and opioid requirements. Journal of Post Anesthesia Nursing 6: 239–245

Gold DT, Smith SD, Bales CW, Lyles KW, Westlund RE, Drezner MK 1991 Osteoporosis in late life: does health locus of control affect psychosocial adaptation? Journal of the American Geriatrics Society 39: 670–675

Graff-Radford SB, Naliboff BD 1988 Age predicts treatment outcome in postherpetic neuralgia. Clinical Journal of Pain 4: 1–4

Green DM, Swets JA 1966 Signal detection theory and psychophysics. Wiley, New York

Guck TP, Meilman PW, Skultety FM, Dowd ET 1986 Prediction of long-term outcome of multidisciplinary pain treatment. Archives of Physical Medicine and Rehabilitation 67: 293–296

Gullo L, Sipahi HM, Pezzilli R 1994 Pancreatitis in the elderly. Journal of Clinical Gastroenterology 19: 64–68

Hall KRL, Stride E 1954 The varying response to pain in psychiatric disorders: a study in abnormal psychology. British Journal of Medical Psychology 27: 48–60

Hallett EC, Pilowsky I 1982 The response to treatment in a multidisciplinary pain clinic. Pain 12: 365–374

Hardy JD, Wolff HG, Goodell H 1943 The pain threshold in man. American Journal of Psychiatry 99: 744–751

Harkins SW 1988 Pain in the elderly. In: Dubner R, Gebhart FG, Bond MR (eds) Proceedings of the 5th World Congress on Pain. Elsevier Science Publisher BV (Biomedical Division), Amsterdam, pp 355–357

Harkins SW, Chapman CR 1976 Detection and decision factors in pain perception in young and elderly men. Pain 2: 253–264

Harkins SW, Chapman CR 1977 The perception of induced dental pain in young and elderly women. Journal of Gerontology 32: 428–435

Harkins SW, Price DD 1992 Assessment of pain in the elderly. In: Turk DC, Melzack R (eds) Handbook of pain assessment. Guilford, New York, pp 315–331

Harkins SW, Price DD, Martelli M 1986 Effects of age on pain perception: thermonociception. Journal of Gerontology 41: 58–63

Harkins SW, Kwentus J, Price DD 1984 Pain and the elderly. In: Benedetti C, Chapman CR, Morieca G (eds) Advances in pain research and therapy, vol 7. Raven, New York, pp 103–121

Harkins SW, Kwentus J, Price DD 1994 Pain and suffering in the elderly. In: Wall PD, Melzack R (eds) Textbook of pain. Churchill Livingstone, Edinburgh, pp 552–560

Harkins SW, Lagua BT, Price DD, Small RE 1995 Geriatric pain. In: Roy R (ed) Chronic pain in old age. University of Toronto Press, Toronto, pp 127–159

Harkins SW, Davis MD, Bush FM, Kasberger J 1996 Suppression of first pain and slow temporal summation of second pain in relation to age. Journal of Gerontology: Medical Sciences 51A: M260–M265

Heft MW, Cooper BY, O'Brien KK, Hemp E, O'Brien R 1996 Aging effects on the perception of noxious and non-noxious thermal stimuli applied to the face. Aging: Clinical and Experimental Research 8: 35–41

Helme RD, McKernan S 1985 Neurogenic flare responses following topical application of capsaicin in humans. Annals of Neurology 18: 505–509

Helme RD, Katz B, Gibson S, Corran T 1989 Can psychometric tools be used to analyse pain in a geriatric population. Clinical and Experimental Neurology 26: 113–117

Herr KA, Mobily PR 1991 Complexities of pain assessment in the elderly: clinical considerations. Journal of Gerontological Nursing 17: 12–19

Herr KA, Mobily PR 1993 Comparison of selected pain assessment tools for use with the elderly. Applied Nursing Research 6: 39–46

Herr KA, Mobily PR, Kohout FJ, Wagenaar D 1998 Evaluation of the faces pain scale for use with the elderly. Clinical Journal of Pain 14: 29–38

Hofland SL 1992 Elder beliefs: blocks to pain management. Journal of Gerontological Nursing 18: 19–24

Horch K, Hardy M, Jimenez S, Jabaley M 1992 An automated tactile tester for evaluation of cutaneous sensibility. Journal of Hand Surgery 17A: 829–837

Hurley AC, Volicer BJ, Hanrahan PA, Houde S, Volicer L 1992 Assessment of discomfort in advanced Alzheimer patients. Research in Nursing, Health 15: 369–377

Huskisson EC 1974 Measurement of pain. Lancet ii: 1127–1131

Jensen MP, Karoly P 1992 Self-report scales and procedures for assessing pain in adults. In: Turk DC, Melzack R (eds) Handbook of pain assessment. Guilford, New York, pp 135–151

Jensen MP, Karoly P, Braver S 1986 The measurement of clinical pain intensity: a comparison of six methods. Pain 27: 117–126

Jonsson CO, Malhammar G, Waldton S 1977 Reflex elicitation thresholds in senile dementia. Acta Psychiatrica Scandinavica 55: 81–96

Kaiko RF 1980 Age and morphine analgesia in cancer patients with post-operative pain. Clinical Pharmacology and Therapeutics 28: 823–826

Katz J, Kavanaugh BP, Sandler AN et al 1992 Preemptive analgesia: clinical evidence of neuroplasticity contributing to postoperative pain. Anesthesiology 77: 439–446

Katz J, Ritvo P, Irvine MJ, Jackson M 1996 Coping with chronic pain. In: Zeidner M, Endler N S (eds) Handbook of coping: theory, research, applications. John Wiley, New York, pp 252–278

Kee WG, Middaugh SJ, Redpath S, Hargadon R 1998 Age as a factor in admission to chronic pain rehabilitation. Clinical Journal of Pain 14: 121–128

Keefe FJ, Williams DA 1990 A comparison of coping strategies in chronic pain patients in different age groups. Journal of Gerontology: Psychological Sciences 45: 161–165

Kenshalo DR 1986 Somesthetic sensitivity in young and elderly humans. Journal of Gerontology 41: 732–742

Kisely S, Tweddle D, Pugh EW 1992 Dementia presenting with sore eyes. British Journal of Psychiatry 161: 120–121

Kremer E, Atkinson JH, Ignelzi RJ 1981 Measurement of pain: patient preference does not confound pain measurement. Pain 10: 241–249

Kwentus JA, Harkins SW, Lignon N, Silverman JJ 1985 Current concepts in geriatric pain and its treatment. Geriatrics 40: 48–57

Lasch H, Castell DO, Castell JA 1997 Evidence for diminished visceral pain with aging: studies using graded intraesophageal balloon distension. American Journal of Physiology 272: G1–G3

Lautenbacher S, Strian F 1991 Similarities in age differences in heat pain perception and thermal sensitivity. Functional Neurology 6: 129–135

Lavsky-Shulan M, Wallace RB, Kohout FJ, Lemke JH, Morris MC, Smith IM 1985 Prevalence and functional correlates of low back pain in the elderly: the Iowa 65+ rural health study. Journal of the American Geriatrics Society 33: 23–28

Lichtenberg PA, McGrogan AJ 1987 Chronic pain in elderly psychiatric inpatients. Clinical Biofeedback and Health 10: 3–7

Lichtenberg PA, Skehan MW, Swensen CH 1984 The role of personality, recent life stress and arthritic severity in predicting pain. Journal of Psychosomatic Research 28: 231–236

Lichtenberg PA, Swensen CH, Skehan MW 1986 Further investigation of the role of personality, lifestyle and arthritic severity in predicting pain. Journal of Psychosomatic Research 30: 327–337

Lipton RB, Pfeffer D, Newman LC, Solomon S 1993 Headaches in the elderly. Journal of Pain and Symptom Management 8: 87–97

Lynch EP, Lazor MA, Gellis JE, Orav J, Goldman L, Marcantonio ER 1998 The impact of postoperative pain on the development of postoperative delirium. Anesthesia and Analgesia 86: 781–785

Macintyre PE, Jarvis DA 1995 Age is the best predictor of postoperative morphine requirements. Pain 64: 357–364

March LM, Brnabic AJM, Skinner JC et al 1998 Musculoskeletal disability among elderly people in the community. Medical Journal of Australia 168: 439–442

Marzinski LR 1991 The tragedy of dementia: clinically assessing pain in the confused, nonverbal elderly. Journal of Gerontological Nursing 17: 25–28

McCaffery M, Beebe A 1989 Pain in the elderly: special considerations. In: McCaffery M, Beebe A (eds) Pain: clinical manual for nursing practice. CV Mosby, St Louis, MO, pp 308–323

McCracken LM, Mosley TH, Plaud JJ, Gross RT, Penzien DB 1993 Age, chronic pain and impairment: results from two clinical samples. Paper presented at the VIIth World Congress on Pain, Paris, France
Melding PS 1997 Coping with pain in old age. In: Mostofsky DI, Lomranz J (eds) Handbook of pain and aging. Plenum, New York, pp 167–184
Melzack R 1975 The McGill Pain Questionnaire: major properties and scoring methods. Pain 1: 277–299
Melzack R 1987 The short-form McGill Pain Questionnaire. Pain 30: 191–197
Melzack R 1988 The tragedy of needless pain: a call for social action. In: Dubner R, Gebhart GF, Bond MR (eds) Proceedings of the Vth World Congress on Pain. Elsevier Science Publishers BV, Amsterdam, pp 1–11
Melzack R, Katz J 1992 The McGill Pain Questionnaire: appraisal and current status. In: Turk DC, Melzack R (eds) Handbook of pain assessment. Guilford, New York, pp 152–168
Melzack R, Wall PD 1988 The challenge of pain. Penguin Books, London
Middaugh SJ, Levin RB, Kee WG, Barchiesi FD, Roberts JM 1988 Chronic pain: its treatment in geriatric and younger patients. Archives of Physical Medicine and Rehabilitation 69: 1021–1025
Miller C, LeLieuvre RB 1982 A method to reduce chronic pain in elderly nursing home residents. Gerontologist 22: 314–317
Monk TG, Parker RK, White PF 1990 Use of PCA in geriatric patients – effect of aging on the postoperative analgesic requirement. Anesthesia and Analgesia 70: S272
Moore AK, Vilderman S, Lubenskyi W, McCans J, Fox GS 1990 Differences in epidural morphine requirements between elderly and young patients after abdominal surgery. Anesthesia and Analgesia 70: 316–320
Moore ME, Berk SN, Nypaver A 1984 Chronic pain: inpatient treatment with small group effects. Archives of Physical Medicine and Rehabilitation 65: 356–361
Mumford JM 1963 Pain perception in man on electrically stimulating the teeth. In: Soulairac A, Cahn J, Charpentier J (eds) Pain. Academic, London, pp 221–229
Mumford JM 1968 Pain perception in man on electrically stimulating the teeth. In: Soulairac A, Cahn J, Charpentier J (eds) Pain. Academic, London, pp 224–229
Nagy VT, Wolfe GR 1984 Cognitive predictors of compliance in chronic disease patients. Medical Care 22: 912–921
Neri M, Agazzani E 1984 Aging and right–left asymmetry in experimental pain measurement. Pain 19: 43–48
Nicholson NL, Blanchard EB 1993 A controlled evaluation of behavioral treatment of chronic headache in the elderly. Behavior Therapy 24: 395–408
Oberle K, Paul P, Wry J, Grace M 1990 Pain, anxiety and analgesics: a comparative study of elderly and younger surgical patients. Canadian Journal on Aging 9: 13–22
Parke B 1992 Pain in the cognitively impaired elderly. Canadian Nurse 88: 17–20
Parker J, Frank R, Beck N et al 1988 Pain in rheumatoid arthritis: relationship to demographic, medical, and psychological factors. Journal of Rheumatology 15: 433–437
Parkhouse N, Le Quesne PM 1988 Quantitative objective assessment of peripheral nociceptive C-fibre function. Journal of Neurology, Neurosurgery and Psychiatry 51: 28–34
Parmelee PA, Katz IR, Lawton MP 1991 The relation of pain to depression among institutionalized aged. Journal of Gerontology: Psychological Sciences 46: 15–21
Parmelee PA, Smith B, Katz IR 1993 Pain complaints and cognitive status among elderly institution residents. Journal of the American Geriatrics Society 41: 517–522
Pasero C, McCaffery M 1996 Postoperative pain management in the elderly. In: Ferrell BR, Ferrell BA (eds) Pain in the elderly. IASP, Seattle, pp 45–68
Politser P, Schneidman D 1990 American College of Surgeons: socio-economic factbook for surgery 1990. American College of Surgeons, Chicago
Popp B, Portenoy RK 1996 Management of chronic pain in the elderly: pharmacology of opioids and other analgesic drugs. In: Ferrell BR, Ferrell BA (eds) Pain in the elderly. IASP, Seattle, pp 21–34
Portenoy RK, Farkash A 1988 Practical management of non-malignant pain in the elderly. Gerontology 43: 29–47
Porter FL, Malhorta KM, Wolf CM, Morris JC, Miller JP, Smith MC 1996 Dementia and the response to pain in the elderly. Pain 68: 413–421
Procacci P, Bozza G, Buzzelli G, Della Corte M 1970 The cutaneous pricking pain threshold in old age. Gerontological Clinics 12: 213–218
Procacci P, Zoppi M, Maresca M 1979 Experimental pain in man. Pain 6: 123–140
Prohaska TR, Keller ML, Leventhal EA, Leventhal H 1987 Impact of symptoms and aging attribution on emotion and coping. Health Psychology 6: 495–514
Puder RS 1988 Age analysis of cognitive-behavioral group therapy for chronic pain outpatients. Psychology and Aging 3: 204–207
Rollman GB 1977 Signal detection theory measurement of pain: a review and critique. Pain 3: 187–211
Ross MM, Crook J 1998 Elderly recipients of home nursing services: pain, disability and functional competence. Journal of Advanced Nursing 27: 1117–1126
Roy R, Thomas M 1986 A survey of chronic pain in an elderly population. Canadian Family Physician 32: 513–516
Roy R, Thomas MR 1987 Elderly persons with and without pain: a comparative study. Clinical Journal of Pain 3: 102–106
Rudy TE, Kerns RD, Turk DC 1988 Chronic pain and depression: toward a cognitive-behavioral mediation model. Pain 35: 129–140
Sandin KJ 1993 Specialized pain treatment for geriatric patients. Clinical Journal of Pain 9: 60
Scapa E, Horowitz M, Waron M, Eshchar J 1989 Duodenal ulcer in the elderly. Journal of Clinical Gastroenterology 11: 502–506
Scapa E, Horowitz M, Avtalion J, Waron M, Eshchar J 1992 Appreciation of pain in the elderly. Israel Journal of Medical Science 28: 94–96
Schludermann E, Zubek JP 1962 Effect of age on pain sensitivity. Perceptual and Motor Skills 14: 295–301
Schumacher GA, Goodell H, Hardy JD, Wolff HG 1940 Uniformity of the pain threshold in man. Science 92: 110–112
Schwartz BS, Stewart WF, Simon D, Lipton RB 1998 Epidemiology of tension-type headache. Journal of the American Medical Association 279: 381–383
Scudds RJ, Robertson JM 1998 Empirical evidence of the association between the presence of musculoskeletal pain and physical disability in community-dwelling senior citizens. Pain 75: 229–235
Segall A, Chappell NL 1991 Making sense out of sickness: lay explanations of chronic illness among older adults. Advances in Medical Sociology 2: 115–133
Sherman ED, Robillard E 1960 Sensitivity to pain in the aged. Canadian Medical Association Journal 38: 944–947
Sigurdsson E, Thorgeirsson G, Sigvaldason H, Sigfusson N 1995 Unrecognized myocardial infarction: epidemiology, clinical characteristics, and the prognostic role of angina pectoris. Annals of Internal Medicine 122: 96–102
Sorkin BA, Turk DC 1995 Pain management in the elderly. In: Roy R (ed) Chronic pain in old age. University of Toronto Press, Toronto, pp 56–80
Sorkin BA, Rudy TE, Hanlon RB, Turk DC, Stieg RL 1990 Chronic pain in old and young patients: differences appear less important than

similarities. Journal of Gerontology: Psychological Sciences 45: 64–68
Sternbach RA 1986 Survey of pain in the United States: the Nuprin pain report. Clinical Journal of Pain 2: 49–53
Takeshima T, Taniguchi R, Kitagawa T, Takahashi K 1990 Headaches in dementia. Headache 30: 735–738
Thorsteinsson G 1987 Chronic pain: use of TENS in the elderly. Gerontology 42: 75–82
Tremblay N 1994 Douleurs du vieillard: revue des connaissances actuelles. In: Roy DJ, Rapin C H (eds) Collection Amaryllis. Les Annales de soins palliatifs. Monographie II: 'Douleur et antalgie'. Institute de Recherche Clinique de Montreal, Montreal, pp 99–112
Tucker MA, Andrew MF, Ogle SJ, Davison JG 1989 Age-associated change in pain threshold measured by transcutaneous neuronal electrical stimulation. Age and Ageing 18: 241–246
Turk DC, Meichenbaum D 1994 A cognitive-behavioural approach to pain management. In: Wall PD, Melzack R (eds) Textbook of pain, 3rd edn. Churchill Livingstone, pp 1337–1348
Turk DC, Okifuji A, Scharff L 1995 Chronic pain and depression: role of perceived impact and perceived control in different age cohorts. Pain 61: 93–101
US Department of Commerce 1991 Global aging: comparative indicators and future trends. US Department of Commerce, Economics and Statistics Administration, Bureau of the Census, Washington, DC
Valkenburg HA 1988 Epidemiological considerations of the geriatric population. Gerontology 34 (suppl 1): 2–10
Wallston FA, Wallston BS, DeVellis R 1978 Development of the Multidimensional Health Locus of Control (MHLC) scales. Health Education Monographs 9: 160–170
Walsh NE, Schoenfeld L, Ramamurthy S, Hoffman J 1989 Normative model for cold pressor test. American Journal of Physical Medicine and Rehabilitation 68: 6–11
Weiner D, Peiper C, McConnell E, Martinez S, Keefe FJ 1996 Pain measurement in elders with chronic low back pain: traditional and alternative approaches. Pain 67: 461–467
Weisenberg M 1994 Cognitive aspects of pain. In: Wall PD, Melzack R (eds) Textbook of pain, 3rd edn. Churchill Livingstone, pp 275–289
Werner P, Cohen-Mansfield J, Watson V, Pasis S 1998 Pain in participants of adult day care centers: assessment by different raters. Journal of Pain and Symptom Management 15: 8–17
Wilke DJ, Savedra MC, Holzemer WL, Tesler MD, Paul SM 1990 Use of the McGill Pain Questionnaire to measure pain: a meta-analysis. Nursing Research 39: 36–41
Wilkieson CA, Madhok R, Hunter JA, Capell HA 1993 Toleration, side-effects and efficacy of sulphasalazine in rheumatoid arthritis patients of different ages. Quarterly Journal of Medicine 86: 501–505
Williamson GM, Schulz R 1992 Pain, activity restriction and symptoms of depression among community-residing elderly adults. Journal of Gerontology 47: 367–372
Williamson GM, Schulz R 1995 Activity restriction mediates the association between pain and depressed affect: a study of younger and older adult cancer patients. Psychology and Aging 10: 369–378
Wolfe F, Ross K, Anderson J, Russell IJ, Hebert L 1995 The prevalence and characteristics of fibromyalgia in the general population. Arthritis and Rheumatism 38: 19–28
Woo J, Ho SC, Lau J, Leung PC 1994 Musculoskeletal complaints and associated consequences in elderly Chinese aged 70 and over. Journal of Rheumatology 21: 1927–1931
Woodrow KM, Friedman GD, Siegelaub AB, Collen MF 1972 Pain tolerance: differences according to age, sex and race. Psychosomatic Medicine 34: 548–556
Wright D, Barrow S, Fisher AD, Horsley D, Jayson MIV 1995 Influence of physical, psychological and behavioural factors on consultations for back pain. British Journal of Rheumatology 34: 156–161
Ysla V, Ysla R, Rosomoff RS, Rosomoff HL 1986 Functional improvement in geriatric chronic pain patients. Archives of Physical Medicine and Rehabilitation 67: 685

Pain in animals

CHARLES E. SHORT

SUMMARY

This chapter will review methods for assessing pain in animals which need healthcare in veterinary hospitals, on farms and ranches, at zoos or wildlife reserves, or in the laboratory. A major purpose is to provide knowledge that can be applied to improve clinical pain management in animals. The concept for pain management in animals and humans is based on similar scientific and ethical considerations. Assessment of the animal patient for the degree of pain management which is needed is complicated by the lack of ability to talk with the patient. How do we know when an animal is expressing pain? Far more reliance on the observations of the animal's behaviour by the healthcare team and the owners or their assistants is necessary than in adult humans. Animal pain recognition and treatment is similar in many concepts to that needed in infants and young children. There is a need to continually improve our understanding of animal pain and to expand our ability to prevent, reduce or minimize their suffering when possible.

INTRODUCTION

The definition of pain in humans as an unpleasant sensory and emotional experience with actual or potential tissue damage (Merskey 1979) may be applied to the animal patient. Bonica (1992) stated that, in man, 50–80% of patients may have inadequate control of pain at some point in their hospital stay. He further noted that animal pain recognition and control are even greater challenges than in the human patient. The assessment of animal pain includes both behavioural and physiological responses (Wall 1992, Livingston 1994). It is generally accepted that animals perceive and react to the sensation termed pain in a manner similar to humans (Flecknell 1994). This is a realistic conclusion because anatomical and biochemical pathways of pain perception in animals and man are similar (Morton & Griffiths 1985, Potthoff & Carithers 1987). Moreover, behavioural similarities can be used to justify the validity of animal research for the benefit of improved pain management in humans (Dubner et al 1976, Vierck & Cooper 1983, Dubner 1985).

It is ethically necessary to minimize clinical pain in animals used for research. Efforts should be made to refine, reduce or replace excessive use of animal models. Carefully designed studies using animal models, especially in the development of new analgesics, can provide objective data for evaluation. This becomes quite apparent if the noxious stimulus applied is of a transient nature, such as the cold pressor test, applied heat for thermal response (Oppel & Hardy 1937, Coderre & Melzack 1985) or cross-clamp of the tail with forceps for mechanical response. The response to tissue injury by chemical substances such as formalin injection or to arthritic models produced by sodium urate crystals (Okuda et al 1984, Coderre & Wall 1987) are of longer duration and not always as adaptable to different experimental designs as protocols without tissue damage.

In the experimental model, it is possible to compare behavioural change evoked by noxious stimuli with control data, and to evaluate the effects of the stimuli on sensory and autonomic function and endocrine secretion. This concept is used to test the effectiveness and duration of pain management in the preclinical development of new analgesics. The animal model has contributed significantly to the understanding of pain and to pain management in both animals and humans.

There is a far greater concern in animal pain management than just the need to address ethical and scientific issues in the research laboratory (Flecknell 1994). The clinical application of pain management in animals to conditions caused by animal-to-animal or human-to-animal injuries, naturally occurring diseases (Amyx 1987) and surgical and diagnostic procedures in all animal species is of global concern. It is recognized that there is no more noble cause in veterinary medicine than the relief of suffering in animals. The veterinarian's oath charges graduates to use their skills and knowledge for the relief of animal suffering. A better understanding of human pain management contributes to greater insight into animal pain. In particular, postoperative pain management in a modern veterinary hospital has benefited greatly from the development of anaesthetic and analgesic drugs to relieve human suffering.

OUTWARD SIGNS OF PAIN IN ANIMALS

As in humans, pain in animals is frequently the health problem which alerts the owner to seek healthcare. Because animals cannot describe pain sensations, initial signs of pain must be identified as the contrast between normal and abnormal behaviour (Laties 1987, Hansen 1997). An understanding of normal behaviour in both natural and unnatural environments is crucial to evaluation. A sudden change in behaviour within the natural environment is often the first indication of an acute tissue injury. The injured animal may attempt to escape from the location where trauma occurred. It may object to return to the scene of trauma. It may lick, bite, scratch or chew at the location of pain sensation. It may walk or run until out of danger, only to be unable to bear weight on the injured part at a later time. Some species or individuals within species will seek cover, hide, lie motionless and become completely silent. Others will vocalize by barking, growling, whimpering, crying, squealing, screaming or hissing. Pain in the silent suffering animal is more difficult to diagnose than in animals who are more expressive.

Changes from normal to abnormal body movements may serve as the primary symptom of pain. The failure to bear weight, kicking, frequent changes in body position, restlessness, rolling, stiffness, abnormal gait, abnormal standing, sitting, lying positions or an unwillingness to move indicates that acute pain may be present. Animals involved in work or sports usually have reduced capability to perform, often proportional to the extent of injury. This can vary from slight modification in performance levels due to sore muscles or inflammation of joints to severe changes where they cannot perform the usual tasks due to cartilage or ligament damage. Fractures or major nerve damage may cause an inability to perform tasks and abnormal physiological function. Comparative evaluation of the responses at rest to those during exercise or manipulation are commonly indicative of the extent of injury and the severity of pain.

The effect of stress or pain on metabolism can be greatly influenced by the duration of pain. In acute pain, tolerance frequently develops before complete tissue healing and the animal returns to normal eating and drinking habits. By contrast, in chronic pain conditions, prolonged symptoms may be observed which include parameters unobserved in acute pain. In some cases, body weight is lost because excessive orthopaedic pain discourages the animal from moving to the source of food or dental pain may prevent it from eating. In other cases, the animal can eat and drink but, due to reduced physical activity, begins to accumulate excessive weight gains.

Errors are made in pain assessment in animals as a result of changes in behaviour which are influenced by factors other than pain. The animal may appear normal in its own environment, yet develop symptoms of pain in an artificial setting. An animal that is forced to return to the site of trauma may have significant behavioural changes. Changes in noise and other environmental conditions may evoke stress even in an animal with no tissue damage to induce pain. Placing a domestic cat in a hospital ward with barking dogs may initiate severe stress even though no physical contact is made. The addition of loud noise, bright lights or major changes in environmental temperature which cause behavioural changes are difficult to categorize into pain or stress, especially in the postoperative recovery period. Pain management is also influenced by the patient's requests. In humans, patient demand influences analgesic selection, dose, interval and methods of administration. In animals, this is subject solely to analysis by an observer.

Facial expressions are often key to the diagnosis of pain: the appearance of the eyes and the position of the ears; is the head erect or drooping; is the animal alert or depressed. Excessive tear formation, dilatation of the pupils, drooping, position of the eyelids, dullness of the eyes and response to changing light or sounds indicate a change from normal pain-free health. Not all animals are outwardly expressive of pain. There are differences in pain tolerance levels among individual animals, just as in humans. The contrast among species, however, creates unique problems in the diagnosis of pain and evaluation of pain management practices. It is difficult to estimate the number of animals that suffered needlessly because they did not vocalize.

Tranquillizers and sedatives calm the animal so that it is less stressed by its environment, although pain relief may not be achieved. Especially in some species, opioid analgesics may increase the stress to environmental noise or bright lights even though the response to tissue damage (pain) is minimized. Injuries may primarily cause somatic pain if superficial. These are frequently observed as fight wounds, especially among dogs and cats. By contrast, the smaller animal attacked by a large dog may suffer deeper wounds with extensive tissue injury. Penetration of the thorax or abdomen may occur. Often injuries to the head and neck regions are present. The tissue damage from these injuries is extensive and readily evident on physical examination. Extensive damage can be coupled with behavioural responses. An aggressive or defensive response of the animal to touch or palpation of the injured area can be expected. Not to be confused in diagnosis are the contrasts between areas of hyperalgesia and allodynia which may be present in spinal injury or other neuropathies (Gilmore 1986, Morgan et al 1993, Sukhiani et al 1996).

Historically, more attention has been given to the control of acute pain related to surgical and diagnostic procedures than to chronic pain. The animal is examined prior to surgery or diagnostic testing for the development of the analgesic–anaesthetic protocol. Physiological responses are recorded before, during and following surgery (Conzemius et al 1997). Differences in responses are evaluated to adjust the administration of medications for pain management. The animal healthcare team has the opportunity to compare objective evaluations in a manner similar to the scientific protocol in experimental animal pain research. The stimuli are the surgery or diagnostic procedures, in contrast to noxious stimuli from a thermal, chemical or mechanical source (Raekallio et al 1997).

Chronic pain states in animals are more difficult to evaluate. A slowly developing chronic condition may not be observed by the owner until it is in an advanced stage. One only has to consider the differences in severe acute visceral pain in equine colic in comparison with cancer pain in animals to realize that in animals as in humans medical treatment of chronic conditions may only occur after much damage and suffering have been endured. Chronic pain in animals, especially involving dental or gastrointestinal deterioration, may be first observed as body weight loss, dull or ungroomed hair, or lethargy.

Arthritic changes in family pets have become an important consideration. All too often in the past, inactivity in an older pet was considered to be a normal part of ageing. As the animal became less active, there was an initial increase in body weight. Body conditions deteriorated. Considerable progress has been made in identifying these symptoms with chronic arthritis. Treatment with anti-inflammatory medications can not only be therapeutic but also contributes to diagnosis, especially in numerous animals where reduction in inflammatory responses of arthritis has restored the animals to a physically active state.

In spite of the advances in understanding animal behaviour, pain scoring is difficult. Visual analogue scores (VAS), numerical rating scales (Conzemius et al 1997, Welsh et al 1993) or any other pain score index usually involves translating subjective assessment values into numbers. Similarly, an evaluation of animal pain and successful management should include both behaviour scoring other and objective measurements. It is not unusual to find significant differences in pain scores among multiple observers. This was recently confirmed in a study utilizing multiple observers evaluating clinical animal pain with the simple descriptive scale (SDS), numerical rating scale (NRS) and VAS. These scales allow human patients to rate the intensity of their pain, but in animals are subject to observer variability (Holton et al 1998). Pain scoring systems can be adapted to special conditions, such as acute, surgical or other types of pain (Table 44.1).

Table 44.1 Pain scores following clinical surgery

Vocalization	*Attention to wound or incision site*	*Mobility*	*Agitation*
0 = no pain-related vocalization	0 = none	0 = unimpaired	0 = calm and/or sleeping
1 = occasional pain-related vocalization	1 = occasional	1 = slightly impaired	1 = mild
2 = frequent pain-related vocalization	2 = frequent	2 = reluctant to position change or frequent position changes	2 = moderate
3 = continuous pain-related vocalization	3 = continuous	3 = resistant to position changes or continuous movement	3 = hysterical or aggressive

Successful pain management = no more than 1 pain criterion with a score of 2 or 3.
Failure of pain management = 2 or more pain criteria scores of 2 or 3.
This system can be adapted for different species or different types of surgery to monitor postoperative pain management.

MEASURABLE RESPONSES INDICATIVE OF PAIN

A careful design to combine subjective behavioural evaluation with objective changes in physiological function provides a more reliable index of the presence of clinical pain and the effectiveness of its management in animals. This, at present, is more predictable with intraoperative and postoperative pain management.

Pain has a significant influence on the autonomic nervous system. Pain stimulation may cause an increase in heart rate, vasoconstriction, an increase in blood pressure and change in blood flow. Respiratory patterns often change, reflective of the site of pain. Endocrine levels also change, and especially indicative of pain are increases in cortisol levels (Benson et al 1991). A comparison of cardiovascular parameters recorded after anaesthetic induction, at the time of skin incision, during surgery and during recovery provides useful information for pain management. Some changes are expected during stimulation unless the animal has received high concentrations of analgesics and anaesthetics, but significant changes in these parameters at the onset of surgery are indicative of inadequate pain management.

These changes are not as easily evaluated in animals with chronic pain. An improved diagnostic approach can be adapted, provided the use of analgesics is included in the evaluation process. A clinical crossover protocol should be used. The animal is evaluated at rest and during stimulation such as during mild exercise. Then it is re-evaluated after receiving analgesics by repeating the same tests. Diagnosis of the level of pain can be accomplished by either evaluating the physiological response to varying doses of analgesic or by increasing the workload. The selective use of medications can be part of the evaluation process. This is especially useful in the use of analgesics for the treatment of chronic pain in performance animals. Furthermore, diagnostic nerve blocks are often used to locate the primary site of pain in animals.

SPECIES CONSIDERATIONS IN ANIMAL PAIN

There are multiple types of pain and differences among species in their response to them. There are also major species differences in the effects of various medications and their dosages for treatment.

A number of parameters are useful in the evaluation of animals with pain or distress. Changes in overall appearance can be an outward sign of discomfort (Conzemius et al 1997). Among all species, the hair coat – such as the loss of the natural healthy appearance, loss of hair or failure to groom – may be an indication of pain and a failure to maintain normal metabolism and body function. The animal may have lost weight and the skin texture may have deteriorated. The eyes may appear sunken, depressed or show evidence of a discharge. Consideration must be given to diagnose the problem relative to chronic pain, infectious disease or metabolic conditions. A reduced food and water intake may be observed. A reduced food intake would contribute to a slower growth rate in younger animals or weight loss at any age. There would also be a reduction in faecal output. An absence of faecal output, failure to eat and signs of visceral pain can be indicative of intestinal blockage.

A reduced fluid intake may be more difficult to detect prior to signs of dehydration in most species. A failure to eat or drink may be associated with orthopaedic pain. It is also commonly associated with dental pain. In some animals, reduced mobility due to pain may result in a failure of proper elimination of urine and faeces, resulting in urine retention and/or constipation, especially among trained indoor pets.

Behavioural patterns are more species specific. Behavioural patterns may also be altered by the site of pain. Species with signs of behaviour indicating pain are listed in Table 44.2. It is recognized that individual animals may exhibit unique patterns. In general, pain induces a behavioural change. Observations of these changes are a subjective means of evaluation in lieu of the animal being able to describe pain to the healthcare team.

Behavioural patterns may vary significantly as a function of animal species as well as the location of tissue damage and the duration of tissue healing. Behavioural patterns alone do not provide a comprehensive evaluation of pain and its management in animals. Perhaps it is even more important in animals than in man to evaluate clinical signs of pain and to determine the extent to which analgesics relieve or manage pain (Johnson 1991).

Of the major farm animal species currently considered in pain management, the horse has received the most attention (Table 44.2). The horse is used for work and sports. Exhaustive work in draft horses and mules may contribute to muscular pain. This can often be diagnosed by soreness of muscles, myositis, inability to move, haematuria and elevated muscle enzyme levels. High-performance events including racing, shows, and other sporting events may contribute to soreness (Klide & Martin 1989) or musculoskeletal breakdown (Eisenmenger et al 1989). Severe tissue damage may contribute to early retirement from

Table 44.2 Species-typical symptoms of pain in animals

Species	*Posture*	*Temperament*	*Vocalization*	*Locomotion*	*Other*
Farm animal					
Horse	Standing with head down, standing on three legs, rolling on ground, recumbency in severe pain, tucked abdomen, arched back, abnormal position of feet and legs, dropped ears	Aggressive, kicking, striking, biting, uncooperative, fighting, defeated, docile, escaping	Quiet, grunting, moaning	Lameness, reduced speed, abnormal gait, non-weight-bearing, reluctance to move, walks on toes or hocks	Self-trauma, significant reduction in performance, dull eyes
Cattle	Prolonged sternal recumbency, head and neck extended or flexed into flank area	Aggressive, kicking, head butting, grinding teeth, docile	Bawling or quiet	Reluctance to move, abnormal gait, lameness, dragging leg, incoordinated, hopping or lunging	Reduced milk production
Sheep	Head and neck dropping, prolonged sternal recumbency	Docile, escaping, grinding teeth	Blatting or quiet	Reluctance to move, abnormal positioning of feet	Defeated outlook
Goat	Head and neck dropping or extended, prolonged sternal recumbency	Docile, escaping, grinding teeth	Blatting or quiet	Reluctance to move, abnormal positioning of feet	Defeated outlook
Pig	Prolonged recumbency, arched back, drooping head	Aggressive, escaping, biting, slashing	Squealing or quiet	Reluctance to move, walking with arched back	Poor growth or loss of weight
Domestic poultry	Prolonged setting on feet, drooping of wings, head and neck, head turned and under wing, hiding	Docile, appears asleep	Excessive noise or quiet	Reluctance to move, no effort to use wings	Reduced egg production
Pets					
Dog	Tail between legs, arched or hunched back, twisted body to protect pain site, drooped head, prolonged sitting position, tucked abdomen, lying in flat, extended position	Aggressive, biting, clawing, attacking, escaping	Barking, howling, moaning, whimpering	Reluctance to move, carrying one leg, lameness, unusual gait, unable to walk, refuses to climb stairs	Unable to perform normal tasks, attacks other animals or people if painful area is touched, chewing painful areas (self-trauma), tearing
Cat	Tucked limbs, arched or hunched head and neck or back, tucked abdomen, lying flat, slumping of the body, drooping of the head	Aggressive, biting, scratching, chewing, attacking, escaping	Crying, hissing, spitting, moaning, screaming	Reluctance to move, carrying one leg, lameness, unusual gait, unable to walk	Attack if painful areas are touched, failure to groom, dilated pupils
Laboratory animals					
Rat	Persistent recumbent posture, hiding	Aggressive or docile	Squealing	Accelerated or depressed movement	Abnormal writhing, eats bedding
Rabbit	Anxious, facing back of cage, hiding	Aggressive, docile, kicking, scratching	Piercing squealing	Accelerated or depressed movement	—
Guinea pig	Anxious, hiding, recumbent	Quiet, terrified, agitated	Repetitive squealing	Drags back legs	—
Subhuman					
Primates	Head forward, arms across body, arms drooping, head and neck sagging, arched back, excessive recumbency	Aggressive, facial grimace, fighting, terrified, agitated, anxious, restlessness	Screaming, crying, whimpering, quiet	Difficult movement, failure to climb, excessive or incoordinated movements	Self-trauma, change in personality
Wild/exotic animals	Recumbency, arched head and neck, hiding	Aggressive, terrified, escaping, fighting	Screaming, squealing, quiet, moaning	Running, flying (escaping), limited movement (hiding), lameness	Refusal or unable to perform trained tasks

high-performance events unless therapy and pain management are successful (Raekallio et al 1997). Diagnosis of the extent of tissue trauma causing pain is essential. The presence of undiagnosed chip fractures or other conditions may be overlooked if pain medications are administered prematurely. Horses encouraged to maintain a high performance during the administration of non-steroidal anti-inflammatory drugs (NSAIDs) can develop chronic pain states.

Abdominal pain due to a range of gastrointestinal anomalies including torsion, blockage, intersusception or rupture presents dramatic symptoms. Although initial symptoms may be mild, untreated visceral pain can result in severe suffering characterized by sweating, restlessness, self-mutilation, elevated heart rates, deterioration of fluid and electrolyte balance, and alteration in blood flow and eventual shock as the stretch and chemoreceptors of the intestines are stimulated (Sanford et al 1986). Often there will be areas of intestinal ischaemia to further contribute to the discomfort (Pascoe et al 1990). Early radiographic or ultrasonographic diagnosis may be helpful in foals or small breeds, but ineffective in larger adult horses (Klohnen et al 1996). The use of systemic analgesics or regional nerve blocks such as epidural morphine may be helpful in diagnosis as well as therapy (Valverde et al 1990).

Cattle are more stoic than horses (Table 44.2). They appear dull and depressed with little interest in their surroundings. Milk production drops in lactating cows. Cows, like other ruminants, may grind their teeth (Sanford et al 1986). Cows may kick at the abdomen during severe intestinal pain. The extremities may be cold, exhibit decreased skin turgor and they may have sunken eyes (Garber & Madison 1991).

Sheep and goats have similar responses. Previously, they received little attention. More recently, concerns for pain management in adult sheep with foot rot or lambs at docking and castration have stimulated efforts for better pain management (Molony & Kent 1997, Molony et al 1997). The use of techniques such as electroacupuncture-induced analgesia (Bossut et al 1986), NSAIDs or opioids (Waterman et al 1991) in sheep have been helpful in defining the signs of pain in sheep and goats, even though they are more likely to vocalize in response to pain than cattle. This is especially true in goats.

Pigs may attempt to escape when handled (McGlone et al 1993). They are prone to vocalize; however, vocalization can be a confusing symptom unless the type of sounds are understood. The farmer is more likely to recognize the difference between pain and other causes of vocalization.

Unusual conditions may become evident in domestic poultry during pain. Acute pain may be present after corrective procedures in chickens (Gentle et al 1990) or after chronic conditions such as degenerative hip disorders in adult male turkeys (Duncan et al 1991). The individual injured or sick bird may fall victim to the flock. Other turkeys or chickens may peck the disabled bird until death unless there is intervention. Signs of pain are head shaking, pecking and beak whipping.

Companion animals have been evaluated more than farm animals (Table 44.2), and signs of pain are usually recognized rapidly by individual owners. Symptoms of pain and pain management methods in dogs and cats are frequently comparable to those in humans. This has been observed in acute injury, postoperative management and chronic pain (Tranquilli et al 1989, Pascoe et al 1990, Nolan & Reid 1993, Popilskis et al 1993, Lascelles et al 1995, Sammarco et al 1996, Smith et al 1996, Conzemius et al 1997). The behavioural patterns of visceral pain have been evaluated by using an intestinal balloon model. The behavioural patterns were altered by analgesics sufficiently to aid in improving the ability to recognize abdominal pain (Sawyer et al 1992).

Species differences in response to pain make it more difficult to have a simple standard scoring system (Morgan & Griffiths 1985, Morton 1986, Benson & Thurmon 1987, Sanford 1992, Morgan et al 1993). However, awareness of the behavioural signs (Table 44.2) contributes to improved diagnosis.

PHYSIOLOGICAL SIGNS OF ANIMAL PAIN

Behavioural signs of pain may be evaluated by observed responses, which may be highly subjective. More objective measurements include obtaining numerical data for comparison between pain and pain-free conditions. This includes recording of physiological parameters before and during pain or during pain without analgesics compared with post-medication. The common physiological signs of pain in animals are described in Table 44.3.

The concept of comparing behavioural patterns with objective measures includes both physical diagnostic skills and more complex measurements with modern instruments.

A neurological system evaluation is indicated if outward peripheral and/or central nervous system symptoms are observed. Upon observing signs of pain, more complex measures of evoked potential analysis, standard EEGs or brain wave analysis by computerized spectral array may be considered. The use of these technologies is especially useful in determining adequate levels of analgesics and anaesthetics in injured animals before, during and following corrective surgery. It has been shown that higher concentrations of medications are necessary to maintain neurological stability

Table 44.3 Common objective signs of animal pain

System	*Signs*	*Measurements*
Neurological	Twitching, tremors, convulsions, paralysis, dilated pupils, hyperaesthesia, reflexes sluggish, absent or exaggerated areas of numbness	Neurological examination, compressed spectral analysis, evoked potential analysis
Cardiovascular	Changes in heart rate, cardiac dysrhythmias, changes in vascular resistance, changes in blood pressure, changes in blood flow, changes in cardiac output	Capillary refill time, palpation of arterial pulse, auscultation, ECG, blood pressure, cardiac output, blood flow measurements
Respiratory	Changes in respiratory rate, changes in minute volume, changes in oxygen saturation, changes in blood gases and pH	Monitor respiratory rate, mucous membrane colour change, pulse oximetry, capnometry, arterial blood gases and pH, mucous membrane colour change
Musculoskeletal	Lameness, unsteady gait, muscle flaccidity, rigidity, reluctance to move, muscle twitching, tetanus, atrophy	Palpation, gait analysis, radiographs, diagnostic nerve blocks, force plate analysis, EMG, CPK
Digestive	Body weight loss or poor growth, faeces altered in volume, colour, amount or consistency, vomiting, jaundice, bleeding	Measure food consumption, blood glucose, insulin levels, total serum protein, serum electrolytes
Urinary	Urine retention, decrease in volume, change in specific gravity	Urinalysis, blood urea nitrogen, serum electrolytes
Endocrine	Hyperactivity, sluggishness, depression	Cortisol, ACTH, catecholamines, endogenous opioid levels
Miscellaneous	Abnormal swelling, protrusion (hernia), changes in body temperature, discoloured skin, crepitation	Physical examination

during corrective surgery in horses compared with elective procedures (Miller et al 1995).

Outward signs of inflammation, increases or decreases in skin temperature, or changes in capillary refill time are simple signs which may be associated with moderate to severe pain. The cardiovascular changes during profound visceral pain reveal increases in heart rate, alteration in vasoconstriction, bloodflow and blood pressure. These changes may be significant as pain influences the autonomic nervous system. Untreated severe pain may ultimately contribute to a shock-like condition. Untreated shock leads to debilitation and, ultimately, death. Severe cardiovascular alterations as a result of extensive visceral pain will more likely show greater correction when the combination of pain management and cardiovascular support are provided.

Measurements of respiratory responses during pain are influenced by both the severity and site of tissue damage. The value of these measurements may be significantly altered by analgesics. An understanding of the influence of analgesics on the cardiopulmonary system is beneficial. While it is known that μ-receptor opioids may contribute to respiratory depression, this is not always observed. The animal with thoracic trauma such as bruises or fractures may have improved ventilation following the use of analgesics. Pain relief allows chest expansion and improved ventilation. This can be both therapeutic and diagnostic. Measurements of arterial blood gases and pH and oxygen saturation may demonstrate improvement.

In non-surgical animals, evaluation of the musculoskeletal system is of great importance. The degree of lameness and the performance levels of many animals are influenced by pain. Pain can be diagnosed by responses during physical examination, however, confirming radiographs or other imaging techniques which provide information on the extent of tissue damage. Further confirmation of pain and its relief can be made by the return towards normal of muscle enzyme levels, positive force plate analysis, or the return to prior exercise performance levels. Pain responses, including cardiopulmonary change, may be present during physical examination of musculoskeletal damage.

Measurements of food and water consumption and the evaluation of laboratory data can provide objective values to indicate the digestive and metabolic state during clinical pain in animals. The failure to recognize the signs of inadequate maintenance of metabolic needs contributes to further discomfort. The conditions enteritis or constipation contribute to visceral pain.

Measurements to evaluate urinary function are helpful in diagnosis. The animal with urethral blockage will initially have pain from an overdistended bladder. Laboratory data are helpful in determining the extent of uraemia. Untreated blockage may eventually lead to severe uraemia with symptoms of neurological depression.

Methods of objective measurement which contribute to recognizing animal pain, and effective pain management, need to be selected to complement the site or duration of injury or disease. These measurements can be influenced by the activity of the patient. The data will often change significantly if the animal becomes more active, in contrast to evaluation at rest.

Clinical pain in animals is of great concern. Extensive efforts have been made to define subjective and objective methods to diagnose the site and extent of pain in multiple species. Pain alters behavioural and physiological parameters from the normal range, and pain management helps to restore these parameters to normal values for the animal patient. These efforts are also necessary to determine the effectiveness of pain management protocols. Pain management has not been addressed in this chapter. All classes of analgesics which are effective in man can be used in most species of animals for the control of clinical pain. Dosages, methods of administration, duration of analgesia and potential side effects usually vary among species. Through the combined scientific efforts of the professions, progress in the management of clinical pain in humans and animals will continue.

REFERENCES

Amayx HL 1987 Control of animal pain and distress in antibody production and infectious disease studies. Journal of the American Veterinary Medical Association 191: 1287–1289

Benson GJ, Thurmon JC 1987 Species difference as a consideration in alleviation of animal pain and distress. Journal of the American Veterinary Medical Association 191: 1227–1230

Benson GJ, Wheaton LG, Thurmon JC et al 1991 Postoperative catecholamine response to onychectomy in isoflurane-anesthetized cats: effects of analgesics. Veterinary Surgery 20: 222–225

Bonica JJ 1992 Pain research and therapy: history, current status, and future goals. In: Short CE, Van Poznak A (eds) Animal pain. Churchill Livingstone, New York, pp 4–5, 20–21

Bossut DFB, Stromberg MW, Malven PV 1986 Electroacupuncture-induced analgesia in sheep: measurement of cutaneous pain thresholds and plasma concentrations of prolactin and β-endorphin immunoreactivity. American Journal of Veterinary Research 47: 669–676

Coderre TJ, Melzack R 1985 Increased pain sensitivity following heat injury involves a central mechanism. Brain Research 15: 259–262

Coderre TJ, Wall PD 1987 Ankle joint urate arthritis (AJUA) in rats: an alternative animal model of arthritis to that produced by Freund's adjuvant. Pain 28: 379–393

Conzemius MG, Hill CM, Sammarco JL, Perkowski SZ 1997 Correlation between subjective and objective measures used to determine severity of post-operative pain in dogs. Journal of the American Veterinary Medical Association 210: 1619–1622

Dubner R 1985 Specialization in nociceptive pathways: sensory discrimination, sensory modulation, and neural connectivity. In: Fields HL, Dubner R, Cervero F (eds) Advances in pain research and therapy, vol 9. Raven, New York, pp 111–137

Dubner R, Beitel RE, Brown FJ 1976 A behavioral animal model for the study of pain mechanisms in primates. In: Weisenberg M, Tursky B (eds) Pain: new perspectives in therapy and research. Plenum, New York, pp 155–170

Duncan IJH, Beatty ER, Hocking PM, Duff SRI 1991 Assessment of pain associated with degenerative hip disorders in adult male turkeys. Research in Veterinary Science 50: 200–203

Eisenmenger E, Kasper I, Eisenmenger M 1989 Bemerkungen zum Schmerz syndrom im leuden-kreuz berich von Pferdes und behandulungsversuch mit neuraltherapie. Pfedeheilkunde 5: 193–199

Flecknell PA 1985 The management of post-operative pain and distress in experimental animals. Animal Tech J Inst Tech 36: 97–103

Flecknell PA 1994 Refinement of animal use in assessment and alleviation of pain and distress. Laboratory Animal 28: 222–231

Garber JL, Madison JB 1991 Signs of abdominal pain caused by disruption of the small intestinal mesentery in three post-parturient cows. Journal of the American Veterinary Medical Association 198: 864–866

Gentle MJ, Waddington D, Hunter LN, Jones RB 1990 Behavioral evidence for persistent pain following partial beak amputation in chickens. Applied Animal Behavioral Science 27: 149–157

Gilmore DR 1986 Lumbosacral pain in the dog. Canine Practice 13: 6–11

Hansen B 1997 Through a glass darkly: using behavior to assess pain. Seminars in Veterinary Medicine and Surgery 12: 61–74

Holton LL, Scott EM, Nolan AM, Reid J, Welsh E, Flaherty D 1998 Comparison of three methods for assessment of pain in dogs. Journal of the American Veterinary Association 212: 61–66

Johnson JM 1991 The veterinarian's responsibility: assessing and managing acute pain in dogs and cats. Part 1. Companion Small Animal 13: 804–808

Klide AM, Martin Jr BB 1989 Methods of stimulating acupuncture points for treatment of chronic back pain in horses. Journal of the American Veterinary Medical Association 195: 1375–1379

Klohnen A, Vachon AM, Fischer Jr AT 1996 Use of diagnostic ultrasonography in horses with signs of acute abdominal pain. Journal of the American Veterinary Medical Association 209: 1597–1601

Laties VG 1987 Control of animal pain and distress in behavioral studies that use food deprivation or aversive stimulation. Journal of the American Veterinary Medical Association 191: 1290–1291

Lascelles BDX, Cripps P, Mirchandani S, Waterman AE 1995 Carprofen as an analgesic for postoperative pain in cats: dose titration and

assessment of efficacy in comparison to pethidine hydrochloride. Journal of Small Animal Practice 36: 535–541
Livingston A 1994 Physiological basis for pain perception in animals. Journal of Veterinary Anaesthesia 21: 15–20
McGlone JJ, Nicholson RI, Hellman JM, Herzog DN 1993 The development of pain in young pigs associated with castration and attempts to prevent castration-induced behavioral changes. Journal of Animal Science 71: 1441–1446
Merskey H 1979 Pain terms: a list with definitions and notes on usage. Pain 6: 249–250
Miller SM, Short CE, Ekström PM 1995 Quantitative EG evaluation to determine the quality of intraoperative analgesia during anesthetic management for equine arthroscopic surgery. American Journal of Veterinary Research 56(3): 374–380
Molony V, Kent JE 1997 Assessment of acute pain in farm animals using behavioral and physiological measurements. Journal of Animal Science 75: 266–272
Molony V, Kent JE, Hosie BD, Graham MJ 1997 Reduction in pain suffered by lambs at castration. Veterinary Journal 153: 205–213
Morgan PW, Parent J, Holmberg DL 1993 Cervical pain secondary to intervertebral disc disease in dogs: radiographic findings and surgical implications. Progress in Veterinary Neurology 4: 76–80
Morton DB 1986 The recognition and assessment of pain distress and discomfort in experimental animals. Zeitschrift fur Versuchstiekunde 28: 215
Morton DB, Griffiths PHM 1985 Guidelines on the recognition of pain, distress, and discomfort in experimental animals and an hypothesis for assessment. Veterinary Record 116: 431–436
Nolan A, Reid J 1993 Comparison of the postoperative analgesic and sedative effects of carprofen and papveretum in the dog. Veterinary Record 133: 240–242
Okuda K, Nakahama H, Miyakawa H, Shima K 1984 Arthritis induced in cats by sodium urate: a possible animal model for chronic pain. Pain 18: 287–297
Oppel TW, Hardy JD 1937 Studies in temperature sensations. I. A comparison of the sensation produced by infrared and visible radiation. II. The temperature changes responsible for the stimulation of the heat end organs. Journal of Clinical Investigation 16: 517–531
Pascoe PJ, Ducharme NB, Ducharme GR, Lumsden JH 1990 A computer derived protocol using recursive partitioning to aid in estimating prognosis of horses with abdominal pain in referral hospitals. Canadian Journal of Veterinary Research 54: 373–378
Popilskis S, Kohn DF, Laurent L, Danilo P 1993 Efficacy of epidural morphine versus intravenous morphine for post-thoracotomy pain in dogs. Journal of Veterinary Anaesthesia 20: 21–25
Potthoff A, Carithers RW 1982 Pain and analgesia in dogs and cats. Companion Small Animal 11: 887–897
Raekallio M, Taylor PM, Bennett RC 1997 Preliminary investigations of pain and analgesia assessment in horses administered phenylbutazone or placebo after arthroscopic surgery. Veterinary Surgery 26: 150–155
Sammarco JL, Conzemius MG, Perkowski SZ et al 1996 Post-operative analgesia for stifle surgery: a comparison of intraarticular bupivacaine, morphine, or saline. Veterinary Surgery 25: 59–69
Sanford J 1992 Guidelines for detection and assessment of pain and distress in experimental animals. In: Short CE, Poznak A (eds) Animal pain. Churchill Livingstone, New York, pp 515–524
Sanford J, Eubank R, Molony V et al 1986 Guidelines for the recognition and assessment of pain in animals. Veterinary Record 118: 334–338
Sawyer DC, Rech RH, Adams T et al 1992 Analgesia and behavioral responses of dogs given oxymorphone-acepromazine and meperidine-acepromazine after methoxyflurane and halothane anesthesia. American Journal of Veterinary Research 53: 1361–1368
Smith JD, Allen SW, Quandt JE, Tachett RL 1996 Indicators of post-operative pain in cats and correlation with clinical criteria. American Journal of Veterinary Research 57: 1674–1678
Sukhiani HR, Parent JM, Atilola MAO, Holmberg DL 1996 Intervertebral disk disease in dogs with signs of back pain done: 25 cases (1986–1993). Journal of the American Veterinary Medical Association 209: 1275–1279
Tranquilli WJ, Fikes LL, Raffe MR 1989 Selecting the right analgesics: indications and dosage requirements. Veterinary Medicine 84: 692–697
Valverde A, Little CB, Dyson DH, Matter CH 1990 Use of epidural morphine to relieve pain in a horse. Canadian Veterinary Journal 31: 211–212
Vierck CJ Jr, Cooper BY, Cohen RH 1983 Human and nonhuman primate reactions to painful electrocutaneous stimuli and to morphine. In: Kitchell RL, Ericson HH (eds) Animal pain: perception and alleviation. American Physiological Society, Bethesda, pp 117–132
Waldmann KH, Otto K, Bollwhan W 1994 Castration of piglets: pain and anaesthesia. Deutsche Tierarztliche Wochenschrift 101: 105–109
Wall PD 1992 Defining 'pain in animals'. In: Short CE, Van Poznak A (eds) Animal pain. Churchill Livingstone, New York, pp 63–80
Waterman AE, Livingston A, Amin A 1991 Further studies on the antinociceptive activity and respiratory effects of buprenorphine in sheep. Journal of Veterinary Pharmacology and Therapeutics 14: 230–234
Welsh EM, Gettinby G, Nolan AM 1993 Comparison of a visual analogue scale and a numerical rating sale for assessment of lameness, using sheep as a model. American Journal of Veterinary Research 54: 976–983

Cancer pain: principles of assessment and syndromes

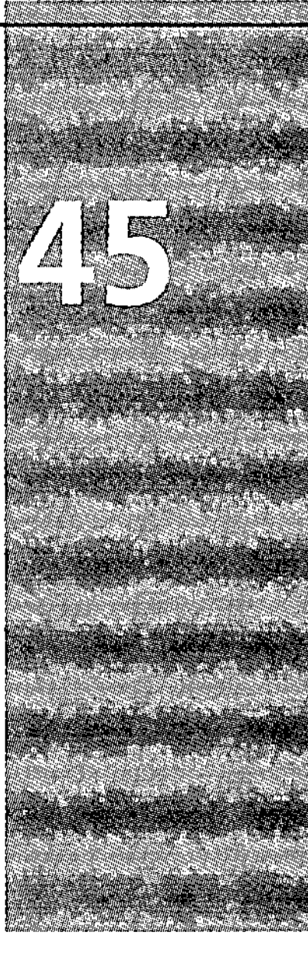

NATHAN I. CHERNY & RUSSELL K. PORTENOY

SUMMARY

Adequate assessment is a necessary precondition for effective pain management. In the cancer population, assessment must recognize the dynamic relationship between the symptom, the illness, and larger concerns related to quality of life. Syndrome identification and inferences about pain pathophysiology are useful elements that may simplify this complex undertaking.

INTRODUCTION

Surveys indicate that pain is experienced by 30–60% of cancer patients during active therapy and more than two-thirds of those with advanced disease (Bonica et al 1990). This has been corroborated in a series of recent studies which identified a pain prevalence of 28% among patients with newly diagnosed cancer (Vuorinen 1993), 50–70% among patients receiving active anticancer therapy (Portenoy et al 1992, 1994a, 1994c, Cleeland et al 1994, Kelsen et al 1995, Larue et al 1995) and 64–80% among patients with far advanced disease (Brescia et al 1992, Tay et al 1994, Donnelly & Walsh 1995). Unrelieved pain is incapacitating and precludes a satisfying quality of life; it interferes with physical functioning and social interaction, and is strongly associated with heightened psychological distress (Ferrell 1995, Ferrell & Dean 1995). Persistent pain interferes with the ability to eat (Feuz & Rapin 1994), sleep (Thorpe 1993, Cleeland et al 1996), think, interact with others (Massie & Holland 1992, Ferrell 1995) and is correlated with fatigue in cancer patients (Burrows et al 1998). The relationship between pain and psychological well-being is complex and reciprocal; mood disturbance and beliefs about the meaning of pain in relation to illness can exacerbate perceived pain intensity (Bond & Pearson 1969, Barkwell 1991) and the presence of pain is a major determinant of function and mood (Daut & Cleeland 1982, Ferrell 1995, Cleeland et al 1996). The presence of pain can provoke or exacerbate existential distress (Strang 1997), disturb normal processes of coping and adjustment (Folkman et al 1986, Fishman 1992, Syrjala & Chapko 1995), and augment a sense of vulnerability, contributing to a preoccupation with the potential for catastrophic outcomes (Fishman 1992, Ferrell 1995).

The relationship between pain and psychological distress among cancer patients has been demonstrated in a range of tumour types (Heim & Oei 1993, Kaasa et al 1993, Lancee et al 1994, Kelsen et al 1995). This relationship is further evidenced by the observations that uncontrolled pain is a major risk factor in cancer-related suicide (Cleeland 1984, Breitbart 1990, Allebeck & Bolund 1991, Baile et al 1993, Van Duynhoven 1994, Goldstein 1997, Henderson & Ord 1997) and that psychiatric symptoms commonly improve with adequate pain relief (Breitbart 1994).

The high prevalence of acute and chronic pain among cancer patients, and the profound psychological and physical burdens engendered by this symptom, oblige all treating clinicians to be skilled in pain management (Edwards 1989, Wanzer 1989, Cherny & Catane 1995, Emanuel 1996, Haugen 1997). The relief of pain in cancer patients is an ethical imperative and it is incumbent upon clinicians to maximize the knowledge, skill and diligence needed to attend to this task.

The undertreatment of cancer pain, which continues to be common (Cherny & Catane 1995, Stjernsward et al. 1996), has many causes, among the most important of which is inadequate assessment (Grossman et al 1991, Von Roenn et al 1993). In a study to evaluate the correlation between patient and clinician evaluation of pain severity, Grossman et al (1991) found that when patients rated their pain as moderate to severe, oncology fellows failed to appreciate the severity of the problem in 73% of cases. In studies of pain relief among cancer patients in the USA (Cleeland et al 1994) and in France (Larue et al 1995), the discrepancy between patient and physician evaluation of the severity of the pain problem was a major predictor of inadequate relief. Surveys indicate that oncology clinicians recognize that suboptimal assessment is one of the most important causes of inadequate pain relief in cancer patients (Von Roenn et al 1993, Cherny et al 1994a, Sapir et al 1997).

APPROACH TO CANCER PAIN ASSESSMENT

Assessment is an ongoing and dynamic process that includes evaluation of presenting problems, elucidation of pain syndromes and pathophysiology, and formulation of a comprehensive plan for continuing care (Coyle 1987, Ventafridda 1989, Shegda & McCorkle 1990, Levy 1991). The objectives of cancer pain assessment include:

1. The accurate characterization of the pain, including the pain syndrome and inferred pathophysiology.
2. The evaluation of the impact of the pain and the role it plays in the overall suffering of the patient.

This assessment is predicated on the establishment of a trusting relationship with the patient in which the clinician emphasizes the relief of pain and suffering as central to the goal of therapy and encourages open communication about symptoms. Clinicians should not be cavalier about the potential for symptom underreporting; symptoms are frequently described as complaints, and there is a common perception that the 'good patient' refrains from complaining (Cleeland 1988, Glajchen et al 1995). The prevalence of pain is so great that an open-ended question about the presence of pain should be included at each patient visit in routine oncological practice. If the patient is either unable or unwilling to describe the pain, a family member may need to be questioned to assess the distress or disability of the patient.

Cancer pain syndromes are defined by the association of particular pain characteristics and physical signs with specific consequences of the underlying disease or its treatment (see below). Syndromes are associated with distinct aetiologies and pathophysiologies, and have important prognostic and therapeutic implications. Pain syndromes associated with cancer can be either acute (Box 45.1) or chronic (Box 45.2). Whereas acute pains experienced by cancer patients are usually related to diagnostic and therapeutic interven-

BOX 45.1

Cancer-related acute pain syndromes

Acute pain associated with diagnostic and therapeutic interventions

Acute pain associated with diagnostic interventions
- Lumbar puncture headache
- Transthoracic needle biopsy
- Arterial or venous blood sampling
- Bone marrow biopsy
- Lumbar puncture
- Colonoscopy
- Myelography
- Percutaneous biopsy
- Thoracocentesis

Acute postoperative pain

Acute pain caused by other therapeutic interventions
- Pleurodesis
- Tumour embolization
- Suprapubic catheterization
- Intercostal catheter
- Nephrostomy insertion
- Cryosurgery-associated pain and cramping

Acute pain associated with analgesic techniques
- Local anaesthetic infiltration pain
- Opioid injection pain
- Opioid headache
- Spinal opioid hyperalgesia syndrome
- Epidural injection pain
- Strontium-89-induced pain flare

Acute pain associated with anticancer therapies

Acute pain associated with chemotherapy infusion techniques
- Intravenous infusion pain
  - Venous spasm
  - Chemical phlebitis
  - Vesicant extravasation
  - Anthracycline-associated flare reaction
- Hepatic artery infusion pain
- Intraperitoneal chemotherapy abdominal pain

Acute pain associated with chemotherapy toxicity
- Mucositis
- Corticosteroid-induced perineal discomfort
- Taxol-induced arthralgias
- Steroid pseudorheumatism
- Painful peripheral neuropathy
- Headache
  - Intrathecal methotrexate meningitic syndrome
  - L-asparaginase associated dural sinuses thrombosis
  - *trans*-retinoic acid headache
- Diffuse bone pain
  - *trans*-retinoic acid

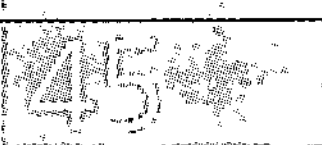

BOX 45.1 (Contd.)

Cancer-related acute pain syndromes

Acute pain associated with anticancer therapies
Acute pain associated with chemotherapy toxicity
  Diffuse bone pain
    Colony stimulating factors
  5-flurouracil-induced anginal chest pain
  Palmar-plantar erythrodysesthesia syndrome
  Postchemotherapy gynaecomastia
  Chemotherapy-induced acute digital ischaemia
Acute pain associated with hormonal therapy
  Leutenizing hormone releasing factor tumour flare in prostate cancer
  Hormone-induced pain flare in breast cancer
Acute pain associated with immunotherapy
  Interferon-induced acute pain
Acute pain associated with growth factors
  Colony-stimulating factor induced musculoskeletal pains
  Erythropoietin injection pain
Acute pain associated with radiotherapy
  Incident pains associated with positioning
  Oropharyngeal mucositis
  Acute radiation enteritis and proctocolitis
  Early-onset brachial plexopathy
  Subacute radiation myelopathy
  Strontium-89-induced pain flare

Acute pain associated with infection
Acute herpetic neuralgia

Acute pain associated with vascular events
Acute thrombosis pain
  Lower-extremity deep venous thrombosis
  Upper-extremity deep venous thrombosis
  Superior vena cava obstruction

tions, chronic pains are most commonly caused by direct tumour infiltration. Adverse consequences of cancer therapy, including surgery, chemotherapy and radiation therapy, account for 15–25% of chronic cancer pain problems, and a small proportion of the chronic pains experienced by cancer patients are caused by pathology unrelated to either the cancer or the cancer therapy (Banning et al 1991, Portenoy et al 1992, 1994a, Miaskowski & Dibble 1995, Grand et al 1996, Twycross et al 1996, Twycross 1997).

PAIN CHARACTERISTICS

The evaluation of pain characteristics provides some of the data essential for syndrome identification. These characteristics include intensity, quality, distribution and temporal relationships.

Intensity

The evaluation of pain intensity is pivotal to therapeutic decision making (Cherny et al 1995, World Health Organization 1996). It indicates the urgency with which relief is needed and influences the selection of analgesic drug, route of administration and rate of dose titration (Cherny et al 1995). Furthermore, the assessment of pain intensity may help characterize the pain mechanism and underlying syndrome. For example, the pain associated with radiation-induced nerve injury is rarely severe; the occurrence of severe pain in a previously irradiated region therefore suggests the existence of recurrent neoplasm or a radiation-induced second primary neoplasm.

Quality

The quality of the pain often suggests its pathophysiology. Somatic nociceptive pains are usually well localized and described as sharp, aching, throbbing or pressure like. Visceral nociceptive pains are generally diffuse and may be gnawing or crampy when caused by obstruction of a hollow viscus, or aching, sharp or throbbing when caused by involvement of organ capsules or mesentery (Cervero 1985, Giamberardino & Vecchiet 1995). Neuropathic pains may be described as burning, tingling or shock like (lancinating).

Distribution

Patients with cancer pain commonly experience pain at more than one site (Portenoy et al, 1992, 1994a, Grond et al 1996). The distinction between focal, multifocal and generalized pain may be important in the selection of therapy, such as nerve blocks, radiotherapy or surgical approaches. The term 'focal' pain, which is used to denote a single site, has also been used to depict pain that is experienced in the region of the underlying lesion. Focal pains can be distinguished from those that are referred to a site remote from the lesion. Familiarity with pain referral patterns is essential to target appropriate diagnostic and therapeutic manoeuvres (Kellgren 1938, Cherny et al 1996). For example, a patient who develops progressive shoulder pain and has no evidence of focal pathology needs to undergo evaluation of the region above and below the diaphragm to exclude the possibility of referred pain from diaphragmatic irritation.

BOX 45.2

Cancer-related chronic pain syndromes

TUMOUR-RELATED PAIN SYNDROMES

Bone pain
Multifocal or generalized bone pain
  Multiple bony metastases
  Marrow expansion
Vertebral syndromes
  Atlantoaxial destruction and odontoid fractures
  C7–T1 syndrome
  T12–L1 syndrome
  Sacral syndrome
Back pain and epidural compression
Pain syndromes of the bony pelvis and hip
  Hip joint syndrome
Acrometastases

Arthritidies
Hypertrophic pulmonary osteoarthropathy
Other polyarthritides

Muscle pain
Muscle cramps
Skeletal muscle tumours

Headache and facial pain
Intracerebral tumour
Leptomeningeal metastases
Base of skull metastases
  Orbital syndrome
  Parasellar syndrome
  Middle cranial fossa syndrome
  Jugular foramen syndrome
  Occipital condyle syndrome
  Clivus syndrome
  Sphenoid sinus syndrome
Painful cranial neuralgias
  Glossopharyngeal neuralgias
  Trigeminal neuralgia
Eye and ear syndromes
  Otalgia
  Eye pain

Tumour involvement of the peripheral nervous system
Tumour-related radiculopathy
  Postherpetic neuralgia
Cervical plexopathy
Brachial plexopathy
  Malignant brachial plexopathy
  Idiopathic brachial plexopathy associated with Hodgkin's disease
Malignant lumbosacral plexopathy
Tumour-related mononeuropathy
Paraneoplastic painful peripheral neuropathy
  Subacute sensory neuropathy
  Sensorimotor peripheral neuropathy

Pain syndromes of the viscera and miscellaneous tumour-related syndromes
Hepatic distention syndrome
Midline retroperitoneal syndrome
Chronic intestinal obstruction
Peritoneal carcinomatosis
Malignant perineal pain
  Malignant pelvic floor myalgia
Adrenal pain syndrome
Ureteric obstruction
Ovarian cancer pain
Lung cancer pain

Paraneoplastic nociceptive pain syndromes
Tumour-related gynaecomastia

CHRONIC PAIN SYNDROMES ASSOCIATED WITH CANCER THERAPY

Postchemotherapy pain syndromes
Chronic painful peripheral neuropathy.
Avascular necrosis of femoral or humeral head
Plexopathy associated with intraarterial infusion
Raynaud's phenomenon

Chronic pain associated with hormonal therapy
Gynaecomastia with hormonal therapy for prostate cancer

Chronic postsurgical pain syndromes
Postmastectomy pain syndrome
Postradical neck dissection pain
Postthoracotomy pain
Postoperative frozen shoulder
Phantom pain syndromes
  Phantom limb pain
  Phantom breast pain
  Phantom anus pain
  Phantom bladder pain
Stump pain
Postsurgical pelvic floor myalgia

Chronic postradiation pain syndromes
Plexopathies
  Radiation-induced brachial and lumbosacral plexopathies
  Radiation-induced peripheral nerve tumour
Chronic radiation myelopathy
Chronic radiation enteritis and proctitis
Burning perineum syndrome
Osteoradionecrosis

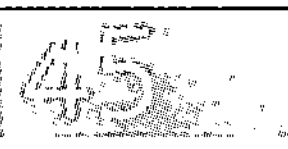

Temporal relationships

Cancer-related pain may be acute or chronic. Acute pain is defined by a recent onset and a natural history characterized by transience. The pain is often associated with overt pain behaviours (such as moaning, grimacing and splinting), anxiety or signs of generalized sympathetic hyperactivity, including diaphoresis, hypertension and tachycardia. Chronic pain has been defined by persistence for 3 months or more beyond the usual course of an acute illness or injury, a pattern of recurrence at intervals over months or years, or by association with a chronic pathological process (Bonica et al 1990). Chronic tumour-related pain is usually insidious in onset, often increases progressively with tumour growth, and may regress with tumour shrinkage. Overt pain behaviours and sympathetic hyperactivity are often absent, and the pain may be associated with affective disturbances (anxiety and/or depression) and vegetative symptoms, such as asthenia, anorexia and sleep disturbance (Reuben et al 1988, McCaffery & Thorpe 1989, Coyle 1990, Ventafridda et al 1990).

Transitory exacerbations of severe pain over a baseline of moderate pain or less are described as 'breakthrough pain' (Portenoy & Hagen 1990). Breakthrough pains are common in both acute or chronic pain states. These exacerbations may be precipitated by volitional actions of the patient (so-called incident pains), such as movement, micturition, cough or defaecation, or by non-volitional events, such as bowel distension. Spontaneous fluctuations in pain intensity can also occur without an identifiable precipitant.

Inferred pain mechanisms

Inferences about the mechanisms that may be responsible for the pain are helpful in the evaluation of the pain syndrome and in the management of cancer pain. The assessment process usually provides the clinical data necessary to infer a predominant pathophysiology.

Nociceptive pain

'Nociceptive pain' describes pain that is perceived to be commensurate with tissue damage associated with an identifiable somatic or visceral lesion. The persistence of pain is thought to be related to the ongoing activation of nociceptors. Nociceptive pain that originates from somatic structures (somatic pain) is usually well localized and described as sharp, aching, burning or throbbing. As previously described, pain that arises from visceral structures (visceral pain) may differ depending on the involved structures. From the clinical perspective, nociceptive pains (particularly somatic pains) usually respond well to opioid drugs (Arner & Meyerson 1988, Jadad et al 1992, Cherny et al 1994b) or to interventions that ameliorate or denervate the peripheral lesion.

Neuropathic pain

The term 'neuropathic pain' is applied when pain is caused by injury to, or diseases of the peripheral or central neural structures or is perceived to be sustained by aberrant somatosensory processing at these sites (Devor et al 1991, Elliott 1994). It is most strongly suggested when a dysaesthesia occurs in a region of motor, sensory or autonomic dysfunction that is attributable to a discrete neurological lesion. The diagnosis can be challenging, however, and is often inferred solely from the distribution of the pain and the identification of a lesion in neural structures that innervate this region.

Although neuropathic pains can be described in terms of the pain characteristics (continuous or lancinating) or site of injury (e.g., neuronopathy or plexopathy), it is useful to distinguish these syndromes according to the presumed site of the aberrant neural activity ('generator') that sustains the pain (Portenoy 1991). Peripheral neuropathic pain is caused by injury to a peripheral nerve or nerve root and is presumably sustained by aberrant processes originating in the nerve root, plexus or nerve. Neuropathic pains believed to be sustained by a central 'generator' include the complex regional pain syndromes (also known as reflex sympathetic dystrophy or causalgia), some of which are sympathetically maintained (sustained by efferent activity in the sympathetic nervous system), and a group of syndromes traditionally known as the deafferentation pains (e.g. phantom pain). A complex regional pain syndrome may occur following injury to soft tissue, peripheral nerve, viscera or central nervous system (Stanton-Hicks et al 1995), and is characterized by focal autonomic dysregulation in a painful region (e.g., vasomotor or pilomotor changes, swelling, or sweating abnormalities) or trophic changes (Simon 1997).

The diagnosis of neuropathic pain has important clinical implications. The response of neuropathic pains to opioid drugs is less predictable and generally less dramatic than the response of nociceptive pains (Jadad et al 1992, Portenoy et al 1990, Cherny et al 1994b, Hanks & Forbes 1997). Optimal treatment may depend on the use of so-called adjuvant analgesics (Lipman 1996, McQuay et al 1996) or other specific approaches, such as somatic or sympathetic nerve blocks (Cherny et al 1996).

Idiopathic pain

Pain that is perceived to be excessive for the extent of identifiable organic pathology can be termed idiopathic, unless the patient presents with affective and behavioural disturbances that are severe enough to infer a predominating psychological pathogenesis, in which case the generic term 'psychogenic pain' or a specific psychiatric diagnosis (somatoform disorder) can be applied (American Psychiatric Association 1994). When the inference of a somatoform disorder cannot be made, however, the label 'idiopathic' should be retained, and assessments should be repeated at appropriate intervals. Idiopathic pain in general, and pain related to a psychiatric disorder specifically, is uncommon in the cancer population, notwithstanding the importance of psychological factors in quality of life.

A STEPWISE APPROACH TO THE EVALUATION OF CANCER PAIN

A practical approach to cancer pain assessment incorporates a stepwise approach that begins with data collection and ends with a clinically relevant formulation.

DATA COLLECTION

A careful review of past medical history and the chronology of the cancer are important to place the pain complaint in context. The pain-related history must elucidate the relevant pain characteristics, as well as the responses of the patient to previous disease-modifying and analgesic therapies. The presence of multiple pain problems is common, and if more than one is reported, each must be assessed independently. The use of validated pain assessment instruments can provide a format for communication between the patient and healthcare professionals, and can also be used to monitor the adequacy of therapy (see below).

The clinician should assess the consequences of the pain, including impairment in activities of daily living; psychological, familial and professional dysfunction; disturbed sleep, appetite and vitality; and financial concerns. The patient's psychological status, including current level of anxiety or depression, suicidal ideation and the perceived meaning of the pain, is similarly relevant. Pervasive dysfunctional attitudes, such as pessimism, idiosyncratic interpretation of pain, self-blame, catastrophizing and perceived loss of personal control, can usually be detected through careful questioning. It is important to assess the patient–family interaction, and to note both the kind and frequency of pain behaviours and the nature of the family response.

Most patients with cancer pain have multiple other symptoms (Coyle et al 1990, Ventafridda et al 1990, Portenoy et al 1994b, Donnelly et al 1995, Vainio & Auvinen 1996). The clinician must evaluate the severity and distress caused by each of these symptoms. Symptom checklists and quality-of-life measures may contribute to this comprehensive evaluation (Bruera et al 1991b, Portenoy et al 1994c).

A physical examination, including a neurological evaluation, is a necessary part of the initial pain assessment. The need for a thorough neurological assessment is justified by the high prevalence of painful neurological conditions in this population (Gonzales et al 1991, Clouston et al 1992). The physical examination should attempt to identify the underlying aetiology of the pain problem, clarify the extent of the underlying disease, and discern the relationship of the pain complaint to the disease.

Careful review of previous laboratory and imaging studies is also essential. This review can provide important information about the cause of the pain and the extent of the underlying disease.

PROVISIONAL ASSESSMENT

The information derived from these data provides the basis for a provisional pain diagnosis, an understanding of the disease status and the identification of other concurrent concerns. This provisional diagnosis includes inferences about the pathophysiology of the pain and an assessment of the pain syndrome.

Additional investigations are often required to clarify areas of uncertainty in the provisional assessment (Gonzales et al 1991). The extent of diagnostic investigation must be appropriate to the patient's general status and the overall goals of care. For some patients, comprehensive evaluation may require numerous investigations, some targeted at the specific pain problem and others needed to clarify the extent of disease or concurrent symptoms. In specific situations, algorithms have been developed to facilitate an efficient evaluation. This is well illustrated by established clinical algorithms for the investigation of back pain in the cancer patient (Portenoy et al 1987, Posner 1987), which provide a straightforward approach for those patients at highest risk for epidural compression of the spinal cord (see below).

The lack of a definitive finding on an investigation should not be used to override a compelling clinical diagnosis. In the assessment of bone pain, for example, plain radiographs provide only crude assessment of bony lesions and further investigation with bone scintigrams, computerized tomography (CT) or magnetic resonance imaging (MRI) may be indicated. To minimize the risk of error, the physician ordering the diagnostic procedures should personally review them with the radiologist to correlate pathological changes with the clinical findings.

Pain should be managed during the diagnostic evaluation. Comfort will improve compliance and reduce the distress associated with procedures. No patient should be inadequately evaluated because of poorly controlled pain.

The comprehensive assessment may also require the additional evaluation of other physical or psychosocial problems identified during the initial assessment. Expert assistance from other physicians, nurses, social workers or others may be essential.

FORMULATION AND THERAPEUTIC PLANNING

The evaluation should enable the clinician to appreciate the nature of the pain, its impact and concurrent concerns that further undermine the quality of life. The findings of this evaluation should be reviewed with the patient and appropriate others. Through candid discussion, current problems can be prioritized to reflect their importance to the patient.

This evaluation may also identify potential outcomes that would benefit from contingency planning. Examples include evaluation of resources for home care, pre-bereavement interventions with the family, and the provision of assistive devices in anticipation of the patient's ambulation decreasing.

MEASUREMENT OF PAIN AND ITS IMPACT ON PATIENT WELL-BEING

Although pain measurement has generally been used by clinical investigators to determine the impact of analgesic therapies, it has become clear that it has an important role in the routine monitoring of cancer patients in treatment settings (Au et al 1994, American Pain Society Quality of Care Committee 1995, Cleeland et al 1997). Because observer ratings of symptom severity correlate poorly with patient ratings and are generally an inadequate substitute for patient reporting (Grossman et al 1991), patient self report is the primary source of information for the measurement of pain.

Pain measures in routine clinical management

Recent guidelines from the Agency for Health Care Policy and Research (1994) and the American Pain Society (American Pain Society Quality of Care Committee 1995) recommend the regular use of pain rating scales to assess pain severity and relief in all patients who commence or change treatments. These recommendations also suggest that clinicians teach patients and families to use assessment tools in the home to promote the continuity of pain management in all settings. The two most commonly used scales for adults are a verbal descriptor scale (i.e. 'Which word best describes your pain; none, mild moderate, severe or excruciating?') or a numerical scale (i.e. 'On a scale from 0 to 10, where 0 indicates no pain and 10 indicates the worst pain you can imagine, how would you rate your pain') (Agency for Health Care Policy and Research 1994).

A recent study demonstrated that the use of a simple verbal pain assessment tool improved the caregiver's understanding of pain status in hospitalized patients (Au et al 1994). Regular pain measurement, using a pain scale to the bedside chart (Fig. 45.1), has been incorporated into a continuous quality improvement strategy at a cancer centre

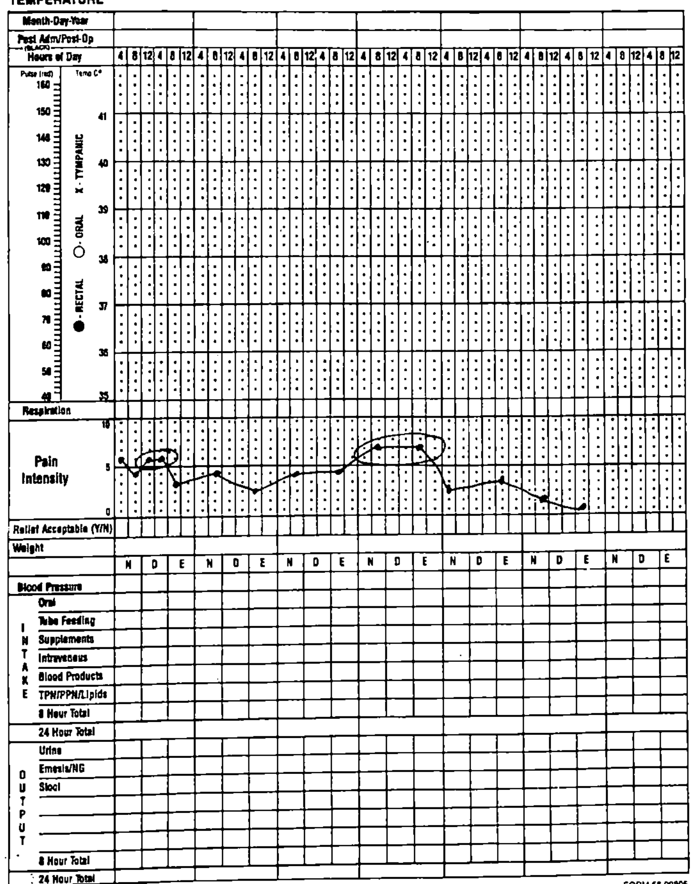
VITAL SIGNS CHART
TEMPERATURE
Month-Day-Year
Post Adm/Post-Op
Hours of Day
4 8 12 4 8 12
Pulse (red) 160 150 140 130 120 110 100 90 80 70 60 50 40
Temp C° 41 40 39 38 37 36 35
● - RECTAL O - ORAL X - TYMPANIC
Respiration
Pain Intensity 10 5 0
Relief Acceptable (Y/N)
Weight
N D E N D E N D E N D E N D E N D E N D E
Blood Pressure
INTAKE: Oral; Tube Feeding; Supplements; Intravenous; Blood Products; TPN/PPN/Lipids; 8 Hour Total; 24 Hour Total
OUTPUT: Urine; Emesis/NG; Stool; 8 Hour Total; 24 Hour Total
TEMP A
FORM 56-09805

Fig. 45.1 Bedside record. Incorporated into the chart is a 10-point pain scale and an item regarding the adequacy of pain control.

(Coyle et al 1993, Bookbinder et al 1996), and preliminary data suggest that nursing knowledge and attitudes regarding the assessment and management of cancer pain have improved as a result. In addition to focusing staff attention on symptom assessment, such measures may be used as a means of reviewing the quality of patient care and ascertaining situation-specific barriers to symptom control (Miaskowski & Donovan 1992, Miaskowski et al 1994).

Instruments for the measurement of pain in research settings

Pain can be measured using unidimensional or multidimensional scales. Unidimensional scales, which generally address intensity or relief, may use visual analogue, numerical and categorical scales. Multidimensional instruments include the Memorial Pain Assessment Card, the McGill Pain Questionnaire and the Brief Pain Inventory.

The Memorial Pain Assessment Card (MPAC) (Fishman et al 1987) is a brief, validated measure that uses 100 mm visual analogue scales (VASs) to characterize pain intensity, pain relief and mood, and an 8-point verbal rating scale (VRS) to further characterize pain intensity (Fig. 45.2). The mood scale, which is correlated with measures of global psychological distress, depression and anxiety, is considered to be a brief measure of global symptom distress (Fishman et al 1987). Although this instrument does not provide detailed descriptors of pain, its brevity and simplicity may facilitate the collection of useful information while minimizing patient burden and encouraging compliance.

The Brief Pain Inventory (BPI; Fig. 45.3) (Daut et al 1983) is a simple and easily administered tool that provides information about pain history, intensity, location and

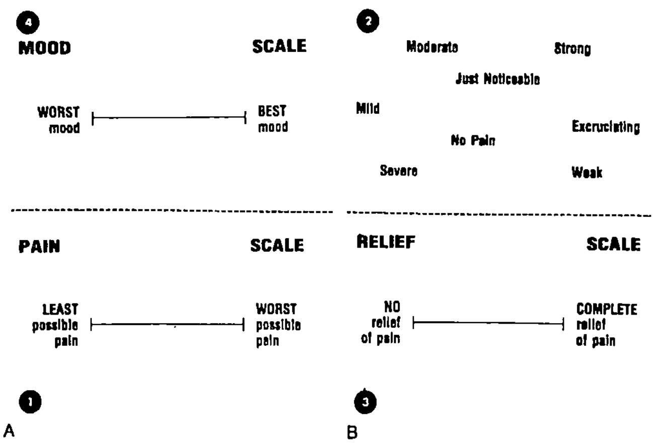

Fig. 45.2 The Memorial Pain Assessment Card (MPAC). (Reproduced with permission Fishman et al 1987)

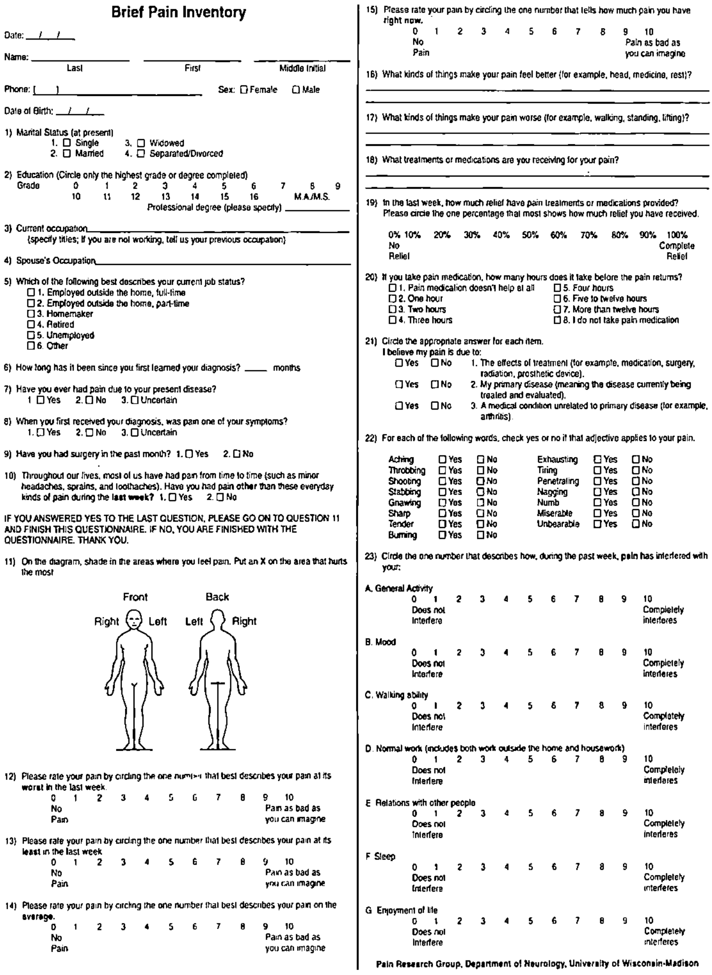

Brief Pain Inventory

Date: __/__/__

Name: ______ Last ______ First ______ Middle Initial

Phone: (   ) ______ Sex: ☐ Female ☐ Male

Date of Birth: __/__/__

1) Marital Status (at present)
1. ☐ Single 3. ☐ Widowed
2. ☐ Married 4. ☐ Separated/Divorced

2) Education (Circle only the highest grade or degree completed)
Grade 0 1 2 3 4 5 6 7 8 9
10 11 12 13 14 15 16 M.A./M.S.
Professional degree (please specify) ______

3) Current occupation ______
(specify titles; if you are not working, tell us your previous occupation)

4) Spouse's Occupation ______

5) Which of the following best describes your current job status?
☐ 1. Employed outside the home, full-time
☐ 2. Employed outside the home, part-time
☐ 3. Homemaker
☐ 4. Retired
☐ 5. Unemployed
☐ 6. Other

6) How long has it been since you first learned your diagnosis? ____ months

7) Have you ever had pain due to your present disease?
1 ☐ Yes 2. ☐ No 3. ☐ Uncertain

8) When you first received your diagnosis, was pain one of your symptoms?
1. ☐ Yes 2. ☐ No 3. ☐ Uncertain

9) Have you had surgery in the past month? 1. ☐ Yes 2. ☐ No

10) Throughout our lives, most of us have had pain from time to time (such as minor headaches, sprains, and toothaches). Have you had pain other than these everyday kinds of pain during the **last week?** 1. ☐ Yes 2. ☐ No

IF YOU ANSWERED YES TO THE LAST QUESTION, PLEASE GO ON TO QUESTION 11 AND FINISH THIS QUESTIONNAIRE. IF NO, YOU ARE FINISHED WITH THE QUESTIONNAIRE. THANK YOU.

11) On the diagram, shade in the areas where you feel pain. Put an X on the area that hurts the most

Front Back
Right Left Left Right

12) Please rate your pain by circling the one number that best describes your pain at its **worst** in the last week.
0 1 2 3 4 5 6 7 8 9 10
No Pain — Pain as bad as you can imagine

13) Please rate your pain by circling the one number that best describes your pain at its **least** in the last week
0 1 2 3 4 5 6 7 8 9 10
No Pain — Pain as bad as you can imagine

14) Please rate your pain by circling the one number that best describes your pain on the **average.**
0 1 2 3 4 5 6 7 8 9 10
No Pain — Pain as bad as you can imagine

15) Please rate your pain by circling the one number that tells how much pain you have **right now.**
0 1 2 3 4 5 6 7 8 9 10
No Pain — Pain as bad as you can imagine

16) What kinds of things make your pain feel better (for example, head, medicine, rest)?

17) What kinds of things make your pain worse (for example, walking, standing, lifting)?

18) What treatments or medications are you receiving for your pain?

19) In the last week, how much relief have pain treatments or medications provided? Please circle the one percentage that most shows how much relief you have received.
0% 10% 20% 30% 40% 50% 60% 70% 80% 90% 100%
No Relief — Complete Relief

20) If you take pain medication, how many hours does it take before the pain returns?
☐ 1. Pain medication doesn't help at all ☐ 5. Four hours
☐ 2. One hour ☐ 6. Five to twelve hours
☐ 3. Two hours ☐ 7. More than twelve hours
☐ 4. Three hours ☐ 8. I do not take pain medication

21) Circle the appropriate answer for each item.
I believe my pain is due to:
☐ Yes ☐ No 1. The effects of treatment (for example, medication, surgery, radiation, prosthetic device).
☐ Yes ☐ No 2. My primary disease (meaning the disease currently being treated and evaluated).
☐ Yes ☐ No 3. A medical condition unrelated to primary disease (for example, arthritis).

22) For each of the following words, check yes or no if that adjective applies to your pain.

Aching	☐ Yes	☐ No	Exhausting	☐ Yes	☐ No
Throbbing	☐ Yes	☐ No	Tiring	☐ Yes	☐ No
Shooting	☐ Yes	☐ No	Penetrating	☐ Yes	☐ No
Stabbing	☐ Yes	☐ No	Nagging	☐ Yes	☐ No
Gnawing	☐ Yes	☐ No	Numb	☐ Yes	☐ No
Sharp	☐ Yes	☐ No	Miserable	☐ Yes	☐ No
Tender	☐ Yes	☐ No	Unbearable	☐ Yes	☐ No
Burning	☐ Yes	☐ No			

23) Circle the one number that describes how, during the past week, **pain** has interfered with your:

A. General Activity
0 1 2 3 4 5 6 7 8 9 10
Does not interfere — Completely interferes

B. Mood
0 1 2 3 4 5 6 7 8 9 10
Does not interfere — Completely interferes

C. Walking ability
0 1 2 3 4 5 6 7 8 9 10
Does not interfere — Completely interferes

D. Normal work (includes both work outside the home and housework)
0 1 2 3 4 5 6 7 8 9 10
Does not interfere — Completely interferes

E. Relations with other people
0 1 2 3 4 5 6 7 8 9 10
Does not interfere — Completely interferes

F. Sleep
0 1 2 3 4 5 6 7 8 9 10
Does not interfere — Completely interferes

G. Enjoyment of life
0 1 2 3 4 5 6 7 8 9 10
Does not interfere — Completely interferes

Pain Research Group, Department of Neurology, University of Wisconsin-Madison

Fig. 45.3 The Brief Pain Inventory. (Reproduced with permission Dact et al 1983)

quality. Numerical scales (range 1–10) indicate the intensity of pain in general, at its worst, at its least and right now. A percentage scale quantifies relief from current therapies. A figure representing the body is provided for the patient to shade the area corresponding to his pain. Seven questions determine the degree to which pain interferes with function, mood and enjoyment of life. The BPI is self administered and easily understood, and has been translated into several languages (Cleeland & Ryan 1994, Caraceni et al 1996, Wang et al 1996).

The McGill Pain Questionnaire (MPQ) (Melzack 1975, 1987) is a self-administered questionnaire that provides global scores and subscale scores that reflect the sensory, affective and evaluative dimensions of pain. The scores are derived from ratings of pain descriptors selected by the patient. A 5-point verbal categorical scale characterizes the intensity of pain and a pain drawing localizes the pain. Further information is collected about the impact of medications and other therapies. The impact of pain on function is not assessed. Although the MPQ has been extensively evaluated in chronic pain patients, the utility of the subscale scores has not been demonstrated for cancer pain (De Conno et al 1994). A short form of the MPQ (SF-MPQ) was developed for use in research settings and has been validated in a palliative care setting (Dudgeon et al 1993).

ACUTE PAIN SYNDROMES

Cancer-related acute pain syndromes are most commonly a result of diagnostic or therapeutic interventions (Stull et al 1996) (Box 45.1) and they generally pose little diagnostic difficulty. Although some tumour-related pains have an acute onset (such as pain from a pathological fracture), most of these will persist unless effective treatment for the underlying lesion is provided. A comprehensive pain assessment in such patients is usually valuable, potentially yielding important information about the extent of disease or concurrent issues relevant to therapy.

ACUTE PAIN ASSOCIATED WITH DIAGNOSTIC AND THERAPEUTIC INTERVENTIONS

Many investigations and treatments are associated with predictable, transient pain. For those patients with a pre-existing pain syndrome, otherwise innocuous manipulations can also precipitate an incident pain.

Acute pain associated with diagnostic interventions

Lumbar puncture headache

Lumbar puncture (LP) headache is the best characterized acute pain syndrome associated with a diagnostic intervention. This syndrome is characterized by the delayed development of a positional headache, which is precipitated or markedly exacerbated by upright posture. The pain is believed to be related to reduction in cerebrospinal fluid volume, which result from ongoing leakage through the defect in the dural sheath and compensatory expansion of the pain-sensitive intracerebral veins (Morewood 1993). The incidence of headache is related to the calibre of the LP needle (0–2% with 27–29-gauge, 0.5–7% with 25–26-gauge, 5–8% with 22-gauge, 10–15% with 20-gauge and 20–30% with 18-guage needles) (Bonica 1953, Tarkkila et al 1994, McConaha et al 1996, Lambert et al 1997). Using a regular bevelled needle, the overall incidence can be reduced by the use of a small gauge needle and by longitudinal insertion of the needle bevel, which presumably induces less trauma to the longitudinal elastic fibres in the dura (Fink 1990, Leibold et al 1993, Morewood 1993, Kempen & Mocek 1997). Recent evidence suggests that the use of a non-traumatic conical tipped needle with a lateral opening spreads the dural fibres, and is associated with a substantially lesser risk of post-LP headaches than regular cannulae (Prager et al 1996, Corbey et al 1997, Lambert et al 1997). The evidence that recumbency after LP reduces the incidence of this syndrome is controversial (Carbaat & van Crevel 1981, Cook et al 1989, Kuntz et al 1992, Martin et al 1994).

LP headache, which usually develops hours to several days after the procedure, is typically described as a dull occipital discomfort that may radiate to the frontal region or to the shoulders (Bonica 1953, Evans 1998, Leibold et al 1993, Morewood 1993). When severe, the pain may be associated with diaphoresis and nausea (Lybecker et al 1995). The duration of the headache is usually 1–7 days (Lybecker et al 1995) and routine management relies on bedrest, hydration and analgesics (Evans 1998). Persistent headache may necessitate the application of an epidural blood patch (Evans 1998). Although a recent controlled study suggested that prophylactic administration of a blood patch may reduce this complication (Martin et al 1994), the incidence and severity of the syndrome do not warrant this treatment. Severe headache has also been reported to respond to treatment with intravenous or oral caffeine (Morewood 1993).

Transthoracic needle biopsy

Transthoracic fine-needle aspiration of an intrathoracic mass is generally a non-noxious procedure. Severe pain has however been associated with this procedure when the underlying diagnosis was a neurogenic tumour (Jones et al 1993).

Transrectal prostatic biopsy

Transrectal ultrasound-guided prostate biopsy is an essential procedure in the diagnosis and management of prostate cancer. In a prospective study, 16% of the patients reported pain of moderate or greater severity (VAS PI ≥ 5) and 19% would not agree to undergo the procedure again without anaesthesia (Irani et al 1997). Transrectal ultrasound-guided prostatic nerve blockade is effective in relieving discomfort associated with this procedure (Nash et al 1996).

Mammography pain

Breast compression associated with mammography can cause moderate, and rarely severe, pain (Leaney & Martin

1992, Aro et al 1996). Unless patients are adequately counselled and treated, occasional patients will refuse repeat mammograms because of pain (Leaney & Martin 1992).

Acute pain associated with therapeutic interventions

Postoperative pain

Acute postoperative pain is universal unless adequately treated. Unfortunately, undertreatment stll occurs despite the availability of adequate analgesic and anaesthetic techniques (Marks & Sachar 1973, Edwards 1990, Agency for Health Care Policy and Research: Acute Pain Management Panel 1992). Guidelines for management have been proposed (Ready 1991, Agency for Health Care Policy and Research: Acute Pain Management Panel 1992). Postoperative pain that exceeds the normal duration or severity should prompt a careful evaluation for the possibility of infection or other complications.

Cryosurgery-associated pain and cramping

Cryosurgery of the cervix in the treatment of intraepithelial neoplasm commonly produces an acute cramping pain syndrome. The severity of the pain is related to the duration of the freeze period and it is not diminished by the administration of prophylactic NSAIDs (Harper 1994).

Other interventions

Invasive interventions other than surgery are commonly used in cancer therapy and may also result in predictable acute pain syndromes. Examples include the pains associated with tumour embolization techniques (Chen et al 1997, Sanz-Altamira et al 1997) and chemical pleurodesis (Walker-Renard et al 1994, Prevost et al 1998).

Acute pain associated with analgesic techniques

Local anaesthetic infiltration pain

Intradermal and subcutaneous infiltration of lidocaine produces a transient burning sensation before the onset of analgesia. This can be modified with the use of buffered solutions (Palmon et al 1998). Other manoeuvres, including warming of the solution (Martin et al 1996) or slowing the rate of injection (Scarfone et al 1998), do not diminish injection pain.

Opioid injection pain

Intramuscular (IM) and subcutaneous (SC) injections are painful. When repetitive dosing is required, the IM route of administration is not recommended (Agency for Health Care Policy and Research: Acute Pain Management Panel 1992, Agency for Health Care Policy and Research 1994). The pain associated with subcutaneous injection is influenced by the volume injected and the chemical characteristics of the injectant. Subcutaneous injection of opioids can produce a painful subdermal reaction; this is infrequently observed with morphine or hydromorphone (Bruera et al 1990) but is common with methadone (Bruera et al 1991a). For this reason, the subcutaneous infusion of methadone is not recommended. There are some data to suggest that the addition of a low concentration of dexamethasone may reduce the likelihood of local irritation (Shvartzman & Bonneh 1994).

Opioid headache

Rarely, patients develop a reproducible generalized headache after opioid administration. Although its cause is not known, speculation suggests that it may be caused by opioid-induced histamine release.

Spinal opioid hyperalgesia syndrome

Intrathecal and epidural injection of high opioid doses is occasionally complicated by pain (typically perineal, buttock or leg) and hyperalgesia. Associated manifestations include segmental myoclonus, piloerection and priapism. This is an uncommon phenomenon that remits after discontinuation of the infusion (Glavina & Robertshaw 1988, De Conno et al 1991, Cartwright et al 1993).

Epidural injection pain

Back, pelvic or leg pain may be precipitated by epidural injection or infusion. The incidence of this problem has been estimated at approximately 20% (De Castro et al 1991). It is speculated that it may be caused by the compression of an adjacent nerve root by the injected fluid (De Castro et al 1991).

Acute pain associated with anticancer therapies

Acute pain associated with chemotherapy infusion techniques

Intravenous infusion pain Pain at the site of cytotoxic infusion is a common problem. Four pain syndromes related to intravenous infusion of chemotherapeutic agents are recognized: venous spasm, chemical phlebitis, vesicant extravasation and anthracycline-associated flare. Venous spasm causes pain that is not associated with inflammation or phlebitis, and which may be modified by the application of a warm compress or reduction of the rate of infusion. Chemical phlebitis can be caused by cytotoxic medications including amasarcine, decarbazine, carmustine (Hundrieser 1988, Mrozek-Orlowski et al 1991) and vinorelbine (Rittenberg et al 1995), and by the infusion of potassium chloride and hyperosmolar solutions (Pucino et al 1988). The pain and linear erythema associated with chemical phlebitis must be distinguished from the more serious complication of a vesicant cytotoxic extravasation (Box 45.3) (Bertelli 1995, Boyle & Engelking 1995). Vesicant extravasation may produce intense pain followed by desquamation and ulceration (Bertelli 1995, Boyle & Engelking 1995). Finally, a brief venous flare reaction is often associated with intravenous administration of the anthracycline, doxorubicin. The flare is typically associated with local urticaria and occasional patients report pain or stinging (Vogelzang 1979, Curran et al 1990).

Hepatic artery infusion pain Cytotoxic infusions into the hepatic artery (for patients with hepatic metastases) are often associated with the development of a diffuse abdominal pain (Kemeny 1991). Continuous infusions can lead to persistent pain. In some patients, the pain is due to the development of gastric ulceration or erosions (Shike et al 1986) or cholangitis (Batts 1998). If the latter complications do not occur, the pain usually resolves with discontinuation of the infusion. A dose relationship is suggested by the observation that some patients will comfortably tolerate reinfusion at a lower dose (Kemeny 1992).

Intraperitoneal chemotherapy pain Abdominal pain is a common complication of intraperitoneal chemotherapy (IPC). A transient mild abdominal pain, associated with sensations of fullness or bloating, is reported by approximately 25% of patients receiving IPC (Almadrones & Yerys 1990). A further 25% of patients report moderate or severe pain necessitating opioid analgesia or discontinuation of therapy (Almadrones & Yerys 1990). Moderate or severe pain is usually caused by chemical serositis or infection (Markman 1986). Drug selection may be a factor in the incidence of chemical serositis; it is a common complication of intraperitoneal anthracyclines, including mitoxantrone (Topuz et al 1997) and doxorubicin (Deppe et al 1991), and with paclitaxel (Francis et al 1995), but it is relatively infrequent with 5-flurouracil or cis-platinum (Schilsky et al 1990). Abdominal pain associated with fever and leukocytosis in blood and peritoneal fluid is suggestive of infectious peritonitis (Kaplan et al 1985).

Intravesical chemotherapy or immunotherapy Intravesical bacillus Calmette-Guerin (BCG) therapy for transitional cell carcinoma of the urinary bladder usually causes a transient bladder irritability syndrome characterized by frequency and/or micturition pain (Kudo et al 1991, Uekado et al 1994). Rarely, treatment may trigger a painful polyarthritis (Kudo et al 1991). Similarly, intravesical doxorubicin often causes a painful chemical cystitis (Matsumura et al 1983, 1992).

Acute pain associated with chemotherapy toxicity

Mucositis Severe mucositis is an almost invariable consequence of the myeloablative chemotherapy and radiotherapy that precedes bone marrow transplantation, but it is less common with standard intensity therapy (Rider 1990, Verdi 1993, Dose 1995). Although the clinical syndrome usually involves the oral cavity and pharynx, the underlying pathology commonly extends to other gastrointestinal mucosal surfaces, and symptoms may occur as a result of involvement of the oesophagus, stomach or intestine (e.g., odynophagia, dyspepsia or diarrhoea). Damaged mucosal surfaces may become superinfected with microorganisms, such as *Candida albicans* and herpes simplex. The latter complication is most likely in neutropenic patients, who are also predisposed to systemic sepsis arising from local invasion by aerobic and anaerobic oral flora. Numerous therapies have been developed to reduce the risk of mucositis, including the use of cryotherapy (Rocke et al 1993, Cascinu et al 1994), surface coating agents (Loprinzi et al 1997), antiviral agents (Redding & Montgomery 1989, Feld 1997) and disinfectant mouthwashes (Spijkervet et al 1990). None are established as effective. Severe mucositis usually requires both local and systemic analgesic therapies. Recently, experience has been reported with patient-controlled analgesia (Chapman & Hill 1989, Chapman et al 1997, Coda et al 1997), tetrachlorodecaoxide (Malik et al 1997) and oral capsaicin (Berger et al 1995a).

Corticosteroid-induced perineal discomfort A transient burning sensation in the perineum is described by some patients following the rapid infusion of large doses (20–100 mg) of dexamethasone (Bell 1988). Patients need to be warned that such symptoms may occur. Clinical experience suggests that this syndrome is prevented by slow infusion.

Steroid pseudorheumatism The withdrawal of corticosteroids may produce a pain syndrome that manifests as diffuse myalgias, arthralgias, and tenderness of muscles and joints. These symptoms can occur with rapid or slow withdrawal (rapid withdrawal appears to be worse) and may occur in patients taking these drugs for long or short periods of time. The pathogenesis of this syndrome is poorly understood, but it has been speculated that steroid withdrawal may sensitize joint and muscle mechanoreceptors and nociceptors (Rotstein & Good 1957). Treatment consists of reinstituting the steroids at a higher dose and withdrawing them more slowly (Rotstein & Good 1957).

Painful peripheral neuropathy The dose-related chemotherapy-induced painful peripheral neuropathy, which is usually associated with vinca alkaloids, cis-platinum and paclitaxel, typically has an acute or subacute course (Postma et al 1995). The vinca alkaloids (particularly vincristine) are also associated with other, presumably neuropathic, acute pain syndromes, including pain in the jaw, legs, arms or abdomen that may last from hours to days (Sandler et al 1969, Rosenthal & Kaufman 1974, McCarthy & Skillings 1992). Vincristine-induced orofacial pain in the distribution of the trigeminal and glossopharyngeal nerves occurs in approximately 50% of patients at the onset of vincristine treatment (McCarthy & Skillings 1992). The pain, which is severe in about half of those affected, generally begins 2–3 days after vincristine administration and lasts for 1–3 days. It is usually self limiting and if recurrence occurs it is usually mild (McCarthy & Skillings 1992).

Headache Intrathecal methotrexate in the treatment of leukaemia or leptomeningeal metastases produces an acute meningitic syndrome in 5–50% of patients (Weiss et al 1974a). Headache is the prominent symptom and may be associated with vomiting, nuchal rigidity, fever, irritability and lethargy. Symptoms usually begin hours after intrathecal treatment and persist for several days. Cerebrospinal fluid (CSF) examination reveals a pleocytosis that may mimic bacterial meningitis. Patients at increased risk for the development of this syndrome include those who have received multiple intrathecal injections and those patients undergoing treatment for proven leptomeningeal metastases (Weiss et al 1974a). The syndrome tends not to recur with subsequent injections.

Systemic administration of L-asparaginase for the treatment of acute lymphoblastic leukaemia produces thrombosis of cerebral veins or dural sinuses in 1–2% of patients (Priest et al 1982). This complication typically occurs after a few weeks of therapy, but its onset may be delayed until after the completion of treatment. It occurs as a result of the depletion of asparagene, which, in turn, leads to the reduction of plasma proteins involved in coagulation and fibrinolysis. Headache is the most common initial symptom, and seizures, hemiparesis, delirium, vomiting or cranial nerve palsies may also occur. The diagnosis may be established by angiography or by gradient echo sequences on MRI scan (Schick et al 1989).

Trans-retinoic acid therapy, which may be used in the treatment of acute promyelocytic leukaemia (APML), can cause a transient severe headache (Visani et al 1996). The mechanism may be related to pseudotumour cerebri induced by hypervitaminosis A.

Diffuse bone pain *Trans*-retinoic acid therapy in patients with APML often produces a syndrome of diffuse bone pain (Castaigne et al 1990, Ohno et al 1993). The pain is generalized, of variable intensity, and closely associated with a transient neutrophilia. The latter observation suggests that the pain may be caused by marrow expansion, a phenomenon that may underlie a similar pain syndrome that occurs following the administration of colony stimulating factors (Hollingshead & Goa 1991).

Paclitaxel-induced arthralgia and myalgia The administration of paclitaxel generates a syndrome of diffuse arthralgias and myalgia in 10–20% of patients (Rowinsky et al 1993, Muggia et al 1995). Diffuse joint and muscle pains generally appear 1–4 days after drug administration and persist for 3–7 days. The pathophysiology of this phenomenon has not been well evaluated.

5-Flurouracil-induced anginal chest pain Patients receiving continuous infusions of 5-flurouracil may develop ischaemic chest pain (Freeman & Costanza 1988). Continuous ambulatory electrocardiographic (ECG) monitoring of patients undergoing 5-FU infusion demonstrated a near threefold increase in ischaemic episodes over pretreatment recordings (Rezkalla et al 1989); these ECG changes were more common among patients with known coronary artery disease. It is widely speculated that coronary vasospasm may be the underlying mechanism (Freeman & Costanza 1988, Rezkalla et al 1989, Eskilsson & Albertsson 1990).

Palmar-plantar erythrodysaesthesia syndrome Protracted infusion of 5-FU can be complicated by the development of a tingling or burning sensation in the palms and soles followed by the development of an erythematous rash. The rash is characterized by a painful, sharply demarcated, intense erythema of the palms and/or soles followed by bulla formation, desquamation and healing. Continuous low dose 5-FU infusion (200–300 mg/m^2/day) will produce this palmar-plantar erythrodysaesthesia syndrome in 40–90% of patients (Lokich & Moore 1984, Leo et al 1994). It occurs rarely with patients undergoing 96–120-h infusions (Bellmunt et al 1988). The pathogenesis is unknown. The eruption is self limiting in nature and it does not usually require the discontinuation of therapy. Symptomatic measures are often required (Bellmunt et al 1988) and treatment with pyridoxine has been reported to induce resolution of the lesions (Fabian et al 1990).

A similar syndrome has recently been reported with liposomal doxorubicin. This drug is thought to be relatively sequested in skin (Uziely et al 1995, Alberts & Garcia 1997). As with 5-FU, this is also a dose-related adverse effect related to repeated dosing.

Postchemotherapy gynaecomastia Painful gynaecomastia can occur as a delayed complication of chemotherapy. Testis cancer is the most common underlying disorder (Trump et al 1982, Aki et al 1996), but it has been reported after therapy for other cancers as well (Glass & Berenberg 1979, Trump et al 1982). Gynaecomastia typically develops after a latency of 2–9 months and resolves spontaneously within a few months. Persistent gynaecomastia is occasionally observed (Trump et al 1982). Cytotoxic-induced disturbance of androgen secretion is the probable cause of this syndrome (Aki et al 1996). In the patient with testicular cancer, this syndrome must be differentiated from tumour-related gynaecomastia, which may be associated with early recurrence (see below) (Trump & Anderson 1983, Saeter et al 1987).

Chemotherapy-induced acute digital ischaemia Raynaud's phenomenon or transient ischaemia of the toes is a common complication of bleomycin, vinblastine and cisplatin (PVB) treatment for testicular cancer (Aass et al 1990). A rare, irreversible digital ischaemia leading to gangrene has been reported after bleomycin (Elomaa et al 1984).

Acute pain associated with hormonal therapy

Lutenizing hormone releasing factor (IHRF) tumour flare in prostate cancer The initiation of LHRF hormonal therapy for prostate cancer produces a transient symptom flare in 5–25% of patients (Chrisp & Goa 1991, Chrisp & Sorkin 1991). The flare is presumably caused by an initial stimulation of leutenizing hormone release before suppression is achieved. The syndrome typically presents as an exacerbation of bone pain or urinary retention; spinal cord compression and sudden death have also been reported (Thompson et al 1990). Symptom flare is usually observed within the first week of therapy, and lasts 1–3 weeks in the absence of androgen antagonist therapy. The co-administration of an androgen antagonist during the initiation of LHRF agonist therapy can prevent this phenomenon (Labrie et al 1987).

Among patients with prostate cancer that is refractory to first-line hormonal therapy, transient tumour flares have been observed with androstenedione (Shearer et al 1990, Davies et al 1992) and medroxyprogesterone (Fossa & Urnes 1986).

Hormone-induced pain flare in breast cancer Any hormonal therapy for metastatic breast cancer can be complicated by a sudden onset of diffuse musculoskeletal pain commencing within hours to weeks of the initiation of therapy (Plotkin et al 1978). Other manifestations of this syndrome include erythema around cutaneous metastases, changes in liver function studies, and hypercalcaemia. Although the underlying mechanism is not understood, this does not appear to be caused by tumour stimulation, and it is speculated that it may reflect normal tissue response (Reddel & Sutherland 1984).

Acute pain associated with immunotherapy

Interferon (IFN)-induced acute pain Virtually all patients treated with IFN experience an acute syndrome consisting of fever, chills, myalgias, arthralgias and headache (Quesada et al 1986). The syndrome usually begins shortly after initial dosing and frequently improves with the continued administration of the drug (Quesada et al 1986). The severity of symptoms is related to type of IFN, route of administration, schedule and dose. Doses of 1–9 million units of interferon-alpha are usually well tolerated, but doses greater than or equal to 18 million units usually produce moderate to severe toxicity (Quesada et al 1986). Acetaminophen pretreatment is often useful in ameliorating these symptoms.

Acute pain associated with growth factors

Colony-stimulating factor-induced musculoskeletal pains. Colony-stimulating factors (CSFs) are haematopoietic growth hormones that stimulate the production, maturation and function of white blood cells. Granulocyte-macrophage CSF (GM-CSF), granulocyte CSF (G-CSF) and interleukin 3 commonly produce mild to moderate bone pain and constitutional symptoms, such as fever, headache and myalgias, during the period of administration (Veldhuis et al 1995, Vial & Descotes 1995).

Erythropoietin (r-HuEPO) injection pain. Subcutaneous administration of r-HuEPO alpha is associated with pain at the injection site in about 40% of cases (Frenken et al 1991). Subcutaneous injection of r-HuEPO alpha is more painful than r-HuEPO beta (Morris et al 1994). r-HuEPO alpha erythropoietin injection pain can be reduced by dilution of the vehicle with benzyl alcohol saline, reduction of the volume of the vehicle to 0.1 ml (Frenken et al 1994), and the addition of lidocaine (Alon et al 1994).

Acute pain associated with radiotherapy

Incident pains can be precipitated by transport and positioning of the patient for radiotherapy. Other pains can be caused by acute radiation toxicity, which is most commonly associated with inflammation and ulceration of skin or mucous membranes within the radiation port. The syndrome depends on the involved field: head and neck irradiation can cause a stomatitis or pharyngitis (Rider 1990), treatment of the chest and oesophagus can cause an oesophagitis (Vanagunas et al 1990), and pelvic therapy can cause a proctitis, cystitis-urethritis or vaginal ulceration.

Oropharyngeal mucositis Radiotherapy-induced mucositis is invariable with doses above 1000 cGy, and ulceration is common at doses above 4000 cGy. Although the severity of the associated pain is variable, it is often severe enough to interfere with oral alimentation. Painful mucositis can persist for several weeks after the completion of the treatment (Rider 1990, Epstein & Stewart 1993).

Acute radiation enteritis and proctocolitis. Acute radiation enteritis occurs in as many as 50% of patients receiving abdominal or pelvic radiotherapy. Involvement of the small intestine can present with cramping abdominal pain associated with nausea and diarrhoea (Yeoh & Horowitz 1988). Pelvic radiotherapy can cause a painful proctocolitis, with tenesmoid pain associated with diarrhoea, mucous discharge and bleeding (Babb 1996). These complications typically resolve shortly after completion of therapy, but may have a slow resolution over 2–6 months (Yeoh & Horowitz 1988, Nussbaum et al 1993, Babb 1996). Acute enteritis is associated with an increased risk of late-onset radiation enteritis (see below).

Early-onset brachial plexopathy A transient brachial plexopathy has been described in breast cancer patients immediately following radiotherapy to the chest wall and adjacent nodal areas. In retrospective studies, the incidence of this phenomenon has been variably estimated as 1.4–20% (Salner et al 1981, Pierce et al 1992); clinical experience suggests that lower estimates are more accurate. The median latency to the development of symptoms was 4.5 months (3–14 months) in one survey (Salner et al 1981). Paraesthesias are the most common presenting symptom, and pain and weakness occur less frequently. The syndrome is self limiting and does not predispose to the subsequent development of delayed-onset progressive plexopathy.

Subacute radiation myelopathy Subacute radiation myelopathy is an uncommon phenomenon that may occur following radiotherapy of extraspinal tumours (Ang & Stephens 1994, Schultheiss 1994). It is most frequently observed involving the cervical cord after radiation treatment of head and neck cancers and Hodgkin's disease. When the cervical cord is involved, patients may develop painful, shock-like pains in the neck that are precipitated by neck flexion (Lhermitte's sign); these pains may radiate down the spine and into one or more extremities. The syndrome usually begins weeks to months after the completion of radiotherapy, and typically resolves over a period of 3–6 months (Ang & Stephens 1994).

Radiopharmaceutical-induced pain flare Strontium-89, rhenium-186 hydroxyethylidene diphosphonate and samarium-153 are systemically administered β-emitting calcium analogues that are taken up by bone in areas of osteoblastic activity. These drugs may help relieve the pain caused by blastic bony metastases (McEwan 1997). A 'flare' response, characterized by transient worsening of pain 1–2 days after administration, occurs in 15–20% of patients (Robinson et al 1995). This flare is usually resolved after 3–5 days and most affected patients subsequently develop a good analgesic response (Robinson et al 1995).

ACUTE PAIN ASSOCIATED WITH INFECTION

Acute herpetic neuralgia

A significantly increased incidence of acute herpetic neuralgia occurs among cancer patients, especially those with haematological or lymphoproliferative malignancies and those receiving immunosuppressive therapies (Portenoy et al 1986, Rusthoven et al 1988). Pain or itch usually precedes the development of the rash by several days and may occasionally occur without the development of skin eruption (Portenoy et al 1986, Galer & Portenoy 1991). The pain, which may be continuous or lancinating, usually resolves within 2 months (Portenoy et al 1986, Galer & Portenoy 1991). Pain persisting beyond this interval is referred to as postherpetic neuralgia (see below). Patients with active tumour are more likely to disseminate the infection (Rusthoven et al 1988). In those predisposed by chemotherapy, the infection usually develops less than 1 month after the completion of treatment. The dermatomal location of the infection is often associated with the site of the malignancy (Rusthoven et al 1988): patients with primary tumours of gynaecological and genitourinary origin have a predilection to lumbar and sacral involvement, and those with breast or lung carcinomas tend to present with thoracic involvement; patients with haematological tumours appear to be predisposed to cervical lesions. The infection also occurs twice as frequently in previously irradiated dermatomes as in non-radiated areas.

ACUTE PAIN ASSOCIATED WITH VASCULAR EVENTS

Acute thrombosis pain

Thrombosis is the most frequent complication and the second cause of death in patients with malignant disease (Donati 1994). Patients with pelvic tumours (Clarke-Pearson & Olt 1989), pancreatic cancer (Heinmoller et al 1995), gastric cancer, advanced breast cancer (Levine et al 1994) and brain tumours (Sawaya & Ligon 1994) are at greastest risk for thrombosis. Thrombotic episodes may precede the diagnosis of cancer by months or years and represent a potential marker for occult malignancy (Agnelli 1997). Postoperative deep vein thrombosis is more frequent in patients operated for malignant diseases than for other disorders, and both chemotherapy and hormone therapy are associated with an increased thrombotic risk (Agnelli 1997).

Tumour cells and their products interact with platelets, clotting and fibrinolytic systems, endothelial cells and tumour-associated macrophages. These interactions may predispose to thrombosis. Cytokine release, acute-phase reaction and neovascularization also may contribute to vivo clotting activation (Donati 1994, Agnelli 1997).

Lower extremity deep venous thrombosis

Pain and swelling are the commonest presenting features of lower extremity deep vein thrombosis (Criado & Burnham 1997). The pain is variable in severity and it is often mild. It is commonly described as a dull cramp, or diffuse heaviness. The pain most commonly affects the calf but may involve the sole of the foot, heel, thigh, groin or pelvis. Pain usually increases on standing and walking. On examination, suggestive features include swelling, warmth, dilatation of superficial veins and tenderness along venous tracts, and pain induced by stretching (Wells et al 1995, Criado & Burnham 1997).

The diagnosis of deep venous thrombosis can usually be confirmed by non-invasive tests, such as ultrasonography or impedance plethysmography, rather than venography. Ultrasonography is sensitive, effectively defines the anatomical extent of the thrombus, and is the diagnostic standard for symptomatic thrombosis (Cogo et al 1998). Impedance plethysmography is a less sensitive alternative (Wells et al 1995). When the findings of these non-invasive approaches are at variance with a strong clinical impression, venography should be considered (Wells et al 1995).

Patients with deep venous thrombosis rarely develop tissue ischaemia or frank gangrene even in the absence of arterial or capillary occlusion. This syndrome is called phlegmasia cerulea dolens. It is most commonly seen in patients with underlying neoplasm (Hirschmann 1987, Lorimer et al 1994) and is characterized by the development of severe pain, extensive oedema and cyanosis of the legs. Gangrene can occur unless the venous obstruction is relieved. When possible optimal therapy is anticoagulation and thrombectomy (Perkins et al 1996). The mortality rate for ischaemic venous thrombosis is about 40%; the cause of death usually is the underlying disease or pulmonary emboli (Hirschmann 1987).

Upper extremity deep venous thrombosis

Only 2% of all cases of deep venous thrombosis involve the upper extremity, and the incidence of pulmonary embolism related to thrombosis in this location is approximately 12% (Nemmers et al 1990). The three major clinical features of upper extremity venous thrombosis are oedema, dilated collateral circulation and pain (Burihan et al 1993). Approximately two-thirds of patients have arm pain. Among patents with cancer, the most common causes are central venous catheterization and extrinsic compression by tumour (Burihan et al 1993). Although thrombosis secondary to intrinsic damage usually responds well to anticoagulation alone and rarely causes persistent symptoms, persistent arm swelling and pain are commonplace when extrinsic obstruction is the cause (Donayre et al 1986).

Superior vena cava obstruction

Superior vena cava (SVC) obstruction is most commonly caused by extrinsic compression from enlarged mediastinal lymph nodes (Escalante 1993). In contemporary series, lung cancer and lymphomas are the most associated conditions. Increasingly, thrombosis of the superior vena cava is caused by intravascular devices (Escalante 1993, Morales et al 1997). This complication is most likely with left-sided ports and when the catheter tip lies in the upper part of the vena (Puel et al 1993). Patients usually present with facial swelling and dilated neck and chest wall veins. Chest pain, headache and mastalgia are less common presentations.

Acute mesenteric vein thrombosis

Acute mesenteric vein thrombosis is most commonly associated with hypercoaguability states. Rarely, it has been associated with extrinsic venous compression by malignant lymphadenopathy (Traill & Nolan 1997), extension of venous thrombosis (Vigo et al 1980) or an iatrogenic hypercoaguable state (Sahdev et al 1985).

CHRONIC PAIN SYNDROMES

Most chronic cancer-related pains are caused directly by the tumour (Box 45.2). Bone pain and compression of neural structures are the two most common causes (Daut & Cleeland 1982, Foley 1987, Banning et al 1991, Grond et al 1996, Twycross et al 1996).

BONE PAIN

Bone metastases are the most common cause of chronic pain in cancer patients (Daut & Cleeland 1982, Foley 1987, Banning et al 1991, Grond et al 1996, Twycross et al 1996). Cancers of the lung, breast and prostate most often metastasize to bone, but any tumour type may be complicated by painful bony lesions. Although bone pain is usually associated with direct tumour invasion of bony structures, more than 25% of patients with bony metastases are pain free (Wagner 1984), and patients with multiple bony metastases typically report pain in only a few sites. The factors that convert a painless lesion to a painful one are unknown. Bone metastases could potentially cause pain by any of multiple mechanisms, including endosteal or periosteal nociceptor activation (by mechanical distortion or release of chemical mediators) or tumour growth into adjacent soft tissues and nerves (Mercadante 1997).

Bone pain due to metastatic tumour needs to be differentiated from less common causes. Non-neoplastic causes in this population include osteoporotic fractures (including those associated with multiple myeloma), focal osteonecrosis, which may be idiopathic or related to chemotherapy, corticosteroids (Socie et al 1997) or radiotherapy (see below), and osteomalacia (Shane et al 1997).

Multifocal or generalized bone pain

Bone pain may be focal, multifocal or generalized. Multifocal bone pains are most commonly experienced by patients with multiple bony metastases. A generalized pain syndrome, which is well recognized in patients with multiple bony metastases, is also rarely produced by the replacement of bone marrow (Jonsson et al 1990, Wong et al 1993). This bone marrow replacement syndrome has been observed in haematogenous malignancies (Golembe et al 1979, Lembersky et al 1988) and, less commonly, solid tumours (Wong et al 1993). This syndrome can occur in the absence of abnormalities on bone scintigraphy or radiography, increasing the difficulty of diagnosis. Rarely, a paraneoplastic osteomalacia can mimic multiple metastases (Shane et al 1997).

Vertebral syndromes

The vertebrae are the most common sites of bony metastases. More than two-thirds of vertebral metastases are located in the thoracic spine; lumbosacral and cervical metastases account for approximately 20% and 10%, respectively (Gilbert et al 1978, Sorensen et al 1990). Multiple level involvement is common, occurring in greater than 85% of patients (Constans et al 1983). The early recognition of pain syndromes resulting from tumour invasion of vertebral bodies is essential, because pain usually precedes compression of adjacent neural structures and prompt treatment of the lesion may prevent the subsequent development of neurological deficits. Accurate diagnosis may be difficult. Referral of pain is common, and the associated symptoms and signs can mimic a variety of other disorders, both malignant (e.g., paraspinal masses) and non-malignant.

Atlantoaxial destruction and odontoid fracture

Nuchal or occipital pain is the typical presentation of destruction of the atlas or fracture of the odontoid process. Pain often radiates over the posterior aspect of the skull to the vertex and is exacerbated by movement of the neck, particularly flexion (Phillips & Levine 1989). Pathological fracture may result in secondary subluxation with compression of the spinal cord at the cervicomedullary junction. This complication is usually insidious and may begin with symptoms or signs in one or more extremity. Typically, there is early involvement of the upper extremities and the occasional appearance of so-called 'pseudo-levels' suggestive of more caudal spinal lesions; these deficits can slowly progress to involve sensory, motor and autonomic function (Sundaresan et al 1981). MRI is probably the best method for imaging this region of the spine (Bosley et al 1985), but clinical experience suggests that CT is also sensitive. Plain radiography, tomography and bone scintigraphy should be viewed as ancillary procedures.

C7–T1 syndrome

Invasion of the C7 or T1 vertebra can result in pain referred to the interscapular region. These lesions may be missed if radiographic evaluation is mistakenly targeted to the painful area caudal to the site of damage. Additionally, visualization of the appropriate region on routine radiographs may be inadequate as a result of obscuration by overlying bone and mediastinal shadows. Patients with interscapular pain should undergo radiography of both the cervical and the thoracic spine. Bone scintigraphy may assist in targeting additional diagnostic imaging procedures, such as CT or MRI. The latter procedures can be useful in assessing the possibility that pain is referred from an extraspinal site, such as the paraspinal gutter.

T12–L1 syndrome

A T12 or L1 vertebral lesion can refer pain to the ipsilateral iliac crest or the sacroiliac joint. Imaging procedures directed at pelvic bones can miss the source of the pain.

Sacral syndrome

Severe focal pain radiating to the buttocks, perineum or posterior thighs may accompany destruction of the sacrum (Hall & Fleming 1970, Feldenzer et al 1989, Porter et al 1994). The pain is often exacerbated by sitting or lying and is relieved by standing or walking. The neoplasm can spread laterally to involve muscles that rotate the hip (e.g., the pyriformis muscle). This may produce severe incident pain induced by motion of the hip, a malignant 'pyriformis syndrome', characterized by buttock or posterior leg pain that is exacerbated by internal rotation of the hip. Local extension of the tumour mass may also involve the sacral plexus (see below).

Back pain and epidural compression

Epidural compression (EC) of the spinal cord or cauda equina is the second most common neurological complication of cancer, occurring in up to 10% of patients (Posner 1987). In the community setting, EC is often the first recognized manifestation of malignancy (Stark et al 1982); at a cancer hospital it is the presenting syndrome in only 8% of cases (Posner 1987). Most EC is caused by posterior extension of vertebral body metastasis to the epidural space (Fig. 45.4). Occasionally, EC is caused by tumour extension from the posterior arch of the vertebra or infiltration of a paravertebral tumour through the intervertebral foramen (Fig. 45.5). Untreated, EC leads inevitably to neurological compromise, ultimately including paraplegia or quadriplegia. Effective treatment can potentially prevent these complications. The most important determinant of the efficacy of treatment is the degree of neurological impairment at the time therapy is initiated. Seventy-five per cent of patients who begin treatment while ambulatory remain so; the efficacy of treatment declines to 30–50% for those who begin treatment while markedly paretic, and is 10–20% for those who are plegic (Gilbert et al 1978, Barcena et al 1984, Portenoy et al 1989, Ruff & Lanska 1989, Rosenthal et al 1992, Maranzano & Latini 1995, Huddart et al 1997, Milross et al 1997).

The treatment of EC generally involves the administration of corticosteroids (see below) and radiotherapy (Maranzano & Latini 1995). Surgical decompression is considered for some patients with radioresistant tumours, those who have previously received maximal radiotherapy

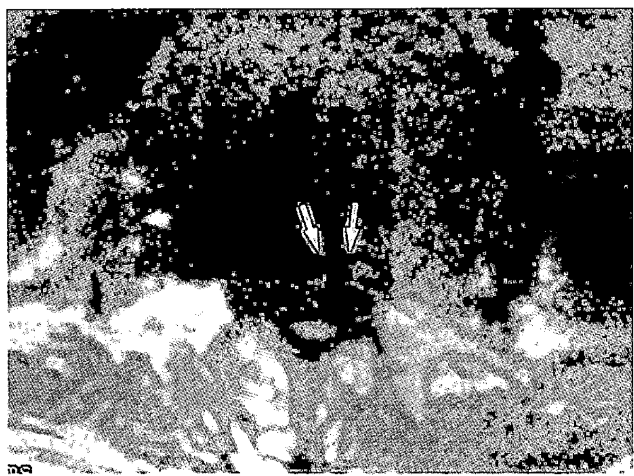

Fig. 45.4 Axial MRI scan of the lumbar spine in a 56-year-old woman with carcinoma of the colon who presented with back pain and L3 radicular pain in the right leg. The scan performed through L3 demonstrates complete obliteration of the epidural space (arrows) and severe compression of the thecal sac.

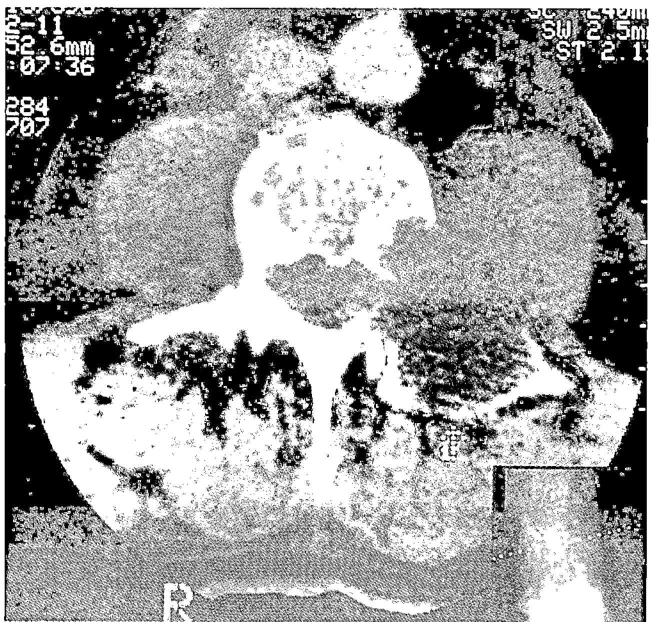

Fig. 45.5 CT scan of lumbar vertebra demonstrating a large metastasis involving the left transverse process, invading into the intervertebral foramen and encroaching into the epidural space.

to the involved field, those with spinal instability or posterior displacement of bony fragments into the spinal canal, and those for whom no other tissue is available for histological diagnosis (Posner 1987, Grant et al 1994, Harris et al 1996). Decompressive laminectomy for posteriorly located lesions and anterior vertebrectomy with spinal stabilization for lesions arising from the vertebral body are the currently recommended procedures (Sundaresan et al 1985, 1996, Tomita et al 1994, Harris et al 1996). Decompressive laminectomy in the setting of vertebral body collapse is not recommended because of the risk of neurological deterioration or spinal instability (22–25%) induced by the procedure (Brice & McKissock 1965, Findlay 1984, Findlay 1987).

Back pain is the initial symptom in almost all patients with EC (Posner 1987), and in 10% it is the only symptom at the time of diagnosis (Greenberg et al 1980). Because pain usually precedes neurological signs by a prolonged period, it should be viewed as a potential indicator of EC, which could lead to treatment at a time that a favourable response is most likely. Back pain, however, is a non-specific symptom that can result from bony or paraspinal metastases without epidural encroachment, from retroperitoneal or leptomeningeal tumour, epidural lipomatosis as a result of steroid administration (Stranjalis et al 1992), or from a large variety of other benign conditions. Because it is infeasible to pursue an extensive evaluation in every cancer patient who develops back pain, the complaint should impel an evaluation that determines the likelihood of EC and thereby selects patients who may be appropriate for definitive imaging of the epidural space. The selection process is based on symptoms and signs and the results of simple imaging techniques.

Clinical features of epidural extension

Some pain characteristics are particularly suggestive of epidural extension (Helweg-Larsen & Sorensen 1994). Rapid progression of back pain in a crescendo pattern is an ominous occurrence (Rosenthal et al 1992). Radicular pain, which can be constant or lancinating, has similar implications (Helweg-Larsen & Sorensen 1994). Radicular pain is usually unilateral in the cervical and lumbosacral regions, and bilateral in the thorax, where it is often experienced as a tight, belt-like band across the chest or abdomen (Helweg-Larsen & Sorensen 1994). The likelihood of EC is also greater when back or radicular pain is exacerbated by recumbency, cough, sneeze or strain (Ruff & Lanska 1989). Other types of referred pain are also suggestive, including Lhermitte's sign (Ventafridda et al 1991) and central pain from spinal cord compression, which usually is perceived some distance below the site of the compression and is typically a poorly localized, non-dermatomal dysaesthesia (Posner 1987).

Weakness, sensory loss, autonomic dysfunction and reflex abnormalities usually occur after a period of progressive pain (Helweg-Larsen & Sorensen 1994). Weakness may begin segmentally if related to nerve root damage or in a multisegmental or pyramidal distribution if the cauda equina or spinal cord, respectively, is injured. The rate of progression of weakness is variable; in the absence of treatment, one-third of patients will develop paralysis within 7 days of the onset of weakness (Barron et al 1959). Patients whose weakness progresses slowly have a better prognosis for neurological recovery with treatment than those who progress rapidly (Helweg-Larsen et al 1990, Helweg-Larsen 1996). Without effective treatment, sensory abnormalities, which may also begin segmentally, may ultimately evolve to a sensory level, with complete loss of all sensory modalities below site of injury. The upper level of sensory findings may correspond to the location of the epidural tumour or be below it by many segments (Helweg-Larsen & Sorensen 1994). Ataxia without pain is the initial presentation of epidural compression in 1% of patients; this finding is presumably a result of early involvement of the spinocerebellar tracts (Gilbert et al 1978). Bladder and bowel dysfunction occur late, except in patients with a

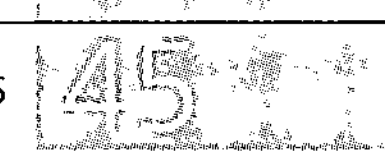

conus medullaris lesion who may present with urinary retention and constipation without preceding motor or sensory symptoms (Helweg-Larsen & Sorensen 1994).

Other features that may be evident on examination of patients with EC include scoliosis, asymmetrical wasting of paravertebral musculature and a gibbus (palpable step in the spinous processes). Spinal tenderness to percussion, which may be severe, often accompanies the pain.

Imaging modalities

Definitive imaging of the epidural space confirms the existence of EC (and thereby indicates the necessity and urgency of treatment), defines the appropriate radiation portals and determines the extent of epidural encroachment (which influences prognosis and may alter the therapeutic approach) (Portenoy et al 1987). The options for definitive imaging include MRI, myelography and CT-myelography. MRI, which is non-invasive and offers accurate soft-tissue imaging and multiplanar views, is generally preferred. A study comparing state-of-the-art MRI techniques with CT-myelography demonstrated equivalent sensitivity and specificity (Helweg-Larsen et al 1992). A 'scanning' mid-sagittal MRI is clearly inadequate (Hagen et al 1989). Myelography or CT-myelography remain appropriate alternatives for patients who lack access to MRI and those unable to undergo the procedure. MRI is relatively contraindicated in patients with severe claustrophobia and absolutely contraindicated for patients with metallic implants, cardiac pacemakers or aneurysm clips. Patients who would benefit from total spinal imaging, such as those with multifocal pain or multiple spinal metastases (who have a 10% chance of EC remote from the symptomatic site (Stark et al 1982)), and those with severe kyphosis or scoliosis, who may not be suitable for MRI scanning because of technical considerations, may also need a different approach. Myelography may also be needed following an MRI scan that is suboptimal or non-diagnostic, particularly if there is neurological deterioration.

Algorithm for the investigation of cancer patients with back pain

Given the prevalence and the potentially dire consequences of EC, and the recognition that back pain is a marker of early (and therefore treatable) EC, algorithms have been developed to guide the evaluation of back pain in the cancer patient. The objective of these algorithms is to select a subgroup who should undergo definitive imaging of the epidural space from among the large number of patients who develop back pain (Portenoy et al 1987). The effective treatment of EC before irreversible neurological compromise occurs is the overriding goal of these approaches.

One such algorithm defines both the urgency and course of the evaluation (Fig. 45.6). Patients with emerging symptoms and signs indicative of spinal cord or cauda equina dysfunction are designated Group 1. The evaluation (and if appropriate, treatment) of these patients should proceed on an emergency basis. In most cases, these patients should receive an intravenous dose of corticosteroid before epidural imaging is performed. Dexamethasone is used customarily. High doses have been advocated on the basis of animal studies (Delattre et al 1989), analgesic efficacy (Greenberg et al 1980) and the dose–response relationship that has been observed during the treatment of intracranial hypertension from mass lesions. One regimen advocates an initial IV bolus of 100 mg followed by 96 mg per day in divided doses, which is tapered over 3–4 weeks. Although a randomized trial failed to identify any difference in neurological outcome between a high (100-mg) and low (10-mg) initial dose (Vecht et al 1989a), these findings must be replicated on a larger sample. High doses can still be recommended on the basis of a favourable clinical experience.

Patients with symptoms and signs of radiculopathy or stable or mild signs of spinal cord or cauda equina dysfunction are designated Group 2. These patients are also usually treated presumptively with a corticosteroid (typically with a more moderate dose) and are scheduled for definitive imaging of the epidural space as soon as possible.

Group 3 patients have back pain and no symptoms or signs suggesting EC. These patients should be evaluated routinely, starting with plain spine radiographs. The presence at the appropriate level of any abnormality consistent with neoplasm indicates a high probability (60%) of EC (Rodichok et al 1986, Hill et al 1993). This likelihood varies, however, with the type of radiological abnormality; for example, one study noted that EC occurred in 87% of patients with greater than 50% vertebral body collapse, 31% with pedicle erosion, and only 7% with tumour limited to the body of the vertebra without collapse (Graus et al 1986). Definitive imaging of the epidural space is thus strongly indicated in patients who have >50% vertebral body collapse, and is generally recommended for patients with pedicle erosion. Some patients with neoplasm limited to the vertebral body can be followed expectantly; imaging should be performed if pain progresses or changes (e.g., become radicular), or if radiographic evidence of progression is obtained.

Among patients with vertebral collapse it is often difficult to distinguish malignant from non-malignant pathol-

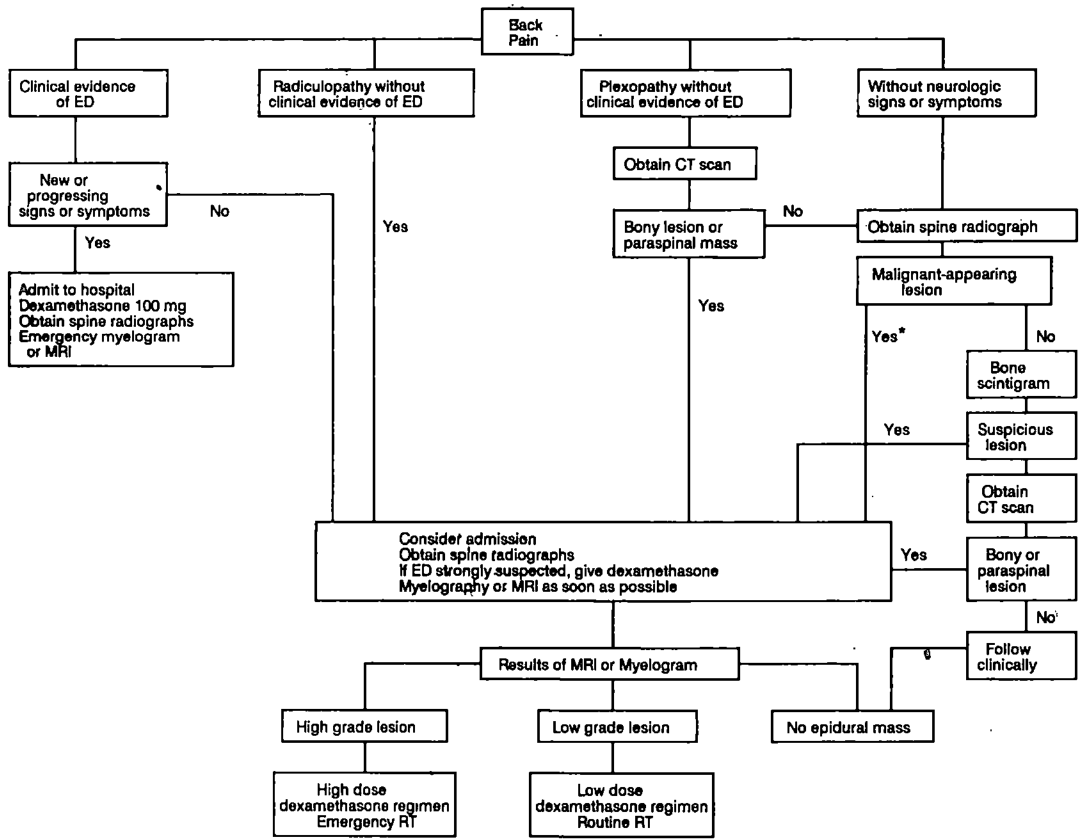

Fig. 45.6 Algorithm for the management of back pain in the cancer patient.

ogy. Vertebral metastases are suggested by destruction of the anterolateral or posterior cortical bone, destruction of the cancellous bone or vertebral pedicle, focal paraspinal soft-tissue mass or an epidural mass. Non-malignant causes are suggested by cortical fractures of the vertebral body without cortical bone destruction, retropulsion of a fragment of the posterior cortex of the vertebral body into the spinal canal, fracture lines within the cancellous bone of the vertebral body, an intravertebral vacuum phenomenon and a thin diffuse paraspinal soft-tissue mass (Laredo et al 1995).

Normal spine radiographs alone are not adequate to ensure a low likelihood of epidural tumour in patients with back pain. The bone may not be sufficiently damaged to change the radiograph or the tumour may involve the epidural space with little or no involvement of the adjacent bone (such as may occur when paraspinal tumour grows through the intervertebral foramen). The latter phenomenon has been most strikingly demonstrated in patients with lymphoma, in whom EC presents with normal radiography more than 60% of the time (Haddad et al 1976, Perry et al 1993). Damage to the vertebra that is not seen on the plain radiograph may potentially be demonstrated by bone scintigraphy. In patients with back pain and normal bone radiography, a positive scintigram at the site of pain is associated with a 12–17% likelihood of epidural disease (O'Rourke et al 1986, Portenoy et al 1989). Although such patients can also be followed expectantly, definitive imaging of the epidural space should be considered, particularly if the pain is progressive.

If both radiography and scintigraphy are normal but the patient has severe or progressive pain, evaluation with CT, or preferably MRI, may still be warranted. If the CT scan demonstrates a bony lesion abutting the spinal canal, a paraspinal mass or a perivertebral soft-tissue collar, imaging of the epidural space is still justified (Portenoy et al 1989, Albertyn et al 1992).

Pain syndromes of the bony pelvis and hip

The pelvis and hip are common sites of metastatic involvement. Lesions may involve any of the three anatomical regions of the pelvis (ischiopubic, iliosacral or periacetabular), the hip joint itself or the proximal femur (Sim 1992). The weight-bearing function of these structures, essential for normal ambulation, contributes to the propensity of disease at these sites to cause incident pain with ambulation.

Hip joint syndrome

Tumour involvement of the acetabulum or head of femur typically produces localized hip pain that is aggravated by weight bearing and movement of the hip. The pain may radiate to the knee or medial thigh, and, occasionally, pain is limited to these structures (Graham 1976, Sim 1992). Medial extension of an acetabular tumour can involve the lumbosacral plexus as it traverses the pelvic sidewall (Fig. 45.7). Evaluation of this region is best accomplished with CT or MRI, both of which can demonstrate the extent of bony destruction and adjacent soft-tissue involvement more sensitively than other imaging techniques (Beatrous et al 1990).

Acrometastases

Acrometastases, metastases in the hands and feet, are rare and often misdiagnosed or overlooked (Healey et al 1986, Leonheart & DiStazio 1994). In the feet, the larger bones containing the higher amounts of red marrow, such as the os calcis, are usually involved (Freedman & Henderson 1995). Symptoms may be vague and can mimic other conditions, such as osteomyelitis, gouty rheumatoid arthritis, Reiter's syndrome, Paget's disease, osteochondral lesions and ligamentous sprains.

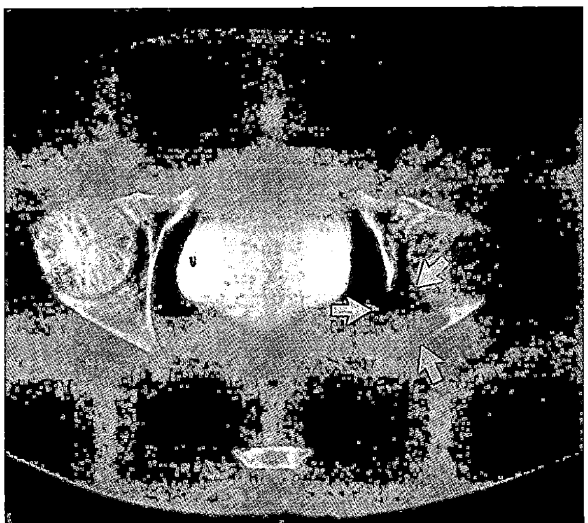

Fig. 45.7 CT scan demonstrating lytic lesion of the right acetabulum with tumour extension into the pelvis (arrows).

ARTHRITIDIES

Hypertrophic pulmonary osteoarthropathy

Hypertrophic pulmonary osteoarthropathy (HPOA) is a paraneoplastic syndrome that includes clubbing of the fingers, periostitis of long bones and, occasionally, a rheumatoid-like polyarthritis (Martinez-Lavin 1997). The syndrome usually causes pain, tenderness and swelling in the knees, wrists and ankles. The onset of symptoms is usually subacute, and it may precede the discovery of the underlying neoplasm by several months. It is most commonly associated with non-small-cell lung cancer. Less commonly, it is associated with benign mesothelioma (Briselli et al 1981), pulmonary metastases from other primary neoplasms (Margolick et al 1982), smooth muscle tumours of the oesophagus (Kaymakcalan et al 1980), breast cancer (Shapiro 1987) and metastatic nasopharyngeal cancer. Effective antitumour therapy is sometimes associated with symptom regression (Shapiro 1987, El-Salhy et al 1998). HPOA is diagnosed on the basis of physical findings, radiological appearance and radionuclide bone scan (Greenfield et al 1967, Sharma 1995, Martinez-Lavin 1997).

Other polyarthritides

Rarely, rheumatoid arthritis, systemic lupus erythematosus and an asymmetrical polyarthritis may occur as paraneoplastic phenomena that resolve with effective treatment of the underlying disease (Pines et al 1984, Rogues et al 1993). A syndrome of palmar and plantar fasciitis and polyarthritis, characterized by pain and polyarticular capsular contractions, has been associated with ovarian (Shiel et al 1985) and breast (Saxman & Seitz 1997) cancers.

MUSCLE PAIN

Muscle cramps

Persistent muscle cramps in cancer patients are usually caused by an identifiable neural, muscular or biochemical abnormality (Siegal 1991). In one series of 50 patients, 22 had peripheral neuropathy, 17 had root or plexus pathology (including six with leptomeningeal metastases), two had polymyositis and one had hypomagnesaemia. In this series, muscle cramps were the presenting symptoms of recognizable and previously unsuspected neurological dysfunction in

64% (27 of 42) of the identified causes (Steiner & Siegal 1989).

Skeletal muscle tumours

Soft-tissue sarcomas arising from fat, fibrous tissue or skeletal muscle are the most common tumours involving the skeletal muscles. Skeletal muscle is one of the most unusual sites of metastasis from any malignancy (Sridhar et al 1987, Araki et al 1994). Lesions are usually painless, but they may cause persistent ache.

HEADACHE AND FACIAL PAIN

Headache in the cancer patient often results from traction, inflammation or infiltration of pain-sensitive structures in the head or neck. Early evaluation with appropriate imaging techniques may identify the lesion and allow prompt treatment, which may reduce pain and prevent the development of neurological deficits (Vecht et al 1992).

Intracerebral tumour

Among 183 patients with new onset chronic headache, as an isolated symptom, investigation revealed underlying tumour in 15 cases (Vazquez-Barquero et al 1994). The prevalence of headache in patients with brain metastases or primary brain tumours is 60–90% (Forsyth & Posner 1993, Suwanwela et al 1994). These headaches are presumably produced by traction on pain-sensitive vascular and dural tissues. Patients with multiple metastases and those with posterior fossa metastases are more likely to report this symptom (Forsyth & Posner 1993). The pain may be focal, overlying the site of the lesion, or generalized. If unilateral, the headache may have lateralizing value, especially in patients with supratentorial lesions (Suwanwela et al 1994). Posterior fossa lesions often cause a bifrontal headache. The quality of the headache is usually throbbing or steady, and the intensity is usually mild to moderate (Suwanwela et al 1994).

Among children, clinical features predictive of underlying tumour include sleep-related headache, headache in the absence of a family history of migraine, vomiting, absence of visual symptoms, headache of less than 6 months duration, confusion and abnormal neurological examination findings (Medina et al 1997).

The headache associated with an intracranial space-occupying lesion is often worse in the morning and exacerbated by stooping, sudden head movement or valsalva manoeuvres (cough, sneeze or strain) (Suwanwela et al 1994). In patients with increased intracranial pressure, these manoeuvres can also precipitate transient elevations in intracranial pressure called 'plateau waves'. These plateau waves, which may also be spontaneous, can be associated with short periods of severe headache, nausea, vomiting, photophobia, lethargy and transient neurological deficits (Matsuda et al 1979; Hayashi et al 1991). Occasionally these plateau waves produce life-threatening herniation syndromes (Matsuda et al 1979, Hayashi et al 1991).

Leptomeningeal metastases

Leptomeningeal metastases, which are characterized by diffuse or multifocal involvement of the subarachnoid space by metastatic tumour, occur in 1–8% of patients with systemic cancer (Grossman & Moynihan 1991). Non-Hodgkin's lymphoma and acute lymphocytic leukaemia both demonstrate a predilection for meningeal metastases (Grossman & Moynihan 1991); the incidence is lower for solid tumours alone. Adenocarcinomas of the breast and lung are the predominant solid tumours (Jayson & Howell 1996).

Leptomeningeal metastases present with focal or multifocal neurological symptoms or signs that may involve any level of the neuraxis (Wasserstrom et al 1982, Grossman & Moynihan 1991). More than one-third of patients presents with evidence of cranial nerve damage, including double vision, hearing loss, facial numbness and decreased vision (Wasserstrom et al 1982). Less common features include seizures, papilloedema, hemiparesis, ataxic gait and confusion (Balm & Hammack 1996). Generalized headache and radicular pain in the low back and buttocks are the most common pains associated with leptomeningeal metastases (Wasserstrom et al 1982, Kaplan et al 1990). The headache is variable and may be associated with changes in mental status (e.g., lethargy, confusion or loss of memory), nausea, vomiting, tinnitus or nuchal rigidity. Pains that resemble cluster headache (DeAngelis & Payne 1987) or glossopharyngeal neuralgia with syncope (Sozzi et al 1987) have also been reported.

The diagnosis of leptomeningeal metastases is confirmed through analysis of the cerebrospinal fluid (CSF). The CSF may reveal elevated pressure, elevated protein, depressed glucose and/or lymphocytic pleocytosis. Ninety per cent of patients ultimately show positive cytology, but multiple evaluations may be required. After a single lumbar punction (LP), the false-negative rate may be as high as 55%; this falls to only 10% after three LPs (Olson et al 1974, Wasserstrom et al 1982, Kaplan et al 1990). Tumour markers, such as lactic dehydrogenase (LDH) isoenzymes (Wasserstrom et al 1982), carcinoembryonic antigen (Twijnstra et al 1987),

β_2-microglobulin (Twijnstra et al 1987) and tissue polypeptide antigen (Bach et al 1991) may help to delineate the diagnosis. Flow cytometry for the detection of abnormal DNA content may be a useful adjunct to cytological examination (Cibas et al 1987). Imaging studies may also be of value. MRI of the cranium and spinal cord with gadolinium enhancement is the most sensitive imaging modality (Fig. 45.8) (Freilich et al 1995). Myelography is abnormal in up to 30% of patients, and CT or MRI of the head may demonstrate enhancement of the dural membranes or ventricular enlargement (Chamberlain et al 1990). Untreated leptomeningeal metastases cause progressive neurological dysfunction at multiple sites, followed by death in 4–6 weeks. Current treatment strategies, which include radiation therapy to the area of symptomatic involvement, corticosteroids, and intraventricular or intrathecal chemotherapy or systemic chemotherapy, have limited efficacy and, in general, patient outlook remains poor (Balm & Hammack 1996, Chamberlain 1997).

Base of skull metastases

Base of skull metastases are associated with well-described clinical syndromes (Greenberg et al 1981), which are named according to the site of metastatic involvement: orbital, parasellar, middle fossa, jugular foramen, occipital condyle, clivus and sphenoid sinus. Cancers of the breast, lung and prostate are most commonly associated with this complication (Greenberg et al 1981), but any tumour type that metastasizes to bone may be responsible.

When base of skull metastases are suspected, axial imaging with CT (including bone window settings) is the usual initial procedure (Fig. 45.9) (Greenberg et al 1981). MRI is more sensitive for assessing soft-tissue extension, and CSF analysis may be needed to exclude leptomeningeal metastases.

Orbital syndrome

Orbital metastases usually present with progressive pain in the retro-orbital and supraorbital area of the affected eye. Blurred vision and diplopia may be associated complaints. Signs may include proptosis, chemosis of the involved eye, external ophthalmoparesis, ipsilateral papilloedema and decreased sensation in the ophthalmic division of the trigeminal nerve. Imaging with MRI or CT scan can delineate the extent of bony damage and orbital infiltration.

Parasellar syndrome

The parasellar syndrome typically presents as unilateral supraorbital and frontal headache, which may be associated with diplopia (Bitoh et al 1985). There may be ophthalmoparesis or papilloedema, and formal visual field testing may demonstrate hemianopsia or quadrantinopsia.

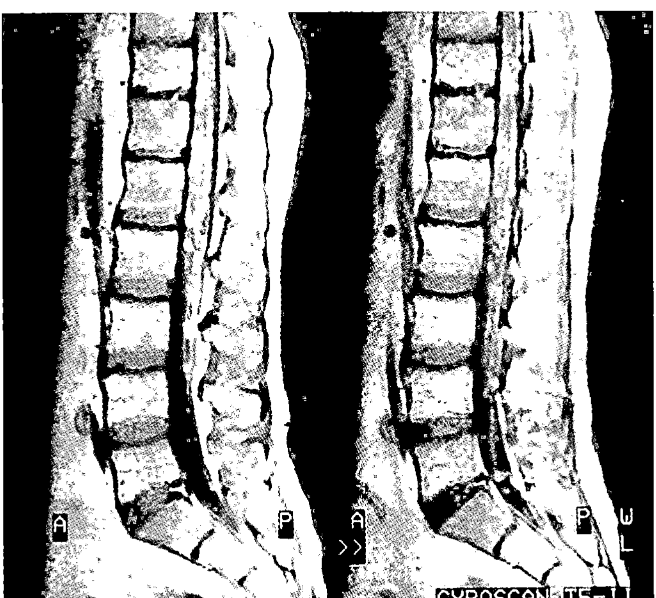

Fig. 45.8 Gadolinium-enhanced MRI scan of the thorocolumbar spine demonstrating multifocal meningeal enhancement consistent with leptomeningeal metastases.

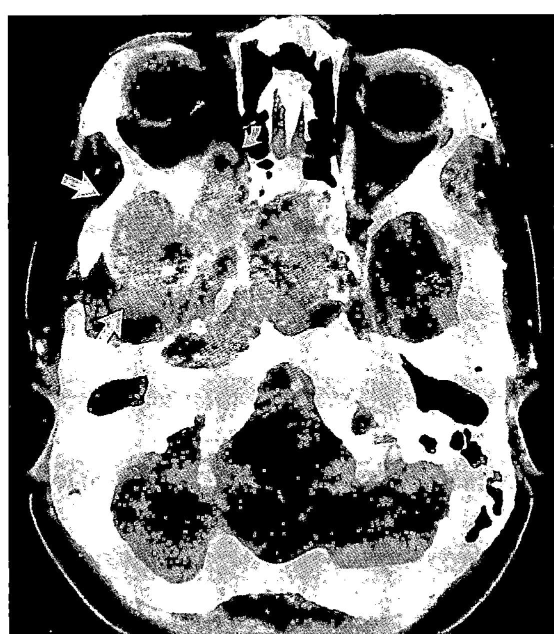

Fig. 45.9 CT scan of the base of skull of a woman with proptosis and right-sided facial pain. There is extensive tumour erosion of the orbital wall, clivus and the floor of the middle cranial fossa.

Middle cranial fossa syndrome

The middle cranial fossa syndrome presents with facial numbness, paraesthesias or pain, which is usually referred to the cheek or jaw (in the distribution of second or third divisions of the trigeminal nerve) (Lossos & Siegal 1992). The pain is typically described as a dull continual ache, but may also be paroxysmal or lancinating. On examination, patients may have hypaesthesia in the trigeminal nerve distribution and signs of weakness in the ipsilateral muscles of mastication. Occasional patients have other neurological signs, such as abducens palsy (Greenberg et al 1981, Bullitt et al 1986).

Jugular foramen syndrome

The jugular foramen syndrome usually presents with hoarseness or dysphagia. Pain is usually referred to the ipsilateral ear or mastoid region and may occasionally present as glossopharyngeal neuralgia, with or without syncope (Greenberg et al 1981). Pain may also be referred to the ipsilateral neck or shoulder. Neurological signs include ipsilateral Horner's syndrome, and paresis of the palate, vocal cord, sternocleidomastoid or trapezius. Ipsilateral paresis of the tongue may also occur if the tumour extends to the region of the hypoglossal canal.

Occipital condyle syndrome

The occipital condyle syndrome presents with unilateral occipital pain that is worsened with neck flexion (Loevner & Yousem 1997, Moris et al 1998). The patient may complain of neck stiffness. Pain intensity is variable, but can be severe. Examination may reveal a head tilt, limited movement of the neck and tenderness to palpation over the occipitonuchal junction. Neurological findings may include ipsilateral hypoglossal nerve paralysis and sternocleidomastoid weakness.

Clivus syndrome

The clivus syndrome is characterized by vertex headache, which is often exacerbated by neck flexion. Lower cranial nerve (VI–XII) dysfunction follows and may become bilateral.

Sphenoid sinus syndrome

A sphenoid sinus metastasis often presents with bifrontal and or retro-orbital pain, which may radiate to the temporal regions (Lawson & Reino 1997). There may be associated features of nasal congestion and diplopia. Physical examination is often unremarkable, although unilateral or bilateral VIth nerve paresis can be present.

Painful cranial neuralgias

As noted, specific cranial neuralgias can occur from metastases in the base of skull or leptomeninges. They are most commonly observed in patients with prostate cancer or lung cancer (Gupta et al 1990). Invasion of the soft tissues of the head or neck, or involvement of sinuses, can also eventuate in such lesions. Each of these syndromes has a characteristic presentation. Early diagnosis may allow effective treatment of the underlying lesion before progressive neurological injury occurs.

Glossopharyngeal neuralgia

Glossopharyngeal neuralgia has been reported in patients with leptomeningeal metastases (Sozzi et al 1987), the jugular foramen syndrome (Greenberg et al 1981), or head and neck malignancies (Dykman et al 1981, Giorgi & Broggi 1984, Metheetrairut & Brown 1993). This syndrome presents as severe pain in the throat or neck, which may radiate to the ear or mastoid region. Pain may be induced by swallowing. In some patients, pain is associated with sudden orthostasis and syncope.

Trigeminal neuralgia

Trigeminal pains may be continual, paroxysmal or lancinating. Pain that mimics classical trigeminal neuralgia can be induced by tumours in the middle or posterior fossa (Bullitt et al 1986, Cheng et al 1993, Barker et al 1996, Hirota et al 1998) or leptomeningeal metastases (De Angelis & Payne 1987). Continual pain in a trigeminal distribution may be an early sign of acoustic neuroma (Payten 1972). All cancer patients who develop trigeminal neuralgia should be evaluated for the existence of an underlying neoplasm.

Ear and eye pain syndromes

Otalgia

Otalgia is the sensation of pain in the ear, while referred otalgia is pain felt in the ear but originating from a non-otologic source. The rich sensory innervation of the ear derives from four cranial nerves and two cervical nerves which also supply other areas in the head, neck, thorax and

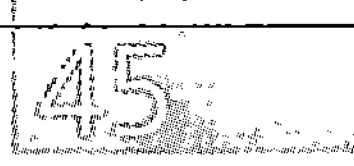

abdomen. Thus, pain referred to the ear may originate in areas far removed from the ear itself. Otalgia may be caused by carcinoma of the orpharynx or hypopharynx (Aird et al 1983, Talmi et al 1997), acoustic neuroma (Morrison & Sterkers 1996), and metastases to the temporal bone or infratemporal fossa (Hill & Kohut 1976, Shapshay et al 1976).

Eye pain

Blurring of vision and eye pain are the two most common symptoms of choridal metastases (Hayreh et al 1982, Servodidio & Abramson 1992, Swanson 1993). More commonly chronic eye pain is related to metastases to the bony orbit, intraorbital structures such as the rectus muscles (Weiss et al 1984, Friedman et al 1990) or optic nerve (Laitt et al 1996).

Uncommon causes of headache and facial pain

Headache and facial pain in cancer patients may have many other causes. Unilateral facial pain can be the initial symptom of an ipsilateral lung tumour (Bongers et al 1992, Schoenen et al 1992, Capobianco 1995, Shakespeare & Stevens 1996). Presumably, this referred pain is mediated by vagal afferents. Facial squamous cell carcinoma of the skin may present with facial pain as a result of extensive perineural invasion (Schroeder et al 1998). Patients with Hodgkin's disease may have transient episodes of neurological dysfunction that have been likened to migraine (Dulli et al 1987). Headache may occur with cerebral infarction or haemorrhage, which may be caused by non-bacterial thrombotic endocarditis or disseminated intravascular coagulation. Headache is also the usual presentation of sagittal sinus occlusion, which may be a result of tumour infiltration, hypercoaguable state or treatment with L-asparaginase therapy (Sigsbee et al 1979). Headache due to pseudotumour cerebri has also been reported to be the presentation of superior vena caval obstruction in a patient with lung cancer (Portenoy et al 1983). Tumours of the sinonasal tract may present with deep facial or nasal pain (Marshall & Mahanna 1997).

NEUROPATHIC PAINS INVOLVING THE PERIPHERAL NERVOUS SYSTEM

Neuropathic pains involving the peripheral nervous system are common and clinically challenging problems in the cancer population. The syndromes include painful radiculopathy, plexopathy, mononeuropathy or peripheral neuropathy.

Painful radiculopathy

Radiculopathy or polyradiculopathy may be caused by any process that compresses, distorts or inflames nerve roots. Painful radiculopathy is an important presentation of epidural tumour and leptomeningeal metastases (see above).

Postherpetic neuralgia

Postherpetic neuralgia is defined solely by the persistence of pain in the region of a zoster infection (Portenoy et al 1986). Although some authors apply this term if pain continues beyond lesion healing, most require a period of weeks to months before this label is used; a criterion of pain persisting beyond 3 months after lesion healing is recommended. One study suggests that postherpetic neuralgia is two to three times more frequent in the cancer population than the general population (Rusthoven et al 1988). In patients with postherpetic neuralgia and cancer, changes in the intensity or pattern of pain, or the development of new neurological deficits, may indicate the possibility of local neoplasm and should be investigated.

Cervical plexopathy

The ventral rami of the upper four cervical spinal nerves join to form the cervical plexus between the deep anterior and lateral muscles of the neck. Cutaneous branches emerge from the posterior border of the sternocleidomastoid. In the cancer population, plexus injury is frequently caused by tumour infiltration or treatment (Jaeckle 1991).

Tumour invasion or compression of the cervical plexus can be caused by direct extension of a primary head and neck malignancy or neoplastic (metastatic or lymphomatous) involvement of the cervical lymph nodes (Jaeckle 1991). Pain may be experienced in the preauricular (greater auricular nerve) or postauricular (lesser and greater occipital nerves) regions, or the anterior neck (transverse cutaneous and supraclavicular nerves). Pain may refer to the lateral aspect of the face or head, or to the ipsilateral shoulder. The overlap in the pain referral patterns from the face and neck may relate to the close anatomical relationship between the central connections of cervical afferents and the afferents carried in cranial nerves V, VII, IX and X in the upper cervical spinal cord. The pain may be aching, burning or lancinating, and is often exacerbated by neck movement or swallowing. Associated features can include ipsilateral Horner's syndrome or hemidiaphragmatic paralysis. The diagnosis must be distinguished from epidural compression of the cervical spinal cord and leptomeningeal metastases. MRI or CT imaging of the neck and cervical spine is usually required to evaluate the aetiology of the pain.

Brachial plexopathy

The two most common causes of brachial plexopathy in cancer patients are tumour infiltration and radiation injury. Less common causes of painful brachial plexopathy include trauma during surgery or anaesthesia, radiation-induced second neoplasms, acute brachial plexus ischaemia and paraneoplastic brachial neuritis.

Malignant brachial plexopathy

Plexus infiltration by tumour is the most prevalent cause of brachial plexopathy. Malignant brachial plexopathy is most common in patients with lymphoma, lung cancer or breast cancer. The invading tumour usually arises from adjacent axillary, cervical and supraclavicular lymph nodes (lymphoma and breast cancer) or from the lung (superior sulcus tumours or so-called Pancoast tumours) (Kori et al 1981, Kori 1995). Pain is nearly universal, occurring in 85% of patients, and often precedes neurological signs or symptoms by months (Kori 1995). Lower plexus involvement (C7, C8, T1 distribution) is typical of Pancoast lesions, and is reflected in the pain distribution, which usually involves the elbow, medial forearm and fourth and fifth fingers. Pain may sometimes localize to the posterior arm or elbow. Severe aching is usually reported, but patients may also experience constant or lancinating dysaesthesias along the ulnar aspect of the forearm or hand. Tumour infiltration of the upper plexus (C5–C6 distribution), which occurs less commonly, is characterized by pain in the shoulder girdle, lateral arm and hand. Seventy-five per cent of patients presenting with upper plexopathy subsequently develop a panplexopathy, and 25% of patients present with panplexopathy (Kori et al 1981).

Cross-sectional imaging is essential in all patients with symptoms or signs compatible with plexopathy (Fig. 45.10). In one study, CT scanning had 80–90% sensitivity in detecting tumour infiltration (Cascino et al 1983); others have demonstrated improved diagnostic yield with a multiplanar imaging technique (Fishman et al 1991). Although there are no comparative data on the sensitivity and specificity of CT and MRI in this setting, MRI does have the theoretical advantage of reliably assessing the integrity of the adjacent epidural space (Sherrier & Sostman 1993, Thyagarajan et al 1995).

Electrodiagnostic studies may be helpful in patients with suspected plexopathy, particularly when neurological examination and imaging studies are normal (Synek 1986). Although not specific for tumour, abnormalities on electromyography (EMG) or somatosensory evoked potentials may establish the diagnosis and thereby confirm the need for additional evaluation.

Patients with malignant brachial plexopathy are at high risk for epidural extension of the tumour (Portenoy et al 1989, Jaeckle 1991). Epidural disease can occur as the neoplasm grows medially and invades vertebrae or tracks along nerve roots through the intervertebral foramina. In the latter case, there may be no evidence of bony erosion on imaging studies. The development of Horner's syndrome, evidence of panplexopathy, or finding of paraspinal tumour or vertebral damage on CT or MRI are highly associated with epidural extension and should lead to definitive imaging of the epidural tumour (Portenoy et al 1989, Jaeckle 1991).

Radiation-induced brachial plexopathy

Two distinct syndromes of radiation-induced brachial plexopathy have been described:

1. Early-onset transient plexopathy (see above).
2. Delayed onset progressive plexopathy.

Delayed-onset progressive plexopathy can occur 6 months to 20 years after a course of radiotherapy that includes the plexus in the radiation portal. In contrast to tumour infiltration, pain is a relatively uncommon presenting symptom (18%) and, when present, is usually less severe than pain accompanying malignant plexopathy (Kori et al 1981). Weakness and sensory changes predominate in the distribution of the upper plexus (C5, C6 distribution) (Mondrup et al 1990, Olsen et al 1990, Vecht 1990).

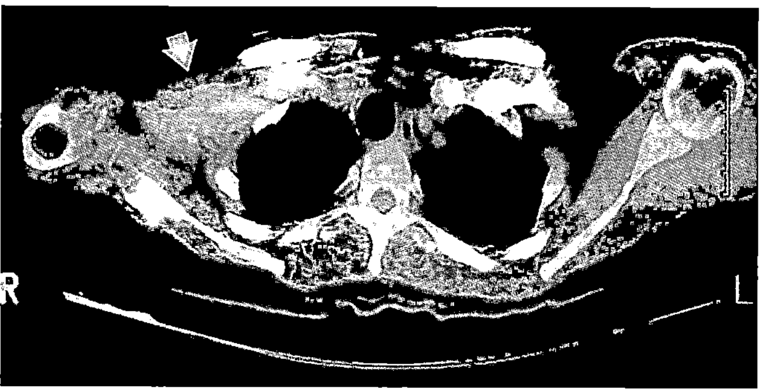

Fig. 45.10 Contrast-enhanced CT scan of the brachial plexus in a 57-year-old woman who has a past history breast cancer and presents with right arm and hand pain. There is a mass in the left brachial plexus (arrow).

 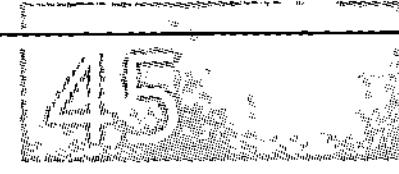

Radiation changes in the skin and lymphoedema are commonly associated. The CT scan usually demonstrates diffuse infiltration that cannot be distinguished from tumour infiltration. On MRI, there may be increased T2 signal in or near the brachial plexus, a finding that is also common in malignant is plexopathy (Thyagarajan et al 1995). Electromyography may demonstrate myokymia (Lederman & Wilbourn 1984, Mondrup et al 1990, Esteban & Traba 1993). Although a careful history, combined with these neurological findings and the results of CT scanning and electrodiagnostic studies can strongly suggest radiation-induced injury, repeated assessments over time may be needed to confirm the diagnosis. Rare patients require surgical exploration of the plexus to exclude neoplasm and establish the aetiology. When due to radiation, plexopathy is usually progressive (Killer & Hess 1990, Jaeckle 1991), although some patients plateau for a variable period of time.

Uncommon causes of brachial plexopathy

Malignant peripheral nerve tumour or a second primary tumour in a previously irradiated site can account for pain recurring late in the patient's course (Richardson et al 1979, Gorson et al 1995). Pain has been reported to occur as a result of brachial plexus entrapment in a lymphoedematous shoulder (Vecht 1990), and as a consequence of acute ischaemia many years after axillary radiotherapy (Gerard et al 1989). An idiopathic brachial plexopathy has also been described in patients with Hodgkin's disease (Lachance et al 1991).

Lumbosacral plexopathy

The lumbar plexus, which lies in the paravertebral psoas muscle, is formed primarily by the ventral rami of L1–4. The sacral plexus forms in the sacroiliac notch from the ventral rami of S1–3 and the lumbosacral trunk (L4–5), which courses caudally over the sacral ala to join the plexus (Chad & Bradley 1987). Lumbosacral plexopathy may be associated with pain in the lower abdomen, inguinal region, buttock or leg (Jaeckle et al 1985). In the cancer population, lumbosacral plexopathy is usually caused by neoplastic infiltration or compression.

Radiation-induced plexopathy also occurs, and occasional patients develop the lesion as a result of surgical trauma, infarction, cytotoxic damage, infection in the pelvis or psoas muscle, abdominal aneurysm or idiopathic lumbosacral neuritis. Polyradiculopathy from leptomeningeal metastases or epidural metastases can mimic lumbosacral plexopathy, and the evaluation of the patient must consider these lesions as well.

Malignant lumbosacral plexopathy

The primary tumours most frequently associated with malignant lumbosacral plexopathy include colorectal, cervical, breast, sarcoma and lymphoma (Jaeckle et al 1985, Jaeckle 1991). Most tumours involve the plexus by direct extension from intrapelvic neoplasm; metastases account for only one-fourth of cases. In one study, two-thirds of patients developed plexopathy within 3 years of their primary diagnosis and one-third presented within 1 year (Jaeckle et al 1985).

Pain is the first symptom reported by most patients with malignant lumbosacral plexopathy. Pain is experienced by almost all patients during the course of the disease, and it is the only symptom in almost 20% of patients. The quality is usually aching, pressure like or stabbing; dysaesthesias appear to be relatively uncommon. Most patients develop numbness, paraesthesias or weakness weeks to months after the pain begins. Common signs include leg weakness that involves multiple myotomes, sensory loss that crosses dermatomes, reflex asymmetry, focal tenderness, leg oedema, and positive direct or reverse straight-leg raising signs.

An upper plexopathy occurs in almost one-third of patients with lumbosacral plexopathy (Jaeckle et al 1985). This lesion is usually caused by direct extension from a low abdominal tumour, most frequently colorectal. Pain may be experienced in the back, lower abdomen, flank or iliac crest or the anterolateral thigh. Examination may reveal sensory, motor and reflex changes in a L1–4 distribution. A subgroup of these patients presents with a syndrome characterized by pain and paraesthesias limited to the lower abdomen or inguinal region, variable sensory loss and no motor findings. CT scan may show tumour adjacent to the L1 vertebra (the L1 syndrome) (Jaeckle et al 1985) or along the pelvic sidewall, where it presumably damages the ilioinguinal, iliohypogastric or genitofemoral nerves. Another subgroup has neoplastic involvement of the psoas muscle and presents with a syndrome characterized by upper lumbosacral plexopathy, painful flexion of the ipsilateral hip, and positive psoas muscle stretch test. This has been termed the malignant psoas syndrome (Stevens & Gonet 1990). Similarly, pain in the distribution of the femoral nerve has been observed in the setting of recurrent retroperitoneal sarcoma (Zografos & Karakousis 1994) and tumour in the iliac crest can compress the lateral cutaneous nerve of the thigh, producing a pain that mimics meralgia paraesthetica (Tharion & Bhattacharji 1997).

A lower plexopathy occurs in just over 50% of patients with lumbosacral plexopathy (Jaeckle et al 1985). This lesion is usually caused by direct extension from a pelvic tumour, most frequently rectal cancer, gynaecological tumours or pelvic sarcoma. Pain may be localized in the buttocks and perineum, or referred to the posterolateral thigh and leg. Associated symptoms and signs conform to an L4–S1 distribution. Examination may reveal weakness or sensory changes in the L5 and S1 dermatomes and a depressed ankle jerk. Other findings include leg oedema, bladder or bowel dysfunction, sacral or sciatic notch tenderness, and a positive straight-leg raising test. A pelvic mass may be palpable.

Sacral plexopathy may occur from direct extension of a sacral lesion or a presacral mass. This may present with predominant involvement of the lumbosacral trunk, which is characterized by numbness of the foot and weakness of knee flexion, ankle dorsiflexion and inversion. Other patients demonstrate particular involvement of the coccygeal plexus, with prominent sphincter dysfunction and perineal sensory loss. The latter syndrome occurs with low pelvic tumours, such as those arising from the rectum or prostate.

A panplexopathy with involvement in a L1–S3 distribution occurs in almost one-fifth of patients with lumbosacral plexopathy (Jaeckle et al 1985). Local pain may occur in the lower abdomen, back, buttocks or perineum. Referred pain can be experienced anywhere in distribution of the plexus. Leg oedema is extremely common. Neurological deficits may be confluent or patchy within the L1–S3 distribution and a positive straight-leg raising test is usually present.

Autonomic dysfunction, particularly anhydrosis and vasodilatation, has been associated with plexus and peripheral nerve injuries. Focal autonomic neuropathy, which may suggest the anatomical localization of the lesion (Evans & Watson 1985), has been reported as the presenting symptom of metastatic lumbosacral plexopathy (Dalmau et al 1989).

Cross-sectional imaging with either CT or MRI is the usual diagnostic procedure to evaluate lumbosacral plexopathy (Fig. 45.11). Scanning should be done from the level of the L1 vertebral body, through the sciatic notch. When using CT scanning techniques, images should include bone and soft-tissue windows. Limited data suggest that MRI may be more sensitive than CT imaging (Taylor et al 1997). Definitive imaging of the epidural space adjacent to the plexus should be considered in patients who have a relatively high risk of epidural extension, including those with bilateral symptoms or signs, unexplained incontinence or a prominent paraspinal mass (Jaeckle et al 1985, Portenoy et al 1989).

Radiation-induced lumbosacral plexopathy

Radiation fibrosis of the lumbosacral plexus is a rare complication that may occur from 1 to over 30 years following

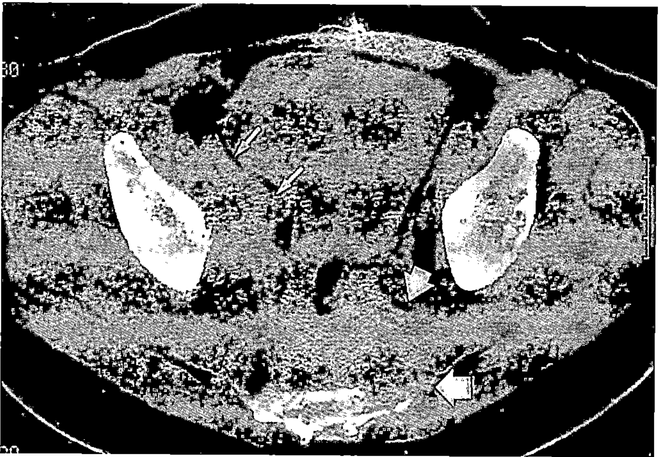

Fig. 45.11 Pelvic CT of a 60-year-old man with unresectable carcinoma of the bladder with severe pain radiating down the posterior aspect of both legs. There is a presacral mass that erodes the sacrum (large arrows) and extends to the pelvic sidewall (small arrows).

radiation treatment. The use of intracavitary radium implants for carcinoma of the cervix may be an additional risk factor (Stryker et al 1990). Radiation-induced plexopathy typically presents with progressive weakness and leg swelling; pain is not usually a prominent feature (Thomas et al 1985, Stryker et al 1990). Weakness typically begins distally in the L5–S1 segments and is slowly progressive. The symptoms and signs may be bilateral (Thomas et al 1985). If CT scanning demonstrates a lesion, it is usually a non-specific diffuse infiltration of the tissues. Electromyography may show myokymic discharges (Thomas et al 1985).

Uncommon causes of lumbosacral plexopathy

Lumbosacral plexopathy may occur following intra-arterial cis-platinum infusion (see below) and embolization techniques. This syndrome has been observed following attempted embolization of a bleeding rectal lesion. Benign conditions that may produce similar findings include haemorrhage or abscess in the iliopsoas muscle (Chad & Bradley 1987), abdominal aortic aneurysms, diabetic radiculoplexopathy, vasculitis and an idiopathic lumbosacral plexitis analogous to acute brachial neuritis (Chad & Bradley 1987).

Painful mononeuropathy

Tumour-related mononeuropathy usually results from compression or infiltration of a nerve from tumour arising in an adjacent bony structure. The most common example of this phenomenon is intercostal nerve injury in a patient with rib metastases. Constant burning pain and other dysaesthesias in the area of sensory loss are the typical clinical presentation. Other examples include the cranial neuralgias previously described, sciatica associated with tumour invasion of the sciatic notch, peroneal nerve palsy associated with primary bone tumours of the proximal fibula, and lateral cutaneous nerve of the thigh neuralgia associated with iliac crest tumours.

Cancer patients also develop mononeuropathies from many other causes. Postsurgical syndromes are well described (see below) and radiation injury of a peripheral nerve occurs occasionally. Rarely, cancer patients develop nerve entrapment syndromes (such as carpal tunnel syndrome) related to oedema or direct compression by tumour (Desta et al 1994).

Painful peripheral neuropathies

Painful peripheral neuropathies have multiple causes, including nutritional deficiencies, other metabolic derangements (e.g., diabetes and renal dysfunction), neurotoxic effects of chemotherapy and, rarely, paraneoplastic syndromes.

Toxic peripheral neuropathy

Chemotherapy-induced peripheral neuropathy is a common problem, which is typically manifested by painful paraesthesias in the hands and/or feet, and signs consistent with an axonopathy, including 'stocking-glove' sensory loss, weakness, hyporeflexia and autonomic dysfunction (McDonald 1991). The pain is usually characterized by continuous burning or lancinating pains, either of which may be increased by contact. The drugs most commonly associated with a peripheral neuropathy are the vinca alkaloids (especially vincristine) (Rosenthal & Kaufman 1974, Forman 1990) and cis-platinum (Mollman et al 1988, Siegal & Haim 1990). Paclitaxel, procarbazine, carboplatinum, misonidazole and hexamethylmelamine have also been implicated as causes for this syndrome (Weiss et al 1974a,b). Data from several studies indicates that the risk of neuropathy associated with cis-platinum can be diminished by the co-administration of the radioprotective agent amifostine at the time of treatment (Spencer & Goa 1995).

Paraneoplastic painful peripheral neuropathy

Paraneoplastic painful peripheral neuropathy can be related to injury to the dorsal root ganglion (also known as subacute sensory neuronopathy or ganglionopathy) or injury to peripheral nerves. These syndromes may be the initial manifestation of an underlying malignancy. Except for the neuropathy associated with myeloma (Kissel & Mendell 1996, Rotta & Bradley 1997), their course is usually independent of the primary tumour (Dalmau & Posner 1997).

Subacute sensory neuropathy is characterized by pain (usually dysaesthetic), paraesthesias, sensory loss in the extremities and severe sensory ataxia (Brady 1996). Although it is usually associated with small-cell carcinoma of the lung (van Oosterhout et al 1996), other tumour types, including breast cancer (Peterson et al 1994), Hodgkin's disease (Plante-Bordeneuve et al 1994) and varied solid tumours, are rarely associated. Both constant and lancinating dysaesthesias occur, typically predate other symptoms, and are usually independent of the primary tumour. Neuropathic symptoms (pain, paraesthesia, sensory loss) may be asymmetrical at onset, with a predilection for the upper limbs. The syndrome, which results from an inflammatory process involving the dorsal root ganglia, may be part of a more diffuse autoimmune disorder that can affect the limbic region, brainstem and spinal cord (Brady 1996, Dalmau & Posner 1997). An antineuronal IgG antibody ('anti-Hu'), which recognizes a low-molecular-weight protein present in most small-cell lung carcinomas, has been associated with the condition (Dalmau & Posner 1997).

A sensorimotor peripheral neuropathy, which may be painful, has been observed in association with diverse neoplasms, particularly Hodgkin's disease and paraproteinaemias (Brady 1996, Dalmau & Posner 1997). The peripheral neuropathies associated with multiple myeloma, Waldenstrom's macroglobulinaemia, small-fibre amyloid neuropathy and osteosclerotic myeloma, are thought to be due to antibodies that cross-react with constituents of peripheral nerves (Kissel & Mendell 1996). Clinically evident peripheral neuropathy occurs in approximately 15% of patients with multiple myeloma, and electrophysiological evidence of this lesion can be found in 40% (Kissel & Mendell 1996). The pathophysiology of the neuropathy that can complicate other neoplasms is unknown.

PAIN SYNDROMES OF THE VISCERA AND MISCELLANEOUS TUMOUR-RELATED SYNDROMES

Pain may be caused by pathology involving the luminal organs of the gastrointestinal or genitourinary tracts, the parenchymal organs, the peritoneum or the retroperitoneal soft tissues. Obstruction of hollow viscus, including intestine, biliary tract and ureter, produces visceral nociceptive syndromes that are well described in the surgical literature (Silen 1983). Pain arising from retroperitoneal and pelvic lesions may involve mixed nociceptive and neuropathic mechanisms if both somatic structures and nerves are involved.

Hepatic distension syndrome

Pain-sensitive structures in the region of the liver include the liver capsule, vessels and biliary tract (Coombs 1990). Nociceptive afferents that innervate these structures travel via the coeliac plexus, the phrenic nerve and the lower right intercostal nerves. Extensive intrahepatic metastases, or gross hepatomegaly associated with cholestasis, may produce discomfort in the right subcostal region, and less commonly in the right mid-back or flank (Coombs 1990, Mulholland et al 1990, De Conno & Polastri 1996). Referred pain may be experienced in the right neck or shoulder, or in the region of the right scapula (Mulholland et al 1990). The pain, which is usually described as a dull aching, may be exacerbated by movement, pressure in the abdomen and deep inspiration. Pain is commonly accompanied by symptoms of anorexia and nausea. Physical examination may reveal a hard irregular subcostal mass that descends with respiration and is dull to percussion. Other features of hepatic failure may be present. Imaging of the hepatic parenchyma by either ultrasound or CT will usually identify the presence of space-occupying lesions or cholestasis (Fig. 45.12).

Occasional patients who experience chronic pain as a result of hepatic distension develop an acute intercurrent subcostal pain that may be exacerbated by respiration. Physical examination may demonstrate a palpable or audible rub. These findings suggest the development of an overlying peritonitis, which can develop in response to some acute event, such as a haemorrhage into a metastasis.

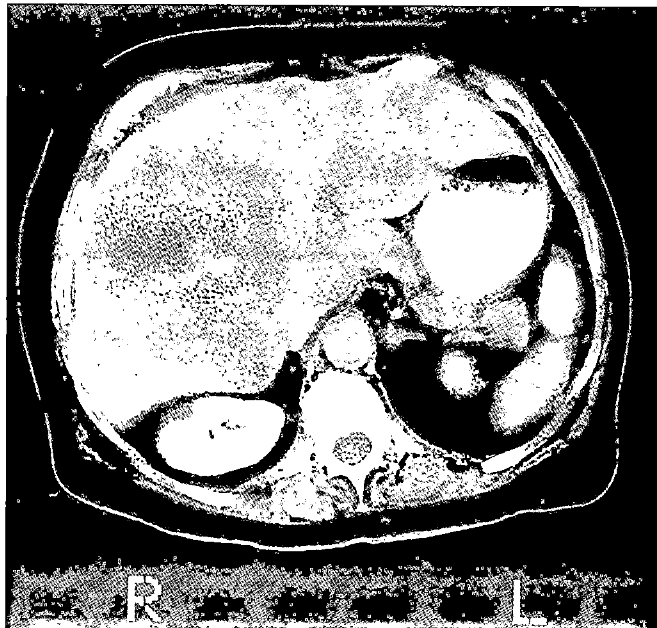

Fig. 45.12 CT scan of the abdomen of a 72-year-old man with metastatic colon cancer and persistent right upper quadrant abdominal pain. The scan demonstrates extensive liver metastases.

Midline retroperitoneal syndrome

Retroperitoneal pathology involving the upper abdomen may produce pain by injury to deep somatic structures of the posterior abdominal wall, distortion of pain-sensitive connective tissue, vascular and ductal structures, local inflammation, and direct infiltration of the coeliac plexus. The most common causes are pancreatic cancer (Kelsen et al 1995, 1997, Grahm & Andren-Sandberg 1997) and retroperitoneal lymphadenopathy (Krane & Perrone 1981, Neer et al 1981, Sponseller 1996), particularly coeliac lymphadenopathy (Schonenberg et al 1991). The pain is experienced in the epigastrium, in the low thoracic region of the back, or in both locations. It is often diffuse and poorly localized. It is usually dull and boring in character, exacerbated with recumbency, and improved by sitting. The lesion can usually be demonstrated by CT, MRI or ultrasound scanning of the upper abdomen (Fig. 45.13). If tumour is identified in the paravertebral space, or vertebral body destruction is identified, consideration should be given to careful evaluation of the epidural space (Portenoy et al 1989).

Chronic intestinal obstruction

Abdominal pain is an almost invariable manifestation of chronic intestinal obstruction, which may occur in patients with abdominal or pelvic cancers (Baines 1994, Ripamonti 1994). The factors that contribute to this pain include smooth muscle contractions, mesenteric tension and mural ischaemia. Obstructive symptoms may be caused primarily by the tumour, or more likely, by a combination of mechanical obstruction and other processes, such as autonomic neuropathy and ileus from metabolic derangements or drugs. Both continuous and colicky pains occur and may be referred to the dermatomes represented by the spinal segments supplying the affected viscera. Vomiting, anorexia and constipation are important associated symptoms. Abdominal radiographs taken in both supine and erect positions may demonstrate the presence of air-fluid levels and

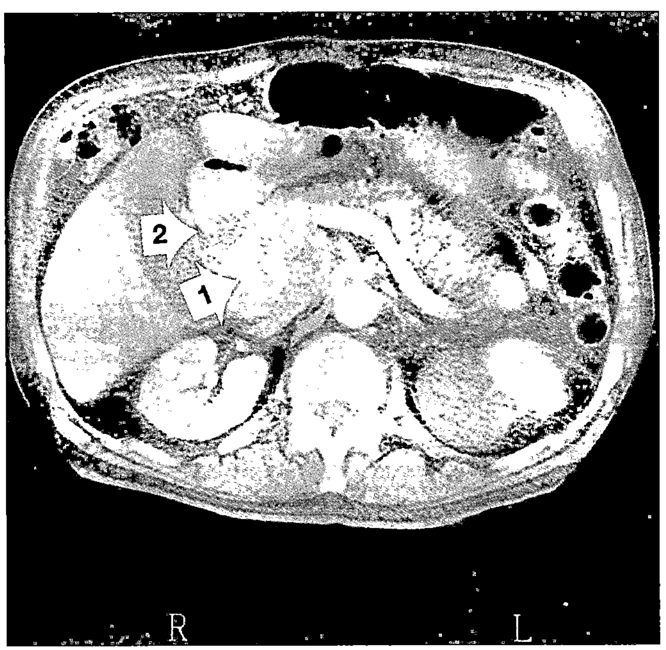

Fig. 45.13 CT scan of the abdomen of a 47-year-old female with epigastric pain and jaundice. The CT shows a large mass in the head of the pancreas (arrow 2) and dilatation of the common bile duct (arrow 1).

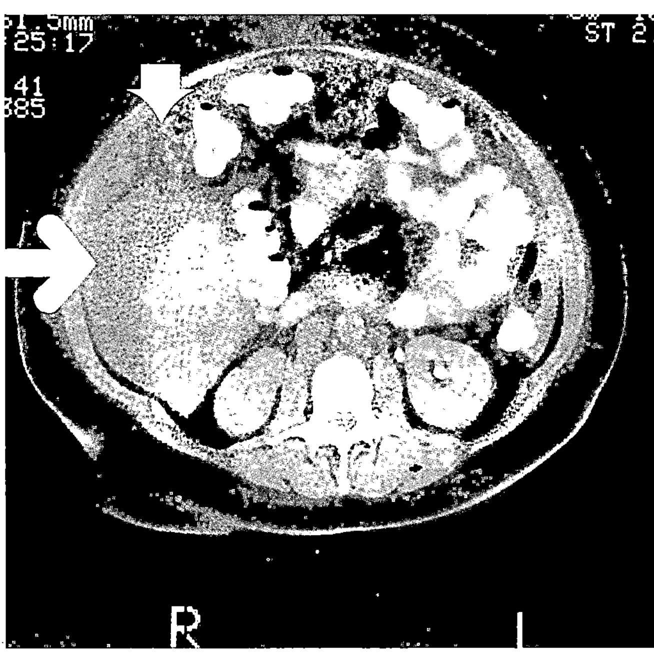

Fig. 45.14 CT scan of the abdomen of a 66-year-old female with stage IV ovarian cancer. The small arrow indicates areas of peritoneal thickening and infiltration. The large horizontal arrow indicates ascitic fluid interposed lateral to the lower lobe of the liver.

intestinal distension. CT or MRI scanning of the abdomen can assess the extent and distribution of intra-abdominal neoplasm, which has implications for subsequent treatment options.

Peritoneal carcinomatosis

Peritoneal carcinomatosis occurs most often by transcoelomic spread of abdominal or pelvic tumour; haematogenous spread of an extra-abdominal neoplasm in this pattern is rare. Carcinomatosis can cause peritoneal inflammation, mesenteric tethering, malignant adhesions and ascites, all of which can cause pain. Pain and abdominal distension are the most common presenting symptoms (Garrison et al 1986, Fromm et al 1990, Ransom et al 1990, Truong et al 1990). Mesenteric tethering and tension appears to cause a diffuse abdominal or low back pain. Tense malignant ascites can produce diffuse abdominal discomfort and a distinct stretching pain in the anterior abdominal wall. Adhesions can also cause obstruction of hollow viscus, with intermittent colicky pain (Averbach & Sugarbaker 1995). CT scanning may demonstrate evidence of ascites, omental infiltration and peritoneal nodules (Archer et al 1996) (Fig. 45.14).

Malignant perineal pain

Tumours of the colon or rectum, female reproductive tract and distal genitourinary system are most commonly responsible for perineal pain (Stillman 1990, Boas et al 1993, Hagen 1993, Miaskowski 1996). Severe perineal pain following antineoplastic therapy may precede evidence of detectable disease and should be viewed as a potential harbinger of progressive or recurrent cancer (Stillman 1990, Boas et al 1993). There is evidence to suggest that this phenomenon is caused by microscopic perineural invasion by recurrent disease (Seefeld & Bargen 1943). The pain, which is typically described as constant and aching, is often aggravated by sitting or standing, and may be associated with tenesmus or bladder spasms (Stillman 1990).

Tumour invasion of the musculature of the deep pelvis can also result in a syndrome that appears similar to the so-called tension myalgia of the pelvic floor (Sinaki et al 1977). The pain is typically described as a constant ache or heaviness that exacerbates with upright posture. When caused by tumour, the pain may be concurrent with other types of perineal pain. Digital examination of the pelvic floor may reveal local tenderness or palpable tumour.

Adrenal pain syndrome

Large adrenal metastases may produce unilateral flank pain and, less commonly, abdominal pain. Pain is of variable severity, and it can be severe (Berger et al 1995b).

Ureteric obstruction

Ureteric obstruction is most frequently caused by tumour compression or infiltration within the true pelvis (Kontturi & Kauppila 1982, Harrington et al 1995). Less commonly, obstruction can be more proximal, associated with retroperitoneal lymphadenopathy, an isolated retroperitoneal metastasis, mural metastases or intraluminal metastases. Cancers of the cervix, ovary, prostate and rectum are most commonly associated with this complication. Non-malignant causes, including retroperitoneal fibrosis resulting from radiotherapy or graft versus host disease, occur rarely (Sklaroff et al 1978, Muram et al 1981, Goodman & Dalton 1982).

Pain may or may not accompany ureteric obstruction. When present, it is typically a dull chronic discomfort in the flank, which may radiate into the inguinal region or genitalia. If pain does not occur, ureteric obstruction may be discovered when hydronephrosis is discerned on abdominal imaging procedures or renal failure develops. Ureteric obstruction can be complicated by pyelonephritis or pyonephrosis, which often present with features of sepsis, flank pain and dysuria. Diagnosis of ureteric obstruction can usually be confirmed by the demonstration of hydronephrosis on renal sonography. The level of obstruction can be identified by pyelography, and CT scanning techniques will usually demonstrate the cause (Greenfield & Resnick 1989).

Pain syndromes associated with specific tumours

Moderate to severe abdominopelvic pain occurs in almost two-thirds of patients with ovarian cancer (Portenoy et al 1994a). Pain often precedes the onset of the disease, and in patients who have been previously treated, it is an important symptom of potential recurrence (Portenoy et al 1994a).

Lung tumours can be associated with visceral pain even in the absence of involvement of the chest wall or parietal pleura. In a large case series of lung cancer patients, pain was unilateral in 80% of the cases and bilateral in 20%. Among patients with hilar tumours the pain was reported in the sternum or the scapula. Upper and lower lobe tumours referred to the shoulder and to the lower chest respectively (Marangoni et al 1993, Marino et al 1986). As previously mentioned, early lung cancers can generate ipsilateral facial pain (Des Prez & Freemon 1983, Schoenen et al 1992, Capobianco 1995, Shakespeare & Stevens 1996). It is postulated that this pain syndrome is generated via vagal afferent neurons.

Other uncommon visceral pain syndromes

The sudden onset of severe abdominal or flank pain may be caused by non-traumatic rupture of a visceral tumour. This has been most frequently reported with hepatocellular cancer (Miyamoto et al 1991). Kidney rupture as a result of renal metastasis from an adenocarcinoma of the colon (Wolff et al 1994) and metastasis-induced perforated appendicitis (Ende et al 1995) also have been reported. Torsion of pedunculated visceral tumours can produce a cramping abdominal pain (Abbott 1990, Reese & Blocker 1994, Andreasen & Poulsen 1997).

Paraneoplastic nociceptive pain syndromes

Tumours that secrete chorionic gonadotrophin (HCG), including malignant and benign tumours of the testis (Tseng et al 1985, Haas et al 1989, Mellor & McCutchan 1989, Cantwell et al 1991) and rarely cancers from other sites (Wurzel et al 1987, Forst et al 1995), may be associated with chronic breast tenderness or gynaecomastia. Approximately 10% of patients with testis cancer have gynaecomastia or breast tenderness at presentation, and the likelihood of gynaecomastia is greater with increasing HCG level (Tseng et al 1985). Breast pain can be the first presentation of an occult tumour (Haas et al 1989, Mellor & McCutchan 1989, Cantwell et al 1991).

CHRONIC PAIN SYNDROMES ASSOCIATED WITH CANCER THERAPY

Most treatment-related pains are caused by tissue-damaging procedures. These pains are acute, predictable and self limited. Chronic treatment-related pain syndromes are associated with either a persistent nociceptive complication of an invasive treatment (such as a postsurgical abscess) or, more commonly, neural injury. In some cases, these syndromes occur long after the therapy is completed, resulting in a difficult differential diagnosis between recurrent disease and a complication of therapy.

Postchemotherapy pain syndromes

Chronic painful peripheral neuropathy

Although most patients who develop painful peripheral neuropathy as a result of cytotoxic therapy gradually improve, some develop a persistent pain. In particular, peripheral neuropathy associated with cis-platinum may continue to progress months after the discontinuation of therapy and may persist for months to years (Rosenfeld &

Broder 1984, LoMonaco et al 1992). This is less common with vincristine or paclitaxel (Hilkens et al 1996).

Avascular (aseptic) necrosis of femoral or humeral head

Avascular necrosis of the femoral or humeral head may occur either spontaneously or as a complication of intermittent or continuous corticosteroid therapy (Ratcliffe et al 1995, Thornton et al 1997). Osteonecrosis may be unilateral or bilateral. Involvement of the femoral head is most common and typically causes pain in the hip, thigh or knee. Involvement of the humeral head usually presents as pain in the shoulder, upper arm or elbow. Pain is exacerbated by movement and relieved by rest. There may be local tenderness over the joint, but this is not universal. Pain usually precedes radiological changes by weeks to months; bone scintigraphy and MRI are sensitive and complementary diagnostic procedures. Early treatment consists of analgesics, a decrease or discontinuation of steroids, and sometimes surgery. With progressive bone destruction, joint replacement may be necessary.

Plexopathy

Lumbosacral or brachial plexopathy may follow cis-platinum infusion into the iliac artery (Castellanos et al 1987) or axillary artery (Kahn et al 1989), respectively. Affected patients develop pain, weakness and paraesthesias within 48 hours of the infusion. The mechanism for this syndrome is thought to be due to small vessel damage and infarction of the plexus or nerve. The prognosis for neurological recovery is not known.

Raynaud's phenomenon

Persistent Raynaud's phenomenon is observed in 20–30% of patients with germ cell tumours treated with cisplatin, vinblastine and bleomycin (Aass et al 1990, Gerl 1994). This effect has also been observed in patients with carcinoma of the head and neck treated with a combination of cisplatin, vincristine and bleomycin (Kukla et al 1982). Pathophysiological studies suggest that a hyperreactivity in the central sympathetic nervous system results in a reduced function of the smooth muscle cells in the terminal arterioles (Hansen et al 1990).

Chronic pain associated with hormonal therapy

Chronic gynaecomastia and breast tenderness are common complications of antiandrogen therapies for prostate cancer. The incidence of this syndrome varies among drugs; it is frequently associated with diethyl stilboesterol (Srinivasan et al 1972) and bicalutamide (Soloway et al 1996), is less common with flutamide (Brogden & Chrisp 1991) and cyproterone (Goldenberg & Bruchovsky 1991), and is uncommon among patients receiving LHRF agonist therapy (Chrisp & Goa 1991, Chrisp & Sorkin 1991). Gynaecomastia in the elderly must be distinguished from primary breast cancer or a secondary cancer in the breast (Olsson et al 1984, Ramamurthy & Cooper 1991).

Chronic postsurgical pain syndromes

Surgical incision at virtually any location may result in chronic pain. Although persistent pain is occasionally encountered after nephrectomy, sternotomy, craniotomy, inguinal dissection and other procedures, these pain syndromes are not well described in the cancer population. By contrast, several syndromes are now clearly recognized as sequelae of specific surgical procedures. The predominant underlying pain mechanism in these syndromes is neuropathic, resulting from injury to peripheral nerves or plexus.

Breast surgery pain syndromes

Chronic pain of variable severity is a common sequela of surgery for breast cancer. In two large surveys, pain, paraesthesias and strange sensations were reported by 30–50% of the patients (Tasmuth et al 1995, 1996). The most common sites of pain were the region of the scar and the ipsilateral arm. The highest incidence of pain was reported by patients who had had both radiotherapy and chemotherapy (Tasmuth et al 1995).

Although chronic pain has been reported to occur after almost any surgical procedure on the breast (from lumpectomy to radical mastectomy), it appears to be more common after breast-conserving treatments than after mastectomy (Tasmuth et al 1995) and is most common after procedures involving axillary dissection (Vecht et al 1989b, Vecht 1990, Hladiuk et al 1992, Maunsell et al 1993). Pain may begin immediately or as late as many months following surgery. The natural history of this condition appears to be variable, and both subacute and chronic courses are possible (International Association for the Study of Pain: Subcommittee on Taxonomy 1986). The onset of pain later than 18 months following surgery is unusual, and a careful evaluation to exclude recurrent chest wall disease is recommended in this setting.

Postmastectomy pain is usually characterized as a constricting and burning discomfort that is localized to the medial arm, axilla and anterior chest wall (Wood 1978, Granek et al 1983, Vecht et al 1989b, Paredes et al 1990, van Dam et al 1993). On examination, there is often an area of sensory loss within the region of the pain (van Dam et al 1993). The aetiology of this pain syndrome is believed to be related to damage to the intercostobrachial nerve, a cutaneous sensory branch of T1,2,3 (Vecht et al 1989b, van Dam et al 1993). There is marked anatomical variation in the size and distribution of the intercostobrachial nerve, and this may account for some of the variability in the distribution of pain observed in patients with this condition (Assa 1974).

In some cases of pain after breast surgery, a trigger point can be palpated in the axilla or chest wall. The patient may restrict movement of the arm, leading to frozen shoulder as a secondary complication.

Postradical neck dissection pain

Several types of postradical neck dissection pain are recognized. A persistent neuropathic pain can develop weeks to months after surgical injury to the cervical plexus. Tightness, along with burning or lancinating dysaesthesias in the area of the sensory loss, are the characteristic symptoms.

A second type of chronic pain can result from musculoskeletal imbalance in the shoulder girdle following surgical removal of neck muscles. Similar to the droopy shoulder syndrome (Swift & Nichols 1984), this syndrome can be complicated by the development of a thoracic outlet syndrome or suprascapular nerve entrapment. The latter syndrome is associated with selective weakness and wasting of the supraspinatus and infraspinatus muscles (Brown et al 1988).

Escalating pain in patients who have undergone radical neck dissection may signify recurrent tumour or soft-tissue infection. These lesions may be difficult to diagnose in tissues damaged by radiation and surgery. Repeated CT or MRI scanning may be needed to exclude tumour recurrence. Empirical treatment with antibiotics should be considered (Bruera & MacDonald 1986, Coyle & Portenoy 1991).

Post-thoracotomy pain

There have been two major studies of post-thoracotomy pain (Kanner et al 1982, 1994). In the first (Kanner et al 1982), three groups were identified: the largest (63%) had prolonged postoperative pain that abated within 2 months after surgery. Recurrent pain, following resolution of the postoperative pain, was usually caused by neoplasm. A second group (16%) experienced pain that persisted following the thoracotomy, then increased in intensity during the follow-up period. Local recurrence of disease and infection were the most common causes of the increasing pain. A final group had a prolonged period of stable or decreasing pain that gradually resolved over a maximum 8-month period. This pain was less likely to represent tumour recurrence. Overall, the development of late or increasing post-thoracotomy pain was a result of recurrent or persistent tumour in more than 95% of patients. This finding was corroborated in the more recent study, which evaluated the records of 238 consecutive patients who underwent thoracotomy and identified recurrent pain in 20 patients, all of whom were found to have tumour regrowth (Keller et al 1994).

Patients with recurrent or increasing post-thoracotomy pain should be carefully evaluated, preferably with a CT scan through the chest (Fig. 45.15). MRI presumably offers a sensitive alternative. Chest radiographs are insufficient to evaluate recurrent chest disease.

Postoperative frozen shoulder

Patients with post-thoracotomy or postmastectomy pain are at risk for the development of a frozen shoulder (Maunsell et al 1993). This lesion may become an independent focus of pain, particularly if complicated by reflex sympathetic dystrophy. Adequate postoperative analgesia and active mobilization of the joint soon after surgery are necessary to prevent these problems.

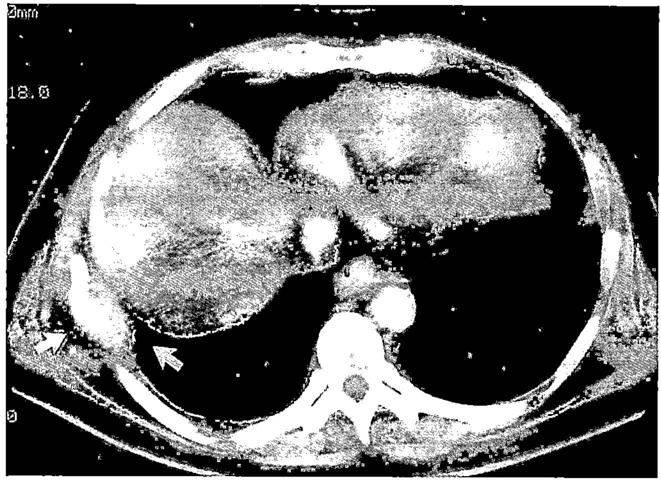

Fig. 45.15 Chest CT scan of a 55-year-old man who had recurrent left-sided chest wall pain 9 months after right upper lobectomy for squamous cell carcinoma of the lung. There is a chest wall recurrence associated with rib destruction and soft-tissue mass (arrow).

Phantom pain syndromes

Phantom limb pain is perceived to arise from an amputated limb, as if the limb were still contiguous with the body. The incidence of phantom pain is significantly higher in patients with a long duration of preamputation pain and those with pain on the day before amputation (Weinstein 1994, Nikolajsen et al 1997b). Patients who had pain prior to the amputation may experience phantom pain that replicates the earlier pain (Katz & Melzack 1990). In a recent study, pain was more prevalent after tumour-related rather than traumatic amputations, and postoperative chemotherapy was an additional risk factor (Smith & Thompson 1995). The pain may be continuous or paroxysmal and is often associated with bothersome paraesthesias. The phantom limb may assume painful and unusual postures and may gradually telescope and approach the stump. Phantom pain may initially magnify and then slowly fade over time. There is growing evidence that preoperative or postoperative neural blockade reduces the incidence of phantom limb pain during the first year after amputation (Pavy & Doyle 1996, Enneking & Morey 1997, Katz 1997, Nikolajsen et al 1997a).

Some patients have spontaneous partial remission of the pain. The recurrence of pain after such a remission, or the late onset of pain in a previously painless phantom limb, suggests the appearance of a more proximal lesion, including recurrent neoplasm (Chang et al 1997).

Phantom pain syndromes have also been described after other surgical procedures. Phantom breast pain after mastectomy, which occurs in 15–30% of patients (Kroner et al 1989, Kwekkeboom 1996, Tasmuth et al 1996), also appears to be related to the presence of preoperative pain (Kroner et al 1989). The pain tends to start in the region of the nipple and then spread to the entire breast. The character of the pain is variable and may be lancinating, continuous or intermittent (Kroner et al 1989). A phantom anus pain syndrome occurs in approximately 15% of patients who undergo abdominoperineal resection of the rectum (Ovesen et al 1991, Boas et al 1993). Phantom anus pain may develop either in the early postoperative period or after a latency of months to years. Late-onset pain is almost always associated with tumour recurrence (Ovesen et al 1991, Boas et al 1993). Rare cases of phantom bladder pain after cystectomy (Brena & Sammons 1979) and phantom eye pain after enucleation (Bond & Wesley 1987, Nicolodi et al 1997) have also been reported.

Stump pain

Stump pain occurs at the site of the surgical scar several months to years following amputation (Davis 1993). It is usually the result of neuroma development. This pain is characterized by burning or lancinating dysaesthesias, which are often exacerbated by movement or pressure and blocked by an injection of a local anaesthetic.

Postsurgical pelvic floor myalgia

Surgical trauma to the pelvic floor can cause a residual pelvic floor myalgia, which like the neoplastic syndrome described previously mimics so-called tension myalgia (Sinaki et al 1977). The risk of disease recurrence associated with this condition is not known, and its natural history has not been defined. In patients who have undergone anorectal resection, this condition must be differentiated from the phantom anus syndrome (see above).

Chronic postradiation pain syndromes

Chronic pain complicating radiation therapy tends to occur late in the course of a patient's illness. These syndromes must always be differentiated from recurrent tumour.

Radiation-induced brachial and lumbosacral plexopathies

Radiation-induced brachial and lumbosacral plexopathies were described previously (see above).

Chronic radiation myelopathy

Chronic radiation myelopathy is a late complication of spinal cord irradiation. The latency is highly variable, but is most commonly 12–14 months. The most common presentation is a partial transverse myelopathy at the cervicothoracic level, sometimes in a Brown–Sequard pattern (Schultheiss & Stephens 1992). Sensory symptoms, including pain, typically precede the development of progressive motor and autonomic dysfunction (Schultheiss & Stephens 1992). The pain is usually characterized as a burning dysaesthesia and is localized to the area of spinal cord damage or below. Imaging studies, particularly MRI, are important to exclude an epidural lesion and demonstrate the nature and extent of intrinsic cord pathology, which may include atrophy, swelling or syrinx. On MRI, the signs associated with radiation-induced injury include high-intensity signal on T2-weighted images or gadolinium enhancement of T1-weighted images (Koehler et al 1996, Alfonso et al 1997). The course of chronic radiation myelopathy is usually characterized by steady progression over months, followed by a subsequent phase of slow progression or stabilization.

Chronic radiation enteritis and proctitis

Chronic enteritis and proctocolitis occur as a late complication in 2–10% of patients who undergo abdominal or pelvic radiation therapy (Yeoh & Horowitz 1987, Nussbaum et al 1993). The rectum and rectosigmoid are more commonly involved than the small bowel, a pattern that may relate to the retroperitoneal fixation of the former structures. The latency is variable (3 months to 30 years) (Yeoh & Horowitz 1987, Nussbaum et al 1993). Chronic radiation injury of the rectum can present as proctitis (with bloody diarrhoea, tenesmus and cramping pain), obstruction due to stricture formation, or fistulae of the bladder or vagina. Small bowel radiation damage typically causes colicky abdominal pain, which can be associated with chronic nausea or malabsorption. Barium studies may demonstrate a narrow tubular bowel segment resembling Crohn's disease or ischaemic colitis. Endoscopy and biopsy may be necessary to distinguish suspicious lesions from recurrent cancer.

Lymphoedema pain

One-third of patients with lymphoedema as a complication of breast cancer or its treatment experience pain and tightness in the arm (Newman et al 1996). Some patients develop entrapment syndromes involving the median nerve in the carpal tunnel or the brachial plexus (Ganel et al 1979, Vecht 1990). Severe or increasing pain in a lymphoedematous arm is strongly suggestive of tumour recurrence or progression (Kori et al 1981, Kori 1995).

Burning perineum syndrome

Persistent perineal discomfort is an uncommon delayed complication of pelvic radiotherapy. After a latency of 6–18 months, burning pain can develop in the perianal region. The pain may extend anteriorly to involve the vagina or scrotum (Minsky & Cohen 1988). In patients who have had abdominoperineal resection, phantom anus pain and recurrent tumour are major differential diagnoses.

Osteoradionecrosis

Osteoradionecrosis is another late complication of radiotherapy. Bone necrosis, which occurs as a result of endarteritis obliterans, may produce focal pain. Overlying tissue breakdown can occur spontaneously or as a result of trauma, such as dental extraction or denture trauma (Epstein 1987, 1997). Delayed development of a painful ulcer must be differentiated from tumour recurrence.

BOX 45.3

Commonly used tissue-vessicant cytotoxic drugs

Amasarcine	Mitomycin-C
BCNU	Mitoxantrone
Cis-platinum	Streptozotocin
Decarbazine	Teniposide
Daunorubicin	Vinblastine
Doxorubicin	Vincristine
Teoposide	Vindesine

REFERENCES

Aass N, Kaasa S, Lund E, Kaalhus O, Heier M S, Fossa S D 1990 Long-term somatic side-effects and morbidity in testicular cancer patients. British Journal of Cancer 61:151–155

Abbott J 1990 Pelvic pain: lessons from anatomy and physiology. Journal of Emergency Medicine 8:441–447

Agency for Health Care Policy and Research 1994 Management of cancer pain: adults. Cancer Pain Guideline Panel. Agency for Health Care Policy and Research. American Family Physician 49:1853–1868

Agency for Health Care Policy and Research: Acute Pain Management Panel 1992 Acute pain management: operative or medical procedures and trauma. Clinical Practice Guideline. US Department of Health and Human Services, Washington

Agnelli G 1997 Venous thromboembolism and cancer: a two-way clinical association. Thrombosis and Haemostasis 78:117–120

Aird D W, Bihari J, Smith C 1983 Clinical problems in the continuing care of head and neck cancer patients. Ear Nose and Throat Journal 62:230–243

Aki F T, Tekin M I, Ozen H 1996 Gynecomastia as a complication of chemotherapy for testicular germ cell tumors. Urology 48:944–946

Alberts D S, Garcia D J 1997 Safety aspects of pegylated liposomal doxorubicin in patients with cancer. Drugs 54(suppl 4):30–35

Albertyn L E, Croft G, Kuss B, Dale B 1992 The perivertebral collar – a new sign in lymphoproliferative malignancies. Australasian Radiology 36:214–218

Alfonso E R, D Gregorio M A, Mateo P et al 1997 Radiation myelopathy in over-irradiated patients: MR imaging findings. European Radiology 7:400–404

Allebeck P, Bolund C 1991 Suicides and suicide attempts in cancer patients. Psychological Medicine 21:979–984

Almadrones L, Yerys C 1990 Problems associated with the administration of intraperitoneal therapy using the Port-A-Cath system. Oncological Nursing Forum 17:75–80

Alon U S, Allen S, Rameriz Z, Warady B A, Kaplan R A, Harris D J 1994 Lidocaine for the alleviation of pain associated with subcutaneous erythropoietin injection. Journal of the American Society of Nephrology 5:1161–1162

American Pain Society Quality of Care Committee 1995 Quality improvement guidelines for the treatment of acute pain and cancer pain. American Pain Society Quality of Care Committee [see comments]. Journal of the American Medical Association 274:1874–1880

American Psychiatric Association 1994 Somatoform disorders. In: Diagnostic and statistical manual of mental disorders (DSM-IV), 4th edn. American Psychiatric Association, Washington, pp 445–471

Andreasen D A, Poulsen J 1997 [Intra-abdominal torsion of the testis with seminoma (see comments).] Ugeskrift fur Laeger 159(14):2103–2104

Ang K K, Stephens L C 1994 Prevention and management of radiation myelopathy. Oncology (Huntingt) 8(11):71–76, 78, 81–82

Araki K, Kobayashi M, Ogata T, Takuma K 1994 Colorectal carcinoma metastatic to skeletal muscle. Hepatogastroenterology 41:405–408

Archer A G, Sugarbaker P H, Jelinek J S 1996 Radiology of peritoneal carcinomatosis. Cancer Treatment Research 82:263–288.

Arner S, Meyerson B A 1988 Lack of analgesic effect of opioids on neuropathic and idiopathic forms of pain. Pain 33:11–23

Aro A R, Absetz Y P, Eerola T, Pamilo M, Lonnqvist J 1996 Pain and discomfort during mammography. European Journal of Cancer. 32A: 1674–9

Assa J 1974 The intercostobrachial nerve in radical mastectomy. Journal of Surgical Oncology 6:123–126

Au E, Loprinzi C L, Dhodapkar M et al 1994 Regular use of a verbal pain scale improves the understanding of oncology inpatient pain intensity. Journal of Clinical Oncology 12:2751–2755

Averbach A M, Sugarbaker P H 1995 Recurrent intraabdominal cancer with intestinal obstruction. International Surgery 80:141–146

Babb R R 1996 Radiation proctitis: a review. American Journal of Gastroenterology 91:1309–1311

Bach F, Soletormos G, Dombernowsky P 1991 Tissue polypeptide antigen activity in cerebrospinal fluid: a marker of central nervous system metastases of breast cancer. Journal of the National Cancer Institute 83:779–784

Baile W F, DiMaggio J R, Schapira D V, Janofsky J S 1993 The request for assistance in dying. The need for psychiatric consultation. Cancer 72:2786–2791

Baines M J 1994 Intestinal obstruction. Cancer Survey 21:147–156

Balm M, Hammack J 1996 Leptomeningeal carcinomatosis. Presenting features and prognostic factors [see comments]. Archives of Neurology 53:626–632

Banning A, Sjogren P, Henriksen H 1991 Pain causes in 200 patients referred to a multidisciplinary cancer pain clinic. Pain 45:45–48

Barcena A, Lobato R D, Rivas J J et al 1984 Spinal metastatic disease: analysis of factors determining functional prognosis and the choice of treatment. Neurosurgery 15:820–827

Barker F G 2nd, Jannetta P J, Babu R P, Pomonis S, Bissonette D J, Jho H D 1996 Long-term outcome after operation for trigeminal neuralgia in patients with posterior fossa tumors. Journal of Neurosurgery 84:818–825

Barkwell D P 1991 Ascribed meaning: a critical factor in coping and pain attenuation in patients with cancer-related pain. Journal of Palliative Care 7:5–14

Barron K D, Hirano A, Araki S et al 1959 Experience with metastatic neoplasms involving the spinal cord. Neurology 9:91–100

Batts K P 1998 Ischemic cholangitis. Mayo Clinic Proceedings 73:380–385

Beatrous T E, Choyke P L, Frank J A 1990 Diagnostic evaluation of cancer patients with pelvic pain: comparison of scintigraphy, CT, and MR imaging [see comments]. American Journal of Roentgenology 155:85–88

Bell A 1988 Preventing perineal burning from i.v. dexamethasone. Oncological Nursing Forum 15:199

Bellmunt J, Navarro M, Hidalgo R, Sole L A 1988 Palmar-plantar erythrodysesthesia syndrome associated with short-term continuous infusion (5 days) of 5-fluorouracil. Tumori 74:329–331

Berger A, Henderson M, Nadoolman W et al 1995a Oral capsaicin provides temporary relief for oral mucositis pain secondary to chemotherapy/radiation therapy [published erratum appears in Journal of Pain and Symptom Management 1996; 11:331]. Journal of Pain and Symptom Management 10:243–248

Berger M S, Cooley M E, Abrahm J L 1995b A pain syndrome associated with large adrenal metastases in patients with lung cancer. Journal of Pain and Symptom Management 10(2):161–166

Bertelli G 1995 Prevention and management of extravasation of cytotoxic drugs. Drug Safety 12:245–255

Bitoh S, Hasegawa H, Ohtsuki H, Obashi J, Kobayashi Y 1985 Parasellar metastases: four autopsied cases. Surgical Neurological 23:41–48

Boas R A, Schug S A, Acland R H 1993 Perineal pain after rectal amputation: a 5-year follow-up. Pain 52:67–70

Bond J B, Wesley R E 1987 Cluster headache after orbital exenteration. Annals of Ophthalmology 19:438

Bond M R, Pearson I B 1969 Psychological aspects of pain in women with advanced cancer of the cervix. Journal of Psychosomatic Research 13:13–19

Bongers K M, Willingers H M, Koehler P J 1992 Referred facial pain from lung carcinoma. Neurology 42:1841–1842

Bonica J J (ed) 1953 Headache and other visceral disorders of the head and neck. In: The management of pain, 1st edn. Lea & Febiger, Philadelphia, pp 1263–1309

Bonica J J, Ventafridda V, Twycross R G 1990 Cancer Pain. In: Bonica J J (ed) The management of pain, vol 1, 2nd edn. Lea & Febiger, Philadelphia, pp 400–460

Bookbinder M, Coyle N, Kiss M et al 1996 Implementing national standards for cancer pain management: program model and evaluation. Journal of Pain and Symptom Management 12(6):334–347

Bosley T M, Cohen D A, Schatz N J et al 1985 Comparison of metrizamide computed tomography and magnetic resonance imaging in the evaluation of lesions at the cervicomedullary junction. Neurology 35:485–492

Boyle D M, Engelking C 1995 Vesicant extravasation: myths and realities. Oncological Nursing Forum 22:57–67

Brady A M 1996 Management of painful paraneoplastic syndromes. Hematology/Oncology Clinics of North America 10:801–809

Breitbart W 1990 Cancer pain and suicide. In: Foley K M, Bonica J J, Ventafridda V (eds) Second International Congress on Cancer Pain. Advances in Pain Research and Therapy, vol 16. Raven, New York, pp 399–412

Breitbart W 1994 Cancer pain management guidelines: implications for psycho-oncology. Psycho Oncology 3:103–108

Brena S F, Sammons E E 1979 Phantom urinary bladder pain – case report. Pain 7:197–201

Brescia F J, Portenoy R K, Ryan M, Krasnoff L, Gray G 1992 Pain, opioid use, and survival in hospitalized patients with advanced cancer. Journal of Clinical Oncology 10(1):149–155

Brice J, McKissock W 1965 Surgical treatment of malignant extradural tumors. British Medical Journal 1:1341–1346

Briselli M, Mark E J, Dickersin G R 1981 Solitary fibrous tumors of the pleura: eight new cases and review of 360 cases in the literature. Cancer 47:2678–2689

Brogden R N, Chrisp P 1991 Flutamide. A review of its pharmacodynamic and pharmacokinetic properties, and therapeutic use in advanced prostatic cancer. Drugs and Aging 1:104–115

Brown H, Burns S, Kaiser C W 1988 The spinal accessory nerve plexus, the trapezius muscle, and shoulder stabilization after radical neck cancer surgery. Annals of Surgery 208:654–661

Bruera E, MacDonald N 1986 Intractable pain in patients with advanced head and neck tumors: a possible role of local infection. Cancer Treatment Report 70(5):691–692

Bruera E, Macmillan K, Selmser P, MacDonald R N 1990 Decreased local toxicity with subcutaneous diamorphine (heroin): a preliminary report. Pain 43:91–94

Bruera E, Fainsinger R, Moore M, Thibault R, Spoldi E, Ventafridda V 1991a Local toxicity with subcutaneous methadone. Experience of two centers. Pain 45:141–143

Bruera E, Kuehn N, Miller M J, Selmser P, Macmillan K 1991b The Edmonton Symptom Assessment System (ESAS): a simple method for the assessment of palliative care patients. Journal of Palliative Care 7:6–9

Bullitt E, Tew J M, Boyd J 1986 Intracranial tumors in patients with facial pain. Journal of Neurosurgery 64:865–871

Burihan E, de Figueiredo L F, Francisco Junior J, Miranda Junior F 1993 Upper-extremity deep venous thrombosis: analysis of 52 cases. Cardiovascular Surgery 1:19–22

Burrows M, Dibble S L, Miaskowski C 1998 Differences in outcomes among patients experiencing different types of cancer-related pain. Oncological Nursing Forum 25:735–741

Cantwell B M, Richardson P G, Campbell S J 1991 Gynaecomastia and extragonadal symptoms leading to diagnosis delay of germ cell tumours in young men [see comments]. Postgraduate Medical Journal 67:675–677

Capobianco D J 1995 Facial pain as a symptom of nonmetastatic lung cancer. Headache 35:581–585

Caraceni A, Mendoza T R, Mencaglia E et al 1996 A validation study of an Italian version of the Brief Pain Inventory (Breve Questionario per la Valutazione del Dolore). Pain 65:87–92

Carbaat P A, van Crevel H 1981 Lumbar puncture headache: controlled study on the preventive effect of 24 hours' bed rest. Lancet ii; 1133–1135

Cartwright P D, Hesse C, Jackson A O 1993 Myoclonic spasms following intrathecal diamorphine. Journal of Pain and Symptom Management 8:492–495

Cascino T L, Kori S, Krol G, Foley K M 1983 CT of the brachial plexus in patients with cancer. Neurology 33:1553–1557

Cascinu S, Fedeli A, Fedeli S L, Catalano G 1994 Oral cooling (cryotherapy), an effective treatment for the prevention of 5-fluorouracil-induced stomatitis. European Journal of Cancer B: Oral Oncology 30B(4):234–6.

Castaigne S, Chomienne C, Daniel M T et al 1990 All-*trans* retinoic acid as a differentiation therapy for acute promyelocytic leukemia. I. Clinical results [see comments]. Blood 76(9):1704–1709

Castellanos A M, Glass J P, Yung W K 1987 Regional nerve injury after intra-arterial chemotherapy. Neurology 37:834–837

Cervero F 1985 Visceral nociception: peripheral and central aspects of visceral nociceptive systems. Philosophical Transactions of the Royal Society London. Series B: Biological Sciences 308:325–337

Chad D A, Bradley W G 1987 Lumbosacral plexopathy. Seminars in Neurology 7:97–107

Chamberlain M C 1997 Pediatric leptomeningeal metastases: outcome following combined therapy. Journal of Child Neurology 12:53–59

Chamberlain M C, Sandy A D, Press G A 1990 Leptomeningeal metastasis: a comparison of gadolinium-enhanced MR and contrast-enhanced CT of the brain. Neurology 40(3 Pt 1):435–438

Chang V T, Tunkel R S, Pattillo B A, Lachmann E A 1997 Increased phantom limb pain as an initial symptom of spinal-neoplasia [published erratum appears in Journal of Pain and Management Symptom 1997;14:135]. Journal of Pain and Management Symptom 13(6):362–364

Chapman C R, Donaldson G W, Jacobson R C, Hautman B 1997 Differences among patients in opioid self-administration during bone marrow transplantation. Pain 71:213–223

Chapman C R, Hill H F 1989 Prolonged morphine self-administration and addiction liability. Evaluation of two theories in a bone marrow transplant unit. Cancer 63:1636–1644.

Chen C, Chen P J, Yang P M et al 1997 Clinical and microbiological features of liver abscess after transarterial embolization for hepatocellular carcinoma. American Journal of Gastroenterology 92(12):2257–2259

Cheng T M, Cascino T L, Onofrio B M 1993 Comprehensive study of diagnosis and treatment of trigeminal neuralgia secondary to tumors. Neurology 43:2298–2302

Cherny N I, Catane R 1995 Professional negligence in the management of cancer pain. A case for urgent reforms [editorial; comment]. Cancer 76:2181–2185

Cherny N I, Ho M N, Bookbinder M, Fahey T J Jr, Portenoy R K, Foley K M 1994a Cancer pain: knowledge and attitudes of physicians at a cancer center (Meeting abstract). Proceedings of the Annual Meeting of the American Society of Clinical Oncologists 13

Cherny N I, Thaler H T, Friedlander-Klar H et al 1994b Opioid responsiveness of cancer pain syndromes caused by neuropathic or nociceptive mechanisms: a combined analysis of controlled, single-dose studies. Neurology 44:857–861

Cherny N J, Chang V, Frager G et al 1995 Opioid pharmacotherapy in the management of cancer pain: a survey of strategies used by pain physicians for the selection of analgesic drugs and routes of administration. Cancer 76:1283–1293

Cherny N I, Arbit E, Jain S 1996 Invasive techniques in the management of cancer pain. Hematology/Oncology Clinics of North America 10(1):121–137

Chrisp P, Goa K L 1991 Goserelin. A review of its pharmacodynamic and pharmacokinetic properties, and clinical use in sex hormone-related conditions. Drugs 41:254–288

Chrisp P, Sorkin E M 1991 Leuprorelin. A review of its pharmacology and therapeutic use in prostatic disorders. Drugs and Aging 1:487–509

Cibas E S, Malkin M G, Posner J B, Melamed M R 1987 Detection of DNA abnormalities by flow cytometry in cells from cerebrospinal fluid. American Journal of Clinical Pathology 88(5):570–577

Clarke-Pearson D L, Olt G 1989 Thromboembolism in patients with Gyn tumors: risk factors, natural history, and prophylaxis. Oncology (Huntington) 3:39–45, 48

Cleeland C S 1984 The impact of pain on the patient with cancer. Cancer 54(11 suppl):2635–2641

Cleeland C S 1988 Clinical cancer: 31. Barriers to the management of cancer pain: the roles of patient and family. Wisconsin Medical Journal 87:13–15

Cleeland C S, Ryan K M 1994 Pain assessment: global use of the Brief Pain Inventory. Annals of the Academy of Medicine Singapore 23:129–138

Cleeland C S, Gonin R, Hatfield A K et al 1994 Pain and its treatment in outpatients with metastatic cancer. New England Journal of Medicine 330:592–596

Cleeland C S, Nakamura Y, Mendoza T R, Edwards K R, Douglas J, Serlin R C 1996 Dimensions of the impact of cancer pain in a four country sample: new information from multidimensional scaling. Pain 67:267–273

Cleeland C S, Gonin R, Baez L, Loehrer P, Pandya K J 1997 Pain and treatment of pain in minority patients with cancer. The Eastern Cooperative Oncology Group Minority Outpatient Pain Study. Annals of Internal Medicine 127:813–816.

Clouston P D, DeAngelis L M, Posner J B 1992 The spectrum of neurological disease in patients with systemic cancer. Annals of Neurology 31:268–273

Coda B A, O'Sullivan B, Donaldson G, Bohl S, Chapman C R, Shen D D

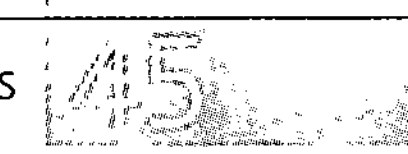

1997 Comparative efficacy of patient-controlled administration of morphine, hydromorphone, or sufentanil for the treatment of oral mucositis pain following bone marrow transplantation. Pain 72:333–346

Cogo A, Lensing A W, Koopman M M et al 1998 Compression ultrasonography for diagnostic management of patients with clinically suspected deep vein thrombosis: prospective cohort study [see comments]. British Medical Journal 316:17–20

Constans J P, de Divitiis E, Donzelli R, Spaziante R, Meder J F, Haye C 1983 Spinal metastases with neurological manifestations. Review of 600 cases. Journal of Neurosurgery 59:111–118

Cook P T, Davies M J, Beavis R E 1989 Bed rest and postlumbar puncture headache. The effectiveness of 24 hours' recumbency in reducing the incidence of postlumbar puncture headache [see comments]. Anaesthesia 44:389–391

Coombs D W 1990 Pain due to liver capsular distention. In: Ferrer-Brechner T (ed) Common problems in pain management. Common problems in anesthesia. Year Book Medical Publishers, Chicago, pp 247–253

Corbey M P, Bach A B, Lech K, Frorup A M 1997 Grading of severity of postdural puncture headache after 27-gauge Quincke and Whitacre needles. Acta Anaesthesiologica Scandinavica 41:779–784

Coyle N 1987 A model of continuity of care for cancer patients with chronic pain. Medical Clinics of North America 71:259–270

Coyle N, Portenoy R K 1991 Infection as a cause of rapidly increasing pain in cancer patients. Journal of Pain and Symptom Management 6:266–269

Coyle N, Adelhardt J, Foley K M, Portenoy R K 1990 Character of terminal illness in the advanced cancer patient: pain and other symptoms during the last four weeks of life. Journal of Pain and Symptom Management 5:83–93

Coyle N, Thaler H, Bookbinder M et al 1993 Implementation of the American Pain Society (APS) standards for cancer pain management: a pilot study at Memorial Sloan-Kettering Cancer Center (MSKCC) (Meeting abstract). Proceedings of the Annual Meeting of the American Society of Clinical Oncologists 12

Criado E, Burnham C B 1997 Predictive value of clinical criteria for the diagnosis of deep vein thrombosis. Surgery 122:578–583

Curran C F, Luce J K, Page J A 1990 Doxorubicin-associated flare reactions. Oncological Nursing Forum 17:387–389

Dalmau J, Graus F, Marco M 1989 'Hot and dry foot' as initial manifestation of neoplastic lumbosacral plexopathy. Neurology 39:871–872

Dalmau J O, Posner J B 1997 Paraneoplastic syndromes affecting the nervous system. Seminars in Oncology 24:318–328

Daut R L, Cleeland C S 1982 The prevalence and severity of pain in cancer. Cancer 50:1913–1918

Daut R L, Cleeland C S, Flanery R C 1983 Development of the Wisconsin Brief Pain Questionnaire to assess pain in cancer and other diseases. Pain 17:197–210

Davies J H, Dowsett M, Jacobs S, Coombes R C, Hedley A, Shearer R J 1992 Aromatase inhibition: 4-hydroxyandrostenedione (4-OHA, CGP 32349) in advanced prostatic cancer. British Journal of Cancer 66:139–142

Davis R W 1993 Phantom sensation, phantom pain, and stump pain. Archives of Physical Medicine and Rehabilitation 74:79–91

DeAngelis L M, Payne R 1987 Lymphomatous meningitis presenting as atypical cluster headache. Pain 30:211–216

De Castro M D, Meynadier M D, Zenz M D 1991 Regional opioid analgesia. Developments in critical care medicine and anesthesiology, vol 20. Kluwer Academic, Dordrecht

De Conno F, Polastri D 1996 [Clinical features and symptomatic treatment of liver metastasis in the terminally ill patient.] Annals Italiani Chirurgia 67(6):819–826

De Conno F, Caraceni A, Martini C, Spoldi E, Salvetti M, Ventafridda V 1991 Hyperalgesia and myoclonus with intrathecal infusion of high-dose morphine. Pain 47:337–339

De Conno F, Caraceni A, Gamba A et al 1994 Pain measurement in cancer patients: a comparison of six methods. Pain 57:161–166

Delattre J Y, Arbit E, Thaler H T, Rosenblum M K, Posner J B 1989 A dose-response study of dexamethasone in a model of spinal cord compression caused by epidural tumor. Journal of Neurosurgery 70:920–926

Deppe G, Malviya V K, Boike G, Young J 1991 Intraperitoneal doxorubicin in combination with systemic cisplatinum and cyclophosphamide in the treatment of stage III ovarian cancer. European Journal of Gynaecological Oncology 12:93–97

Des Prez R D, Freemon F R 1983 Facial pain associated with lung cancer: a case report. Headache 23:43–44

Desta K, O'Shaughnessy M, Milling M A 1994 Non-Hodgkin's lymphoma presenting as median nerve compression in the arm. Journal of Hand Surgery 19:289–291

Devor M, Basbaum A I, Bennett G J et al 1991 Group Report: mechanisms of neuropathic pain following peripheral injury. In: Basbaum A, Besson J-M (eds) Towards a new pharmacotherapy of pain. John Wiley, New York, pp 417–440

Donati M B 1994 Cancer and thrombosis. Haemostasis 24:128–131

Donayre C E, White G H, Mehringer S M, Wilson S E 1986 Pathogenesis determines late morbidity of axillosubclavian vein thrombosis. American Journal of Surgery 152:179–184

Donnelly S, Walsh D 1995 The symptoms of advanced cancer. Seminars in Oncology 22(2 suppl 3):67–72

Donnelly S, Walsh D, Rybicki L 1995 The symptoms of advanced cancer: identification of clinical and research priorities by assessment of prevalence and severity. Journal of Palliative Care 11:27–32

Dose A M 1995 The symptom experience of mucositis, stomatitis, and xerostomia. Seminars in Oncological Nursing 11:248–255

Dudgeon D, Raubertas R F, Rosenthal S N 1993 The short-form McGill Pain Questionnaire in chronic cancer pain. Journal of Pain and Symptom Management 8:191–195

Dulli D A, Levine R L, Chun R W, Dinndorf P 1987 Migrainous neurologic dysfunction in Hodgkin's disease [letter]. Archives of Neurology 44:689

Dykman T R, Montgomery E B Jr, Gerstenberger P D, Zeiger H E, Clutter W E, Cryer P E 1981 Glossopharyngeal neuralgia with syncope secondary to tumor. Treatment and pathophysiology. American Journal of Medicine 71:165–170

Edwards R B 1989 Pain management and the values of health care providers. In: Hill C S, Fields W S (eds) Drug treatment of cancer pain in a drug oriented society. Advances in pain research and therapy, vol 11. Raven, New York, pp 101–112

Edwards W T 1990 Optimizing opioid treatment of postoperative pain. Journal of Pain and Symptom Management 5(1 suppl):S24–36

Elliott K J 1994 Taxonomy and mechanisms of neuropathic pain. Seminars in Neurology 14(3):195–205

Elomaa I, Pajunen M, Virkkunen P 1984 Raynaud's phenomenon progressing to gangrene after vincristine and bleomycin therapy. Acta Medica Scandinavica 216:323–326

El-Salhy M, Simonsson M, Stenling R, Grimelius L 1998 Recovery from Marie–Bamberger's syndrome and diabetes insipidus after removal of a lung adenocarcinoma with neuroendocrine features. Journal of International Medicine 243:171–175

Emanuel E J 1996 Pain and symptom control. Patient rights and physician responsibilities. Hematology/Oncology Clinics of North America 10(1):41–56

Ende D A, Robinson G, Moulton J 1995 Metastasis-induced perforated appendicitis: an acute abdomen of rare aetiology. Australian and New Zealand Journal of Surgery 65(1):62–63

Enneking F K, Morey T E 1997 Continuous postoperative infusion of a regional anesthetic after an amputation of the lower extremity. A randomized clinical trial [letter]. Journal of Bone and Joint Surgery [Am] 79:1752–1753

Epstein J, van der Meij E, McKenzie M, Wong F, Lepawsky M, Stevenson-Mooc P. 1997. Postradiation osteoneorosis of the mandible: a long-term follow-up study. Oral Surg Oral Med Oral Pathol Oral Radiol Endod 83: 657–62

Epstein JB, Rea G, Wong FL, Spinelli J, Stevenson-Moore P 1987. Osteonecrosis; study of the relationship of dental extractions in patients receiving radiotherapy. Head, Neck Surgery 10: 48–54

Epstein J B, Stewart K H 1993 Radiation therapy and pain in patients with head and neck cancer. European Journal of Cancer B: Oral Oncology 29B:191–199

Escalante C P 1993 Causes and management of superior vena cava syndrome. Oncology (Huntingt) 7:61–68, 71–72, 75–77

Eskilsson J, Albertsson M 1990 Failure of preventing 5-fluorouracil cardiotoxicity by prophylactic treatment with verapamil. Acta Oncologica 29:1001–1003

Esteban A, Traba A 1993 Fasciculation-myokymic activity and prolonged nerve conduction block. A physiopathological relationship in radiation-induced brachial plexopathy. Electroencephalography and Clinical Neurophysiology 89:382–391

Evans R J, Watson C P N 1985 Lumbosacral plexopathy in cancer patients. Neurology 35:1392–1393

Evans R W 1998 Complications of lumbar puncture. Neurologic Clinics 16:83–105

Fabian C J, Molina R, Slavik M, Dahlberg S, Giri S, Stephens R 1990 Pyridoxine therapy for palmar-plantar erythrodysesthesia associated with continuous 5-fluorouracil infusion. Investigational New Drugs 8:57–63

Feld R 1997 The role of surveillance cultures in patients likely to develop chemotherapy-induced mucositis. Supportive Care in Cancer 5:371–375

Feldenzer J A, McGauley J L, McGillicuddy J E 1989 Sacral and presacral tumors: problems in diagnosis and management. Neurosurgery 25:884–891

Ferrell B R 1995 The impact of pain on quality of life. A decade of research. Nursing Clinics of North America 30:609–624

Ferrell B R, Dean G 1995 The meaning of cancer pain. Seminars in Oncological Nursing 11:17–22

Feuz A, Rapin C H 1994 An observational study of the role of pain control and food adaptation of elderly patients with terminal cancer. Journal of the American Dietetic Association 94(7):767–770

Findlay G F 1984 Adverse effects of the management of malignant spinal cord compression. Journal of Neurology, Neurosurgery and Psychiatry 47:761–768

Findlay G F 1987 The role of vertebral body collapse in the management of malignant spinal cord compression. Journal of Neurology, Neurosurgery and Psychiatry 50:151–154

Fink B R 1990 Postspinal headache [letter]. Anesthesia and Analgesia 71:208–209

Fishman B 1992 The cognitive behavioral perspective on pain management in terminal illness. Hospital Journal 8:73–88

Fishman B, Pasternak S, Wallenstein S L, Houde R W, Holland J C, Foley K M 1987 The Memorial Pain Assessment Card. A valid instrument for the evaluation of cancer pain. Cancer 60:1151–1158

Fishman E K, Campbell J N, Kuhlman J E, Kawashima A, Ney D R, Friedman N B 1991 Multiplanar CT evaluation of brachial plexopathy in breast cancer. Journal of Computer Assisted Tomography 15:790–795

Foley K M 1987 Pain syndromes in patients with cancer. Medical Clinics of North America 71:169–184

Folkman S, Lazarus R S, Dunkel-Schetter C, DeLongis A, Gruen R J 1986 Dynamics of a stressful encounter: cognitive appraisal, coping, and encounter outcomes. Journal of Personality and Social Psychology 50:992–1003

Forman A 1990 Peripheral neuropathy in cancer patients: clinical types, etiology, and presentation. Part 2. Oncology (Huntingt) 4:85–89

Forst T, Beyer J, Cordes U et al 1995 Gynaecomastia in a patient with a hCG producing giant cell carcinoma of the lung. Case report. Experimental and Clinical Endocrinology and Diabetes 103:28–32

Forsyth P A, Posner J B 1993 Headaches in patients with brain tumors: a study of 111 patients. Neurology 43:1678–1683

Fossa S D, Urnes T 1986 Flare reaction during the initial treatment period with medroxyprogesterone acetate in patients with hormone-resistant prostatic cancer. European Urology 12:257–279

Francis P, Rowinsky E, Schneider J, Hakes T, Hoskins W, Markman M 1995 Phase I feasibility and pharmacologic study of weekly intraperitoneal paclitaxel: a Gynecologic Oncology Group pilot Study. Journal of Clinical Oncology 13:2961–2967

Freedman D M, Henderson R C 1995 Metastatic breast carcinoma to the os calcis presenting as heel pain. Southern Medical Journal 88:232–234

Freeman N J, Costanza M E 1988 5-Fluorouracil-associated cardiotoxicity. Cancer 61:36–45

Freilich R J, Krol G, DeAngelis L M 1995 Neuroimaging and cerebrospinal fluid cytology in the diagnosis of leptomeningeal metastasis. Annals of Neurology 38:51–57

Frenken L A, van Lier H J, Gerlag P G, den Hartog M, Koene R A 1991 Assessment of pain after subcutaneous injection of erythropoietin in patients receiving haemodialysis. British Medical Journal 303:288

Frenken L A, van Lier H J, Koene R A 1994 Analysis of the efficacy of measures to reduce pain after subcutaneous administration of epoetin alfa [see comments]. Nephrology, Dialysis, Transplantation 9:1295–1298

Friedman J, Karesh J, Rodrigues M, Sun C C 1990 Thyroid carcinoma metastatic to the medial rectus muscle. Opthalamic Plastic and Reconstructive Surgery 6:122–125

Fromm G L, Gershenson D M, Silva E G 1990 Papillary serous carcinoma of the peritoneum. Obstetrics and Gynecology 75:89–95

Galer B S, Portenoy R K 1991 Acute herpetic and postherpetic neuralgia: clinical features and management. Mount Sinai Medical Journal 58:257–266

Ganel A, Engel J, Sela M, Brooks M 1979 Nerve entrapments associated with postmastectomy lymphedema. Cancer 44:2254–2259

Garrison R N, Kaelin L D, Galloway R H, Heuser L S 1986 Malignant ascites. Clinical and experimental observations. Annals of Surgery 203:644–651

Gerard J M, Franck N, Moussa Z, Hildebrand J 1989 Acute ischemic brachial plexus neuropathy following radiation therapy. Neurology 39:450–451

Gerl A 1994 Vascular toxicity associated with chemotherapy for testicular cancer. Anticancer Drugs 5:607–614

Giamberardino M A, Vecchiet L 1995 Visceral pain, referred hyperalgesia and outcome: new concepts. European Journal of Anaesthesiology. Supplement 10:61–66

Gilbert R W, Kim J H, Posner J B 1978 Epidural spinal cord compression from metastatic tumor: diagnosis and treatment. Annals of Neurology 3:40–51

Giorgi C, Broggi G 1984 Surgical treatment of glossopharyngeal neuralgia and pain from cancer of the nasopharynx. A 20-year experience. Journal of Neurosurgery 61:952–955

Glajchen M, Blum D, Calder K 1995 Cancer pain management and the role of social work: barriers and interventions. Health and Social Work 20:200–206

Glass A R, Berenberg J 1979 Gynecomastia after chemotherapy for lymphoma. Archives of Internal Medicine 139:1048–1049

Glavina M J, Robertshaw R 1988 Myoclonic spasms following intrathecal morphine. Anaesthesia 43:389–390

Goldenberg S L, Bruchovsky N 1991 Use of cyproterone acetate in prostate cancer. Urologic Clinics of North America 18(1):111–122

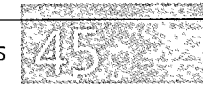

Goldstein F J 1997 Inadequate pain management: a suicidogen (Dr Jack Kevorkian: friend or foe?). Journal of Clinical Pharmacology 37:1–3

Golembe B, Ramsay N K, McKenna R, Nesbit M E, Krivit W 1979 Localized bone marrow relapse in acute lymphoblastic leukemia. Medical and Pediatric Oncology 6:229–234

Gonzales G R, Elliott K J, Portenoy R K, Foley K M 1991 The impact of a comprehensive evaluation in the management of cancer pain. Pain 47:141–144

Goodman M, Dalton J R 1982 Ureteral strictures following radiotherapy: incidence, etiology and treatment guidelines. Journal of Urology 128:21–24

Gorson K C, Musaphir S, Lathi E S, Wolfe G 1995 Radiation-induced malignant fibrous histiocytoma of the brachial plexus. Journal of Neurooncology 26:73–77

Graham D F 1976 Hip pain as a presenting symptom of acetabular metastasis. British Journal of Surgery 63:147–148

Grahm A L, Andren-Sandberg A 1997 Prospective evaluation of pain in exocrine pancreatic cancer. Digestion 58:542–549

Granek I, Ashikari R, Foley K M 1983 Postmastectomy pain syndrome: clinical and anatomic correlates. Proceedings of the American Society of Clinical Oncology 3: abstract 122

Grant R, Papadopoulos S M, Sandler H M, Greenberg H S 1994 Metastatic epidural spinal cord compression: current concepts and treatment. Journal of Neurooncology 19:79–92

Graus F, Krol G, Foley K 1986 Early diagnosis of spinal epidural metastasis: correlation with clinical and radiological findings. Proceedings of the American Society of Clinical Oncology 5:abstract 1047

Greenberg H S, Kim J H, Posner J B 1980 Epidural spinal cord compression from metastatic tumor: results with a new treatment protocol. Annals of Neurology 8:361–366

Greenberg H S, Deck M D, Vikram B, Chu F C, Posner J B 1981 Metastasis to the base of the skull: clinical findings in 43 patients. Neurology 31:530–537

Greenfield A, Resnick M I 1989 Genitourinary emergencies. Seminars in Oncology 16:516–520

Greenfield G B, Schorsch H A, Shkolnik A 1967 The various roentgen appearances of pulmonary hypertrophic osteoarthropathy. American Journal of Roentgenology Radium Therapy and Nuclear Medicine 101:927–931

Grond S, Zech D, Diefenbach C, Radbruch L, Lehmann K A 1996 Assessment of cancer pain: a prospective evaluation in 2266 cancer patients referred to a pain service. Pain 64:107–114

Grossman S A, Moynihan T J 1991 Neoplastic meningitis. Neurologic Clinics 9:843–856

Grossman S A, Sheidler V R, Swedeen K, Mucenski J, Piantadosi S 1991 Correlation of patient and caregiver ratings of cancer pain. Journal of Pain and Symptom Management 6:53–57

Gupta S R, Zdonczyk D E, Rubino F A 1990 Cranial neuropathy in systemic malignancy in a VA population [see comments]. Neurology 40:997–999

Haas G P, Pittaluga S, Gomella L et al 1989 Clinically occult Leydig cell tumor presenting with gynecomastia. Journal of Urology 142:1325–1327

Haddad P, Thaell J F, Kiely J M, Harrison E G, Miller R H 1976 Lymphoma of the spinal extradural space. Cancer 38:1862–1866

Hagen N, Stulman J, Krol G et al 1989 The role of myelography and magnetic resonance imaging in cancer patients with symptomatic and asymptomatic epidural disease. Neurology 39:309

Hagen N A 1993 Sharp, shooting neuropathic pain in the rectum or genitals: pudendal neuralgia. Journal of Pain and Symptom Management 8:496–501

Hall J H, Fleming J F 1970 The 'lumbar disc syndrome' produced by sacral metastases. Canadian Journal of Surgery 13:149–156

Hanks G W, Forbes K 1997 Opioid responsiveness. Acta Anaesthesiologica Scandinavica 41 (1 pt 2):154–158

Hansen S W, Olsen N, Rossing N, Rorth M 1990 Vascular toxicity and the mechanism underlying Raynaud's phenomenon in patients treated with cisplatin, vinblastine and bleomycin [see comments]. Annals of Oncology 1:289–292

Harper D M 1994 Pain and cramping associated with cryosurgery. Journal of Family Practice 39:551–557

Harrington K J, Pandha H S, Kelly S A, Lambert H E, Jackson J E, Waxman J 1995 Palliation of obstructive nephropathy due to malignancy. British Journal of Urology 76:101–107

Harris J K, Sutcliffe J C, Robinson N E 1996 The role of emergency surgery in malignant spinal extradural compression: assessment of functional outcome. British Journal of Neurosurgery 10:27–33

Haugen P S 1997 Pain relief. Legal aspects of pain relief for the dying. Minnesota Medicine 80:15–18

Hayashi M, Handa Y, Kobayashi H, Kawano H, Ishii H, Hirose S 1991 Plateau-wave phenomenon (I). Correlation between the appearance of plateau waves and CSF circulation in patients with intracranial hypertension. Brain 114(pt 6):2681–2691

Hayreh S S, Blodi F C, Silbermann N N, Summers T B, Potter P H 1982 Unilateral optic nerve head and choroidal metastases from a bronchial carcinoma. Ophthalmologica 185:232–241

Healey J H, Turnbull A D, Miedema B, Lane J M 1986 Acrometastases. A study of twenty-nine patients with osseous involvement of the hands and feet. Journal of Bone and Joint Surgery [Am] 68(5):743–746

Heim H M, Oei T P 1993 Comparison of prostate cancer patients with and without pain. Pain 53:159–162

Heinmoller E, Schropp T, Kisker O, Simon B, Seitz R, Weinel R J 1995 Tumor cell-induced platelet aggregation in vitro by human pancreatic cancer cell lines. Scandinavian Journal of Gastroenterology 30:1008–1016

Helweg-Larsen S 1996 Clinical outcome in metastatic spinal cord compression. A prospective study of 153 patients. Acta Neurologica Scandinavica 94:269–275

Helweg-Larsen S, Sorensen P S 1994 Symptoms and signs in metastatic spinal cord compression: a study of progression from first symptom until diagnosis in 153 patients. European Journal of Cancer 30A:396–398

Helweg-Larsen S, Rasmusson B, Sorensen P S 1990 Recovery of gait after radiotherapy in paralytic patients with metastatic epidural spinal cord compression. Neurology 40:1234–1236

Helweg-Larsen S, Wagner A, Kjaer L et al 1992 Comparison of myelography combined with postmyelographic spinal CT and MRI in suspected metastatic disease of the spinal canal. Journal of Neurooncology 13:231–237

Henderson J M, Ord R A 1997 Suicide in head and neck cancer patients. Journal of Oral and Maxillofacial Surgery 55:1217–1222

Hilkens P H, Verweij J, Stoter G, Vecht C J, van Putten W L, van den Bent M J 1996 Peripheral neurotoxicity induced by docetaxel [see comments]. Neurology 46:104–108

Hill B A, Kohut R I 1976 Metastatic adenocarcinoma of the temporal bone. Archives of Otolaryngology 102(9):568–71

Hill M E, Richards M A, Gregory W M, Smith P, Rubens R D 1993 Spinal cord compression in breast cancer: a review of 70 cases. British Journal of Cancer 68:969–973

Hirota N, Fujimoto T, Takahashi M, Fukushima Y 1998 Isolated trigeminal nerve metastases from breast cancer: an unusual cause of trigeminal mononeuropathy [in process citation]. Surgical Neurology 49:558–561

Hirschmann J V 1987 Ischemic forms of acute venous thrombosis. Archives of Dermatology 123:933–936

Hladiuk M, Huchcroft S, Temple W, Schnurr B E 1992 Arm function after axillary dissection for breast cancer: a pilot study to provide parameter estimates. Journal of Surgical Oncology 50:47–52

Hollingshead L M, Goa K L 1991 Recombinant granulocyte colony-stimulating factor (rG-CSF). A review of its pharmacological properties and prospective role in neutropenic conditions. Drugs 42:300–330

Huddart R A, Rajan B, Law M, Meyer L, Dearnaley D P 1997 Spinal cord compression in prostate cancer: treatment outcome and prognostic factors. Radiotherapy and Oncology 44:229–236

Hundrieser J 1988 A non-invasive approach to minimizing vessel pain with DTIC or BCNU. Oncological Nursing Forum 15:199

International Association for the Study of Pain: Subcommittee on taxonomy 1986 Classification of chronic pain. Pain 3(suppl):135–138

Irani J, Fournier F, Bon D, Gremmo E, Dore B, Aubert J 1997 Patient tolerance of transrectal ultrasound-guided biopsy of the prostate. British Journal of Urology 79:608–610

Jadad A R, Carroll D, Glynn C J, Moore R A, McQuay H J 1992 Morphine responsiveness of chronic pain: double-blind randomised crossover study with patient-controlled analgesia [see comments]. Lancet 339:1367–1371

Jaeckle K A 1991 Nerve plexus metastases. Neurologic Clinics 9:857–866

Jaeckle K A, Young D F, Foley K M 1985 The natural history of lumbosacral plexopathy in cancer. Neurology 35:8–15

Jayson G C, Howell A 1996 Carcinomatous meningitis in solid tumours. Annals of Oncology 7:773–786

Jones H M, Conces D J Jr, Tarver R D 1993 Painful transthoracic needle biopsy: a sign of neurogenic tumor. Journal of Thoracic Imaging 8:230–232

Jonsson O G, Sartain P, Ducore J M, Buchanan G R 1990 Bone pain as an initial symptom of childhood acute lymphoblastic leukemia: association with nearly normal hematologic indexes. Journal of Pediatrics 117(2 pt 1):233–237

Kaasa S, Malt U, Hagen S, Wist E, Moum T, Kvikstad A 1993 Psychological distress in cancer patients with advanced disease. Radiotherapy and Oncology 27:193–197

Kahn C E Jr, Messersmith R N, Samuels B L 1989 Brachial plexopathy as a complication of intraarterial cisplatin chemotherapy. Cardiovascular and Interventional Radiology 12:47–49

Kanner R, Martini N, Foley K M 1982 Nature and incidence of postthoracotomy pain. Proceedings of the American Society of Clinical Oncology 1:abstract 590

Kaplan J G, DeSouza T G, Farkash A et al 1990 Leptomeningeal metastases: comparison of clinical features and laboratory data of solid tumors, lymphomas and leukemias. Journal of Neurooncology 9:225–229

Kaplan R A, Markman M, Lucas W E, Pfeifle C, Howell S B 1985 Infectious peritonitis in patients receiving intraperitoneal chemotherapy. American Journal of Medicine 78:49–53

Katz J 1997 Prevention of phantom limb pain by regional anaesthesia. Lancet 349:519–520

Katz J, Melzack R 1990 Pain 'memories' in phantom limbs: review and clinical observations. Pain 43:319–336

Kaymakcalan H, Sequeria W, Barretta T, Ghosh B C, Steigmann F 1980 Hypertrophic osteoarthropathy with myogenic tumors of the esophagus. American Journal of Gastroenterology 74:17–20

Keller S M, Carp N Z, Levy M N, Rosen S M. 1994 Chronic post thoracotomy pain. Journal of Cardiovascular Surgery (Torino) 35(6 suppl 1):161–164

Kellgren J G 1938 On distribution of pain arising from deep somatic structures with charts of segmental pain areas. Clinical Science 4:35–46

Kelsen D P, Portenoy R K, Thaler H T et al 1995 Pain and depression in patients with newly diagnosed pancreas cancer. Journal of Clinical Oncology 13:748–755

Kelsen D P, Portenoy R, Thaler H, Tao Y, Brennan M 1997 Pain as a predictor of outcome in patients with operable pancreatic carcinoma. Surgery 122:53–59

Kemeny M M 1991 Continuous hepatic artery infusion (CHAI) as treatment of liver metastases. Are the complications worth it? Drug Safety 6:159–165

Kemeny N 1992 Review of regional therapy of liver metastases in colorectal cancer. Seminars in Oncology 19(2 suppl 3):155–162

Kempen P M, Mocek C K 1997 Bevel direction, dura geometry, and hole size in membrane puncture: laboratory report. Regional Anesthesia 22(3):267–272

Killer H E, Hess K 1990 Natural history of radiation-induced brachial plexopathy compared with surgically treated patients. Journal of Neurology 237:247–250

Kissel J T, Mendell J R 1996 Neuropathies associated with monoclonal gammopathies. Neuromuscular Disorders 6:3–18

Koehler P J, Verbiest H, Jager J, Vecht C J 1996 Delayed radiation myelopathy: serial MR-imaging and pathology. Clinical Neurology and Neurosurgery 98:197–201

Kontturi M, Kauppila A 1982 Ureteric complications following treatment of gynaecological cancer. Annals Chirurgiae et Gynaecologiae 71:232–238

Kori S H 1995 Diagnosis and management of brachial plexus lesions in cancer patients. Oncology (Huntingt) 9:756–760, 765

Kori S H, Foley K M, Posner J B 1981 Brachial plexus lesions in patients with cancer: 100 cases. Neurology 31:45–50

Krane R J, Perrone T L 1981 A young man with testicular and abdominal pain. New England Journal of Medicine 305:331–336

Kroner K, Krebs B, Skov J, Jorgensen H S 1989 Immediate and long-term phantom breast syndrome after mastectomy: incidence, clinical characteristics and relationship to pre-mastectomy breast pain. Pain 36:327–334

Kudo S, Tsushima N, Sawada Y et al 1991 [Serious complications of intravesical bacillus Calmette-Guerin therapy in patients with bladder cancer.] Nippon Hinyokika Gakkai Zasshi 82:1594–1602

Kukla L J, McGuire W P, Lad T, Saltiel M 1982 Acute vascular episodes associated with therapy for carcinomas of the upper aerodigestive tract with bleomycin, vincristine, and cisplatin. Cancer Treatment Reports 66(2):369–370

Kuntz K M, Kokmen E, Stevens J C, Miller P, Offord K P, Ho M M 1992 Post-lumbar puncture headaches: experience in 501 consecutive procedures. Neurology 42:1884–1887

Kwekkeboom K 1996 Postmastectomy pain syndromes. Cancer Nursing 19:37–43

Labrie F, Dupont A, Belanger A, Lachance R 1987 Flutamide eliminates the risk of disease flare in prostatic cancer patients treated with a luteinizing hormone-releasing hormone agonist. Journal of Urology 138:804–806

Lachance D H, O'Neill BP, Harper C M Jr, Banks P M, Cascino T L 1991 Paraneoplastic brachial plexopathy in a patient with Hodgkin's disease. Mayo Clinic Proceedings 66:97–101

Laitt R D, Kumar B, Leatherbarrow B, Bonshek R E, Jackson A 1996 Cystic optic nerve meningioma presenting with acute proptosis. Eye 10(pt 6):744–746

Lambert D H, Hurley R J, Hertwig L, Datta S 1997 Role of needle gauge and tip configuration in the production of lumbar puncture headache. Regional Anesthesia 22:66–72

Lancee W J, Vachon M L, Ghadirian P, Adair W, Conway B, Dryer D 1994 The impact of pain and impaired role performance on distress in persons with cancer. Canadian Journal of Psychiatry 39:617–622

Laredo J D, Lakhdari K, Bellaiche L, Hamze B, Janklewicz P, Tubiana J M 1995 Acute vertebral collapse: CT findings in benign and malignant nontraumatic cases. Radiology 194:41–48

Larue F, Colleau S M, Breasseur L, Cleeland C S 1995 Multicentre study of cancer pain and its treatment in France. British Medical Journal 310:1034–1037

Lawson W, Reino A J 1997 Isolated sphenoid sinus disease: an analysis of 132 cases. Laryngoscope 107(12 pt 1):1590–1595

Leaney B J, Martin M 1992 Breast pain associated with mammographic compression. Australasian Radiology 36:120–123
Lederman R J, Wilbourn A J 1984 Brachial plexopathy: recurrent cancer or radiation? Neurology 34:1331–1335
Leibold R A, Yealy D M, Coppola M, Cantees K K 1993 Post-dural-puncture headache: characteristics, management, and prevention. Annals of Emergency Medicine 22:1863–1870
Lembersky B C, Ratain M J, Golomb H M 1988 Skeletal complications in hairy cell leukemia: diagnosis and therapy. Journal of Clinical Oncology 6:1280–1284
Leo S, Tatulli C, Taveri R, Campanella G A, Carrieri G, Colucci G 1994 Dermatological toxicity from chemotherapy containing 5-fluorouracil. Journal of Chemotherapy 6(6):423–426
Leonheart E E, DiStazio J 1994 Acrometastases. Initial presentation as diffuse ankle pain. Journal of the American Podiatric Medical Association 84:625–627
Levine M, Hirsh J, Gent M et al 1994 Double-blind randomised trial of a very-low-dose warfarin for prevention of thromboembolism in stage IV breast cancer [see comments]. Lancet 343:886–889
Levy M H 1991 Effective integration of pain management into comprehensive cancer care. Postgraduate Medical Journal 67(suppl 2):S35–43
Lipman A G 1996 Analgesic drugs for neuropathic and sympathetically maintained pain. Clinics in Geriatric Medicine 12:501–515
Loevner L A, Yousem D M 1997 Overlooked metastatic lesions of the occipital condyle: a missed case treasure trove. Radiographics 17:1111–1121
Lokich J J, Moore C 1984 Chemotherapy-associated palmar-plantar erythrodysesthesia syndrome. Annals of Internal Medicine 101:798–799
LoMonaco M, Milone M, Batocchi A P, Padua L, Restuccia D, Tonali P 1992 Cisplatin neuropathy: clinical course and neurophysiological findings. Journal of Neurology 239:199–204
Loprinzi C L, Ghosh C, Camoriano J et al 1997 Phase III controlled evaluation of sucralfate to alleviate stomatitis in patients receiving fluorouracil-based chemotherapy. Journal of Clinical Oncology 15:1235–1238
Lorimer J W, Semelhago L C, Barber G G 1994 Venous gangrene of the extremities [see comments]. Canadian Journal of Surgery 37:379–384
Lossos A, Siegal T 1992 Numb chin syndrome in cancer patients: etiology, response to treatment, and prognostic significance [see comments]. Neurology 42:1181–1184
Lybecker H, Djernes M, Schmidt J F 1995 Postdural puncture headache (PDPH): onset, duration, severity, and associated symptoms. An analysis of 75 consecutive patients with PDPH. Acta Anaesthesiologica Scandinavica 39:605–612
McCaffery M, Thorpe D M 1989 Differences in perception of pain and the development of adversarial relationships among health care providers. In: Hill C S, Fields W S (eds) Drug treatment of cancer pain in a drug oriented society. Advances in pain research and therapy, vol 11. Raven, New York, pp 19–26
McCarthy G M, Skillings J R 1992 Jaw and other orofacial pain in patients receiving vincristine for the treatment of cancer. Oral Surgery, Oral Medicine, Oral Pathology 74:299–304
McConaha C, Bastiani A M, Kaye W H 1996 Significant reduction of post-lumbar puncture headaches by the use of a 29-gauge spinal needle. Biological Psychiatry 39:1058–1060
McDonald D R 1991 Neurological complications of chemotherapy. Neurology Clinics 9:955–967
McEwan A J 1997 Unsealed source therapy of painful bone metastases: an update. Seminars in Nuclear Medicine 27:165–182
McQuay H J, Tramer M, Nye B A, Carroll D, Wiffen P J, Moore R A 1996 A systematic review of antidepressants in neuropathic pain. Pain 68:217–227
Malik I A, Moid I, Haq S, Sabih M 1997 A double-blind, placebo-controlled, randomized trial to evaluate the role of tetrachlorodecaoxide in the management of chemotherapy-induced oral mucositis. Journal of Pain and Symptom Management 14:82–87
Marangoni C, Lacerenza M, Formaglio F, Smirne S, Marchettini P 1993 Sensory disorder of the chest as presenting symptom of lung cancer. Journal of Neurology, Neurosurgery and Psychiatry 56:1033–1034
Maranzano E, Latini P 1995 Effectiveness of radiation therapy without surgery in metastatic spinal cord compression: final results from a prospective trial [see comments]. International Journal of Radiation Oncology and Biological Physics 32:959–967
Margolick J, Bonomi P, Fordham E, Yordan E, Slayton R, Wilbanks G 1982 Hypertrophic osteoarthropathy associated with endometrial carcinoma. Gynecologic Oncology 13:399–404
Marino C, Zoppi M, Morelli F, Buoncristiano U, Pagni E 1986 Pain in early cancer of the lungs. Pain 27:57–62
Markman M 1986 Cytotoxic intracavitary chemotherapy. American Journal of the Medical Sciences 291:175–179
Marks R M, Sachar E J 1973 Undertreatment of medical impatients with narcotic analgesics. Annals of Internal Medicine 78:173–181
Marshall J A, Mahanna G K 1997 Cancer in the differential diagnosis of orofacial pain. Dental Clinics of North America 41:355–365
Martin R, Jourdain S, Clairoux M, Tetrault J P 1994 Duration of decubitus position after epidural blood patch. Canadian Journal of Anaesthesia 41:23–25
Martin S, Jones J S, Wynn B N 1996 Does warming local anesthetic reduce the pain of subcutaneous injection? American Journal of Emergency Medicine 14:10–12
Martinez-Lavin M 1997 Hypertrophic osteoarthropathy. Current Opinions in Rheumatology 9:83–86
Massie M J, Holland J C 1992 The cancer patient with pain: psychiatric complications and their management. Journal of Pain and Symptom Management 7:99–109
Matsuda M, Yoneda S, Handa H, Gotoh H 1979 Cerebral hemodynamic changes during plateau waves in brain-tumor patients. Journal of Neurosurgery 50:483–488
Matsumura Y, Ozaki Y, Ohmori H. 1983 Intravesical adriamycin chemotherapy in bladder cancer. Cancer Chemotherapy and Pharmacology 11 (Suppl):S69–73
Matsumura Y, Akaza H, Isaka S et al 1992 The 4th study of prophylactic intravesical chemotherapy with adriamycin in the treatment of superficial bladder cancer: the experience of the Japanese Urological Cancer Research Group for Adriamycin. Cancer Chemotherapy and Pharmacology 30(suppl):S10–14
Maunsell E, Brisson J, Deschenes L 1993 Arm problems and psychological distress after surgery for breast cancer. Can J Surg 36(4):315–320
Medina L S, Pinter J D, Zurakowski D, Davis R G, Kuban K, Barnes P D 1997 Children with headache: clinical predictors of surgical space-occupying lesions and the role of neuroimaging. Radiology 202:819–824
Mellor S G, McCutchan J D 1989 Gynaecomastia and occult Leydig cell tumour of the testis. British Journal of Urology 63:420–422
Melzack R 1975 The McGill Pain Questionnaire: major properties and scoring methods. Pain 1:277–299
Melzack R 1987 The short-form McGill Pain Questionnaire. Pain 30:191–197
Mercadante S 1997 Malignant bone pain: pathophysiology and treatment. Pain 69:1–18
Metheetrairut C, Brown D H 1993 Glossopharyngeal neuralgia and syncope secondary to neck malignancy. Journal of Otolaryngology 22:18–20
Miaskowski C 1996 Special needs related to the pain and discomfort of

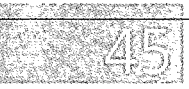

patients with gynecologic cancer. Journal of Obstetrics, Gynecologic and Neonatal Nursing 25:181–188
Miaskowski C, Dibble S L 1995 The problem of pain in outpatients with breast cancer. Oncologic Nursing Forum 22:791–797
Miaskowski C, Donovan M 1992 Implementation of the American Pain Society Quality Assurance Standards for Relief of Acute Pain and Cancer Pain in oncology nursing practice. Oncologic Nursing Forum 19:411–415
Miaskowski C, Nichols R, Brody R, Synold T 1994 Assessment of patient satisfaction utilizing the American Pain Society's Quality Assurance Standards on acute and cancer-related pain. Journal of Pain and Symptom Management 9:5–11
Milross C G, Davies M A, Fisher R, Mameghan J, Mameghan H 1997 The efficacy of treatment for malignant epidural spinal cord compression. Australasian Radiology 41:137–142
Minsky B D, Cohen A M 1988 Minimizing the toxicity of pelvic radiation therapy in rectal cancer. Oncology (Huntingt) 2:21–25, 28–29
Miyamoto M, Sudo T, Kuyama T 1991 Spontaneous rupture of hepatocellular carcinoma: a review of 172 Japanese cases. American Journal of Gastroenterology 86(1):67–71
Mollman J E, Hogan W M, Glover D J, McCluskey L F 1988 Unusual presentation of cis-platinum neuropathy. Neurology 38:488–490
Mondrup K, Olsen N K, Pfeiffer P, Rose C 1990 Clinical and electrodiagnostic findings in breast cancer patients with radiation-induced brachial plexus neuropathy. Acta Neurologica Scandinavica 81(2):153–158
Morales M, Llanos M, Dorta J 1997 Superior vena cava thrombosis secondary to hickman catheter and complete resolution after fibrinolytic therapy. Support Care Cancer 5:67–69
Morewood G H 1993 A rational approach to the cause, prevention and treatment of postdural puncture headache [see comments]. Canadian Medical Association Journal 149:1087–1093
Moris G, Roig C, Misiego M, Alvarez A, Berciano J, Pascual J 1998 The distinctive headache of the occipital condyle syndrome: a report of four cases. Headache 38:308–311
Morris K P, Hughes C, Hardy S P, Matthews J N, Coulthard M G 1994 Pain after subcutaneous injection of recombinant human erythropoietin: does Emla cream help? Nephrology, Dialysis, Transplantatian 9:1299–1301
Morrison G A, Sterkers J M 1996 Unusual presentations of acoustic tumours. Clinics in Otolaryngology 21:80–83
Mrozek-Orlowski M, Christie J, Flamme C, Novak J 1991 Pain associated with peripheral infusion of carmustine. Oncologic Nursing Forum 18:942
Muggia F M, Vafai D, Natale R et al 1995 Paclitaxel 3-hour infusion given alone and combined with carboplatin: preliminary results of dose-escalation trials. Seminars in Oncology 22(4 suppl 9):63–66
Mulholland M W, Debas H, Bonica J J 1990 Diseases of the liver, biliary system and pancreas. In: Bonica J J (ed) The management of pain. vol. 2. Lea & Febiger, Philadelphia, pp 1214–1231
Muram D, Oxorn H, Curry R H, Drouin P, Walters J H 1981 Postradiation ureteral obstruction: a reappraisal. American Journal of Obstetrics and Gynecology 139:289–293
Nash P A, Bruce J E, Indudhara R, Shinohara K 1996 Transrectal ultrasound guided prostatic nerve blockade eases systematic needle biopsy of the prostate. Journal of Urology 155:607–609
Neer R M, Ferrucci J T, Wang C A, Brennan M, Buttrick W F, Vickery A L 1981 A 77-year-old man with epigastric pain, hypercalcemia, and a retroperitoneal mass. New England Journal of Medicine 305:874–883
Nemmers D W, Thorpe P E, Knibbe M A, Beard D W 1990 Upper extremity venous thrombosis. Case report and literature review. Orthopedic Review 19:164–172
Newman M L, Brennan M, Passik S 1996 Lymphedema complicated by pain and psychological distress: a case with complex treatment needs. Journal of Pain and Symptom Management 12:376–379
Nicolodi M, Frezzotti R, Diadori A, Nuti A, Sicuteri F 1997 Phantom eye: features and prevalence. The predisposing role of headache. Cephalalgia 17:501–504
Nikolajsen L, Ilkjaer S, Christensen J H, Kroner K, Jensen T S 1997a Randomised trial of epidural bupivacaine and morphine in prevention of stump and phantom pain in lower-limb amputation [see comments]. Lancet 350:1353–1357
Nikolajsen L, Ilkjaer S, Kroner K, Christensen J H, Jensen T S 1997b The influence of preamputation pain on postamputation stump and phantom pain. Pain 72:393–405
Nussbaum M L, Campana T J, Weese J L 1993 Radiation-induced intestinal injury. Clinics in Plastic Surgery 20:573–580
Ohno R, Yoshida H, Fukutani H et al 1993 Multi-institutional study of all-*trans*-retinoic acid as a differentiation therapy of refractory acute promyelocytic leukemia. Leukaemia Study Group of the Ministry of Health and Welfare. Leukemia 7:1722–1727
Olsen N K, Pfeiffer P, Mondrup K, Rose C 1990 Radiation-induced brachial plexus neuropathy in breast cancer patients. Acta Oncologica 29:885–890
Olson M E, Chernik N L, Posner J B 1974 Infiltration of the leptomeninges by systemic cancer. A clinical and pathologic study. Archives of Neurology 30:122–137
Olsson H, Alm P, Kristoffersson U, Landin-Olsson M 1984 Hypophyseal tumor and gynecomastia preceding bilateral breast cancer development in a man. Cancer 53:1974–1977
O'Rourke T, George C B, Redmond J D et al 1986 Spinal computed tomography and computed tomographic metrizamide myelography in the early diagnosis of metastatic disease. Journal of Clinical Oncology 4:576–583
Ovesen P, Kroner K, Ornsholt J, Bach K 1991 Phantom-related phenomena after rectal amputation: prevalence and clinical characteristics. Pain 44:289–291
Palmon S C, Lloyd A T, Kirsch J R 1998 The effect of needle gauge and lidocaine pH on pain during intradermal injection. Anesthesia and Analgesia 86:379–381
Paredes J P, Puente J L, Potel J 1990 Variations in sensitivity after sectioning the intercostobrachial nerve. American Journal of Surgery 160:525–528
Pavy T J, Doyle D L 1996 Prevention of phantom limb pain by infusion of local anaesthetic into the sciatic nerve [see comments]. Anaesthesia and Intensive Care 24:599–600
Payten R J 1972 Facial pain as the first symptom in acoustic neuroma. Journal of Laryngology and Otology 86:523–534
Perkins J M, Magee T R, Galland R B 1996 Phlegmasia caerulea dolens and venous gangrene [see comments]. British Journal of Surgery 83:19–23
Perry J R, Deodhare S S, Bilbao J M, Murray D, Muller P 1993 The significance of spinal cord compression as the initial manifestation of lymphoma. Neurosurgery 32:157–162
Peterson K, Forsyth P A, Posner J B 1994 Paraneoplastic sensorimotor neuropathy associated with breast cancer. Journal of Neurooncology 21:159–170
Phillips E, Levine A M 1989 Metastatic lesions of the upper cervical spine. Spine 14:1071–1077
Pierce S M, Recht A, Lingos T I et al 1992 Long-term radiation complications following conservative surgery (CS) and radiation therapy (RT) in patients with early stage breast cancer [see comments]. International Journal of Radiation Oncology and Biological Physics 23(5):915–923
Pines A, Kaplinsky N, Olchovsky D, Frankl O 1984 Rheumatoid arthritis-like syndrome: a presenting symptom of malignancy. Report of 3 cases and review of the literature. European Journal of Rheumatology and Inflammation 7:51–55

Plante-Bordeneuve V, Baudrimont M, Gorin N C, Gherardi R K 1994 Subacute sensory neuropathy associated with Hodgkin's disease. Journal of the Neurological Sciences 121:155–158

Plotkin D, Lechner J J, Jung W E, Rosen P J 1978 Tamoxifen flare in advanced breast cancer. Journal of the American Medical Association 240:2644–2660

Portenoy R K 1991 Issues in the management of neuropathic pain. In: Basbaum A, Besson J-M (eds) Towards a new pharmacotherapy of pain. John Wiley, New York, pp 393–416

Portenoy R K, Hagen N A 1990 Breakthrough pain: definition, prevalence and characteristics [see comments]. Pain 41:273–281

Portenoy R K, Abissi C J, Robbins J B 1983 Increased intracranial pressure with normal ventricular size due to superior vena cava obstruction [letter]. Archives of Neurology 40:598

Portenoy R K, Duma C, Foley K M 1986 Acute herpetic and postherpetic neuralgia: clinical review and current management. Annals of Neurology 20:651–664

Portenoy R K, Lipton R B, Foley K M 1987 Back pain in the cancer patient: an algorithm for evaluation and management. Neurology 37:134–138

Portenoy R K, Galer B S, Salamon O et al 1989 Identification of epidural neoplasm. Radiography and bone scintigraphy in the symptomatic and asymptomatic spine. Cancer 64:2207–2213

Portenoy R K, Foley K M, Inturrisi C E 1990 The nature of opioid responsiveness and its implications for neuropathic pain: new hypotheses derived from studies of opioid infusions [see comments]. Pain 43:273–286

Portenoy R K, Miransky J, Thaler H T et al 1992 Pain in ambulatory patients with lung or colon cancer. Prevalence, characteristics, and effect. Cancer 70:1616–1624

Portenoy R K, Kornblith A B, Wong G et al 1994a Pain in ovarian cancer patients. Prevalence, characteristics, and associated symptoms. Cancer 74:907–915

Portenoy R K, Thaler H T, Kornblith A B et al 1994b Symptom prevalence, characteristics and distress in a cancer population. Quality of Life Research 3:183–189

Portenoy R K, Thaler H T, Kornblith A B et al 1994c The Memorial Symptom Assessment Scale: an instrument for the evaluation of symptom prevalence, characteristics and distress. European Journal of Cancer 30A:1326–1336

Porter A D, Simpson A H, Davis A M, Griffin A M, Bell R S 1994 Diagnosis and management of sacral bone tumours [see comments]. Canadian Journal of Surgery 37:473–478

Posner J B 1987 Back pain and epidural spinal cord compression. Medical Clinics of North America 71:185–205

Postma T J, Vermorken J B, Liefting A J, Pinedo H M, Heimans J J 1995 Paclitaxel-induced neuropathy. Annals of Oncology 6:489–494

Prager J M, Roychowdhury S, Gorey M T, Lowe G M, Diamond C W, Ragin A 1996 Spinal headaches after myelograms: comparison of needle types. American Journal of Roentgenology 167:1289–1292

Prevost A, Nazeyrollas P, Milosevic D, Fernandez-Valoni A 1998 Malignant pleural effusions treated with high dose intrapleural doxycycline: clinical efficacy and tolerance. Oncology Report 5:363–366

Priest J R, Ramsay N K, Steinherz P G et al 1982 A syndrome of thrombosis and hemorrhage complicating L-asparaginase therapy for childhood acute lymphoblastic leukemia. Journal of Pediatrics 100:984–989

Pucino F, Danielson B D, Carlson J D et al 1988 Patient tolerance to intravenous potassium chloride with and without lidocaine. Drug Intelligence and Clinical Pharmacology 22:676–679

Puel V, Caudry M, Le Metayer P et al 1993 Superior vena cava thrombosis related to catheter malposition in cancer chemotherapy given through implanted ports. Cancer 72:2248–2252

Quesada J R, Talpaz M, Rios A, Kurzrock R, Gutterman J U 1986 Clinical toxicity of interferons in cancer patients: a review. Journal of Clinical Oncology 4:234–243

Ramamurthy L, Cooper R A 1991 Metastatic carcinoma to the male breast. British Journal of Radiology 64:277–278

Ransom D T, Patel S R, Keeney G L, Malkasian G D, Edmonson J H 1990 Papillary serous carcinoma of the peritoneum. A review of 33 cases treated with platin-based chemotherapy. Cancer 66:1091–1094

Ratcliffe M A, Gilbert F J, Dawson A A, Bennett B 1995 Diagnosis of avascular necrosis of the femoral head in patients treated for lymphoma. Hematological Oncology 13:131–137

Ready L B 1991 The treatment of post operative pain. In: Bond M R, Charlton J E, Woolf C J (eds) Proceedings of the VIth World Congress on Pain. Pain research and clinical management, vol 4. Elsevier, Amsterdam, pp 53–58

Reddel R R, Sutherland R L 1984 Tamoxifen stimulation of human breast cancer cell proliferation in vitro: a possible model for tamoxifen tumour flare. European Journal of Cancer and Clinical Oncology 20:1419–1424

Redding S W, Montgomery M T 1989 Acyclovir prophylaxis for oral herpes simplex virus infection in patients with bone marrow transplants. Oral Surgery, Oral Medicine, Oral Pathology 67:680–683

Reese J A, Blocker S H 1994 Torsion of pedunculated hepatocellular carcinoma. Report of a case in a young woman presenting with abdominal pain. Missouri Medicine 91:594–595

Reuben D B, Mor V, Hiris J 1988 Clinical symptoms and length of survival in patients with terminal cancer. Archives of Internal Medicine 148:1586–1591

Rezkalla S, Kloner R A, Ensley J et al 1989 Continuous ambulatory ECG monitoring during fluorouracil therapy: a prospective study. Journal of Clinical Oncology 7:509–514

Richardson R R, Siqueira E B, Oi S, Nunez C 1979 Neurogenic tumors of the brachial plexus: report of two cases. Neurosurgery 4(1):66–70

Rider C A 1990 Oral mucositis. A complication of radiotherapy. New York State Dental Journal 56:37–39

Ripamonti C 1994 Management of bowel obstruction in advanced cancer. Current Opinions in Oncology 6:351–357

Rittenberg C N, Gralla R J, Rehmeyer T A 1995 Assessing and managing venous irritation associated with vinorelbine tartrate (Navelbine). Oncologic Nursing Forum 22:707–710

Robinson R G, Preston D F, Schiefelbein M, Baxter K G 1995 Strontium 89 therapy for the palliation of pain due to osseous metastases. Journal of the American Medical Association 274:420–424

Rocke L K, Loprinzi C L, Lee J K et al 1993 A randomized clinical trial of two different durations of oral cryotherapy for prevention of 5-fluorouracil-related stomatitis. Cancer 72:2234–2238

Rodichok L D, Ruckdeschel J C, Harper G R et al 1986 Early detection and treatment of spinal epidural metastases: the role of myelography. Annals of Neurology 20:696–702

Rogues A M, Vidal E, Boudinet F, Loustaud V, Arnaud M, Liozon F 1993 Breast cancer with systemic manifestations mimicking Still's disease. Journal of Rheumatology 20:1786–1787

Rosenfeld C S, Broder L E 1984 Cisplatin-induced autonomic neuropathy. Cancer Treatment Reports 68:659–660

Rosenthal M A, Rosen D, Raghavan D et al 1992 Spinal cord compression in prostate cancer. A 10-year experience. British Journal of Urology 69:530–533

Rosenthal S, Kaufman S 1974 Vincristine neurotoxicity. Annals of Internal Medicine 80:733–737

Rotstein J, Good R A 1957 Steroid pseudorheumatism. Archives of Internal Medicine 99:545–555

Rotta F T, Bradley W G 1997 Marked improvement of severe polyneuropathy associated with multifocal osteosclerotic myeloma following surgery, radiation, and chemotherapy. Muscle and Nerve 20:1035–1037

Rowinsky E K, Chaudhry V, Cornblath D R, Donehower R C 1993 Neurotoxicity of Taxol. Journal of the National Cancer Institute Monographs (15):107–15

Ruff R L, Lanska D J 1989 Epidural metastases in prospectively evaluated veterans with cancer and back pain. Cancer 63:2234–2241

Rusthoven J J, Ahlgren P, Elhakim T et al 1988 Varicella-zoster infection in adult cancer patients. A population study. Archives of Internal Medicine 148:1561–1566

Saeter G, Fossa S D, Norman N 1987 Gynaecomastia following cytotoxic therapy for testicular cancer. British Journal of Urology 59:348–352

Sahdev P, Wolff M, Widmann W D 1985 Mesenteric venous thrombosis associated with estrogen therapy for treatment of prostatic carcinoma. Journal of Urology 134:563–564

Salner A L, Botnick L E, Herzog A G et al 1981 Reversible brachial plexopathy following primary radiation therapy for breast cancer. Cancer Treatment Reports 65:797–802

Sandler S G, Tobin W, Henderson E S 1969 Vincristine-induced neuropathy. A clinical study of fifty leukemic patients. Neurology 19:367–374

Sanz-Altamira P M, Spence L D, Huberman M S et al 1997 Selective chemoembolization in the management of hepatic metastases in refractory colorectal carcinoma: a phase II trial. Diseases of the Colon and Rectum 40:770–775

Sapir R, Catane R, Cherny N I 1997 Cancer pain: knowledge and attitudes of physicians in Israel (Meeting abstract). Proceedings of the Annual Meeting of the American Society of Clinical Oncologists 16

Sawaya R E, Ligon B L 1994 Thromboembolic complications associated with brain tumors. Journal of Neurooncology 22:173–181

Saxman S B, Seitz D 1997 Breast cancer associated with palmar fasciitis and arthritis. Journal of Clinical Oncology 15:3515–3516

Scarfone R J, Jasani M, Gracely E J 1998 Pain of local anesthetics: rate of administration and buffering. Annals of Emergency Medicine 31:36–40

Schick R M, Jolesz F, Barnes P D, Macklis J D 1989 MR diagnosis of dural venous sinus thrombosis complicating L-asparaginase therapy. Computerized Medical Imaging and Graphics 13:319–327

Schilsky R L, Choi K E, Grayhack J, Grimmer D, Guarnieri C, Fullem L 1990 Phase I clinical and pharmacologic study of intraperitoneal cisplatin and fluorouracil in patients with advanced intraabdominal cancer. Journal of Clinical Oncology 8:2054–2061

Schöenen J, Broux R, Moonen G 1992 Unilateral facial pain as the first symptom of lung cancer: are there diagnostic clues? Cephalalgia 12:178–179

Schonenberg P, Bastid C, Guedes J, Sahel J 1991 [Percutaneous echography-guided alcohol block of the celiac plexus as treatment of painful syndromes of the upper abdomen: study of 21 cases. Schweizerische Medizinische Wochenschrift 121:528–531

Schroeder T L, Farlane D F, Goldberg L H 1998 Pain as an atypical presentation of squamous cell carcinoma. Dermatologic Surgery 24:263–266

Schulthesis T E 1994 Spinal cord radiation tolerance [editorial]. International Journal of Radiation Oncology and Biological Physics 30:735–736

Schultheiss T E, Stephens L C 1992 Invited review: permanent radiation myelopathy. British Journal of Radiology 65:737–753

Seefeld P H, Bargen J A 1943 The spread of carcinoma of the rectum: invasion of lymphatics, veins and nerves. Annals of Surgery 118:76–90

Servodidio C A, Abramson D H 1992 Presenting signs and symptoms of choroidal melanoma: what do they mean? Annals of Ophthalmology 24:190–194

Shakespeare T P, Stevens M J 1996 Unilateral facial pain and lung cancer. Australasian Radiology 40:45–46

Shane E, Parisien M, Henderson J E et al 1997 Tumor-induced osteomalacia: clinical and basic studies. Journal of Bone and Mineral Research 12(9):1502–1511

Shapiro J S 1987 Breast cancer presenting as periostitis. Postgraduate Medicine 82:139–140

Shapshay S M, Elber E, Strong M S 1976 Occult tumors of the infratemporal fossa: report of seven cases appearing as preauricular facial pain. Archives of Otolaryngology 102:535–538

Sharma O P 1995 Symptoms and signs in pulmonary medicine: old observations and new interpretations. Disease-a-Month 41:577–638

Shearer R J, Davies J H, Dowsett M et al 1990 Aromatase inhibition in advanced prostatic cancer: preliminary communication. British Journal of Cancer 62:275–276

Shegda L M, McCorkle R 1990 Continuing care in the community. Journal of Pain and Symptom Management 5:279–286

Sherrier R H, Sostman H D 1993 Magnetic resonance imaging of the brachial plexus. Journal of Thoracic Imaging 8:27–33

Shiel W C Jr, Prete P E, Jason M, Andrews B S 1985 Palmar fasciitis and arthritis with ovarian and non-ovarian carcinomas. New syndrome. American Journal of Medicine 79:640–644

Shike M, Gillin J S, Kemeny N, Daly J M, Kurtz R C 1986 Severe gastroduodenal ulcerations complicating hepatic artery infusion chemotherapy for metastatic colon cancer. American Journal of Gastroenterology 81:176–179

Shvartzman P, Bonneh D 1994 Local skin irritation in the course of subcutaneous morphine infusion: a challenge. Journal of Palliative Care 10:44–45

Siegal T 1991 Muscle cramps in the cancer patient: causes and treatment. Journal of Pain and Symptom Management 6:84–91

Siegal T, Haim N 1990 Cisplatin-induced peripheral neuropathy. Frequent off-therapy deterioration, demyelinating syndromes, and muscle cramps. Cancer 66:1117–1123

Sigsbee B, Deck M D, Posner J B 1979 Nonmetastatic superior sagittal sinus thrombosis complicating systemic cancer. Neurology 29:139–146

Silen W 1983 Cope's early diagnosis of the acute abdomen, 16th edn. Oxford, New York.

Sim F H 1992 Metastatic bone disease of the pelvis and femur. Instructional Course Lectures 41:317–327

Simon D L 1997 Algorithm for timely recognition and treatment of complex regional pain syndrome (CRPS): a new approach for objective assessment [letter]. Clinical Journal of Pain 13:264–272

Sinaki M, Merritt J L, Stillwell G K 1977 Tension myalgia of the pelvic floor. Mayo Clinic Proceedings 52:717–722

Sklaroff D M, Gnaneswaran P, Sklaroff R B 1978 Postirradiation ureteric stricture. Gynecologic Oncology 6:538–545

Smith J, Thompson J M 1995 Phantom limb pain and chemotherapy in pediatric amputees. Mayo Clinic Proceedings 70:357–364

Socie G, Cahn J Y, Carmelo J et al 1997 Avascular necrosis of bone after allogeneic bone marrow transplantation: analysis of risk factors for 4388 patients by the Societe Francaise de Greffe de Moelle (SFGM). British Journal of Haematology 97:865–870

Soloway M S, Schellhammer P F, Smith J A, Chodak G W, Kennealey G T 1996 Bicalutamide in the treatment of advanced prostatic carcinoma: a phase II multicenter trial. Urology 47(1A suppl):33–37, 48–53

Sorensen S, Borgesen S E, Rohde K et al 1990 Metastatic epidural spinal cord compression. Results of treatment and survival. Cancer 65:1502–1508

Sozzi G, Marotta P, Piatti L 1987 Vagoglossopharyngeal neuralgia with syncope in the course of carcinomatous meningitis. Italian Journal of Neurological Sciences 8(3):271–275

Spencer C M, Goa K L 1995 Amifostine. A review of its pharmacodynamic and pharmacokinetic properties, and therapeutic

potential as a radioprotector and cytotoxic chemoprotector. Drugs 50:1001–1031
Spijkervet F K, van Saene H K, van Saene J J, Panders A K, Vermey A, Mehta D M 1990 Mucositis prevention by selective elimination of oral flora in irradiated head and neck cancer patients.Journal of Oral Pathology 19(10):486–489
Sponseller P D 1996 Evaluating the child with back pain. Journal of Oral Pathology American Family Physician 54:1933–1941
Sridhar K S, Rao R K, Kunhardt B 1987 Skeletal muscle metastases from lung cancer. Cancer 59:1530–1534
Srinivasan V, Miree J Jr, Lloyd F A 1972 Bilateral mastectomy and irradiation in the prevention of estrogen induced gynecomastia. Journal of Urology 107:624–625
Stanton-Hicks M, Janig W, Hassenbusch S, Haddox J D, Boas R, Wilson P 1995 Reflex sympathetic dystrophy: changing concepts and taxonomy [see comments]. Pain 63:127–133
Stark R J, Henson R A, Evans S J 1982 Spinal metastases. A retrospective survey from a general hospital. Brain 105(pt 1):189–213
Steiner I, Siegal T 1989 Muscle cramps in cancer patients. Cancer 63:574–577
Stevens M J, Gonet Y M 1990 Malignant psoas syndrome: recognition of an oncologic entity. Australasian Radiology 34:150–154
Stillman M 1990 Perineal pain: diagnosis and management, with particular attention to perineal pain of cancer. In: Foley K M, Bonica J J, Ventafrida V (eds) Second international congress on cancer pain. Advances in pain research and therapy, vol 16. Raven, New York, pp 359–377
Stjernsward J, Colleau S M, Ventafridda V 1996 The World Health Organization Cancer Pain and Palliative Care Program. Past, present, and future. Journal of Pain and Symptom Management 12:65–72
Strang P 1997 Existential consequences of unrelieved cancer pain. Palliative Medicine 11:299–305
Stranjalis G, Jamjoom A, Torrens M 1992 Epidural lipomatosis in steroid-treated patients. Spine 17:1268
Stryker J A, Sommerville K, Perez R, Velkley D E 1990 Sacral plexus injury after radiotherapy for carcinoma of cervix. Cancer 66:1488–1492
Stull D M, Hollis L S, Gregory R E, Sheidler V R, Grossman S A 1996 Pain in a comprehensive cancer center: more frequently due to treatment than underlying tumor (Meeting abstract). Proceedings of the Annual Meeting of the American Society of Clinical Oncologists 15:abstract 1717
Sundaresan N, Galicich J H, Lane J M, Greenberg H S 1981 Treatment of odontoid fractures in cancer patients. Journal of Neurosurgery 54:187–192
Sundaresan N, Galicich J H, Lane J M, Bains M S, McCormack P 1985 Treatment of neoplastic epidural cord compression by vertebral body resection and stabilization. Journal of Neurosurgery 63:676–684
Sundaresan N, Steinberger A A, Moore F et al 1996 Indications and results of combined anterior-posterior approaches for spine tumor surgery. Journal of Neurosurgery 85:438–446
Suwanwela N, Phanthumchinda K, Kaoropthum S 1994 Headache in brain tumor: a cross-sectional study. Headache 34:435–438
Swanson M W 1993 Ocular metastatic disease. Optometry Clinics 3:79–99
Swift T R, Nichols F T 1984 The droopy shoulder syndrome. Neurology 34:212–215
Synek V M 1986 Validity of median nerve somatosensory evoked potentials in the diagnosis of supraclavicular brachial plexus lesions. Electroencephalography and Clinical Neurophysiology 65:27–35
Syrjala K L, Chapko M E 1995 Evidence for a biopsychosocial model of cancer treatment-related pain. Pain 61:69–79
Talmi Y P, Waller A, Bercovici M et al 1997 Pain experienced by patients with terminal head and neck carcinoma. Cancer 80:1117–1123
Tarkkila P, Huhtala J, Salminen U 1994 Difficulties in spinal needle use. Insertion characteristics and failure rates associated with 25-, 27- and 29-gauge Quincke-type spinal needles. Anaesthesia 49:723–725
Tasmuth T, von S K, Hietanen P, Kataja M, Kalso E 1995 Pain and other symptoms after different treatment modalities of breast cancer. Annals of Oncology 6:453–459
Tasmuth T, von Smitten K, Kalso E 1996 Pain and other symptoms during the first year after radical and conservative surgery for breast cancer. British Journal of Cancer 74:2024–2031
Tay W K, Shaw R J, Goh C R 1994 A survey of symptoms in hospice patients in Singapore. Annals of the Academy of Medicine Singapore 23:191–196
Taylor B V, Kimmel D W, Krecke K N, Cascino T L 1997 Magnetic resonance imaging in cancer-related lumbosacral plexopathy. Mayo Clinic Proceedings 72:823–829
Tharion G, Bhattacharji S 1997 Malignant secondary deposit in the iliac crest masquerading as meralgia paresthetica. Archives of Physical Medicine and Rehabilitation 78:1010–1011
Thomas J E, Cascino T L, Earle J D 1985 Differential diagnosis between radiation and tumor plexopathy of the pelvis. Neurology 35:1–7
Thompson I M, Zeidman E J, Rodriguez F R 1990 Sudden death due to disease flare with luteinizing hormone-releasing hormone agonist therapy for carcinoma of the prostate [see comments]. Journal of Urology 144:1479–1480
Thornton M J, O'Sullivan G, Williams M P, Hughes P M 1997 Avascular necrosis of bone following an intensified chemotherapy regimen including high dose steroids. Clinical Radiology 52:607–612
Thorpe D M 1993 The incidence of sleep disturbance in cancer patients with pain. In: 7th World Congress on Pain: Abstracts. IASP Publications, Seatle, abstract 451
Thyagarajan D, Cascino T, Harms G 1995 Magnetic resonance imaging in brachial plexopathy of cancer. Neurology 45(3 pt 1):421–427
Tomita K, Toribatake Y, Kawahara N, Ohnari H, Kose H 1994 Total en bloc spondylectomy and circumspinal decompression for solitary spinal metastasis. Paraplegia 32:36–46
Topuz E, Aydiner A, Saip P, Bengisu E, Berkman S, Disci R 1997 Intraperitoneal cisplatin-mitoxantrone in ovarian cancer patients with minimal residual disease. European Journal of Gynaecological Oncology 18:71–75
Traill Z C, Nolan D J 1997 Metastatic oesophageal carcinoma presenting as small intestinal ischaemia: imaging findings. European Radiology 7:341–343
Trump D L, Anderson S A 1983 Painful gynecomastia following cytotoxic therapy for testis cancer: a potentially favorable prognostic sign? Journal of Clinical Oncology 1:416–420
Trump D L, Pavy M D, Staal S 1982 Gynecomastia in men following antineoplastic therapy. Archives of Internal Medicine 142:511–513
Truong L D, Maccato M L, Awalt H, Cagle P T, Schwartz M R, Kaplan A L 1990 Serous surface carcinoma of the peritoneum: a clinicopathologic study of 22 cases. Human Pathology 21:99–110
Tseng A Jr, Horning S J, Freiha F S, Resser K J, Hannigan J F Jr, Torti F M 1985 Gynecomastia in testicular cancer patients. Prognostic and therapeutic implications. Cancer 56:2534–2538
Twijnstra A, Ongerboer de Visser B W, van Zanten A P 1987 Diagnosis of leptomeningeal metastasis. Clinical Neurology and Neurosurgery 89:79–85
Twycross R 1997 Cancer pain classification. Acta Anaesthesiologica Scandinavica 41(1 pt 2):141–145
Twycross R, Harcourt J, Bergl S 1996 A survey of pain in patients with advanced cancer. Journal of Pain and Symptom Management 12:273–282
Uekado Y, Hirano A, Shinka T, Ohkawa T 1994 The effects of intravesical chemoimmunotherapy with epirubicin and bacillus Calmette–Guerin for prophylaxis of recurrence of superficial bladder

cancer: a preliminary report. Cancer Chemotherapy and Pharmacology 35(suppl): S65–68
Uziely B, Jeffers S, Isacson R et al 1995 Liposomal doxorubicin: antitumor activity and unique toxicities during two complementary phase I studies. Journal of Clinical Oncology 13(7):1777–1785
Vainio A, Auvinen A 1996 Prevalence of symptoms among patients with advanced cancer: an international collaborative study. Symptom Prevalence Group. Journal of Pain and Symptom Management 12:3–10
van Dam M S, Hennipman A, de Kruif J T, van der Tweel I, de Graaf P W 1993 [Complications following axillary dissection for breast carcinoma (see comments)]. Nederlands Tijdschrift voor Geneeskunde 137:2395–2398
Van Duynhoven V 1994 Patients need compassionate pain control. An alternative to physician-assisted suicide. Oregon Nurse 59:11
van Oosterhout A G, van de Pol M, ten Velde G P, Twijnstra A 1996 Neurologic disorders in 203 consecutive patients with small cell lung cancer. Results of a longitudinal study. Cancer 77:1434–1441
Vanagunas A, Jacob P, Olinger E 1990 Radiation-induced esophageal injury: a spectrum from esophagitis to cancer. American Journal of Gastroenterology 85:808–812
Vazquez-Barquero A, Ibanez F J, Herrera S, Izquierdo J M, Berciano J, Pascual J 1994 Isolated headache as the presenting clinical manifestation of intracranial tumors: a prospective study [see comments]. Cephalalgia 14:270–272
Vecht C J 1990 Arm pain in the patient with breast cancer. Journal of Pain and Symptom Management 5:109–117
Vecht C J, Haaxma-Reiche H, van Putten W L, de Visser M, Vries E P, Twijnstra A 1989a Initial bolus of conventional versus high-dose dexamethasone in metastatic spinal cord compression. Neurology 39:1255–1257
Vecht C J, Van de Brand H J, Wajer O J 1989b Post-axillary dissection pain in breast cancer due to a lesion of the intercostobrachial nerve. Pain 38:171–176
Vecht C J, Hoff A M, Kansen P J, de Boer M F, Bosch D A 1992 Types and causes of pain in cancer of the head and neck. Cancer 70:178–184
Veldhuis G J, Willemse P H, van Gameren M M et al 1995 Recombinant human interleukin-3 to dose-intensify carboplatin and cyclophosphamide chemotherapy in epithelial ovarian cancer: a phase I trial. Journal of Clinical Oncology 13:733–740
Ventafridda V 1989 Continuing care: a major issue in cancer pain management. Pain 36:137–143
Ventafridda V, Ripamonti C, De Conno F, Tamburini M, Cassileth B R 1990 Symptom prevalence and control during cancer patients' last days of life. Journal of Palliative Care 6:7–11
Ventafridda V, Caraceni A, Martini C, Sbanotto A, De Conno F 1991 On the significance of Lhermitte's sign in oncology. Journal of Neurooncology 10:133–137
Verdi C J 1993 Cancer therapy and oral mucositis. An appraisal of drug prophylaxis. Drug Safety 9:185–195
Vial T, Descotes J 1995 Clinical toxicity of cytokines used as haemopoietic growth factors. Drug Safety 13:371–406
Vigo M, De Faveri D, Biondetti P R Jr, Benedetti L 1980 CT demonstration of portal and superior mesenteric vein thrombosis in hepatocellular carcinoma. Journal of Computed Assisted Tomography 4:627–629
Visani G, Bontempo G, Manfroi S, Pazzaglia A, D'Alessandro R, Tura S 1996 All-*trans*-retinoic acid and pseudotumor cerebri in a young adult with acute promyelocytic leukemia: a possible disease association [see comments]. Haematologica 81:152–154
Vogelzang N J 1979 'Adriamycin flare': a skin reaction resembling extravasation. Cancer Treatment Report 63:2067–2069
Von Roenn J H, Cleeland C S, Gonin R, Hatfield A K, Pandya K J 1993 Physician attitudes and practice in cancer pain management. A survey from the Eastern Cooperative Oncology Group. Annals of Internal Medicine 119(2):121–126
Vuorinen E 1993 Pain as an early symptom in cancer. Clinical Journal of Pain 9:272–278
Wagner G 1984 Frequency of pain in patients with cancer. Recent Results in Cancer Research 89:64–71
Walker-Renard P B, Vaughan L M, Sahn S A 1994 Chemical pleurodesis for malignant pleural effusions [see comments]. Annals of Internal Medicine 120:56–64
Wang X S, Mendoza T R, Gao S Z, Cleeland C S 1996 The Chinese version of the Brief Pain Inventory (BPI-C): its development and use in a study of cancer pain. Pain 67:407–416
Wanzer S H, Federman D D, Adelstein S J et al 1989. The Physicians responsibility toward hopelessly ill patients. A second look. N Engl J Med 320: 844–9
Wasserstrom W R, Glass J P, Posner J B 1982 Diagnosis and treatment of leptomeningeal metastases from solid tumors: experience with 90 patients. Cancer 49:759–772
Weinstein S M 1994 Phantom pain. Oncology (Huntingt) 8:65–70, 73–74
Weiss H D, Walker M D, Wiernik P H 1974a Neurotoxicity of commonly used antineoplastic agents (first of two parts). New England Journal of Medicine 291:75–81
Weiss H D, Walker M D, Wiernik P H 1974b Neurotoxicity of commonly used antineoplastic agents (second of two parts). New England Journal of Medicine 291:127–133
Weiss R, Grisold W, Jellinger K, Muhlbauer J, Scheiner W, Vesely M 1984 Metastasis of solid tumors in extraocular muscles. Acta Neuropathologica (Berlin) 65:168–171
Wells P S, Hirsh J, Anderson D R et al 1995 Comparison of the accuracy of impedance plethysmography and compression ultrasonography in outpatients with clinically suspected deep vein thrombosis. A two centre paired-design prospective trial. Thrombosis and Haemostasis 74:1423–1427
Wolff J M, Boeckmann W, Jakse G 1994 Spontaneous kidney rupture due to a metastatic renal tumour. Case report. Scandinavian Journal of Urology and Nephrology 28:415–417
Wong K F, Chan J K, Ma S K 1993 Solid tumour with initial presentation in the bone marrow – a clinicopathologic study of 25 adult cases. Hematological Oncology 11:35–42
Wood K M 1978 Intercostobrachial nerve entrapment syndrome. Southern Medical Journal 71:662–623
World Health Organization 1996 Cancer pain relief, 2nd edn. World Health Organization, Geneva
Wurzel R S, Yamase H T, Nieh P T 1987 Ectopic production of human chorionic gonadotropin by poorly differentiated transitional cell tumors of the urinary tract. Journal of Urology 137:502–504
Yeoh E K, Horowitz M 1987 Radiation enteritis. Surgery, Gynecology and Obstetrics 165:373–379
Yeoh E, Horowitz M 1988 Radiation enteritis. British Journal of Hospital Medicine 39:498–504
Zografos G C, Karakousis C P 1994 Pain in the distribution of the femoral nerve: early evidence of recurrence of a retroperitoneal sarcoma. European Journal of Surgical Oncology 20:692–693

Cancer, mind and spirit

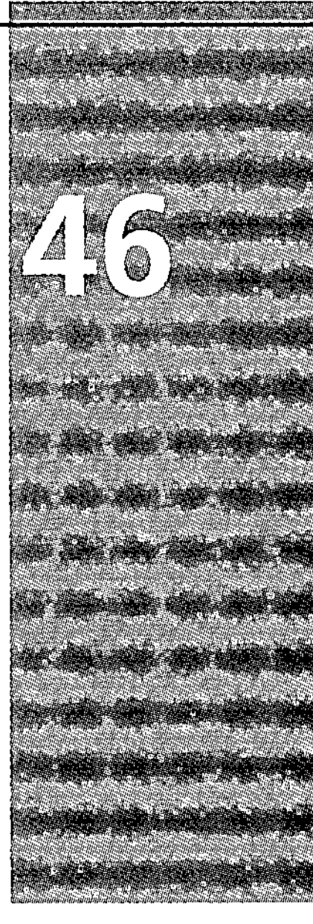

WILLIAM BREITBART, STEVEN D. PASSIK &
BARRY D. ROSENFELD

SUMMARY

Unfortunately, cancer patients with pain are most vulnerable to such psychiatric complications of cancer as depression, anxiety and delirium. The clinician who wants to provide comprehensive management of cancer pain must be familiar with or have available expertise in psychiatric assessment and intervention in the cancer patient. Knowledge of the indications and usefulness of psychotropic drugs in the cancer pain population will be most rewarding, particularly because these drugs are useful not only in the treatment of psychiatric complications of cancer, but also as adjuvant analgesic agents in the management of cancer pain. Psychotherapy and cognitive-behavioural techniques have also been shown to decrease psychological distress in cancer pain patients and provide useful tools for regaining a sense of control and reducing cancer pain. Psychopharmacological, psychotherapeutic and cognitive-behavioural interventions are all powerful psychiatric contributions to a multidisciplinary approach to the management of cancer pain. The mainstay of pharmacological interventions for cancer pain continues to be the appropriate use of narcotic analgesics. There is, however, growing awareness and acceptance of the benefits for cancer pain patients derived from psychiatric contributions to pain control. These same principles may be applied to patients with HIV infection and pain with beneficial results.

INTRODUCTION

The cancer patient faces a wide range of psychological and physical stressors throughout the course of illness. These stressors include fears of a painful death, physical disability, disfigurement and growing dependency on others. Although such fears exist in most if not all cancer patients, the degree of psychological distress experienced varies greatly between individuals and depends in part on the patient's personality style, coping abilities, available social supports and medical factors (Holland & Rowland 1989). One of the most feared consequences of cancer, however, is the potential for pain. Pain has a profound impact on a patient's level of emotional distress and psychological factors such as mood, anxiety and the meaning attributed to pain can intensify a patient's experience of cancer pain (Ahles et al 1983). Because of the relationship between psychological factors and pain experience, clinicians who treat patients with cancer pain face complex diagnostic and therapeutic challenges. The appropriate management of cancer pain therefore requires a multidisciplinary approach, recognizing the importance of accurate diagnosis and treatment of concurrent psychological symptoms and psychiatric syndromes (Breitbart 1989a). This chapter reviews the common psychological issues and psychiatric complications (e.g., anxiety, depression, delirium) seen in cancer pain patients and provides guidelines for their assessment and management. In addition, psychiatric and psychological interventions in cancer pain management are reviewed. Finally, the problem of pain in AIDS is addressed with special focus on psychiatric issues in pain assessment and management.

PSYCHOLOGICAL IMPACT OF CANCER AND THE ROLE OF PAIN

Patients diagnosed with cancer often demonstrate a consistent pattern of emotional responses that have been described by Holland, Massie and others (Massie & Holland 1987, Breitbart & Holland 1988, Breitbart 1989a). These responses usually consist of an initial period of shock, denial and disbelief, followed by a period of anxiety and/or depression. Disturbed sleep, diminished appetite and concentration, irritability, pervasive thoughts about cancer and fears about the future often interfere with normal daily activities. These 'stress responses' generally occur at specific points in the course of cancer and its treatment: after diagnosis, with relapse, prior to diagnostic tests, surgery, radiation and chemotherapy, as well as after treatment has concluded and patients enter the phase of survivorship. Distress usually resolves slowly over a period of several weeks and patients gradually return to their prior level of homeostasis once a treatment plan has been agreed upon and emotional supports arise. Psychiatric intervention is not typically necessary for most cancer patients, although anxiolytic or sedative medications and relaxation techniques may be helpful in restoring sleep patterns and minimizing emotional distress in many cancer patients and/or their family members. The support of family and friends, social workers, clergy and hospital staff are usually sufficient to help patients cope with these brief crisis periods.

The degree of psychological distress observed in cancer patients also varies considerably between individuals. Some patients experience persistently high levels of anxiety and depression for weeks or months which significantly hinder their ability to function independently, or even comply with cancer treatment. Others experience only mild or transient symptoms, which remit rapidly without intervention. This variability is influenced by a number of different factors, most notably medical variables (the presence and degree of pain, stage of disease) and psychological issues (pre-existing psychiatric disorders, coping abilities, level of emotional development). Such significant levels of distress generally require psychiatric intervention and are often the result of psychiatric disorders that have developed as a complication of cancer. For the most part, however, physicians treating cancer patients are confronted with psychologically healthy individuals who are reacting to the stresses imposed by cancer and its treatment. Nearly 90% of the psychiatric disorders observed in cancer patients are reactions to or manifestations of the disease or treatments (Derogatis et al 1983, Massie & Holland 1987). Along with an expectation of psychological distress associated with cancer, the public perceives cancer as an extremely painful disease, and pain is one of the most feared consequences of the disease process (Levin et al 1985). Approximately 15% of all cancer patients without metastatic disease report significant pain (Kanner & Foley 1981, Daut & Cleeland 1982). In patients with advanced disease, between 60 and 90% of all patients report debilitating pain and as many as 25% of all cancer patients die while still experiencing considerable pain (Foley 1975, 1985, Twycross & Lack 1983, Cleeland 1984). These findings highlight the importance of understanding the factors which influence the experience of pain for effective management of cancer pain.

Not only does pain have a profound impact on psychological distress in cancer patients, but psychological factors appear to influence the experience and intensity of cancer pain. Psychological variables such as perceived control, meaning attributed to the pain experience, fear of death, hopelessness and anxious or depressed mood all appear to contribute to the experience of cancer pain and suffering (Bond 1979, Spiegel & Bloom 1983a, Ahles et al 1983). These interrelationships have been supported by considerable psychosocial research exploring the relationship between psychological variables and cancer pain. In a study of women with metastatic breast cancer, Spiegel and Bloom (1983a) found that although the site of metastasis did not predict the intensity of pain report, greater depression and the belief that pain represented the spread of disease (e.g., the meaning attributed to the pain) did significantly predict a greater degree of pain experienced. Daut and Cleeland (1982) also found that cancer patients who believed that their pain represented disease progression reported significantly more interference with their ability to function and enjoy daily activities than did patients who attributed their pain to a benign cause. Other research has demonstrated that patients with advanced disease who report high levels of emotional disturbance also report more pain (McKegney et al 1981), as do patients with more anxiety and depression (Bond & Pearson 1969, Bond 1973).

Current conceptual models of cancer pain emphasize the multidimensional nature of the pain experience, incorporating the contribution of cognitive, motivational, behavioural and affective components, as well as sensory (nociceptive) phenomena. This multidimensional formulation of cancer pain has opened the door to psychiatric and psychological participation in pain research, assessment and treatment (Melzack & Wall 1983, Lindblom et al 1986). Pain is no longer considered simply as a nociceptive event, but is widely recognized and accepted as a psychological process involving nociception, perception and expression. Because of the important role played by psychological variables in the experience and intensity of cancer pain, appropriate and effective management of cancer pain requires a multidisciplinary approach that incorporates neurology, neurosurgery, anaesthesiology and rehabilitative medicine, in addition to a considerable reliance on the input of psychiatrists or psychologists (Foley 1975, 1985, Breitbart 1989a). The challenge of untangling and addressing both the physical and psychological issues involved in cancer pain is essential to developing a rational and effective management strategy. Psychosocial therapies directed primarily at psychological variables have a profound impact on nociception, while somatic therapies directed at nociception have beneficial effects on psychological sequelae of cancer pain. Ideally such somatic and psychosocial therapies are used simultaneously in a multidisciplinary approach to cancer pain management (Breitbart 1989a, Breitbart & Holland 1990, Ahles & Martin 1992).

Unfortunately, psychological variables are too often proposed as the sole explanation for continued pain or lack of response to conventional therapies, when in fact medical factors have not been adequately appreciated or examined. The psychiatrist or psychologist is often the last member of the treatment team to be asked to consult on a cancer patient with unrelieved pain and, in that role, must be vigilant that an accurate pain diagnosis is made. They also must be capable of assessing the adequacy of the medical analgesic management provided. Psychological distress in patients with cancer pain should be initially assumed to be the consequence of uncontrolled pain. Personality factors may appear distorted or exaggerated by the presence of pain and the relief of pain often results in the disappearance of a perceived psychiatric disorder (Marks & Sachar 1973, Cleeland 1984).

Table 46.1. Rates of DSM-III psychiatric disorders and prevalence of pain observed in 215 cancer patients from three cancer centres[1]

Diagnostic category	*Number in diagnostic class*	*Psychiatric diagnoses (%)*	*Number with significant pain[2]*
Adjustment disorders	69 (32%)	68	
Major affective disorders	13 (6%)	13	
Organic mental disorders	8 (4%)	8	
Personality disorders	7 (3%)	7	
Anxiety disorders	4 (2%)	4	
Total with DSM III psychiatric disorder diagnosis	101 (47%)		39 (39%)
Total without DSM III psychiatric disorder diagnosis	114 (53%)		21 (19%)
Total patient population	215 (100%)		60 (28%)

[1] Adapted from Derogatis et al 1983.
[2] Score greater than 50 mm on a 100-mm VAS for pain severity.

PSYCHIATRIC DISORDERS IN CANCER PAIN PATIENTS: ASSESSMENT AND MANAGEMENT

While recognizing the potential for psychological disturbance as the result of uncontrolled cancer pain, research has suggested an increased frequency of psychiatric disorders in cancer patients with pain. The Psychosocial Collaborative Oncology Group, which described the prevalence of psychiatric disorders in cancer patients (Table 46.1), noted that 39% of patients with a psychiatric diagnosis also reported experiencing significant pain, while only 19% of patients without a psychiatric diagnosis reported significant pain (Derogatis et al 1983). The most frequent psychiatric diagnoses seen in cancer patients with pain include adjustment disorder with depressed or anxious mood and major depression. In a specific cancer-related painful condition, epidural spinal cord compression (ESCC), the prevalence of psychiatric disorders is as high as 52% (Breitbart et al 1993). ESCC is a common neurological complication of cancer that occurs in 5–10% of cancer patients and often presents initially as severe pain. These patients are typically treated with a combination of high-dose dexamethasone and radiotherapy, receiving as much as 96 mg/day of dexamethasone for up to a week, with gradually tapering doses for up to 3–4 weeks. Such treatments for ESCC are reported to be complicated by significantly high rates of both depression and delirium (Stiefel et al 1989, Breitbart et al 1993). A diagnosis of a major depressive episode was warranted in 22% of all patients undergoing this treatment regimen, compared with only 4% so diagnosed in a control sample of cancer patients. Delirium was diagnosed during the course of treatment in 24% of the ESCC patients compared to 10% of a comparison sample. These findings of increased frequency of psychiatric disturbances in cancer patients with pain have been supported by a number of other researchers (e.g., Woodforde & Fielding 1970, Ahles et al 1983).

Because of the confounding influence of pain on a patient's psychological condition, it is imperative that the patient's mental state be reassessed after pain has been adequately controlled in order to determine whether a psychiatric disorder is indeed present. Psychiatric complications of cancer pain can result in increased morbidity and mortality. The management of psychiatric complications of cancer pain is essential for patients to maintain an optimal quality of life. For cancer pain patients, interventions that help decrease mood disturbance also help to reduce pain. A multidisciplinary approach, incorporating psychotherapeutic, behavioural and psychopharmacological interventions, is the optimal method for treating psychiatric complications in cancer pain patients. Treatment decisions, however, are predicated on the assumption that a thorough medical and psychiatric assessment has led to an accurate diagnosis, thus allowing specific and effective intervention. The management of specific psychiatric disorders such as depression, delirium and anxiety in cancer patients (including those with pain) has been reviewed in detail in the 'Handbook of psychooncology' edited by Holland and Rowland (1989), as well as in other sources (Massie & Holland 1987, Breitbart & Holland 1988, Holland 1989b, Massie & Holland 1990). A brief guide to the diagnosis and management of these disorders is presented below.

DEPRESSION IN CANCER PAIN PATIENTS

Depression occurs in roughly 20–25% of all cancer patients and the prevalence increases with higher levels of disability, advanced illness and pain (Plumb & Holland 1977, Bukberg et al 1984, Massie & Holland 1990). The somatic symptoms of depression (e.g., anorexia, insomnia, fatigue and weight loss) are unreliable and lack specificity in the cancer patient (Endicott 1983). Thus, the psychological symptoms of depression take on greater diagnostic value and include the following: dysphoric mood, hopelessness, worthlessness, guilt and suicidal ideation (Plumb & Holland 1977, Endicott 1983, Bukberg et al 1984, Massie & Holland 1990). A family history of depression and a history of previous depressive episodes further support the reliability of a diagnosis. A number of specific types of cancer are also associated with higher rates of depression; for example, patients with pancreatic cancer are more likely to develop depression than patients with other types of intra-abdominal malignancy (Holland et al 1986). Once the presence of depressive symptomatology has been established, evaluation of potential organic aetiologies such as corticosteroids (Stiefel et al 1989), chemotherapeutic agents (vincristine, vinblastine, asparaginase, intrathecal methotrexate, interferon, interleukin) (Holland et al 1974, Young 1982, Adams et al 1984, Denicoff et al 1987), amphotericin (Weddington 1982), whole-brain radiation (DeAngelis et al 1989), central nervous system metabolic–endocrinological complications (Breitbart 1989b) and paraneoplastic syndromes (Posner 1988, Patchell & Posner 1989) that can present as depression must precede initiation of treatment.

TREATMENT OF DEPRESSION

Depressed cancer-pain patients are usually treated with a combination of antidepressant medications, supportive psychotherapy and cognitive-behavioural techniques (Massie & Holland 1990). Many of these techniques are useful in the management of psychological distress in cancer patients and have been applied to the treatment of depressive and anxious symptoms related to cancer and cancer pain. Psychotherapeutic interventions, either in the form of individual or group therapy, have been shown to effectively reduce psychological distress and depressive symptoms in cancer pain patients (Spiegel et al 1981, Spiegel & Bloom 1983a, b, Massie et al 1989). Cognitive-behavioural interventions, such as relaxation, distraction with pleasant imagery, and cognitive restructuring, also appear to be effective in reducing symptomatology in patients with mild to moderate levels of depression (Holland et al 1991).

Psychopharmacological interventions (i.e., antidepressant medications), however, are the mainstay of symptom management in cancer patients with severe depressive symptoms (Massie & Holland 1990). The efficacy of antidepressants in the treatment of depression in cancer patients, including those with or without pain, has been well established in case observations and clinical trials (Purohit et al 1978, Costa et al 1985, Popkin et al 1985, Rifkin et al 1985, Massie & Holland 1987, 1990, Breitbart & Holland 1988, Breitbart 1989a). Antidepressant medications used in cancer pain patients are listed in Table 46.2.

Tricyclic antidepressants

Among the multitude of available antidepressant medications, tricyclic antidepressants (TCAs) are the most frequently used in the cancer setting. Treatment is initiated at low dose (10–25 mg at bedtime), particularly with debilitated patients, and slowly increased by 10–25 mg every 1–2 days until a therapeutic effect has been achieved. Depressed cancer patients often respond to doses considerably lower (25–125 mg orally) than those typically required by the physically healthy (150–300 mg o.d.) (Massie & Holland 1990). The choice of TCA depends on the side-effects profile, existing medical problems, the nature of depressive symptoms and past response to specific antidepressants. Sedating TCAs like amitriptyline or doxepin are prescribed for the agitated, depressed patient with insomnia. Doxepin is highly antihistaminic and as such is useful in improving appetite. Desipramine and nortriptyline are relatively non-anticholinergic and are therefore used when concerns about urinary retention, decreased intestinal motility or stomatitis exist. Patients receiving multiple drugs with anticholinergic properties (e.g., meperidine, atropine, diphenhydramine, phenothiazines) are at risk for developing an anticholinergic delirium, and so TCAs with potent anticholinergic properties should be avoided or used with caution. Amitriptyline, imipramine and doxepin can be given intramuscularly in patients unable to use an oral

Table 46.2. Antidepressant medications used in cancer pain patients. (Adapted from Massie & Holland 1990)

Generic name	*Approximate daily dosage range (mg)*[1]	*Route*[1]
Tricyclic antidepressants		
Amitriptyline	10–150	PO, IM, PR
Doxepin	12.5–150	PO, IM
Imipramine	12.5–150	PO, IM
Desipramine	12.5–150	PO, IM
Nortriptyline	10–125	PO
Clomipramine	10–150	PO
Second-generation antidepressants		
Buproprion	200–450	PO
Trazodone	25–300	PO
Serotonin specific re-uptake inhibitors		
Fluoxetine	20–60	PO
Sertraline	50–200	PO
Paroxetine	10–40	PO
Nefazodone	50–500	PO
Serotonin/noradrenaline re-uptake inhibitors		
Venlafaxine	37.5–450	PO
Heterocyclic antidepressants		
Maprotiline	50–75	PO
Amoxapine	100–150	PO
Monoamine oxidase inhibitors		
Isocarboxazid	20–40	PO
Phenelzine	30–60	PO
Tranylcypromine	20–40	PO
Psychostimulants		
Dextroamphetamine	2.5–20 b.i.d.	PO
Methylphenidate	2.5–20 b.i.d.	PO
Pemoline	37.5–75 b.i.d.	PO, SL[2]
Benzodiazepines		
Alprazolam	0.25–2.0 t.i.d.	PO
Lithium carbonate	600–1200	PO

[1] PO = peroral; IM = intramuscular; PR = per rectum; SL = sublingual; b.i.d. = two times a day; t.i.d. = three times a day; intravenous infusions of a number of tricyclic antidepressants are utilized outside of the USA; this route is however not FDA approved.
[2] Available in chewable tablet form that can be absorbed without swallowing.

route. Rectal suppositories containing amitriptyline or other TCAs can also be used. Although not approved for use in the USA, TCAs such as amitriptyline have been used safely by the intravenous route as a slow infusion (Breitbart & Holland 1988, Massie & Holland 1990).

Second-generation antidepressants

If a patient does not respond to a TCA, or cannot tolerate its side effects, a second-generation (buproprion, trazodone), heterocyclic (maprotiline, amoxapine), serotonin-specific re-uptake inhibitors (SSRIs, fluoxetine, sertraline, paroxetine, nefazodone and fluvoxamine), or serotonin–noradrenaline re-uptake inhibitors (SNRIs – venlafaxine) antidepressants can be used. The second-generation antidepressants are generally considered to be less cardiotoxic than the TCAs (Glassman 1984). Trazodone is highly sedating and, in low doses (100 mg at bedtime), is particularly helpful for treating depressed cancer patients with insomnia. Trazodone has been associated with priapism and should, therefore, be used with caution in male patients (Sher et al 1983). Buproprion is a relatively new drug in the USA and its efficacy in cancer patients is unclear. At present, it is not the first drug of choice for depressed patients with cancer; however, buproprion may be considered if patients have a poor response to a reasonable trial of other antidepressants. Buproprion may be somewhat activating in medically ill patients. It should be avoided in patients with seizure disorders and brain tumours and in those who are malnourished (Peck et al 1983).

Selective serotonin re-uptake inhibitors

The SSRIs are a recent important addition to the available antidepressant medications. They have been found to be as effective in the treatment of depression as the tricyclics (Mendels 1987) and have a number of features which may be particularly advantageous for the terminally ill. The SSRIs have a very low affinity for adrenergic, cholinergic and histamine receptors, thus accounting for negligible orthostatic hypotension, urinary retention, memory impairment, sedation or reduced awareness (Cooper 1988). They have not been found to cause clinically significant alterations in cardiac conduction and are generally favourably tolerated along with a wider margin of safety than the TCAs in the event of an overdose. They do not therefore require therapeutic drug level monitoring.

Most of the side effects of SSRIs result from their selective central and peripheral serotonin re-uptake. These include increased intestinal motility (loose stools, nausea, vomiting, insomnia, headaches and sexual dysfunction). Some patients may experience anxiety, tremor, restlessness and akathisia (the latter is relatively rare but it can be problematical for the terminally ill patient with Parkinson's disease) (Preskorn & Burke 1992). These side effects tend to be dose related and may be problematical for patients with advanced disease.

There are five SSRIs currently being marketed, including sertraline, fluoxetine, paroxetine, nefazodone and fluvoxamine. With the exception of fluoxetine, whose elimination half-life is 2–4 days, the SSRIs have an elimination half-life of about 24 hours. Fluoxetine is the only SSRI with a potent active metabolite – norfluoxetine – whose elimination half-life is 7–14 days. Fluoxetine can cause mild nausea and a brief period of increased anxiety as well as appetite suppression that usually lasts for a period of several weeks. Some patients can experience transient weight loss, but weight usually returns to baseline level. The anorectic properties of fluoxetine has not been a limiting factor in the use of this drug in cancer patients. Fluoxetine and norfluoxetine do not reach a steady state for 5–6 weeks, compared with 4–14 days for paroxetine, fluvoxamine and sertraline. These differences are important, especially for the terminally ill patient in whom a switch from as SSRI to another antidepressant is being considered. If a switch to a monamine oxidase inhibitor is required, the washout period for fluoxetine will be at least 5 weeks, given the potential drug interactions between these two agents. Since fluoxetine has entered the market, there have been several reports of significant drug–drug interactions. (Ciraulo & Shader 1990, Pearson 1990). Until it has been studied further in the medically ill, it should be used cautiously in the debilitated dying patient. Paroxetine, fluvoxamine and sertraline on the other hand require considerably shorter washout periods (10–14 days) under similar circumstances.

All the SSRIs have the ability to inhibit the hepatic isoenzyme P450 11D6, with sertraline (and according to some sources, luvox) being least potent in this regard. This is important with respect to dose/plasma level ratios and drug interactions, because the SSRIs are dependent on hepatic metabolism. For the elderly patient with advanced disease, the dose–response curve for sertraline appears to be relatively linear. On the other hand, particularly for paroxetine (which appears to most potently inhibit cytochrome P450 11D6), small dosage increases can result in dramatic elevations in plasma levels. Paroxetine, and to a somewhat lesser extent fluoxetine, appear to inhibit the hepatic enzymes responsible for their own clearance (Preskorn 1993). The co-administration of these medications with other drugs that are dependent on this enzyme system for their catabolism (e.g., tricyclics, phenothiazines, type IC antiarrhythmics and quinidine) should be carried out cautiously. Luvox has been shown in some instances to elevate the blood levels of propranolol and warfarin by as much as twofold, and should thus not be prescribed together with these agents.

SSRIs can generally be started at their minimally effective doses. For the terminally ill, this usually means initiating therapy at approximately half the usual starting dose used in an otherwise healthy patient. For fluoxetine, patients can begin on 5 mg (available in liquid form) given

 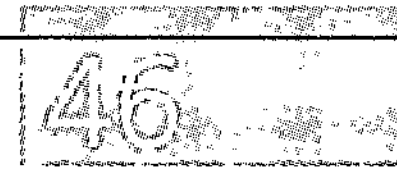

once daily (preferably in the morning) with a range of 10–40 mg per day; given its long half-life, some patients may only require this drug every second day. Paroxetine can be started at 10 mg once daily (either morning or evening) for the patient with advanced disease, and has a therapeutic range of 10–40 mg per day. Fluvoxamine, which tends to be somewhat more sedating, can be started at 25 mg (in the evenings) and has a therapeutic range of 50–300 mg. Sertraline can be initiated at 50 mg, morning or evening, and titrated within a range of 50–200 mg per day. Nefazodone can be started at 50 mg bid and titrated within a range of 100–500 mg per day. If patients experience activating effects on SSRIs, they should not be given at bedtime but rather moved earlier into the day. Gastrointestinal upset can be reduced by ensuring the patient does not take medication on an empty stomach.

Serotonin-noradrenaline re-uptake inhibitor

Venlafaxine (Effexor) is the only antidepressant in this class and was just recently released on the market. It is a potent inhibitor of neuronal serotonin and noradrenaline re-uptake and appears to have no significant affinity for muscarinic, histamine or α_1-adrenergic receptors. Some patients may experience a modest sustained increase in blood pressure, especially at doses above the recommended initiating dose. Compared with the SSRIs, its protein binding (<35%) is very low. Few protein binding-induced drug interactions are thus expected. Like other antidepressants, venlafaxine should not be used in patients receiving monamine oxidase inhibitors. Its side-effect profile tends to generally be well tolerated with few discontinuations. While there is currently no data addressing its use in the terminally ill depressed patient, its pharmacokinetic properties and side-effect profile suggest it may have a role to play.

Trazodone

If given in sufficient doses (100–300 mg/day), trazodone can be an effective antidepressant. Although its anticholinergic profile is almost negligible, it has considerable affinity for α_1 adrenoceptors and may thus predispose patients to orthostatic hypotension and its problematical sequelae (i.e., falls, fractures, head injuries). Trazedone is very sedating and in low doses (100 mg q.h.s.) is helpful in the treatment of the depressed cancer patient with insomnia. It is highly serotonergic and its use should be considered when the patient requires adjunct analgesics effect in addition to antidepressant effects. Trazodone has little effect on cardiac conduction but can cause arrhythmias in patients with premorbid cardiac disease (Rudorfer & Potter 1989). Trazodone has also been associated with priapism and should thus be used with caution in male patients (Sher et al 1983). It is highly sedating, with drowsiness being its most common adverse side effect. In smaller doses it can thus be used as an effective sedative hypnotic.

Bupropion

Bupropion is a relatively new drug in the USA and there has not been much experience with its use in the medically ill. At present, it is not the first drug of choice for depressed patients with cancer. However, one might consider prescribing bupropion if patients have a poor response to a reasonable trial of other antidepressants. Bupropion may have a role in the treatment of the psychomotor-retarded depressed terminally ill patient, as it has energizing effects similar to the stimulant drugs (Peck et al 1983, Shopsin 1983). However, because of the increased incidence of seizures, in patients with CNS disorders bupropion has a limited role in the oncology population.

Heterocyclic antidepressants

The heterocyclic antidepressants have side-effect profiles similar to those of the TCAs. Maprotiline should be avoided in patients with brain tumours and in those with seizures, because the incidence of seizures is increased by this medication (Lloyd 1977). Amoxapine has mild dopamine blocking activity. Hence, patients who are taking other dopamine blockers (e.g., antiemetics) have an increased risk of developing extrapyramidal symptoms and dyskinesias (Ayd 1979). Mianserin (not available in the USA) is a serotonergic antidepressant with adjuvant analgesic properties that is used widely in Europe and Latin America. Costa and colleagues (1985) found mianserin to be a safe and effective drug for the treatment of depression in cancer patients.

Psychostimulants

The psychostimulants (dextroamphetamine, methylphenidate and pemoline) have been shown to be effective antidepressants in cancer patients with and without pain as well as other medically ill populations (Katon & Raskind 1980, Kaufmann et al 1982, Fisch 1985, Chiarillo & Cole 1987, Fernandez et al 1987b). They are most helpful in the treatment of depression in cancer patients with pain and advanced disease and in those cases where dysphoric mood is associated with psychomotor retardation, aesthenia and mild cognitive impairment. Psychostimulants have been shown to improve attention, concentration and overall performance on neuropsychological testing in the medically ill (Fernandez et al 1988). In relatively low dose, psychostimulants can increase appetite, promote a sense of well-being and decrease weakness and fatigue in cancer pain patients. Treatment with dextroamphetamine or methylphenidate is usually initiated with a dose of 2.5 mg at 8.00 a.m. and at noon, and gradually increased over several days until a desired effect is achieved or side effects (overstimulation, anxiety, insomnia, paranoia, confusion) intervene. Most patients respond to doses of 30 mg or less per day, although occasionally patients require up to 60 mg per day. Patients are usually maintained on psychostimulants for 1–2 months, and approximately two-thirds will be able to be withdrawn from this medication without a recurrence of depressive symptoms. Patients whose symptoms re-emerge after treatment has been withdrawn can be maintained on a psychostimulant for up to 1 year without significant abuse problems (although tolerance will develop and dose adjustments may be necessary). An additional benefit of such stimulants as methylphenidate and dextroamphetamine is that they have been shown to reduce sedation secondary to opioid analgesics and provide adjuvant analgesia in cancer pain patients (Bruera et al 1987). See the section on 'Psychotropic adjuvant analgesics for cancer pain' below.

Pemoline is a unique psychostimulant chemically unrelated to amphetamine. It is a less potent stimulant with little abuse potential (Chiarillo & Cole 1987). Advantages of pemoline as a psychostimulant in cancer pain patients include the lack of abuse potential, the lack of governmental regulation (in the USA) through special triplicate prescriptions, milder sympathomimetic effects as compared to other psychostimulants and, most importantly, availability in chewable tablet form that can be absorbed through the buccal mucosa and can therefore be used by cancer patients who have difficulty swallowing or have intestinal obstruction. In our clinical experience, pemoline is as effective as methylphenidate or dextroamphetamine in the treatment of depressive symptoms in cancer pain patients (Breitbart & Mermelstein 1992). Pemoline is usually started at a dose of 18.75 mg at 8.00 a.m. and noon, and increased gradually over the next several days. Typically, patients require 75 mg a day or less. Pemoline should be used with caution in patients with liver impairment and liver function tests should be monitored periodically with longer-term treatment (Nehra et al 1990).

Monamine oxidase inhibitors

In the cancer pain patient, use of a monamine oxidase inhibitor (MAOI) must be accompanied by caution. Dietary restrictions, such as the avoidance of tyramine-containing foods while on an MAOI, are often unpopular among cancer patients who may already have dietary and nutritional restrictions. Narcotic analgesics may also be problematical or even dangerous in patients taking MAOIs, because myoclonus and delirium have been reported (Breitbart & Holland 1988), thus limiting the utility of these agents in cancer patients with pain. The use of meperidine in patients taking an MAOI is absolutely contraindicated and can lead to hyperpyrexia and cardiovascular collapse.

Sympathomimetic drugs and other less obvious monoamine oxidase inhibitors such as the chemotherapeutic agent procarbazine can cause a hypertensive crisis in patients taking an MAOI. If a patient has responded well to an MAOI for depression in the past, its continued use is warranted, but again with extreme caution.

Lithium carbonate

Patients who have been treated with lithium carbonate prior to a cancer illness can be maintained on it throughout cancer treatment, although close monitoring is necessary, especially in preoperative and postoperative periods when fluids and salt may be restricted and fluid balance shifts can occur. Maintenance doses of lithium may need reduction in seriously ill patients. Lithium carbonate is primarily eliminated through renal excretion and so should be prescribed with caution in patients receiving cisplatinum and other nephrotoxic agents. Several authors have reported possible beneficial effects from the use of lithium in neutropenic cancer patients; however, the functional capabilities of these leucocytes have not been determined. This leucocyte stimulation effect appears to be transient (Stein et al 1980).

Benzodiazepines

The triazolobenzodiazepine alprazolam has been shown to be a mildly effective antidepressant as well as an anxiolytic. Alprazolam is particularly useful in cancer patients who have mixed symptoms of anxiety and depression (i.e., adjustment disorder with anxious and depressed mood). Alprazolam alone is probably not adequate in the treatment of major depressive syndromes. The starting dose is 0.25 mg three times a day, although therapeutic effects may require 4–6 mg daily (Holland et al 1991).

Electroconvulsive therapy

Occasionally, it is necessary to consider electroconvulsive therapy (ECT) for severely depressed cancer pain patients such as those whose depression includes psychotic features or patients for whom treatment with antidepressants pose unacceptable side effects. The safe, effective use of ECT in depressed cancer patients has been reviewed by others (Massie & Holland 1990) and will not be elaborated here, although this alternative may yield secondary analgesic benefits for the depressed patient with otherwise unrelieved pain.

ANXIETY IN CANCER PAIN PATIENTS

A number of different types of anxiety syndrome commonly appear in cancer patients with and without pain, including:

1. Reactive anxiety related to the stresses of cancer and its treatment.
2. Anxiety that is a manifestation of a medical or physiological problem related to cancer, such as uncontrolled pain (organic anxiety disorder).
3. Phobias, panic and chronic anxiety disorders that predate the cancer diagnosis but are exacerbated during illness (Massie & Holland 1987, Holland 1989b).

REACTIVE ANXIETY

Although many, if not all, patients experience some anxiety at critical moments during the evaluation and treatment of cancer (i.e., while waiting to hear of diagnosis or possible recurrence, before procedures, diagnostic tests, surgery or while awaiting test results), such anxiety may disrupt a patient's ability to function normally, interfere with interpersonal relationships and even impact upon the ability to understand or comply with cancer treatments. In such cases, anxiety can be effectively treated pharmacologically with benzodiazepines such as alprazolam, oxazepam or lorazepam. In patients whose level of anxiety is relatively mild, and when sufficient time exists for the patient to learn a behavioural technique, relaxation and imagery exercises or cognitive restructuring can be useful in reducing levels of distress (Holland et al 1991). The optimal treatment of anxiety generally incorporates both a benzodiazepine and relaxation exercises or other behavioural interventions.

ORGANIC ANXIETY

The diagnosis of organic anxiety disorder assumes that a medical factor is the aetiological agent in the production of anxious symptoms. Cancer patients with pain are exposed to multiple potential organic causes of anxiety, including medications, uncontrolled pain, infection, metabolic derangements, etc. Patients in acute pain and those with acute or chronic respiratory distress often appear anxious. The anxiety that accompanies acute pain is best treated with analgesics; the anxiety that accompanies severe respiratory distress is usually relieved by oxygen and the judicious use of morphine and/or antihistamines. Many patients receiving corticosteroids experience insomnia and anxiety symptoms which vary from mild to severe. Because steroids prescribed as part of cancer therapy usually cannot be discontinued, anxiety symptoms are often relieved with benzodiazepines or low-dose antipsychotics (Stiefel et al 1989). Patients developing an encephalopathy (delirium) or who are in the early stages of dementia can also appear restless or anxious. Symptoms of anxiety are also frequent sequelae of a withdrawal from narcotics, alcohol, benzodiazepines and barbiturates. Because patients who abuse alcohol often inaccurately report alcohol intake before admission, the physician needs to consider alcohol withdrawal in all patients who develop otherwise unexplained anxiety symptoms during early days of admission to the hospital. Other medical conditions that may have anxiety as a prominent or presenting symptom include hyperthyroidism, phaeochromocytoma, carcinoid, primary and metastatic brain tumour and mitral valve prolapse (Breitbart 1989b, Holland 1989b).

PHOBIAS AND PANIC

Occasionally, patients have their first episode of panic or phobia while in the cancer setting. Approximately 20% of Memorial Hospital patients scheduled to have an MRI scan examination developed anxiety (typically claustrophobia) of such intensity that they were unable to complete the procedure (Brennan et al 1988). A number of variants of anxiety disorders (e.g., panic attack, needle phobia or claustrophobia) can complicate treatment and thus a prompt psychiatric consultation is recommended. The techniques available to treat these disorders include both behavioural interventions (such as relaxation training, systematic desensitization and in vivo or imaginative exposure for specific phobias) and more rapid pharmacological approaches for both phobias and panic. If there is the luxury of time (days to weeks) and the patient will have to face the stress (venipunctures, bone marrow aspirations) repeatedly, behavioural interventions may be advisable in order to enable the patient to gain some control over such fear. Often, however, the need for anxiety relief is immediate because of the urgency of many medical procedures and benzodiazepines (e.g., alprazolam 0.25–1.0 mg PO), in addition to providing emotional support, are used to help the phobic patient undergo necessary procedures.

PHARMACOLOGICAL TREATMENT OF ANXIETY SYMPTOMS AND DISORDERS

The most commonly used drugs for the treatment of anxiety are the benzodiazepines (Massie & Holland 1987, Holland 1989b). Other medications used to alleviate anxiety include buspirone, antipsychotics, antihistamines, betablockers and antidepressants (Table 46.3).

Benzodiazepines

For cancer pain patients, the preferred benzodiazepines are those with shorter half-lives (i.e., alprazolam, lorazepam and oxazepam). These medications are better tolerated and are complicated less frequently by toxic accumulation of active metabolites when combined with other sedating medications (e.g., analgesics, diphenhydramine). Determining the optimal starting dose depends on a number of factors, including the severity of the anxiety, the patient's physical state (respiratory and hepatic impairment), estimated tolerance to benzodiazepines and the concurrent use of other medications (antidepressants, analgesics, antiemetics). The dose schedule also depends on the half-life of the drug; shorter-acting benzodiazepines must be given three to four times a day, while longer-acting diazepam can be used on a twice-daily schedule. Anxiolytic medications are often prescribed only on an as needed basis for patients whose anxiety is limited to specific events such as medical procedures or chemotherapy treatments. However, patients with chronic anxiety should be treated with anxiolytics on an around-the-clock schedule as with analgesics for chronic pain. The most common side effects of the benzodiazepines are drowsiness and motor incoordination. Physicians must be aware of synergistic effects when they are used with other CNS depressants and the possibility of resulting confusional states. If these occur, the dose should be lowered. If side effects persist, the anxiolytic should be discontinued and another class of medication used. In patients taking benzodiazepines chronically (for periods of several weeks), abrupt discontinuation can lead to a serious withdrawal syndrome similar to alcohol withdrawal.

Midazolam (Versed) is a very short-acting benzodiazepine that is administered, usually as an intravenous infusion, in critical care settings where sedation is the goal in an agitated or anxious patient on a respirator. Clonazepam, a long-acting benzodiazepine, has been found to be extremely useful in cancer patients for a multitude of symptoms and treatment needs. Symptoms of anxiety and depersonalization or derealization, particularly in the presence of seizure disorders, brain tumours and mild organic mental disorders, are often successfully treated with clonazepam. Patients who experience end-of-dose failure with breakthrough anxiety on shorter-acting drugs also find clonazepam helpful, as do patients with organic mood disorders who have symptoms of mania and as an adjuvant analgesic in patients with neuropathic pain (Chouinard et al 1983, Walsh 1990). Clonazepam is also frequently used when attempting to taper off a shorter-acting benzodiazepine such as alprazolam and in the treatment of panic disorder.

Table 46.3 Anxiolytic medications used in cancer-pain patients

Generic name	*Approximate daily dosage range (mg)*	*Route*[1]
Benzodiazepines		
Very short acting		
Midazolam	10–60 per 24 h	IV, SC
Short acting		
Alprazolam	0.25–2.0 t.i.d.–q.i.d.	PO, SL
Oxazepam	10–15 t.i.d.–q.i.d.	PO
Lorazepam	0.5–2.0 t.i.d.–q.i.d.	PO, SL, IV, IM
Intermediate acting		
Chlordiazepoxide	10–50 t.i.d.–q.i.d.	PO, IM
Long acting		
Diazepam	5–10 b.i.d.–b.i.d.	PO, IM, IV, PR
Clorazepate	7.5–15 b.i.d.–q.i.d.	PO
Clonazepam	0.5–2 b.i.d.–q.i.d.	PO
Non-benzodiazepines		
Buspirone	5–20 t.i.d.	PO
Neuroleptics		
Haloperidol	0.5–5 q 2–12 h	PO, IV, SC, IM
Methotrimeprazine	10–20 q 4–8 h	PO, IV, SC
Thioridazine	10–75 t.i.d.–q.i.d.	PO
Chlorpromazine	12.5–50 q 4–12 h	PO, IM, IV
Antihistamine		
Hydroxyzine	25–50 q 4–6 h	PO, IV, SC
Tricyclic antidepressants		
Imipramine	12.5–150 h	PO, IM
Clomipramine	10–150 h	PO

[1] PO = per oral; IM = intramuscular; PR = per rectum; IV = intravenous; SC = subcutaneous; SL = sublingual; b.i.d. = two times a day; t.i.d. = three times a day; q.i.d. = four times a day; q (2–12) h, every (2–12) hours.
Parenteral doses are generally twice as potent as oral doses; intravenous bolus injections or infusions should be administered slowly.

Non-benzodiazepine anxiolytics

Buspirone is a non-benzodiazepine anxiolytic that is useful, along with psychotherapy, in patients with chronic anxiety or anxiety related to adjustment disorders. The onset of anxiolytic action is delayed relative to a benzodiazepine, taking 5–10 days for the relief of anxiety to begin. Because buspirone is not a benzodiazepine, it is not useful in preventing benzodiazepine withdrawal, and so one must be cautious when switching from a benzodiazepine to buspirone. The effective dose of buspirone is 10–20 mg PO t.i.d. (Robinson et al 1988).

Antipsychotics such as thioridazine are useful in treating severe anxiety unresponsive to high doses of benzodiazepines and in treating anxiety in patients with cognitive impairment (e.g., encephalopathy or dementia) in whom benzodiazepines may worsen an organic mental syndrome. Thioridazine can be started at a low dose (10–20 mg PO two to three times per day) and increased, if necessary, up to 100 mg three times per day. Antihistamines are infrequently prescribed for anxiety because of their low efficacy; hydroxyzine can be useful for anxious patients with respiratory impairment in whom benzodiazepines are relatively contraindicated. Acute panic is best treated with alprazolam or clonazepam. For maintenance treatment of panic disorder, the tricyclic antidepressant imipramine (used in doses comparable to those for the treatment of depression), alprazolam, clonazepam and the monamine oxidase inhibitors (e.g., phenalzine) all have demonstrated antipanic effects. Propranolol can be a helpful adjunct in blocking the physiological manifestations of anxiety in patients with panic disorders (Holland 1989b).

DELIRIUM (ORGANIC MENTAL DISORDERS)

Delirium and other organic mental disorders occur in roughly 15–20% of hospitalized cancer patients (Levine et al 1978, Posner 1979) and are the second most common group of psychiatric diagnoses ascribed to cancer patients. Delirium and other organic mental disorders are an even more common occurrence in patients with advanced illness. Massie et al (1983) found delirium in more than 75% of terminally ill cancer patients they studied. The 'Diagnostic and statistical manual of mental disorders', 3rd edn (revised) (DSM-III-R) (Spitzer & Williams 1987) divides organic mental disorders and syndromes into the subcategories of delirium, dementia, amnestic disorder, organic delusional disorder, organic hallucinosis, organic mood disorder, organic anxiety disorder, organic personality disorder, intoxications and withdrawal states. Lipowski (1987) has grouped these different disorders into those characterized by general cognitive impairment (i.e., delirium and dementia), and those in which cognitive impairment is selective, limited or non-existent (i.e., amnestic disorder, organic hallucinosis, organic mood disorder, etc.). In organic mental disorders where cognitive impairment is selective, limited or not observable, prominent symptoms tend to consist of anxiety, mood disturbance, delusions, hallucinations or personality change.

Delirium has been described as an aetiologically non-specific, global cerebral dysfunction characterized by concurrent disturbances in any of a number of different functions, including level of consciousness, attention, thinking, perception, emotion, memory, psychomotor behaviour and sleep–wake cycle. Disorientation, fluctuation, or waxing and waning of the above symptoms, as well as acute or abrupt onset of such disturbances, are critical features of a delirium. Delirium is also conceptualized as a reversible process (e.g., as compared to dementia), even in patients with advanced illness. Delirium, however, may not be reversible in the last 24–48 hours of life. This is most likely to be due to the influence of irreversible processes such as multiple organ failure occurring in the final hours of life. Delirium in these last days of life is often referred to as 'terminal restlessness' or 'terminal agitation' in the palliative care literature.

Early symptoms of delirium or other organic syndromes are often misdiagnosed as anxiety, anger, depression or psychosis. Because of the potential for diagnostic error, the diagnosis of an organic mental disorder should be considered in *any* medically ill patient demonstrating an acute onset of agitation or uncooperative behaviour, impaired cognitive function, altered attention span, a fluctuating level of consciousness or intense, uncharacteristic anxiety or depression (Lipowski 1987). A common error among medical and nursing staff is to conclude that a new psychological symptom represents a functional psychiatric disorder without adequately considering, evaluating and/or eliminating possible organic aetiologies. For example, the patient with mood disturbance meeting DSM-III-R criteria for major depression, who is severely hypothyroid or on high-dose corticosteroids, may be more accurately diagnosed as having an organic mood disorder, depressed type (if organic factors are judged to be the primary aetiology related to the mood disturbance). Similarly, the patient with hyponatraemia, or the patient on acyclovir for CNS herpes, who is experiencing visual hallucinations but has an intact sensorium with minimal cognitive deficits, is more accurately diagnosed as having an organic hallucinosis rather than a psychotic disorder.

In many cases, differentiating between delirium and dementia can be extremely difficult, because they frequently share clinical features such as impaired memory, thinking, judgement and disorientation. Dementia, however, typically appears in relatively alert individuals with little or no clouding of consciousness. The temporal onset of symptoms in dementia is also less acute (i.e., chronically progressive) and the sleep–wake cycle appears less impaired. Most prominent in dementia are difficulties in short- and long-term memory, impaired judgement and abstract thinking as well as disturbed higher cortical functions (e.g., aphasia, apraxia). Occasionally one will encounter delirium superimposed on an underlying dementia, particularly in elderly patients or patients with AIDS or a paraneoplastic syndrome. A number of different clinical scales or instruments have also been developed to facilitate the diagnosis of delirium, dementia or other cognitive impairments. The delirium rating scale (DRS) developed by Trzepacz et al (1988) is a 10-item clinician-rated symptom measure assessing delirium. The scale is based on DSM-III-R diagnostic criteria for delirium and is designed to be used by the clinician to identify delirium and reliably distinguish it from dementia or other neuropsychiatric disorders. Each item consists of a series of descriptive statements or behaviours, each weighted with a numerical value reflecting the similarity of that feature with the phenomenology of delirium. The scale is completed by clinicians and the weighted statements are summed to generate a DRS score. A cut-off score of 12 or greater differentiates delirious from non-delirious patients. The mini-mental-state examination (MMSE) (Folstein et al 1975) is also a useful tool for the screening of cognitive deficits, but does not distinguish between delirium and dementia. The MMSE is a series of questions and tasks which assess five general cognitive areas, including orientation, registration, attention and calculation, recall and language. The MMSE quantifies the patient's level of cognitive impairment and is more sensitive to cortical dementias such as Alzheimer's disease than it is in detecting subcortical deficits such as those found in AIDS dementia.

Organic mental disorders can be caused either by the direct effects of cancer on the central nervous system (CNS), or the indirect CNS effects of the disease or treatments (medications, electrolyte imbalance, failure of a vital organ or system, infection, vascular complications and pre-existing cognitive impairment or dementia). Given the large numbers of medications cancer pain patients require, and their fragile physiological state, even routinely ordered hypnotics may engender an episode of delirium. Perhaps most relevant to cancer pain management is the role that narcotic analgesics play in the development of delirium. Certainly opioid analgesics such as meperidine, morphine sulphate hydromorphone and levorphanel have been reported to cause confusional states, particularly in the elderly cancer patient and in the terminally ill patient (Bruera et al 1989b, 1990b). The toxic accumulation of meperidine's metabolite, normeperidine, is associated with florid delirium accompanied by myoclonus and possible seizures. The routine use of stable regimens of oral narcotic analgesics for the control of cancer pain is rarely complicated by overt delirium or confusional states (Liepzig et al 1987); in fact, most patients have minimal functional or cognitive impairment. There have been reports of organic hallucinosis, complicating standard regimens of oral opioids (Jellema 1987). Significant cognitive impairment as well as delirium can, however, occur during periods of rapid opioid dosage escalation, especially in older patients receiving intravenous infusions of opioids (Portenoy 1987, Bruera et al 1989b, Eller et al 1992). Eller et al (1992) recently studied the incidence of acute confusional states in 94 adult cancer patients receiving continuous intravenous morphine infusion for pain control. In this retrospective review, 68% exhibited some alteration in mental status and 53% had symptoms suggestive of delirium. Factors that increased the risk of developing delirium included opioid dosage (higher dosage) age (over 65) and impaired renal function (creatinine >1.5 mg/100 ml).

Chemotherapeutic agents known to cause delirium (Table 46.4) include methotrexate, fluorouracil, vincristine, vinblastine, bleomycin, BCNU, cis-platinum, asparaginase, procarbazine and the glucocorticosteroids (Holland et al 1974, Weddington 1982, Young 1982, Adams et al 1984, Denicoff et al 1987, Stiefel et al 1989). With the exception of steroids, however, most patients receiving chemotherapeutic agents do not develop prominent CNS effects. The spectrum of mental disturbances caused by corticosteroids ranges from minor mood lability to mania or depression, cognitive impairment (reversible dementia) to delirium (steroid psychosis). The incidence of these disorders varies greatly, with 3–57% of non-cancer patients developing an organic mental disorder. Although these disturbances are most common with higher doses and usually develop within the first 2 weeks of steroid use, they can occur at any time, on any dose, even during the tapering phase (Stiefel et al 1989). Prior psychiatric illness or prior mental disturbance due to steroid use does not predict susceptibility to, or the nature of, subsequent mental disturbance with steroids. These disorders often reverse rapidly upon dose reduction or discontinuation (Stiefel et al 1989).

Table 46.4 Neuropsychiatric side effects of chemotherapeutic drugs

Drug	*Neuropsychiatric symptoms*
Methotrexate (intrathecal)	Delirium, dementia, lethargy, personality change
Vincristine, vinblastine	Delirium, hallucinations, lethargy, depression
Asparaginase	Delirium, hallucinations, lethargy, cognitive dysfunction
BCNU	Delirium, dementia
Bleomycin	Delirium
Fluorouracil	Delirium
Cis-platinum	Delirium
Hydroxyurea	Hallucinations
Procarbazine	Depression, mania, delirium, dementia
Cytosine arabinoside	Delirium, lethargy cognitive dysfunction
Hexylmethylamine	Hallucinations
Isophosphamide	Delirium, lethargy, hallucinations
Prednisone	Depression, mania, delirium, psychoses
Interferon	Flu-like syndrome, delirium, hallucinations, depression
Interleukin	Cognitive dysfunction, hallucinations

MANAGEMENT OF DELIRIUM

The appropriate approach in the management of delirium in the cancer pain patient includes interventions that are directed both at the underlying causes and symptoms of delirium. Identification and correction of the underlying cause(s) for delirium must take place while symptomatic and supportive therapies are initiated (Lipowski 1987, Fleishman & Lesko 1989). In the case of the cancer patient in pain who develops delirium while on a high-dose opioid infusion, often the mere reduction of dose or infusion rate (if pain is controlled) will begin to resolve symptoms of delirium within hours. Other strategies include switching from one opioid (e.g., morphine) to another (e.g., hydromorphone). Often, delirium will occur or persist even after such manoeuvres or pain may require continued high-dose infusion. The use of a concomitant neuroleptic drug (e.g., haloperidol) is indicated. Symptomatic treatment measures include support for and communication with the patient and family, reassurance, manipulation of the environment to provide a reorienting, safe milieu and then appropriate use of pharmacotherapies. Measures to help reduce anxiety and disorientation (i.e., increased structure and familiarity) may include a quiet, well-lit room with familiar objects, a visible clock or calendar and the presence of family. Judicious use of physical restraints, along with one-to-one nursing observation, may also be necessary and useful. Often, these supportive techniques alone are not effective and symptomatic treatment with neuroleptic or sedative medications is necessary (Table 46.5).

Table 46.5 Medications useful in managing delirium in cancer pain patients

Generic name	*Approximate daily dosage range (mg)*	*Route*[1]
Neuroleptics		
Haloperidol	0.5–q2–12 h	PO, IV, SC, IM
Thioridazine	10–75 q 4–8 h	PO
Chlorpromazine	12.5–50 q 4–12 h	PO, IV, IM
Methotrimeprazine	12.5–50 q 4–8 h	PO, IV, SC
Molindone	10–50 q 8–12 h	PO
Droperidol	0.5–5 q 12 h	IV, IM
Novel antipsychotics		
Risperadone	1–3 q 12 h	PO
Olanzipine	2.5–5 q 12 h	PO
Benzodiazepines		
Lorazepam	0.5–20 q 1–4 h	PO, IV, IM
Anaesthetics		
Propofol	10–50 q 1 h	IV
Midazolam	30–100 per 24 h	IV, SC

[1] Parenteral doses are generally twice as potent as oral doses; IV = intravenous infusions or bolus injections should be administered slowly; IM = intramuscular injections should be avoided if repeated use becomes necessary; PO = oral forms of medication are preferred; SC = subcutaneous infusions are generally accepted modes of drug administration in the terminally ill; q (2–12) h = every (2–12) hours.

Neuroleptic medications in the management of delirium

Neuroleptic medications vary in their sedating properties and in their potential for producing orthostatic hypotension, neurological side effects (acute dystonia, extrapyramidal symptoms) and anticholinergic effects. The acutely agitated cancer patient requires a sedating medication; the patient with hypotension requires a drug with the least effect on blood pressure; the delirious postoperative patient who has an ileus or urinary retention should receive an antipsychotic with the least anticholinergic effects.

Haloperidol, a neuroleptic agent that is a potent dopamine blocker, is the drug of choice for the treatment of delirium in the cancer pain patient because of its useful sedating effects and low incidence of cardiovascular and anticholinergic effects (Adams et al 1986, Lipowski 1987, Murray 1987). Relatively low doses of haloperidol (1–3 mg/day) are usually effective in targeting agitation, paranoia and fear. Typically 0.5–1.0 mg haloperidol (PO, IV, IM, SC) is administered initially, with repeat doses every 45–60 minutes titrated against symptoms (Massie et al 1983, Fleishman & Lesko 1989). Peak plasma concentrations are achieved in 2–4 hours after an oral dose and measurable plasma concentrations occur 15–30 minutes after intramuscular administrations. Although not yet approved by the Food and Drug Administration for intravenous use, haloperidol is commonly and safely administered by this route. The intravenous route is preferable in agitated or paranoid patients as it facilitates rapid onset of medication effects (Lipowski 1987, Adams 1988, Fleischman & Lesko 1989). If intravenous access is unavailable, we suggest starting with intramuscular or subcutaneous administration and switching to the oral route when possible. The majority of delirious patients can be managed with oral haloperidol. Parenteral doses are roughly twice as potent as oral doses. Delivery of haloperidol by the subcutaneous route is utilized by many palliative care practitioners (Fainsinger & Bruera 1992). Although our experience has been that most patients respond to doses of less than 20 mg of haloperidol in a 24-hour period, others advocate high doses (up to 250 mg/24 hour of IV haloperidol) in selected cases (Adams et al 1986, Murray 1987, Fernandez et al 1989).

A drawback to the use of haloperidol is the potential for causing extrapyramidal side effects and movement disorders. Acute dystonias and extrapyramidal side effects can generally be controlled by the use of antiparkinsonian medications (e.g., diphenhydramine, benztropine, trihexyphenidyl); akathisia responds either to low doses of a propranolol (e.g., 5 mg two to three times per day), lorazepam (0.5–1.0 mg two to three times per day) or benztropine (1–2 mg once to twice per day). A rare but at times fatal complication of antipsychotics is the neuroleptic malignant syndrome (NMS). NMS usually occurs after prolonged high-dose administration of neuroleptics and is characterized by hyperthermia, increased mental confusion, leucocytosis, muscular rigidity, myoglobinuria and high serum creatine phosphokinase (CPK). Treatment consists of discontinuing the neuroleptic and use of dantrolene sodium (0.8–10 mg per kilogram per day) or bromocriptine mesylate (2.5–10 mg three times per day) (Fleishman & Lesko 1989).

Benzodiazepines in the management of delirium

A common strategy in the management of agitated delirium is to add parenteral lorazepam to a regimen of haloperidol (Adams et al 1986, Murray 1987, Fernandez et al 1989). Lorazepam (0.5–1.0 mg every 1–2 hours PO or IV) along with haloperidol, may be more effective in rapidly sedating the agitated delirious patient. Despite these clinical observations suggesting lorazepam as an effective adjunct to antipsychotic medications, benzodiazepines alone have limited benefit in the treatment of delirium. In a double-blind, randomized comparison trial of haloperidol versus chlorpromazine versus lorazepam, it was demonstrated that lorazepam alone, in doses up to 8 mg in a 12-hour period, was ineffective in the treatment of delirium and in fact contributed to worsening delirium and cognitive impairment (Breitbart et al 1996c). Both neuroleptic drugs, however, in low doses (approximately 2 mg of haloperidol equivalent/24 h), were highly effective in controlling the symptoms of delirium (dramatic improvement in DRS scores) and improving cognitive function (dramatic improvement in MMSE scores). In addition, haloperidol and chlorpromazine have both been found effective in improving the symptoms of both hypoactive as well as hyperactive delirium (Platt et al 1994). Perhaps the only setting in which benzodiazepines alone have an established role is in the management of delirium in the dying patient.

Several newer, novel antipsychotic agents may be useful in the management of delirium. These agents, which include risperdone and olanzapine, have fewer neurological side effects (e.g., extrapyramidal side effects, or tardive dyskinesia), but typically are only available by the oral route. Risperdal has been shown to be useful in the treatment of dementia and psychosis in AIDS patients at doses of 1–6 mg per day, suggesting safe use in patients with delirium (Singh 1996). Olanzapine, in doses from 1.5 to 20 mg per day, has been demonstrated to improve the symptoms of delirium in an open trial of 11 medically ill patients with delirium (Sipahimalani & Masand 1998).

Management of delirium in the dying cancer pain patient

The treatment of delirium in the dying cancer pain patient is unique for the following reasons:

1. Most often, the aetiology of terminal delirium is multifactorial or may not be found; Bruera et al (1990b) reported that an aetiology was discovered in less than 50% of terminally ill patients with cognitive dysfunction.
2. When a distinct cause is found, it is often irreversible (such as hepatic failure or brain metastases).
3. Work-up may be limited by the setting (home, hospice).
4. The consultant's focus is usually on the patient's comfort and ordinarily helpful diagnostic procedures that are unpleasant or painful (i.e. CT scan, lumbar puncture) may be avoided.

When confronted with a delirium in the terminally ill or dying cancer patient, a differential diagnosis should always be formulated; however, studies should be pursued only when a suspected factor can be identified easily and treated effectively.

The use of medications in the management of delirium in the dying patient remains controversial in some circles. Some have argued that pharmacological interventions with neuroleptics or benzodiazepines are inappropriate in the dying patient. Delirium is viewed as a natural part of the dying process that should not be altered. Another rationale that is often raised is that these patients are so close to death that aggressive treatment is unnecessary. Parenteral neuroleptics or sedatives may be mistakenly avoided because of exaggerated fears that they might hasten death through hypotension or respiratory depression. Many clinicians are unnecessarily pessimistic about the possible results of neuroleptic treatment for delirium. They argue that because the underlying pathophysiological process often continues unabated (such as hepatic or renal failure), no improvement can be expected in the patient's mental status. There is concern that neuroleptics or sedatives may worsen a delirium by making the patient more confused or sedated. Clinical experience in managing delirium in dying cancer patients suggests that the use of neuroleptics in the management of agitation, paranoia, hallucinations and altered sensorium is safe, effective and quite appropriate. Management of delirium on a case-by-case basis is always the most logical course of action. The agitated, delirious dying patient should probably be given neuroleptics to help restore calm. A 'wait and see' approach, prior to using neuroleptics, may be most appropriate with patients who have a lethargic or somnolent presentation of delirium. The consultant must educate staff and patients and weigh each of these issues in making the decision about whether or not to use pharmacological interventions for the dying patient who presents with delirium.

Methotrimeprazine (IV or SC) is often utilized to control confusion and agitation in terminal delirium (Oliver 1985). Dosages range from 12.5 to 50 mg every 4–8 hours up to 300 mg per 24 hours for most patients. Hypotension and excessive sedation are problematical limitations of this drug. Midazolam, given by subcutaneous or intravenous infusion in doses ranging from 30 to 100 mg/24 h, are also used to control agitation related to delirium in the terminal stages (de Sousa & Jepson 1988, Bottomley & Hanks 1990). Propofol, a short-acting anaesthetic agent, has also begun to be utilized primarily as a sedating agent for the control of agitated patients with 'terminal' delirium. In several case reports of propofol's use in terminal care, an intravenous loading dose of 20 mg of propofol was followed by a continuous infusion of propofol, with initial doses ranging from 10 mg/h to 70 mg/h, and with titration of doses up to as high as 400 mg/h over a period of hours to days in several agitated patients. (Mercandante et al 1995, Moyle 1995, DeSousa & Jepson 1998). The goal of treatment with midazolam, propofol and to some extent with methotrimeprazine, is quiet sedation only. As opposed to neuroleptic drugs such as haloperidol, a midazolam infusion does not clear a delirious patient's sensorium or improve cognition. These clinical differences may be caused by the underlying pathophysiology of delirium. One hypothesis postulates that an imbalance of central cholinergic and adrenergic mechanisms underlies delirium and so a dopamine blocking drug may initiate a rebalancing of these systems (Itil & Fink 1966). While neuroleptic drugs such as haloperidol are most effective in achieving the goals of diminishing agitation, clearing the sensorium and improving cognition in the delirious patient, this is not always possible in the last days of life. Processes causing delirium may be ongoing and irreversible during the active dying phase. Ventafridda et al (1990a) and Fainsinger et al (1991) have reported that a significant group (10–20%) of terminally ill patients experience delirium that can be controlled only by sedation to the point of a significantly decreased level of consciousness.

CANCER PAIN AND SUICIDE PHYSICIAN-ASSISTED SUICIDE, EUTHANASIA

Uncontrolled pain is a major factor in cancer suicide (Breitbart 1987, 1990b). Cancer is perceived by the public as an extremely painful disease compared to other medical conditions. In Wisconsin, a study revealed that 69% of the public agreed that cancer pain could cause a person to consider suicide (Levin et al 1985). The majority of suicides were observed among patients with cancer who had severe pain, which was often inadequately controlled or tolerated poorly (Bolund 1985). Although relatively few cancer patients commit suicide, they are at increased risk (Farberow et al 1963, Breitbart 1987). Factors associated with an increased risk of suicide in cancer patients are listed in Box 46.1. Patients with advanced illness are at highest risk and are the most likely to have the complications of pain, depression, delirium and deficit symptoms. Psychiatric disorders are frequently present in hospitalized cancer patients who attempt suicide. A review of the psychiatric consultation data at Memorial Sloan-Kettering Cancer Center (MSKCC) showed that one-third of cancer patients who were seen for evaluation of suicide risk received a diagnosis of major depression; approximately 20% met criteria for delirium and more than 50% were diagnosed with an adjustment disorder (Breitbart 1987).

Thoughts of suicide probably occur quite frequently, particularly in the setting of advanced cancer, and seem to act as a steam valve for feelings often expressed by patients as 'If it gets too bad, I always have a way out'. It has been our experience in working with cancer pain patients that once a trusting and safe relationship develops, patients almost universally reveal that they have occasionally had persistent thoughts of suicide as a means of escaping the threat of being overwhelmed by pain. Recent published reports, however, suggest that suicidal ideation is relatively infrequent in cancer and is limited to those who are significantly depressed. Silberfarb et al (1980) found that only three of 146 breast cancer patients had suicidal thoughts, whereas none of the 100 cancer patients interviewed in a Finnish study expressed suicidal thoughts (Achte & Vanhkouen 1971). A study conducted at St Boniface Hospice in Winnipeg, Canada, demonstrated that only 10 of 44 terminally ill cancer patients were suicidal or desired an early death and all 10 were suffering from clinical depression (Brown et al 1986). At the MSKCC, suicide risk evaluation accounted for 8.6% of psychiatric consultations, usually requested by staff in response to patients verbalizing suicidal wishes (Breitbart 1987). In the 71 cancer patients who had suicidal ideation with serious intent, significant pain was a factor in only 30% of cases. In striking contrast, virtually all 71 suicidal cancer patients had a psychiatric disorder (mood disturbance or organic mental disorder) at the time of evaluation (Breitbart 1987).

BOX 46.1

Cancer pain suicide vulnerability factors

Pain; suffering aspects
Multiple physical symptoms
Advanced illness; poor prognosis
Depression; hopelessness
Delirium; disinhibition
Control; helplessness
Preexisting psychopathology
Suicide history; family history
Inadequate social support

We recently examined the role of cancer pain in suicidal ideation by assessing 185 cancer pain patients involved in ongoing research protocols of the MSKCC Pain and Psychiatry Services (Saltzburg et al 1989). Suicidal ideation occurred in 17% of the study population, with the majority reporting suicidal ideation without intent to act. Interestingly, in this population of cancer patients who all had significant pain, suicidal ideation was not directly related to pain intensity, but was strongly related to degree of depression and mood disturbance. Pain was related to suicidal ideation indirectly in that patients' perception of poor pain relief was associated with suicidal ideation. Our group at Memorial (Breitbart et al 1991) examined these same issues in an AIDS population and found similar relationships between pain, mood and suicidal ideation. Perceptions of pain relief may have more to do with aspects of hopelessness than pain itself. Pain plays an important role in vulnerability to suicide; however, associated psychological distress and mood disturbance seem to be essential cofactors in raising the risk of suicide in cancer patients. Pain has adverse effects on patients' quality of life and sense of control and impairs the family's ability to provide support. Factors other than pain, such as mood disturbance, delirium, loss of control and hopelessness, contribute to cancer suicide risk (Breitbart 1990b).

Chochinov et al (1995) found that of 200 terminally ill patients in a palliative care facility, 44.5% acknowledged at least a fleeting desire to die. However 17 patients (8.5%) reported an unequivocal desire for death to come soon and indicated that they held this desire consistently over time. Among this group, 10 (58.8%) met criteria for a diagnosis of depression, compared to a prevalence of depression of only 7.7% in patients who did not endorse a genuine, consistent desire for death. Patients with a desire for death were also found to have significantly more severe intensity pain and less social support than those patients without a desire for death.

In a study of cancer patients by Emanuel and colleagues (1996), 25% reported that they had seriously thought about euthanasia, and 12% had discussed this option with their physicians. Patients in this study who either thought about euthanasia or discussed this option with their physician were significantly more likely to be depressed. In a follow-up multicentre study of 988 terminally ill cancer patients, 11.6% had thoughts of ending their life or asking a physician to end their life and 3.7% had discussed it with someone (Fairclough et al 1998). Again, depression was the strongest single predictor of thoughts about ending their life.

In a 1988 survey of Californian physicians, 57% of those responding reported that they had been asked by terminally ill patients to hasten death. Persistent pain and terminal illness were the primary reasons for those requests for physician-assisted suicide (Helig 1988).

EUTHANASIA AND ASSISTED SUICIDE IN CLINICAL PRACTICE

A number of surveys have been published documenting the practice of euthanasia and assisted suicide among healthcare professionals. For example, an anonymous survey of Washington physicians conducted in 1995 found that 26% of responding physicians had received at least one request for assisted suicide, and two-thirds of those physicians had granted such requests (Back et al 1996). Thus, roughly one in six Washington physicians acknowledged having granted a patient's request for assisted suicide or euthanasia. Of course, because this study was a survey it is not possible to determine whether responding physicians were an accurate representation of all Washington physicians (e.g., physicians less interested in or more opposed to assisted suicide may have been more likely to refuse to return the surveys), let alone for the larger USA, yet these statistics suggest that assisted suicide is not a rare event, despite the illegal status. (It is also possible that, despite the anonymous nature of the survey, some physicians who had in fact carried out these requests were unwilling to acknowledge their actions for fear of repercussions.)

Even more striking results were reported in a survey of San Francisco area AIDS physicians. Slome and colleagues (1997) found that 98% of respondents had received requests for assisted suicide and more than half of all responding physicians reported having granted at least one patient's request for assisted suicide. The average number of times that responding physicians had granted requests for assisted suicide was 4.2, with some physicians fulfilling dozens of such requests. Moreover, in response to a hypothetical vignette, nearly half of the sample (48%) indicated that they would be likely to grant a hypothetical patient's *initial* request for assisted suicide.

A more recent national survey sampled nearly two thousand physicians from those discliplines most likely to recieve requests for assisted suicide or euthanasia (Meier et al 1998). Meier and colleagues found that more than 18% of responding physicians reported having received at least one request for assisted suicide and more than 11% had received requests for 'lethal injection' (the author's definition of euthanasia). Only 6.4% of the total sample, however, reported having acceded to a request for hastened death (3.3% reported having prescribed medications to be used for this purpose and 4.7% reported having provided lethal injection), roughly one-quarter of those who reported having received one. The most common reasons for these requests for hastened death (according to physicians) included 'discomfort other than pain' (present in 79% of cases), 'loss of dignity' (53% of cases), 'fear of uncontrollable symptoms' (52% of cases), pain (50% of cases) and 'loss of meaning in their lives' (47% of cases). Although most physicians responded to requests for hastened death with either more aggressive palliative care (i.e., increased analgesic medications) or less aggressive life-prolonging treatments, 25% of physicians reported having prescribed antidepressant medications. Despite this seeming acknowledgment of the possible role of depression in patient requests for hastened death, only 2% of physicians reported having sought psychiatric consultation for their patients who requested assistance in dying.

Perhaps the most striking research to date regarding the use of assisted suicide and euthanasia was a study of critical care nurses conducted by David Asch (1996). This study, based on the results of an anonymous survey, found that 17% of respondents reported having received at least one request for assisted suicide and 11% had granted such a request. Aproximately 5% of responding nurses acknowledged having hastened a patient's death at the request of the physician, but without the request of the patient or the family (termed 'involuntary euthanasia' by some writers). Moreover, 4.7% of the sample indicated that they had hastened a patient's death without the knowledge of or request by the physician. Respondents described having stopped oxygen therapy or increased pain medication in order to hasten death (Asch 1996). Asch suggested, based on the reports of respondent nurses, that these actions were done in order to ease the suffering of the patients, and cited the traditional role of nursing in palliative care as the basis for these results. It should also be noted that Asch's controversial study generated considerable response, including many suggestions that methodological issues such as vague wording of questions may make these data unreliable (e.g., Scanlon 1996). Nevertheless, while these data may not accurately indicate the true prevalence of assisted suicide or euthanasia in the USA, requests for assistance in dying are clearly not rare events and physicians occasionally grant such requests despite legal prohibitions. Furthermore, because legal restrictions limit the ability of physicians to consult with colleagues regarding how to react to a request for assisted suicide, the appropriateness of patient requests and physician responses is unknown.

In the Netherlands, however, where physician-assisted suicide and euthanasia have been practised regularly for more than 10 years, data regarding the frequency of requests for assistance in dying and the proportion of terminally ill patients whose lives end in this manner are available. Euthanasia was granted its current status in 1984 after a Dutch supreme court decision authorized this practice, provided a number of conditions were met. Specifically, the patient's request for assisted suicide must be considered free, conscious, explicit and persistent. Both the physician and patient must agree that the patient's suffering is intolerable and other measures for relief must have been exhausted. A second physician must be consulted, and must concur with the decision to assist in ending the patient's life. Finally all of these conditions must be adequately documented and reported to the governmental body supervising the practice of euthanasia. Because of the availability of such records, several studies have documented the proportion of deaths in the Netherlands in which euthanasia/assisted suicide are implicated (these estimates were adjusted to account for the under-reporting of euthanasia acknowledged by many Dutch physicians). In reporting on euthanasia and assisted suicide practices in the Netherlands from 1990 to 1995, van der Maas and colleagues (1996) incorporated both official reports of euthanasia as well as responses to anonymous surveys to estimate the rates of euthanasia and assisted suicide. They concluded that euthanasia and assisted suicide were involved in roughly 4.7% of all deaths in the Netherlands during 1995, a substantial increase over the 2.7% of deaths involving medical assistance reported in a 1991 study.

Supporters of assisted suicide point to the Netherlands data as evidence that legalization has not led to widespread abuse or overuse of euthanasia/assisted suicide. Critics, however, suggest that the 75% increase in deaths involving euthanasia or assisted suicide (from 2.7% to 4.7%) demonstrates a growing tendency towards more frequent, and therefore a greater number, of potentially inappropriate cases of euthanasia. Such concerns are clearly reflected in a 1994 Dutch supreme court decision in which the right to euthanasia/assisted suicide was extended to include patients suffering from chronic illnesses that are not terminal, including mental disorders such as depression, provided the illness is refractory to treatment and causes intolerable suffering. Although the vast majority of requests for assisted suicide from mentally ill individuals have been denied, isolated cases have occurred in which mentally ill Dutch adults have been allowed to receive physician-assisted suicide or euthanasia as a result of this court ruling. This experience has been identified as evidence of the 'slippery slope' argument (e.g., Hendin et al 1997), in which legalization of assisted suicide is presumed to lead to a gradual widening of the group of patients eligible for this 'intervention', many of whom may not be appropriate (e.g., physically healthy but clinically depressed individuals).

What is the appropriate response to such a request? The clinician in the oncology setting faces a dilemma when confronting the issue of assisted suicide or euthanasia in the cancer patient. From the medical perspective, professional training reinforces the view of suicide as a manifestation of psychiatric disturbance to be prevented at all costs. However, from the philosophical perspective, many in our society view suicide in those who face the distress of an often fatal and painful disease like cancer as 'rational' and a means to regain control and maintain a 'dignified death'. An internal debate thus often takes place within the cancer care professional that is not dissimilar to the public debate that surrounds celebrated cases in which the rights of patients to terminate life-sustaining measures or receive active euthanasia are at issue.

The term 'euthanasia' encompasses a number of concepts, all of which have become controversial but important issues in the care of terminally ill patients. Active euthanasia refers to the intentional termination of a patient's life by a physician. Physician-assisted suicide is the provision by a physician of the means by which patients can end their own lives. Passive euthanasia refers to the withholding or withdrawal of life-sustaining measures and is viewed as acceptable in many societies (Pellegrino 1991). Active euthanasia and physician-assisted suicide, however, are perhaps the most intensely and bitterly debated issues in medical ethics today.

Active euthanasia has been taking place in the Netherlands for a decade (de Wachter 1989, van der Maas et al 1991). While still illegal, the active termination of a patient's life by a physician is tolerated under the condition that:

1. The patient's consent is free, conscious, explicit and persistent.
2. The patient and physician agree that the suffering is intolerable.

3. Other measures for relief have been exhausted.
4. A second physician must concur.
5. These facts must be documented.

A best estimate is that 1.8% of deaths in the Netherlands are the result of euthanasia with physician involvement (van der Maas et al 1991). Common reasons for requesting euthanasia included: loss of dignity (57%), pain (46%), unworthy dying (sic) (46%), being dependent on others (33%) and tiredness of life (sic) (23%) (van der Mass et al 1991). Recently, the states of California and Washington have considered initiatives that would allow active euthanasia along the Netherlands model. Physician opponents of Washington State's recent referendum on euthanasia (Initiative 119) agreed that the vote was as much about pain control as it was about dying, and proposed that the state require physicians to take pain management courses in order to maintain licenses. Many supporters of Initiative 119 voted for the measure because of fear that their death would be painful (American Medical News 1992). The case of 'Debbie', published in the 'Journal of the American Medical Association' in 1988, forced a debate on active euthanasia in the USA that is ongoing (Gaylin et al 1988, Wanzer et al 1989, Singer 1990).

Physician-assisted suicide has also become a topic of public debate, following the dramatic case in 1990 of a woman with Alzheimer's disease who utilized Dr Kevorkian's 'suicide machine'. Dr Kevorkian was acquitted by a Michigan Court of any wrongdoing. Dr Timothy E. Quill, a physician who assisted a leukaemia patient in committing suicide, was not indicted by a Rochester grand jury in July 1991. Dr Quill's account of his participation in his patient's suicide was published in the 7 March 1991 issue of the 'New England Journal of Medicine' (Quill 1991) and sparked a continuing debate regarding the physician's role in aiding dying patients. In interviews after he published this article, Dr Quill said he had decided to go public in order to present an alternative to Dr Kevorkian's approach, using a machine in the death of a patient whom Dr Kevorkian did not know well. In contrast to the Kevorkian case, Dr Quill had been treating the patient with leukaemia for 8 years and knew her quite well. In his article, Dr Quill described the process which he and the patient undertook, exploring her choice actively to take her life. He also described recommending that the patient contact the Hemlock Society and prescribing barbiturates for sleep 1 week later at the patient's request. While Dr Quill's patient was not suffering with uncontrolled pain, many physicians who care for cancer pain patients report interactions with patients where requests for assistance in suicide are expressed. Foley (1991) reports that, in a large cancer centre pain clinic, patients not uncommonly consider suicide or request hastened death or physician-assistance, but change their minds once adequate pain control has been provided.

'The Humane and Dignified Death Act', a proposed law that would free doctors from criminal and civil liability if they participated in voluntary active euthanasia, did not appear on the 1988 California ballot because the sponsoring group (Americans Against Human Suffering) failed to obtain the required number of signatures. That group, an affiliate organization of the National Hemlock Society, did however undertake a survey of Californian physicians, as part of their efforts to build up support for the act, that was quite revealing (Helig 1988). Of the physicians who responded, 70% agreed that patients should have the option of active euthanasia in terminal illness. More than half of the physicians said that they would practise active voluntary euthanasia if it were legal. Some 23% revealed that they had already practised active euthanasia at least once in their careers. Of the 60% of physicians who indicated that they had been asked by patients with terminal illness to hasten death, nearly all agreed that such requests from patients can be described as 'rational'. Public support for the 'right to die' has been growing as well. Of the general population, 65–85% support a change in the law to permit physicians to help patients die and there is greater acceptance by the public of suicide when pain and suffering coexist with terminal illness.

Those of us who provide clinical care for cancer patients with pain and advanced illness are sympathetic to the goals of symptom control and relief of suffering, but are also obviously influenced by those who view suicide or active voluntary euthanasia as rational alternatives for those already dying and in distress. Ironically, while inadequate pain control seems to be a factor in driving patients towards suicide or assisted suicide/euthanasia, an obstacle to adequate pain control is the concern by many that aggressive pain control (e.g., opioid infusions) is a form of euthanasia. Many have argued that adequate pain control is not physician-assisted suicide or euthanasia (Wanzer et al 1989, Foley 1991, Pellegrino 1991). Danger lies in the premature assumption that suicidal ideation or a request to hasten death in the cancer patient represents a 'rational act' that is unencumbered by psychiatric disturbance. Accepted criteria for 'rational suicide' (Siegel 1982, Siegel & Tuckel 1984) include the following:

1. The person must have clear mental processes that are unimpaired by psychological illness or severe emotional distress, such as depression.

2. The person must have a realistic assessment of the situation.
3. The motives for the decision of suicide are understandable to most uninvolved observers.

Clearly there are suicides that occur in the cancer setting that meet these criteria for rationality; however, a significant percentage, possibly the majority, do not, by virtue of the fact that significant psychiatric comorbidity exists. By reviewing the current research data on cancer suicide and the role of such factors as pain, depression and delirium, we hope to provide a factual framework on which to base guidelines for the management of this vulnerable group of patients.

ASSESSMENT ISSUES IN THE TREATMENT OF CANCER PAIN: OBSTACLES TO ADEQUATE PAIN CONTROL

Cancer pain is often inadequately managed. Cleeland and colleagues (1994) estimate that roughly 40% of cancer pain patients receive inadequate analgesic therapy. A survey of 1177 oncologists who participate in the Eastern Cooperative Oncology Group (ECOG) was undertaken to assess cancer pain management (von Roenn et al 1993). Over 85% reported that they felt the majority of cancer patients are undermedicated for pain. Only 51.4% believed that pain control in their own setting was good or very good. Barriers to adequate pain management described by this survey of oncologists included:

1. Patient reluctance to report pain (62%).
2. Patient reluctance to take medications (62%).
3. Physician reluctance to prescribe pain medication (61%).
4. Most importantly, poor pain assessment knowledge and skills (61%).

Inadequate management of cancer pain is often due to a lack of ability to properly assess pain in all its dimensions (Marks & Sachar 1973, Foley 1985, Breitbart 1989a). All too frequently, psychological variables are proposed to explain continued pain or lack of response to therapy, when in fact medical factors have not been adequately appreciated. Other causes of inadequate cancer pain management include:

1. Lack of knowledge of current therapeutic approaches.
2. Focus on prolonging life and cure versus alleviating suffering.
3. Inadequate physician–patient relationship.
4. Limited expectations of patients.
5. Unavailability of narcotics.
6. Fear of respiratory depression.
7. Most important, fear of addiction.

Fear of addiction affects both patient compliance and physician management of narcotic analgesics leading to undermedication of cancer pain (Marks & Sachar 1973, Macaluso et al 1988a). Studies of the patterns of chronic narcotic analgesic use in patients with cancer have demonstrated that, although tolerance and physical dependence commonly occur, addiction (psychological dependence) is rare and almost never occurs in an individual without a history of drug abuse prior to cancer illness (Kanner & Foley 1981). Passik (1992) reviewed the requests for psychiatric consultation at Memorial Sloan-Kettering Cancer Centre for a 1-year period. In only 36 of 1200 (3%) requests for psychiatric consultation was substance abuse cited as the primary reason for the request. Interestingly, in one-third of these cases the psychiatry service consultant did not go on to concur with the labelling of the patient as a substance abuser (usually citing uncontrolled pain as the reason for the supposedly aberrant behaviour on the part of the patient). Fears of iatrogenic addiction result largely from the erroneous assumption that the opioids are highly addictive drugs and that the problem of addiction resides in the drugs themselves. Cancer patients allowed to self-administer morphine for several weeks during an episode of painful mucositis do not demonstrate escalating use (Chapman 1989). Of 11 882 inpatients surveyed in the Boston Collaborative Drug Surveillance Project, who had no prior history of addiction and were administered opioids, only four cases of psychological dependence could be documented (Porter & Jick 1980). A survey of burn centers identified no cases of iatrogenic addiction in a sample of over 10 000 patients without prior drug abuse history, who were administered opioids for pain (Perry & Heidrich 1982). A study of opioid use in headache patients identified opioid abuse in only three of 2369 patients prescribed opioids (Medina & Diamond 1977). These data suggest that patients without a prior history of substance abuse are highly unlikely to become addicted following the administration of opioid drugs as part of their medical treatment.

Escalation of narcotic analgesic use by cancer pain patients is usually a result of the progression of cancer or the development of tolerance. Tolerance means that a larger dose of narcotic analgesic is required to maintain an original analgesic effect. Physical dependence is characterized by the onset of signs and symptoms of withdrawal if the narcotic is suddenly stopped or a narcotic antagonist is administered. Tolerance usually occurs in association with physical dependence, but does not imply psychological dependence or addiction, is not equivalent to physical dependence or tolerance and is a behavioural pattern of compulsive drug abuse characterized by a craving for the drug and overwhelming involvement in obtaining and using it for effects other than pain relief. The cancer pain patient with a history of intravenous opioid abuse presents an often unnecessarily difficult management problem. Macaluso et al (1988a) reported on their experience in managing cancer pain in such a population. Of 468 inpatient cancer pain consultations, only eight (1.7%) had a history of intravenous drug abuse, but none had been actively abusing drugs in the previous year. All eight of these patients had inadequate pain control and more than half were intentionally undermedicated because of concern by staff that drug abuse was active or would recur. Adequate pain control was ultimately achieved in these patients by using appropriate analgesic dosages and intensive staff education. Refer to the section below on 'Psychotherapy and cancer pain' for a more extensive review of the management of substance abuse problems in cancer pain patients.

The risk of inducing respiratory depression is too often overestimated and can limit the appropriate use of narcotic analgesics for pain and symptom control. Bruera et al (1990a) demonstrated that, in a population of terminally ill cancer patients with respiratory failure and dyspnoea, administration of subcutaneous morphine actually improved dyspnoea without causing a significant deterioration in respiratory function. The adequacy of cancer pain management can be influenced by the lack of concordance between patient ratings or complaints of their pain and those made by caregivers. Persistent cancer pain is often ascribed to a psychological cause when it does not respond to treatment attempts. In our clinical experience we have noted that patients who report their pain as 'severe' are quite likely to be viewed as having a psychological contribution to their complaints. Staff members' ability to empathize with a patient's pain complaint may be limited by the intensity of the pain complaint. Grossman et al (1991) found that while there is a high degree of concordance between patient and caregiver ratings of patient pain intensity at the low and moderate levels, this concordance breaks down at high levels. Thus, a clinician's ability to assess a patient's level of pain becomes unreliable once a patient's report of pain intensity rises above 7 on a visual analogue rating scale of 0–10. Physicians must be educated as to the limitations of their ability objectively to assess the severity of a subjective pain experience. Additionally, patient education is often a useful intervention in such cases. Patients are more likely to be believed and adequately treated if they are taught to request pain relief in a non-hysterical business-like fashion.

The optimal treatment of cancer pain is multimodal and includes pharmacological, psychotherapeutic, cognitive-behavioural, anaesthetic, stimulatory and rehabilitative approaches. Psychiatric participation in cancer pain management involves the use of psychotherapeutic, cognitive-behavioural and psychopharmacological interventions which are described below.

PSYCHOTHERAPY AND CANCER PAIN

The goals of psychotherapy with cancer pain patients are to provide support, knowledge and skills (Table 46.2). Utilizing short-term supportive psychotherapy based on a crisis intervention model, the therapist provides emotional support, continuity, information and assists in adaptation to the crisis. The therapist has a role in emphasizing past strengths, supporting previously successful coping strategies, and teaching new coping skills such as relaxation, cognitive restructuring, use of analgesics, self observation, assertiveness and communication skills. Communication skills are of paramount importance for both patient and family, particularly around pain and analgesic issues. The patient and family are the unit of concern, and often require a more general long-term, supportive relationship within the healthcare system, in addition to specific psychological approaches dealing with pain that a psychiatrist, psychologist, social worker or nurse can provide.

Group interventions with individual patients, spouses, couples and families are a powerful means of sharing experiences and identifying successful coping strategies. Utilizing psychotherapy to decrease symptoms of anxiety and depression, factors that can intensify pain, has been empirically demonstrated to have beneficial effects on cancer pain and overall quality of life. Spiegel and Bloom (1983b) demonstrated, in a controlled randomized prospective study, the effect of both supportive group therapy for metastatic breast cancer patients in general and, in particular, the effect of hypnotic pain control exercises. Patients were divided into either a support group focused on the practical and existential problems of living with cancer, a self-hypnosis exercise group or a control group. Results indicated that the patients receiving treatment experienced significantly less pain than the control patients. Passik et al (1991) described the efficacy of a psychoeducational group for the spouses of brain tumour patients. They have demonstrated the importance of addressing bereavement issues at an early stage in the patient's illness. The group members reported considerable benefit from one another's emotional support into widowhood and described improved quality of patient care (including pain management and all forms of nursing care) as a result of the support group.

Psychotherapeutic interventions that have multiple foci may be most useful. Based upon a prospective study of cancer pain, cognitive behavioural and psychoeducational techniques based upon increasing support, self efficacy and providing education may prove to be helpful in assisting patients in dealing with increased pain (Syrajala et al 1992). The results of an evaluation of patients with cancer pain indicate psychological and social variables are significant predictors of pain. More specifically, distress specific to the illness, self-efficacy and coping styles were predictors of increased pain.

Utilizing psychotherapy to diminish symptoms of anxiety and depression, factors that can intensify pain, has beneficial effects on the experience of cancer pain. Speigel and Bloom (1983b) demonstrated, in a controlled randomized prospective study, the effect of both supportive group therapy for metastatic breast cancer patients in general and, in particular, the effect of hypnotic pain control exercises. Their support group focused not on interpersonal processes or self exploration, but rather on a series of themes related to the practical and existential problems of living with cancer. Patients were divided into two treatment groups and a control group. The treatment group patients experienced significantly less pain than the control patients, and the control group showed a large increase in pain.

While psychotherapy in the cancer pain setting typically focuses on more current issues around illness and treatment (rather than psychoanalytical or insight-oriented approaches), the exploration of reactions to cancer often facilitates an insight into more pervasive life issues. Some patients opt to continue with exploratory psychotherapy during extended illness-free periods or survivorship. Theoretical constructs derived from psychotherapy with chronic non-cancer pain patients can be helpful in guiding psychotherapy with the cancer-pain patient. Alexithymia and pain-induced dissociative symptoms (remnants of early life trauma) have proven to be useful adjuncts to the psychotherapeutic treatment of many cancer pain patients and are discussed in detail below. Psychiatric observations of chronic non-cancer pain patients may have relevance to a subset of cancer pain patients, although the degree of overlap between these two populations has received little empirical investigation.

Alexithymia, or the inability to express and articulate emotional experiences, is considered a personality trait associated with chronic pain and somatization. Recent research has demonstrated the utility of this construct in understanding the cancer pain patient as well. Dalton and Feuerstein (1989), for example, demonstrated that patients who reported more prolonged and severe pain also scored higher on a measure designed to assess alexithymia when compared to patients experiencing sporadic or less intense pain. The cancer setting is characterized by highly emotionally charged issues revolving around loss, disability, disfigurement and death (Massie & Holland 1987). Patients are faced with intense emotions that can be threatening or difficult to articulate. Therapists can be quite helpful to alexithymic patients by acknowledging such feelings and allowing for their verbalization. In many instances, the therapist must actually provide the patient with a lexicon for their expression (Passik & Wilson 1987). Analogously, the meaning patients attribute to their pain can influence the amount of pain they report. Therapists can help to correct misperceptions about pain when appropriate and allow for the open discussion of issues and fears that might prolong or intensify a pain experience.

Increased awareness of the impact of traumatic events on psychological functioning and, in particular, on the development of dissociative states and disorders (psychogenic amnesia, fugue states, multiple personality disorder, conversion, post-traumatic stress disorder), has led to a growing acknowledgment of the traumatic impact of pain. Patients with dissociative disorders suffer from a wide variety of transient physical problems such as dysaesthesias, anaesthesias and pain (Terr 1991). In the chronic non-malignant pain population there has also been growing empirical support for the existence of such sequelae of chronic pain. Patients with chronic pelvic pain and premenstrual syndrome, for example (Walker et al 1988, Paddison et al 1990), were found to have an unusually high prevalence of early sexual abuse. The prevalence of such phenomena in the cancer pain population is unknown. However, the cancer setting, with its life-threatening backdrop, toxic and disfiguring treatments and invasive procedures, can reawaken long-dormant traumata in even high-functioning patients with abuse histories. Inquiry into such issues can be essential to the evaluation and treatment of such patients. Although not generally a part of a routine psychiatric assessment in the medical setting, the recognition of the need to inquire into these areas requires attentive listening with the 'third ear' (Reik 1948).

THE SUBSTANCE-ABUSING PATIENT

Substance abuse is increasingly prevalent in the population at large and so will be encountered in the care of cancer pain patients. The management of cancer pain in the active abuser and in the patient with a history of substance abuse is a particularly difficult and challenging problem (Payne 1989, McCaffery & Vourakis 1992). Portenoy and Payne (1992) have outlined a range of aberrant drug-taking behaviours that help to identify the substance-abusing cancer pain patient. When patients obtain and use street drugs, purchase opioids from non-medical sources or engage in illegal behaviours such as forging prescriptions or selling their prescription medications, a diagnosis of substance abuse is clear. More subtle and difficult to interpret are behaviours such as dose escalation without contact with the physician, contacting multiple physicians to obtain opioids, making frequent visits to emergency rooms, hoarding medications and using medications to relieve symptoms other than pain. What renders these behaviours difficult to interpret (though many physicians might feel that they are uniformly aberrant regardless of mitigating circumstances) is that such behaviours usually arise in the setting of an evolving pain complaint with fluctuating intensity and degree of relief. Many behaviours that are used to define addiction in the physically healthy have limited utility when assessing the cancer pain patient. Relapse after withdrawal from a substance is a common feature in definitions of addiction (Jaffe 1985). However, relapse of pain complaints after decrease or withdrawal from a particular medication in a cancer pain patient may simply signal the return to the baseline level of the underlying pain and may reflect the need for continued treatment with opioids. Furthermore, the need for chronic use of an opioid presupposes that the patient will become tolerant and physiologically dependent. The fact that the patient develops an abstinence syndrome upon abrupt discontinuation of the drug, or requires higher doses for continued pain control, has little bearing upon the diagnosis of drug abuse.

Psychological dependence is generally accepted as central to the definition of addiction and can be inferred from such behaviours as loss of control over the drug, compulsive use or use despite harm. Patients may directly state that they have lost control over their pain medicines or have become overly concerned with acquisition of these drugs. They may even be aware that their behaviour in seeking pain medicines has alienated their healthcare team and jeopardized their cancer treatment. Pain, psychological distress, the adequacy and duration of pain relief and the patient's prior cancer pain experience must be taken into account when assessing the 'drug-seeking' patient. What appears to be highly aberrant drug-seeking behaviour (obsessive preoccupation with the availability of opioids) may simply be a reflection of inadequate pain control. The term 'pseudoaddiction' (Weissman & Haddox 1989) has been coined to describe the phenomenon in which the highly preoccupied and apparently out-of-control patient ceases to act in an aberrant fashion upon the provision of adequate pain control. Drug-taking behaviours that are unsanctioned by the physician and that fall in the less severe end of the range of these behaviours should be given the benefit of the doubt and seen as reflections of inadequate pain control, especially if the physician's expectations about the patient's responsibility for communication about dose escalation has not been made explicit. Some patients, such as those with a prior history of drug abuse (but not actively abusing), may require more explicit discussions of the rules for treatment than that given to other patients being started on opioid therapy. Paradoxically, such an explicit outline of the parameters of opioid therapy will provide structure as well as comfort to patients who are concerned about relapsing into active abuse.

The psychiatrist or psychologist in the oncology setting who consults in the care of the active substance-abusing patient is faced with many obstacles. Foremost among them is the limited access patients with serious medical illnesses have to traditional modes of treatment for drug and alcohol problems. The demands of cancer treatment are not generally accommodated by inpatient drug treatment centres. Twelve-step and methadone maintenance programmes can be rigid in their approach to the cancer patient's use of opioids and psychiatric medications for symptom control. Hospital staff members are often resentful and frightened of the substance-abusing patient and this can detract from the psychiatrist's or psychologist's ability to create a caretaking environment and alliance with the patient. The addict, frightened and regressed in the face of potentially life-threatening illness, can be tremendously distrustful of the staff and may attempt to cope through drug use, guile and manipulation rather than trusting in the staff's competence and goodwill. At Memorial Hospital we have established several guidelines for the inpatient treatment of the active substance-abusing cancer pain patient (in concert with hospital administration and security) that have allowed us to provide surveillance of illicit drug use and control over manipulation. The structured treatment guidelines set clear limits, help avoid medications appropriately used for pain and symptom control from becoming a focus of conflict and communicate knowledge about pain and substance-abuse management. In return for compliance, the patient, through the collaborative efforts of staff, is afforded a consistent and caring approach to pain and symptom control. In extreme cases, patients are informed that they will receive cancer treatment at our facility only if they comply with the recommendations of the pain/psychiatry team.

The active substance abuser is, when possible, admitted to the hospital with forewarning of the type of management he will receive. The patient admitted for a surgical procedure is brought into the hospital earlier to allow for stabilization of drug regimens and to avoid the development of withdrawal syndromes. The patient is admitted to a private room as close to the nursing station as possible to allow for monitoring and is informed that a search of his possessions will be conducted. Drugs, alcohol and previously prescribed medications are removed from the patient's possession. The patient is restricted to his room or floor until the danger of withdrawal or illicit drug use has been judged to be diminished. The patient is required to wear hospital pyjamas in an effort to render less likely his leaving the hospital to buy drugs. The patient's visitors are restricted to family and friends who are known to be drug free (the psychiatry service consultant interviews those whom the patient would like to have visit). Packages brought to the hospital by family members and friends are searched by members of hospital security to ensure that they do not contain contraband. The patient is instructed to produce a urine specimen daily and more frequently if deemed necessary because of unconventional behaviour. Most laboratories in general hospitals are like our own in that they cannot return results of urine toxicology screens in a timely fashion. Thus, we collect daily specimens (for surveillance) and have them sent to the laboratory when clinically indicated.

Once these parameters are established, the patient is assessed several times daily for the adequacy of pain and other physical and psychological symptom control. Medications are prescribed in a manner that takes the patient's tolerance into account. Furthermore, medications are given on an around-the-clock basis so as to avoid frequent encounters with floor staff that centre upon obtaining medications. Through the use of these guidelines, we have assisted in the management of patients who might otherwise have difficulty in rendering themselves 'treatable'. The plan also helps to contain staff sentiments such as anger and mistrust that might otherwise become a self-fulfilling prophecy in which the undertreated substance-abusing cancer pain patient acts in an aberrant fashion that compromises treatment.

THE DYING CANCER PAIN PATIENT

Psychotherapy with the dying patient in pain consists of active listening with supportive verbal interventions and the occasional interpretation (Cassem 1987). Despite the seriousness of the patient's plight, it is not necessary for the psychiatrist or psychologist to appear overly solemn or emotionally restrained. Often, it is only the psychotherapist, of all the patient's caregivers, who is comfortable enough to converse lightheartedly and allow the patient to talk about his life and experiences, rather than focus solely on impending death. The dying patient who wishes to talk or ask questions about death and pain and suffering should be allowed to do so freely, with the therapist maintaining an interested interactive stance. It is not uncommon for the dying patient to benefit from pastoral counselling. If a chaplaincy service is available, it should be offered to the patient and family. As the dying process progresses, psychotherapy with the individual patient may become limited by cognitive and speech deficits. It is at this point that the focus of supportive psychotherapeutic interventions shifts primarily to the family. In our experience, a very common issue for family members at this point is the level of alertness of the patient. Attempts to control pain are often accompanied by sedation that can limit communication between patient and family. This can sometimes become a source of conflict, with some family members disagreeing among themselves or with the patient about what constitutes an appropriate balance between comfort and alertness. It can be helpful for the physician to clarify the patient's preferences as they relate to these issues early, so that conflict can be avoided and work related to bereavement can begin.

CANCER PAIN AND THE FAMILY

The many stressors faced by the families of cancer patients have prompted mental health professionals who work with such patients to refer to them as 'second-order patients' (Rait & Lederberg 1990). Family members face a difficult and ongoing process of adjustment throughout the stages of the cancer patient's illness. They are called upon to perform the sometimes onerous tasks of providing emotional support, meeting basic caretaking needs, sharing the responsibility for medical decision making, weathering financial and social costs and maintaining stability in the midst of the changes caused by cancer. Cancer pain can impact upon the performance of each of these tasks and the presence of pain has been found to be associated with increased emotional and financial burden in the family (Mor et al 1987). Pain is viewed as a major concern by family members of cancer patients and, perhaps more than other physical symptoms, it is perceived as a powerful threat to the ongoing ability to manage the disease (Ferrell 1991). Many studies have documented the concern family members have about cancer pain and the priority families place upon patient comfort (Hinds 1985, Rowat 1985, Kristjanson 1986, Blank et al 1989, Hull 1989). The management of cancer pain should provide for the inclusion of family members. A programme for family members should include education in pain management issues (i.e., the assessment of pain, proper administration and scheduling of medications, addiction), emotional support and stress management skills and structured opportunities for respite from caregiving responsibilities (Warner 1992).

As was noted above, cancer patients with pain are more likely to develop psychiatric disorders than are patients without pain. The presence of serious depression or organic mental syndromes can seriously disrupt family–patient relationships and render the provision of ongoing emotional support for the patient difficult if not impossible. Family members themselves are vulnerable to developing stress-related emotional disorders which can further break down the support they can afford the patient. Ferrell et al (1991) examined patients with pain and its effects upon caregivers. Caregivers consistently described the patient's pain as highly distressing to themselves. They rated the patient's pain as more intense than did the patient and viewed the patient as extremely distressed by the pain. Thus pain heightened the burden of caregiving, especially in the areas of sleep disturbance, physical strain and emotional adjustment. In the advanced cancer patient, whose pain may be difficult to relieve without some sacrifice of mental clarity, family members may come into conflict with the patient or among one another if there is disagreement about the goals of pain treatment (mental clarity with residual pain versus greater comfort even if accompanied by sedation). Discussions of the patient's and family members' goals for treatment should be held early in the disease course, so that the patient and family can resolve conflicts with the full participation of the patient. Another issue which can lead to difficulty in the provision of emotional support are misconceptions harboured by family members about drug tolerance, dependence and addiction. Family members often become alarmed at the patient's increasing need for opioids and can withold treatment or their advocacy for the patient for fear that the patient will become addicted or 'use up' the drug's ability to relieve pain. Education about addiction, tolerance and the meaning of physiological dependence is crucial in the avoidance of such unnecessary conflicts. As described earlier in this chapter, some family members may view aggressive pain control as a form of euthanasia, and so may become quite distressed and act to prevent adequate pain control in a dying patient.

The family's tasks of providing basic caregiving and weathering the financial and social strains are also complicated by the presence of cancer pain. New technologies in pain treatment necessitate that family members become skilled in increasingly complex pain regimens, including the administration of medications and the coordination of multiple drug regimens. Learning how to assess pain and the side effects of pain treatment can vastly complicate the caregiver's burden. These advances can also dramatically increase the financial and social costs of cancer care for the family. The prescription of various modalities for pain control needs to take into account family resources, so as to avoid overburdening the family emotionally and financially.

Finally, the family's ability to provide the patient with continuity in the midst of change can be seriously threatened by the development of or changes in cancer pain. To provide for such continuity, family members need to feel as if they are able to predict or exert some control over the disease course. Cancer pain is often viewed as a harbinger of disease progression and as such can be a signal for the patient and family that they are about to enter a new phase of the disease. When cancer pain is continually unrelieved, it can confuse such signals and sacrifice family members' sense of control. The ability to maintain stability and provide the patient with a safe and supportive family environment can thus be disrupted.

CANCER PAIN AND STAFF STRESS

Those of us who work intensively with cancer patients have chosen a rewarding but stressful occupation. The painful nature of cancer and cancer treatment, difficult ethical dilemmas in treatment decision making, emotional reactions of patients and staff to cancer pain, and poor staff communication or conflict all contribute to the stressful cancer work environment.

Vachon (1987) described the stressors that are regularly encountered by oncologists and oncology nurses. These include caring for the patient who is extremely ill, dealing with the deaths of patients of all ages, poor staff communications, being intensely involved with patients and their families, conflicts between research and clinical care goals and the workload imposed by the complicated and taxing work of palliative care.

A survey conducted by Schmale and colleagues (1987) of 147 physicians who were members of the American Society of Clinical Oncology indicated that oncologists felt challenged by oncology but, nevertheless, they felt pressured, suffering from the negative responses and emotional problems of patients and families, the burden of dealing with dying patients, the frustration of ineffective treatments and the impact of negative personal life events. They identified a need for more emotional support for themselves as well as their patients. In a study carried out at Dana-Farber

Cancer Institute (Peteet et al 1989), the greatest source of stress for physicians was their inability to help patients. Nurses felt that ethical issues, particularly as they revolve around 'do not resuscitate' (DNR) status, and competing research and clinical goals were the most stressful. von Roenn and colleagues (1993) found that the majority of oncologists felt they were inadequately trained in pain assessment and management. Thus, dealing with cancer patients who have difficult pain problems can increase this sense of inability to help and can intensify physician and nurse stress.

Intense medical involvement with cancer pain patients tends to elicit common reactions which are well known to healthcare workers in the field. The first is the need to try to 'save' patients from their cancer illness or death. The healthcare worker may wish to rescue patients from their dreadful plight. Unfortunately, disease often progresses, and failure to save or rescue patients provokes feelings of helplessness, impotence and a sense of futility. Low self-esteem and depression may result and sometimes lead to a sense of resentment towards the patient. In an attempt to deal with these feelings of helplessness and futility, the physician or nurse may become overinvolved in the patient's medical care, encouraging or demanding inappropriately aggressive or unrealistic interventions. Staff members often find the transition from active treatment to palliative care difficult. Accepting altered treatment goals and relinquishing the hope of survival for a special patient can be very painful (Spikes & Holland 1975). The inability to recognize that such a transition in care is necessary can lead to a delay in dealing with issues such as DNR orders or other practical issues. Unaware of such reactions, a nurse or physician with a cancer patient may develop an adversarial relationship with other health professionals involved in that individual's care. A grandiose or self-serving attitude may develop in which the nurse or physician feels that only he or she understands the patient and knows how best to care for him medically. Unchecked, such attitudes can lead to staff conflict. More commonly, such an attitude reflects an over-inflated sense of responsibility for the patient's fate, which can result in enormous guilt once the patient's condition ultimately worsens. An alternative response to feelings of helplessness and futility involve avoidance of or premature withdrawal from the patient. Such avoidance or withdrawal is often based on unrecognized angry feelings that reflect the impotence felt in dealing with a patient whose condition progresses and deteriorates despite all efforts (Massie et al 1989).

A second common reaction is the need to 'protect' the patient. This often takes the form of an avoidance to confront or bring up for discussion, even when appropriate, topics that may be painful or emotionally distressing to the patient. Consequently, important issues may go unaddressed, such as the patient's feelings about pain, suffering and death, practical issues such as a will, DNR status and tying up financial loose ends. It is also important for the health professional to confront extreme denial and other maladaptive defenses on the part of the patient, especially when they interfere with treatment compliance. Recognition of our human limitations and personal vulnerabilities to loss are as important as being aware of these common countertransference reactions. Hopefully such awareness can benefit our patients, colleagues and ourselves.

A third common reaction is the tendency to blame the patients for their continued complaints of pain and discomfort. Ignoring the fact that cancer pain management is complex, this reaction takes the form of interpreting the patients' failure to respond to efforts at pain and symptom control as a desire on their part to perpetuate their symptomatology. Patients who have failed to respond to efforts at pain control are seen as 'needing their pain', 'communicating through pain' or drug seeking. In an effort to protect oneself from feelings of inadequacy, healthcare workers can displace their anger upon patients and withhold appropriate diagnostic tests or interventions.

The consequences of stress in the cancer work environment include the development of physical symptoms, psychological symptoms, 'burnout' or even more serious psychiatric impairment (e.g., alcoholism, drug abuse or depression). The most frequent physical symptoms of chronic stress include tension headache, exhaustion, fatigue, insomnia, gastrointestinal disturbances (with increase or decrease in appetite) when no medical explanation can be found and minor aches and pains (often questioned as signs of leukaemia or cancer). Psychological symptoms of stress in cancer staff include loss of enthusiasm for work, depression, irritability and frustration and a cynical view of medicine and colleagues (Hall et al 1979, Maslach 1979, Holland & Holland 1985, Mount 1986). Physicians and nurses can become overinvolved in their work, with excessive dedication and commitment, spend longer hours with less productivity and show decreased sensitivity to the emotional needs of patients and others; conversely, they may become detached and disinterested in medical practice. These two presentations of burnout in oncologists and oncology nurses have been described as the 'I must do everything' syndrome and the 'I hate medicine' syndrome. Potential outcomes of both of these syndromes, if allowed to progress, include alcoholism, substance abuse, depression and even suicide (Hall et al 1979, Holland & Holland 1985, Mount 1986).

The burnout syndrome, described by Maslach (1979), is characterized by emotional exhaustion, depersonalization and lack of a sense of personal accomplishment. Emotional exhaustion is experienced as being emotionally overextended and exhausted by work. Depersonalization is a poor term to describe the sense of distance and reduced empathy that the person usually feels toward patients. Lack of personal accomplishment is expressed by such comments as 'What do I ever accomplish anyway?' Staff begin to feel that all treatment is futile in cancer, so why bother at all. Millerd (1977) conceptualized these problems as a form of survivor syndrome, as post-traumatic stress disorder, in health caregivers who have dealt repeatedly with losses from death; some of the adverse symptoms are the same as those seen in survivors of natural disasters.

A variety of coping methods can be introduced at both the personal and organizational levels and can be useful in the prevention and management of burnout (Hartl 1979, Koocher 1979, Mount 1986). One of the most important strategies is to be able to recognize the physical and psychological symptoms of stress in oneself. It is additionally important to identify them in colleagues and point out that such symptoms are common, transient and reversible when dealt with early. Discomfort in pointing out emotional distress in a colleague should not be any greater than suggesting a consultation for a medical symptom. In the cancer centre, having the support of one's peers helps to decrease feelings of demoralization (Kash & Holland 1990). Providing ongoing education in pain management can help reduce stress and feelings of inadequacy for staff members.

Mental health professionals can perform several staff support roles in the oncology setting. Lederberg (1989) categorizes these roles into two: (i) support and backup to unit leaders, and (ii) facilitator of communications. Fulfilling such roles can be accomplished with activities that range from providing support to colleagues or helping identify and deal with troubled staff, to leading groups and conferences or participating in daily rounds. Ideally, an active role on the unit makes the liaison psychiatrist most familiar with the problems of the unit. The mental health consultant can be an outsider, but this usually limits one's effectiveness.

COGNITIVE-BEHAVIOURAL INTERVENTIONS IN CANCER PAIN

Cognitive-behavioural interventions are effective in the management of acute procedure-related cancer pain and as an adjunct in the management of chronic cancer pain (Table 46.6). Hypnosis, biofeedback and multicomponent cognitive-behavioural interventions have been used to provide comfort and minimize pain in adults, children and adolescents undergoing bone marrow aspirations, spinal taps and other painful procedures (Hilgard & LeBaron 1982, Redd et al 1982, Zeltzer & LeBaron 1982, Kellerman et al 1983, Jay et al 1986). In chronic cancer pain, cognitive-behavioural techniques are most effective when they are employed as part of a multimodal, multidisciplinary approach that has assured adequate medical assessment and management, including the appropriate use of opioid and non-opioid analgesics (Breitbart & Holland 1990). Cognitive-behavioural intervention in chronic cancer pain has included such techniques as biofeedback, group therapy and self hypnosis, music therapy, relaxation, imagery–distraction, behavioural rehearsal and positive reinforcement (occasionally as part of a multicomponent study) (Fotopoulos et al 1979, Turk & Rennert 1981, Spiegel & Bloom 1983b, Graffam & Johnson 1987, Zimmerman et al 1989, Beck 1991). Syrjala and colleagues (1992) tested the efficacy of psychological techniques for reducing pain related to oral mucositis in patients receiving bone marrow transplantation. This controlled clinical trial compared four interventions:

1. Hypnosis training – combined relaxation and imagery.
2. Cognitive-behavioural coping skills training – relaxation, cognitive restructuring, information, short-term goal-setting, exploration of meaning of pain.
3. Therapist contact control.
4. Treatment as usual.

Patients in these groups met the psychologist twice pre-transplant and then had 10 inhospital sessions during the course of transplantation. All patients received opioids for their pain and opioid use was monitored. Interestingly, hypnosis was the most effective technique in reducing reported oral pain, even more effective than cognitive-behavioural training.

Cognitive-behavioural techniques useful in cancer pain (Box 46.2) include passive relaxation with mental imagery, cognitive distraction or focusing, cognitive restructuring, progressive muscle relaxation, biofeedback, hypnosis, systematic desensitization and music therapy (Cleeland & Tearnan 1986, Cleeland 1987, Fishman & Loscalzo 1987). Some techniques are primarily cognitive in nature, focusing on perceptual and thought processes, and others are directed at modifying patterns of behaviour that help cancer patients cope with pain. Behavioural techniques include methods of modifying physiological pain reactions, respon-

Table 46.6 Selected studies demonstrating efficacy of cognitive-behavioural interventions in cancer pain

Study	*Type of pain*	*Intervention*	*Outcome*
Hilgard & LeBaron (1982)	Bone marrow aspiration in children	Hypnosis	↓pain
Kellerman et al (1983)	Bone marrow aspiration; lumbar puncture in adolescents	Hypnosis	↓pain
Zeltzer & LeBaron (1982)	Bone marrow aspiration; lumbar puncture in adolescents	Hypnosis	↓pain
Redd et al (1982)	Hyperthermia adults	Hypnosis	↓pain
Jay et al (1986)	Bone marrow aspiration; lumbar puncture	Cognitive[2]-behavioural multicomponent programme	↓pain
Spiegel and Bloom (1983b)[1]	Chronic pain breast cancer	Group therapy and self-hypnosis	↓pain
Fotopoulos et al (1979)	Chronic cancer pain	EMG, EEG, biofeedback	↓pain
Turk & Rennert (1981)	Chronic cancer pain; terminally ill	Cognitive-behavioural multicomponent programme	↓pain
Syrjala et al (1992)[1]	Oral mucositis in BMT patients	Hypnosis versus cognitive-behavioural training versus control	↓pain with hypnosis

[1] Controlled study.
[2] Filmed modelling, breathing training, imagery/distraction, behavioural rehearsal, positive reinforcement.
BMT = bone marrow transplant.

dent pain behaviours and operant pain behaviours. The most fundamental technique is self-monitoring. The development of the ability to monitor one's behaviours allows a person to notice dysfunctional reactions and learn to control them. Systematic desensitization is useful in extinguishing anticipatory anxiety that leads to avoidant behaviours and in remobilizing inactive patients. Graded task assignment is analogous to in vivo systematic desensitization, in which patients are encouraged to delineate and then execute a series of small steps towards an ultimate goal. Contingency management, a behavioural intervention in which healthy or adaptive behaviours are reinforced, has also been applied to the management of chronic pain as a method for modifying dysfunctional operant pain behaviours associated with secondary gain (Cleeland 1987, Loscalzo & Jacobsen 1990). Primarily cognitive techniques for coping with pain are aimed at increasing relaxation and reducing the intensity and emotional distress that accompany the pain experience. Cognitive restructuring, a technique often used in the treatment of depression or anxiety, is an effective method of altering a patient's interpretation of events and bodily sensations. Because many patients are plagued by disturbing and maladaptive thoughts or beliefs, identifying and modifying these beliefs can allow for more accurate assessment of the situation and thereby decrease subjective distress (Fishman & Loscalzo 1987).

Most cancer patients with pain are appropriate candidates for useful application of cognitive and behavioural techniques; the clinician, however, should take into account the intensity of pain and the mental clarity of the patient. Ideal candidates have mild to moderate pain and can benefit from these interventions, whereas patients with severe pain can expect limited benefit from psychological interventions unless somatic therapies can lower the level of pain to some degree. Confusional states also interfere dramatically with a patient's ability to focus attention and thus limit the

BOX 46.2

Cognitive-behavioural techniques used for cancer pain patients

Psychoeducation
Preparatory information

Relaxation
Passive breathing
Progressive muscle relaxation

Distraction
Focusing
Controlled mental imagery
Cognitive distraction
Behavioural distraction

Combined relaxation and distraction techniques
Passive relaxation with mental imagery
Progressive muscle relaxation with imagery
Systematic desensitization
Meditation
Hypnosis
Biofeedback
Music therapy

Cognitive therapies
Cognitive restructuring

Behavioural therapies
Self-monitoring
Modelling
Behavioural rehearsal
Graded task management
Contingency management

usefulness of these techniques (Loscalzo & Jacobsen 1990). Occasionally these techniques can be modified to enable patients with mild cognitive impairments to benefit. This often involves the therapist taking a more active role by orienting the patient, creating a safe and secure environment and evoking a conditioned response to the therapist's voice or presence.

Cancer patients are usually highly motivated to learn and practise cognitive-behavioural techniques because they are often effective not only in symptoms control, but in restoring a sense of self control, personal efficacy and active participation in their care. It is important to note that these techniques must not be used as a substitute for apropriate analgesic management of cancer pain but rather as part of a comprehensive multimodal approach. The lack of side effects associated with psychological interventions makes them particularly attractive in the oncology setting as a supplement to already complicated medication regimens. The successful use of these techniques should never lead to the erroneous conclusion that the pain was of psychogenic origin and therefore not 'real'. Although the specific mechanisms by which these cognitive and behavioural techniques relieve pain vary, most share the elements of relaxation and distraction. Distraction or redirection of attention helps reduce awareness of pain and relaxation reduces muscle tension and sympathetic arousal (Cleeland 1987).

RELAXATION TECHNIQUES

Several techniques are used to achieve a mental and physical state of relaxation. Muscular tension, autonomic arousal and mental distress exacerbate pain (Cleeland 1987, Loscalzo & Jacobsen 1990). Some specific relaxation techniques include: (i) passive relaxation, (ii) progressive muscle relaxation and (iii) meditation. Other methods that employ both relaxation and cognitive techniques include hypnosis, biofeedback and music therapy, and are discussed later in this chapter. Passive relaxation, focused breathing and passive muscle relaxation exercises involve the focusing of attention systematically on one's breathing, on sensations of warmth and relaxation or on release of muscular tension in various body parts. Verbal suggestions and imagery are used to help promote relaxation. Muscle relaxation is an important component of the relaxation response and can augment the benefits of simple focused breathing exercises, leading to a deeper experience of relaxation and self control. Progressive or active muscle relaxation involves the active tensing and relaxing of various muscle groups in the body, focusing attention on the sensations of tension and relaxation. Clinically, in the hospital setting, relaxation is most commonly achieved through the use of a combination of focused breathing and progressive muscle relaxation exercises. Once patients are in a relaxed state, imagery techniques can then be used to induce deeper relaxation and facilitate distraction from or manipulation of a variety of cancer-related symptoms. Scripts that can be utilized by therapists to aid in teaching patients passive and/or active relaxation techniques are available in the literature (McCaffery & Beebe 1989, Loscalzo & Jacobsen 1990, Horowitz & Breitbart 1993).

IMAGERY/DISTRACTION TECHNIQUES

Clinically, relaxation techniques are most helpful in managing pain when combined with some distracting or pleasant imagery. The use of distraction or focusing involves control over the focus of attention. Imagery refers to the use of one's imagination, usually during a relaxed state or hypnotic trance, to manipulate some aspect of the pain experience or enhance distraction. Once in a relaxed state, the cancer patient with pain can use a variety of imagery techniques, including: (i) pleasant distracting imagery; (ii) transformational imagery and (iii) dissociative imagery (Breitbart 1987, Fishman & Loscalzo 1987, Breitbart & Holland 1990, Loscalzo & Jacobsen 1990). Transformational imagery involves the imaginative transformation of either the painful sensation itself, or the context of pain, or both. Patients can imaginatively transform a sensation of pain in their arm, for instance, into a sensation of warmth or cold. They can use such imagery as 'dipping their arm into a bucket of cold spring water', or into a 'vat of warm honey'. Such techniques can also be used to alter the context of the pain. Dissociative imagery or dissociated somatization refers to the use of one's imagination to disconnect or dissociate from the pain experience. Specifically, patients can sometimes imagine that they leave their pain-racked body in bed and walk about for 5 or 10 minutes pain free. Patients can also imagine that a particularly painful part of their body becomes disconnected or dissociated from the rest of them, resulting in a period of freedom from pain. These techniques can provide much-needed respite from pain. Even short periods of relief from pain can break the vicious pain cycle that entraps many cancer patients. Again, scripts for imagery exercises are available in the literature (McCaffery & Beebe 1989, Loscalzo & Jacobsen 1990, Horowitz & Breitbart 1993).

HYPNOSIS

Hypnosis is efficacious in the treatment of some cancer pain (Barber & Gitelson 1980, Redd et al 1982, Spiegel & Bloom 1983b, Spiegel 1985). The hypnotic trance is essentially a state of heightened and focused concentration and thus it can be used to manipulate the perception of pain. The depth of hypnotizability may determine the effectiveness as well as the strategies employed during hypnosis. One-third of cancer patients are not hypnotizable and it is recommended that other techniques be employed for them. Of the two-thirds of patients who are identified as being less, moderately and highly hypnotizable, three principles underlie the use of hypnosis in controlling pain (Spiegel 1985): (i) use self-hypnosis; (ii) relax, do not fight the pain and (iii) use a mental filter to ease the hurt in pain. Patients who are moderately or highly hypnotizable can often alter sensations in a painful area by changing temperature sensation or experiencing tingling. Patients who are hypnotizable to a lesser degree can still utilize techniques that distract attention, such as concentrating on a mental image of a pleasant scene.

BIOFEEDBACK

Fotopoulos et al (1979) noted significant pain relief in a group of cancer patients who were taught electromyographic (EMG) and electroencephalographic (EEG) biofeedback-assisted relaxation. Only two of 17 were able to maintain analgesia after the treatment ended. A lack of generalization of effect can be a problem with biofeedback techniques. Although physical condition may make a prolonged training period impossible, especially for the terminally ill, most cancer patients can utilize EMG and temperature biofeedback techniques for learning relaxation-assisted pain control (Cleeland 1987).

MUSIC THERAPY

Munro and Mount (1978) have written extensively on the use of music therapy with cancer patients, documenting clinical examples and suggesting mechanisms of action. Music can often capture the focus of attention like no other stimulus and helps patients distract their attention away from pain, while expressing themselves in meaningful ways. Several studies have demonstrated beneficial effects of pain experience through the use of patient-selected instrumental audiotapes, and by listening to music or humming sounds (Zimmerman et al 1989, Beck 1991).

AROMA THERAPY

Aromas have been shown to have innate relaxing and stimulating qualities. Our colleagues at Memorial Hospital have recently begun to explore the use of aroma therapy for the treatment of procedure-related anxiety (i.e., anxiety related to MRI scans). Utilizing the scent of heliotropin, Manne et al (1991) reported that two-thirds of the patients found the scent especially pleasant and reported much less anxiety than those who were not exposed to the scent during MRI. As a general relaxation technique, aroma therapy may have an application for pain management, but this is as yet unstudied.

PSYCHOTROPIC ADJUVANT ANALGESICS FOR CANCER PAIN

While the mainstay of pharmacological management of cancer pain is the aggressive use of narcotic analgesics, there is a growing appreciation for the role of adjuvant analgesic drugs in providing maximal comfort (Breitbart 1989a, Breitbart & Holland 1990, Walsh 1990). Psychotropic drugs, particularly antidepressants, psychostimulants, neuroleptics and anxiolytics, are useful as adjuvant analgesics in the pharmacological management of cancer pain. Psychiatrists are often the most experienced in the clinical use of these drugs and so can play an important role in assisting pain control. Table 46.7 lists the various psychotropic medications with their analgesic properties, routes of administration and approximate daily doses. These medications have been shown earlier (see Tables 46.2, 46.3) to be effective in managing symptoms of depression, anxiety or delirium that commonly complicate the course of cancer patients with pain. They also potentiate the analgesic effects of opioid drugs and often have analgesic properties of their own.

ANTIDEPRESSANTS

The current literature supports the use of antidepressants as adjuvant analgesic agents in the management of a wide

Table 46.7 Psychotropic adjuvant analgesic drugs for cancer pain

Generic name	*Trade name*	*Approximate daily dosage range (mg)*	*Route*
Tricyclic antidepressants			
Amitriptyline	Elavil	10–150	PO, IM, PR
Nortriptyline	Pamelor, Aventyl	10–150	PO
Imipramine	Tofranil	12.5–150	PO, IM
Desipramine	Norpramin	10–150	PO
Clomipramine	Anafranil	10–150	PO
Doxepin	Sinequan	12.5–150	PO, IM
Heterocyclic and non-cyclic antidepressants			
Trazodone	Desyrel	25–300	PO
Maprotiline	Ludiomil	50–300	PO
Serotonin specific re-uptake inhibitors			
Fluoxetine	Prozac	20–60	PO
Paroxetine	Paxil	10–40	PO
Amine precursors			
L-Tryptophan		500–3000	PO
Psychostimulants			
Methylphenidate	Ritalin	2.5–20 b.i.d.	PO
Dextroamphetamine	Dexedrine	2.5–20 b.i.d.	PO
Phenothiazines			
Fluphenazine	Prolixin	1–3	PO, IM
Methotrimeprazine	Levoprome	10–20 q 6 h	IM, IV
Butyrophenones			
Haloperidol	Haldol	1–3	PO, IM, IV
Pimozide	Orap	2–6 b.i.d.	PO
Antihistamines			
Hydroxyzine	Vistaril	50 q 4–6 h	PO, IM, IV
Steroids			
Dexamethasone	Decadron	4–16	PO, IV
Benzodiazepines			
Alprazolam	Xanax	0.25–2.0 t.i.d.	PO
Clonazepam	Klonopin	0.5–4 b.i.d.	PO

PO = per oral; IM = intramuscular; PR = parenteral; IV = intravenous; q 6 h = every 6 hours; b.i.d. = two times a day, t.i.d. = three times a day.

variety of chronic pain syndromes, including cancer pain (Walsh 1983, 1990, Butler 1986, France 1987, Getto et al 1987, Magni et al 1987, Ventafridda et al 1987). There is substantial evidence (see Ch. 50) that the tricyclic antidepressants, in particular, are analgesic and useful in the management of such chronic pain syndromes as postherpetic neuralgia, diabetic neuropathy, fibromyalgia, headache and low-back pain. Amitriptyline is the tricyclic antidepressant most studied, and proven effective as an analgesic, in a large number of clinical trials, addressing a wide variety of chronic pain syndromes (Pilowsky et al 1982, Watson et al 1982, Max et al 1987, 1988, Sharav et al 1987). Other tricyclic antidepressants that have been shown to have efficacy as analgesics include imipramine (Kvindesal et al 1984, Young & Clarke 1985, Sindrup et al 1989), desipramine (Kishore-Kumar et al 1990, Max et al 1991), nortriptyline (Gomez-Perez et al 1985), clomipramine (Langohr et al 1982, Tiengo et al 1987) and doxepin (Hammeroff et al 1982).

The heterocyclic and non-cyclic antidepressant drugs such as trazodone, minserin, maprotiline and the newer serotinin-specific re-uptake inhibitors (SSRIs) fluoxetine and paroxetine may also be useful as adjuvant analgesics for chronic pain syndromes, including cancer pain. Trazodone has been found to be analgesic in a cancer pain population; however, a trial for dysaesthetic pain in patients with traumatic myelopathy failed to show efficacy (Davidoff et al 1987, Magni et al 1987, Ventafridda et al 1987). Mianserin (removed from the marketplace) was a potent serotonin re-uptake blocker with few adverse side effects, thus making it an attractive choice as an antidepressant or adjuvant analgesic in the cancer pain patient (Costa et al 1985). Maprotiline, a noradrenaline re-uptake blocker, demonstrated moderate analgesic properties in a controlled comparison study against clomipramine (Eberhard et al 1988). In a double-blind crossover trial, maprotiline relieved pain related to postherpetic neuralgia, but was not as effective as amitriptyline (Watson et al 1992).

Fluoxetine, a potent antidepressant with SSRI activity (Feighner 1985) has been shown to have analgesic properties in experimental animal pain models (Hynes et al 1985) but failed to show analgesic effects in a clinical trial for neuropathy (Max 1992). Several case reports suggest fluoxetin may be a useful adjuvant analgesic in the management of headache (Diamond & Frietag 1989) and fibrositis (Geller 1989). Paroxetine, a newer SSRI, is the first antidepressant of this class shown to be a highly effective analgesic in a controlled trial for the treatment of diabetic neuropathy (Sindrup et al 1990). Newer antidepressants such as sertraline, venlafaxine and nefazodone may also eventually prove to be clinically useful as adjuvant analgesics. Nefazodone, for instance, has been demonstrated to potentiate opioid analgesics in an animal model (Pick et al 1992).

Tryptophan, a serotonin precursor, has been generally removed from the marketplace, but was used for chronic pain (King 1980, Seltzer et al 1983) in doses of 2–4 g; however, nausea is a common side effect with higher doses, thus limiting usefulness in debilitated cancer patients. Monoamine oxidase inhibitors (MAOIs) are also less useful in the cancer setting because of dietary restriction and potentially dangerous interactions between MAOIs and narcotics such as meperidine. Among the MAOI drugs available, phenelzine has been shown to have adjuvant analgesic properties in patients with atypical facial pain and migraine (Lascelles 1966, Anthony & Lance 1969).

Table 46.8 is a compilation of the studies, both controlled and uncontrolled, that demonstrate adjuvant analgesic efficacy of antidepressants for cancer pain. The antidepressants most commonly used in clinical studies on the management of cancer pain include amitriptyline, imipramine, clomipramine, trazodone and doxepin (Walsh 1986, Magni et al 1987, Ventafridda et al 1987). In a placebo-controlled double-blind study of imipramine in chronic cancer pain, Walsh (1986) demonstrated that imipramine had analgesic effects independent of its mood effects and was a potent coanalgesic when used along with morphine. In general, the antidepressants are utilized in cancer pain as adjuvant analgesics, potentiating the effects of opioid analgesics, and are rarely used as the primary analgesic (Botney & Fields 1983, Walsh 1986, Ventafridda et al 1987). Ventafridda et al (1987) reviewed a multicentre clinical study with antidepressant agents (trazodone and amitriptyline) in the treatment of chronic cancer pain that included a deafferentation or neuropathic component. Almost all of these patients were already receiving weak or strong opioids and experienced improved pain control. A subsequent randomized double-blind study showed both amitriptyline and trazodone (a triazolo pyridine) to have similar therapeutic analgesic efficacy (Ventafridda et al 1987). Magni et al (1987) reviewed the use of antidepressants in Italian cancer centres and found that a wide range of antidepressants were used for a variety of cancer pain syndromes, with anitriptyline being the most commonly prescribed, for a variety of cancer pains. In nearly all cases, antidepressants were used in association with opioids. Good or fair analgesic results were reported in 51% of patients and the inclusion of all worthwhile responses (improved sleep, etc.) raised the proportion with benefit to 98%.

Table 46.8 Studies of antidepressants for cancer pain

Study	*Drug*	*Efficacy of pain relief (%)*
Gebhardt et al (1969)	Clomipramine	67
Adjan (1970)	Clomipramine	90
Bernard & Scheuer (1972)	Clomipramine + neuroleptic	87
Adjan (1970)	Imipramine	80
Monkemeier & Steffen (1970)	Imipramine	75
Barjou (1971)	Imipramine	70–80
Deutschmann (1971)	Imipramine	80
Hughes et al (1963)	Imipramine	70
Fiorentino (1969)	Imipramine[1]	p
Walsh (1986)	Imipramine[1]	p
Ventafridda et al (1987)	Amitriptyline[1]	p
	vs trazodone	p
Magni et al (1987)	Amitriptyline, Imipramine, Clomipramine, Trazodone, Doxepin	51–98
Breivik & Rennemo (1982)	Amitriptyline	67
Bourhis et al (1978)	Amitriptyline	0
	Trimipramine	0
Carton et al (1976)	Amitriptyline	70–80
Fernandez et al (1987a)	Alprazolam	75
Bruera et al (1989a)	Methylphenidate[a]	p

[1] Controlled study.
p = Drug more effective than placebo.

MECHANISMS OF ANTIDEPRESSANT ANALGESIA

The antidepressants are effective as adjuvants in cancer pain through a number of mechanisms that include: (i) antidepressant activity (France 1987); (ii) potentiation or enhancement of opioid analgesia (Malseed & Goldstein 1979, Botney & Fields 1983, Ventafridda et al 1990b); and (iii) direct analgesic effects (Spiegel et al 1983). The relief of depression in patients with chronic pain has been demonstrated to result in reported pain relief (Bradley 1963); thus, the antidepressant effects of the tricyclics and other antidepressants probably make an important contribution to the analgesic properties of this class of drugs. Antidepressants, however, also potentiate the analgesic effects of the opioid drugs. This occurs through direct action of the antidepressants on the central nervous system (CNS) that is likely to be mediated through serotonergic, catecholaminergic and anticholinergic effects (Botney & Fields 1983). Manipulation of CNS serotonin can dramatically influence the degree of analgesia produced by an opioid analgesic such as morphine. Increasing levels of CNS serotonin result in greater degrees of analgesia produced by an opioid drug, while depletion of CNS serotonin results in decreased opioid analgesia (Botney & Fields 1983). Serotonin is an important neurotransmitter mediator of opioid analgesia. The modulation of the noradrenergic and cholinergic systems in the brain also has profound effects on opioid analgesia (Basbaum & Fields 1978, Botney & Fields 1983, Gram 1983). Additionally, antidepressants can potentiate the analgesic effects of opioids through pharmacokinetic mechanisms. Imipramine, orally administered, can increase the bioavailability of morphine by reducing its rate of elimination (Feinman 1985). Desipramine can elevate methadone levels in serum (Liu & Wang 1975).

Antidepressants have direct analgesic properties of their own, independent of their effects on mood or potentiation of opioid analgesia (Gram 1983, Fields & Basbaum 1984). A leading hypothesis is that mechanisms involving serotonin and noradrenaline mediate clinical analgesia via descending systems originating in the brainstem and influencing the dorsal horn of the spinal cord (Basbaum & Fields 1978, Fields & Basbaum 1984, Watson et al 1992). The various tricyclic, heterocyclic and non-cyclic antidepressants have effects on a number of neurotransmitters and their receptors (Charney et al 1981). A drug like amitriptyline acts to elevate levels of serotonin and noradrenaline in the nervous system by blocking the synaptic reuptake of both catecholamines (Basbaum & Fields 1978, Dubner & Bennett 1983). Other antidepressants have been demonstrated to have more specific serotonergic or noradrenergic properties. Many antidepressants with mixed or predominantly serotonergic properties such as amitriptyline, imipramine, nortriptyline, clomipramine, doxepin and trazadone have been shown to have direct analgesic effects. However, newer more selective serotonin reuptake inhibitors such as zimelidine and fluoxetine, as well as serotonin antagonists such as buspirone, have proven disappointing in clinical studies of neuropathic pain (Watson & Evans 1985, Kishore-Kumar et al 1989). Maprotiline and desipramine, both rather selective noradrenergic agents, have now been demonstrated to have direct analgesic properties (Kishore-Kumar et al 1990, Watson et al 1992). Given these findings, the mechanisms of analgesia shared universally by all antidepressants are still not agreed upon. Variation among individuals in pain (as to the status of their own neurotransmitter systems) is an important variable (Watson et al 1992). Other possible mechanisms of antidepressant analgesic activity have been proposed (see Ch. 50).

RECOMMENDATIONS FOR CLINICAL USE

At this point, it is clear that many antidepressants have analgesic properties. There is no definite indication that any one drug is more effective than the others, although the most experience has been accrued with amitriptyline which remains the drug of first choice. What is the appropriate dose of tricyclic antidepressant when the drug is utilized as an analgesic and not as an antidepressant? Sharav et al (1987) argued that a low dose (10–30 mg) of amitriptyline is as analgesic as a high dose (75–150 mg). Zitman et al (1990), however, demonstrated only modest analgesic results from low-dose amitriptyline. More recently, Max et al (1987, 1988) presented compelling evidence that the therapeutic analgesic effects of amitriptyline are correlated with serum levels just as the antidepressant effects are, and analgesic treatment failure is caused by low serum levels. A high-dose regimen of up to 150 mg of amitriptyline or higher is suggested (Kvindesal et al 1984, Watson & Evans 1985). The time course of onset of analgesia appears to be a biphasic process. There are immediate or early analgesic effects occurring within hours or days that are probably mediated by inhibition of synaptic reuptake of catecholamines (Botney & Fields 1983, Spiegel et al 1983, Tiengo et al 1987). Additionally, there are later longer analgesic effects that peak over a 4–6-week period that are likely to be due to receptor effects of the antidepressants (Pilowsky et al 1982, Max et al 1987, 1988).

Treatment should be initiated with a small dose of amitriptyline (i.e., 10–25 mg at bedtime), especially in debilitated patients, and increased slowly by 10–25 mg every 2–4 days towards 150 mg, with frequent assessment of pain and side effects until a beneficial effect is achieved. Maximal effect as an adjuvant analgesic may require continuation of the drug for 2–6 weeks. Serum levels of antidepressant drug, when available, may also help in management to assure that therapeutic levels are being achieved. Both pain and depression in cancer patients often respond to lower doses (25–100 mg) of antidepressant than are usually required in the physically healthy (100–300 mg), most likely because of impaired metabolism of these drugs. The choice of drug often depends on the side effect profile, existing medical problems, the nature of depressive symptoms if present and past response to specific antidepressants. Sedating drugs like amitriptyline are helpful when insomnia complicates the presence of pain and depression in a cancer patient. Anticholinergic properties of some of these drugs should also be kept in mind. Occasionally, in patients who have limited analgesic response to a tricyclic, potentiation of analgesia can be accomplished with the addition of lithium augmentation (Tyler 1974).

PSYCHOSTIMULANTS

The psychostimulants, dextroamphetamine and methylphenidate, are useful agents prescribed selectively for medically ill cancer patients with depression (Kaufmann et al 1982, Fernandez et al 1987b). Psychostimulants are also useful in diminishing excessive sedation secondary to narcotic analgesics and are potent adjuvant analgesics. Bruera et al (1987, 1989a) demonstrated that a regimen of 10 mg methylphenidate with breakfast and 5 mg with lunch significantly decreased sedation and potentiated the analgesic effect of narcotics in patients with cancer pain. Methylphenidate has also been demonstrated to improve functioning on a number of neuropsychological tests, including tests of memory, mental speed and concentration, in patients receiving continuous infusions of opioids for cancer pain (Bruera et al 1992).

Dextroamphetamine has also been reported to have additive analgesic effects when used with morphine to control postoperative pain (Forrest et al 1977). In relatively low dose, psychostimulants stimulate appetite, promote a sense of well-being, and improve feelings of weakness and fatigue in cancer patients. Treatment with dextroamphetamine or methylphenidate usually begins with doses of 2.5 mg at 8.00 a.m. and at noon. The dosage is slowly increased over several days until a desired effect is achieved or side effects (overstimulation, anxiety, insomnia, paranoia, confusion) intervene. Typically, a dose greater than 30 mg per day is not necessary, although occasionally patients require up to 60 mg per day. Patients usually are maintained on methylphenidate for 1–2 months and approximately two-thirds will-be able to be withdrawn from the drug without a recurrence of depressive symptoms. If symptoms recur, patients can be maintained on a psychostimulant for up to 1 year without significant abuse problems. Tolerance can develop and adjustment of the dose may be necessary.

NEUROLEPTICS

Methotrimeprazine is a phenothiazine that is equianalgesic to morphine, has none of the opioid effects on gut motility and probably produces analgesia through α-adrenergic blockade (Beaver et al 1966). In patients who are opioid tolerant, it provides an alternative approach to providing analgesia by a non-opioid mechanism. It is a dopamine blocker and so has antiemetic as well as anxiolytic effects. Methotrimeprazine can produce sedation, anticholinergic symptoms and hypotension, and should be given cautiously by slow intravenous infusion, or subcutaneous infusion. Dosages for methotrimeprazine range from 12.5 to 50 mg every 4–8 hours up to 300 mg over 24 hours for most patients. In addition to its analgesic effects, methotrimeprazine is used as an anxiolytic and in the management of agitation and confusion in the terminally ill (Oliver 1985). Other phenothiazines such as chlorpromazine and prochlorperazine (Compazine) are useful as antiemetics in cancer patients, but probably have limited use as analgesics (Houde & Wallenstein 1966). Fluphenazine in combination with TCAs has been shown to be helpful for neuropathic pains (Gomez-Perez et al 1985). Haloperidol is the drug of choice in the management of delirium or psychoses in cancer patients and has clinical usefulness as a coanalgesic for cancer pain (Maltbie et al 1979). Both fluphenazine and haloperidol are most commonly used in low doses (2–8 mg per day) for neuropathic pain. The benefits of prolonged use of neuroleptics for analgesia must be weighed against the risk of developing tardive dyskinesia, particularly in the young patient with good long-term prognosis. Pimozide (Orap), a butyrophenone, has been shown to be effective as an analgesic in the management of trigeminal neuralgia at doses of 4–12 mg per day (Lechin et al 1989).

ANXIOLYTICS

Hydroxyzine is a mild anxiolytic with sedating and analgesic properties that are useful in the anxious cancer patient with pain (Beaver & Feise 1976). This antihistamine has antiemetic activity as well. Parenteral hydroxyzine at 100 mg has analgesic activity approaching 8 mg of morphine and has additive analgesic effects when combined with morphine. Adding 25 mg to 50 mg of hydroxyzine every 4–6 hours orally, intravenously or subcutaneously to a regimen of opioids often helps relieve anxiety as well as providing adjuvant analgesia. Benzodiazepines have not been felt to have specific analgesic properties, although they are potent anxiolytics and anticonvulsants. Some authors have suggested that their anticonvulsant properties make certain benzodiazepine drugs useful in the management of neuropathic pain. Recently, Fernandez et al (1987b) showed that alprazolam, a unique benzodiazepine with mild antidepressant properties, was a helpful adjuvant analgesic in cancer patients with phantom limb pain or deafferentation (neuropathic) pain. Clonazepam (Klonopin) may also be useful in the management of lancinating neuropathic pains in the cancer setting, and has been reported to be an effective analgesic for patients with trigeminal neuralgia, headache and post-traumatic neuralgia (Caccia 1975, Swerdlow & Cundill 1981).

PSYCHIATRIC ASPECTS OF PAIN IN AIDS

Studies conducted between 1990 and 1995 have documented that pain in individuals with HIV infection or AIDS is highly prevalent, diverse and varied in syndromal presentation; associated with significant psychological and functional morbidity; and alarmingly undertreated (Lebovits et al 1989, McCormack et al 1993, O'Neill & Sherrard 1993, Singer et al 1993, Breitbart 1996, 1997, Breitbart et al 1996a,b, Rosenfeld et al 1996, Hewitt et al 1997). With the introduction of highly active antiretroviral therapies (i.e., combination therapies including protease inhibitors), the face of the AIDS epidemic, particularly for those who can avail themselves of and/or tolerate these new therapies, is indeed changing. Death rates from AIDS in the USA have dropped dramatically in the last 18 months, and rates of serious opportunistic infections and cancers are declining. Despite these hopeful developments, the future is still unclear, and millions of patients with HIV disease worldwide will continue to die of AIDS and suffer from the enormous burden of physical and psychological symptoms. Even with the advances in AIDS therapies, pain continues to be an issue in the care of patients with HIV disease. As the epidemiology of the AIDS epidemic changes in the USA, managing pain in AIDS patients with a history of substance abuse is becoming an ever-growing challenge. Pain management needs to be more integrated into the total care of patients with HIV disease.

PREVALENCE OF PAIN IN HIV DISEASE

Estimates of the prevalence of pain in HIV-infected individuals have been reported to range from 30% to over 90%, with the prevalence of pain increasing as disease progresses (Lebovits et al 1989, Schofferman & Brody 1990, Breitbart et al 1991, 1996a,b, Singer et al 1993, Kimball & McCormick 1996, Larue et al 1997), particularly in the latest stages of illness.

Studies suggest that approximately 30% of ambulatory HIV-infected patients in the early stages of HIV disease (pre-AIDS; Category A or B disease) experience clinically significant pain, and as many as 56% have had episodic painful symptoms of less clear clinical significance (Singer et al 1993, Breitbart et al 1996b, Larue et al 1997). In a prospective cross-sectional survey of 438 ambulatory AIDS patients in New York City, 63% reported 'frequent or persistent pain of at least two weeks duration' at the time of assessment (Breitbart et al 1996b). The prevalence of pain in this large sample increased significantly as HIV disease progressed, with 45% of AIDS patients with Category A3 disease reporting pain, 55% of those with Category B3 and 67% of those with Category C1, 2 or 3 disease reporting pain. Patients in this sample of ambulatory AIDS patients also were more likely to report pain if they had other con-

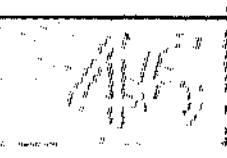

current HIV- related symptoms (e.g., fatigue, wasting), had received treatment for an AIDS-related opportunistic infection or if they had not been receiving antiretroviral medications (e.g., AZT, ddl, ddC, d4t).

In a study of pain in hospitalized patients with AIDS in a public hospital in New York City, over 50% of patients required treatment for pain, with pain being the presenting complaint in 30% and the second most common presenting problem after fever (Lebovits et al 1989). In a French multicentre study, 62% of hospitalized patients with HIV disease had clinically significant pain (Larue et al 1997). Schofferman and Brody (1990) reported that 53% of patients with far-advanced AIDS cared for in a hospice setting had pain, while Kimball and McCormack (1996) reported that up to 93% of AIDS patients in their hospice experienced at least one 48-hour period of pain during the last 2 weeks of life.

Larue and colleagues (1994) demonstrated that patients with AIDS being cared for in a hospice or at home had prevalence rates and intensity ratings for pain that were comparable to and even exceeded those of cancer patients. Breitbart and colleagues (1996a) reported that ambulatory AIDS patients in their New York City sample reported a mean pain intensity 'on average' of 5.4 (on the 0–10 numerical rating scale of the Brief Pain Inventory) and a mean pain 'at its worst' of 7.4. In addition, as with pain prevalence, the intensity of pain experienced by patients with HIV disease increases significantly as disease progresses. AIDS patients with pain, like their counterparts with cancer pain, typically describe an average of 2.5 to 3 concurrent pains at a time (Breitbart et al 1996a, Hewitt et al 1997).

PAIN SYNDROMES IN HIV/AIDS: AETIOLIOGIES AND CLASSIFICATION

Pain syndromes encountered in AIDS are diverse in nature and aetiology. The most common pain syndromes reported in studies to date include painful sensory peripheral neuropathy, pain due to extensive Karposi's sarcoma, headache, oral and pharyngeal pain, abdominal pain, chest pain, arthralgias and myalgias, as well as painful dermatological conditions (Lebovits et al 1989, Schofferman & Brody 1990, Breitbart et al 1991, 1996b, Penfold & Clark 1992, O'Neill & Sherrard 1993, Singer et al 1993, Larue et al 1994, Hewitt et al 1997). In a sample of 151 ambulatory AIDS patients who underwent a research assessment which included a clinical interview, neurological examination and review of medical records (Hewitt et al 1997), the most common pain diagnoses included headaches (46% of patients; 17% of all pains), joint pains (arthritis, arthralgias, etc. – 31% of patients; 12% of pains), painful polyneuropathy (distal symmetrical polyneuropathy – 28% of patients; 10% of pains), and muscle pains (myalgia, myositis – 27% of patients; 12% of pains). Other common pain diagnoses included skin pain (Kaposi's sarcoma, infections – 25% of patients; 30% of homosexual males in the sample had pain from extensive KS lesions), bone pain (20% of patients), abdominal pain (17% of patients), chest pain (13%) and painful radiculopathy (12%). Patients in this sample had a total of 405 pains (averaging 3 concurrent pains), with 46% of patients diagnosed with neuropathic-type pain, 71% with somatic pain, 29% with visceral pain and 46% with headache (classified separately because of controversy as to pathophysiology). When pain type was classified by pains (as opposed to patients) 25% were neuropathic pains, 44% were nociceptive-somatic, 14% were nociceptive-visceral and 17% were idiopathic-type pains. Patients in this study with lower CD4 + cell counts were significantly more likely to be diagnosed with polyneuropathy and headache. Hewitt and colleagues (1997) demonstrated that while pains of a neuropathic nature (e.g., polyneuropathies, radiculopathies) certainly comprise a large proportion of pain syndromes encountered in AIDS patients, pains of a somatic and/or visceral nature are also extremely common clinical problems.

Pain syndromes seen in HIV disease can be categorized into three types (Box 46.3):

1. Those directly related to HIV infection or consequences of immunosuppression.
2. Those due to AIDS therapies.
3. Those unrelated to AIDS or AIDS therapies (Breitbart 1997, Hewitt et al 1997).

In studies to date, approximately 45% of pain syndromes encountered are directly related to HIV infection or consequences of immunosuppression; 15–30% are caused by therapies for HIV- or AIDS-related conditions, as well as diagnostic procedures, and the remaining 25–40% are unrelated to HIV or its therapies (Hewitt et al 1997).

Our group at Memorial has reported on the experience of pain in women with AIDS (Breitbart et al 1995, Hewitt et al 1997). While preliminary in nature, our studies suggest that women with HIV disease experience pain more frequently than men with HIV disease and report somewhat higher levels of pain intensity. This may in part be a reflection of the fact that women with AIDS-related pain are twice as likely to be undertreated for their pain compared to men (Breitbart et al 1996a). Women with HIV disease have unique pain syndromes of a gynaecological

BOX 46.3

Pain related to HIV/AIDS infection or consequences of infection
HIV neuropathy
HIV myelopathy
Kaposi's sarcoma
Secondary infections (intestines, skin)
Organomegaly
Arthritis/vasculitis
Myopathy/myositis

Pain related to HIV/AIDS therapy
Antiretrovirals, antivirals
Antimyocobacterials, pneumocystis carinii
Pneumonia prophylaxis
Chemotherapy (vincristine)
Radiation
Surgery
Procedures (bronchoscopy, biopsies)

Pain unrelated to AIDS or AIDS therapy
Disc disease
Diabetic neuropathy

nature specifically related to opportunistic infectious processes and cancers of the pelvis and genitourinary tract (Marte & Allen 1991). Women with AIDS were significantly more likely to be diagnosed with radiculopathy and headache in one survey (Hewitt et al 1997).

Children with HIV infection also experience pain (Strafford et al 1991). HIV-related conditions in children that are observed to cause pain include: meningitis and sinusitis (headaches); otitis media; shingles; cellulitis and abscesses; severe candida dermatitis; dental caries; intestinal infections, such as *Mycobacterium avium intracellular* (MAI) and cryptosporidium; hepatosplenomegaly; oral and oesophageal candidiasis; and spasticity associated with encephalopathy that causes painful muscle spasms.

IMPACT OF PAIN: PSYCHOLOGICAL DISTRESS

Pain in patients with HIV disease has a profound negative impact on physical and psychological functioning, as well as overall quality of life (Rosenfeld et al 1996, Larue et al 1997). In a study of the impact of pain on psychological functioning and quality of life in ambulatory AIDS patients (Rosenfeld et al 1996), depression was significantly correlated with the presence of pain. In addition to being significantly more distressed, depressed and hopeless, those with pain were twice as likely to have suicidal ideation (40%) as those without pain (20%). HIV-infected patients with pain were more functionally impaired (Rosenfeld et al 1996). Such functional interference was highly correlated to levels of pain intensity and depression. Patients with pain were more likely to be unemployed or disabled and reported less social support. Larue and colleagues (1997) reported that HIV-infected patients with pain intensities greater than 5 (on a 0–10 numerical rating scale (NRS)) reported significantly poorer quality of life during the week preceding their survey than patients without pain. Pain intensity had an independent negative impact on HIV patients' quality of life, even after adjustment for treatment setting, stage of disease, fatigue, sadness and depression. Singer and colleagues (1993) also reported an association between the frequency of multiple pains, increased disability and higher levels of depression. Psychological variables, such as the amount of control people believe they have over pain; emotional associations and memories of pain; fears of death; depression; anxiety; and hopelessness, contribute to the experience of pain in people with AIDS and can increase suffering (Breitbart 1993, Rosenfeld et al 1996). Our group also reported (Payne et al 1994) that negative thoughts related to pain were associated with greater pain intensity, psychological distress and disability in ambulatory patients with AIDS. Those AIDS patients who felt that pain represented a progression of their HIV disease reported more intense pain than those who did not see pain as a threat.

UNDERTREATMENT OF PAIN IN AIDS

Reports of dramatic undertreatment of pain in AIDS patients have appeared in the literature (Lebovits et al 1989, McCormack et al 1993, Breitbart et al 1996a, Larue et al 1997). These studies suggest that all classes of analgesics, particularly opioid analgesics, are underutilized in the treatment of pain in AIDS. Our group has reported (Breitbart et al 1996b) that less than 8% of individuals in our cohort of ambulatory AIDS patients reporting pain in the severe range (8–10 on a NRS of pain intensity) received a strong opioid, such as morphine, as recommended by published guidelines (i.e., the WHO Analgesic Ladder). In addition, 18% of patients with 'severe' pain were prescribed no anagesics whatsoever, 40% were prescribed a non-opioid analgesic (e.g., NSAID), and only 22% were prescribed a 'weak' opioid' (e.g., acetaminophen in combination with oxycodone). Utilizing the Pain Management Index (PMI) (Zelman et al 1987), a measure of adequacy of analgesic therapy derived from the Brief Pain Inventory's (BPI) record of pain intensity and strength of analgesia prescribed, we further examined adequacy of pain treatment. Only 15% of our sample received adequate analgesic therapy based on the PMI. This degree of undermedication of pain in AIDS (85%) far exceeds published reports of undermedication of pain (using the PMI) in cancer populations of 40% (Cleeland et al 1994). Larue and colleagues (1997) report that in France, 57% of patients with HIV disease reporting moderate to severe pain did not receive any analgesic treatment at all, and only 22% received a 'weak' opioid.

While opioid analgesics are underutilized, it is also clear that adjuvant analgesic agents, such as the antidepressants, are also dramatically underutilized (Lebovits et al 1989, McCormack et al 1993, Breitbart et al 1996a, Larue et al 1997). Breitbart and colleagues (1996a) report that less than 10% of AIDS patients reporting pain received an adjuvant analgesic drug (e.g., antidepressants, anticonvulsants), despite the fact that approximately 40% of the sample had neuropathic-type pain. This class of analgesic agents is a critical component of the WHO Analgesic Ladder, particularly in managing neuropathic pain, and is vastly underutilized in the management of HIV-related pain.

A number of different factors have been proposed as potential influences on the widespread undertreatment of pain in AIDS, including patient, clinician and healthcare system-related barriers (Passik et al 1994, Breitbart et al 1996a, 1998, 1999). Sociodemographic factors which have been reported to be associated with undertreatment of pain in AIDS include gender, education and substance abuse history (Breitbart et al 1996b). Women, less educated patients, and patients who reported injection drug use as their HIV risk transmission factor are significantly more likely to receive inadequate analgesic therapy for HIV-related pain.

Breitbart and colleagues (1998) surveyed 200 ambulatory AIDS patients, utilizing a modified version of the Barriers Questionnaire (BQ; Ward et al 1993) which assesses a variety of patient-related barriers to pain management (resulting in patient reluctance to report pain or take opioid analgesics). Results of this study demonstrated that patient-related barriers (as measured by BQ scores) were significantly correlated with the undertreatment of pain (as measured by the PMI) in AIDS patients with pain. Additionally, BQ scores were significantly correlated with higher levels of psychological distress and depression, indicating that patient-related barriers contributed to the undertreatment of pain and poorer quality of life. The most frequently endorsed BQ items were those concerning the addiction potential of opioids, side effects and discomfort related to opioid administration, and misconceptions about tolerance. While there were no age, gender or HIV risk transmission factor associations with BQ scores, non-white and less educated patients scored higher on the BQ. Several additional 'AIDS-specific' patient-related barriers examined (Passik et al 1994, Breitbart et al 1998) reveal that 66% of patients are trying to limit their overall intake of medications (i.e., pills) or utilize non-pharmacological interventions for pain, 50% of patients cannot afford to fill a prescription for analgesics or have no access to pain specialists, and about 50% are reluctant to take opioids for pain out of a concern that family/friends/physicians will assume they are misusing or abusing these drugs.

In a survey of approximately 500 AIDS care providers (Breitbart et al 1999), clinicians (primarily physicians and nurses) rated the barriers to AIDS pain management they perceived to be the most important in the care of AIDS patients. The most frequently endorsed barriers were those regarding lack of knowledge about pain management or access to pain specialists, and concerns regarding the use and addiction potential of opioid drugs in the AIDS population. The top five barriers endorsed by AIDS clinicians included: lack of knowledge regarding pain management (51.8%); reluctance to prescribe opioids (51.5%); lack of access to pain specialists (50.9%); concern regarding drug addiction and/or abuse (50.5%); and lack of psychological support/drug treatment services (43%). Patient reluctance to report pain and patient reluctance to take opioids were less commonly endorsed barriers, with about 24% of respondents endorsing those barriers. By contrast, past surveys of oncologists (von Roenn et al 1993) rated patient reluctance to report pain or take opioids as two of the top four barriers. Like AIDS care providers, oncologists also endorsed highly a reluctance to prescribe opioids, even to a population of cancer patients with a significantly lower prevalence of past or present substance abuse disorders. Both oncologists and AIDS care providers report they have inadequate knowledge of pain management and pain assessment skills.

Pain management and substance abuse in AIDS

Individuals who inject drugs are among the AIDS exposure categories with the highest rate of increase over the past 5 years, especially in large urban centres. Pain management in the substance-abusing AIDS patient is perhaps the most challenging of clinical goals. Fears of addiction and concerns regarding drug abuse affect both patient compliance and physician management of pain and use of narcotic analgesics, often leading to the undermedication of HIV-infected patients with pain.

Studies of patterns of chronic narcotic analgesic use in patients with cancer, burns and postoperative pain, however, have demonstrated that although tolerance and physical dependence commonly occur, addiction, i.e., psychological dependence and drug abuse, are rare and almost never occur in individuals who do not have histories of drug abuse (Porter & Jick 1980, Kanner & Foley 1981, Perry & Heidrich 1982). More relevant to the clinical problem of pain management in AIDS patients, however, is the issue of managing pain in the growing segment of HIV-infected patients who have a history of substance abuse or who are actively abusing drugs. The use specifically of opioids for pain control in patients with HIV infection and a history of substance abuse, raises several difficult pain treatment questions, including: how to treat pain in people who have a high tolerance to narcotic analgesics; how to mitigate this population's drug-seeking and potentially manipulative behaviour; how to deal with patients who may offer unreliable medical histories or who may not comply with treatment recommendations; and how to counter the risk of patients spreading HIV while high and disinhibited.

Perhaps of greatest concern to clinicians is the possibility that they are being lied to by a substance-abusing AIDS patient complaining of pain. Clinicians must rely on a patient's subjective report, which is often the best or only indication of the presence and intensity of pain, as well as the degree of pain relief achieved by an intervention. Physicians who believe they are being manipulated by drug-seeking patients often hesitate to use appropriately high doses of narcotic analgesics to control pain. The fear is that the clinician is being 'duped' into prescribing narcotic analgesics which will then be abused or sold. Clinicians do not want to contribute to or help sustain addiction. This leads to an immediate defensiveness on the part of the clinician, and an impulse to avoid prescribing opioids and even to avoid full assessment of a pain complaint.

Because concerns are often raised regarding the credibility of AIDS patients' report of pain, particularly where there is a history of injection drug use, Breitbart and colleagues (1997) conducted a study of 516 ambulatory AIDS patients, in which they compared the report of pain experience and the adequacy of pain management among patients with and without a history of substance abuse. This study found that there were no significant differences in the report of pain experience (i.e., pain prevalence, pain intensity and pain-related functional interference) among patients who reported injection drug use (IDU) as their HIV transmission risk factor and those who reported other transmission factors (non-IDU). Furthermore, there were no differences in the report of pain experience among patients who acknowledged current substance abuse, those in methadone maintenance and those who were in drug-free recovery. The description of HIV-related pain was comparable among IDU and non-IDU groups. What was different was the treatment received by these two groups. Patients in the IDU group were significantly more undermedicated for pain compared to the non-IDU group. In addition, clinicians did not distinguish among various types of patients in the IDU group (i.e., active users, those in drug-free recovery and those in methadone maintenance), and withheld the use of opioids in all patients, resulting in only 8–10% of IDU patients receiving adequate analgesia based on the Pain Management Index (Breitbart et al 1997).

Unfortunately the existence or severity of pain cannot be objectively proven. The clinician must accept and respect the report of pain in spite of the possibility of being duped and proceed in the evaluation, assessment and management of pain. Experience from the cancer pain literature suggests that it is possible to adequately manage pain in substance abusers with life-threatening illness and to do so safely and responsibly utilizing opioid analgesics and several sound principles of pain management outlined here (Table 46.9) (Macaluso et al 1988, McCaffery & Vourakis 1992, Portenoy & Payne 1992). Most clinicians experienced in working with this population of patients recommend that practitioners set clear and direct limits. While this is an important aspect of the care of intravenous drug-using people with HIV disease, it is by no means the whole answer. As much as possible, clinicians should attempt to eliminate the issue of drug abuse as an obstacle to pain management by dealing directly with the problems of opiate withdrawal and drug treatment. Clinicians should err on the side of believing patients when they complain of pain, and should utilize knowledge of specific HIV-related pain syndromes to corroborate the report of a patient perceived as being unreliable.

The clinician must be familiar with, and understand, the current terminology relevant to substance abuse and addiction. It is important to distinguish between the terms 'tolerance', 'physical dependence', and 'addiction' or 'abuse' (psychological dependence). Tolerance is a pharmacological property of opioid drugs defined by the need for increasing doses to maintain an (analgesic) effect. Physical dependence is characterized by the onset of signs and symptoms of withdrawal if narcotic analgesics are abruptly stopped or a narcotic antagonist is administered. Tolerance usually occurs in association with physical dependence. Addiction or abuse (also often termed psychological dependence) is a psychological and behavioural syndrome in which there is drug craving, compulsive use (despite physical, psychological or

Table 46.9 An approach to pain management in substance abusers with HIV disease

1.	Substance abusers with HIV disease deserve pain control; we have no obligation to treat pain and suffering in all our patients.
2.	Accept and respect the report of pain.
3.	Be careful about the label 'substance abuse'; distinguish between tolerance, physical dependence, and 'addiction' (psychological dependence or drug abuse).
4.	Not all 'substance abusers' are the same; distinguish between active users, persons in methadone maintenance, and those in recovery.
5.	Individualize pain treatment.
6.	Use the principles of pain management outlined for all patients with HIV disease and pain (WHO Ladder).
7.	Set clear goals and conditions for opioid therapy: set limits, recognize drug abuse behaviours, make consequences clear, use written contracts, establish a single prescriber.
8.	Use a multidimensional approach: pharmacologic and nonpharmacologic interventions, attention to psychosocial issues, team approach.

from Breitbart (May 1999).

social harm to user), other aberrant drug-related behaviours and relapse after abstinence (American Pain Society 1992). The term 'pseudo-addiction' has been coined to describe the patient who exhibits behaviour that clinicians associate with addiction, such as requests for higher doses of opioid, but which is in fact caused by uncontrolled pain and inadequate pain management (Weissman & Haddox 1989).

The clinician must also distinguish between the 'former' addict who has been drug free for years, the addict in a methadone maintenance programme and the addict who is actively abusing illicit and/or prescription drugs. Actively using addicts and those on methadone maintenance with pain must be assumed to have some tolerance to opioids and may require higher starting and maintenance doses of opioids. Preventing withdrawal is an essential first step in managing pain in this population. In addition, 'active' addicts with AIDS will understandably require more in the way of psychosocial support and services to adequately deal with the distress of their pain and illness. Former addicts may pose the challenge of refusing opioids for pain because of fears of relapse. Such patients can be assured that opioids, when prescribed and monitored responsibly, may be an essential part of pain management, and the use of the drug for pain is quite different from its use when they were abusing similar drugs. Some authorities emphasize the importance of conducting a comprehensive pain assessment in order to define the pain syndrome. Specific pain syndromes often respond best to specific interventions (i.e., neuropathic pains respond well to antidepressants or anticonvulsants). Adequate assessment of the cause of pain is essential in all AIDS patients, and particularly in the substance abuser. It is critical that adequate analgesia be provided while diagnostic studies are underway. Often treatments directed at the underlying disorder causing pain are very effective as well. For example, headache from CNS toxoplasmosis responds well to primary treatments and steroids.

When deciding on an appropriate pharmacological intervention in the substance abuser, it is advisable to follow the WHO Analgesic Ladder. This approach advocates selection of analgesics based on severity of pain; however clinicians also often take into account the nature of the pain syndrome in selecting analgesics. For mild to moderate pain, NSAIDs are indicated. The NSAIDs are continued with adjuvant analgesics (antidepressants, anticonvulsants, neuroleptics, steroids) if a specific indication exists. Patients with moderate to severe pain, or those who do not achieve relief from NSAIDs, are treated with a 'weak' opioid, often in combination with NSAIDs and adjuvant drugs, if indicated.

It has been pointed out that it is critical to apply appropriate pharmacological principles for opioid use. One should avoid using agonist-antagonist opioid drugs. The use of p.r.n. dosing often leads to excessive drug-centred interactions with staff that are not productive. While patients should not necessarily be given the specific drug or route they want, every effort should be made to give patients more of a sense of control and a sense of collaboration with the clinician. Often a patient's report of beneficial or adverse effects of a specific agent are useful to the clinician.

The management of pain in substance-abusing AIDS patients requires a team approach. Early involvement of pain specialists, psychiatric clinicians and substance abuse specialists is critical. Non-pharmacological pain interventions should be appropriately applied, not as a substitute for opioids but as an important adjunct. Realistic goals for treatment must be set, and problems related to inappropriate behaviour around the handling of prescription and interactions with staff should be anticipated.

Hospital staff must be educated and made aware that such difficult patients evoke feelings that if acted on could interfere with providing good care. Clear limit setting is helpful for both the patient and treating staff. Sometimes written rules about what behaviours are expected and what behaviours are not tolerated and the consequence should be provided. The use of urine toxicology monitoring, restrictions of visitors, strict limits on amount of drug per prescription can all be very useful. It is important to also remember that rehabilitation or detoxification from opioids is not appropriate during an acute medical crisis and should not be attempted at that time. Once more stable medical conditions exist, referral to a drug rehabilitation programme may be very useful. Constant assessment and re-evaluation of the effects of pain interventions must also take place in order to optimize care. Special attention should be given to points in treatment where routes of administration are changed or where opioids are being tapered. It must be made clear to patients what drugs and/or regimen would be introduced to control pain when opioids are tapered or withdrawn, and what options are available if that non-opioid regimen is ineffective.

Finally, it is important to recognize that substance abusers with AIDS are quite likely to have co-morbid psychiatric symptoms as well as multiple other physical symptoms, which can all contribute to increased pain and suffering. Adequate attention must be paid to these physical and psychological symptoms for pain management to be optimized.

PSYCHIATRIC MANAGEMENT OF PAIN IN AIDS

The psychiatric management of HIV-related pain involves the use of psychotherapeutic, cognitive-behavioural and psychopharmacological techniques. Psychotherapists can offer short-term supportive psychotherapy, based on a crisis –intervention model, and provide emotional support, continuity of care, information about pain management and assistance to patients in adapting to their crises. This often involves working with 'families' that are not typical and that may consist of gay lovers, estranged spouses or parents, and fragmented or extended families. People with HIV disease may also require treatment for substance abuse.

Cognitive-behavioural techniques for pain control, such as relaxation, imagery, hypnosis and biofeedback, are effective as part of a comprehensive multimodal approach, particularly among patients with HIV disease who may have an increased sensitivity to the side effects of medications. Non-pharmacological interventions, however, must never be used as a substitute for the appropriate analgesic management of pain. The mechanisms by which these non-pharmacological techniques work are not known; however, they all seem to share the elements of relaxation and distraction. Additionally, patients often feel a sense of increased control over their pain and their bodies. Ideal candidates for the application of these techniques are mentally alert and have mild to moderate pain. Confusion interferes significantly with a patient's ability to focus attention and so limits the usefulness of cognitive-behavioural interventions.

Psychiatric disorders, particularly organic mental disorders such as AIDS–dementia complex, can occasionally interfere with adequate pain management in patients with HIV disease. Opiate analgesics, the mainstay of treatment for moderate to severe pain, may worsen dementia or cause treatment-limiting sedation, confusion or hallucinations in patients with neurological complications of AIDS. The judicious use of psychostimulants to diminish sedation and neuroleptics to clear confusion can be quite helpful.

Psychotropic drugs, particularly the TCAs and the psychostimulants, are useful in enhancing the pain-blocking properties of analgesics in pharmacological management of HIV-related pain. The tricyclic antidepressants (amitriptyline, nortriptyline, imipramine, desipramine, doxepin) and some of the newer non-cyclic antidepressants (trazodone and fluoxetine) have potent analgesic properties and are widely used to treat a variety of chronic pain syndromes. They may have their most beneficial effect in the treatment of neuropathic pain, that is, pain due to nerve damage, such as the peripheral neuropathies seen commonly in people with HIV infection. Antidepressants have direct analgesic effects and the capacity to enhance the analgesic effects of morphine.

Psychostimulants such as dextroamphetamine or methylphenidate are useful antidepressants in people with HIV disease who are cognitive impaired and are also helpful in diminishing sedation secondary to narcotic analgesics. Psychostimulants also enhance the analgesic effects of opiate analgesics.

The inadequate management of pain is often caused by the inability to properly assess pain in all its dimensions. All too frequently, physicians presume that psychological variables are the cause of continued pain or lack of response to medical treatment, when in fact they have not adequately appreciated the role of medical factors. Other causes of inadequate pain management include: lack of knowledge of current pharmaco- or psychotherapeutic approaches; a focus on prolonging life rather than alleviating suffering; lack of communication or unsuccessful communication between doctors and patients; limited expectations of patients to achieve pain relief; limited capacity of patients impaired by organic mental disorders to communicate; unavailability of narcotics; doctors' fear of causing respiratory depression; and, most importantly, doctors' fear of amplifying addiction and drug abuse.

REFERENCES

Achte KA, Vanhkouen ML 1971 Cancer and the psyche. Omega 2: 46–56

Adams F 1988 Neuropsychiatric evaluation and treatment of delirium in cancer patients. Advances in Psychosomatic Medicine 18: 26–36

Adams F, Quesada JR, Gutterman JU 1984 Neuropsychiatric manifestations of human leukocyte interferon therapy in patients with cancer. Journal of the American Medical Association 252: 938–941

Adams F, Fernandez F, Andersson BS 1986 Emergency pharmacotherapy of delirium in the critically ill cancer patient. Psychosomatics 27: 36–37

Adjan M 1970 Uber therapeutischen beeinflussung des schmerzsmptoms bei unheilboren tumorkranken. Therapie der Hergenwart 10: 1620–1627

Ahles TA, Martin JB 1992 Cancer pain: a multidimensional perspective. Hospice Journal 8: 25–48

Ahles TA, Blanchard EB, Ruckdeschel JC 1983 The multidimensional nature of cancer related pain. Pain 17: 277–288

American Medical News 1992 20 January 1992, p 9

American Pain Society 1992 Principles of analgesic use in the treatment of acute pain and cancer pain, 3rd edn. American Pain Society, Skokie, IL

Anthony M, Lance JW 1969 MAO inhibition in the treatment of migraine. Archives of Neurology 21: 263

Asch D 1996 The role of critical care nurses in euthanasia and assisted suicide. New England Journal of Medicine 334: 1374–1379

Ayd F 1979 Amoxapine: a new tricyclic antidepressant. International Drug Therapy Newsletter 14: 33–40

Back AL, Wallace JI, Starks HE, Pearlman RA 1996 Physician-assisted suicide and euthanasia in Washington State. Journal of the American Medical Association 275: 919–925

Barber J, Gitelson J 1980 Cancer pain: psychological management using hypnosis. CA: a Cancer Journal for Clinicians 3: 130–136

Barjou B 1971 Etude du Tofranil sules douleurs en chirugie. Revue de Medecine de Tours 6: 473–482

Basbaum AI, Fields HL 1978 Endogenous pain control mechanisms: review and hypothesis. Annals of Neurology 4: 451–462

Beaver WT, Feise G 1976 Comparison of the analgesic effects of morphine, hydroxyzine and their combination in patients with postoperative pain. In: Bonica JJ, Albe-Fessard D (eds) Advances in pain research and therapy. Raven, New York, pp 533–557

Beaver WT, 'Wallenstein SL, Houde RW et al 1966 A comparison of the analgesic effect of methotrimeprazine and morphine in patients with cancer. Clinical Pharmacology and Therapeutics 7: 436–446

Beck SL 1991 The therapeutic use of music for cancer-related pain. Oncology Nursing Forum 18: 1527–1537

Bernard A, Scheuer H 1972 Action de la clomipramine (Anafranil) sur la douleur des cancers en pathologie cervico-faciale. Journal Francais d'Oto Rhino Laryngologie 21: 723–728

Blank SS, Clark L, Longman AJ, Atwood JR 1989 Perceived home care needs of cancer patients and their caregivers. Cancer Nursing 12: 78–84

Bolund C 1985 Suicide and cancer: II. Medical and care factors in suicide by cancer patients in Sweden. 1973–1976. Journal of Psychosocial Oncology 3: 17–30

Bond MR 1973 Personality studies in patients with pain secondary to organic disease. Journal of Psychosomatic Research 17: 257–263

Bond MR 1979 Psychological and emotional aspects of cancer pain. In: Bonica JJ, Ventafridda V (eds) Advances in pain research and therapy, vol 2. Raven, New York, pp 81–88

Bond MR, Pearson IB 1969 Psychological aspects of pain in women with advanced cancer of the cervix. Journal of Psychosomatic Research 13: 13–19

Botney M, Fields HC 1983 Amitriptyline potentiates morphine analgesia by direct action on the central nervous system. Annals of Neurology 13: 160–164

Bottomley DM, Hanks GW 1990 Subcutaneous midazolam infusion in palliative care. Journal of Pain Symptom Management 5: 259–261

Bourhis A, Boudouresue G, Pellet W, Fondarai J, Ponzio J, Spitalier JM 1978 Pain, infirmity and psychotropic drugs in oncology. Pain 5: 263–274

Bradley JJ 1963 Severe localized pain associated with the depressive syndrome. British Journal of Psychiatry 109: 741–745

Breitbart W 1987 Suicide in cancer patients. Oncology 1: 49–53

Breitbart W 1989a Psychiatric management of cancer pain. Cancer 63: 2336–2342

Breitbart WB 1989b Endocrine-related psychiatric disorder. In: Holland J, Rowland J (eds) The handbook of psychooncology: the psychological care of the cancer patient. Oxford University Press, New York, pp 356–366

Breitbart W 1990a Psychiatric aspects of pain and HIV disease. Focus, a Guide to AIDS Research and Counselling 5: 1–3

Breitbart W 1990b Cancer pain and suicide. In: Foley KM et al (eds) Advances in pain research and therapy, vol 16. Raven, New York, pp 399–412

Breitbart W 1993 Suicide risk and pain in cancer and AIDS patients. In: Chapman R, Foley KM (eds) Current emerging issues in cancer pain: research and practice. Raven, New York, pp 49–65

Breitbart W 1996 Pharmacotherapy of pain in AIDS. In: Wormser G (ed) A clinical guide to AIDS and HIV. Lippencott-Raven, Philadelphia, pp 359–378

Breitbart W 1997 Pain in AIDS. In: Jensen J, Turner J, Wiesenfeld-Hallin Z (eds) Proceedings of the 8th World Congress on Pain, Progress in Pain Research and Management, vol. 8. IASP Press, Seattle, pp 63–100

Breitbart W, Holland JC 1988 Psychiatric complications of cancer. In: Brain MC, Carbone PP (eds) Current therapy in hematology oncology, vol 3. BC Decker, Toronto, pp 268–274

Breitbart W, Holland J 1990 Psychiatric aspects of cancer pain. In: Foley KM et al (eds) Advances in pain research and therapy, vol 16. Raven, New York, pp 73–87

Breitbart W, Mermelstein H 1992 Pemoline: an alternative psychostimulation in the management of depressive disorders in cancer patients. Psychosomatics 33: 352–356

Breitbart W, Passik S, Bronaugh T et al 1991 Pain in the ambulatory AIDS patient: prevalence and psychosocial correlates. 38th Annual

Meeting, Academy of Psychosomatic Medicine, October 17–20, Atlanta, Georgia (abstract)
Breitbart W, Stiefel F, Pannulo S, Kornblith A, Holland JC 1993 Neuropsychiatric cancer patients with epidural spinal cord compression receiving high dose corticosteroids: a prospective comparison study. Psycho-oncology 2: 233–245
Breitbart W, McDonald M, Rosenfeld B et al 1995 Pain in women with AIDS. Proceeding of the 14th Annual Meeting of the American Pain Society, Los Angeles, CA (abstract)
Breitbart W, Rosenfeld B, Passik S, McDonald M, Thaler H, Portenoy R 1996a The undertreatment of pain in ambulatory AIDS patients. Pain 65: 239–245
Breitbart W, McDonald MV, Rosenfeld B et al 1996b Pain in ambulatory AIDS patients – I: Pain characteristics and medical correlates. Pain 68: 315–321
Breitbart W, Marotta R, Platt M et al 1996c A double blind trial of haloperidol, chlorpromazine and lorazepam in the treatment of delirium in hospitalized AIDS patients. American Journal of Psychiatry 153: 231–237
Breitbart W, Passik S, McDonald M et al 1998 Patient-related barriers to pain management in ambulatory AIDS patients. Pain 76: 9–16
Breitbart W, Rosenfeld B, Kaim M 1999 Clinician related barriers to pain management in AIDS. Pain (in press)
Breivik H, Rennemo F 1982 Clinical evaluation of combined treatment with methadone and psychotropic drugs in cancer patients. Acta Anaesthesiologica Scandinavica 74 (suppl): 135–140
Brennan SC, Redd WH, Jacobsen PB et al 1988 Anxiety and panic during magnetic resonance scans. Lancet ii: 512
Brown JH, Henteleff P, Barakat S, Rowe JR 1986 Is it normal for terminally ill patients to desire death. American Journal of Psychiatry 143: 208–211
Bruera E, Chadwick S, Brennels C, Hanson J, MacDonald RN 1987 Methylphenidate associated with narcotics for the treatment of cancer pain. Cancer Treatment Reports 71: 67–70
Bruera E, Brenneis C, Paterson AH, MacDonald RN 1989a Use of methylphenidate as an adjuvant to narcotic analgesics in patients with advanced cancer: Journal of Pain Symptom Management 4: 3–6
Bruera E, MacMillan K, Kuehn N et al 1989b The cognitive effects of the administration of narcotics. Pain 39: 13–16
Bruera E, MacMillan K, Pither J, MacDonald RN 1990a Effects of morphine on the dyspnea of terminal cancer patients. Journal of Pain Symptom Management 5: 341–344
Bruera E, Miller L, McCalion S 1990b Cognitive failure in patients with terminal cancer: a prospective longitudinal study. Psychosocial Aspects of Cancer 9: 308–310
Bruera E, Miller MJ, MacMillan K, Kuehn N 1992 Neuropsychological effects of methylphenidate in patients receiving a continuous infusion of narcotics for cancer pain. Pain 48: 163–166
Bukberg J, Penman D, Holland J 1984 Depression in hospitalized cancer patients. Psychosomatic Medicine 43: 122–199
Butler S 1986 Present status of tricyclic antidepressants in chronic pain therapy. In: Benedetti C et al (eds) Advances in pain research and therapy, vol 7. Raven, New York, pp 173–196
Caccia MR 1975 Clonazepam in facial neuralgia and cluster headache: clinical and electrophysiological study. European Neurology 13: 560–563
Carton M, Cabarrot E, Lafforque C 1976 Interest de L'amitriptyline utilisee comme antalgique en cancerologie. Gazette Medicale de France 83: 2375–2378
Cassem NH 1987 The dying patient. In: Hacket TP, Cassem NH (eds) Massachusetts General Hospital handbook of general hospital psychiatry, 2nd edn. PSG Publishing, Littleton, MA, pp 332–352
Chapman CR 1989 Giving the patient control of opioid analgesic administration. In: Hill CS, Fields WS (eds) Advances in pain research and therapy, vol 11. Raven, New York, pp 339–352
Charney DS, Meukes DB, Heniuger PR 1981 Receptor sensitivity and the mechanism of action of antidepressant treatment: Archives of General Psychiatry 38: 1160–1180
Chiarillo RJ, Cole JO 1987 The use of psychostimulants in general psychiatry. A reconsideration. Archives of General Psychiatry 44: 286–295
Chochinov HM, Wilson LG, Enns M 1995 Desire for death in the terminally ill. American Journal of Psychiatry 152: 1185–1191
Chouinard G, Young SN, Annable L 1983 Antimanic effect of clonazepam. Biological Psychiatry 18: 451–466
Ciraulo DA, Shader RI 1990 Fluoxetine drug–drug interactions: I. Antidepressants and antipsychotics. Journal of Clinical Psychopharmacology 10: 48–50
Cleeland CS 1984 The impact of pain on the patient with cancer. Cancer 54: 2635–2641
Cleeland CS 1987 Nonpharmacologic management of cancer pain. Journal of Pain and Symptom Control 2: 523–528
Cleeland CS, Tearnan BH 1986 Behavioral control of cancer pain. In: Holzman D, Turk DC (eds) Pain management. Pergamon, New York, pp 193–212
Cleeland CS, Gonin R, Hatfield AK et al 1994 Pain and its treatment in outpatients with metastatic cancer: the Eastern Cooperative Oncology Group's outpatients study. New England Journal of Medicine 330: 592–596
Costa D, Mogos I, Toma T 1985 Efficacy and safety of mianserin in the treatment of depression of women with cancer. Acta Psychiatrica Scandinavica 72: 85–92
Dalton JA, Feuerstein M 1989 Fear, alexithymia and cancer pain. Pain 38: 159–170
Daut RL, Cleeland CS 1982 The prevalence and severity of pain in cancer. Cancer 50: 1913–1918
Davidoff G, Guarracini M, Roth E et al 1987 Trazodone hydrochloride in the treatment of dysesthetic pain in traumatic myelopathy: a randomized, double-blind, placebo-controlled study. Pain 29: 151–161
de Sousa E, Jepson A 1988 Midazolam in terminal care. Lancet i: 67–68
de Wachter MAH 1989 Active euthanasia in the Netherlands. Journal of the American Medical Association 262: 3316–3319
DeAngelis LM, Delattre J, Posner JB 1989 Radiation-induced dementia in patients cured of brain metastases. Neurology 39: 789–796
Denicoff KD, Rubinow DR, Papa MZ et al 1987 The neuropsychiatric effects of treatment with interleukin-w and lymphokine-activated killer cells. Annals of Internal Medicine 107: 293–300
Derogatis LR, Morrow GR, Fetting J et al 1983 The prevalence of psychiatric disorders among cancer patients. Journal of the American Medical Association 249: 751–757
Deutschmann W 1971 Tofranil ider schmerzbehandlung de krebskranken. Medizinische Welt 22: 1346–1347
Dubner R, Bennett GJ 1983 Spinal and trigeminal mechanisms of nociception. Annual Review of the Neurosciences 6: 381–418
Eberhard G et al 1988 A double-blind randomized study of clomipramine versus maprotiline in patients with idiopathic pain syndromes. Neuropsychobiology 19: 25–32
Eller KC, Sison AC, Breitbart W, Passik S 1992 Morphine-induced acute confusional states: a retrospective analysis (abstract). Academy of Psychosomatic Medicine 39th Annual Meeting, San Diego, CA
Emanuel EJ, Fairclough DL, Daniels ER, Clarridge BR 1996 Euthanasia and physician assisted suicide. Attitudes and experiences of oncology patients, oncologists and the public. Lancet 347: 1805–1810
Endicott J 1983 Measurement of depression in patients with cancer. Cancer 53: 2243–2248
Fainsinger R, Bruera E 1992 Treatment of delirium in a terminally ill patient. Journal of Pain Symptom Management 7: 54–56
Fainsinger R, MacEachern T, Hanson J et al 1991 Symptom control

during the last week of life in a palliative care unit. Journal of Palliative Care 7: 5–11
Fairclough D, Slutsman J, Omandsun LL, Emanuel EJ 1998 Interest in euthanasia and physician assisted suicide among terminally ill oncology patients: results from Commonwealth–Cummings Project. Proceedings of American Society of Clinical Oncology Annual Meeting. V17: abstract no 186, p 48a
Farberow NL, Schneidman ES, Leonard CV 1963 Suicide among general medical and surgical hospital patients with malignant neoplasms. Medical Bulletin 9, US Veterans Administration, Washington DC
Feinman C 1985 Pain relief by antidepressants: possible modes of actions. Pain 23: 1–8
Fernandez F, Adams F, Holmes VF 1987a Analgesic effect of alprazolam in patients with chronic, organic pain of malignant origin. Journal of Clinical Psychopharmacology 3: 167–169
Fernandez F, Adams F, Holmes VF et al 1987b Methylphenidate for depressive disorders in cancer patients. Psychosomatics 28: 455–461
Fernandez F, Adams F, Levy J et al 1988 Cognitive impairment due to AIDS related complex and its response to psychostimulants. Psychosomatics 29: 38–46
Fernandez F, Levy JK, Mansell PWA 1989 Management of delirium in terminally ill AIDS patients. International Journal of Psychiatry in Medicine 19: 165–172
Ferrell B 1991 Pain as a metaphor for illness: impact of cancer pain on family caregiver. Oncology Nursing Forum 18: 1303–1308
Ferrell BR, Ferrell BA, Rhiner M, Grant M 1991 Family factors influencing cancer. Pain Management Postgraduate Medical Journal 67: 564–569
Fields HL, Basbaum AI 1984 Endogenous pain control mechanisms. In: Wall PD, Melzack R (eds) Textbook of pain. Churchill Livingstone, Edinburgh, pp 142–152
Fiorentino M 1969 Sperimentazione controllata dell' Imipramina come analgesico maggiore in oncologia. Revista Medica de Trentina 5: 387–396
Fisch R 1985–1986 Methylphenidate for medical inpatients. International Journal of Psychiatry in Medicine 15: 75–79
Fishman B, Loscalzo M 1987 Cognitive-behavioral interventions in the management of cancer pain: principles and applications. Medical Clinics of North America 71: 271–287
Fleishman SB, Lesko LM 1989 Delirium and dementia. In: Holland J, Rowland J (eds) The handbook of psychooncology: psychological care of the cancer patient. Oxford University Press, New York, pp 342–355
Foley KM 1975 Pain syndromes in patients with cancer. In: Bonica JJ, Ventafridda V, Fink RB, Jones LE, Loeser JD (eds) Advances in pain research and therapy, vol 2. Raven, New York, pp 59–75
Foley KM 1985 The treatment of cancer pain. New England Journal of Medicine 313: 845
Foley KM 1991 The relationship of pain and symptom management to patient requests for physician-assisted suicide. Journal of Pain and Symptom Management 6: 289–295
Folstein MF, Folstein SE, McHugh PR 1975 Mini-mental state. Journal of Psychiatric Research 12: 189–198
Forrest WH, Brown BW, Brown CR et al 1977 Dextroamphetamine with morphine for the treatment of post-operative pain. New England Journal of Medicine 296: 712–715
Fotopoulos SS, Graham C, Cook MR 1979 Psychophysiologic control of cancer pain. In: Bonica JJ, Ventafridda, V (eds) Advances in pain research and therapy, vol 2. Raven, New York, pp 231–244
France RD 1987 The future for antidepressants: treatment of pain. Psychopathology 20: 99–113
Gaylin W, Kass LR, Pellegrino ED, Siegler M 1988 Doctors must not kill. JAMA 259: 2139–2140
Gebhardt KH, Beller J, Nischk R 1969 Behandlung des karzinomschmerzes mit chlorimipramin (Anafrani). Mediziniche Klinik 64: 751–756
Getto CJ, Sorkness CA, Howell T 1987 Antidepressants and chronic nonmalignant pain: a review. Journal of Pain Symptom Control 2: 9–18
Glassman AH 1984 The newer antidepressant drugs and their cardiovascular effects. Psychopharmacology Bulletin 20: 272–279
Gomez-Perez FJ, Rull JA, Dies H et al 1985 Nortriptyline and fluphenazine in the symptomatic treatment of diabetic neuropathy. A double-blind cross-over study. Pain 23: 395–400
Graffam S, Johnson A 1987 A comparison of two relaxation strategies for the relief of pain and its distress. Journal of Pain and Symptom Management 2: 229–231
Gram LF 1983 Antidepressants: receptors, pharmacokinetics and clinical effects. In: Burrows GD et al (eds) Antidepressants. Elsevier, Amsterdam, pp 81–95
Grossman SA, Sheidler VR, Swedeon K et al 1991 Correlations of patient and caregiver ratings of cancer pain. Journal of Pain and Symptom Management 6: 53–57
Hall RCW, Gardner ER, Perl M, Stickney SK, Pfefferbaum B 1979 The professional burnout syndrome. Psychiatric Opinion 16: 12–17
Hammeroff SR, Cork RC, Scherer K et al 1982 Doxepin effects on chronic pain, depression and plasma opioids. Journal of Clinical Psychiatry 2: 22–26
Hartl DE 1979 Stress management and the nurse. In: Sutterley DC, Donnelly GF (eds) Stress management. Aspen, Germantown MD, pp 163–172
Helig S 1988 The San Francisco Medical Society euthanasia survey. Results and analysis. San Francisco Medicine 61: 24–34
Hendin H, Rutenfrans C, Zylicz Z 1997 Physician-assisted suicide in the Netherlands: lessons from the Dutch. Journal of the American Medical Association 277: 1720–1722
Hewitt D, McDonald M, Portenoy R, Rosenfeld B, Passik S, Breitbart W 1997 Pain syndromes and etiologies in ambulatory AIDS patients. Pain 70: 117–123
Hilgard E, LeBaron S 1982 Relief of anxiety and pain in children with cancer: quantitative measures and clinical observations. International Journal of Clinical and Experimental Hypnosis 30: 417–422
Hinds C 1985 The needs of families who care for patients with cancer at home: are we meeting them? Journal of Advanced Nursing 10: 575–585
Holland JC 1989b Anxiety and cancer: the patient and family. Journal of Clinical Psychiatry 50: 20–25
Holland JC, Holland JF 1985 A neglected problem: the stresses of cancer care on physicians. Primary Care and Cancer 5: 16–22
Holland JC, Rowland J (eds) 1989 Handbook of psychooncology. Psychological care of the patient with cancer. Oxford University Press, New York
Holland JC, Fassanellos, Ohnuma T 1974 Psychiatric symptoms associated with L-asparaginase administration. Journal of Psychiatric Research 10: 165
Holland JC, Hughes Korzun A, Tross S et al 1986 Comparative psychological disturbance in pancreatic and gastric cancer. American Journal of Psychiatry 143: 982–986
Holland JC, Morrow G, Schmale A et al 1991 A randomized clinical trial of alprazolam versus progressive muscle relaxation in cancer patients with anxiety and depressive symptoms. Journal of Clinical Oncology 9: 1004–1011
Horowitz SA, Breitbart W 1993 Relaxation and imagery for symptom control in cancer patients. In: Breibart W, Holland JC (eds) Psychiatric aspects of symptom management in cancer patients. American Psychiatric Press, Washington DC, pp 147–172
Houde RW, Wallenstein SL 1966 Analgesic power of chlorpromazine alone and in combination with morphine (abstract). Federation Proceedings 14: 353

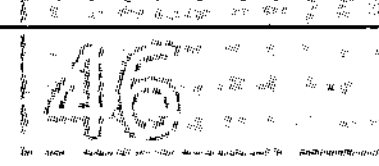

Hughes A, Chauverghe J, Lissilour T, Lagarde C 1963 L'imipramine utilisee comme antalgique majeur en carcinologie: Etude de 118 cas. Presse Medicale 71: 1073–1074
Hull MM 1989 Family needs and supportive nursing behaviors during terminal cancer: a review. Oncology Nursing Forum 16: 787–792
Itil T, Fink M 1966 Anticholinergic drug-induced delirium: experimental modification, quantitative EEG and behavioral correlations. Journal of Nervous and Mental Disease 143: 492–507
Jaffe JH 1985 Drug addition and drug abuse. In: Gilman AG, Goodman LS, Rall TW, Murad F (eds) The pharmacological basis of therapeutics, 7th edn. Macmillan, New York, pp 532–581
Jay S, Elliott C, Varnis J 1986 Acute and chronic pain in adults and children with cancer. Journal of Consulting and Clinical Psychology 54: 601–607
Jellema JC 1987 Hallucinations during sustained-release opioid and methadone administration. Lancet ii: 392
Kanner RM, Foley KM 1981 Patterns of narcotic use in a cancer pain clinic. Annals of the New York Academy of Sciences 362: 161–172
Kash KM, Holland JC 1990 Reducing stress in medical oncology house officers: a preliminary report of a prospective intervention study. In: Hendrie HC, Lloyd C (eds) Educating competent and humane physicians. Indiana University Press, Bloomington, pp 183–195
Katon W, Raskind M 1980 Treatment of depression in the medically ill elderly with methylphenidate. American Journal of Psychiatry 137: 963–965
Kaufmann MW, Murray GB, Cassem NH 1982 Use of psychostimulants in medically ill depressive patients. Psychosomatics 23: 817–819
Kellerman J, Zetter L, Ellenberg L et al 1983 Adolescents with cancer: hypnosis for the reduction of acute pain and anxiety associated with medical procedures. Journal of Adolescent Health Care 4: 85–90
Kimball LR, McCormick WC 1996 The pharmacologic management of pain and discomfort in persons with AIDS near the end of life: use of opioid analgesia in the hospice setting. Journal of Pain and Symptom Management 11: 88–94
King RB 1980 Pain and tryptophan. Journal of Neurosurgery 53: 44–52
Kishore-Kumar R, Schafer SC, Lawlow BA, Murphy DL, Max MB 1989 Single doses of the serotonin agonists buspirone and chlorophenylpiperazine do not relieve neuropathic pain. Pain 37: 227–233
Kishore-Kumar R, Max MB, Schafer SC et al 1990 Desipramine relieves postherpetic neuralgia. Clinical Pharmacology and Therapeutics 47: 305–312
Koocher GP 1979 Adjustment and coping strategies among the caretakers of cancer patients. Social Work in Health Care 5: 145–150
Kristjanson LJ 1986 Indications of quality of palliative care from a family perspective. Journal of Palliative Care 1: 8–17
Kvindesal B, Molin J, Froland A, Gram LF 1984 Imipramine treatment of painful diabetic neuropathy. Journal of the American Medical Association 251: 1727–1730
Langohr HD, Stohr M, Petruch F 1982 An open and double-blind crossover study on the efficacy of clomipramine (anafranil) in patients with painful mono- and polyneuropathies. European Neurology 21: 309–315
Larue F, Brasseur L, Musseault P, Demeulemeester R, Bonifassi L, Bez G 1994 Pain and HIV infection: a French national survey [abstract]. Journal of Palliative Care 10: 95
Larue F, Fontaine A, Colleau S 1997 Underestimation and undertreatment of pain in HIV disease: multicentre study. British Medical Journal 314: 23–28
Lascelles RG 1966 Atypical facial pain and depression. British Journal of Psychology 122: 651
Lechin F et al 1989 Pimozide therapy for trigeminal neuralgia. Archives of Neurology 9: 960–964
Lederberg M 1989 Psychological problems of staff and their management. In: Holland JC, Rowland J (eds) Handbook of psychooncology: psychological care of the patient with cancer. Oxford University Press, New York, pp 678–682
Levin DN, Cleeland CS, Dan R 1985 Public attitudes toward cancer pain. Cancer 56: 2337–2339
Levine PM, Silverfarb PM, Lipowski ZJ 1978 Mental disorders in cancer patients: a study of 100 psychiatric referrals. Cancer 42: 1385–1391
Liepzig RM, Goodman H, Gray P et al 1987 Reversible narcotic-associated mental status impairment in patients with metastatic cancer. Pharmacology 53: 47–57
Lindblom U, Merskey H, Mumford JM et al 1986 Pain terms: a current list with definitions and notes on usage. Pain 3: 5215–5221
Lipowski ZJ 1987 Delirium (acute confusional states). Journal of the American Medical Association 285: 1789–1792
Liu SF, Wang RIH 1975 Increased analgesia and alterations in distribution and metabolism of methadone by desipramine in the rat. Journal of Pharmacology and Experimental Therapeutics 195: 94–104
Lloyd AH 1977 Practical consideration in the use of maprotiline (ludiomil) in general practice. Journal of International Medical Research 5: 122–125
Loscalzo M, Jacobsen PB 1990 Practical behavioral approaches to the effective management of pain and distress. Journal of Psychosocial Oncology 8: 139–169
Macaluso C, Weinberg D, Foley KM 1988a Opiod abuse and misuse in a cancer pain population. Second International Congress on Cancer Pain, July 14–17, Rye, New York (abstract)
Macaluso C, Weinberg D, Foley KM 1988b Opioid abuse and misuse in a cancer pain population. Journal of Pain and Symptom Management 3: 54
McCaffrey M, Beebe A 1989 Pain: clinical manual for nursing practice. CV Mosby, Philadelphia, pp 353–360
McCaffrey M, Vourakis C 1992 Assessment and relief of pain in chemically dependent patients. Orthopaedic Nursing 11: 13–27
McCormack JP, Li R, Zarowny D, Singer J 1993 Inadequate treatment of pain in ambulatory HIV patients. Clinical Journal of Pain 9: 247–283
McKegney FP, Bailey CR, Yates JW 1981 Prediction and management of pain in patients with advanced cancer. General Hospital Psychiatry 3: 95–101
Magni G, Arsie D, DeLeo D 1987 Antidepressants in the treatment of cancer pain. A survey in Italy. Pain 29: 347–353
Malseed RT, Goldstein FJ 1979 Enhancement of morphine analgesics by tricyclic antidepressants. Neuropharmacology 18: 827–829
Maltbie AA, Cavenar JO, Sullivan JL et al 1979 Analgesia and haloperidol: a hypothesis. Journal of Clinical Psychiatry 40: 323–326
Manne S, Redd W, Jacobsen P, Georgiades I 1991 Aroma for treatment of anxiety during MRI scan. American Psychiatric Association Annual Meeting, 7–12 May, New Orleans (abstract)
Marks RM, Sachar EJ 1973 Undertreatment of medical inpatients with narcotic analgesics. Annals of Internal Medicine 78: 173–181
Marte C, Allen M 1991 HIV-related gynecologic conditions: overlooked complications. Focus: A Guide to AIDS Research and Counseling 7: 1–3
Maslach C 1979 The burnout syndrome and patient care. In: Garfield CA (ed) Stress and survival, the emotional realities of life-threatening illness. Mosby, St Louis, pp 89–96
Massie MJ, Holland JC 1987 The cancer patient with pain: psychiatric complications and their management. Medical Clinics of North America 71: 243–258
Massie MJ, Holland JC 1990 Depression and the cancer patient. Journal of Clinical Psychiatry 51: 12–17
Massie MJ, Holland JC, Glass E 1983 Delirium in terminally ill cancer patients. American Journal of Psychiatry 140: 1048–1050

Massie MJ, Holland JC, Straker N 1989 Psychotherapeutic interventions. In: Holland JC, Rowland J (eds) Handbook of psychooncology: psychological care of the patient with cancer. Oxford University Press, New York, pp 455–469

Max MB 1992 Effects of desipramine, amitryptyline, and fluoxetine on pain and diabetic neuropathy. New England Journal of Medicine 326: 1250–1256

Max MB, Culnane M, Schafer SC et al 1987 Amitriptyline relieves diabetic-neuropathy pain in patients with normal and depressed mood. Neurology 37: 589–596

Max MB, Schafer SC, Culnane M, Smollen B, Dubner R, Gracely RH 1988 Amitriptyline, but not lorazepam, relieves postherpetic neuralgia. Neurology 38: 1427–1432

Max MB, Kishore-Kumar R, Schafer SC et al 1991 Efficacy of desipramine in painful diabetic neuropathy: a placebo-controlled trial. Pain 45: 3–10

Medina, Diamond 1977 Drug dependency in patients with chronic headaches. Headache 17(1): 12–74

Meier DE, Emmons C, Wallenstein S, Quill T, Morrison RS, Cassel CK 1998 A national survey of physician-assisted suicide and euthanasia in the United States. New England Journal of Medicine 338: 1193–1201

Melzack R, Wall PD 1983 The challenge of pain. Basic Books, New York

Mendels J 1987 Clinical experience with serotonin reuptake inhibiting antidepressants. Journal of Clinical Psychiatry 48(suppl): 26–30

Mercadante S, DeConno F, Ripamonti 1995 Propofol in terminal care. Journal of Pain and Symptom Management 10: 639–642

Millerd EJ 1977 Health professionals as survivors. Journal of Psychiatric Nursing and Mental Health Services 15: 33–36

Monkemeir D, Steffen U 1970 Zur schmerzbehandlung mit Imipramin bei krebserkrankungen. Medizinische Klinik 65: 213–215

Mor V, Guadagnoli E, Wool M 1987 An examination of the concrete service needs of advanced cancer patients. Journal of Psychosocial Oncology 5: 1–17

Mount BM 1986 Dealing with our losses. Journal of Clinical Oncology 4: 1127–1134

Moyle J 1995 The use of propofol in palliative medicine. Journal of Pain and Symptom Management 10: 643–646

Munro SM, Mount B 1978 Music therapy in palliative care. Canadian Medical Association Journal 119: 1029–1034

Murray GB 1987 Confusion, delirium, and dementia. In: Hackett TP, Cassem NH (eds) Massachusetts General Hospital handbook of general hospital psychiatry, 2nd edn. PSG Publishing, Littleton, MA, pp 84–115

Nehra A, Mullick F, Ishak KG, Zimmerman AJ 1990 Pemoline associated hepatic injury. Gastroenterology 99: 1517–1519

Oliver OJ 1985 The use of methotrimeprazine in terminal care. British Journal of Clinical Practice 39: 339–340

O'Neill WM, Sherrard JS 1993 Pain in human immunodeficiency virus disease: a review. Pain 54: 3–14

Paddison PL, Gise LH, Lebovits A et al 1990 Sexual abuse and premenstrual syndrome: comparison between a lower and higher socioeconomic group. Psychosomatics 31: 265–272

Passik S 1992 Psychotherapy of the substance abusing cancer patient. American Psychiatric Association Annual Meeting, 4–10 May, Washington, DC (abstract)

Passik S, Wilson A 1987 Technical considerations of the frontier of supportive and expressive modes in psychotherapy. Dynamic Psychotherapy 5: 51–62

Passik S, Horowitz S, Malkin M, Gargan R 1991 A psychoeducational support group for spouses of brain tumor patients. American Psychiatric Association Annual Meeting, 7–12 May, New Orleans (abstract)

Passik S, Breitbart W, Rosenfeld B et al 1994 AIDS specific patient-related barriers to pain management. American Pain Society, 13th Annual Meeting, Miami, FL, 10–13 November (abstract)

Patchell RA, Posner JB 1989 Cancer and the nervous system. In: Holland J, Rowland J (eds) The handbook of psychooncology: the psychological care of the cancer patient. Oxford University Press, New York, pp 327–341

Payne RM 1989 Pain in the drug abuser. In: Foley KM, Payne RM (eds) Current therapy of pain. BC Decker, Philadelphia, pp 46–54

Payne D, Jacobsen P, Breitbart W, Passik S, Rosenfeld B, McDonald M 1994 Negative thoughts related to pain are associated with greater pain, distress and disability in AIDS pain. American Pain Society, 13th Scientific Meeting, Miami, FL, November (abstract)

Pearson HJ 1990 Interaction of fluoxetine with carbamazepine. Journal of Clinical Psychiatry 51: 126

Peck AW, Stern WC, Watkinson C 1983 Incidence of seizures during treatment with tricyclic antidepressant drugs and buproprion. Journal of Clinical Psychiatry 44: 197–201

Pellegrino ED 1991 Ethics. Journal of the American Medical Association 265: 3188

Penfold R, Clark AJM 1992 Pain syndromes in HIV infection. Canadian Journal of Anesthesia 39: 724–730

Perry S, Heidrich G 1982 Management of pain during debridement: a survey of US burn units. Pain 13: 267–280

Peteet JR, Murrary-Ross D, Medeiros C et al 1989 Job stress and satisfaction among the staff members at a cancer center. Cancer 64: 975–982

Pick CG, Paul D, Eison MS, Pasternak G 1992 Potentiation of opioid analgesia by the antidepressant nefazodone. European Journal of Pharmacology 2: 375–381

Pilowsky I, Hallett EC, Bassett DL, Thomas PG, Penhall RK 1982 A controlled study of amitriptyline in the treatment of chronic pain. Pain 14: 169–179

Platt M, Breitbart W, Smith M, Marotta R, Weisman H, Jacobsen P 1994 Efficacy of neuroleptics for hypoactive delirium [letter]. Journal of Neuropsychiatry and Clinical Neurosciences 6: 66–67

Plumb MM, Holland JC 1977 Comparative studies of psychological function in patients with advanced cancer. Psychosomatic Medicine 39: 264–276

Popkin MK, Callies AL, Mackenzie TB 1985 The outcome of antidepressant use in the medically ill. Archives of General Psychiatry 42: 1160–1163

Portenoy RK 1987 Continuous intravenous infusion of opioid drugs. Medical Clinics of North America 71: 233–241

Portenoy RK, Payne R 1992 Acute and chronic pain. In: Lowinson JH, Ruiz P, Millman RB (eds) Comprehensive textbook of substance abuse. Williams & Wilkins, Baltimore, pp 691–721

Porter J, Jick H 1980 Addiction rate in patients treated with narcotics. New England Journal of Medicine 302: 123

Posner JB 1979 Delirium and exogenous metabolic brain disease. In: Beeson PB et al (eds) Cecil's textbook of medicine. WB Saunders, Philadelphia, pp 644–651

Posner JB 1988 Nonmetastatic effects of cancer on the nervous system. In: Wyngaarden JB et al (eds) Cecil's textbook of medicine. WB Saunders, Philadelphia, pp 1104–1107

Preskorn SH 1993 Recent pharmacologic advances in antidepressant therapy for the elderly. American Journal of Medicine 94(suppl 5A): 2S–12S

Preskorn S, Burke M 1992 Somatic therapy for major depressive disorder: selection of an antidepressant. Journal of Clinical Psychiatry 53(suppl): 1–14

Purohit DR, Navlakha PL, Modi RS et al 1978 The role of antidepressants in hospitalized cancer patients. Journal of the Association of Physicians of India 26: 245–248

Quill TE 1991 Sounding board: death and dignity: a case of individualized decision making. New England Journal of Medicine 324: 691–694

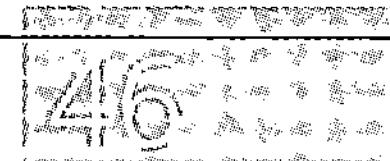

Rait D, Lederberg M 1990 The family of the cancer patient. In: Holland J, Rowland J (eds) The handbook of psychooncology. Oxford University Press, New York, pp 585–598

Redd WB, Reeves JL, Storm FK, Minagawa RY 1982 Hypnosis in the control of pain during hyperthermia treatment of cancer. In: Bonica JJ et al (eds) Advances in pain research and theory, vol 5. Raven, New York, pp 857–861

Reik T 1948 Listening with a third ear. Farrar Straus, New York

Rifkin A, Reardon G, Siris S et al 1985 Trimipramine in physical illness with depression. Journal of Clinical Psychiatry 46: 4–8

Robinson D, Napoliello MJ, Schenk J 1988 The safety and usefulness of buspirone as an anxiolytic drug in elderly versus young patients. Clinical Therapeutics 10: 740–746

Rosenfeld B, Breitbart W, McDonald MV, Passik SD, Thaler H, Portenoy RK 1996 Pain in ambulatory AIDS patients – II: Impact of pain on psychological functioning and quality of life. Pain 68: 323–328

Rowat K 1985 Chronic pain: a family affair. In: King K (ed) Recent advances in nursing long term care. Churchill Livingstone, Edinburgh, pp 259–271

Rudorfer MV, Potter WZ 1989 Anti-depressants. A comparative review of the clinical pharmacology and therapeutic use of the 'newer' versus the 'older' drugs. Drugs 37: 713–738

Saltzburg D, Breitbart W, Fishman B et al 1989 The relationship of pain and depression to suicidal ideation in cancer patients (abstract). ASCO Annual Meeting, 21–23 May, San Francisco

Scanlon C 1996 Euthanasia and nursing practice: right question, wrong answer. New England Journal of Medicine 324: 1401–1402

Schmale J, Weinberg N, Pieper S 1987 Satisfactions, stresses, and coping mechanisms of oncologists in clinical practice (abstract). Proceedings of the American Society of Clinical Oncology 6: 255

Seltzer S, Dewart D, Pollack RL, Jackson E 1983 The effects of dietary tryptophan on chronic maxillofacial pain and experimental pain tolerance. Journal of Psychiatric Research 17: 181–186

Sharav Y, Singer E, Schmidt E, Dione RA, Dubner R 1987 The analgesic effect of amitriptyline on chronic facial pain. Pain 31: 199–209

Sher M, Krieger JN, Juergen S 1983 Trazodone and priapism. American Journal of Psychiatry 140: 1362–1364

Shopsin B 1983 Buproprion: a new clinical profile in the psychobiology of depression. Journal of Clinical Psychiatry 44: 140–142

Siegel K 1982 Rational suicide: considerations for the clinician. Psychiatric Quarterly 54: 77–83

Siegel K, Tuckel P 1984 Rational suicide and the terminally ill cancer patient. Omega 15: 263–269

Silberfarb PM, Manrer LH, Cronthamel CS 1980 Psychological aspects of neoplastic disease. I: Functional status of breast cancer patients during different treatment regimens. American Journal of Psychiatry 137: 450–455

Sindrup SH, Ejlertsen B, Froland A et al 1989 Imipramine treatment in diabetic neuropathy: relief of subjective symptoms without changes in peripheral and autonomic nerve function. European Journal of Clinical Pharmacology 37: 151–153

Singer PA 1990 Euthanasia: a critique. New England Journal of Medicine 322: 1881–1883

Singer EJ, Zorilla C, Fahy-Chandon B et al 1993 Painful symptoms reported for ambulatory HIV-infected men in a longitudinal study. Pain 54: 15–19

Singh A 1996 Safety of Risperidone in Patients with HIV and AIDS. Proceedings of the 149th Annual Meeting, American Psychiatric Association. 4–9 May, p 126 (abstract)

Sipahimalarni A, Masand PS 1998 Olanzapine in the treatment of delirium. Psychosomatics 39: 422–430

Slome LR, Mitchell TF, Charlebois E, Benevedes JM, Abrams DI 1997 Physician-assisted sucide and patients with human immunodeficiency virus disease. New England Journal of Medicine 336: 417–421

Spiegel D 1985 The use of hypnosis in controlling cancer pain. CA: A Cancer Journal for Clinicians 4: 221–231

Spiegel D, Bloom JR 1983a Pain in metastatic breast cancer. Cancer 52: 341–345

Spiegel D, Bloom JR 1983b Group therapy and hypnosis reduce metastatic breast carcinoma pain. Psychosomatic Medicine 4: 333–339

Spiegel D, Bloom JR, Yalom ID 1981 Group support for patients with metastatic cancer: a randomized prospective outcome study. Archives of General Psychiatry 38: 527–533

Spiegel K, Kalb R, Pasternak GW 1983 Analgesic activity of tricyclic antidepressants. Annals of Neurology 13: 462–465

Spikes J, Holland J 1975 The physician's response to the dying patient. In: Strain JJ, Grossman S (eds) Psychological care of the medically ill. Appleton-Century-Crofts, New York, pp 138–148

Spitzer RL, Williams JBW (eds) 1987 American Psychiatric Association Diagnostic and statistical manual of mental disorders, 3rd edn (revised). American Psychiatric Association, Washington

Stein RS, Flexner JH, Graber SE 1980 Lithium and granulocytopenia during induction therapy of acute myelogenous leukemia: update of an ongoing trial. Advances in Experimental Medicine and Biology 127: 187–198

Stiefel FC, Breitbart W, Holland JC 1989 Corticosteroids in cancer: neuropsychiatric complications. Cancer Investigation 7: 479–491

Strafford M, Cahill C, Schwartz T et al 1991 Recognition and treatment of pain in pediatric patients with AIDS. Journal of Pain and Symptom Management 6: 146 (abstract)

Swerdlow M, Cundill JG 1981 Anticonvulsant drugs used in the treatment of lancinating pains: a comparison. Anesthesia 36: 1129–1134

Syrjala KL, Cummings C, Donald GW 1992 Hypnosis or cognitive behavioral training for the reduction of pain and nausea during cancer treatment: a controlled clinical trial. Pain 48: 137–146

Terr L 1991 Childhood traumas: an outline and overview. American Journal of Psychiatry 148: 10–20

Tiengo M, Pagnoni B, Calmi A, Rigoli M, Braga PC, Panerai AE 1987 Chlorimipramine compared to pentazocine as a unique treatment in post-operative pain. International Journal of Clinical Pharmacology Research 7: 141–143

Trzepacz PT, Baker RW, Greenhouse J 1988 A symptom rating scale for delirium. Psychiatric Research 23: 89–97

Turk D, Rennert K 1981 Pain and the terminally ill cancer patient: a cognitive–social learning perspective. In: Sobel H (ed) Behavior therapy in terminal care. Ballinger, Cambridge

Twycross RG, Lack SA 1983 Symptom control in far advanced cancer: pain relief. Pitman Books, London

Tyler MA 1974 Treatment of the painful shoulder syndrome with amitriptyline and lithium carbonate. Canadian Medical Association Journal 111: 137–140

Vachon MLS 1987 Occupational stress in the care of the critically ill, the dying, and the bereaved. Hemisphere, Washington DC

van der Maas PJ, van Delden JJM, Piznenborg L, Looman CWN 1991 Euthanasia and other medical decisions concerning the end of life. Lancet 338: 669–674

van der Maas PJ, van der Wal G, Haverkate I et al 1996 Euthanasia, physician assisted suicide and other medical practices involving the end of life in the Netherlands, 1990–1995. New England Journal of Medicine 335: 1699–1705

Ventafridda V, Bonezzi C, Caraceni A et al 1987 Antidepressants for cancer pain and other painful syndromes with deafferentation component: comparison of amitriptyline and trazodone. Italian Journal of Neurological Sciences 8: 579–587

Ventafridda V, Ripamonti C, DeConno F et al 1990a Symptom prevalence and control during cancer patients' last days of life. Journal of Palliative Care 6: 7–11

Ventafridda V, Bianchi M, Ripamonti C et al 1990b Studies on the effects of antidepressant drugs on the antinociceptive action of morphine and on plasma morphine in rat and man. Pain 43: 155–162

von Roenn JH, Cleeland CS, Gonin R et al 1993 Physicians' attitudes toward cancer pain management survey: results of the Eastern Cooperative Oncology Group survey. Annals of Internal Medicine 119: 121–126

Walker E, Katon W, Griffins JH et al 1988 Relationship of chronic pelvic pain to psychiatric diagnosis and childhood sexual abuse. American Journal of Psychiatry 145: 75–80

Walsh TD 1983 Antidepressants and chronic pain. Clinical Neuropharmacology 6: 271–295

Walsh TD 1986 Controlled study of imipramine and morphine in chronic pain due to advanced cancer. ASCO, 4–6 May, Los Angeles (abstract)

Walsh TD 1990 Adjuvant analgesic therapy in cancer pain. In: Foley KM et al (eds) Advances in pain research and therapy, vol 16. Second International Congress on Cancer Pain. Raven Press, New York, pp 155–166

Wanzer SH, Federman DD, Edelstein ST et al 1989 The physician's responsibility toward hopelessly ill patients: a second look. New England Journal of Medicine 320: 844–849

Ward SE, Goldberg N, Miller-McCauley C, Mueller C et al 1993 Patient-related barriers to management of cancer pain. Pain 52: 319–324

Warner MM 1992 Involvement of families in pain control of terminally ill patients. Hospice Journal 8: 155–170

Watson CP, Evans RJ 1985 A comparative trial of amitriptyline and zimelidine in postherpetic neuralgia. Pain 23: 387–394

Watson CP, Evans RJ, Reed K, Merskey H, Goldsmith L, Warsh J 1982 Amitriptyline versus placebo in postherpetic neuralgia. Neurology 32: 671–673

Watson CP, Chipman M, Reed K, Evans RJ, Birkett N 1992 Amitriptyline versus maprotiline in postherpetic neuralgia: a randomized, double-blind, cross over trial. Pain 48: 29–36

Weddington WW 1982 Delirium and depression associated with amphotericin B. Psychosomatics 23: 1076–1078

Weissman DE, Haddox JD 1989 Opioid pseudoaddiction – an iatrogenic syndrome. Pain 36: 363–366

Woodforde JM, Fielding JR 1970 Pain and cancer. Journal of Psychosomatic Research 4: 365–370

Young DF 1982 Neurological complications of cancer chemotherapy. In: Silverstein A (ed) Neurological complications of therapy: selected topics. Futura Publishing, New York, pp 57–113

Young RJ, Clarke BF 1985 Pain relief in diabetic neuropathy: the effectiveness of imipramine and related drugs. Diabetic Medicine 2: 363–366

Zelman D, Cleeland C, Howland EB 1987 Factors in appropriate pharmacological management of cancer pain: a cross-institutional investigation. Pain (suppl): S136

Zeltzer L, LeBaron S 1982 Hypnosis and non-hypnotic techniques for reduction of pain and anxiety in painful procedures in children and adolescents with cancer. Journal of Pediatrics 101: 1032–1035

Zimmerman L, Porzehl B, Duncan K, Schmitz R 1989 Effects of music in patients who had chronic cancer pain. Western Journal of Nursing Research 11: 298–309

Zitman FG, Linssen ACG, Edelbroek PM, Stijnen T 1990 Low dose amitriptyline in chronic pain: the gain is modest. Pain 42: 35–42

Pain and impending death

CICELY M. SAUNDERS & MICHAEL PLATT

When people take a positive interest in the welfare of the dying, their last days on earth need not be distressful.
(Hinton 1967)

Fear of pain in dying is still common and was the reason for the majority of requests for euthanasia in one study from a hospice in the Netherlands, which not only cares for inpatients but also consults with a large number of family doctors. However, once reassured by effective consultation and/or treatment, few requests were repeated and the patients died peacefully from their illness (Zylicz 1997).

A recent survey revealed that only a small percentage of those questioned ('61 palliative care experts') had to induce sedation in intractable distress in the dying (Chater et al 1998).

Other studies reported later in this chapter document the fact that pain at the end of life can be controlled, usually without such sedation, by teams experienced in the multiprofessional practice of palliative medicine presented in detail in the *Oxford Textbook of Palliative Medicine* (1996). It is sadly true that not all patients benefit from this experience. In some developing countries, this is because of lack of resources, but it is not only in such deprived conditions that patients suffer relievable terminal distress. Myths concerning the use of narcotics still abound (Wall 1997).

The Support Study (SUPPORT Principal Investigators 1995) has been the most extensive report published, with a total of 9105 adults hospitalized with one or more of nine life-threatening diagnoses and an overall 6-month mortality rate of 47%. The second phase of this study documented the results of the intervention of specially trained nurses in an attempt to improve communication and care, and found that there was no overall improvement, including the level of reported pain. Half of the patients who died had moderate or severe pain during most of their final 3 days of life in the intervention group of 2652 patients, and there was no difference in their experience compared with the control group. An Editorial (Lo 1995) notes that 'apparently no component of the SUPPORT intervention directly addressed the problem of inadequate pain control'. Communication between physicians and patients remained poor; for example, the former failed to implement patients' refusal of CPR (cardiopulmonary resuscitation) intervention, while they misunderstood patients' preferences regarding CPR in 80% of cases. These results have led to a number of calls to address education, leading to better practice in decision making and the control of distress (Foley 1997).

Some earlier studies of the last days of life (Hinton 1963, Parkes 1978, Keane et al 1983, Wilkes 1984) showed that while the majority of patients die peacefully at the end, sufficient attention was not always given earlier to what had by then become a multisystem disease or deterioration. Hinton's report was a uniquely detailed study, comparing the physical discomfort and mental state of 102 dying patients with 102 patients in the same wards with diseases in the same systems that were serious but not fatal. He found that while pain was adequately controlled in 82% of 82 patients with malignant disease, vomiting and nausea were relieved in 63% and dyspnoea in only 18%. These symptoms were more common in patients dying with renal or cardiac failure – a total of 14 patients in all. Eleven per cent of his patients were unrousable for the last week of life, 34% were unconscious for at least 24 hours and 60% for 6 or 9 hours before death; only 6% were conscious just before they died. The act of dying itself was rarely distressful. Hinton noticed a significant degree of depression in 46%, with a rise in the last week or two of life. This contrasts with the group of 77 patients in his later home-care study, where he found only 5% of serious depression among the patients with a decrease as death approached (Hinton 1994). Many of his patients were eventually admitted to St Christopher's Hospice, but the families afterwards felt that this was an extension of home care and were satisfied with what they themselves had achieved and the way the patients finally died. A further study of their retrospective observations showed they tended to overestimate pain as compared to their reports to him during the patient's illness (Hinton 1996).

Long before the possibilities of intensive care were widely practised, the first clinical study of the way patients die was reported by Sir William Osler in his lecture 'Science and immortality' (Osler 1906). Cards were completed in his wards in the Johns Hopkins Hospital by the nurses and they are preserved in the Osler Library at McGill University, Montreal (Fig. 47.1).

Osler states:

> *In our modern life the educated man dies ... generally unconscious and unconcerned. I have careful records of about 500 death bed studies, particularly with reference to the modes of death and the sensations of the dying. The latter alone concerns us here. 90 suffered bodily pain or distress of one sort or another, 11 showed mental apprehension, 2 positive terror, 1 expressed spiritual exaltation, 1 bitter remorse. The great majority gave no signs one way or the other; like their birth, their death was a sleep and a forgetting.* (Osler 1906)

A STUDY OF THE ACT OF DYING
JOHNS HOPKINS HOSPITAL

Age 35 Nationality U.S.A. Religion P. C. H.

Length of illness. Hysterectomy June 2nd Did well until June 8th, when peritonitis set in. Died in 17 hrs.

The act of dying:

If sudden.

Did respiration stop before pulse — how long ? Radial pulse not palpable for ½ hr before respiration ceased.

Coma or unconsciousness before death — how long ? Irrational for about 8 hours, Completely unconscious for 4 hours before death

If any fear or apprehension, of what nature None whatever

Bodily, i.e. pain. Slight, abdominal pain.

Mental. None. Was calm as long as she remained rational

Spiritual — remorse, etc. None whatever

This card is not to be filled out unless done within twenty-four hours of the death of the individual.

N. B. The object of this investigation is to ascertain, the relative proportion of cases in which (1) the death is sudden ; (2) accompanied by coma or unconsciousness ; (3) by pain, dread or apprehension. Prof. Osler requests the intelligent co-operation of the members of the medical and nursing staff. Please note fully any other special circumstances connected with the act of dying.

Fig. 47.1 A study of the act of dying.

Death was likely then to have come at an earlier age than most deaths today, often of infections and certainly without all the interventions of the intensive care unit. Perhaps a somewhat comparable study would be that of the home-care patients receiving hospice care during admissions to St Christopher's Hospice for the last 48 hours of life (Boyd 1993). This included 9.8% of admissions over a 6-month period, with 34 patients admitted from home and 13 transferred from local hospitals. Most of the patients from home were being visited by the hospice's own team of specialist nurses and were being cared for by family and friends; admission was arranged for symptom control and nursing or because carers (often elderly) had become exhausted.

All but three of the patients required an opioid, most receiving it parenterally in the last few hours. In general, low doses gave rapid control of symptoms and only one patient needed escalating doses. Dyspnoea presented more of a problem than pain. That most of these very sick patients were at home so late in their illness makes them a different group compared to those in acute wards or, still more, intensive care beds.

Of Boyd's patients in the hospice all were reported as having died peacefully, but 16 (34%) needed intervention for one or more problems in the 3 hours before death (Boyd 1993). For none of these was the problem one of pain. It would seem that the main problem is one of changing gear, of ceasing to try and prolong life and accepting that death is now inevitable and that the duty of the physician and the whole multiprofessional team is to relieve the patient's suffering and support the family. This has become more difficult as technology has developed and as people have sometimes seemed to believe that death must be from a failure of medicine to preserve life.

Most palliative-care studies give similar figures. However, Ventafridda et al (1990) carried out a prospective study of 120 patients at home and found that more than 50% had suffering which they considered unendurable during their last days, which were controlled only by means of sedation. Pain was the problem for 31 patients, dyspnoea 33, delirium 11 and vomiting five. In a guest editorial, Mount (1990) asks whether this may be a different population (or culture?) and points out that many hospices are able to admit when control at home breaks down (often through carer exhaustion, as reported by Boyd (1993). By contrast, Lichter and Hunt (1990) followed 200 consecutive patients in an integrated hospice inpatient and home-care programme. Around 40% died in their own homes but, in identifying and treating the same symptoms as in the Boyd study, they found that with a ready awareness of the problems that may arise in the last 48 hours of life, it was possible to keep their patients comfortable to the end. Thirty per cent of their patients were conscious until death, 38% became unconscious from 12 to 24 hours before death, 7% became unconscious 24–48 hours prior to death and 10% for over 48 hours. He writes in some detail of the organic brain disorder which may present as delirium but notes that this did not follow a rapid escalation in the use of analgesics or other drugs. As he says, in its management all unnecessary drugs should be discontinued but that sedation and antispasmodic treatment may be needed and a combination of a neuroleptic and a benzodiazepine is indicated (Lichter & Hunt 1990).

A more recent study by Turner et al (1996) of an integrated palliative-care service looked at the last 3 days of life of 50 consecutive patients, with particular concern for what they defined as 'dignity in dying'. Personal function was maintained at least in a moderate degree in the majority of patients. Of the 28 with pain, it was estimated that 15 had good control, 12 moderate and two only poor. Dose escalation did not generally occur. The same team has repeated this study with 132 consecutive patients. Here pain was the most common major symptom with good relief achieved in 58.5%, moderate control in 42% and poor relief in 1.5%. Escalating doses of morphine or sedative were not required and nearly 80% were able to recognize family or friends (personal communication).

The efficacy of the World Health Organization guidelines for cancer pain relief (World Health Organization 1990), which has been translated into many languages, was examined in 401 dying patients by Grond et al (1991). They report that at the time of death, only 3% of patients experienced severe or very severe pain, whereas 52% had no pain at all, 24% only mild or moderate pain and 20% were unable to rate pain intensity. Forty-four per cent of patients required parenteral drugs. Additional adjuvant drugs were used in 90% of patients. This study was carried out by a department of anaesthesiology and a pain clinic with 45% of the patients treated in a general ward.

From this selection of recent evidence it would seem that in experienced hands adequate pain relief can be achieved in the great majority of patients. However the SUPPORT study and reports of patients with diseases other than cancer show that there is much to be done before it will be possible to say that all dying patients are given the relief that has been shown to be possible (Addington-Hall & McCarthy 1995). Better community care and a readiness in all settings to appreciate that death is both inevitable and imminent are called for if we are to be satisfied that 'Competent care for the dying' is responding to need and can counter demands for euthanasia and physician-assisted suicide (Foley 1997). Dependence and loss of dignity are also cited as reason for such requests, but the relief of pain that has been shown to be possible can make a difference here too and needs to be taught widely. The research summarized by the UK's National Council for Hospice and Specialist Palliative Care Services (Higginson et al 1997) is available from the address given in the Appendix at the end of this chapter, and is the basis of their booklet 'Changing gear – guidelines for managing the last days of life' which gives clear guidance for recognition, assessment and treatment (National Council for Hospice and Specialist Palliative Care Services 1997). It recognizes relatives' needs and calls for the collaborative multiprofessional approach that is needed, especially for the rare intractable situation. Rehydration with intravenous or subcutaneous fluids has been shown not to be of any benefit at this stage and may cause peripheral and pulmonary oedema in patients with severe hypoalbumionaemia (Ellershaw et al 1995). This may be difficult to explain to relatives, who fear their loved one is dying, or being allowed to die, of dehydration.

Recognizing that death is approaching may not be easy, but experienced nurses usually make more reliable predictions than other professionals because of their closer contact with the patient. They note a deepening feeling of profound weakness and an increasing irritability of mood and sensitivity to 'minor' discomforts. Patients may become increasingly apprehensive and need continual contact and reassurance. Terminal restlessness may be caused by various factors such as pain, dyspnoea, metabolic disturbances leading to confusion, retention or the inability to move any longer without assistance. Some of this can be corrected and causes should be sought and treated. However, in many it may be that earlier irritability simply escapes self-control. Families are understandably concerned if these symptoms are not controlled and need an explanation that this is not a new mental illness but a common part of severe illness. Nurses (and others) are anxious that their patients should not be sedated to the point where they cannot recognize or speak to their families, and a careful balance must be kept between an individual's need and the drugs and dosages used. Although it can sometimes be difficult to achieve symptom control without causing drowsiness (which in many cases is a consequence of increasing weakness), it is important to keep families informed at all times.

Only medications which will control or prevent distressing symptoms should be used at this time and considerable skill and tact are often needed when explaining this to relatives. As a general rule, the only drugs needed in the final days of life are one or more of those listed in Appendix 47.1. At this time the skilled communication essential to all palliative care must be prompt. In less urgent situations, both patient and family must be encouraged to express fears and anxieties, sometimes elicited by direct questioning. This is especially important when the family comes from a different culture. For a peaceful and supported home death a back-up plan is vital. Telephone numbers for a 24-hour call response are rarely abused and families often find bereavement eased by the satisfaction of their achievements in care during the final hours.

The change from oral medication to injections occurs for most hospice patients only during the last 48 hours. A balance has to be struck between giving extra responsibility for this decision to a nurse or leaving a patient in distress until a doctor is available. Sometimes heroic efforts are made to help a patient to swallow in order to avoid the change to injections, because such responsibility can be given only to the experienced person. Setting up a syringe driver may solve this problem, especially in home care. The family also needs an explanation if this necessary changeover is not to become threatening or misunderstood. Even then, difficulty in distinguishing between post hoc and propter hoc may cause distress. Every time a patient dies within a short time of an injection, many families (and indeed many nurses) need reassurance that this was not the cause of death, and that 'the proper medical treatment that is administered and that has an incidental effect on determining the exact moment of death is not the cause of death in any sensible use of the term' (Devlin 1985).

FEAR AND IMPENDING DEATH

Fear is an occasionally overwhelming symptom of impending death and calls for physical contact and adequate medication. All the common fears of dying, of separation from loved people, of uncompleted responsibilities, of dependence which may be stronger than that of pain or mutilation or even an unfocused fear of the mystery of death may be exacerbated (Parkes 1973). As Parkes suggests, although one cannot deal effectively with everyone's fear, 'there are no cases for whom nothing can be done'. Fears of separation and loss are proper causes of grief, but if expressions of appropriate sorrow are encouraged, the patient can often move on to a deeper enjoyment of the life left to him. Fear of failure may lead to what has been termed 'the life review', in which problems of longstanding are sometimes worked through at surprising speed (Butler 1963). Crises of all kinds can lead to different forms of acceleration. Fears for dependents are frequently realistic and instituting or planning practical arrangements can bring comfort to all who are involved. Fears of losing physical function 'seem to derive mainly from fantasies of the effects of this loss of control on those around'. This is an obvious component of the widespread fear of incontinence. Parkes also found that patients who had been in pain were often more afraid of disgracing themselves by crying aloud than they were of the pain itself. This fear of physical pain is often unrealistic, or should be made so by effective treatment both for the patient and others around him. Such fear should be listened to and the possibilities of relief explained and given.

Fear of mutilation or physical deterioration may be helped by the attitude of the staff towards the weakening body. This attitude is reflected in verbal reassurances that the essence of this person still remains and is recognized and respected. Fear of the unknown is helped when the known, as seen by the patient, is rendered attentive and reassuring. Trust and faith in life and death are interwoven and both are enhanced by the attitude of those around. It is most important that the staff should be at ease, with some confidence that both life and death are meaningful and that death is a necessary and fitting end to the accomplishment of living. A supportive atmosphere is best created with few if any words.

THE NEED FOR RESEARCH INTO SYMPTOM CONTROL OF THE DYING

Hinton suggested that if comparison of the distress of dying after different treatments were available, it would add another factor to decisions made at an earlier stage (Hinton 1964). Such assessments have been made in combined pathological (clinical and therapeutic) studies. Of 18 patients with head and neck cancer submitted to salvage surgery, there were no significant differences in terminal pain or in difficulty of speech and swallowing. These symptoms were all common but success was achieved in terms of pain relief and a 'quiet' death in the special units in which these patients died. The results in this study suggest that a decision not to operate on older patients with advanced tumours would not condemn them to a more unpleasant death and would avoid the added trauma of unsuccessful major surgery (Pittam 1992).

A clinical and pathological study was made of 40 patients with intestinal obstruction caused by far-advanced abdominal and/or pelvic malignant disease. Surgical intervention was feasible in only two cases. The remaining 38 patients were managed medically without intravenous fluids and nasogastric suction. Obstructive symptoms such as intestinal colic, vomiting and diarrhoea were effectively controlled by drugs (Baines et al 1985).

Recent discussion on 'necessary sustenance' when a patient is dying tends to ignore the fact that patients gradually lose their urge to eat and that feelings of thirst are better helped by the slow giving of normal fluids and of ice to suck, and by scrupulous mouth care, than by intravenous fluids. Such intravenous infusions are often continued until death in seriously ill patients because it is thought that electrolyte imbalance and dehydration may cause distress. However, the infusion may cause discomfort and distress to the patient, act as a barrier to relatives and divert the attending medical and nursing personnel from the care of the patient to that of the electrolyte and fluid balance.

EXPERIENCES OF 'DEATH'

Books have been written about patients who, in accident or illness, have 'died' and returned to life with clear memories of 'out-of-body experiences'. The fact that fear and pain seem to have been entirely absent, and that these experiences have been full of peace and light, has evidently comforted many people. Whether these are in fact experiences of 'death' rather than of some form of altered consciousness appears unproven, indeed unprovable.

Among many thousands of patients I have known as they faced their death, only one, a former nurse in her mid-40s with multiple sclerosis, had told me such a story. These stories, as they stand, have helped some patients to lose their fear of death. In no way are they proof of immortality; that seems to remain a matter of faith.

PAIN AND SUDDEN DEATH

Death from injury in an accident is remembered by several witnesses as apparently painless. Worcester (1935) pointed out that those who have been rescued from death by drowning, even after apparently hopeless hours of artificial respiration, always say that before losing consciousness they experienced no suffering whatever. Melzack and Wall (1982) reported that, of patients admitted to an emergency room, 37% had no pain in the initial phase of injury, although they point out that 40% reported very severe pain.

Sudden death from coronary occlusion may also be painless, although some of those who survive for long enough to speak may refer to most severe pain. An elderly nurse died after a series of myocardial infarcts. Talking with a friend, she suddenly interrupted her to say, quite calmly, 'I need one of my pills', and died without another breath or sign of distress. The same evidently happens after some cerebrovascular accidents. Many would choose this way of dying, although research on bereavement suggests that it is more difficult for the survivors to come to terms with than the slower, expected death when there has been opportunity to bid farewell and resolve outstanding difficulties.

Lewis Thomas (1980) discussed the apparent painlessness of some traumatic deaths in his essay, 'On natural death'. He writes:

> *Pain is useful for avoidance, for getting away when there's time to get away, but when it is endgame, and no way back, pain is likely to be turned off, and the mechanisms for this are wonderfully precise and quick. If I had to design an ecosystem in which creatures had to live off each other and in which dying was an indispensable part of living, I could not think of a better way to manage.*

THERAPY IN INTENSIVE CARE UNITS

The intensive care environment is a place where aggressive life-saving techniques are used with the latest high-technology medicine and pharmacology. It is inevitable that pain and death occur frequently, neither of which are handled well in such an environment (Hall et al 1994, Hanson et al 1997). Advanced surgical techniques, improved resuscitation and trauma life support, together with greater media and public awareness of resuscitation techniques, are causing increased demands for intensive care beds. The general ageing of the population at one end and the increasing survival of premature neonates at the other, are also driving this demand. To counter this, it has been recognized that not all admissions to intensive care are necessarily appropriate and intensivists are examining how best to decide which patients in need of critical care are appropriate for admission (Campbell & McHaffie 1995, 'SUPPORT' Principal Investigators 1995). A decision of 'futility of further medical management' needs to be made either prior to admission to intensive care or during the intensive care management when it is realized that further therapy is indeed futile (Sanders & Raffin 1993, Campbell & McHaffie 1995, Robb 1997, Yu 1997). Whatever decision is made, adequate management of pain and suffering is mandatory for both the patient and the relatives. It is, however, often difficult for medical staff to make a decision of 'futility' in deciding on the further management of patients with severely life-limiting injuries or disease in the acute situation, especially after major surgery. This may be due to a combination of factors, which include lack of evidence-based criteria in the triaging of patients, pressure from relatives to do as much as possible for the loved one and fear of medicolegal complications. As medicine and technology enable the potentiation of life through previously fatal diseases and trauma, the intensive care unit contains a microcosm of ethical and social issues which include withdrawal of medical treatment, 'euthanasia' and the management of the dying patient on life support. Several recent papers highlight some of the issues affecting the medical care of patients in intensive care, especially in the area of care of the dying patient on life support therapy. This encompasses a large age range of patients, from the 20-week-old premature neonate to the very elderly.

The patient in intensive care is often artificially ventilated, requiring sedation and sometimes paralysis. However, they may be aware, particularly of pain and discomfort, and may also be very distressed about family, financial and other worries (Cherny et al 1994). The normal indications of pain and distress in a patient who is sedated or anaesthetized consist of increased sympathetic activity such as sweating, lacrimation, increased blood pressure and tachycardia. However, in the critically ill patient, cardiac support drugs, sedative and anaesthetic drugs and pathophysiological states such as septic shock and cerebral injury, may mask or confuse these signs. Additionally, the use of pharmacological paralysing agents prevent the patient from moving in response to pain. Recently, several centres have set out to investigate the objective measurement of pain in unresponsive patients, often particularly focusing on the dying patient. These include studies in children on paediatric intensive care units, in addition to critically ill adults on ventilators. ('SUPPORT' Principal Investigators 1995, Chambliss & Anand 1997, Puntillo et al 1997).

The sources of pain are often multiple, with combinations of neuropathic and acute physiological pain – from the primary pathology, from treatment modalities such as radiation, from bedsores and skin ulcers, from pre-existing concurrent disease, or simply the discomfort of an endotracheal tube or intravenous line. Pain may be considered as contributing significantly to an overall sense of suffering. Cherny devised a model of suffering which incorporates pain and the various factors which affect quality of life (Cherny et al 1994). This model also includes the importance of family and social stresses, emphasizing the importance of adequate communication and counselling with close family and friends – especially once the decision of futility of further treatment has been made (Jones 1997). Psychosocial and spiritual processes strongly influence the impact and expression of pain and these need to be taken into account in the assessment and treatment of pain in intensive care. This needs a holistic approach to the patient (Kolcaba & Fisher 1996), as well as some novel approaches to the treatment of pain.

The data used by critical care nurses in assessing pain appears to be a combination of facial appearances (grimacing, etc.), movements of the patient and the sympathetic activity mentioned above. Studies assessing the use of pain measurement scores using this sort of data (behavioural and physiological) suggest that pain is better managed this way (Puntillo et al 1997). Many units are now using pain and sedation scores to assess the adequacy of pain control in

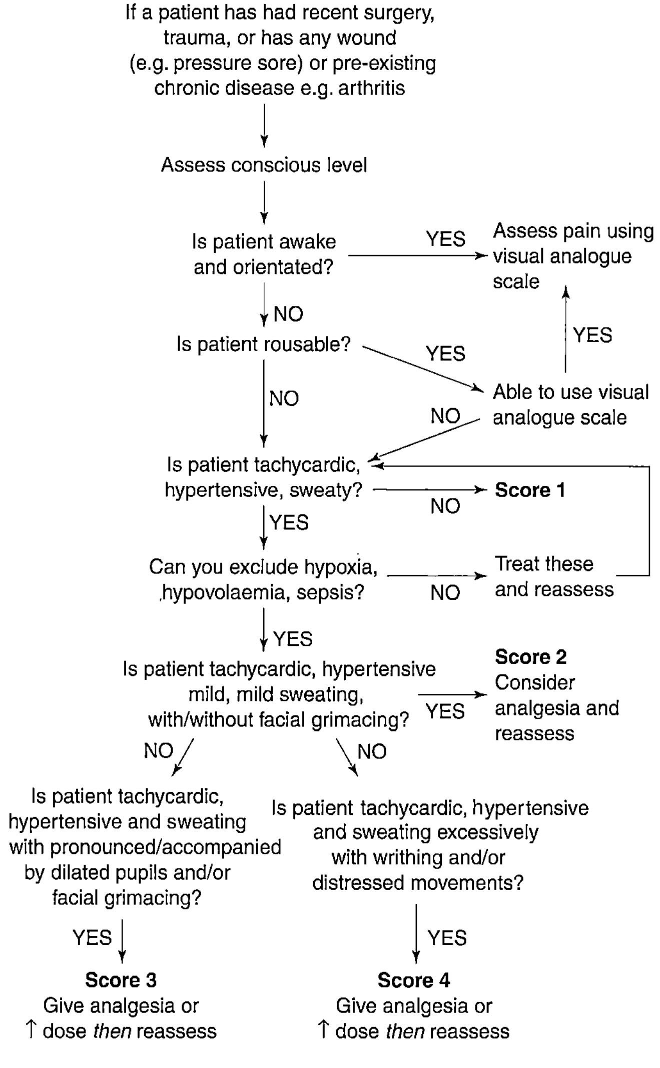

Fig. 47.2 Action flow chart used for patients in an intensive care unit.

patients on life support in intensive care. The intensive care unit at St Mary's Hospital in London uses a scoring system for pain and sedation (appended to the Glasgow Coma Scale) with an action flow chart which is currently in trial operation (Fig. 47.2).

Once a decision is made to withdraw active treatment from a clinically ill patient (which should be seen as a positive decision), adequate pain control and sedation continue to be of paramount importance. The close relatives of the patient also need to be properly consulted and counselled as necessary, and in many cases involved in the decision-making process. It should be noted that a withdrawal of active treatment is not the same as euthanasia, and patients die of the disease processes for which they were being treated. The use of adequate analgesia does not of itself cause death, which should be as pain free and dignified as possible, with the wishes of the patient, who should be as informed as possible (Harton 1996), and the relatives being respected. The diagnosis of brain death and the harvesting of organs for transplantation are no excuse for inadequate sedation and analgesia. Ultra-short-acting drugs such as the opioid remifentanil and intravenous anaesthetic agents such as propofol can be used to prevent the accumulation of sedative drugs to allow for the diagnosis of brain-stem death. The patient should always be appropriately anaesthetized for organ harvest and good analgesia and sedation must always be assured. There are many modern potent opioids that can be used to provide profound analgesia which do not affect cardiac output and help to maintain adequate tissue perfusion.

When life support for a ventilator-dependent patient is to be withdrawn, rather than actually having to cease artificial ventilation prior to death, the reduction of inspired oxygen concentration to that of room air, together with the removal of adjunctive ventilatory support such as PEEP (positive end-expiratory pressure), is usually sufficient before death ensues. At all stages, adequate analgesia and sedation for the patient must be provided (Edwards & Ueno 1991). A recent study showed that 10% of relatives of patients who died in hospital felt that pain could have been better managed (Hanson et al 1997). The relatives and close friends must not be forgotten, and they should be fully informed on the decisions that are made and the reasons for this.

The development of 'living wills' is inevitably going to contribute to the debate on end-of-life issues, especially in the intensive care environment. However, patients should never have to fear that pain will not be treated or that their lives will end in undignified pain and terror. Whatever the situation, even at life's end on a 'life support machine,' we have the pharmacology and the technology to treat pain and distress (although not always the means to treat spiritual distress), without recourse to euthanasia.

APPENDIX 47.1

The Appendix to the National Council's booklet 'Changing gear – guidelines for managing the last days of life in adults' gives help in the control of all likely symptoms. The following suggestions are clear and direct:

1. Pain

Pain (non-neuropathic)

NSAIDs:

- Indicated for superficial or deep somatic pain and pain of bone secondaries should be continued in patients already taking NSAIDs.
- Suppositories, e.g. diclofenac 100 mg b.d.
- Injections, e.g. ketorolac 30 mg per 24 hours.
- Gel, e.g. diclofenac, may be used for painful decubitus ulcers.

Opioids:

- Diamorphine is the drug of choice for parenteral administration (other opioids of high solubility may be used).
- Regular 4-hourly injections.
- Continuous subcutaneous infusion by syringe driver.

2. Dose conversion from oral morphine to parenteral diamorphine

1. Calculate total daily dose of oral morphine.
2. Divide total oral dose by 3 to give equivalent daily dose of parenteral diamorphine.
3. Increase diamorphine dose by 50% if pain is not controlled.
4. Infuse total daily dose in 24 hours by syringe driver.
   OR
   Divide total daily dose by 6 to calculate dose for 4 hourly injection.

3. Use of portable infusion devices

Portable infusion devices, commonly known as syringe drivers, allow continuous infusion of medications to be given subcutaneously. This prevents the need for multiple injections and maintains a smooth delivery of medication. There are a number of such devices currently available. It is always important to follow the manufacturers instructions for safe administration of drugs.

Drugs commonly given by this method include:
diamorphine
midazolam
hyoscine hydrobromide or butylbromide
glycopyrronium
haloperidol
cyclizine (may precipitate in combination with other drugs)
metoclopramide
methotrimeprazine

Only one of these may be combined with diamorphine at one time.

4. Management of specific symptoms

Pain (neuropathic)

Anticonvulsants:

- Indicated for treatment of burning or shooting pains when patient unable to take oral anticonvulsants.
- Midazolam 5–10 mg 4 hourly SC.
- Clonazepam 0.25–1 mg 4 hourly SC.

Phenothiazines
methotrimeprazine:

- Also has sedative and antiemetic properties.
- Indicated for pain when sedation is also required.
- 20–25 mg t.d.s. by SC injection.
- Local reaction can occur at the injection site.

Breathlessness

- May be more distressing than pain.
- Some patients have a fast respiratory rate but are not distressed by this.

Opioids:

- Diamorphine is the opioid of choice (or another opioid of high solubility may be used).
- 2.5–5 mg 4 hourly by SC injection for opioid-naïve patients.

Benzodiazepines:

- Indicated for breathlessness associated with anxiety.
- Lorazepam 0.5–1 mg sublingually.
- Midazolam 2.5–5 mg by SC injection 4 hourly or via syringe driver.

Phenothiazines:

- Indicated for breathlessness associated with anxiety or extreme agitation.
- Less commonly used since introduction of water-soluble benzodiazepines.
- Methotrimeprazine 25–50 mg 6–8 hourly.

Oxygen therapy:

- Several studies have shown that oxygen is more effective than air at relieving dyspnoea when given acutely, even in patients with normal oxygen saturation.
- Should be administered in least obtrusive way, via nasal prongs.
- Humidifaction is needed to minimize drying out mucous membranes.
- Often not needed if dyspnoea is relieved by other measures.

Cough/noisy respirations

- Cough and 'rattly' breathing usually herald tracheobronchitis or bronchopneumonia as a terminal event because the patient is too weak to clear secretions.
- Antibiotics are rarely appropriate.
- Appropriate positioning of patient by nurse.

Anticholinergics reduce the volume of secretions:

- Hyoscine hydrobromide 0.2–0.4 mg hourly SC.
- Indicated if sedation is also required.
- Compatible with diamorphine in syringe driver.

This may cause agitated confusion in the elderly, in which case change to:

- Glycopyrronium 0.2 mg 4 hourly.
- Less likely to cause confusion/agitation

Local anaesthetics suppress distressing cough when patient is too weak to clear secretions:

- Bupivacaine 2.5 ml 0.25% via nebulizer 6 hourly.

Terminal restlessness

Exclude correctable causes such as urinary retention (catheterize) or steroid therapy (discontinue).

Benzodiazepines:

- midazolam 5–20 mg 4 hourly SC or via syringe driver has become the treatment of choice.

Agitation/delirium

Major tranquillizers:

- Methotrimeprazine 25–50 mg 6–8 hourly by SC injection.
- Haloperidol 5–20 mg 4–6 hourly by SC injection.

Benzodiazepines:

- Midazolam 5–20 mg 4 hourly SC as an adjunct to major tranquillizer.

Myoclonic jerking:

Usually due to rapid escalation of opioid dose.

Benzodiazepines:

- Midazolam 5–10 mg SC.

From: 'Changing gear – guidelines for managing the last days of life in adults' published by the National

Council for Hospice and Specialist Palliative Care Services, 7th Floor, 1 Great Cumberland Place, London W1H 7AL.

The selection of these drugs needs to be individualized. A blanket ordering of what may be an overdose for a particular patient would hardly seem to be the way to end a long-term commitment to a patient's care on the part of his doctors and nurses. Drugs are used as fine instruments and to turn to their use as a blunderbuss at the end would intimate a final attitude tantamount to 'writing off the patient'. Clinical assessment and response to the needs of the patient cease only at death and support for the family afterwards depends on the doctor's presence and interest throughout the illness she has committed herself to manage.

REFERENCES

Addington-Hall J, McCarthy M 1995 Dying from cancer: results of a national population-based investigation. Palliative Medicine 9: 295–305

Baines MB, Oliver DJ, Carter RL 1985 Medical management of intestinal obstruction in patients with advanced malignant disease. Lancet ii: 990–993

Boyd KJ 1993 Short terminal admissions to a hospice. Palliative Medicine 7: 289–294

Butler RN 1963 The life review. An interpretation of reminiscence in the aged. Psychiatry 26: 65–76

Campbell AGM, McHaffie HE 1995 Prolonging life and allowing death: infants. Journal of Medical Ethics 21: 339–344

Chambliss CR, Anand KJ 1997 Pain management in the pediatric intensive care unit. Current Opinions in Pediatrics 9: 246–253

Chater S, Viola R, Paterson J, Jarvis V 1998 Sedation for intractable distress in the dying a survey of experts. Palliative Medicine 12: 255–269

Cherny NI, Coyle N, Foley KM 1994 Suffering in the advanced cancer patient: a definition and taxonomy. Journal of Palliative Care 10: 57–70

Devlin P 1985 Easing the passing. Bodley Head, London

Edwards BS, Ueno WM 1991 Sedation before ventilator withdrawal (Case presentation). Journal of Clinical Ethics 2: 118–122

Ellershaw JE, Sutcliffe JM, Saunders CM 1995 Dehydration and the dying patient. Journal of Pain and Symptom Management 10: 192–197

Foley K 1997 Competent care for the dying instead of physician-assisted suicide. New England Journal of Medicine 336: 54–58

Grond S, Zech D, Schug A et al 1991 Validation of World Health Organization guidelines for cancer pain relief during the last days and hours of life. Journal of Pain and Symptom Management 6: 411–422

Hall Lord ML, Larsson G, Bostrom I 1994 Elderly patients' experiences of pain and distress in intensive care: a grounded theory study. Intensive Critical Care and Nursing 10: 133–141

Hanson LC, Danis M, Garrett J 1997 What is wrong with end-of-life care? Opinions of bereaved family members. Journal of the American Geriatric Society 45: 1339–1344

Higginson IJ, Sen-Gupta G, Dunlop R 1997 Changing gear – guidelines for managing the last days of life in adults – the research evidence. Proceedings of a Working Party on Clinical Guidelines in Palliative Care. The National Council for Hospice and Specialist Palliative Care Services, London

Hinton JM 1963 The physical and mental distress of the dying. Quarterly Journal of Medicine 32: 1–21

Hinton JM 1964 Editorial: problems in the care of the dying. Journal of Chronic Diseases 17: 201–205

Hinton J 1967 Dying. Penguin Books, Middlesex

Hinton JM 1994 Can home care maintain an acceptable quality of life for patients with terminal cancer and their relatives? Palliative Medicine 8: 183–196

Hinton JM 1996 How reliable are relatives' retrospective reports of terminal illness? Patients' and relatives' accounts compared. Social Science and Medicine 43: 1229–1236

Horton S 1996 Imparting the knowledge of impending death to the intensive care patient who is unable to respond. Nursing in Critical Care 1: 250–253

Jones A 1997 Family therapy in a critical care unit. Nursing Standard 11: 40–42

Keane WG, Gould JH, Millard PH 1983 Death in practice. Journal of the Royal College of General Practitioners 1: 347–351

Kolcaba KY, Fisher EM 1996 A holistic perspective on comfort care as an advance directive. Critical Care in Nursing Quarterly 18: 66–76

Lichter I, Hunt E 1990 The last 48 hours of life. Journal of Palliative Care 6: 7–15

Lo B 1995 Improving care near the end of life – why is it so hard? Journal of the American Medical Association 274: 1634–1636

Melzack R, Wal PD 1982 Acute pain in an emergency clinic: latency of onset and description patterns related to different injuries. Pain 14: 33–43

Mount B 1990 Editorial – A final crescendo of pain? Journal of Palliative Care 6: 5–6

National Council for Hospice and Specialist Palliative Care Services 1997 Changing gear – guidelines for managing the last days of life in adults. Proceedings of a Working Party on Clinical Guidelines in Palliative Care. National Coucil for Hospice and Specialist Palliative Care Services, London

Osler W 1906 Science and immortality. Constable, London

Oxford Textbook of Palliative Medicine, 2nd edn 1996 Oxford University Press, Oxford

Parkes CM 1973 Attachment and autonomy at the end of life. In: Gosling R (ed) Support, innovation and autonomy. Tavistock, London, pp 151–166

Parkes CM 1978 Home or hospital? Terminal care as seen by surviving spouses. Journal of the Royal College of General Practitioners 28: 19–30

Pittam MR 1992 Does unsuccessful salvage surgery modify the terminal course of patients with squamous carcinomas of head and neck? Clinical Oncology 8: 195–200

Puntillo KA, Miaskowski C, Kehrle K et al 1997 Relationship between behavioural and physiological indicators of pain, critical care patients' self-reports of pain, and opioid administration. Critical Care Medicine 25: 1159–1166

Robb YA 1997 Ethical considerations relating to terminal weaning in intensive care. Intensive Critical Care Nursing 13: 156–162

Sanders LM, Raffin TA 1993 The ethics of withholding and withdrawing critical care. Cambridge Quarterly of Healthcare Ethics 2: 175–184

'SUPPORT' Principal Investigators 1995 A controlled trial to improve care for seriously ill hospitalized patients. The study to understand prognoses and preferences for outcomes and risks of treatments (SUPPORT). Journal of the American Medical Association 274: 1591–1598

Thomas L 1980 On natural death. In: Thomas L (ed) The medusa and the snail – more notes of a biology watcher. Allen Lane, London, pp 102–105

Turner K, Chye R, Aggarwal G et al 1996 Dignity in dying: a preliminary study of patients in the last three days of life. Journal of Palliative Care 12: 7–13

Ventafridda V, Ripamonti C, De Conno F, Tamburini M 1990 Symptom prevalence and control during cancer patients' last days of life. Journal of Palliative Care 6: 7–11

Wall PD 1997 The generation of yet another myth on the use of narcotics. Pain 73: 121–122

Wilkes E 1984 Occasional survey: dying now. Lancet i: 950–952

Worcester A 1935 The care of the aged, the dying and the dead. CC Thomas, Springfield, Illinois

World Health Organization 1990 Cancer pain relief. World Health Organization, Geneva

Yu VY 1997 Ethical decision-making in newborn infants. Acta Medica Portuguesa 10: 197–204

Zylicz Z 1997 Dealing with people who want to die. Palliative Care Today 6: 54–56

SECTION 3

THERAPEUTIC ASPECTS

- Pharmacology
- Surgery
- Stimulation
- Physiotherapy
- Psychotherapy
- Special cases

48

Methods of therapeutic trials

HENRY J. McQUAY & R. A. MOORE

Clinical trials are used to show that our analgesic interventions, be they drugs, injections, operations, psychological or physical manoeuvres, or even prayer, are effective and safe. Clinical trials need to produce credible results. To make the results credible it is vital to design, conduct and analyse trials in such a way as to minimize bias. Then the credibility which is needed can be achieved.

The efficacy of analgesic interventions is judged by the change they bring about in the patient's report of pain. A brief description of methods of pain measurement is followed by sections on trial design and pain models.

PAIN MEASUREMENT FOR TRIALS

Pain is a personal experience, which makes it difficult to define and measure. It includes both the sensory input and any modulation by physiological, psychological and environmental factors. Not surprisingly there are no objective measures – there is no way to measure pain directly by sampling blood or urine or by performing neurophysiological tests. Measurement of pain must therefore rely on recording the patient's report. The assumption is often made that because the measurement is subjective it must be of little value. The reality is that if the measurements are done properly, remarkably sensitive and consistent results can be obtained. There are contexts, however, when it is not possible to measure pain at all, or when reports are likely to be unreliable. These include impaired consciousness, young children, psychiatric pathology, severe anxiety, unwillingness to cooperate, and inability to understand the measurements. Such problems are deliberately avoided in trials. Most analgesic studies include measurements of pain intensity and/or pain relief, and the commonest tools used are categorical and visual analogue scales.

CATEGORICAL AND VISUAL ANALOGUE SCALES (FIG. 48.1)

Categorical scales use words to describe the magnitude of the pain. They were the earliest pain measure (Keele 1948). The patient picks the most appropriate word. Most research groups use four words (none, mild, moderate, severe). Scales to measure pain relief were developed later. The commonest is the five-category scale (none, slight, moderate, good or lots, complete).

For analysis numbers are given to the verbal categories (for pain intensity: none=0, mild=1, moderate=2 and

Categorical verbal rating scale

Pain intensity	
severe	3
moderate	2
slight	1
none	0

Pain relief	
complete	4
good	3
moderate	2
slight	1
none	0

Visual analogues

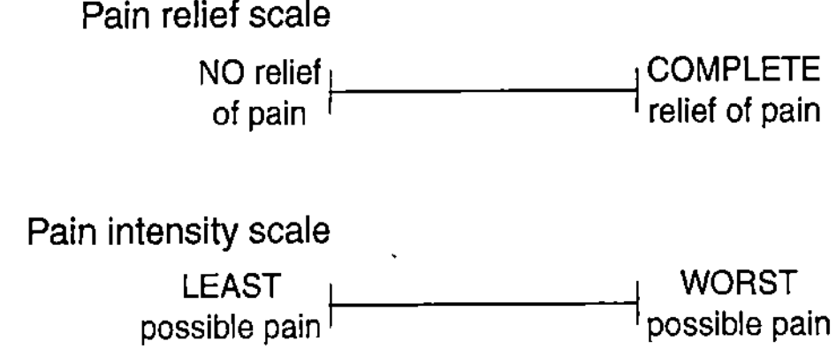

Fig. 48.1 Categorical and visual analogue scales.

severe=3; for relief: none=0, slight=1, moderate=2, good or lots=3, complete=4). Information from different subjects is then combined to produce means (rarely medians) and measures of dispersion (usually standard errors of means). The validity of converting categories into numerical scores was checked by comparison with concurrent visual analogue scale measurements. Good correlation was found, especially between pain relief scales using cross-modality matching techniques (Scott & Huskisson 1976, Wallenstein et al 1980, Littman et al 1985). Results are usually reported as continuous data, mean or median pain relief or intensity. Few studies present results as discrete data, giving the number of participants who report a certain level of pain intensity or relief at any given assessment point. The main advantages of the categorical scales are that they are quick and simple. The small number of descriptors may force the scorer to choose a particular category when none describes the pain satisfactorily.

Visual analogue scales (VAS), lines with the left end labelled 'no relief of pain' and the right end labelled 'complete relief of pain', seem to overcome this limitation. Patients mark the line at the point that corresponds to their pain. The scores are obtained by measuring the distance between the no relief end and the patient's mark, usually in millimetres. The main advantages of VAS are that they are simple and quick to score, avoid imprecise descriptive terms and provide many points from which to choose. More concentration and coordination are needed, which can be difficult postoperatively or with neurological disorders.

Pain relief scales are perceived as more convenient than pain intensity scales, probably because patients have the same baseline relief (zero) whereas they could start with different baseline intensity. A patient with severe initial pain intensity has more scope to show improvement than one who starts with mild pain. Relief scale results are thus easier to compare across patients. They may also be more sensitive than intensity scales (Sriwatanakul et al 1982, Littman et al 1985). A theoretical drawback of relief scales is that the patient has to remember what the pain was like to begin with. The evidence we have (Edwards et al 1999b) is that, within limits, the choice of pain measurement scale is not crucial.

One point about scales is that we rarely know how much movement on a particular scale equates to a clinically meaningful change. Even using the binary outcome of pain 50% relieved we do not know if this degree of relief is adequate for the patient. Determining the significance of any differences observed is important for patients and for clinicians who will be applying the trial results.

One example of where scale change and clinical importance were tested comes from McMaster. They used seven-point Likert scales measuring dyspnoea, fatigue and emotional function in patients with chronic heart and lung disease to determine how much change constituted a minimal clinically important difference (MCID). The answer was that the MCID was a mean change in score of approximately 0.5 per item on the seven-point scale (Jaeschke et al 1989). The same 'spadework' is needed for our pain scales.

OTHER TOOLS

Verbal numerical scales and global subjective efficacy ratings are also used. Verbal numerical scales are regarded as an alternative or complementary to the categorical and VAS scales. Patients give a number to the pain intensity or relief (for pain intensity 0 usually represents no pain and 10 the maximum possible, and for pain relief 0 represents none and 10 complete relief). They are very easy and quick to use, and correlate well with conventional VASs (Murphy et al 1988).

Global subjective efficacy ratings, or simply global scales, are designed to measure overall treatment performance. Patients are asked questions like 'How effective do you think the treatment was?' and answer using a labelled numerical or a categorical scale. Although these judgements probably include adverse effects, they can be the most sensitive discriminant between treatments. One of the oldest scales was the binary question 'Is your pain half gone?'. Its advantage is that it has a clearer clinical meaning than a 10-mm shift on a VAS. The disadvantage, for the small trial intensive measure pundits at least, is that all the potential intermediate information (1–49% or greater than 50%) is discarded.

Analgesic requirements (including patient-controlled analgesia, PCA), special paediatric scales and questionnaires like the McGill are also used. The limitation to guard against is that they usually reflect other experiences as well as or instead of pain (Jadad & McQuay 1993). PCA in particular is a fraught pain outcome. Individual variation is huge, so that a large trial group size is necessary to show any difference. If PCA is used with a pain scale, then any difference between trial groups in PCA consumption is only valid at similar pain scale values.

Judgement by the patient rather than by the carer is the ideal. Carers overestimate the pain relief compared with the patient's version.

RESTRICTING TO MODERATE AND SEVERE INITIAL PAIN INTENSITY

The trail blazers of analgesic trial methodology found that if patients had no pain to begin with, it was impossible to assess analgesic efficacy, because there was no pain to relieve. To optimize trial sensitivity a rule developed, which was that only those patients with moderate or severe pain intensity at baseline would be studied. Those with mild or no pain would not. For those using VASs, we know from individual patient data that if a patient records a baseline VAS pain intensity score in excess of 30 mm they would probably have recorded at least moderate pain on a four-point categorical scale (Collins et al 1997).

This, the requirement that only patients with moderate or severe baseline pain intensity should be studied, presents particular problems for pre-emptive techniques and local anaesthetic blocks. With pre-emptive techniques the whole idea is that there is no pain when the intervention is made. The sensitivity of the subsequent measurements, such as time to further analgesic requirement, is then of supreme importance. The same applies to local anaesthetic blocks given during surgery, because we cannot be sure that the patient would have had any pain. It is known that a proportion of patients (6% after minor orthopaedic operations (McQuay et al 1982)), have little or no analgesic requirement after surgery.

OUT-OF-HOSPITAL STUDIES

Reduced length of stay in hospital has forced acute pain investigators to develop methods which work out of hospital. For chronic pain outpatients this has always been necessary. Most investigators use patient diaries, supplemented by telephone calls. There is little empirical information to help choose between particular scales and methods of presentation, just examples of particular trials which proved to be sensitive. Over the years our diaries have become simpler, and an example is shown in Figure 48.2. For chronic long-term use patients are asked to complete the diary just before bed, noting their current pain intensity and their typical pain intensity for the day. In such long-term studies the average weekly typical pain intensity is a useful outcome.

ANALYSIS OF PAIN-SCALE RESULTS – SUMMARY MEASURES

In the research context pain is usually assessed before the intervention is made and then on multiple occasions. Ideally the area under the time–analgesic effect curve for the intensity (sum of pain intensity differences; *SPID*) or relief (total pain relief; *TOTPAR*) measures is derived.

$$SPID = \sum_{t=0-6}^{n} PID_t \quad TOTPAR = \sum_{t=0-6}^{n} PR_t$$

where at the *t*th assessment point (t= 0, 1, 2, n), P_t and PR_t are pain intensity and pain relief measured at that point respectively, P_0 is pain intensity at t=0 and PID_t is the pain intensity difference calculated as $(P_0–P_t)$ (Fig. 48.3).

Name .... **Oxford Pain Chart** Treatment Week ....

Please fill in this chart each evening before going to bed. Record your pain intensity and the amount of pain relief. If you have any side effects please note them in the side effects box.

	Date							
Pain Intensity How bad has your pain been today?	severe							
	moderate							
	mild							
	none							
Pain Relief How much pain relief have the tablets given today?	complete							
	good							
	moderate							
	slight							
	none							
Side effects Has the treatment upset you in any way?								

How effective was the treatment this week? *poor fair good very good excellent* Please circle your choice

Fig. 48.2 Oxford Pain Chart.

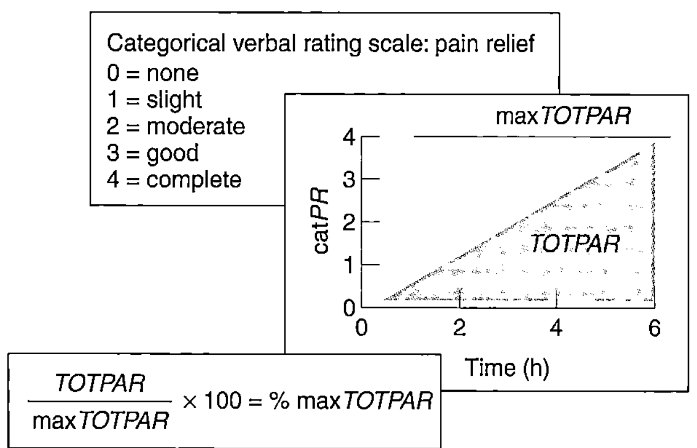

Categorical verbal rating scale: pain relief
0 = none
1 = slight
2 = moderate
3 = good
4 = complete
maxTOTPAR
TOTPAR
catPR
Time (h)
TOTPAR / maxTOTPAR × 100 = % maxTOTPAR

Fig. 48.3 Calculating percentage of maximum possible pain relief score.

These summary measures reflect the cumulative response to the intervention. Their disadvantage is that they do not provide information about the onset and peak of the analgesic effect. If onset or peak are important, then time to maximum pain relief (or reduction in pain intensity) or time for pain to return to baseline are necessary.

OUTCOMES OTHER THAN PAIN

Currently there is growing awareness that we should not focus on pain to the exclusion of other outcomes. Mobility, satisfaction and length of stay are important in the acute context, mobility or disability (function) and satisfaction are important in the chronic context. In chronic pain an analgesic intervention which improves pain by as little as 10% may be very important to the patient, because this small shift in pain allows an important shift in function. Measured solely as pain reduction this might be missed. However, still it is not known if 'global' quality of life scales such as the SF36 are adequate to pick up these niceties – one suspects not.

For function (disability) the researcher often has the choice of off-the-shelf validated scales developed in other clinical contexts or to develop their own. In chronic pain we have found that the small shifts in function which matter to patients are picked up poorly (if at all) by scales developed for advanced cancer. A fruitful approach may be to determine which outcomes matter to patients, for instance by using patient focus groups. Given adequate consensus the output may then be used to fashion a function outcome scale for the trial, with minimal clinically important difference predetermined. This will take time to develop and validate.

OUTPUTS FROM TRIALS

There are a number of statistical ways to examine the results of clinical trials, which include *P* values, odds ratios, relative risk, relative risk reduction or increase and so on. All may have their place, but they are difficult outputs for the non-specialist to interpret. In order to overcome this, we use the number needed to treat (NNT). The NNT, as the name implies, is an estimate of the number of patients that would need to be given a treatment for one of them to achieve a desired outcome. The NNT should specify the patient group, the intervention and the outcome. Using postoperative pain as the example, the NNT describes the number of patients who have to be treated with an analgesic intervention for one of them to have at least 50% pain relief over 4–6 hours who would not have had pain relief of that magnitude with placebo. That does not mean that pain relief of a lower intensity will not occur.

For an analgesic trial, the NNT is calculated very simply as:

NNT = 1/(proportion of patients with at least 50% pain relief with analgesic – proportion of patients with at least 50% pain relief with placebo)

Taking a hypothetical example from a randomized trial:

50 patients were given placebo, and 10 of them had more than 50% pain relief over 6 hours

50 patients were given ibuprofen, and 27 of them had more than 50% pain relief over 6 hours.

The NNT is therefore:

$$\text{NNT} = 1/(27/50) - (10/50)$$
$$= 1/0.54 - 0.20 = 1/0.34 = 2.9$$

The best NNT would, of course, be 1, when every patient with treatment benefited, but no patient given control. Generally NNTs between 2 and 5 are indicative of effective analgesic treatments. Figure 48.4 shows a league table for single-dose postoperative NNTs, using the criterion of at least 50% pain relief over 4–6 hours in patients with moderate to severe pain (McQuay & Moore 1998).

For adverse effects, we can calculate a number needed to harm (NNH), in exactly the same way as an NNT. For an NNH, large numbers are obviously better than small numbers.

Questions have been raised in the past about the wisdom of combining information gathered in analgesic trials using different pain models (dental versus postoperative or episiotomy pain), or different pain measurements, or different durations of observation. Analysis of the great mass of information on aspirin has shown that none of these variables has any effect on the magnitude of the analgesic effect (Edwards et al 1999b).

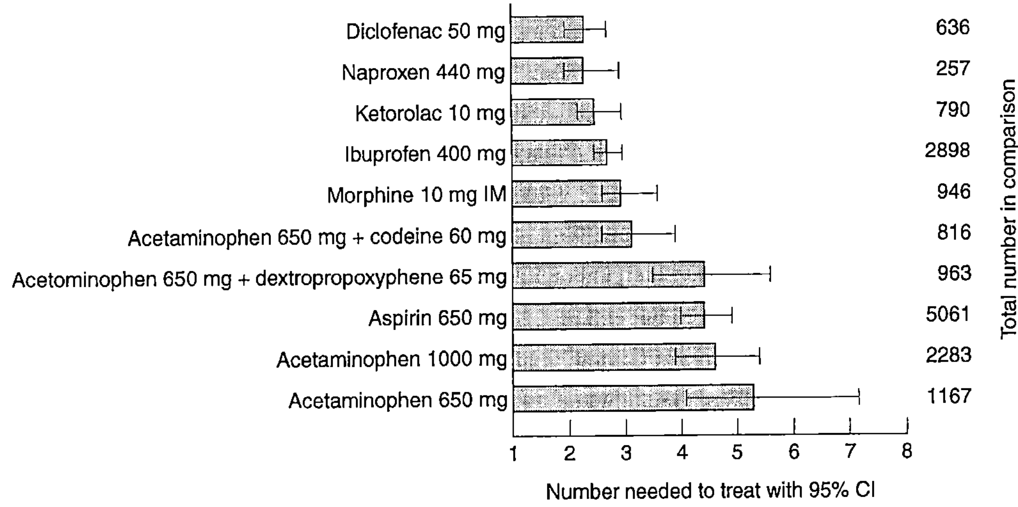

Fig. 48.4 League table of number needed to treat (NNT) for postoperative pain. NNT for at least 50% pain relief over 4–6 hours in patients with moderate to severe pain, all oral analgesics except IM morphine, all single-dose studies.

STUDY DESIGN AND VALIDITY

Pain measurement is one of the oldest and most studied of the subjective measures, and pain scales have been used for over 40 years. Even in the early days of pain measurement there was understanding that the design of studies contributed directly to the validity of the result obtained. Trial designs which lack validity produce information that is at best difficult to use, and which much of the time will be useless, and therefore unethical.

PLACEBO

People in pain respond to placebo treatment. Some patients given placebo obtain 100% pain relief. The effect is reproducible, and some work has been done to try and assess the characteristics of the 'placebo responder', by sex, race and psychological profile. Older women, church attending but not necessarily God believing, reputedly are more likely to respond to placebo (Beecher 1955).

Two common misconceptions are that a fixed fraction (one-third) of the population responds to placebo, and that the extent of the placebo reaction is also a fixed fraction (again about one-third of the maximum possible (Wall 1992)). As Wall points out, these ideas stem from a misreading of Beecher's work of 40 years ago (Wall 1994). In Beecher's five acute pain studies, 139 patients (31%) of 452 given placebo had 50% or more relief of postoperative pain at two checked intervals (Beecher 1955). The proportion of patients who had 50% or more relief of pain varied across the studies, ranging from 15 to 53%. There was neither a fixed fraction of responders, nor a fixed extent of response.

Placebo responses have also been reported as varying systematically with the efficacy of the active analgesic medicine. Evans pointed out that in seven studies the placebo response was always about 55% of the active treatment, whether that was aspirin or morphine: the stronger the drug, the stronger the placebo response (Evans 1974), and this observation suggests that significant observer bias (see below) occurs. We believe that the idea that there is a constant relationship between active analgesic and placebo response is an artefact of using an inappropriate statistical description (using a mean when the distribution is not normal) (McQuay et al 1996). Gøtzsche has confirmed similar magnitudes of effect for non-steroidal anti-inflammatory drugs in active and placebo-controlled studies (Gøtzsche 1993), showing that the presence of a placebo does not affect the active treatment.

For many investigators the issue of whether or not to include a placebo group in pain trials causes great angst, personal or institutional. The mechanics of using placebo are important here. A patient is not left to suffer for an indeterminate time. An 'escape' analgesic is given after a set time if the patient has no relief. This interval is usually an hour in oral postoperative studies. The patient is also free to withdraw from the trial at any time. This is workable and necessary in circumstances where the variation in response to a pain is large (McQuay & Moore 1996). When placebos are not possible, then great care must be taken in the trial design to provide indices of validity and sensitivity. Many times placebo can be incorporated in contexts where

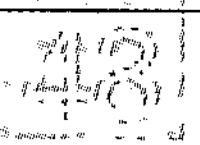

it initially seems unthinkable by using an add-on design, with existing medication providing 'cover' and a new drug (or placebo control) being added on. An additional level of sophistication may be achieved by using an 'active' placebo which mimics any adverse effect of the active treatment (Max et al 1994).

RANDOMIZED CONTROLLED TRIALS

Because the placebo response was an established fact in analgesic studies, randomization was used from the early 1950s to try to avoid any possibility of bias from placebo responders, and to equalize their numbers in each treatment group. Randomization is necessary even in studies without placebo, because an excess of placebo responders in an active treatment arm of a study might inflate the effects of an analgesic.

The randomized controlled trial (RCT) is the most reliable way to estimate the effect of an intervention. The principle of randomization is simple. Patients in a randomized trial have the same probability of receiving any of the interventions being compared. Randomization abolishes selection bias because it prevents investigators influencing who has which intervention. Randomization also helps to ensure that other factors, such as age or sex distribution, are equivalent for the different treatment groups. Inadequate randomization, or inadequate concealment of randomization, lead to exaggeration of therapeutic effect (Schulz et al 1994). In broad terms methods of randomization which do not give each patient the same probability of receiving any of the interventions being compared, such as allocation by date of birth, day of the week or hospital number, are bad, whereas tossing a coin, tables of random numbers or the computer variant, which do give the same probability to each patient, are good.

An example of the impact of randomization on the conclusions one draws is the use of transcutaneous electrical nerve stimulation (TENS) in postoperative pain. In a systematic review 17 reports on 786 patients could be regarded unequivocally as RCTs in acute postoperative pain. Fifteen of these 17 RCTs demonstrated no benefit of TENS over placebo. Nineteen reports had pain outcomes but were not RCTs; in 17 of these 19, TENS was considered by their authors to have had a positive analgesic effect (Carroll et al 1996).

Stratification, deliberately making sure that patients with factors known or suspected to influence the outcome are equally distributed (randomized) into the trial groups, may be incorporated (see Senn (1997) for discussion). The randomization may be organized in blocks, which is helpful where multiple institutions are involved in a study, or where there are multiple observers. Each institution or observer works their way through a particular block(s).

DOUBLE-BLINDING

Double-blinding means that neither the investigating team nor the patient know which of the interventions under test the patient is actually receiving. Double-blinding is relatively easy to organize for drug trials. With non-drug interventions it may be difficult or impossible. While people have struggled to blind TENS or acupuncture it is hard to see how twice-a-day versus once-a-day physiotherapy can be blinded. Does it matter? We know that studies which are not blinded overestimate treatment effects by some 17% (Schulz et al 1995). With a subjective outcome like pain the ideal is clearly that the study should be both randomized and double-blind. If the intervention cannot be blinded then the study should be randomized and open. The study size will in all likelihood have to be increased for the open condition compared with the double blind. Precisely how much bigger it will need to be will depend on the intervention and on the outcome.

TRIAL DESIGNS

The two classic clinical trial designs used in pain are the parallel group and the crossover (Fig. 48.5). Max and Laska provide a good review of these classic designs as they apply to single-dose trials (Max & Laska 1991).

Parallel group and crossover

The advantage of the parallel group is its simplicity. Whereas the crossover design assumes that the underlying

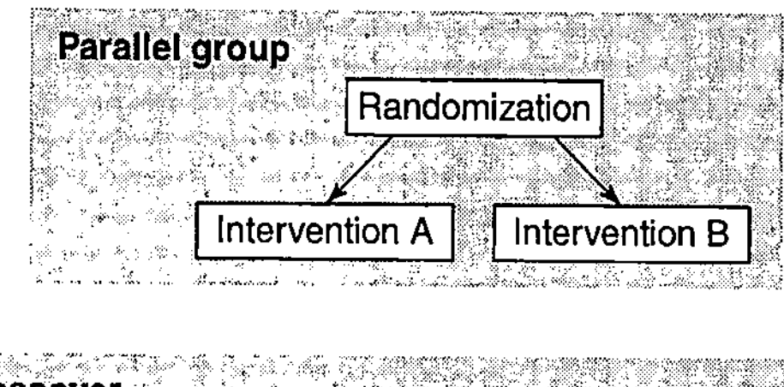

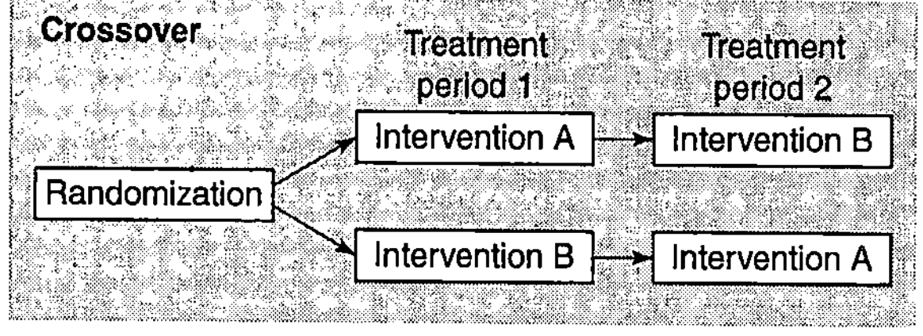

Fig. 48.5 Parallel and crossover trial designs.

pain will not change from treatment period 1 to period 2, no such assumption is required for a parallel group design. A second assumption of the crossover design is that it assumes that there is negligible treatment carryover effect from treatment period 1 to period 2. A relative disadvantage of parallel group compared with crossover is that more patients are needed for parallel group. James et al (1985) argued that 2.4 times as many subjects would have to be recruited in a non-crossover design to obtain precision equivalent to that of the crossover design, given a negligible treatment carryover effect. These arguments are dealt with in detail in Senn (1993).

Parallel group designs may be used in both acute and chronic pain, but it is unusual to find crossover designs in acute pain, because patients go home much earlier than they did and because postoperative pain wanes, so that there may be a decrease in pain intensity in period 2 compared with period 1. Crossover designs are attractive in chronic pain because fewer patients are necessary, and this is particularly important for the study of homogeneous groups with rare syndromes.

N of 1

Single-patient of N of 1 designs are really crossover designs in single patients (McQuay 1991). Each patient has multiple 'pairs' of treatments, for instance dextromethorphan and placebo, with the order of the pairs randomized (McQuay et al 1994). If five pairs are used some sort of statistical significance can be adduced. If multiple patients are used then the trial can be analysed like a normal crossover design. Examples are trials of amitriptyline in fibromyalgia (Jaeschke et al 1991) and of paracetamol in osteoarthritis (March et al 1994). In reality while this may be a better way of doing early testing than open studies, and while it may be helpful for single-patient therapeutic decisions, it is more onerous and no more informative than conventional crossover designs for 'formal' trials.

AUDIT

Most of us use a form of before-and-after audit to introduce new proven interventions, and hopefully all of us use audit as part of quality control on the care we deliver. Such audits can also help to generate hypotheses, but the problems of case-mix (you treat worse cases than I do) and selection and observer bias mean that audit results are not generalizable in the way that RCT results should be. Their value lies in telling us how well-established treatment protocols work, and in control of quality of care (Haynes et al 1995).

SENSITIVITY

Particularly for a new analgesic, a trial should prove its internal sensitivity – that the study was an adequate analgesic assay. This can be carried out in several ways. For instance, if a known analgesic (acetaminophen) can be shown to have statistical difference from placebo, then the analgesic assay should be able to distinguish another analgesic of similar effectiveness. Alternatively, two different doses of a standard analgesic (e.g. morphine) could be used – showing the higher dose to be statistically superior to the lower dose again provides confidence that the assay is sensitive.

EQUIVALENCE: A VERSUS B DESIGNS

Studies of analgesics of an A versus B design are notoriously difficult to interpret. If there is a statistical difference, then that suggests sensitivity. Lack of a significant difference means nothing – there is no way to determine whether there is an analgesic effect which is no different between A and B, or whether the assay lacks the sensitivity to measure a difference that is actually present.

This is not just a problem for pain studies (Jones et al 1996, McQuay & Moore 1996, Senn 1997). Designs which minimize these problems include using placebo or using two doses of a standard analgesic (Fig. 48.6). In the latter case simple calculations could show what dose of the new analgesic was equivalent to the usual dose of the standard analgesic.

CHOICE OF STANDARD ANALGESIC

For drug trials in acute pain the standard injectable drug is morphine. Current standard oral drugs include paracetamol, ibuprofen and aspirin. This oversimplification conceals problems of opioid versus non-steroidal anti-inflammatory drug (NSAID), and of the sensitivity of the pain model used. If there is a conflict it is between the pragmatic and the explanatory (Schwartz & Lellouch 1967). The pragmatic is the clinical need to know whether the new drug is better than the standard (or as good with fewer adverse effects). The explanatory is to know whether the intervention works at all. For the pragmatic mode the standard analgesic needs to be current standard treatment or a close relation. For the explanatory mode the control may be placebo (negative control) or active drug (see Fig. 48.5 bottom panel). Clever pain trial designs can combine the pragmatic and the explanatory.

For drug trials in chronic nociceptive pain the same standards apply. In chronic neuropathic pain life is more complicated, because in some pain syndromes there is as yet no

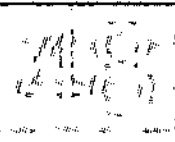

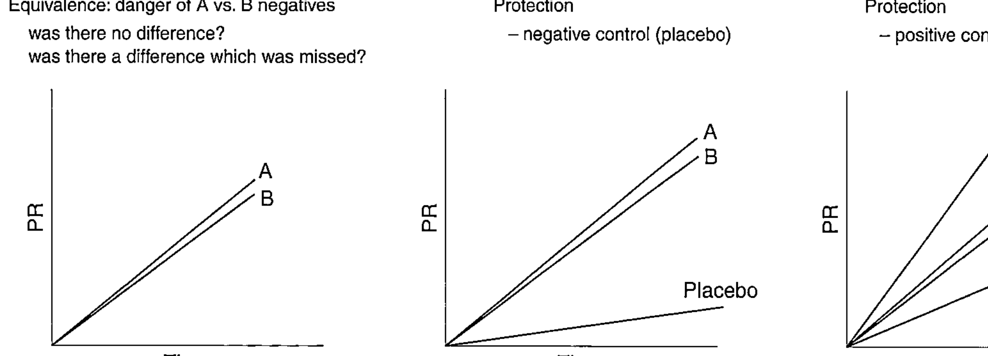

Fig. 48.6 Using placebo or active comparators to protect against A versus B negative results.

gold standard, although tricyclic antidepressants or carbamazepine are achieving that status.

For non-drug trials in both acute and chronic pain life is more complicated. Again the pragmatic need is to show how the new intervention performs against the current standard treatment. If that means a trial of drug versus non-drug then that is what the randomization should be, and if blinding is not feasible the trial should be randomized and open.

PROBLEMS

The correct design of an analgesic trial is situation dependent. In some circumstances very complicated designs have to be used to ensure sensitivity and validity.

No gold standard

There may be circumstances in chronic pain when there is no established analgesic treatment of sufficient effectiveness to act as the gold standard against which to measure a new treatment. A negative (no difference) equivalence study of one useless treatment against the new treatment would not help, because we would not know if both were good or both were bad. In this context placebo or no-treatment controls may be vital, especially when effects are to be examined over prolonged periods of weeks or months. But paradoxically it is often precisely these circumstances in which ethical constraints act against using placebo or non-treatment controls because of the need to do *something.* Add-on designs provide one solution.

When there is no pain to begin with

As suggested above when there is no pain it is difficult to measure an analgesic response. Yet a number of studies seek to do this by pre-empting pain, or by intervening when there is no pain (intraoperatively, for instance) to produce analgesia when pain is to be expected. These are difficult, but not impossible, circumstances in which to conduct research. Meticulous attention to trial design is necessary to be able to show differences. A current example of this dilemma is intra-articular morphine (Kalso et al 1997).

PAIN MODELS

The word model here is used as a shorthand for the patient population to be studied. Often there is much agonizing over which is the most appropriate population for study (Fig. 48.7). In reality in nociceptive pain a drug which is an analgesic in one population will also be an analgesic in other populations. This is a splitter versus lumper argument. Splitters believe that pain in the foot cannot be managed with a drug which is good for treating pain in the arm. Lumpers hold that a drug which works as an analgesic at one site will work at other sites. We side with the lumpers, and the choice of pain model should be made on the basis of the question you want to answer, again using the explanatory/pragmatic yardstick. If the question is pragmatic, such as which is the best treatment in a particular setting, then there is no point in running the trial in a diametrically opposed population. The evidence we have (Edwards et al 1999b) is that choice of pain model makes no difference to the measured efficacy of an analgesic (but see the caveat for opioids below).

In acute pain over recent years the removal of lower third molars has proved a sensitive and reliable testbed for the investigation of oral analgesics, and would be our model of choice for an explanatory trial of an oral analgesic. The

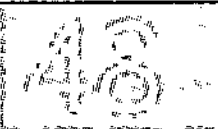

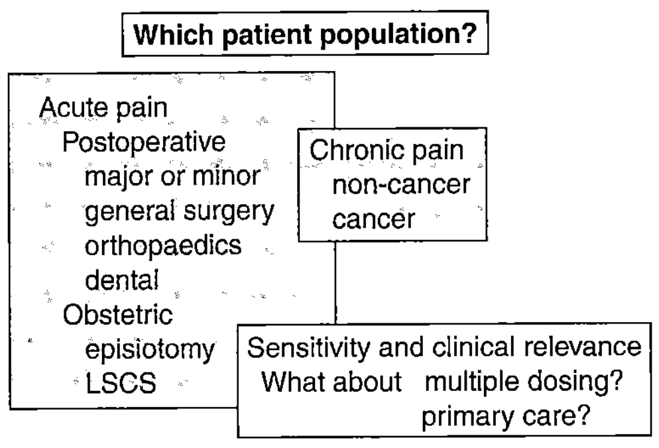

Fig. 48.7 Which patient population?

splitters do have an argument in this context, because opioids perform slightly less well relative to NSAIDs in oral surgery compared with other models (Moore & McQuay 1997). It is becoming increasingly difficult to test injectable drugs as hospital length of stay shrinks, but injections are still given on the day of surgery to major abdominal and orthopaedic surgery patients.

In chronic pain (as usual) life is more complicated. Firstly patients take drugs long term. Most analgesics are proven in acute pain, because trials are easier in acute pain, and the drugs are then used in chronic pain. Single-dose trial results by and large do extrapolate to multiple dosing, but single-dose trials may underestimate efficacy in multiple dosing, particularly for opioids, and may underestimate the incidence of adverse effects. Secondly there is the conundrum of neuropathic pain. The problem with neuropathic pain is that putative remedies cannot be tested in the nociceptive pain, which would be much easier. Drugs such as antidepressants and anticonvulsants, which have proven efficacy in neuropathic pain, have been shown to be ineffective in nociceptive pain. A negative trial result in acute (or chronic) nociceptive pain does not therefore mean that the drug will not work in neuropathic pain.

Our remedies for neuropathic pain have to be tested in neuropathic pain. The constraints here are limited numbers of patients in any one centre, and continuing uncertainty about the generalizability of results in one neuropathic pain syndrome to others. Again drugs such as antidepressants and anticonvulsants have proven efficacy in a variety of pain syndromes, but systemic local anaesthetics appear to work in some syndromes but not in others (Kalso et al 1998). The likelihood is that lumping all chronic neuropathic syndromes together is naive, and increasingly we shall need to subdivide as the years pass. The problem for the current researcher is knowing if a result, positive or negative, in one syndrome is predictive for the others. This may be a context in which the N of 1 designs are useful, because the intervention can be tested on patients with different neuropathic pain syndromes in an explanatory design (McQuay et al 1994).

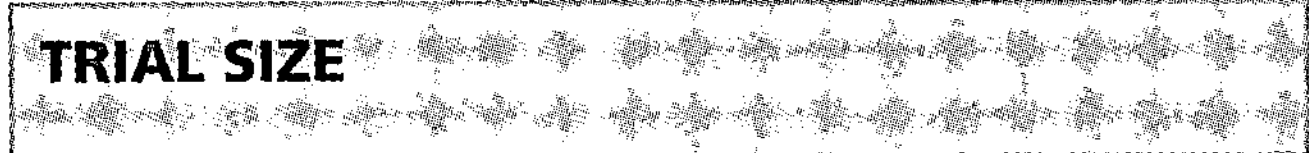

TRIAL SIZE

The variability in patients' response to interventions, seen in both acute pain and chronic pain, may have a huge impact on trial results. Many explanations such as trial methods, environment or culture have been proposed, but we believe that the main cause of the variability may be random chance, and that if trials are small their results may be incorrect, simply because of the random play of chance. This is highly relevant to the questions of 'How large do trials have to be for statistical accuracy?' and 'How large do trials have to be for clinical accuracy?'.

Words can be confusing. We are talking here about the variability in patients' response to an intervention, whether the intervention is an experimental treatment or control, which could be a placebo. If we decide on some indication of success of the treatment, such as relief of at least 50% of a symptom, then a proportion of patients will achieve success with the experimental treatment, and a proportion of patients will achieve success with the control. We use the phrase experimental event rate (EER) to describe the proportion of patients achieving success (the event) with the experimental treatment, and the phrase control event rate (CER) to describe the proportion of patients achieving success (the event) with the control treatment. Clinical efficacy of the intervention is then analysed as the number needed to treat (NNT) (Cook & Sackett 1995).

THE OBSERVATION – SUCCESS (EVENT) RATES VARY

The medical literature contains many examples of clinical trials which reach different conclusions about how successful an intervention may be, or whether it works at all. In pain research, for instance, one study with tramadol concluded that it was an excellent analgesic (Sunshine et al 1992) and another that it had no analgesic effect at all (Stubhaug et al 1995). The reality is that the proportion of patients who respond to treatment, either with placebo or active therapy, varies, and the extent of that response also varies. Which of the tramadol papers was correct? What follows is concerned with the impact that this variation may have on trial results, about the causes of the variation, and about how the variation can be explained.

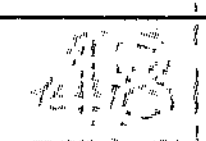

This variation is seen in both acute pain and chronic pain, and also in other areas of medicine, but here the examples are taken from acute pain. For example, with ibuprofen, there was a huge range in response rates for placebo and ibuprofen 400 mg in randomized, double-blind studies in patients with moderate or severe postoperative pain (Fig. 48.8). In individual trials between 0 and 60% of patients achieved at least 50% pain relief with placebo, and between about 10 and 100% with ibuprofen 400 mg.

What is going on? Attempts have been made to try to understand or explain this variability (Cooper 1991), especially the variability in control event rate (Evans 1974, McQuay et al 1996), but it is important to recognize that the variability is not unique to pain. Variation in event rates is also seen in trials of antiemetics in postoperative vomiting (Tramer et al 1995), of antibiotics in acute cough (Ali & Goetz 1997), and in trials of prophylactic natural surfactant for preterm infants the control event rate with placebo for bronchopulmonary dysplasia varied between 24 and 69% (Soll & McQueen 1992).

IMPLICATIONS OF EVENT-RATE VARIABILITY

The importance of event-rate variability is that it undermines the credibility of trial results, particularly results from single trials or from small trials.

Implications for interpretation

There is a danger that we seize on the latest report of an RCT and, acting on its findings, change our practice. A pain

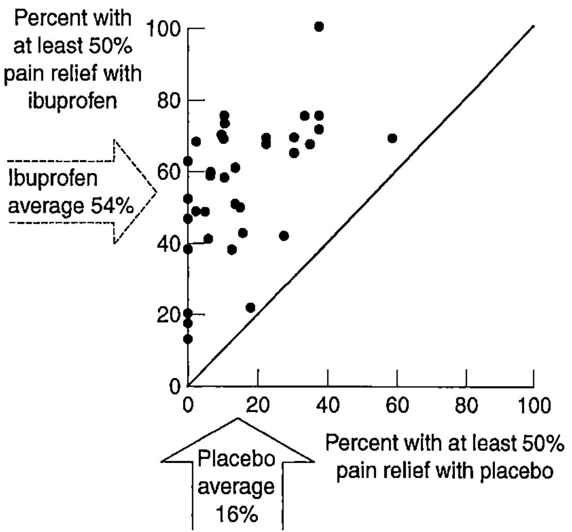

Fig. 48.8 L'Abbé plot of percentage of patients with at least 50% pain relief with placebo or ibuprofen 400 mg in randomized double-blind trials.

example might be nitroglycerin (NTG) patches for shoulder pain (Berrazueta et al 1996). Randomization was between a daily 5 mg NTG transdermal patch and an identical placebo applied in the most painful area. At the start, and after 24 and 48 hours, pain intensity was measured on a 10-point scale. At 48 hours, pain intensity was 2 or less (out of 10) in 9/10 patients given NTG compared with 0/10 given placebo. There was no reduction in pain intensity in placebo patients. The NNT for pain intensity of 2 or less for NTG compared with placebo was 1.1 (0.9–1.4).

This near-perfect result in a small (10 patients per group) randomized trial is so good because 9 of 10 patients did well on treatment and none did well on control (placebo). If some of the controls (three more) had improved and a few of those with NTG (two fewer) did not, then the NTG would look much less impressive, with confidence intervals indicating no benefit of treatment over placebo. Success comes down to the results in a few patients. Knowing that event rates vary, how safe is the published trial result? Could it just be a fluke that in this small trial none of the control patients responded?

SOURCE OF EVENT-RATE VARIABILITY

Trial design

One obvious source is trial design. Could there be undiscovered bias despite randomization and the use of double-blind methods, which if true would undermine the confidence placed in analgesic trial results?

Randomization controls for selection bias, and the double-blind design is there to control observer bias. Patients may know a placebo was one possible treatment, and investigators know the study design and active treatments; it has been suggested that this can modify patients' behaviour in trials (Gracely et al 1985, Wall 1993). Patients may have opportunities to communicate with each other. Doctors know the trial design when recruiting patients, which may be a source of bias (Bergmann et al 1994). Nurse observers spend most time with patients, and the nurse might be able to influence a patient's response by his/her demeanour based on experience of other patients' reactions. That would produce time-dependent changes in study results, as has been seen before (Shapiro et al 1954).

Population

The reason for large variations in control event rates with placebo may have something to do with the population studied – Scottish stoics versus Welsh wimps. There is little evidence for this, but there may be differences between men and women, or in response in different pain models (Moore & McQuay 1997).

Environmental

Another explanation is the environmental situation in which a trial is conducted. Inpatients in a nice hospital with a charming nurse might have a good response, while outpatients filling in diaries alone at home might not (Dahlstrom & Paalzaw 1977). Other clinical or societal factors which we have yet to recognize may influence event rates.

Random effects

An individual patient can have no pain relief or 100% pain relief. That is true whether they get control (placebo) or active treatment (Fig. 48.9) (McQuay et al 1996). Clearly if we choose only one patient to have placebo and only one patient to have treatment, either or both could pass or fail to reach the dichotomous hurdle of at least 50% pain relief. The more patients who have the treatment or placebo, the more likely we are to have a result that reflects the true underlying distribution. But how many is enough for us to be comfortable that random effects can be ignored?

Until the full effects of the random play of chance are appreciated, we cannot begin to unravel the effects of trial design, or population or environmental effects. Here we discuss the effects of random chance in trials of single doses of analgesics in acute pain of moderate or severe intensity. The next section describes the origin of the data used to determine real control event rate (CER) in acute pain trials and the questions to be addressed by the calculations and simulations.

INVESTIGATING VARIABILITY

The true underlying control event rate (CER) and experimental event rate (EER) were determined from single-dose acute pain analgesic trials in over 5000 patients (Moore et al 1998). Trial group size required to obtain statistically significant and clinically credible (0.95 probability of NNT within ± 0.5 of its true value) results were computed using these values. Ten thousand trials using these CER and EER values were then simulated, using varying trial group sizes, to investigate the variation in observed CER and EER as a result of random chance alone (Fig. 48.10).

Most common analgesics have EERs in the range 0.4–0.6 and CER of about 0.19. With such efficacy, to have a 90% chance of obtaining a statistically significant result in the correct direction requires group sizes in the

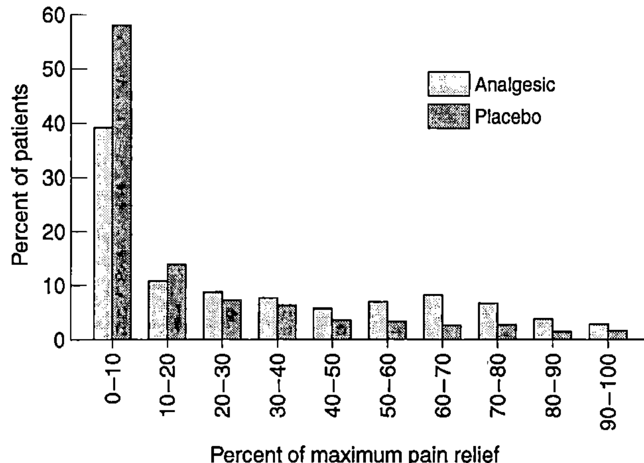

Fig. 48.9 Percentage of maximum pain relief obtained in single-dose randomized double-blind trials in postoperative pain for 826 patients given placebo and 3157 patients given analgesics. The percentage of patients achieving different degrees of success (percentage of maximum possible pain relief) with placebo and with active oral analgesics. The skewed distribution, with a greater proportion of placebo patients achieving minimal relief, is to be expected (McQuay et al 1996).

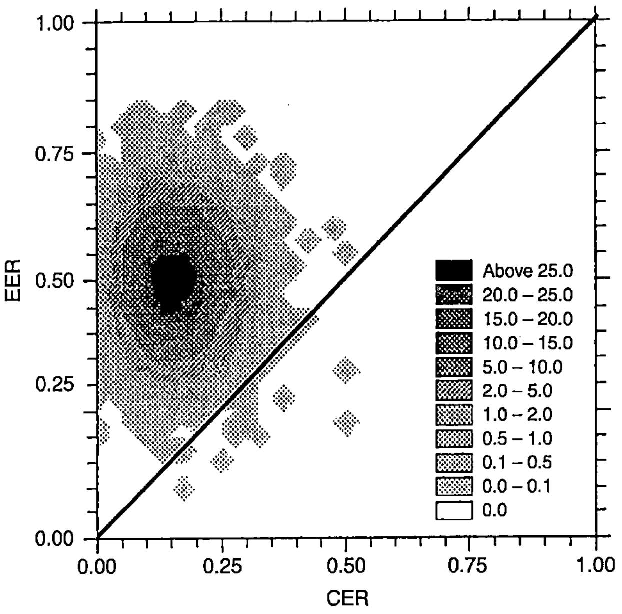

Fig. 48.10 Two-dimensional L'Abbé plot of the probability density for trials in acute postoperative pain. Simulated information for trials of different group size (minimum 10 patients), with an underlying 16% of patients achieving at least 50% pain relief with placebo, and 50% achieving at least 50% pain relief with active treatment. The scale represents the percentage density per unit area obtained with the 10 000 simulations, where the unit of area has been chosen as a square of side 0.1. The scale can therefore be interpreted as the percentage of trials that are likely to fall into a square of side 0.1 on any of the plots, so that the maximum density of just over 25% occurs only in a region of about three-quarters of a unit area, centred over the point (0.16, 0.5) that corresponds to the true CER and EER (i.e. approximately 0.75 × 0.25 × 10 000 = 1875 of the 10 000 simulated trials fell within this small area very close to the true value of the EER and CER).

range 30–60. For clinical credibility nearly 500 patients are required in each group. Only with an extremely effective drug (EER > 0.8) will we be reasonably sure of obtaining a clinically credible NNT with commonly used group sizes of around 40 patients per treatment arm. The simulated trials showed substantial variation in CER and EER, with the probability of obtaining the correct values improving as group size increased.

SO WHERE DOES THAT LEAVE US?

We contend that much of the variability in control and experimental event rates is due to random chance alone. Single small trials are unlikely to be correct. To be sure of getting correct (clinically credible) results in clinical trials, we must study more patients than the conventional 40 patients per group. Acute pain trials with 1000 patients are rare, so that credible estimates of clinical efficacy are only likely to come from large trials or from pooling multiple trials of conventional (small) size.

Size is everything. The variability in the response rates to both placebo and active treatments means that if we want to be sure of getting the correct (clinically credible) result in clinical trials, more patients must be studied than the conventional 40 patients per group, a number chosen to be sure (statistically) of not getting the wrong answer.

This variability in the response rates to both placebo and active treatments has been recognized before, and was blamed on either flaws in trial design and conduct or on non-specific effects of placebo (Evans 1974). We contend that much of this variability is a result of random chance alone, and abstruse causes need not be searched for. This variability is the likely cause of the two discordant reports of tramadol's efficacy (Sunshine et al 1992, Stubhaug et al 1995). It also justifies clinical conservatism, the caution necessary before taking the results of a single (small) trial into practice. Such a single small trial is unlikely to be correct. A trial with group sizes of 40 could have NNT values between 1 and 9 just by chance, when the true value was 3. The variability is not a pain-specific problem (Soll et al 1992, Tramer et al 1995, Ali & Goetz 1997).

Most clinical trials of analgesics are performed to demonstrate statistical superiority over placebo, and are powered to be sure (statistically) of not getting the wrong answer. To achieve this, group sizes of about 40 patients are used; 95% of the time this will yield the desired statistical superiority over placebo, given a useful intervention like 400 mg of ibuprofen (Moore et al 1998). But to reach a clinically credible estimate of efficacy, defined as a NNT within ± 0.5 of the true value, we need ten times as many patients (Moore et al 1998).

Acute pain trials with 1000 patients do not happen. This means that credible estimates of clinical efficacy are only likely to come by doing such large trials, or from pooling multiple trials of conventional (small) size. Those estimates also need data on 1000 patients to achieve this credibility.

Comparing Figures 48.8 and 48.10, all the points on Figure 48.8 fall within the variability predicted due to random chance alone. No other explanation is necessary. Only when we have substantial data should we investigate other possible influences such as pain model (Moore & McQuay 1997), population studied and nebulous environmental factors.

Powering trials for statistical significance is arguably not good enough, because the true size of the clinical effect will still be uncertain. Clinically useful trials also need clinically useful outcomes, as well as a trial size big enough to allow us to be confident about effect size. We need to know what degree of improvement on a particular scale matters to the patient (Guyatt et al 1998). This is quite a challenge to the way clinical trials are carried out at present, where the focus is on the minimum size necessary for statistical significance.

ADVERSE EFFECTS

Clinical trials concentrate on efficacy (Beaver 1983) and adverse effects are reported almost as an afterthought, even though good information was collected. However adverse effects are often the reason why patients stop taking the drug, or cannot tolerate an effective dose. In single-dose analgesic studies adverse effects of any severity are rare, and statistical power is calculated for efficacy and not adverse effects. Multiple-dose studies are more representative of clinical practice, and can yield dose–response relationships for both efficacy and adverse effects (McQuay et al 1993).

There are some obvious distinctions between the various ways of assessing adverse effects, and some more subtle ones. Perhaps the most important is whether or not a checklist is used. This could be presented verbally or on paper, and of course begs the question of how extensive a checklist. The alternative is a more open question(s), such as 'Have you had any problem with the drugs?'. The open question might result in lower reported adverse effect incidence than the checklist, and verbal lower than paper (Huskisson & Wojtulewski 1974, Myers et al 1987). The significance of any differences in incidence using the different methods is not clear. These complexities are often forgotten. The CONSORT guidelines for the reporting of clinical trials did include adverse effects (Begg et al 1996). Their recommendation was that trialists should 'define what constituted adverse events and how they were monitored by intervention group'.

In a systematic review of adverse effect reporting (Edwards et al 1999b), information on adverse effect assessment and reported results was extracted from 52 randomized single-dose postoperative trials of paracetamol or ibuprofen compared with placebo. Only two of the 52 trials made no mention of adverse effects. No method of assessment was given in 19 trials, patient diaries were used in 18, spontaneous reporting in seven and direct questioning in six. Clearly the standard of reporting could be improved. Studies which used patient diaries yielded a significantly higher incidence of adverse effects than those which used other forms of assessment.

In that review the single-dose studies were able to detect a difference between ibuprofen 400 mg and placebo for somnolence/drowsiness with ibuprofen 400 mg (number needed to harm 19 (95% confidence interval 12–41)). Nine out of the 10 trials reporting somnolence/drowsiness with ibuprofen 400 mg were in dental pain. Similarly in a review of 72 randomized single-dose trials of postoperative aspirin versus placebo, single-dose aspirin 600/650 mg produced significantly more drowsiness and gastric irritation than placebo, with numbers needed to harm of 28 (19–52) and 38 (22–174) respectively (Edwards et al 1999b).

The recommendations of the adverse effect review (Edwards et al 1998a) were that reports of trials should provide:

- Details of the type of anaesthetic used (if relevant).
- A description of the format of questions and/or checklists used in the assessment of adverse effects.
- Details of how the severity of adverse effects was assessed.
- Full details of the type and frequency of adverse effects reported for active drug and for placebo.
- Details of the severity of the reported adverse effects.
- Full details of adverse effect-related patient withdrawals.
- Where possible, the likely relationship between the adverse effect and the study drug.

CONCLUSION

Clinical trials in acute and chronic pain can achieve high levels of precision if they adhere to some simple rules. What current trials cannot give us is an accurate picture of the clinical effectiveness of an analgesic intervention, or a fair representation of the harm that may be caused. These both need much larger numbers of patients, and in future trial design may have to change to take this into account.

REFERENCES

Ali MZ, Goetz MB 1997 A meta-analysis of the relative efficacy and toxicity of single daily dosing versus multiple daily dosing of aminoglycosides. Clinical Infectious Diseases 24: 796–809

Beaver WT 1983 Measurement of analgesic efficacy in man. In: Bonica JJ, Lindblom U, Iggo A (ed) Advances in pain research and therapy, vol 5. Raven, New York, pp 411–434

Beecher HK 1955 The powerful placebo. Journal of the American Medical Association 159: 1602–1606

Begg C, Cho M, Eastwood S et al 1996 Improving the quality of reporting of randomized controlled trials. The CONSORT statement. Journal of the American Medical Association 276: 637–639

Bergmann J-F, Chassany O, Gandiol J et al 1994 A randomised clinical trial of the effect of informed consent on the analgesic activity of placebo and naproxen in cancer pain. Clinical Trials and Meta-Analysis 29: 41–47

Berrazueta JR, Losada A, Poveda J et al 1996 Successful treatment of shoulder pain syndrome due to supraspinatus tendinitis with transdermal nitroglycerin. A double blind study. Pain 66: 63–67

Carroll D, Tramer M, McQuay H, Nye B, Moore A 1996 Randomization is important in studies with pain outcomes: systematic review of transcutaneous electrical nerve stimulation in acute postoperative pain. British Journal of Anaesthesia 77: 798–803

Collins SL, Moore RA, McQuay HJ 1997 The visual analogue pain intensity scale: what is moderate pain in millimetres? Pain 72:95–97

Cook RJ, Sackett DL 1995 The number needed to treat: a clinically useful measure of treatment effect. British Medical Journal 310: 452–454

Cooper SA 1991 Single-dose analgesic studies: the upside and downside of assay sensitivity. The design of analgesic clinical trials. In: Max MB, Portenoy RK, Laska EM (eds) Advances in pain research and therapy, vol 18. Raven, New York, pp 117–124

Dahlstrom BE, Paalzow LK 1977 Pharmacokinetic interpretation of the enterohepatic recirculation and first-pass elimination of morphine in the rat. Journal of Pharmacokinetics and Biopharmaceutics 6: 505–519

Edwards JE, McQuay HJ, Moore RA, Collins SL 1999a Guidelines for reporting adverse effects in clinical trials should be improved – lessons from acute pain Journal of Pain and Symptom Management (in press)

Edwards JE, Oldman A, Smith L, Carroll D, Wiffen PJ et al 1999b Oral aspirin in postoperative pain: a quantitative systematic review Pain (in press)

Evans FJ 1974 The placebo response in pain reduction. In: Bonica JJ (ed) Advances in neurology, vol 4. Raven, New York, pp 289–296

Gøtzsche PC 1993 Meta-analysis of NSAIDs: contribution of drugs, doses, trial designs, and meta-analytic techniques. Scandinavian

Journal of Rheumatology 22: 255–260
Gracely RH, Dubner R, Deeter WR, Wolskee PJ 1985 Clinicians' expectations influence placebo analgesia. Lancet i: 43
Guyatt GH, Juniper EF, Walter SD, Griffith LE, Goldstein RS 1998 Interpreting treatment effects in randomised trials. British Medical Journal 316: 690–693
Haynes TK, Evans DEN, Roberts D 1995 Pain relief after day surgery: quality improvement by audit. Journal of One-day Surgery Summer: 12–15
Huskisson EC, Wojtulewski JA 1974 Measurement of side effects of drugs. British Medical Journal 2: 698–699
Jaeschke R, Singer J, Guyatt GH 1989 Measurement of health status: ascertaining the minimal clinically important difference. Controlled Clinical Trials 10: 407–415
Jaeschke R, Adachi J, Guyatt G, Keller J, Wong B 1991 Clinical usefulness of amitriptyline in fibromyalgia: the results of 23 N-of-1 randomized controlled trials. Journal of Rheumatology 18: 447–451
Jadad AR, McQuay HJ 1993 The measurement of pain. In: Pynsent P, Fairbank J, Carr A (eds) Outcome measures in orthopaedics. Butterworth Heinemann, Oxford pp 16–29
James KE, Forrest WH, Rose RL 1985 Crossover and noncrossover designs in four-point parallel line analgesic assays. Clinical Pharmacology and Therapeutics 37: 242–252
Jones B, Jarvis P, Lewis JA, Ebbutt AF 1996 Trials to assess equivalence: the importance of rigorous methods. British Medical Journal 313: 36–39
Kalso E, Tramer M, Carroll D, McQuay H, Moore RA 1997 Pain relief from intra-articular morphine after knee surgery: a qualitative systematic review. Pain 71: 642–651
Kalso E, Tramèr MR, Moore RA, McQuay HJ 1998 Systemic local anaesthetic type drugs in chronic pain: a qualitative systematic review. European Journal of Pain 2: 3–14
Keele KD 1948 The pain chart. Lancet ii: 6–8
Littman GS, Walker BR, Schneider BE 1985 Reassessment of verbal and visual analogue ratings in analgesic studies. Clinical Pharmacology and Therapeutics 38: 16–23
March L, Irwig L, Schwarz J et al 1994 N of 1 trials comparing a non-steroidal anti-inflammatory drug with paracetamol in osteoarthritis. British Medical Journal 309: 1041–1046
Max MB, Laska EM 1991 Single-dose analgesic comparisons. The design of analgesic clinical trials. In: Max MB, Portenoy RK, Laska EM (eds) Advances in pain research and therapy, vol 18. Raven, New York, pp 55–95
Max MB, Culnane M, Schafer SC et al 1987 Amitriptyline relieves diabetic neuropathy pain in patients with normal or depressed mood. Neurology 37: 589–596
McQuay HJ 1991 N of 1 trials. The design of analgesic clinical trials. In: Max MB, Portenoy RK, Laska EM (eds) Advances in pain research and therapy, vol 18. Raven, New York, pp 179–192
McQuay H, Moore A 1996 Placebos are essential when extent and variability of placebo response are unknown. British Medical Journal 313: 1008
McQuay HJ, Moore RA 1998 An evidence-based resource for pain relief. Oxford University Press, Oxford
McQuay HJ, Bullingham RE, Moore RA, Evans PJ, Lloyd JW 1982 Some patients don't need analgesics after surgery. Journal of the Royal Society of Medicine 75: 705–708
McQuay HJ, Carroll D, Guest PG et al 1993 A multiple dose comparison of ibuprofen and dihydrocodeine after third molar surgery. British Journal of Oral and Maxillofacial Surgery 31: 95–100
McQuay HJ, Carroll D, Jadad AR et al 1994 Dextromethorphan for the treatment of neuropathic pain: a double-blind randomised controlled crossover trial with integral n-of-1 design. Pain 59: 127–133
McQuay H, Carroll D, Moore A 1996 Variation in the placebo effect in randomised controlled trials of analgesics: all is as blind as it seems. Pain 64: 331–335
Moore RA, McQuay HJ 1997 Single-patient data meta-analysis of 3453 postoperative patients: oral tramadol versus placebo, codeine and combination analgesics. Pain 69: 287–294
Moore RA, Collins S, Gavaghan D, Tramèr M, McQuay HJ 1998 Size is everything – large amounts of information are needed to overcome random effects in estimating direction and magnitude of treatment effects. Pain 78: 209–216
Murphy DF, McDonald A, Power C, Unwin A, MacSullivan R 1988 Measurement of pain: a comparison of the visual analogue with a nonvisual analogue scale. Clinical Journal of Pain 3: 197–199
Myers MG, Cairns JA, Singer J 1987 The consent form as a possible cause of side effects. Clinical Pharmacology and Therapeutics 42: 250–253
Schulz KF, Chalmers I, Hayes RJ, Altman DG 1994 Failure to conceal treatment allocation schedules in trials influences estimates of treatment effects. Controlled Clinical Trials 15: 63S–64S
Schulz KF, Chalmers I, Hayes RJ, Altman DG 1995 Empirical evidence of bias: dimensions of methodological quality associated with estimates of treatment effects in controlled trials. Journal of the American Medical Association 273: 408–412
Schwartz D, Lellouch J 1967 Explanatory and pragmatic attitudes in therapeutic trials. Journal of Chronic Disease 20: 637–648
Scott J, Huskisson EC 1976 Graphic representation of pain. Pain 2: 175–184
Senn S (ed) 1993 Cross-over trials in clinical research. Wiley, Chichester
Senn S (ed) 1997 Statistical issues in drug development. Wiley, Chichester
Shapiro AP, Myers T, Reiser MF, Ferris EB 1954 Comparison of blood pressure response to veriloid and to the doctor. Psychosomatic Medicine 16: 478–488
Soll JC, McQueen MC 1992 Respiratory distress syndrome. In: Sinclair JC, Bracken ME (eds) Effective care of the newborn infant. Oxford University Press, Oxford, pp 333
Sriwatanakul K, Kelvie W, Lasagna L 1982 The quantification of pain: an analysis of words used to describe pain and analgesia in clinical trials. Clinical Pharmacology and Therapeutics 32: 141–148
Stubhaug A, Grimstad J, Breivik H 1995 Lack of analgesic effect of 50 and 100 mg oral tramadol after orthopaedic surgery: a randomized, double-blind, placebo and standard active drug comparison. Pain 62: 111–118
Sunshine A, Olson NZ, Zighelboim I, DeCastro A, Minn FL 1992 Analgesic oral efficacy of tramadol hydrochloride in postoperative pain. Clinical Pharmacology and Therapeutics 51: 740–746
Tramer M, Moore A, McQuay H 1995 Prevention of vomiting after paediatric strabismus surgery: a systematic review using the numbers-needed-to-treat method. British Journal of Anaesthesia 75: 556–561
Wall PD 1992 The placebo effect: an unpopular topic. Pain 51: 1–3
Wall PD 1993 Pain and the placebo response. Experimental and theoretical studies of consciousness. Wiley, Chichester, pp 187–216
Wall PD 1994 The placebo and the placebo response In: Wall PD, Melzack R (eds) Textbook of pain. Churchill Livingstone, Edinburgh, pp 1297–1308
Wallenstein SL, Heidrich IIIG, Kaiko R, Houde RW 1980 Clinical evaluation of mild analgesics: the measurement of clinical pain. British Journal of Clinical Pharmacology 10: 319S–327S

Antipyretic (non-narcotic) analgesics

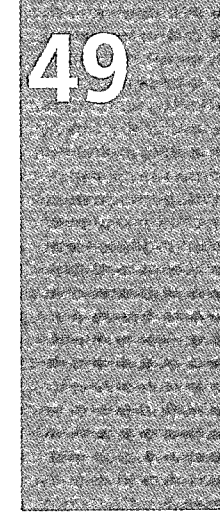

KAY BRUNE & HANNS ULRICH ZEILHOFER

INTRODUCTION

HISTORICAL REMARKS

Fever was the cardinal symptom of disease in hypocratic medicine. It was assumed to result from an imbalance of body fluids. Therefore it was the aim of hypocratic medicine to correct the balances of fluids by either bloodletting, purgation, sweating or, above all, applying drugs which normalize body temperature.

The main compound in the eighteenth and nineteenth century for that purpose was quinine, which became scarce in continental Europe during and after the Napoleonic wars as a result of the continental blockade. The emerging synthetic chemistry and drug industry concentrated on producing chemical analogues of quinine and its derivative quinoline as substitutes of the natural products. Also, pharmaceutical chemists attempted to isolate substances with similar antipyretic activity from other plants. The results of these efforts were the three prototypes of antipyretic non-narcotic analgesic drugs still in use. Building on the work of Piria in Italy, Kolbe synthesized salicylic acid as an antipyretic agent in 1874. In 1897 it was acetylated by Hoffmann to form aspirin. In 1882, Knorr and Filene, in Erlangen, synthesized and tested an analogue of, as they believed, quinoline, antipyrine which proved effective in the clinic. Almost at the same time Cahn and Hepp in Strassbourg found that acetanilide also reduced fever. They called it antifebrin and introduced it into therapy. Its less toxic derivatives phenacetin and paracetamol (acetaminophen) are still cornerstones of pain treatment worldwide.

In conclusion, it can be stated that the enthusiasm for antipyretic therapy resulted in the discovery of the three prototypes of antipyretic analgesics, which are still in use throughout the world and make up the millions of daily doses presented or bought over the counter (for details see Brune 1997).

For more than hundred a years little was known about the mode of action of these compounds. With the emergence of scientific (evidence based) medicine many puzzling results were obtained. It appeared as if salicylates, for example, were active in almost every system tested. They were found to interfere with the release of histamine, serotonin and adrenaline. They activated complement, induced the release of cytokines and the activation of leukocytes (Brune et al 1976). Only recently has a sufficient explanation of the mode of action of the antipyretic analgesics been made.

Experimental and clinical findings within the last 30 years have added to our understanding, so that a coherent pharmacological explanation of the effects and major side effects of the antipyretic analgesics may now be given. It started with the pioneering discovery of Sir John Vane and his co-workers that aspirin blocks the production of prostaglandins (Vane 1971). This simple monocausal explanation, however, could not reconcile all experimental findings (for a review see McCormack & Brune 1991, Brune & McCormack, 1994). For example, salicylic acid and paracetamol (acetaminophen) do not inhibit prostaglandin production in inflamed tissue at meaningful concentrations.

THE MODE OF ACTION

BIODISTRIBUTION OF ANTIPYRETIC ANALGESICS – EFFECTS

Following the discovery by Vane and co-workers of the inhibition of prostaglandin synthesis by aspirin-like drugs

(Vane 1971), we wondered why aspirin and its pharmacological relatives, the (acidic) non-steroidal anti-inflammatory drugs (NSAIDs, Table 49.1), exerted anti-inflammatory activity and analgesic effects, while the non-acidic drugs, phenazone and acetaminophen, were analgesic only (Graf et al 1975). It was speculated that all acidic anti-inflammatory analgesics, which are highly bound to plasma proteins and show a similar degree of acidity (pK_a values between 3.5 and 5.5), should lead to a specific drug distribution within the body of man or animals (Fig. 49.1). High concentrations of these compounds are reached in the bloodstream, the liver, spleen and bone marrow (due to high protein binding and an open endothelial layer of the vasculature), but also in body compartments with acidic extracellular pH values (Brune et al 1976). The latter type of compartments includes inflamed tissue, the wall of the upper GI tract and the collecting ducts of the kidneys. By contrast (Fig. 49.1) acetaminophen and phenazone, compounds with almost neutral pK_a values which are only scarcely bound to plasma proteins, should distribute almost homogeneously (and quickly) throughout the body, because of their ability to permeate barriers such as the blood–brain barrier easily (Brune et al 1980). It is obvious that the degree of inhibition of prostaglandin production because of inhibition of the responsible enzymes (the cyclooxygenases, Fig. 49.2) would depend on the potency of the drug and the local concentrations.

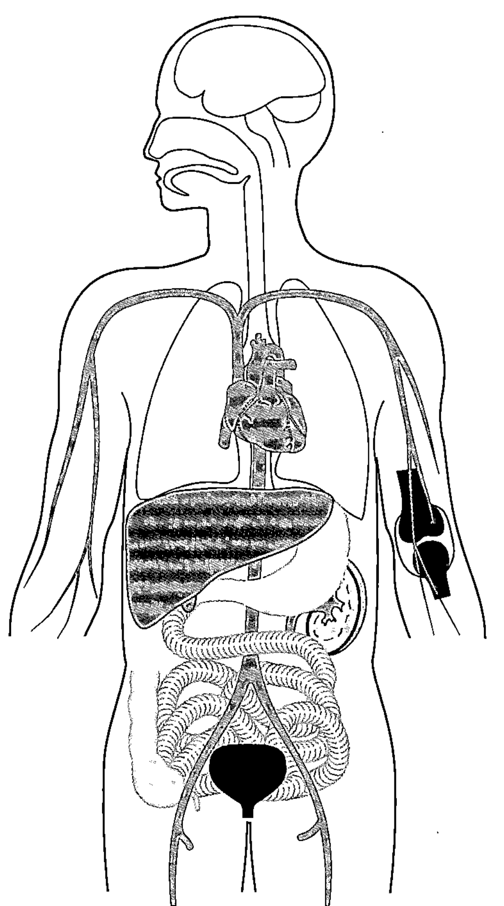

Fig. 49.1 Schematic representation of the distribution of acidic antipyretic analgesics in the human body (transposition of the data from animal experiments to human conditions). Dark areas indicate high concentrations of the acidic antipyretic analgesics, i.e. stomach and upper gastrointestinal-tract wall, blood, liver, bone marrow, spleen (not shown), inflamed tissue (e.g. joints), as well as the kidney (cortex > medulla). Some acidic antipyretic analgesics are excreted in part unchanged in urine and achieve high concentrations in this body fluid, others encounter enterohepatic circulation and are found in high concentrations as conjugates in the bile.

BIODISTRIBUTION OF ANTIPYRETIC ANALGESICS – SIDE EFFECTS

High drug concentrations as a result of drug accumulation (NSAIDs) should lead to an almost complete inhibition of cyclooxygenases in some body compartments, for example the inflamed tissue, bloodstream, stomach wall and the kidney, while equal distribution throughout the body might

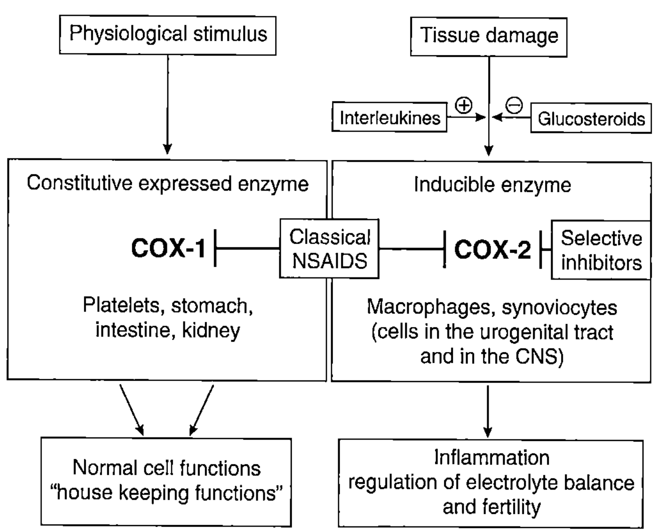

Fig. 49.2 Simplified description of the physiological and pathophysiological roles of COX 1 and 2. The COX 1 is expressed constitutively in most tissues and fulfills housekeeping functions by producing prostaglandins. The COX 2 is an inducible isoenzyme, which becomes expressed in inflammatory cells (e.g. macrophages and synoviocytes) after exposure to proinflammatory cytokines, and is downregulated by glucocorticoids. In the kidney (macula densa) and in other areas of the urogenital tract and in the CNS, COX 2 is already significantly expressed even in the absence of inflammation. The induction in peripheral and central nervous tissues of its expression appears most prominent in connection with inflammatory painful reactions. Both enzymes are blocked by classical acidic antipyretic analgesics (NSAIDs).

lead to some inhibition throughout. These observations and contentions did explain the fact that only the acidic, antipyretic analgesics (NSAIDs, Table 49.1) are anti-inflammatory and cause acute side effects in the GI tract (ulcerations), the bloodstream (inhibition of platelet aggregation) and the kidney (fluid and potassium retention), while the non-acidic drugs acetaminophen and phenazone, as well as their derivatives with similar physicochemical characteristics (Table 49.2), should be devoid of both the anti-inflammatory activity and the gastric and the (acute) renal toxicity. Finally, chronic inflammation of the upper respiratory tract, as in asthma, nasal polyps, etc., would lead to the accumulation of inflammatory prostaglandin-producing cells in the respiratory mucosa. Inhibition of cyclooxygenases shifts part of the metabolism of the prostaglandin precursor arachidonic acid into the production of leukotrienes (Fig. 49.3) which induce pseudoallergic reaction (aspirin asthma). These patients comprise a well-defined risk group (Hoigné & Szczeklik 1992) and should receive antipyretic analgesics, particularly acidic NSAIDs, only under the control of a physician. A couple of questions still remained unresolved for decades; these may be now answered by recent findings arising from molecular biological approaches. New aspects of the mode of action of the antipyretic analgesic drugs arose from two discoveries: one from molecular biology and another one from (molecular) neuropharmacology.

DIFFERENT CYCLOOXYGENASES

A couple of years ago molecular biology discovered that two different genes code for the enzymes comprising the so-called cyclooxygenases COX 1 and COX 2 (Fig. 49.2). They appear on different chromosomes and their expression is different. These enzymes were sequenced, cloned, expressed and investigated by crystallography (Kujubu et al 1991, O'Banion et al 1991). After the enzymes had been characterized and had become available, new compounds

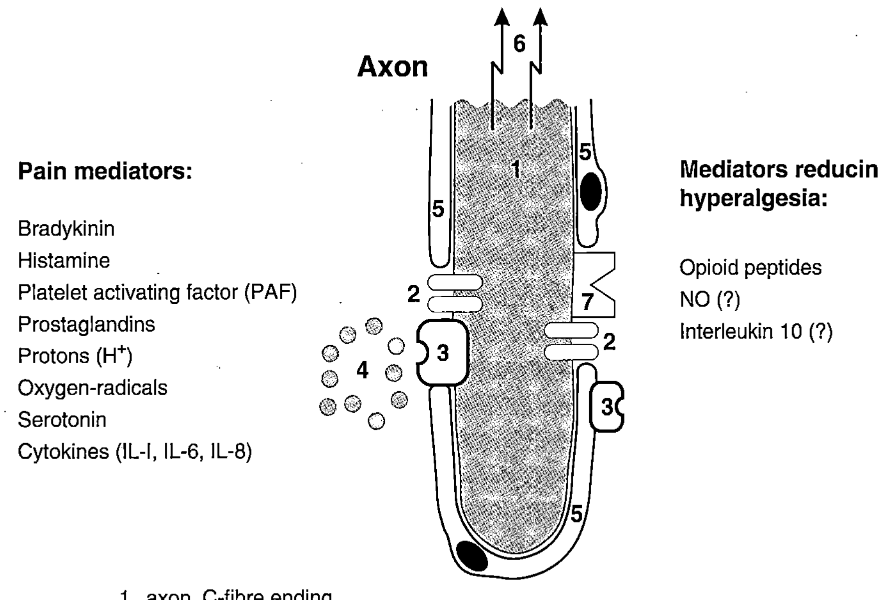

Fig. 49.3 Schematic representation of a polymodal (nociceptive) C-fibre ending. It is attempted to visualize the increase of sensitivity of a polymodal nociceptor due to proinflammatory (hyperalgetic) mediators. It is assumed that proalgetic (hyperalgetic) mediators either increase the sensitivity of receptor-coupled ion channels or influence the coverage of the C-fibre ending by, for example, contracting the covering Schwann cells. In addition, it has recently been shown that nociceptors may develop new (μ) receptors under the influence of cytokines. (Adapted from Heppelmann et al 1990.)

were investigated to determine their ability to selectively inhibit either enzyme (Patrignani et al 1994). It turned out that both enzymes insert as homodimers in the membranes of the endoplasmic reticulum (including the nuclear membrane) of most cells (Smith & De Witt 1996). The enzymes form a hydrophilic groove or channel opening through the membrane. The substrate (arachidonic acid) or a substrate inhibitor inserts into this groove. Interestingly, the COX 2 enzyme displays a slightly more roomy space than the COX 1, which makes a selective inhibition of COX 2 possible (Kurumball et al 1996). Nevertheless, most clinically useful antipyretic analgesics turned out finally to be rather unspecific inhibitors of both enzymes, although divergent claims may be found in the literature (Riendeau et al 1997, Tegeder et al 1998). However, some experimental compounds proved selective (Masferrer et al 1994, Riendeau et al 1997).

Using specific detection methods for both enzymes and these selective compounds, it was possible to show that both enzymes are differentially distributed throughout the body and that both enzymes are regulated differently. They may also serve different functions in health and disease (Vane 1994, Lipsky 1997). Summarizing these observations, it may be concluded that COX 1 is constitutively present in almost all tissues. It appears to produce more or less constant amounts of eicosanoids (prostaglandins and related substances, Fig. 49.3) maintaining homeostasis in many organs, for example stomach, lung, kidney and others. In some organs however (e.g. the female genital tract), the activity of both COX 1 and COX 2 appears to be regulated by steroid hormones (oestrogens and gestagens, Lim et al 1997, Deysk personal communication). On the other hand, COX 2 appears to be expressed constitutively in the central nervous system and the urogenital tract. During inflammatory disease states COX 2 becomes expressed in macrophages and other cells in inflamed tissue (Harris et al 1994, Seibert et al 1994, Beiche et al 1996). In the two organ systems and the inflamed tissue the expression of the enzyme is suppressed by glucocorticoids (Masferrer et al 1992, Yamagata et al 1993). From this observation it was concluded that a selective inhibition of COX 2 may be sufficient to achieve analgesic/anti-inflammatory effects but would spare the GI tract and most organ systems. This concept is presently being tested by both enzyme-selective inhibitors as well as so-called knock-out (k.o.) mice (see below).

ANIMALS LACKING CYCLOOXYGENASES

Soon after the discovery of the genes of the two cyclooxygenases mice were generated which were deficient in one of the enzymes coding for COX 1 or COX 2, the so-called k.o. mice. Eliminating the gene in fertilized oocytes leads to viable animals which lack the enzyme and may be tested in physiological and pharmacological experiments. Finally it was possible to create so-called double k.o. cells (the corresponding animals did not survive outside the uterus) which lack COX 1 and COX 2. These animals are presently also used for physiological and pharmacological experiments (Kirtikara et al 1998). The most important results of these experiments are briefly described. COX 1 k.o. mice show no major functional deficits. They show nociceptive reflexes and fever as well as inflammation. Interestingly, these animals get ulcers when treated with NSAIDs (Langenbach et al 1995). COX 2 k.o. mice are born with severe renal dysfunctions and usually die within 2–3 months after birth. Their nociceptive reflexes are apparently impaired and they do not develop fever (Dinchuck et al 1995, Morham et al 1995, SG Morham, personal communication, 1998), but inflammatory responses are normal in several standard models. Female COX 2 k.o. mice are infertile (Dinchuck et al 1995, Lim et al 1997).

These astonishing observations may explain some facets of the mode of action of classical antipyretic analgesics. The possibility of blocking COX 2 specifically has led to new drugs which are currently being introduced into clinical use (Table 49.2). They have definitely been shown to exert analgesic effects in osteoarthritis (Lane 1997).

MECHANISMS OF HYPERALGESIA

Before discussing these new insights some neurobiological observations shall also be described. Recent findings shed light on the molecular basis of sensitizations to painful stimuli. It could be shown that prostaglandins regulate the sensitivity of so-called polymodal nociceptors. These receptors are present in almost all tissues throughout the body. A significant portion of these nociceptors cannot easily be activated by physiological stimuli as (mild) pressure or (some) increase of temperature (Schaible & Schmidt 1988, Kress et al 1992). Following tissue trauma and the release of prostaglandins, these 'silent' polymodal nociceptors become responsive (Neugebauer et al 1995). They change their characteristics and become excitable to pressure, temperature changes and tissue acidosis (Weissmann 1993). This process results in a phenomenon called hyperalgesia – in some instances allodynia (for details see Ch. 10).

It has recently been shown that prostaglandin E2 and other inflammatory mediators facilitate the activation of tetrodotoxin-resistant Na^+ channels in dorsal root ganglion neurons (England et al 1996, Gold et al 1996). A certain type of TTX-resistant Na^+ channel has recently been cloned (Akopian et al 1996) and it appears to be selectively expressed in small- and medium-sized dorsal root ganglion neurons. Compelling evidence indicates that these small DRG neurons are the somata which give rise to thinly and unmyelinated C and Aδ nerve fibres, which mainly conduct nociceptive stimuli. Modulation of these Na^+ channels involves activation of adenylate cyclase and increases in c-AMP, possibly leading to protein kinase A-dependent phosphorylation of the channels. By this or a similar mechanism prostaglandins produced during inflammatory responses may significantly increase the excitability of nociceptive nerve fibres and this or a similar mechanism may also contribute to the activation of 'sleeping nociceptors'. It appears reasonable that at least part of the peripheral antinociceptive action of antipyretic analgesics arises from prevention of this sensitization. Figure 49.3 summarizes mechanisms of activation and sensitization of the nociceptive primary afferent terminal.

Besides this sensitization of peripheral nociceptors, prostaglandins may also act in the central nervous system (CNS) to produce hyperalgesia in the spinal cord dorsal horn (Neugebauer et al 1995). Some of these central forms of hyperalgesia seem to be reversed by inhibition of prostaglandin synthesis. The role of cyclooxygenase in the CNS is not yet entirely clear. It has, however, been shown that COX 2 expression is induced in the hippocampus during epileptiform activity (Yamagata et al 1993). It appears likely that COX 2 expression is increased via NMDA receptor-activation and a calcium-dependent mechanism in the CNS. Activity-dependent increases in COX 2 mRNA have been demonstrated in the spinal cord which by a so far unknown mechanism might facilitate transmission of nociceptive input (Beiche et al 1996). COX 1 and 2 are expressed constitutively there. COX 2 becomes upregulated briefly after damage of, for example, a paw (limb) trauma in the corresponding sensory segments of the spinal cord (Beiche et al 1996). There is now also evidence that the analgesic action of antipyretic analgesics in the spinal cord might be not only a result of reduced prostaglandin levels, but also an increase of other arachidonic acid metabolites (Vaughan et al 1997). Production of 12-HPETEs appears to be a mediator of opioid-induced analgesia in the midbrain and these recent findings may provide a molecular basis for the purported clinical potentiation of opioid action by antipyretic analgesics (Williams 1997) (Fig. 49.4). Moreover, it could be shown that the non-acidic antipyretic analgesic of the phenazone type exerts its analgesic effects predominantly in the spinal cord, which is easily accessible to these compounds because of the physicochemical characteristics allowing for fast passage through the blood–brain barrier (Neugebauer et al 1995). Finally, there are findings suggesting that new selective non-acidic COX 2 inhibitors (Table 49.2) may be weaker analgesics than the conventional drugs. This may be caused by their high degree of lipophilicity in concert with negligible solubility in aqueous solutions, leading to limited diffusion into the CNS after oral administration. It may also indicate that inhibition of both COX 2 and COX 1 is necessary for the treatment of acute pain (Dirig et al 1997, 1998).

ACIDIC ANTIPYRETIC ANALGESICS IN CLINICAL USE

Based on the finding that aspirin at high doses (> 3 g/day) not only inhibits fever and pain but also interferes with inflammation, i.e. swelling, redness and warming of the tissues. Winter in the USA developed an assay to search for drugs with a similar profile of activity (Winter et al 1962, Otterness & Bliven 1985). Within the past 40 years hundreds of those compounds were discovered. Amazingly, all which survived the test of experimental pharmacology and clinical trials turned out to be acids with a high degree of lipophilic-hydrophilic polarity, similar pK_a values and, in vivo, a high degree of plasma protein binding (Table 49.1). Suggestions for their clinical use may be found in Tables 49.3 and 49.4.

Apart from aspirin, all these compounds differ in two characteristics, their potency, i.e. the single dose necessary to achieve a certain degree of effect, ranging between a few milligrams (lornoxicam) to about 1 g (e.g. salicylic acid). They may also differ in their pharmacokinetic characteristics, i.e. the speed of absorption (time to peak, t_{max}; which may also depend heavily on the galenic formulation used), the maximal plasma concentrations (c_{max}), the elimination half-life ($t_{1/2}$) and the oral bioavailability (AUC_{rel}). Interestingly, all the widely used drugs lack a relevant degree of so-called COX 2 selectivity, in other words, an inhibition of COX 2 at concentrations (doses) which do not block COX 1. This is surprising, because they have all been selected on the basis of their high anti-inflammatory potency and low gastrotoxicity (which is believed to depend on COX 1 inhibition). The key characteristics of the most important NSAIDs have been compiled in Table 49.1

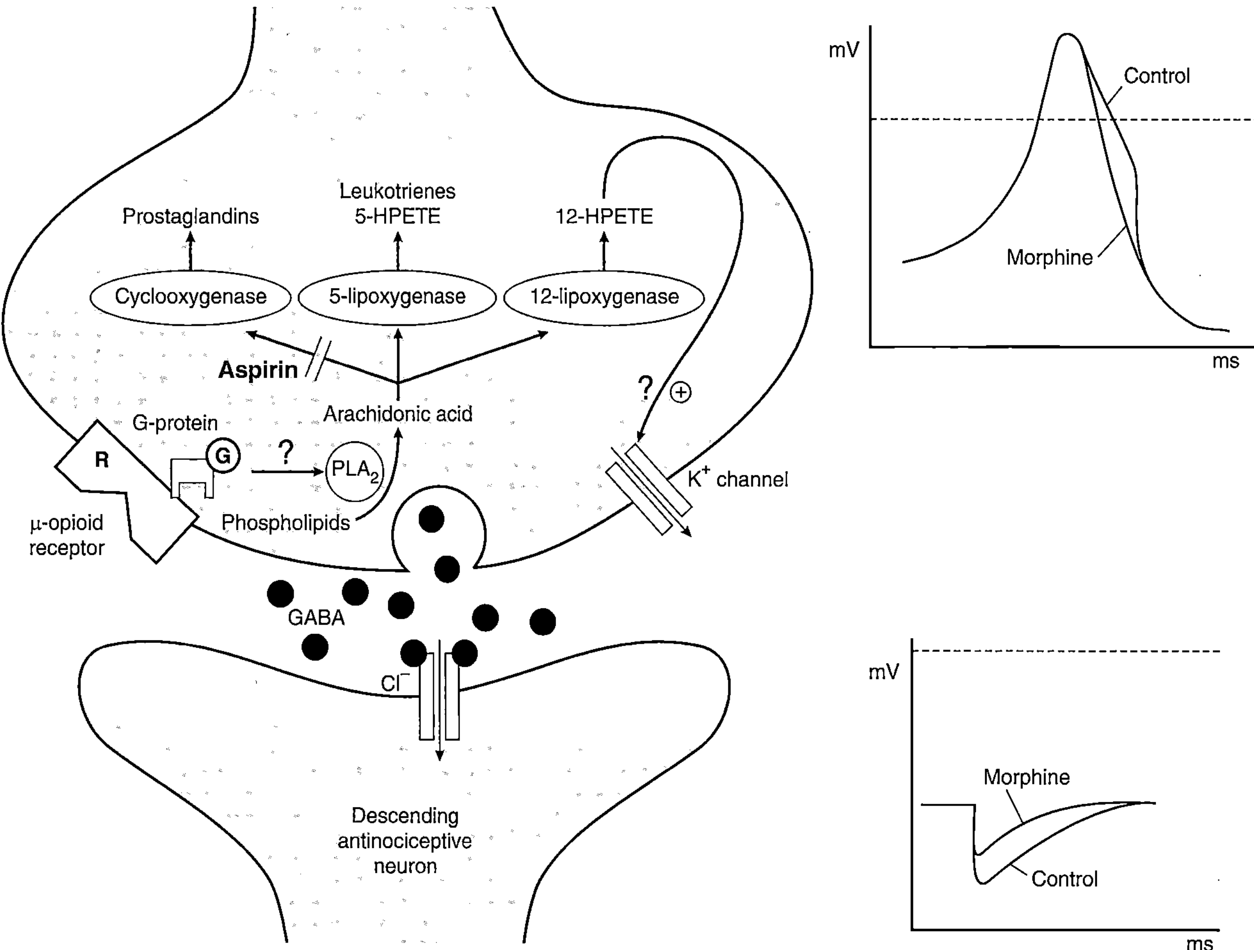

Fig. 49.4 Some of the antinociceptive actions of opioid peptides are located in the midbrain. In this brain region, μ-opioid agonists located at the presynaptic terminals of inhibitory GABAergic interneurons activate phospholipase A_2 (PLA_2) via a so far unknown mechanism. This in turn leads to an increase in intracellular concentration of arachidonic acid, the substrate of at least three enzymes: the cyclooxygenases, 5-lipoxygenase and 12-lipoxygenase. Among the products of the 12-lipoxygenase are the 12-HPETEs, which according to the model presented here activate a potassium conductance and thereby shorten action potential duration (the inset shows an action potential under control conditions and in the presence of opioids). Shortening of the action potential leads to a decrease in the amount of GABA released into the synaptic cleft. The reduction in GABA concentration may cause a 'disinhibition' of a descending 'antinociceptive' neuron. Inhibitory postsynaptic potentials become smaller due to the presynaptic action of opioids. Inhibitors of the cyclooxygenases like aspirin may facilitate the action of opioids in this model by enhancing the concentration of arachidonic acid and thereby increase the production of 12-HPETEs at the expense of prostaglandin formation.

(most data are from Herzfeldt & Kümmel 1983, Verbeck et al 1983, Brune & Lanz 1985).

Table 49.1 also contains the data on aspirin, which differs in many respects from the other NSAIDs and should, because of its historical and actual importance, be discussed at the end of this chapter in detail. Otherwise the drugs can be categorized into four different groups:

(a) NSAIDs with low potency and short elimination half-life.
(b) NSAIDs with high potency and short elimination half-life.
(c) NSAIDs with intermediate potency and intermediate elimination half-life.
(d) NSAIDs with high potency and long elimination half-life.

These differences, in contrast to the chemical heterogeneity, have some bearing on the optimal clinical use (Tables 49.3, 49.4).

Table 49.1 Acidic antipyretic analgesics (anti-inflammatory antipyretic analgesics, NSAIDs): chemical classes, structures, physicochemical and pharmacological data, therapeutic dosage

Chemical/pharmacokinetic subclasses	*Structure (prototype)* *Lipophil* *Hydrophil*	*pK$_a$(binding to plasma proteins) (%)*	*t_{max}[1] time to peak plasma concentration*	*$t_{1/2}$[2] elimination half-line*	*Oral bioavailability (%)*	*Single dose (range)/ Daily dose (max) In adults*
a) *Low potency/fast elimination:*	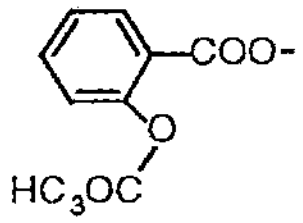 aspirin					
Salicylates						
Aspirin[1]		3.5(>80)	~0.25 h[3]	~20 min[3]	20–70	(0.05–0.1 g)/~6 g[2]
Salicylic acid		2.9(>90)	(0.5–2 h)[4]	2.5–7 h[5]	80–100	(0.5–1 g)/6 g
Arylpropionic acids	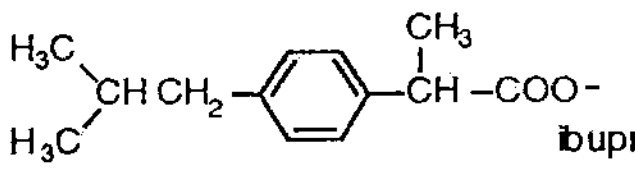 ibuprofen					
Ibuprofen		4.4(99)	0.5–2 h	2–4 h	80–100	(0.2–0.4 g)/3.2 g
Anthranilic acids						
Mefenamic acid		4.2(>90)	2–4 h	1–2 h		(0.25–0.5 g)/1.25 g
b) *High potency/fast elimination:*	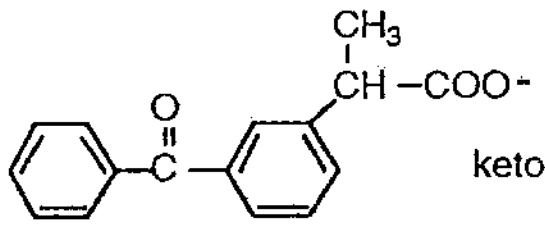 ketoprofen					
Arylpropionic acids						
Flurbiprofen						
Ketoprofen		4.2(99)	0.5–2 h	1.1–4 h	~90	(15–100 mg)/300 mg
Arylacetic acids	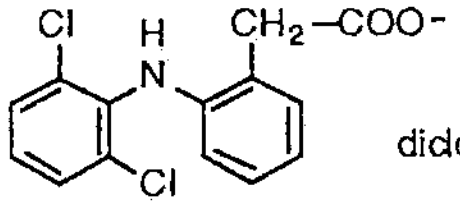 diclofenac					
Diclofenac		4(99)	0.5–24 h[6]	1–2 h	30–80[5]	(25–75 mg)/200 mg
		4.5(99)	0.5–2 h	2.6-(11.2 h)[7]	90–100	(25–75 mg)/200 mg
Indomethacin						
Ketorolac						
Oxicam		4.9(99)	0.5–2 h	4–10 h	~100	(4–12 mg)/16 mg
Lornoxicam	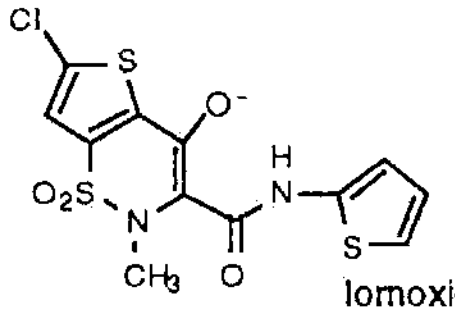 lornoxicam					
c) *Intermediate potency/ intermediate elimination speed:*	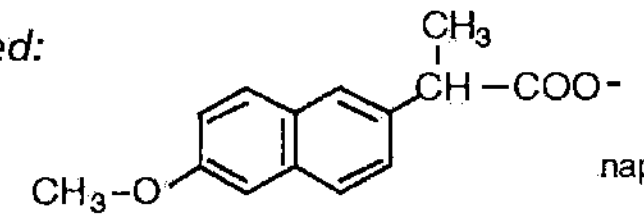 naproxen					
Salicylates						
Diflunisal		3.8(98–99)	2–3 h	8–12 h	80–100	(250–500 mg)/1 g
Arylpropionic acids						
Naproxen	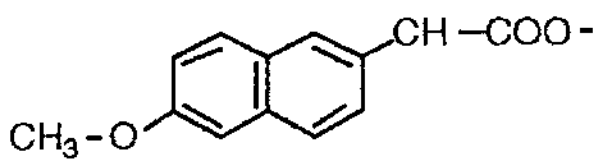 6MNA	4.15(99)	2–4 h	13–15 h[7]	~95	(0.5–1 g)/2 g
Arylacetic acids						
6 MNA (from Nabumetone)[8]		4.2	3–6 h	20–24 h	20–50 h	(0.5–1 g)/1.5 g

[1] Time to reach maximum plasma concentration after oral administration.
[2] Terminal half-life of elimination.
[3] Of aspirin the prodrug of salicylic acid.
[4] Depending on galenic formulation.
[5] Dose dependent.
[6] Monolithic acid-resistant tablet or similar form.
[7] Enterohepatic circulation.
[8] 6MNA, active metabolite of nabumetone.

Data from Brune and Lanz, 1985; Herzfeld and Kümmel, 1983; Verbeeke et al., 1983.

Table 49.1 (Contd.)

Chemical/pharmacokinetic subclasses	*Structure (prototype)* *Lipophil* *Hydrophil*	pK_a*(binding to plasma proteins) (%)*	t_{max}[1] *time to peak plasma concentration*	$t_{1/2}$[2] *elimination half-line*	*Oral bioavailability (%)*	*Single dose (range)/ Daily dose (max) In adults*
d) ***High potency/slow elimination*** **Oxicams** Meloxicam Piroxicam	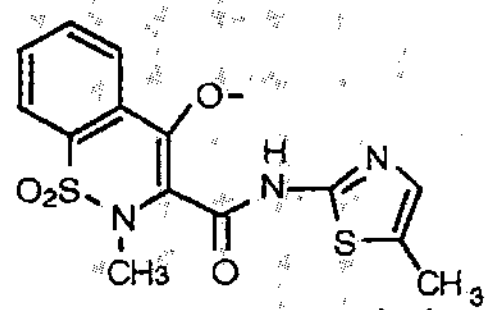 meloxicam	5.1>(99)	3–5 h	14–160 h[7]	~100	(20–40 mg)/initially: 40 mg
Tenoxicam	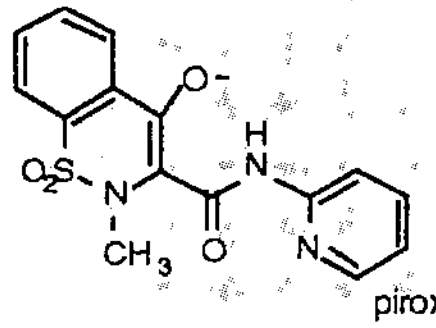 piroxicam	5.0>(99)	3–5 h	25–175 h[7]	~100	(20–40 mg)/initially: 40 mg

[1] Time to reach maximum plasma concentration after oral administration.
[2] Terminal half-life of elimination.
[3] Of aspirin the prodrug of salicylic acid.
[4] Depending on galenic formulation.
[5] Dose dependent.
[6] Monolithic acid-resistant tablet or similar form.
[7] Enterohepatic circulation.
[8] 6MNA, active metabokite of nabumetone.

Data from Brune and Lanz, 1985; Herzfeld and Kümmel, 1983; Verbeeke et al., 1983.

Table 49.2 Non-acidic antipyretic analgesics: chemical classes, structures, pharmacokinetic data, therapeutic dosage

Chemical pharmacological class monosubstance	*Structure*	*Fraction bound to plasma proteins (%)*	t_{max}[1]	$t_{1/2}$[2]	*Oral bioavailability (%)*	*Daily dose (single dose) In adults*
Aniline derivatives Paracetamol (acetaminophen)	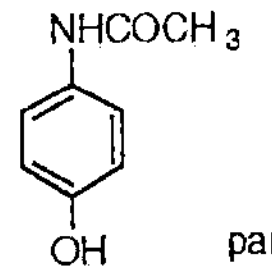 paracetamol	5–50 dose dependent	0.5–1.5 h	1.5–2.5 h	70–100	1–6 g/(0.5–1 g)
Phenazonderivatives (pyrazolinone[3]) Phenazone (antipyrine)	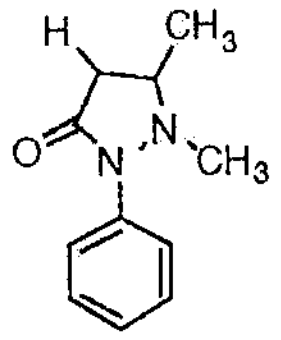 phenazone	<10	0.5–2 h	5–24 h	~100	1–6 g/(0.5–2 g)
Propyphenazone (isopropylantipyrine)	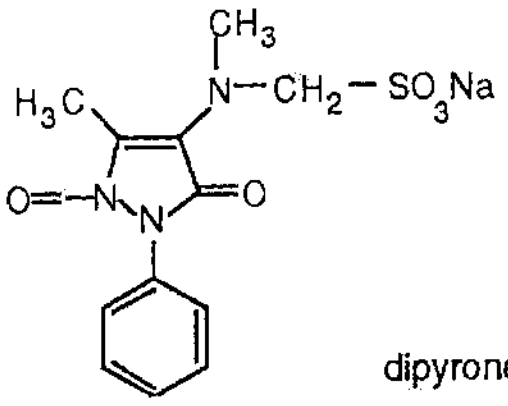	~10	0.5–1.5 h	1–2.5 h	~100	1–6 g/(0.5–1 g)
Metamizole-Na (dipyrone-Na)[4]	dipyrone	<20	—	—	—	1–6 g/(0.5–2 g)
4-MAP[5]		~50	1–2 h	2–4 h	~100	—
4-AP[6] (active metabolites)		~50		4–5.5 h		—
Selective COX-2 inhibitors[7] Celecoxib (Celebra®)[8]	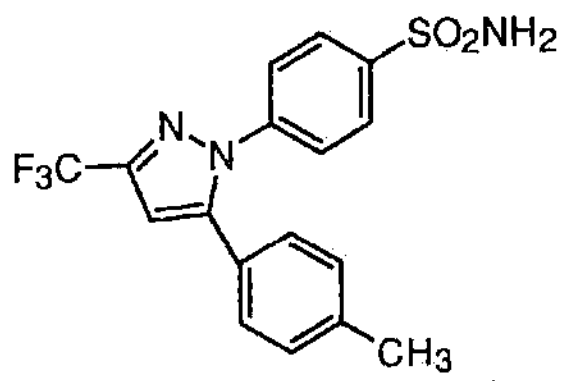 celecoxib	~97	2–4 h	9–15 h	70–80	400 mg/ (100–200 mg)
Rofecoxib (Vioxx®)[9]	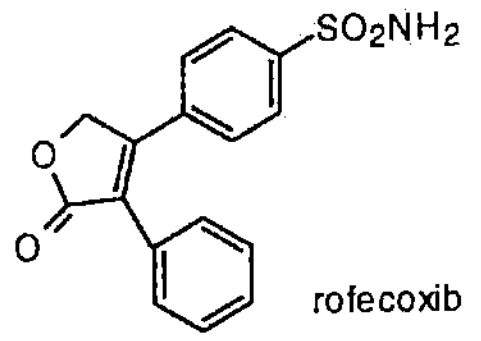 rofecoxib	?	2–4 h	~12 h	?	50 mg/ (12.5–25 mg)

[1] Time to reach maximum plasma concentration after oral administration.
[2] Terminal half-life of elimination, dependent on liver function with phenazone.
[3] Terms like pyrazole and, incorrectly, pyrazolone are also in use.
[4] Noraminopyrinemethanosulfonate-Na.
[5] 4-MAP=4-methylaminophenazone.
[6] 4-AP=4-aminophenazone.
[7] Other antipyretic analgesics (exception: acetaminophen) block both COXs at therapeutic concentrations.
[8] Launch expected in 1998, data with permission of Searle, proven effect in osteoarthritis.
[9] Launch expected in 1999, data with permission of MSD, proven effect in osteoarthitis.

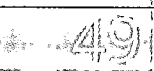

NSAIDS WITH LOW POTENCY AND SHORT ELIMINATION HALF-LIFE

The prototype of a type (a) compound is ibuprofen. Depending on the galenic formulation, fast or slow absorption may be achieved (Laska et al 1986). Fast absorption is seen for example when it is given as lysin salt (Geisslinger et al 1993). The bioavailability of ibuprofen is close to 100% and the elimination is always fast, even in patients suffering from mild or severe impairment of the liver (metabolism) or kidney function (Brune & Lanz 1985). Therefore, ibuprofen is used in single doses between 200 mg and 1 g. A maximum dose of 3.2 g per day (USA) or 2.4 g (Europe) for rheumatoid arthritis is possible. Ibuprofen (at low doses) appears particularly useful for the treatment of acute occasional inflammatory pain. It may also be used, although with less benefit, in chronic rheumatic diseases (high doses). At high doses the otherwise harmless compound increases in toxicity (Kaufman et al 1993). Ibuprofen is also used as a pure *S*-enantiomer because only this enantiomer is a (direct) COX inhibitor. On the other hand, the *R*-enantiomer, comprising 50% of the usual racemic mixture, is converted to the *S*-enantiomer in the human body (Rudy et al 1991). Therefore, it has not been proven but it is possible that the use of the pure *S*-enantiomer offers any therapeutic or toxicological benefit (Mayer & Testa 1997). Other drugs of this group are salicylates and *some* mefenamic acid. The latter does not appear to offer major advantages; on the contrary, this compound and other fenamates are rather toxic at overdosage (CNS). The drugs of this group are particularly useful for blocking occasional mild inflammatory pain.

NSAIDS WITH HIGH POTENCY AND SHORT ELIMINATION HALF-LIFE

The drugs of group (b) are prevailing in the therapy of rheumatic (arthritic) pain. The most widely used compound worldwide is diclofenac, which appears to be slightly less active on COX 1 when compared to COX 2 (Tegeder et al 1998). This is taken as a reason for the relatively low incidence of gastrointestinal side effects (Henry et al 1996). The limitations of diclofenac result from the usual galenic formulation, consisting of a monolythic acid-resistant encapsulation. This may cause retarded absorption of the active ingredient, due to retention of such monolythic formulations in the stomach for hours or even days (Brune & Lanz 1985). Moreover, diclofenac encounters a considerable first-pass metabolism which causes limited (about 50%) oral bioavailability. Consequently lack of therapeutic effect may require adaptation of dosage or change of the drug. New galenic formulations (microencapsulations, salts, etc.) remedy some of these deficits. The slightly higher incidences of liver toxicity with diclofenac may result from the high degree of first-pass metabolism, but other interpretations appear feasible. Group (b) contains important drugs such as lornoxicam, flubiprofen and indomethacin (very potent), but also ketoprofen and fenoprofen (less active). All of them show a high oral bioavailability and good effectiveness, but also a relatively high risk of unwanted drug effects (Henry et al 1996). The drugs of this group are widely used in arthritis and osteoarthritis.

NSAIDS WITH INTERMEDIATE POTENCY AND INTERMEDIATE ELIMINATION HALF-LIFE

The third group is intermediate in potency and speed of elimination. Some form of migraine and menstrual cramps appear adequate indications for diflunisal and, a drug which has been better investigated, naproxen.

NSAIDS WITH HIGH POTENCY AND LONG ELIMINATION HALF-LIFE

The fourth group (d) consists of the oxicams (meloxicam, piroxicam and tenoxicam). These compounds owe their slow elimination to slow metabolism together with a high degree of enteropathic circulation (Brune & Lanz 1985, Schmid et al 1995). The long half-life (days) does not make these oxicams drugs of first choice for acute pain of (probably) short duration. Their main indication is inflammatory pain which is likely to persist for days, i.e. pain resulting from chronic polyarthritis or even cancer (bone metastases). The high potency and long persistence in the body may be the reason for the *somewhat* higher incidence of serious adverse drug effects in the gastrointestinal (GI) tract and the kidney (Henry et al 1996).

COMPOUNDS OF SPECIAL INTEREST

A few compounds deserve special discussion. The most popular one is aspirin (Table 49.1). Aspirin actually comprises two active compounds, acetic acid which is released before, during and after absorption and salicylic acid (the residue). Acetylsalicylic acid is about hundred times more potent as inhibitor of cyclooxygenases than salicylic acid, which is practically devoid of this effect at analgesic doses. The acetate released from aspirin acetylates a serin residue in the active centre(s) of COX 1 (highly effective) and COX

2 (less effective). Consequently, aspirin inactivates both cyclooxygenases permanently. (Building on this knowledge bulkier aspirin analogues, acetylating exclusively COX 2, are being investigated at present (Kalgutkar et al 1998).) However, most cells compensate for this enzyme loss by the production of a new enzyme with the exception of blood platelets. Therefore a single dose of aspirin blocks the platelet COX 1 and therefore thromboxane synthesis for many days. When low doses are applied, absorbed aspirin acetylates the COX 1 of platelets passing through the capillary bed of the gastrointestinal tract but not the cyclooxygenase of endothelial cells (prostacyclin synthetase) outside the gut. This is because of the rapid cleavage of aspirin leaving little if any unmetabolized aspirin after primary liver passage. These latter cells continue to release prostacyclin and maintain their antithrombotic activity. Thus low-dose aspirin has its only indication in the prevention of thrombotic and embolic events. It may cause bleeding from existing ulcers due to its long-lasting platelet effect and topical irritation of the gastrointestinal mucosa.

Aspirin may be used as solution (effervescent) or as (lysine-) salt, allowing for very fast absorption, distribution and fast pain relief. The inevitable irritation of the gastric mucosa may be acceptable in otherwise healthy patients. It may be added that the old claims that aspirin is less toxic to the GI tract than salicylic acid are not based on scientific evidence but dates from a letter by the father of the discoverer, Hoffmann. He found his daily dose of 10 g of aspirin much more palatable than the same amount of sodium salicylate.

Aspirin should not be used in pregnant women (premature bleeding, closure of ductus arteriosus) or children before puberty (Reye's syndrome).

Recently it has been claimed that the relatively new drugs nabumetone, etodolac and meloxicam are particularly well tolerated by the Gl tract because they inhibit predominantly the COX 2. These results are not fully accepted. The active metabolite of nabumetone shows no selectivity for COX 2, the selectivity of etodolac and meloxicam is not superior to that of diclofenac when tested ex vivo in humans (Patrignani et al 1994, Riendeau et al 1997).

New hopes rest on some acidic, highly protein-bound selective COX 2 inhibitors which are in the 'pipeline' in several companies. It will have to be shown if these compounds are equally effective but devoid of important unwanted drug effects when compared to the well-known drugs that have been used in large quantities for years.

Two of the COX 2 selective inhibitors, which will probably be used clinically soon, are listed in Table 49.2. Their pharmacokinetic characteristics (slow absorption, slow elimination) makes them unlikely candidates for acute pain of short duration. They have, however, both been shown to work in osteoarthritic pain (Lane 1997). As in all non-acidic compounds, but also in line with the COX 2 concept, these compounds appear devoid of GI toxicity. They appear, however, to influence water and salt excretion by the kidneys.

NON-ACIDIC ANTIPYRETIC ANALGESICS

ANILINE DERIVATIVES

The remaining representative of this group which was discovered at the same time as aspirin is acetaminophen. The pharmacokinetic and pharmacodynamic data are compiled in Table 49.2. It may be stated that acetaminophen is a very weak, possibly indirect, inhibitor of cyclooxygenases. Evidence that acetaminophen, which is clearly antipyretic and (weakly) analgesic, is indeed working through cyclooxygenase inhibition, comes from COX 2 k.o. mice which do not develop fever (SG Morham, personal communication). Induction of fever is clearly blocked by acetaminophen in several species. The major advantage of acetaminophen consists of its relative lack of (serious) side effects provided that the dose limits (approximately 1 g/10 kg body weight per day) are obeyed, yet serious events were observed with low doses in a few cases (Bridger et al 1998). Acetaminophen is metabolized to highly toxic nucleophilic benzoquinones which bind covalantly to DNA and structural proteins in parenchymal cells as, for example liver and kidney, where these reactive intermediates are produced (Fig. 49.5) (for a review see Seeff et al 1986). The consequence is cell death and death of the whole organism as a result of liver necrosis. Early detection of overdosage can be antagonized (within the first 12 hours after intake). The administration of an *N*-acetylcysteine or glutathion regenerates the detoxifying mechanisms (Fig. 49.5). The predominant indication of paracetamol is fever and mild forms of pain seen in the context of viral infections but not in, for example, postoperative pain (Fig. 49.5). Many patients with recurrent headache also benefit from acetaminophen and its low toxicity. Acetaminophen is also used in children, but because of its somewhat lower toxicity in juvenile patients lethal effects from (unvoluntary) overdosage are seen.

To what extent acetaminophen in combination with aspirin and caffeine acts synergistically (Laska et al 1984), but also causes so-called analgesic nephropathy, is unclear (Porter 1996). Also, claims that such combinations are more frequently abused than single-entity analgesics are supported only by (weak) epidemiological data. The mech-

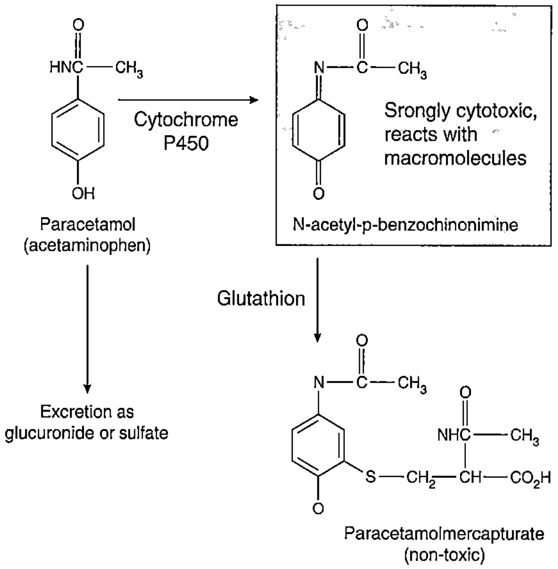

Paracetamol (acetaminophen)

Cytochrome P450

Srongly cytotoxic, reacts with macromolecules

N-acetyl-p-benzochinonimine

Glutathion

Excretion as glucuronide or sulfate

Paracetamolmercapturate (non-toxic)

Fig. 49.5 Schematic diagram of the metabolism of paracetamol (acetaminophen). At therapeutic doses most of the paracetamol is metabolized in the liver in a phase II reaction and excreted as glucuronide or sulfate. At higher doses the responsible enzymes become saturated and paracetamol is metabolized in the liver via a P450-dependent mechanism, which leads to the formation of *N*-acetyl-*p*-benzochinonimine, a highly cell toxic metabolite. This metabolite can initially be detoxified via a glutathion-dependent step to paracetamolmercapturate. At doses beyond 100 mg/kg the glutathion becomes exhausted and *N*-acetyl-*p*-benzochinonimine now reacts with macromolecules in hepatocytes, leading to cell death and acute liver failure.

anism appears uncertain (Elseviers & De Broe 1996). Acetanilide and phenacetine, the precursors of acetaminophen, have definitely been banned because of their higher toxicity. Acetaminophen should not be given to patients with seriously impaired liver function.

PHENAZONE AND ITS DERIVATIVES

Following the discovery of phenazone 120 years ago, the drug industry has tried to improve three aspects of this compound. It has been: (i) chemically modified to produce a more potent compound; (ii) to yield a water-soluble derivative to be given parenterally; (iii) to find a compound which is eliminated faster than and more reliably than phenazone in all patients. The best-known results of these attempts are aminophenazone, dipyrone and propyphenazone (Tables 49.3, 49.4). Aminophenazone is not in use anymore because it might lead to the formation of nitrosamines, which are known to increase the risk of stomach cancer. The other two compounds differ from phenazone in their potency and elimination half-life (Levy et al 1995), their water solubility (dipyrone is a water-soluble prodrug of methylaminophenazone) and their general toxicity (propyphenazone and dipyrone do not lead to nitrosamines in the acidic environment of the stomach).

Phenazone, propyphenazone and dipyrone are used in many countries worldwide as the dominant antipyretic analgesics (Latin America, many countries in Asia, Eastern Europe and Central Europe). Dipyrone has been accused of causing agranulocytosis. Although there appears to be a statistically significant link, the incidence is extremely rare (1 case per million treatment periods) (The International Agranulocytosis and Aplastic Anemia Study 1986, Kaufman et al 1991).

All antipyretic analgesics have also been claimed to cause Stevens–Johnson's syndrome and Lyell's syndrome as well as shock reactions. New data indicate that the incidence of these events is in the same order of magnitude as, for example, with penicillins (Roujeau et al 1995, Mockenhaupt et al 1996, The International Collaborative Study of Severe Anaphylaxis 1998). All non-acidic phenazone derivatives lack anti-inflammatory activity, they are devoid of gastrointestinal and (acute) renal toxicity. Dipyrone is safe at overdosage, which is in contrast to paracetamol (Wolhoff et al 1983). If one compares aspirin, acetaminophen and propyphenazone when used for the same indication (e.g. occasional headache), it is obvious that aspirin is more dangerous than either propyphenazone or acetaminophen. But as always with old compounds a rational discussion of its pros and cons is put aside in favour of new developments which appear on the horizon. Perhaps the new pure enantiomers of arylpropionic acids (Lötsch et al 1995, Szelenyi et al 1998) or, more likely, the COX 2-specific inhibitors (Vane 1994) of cyclooxygenases, will soon substitute acetaminophen, aspirin and dipyrone (Jonzeau et al 1997).

 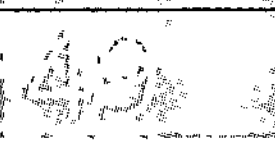

Table 49.3 Indications for acidic antipyretic analgesics (anti-inflammatory antipyretic analgesics, NSAIDs)[1]

Acute and chronic pain, produced by inflammation of different aetiology	*High dose*	*Middle dose*	*Low dose*
Arthritis: chronic polyarthritis (rheumatoid arthritis ankylosing spondilytis (Morbus Bechterew) acute gout (gout attack)	Diclofenac, indomethacin, ibuprofen, piroxicam, (phenylbutazone)[2]	Diclofenac, indomethacin, ibuprofen, piroxicam, (phenylbutazone)[2]	no
Cancer pain (e.g. bone metastasis)	(Indomethacin[3]), diclofenac[3], ibuprofen[3], piroxicam[3])	(Indomethacin[3]), diclofenac[3], ibuprofen[3], piroxicam[3]	Acetylsalicylic acid[4], ibuprofen[3]
Active arthritis (acute pain – inflammatory episodes)	No	Diclofenac, indomethacin, ibuprofen, piroxicam	Ibuprofen, ketoprofen
Myofascial pain syndromes (antipyretic analgesic are often prescribed but of limited value)	No	Diclofenac, ibuprofen, piroxicam	Ibuprofen, ketoprofen
Post-traumatic pain, swelling	No	(Indomethacin), diclofenac, ibuprofen	Acetylsalicylic acid, ibuprofen[3]
Postoperative pain, swelling	No	(Indomethacin), diclofenac, ibuprofen	Ibuprofen

[1] Dosage range of NSAIDs and example of monosubstances (but note dosage prescribed for each agent).
[2] Indicated only in gout attacks.
[3] Compare the sequence staged scheme of WHO for cancer pain.
[4] Blood coagulation and renal function must be normal.

Table 49.4 Indications for non-acidic antipyretic analgesics

Acute pain and fever	*Pyrazolinones (high dose)*	*Pyrazolinones (low dose)*	*Anilines (high dose is toxic)*
Spastic pain (colics)	Yes	Yes	No
Conditions associated with high fever	Yes	Yes	No
Cancer pain	Yes	Yes	Yes
Headache, migraine	No	Yes	Yes[2]
General disturbances associated with viral infections	No	Yes[1]	Yes

[1] If other analgesics and antipyretics are contraindicated, e.g. gastroduodenal ulcer, blood coagulation disturbances, asthma.
[2] In particular patients.

REFERENCES

Akopian AN, Sivilotti L, Wood JN 1996 A tetrodotoxin-resistant voltage-gated sodium channel expressed by sensory neurons. Nature 379: 257–262

Beiche F, Scheuerer S, Brune K, Geisslinger G, Goppelt-Struebe M 1996 Upregulation of cyclooxygenase-2 mRNA in the rat spinal cord following peripheral inflammation. FEBS Letters 390: 165–169

Brune K 1997 The early history of non-opioid analgesics. Acute Pain 1: 33–40

Brune K, Lanz R 1985 Pharmacokinetics of non-steroidal anti-inflammatory drugs. In: Bonta IL, Bray MA, Parnham MJ (eds) Handbook of inflammation, vol 5, the pharmacology of inflammation Elsevier, Amsterdam. pp 413–449

Brune K, McCormack K 1994 The over-the-counter use of nonsteroidal anti-inflammatory drugs and other antipyretic analgesics. In: Lewis AJ, Furst DE (eds) Nonsteroidal anti-inflammatory drugs: mechanisms and clinical uses, 2nd edn. Marcel Dekker, New York pp 97–126

Brune K, Glatt M, Graf P 1976 Mechanism of action of anti-inflammatory drugs. General Pharmacology 7: 27–33

Brune K, Rainsford KD, Schweitzer A 1980 Biodistribution of mild analgesics. British Journal of Clinical Pharmacology 10(suppl 2): 279–284

Bridger S, Henderson K, Glucksman E, Ellis AJ, Henry JA, Williams R 1998 Deaths from low dose paracetamol poisoning. American Medical Journal 316: 1724–1725

Dinchuk JE, Car BD, Focht RJ et al 1995 Renal abnormalities and an altered inflammatory response in mice lacking cyclooxygenase II. Nature 378: 406–409

Dirig DM, Konin GP, Isakson PC, Yaksh TL 1997 Effect of spinal cyclooxygenase inhibitors in rat using the formalin test and in vitro prostaglandin E2 release. European Journal of Pharmacology 331: 155–160

Dirig DM, Isakson PC, Yaksh TL 1998 Effect of COX-1 and COX-2 inhibition on induction and maintenance of carrageenan-evoked thermal hyperalgesia in rats. Pharmacology and Experimental Therapeutics 285: 1031–1038

Elseviers MM, De Broe ME 1996 Combination analgesic involvement in the pathogenesis of analgesic nephropathy: the European perspective. American Journal of Kidney Disease 28(suppl 1): 48–55

England S, Bevan S, Docherty RJ 1996 PGE2 modulates the tetrodotoxin-resistant sodium current in neonatal rat dorsal root ganglion neurones via the cyclic AMP-protein kinase A cascade. Journal of Physiology (London) 495: 429–440

Geisslinger G, Menzel S, Wissel K, Brune K 1993 Single dose pharmacokinetics of different formulations of ibuprofen and aspirin. Drug Investigation 5: 238–242

Gold MS, Reichling DB, Shuster MJ, Levine JD 1996 Hyperalgesic agents increase a tetrodotoxin-resistant Na^+ current in nociceptors. Proceedings of the National Academy of Sciences USA 93: 1108–1112

Graf P, Glatt M, Brune K 1975 Acidic nonsteroid anti-inflammatory drugs accumulating in inflamed tissue. Experientia 31: 951–954

Harris RC, McKanna JA, Aiai Y, Jacobson HR, DuBois RN, Breyer MD 1994 Cyclooxygenase-2 is associated with the macula densa of rat kidney and increases with salt restriction. Journal of Clinical Investigation 94: 2504–2510

Henry D, Lim LL, Garcia Rodriguez LA et al 1996 Variability in risk of gastrointestinal complications with individual non-steroidal anti-inflammatory drugs: results of a collaborative meta-analysis. British Medical Journal 312: 1563–1566

Heppelmann B, Messlinger K, Neiss WF, Schmidt RF 1990 Ultrastructural three-dimensional reconstruction of group III and group IV, sensory nerve endings ('free nerve endings') in the knee joint capsule of the cat: evidence for multiple receptive sites. Journal of Comparative Neurology 292: 103–116

Herzfeldt CD, Kümmel R 1983 Dissociation constants, solubilities and dissolution rates of some selected nonsteroidal anti-inflammatories. Drug Development and Industrial Pharmacy 9: 767–793

Hoigne RV, Szczeklik A 1992 Allergic and pseudoallergic reactions associated with nonsteroidal anti-inflammatory drugs. In: Borda IT, Koff RS (eds) NSAIDs: a profile of adverse effects. Hanley & Belfus, Philadelphia/Mosby-Yearbook, St Louis, pp 57–184

The International Agranulocytosis and Aplastic Anemia Study 1986 Risks of agranulocytosis and aplastic anemia: a first report of their relation to drug use with special reference to analgesics. Journal of the American Medical Association 256: 1749–1757

The International Collaborative Study of Severe Anaphylaxis 1998 Epidemiology 9: 141–146

Jouzeau J-Y, Terlain B, Abid A, Nédélec E, Netter P 1997 Cyclo-oxygenase isoenzymes: how recent findings affect thinking about nonsteroidal anti-inflammatory drugs. Drugs 53: 563–582

Kalgutkar AS, Crews BC, Rowlinson SW, Garner C, Seibert K, Marnett LJ 1998 Aspirin-like molecules that covalently inactivate cyclooxygenase-2. Science 280: 1268–1270

Kaufman DW, Kelly JP, Levy M, Shapiro S 1991 The drug etiology of agranulocytosis an aplastic anemia. Monographs in epidemiology and biostatistics 18. Oxford University Press, Oxford

Kaufman DW, Kelly JP, Sheehan JE et al 1993 Nonsteroidal anti-inflammatory drug use in relation to major upper gastrointestinal bleeding. Clinical Pharmacology and Therapeutics 53: 485–494

Kirtikara K, Morham SG, Raghow R et al 1998 Compensatory prostaglandin E_2 biosynthesis in cyclooxygenase 1 or 2 null cells. Journal of Experimental Medicine 187: 517–523

Kress M, Koltzenburg M, Reeh PW, Handwerker HO 1992 Responsiveness and functional attributes of electrically localized terminals of cutaneous C-fibers in vivo and in vitro. Journal of Neurophysiology 68: 581–595

Kujubu DA, Fletcher BS, Varnum BC, Lim RW, Herschman HR 1991 TIS 10, a phorbol ester tumor promoter-inducible mRNA from Swiss 3T3 cells, encodes a novel prostaglandin synthase/cyclooxygenase homologue. Journal of Biological Chemistry 266: 12866–12872

Kurumball RG, Stevens AM, Gierse JK et al 1996 Structural basis for the selective inhibition of cyclooxygenase-2 by anti-inflammatory agents. Nature 384: 644–648

Lane NE 1997 Pain management in osteoarthritis: the role of COX-2 inhibitors. Journal of Rheumatology 24(suppl 49): 20–24

Langenbach R, Morham SG, Tiana HI et al 1995 Prostaglandin synthase 1 gene disruption in mice reduces arachidonic acid-induced inflammation and indomethacin-induced gastric ulceration. Cell 83: 483–492

Laska EM, Sunshine A, Mueller F, Elvers WB, Siegel C, Rubin A 1984 Caffeine as an analgesic adjuvant. Journal of the American Medical Association 251: 1711–1718

Laska EM, Sunshine A, Marrero I, Olson N, Siegel C, McCormick N 1986 The correlation between blood levels of ibuprofen and clinical analgesic response. Journal of the American Medical Association 40: 1–7

Levy M, Zylber-Katz E, Rosenkranz B 1995 Clinical pharmacokinetcs of dipyrone and its metabolites. Clinical Pharmacokinetics 28: 216–234

Lim H, Paria BC, Das SK et al 1997 Multiple female reproductive failures in cyclooxygenase 2-deficient mice. Cell 91: 197–208

Lipsky PE 1997 Progress toward a new class of therapeutics: selective COX-2 inhibition: introduction and course description. Journal of Rheumatology 24(suppl 49): 1–5

Lötsch J, Geisslinger G, Mohammadian P, Brune K, Kobal G 1995 Effects of flurbiprofen enantiomers on pain-related chemosomatosensory evoked potentials in human subjects. British Journal of Clinical Pharmacology 40: 339–346

McCormack K, Brune K 1991 Dissociation between the antinociceptive and anti-inflammatory effects of the nonsteroidal anti-inflammatory drugs. A survey of their analgesic efficacy. Drugs 41: 533–547

Masferrer JL, Seibert K, Zweifel BS, Needleman P 1992 Endogenous glucocorticoids regulate an inducible cyclooxygenase enzyme. Proceedings of the National Academy of Sciences, USA 89: 3917–3921

Masferrer J, Zweifel B, Manning PT et al 1994 Selective inhibition of inducible cyclooxygenase 2 in vivo is anti-inflammatory and non-ulcerogenic. Proceedings of the National Academy of Sciences, USA 91: 3228–3232

Mayer JM, Testa B 1997 Pharmacodynamics, pharmacokinetics and toxicity of ibuprofen euanhoners. Drugs of the Future 22: 1347–66

Mockenhaupt M, Schlingmann J, Schroeder W, Schoepf E 1996 Evaluation of non-steroidal anti-inflammatory drugs (NSAIDs) and muscle relaxants as risk factors for Stevens–Johnson syndrome (SJS) and toxic epidermal necrolysis (TEN). Pharmacoepidemiology and Drug Safety 5: 116

Morham SG, Langenbach R, Loftin CD et al 1995 Prostaglandin synthase 2 gene disruption causes severe renal pathology in the mouse. Cell 83: 473–482

Neugebauer V, Geisslinger G, Rümenapp P et al 1995 Antinociceptive effects of R(−)- and S(+)-flurbiprofen on rat spinal dorsal horn neurons rendered hyperexcitable by an acute knee joint inflammation. Journal of Pharmacology and Experimental Therapeutics 275: 618–628

O'Banion MK, Sadowski HB, Winn V, Young DA 1991 A serum- and glucocorticoid regulated 4-kilobase mRNA encodes a cyclooxygenase-related protein. Journal of Biological Chemistry 266: 23261–23267

Otterness IG, Bliven ML 1985 Laboratory models for testing nonsteroidal anti-inflammatory drugs. In: Lombardino J (ed) Nonsteroidal anti-inflammatory drugs. John Wiley, New York, pp 111–252

Patrignani P, Panara MR, Greco A et al 1994 Biochemical and pharmacological characterization of the cyclooxygenase activity of human blood prostaglandin endoperoxide synthase. Journal of Pharmacology and Experimental Therapeutics 271: 1705–1712

Porter GA 1996 Acetaminophen/aspirin mixtures: experimental data. American Journal of Kidney Disease 28(suppl 1): 30–33

Roujeau JC, Kelly JP, Naldi L et al 1995 Drug etiology of Stevens–Johnson syndrome and toxic epidemal necrolysis, first results from an international case-control study. New England Journal of Medicine 333: 1600–1609

Riendeau D, Charleson S, Cromslish W, Mancini JA, Wong E, Guay J 1997 Comparison of the cyclooxygenase-1 inhibitory properties of nonsteroidal anti-inflammatory drugs (NSAIDs) and selective COX-2 inhibitors, using sensitive microsomal and platelet assays. Canadian Journal of Physiology and Pharmacology 75: 1088–1095

Rudy AC, Knight PM, Brater DC, Hall SD 1991 Stereoselective metabolism of ibuprofen in humans: administration of *R*-, *S*- and racemic ibuprofen. Journal of Pharmacology and Experimental Therapeutics 259: 1133–1139

Schaible HG, Schmidt RF 1988 Time course of mechanosensitivity changes in articular afferents during a developing experimental arthritis. Journal of Neurophysiology 60: 2180–2195

Schmid J, Buisch U, Heinzel G Bozler G, Kaschke S, Kummer M 1995 Meloxicam: pharmacokinetics and metabolic pattern after intravenous infusion and oral administration to healthy subjects. Drug Metabolism and Disposition 23: 1206–1213

Seeff LB, Cuccherini BA, Zimmerman HJ, Adler E, Benjamin SB, 1986 Acetaminophen hepatotoxicity in alcoholics. Annals of Internal Medicine 104: 399–404

Seibert K, Zhang Y, Leahy K et al 1994 Pharmacological and biochemical demonstration of the role of cyclooxygenase (COX)-2 in inflammation and pain. Proceedings of the National Academy of Sciences USA 91: 12013–12017

Smith WL, De Witt DL 1996 Prostaglandin endoperoxide H synthases (cyclooxygenases)-1 and -2. Advances in Immunology 62: 167–215

Szelenyi I, Geisslinger G, Polymeropoulos E, Paul W, Herbst M, Brune K 1998 The real gordian knot: racemic mixtures versus pure enantiomers. Drug News Perspectives 11: 139–160

Tegeder I, Krebs S, Muth-Selbach U, Lötsch J, Brune K, Geisslinger G 1998 Comparison of inhibitory effects of meloxicam and diclofenac on human thromboxane biosynthesis after single doses and at steady state. Clinical Pharmacology and Therapeutics (in press).

Vane J R 1971 Inhibition of prostaglandin synthesis as a mechanism of action of aspirin-like drugs. Nature New Biology 231: 232–235

Vane J 1994 Towards a better aspirin. Nature 367: 215–216

Vaughan CW, Ingram SL, Connor MA, Christie MJ 1997 How opioids inhibit GABA-mediated neurotransmission. Nature 390: 611–614

Verbeck RK, Blackburn JL, Loewen GR 1983 Clinical pharmacokinetics of non-steroidal anti-inflammatory drugs. Clinical Pharmacokinetics 8: 297–331

Weissmann G 1993 Prostaglandins as modulators rather than mediators of inflammation. Journal of Lipid Medicine 6: 275–286

Williams JT 1997 The painless synergism of aspirin and opium. Nature 390: 557

Winter CA, Risley EA, Nuss GW 1962 Carrageenin-induced edema in hind paw of the rat as an assay for anti-inflammatory drugs. Proceedings of the Society of Experimental Biology New York 111: 544–552

Wolhoff H, Altrogge G, Pola W, Sistovaris N 1983 Metamizol – akute Überdosierung in suizidaler Absicht. Deutsche Medizinische Wochenschrift 108: 1761–1764

Yamagata K, Andreasson KI, Kaufmann WE, Barnes CA, Worley PF 1993 Expression of a mitogen-inducible cyclooxygenase in brain neurons: regulation by synaptic activity and glucocorticoids. Neuron 11: 371–386

Psychotropic drugs

RICHARD MONKS & HAROLD MERSKEY

INTRODUCTION

The aim of this chapter is to describe the clinical use of various psychotropic drugs in the treatment of pain states, especially those of chronic duration. Because human pain is an experience with an affective element, it is not surprising that these substances have been used as part of the therapeutic approach to this complex problem. However, there is also reason to believe that some of them have analgesic properties which are independent of their psychological effects. In this chapter the rationale and indications for use, effectiveness and adverse effects of antidepressants, neuroleptics, lithium carbonate and the antianxiety drugs will be discussed.

RATIONALE FOR TREATMENT

ANTIDEPRESSANTS

Tricyclic-type antidepressants, selective serotonin reuptake inhibitors, serotonin-noradrenaline reuptake inhibitors and monoamine oxidase inhibitors

A number of different but related mechanisms have been suggested to explain the presumed efficacy of tricyclic and heterocyclic antidepressants (TCAD), selective serotonin reuptake inhibitors (SSRI), serotonin-adrenaline reuptake inhibitors (SNRI) and monoamine oxidase inhibitors (MAOI) in pain conditions.

Antidepressant action

Analgesic effects of these drugs may result from their antidepressant action. Paoli et al (1960) were the first to report TCAD therapy of chronic pain states, nothing that they had intended to improve the 'reactive' depression which was often present.

Various studies have shown that a substantial minority of chronic pain patients are clinically depressed and, compared with non-depressed pain controls, show an increased incidence of familial affective disorders, biological markers of depression and response to TCAD (Blumer et al 1982, Krishnan et al 1985, Atkinson et al 1986, France et al 1986, Magni et al 1987, Mellerup et al 1988).

In clinical trials with adequate data, the vast majority of patients with coexisting chronic pain and depression obtained relief from both disorders when responding to MAOI or TCAD therapy (Okasha et al 1973, Couch et al 1976, Jenkins et al 1976, MacNeill & Dick 1976, Ward et al 1979, Turkington 1980, Lindsay & Wyckoff 1981, Watson et al 1982, Hameroff et al 1984, Magni et al 1987, Puttini et al 1988, Saran 1988, Loldrup et al 1989, Nappi et al 1990). Also, the onset of a depressive disorder preceding or coinciding with the onset of a chronic atypical pain complaint predicted a much better response to TCAD or MAOI than if the depression followed the pain onset (Bradley 1963).

Separate analgesic effect

There is evidence to suggest the existence of an analgesic action of TCAD and MAOI that is not mediated by any measurable antidepressant action. The onset of analgesia with TCAD in chronic pain states is more rapid than the usual onset of an antidepressant effect in some clinically depressed patients (3–7 days vs 14–21 days) (Langohr et al 1982, Mitas et al 1983, Hameroff et al 1984, Smoller 1984, Montastruc et al 1985, Gourlay et al 1986, Levine et al 1986).

Also, chronic pain relief with TCAD, SSRI and MAOI has been reported despite a lack of antidepressant response (Lascelles 1966, Couch & Hassanein 1976, Alcoff et al 1982, Watson et al 1982, Ward et al 1984, Fogelholm & Murros 1985, Gourlay et al 1986, Macfarlane et al 1986, Goldenberg et al 1996). Similar improvements have been obtained in patients without detectable depression (Lance & Curran 1964, Couch et al 1976, Jenkins et al 1976, Watson et al 1982, Feinmann et al 1984, Kvinesdal et al 1984, Montastruc et al 1985, Watson & Evans 1985, Zeigler et al 1987, Puttini et al 1988, Bendtsen et al 1996, Vrethem et al 1997).

Neurotransmitter alteration

It has been suggested that both the analgesic and antidepressant action of TCAD, SSRI, SNRI and MAOI are caused by their action on central neurotransmitter functions, particularly those mediated by the catecholamine and indolamine systems (Sternbach et al 1976, Lee & Spencer 1977, Messing & Lytle 1977, Basbaum & Fields 1978, Murphy et al 1978, Schildkraut 1978). Also, increased synaptic monoamines may inhibit nociception at the thalamic (Andersen & Dafny 1983), brainstem (Roberts 1984) and spinal cord levels (Dubner & Bennett 1983, Hammond 1985, Hwang & Wilcox 1987, Proudfit 1988). Given acutely (minutes to hours), TCAD and MAOI increase synaptic levels of dopamine, noradrenaline or serotonin. Chronic administration (days to weeks) probably stabilizes acute changes by regulating central and peripheral monoamine receptors or altering the activities of cerebral and spinal cord monoamine comodulators, such as substance P, thyrotropin-releasing hormone-like peptides and gamma amino-butyric acid (GABA) (Fuxe et al 1983, Sugrue 1983, Lloyd & Pile 1984, Willner 1985).

Animal experiments on acute pain suggest the existence of both serotonin and noradrenaline bulbospinal and central antinociceptive pathways, which interact in a complex way (Basbaum & Fields 1978, Soja & Sinclair 1983, Barber et al 1989, Ardid et al 1995, Cerda et al 1997). The analgesic effects observed with TCAD and with SSRI in such studies seem to depend on monoamine neurotransmission and, to a lesser extent, opiate (Biegon & Samuel 1980, Eschalier et al 1981, Schreiber et al 1996) and possibly adenosine (Sierralta et al 1995) receptors. G-proteins may represent an important transduction step in central analgesia induced by TCAD (Galeotti et al 1996).

Similar findings in some human acute and chronic pain studies suggest that analgesic properties of TCAD depend on interrelated central serotonergic and opiate mechanisms (Sternbach et al 1976, Johansson & Von Knorring 1979, Willer et al 1984). Human acute pain studies with the newer antidepressants fluoxetine (SSRI) and ritanserin (a $5HT_2$ antagonist) reveal antinociceptive properties that are likely to occur centrally and are not blocked by naloxone (Messing et al 1975, Sandrini et al 1986). Drug trials comparing various TCAD used for patients with chronic pain tend to favour more serotonergic drugs (Sternbach et al 1976, Carasso 1979, Ward et al 1984, Eberhard et al 1988, Sindrup et al 1990a, Bendtsen et al 1996, McQuay et al 1996, Vrethem et al 1997). However, there is evidence that noradrenergic mechanisms also may be involved, both in acute pain (Taniguchi et al 1995) and in chronic pain with depression (Ward et al 1983). Also, antidepressants with predominantly noradrenergic effects have been shown to be effective in adequate controlled trials (Fogelholm & Murros 1985, Loldrup et al 1989, Kishore-Kumar et al 1990, Sindrup et al 1990a, Max et al 1991, Vrethem et al 1997).

Further, most controlled clinical trials with antidepressants, such as citalopram, femoxetine, fluoxetine, paroxetine, trazodone and zimelidine, that are selectively serotonergic in their effects, have shown results that are no better than those of a placebo (Johansson & Von Knorring 1979, Gourlay et al 1986, Lynch et al 1990, Bendtsen et al 1996) or are inferior to those of a less selective antidepressant (Sjaastad 1983, Watson & Evans 1985, Frank et al 1988, Sindrup et al 1990b, McQuay et al 1996). Trazodone, ritanserin and fluoxetine, respectively, provided pain relief equal to that of low-dose amitriptyline in two non-placebo-controlled trials and one placebo-controlled trial, which were the exceptions (Ventafridda et al 1987, Nappi et al 1990, Rani et al 1996). In keeping with the former findings, a recent meta-analysis of 39 placebo-controlled studies of antidepressant analgesia in chronic pain found that antidepressants with mixed serotonergic and noradrenergic properties had a larger effect size than that of drugs with more specific properties when other patient disorders and study variable were eliminated (Onghena & Van Houdenhove 1992).

Opiate effects

The analgesic effect of the opiates, like TCAD and MAOI, appears to be modulated by central biogenic amines, at least in animal acute pain trials (Lee & Spencer 1977). TCAD, SSRI and MAOI enhance opiate analgesia and may induce tolerance in animal experiments (Contreras et al 1977, Fuentes et al 1977, Lee & Spencer 1977, Tofanetti et al 1977, Gonzalez et al 1980, Botney & Fields 1983, Paul &

Hornby 1995, Sierralta et al 1995, Schreiber et al 1996). These effects may be mediated by changes in catecholamine neurotransmitters and/or serotonin, but TCAD may also bind directly to opiate receptors (Biegon & Samuel 1980).

Endogenous morphine-like substances (endorphins) seem to have a role in acute and chronic pain in animals and man (Terenius 1978, 1979). Preliminary work with an SSRI-type drug, zimelidine, found therapeutic efficacy to be correlated with changes in cerebrospinal fluid (CSF) endorphin and indolamine activity in human chronic pain (Johansson et al 1980). However, more recent clinical trials did not show a correlation of TCAD-induced improvement with changes in CSF beta endorphin (Ward et al 1984, France & Urban 1991) or with plasma β-endorphin and enkephalin-like activity (Hameroff et al 1984).

Miscellaneous effects

Analgesic properties of antidepressants also have been attributed to non-specific physiological effects such as sedation, diminished anxiety, muscle relaxation and restored sleep cycles. These effects alone do not seem adequate to explain the superiority of TCAD to more powerful anxiolytics such as the benzodiazepines in relieving chronic pain. Also, changes in anxiety, depression and chronic pain with TCAD treatment were not found to be significantly correlated with each other in one double-blind controlled trial (Ward et al 1984).

Other specific TCAD effects, which have been invoked to explain their analgesic effects, include: central or peripheral histamine receptor blockade (Rumore & Schlichting 1986), inhibition of prostaglandin synthetase (Krupp & Wesp 1975) and a calcium-channel blocking effect (Peroutko et al 1984). Anti-inflammatory effects of TCAD have been demonstrated in two chronic pain experiments using arthritic rats (Butler et al 1985, Godefroy et al 1986).

NEUROLEPTICS

Neuroleptics commonly used for pain include the phenothiazines, thioxanthenes and butyrophenones. Of current interest are atypical neuroleptics such as clozapine and risperidone. Mechanisms of action responsible for any analgesic effects of these drugs are unknown. However, various possibilities have been considered.

Antipsychotic action

The vast majority of clinical pain syndromes relieved by neuroleptics are not delusional in nature and do not occur in the presence of a psychotic disorder.

Neurotransmitter alteration

Neuroleptic drugs show a wide range of actions on neurotransmitter systems centrally and peripherally. Based on results from acute animal pain studies, it has been suggested that neuroleptic analgesia might be mediated by inhibition of dopamine, noradrenaline, serotonin or histamine neurotransmission (Malec & Langwinski 1981, Tricklebank et al 1984, Rumore & Schlichting 1986). The limited data from human clinical trials do not suggest a correlation of analgesic effectiveness with adrenergic or muscarine blocking effects of specific neuroleptics.

Opiate effects

Haloperidol shows isomorphic similarity to meperidine and morphine (Maltbie et al 1979). The antinociceptive effect of risperidone in acute pain in mice is antagonized by naloxone and selective μ- and κ-opioid receptor antagonists (Schreiber et al 1997). Various neuroleptics inhibit naloxone or met-enkephalin binding to opiate receptors (Creese et al 1976, Somoza 1978). These observations have been cited to explain neuroleptic analgesia effects, synergistic action with narcotics and amelioration of narcotic withdrawal.

Miscellaneous effects

Sedation may explain single-dose analgesic effects of more sedating neuroleptics, although sedation alone does not guarantee pain relief (Petts & Pleuvry 1983). Additionally, high-potency alerting neuroleptics diminish chronic pain. Anxiolytic properties of neuroleptics in chronic pain patients have been reported (Hackett et al 1987), but are insufficient to explain their analgesic effects in patients who have not responded to benzodiazepines. Local anaesthetic and skeletal muscle relaxant effects of neuroleptics only occur at higher concentrations of these drugs than are obtained at usual clinical doses.

Combined neuroleptic–antidepressant regimens might provide superior analgesic effectiveness because neuroleptics inhibit TCAD degradation and enhance TCAD plasma levels (Hirschowitz et al 1983). Similarly, carbamazepine may augment TCAD levels in combined antidepressant–anticonvulsant regimens (Gerson et al 1977).

LITHIUM CARBONATE

Ekbom's initial use of lithium in cluster headache was based on the observation that this disorder, like bipolar affective disorders, is cyclic in nature (Ekbom 1974). However, analgesic effects of lithium in cluster headache occur in the absence of depression or antidepressant effect and at lower serum levels than in bipolar affective disorders (Kudrow 1977, Mathew 1978, Pearce 1980). Lithium has complex acute and chronic effects on neurotransmission which may influence pain. It enhances serotonin availability in the brain, diminishes catecholamine neurone activity, alters central adrenergic, dopaminergic, GABA and opiate receptor binding and inhibits central and peripheral adenylate cyclase-mediated cyclic adenosine monophosphate production, including that induced by prostaglandin E (Gold & Byck 1978, Bunney & Garland 1984).

ANTIANXIETY DRUGS

The benzodiazepines (BDZ) and buspirone, a nonBDZ with D2 dopamine antagonist/agonist and 5-HT1A receptor agonist properties, are reported to have antinociceptive properties.

Anxiolytic and miscellaneous effects

BDZ usually are given to pain sufferers in an attempt to diminish anxiety, excessive muscle tension and insomnia thought to worsen acute and chronic pain states (Shimm et al 1979, Hollister et al 1981). One benzodiazepine, alprazolam, also has demonstrated antidepressant properties (Feighner et al 1983, Fernandez et al 1987). Another, clonazepam, may achieve analgesic effects by its anticonvulsant properties (Swerdlow & Cundill 1981).

Neurotransmitter/receptor activites

The stimulation of BDZ receptors affects noradrenaline, serotonin, dopamine and GABA neurotransmission (Hamlin & Gold 1984). In animal studies of acute pain intrathecally administered BDZ, analgesic effects and enhancement of morphine appear to be mediated by opioid, *N*-methyl-D-aspartate (NMDA) and, to a lesser extent, BDZ receptors (Wüster et al 1980, Luger et al 1995, Pick 1996, 1997). On the other hand, intracranially administered BDZ appeared not to have analgesic effects (Pick 1996, 1997), abolished conditioned hypoalgesia (Harris & Westbrook 1995) and antagonized morphine antinociception, possibly through the activation of GABA-A and NMDA receptors (Luger et al 1995). Of relevance is the finding that flumazenil, a BDZ receptor antagonist, appears to block preoperative diazepam inhibition of morphine analgesia in human dental pain (Gear et al 1997). Possible long-term BDZ administration effects on serotonin turnover and BDZ receptor function are a concern (Snyder et al 1977, Hamlin & Gold 1984).

A mechanism of action for possible buspirone analgesic effects is unknown; however, its known serotonergic properties may provide a clue for further exploration.

INDICATIONS FOR USE

It is important to recognize that the use of psychotropic drugs is only one of the adjunctive measures available in the comprehensive approach required for many pain problems, especially those of more chronic duration. A careful evaluation of some of the psychological and social factors contributing to the pain complaint is necessary to prescribe these drugs rationally (Bonica 1977).

The antidepressants, neuroleptics and benzodiazepines are often used for the initial control of target symptoms such as depression, anxiety, abnormal muscle tension, insomnia and fatigue. TCAD and occasionally neuroleptics are also used for withdrawal/detoxication from narcotics, other analgesics, minor tranquillizers and alcohol (Khatami et al 1979, Halpern 1982). Combinations of TCAD and narcotics are used for some pain disorders refractory to either alone (Urban et al 1986).

TREATMENT INDICATIONS FOR EACH PSYCHOTROPIC GROUP

A review of the pain literature was used to delineate specific treatment indications for each psychotropic drug group.

ANTIDEPRESSANTS (TCAD, SSRI, SNRI AND MAOI)

Depression

A trial of antidepressants is usually indicated if the patient with acute or chronic pain is clinically depressed (Bradley 1963, Lascelles 1966, Merskey & Hester 1972, Ward et al 1979, Lindsay & Wyckoff 1981, Hameroff et al 1984, Smoller 1984, Magni et al 1987, Max et al 1991). This is particularly so if the onset of depression preceded or coincided with the onset of pain (Bradley 1963), if there is a past history of favourable response of depression or pain to antidepressants, or if the current episode of depression is 'endogenous' in nature (anorexia, early morning awakening, psychomotor changes or anhedonia).

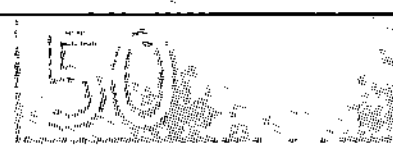

Biological markers of depression such as dexamethasone non-suppression, shortened rapid eye movement sleep latency and level of urinary 3-methoxy-4-hydroxyphenethylene glycol (MHPG) have been noted to predict pain relief with TCAD in depressed patients (Blumer et al 1982, Ward et al 1983, Smoller 1984). Also, [^{3}H]imipramine platelet-binding site density was found to be diminished in chronic idiopathic pain patients without major depression. Binding site density, pain scores and depression ratings were all improved after TCAD treatment in patients with a family history of depressive spectrum disorder (Magni et al 1987).

Tricyclic-type antidepressants

Acute pain

Only two papers were found in which TCAD were used to treat acute clinical pain. In the first, neither amitriptyline nor desipramine given for 7 days was found to be superior to placebo in alleviating postoperative dental pain. However, desipramine significantly enhanced morphine analgesia in these patients (Levine et al 1986). In the second, amitriptyline was found to be more effective than acetaminophen in reducing acute low back pain intensity after 2 weeks in a 5-week double-blind controlled trial (Stein et al 1996). Although TCAD have been found to be effective in treating migraine headache, the papers listed in Table 50.1 reported on patients suffering chronic high-frequency attacks of this disorder. In short, there is little well-substantiated indication for TCAD use for acute pain alone.

Chronic pain

Table 50.1 lists the 106 papers with 124 trials of TCAD for chronic pain that could be found. Although pain relief was demonstrated for all listed disorders, not all trials were successful (see Table 50.1 and section on 'Effectiveness' below). Pain of 'psychological origin' refers to disorders in which structural damage was not found and in which anxiety and depression were obvious and antedated or coincided with the onset of atypical pain. 'Mixed' pain refers to various non-neoplastic chronic pain disorders grouped together to compare treatment groups in those papers reviewed.

Unfortunately, most of the trials reviewed suffered from inadequacies of various sorts. However, Table 50.2 details the results of adequately controlled trials using TCAD for chronic pain. In 46 out of 48 trials, TCAD produced pain relief which was statistically and clinically superior to that obtained with placebo ('positive'). In two low back pain studies and one rheumatoid arthritis study, the TCAD and comparison placebo both produced clinically important pain relief which did not differ statistically in the two groups ('tie'). In one 'mixed' pain study, neither TCAD nor placebo were found to change pain or depression ratings ('negative').

The clinical use of amitriptyline and imipramine for chronic osteoarthritis and rheumatoid arthritis; amitriptyline for fibromyalgia; amitriptyline and imipramine for diabetic neuropathy; amitriptyline for migraine; amitriptyline for postherpetic neuralgia, and amitripyline and mianserin for chronic tension headaches is supported by at least two adequately controlled studies for each indication.

SSRI antidepressants

Chronic pain

Table 50.1 lists the 20 papers with 20 trials of SSRI antidepressants given for chronic pain. Although analgesia was reported for each disorder, many trials did not support the clinical use of these drugs. Table 50.2 lists all adequately controlled trials that could be found. Of 10 trials only five showed pain relief statistically and clinically superior to that obtained by placebo. No single SSRI drug had more than one trial supporting its use for a specific pain disorder.

SNRI antidepressants

Table 50.1 lists the two trials of the SNRI-type antidepressant venlafaxine given for chronic pain. One case study reported the relief of chronic low back pain followed by improvement in major depression (Songer & Schulte 1996). The second paper reported pain relief in a small series of case studies of persons with mixed neurological disorders (Taylor & Rowbotham 1996).

Monoamine oxidase inhibitor

Chronic pain

MAOI drugs, usually phenelzine, have been found to be successful in diminishing pain in each of the eight papers describing nine trials listed in Table 50.1. Only two adequately controlled trials were found, both with phenelzine, one in chronic fatigue syndrome and one in facial pain of psychological origin. In one non-placebo-controlled trial, MAOI drugs with 5-hydroxytryptophan proved superior to MAOI and to amitriptyline for fibromyalgia (Nicolodi & Sicuteri 1996).

Table 50.1 Chronic pain disorders treated with antidepressants

Disorder	Total trials	References (number of trials)
Tricyclic-type drugs		
Arthritis	13	Kuipers 1962(3), McDonald Scott 1969, Thorpe & Marchant-Williams 1974, Gingras 1976, MacNeill & Dick 1976, Ganvir et al 1980, Macfarlane et al 1986, Frank et al 1988(2), Puttini et al 1988, Rani et al 1996
Central poststroke	1	Leijon & Boivie 1989
Fibromyalgia	5	Carette et al 1986, Bibolotti et al 1988, Goldenberg et al 1986, Caruso et al 1987, Goldenberg et al 1996
Low back pain	6	Kuipers 1962, Jenkins et al 1976, Sternbach et al 1976, Alcoff et al 1982, Ward et al 1984(2)
Migraine	9	Gomersall & Stuart 1973, Couch & Hassanein 1976, Couch et al 1976, Noone 1977, Mørland et al 1979, Langohr et al 1985, Martucci et al 1985, Monro et al 1985, Zeigler et al 1987
Mixed	15	Rafinesque 1963, Adjan 1970, Desproges-Gotteron et al 1970, Radebold 1971, Evans et al 1973, Kocher 1976, Duthie 1977, Pilowsky et al 1982, Hameroff et al 1984, Zitman et al 1984, Edelbröck et al 1986, Sharav et al 1987(2), Nappi et al 1990, Pilowsky et al 1995
Mixed neurological	6	Paoli et al 1960, Laine et al 1962, Merskey & Heseter 1972, Castaigne et al 1979, Montastruc et al 1985, Ventafridda et al 1987
Myofascial dysfunction	2	Gessel 1975, Smoller 1984
Neoplastic	7	Hugues et al 1963, Parolin 1966, Fiorentino 1967, Gebhardt et al 1969, Adjan 1970, Bernard & Scheuer 1972, Bourhis et al 1978
Neuralgia postherpetic	9	Woodforde et al 1965, Taub 1973, Hatangdi et al 1976, Carasso 1979(2), Watson et al 1982, Watson & Evans 1985, Max et al 1988, Kishore-Kumar et al 1990
Neuralgia trigeminal	2	Carasso 1979(2)
Neurological perineal	1	Magni et al 1982
Neuropathy		
diabetic	16	Davis et al 1977, Gade et al 1980, Turkington 1980(2), Mitas et al 1983, Kvinesdal et al 1984, Max et al 1987, Sindrup et al 1989, Lynch et al 1990(2), Sindrup et al 1990a(2), 1990b, Max et al 1991, Vrethem et al 1997(2)
mononeuropathy	1	Langohr et al 1982
Postsurgical	1	Eija et al 1996
Painful shoulder syndrome	1	Tyber 1974
Phantom limb	1	Urban et al 1986
Psychological origin	13	Bradley 1963, Singh 1971(2), Okasha et al 1973(2), Ward et al 1979, Lindsay & Wyckoff 1981, Feinmann et al 1984, Magni et al 1987, Eberhard et al 1988(2), Saran 1988, Valdes et al 1989
Tension headache	15	Lance & Curran 1964(2), Diamond & Baltes 1971, Carasso 1979(2), Kudrow 1980, Sjaastad 1983, Fogelholm & Morros 1985, Martucci et al 1985, Llodrup et al 1989(2), Boline et al 1995, Bendtsen et al 1996, Mitsikostas et al 1997, Cohen 1997
SSRI-type drugs		
Arthritis	2	Frank et al 1988, Rani et al 1996
Fibromyalgia	2	Lynch et al 1990, Goldenberg et al 1996
Low back pain	1	Goodkin et al 1990
Migraine	3	Adly et al 1992, Saper et al 1994, Black & Sheline 1995
Mixed	3	Johansson & Von Knorring 1979, Gourlay et al 1986, Nappi et al 1990
Mixed neurological	2	Davidoff et al 1987, Ventafridda et al 1987
Neuralgia		
diabetic	3	Khurana 1983, Theesen & Marsh 1989, Sindrup et al 1990b
postherpetic	1	Watson & Evans 1985
Tension headache	3	Sjaastad 1983, Norregaard et al 1995, Bendtsen et al 1996

Table 50.1 (Contd.)

Disorder	Total trials	References (number of trials)
SNRI-type drugs		
Low back pain	1	Songer & Schulte 1996
Mixed	1	Taylor & Rowbotham 1996
MAOI-type drugs		
Chronic fatigue syndrome	1	Natelson et al 1996
Facial pain of psychological origin	2	Lascelles 1966(2)
Fibromyalgia	1	Nicolodi & Sicuteri 1996
Migraine	2	Anthony & Lance 1969, Merikangas & Merikangas 1995
Psychological origin	3	Bradley 1963, Lindsay & Wyckoff 1981, Raskin 1982

Table 50.2 Antidepressants: adequately controlled trials in chronic pain

Disorder	Drug	Positive	Tie	Negative	References
TCAD-type drugs					
Arthritis	Amitriptyline	2	–	–	Frank et al 1988, Rani et al 1996
	Desipramine	–	1	–	Frank et al 1988
	Dibenzepin	1	–	–	Thorpe & Marchant-Williams 1974
	Dothiepin	1	–	–	Puttini et al 1988
	Imipramine	2	–	–	McDonald Scott 1969, Gingras 1976
	Trimipramine	1	–	–	Macfarlane et al 1986
Central poststroke	Amitriptyline	2	–	–	Leijon & Boivie 1989
Fibromyalgia	Amitriptyline	2	–	–	Goldenberg et al 1986, 1996
	Dothiepin	1	–	–	Caruso et al 1987
Low back pain	Amitriptyline	–	1	–	Sternbach et al 1976
	Clomipramine	1	–	–	Sternbach et al 1976
	Imipramine	1	1	–	Jenkins et al 1976, Alcoff et al 1982
Migraine	Amitriptyline	3	–	–	Gomersall & Stuart 1973 Couch et al 1976, Zeigler et al 1987
Mixed	Mianserin	1	–	–	Monro et al 1985
	Amitriptyline	2	–	1	Pilowsky et al 1982, Sharav et al 1987(2)
	Doxepin	1	–	–	Hameroff et al 1984
Neoplastic	Imipramine	1	–	–	Fiorentino 1967
Neuropathy diabetic	Amitriptyline	3	–	–	Turkington 1980, Max et al 1987, Vrethem et al 1997
	Clomipramine	1	–	–	Sindrup et al 1990a
	Desipramine	1	–	–	Max et al 1991
	Imipramine	4	–	–	Turkington 1980, Kvinesdal et al 1984, Sindrup et al 1989, 1990b
	Maprotyline	1	–	–	Vrethem et al 1997
mononeuropathy	Clomipramine	1	–	–	Langohr et al 1982
Neuralgia	Amitriptyline	2	–	–	Watson et al 1982, Max et al 1988
postherpetic	Desipramine	1	–	–	Kishore-Kumar et al 1990
Psychological	Amitriptyline	1	–	–	Okasha et al 1973
origin	Dothiepin	1	–	–	Feinmann et al 1984
	Doxepin	1	–	–	Okasha et al 1973
Tension headache	Amitriptyline	3	–	–	Lance & Curran 1964, Diamond & Baltes 1971, Bendtsen et al 1996
	Clomipramine	1	–	–	Loldrup et al 1989
	Maprotyline	1	–	–	Fogelholm & Murros 1985
	Mianserin	2	–	–	Martucci et al 1985, Loldrup et al 1989

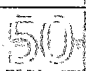

Table 50.2 (Contd.)

Disorder	Drug	Positive	Tie	Negative	References
SSRI-type drugs					
Arthritis	Trazodone	–	1	–	Frank et al 1988
	Fluoxetine	1	–	–	Rani et al 1996
Fibromyalgia	Fluoxetine	1	–	–	Goldenberg et al 1996
Low back pain	Trazodone	–	–	1	Goodkin et al 1990
Migraine	Fluoxetine	–	1	–	Saper et al 1994
Mixed	Zimelidine	1	–	–	Gourlay et al 1986
Neuropathy					
diabetic	Paroxetine	1	–	–	Sindrup et al 1990b
Tension headache	Citalopram	–	2	–	Norregaard et al 1995, Bendtsen et al 1996
	Femoxetine	1	–	–	Sjaastad 1983
MAOI-type drugs					
Chronic fatigue					
syndrome	Phenelzine	1	–	–	Natelson et al 1996
Psychological	Phenelzine	1	–	–	Lascelles 1966

NEUROLEPTICS

Psychosis

Neuroleptics are indicated for those psychiatric disorders which are associated with delusional or hallucinatory pain such as schizophrenia, delusional depressions and monosymptomatic hypochondriacal psychosis (Munro & Chmara 1982).

Pain-associated problems

Overwhelming pain characterized by anxiety, psychomotor agitation and insomnia, which does not respond to benzodiazepines in acute pain or TCAD in chronic pain, may be treated, at least on a short-term basis, by neuroleptics. In patients with neoplastic pain, neuroleptics are useful in managing nausea, vomiting, bladder or rectal tenesmus and ureteral spasm (Twycross 1979).

Acute pain

In 14 papers describing 21 trials in which neuroleptics alone were given for acute pain (Table 50.3), the most common indication for use in the mixed and postoperative group was abdominal, dental or postpartum pain.

Only five of these trials were judged to be adequate. In two studies of acute postoperative pain (Taylor & Doku 1967, Fazio 1970) and one of acute myocardial infarction (Davidson et al 1979), methotrimeprazine 10–20 mg intramuscularly (IM) gave analgesic results equivalent to meperidine 50 mg intramuscularly. In one study chlorpromazine 25 mg intravenously (IV) was found to be as markedly successful as ketorolac 60 mg IM in acute migraine headache (Shrestha et al 1996). In the remaining trial, premedication with haloperidol 5 or 10 mg orally was no better than placebo in diminishing analgesic requirements or providing pain relief. However, a potent antiemetic effect of haloperidol was demonstrated (Judkins & Harmer 1982).

Chronic pain

In 26 papers describing 31 trials of neuroleptics alone administered for chronic pain (Table 50.3), the main indication for the use of neuroleptics in chronic pain was for patients with recognizable organic lesions which were not treatable by more conservative means. Because of their adverse effects, neuroleptics should only be given after transscutaneous electrical nerve stimulation, other benign local measures and regular non-narcotic analgesics at fixed times have been tried. Neuroleptics may be strongly indicated in the management of pain which wakes patients from sleep (e.g. cluster headache or persistent early-morning migraine). They are most commonly employed with a variety of neurological disorders which are notoriously resistant to other forms of intervention. They may be used for thalamic or similar central pain which does not respond to antidepressants, carbamazepine or clonazepam. They are often helpful in nerve lesions including causalgias, neuralgias, neuropathies, traumatic avulsion of the brachial plexus and some instances of back pain, particularly if there is clear evidence of associated damage to nerves or nerve roots. Often

Table 50.3 Disorders treated with neuroleptics

Disorder	*Total trials*	*References*
Acute pain		
Mixed	1	Montilla et al 1963
Herpes zoster	3	Sigwald et al 1959(2), Farber & Burks 1974
Postoperative	14	Jackson & Smith 1956(3), Lasagna & DeKornfeld 1961(3) Bronwell et al 1966, Stirman 1967, Taylor & Doku 1967, Fazio 1970, Minuck 1972(2), Judkins & Harmer 1982(2)
Migraine	2	Iserson 1983, Shrestha et al 1996
Myocardial infarction	1	Davidson et al 1979
Chronic pain		
Arthritis	1	Breivik & Slørdahl 1984
Migraine	1	Polliack 1979
Mixed	6	Sadove et al 1955, Bloomfield et al 1964, Kast 1966, Cavenar & Maltbie 1976, Kocher 1976, Langohr et al 1982
Mixed neurological	1	Merskey & Hester 1972
Myofascial dysfunction	1	Raft et al 1979
Neoplastic	10	Beaver et al 1966(2), Maltbie & Cavenar 1977, Bourhis et al 1978, Schick et al 1979(2), Breivik & Rennemo 1982, Hanks et al 1983(2), Landa et al 1984
Neuralgia postherpetic	5	Sigwald et al 1959(2), Nathan 1978(2), Duke 1983
Neuropathy diabetic	2	Davis et al 1977, Mitas et al 1983
Radiation fibrosis	1	Daw & Cohen-Cole 1981
Tension headache (chronic)	2	Hakkarainen 1977, Hackett et al 1987
Thalamic pain	1	Margolis & Gianascol 1956

they are of value as an adjunct in the treatment of painful neoplasms, allowing decreased doses or discontinuation of narcotics in some patients (Parolin 1966, Cavenar & Maltbie 1976, Schick et al 1979, Breivik & Rennemo 1982).

Only five adequate controlled trials of neuroleptic therapy for chronic pain were found. Single doses of methotrimeprazine 15 mg were found to have analgesic properties equal to 8–15 mg of morphine in patients with mixed sources of chronic pain (Bloomfield et al 1964, Kast 1966) and in patients with chronic pain of neoplastic origin (Beaver et al 1966). Fluphenazine and flupenthixol each at 1 mg orally per day were both clinically and statistically superior to placebo in the treatment of chronic tension headache in trials of 2 months and 6 weeks respectively (Hakkarainen 1977, Hackett et al 1987). Preliminary reports of two placebo-controlled crossover trials of flupenthixol for severe cancer pain (Landa et al 1984) and for chronic osteoarthritic hip pain (Breivik & Slørdahl 1984) suggest that this neuroleptic may exhibit significant analgesic and antidepressant properties.

COMBINED DRUG THERAPY

Antidepressant and anticonvulsant

A combination of TCAD and an anticonvulsant may be useful for neuralgias which are resistant to either drug alone. Three clinical trials were found describing the successful treatment of chronic postherpetic neuralgia with combinations of TCAD with carbamazepine or with diphenylhydantion (Hatangdi et al 1976, Gerson et al 1977) or with valproic acid (Raferty 1979).

Antidepressant and neuroleptic

No evidence was found to support the use of TCAD–neuroleptic combined therapy for acute pain, but such therapy was used for chronic pain in the 18 trials listed in Table 50.4. Combined therapy is usually indicated when either drug group alone is indicated but has not proven efficacious and adverse effects are not a contraindication. The best results seem to occur with arthritic pain, treatment-resistant headaches, neoplastic pain and a variety of neurological pain disorders such as causalgias, de-afferentation syndromes, neuralgias and neuropathies.

Table 50.4 Disorders treated with antidepressant and neuroleptic combination

Disorder	Total trials	References
Head pain of psychological origin	1	Sherwin 1979
Mixed	3	Kocher 1976(2), Duthie 1977
Mixed neurological	2	Merskey & Hester 1972, Langohr et al 1982
Neoplastic	3	Bernard & Scheuer 1972, Bourhis et al 1978, Breivik & Rennemo 1982
Neuralgia postherpetic	3	Taub 1973, Langohr et al 1982, Weis et al 1982
Neuropathy diabetic	6	Davis et al 1977, Gade et al 1980, Khurana 1983, Mitas et al 1983, Gomez-Perez et al 1985, 1996

Only two adequately controlled trials of TCAD–neuroleptic treatment were found. A nortriptyline and fluphenazine combination was found to be clearly superior to placebo in decreasing pain and paraesthesias in patients with diabetic polyneuropathy in one study (Gomez-Perez et al 1985), and equally efficacious and superior to placebo when compared to carbamazapine for diabetic polyneuropathy pain (Gomez-Perez et al 1996).

LITHIUM

Lithium alone has been reported to be useful in episodic and chronic cluster headaches (Ekbom 1974, 1981, Kudrow 1977, 1978, Mathew 1978, Bussone et al 1979, Pearce 1980) and, when combined with amitriptyline, in the treatment of painful shoulder syndrome (Tyber 1974). Lithium alone or combined with TCAD or with neuroleptics may be useful for pain syndromes which are associated with bipolar affective disorders and some recurrent unipolar depressions. No controlled adequate trials of lithium therapy for acute or chronic pain were found.

ANTIANXIETY DRUGS

Anxiety

The benzodiazepines may be useful in the short-term (4 weeks or less) management of anxiety, muscle spasm and insomnia which are frequently associated with acute pain and which may occur during acute exacerbations of chronic pain disorders. Non-drug psychological management techniques for these pain-related problems should be tried first where time and available resources permit.

Acute pain

There is suggestive evidence that short-term BDZ use may diminish the acute pain associated with myocardial infarction (Monks 1981), anxiety-related gastrointestinal disorders (Lasagna 1977) and acute and chronic intervertebral disc problems with skeletal muscle spasm (Lasagna 1977, Hollister et al 1981). Only two adequately controlled trials were found. In the first, lorazepam was superior to placebo when added to opioids for procedural pain in major burn injuries but only for those persons with high baseline pain and high state anxiety (Patterson et al 1997). In the second, alprazolam was superior to progesterone and to placebo in providing pain relief when used cyclically in severe premenstrual syndrome (Freeman et al 1995).

Chronic pain

In general, reservations must be expressed about the use of BDZ for chronic pain. Benzodiazepines cause dependency and cognitive impairment, thus promoting the complaint of chronic pain (see 'Adverse effects' below). Although it may be necessary to continue established use of benzodiazepines for certain patients, initiation of their use in chronic pain is seldom indicated.

Two uncontrolled studies were found reporting important BDZ analgesic effects on chronic pain. In the first, alprazolam was found to be very effective in relieving causalgic but not other types of neoplastic pain (Fernandez et al 1987). In the second, clonazepam provided effective relief for more than 6 months in two patients with lancinating phantom limb pain (Bartush et al 1996). Clonazepam, a BDZ with sedative and anticonvulsant properties, has shown some promise in the treatment of neuralgias (Swerdlow & Cundill 1981) and deserves further investigation in view of its relative freedom from adverse effects as compared with other anticonvulsants.

Seven adequate controlled trials of BDZ in chronic pain were found. Three trials reported on the treatment of chronic tension headache. Diazepam was found to be equal to flupenthixol (a neuroleptic) and superior to placebo in diminishing chronic tension headache pain and analgesic use (Hackett et al 1987). Alprazolam was superior to placebo in decreasing headache severity and analgesic use (Shukla et al 1996). Chlordiazepoxide was effective but definitely inferior to a comparison TCAD (Lance & Curran 1964). Of the remaining four trials, two showed some analgesic effect with diazepam for pain of psychological origin but again two comparison TCAD were clearly superior (Okasha et al 1973). Three trials showed either no analgesia (Turkington 1980) or results equivalent to those of placebo controls (Max et al 1988, Quijada-Carrera & Garcia-Lopez 1996).

One controlled trial found buspirone to have analgesic effects comparable to amitriptyline in the treatment of chronic tension headache (Mitsikostas et al 1997).

EFFECTIVENESS

ANTIDEPRESSANTS

Tricyclic antidepressants

Chronic pain

The outcome of the 124 TCAD trials for chronic pain listed in Table 50.1 may be summarized. Although only one of these directly compared TCAD with non-drug therapies, nearly one-half of the trials reported failure of previous analgesic and/or non-drug therapy. Only 5/122 trials failed to show clinically important analgesia and, in controlled trials, pain relief superior to that with placebo. In one uncontrolled trial, amitriptyline and subsequently phenelezine (a MAOI) showed mild antidepressant action, but not analgesia, in a small (n=10) uncontrolled study of chronic headache after closed head injury (Saran 1988). The outcome of adequately controlled trials (Table 50.2) has been presented (see 'indications for use' above).

In three controlled trials TCAD were compared with non-placebo control drugs commonly used in the disorder studied. Amitriptyline and propranolol proved equally effective and clearly superior to placebo in decreasing the pain associated with high-frequency chronic migraine (Zeigler et al 1987). Low-dose amitriptyline was superior to naproxen and to placebo in alleviating the pain and fatigue associated with fibromyalgia (Goldenberg et al 1986). Amitriptyline provided greater pain relief than carbamazepine and placebo and was better tolerated than carbamazepine in the treatment of persons with central poststroke pain (Leijon & Boivie 1989).

Two TCAD trials examined non-drug treatment effects. In one non-blinded trial amitriptyline was compared to spinal manipulation for chronic tension headache. While the amitriptyline was slightly more effective after 6 weeks of treatment, the drug group relapsed 4 weeks post-treatment while the non-drug group showed continued benefit (Boline et al 1995). In the other open trial patients with chronic non-neoplastic pain received amitriptyline with either cognitive-behavioural therapy (CBT) or supportive therapy. There was no statistical difference between the groups despite a trend favouring the CBT group at 6 month follow-up (Pilowsky et al 1995).

In 59 of the 75 trials giving details, ≥50% of patients obtained moderate to total pain relief. Analgesic use was significantly diminished in those studies giving information. A variety of measures indicated acceptable patient compliance with TCAD regimens. In the vast majority of trials, drop-out rates were less than 10%, no different from the rates for comparison placebos. TCAD blood levels, where measured, were in the expected range for doses employed. When asked, patients and physicians preferred TCAD to placebo.

Unfortunately, the length of follow-up on TCAD was rather limited in the trials (80% ≤3 months). However, two recent papers have reported on longer-term treatment. One questionnaire follow-up study reported on 104 patients with chronic non-neoplastic pain who were treated with a variety of TCAD (Blumer & Heilbronn 1981). At 9–16 months, 57% were significantly improved but still on TCAD and 31% had dropped out. At 21–28 months, about one-quarter of the 104 patients were improved or were free of pain and still on TCAD, while an additional one-tenth were able to discontinue TCAD with sustained relief. It was noted that some patients only began to improve after months of TCAD therapy. The other study concerned 93 patients with chronic facial pain of psychological origin treated with dothiepin (Feinmann et al 1984). At 12 months, 73% were pain free; 38% of the pain-free group were still obliged to take dothiepin to prevent the relapse of pain. An additional 8% continued to take dothiepin with partial relief and 9% were lost to follow-up.

A number of clinical and laboratory factors may predict increased TCAD analgesic effect in chronic pain disorders. The presence of clinically important depression (Bradley 1963, Rafinesque 1963, Lascelles 1966, Radebold 1971, Gessel 1975, Loldrup et al 1989), a family history of depressive spectrum disorders (Magni et al 1987), an absence of previous analgesic use (Bourhis et al 1978, Kudrow 1980), dexamethasone non-suppression (Smoller 1984) and increased MHPG levels in CSF associated with increased anxiety scores (Ward et al 1983) have all been noted to correlate with TCAD-induced pain relief.

Newer studies have reported conflicting evidence on the value of the dexamethasone suppression test (DST) results (Valdes et al 1989, Nappi et al 1990).

Head pain, except that from closed head injury, is more likely to be associated with good outcome than that with other body sites (Lodrup et al 1989, Onghena & van Houdenhove 1992). Blood levels of TCAD and their metabolites have been positively correlated with analgesic response in some studies (Johansson & Von Knorring 1979, Lindsay & Wyckoff 1981, Watson et al 1982, Hameroff et al 1984, Kvinesdal et al 1984, Zitman et al 1984, Montastruc et al 1985, Max et al 1987, 1988, Leijon & Boivie 1989) but not in others (Loldrup et al 1989, Kishore-Kumar et al 1990, Sindrup et al 1990a, Max et al 1991). Specific therapeutic blood levels for analgesic response to amitriptyline (Watson et al 1982, Max et al 1987), imipramine (Sindrup et al 1990b) and clomipramine (Montastruc et al 1985) have been suggested.

Poorer outcomes with TCAD for chronic pain have been reported with certain Minnesota Multiphasic Personality Inventory profiles (Pheasant et al 1983), dexamethasone suppression test (DST) non-suppression (Nappi et al 1990), increased analgesic use (Nappi et al 1990), a family history of pain disorders (Valdes et al 1989) and increased levels of E-10-hydroxy nortriptyline, an inactive metabolite of amitriptyline (Edelbroek et al 1986).

Evidence for specific predictors which are clinically useful is still sparse and most of the work cited above requires replication.

SSRI antidepressants

Chronic pain

Of the 20 studies listed in Table 50.1, 12 found clinically important pain relief. These included five out of 10 adequately controlled trials (Table 50.2), one placebo-controlled trial (Johansson & Von Knorring 1979), three TCAD-controlled trials (Watson & Evans 1985, Ventafridda et al 1987, Nappi et al 1990), one small uncontrolled trial (Khurana 1983) and two case studies (Theeson & Marsh 1989, Black & Sheline 1995).

Of the remaining seven studies, five adequate (Table 50.2) and two other controlled trials (Lynch et al 1990, Adly et al 1992) found the SSRI equally as effective as placebo and two controlled studies found little or no analgesic effect (Davidoff et al 1987, Goodkin et al 1990).

Six of nine trials with relevant data showed >50% of patients with moderate to marked pain relief. Analgesic use was seldom documented. Compliance, as indicated by blood levels and a low drop-out rate (average 4%), was excellent. About 70% of studies lasted 3 months or less. Outcomes did not seem to be predicted by specific variables.

In general, as discussed under 'Rationale for treatment' above, SSRI tend to be less efficacious but better tolerated than TCAD-type drugs. For example, in four out of six adequate trials TCAD were superior to their SSRI controls (Sjaastad 1983, Frank et al 1988, Sindrup et al 1990b, Bendtsen et al 1996). Of the remaining controlled trials one favoured the TCAD (Watson & Evans 1985) and two found low-dose amitriptyline equal to an SSRI control (Ventafridda et al 1987, Nappi et al 1990).

SNRI antidepressants

No adequate controlled trials of venlafaxine were found. In the two papers listed in Table 50.1, about one-half those treated experienced >50% pain relief. The vast majority of those studied had inadequate pain relief or intolerable side effects with previous trials of at least one other antidepressant. The drop-out rate was 23% overall. The treatment duration was 1–7 months.

Monoamine oxidase inhibitors

Chronic pain

The only two controlled trials both reported analgesic effects clearly superior to those of placebo (Table 50.2). A majority of patients experienced ≥50% pain relief in those MAOI trials listed in Table 50.1. In most instances, depression and pain were alleviated at the same time. Substantial previous therapies had not been helpful for a majority of patients. Patient compliance was acceptable; drop-out rates averaged 4%. The length of follow-up was <3 months in 70% of studies. Decreased pretreatment plasma 5-hydroxytryptamine during an attack was correlated with successful treatment of migraine headaches using phenelzine (Anthony & Lance 1969).

The efficacy of MAOI for chronic pain remains unestablished in view of the small number of patient studies. Unfortunately, little data is available to compare directly the analgesic effects of MAOI with other drug or non-drug therapy.

NEUROLEPTICS

Acute pain

Of the 21 trials listed in Table 50.3, 20 reported clinically important analgesic effects of neuroleptics in patients with acute pain. In 15 of these trials, a single dose of methotrimeprazine was found to compare favourably with a narcotic control and/or to be superior to placebo in postoperative pain (see 'Indications for use' above). In one other paper the authors found no significant difference in postoperative pain scores or narcotic use among patients premedicated with haloperidol 5 or 10 mg or placebo (Judkins & Harmer 1982). Two additional studies, one single group outcome (Iserson 1983), and one controlled trial (Shrestha et al 1996) respectively reported 93 and 96% marked to total relief from migraine attacks following a single IM or IV dose of chlorpromazine.

The remaining three trials were concerned with ongoing regimens of neuroleptic therapy for acute herpes zoster neuralgia. Treatment with chlorpromazine, chlorprothixene or methotrimeprazine (one trial each) produced total relief in 92–100% of patients within 1–5 days if the therapy was started within 3 months of the onset of the disorder (Sigwald et al 1959, Farber & Burks 1974). These trials were uncontrolled and did not detail previous failed therapies.

Chronic pain

Twenty-nine of the 31 trials listed in Table 50.3 reported clinically important analgesic effects of neuroleptics given for chronic pain. In one retrospective study, haloperidol 5 and 10 mg did not decrease narcotic use in patients with neoplastic pain (Hanks et al 1983), but in an adequate controlled trial minor analgesic use was significantly more diminished with flupenthixol than with placebo in patients with chronic tension headache (Hackett et al 1987). Four of the 31 trials were single-dose experiments or therapy. Methotrimeprazine compared favourably with narcotic controls in mixed or neoplastic chronic pain in three trials (see 'Indications for use' above). One uncontrolled trial reported 'success' in treating chronic recurrent headaches with one dose of trifluoperazine combined with a nonsteroidal anti-inflammatory agent (Polliack 1979). In the remaining 27 trials, longer-term continuous neuroleptic regimens were used to manage various chronic pain disorders. In 16 of the 20 trials with relevant data, the majority of patients experienced moderate to total pain relief with neuroleptics.

Unfortunately, the majority of trials lasted less than 3 months. The importance of this limitation is demonstrated in the case of chronic postherpetic neuralgia, where two trials lasting more than 6 months reported almost total failure after initial impressive relief (Nathan 1978). On the other hand, in another trial, 75% of patients with this disorder maintained their initial pain-free state for 10–20 months following the inception of neuroleptic therapy (Duke 1983).

The duration of the disorder may be of importance. In herpes zoster neuralgia, if neuroleptic therapy was started within 3 months of onset, more than 90% of patients experienced total pain relief, whereas less than 20% of patients obtained good or total pain relief if the condition had been of longer duration (Sigwald et al 1959).

In addition to the controlled trials already mentioned (see 'Indications for use' above), the evidence for neuroleptic-induced pain relief is supported by a series of anecdotal single-patient experiments and uncontrolled group reports of patients with diabetic neuropathy, neoplastic pain, postherpetic neuralgia and thalamic pain (Margolis & Gianascol 1956, Sigwald et al 1959, Cavenar & Maltbie 1976, Davis et al 1977, Maltbie & Cavenar 1977, Daw & Cohen-Cole 1981, Duke 1983). Patients with very chronic stable baseline pain disorders, refractory to many interventions, responded rapidly (≤4 days), frequently had total pain relief and suffered relapse rapidly with placebo substitution or stopping the neuroleptic.

Treatment acceptability in all but one trial was good (≤10% drop-out). In the remaining study, a moderate-dose chlorprothixene (50–100 mg/day orally) regimen was associated with a 35% patient refusal to take the drug for more than 2 weeks despite significant analgesic effects.

In one other trial, the addition of haloperidol to relaxation training led to important pain relief in a group of patients with chronic myofascial dysfunction who were previously unresponsive to this and other forms of behaviour therapy (Raft et al 1979).

COMBINED DRUG THERAPY

TCAD and anticonvulsant

In three trials 72–89% of patients with chronic postherpetic neuralgia experienced moderate to complete relief. Follow-up ranged from 1 to 18 months with a mean of 3 months. In two of the three trials drop-out rates were similar to those noted for TCAD alone, i.e. with nortriptyline plus diphenylhydantoin or carbamazepine, the rate was 12% (Hatangdi et al 1976) and with amitriptyline plus valproic acid 8% (Raferty 1979). In the third trial, patients were entered into a limited cross-over non-blind study in which a regimen of clomipramine plus carbamazepine was compared with transcutaneous nerve stimulation, with each being given for 8 weeks. The drop-out rate for the drug group was 50%, while that for transcutaneous nerve stimulation was 70%. Clearly superior analgesic results were reported for the drug group (Gerson et al 1977).

TCAD and neuroleptic

Seventeen of the 18 combined TCAD and neuroleptic trials for chronic pain listed in Table 50.4 reported good to total pain relief in the majority of patients. Follow-up was ≤3 months in six trials and 6–36 months in five further trials. The average drop-out rate in 13 trials with information was 12%. Most patients had received extensive previous therapy and those disorders treated tended to be resistant to other forms of therapy.

There is evidence to suggest that combined therapy may be more efficacious than TCAD or neuroleptic therapies alone for a significant group of patients. In three trials with flexible drug schedules, about one-third of patients responded to the combined regimen but not TCAD or neuroleptics alone (Davis et al 1977, Khurana 1983, Mitas et al 1983). One controlled trial, comparing clomipramine plus neuroleptic to neuroleptic therapy alone for mixed neurological chronic pain, found 67% compared with 47% good to total relief in the combined and neuroleptic groups respectively, with the drop-out rate being lower in the combined therapy group (Langohr et al 1982). Another controlled trial found the TCAD–neuroleptic combination (nortriptyline with fluphenazine) equally markedly effective as carbamazepine for pain with diabetic polyneuropathy (Gomez-Perez et al 1996).

LITHIUM

Most evidence for the use of lithium in the management of pain is derived from studies with cluster headache. Combining the results of six trials, about one-third of the 69 patients treated with lithium for episodic cluster headache experienced good to total control of pain during a 1-month treatment period (Mathew 1978, Ekbom 1981). In 10 trials of lithium given for chronic cluster headache, more than two-thirds of 118 patients obtained good to total pain relief for periods of up to 6 months or longer (Ekbom 1974, 1981, Kudrow 1977, Mathew 1978, Bussone et al 1979, Pearce 1980). Although no adequate controlled trials were found, the evidence that lithium helped to relieve chronic cluster headache is compelling, given the natural history of the disorder and its non-response to other treatments. Also, one open controlled trial reported lithium to be strikingly superior to methysergide and to prednisone in the treatment of this disorder (Kudrow 1978). Unfortunately no trials were found to compare lithium with verapamil treatment (Lewis & Solomon 1996).

In one uncontrolled trial of lithium and amitriptyline for painful shoulder syndrome, 40% of patients experienced complete pain relief and increased range-of-motion of the joint, while 20% showed resolution of radiographic abnormalities (Tyber 1974).

Lithium therapy was well tolerated in all but one trial, with drop-out rates being ≤3%.

ANTIANXIETY DRUGS

Acute pain

The results of the only two adequate controlled trials have been summarized under 'Indications for use' above. Three addition controlled trials reported clinically important analgesic effects during the first week postmyocardial infarction (Hackett & Cassem 1972, Melsom et al 1976, Dixon et al 1980). In these trials one-third to a majority of patients experienced moderate or good pain relief, and in one study analgesic use was diminished. Compliance was excellent with very few drop-outs (0–2%).

Chronic pain

Of the seven adequate controlled trials and two uncontrolled BDZ trials presented in the section on indications, only three reported >50% patients with moderate to marked relief. Analgesic use was diminished in one study reporting this data. Drop-out rates averaged 5%. BDZ were inferior to TCAD in all four trials where comparison was possible.

Given these results it is not possible to recommend BDZ as first-line treatment for chronic pain.

In one controlled trial 54.4% and 60.7% of buspirone and amitriptyline patients respectively obtained >50% reduction in chronic tension headache pain, although patient opinion of treatment and analgesic use statistics favoured amitriptyline. Drop-outs were comparable (15% buspirone, 16% amitriptyline) in this 12-week study (Mitsikostas et al 1997).

ADVERSE EFFECTS

Extensive reviews of the adverse effects of psychotropic drugs are available elsewhere (Hollister 1978, Baldessarini 1990). In this section, discussion is directed towards those problems more specifically encountered in the treatment of patients with pain disorders.

ANTIDEPRESSANTS

Tricyclic-type antidepressants

Adverse effects with TCAD include anticholinergic autonomic effects, allergic and hypersensitivity reactions, cardio-

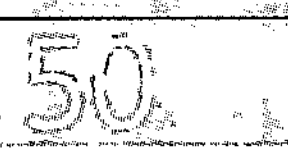

vascular and central nervous system problems, drug interactions, overdoses, drug withdrawal effects and weight gain. The safety of TCAD during pregnancy and lactation has not been established.

Anticholinergic autonomic effects are usually transient and irritating at worst (dry mouth, palpitations, decreased visual accommodation, constipation and oedema) but may occasionally be more serious (postural hypotension, loss of consciousness, aggravation of narrow-angle glaucoma, urinary retention and paralytic ileus). There is more risk in the elderly or those on other anticholinergic drugs (e.g. neuroleptics, antiparkinsonian drugs). Slowing initial administration, lowering TCAD doses, discontinuing other drugs or using a less anticholinergic drug (Table 50.5) may be necessary. TCAD may cause sexual dysfunctions such as loss of libido, impotence and ejaculatory problems. Trazodone may cause priapism and permanent impotence.

Allergic/hypersensitivity reactions such as cholestatic jaundice, skin reactions and agranulocytosis are quite uncommon but require giving the patient adequate precautions. Zimelidine was withdrawn from use because of hepatotoxicity and haemolytic anaemia associated with its use.

Anticholinergic and quinidine-like cardiac effects of tricyclic antidepressants cause serious reservations about their use in patients with pre-existing conduction defects and/or cardiac ischaemia, particularly postmyocardial infarction (Roose & Glassman 1994).

Orthostatic hypotension is common with TCAD which block adrenergic receptors (Table 50.5). Imipramine is more hazardous for the elderly and others vulnerable to falls or hypotension. Those at risk require safer drugs and measurement of orthostatic change before and after an initial test dose. Possible interventions include patient education, use of a bedside commode and night light, surgical support stockings and, in severe cases, 9-α-fluorohydrocortisone 0.025–0.05 mg orally twice a day.

Various central nervous system (CNS) adverse effects have been reported (sedation, tremor, seizures, insomnia, exacerbation of schizophrenia or mania and atropine-like delirium). The elderly are at particular risk, especially if there is previous brain damage or when combinations of drugs with anticholinergic properties are used.

TCAD potentiate CNS depressants (alcohol, anxiolytics, narcotics), potentiate other anticholinergics, antagonize certain antihypertensives (α-methyldopa, guanethidine) and may produce lethal hypertensive episodes with MAOI.

Table 50.5 Antidepressant drugs used in the management of chronic pain

Drug	*Oral dosage range (mg/day)*	*Anticholinergic potency*	*Orthostatic hypotension*	*Sedation*
Tricyclic-type antidepressants				
Amitriptyline	10–300	High	Moderate	High
Clomipramine	20–300	Moderate	Moderate	Moderate
Desipramine	25–300	Low	Low	Low
Doxepin	30–300	Moderate	Moderate	High
Imipramine	20–300	High	High	Moderate
Maprotiline	50–300	Low	Low	High
Nortriptyline	50–150	Moderate	Low	Moderate
Ritanserin	10	Nil	Nil	Nil
Trazodone	50–600	Low	Moderate	High
Trimipramine	50–300	Moderate	?Moderate	High
SSRI-type antidepressants				
Fluoxetine	5–40	Nil	Nil	Nil
Paroxetine	20–40	Low	Nil	Nil
Ritanserin	10	Nil	Nil	Nil
Trazodone	50–600	Low	Moderate	High
SNRI antidepressant				
Venlafaxine	37.5–300	Nil	Nil	Low
Monoamine oxidase inhibitors				
Phenelzine	30–90	Low	High	None
Tranylcypromine	10–40	Low	?Moderate	None

Acute overdoses of TCAD in excess of 2000 mg can be fatal. Initial prescriptions of greater than 1 week's supply are unwise for the depressed patient.

There are no well-controlled studies of TCAD use in pregnancy. If not essential, TCAD use during the first trimester is best avoided.

Mild withdrawal reactions have been observed after the abrupt cessation of imipramine 300 mg/day given for 2 months. Gradual termination of TCAD seems prudent.

In considering TCAD trials listed in Table 50.1, severe adverse effects were rare. Delirium (8–13% of patients in papers with data) and drowsiness (3–28%) were the most common reasons for discontinuing therapy and were usually noted with high doses and drug combinations (TCAD with neuroleptics or with anticonvulsants), especially in the elderly. Delirium (2%) and dissociative reactions (5%) were noted with TCAD–lithium combined therapy (Tyber 1974). One case of myocardial infarction and one case of suicide occurred in trials of TCAD alone; both patients were suffering from advanced neoplastic conditions. One other death occurred in a 80-year-old male with pre-existing 'severe cardiac decompensation' within 1 month of starting amitriptyline and valproic acid for postherpetic neuralgia (Raferty 1974).

Adverse effects and drop-out rates were correlated with higher plasma levels of TCAD and their metabolites in at least two studies (Gerson et al 1977, Kvinesdal et al 1984).

Although little is known about adverse effects of long-term TCAD administrations, one study reported on 46 depressed patients treated with doxepin for 2–10 years (Ayd 1979). No patients were noted to have any serious side effects or any drug-caused impairment of intellectual, social or other functions.

SSRI antidepressants

Although the selective serotonin reuptake blockers such as paroxetine and fluoxetine require further study to demonstrate any analgesic properties in human chronic pain, they appear attractive for persons at risk of adverse effects from tricyclic antidepressants. Most are free of anticholinergic, adrenergic and histaminergic receptor action and thus are relatively unlikely to produce anticholinergic autonomic, cardiac, orthostatic hypotension, sedation or weight gain problems. Overdosage with these drugs are less dangerous than those with tricyclic antidepressants.

On the other hand, their use may be associated with increased insomnia, diarrhoea, nausea, agitation, anxiety, exacerbation of mania or psychosis, sexual disturbances, headache and tremor. Akathisia, other extrapyramidal effects, anorgasmia and a serum sickness-like illness have been reported with fluoxetine. A central hyperserotonergic syndrome, including autonomic instability, hyperthermia, rigidity, myoclonus and delirium, may occur when these drugs are prescribed with other serotonergic drugs like lithium and/or monoamine oxidase inhibitors (Sternback 1991). Other more recently noted adverse effects include increased body sway and potential for falls, sinus node slowing, weight loss and hyponatraemia.

The SSRI antidepressants are metabolized by and inhibit cytochrome 450 isoenzymes. Individual SSRI have widely differing drug interaction potential across isoenzyme systems. Important interactions can occur with other psychotropic agents, antiarrythmics, anticonvulsants, terfenadine, astemizote, cisapride, tolbutamide and anticoagulants (Nemeroff et al 1996).

In the SSRI trials listed in Table 50.1 there were very few serious adverse effects, with the exception of one patient on zimelidine who developed increased levels of liver enzymes and fever. This drug has since been withdrawn from the market for similar problems. Gastrointestinal adverse effects were most common (46% of patients in studies with details). Drop-out rates averaged 10% but varied widely (0–33%).

SNRI antidepressants

Venlafaxine blocks neuronal reuptake of serotonin and norepinephrine but is relatively free of muscarinic cholinergic, histaminic and α-adrenergic receptor effects. It has little potential for drug interaction. However, venlafaxine may increase hypertensive problems, exacerbate existing seizure disorders and trigger mania. More common complaints include nausea, asthenia, sweating, anorexia, somnolence, dizziness and dry mouth. In the only clinical trials found, two out of 14 patients dropped out because of adverse effects, one for nausea and one for hypertension, ataxia and drowsiness (Songer & Schulte 1996, Taylor & Rowbotham 1996).

Monoamine oxidase inhibitors

Although relatively free of anticholinergic side effects, MAOI may cause urinary retention, orthostatic hypotension, severe parenchymal hepatotoxic reactions, CNS effects (insomnia, agitation, exacerbation of mania or schizophrenia), hypertensive crises and drug interactions.

Fortunately, serious adverse effects are rare if medications, foods and beverages with sympathomimetic activities are avoided (Tyrer 1976, Baldessarini 1990). In pain patients, narcotics, especially meperidine, should be avoided and anaesthetics used with great caution (Janowski & Janowski 1985). Hypertensive crises resulting from enhanced sympathomimetic action are best treated with immediate but slow intravenous injection of phentolamine 5 mg or, in an emergency, chlorpromazine 50–100 mg intramuscularly.

In those trials in which MAOI were used to treat pain disorders, phenelzine was discontinued because of jaundice in 4%, impotence in 4% and insomnia in 16% of patients in one study (Anthony & Lance 1969), while orthostatic hypotension was found in 6% and headache in 3% of patients in another (Lascelles 1966).

Long-term MAOI use in chronic pain is unreported, but efficacious and acceptably safe use has been described for up to several years in patients with anxiety disorders (Tyrer 1976).

A new class of compounds, the reversible inhibitors of MAO type A (RIMA), such as moclobemide, brofaromine and toloxatone, appear to be effective antidepressants and are reported to be virtually free of the hepatotoxicity, hypertensive crises and orthostatic hypotension encountered with the older irreversible mixed MAO-A and MAO-B inhibitors reported on in this chapter (Da Prada et al 1990). However, it is prudent to observe the same precautions for use, especially regarding drug–drug interactions, given mixed enzyme inhibition at higher RIMA doses. Unfortunately, it is not known whether RIMA have any analgesic properties.

NEUROLEPTICS

Neuroleptics may also cause anticholinergic effects, orthostatic hypotension, quinidine-like cardiac effects and sedation (Table 50.6). These side effects are more prominent with the low-potency phenothiazines and thiothixenes, particularly when they are combined with TCAD or carbamazepine.

CNS effects are a frequent source of patient non-compliance. Patients may note malaise, dysphoria (boring, 'unpleasant' or 'wretched' feelings) or even overt depression. Acute extrapyramidal syndromes (parkinsonism, akathisia and dystonia) usually occur early in treatment, especially with high-potency drugs (Table 50.6).

Other neurological syndromes include neuroleptic malignant syndrome, perioral tremor (relatively benign and responsive to anticholinergic drugs) and tardive dyskinesia (TD). Tardive dyskinesia may occur in up to 40% of those who have taken neuroleptics regularly over periods of 12 months or more. The likelihood of developing TD seems to be proportional to the total quantity of neuroleptic taken over time but occasionally may occur even with low doses taken over several months (Monks 1980). It is more likely to occur in elderly females and in those with previous brain damage and may be more frequent in those who have also received antiparkinsonian drugs. TD is best managed by prevention (adequate indication for use, alternative regimen if possible), informed consent (patient and

Table 50.6 Neuroleptic drugs used in the management of chronic pain

Drug	*Oral dosage range (mg/day)*	*Anti cholinergic potency*	*Orthostatic hypotension*	*Sedative potency*	*Extra pyramidal effects*
Phenothiazines					
Chlorpromazine	25–500	High	High	High	Low
Fluphenazine	1–10	Low	Low	Low	High
Methotrimeprazine	15–100	High	High	High	Moderate
Pericyazine	5–200	High	High	High	Low
Perphenazine	8–64	Moderate	Moderate	Moderate	Moderate
Thioridazine	10–200	High	High	High	Low
Trifluoperazine	3–20	Low	Low	Low	High
Thioxanthenes					
Chlorprothixene	50–200	High	High	High	Low
Flupenthixol	0.5–2	Low	?None	Absent	High
Miscellaneous					
Haloperidol	0.5–30	Low	Low	Moderate	High

family adequately informed and vigilant regarding the emergence of TD), regular examination for TD by the physician at follow-up visits and the use of low-dose short-term therapy with regular attempts to decrease or discontinue the neuroleptic should it no longer be necessary (American Psychiatric Association 1980). If neuroleptics are stopped at the first sign of TD, the symptoms become worse but gradually fade over a period of 2 or 3 months in most cases.

Novel neuroleptics, such as clozapine and risperidone, have dopamine and serotonin receptor blocking activity and may have decreased risk for extrapyramidal symptoms (EPS) and TD (Andrew 1994). These newer drugs may offer a means to prevent TD or, where treatment with neuroleptics is essential, to continue their use for those with TD. Given their relatively better risk profile and their serotonergic activities the novel neuroleptics would seem of interest for use in chronic pain. Unfortunately no human clinical trials could be found.

Other adverse effects of neuroleptics include weight gain, sexual dysfunction, endocrine disorders, exacerbation of epileptic disorders, photosensitivity, blood dyscrasias (agranulocytosis, leucopenia), cholestatic jaundice and ocular and skin pigmentation. The neuroleptics also increase the effects of CNS depressants and block the action of guanethidine.

In the trials of neuroleptics alone or in combination with TCAD, the commonest problems were somnolence and delirium, with a higher incidence of these problems occurring with high-dose chlorprothixene or methotrimeprazine therapy. Myoclonus and TD were both noted in a single patient in these predominantly short-term trials (Sigwald et al 1959). In one placebo-controlled trial adverse effects were mild but more common with a TCAD–neuroleptic combination (nortriptyline and fluphenazine) than with an anticonvulsant (carbamazepine) alone (Gomez-Perez et al 1996).

LITHIUM

Reported hazards of lithium administration include intoxication and the development of renal, thyroid, cardiac, neuromuscular, neurotoxic, dermatological and birth abnormalities (Klein et al 1980, Bendz 1983, Baldessarini 1990). With careful monitoring of clinical symptoms and blood levels of the drug, short-term lithium use is reasonably safe. The issue of renal morphological changes (interstitial fibrosis and nephron atrophy) with longer-term use is still a cause of concern and preventive measures should include using the lowest dose of lithium for the least time possible, using a single daily maintenance dose and monitoring renal function (Amdisen & Grof 1980, Bendz 1983). Lithium-induced goitre and hypothyroidism usually respond to thyroid hormone.

In studies of lithium use for cluster headaches, the drug had to be discontinued because of lithium headaches (3%), severe nausea and vomiting (6%), lethargy, general weakness (6%) or severe tremor (1%). The most common minor symptom was tremor, which was treatable by propranolol (Kudrow 1977, Mathew 1978, Pearce 1980). Long-term lithium use in pain patients has yet to be reported in detail.

ANTIANXIETY DRUGS

Although physical dependency and withdrawal may occur with prolonged (≥6 weeks) moderate to high dosage use of BDZ, such problems are rarely encountered at therapeutic doses (Marks 1980).

Daytime sedation, impaired coordination and judgement, and other forms of cognitive impairment, have been reported to be common, with prolonged steady use of these drugs for chronic pain (Hendler et al 1980, McNairy et al 1984). These adverse effects are more likely if the patient is elderly or brain damaged, if longer-acting BDZ are used or if other central-depressant drugs are given at the same time (Committee on the Review of Medicine 1980, Marks 1980). Other reported adverse effects include depression, suicidal thoughts, impulsivity and rebound insomnia.

Studies of patients treated in pain centres suggest that global and specific neuropsychological test impairments and electroencephalogram abnormalities occur more often in patients on BDZ than in comparable controls (Hendler et al 1980, McNairy et al 1984). However, in the general population, 15% of all BDZ users continue these drugs on a daily long-term basis. Most claim continued benefit without tolerance to the drugs developing. A similar result was reported in one study of long-term diazepam use (1 month to 16 years) in a neurosurgical clinic for patients with chronic pain and muscle spasm (Hollister et al 1981). Despite daily use, an older population and concomitant use of other drugs, 77% of patients felt that diazepam benefited them. Only a small number (10 out of 108) reported any side effects (usually oversedation). Side effects could not be correlated with plasma levels of diazepam or nordiazepam and the values did not suggest abuse of the drug. Unfortunately, neuropsychological testing of these patients was not reported. In those BDZ trials described under 'indications for use' above, initial sedation and dizziness were the commonest adverse effects. Acute depressive mood changes occurred in 18% of patients in one trial (Max et al 1988). Drop-out rates due to BDZ effects were usually less than 5%.

Buspirone is usually well tolerated with drop-out rates from non-pain trials averaging 10%. More frequent adverse effects include dizziness, headache, nausea and, less frequently, insomnia. Dystonias and cogwheel rigidity have been reported.

DESCRIPTION OF TREATMENT

GENERAL CONSIDERATIONS

Certain principles of psychotropic drug use are worth mentioning:

1. There must be adequate indications for the use of these drugs. Moreover, this symptomatic management must not delay the discovery of treatable causes of pain.
2. Every effort must be made to establish a working alliance with the patient and his support system (family, other health professionals). A clear explanation of indications, goals, methods, alternative management and risk of intervention and non-intervention is essential in this regard.
3. Management should begin with the most benign efficacious intervention and a more hazardous regimen used only if treatment fails and informed consent is given (e.g. transcutaneous nerve stimulation then TCAD and neuroleptic therapy). Figures 50.1 and 50.2 depict one possible protocol based on this approach.
4. The therapeutic trial must be at an adequate dose for a sufficient length of time.
5. Other drugs should be reduced or eliminated, if at all feasible, as soon as possible. Detoxification from narcotics, alcohol, hypnotics and antianxiety drugs is often necessary to obtain a therapeutic response (Halpern 1982, Buckley et al 1986).
6. The physician must be available during the initiation of therapy and during changes in regimen.
7. Elderly patients usually require only one-third to one-half of the usual adult daily doses. Cumulative increases in psychotropics and their metabolites occur over a much longer period and maximum adverse effects may not be seen for weeks.

ANTIDEPRESSANTS

Tricyclic-type, SSRI and SNRI, antidepressants

Table 50.5 lists the generic names and approximate dosage ranges of some of the tricyclic-type antidepressants (bicyclic, tricyclic, tetracyclic and similar drugs). Figures 50.1 and 50.2 illustrate the approach to antidepressant use outlined below.

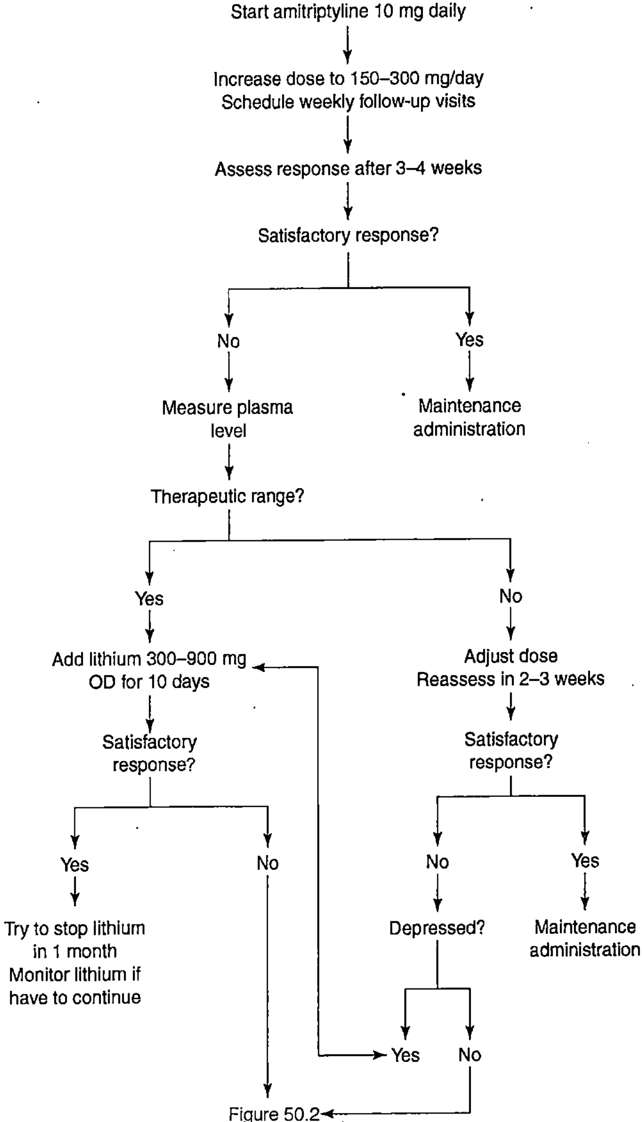

Fig. 50.1 Suggested sequence of psychotropic drug use in chronic pain disorders listed in Table 50.1.

Precautions

Baseline blood studies (liver function, haemoglobin measurement and blood count) are performed. An electrocardiogram is obtained in all elderly patients and those with cardiovascular problems. Patients at risk from possible hypotension may have lying and sitting blood pressure determination before and 1–2 hours following an initial oral 10–50 mg test dose.

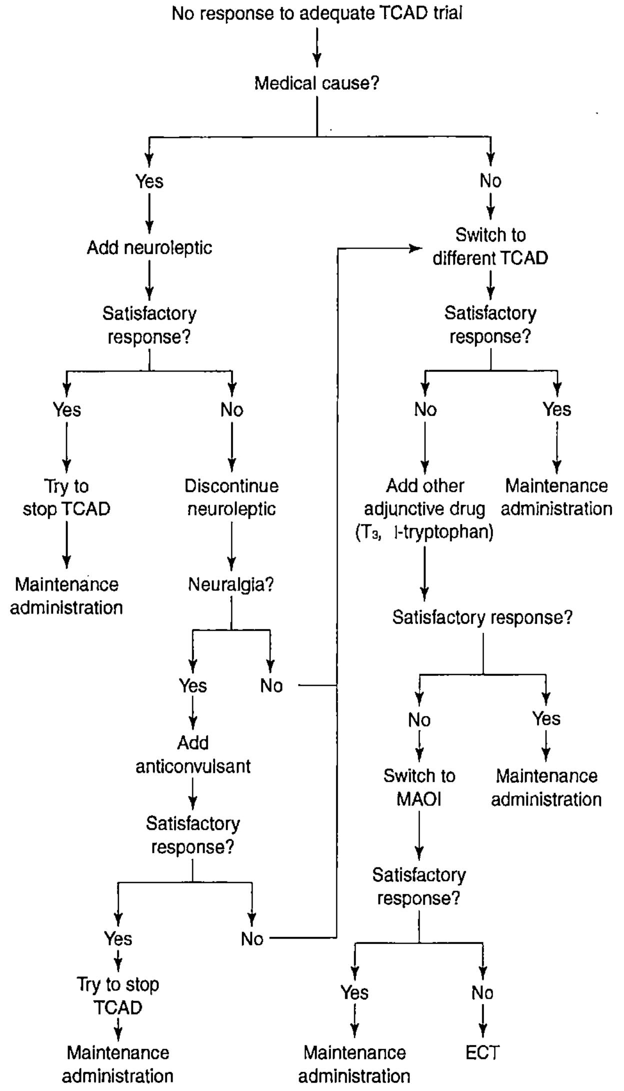

Fig. 50.2 Suggested sequence of psychotropic drug use in chronic pain disorders listed in Table 50.1 (continued from Fig 50.1).

Choice of drugs

There is little evidence to support the use of one TCAD over any other. However, a past positive response of pain or depression in the patient or his blood relatives to a particular TCAD would favour its use. A history of therapeutic failure or adverse effects with a TCAD requires further information. These difficulties are usually a result of inadequate trials, non-compliance or avoidable adverse effects. If the drug history is not helpful, patients with disorders listed in Table 50.2 should start one of the drugs proven effective in these adequately controlled trials. As already discussed under 'Rationale for treatment' above, for most chronic pain disorders there appears to be an advantage to initiating therapy with a tricyclic antidepressant with mixed neurotransmitter properties (e.g. amitriptyline, imipramine, clomipramine or doxepin) unless the potential side effects of these drugs dictate otherwise. Overall, amitriptyline is a reasonable choice for most younger persons.

Drug side effects may be exploited (e.g. by the use of a more sedating TCAD such as amitriptyline, doxepin or trimipramine for patients with marked sleep disturbance or high daytime arousal). For example, a single dose of 50–75 mg of one of these TCAD at bedtime is often used in substitution–detoxification programmes during the initial 1–2 months of treatment to obtain rapid symptomatic relief, prevent the exacerbation of anxiety and depression and to facilitate optimal levels of function (Halpern 1982).

TCAD may be taken to minimize adverse effects. For example, there are fewer anticholinergic effects with desipramine or maprotiline as discussed under 'Adverse effects' below (Table 50.5). Despite the preliminary nature of evidence supporting its use, venlafaxine may be a reasonable initial choice in patients at high risk of anticholinergic, hypotensive or drug interaction adverse events.

Initial administration

In dealing with chronic pain, schedules and doses of TCAD are best arranged to increase compliance and decrease adverse effects. For example, with amitriptyline, the patient is instructed to start with 10 mg orally 1–2 hours before bedtime. The next day this dose is increased to 25 mg, subsequently, the dose is increased by 25 mg/day every several days as tolerated. This is continued until a therapeutic response is obtained or a total daily dose of 150 mg/day is reached. If undue side effects supervene, a lower dose should be employed than the dose at which these effects appeared. If there is no response after 150 mg/day for 1 week and there are no medical contraindications or serious adverse effects, the dose may be increased by 25 mg/day to the maximum dose indicated in Table 50.5. If there is no therapeutic effect after a further 3 weeks, a TCAD blood level should be performed (Fig. 50.1). If plasma levels are lower than usual antidepressant levels, i.e. amitriptyline plus nortriptyline metabolite >120 ng/ml, imipramine >225 ng/ml or nortriptyline between 50 and 150 ng/ml (Perry et al 1987), check for non-compliance and attempt to achieve these plasma levels for at least 3–4 weeks. If there is no direct response in spite of adequate levels or if it is not possible to achieve these levels through discussion and regimen alterations to improve side effects and compliance, either discontinue the drug by 25 mg/day decrements or move to one of the alternative strategies outlined for non-response below.

In the majority of reported clinical trials and in clinical practice, the therapeutic dose of TCAD like amitriptyline, even in the initial phase, is between 50 and 150 mg/day orally (average 75 mg). There is some evidence that head pain (migraine, psychogenic head and face pain and chronic tension headache) may respond at lower doses such as 25–75 mg/day (Lance & Curran 1964, Diamond & Baltes 1971, Okasha et al 1973, Gessel 1975, Carasso 1979, Kudrow 1980, Sharav et al 1987).

Lower doses and slower rates of administration of TCAD are necessary in patients over 60 years old (Nies et al 1977). Treatment is usually initiated at 20–30 mg/day and increased by 10 mg, with total daily doses of 50–150 mg/day usually being adequate.

Initial parenteral TCAD administration for pain patients has been advocated by some authors (Fiorentino 1967, Gebhardt et al 1969, Adjan 1970, Desproges-Gotteron et al 1970, Radebold 1971, Bernard & Scheuer 1972, Monstastruc et al 1985). A typical regimen would be clomipramine 25–50 mg/day intravenously for 3–5 days in hospital, then switching to usual oral doses.

Maintenance administration

There are several clinical reports of TCAD pain therapy lasting more than 3 months (Kuipers 1962, Gade et al 1980, Blumer & Heilbronn 1981, Feinmann et al 1984, Urban et al 1986, Valdes et al 1989). Despite the lack of detail in many of these reports, certain patients require maintenance TCAD for months to years, and in most instances the daily dose approximated the initial dose (20–75 mg). In usual clinical practice, especially with higher initial doses, some slow reduction to lower maintenance levels is possible 1 month after maximum therapeutic response has been obtained. After a further 3–6 months of remission, slow discontinuation of the drug may be tried as the patients are closely watched for relapse of pain and for depressive symptoms.

During maintenance therapy, a single daily evening dose of the more sedating TCAD may be used to improve compliance, decrease daytime adverse effects and provide hypnotic effect. Patients vulnerable to nocturnal disorientation or postural hypotensive episodes may require continued divided doses.

Non-response or relapse

Many instances of non-response are a result of poor compliance or an inadequate regimen. Careful preparation of patients, close initial follow-up, simplified, typed drug schedules, and the support of the family and of the primary physician are all important in increasing compliance.

In the case of non-response to an adequate trial of TCAD and where an alternative drug or non-drug therapy is unhelpful or unavailable, other strategies may be used:

1. Lithium potentiation If depression and chronic pain are present, lithium carbonate 300–900 mg/day may be added to the TCAD (Fig. 50.1). If an antidepressant response is not seen within 10 days, lithium should be stopped and further alternatives considered (Fig. 50.1). If there is a satisfactory response, lithium may be discontinued after another month of therapy in a majority of persons (De Montigny et al 1981). Where there is an antidepressant but no analgesic response, additional therapy may be attempted (Fig. 50.2).

2. Alternate TCAD, SSRI or other antidepressant In the obviously depressed patient, especially when depression is felt to be the primary disorder, a second therapeutic trial with a TCAD with different monoamine properties is initiated after tapering off the first TCAD over a period of 7–10 days. For example, if a more serotonergic drug was used first and failed, a drug with stronger noradrenergic effects (desipramine, imipramine, nortriptyline or maprotiline) would be substituted and a second adequate trial instituted. If adverse effects prevent the use of the less selective TCAD, a selective SSRI (fluoxetine, paroxetine) or SNRI (venlafaxine) may be tried.

3. TCAD–neuroleptic combination For the patient with milder or no depressive symptoms, or where an obvious medical cause is present, an alternative approach would be to add a neuroleptic to the first TCAD regimen instead of switching to a second TCAD (Fig. 50.2, Table 50.4). In order to decrease adverse effects (Table 50.6), oral doses of haloperidol 0.5–5 mg/day (Bernard & Scheuer 1972, Kocher 1976), fluphenazine 1–3 mg/day (Hatangdi et al 1976, Gomez-Perez et al 1985, 1996) or perphenazine 4–16 mg/day (Taub 1973, Duthie 1977, Weis et al 1982) are used. If one of these drugs is ineffective, if extrapyramidal adverse effects are a problem, or if more sedation is required, a low-potency neuroleptic such as methotrimeprazine 5–100 mg/day, chlorpromazine 25–100 mg/day or pericyazine 5–100 mg/day may be used (Sigwald et al 1959, Merskey & Hester 1972).

The neuroleptic is started at the lowest dose listed above and stepped up by increments of this dose daily until a clear therapeutic effect or the maximum recommended dose is reached. If no therapeutic response is obvious by 2 weeks, the neuroleptic and then the TCAD are tapered off over 7–10 days each and discontinued. A different TCAD may then be tried (Fig. 50.2).

If the combination is effective, an attempt should be made to taper off the TCAD, as the neuroleptic alone may be adequate. If both drugs are necessary, it is worth trying to taper off the neuroleptic after 3 months of stable response as it may no longer be necessary (Khurana 1983). Otherwise, maintenance administration guidelines are those described for each drug group used alone.

4. TCAD–anticonvulsant combination Patients with neuralgias that are resistant to TCAD or a TCAD–neuroleptic combination may be aided by the addition of clonazepam 1.5–10 mg/day (Swerdlow & Cundhill 1981), carbamazepine 150–1000 mg/day (Hatangdi et al 1976, Gerson et al 1977) or valproic acid 200–600 mg/day (Raferty 1979) to an adequate TCAD regimen. Because of frequent adverse effects, especially with TCAD–carbamazapine combinations, blood level monitoring of both drugs is advisable. Hospitalization of frail elderly patients during the initiation of therapy is advisable. If the combination is effective, attempt to taper off the TCAD after 3 months of stable response. Further maintenance administration guidelines are those for each drug group used alone. If there is no response, a different TCAD may be tried (Fig. 50.2).

5. Other alternatives The addition of an adjunctive drug, such as triiodothyronine (25–50 μg/day) to an adequate TCAD regimen, may produce an antidepressant response in a minority of depressives not responding to TCAD alone (Goodwin et al 1982). L-Tryptophan (2–4 g/day) may have some analgesic properties when used alone or with TCAD but further studies are needed (France & Krishnan 1988).

TCAD–SSRI combinations are occasionally used for the treatment of refractory depressions and one pain trial found an amitriptyline–fluoxetine regimen superior to either drug alone for fibromyalgia (Goldenberg et al 1996). High plasma levels of the TCAD with increased risk for adverse effects may occur in such regimens.

For a patient with pain of psychological origin, especially in the presence of depressive symptoms, a trial with MAOI would be warranted following failed treatment with adequate trials of two different TCADs. Also, atypical depressive symptoms such as hypersomnia, increased appetite and weight, panics, phobias and depersonalization may respond preferentially to MAOI (Liebowitz et al 1988). A wash-out period of 2 weeks between TCAD and MAOI trials is essential.

Finally, electroconvulsvie therapy has been used successfully in a small number of drug-refractory pain patients with or without TCAD therapy (Lascelles 1966, Mandel 1975). It is likely this treatment is not indicated unless warranted by the clinical depression alone.

SSRI antidepressants

SSRI drugs and usual doses are listed in Table 50.5.

Precautions

Baseline blood studies would include a haemogram and electrolytes. An electrocardiogram and liver function studies are prudent in patients with a history of cardiac or liver abnormalities. A baseline weight is advisable in the elderly.

Choice of drugs

The same approach to choice as outlined under TCAD antidepressants is reasonable. Fluoxetine is helpful in lethargic patients, while paroxetine might offer some initial advantage in those with anxiety or psychomotor agitation.

Initial administration

Fluoxetine is usually started at 10 mg (5 mg in the elderly) each morning to avoid insomnia. It is increased to 20 mg per day after 1–2 weeks if well tolerated and may be increased to 40 mg per day after a further 3 weeks if the results are inadequate and the drug is still tolerated. Higher doses often are required if obsessive-compulsive symptoms are prominent. Paroxetine doses and increases are similar, but the drug can be given any time of day. The speed of administration may have to be slowed if there is an increase in anxiety or jitteriness in the first 1–2 weeks. These usually diminish thereafter.

Non-response

Alternative and augmentation strategies are outlined under 'Antidepressants' above and in Figures 50.1 and 50.2. SSRI should be tapered off over 1 week or so.

Maintenance

The maintenance and initial doses are usually the same.

Monamine oxidase inhibitors

The characteristics of the irreversible mixed type MAO-A and MAO-B inhibitors, phenelzine and tranylcypromine, are listed in Table 50.5. The newer RIMA drugs are not described here as their analgesic properties are unknown.

Precautions

Because of potential adverse reactions and a narrower spectrum of antidepressant action, MAOI are usually reserved for TCAD-resistant chronic pain disorders. The MAOI should only be used with patients capable of following stringent restrictions of foods, beverages and other medications, and not suffering from a variety of medical ailments (see 'Adverse effects' above; Baldessarini 1977, 1990). The patient should be given a list of potentially dangerous items and a card to carry which details the drug and specific countermeasures for medical emergencies. Patients at risk of orthostatic hypotension should have lying and standing blood pressure monitored before and during initial treatment.

Maintenance administration

Despite the absence of published data concerning MAOI and chronic pain, clinical experience suggests that the initial therapeutic and maintenance doses are of the same magnitude.

Non-response or relapse

Measures of platelet MAOI may be used to determine adequate dosage and patient compliance (Baldessarini 1990). Although only anecdotal evidence exists, it is possible that the compliance and therapeutic outcome may be enhanced by the addition of minor tranquillizers or small-dose neuroleptics to the MAOI (Bradley 1963, Lascelles 1966).

L-Tryptophan 0.5–1.0 g three times a day may be added to phenelzine in order to obtain improvement in patients with depression who have not responded sufficiently to the MAOI. There is evidence that this combination has a very potent antidepressant effect (Coppen 1972). One controlled trial found this combination superior to phenelzine or amitriptyline alone for fibromyalgia pain (Nicholodi & Sicuteri 1996). Once improvement appears, some side effects such as sluggish behaviour, slurred speech and ataxia may also develop. These are easily dealt with by reduction of the dose of each drug (usually by about one-third).

NEUROLEPTICS

Dosages for neuroleptics used in the treatment of chronic pain are listed in Table 50.6.

Precautions

As indicated, neuroleptics are best employed for pain associated with physical causes. In general, antidepressants should be considered before neuroleptics because, for the most part, they are better tolerated by patients and are much less prone to be associated with long-term complications such as TD. Baseline laboratory tests are identical to those for TCAD. A written informed consent is advisable, especially regarding the risk of TD.

Initial administration

The physician should familiarize herself with one or two of the neuroleptics and use them preferentially. There is no convincing evidence that one neuroleptic is more effective than another.

Among the low-potency neuroleptics, methotrimeprazine is a reasonable choice. This drug is started at 5–10 mg about 2–3 hours before bedtime. This often enables a reduction to be made in the use of other night sedatives. If the medication is taken too near bedtime, the hypnotic effect will not occur for several hours and there may be morning drowsiness. If proven acceptable in the evening, enabling good sleep without waking from pain, the use of the medication may be extended to daytime with 2.5 mg taken three times a day. In general, it is not advisable to exceed 75–100 mg/day of methotrimeprazine. Most adverse effects seem to occur above the 50 mg daily level. The same pattern of use may be applied with any of the other sedative phenothiazines, such as chlorpromazine or pericyazine, varying the dose with the potency of the individual medication.

High-potency neuroleptics are utilized for patients at risk from autonomic, anticholinergic or sedative adverse effects, especially those on TCAD–neuroleptic combinations. Neuroleptics such as haloperidol or fluphenazine are started with a 1-mg oral test dose (0.25–0.5 mg in elderly) and, if tolerated, increased by 1 mg/day to the usual effective dose of 3–5 mg/day (0.5–2 mg/day in the elderly). If there is no response after 1 week, the drug is further increased by 1 mg/day, as tolerated, to effective or maximum dosage.

With either high- or low-potency neuroleptics, a therapeutic response should be seen within 2 weeks of maximum tolerable dosage; if not, the drug is tapered off and discontinued.

Maintenance administration

It is important to emphasize that the dose of any psychotropic drug must be tailored to the individual's response and his needs. As with TCAD–neuroleptic combinations, intermittent (3-monthly) attempts should be made to lower and discontinue the neuroleptic in view of the risk of TD.

A careful clinical examination and chart notation regarding involuntary movements should be made at each follow-up visit.

LITHIUM CARBONATE

Lithium salts are given orally, usually in the form of lithium carbonate.

Precautions

Lithium use for pain is contraindicated in the presence of certain medical conditions (renal tubular disease, myocardial infarction, myasthenia gravis and cardiac conduction defects) and in early pregnancy (Klein et al 1980). Patients must cooperate with regular blood tests and be capable of recognizing early signs of intoxication. Baseline investigations include serum creatinine and electrolytes, thyroid tests, haemogram, pregnancy test, urinalysis, 24-hour urine volume and creatinine clearance. Close monitoring of lithium blood levels is necessary for patients who are also taking drugs that may increase lithium levels, such as diuretics, carbamazepine and various non-steroidal anti-inflammatory agents.

Initial administration

In studies reporting on the treatment of cluster headaches, lithium carbonate 300 mg was given orally on the first day and increased to 300 mg two or three times per day by the end of the first week (Ekbom 1974, Kudrow 1977, Mathew 1978). The dosage was adjusted according to clinical response, severity of side effects and in order to keep weekly serum lithium levels between 0.5 and 1.2 mmol/l.

Maintenance therapy

Little data are available for episodic cluster headache beyond 2 weeks' administration (Mathew 1978). In the chronic cluster group, maintenance periods of 16–32 weeks are reported with continuing improvement, despite lowered lithium dosages and mean serum levels (0.3–0.4 mmol/l; Kudrow 1977, Mathew 1978). In another report even lower lithium levels were possible (0.3–0.4 mmol/l; Pearce 1980).

Once maintenance dosage is achieved, lithium determinations may be performed less frequently (monthly, then 3 monthly). Serum creatinine and thyroid stimulating hormone levels are repeated 6 monthly. Creatinine clearance and 24-hour urine volume are repeated each year. Other tests are undertaken if clinically indicated. After a 3–6-month symptom-free interval, lithium dosage may be tapered off and, if possible, discontinued.

Non-response or relapse

Most treatment failures were a result of intolerable adverse effects, despite serum lithium levels less than 1.2 mmol/l. Some patients were able to continue with lower doses of lithium (Kudrow 1977) and others with incapacitating tremor were helped by propranolol (Mathew 1978).

ANTIANXIETY DRUGS

Benzodiazepine preparations used in the management of anxiety and pain are listed in Table 50.7.

Precautions

Patients should be educated to expect only short-term BDZ use. Alternative therapies for anxiety and muscle tension, such as behavioural-cognitive techniques, should be started as soon as possible. Benzodiazepines should not be used for those subjects who are dependent on alcohol or other drugs. Baseline tests are only performed if clinically indicated, except for clonazepam, where a complete haemogram should be done.

Initial administration

Benzodiazepine choice, dose and administration schedules are those used in the treatment of anxiety and are well described elsewhere (Hollister et al 1981, Monks 1981, Greenblatt et al 1983, Baldessarini 1990). Doses of BDZ in excess of diazepam 10–15 mg/day orally or its equivalent are seldom indicated.

After 3–4 weeks of therapy, BDZ are tapered off and withdrawn over 1–2 weeks. A longer period of withdrawal may be necessary for alprazolam, i.e. decrease by 0.125–0.25 mg each 4–7 days. Further brief, intermittent courses of BDZ may be used for exacerbations of the pain disorder.

In the rare instance where longer-term treatment is essential (e.g. phantom pain or chronic musculoskeletal pain unresponsive to other drug and non-drug approaches), BDZ use should be carefully monitored for the development of tolerance, cognitive disturbance, ataxia, depression or unexpected escalation in pain complaints.

Table 50.7 Antidepressant drugs used in the management of chronic pain

Drug	*Oral dosage range (mg/day)*	*Main indications*
Alprazolam	0.75–6.0	Panics, anxiety-depression
Chlordiazepoxide	10–100	Generalized anticipatory anxiety
Clonazepam	0.5–10	Panics, seizures, neuralgias, phantom pain
Clorazepate	7.5–60	Generalized anticipatory anxiety
Diazepam	4–40	Generalized anticipatory anxiety, muscle spasm
Lorazepam	1–6	Generalized anticipatory anxiety
Oxazepam	30–120	Generalized anticipatory anxiety

CONCLUSIONS

Additional adequate clinical trials are required to establish psychotropic efficacy in most pain disorders. There is a particular need for psychotropic regimens to be compared or combined with other somatic therapies (TENS, nerve blocks) and various non-drug interventions. One relevant study in persons with psychogenic pain disorder found that the combination of amitriptyline and psychotherapy was superior to either treatment alone (Pilowsky & Barrow 1990).

Antidepressants are indicated in most pain patients with clinically detectable depression. They may be useful in relieving pain-related problems such as anxiety, panics and insomnia. They may help in the early stages of detoxification from narcotics and antianxiety–sedative drugs. They appear to have an analgesic effect in specific chronic pain states such as chronic osteo- and rheumatoid arthritis, diabetic neuropathy, fibromyalgia, migraine, head and face pain of psychological origin, postherpetic neuralgia and chronic tension headaches. Further studies are needed comparing antidepressants and anticonvulsants in neuropathic pain (McQuay et al 1996) and in chronic high-frequency migraine headache (Silbertstein 1996). Tricyclic-type drugs remain the antidepressants of first choice for chronic pain. SSRI and MAOI may be useful where TCAD fail or are not advisable because of adverse effects. The SNRI antidepressant, venlafaxine, is a promising agent given some initial successes and a relatively benign adverse effect/drug interaction profile. More evidence is desirable.

Neuroleptics are the treatment of choice for delusional pain. They may be efficacious alone or in combination with TCAD for some types of chronic pain which are often resistant to other forms of therapy, i.e. arthritic pain, causalgias, neuralgias, neuropathies, phantom pain and thalamic pain. Studies examining the use of novel neuroleptics in chronic pain are strongly recommended.

Lithium carbonate is effective in relieving chronic cluster headache and may prevent episodic cluster headache. Studies are needed to compare its use with calcium-channel blockers such as verapamil.

The benzodiazepines may be useful in the short-term management of acute or chronic pain which is closely related to anxiety. Continuous benzodiazepine use for chronic pain is not recommended.

In general, with reasonable precautions, psychotropic regimens are well tolerated and acceptably free from important adverse effects.

Acknowledgements

The authors wish to express their gratitude to Ms Bev Nickless for her patience and skill.

REFERENCES

Adjan M 1970 Uber therapeutischen Beeinflussung des Schmerzsumptoms bei unheilbaren Tumorkranken. Therapie der Gegenwart 10: 1620–1627

Adly C, Straumanis J, Chesson A 1992 Fluoxetine prophylaxis of migraine. Headache 32: 101–104

Alcoff J, Jones E, Rust P, Newman R 1982 Controlled trial of imipramine for chronic low back pain. Journal of Family Practice 14: 841–846

Amdisen A, Grof P 1980 Lithium and the kidneys. International Drug Therapy News 15: 3–4

American Psychiatric Association 1980 Task force on late neurological effects of antipsychotic drugs. Tardive dyskinesia. American Journal of Psychiatry 137: 1163–1172

Andersen E, Dafny N 1983 An ascending serotonergic pain modulation pathway from the dorsal raphe nucleus to the parafascicularis nucleus of the thalamus. Brain Research 269: 57–67

Andrew HG 1994 Clinical relationship of extrapyramidal symptoms and tardive dyskinesia. Canadian Journal of Psychiatry 39(suppl 2): S76–S80

Anthony M, Lance JW 1969 Monoamine oxidase inhibitors in the treatment of migraine. Archives of Neurology 21: 263–268

Ardid D, Eschalier A, LeBars D et al 1995 Involvement of bulbospinal pathways in the antinociceptive effect of clomipramine in the rat. Brain Research 695: 253–256

Atkinson JH, Kremer EF, Risch SC, Jankowsky DS 1986 Basal and post-dexamethasone cortisol and prolactin concentrations in depressed and non-depressed patients with chronic pain syndromes. Pain 25: 23–24

Ayd FJ 1979 Continuation and maintenance doxepin therapy: 10 years' experience. International Drug Therapy News 14: 9–16

Baldessarini RJ 1977 Chemotherapy in psychiatry. Harvard University Press, Cambridge, Massachusetts, pp 101–121

Baldessarini RJ 1990 Drugs and the treatment of psychiatric disorders. In: Goodman Gilman A, Rall TTW, Nies AS, Taylor P (eds) The pharmacological basis of therapeutics, vol 8. Pergamon, New York, pp 383–435

Barber A, Harting S, Wolf HP 1989 Antinociceptive effects of the $5HT_2$ antagonist ritanserin in rats: evidence for an activation of descending monoaminergic pathways in the spinal cord. Neuroscience Letters 99: 234–238

Bartusch SL, Jernigan JR, D'Alessio JG, Sanders BJ 1996 Clonazepam for the treatment of lancinating phantom limb pain. Clinical Journal of Pain 12: 59–62

Basbaum AI, Fields HL 1978 Endogenous pain control mechanisms: review and hypothesis. Annals of Neurology 4: 451–462

Beaver WT, Wallenstein SL, Houde RW et al 1966 A comparison of the analgesic effect of methotrimeprazine and morphine in patients with cancer. Clinical Pharmacology and Therapeutics 7: 436–446

Bendz H 1983 Kidney function in lithium-treated patients. A literature survey. Acta Psychiatrica Scandinavica 68: 303–324

Bendtsen L, Olesen J, Jensen R 1996 A non-selective (amitriptyline), but not a selective (citalopram), serotonin reuptake inhibitor is effective in the prophylactic treatment of chronic tension-type headache. Journal of Neurology, Neurosurgery and Psychiatry 61: 285–290

Bernard A, Scheuer H 1972 Action de la clomipramine (Anafranil) sur la douleur des cancers en pathologie cervico-faciale. Journal Francais d'Oto-rhino-laryngologie 21: 723–728

Bibolotti E, Borghi C, Pasculli E et al 1986 The management of fibrositis: a double blind comparison of maprotyline (Ludiomil chlorimipramine and placebo. Clinical Trials Journal 23: 269–280

Biegon A, Samuel D 1980 Interaction of tricyclic antidepressants with opiate receptors. Biochemical Pharmacology 29: 460–462

Black KJ, Sheline YI 1995 Paroxetine as migraine prophylaxis. Journal of Clinical Psychiatry 56: 330–331

Bloomfield S, Simard-Savoie S, Bernier J, Tétreault L 1964 Comparative analgesic activity of levomepromazine and morphine in patients with chronic pain. Canadian Medical Association Journal 90: 1156–1159

Blumer D, Heilbronn M 1981 Second-year follow-up study on systematic treatment of chronic pain with antidepressants. Henry Ford Hospital Medical Journal 29: 67–68

Blumer D, Zorick F, Heilbronn M, Roth T 1982 Biological markers for depression in chronic pain. Journal of Nervous and Mental Disease 170: 425–428

Boline PD, Anderson AV, Nelson C et al 1995 Spinal manipulation vs amitriptyline for the treatment of chronic tension-type headaches: a randomized clinical trial. Journal of Manipulative Physiological Therapeutics 18: 148–154

Bonica JJ 1977 Basic principles in managing chronic pain. Archives of Surgery 112: 783–788

Botney M, Fields HL 1983 Amitriptyline potentiates morphine analgesia in a direct action on the central nervous system. Annals of Neurology 13: 160–164

Bourhis A, Boudouresque G, Pellet W et al 1978 Pain infirmity and psychotropic drugs in oncology. Pain 5: 263–274

Bradley JJ 1963 Severe localized pain associated with the depressive syndrome. British Journal of Psychiatry 109: 741–745

Breivik H, Rennemo F 1982 Clinical evaluation of combined treatment with methadone and psychotropic drugs in cancer patients. Acta Anaesthetica Scandinavica 74: 135–140

Breivik H, Slørdahl J 1984 Beneficial effects of flupenthixol for osteoarthritic pain of the hip: a double blind cross-over comparison with placebo. Pain 2(suppl): 5254

Bronwell AW, Rutledge R, Dalton ML 1966 Analgesic effect of methotrimeprazine and morphine. Archives of Internal Medicine 111: 725–728

Buckley FP, Sizemore WA, Charlton JE 1986 Medication management in patients with chronic non-malignant pain: a review of the use of a drug withdrawal protocol. Pain 26: 153–165

Bunney WE, Garland MA 1984 Lithium and its possible modes of action. In: Post RM, Ballenger JC (eds) Neurobiology of mood disorders. Williams & Wilkins, London, pp 731–743

Bussone G, Boiardi A, Merati B, Crenna P, Picco A 1979 Chronic cluster headache: response to lithium treatment. Journal of Neurology 221: 181–185

Butler SH, Weil-Fugazza J, Godefroy F, Besson JM 1985 Reduction of arthritis and pain behavior following chronic administration of amitriptyline or imipramine in rats with adjuvant-induced arthritis. Pain 23: 159–175

Carasso RL 1979 Clomipramine and amitriptyline in the treatment of severe pain. International Journal of Neuroscience 9: 191–194

Carette S, McCain GA, Bell DA, Fam AG 1986 Evaluation of amitriptyline in primary fibrositis: a double blind, placebo controlled trial. Arthritis and Rheumatism 29: 655–659

Caruso I, Sarzi Puttini PC, Boccassini L et al 1987 Double blind study of dothiepin versus placebo in the treatment of primary fibromyalgia syndrome. Journal of International Medical Research 15: 154–159

Castaigne P, Laplane D, Morales R 1979 Traitement par la clomipramine des douleurs des neuropathies périphériques. Nouvelle Presse Médicale 8: 843–845

Cavenar JO, Maltbie AA 1976 Another indication for haloperidol. Psychosomatics 17: 128–130

Cerda SE, Eisenach JC, Deal DD, Tong C 1997 A physiologic assessment of intrathecal amitriptyline in sheep. Pain 69: 161–169

Cohen GL 1997 Protriptyline, chronic tension-type headaches, and weight loss in women. Headache 37: 433–436

Committee on the Review of Medicine 1980 Systematic review of the benzodiazepines. Guidelines for data sheets on diazepam,

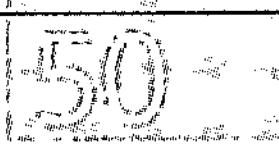

chlordiazepoxide, medazepam, clorazepate, lorazepam, oxazepam, temazepam, trazolam, nitrazepam and flurazepam. British Medical Journal 280: 910–912

Contreras E, Tamayo L, Quijada L 1977 Effects of tricyclic compounds and other drugs having a membrane stabilising action on analgesia, tolerance to and dependence on morphine. Archives of Internal Psychodynamics 228: 293–299

Coppen A 1972 Indoleamines and affective disorders. Journal of Psychiatric Research 9: 163–171

Couch JR, Hassanein RS 1976 Migraine and depression: effect of amitriptyline prophylaxis. Transactions of the American Neurological Association 101: 1–4

Couch JR, Ziegler DK, Hassanein R 1976 Amitriptyline in the prophylaxis of migraine. Effectiveness and relationship of antimigraine and anti-depressant effects. Neurology 26: 121–127

Creese I, Feinberg AP, Snyder SH 1976 Butyrophenone influences on the opiate receptor. European Journal of Pharmacology 36: 231–235

Da Prada M, Kettler R, Burkard WP, Lorez HP, Haefely W 1990 Some basic aspects of reversible inhibitors of monoamine oxidase-A. Acta Psychiatrica Scandinavia (suppl 360): 7–12

Davidoff G, Guarracini M, Roth E, Sliwa J, Yarkony G 1987 Trazodone hydrochloride in the treatment of dysesthetic pain in traumatic myelopathy: a randomized double-blind placebo controlled study. Pain 29: 151–161

Davidson O, Lindeneg O, Walsh M 1979 Analgesic treatment with levomepromazine in acute myocardial infarction. Acta Medica Scandinavica 205: 191–194

Davis JL, Lewis SB, Gerich JE, Kaplan RA, Schultz TA, Wallin JD 1977 Peripheral diabetic neuropathy treated with amitriptyline and fluphenazine. Journal of the American Medical Association 238: 2291–2292

Daw JL, Cohen-Cole SA 1981 Haloperidol analgesia. Southern Medical Journal 74: 364–365

De Montigny C, Grunberg F, Mayer A, Deschenes JP 1981 Lithium induces rapid relief of depression in tricyclic antidepressant drug non-responders. British Journal of Psychiatry 138: 252–256

Desproges-Gotteron R, Abramon JY, Borderie J, Lathelize H 1970 Possibilités thérapeutiques actuelles dans les lombalgies d'origine névrotique. Rheumatologie 22: 45–48

Diamond S, Baltes BJ 1971 Chronic tension headache – treatment with amitriptyline – double blind study. Headache 11: 110–116

Dixon RA, Edwards RI, Pilcher J 1980 Diazepam in immediate post myocardial infarct period. A double blind trial. British Heart Journal 43: 535–540

Dubner R, Bennett GJ 1983 Spinal and trigeminal mechanisms of nociception. Annual Review of Neuroscience 6: 381–418

Duke EE 1983 Clinical experience with pimozide: emphasis on its use in post herpetic neuralgia. Journal of the American Academy of Dermatology 8: 845–850

Duthie AM 1977 The use of phenothiazines and tricyclic antidepressants in the treatment of intractable pain. South African Medical Journal 51: 246–247

Eberhard G, Von Knorring L, Nilsson HL et al 1988 A double-blind randomized study of clomipramine versus maprotyline in patients with idiopathic pain syndromes. Neuropsychobiology 19: 25–34

Edelbroek PM, Linssen CG, Zitman FG et al 1986 Analgesic and antidepressant effects of amitryptyline in relation to its metabolism in patients with chronic pain. Clinical Pharmacology and Therapeutics 39: 156–162

Eija K, Pertti NJ, Tiina T 1996 Amitriptyline effectively relieves neuropathic pain following treatment of breast cancer. Pain 64: 293–302

Ekbom K 1974 Lithium vid kroniska symptom av cluster headache. Preliminart Meddelande Opuscula Medica (Stockholm) 19: 148–158

Ekbom K 1981 Lithium for cluster headache: review of the literature and preliminary results of long-term treatment. Headache 21: 132–139

Eschalier A, Montastruc JL, Devoice JL, Rigal F, Gaillard-Plaza G, Pechadre JC 1981 Influence of naloxone and methylsergide on the analgesic effect of clomipramine in rats. European Journal of Pharmacology 74: 1–7

Evans W, Gensler F, Blackwell B, Galbrecht C 1973 The effects of anti-depressant drugs on pain relief and mood in the chronically ill. Psychosomatics 14: 214–219

Farber GA, Burks JW 1974 Chlorprothixene therapy for herpes zoster neuralgia. Southern Medical Journal 67: 808–812

Fazio AN 1970 Control of postoperative pain: a comparison of the efficacy and safety of pentazocine, methotrimeprazine, meperidine and placebo. Current Therapeutic Research and Clinical Experimentation 12: 73–77

Feighner JP, Aden GC, Fabre LF, Rickels K, Smith WT 1983 Comparison of alprazolam, imipramine, and placebo in the treatment of depression. Journal of the American Medical Association 249: 3057–3064

Feinmann C, Harris M, Cawley R 1984 Psychogenic facial pain: presentation and treatment. British Medical Journal 288: 436–438

Fernandez F, Frank A, Holmes VF 1987 Analgesic effect of alprazolam in patients with chronic organic pain of malignant origin. Journal of Clinical Psychopharmacology 7: 167–169

Fiorentino M 1967 Sperimentazione controllata dell'imipramina come analgesico maggiore in oncologia. Rivista Medica Trentina 5: 387–396

Fogelholm R, Murros K 1985 Maprotyline in chronic tension headaches: a double blind crossover study. Headache 25: 273–275

France RM, Krishnan KRR 1988 Psychotropic drugs in chronic pain. In: France RD, Krishnan KRR (eds) Chronic pain. American Psychiatric Press, Washington DC, pp 343–346

France RD, Urban BJ 1991 Cerebrospinal fluid concentrations of beta-endorphin in chronic low back pain patients. Influence of depression and treatment. Psychosomatics 32: 72–77

France RD, Krishnan KRR, Trainor M 1986 Chronic pain and depression. III. Family history studies of depression and alcoholism in chronic low back pain patients. Pain 24: 185–190

Frank RG, Kashani JH, Parker JC et al 1988 Antidepressant analgesia in rheumatoid arthritis. Journal of Rheumatology 15: 1632–1638

Freeman GW, Polansky M, Sondheimer SJ, Rickels K 1995 A double blind trial of oral progresterone, alprazolam, and placebo in the treatment of severe premenstrual syndrome. Journal of the American Medical Association 274: 51–57

Fuentes JA, Garzon J, Del Rio J 1977 Potentiation of morphine analgesia in mice after inhibition of brain type B monoamine oxidase. Neuropharmacology 16: 857–862

Fuxe K, Ogren SO, Agnati LF et al 1983 Chronic antidepressant treatment and central 5-HT synapses. Neuropharmacology 22: 389–400

Gade GN, Hofeldt FD, Treece GL 1980 Diabetic neuropathic cachexia. Journal of the American Medical Association 243: 1160–1161

Galeotti N, Bartolini A, Ghelardini C 1996 Effect of pertussis toxin on morphine, diphenhydramine, baclofen, clomipramine and physotigmine antinociception. European Journal of Pharmacology 308: 125–133

Ganvir P, Beaumont G, Seldrup J 1980 A comparative trial of clomipramine and placebo as adjunctive therapy in arthralgia. Journal of International Medical Research 8(suppl 3): 60–66

Gear RW, Levine JD, Gordon NC et al 1997 Benzodiazepine mediated antagonism of opioid analgesia. Pain 71: 25–29

Gebhardt KH, Beller J, Nischik R 1969 Behandlung des Karzinomschmerzes mit Chlorimipramin (Anafranil). Medizinische Klinik 64: 751–756

Gerson GR, Jones RB, Luscombe DK 1977 Studies on the concomitant use of carbamazepine and clomipramine for the relief of post-herpetic neuralgia. Postgraduate Medical Journal 53(suppl 4): 104–109

Gessel AH 1975 Electromyographic biofeedback and tricyclic anti-depressant in myofascial pain-dysfunction syndrome: psychological predictors of outcome. Journal of the American Dental Association 91: 1048–1052

Gingras M 1976 A clinical trial of Tofranil in rheumatic pain in general practice. Journal of International Medical Research 4(suppl 2): 41–49

Godefroy F, Butler SH, Weil-Fugazza J, Besson JM 1986 Do acute or chronic tricyclic antidepressants modify morphine antinociception in arthritic rats? Pain 25: 233–244

Gold MS, Byck R 1978 Endorphins, lithium and naloxone: their relationship to pathological and drug induced manic euphoric states. In: Petersen RC (ed) The international challenge of drug abuse. National Institute on Drug Abuse, Rockville, p 192

Goldenberg DL, Felson DT, Dinerman H 1986 A randomized controlled trial of amitriptyline and naproxen in the treatment of patients with fibromyalgia. Arthritis and Rheumatism 29: 1371–1377

Goldenberg D, Schmid C, Ruthazer R et al 1996 A randomized double-blind crossover trial of fluoxetine and amitriptyline in the treatment of fibromyalgia. Arthritis and Rheumatism 39: 1852–1859

Gomersall JD, Stuart A 1973 Amitriptyline in migraine prophylaxis. Changes in pattern of attacks during a controlled clinical trial. Journal of Neurology, Neurosurgery and Psychiatry 36: 684–690

Gomez-Perez FJ, Riell JA, Dies H et al 1985 Nortriptyline and fluphenazine in the symptomatic treatment of diabetic neuropathy. A double-blind cross-over study. Pain 23: 395–400

Gomez-Perez FJ, Rull JA, Aquilar CA et al 1996 Nortriptyline-fluphenazine vs carbamazepine in the symptomatic treatment of diabetic neuropathy. Archives of Medical Research 27: 525–529

Gonzalez JP, Sewell RDE, Spencer PS 1980 Antinociceptive activity of opiates in the presence of the antidepressant agent nomifensine. Neuropharmacology 19: 613–618

Goodkin K, Gullion CM, Agras WS 1990 A randomized double-blind placebo controlled trial of trazodone hydrochloride in chronic low back pain syndrome. Journal of Clinical Psychopharmacology 10: 269–278

Goodwin RK, Prange AJ, Post RM, Muscettola G, Lipton MA 1982 Potentiation of antidepressant effect by L-triiodothyronine in tricyclic nonresponders. American Journal of Psychiatry 139: 34–38

Gourlay GK, Cherry DA, Cousins MF, Love BL, Graham JR, McLachlan MO 1986 A controlled study of a serotonin reuptake blocker, zimelidine, in the treatment of chronic pain. Pain 25: 35–52

Greenblatt DJ, Shader RI, Abernathy DR 1983 Current status of benzodiazepines, Parts I and II. New England Journal of Medicine 309: 354–358, 410–416

Hackett G, Boddie HG, Harrison P 1987 Chronic muscle contraction headache: the importance of depression and anxiety. Journal of the Royal Society of Medicine 80: 689–691

Hackett TP, Cassem NH 1972 Reduction of anxiety in the coronary care unit: a controlled double blind comparison of chlordiazepoxide and amobarbital. Current Therapeutic Research 14: 649–656

Hakkarainen H 1977 Brief report, fluphenazine for tension headache; double blind study. Headache 17: 216–218

Halpern L 1982 Substitution-detoxification and the role in the management of chronic benign pain. Journal of Clinical Psychiatry 43: 10–14

Hameroff SR, Weiss JL, Lerman JC et al 1984 Doxepin effects on chronic pain and depression: a controlled study. Journal of Clinical Psychiatry 45: 45–52

Hamlin C, Gold MS 1984 Anxiolytics: predicting response/maximizing efficacy. In: Gold MS, Lydiard RB, Carman JS (eds) Advances in psychopharmacology: predicting and improving treatment response. CRC Press, Boca Raton, pp 238–244

Hammond DL 1985 Pharmacology of central pain-modulating networks (biogenic amines and nonopioid analgesics). In: Field HL, Dubner R, Cervero F (eds) Advances in pain research and therapy. Raven, New York, pp 499–511

Hanks GW, Thomas PJ, Trueman T, Weeks E 1983 The myth of haloperidol potentiation. Lancet ii: 523–524

Harris JA, Westbrook RF 1995 Effects of benzodiazepine microinjection into the amygdala or periaqueductal gray on the expression of conditioned fear and hypoalgesia in rats. Behavioural Neuroscience 109: 295–304

Hatangdi VS, Boa RA, Richards EG 1976 Post herpetic neuralgia: management with antiepileptic and tricyclic drugs. In: Bonica JJ, Albe Fessard D (eds) Advances in pain research and therapy, vol 1. Raven, New York, pp 583–587

Hendler N, Cimini A, Terence MA, Long D 1980 A comparison of cognitive impairment due to benzodiazepines and to narcotics. American Journal of Psychiatry 137: 828–830

Hirschowitz J, Bennett JA, Zemlan FP, Garrer DL 1983 Thioridazine effect on desipramine plasma levels. Journal of Clinical Psychopharmacology 3: 376–379

Hollister LE 1978 Drug therapy, tricyclic antidepressants. Part I and II. New England Journal of Medicine 229: 1106–1109, 1168–1171

Hollister LE, Conley FK, Britt RH, Shuer L 1981 Long-term use of diazepam. Journal of the American Medical Association 246: 1568–1570

Hugues A, Chauvergne J, Lissilour T, Lagarde C 1963 L'imipramine utilisée comme antalgique majeur en carcinologie. Etude de 118 cas. Presse Médicale 71: 1073–1074

Hwang SA, Wilcox GL 1987 Analgesic properties of intrathecally administered heterocyclic antidepressants. Pain 28: 343–355

Iserson KV 1983 Parenteral chlorpromazine treatment of migraine. Annals of Emergency Medicine 12: 756–758

Jackson GL, Smith DA 1956 Analgesic properties of mixtures of chlorpromazine with morphine and meperidine. Annals of Internal Medicine 45: 640–652

Janowski EC, Janowski DS 1985 What precautions should be taken if a patient on an MAOI is scheduled to undergo anaesthesia? Journal of Clinical Psychopharmacology 5: 128–129

Jenkins DG, Ebbutt AF, Evans CD 1976 Imipramine in treatment of low back pain. Journal of International Medical Research 4(suppl 2): 28–40

Johansson F, Von Knorring L 1979 A double-blind controlled study of a serotonin uptake inhibitor (zimelidine) versus placebo in chronic pain patients. Pain 7: 69–78

Johansson F, Von Knorring L, Sedvall G, Terenius L 1980 Changes in endorphins and 5-hydroxyindoleacetic acid in cerebrospinal fluid as a result of treatment with a serotonin reuptake inhibitor (zimelidine) in chronic pain patients. Psychiatry Research 2: 167–172

Judkins KC, Harmer M 1982 Haloperidol as an adjunct analgesic in the management of postoperative pain. Anaesthesia 37: 1118–1120

Kast EC 1966 An understanding of pain and its measurement. Medical Times 94: 1501–1513

Khatami M, Woody G, O'Brien C 1979 Chronic pain and narcotic addiction: a multitherapeutic approach – a pilot study. Comprehensive Psychiatry 20: 55–60

Khurana RC 1983 Treatment of painful diabetic neuropathy with trazodone. Journal of the American Medical Association 250: 1392

Kishore-Kumar R, Max MB, Schafer SC et al 1990 Desipramine relieves posherpetic neuralgia. Clinical Pharmacology and Therapeutics 47: 305–312

Klein DT, Gittlemann K, Quitkin F, Ripkin A 1980 Diagnosis and drug treatment of psychiatric disorders. Williams & Wilkins, Baltimore, pp 470–486

Kocher R 1976 Use of psychotropic drugs for treatment of chronic severe pain. In: Bonica JJ, Albe Fessard D (eds) Advances in pain research and therapy, vol 1. Raven, New York, pp 579–582
Krishnan KRR, France RD, Pelton S, McCann UD, Davidson J, Urban BJ 1985 Chronic pain and depression. I. Classification of depression in chronic low back pain patients. Pain 22: 279–287
Krupp P, Wesp M 1975 Inhibition of prostaglandin synthetase by psychotropic drugs. Experientia 31: 330–331
Kudrow L 1977 Lithium prophylaxis for chronic cluster headache. Headache 17: 15–18
Kudrow L 1978 Comparative results of prednisone, methylsergide and lithium therapy in cluster headache. In: Greene R (ed) Current concepts in migraine research. Raven, New York, pp 159–163
Kudrow L 1980 Analgesics and headache. In: The use of analgesics in the management of mild to moderate pain. Postgraduate Medical Communications, Riker Laboratories, Northridge, California, pp 60–62
Kuipers RKW 1962 Imipramine in the treatment of rheumatic patients. Acta Rheumatologica Scandinavica 8: 45–51
Kvinesdal B, Molin J, Frøland A, Gram LF 1984 Imipramine treatment of painful diabetic neuropathy. Journal of the American Medical Association 251: 1727–1730
Laine E, Linguette M, Fossati P 1962 Action de l'imipramine injectable dans les symptômes douloureux. Lille Médicale 7: 711–716
Lance JW, Curran DA 1964 Treatment of chronic tension headache. Lancet i: 1236–1239
Landa L, Breivik H, Husebo S, Elgen A, Rennemo F 1984 Beneficial effects of flupenthixol on cancer pain patients. Pain 2(suppl): S253
Langohr HD, Stöhr M, Petruch F 1982 An open and double-blind cross-over study on the efficacy of clomipramine (Anafranil) in patients with painful mono- and polyneuropathies. European Neurology 2: 309–317
Langohr HD, Gerber WD, Koletzki E, Mayer K, Schroth G 1985 Clomipramine and metoprolol in migraine prophylaxis: a double blind crossover study. Headache 25: 107–113
Lasagna I 1977 The role of benzodiazepines in nonpsychiatric medical practice. American Journal of Psychiatry 134: 656–658
Lasagna RG, DeKornfeld TJ 1961 Methotrimeprazine. A new phenothiazine derivative with analgesic properties. Journal of the American Medical Association 178: 887–890
Lascelles RG 1966 Atypical facial pain and depression. British Journal of Psychiatry 122: 651–659
Lee R, Spencer PSJ 1977 Antidepressants and pain: a review of the pharmacological data supporting the use of certain tricyclics in chronic pain. Journal of International Medical Research 5(suppl 1): 146–156
Leijon G, Boivie J 1989 Control post-stroke pain: a controlled trial of amitriptyline and carbamazepine. Pain 36: 27–36
Levine JD, Gordon NC, Smith R, McBryde R 1986 Desipramine enhances opiate postoperative analgesia. Pain 27: 45–49
Lewis TA, Solomon GD 1996 Advances in cluster headache management. Cleveland Clinic Journal of Medicine 63: 237–244
Liebowitz MR, Quitkin FM, Stewart JW et al 1988 Antidepressant specificity in atypical depression. Archives of General Psychiatry 45: 129–137
Lindsay PG, Wyckoff M 1981 The depression–pain syndrome and its response to antidepressants. Psychosomatics 22: 571–577
Lloyd KG, Pile A 1984 Chronic antidepressants and GABA synapses. Neuropharmacology 23: 841–842
Loldrup D, Langemark M, Hansen HJ, Olesen J, Bech P 1989 Clomipramine and mianserin in chronic idiopathic pain syndrome. Psychopharmacology 99: 1–7
Luger TJ, Hayashi T, Grabner-Weiss C, Lorenz IH 1995 Effects of the NMDA-antagonist, MK 801, on benzodiazepine-opiod interactions at the spinal and supraspinal level in rats. British Journal of Pharmacology 114: 1097–1103
Lynch SA, Max MB, Muir J, Smoller B, Dubner R 1990 Efficacy of antidepressants in relieving diabetic neuropathy pain: amitriptyline vs desipramine, and fluoxetine vs placebo. Neurology 40(suppl 1): 437
McDonald Scott WA 1969 The relief of pain with an antidepressant in arthritis. Practitioner 202: 802–807
Macfarlane JG, Jalali S, Grace EM 1986 Trimipramine in rheumatoid arthritis: a randomized double-blind trial in relieving pain and joint tenderness. Current Medical Research and Opinion 10: 89–93
McNairy SL, Maruta T, Ivnik RJ, Swanson DW, Ilstrup DM 1984 Prescription medication dependence and neuropsychologic function. Pain 18: 169–178
MacNeill AL, Dick WC 1976 Imipramine and rheumatoid factor. Journal of Internal Medicine Research 4(suppl 2): 23–27
McQuay HJ, Moore RA, Wissen PJ et al 1996 A systematic review of antidepressants in neuropathic pain. Pain 68: 217–227
Magni G, Andreoli F, Arduino C et al 1987 Modifications of [^{3}H] imipramine binding sites in platelets of chronic pain patients treated with mianserin. Pain 30: 311–320
Magni G, Bertolini C, Dodi G 1982 Treatment of perineal neuralgia with antidepressants. Journal of the Royal Society of Medicine 75: 214–215
Malec D, Langwinski R 1981 Central action of narcotic analgesics. VIII. The effect of dopaminergic stimulants on the action of analgesics in rats. Polish Journal of Pharmacologic Pharmacology 33: 243–282
Maltbie AA, Cavenar JO 1977 Haloperidol and analgesia: case reports. Military Medicine 142: 946–948
Maltbie AA, Cavenar JO, Sullivan JL, Hammett XX, Zung WWK 1979 Analgesia and haloperidol: a hypothesis. Journal of Clinical Psychiatry 40: 323–326
Mandel MR 1975 Electroconvulsive therapy for chronic pain associated with depression. American Journal of Psychiatry 132: 632–636
Margolis LH, Gianascol AJ 1956 Chlorpromazine in thalamic pain syndrome. Neurology 6: 302–304
Marks J 1980 The benzodiazepines – use and abuse. Arzneimittel Forschung/Drug Research 30(I)(5a): 889–891
Martucci N, Manna V, Porto C, Agnoli A 1985 Migraine and the noradrenergic control of vasomotricity: a study with alpha-2 stimulated and alpha-2 blocker drugs. Headache 25: 95–100
Mathew NT 1978 Clinical subtypes of cluster headache and response to lithium therapy. Headache 18: 26–30
Max MB, Culnane M, Schafer SC et al 1987 Amitriptyline relieves diabetic neuropathy pain in patients with normal or depressed mood. Neurology 37: 589–596
Max MB, Schafer SC, Culnane M, Smoller B, Dubner R, Gracely RH 1988 Amitriptyline, but not lorazepam, relieves postherpetic neuralgia. Neurology 38: 1427–1432
Max MB, Kishore-Kumar R, Schafer SC et al 1991 Efficacy of desipramine in painful diabetic neuropathy: a placebo-controlled trial. Pain 45: 3–9
Mellerup ET, Bech P, Hansen HJ, Langemark M, Loldrup D, Plenge P 1988 Platelet ^{3}H-imipramine binding in psychogenic pain disorders. Psychiatry Research 29: 149–156
Merikangas KR, Merikangas JR 1995 Combination monoamine oxidase inhibitor and beta blocker treatment of migraine, with anxiety and depression. Biological Psychiatry 38: 603–610
Melsom M, Andreassen P, Melsom H 1976 Diazepam in acute myocardial infarction: clinical effects and effects on catecholamine, free fatty acids and cortisol. British Heart Journal 38: 804–810
Merskey H, Hester RN 1972 The treatment of chronic pain with psychotropic drugs. Postgraduate Medical Journal 48: 594–598
Messing RB, Lytle LD 1977 Serotonin-containing neurons: their possible role in pain and analgesia. Pain 4: 1–21
Messing RB, Phebus L, Fisher LA, Lytle LD 1975 Analgesic effect of fluoxetine hydrochloride (Lilly 110140), a specific inhibitor of

serotonin uptake. Psychopharmacology Communications 1: 511–521

Minuck R 1972 Postoperative analgesia – combination of methotrimeprazine and meperidine as postoperative analgesic agents. Canadian Medical Association Journal 90: 1156–1159

Mitas JA, Mosley CA, Drager AM 1983 Diabetic neuropathic pain: control by amitriptyline and fluphenazine in renal insufficiency. Southern Medical Journal 76: 462–467

Mitsikostas DD, Ilias A, Thomas A, Gatzonis S 1997 Buspirone vs amitriptyline in the treatment of chronic tension-type headache. Acta Neurologica Scandinavica 96: 247–251

Monks RC 1980 Tardive dyskinesia with low dose neuroleptic therapy. Modern Medicine 35: 519

Monks RC 1981 Psychopharmacological management of post myocardial depression and anxiety. Canadian Family Physician 27: 1117–1121

Monro D, Swade C, Coppen A 1985 Mianserin in the prophylaxis of migraine: a double-blind study. Acta Psychiatrica Scandinavica S320: 98–103

Montastruc JL, Tran MA, Blanc M et al 1985 Measurement of plasma levels of clomipramine in the treatment of chronic pain. Clinical Neuropharmacology 8: 78–82

Montilla E, Fredrik WS, Cass LJ 1963 Analgesic effect of methotrimeprazine and morphine. Archives of Internal Medicine 111: 91–94

Mørland TJ, Storli OV, Mogstead TE 1979 Doxepin in the prophylactic treatment of mixed 'vascular' and tension headache. Headache 19: 382–383

Munro A, Chmara J 1982 Monosymptomatic hypochondriacal psychoses. A diagnostic checklist based on 50 cases of the disorder. Canadian Journal of Psychiatry 27: 374–376

Murphy DL, Campbell I, Costa JL 1978 Current status of the indoleamine hypothesis of the effective disorders. In: Lipton MA, Mascio AD, Killam KF (eds) Psychopharmacology: a generation of progress. Raven, New York, pp 1235–1247

Nappi G, Sandrini G, Granella F et al 1990 A new 5-HT_2 antagonist (ritanserin) in the treatment of chronic headache with depression. A double-blind study vs amitriptyline. Headache 30: 439–444

Natelson BH, Findley TW, Policastro T et al 1996 Randomized double blind, controlled placebo-phase in trial of low dose phenelzine in the chronic fatigue syndrome. Psychopharmacology (Berlin) 124: 226–230

Nathan PW 1978 Chlorprothixene (Taractan) in post herpetic neuralgia and other severe chronic pain. Pain 5: 367–371

Nemeroff CB, DeVane CL, Pollack BG 1996 Newer antidepressants and the cytochrome P450 system. American Journal of Psychiatry 153: 331–320

Nicolodi M, Sicuteri F 1996 Fibromyalgia and migraine, two faces of the same mechanism, serotonin as the common clue for pathogenesis and therapy. Advances in Experimental Medicine and Biology 398: 373–379

Nies A, Robinson DS, Friedman MJ et al 1977 Relationship between age and tricyclic antidepressant levels. American Journal of Psychiatry 134: 790–793

Noone JF 1977 Psychotropic drugs and migraine. Journal of International Medical Research 5(suppl 1): 66–71

Norregaard J, Danneskiold-Samsoe B, Volkmann H 1995 A randomized controlled trial of citalopram in the treatment of fibromyalgia. Pain 61: 445–449

Okasha A, Ghaleb HA, Sadek A 1973 A double-blind trial for the clinical management of psychogenic headache. British Journal of Psychiatry 122: 181–183

Onghena P, van Houdenhove B 1992 Antidepressant-induced analgesia in chronic non-malignant pain: a meta-analysis of 39 placebo controlled studies. Pain 49: 205–219

Paoli F, Darcourt G, Cossa P 1960 Note préliminaire sur l'action de l'imipramine dans les états douloureux. Revue Neurologique 102: 503–504

Parolin AR 1966 El tratamiento del dolor y la ansiedad en el carcinoma avanzado. El Medico Practico 21: 3–4

Patterson DR, Sharar SR, Carrougher GJ, Ptaceck JT 1997 Lorazepam as an adjunct to opioid analgesics in the treatment of burn pain. Pain 72: 367–374

Paul D, Hornby PJ 1995 Potentiation of intathecal DAMGO antinociception, but not gastrointestinal transit inhibition, by 5-hydroxytryptamine and norepinephrine uptake blockage. Life Sciences 56: PL83–87

Pearce JMS 1980 Chronic migraneous neuralgia, a variant of cluster headache. Brain 103: 149–159

Peroutko SJ, Banghart SB, Allen GS 1984 Relative potency and selectivity of calcium antagonists used in the treatment of migraine. Headache 24: 55–58

Perry PJ, Pfohl BM, Holstad G 1987 The relationship between antidepressant response and tricyclic antidepressant plasma concentration. A retrospective analysis of the literature using logistic regression analysis. Clinical Pharmacokinetics 13: 381–392

Petts HV, Pleuvry BJ 1983 Interactions of morphine and methotrimeprazine in mouse and man with respect to analgesia, respiration and sedation. British Journal of Anaesthesia 55: 437–441

Pheasant H, Bursk A, Goldfarb J et al 1983 Amitriptyline and chronic low back pain: a randomized double blind cross over study. Spine 8: 552–557

Pick CG 1996 Strain differences in mice antinociception: relationship between alprazolam and opioid receptor subtypes. European Neuropsychopharmacology 6: 201–205

Pick CG 1997 Antinociceptive interaction between alprazolam and opioids. Brain Research Bulletin 42: 239–243

Pilowsky I, Barrow CG 1990 A controlled study of psychotherapy and amitriptyline individually and in combination in the treatment of chronic intractable 'psychogenic' pain. Pain 40: 3–19

Pilowsky I, Hallett EC, Bassett DL, Thomas PG, Penhall RK 1982 A controlled study of amitriptyline in the treatment of chronic pain. Pain 14: 169–179

Pilowsky I, Soda J, Forsten C et al 1995 Out-patient cognitive-behavioural therapy with amitriptyline for chronic non-malignant pain: a comparative study with 6-month follow-up. Pain 60: 49–54

Polliack J 1979 Chronic recurrent headaches. South African Medical Journal 56: 980

Proudfit HK 1988 Pharmacological evidence for the modulation of nociception by noradrenergic neurons. In: Field HL, Besson JM (eds) Pain modulation. Progress in brain research. Elsevier, Amsterdam, pp 357–370

Puttini PS, Cazzola M, Boccasini L et al 1988 A comparison of dothiepin versus placebo in the treatment of pain in rheumatoid arthritis and the association of pain with depression. Journal of International Medical Research 16: 331–337

Quijada-Carrera J, Garcia-Lopez A 1996 Comparison of tenoxicam and bromazepam in the treatment of fibromyalgia: a randomized double-blind, placebo-controlled trial. Pain 65: 221–225

Radebold H 1971 Behandlung chronischer Schmerzzustande mit Anafranil. Medizinische Welt 22: 337–339

Raferty H 1979 The management of post herpetic pain using sodium valproate and amitriptyline. Journal of the Irish Medical Association 72: 399–401

Rafinesque J 1963 Emploi du Tofranil à titre antalgique dans les syndromes douloureux de diverses origines. Gazette Médicale de France 1: 2075–2077

Raft D, Toomey T, Gregg JM 1979 Behavior modification and haloperidol in chronic facial pain. Southern Medical Journal 72: 155–159

Rani PU, Shobha JC, Rao TR et al 1996 an evaluation of antidepressants in rheumatic pain conditions. Anesthesia and Analgesia 83: 371–375

 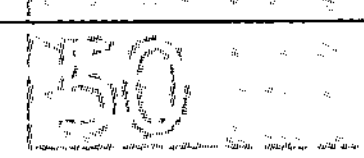

Raskin DE 1982 MAO inhibitors in chronic pain and depression. Journal of Clinical Psychiatry 43: 122

Roberts MHT 1984 5-Hydroxytryptamine and antinociception. Neuropharmacology 23: 1529–1536

Roose SP, Glassman AH 1994 Antidepressant choice in the patient with cardiac disease: lessons from the Cardiac Arrhythmia Suppression Trial (CAST) Studies. Journal of Clinical Psychiatry (suppl A): 83–87

Rumore MM, Schlichting DA 1986 Clinical efficacy of antihistamines as analgesics. Pain 25: 7–22

Sadove MS, Rose RF, Balagot RC, Reyes R 1955 Chlorpromazine in the management of pain. Modern Medicine 23: 117–120

Sandrini G, Alfonsi E, DeRysky C, Marini S, Facchinetti F, Nappi G 1986 Evidence for serotonin-S_2 receptor involvement in analgesia in human. European Journal of Pharmacology 130: 311–314

Saper JR, Silberstein SD, Lake AE III, Winters ME 1994 Double-blind trial of fluxetine: chronic daily headache and migraine. Headache 34: 497–502

Saran A, 1988 Antidepressants not effective in headache associated with minor closed head injury. International Journal of Psychiatry in Medicine 18: 75–83

Schick E, Wolpert E, Reichert A, Queisser W 1979 Neuroleptanalgesie mit einen hechpotenten Depotneuroleptikum zur Schmerztherapie bei metastasierenden Malignomen. Verhandlungen der Deutschen Gesellschaft fur Innere Medizin 85: 1113–1114

Schildkraut JN 1978 Current status of the catecholamine hypotheses of affective disorders. In: Lipton MA, Mascio AD, Killam KF (eds) Psychopharmacology: a generation of progress. Raven, New York, pp 1223–1234

Schreiber S, Pick CG, Yanai J, Becker MM 1996 The antinociceptive effect of fluvoxamine. European Neuropsychopharmacology 6: 281–284

Schreiber S, Pick CG, Weizman R, Becker MM 1997 Augmentation of opioid induced antinociception by the atypical drug risperidone in mice. Neuroscience Letters 228: 25–28

Sharav Y, Singer E, Schmidt E, Dionne RA, Dubner R 1987 The analgesic effect of amitriptyline on chronic facial pain. Pain 31: 199–209

Sherwin D 1979 A new method for treating 'headaches'. American Journal of Psychiatry 136: 1181–1183

Shimm DS, Logue GL, Maltbie AA, Dugan S 1979 Medical management of chronic cancer pain. Journal of the American Medical Association 241: 2411

Shrestha M, Hayes TE, Moreden J, Singh R 1996 Ketorolac vs chlorpromazine in the treatment of acute migraine without aura – a prospective randomized, double-blind trial. Archives of Internal Medicine 156: 1725–1728

Shukla R, Ahuja RC, Nag D 1966 Alprazolam in chronic tension type headache. Journal of the Association of Physicians of India 44: 641–644

Silberstein SD 1996 Divalproex sodium in headache: literature review and clinical guidelines. Headache 36: 547–555

Sierralta F, Miranda HF, Mendez M, Pinardi G 1995 Interaction of opioids with antidepressant-induced antinociception. Psychopharmacology 122: 374–378

Sigwald J, Bouttier D, Caille F 1959 Le traitement du zona et des algies zostériennes. Etude des résultats obtenus avec la levomepromazine. Thérapie 14: 818–824

Sindrup SH, Ejlertsen B, Frøland A, Sindrup EH, Brøsen K, Gram LF 1989 Imipramine treatment in diabetic neuropathy: relief of subjective symptoms without changes in peripheral and autonomic nerve function. European Journal of Clinical Pharmacology 37: 151–153

Sindrup SH, Gram CF, Skjold T et al 1990a Clomipramine vs desipramine vs placebo in the treatment of diabetic neuropathy symptoms: a double-blind crossover study. British Journal of Clinical Pharmacology 30: 683–691

Sindrup SH, Gram LF, Brosen K, Eshoj O, Mogensen EF 1990b. The selective serotonin reuptake inhibitor paroxetine is effective in the treatment of diabetic neuropathy symptoms. Pain 42: 135–144

Singh G 1971 Drug treatment of chronic intractable pain in patients referred to a psychiatry clinic. Journal of the Indian Medical Association 56: 341–345

Sjaastad O 1983 So-called 'tension headache' – the response to a 5-HT uptake inhibitor: femoxetine. Cephalgia 3: 53–60

Smoller B 1984 The use of dexamethasone suppression test as a marker of efficacy in the treatment of a myofascial syndrome with amitriptyline. Pain (suppl) 2: S250

Snyder S, Enna JJ, Young AB 1977 Brain mechanisms associated with the therapeutic actions of benzodiazepines: focus on neurotransmitters. American Journal of Psychiatry 134: 662–664

Soja PF, Sinclair JG 1983 Evidence that noradrenaline reduces tonic descending inhibition of cat spinal cord nociceptor-driven neurones. Pain 15: 71–81

Somoza E 1978 Influence of neuroleptics on the binding of metenkephalin, morphine and dihydromorphine to synaptosome-enriched fractions of rat brain. Neuropharmacology 17: 577–581

Songer DA & Schulte H 1996 Venlafaxine for the treatment of chronic pain. American Journal of Psychiatry 153: 737

Stein D, Floman Y, Elizur A et al 1996 The efficacy of amitriptyline and acetaminophen in the management of acute low back pain. Psychosomatics 37: 63–70

Sternbach RA, Janowsky DS, Huey IY, Segal DS 1976 Effects of altering brain serotonin activity on human chronic pain. In: Bonica JJ, Albe Fessard D (eds) Advances in pain research and therapy, vol 1. Raven, New York, pp 601–606

Sternback H 1991 The serotonin syndrome. American Journal of Psychiatry 148: 705–713

Stirman J 1967 A comparison of methotrimeprazine and meperidine as analgesic agents. Anesthesia and Analgesia 46: 176–180

Sugrue MF 1983 Chronic antidepressant therapy and associated changes in central monoaminergic receptor functioning. Pharmacology and Therapeutics 21: 1–33

Swerdlow M, Cundill JG 1981 Anticonvulsant drugs used in the treatment of lancinating pain. A comparison. Anaesthesia 36: 1129–1132

Taniguchi K, Oyama T, Honda N et al 1995 The effect of imipramine, amitriptyline and clondine administered by iontophoresis on the pain threshold. Acta Anaesthesiologica Belgica 46: 121–125

Taub A 1973 Relief of post herpetic neuralgia with psychotropic drugs. Journal of Neurosurgery 39: 235–239

Taylor K, Rowbotham MC 1996 Venlafaxine hydrochloride and chronic pain. Western Journal of Medicine 165: 147–148

Taylor RG, Doku HC 1967 Methotrimeprazine: evaluated as an analgesic following oral surgery. Journal of Oral Medicine 22: 141–144

Terenius L 1978 Endogenous peptides and analgesia. Annual Review of Pharmacology 18: 189

Terenius L 1979 Endorphins in chronic pain. In: Bonica JJ, Liebeskind JC, Albe Fessard D (eds) Advances in pain research and therapy, vol 3. Raven, New York, pp 458–471

Theesen KA, Marsh WR 1989 Relief of diabetic neuropathy with fluoxetine. DICP, The Annals of Pharmacotherapy 23: 572–574

Thorpe P, Marchant-Williams R 1974 The role of an antidepressant, dibenzepin (Noveril), in the relief of pain in chronic arthritic states. Medical Journal of Australia 1: 264–266

Tofanetti O, Albiero L, Galatulas I, Genovese E 1977 Enhancement of propoxyphene-induced analgesia by doxepin. Psychopharmacology 51: 213–215

Tricklebank MD, Huston PH, Curzon G 1984 Involvement of dopamine in the antinociceptive response to footshock. Psychopharmacology 82: 185–188

Turkington RW 1980 Depression masquerading as diabetic neuropathy. Journal of the American Medical Association 243: 1147–1150
Twycross RG 1979 Non-narcotic, corticosteroid and psychotropic drugs. In: Twycross RG, Ventafridda V (eds) The continuing care of terminal cancer patients. Pergamon, Oxford, pp 126–128
Tyber MA 1974 Treatment of the painful shoulder syndrome with amitriptyline and lithium carbonate. Canadian Medical Association Journal 111: 137–140
Tyrer P 1976 Towards rational therapy with monoamine oxidase inhibitors. British Journal of Psychiatry 128: 354–360
Urban BJ, France RD, Steinberger EK, Scott DL, Maltbie AA 1986 Long term use of narcotic/antidepressant medication in the management of phantom limb pain. Pain 24: 191–196
Valdes M, Garcia L, Treserra J, De Pablo J, De Flores T 1989 Psychogenic pain and depressive disorders: an empirical study. Journal of Affective Disorders 16: 21–25
Ventafridda V, Bonezzi C, Caraceni A et al 1987 Antidepressants for cancer pain and other painful syndromes with deafferentation component: comparison of amitriptyline and trazodone. Italian Journal of Neurological Sciences 8: 579–587
Vrethem M, Thorell LH, Lindstrom T et al 1997 A comparison of amitriptyline and maprotiline in the treatment of painful polyneuropathy in diabetics and nondiabetics. Clinical Journal of Pain 13: 313–323
Ward NG, Bloom VL, Friedel RO 1979 The effectiveness of tricyclic antidepressants in the treatment of coexisting pain and depression. Pain 7: 331–341
Ward NG, Bloom VL, Fawcett J, Friedel RP 1983 Urinary 3-methoxy-4-hydroxyphenethylene glycol in the prediction of pain and depression relief with doxepin: preliminary findings. Journal of Nervous and Mental Disease 171: 55–58
Ward N, Bokan JA, Phillips M, Benedetti C, Butler S, Spengler D 1984 Antidepressants in concomitant chronic back pain and depression: doxepin and desipramine compared. Journal of Clinical Psychiatry 45: 54–59
Watson CPN, Evans RJ 1985 A comparative trial of amitriptyline and zimelidine in post-herpetic neuralgia. Pain 23: 387–394
Watson CPN, Evans RJ, Reed K, Merskey H, Goldsmith L, Warsh J 1982 Amitriptyline versus placebo in postherpetic neuralgia. Neurology 32: 671–673
Weis O, Sriwatanakul K, Weintraub M 1982 Treatment of post-herpetic neuralgia and acute herpetic pain with amitriptyline and perphenazine. South African Medical Journal 62: 274–275
Willer JC, Roby A, Maulet C, Gerard A 1984 Possible tryptaminergic involvement of pain and of endogenous opiate activity in man. Pain 2(suppl): 251
Willner P 1985 Antidepressants and serotonergic neurotransmission: an integrative review. Psychopharmacology 85: 387–404
Woodforde JM, Dwyer B, McEwen BW et al 1965 Treatment of post-herpetic neuralgia. Medical Journal of Australia 2: 869–872
Wüster M, Duka T, Herz A 1980 Diazepam effects on striatal metenkephalin levels following long-term pharmacological manipulation. Neuropharmacology 19: 501–505
Zeigler DK, Hurwitz A, Hassanein RS, Kodanaz HA, Preskorn SH, Mason J 1987 Migraine prophylaxis. A comparison of popranolol and amitriptyline. Archives of Neurology 44: 486–489
Zitman FG, Linssen ACG, Edelbroek PM 1984 Amitriptyline versus placebo in chronic benign pain: a double blind study. Pain 2(suppl): S250

Opioids

ROBERT G. TWYCROSS

INTRODUCTION

The emphasis in this chapter is on the use of strong opioids for the relief of cancer pain. Opioids have been described as 'the mainstay of cancer pain management' (WHO 1986) but in many countries morphine and codeine are not available for medicinal use or, if available, are underused (WHO 1990, 1996). The main reason for unavailability and underuse appears to be 'opiophobia' (Zenz & Willweber-Strumpf 1993). This cultural phenomenon varies in intensity from country to country and is reflected in widely divergent medicinal morphine use (Fig. 51.1).

Opiophobia relates to fears concerning diversion/addiction and respiratory depression. One tangible manifestation, for example, is the need to use special prescription forms or books in most countries in Western Europe (Zenz & Willweber-Strumpf 1993). In Italy, Portugal and Spain, doctors have to apply personally to the authorities to obtain the special forms and, in Portugal and Spain, have to pay for them. In Italy and Spain, the patient needs a special identity card before the doctor is allowed to prescribe a strong opioid. In Spain, the card is valid for only 3 months. Further, if the dose is changed within 1 month, the patient must obtain a new card. The period for which a prescription remains valid varies

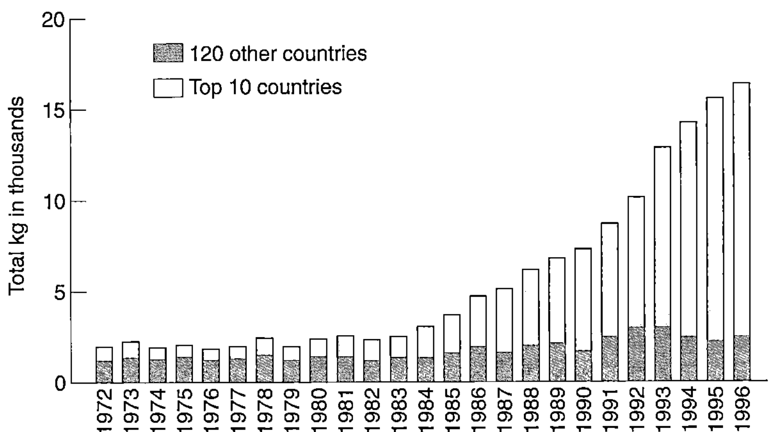

Fig. 51.1 World consumption of morphine 1972–1996. □ = 10 top countries (Australia, Canada, Denmark, Iceland, Ireland, New Zealand, Norway, Sweden, UK, USA); ■ = 120 other countries. Data from International Narcotics Control Board; figure prepared by University of Wisconsin Pain and Policy Studies Group/WHO Collaborating Center, 1998.

(Table 51.1). A short period may prevent a patient from taking an extended holiday.

National legislation in this area often dates back to before the Second World War when the main concern was to prevent drug trafficking and abuse and cancer was not as common. The regulations, however, now commonly obstruct the provision of strong opioids to cancer and other patients. This is disturbing, not least because it contravenes the spirit and the letter of the United Nations' Single Convention on Narcotic Drugs 1961 which states in its preamble that 'The medical use of narcotic drugs continues to be indispensable for the relief of pain and suffering and ... adequate provision must be made to ensure the availability of narcotic drugs for such purposes'.

Opioids have innumerable actions which vary according to drug, dose and circumstances (Table 51.2). The key to a balanced view about them lies in the realization that there are significant differences in man between opioid *clinical* pharmacology (patients) and opioid *laboratory* pharmacology (healthy volunteers). These differences relate to the presence or absence of pain. Thus, in the absence of pain, respiratory depression and tolerance may well occur but, in patients with pain, these phenomena are rarely of clinical importance.

There is, however, a growing realization by pharmaceutical companies that promoting cancer pain management can create significant profits. Physicians are therefore being increasingly exposed to commercial pressures in relation to the choice of opioid and formulation. The danger is that opioid use will become more influenced by commercial interests than by scientific and humane considerations. Now as never before, there is a need for physicians to be aware of the differences between various opioids (where they exist) so as to ensure that patients receive what is truly best for them at an affordable price.

RISK OF DIVERSION

The diversion of medicinal opioids for illicit use by other people is a rightful concern of governments and law enforcement agencies. However, only a very small percentage of illicit drugs comes from healthcare sources. Further, orally administered morphine is generally not a drug of choice for opioid-dependent persons. The experience in Sweden in this respect is encouraging. There, the medicinal use of morphine and methadone increased 17 times between 1975 and 1982 because of the increasing use of oral strong opioids to control cancer pain, but there was no associated increase in illicit drug use or diversion of strong opioids to established addicts (Agenas et al 1982). On the other hand, some years ago in one country, some doctors were conned into prescribing modified-release morphine

Table 51.1 Prescribing regulations in Western Europe in 1992 for morphine tablets (from Zenz & Willweber-Strumpf (1993) and Sohn & Zenz (1998))

Country	*Special prescription form or book*	*Maximum amount prescribable (days)*	*Prescription validity*
Austria	+	No information	14 days
Belgium	–	No regulations	No regulations
Denmark	+	No regulations	No regulations
France	+	14	No information
Germany	+	28	7 days
Greece	+	1–2	No information
Ireland	–	Unlimited	No information
Italy	+	8	10 days
Netherlands	–	Unlimited	No information
Portugal	+	No information	10 days
Spain	+	30	No information
Switzerland	+	No information	No information
United Kingdom	–	No information	No information

Table 51.2 Opioid pharmacodynamics[1]

Central nervous system	**Gastrointestinal tract**
Analgesia	Delayed gastric emptying
Nausea and vomiting	Increased tone of sphincter of Oddi
Sedation	Increased intestinal tone (hypersegmentation) } Constipation[2]
Euphoria/dysphoria	Decreased intestinal propulsive contractions } Constipation[2]
Respiratory system	**Urogenital tract**
Decreased rate and tidal volume	Inhibition of voiding reflex
CO_2 response curve shifted to right	Increased detrusor muscle tone
Decreased response to hypoxia	
Bronchoconstriction	
Cardiovascular system	**Miscellaneous**
Hypotension (decreased venous return)	Histamine release
Bradycardia	Pruritus
	Muscle rigidity

[1]Effects vary with individual opioids, dose, circumstances and subject sensitivity.
[2]Constipation is also partly a CNS effect.

tablets to 'patients' claiming to have chronic pain for which they needed strong opioids. This is clearly an ongoing potential problem but is distinct from the theft of morphine from cancer patients.

Collective global experience indicates, however, that it is extremely rare for a patient's supply of morphine to be misappropriated by another person. One patient who was short of money sold his 'Brompton Mixture' to a group of addicts who found it cheaper and longer lasting in its effects than street heroin (Fischbeck et al 1980). In another case, a family member misappropriated a patient's medication for personal use. Such anecdotes, although important, must be put in perspective and should not disproportionately dominate thinking, policy and practice.

RISK OF ADDICTION

Drug addiction or, more properly, drug dependence is defined as a state, psychological and sometimes also physical, characterized by behavioural and other responses that always include a compulsion to take the drug on a continuous or periodic basis in order to experience its psychic effects and sometimes to avoid the discomfort of its absence (WHO 1969). Tolerance may or may not be present. The fear of causing psychological dependence is a potent cause of underprescription and underuse of strong opioid analgesics (Hill 1987). Published data indicate, however, that this fear is unfounded and unnecessary.

Among nearly 12 000 hospital patients who received strong opioids, there were only four reasonably well-documented cases of addiction in patients who had no history of drug abuse (Porter & Jick 1980). The dependence was considered major in only one instance. Studies of chronically ill patients have shown that abuse of non-opioid analgesics or combinations of weak opioids and non-opioids is more common than the abuse of strong opioids (Maruta et al 1979, Tennant & Rawson 1982, Tennant & Uelman 1983). In patients with non-malignant chronic pain, long-term opioid use is not associated with psychological dependence (Taub 1982, Portenoy & Foley 1986). It would seem, therefore, that drug use alone is not a major factor in the development of psychological dependence. Support for this view comes from studies of USA military personnel addicted to strong opioids in Vietnam (Robins et al 1974). In this group, drug abuse was strongly dependent on factors such as personality, social environment and the availability of money.

From time to time, a patient is encountered who appears to be addicted because of demands for 'an injection' every 2–3 hours. Typically, such a patient has a long history of poor pain control and for several weeks will have been receiving repeated ('4-hourly as needed') but inadequate opioid injections. However, after the institution of regular oral medication and the establishment of satisfactory pain relief, the clock watching and demanding behaviour stop. This situation has been called 'pseudoaddiction (Weissman & Haddox 1989). It is not true psychological dependence because the patient is not demanding an opioid in order to experience its psychological effects but to obtain relief from pain for a few hours.

More difficult to deal with is the rare patient, usually young, who was a 'street addict' before becoming ill. Usually one of two errors will be made. On the one hand, his pain is discounted by the professional staff and requests for strong opioids are resisted ('After all, he's an addict'). Alternatively, the patient is treated as a non-addict and allowed to escalate his opioid intake far beyond reasonable estimates of what is needed to control the pain. This is one situation in which the patient's statements about what hurts must be carefully balanced by the judgement of an experienced and compassionate physician (Passik et al 1998a,b). Comparable wisdom needs to be exercised in addicts who are cured of cancer but who continue to request opioids for pain relief. One such person extracted morphine from modified-release tablets and injected intravenously up to 12 times a day (Bloor & Smalldridge 1990).

TOLERANCE

In the past, predictions about tolerance were made on the basis of animal and volunteer studies. The subjects were not in pain and the emphasis was on inducing tolerance and physical dependence as rapidly as possible by using maximum tolerated doses rather than by administering the drugs in doses and at intervals comparable to a clinical regimen. Although such studies may be useful in predicting abuse liability, they are irrelevant to clinical practice. Several studies which review the long-term opioid requirements of cancer patients have demonstrated that the longer the duration of treatment:

1. the slower the rate of rise in dose
2. the longer the periods without a dose increase
3. the greater the likelihood of a dose reduction
4. the greater the likelihood of stopping opioid medication altogether (Twycross 1974, Twycross & Wald 1976, Twycross & Lack 1983).

Of nearly 1000 advanced cancer patients who received opioids, only 5% required an average daily increase of more than 10% of the previous dose; 81% had a stable dose and 14% discontinued opioids (Brescia et al 1992). The main reason for increasing the dose is not tolerance but progression of the disease (Twycross 1974, Kanner & Foley 1981, Brescia et al 1992), and 'tolerance should not be said to exist if ... the need for higher doses to maintain an effect appears to result from increasing pathology rather than exposure to the drug' (Portenoy 1994). Thus, within the context of continuing comprehensive biopsychosocial care, morphine may be used for long periods in cancer patients without concern about tolerance (Table 51.3). Further, even if physical dependence develops after several weeks of continuous treatment, this does not prevent a downward adjustment of dose if the pain is relieved by non-drug measures (e.g. radiation therapy or neurolytic block).

With the exception of constipation and miosis, tolerance to the adverse effects of morphine develops more readily than tolerance to analgesia (Bruera et al 1989, Ling et al 1989). Should tolerance develop, an upward adjustment of dose is all that is necessary to regain pain control. Tolerance does occur, however, in other contexts. Street addicts who use opioids in the absence of pain develop tolerance and may need increasing doses to obtain the same effect. Acute tolerance in the absence of pain has also been shown in animals (Colpaert et al 1980).

RESPIRATORY DEPRESSION

The respiratory depressant effect of opioids has been demonstrated in volunteer studies (Rigg 1978). If volunteers are subjected to a painful stimulus, however, respiratory depression does not occur (Borgbjerg et al 1996). In other words, *pain is a physiological antagonist to the central depressant effects of morphine.* Yet, as is well known, respiratory depression may occur postoperatively (Longnecker et al 1973). This stems from both postanaesthetic pulmonary and drug-related factors (Brismar et al 1985, Heneghan & Jones 1985, Jones & Jordan 1987). For example, postoperatively, patients commonly receive a standard dose of morphine by injection which, inevitably for some, will be excessive. In contrast, cancer patients with pain:

1. have previously been receiving a weak opioid (i.e. are not opioid naïve)

Table 51.3 Possible causes of pseudotolerance[1] (from Pappagallo 1998)

Progression of underlying disease
Onset of second new disorder
Increased physical activity
Lack of compliance
Change in opioid formulation
Drug interaction

[1]Reasons for opioid dose escalation other than tolerance.

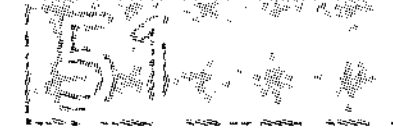

2. take opioid medication by mouth (slower absorption, lower peak concentration)
3. titrate the dose upwards step by step (less likelihood of an excessive dose being given).

Hence, in cancer patients, when the dose of morphine is titrated against the patient's pain, clinically important respiratory depression does not occur (Walsh 1984). Indeed, a review of the time of death of cancer patients showed that a double dose of morphine at bedtime caused no excess nocturnal mortality (Regnard & Badger 1987). There is therefore a broad margin of safety, with sedation occurring at doses significantly lower than those causing respiratory depression.

Respiratory depression may well occur, however, if the underlying pain is suddenly removed and the dose of morphine is not reduced. A 76-year-old man with a pleural mesothelioma needed oral morphine 90 mg every 4 hours to relieve severe chest pain (Hanks et al 1981). Several hours after a successful nerve block with intrathecal chlorocresol, the patient became drowsy, confused and cyanosed with a respiratory rate of 3–4/min. He required naloxone on two occasions to correct this (Fig. 51.2). There is need for caution, therefore, if the level of pain is suddenly altered as a result of non-drug measures, particularly in those with limited respiratory reserve. Thus, if a patient's pain is relieved by neurolysis or neurosurgery, the dose of morphine should be immediately reduced to 25% of the previous analgesic dose. If the nerve block is totally successful, the rest of the morphine can be phased out gradually over the next 1–2 weeks. If only partly successful, however, it may be necessary to increase the dose again to 50–60% of the original dose or even more.

Respiratory depression may occur with spinal opioids. This is more likely in opioid-naive patients (Writer et al 1985). Guidance about appropriate monitoring over the first 24 hours is available (Etches et al 1989). In advanced cancer, because patients have invariably already been receiving opioids regularly by mouth or injection, serious respiratory depression is rare. Rightly used, morphine is a safe drug for cancer pain management.

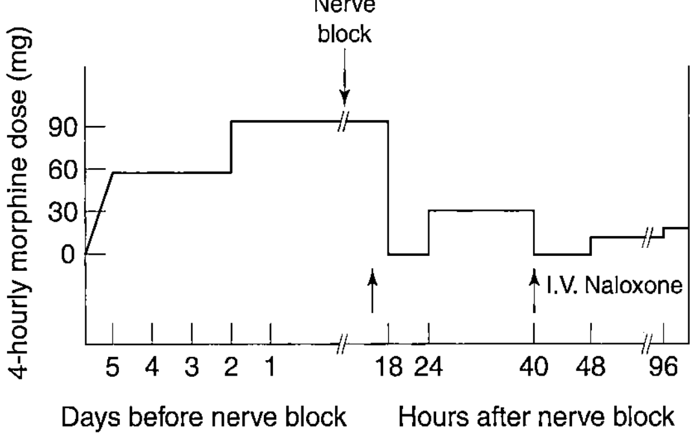

Fig. 51.2 Morphine requirements in a 76-year-old man with a pleural mesothelioma before and after intrathecal chlorocresol nerve block.

Further, morphine is used to relieve breathlessness in both advanced chronic obstructive pulmonary disease ('pink puffers') and advanced cancer (Woodcock et al 1981, Light et al 1989, Bruera et al 1990). Benefit comes partly by reducing the rate of exercise-induced tachypnoea. Doses are generally smaller than for pain control (Twycross 1994).

OPIOIDS AND SURVIVAL

Many people believe that using opioids for pain relief inevitably 'advances death'. Although this view is obviously false (consider acute and postoperative pain management), the suspicion remains in the minds of the general public that opioids are nothing more than a polite way to kill terminally ill patients. Regrettably, this view finds expression in the press. For example, the *New York Times* carried an article in 1997 entitled 'When morphine fails to kill' (Wall 1997). There are obvious dangers if physicians are portrayed as beneficent executioners, not least because many patients will decline opioids and suffer unnecessary pain instead.

Whether a patient dies shortly after the prescription of morphine depends on when morphine is started. Obviously, if a patient is already near to death when prescribed morphine, he will die soon afterwards, particularly if exhausted by long-continued pain and insomnia. Circumstantial evidence suggests, however, that the correct use of morphine prolongs the life of a cancer patient because of:

1. freedom from pain
2. improved rest and sleep
3. increased appetite and strength
4. increased physical activity.

Data on file indicate that one-third of patients survive more than 4 weeks and 10% for more than 3 months (Fig. 51.3). These figures are underestimates because the duration of treatment was measured only from the first inpatient admission and many had been taking morphine for several weeks before this. 'We must help the patients to be absolutely clear that their treatment for pain is just that and that it is not an alternative route to an early grave' (Wall 1997).

On the other hand, it has been claimed that, in the Netherlands, doctors frequently use morphine in doses

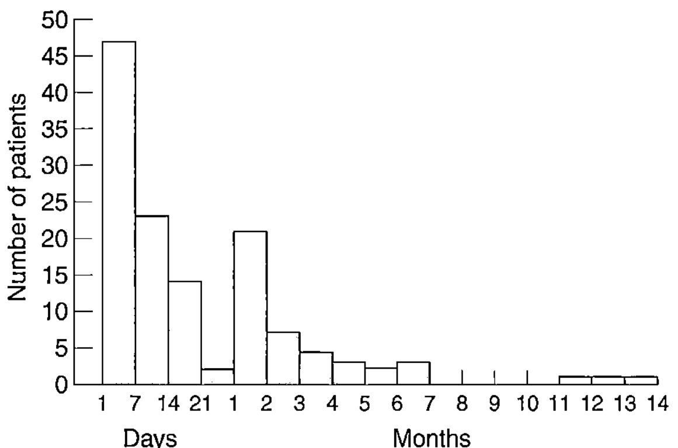

Fig. 51.3 Histogram showing survival after commencing treatment with morphine sulphate in 129 patients admitted to Sobell House in 1978. Median duration of treatment = 13 days; 33% of patients survived for more than 4 weeks; 12% for more than 3 months.

higher than necessary for pain relief. It has been estimated that 16% of all deaths in the Netherlands (>20 000 annually) are related to opioid doses which have been increased not because of pain but with the intention of hastening death (Van der Mass et al 1991). Because morphine is so often used in this way, many patients are afraid to take morphine even though they would benefit by it. Indeed, one study revealed that 30% of patients decreased the dose or discontinued opioid drugs immediately after discharge from hospital (Dorrepaal 1989, Zylicz 1993).

OPIOIDS AND PSYCHOMOTOR FUNCTION

It is also widely believed that taking medicinal morphine regularly will turn the patient into a zombie. However, in one controlled study of the psychomotor impact of morphine on cancer patients, it was not possible to demonstrate a significant negative impact on function such as would impair driving (Vainio et al 1995). In two tests of high-level concentration, a significant dose-dependent relationship was observed between plasma concentrations of morphine and its glucuronide metabolites and poor performance. Even so, overall results in the cancer patients (with and without morphine) showed no differences from those seen in physically healthy adults of similar age.

Other studies have reported similar results (Hanks et al 1995, O'Neill et al 1995). A few patients, however, are adversely affected. Work still needs to be done to elucidate the possible role of psychostimulants (such as dexamphetamine or methylphenidate) in these patients (O'Neill 1994). In patients most susceptible to morphine-induced cognitive failure (delirium), it may well be necessary to switch to another opioid.

OPIOID CLASSIFICATION

In the past, opioids were classified as:

1. opium and opium alkaloids (codeine, morphine, etc.)
2. opiates (semisynthetic derivatives of an opium alkaloid, e.g. diamorphine, buprenorphine)
3. opioids (synthetic drugs, e.g. pethidine, methadone).

The synthetic opioids were subdivided according to chemical structure. Now, opioid is used as a generic term and includes all drugs with morphine-like actions. In the Revised Method for Relief of Cancer Pain (WHO 1996), the following classification was adopted:

1. opioids for mild to moderate pain
2. opioids for moderate to severe pain.

These terms have little to commend them and are too clumsy for everyday clinical use. In practice, the terms 'weak opioid' (codeine, etc.) and 'strong opioid' (morphine, etc.) continue to have wide currency and are used here. It must be remembered, however, that within any class of drugs, efficacy comprises a spectrum and individual drugs cannot always be rigidly pigeon-holed into one particular subclass.

The use of the terms 'mild analgesics' for non-opioids and 'strong analgesics' for opioids, although still sometimes used, must be discouraged. There are occasions when morphine (a 'strong analgesic') does not relieve pain which aspirin (a 'mild analgesic') does. Further, parenteral NSAIDs are frequently used to relieve biliary and ureteric colic (Broggini et al 1984, Lundstam et al 1985, Hetherington & Philip 1986, Thompson et al 1989) and postoperative pain (Nuutinen et al 1986) because they are as effective as or better than opioids.

OPIOID RECEPTORS

The nomenclature for opioid receptors has been revised (Table 51.4). The endogenous ligands for each receptor are known, together with exogenous agonists and antagonists (Dickenson 1991, Vaught 1991). Naloxone is an antagonist at all three receptors. Recently, genetically modified mice have been produced without one or other opioid receptor (knockout mice). Studies with such mice will clarify our knowledge of the various opioids in clinical use. Thus, morphine exerts no analgesic action in OP_3 (μ) receptor knockout mice (Matthes et al 1996, Sora et al 1997) nor does it inhibit gastrointestinal transit (Roy et al

Table 51.4 Classification of opioid receptors (from Dhawan et al 1996)

Preferential endogenous opioid ligands	*Opioid receptors*		
	IUPHAR recommendation	*Pharmacology nomenclature*	*Molecular biology nomenclature*
Enkephalins	OP_1	δ	DOR
Dynorphins	OP_2	κ	KOR
β-endorphin	OP_3	μ	MOR

IUPHAR = International Union of Pharmacology; DOR refers to mouse vas **d**eferens; KOR to **k**etocyclazocine; MOR to **m**orphine.

1998). The ability of morphine to kill mice is also dramatically reduced (Loh et al 1998). In contrast, a highly selective OP_1 (δ) agonist is analgesic in such mice (Vaught et al 1998).

In OP_2 (κ) receptor knockout mice, morphine analgesia is unaffected (Simonin et al 1988). The OP_2 receptor, however, is involved in some way in the perception of visceral chemical pain and in the expression of morphine abstinence (Simonin et al 1988). Although one school of thought subdivides the OP_3 receptor into μ_1 and μ_2 receptors (Kamei et al 1993), the current general opinion is that subtypes of the three main opioid receptors do not exist.

During the process of identifying and cloning the three traditional opioid receptors, a new opioid-like receptor was identified. This was nicknamed the orphan receptor because at first it had no known ligand. The ligand was subsequently identified simultaneously by two groups who named it orphanin and (erroneously) nociceptin. Agonists at the new receptor produce analgesia at the spinal level. The receptor has been named opioid receptor like type 1 (ORL_1) and its ligand orphanin FQ (Meunier 1997). Early work suggest that this receptor is widespread and it will be interesting to see which currently available opioids are ORL_1 agonists.

Conventional views about full agonists and partial agonists are also undergoing revision. Depending on the local density of the receptor population, some opioids behave either as full agonists or as partial agonists.

MECHANISM OF ACTION

Opioid receptors are synthesized in the cell body of the sensory neuron and are transported in both central and peripheral directions. Thus, in the spinal cord, opioid receptors are found in the dorsal horn in the terminal zones of C fibres, primarily in lamina I of the substantia gelatinosa. OP_3 receptors predominate (in the rat, 70% OP_3, 24% OP_1 and 6% OP_2). Stimulation of the presynaptic OP_1 and OP_3 receptors is associated with hyperpolarization of the terminal and reduced excitatory neurotransmitter release. This relates primarily to inhibition of voltage-gated calcium channels. Postsynaptic membranes contain opioid receptors which are linked to potassium channels. Stimulation of the receptor enhances the outward flow of potassium, thereby stabilizing the membrane and making it less sensitive to neurotransmitters. The action of morphine at opioid receptors is carried forward by a second messenger G-protein (Traynor 1996). Opioid receptors are also linked by an inhibitory G-protein to adenyl cyclase (Satoh & Minami 1995).

Peripherally, neural opioid receptors are silent until activated by inflammatory substances (Stein 1993, Andreev et al 1994). This results in an enhanced response to opioids (Stanfa et al 1994), which is probably related to reduced release of an antianalgesic substance, cholecystokinin (CCK) (Wiertelak et al 1992). CCK is found predominantly in intrinsic dorsal horn neurons and interferes with morphine analgesia via the CCK_B receptor. Knowledge of these peripheral receptors has led to the intra-articular use of small doses of morphine (0.5–0.6 mg) during knee surgery – with analgesic benefit lasting up to 48 hours (Khoury et al 1992, Joshi 1993) – and injection into the mesosalpinx at the time of tubal occlusion surgery (Snyder 1993).

Opioid receptors have also been identified on the surface of immune cells (Stein et al 1990). T and B lymphocytes, monocytes and macrophages contain propiomelanocortin-mRNA and proenkephalin-mRNA in abundance, suggesting synthesis of opioid peptides by these cells (Przewlocki et al 1992).

In contrast, reduced response to opioids occurs with some neuropathic pains. This parallels the induction of CCK production in afferent fibres which occurs after nerve section. Opioid responsiveness is restored by CCK receptor antagonists (Stanfa et al 1994). Other relevant factors include:

1. degeneration of the C-fibre afferents and loss of the presynaptic opioid receptors

2. pathological transmission of pain by large-diameter A fibres which do not possess opioid receptors
3. the inability of opioids to overcome the increased activity in second-order spinal neurons which occurs with dorsal horn excitation (Dickenson & Sullivan 1986).

This latter phenomenon is associated with activation of the N-methyl D-aspartate (NMDA) receptor-channel complex by the excitatory amino acid glutamate.

Clinical experience suggests that, in inflammatory pain also, an acute enhanced response to opioids may subsequently give way to a reduced chronic response. Studies in animals with experimentally induced arthritis indicate that this is associated with dorsal horn excitation, i.e. activation of the NMDA receptor-channel complex (Sorkin et al 1992, Sluka & Westlund 1993).

New discoveries continue to reveal even greater complexities surrounding nociception and antinociception. For example, it has been known for many years that tricyclic antidepressants are analgesic in certain circumstances. It has recently been shown, however, that naloxone shifts the dose-response relationships to the right for such drugs (Gray et al 1998). Data are consistent with the view that antidepressants induce endogenous opioid peptide release and that the principal effect is via the OP_1 (δ) receptor.

In recent years, attention has been directed towards pulmonary opioid receptors. In addition to the high-affinity receptors in C fibre peripheral nerve endings, there is a high concentration of low-affinity receptors adjacent to the pulmonary J receptors (Cabot et al 1996). This has led to speculation about the possible benefits of nebulized morphine in breathlessness. In one study in patients with severe chronic pulmonary disease, nebulized morphine 5 mg (with a lung bioavailability of about one-third) increased exercise tolerance by a mean of 65 seconds compared with 9 seconds for placebo (Young et al 1989). In a second study, however, results were not clearcut (Beauford et al 1993). Likewise, in cancer patients, a controlled study comparing nebulized morphine with saline failed to demonstrate definite benefit, even with much higher doses (up to 50 mg) (Davis et al 1996).

OPIOIDS AND CANCER PAIN

Opioids are not the panacea for cancer pain management (Woolf & Wall 1986, Schulze et al 1988, McQuay et al 1990, Hanks 1991). Indeed, analgesics generally should be regarded as just one part of a multimodal strategy (Twycross 1994). Even so, with cancer pain, drugs generally provide satisfactory relief if the right drugs are administered in the right doses at the right time intervals (WHO 1986, 1996, Grond et al 1996).

Analgesics can conveniently be divided into three classes:

1. non-opioid (paracetamol and non-steroidal anti-inflammatory drugs)
2. opioid (weak and strong)
3. adjuvant (corticosteroids, antidepressants, anticonvulsants, muscle relaxants, etc.).

The principles governing their use have been summarized as 'by the mouth', 'by the clock', 'by the ladder' (Fig. 51.4), 'individualized treatment' and 'attention to detail' (WHO 1986, Twycross 1994, Hanks et al 1996). The concept behind the analgesic ladder is 'broad-spectrum analgesia', i.e. drugs from each class of analgesics are used appropriately either singly or in combination so as to maximize their analgesic impact (Fig. 51.5). Thus, non-opioids as well as opioids are generally necessary for severe bone or soft tissue pain. In cancer-related neuropathic pain, the benefits of both non-opioids and opioids should be exploited before introducing or substituting adjuvant analgesics. Adjuvant analgesics, however, are necessary to relieve many neuropathic pains (Fig. 51.6). In addition, a laxative is almost always necessary to relieve opioid-induced constipation and about 50% of patients need an antiemetic (Twycross 1994). Appropriate psychotropic medication is necessary for both highly anxious and clinically depressed patients.

Persistent pain requires preventive therapy. This means that analgesics should be given regularly and prophylactically; p.r.n. medication is irrational and inhumane (Fig. 51.7). The right dose of an analgesic is the dose which

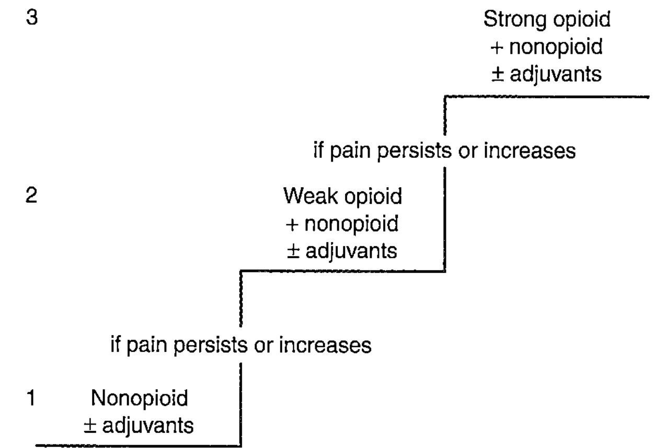

Fig. 51.4 The WHO analgesic ladder for cancer pain management.

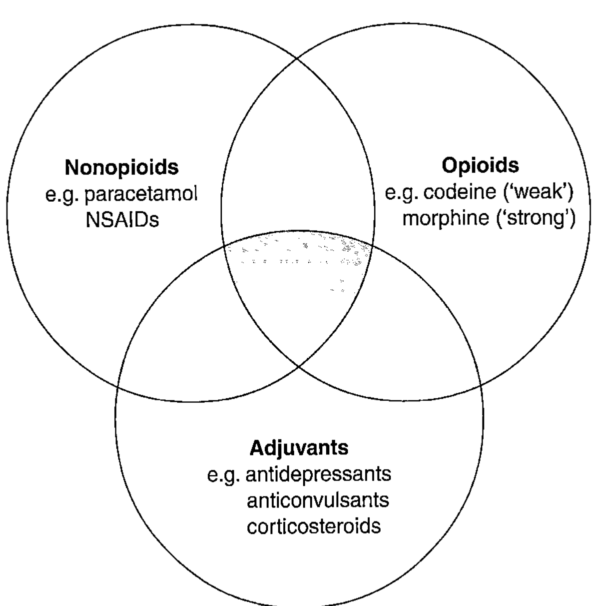

Fig. 51.5 Broad-spectrum analgesia; analgesics from different classes are used in various combinations to maximize pain relief.

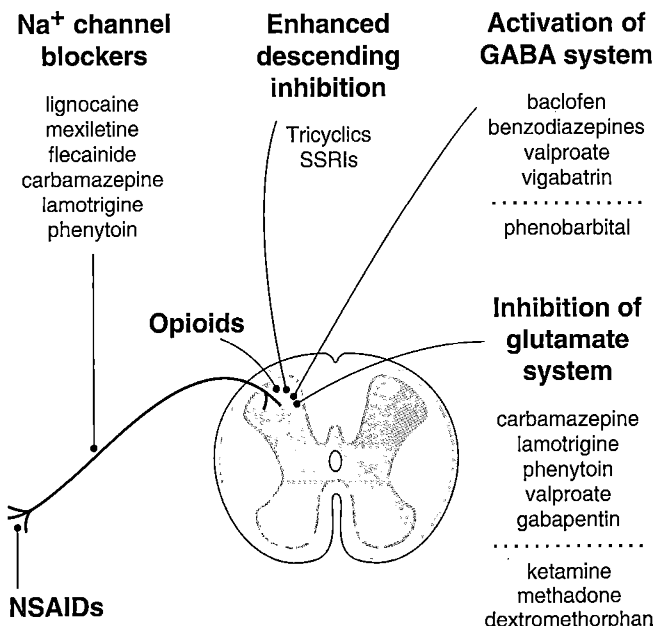

Fig. 51.6 Cross-section of spinal cord to illustrate main sites of action of conventional and adjuvant analgesics.

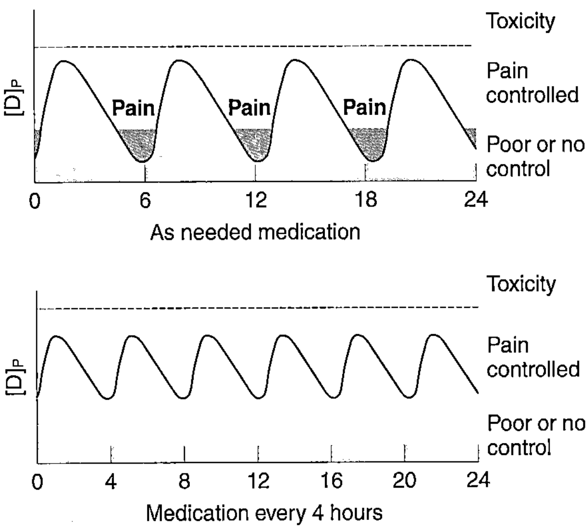

Fig. 51.7 Comparison of morphine p.r.n. with regular morphine q4h. [D]p = plasma concentration of drug.

relieves the pain. Ceiling doses exist for all analgesics, however, either in absolute terms (an increased dose yield no more pain relief) or relative terms (an increased dose yields more adverse effects than pain relief). In practice, doses of oral morphine typically range from as little as 30 mg daily (i.e. 5 mg q4 h) up to 1200 mg daily (normal release 200 mg q4 h or modified release 600 mg q12 h, 1200 mg o.d.) and occasionally much more (Twycross 1994).

The use of morphine is determined by analgesic need and not, for example, by the doctor's estimate of life expectancy – which is often wrong. The right dose of morphine is the one which gives adequate relief for 4 hours without unacceptable adverse effects. 'Maximum' or 'recommended' doses, derived mainly from postoperative parenteral single-dose studies, are not applicable for cancer pain (Brescia et al 1992, McCormack et al 1992). The following points should be noted.

1. It is pharmacological nonsense to prescribe simultaneously two weak opioids or two strong opioids.
2. For breakthrough pain, patients should be advised to take an extra dose of their regular opioid (normal-release formulation), although it is sometimes necessary for patients to supplement with a second opioid (e.g. morphine p.r.n. in addition to transdermal fentanyl).
3. For regular use, avoid short-acting drugs such as dextromoramide, pentazocine and pethidine.

All cancer patients receiving analgesics need close supervision to achieve maximum comfort with minimal adverse effects. Review is sometimes necessary within hours of starting treatment; it is certainly required after 1–2 days and at the end of the first week. Subsequently, new pains may develop and old pains re-emerge. A fresh complaint of pain demands re-evaluation, not just a message to increase pain medication, although this may be an important short-term measure.

As noted above, with a given patient population, the dose of morphine to relieve cancer pain varies considerably. In addition to this well-recognized interpatient variation, there appears to be wide intercentre variation (Boisvert & Cohen 1995). Reasons for this are not always obvious but probably include:

1. reports based on small or atypical samples (Twycross 1997)
2. use of *mean* rather than *median* maximum doses (the mean is often much higher)
3. differences in the concurrent use of non-opioid and adjuvant analgesics (Ferris et al 1990, Schug et al 1992)
4. differences in psychological support and in the use of non-drug treatments, e.g. relaxation, massage.

An agreed protocol for reporting morphine requirements is needed to facilitate crosstalk between centres (Bruera et al 1995).

OPIOIDS AND POSTOPERATIVE PAIN

In the past, postoperative pain has been managed badly and scandal avoided only because patients did not expect any better and it is by definition short-lived. Rather like parturition pain, postoperative pain tends to be forgotten in the joy of new life. In recent years, however, considerable effort has been put into better postoperative pain management (RCS 1990). IV patient-controlled analgesia (PCA) is increasingly used.

OPIOIDS AND CHRONIC PAIN OF NON-MALIGNANT ORIGIN

While there is a clear consensus about the use of morphine and other strong opioids for severe pain in cancer, its use for non-malignant chronic pain is still controversial. Clinical experience, however, demonstrates that some chronic pain patients derive considerable benefit from opioids (Knight 1989, Portenoy 1990, Zenz et al 1992). Controlled data confirm this (Rowbotham et al 1991, Jadad et al 1992).

The situation is comparable to cancer pain in that it is important to identify which pains respond well to opioids and which do not. On the other hand, the situation differs in as much as the chronic use of opioids in non-terminal conditions could well mean 10–30 years, compared with weeks or months. The use of IV PCA to compare morphine with placebo is the best way to test for opioid responsiveness in chronic pain patients (Jadad et al 1992), but will not always be feasible. Guidelines for strong opioid use in non-malignant chronic pain are available (Box 51.1).

ROUTES OF ADMINISTRATION

Although other routes of administration are sometimes used, oral, sublingual, rectal, conventional parenteral (SC, IM, IV) and spinal (epidural and intrathecal) routes generally suffice. For cancer pain, the oral route remains the norm for patients who can swallow. For acute pain (e.g. postoperative), a conventional parenteral route is the norm. In wealthier countries, given the availability of syringes, portable syringe drivers and PCA devices, injections are likely to be used in preference to suppositories. The oral to parenteral potency ratio varies from opioid to opioid (see below).

SUBLINGUAL

Sublingual preparations are particularly useful when strong opioids are necessary but cannot be taken by mouth and injections are problematic, e.g. in children, haemophiliacs and home care. However, opioids like methadone with a high oral bioavailability do not demonstrate significant gain in bioavailability when taken sublingually (McQuay et al 1986b). The same is true for morphine (Pannuti et al 1982,

BOX 51.1

Strong opioids in the management of chronic pain of non-malignant origin (from Gourlay & Cherry 1991)

1. There must be a clear understanding that opioids are to be used for a limited term in the first instance.
2. Their use is contingent upon certain obligations or goals being met by the patient, e.g. increased mobilization, return to work, no unauthorized demands for emergency injectable opioids from locum services and changes in unacceptable or non-productive behaviours, i.e. a contractual arrangement (which can be in the form of a written document) that opioids will be supplied for a limited term in exchange for agreed goals.
3. Extension of the initial term can be contemplated only upon agreed improvements being met by patients.
4. The patient understands that there will be regular and random blood samples collected to ensure compliance with dosing schedule and that other opioid drugs are not being consumed.

McQuay et al 1986b). In contrast, buprenorphine is given sublingually because of the considerable gain in bioavailability compared to the oral route. Postoperatively, 0.4 mg sublingually produces analgesia equivalent to 0.3 mg intramuscularly. Sublingual systemic availability is 55% (range 16–94%), compared with 15% after oral administration (McQuay et al 1986a).

RECTAL

Rectally, morphine bypasses the portal circulation to a variable extent according to how much is absorbed into the middle and inferior rectal veins (systemic circulation) compared with the superior rectal vein (portal circulation). This results in variable rectal bioavailability, ranging from 70% to 120% of the oral (Kaiko et al 1989). In practice, however, the same dose is given rectally as orally. Clearly, after any change of route, there may be need to adjust the initial conversion dose up or down in order to either regain pain relief or reduce sedation and other adverse effects caused by overdosage.

Absorption per colostomy differs considerably from rectal absorption. In one study, mean relative availability was only 43%, ranging from 0% to 127% (Hojsted et al 1990). Reasons for poor availability probably include:

1. poor vascularity
2. insertion of tablets into faeces
3. hepatic first-pass metabolism.

CONVENTIONAL INJECTIONS

Terminally ill cancer patients often receive parenteral medication for several days or even weeks. Portable battery-driven syringe drivers are increasingly used to deliver a continuous SC infusion of morphine or diamorphine together with an antiemetic (Walsh et al 1992). Other drugs may also be included provided they are miscible and stable in combined solution (Twycross et al 1998).

Some cancer patients have a permanent central venous catheter to facilitate chemotherapy and repeated blood sampling. Catheters have been kept in situ for periods of up to 3 years, with a median duration of 40 days (McCredie & Lawson 1984). These catheters can be used for morphine (and other symptom-control drugs) by either continuous infusion or intermittent bolus (Portenoy et al 1986). As IV administration limits the mobility of the patient, it is generally not preferable to the oral, rectal or SC routes. Acute tolerance to the analgesic effect of repeat IV bolus injections of diamorphine hydrochloride has been reported (Hanks & Thomas 1985). On the other hand, continuous IV infusions of morphine have been used successfully in children for long periods (Miser et al 1980).

SPINAL OPIOIDS

The presence of opioid receptors in high density in the dorsal horn of the spinal cord (Pert & Snyder 1973) provides the logical basis for spinal opioid use (Sabbe & Yaksh 1990). Compared with conventional routes, extradural and intrathecal administration carry a potentially higher morbidity. The use of the spinal route can therefore be justified only if it results in equal or greater pain relief with less troublesome or fewer adverse effects than conventional routes (Hogan et al 1991, Sjoberg et al 1991).

Duration of analgesic effect after spinal opioids is considerably longer than after IM injection. In patients having cardiac surgery, analgesia of about 36 hours duration was achieved by lumbar intrathecal injection of 2–4 mg of morphine (Mathews & Abrams 1980). In patients having total hip replacement, lower doses gave 24–48 hours analgesia (Kalso 1983, Paterson et al 1984). Diamorphine provides the same duration of analgesia as morphine at the same dose. Opioids which are highly lipid soluble are relatively less potent when given intrathecally because of their ability easily to diffuse away from the subarachnoid space and therefore from the sites of action in the dorsal horn (McQuay et al 1989).

The advantage of the epidural route is the potentially lower morbidity, notably headache and infection. On the other hand, in chronic use the catheter tip may occlude (it is not bathed in CSF) or migrate intrathecally. Further, spinal opioid availability is less certain than with the intrathecal route. Systemic absorption adds another dimension to both pharmacokinetic and pharmacodynamic considerations. Only 10–20% of an epidural dose of morphine (low lipid solubility) crosses the dura into the CSF. This is reflected in the higher doses used by this route. Extradural morphine 5 mg twice daily is equivalent to intrathecal morphine 1 mg once a day, a potency ratio of 1:10 (Watson et al 1984). Postoperatively, epidural morphine 5 mg gives a median duration of relief of 10 hours (Watson et al 1984). Doses used with infusions have been as low as 0.3 mg/h (Cullen et al 1985). This suggests that the dose response for morphine is different with a bolus compared with an infusion. Standard anaesthetics textbooks and other accounts (e.g. Swarm & Cousins 1997) should be used for more detail.

Adverse effects vary according to dose, whether the opioid is given intrathecally or epidurally and whether usage is acute or chronic. Troublesome adverse effects are generally less with chronic compared with acute use. The incidence of adverse effects and complications after postoperative epidural morphine is shown in Table 51.5. IM naloxone reverses the adverse effects associated with epidural morphine, notably respiratory depression, urinary retention and pruritus, without reducing analgesia (Korbon et al 1985, Ueyama et al 1992). However, rectovaginal muscle spasms seen in one patient receiving intrathecal morphine necessitated the ongoing use of midazolam by PCA (Littrell et al 1992).

Tolerance to spinal opioids may occur with chronic use; it is a predictable consequence of the very high local concentrations of opioid in the cerebrospinal fluid. Tolerance develops more rapidly with infusions than with p.r.n. bolus injections (Erickson et al 1984). It is not an insuperable problem, as increasing the dose corrects the reduced response. Abstention for about a week leads to a reversal of tolerance.

Spinal opioids have a definite place in the relief of pain after major surgery and after injuries such as multiple rib fractures (Ullman et al 1989). In these situations the use is self-limiting and is unlikely to exceed 14 days. With chronic pain, until the promise of higher quality pain relief is realized, the spinal route should be used only after systemically administered opioids have been found to be ineffective or associated with intolerable adverse effects (Sjostrand & Rawal 1986).

A safe method of converting from conventional parenteral routes to intrathecal administration is to use 1% of the former total daily dose (Coombs 1986). Practices differ, however, and some centres use 2%. Likewise, when converting directly from oral to epidural, recommended dose ratios vary between 30 and 50 and from IV or SC to epidural, between 5 and 10. Generally, lower doses should be used if bupivacaine is administered, concurrently (Hogan et al 1991, Sjoberg et al 1991). Combined therapy is perhaps one reason for the different recommendations.

Table 51.5 Incidence of complications in opioid-naïve patients after 5 mg epidural morphine (*n* = 128) (from Writer et al 1985)

Complications	*Incidence (%)*
Nausea	48
Vomiting	30
Pruritus	41
Urinary retention	34
Hypotension	4
Respiratory depression	4

WEAK OPIOIDS

The division of opioids into 'weak' and 'strong' is to a certain extent arbitrary. By IM injection, all the weak opioids can provide analgesia equivalent, or nearly equivalent, to morphine 10 mg. In practice, however, dextropropoxyphene and dihydrocodeine are not used parenterally and codeine infrequently.

Weak opioids are said to have a ceiling effect for analgesia. This is an oversimplification. Whereas mixed agonist-antagonists such as pentazocine have a true ceiling effect (Martin 1979), the maximum effective dose of weak opioid agonists is arbitrary. At higher doses there are progressively more adverse effects, notably nausea and vomiting, which outweigh any additional analgesic effect. For example, the amount of dextropropoxyphene in compound tablets was chosen so that only a small minority of patients would experience nausea and vomiting with two tablets. This adds a further constraint; in practice the upper dose limit is set by the number of tablets which a patient will accept, possibly only 2–3 of any preparation. There is little to choose between the weak opioids in terms of efficacy (Table 51.6). Codeine and dihydrocodeine are more constipating and, for this reason, co-proxamol is preferred at most palliative care units in the UK. The following general rules should be observed.

1. A weak opioid should be *added to*, not substituted for, a non-opioid.
2. Do not 'kangaroo' from weak opioid to weak opioid.
3. If a weak opioid is inadequate when given regularly, change to morphine or an alternative strong opioid.

CODEINE PHOSPHATE

Codeine (methylmorphine) is an opium alkaloid, about one-tenth as potent as morphine. An increasing analgesic response has been reported with IM doses up to 360 mg (Beaver 1966). In practice, however, codeine is used orally in doses of 20–60 mg, generally in combination with a non-opioid. Its oral to parenteral potency ratio is 2:3, about double that of morphine. The main metabolite is codeine-6-glucuronide (which has comparable weak binding to the μ receptor), together with small amounts of norcodeine, morphine, morphine-3-glucuronide and morphine-6-glucuronide. It has been suggested that codeine is a pro-drug of morphine because codeine lacks significant analgesic activity in animals if demethylation is blocked (Cleary et al 1994) and in humans who are CYP2D6 poor

Table 51.6 Weak opioids

Drug	*Bioavailability (%)*	*Time to maximum concentration (h)*	*Plasma half-life (h)*	*Duration of analgesia (h)*[1]	*Potency ratio with codeine*
Codeine	40 (12–84)	1–2	2.5–3.5	4–5	1
Dextropropoxyphene	40	2–2.5	6–12[2]	6–8	7/8[3]
Dihydrocodeine	20	1.6–1.8	3.5–4.5	3–4	4/3
Meptazinol	<10	0.5–2	3.5–5[4]	3–4	2/5[5]
Pentazocine	20	1	3	2–3	1[5]
Tramadol	70	2	6	4–6	2[5]

[1]When used in usual doses for moderate pain.
[2]Increased >50% in elderly.
[3]Multiple doses; single dose = 1/2–2/3.
[4]Multiple doses in elderly; single dose = 2 h.
[5]Estimated on basis of potency ratio with morphine.

metabolizers (Eckhardt et al 1998). The adverse effects of codeine are identical in both extensive and poor metabolizers, even though the latter experience no compensatory beneficial analgesia. The amount of codeine biotransformed to morphine varies from 2% to 10% (Hanks & Cherry 1997). In another human study, however, at least part of the analgesic effect of codeine appeared to be direct (Quiding et al 1993).

DEXTROPROPOXYPHENE

Propoxyphene is a synthetic derivative of methadone. Its analgesic properties reside in the dextroisomer, dextropropoxyphene. It is a μ agonist with receptor affinity similar to that of codeine. It is also a weak NMDA receptor-channel blocker (Ebert et al 1995). Dextropropoxyphene undergoes extensive first-pass hepatic metabolism; this is dose dependent and systemic availability increases with increasing doses (Perrier & Gibaldi 1972). The principal metabolite, norpropoxyphene, is also analgesic but crosses the blood–brain barrier to a much lesser extent. Both dextropropoxyphene and norpropoxyphene achieve steady-state plasma concentrations 5–7 times greater than those after the first dose. Randomized controlled trials in patients with postsurgical pain, arthritis and musculoskeletal pain collectively show no added benefit when dextropropoxyphene is combined with paracetamol compared with paracetamol alone (Li Wan Po & Zhang 1997). Such reports have led to doubts about the general efficacy of dextropropoxyphene. However, dextropropoxyphene 65 mg has been shown to have a definite analgesic effect in several placebo-controlled trials and a dose-response curve has been established (Fig. 51.8), thereby confirming its efficacy (Beaver 1984). Dextropropoxyphene causes less nausea and vomiting, drowsiness and dry mouth than low-dose morphine, particularly during initial treatment (Mercadante et al 1998).

DIHYDROCODEINE

Dihydrocodeine is a semisynthetic analogue of codeine. Like codeine, it is analgesic, antitussive and antidiarrhoeal. Its potency to SC morphine 10 mg varies from 30 to 70 mg (Palmer et al 1966). By injection 60 mg provides significantly more analgesia than 30 mg but 90 mg provides little more than 60 mg. Dihydrocodeine is approximately twice as potent as codeine parenterally but, because its oral

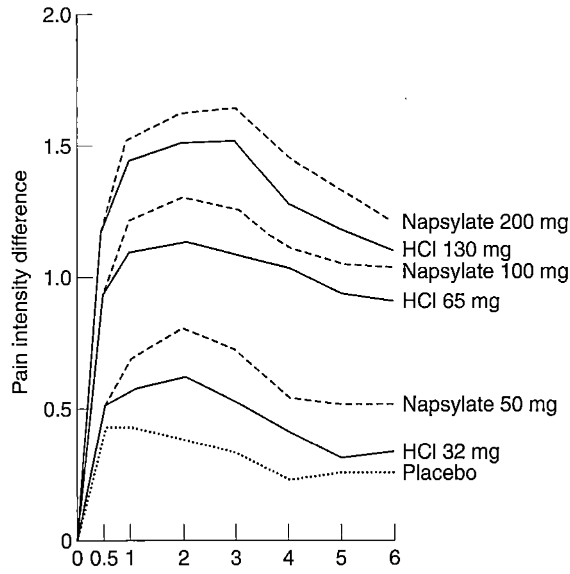

Fig. 51.8 Dose-response data for dextropropoxyphene hydrochloride and dextropropoxyphene napsilate. A placebo would not manifest a dose-response curve. (From Beaver 1984 with permission.)

bioavailability is low, the two drugs are essentially equipotent by mouth (Anonymous 1991).

TRAMADOL

Tramadol is a synthetic, centrally acting analgesic. It has both opioid and non-opioid properties (Raffa et al 1992, Lee et al 1993). The latter are related to stimulation of neuronal serotonin release and inhibition of presynaptic reuptake of norepinephrine (noradrenaline) and serotonin. Naloxone only partially reverses the analgesic effect of tramadol (Raffa et al 1992). Tramadol is converted in the liver to O-desmethyltramadol which is itself an active substance, 2–4 times more potent than tramadol. Further biotransformation results in inactive metabolites which are excreted by the kidneys. A comparison of receptor site affinities and monoamine reuptake inhibition illustrates the unique combination of properties which underlie the action of tramadol (Tables 51.7, 51.8); it is necessary to invoke synergism to explain its analgesic effect. Tramadol causes much less constipation and respiratory depression than equianalgesic doses of morphine (Wilder-Smith & Bettiga 1997). Its dependence liability is also considerably less (Preston et al 1991) and it is not a controlled (Schedule 2) drug (Radbruch et al 1996). By injection, tramadol is one-tenth as potent as morphine. By mouth, because of much better bioavailability, it is one-fifth as potent; it can be regarded as double-strength codeine.

Table 51.7 Opioid receptor affinities: K_i (μM) values[1] (from Raffa et al 1992 with permission)

	OP_1 (δ)	OP_2 (κ)	OP_3 (μ)
Morphine	0.09	0.6	0.0003
Dextropropoxyphene	0.38	1.2	0.03
Codeine	5	6	0.2
Tramadol	58	43	2

[1]The lower the K_i value, the greater the receptor affinity.

Table 51.8 Inhibition of monoamine uptake: K_i (μM) values[1] (from Raffa et al 1992 with permission)

	Norepinephrine	Serotonin
Imipramine	0.0066	0.021
Tramadol	0.78	0.99
Dextropropoxyphene	IA[2]	IA[2]
Codeine	IA[2]	IA[2]
Morphine	IA[2]	IA[2]

[1]The lower the K_i value, the greater the receptor affinity.
[2]IA = inactive at 10 μM.

STRONG OPIOIDS

Globally, morphine remains the strong opioid of choice (WHO 1986); other strong opioids are used mainly when morphine is not readily available or when a patient has intolerable adverse effects with morphine. Differences between opioids relate, inter alia, to differences in receptor affinity, lipid solubility and plasma half-lives. Strong opioids tend to cause the same range of adverse effects (Table 51.9), although to a varying degree. As already noted, with individualized treatment, strong opioids do not cause respiratory depression in patients in pain. However, because of the possibility of an additive sedative effect, care should be taken when strong opioids and psychotropic drugs are used concurrently. Several important drug interactions occur (Table 51.10). For example, cimetidine inhibits the metabolism of methadone, which may lead to increasing drowsiness or even coma (Sorkin & Ogawa 1983). Rifampicin accelerates methadone metabolism by induction of a phase I drug metabolizing enzyme (CYP3A4) and has on occasion precipitated opioid withdrawal symptoms (Kreek et al 1976, Holmes 1990). Rifampicin also reduces morphine analgesia by induction of a phase II drug metabolizing enzyme (UDP-glucuronyltransferase) (Fromm et al 1997).

There is little to choose between the various opioids in terms of speed of onset of action. Most begin to take effect about 20–30 minutes after oral administration. If a rapid onset of action is desirable, the IV route should be used. Speed of absorption after IM injection varies according to the vascularity of the muscle. Uptake from the gluteal muscles is slower in females than in males and uptake from deltoid is faster than from the gluteal muscles (Kaiko 1986).

Table 51.9 Adverse effects of opioid analgesics

Common initial	**Occasional**
Nausea and vomiting	Dry mouth
Drowsiness	Sweating
Unsteadiness	Pruritus
Delirium (confusion)	Hallucinations
	Myoclonus
Common ongoing	**Rare**
Constipation	Respiratory depression
Nausea and vomiting	Psychological dependence

Table 51.10 Drug-induced alterations in opioid pharmacokinetics and/or pharmacodynamics

Opioid	*Interaction*	*Result*	*Reference*
Any opioid	Alcohol or other CNS depressants	Enhanced depressant effects	Inturrisi 1990
Methadone	Phenytoin	Increased biotransformation → reduced effect	Tong et al 1981
Methadone	Rifampicin	Increased biotransformation → reduced effect	Kreek et al 1976
Morphine	Amitriptyline	Increased bioavailability	Ventafridda et al 1987
Morphine	Clomipramine	Increased bioavailability	Ventafridda et al 1987
Morphine	Rifampicin	Increased biotransformation → reduced effect	Fromm et al 1997
Pethidine	Monoamine oxidase inhibitors	Agitation, delirium, hyperpyrexia, myoclonus, convulsions (serotonin syndrome)	Inturrisi 1990 Sporer 1995
Pethidine	Phenobarbital	Increased biotransformation → accumulation of norpethidine	Stambaugh et al 1977
Pethidine	Phenytoin	Increased biotransformation → accumulation of norpethidine	Pond & Kretschzmar 1981

Rapid onset is not a critical factor, however, for patients receiving regular medication by the clock.

A longer duration of action means that fewer doses are needed each day. The advent of modified-release formulations of morphine means, however, that there is now less reason for choosing an opioid other than morphine on the grounds of longer duration of effect. Opioids that last longer than morphine include buprenorphine, levorphanol, methadone and phenazocine.

Dextromoramide and pethidine have short durations of action and are not recommended for regular prophylactic analgesia. Because of its rapid onset of action, some centres use dextromoramide for breakthrough pain in patients taking regular morphine or as prophylactic additional analgesia before a painful dressing or other procedure. However, at other centres, such procedures are timed to coincide with the peak plasma concentration after a regular or p.r.n. dose of morphine. Pentazocine should not be used; it is a weak opioid by mouth and often causes psychotomimetic effects (dysphoria, depersonalization, frightening dreams, hallucinations). When converting from an alternative strong opioid to oral morphine, the initial dose depends on the relative potency of the two drugs (Table 51.11).

OPIOID HYPEREXCITABILITY AND OPIOID SUBSTITUTION

In patients who have intolerable adverse effects with morphine (Table 51.12), it may be necessary to substitute an alternative strong opioid. For adverse effects such as cognitive failure, hallucinations or myoclonus, hydromorphone and oxycodone have been used. However, for patients experiencing opioid-induced hyperexcitability (Sjogren et al 1993, 1994, Hagen & Wanson 1997), methadone is preferable. Methadone is considered by some also to be the opioid of choice for patients with neuropathic pain (Morley & Makin 1998).

Animal studies have demonstrated that behavioural features suggestive of allodynia and hyperalgesia occur when morphine, morphine-3-glucuronide or morphine-6-glucuronide is injected into the cerebral ventricles (Labella et al 1979). However, M3G is several hundred times more potent than morphine in this respect even though it is inactive at opioid receptors. Generally, the more potent an opioid is as an analgesic, the less likely it is to cause hyperexcitability (Smith & Smith 1995). Further, naloxone exaggerates the abnormal behaviour, strongly suggesting that a non-opioid receptor system is primarily responsible for opioid hyperexcitability (Smith & Smith 1995). In humans, normorphine has also been implicated (Glare et al 1990) and, in relation to hydromorphone, hydromorphone-3-glucuronide (MacDonald et al 1993).

Animal studies show that high doses of methadone, fentanyl, alfentanil and sufentanil do not cause opioid hyperexcitability (Frenk et al 1984, Hagen & Wanson 1997). This has led some to conclude that these drugs are free from comparable effects in humans. Unfortunately, although probably less neurotoxic than other opioids, this may well not be the case. For example, bilateral synchronous myoclonic jerks involving the extremities and trunk have been reported in an 87-year-old woman treated with transdermal fentanyl 75 μg/h (Adair & El-Nachef 1994).

Strychnine, a glycine antagonist, can produce similar behaviour (Hagen & Wanson 1997). Glycine mediates postsynaptic inhibition on dorsal horn neurons. It is possible, therefore, that opioids and/or their metabolites act via spinal antiglycinergic effect. Sodium bisulphite, a preservative in ampoules of morphine sulphate, may be responsible in some cases (Gregory et al 1992).

Table 51.11 Approximate oral analgesic equivalence to morphine[1] (from Twycross et al 1998 with permission

Analgesic	*Potency ratio with morphine*	*Duration of action (hours)[2]*	*Plasma half-life (hours)*
Codeine Dihydrocodeine	1/10	3–6	2.5–3.5 3.5–4.5
Pethidine	1/8	2–4	3–4
Tramadol	1/5[3]	4–6	6
Dipipanone (in Diconal UK)	1/2	4–6	?
Papaveretum	2/3[4]	3–5	1.5–4.5
Oxycodone	1.5–2[3]	3–4	3.5
Dextromoramide	[2][5]	2–3	7
Levorphanol	5	4–6	12–16
Phenazocine	5	6–8	?
Methadone	5–10[6]	8–12	8–75
Hydromorphone	7.5	4–5	2.5
Buprenorphine (sublingual)	60	6–8	3
Fentanyl (transdermal)	150	72	22[7]

[1]Multiply dose of opioid by its potency ratio to determine the equivalent dose of morphine sulphate.
[2]Dependent in part on severity of pain and on dose; often longer lasting in very elderly and those with renal dysfunction.
[3]Tramadol and oxycodone are both relatively more potent by mouth because of high bioavailability; parenteral potency ratios with morphine are 1/10 and 3/4 respectively.
[4]Papaveretum (strong opium) is standardized to contain 50% morphine base; potency expressed in relation to morphine sulphate.
[5]Dextromoramide: a single 5 mg dose is equivalent to morphine 15 mg in terms of peak effect but is shorter acting; overall potency ratio adjusted accordingly.
[6]Methadone: a single 5 mg dose is equivalent to morphine 7.5 mg. However, its long plasma half-life and broad-spectrum of action result in a much higher than expected potency ratio when given repeatedly (Bruera et al 1996).
[7]After removal of skin patch; single dose IV = 3–4 h.

Table 51.12 Potential intolerable effects of morphine

Type	*Effects*	*Initial action*	*Comment*
For general adverse effects of opioid analgesics see Table 51.9			
Gastric stasis	Epigastric fullness, flatulence, anorexia, hiccup, persistent nausea	Metoclopramide 10–20 mg q4h; cisapride 10–20 mg b.d.	If the problem persists, change to an alternative opioid
Sedation	Intolerable persistent sedation	Reduce dose of morphine; consider methylphenidate 10 mg once to twice a day	Sedation may be caused by other factors; stimulant rarely appropriate
Cognitive failure	Agitated delirium with hallucinations	Reduce dose of morphine and/or prescribe haloperidol 3–5 mg at once and at bedtime; if necessary switch to an alternative opioid	Some patients develop intractable delirium with one opioid but not with an alternative opioid
Myoclonus	Multifocal twitching +/– jerking of limbs	Reduce dose of morphine but revert to former dose if pain recurs; consider a benzodiazepine	Unusual with typical oral doses; more common with high-dose IV and spinal morphine
Hyperexcitability	Abdominal muscle spasms and symmetrical jerking of legs; whole-body allodynia and hyperalgesia manifesting as excruciating pain	Reduce dose of morphine; consider changing to an alternative opioid	A rare syndrome in patients receiving intrathecal or high-dose IV morphine; occasionally seen with typical SC and oral doses
Vestibular stimulation	Incapacitating movement-induced nausea and vomiting	Cyclizine or dimenhydrinate or promethazine 25–50 mg q8h–q6h	Rare. Try an alternative opioid or levomepromazine (methotrimeprazine)
Histamine release			
• cutaneous	Pruritus	Oral antihistamine (e.g. chlorphenamine 4 mg b.d.–t.d.s.)	If the pruritus does not settle in a few days, prescribe an alternative opioid
• bronchial	Bronchoconstriction → dyspnoea	IV/IM antihistamine (e.g. chlorphenamine 5–10 mg) and a bronchodilator	Rare. Change to a chemically distinct opioid immediately, e.g. methadone or phenazocine

Unfortunately, 'opioid rotation' has become the 'flavour of the month' in certain quarters (Fallon 1997). At one centre in Edmonton, Canada, the incidence of opioid substitution is 40% (De Stoutz et al 1995). In the UK it is 5–10% at most (data on file). In Edmonton, however, it appears that the opioid is changed if the patient develops signs of cognitive failure (confusion, delirium) rather than reducing the dose of the opioid and reviewing medication and other factors generally. There also seems to be less concurrent use of non-opioids and adjuvant analgesics (see Fig. 51.5). This is likely to result in higher doses of opioids being used – sometimes much higher – with a corresponding likelihood of a greater incidence of intolerable adverse effects.

MORPHINE

Morphine is the main pharmacologically active constituent of opium. It is readily absorbed by all routes of administration. It is effective by mouth (Box 51.2). When given regularly, the oral to SC potency ratio is normally between 1:2 and 1:3; the same ratio holds true for IM and IV injections (Max & Payne 1992, Hanks et al 1996). The liver is the principal site of morphine metabolism (Hasselstrom et al 1986). Metabolism also occurs in other organs (Mazoit et al 1987), notably the CNS (Sandouk et al 1991). Glucuronidation is rarely impaired in hepatic failure (Hasselstrom et al 1986) and morphine is well tolerated in most patients with hepatic impairment, although with impairment severe enough to prolong the prothrombin time, the plasma half-life of morphine may increase (Mazoit et al 1987) and the dose of morphine may need to be reduced or given less often, i.e. q6h–q8h.

Morphine-3-glucuronide (M3G) and morphine-6-glucuronide (M6G) are the major metabolites of morphine in man (McQuay et al 1990). M6G binds to opioid receptors whereas M3G does not. In rats, M6G is 45 times more potent than morphine intracerebrally and nearly four times more potent subcutaneously (Shimomura et al 1971). M6G contributes substantially to the analgesic effect of morphine in humans, can cause nausea and vomiting (Thompson et al 1992) and respiratory depression (Osborne et al 1986).

M3G and M6G are far more lipophilic than expected (Carrupt et al 1991). Glucuronides are normally highly polar hydrophilic compounds which are unable to cross the blood–brain barrier. M3G and M6G, however, exist in equilibrium between extended and folded forms. Whereas the extended form is highly hydrophilic, the folded form is almost as lipophilic as morphine itself. This form may well predominate in biological membranes, thereby facilitating movement into the CNS.

BOX 51.2

Starting a patient on oral morphine

Morphine is indicated in patients with pain which does not respond to the combined optimized use of a non-opioid and a weak opioid. The starting dose of oral morphine is calculated to give a greater analgesic effect than the medication already in use.

1. If the patient was previously receiving a weak opioid, give 10 mg q4h or modified-release 30 mg q12h
2. If changing from an alternative strong opioid (e.g. fentanyl, methadone), a much higher dose of morphine may be needed (see Table 51.11).

With frail elderly patients, however, consider starting on a lower dose (e.g. 5 mg q4h) in order to reduce initial drowsiness, confusion and unsteadiness.

Upward titration of the dose of morphine stops when either the pain is relieved or intolerable adverse effects supervene. In the latter case, it is generally necessary to consider alternative measures. The aim is to have the patient free of pain and mentally alert.

Modified-release morphine may not be satisfactory in patients troubled by frequent vomiting or those with diarrhoea or an ileostomy

Scheme 1: ordinary (normal-release) morphine tablets or solution

1. Morphine given q4h 'by the clock' with p.r.n. doses of equal amount.
2. After 1–2 days, recalculate q4h dose based on total used in the previous 24 hours (i.e. regular + p.r.n. use).
3. Continue q4h and p.r.n. doses.
4. Increase the regular dose until treatment gives adequate relief from pain, maintaining availability of p.r.n. doses.
5. *A double dose at bedtime obviates the need to wake the patient for treatment during the night.*

Scheme 2: ordinary (normal-release) morphine and modified-release morphine

1. Begin as for Scheme 1.
2. When the q4h dose is stable, it is replaced with modified-release morphine q12h, or o.d. if a 24-hour preparation is prescribed.
3. The q12h dose will be *three times* the previous q4h dose; an o.d. dose will be *six times* the previous q4h dose, rounded to a convenient number of tablets.
4. Continue to provide ordinary (normal-release) morphine tablets or solution for p.r.n. use.

Scheme 3: modified-release morphine when ordinary (normal-release) morphine is unavailable

In some countries, q12h modified-release morphine is available but ordinary morphine preparations are not.

BOX 51.2

Starting a patient on oral morphine (Contd.)

Scheme 3: modified-release morphine when ordinary (normal-release) morphine is unavailable (Contd.)

1. Starting dose generally modified-release morphine 20–30 mg b.d.
2. Use a weak opioid or an alternative strong opioid for p.r.n. medication.
3. Dose of modified-release morphine adjusted every 48h until adequate relief throughout each 12-hour period.
4. If of benefit, maintain the availability of p.r.n. doses of a weak opioid or an alternative strong opioid.

In patients with severely impaired renal function, morphine and its active congeners have an increased and prolonged effect (McQuay & Moore 1984, Barnes et al 1985). A series of case reports confirm this observation (Mostert et al 1971, Don et al 1975, Barnes & Goodwin 1983, Redfern 1983). Cumulation of the active metabolite M6G is the probable explanation of this phenomenon, as elimination of morphine itself is unimpaired in renal failure, even in anephric patients (Aitkenhead et al 1984, Sawe et al 1985, Woolner et al 1986).

Morphine is available in an increasing number of formulations, both normal release (q4h) and modified release (q12h, o.d.). Once-daily formulations of morphine have been shown to be as efficacious as twice-daily formulations (Kerr 1995, O'Brien et al 1997).

BUPRENORPHINE

Buprenorphine is a potent partial OP_3 (μ) agonist, OP_2 (κ) antagonist and OP_1 (δ) agonist (Hill 1992, Corbett et al 1993). It is an alternative to oral morphine in the low to middle part of morphine's dose range. Subjective and physiological effects are generally similar to morphine. Buprenorphine is available as a sublingual tablet; ingestion markedly reduces bioavailability. Vomiting is more common after sublingual administration than after IM injection. Unlike most opioids, buprenorphine does not increase pressure within the biliary and pancreatic ducts (Staritz et al 1985). Buprenorphine does slow intestinal transit (Anonymous 1979), but probably less so than morphine. In low doses, buprenorphine and morphine are additive in their effects; at very high doses, antagonism by buprenorphine may occur. There is no need, however, to prescribe both; use one or the other. In standard doses, naloxone does not reverse the effects of buprenorphine. The manufacturers recommend doxapram, a non-specific respiratory stimulant, in the event of difficulties following massive self-poisoning. It is generally considered that there is an analgesic ceiling at a daily dose of 3–5 mg, equivalent to 180–300 mg of oral morphine/24 h. In some countries, 1.6 mg is regarded as the ceiling daily dose. Whether this represents genetic differences or local custom is not clear.

DIAMORPHINE

Diamorphine (diacetylmorphine, heroin) is available for medicinal use only in the UK. It is a prodrug without intrinsic activity (Inturrisi et al 1984). In vivo or in solution, it is rapidly deacetylated to monoacetylmorphine and then more slowly to morphine itself (Barrett et al 1992). It is well absorbed by all routes of administration. Because of greater lipid solubility, diamorphine and monoacetylmorphine cross the blood–brain barrier more readily than morphine. This accounts for the observed potency difference between parenteral diamorphine and morphine. IM diamorphine is more than twice as potent as morphine; orally, however, the two opioids are almost equipotent. In terms of analgesic efficacy and effect on mood, diamorphine has no clinical advantage over morphine by oral or IM routes (Twycross 1977, Beaver et al 1981, Kaiko et al 1981). Diamorphine hydrochloride is much more soluble than morphine sulphate/hydrochloride and is the strong opioid of choice for parenteral use in the UK because large amounts can be given in very small volumes (Table 51.13).

Diamorphine IM is 2–2.5 times more potent than morphine IM (Reichle et al 1962, Beaver et al 1981, Kaiko et al 1981, Hanks & Hoskin 1987). If diamorphine is only a prodrug, this is perhaps surprising. The following points provide an explanation.

1. Diamorphine is a prodrug for monoacetylmorphine as well as morphine.

Table 51.13 Solubility of selected opioids

Preparation	*Amount of water needed to dissolve 1 g at 25°C (ml)*
Morphine	5000
Morphine hydrochloride	24
Morphine sulphate	21
Diamorphine hydrochloride	1.6[1]
Hydromorphone	3

[1] 1 g of diamorphine hydrochloride dissolved in 1.6 ml has a volume of 2.4 ml.

2. Monoacetylmorphine may be more potent than morphine (Wright & Barbour 1935).
3. By injection, hepatic first-pass metabolism is circumvented and more monoacetylmorphine will be available.
4. Diamorphine is highly lipophilic and crosses the blood–brain barrier more readily than morphine.

The following conversion ratios are approximate but serve as a general guide:

1. oral morphine to SC diamorphine – give one-third of the oral dose
2. oral diamorphine to SC diamorphine – give half the oral dose.

FENTANYL

Fentanyl, like morphine, is a strong OP_3 (μ) agonist. It is widely used IV as an perioperative analgesic. Transdermal patches are available for cancer pain management (Box 51.3). Steady-state plasma concentrations of fentanyl are achieved after 36–48 hours (Gourlay et al 1989). Time to reach a minimal effective plasma concentration ranges from 3 to 23 hours (Gourlay et al 1989). After removal of a patch, the elimination plasma half-life is almost 24 hours (Portenoy et al 1993). Rescue medication will be necessary during the first 24 hours. If effective analgesia does not last for 3 days, the correct response is to increase the patch strength. Even so, some patients do best if the patch is changed every 2 days (Donner et al 1998). The manufacturer recommends a conversion ratio for morphine and fentanyl of 150:1 but some centres use a ratio conversion of 100:1 when deciding the initial patch strength (Donner et al 1996).

Transdermal fentanyl is less constipating than morphine (Ahmedzai & Brooks 1997, Grond et al 1997, Donner et al 1998, Megens et al 1998). Thus, when converting from morphine to fentanyl, the dose of laxative should be halved and subsequently adjusted according to need. Some patients experience withdrawal symptoms when changed from oral morphine to transdermal fentanyl despite satisfactory pain relief, e.g. intestinal colic, diarrhoea, nausea, sweating and restlessness. These symptoms are easily treatable by using rescue doses of morphine until they resolve after a few days.

Transdermal fentanyl can be continued until the death of the patient and the dose varied as necessary. Rescue medication will continue to be ordinary morphine tablets or solution (or an alternative normal-release strong opioid preparation). If a patient is unable to swallow, it is impor-

BOX 51.3

Guidelines for the use of transdermal fentanyl patches

1. Transdermal fentanyl is an alternative strong opioid which can be used in place of both oral morphine and SC morphine/diamorphine in the management of cancer pain.
2. Indications for using transdermal fentanyl include:
   - intractable morphine-induced constipation
   - intolerable adverse effects with morphine, e.g. nausea and vomiting (despite the appropriate use of antiemetics) and/or hallucinations (despite the use of haloperidol)
   - 'tablet phobia' or difficulty swallowing oral preparations
   - poor compliance with oral medication.
3. Transdermal fentanyl is *contra-indicated* in patients who need rapid titration of their medication for severe uncontrolled pain.
4. *Warning*: pain not relieved by morphine will *not* be relieved by fentanyl. If in doubt, seek specialist advice before prescribing transdermal fentanyl.
5. Transdermal fentanyl patches are available in four strengths: 25, 50, 75 and 100 μg/h *for 3 days*:
   - patients with inadequate relief from *codeine*, *dextropropoxyphene* or *dihydrocodeine* ≥ 240 mg/day should start on 25 μg/h
   - patients on *oral morphine*: divide 24-h dose in mg by 3 and choose nearest patch strength in μ g/h
   - patients on *SC diamorphine*: choose nearest patch strength in μg/h.

   Note: these doses are slightly higher than the manufacturer's recommendations.
6. Apply the transdermal fentanyl patch to *dry, non-inflamed, non-irradiated, unshaven, hairless skin* on the upper arm or trunk; body hair may be clipped but not shaved. Some patients need Micropore around the edges to ensure adherence.
7. Systemic analgesic concentrations are generally reached within 12 h, so:
   - if converting from *4-hourly oral morphine*, continue to give regular doses for 12 hours
   - if converting from *12-hourly morphine preparations*, apply the fentanyl patch at the same time as giving the final 12-hourly dose
   - if converting from a *syringe driver*, maintain the syringe driver for about 12 hours after applying the first patch.
8. Steady-state plasma concentrations of fentanyl are achieved only after 36–48 h; the patient should use 'rescue doses' liberally during the first 3 days, particularly during the first 24 hours. Rescue doses should be approximately half the fentanyl patch strength given as normal-release morphine in mg. [Example: with fentanyl 50 μg/h, use morphine 20–30 mg p.r.n.]

BOX 51.3

Guidelines for the use of transdermal fentanyl patches (Contd.)

9. After the first 48 h, if a patient continues to need two or more rescue doses of morphine, the patch strength should be increased by 25 μg/h. When using the manufacturer's recommended starting doses, about 50% of patients need to increase the patch strength after the first 3 days.
10. If the patient continues to experience breakthrough pain on the third day after patch application, increase the patch strength and review.
11. About 10% of patients experience opioid withdrawal symptoms when changed from morphine to transdermal fentanyl. Patients should be warned that they may experience symptoms 'like gastric flu' for a few days after the change and to use rescue doses of morphine for these symptoms.
12. Fentanyl is less constipating than morphine; halve the dose of laxatives when starting fentanyl and titrate according to need. Some patients develop diarrhoea; if troublesome, use rescue doses of morphine to control it and completely stop laxatives.
13. Fentanyl probably causes less nausea and vomiting than morphine but, if necessary, prescribe haloperidol 1.5 mg stat and nocte.
14. In febrile patients, the rate of absorption of fentanyl increases and occasionally causes toxicity, principally drowsiness. Absorption may also be enhanced by an external heat source over the patch, e.g. electric blanket or hot-water bottle; patients should be warned about this. Patients may shower with a patch but should not soak in a hot bath.
15. Remove patches after 72 h; change the position of the new patches so as to rest the underlying skin for 3–6 days.
16. A reservoir of fentanyl accumulates in the skin under the patch and significant blood levels persist for 24 h, sometimes more, after removing the patch. This only matters, of course, if transdermal fentanyl is discontinued.
17. In moribund patients, it is best to continue transdermal fentanyl and give rescue doses of SC diamorphine based on the 'rule of 5', i.e. divide the patch strength by 5 and give as *mg of diamorphine*. [Example: with fentanyl 100 μg/h, use diamorphine 20 mg p.r.n.]
18. In moribund patients, should it be decided to replace the patch by *continuous SC diamorphine*:
    - give *half the patch strength as mg/24 h* rounded up to a convenient ampoule size
    - after 24 h, give the *whole of the previous patch strength as mg/24 h* rounded up to a convenient ampoule size.

(Contd.)

19. Transdermal fentanyl patches are unsatisfactory in some patients, generally because of failure to remain adherent or allergy to the silicone medical adhesive.
20. Used patches still contain fentanyl. After removal, fold the patch with the adhesive side inwards and discard in a sharps container (hospital) or dustbin (home); wash hands. Ultimately, any unused patches should be returned to a pharmacy.

tant to give adequate rescue doses of an alternative strong opioid by injection (Box 51.4).

FENTANYL DERIVATIVES

Alfentanil is less potent than fentanyl and has a shorter half-life (Table 51.14). Despite being less lipid soluble than fentanyl, alfentanil has a more rapid onset of action because, at pH 7.4, about 90% of the unbound drug in plasma is unionized. This generates a large concentration gradient for diffusion across the blood–brain barrier. As with fentanyl, alfentanil accumulates during infusion and the plasma half-life increases accordingly. Alfentanil has no active metabolites. Alfentanil has also been used successfully in cancer patients with renal failure who became agitated on SC diamorphine (Kirkham & Pugh 1995). The starting dose for alfentanil was one-tenth that of the diamorphine.

Remifentanil is a fentanyl derivative with an ester bond which is broken down by plasma and tissue esterases (Editorial 1996). Remifentanil therefore has an extremely short and predictable half-life which is not affected by hepatic or renal function (Table 51.14). No matter how long the drug is infused, the half-life remains the same. This contrasts with alfentanil and fentanyl whose half-lives are

BOX 51.4

Rescue medication for patients receiving transdermal fentanyl

Divide the delivery rate ('patch size') of transdermal fentanyl (μg/h):

1. by 2 and give as oral morphine (mg)
2. by 3 and give as SC morphine (mg)
3. by 5 and give as SC diamorphine (mg)
4. by 15 and give as SC hydromorphone (mg)

Table 51.14 Pharmacokinetic values of fentanyl and its congeners

	Volume of distribution (litre/kg)	*Clearance (ml/min/kg)*	*Plasma half-life (hours)*
Alfentanil	0.8	6	1.6
Fentanyl	4.0	13	3.5
Remifentanil	0.4	40	0.05
Sufentanil	1.7	12.7	2.7

prolonged significantly when infused. The main metabolic product of ester hydrolysis is a carboxylic acid derivative which is excreted by the kidneys (plasma half-life about 90–140 minutes). Although elimination is delayed in renal failure, significant pharmacological effects are unlikely as its potency relative to remifentanil is only 0.1–0.3%. Remifentanil is formulated in glycine which makes it unsuitable for intrathecal use.

Sufentanil is more potent than remifentanil and its half-life is between that of alfentanil and fentanyl (Table 51.14). Although used extensively elsewhere, it is not available in the UK.

HYDROMORPHONE

Hydromorphone is an analogue of morphine with similar pharmacokinetic and pharmacodynamic properties. By mouth and by injection, it is about 7.5 times more potent than morphine (McDonald & Miller 1997). Hydromorphone provides useful analgesia for about 4 hours. As with morphine, there is wide interpatient variation in bioavailability. The main metabolite is hydromorphone-3-glucuronide; hydromorphone-6-glucuronide is not formed (Babul & Darke 1992). Two minor metabolites, dihydroisomorphine and dihydromorphine, are pharmacologically active and are metabolized to 6-glucuronides. By the spinal route in opioid-naive subjects, hydromorphone causes much less pruritus than morphine, 11% compared with 44% (Chaplan et al 1992). Hydromorphone is available in many countries in a range of preparations for oral and parenteral administration. It is available in some countries in high-potency ampoules containing 10 mg/ml and 20 mg/ml to facilitate use in continuous SC infusions.

METHADONE

Methadone is an OP_3 (μ) agonist and a NMDA receptor-channel blocker (Gorman et al 1997). It also blocks the presynoptic reuptake of serotonin (Codd et al 1995). Methadone is a racemic mixture; L-methadone is responsible for almost all the analgesic effect, whereas D-methadone is a useful antitussive. Methadone is a basic and lipophilic drug which is absorbed well from all routes of administration. There is a high volume of distribution with only about 1% of the drug in the blood. Methadone accumulates in tissues when given repeatedly, creating an extensive reservoir (Robinson & Williams 1971). Protein binding (principally to a glycoprotein) is 60–90% (Eap et al 1990); this is double that of morphine. Both volume of distribution and protein binding contribute to the long plasma half-life and accumulation is a potential problem. Methadone is metabolized chiefly in the liver to several metabolites (Fainsinger et al 1993). About half of the drug and its metabolites are excreted by the intestines and half by the kidneys (Inturrisi & Verebely 1972); one-third is excreted unchanged by the kidneys. Renal and hepatic impairment, however, do not affect methadone clearance (Kreek et al 1980, Novick et al 1981).

In single oral doses, methadone is about half as potent as IM (Beaver et al 1967) and a single IM dose is marginally more potent than morphine. With repeated doses, methadone is several times more potent. It is also longer acting; with chronic administration, analgesia lasts 6–12 hours and sometimes more. Patients who obtain only poor relief with morphine but have severe adverse effects (drowsiness, delirium, nausea and vomiting) often obtain good relief with relatively (sometimes incredibly) low-dose methadone with few or no adverse effects (Box 51.5). Methadone may be particularly beneficial for neuropathic pain because of its NMDA antagonism (Morley & Makin 1998). Methadone can also be used in small doses

BOX 51.5

Calculating the starting dose of oral methadone (based on Morley & Makin 1998)

1. Stop morphine (or other strong opioid).
2. Give a fixed dose of methadone that is 1/10 of the 24h oral morphine dose when the 24h dose is <300 mg.
3. When the 24h morphine dose is >300 mg, the fixed methadone dose should be 30 mg.
4. The fixed dose is taken orally p.r.n. *but not more frequently than q3h.*
5. On day 6, the amount of methadone taken over the previous 2 days is noted and converted into a regular q12h dose (and q3h p.r.n.).
6. If p.r.n. medication continues to be needed, increase the dose of methadone by 1/2–1/3 every 4–6 days (e.g. 10 mg b.d. → 15 mg b.d.; 30 mg b.d. → 40 mg b.d.).

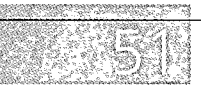

(e.g. 5–10 mg) in patients with chronic renal failure who have developed excessive drowsiness and/or delirium with morphine because of accumulation of morphine-6-glucuronide.

OXYCODONE

Oxycodone is an OP_2 (κ) and OP_3 (μ) agonist with similar properties to morphine (Poyhia & Kalso 1992, Ross & Smith 1997). The analgesic effect of oxycodone is mediated via the parent compound and not, as has been suggested, by oxymorphone, a highly potent minor metabolite (Heiskanen & Kalso 1997). The maximum plasma concentration of oxycodone increases by 50% in renal failure, causing more sedation (Kaiko et al 1996a). Parenterally, it is about three-quarters as potent as morphine (Kaiko et al 1996b). However, oral bioavailability is two-thirds or more, compared with about one-third for morphine, and is less variable. This means that by mouth oxycodone is about 1.5–2 times more potent than morphine (Heiskanen et al 1996, Kaiko et al 1996a).

PETHIDINE

Pethidine (meperidine) is a synthetic opioid analgesic. It is included because globally it is still widely used. For cancer pain, however, it is a third-rate analgesic and its use should be discouraged. Pethidine differs in several ways from morphine, not least because it manifests antimuscarinic effects (Box 51.6). It is about one-third as potent by mouth as by SC or IM injection. Peak plasma concentrations occur 1–2 hours after ingestion. Absorption from the alimentary canal is more variable than with morphine.

BOX 51.6

How pethidine differs from morphine

Shorter duration of action
Antimuscarinic effects
Pupils not constricted
Not antitussive
Less constipating
Less smooth muscle spasm (e.g. biliary tract, sphincter of Oddi)
More vomiting
Metabolized to norpethidine (may cause tremors, multifocal myoclonus, agitation, convulsions)
Interactions with:

1. phenobarbitone } increase production of norpethidine
2. chlorpromazine } increase production of norpethidine
3. monoamine oxidase inhibitors → serotonin syndrome (Sporer 1995)

Pethidine is hydrolysed to pethidinic acid which, in turn, is partially conjugated. It is also N-demethylated to norpethidine which may then be hydrolysed to norpethidinic acid and conjugated. Norpethidine is a CNS stimulant and causes agitation, tremor, multifocal myoclonus and convulsions. This limits the amount of pethidine which can safely be given on a regular basis. About one-third of administered pethidine can be accounted for in the urine as N-demethylated derivatives. Little is excreted unchanged, but more if the urine is acid. Pethidine is about one-eighth as potent as morphine. Despite a plasma half-life of 3–4 hours, pethidine is generally shorter acting than morphine, useful analgesia lasting only 2–4 hours.

A potentially fatal interaction – the serotonin syndrome – occurs between pethidine and MAOIs (Inturrisi 1990, Sporer 1995). This is associated with an increased brain serotonin concentration. The serotonin syndrome is not seen with morphine or other strong opioids (Twycross et al 1998). There is, however, a case report which links tramadol and sertraline as co-causal agents (Mason & Blackburn 1997).

NALOXONE

Naloxone is a potent pure opioid antagonist. It has a high affinity for morphine receptor sites and reverses the effect of opioid analgesics by displacement. The degree of displacement is dose related. Partial antagonism may be obtained by using small doses. Activity after oral administration is low; it is one-fifteenth as potent by mouth as by injection. Naloxone is rapidly metabolized by the liver, primarily to naloxone glucuronide which is excreted by the kidneys.

The most important clinical property of naloxone is reversal of opioid-induced respiratory depression (and other opioid effects) caused by either an overdose of an opioid (including codeine and dextropropoxyphene) or an exaggerated response to conventional doses. Naloxone also reverses the opioid effects of pentazocine and other mixed agonist-antagonists; antagonism of buprenorphine is less complete because of the latter's high receptor affinity. Naloxone is not effective against respiratory depression caused by non-opioids such as barbiturates.

Naloxone has also been shown to be of benefit in patients with chronic idiopathic constipation (Kreek et al 1983), in septic shock (Peters et al 1981), morphine-induced peripheral vasodilatation (Cohen & Coffman

1980), ischaemic central neurological deficits (Baskin & Hosobuchi 1981, Bousigue et al 1982) and poststroke central pain (Ray & Tai 1988).

Naloxone should not be used for drowsiness and/or delirium which is not life-threatening because of the danger of totally reversing the opioid analgesia and precipitating severe/agonizing pain and a major physical withdrawal syndrome (Box 51.7). With epidural morphine, however, naloxone 400 μg reverses respiratory depression without reversing analgesia (Korbon et al 1985). Oral naloxone has been used to treat opioid-induced constipation (Sykes 1996).

BOX 51.7

Naloxone for iatrogenic opioid overdose (based on the recommendations of the American Pain Society (Max & Payne 1992))

If respiratory rate ≥ 8/min and the patient is easily rousable and not cyanosed, adopt a policy of 'wait and see'; consider reducing or omitting the next regular dose of morphine.

If respiratory rate <8/min and the patient is barely rousable/unconscious and/or cyanosed:

1. dilute a standard ampoule containing naloxone 400 μg to 10 ml with saline for injection
2. administer 0.5 ml (20 μg) IV every 2 min until the patient's respiratory status is satisfactory
3. further boluses may be necessary because naloxone is shorter acting than morphine (and other opioids).

REFERENCES

Adair JC, El-Nachef A 1994 Fentanyl neurotoxicity. Annals of Emergency Medicine 27: 791–792

Agenas I, Gustafsson L, Rane A, Sawe J 1982 Analgetikaterapi for cancerpatienter. Lakartidningen 79: 287–289

Ahmedzai S, Brooks D 1997 Transdermal fentanyl versus sustained-release oral morphine in cancer pain: preference, efficacy and quality of life. Journal of Pain and Symptom Management 13: 254–261

Aitkenhead AR, Vater M, Achola K, Cooper CMS, Smith G 1984 Pharmacokinetics of single dose IV morphine in normal volunteers and patients with end-stage renal failure. British Journal of Anaesthesia 56: 813–819

Andreev N, Urban L, Dray A 1994 Opioids suppress spontaneous activity of polymodal nociceptors in rat paw skin induced by ultraviolet irradiation. Neuroscience 58: 793–798

Anonymous 1979 Buprenorphine injection (Temgesic). Drug and Therapeutics Bulletin 17: 17–19

Anonymous 1991 Dihydrocodeine (tartrate). In: Dollery C (ed) Therapeutic Drugs. Churchill Livingstone, Edinburgh, pp 133–136

Babul N, Darke AC 1992 Putative role of hydromorphone metabolites in myoclonus. Pain 51: 260–261

Barnes JN, Goodwin FJ 1983 Dihydrocodeine narcosis in renal failure. British Medical Journal 286: 438–439

Barnes JN, Williams A, Tomson M, Toseland P, Goodwin F 1985 Dihydrocodeine in renal failure: further evidence for an important role in the kidney in the handling of opioid drugs. British Medical Journal 290: 740–742

Barrett DA, Dyssegaard ALP, Shaw N 1992 The effect of temperature and pH on the deacetylation of diamorphine in aqueous solution and in human plasma. Journal of Pharmacy and Pharmacology 44: 606–608

Baskin DS, Hosobuchi Y 1981 Naloxone reversal of ischaemic neurological deficits in man. Lancet ii: 272–275

Beauford W, Stansbury D, Light R 1993 Effects of nebulized morphine sulfate on the exercise tolerance of the ventilatory limited COPD patient. Chest 104: 175–178

Beaver WT 1966 Mild analgesics: a review of their clinical pharmacology (part II). American Journal of Medical Science 251: 576–599

Beaver WT 1984 Analgesic efficacy of dextropropoxyphene and dextropropoxyphene-containing combinations: a review. Human Toxicology 3(suppl): 191–220

Beaver WT, Wallenstein SL, Houde RW, Rogers A 1967 A clinical comparison of the analgesic effects of methadone and morphine administered intramuscularly, and of orally and parenterally administered methadone. Clinical Pharmacology and Therapeutics 8: 415–426

Beaver WT, Schein PS, Hext M 1981 Comparison of the analgesic effect of intramuscular heroin and morphine in patients with cancer pain. Clinical Pharmacology and Therapeutics 29: 232–233

Bloor RN, Smalldridge NJF 1990 Intravenous use of slow release morphine sulphate tablets. British Medical Journal 300: 640–641

Boisvert M, Cohen SR 1995 Opioid use in advanced malignant disease: why do different centers use vastly different doses? A plea for standardized reporting. Journal of Pain and Symptom Management 10: 632–638

Borgbjerg FM, Nielsen K, Franks J 1996 Experimental pain stimulates respiration and attenuates morphine-induced respiratory depression: a controlled study in human volunteers. Pain 64: 123–128

Bousigue J-Y, Giraud L, Fournie D, Tremoulet M 1982 Naloxone reversal of neurological deficit. Lancet ii: 618–619

Brescia F, Portenoy R, Ryan M, Krasnoff L, Gray G 1992 Pain, opioid use, and survival in hospitalized patients with advanced cancer. Journal of Clinical Oncology 10: 149–155

Brismar B, Hedenstierna G, Lundquist H, Strandberg A, Svensson L, Tokics L 1985 Pulmonary densities during anesthesia with muscular relaxation: a proposal of atelectasis. Anaesthesiology 62: 422–428

Broggini M, Corbetta E, Grossi E, Borghi C 1984 Diclofenac sodium in biliary colic: a double blind trial. British Medical Journal 288: 1042

Bruera E, Macmillan K, Hanson J, MacDonald R 1989 The cognitive effects of the administration of narcotic analgesics in patients with cancer pain. Pain 39: 13–16

Bruera E, Macmillan K, MacDonald RN 1990 Effects of morphine on the dyspnea of terminal cancer patients. Journal of Pain and Symptom Management 5: 341–344

Bruera E, Schoeller T, Wenk R et al 1995 A prospective multicenter assessment of the Edmonton Staging System for cancer pain. Journal of Pain and Symptom Management 10: 348–355

Bruera E, Pereira J, Watanabe S, Belzile M, Kuehn N, Hanson J 1996 Opioid rotation in patients with cancer pain. Cancer 78: 852–857

Cabot P, Cramond T, Smith M 1996 Quantitative autoradiography of peripheral opioid binding sites in rat lung. European Journal of Pharmacology 310: 47–53

Carrupt P, Testa B, Bechalany A, El-Tayar N, Descas P, Perrissoud D 1991 Morphine-6-glucuronide and morphine-3-glucuronide as molecular chameleons with unexpected lipophilicity. Journal of Medicinal Chemistry 34: 1272–1275
Chaplan SR, Duncan SR, Brodsky JB, Brose WG 1992 Morphine and hydromorphone epidural analgesia. Anesthesiology 77: 1090–1094
Cleary J Mikus G, Samagyi A, Bochner F 1994 The influence of pharmacogenetics on opioid analgesia: studies with codeine and oxycodone in the Sprague-Dawley/Dark Agouti rat model. Journal of Pharmacology and Experimental Therapeutics 271: 1528–1534
Codd EE, Shank RP, Schupsky RB 1995 Serotonin and norepinephrine uptake inhibiting activity of centrally acting analgesics: Structural determinants and role in antinociception. Journal of Pharmacology and Experimental Therapeutics 274: 1263–1270
Cohen RA, Coffman JD 1980 Naloxone reversal of morphine-induced peripheral vasodilatation. Clinical Pharmacology and Therapeutics 28: 541–544
Colpaert FC, Niemegeers CJE, Janssen PAJ, Maroli AN 1980 The effects of prior fentanyl administration and of pain on fentanyl analgesia: tolerance to and enhancement of narcotic analgesia. Journal of Pharmacology and Experimental Therapeutics 213: 418–426
Coombs D 1986 Management of chronic pain by epidural and intrathecal opioids: newer drugs and delivery systems. In: Sjostrand U, Rawal N (eds) International anaesthesiology clinics. Little, Brown, Boston, pp 59–74
Corbett AD, Paterson SJ, Kosterlitz HW 1993 Selectivity of ligands for opioid receptors. In: Herz A (ed) Opioids. Springer-Verlag, London, pp 657–672
Cullen M, Staren E, El-Ganzouri A, Logas W, Ivkanovich A, Economou S 1985 Continuous epidural infusion for analgesia after major abdominal operations: a randomized prospective double-blind study. Surgery 98: 718–726
Davis C, Penn K, A'Hern R, Daniels J, Slevin M 1996 Single dose randomized controlled trial of nebulized morphine in patients with cancer related breathlessness. Palliative Medicine 10: 64–65
De Stoutz N, Bruera E, Suarez-Almazor M 1995 Opioid rotation for toxicity reduction in terminal cancer patients. Journal of Pain and Symptom Management 10: 378–384
Dhawan B, Cesselin F, Raghubir R et al 1996 International Union of Pharmacology. XII. Classification of opioid receptors. Pharmacological Reviews 48: 567–593
Dickenson AH 1991 Mechanisms of the analgesic actions of opiates and opioids. British Medical Bulletin 47: 690–702
Dickenson AH, Sullivan AF 1986 Electrophysiological studies on the effects of intrathecal morphine on nociceptive neurones in the rat dorsal horn. Pain 24: 211–222
Don HF, Dieppa RA, Taylor P 1975 Narcotic analgesics in anuric patients. Anaesthesiology 42: 745–747
Donner B, Zenz M, Tryba M, Strumpf M 1996 Direct conversion from oral morphine to transdermal fentanyl: a multicenter study in patients with cancer pain. Pain 64: 527–534
Donner B, Zenz M, Strumpf M, Raber M 1998 Long-term treatment of cancer pain with transdermal fentanyl. Journal of Pain and Symptom Management 15: 168–175
Dorrepaal K 1989 Pijn bij patienten met kanker. University of Amsterdam, Amsterdam
Eap CB, Cuendet C, Baumann P 1990 Binding of D-methadone, L-methadone and DL-methadone to proteins in plasma of healthy volunteers: role of variants of X1-acid glycoprotein. Clinical Pharmacology and Therapeutics 47: 338–346
Ebert B Tharkildsen C, Anderson S et al 1998 Opioid analgesics as noncompetitive N-Methyl-D-Aspartate (NMDA) antagonists. Biochemical Pharmacology 56: 553–559
Eckhardt K, Li S, Ammon S, Schanzle G, Mikus G, Eichelbaum M 1998 Same incidence of adverse drug events after codeine administration irrespective of the genetically determined differences in morphine formation. Pain 76: 27–33
Editorial 1996 Remifentanil – an opioid for the 21st century. British Journal of Anaesthesia 76: 341–343
Erickson D, Lo J, Michaelson M 1984 Intrathecal morphine for treatment of pain due to malignancy. Pain 2: 19
Etches R, Sandler A, Daley M 1989 Respiratory depression on spinal opioids. Canadian Journal of Anaesthesiology 36: 165–185
Fainsinger R, Schoeller T, Bruera E 1993 Methadone in the management of cancer pain: clinical review. Pain 52: 137–147
Fallon M 1997 Opioid rotation: does it have a role? Palliative Medicine 11: 177–178
Ferris FD, Kerr IG, De Angelis C, Sone M, Hume S 1990 Inpatient narcotic infusions for patients with cancer pain. Journal of Palliative Care 6: 51–59
Fischbeck KH, Mata M, D'Aquisto R, Caronna JJ 1980 Brompton mixture taken intravenously by a heroin addict. Western Journal of Medicine 133: 80
Frenk H, Watkins LR, Mayer DJ 1984 Differential behavioral effects induced by intrathecal microinjection of opiates: comparison of convulsive and cataleptic effects produced by morphine, methadone, and D-ala^2-methionine-enkephalinamide. Brain Research 299: 31–42
Fromm M, Eckhardt K, Li S, Schanzle G, Hofmann U, Mikus G, Eichelbaum M 1997 Loss of analgesic effect of morphine due to coadministration of rifampin. Pain 72: 261–267
Glare PA, Walsh TD, Pippenger CE 1990 Normorphine, a neurotoxic metabolite. Lancet 335: 725–726
Gorman A, Elliott K, Inturrisi C 1997 The d- and l- isomers of methadone bind to the non-competitive site on the N-methyl-D-aspartate (NMDA) receptor in rat forebrain and spinal cord. Neuroscience Letters 223: 5–8
Gourlay GK, Cherry D 1991 Response to controversy corner: 'Can opioids be successfully used to treat severe pain in nonmalignant conditions?'. Clinical Journal of Pain 7: 347–349
Gourlay GK, Kowalski SL, Plummer JL, Cherry DA, Gaukroger P, Cousins MJ 1989 The transdermal administration of fentanyl in the treatment of post-operative pain: pharmacokinetics and pharmacodynamic effects. Pain 37: 193–202
Gray A, Spencer P, Sewell R 1998 The involvement of the opioidergic system in the antinociceptive mechanism of action of antidepressant compounds. British Journal of Pharmacology 124: 669–674
Gregory RE, Grossman S, Sheidler VR 1992 Grand mal seizures associated with high-dose intravenous morphine infusions: incidence and possible etiology. Pain 51: 255–258
Grond S, Zech D, Diefenbach C, Radbruch L, Lehmann KA 1996 Assessment of cancer pain: a prospective evaluation in 2266 cancer patients referred to a pain service. Pain 64: 107–114
Grond S, Zech D, Lehmann K, Radbruch L, Breitenbach H, Hertel D 1997 Transdermal fentanyl in the long-term treatment of cancer pain: a prospective study of 50 patients with advanced cancer of the gastrointestinal tract or the head and neck region. Pain 69: 191–198
Hagen N, Wanson R 1997 Strychnine-like multifocal myoclonus and seizures in extremely high-dose opioid administration: treatment strategies. Journal of Pain and Symptom Management 14: 51–58
Hanks GW 1991 Opioid responsive and opioid non-responsive pain in cancer. British Medical Bulletin 47: 718–731
Hanks GW, Cherry N 1997 Opioid analgesic therapy. In: Doyle D, Hanks G W, MacDonald N (eds) Oxford textbook of palliative medicine. Oxford University Press, Oxford, pp 331–355
Hanks GW, Hoskin PJ 1987 Opioid analgesics in the management of pain in patients with cancer: a review. Palliative Medicine 1: 1–25
Hanks GW, Thomas EA 1985 Intravenous opioids in chronic cancer pain. British Medical Journal 291: 1124–1125

Hanks GW, Twycross RG, Lloyd JW 1981 Unexpected complication of successful nerve block. Anaesthesia 36: 37–39
Hanks GW, O'Neill WM, Simpson P, Wesnes K 1995 The cognitive and psychomotor effects of opioid analgesics: II. A randomized controlled trial of single doses of morphine, lorazepam and placebo in healthy subjects. European Journal of Clinical Pharmacology 48: 455–460
Hanks GW, De Conno F, Ripamonti C et al 1996 Morphine in cancer pain: modes of administration. British Medical Journal 312: 823–826
Hasselstrom J, Eriksson L, Persson A, Rane A, Svensson J, Sawe J 1986 Morphine metabolism in patients with liver cirrhosis. Acta Pharmacologica Toxicologica
Heiskanen T, Kalso E 1997 Controlled-release oxycodone and morphine in cancer related pain. Pain 73: 37–45
Heiskanen T, Ruismaki P, Kalso E 1996 Double-blind, randomised, repeated dose, crossover comparison of controlled-release oxycodone and controlled-release morphine in cancer pain 1: pharmacodynamic profile. Abstracts of 8th World Congress on Pain. IASP Press, Seattle, pp 17–18
Heneghan CPH, Jones JG 1985 Pulmonary gas exchange and diaphragmatic position. British Journal of Anaesthesia 57: 1161–1166
Hetherington JW, Philip NH 1986 Diclofenac sodium versus pethidine in acute renal colic. British Medical Journal 92: 237–238
Hill RG 1992 Multiple opioid receptors and their ligands. Frontiers of Pain 4: 1–4
Hill SC 1987 Painful prescriptions. Journal of the American Medical Association 257: 2081–2083
Hogan Q, Haddox J, Abram S, Weissman D, Taylor M, Janjan N 1991 Epidural opiates and local anaesthetics for the management of cancer pain. Pain 46: 271–279
Hojsted J, Rubeck-Petersen K, Raik H, Bigler D, Broem-Christiansen C 1990 Comparative bioavailability of a morphine suppository given rectally and in a colostomy. European Journal of Clinical Pharmacology 39: 49–50
Holmes V 1990 Rifampin-induced methadone withdrawal in AIDS. Journal of Clinical Psychopharmacology 10: 443
Inturrisi CE 1990 Effects of other drugs and pathologic states on opioid disposition and response. In: Benedetti C, Giron G, Chapman C (eds) Advances in pain research and therapy, 14. Raven Press, New York, pp 171–180
Inturrisi CE, Verebely K 1972 The levels of methadone in the plasma in methadone maintenance. Clinical Pharmacology and Therapeutics 13: 633–637
Inturrisi CE, Max MB, Foley KM, Schultz M, Shin SU, Houde RW 1984 The pharmacokinetics of heroin in patients with chronic pain. New England Journal of Medicine 310: 1213–1217
Jadad A, Carroll D, Glynn C, Moore R, McQuay H 1992 Morphine sensitivity of chronic pain: a double-blind randomized crossover study using patient-controlled analgesia. Lancet 1: 1367–1371
Jones JG, Jordan C 1987 Postoperative analgesia and respiratory complications. Hospital Update 13: 115–124
Joshi G 1993 Peripheral analgesia. Lancet 342: 320
Kaiko RF 1986 Discussion. In: Foley K M (ed) Advances in pain research and therapy, vol 8. Raven Press, New York, pp 235–237
Kaiko RF, Wallenstein SL, Rogers AG, Grabinski PY, Houde RW 1981 Analgesic and mood effects of heroin and morphine in cancer patients with postoperative pain. New England Journal of Medicine 304: 1501–1505
Kaiko R F, Healy W, Pav J, Thomas G B, Goldenheim P D 1989 The comparative bioavailability of MS Contin tablets (controlled release oral morphine) following rectal and oral administration. In: Twycross R G (ed) The Edinburgh Symposium on Pain Control and Medical Education. Royal Society of Medicine, London, pp 235–241
Kaiko RF, Benziger D, Chang C, Hou Y, Grandy R 1996a Clinical pharmacokinetics of controlled-release oxycodone in renal impairment. Clinical Pharmacology and Therapeutics 59: 130
Kaiko RF, Laccuture P, Hopf K, Brown J, Goldenheim P 1996b Analgesic onset and potency of oral controlled-release (CR) oxycodone and controlled-release morphine. Clinical Pharmacology and Therapeutics 59: 130
Kalso E 1983 Effects of intrathecal morphine injected with bupivacaine on pain after orthopaedic surgery. British Journal of Anaesthesia 55: 415–422
Kamei J, Iwamoto Y, Suzuki T, Misawa M, Nagase H, Kasuya Y 1993 The role of the mu 2-opioid receptor in the antitussive effect of morphine in mu 1-opioid receptor-deficient CXBK mice. European Journal of Pharmacology 240: 99–101
Kanner RM, Foley KM 1981 Patterns of narcotic drug use in cancer pain clinic. Annals of the New York Academy of Science 362: 162–172
Kerr R 1995 Clinical experience with 12–24 hourly kapanol. Pain Control – Current Practice and New Developments (Amsterdam) October: 15–18
Khoury G, Chen C, Garland D, Stein C 1992 Intraarticular morphine, bupivacaine and morphine/bupivacaine for pain control after knee videoarthroscopy. Anaesthesiology 77: 263–266
Kirkham SR, Pugh R 1995 Opioid analgesia in uraemic patients. Lancet 345: 1185
Knight C 1989 The use of opioids in chronic low back pain. In: Twycross RG (ed) The Edinburgh Symposium on Pain Control and Medical Education. Royal Society of Medicine, London, pp 201–204
Korbon G, James D, Verlander J, DiFazio C, Rosenbaum S, Levy S, Perry P 1985 Intramuscular naloxone reverses the side effects of epidural morphine while preserving analgesia. Regional Anaesthesia 10: 16–20
Kreek MJ, Garfield JW, Gutjahr CL, Giusti LM 1976 Rifampin-induced methadone withdrawal. New England Journal of Medicine 294: 1104–1106
Kreek MJ, Schecter AJ, Gutjahr CL, Hecht M 1980 Methadone use in patients with chronic renal disease. Drug and Alcohol Dependence 5: 197–205
Kreek MJ, Schaefer RA, Hahn EF, Fishman J 1983 Naloxone, a specific opioid antagonist, reverses chronic idiopathic constipation. Lancet i: 261–262
Labella FS, Pinksy C, Havlicek V 1979 Morphine derivatives with diminished opiate receptor potency show enhanced central excitatory activity. Brain Research 174: 263–271
Lee C, McTavish D, Sorkin E 1993 Tramadol: a preliminary review of its pharmacodynamic and pharmacokinetic properties, and therapeutic potential in acute and chronic pain states. Drugs 46: 313–340
Light RW, Muro JR, Sato RJ, Stansbury DW, Fischer CE, Brown SE 1989 Effects of oral morphine on breathlessness and exercise tolerance in patients with chronic obstructive pulmonary disease. American Review of Respiratory Diseases 139: 126–133
Ling GSF, Paul D, Simantov R, Pasternak GW 1989 Differential development of acute tolerance to analgesia, respiratory depression, gastrointestinal transit and hormone release in a morphine model. Life Science 45: 1627–1636
Littrell R, Kennedy L, Birmingham W, Leak W 1992 Muscle spasms associated with intrathecal morphine therapy: treatment with midazolam. Clinical Pharmacy 11: 57–59
Li Wan Po A, Zhang W 1997 Systematic overview of co-proxamol to assess analgesic effects of addition of dextropropoxyphene to paracetamol. British Medical Journal 315: 1565–1571
Loh H, Liu H, Cavalli A, Yang W, Chen Y, Wei L 1998 mu opioid receptor knockout in mice: effects on ligand-induced analgesia and morphine lethality. Brain Research Molecular Brain Research 54: 321–326
Longnecker D, Grazis P, Eggers G 1973 Naloxone for antagonism of

morphine-induced respiratory depression. Anesthesia and Analgesia 52: 447–452

Lundstam S, Ivarsson L, Lindblad L, Kral J 1985 Treatment of biliary pain by prostaglandin synthetase inhibition with diclofenac sodium. Current Therapeutic Research 37: 435–439

MacDonald N, Der L, Allan S, Champion P 1993 Opioid hyperexcitability: the application of alternate opioid therapy. Pain 53: 353–355

Martin W 1979 History and development of mixed opioid agonists, partial agonists and antagonists. British Journal of Clinical Pharmacology 7: 2735–2795

Maruta T, Swanson DW, Finlayson RE 1979 Drug abuse and dependency in patients with chronic pain. Mayo Clinic Proceedings 54: 241–244

Mason B, Blackburn J 1997 Possible serotonin syndrome associated with tramadol and sertraline coadministration. Annals of Pharmacotherapy 31: 175–177

Mathews ET, Abrams LD 1980 Intrathecal morphine in open heart surgery. Lancet 1: 543

Matthes H, Maldonado R, Simonin F et al 1996 Loss of morphine-induced analgesia, reward effect and withdrawal symptoms in mice lacking the mu-opioid-receptor gene. Nature 383: 819–823

Max MB, Payne R (co-chairs) 1992 Principles of analgesic use in the treatment of acute pain and cancer pain. American Pain Society, Skotie, Illinois, USA

Mazoit J-X, Sandouk P, Zetlaoui P, Scherman J-M 1987 Pharmacokinetics of unchanged morphine in normal and cirrhotic subjects. Anesthesia and Analgesia 66: 293–298

McCormack A, Hunter-Smith D, Piotrowski ZH, Grant M, Kubik S, Kessel K 1992 Analgesic use in home hospice cancer patients. Journal of Family Practice 34: 160–164

McCredie K, Lawson M 1984 Percutaneous insertion of silicone central venous catheters for long term intravenous access in cancer patients. Internal Medicine 5: 100–105

McDonald C, Miller A 1997 A comparative potency study of a controlled release tablet formulation of hydromorphone with controlled release morphine in patients with cancer pain. Abstracts of the Fifth Congress. European Journal of Palliative Care. p 37

McQuay HJ, Moore RA 1984 Be aware of renal function when prescribing morphine. Lancet 2: 284–285

McQuay HJ, Moore RA, Bullingham RES 1986a Buprenorphine kinetics. In: Foley KM, Inturrisi CE (eds) Advances in pain research and therapy, vol 8. Raven Press, New York, pp 271–278

McQuay HJ, Moore RA, Bullingham RES 1986b Sublingual morphine, heroin, methadone and buprenorphine. Kinetics and effects. In: Foley K M, Inturrisi CE (eds) Advances in pain research and therapy, vol 8. Raven Press, New York, pp 407–412

McQuay HJ, Sullivan A, Smallman K, Dickenson A 1989 Intrathecal opioids, potency and lipophilicity. Pain 36: 111–115

McQuay HJ, Carrol D, Faura CC, Gavaghan DJ, Hand CW, Moore RA 1990 Oral morphine in cancer pain: influences on morphine and metabolite concentration. Clinical Pharmacology and Therapeutics 48: 236–244

Megens A, Artois K, Vermiere J, Meert T, Awouters F 1998 Comparison of the analgesic and intestinal effects of fentanyl and morphine in rats. Journal of Pain and Symptom Management 15: 253–257

Mercadante S, Salvaggio L, Dardanoni G, Agnello A, Garofalo S 1998 Dextropropoxyphene versus morphine in opioid-naive cancer patients with pain. Journal of Pain and Symptom Management 15: 76–81

Meunier J-C 1997 Nociceptin/orphanin FQ and the opioid receptor-like ORL 1 receptor. European Journal of Pharmacology 340: 1–15

Miser AW, Miser JS, Clark BS 1980 Continuous intravenous infusion of morphine sulphate for control of severe pain in children with terminal malignancy. Journal of Paediatrics 96: 930–932

Morley J, Makin M 1998 The use of methadone in cancer pain poorly responsive to other opioids. Pain Reviews 5: 51–58

Mostert JW, Evers JL, Hobika GH, Moore RH, Ambrus JL 1971 Cardiorespiratory effects of anaesthesia with morphine or fentanyl in chronic renal failure and cerebral toxicity after morphine. British Journal of Anaesthesia 43: 1053–1060

Novick DM, Kreek MJ, Fanizza AM, Yancovitz SR, Gelb AM, Stenger RJ 1981 Methadone disposition in patients with chronic liver disease. Clinical Pharmacology and Therapeutics 30: 353–362

Nuutinen LS, Wuolijoki F, Pentikainen T 1986 Diclofenac and oxycodone in treatment of postoperative pain: a double-blind trial. Acta Anaesthesiologica Scandinavica 30: 620–624

O'Brien T, Mortimer P, McDonald C, Miller A 1997 A randomised crossover study comparing the efficacy and tolerability of a novel once-daily morphine preparation (MXL capsules) and MST Continus tablets in cancer patients with severe pain. Palliative Medicine 11: 475–482

O'Neill WM 1994 The cognitive and psychomotor effects of opioid drugs in cancer pain management. Cancer Surveys 21: 67–84

O'Neill WM, Hanks GW, White L, Simpson P, Wesnes K 1995 The cognitive and psychomotor effects of opioid analgesics: I. A randomized controlled trial of single doses of dextropropoxyphene, lorazepam and placebo in healthy subjects. European Journal of Clinical Pharmacology 48: 447–453

Osborne RJ, Joel SP, Slevin ML 1986 Morphine intoxication in renal failure: the role of morphine-6-glucuronide. British Medical Journal 292: 1548–1549

Palmer RN, Eade OE, O'shea PJ, Cuthbert MF 1966 Incidence of unwanted effects of dihydrocodeine bitartrate in healthy volunteers. Lancet 2: 620–621

Pannuti F, Rossi AP, Iafelice G et al 1982 Control of chronic pain in very advanced cancer patients with morphine hydrochloride administered by oral, rectal and sublingual route. Clinical report and preliminary results on morphine pharmacokinetics. Pharmacology Research Communications 14: 369–380

Pappagallo M 1998 The concept of pseudotolerance to opioids. Journal of Pharmaceutical Care in Pain and Symptom Control 6: 95–98

Passik S, Portenoy R, Ricketts P 1998a Substance abuse issues in cancer patients. Part 1: prevalence and diagnosis. Oncology 12: 517–521

Passik S, Portenoy R, Ricketts P 1998b Substance abuse issues in cancer patients. Part 2: evaluation and treatment. Oncology 12: 729–734

Paterson GMC, McQuay HJ, Bullingham RES, Moore RA 1984 Intradural morphine and diamorphine dose-response studies. Anaesthesia 39: 113–117

Perrier D, Gibaldi M 1972 Influence of first-pass effect on the systemic availability of propoxyphene. Journal of Clinical Pharmacology Nov/Dec: 449–452

Pert CB, Snyder SH 1973 Opiate receptor: demonstration in nervous tissue. Science 179: 1011–1014

Peters WP, Johnson MW, Friedman PA, Mitch WE 1981 Pressor effect of naloxone in septic shock. Lancet i: 529–532

Pond SM, Kretschzmar KM 1981 Effect of phenytoin on meperidine clearance and normeperidine formation. Clinical Pharmacology and Therapeutics 30: 680–686

Portenoy RK 1990 Chronic opioid therapy in nonmalignant pain. Journal of Pain and Symptom Management 5: 46–62

Portenoy RK 1994 Tolerance to opioid analgesics: clinical aspects. Cancer Surveys 21: 49–65

Portenoy RK, Foley KM 1986 Chronic use of opioid analgesics in non-malignant pain: report of 38 cases. Pain 25: 171–186

Portenoy RK, Moulin D, Rogers A, Inturrisi C, Foley K 1986 Intravenous infusion of opioids for cancer pain: clinical review and guidelines for use. Cancer Treatment Reports 70: 575–581

Portenoy RK, Southam MA, Gupta SK et al 1993 Transdermal fentanyl for cancer pain. Anesthesiology 78: 36–43

Porter J, Jick J 1980 Addiction rare in patients treated with narcotics. New England Journal of Medicine 302: 123

Poyhia R, Kalso E 1992 Antinociceptive effects and central nervous system depression caused by oxycodone and morphine in rats. Pharmacology and Toxicology 70: 125–130

Preston K, Jasinski D, Testa M 1991 Abuse potential and pharmacological comparison of tramadol and morphine. Drug and Alcohol Dependency 27: 7–18

Przewlocki R, Hassan A, Lason W, Epplen C, Herz A, Stein C 1992 Gene expression and localization of opioid peptides in immune cells of inflamed tissue; functional role in antinociception. Neuroscience 48: 491–500

Quiding H, Lundqvist G, Boreus L, Bondesson U, Ohrvik J 1993 Analgesic effect and plasma concentrations of codeine and morphine after two dose levels of codeine following oral surgery. European Journal of Clinical Pharmacology 44: 319–323

Radbruch L, Grond S, Lehmann K 1996 A risk-benefit assessment of tramadol in the management of pain. Drug Safety 15: 8–29

Raffa RB, Friderichs E, Reimann W, Shank RP, Codd EE, Vaught JL 1992 Opioid and nonopioid components independently contribute to the mechanism of action of tramadol, an 'atypical' opioid analgesic. Journal of Pharmacology and Therapeutics 260: 275–285

Ray D, Tai Y 1988 Infusions of naloxone in thalamic pain. British Medical Journal 296: 969–970

Redfern N 1983 Dihydrocodeine overdose treated with naloxone infusion. British Medical Journal 287: 751–752

Regnard CFB, Badger C 1987 Opioids, sleep and the time of death. Palliative Medicine 1: 107–110

Reichle CW, Smith GM, Gravenstein JS, Macris SG, Beecher HK 1962 Comparative analgesic potency of heroin and morphine in postoperative patients. Journal of Pharmacology and Experimental Therapeutics 136: 43–46

Rigg J 1978 Ventilatory effects and plasma concentration of morphine in man. British Journal of Anaesthesia 50: 759–760

Robins LN, Davis DH, Nurco DN 1974 How permanent was Vietnam drug addiction? American Journal of Public Health 64: 38–43

Robinson AE, Williams FM 1971 The distribution of methadone in man. Journal of Pharmacy and Pharmacology 23: 353–358

Ross F, Smith M 1997 The intrinsic antinociceptive effects of oxycodone appear to be kappa-opioid receptor mediated. Abstracts of the 20th Annual Meeting of Scandinavian Association for the Study of Pain, IASP Press, Seattle, USA p. 461

Rowbotham M, Reisner-Keller L, Fields H 1991 Both intravenous lidocaine and morphine reduce the pain of postherpetic neuralgia. Neurology 41: 1024–1028

Roy S, Liu H, Loh H 1998 Mu-opioid receptor-knockout mice: the role of mu-opioid receptor in gastrointestinal transit. Brain Research Molecular Brain Research 56: 281–283

Royal College of Surgeons 1990 Pain after surgery. Royal College of Surgeons, London

Sabbe M, Yaksh T 1990 Pharmacology of spinal opioids. Journal of Pain and Symptom Management 5: 191–203

Sandouk P, Serrie A, Scherrmann J, Langlade A, Bourre J 1991 Presence of morphine metabolites in human cerebrospinal fluid after intracerebroventricular administration of morphine. European Journal of Drug Metabolism and Pharmacology 16: 166–171

Satoh M, Minami M 1995 Molecular pharmacology of the opioid receptors. Pharmacology and Therapeutics 68: 343–364

Sawe J, Svensson JO, Odar-Cederlof I 1985 Kinetics of morphine in patients with renal failure. Lancet 1: 211–214

Schug SA, Zech D, Grond S, Jung H, Meuser T, Stobbe B 1992 A long-term survey of morphine in cancer pain patients. Journal of Pain and Symptom Management 7: 259–266

Schulze S, Roikjaer O, Hasselstrom L, Jensen N, Kehlet H 1988 Epidural bupivacaine and morphine plus systemic indomethacin eliminates pain but not systemic response and convalescence after cholecystectomy. Surgery 103: 321–327

Shimomura K, Kamata O, Ueki S, Ida S, Oguri K 1971 Analgesic effect of morphine glucuronides. Tohoku Journal of Experimental Medicine 105: 45–52

Simonin F, Valverde O, Smadja C et al 1988 Disruption of the kappa-opioid receptor gene in mice enhances sensitivity to chemical visceral pain, impairs pharmacological actions of the selective kappa-agonist U50,488H and attenuates morphine withdrawal. EMBO Journal 17: 886–897

Sjoberg M, Appelgren L, Einarsson S et al 1991 Long-term intrathecal morphine and bupivacaine in 'refractory' cancer pain. Results from the first series of 52 patients. Acta Anaesthesiologica Scandinavica 35: 30–43

Sjogren P, Jonsson T, Jensen NH, Drenck NE, Jensen TS 1993 Hyperalgesia and myoclonus in terminal cancer patients treated with continuous intravenous morphine. Pain 55: 93–97

Sjogren P, Jensen N-H, Jensen TS 1994 Disappearance of morphine-induced hyperalgesia after discontinuing or substituting morphine with other opioid antagonists. Pain 59: 313–316

Sjostrand UH, Rawal N 1986 International anaesthesiology clinics 24. Regional opioids in anaesthesiology and pain management. Little, Brown, Boston

Sluka K, Westlund K 1993 An experimental arthritis model in rats: the effects of NMDA and non-NMDA antagonists on aspartate and glutamate release in the dorsal horn. Neuroscience Letters 149: 99–102

Smith GD, Smith MT 1995 Morphine-3-glucuronide: evidence to support its putative role in the development of tolerance to the antinociceptive effects of morphine in the rat. Pain 62: 51–60

Snyder D 1993 Low-dose morphine injected into the mesosalpinx may provide analgesia for outpatient laparoscopic tubal occlusion. Anaesthesiology 79: A27

Sohn W, Zenz M (eds) 1998 Morphinverschreibung in Europa. Springer Verlag, Berlin

Sora I, Takahashi N, Funada M et al 1997 Opiate receptor knockout mice define mu receptor roles in endogenous nociceptive responses and morphine-induced analgesia. Proceedings of the National Academy of Science USA 94: 1544–1549

Sorkin E, Ogawa C 1983 Cimetidine potentiation of narcotic action. Drug Intelligence and Clinical Pharmacy 17: 60–61

Sorkin L, Westlund K, Sluka K, Dougherty P, Willis W 1992 Neural changes in acute arthritis in monkeys, IV: time-course of amino acid release into the lumbar dorsal horn. Brain Research Reviews 17: 39–50

Sporer K 1995 The serotonin syndrome: implicated drugs, pathophysiology and management. Drug Safety 13: 94–104

Stambaugh JE, Wainer IW, Hemhill DM, Schwartz I 1977 A potentially toxic drug interaction between pethidine (meperidine) and phenobarbitone. Lancet 1: 398–399

Stanfa L, AH D, Xu X, Wiesenfeld-Hallin Z 1994 Cholecystokinin and morphine analgesia: variations on a theme. Trends in Pharmacological Sciences 15: 65–66

Staritz M, Poralla T, Manns M, Ewe K, Meyer zum Buschenfelde K 1985 Pentazocine hampers bile flow. Lancet 1: 573–574

Stein C 1993 Peripheral mechanisms of opioid analgesia. Anesthesia and Analgesia 76: 182–191

Stein C, Hassan A, Przewlocki R, Gramsch C, Peter K, Herz A 1990 Opioids from immunocytes interact with receptors on sensory nerves to inhibit nociception in inflammation. Proceedings of the National Academy of Science USA 87: 5935–5939

Swarm R, Cousins M 1997 Anaesthetic techniques for pain control. In: Doyle D, Hanks GW, MacDonald N (eds) Oxford textbook of palliative medicine. Oxford Medical Publications, Oxford, pp 390–414

Sykes N 1996 Current management of constipation in cancer pain. Progress in Palliative Care 4: 170–177

Taub A 1982 Opioid analgesics in the treatment of chronic intractable pain of non-neoplastic origin. In: Kitahata L M, Collins J D (eds) Narcotic analgesics in anaesthesiology. Williams and Wilkins, Baltimore, pp 199–208

Tennant FS, Rawson RA 1982 Outpatient treatment of prescription opioid dependence. Archives of Internal Medicine 142: 1845–1847

Tennant FS, Uelman GF 1983 Narcotic maintenance for chronic pain: medical and legal guidelines. Postgraduate Medicine 73: 81–94

Thompson JF, Pike JM, Chumas PD, Rundle JSH 1989 Rectal diclofenac compared with pethidine injection in acute renal colic. British Medical Journal 299: 1140–1141

Thompson P, Bingham S, Andrews P, Patel N, Joel S, Slevin M 1992 Morphine-6-glucuronide: a metabolite of morphine with greater emetic potency than morphine in the ferret. British Journal of Pharmacology 106: 3–8

Tong T, Pond S, Kreek M, Jaffery N, Benowitz N 1981 Phenytoin-induced methadone withdrawal. Annals of Internal Medicine 94: 349–351

Traynor J 1996 The mu-opioid receptor. Pain Reviews 3: 221–248

Twycross RG 1974 Clinical experience with diamorphine in advanced malignant disease. International Journal of Clinical Pharmacology, Therapy and Toxicology 9: 184–198

Twycross RG 1977 Choice of strong analgesic in terminal cancer: diamorphine or morphine? Pain 3: 93–104

Twycross RG 1994 Pain relief in advanced cancer. Churchill Livingstone, Edinburgh

Twycross RG 1997 Update on analgesics. In: Kaye P (ed) Tutorials in palliative medicine. EPL Publications, Northampton, pp 94–131

Twycross RG, Lack S 1983 Symptom control in far advanced cancer: pain relief. Pitman, London

Twycross RG, Wald SJ 1976 Longterm use of diamorphine in advanced cancer. In: Bonica J J, Albe-Fessard D A F (eds) Advances in pain research and therapy, vol 1. Raven Press, New York, pp 653–661

Twycross RG, Wilcock A, Thorp S 1998 Palliative care formulary. Radcliffe Medical Press, Oxford

Ueyama H, Nishimura M, Tashiro C 1992 Naloxone reversal of nystagmus associated with intrathecal morphine administration (letter). Anesthesiology 76: 153–155

Ullman D, Fortune J, Greenhouse B, Wimpy R, Kennedy T 1989 The treatment of patients with multiple rib fractures using continuous thoracic epidural narcotic infusion. Regional Anesthesia 14: 43–47

Vainio A, Ollila J, Matikainen E, Rosenberg P, Kalso E 1995 Driving ability in cancer patients receiving longterm morphine analgesia. Lancet 346: 667–670

Van der Mass P, Van Delden J, Pijnenborg L 1991 Medische beslissingen rond het levenseinde. S D U, The Hague, pp 57–62

Vaught J 1991 What is the relative contribution of mu, delta and kappa opioid receptors to antinociception and is there cross-tolerance? In: Basbaum A, Besson J-M (eds) Towards a new pharmacotherapy of pain. John Wiley, Chichester, pp 121–136

Vaught J, Mathiasen J, Raffa R 1998 Examination of the involvement of supraspinal and spinal mu and delta opioid receptors in analgesia using the mu receptor deficient CXBR mouse. Journal of Pharmacology and Experimental Therapeutics 245: 13–16

Ventafridda V, Ripamonti C, Conno F D, Bianchi M, Pazzuconi F, Panerai A 1987 Antidepressants increase bioavailability of morphine in cancer patients (letter). Lancet i: 204

Wall P 1997 The generation of yet another myth on the use of narcotics. Pain 73: 121–122

Walsh T 1984 Opiates and respiratory function in advanced cancer. Recent Results in Cancer Care 89: 115–117

Walsh T, Smyth E, Currie K, Glare P, Schneider J 1992 A pilot study, review of the literature, and dosing guidelines for patient-controlled analgesia using subcutaneous morphine sulphate for chronic cancer pain. Palliative Medicine 6: 217–226

Watson PJQ, Moore RA, McQuay HJ et al 1984 Plasma morphine concentrations and analgesic effects of lumbar extradural morphine and heroin. Anesthesia and Analgesia 63: 629–634

Weissman D, Haddox J 1989 Opioid pseudoaddiction: an iatrogenic syndrome. Pain 36: 363–366

Wiertelak E, Maier S, Watkins L 1992 Cholecystokinin antianalgesia: safety cues abolish morphine analgesia. Science 256: 830–833

Wilder-Smith C, Bettiga A 1997 The analgesic tramadol has minimal effect on gastrointestinal motor function. British Journal of Clinical Pharmacology 43: 71–75

Woodcock A, Gross E, Gellert A, Shah S, Johnson M, Geddes D 1981 Effects of dihydrocodeine alcohol, and caffeine on breathlessness and exercise tolerance in patients with chronic obstructive lung disease and normal blood gases. New England Journal of Medicine 305: 1611–1616

Woolf C, Wall P 1986 Morphine sensitive and morphine insensitive actions of C-fibre input on the rat spinal cord. Neuroscience Letters 64: 221–225

Woolner DF, Winter D, Frendin TJ, Begg EJ, Lynn KL, Wright G 1986 Renal failure does not impair the metabolism of morphine. British Journal of Clinical Pharmacology 22: 55–59

World Health Organization 1969 Expert Committee on Drug Dependence, 16th report. Technical report series no. 407. WHO, Geneva

World Health Organization 1986 Cancer pain relief. WHO, Geneva

World Health Organization 1990 Cancer pain relief and palliative care. Technical report series no. 804. W H O, Geneva

World Health Organization 1996 Cancer pain relief: with a guide to opioid availability. WHO, Geneva

Wright CI, Barbour FA 1935 The respiratory effects of morphine, codeine and related substances. Journal of Pharmacology and Experimental Therapeutics 54: 25–33

Writer WDR, Hurtig JB, Evans D, Reed RE, Hope CE, Forrest JBN 1985 Epidural morphine prophylaxis of postoperative pain: report of a double-blind multicentre study. Canadian Medical Association Journal 32: 330–338

Young IH, Daviskas E, Keena VA 1989 Effect of low dose nebulized morphine on exercise advance in patients with chronic lung disease. Thorax 44: 387–390

Zenz M, Willweber-Strumpf A 1993 Opiophobia and cancer pain in Europe. Lancet 341: 1075–1076

Zenz M, Strumpf M, Tryba M 1992 Long-term opioid therapy in patients with chronic non-malignant pain. Journal of the Royal Society of Medicine 7: 69–77

Zylicz Z 1993 Opiophobia and cancer pain. Lancet 341: 1473–1474

Local anaesthetics and epidurals

H. J. McQUAY & R. A. MOORE

Local anaesthetics are amazing drugs. Injected into tissue, around a nerve or for a regional block, they produce reversible block. An old advertisement from a travelling dentist (1920s) says 'Teeth carefully extracted – Adults, 6d each – With Cocaine, 6d extra'. The moral for acute pain is that local anaesthesia is a luxury rather than a necessity. At least, that was the moral. The ground is now shifting. Asking radical questions about acute postoperative management, such as 'Why are all operations not ambulatory, pain-free and risk-free?' or, more familiar, 'Why is this patient still in hospital?', is forcing a reconsideration of the role of combined (local or regional plus general anaesthesia) approaches. Instead of asking questions such as 'Is regional better than general anaesthesia', we need to look at the whole episode, before, during and after surgery, not just the operative period. Henrik Kehlet (1994, 1997), the Danish surgeon, has been the major force provoking these ideas, refreshingly from professional rather than cost-cutting motives. Costs of each care episode should, however, fall if the hospital stay is reduced and a healthy patient returned home will cost the community less than a sick patient requiring considerable input from the primary care team. These issues are relevant to this chapter because the radical changes depend on the use of nerve blocks or regional techniques using local anaesthetics.

Another Scandinavian pioneer, Staffan Arnér from Stockholm, has tackled one of the conundrums of local anaesthetic use in chronic pain, which is why pain relief from local anaesthetics can far outlast the duration of action of the local anaesthetic (Arner et al 1990).

This chapter will discuss these important aspects of local anaesthetics and will also cover epidural use of opioids alone and in combination with local anaesthetics. The aim is not to cover the mechanics of particular blocks, which is done well in a variety of books, but rather to look into the crystal ball – in which areas does current evidence suggest we could use local anaesthetics more and which areas need greater research focus?

ACUTE PAIN

A SIMPLE OPERATION

The first example is of a common operation, inguinal hernia repair, which can be done under local anaesthetic alone. Outcomes which need to be considered include the choice of anaesthesia and analgesia, postherniorrhaphy pain and convalescence, postoperative morbidity (predominantly urinary retention) and choice of surgical technique and recurrence rate. In a randomized double-blind double-dummy study (Nehra et al 1995) of 200 men, Nehra and colleagues compared 0.5% bupivacaine ilioinguinal field block plus oral papaveretum-aspirin tablets with bupivacaine plus oral placebo, saline plus papaveretum-aspirin or saline plus oral placebo to assess pain relief after hernia surgery. Patients were prescribed postoperative opioids to be given on demand. Pain levels and mobility were assessed 6 and 24 hours after operation. The combination of bupivacaine plus papaveretum-aspirin provided the best results, producing (not surprisingly) significantly less pain and requiring less additional opioid and with better mobility than saline plus oral placebo. A similar trial nearly 20 years ago (Teasdale et al 1982) randomized 103 patients to either local or general anaesthesia; those patients having local anaesthesia were able to walk, eat and pass urine significantly earlier than those having general anaesthesia, who experienced more nausea, vomiting, sore throat and headache.

An audit of inguinal hernia repair under local anaesthesia in an ambulatory set-up provides confirmation that these results may be generalized. Prospective data were collected from 400 consecutive elective ambulatory operations for inguinal hernia (29 operations in ASA group III patients) under unmonitored local anaesthesia (Callesen et al 1998). Median postoperative hospital stay was 85 minutes. Two patients needed general anaesthesia and nine patients (2%) needed overnight admission. One-week postoperative morbidity was low, with one patient with transient cerebral ischaemia and one with pneumonia, but none with urinary retention. The high satisfaction (88%) on follow-up makes this a triumph for local anaesthesia, but the variation in general practitioners' recommendations for convalescence, such as between 1 and 12 weeks off work, may need to be changed if the full benefit to the individual and to the society is to be harnessed (Kehlet & Callesen 1998).

A COMPLEX OPERATION – WHAT IS THE QUESTION? IS IT STILL GENERAL VERSUS REGIONAL?

Our old question was whether regional or regional-supplemented general anaesthesia could produce major reductions in morbidity and mortality – the general versus regional anaesthesia question. An example is vascular surgery. The Yeager et al study (1987) did suggest improvement with regional anaesthesia in patients undergoing abdominal aortic aneurysm or lower extremity vascular surgery. A feature of subsequent studies which showed no difference between regional and general anaesthesia was an increasing extent of control over all aspects of postoperative care (Christopherson et al 1993, Bode et al 1996). The effect of the detailed protocols was that bad outcomes were reduced in all groups (Beattie et al 1996). The implication is that even if there was a difference, it would take a very large study to show it using the morbidity and mortality outcomes (Rigg & Jamrozik 1998). But the suggestion is that only if the postoperative protocols allow any advantage to be expressed, such as advantage in time to feeding or time to walking, will we see a difference between regional and general anaesthesia. Epidural local anaesthetic may well allow bowel function to return earlier (Liu et al 1995), but only if protocol allows it will we see patients going home 2 days after major surgery (Bardram et al 1995). The point is that this radical change is only possible if the procedure is done under an epidural, because the epidural makes it possible for the patient to mobilize early and for bowel function to return earlier.

For some operations there is proven advantage of regional over general anaesthesia. For hip (Sharrock & Salvati 1996) and knee (Williams-Russo et al 1996) replacements, 'solid' epidural anaesthesia with sedation during surgery followed by postoperative epidural can produce reduced blood loss, faster surgery, reduced morbidity and faster rehabilitation. In this context change has been gradual rather than radical but again the key is the epidural, both for the operation and afterwards.

Returning to the old question, general versus regional anaesthesia, a recent set of meta-analyses looked at randomized, controlled trials (RCTs) to assess the effects of seven different interventions on postoperative pulmonary function after a variety of procedures (Ballantyne et al 1998). The seven were epidural opioid, epidural local anaesthetic, epidural opioid with local anaesthetic, thoracic versus lumbar epidural opioid, intercostal nerve block, wound infiltration with local anaesthetic and intrapleural local anaesthetic. Compared with systemic opioids, epidural opioids decreased the incidence of atelectasis significantly. Epidural local anaesthetics compared with systemic opioids increased PaO_2 significantly and decreased the incidence of pulmonary infections and pulmonary complications overall. Intercostal nerve blockade did not produce significant improvement in pulmonary outcome measures.

Interestingly, on the surrogate measures of pulmonary function (FEV_1, FVC and PEFR), there were no clinically or statistically significant differences, showing again the importance of choice of outcome measure. The results do confirm that postoperative epidural pain control can significantly decrease the incidence of pulmonary morbidity (Ballantyne et al 1998).

WHAT ARE THE IMPLICATIONS FOR LOCAL ANAESTHETICS?

With the local anaesthetics, we now have the so-called multimodal approach for the postoperative period, using NSAIDs and paracetamol (Kehlet 1997, McQuay et al 1997). Slow-release or very long-acting local anaesthetics may deliver further radical improvement by improving the postoperative period. Long-acting local anaesthetics are not new (Scurlock & Curtis 1981, King 1984) and the problem is to be sure that the block is indeed reversible and that the extended duration is not due to a toxic effect (Lipfert et al 1987). The new thought is that instead of focusing exclusively on a particular block or a particular local anaesthetic, we need to think of the wider context and choose our outcomes accordingly. New drug features and new ways of doing particular blocks are obviously important, but should not preclude answering the bigger question.

CHOOSING A BLOCK FOR A PARTICULAR PROCEDURE

An example, albeit a special case, of how to determine the most effective local anaesthetic technique is the RCT of 52 babies which compared ring block, dorsal penile nerve block, a topical eutectic mixture of local anaesthetics (EMLA) and topical placebo for neonatal circumcision (Lander et al 1997). The authors used placebo because it represented current practice, with no anaesthetic for neonatal circumcision. The three treatment groups all had significantly less crying and lower heart rates during and following circumcision compared with the untreated group. The ring block was equally effective through all stages of the circumcision, whereas the dorsal penile nerve block and EMLA were not effective during foreskin separation and incision.

Many of the recent comparisons, for instance in thoracic anaesthesia, of one block against another are designed as A versus B comparisons. Unless the trials are very big, which most are not, one ends up concluding that the trial showed no difference and we do not know if the trial was capable of revealing a difference if in fact there was one (McQuay & Moore 1996a). Choice of block also involves comparing the morbidity of the contenders. Again, size of trial is crucial. Rare events will not be picked up in small trials.

PROBLEMS WITH LOCAL BLOCKS

One important question is whether using nerve blocks or powerful epidural techniques has deleterious consequences. For most nerve blocks, for instance axillary brachial plexus block, we just do not know the incidence of long-term nerve problems. In all likelihood, it is vanishingly small. In a 1-year prospective survey of the French-Language Society of Paediatric Anaesthesiologists, Giaufre et al reported that 38% of the 24 409 local anaesthetic procedures were peripheral nerve blocks and local anaesthesia techniques. These were reported as 'generally safe' (Giaufre et al 1996).

In the same survey, 'central blocks' (15 013), most of which were caudals, accounted for more than 60% of all local anaesthetic procedures. Their complication rate for central blocks works out at 15 per 10 000 (25 incidents involving 24 patients). These were rated as minor and did not result in any sequelae or medicolegal action.

In adults, a report from Finland (Aromaa et al 1997) reviewed all claims (1987–1993) about severe complications associated with epidural and spinal anaesthesia. Eighty-six claims were associated with spinal and/or epidural anaesthesia. There were 550 000 spinals and 170 000 epidurals. With spinals, there were 25 serious complications: cardiac arrests (2), paraplegia (5), permanent cauda equina syndrome (1), peroneal nerve paresis (6), neurological deficits (7) and bacterial infections (4). With epidurals, there were nine serious complications: paraparesis (1), permanent cauda equina syndrome (1), peroneal nerve paresis (1), neurological deficit (1), bacterial infections (2), acute toxic reactions related to the anaesthetic solution (2) and overdose of epidural opioid (1). This gives an overall incidence of serious complications of 0.45 per 10 000 for spinal and 0.52 per 10 000 for epidural.

Again in adults, a French survey (Auroy et al 1997) reported on 40 640 spinals and 30 413 epidurals. Of the 98 severe complications, 89 were attributed fully or partially to the regional anaesthesia. There were 26 cardiac arrests with spinals (6.4 ± 1.2 per 10 000 patients) and six were fatal. There were three arrests with epidurals. Of 34 neurological complications (radiculopathy, cauda equina syndrome, paraplegia), 21 were associated either with paraesthesia during puncture (n = 19) or with pain during injection (n = 2), suggesting nerve trauma or intraneural injection. Neurological sequelae were significantly more common after spinal anaesthesia (6 ± 1 per 10 000) than after each of the other types of regional procedures (1.6 ± 0.5 per 10 000).

Yuen et al (1995) described 12 patients (out of an estimated 13 000) with complications after lumbar epidurals. Eleven patients had lumbosacral radiculopathy or polyradiculopathy, 10 after epidural and one after subarachnoid injection of medication during intended epidural. One patient had a thoracic myelopathy after an unintended spinal. From their data, one may estimate the incidence of short-term (persisting less than 1 year) neurological sequelae after an epidural as nine per 10 000 and for longer term (persisting more than 1 year), two per 10 000. As the authors point out, these incidences appear to have changed little from previous case series (Yuen et al 1995).

An important RCT looked at the question of whether there was any difference in long-term cognitive dysfunction after total knee replacement surgery in 262 older adults (median age 69 years; 70% women) after epidural or general anaesthesia (Williams-Russo et al 1995). This is the largest trial to date of the effects of general versus regional anaesthesia on cerebral function, with more than 99% power to detect a clinically significant difference on any of the neuropsychological tests. Preoperative neuropsychological assessment was repeated postoperatively at 1 week and 6 months. Cognitive outcome was assessed by within-patient change on 10 tests of memory, psychomotor and language skills. There were no significant differences between the epidural and general anaesthesia groups on any of the 10 cognitive tests at either 1 week or 6 months. Overall, 5% of patients showed a long-term clinically significant deterioration in cognitive function.

The difficulty in establishing whether a putative risk really is a risk is apparent in the controversy about backache after childbirth epidural.

CHRONIC PAIN

Two aspects of local anaesthetic use in chronic pain are featured because they are of current interest: why blocks last a long time, and the use of epidural corticosteroids for sciatica.

WHY DO BLOCKS LAST A LONG TIME?

Many of us do peripheral nerve blocks with local anaesthetic for pain due to trauma or surgery and the dogma is that the local anaesthetic block alone can occasionally produce a cure and more often reduces pain for a duration which far outlasts the duration of the local anaesthetic. In a descriptive study, Arner et al (1990) reported on 38 consecutive patients with neuralgia after peripheral nerve injury, treated with one or two series of peripheral local anaesthetic blocks. The blocks were technically successful, with all patients experiencing an initial total relief of ongoing pain between 4 and 12 hours. In the 17 patients who had evoked pain (hyperalgesia or allodynia), it was blocked together with the spontaneous pain. In 18 patients the analgesia outlasted the conduction block. Thirteen patients had complete pain relief for 12–48 hours and in five, pain relief was complete for 2–6 days. Eight patients had a second phase of analgesia, varying from 4 hours to 6 days and coming on within 12 hours of the pain recurring.

Arner et al chose to concentrate on complete pain relief and, using this yardstick, mono- or biphasic prolonged complete analgesia occurred in 25 out of 38 patients. A tantalizing further result is that for 15 of the 20 patients who had complete analgesia initially but lasting less than 12 hours, partial improvement lasting weeks to months was noted. Conversely, only one of the 18 patients who had more than 12 hours initial relief reported prolonged partial improvement. Their paper provides some empirical support for the (common) clinical use of local anaesthetic blocks in this context and also reopens the interesting question of why a block can reduce pain for far longer than the local anaesthetic should work.

Arner et al discuss systemic uptake and axoplasmic transport of local anaesthetic as putative mechanisms, but their experiments showed little evidence of transport. The explanation may lie in 'breaking the cycle'. The peripheral pain input is blocked and system can then reset itself. This suggests many questions. For how long does the input have to be blocked to allow the system to reset? For which types of pain is this true? Their study provides clinical legitimacy for further investigation.

EPIDURAL CORTICOSTEROIDS FOR SCIATICA

Two systematic reviews have addressed the effectiveness of epidural steroid injections for sciatica and back pain. Both examined the RCTs published up to the end of 1994.

The analysis by Koes and colleagues (1995) from Amsterdam goes into great depth examining methodological quality of the trials and how this has been scored by the reviewers. This type of review is, frankly, disappointing and does not produce any meta-analytic judgements on which to work and few enlightening ideas about the future research agenda other than some anodyne comments about possible trial design.

The most that this review can tell us is that, of the four studies with the highest methodological quality assessed by their particular scoring system, two had positive outcomes for epidural steroids (judged by their authors) and two had negative outcomes.

In contrast, a meta-analysis of the same trials by Watts and Silagy (1995) is an important step forward in showing that epidural corticosteroids have an analgesic effect on sciatica compared with control. Their analysis, using odds ratios, answered the question 'Do epidural steroids work?'.

We wished to address the question 'How well do they work?', to try to assess the extent of the benefit given by the steroids. To do this, we reanalysed their data and, adding a new trial (Carette et al 1997), used NNT (McQuay & Moore 1998) as the measure of clinical benefit (Table 52.1), using the outcome of at least 75% pain relief for short-term outcomes (1–60 days) and at least 50% pain relief for long-term outcomes (12 weeks to 1 year). When the number of patients entered into individual studies is small, this approach is most likely to produce a reliable indication of the clinically relevant outcomes needed by patients, providers and purchasers in making decisions about a technique which carries small but finite risk (see above).

Short-term relief

There were 11 trials which gave short-term relief data (more than 75% pain relief), with 319 patients given

Table 52.1 Epidural corticosteroids for sciatica

Trial	*Improved on epidural steroid*	*Improved on control*	*Relative benefit (95%CI)*	*NNT (95%CI)*
Short-term relief (1–60 days)				
Beliveau 1971	18/24	16/24	1.1 (0.8–1.6)	12 (3–∞)
Breivik et al 1976	9/16	5/19	2.1 (0.9–5.1)	3.3 (1.6–∞)
Bush & Hillier 1991	8/12	2/11	3.7 (0.98–13.7)	2.1 (1.2–7.5)
Carette et al 1997	25/76	23/78	1.1 (0.5–2.4)	29 (5.5–∞)
Cuckler et al 1985	12/19	8/31	1.1 (0.5–2.4)	33 (4–∞)
Dilke et al 1973	21/35	11/36	2.0 (1.1–3.4)	3.5 (1.9–14)
Klenerman et al 1984	15/19	32/44	1.1 (0.8–1.5)	17 (3–∞)
Mathews et al 1987	14/21	18/32	1.2 (0.8–1.8)	10 (3–∞)
Popiolek et al 1991	18/28	8/30	2.4 (1.3–4.6)	2.6 (1.6–7.2)
Ridley et al 1988	17/19	3/16	4.8 (1.7–13)	1.4 (1.1–2.1)
Snoek et al 1977	8/27	5/24	1.4 (0.5–3.8)	11 (3–∞)
Combined short term (>75%)	**165/319**	**131/345**	**1.5 (1.2–1.9)**	**7.3 (4.7–16)**
Long-term relief (12–52 weeks)				
Bush & Hillier 1991	10/12	7/11	1.3 (0.8–2.2)	5.0 (1.8–∞)
Carette et al 1997	41/74	43/77	1.0 (0.7–1.3)	∞
Cuckler et al 1985	11/46	4/27	1.6 (0.6–4.6)	10.99 (3.66–∞)
Dilke et al 1973	16/43	8/38	1.8 (0.9–3.7)	6.3 (2.8–∞)
Mathews et al 1987	9/23	14/34	0.95 (0.5–1.8)	∞
Swerdlow & Sayle-Creer 1969	76/117	98/208	1.4 (1.1–1.7)	5.6 (3.5–14)
Combined long term	**163/315**	**174/395**	**1.3 (1.1–1.5)**	**13 (6.6–314)**

Relative benefit and NNT were calculated for this table

epidural steroids and 345 given placebo. Only three of these studies were themselves statistically significant (Dilke et al 1973, Ridley et al 1988, Popiolek et al 1991), but overall there was a statistically significant benefit (1.5 with 95% CI 1.2–1.9).

The NNT for short-term (1–60 days) greater than 75% pain relief from the 10 trials, with short-term outcomes combined, was just under 7.3, with 95% CI from 4.7 to 16. This means that for seven patients treated with epidural steroid, one will obtain more than 75% short-term pain relief who would not have done had they received the control treatment (placebo or local anaesthetic).

Long-term relief

There were six trials which gave long-term relief data, with 315 patients given epidural steroids and 395 given placebo. Only one of these studies was itself statistically significant (Swerdlow & Sayle-Creer 1969), but overall there was a statistically significant benefit (1.3 with 95% CI 1.1–1.5).

The NNT for long-term (12 weeks up to 1 year) improvement from the six trials combined was about 13 for 50% pain relief, with 95% CI from 6.6 to 314. This means that for 13 patients treated with epidural steroid, one will obtain more long-term pain relief who would not have done had they received the control treatment (placebo or local anaesthetic).

Conclusion

These NNT values at first sight appear disappointing. Here is an intervention which shows statistically significant improvement compared with control and yet the clinical benefit, the number needed to treat for one patient to reach the chosen endpoint, is 7 for short-term benefit and 13 for long term. The short-term endpoint, however, is quite a high hurdle. Using an easier hurdle of 50% relief rather than 75%, the 'best' NNT achieved by drug treatment of neuropathic pain was just under 3. Patients may choose the epidural if it means they do not have to take medication, particularly if it gives a higher level of relief, even though there is a 1 in 7 chance of this level of response.

The long-term NNT of 13 is perhaps not surprising. Occasional patients in most clinics report a 'cure' as a result of a steroid epidural, but the majority of epidural steroid successes return for repeat epidurals. That one patient has relief lasting between 12 weeks and a year for 12 treated with epidural steroid fits with experience.

The message is that we will inevitably have to expose our practice to the searching type of analysis which Watts and Silagy (1995) have used for epidural steroid. This intervention has shown a statistically significant benefit over control. Others will not and will be discarded. For those interventions which do show statistically significant benefit over control, there is then a further stage, which is to define the clinical benefit of the intervention. The NNTs for effectiveness are one possible definition, particularly when coupled with NNTs for minor and major harm (NNT of about 40 for dural tap in Watts & Silagy 1995).

For patients with chronic disease, and in this case chronic painful disease, interventions may be attractive even if their success rate is far lower than would be acceptable in, say, the management of postoperative pain. This means that the interpretation of measures of clinical benefit, such as NNTs, has to be context dependent. For the moment, we need the best possible analysis, as Watts and Silagy have demonstrated, of the data available. If the data are poor then that establishes the clinical research agenda. If the data are reasonable then we can try to define measures of clinical benefit. The art of clinical practice will then come into play, as patient and doctor juggle the risk and benefit of the alternatives, albeit with better data than we have at present.

MORE ON EPIDURALS – LOCAL ANAESTHETIC AND OPIOID

For over 20 years we have known that opioids applied to the spinal cord have analgesic effect. It has proved surprisingly difficult to define a clinical role for spinal (epidural and intrathecal) opioids, maximizing the analgesic benefit while minimizing the risk. The original question addressed was the advantage of spinal opioids over spinal local anaesthetics. The next question was the advantage of spinal opioids over intramuscular, oral or subcutaneous opioids. Now we have come full circle because it is the use of spinal combinations of local anaesthetic and opioid which promises the greatest clinical benefit.

It is ironic that these questions are being addressed for spinal opioids while our ignorance about the conventional routes of administration for opioids, whether oral, subcutaneous, intramuscular or intravenous, remains profound. The single most important point is to distinguish between the fact that it can be done and the clinical questions of whether it should be done and if so, when and to whom? New routes often have a high profile so that it may be very difficult to determine their real clinical role. The ultimate arbiter of the clinical role is the risk:benefit ratio. The aim is better analgesia with fewer adverse effects and no increase in morbidity. For instance, in chronic pain oral opioids can provide good relief with manageable adverse effects for the majority of patients. New routes must be considered as replacements, adjuncts or alternatives to the oral route.

Well-designed RCTs which compared the new route with the established routes would give us the answers. There are still few such trials available. They are difficult to do well, particularly in chronic and cancer pain.

The underlying issues for new routes are kinetic and clinical logic. The spinal routes have the kinetic logic of applying the opioid directly to opioid receptors in the cord. The clinical advantage sought is better analgesia without the problems of systemic opioid use or even the same analgesia with fewer adverse effects. Proposed alternatives must provide an improved risk:benefit ratio and be logistically feasible.

UNDERLYING ISSUES

THE EPIDURAL SPACE

The spinal epidural space extends from the sacral hiatus to the base of the skull. Drugs injected into the epidural space can then block or modulate afferent impulses and cord processing of those impulses. The way in which they block and modulate impulses and processing is probably the same as the mechanism which operates when the same drugs are injected intrathecally. There are some important differences between the epidural and intrathecal spaces, however, which affect clinical practice. The fact that the epidural space is a relatively indirect method of access compared with the intrathecal provides potential clinical advantage compared with the intrathecal route, but also complicates matters.

The epidural space provides access for drugs to the neuraxis, as does intrathecal injection. The potential clinical advantage of an epidural is the fact that the meninges are not physically breached, so that headache from cerebrospinal fluid (CSF) leakage does not occur and the danger of meningitis is also reduced. Chronic administration through catheters should therefore be safer by the epidural route than by the subarachnoid route. The first disadvantage is that the epidural space is vascular and contains fat. A large proportion of the epidural dose is taken up by extradural fat and by vascular absorption and so less drug is immediately available for neural blocking action. The second disadvantage is that the epidural tissues react to foreign bodies more than the sheltered subarachnoid space.

Epidural catheters often become walled off by fibrous tissue within days to weeks, whereas intrathecal catheters are much less prone to blockage (Durant & Yaksh 1986); this problem is in part overcome by using continuous infusion rather than intermittent bolus.

REACHING THE SITE OF ACTION

It used to be thought that the dura mater was impermeable to local anaesthetics and that epidural block with local anaesthetic occurred at the mixed nerve and dorsal root ganglia beyond the dural sleeves surrounding each pair of anterior and posterior spinal roots. Radioactive tracer studies have shown that the dura matter is not impermeable and that subarachnoid and epidural local anaesthetics act at precisely the same sites, namely the spinal roots, mixed spinal nerves and the surface of the spinal cord to a depth of 1 mm or more, depending on the lipid solubility of the anaesthetic (Bromage et al 1963). With both epidural and subarachnoid injection, the local anaesthetic drug entered the CSF and remained there until taken up by the lipids of the cord and spinal roots or until 'washed out' by vascular uptake into the blood vessels of the region.

Opioids have to reach the opioid receptors in the substantia gelatinosa of the cord in order to have spinal effect. Some of the opioid injected into the epidural space will reach the CSF and then the cord. Some will be absorbed into the bloodstream and some will be bound by fatty tissue in the epidural space. The proportion of the dose injected which goes in each of these directions depends on lipid solubility and on molecular weight (Moore et al 1982). Lipid-soluble opioids will be subject to greater vascular uptake from the epidural space than lipid-insoluble opioids. High molecular weight drugs diffuse across the dura with less ease than drugs of low molecular weight. Once across the dura, drugs which have low lipid solubility may maintain high concentrations in the CSF for long periods of time and so can spread rostrally. Sampling at cisternal level after lumbar intrathecal injection of morphine confirmed that high concentrations are found within an hour (Moulin et al 1986). Drugs with high lipid solubility will be bound much faster in the cord, leaving lower concentrations of drug in the CSF available to spread rostrally.

There is a similar range of lipophilicity and molecular size for the two drug classes, local anaesthetics and opioids, so that the journey from the injection site to the target sites is likely to be accomplished in roughly the same timespan for both classes of drug and proportional losses by vascular absorption and uptake into neighbouring fat depots are also likely to be similar. With both local anaesthetics (Burm et al

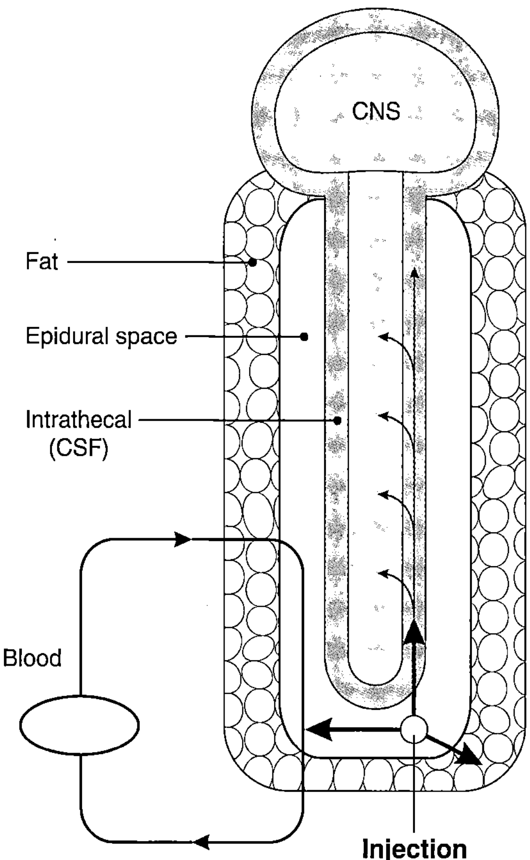

Fig. 52.1 The epidural space and the fate of injected drugs, which may go into fat, blood or CSF and then into the spinal cord.

1986) and opioids (Jamous et al 1986), vascular uptake is slowed and neural blockade increased by adding a dilute concentration of adrenaline (3–5 μg/ml) to the injected agent.

LIPOPHILICITY AND POTENCY

Within each class of drug, however, there is a wide range of lipophilicity and this may have considerable influence on the relative potencies of the drugs within a class. Using an electrophysiological model, single unit recordings were made in the lumbar dorsal horn in the intact anaesthetized rat from convergent, multireceptive neurons. Activity was evoked by Aβ and C-fibre transcutaneous electrical stimulation of hindpaw receptive fields. With intrathecal application of opioids, the effect of lipid solubility in determining relative intrathecal potency was measured. Initially four μ opioid receptor agonists were used – morphine, pethidine, methadone and normorphine – because all four drugs had relatively high affinity for μ and little for δ and κ, precluding receptor affinity to other receptor subtypes as a complicating factor. The

ED_{50} values from the dose–response curves were expressed against the partition coefficients. A significant correlation was found between the log ED_{50} and lipophilicity but this was an inverse relationship, so that the least lipid-soluble agonists, morphine and normorphine, were the most potent and the highly lipid-soluble methadone was considerably the least potent.

The same approximate order of potency – morphine=normorphine>pethidine>methadone – was seen in behavioural hot plate and tail flick tests, although the cut-off maxima necessary in those tests made it difficult to determine an ED_{50} for the more lipophilic and hence less potent compounds (Yaksh & Noueihed 1985). In a second study (Dickenson et al 1990), three opioids – fentanyl, etorphine and buprenorphine – all highly potent by the systemic route in man and animals, were applied either intrathecally or intravenously. Figure 52.2 shows the relationship between intrathecal potency and lipophilicity for the seven opioids tested in these two studies. For fentanyl and buprenorphine, potency correlated well with lipophilicity. The potency of etorphine, however, was considerably greater than would be expected if lipophilicity were the only determinant.

Non-specific binding is the probable explanation of the inverse correlation between intrathecal potency and lipid solubility. When radiolabelled opioid distribution was visualized by autoradiography (Herz & Teschemacher 1971), the highly lipid-soluble opioids were found to be restricted largely to fibre tracts and penetrated the grey matter poorly. The thickly myelinated large A fibres cap the spinal cord grey matter. They pass medially over the dorsal horn before penetrating the grey matter. This means that the lipid-rich A fibres come between the injection site and the opioid receptors in the grey matter. Lipid-soluble opioids will be taken up rapidly but preferentially in this lipid-rich tissue. Drug bound in this non-specific way cannot then go on to bind to the receptors.

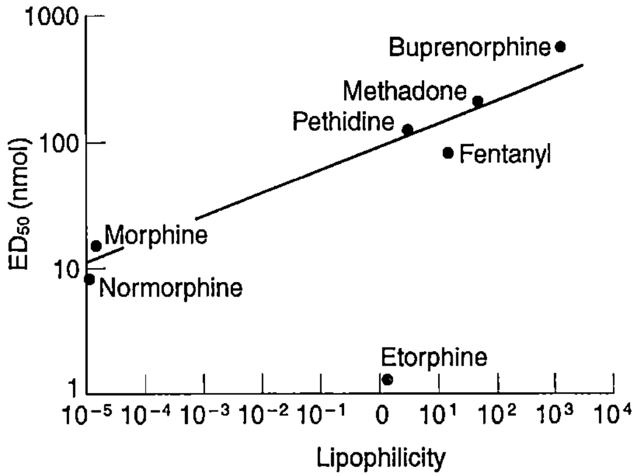

Fig. 52.2 Relationship between lipophilicity and potency.

Systemic potency ratios in man are thus unlikely to be accurate guides to spinal effectiveness, which makes it difficult to choose the dose of intrathecal (or extradural) opioid necessary to produce the same analgesia as a given dose of morphine. Many of the epidural opioid studies which used opioids other than morphine have used the systemic potency ratio to morphine as the guide for spinal potency. Extrapolation from the animal data suggests that for drugs with high lipophilicity, the intrathecal dose required to give analgesia equivalent to that produced by a 0.5 mg bolus dose of intrathecal morphine is likely to be of the order of 5 mg for pethidine and close to 8.5 mg for methadone.

Clinical studies support this argument. Systemically, methadone is equipotent to morphine. From the animal work, intrathecal methadone was approximately 18-fold less potent than intrathecal morphine (McQuay et al 1989). An intrathecal dose of 0.5 mg of morphine provided significantly superior analgesia to 20 mg of methadone (Jacobson et al 1990).

For extradural use, life is even less straightforward. Previous calculations showed that the proportion of an extradural dose transferred across the dura could vary from up to 20% for morphine (low lipid solubility) to 0.2% for buprenorphine (high lipid solubility) (Moore et al 1982). Because of the significant inverse correlation between lipid solubility and potency shown for the drug once in the cerebrospinal fluid, the extradural dose of highly lipid-soluble drugs may have to be surprisingly high to give effect equianalgesic to that of 5 mg of extradural morphine.

The clinical results around this theory remain conflicting. No clinical advantage was seen with extradural fentanyl compared with intravenous injection of the same dose, either in postoperative orthopaedic pain (Loper et al 1990) or after Caesarean section (Ellis et al 1990). After laparotomy, intravenous alfentanil (0.36 mg/h), combined with epidural bupivacaine 0.125%, was as effective as epidural alfentanil (0.36 mg/h) (Van den Nieuwenhuyzen et al 1998). The classic danger, of course, is that these are A versus B trial designs, often with small numbers of patients, and may be insensitive to real differences. Others have found epidural fentanyl to provide superior analgesia compared with intravenous fentanyl, after thoracotomy (Salomäki et al 1991), during childbirth (D'Angelo et al 1998) and after Caesarean section (Cooper et al 1995). These trials are also small, with maximum group size of 20. The trials in childbirth and after Caesarean section really investigated epidural fentanyl plus local anaesthetic rather than fentanyl alone. We would conclude that this controversy shows the necessity of systemic controls in extradural studies, because the vascular uptake of a lipophilic drug from the epidural space will in itself result in analgesia and is similar in its time course and extent to the uptake seen after the same dose given parenterally.

We would also contend that lipophilic opioids on their own (not combined with local anaesthetic) are a poor choice for epidural use; non-specific binding means that they have low spinal potency and substantial systemic analgesic effect makes it difficult to determine any spinal action. In practice, bolus injection of epidural opioid is often given with, or soon after, injection of epidural local anaesthetic. Clinical impressions of good analgesia after epidural injection of lipophilic opioid may reflect synergism between the opioid and the local anaesthetic and systemic effect of the opioid.

COMBINATIONS OF LOCAL ANAESTHETIC AND OPIOID

Epidural opioids on their own did not provide reliable analgesia in several pain contexts (Husemeyer et al 1980, Hogan et al 1991). Empirically, combinations of local anaesthetic and opioid were found to work well and extradural infusions of these combinations are now widely used for postoperative pain. The benefit is analgesia with minimal motor block and hypotension.

Two experimental studies have confirmed synergism between local anaesthetic and opioid (Fig. 52.3). Using visceral as well as conventional behavioural tests, Maves and Gebhart (1992) did an isobolographic analysis for morphine and lignocaine. They showed that the analgesic effect of the intrathecal combination was greater than would be expected for a simply additive relationship. Using an electrophysiological model, Fraser et al (1992) compared the dose-response curve for lignocaine combined with a dose of morphine with the dose-response curve for lignocaine alone. Adding morphine, at a dose well below the ED_{50}, produced a 10-fold leftward shift in the lignocaine dose-response curve.

These studies support what has been observed clinically, that doses of local anaesthetic and opioid, doses which might be regarded as homeopathic for either drug independently, can produce good analgesia. Neither study was designed to answer the important question of the minimal effective doses of the combination components. While the minimum effective doses will vary with pain context, studies answering the question for one type of pain may tell us which component is the prime mover. The mechanism of the synergy is not known. It may be that the local anaesthetic, by reducing the afferent input, is moving the opioid dose-response to the right. Such explanations, however, only account for one direction of synergy and the evidence suggests that the synergy is bidirectional (see Fig. 52.3). Clinical observations suggest that chronic infusion of the combination can produce selective blockade, blocking pain fibres while leaving other sensory input (and motor function) intact. These contradict the observation that block of pain by epidural opioid alone is associated with blunting of sensitivity to cold and pin-scratch sufficient for a segmental effect on cutaneous sensation to be detectable (Bromage et al 1982a). Such selectivity may, of course, be dose dependent.

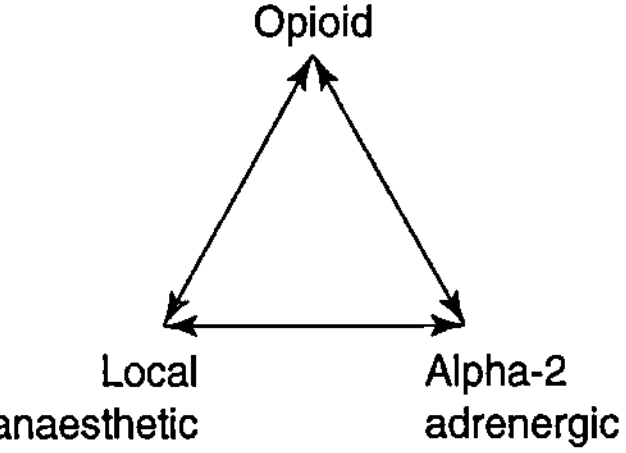

Fig. 52.3 Interactions between epidural local anaesthetic, opioid and α_2-adrenergic agonists.

OTHER DRUGS

Many drugs have been given as analgesics via the epidural route. Steroids given for the management of back pain have already been mentioned. Caveats about toxicity are necessary.

α_2-Adrenergic agonists

In both electrophysiological (Sullivan et al 1987) and behavioural studies, α_2-adrenergic agonists have an antinociceptive effect. Much of the early work was with clonidine and this may have been misleading in terms of the properties of purer α_2-adrenergic agonists. Intrathecal clonidine showed a plateau at 50% of maximum effect. The newer drug, dexmedetomidine, is considerably more potent than clonidine and did not show such a ceiling to antinociception (Sullivan et al 1992a).

α_2-Adrenergic agonists have synergistic effect with both spinal opioid (Sullivan et al 1987, 1992b, Ossipov et al 1989) and spinal local anaesthetic (see Fig. 52.3). The evidence for the local anaesthetic interaction comes mainly from clinical studies (Racle et al 1988, Bonnet et al 1989b, 1990, Carabine et al 1992, Huntoon et al 1992).

Midazolam

Midazolam on its own has a very limited antinociceptive effect in standard behavioural or electrophysiological models (Clavier et al 1992, Dirig & Yaksh 1995), although effects have been found in other models (Niv et al 1983, Goodchild & Serrao 1987). Midazolam may have effects on A∂ fibres (Clavier et al 1992) and may interact when combined with opioid (Moreau & Pieri 1988).

THERAPEUTIC ASPECTS

Both epidural local anaesthetics and epidural opioids can produce analgesia. The adverse effects of the two drug classes are different. Epidural local anaesthetics can produce hypotension because of sympathetic blockade and carry the risks of local anaesthetic toxicity for which there is no specific antagonist. Epidural local anaesthetics produce motor block in a dose-dependent way. Epidural opioids can produce delayed respiratory depression, urinary retention, pruritus and nausea and vomiting, particularly in the opioid-naive patient. Naloxone is a specific antagonist. Epidural opioids do not produce a motor block. The combination of epidural local anaesthetic and opioid can also produce pain relief and the synergism between the drug classes offers the potential of effective analgesia at low doses of the components, minimizing the adverse effects of both. These features are summarized in Table 52.2.

Analgesic effect of epidural analgesics can be measured by a number of techniques, directly by measuring decrease in intensity or increase in pain relief or indirectly via decreased need for other (parenteral) analgesics. Comparison with other, non-epidural methods of pain relief has also involved indirect measures, such as the relative effects on respiration, time for patients to recover and effects on stress hormones. The ultimate arbiter has to be analgesic effect because indirect measures, such as reduction of the expected rise of stress hormones, do not have a direct relationship with analgesia.

For many years, RCTs which compared the analgesia and adverse effects of oral or parenteral analgesics used the rule that sensible comparisons of adverse effect incidence can only be made when the study drugs are compared at equianalgesic dosage. Very few RCTs which compare the adverse effects of different epidural opioids (or, indeed, epidural opioids with other techniques) have made equianalgesia the key criterion. Pronouncements about relative incidence of adverse effects can carry little weight unless the disparity in incidence or severity is measured at doses which produce equivalent analgesic effect.

The clinical decision to use epidural analgesia for pain relief is just that, a clinical decision. It presupposes that the analgesia is as good or better than analgesia from lower

Table 52.2 Effects of local epidural anaesthetics and epidural opioids and of the combination

	Local anaesthetics	*Opioids*	*Combination*
Quality of blockade			
Sensory block	All modalities, dose dependent	Mainly pain	Mainly pain
LA dose-dependent sympathetic block	Yes, dose dependent	None	LA dose dependent
Motor block	Slight to complete, dose dependent	None	LA dose dependent
Vascular uptake	Dose dependent and reduced by adrenaline	Reduced by adrenaline 1:200 000	
Possible to limit segmental blockade	Yes	Yes, but may spread rostrally	
Duration of action	Short	Variable, drug dependent	(Infusion)
Adverse effects			
Central respiratory depression	No	Yes, dose dependent	Minimal (low doses)
Urinary retention	Yes, relatively short	Yes, may be very prolonged	Minimal (low doses)
Pruritus	No	Yes	Minimal (low doses)
Nausea and vomiting	No	Yes	Minimal (low doses)

LA = local anaesthetic

technology methods, that the potentially higher risk of adverse effects is worthwhile and that the facilities exist to deliver the epidural analgesia effectively and safely. Combination techniques are superseding the use of epidural opioids on their own and the RCTs to define the clinical role are still emerging.

ACUTE PAIN

Analgesia

Although both epidural local anaesthetics and epidural opioids can produce analgesia, there is some doubt about the ability of epidural opioids to produce analgesia as good (Husemeyer et al 1980) as epidural local anaesthetics in severe pain states. In childbirth, the degree of analgesia was inadequate to relieve the pain of second-stage labour (Husemeyer et al 1980, Hughes et al 1984), although satisfactory relief of first-stage pain could be achieved. No such doubt is seen with the epidural combination of local anaesthetics and opioids. The difference between the pain severity of different pain states should be emphasized, because it also means that categoric prescriptions for the doses to be used in combination infusions are likely to be valid only for a particular pain state or set of circumstances. Indeed, the dynamic nature of postoperative pain means that the dosage required on the day of surgery may be much higher than the dosage required on subsequent days.

A clear demonstration of the advantage of the combination of local anaesthetic and opioid was seen in a comparison of 0.125% bupivacaine in saline, diamorphine 0.5 mg in 15 ml and diamorphine mixed with 0.125% bupivacaine (0.5 mg in 15 ml) infused at a rate of 15 ml/h for pain after major gynaecological surgery. The combination produced analgesia significantly superior to either of its components alone, without major adverse effects (Lee et al 1988). Giving the diamorphine intravenously with epidural bupivacaine was significantly less effective than giving the same dose epidurally in combination with epidural bupivacaine (Lee et al 1991).

Many important questions are still to be answered. One practical issue is the ability of combination infusions to control pain remote from the catheter site, as with thoracic pain and a lumbar catheter. Another is whether there is any difference in efficacy or adverse effects if the drugs are given continuously rather than intermittently. For local anaesthetic alone, there was little difference (Duncan et al 1998).

Combination dosage

Three strategies in dosage are discernible, the low (Cullen et al 1985, Logas et al 1987, Lee et al 1988), the intermediate (Bigler et al 1989, Seeling et al 1990) and the high (Hjortso et al 1985, Schulze et al 1988, Scott et al 1989). High doses (bupivacaine 0.5% 25 mg/h and morphine 0.5 mg/h) were used to produce analgesia immediately after upper abdominal surgery but at some risk (Scott et al 1989). The stress response was not blocked. Lower doses (bupivacaine 0.1% 4 mg/h and morphine 0.4 mg/h) did not provide total pain relief after thoracotomy (Logas et al 1987). The issue of the minimum effective dose is of great importance and, unfortunately, may have to be defined for particular circumstances. It is too early (and too circumstance dependent) for consensus to emerge but an intermediate dose, 0.25% bupivacaine 10 mg/h with morphine 0.2 mg/h, has its advocates for use in pain after major surgery.

Other analgesics

α_2-Adrenergic agonists The rôle of these drugs as analgesics on their own remains unclear. It is very difficult to preserve the double blinding in studies of α_2-adrenergic agonists because of the hypotensive and sedative effects of the drugs. Comparisons of epidural clonidine with epidural placebo for postoperative pain relief are all marred by this fault because significant hypotension was a feature (Gordh 1988, Bonnet et al 1989a, Bernard et al 1991). No analgesic dose-response curve could be defined for clonidine (Mendez et al 1990).

There is clear evidence, however, for both enhancement of the effect of local anaesthetics (Racle et al 1988, Bonnet et al 1989b, 1990, Carabine et al 1992, Huntoon et al 1992) and enhancement of the effect of opioids. With fentanyl (Rostaing et al 1991) and sufentanil (Vercauteren et al 1990) duration of effect was extended; with morphine Motsch et al (1990) found that adding clonidine produced significantly better pain scores. There may thus be an adjuvant rôle for α_2-adrenergic agonists.

Midazolam Midazolam is reported to have analgesic effect in postoperative pain (see Serrao et al 1992) but this is hard to understand in view of the drug's failure in animal nociceptive pain models.

Adverse effects

Toxicity

Epidural delivery necessarily places drugs at the neuraxis. Toxicity is therefore a real risk. Standard epidural analgesics, specifically local anaesthetics and opioids, have not produced toxicity to date and clonidine was tested before it was used.

Perhaps the major worry is that new analgesics without toxicology will be introduced.

Motor block

Techniques of epidural local anaesthesia have been refined to a point where the neural pathways conducting pain can be blocked with a high degree of anatomical selectivity, but motor block is an inevitable accompaniment if large doses of local anaesthetic are needed to stop the pain. In labour pain, the motor block results in a higher incidence of instrumental delivery compared with non-epidural pain relief (Howell & Chalmers 1991) and perhaps in a higher incidence of Caesarean section (Morton et al 1994). This motor block is not seen with epidural opioids alone or when low doses of local anaesthetic are combined with opioid.

Vasodilatation and hypotension

Vasodilatation in the lower parts of the body from blockade of sympathetic vasomotor nerves in the segments involved is another inevitable accompaniment of epidural local anaesthetic. In labour, this requires prophylaxis. Hypotension also occurs with α_2-adrenergic agonists and their use in combination with local anaesthetics could accentuate the risk. Again, the risk is minimized with epidural opioids alone or with the low doses of local anaesthetic used when combined with opioid.

Respiratory depression

Epidural block with local anaesthetics of intercostal and abdominal muscles is unlikely to cause significant impairment of respiratory function unless the phrenic segments (C3, C4 and C5) are also blocked. Respiratory depression after epidural opioids in opioid-naive subjects is much more subtle, more delayed in onset and longer lasting. The epidural opioids all reach the CSF by diffusion through the meninges and variable degrees of cephalad spread occur within the CSF. Morphine, being relatively less lipid soluble, will maintain substantial CSF concentrations to a greater extent than more lipid-soluble drugs, increasing the chance of drug reaching opioid receptors in the brain and so increasing the chance of respiratory depression. In volunteers, 10 mg of epidural morphine produced a depression of the CO_2 response curve far greater than that seen after intravenous administration, with the nadir of depression between the sixth and 12th hours after administration (Camporesi et al 1983).

Profound respiratory depression may be precipitated if other opioids are given parenterally during this danger period. Precautions must be taken to see that this mixed type of medication is avoided and that patients are under appropriate surveillance, so that any case of delayed respiratory depression can be treated promptly (Ready et al 1988). Life-threatening apnoeic intervals can also arise abruptly after small doses of epidural opioids alone, with little warning. Theoretically, highly lipid-soluble opioids such as fentanyl and sufentanil should be less prone to rostral spread in the CSF. In practice, volunteer studies suggest that although apnoeic intervals after epidural sufentanil were less frequent and less prolonged than after morphine (Klepper et al 1987), at equianalgesic doses of the drugs the CO_2 response curve was depressed and displaced equally severely.

Epidural opioids given on their own for relief of acute pain in opioid-naive subjects are only as safe as the quality of surveillance that is given. Whether the lower doses used in combination with local anaesthetics reduce the risk has still to be established.

Systemic effects

With epidural opioids, systemic effects of the opioid are to be expected. Vascular uptake from the epidural space is appreciable, with blood concentration curves of opioid which are almost indistinguishable from those after intramuscular or intravenous administration (see, for morphine, Bromage et al 1982a, Chauvin et al 1982, Nordberg et al 1983). All the adverse effects of systemic opioids should therefore be expected. Placental transfer of opioid to the fetus and subsequent neonatal respiratory depression are thus not prevented by changing from parenteral opioid to epidural opioid.

Bladder function

Urinary retention is a common complication of epidural analgesic techniques after either local anaesthetics or opioids. The incidence appears to be dose related and in the case of local anaesthetics, retention is probably due to bladder deafferentation because the distended bladder does not give rise to discomfort. With epidural opioids, the mechanism seems to be more complicated because retention and bladder distension to volumes above 800 ml in volunteers gave rise to marked discomfort and distress (Bromage et al 1982b).

Urodynamic and electromyographic studies in male volunteers indicated that the cause was detrusor muscle relaxation and not increased motor activity in the pelvic floor muscles (Rawal et al 1983). The origin of this detrusor relaxation is unclear, but the time sequence mirrors that of antinociception, beginning within 15 minutes but taking about 60 minutes to reach peak effect and then lasting 14–16 hours. The overall intensity and duration of bladder relaxation appears to be independent of dose within the range of 2–10 mg. Retention with epidural opioids, like all the other adverse effects of epidural opioids, can be relieved by naloxone, although repeated doses may be needed to ensure complete evacuation of the bladder (Bromage et al 1982b).

The high incidence of retention from either local anaesthetic or opioid blockade is a factor in the clinical decision to use epidural analgesia.

Pruritus

Pruritus is not seen after epidural local anaesthetics, but it is a frequent adverse effect of epidural opioids in the opioid-naive patient. The itching is usually generalized but can be in the analgesic segments. The cause of the pruritus is unclear. The onset is often hours after analgesic effect is established, perhaps suggesting modulation of cutaneous sensation in the cord. Pruritus can be a major problem in acute pain management with epidural opioids, severe enough to cause distress. It can be reversed by naloxone, but then the analgesia is likely to be reversed.

Long-term risks

Argument continues about whether or not epidural local anaesthetics in childbirth can cause chronic backache (MacArthur et al 1990, McQuay & Moore 1996b). We still need a true RCT to clarify the issue; difficult labours are more likely to need epidural block and may be associated with a higher risk of backache. If motor block with local anaesthetic is indeed the cause, rather than the delivery or the epidural procedure per se, then the use of opioids or combinations should be preferred.

CHRONIC PAIN

Epidural analgesics have roles in both chronic non-malignant pain and cancer pain.

Chronic non-malignant pain

In chronic non-malignant pain the primary role for epidural local anaesthetics is their injection combined with steroid for the management of back pain with the object of reducing local oedema and nerve root compression, although block of C-fibre transmission (Johannson et al 1990) may be the mechanism of the analgesia claimed. The trials have been mentioned above.

Epidural opioids alone have little place in the long-term management of ongoing non-malignant pain (but see Plummer et al 1991), although acute exacerbations may be handled on a one-off basis.

The rôle of epidural clonidine is contentious. Apart from its ability to extend the duration of local anaesthetics, it may also be able to relieve some forms of neuropathic or deafferentation pain. Glynn et al (1988) found epidural clonidine to be as effective as epidural morphine in 20 chronic pain patients using a crossover design. As in earlier studies, there was a suggestion that clonidine was more effective than morphine for neuropathic pain and it may be that α_2-adrenergic drugs find a place as adjuvants in local anaesthetic and opioid combinations for resistant neuropathic pain. This suggestion is supported by the findings in neuropathic cancer pain (Eisenach et al 1995).

Epidural midazolam was found in one RCT to be as effective as epidural steroid in the management of chronic back pain (Serrao et al 1992). Experience is limited, so that more studies are needed to clarify whether there is a clinical rôle.

Cancer pain

Epidural opioids are used in chronic cancer pain as an alternative to other (oral or subcutaneous) routes (Plummer et al 1991). There has been little evidence from RCTs to support the argument that better analgesia is provided at lower incidence of adverse effects. Indeed, one trial found that subcutaneous opioid was just as good as epidural opioid alone (Kalso et al 1996).

Long-term administration, either as intermittent bolus or by infusion, is technically feasible. The choice of delivery system lies between the low technology percutaneous exterior epidural catheter and micropore filter, tunnelled subcutaneous catheter with external injection port and micropore filter, high technology totally implanted system with small subcutaneous reservoir and injection port, totally implanted system with large internal reservoir and automatic metered or manually controlled dosing device. Implanted systems are more likely to maintain hygiene and convenience, in theory protecting from infection and mechanical displacement. Implanted devices have high initial costs compared with simple percutaneous approaches, but over a period of months this may even out because of the higher costs of maintaining or replacing percutaneous catheters.

These technical approaches for administering small

metered doses of spinal morphine over periods of weeks or months have proved to be well suited to home management and highly appreciated by the patients and their families. The problems include blockage, infection, pain on injection and leaks (Plummer et al 1991). It is important to be sure that the patient's pain cannot be controlled by simpler routes and that it can indeed be controlled by this method before embarking on what is a substantial undertaking (Jadad et al 1991). Preliminary trials with a percutaneous catheter to assess the effectiveness and the acceptability of adverse effects are necessary.

The main argument against the use of the epidural route as (merely) an alternative way to deliver opioid is that the opioid, whether given orally or spinally, must in the end be working at the opioid receptor. Failed management with oral opioid, failed because the pain was not responsive (Arner & Meyerson 1988, Jadad et al 1992) rather than because the opioid was not absorbed, is thus a questionable indication for epidural opioid. The protagonists can point to many thousands of patients treated. Epidural opioids alone, however, are not a universal panacea in cancer pain (Hogan et al 1991); if conventional routes for opioids do not relieve the pain, combinations of local anaesthetic and opioid appear to have a higher success rate than opioid alone.

A systematic review (Ballantyne et al 1996) compared the efficacy of epidural, subarachnoid and intracerebroventricular opioids in cancer. Intracerebroventricular therapy appeared at least as effective against pain as other approaches and was the only fixed system associated with fewer technical problems than the use of simple percutaneous epidural catheters.

Combination of Local Anaesthetic and Opioid

The situation is changing with the advent of epidural infusion of combination of local anaesthetics and opioid. Intrathecal use of such combinations in cancer pain is described by Sjöberg et al (1991). Most cancer pain, some 80%, responds to simple management with oral opioid and other analgesics. The two kinds of pain which respond badly to simple management are movement-related pain and neuropathic pain.

Movement-related pain can theoretically be controlled with oral opioid. In practice, the dose of opioid required to control the patient's pain on movement is such that the patient is soundly sedated when not moving (not in pain). Conventional wisdom is that NSAIDs should be added if they have been omitted. In practice, this often has little impact. Some such pains, for instance due to vertebral metastases, can be helped by extradural steroid. The final resort is to use continuous epidural infusion of a combination of local anaesthetic and opioid. The synergy between the local anaesthetic and the opioid means that low doses can provide analgesia with little loss of mobility. There are few RCTs of this usage. The need for greater volume means that few of the devices available for implanted infusion of opioid alone are suitable, so that percutaneous catheters and external syringe drivers may be necessary. This method appears to produce analgesia for pains poorly responsive to opioids alone. The logic, then, is that pains poorly responsive to opioid orally are unlikely to improve simply by changing the route by which the opioid is given. Epidural use of local anaesthetic and opioid can produce the necessary analgesia.

The management of neuropathic cancer pain is often not straightforward. If such pain cannot be controlled by opioid, antidepressant or anticonvulsant and steroids are inappropriate, then again epidural infusion of a combination of local anaesthetic and opioid should be considered. An RCT of 85 patients comparing 30 μg/h epidural clonidine with placebo for 14 days showed successful analgesia was commoner with epidural clonidine (45%) than with placebo (21%) and more so in neuropathic pain (56% vs 5%) (Eisenach et al 1995).

CONCLUSION

Epidural local anaesthetics have been used for many years in the management of acute pain in trauma, surgery and obstetrics, as well as in chronic pain, and their limitations and capabilities are well understood in these clinical areas. Opioids by this route are a new departure and our short experience in human subjects dates from as recently as 1979. Early enthusiasm in this field has been tempered by RCTs and the field remains dynamic, with a switch from the use of either local anaesthetics or opioids on their own to the combination of the two. The α_2-adrenergic agonists in existing forms may also have a limited rôle on their own but may interact with local anaesthetics and opioids to provide a clinical advantage. Their importance is that they suggest that other beneficial interactions may emerge.

The fact that the field is dynamic, with a recent switch to the combination of local anaesthetics and opioids, means that we do not yet have the necessary information as to minimal effective dose. Randomized controlled trials are thus required to define the clinical role of epidural combinations versus non-epidural pain relief in all the various pain contexts. There is still major concern that these powerful analgesic tools should be used effectively, safely and economically. The dream of attaining prolonged and powerful analgesia without adverse effects has not yet been realized and as far as these epidural techniques are concerned, pain relief must still be bought at the cost of some risk. In some areas of pain management, however, these techniques are radically changing the quality of the service we deliver.

REFERENCES

Arner S, Lindblom U, Meyerson BA, Molander C 1990 Prolonged relief of neuralgia after regional anesthetic blocks. A call for further experimental and systematic clinical studies. Pain 43:287–297

Arner S, Meyerson BA 1988 Lack of analgesic effect of opioids on neuropathic and idiopathic forms of pain. Pain 33:11–23

Aromaa U, Lahdensuu M, Cozanitis DA 1997 Severe complications associated with epidural and spinal anaesthesias in Finland 1987–1993. A study based on patient insurance claims. Acta Anaesthesiologica Scandinavica 41:445–452

Auroy Y, Narchi P, Messiah A et al 1997 Serious complications related to regional anesthesia: results of a prospective survey in France. Anesthesiology 87:479–486

Ballantyne JC, Carr DB, Berkey CS, Chalmers TC, Mosteller F 1996 Comparative efficacy of epidural, subarachnoid, and intracerebroventricular opioids in patients with pain due to cancer. Regional Anesthesia 21:542–556

Ballantyne JC, Carr DB, DeFerranti S et al 1998 The comparative effects of postoperative analgesic therapies on pulmonary outcome: cumulative meta-analyses of randomized, controlled trials. Anesthesia and Analgesia 86:598–612

Bardram L, Funch-Jensen P, Jensen P, Crawford ME, Kehlet H 1995 Recovery after laparoscopic colonic surgery with epidural analgesia, and early oral nutrition and mobilisation. Lancet 345:763–764

Beattie C, Roizen MF, Downing JW 1996 Cardiac outcomes after regional or general anesthesia: do we know the question? Anesthesiology 85:1207–1209

Beliveau P 1971 A comparison between epidural anaesthesia with and without corticosteroid in the treatment of sciatica. Rheumatology and Physical Medicine 11:40–43

Bernard J-M, Hommeril J-L, Passuti N, Pinaud M 1991 Postoperative analgesia by intravenous clonidine. Anesthesiology 75:577–582

Bigler D, Dirkes W, Hansen R, Rosenberg J, Kehlet H 1989 Effects of thoracic paravertebral block with bupivacaine versus combined thoracic epidural block with bupivacaine and morphine on pain and pulmonary function after cholecystectomy. Acta Anaesthesiologica Scandinavica 33:561–564

Bode RH Jr, Lewis KP, Zarich SW et al 1996 Cardiac outcome after peripheral vascular surgery. Comparison of general and regional anesthesia. Anesthesiology 84:3–13

Bonnet F, Boico O, Rostaing S et al 1989a Postoperative analgesia with extradural clonidine. British Journal of Anaesthesia 63:465–469

Bonnet F, Buisson VB, Francois Y, Catoire P, Saada M 1990 Effects of oral and subarachnoid clonidine on spinal anesthesia with bupivacaine. Regional Anesthesia 15:211–214

Bonnet F, Diallo A, Saada M et al 1989b Prevention of tourniquet pain by spinal isobaric bupivacaine with clonidine. British Journal of Anaesthesia 63:93–96

Breivik H, Hesla PE, Molnar I, Lind B 1976 Treatment of chronic low back pain and sciatica: comparison of caudal epidural injections of bupivacaine and methylprednisolone with bupivacaine followed by saline. In: Bonica J J, Albe-Fessard D (eds) Advances in pain research and therapy, vol 1. Raven Press, New York, pp 927–932

Bromage PR, Camporesi EM, Durant PAC , Nielson CH 1982a Rostral spread of epidural morphine. Anesthesiology 56:431–436

Bromage PR, Camporesi EM, Durant PAC, Nielson CH 1982b Nonrespiratory side effects of epidural morphine. Anesthesia and Analgesia 61:490–495

Bromage PR, Joyal AC, Binney JC 1963 Local anaesthetic drugs: penetration from the spinal extradural space into the neuraxis. Science 140:392–393

Burm AGL, Van Kleef JW, Gladines MPRR, Olthof G, Spierdijk J 1986 Epidural anesthesia with lidocaine and bupivacaine: effects of epinephrine on the plasma concentration profiles. Anesthesia and Analgesia 65:1281–1284

Bush K, Hillier S 1991 A controlled study of caudal epidural injections of triamcinolone plus procaine for the management of intractable sciatica. Spine 16:572–575

Callesen T, Bech K, Kehlet H 1998 The feasibility, safety and cost of infiltration anaesthesia for hernia repair. Hvidovre Hospital Hernia Group. Anaesthesia 53:31–35

Camporesi EM, Nielson CH, Bromage PR, Durant PAC 1983 Ventilatory CO_2 sensitivity following intravenous and epidural morphine in volunteers. Anesthesia and Analgesia 62:633–640

Carabine UA, Milligan KR, Moore J 1992 Extradural clonidine and bupivacaine for postoperative analgesia. British Journal of Anaesthesia 68:132–135

Carette S, Leclaire R, Marcoux S et al 1997 Epidural corticosteroid injections for sciatica due to herniated nucleus pulposus. New England Journal of Medicine 336:1634–1640

Chauvin M, Samii K, Schermann JM et al 1982 Plasma pharmacokinetics of morphine after i.m. extradural and intrathecal administration. British Journal of Anaesthesia 54:843–847

Christopherson R, Beattie C, Frank S M et al 1993 Perioperative morbidity in patients randomized to epidural or general anesthesia for lower extremity vascular surgery. Perioperative Ischemia Randomized Anesthesia Trial Study Group. Anesthesiology 79:422–434

Clavier N, Lombard M-C, Besson J-M 1992 Benzodiazepines and pain: effects of midazolam on the activities of nociceptive non-specific dorsal horn neurons in the rat spinal cord. Pain 48:61–71

Cooper DW, Ryall DM, Desira WR 1995 Extradural fentanyl for postoperative analgesia: predominant spinal or systemic action? British Journal of Anaesthesia 74:184–187

Cuckler JM, Bernini PA, Wiesel SW et al 1985 The use of epidural steroids in the treatment of lumbar radicular pain. Journal of Bone and Joint Surgery 67A:63–66

Cullen ML, Staren ED, El-Ganzouri A et al 1985 Continuous epidural infusion for analgesia after major abdominal operations: a randomised, prospective, double-blind study. Surgery 10:718–728

D'Angelo R, Gerancher JC, Eisenach JC, Raphael BL 1998 Epidural fentanyl produces labor analgesia by a spinal mechanism. Anesthesiology 88:1519–1523

Dickenson AH, Sullivan AF, McQuay HJ 1990 Intrathecal etorphine, fentanyl and buprenorphine on spinal nociceptive neurones in the rat. Pain 42:227–234

Dilke TFW, Burry HC, Grahame R 1973 Extradural corticosteroid injection in management of lumbar nerve root compression. British Medical Journal 2:635–637

Dirig DM, Yaksh TL 1995 Intrathecal baclofen and muscimol, but not midazolam, are antinociceptive using the rat-formalin model.

Journal of Pharmacology and Experimental Therapeutics 275:219–227

Duncan LA, Fried MJ, Lee A, Wildsmith JA 1998 Comparison of continuous and intermittent administration of extradural bupivacaine for analgesia after lower abdominal surgery. British Journal of Anaesthesia 80:7–10

Durant PAC, Yaksh TL 1986 Distribution in cerebrospinal fluid, blood, and lymph of epidurally injected morphine and inulin in dogs. Anesthesia and Analgesia 65:583–592

Eisenach JC, DuPen S, Dubois M, Miguel R, Allin D 1995 Epidural clonidine analgesia for intractable cancer pain. The Epidural Clonidine Study Group. Pain 61:391–399

Ellis DJ, Millar WL, Reisner LS 1990 A randomised double-blind comparison of epidural versus intravenous fentanyl infusion for analgesia after Cesarian section. Anesthesiology 72:981–986

Fraser HM, Chapman V, Dickenson AH 1992 Spinal local anaesthetic actions on afferent evoked responses and wind-up of nociceptive neurones in the rat spinal cord: combination with morphine produces marked potentiation of nociception. Pain 49:33–41

Giaufre E, Dalens B, Gombert A 1996 Epidemiology and morbidity of regional anesthesia in children: a one-year prospective survey of the French-Language Society of Pediatric Anesthesiologists. Anesthesia and Analgesia 83:904–912

Glynn C, Dawson D, Sanders R 1988 A double blind comparison between epidural morphine and epidural clonidine in patients with chronic non cancer pain. Pain 34:123–128

Goodchild CS, Serrao JM 1987 Intrathecal midazolam in the rat: evidence for spinally-mediated analgesia. British Journal of Anaesthesia 59:1563–1570

Gordh T Jr 1988 Epidural clonidine for treatment of postoperative pain after thoracotomy. A double blind placebo controlled study. Acta Anaesthesiologica Scandinavica 32:702–709

Herz A, Teschemacher H J 1971 Activities and sites of antinociceptive action of morphine like analgesics. Advances in Drug Research 6:79–119

Hjortso NC, Neumann P, Frosig F et al 1985 A controlled study on the effect of epidural analgesia with local anaesthetics and morphine on morbidity after abdominal surgery. Acta Anaesthesiologica Scandinavica 29:790–796

Hogan Q, Haddox JD, Abram S et al 1991 Epidural opiates and local anaesthetics for the management of cancer pain. Pain 46:271–279

Howell CJ, Chalmers I 1991 A review of prospectively controlled comparisons of epidural forms of pain relief during labour. International Journal of Obstetric Anesthesia 2:1–17

Hughes SC, Rosen MA, Shnider SM et al 1984 Maternal and neonatal effects of epidural morphine for labor and delivery. Anesthesia and Analgesia 63:319–324

Huntoon M, Eisenach JC, Boese P 1992 Epidural clonidine after cesarian section. Anesthesiology 76:187–193

Husemeyer RP, O'Connor MC, Davenport HT 1980 Failure of epidural morphine to relieve pain in labour. Anaesthesia 35:161–163

Jacobson L, Chabal C, Brody MC, Ward RJ, Wasse L 1990 Intrathecal methadone: a dose-response study and comparison with intrathecal morphine 0.5 mg. Pain 43:141–148

Jadad AR, Carroll D, Glynn CJ, Moore RA, McQuay HJ 1992 Morphine responsiveness of chronic pain: double-blind randomised crossover study with patient-controlled analgesia. Lancet 339:1367–1371

Jadad AR, Popat MT, Glynn CJ, McQuay HJ 1991 Double-blind testing fails to confirm analgesic response to extradural morphine. Anaesthesia 46:935–937

Jamous MA, Hand CW, Moore RA, Teddy PJ, McQuay HJ 1986 Epinephrine reduces systemic absorption of extradural diacetylmorphine. Anesthesia and Analgesia 65:1290–1294

Johannson A, Hao J, Sjölund B 1990 Local corticosteroid application blocks transmission in normal nociceptive C-fibres. Acta Anaesthesiologica Scandinavica 34:335–338

Kalso E, Heiskanen T, Rantio M, Rosenberg PH, Vainio A 1996 Epidural and subcutaneous morphine in the management of cancer pain: a double-blind cross-over study. Pain 67:443–449

Kehlet H 1994 Postoperative pain relief – what is the issue? British Journal of Anaesthesia 72:375–378

Kehlet H 1997 Multimodal approach to control postoperative pathophysiology and rehabilitation. British Journal of Anaesthesia 78:606–617

Kehlet H, Callesen T 1998 Recommendations for convalescence after hernia surgery. A questionnaire study. Ugeskrift for Laeger 160:1008–1009

King JS 1984 Dexamethasone – a helpful adjunct in management after lumbar discectomy. Neurosurgery 14:697–700

Klenerman L, Greenwood R, Davenport HT, White DC, Peskett S 1984 Lumbar epidural injections in the treatment of sciatica. British Journal of Rheumatology 23:35–38

Klepper ID, Sherrill DL, Boetger CL, Bromage PR 1987 The analgesic and respiratory effects of epidural sufentanil and the influence of adrenaline as an adjuvant. Anesthesiology 59:1147–1159

Koes BW, Scholten RPM, Mens JMA, Bouter LM 1995 Efficacy of epidural steroid injections for low-back pain and sciatica: a systematic review of randomized clinical trials. Pain 63:279–288

Lander J, Brady-Fryer B, Metcalfe JB, Nazarali S, Muttitt S 1997 Comparison of ring block, dorsal penile nerve block, and topical anesthesia for neonatal circumcision: a randomized controlled trial. Journal of the American Medical Association 278:2157–2162

Lee A, McKeown D, Brockway M, Bannister J, Wildsmith JAW 1991 Comparison of extradural and intravenous diamorphine as a supplement to extradural bupivacaine. Anaesthesia 46:447–450

Lee A, Simpson D, Whitfield A, Scott DB 1988 Postoperative analgesia by continuous extradural infusion of bupivacaine and diamorphine. British Journal of Anaesthesia 60:845–850

Lipfert P, Seitz RJ, Arndt J O 1987 Ultralong-lasting nerve block: triethyldodectyl ammonium bromide is probably a neurotoxin rather than a local anesthetic. Anesthesiology 67:896–904

Liu SS, Carpenter RL, Mackey DC et al 1995 Effects of perioperative analgesic technique on rate of recovery after colon surgery. Anesthesiology 83:757–765

Logas WG, El Baz N, El Ganzouri A et al 1987 Continuous thoracic epidural analgesia for postoperative pain relief following thoracotomy: a randomized prospective study. Anesthesiology 67:787–791

Loper KA, Ready BL, Downey M et al 1990 Epidural and intravenous fentanyl infusions are clinically equivalent after knee surgery. Anesthesia and Analgesia 70:72–75

MacArthur C, Lewis M, Knox EG, Crawford JS 1990 Epidural analgesia and long term backache after childbirth. British Medical Journal 301:9–12

Mathews JA, Mills SB, Jenkins VM et al 1987 Back pain and sciatica: controlled trials of manipulation, traction, sclerosant and epidural injections. British Journal of Rheumatology 26:416–423

Maves TJ, Gebhart GF 1992 Antinociceptive synergy between intrathecal morphine and lidocaine during visceral and somatic nociception in the rat. Anesthesiology 76:91–99

McQuay HJ, Justins D, Moore RA 1997 Treating acute pain in hospital. British Medical Journal 314:1531–1535

McQuay HJ, Moore RA 1998 An evidence-based resource for pain relief. Oxford University Press, Oxford

McQuay HJ, Sullivan A F, Smallman K, Dickenson AH 1989 Intrathecal opioids, potency and lipophilicity. Pain 36:111–115

McQuay H, Moore A 1996a Placebos are essential when extent and variability of placebo response are unknown. British Medical Journal 313:1008

McQuay H, Moore A 1996b Epidural anaesthesia and low back pain after delivery. British Medical Journal 312:581

Mendez R, Eisenach JC, Kashtan K 1990 Epidural clonidine analgesia after cesarean section. Anesthesiology 73:848–852

Moore RA, Bullingham RE, McQuay H J et al 1982 Dural permeability to narcotics: in vitro determination and application to extradural administration. British Journal of Anaesthesia 54:1117–1128

Moreau J-L, Pieri L 1988 Effects of an intrathecally administered benzodiazepine receptor agonist, antagonist and inverse agonist on morphine-induced inhibition of a spinal nociceptive reflex. British Journal of Pharmacology 93:964–968

Morton SC, Williams MS, Keeler EB, Gambone JC, Kahn KL 1994 Effect of epidural analgesia for labor on the cesarean delivery rate. Obstetrics and Gynecology 83:1045–1052

Motsch J, Graber E, Ludwig K 1990 Addition of clonidine enhances postoperative analgesia from epidural morphine: a double blind study. Anesthesiology 73:1067–1073

Moulin DE, Inturrisi CE, Foley KM 1986 Epidural and intrathecal opioids: cerebrospinal fluid and plasma pharmacokinetics in cancer pain patients. Opioid analgesics in the management of cancer pain. In: Foley K M, Inturrisi C E (eds) Advances in pain research and therapy, vol 8. Raven Press, New York, pp 369–383

Nehra D, Gemmell L, Pye JK 1995 Pain relief after inguinal hernia repair: a randomized double-blind study. British Journal of Surgery 82:1245–1247

Niv D, Whitwam JG, Loh L 1983 Depression of nociceptive sympathetic reflexes by the intrathecal administration of midazolam. British Journal of Anaesthesia 55:541–547

Nordberg G, Hedner T, Mellstrand T, Dahlstrom B 1983 Pharmacokinetic aspects of epidural morphine analgesia. Anesthesiology 58:545–551

Ossipov MH, Suarez LJ, Spaulding TC 1989 Antinociceptive interactions between alpha2-adrenergic and opiate agonists at the spinal level in rodents. Anesthesia and Analgesia 68:194–200

Plummer JL, Cherry DA, Cousins MJ et al 1991 Long term spinal administration of morphine in cancer and non-cancer pain: a retrospective study. Pain 44:215–220

Popiolek A, Domanik A, Mazurkiewicz G 1991 Leczenie sterydowymi ostrzknieciami nadopow owymi chorychz prewlekla rwa kulszowa w przebiegu dyskopatti. [Epidural injections of steroids in the treatment of patients with chronic sciatica in discopathy.] Neurologia i Neurochirurgia Polska 25(5): 640–646

Racle JP, Poy JY, Benkhadra A, Jourdren L, Fockenier F 1988 Prolongation of spinal anesthesia with hyperbaric bupivacaine by adrenaline and clonidine in the elderly. Annales Francaises d'Anesthesie et de Reanimation 7:139–144

Rawal N, Möllefors K, Axelsson K, Lingårdh G, Widman B 1983 An experimental study of urodynamic effects of epidural morphine and naloxone reversal. Anesthesia and Analgesia 62:641–647

Ready LB, Oden R, Chadwick HS et al 1988 Development of an anaesthesiology based postoperative pain management service. Anesthesiology 68:100–106

Ridley MG, Kingsley GH, Gibson T, Grahame R 1988 Outpatient lumbar epidural corticosteroid injection in the management of sciatica. British Journal of Rheumatology 27:295–299

Rigg JRA, Jamrozik K 1998 Outcome after general or regional anaesthesia in high-risk patients. Current Opinion in Anaesthesiology 11:327–331

Rostaing S, Bonnet F, Levron JC et al 1991 Effect of epidural clonidine on analgesia and pharmacokinetics of epidural fentanyl in postoperative patients. Anesthesiology 75:420–425

Salomäki TE, Laitinen JO, Nuutinen LS 1991 A randomised double-blind comparison of epidural versus intravenous fentanyl infusion for analgesia after thoracotomy. Anesthesiology 75:790–795

Schulze S, Roikjaer O, Hasselstrom L, Jensen NH, Kehlet H 1988 Epidural bupivacaine and morphine plus systemic indomethacin eliminates pain but not systemic response and convalescence after cholecystectomy. Surgery 103:321–327

Scott NB, Mogensen T, Bigler D, Lund C, Kehlet H 1989 Continuous thoracic extradural 0.5% bupivacaine with or without morphine: effect on quality of blockade, lung function and the surgical stress response. British Journal of Anaesthesia 62:253–257

Scurlock JE, Curtis BM 1981 Tetraethylammonium derivatives: ultralong-acting local anesthetics. Anesthesiology 54:265–269

Seeling W, Bruckmooser KP, Hufner C et al 1990 No reduction in postoperative complications by the use of catheterized epidural analgesia following major abdominal surgery. Anaesthesist 39:33–40

Serrao JM, Marks RL, Morley SJ, Goodchild CS 1992 Intrathecal midazolam for the treatment of chronic mechanical low back pain: a controlled comparison with epidural steroid in a pilot study. Pain 48:5–12

Sharrock NE, Salvati EA 1996 Hypotensive epidural anesthesia for total hip arthroplasty: a review. Acta Orthopaedica Scandinavica 67:91–107

Sjöberg M, Applegren L, Einarsson S et al 1991 Long-term intrathecal morphine and bupivacaine in 'refractory' cancer pain. I. Results from the first series of 52 patients. Acta Anaesthesiologica Scandinavica 35:30–43

Snoek W, Weber H, Jorgenson B 1977 Double blind evaluation of extradural methyl prednisolone for herniated lumbar discs. Acta Orthopaedica Scandinavica 48:635–641

Sullivan AF, Dashwood MR, Dickenson AH 1987 Alpha adrenoceptor modulation of nociception in rat spinal cord: location, effects and interactions with morphine. European Journal of Pharmacology 138:169–177

Sullivan AF, Kalso EA, McQuay HJ, Dickenson AH 1992a The antinociceptive actions of dexmedetomidine on dorsal horn neuronal responses in the anaesthetized rat. European Journal of Pharmacology 215:127–133

Sullivan AF, Kalso EA, McQuay HJ, Dickenson AH 1992b Evidence for the involvement of the mu but not delta opioid receptor subtype in the synergistic interaction between opioid and alpha 2 adrenergic antinociception in the rat spinal cord. Neuroscience Letters 139:65–68

Swerdlow M, Sayle-Creer W 1969 A study of extradural medication in the relief of lumbosciatic syndrome. Anaesthesia 23:341–345

Teasdale C, McCrum AM, Williams NB, Horton RE 1982 A randomised controlled trial to compare local with general anaesthesia for short-stay inguinal hernia repair. Annals of the Royal College of Surgeons of England 64:238–242

Van den Nieuwenhuyzen MC, Stienstra R, Burm AG, Vletter AA, Van Kleef J W 1998 Alfentanil as an adjuvant to epidural bupivacaine in the management of postoperative pain after laparotomies: lack of evidence of spinal action. Anesthesia and Analgesia 86:574–578

Vercauteren M, Lauwers E, Meert T, De Hert S, Adriaensen H 1990 Comparison of epidural sufentanil plus clonidine with sufentanil alone for postoperative pain relief. Anaesthesia 45:531–534

Watts RW, Silagy CA 1995 A meta-analysis on the efficacy of epidural corticosteroids in the treatment of sciatica. Anaesthesia and Intensive Care 23:564–569

Williams-Russo P, Sharrock NE, Haas SB et al 1996 Randomized trial of epidural versus general anesthesia: outcomes after primary total knee replacement. Clinical Orthopaedics 199–208

Williams-Russo P, Sharrock NE, Mattis S, Szatrowski TP, Charlson ME 1995 Cognitive effects after epidural vs general anesthesia in older adults. A randomized trial. JAMA 274:44–50

Yaksh TL, Noueihed R 1985 The physiology and pharmacology of spinal opiates. Annual Review of Pharmacology and Toxicology 25:433–462

Yeager MP, Glass DD, Neff RK, Brinck-Johnsen T 1987 Epidural anaesthesia and analgesia in high risk surgical patients. Anesthesiology 66:729–736

Yuen EC, Layzer RB, Weitz SR, Olney RK 1995 Neurologic complications of lumbar epidural anesthesia and analgesia. Neurology 45:1795–1801

Other drugs including sympathetic blockers

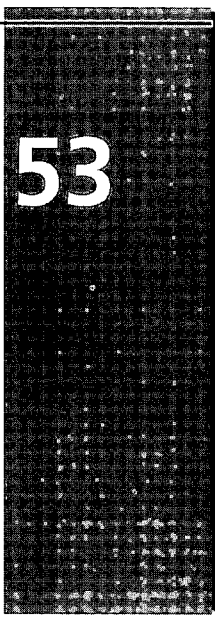

R. MUNGLANI & R. G. HILL

INTRODUCTION

The understanding of the physiology and pharmacology of pain is increasing at a rapid rate. This is making new therapeutic strategies increasingly accessible. This chapter deals with some of the new developments and also attempts to deal with the mechanisms and utility of drugs originally introduced for other therapeutic targets but which have been found empirically to have a place in the treatment of pain. We also try to put the established techniques of sympathetic block in their proper context following the lead set by Hannington Kiff (1994) in his contributions to earlier editions of this book. Although there is inevitably some overlap with other chapters dealing with the preclinical pharmacology of analgesia the emphasis here is on drugs which have been evaluated in the clinic or are in routine clinical use but have as yet an incompletely explained mechanism of action.

ATYPICAL ANALGESIC DRUGS

ADRENOCEPTOR AGONISTS FOR SPINAL ANALGESIA

It has been known for some time that the α_2 adrenoceptor agonist clonidine has distinct analgesic properties when given either systemically or spinally, which are separable from its other pharmacology. The use of this drug as an analgesic is limited by the sedative and vasodepressor properties which are produced by similar doses. The ratio of unwanted to wanted effects can be maximized by giving clonidine intrathecally and it also works well when given epidurally. It has been claimed to be effective against acute and chronic pains, including cancer pain (Coombs et al 1985, Eisenach et al 1989, 1995) and may be effective in patients who have become tolerant to opioids or are suffering neuropathic pain. In a multicentre double-blind trial, epidural clonidine given concomittantly with epidural morphine improved pain relief in patients with severe cancer pain (Eisenach et al 1995). Only those patients with neuropathic pain benefitted from this treatment. Falls in systemic blood pressure after epidural clonidine were rated as severe in only two patients out of 38 studied and incidence of dry mouth and sedation was similar to that seen on morphine alone.

Clonidine is used on occasion as an adjunct to other analgesic drugs and has been shown to potentiate the action of opioids and local anaesthetics. Related drugs have similar properties, e.g. xylazine and dexmedetomidine. The postsynaptic mechanism of the analgesic effect is similar to that of morphine and is exerted via postsynaptic receptors on central sensory neurones that are coupled to a K^+ channel, such that increasing outward K^+ conductance reduces cellular excitability.

Recent studies using selective antibodies to identify the localization of the $_{A,B}$ and $_C$ subtypes of α_2 receptor within the dorsal horn of the spinal cord suggest that the α_{2A} receptor is responsible for the analgesic properties (Stone et al 1998). This conclusion is supported by the observation that in mice with the gene for the α_{2A} receptor mutated to substitute the vital aspartate residue at position 79 with arginine, dexmedetomidine and clonidine are no longer capable of producing analgesia, anaesthesia sparing or hyperpolarization of locus ceruleus neurons (Lakhlani et al 1997). This is unfortunate as in these mutant mice rotarod performance impairment and loss of righting reflex effects of clonidine are also lost, suggesting that the same receptor produces the sedative and vasodepressor effects and thus it is unlikely that an improved α_2 agonist analgesic will be discovered. There is some suggestion that a family of related imidazoline receptors exist which are responsible for some of the pharmacology of clonidine and its analogues but these have not yet been cloned and thus cannot be considered as viable drug discovery targets. An extensive review of the role of monoamines and their receptors in the control of nociception can be found in Millan (1997).

SEROTONIN RECEPTOR LIGANDS

Serotonin or 5-hydroxytryptamine (5HT) has been implicated in the control of pain sensation as a result of physiological studies on the descending inhibition of dorsal horn nociception by stimulation of 5HT-containing pathways originating in the vicinity of the midbrain raphe nuclei. The use of 5HT receptor agonists as analgesics has been very limited to date due to the lack of agents which are selective for the different receptor subtypes (14 to date) and also to limiting side effects (nausea, sedation, decreased blood pressure) that have been seen with the agents which have been evaluated in man. It is unlikely that the analgesic properties of tricyclic antidepressants are due to effects on 5HT as the selective 5HT uptake blockers such as fluoxetine and paroxetine appear less useful for the treatment of pain than the non-selective agents such as amitriptyline. It has recently been suggested, however, that the novel analgesic DUP-631 works by blocking uptake of both 5HT and noradrenaline (Cook & Schmidt 1997) and this has also been suggested as the underlying factor behind the analgesic actions of tricyclic antidepressants (Godfrey 1996) although other mechanisms such as ion channel blockade have been suggested (see below).

The $5HT_{1B/D}$ agonists such as sumatriptan, zolmitriptan, naratriptan and rizatriptan are extremely effective in the treatment of migraine headache but do not appear to be generally analgesic. This is likely to be attributable to a selective regional distribution of these receptors such that, for example, sensory input within the dorsal horn of the spinal cord originating in the occipital division of the trigeminal nerve can be attenuated by agents of this class (Storer & Goadsby 1997) but that from lumbar dorsal roots cannot (Cumberbatch et al 1998). Activation of meningeal $5HT_{2B}$ receptors has been suggested to be an early stage in the generation of migraine headache (Schmuck et al 1996) and blockade of $5HT_2$ receptors will reduce c-fos expression in the rat trigeminal complex following noxious peripheral stimuli (Ebersberger et al 1995).

Many different 5HT receptors have been found on sensory neurons, including $5HT_{1A}$, $5HT_2$, $5HT_3$ and $5HT_4$. It is interesting to note that $5HT_4$ receptors have been shown to couple positively to tetrodotoxin-insensitive sodium channels in a subpopulation of capsaicin-sensitive rat sensory neurons (Cardenas et al 1997). This is consistent with previous observations showing that 5HT and PGs together powerfully excite peripheral nociceptors and raises the possibility of using $5HT_4$ antagonists as analgesics. It has also been suggested that $5HT_{2A}$ receptors are involved in the peripheral mechanisms leading to thermal hyperalgesia, however (Tokunaga et al 1998).

EXCITATORY AMINO ACID RECEPTOR ANTAGONISTS

Glutamate is the most widely distributed excitatory neurotransmitter in the central nervous system and is probably released by all primary afferent fibres synapsing with secondary sensory neurons in the dorsal horn of the spinal cord (see Salt & Hill 1983 for historical review). It is now known that glutamate can act at two families of ionotropic receptors, for convenience referred to as NMDA and non-NMDA receptors, and at a group of G-protein coupled receptors known as the metabotropic glutamate receptors. The majority of studies in man have used agents that act at NMDA receptors and thus this will be focus of the work described here but there is a strong theoretical rationale, supported by much preclinical and a small body of clinical studies, for believing that analgesic effects could be produced by drugs acting at other glutamate receptors also.

NMDA receptors

The dissociative anaesthetics phencyclidine and ketamine have long been known to have pronounced analgesic actions at subanaesthetic doses but it is only comparatively recently that this action was explained as being due to blockade of glutamate action at NMDA receptors. The utility of these agents is limited by the production of hallucinations and ataxia at doses only slightly higher than those needed to produce analgesia, but nevertheless ketamine in particular has been shown to have an application in controlling pain that may not be sensitive to other analgesic agents. Postsurgically it has been shown that ketamine will suppress the central sensitization expressed as punctate hyperalgesia around a surgical incision (Stubhaug et al 1997) and the secondary hyperalgesia in man following an experimental burn (Warnke et al 1997). Interestingly, in this latter study, the wind-up of pain caused by repeated stimulation with a

Von Frey hair in the region of secondary analgesia was suppressed by ketamine but not by morphine. In patients with the usually intractable pain of postherpetic neuralgia, subcutaneous ketamine was found to give relief (Eide et al 1995). Ketamine, although usually administered by injection as part of anaesthetic practice, has reasonable oral bioavailability and will relieve the pain of glossopharyngeal neuralgia (Eide & Stubhaug 1997) or postamputation stump pain (Nikolajsen et al 1997) when given by this route.

This is an active area for drug discovery and other ligands with a similar mechanism of action to ketamine (i.e. producing use-dependent block of the receptor-coupled ion channel) are in clinical trial. Amantidine, better known as an antiviral and dopamine receptor ligand, will block NMDA receptor ion channels and in a double-blind trial was found to give pain relief in cancer patients suffering from neuropathic pain (Pud et al 1998). Cambridge Neuroscience have reported that CNS-5161 was effective at reducing pain in volunteers and Neurobiological Technologies have reported that diabetic patients treated with memantine experienced a 30% reduction of night-time pain and a 18% reduction in daytime pain and a variety of studies with dextromethorphan indicate that this compound has weak but reproducible analgesic effects (company communications, 1998).

There is evidence from experiments in animals that agents acting at the glycine-coagonist site on the NMDA receptor complex may offer a better side effect profile than the ion channel-blocking drugs referred to above. This may be most evident when a partial agonist for the receptor is used (see Laird et al 1996).

ANTAGONISTS OF THE ACTION OF SUBSTANCE P AND OTHER EXCITATORY NEUROPEPTIDES

There has been extensive interest in the putative role of substance P in nociceptive processes ever since the first suggestion that this peptide was concentrated in dorsal roots (see Salt & Hill 1983 for historical review). Recent studies have shown that mice in which the gene for the NK_1 receptor had been deleted showed deficiencies in spinal wind-up and intensity coding of spinal reflexes, although baseline nociception was unaffected (De Felipe et al 1998). In mice where the gene encoding the synthesis of the precursor for substance P, preprotachykinin, had been deleted, again responses to mildly painful stimuli were intact but the response to more intense stimuli was attenuated (Cao et al 1998, Zimmer et al 1998). The discovery of non-peptide antagonists of the NK_1 receptor at which this peptide exerts its effects (for review, see Longmore et al 1995) has allowed rigorous testing of the hypothesis that antagonism of the effects of substance P might lead to analgesia. In animal experiments, convincing evidence has been obtained for antinociceptive effects with these compounds, especially in inflammatory hyperalgesia (Rupniak et al 1995) or hypersensitivity induced by experimental diabetes (Field et al 1998), yet investigations in man have failed to demonstrate convincing analgesic properties in most studies so far published (see, for example, Reinhardt et al 1998, Block et al 1998).

Although there are many other peptides in primary afferent nociceptors that might be candidates for a role in nociceptive transmission, as yet there are few non-peptide antagonists that might be investigated clinically. This field is moving rapidly and our increased understanding of the complexities of the molecular biology of receptors, such as that for calcitonin gene-related peptide (CGRP) (McLatchie et al 1998), make it likely that increased numbers of such antagonists will be produced as potential analgesics.

ION CHANNEL BLOCKERS

Ever since the introduction of local anaesthetics, it has been common for clinicians to use drugs which block ion channels in order to control pain. This approach has expanded recently with the use of membrane-stabilizing anticonvulsant drugs to treat various intractable pain conditions. It is only in the last few years, however, that the molecular biology of ion channels has been sufficiently well understood to allow the rational design of agents that block a single channel type or subtype. Many established drugs, such as morphine, exert their effects by influencing the activity of ion channels indirectly by activating receptors that are coupled to ion channels by second messenger systems. This section is not concerned with such drugs but rather with those that directly influence the activity of voltage-gated ion channels. Recent reviews of this area can be found in McClure and Wildsmith (1991) and Fields et al (1997).

Na channels

There is now evidence that Na channels are overexpressed in biopsies taken from painful neuromas (England et al 1996). It has been suggested that the slow, tetrodotoxin-resistant Na current is the best target for a drug that will relieve pain but have minimal side effects (Rizzo et al 1996). This channel is overexpressed in the presence of inflammation and is only found on NGF-dependent unmyelinated nociceptive afferent fibres (Akopian et al 1996, Friedel et al 1997). It has been found in unmyelinated fibres of biopsied human sural nerve (Quasthoff et al 1995). No compound that will block the TTX-resistant Na sodium current in a selective way is available at present but the recent cloning and expression of the channel (Akopian et al 1997) make this an achievable objective.

Those agents that are currently available, though widely used, are suboptimal. For example, lignocaine does not select between Na channels in neurons and those in other tissues and in molar terms it is a rather weak blocker. It has a higher affinity for the TTX-sensitive current in myelinated fibres than for the TTX-resistant current in nociceptors (Scholz et al 1998). Only its use-dependent mechanism of action has allowed its safe application as a local anaesthetic (see Murdoch Ritchie 1994). When given intravenously, it has been found to be effective in the treatment of a number of neuropathic pain states whereas efficacy against other pains is the subject of debate, with positive and negative studies being reported. If infusion rate is limited to 5 mg/kg/h (Fields at al 1997) then side effects are mild with minimal cardiovascular changes. Pain relief after a 1-hour infusion lasts several hours and on occasion very much longer than this. It has also been found to be effective against migraine headache when given intranasally (Maizels et al 1996).

The anticonvulsants phenytoin and carbamazepine also inhibit both TTX-resistant and TTX-sensitive currents in rat DRG cells (Rush & Elliot 1997) and this may explain the clinical effectiveness of these agents in treating pain (McQuay et al 1995). Lamotrigine, a more recently introduced Na channel-blocking anticonvulsant, is also proving useful in the treatment of neuropathic pain and the recent demonstration that it reduces cold-induced pain in volunteer subjects may indicate a wider utility in treating other pains (Webb & Kamali 1998). It is also relevant to note that tricyclic antidepressants have been shown to block neuronal Na channels and this may account for some of the analgesic activity of this class of compound (Pancrazio et al 1998).

Ca channels

The neuronal Ca channels are now a large and complex family with L, N, P, Q, R and T type currents being found in brain and other neuronal tissues (Birnbaumer et al 1994, Perez-Reyes et al 1998). This diversity, although confusing, provides a number of alternative targets for the design of new analgesic drugs. Blockers of L-type Ca currents are the most accessible, having been used to treat cardiovascular disorders for many years. Although the cardiovascular effects may limit their utility it has recently been shown that nimodipine will reduce the daily dose of morphine needed to provide pain relief in a group of cancer patients (Santillan et al 1998) and that this effect is not due to a pharmacokinetic interaction of the drugs. Epidural verapamil has been shown to reduce analgesic consumption in patients after lower abdominal surgery (Choe et al 1998). In animal experiments it is readily demonstrable that L-channel blockers (such as nimodipine, verapamil and diltiazem) have antinociceptive properties (Rupniak et al 1993, Neugebauer et al 1996) and it is important to consider the presence of this type of activity when evaluating a novel agent as an analgesic (Rupniak et al 1993).

N, P and Q type Ca currents have all been implicated in pain perception on the basis of anatomical location and animal experiments with inverterbrate toxins which show some specificity for the individual channels. The best studied is the N channel, which has been located on the terminals of sensory nerve fibres, and blockade of this channel with the *Conus* toxin ω-conotoxin GV1A can be shown to reduce sensory transmitter release and cause antinociception in experimental animals (Bowersox et al 1994). As these toxins are peptides, it is necessary to apply them intrathecally (Malmberg & Yaksh 1995) but they produce striking effects at extremely low doses in a variety of tests, including formalin and hot plate, and continuous infusion for 7 days results in a maintained elevation of nociceptive threshold. This was not seen in similar experiments with L- or P- channel blockers (Miljanich & Ramachandran 1995 but see below). Spinal cord neuronal recordings in the presence and absence of inflammatory stimuli suggest that the N channel may be important in the development of spinal cord hyperexcitability and hyperalgesia (Neugebauer et al 1996, Nebe et al 1998). Studies on cerebral ischaemia, in which the conotoxin SNX-111 (or ziconotide) was given intravenously to man, show that such agents can be tolerated although there was evidence of orthostatic hypotension caused by sympatholysis (Miljanich & Ramachandran 1995). Intrathecal studies in man with ziconotide have indicated that it produces profound pain relief in patients with severe cancer pain (company communication, Wall St Journal, 13 January 1998) without unacceptable side effects, although these data are yet to be published.

Peptide blockers of P-type channels have also been studied for their antinociceptive effects in animals. They appear to be most effective in the presence of inflammation (Nebe et al 1997) and have a different effect to N-channel blockers in that they attenuate the late but not the early phase of the formalin response (Diaz & Dickenson 1997). No information is yet available about the action of P-channel blockers in man but it is relevant to note that mutation of P/Q type calcium channels has been associated with the occurrence of familial hemiplegic migraine (Ophoff et al 1996), suggesting one logical therapeutic use for blockers of this channel.

Gabapentin is a novel agent that is proving useful for the treatment of neuropathic pain (Rosner et al 1996, Rosenberg et al 1997), especially for postherpetic neuralgia. It has also been suggested to be useful in treating the pain of multiple sclerosis (Houtchens et al 1997). The precise mode of action of this drug is obscure but it binds with high affinity to the $\alpha2\delta$ subunit of calcium channels (Gee et al 1996), although this may not be its only mechanism. It will reduce transmitter release and is active in a number of animal nociception assays (Taylor 1998). A more potent analogue, S-(+)-3-isobutylgaba, is currently in development for the treatment of pain (Field et al 1997).

NICOTINIC AGONISTS

There is a rich literature on the antinociceptive effects of cholinergic agonists in animals but the clinical exploitation of these effects has been limited by the severe side effects produced by non-specific activation of cholinergic systems. Recent detailed knowledge of the molecular biology of cholinoceptors makes it possible to design agents which are receptor subtype selective and thus may have an improved ratio of wanted to unwanted effects. A number of agents have been evaluated preclinically but there are as yet no clinical data.

The cholinergic analgesia story was revived following the anouncement by Daly and his colleagues (Spande et al 1992) that epibatidine, an alkaloid extracted from the skin of an Ecuadorean frog, was a more potent analgesic than morphine. This compound was subsequently shown to be a potent nicotinic agonist (Badio & Daley 1994) but was too toxic to be developed as a clinical analgesic (Rupniak et al 1994). An analogue of epibatidine, ABT-594, has recently been reported as an analgesic development candidate with an improved therapeutic ratio. This agent, in contrast to epibatidine, does not act at neuromuscular junction nicotinic receptors and has low affinity at some CNS nicotinic sites ($\alpha7$) but high affinity at others ($\alpha4\beta2$). It has moderate affinity at autonomic and sensory ganglion ($\alpha3$-containing) receptors (Donelly-Roberts et al 1998). In vivo, ABT 594 showed antinociceptive activity in thermal and chemical (formalin) tests that was reversed by the brain penetrant nicotinic antagonist mecamylamine and analgesia persisted after chronic dosing of drug (Bannon et al 1998). Acute dosing caused a decrease in locomotor activity, a decrease in body temperature and loss of balance but these effects, unlike the antinociception, showed tolerance on repeated dosing. A part of the analgesia produced by ABT-594 may be due to activation of descending inhibitory pathways originating in the nucleus raphe magnus (Bitner et al 1998).

It remains to be demonstrated whether agents of this type will be clinically useful and it is noteworthy that although our knowledge of the molecular biology of nicotinic receptors is now extensive, we do not know which receptor type is most important in nociceptive processing. One limitation may be the ability of such drugs to interact with brain reward systems and thus produce dependence (Epping-Jordan et al 1998).

CAPSAICIN (VR-1) RECEPTOR ACTIVATORS AND BLOCKERS

The use of capsaicin as a rubefacient in treatment of painful disorders is traditional but it is only in the last 20 years that the pharmacology of the active principle, capsaicin, has become well understood. The early work of the Janscos in Hungary (see Salt & Hill 1983 for background) showed that systemic administration to rodents would deplete peptides from small primary afferent fibres without affecting CNS neurons, large sensory fibres or autonomic fibres. Such administration produced initial nociceptive behaviour, consistent with the pain seen when capsaicin is injected or applied topically in man, followed by prolonged elevation of nociceptive thresholds.

Preparations containing capsaicin for topical application are now widely available and are sometimes effective in painful conditions involving unmyelinated fibre dysfunction. These include postherpetic neuralgia, postmastectomy pain and diabetic neuropathy (Szallasi 1997). Commercial preparations generally contain only low concentrations of capsaicin (<1%) and even at this dose compliance can be low because of the burning sensation experienced on application. Recently a trial has been made of high-dose (5–10%) topical capsaicin applied under regional anaesthetic cover in patients with refractory pain (Robbins et al 1998). Even with regional anaesthesia, burning pain due to the capsaicin was experienced by some patients and had to be treated with IV fentanyl. Marked temporary pain relief was obtained in nine of 10 patients, with seven of these achieving significant and prolonged pain relief on repeated application. Capsaicin is not suitable for oral administration to man as it is poorly absorbed from and highly irritant to the GI tract. It is not yet clear whether it is necessary to first stimulate the receptor to desensitize it (causing the patient discomfort) or whether it might be possible to block the receptor painlessly with a silent antagonist or partial agonist yet still give clinical pain relief.

Workers at Novartis have produced analogues of capsaicin which are not pain producing yet still have antinociceptive properties in animals and are free of unwanted bronchoconstrictor activity. One of these drugs has entered clinical development as a potential analgesic (Wrigglesworth et al 1996). Recently a specific receptor (VR-1) for capsaicin-like compounds has been expression cloned (Caterina et al 1997) from a DRG library. It is likely that this discovery will rapidly lead to further novel agonists and antagonists of this receptor which can be clinically evaluated for treatment of pain.

SYMPATHETIC BLOCKS: PRESENT AND FUTURE ROLES

The association in some patients of severe pain with sympathetic end-organ dysfunction such as sweating, blood flow and temperature has led to the attempt to treat these pains with sympatholytic techniques (Leriche 1916, Livingstone 1943, Loh & Nathan 1978). It has been shown that electrical stimulation of sympathetic ganglia by intraoperatively placed electrodes in patients who had undergone preganglionic sympathetectomy for causalgia would cause reproduction of the patients' pain (Walker & Nulsen 1974). Despite observations such as these, the dichotomy between observations made in basic research studies and in clinical practice is rarely as extreme as in the area of sympathetic blocks.

The last 15 years have has seen major advances in the understanding of the role of the sympathetic nervous system in pain states, as illustrated by the development of a variety of models and experimental preparations. In contrast, with the recent emphasis on meta-analysis of outcome studies in the field of pain, the clinical results of sympathetic block have been the subject of controversy. The introduction of the complex regional pain syndrome (CRPS) classification attempts to bring some sort of coherent thought to the variety of clinical syndromes but it does not solve the fundamental difficulty of relating the clinical picture to pathophysiology. More importantly, the CRPS classification has little value in predicting response of clinical pain states to a variety of sympathetic blocks and little prognostic value in determing long-term pain experience or disability. This has led to a number of papers and editorials questioning the whole concept of the role of the sympathetic system in pain states and dismissing the short- and long-term results of sympathetic blocks in clinical practice (Ochoa & Verdugo 1993, Verdugo & Ochoa 1994, Schott 1994, 1995, 1998). We know that the interaction between activity in the sympathetic system and the rest of the patient's pain state may be mediated at a number of neuroanatomical locations. Thus it is very likely that the apparently clinically uniform group of patients chosen for a particular study will have a range of contributing pathophysiologies on presentation, which will also change with time since onset of condition. Even more importantly, the sensitivity of the pain state to sympathetic block will change with time. Since clinicians treat on the basis of clinical picture, we are likely to see a wide range of responses to, say, intravenous regional blockade (IVRB) with guanethidine, ranging from virtually no response to almost miraculous and long-term alleviation of symptoms. Thus general pronouncements about the usefulness (or usually the lack of it!) of some treatment modality in, for example, algodystrophy, RSD or CRPS type 1 only serve to illustrate our failure to understand the complexity of the system we are dealing with and the lack of predictive clinical signs, symptoms and investigations to help us determine pathophysiologically a homogeneous group of patients for treatment (see also Chaplan 1996, Tanelian 1996a, b). The wide range of responses in patients treated with sympathetic blocks for pain should not make us question the very role of the sympathetic system in pain states when the basic science evidence for its involvement is so very clearly there. Instead, it should encourage us into further attempting to understand the pathophysiology and pharmacological sensitivity within an individual patient.

The ordinary clinician has to attempt to treat patients and in response, this section will briefly outline the increasing understanding of the pathophysiology of sympathetic related pain disorders and attempt to relate this to clinical pain conditions, followed by a short description of techniques and indications, long-term results and complications of the most common sympathetic blocks. This section will not attempt to give techniques of such procedures in any great detail, as these are now elegantly covered in recently produced and sometimes colourful texts (Hahn et al 1996, Prithvi Raj et al 1996, Waldman & Winnie 1996, Cousins & Bridenbaugh 1998).

BASIC SCIENTIFIC EVIDENCE FOR THE ROLE OF THE SYMPATHETIC NERVOUS SYSTEM IN PAIN

It is surprising to find that the sympathetic nervous system has very little effect on the function of normal nociceptors and prolonged periods of high-intensity sympathetic fibre stimulation are required to show any changes. Where these effects have been observed, it may have been by way of sympathetic effector organ activity causing cooling of the skin, piloerection, etc. In fact, as noted in the comprehensive review by Koltzenburg (1997), many of the effects of sympathetic stimulation were mimicked by occlusion of the vascular supply and the weak effects of sympathetic stimulation were often blocked by α adrenoreceptor antagonists.

After nerve injury, however, the situation is different and interactions have been shown to occur between the sensory system and the sympathetic system at the level of the dorsal root ganglion, at the end of regenerating nerves and also in undamaged fibres running in partially injured nerves. It has been shown experimentally that there is cross-excitation between nerves of all sizes after injury via ephapses (which are rare on undamaged nerves). Though sympathetic fibres may not contribute to this crosstalk, the end of individual sensory nerve fibres, as well as being exquisitely sensitive to mechanical and thermal stimuli, are also excited by electrical stimulation of postganglionic sympathetic neurons and by local or systemic administration of catecholamines. The sympathetic facilitation appears to be working via catecholamines working at α_1 or α_2 receptors and via neuropeptide Y (NPY), which coexists with catecholamines in sympathetic fibres, working via Y_1 and Y_2 receptors (Tracey et al 1995), but see also Coughnon et al (1997) and Munglani et al (1998) for reviews.

After nerve injury, adjacent functioning nerves also become weakly sensitive to circulating catecholamines and it has also been shown that the discharges of some mechanoreceptors can be reduced by sympathetic blockade. In animal models of partial nerve injury the adrenergic excitation of neurons can be shown to peak at 2 weeks before disappearing. This particular feature is reminiscent of the development of CRPS where early on in the syndrome, the sympathetic contribution to the pain state is much greater than later on (Sato & Perl 1991, Na et al 1993, Koltzenburg 1997). After nerve injury in the dorsal root ganglion (DRG), spontaneous discharges start within a few days (Devor & Wall 1990). There is also cross-excitation between the DRG neurons, mainly in myelinated neurons, mediated by an increase in extracellular potassium concentration (Utzschneider et al 1992). There is a profuse growth of sympathetic fibres into the dorsal root ganglion and postganglionic sympathetic fibres form baskets, mainly around the large myelinated afferents (McLachlan et al 1993). Nerve growth factor (NGF) overexpression in mice duplicates this response, suggesting a possible mechanism (Davis et al 1994; see also McMahon & Bennett 1997).

Despite the preclinical evidence for pronounced effects of the sympathetic system on the somatosensory nerves, it is clear that the sympathetic system itself may even show a decreased level of activity after nerve damage. Reduced levels of circulating adrenaline in the venous outflow of the symptomatic limb suggest that the main problem may be a denervation supersensitivity (Arnold et al 1993). Experiments in animals suggest that after a peripheral nerve lesion, there is atrophy of the sympathetic cell bodies and fibres which may predispose to such denervation supersensitivity of receptors on the blood vessels. This may account for the observation of disturbances of thermoregulatory control, leading to an affected limb which is cooler than normal and which may show further decreases in temperature in response to circulating catecholamines and perhaps to stress. The cooling of the limb may also be consistent with the phenomenon of cold allodynia (Janig 1988, Magerl et al 1996).

Inflammation-related pain may also receive a contribution from the sympathetic system. Anecdotally, some patients with rheumatoid arthritis have been reported to show a significant response to IVRB with guanethidine (Hannington-Kiff 1994) and a small overall response was found in another independent study (Levine et al 1986a). Capsaicin (but not bradykinin) induced hyperalgesia can be slightly enhanced by coadministration of noradrenaline whilst phentolamine slightly decreases it (Meyer et al 1992, Drummond 1995, Liu et al 1996). There is more evidence for the role of the sympathetic system in mediating inflammation per se. Preceding surgical or chemical sympathectomy (but not local anaesthetic block) will reduce plasma extravasation induced by bradykinin or serotonin and has been reported to reduce joint destruction in experimental Freund's adjuvant arthritis. Destruction of the postganglionic sympathetic nerve fibres (PGSN) by the selective neurotoxin 6-hydroxy-dopamine shows that the presence but not activity of these PGSN also seems to be vital to inflammation (Levine et al 1986b, Levine & Taiwo 1994). Other studies suggest that the sympathetic contribution to cutaneous hyperalgesia is mediated by activation of α_2 but not α_1 receptors, which then releases prostaglandins such as prostaglandin E_2 which sensitize cutaneous nociceptors. Indeed, there are clinical reports of IVRB with ketorolac (a cyclo-oxygenase inhibitor) being effective in sympathetically maintained pain (SMP). Other tissue mediators which may be involved include interleukin-8 (IL-8) and NGF since, in animal experiments, the effects they produce can be diminished by sympathectomy and perhaps also by IL-1 and TNFα (Cuhna et al 1992a,b, Safieh-Garabedian et al 1995, Andreev et al 1995, Woolf et al 1996). However, the relevance of these studies to man has been questioned and, for example, sympathectomy does not abolish hyperalgesia in man (Meyer et al 1992).

DIAGNOSIS AND TREATMENT OF SYMPATHETICALLY MAINTAINED PAIN

The diagnosis of SMP is quite simple: if at any stage of the pain history, a placebo-controlled block of the sympathetic system causes relief of symptoms then that patient has a SMP. Failure to relieve symptoms leads to the diagnosis of SIP (sympathetically independent pain). Causalgia refers to a burning pain usually associated with nerve injury, whilst reflex sympathetic dystrophy refers to a collection of symptoms and signs including pain, temperature change and oedema in an affected limb but which may or may not have a significant contribution from the sympathetic nervous system. Unfortunately history, symptoms and signs are no predictors of whether a particular case is likely to be a SMP, though a few conditions are more likely to be associated with it (Table 53.1).

It has also been reported in one study that cold allodynia as a feature is present in 50% of SIP and all SMP patients (Frost et al 1988, Campbell et al 1994). The response to IVRB with guanethidine has also been used as a test of SMP, though this is not recommended. A positive response to a block has been suggested to mean relief of symptoms lasting weeks to months whilst a negative response would be little or no pain relief or relief lasting less than a week (Wahren et al 1991). How to interpret intense but short-lived responses is not clear but the CRPS concept may be of use (see below). Local anaesthetic blocks of the sympathetic chain may also be useful but it has been suggested that even small amounts of local anaesthetic diffusing onto somatosensory nerve roots may cause relief and hence give a false-positive response. Furthermore, a non-specific systemic action may be present, especially with higher doses of local anaesthetic (Charlton 1986). Other cautionary notes on the interpretation of the results of blocks are given in Hogan (1997) and Stolker et al (1994).

Table 53.1 Conditions associated with Sympathetically Mediated Pain (SMP)

Acute shingles (herpes zoster)
Neuralgias including postherpetic neuralgia
Painful metabolic neuropathies
Phantom pain
Traumatic nerve injuries
Soft tissue injury

Using the knowledge that α adrenoceptors may be involved in SMP, an intravenous infusion of phentolamine (α-adrenergic antagonist) has been tried as a diagnostic (Arner 1991, Raja et al 1991). The emerging consensus is that these investigations must be placebo controlled and that the information gained is similar to but not identical with that obtained from other blocks. As well as the factors mentioned above, differences between the results of sympathetic ganglion blockade and IV phentolamine administration have been suggested to be due to non-adrenergic sympathetic activity and to an insufficient dose of phentolamine (0.5 mg/kg used initially but 1 mg/kg may be required to fully block sympathetically mediated vasoconstriction and other reflexes) (Campbell et al 1994). Possible sympatholytic treatments for SMP are listed in Table 53.2.

What is known about the clinical outcomes after sympathetic block is discussed later in this chapter but the conceptual problem is to find a place for SMP, diagnostic and therapeutic sympathetic blocks in the new classification of CRPS (Stanton-Hicks et al 1995). The new classification arose out of the 1993 Orlando conference on the subject where it was decided that the term RSD described a symptom complex of spontaneous pain, allodynia/hyperalgesia, motor dysfunction, abnormal sweating and abnormal vascular reactivity followed by trophic changes in the limb,

Table 53.2 Interventional techniques for therapeutic sympatholysis (adapted from Campbell et al 1994)

Percutaneous techniques
Sympathetic ganglion block
Epidural nerve block with or without clonidine
Peripheral nerve block
Phenol or alcohol block of the sympathetic chain
Pulsed or continuous radiofrequency sympathectomy
Intravenous techniques
Regional (e.g. guanethidine, bretylium, ketorolac, phentolamine, clonidine, reserpine, ketanserin with or without local anaesthesia)
Systemic (e.g. phentolamine, pamimdronate)
Surgery
Oral therapy
Prazosin
Phenoxybenzamine
Nifedipine
Clonidine
Topical
Clonidine

References: Breivik et al 1998, Shir et al 1993, Rauck et al 1993, Blanchard et al 1990, Hanna & Peat 1989, Ghostine et al 1984, Tabira et al 1983, Abram & Lightfoot 1981, Hannington-Kiff 1977 and see text for further references.

all in a non-dermatomal distribution. This syndrome often followed injury but unfortunately, not all patients responded to sympathetic blocks with relief of symptoms in either the short or long term. Hence, RSD was thought to be a misleading name.

CRPS taxonomy therefore recognized the SIP component of the pain state. More importantly, it recognized that a particular pain state may be predominantly a SMP but with time become predominantly SIP. CRPS type 1 was described as similar to the old RSD whilst CRPS type 2 usually followed nerve injury (causalgia). Therefore the diagnosis of SMP and hence the rationale for diagnostic and therapeutic sympatholytic procedures is not automatic when a diagnosis of CRPS is made. It is recognized that the CRPS complex may include a sympathetic component but also sensory, autonomic, inflammatory, psychological and motor components, all of which may need treatment. Sympatholytic blocks play only a part in the overall treatment strategy in patients with CRPS. Furthermore, despite aggressive treatment and initial resolution in 66% of patients (Weil 1992), the symptoms may recur, with an incidence in one study of 1.8% per year (Veldman & Goris 1996). The reader is referred to Scadding (Ch. 35) and especially to Boas (1996), Janig and Stanton-Hicks (1996) and Wilson et al (1996) for further discussion of CRPS and diagnostic algorithms. It is useful to include the criteria for diagnosis of sympathetic dysfunction within the diagnostic algorithm for CRPS (Table 53.3).

Table 53.3 Algorithm for diagnosis of CRPS and sympathetic dysfunction (adapted from Wilson et al 1996)

Pain
CRPS is a pain syndrome. The characteristics of the pain may vary

History
Usually precipitated by noxious event or immobilization
Usually unilateral though may spread
Identifiable nerve lesion as a cause is defined as a CRPS type 2
Other anatomic, physiological or psychological cause which would fully account for the degree of pain and dysfunction excludes a diagnosis of CRPS

Symptoms (patient report)
A Pain (spontaneous or evoked)
  Burning
  Aching, throbbing
B Hyperalgesia or allodynia at some stage to light touch or joint movement
C Associated symptoms (minor)
  Swelling
  Temperature and colour: asymmetry and instability
  Sweating: asymmetry and instability
  Trophic changes: hair, nails and skin

Signs (observed)
Hyperalgesia or allodynia
Oedema (usually unilateral)
Vasomotor changes: colour, temperature instability, asymmetry
Sudomotor changes
Trophic changes in skin, joint nail, hair
Impaired motor function

Criteria required for diagnosis of CRPS 1
History of pain
  plus allodynia, hyperalgesia or hyperaesthesia
  plus two other signs from the above list
Characteristics of spontaneous pain
  SMP or SIP or mixture

Criteria for diagnosis of sympathetic dysfunction
Non-invasive tests
  Spontaneous or provoked surface temperature difference by ≥1°C
  Resting evoked sudomotor asymmetry
Invasive tests
  Up to three sympathetic ganglion blocks demonstrating inhibition of sympathetically mediated vasoconstriction
  Placebo-controlled systemic infusion of α-adrenergic antagonist
  Neuraxial blockade may provide further information
Tests of unknown pathophysiological significance
  Three-phase bone scan
  Radiographic patchy demineralization
  Tourniquet ischaemia test
Tests requiring further study and utility not yet demonstrated
  Laser-cutaneous blood flow measurement
  Percutaneous oxygen partial pressure differences
  Computer-assisted sensory examination
  Somatosensory evoked potential
Regional sympathetic blockade is not recommended for diagnostic use due to multiple physiological actions

SYMPATHETIC BLOCKS

The rest of this chapter will be devoted to describing the indications, complications and the evidence for the efficacy of some of the sympatholytic procedures. Technical details will be kept to a minimum here due to lack of space and the recent publication of some excellent books on neural blockade to which the reader is referred (Hahn et al 1996, Prithvi Raj et al 1996, Waldman & Winnie 1996, Cousins & Bridenbaugh 1998).

A list of common sympathetic nerve blocks is given in Table 53.4.

SPHENOPALATINE GANGLION BLOCK

This ganglion is one of four within the head and is located posterior to the middle turbinate and 1–9 mm deep to the lateral mucosa. Within the 5–7 mm triangular ganglion are cells which communicate with the first and second division

Table 53.4 Types of autonomic blocks

Sphenopalatine block
Stellate ganglion block
Thoracic sympathetic block
Coeliac plexus block
Splanchnic nerve block
Lumbar sympathetic block
Superior hypogastric nerve block
Ganglion of Impar block

of the trigeminal nerve, facial nerve and carotid plexus and through which there is a direct communication with the cervical sympathetic ganglion chain and parasympathetic fibres via the superficial petrosal nerve. Because of the proximity of the ganglion to the nasal mucosa, blockade may be achieved by topical cocaine or local anaesthetic or else by a lateral approach under fluoroscopy under the zygoma lateral to the mandible and passing the mandibular branch of the trigeminal nerve before entering the sphenopalatine fossa. Local anaesthetic and radiofrequency procedures have been described. This block may be useful in Sluder's neuralgia, cluster headaches and migraine. Side effects include nose bleeds and numbness of the hard palate and teeth. See Prithvi Raj et al (1996) and also Waldman and Winnie (1996) for further details.

STELLATE GANGLION BLOCK

For the head and neck, sympathetic fibres originate in the anterolateral horn of the spinal cord at T1–2, whilst for the upper extremity they originate from T8–9 and travel as white rami to join the sympathetic chain and synapse at the stellate, middle or superior cervical ganglion. The stellate (often fused to the first thoracic ganglion) is approximately 2.5 cm long × 1 cm wide × 0.5 cm thick and lies over C7–T1. T2–3 grey rami may also supply the upper limb ('Kuntz's nerves') without passing through the stellate and may be blocked via a posterior approach. Two techniques for blockade of the stellate are described. One uses the transverse process of C6 (Chaussignac's tubercle) and the other uses a more medial approach to the anterolateral border of C7 (Leriche & Fontain 1934; Moore 1954, Stanton-Hicks 1986, Stanton-Hicks et al 1996, Prithvi Raj et al 1996).

The patient is placed supine with a hyperextended neck. Chaussignac's tubercle is found medial to the sternocleidomastoid muscle and the carotid artery is pushed laterally (Fig. 53.1). The tubercle is usually at a depth of 2–2.5 cm. If the needle is placed more medially it will penetrate deeper before hitting the medial part of the transverse process and

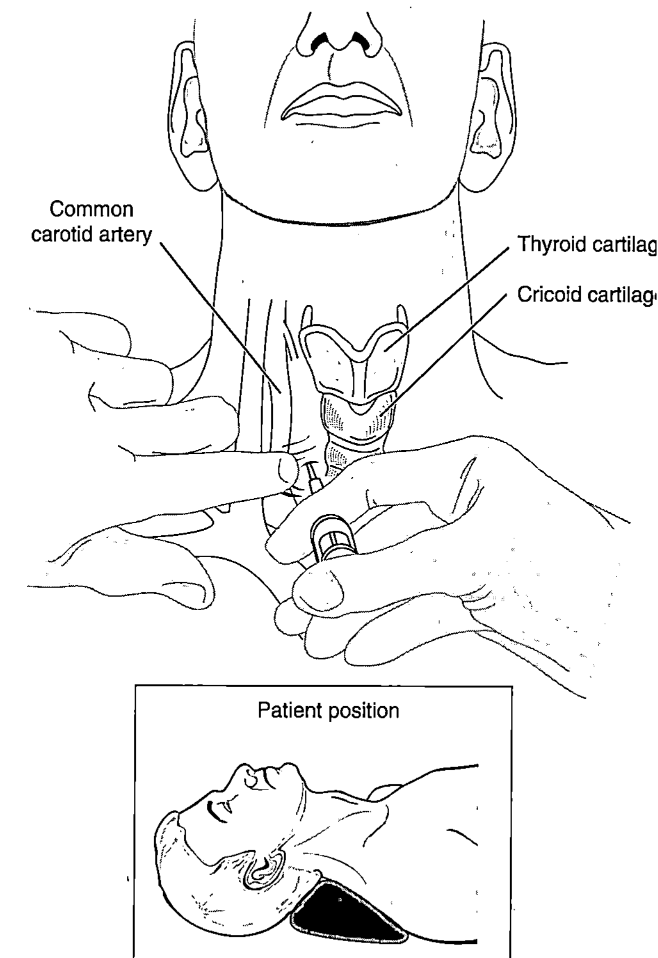

Fig. 53.1 Stellate ganglion block.

the lateral part of the vertebral body, which are both covered by longus colli muscle. In this event, the operator must withdraw the needle up to 0.5 cm to avoid injecting into the substance of the muscle (which will limit caudad spread and may also predispose to a somatosensory block by lateral diffusion). Stellate ganglion blockade attempted at the body of C7 (two finger breadths below C6) avoids the problems of injection into vertebral artery, dural sheath and the belly of longus colli. Solution placed at this level may also diffuse from the periosteum of the vertebral body to the stellate ganglion and upper thoracic sympathetic ganglia. Careful aspiration must be performed before injection of a test dose of less than 1 ml of 0.25% bupivacaine due to the possibility of intravertebral artery injection; 10 ml of local anaesthetic is typically enough to block the plexus and outflow to the upper limb (Bonica et al 1979). Successful blockade of the preganglionic fibres that pass through the stellate produces a Horner's syndrome: miosis, ptosis and enopthalmos as well as conjunctival injection, nasal congestion and facial anhydrosis. In the arm a rise of temperature, venous engorgement and dryness of the skin will be observed and represents a 95% blockade of fibres. Stanton-Hicks suggests that even an experienced operator may not achieve more than a 70–75% block (Stanton-Hicks et al 1996). Side effects include recurrent laryngeal nerve or, less commonly, phrenic nerve blockade. Obviously, a neurolytic stellate ganglion block may produce permanent complications or side effects. Blockade of the brachial plexus may also occur as well as pneumothorax if a too lateral approach is used at the C7 level. Objective tests of efficacy of sympathetic block are listed in Table 53.5 and apply to most of the blocks of autonomic function described here.

Indications for stellate ganglion blockade are many and are listed in Table 53.6.

THORACIC SYMPATHETIC BLOCK

The thoracic sympathetic chain lies near the somatic nerves as they emanate from the intravertebral foramen. There is a 4% incidence of pneumothorax during blockade even in experienced hands (Prithvi Raj et al 1996). Permanent neurolysis of the sympathetic chain may be indicated in some cancer pains with a strong SMP component.

COELIAC PLEXUS BLOCK

Preganglionic fibres originate in the anterolateral dorsal horn from T5 to T12, leaving with the ventral spinal routes to join the white rami, and do not synapse in the sympathetic trunks but pass through as the splanchnic nerves to synapse in the coeliac, aortic, renal and mesenteric ganglia. These are efferent nerve fibres but afferent sympathetic nerve fibres also exist within the spinal nerves. The coeliac plexus lies anterior and lateral to the aorta and crus of the diaphragm and contains within it fibres from the preganglionic splanchnic nerves, preganglionic parasympathetic vagal fibres, fibres from the phrenic and sympathetic postganglionic. Three pairs of ganglia have been identified within the plexus – coeliac, superior mesenteric and aortic – which will innervate all the abdominal viscera apart from part of the transverse colon, descending colon, rectum and pelvic viscera (Prithvi Raj et al 1996).

Upper abdominal malignancy pain, including that from pancreas, liver, gallbladder, etc., may respond to blockade. Local anaesthetic, with or without steroid, and neurolytic blocks have been described. In non-malignant pain, coeliac plexus block and intercostal blocks may help distinguish anterior abdominal wall from visceral pain syndromes. Neurolytic coeliac plexus block may work for 6–12 months before pain, perhaps caused by regeneration of nerve fibres or else the onset of deafferentation pain, returns (also see references in Prithvi Raj et al 1996). The block is performed using 15 cm 22 G needles under fluoroscopic guidance.

Table 53.5 Tests for efficacy of sympathetic block (from Stanton-Hicks et al 1996)

Sympathetic function
Skin plethysmography and ice response
Skin conductance response (SCR) or sympathogalvanic response (SGR) – a simple measure of sudomotor response
Skin potential response (SPR) – reflects activity in sudomotor neurons, requires a modified ECG
The cobalt blue test – a colour change of cobalt blue-soaked filter paper from blue to pink indicates sweating
Cold pressor test – using telethermography, the response to dipping of the affected and unaffected limbs in ice-cold water is observed and is usually followed by rewarming in 20–25 minutes in the unaffected limb and 45 minutes or longer in the limb with dysautonomia

Blood flow measurements
Occlusion skin plethysmography
Temperature measurement – contact or non-contact, adequate sympatholysis is associated with a temperature of ≥34°C at fingertips
Laser Doppler flowmetry

Table 53.6 Indications for stellate ganglion block (from Prithvi Raj et al 1996)

Pain
SMP in CRPS type 1 and type 2
Herpes zoster
Early postherpetic neuralgia
Phantom limb pain
Paget's disease
Neoplasm
Postradiation neuritis
Pain from CNS lesions
Intractable angina pectoris

Vascular insufficiency
Raynauds's disease
Frostbite
Vasospasm
Occlusive vascular disease
Embolic vascular disease
Scleroderma

Other
Hyperhydrosis
Ménière's disease
Shoulder hand syndrome
Stroke
Sudden blindness
Vascular headaches

A point 7–8 cm lateral to L1 but below the 12th rib is identified on the prone patient. The needles are inserted in a medial anterior and cephalad direction, usually hitting the vertebral body before advancing further. Many variations exist, including transdiscal and transaortic approaches. Complications include a reported incidence of paraplegia of 0.15%, despite the use of fluoroscopy and contrast media, and this may be mediated via damage to the artery of Adamquicz. Impotence has also been reported at an incidence of 3% (Black 1973, Davies 1993) and other complications are listed in Table 53.7.

LUMBAR SYMPATHETIC BLOCK

The cell bodies of the preganglionic sympathetic neurons lie in the anterolateral dorsal horn from T10 to L2–3 and pass through the white rami and sympathetic trunk to the sympathetic and sacral ganglia and then usually join the L1–5 and S1–3 spinal nerves by way of the grey rami or form a diffuse plexus around the iliac arteries. Preganglionic fibres for the visceral structures synapse commonly in T10–12 and L1 ganglia and then join the aortic and hypogastric plexus to supply the kidney, ureter, bladder, distal transverse colon, rectum, prostate, testicle, cervix and uterus. Reported indications for lumbar sympathetic block (LSB) include diagnosis of SMP, treatment of vascular insufficiency, deafferentation pains, neuropathic pain, acute herpes zoster (HZ) and cancer pains. The realization that the intravertebral discs have a dual nerve supply, i.e. both somatosensory and sympathetic, has led to the increasing use of diagnostic, neurolytic and radiofrequency lesions of the chain in the treatment of otherwise intractable back pain (Jinkins et al 1988, Nakamura et al 1996, Takahashi et al 1996, Munglani 1997). Often this is combined with facet denervation (Erdmann et al 1995) and the results can be quite remarkable (Munglani 1997 and unpublished observations). Radiofrequency lesions of the sympathetic chain may work where neurolytic block has failed (Hogan 1997). Further research is needed to explain why patients often respond to diagnostic local anaesthetic block of the sympathetic chain and yet subsequent neurolytic block seems to work in only about 30%, with a duration of action that may only be 6–12 months. One possibility is that pain relief by the use of local anaesthetic LSB may also involve spread of solution to the somatosensory nerves and there may be some systemic absorption, leading to false-positive results (Stanton-Hicks et al 1996).

The lateral and the paramedian approaches to the lumbar sympathetic plexus have both been described. Bonica recommended blocking at T12–L1 to achieve a total interruption of sympathetic outflow to the lower limb but often the block is made at L3 (Stanton-Hicks et al 1996). The lateral approach is more direct and causes less discomfort. The entry site is made 7–8 cm opposite the spinous processes of L2–4. Using fluoroscopy, the needle is advanced until it is in contact with the anterolateral border of the vertebral body, anterior to the psoas and the position is confirmed with contrast medium; 15–20 ml of local anaesthetic has been recommended to ensure spread over three vertebral bodies (Fig. 53.2).

Sympatholysis is confirmed by increasing temperature of the toes, dilatation of the veins and dryness of the skin. Side effects include backache, intravascular injection, trauma to kidney or ureter and neurolytic blockade of genitofemoral nerve which will lead to groin soreness though a new transdiscal approach is claimed to lower this (Ohno & Oshita 1997). Other complications are discussed in more detail in Charlton and Macrae (1998).

Table 53.7 Some possible side effects and complications of coeliac axis blockade (from Plancarte et al 1996)

Procedure-related pain
Failure to relieve pain
Hypotension
Diarrhoea
Paraesthesia or deficit of lumbar somatic nerves
Subarachnoid or epidural injection
Intrapsoas muscle injection
Intravascular injection
Thrombosis or embolism
Retroperitoneal haematoma
Pneumothorax
Chylothorax
Renal injury
Abscess
Peritonitis
Perforation of cyst or tumour
Paraplegia
Lower chest pain
Impotence
Lower extremity warmth or fullness
Urinary abnormalities

HYPOGASTRIC PLEXUS BLOCK (PRESACRAL SYMPATHETIC BLOCK)

The superior hypogastric plexus lies anterior to the fifth lumbar vertebrae just inferior to the aortic bifurcation. This block was highlighted by Plancarte (1989) and shows promise as a useful treatment for pelvic malignant pain as well as possibly other non-malignant conditions. Theoretically, problems with rectal, bladder and erectile

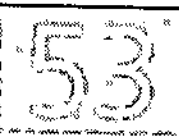

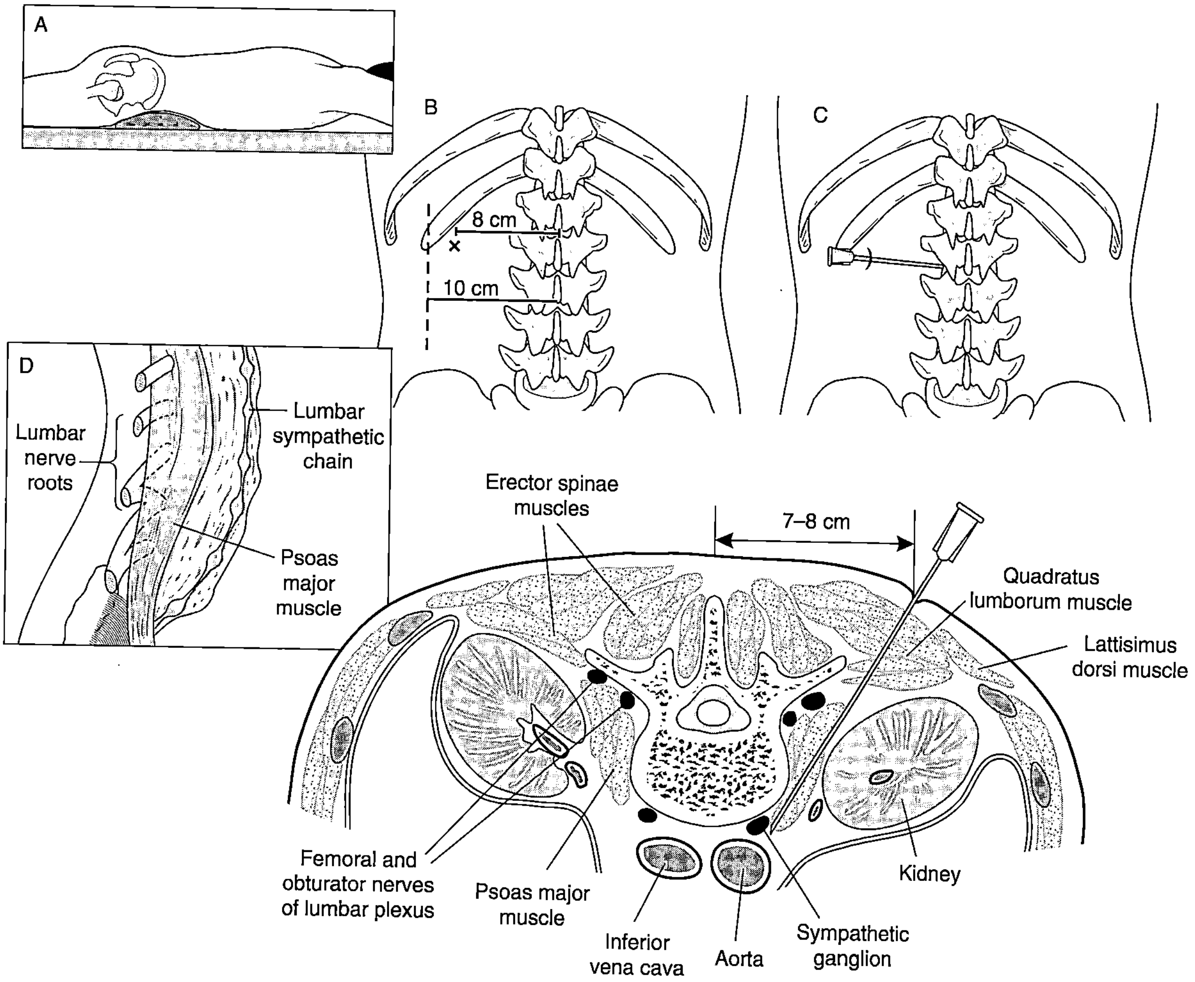

Fig. 53.2 Lumbar sympathetic block.

function may all occur though initial reported experience has not confirmed this (De Leon-Casasola et al 1993, Plancarte et al 1996, Prithvi Raj et al 1996).

GANGLION OF IMPAR BLOCK

This has recently been described for the treatment of intractable neoplastic perineal pain of sympathetic origin (Plancarte et al 1996). The ganglion of Impar is a solitary retroperitoneal structure at the level of the sacrococcygeal junction which may be reached by a bent needle round the coccyx or else through the sacrococcygeal membrane. In a pilot study, 16 patients with advanced cancer of the cervix, colon, bladder or rectum experienced relief of symptoms with local anaesthetic test block. Eight patients experienced 100% relief with 4–6 ml of phenol and the rest experienced at least 50% relief. This block has also been tried in the treatment of benign coccidynia with good effect (Munglani, unpublished observations).

INTRAVENOUS REGIONAL ANAESTHESIA

Pharmacological end-organ manipulation can be used to both diagnose (now controversially) and treat SMP. Hannington-Kiff (1977) introduced the technique using guanethidine, but subsequently its use has been described with many other drugs including bretylium, ketorolac, phentolamine, reserpine and ketanserin. Guanethidine depletes nerve endings of noradrenaline stores as well as preventing reuptake. Bretylium may last longer. Advantages of the technique include the ease with which it can be performed and that it can be used in the presence of systemic anticoagulation. Complications include delayed hypotension and possible neuropraxia and one case of pulmonary embolism on deflation of the leg cuff after IVRB has been seen personally (Munglani, unpublished observations). The results of IVRB with guanethidine in a proportion of patients can be quite remarkable (Ramamurthy et al 1995) and this conclusion was supported by many studies (e.g. Wahren et al 1995). Recent randomized, controlled trials failed to show any benefit, suggesting either a placebo response, an effect of the inflated cuff itself or, as discussed above, failure to understand the complex nature of CRPS in patients (in particular the varying proportion of SMP which may reduce with time within a patient) (Jadad et al 1995, Kaplan et al 1996). For further details and discussion of the technique of IVRB, see Hannington-Kiff (1994), Holmes (1998) and Stanton-Hicks et al (1996).

SYMPATHETIC BLOCKS: DEFINING A FUTURE ROLE IN THERAPY

Whilst there may be little doubt as to the role of sympathetic (especially neurolytic) blocks in the management of vascular insufficiency and cancer-related pains (Plancarte et al 1996, Boas 1998), randomized controlled trials have cast doubt on the usefulness of such autonomic blocks (and IVRB with guanethidine) in changing long-term outcome in other conditions including postherpetic neuralgia, low back pain and CRPS of limbs. An excellent review is provided by Boas (1998) and some of the points raised therein will be summarized here.

Whilst dramatic changes are often seen when autonomic blocks are first performed, Boas points out that evidence is lacking that early treatment changes outcome. An example given is the treatment of postherpetic neuralgia (PHN). One possibility is that although PHN is predominantly a SMP initially, with time it becomes a SIP. Further, attempting to treat the mechanisms maintaining a pain initially may not delay or prevent the development of subsequent alternative neurobiological mechanisms maintaining the pain over a longer period (Munglani et al 1996, Munglani 1997). Turning to the management of CRPS, Boas emphasizes that treatment of the SMP is but one part of the picture and adjuvant drugs such as antidepressants and anticonvulsants, physiotherapy and addressing the psychological issues are all important in changing long-term outcome. Novel treatments such as epidural clonidine (Rauck et al 1993 and see above), as well as more established therapies, will have to run the imperfect gauntlet of our changing understanding of SMP within the taxonomy of CRPS and randomized controlled trials to gain a place in the clinical armamentarium of pain clinic procedures.

CONCLUSION

There is a growing realization that not all drugs used to treat pain, in particular intractable pain, are simple analgesics in the conventional sense. The use of ion channel blockers in particular seems likely to increase, especially as non-peptide agents selective for particular calcium channel subtypes become available. The adrenergic system can be modulated to relieve pain by attenuating its peripheral effects or by using α_2 agonist drugs to activate central inhibitory receptors but the possibility for future development of drugs in this area seems limited. Clinical studies currently in progress will reveal the potential utility of agents that act at NMDA, capsaicin and nicotinic receptors and it is likely that at least one of these approaches will produce a drug that will be of lasting benefit.

REFERENCES

Abram SE, Lightfoot RW 1981 Treatment of long standing causalgia with prazosin. Regional Anesthesia 6: 79–81

Akopian AN, Sivlotti L, Wood JN 1996 A tetrodotoxin resistant voltage gated sodium channel expressed by sensory neurones. Nature 379: 257–262

Andreev NY, Dimitrieva N, Koltzenburg M, McMahon SB 1995 Peripheral administration of nerve growth factor in the adult rat produces a thermal hyperalgesia that requires the presence of sympathetic post-ganglionic neurones. Pain 63: 109–115

Arner S 1991 Intravenous phentolamine test: diagnostic, prognostic use in reflex sympathetic dystrophy. Pain 46: 17–22

Arnold J, Teasell RW, Macleod AP, Brown JE, Carruthers SG 1993 Increased venous alpha-adrenoreceptor responsiveness in patients with reflex sympathetic dystrophy. Annals of Internal Medicine 118: 619–621

Badio B, Daley JW 1994 Epibatidine, a potent analgesic and nicotinic agonist. Molecular Pharmacology 45: 563–569

Bannon AW, Decker MW, Curzon P et al 1998 ABT-594 [(R)-5-(2-azetidinylmethoxy)-2-chloropyridine]: a novel, orally effective antinociceptive agent acting via neuronal nicotinic acetylcholine receptors: II. In vivo characterisation. Journal of Pharmacology and Experimental Therapeutics 285: 787–794

Birnbaumer L, Campbell KP, Catterall WA et al 1994 The naming of voltage gated calcium channels. Cell 13: 505–506

Bitner RS, Nikkel AL, Curzon P, Arneric SP, Bannon AW, Decker MW 1998 Role of the nucleus raphe magnus in antinociception produced by ABT-594: immediate early gene responses possibly linked to neuronal nicotinic acetylcholine receptors on serotoninergic neurons. Journal of Neuroscience 18: 5426–5432

Black A 1973 Coeliac plexus block. Anaesthesia and Intensive Care 1: 315–318

Blanchard J, Ramamurthy S, Walsh N 1990 Intravenous regional sympatholysis: a double blind comparison of guanethidine, reserpine and normal saline. Journal of Pain and Symptom Management 5: 357

Block G, Rue D, Panebianco D, Reines S 1998 The substance P antagonist L-754,030 is ineffective in the treatment of postherpetic neuralgia. American Academy of Neurology, Annual Meeting, Minneapolis, April

Boas RA 1996 Complex regional pain syndromes: symptoms, signs, differential diagnosis. In: Janig W, Stanton-Hicks M (eds) Reflex sympathetic dystrophy: a reappraisal. IASP Press, Seattle, pp 93–105

Boas RA 1998 Sympathetic nerve blocks: in search of a role. Regional Anaesthesia and Pain Management 23: 292–305

Bonica JJ, Liebeskind JC, Albe-Fessard LB 1979 Advances in pain research and therapy. Raven, New York

Bowersox SS, Valentino KL, Luther RR 1994 Neuronal voltage-sensitive calcium channels. Drug News and Perspectives 7: 261–268

Breivik H, Cousins MJ, Lofstrom JB 1998 Sympathetic neural blockade of upper and lower extremity. In: Cousins MJ, Bridenbaugh PO (eds) Neural blockade. Lippincott-Raven, Philadelphia, pp 411–450

Campbell JN, Raja SN, Selig DK, Belzberg AJ, Meyer RA 1994 Diagnosis and management of sympathetically maintained pain. In: Fields HL, Liebskind JC (eds) Pharmacological approaches to the treatment of chronic pain: new concepts and critical issues. IASP Press, Seattle, pp 85–100

Cao YQ, Mantyh PW, Carlsson EJ, Gillespie A-M, Epstein CJ, Basbaum AI 1998 Primary afferent tachykinins are required to experience moderate to intense pain. Nature 392: 390–394

Cardenas CG, Del Mar LP, Cooper BY, Scroggs RS 1997 5-HT_4 receptors couple positively to tetrodotoxin-insensitive sodium channels in a subpopulation of capsaicin-sensitive rat sensory neurons. Journal of Neuroscience 17: 7181–7189

Caterina MJ, Schumacher MA, Tominaga M, Rosen TA, Levine JD, Julius D 1997 The capsaicin receptor: a heat activated ion channel in the pain pathway. Nature 389: 816–824

Chaplan SR 1996 Rethinking reflex sympathetic dystrophy. Pain Forum 5: 257–261

Charlton JE 1986 Current views on the use of nerve blocking in the relief of chronic pain. In: Swerdlow M (ed) The therapy of pain. MTP, Lancaster, pp 133–164

Charlton JE, Macrae WA 1998 Complications of neurolytic neural blockade. In: Cousins M, Bridenbaugh PO (eds) Neural blockade. Lippincott-Raven, Philadelphia, pp 663–672

Choe H, Kim J-S, Ko S-H, Kim D-C, Han Y-J, Song H-S 1998 Epidural verapamil reduces analgesic consumption after lower abdominal surgery. Anesthesia and Analgesia 86: 786–790

Cook L, Schmidt WK 1997 DUP-631: unique analgesia and biochemical profile of a serotonin-norepinephrine uptake inhibitor. ACNP 36th Annual Meeting Abstracts

Coombs DW, Saunders RL, LaChance D, Savage S, Ragnarsson TS, Jensen LE 1985 Intrathecal morphine tolerance: use of intrathecal clonidine, DADLE and intraventricular morphine. Anesthesiology 62: 357–363

Coughnon N, Hudspith M, Munglani R 1997 The therapeutic potential of NPY in central nervous system disorders with special reference to pain and sympathetically maintained pain. Expert Opinion in Investigational Drugs 6: 759–769

Cousins MJ, Bridenbaugh PO 1998 Neural blockade. Lippincott-Raven, Philadelphia

Cuhna FQ, Lorenzetti BB, Ferreira SH 1992a Interleukin-8 as a mediator of sympathetic pain. British Journal of Pharmacology 107: 660–664

Cuhna FQ, Poole S, Lorenzetti BB, Ferreira SH 1992b The pivotal role of tumour necrosis factor alpha in the development of inflammatory hyperalgesia. British Journal of Pharmacology 107: 660–664

Cumberbatch MJ, Hill RG and Hargreaves RJ 1998. Differential effects of the 5-HT ID/IB receptor agonist naratriptan on trigeminal versus spinal nociceptive responses. Cephalalgia 18: 659–663

Davies D 1993 Incidence of major complications of coeliac plexus block. Journal of the Royal Society of Medicine 86: 264–266

Davis BM, Albers KM, Seroogy KB, Katz DM 1994 Over expression of nerve growth factor in transgenic mice induces novel sympathetic projections to primary sensory neurones. Journal of Comparative Neurology 349: 464–474

De Felipe C, Herrero JF, O'Brien JA et al 1998 Altered nociception, analgesia and aggression in mice lacking the receptor for substance P. Nature 329: 394–397

De Leon-Casasola OA, Kent E, Lema MJ 1993 Neurolytic superior hypogastric plexus block for chronic pelvic pain associated with cancer. Pain 64: 145–151

Devor M, Wall PD 1990 Cross-excitation in dorsal root ganglia of nerve-injured and intact rats. Journal of Neurophysiology 64: 1733–1746

Diaz A, Dickenson AH 1997 Blockade of spinal N- and P-type, but not L-type, calcium channels inhibits the excitability of rat dorsal horn neurones produced by subcutaneous formalin inflammation. Pain 69: 93–100

Donelly-Roberts DL, Puttfarken PS, Kuntzweiler TA et al 1998 ABT-594 [(R)-5-(2-azetidinylmethoxy)-2-chloropyridine]: a novel, orally effective antinociceptive agent acting via neuronal nicotinic acetylcholine receptors: I in vitro characterisation. J Pharmacol Exp Ther 285: 777–786

Drummond PD 1995 Noradrenaline increases hyperalgesia to heat in skin sensitized by capsaicin. Pain 60: 311–315

Ebersberger A, Anton F, Tolle TR, Zieglgansberger W 1995 Morphine, 5-HT_2 and 5-HT_3 receptor antagonists reduce c-fos expression in the trigeminal nuclear complex following noxious chemical stimulation of the rat nasal mucosa. Brain Research 676: 336–342

Eide PK, Stubhaug A 1997 Relief of glossopharyngeal neuralgia by ketamine-induced N-methyl aspartate receptor blockade. Neurosurgery 41: 505–508

Eide PK, Stubhaug A, Oye I, Breivik H 1995 Cutaneous subcutaneous administration of the N-methyl-D-aspartic acid (NMDA) receptor antagonist ketamine in the treatment of post-herpetic neuralgia. Pain 61: 221–228

Eisenach JC, Rauck RL, Buzzanell C, Lysak SZ 1989 Epidural clonidine analgesia for intractable cancer pain: phase I. Anesthesiology 71: 647–652

Eisenach JC, DuPen S, Dubois M, Miguel R, Allin D and the Epidural Clonidine Study Group 1995 Epidural clonidine analgesia for intractable cancer pain. Pain 61: 391–399

England JD, Happel LT, Kline DG et al 1996 Sodium channel accumulation in humans with painful neuromas. Neurology 47: 272–276

Epping-Jordan MP, Watkins SS, Koob GF, Markou A 1998 Dramatic decreases in brain reward function during nicotine withdrawal. Nature 393: 76–79

Erdmann W, Pernak J, Grosveld WMJH 1995 Results of radio frequency sympathectomy in post laminectomy pain syndrome in the Netherlands. Pain Clinic 8: 127–131

Field MJ, Oles RJ, Lewis AS, McCleary S, Singh L 1997 Gabapentin (neurontin) and 3-(+)-isobutylgaba represent a novel class of selective antihyperalgesic agent. British Journal of Pharmacology 121: 1513–1522

Field MJ, McLeary S, Boden P, Suman-Chauhan N, Hughes J, Singh L 1998 Involvement of the central tachykinin NK_1 receptor during maintenance of mechanical hypersensitivity induced by diabetes in the rat. J Pharmacol Exp Ther 285: 1226–1232

Fields HL, Rowbotham MC, Devor M 1997 Excitability blockers: anticonvulsants and low concentration local anaesthetics in the treatment of chronic pain. In: Dickenson A, Besson J-M (eds) The pharmacology of pain. Springer, Berlin, pp 93–116

Friedel RH, Schnurch H, Stubbusch J, Barde Y-A 1997 Identification of genes differentially expressed by nerve growth factor- and neurotrophin-3-dependent sensory neurons. Proceedings of the National Academy of Sciences of the USA 94: 12670–12675

Frost SA, Raja SN, Campbell JN, Meyer RA, Khan AA 1988 Does

hyperalgesia to cooling stimuli characterise patients with sympathetically maintained pain? In: Dubner GF, Gebhart J, Bond MR (eds) Proceedings of the Vth World Congress on Pain. Elsevier, Amsterdam, pp 151–156

Gee NS, Brown JP, Dissanayake VUK, Offord J, Thurlow R, Woodruff GN 1996 The novel anticonvulsant drug, gabapentin (Neurontin), binds to the $\alpha 2\delta$ subunit of a calcium channel. Journal of Biological Chemistry 271: 5768–5776

Ghostine SY, Comair YG, Turner DM, Kassell NF, Azar CG 1984 Phenoxybenzamine in the treatment of causalgia. Journal of Neurosurgery 60: 1263–1268

Godfrey RG 1996 A guide to the understanding and use of tricyclic antidepressants in the overall management of fibromyalgia and other chronic pain syndromes. Archives of Internal Medicine 156: 1047–1052

Hahn MB, McQuillan PM, Sheplock GJ 1996 Regional anesthesia. Mosby, St Louis

Hanna MH, Peat SJ 1989 Ketanserin in reflex sympathetic dystrophy: a controlled randomised double blind cross-over study. Clinical Journal of Pain 5: 205–209

Hannington-Kiff JG 1977 Relief of Sudeck's atrophy by regional intravenous guanethidine. Lancet 1: 1132–1133

Hannington-Kiff JG 1994 Sympathetic nerve blocks in painful limb disorders. In: Wall PD, Melzack R (eds) Textbook of pain, 3rd edn. Churchill Livingstone, Edinburgh, pp 1035–1052

Hogan QH 1997 Neural blockade for diagnosis and prognosis. Anesthesiology 86: 216–241

Holmes CM 1998 Intravenous regional blockade. In: Cousins M, Bridenbaugh PO (eds) Neural blockade. Lippincott-Raven, Philadelphia, pp 395–410

Houtchens MK, Richert JR, Sami A, Rose JW 1997 Open label gabapentin treatment for pain in multiple sclerosis. Multiple Sclerosis 3: 250–253

Jadad AR, Carroll D, Glynn CJ, McQuay HJ 1995 Intravenous sympathetic blockade for pain relief in reflex sympathetic dystrophy: a review and a randomized double blind crossover study. J Pain Symp Man 10: 13–20

Janig W 1988 Pathophysiology following nerve injury. In: Dubner GF, Gebhart J, Bono MR (eds) Proceedings of the 5th World Congress on Pain. Elsevier, Amsterdam, p 89

Janig W, Stanton-Hicks M 1996 Reflex sympathetic dystrophy: a reappraisal. IASP Press, Seattle

Jinkins JR, Whittemore AR, Bradley WG 1988 The anatomic basis of vertebrogenic pain and the autonomic syndrome associated with lumbar disc extrusion. American Journal of Neuroradiology 10: 219–231

Kaplan R, Claudio M, Kepes E, Gu XF 1996 Intravenous guanethidine in patients with reflex sympathetic dystrophy. Acta Anaesthesiologica Scandinavica 40: 1216–1222

Koltzenburg M 1997 The sympathetic nervous system and pain. In: Dickenson A, Besson J-M (eds) The pharmacology of pain. Springer, Berlin, pp 61–82

Laird JMA, Mason GS, Webb J, Hill RG, Hargreaves RJ 1996 Effects of a partial agonist and a full antagonist acting at the glycine site of the NMDA receptor on inflammation-induced mechanical hyperalgesia in rats. British Journal of Pharmacology 117: 1487–1492

Lakhlani PP, MacMillan LB, Guo TZ et al 1997 Substitution of a mutant α_{2A}-adrenergic receptor via 'hit and run' gene targeting reveals the role of this subtype in sedative, analgesic, and anesthetic-sparing responses *in vivo*. Proc Natl Acad Sci USA 94: 9950–9955

Leriche R 1916 De la causalgie envisagee comme une nevrite du sympathique et des son traitment par la dendation et l'excision des plexus nerveux periarterials. Presse Medicale 24: 178–180

Leriche R, Fontain RL 1934 Anaesthesie isolee du ganglion etoile: sa technique, ses indications, ses results. Presse Medicale 42: 846

Levine J, Taiwo Y 1994 Inflammatory pain. In: Wall PD, Melzack R (eds) Textbook of pain, 3rd edn. Churchill Livingstone, Edinburgh, pp 45–56

Levine JD, Fye K, Heller P, Basbaum AI, Whiting OK 1986a Clinical response to regional intravenous guanethidine in patients with rheumatoid arthritis. Journal of Rheumatology 13: 1040–1043

Levine JD, Taiwo YO, Collins SD, Tam JK 1986b Noradrenaline hyperalgesia is mediated through interaction with sympathetic postganglionic neurons rather than activation of primary afferent nociceptors. Nature 323: 158–160

Liu M, Max MB, Parada S, Robinovitz E, Bennett GJ 1996 Sympathetic blockade with intravenous phentolamine inhibits capsaicin evoked allodynia in humans. Abstracts of the 8th World Congress on Pain, Vancouver

Livingstone WK 1943 Pain mechanisms: a physiological interpretation of causalgia and its related states. MacMillan, New York

Loh L, Nathan PW 1978 Painful peripheral states and sympathetic blocks. Journal of Neurology, Neurosurgery and Psychiatry 41: 664–671

Longmore J, Swain CJ, Hill RG 1995 Neurokinin receptors. Drug News and Perspectives 8: 5–23

Magerl W, Koltzenburg M, Schmitz J, Handwerker HO 1996 Asymmetry and time course of cutaneous sympathetic reflex responses following sustained excitation of the chemosensitive nociceptors in humans. Journal of the Autonomic Nervous System 57: 63–72

Maizels M, Scott B, Cohen W, Chen W 1996 Intranasal lidocaine for treatment of migraine. Journal of the American Medical Association 276: 319–321

Malmberg AB, Yaksh TL 1995 Effect of continous intrathecal infusion of ω-conopeptides, N-type calcium channel blockers, on behaviour and antinociception in the formalin and hotplate tests in rats. Pain 60: 83–90

McClure JH, Wildsmith JAW 1991 Conduction blockade for postoperative analgesia. Edward Arnold, London, p 230

McLachlan EM, Janig W, Devor M, Michaelis M 1993 Peripheral nerve injury triggers noradrenergic sprouting within dorsal root ganglia. Nature 363: 543–545

McLatchie LM, Fraser NJ, Main MJ et al 1998 RAMPs regulate the transport and ligand specificity of the calcitonin-receptor-like receptor. Nature 393: 333–339

McMahon SB, Bennett DHL 1997 Growth factors and pain. In: Dickenson A, Besson J-M (eds) The pharmacology of pain. Springer, Berlin, pp 135–165

McQuay H, Carroll D, Jadad AR, Wiffen P, Moore A 1995 Anticonvulsant drugs for management of pain: a systematic review. British Medical Journal 311: 1047–1052

Meyer RA, Davis KD, Raja SN, Campbell JN 1992 Sympathectomy does not abolish bradykinin induced cutaneous hyperalgesia in man. Pain 51: 323–327

Miljanich GP, Ramchandran J 1995 Antagonists of neuronal calcium channels: structure, function and therapeutic implications. Annual Review of Pharmacology and Toxicology 35: 707–734

Millan MJ 1997 The role of descending noradrenergic and serotoninergic pathways in the modulation of nociception: focus on receptor multiplicity. In: Dickenson A, Besson J-M (eds) The pharmacology of pain. Springer-Verlag, Berlin, pp 385–446

Moore DC 1954 Stellate ganglion block. Charles C Thomas, Springfield

Munglani R 1997 Advances in chronic pain therapy with special reference to back pain. In: Ginsburg R, Kaufmann L (eds) Anaesthesia review 14. Churchill Livingstone, Edinburgh pp 153–174

Munglani R, Fleming B, Hunt SP 1996 Remembrance of times past: the role of c-fos in pain. British Journal of Anaesthesia 76: 1–4

Munglani R, Hudspith M, Hunt SP 1998 Therapeutic potential of NPY. Drugs 52: 371–389

Murdoch Ritchie JM 1994 Mechanism of action of local anaesthetics. In:

Fields HL, Liebeskind JC (eds) Progress in pain research and management. IASP Press, Seattle, pp. 189–204

Na HS, Leem JW, Chung JM 1993 Abnormalities of mechanoreceptors in a rat model of neuropathic pain: possible involvement in mediating mechanical allodynia. Journal of Neurophysiology 70: 522–528

Nakamura SI, Takahashi K, Takahashi Y, Yamagata M, Moriya H 1996 The afferent pathways of discogenic low-back pain. Evaluation of L2 spinal nerve infiltration. Journal of Bone and Joint Surgery 78: 606–612

Nebe J, Vanegas H, Neugebauer V, Schaible H-G 1997 ω-agatoxin IVA, a P-type calcium channel antagonist, reduces nociceptive processing in spinal cord neurons with input from the inflamed but not from the normal knee joint – an electrophysiological study in the rat in vivo. European Journal of Neuroscience 9: 2193–2201

Nebe J, Vanegas H, Scaible H-G 1998 Spinal application of ω-conotoxin GIVA, an N-type calcium channel antagonist, attenuates enhancement of dorsal spinal neuronal responses caused by intra-articular injection of mustard oil in the rat. Experimental Brain Research 120: 61–69

Neugebauer V, Vanegas H, Nebe J, Rumenapp P, Schaible H-G 1996 Effects of N-, L-type calcium channel antagonists on the responses of spinal cord neurons to mechanical stimulation of the normal and the inflamed knee joint. J Neurophysiol 76: 3740–3749

Nikolajsen L, Hansen PO, Jensen TS 1997 Oral ketamine therapy in the treatment of postamputation stump pain. Acta Anaesth Scand 41: 427–429

Ochoa JL, Verdugo RJ 1993 Reflex sympathetic dystrophy: definitions and history of ideas with critical review of human studies. In: Low P (ed) Clinical autonomic disorders. Little, Brown, Boston, p 473

Ohno K, Oshita S 1997 Transdiscal lumbar sympathetic block: a new technique for a chemical sympathectomy. Reg Anaesth Pain Man 85: 1312–1316

Ophoff RA, Terwindt GM, Vergouwe MN et al 1996 Familial hemiplegic migraine and episodic ataxia type-2 are caused by mutations in the Ca^{++} channel gene CACNL1A4. Cell 87: 543–552

Pancrazio JJ, Kamatchi GL, Roscoe AK, Lynch C 1998 Inhibition of neuronal Na^+ channels by antidepressant drugs? J Pharm Exp Ther 284: 208–214

Perez-Reyes E, Cribbs LL, Daud A et al 1998 Molecular characterisation of a neuronal low-voltage-activated T-type calcium channel. Nature 391: 896–900

Plancarte R 1989 Hypogastric block: retroperitoneal approach. Anaesthesiology 71: A739

Plancarte R, Velazquez R, Patt RB 1996 Neurolytic blocks of the sympathetic axis. In: Patt RB (ed) Cancer pain JB Lippincott, Philadelphia

Prithvi Raj P, Rauck RL, Racz GB 1996 Autonomic blocks. In: Prithvi Raj P (ed) Pain medicine. Mosby, St Louis, pp 227–258

Pud D, Eisenberg E, Spitzer A, Adler R, Fried G, Yarnitsky D 1998 The NMDA receptor antagonist amantadine reduces surgical neuropathic pain in cancer patients: a double blind, randomized, placebo controlled trial. Pain 75: 349–354

Quasthoff S, Grosskreutz J, Schroder JM, Schneider U, Grafe P 1995 Calcium potentials and tetrodotoxin resistant sodium potentials in unmyelinated C fibres of biopsied human sural nerve. Neuroscience 69: 955–965

Raja SN, Treede RD, Davis KD, Campbell JN 1991 Systemic alpha adrenergic blockade with phentolamine: a diagnostic test for sympathethetically maintained pain. Anesthesiology 74: 691–698

Ramamurthy S, Hoffman J and Guanethidine Study Group 1995 Intravenous regional guanethidine in the treatment of reflex sympathetic dystrophy/causalgia: a randomised double blind study. Anaesth Analg 81: 718–723

Rauck R, Eisenach JC, Young LD 1993 Epidural clonidine treatment for refractory reflex sympathetic dystrophy. Anesthesiology 79: 1163–1169

Reinhardt RR, Laub JB, Fricke J, Polis AB, Gertz BJ 1998 Comparison of a neurokinin-1 antagonist, L-754,030, to placebo, acetaminophen and ibuprofen in the dental pain model. American Society of Clinical Pharmacology and Therapeutics, New Orleans

Rizzo MA, Kocsis JD, Waxman SG 1996 Mechanisms of paresthesiae, dysesthesiae and hyperesthesiae: role of Na^+ channel heterogeneity. European Neurology 36: 3–12

Robbins WR, Staats PS, Levine J et al 1998 Treatment of intractable pain with topical large-dose capsaicin; preliminary report. Anesth Analg 86: 579–583

Rosenberg JM, Harrell C, Ristic H, Werner RA, De Rosayro AM 1997 The effect of gabapentin on neuropathic pain. Clin J Pain 13: 251–255

Rosner H, Rubin L, Kestenbaum A 1996 Gabapentin adjunctive therapy in neuropathic pain states. Clin j pain 12: 56–58

Rupniak NMJ, Boyce S, Williams AR et al 1993 Antinociceptive activity of NK1 receptor antagonists: non-specific effects of racemic RP-67580. British Journal of Pharmacology 110: 1607–1613

Rupniak NMJ, Patel S, Marwood R et al 1994 Antinociceptive and toxic effects of (+) epibatidine oxalate attributable to nicotinic agonist activity. British Journal of Pharmacology 113: 1487–1493

Rupniak NMJ, Carlson E, Boyce S, Webb JK, Hill RG 1995 Enantioselective inhibition of the formalin paw late phase by the NK1 receptor antagonist L-733,060 in gerbils. Pain 67: 188–195

Rush AM, Elliot JR 1997 Phenytoin and carbamazepine: differential inhibition of sodium currents in small cells from adult rat dorsal root ganglia. Neuroscience Letters 226: 95–98

Safieh-Garabedian B, Poole S, Allchorne A, Winter J, Woolf CJ 1995 Contribution of interleukin-1 beta to the inflammation-induced increase in nerve growth factor levels and inflammatory hyperalgesia. British Journal of Pharmacology 115: 1265–1275

Salt TE, Hill RG 1983 Transmitter candidates of somatosensory primary afferent fibres. Neuroscience 10: 1083–1103

Santillan R, Hurle MA, Armijo JA, De Los Mozos R, Florez J 1998 Nimodipine-enhanced opiate analgesia in cancer patients requiring morphine dose escalation: a double blind placebo-controlled study. Pain 76: 17–26

Sato J, Perl ER 1991 Adrenergic excitation of cutaneous pain receptors induced by peripheral nerve injury. Science 251: 1608–1610

Schmuck K, Ullmer C, Kalkman O, Probst A, Lubbert H 1996 Activation of meningeal 5-HT_{2B} receptors: an early step in the generation of migraine headache? European Journal of Neuroscience 8: 959–967

Scholz A, Kuboyama N, Hempelmann G, Vogel W 1998 Complex block of TTX-resistant Na^+ currents by lidocaine and bupivicaine reduce firing frequency in DRG neurons. J Neurophysiol 79: 1746–1754

Schott GD 1994 Visceral afferents and their contribution to 'sympathetic dependent' pain. Brain 117: 397–413

Schott GD 1995 An unsympathetic view of pain. Lancet 345: 634–635

Schott GD 1998 Interrupting the sympathetic outflow in causalgia and reflex sympathetic dystrophy. Br Med J 316: 1

Shir Y, Cameron LB, Raja SN, Bourke DL 1993 The safety of intravenous phentolamine administration in patients with neuropathic pain. Anaesthes Analg 76: 1008–1011

Spande TF, Garraffo HM, Edwards MW, Yeh HJC, Pannell L, Daley JW 1992 Epibatidine: a novel (chloropyridyl) azabicycloheptane with potent analgesic activity from an Ecuadorian poison frog. Journal of the American Chemical Society 114: 3475–3478

Stanton-Hicks M 1986 Blocks of the sympathetic nervous system. In: Prithvi Raj P (ed) Practical management of pain. Year Book Medical, Chicago, pp 661–681

Stanton-Hicks M, Janig W, Hassenbusch S, Haddox JD, Boas R, Wilson

P 1995 Reflex sympathetic dystrophy: changing concepts and taxonomy. Pain 63: 127–133

Stanton-Hicks M, Prithvi Raj P, Racz GB 1996 Use of regional anaesthetics in the diagnosis of reflex sympathetic dystrophy and sympathetically maintained pain. In: Janig W, Stanton-Hicks M (eds) Reflex sympathetic dystrophy: a reappraisal. IASP Press, Seattle, pp 217–237

Stolker RJ, Vervest ACM, Groen GJ 1994 The management of chronic spinal pain by blockades: a review. Pain 58: 1–20

Stone LS, Broberger C, Vulchanova L et al 1998 Differential distribution of α_{2A} and α_{2C} adrenergic receptor immunoreactivity in the rat spinal cord. J. Neurosci. 18: 5928–5937

Storer RJ, Goadsby PJ 1997 Microiontophoretic application of serotonin 5-$HT_{1B/1D}$ agonists inhibits trigeminal cell firing in the cat. Brain 120: 2171–2177

Stubhaug A, Breivik H, Eide PK, Kreunen M, Foss A 1997 Mapping of punctate hyperalgesia around a surgical incision demonstrates that ketamine is a powerful suppressor of central sensitization to pain following surgery. Acta Anaesthes. Scand 41: 1124–1132

Szallasi A 1997 Perspectives on vanilloids in clinical practice. Drug News and Perspectives 10: 522–527

Tabira T, Shibasaki H, Kuroiwa Y 1983 Reflex sympathetic dystrophy (causalgia) treatment with guanethidine. Archives of Neurology 40: 430–432

Takahashi H, Yanagida H, Morita S 1996 Analysis of the underlying mechanism of sympathetically maintained pain in the back and leg due to lumbar impairment: pain relieving effect of lumbar chemical sympathetectomy. Pain Clinic 9: 251–258

Tanelian DL 1996a Further comments regarding RSD studies. Pain Forum 5: 265–266

Tanelian DL 1996b Reflex sympathetic dystrophy. Pain Forum 5: 247–256

Taylor CP 1998 Mechanisms of action of gabapentin. Drugs of Today 34: 3–11

Tokunaga A, Saika M, Senba E 1998 5-HT_{2A} receptor subtype is involved in the thermal hyperalgesic mechanisms of serotonin in the periphery. Pain 76: 349–355

Tracey DJ, Romm MA, Yao NNL 1995 Peripheral hyperalgesia in experimental neuropathy: exacerbation by neuropeptide Y. Brain Res 669: 245–254

Utzschneider D, Kocsis J, Devor M 1992 Mutual excitation among dorsal root ganglion neurons in the rat. Neuroscience Letters 146: 53–56

Veldman PH, Goris RJ 1996 Multiple reflex sympathetic dystrophy. Which patients are at risk of developing a recurrence of reflex sympathetic dystrophy in the same or another limb? Pain 64: 463–466

Verdugo RJ, Ochoa JL 1994 Sympathetically mediated pain. Phentolamine block questions the concept. Neurology 44: 1003–1009

Wahren LK, Torebjork HE, Nystrom B 1991 Quantitative sensory testing before and after regional guanethidine block in patients with neuralgias of the hand. Pain 46: 24–30

Wahren LK, Gordh T, Torebjork E 1995 Effects of regional intravenous guanethidine in patients with neuralgias in the hand: a follow up study over a decade. Pain 62: 379–385

Waldman SD, Winnie AP 1996 Interventional pain management. WB Saunders, Philadelphia

Walker AE, Nulsen F 1974 Electrical stimulation of the upper thoracic portion of the sympathetic chain in man. Archives of Neurology and Psychiatry 59: 559–560

Warnke T, Stubhaug A, Jorum E 1997 Ketamine, an NMDA receptor antagonist, suppresses spatial and temporal properties of burn-induced hyperalgesia in man: a double blind, cross over comparison with morphine and placebo. Pain 72: 99–106

Webb J, Kamali F 1998 Analgesic effects of lamotrigine and phenytoin on cold induced pain: a cross over, placebo controlled study in healthy volunteers. Pain 76: 357–363

Weil SM 1992 Reflex sympathetic dystrophy. In: Evans RW, Bashin DS, Yatso FM (eds) Prognosis in neurological disorders. Oxford University Press, Oxford

Wilson PR, Low PA, Bedder MD, Covington EC, Rauck RL 1996 Diagnostic algorithm for complex regional pain syndromes. In: Janig W, Stanton-Hicks M (eds) Reflex sympathetic dystrophy: a reappraisal. IASP Press, Seattle, pp 93–105

Woolf CJ, Ma QP, Allchorne A, Poole S 1996 Peripheral cell types contributing to the hyperalgesic action of nerve growth factor in inflammation. J Neurosci 16: 2716–2723

Wrigglesworth R, Walpole CSJ, Bevan S et al 1996 Analogues of capsaicin with agonist activity as novel analgesic agents: structure activity studies. 4. Potent, orally active analgesics. Journal of Medicinal Chemistry 39: 4942–4951

Zimmer A, Zimmer AM, Baffi J et al 1998 Hypoalgesia in mice with a targeted deletion of the tachykinin I gene. Proc Natl Acad Sci USA 95: 2630–2635

Root and ganglion surgery

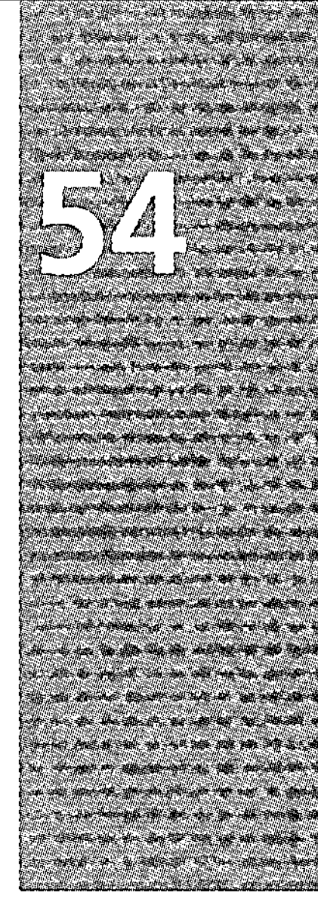

DAVID DUBUISSON

INTRODUCTION

Surgery of the spinal and cranial nerve roots has now evolved over more than a century. When sectioning of spinal roots was introduced by Bennett (1889) and Abbe (1889), anatomical principles suggested that pain could be selectively abolished by ablating segmental sensory inputs while sparing motor function. The technical difficulties and operative risks were considerable. In recent times, the use of binocular operating microscopes, microsurgical instrumentation, neural monitoring and improved anaesthesiology has made a variety of root operations feasible at both spinal and cranial levels. The risks are diminishing but still not negligible. Of greater concern is the frequent failure of nerve root surgery to provide relief. Although certain pain syndromes such as trigeminal, vagoglossopharyngeal and occipital neuralgia do respond favourably to root surgery most of the time, surgical outcome statistics accumulated over many decades demonstrate that some other common conditions such as postherpetic neuralgia and nerve root scarring after failed back surgery are much less likely to be relieved. Moreover, the sensory consequences of rhizotomy can include not only loss of cutaneous sensation with numbness but also dysaesthesias, loss of proprioception and anaesthesia dolorosa. A variety of neuroactive peptides and other chemical substances are depleted from the dorsal horn after rhizotomy. The physiological consequences of this, and the implications for further treatment if rhizotomy fails, are not fully understood. In theory, loss of opiate receptors in the dorsal horn following rhizotomy (Lamotte et al 1976) might limit the effectiveness of opiate analgesics after rhizotomy. North et al (1991) point out that root ablation destroys primary afferent fibres ascending in the dorsal columns, which may alter the neural substrate for electrical spinal cord stimulation. It is not clear whether modifications of root ablation such as percutaneous radiofrequency technique or microsurgical partial dorsal rootlet section can prevent or limit these untoward sequelae.

Recognition of the anatomical factors causing painful root or cranial nerve compression can in some cases lead to alternative treatments that spare the roots. Examples include microsurgical foramenotomy to relieve spinal roots constricted by bone and ligamentous hypertrophy; microvascular decompression to treat neuralgias of the cranial nerves; and electrical spinal cord stimulation to treat limb pain associated with epidural fibrosis and arachnoiditis. Magnetic resonance imaging (MRI) and computed tomography (CT) now routinely demonstrate sites of root compression that might have gone unrecognized 20 years ago. Decompression is increasingly a viable alternative to root or ganglion ablation, though not in all cases. There is no unanimous agreement as to which procedure is best for each patient, but the emphasis is changing from complete root ablation to minimal root lesioning or decompression when possible. This chapter reviews the techniques and outcomes of various types of root surgery (Fig. 54.1) at spinal and cranial levels. The subject of trigeminal neuralgia is also covered in Chapter 32. The topic of dorsal root entry zone (DREZ) lesions is discussed in Chapter 37.

DESCRIPTION

CRANIAL NERVE SECTION

Since the time of Dandy (1927), the most widely used approach to cranial nerves 5, 7, 9 and 10 has been posterior

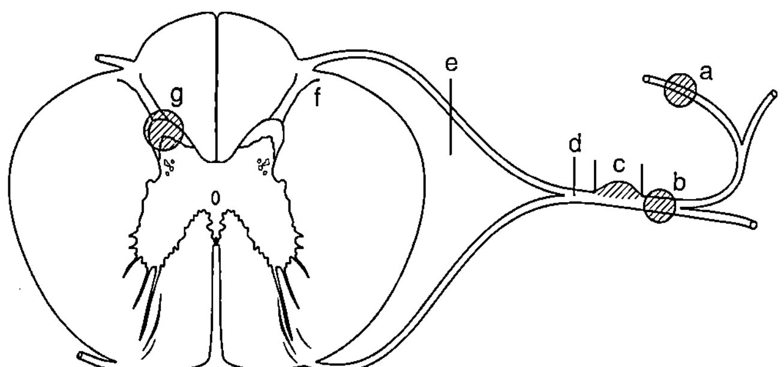

Fig. 54.1 Targets of spinal root and ganglion surgery. **a** percutaneous radiofrequency lesion of medial branch of posterior primary ramus; **b** percutaneous radiofrequency lesion of spinal nerve or dorsal root ganglion at the intervertebral foramen; **c** dorsal root ganglionectomy; **d** extradural rhizotomy; **e** intradural rhizotomy; **f** microsurgical partial posterior rhizotomy; **g** radiofrequency dorsal root entry zone (DREZ) lesion.

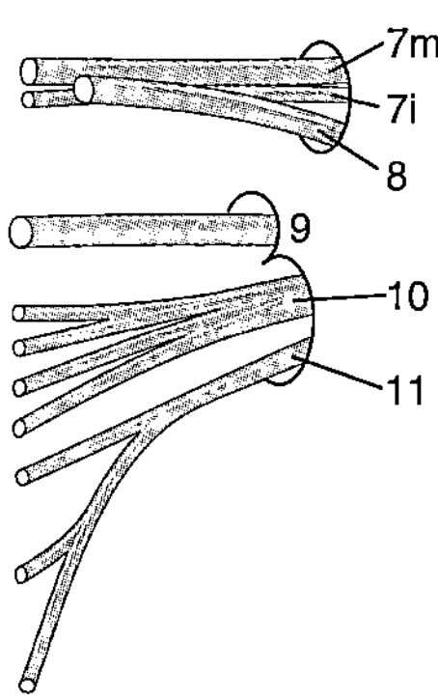

Fig. 54.2 A simplified schematic of the relationships of the lower cranial nerves in the posterior fossa. **7m** Motor division of facial nerve; **7i** sensory division of facial nerve (nervus intermedius); **8** vestibular component of eighth cranial nerve; **9** glossopharyngeal nerve; **10** vagus nerve; **11** accessory nerve. Note that the nervus intermedius is actually hidden from view by the superior and inferior vestibular nerves (not shown) and may consist of short anastomotic segments leaving the eighth nerve to join the seventh as they enter the internal auditory meatus. The cochlear (auditory) nerve, not shown, is anterior and inferior to the nervus intermedius. The ninth nerve enters the pars nervosa of the jugular foramen where it is separated from the 10th nerve by a dural septum.

fossa craniectomy. White and Kjellberg (1973) described the use of 'wake-up anaesthesia' to observe the patient's response to electrical stimulation of individual cranial nerve rootlets. However, difficulties in managing the airway of a heavily sedated patient and a preference for immobilization of the head during microsurgery have led most neurosurgeons to favour general anaesthesia for these procedures. Cranial nerves 5–10 are all accessible by a retromastoid craniectomy. The root of the trigeminal nerve is exposed high in the posterior fossa by gentle retraction of the tentorial surface of the cerebellum. The nervus intermedius is accessible in or near the internal auditory meatus. In cases of glossopharyngeal neuralgia or other throat pain, the ninth and 10th nerves are identified at the jugular foramen (Fig. 54.2).

Partial trigeminal root section is not widely used as the initial surgical treatment for facial pain, because alternatives emphasizing preservation of sensation are available. Tytus (1982) and Adams et al (1982) favoured partial rhizotomy to treat trigeminal neuralgia, but most other neurosurgeons who perform open microsurgery for this condition reserve partial rhizotomy of the fifth nerve for cases in which exploration fails to identify blood vessels or other anatomical features amenable to microsurgical decompression or for cases in which such vessels cannot safely be moved. Partial rhizotomy may also be appropriate in some rare cases of skull base malignancy in which tumour invasion precludes safe access to the trigeminal ganglion for a percutaneous lesioning procedure. When partial rhizotomy of the trigeminal nerve is employed, it is customary to spare the rostromedial portion of the sensory root, which is most likely to subserve corneal sensation. Despite the presence of numerous anastomoses between rootlets posterior to the Gasserian ganglion (Gudmundsson et al 1971), there is a fairly well-maintained somatotopic representation of the three trigeminal divisions near the root entry zone, with the first division located rostromedially and the third division caudolaterally (Rhoton 1993). Some variation in the orientation of the main sensory root and in the location and number of accessory rootlets near the pons is common. The presence of unmyelinated axons in the trigeminal 'motor' root has been documented. Axonal transport from a purely sensory branch of the nerve provided indirect evidence for the afferent function of these fibres. While it is not recommended that the portio minor of the trigeminal root be divided surgically, these data may help to explain failures of pain control after rhizotomy of the portio major.

In cases of glossopharyngeal neuralgia or other throat pain, the ninth and 10th nerves are identified at the jugular foramen, where they are separated by a dural septum. In cases of this type, all of the glossopharyngeal rootlets and one to three rostral filaments of the vagus are sectioned. Adson (1924) recommended section of the ninth nerve proximal to its superior (petrous) ganglion. Dandy (1927) found that intracranial section of the ninth nerve alone could be ineffective for controlling glossopharyngeal neuralgia and advocated inclusion of 1/8 to 1/6 of the vagus filaments. However, partial section of vagal rootlets can in some patients cause dysphagia, vocal cord paralysis or intractable coughing (Taha et al 1994). Robson and Bonica

(1950) recommended a preoperative trial of topical anaesthesia of the tonsillar fossa; persisting pain in the ear relieved by nerve block at the jugular foramen was felt to be evidence of a vagal contribution. However, this fails to take into consideration the recurrent course of the tympanic branch of the ninth nerve, which might also be blocked by local anaesthetic at the jugular foramen. Rhoton (1993) favoured sectioning of fewer rostral vagal rootlets if the diameters of the upper rootlets appeared relatively large. In an effort to reduce the risk of dysphonia, White and Sweet (1969) used 'wake-up' anaesthesia and stimulated individual vagus filaments to reproduce the patient's pain, avoiding filaments that did not contribute. Taha et al (1994) monitored vagal motor function during general anaesthesia by inserting an electrode in the ipsilateral false vocal cord as the patient was intubated. Individual rostral vagal rootlets were then stimulated electrically during surgery with currents of 0.05–0.1 mA, avoiding section of a rootlet when laryngeal motor responses were recorded at low threshold.

Haemostasis must be especially thorough and brain retraction delicate during these operations. Interruption of carotid sinus afferents may lead to a substantial and sometimes prolonged rise of blood pressure and the tight confines of the posterior fossa create an unforgiving environment if haematoma or cerebellar contusion should occur. Prior to rootlet section, manipulation of ninth and 10th nerve rootlets may cause sudden tachycardia or drop in blood pressure (Nagashima et al 1976, Rushton et al 1981). Cardiovascular instability at the time of rhizotomy may be damped to some extent by applying a small cotton wick soaked in local anaesthetic before cutting the rootlets. Continuous electrocardiographic and intra-arterial blood pressure monitoring are essential.

If it is necessary to section the intermedius component of the seventh nerve in the treatment of geniculate neuralgia, attention is directed to the internal auditory meatus and the seventh–eighth nerve complex. The nervus intermedius is hidden from view by the vestibular nerves, which must be separated from it by microdissection. Electromyographic monitoring of facial nerve function and monitoring of brainstem auditory evoked potentials may help to identify neural structures and to reduce the incidence of permanent neurological deficits (Moller 1993). The anatomy of the nervus intermedius is highly variable. The sensory component of the seventh nerve may consist of up to four tiny filaments which leave the eighth nerve to join the seventh nerve with short free segments as they approach the internal auditory meatus. In some instances, these free segments may all be located within the meatus (Rhoton 1993). White and Sweet (1969) sectioned the vestibular component of the eighth nerve when a distinct nervus intermedius could not be identified. Pulec (1976) preferred excision of the geniculate ganglion to treat geniculate neuralgia. Other authors recommend a combination of nervus intermedius section plus microvascular decompression of the fifth, ninth and 10th cranial nerves to treat primary otalgia (Rupa et al 1991, Lovely & Jannetta 1997).

MICROVASCULAR DECOMPRESSION OF THE TRIGEMINAL ROOT

In patients with trigeminal neuralgia, the root of the fifth cranial nerve near its root entry zone in the pons is commonly found to be indented by or in contact with an artery, vein, arachnoidal adhesions, tumour or some combination of these. Dandy (1932) described this type of compression in the course of operations for partial root section. Later, Gardner (1962) devised a technique of inserting a gelatin sponge between the root and an impinging vessel. This method was improved by use of the operating microscope (Jannetta 1967). The operation, known as microvascular decompression (MVD), has in recent years become one of the most widely practised surgical procedures to treat trigeminal neuralgia, although not without risk and controversy (Jannetta 1976, Apfelbaum 1977, Burchiel et al 1981, Breeze & Ignelzi 1982, Van Loveren et al 1982, Swanson & Farhat 1982, Barba & Alksne 1984, Piatt & Wilkins 1984, Bederson & Wilson 1989, Zakrzewska & Thomas 1993, Cho et al 1994, Linskey et al 1994, Sun et al 1994, Mendoza & Illingworth 1995, Barker et al 1996, 1997, Melvill & Baxter 1996, Rath et al 1996, Resnick et al 1996, Kondo 1997, Liao et al 1997, Miles et al 1997). There is an implicit or sometimes explicit assumption that the operation addresses the primary aetiology of neuralgic pain, but this is not the only advantage claimed by practitioners of MVD. The operation also has the goal of preserving the integrity of the nerve, thereby reducing risks of unpleasant dysaesthetic complications and loss of corneal sensation. In this regard, the operation may be especially useful in the management of first division neuralgia.

Published rates of neurovascular compression confirmed at surgical exploration vary from 10% (Adams et al 1982) to 100% (Sun et al 1994). There is some controversy about what constitutes a 'significant' amount of neurovascular contact (see Results). Based on a review of prior literature, Rohrer and Burchiel (1993) estimated that, with the exception of patients with multiple sclerosis, 62–64% of patients with trigeminal neuralgia have an artery impinging on the nerve, 12–24% have a vein, 13–14% have a combination of artery and vein and 8% have a tumour or vascular malformation. Some authors have studied neurovascular relationships of the trigeminal root by preoperative MRI or MR angiography (Tash et al 1989, Wong et al 1989, Hutchins et al 1990, Korogi et al 1995, Masur et al 1995, Meaney et al 1995, Boecher-Schwarz et al 1998). While the best available radiological techniques are reasonably sensitive, they often demonstrate neurovascular contacts on the asymptomatic side, sometimes fail to predict the specific neurovascular anatomy later found at operation and occasionally predict vascular compression that cannot be confirmed at surgery. Regardless of one's extent of reliance on this information, it is undoubtedly worthwhile to use MR imaging to rule out tumour, vascular malformation, aneurysm and demyelinating plaques before proceeding with MVD or any other posterior fossa surgery.

When vascular compression is found, the vessel involved is most often the superior cerebellar artery or the caudal and rostral trunks into which it bifurcates near the pons, along the superior and medial aspect of the root (Rhoton 1993). Less frequently, the anterior inferior cerebellar artery and its branches, or venous structures, may adhere to the nerve. Only about 2% of cases involve the vertebral or basilar arteries (Linskey et al 1994). Adequate exposure of the root entry at the pons may require retraction of an overhanging portion of the cerebellar hemisphere. The safest approach is along the superolateral surface of the cerebellum near the tentorium, so that retraction does not stretch the nearby auditory and facial nerve complex or bands of arachnoid attached to it. It may be necessary to coagulate the superior petrosal vein or a portion of its tributaries in order to gain adequate access. Veins indenting the trigeminal root are usually cauterized and divided, while arteries are moved away from the root and kept separate from it by prosthetic material (muscle, polyvinyl chloride sponge, shredded Teflon felt), a small fascial sling (Melvill & Baxter 1996) or tissue adhesive (Kondo 1997). To minimize postoperative fibrosis around the nerve, it is wise to position Teflon or other prosthetic material so that it displaces the vessel without directly contacting the nerve (Premsagar et al 1997). If no source of trigeminal root compression can be identified or if MVD cannot safely be completed, partial rhizotomy can be carried out as an alternative. Patients are usually maintained on gradually tapering doses of anticonvulsant medication following surgery.

MICROVASCULAR DECOMPRESSION OF LOWER CRANIAL NERVES

In cases of neuralgic pain involving the throat or auditory canal, the ninth and 10th cranial nerves may be found to be compressed by vascular structures such as the posterior inferior cerebellar artery, the vertebral artery or, less commonly, the anterior inferior cerebellar artery. Microvascular decompression of the ninth and 10th nerves was first proposed by Laha and Jannetta (1977) as a treatment for vagoglossopharyngeal neuralgia. Several neurosurgical centres have now reported use of MVD with or without section of nerve rootlets as a treatment for this condition (Laha & Jannetta 1977, Morales et al 1977, Tsuboi et al 1985, Panagopoulos et al 1987, Fraioli et al 1989, Sindou et al 1991, Sindou & Mertens 1993, Ferrante et al 1995, Taha & Tew 1995, Resnick et al 1995, Kondo 1998). Taha and Tew (1995) favoured intradural rhizotomy but considered microvascular decompression to be a helpful adjunct to sectioning of ninth and 10th nerve rootlets in cases where there was severe cross-compression of caudal vagal rootlets by vessels. These authors also recommended MVD instead of rootlet section in cases with pre-existing contralateral vocal cord paralysis and for rare cases of bilateral vagoglossopharyngeal neuralgia. Sindou et al (1991), Resnick et al (1995), Kondo (1998) and others have reported satisfactory long-term results in sizable numbers of cases when MVD was used as the sole treatment.

Techniques for MVD of the ninth and 10th nerves vary. Some surgeons use prosthetic implants consisting of small pieces of polyvinyl chloride sponge or shredded Teflon, but this is sometimes problematic. Lack of mobility of the offending vessels, often stiffened by atherosclerosis, may make it impossible to place these materials safely without compressing the brainstem or traumatizing delicate arterial branches. The lower cranial nerves are surrounded by tiny perforating end-arterioles, disturbance of which may lead to brainstem infarction. Also, most of the rootlets of the ninth and 10th nerves are quite small and fragile, so that they are easily damaged by dissection. Kondo (1998) recommends use of Biobond adhesive to reposition the vertebral or posterior inferior cerebellar artery away from the rootlets, attaching the vessel to the nearby dura of the petrous bone without any use of a prosthetic cushion. This method not only avoids the problem of compressing small neural and vascular structures, but also that of pain recurrence due to fibrosis or formation of a granuloma around the implant. If repositioning of vessels appears too risky, it is wise to proceed with root section instead.

PERCUTANEOUS LESIONS OF THE TRIGEMINAL GANGLION

Three percutaneous methods directed at the Gasserian ganglion or the trigeminal root just behind it are currently used to treat trigeminal neuralgia: RF rhizotomy, glycerol rhizotomy and balloon microcompression. These procedures require unimpeded access through the foramen ovale, which may not be the case in patients with skull base tumours or in those with scarring from prior alcohol injection in the area. The percutaneous approach for each of these procedures is similar. Following local anaesthetic in the skin, a needle is introduced through a point on the cheek just lateral to the corner of the mouth and guided, by fluoroscopic imaging of the skull base, into the foramen ovale. The depth of insertion of the needle is confirmed and adjusted if necessary by lateral fluoroscopy.

For percutaneous RF lesioning of the trigeminal root near the Gasserian ganglion (Sweet & Wepsic 1974, Nugent & Berry 1974, Siegfried 1981, Tew & Van Loveren 1988, Frank & Fabrizi 1989, Broggi et al 1990, Sweet 1990, Taha & Tew 1998), a temperature-monitoring electrode is inserted and the patient, if sedated during needle insertion, is awakened and brief trains of electrical stimulation are carried out. The electrode tip is further adjusted until the patient reports paraesthesias in the appropriate portion of the face, preferably at stimulation voltages around 0.2 V. Usually a straight electrode will pass sequentially through the third, second and first trigeminal divisions, but use of a curved electrode emerging beyond the tip of the guide needle can be helpful to gain access to the different divisions of the nerve (Tobler et al 1983). The patient is then heavily sedated with a short-acting agent and a heat lesion created at 60°C for 60 seconds. This can be enlarged if necessary, by moving the electrode tip or by using a slightly hotter temperature, after re-examining the patient for sensory loss or possible loss of the corneal reflex. Further details regarding percutaneous RF rhizotomy are given in Gybels and Sweet (1989) and in Taha and Tew (1998).

Percutaneous glycerol rhizotomy (Håkanson 1981, 1983, Sweet & Poletti 1985, Arias 1986a, Beck et al 1986, Saini 1987, Young 1988, Burchiel 1988, Waltz et al 1989, Ischia et al 1990, Fujimaki et al 1990, North et al 1990, Slettebo et al 1993, Bergenheim & Hariz 1995) is performed by a similar approach through the foramen ovale with fluoroscopy, using a spinal needle. When the trigeminal cistern is punctured via the foramen ovale, CSF usually emerges. A water-soluble radiographic contrast material is injected to outline the cistern. The contrast material is drained out, then 0.2–0.35 ml of sterile glycerol is injected in small increments of 0.05 ml, with the patient in a seated position and the neck flexed. The patient may experience paraesthesias or pain at the time of glycerol injection and this response may be used to further confirm needle placement. The patient must remain in the head-down, sitting position for about an hour afterward to prevent the liquid glycerol from escaping into the posterior fossa. Additional technical details of the procedure may be found in Håkanson and Linderoth (1998).

Percutaneous balloon microcompression (Mullan & Lichtor 1983, Belber & Rak 1987, Fraioli et al 1989, Lichtor & Mullan 1990, Lobato et al 1990, Brown et al 1993, Gerber & Mullan 1998) is performed with brief general anaesthesia. The foramen ovale is penetrated with a 14-gauge needle. The needle should not advance beyond the foramen, but should be engaged securely for introduction of a #4 French Fogarty catheter filled with radiographic contrast. A catheter depth stop may be used to limit emergence of the balloon into the trigeminal cistern. The balloon is inflated with 0.5–1.0 ml of contrast, forming a pear-shaped outline on fluoroscopy, and this is held for 60 seconds. Careful electrocardiographic monitoring is essential because profound bradycardia may occur during needle insertion or balloon inflation. The balloon catheter and guide needle are withdrawn together in order to prevent shearing of the catheter tip. The patient is not awakened for sensory testing during the procedure and repeated or prolonged balloon inflation is not recommended. Balloon microcompression is not as selective as RF lesioning for treatment of neuralgia restricted to one division of the trigeminal territory. Moreover, it may be less effective than RF lesioning for treatment of isolated third division neuralgia (Fraioli et al 1989).

PERCUTANEOUS THERMOCOAGULATION OF THE GLOSSOPHARYNGEAL NERVE

A percutaneous thermocoagulation technique for rhizotomy of the ninth nerve is available to treat pain due to oropharyngeal cancer or idiopathic glossopharyngeal neuralgia (Lazorthes & Verdie 1979, Isamat et al 1981, Arbit & Krol 1991, Tew 1982, Pagura et al 1983, Giorgi & Broggi 1984, Salar et al 1986, Arias 1986b, Tew & Van Loveren 1988, Gybels & Sweet 1989, Taha & Tew 1995). The target of the lesion is the glossopharyngeal nerve or its superior ganglion, at the pars nervosa of the jugular foramen. Because the superior ganglion of the ninth nerve lies within or below the level of the foramen in 68% of cases (Rhoton & Buza 1975), lesions of this type will not always interrupt afferent fibres proximal to the ganglion. The approach is generally similar to that used to reach the trigeminal ganglion, except that the needle trajectory is about 14° caudal to the trajectory into the foramen ovale and the electrode does not actually penetrate intracranially through the jugular foramen. Further technical details are given elsewhere (Gybels & Sweet 1989, Van Loveren et al 1990). A lateral approach starting below the external auditory canal has also been described (Ori et al 1985). Use of intraoperative fluoroscopy or CT guidance (Arbit & Krol 1991) is essential to locate the pars nervosa of the jugular foramen. Final adjustments of the electrode position are determined in the awake patient by responses to low-voltage electrical stimulation, seeking paraesthesias in the throat or ear without vagal cardiovascular responses, coughing or reaction of muscles innervated by the spinal accessory nerve. Because bradycardia and hypotension can occur in response to stimulation of afferents from the carotid sinus or vagal motor efferents, it is important to monitor the electrocardiogram and intra-arterial blood pressure continuously. At the time of lesioning, the patient must be adequately sedated. Unwanted neurological deficits such as hoarseness and dysphagia can be minimized by heating the electrode tip in small increments with temperature monitoring and frequent neurological examination.

INTRADURAL SPINAL ROOT SECTION

There are few clinical conditions for which intradural rhizotomy is the treatment of choice today, because less invasive alternatives are available. Root section in the subarachnoid space has been used mainly at cervical and thoracic levels where the roots exit from the spinal canal in close proximity to the corresponding cord segments. In the lumbosacral region, the nerve roots exit far caudal to the cord, which usually ends around the level of the L1–2 disc. Intradural section of posterior rootlets near the conus medullaris is feasible if stimulation is used to identify the pertinent rootlets, but since it is rarely desirable to section completely more than one or two lumbosacral roots, a smaller extradural exposure of the root sheaths near the intervertebral foramina is usually preferred. For intradural root section, the correct vertebral level must first be identified by suitable radiological technique. The operation is usually performed under general anaesthesia, but White and Kjellberg (1973) found it advantageous to wake the patient during the procedure in order to choose roots for sectioning. Stimulation of dorsal roots was used to confirm the contribution of individual roots to the patient's pain. Posterior rootlets leave their parent root to enter the cord as a fan-shaped array (Fig. 54.3). The appropriate rootlets are freed of accompanying blood vessels by microdissection before dividing them. It is sometimes necessary to divide anastomotic connections with rootlets of adjacent cord segments (Schwartz 1956).

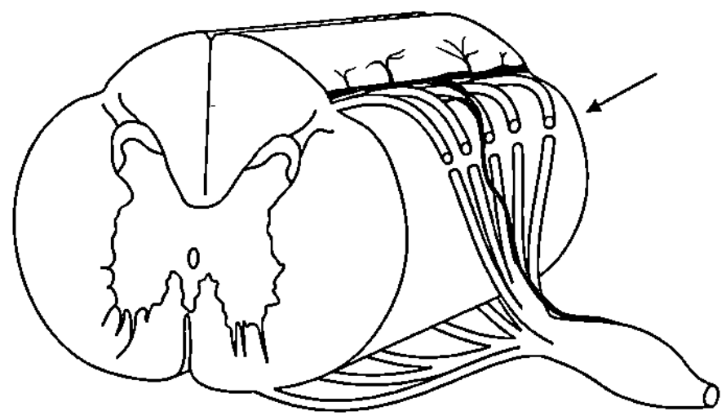

Fig. 54.3 Intradural rhizotomy. Individual posterior rootlets fan apart to enter the cord. Note sparing of the radicular artery. Arrow marks point at which rootlets have been sectioned.

To treat truncal pain, posterior rootlets in the cord segment corresponding to the painful area are sectioned along with one or two roots below and above that level. For intradural root section, this requires a series of laminectomies or hemilaminectomies, so that an extradural approach with multiple ganglionectomies may be easier (see below). Six or more consecutive thoracic dorsal roots can be sectioned without important loss of function. In the cervical and lumbosacral regions, the number of roots which can safely be sacrificed is limited by loss of function in the limb. White and Kjellberg (1973) found minimal hypoaesthesia and no proprioceptive deficit after section of a single dorsal root of the brachial or lumbosacral plexus. Section of two major plexus roots did not result in serious loss of function provided the second and third sacral roots were spared. These authors also recommended preserving at least C6 or C7 or else both C5 and C8 to protect proprioception in the upper limb in cases of extensive brachial rhizotomy and at least one root of the L2–L3–L4 group in cases of extensive lumbosacral rhizotomy. Section of both L5 and S1 may be done at some risk of interfering with proprioception in the ankle and foot. Combined cranial and upper cervical rhizotomies are occasionally undertaken in cases of head and neck cancer, but in most cases of this type, use of an intrathecal narcotic delivery system would be more easily tolerated.

EXTRADURAL ROOT SECTION

In the lumbosacral region where roots do not exit at the level of the corresponding cord segments, it is preferable to identify the dorsal roots near the intervertebral foramina. This can be done by opening the subarachnoid space, but most surgeons (e.g. Scoville 1966, White & Kjellberg 1973, Bertrand 1975, Strait & Hunter 1981) prefer an extradural approach (Fig. 54.4). If previous discectomy or other spinal surgery has been done, the presence of epidural

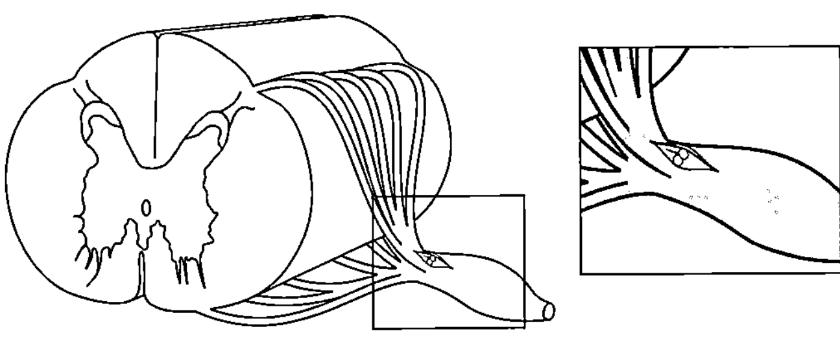

Fig. 54.4 Extradural rhizotomy. The root sheath is opened proximal to the dorsal root ganglion. The dorsal root, bifid at that point, is sectioned, sparing the motor fibres in the ventral compartment of the root sheath. For dorsal root ganglionectomy, the opening in the root sheath is extended and the ganglion is excised, dividing its connections to the sympathetic chain and ventral root.

fibrosis may obscure the root, making it necessary to remove additional bone from the laminae and articular facets for adequate exposure. Two distinct dorsal root fascicles are usually present, posterior to the ventral root bundle (Osgood et al 1976). Electrical stimulation can be used to distinguish ventral root filaments but in chronically damaged roots the threshold for excitation of motor responses is higher than usual and in some cases it may be impossible to produce muscle contractions (Bertrand 1975). Leakage of cerebrospinal fluid (CSF) is seldom a problem if section is carried out close to the dorsal root ganglion. Scoville (1966) described a similar approach for extradural section of cervical dorsal roots but he recommended a slightly different technique for extradural section of thoracic roots. He exposed the dorsal root ganglion laterally by removing a small amount of bone from the outer edge of the lamina just caudal to the transverse process. The sensory portion of the root was divided just proximal to the ganglion.

For the treatment of certain cases of intractable perineal and perianal pain due to advanced malignancy, a simplified extradural method of sectioning the lower sacral roots has been advocated (Crue & Todd 1964, Felsoory & Crue 1976). The dural tube is exposed by a laminectomy of the upper sacrum. The dural tube and its contents are ligated and divided caudal to the S1 root sheaths when bladder function is no longer important. In occasional patients whose pain extends to the leg, the S1 root is included on the painful side. In patients with residual bladder function, the S2 root on the least painful side is excluded from section.

DORSAL ROOT GANGLIONECTOMY

Concern about possible afferent connections to the cord from dorsal root ganglion cells via ventral roots or sympathetic communicating rami has led some surgeons to use dorsal root ganglion removal in preference to root section proximal to the ganglion. Subsequent to the description by Scoville (1966) of extradural dorsal rhizotomy by a posterolateral approach to the foramen, Smith (1970) reported isolation of the ganglion by a combination of dorsal rhizotomy, distal section and division of sympathetic rami to treat intercostal neuralgia. Additional small series of cases treated by dorsal root ganglionectomy are now available (Osgood et al 1976, Hosobuchi 1980, Pawl 1982, Gybels & Sweet 1989, Young 1990, North et al 1991, Taub et al 1995). Microsurgical technique for ganglionectomy and its application to lumbosacral dorsal root ganglia was introduced by Osgood et al (1976). The dural sleeve over the ganglion is incised from the bifid sensory root proximally to the division of the spinal nerve into anterior and posterior primary rami. With magnification, the yellow ganglion tissue can be dissected free and excised, sparing the ventral root compartment. The ganglia may be submitted to a pathologist for confirmation if desired. Spinal fluid leakage is usually minimal and can be controlled by a few microsutures. Lozano and colleagues (Lozano 1998, Lozano et al 1998) have described methods for extradural exposure and removal of the C2 dorsal root ganglion to treat occipital neuralgia. The C2 ganglion is accessible behind the C1–C2 facet joint and can be approached with little or no bone removal.

Apart from its recent use in treating occipital neuralgia, dorsal root ganglionectomy has been used for two broad categories of chronic pain. Truncal neuralgias and post-thoracotomy pain constitute one category, typically treated by ganglionectomies at multiple consecutive levels of the thoracic spine. Another category consists of patients with lumbosacral radiculopathy, treated by ganglionectomy at one or two levels. As noted previously, ablative root surgery can be carried out with relative impunity at six thoracic levels whereas multiple rhizotomies or ganglionectomies would produce disabling proprioceptive deficits in the limb if performed at cervical and lumbar levels.

PARTIAL POSTERIOR RHIZOTOMY

The term 'partial posterior rhizotomy' as used here refers to partial microsurgical sectioning of individual posterior rootlets at their junction with the spinal cord. Other terms for this procedure include 'selective posterior rhizotomy', 'selective posterior rhizidiotomy' and 'microsurgical DREZ-otomy'. This partial rootlet sectioning technique, developed by Sindou and his colleagues (Sindou et al 1974a,b,c, 1976, 1981), postulates an anatomical separation of large and small primary afferent axons within each rootlet at the dorsal root entry zone. It is suggested that small-diameter afferents cluster in the lateral aspect of each rootlet and penetrate the Lissauer tract where they can be divided selectively by a shallow microsurgical incision (Fig. 54.5). This microlesion along the ventrolateral aspect of individual dorsal rootlets presumably enters the lateral division of the Lissauer tract. However, the term 'Lissauer tractotomy' refers to an older procedure devised by Hyndman (1942) in which transverse sections were made in the tract.

The approach for partial posterior rhizotomy is similar to that used for intradural dorsal root section but the rootlets are not completely divided. Near the cord, the individual rootlets are dissected free of blood vessels and arachnoid under high magnification with an operating microscope. Each rootlet is then lifted medially with a blunt microsurgical hook. Underlying pial vessels are dissected away or lightly coagulated with a bipolar forceps. A microsurgical blade is used to make an incision 1–2 mm deep in the ventrolateral aspect of the rootlet–cord junction at an angle of about 45° from the sagittal plane (Fig. 54.6). A similar incision is made along each rootlet of the involved segments. There are no strict limitations to the number and levels of rootlets treated. Since the points of entry of the lumbosacral rootlets are nearly continuous, it may be easier in this region to retract all of the selected rootlets medially and, after moving or coagulating pial vessels, to make a continuous 1–2 mm incision along the posterolateral sulcus of the cord (Sindou et al 1976). Identification of lumbar and sacral rootlets is aided by electrical stimulation of corresponding ventral rootlets looking for muscle contractions, and by measurements. The dorsal rootlets of S2 and S3

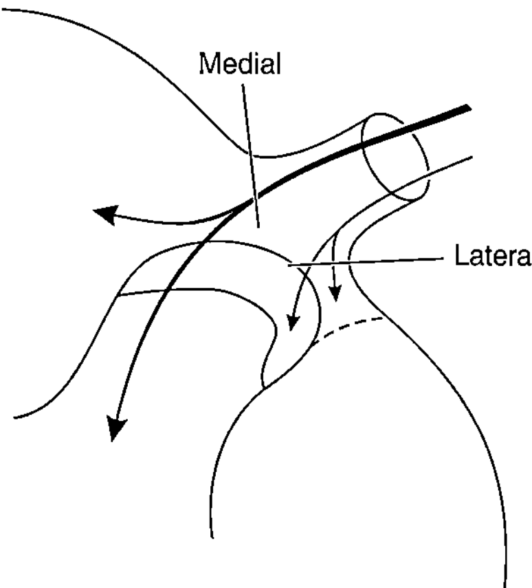

Fig. 54.5 The parcellation of primary afferent fibres postulated by Sindou et al (1976). Small-diameter primary afferents are preferentially destroyed by a lesion placed in the Lissauer tract on the ventrolateral aspect of the posterior rootlet. Mainly large-diameter afferents would be interrupted by lesioning the medial aspect of the root entry point.

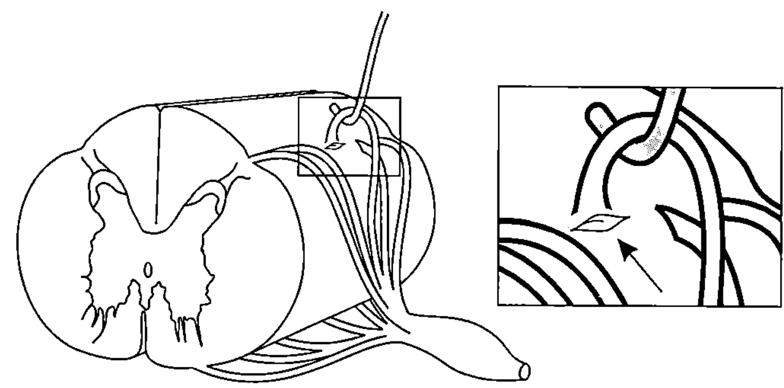

Fig. 54.6 Partial posterior rhizotomy (after Sindou et al 1976). Each posterior rootlet is lifted with a microsurgical hook to permit access to its ventrolateral aspect. An incision 1–2 mm deep is made at the cord–rootlet junction (inset).

spread rostrally 20–35 mm from the coccygeal root entry zone (Sindou et al 1976). Stimulation of ventral rootlets arising from the second, third and fourth sacral segments may produce contractions of the urinary bladder (Rockswold et al 1974).

Partial posterior rhizotomy has been used mainly to treat limb pain, where preservation of proprioceptive and tactile sensation is critical and complete dorsal rhizotomy at multiple levels would not be feasible. Because complete rhizotomy in the upper cervical region can lead to unpleasant scalp numbness and sometimes vertigo, the author has used partial posterior rhizotomy at these levels to treat severe occipital pain. Dorsal rootlets of the C1 through upper C3 cord segments are accessible through laminectomy of C1 and limited laminotomy of C2. The rootlets at upper cervical levels are much less freely mobile than rootlets at other levels of the cord and dorsal rootlets at C1 are absent in about half the cases. Cervical proprioception and scalp sensation are almost entirely spared by partial posterior rhizotomy at upper cervical levels (Dubuisson 1995).

MICROSURGICAL DECOMPRESSION OF SPINAL ROOTS

Spine surgery commonly involves decompression of nerve roots to treat varying combinations of weakness, sensory loss, pain and restriction of motion. The techniques chosen for root decompression should be dictated by specific anatomical features of the case. Single or multiple roots may be decompressed by removal of herniated discs and osteophytes; partial excision of hypertrophic zygapophyseal joints ('facetectomy') and thickened ligaments; laminectomy; and foramenotomy. A comprehensive review of these techniques would be beyond the scope of this chapter. Here we are concerned with surgical techniques designed to decompress individual spinal nerve roots and ganglia at the intervertebral foramina and their use in the treatment of radicular pain syndromes. These procedures offer a non-destructive alternative to root section in selected cases.

Foramenotomy, meaning surgical enlargement of the intervertebral foramen around a constricted nerve root, has been used effectively to treat root compression in the cervical region (Henderson et al 1983, Williams 1983, Krupp et al 1990, Jho 1996, 1998, Silveri et al 1997). Foramenotomy requires careful preoperative correlation of the clinical features of the radicular syndrome with detailed preoperative MRI or CT imaging. Foramenotomy for cervical radicular pain is not without risk, as the entrapped cervical roots are relatively small and easily damaged. In this author's opinion, cervical foramenotomy is most safely performed under high magnification with an operating microscope. When the procedure is done by a posterior approach, bone is gradually removed from the medial aspect of the facet complex using a high-speed air drill and continuous cool irrigation to prevent overheating of the root. Usually an opening about 5–7 mm in diameter will suffice to expose the foramen, leaving a thin shell of bone directly behind the root sleeve. Miniature curettes and bone punches are then used to remove the remaining bone with minimal disturbance to the root and its vasculature. Foramenotomy can typically be accomplished without affecting the strength of the joints, but biomechanical data suggest that removal of more than 50% of the transverse diameter of the facet complex may lead to spinal instability.

Posterior foramenotomy as an exclusive treatment for radiculopathy does not remove disc material and osteophytes impinging on the root from an anterior direction. Some surgeons combine posterior cervical foraminotomy with discectomy (Scoville et al 1976, Fager 1976, Aldrich 1990). As an alternative, a technique of microsurgical cervical foramenotomy by anterolateral, transforaminal approach has been developed (Jho 1996, 1998). Although this controversial technique requires microsurgical drilling in close proximity to the vertebral artery, it does effectively remove osteophytes and disc material from the foramen, decompressing the root and dorsal root ganglion.

Poletti has described microsurgical decompression techniques to treat occipital, neuralgia and cervical pain caused by C2 or C3 root constriction (Poletti 1983, 1996, Poletti & Sweet 1990). Cases managed in this way were carefully studied by preoperative radiological imaging demonstrating the sites of root constriction and by confirmatory local anaesthetic blocks.

PERCUTANEOUS RADIOFREQUENCY LESIONS OF SPINAL ROOTS AND GANGLIA

Radiofrequency lesions of the spinal nerve roots and ganglia can be performed by a percutaneous technique using local anaesthesia with monitored sedation (Uematsu et al 1974, Lazorthes et al 1976, Sluijter & Mehta 1981, Pagura 1983, Nash 1986, Garcia Cosamalon et al 1991, Van Kleef et al 1993, 1996, Stolker et al 1994a). To reach spinal roots or ganglia at cervical, thoracic or lumbar levels, a guide needle is introduced through the skin and paraspinal muscles and positioned at the intervertebral foramen by radiological guidance using intermittent fluoroscopy. CT imaging has also been used to guide percutaneous rhizotomy (Garcia Cosamalon et al 1991), but anatomical studies by Stolker et al (1994a) found that needle control was as accurate or more so with fluoroscopic imaging. Needle trajectories that penetrate the foramen almost parallel to the root carry increased risk of CSF leak or even cord injury. Needle entry into the foramen by a sagittal approach will at most levels give access to the dorsal root ganglion but at thoracic levels above T9, a straight posterior percutaneous approach to the ganglion may be hindered by the overlying lateral border of the lamina. A more lateral trajectory to the foramen risks pleural puncture, so that it may be necessary to place a drill hole through the bone with a Kirschner wire under fluoroscopic guidance (Stolker et al 1994a,b). The hole is centred mediolaterally at mid-pedicle and placed just caudal to the transverse process. When the foramen is entered, the patient, if awake, will usually experience some discomfort in the territory of the root. An electrode is inserted through the guide needle and low-intensity electrical stimulation is used to verify that the root innervates the region of chronic pain. A tingling sensation should be elicited in the corresponding dermatome with stimulation at 50 Hz and 0.4–1.2 V. A response to stimulation at 0.3 V or less may indicate actual contact or penetration of the ganglion, risking excessive destruction of the root if the lesion is made in this location. Also, in order to avoid lesioning of ventral root fibres, repetitive stimulation at 2 Hz should not elicit rhythmic muscle contractions at less than 1.5 times the threshold for sensory paraesthesias (Van Kleef & Sluijter 1998). Further confirmation of root level and extent of involvement of a given root in the patient's pain disorder can sometimes be indicated by the pattern of muscle contractions induced by stimulation. The patient is then sedated and the root is lesioned with a radiofrequency current generator. The use of a temperature-monitoring electrode and timer helps to limit the size of the lesion. The initial lesion is usually made for 60 seconds at 67°C.

Percutaneous lesioning of an individual root can be carried out in a stepwise fashion if desired, sedating the patient during the lesion and waking the patient to test for reduced sensitivity in the painful area. If the lesion is inadequate, the electrode may be repositioned or the lesion repeated at slightly higher temperature. With careful technique, motor function can usually be preserved along with some cutaneous sensation.

Percutaneous radiofrequency rhizotomy is helpful in cases of segmental cancer pain, particularly when the patient is debilitated and unable to undergo an open procedure under general anaesthesia. However, tumour invasion of the root or foramen may present an obstacle to safe performance of the procedure. Another situation in which percutaneous rhizotomy has been useful is truncal pain following thoracotomy or trauma, where avoidance of additional open incisions in the thoracic region may be attractive to the patient.

PERCUTANEOUS RADIOFREQUENCY MEDIAL BRANCH NEUROTOMY

Percutaneous radiofrequency thermocoagulation of nerves innervating the spinal zygapophyseal joints has been used in the treatment of cervical and lumbar pain (Shealy 1975, 1976, Burton 1976, Lazorthes et al 1976, Lora & Long 1976, Ogsbury et al 1977, McCulloch & Organ 1977, Mehta & Sluijter 1979, Oudenhoven 1979, Bogduk & Long 1980, Sluijter & Mehta 1981, Verdie & Lazorthes 1982, Rashbaum 1983, Andersen et al 1987, Ignelzi 1990, North et al 1994, Lord et al 1995, 1996). Because low back pain, neck pain and sometimes referred arm, leg or sacrococcygeal pain were known to originate in some cases from arthritic or spondylotic facet joints (Ayers 1935, Badgely & Arbor 1941, Harris & McNab 1954), techniques were devised which attempted to denervate the joints. Rees (1976) described a 'facet rhizolysis' in which he claimed to sever the articular branches of posterior primary rami using a long, thin blade. This method was criticized by King (1976), who demonstrated that in an average patient the lumbosacral joints could not in fact be denervated by the Rees procedure because the blade was not long enough to reach them. Shealy (1975) introduced percutaneous radiofrequency technique with fluoroscopic guidance of a hollow guide needle to contact the lumbar zygapophyseal joints. A temperature-monitoring electrode was passed through the guide needle and radiofrequency current passed to generate a heat lesion. This procedure, performed with local anaesthesia or light sedation, could be repeated at multiple levels during the same operative session if necessary. Fluoroscopically guided radiofrequency neurotomy of the medial branches of posterior primary rami (Fig. 50.1) has been further refined by anatomical studies of these nerve levels (Bogduk & Long 1979, Bogduk et al 1982, 1987, Lord et al 1995). Although the procedure is strictly speaking not a type of rhizotomy, the technical similarities and anatomical proximity of these lesioning methods make it convenient to discuss medial branch neurotomy as a variant of root surgery.

Local anaesthetic blocks directed at the zygapophyseal joints are recommended as a preliminary means of identifying levels concerned in the patient's pain. These blocks should be performed with fluoroscopy, using small volumes of 0.5% bupivacaine or 2% lidocaine. In the lumbar region, this typically requires injection of 1–3 ml per target around joints from L4 through S1 on the symptomatic side or bilaterally when necessary. In patients responding consistently to temporary blocks, lesioning is subsequently carried out at the effective levels, using a radiofrequency electrode with temperature-monitoring tip and fluoroscopic guidance. The articular branches lie rostral and caudal to the joint, not directly lateral to it (Bogduk & Long 1979). Needle placements by a true sagittal, posteroanterior approach in the lower lumbar region often fail to make contact with the medial branches because the bony joint structures bulge laterally to overhang and shield the bony recess where the medial branch is located. A somewhat oblique trajectory is preferable because this places the uninsulated lesioning tip parallel to the nerve branch, maximizing effective spread of current (Bogduk et al 1987). Electrical stimulation through the electrode tip is used to search for targets that reproduce the patient's pain at minimal threshold. Individual radiofrequency lesions are made at 80°C for 60–90 seconds. Oudenhoven (1977) found that electromyographic evidence of denervation in the multifidus muscles after percutaneous medial branch lesioning tended to correlate with good clinical outcomes.

Techniques to treat cervical zygapophyseal joint pain have been developed by Lord et al (1995, 1996). Preliminary local anaesthetic blocks are performed by a lateral approach under fluoroscopic control, using 0.5 ml of 2% lidocaine or 0.5% bupivacaine near the medial branches of the two posterior rami supplying the putatively symptomatic joint. For lesioning, both parasagittal and oblique passes of the electrode are used at each level.

RATIONALE

The basic purpose of spinal dorsal root section and of cranial nerve section is to denervate the area in which pain

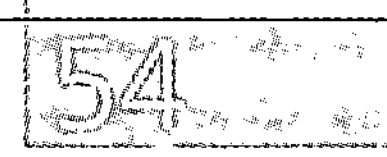

is felt, without compromising the spinal cord or brainstem. It might be assumed that root section would be of greatest benefit in pain due to intrinsic lesions of the sensory ganglion or root itself where the underlying disturbance is thought to be disordered or excessive activity of primary afferent fibres. It might also be assumed that root section should effectively relieve pain which is peripheral, circumscribed and radicular in quality, because the afferent territory of a small number of roots might encompass the painful region. Judging from the long-term results of root section, however, neither of these assumptions seems entirely accurate.

Some of the reasons for failure are already known or suspected. For instance, herpes zoster produces segmental pain with involvement of sensory ganglia, yet root section usually fails to provide relief (White & Sweet 1969, Onofrio & Campa 1972). This might be due to additional herpetic lesions of adjacent ganglia or of the spinal cord. The results of dorsal root section for pain associated with chronic mechanical damage and scarring of roots are also poor in the long term. We know from the work of Howe et al (1977) that chronic nerve and ganglion compression in animals leads to the development of mechanosensitivity of primary afferents. Wall and Devor (1983) showed that dorsal root ganglia may also be sites of ectopic impulse generation. The development of mechanosensitivity and ectopic discharge in dorsal root ganglion cells is a likely explanation for the appearance of chronic radicular pain in failed back surgery syndrome. Further evidence for ectopic discharge in human dorsal root afferents was provided by Nordin et al (1984), who used percutaneous microneurography to correlate this type of neuronal activity with the dysaesthesias referred to the foot during straight leg raising in a patient with persistent radicular pain following disc surgery. Dorsal root section for postlaminectomy radicular pain might reasonably be expected to interrupt abnormal trains of nerve impulses from the damaged sites, yet in most reported series, the long-term success rate is poor (Loeser 1972, Onofrio & Campa 1972, Bertrand 1975). Failure of dorsal rhizotomy to relieve sciatica may be partly related to sparing of ventral root afferents which would be eliminated by dorsal root ganglionectomy. However, not all authors agree that chronic sciatica responds well to ganglionectomy (see Gybels & Sweet 1989, North et al 1991). Moreover, due to involvement of multiple roots and other limiting factors, only about 2–3% of patients with chronic back pain and sciatica associated with disc problems are felt to be suitable candidates for ganglionectomy (Taub et al 1995). Long-term failure of either rhizotomy or ganglionectomy might be explained by spontaneous activity of chronically deafferented transmission neurons in the cord (Loeser & Ward 1967, Loeser et al 1968) or at higher levels of the nervous system (Rinaldi et al 1991). There are reasons to suspect that further deafferentation might even aggravate the problem. Following partial deafferentation of the dorsal horn in cats, initially unresponsive dorsal horn cells later became responsive to new afferent inputs (Basbaum & Wall 1976). Ovelmen-Levitt et al (1984) reported that receptive fields of deep dorsal horn neurons expanded to the flank and thoracic dermatomes after lumbar dorsal rhizotomies or root avulsions. These altered synaptic relationships within the cord, with afferent drive assumed by previously ineffective synapses or by newly formed synapses, may account for late failures of rhizotomy.

MULTIPLE ROOT SECTION

Some peripheral sources of pain fail to respond to root section, but it can often be argued that too few roots were divided. It has been known since the time of Sherrington that each cutaneous region is innervated by at least three consecutive roots (Sherrington 1898, Foerster 1933). Studies in primates (Dykes & Terzis 1981) make it clear that the full extent of dermatomal overlap is more extensive than this. Anatomical and physiological studies stress the presence of long-ranging primary afferent fibres within the spinal cord, which in some species may travel six or more segments to contact distant cord neurons (Imai & Kusuma 1969, Wall & Werman 1976). We know that some dorsal horn neurons, deprived of their most direct primary afferent contacts by multiple root section, begin to respond to these long-ranging afferents, taking on new and 'distant' receptive fields (Wall 1977). These facts may partly explain the recurrence of some types of pain after section of a limited number of dorsal roots. Also, root section may provide initial relief of pain from a small region of infection or malignancy yet a recurrence of pain could result from spread of the disease to involve intact neighbouring afferent dermatomes and sclerotomes. Also, peripheral nerve fibres may sprout into denervated areas of skin (Wedell et al 1941). Division of larger numbers of roots might compensate for these factors.

Some of the limitations of rhizotomy and ganglionectomy could be related to the levels of the spine involved. For example, chronic radiculopathy after failed disc surgery typically involves roots at cervical or lumbar levels where there are strict practical limitations on the number of roots sectioned. Loeser (1972) found no relationship between the success of dorsal rhizotomy and the number of roots sectioned. However, available literature on dorsal rhizotomy tends to show better results for truncal pain than for lumbar radiculopathies and this may be related to the larger number of roots sectioned at thoracic levels (North et al 1991). Extradural microsurgical techniques for thoracic ganglionectomy do not require conventional laminectomies and may further encourage root surgery at multiple levels. Results of ganglionectomy at three or more levels to treat thoracic pain (Hosobuchi 1980, Young 1996) are generally encouraging. The necessity to preserve limb proprioception makes it impossible to determine the effects of ganglionectomy at three or more lumbosacral levels.

PARTIAL DORSAL ROOTLET SECTION

The rationale of conserving some important dorsal roots of the brachial or lumbosacral plexus is that a completely deafferented limb is useless. Obviously this could limit the success of multiple rhizotomy for processes such as lung apex tumours or tumours of the pelvic region because not all roots innervating the region can be sectioned. Sindou's technique of microsurgical partial dorsal rootlet section largely circumvents this problem because it leaves intact at least some of the large proprioceptive and low-threshold mechanoreceptive axons in the medial portion of the root entry zone. Because some patients experience disabling vertigo as well as unpleasant numbness in the scalp after complete rhizotomy at upper cervical levels, partial posterior rhizotomy may be preferable at these levels also (Dubuisson 1995). Sindou et al (1974b) have used partial posterior rhizotomy to relieve pain in the arm associated with severe spasticity in hemiplegic patients. Prolonged or spasmodic muscle contraction might contribute to other types of pain such as chronic low back pain, post-thoracotomy pain, postlaparotomy pain and postherpetic neuralgia. The extent and importance of disordered muscle activity in these syndromes are unknown.

Some disruption of pial arteries and veins occurs during surgical procedures around the dorsal root entry zone, particularly when bipolar cautery is used for haemostasis. Vascular compromise of the dorsal horn might create a functionally more extensive lesion than the one visible to the surgeon. Wall (1962) carried out physiological and anatomical studies of the dorsal horn and ascending sensory tracts following tiny lesions of the ventrolateral cord–rootlet junction in cats. Using a dye perfusion technique, he detected a substantial decrease in perfusion of the entire dorsal horn after seemingly minor interference with the pial vessels. It is not known whether this occurs during partial posterior rhizotomy in humans. The larger overall size of the cord in humans probably makes it safer to coagulate a few tiny arterioles around the root entry zone, but the possibility of dorsal horn infarction is still present.

Not all authors find a distinct lateral separation of small afferents at the cord–rootlet junction. Wall (1962) felt that the longitudinally directed fibres of the Lissauer tract might be deflected by entering rootlets so as to create a false impression of large numbers of fine primary afferents entering laterally. Snyder (1977) failed to find a lateral subdivision of the dorsal rootlet in the cat, but he agreed that such a parcellation of small and large afferents was present in the monkey. Kerr (1975) studied thin sections of rootlets cut tangential to the root entry zone of monkey and cat cord and concluded that the distribution of large and small fibres within the rootlet was random until they were within 1 mm of the cord and then fine afferents tended laterally. While such an arrangement appears to exist in man, Sindou et al (1976) admit that other patterns may sometimes be present. Lack of fibre subdivisions within rootlets could limit the effectiveness of partial posterior rhizotomy.

PERCUTANEOUS PROCEDURES

An obvious advantage of percutaneous root lesions is that they are minimally invasive, with no need for general anaesthesia. Operating time is usually reduced in comparison to open rhizotomy or ganglionectomy and postoperative pain is less. The risk of death from an operative complication is close to zero for percutaneous procedures of all types. In most cases, percutaneous procedures are performed on an outpatient basis. These factors are considered to be more critical in elderly or debilitated patients and in patients who are poor candidates for general anaesthesia. However, such patients may also be poor candidates for monitored sedation or for procedures done with local anaesthetic due to limited respiratory function, pain preventing the patient from lying still and confusion from drugs or central nervous system involvement by the underlying disease.

Radiofrequency thermocoagulation of roots, dorsal root ganglia and root branches is based on the assumption that heat lesions preferentially destroy small myelinated and unmyelinated fibres, including the bulk of known nociceptive afferents, but leave intact the majority of innocuous mechanoreceptors and proprioceptors (Letcher & Goldring 1968). This concept is disputed by other authors who find that large and small fibres are destroyed indiscriminately (Uematsu 1977, Smith et al 1981, Hamann & Hall 1992). Widespread experience with thermocoagulation of the trigeminal ganglion supports the view that sparing of at least some innocuous mechanoreceptive afferents can be achieved by careful control of temperature. This is not necessarily true of spinal dorsal root and ganglion thermocoagulations. One obvious difference is that the trigeminal ganglion lies within a small cistern where it is surrounded by CSF. Nevertheless, percutaneous spinal dorsal root ganglion lesions have been accomplished safely even at mid-cervical levels, without loss of motor function in the arms or development of deafferentation syndrome (Van Kleef et al 1993).

It is not unreasonable to think that some of the success of thermocoagulation procedures might be due to destruction of large-diameter afferents, which might contribute to pain in many of the cases treated. The pain of cranial neuralgias is known to be triggered by innocuous stimuli. Myelinated afferent fibres, presumed to be responsible for transmission of these normally innocuous stimuli, have been shown to be responsible for hyperalgesia associated with nerve injury (Campbell et al 1988). Since the altered synaptic relationships and physiology of partially deafferented cord and brainstem neurons are not fully understood, it seems premature to interpret the results of root or ganglion thermocoagulation solely in terms of large and small afferent fibre spectra.

Open root surgery usually has the goal of sectioning primary afferents between their ganglion cells and the cord or brainstem, thereby preventing regeneration. Carefully placed percutaneous lesions of the ninth cranial nerve at the jugular foramen may sometimes accomplish the same goal, but with less certainty because the location of the superior glossopharyngeal ganglion is variable (Rhoton & Buza 1975) and the final lesion is not directly visible to the surgeon. Percutaneous rhizotomy at spinal levels can probably also limit effective regeneration by virtue of destroying dorsal root ganglion cells, but this requires considerable accuracy of needle placement and the completeness of root ablation is certainly less than that of an open procedure. In fact, direct lesioning of dorsal root ganglia may not provide better results than placement of RF lesions adjacent to the ganglia (Van Kleef et al 1996).

DIAGNOSTIC NERVE ROOT BLOCKS PRIOR TO SURGERY

There continues to be controversy in the use of selective nerve root blocks with local anaesthetics to predict the result of ablative root surgery. Many surgeons rely on preliminary root blocks to determine the segmental level involved, to decide whether a permanent root lesion might relieve the patient's pain and to give the patient some warning of what to expect should section be carried out. Some patients cannot tolerate numbness and should not be subjected to rhizotomy. Some reports (Loeser 1972, Onofrio & Campa 1972) indicate that an effective root block does not reliably predict a good response to subsequent root section. It is probably unwise to carry out root section or ganglionectomy if a series of accurately placed root blocks gives consistent lack of relief, but when preliminary root blocks show inconsistent results or the duration of pain relief is shorter than expected, it is not always clear that root surgery will fail. It is difficult to eliminate the possibility that spread of the local anaesthetic agent might reach adjacent roots. Small volumes of relatively concentrated local anaesthetic help to limit the territory of the block. In some cases, local anaesthetic may enter periradicular blood vessels or the subarachnoid space, leading to spurious results.

Dorsal horn neurons in a given cord segment receive afferent inputs not only from the dorsal root at the same segmental level but from many neighbouring roots, as noted above. From a physiological viewpoint, blocking one root should reduce the total afferent drive of dorsal horn neurons in several neighbouring cord segments, possibly reducing the patient's subjective experience of pain even when activity in another root was the primary cause. Moreover, root blocks undertaken with the preconceived notion that pain is monoradicular may be difficult to interpret if afferents in several roots are involved, as is often the case with arachnoiditis, epidural fibrosis, post-thoracotomy pain, postherpetic neuralgia and other conditions. Bonica (1974) argued that three or more selective root blocks of differing duration may be needed to predict the result of root section with any accuracy. In some cases, use of saline placebo for at least one of the blocks may be necessary. Lord et al (1996) used three blocks prior to cervical medial branch neurotomy: a short-acting local anaesthetic, a long-acting agent and placebo. However, despite this time-consuming process, some patients experienced an apparent placebo reaction following sham neurotomy. These responses were not reliably predicted by the preliminary blocks. Individual considerations should be given regarding the interpretation of diagnostic blocks. Johnson et al (1974) used intercostal nerve conduction studies to investigate level of involvement prior to thoracic root section. These studies were felt to increase the likelihood of pain relief in patients chosen to have surgery.

DORSAL ROOT GANGLIONECTOMY

Dorsal root ganglionectomy has practical and theoretical advantages over dorsal rhizotomy. The practical advantage is that ganglionectomy at thoracic levels can be carried out by an extradural approach requiring minimal bone removal.

This is less advantageous in the lower lumbar region where extensive bone removal is needed. Multiple laminectomies and a long dural opening make dorsal rhizotomy at more than a few levels unattractive for surgeon and patient, but ganglionectomy can be done at five or six levels if the patient is willing to tolerate significant incisional discomfort during the recovery period (Young 1996).

Ganglionectomy has some putative benefits in terms of eliminating afferent fibre connections to the ventral root and sympathetic chain. The presence of unmyelinated afferent fibres in ventral roots has been documented in anatomical studies (Coggeshall et al 1974, 1975). Physiological studies have shown nociceptive sensory receptive fields for unmyelinated ventral root fibres (Clifton et al 1976, Coggeshall & Ito 1977, Azerad et al 1986). These fibres originate from dorsal root ganglion cells and many of them loop into the ventral root but return to the ganglion to enter the cord via the dorsal root (Risling & Hildebrand 1982). Some have been shown to enter the cord directly through the ventral root and to form terminal arborizations in the dorsal horn (Light & Metz 1978). Myelinated afferents have also been identified in the ventral roots (Loeb 1976, Longhurst et al 1980).

Hosobuchi (1980) reported three patients who underwent dorsal root ganglionectomies for chest wall pain not adequately relieved by prior dorsal rhizotomy. Two of the patients had improved pain control after ganglionectomy, suggesting that some persistent ventral root afferents might have been eliminated. Several surgeons have reported encouraging results of thoracic ganglionectomies. Young (1996) reported excellent results in a series of patients undergoing dorsal root ganglionectomy at multiple levels. Results of multiple ganglionectomy in various reported series seem slightly better than those of dorsal rhizotomy, but direct comparison is hampered by incomplete data on follow-up time intervals, exact number and level of roots involved and conditions treated.

MICROVASCULAR DECOMPRESSION

Proponents of microvascular decompression of cranial nerves for trigeminal and vagoglossopharyngeal neuralgia hold that decompression preserves function in the nerves which would otherwise be lost during rhizotomy. However, in some cases, deficits may occur from root dissection during these procedures. Also, significant vascular compression will not be found in all cases and in some it may be impossible to separate vascular structures safely from the rootlets so that rhizotomy must be carried out anyway. Some neurosurgeons continue to favour intradural rhizotomy of the lower cranial nerves over microvascular decompression, on the grounds that rhizotomy is equally safe and has a well-established long-term success rate. Nevertheless, some recent series of cases of vagoglossopharyngeal neuralgia treated by microvascular decompression without rhizotomy show convincing long-term pain control. It might be thought that the decompression procedure succeeds because of subtle pressure on the rootlets by prosthetic materials used during the operation, yet Kondo (1998) achieved excellent results without prosthetic materials except a tissue adhesive holding the vessel to the dura. It might be argued that even delicate microdissection around the nerves could cause some direct injury and that the effect of MVD is due to this mild lesioning effect. However, postoperative sensory deficits are typically minimal or undetectable and when seen at all, they tend to be transient while pain relief continues, implying that neural damage is not the ingredient essential for pain relief (Miles et al 1997). In a survey of 1204 patients who underwent MVD for trigeminal neuralgia, Barker et al (1997) found no evidence that postoperative trigeminal numbness predicted relief of typical tic pain, although numbness was related to the type of operative findings and to the appearance of postoperative dysaesthesias.

Vascular contacts with the trigeminal nerve root were noted in 60% of 50 cadaveric roots in 25 cadavers, none with a prior history of trigeminal neuralgia (Hardy & Rhoton 1978). This information and similar reports of asymptomatic neurovascular contacts seen by MR angiography studies have been used in an effort to refute the concept of a vascular compressive aetiology for trigeminal neuralgia. However, it can also be argued that the frequency of such contacts in the general population might explain why trigeminal neuralgia is such a common condition. If one believes that the entire cause of cranial neuralgias is vascular compression near the brainstem, it is easy to understand how decompression would help but more difficult to explain how percutaneous procedures can give relief. Possibly, MVD would provide relief by eliminating a source of ectopic impulse generation in chronically compressed, demyelinated and mechanosensitive afferent fibres, whereas percutaneous procedures would reduce this type of impulse generation by simply destroying the same fibres.

INDICATIONS

Despite its many irrational aspects, root surgery is still useful in carefully selected cases to reduce noxious inputs from a circumscribed part of the body. With careful attention to technique, it is possible to spare motor and proprioceptive fibres. There are some potential adverse consequences of extensive denervation (see Complications and side effects, below), but in general the zone of sensory loss produced by rhizotomy is more stable than that produced by cordotomy (Loeser 1982).

The indications for cranial nerve surgery are better defined than those for spinal root surgery. Trigeminal, glossopharyngeal or geniculate neuralgia refractory to medical management is a suitable indication for root surgery provided the patient is in good enough health to undergo an operation safely. The choice of operation will depend on several factors, including the surgeon's expertise and level of comfort with the various procedures and the patient's tolerance of risk. When MVD is contemplated, even with preoperative MR imaging it will not be possible to predict with certainty that the surgeon will find vessels or other abnormalities amenable to microsurgical decompression and some back-up plan should be agreed upon before embarking on posterior fossa exploration. Partial rhizotomy of the trigeminal nerve or standard rhizotomy of the ninth and upper 10th nerves can be carried out during the same operation. In cases of trigeminal neuralgia, partial rhizotomy is customarily offered as a back-up procedure, but it does not seem unreasonable to offer a subsequent percutaneous procedure instead, if MVD cannot be completed. Percutaneous lesioning procedures are often recommended as the initial surgical choice in the treatment of cranial neuralgias because they can be carried out on an outpatient basis and they are felt to carry less risk. However, these procedures are by no means free of risks (see Complications and side effects). Also, not all patients can tolerate percutaneous lesion procedures, which require intermittent sedation and awakening and a high level of co-operation during awake testing. Risk of corneal sensory loss and keratitis after open or percutaneous rhizotomy may be unacceptable to some patients, especially those with poor vision in the contralateral eye and those with first division trigeminal pain. Microvascular decompression is probably the best option to preserve fifth nerve function. In cases of idiopathic vagoglossopharyngeal neuralgia, percutaneous RF lesions can be effective for pain control but some surgeons find the rate of complications, such as vocal cord paralysis and dysphagia, to be unacceptably high and prefer open root surgery to treat this condition unless the patient is too elderly or infirm to tolerate it (Taha & Tew 1998). Geniculate neuralgia is amenable to treatment by nervus intermedius section or excision of the geniculate ganglion but if posterior fossa exploration reveals adhesions, vessels or other abnormalities that might cause otalgia, MVD of the fifth, ninth and 10th nerves may be a beneficial adjunct (Rupa et al 1991, Lovely & Jannetta 1997).

Pain associated with ear and throat cancer, when increasingly refractory to narcotic medications and especially when unilateral, may be a suitable indication for percutaneous RF lesioning of the glossopharyngeal nerve (Gybels & Sweet 1989, Taha & Tew 1998). Cancer of the head and neck associated with intractable pain in the face, neck, throat or ear may occasionally justify section of some combination of cranial and upper cervical roots (Sindou et al 1976). This type of extensive root surgery does not carry a high success rate and is seldom performed today. In general, open root surgery for cancer pain is only warranted in a patient who is markedly refractory to narcotics, whose overall health does not preclude general anaesthesia and whose life expectancy is substantially greater than the time required for hospitalization and postoperative recovery. This also applies to multiple root section or ganglionectomy to treat pain of malignancy elsewhere in the body, especially when another treatment such as a spinal narcotic delivery system might be equally effective. In most cases of truncal or lower extremity cancer pain, it seems preferable to choose percutaneous root lesioning or cordotomy, which may require a brief stay in the hospital or may be tolerated as an outpatient procedure, than to choose an open surgical procedure which might lead to prolonged hospitalization for an already debilitated patient.

Spinal root surgery is often useful for pain associated with tumours of the lung apex and brachial plexus region. Here, microsurgical partial posterior rhizotomy can be used to prevent total denervation of the arm. The same principle can be applied to malignancy involving the lumbosacral plexus and causing leg pain, but cordotomy will often provide a simpler solution. For pain due to malignant perineal and sacral tumours, bilateral section of the third, fourth and fifth sacral and of the coccygeal roots can be effective. The method of Crue and Todd (1964) is probably the simplest way to achieve this but concern for remaining bladder function may demand a more restricted approach with intraoperative stimulation of individual roots. Pain limited to the superficial anococcygeal region may require section of only S4, S5 and the coccygeal roots. Obviously, when previous colostomy and urinary diversion have been done, bilateral section of sacral roots can be undertaken with greater impunity. Pain associated with chest wall malignancies may also respond well to multiple root section or ganglionectomy, particularly when it is feasible to divide one or two roots above and below the painful segments.

Root surgery for pain associated with benign conditions at spinal levels has widely varying success rates that appear to depend partly on the underlying disease process and partly on the location of pain. Occipital neuralgia refractory to medications and to repeated nerve blocks with local anaesthetic and steroids can usually be relieved by C2 ganglionectomy (Lozano et al 1998) or by intradural sectioning of the C1 through upper C3 roots, if the patient is willing to undergo general anaesthesia. To preserve scalp sensation and cervical proprioception, the author prefers microsurgical partial posterior rhizotomy for this condition (Dubuisson 1995). Refractory occipital neuralgia is one of the best indications for root surgery because of the high likelihood of relief and the low incidence of complications. Good initial results of rhizotomy for occipital neuralgia tend to be permanent, especially in post-traumatic cases (Hunter & Mayfield 1949). Cases of occipital pain in which discrete construction of the C2 or C3 root can be demonstrated radiologically may be considered for microsurgical decompression (Poletti 1983, 1996, Poletti & Sweet 1990). A technique has also been developed for treatment of pain in the occipital region by electrical spinal cord stimulation (Barolat 1998). This requires general anaesthesia and an open exposure of the epidural space but has the advantage of preserving root function. Although the long-term results of cord stimulation for occipital neuralgia are not yet known, some patients may prefer to explore this option before committing to ablative root surgery.

In the small number of cases reported, postherpetic neuralgia was seldom adequately relieved by dorsal rhizotomy (White & Sweet 1969, Loeser 1972, Onofrio & Campa 1972). Smith (1970) reported success in two cases of thoracic postherpetic neuralgia treated by an extensive disconnection of the dorsal root ganglia. More recent literature is inconclusive regarding the use of multiple thoracic ganglionectomy for this condition. Multiple ganglionectomy has been used with reasonably good outcomes to treat other truncal pain disorders (Hosobuchi 1980, North et al 1991, Young 1996). The procedure has the advantage that laminectomies are not required, although there may still be considerable incisional discomfort due to disruption of the paraspinal muscles. Also, multiple rhizotomies or ganglionectomies at truncal level can be followed at least transiently by dysaesthesias in neighbouring dermatomes, as discussed later in this chapter. Thoracic segmental pain syndromes can also be managed effectively by percutaneous radiofrequency lesions of the roots or ganglia (Garcia Cosamalon et al 1991, Stolker et al 1994b). A conservative approach for cases of truncal pain refractory to medications, nerve blocks and transcutaneous electrical stimulation would be to offer trials of electrical spinal cord stimulation next. If stimulation were ineffective or intolerable, percutaneous RF lesions could be tried after preliminary root blocks and multiple dorsal root ganglionectomy would be considered as a more radical solution if needed.

Multilevel percutaneous 'facet denervation' is practised mainly in cases of refractory low back and neck pain. There is no indisputable indication for the procedure. The concept of a 'facet syndrome' has considerable merit on clinical grounds. Nevertheless, diagnosis of this syndrome can be confounded by the multiplicity of anatomical and physiological variables involved in back and neck pain and lack of objective radiological criteria to identify patients who might be helped by lesioning nerve branches to the joints. Scepticism about the procedure began during the era in which 'facet denervation' practised with a percutaneous scalpel was criticized when the blade was later shown to be too short to reach the zygapophyseal joints (King 1976). Efforts to re-establish the procedure as a percutaneous RF medial branch neurotomy with radiological guidance placed it on somewhat more objective ground. According to recent literature, the appropriate indication for RF medial branch neurotomy is a consistent response to highly selective local anaesthetic blocks, radiologically guided toward the medial branches of posterior primary rami innervating the targeted joints (Lord et al 1996, Van Kleef & Sluijter 1998). However, the presumption that nerve blocks will accurately and reliably predict a response to RF lesioning is not justified, as noted earlier.

RESULTS

The success of root and ganglion surgery seems to depend less on the exact technique employed than on the problem treated. Long-term results sampled at least 3 months after the procedure are invariably worse than immediate results. Table 54.1 shows the percentages of patients who reported either substantial relief or complete relief of their pain after open root section or dorsal root ganglionectomy for various conditions. These percentages were derived by adding patients from several series of intradural or extradural rhizotomies or ganglionectomies for which some useful data were given concerning follow-up. Results of dorsal root ganglionectomy have not been analysed separately because the available literature does not allow any kind of statistically meaningful comparison that might establish a difference between outcomes of ganglionectomy and outcomes of rhizotomy. Much of the data in Table 54.1 is derived from the era prior to binocular operating microscopes and microsurgical techniques and the appearance of CT and

Table 54.1 Results of open rhizotomy or ganglionectomy at spinal and lower cranial levels.

Condition	*Levels*	*Immediate relief (%)*	*Relief after 3 mos. (%)*	*No. of cases*	*Authors*
Geniculate neuralgia	Nervus intermedius (*)	87	80	49	Cases cited in White & Sweet 1969, Pulec 1976, Rupa et al 1991, Lovely & Jannetta 1997
Vagoglossopharyngeal neuralgia	IX+ upper X	84	79	178	Robson & Bonica 1950, Bohm & Strang 1962, Walker 1966, White & Sweet 1969, Laha & Jannetta 1977, Rushton et al 1981, Taha & Tew 1995
Occipital neuralgia	C1–3 or C2 ganglion	78	70	104	Hunter & Mayfield 1949, Chambers 1954, Cusson & King 1960, Scoville 1966, White & Sweet 1969, Echols 1970, Onofrio & Campa 1972, Dubuisson 1995, Lozano et al 1998
Postherpetic neuralgia	Multiple spinal roots	36	29	11	White & Sweet 1969, Smith 1970, Loeser 1972, Onofrio & Campa 1972
Truncal postsurgical, post-traumatic, idiopathic	Multiple spinal roots or ganglia	81	65	106	Scoville 1966, Echols 1970, Smith 1970, Loeser 1972, Onofrio & Campa 1972, White & Kjellberg 1973, Osgood et al 1976, Dubuisson (this chapter)
Chronic sciatica (failed back surgery)	Lumbosacral roots	73	42	273	Loeser 1972, Onofrio & Campa 1972, White & Kjellberg 1973, Jain 1974, Bertrand 1975, Osgood et al 1976, Strait & Hunter 1981, Pawl 1982, Gybels & Sweet 1989, North et al 1991, Taub et al 1995
Coccygodynia	S3–C1	79	58	52	Bohm 1962, Echols 1970, Albrektsson 1981, Saris et al 1986
Cancer	Multiple spinal +/– cranial	59	47	585	Cases cited in Sindou et al 1976, including 153 cases with long-term follow-up

*Includes MVD of other cranial nerves in some cases

MRI imaging. Careful descriptions of both immediate and long-term results are seldom given in these series. Especially in older series, the criteria for good results are either not specified by the authors or, if specified, not always objective. Despite these limitations, it is apparent that the most consistent short- and long-term pain relief is reported for idiopathic cranial neuralgias, occipital neuralgia, coccygodynia and certain benign truncal pain conditions. The least satisfactory results of open root surgery are reported for postherpetic neuralgia (29% of patients reporting long-term relief) and failed lumbar spine surgery (42% incidence of long-term pain relief). Results of percutaneous radiofrequency root and ganglion lesions, in a more limited variety of conditions, are summarized in Table 54.2.

The topic of trigeminal neuralgia is also discussed in Chapter 32. Surgical treatment of this condition is enormously controversial, partly because so many options are available. For the purposes of this chapter, results of the currently popular root and ganglion procedures can be summarized as follows. In the treatment of trigeminal neuralgia, percutaneous RF lesions carry approximately 82–100% initial success rates, with 5–42% of patients experiencing recurrences after 2 years and about 50% having recurrences after 5 years (Gybels & Sweet 1989, Rohrer &

Table 54.2 Results of percutaneous radiofrequency lesions of spinal and lower cranial nerve roots or ganglia (selected series).

Level (condition)	*Immediate relief(%)*	*Relief after 3 mos. (%)*	*No. of cases*	*Authors*
Spinal roots or ganglia	72	61	124	Uematsu et al 1974, Lazorthes et al 1976, Nash 1986, Van Kleef et al 1993, Stolker 1994b
Ninth nerve (vagoglossopharyngeal neuralgia)	95	75	22	Lazorthes & Verdie 1979, Isamat et al 1980, Giorgi & Broggi 1984, Arias 1986b, Salar et al 1986, Tew & Van Loveren 1988, Gybels & Sweet 1989, Arbit & Krol 1991
Ninth nerve (orofacial cancer)	64	64	42 (25 with long-term follow-up)	Lazorthes & Verdie 1979, Pagura et al 1983, Giorgi & Broggi 1984, Tew & Van Loveren 1988, Gybels & Sweet 1989

Burchiel 1993). Success of the procedure is associated with production of facial numbness, particularly in areas including the cutaneous trigger zones. Nevertheless, Nugent reported excellent results with a low incidence of dysaesthesias when lesser degrees of sensory loss, short of full analgesia, were accepted. Percutaneous trigeminal glycerol rhizotomy carries approximately 67–96% initial success rates, with early recurrences in about 20% of patients and recurrences within 5–10 years in about 50% (Håkanson & Linderoth 1998). Percutaneous balloon microcompression of the trigeminal ganglion has approximately 93–100% initial success rate and recurrences in about 20–30% of patients at 5 years (Abdennebi et al 1995, Gerber & Mullan 1998). Far smaller numbers of patients have been reported for balloon microcompression than for the other trigeminal root and ganglion procedures mentioned here. Partial rhizotomy of the trigeminal root in the posterior fossa carries an approximately 80–90% rate of long-term pain relief (Rohrer & Burchiel 1993), but with troublesome facial paraesthesias and dysaesthesias in many cases. Microvascular decompression surgery has an initial success rate as high as 96–98% and significant pain recurrence over several years in 12–29% of cases (Rohrer & Burchiel 1993). Most authors find that the success rate of MVD is less when the neurovascular contacts do not include an artery. Piatt and Wilkins (1984) noted an 83% success rate when an artery was embedded in the root entry zone or otherwise distorted the root. There was a 62% success rate with lesser degrees of arterial contact and only 42% success rate in cases with venous contacts or no vascular impingement. In the series of Jannetta and his colleagues, 1185 patients undergoing MVD were reported (Barker et al 1996), with 70% said to be pain free off medications 10 years after surgery. Patients with strictly paroxysmal pain have higher success rates than those with constant background pain (Szapiro et al 1985). Although some sensory loss may follow MVD for trigeminal neuralgia, the procedure appears to carry a very low incidence of dysaesthesias and anaesthesia dolorosa (Rohrer & Burchiel 1993). Microvascular decompression is not an appropriate choice for most patients with multiple sclerosis, because the procedure does not provide reliable pain relief in this population (Resnick et al 1996).

Vagoglossopharyngeal neuralgia can be controlled in most patients by either percutaneous or open procedures. Gybels and Sweet (1989), citing the increased risk of death associated with cardiovascular instability during intracranial 9th–10th nerve surgery, recommended percutaneous lesioning as the initial procedure of choice. Taha and Tew (1998) reported good or excellent results in all 12 of their patients who underwent intracranial root section for idiopathic vagoglossopharyngeal neuralgia, with no mortality and minimal permanent morbidity. These authors felt that the use of percutaneous ninth nerve lesioning should be limited to cases of cancer pain because of the high incidence of postoperative hoarseness, vocal cord paralysis and dysphagia. The numbers of reported cases are relatively small, so it is difficult to be dogmatic about the choice of treatment. Open section of the ninth and upper 10th nerves carries approximately 84% initial success rate, versus 95% initial success rate for the percutaneous procedure; however, there appears to be little difference in long-term results. Microvascular decompression of the ninth and 10th nerves has been shown to have an initial success rate of 89–95% (Resnick et al 1995, Kondo 1998), with little or no risk of pain recurrence in the long term but with a 5% perioperative mortality rate.

Several types of root and ganglion operations have been used effectively to treat medically refractory occipital neuralgia. The choice of operation depends on the surgeon's preference and on the range of conditions included in the term 'occipital neuralgia'. Aetiologies and locations of pain are certainly not uniform for this diagnostic category. White and Sweet (1969) cited literature and personal experience to support their contention that the results of combined C2 and C3 rhizotomy were better than those of C2 rhizotomy alone. Dubuisson (1995) reported that partial posterior rhizotomy at C1-upper C3 levels gave long-term pain relief in about 70% of patients with refractory occipital neuralgia, almost entirely sparing scalp sensation. Some patients in this series experienced pain in the temporal and periorbital regions, which was sometimes eliminated by the procedure but more often not helped. Nevertheless, pain within the C2 dermatomal territory was relieved or reduced by more than 50% in all cases. Selective C2 ganglionectomy was said to relieve occipital neuralgia or reduce its intensity by more than 50% in 26 of 39 cases (Lozano et al 1998), with a higher success rate for post-traumatic occipital pain than for idiopathic neuralgia. This is a simpler procedure than partial posterior rhizotomy because ganglionectomy does not require an intradural exposure. Surgeons with special interest in C2 and C3 root compression syndromes may be able to select a subgroup of patients who will gain relief from microsurgical root decompression.

Root surgery has not been conspicuously successful in the treatment of widespread arachnoiditis or postoperative epidural fibrosis, although occasional cases of localized intradural scarring may benefit (Jain 1974). Dorsal rhizotomy for cases of 'battered root' syndrome following lumbar disc surgery or spinal fusion has a very poor success rate with essentially all patients reporting eventual failure, and most describing troublesome dysaesthesias as a complication, according to Bertrand (1975). Only a third of the 47 patients reported by Strait and Hunter (1981) were able to increase their physical activities following extradural rhizotomy. Dorsal root ganglionectomy to treat persistent sciatica that could be relieved by local anaesthetic block of one or two lumbosacral roots was studied in a group of 61 patients (Taub et al 1995), with the conclusion that sciatica was markedly reduced or eliminated in 59%. Postoperative dysaesthesias were noted in 60% of this group, however, and often required additional measures for control. North et al (1991) and Sweet (in Gybels & Sweet 1989) reported less enthusiastic results of lumbosacral ganglionectomy for limb pain in failed back surgery syndrome, citing failure in most cases and appearance of troubling dysaesthesias in many. Pain associated with failed disc surgery and nerve root damage would therefore appear to be a poor indication for any type of dorsal root surgery because of its high failure rate and the likelihood of dysaesthesias or anaesthesia dolorosa. It seems likely that the underlying root damage in these cases has already led to disordered afferent impulse generation and perhaps irreversible patterns of neuronal transmission within the central nervous system, so that further deafferentation by rhizotomy or ganglionectomy will often be futile or detrimental. Because alternatives such as electrical spinal cord stimulation are available to treat this condition, few surgeons would now opt for ablative root surgery.

Root surgery for postherpetic neuralgia cannot be strongly endorsed, as it carries only a 29% long-term success rate. As noted earlier, there are some reasons to suspect that multiple dorsal root ganglionectomy might fare better, but the literature is inconclusive on this point. Open rhizotomy and dorsal root ganglionectomy at multiple levels have been used with respectable success rates in the treatment of non-herpetic truncal pain due to trauma, surgical scars and idiopathic intercostal neuralgia (Table 54.1). As noted earlier, the extradural approach and relative lack of disabling neurological deficits from multiple thoracic dorsal root ganglionectomies may make it feasible to encompass the area of pain more widely at these levels. Encouraging results of percutaneous RF partial rhizotomy for segmental thoracic pain syndromes were reported in 45 patients with 86% of patients reporting good or excellent pain control at follow-ups of 13–46 months (Stolker et al 1994b).

Root surgery for cancer pain has a modest overall success rate (47% late pain relief), but the results are still discouraging and management of cancer pain has shifted overwhelmingly toward use of oral and intrathecal narcotics. In patients who require further measures, patient selection is a critical issue. Some of the best published results pertain to partial posterior rhizotomy for tumours of the brachial and lumbosacral plexus regions, where initial relief can be as high as 87–100% of cases (Vlahovitch & Fuentes 1975, Sindou et al 1981). Relief is generally sustained over the survival period of the patient. Unfortunately, only a minority of patients with metastatic cancer can safely undergo open root surgery of this type. If root surgery is contemplated, it is probably best that it be carried out relatively early in the course of treatment while the patient's overall health permits a safer perioperative course and the extent of tolerance to narcotics is not so great as to impede adequate treatment of postoperative incisional pain. Percutaneous RF lesioning of spinal roots and ganglia, and of cranial nerves, provides respectable early relief of pain due to malignancy (Table 54.2). Late results of spinal RF lesions are hard to judge because the technique is often used as a minimally invasive means of treating pain in debilitated, terminally ill patients. In general, long-term results of percutaneous RF lesions, cranial or spinal, are similar to those of open root surgery for cancer pain.

Percutaneous medial branch neurotomy ('facet denervation') in the lumbar region has met with mixed reviews, with more than 50% pain relief for follow-up periods averaging 8–27 months reported in 17–82% of patients. Many authors have reported a substantially higher rate for the procedure in patients with prior back surgery (Shealy 1975, McCulloch & Organ 1977, Ignelzi & Cummings 1980, Long 1982), but North et al (1994) found RF lumbar facet denervation to have moderate long-term benefit and prior back surgery was not a significant prognostic factor. In a randomized, double-blind trial of percutaneous RF neurotomy for chronic cervical pain, Lord et al (1996) reported that nine of 12 patients in the active treatment group (electrode temperature 80°C) and six of 12 patients in the control group (electrode temperature 37°C) were relieved of pain during the period immediately after operation. However, seven patients in the active treatment group and one in the control group remained free of pain at 27 weeks. The apparent placebo response immediately after the control procedure, in which the electrode was not heated at all, was observed in 50% of patients. This was noted even among patients who had been tested beforehand with placebo-controlled diagnostic blocks, a finding described by the authors as 'a sobering reminder of the complex and inconstant dynamics of placebo phenomena'.

COMPLICATIONS AND SIDE EFFECTS

Some of the risks of root and ganglion surgery have been mentioned in the preceding discussion and may be obvious to the clinician on anatomical grounds, although not always so apparent to the patient. As a generality, all root and ganglion procedures, whether cranial or spinal, open or percutaneous, share two broad categories of risk. The first is failure to achieve adequate pain relief. The second is excessive or unwanted loss of sensation.

Failure to achieve pain relief after root surgery may sometimes be due to an inadequate number of roots divided or ganglia excised or, in the case of percutaneous lesions, inaccurate targeting or incomplete thermocoagulation. When no pain relief is seen immediately following spinal root surgery, there is the unfortunate possibility that the wrong root was sectioned, either because of misleading preoperative blocks with local anaesthetic or because of an error identifying the correct level of the spine with intraoperative X-ray films or fluoroscopy. Levels of thoracic and lumbar vertebrae and roots can frequently be difficult to confirm in the operating room because of variations in the number of ribs and variable sacralization of lower lumbar vertebrae. In obese patients, these factors become even more problematic as intraoperative X-ray films and fluoroscopy yield technically inferior images. Particularly in the thoracic region, preoperative CT and MRI may demonstrate only a portion of the spine, so that intraoperative counting of vertebrae is inconclusive. It can be very helpful to insist that a preoperative sagittal MRI scout image be obtained, demonstrating all the vertebrae between the level of intended surgery and either the skull base or the sacrum. Surgeons planning root or ganglion surgery should take care to understand the idiosyncrasies of each patient's spine before embarking on the surgical procedure. Also, when diagnostic nerve root blocks were not performed by the surgeon, it is always worth enquiring as to how the levels of the blocks were ascertained in the clinic.

Adverse outcomes involving excessive loss of sensation depend partly on the segmental levels involved and partly on the likelihood of deafferentation phenomena following a given procedure. Loss of cutaneous sensation with numbness is seldom a disabling problem after root surgery, but some patients who have not been exposed to this feeling by prior anaesthetic root block may find it as disturbing as their original pain. This seems especially true for loss of sensation in the face and mouth after trigeminal surgery and for numbness in the genitalia after root surgery at the level of the thoracolumbar junction or sacrum. The latter may lead to sexual dysfunction. Some patients will experience severe pain in the deafferented dermatomes ('denervation dysaesthesia' or anaesthesia dolorosa) following rhizotomy or ganglionectomy. It might be thought that this would be more of a problem after ablation of multiple roots, but the condition is frequent after rhizotomy or ganglionectomy of one or two roots to treat radicular pain in failed back surgery syndrome (Bertrand 1975, Gybels & Sweet 1989, Taub et al 1995) and is troublesome in about 8% of patients after partial rhizotomy of the trigeminal nerve in the posterior fossa (Rohrer & Burchiel 1993). Young (1996) found anaesthesia dolorosa after dorsal root ganglionectomies, mostly at truncal levels, to be an uncommon phenomenon. Osgood et al (1976) noted dysaesthesias in four of 18 patients undergoing ganglionectomy. Sweet (1984) noted that the unpleasant sensations were often referred to the margins of the denervated zone following rhizotomies. Hosobuchi (1980) also described this phenomenon in patients undergoing multiple thoracic dorsal root ganglionectomies. In the series of patients undergoing dorsal root ganglionectomy at lumbosacral levels (Taub et al 1995), spontaneous and evoked dysaesthesias in the dermatomal distribution of resected dorsal root ganglia were seen in 36 of 61 patients and were rated as mild to moderate in 33 (72%), marked in 11 and severe in one case. These dysaesthesias were more frequent after resection of more than one ganglion and were usually relieved by systemic lidocaine.

Young (1996) described cases of troublesome bulging of the abdominal wall following multiple dorsal root ganglionectomies at truncal levels, presumably due to denervation in the abdominal wall musculature. Extradural and intradural root surgery at multiple levels can be followed by a prolonged period of postoperative incisional pain due to the extent of paraspinal muscle disturbance. Other risks of spinal intradural root surgery include CSF leak, aseptic or bacterial meningitis and cord damage from haematoma or disturbance of radicular arteries.

Percutaneous cranial nerve lesioning procedures carry very low mortality rates, approximating zero. Possible complications of these procedures include injury to the optic nerve or other cranial nerves due to incorrect needle positioning; infections; intracranial haemorrhages (occasionally fatal); trigeminal motor weakness; loss of corneal sensation with risk of keratitis; facial dysaesthesias and anaesthesia dolorosa. Percutaneous trigeminal glycerol rhizotomy may carry a greater risk of postoperative dysaesthesias than RF lesioning (Gybels & Sweet 1989). An advantage claimed by proponents of balloon microcompression for trigeminal neuralgia is that postoperative dysaesthesias and corneal sensory loss are less than with other percutaneous procedures (Gerber & Mullan 1998). In a study comparing RF thermocoagulation, glycerol injection and balloon microcompression (Fraioli et al 1989), there was a higher incidence of unwanted sensory loss after RF rhizotomy, but the incidence of corneal sensory loss was similar for the three procedures. Keratitis was not seen after balloon microcompression in this study. Rare cases of carotid-cavernous fistula have resulted from balloon microcompression procedures (Kuether et al 1996, Gerber & Mullan 1998). Percutaneous RF lesioning of the ninth nerve can be complicated by hoarseness or frank vocal cord paralysis, intractable coughing and dysphagia, as noted earlier.

Deaths have been associated with posterior fossa procedures for trigeminal neuralgia, including MVD, often as a result of postoperative cerebellar or brainstem infarction, and sometimes occurring after seemingly uneventful surgery by experienced surgeons. The operative mortality rate for MVD of the fifth nerve may vary from about 0.2% to 5%, depending on the size of the series reported and presumably the degree of experience of the surgeons (Gybels & Sweet 1989, Rohrer & Burchiel 1993, Barker et al 1996). Posterior fossa procedures for vagoglossopharyngeal neuralgia, including rhizotomy and MVD, carry a 5% mortality rate in most of the available literature. This may be partly related to cardiovascular instability caused by the procedure, including bouts of sudden arterial hypotension or hypertension, cardiac arrhythmias or cardiac arrest, and partly due to infarction in the brainstem or cerebellum or thrombosis of a major venous sinus. Dysaesthesias and loss of corneal sensation are not common after MVD of either the fifth or ninth and 10th nerves, as might be expected because the operation has a goal of preserving the integrity of the nerves. However, deficits of these and other cranial nerves have been described, the commonest of which is probably hearing loss, a problem occurring in 1–19% of cases depending on the studies quoted (Rohrer & Burchiel 1993, Barker et al 1996). Delayed hearing loss has been reported after MVD (Fuse & Moller 1996) and was felt to be due to fibrotic reaction around the auditory nerve. Granulomas forming around shredded Teflon material have also been described and may be related to recurrences of pain (Premsagar et al 1997). Nervus intermedius section is expected to result in decreased lacrimation, salivation and taste but may be complicated by hearing loss, facial paresis and vertigo (Rupa et al 1991). Other potential complications of posterior fossa operations include vertigo, ataxia, CSF leak and aseptic or bacterial meningitis, all either transient or amenable to treatment in most instances.

Percutaneous rhizotomy, ganglion lesions and medial branch neurotomy are relatively free of serious complications. Van Kleef et al (1993) reported transient burning sensations, lasting 6 weeks or less, in 12 of 20 patients who underwent percutaneous RF lesions of the cervical dorsal root ganglia. Dysaesthesias are said to be less frequent with small-diameter RF electrodes and with avoidance of direct penetration of the root or ganglion (Van Kleef et al 1993, Van Kleef & Sluijter 1998). A neuralgic pain syndrome ('lumbar lateral branch neuralgia'), with burning pain and hyperaesthesia in the iliac region, has been described as a complication of RF medial branch neurotomy (Bogduk 1981). Spinal cord injury has been reported as a complication of percutaneous RF rhizotomy (Koning et al 1991). Possible explanations include damage to radicular vessels or direct injury from the needle or heat from the electrode, a notion which has led most practitioners of percutaneous RF lesioning to approach the targets in the sagittal plane.

REFERENCES

Abbe R 1889 A contribution to the surgery of the spine. Medical Record 35: 149–152

Abdennebi B, Bouatta F, Chitti M, Bougatene B 1995 Percutaneous balloon compression of the Gasserian ganglion in trigeminal neuralgia. Long-term results in 150 cases. Acta Neurochirurgica 136: 72–74

Adams CBT, Kaye AH, Teddy PJ 1982 The treatment of trigeminal neuralgia by posterior fossa microsurgery. Journal of Neurology, Neurosurgery and Psychiatry 45: 1020–1026

Adson AW 1924 The surgical treatment of glossopharyngeal neuralgia. Archives of Neurology and Psychiatry 12: 487–506

Albrektsson B 1981 Sacral rhizotomy in cases of anococcygeal pain. Acta Orthopaedica Scandinavica 52: 187–190

Aldrich F 1990 Posterolateral microdiscectomy for cervical monoradiculopathy caused by posterolateral soft cervical disc sequestration. Journal of Neurosurgery 72: 370–377

Andersen KH, Mosdal C, Vaernet K 1987 Percutaneous radiofrequency facet denervation in low-back and extremity pain. Acta Neurochirurgica 87: 48–51

Apfelbaum RI 1977 A comparison of percutaneous radiofrequency trigeminal neurolysis and microvascular decompression of the trigeminal nerve for the treatment of tic douloureux. Neurosurgery 1: 16–21

Arbit E, Krol G 1991 Percutaneous radiofrequency neurolysis guided by computed tomography for the treatment of glossopharyngeal neuralgia. Neurosurgery 29: 580–582

Arias MJ 1986a Percutaneous retrogasserian glycerol rhizotomy for trigeminal neuralgia: a prospective study of 100 cases. Journal of Neurosurgery 65: 32–36

Arias MJ 1986b Percutaneous radiofrequency thermocoagulation with low temperature in the treatment of essential glossopharyngeal neuralgia. Surgical Neurology 25: 94–96

Ayers CE 1935 Further case studies of lumbo-sacral pathology with consideration of involvement of intervertebral discs and articular facets. New England Journal of Medicine 213: 716–721

Azerad J, Hunt CC, Laporte Y, Pollin B, Thiesson D 1986 Afferent fibers in cat ventral roots: electrophysiological and histological evidence. Journal of Physiology 379: 229–243

Badgely CE, Arbor A 1941 The articular facets in relation to low back pain and sciatic radiation. Journal of Bone and Joint Surgery 23: 481–496

Barba D, Alksne JF 1984 Success of microvascular decompression with and without prior surgical therapy for trigeminal neuralgia. Journal of Neurosurgery 60: 104–107

Barker FG 2nd, Jannetta PJ, Bissonette DJ, Larkins MV, Jho HD 1996 The long-term outcome of microvascular decompression for trigeminal neuralgia. New England Journal of Medicine 334: 1077–1083

Barker FG 2nd, Jannetta PJ, Bissonette DJ, Jho HD 1997 Trigeminal numbness and tic relief after microvascular decompression for typical trigeminal neuralgia. Neurosurgery 40: 39–45

Barolat G 1998 Spinal cord stimulation for persistent pain management. In: Gildenberg PL, Tasker RR (eds) Textbook of stereotactic and functional neurosurgery. McGraw-Hill, New York, pp 1519–1537

Basbaum AI, Wall PD 1976 Chronic changes in the response of cells in adult cat dorsal horn following partial deafferentation: the appearance of responding cells in a previously non-responsive region. Brain Research 116: 181–204

Beck DW, Olson JJ, Urig EJ 1986 Percutaneous retrogasserian glycerol rhizotomy for treatment of trigeminal neuralgia. Journal of Neurosurgery 65: 28–31

Bederson JB, Wilson CB 1989 Evaluation of microvascular decompression and partial sensory rhizotomy in 252 cases of trigeminal neuralgia. Journal of Neurosurgery 71: 359–367

Belber CJ, Rak RA 1987 Balloon compression rhizolysis in the surgical management of trigeminal neuralgia. Neurosurgery 20: 908–913

Bennett WH 1889 A case in which acute spasmodic pain in the left lower extremity was completely relieved by subdural division of the posterior roots of certain spinal nerves. Medico-Chirurgical Transactions 72: 329–348

Bergenheim T, Hariz M 1995 Influence of previous treatment on outcome after glycerol rhizotomy for trigeminal neuralgia. Neurosurgery 36: 303–310

Bertrand G 1975 The 'battered' root problem. Orthopedic Clinics of North America 6: 305–310

Boecher-Schwarz HG, Bruehl K, Kessel G, Guenthner M, Perneczky A, Stoeter P 1998 Sensitivity and specificity of MRA in the diagnosis of neurovascular compression in patients with trigeminal neuralgia. A correlation of MRA and surgical findings. Neuroradiology 40: 88–95

Bogduk N 1981 Lumbar lateral branch neuralgia: a complication of rhizolysis. Medical Journal of Australia 1: 242–243

Bogduk N, Long DM 1979 The anatomy of the so-called 'articular nerves' and their relationship to facet denervation in the treatment of low back pain. Journal of Neurosurgery 51: 172–177

Bogduk N, Long DM 1980 Percutaneous lumbar medial branch neurotomy. Spine 5: 193–200

Bogduk N, Wilson AS, Tynan W 1982 The human lumbar dorsal rami. Journal of Anatomy 134: 383–397

Bogduk N, McIntosh J, Marsland A 1987 Technical limitations to the efficacy of radiofrequency neurotomy for spinal pain. Neurosurgery 20: 529–535

Bohm E 1962 Late results of sacral rhizotomy in coccygodynia. Acta Chirurgica Scandinavica 123: 6–8

Bohm E, Strang RR 1962 Glossopharyngeal neuralgia. Brain 85: 371–388

Bonica JJ 1974 Floor discussion: dorsal rhizotomy. In: Bonica JJ (ed) Pain. Advances in neurology, vol.4. Raven Press, New York, p 626

Breeze R, Ignelzi RJ 1982 Microvascular decompression for trigeminal neuralgia: results with special reference to the late recurrence rate. Journal of Neurosurgery 57: 487–490

Broggi G, Franzini A, Lasio G, Giorgi C, Servello D 1990 Long term results of percutaneous retrogasserian thermorhizotomy for 'essential' trigeminal neuralgia: considerations in 1000 patients. Neurosurgery 26: 783–786

Brown JA, McDaniel MD, Weaver MT 1993 Percutaneous trigeminal nerve compression for treatment of trigeminal neuralgia: results in 50 patients. Neurosurgery 32: 570–573

Burchiel KJ 1988 Percutaneous retrogasserian glycerol rhizolysis in the management of trigeminal neuralgia. Journal of Neurosurgery 69: 361–366

Burchiel KJ, Steege TD, Howe JF, Loeser JD 1981 Comparison of percutaneous radiofrequency gangliolysis and microvascular decompression for the surgical management of tic douloureux. Neurosurgery 9: 111–119

Burton CV 1976 Percutaneous radiofrequency facet denervation. Applied Neurophysiology 39: 80–86

Campbell JN, Raja SN, Meyer RA, MacKinnon SE 1988 Myelinated afferents signal the hyperalgesia associated with nerve injury. Pain 32: 89–94

Chambers WR 1954 Posterior rhizotomy of the second and third cervical nerves for occipital pain. Journal of the American Medical Association 155: 431–432

Cho DY, Chang CG, Wang YC, Wang FH, Shen CC, Yang DY 1994 Repeat operations in failed microvascular decompression for trigeminal neuralgia. Neurosurgery 35: 665–669

Clifton GL, Coggeshall RE, Vance WH, Willis WD 1976 Receptive fields of unmyelinated ventral root afferent fibres in the cat. Journal of Physiology 256: 573–600

Coggeshall RE, Ito H 1977 Sensory fibres in ventral root L7 and S1 in the cat. Journal of Physiology 267: 215–235

Coggeshall RE, Coulter JD, Willis WD 1974 Unmyelinated fibers in the ventral roots of the cat lumbosacral enlargement. Journal of Comparative Neurology 153: 39–58

Coggeshall RE, Applebaum ML, Fazen M, Stubbs TB 3rd, Sykes MT 1975 Unmyelinated axons in human ventral roots: a possible explanation for the failure of dorsal rhizotomy to relieve pain. Brain 98: 157–166

Crue BL, Todd EM 1964 A simplified technique of sacral rhizotomy for pelvic pain. Journal of Neurosurgery 21: 835

Cusson DL, King AB 1960 Cervical rhizotomy in the management of some cases of occipital neuralgia. Guthrie Clinic Bulletin 29: 198–208

Dandy WE 1927 Glossopharyngeal neuralgia (tic douloureux): its diagnosis and treatment. Archives of Surgery 15: 198–214

Dandy WE 1932 Treatment of trigeminal neuralgia by the cerebellar route. Annals of Surgery 96: 787–795

Dubuisson D 1995 Treatment of occipital neuralgia by partial posterior rhizotomy at C1-3. Journal of Neurosurgery 82: 581–586

Dykes RW, Terzis JK 1981 Spinal nerve distributions in the upper limb: the organization of the dermatome and afferent myotome. Philosophical Transactions of the Royal Society of London Series B: Biological Sciences 293: 509–554

Echols DH 1970 The effectiveness of thoracic rhizotomy for chronic pain. Neurochirurgia 13: 69–74

Fager CA 1976 Management of cervical disc lesions and spondylosis by posterior approaches. Clinical Neurosurgery 24: 488–507

Felsoory A, Crue BL 1976 Results of 19 years' experience with sacral rhizotomy for perineal and perianal cancer pain. Pain 2: 431–433

Ferrante L, Artico M, Nardacci B, Fraioli B, Cosentino F, Fortuna A 1995 Glossopharyngeal neuralgia with cardiac syncope. Neurosurgery 36: 58–63

Foerster O 1933 The dermatomes in man. Brain 56: 1–39

Fraioli B, Esposito V, Ferrante L, Trubiani L, Lunardi P 1989 Microsurgical treatment of glossopharyngeal neuralgia. Case report. Neurosurgery 25: 630–632

Frank F, Fabrizi A 1989 Percutaneous treatment of trigeminal neuralgia. Acta Neurochirurgica 97: 128–130

Fujimaki T, Fukushima T, Miyazaki S 1990 Percutaneous retrogasserian glycerol injection in the management of trigeminal neuralgia: long-term followup results. Journal of Neurosurgery 73: 212–216

Fuse T, Moller MB 1996 Delayed and progressive hearing loss after microvascular decompression of cranial nerves. Annals of Otology, Rhinology and Laryngology 105: 158–161

Garcia Cosamalon PJ, Mostaza A, Fernandez J et al 1991 Dorsal percutaneous radiofrequency rhizotomy guided with CT scan in intercostal neuralgias. Acta Neurochirurgica 109: 140–141

Gardner WJ 1962 Concerning the mechanism of trigeminal neuralgia and hemifacial spasm. Journal of Neurosurgery 19: 947–958

Gerber AM, Mullan SF 1998 Trigeminal nerve compression for neuralgia. In: Gildenberg PL, Tasker RR (eds) Textbook of stereotactic and functional neurosurgery. McGraw-Hill, New York, pp 1707–1713

Giorgi C, Broggi G 1984 Surgical treatment of glossopharyngeal neuralgia and pain from cancer of the nasopharynx. A 20 year experience. Journal of Neurosurgery 61: 952–955

Gudmundsson K, Rhoton AL Jr, Rushton JG 1971 Detailed anatomy of the intracranial portion of the trigeminal nerve. Journal of Neurosurgery 35: 592–600

Gybels JM, Sweet WH 1989 Neurosurgical treatment of persistent pain. Physiological and pathological mechanisms of human pain. Karger, New York

Håkanson S 1981 Trigeminal neuralgia treated by the injection of glycerol into the trigeminal cistern. Neurosurgery 9: 638–646

Håkanson S 1983 Retrogasserian glycerol injection as a treatment of tic douloureux. Advances in Pain Research and Therapy 5: 927–933

Håkanson S, Linderoth B 1998 Injection of glycerol into the Gasserian cistern for treatment of trigeminal neuralgia. In: Gildenberg PL, Tasker RR (eds) Textbook of stereotactic and functional neurosurgery. McGraw-Hill, New York, pp 1697–1706

Hamann W, Hall S 1992 Acute effect and recovery of primary afferent fibres after graded RF lesions in anaesthetized rats. British Journal of Anaesthesia 68: 443

Hardy DG, Rhoton AL Jr 1978 Microsurgical relationships of the superior cerebellar artery and the trigeminal nerve. Journal of Neurosurgery 49: 669–678

Harris RI, McNab I 1954 Structural changes in the intervertebral discs: their relationship to low back pain and sciatica. Journal of Bone and Joint Surgery 36B: 304–322

Henderson CM, Hennessy RG, Shuey HM, Shackleford EG 1983 Posterior-lateral foraminotomy as an exclusive operative technique for cervical radiculopathy: a review of 846 consecutively operated cases. Neurosurgery 13: 504–512

Hosobuchi Y 1980 The majority of unmyelinated afferent axons in human ventral roots probably conduct pain. Pain 8: 167–180

Howe JF, Loeser JD, Calvin WH 1977 Mechanosensitivity of dorsal root ganglia and chronically injured axons: a physiological basis for the radicular pain of nerve root compression. Pain 3: 25–41

Hunter CR, Mayfield FH 1949 Role of the upper cervical roots in the production of pain in the head. American Journal of Surgery 78: 743–751

Hutchins LG, Harnsberger HR, Jacobs JM, Apfelbaum RI 1990 Trigeminal neuralgia (tic douloureux): M R imaging assessment. Radiology 175: 837–841

Hyndman OR 1942 Lissauer's tract section. Journal of the International College of Surgeons 5: 394–400

Ignelzi RJ 1990 Radiofrequency lesions in the treatment of lumbar spinal pain. Contemporary Neurosurgery 12: 1–5

Ignelzi RJ, Cummings TW 1980 A statistical analysis of percutaneous radiofrequency lesions in the treatment of chronic low back pain and sciatica. Pain 8: 181–187

Imai Y, Kusama T 1969 Distribution of the dorsal root fibres in the cat. Brain Research 13: 338–359

Isamat F, Ferran E, Acebes JJ 1981 Selective percutaneous thermocoagulation rhizotomy in essential glossopharyngeal neuralgia. Journal of Neurosurgery 55: 575–580

Ischia S, Luzzani A, Polati E 1990 Retrogasserian glycerol injection: a retrospective study of 112 patients. Clinical Journal of Pain 6: 291–296

Jain KK 1974 Nerve root scarring and arachnoiditis as a complication of lumbar intervertebral disc surgery: surgical treatment. Neurochirurgia 17: 185–192

Jannetta PJ 1967 Arterial compression of the trigeminal nerve at the pons in patients with trigeminal neuralgia. Journal of Neurosurgery 26: 159–162

Jannetta PJ 1976 Microsurgical approach to the trigeminal nerve for tic douloureux. Progress in Neurological Surgery 7: 180–200

Jho H-D 1996 Microsurgical anterior cervical foraminotomy for radiculopathy: a new approach to cervical disc herniation. Journal of Neurosurgery 84: 155–160

Jho H-D 1998 Anterior cervical microforaminotomy: a disc preservation technique. Operative Techniques in Orthopaedics 8: 46–52

Johnson ER, Powell J, Caldwell J, Crane C 1974 Intercostal nerve conduction and posterior rhizotomy in the diagnosis and treatment of thoracic radiculopathy. Journal of Neurology, Neurosurgery and Psychiatry 37: 330–332

Kerr FWL 1975 Neuroanatomical substrates of nociception in the spinal cord. Pain 1: 325–356

Kings JS 1976 Randomized trial of the Rees and Shealy methods for the treatment of low back pain. In: Morley TP (ed) Current controversies in neurosurgery. W B Saunders, Philadelphia, pp 89–94

Kondo A 1997 Follow-up results of microvascular decompression in trigeminal neuralgia and hemifacial spasm. Neurosurgery 40: 46–51

Kondo A 1998 Follow-up results of using microvascular decompression for treatment of glossopharyngeal neuralgia. Journal of Neurosurgery 88: 221–225

Koning HM, Koster HG, Niemeijer RPE 1991 Ischaemic spinal cord lesion following percutaneous radiofrequency spinal rhizotomy. Pain 45: 161–166

Korogi Y, Nagahiro S, Du C et al 1995 Evaluation of vascular compression in trigeminal neuralgia by 3D time-of-flight M R A. Journal of Computer Assisted Tomography 19: 879–884

Krupp W, Schattke H, Muke R 1990 Clinical results of the foraminotomy as described by Frykholm for the treatment of lateral cervical disc herniation. Acta Neurochirurgica 107: 22–29

Kuether TA, O'Neill OR, Nesbit GM, Barnwell SL 1996 Direct carotid cavernous fistula after trigeminal balloon microcompression gangliolysis: case report. Neurosurgery 39: 853–855

Laha RK, Jannetta PJ 1977 Glossopharyngeal neuralgia. Journal of Neurosurgery 47: 316–320

Lamotte C, Pert CB, Snyder SH 1976 Opiate receptor binding in primate spinal cord: distribution and changes after dorsal root section. Brain Research 112: 407–412

Lazorthes Y, Verdie JC 1979 Radiofrequency coagulation of the petrous ganglion in glossopharyngeal neuralgia. Neurosurgery 4: 512–516

Lazorthes Y, Verdie JC, Lagarrigue J 1976 Thermocoagulation percutanee des nerfs rachidiens a visee analgesique. Neurochirurgie 22: 445–453

Letcher FS, Goldring S 1968 The effect of radiofrequency current and heat on peripheral nerve action potential in the cat. Journal of Neurosurgery 29: 42–47

Liao JJ, Cheng WC, Chang CN et al 1997 Reoperation for recurrent trigeminal neuralgia after microvascular decompression. Surgical Neurology 47: 562–568

Lichtor T, Mullan JF 1990 A 10-year follow-up review of percutaneous microcompression of the trigeminal ganglion. Journal of Neurosurgery 72: 49–54

Light AR, Metz CB 1978 The morphology of the spinal cord efferent and afferent neurons contributing to the ventral roots of the cat. Journal of Comparative Neurology 179: 501–515

Linskey ME, Jho HD, Jannetta PJ 1994 Microvascular decompression for trigeminal neuralgia caused by vertebrobasilar compression. Journal of Neurosurgery 81: 1–9

Lobato RD, Rivas JJ, Sarabia R, Lamas E 1990 Percutaneous microcompression of the Gasserian ganglion for trigeminal neuralgia. Journal of Neurosurgery 72: 546–553

Loeb GE 1976 Ventral root projections of myelinated dorsal root ganglion cells in the cat. Brain Research 106: 159–165

Loeser JD 1972 Dorsal rhizotomy for the relief of chronic pain. Journal of Neurosurgery 36: 745–750

Loeser JD 1982 Dorsal rhizotomy. In: Youmans JR (ed) Neurological surgery, 2nd edn. WB Saunders, Philadelphia, pp 3664–3671

Loeser JD, Ward AA 1967 Some effects of deafferentation on neurons of the cat spinal cord. Archives of Neurology 17: 629–636

Loeser JD, Ward AA, White LE 1968 Chronic deafferentation of human spinal cord neurons. Journal of Neurosurgery 29: 48–50

Long DM 1982 Pain of spinal origin. In: Youmans JR (ed) Neurological surgery, 2nd edn. WB Saunders, Philadelphia, pp 3613–3626

Longhurst JC, Mitchell JH, Moore MB 1980 The spinal ventral root: an afferent pathway of the hind-limb pressor reflex in cats. Journal of Physiology 301: 467–476

Lora J, Long DM 1976 So-called facet denervation in the management of intractable back pain. Spine 1: 121–126

Lord SM, Barnsley L, Bogduk N 1995 Percutaneous radiofrequency neurotomy in the treatment of cervical zygapophyseal joint pain: a caution. Neurosurgery 36: 732–739

Lord SM, Barnsley L, Wallis BJ, McDonald GJ, Bogduk N 1996 Percutaneous radio-frequency neurotomy for chronic cervical zygapophyseal joint pain. New England Journal of Medicine 335: 1721–1726

Lovely TJ, Jannetta PJ 1997 Surgical management of geniculate neuralgia. American Journal of Otolaryngology 18: 512–517

Lozano AM 1998 Treatment of occipital neuralgia. In: Gildenberg P L, Tasker R R (eds) Textbook of stereotactic and functional neurosurgery. McGraw-Hill, New York, pp 1729–1733

Lozano AM, Vanderlinden G, Bachoo R, Rothbart P 1988 Microsurgical C-2 ganglionectomy for chronic intractable occipital pain. Journal of Neurosurgery 89: 359–365

Masur H, Papke K, Bongartz G, Vollbrecht K 1995 The significance of three-dimensional MR-defined neurovascular compression for the pathogenesis of trigeminal neuralgia. Journal of Neurology 242: 93–98

McCulloch JA, Organ LW 1977 Percutaneous radiofrequency lumbar rhizolysis (rhizotomy). Canadian Medical Association Journal 116: 30–32

Meaney JF, Eldridge PR, Dunn LT, Nixon TE, Whitehouse GH, Miles JB 1995 Demonstration of neurovascular compression in trigeminal neuralgia with magnetic resonance imaging. Comparison with surgical findings in 52 consecutive operative cases. Journal of Neurosurgery 83: 799–805

Mehta M, Sluijter ME 1979 The treatment of chronic back pain: a preliminary survey of the effect of radiofrequency denervation of the posterior vertebral joints. Anesthesia 34: 768–775

Melvill RL, Baxter BL 1996 A tentorial sling in microvascular decompression for trigeminal neuralgia. Technical note. Journal of Neurosurgery 84: 127–128

Mendoza N, Illingworth RD 1995 Trigeminal neuralgia treated by microvascular decompression: a long-term follow-up study. British Journal of Neurosurgery 9: 13–19

Miles JB, Eldridge PR, Haggett CE, Bowsher D 1997 Sensory effects of microvascular decompression in trigeminal neuralgia. Journal of Neurosurgery 86: 193–196

Moller AR 1993 Intraoperative neurophysiologic monitoring of cranial nerves. In: Barrow DL (ed) Surgery of the cranial nerves of the posterior fossa. American Association of Neurological Surgeons, pp 175–199

Morales F, Albert P, Alberca R, De Valle B, Narros A 1977 Glossopharyngeal and vagal neuralgia secondary to vascular compression of the nerves. Surgical Neurology 8: 431–433

Mullan S, Lichtor T 1983 Percutaneous microcompression of the trigeminal ganglion for trigeminal neuralgia. Journal of Neurosurgery 59: 1007–1012

Nagashima C, Sakaguchi A, Kamisawa A, Kawanuma S 1976 Cardiovascular complications on upper vagal rootlet section for glossopharyngeal neuralgia. Case report. Journal of Neurosurgery 44: 248–253

Nash TP 1986 Percutaneous radiofrequency lesioning of dorsal root ganglia for intractable pain. Pain 24: 67–73

Nordin M, Nystrom B, Wallin U, Hagbarth K-E 1984 Ectopic sensory discharges and paresthesiae in patients with disorders of peripheral nerves, dorsal roots and dorsal columns. Pain 20: 231–245

North RB, Kidd DH, Piantadosi S, Carson BS 1990 Percutaneous retrogasserian glycerol rhizotomy. Journal of Neurosurgery 72: 851–856

North RB, Kidd DH, Campbell JN, Long DM 1991 Dorsal root ganglionectomy for failed back surgery syndrome: a 5-year follow-up study. Journal of Neurosurgery 74: 236–242

North RB, Han M, Zahurak M, Kidd DH 1994 Radiofrequency lumbar facet denervation: analysis of prognostic factors. Pain 57: 77–83

Nugent GR, Berry B 1974 Trigeminal neuralgia treated by percutaneous radiofrequency coagulation of the Gasserian ganglion. Journal of Neurosurgery 40: 517–523

Ogsbury JS, Simon RH, Lehman RAW 1977 Facet denervation in the treatment of low back syndrome. Pain 3: 257–263

Onofrio BM, Campa HK 1972 Evaluation of rhizotomy. Review of 12 years' experience. Journal of Neurosurgery 36: 751–755

Ori C, Salar G, Giron GP 1985 Cardiovascular and cerebral complications during glosopharyngeal nerve thermocoagulation. Anesthesia 40: 433–437

Osgood CP, Dujovny M, Faille R, Abassy M 1976 Microsurgical ganglionectomy for chronic pain syndromes. Journal of Neurosurgery 45: 113–115

Oudenhoven RC 1977 Paraspinal electromyography following facet rhizotomy. Spine 2: 299–304

Oudenhoven RC 1979 The role of laminectomy, facet rhizotomy and epidural steroids. Spine 4: 145–147

Ovelmen-Levitt J, Johnson B, Bedenbaugh P, Nashold BS 1984 Dorsal root rhizotomy and avulsion in the cat: a comparison of long term effects on dorsal horn neuronal activity. Neurosurgery 15: 921–927

Pagura JR 1983 Percutaneous radiofrequency spinal rhizotomy. Applied Neurophysiology 46: 138–146

Pagura JR, Schnapp M, Passarelli P 1983 Percutaneous radiofrequency glossopharyngeal rhizotomy for cancer pain. Applied Neurophysiology 46: 154–159

Panagopoulos K, Chakraborty M, Deopujari CE, Sengupta RP 1987 Neurovascular decompression for cranial rhizopathies. British Journal of Neurosurgery 1: 235–241

Pawl RP 1982 Microsurgical ganglionectomy for treatment of arachnoiditis-related unilateral sciatica. Presented to the American Pain Society, Miami, 1982.

Piatt JH, Wilkins RH 1984 Treatment of tic douloureux and hemifacial spasm by posterior fossa exploration: therapeutic implications of various neurovascular relationships. Neurosurgery 14: 462–471

Poletti CE 1983 Proposed operation for occipital neuralgia: C2 and C3 root decompression. Case report. Neurosurgery 12: 221–224

Poletti CE 1996 Third cervical nerve root and ganglion compression: clinical syndrome, surgical anatomy, and pathology findings. Neurosurgery 39: 941–948

Poletti CE, Sweet WH 1990 Entrapment of the C2 root and ganglion by the atlanto-apostrophic ligament: clinical syndrome and surgical anatomy. Neurosurgery 27: 288–291

Premsagar IC, Moss T, Coakham HB 1997 Teflon-induced granuloma following treatment of trigeminal neuralgia by microvascular decompression. Report of two cases. Journal of Neurosurgery 87: 454–457

Pulec JL 1976 Geniculate neuralgia: diagnosis and surgical management. Laryngoscope 86: 955–964

Rashbaum RF 1983 Radiofrequency facet denervation. Orthopedic Clinics of North America 14: 569–575

Rath SA, Klein HJ, Richter HP 1996 Findings and long-term results of subsequent operations after failed microvascular decompression for trigeminal neuralgia. Neurosurgery 39: 933–938

Rees S 1976 Disconnective neurosurgery: multiple bilateral percutaneous rhizolysis (facet rhizotomy). In: Morley TP (ed) Current controversies in neurosurgery. W B Saunders, Philadelphia, pp 80–88

Resnick DK, Jannetta PJ, Bisonette D, Jho HD, Lanzino G 1995 Microvascular decompression for glossopharyngeal neuralgia. Neurosurgery 36: 64–69

Resnick DK, Jannetta PJ, Lunsford LD, Bissonette DJ 1996 Microvascular decompression for trigeminal neuralgia in patients with multiple sclerosis. Surgical Neurology 46: 358–361

Rhoton AL Jr 1993 Microsurgical anatomy of posterior fossa cranial nerves. In: Barrow DL (ed) Surgery of the cranial nerves of the posterior fossa. American Association of Neurological Surgeons, pp 1–103

Rhoton AL Jr, Buza R 1975 Microsurgical anatomy of the jugular foramen. Journal of Neurosurgery 42: 541–550

Rinaldi PC, Young RF, Albe-Fessard D, Chodakiewitz J 1991 Spontaneous neuronal hyperactivity in the medial and intralaminar thalamic nuclei of patients with deafferentation pain. Journal of Neurosurgery 74: 415–421

Risling M, Hildebrand C 1982 Occurrence of unmyelinated axon profiles at distal, middle and proximal levels in the ventral root L7 of cats and kittens. Journal of Neurological Sciences 56: 219–231

Robson JT, Bonica J 1950 The vagus nerve in surgical consideration of glossopharyngeal neuralgia. Journal of Neurosurgery 7: 482–484

Rockswold GL, Bradley WE, Chou SN 1974 Effect of sacral nerve blocks on the function of the urinary bladder in humans. Journal of Neurosurgery 40: 83–89

Rohrer DC, Burchiel KJ 1993 Trigeminal neuralgia and other trigeminal dysfunction syndromes. In: Barrow DL (ed) Surgery of the cranial nerves of the posterior fossa. American Association of Neurological Surgeons, pp 201–219

Rupa V, Saunders RL, Weider DJ 1991 Geniculate neuralgia: the surgical management of primary otalgia. Journal of Neurosurgery 75: 505–511

Rushton JG, Stevens JC, Miller RH 1981 Glossopharyngeal (vagoglossopharyngeal) neuralgia. Archives of Neurology 38: 201–205

Salar G, Iob I, Ori C 1986 Combined thermocoagulation of the 5th and 9th cranial nerves for oral pain of neoplastic aetiology. Journal of Maxillofacial Surgery 14: 1–4

Saris SC, Silver JM, Vieira JFS, Nashold BS 1986 Sacrococcygeal rhizotomy for perineal pain. Neurosurgery 19: 789–793

Schwartz HG 1956 Anastomoses between cervical nerve roots. Journal of Neurosurgery 13: 190–194

Scoville WB 1966 Extradural spinal sensory rhizotomy. Journal of Neurosurgery 25: 94–95

Scoville WB, Dohrman GJ, Corkill G 1976 Late results of cervical disc surgery. Journal of Neurosurgery 45: 203–210

Shealy CN 1975 Percutaneous radiofrequency denervation of spinal facets. Journal of Neurosurgery 43: 448–451

Shealy CN 1976 Facet denervation in the management of back and sciatic pain. Clinical Orthopedics 115: 157–164

Sherrington CS 1898 Experiments in the examination of the peripheral distribution of the fibres of the posterior roots of some spinal nerves. Part II. Philosophical Transactions of the Royal Society of London Series B: Biological Sciences 190: 45–186

Siegfried J 1981 Percutaneous controlled thermocoagulation of Gasserian ganglion in trigeminal neuralgia. Experience with 1000 cases. In: Samii M, Jannetta P (eds) The cranial nerves. Springer-Verlag, Berlin, pp 322–330

Silveri CP, Simpson JM, Simeone FA, Balderston RA 1997 Cervical disk disease and the keyhole foraminotomy: proven efficacy at extended long-term follow up. Orthopedics 20: 687–692

Sindou M, Mertens P 1993 Microsurgical vascular decompression (MVD) in trigeminal and glosso-vago-pharyngeal neuralgias. A twenty year experience. Acta Neurochirurgica 58 (suppl): 168–170

Sindou M, Fischer G, Goutelle A, Mansuy L 1974a La radicellotomie postérieure sélective. Premiers résultats dans la chirurgie de la douleur. Neurochirurgie 20: 391–408

Sindou M, Fischer G, Goutelle A, Schott B, Mansuy L 1974b La radicellotomie postérieure sélective dans le traitement des spasticités. Revue Neurologique 130: 201–215

Sindou M, Quoex C, Baleydier C 1974c Fiber organization at the posterior spinal cord-rootlet junction in man. Journal of Comparative Neurology 153: 15–26

Sindou M, Fischer G, Mansuy L 1976 Posterior spinal rhizotomy and selective posterior rhizidiotomy. Progress in Neurological Surgery 7: 201–250
Sindou M, Fischer G, Goutelle A, Allegre GE 1981 Microsurgical selective posterior rhizotomy. Pain 1 (suppl): 354
Sindou M, Mifsud JJ, Boisson D, Goutelle A 1986 Selective posterior rhizotomy in the dorsal root entry zone for treatment of hyperspasticity and pain in the hemiplegic upper limb. Neurosurgery 18: 587–595
Sindou M, Henry JF, Blanchard P 1991 Névralgie essentielle du glossopharyngien: Étude d'une série de 14 cas et revue de la littérature. Neurochirurgie 37: 18–25
Slettebo H, Hirschberg H, Lindegaard KF 1993 Long-term results after percutaneous retrogasserian glycerol rhizotomy in patients with trigeminal neuralgia. Acta Neurochirurgica 122: 231–235
Sluijter ME, Mehta M 1981 Treatment of chronic back and neck pain by percutaneous thermal lesions. In: Lipton S, Miles JK (eds) Persistent pain: modern methods of treatment. Academic Press, London, pp 141–179
Smith FP 1970 Trans-spinal ganglionectomy for relief of intercostal pain. Journal of Neurosurgery 32: 574–577
Smith HP, McWhorter JM, Challa VR 1981 Radiofrequency neurolysis in a clinical model. Neuropathological correlation. Journal of Neurosurgery 55: 246–253
Snyder R 1977 The organization of the dorsal root entry zone in cats and monkeys. Journal of Comparative Neurology 174: 47–70
Stolker RJ, Vervest AC, Ramos LM, Groen GJ 1994a Electrode positioning in thoracic percutaneous partial rhizotomy: an anatomical study. Pain 57: 241–251
Stolker RJ, Vervest AC, Groen GJ 1994b The treatment of chronic thoracic pain by radiofrequency percutaneous partial rhizotomy. Journal of Neurosurgery 80: 986–992
Strait TA, Hunter SE 1981 Intraspinal extradural sensory rhizotomy in patients with failure of lumbar disc surgery. Journal of Neurosurgery 54: 193–196
Sun T, Saito S, Nakai O, Ando T 1994 Long-term results of microvascular decompression for trigeminal neuralgia with reference to probability of recurrence. Acta Neurochirurgica 126: 144–148
Swanson SE, Farhat 1982 Neurovascular decompression with selective partial rhizotomy of the trigeminal nerve for tic douloureux. Surgical Neurology 18: 3–6
Sweet WH 1984 Deafferentation pain after posterior rhizotomy, trauma to a limb, and herpes zoster. Neurosurgery 15: 928–932
Sweet WH 1990 Treatment of trigeminal neuralgia by percutaneous rhizotomy. In: Youmans J (ed) Neurological surgery, 3rd edn. WB Saunders, Philadelphia, pp 3888–3921
Sweet WH, Poletti CE 1985 Problems with retrogasserian glycerol in the treatment of trigeminal neuralgia. Applied Neurophysiology 48: 252–257
Sweet WH, Wepsic JG 1974 Controlled thermocoagulation of the trigeminal ganglion and rootlets for differential destruction of pain fibers. 1. Trigeminal neuralgia. Journal of Neurosurgery 39: 143–156
Szapiro J Jr, Sindou M, Szapiro J 1985 Prognostic factors in microvascular decompression for trigeminal neuralgia. Neurosurgery 17: 920–929
Taha JM, Tew JM Jr 1995 Long-term results of surgical treatment of idiopathic neuralgias of the glossopharyngeal and vagal nerves. Neurosurgery 36: 926–931
Taha JM, Tew JM Jr 1998 Radiofrequency rhizotomy for trigeminal and other cranial neuralgias. In: Gildenberg PL, Tasker RR (eds) Textbook of stereotactic and functional neurosurgery. McGraw-Hill, New York, pp 1687–1696
Taha JM, Tew JM Jr, Keith RW, Payner TD 1994 Intraoperative monitoring of the vagus nerve during intracranial glossopharyngeal and upper vagal rhizotomy: technical note. Neurosurgery 35: 775–777
Tash RR, Sze G, Leslie DR 1989 Trigeminal neuralgia: MR imaging features. Radiology 172: 767–770
Taub A, Robinson F, Taub E 1995 Dorsal root ganglionectomy for intractable monoradicular sciatica. In: Schmidek HH, Sweet WH (eds) Operative neurosurgical techniques, 3rd edn. WB Saunders, Philadelphia, pp 1585–1593
Tew JM 1982 Treatment of pain of glossopharyngeal and vagus nerve by percutaneous rhizotomy. In: Youmans JR (ed) Neurological surgery, 2nd edn. WB Saunders, Philadelphia, pp 3609–3612
Tew JM, Van Loveren HR 1988 Percutaneous rhizotomy in the treatment of intractable facial pain (trigeminal, glossopharyngeal, and vagal nerves). In: Schmidek HH, Sweet WH (eds) Current techniques in operative neurosurgery, 2nd edn. Grune & Stratton, Orlando, Florida, pp 1111–1123
Tobler WD, Tew JM, Cosman E, Keller JT, Quallen B 1983 Improved outcome in the treatment of trigeminal neuralgia by percutaneous stereotactic rhizotomy with a new, curved tip electrode. Neurosurgery 12: 313–317
Tsuboi M, Suzuki K, Nagao S, Nishimoto A 1985 Glossopharyngeal neuralgia with cardiac syncope. A case successfully treated by microvascular decompression. Surgical Neurology 24: 279–283
Tytus JS 1982 Treatment of trigeminal neuralgia through temporal craniotomy. In: Youmans JR (ed) Neurological surgery, 2nd edn. WB Saunders, Philadelphia, pp 3580–3585
Uematsu S 1977 Percutaneous electrothermocoagulation of spinal nerve trunk, ganglion and rootlets. In: Schmidek HH, Sweet WH (eds) Current techniques in operative neurosurgery. Grune & Stratton, New York, pp 469–490
Uematsu S, Udvarhelyi GB, Benson DW, Siebens AA 1974 Percutaneous radiofrequency rhizotomy. Surgical Neurology 2: 319–325
Van Kleef M, Sluijter ME 1998 Radiofrequency lesions in the treatment of pain of spinal origin. In: Gildenberg PL, Tasker RR (eds) Textbook of stereotactic and functional neurosurgery. McGraw-Hill, New York, pp 1585–1599
Van Kleef M, Spaans F, Dingemans A, Barendse GAM, Floor E, Sluijter ME 1993 Effects and side effects of a percutaneous thermal lesion of the dorsal root ganglion in patients with cervical pain syndrome. Pain 52: 49–53
Van Kleef M, Liem L, Lousberg R, Barendse G, Kessels F, Sluijter M 1996 Radiofrequency lesion adjacent to the dorsal root ganglion for cervicobrachial pain: a prospective double-blind randomized study. Neurosurgery 38: 1127–1132
Van Loveren H, Tew JM Jr, Keller JT, Nurre MA 1982 A ten-year experience in the treatment of trigeminal neuralgia. Comparison of percutaneous stereotaxic rhizotomy and posterior fossa exploration. Journal of Neurosurgery 57: 757–764
Van Loveren H, Tew JM, Thomas GM 1990 Vagoglossopharyngeal and geniculate neuralgias. In: Youmans JR (ed) Neurological surgery, 3rd edn. WB Saunders, Philadelphia, pp 3943–3949
Verdie JC, Lazorthes Y 1982 Thermocoagulation percutanee analgesique des racines rachidiennes. 218 cas. Nouvelle Presse Medicale 11: 2131–2134
Vlahovitch B, Fuentes JM 1975 Resultats de la radicellotomie selective posterieure a l'etage lombaire et cervicale. Neurochirurgie 21: 29–42
Walker AE 1966 Neuralgias of the glossopharyngeal, vagus and intermedius nerves. In: Knighton RS, Dumke PR (eds) Pain. Little, Brown, Boston, pp 421–429
Wall PD 1962 The origin of a spinal cord slow potential. Journal of Physiology 164: 508–526
Wall PD 1977 The presence of ineffective synapses and the circumstances which unmask them. Philosophical Transactions of the Royal Society of London 278: 361–372
Wall PD, Devor M 1983 Sensory afferent impulses originate from dorsal root ganglia as well as from the periphery in normal and nerve injured rats. Pain 17: 321–339

Wall PD, Werman R 1976 The physiology and anatomy of long-ranging afferent fibres within the spinal cord. Journal of Physiology 255: 321–334

Waltz TA, Dalessio DJ, Copeland B, Abbott G 1989 Percutaneous injection of glycerol for the treatment of trigeminal neuralgia. Clinical Journal of Pain 5: 195–198

Wedell G, Guttmann L, Guttmann E 1941 Local extension of nerve fibers into denervated areas of skin. Journal of Neurology, Neurosurgery and Psychiatry 4: 206–224

White JC, Kjellberg RN 1973 Posterior spinal rhizotomy: a substitute for cordotomy in the relief of localized pain in patients with normal life expectancy. Neurochirurgia 16: 141–170

White JC, Sweet WH 1969 Pain and the neurosurgeon. Charles C Thomas, Springfield, Illinois

Williams RW 1983 Microcervical foraminotomy: a surgical alternative for intractable radicular pain. Spine 8: 708–716

Wong BY, Steinberg GK, Rosen L 1989 Magnetic resonance imaging of vascular compression in trigeminal neuralgia: case report. Journal of Neurosurgery 70: 132–134

Young RF 1988 Glycerol rhizolysis for treatment of trigeminal neuralgia. Journal of Neurosurgery 69: 39–45

Young RF 1990 Dorsal rhizotomy and dorsal root ganglionectomy. In: Youmans JR (ed) Neurological surgery, 3rd edn. WB Saunders, Philadelphia, pp 4026–4035

Young RF 1996 Dorsal rhizotomy and dorsal root ganglionectomy. In: Youmans JR (ed) Neurological surgery, 4th edn. WB Saunders, Philadelphia, pp 3442–3451

Zakrzewska JM, Thomas DG 1993 Patients' assessment of outcome after three surgical procedures for the management of trigeminal neuralgia. Acta Neurochirurgica 122: 225–230

Disc surgery

55

ERIK SPANGFORT

THE DEVELOPMENT OF DISC SURGERY

Although ruptured intervertebral discs had been described and operated on previously, the era of disc surgery unquestionably began in September 1933, when Mixter and Barr presented a series of successful operations for disc herniation, or ruptured disc as they called it, to the New England Surgical Society in Boston (Mixter & Barr 1934).

The original series presented by Mixter and Barr included disc ruptures in the cervical and thoracic spine. Surgical treatment of disc herniations in the cervical and especially the thoracic spine is, however, rare compared with herniations of the lower lumbar discs and is not discussed in detail in this chapter.

The simplistic concept that low back pain with or without sciatica was usually caused by a disc herniation and cured by a fairly simple operation was readily and rapidly accepted all over the world and maintained an overwhelming dominance over lay and medical minds for the next 40 years.

Throughout these years a vast number of papers dealing with all aspects of the disc problem were published and when the results of disc surgery were compiled, it became obvious that discectomy was not always a successful procedure.

The reported rate of surgical failures was usually 5–10%, but there were large variations among the reports and some claimed more than 50% failures. A growing number of unfortunate, severely disabled patients with 'failed back surgery syndrome' became a highly complex challenge and a heavy burden to the medical profession. Distrust of discectomy was spreading widely (Wilson 1967). Evidently, some pertinent questions concerning disc surgery had to be answered.

Studies to identify the causes of surgical failures revealed that inaccuracy of diagnosis and a poor selection of patients for initial lumbar disc operation were more important factors than technical errors during the operation itself (Macnab 1971, Nachemson 1976, Finneson 1978, Spengler & Freeman 1979). The operation, discectomy, was used inappropriately on loose and wide indications.

It was shown that the single most important factor for prediction of a successful discectomy is the degree of herniation found by the operation (Spangfort 1972, Vucetic 1997). In patients with complete herniations, i.e. rupture of the annulus and extrusion of fragments of disc tissue into the spinal canal, complete relief of sciatic pain was achieved in more than 90% of the patients, independent of age, sex, level of herniation and other variables (Fig. 55.1). As the degree of herniation decreases, the rate of failure increases significantly and the majority of patients with a 'negative exploration' do not benefit from the operation.

Obviously, improvement of surgical results was crucially dependent on accurate preoperative diagnosis and a strict selection of patients with high-grade herniations for discectomy.

In the last 20 years the development in this field has been intensive and interesting. A basic feature is, no doubt, a growing awareness among low back specialists of the fact that the damage caused by a disc herniation depends not only on the volume of disc tissue protruding or extruding into the spinal canal, but also on the space available for herniated disc tissue in the individual spinal canal.

In this broader context, disc herniation is only one of several pathomechanisms causing mechanical compression syndromes in the lumbar spine.

Reduction of the space available for the neural elements, generally called spinal stenosis of developmental, post-

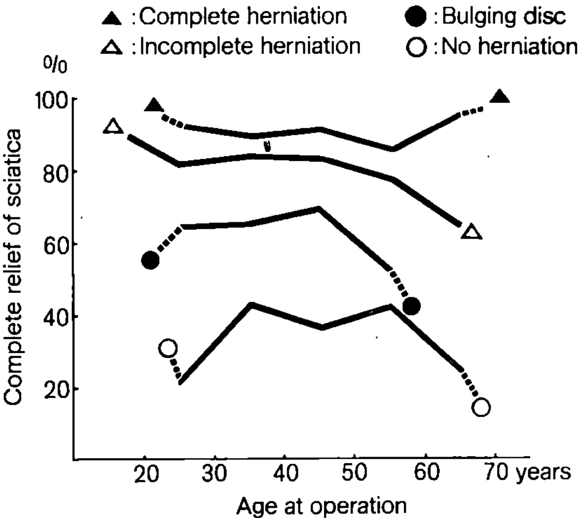

Fig. 55.1 The rate of complete relief of sciatica by age at operation and degree of herniation in 2503 operations. (From Spangfort 1972.)

traumatic or degenerative type, is recognized as a nosological entity which, alone or in combination with disc herniation, may produce disabling symptoms from the spine. It is also recognized that when stenosis is involved in a disc syndrome, the results of surgical treatment with traditional discectomy are usually unsatisfactory. Spinal stenosis requires a radical change in surgical technique.

As well as growing awareness of clinical problems attributed to spinal stenosis, several other changes have recently influenced the surgical treatment of spinal disorders.

Diagnostic methods necessary to analyse the pathological anatomy of the diseased spine have been highly amplified by the advent of safer water-soluble contrast agents, epidural venography and, in particular, computed tomography (CT) and magnetic resonance imaging (MRI).

In spite of this impressive development of technological investigative methods, it may still be extremely difficult to supply the necessary diagnostic foundation for decisions about proper surgical treatment in individual cases of lumbar pain syndromes. Surgical management of these conditions cannot be satisfactorily improved without a better clinical analysis and interpretation of the main symptom, i.e. pain.

DISC OPERATION

SURGICAL TECHNIQUE

The earliest cases of disc herniation were classified as tumours and removed by a neurosurgical approach with complete laminectomy on at least two vertebrae and transdural extirpation of the herniated disc tissue.

In 1939, Love described the unilateral interlaminar approach, which is still the routine technique in most quarters. The laminae of the two vertebrae between which the herniation has occurred are exposed by subperiosteal dissection and the strong ligamentum flavum is resected, if necessary together with some part of the adjacent lamina. In most cases this exposure allows identification of the underlying nerve root, inspection of the surface of the intervertebral disc after medial retraction of the root and removal of the possible herniation. Occasionally more bone has to be removed and in some cases a hemilaminectomy and/or a partial resection of the posterior facet joint is performed to obtain an adequate exposure.

Bilateral exposure is usually not necessary in typical cases of disc herniation.

EXTENT OF EXPOSURE

It is, of course, desirable to minimize surgical damage to the anatomical structures as much as possible, even if it is still unproven that the extent of exposure has any major effect on the results of disc operation (Busch et al 1950, Eyre-Brook 1952, Naylor 1974, Fager & Freidberg 1980, Weber 1983). Inadequate exposure, on the other hand, increases the risk of surgical injuries to the nerve roots, the dura and the vessels and also the risk of failure to locate displaced and migrating fragments extruded from a ruptured disc.

We do not share the opinion that the lower two or three disc spaces should always be explored during a disc operation. With modern diagnostic methods applied in a meticulous preoperative investigation, the extent and type of appropriate exposure should be clearly defined before the operation.

The development of microsurgical technique facilitates the procedure and implies less surgical trauma, but early expectations of considerably better results by microsurgery have not been confirmed (Tullberg et al 1993, McCulloch 1996).

Percutaneous lumbar discectomy (nucleotomy) was introduced with the aim of decompressing the disc. Discography is performed before or during the operation, as the method is not suitable for patients with rupture of the annulus (complete herniations). It is possible that the method is useful in a small group of strictly selected patients, but the proper indications are not yet established (Onik et al 1997).

VOLUME OF TISSUE REMOVED

Free fragments and disc tissue protruding into the spinal canal must be removed for a good operative result. There is, however, no general agreement about the need to remove as much tissue as possible from the interior of the disc space. It has been presumed by many that a radical excision of the disc improves surgical results and reduces the rate of recurrence, but so far there is no evidence in support of this assumption (Hirsch & Nachemson 1963, Mochida et al 1996). We have followed the principle expressed by Busch et al (1950) that the disc space should be evacuated 'but without fanaticism'.

In several reports the specimens of disc tissue removed by operation are measured by weight and the reported mean values range from 0.79 g (Boemke 1951) to 9.88 g (Hanraets 1959). O'Connell (1951) found a mean weight of 1.95 g; he also reported that the mean weight of lumbar discs excised at autopsy was 24.6 g. He concluded that only exceptionally does the specimen removed at operation represent more than 20% of the average normal intervertebral disc by weight.

Capanna et al (1981), applying a technique of intraoperative discography, estimated the percentage of disc volume removed by disc surgery. The average volume removed was found to equal only 6% of the total disc volume. There was little difference in the percentage of disc removal when different operative approaches were used or when more or less 'extensive' disc extirpation was performed.

In my study of the lumbar disc operation (Spangfort 1972), the volume of disc tissue removed was analysed in 645 cases (unpublished). The volume was measured by replacement of water in a graded tube immediately after removal and the total mean in this series was 2.14 (s.d. 1.04) ml, with no single specimen larger than 7 ml. The mean volume was correlated with the degree of herniation and increased from 1.25 ml in negative explorations to 1.52 ml in 'bulging discs', 2.01 ml in incomplete herniations and 2.36 ml in ruptured discs. In 90 reoperations, where a disc herniation was found, the mean volume was almost the same (2.09 ml).

These studies all indicate that the average volume of disc tissue removed by discectomy represents only 6–8% of the total disc volume and apparently it is not easy to excise disc tissue with the instruments usually applied for this purpose (rongeur and curette) unless the disc is already in a certain condition of degeneration and fragmentation.

THE 'COMBINED OPERATION'

Since 1940 it has become increasingly common to advocate concomitant discectomy and some type of fusion operation as a standard procedure in an attempt to improve the results of disc surgery. Arthrodesis of the spine (or fusion) was already an established and approved operation, based on the principles of Albee and Hibbs, in the treatment of an unstable spine. Compared with simple discectomy, fusion is a surgical procedure of considerable magnitude with prolonged convalescence and more serious postoperative complications.

Most studies comparing discectomy with and without concomitant fusion indicate that the results after the 'combination operation' are 5–10% better than after simple discectomy (Nachlas 1952, Van Hoytema & Oostrom 1961, White 1966). The issue is still controversial, but the dominating conclusion has been that the advantage of the 'combined operation' is too small to warrant the use of this method as a routine in patients with typical lumbar disc herniations. The surgical indications for discectomy and spine fusion are different. The special indications for fusion should be considered separately in each individual case when disc surgery is planned (Symposium 1981).

REOPERATION AFTER DISCECTOMY

The rate of reoperations after a first disc operation is usually reported as 10–15% and the risk of acquiring a new disc herniation is probably considerably increased in patients with a verified herniation in their medical history.

Recurrences occur both on the same side and level and at other locations, but rarely within the first year after a discectomy. The mean interval between the first and second operation for true disc herniation is 5–6 years in our experience, but a true recurrence from the same disc may occur more than 20 years after the first operation.

The pathological process, which in some patients results in a true disc herniation, tends to begin at the lumbosacral level and proceed in the cranial direction with age. The mean age at operation for verified ruptures at the level L5–S1 was found to be 38 years, at the level L4–5 42 years and in the unusual herniations at the three higher levels, 47 years (Spangfort 1972). Simultaneous complete ruptures of two different discs were never found during the same operation in this series and seem to be rare.

Thus, symptoms of a recurrent disc herniation may be expected with a certain degree of probability approximately 5 years after a first operation, although not necessarily severe enough to motivate a reoperation. In this situation there is no reason to classify the first operation as a failure.

In patients without relief of pain for at least 6 months after a first operation, the operation has usually been a failure, in some cases caused by technical errors during the operation, e.g. failure to locate an offending fragment or exposure at a wrong level, but in the majority caused by an incomplete or wrong preoperative diagnosis: another type of operation should have been performed or the patient should not have been exposed to surgical treatment at all. In the latter group the probability of a successful reoperation with the same technique is low. If the first operation was a negative exploration, the risk of a second negative exploration is about 50%.

The results of reoperations are generally less favourable than those of first operations. This is partly due to a higher rate of surgical complications at reoperation, but the main reason is diagnostic difficulties in patients assessed for repeat surgery, which results in high rates of negative explorations in this group. When the degree of herniation found by reoperation is considered, the results are, however, almost as good.

In my study of disc operations, the rate of excellent results (i.e. complete relief of both low back pain and sciatica) decreased from 62.0% after first operations to 43.1% after second operations and 28.6% after third operations. If a disc herniation was found by reoperation (161 cases) the rate of excellent results was still 53.4%, but if the reoperation was a negative exploration (69 cases) the rate was as low as 14.5%. Again, preoperative diagnosis is crucial for the result of operation. Proper selection of patients for reoperation is, however, often a difficult task even for the experienced low back specialist.

The multioperated low back patient with a 'failed back surgery syndrome', who seldom achieves satisfactory relief of pain by any combination of measures, should be carefully examined by a qualified investigation, preferably in a centre specializing in assessing these highly complicated patients, before further 'salvage surgery' is attempted: 'No matter how severe or how intractable the pain, it can always be made worse by surgery' (Finneson 1978).

EPIDURAL SCAR FORMATION

The prevalent pathological condition found in reoperations for recurrent pain after disc surgery is often a dense fibrous scar formation strangling the dura and nerve roots. This scar formation is considered a major cause of recurrent symptoms after discectomy; it also complicates correct diagnosis and reoperation of a true recurrent disc herniation. Excision of the scar tissue (neurolysis) is difficult and the results are usually poor.

LaRocca and Macnab (1974) called this excessive fibrosis 'the laminectomy membrane' and showed that the main source is fibrous tissue from traumatized surrounding muscles. Langenskiöld and Kiviluoto (1976) reported efficient prevention of epidural scar formation by the use of free grafts of subcutaneous fat tissue placed outside the spinal canal.

It has been confirmed that covering raw bone, muscles and nerve roots with free fat grafts effectively prevents epidural scar formation (Yong-Hing et al 1980, Quist et al 1998).

URGENT DISC SURGERY

The only indication for immediate disc surgery is acute compression of the cauda equina by a large herniation causing a sacral syndrome with neurological signs from the second and lower sacral roots, i.e. dysfunction of the bladder and bowel with loss of sphincter control, impairment of sexual function and saddle-shaped loss of sensation in the sacral dermatomes. In most cases the herniation is large, situated in the midline and ruptured. The condition is rare, probably less than one case per year in a population of 200 000.

In patients with symptoms of acute cauda equina compression a qualified examination, including cystometry and myelography, CT or MRI, is urgent. Bladder dysfunction is, however, a common symptom in patients with severe low back pain and not necessarily caused by a large disc herniation. Immediate surgical decompression is generally considered mandatory when an acute disc herniation is identified as the cause of the syndrome. Severe impairment of bladder function, bilateral saddle anaesthesia and a preoperative duration of more than 2 days appear to imply a poor prognosis for satisfactory neurological recovery after surgical decompression (Aho et al 1969).

SURGICAL INDICATIONS AND SELECTION OF PATIENTS

Except for the rare cases of acute cauda equina syndrome, the purpose of discectomy is relief of pain, in particular severe sciatic pain, caused by a disc herniation, i.e. by dislocated (protruding or extruding) disc tissue. The disc herniation is a special lesion occurring sometimes in the course of disc degeneration. However, disc degeneration in itself is not an indication for discectomy.

Complete relief of sciatic pain after discectomy is correlated primarily with the degree of herniation (Fig. 55.2). The rate of complete relief is excellent in patients with high-grade herniations and the ideal indications for discectomy

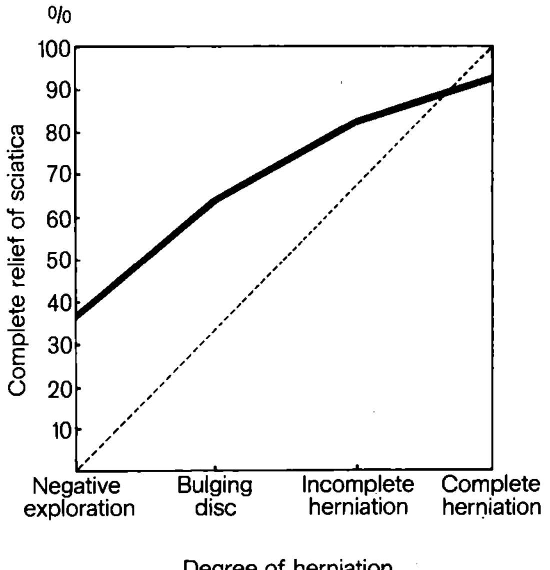

Fig. 55.2 The correlation between complete relief of sciatica and the degree of herniation in 2503 operations. (From Spangfort 1972.)

are recently ruptured herniations and large incomplete herniations in the process of rupturing or dissecting beneath the posterior longitudinal ligament. Only by meticulous selection of patients with high-grade herniations is it possible to improve the results of discectomy and avoid a growing number of disastrous failures.

Disc surgery is pain surgery: the first condition for considering the possibility of discectomy is that the pain is severe enough to motivate surgical treatment. The next condition is that the pain is caused predominantly by a high-grade herniation. These conditions must be strictly respected. The point is to establish the presence and location of an offending disc herniation and, unfortunately, surgical exposure is still the only way to do so with complete certainty.

The decision to advise discectomy must therefore be based on a systematic and comprehensive diagnostic investigation, comprising a detailed history and an adequate analysis of the pain syndrome, disentangling in each case debut and duration of pain, temporal pattern, activities and circumstances affecting the pain, anatomical and topographical patterns, sensory modalities and an assessment of the intensity of the pain. Furthermore, a complete physical examination is necessary, including the recording of posture and gait, degree of lordosis, range and pattern of spinal motion, pattern of pain by rest, motion and weight bearing and a neurological examination, as well as psychological assessment, routine laboratory tests and plain radiographs of the spine and pelvis.

In detailed analyses of the pain syndrome – particularly of the topographical pattern and sensory modalities, which are of fundamental importance in diagnosing a disc herniation – we have found diagnostic thermography of little value. To achieve this information, in our experience, a pain-drawing method is definitely superior, as well as being cheap and convenient. Our present pain-drawing system (Fig. 55.3) was developed from the model published by Ransford et al (1976) and has become indispensable in our preoperative investigation (Brismar et al 1996).

Progressive neurological deficits are usually listed as an indication for disc surgery. Strictly speaking, we do not agree with this. We consider neurological deficits important diagnostic signs but not an independent indication for discectomy, as surgical treatment has not been shown to improve the average prognosis of peripheral neurological deficits. If surgical treatment of a disc herniation cures neurological deficits, which is most likely in some cases, we

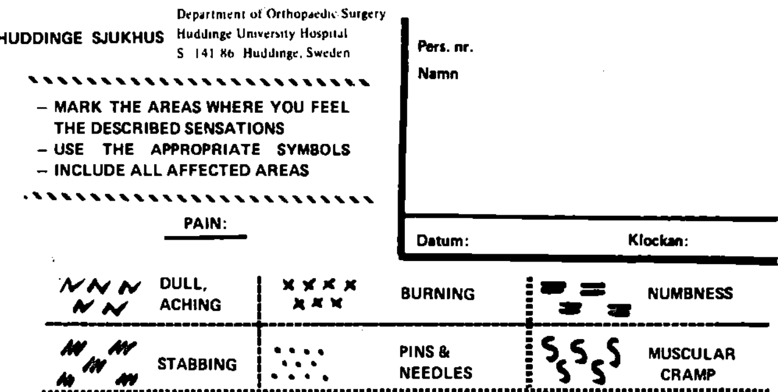
HUDDINGE SJUKHUS Department of Orthopaedic Surgery Huddinge University Hospital S 141 86 Huddinge, Sweden

Pers. nr.
Namn

– MARK THE AREAS WHERE YOU FEEL THE DESCRIBED SENSATIONS
– USE THE APPROPRIATE SYMBOLS
– INCLUDE ALL AFFECTED AREAS

PAIN:

Datum: Klockan:

DULL, ACHING | BURNING | NUMBNESS
STABBING | PINS & NEEDLES | MUSCULAR CRAMP

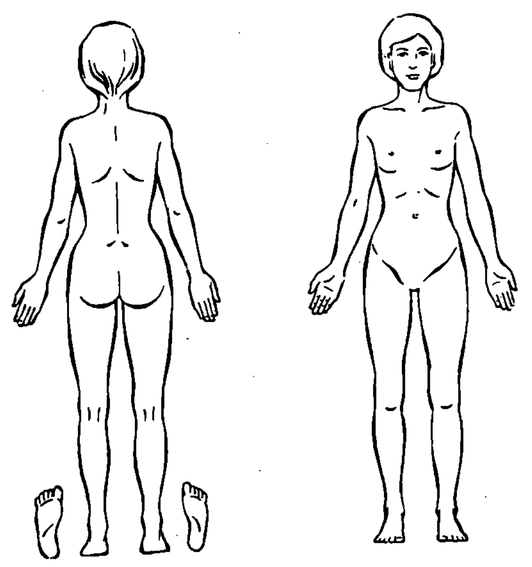

Fig. 55.3 Main form for pain drawing used for patients with low back pain. (Modified from Ransford et al 1976.)

still cannot identify the subgroup of patients who will benefit from discectomy in this respect.

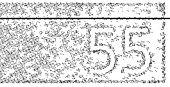

The rupture of a disc herniation into the spinal canal is an anatomical disaster and surgical measures against it are widely independent of the patient's general psychological status. Certainly, individual psychological experience of pain and suffering is the main indication for discectomy and inappropriate or incomprehensible description of the symptoms and unusual or pathological pain behaviour may seriously complicate the objective diagnostic interpretation and assessment, but in the case of an unequivocal diagnosis of disabling disc herniation we do not deny the patient surgical relief for psychological reasons. The emotionally unstable patient may, indeed, be in greater need of immediate pain relief than the stable one.

The situation is somewhat different in other types of low back surgery, especially 'salvage surgery', in which the psychological variables apparently play a more dominant role in surgical treatment.

It is generally recognized that, with the exceptions already mentioned, surgical treatment of a disc herniation should be advised only if non-surgical treatment fails. A reasonable trial period is 1–3 months in many cases, but we hesitate to accept rigid rules, as a wide variety of circumstances necessitates individual evaluation and decision in every case.

NON-SURGICAL VERSUS SURGICAL TREATMENT

So far, it has not been possible to design a clinical trial of the differences between non-surgical and surgical treatment which completely fulfils scientific criteria. One problem is that a disc herniation can be definitely confirmed and classified only by surgical exposure. Another obstacle is the fact that, when patients with a convincing clinical diagnosis of disc herniation are randomized to comparable groups for one of the two treatment modalities, there are always some patients allocated to non-surgical treatment in whom the pain becomes so excruciating that they cannot reasonably be denied surgical relief. This important group is therefore lost for comparison.

A few studies from which it is possible to draw tentative conclusions (e.g. Hakelius 1970, Nashold & Hrubec 1971, Hasue & Fujiwara 1979) do, however, indicate that surgical treatment does not necessarily improve the prognosis in the long term, as regards either pain or the risk of persistent neurological deficits.

Weber (1983), in his controlled prospective study, allocated 126 patients with questionable indications for discectomy to either operation or physiotherapy and then compared the groups for 10 years. After 1 year the results were significantly better after surgical treatment than after non-surgical treatment. After 4 years the operated patients still showed better results, but the difference was no longer significant. Only minor changes occurred throughout the last 6 years of observation. After 10 years no patients in the two groups complained of sciatic pain and the rates of persistent low back pain were equal in the groups. The severity of low back pain decreased over the last 6 years in both groups.

If the clinical situation allows a choice between non-surgical and surgical treatment, the patient should be informed that the benefit expected from the operation is immediate relief of sciatic pain and not necessarily an improvement of the long-range prognosis, which is fairly good anyway.

NUCLEOLYSIS

Chemonucleolysis was introduced as a non-surgical treatment, a last alternative to surgical treatment. Considering the invasive procedure and the complications, chemonucleolysis should, however, be classified as surgery.

After 30 years of controversy the efficacy of chemonucleolysis has now been shown in controlled trials and the method is recommended subject to strict selection of patients (Nordby et al 1996, Brown 1996). Still, in some countries the method is seldom or never used.

Recently nucleolysis has been achieved by percutaneous laser disc decompression, by which a portion of the nucleus is vaporized by laser energy. The method is still at an experimental stage (Quigley & Maroon 1994).

COMPLICATIONS OF DISC SURGERY

MORTALITY RATE

The mortality rate associated with disc surgery is low. In a survey of 54 reports from the period 1937–72 with a total of 25 392 operations, the mean rate was 0.3% and constantly decreasing over the years. Pulmonary embolism and postoperative infections were the most frequent causes of death (Spangfort 1972).

INJURY TO VESSELS AND VISCERA

Injury to abdominal vessels is an uncommon but extremely dangerous complication in disc surgery. Not all cases are

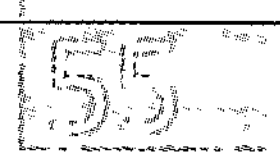

reported in the literature, but an estimated incidence of this complication is less than one case in 2000 operations (DeSaussure 1959, Birkeland & Taylor 1969).

The disaster usually occurs when the instrument used for evacuating tissue from the interior of the disc space accidentally and without the surgeon being aware of it passes through the anterior wall of the disc. The major vessels (the abdominal aorta, the inferior vena cava and the common iliac vessels) are in close proximity to the anterior surface of the lumbar discs and easily within range of the biting rongeur (Nilsonne & Hakelius 1965). Laceration of these vessels may cause a dramatic retroperitoneal haemorrhage, which is detectable in the surgical field in only half of the cases: the first warning of a vascular catastrophe may be symptoms of severe hypovolaemic shock during or after surgery. Immediate laparotomy and repair of the injured vessel is imperative.

Arteriovenous fistula is another type of vascular injury, which may produce complex circulatory impairment and cardiac failure. The diagnosis is often delayed for months or years, but the mortality rate is lower.

Injuries to the bowel, the ureter and the sympathetic trunk may occur by the same mechanism, but are less commonly reported in the literature.

In 95% of all disc operations the total loss of blood is less than 500 ml. Damage to the epidural veins is the usual cause of more extensive bleeding and, although this type of haemorrhage is almost always well within safe limits, the bleeding may cause troublesome difficulties, at least in the narrow field exposed by the interlaminar approach.

INJURIES TO NEURAL STRUCTURES

Injuries to the nerve roots, and even to the cauda equina, may occur during the operation in spite of careful surgical technique. Surgical damage to nerve roots is reported by surgeons in 0.5–3% of all operations; in reoperations the rate is two or three times higher. Verified damage to a nerve root is not always followed by significant clinical symptoms. Motor weakness in the leg, obviously caused by the operation, occurs in at least 5% of all operations, but in the majority the paresis is partial and recovers satisfactorily with time.

DURA LESIONS

Minor surgical lesions to the dura are not uncommon and are often revealed by leakage of cerebrospinal fluid during the operation. If the lesion is located and closed with fine sutures, the complication is usually harmless. In rare cases a dura lesion results in the formation of an extradural pseudocyst or a fistula leaking cerebrospinal fluid, which requires secondary surgery.

THROMBOEMBOLISM

Postoperative thromboembolism is reported to average 2% in the literature. The complication is usually diagnosed between the fourth and 12th day after the operation and is rare in patients below 40 years. A period of immobilization before surgery is probably a pathogenetic factor.

POSTOPERATIVE INFECTIONS

With modern surgical technique and facilities, the mean rate of postoperative wound infections after discectomy should not exceed a total of 2–3%, with severe infections accounting for less than 0.5%.

Septic meningitis, epidural abscess and frank pyogenic spondylitis are rare and major complications.

POSTOPERATIVE DISCITIS

This condition is now recognized as a complication to disc surgery. Most cases are caused by a low-grade infection of the disc space, but an aseptic or 'mechanical' type of postoperative discitis also seems to occur (Fouquet et al 1992). The true incidence is unknown, but probably does not exceed 1–2%.

The most typical symptom, almost pathognomonic, is violent, spasmodic pain in the back precipitated by the slightest movement and in most cases appearing during the first or second week after an otherwise uneventful postoperative course. The pain is referred to the lower abdomen, the groins, hips or upper thighs. True root pain is unusual and the patient often describes the pain as a new and terrible experience.

Systemic reactions are scarce. Some patients have a moderate fever and/or infection of the surgical wound. The sedimentation rate (ESR) is usually elevated and a second rise of the postoperative ESR, which normally reaches its peak 3–4 days after the operation, is a significant warning.

Early radiological changes may appear 3–4 weeks after the onset of pain and the main features are fuzziness and irregular defects of the endplates, cavitations into one or both of the adjacent vertebrae, marked narrowing of the intervertebral disc space and vertebral sclerosis. Later, there is abundant new bone formation, which often results in solid bony fusion. MRI is now considered the best method for diagnosing the condition.

The acute pain syndrome lasts between 6 and 12 weeks in most cases and complete immobilization is the most effective management. Adequate treatment with antibiotics until the ESR is normal is recommended. There is no indication for surgical intervention when the clinical picture is typical. The course is always prolonged and the pain may be a frightening experience for the patient. The complication seems to increase the risk of chronic low back pain and vocational disability, but otherwise many studies indicate a fairly good long-term prognosis (Iversen et al 1992, Rohde et al 1998).

SPINAL ARACHNOIDITIS

An association between lumbar disc disease and arachnoiditis, a progressive inflammatory reaction of the pia arachnoid, was suspected long ago (French 1946) but the condition is difficult to diagnose, the more so because intradural exploration is seldom performed during a disc operation, and the complication has been considered rare. Recent studies indicate, however, that some degree of arachnoiditis is common, at least in patients with severe pain and disability secondary to disc surgery. Arachnoiditis may be clinically silent and the correlation between the pathology and pain is still poorly defined (Symposium 1978).

Many aetiological factors are apparently involved in the development of arachnoiditis: injection of contrast media, anaesthetics and other agents into the subarachnoid space, infection, the presence of blood, trauma, disc lesions and spinal stenosis, surgical injuries and unknown individual factors (Ransford & Harries 1972).

Symptoms vary considerably and mild cases are probably often overlooked. In severe cases, the condition is extremely distressing. The pain is constant in the back and radiates to one or both legs, often in a well-defined distribution of more than one root. The pain is described as burning or cramping – painful muscle cramps and violent spasms of the legs are usual. The cauda equina may be involved. Pain is unrelieved by rest and poorly correlated to weight bearing and motion.

Treatment of this neuralgic pain syndrome is extremely difficult, but the condition is not inevitably progressive – a slow recovery over the years occurs in some patients. Severe psychological complications in response to the constant torturing pain are, however, the rule.

REFERENCES

Aho AJ, Auranen A, Pesonen K 1969 Analysis of cauda equina symptoms in patients with lumbar disc prolapse. Acta Chirurgica Scandinavica 135: 413–420

Birkeland IW Jr, Taylor TKF 1969 Major vascular injuries in lumbar disc surgery. Journal of Bone and Joint Surgery 51B: 4–19

Boemke F 1951 Feingewebliche Befunde beim Bandscheibenvorfall. Langenbecks Archiv 267: 484–492

Brismar H, Vucetic N, Svensson O 1996 Pain patterns in lumbar disc hernia. Drawings compared to surgical findings in 159 patients. Acta Orthopaedica Scandinavica 67: 470–472

Brown MD 1996 Update on chemonucleolysis. Spine 21 (suppl 24S): 62S–68S

Busch E, Andersen A, Broager B et al 1950 Le prolapsus discal lombaire. Acta Psychiatrica et Neurologica 25: 443–500

Capanna AH, Williams RW, Austin DC et al 1981 Lumbar discectomy – percentage of disc removal and detection of anterior annulus perforation. Spine 6: 610–614

DeSaussure RL 1959 Vascular injury coincident to disc surgery. Journal of Neurosurgery 16: 222–229

Eyre-Brook AL 1952 A study of late results from disc operations. British Journal of Surgery 39: 289–296

Fager CA, Freidberg SR 1980 Analysis of failures and poor results of lumbar spine surgery. Spine 5: 87–94

Finneson BE 1978 A lumbar disc surgery predictive score card. Spine 3: 186–188

Fouquet B, Goupille P, Jattiot F et al 1992 Discitis after lumbar disc surgery. Features of 'aseptic' and 'septic' forms. Spine 17: 356–358

French JD 1946 Clinical manifestations of lumbar spinal arachnoiditis. Surgery 20: 718–729

Hakelius A 1970 Prognosis in sciatica. Acta Orthopaedica Scandinavica 129 (suppl): 1–76

Hanraets PRMJ 1959 The degenerative back and its differential diagnosis. Elsevier, Amsterdam

Hasue M, Fujiwara M 1979 Epidemiologic and clinical studies of long-term prognosis of low-back pain and sciatica. Spine 4: 150–155

Hirsch C, Nachemson A 1963 The reliability of lumbar disk surgery. Clinical Orthopaedics and Related Research 29: 189–195

Iversen E, Herss Nielsen VA, Gadegaard Hansen L 1992 Prognosis in postoperative discitis. A retrospective study of 111 cases. Acta Orthopaedica Scandinavica 63: 305–309

Langenskiöld A, Kiviluoto O 1976 Prevention of epidural scar formation after operations on the lumbar spine by means of free fat transplants. Clinical Orthopaedics and Related Research 115: 92–95

LaRocca H, Macnab I 1974 The laminectomy membrane. Journal of Bone and Joint Surgery 56B: 545–550

Love JG 1939 Removal of protruded intervertebral disks without laminectomy. Proceedings of the Staff Meetings of the Mayo Clinic 14: 800 (1940, 15: 4)

Macnab I 1971 Negative disc exploration. Journal of Bone and Joint Surgery 53A: 891–903

McCulloch JA 1996 Focus issue on lumbar disc herniation: macro- and microdiscectomy. Spine 21 (suppl 24S) 45S–56S

Mixter WJ, Barr JS 1934 Rupture of the intervertebral disc with involvement of the spinal canal. New England Journal of Medicine 211: 210–215

Mochida J, Nishimura K, Nomura T et al 1996 The importance of preserving disc structure in surgical approaches to lumbar disc herniation. Spine 21: 1556–1564

Nachemson AL 1976 The lumbar spine – an orthopaedic challenge. Spine 1: 59–71

Nachlas W 1952 End-result study of the treatment of herniated nucleus

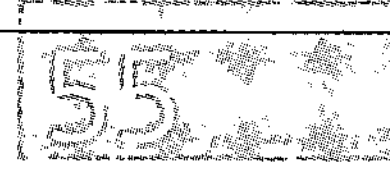

pulposus by excision with fusion and without fusion. Journal of Bone and Joint Surgery 34A: 981–988

Nashold BS, Hrubec Z 1971 Lumbar disc disease. A 20-year clinical follow-up study. C V Mosby, St Louis

Naylor A 1974 The late results of laminectomy for lumbar disc prolapse. Journal of Bone and Joint Surgery 56B: 17–29

Nilsonne U, Hakelius A 1965 On vascular injury in lumbar disc surgery. Acta Orthopaedica Scandinavica 35: 329–337

Nordby EJ, Fraser RD, Javid MJ 1996 Spine update. Chemonucleolysis. Spine 21: 1102–1105

O'Connell JEA 1951 Protrusions of the lumbar intervertebral discs. Journal of Bone and Joint Surgery 33B: 8–30

Onik GM, Kambin P, Chang MK 1997 Controversy. Minimally invasive disc surgery. Nucleotomy *versus* fragmentectomy. Spine 22: 827–830

Quigley MR, Maroon JC 1994 Laser discectomy: A review. Spine 19: 53–56

Quist JJ, Dhert WJA, Meij BP et al 1998 The prevention of peridural adhesions. A comparative long-term histomorphometric study using a biodegradable barrier and a fat graft. Journal of Bone and Joint Surgery 80B: 520–526

Ransford AO, Harries BJ 1972 Localised arachnoiditis complicating lumbar disc lesions. Journal of Bone and Joint Surgery 54B: 656–665

Ransford AO, Cairns D, Mooney V 1976 The pain drawing as an aid to the psychologic evaluation of patients with low back pain. Spine 1: 127–134

Rohde V, Meyer B, Schaller C, Hassler WE 1998 Spondylodiscitis after lumbar discectomy. Incidence and a proposal for prophylaxis. Spine 23: 615–620

Spangfort EV 1972 The lumbar disc herniation. A computer-aided analysis of 2504 operations. Acta Orthopaedica Scandinavica 142 (suppl): 1–95

Spengler DM, Freeman CW 1979 Patient selection for lumbar discectomy – an objective approach. Spine 4: 129–134

Symposium 1978 Lumbar arachnoiditis: nomenclature, etiology, and pathology. Spine 3: 21–92

Symposium 1981 The role of spine fusion for low-back pain. Spine 6: 277–314

Tullberg T, Isacson J, Weidenhielm L 1993 Does microscopic removal of lumbar disc herniation lead to better results than the standard procedure? Spine 18: 24–27

Van Hoytema G, Oostrom J 1961 The operation for herniation of the nucleus pulposus with intervertebral body fusion. Archivum Chirurgicum Neerlandicum 13: 71–80

Vucetic N 1997 Clinical diagnosis of lumbar disc herniation. Outcome predictors for surgical treatment. Thesis, Karolinska Institute, Stockholm

Weber H 1983 Lumbar disc herniation – a controlled, prospective study with 10 years of observation. Spine 8: 131–140

White JC 1966 Results in surgical treatment of herniated lumbar intervertebral discs. Clinical Neurosurgery 13: 42–51

Wilson JC Jr 1967 Low back pain and sciatica – a plea for better care of the patient. Journal of the American Medical Association 200: 705–712

Yong-Hing K, Reilly J, de Korompay V, Kirkaldy-Willis WH 1980 Prevention of nerve root adhesions after laminectomy. Spine 5: 59–64

Orthopaedic surgery

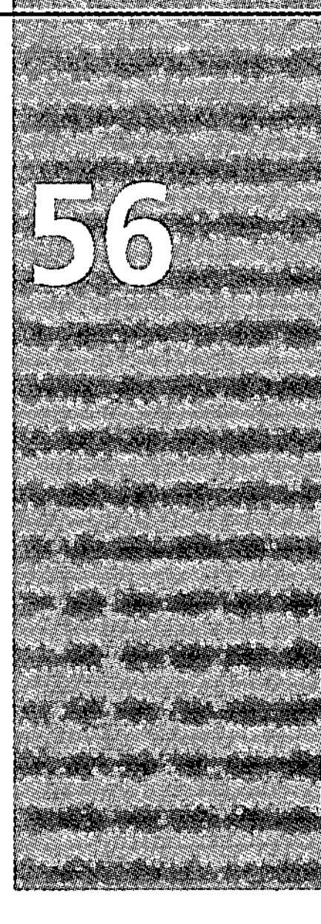

ROBERT F. McLAIN & JAMES N. WEINSTEIN

INTRODUCTION

The orthopaedist is called on to treat a wide variety of musculoskeletal disorders, among which pain is often the common denominator. These disorders are exceptionally diverse in nature, arising out of neoplastic, inflammatory, developmental, metabolic or traumatic conditions, and so are the mechanisms by which they produce pain. Pain is the symptom that most often drives the patient to seek treatment; it is, however, a non-specific symptom and provides little insight, by itself, as to the serious or benign nature of the underlying malady. Whether the pain source is a life-threatening tumour or an ankle sprain, one of the patient's key concerns is the alleviation of pain; it is, therefore, the physician's responsibility to formulate a plan that offers the best treatment of the underlying disease while effectively limiting or eliminating the symptom of pain.

When the physician encounters the patient complaining of musculoskeletal pain, his initial task is to identify the true nature of the patient's problem: is the pain severe and debilitating in and of itself or does it simply trigger the patient's fear of a possible malignant cause? Is it a manifestation of underlying psychological turmoil or is it physiologically normal pain interfering with an active, functional patient? The next task is to seek out the source and cause of the pain, if possible, and to exclude the possibility of an underlying systemic or malignant process that may threaten the patient's life. Finally, the orthopaedic surgeon reviews the treatment options and formulates a treatment plan suited to the individual patient and the specific disorder. The physician's objectives in treating the orthopaedic patient are to reduce the patient's pain, to correct the underlying musculoskeletal disorder and to improve overall function and he or she may take advantage of a wide variety of modalities to accomplish these goals.

MECHANISMS OF MUSCULOSKELETAL PAIN

The musculoskeletal system consists of the bones and articulations of the skeleton and the ligaments, muscles and tendons that connect and mobilize them. The system is made up of diverse tissues with radically different characteristics. Injuries or disorders of the musculoskeletal system may directly affect muscle, bone, tendon, ligament, articular cartilage, periosteum, synovium or articular capsule and may directly or indirectly affect the overlying integument, the indwelling haematopoietic tissues or neural elements associated with or contained within the skeletal framework. These tissues are richly innervated by a variety of neural receptors (transducers) that inform, modulate and co-ordinate their individual and collective musculoskeletal functions.

JOINT PAIN

The articulations of the appendicular skeleton are specialized to bear loads and allow motion through specific, proscribed arcs of excursion. In the extremities and in the posterior elements of the spine, these are synovial joints. The components of these joints are specialized to meet specific demands of function: articular cartilage absorbs and distributes loads; subchondral bone resists deformation and supports and nourishes the cartilage; ligaments maintain alignment and constrain joint excursion; musculotendinous units flex, extend and stabilize the joint. Derangement of the joint may result in destruction of the articular cartilage, fracture of the subchondral bone, attenuation or disruption of the ligaments and excessive strains and inflammation of the muscles. Nerve endings in these or other tissues may signal the presence of ongoing or incipient tissue damage, producing the sensation of pain.

Synovial joints enjoy a dual pattern of innervation: *primary articular nerves* are independent branches from larger peripheral nerves, which specifically supply the joint capsule and ligaments; *accessory articular nerves* reach the joint after passing through muscular or cutaneous tissues to which they provide primary innervation (Wyke 1972). These muscular tissues may overlie or run adjacent to the joint in question and the musculotendinous insertion often ramifies with connective tissues of the joint capsule, allowing intramuscular nerves embedded in the intrafascicular connective tissue to extend branches that reach the joint (Gardner 1944, 1948). Both primary and accessory articular nerves are mixed afferent nerves, containing proprioceptive and nociceptive fibres. These fibres supply innervation to virtually all of the periarticular soft tissues, though some structures are more heavily innervated than others.

Freeman and Wyke (1967) have described four basic types of afferent nerve endings in articular tissues and have documented the presence of those endings in a wide variety of joints. While the type 4 receptors (free nerve endings) are the only ones thought to be exclusively nociceptive, it is known that the proprioceptive endings of groups 1–3 are capable of responding to excessive joint excursion as a noxious stimulus and that they play an important role in mediating protective muscular reflexes that maintain joint stability (Palmer 1958, Eckholm et al 1960). Deandrade et al (1965) and Kennedy et al (1982) have both demonstrated that the presence of a joint effusion, a common finding in patients with inflammatory, traumatic or degenerative joint disease, can produce significant reflex inhibition of the quadriceps mechanism. Histological studies have demonstrated receptors in ligaments (Gardner 1948, O'Connor & Gonzales 1979, De Avila et al 1989), capsule (Freeman & Wyke 1967, Grigg et al 1982) and meniscal tissues (O'Connor & McConnaughey 1978), as well as periarticular fat and muscle (Freeman & Wyke 1967, Dee 1978). Giles and Harvey (1987) have demonstrated nociceptive free nerve endings in capsular tissue from human facets and reported similar endings in the apophyseal synovium. These nociceptive endings are supplied by small myelinated type 3 nerve fibres and small unmyelinated type 4 fibres.

While capsule, fat and muscle are richly supplied with nociceptive free nerve endings, investigators have previously reported a relative paucity of these receptors in the synovium, ligaments and menisci. In most situations the neural impulses that signal joint pain have been thought to be generated by receptors in tissue surrounding the joint and not by the tissues directly exposed to mechanical stresses or trauma. The stimuli that these periarticular receptors respond to may be either mechanical (capsular distension, ligamentous instability, direct trauma) or chemical (Wyke 1981).

The role of the synovium in producing and releasing kinins, prostaglandins and other chemical irritants has been suggested to explain why joints with synovitis are frequently painful, even though the synovium has long been thought to have few receptors. However, it now appears that the synovial tissues may produce joint pain by both direct and indirect mechanisms. Using antisera against specific neuronal markers, investigators re-examining synovial innervation have found vastly greater numbers of small-diameter nerve fibres than were previously reported using standard histological methods (Gronblad et al 1988, 1991, Weinstein et al 1988a, Kidd et al 1990). Nearly all of these fibres have been immunoreactive for vasoactive and pain-related neuropeptides. Substance P (sP) has been shown to accumulate in articular fluid following capsaicin injection and is known to produce plasma extravasation and vasodilatation (Yaksh 1988, Lam & Ferrell 1989, 1991). Levels of sP are higher in joints with more severe arthritis and infusion of the neuropeptide into joints with mild disease has been shown to accelerate the degenerative process (Levine et al 1984). Calcitonin gene-related peptide (CGRP) has also been implicated as a mediator in the early stages of arthritis (Konttinen et al 1990). Whether sP plays a direct role in the stimulation or sensitization of intra-articular pain receptors is not established, but sensitization is important and several mechanisms have been confirmed experimentally. Grigg et al (1986) have shown that the induction of experimental arthritis results in sensitization of free nerve endings in the joint capsule. When acute inflammation is induced, afferent receptors which are normally silent during joint motion become responsive to previously innocuous stimuli, including motion in the normal range. A similar sensitizing effect is produced by intra-articular infusion of prostaglandins or bradykinin (Schaible et al 1987, Neugebauer et al 1989), providing further evidence that local sensitization is at least partly responsible for the pain felt in arthritic or inflamed joints. There is also strong evidence of a central nervous system component in sensitizing spinal cord neurons that receive input from these joint afferents, a means of further amplifying the nociceptive discharges from the joint (Neugebauer & Schaible 1990).

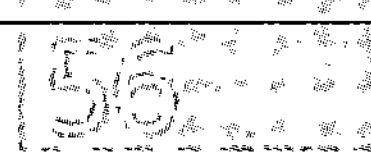

BONE AND PERIOSTEUM

Bone is a dynamic composite tissue involved in a variety of physiological processes and capable of a number of biological responses to injury or stress. It is the one tissue in the body able to repair itself after injury without forming scar. It responds to minute pezoelectric currents generated by stresses by increasing its mass in areas of increased load and by removing support from areas seeing little load. It is sensitive to pressure internally and to direct injury externally.

The external covering of the bone is the periosteum. This tough fibrous sheath adheres to the outer cortex of the bone and contains the pluripotent mesenchymal cells necessary for bone growth and fracture healing. The periosteum is highly vascular and copiously supplied with both free nerve endings and encapsulated endings; the complex free nerve endings are thought to generate painful discharges, while the encapsulated endings are thought to be sensitive to pressure (Ralston et al 1960, Cooper 1968). In periosteal tissue, Hill and others have documented the presence of nerves immunoreactive to a wide variety of pain-related and vasoactive neuropeptides (Hill & Elde 1991). Gronblad et al (1984) have demonstrated an extensive ramification of sP-reactive nerve fibres in both the superficial and deep layers of the periosteal sheath. They also reported the presence of sP immunoreactivity in some encapsulated, glomerular-type receptors from the same tissue. Encapsulated sP-reactive nerve endings have previously been reported in the posterior longitudinal ligament of the spine, implicating that structure as a source of low back pain (Liesi et al 1983).

Bjurholm et al (1988a) have demonstrated both sP- and CGRP-containing nerves in the marrow, periosteum and cortex of long bones, as well as the associated muscles and ligaments. They noted a higher density of sP- and CGRP-immunoreactive fibres in epiphyseal rather than diaphyseal marrow and saw that some fibres from the abundantly innervated periosteum penetrated the cortex and entered the marrow space by way of the Volkmann's canals. These two neuropeptides, sP and CGRP, have been associated with nociceptor transmission (Skofitsch & Jacobowitz 1985, Badalamente et al 1987) as well as an acceleration of experimental arthritis and an increase in its severity following local infusion (Colpaert et al 1983, Levine et al 1984).

Vasoactive intestinal peptide (VIP), and a number of other vasoactive neuropeptides, have also been localized to fine nerve fibres predominantly found in cancellous bone of the epiphysis and in the periosteum (Bjurholm et al 1988b). The vasodilatory effect of VIP has been clearly demonstrated (Said & Mutt 1970), while neuropeptide Y (NPY) has been shown to be a powerful vasoconstrictor (Lundberg et al 1982). Fibres containing these neuropeptides tend to congregate at the osteochondral junction of the epiphyseal plate, with VIP fibres running in the marrow spaces while NPY fibres follow the small vessels nourishing the epiphysis. Although the primary role of these peptides is likely to be related to the regulation of growth, it is possible that these or similar peptides might also play a role in the production or prevention of intraosseous hypertension, a proposed cause of bone and joint pain.

As a result, bone is a tissue capable of responding to both internal and external pressure changes, physical distortion, inflammation and periosteal injury by transmitting pain signals proximally. Bone pain may be produced by microfracture and subsidence in osteoarthritis, by periosteal elevation and distortion in infection or tumour, by vascular congestion and infarction in sickle cell crisis and by mechanical disruption in fractures and other traumatic conditions.

MUSCULOTENDINOUS PAIN

The nociceptive innervation of muscle has been discussed previously (Ch. 1). The primary nociceptive endings in muscle are unencapsulated free nerve endings similar to those seen in periarticular tissues, which transmit their impulses centrally by way of type III and IV afferent fibres. Intramuscular mechanoreceptors may also produce pain impulses when exposed to noxious stimuli. Muscular pain receptors may be either chemonociceptive or mechanonociceptive and may respond to stimuli as either specific or polymodal receptors. Chemonociceptive endings may respond to metabolites that accumulate during anaerobic metabolism, to products of cell injury produced by trauma or ischaemia or to chemical irritants such as bradykinin, serotonin or potassium. Mechanonociceptive units may respond to stretch, pressure or disruption. Some receptors may also respond to thermal stimuli (Kumazawa & Mizumura 1977, Mense & Schmidt 1977). Recent studies have demonstrated that intramuscular injection of CGRP in combination with either sP or neurokinin A elicits a significant pain sensation though, when injected alone, none of the neuropeptides produces muscular pain (Pedersen-Bjergaard et al 1989, 1991). It is thought that the neurogenic inflammatory response produced by CGRP, which results in persistent vasodilatation, erythema and oedema formation, may also serve to sensitize nociceptors to the presence of other pain-related neuropeptides (Piotrowski & Foreman 1986, Fuller et al 1987). This receptor sensitization, as well as the increase in intramuscular blood flow and interstitial oedema, may represent a primary mechanism of muscular pain.

Muscular pain may be the result of a direct injury, such as a blow or puncture, which disrupts or damages the muscle tissue and its intrafascicular nerve fibres, or the distension and pressure produced by the ensuing haematoma and oedema. Pain also results from indirect trauma, such as athletic injuries, where the muscle is torn or ruptured as it strains against an excessive resistance force. Inflammation and oedema, components of the normal healing process, play a role in the mediation of pain symptoms. In major musculoskeletal injuries persistent spasm may occur, resulting in severe muscle pain as well as further trauma to the muscle and other tissues of the soft tissue envelope.

A more ominous type of muscle pain occurs when excessive pressure in or around the muscle results in ischaemia. Compartment syndromes occur in patients with bleeding disorders, vascular injuries, musculoskeletal trauma and systemic infections and can result from constrictive dressings or casts. They are also a common finding in patients with stroke, intoxication, metabolic disorders or head injuries; patients with these conditions are often 'found down' and have lain in one position for so long that the blood supply to an extremity has been compromised. Pain in compartment syndrome is severe and unremitting and out of proportion to the injury sustained. The clinical condition mimics the symptoms produced by experimental tourniquet pain and it is likely that the pathophysiology of the two conditions is the same (Smith et al 1966, Sternbach et al 1974). Like tourniquet pain, compartment syndrome pain is progressive in intensity and rapidly resolves if pressure is released in a timely fashion, either by removing the constricting dressing or by performing a surgical release of the compartment fascia (Matsen 1975, Mubarak & Owen 1977).

NEURAL ELEMENTS

Nerves are subject to injury and irritation as they pass through the muscular compartments and around the bony articulations of the extremities. Several recent studies have shown that environmental stimuli can produce histological changes in dorsal root ganglion neurons similar to those seen following injury and can induce marked changes in the levels of pain-related neuropeptides contained within the ganglion (Weinstein 1986, Weinstein et al 1988b, McLain & Weinstein 1991, 1992). Compression and injury to the spinal nerves and dorsal root ganglion are discussed in detail in Chapters 37 and 54.

TREATMENT MODALITIES – PRINCIPLES AND APPLICATION

The goals of orthopaedic treatment are to reduce pain, correct deformity and improve function. To accomplish these goals, the surgeon may employ any of a number of different treatment modalities, both surgical and non-surgical. These modalities can be roughly segregated into four different levels:

1. immobilization
2. fusion
3. resection
4. reconstruction.

In addition, the orthopaedist routinely uses a number of tools available to the primary care physician – injections, physical therapy, non-steroidal anti-inflammatory medications and oral analgesics – to supplement or augment the pain relief provided by these modalities.

IMMOBILIZATION

The immobilization of injured extremities and joints is among the oldest and most effective means of controlling musculoskeletal pain. Archaic splints have been discovered among the burial trappings of Egyptian mummies and are described throughout medieval writings (Colton 1992). In modern orthopaedic care the splint is only the simplest of the many forms of immobilization available to the patient.

Immobilization of an injured extremity can be accomplished by either direct or indirect means, using internal splints, external splints or traction. Splinting effectively reduces pain in both soft tissue and bony trauma, inflammatory conditions, infections of the soft tissues or joints, joint instability, intra-articular derangements and a variety of other musculoskeletal conditions. By preventing joint excursion, muscle contraction and displacement of bony fractures, splinting ensures appropriate immobilization and enforces rest on the injured tissues, eliminating many of the stimuli that trigger local nociceptors.

In the fractured limb, pain is initially produced by the distortion or disruption of intramedullary nerve fibres and receptors in the broken bone, by stretched or disrupted receptors in the torn periosteum and by injury or pressure on receptors in the muscle and soft tissue overlying the fracture (Fig. 56.1). A haematoma rapidly accumulates and expands until the pressure within the compartment is significantly elevated; distension of the fascia and soft tissue triggers further pain receptors. Damaged tissues release bradykinin, histamine, potassium and neurotransmitters which sensitize local nociceptors, alter vascular permeability and mediate the influx of inflammatory cells. The result is oedema, inflammation and irritation of the injured muscle, triggering muscle spasms and involuntary contractions. This produces further tissue damage and increasing defor-

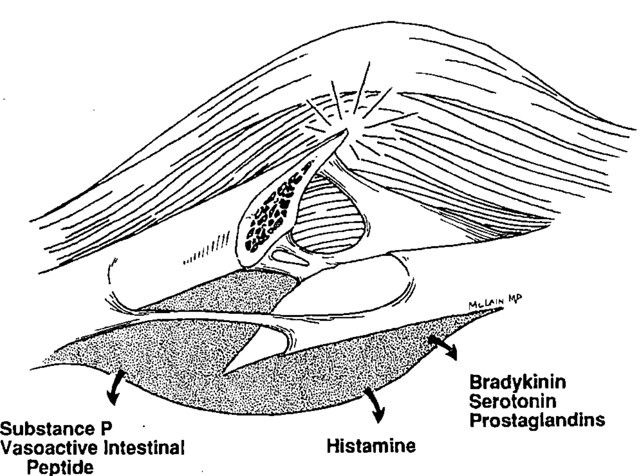

Fig. 56.1 Pain in musculoskeletal trauma. Fractures, dislocations and sprains elicit pain through a variety of inter-related and independent mechanisms which act locally and systemically to generate and mediate the pain sensation: fine nerve endings in the cancellous bone and periosteal lining are triggered by the physical disruption of the bone and the tearing and stretching of the periosteum; nerve endings in the surrounding muscle and soft tissue may be damaged directly or subjected to pressure or stretch by the displaced fracture fragments or the expanding haematoma; inflamed muscle may be triggered to spasm, producing pain and further distortion of tissues; damaged cells, nerve endings and inflammatory cells elaborate a variety of neurochemical mediators, including neuropeptides, algesic chemicals and inflammatory components.

mity, as well as uncontrolled pain. In a patient with multiple fractures this may lead to life-threatening haemorrhage and systemic shock (Chapman 1989). A variety of splinting techniques may be needed to manage such a patient through the course from initial resuscitation to definitive fixation (Fig. 56.2). External splints are the simplest of orthopaedic interventions, yet provide satisfactory treatment for injuries ranging from ligamentous sprains to long bone fractures. By preventing motion, the splint reduces the stimulation of nociceptors in injured tissues and lowers tension on irritated muscles, alleviating spasm and promoting rest.

In conditions of joint inflammation, haemarthrosis or pyarthrosis, pain is produced by the distension of the joint capsule. Chemical pain mediators which sensitize receptors in the fat pads and joint capsule directly stimulate chemonociceptors (Heppelmann et al 1985, 1986). Irritation of the synovium results in secondary oedema, synovial hypertrophy and an effusion, which stretch and distort the capsule. Any motion of the joint serves to increase the tension on the capsule and mechanically distorts the inflamed tissues, resulting in increased pain. What is ordinarily benign movement is now extremely painful. Joint motion in this inflamed state causes further release of noxious neuropeptides, kinins and inflammatory agents which act to stimulate receptors in the capsule and surrounding periosteum. Inflammation results in the appearance or increase in spontaneous activity of fine joint afferents and an increase in sensitivity to movement (Schaible & Schmidt 1985). By immobilizing the joint in a splint, these mechanisms can be attenuated. An appropriately applied splint will control joint motion while healing occurs and, by immobilizing the irritated tissues, can be instrumental in treating soft tissue inflammation such as occurs in tendonitis. The period of immobilization depends not only on pain and swelling, but also on the aetiology of the problem as well as the specific tissues involved. Bony injuries heal well with rigid immobilization, while ligamentous injuries often heal better with early motion despite pain.

Traction has long been recognized as an effective means of obtaining and maintaining a reduction in fractures of long bones (Charnley 1961a). By applying persistent longitudinal traction, muscle spasm can often be overcome and bony alignment restored. This prevents further tissue damage and reduces pain caused by distortion of soft tissues and movement of the ends of the fractured bone. Once the muscle fatigues and the spasm is overcome, muscle pain quickly subsides. Traction is typically used by emergency personnel for the transport of injured patients or as temporary treatment prior to casting or internal fixation. In patients who cannot tolerate surgery, skeletal traction remains a viable method of treating fractures. The complications of traction and prolonged immobilization (deep venous thrombosis, pulmonary embolus, pneumonia, infection) must be weighed against the risk of operative treatment or the disability associated with a poorly aligned fracture should neither traction nor surgery be employed.

Internal fixation or 'internal splintage' provides all the benefits of fracture reduction, tissue immobilization and protection from additional injury, but offers the additional benefit of early functional return. Because the bone is fixed internally, the adjacent joints can be left free for early range of motion. This reduces the complications of joint stiffness, muscular adhesions and atrophy which commonly accompany treatment with external casts, splints or traction. Rigid fixation of fractures eliminates motion at the injured bone ends and hence the pain caused by the abrading fracture surfaces. Immobilization limits the extent of subsequent muscle and periosteal damage, reducing the quantity of noxious metabolites, kinins and debris produced at the site of injury.

Depending on the location and the comminution of a fracture, the surgeon may elect to stabilize it using either plates and screws or an intramedullary device. In applying a

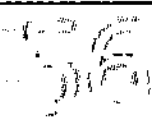

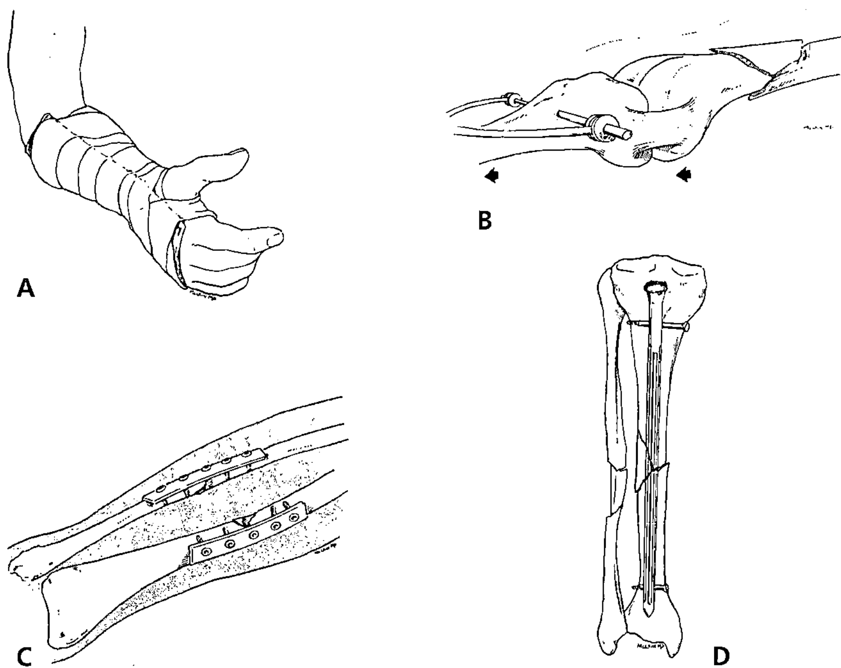

Fig. 56.2 Immobilization of musculoskeletal injuries: methods of immobilizing injured limbs range from passive, non-invasive techniques to sophisticated methods of internal fixation. **A** Splint immobilization can be applied to any extremity. The external splint is easy to apply, prevents excessive motion of joints and stabilizes soft tissues and allows the patient to return to limited function. **B** Skeletal traction is applied primarily in fractures of the femur, but can be used in any long bone fracture. The longitudinal traction overcomes powerful muscle spasm and controls alignment in injuries which cannot be splinted. **C** Internal fixation, using plates and screws, allows the surgeon to reduce anatomically the fracture fragments and rigidly fix the fracture. This ensures the best possible result in terms of alignment, joint congruency and anatomical relationships and also permits the patient to start range-of-motion exercises before the fracture has healed. **D** Intramedullary fixation restores alignment without exposing the fractures site, thereby reducing the risk of infection. By sharing the load applied to the limb, the intramedullary device minimizes the risk of non-union and allows early mobilization.

plate to the fracture, the surgeon opens the fracture site and reduces the fragments under direct vision. The plate is then applied so that it compresses the fracture fragments and promotes healing. Additional screws may be used to reduce and fix additional fragments which have broken off from the main segments of bone (Fig. 56.2). In this way complex fractures may be fixed rigidly enough to allow beneficial early motion of the adjacent joints and active movement of the muscles and tendons overlying the injury. This is particularly important in fractures of the upper extremity where malalignments are poorly tolerated and joint and muscle contractures result in persistent pain and permanent disability. In fractures of the forearm, for instance, cast treatment requires prolonged immobilization of the elbow, the wrist and the hand; this form of treatment is rarely adequate to control the position of the broken bones. The result is stiffness and pain in the joints, adhesions of the finger flexor muscles and loss of forearm rotation because of bony malalignment. Rehabilitation may be prolonged and painful and the patient's final function is often compromised. Open reduction and internal fixation of this injury are universally recommended; the patient is able to begin elbow motion the day after surgery and begins active finger motion and grip within a few days. Range of motion is restored to nearly normal and pain is a rare complication.

Intramedullary fixation of long bone fractures has become the standard of care in most trauma centres around the world. The technique involves opening a portal into the medullary canal at a site remote to the actual fracture. A rod is then passed down the medullary canal, across the fracture, and into the canal of the far fragment. Locking screws can be placed proximally and distally to control shortening and rotation (Küntscher 1968, Winquist & Hanson 1978). The use of intramedullary rods has two advantages over plate fixation. Firstly, the surgeon does not have to open the fracture site to fix the fracture, thus reducing the risk of infection. Secondly, the device allows the natural forces of gravity and muscle contraction to compress the fracture, stimulating the healing process. Intramedullary fixation is most commonly used in femur fractures, but can be applied to injuries of the tibia, humerus and ulna as well (Fig. 56.3).

Specialized fixation devices have been developed for fractures which have proven to be particularly difficult to treat by conservative means. Hip fractures, for example, are common injuries among elderly patients. In 1931 Smith-Peterson demonstrated a reduction in mortality from 75% to 25% and an increase in union rate from 30% to 70% when femoral neck fractures were internally fixed (Smith-Peterson et al 1931). Intertrochanteric hip fractures are particularly serious injuries and even as late as 1966, Horowitz reported a 35% mortality rate in patients treated non-operatively. In more than half of the patients that survive, the residual pain, deformity, prolonged recumbency and high rate of non-union result in a significant loss of independence. For this reason, open treatment of intertrochanteric fractures is the treatment of choice for most patients. Although a number of devices have been developed to address the unique anatomy of the proximal femur, since the mid 1970s the sliding hip screw and side plate have been the gold standard for internal fixation (Fig. 56.4). The biomechanical principles of this fixation system allow the patient to bear weight on the injured limb immediately postoperatively, permitting rehabilitation of muscles and avoiding recumbency and contractures. Failure rates have been reduced to around 4% (Rao et al 1983) and 70% will regain good to excellent function (Miller 1978). Most patients are able to ambulate with a walker or crutches, using only oral analgesics for pain, within the first week after their operation.

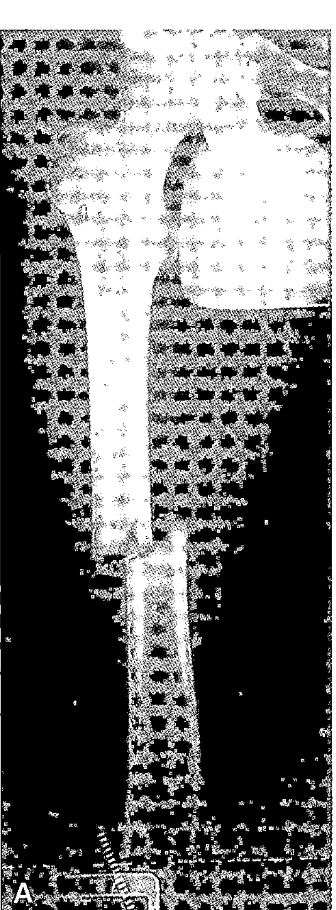

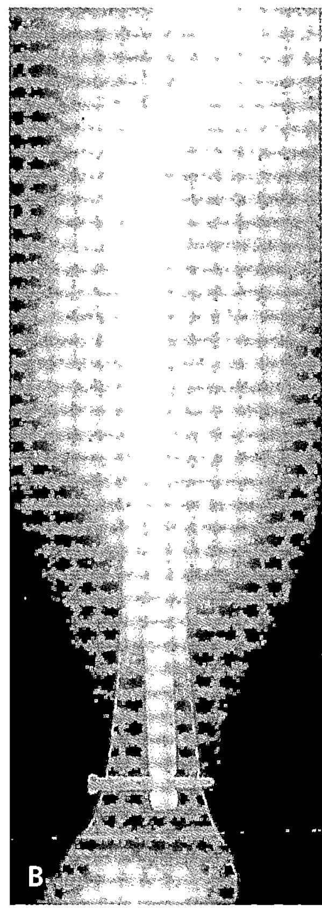

Fig. 56.3 Intramedullary fixation of a femur fracture. Intramedullary rodding allows the surgeon to restore length and axial alignment of this long bone fracture without opening the fracture site or damaging the massive muscular sheath that surrounds the femur. **A** AP radiograph of transverse femur fracture sustained in an auto accident; alignment and length are being maintained by longitudinal skeletal traction. **B** Same extremity after intramedullary fixation. Locking screws have been placed proximally and distally to prevent rotational or angular displacement. This patient was able to walk with crutches within 48 hours of surgery and was fully weight bearing at 3 weeks.

FUSION

Joint fusion represents a permanent form of musculoskeletal immobilization. Fusions are carried out in patients with pain secondary to joint infections, severe degenerative disease, severe articular trauma or disabling ligament instability, with the goal of restoring maximum function while eliminating pain. Although fusion is unglamorous and modern technology has provided us with so many options as to make fusion seem like a last resort for most patients, joint arthrodesis is still a highly successful operation for young patients with rugged functional demands. Patients who are younger than 40 years, weigh in excess of 200 lbs and/or have excessive activity requirements are at high risk for failure when treated with a conventional total joint prosthesis. In these patients a hip or knee fusion may be the right choice. Callaghan et al (1985) reviewed 28 patients with hip fusions, followed up for an average of 35 years. Although most patients eventually developed some degree of pain in the ipsilateral knee or low back, these patients had enjoyed years to decades of physical activity before developing symptoms. Over half these patients had returned to manual labour occupations, which would have been discouraged even with modern arthroplasty techniques. Approximately one-quarter of the patients underwent a late conversion to a total hip arthroplasty, with subsequent relief of their pain. Arthrodesis has been shown in this study and others reliably to relieve hip pain and improve function in selected, physically active patients (Sponseller et al 1984).

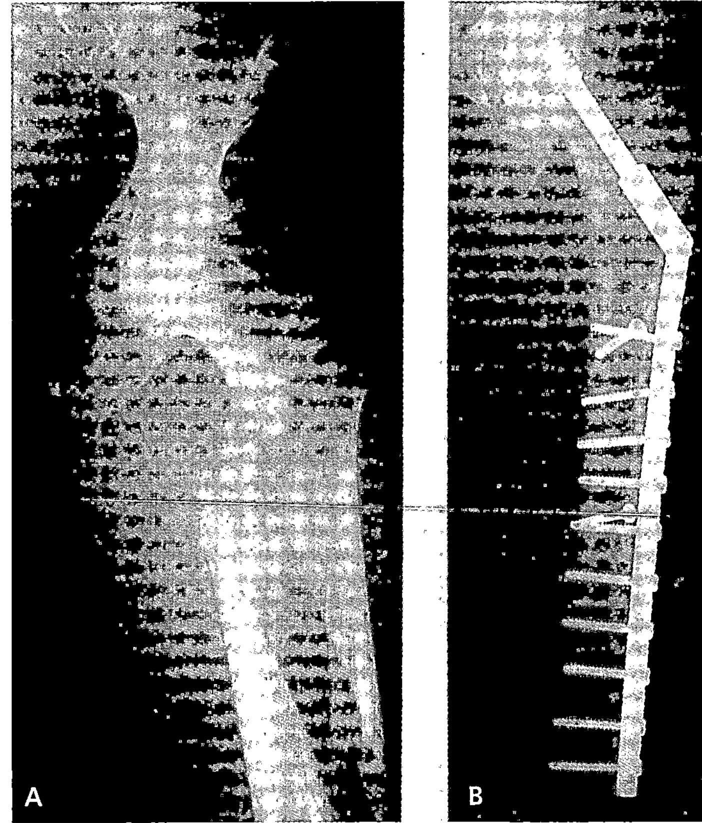

Fig. 56.4 Hip screw and side plate. **A** Severely comminuted fracture of the proximal femur in a middle-aged patient. Non-operative management is likely to result in non-union, deformity and pain. **B** Specially designed hip screw provides fixation of long spiral fracture of the femoral shaft while maintaining alignment of the femoral head and neck. The screw placed in the femoral head is designed to slide through the barrel of the side plate, allowing this fragment to collapse down on the shaft fragments during weight bearing while maintaining an appropriate angle between the neck and the shaft.

Another area in which fusion is often the best choice for pain relief and improved function is the wrist. Wrist arthrodesis has long enjoyed a reputation for reliable and satisfactory reconstruction in patients suffering severe trauma, infection, inflammatory disease or tumour. Steindler recommended the procedure for patients with polio or spastic hemiparesis (Steindler 1918) and later for tuberculosis (Steindler 1921) and others have described the procedures and outcomes for rheumatoid arthritis, post-traumatic arthritis and infections (Abbott et al 1942, Haddad & Riordan 1967, Millender & Nalebuff 1973). In these patients, end-stage joint destruction results in chronic resting pain, severe pain with activity, wrist deformity and loss of grip strength. Arthrodesis removes the painful joint tissues, eliminates motion and restores alignment and power grip. For patients with limited areas of joint disease within the wrist, a variety of intercarpal fusions have been described which maintain some joint motion while relieving pain and instability (Watson & Hempton 1980). Arthrodesis is performed by removing the articular cartilage and preparing the bone ends so that broad areas of bleeding, cancellous bone can be approximated and held firmly in place. Either internal or external fixation may be applied to ensure compression of the surfaces until fusion occurs. The surgical technique used is designed to maximize both the potential for fusion and the function of the limb after fusion. This means that the positioning of the limb at the time of surgery is critical to the patient's ability to use the extremity productively and painlessly. Optimal positions of function have been described for the wrist, hip, knee, shoulder, elbow and ankle, as well as the digits of both feet and hands. A patient with a solid arthrodesis in a position of function will consistently demonstrate greater function and satisfaction than a patient with a mobile but painful joint.

RESECTION

The ability surgically to remove the pathological tissue, segment or limb from a patient provides the orthopaedist with a variety of options in palliating painful musculoskeletal conditions. The simplest resections may require only the removal of a small piece of tissue, as in the patient with a torn meniscal cartilage, while the most complex of procedures may result in the internal resection of an entire long bone and its muscular envelope, for the patient with a primary bone tumour. Modern techniques allow us to consider limb-salvaging operations where terminal amputations are a viable but less satisfactory option. Modern prosthetics provide superior function and cosmesis where amputation is the logical and preferred choice.

Removal of pathological tissue from within a joint is a commonly performed procedure in patients with post-traumatic or inflammatory problems involving the articular cartilage, menisci or synovium. Arthroscopic surgery now allows surgeons to perform many of these procedures without opening the joint and, although most commonly performed in the knee, arthroscopy can be used in the shoulder, hip, wrist or ankle. In some situations, as with meniscal tears, arthroscopy actually provides better visualization and easier access to the damaged tissue than can be obtained through open methods.

Osteochondral loose bodies can occur in any joint, but are most common within the knee. These fragments usually result from previous cartilage injuries and may produce pain by impinging between the joint surfaces, compressing the synovial lining or irritating the capsular tissues (O'Connor & Shahriaree 1984). Simply removing the loose bodies and lavaging the joint can result in significant pain relief, particularly if there is a component of crystal-induced synovitis (O'Connor 1973). Meniscal tears are very common problems, resulting in pain and dysfunction in the most active and productive segment of our population. Depending on the size and pattern of a tear, the patient may present with persistent, nagging pain, occasional, severe pain or an acutely 'locked' knee, in which the torn meniscal tissue is found incarcerated within the joint, preventing flexion or extension. Through the arthroscope the orthopaedist is able to diagnose and access the injury and, as indicated, partially or completely resect the torn meniscus or repair it when possible. Since total meniscectomy has been shown to precipitate degenerative changes in the knee, partial meniscectomy or repair is widely recommended (Dandy & Jackson 1975, Jackson & Rouse 1982).

Synovial inflammation and hypertrophy may occur with any chronic inflammatory process, but are particularly prominent in rheumatoid and tuberculous arthritis, haemophilic arthritis and in pigmented villonodular synovitis (Wilkinson 1969, Montane et al 1986). It has previously been reported that the synovium is a relatively insensitive tissue (Kellgren & Samuel 1950) and that the pain of synovitis was produced by distortion of the capsule and the elaboration of inflammatory factors. As noted above, more recent techniques have demonstrated free nerve endings and neuropeptide-containing nerve fibres within the synovium which suggest a much greater role in pain sensation and mediation than previously thought (Kidd et al 1990, Konttinen et al 1990).

Synovectomy, either open or arthroscopic, has been shown to be effective in reducing pain and disability in patients with persistent synovitis due to haemophilia. Montane et al (1986) demonstrated that open synovectomy was able to eliminate recurrent haemarthroses, reduce pain and arrest the progressive arthrosis in 12 of 13 patients with haemophilic synovitis. Although some studies have questioned the efficacy of synovectomy in treating clinical symptoms of rheumatoid arthritis (Arthritis Foundation 1977), others have shown significant benefit to function and pain relief when carried out in early stages of the disease (Ishikawa et al 1986).

Resection of tumours of bone or soft tissue, and of destructive infections of bone, is often necessary for patient welfare as well as pain relief. Tumours produce pain as they displace normal tissues during growth. Expansile lesions, whether tumour or infection, may elevate the periosteum away from the bone, producing local pressure and disrupting nerve endings. Destructive lesions may weaken bone to the point of fracture or impending fracture and pathological fractures may prove very reluctant to heal. Compression of vascular structures may produce ischaemia or venous congestion, and of nerves, paralysis, paraesthesias or pain. Some neoplastic lesions, such as osteoid osteomas and osteoblastomas, may elaborate factors which produce pain directly (Sherman & McFarland 1965, Marsh et al 1975). Pain relief can be obtained by any means that reduces the distension of the soft tissues or compression of neurovascular structures. In cases of soft tissue infection, simple drainage of the abscess provides prompt and dramatic pain relief. Antibiotic therapy also provides rapid pain relief as the infection subsides and swelling is reduced. Pain due to expanding tumour mass can be reduced or eliminated by radiotherapy or chemotherapy; necrosis and shrinkage of the tumour relieves pressure on surrounding structures. While medical management is often able to control pain or slow the progress of disease, in many cases surgery is needed to ensure the best chance of curing the patient. In infections, debridement or resection of infected bone is necessary to prevent recurrence and in tumours, removal of the tumour, the surrounding soft tissues and sometimes all of the associated musculature may be necessary to provide local tumour control, depending on the tumour type. In any case, the type of resection chosen is determined on the basis of the location and nature of the lesion involved and the health and prognosis of the patient. Quality of life issues must always be considered – in some cases surgical resection may be the safest and most efficacious treatment available to the patient, while in others it may provide little benefit despite an extensive, debilitating operation.

The oldest and most straightforward form of resection is amputation, until this century the only rational treatment of tumours, infections, open fractures or other severely painful or potentially lethal lesions of the extremities. Although modern antibiotics, chemotherapeutic agents and surgical techniques have made it possible to salvage the vast majority of infected and injured limbs and many of those affected by tumour, amputation is still indicated in a number of clinical situations. Diabetic patients, with poor sensation, poor circulation and impaired healing potential, often require amputation to eliminate chronic and recurrent infections, non-healing wounds and neuropathic pain (Ecker & Jacobs 1970, Wagner 1986). Vascular insufficiency, whether associated with atherosclerosis or diabetes mellitus, accounts for nearly 80% of all lower extremity amputations (Glatty 1964, Mazet 1968). Tumours requiring a wide resection distal to the mid-tibia are still best treated by amputation, as reconstruction of this area is very difficult and the results somewhat unreliable.

Amputation remains an appropriate alternative in the care of some traumatic injuries. Advances in surgical technique, microvascular repair and soft tissue transfers have made it possible to 'save' almost any extremity; the decision to do so may be a disservice to some patients, however (Lange et al 1985). Patients with severe injuries to the lower leg, with open fractures and significant muscle and soft tissue damage, often require extensive reconstruction and multiple surgeries to repair the damage. These patients who, in the past, would have lost their legs, can now retain their limb and obtain a good outcome in terms of pain and long-term disability (Chapman & Mahoney 1979, Cierny et al 1983). However, patients with prolonged ischaemia of the limb, disruption of major nerves or mangling injuries of hand or foot have a poor prognosis; the patient is often left with a viable but functionless extremity, prone to infection and often painful. In these patients primary amputation offers the best likelihood of rapid return to painless activity and function (Hansen 1987, Caudle & Stern 1987).

Limb salvage surgery has made tremendous advances in the past decade. Limb salvage resections amount to 'internal amputations' and their success depends on the surgeon's ability to replace adequately the resected tissue elements with something that will function in an acceptably similar way. Likewise, the segment of the limb being salvaged has to be of enough importance to warrant a highly technical and demanding operation and extensive rehabilitation. Below-knee prostheses provide excellent, pain-free function with few problems in terms of fit, cosmesis or activity restrictions. Reconstructions of the foot and ankle often function poorly; stiffness and pain are frequent complications which may severely limit the patient. Hence, salvage of the foot and ankle is rarely warranted. On the other hand, patients with above-knee amputations expend significantly more energy in walking than do those with below-knee amputations. The fitting of above-knee prostheses can be more difficult and, when the amputation is performed high up on the thigh, the fit becomes more difficult and the function poorer; these patients have a greater tendency to become wheelchair bound than patients with below-knee amputations (Volpicelli et al 1983). For this reason, a tumour of the femur or knee in a young, active individual is one of the most common indications for limb salvage surgery (Fig. 56.5).

RECONSTRUCTION

Of all procedures performed by the orthopaedic surgeon, joint reconstruction can have the most dramatic impact on the patient's function and satisfaction with life.

Regardless of the initial insult (trauma, rheumatic disease, osteoarthritis, ligamentous instability, metabolic disorders, neoplasia or infection) the fundamental problem in end-stage joint disease is the erosion or destruction of the articular surfaces. Operative treatment seeks to remedy this problem by accomplishing one or more of the following.

1. Eliminating the contact between the two damaged joint surfaces. Excisional arthroplasty and interpositional arthroplasty are techniques used to either remove the damaged joint surfaces or place tissue between them to reduce contact.
2. Transferring contact from the damaged articular surface to areas of healthy cartilage. Osteotomies alter joint contact by changing the alignment of the limb or the orientation of the joint surfaces.
3. Replacing the joint surfaces. Total joint arthroplasty can be performed in virtually any joint of the appendicular skeleton, but has had its most profound effect on the treatment of disorders of the hip, knee and shoulder.

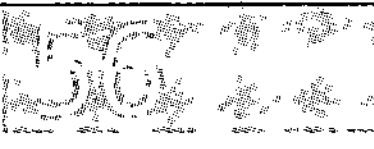

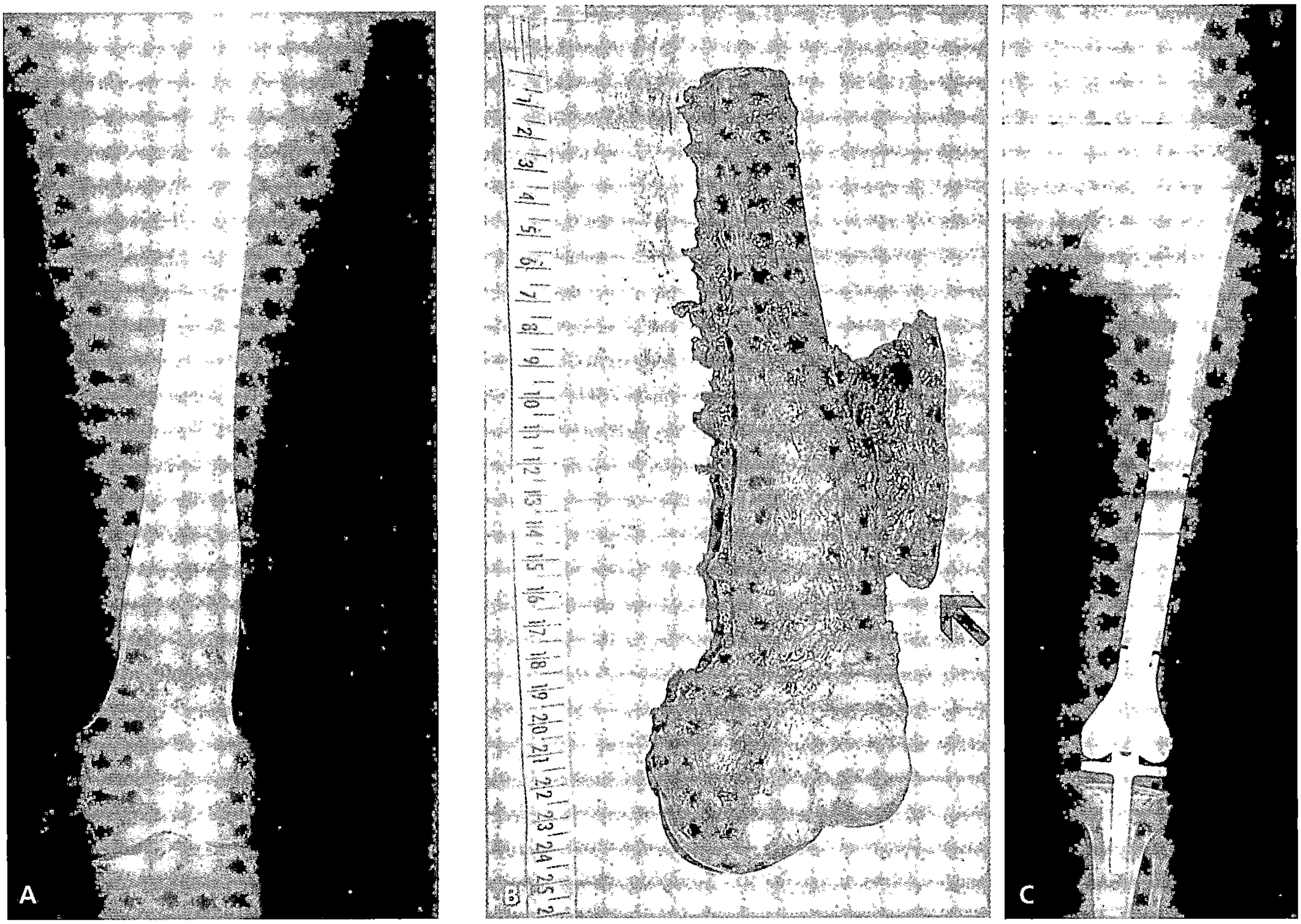

Fig. 56.5 Limb salvage surgery. **A** Grade I chondrosarcoma of the distal femur in a 40-year-old man; the tumour is confined to the medullary canal but has extended well up the shaft. The prognosis for this lesion, which has a tendency to recur locally, is good if local control can be obtained. Traditional treatment would have been a high thigh amputation. **B** Resection of the tumour involves removal of the entire distal femur, with a suitable margin of normal bone at the proximal end. The biopsy tract has also been excised en bloc with the specimen to limit the chances of local recurrence (arrow). **C** A custom endoprosthesis was implanted to salvage the limb. This prosthesis has a long proximal stem which is cemented into the amputated end of the femur and an artificial knee joint which replaces both the femoral and tibial side of the articulation. Pain relief is excellent with this implant and the patient has near-normal function despite the wide resection of this tumour.

Excisional arthroplasty

One of the earliest forms of joint reconstruction was the excisional arthroplasty, performed by excising the joint surfaces and surrounding bone and allowing a pseudarthrosis to form which might allow reasonable motion and function with tolerable pain. This procedure is still used, primarily in patients who cannot tolerate a total joint arthroplasty or in joints unsuitable for that procedure.

The Girdlestone excision of the hip remains a viable option for the treatment of hip fractures or infections in elderly or feeble patients whose primary goal is to be able to sit or transfer comfortably (Girdlestone 1943). It may be the only option in patients with infections of the hip joint or those who have failed previous total joint arthroplasty. The cost to the patient is significant shortening of the limb and instability; patients are able to walk on a Girdlestone hip, but usually have a significant limp and require some assistive device. The quality of the outcome depends on the formation of a tough scar around the proximal end of the femur. Prolonged traction and bracing may be required to allow that scar to mature between the femur and acetabulum, providing enough stability to walk on. Girdlestone patients treated for infection appear to have somewhat better results than those treated for fracture or degenerative disease and it is thought that the presence of infection, by producing a more intense scarring response, may actually lead to a stronger pseudarthrosis (Parr et al 1971). Nonetheless, few patients are very satisfied with the long-term results of resection arthroplasty (Petty & Goldsmith 1980).

Interpositional arthroplasty

Soft tissue arthroplasties are performed by interposing adjoining soft tissues between the joint's ends to provide a resilient, biologically active gliding surface where the original articular surface has been worn away. Interposition of deep fascia has been tried in large weight-bearing joints, such as the hip, with limited success and has largely been abandoned in favour of fusion or joint replacement. In smaller joints, however, fascial interposition remains a successful operation, providing excellent symptomatic relief and good function in the joints of the elbow, wrist and thumb (Smith-Peterson et al 1943, Froimson 1970, Beckenbaugh & Linscheid 1982).

Osteotomy

Osteotomy is a commonly applied procedure in orthopaedics and is primarily used in one of two scenarios: cases in which deformity or malalignment result in poor function and predispose to early joint degeneration, and cases in which degenerative disease has damaged one area of weight-bearing cartilage while sparing the rest. Congenital and acquired deformities of the lower extremity (Blount's disease, congenital coxa vara, rickets) may sufficiently derange the weight-bearing axis of the limb so as to assure progressive deformity and early joint destruction (Langenskiold & Riska 1964, Schoenecker et al 1985). In these patients, corrective osteotomies, performed at the right age, may restore alignment, height and function, with relatively little risk (Deitz & Weinstein 1988). In children with congenital dislocation of the hip, osteotomy may be necessary to correct the rotational deformity of the proximal femur and to allow reduction of the coxa-femoral joint without applying excessive pressure to the femoral head.

Osteotomies are sometimes needed for post-traumatic malunion, particularly when the deformity is in a plane other than that of the joint's motion. Injuries resulting in a varus or valgus deformity of the lower extremity force the weight-bearing joints to be loaded eccentrically, causing pain and early joint destruction. Corrective osteotomies are designed to return the limb to its natural alignment and restore normal joint mechanics. For instance, malunion of a distal radius fracture (Colles' fracture) can be satisfactorily corrected with a distal radius osteotomy to restore joint alignment and stability, grip strength and pain-free function (Fernandez 1988) (Fig. 56.6).

Proximal tibial osteotomy (Fig. 56.7) remains the most successful operation for osteoarthritis of the knee, short of joint replacement (Jackson & Waugh 1961). In younger patients with greater functional demands this procedure is the treatment of choice, allowing the patient unrestricted activity without lifting limits or restrictions of sports or recreation. By transferring contact forces from the side of the joint with advanced degenerative disease to the side with residual healthy cartilage, tibial osteotomy may provide the patient with years of unrestricted function before replacement arthroplasty is necessary, which, for many patients, translates to additional years of gainful employment, recreation and fitness (Holden et al 1988). Although results do deteriorate over time, 40% of patients with a high tibial osteotomy remain pain free more than 9 years after their operation (Insall et al 1984). A variety of osteotomies have been described for treatment of disorders of the hip joint, but are no longer commonly used. With consistently excellent results, total hip arthroplasty has largely displaced hip osteotomies as a treatment of osteoarthritis. A proximal femoral osteotomy requires a longer convalescence than a total hip arthroplasty and greater patient compliance is required for success. Also, since the range of motion of the hip is not improved by osteotomy, patients with contractures or limited motion are poor candidates. Nonetheless, in young, active patients at risk for early total joint failure, osteotomies of the hip provide a valuable treatment alternative and may provide definitive correction in 15–20% of cases (Fortune 1990).

Total joint arthroplasty

There are few, if any, operations as successful for managing pain and restoring function as joint replacement arthroplasty. Since Charnley first reported his hip replacement procedure (Charnley 1961b), total joint arthroplasty has become the most frequently performed reconstructive procedure in orthopaedic surgery. Replacement joints are now available for most joints of the extremities and are routinely applied in the treatment of arthrosis of the hip, knee and shoulder. Technical advances now allow the surgeon to choose between cemented and bone ingrowth methods of fixation and modular implants allow the surgeon to customize implants to fit the needs of individual patients. Total hip arthroplasty can provide dramatic and long-lasting pain relief in patients with osteoarthritis, rheumatoid arthritis, avascular necrosis of the femoral head, non-unions of the femoral neck, post-traumatic degenerative disease and a number of other congenital or acquired maladies of the hip joint. Total hip arthroplasty can also be performed in patients with previous fusions or osteotomies and in patients with previous arthroplasties which have loosened. Relative contraindications to arthroplasty include obesity,

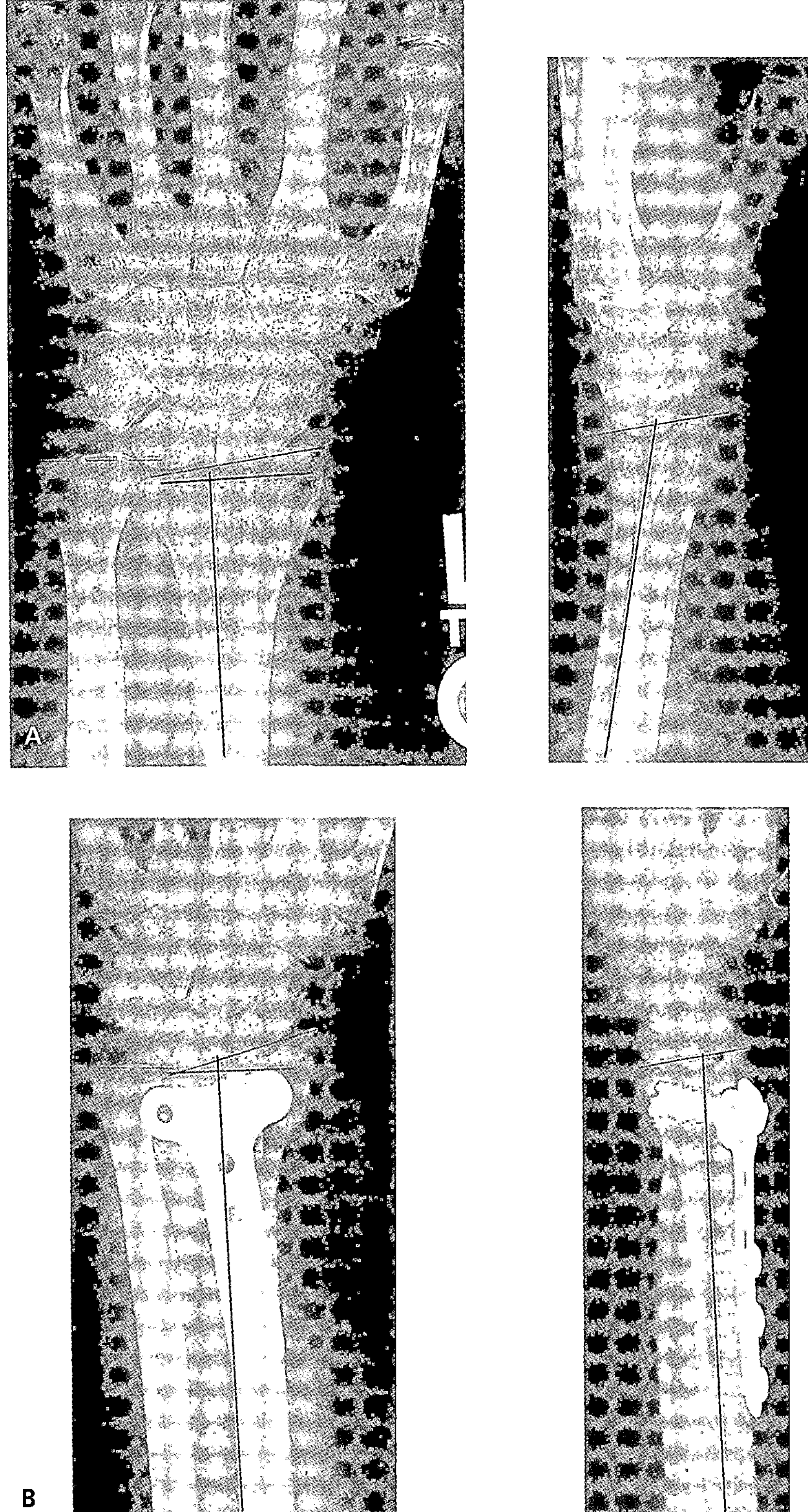

Fig. 56.6 Distal radial osteotomy. **A** AP and lateral views show malunion of wrist. Note on the AP view that radial inclination is reduced to 5° (normal, 20–25°) and that the radius is considerably shortened relative to the ulna. On the lateral view, the wrist is ***dorsally*** angulated 18°, compared to a normal ***palmar*** tilt of 10–25°, resulting in derangement of the radiocarpal articulation. This patient has chronic pain, weakness and a predisposition to severe degenerative disease. **B** A distal radial osteotomy was performed using an iliac crest bone graft to restore the normal orientation of the radiocarpal joint. Following the corrective osteotomy, the radial inclination is improved and length restored. The normal volar tilt has also been restored.

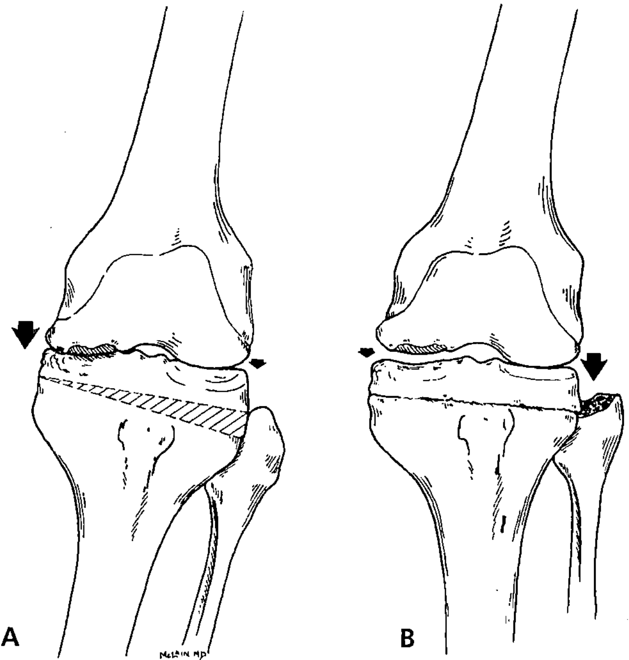

Fig. 56.7 Proximal tibial osteotomy. Osteotomy to correct deformity of the knee and reduce stress on a joint compartment with severe arthritis is an effective and commonly used operation. **A** Patients with severe medial compartment osteoarthritis develop genu valgum, which result in a progressive shift of loads onto the injured side (large arrow). As weight is shifted to the diseased compartment, the healthy cartilage in the lateral compartment sees less load and remains intact. A corrective osteotomy performed through the cancellous bone of the proximal tibia (cross-hatched area) corrects the valgus deformity, shifting weight away from the damaged medial cartilage and on to the healthy lateral cartilage. **B** By restoring the normal alignment of the knee, ligament and muscle stresses are normalized. An osteotomy performed through the vascular cancellous bone of the tibial metaphysis heals reliably.

youth, high functional demands and active or chronic infection in the joint (Salvati et al 1991). The use of bone ingrowth (cementless) prostheses promises improved success even in these difficult patients.

Although modern implants are the product of significant technological evolution, the basic concept behind the original plastic and metal prosthesis of Charnley still pertains: a small-diameter, polished metal head, mounted on a femoral stem, articulates with a metal-backed high-density polyethylene socket embedded in the acetabulum, with both components fixed so as to restore anatomical alignment and range of motion (Fig. 56.8). Because the longevity of the device is determined, in part, by the positioning and fixation of the components, attention to surgical technique is critical to the survival of the implant and the duration of symptomatic relief. Failure of the arthroplasty usually occurs because of loosening or infection or a combination of the two. The earliest symptom of failure is recurrence of groin or thigh pain, usually worse with weight bearing, which may appear before any radiographic evidence of loosening can be detected.

In performing a total hip arthroplasty, the hip joint may be exposed through one of several surgical approaches. The capsule of the joint is excised and the femoral head dislocated from the acetabulum. The femoral neck is transected and the femoral head discarded. The acetabulum is prepared by removing the remaining articular cartilage and any medial osteophytes with a domed reamer, and the femoral shaft by the insertion of a broach contoured to match the femoral implant being used. The implant is then inserted and either fixed in place with polymethylmethacrylate (PMMA) cement or press-fit in the case of bone ingrowth components. The patient is usually out of bed on the first postoperative day and ambulating independently within the week. In patients with severe degenerative disease pain relief is often immediate and range of motion improved. Although long-term results are not yet available for cementless prostheses, cemented prostheses have provided good to excellent results in the majority of patients in long-term follow-up studies (Charnley & Cupic 1973). A review of Charnley low-friction arthroplasties at 15–21-year follow-up showed that less than 4% had become painful, 11% produced occasional discomfort and 85% were still functioning painlessly (Wroblewski 1986). McCoy et al (1988) reported good to excellent results in 88% of Charnley hips followed for 15 years or more. Improvements in cement technique promise even greater longevity for the hips currently being implanted (Harris & McGann 1986, Russoti et al 1988).

Total knee arthroplasty has enjoyed a similar rise in popularity as component design has evolved and implant technology has been refined; the clinical success of knee arthroplasty now equals or exceeds that of total hip arthroplasty with respect to pain relief, functional restoration and survival of the implant at 10 years (Insall et al 1983, Ewald et al 1984). Modern implant designs simulate the geometry of the normal knee, providing eccentric femoral condylar surfaces, broad, non-conforming tibial surfaces of high-density polyethylene and a replacement surface for the patella. Failure to replace the patellar surface was a source of clinical failure in the past, while attempts to increase implant stability by constraining the femoral and tibial components led to loosening and mechanical failure. Currently, most knee implants are cemented in place with PMMA, as bone ingrowth implants have proven less reliable in knee surgery than in the hip.

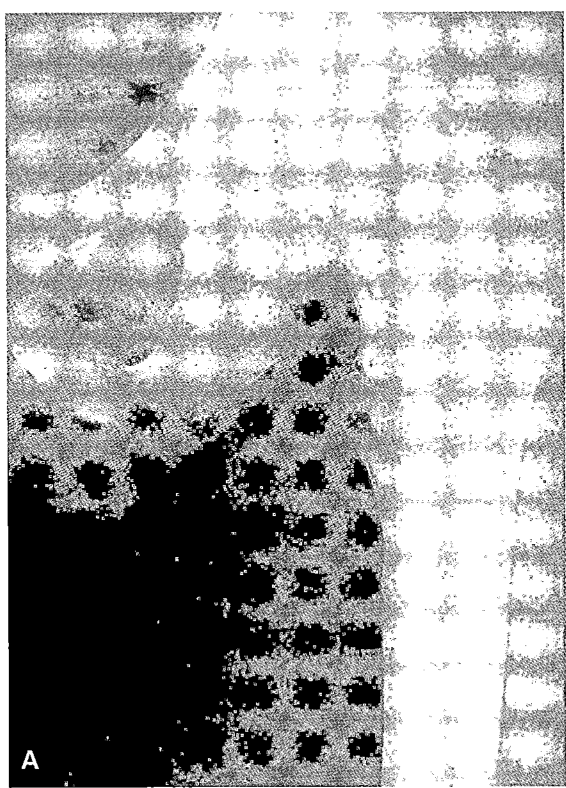

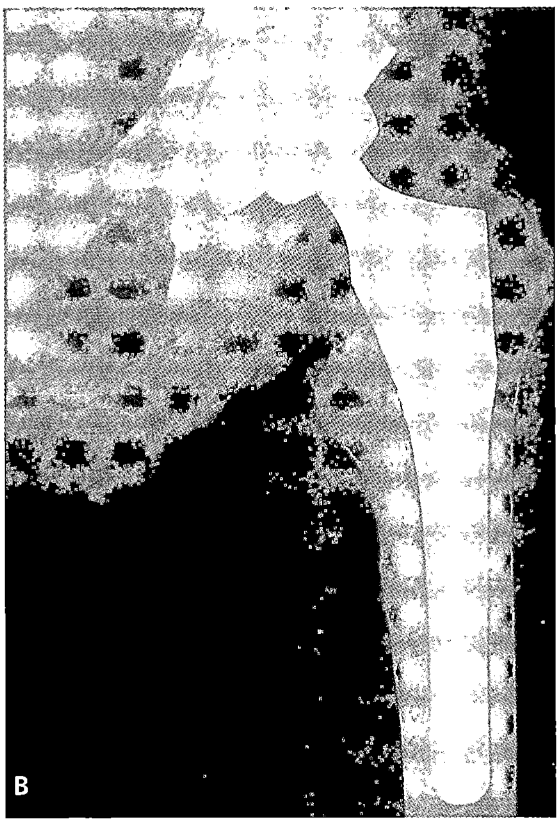

Fig. 56.8 Total hip arthroplasty. **A** AP view of the pelvis, showing severe, unilateral degenerative disease of the hip. Loss of the joint space is apparent, while several signs of DJD (sclerosis of the subchondral bone, formation of subchondral cysts, osteophyte formation) are also seen. **B** A total hip arthroplasty, with a metal-backed acetabular cup and an uncemented femoral component. Pain relief is reliably excellent.

SUMMARY

The orthopaedic surgeon has a wide variety of techniques and a vast array of technology available for the treatment of musculoskeletal disorders. The rational treatment of musculoskeletal problems requires that the surgeon match the treatment to the disease and that options be tried in the order of their invasiveness and potential risk. Likewise, the natural history of the disorder must be considered in order to weigh the risks of intervention against those of observation and supportive therapy. As many interventions provide only transient pain relief, the patient may require a series of procedures over the course of his or her lifetime and the physician must use good judgement early on to avoid 'burning bridges' with respect to later procedures. The majority of patients will be well cared for with a judicious combination of medical management and an occasional surgical intervention, well timed and tailored to the patient's needs. The injudicious application of technology to orthopaedic problems can lead to unmanageable problems in later life; cementing a total hip implant into a young, non-compliant patient is bound to lead to early failure, repeated revisions and, in the end, an excisional arthroplasty before the patient reaches middle age. On the other hand, a patient with a traumatic injury to the knee might undergo an acute ligament or meniscal repair as a young man, arthroscopic debridement or synovectomy to control symptoms in middle age, a high tibial osteotomy for unicompartmental degenerative disease at 50, a hemiarthroplasty at 60 and a total condylar knee replacement at the age of 70, at which time that arthroplasty could be expected to provide excellent function for another 15–20 years. The goal of such a treatment hierarchy, as aggressive as it may appear, is to keep the patient functioning at the highest possible level throughout his life, with a minimal or acceptable level of pain; such a patient is pleased with his care and an asset to his family and community rather than a burden. Regardless of the nature of the disorder, the orthopaedist's challenge is to maintain the patient as an independent, productive member of society, capable of enjoying and participating in life; if this can be accomplished both the physician and the patient will be well satisfied.

Despite the great advances made over past decades in the diagnosis and treatment of most common orthopaedic disorders, the source of musculoskeletal pain is often an enigma to the treating physician. With proper education, appropriate expectations and a comprehensive approach to orthopaedic disease and pain management, the majority of our patients can expect successful outcomes. Still, in many cases, residual pain must be expected and dealt with. It is only through a better understanding of pain itself – the pathophysiology, neurochemistry, anatomy and psychology of pain – that we as treating physicians can continue to offer our patients more efficacious and responsible therapy. We hope this chapter has effectively touched on many of the common orthopaedic disorders that produce musculoskeletal pain and has provided some insight into the current principles of orthopaedic management.

REFERENCES

Abbott LC, Saunders JB de CM, Bost FC 1942 Arthrodesis of the wrist with the use of grafts of cancellous bone. Journal of Bone and Joint Surgery 24: 883–898

Arthritis Foundation Committee on Evaluation of Synovectomy 1977 Multicenter evaluation of synovectomy in the treatment of rheumatoid arthritis. Report of results at the end of three years. Arthritis and Rheumatology 20: 765–771

Badalamente MA, Dee R, Ghillani R, Chien PF, Daniels K 1987 Mechanical stimulation of dorsal root ganglia induces increased production of substance P: a mechanism of pain following nerve root compromise? Spine 12: 552–555

Beckenbaugh RD, Linscheid RL 1982 Arthroplasty in the hand and wrist. In: Green DP (ed) Operative hand surgery. Churchill Livingstone, New York, pp 141–184

Bjurholm A, Kreicbergs A, Brodin E, Schultzberg M 1988a Substance P and CGRP immunoreactive nerves in bone. Peptides 9: 165–171

Bjurholm A, Kreicbergs A, Terenius L, Goldstein M, Schultzberg M 1988b Neuropeptide Y-, tyrosine hydroxylase-, and vasoactive intestinal peptide-immunoreactive nerves in bone and surrounding tissues. Journal of the Autonomic Nervous System 25: 119–125

Callaghan JJ, Brand RA, Petersen DR 1985 Hip arthrodesis. Journal of Bone and Joint Surgery 67A: 1328–1335

Caudle RJ, Stern PJ 1987 Severe open fractures of the tibia. Journal of Bone and Joint Surgery 69A: 801–807

Chapman MW 1989 Orthopaedic management of the multiply injured patient. In: Evarts CM (ed) Surgery of the musculoskeletal system, 2nd edn. Churchill Livingstone, New York, pp 19–35

Chapman MW, Mahoney M 1979 The role of early internal fixation in the management of open fractures. Clinical Orthopaedics and Related Research 138: 120–131

Charnley J 1961a The closed treatment of common fractures. Churchill Livingstone, Edinburgh, pp 1–67

Charnley J 1961b Arthroplasty of the hip. Lancet 1: 1129–1132

Charnley J, Cupic Z 1973 The nine and ten year results of the low-friction arthroplasty of the hip. Clinical Orthopaedics and Related Research 95: 9–25

Cierny G, Byrd HS, Jones RE 1983 Primary versus delayed soft tissue coverage for severe open tibial fractures. A comparison of results. Clinical Orthopaedics and Related Research 178: 54–63

Colpaert FC, Donnerer J, Lembeck F 1983 Effects of capsaicin on inflammation and on the substance P content of nervous tissues in rats with adjuvant arthritis. Life Sciences 32: 1827–1834

Colton CL 1992 The history of fracture treatment. In: Browner BD, Jupiter JB, Levine AM, Trafton PG (eds) Skeletal trauma. WB Saunders, Philadelphia, pp 3–30

Cooper RR 1968 Nerves in cortical bone. Science 160: 327–328

Dandy DJ, Jackson RW 1975 The diagnosis of problems after meniscectomy. Journal of Bone and Joint Surgery 57B: 349–352

Deandrade JR, Grant C, Dixon A 1965 Joint distension and reflex muscle inhibition in the knee. Journal of Bone and Joint Surgery 47A: 313–332

De Avila GA, O'Connor BL, Visco DM, Sisk TD 1989 The mechanoreceptor innervation of the human fibular collateral ligament. Journal of Anatomy 162: 1–7

Dee RM 1978 The innervation of joints. In: Sokoloff L (ed) Joints and synovial fluid. Academic Press, New York

Dietz FR, Weinstein SL 1988 Spike osteotomy for angular deformities of the long bones Journal of Bone and Joint Surgery 70A: 848–852

Ecker MD, Jacobs BS 1970 Lower extremity amputations in diabetic patients. Diabetes 19: 189–195

Eckholm J, Eklund G, Skoglund S 1960 On the reflex effects from the knee joint of the cat. Acta Physiologica Scandinavica 50: 167–174

Ewald FC, Jacobs MA, Miegel RE, Walker PS, Poss R, Sledge CB 1984 Kinematic total knee replacement. Journal of Bone and Joint Surgery 66A: 1032–1040

Fernandez DL 1988 Radial osteotomy and Bowers arthroplasty for malunited fractures of the distal end of the radius. Journal of Bone and Joint Surgery 70A: 1538–1551

Fortune WP 1990 Hip osteotomies. In: Evarts CM (ed) Surgery of the musculoskeletal system, vol 3. Churchill Livingstone, New York, pp 2795–2832

Freeman MAR, Wyke BD 1967 The innervation of the knee joint. An anatomical and histological study in the cat. Journal of Anatomy 101: 505–532

Froimson AI 1970 Tendon arthroplasty of the trapeziometacarpal joint. Clinical Orthopaedics and Related Research 70: 191–199

Fuller RW, Conradson TB, Dixon CMS, Crossman DC, Barnes PJ 1987 Sensory neuropeptide effects in human skin. British Journal of Pharmacology 92: 781–788

Gardner E 1944 The distribution and termination of nerves in the knee joint of the cat. Journal of Comparative Neurology 80: 11–32

Gardner E 1948 The innervation of the knee joint. Anatomical Record 101: 109–130

Giles LGF, Harvey AR 1987 Immunohistochemical demonstration of nociceptors in the capsule and synovial folds of human zygapophyseal joints. British Journal of Rheumatology 26: 362–364

Girdlestone GR 1943 Acute pyogenic arthritis of the hip. An operation giving free access and effective drainage. Lancet 1: 419–421

Glatty H 1964 A statistical study of 12 000 new amputees. Southern Medical Journal 57: 1373–1378

Grigg P, Hoffman AH, Fogarty KE 1982 Properties of Golgi–Mazzoni afferents in cat knee joint capsule as revealed by mechanical studies in isolated joint capsule. Journal of Neurophysiology 47: 31–40

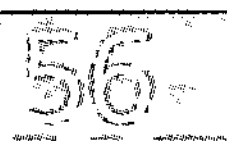

Grigg P, Schaible HG, Schmidt RF 1986 Mechanical sensitivity of group III and IV afferents from posterior articular nerve in normal and inflammed cat knee. Journal of Neurophysiology 55: 635–643

Gronblad M, Liesi P, Korkala O, Karaharju E, Polak J 1984 Innervation of human bone periosteum by peptidergic nerves. Anatomical Record 209: 297–299

Gronblad M, Konttinen Y, Korkala O, Liesi P, Hukkanen M, Polak J 1988 Neuropeptides in synovium of patients with rheumatoid arthritis and osteoarthritis. Journal of Rheumatology 15: 1807–1810

Gronblad M, Weinstein JN, Santavirta S 1991 Immunohistochemical observations on spinal tissue innervation. Acta Orthopaedica Scandinavica 62: 614

Haddad RJ, Riordan DC 1967 Arthrodesis of the wrist. A surgical technique. Journal of Bone and Joint Surgery 49A: 950–954

Hansen ST 1987 The type-IIIC tibial fracture. Salvage or amputation? Journal of Bone and Joint Surgery 69A: 799–800

Harris WH, McGann WA 1986 Loosening of the femoral component after use of the medullary plug cementing technique. Journal of Bone and Joint Surgery 68A: 1064–1066

Heppelmann B, Schaible HG, Schmidt RF 1985 Effects of prostaglandin E1 and E2 on the mechanosensitivity of group III afferents from normal and inflamed cat knee joints. In: Fields HL, Dubner R, Cervero F (eds) Advances in pain research and therapy. Raven Press, New York, pp 91–101

Heppelmann B, Pfeffer A, Schaible HG, Schmidt RF 1986 Effects of acetylsalicylic acid and indomethacin on single group III and IV sensory units from acutely inflamed joints. Pain 26: 337–351

Hill EL, Elde R 1991 Distribution of CGRP-, VIP-, DβH-, SP-, and NPY-immunoreactive nerves in the periosteum of the rat. Cell and Tissue Research 264: 469–480

Holden DL, Stanley LJ, Larson RL, Slocum DB 1988 Proximal tibial osteotomy in patients who are fifty years old or less. Journal of Bone and Joint Surgery 70A: 977–982

Horowitz BG 1966 Retrospective analysis of hip fractures. Surgery, Gynecology and Obstetrics 123: 565–570

Insall JN, Hood RW, Flawn LB, Sullivan DJ 1983 The total condylar knee prosthesis in gonarthrosis. A five to nine year follow-up of the first one hundred consecutive replacements. Journal of Bone and Joint Surgery 65A: 619–628

Insall JN, Joseph DM, Msika C 1984 High tibial osteotomy for varus gonarthrosis. Journal of Bone and Joint Surgery 66A: 1040–1048

Ishikawa H, Ohno O, Hirohata K 1986 Long-term results of synovectomy in rheumatoid patients. Journal of Bone and Joint Surgery 68A: 198–205

Jackson RW, Rouse DW 1982 The results of partial arthroscopic meniscectomy in patients over 40 years of age. Journal of Bone and Joint Surgery 64B: 481–486

Jackson JP, Waugh W 1961 Tibial osteotomy for osteoarthritis of the knee. Journal of Bone and Joint Surgery 43B: 746–751

Kellgren JH, Samuel EP 1950 Sensitivity and innervation of the articular cartilage. Journal of Bone and Joint Surgery 32B: 84–92

Kennedy JC, Alexander IJ, Hayes KC 1982 Nerve supply of the human knee and its functional importance. American Journal of Sports Medicine 10: 329–335

Kidd BL, Mapp PI, Blake DR, Gibson SJ, Polak JM 1990 Neurogenic influences in arthritis. Annals of the Rheumatic Diseases 49: 649–652

Konttinen Y, Rees R, Hukkanen M et al 1990 Nerves in inflammatory synovium: immunohistochemical observations on the adjuvant arthritic rat model. Journal of Rheumatology 17: 1586–1591

Kumazawa T, Mizumura K 1977 Thin fiber receptors responding to mechanical, chemical and thermal stimulation in the skeletal muscle of the dog. Journal of Physiology 273: 179–194

Küntscher G 1968 The intramedullary nailing of fractures. Clinical Orthopaedics and Related Research 60: 5–12

Lam FY, Ferrell WR 1989 Inhibition of carrageenan-induced inflammation in the rat knee joint. Annals of the Rheumatic Diseases 48: 928–932

Lam FY, Ferrell WR 1991 Neurogenic component of different models of acute inflammation in the rat knee model. Annals of the Rheumatic Diseases 50: 747–751

Lange RH, Bach AW, Hansen ST, Johansen KH 1985 Open tibial fractures with associated vascular injuries. Prognosis for limb salvage. Journal of Trauma 25: 203–208

Langenskiold A, Riska EB 1964 Tibia vara (osteochondrosis deformans tibia). A survey of seventy-one cases. Journal of Bone and Joint Surgery 46A: 1405–1420

Levine JD, Clark R, Devor M, Helms C, Moskowitz M, Basbaum AI 1984 Interneuronal substance P contributes to the severity of experimental arthritis. Science 226: 547–549

Liesi P, Gronblad M, Korkala O, Karaharju E, Rusanen M 1983 Substance P. A neuropeptide involved in low back pain? Lancet 1: 1328–1329

Lundberg JM, Terenius L, Hokfelt T et al 1982 Neuropeptide Y (NPY)-like immunoreactivity in peripheral noradrenergic neurons and effects of NPY on sympathetic function. Acta Physiologica Scandinavica 116: 477–480

Marsh BW, Bonfiglio M, Brady LP, Enneking WF 1975 Benign osteoblastoma: range of manifestations. Journal of Bone and Joint Surgery 57A: 1–9

Masten FA 1975 Compartmental syndrome: a unifying concept. Clinical Orthopaedics and Related Research 113: 8–14

Mazet R 1968 Syme's amputation. A follow-up study of fifty-one adults and thirty-two children. Journal of Bone and Joint Surgery 50A: 1549–1563

McCoy TH, Salvati EA, Ranawat CS 1988 A fifteen year follow-up study of one hundred Charnley low-friction arthroplasties. Orthopedic Clinics of North America 19: 467–476

McLain RF, Weinstein JN 1991 Ultrastructural changes in the dorsal root ganglion associated with whole body vibration. Journal of Spinal Disorders 4: 142–148

McLain RF, Weinstein JN 1992 Nuclear clefting in dorsal root ganglion neurons. A response to whole body vibration. Journal of Comparative Neurology, 322: 538–547

Mense S, Schmidt RF 1977 Muscle pain. Which receptors are responsible for the transmission of noxious stimuli? In: Clifford Rose (ed) Physiological aspects of clinical neurology. Blackwell, Oxford, pp 265–278

Millender LH, Nalebuff EA 1973 Arthrodesis of the rheumatoid wrist. An evaluation of sixty patients and a description of a different surgical technique. Journal of Bone and Joint Surgery 55A: 1026–1034

Miller CW 1978 Survival and ambulation following hip fracture. Journal of Bone and Joint Surgery 60A: 930–934

Montane I, McCollough NC, Lian EC-Y 1986 Synovectomy of the knee for hemophilic arthropathy. Journal of Bone and Joint Surgery 68A: 210–216

Mubarak SJ, Owen CA 1977 Double incision fasciotomy of the leg for decompression of compartment syndromes. Journal of Bone and Joint Surgery 59A: 184–187

Neugebauer V, Schaible HG 1990 Evidence for a central component in the sensitization of spinal neurons with joint input during development of acute arthritis in cat's knee. Journal of Neurophysiology 64: 299–311

Neugebauer V, Schaible HG, Schmidt RF 1989 Sensitization of articular afferents to mechanical stimuli by bradykinin. Pflügers Archiv 415: 330–335

O'Connor BL, Gonzales J 1979 Mechanoreceptors of the medial collateral ligament of the cat knee joint. Journal of Anatomy 129: 719–729

O'Connor BL, McConnaughey JS 1978 The structure and innervation of the cat knee menisci and their relation to a 'sensory hypothesis' of meniscal function. American Journal of Anatomy 153: 431–442

O'Connor RL 1973 The arthroscope in the management of crystal-induced synovitis of the knee. Journal of Bone and Joint Surgery 55A: 1443–1449

O'Connor RL, Shahriaree H 1984 Arthroscopic technique and normal anatomy of the knee. In: Shahriaree H, O'Connor RL (eds) O'Connor's textbook of arthroscopic surgery. JB Lippincott, Philadelphia

Palmer I 1958 Pathophysiology of the medial ligament of the knee joint. Acta Chirurgica Scandinavica 115: 312–318

Parr PL, Croft C, Enneking WF 1971 Resection of the head and neck of the femur with and without angular osteotomy. Journal of Bone and Joint Surgery 53A: 935–944

Pedersen-Bjergaard U, Nielsen LB, Jensen K, Edvinsson L, Jansen I, Olesen J 1989 Algesia and local responses induced by neurokinin A and substance P in human skin and temporal muscle. Peptides 10: 1147–1152

Pedersen-Bjergaard U, Nielsen LB, Jensen K, Edvinsson L, Jansen I, Olesen J 1991 Calcitonin gene-related peptide, neurokinin A, and substance P. Effects on nociception and neurogenic inflammation in human skin and temporal muscle. Peptides 12: 333–337

Petty W, Goldsmith S 1980 Resection arthroplasty following infected total hip arthoplasty. Journal of Bone and Joint Surgery 62A: 889–896

Piotrowski W, Foreman JC 1986 Some effects of calcitonin gene-related peptide in human skin and on histamine release. British Journal of Dermatology 114: 37–46

Ralston HJ, Miller MR, Kasahara M 1960 Nerve endings in human fasciae, tendons, ligaments, periosteum, and joint synovial membrane. Anatomical Record 136: 137–148

Rao JP, Banzon MT, Weiss AB, Raychack J 1983 Treatment of unstable intertrochanteric fractures with anatomic reduction and compression hip screw fixation. Clinical Orthopaedics and Related Research 175: 65–71

Russoti GM, Coventry MB, Stauffer RN 1988 Cemented total hip arthroplasty with contemporary techniques. A five-year minimum follow-up study. Clinical Orthopaedics and Related Research 235: 141–147

Said SI, Mutt V 1970 Polypeptide with broad biological activity isolation from small intestine. Science 169: 1217–1218

Salvati EA, Huo MH, Buly RL 1991 Cemented total hip replacement: long-term results and future outlook. In: Tullos HS (ed) Instructional course lectures, vol XL. AAOS, pp 121–134

Schaible HG, Schmidt RF 1985 Effects of an experimental arthritis on the sensory properties of fine articular afferent nerves. Journal of Physiology 54: 1109–1122

Schaible HG, Schmidt RF, Willis WD 1987 Spinal mechanisms in arthritis pain. In: Schaible HG, Schmidt RF, Vahle-Hinz C (eds) Fine afferent nerve fibers and pain. VCH Publishers, Weinheim, pp 399–409

Schoenecker PL, Meade WC, Pierron RL, Sheridan JJ, Capelli AM 1985 Blount's disease. A retrospective review and recommendations for treatment. Journal of Pediatric Orthopedics 5: 181–186

Sherman MS, McFarland G 1965 Mechanism of pain in osteoid osteomas. Southern Medical Journal 58: 163

Skofitsch G, Jacobowitz DM 1985 Calcitonin gene-related peptide co-exists with substance P in capsaicin sensitive neurons and sensory ganglia of the rat. Peptides 6: 747–754

Smith GM, Egbert LD, Markowitz RA, Mosteller F, Beecher HK 1966 An experimental pain method sensitive to morphine in man. The submaximal effort tourniquet technique. Journal of Pharmacology and Experimental Therapeutics 154: 324–332

Smith-Peterson MN, Cave EF, Vangorder GW 1931 Intracapsular fractures of the femoral neck – treatment by internal fixation. Archives of Surgery 23: 715–759

Smith-Peterson MN, Aufranc OE, Larson CB 1943 Useful surgical procedures for rheumatoid arthritis involving joints of the upper extremity. Archives of Surgery 46: 764–770

Sponseller PD, McBeath AA, Perpich M 1984 Hip arthrodesis in young patients. A long-term follow-up study. Journal of Bone and Joint Surgery 66A: 853–859

Steindler A 1918 Orthopaedic operations on the hand. Journal of the American Medical Association 71: 1288–1291

Steindler A 1921 Operative methods and end-results of disabilities of the shoulder and arm. Journal of Orthopaedic Surgery 3: 652–658

Sternbach RA, Murphy RW, Zimmermans G, Greenhoot JH, Akeson WH 1974 Measuring the severity of clinical pain. In: Bonica JJ (ed) Advances in neurology, vol 4. Raven Press, New York

Volpicelli LJ, Chambers RB, Wagner FW 1983 Ambulation levels of bilateral lower extremity amputees. Journal of Bone and Joint Surgery 65A: 599–604

Wagner FW Jr 1986 Amputations of the foot. In: Chapman MW (ed) Operative orthopaedics. JB Lippincott, Philadelphia, pp 1777–1797

Watson HK, Hempton RF 1980 Limited wrist arthrodeses I: the triscaphoid joint. Journal of Hand Surgery 5: 320–327

Weinstein JN 1986 Mechanisms of spinal pain. The dorsal root ganglion and its role as a mediator of low-back pain. Spine 11: 999–1001

Weinstein JN 1988 New perspectives on low back pain. Workshop at Airlie, Virginia, supported by the AAOS/NIH/NASS. AAOS, pp 35–130

Weinstein JN 1991 Anatomy and neurophysiologic mechanisms of spinal pain. In: Frymoyer JW (ed) The adult spine: principles and practice. Raven Press, New York, Ch 30

Weinstein JN 1992 The role of neurogenic and non neurogenic mediators as they relate to pain and the development of osteoarthritis. A clinical review. Spine 17: S356–S361

Weinstein JN, Claverie J, Gibson S 1988a The pain of discography. Spine 13: 1444–1448

Weinstein JN, Pope M, Schmidt R, Serroussi R 1988b Neuropharmacological effects of vibration on the dorsal root ganglion. An animal model. Spine 13: 521–525

Wilkinson MC 1969 Tuberculosis of the hip and knee treated by chemotherapy, synovectomy, and debridement. Journal of Bone and Joint Surgery 51A: 1343–1359

Winquist RA, Hanson ST 1978 Segmental fractures of the femur treated by closed intramedullary nailing. Journal of Bone and Joint Surgery 60A: 934–993

Wroblewski BM 1986 15–21 year results of the Charnley low-friction arthroplasty. Clinical Orthopaedics and Related Research 211: 30–35

Wyke B 1972 Articular neurology – a review. Physiotherapy 58: 94–99

Wyke B 1981 The neurology of joints. A review of general principles. Clinics in Rheumatology 7: 233–239

Yaksh TL 1988 Substance P release from knee joint afferent terminals: modulation by opioids. Brain Research 458: 319–324

Yamashita T, Cavanaugh JM, El-Bohy A, Getchell TV, King AI 1990 Mechanosensitive afferent units in the lumbar facet joint. Journal of Bone and Joint Surgery 72A: 865–870

Central neurosurgery

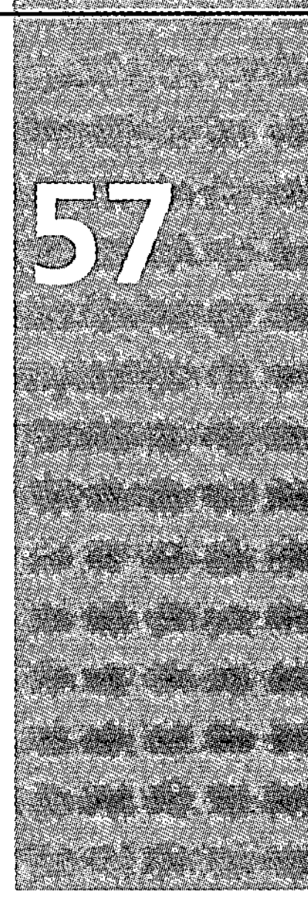

JAN M. GYBELS & RON R. TASKER

INTRODUCTION

It is now 50 years since the birth of stereotactic surgery and 35 years since the first percutaneous cordotomy. Over this time an extensive literature has accumulated dealing with the usefulness of destructive lesions in the central nervous system for the relief of chronic pain. However, much of these data are of questionable value in, firstly, assessing the efficacy of these procedures themselves and, secondly, comparing them with other pain treatment modalities. It is the authors' opinion that it is time for a change in the way we document outcomes for all pain treatment strategies. Not only do we need to answer specific questions – Does destructive surgery for pain relief still have a role? Is the current virtual replacement of such destructive procedures by modulatory and non-surgical strategies preferable? – but also we must look ahead, in a general way.

New techniques are being developed which, with new understandings of pain physiology, will lead to a re-examination of old treatments and, from time to time, development of new ones. We must make it possible to decide if innovations are worth pursuing and to effectively compare different treatment strategies. In short, we must enter the realm of evidence-based practice. Outcome data for surgical and non-surgical treatments alike must be obtained in the following way. The selection of patients for a particular treatment modality must follow an identified and consistent algorithm. All patients in a therapy group should suffer from the same problem and be treated identically with the same length of follow-up. Ideally, randomized crossover or parallel group designed studies should be used and before patients are entered into these streams, narcotic management must be standardized. To collect meaningful data concerning success of any form of treatment, multiple assessments are necessary, preferably done by a disinterested, ideally blinded, third party using semiquantitative measures over a prolonged period of time. In addition to the simple rating by the patient of his level of pain, drug intake, lifestyle, quality of life and physical and work capabilities must be taken into account along with cost–benefit analyses, including review of complications. And every effort should be made to incorporate the resulting outcome data into a consensus conference such as that published by North and Levy (1994). Only with these guidelines can two different therapies, or the same therapy applied in different centres, be compared.

When it is obvious that the outcome statistics of a given study are favourable and a consensus can be reached to that effect, the healthcare community should support that treatment; in the reverse situation, it should not do so. When a given outcome statistic, favourable or otherwise, disagrees with current consensus or is derived from a new approach, the procedure must be carefully re-examined in multiple centres using standardized techniques and the treatment supported or withheld only after consensus has been reached. Only then will we be in a position to intelligently advise patients concerning choice of treatment with the decision to replace one treatment with another.

In the course of this chapter we will address the various destructive procedures performed on the spinal cord and brain for the relief of chronic pain, citing available outcome data. With few exceptions, these will not have been obtained using the criteria outlined above; we will be forced to make do with what data we have in defining the overall usefulness of each procedure. It is currently difficult to find accurate outcome statistics for pain surgery with which to guide patients (Gybels 1991a,b). There is no generally agreed method for measuring pain, the need for which is all the more important because pain surgery may reduce but rarely abolish a patient's pain. Pain gradually recurs after surgery (Tasker 1994) so that outcome is linked to the length of follow-up which is variable across reported series or else not adequately defined. The pathophysiology of different pain syndromes varies, each requiring a specific surgical procedure. In some patients the pathophysiology may be unclear and in some reported series it may be variable or undefined. No one procedure can be successful in multiple pain syndromes so that meaningful outcome statistics for a particular procedure can only be obtained if all the patients in a reported series have pain with the same pathophysiology and undergo the same procedure. Finally, patient selection must be uniform; exclusion of subjects from the final outcome statistics based upon some particular diagnostic test needs to be uniform.

EXPECTATIONS OF PAIN SURGERY

As understanding of physiological neuroanatomy advanced, the expectation began to be realized of abolishing chronic pain by suitable functional neurosurgical procedures aimed at manipulating the somatosensory pathways carrying pain signals through the central nervous system (Willis 1985). Unfortunately, despite the fact that destructive and, later, modulating strategies were aimed at the peripheral and central nervous system (see Chapters 51 and 56), dramatic success in relieving chronic pain still eludes the surgeon, as it does the practitioner of more conservative therapy (Tasker 1994). The initial success rate of surgical procedures used to relieve pain is often limited and pain recurs steadily through the postoperative years. For example, in the University of Washington experience with the treatment of tic douloureux (Loeser 1994), the chronic pain syndrome for which the most successful treatment is available, 80% of patients enjoyed pain relief 1 year after radiofrequency coagulation, 50% at 5 years; after microvascular decompression 85% were painfree after 1 year, 80% after 5 years, while after 15 years tic had recurred in half the patients in the study.

Failure of pain surgery depends on multiple factors implicating the surgeon, his technique, the patient, the patient's disease and the nervous system (Tasker 1994). Some patients are not appropriate candidates for any neurosurgical procedure by virtue of multiple factors. Most pain operations are designed to correct a particular pathophysiological process causing pain. The wrong procedure may be chosen for the pathophysiology at hand through lack of knowledge by the scientific community at large or by the particular treatment team. Or else the procedure may be performed suboptimally. On the other hand, once pain is relieved it may recur by virtue of the placebo effect or by progress of the disease causing the pain, producing new pain syndromes not present at the time of the original surgery. An example is a cancer patient who originally suffered from nociceptive pain down a leg caused by neural compression. As disease progresses it actually destroys the lumbosacral plexus to produce neuropathic pain (Tasker 1987). And pain may be produced by the very surgery done to relieve pain, as is the case with postcordotomy dysaesthesia or iatrogenic anaesthesia dolorosa. Finally, pain may recur through rearrangement in the nervous system through neuroplasticity or regeneration.

Expectations for any surgical procedure advocated for the relief of chronic pain must be realistic. Each patient has an individual tolerance for balancing the relatively low success rate of pain surgery and the inevitability of pain recurrence over time against the magnitude and likely complications of the procedure.

Destructive procedures were originally aimed at interrupting somatosensory pathways thought to transmit pain signals from a particular bodily part, traditionally considered to include the somatotopographically specific spinothalamic tract and the somatotopographically nonspecific spinoreticulothalamic pathway discussed in Section 1 of this book. These lesional procedures, though once popular, are now seldom performed in most neurosurgical centres for a variety of reasons. The limited initial success rate and propensity for recurrence with time discourage patients and surgeons alike from embarking on a complex procedure and from accepting its risks. The increasing role of comprehensive pain clinics has spread decision making about therapeutic strategies amongst a wide spectrum of healthcare professionals other than neurosurgeons. The growth of interest in chronic infusion of morphine by whatever route, discussed in Chapter 48, has probably had the greatest influence of all in steering patients away from destructive neurosurgical procedures but careful studies have not been done to establish its long-term efficacy, particularly in non-cancerous disease, and to compare its cost effectiveness with other means of treatment.

INDICATIONS

Neurosurgical procedures to treat pain should be considered only after more conservative measures have failed. The simplest, least invasive, appropriate procedure should then be considered first and only when there are no absolute contraindications to surgery such as a bleeding diathesis or illness so terminal that surgery is impractical. The diagnosis should be known and the pathophysiology of the pain understood to allow tailoring of the procedure to the patient's needs.

Gybels (1991) has attempted to draw up guidelines for the selection of procedures for the relief of cancer pain based on the expected length of the patient's survival. He felt that if life expectancy was 1–2 months, cerebrospinal fluid opiate infusions and percutaneous neurolytic procedures were in order. If survival was anticipated to be 2–5 months and the above methods failed, cordotomy or other destructive procedures could be considered. For patients likely to survive over 5 months periventricular grey stimulation could also be done. Hassenbusch (1995) felt that severity of pain, expected survival time, the presence of focal versus diffuse pain and the preference for ablative or modulatory options were important factors in decision making. Simple ablative or neuroaugmentative techniques were feasible in patients with a longer life expectancy; more complex destructive procedures could be considered if these strategies failed. He felt that there were no generally accepted guidelines for treating patients with severe pain and short life expectancy.

Sindou and Mertens (1997) offered the algorithm shown in Figure 57.1 for the significant treatment of neuropathic pain which is in general agreement with the principles this chapter will develop. However, the authors are unaware of outcome data for the use of morphine infusions for the treatment of the various neuropathic pain syndromes.

PROCEDURES ON THE SPINAL CORD

CORDOTOMY

Introduction

The concept of a pain pathway in the spinal cord arose from clinical pathological studies of patients with cord lesions (Spiller 1905) and led to the first pain tract section by open means by Spiller and Martin (1912). Open cordotomy, usually done simultaneously bilaterally at T1 and T2, then became a standard operation, particularly for pain caused by cancer. As time went on, Mullan and his colleagues introduced the concept of percutaneous cervical cordotomy using a radiosurgical source (Mullan et al 1963) and later an anodal electrolytic system (Mullan et al 1965), thus sparing sick patients the risks of open operation. Though the controversy (Tasker 1976a, 1977, Poletti 1988) over open versus percutaneous cordotomy continues, the only argument in favour of the former in our opinion is unavailability of a surgeon capable of doing the percutaneous operation. The open procedure does not offer greater accuracy and prevents the physiological corroboration of the target site so easily accomplished with the percutaneous procedure. When it is impossible to rely on patient communication, the percutaneous procedure can be done under general anaesthesia (Izumi et al 1992, Tasker 1995), sacrificing only the patient's description of the effects of stimulation. Congenital or pathological abnormalities (Morley 1953, Voris 1957a,b) that might interfere with or render dangerous the percutaneous procedure have not been a problem in the authors' experience but could account for occasional failure to produce adequate analgesia.

Percutaneous cordotomy was perfected by the contributions of many. Neurolept analgesia made the procedure feasible. Myelography with the image intensifier to identify cord and the location of the spinothalamic tract (Onofrio 1971) and later online CT imaging (Izumi et al 1992, Kanpolat et al 1993, 1995, Fenstermaker et al 1995 advanced it). Intradural impedance monitoring tracked penetration of the cord with a cordotomy electrode (Gildenberg et al 1969) and extradural impedance monitoring and surface stimulation (Meyerson & Von Holst 1990) are also helpful. Detailed physiological corroboration of target site (Taren et al 1969, Taren 1971, Tasker & Organ 1973, Tasker et al 1974) and radiofrequency current for lesion making (Sweet et al 1960, Rosomoff et al 1965) made the procedure precise.

Although three different percutaneous techniques have been described – the high dorsal approach usually in the C1–C2 interspace (Crue et al 1968, Hitchcock 1970) requiring a stereotactic frame (Hitchcock 1969), the free-hand, low anterior cervical approach, usually at C5–6 (Lin et al 1966) and the free-hand high lateral cervical approach at C1–2 or occiput–C1 interspace (Mullan et al 1963) – the latter has been most commonly employed. The advantage of the low cervical approach is that the lesion is made below the level of the ipsilaterally distributed reticulospinal respiratory outflow, avoiding respiratory complications (Nathan 1963, Belmusto et al 1965, Hitchcock & Leece 1967, Mullan & Hosobuchi 1968, Fox 1969). The disadvantages include the lower level of analgesia achieved and the difficulty of making small readjustments in the electrode position since the disc and the cord must first be traversed before entering the spinothalamic tract.

Indications and contraindications

Percutaneous cordotomy should be considered for the relief of pain dependent upon transmission of signals in the

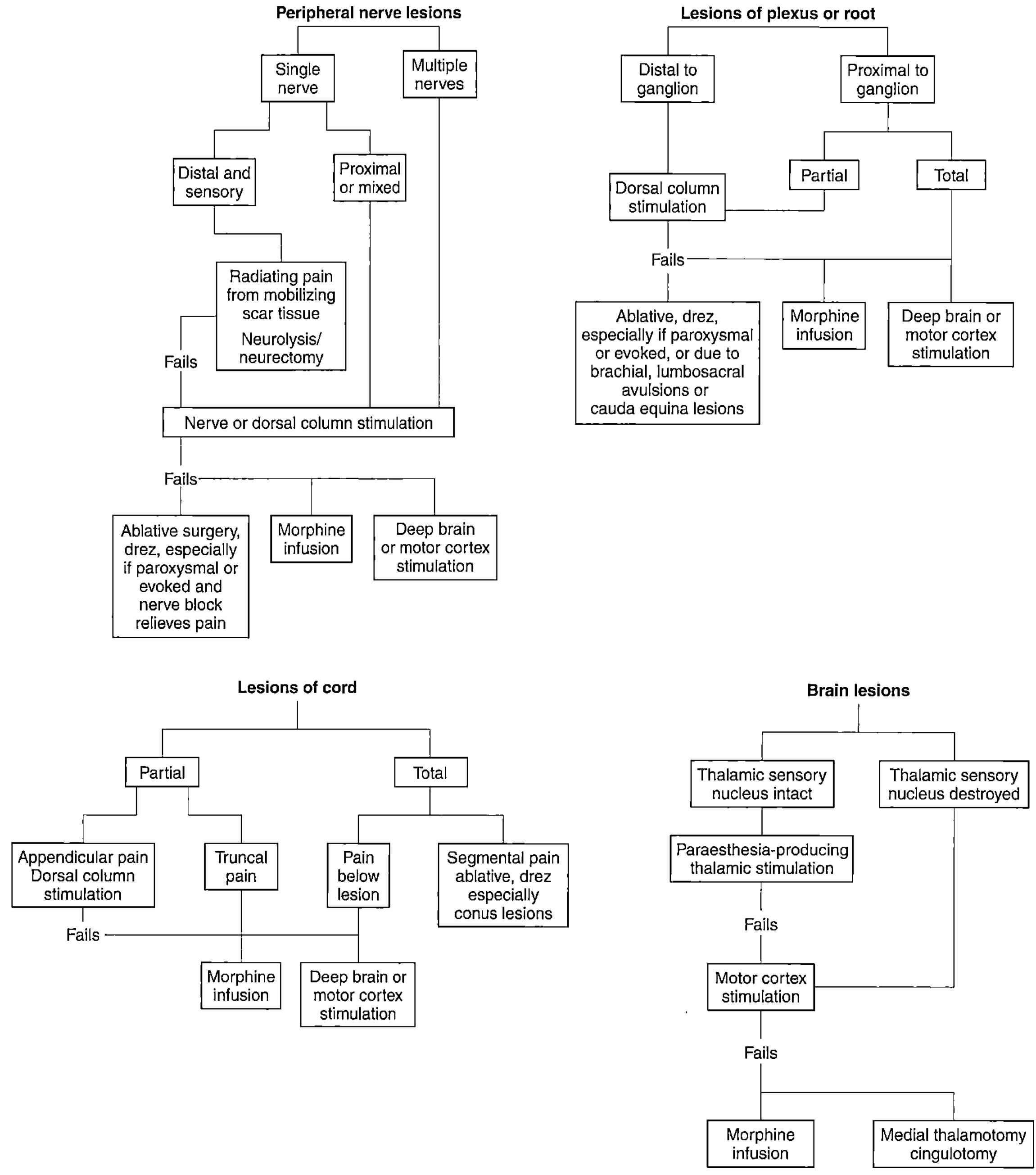

Fig. 57.1 Algorithm for the surgical treatment of neuropathic pain. (Modified from Sindou & Mertens 1997.)

somatotopographically organized spinothalamic tract and possibly the non-somatotopographically organized spinoreticulothalamic tract from below the level of the intervention. The commonest indication has been the relief of pain caused by cancer, particularly through invasion of the lumbosacral plexus by cervical and colorectal disease. In cancer patients midline pelvic and perineal pain responds less well than primarily unilateral leg pain (Meyerson et al 1984), not only because of the need for bilateral intervention but also probably because of the fact that such midline pain may include a major neuropathic element.

It has been traditionally stated that cordotomy is more effective for 'malignant' than 'benign' pain but there is no physiological reason to expect any such difference as long as the pain syndrome is nociceptive. Perhaps the fact that benign pain is often neuropathic in origin and that the commonest type of neuropathic pain is steady burning pain, which in our opinion responds poorly to pain tract section, accounts for this bias (Tasker & Dostrovsky 1989). Additionally, patients with pain not caused by cancer survive longer and pain tends to recur steadily with time after pain surgery.

Somatotopographic level of pain is another limiting factor in the use of cordotomy. It has been mentioned that nociceptive signals must enter the cord below the level of the cordotomy for the procedure to relieve the pain. In fact, since spinothalamic fibres decussate over several dermatomes before entering the spinothalamic tract the highest level of persistently attainable analgesia with percutaneous cordotomy at the C1, C2 level is about C5.

The major contraindications to cordotomy are respiratory. Unconscious breathing, in contradistinction to taking voluntary breaths on command presumably dependent on the corticospinal tract, is maintained by strictly ipsilaterally distributed reticulospinal fibres that lie alongside the cervical fibres of the spinothalamic tract. A cordotomy lesion at the occiput–C1 or C1–2 interspaces that achieves analgesia into the cervical dermatomes is likely to interrupt this pathway, abolishing ipsilateral unconscious respiration whether during sleep or wakefulness. If both lungs are healthy and innervated, such a unilateral lesion is not dangerous, but the patient may suffer respiratory insufficiency if both lungs are diseased or if the lung contralateral to the cordotomy has been rendered ineffective through disease, surgery or diaphragmatic denervation. This latter denervation may be the result of Pancoast's syndrome or cordotomy on the other side.

Indications for cordotomy include a consideration of the pathophysiology of the pain. One would expect relief of nociceptive pain dependent on transmission in pain pathways. Neuropathic pain, on the other hand, may have at least three components (Tasker et al 1980, 1992, Tasker & Dostrovsky 1989): a steady, often dysaesthetic causalgic, a neuralgic and an evoked element, the latter including allodynia and hyperpathia. There is clinical evidence (Tasker and Carvalho 1990, Tasker et al 1992) to suggest that the evoked and neuralgic elements depend upon transmission in pain fibres just as nociceptive pain does. The explanation for the fact that the neuralgic element of neuropathic pain is dependent upon transmission in pain tracts might be that it depends upon ectopic impulse generation at a lesion site in the nervous system discharging into the spinothalamic tract. Allodynia results from garbled programming in the dorsal horn (Woolf 1992) leading to transmission in the spinothalamic tract. Hyperpathia would be expected to implicate the spinothalamic tract as well. Thus, interrupting spinothalamic tract or transecting the spinal cord should relieve neuralgic or evoked but not steady burning dysaesthetic pain in the distribution of damaged sensory fibres even if it is the result of cancer (Tasker 1987) (Table 57.1).

Indications for percutaneous cordotomy in the author's series (Tasker 1995) were: cancer of the cervix (22%), cancer of the rectum (16%), cancer of the colon (10%), cancer of the lung (7%), cancer of the breast (4%), cancer at other sites (29%), central pain caused by cord lesions (7%) and other non-cancerous disorders (5%).

The target of cordotomy

Much has been written about the anatomical site for and the clinical results of satisfactory cordotomy. Mayer et al (1975) related success to the thresholds for inducing pain at the cordotomy lesion site by anterolateral cord stimulation but in our experience such cord stimulation rarely induces pain (Tasker & Organ 1973, Tasker et al 1974). Noordenbos and Wall (1976) felt that section of the cord restricted to the location of the spinothalamic tract resulted in incomplete analgesia; section of the entire anterolateral quadrant was needed for the greatest degree of analgesia which even then was incomplete. Such a lesion resulted in

Table 57.1 Percentage relief of three common components of central pain of cord origin by neurosurgery

Pain type	*Destructive procedures**			*Chronic stimulation***		
	n	Good	Fair	*n*	Good	Fair
Diffuse steady	47	4	22	34	20**	16***
Intermittent neuralgic	27	56	33	11	0	0
Allodynia, hyperpathia	19	58	26	19	0	16

* Cordotomy, DREZ, cordectomy
** Dorsal column, paraesthesiae-producing deep brain stimulation
*** 26% good, 15% fair if complete lesions excluded

inability to evoke pain or cold contralaterally below the lesion and increased touch threshold contralaterally as well. Nathan (1990) reported that adequate cordotomy also abolished itch contralaterally but that it did not affect mechanoreception, graphaesthesia, position or vibration sense; tactile sensibility was rarely affected.

Noordenbos and Wall (1976) concluded that the effective cordotomy divided spinothalamic, spinotectal, spinoreticular and dorsal and ventral spinocerebellar pathways leading to degeneration in nucleus ventralis posterior lateralis, parafascicularis, centralis lateralis, cuneiformis, as well as in periaqueductal grey and lower brainstem reticular nuclei. Lahuerta et al (1990, 1994) carefully documented the sensory deficits incurred by successful cordotomy, implicating both A δ and C fibres though the modalities involved in the sensory loss were rather variable. They concluded that the effective lesion need only encompass the anterolateral funiculus between the level of the dentate ligament and a line drawn perpendicularly from the medial angle of the ventral grey matter or the dorsal horn to the surface of the cord destroying 20% of the hemicord. Such lesions do not necessarily abolish the flexion reflex in response to pain (Garciá-Larrea et al 1993) which appears to depend on descending reticulospinal pathways. Di Piero et al (1991) studied five patients with unilateral cancer pain using PET scanning, demonstrating reduced blood flow in three out of four patients in the hemithalamus contralateral to the pain, an abnormality that was abolished by successful cordotomy. When patient studies were compared pre- and postcordotomy, a significant increase in cerebral blood flow occurred only in dorsal anterior thalamus.

Technique

High cervical lateral percutaneous cordotomy is usually accomplished under local anaesthesia with intravenous sedation. A sharpened stainless steel electrode insulated with shrink-fit Teflon tubing leaving a 2 mm bare tip is introduced through a # 19 thin wall lumbar puncture needle at the C1–2 interspace to penetrate the spinal cord at the level of the dentate ligament to a depth of 2 mm, when further advancement of the electrode is resisted by the cuff of the Teflon tubing. This is facilitated with positive contrast myelography, image intensification and impedance monitoring. Recordings of 400 ohms are made when the tip is in spinal fluid, up to 1200 ohms in the cord. Location in spinothalamic tract is confirmed by electrical stimulation with electronic back-up provided by a suitable instrument such as the OWL Universal Radiofrequency System (available from Diros Technology, 965 Pape Ave, Toronto, Canada M4K 3V6) or that provided by the Radionics Corporation (Box 438, 76 Cambridge St, Burlington, MA). Table 57.2 lists the possible responses from stimulating the electrode at 2 Hz (Tasker 1995). If the electrode lies in the spinothalamic tract, muscle contractions in time with the stimulation should appear in the ipsilateral trapezius or shoulder girdle and sometimes in the upper limb, but not in the lower limb, at 2–6 volts. In our series, contrac-

Table 57.2 Responses to cord stimulation at 2 Hz

Response	*Significance*
No motor response 0–10 V	Defects in equipment Stimulator not turned on Patient's muscles paralysed Gross misplacement of needle, probably not in subarachnoid space or at least outside cord
Response in contralateral side of neck or stronger in contralateral than ipsilateral side	Electrode advanced too far
Responses in ipsilateral side of neck or accompanied by only weak response in contralateral side, often in trapezius, sternomastoid or posterior nuchal muscles	Compatible with location either in anterior horn (especially if threshold <1 V) or in spinothalamic tract (1–3 V) when contralateral sensory effects may be reported as well in 1 patient of 4
Responses in ipsilateral neck and upper limb	Compatible with location either in anterior horn (especially if threshold <1 volt) or in spinothalamic tract (1–3 V) when contralateral sensory effects may be reported as well
Responses in ipsilateral upper limb or, especially, trunk or lower limb	Electrode probably in corticospinal tract

tions occurred in trapezius alone in 40% of patients, in trapezius plus other upper limb muscles in a further 19%, in other neck muscles in 27.6%, in upper limb alone in 9.6%; no motor contractions occurred in 3.6%.

Table 57.3 lists similar data for 100 Hz stimulation (Tasker 1995). An ideal response should include a warm or cold feeling somewhere in the contralateral body with a threshold below 1 volt (average 0.4 volts) without tetanization anywhere. Ipsilateral tetanization suggests that the electrode is too close to the corticospinal tract whose location in cordotomy patients is carefully reviewed by Nathan (1994).

In our series, contralateral hot feelings were elicited in 27.4%, warmth in 7.7%, burning in 28.2%, cold or cool sensations in 16.2%, non-specific paraesthesiae in 1.7%, pain in 6.8%. In 12% of patients the exact sensation elicited was not recorded. Once a sensory response occurs, it is wise to stimulate suprathreshold to search for ipsilateral tetanization and to avoid lesion making if motor responses occur near the sensory threshold, especially if the induced response is one of ipsilateral paraesthesiae. Rarely, ipsilateral facial paraesthesiae identify stimulation of the trigeminal complex.

When the electrode position is deemed satisfactory, graded 60-second radiofrequency lesions are made with serial testing of ipsilateral leg and arm power as well as of level and depth of contralateral analgesia. A minimal lesion is first made at 35 mA at a temperature of 60–75°C. If no untoward effects occur, the lesion is then enlarged in 10 mA increments to a maximum of 50 mA with a temperature of about 90°C. In our experience a single lesion sufficed in 84% of cases. A successful lesion typically greatly increases the threshold for inducing painful sensation, using superficial or deep contralateral stimuli with little change in tactile threshold. Particularly if the patient's pain is located in the lower quarter of the body, sacral sparing should be avoided. Though appreciation of temperature is usually reduced or abolished in a similar part of the body as that of pinprick, there are frequent small mismatches and accumulated evidence suggests dissociation of the pain and temperature pathways (Stookey 1929, Sherman & Arieff 1948, Friehs et al 1995). Frequently, ipsilateral ptosis from sympathetic tract damage is seen though it is often transient and, for a short time postoperatively, ipsilateral respiratory excursion may be lessened from encroachment on the reticulospinal tract. In the operating room, examination may reveal paresis in the ipsilateral lower limb but in our experience, any patient who can still elevate the limb off the table, however weakly, will recover and not suffer significant persistent disability.

Table 57.3 Responses to cord stimulation at 100 Hz

Response	*Significance*
No motor or sensory response	Defects in equipment Stimulator not turned on Patient's muscles paralysed Gross misplacement of needle, probably not in subarachnoid space or at least outside cord
Tetanization of ipsilateral neck	Electrode in anterior horn
Tetanization of contralateral neck or contralateral body below neck	Electrode has penetrated too deeply
Tetanization of ipsilateral side below neck	Electrode in corticospinal tract
No tetanization at threshold, possibly slight tetanization in ipsilateral leg stimulation suprathreshold for contralateral sensory responses yielding a sensation of contralateral warmth, cold, rarely burning, pain or paraesthesias referred usually to lower limb	Electrode is located in caudal dermatomes of spinothalamic tract where lesion tends to affect more caudal dermatomes of tract; slight risk of ipsilateral leg paresis
No tetanization, even suprathreshold, with contralateral sensory responses as above that are referred to hand	Electrode located centrally in spinothalamic tract and lesion likely to produce extensive analgesia
No tetanization but contralateral sensory response as above in neck or upper trunk	Electrode located in most rostral dermatomes of spinothalamic tract and not likely to produce sufficient analgesia but, rather, suspended analgesia
No tetanization but ipsilateral responses only	Explanation uncertain; may be subthreshold corticospinal responses; test suprathreshold stimulation
No tetanization but ipsilateral and contralateral sensory responses as above	Electrode position acceptable if suprathreshold stimulation does not induce tetanization and all other criteria are met

Results

Published data suggest a range of 63–77% complete, 68–96% significant pain relief after unilateral percutaneous cordotomy (Tasker 1982a, 1988, 1993, 1995) based on differing patient samples, lengths of follow-up and methods of pain assessment. In a highly significant study, Rosomoff et al (1990) found complete pain relief in 90% of patients immediately after surgery, 84% at 3 months, 61% at 1 year, 43% between 1 and 5 years and 37% between 5 and 10 years, clearly documenting pain recurrence with time. Obviously their long surviving patients did not suffer from cancer, the usual indication for most cordotomies. In our own experience with 244 percutaneous cordotomies, nearly all done in patients with cancer, significant pain relief occurred in 94.4% immediately postoperatively, 82.3% at latest follow-up (1–3 months). In eight patients with neuropathic pain caused by spinal cord injury and one with cerebral palsy, pain recurred after 1, 1.1, 4, 4, 5, 6, 7, 13 and 21 years respectively. Repetition of cordotomy in six patients after 4, 4, 5, 6, 7 and 21 years respectively restored the level of analgesia in all but pain relief in only three.

Complications

The chief complications of unilateral cordotomy (Tasker 1982a, 1988, 1993, 1995) are: death (nearly always from respiratory complications) (0–5%), significant reversible respiratory complications (up to 10%), significant persistent paresis or ataxia (up to 10%), significant worsening of control of micturition (up to 15%), significant postcordotomy dysaesthesia (less than 10%). Respiratory complications can be avoided by attention to the factors mentioned under 'Indications'. Paresis and ataxia can be minimized by careful attention to physiological monitoring of the lesion site. However, postcordotomy dysaesthesia cannot be anticipated or avoided, being an example of idiosyncratic central pain caused by an iatrogenic spinal cord lesion. The pathways for control of micturition lie adjacent to the spinothalamic tract where they are vulnerable to damage with a correctly placed cordotomy lesion. However, if the pathway on the opposite side of the cord to that on which the cordotomy is being done is intact and micturition is not grossly defective to start with, damage to the pathway by unilateral cordotomy usually does not worsen bladder control.

'Mirror pain' (Nathan 1956, Bowsher 1988, Nagaro et al 1987, 1993a,b, Ischia & Ischia 1988) is a curious complication of cordotomy seen in about 40% of the author's patients and reported in 9–63.3% of patients in series in the literature (Tasker 1982a, 1988, 1993, 1995). Essentially, the patient develops new pain or aggravation of pre-existing but minor pain in much the same location somatotopographically as that of the pain for which the cordotomy was done but on the other side of the body. This may be associated with allochiria, the induction of mirror image pain by application of, say, pinch below the level of the analgesia induced by the cordotomy. These phenomena are thought to be the result of opening up after the cordotomy of previously inactive synapses since they may appear immediately postoperatively and are abolished by epidural blockade below the level of the analgesia (Nagaro et al 1993a).

BILATERAL CORDOTOMY

It is rare for cancer pain to be unilateral, though often after relief of the pain on the worst side, that on the other can be managed conservatively. Thus the bilateral procedure must sometimes be considered and it is best to separate the procedures on the two sides by at least 1 week. Although the same indications and techniques apply for cordotomy on the second side as on the first, it must be remembered that, if the expected rate of significant pain relief with unilateral cordotomy is, say, 80%, that after bilateral surgery is 80% × 80% or 64%; similar calculations apply to the complications except for respiratory and micturitional problems. If the first cordotomy has interfered with automatic respiration ipsilaterally, usually associated with high levels of analgesia into the cervical dermatomes, then it is probably unwise to do a high cervical cordotomy on the other side unless high levels of analgesia into the cervical origin can be avoided, for doing so will abolish unconscious respiration on both sides and risk death from respiratory insufficiency. Although it is unusual to have micturitional complications from unilateral cordotomy, they are very likely after the bilateral procedure since the bladder pathways are so close to the ideal cordotomy lesion that they are readily damaged; bilateral damage results in loss of control of voiding. Permanent worsening of micturition was reported in up to 20% of patients undergoing bilateral cordotomy (Tasker 1982a, 1988, 1993, 1995).

Some authors have minimized the risks of the bilateral operation. Amano et al (1991) have suggested that the bilateral operation is not only more effective than the unilateral for pain relief but also carries little added risk though Sanders and Zuurmond (1995), in a recent review, found the bilateral procedure exposed the patient to too great a risk for them to recommend it.

Since cordotomy outcome data are now so seldom reported it is of interest to mention these latter authors' results (Sanders & Zuurmond 1995) in 62 patients, 18 of whom underwent bilateral surgery. In all cases pain was caused by cancer with 80% of the unilateral and 50% of the bilateral group enjoying 'satisfactory' results, 10% and 33% respectively 'partial' results. Urinary retention occurred in 6.5% of the unilateral, 11.1% of the bilateral group, hemiparesis in 8.1% and 11.1% respectively, mirror pain in 6.5% and 5.6% respectively. There were no respiratory complications.

CT-GUIDED PERCUTANEOUS CORDOTOMY

Izumi et al (1992) and particularly Kanpolat et al (1993, 1995) have pioneered the use of CT guidance for cordotomy. Kanpolat et al (1995) report 97% complete pain control in a series of 67 patients with cancer, operated on between 1987 and 1995. In 45 cases analgesia was tailored so as to affect only the painful portion of the body. Complications may be reduced using CT guidance for they reported only one case of transient hemiparesis and one of ataxia in a series of 54 procedures.

LESIONS OF THE DORSAL ROOT ENTRY ZONE

Introduction

Lesioning of the dorsal root entry zone (DREZ) for pain relief has an interesting history. Capitalizing on the anatomical segregation of pain-conducting fibres from other somatosensory fibres in the DREZ area into Lissauer's tract (Hyndman 1942, Denny-Brown et al 1973), Hyndman advocated sectioning of Lissauer's tract during open cordotomy to interrupt pain fibres prior to their decussation in the hope of eliminating the usual 4–5-dermatome gap between the level of an open cordotomy lesion and that of the analgesia produced. In more recent times Sindou, after completion of his dissertation on the dorsal horn in which he demonstrated convergence of fine group III and IV afferents in the ventrolateral part of the DREZ (Sindou 1972, Sindou et al 1974b), developed a microsurgical procedure in which the pain-related, small myelinated and unmyelinated afferent fibres and the median pain activating part of Lissauer's tract were severed with a blade for relief of chronic pain in the dermatomes related to the section (Sindou et al 1974a, 1976, 1986, 1991, Sindou & Goutelle 1983, Sindou & Daher 1988, Sindou & Jeanmonod 1989, Sindou 1995). At the same time, Nashold and Ostdahl (1979) and Nashold et al (1976) developed a related procedure in which multiple radiofrequency lesions were made under direct vision in the DREZ.

Sindou's procedure appears to have been used initially to treat nociceptive pain, having the advantage of inducing analgesia in the cervical as well as lower dermatomes without risk to the respiratory fibres in the reticulospinal tract. Nashold's procedure was directed towards the control of neuropathic pain syndromes, possibly stimulated by the notion that it destroyed bursting cells in the dorsal horn (Loeser et al 1968) which Albe-Fessard and Lombard (1983) had demonstrated in the laboratory to be related to denervation and which were candidate generators of neuropathic pain. Though we are unaware of any comparative study of the two procedures, they appear similar except for the method of lesion making. The Nashold DREZ operation appears to have been much more widely adopted, particularly for controlling the pain associated with brachial plexus avulsion as well as other deafferentation syndromes. Unlike cordotomy, the DREZ procedure continues to occupy an important role in current neurosurgery.

Indications

Sindou and his colleagues (Sindou et al 1974a, 1976, 1986, 1991, Sindou & Goutelle 1983, Sindou & Daher 1988, Sindou & Jeanmonod 1989, Sindou 1995, Emery et al 1997) used his procedure to treat the pain of cancer, pain and spasticity in patients with central nervous lesions and neuropathic pain. The Nashold procedure (Nashold et al 1976, 1990, Powers et al 1984, 1988, Richter & Seitz 1984, Samii & Moringlane 1984, Thomas & Jones 1984, Saris et al 1985, Wiegand & Winkelmüller 1985, Friedman & Nashold 1986, 1990, Moossy et al 1987, Campbell et al 1988, Friedman & Bullitt 1988, Friedman et al 1988, 1996, Ishijima et al 1988, Bronec & Nashold 1990, Sampson et al 1995, Roth et al 1997) was advocated for a variety of neuropathic syndromes in addition to its primary indication in the pain of brachial plexus avulsion and the rarely encountered lumbosacral plexus avulsion, including postherpetic neuralgia, pain associated with amputations and central pain of spinal cord origin. The longer term efficacy in postherpetic neuralgia now appears questionable. In patients with cord central pain, the operation appears most effective in 'end-zone pain' according to the Nashold group.

The pathophysiology of the DREZ procedure remains unclear. In interrupting Lissauer's tract, it would be expected to relieve nociceptive pain, as reported by Sindou, but Nashold's procedure has been used mostly to treat neuropathic pain. Some authors would maintain that it does so by destroying deafferented bursting cells that somehow serve as triggers for neuropathic pain. Sindou's group (Jeanmonod et al 1989a) have recorded with microelectrodes during DREZ procedures for neuropathic pain, finding hyperactive, deafferented units mostly in lamina IV or V, though one was found more superficial. It is our opinion, however, that bursting cells are markers of deafferentation, not of pain, and a closer study of neuropathic pain syndromes leads to a possible alternative explanation for the success of the DREZ operation. As mentioned under 'Indications' for cordotomy, neuropathic pain consists of three common components: spontaneous, steady, often burning or dysaesthetic pain, neuralgic pain and allodynia and hyperpathia. Clinical evidence (Tasker et al 1992) suggests that destructive cord surgery (cordotomy, the DREZ procedure and cord transection) in patients with central pain caused by cord damage is effective only for the relief of the two latter components but not of the steady component. The Nashold group's conclusion (Nashold & Bullitt 1981, Friedman & Bullitt 1988, Nashold 1991, Sampson et al 1995), that the DREZ operation tends to relieve 'end-zone pain' (Nashold et al 1990) by which they mean locally appreciated allodynia and spontaneous neuralgic pain but not diffuse steady pain, seems to agree with these findings. In pain after brachial plexus avulsion, neuralgic components are usually a major component but there is anecdotal evidence that associated steady pain may also be relieved.

Technique

Both the Sindou and the Nashold procedure require identification of the dermatomes in which the pain is located and the exposure at laminectomy of the corresponding dorsal root entry zones. In cases of plexus avulsion, this may be helped by identifying the avulsed roots with magnetic resonance imaging (MRI). Nashold and his co-workers (Nashold et al 1985, Makachinas et al 1988) have identified the correct level by searching for the largest amplitude spinal cord-evoked potentials in response to stimulation of peripheral nerves or roots serving the painful area. Obviously, this technique could be used only to mark the boundaries of lesion making in brachial plexus avulsion and would be of questionable benefit in spinal cord injury. Fazl's group (Fazl & Houlden 1995, Fazl et al 1995) have used intrathecal spinal cord stimulation with subdural recording to differentiate dorsal column and DREZ pathways from dorsolateral cord pathways to reduce the complications of the DREZ operation. They found evoked potentials absent from the DREZ and latencies longer from the dorsal and the dorsolateral cord. Sindou's group (Jeanmonod et al 1989a, 1991) localized the lesion with motor responses to stimulation and evoked electrospinographic recordings.

In Sindou's operation a cut is made under the surgical microscope at a 45° angle at each affected dermatome to a depth of 2 mm (3–4 in cases of root avulsion) into the substance of the cord at the line of entry of the dorsal rootlets.

With Nashold's procedure a sharpened 1.7–2.0 mm diameter electrode, with a 0.25 mm diameter tip insulated except for its terminal 2 mm, is inserted to a depth of 2 mm at a 25–45° lateral to medial angle at the dorsal root line. Fifteen 30-second, 70–80°C radiofrequency lesions are made every millimetre over the extent of cord related to the pain, totalling 10–15 lesions per spinal cord segment. In the case of plexus avulsion lesions are extended into the domain of the uninjured rootlets above and below the avulsion. A technique for making lesions with laser has also been described but has not been widely accepted (Powers et al 1984, 1988, Young 1986, Young et al 1994).

Yoshida et al (1992) have examined DREZ lesions with MRI, comparing their results with those reported in the literature in two autopsy studies. In cases with brachial plexus avulsion, the cord is enlarged at the site of the avulsion prior to the DREZ procedure. Lesions made there are extensive and involve the hemicord with high signal on T2 and proton density scans superimposed on a preoperative picture of cord atrophy associated with a high signal in T2 or T2 plus proton density scans in the dorsal horn and sometimes also in the vicinity of the ventral horn. In patients who did not have brachial plexus avulsion, the lesion made with similar parameters was discrete and localized to the dorsal horn; the significance of these findings is unclear.

Results

The Sindou Procedure

Sindou (1995) reports 83% good results with the DREZ procedure in cancer pain. Whereas in neuropathic pain allodynia was relieved in 88.2%, spontaneous steady pain responded less well unless it was lancinating. Jeanmonod & Sindou (1991) found muscle tone and stretch reflexes were reduced at sites somatotopographically related to the lesion and their operation produced analgesia or severe hypalgesia, moderate hypaesthesia but only slight diminution of proprioception and cutaneous spatial discrimination in affected dermatomes. There was moderate reduction of presynaptic action potentials recorded from the cord (N11 and N21), a partial short-term reduction of the cortical postcentral N20 potential, moderate reduction of the postsynaptic dorsal horn waves (N13 and N24) and disappearance of dorsal horn waves related to fine afferents (N2 and possibly N3) in evoked electrospinographic recording. These electrodiagnostic studies were used online to help localize lesion sites.

In a small series of 20 patients undergoing electrophysiologically guided procedures (Jeanmonod & Sindou 1991), three patients developed minimal and two reversible lower limb weakness, one urinary retention. In a review of 220 patients with pain (139 neuropathic, 81 cancerous origin) operated on over 20 years, Sindou (1995) found that the best results occurred in well-localized cancer pain, brachial plexus avulsion, pain caused by injury to the cauda equina and cord, peripheral nerve injury, amputation-related pain and herpes zoster, especially when the pain was neuralgic, allodynic or hyperpathic.

Emery et al (1997), using the Sindou technique, reported that 79% of their 37 patients enjoyed over 75% pain relief, while 22% had 50–75% relief. In the patients followed longer term (1–10 years), 70% still reported over 50% pain relief, with 13% under 50% pain relief.

The Nashold Procedure

Brachial Plexus Avulsion The extensive literature attests to the importance of the operation in the treatment of pain of brachial plexus avulsion (Nashold & Ostdahl 1979, Samii & Moringlane 1984, Thomas & Jones 1984, Wiegand & Winkelmüller 1985, Campbell et al 1988, Friedman & Bullitt 1988, Friedman et al 1988, 1996, Bronec & Nashold 1990, Nashold & El Naggar 1992, Roth et al 1997) and the much rarer lumbosacral avulsions (Moossy et al 1987), making it one of the few destructive procedures still in regular use for the relief of chronic pain. According to Gybels and Sweet (1989), Nashold operated on 39 cases of pain from brachial plexus avulsion with 54% good (no analgesics, no limitations imposed by pain) and 13% fair results, a result that improved to 82% good as further technical refinements were introduced. Thomas and Jones (1984) reported 59% of patients with 75–100% pain relief; 12% of patients suffered new neurological deficits. Gybels and Sweet (1989) summarized the results of 98 other DREZ operations for pain from brachial plexus avulsion from the literature, 67% of which gave more than 70% pain relief.

In a more recent review, Friedman et al (1996) noted variation in published results from 29–100% pain relief in a total of 341 cases averaging 72% good results. In their own series, there were 59% good, 12% fair results; 40% suffered increased neurological deficit postoperatively including 25% with sensory changes and 27% clumsiness, fatigue or hyperreflexia in the ipsilateral lower limb. Roth et al (1997) reported 68% permanent good or fair results in 22 patients over a mean 52-month follow-up. In their whole series of 63 patients which included patients with other than brachial plexus avulsion, there were three deaths from pulmonary embolism and myocardial infarction, a 9% incidence of permanent ataxia and 14% of minor neurological deficits; 22% of procedures had to be repeated.

Pain from spinal cord lesions

The DREZ procedure has also been used extensively to treat cord central pain (Nashold & Bullitt 1981, Richter & Seitz 1984, Wiegand & Winkelmüller 1985, Friedman & Nashold 1986, 1990, Friedman & Bullitt 1988, Bronec & Nashold 1990, Nashold et al 1990, Nashold 1991, Nashold & El-Naggar 1992, Sampson et al 1995, Friedman et al 1996, Roth et al 1997). It is, however, very effective only in certain elements of cord central pain, which we believe are often similar to those responding to cordotomy (discussed above) and cordectomy (reviewed below).

Sampson et al (1995) reviewed 39 patients over a mean 3-year follow-up, 12 suffering from steady burning pain, 12 from electrical intermittent pain, seven from both types. In 16 patients pain was diffuse below the level and in 23 it was present only in a hyperesthetic end zone just above their level. Fifty-four per cent of these patients enjoyed a good result, which meant that they required no narcotics; 20% reported a fair result, meaning that pain was reduced and narcotics were not necessary. Patients with incomplete lesions, end-zone and electrical pain and those injured by blunt trauma did best. Friedman and Bullitt (1988) found, in a review of 31 cases, that end-zone pain, whether it was burning or neuralgic in nature, was relieved in 80% of cases, diffuse pain in 32%; three patients suffered additional weakness postoperatively that had not been present before. Wiegand and Winkelmüller (1985) reported that 45% of 20 patients gained 100% pain relief and 5% had 80% relief with one patient developing new paresis in addition to what had been present before. Friedman et al (1996) reported pain relief in 54% of patients with cord central pain, relief being most readily achieved when the pain extended into dermatomes immediately caudal to the injury (described as root, radicular or end-zone pain), rather than into remotely distal dermatomes when it tended to be diffuse and burning. Roth et al (1997) reported 52% good or fair pain relief in 23 patients with cord central pain over a mean 53-month follow-up, noting that diffuse distal pain was poorly relieved.

Postherpetic neuralgia

The DREZ operation was used initially for the relief of postherpetic neuralgia (Friedman & Bullitt 1988, Gybels & Sweet 1989, Friedman et al 1996, Roth et al 1997) but results have been disappointing. Gybels and Sweet's review (1989) of the Duke experience with 32 patients with this condition records 90% early pain relief, 50% at 6 months postoperatively and eventual recurrence in 66%, only 25% of patients enjoying excellent extended relief. Ten of those with recurrent pain postoperatively developed a pain that was different in type from that present preoperatively and 69% developed significant gait disturbance postoperatively. Roth et al (1997) reported 20% of 10 patients with post-herpetic neuralgia relieved. Friedman et al (1996) noted 34% relief with gradual recurrence.

Amputation-related pain

The usefulness of the DREZ operation in amputation-related pain appears restricted to amputations carried out after brachial or lumbosacral plexus avulsion (Nashold et al 1976, Saris et al 1985, 1988a,b, Sindou 1995). Saris et al (1988a), reviewing 22 Duke patients, found that results were better in phantom pain than in stump or combined stump/phantom pain. Six out of nine of their cases of phantom pain enjoyed good pain relief but five of these six had had their amputations because of brachial plexus avulsion. Stump pain was not relieved in any of their nine cases and results were poor (two out of seven relieved) in combinations of stump and phantom pain together. Miscellaneous authors quoted by Gybels and Sweet (1989) contributed 17 cases with amputation-related pain, 35% of whom enjoyed total relief, 12% more than 50% relief. Saris et al (1988b) found 14% of patients with amputation-related pain did well if the amputation was unrelated to brachial plexus avulsion.

Miscellaneous neuropathic pain

The Nashold DREZ procedure has little success in conditions other than plexus avulsion and cord injury; 18% of 12 patients operated on by the Nashold group for intractable sciatica enjoyed good relief (Saris et al 1988b). Gybels and Sweet (1989) concluded the procedure was ineffective in this condition. Roth et al (1997) reported 13% relief in a group of eight patients with various other neuropathic syndromes (one with syringomyelia, two with radiation plexitis, two with pain following surgery on the brachial plexus, one with pain from carcinoma in the brachial plexus, one with obstetrical plexus palsy and one with phantom pain).

Complications

Fazl et al (1995), in a literature review, found a 0–60% (mean 38%) reported complication rate after the Nashold DREZ procedure. In the series of patients with cord central pain described by Nashold's group (Nashold & Ostdahl 1979), 10% suffered from permanent weakness, 8% bladder or sexual dysfunction, 3% paraesthesiae.

CORDECTOMY

Introduction and indications

Cordectomy is rarely performed today, the DREZ procedure probably being preferable. Though percutaneous cordotomy achieves the same result and has less impact, it exposes the patient to the risk of paresis in the upper limbs and requires special expertise that cordectomy does not demand. The concept of cordectomy, first performed by Armour (1927), was a simple one. The neurosurgeon faced with the problem of pain related to spinal cord injury surmised that transection or excision of the spinal cord just above the level of injury should eliminate pain transmission from the area of pain and hopefully relieve it. If the degree of existing deficit from cord injury was severe enough, such a procedure would add only a mild extra deficit consisting of a segment or two's elevation of sensory loss.

A considerable experience with very small series of patients accumulated, with somewhat conflicting results. The most useful information comes from the work of Jefferson (1983), who showed that cordectomy relieved the pain of spinal cord injury when the level of cord injury was near the termination of the spinal cord and the pain was referred to knees and legs. Our study (Tasker et al 1992) of the same phenomenon discussed above suggested that, like cordotomy and the DREZ operation, cordectomy was capable of relieving the neuralgic elements of cord injury pain that usually radiated down the legs like sciatica, presumably dependent upon ectopic impulse generation at an injury site in the roots of the cauda equina with projection over the spinothalamic tract (Fig. 57.2). The procedure also relieved allodynia which is known to result from garbled processing in somatosensory input at the dorsal horn level with transmission in the spinothalamic tract.

Technique

Though termed cordectomy, the usual procedure is a simple transection of the cord exposed by laminectomy 1–2 segments above the lesion responsible for the pain.

Results

Reported series are usually small except for the 19 patients reported by Jefferson (1983). With pain referred to the

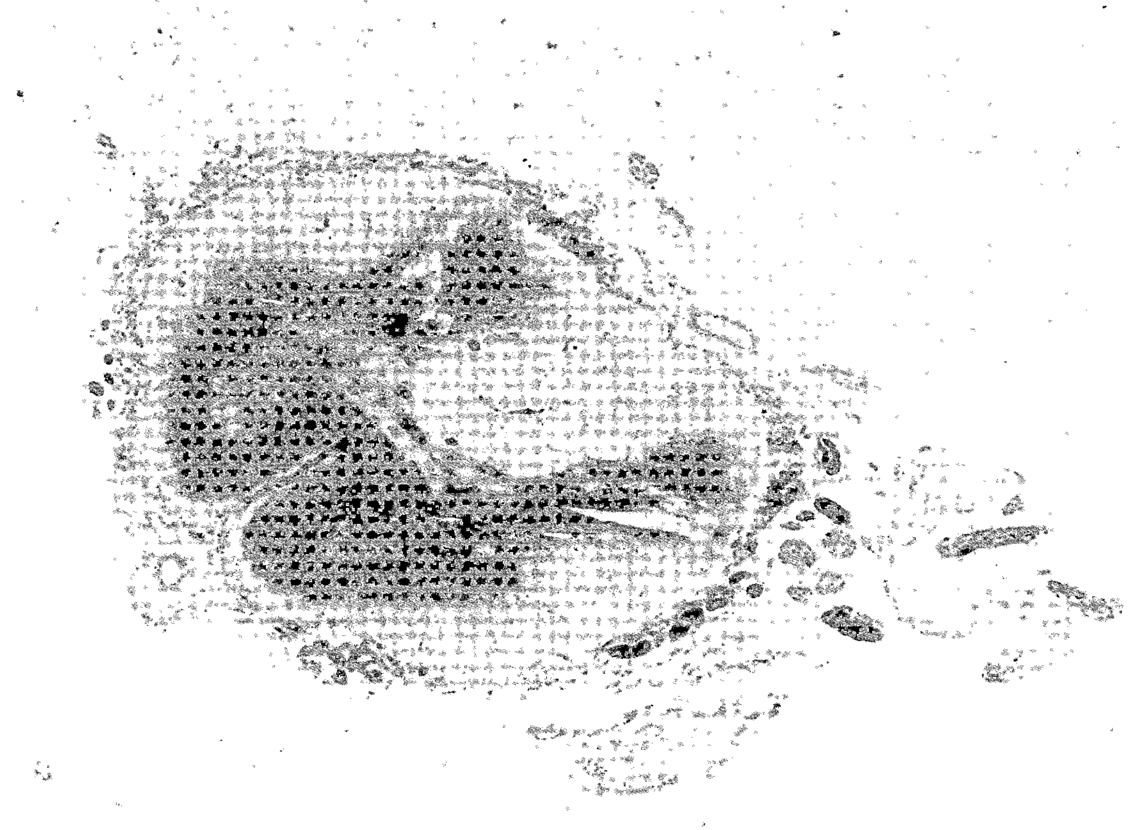

Fig. 57.2 Surgical specimen after cordectomy at TID for pain caused by a complete post-traumatic cord lesion at T12. Cordectomy relieved the patient's neuralgic pain shooting down his legs but not the steady burning pain felt diffusely below his lesion.

lower limbs, cordectomy at or below T11 reduced pain by a factor of 70–100% in 93% of the patients. The one patient in this group not relieved enjoyed 50% relief. In patients with pain in the upper thighs, lower abdomen, buttocks and rectum and in those with cordectomies at T10, T10–11 or above, pain was not relieved.

COMMISSURAL MYELOTOMY, STEREOTACTIC C_1, CENTRAL MYELOTOMY AND LIMITED (PUNCTUATE) MIDLINE MYELOTOMY

Historical note and surgical variants in location

Inspired by Greenfield, Armour in 1926 performed the first commissural myelotomy (Armour 1927). The rationale was that in cases of bilateral topographically relatively limited bilateral pain, a single cut through the decussation of the spinothalamic tract could avoid the drawbacks of bilateral anterolateral cordotomy. The depth of the cut has been a matter of controversy. Some authors limited the incision to a depth of 2–3 mm, thereby just reaching the grey substance (Mansuy et al 1944); some did not exceed 4 mm, thereby seeking to limit the incision to the posterior commissure (Wertheimer & Lecuire 1953) while some cut deeper ventral to the central canal (Guillaume et al 1945).

As side effect, a girdle-shaped hypalgesia is usually seen in cases of complete commissural myelotomy, while less consistent configuration of the hypalgesia is often reported in posterior commissural myelotomy. Paraesthesias and dysasthesias in the legs, usually transient, are frequently seen. It is of particular interest that the clinical pain is often relieved even when there is a slight or no hypalgesia (Cook et al 1984). There may also be loss of pain and temperature sensibility far caudal or more cranial than would be expected from the level and length of the commissurotomy. Probably of interest for this discussion are the findings of stereotactic C_1 central myelotomy as pioneered by Hitchcock (1974). His type of 'central myelotomy' differs from commissural myelotomy by the larger spatial extension of the lesion, its location limited to the single C_1 level in the spinal cord not determined by the metameric distribution of the pain and the minimal injury to the dorsal columns. There again, the sensory findings in man point to the existence of a central pathway for pain in the human spinal cord, the destruction of which diminishes or even eliminates the conscious awareness of clinical persistent pain with modest, if any, loss of pain from discrete noxious stimuli. The results of stereotactic C_1 central myelotomy, shown in Table 57.4, led Gildenberg and Hirshberg (1984) to carry out open lower one level lesions near the central canal at vertebral levels T9 or T10.

Human surgical cases with, in one case, histological verification (Fig. 57.3), along with neuroanatomical and neurophysiological findings in animal experiments (Fig. 57.4) have led to a further investigation of the question whether there is a pathway in the posterior funiculus that signals visceral pain (Hirshberg et al 1996), to a modified midline myelotomy with the specific intent of interrupting only the midline posterior column visceral pathway (Nauta et al 1997) and to the publication of two editorials in the journal *Pain* (Gybels 1997, Berkley 1997). In one of these (Berkley 1997), it was emphasized:

> *With a simplistic fascicular view that the dorsal columns convey visceral pain, we might be misleadingly encouraged to try the relatively simple surgery of limited myelotomy for many types of pelvic visceral pain. In contrast, with the holistic view that perceptions arise out of the cooperative balance of information flowing through all systems into a dynamic brain, we would be concerned that this irreversible surgery might have unanticipated iatrogenic effects (e.g. new pains, spatiotemporal dysfunctions, visceral dysfunctions in actions that depend on the recognition of visceral distension, less pleasure in massage or touch, etc...).*

Results

Tables 57.4 and 57.5 summarize the latest results of the different types of 'central' myelotomy.

It is difficult to estimate the real success of these interventions but in eight articles reporting on 175 cases of complete commissural myelotomy, early complete relief of pain was achieved in an average of 92% of the cases, but with time the outcome decays. In the cases where follow-up was longer and up to 11 year, 59% of 63 patients with malignant tumours and 48% of 21 patients with other than malignant causes had a 'good' outcome at the latest follow-up.

SUMMARY: DESTRUCTIVE PROCEDURES IN THE SPINAL CORD FOR THE RELIEF OF CHRONIC PAIN

Percutaneous cordotomy is one of the most effective surgical procedures for the relief of nociceptive pain, particularly that caused by cancerous invasion of the lumbosacral plexus. It still ought to be employed, as the DREZ operation still is, in properly selected patients. Unfortunately, in many centres all cancer patients, and many others, are indiscriminately treated with morphine infusions, some of whom would be more effectively managed by percutaneous cordotomy. Because of the lack of referral of suitable candidates, it is a concern that the special skill required to perform this useful operation is gradually being lost.

The DREZ procedure, by whatever technique, remains one of the few destructive procedures still regularly performed in the central nervous system for the relief of pain. It is admirably effective in patients with pain from brachial plexus avulsion and with neuralgic or 'end-zone' pain associated with lesions of the conus and cauda equina. It is one of the great recent contributions to pain surgery.

'The extent to which both commissural and central myelotomy should be utilized at present is unclear' (Gybels

Table 57.4 Late results of stereotactic C_1 central myelotomy (from Van Roost & Gybels 1989) and limited (punctate) midline myelotomy (Gildenberg & Hirshberg 1984, Nauta et al 1997)

Author	*Year*	*Operation level*	*Late success* %	*n*	*Malignant* %	*n*
Hitchcock	1970b	Centr. C0–1	43	7	43	7
Papo and Luongo	1976	Centr. C2–4	40	10	33	9
Hitchcock	1977	Centr. C0–1	80	25		
Schvarcz	1978	Centr. C0–1	78	75	79	61
Eiras et al	1980	Centr. C0–1	58	12	58	12
Sourek	1985 1987	Centr. C0–1	57	30	Minority	
Gildenberg & Hirshberg	1984	Compl. + centr. T9–10	66	12	66	12
Nauta et al	1997	Centr. T8	(4 months)	1		1

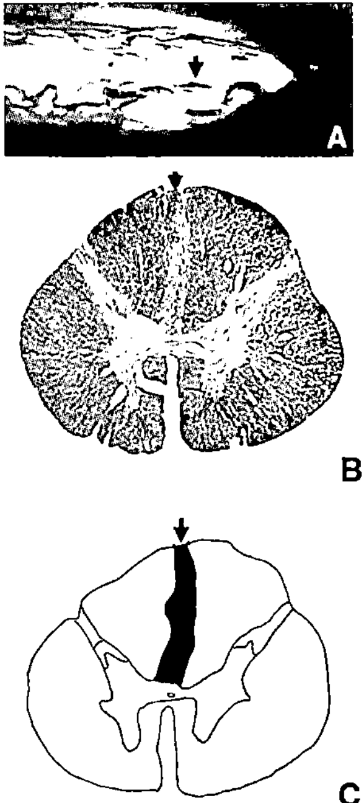

Fig. 57.3 A Photograph of the spinal cord of case I as viewed through the operating microscope just after a limited posterior midline myelotomy was done at T10. The entry line of the mechanical microdissector is indicated by the arrow. The spinal cord of the patient was removed postmortem and fixed in 10% neutral formalin. B Photomicrograph of a histological section stained for myelin through the spinal cord of case I rostral to the lesion. The vertical, linear area of demyelination indicated by the arrow just to the left of the midline defines the part of the fasciculus gracilis that was interrupted by the lesion. The tissue section was stained with luxol fast blue, hematoxylin and eosin. C Composite drawing of the lesion made by projecting a series of sections through the lesioned area. The diameter of the human spinal cord at T10 is 8 mm. (Reproduced from Hirshberg et al 1996 with permission.)

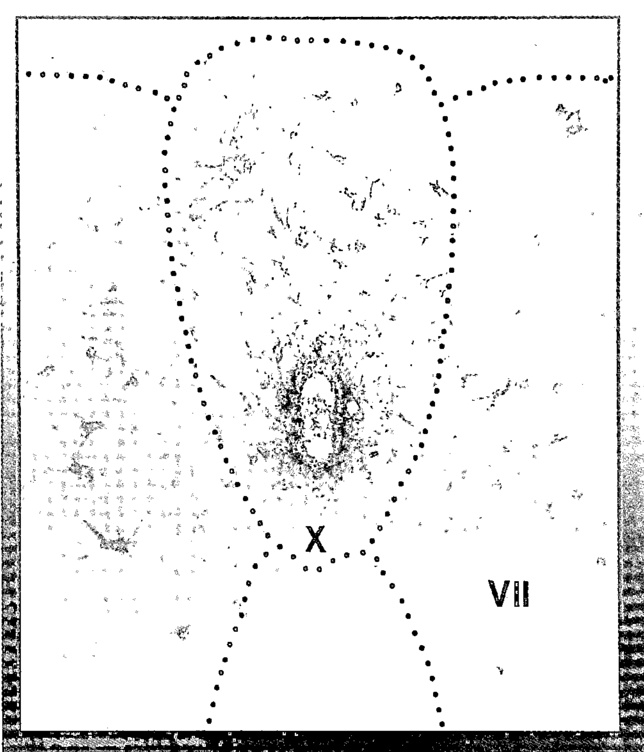

Fig. 57.4 The photomicrograph shows the central portion of a rat spinal cord section taken through the S2 segment that had had a bilateral injection of WGA-HRP into the dorsal columns at the C5–6 level 7 days prior to sacrificing the animal. Note the numerous retrogadely labelled neurons around the central canal (lamina X), especially dorsally, and in the adjacent grey matter (lamina VII). (Reproduced from Hirshberg et al 1996 with permission.)

1997). New interest in the operation, taking advantage of new knowledge and new techniques, should be moderated by a need to re-evaluate it and compare it with alternative strategies using the guidelines listed in the Introduction.

Cordectomy appears to be largely of historical interest.

OPERATIONS ON THE BRAIN

INTRODUCTION

After the introduction of cordotomy, it seemed logical to extend the principle of pain tract interruption cephalad for the relief of, particularly, cancer pain of the upper portion of the body, especially of the head and neck. First by open means, section of the medullary and mesencephalic spinothalamic tracts and of the trigeminal thalamic pathways was undertaken, the former often in conjunction with multiple upper cervical and lower cranial sections. With the advent of stereotactic techniques (Spiegel & Wycis 1949), it became possible to perform the same procedures more precisely with less impact on the patient, using a greater range of targets than had been possible by open means. An unexplained bonus in the case of mesencephalic tractotomy was the much lower incidence of iatrogenic neuropathic pain after the stereotactic procedure than had been seen when the operation was done by open means.

Attention was initially applied to stereotactic interruption of the spinothalamic pathway, first in the mesencephalon (Spiegel & Wycis 1962) and then in Hassler's ventrocaudal somatosensory relay nucleus (Schaltenbrand & Bailey 1959, Schaltenbrand & Wahren 1977) by Hécaen et al (1949), Hassler and Riechert (1959) and Monnier and Fischer (1951). However, lesioning this structure interfered with proprioception, carried a high incidence of postoperative neuropathic pain and, according to Mark and his group, was less effective in relieving pain than was lesioning of the medial thalamic structures (Mark et al 1960, 1961,

Table 57.5 Late results of commissural myelotomy (from Van Roost & Gybels 1989)

Author, year	*Operation level*	*Late success*		*Malignant*		*Benign*	
		%	*n*	%	*n*	%	*n*
Arutjunov 1952	Compl. C-T/T-L	87	15	87	15		
Wertheimer & Lecuire 1953	Post. T4–6	65	80				
Lembcke 1964	Compl. C2–5-T1	86	7	0	1	100	6
Sourek 1969, 1977	Compl. C4–7/T7-L1	84	38				
Grunert et al 1970	Compl. C3–T1/T-L	55	11	56	9	50	2
Broager 1974	Compl. T9–11	58	33				
Cook & Kawakami 1977	Compl. C4–T1/5-L1	20	10	67	3	0	7
King 1977	Compl. T9–11-S1	70	10	86	7	33	3
Fascendini et al 1979	Compl. T6–8-L1			17	6		
Adams et al 1982b	Compl. T2–4/low T-L-S	63	24	62	21	67	3
Goedhart et al 1984	Compl. S2–5	37.5	8	37.5	8		
Sweet & Poletti 1984a	Compl. conus	33	9	33	9		

1963, Ervin & Mark 1960, Mark & Ervin 1965). The alternatives of pontine spinothalamic section (Hitchcock 1973, 1988, Hitchcock et al 1985a,b,c) and of lesioning of the specific pain relay in the posteroinferior shell of the sensory thalamus (Hassler & Riechert 1959, Siegfried & Krayenbühl 1972, Halliday & Logue 1972, Hitchcock & Teixeira 1981, Ralston & Ralston 1992), including Hassler's parvocellular ventrocaudal nucleus (Hassler 1972), were also introduced though apparently little used.

With growing experience in stereotactic surgery, attention moved away from the specific spinothalamic tract to the non-specific pain pathway, particularly following the publications of Mark and his group (Mark et al 1960, 1961, 1963, Ervin & Mark 1960, Mark & Ervin 1965). Though Wycis and Spiegel (1962) had done a dorsomedian thalamotomy in 1947 to optimize the effect of a mesencephalic tractotomy, Hécaen et al (1949) apparently performed the first medial thalamotomy in 1949. The non-specific pathway is positioned medial to the spinothalamic tract in the midbrain, but lateral to the periaqueductal grey and has been thought at different times to relay in such medial thalamic nuclei as centrum medianum, parafascicular, intralaminar and centrolateral. The pulvinar also was used as a target, first by Kudo et al (1968) and later by others (Richardson & Zorub 1970, Fraioli & Guidette 1975, Mayanagi & Bouchard 1976/1977, Laitinen 1977).

Meanwhile, growing experience with mesencephalic tractotomy suggested that lesioning of the non-specific part of the pain pathway in the upper midbrain was most important for pain relief (Pagni 1974, Nashold et al 1974, Nashold 1982, Amano et al 1986). It was also appreciated that the non-specific part of the pain pathway projected to the hypothalamus and the limbic system (Spiegel et al 1954a,b, Willis 1985), explaining some subsequent clinical observations. As a result, the hypothalamus was identified as a target for stereotactic surgery and first used by Fairman (1972, 1973, 1976) and soon after by Sano and his colleagues (Sano 1977, 1979, Mayanagi et al 1978, Mayanagi & Sano 1988), in addition to cingulotomy.

Initially, most stereotactic pain procedures were used to treat the pain of cancer but as time went on they were also used to treat various deafferentation syndromes, raising questions as to whether the same procedures were effective in both cancer and neuropathic pain and whether it was preferable to lesion the specific or the non-specific pain pathways. However, the numbers of destructive brain operations were always smaller than in the cord, making outcome data difficult to obtain, their success less and risks greater. The frequency with which they are used was further diminished (Gybels et al 1993) by the advent of chronic stimulation of the brain (so-called deep brain stimulation (DBS)), discussed in Chapter 56, and morphine infusion discussed in Chapter 48.

INDICATIONS

Gybels and Sweet (1989) have tried to answer the question of whether there are still indications for destructive brain lesioning for the relief of pain, with the following conclusions.

1. Trigeminal nucleotomy, at either one or many levels, needs further critical evaluation before its place can be decided.
2. Published experience with bulbar and pontine spinothalamic tractotomy is limited but they may offer deep sustained high-level analgesia at a lesser risk than many other procedures.
3. Two recent long-term follow-ups from Tokyo and Duke University describe satisfactory relief of central neurogenic pain by mesencephalotomies in about two-thirds of 55 patients. The most widespread use of the procedure is pain of malignancies involving the head and neck. It competes with brain stimulation and intraventricular morphine.
4. The risks of failure and complications are significantly greater for thalamotomies than for more peripheral operations so that these should usually be reserved for patients with cancer in the head and neck and certain other selected cases.
5. Such important structures are concentrated in the hypothalamus that hypothalamotomy has little appeal to most neurosurgeons as a stereotactic target, despite the low complication rate described.
6. Appropriately placed and circumscribed frontal lobe lesions may be gratifyingly beneficial.
7. Three cases of pre- and postcentral gyrectomy for pain relief are encouraging but too few.

Gybels and Nuttin (1995) sent 215 questionnaires to the members of the European Society for Stereotactic and Functional Neurosurgery in 1994, 54 of which were completed. For cancer pain, 63 supraspinal destructive lesions were done in 1993, 51 for neuropathic pain, compared with 836 spinal procedures. Overall, they concluded: '... for the time being there are only very few indications for destructive neurosurgery at supraspinal levels for the relief of pain'.

However, the field of stereotactic surgery is constantly evolving and new and better techniques for destructive surgery are to be expected. Just as stereotactic lesion making replaced open surgery, the use of radiosurgery has the potential to make lesion making non-invasive once functional imaging becomes sufficiently accurate and the necessary equipment for radiosurgery sufficiently available. Although many functional procedures have already been done with the gamma-knife (Leksell et al 1972, Steiner et al 1980, Young et al 1994, 1995) there is still concern in the minds of most experienced functional stereotactic surgeons that physiological corroboration is necessary for optimal results and that sufficiently accurate physiological localization still depends on invasive studies.

The general principles for considering stereotactic operations for pain relief are similar to those discussed in the Introduction and under Spinal Procedures. One of the main indications is cancer pain that cannot be treated by less complex procedures, especially percutaneous cordotomy, particularly pain that is widespread or located in the upper quarter of the body, especially the head and neck. The other major indications are the central pain syndromes caused by spinal cord injury and stroke that are usually refractory to simpler measures, as well as a difficult group of conditions such as phantom and stump pain, postherpetic neuralgia and anaesthesia dolorosa.

We have seen in the discussion of indications for operations on the spinal cord that interrupting pain pathways (cordotomy, DREZ procedures, cordectomy) is useful for the relief of nociceptive pain caused by cancer and of the allodynia, hyperpathia and neuralgic pain of neuropathic syndromes, while the diffuse, steady, burning, dysaesthetic pain of neuropathic syndromes responds better to chronic stimulation that induces paraesthesiae in the area of pain. The same appears to be true, based on our experience, for destructive procedures and chronic stimulation in the brain performed for the relief of central pain of brain origin (Table 57.6), though numbers are small. In four of our patients (Parrent et al 1992) periventricular grey stimulation, which is thought to act by blocking entry of nociceptive impulses into the spinothalamic tract, suppressed allodynia and hyperpathia in stroke-induced pain while Nashold and Wilson (1966) have documented the relief of intermittent lancinating bouts of neuropathic pain caused by stroke by mesencephalic lesions. Bendok and Levy (1998) (Table 57.7), in their review of published outcome data for DBS, found that paraesthesiae-producing DBS was more effective for the relief of neuropathic pain of unspecified type, steady, diffuse pain being commonest, while DBS in periventricular or periaqueductal grey was more effective for relieving nociceptive pain.

Table 57.6 Percentage relief of three common components of central pain of brain origin by neurosurgery

Pain type	*Destructive**		*Chronic stimulation***	
	n		*n*	
Diffuse steady	10	30	18	50
Intermittent neuralgic	1	(0)	1	(100)
Allodynia, hyperpathia	12	25	5	60

* Mesencephalic tractotomy, medial thalamotomy
** Trigeminal and paraesthesiae-producing deep brain stimulation

Table 57.7 Percentage pain relief with DBS by pain type (from Bendok & Levy 1998)

Pain type	*n*	*DBS site* *PVG/PAG*	*n*	*Paraesthesiae-producing*
Nociceptive	291	59	51	0
Neuropathic	155	23	409	56

PVG/PAG = periventricular, periaqueductal grey stimulation

We interpret these observations in the following way: destructive stereotactic procedures such as mesencephalotomy and thalamotomy at various sites that interrupt pain pathways, as well as PVG/PAG DBS, relieve nociceptive pain and the allodynia, hyperpathia and neuralgic elements of neuropathic syndromes because all of these depend on transmission in pain pathways. Paraesthesiae-producing DBS is preferable for the relief of steady diffuse neuropathic pain which behaves as if it is not dependent on conduction in pain pathways (Tasker et al 1980, 1992, Tasker & Dostrovsky 1989).

LESIONS IN THE BRAINSTEM AND DIENCEPHALON

Bulbar trigeminal tractotomy and nucleotomy

The central connections of the afferent trigeminal fibres to their central sensory nuclei differ from those of any other posterior roots in that they consist of five different components extending continuously through the brainstem from the second cervical segment of the cord upward through the mesencephalon. In a caudorostral direction, these are the three nuclei of the spinal tract, the main or principal sensory nucleus and the mesencephalic sensory nucleus (Fig. 57.5). The fibres of the sensory root, upon entering the pons, traverse its basilar portion and cross dorsomedially in the direction of the main sensory nucleus. Many of the fibres then bifurcate into ascending and descending branches. Many of the latter are very long, descending as a distinct bundle, the spinal tract of the trigeminal nerve, to below the caudal end of the medulla oblongata where it merges with the dorsolateral tract of Lissauer in the spinal cord. As the fibres descend, each gives off many collaterals and finally terminals to a long small-celled nucleus, lying immediately medial to the tract, the nucleus of the spinal tract which is continuous with the gelatinous substance of the dorsal horn of the cord. The rostral parts of the tract are covered by the fibres of the brachium pontis. It is plausible to regard the main sensory nucleus as being partially homologous to the nuclei of the dorsal funiculi of the cord, concerned with tactile sensibility. The mesencephalic nucleus has been assumed to mediate proprioceptive impulses from the muscles of the jaw. Olszewski (1950) subdivides the nucleus of the spinal tract into three architectonically different portions, called the n. caudalis, interpolaris and oralis, respectively. His nucleus caudalis includes the subnucleus gelatinosus, homologous to the cord's nucleus of similar name, and he finds that it extends in man only up to 1–2 mm below the obex.

Lesions have been placed at different levels in this trigeminal complex by making a cut, originally at the level between the middle and inferior thirds of the eminentia olivaris, 8–10 mm cranial to the inferior end of the fourth ventricle, 3–3.5 mm deep (Sjögvist 1938), but it is not clear as to how far rostrally in man one may need to extend trigeminal tractotomy and nucleotomy in order to destroy the all-important substantia gelatinosa of the n. caudalis.

Hitchcock and Schvarcz (Hitchcock & Schvarcz 1972) were the neurosurgeons who first described making stereotactically placed RF lesions in the secondary afferent neurons of the descending cephalic pain pathway in the nucleus caudalis. The discussion about this intervention is nicely illustrated by a case history which was discussed in the 1996 issue of *Controversies in neurosurgery*.

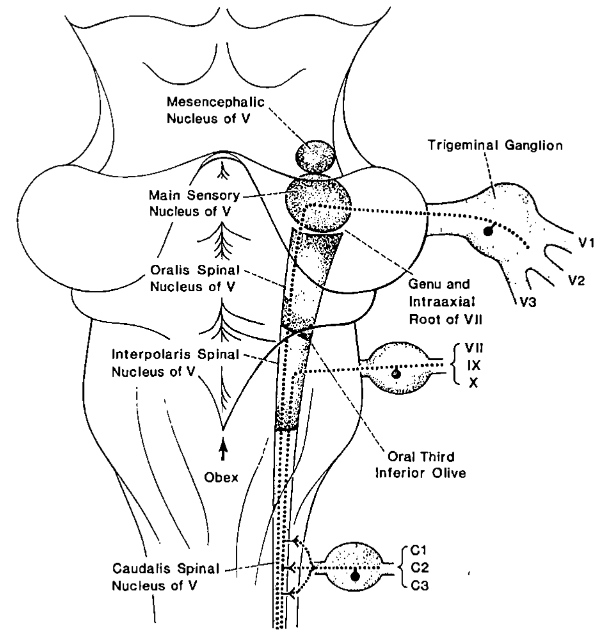

Fig. 57.5 Topography of brainstem trigeminal nuclei. Levels of boundary zones of subnuclei are indicated. (Reproduced from Gybels & Sweet 1989 with permission.)

The case (Gybels 1996) A 50-year-old man underwent resection of a petroclival meningioma. Three months after surgery, he began to have facial pain, which was persistent and increasing, associated with dysaesthesia and intractable to all forms of medical treatment. This pain deeply affected his life and performance.

Surgeon A (J. Schvarcz) What should not be done in this case? No further peripheral denervation. My first choice of neurosurgical treatment would be radiofrequency lesions stereotactically placed in the nucleus caudalis of the trigeminal system. I have performed over 200 nucleotomies. In a consecutive series of 141 patients with deafferentation pain, with follow-up from 1 to 16 years, abolition of the allodynia and a significant reduction or, less frequently, a complete abolition of the deep background pain was obtained in 72.6% of the cases without lasting side effects.

Surgeon B (K. Burchiel) It is very unlikely that this pain will respond to further peripheral denervation. Overall, the chance of a tractotomy or caudalis nucleotomy producing satisfactory relief is about 75%. Almost 100% of the patients will experience an undesired deficit of some sort, with debilitating limb ataxia in 10% and disabling contralateral limb sensory loss in 15% of the patients. One of the guiding principles for the management of difficult pain problems has to do with the Hippocratic oath: *Primum non nocere*. For all these reasons, this man should have a trial of deep brain stimulation, prior to consideration of an ablative operation. The probability that deep brain stimulation will help his pain is 50% and the risk to him is about 15%.

Multiple lesions of descending cephalic pain tract and nucleus caudalis DREZ lesions

Nashold (Bernard et al 1987) performed the first nucleus caudalis DREZ in 1982 by making a row of lesions in the axis of the spinal grey column and Lissauer's tract extending from the uppermost C_2 dorsal root up to or slightly above the level of the obex. The lesions are of course distant from the entry zones of the roots V, VII, IX and X and referring to them as DREZ lesions perhaps obscures the difference between them and the truly DREZ lesions in the spinal cord. The Duke experience, with 46 nucleus caudalis DREZ coagulations performed during the preceding 5 years with a mean follow-up of 32 months, was reviewed retrospectively (Gorecki et al 1995). It turned out that:

> *Nucleus caudalis DREZ coagulation eliminates pain in the long term in a small number of patients with neural injury pain. Fewer than half of the patients who underwent this procedure indicated that they had obtained enough benefit to do it again. A similar number described improved quality of life. Patients must understand the risk of complications, which affect nearly half of the patients. The complications can be more disturbing to the patient than is immediately apparent on physical testing, particularly since most patients are seeking the elimination of discomfort. Although side effects diminish with time, there is a high incidence of persisting deficit, at least as perceived and described by the patients.*

Bulbar and pontine spinothalamic tractotomy

In the medulla oblongata the spinothalamic tract runs relatively superficially between the dorsolateral surface of the inferior olive ventrally and the descending or trigeminal cephalic pain tract dorsally. It courses more deeply in the pons until the anterior border of the brachium pontis is reached; at this point it runs dorsally to occupy a more superficial position in the mesencephalon.

Only a limited number of open bulbar spinothalamic tractotomies have been reported (White & Sweet 1969). Cassinari and Pagni (1969) collected about 60 cases in the literature, mostly cancer cases with a short life expectancy, and commented that it was rare for central pain to occur after bulbar spinothalamic tractotomy. They suggested this low incidence of central pain might be due to the fact that the surgical incision interrupts the spinoreticular fibres which run intermingled with the spinothalamic fibres before the spinoreticular fibres reach the nucleus gigantocellularis of Olszewski in the bulbar reticular formation.

In 1973 Hitchcock introduced stereotactic spinothalamic tractotomy at the pontine level. He chose this level reasoning that a lesion of the spinothalamic tract here should provide a high level of analgesia without too great a risk to respiration, micturition and upward gaze. Published experience with this procedure is limited but according to Hitchcock et al (1985a), it may offer deep, sustained, high-level analgesia at lesser risk than many other procedures.

Stereotactic mesencephalic tractotomy and thalamotomy

Destructive lesioning of the mesencephalic pain tract and of various nuclei in the thalamus has been used almost interchangeably in the treatment of chronic pain using the indications outlined under Introduction and under Indications for this portion of the chapter. Most published experience relates to mesencephalic tractotomy and medial thalamotomy. Frank et al (1987) compared the two procedures for the relief of cancer pain. In their hands, mesencephalotomy achieved 83.5% relief at the expense of a 1.8% mortality and a 10.1% complication rate, while medial thalamotomy yielded 57.9% pain relief, with a tendency towards pain recurrence, with no mortality and a low morbidity mainly in the form of transient cognitive problems.

Technique for stereotactic brain operations

Conventional destructive stereotactic surgery employs the same principles whatever the target. A suitable stereotactic frame, preferably MRI compatible, is applied to the patient's head and the three-dimensional co-ordinates of anterior and posterior commissures are determined using the scanner software. The location of the target is then extrapolated from these landmarks using suitable sagittal atlas plates such as those from the Schaltenbrand and Bailey (1959) and the Schaltenbrand and Wahren (1977) atlases. It is convenient to use a computer software program adaptable to a personal computer to shrink or expand the atlas plates until they match the anterior commissure–posterior commissure distance of the patient being operated on (Tasker & Dostrovsky 1992). The stereotactic co-ordinates are then read off the modified atlas diagram and applied to the stereotactic frame. In some situations, landmarks other than the two commissures may be used as in pontine spinothalamic tractotomy while the cingulumotomy target is clearly visible on the MR scan so that its co-ordinates can be determined directly as they are for stereotactic biopsy. The target is then approached through a burr or twist-drill hole made in the same sagittal plane as the target so that all electrode trajectories and physiological data collected can be plotted on the same sagittal diagram, facilitating their evaluation. The physiological data collected depend on the target.

Mesencephalic tractotomy

Technique

For mesencephalic tractotomy, the three-dimensional co-ordinates of the mesencephalic spinothalamic tract are read off the computer-revised 9 mm sagittal atlas diagram and a twist-drill or burr hole is made 9 mm from the midline, followed by either macro- or microstimulation carried out sequentially as the electrode is introduced towards the expected location of the spinothalamic tract. Though Amano et al (1978) have reported recording of nociceptive neurons in the area, this is a difficult undertaking and we have relied on the identification of the spinothalamic tract, which lies 6–9 mm from the midline, and of the medial lemniscus, which lies 10–12 mm from the midline, in dorsal mesencephalon by the differential effects of stimulation (Tasker 1976). Stimulating the medial lemniscus at threshold evokes a somatotopographically organized sensation of contralateral paraesthesiae while stimulating the spinothalamic tract evokes similarly disposed feelings of warmth or cold. Stimulating, presumably, the spinoreticulothalamic tract lying between the 6 mm sagittal plane and the periaqueductal grey does not evoke conscious effects except by volume conduction.

Once the spinothalamic tract is outlined one or more radiofrequency lesions are made to encompass it using an electrode 1.1 mm in diameter with a 3 mm bare tip, beginning at 25 mA achieving temperatures below 70°C and gradually increasing to about 65 mA and 90°C. Degree of analgesia produced and neurological function are monitored continually. The lesion is extended medially to the acqueduct, sparing the medial lemniscus (Nashold et al 1977). Analgesia should be expected in the contralateral half of the body, particularly in its upper portion. Although initially the patient may exhibit difficulty in moving the contralateral limbs, this deficit disappears within hours. Figure 57.6 demonstrates left mesencephalic tractotomy as shown in MRI scanning and Figure 57.7 shows a mesencephalotomy (in a different patient) and medial thalamotomy lesion at autopsy, the physiological localization data and the sensory loss produced. Mesencephalic tractotomy is more effective for the relief of nociceptive pain caused by cancer than of neuropathic pain in most authors' experience, as shown in Table 57.8, though our own experience (see Table 57.6) suggests that destructive surgery, including mesencephalic tractotomy, may be effective for the neuralgic and evoked elements of neuropathic pain. Table 57.8 also suggests that mesencephalic tractotomy is more effective than medial thalamotomy.

Results

Table 57.8 reviews published outcome data for mesencephalic tractotomy with 80–85% reported relief of nociceptive (mostly cancer) pain compared with 27–36% of neuropathic pain at the expense of a 5–10% mortality and a 15–20% incidence of dysaesthesiae and oculomotor deficits. A recent report by Amano et al (1992) underlines the safety of the procedure in their hands, as does the recent report of Frank et al (1987) and Frank and Fabrizi (1997) listing 40 cases operated on between 1990 and 1996, six bilaterally, in whom only five incidences of Parinaud's syndrome and two of mild dysaesthesia occurred.

In contrast to our poorer results and those of others in the treatment of neuropathic pain, Amano et al (1986)

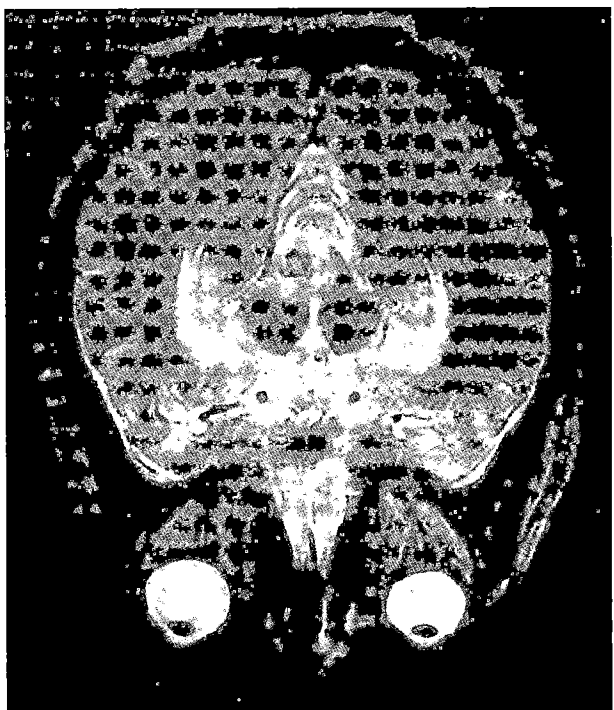

Fig. 57.6 MRI scan on the same day as a left stereotactic radiofrequency mesencephalic tractotomy in a young woman with recurrent neurofibrosarcoma of the right brachial plexus. She suffered from excruciating pain chiefly in the right upper extremity, mostly of a nociceptive type but with some elements of neuropathic pain associated with the sensory loss from her lesion. She was desperate despite 100 MS-Contin hourly plus Dilaudid infusion of 75 mg an hour plus boluses as necessary. The mesencephalic tractotomy initially relieved her pain and induced cold analgesia and pinprick hypalgesia of the right half of the body except for the head and neck; there was slight reduction of appreciation of pinprick in the right first division trigeminal territory. She survived 8 months after having required a ventriculoperitoneal shunt for hydrocephalus of unknown origin 1 month after her operation and developing cord compression from recurrent sarcoma 4 months after her tractotomy. Her pain gradually recurred but was well controlled with Dilaudid infusion reaching 60 mg per hour 4 months postoperatively.

found 64% good long-term results in 28 patients with this type of pain while Shieff and Nashold (1987, 1988) were successful in relieving 67% of 27 patients with stroke-induced pain with an 8% mortality (see Table 57.8). We do not have descriptions of the types of pain syndromes involved in these patients and the explanation for the discrepancy is unclear. We must await further evidence supporting this encouraging experience in a most refractory condition.

Medial thalamotomy

Technique

The 'non-specific' medial thalamic nuclei targeted in pain surgery cannot be easily identified by physiological means,

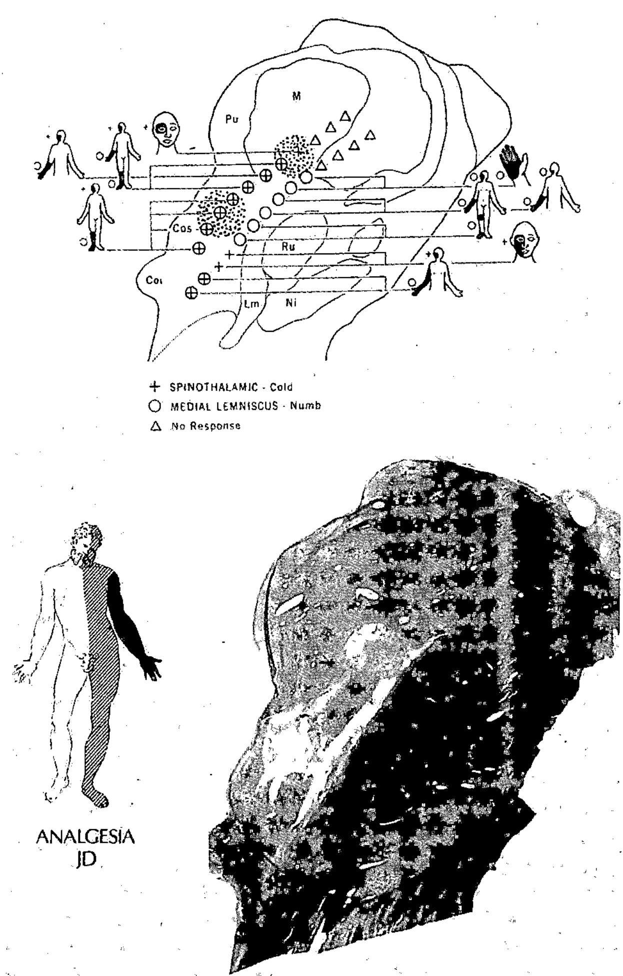

Fig. 57.7 Lower right Sagittal section 9 mm from midline made at autopsy of the midbrain and thalamus of a man with recurrent carcinoma of the lower posterior gingiva initially treated by X-ray therapy. There was local recurrence with invasion of lymph nodes and excruciating pain of the left mandible, ear, temple, throat, tongue and neck associated with dysphagia and trismus. Radiofrequency lesions were made stereotactically in the right mesencephalic spinothalamic tract and the junction of the right centrum medianum and parafascicular nucleus. He survived 4 months during which time he complained only of mild ache on the vertex of the skull and over the cervical thoracic spine. The figurine at lower left demonstrates the sensory loss produced, which consisted of incomplete left hemianalgesia and hemithermanalgesia except for the left upper extremity where the sensory loss was complete to clinical testing. There was no interference with appreciation of touch, position or vibration sense. The upper portion of the diagram plots a reconstruction of the physiological data obtained by macrostimulation for corroboration of the target sites. The hatched areas represent the lesions, the triangles, crosses and circles the sites stimulated every 2.0 mm along two parasagittal trajectories. Empty circles represent sites where contralateral paraesthesiae were produced, crosses sites where contralateral cold sensations were induced. Circles with crosses indicate sites where both responses occurred; triangles indicate sites where no response was reported with up to 3 volts stimulation. The small figurine charts plot the projected fields of these responses. Pu = pulvinar; M = dorsomedian nucleus; Cos, Coi = superior and inferior colliculi; Lm = medial lemniscus; Ru = red nucleus; Ni = substantia nigra.

Table 57.8 Percentage useful pain relief and complications after stereotactic destructive brain lesions for relief of chronic pain

Lesion site	Neuropathic pain (unspecified) No. of cases	Pain relief	Complications	Nociceptive pain No. of cases	Pain relief	Complications
Ventrocaudal ± medial thalamic nuclei, unilateral	56*	32	32	31	77	32
Medial thalamus						
Uni- or bilateral	47**	29	4–21	175	46	7
	69***	67				
Pulvinar						
Uni- or bilateral	18*	22	5	26	88	21
Hypothalamus						
Uni- or bilateral	5*	0	0	12	67	0
Mesencephalic tractotomy	****	27		****	80	5–10% mortality 15–20% dysaesthesia 15–20% oculomotor for all 92 cases
	150*****	36		270	85	0–8% mortality 27% complications for all 420 cases
	28******	64				
	27*******	67				8% mortality

* Tasker 1982b
** Tasker 1984
*** Jeanmonod et al 1994
**** 92 cases overall (Tasker 1984)
***** Gybels & Sweet 1989
****** Amano et al 1986
******* Shieff and Nashold 1988

though Sano et al (1970) were able to record nociceptive neurons in the internal thalamic lamina. In most centres localization depends on mapping the position of these nuclei relative to the commissures or to the ventrocaudal nucleus, as discussed below. Lesions are made as in mesencephalotomy. There is, however, little consensus upon which of the various medial thalamic nuclei constitute the optimal target. Figure 57.7 illustrates a combined medial thalamotomy-mesencephalic tractotomy lesion. The triangles illustrate sites where stimulation induced no response in the medial thalamus, though some responses occurred inferiorly from volume conduction to the medial lemniscus and the spinothalamic tract, current spread being estimated to be up to 2–3 mm radius with the microstimulation used. Figure 57.8 illustrates a medial thalamotomy in sagittal MRI scan 3 days postoperatively.

Results

Medial thalamotomy presumably interrupts pain transmission in the non-specific spinoreticulothalamic tract and would therefore be expected to relieve nociceptive pain, particularly that caused by cancer, but not the diffuse, steady, burning dysaesthetic element of neuropathic pain felt in a part of the body where sensation has been altered. Literature reviews support this notion, as shown in Table 57.8, with a 46% incidence of useful relief of nociceptive pain compared with 29% of neuropathic pain. This is considerably less successful than the 80–85% relief reported after mesencephalotomy but the poorer outcome is compensated for by the lower complication rate: 4–21% of usually transient problems after medial thalamotomy compared with the 5–10% mortality and 15–27% incidence of dysaesthesia and also of oculomotor dysfunction after mesencephalotomy.

Against these older sobering data, Jeanmonod et al (1993, 1994) (see Table 57.8) have recently reported that 67% of patients in two series of 45 and 69 individuals respectively suffering from neuropathic pain enjoyed 50–100% relief after lesioning of the centrolateral nucleus. The explanation for this discrepancy is unclear. Choice of target, more modern technique, different selection of patients could all be factors. For example, if a patient with neuropathic pain had a large component of neuralgic or allodynic pain, one would expect a better result than for diffuse steady pain. They do state that they guide their lesioning by targeting bursting cells in the medial thalamus which they

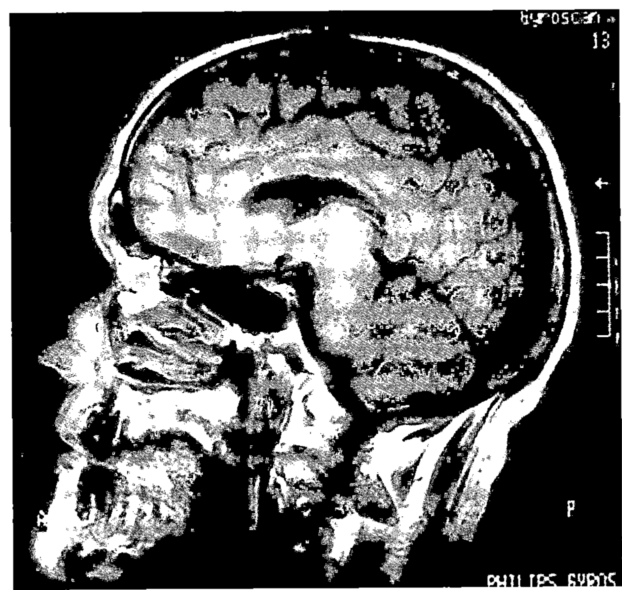

Fig. 57.8 Sagittal MRI scan of a man who had undergone a right medial thalamotomy for intractable pain in the left leg and abdomen of uncertain origin 3 days before. No neurological including somatosensory deficit ensued and the pain was not relieved.

regard as markers of deafferentation neuronal hypersensitivity and pain generators.

The issue of bursting cells

Jeanmonod et al (1994, 1996) and Rinaldi et al (1991) have drawn attention to the presence of bursting cells in the medial thalamus, considering them markers of neuropathic pain (see the discussion under the DREZ procedure). However, different interpretations can be put on their observations. We have found bursting cells frequently in the thalamus in deafferented patients whether or not neuropathic pain is also present and consider them to be markers not of pain but of deafferentation. Moreover, bursting cells occur normally in the awake state in the medial thalamus as well as more extensively during sleep.

Our own personal experience with the results of medial thalamotomy and mesencephalotomy in both nociceptive and neuropathic pain is less encouraging than the reports of many authors (see Table 57.8).

Gamma-knife medial thalamotomy

Young et al (1995) report 24 gamma-knife thalamotomies for intractable pain, 15 of whom have been followed for an average of 12 months; 27% were virtually pain free at follow-up and 33% enjoyed more than 50% relief. In another publication (Young et al 1994) concerning 10 patients, four of whom suffered from pain caused by spinal disorders, two with postherpetic neuralgia, one with spinal cord injury, one with 'thalamic syndrome', one with facial anaesthesia dolorosa and one with brainstem infarction, three enjoyed excellent and four good pain relief without complications. Particularly careful evaluations of radiothalamotomy will be necessary in order to compare efficacy and safety with that of conventional techniques in view of the current inadequacies of imaging studies.

Basal thalamotomy

The tactile relay of the thalamus in the ventrocaudal nucleus, which also relays nociceptive information, is no longer lesioned in attempts to relieve pain because of the associated high complication rate (see Table 57.8); rather, it is a prime target for insertion of DBS electrodes. Tantalizingly, however, the 'microthalamotomy' effect of implanting a DBS electrode temporarily may abolish the pain where formal thalamotomy and even DBS may fail. This nucleus is readily identified by either macrostimulation, microstimulation or microelectrode recording (Tasker et al 1987, Lenz et al 1988) and its location used to determine the site of adjacent non-responsive structures such as the medial thalamus. Stimulation elicits contralateral specifically somatotopographically organized paraesthesiae (projected fields (PFs)) while recording identifies neurons with receptive tactile fields (RFs) in the same area as the PFs.

The body is represented in the tactile relay nucleus in a medial to lateral homunculus with intraoral representation abutting against the medial thalamic nuclei about 11–12 mm from the midline, the foot against the internal capsule about 18 mm from the midline. In the posteroinferior corner of ventrocaudal nucleus, particularly in the 14–16 mm sagittal plane, a parasagittally directed electrode passing from anterodorsally to posteroinferiorly will encounter an abrupt change in the quality of the PFs from paraesthesiae to ones with hot, cold or sometimes painful sensations. The somatotopographic organization changes just as abruptly. Often as the electrode progresses through the ventrocaudal nucleus, paraesthetic responses are typically found over long distances referred to the contralateral upper limb until the basal area is reached, when they may abruptly switch to the contralateral lower limb. It is in this posteroinferior rim region (Tasker 1976b) that lesions produce contralateral dissociated sensory loss and may be effective for the relief of chronic pain (Hassler & Riechert 1959, Hassler 1972, Siegfried & Krayenbühl 1972, Halliday & Logue 1972, Hitchcock & Teixeira 1981, Tasker et al 1982). Though the results are encouraging, numbers are small so that conclusions concerning the usefulness of this procedure are difficult to make.

Pulvinarotomy

The pulvinar is an enigmatic nucleus whose involvement in pain perception is unclear; Willis (1985) does not include it in his monograph reviewing the pathophysiology of pain. In general, reported experience is limited (Kudo et al 1968, Richardson & Zorub 1970, Laitinen 1977, Yoshii et al 1980, 1990, Tasker 1982b, Gybels & Sweet 1989, Whittle and Jenkinson 1995) and suggests that pulvinarotomy is more effective for the relief of cancer than of neuropathic pain and that the pain relief tends to be short-lived. Autopsy studies (Tasker 1982b) suggest that the supranucleus of the pulvinar is the preferable target choice. A personal literature review (see Table 57.8) suggested 81% of patients with cancer pain enjoyed short-term relief whereas only 22% of those with neuropathic pain did so.

Hypothalamotomy

Spiegel et al (1954b) suggested that the hypothalamus played a role in pain processing. The hypothalamic target is located 2–5 mm lateral to the third ventricle wall in the triangle defined by the mid-point of the anterior commissure–posterior commissure line, mamillary body and posterior commissure where stimulation causes elevation of the blood pressure and pulse rate, dilatation of pupils and may cause neck tilting and EEG desynchronization (Sano 1977, 1979).

Fairman (1972, 1973, 1976) reported relief of pain in 76% of 54 patients with cancer following hypothalamotomy with only 10% transient complications. Sano (1977) operated on 20 patients. None of the seven with neuropathic pain did well, but nine of the 13 with cancer pain (69%) did so. Other published experience is similar (Mayanagi et al 1978, Sano 1979, Moser et al 1980, Tasker 1982b, Mayanagi & Sano 1988, Levin 1993). A personal literature review (see Table 57.8) suggested a two-thirds chance of relief of cancer pain but a tendency for postoperative pain recurrence. Sano's target (144) was thought to be the projection site of A∂ fibres and subsequent studies have confirmed a spinohypothalamic pain pathway.

Pituitary ablation

Hypophyseal ablation has long been used in the treatment of hormone-dependent cancer and the pain that accompanies it. The introduction of alcohol into the pituitary gland (Moricca 1974, 1976) has greatly simplified the procedure and reduced its impact on sick patients. A cannula is introduced through one nasal passage across the sphenoid sinus and through the anterior wall or floor of the sella turcica until it is confirmed radiologically to lie in the hypophysis. The procedure can also be done stereotactically (Levin 1988). Increments of 0.1 ml of absolute alcohol to a total of 2.0 ml are injected at one or multiple sites while neurological responses are monitored. Not only is the pain of hormone-dependent cancer relieved (41–95% short-term) but also that of non-hormone dependent cancer (69%). Pain tends to recur after 3–4 months and complications include: mortality (2–6.5%), CSF rhinorrhoea (3–20%), meningitis (0.3–1%), visual and oculomotor deficits (2–10%), diabetes insipidus (5–60%).

Levin (1988) found a 75–94% incidence of relief of cancer pain in a literature review while in his own 110 patients, 73–97% were relieved depending on the type of cancer being treated. Pain tended to recur and even in those patients enjoying relief, pain exacerbations occurred frequently postoperatively. There was only one incidence of CSF rhinorrhoea in his series, six of oculomotor palsies with or without visual field defects.

Various studies have failed to reveal a mechanism of pain relief from this procedure.

LESIONS IN THE TELENCEPHALON

Pre- and postcentral gyrectomy

White and Sweet summarized results of postcentral gyrectomy up to 1969 in their classic treatise on pain. Of 30 early successes in 38 cases from 23 centres, only seven persisted with pain relief at 10 or more months. Since that time, only a few cases have been reported. Three have been published in which pre- and postcentral gyrectomy was performed with pain relief without disfiguring motor deficit in the face in two cases (Lende et al 1971) or further sensory or motor deficit (Sano 1977). Longest follow-up was 20 months. With this limited evidence, pre- and postcentral gyrectomy has to be considered as experimental neurosurgery.

Limbic surgery

In this section, the emphasis will be placed on cingulotomy for the following reasons: important series with long-term follow-up and quantitative outcome data are available and the procedure is actually being used. However, there are other approaches to the limbic system such as subcaudate tractotomy and anterior capsulotomy. Their efficacy and safety in psychiatric disease, and in particular obsessive compulsive disorder, has been well established (Cosyns et al 1994), but there are not enough long-term data to substantiate their role in the treatment of pain. The interested reader can find much information in Gybels and Sweet (1989) and Bouckoms (1994).

Following early interventions of removal of the anterior 4 cm in the cingulate gyri on each side, Foltz and White (1962) began in 1955 to make stereotactically electrical lesions in the white matter of the anterior cingulum in patients with a primary complaint of severe pain but with superimposed major anxiety, depression or emotional lability. By 1966 they could report in 26 patients 22 excellent and good results, i.e. no or only occasional mention of pain.

Ballantine began in 1962 to use stereotactic methods to make similar lesions. This he has since developed into one of the largest series in the world of 485 patients treated by limited frontal white matter lesions for affective psychoses and/or pain. Because of the controversy in the late 1960s and early 1970s with respect to psychosurgery, he enlisted the interest of the world-famous psychologists at the MIT under the leadership of Teuber (Teuber et al 1977). They studied patients in an MIT clinical research centre which was geographically, administratively and financially independent of the psychiatrists, neurologists and neurosurgeons who were clinically responsible for the patients. They studied patients intensively before and after operation, each patient serving as his own control. In addition, a psychiatrist and a neurologist not involved in the patient's care assessed the patient's status and the adequacy of the previous therapies as one of the prerequisites to the cingulotomy. Patients, relatives and close friends were interviewed and a full day was devoted to psychological and other testing in the week before the operation. The follow-up assessments were even more extensive, involving a 3- or 4-day admission to the MIT centre. A substantial series of reports describes the results of 85 exhaustively studied cingulotomy patients – 26 of them for pain. In an initial group of 16 patients, the late result was of marked improvement in nine and moderate in three. The most striking result is that for some years not one of the extensive battery of performance tests and other studies revealed any postoperative 'visible impairment of the patient's capacity to perform a wide variety of tasks in the laboratory or in real life' (Teuber et al 1977). Recently two esoteric tests have revealed small postoperative deficits only in those over 30 years of age. Corkin (1980) has provided a summary of this massive documentation.

In the 23 years ending September 1987, Ballantine et al (1987) had carried out their bilateral cingulotomy in 139 patients for the treatment of chronic pain. Their RF lesions in the anterior supracollosal white matter, as assessed by postoperative CT scans, are in the coronal plane 2.5 cm posterior to the anterior tips of the lateral ventricles. Each lesion is a cylinder about 2 cm high and 1 cm in diameter, made by a temperature of 80–85°C for 100 seconds (Figs 57.9, 57.10).

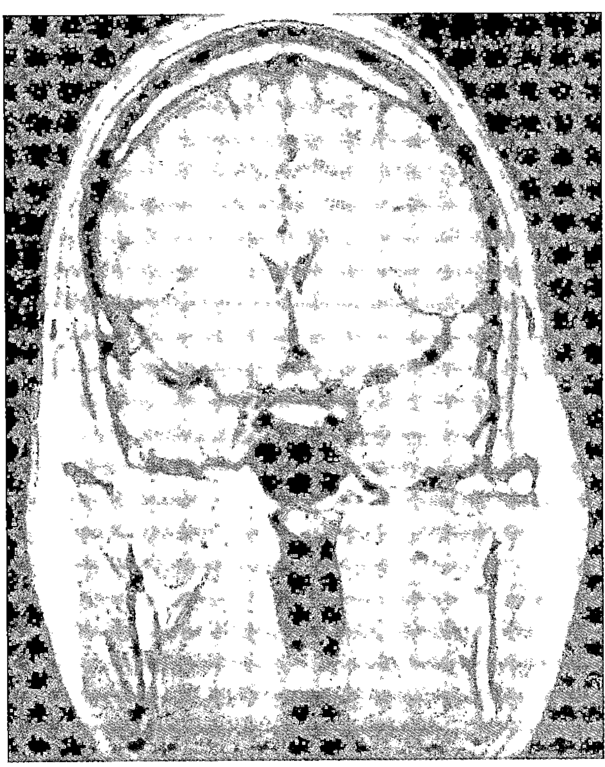

Fig. 57.9 Coronal MRI view of bilateral radiofrequency cingulotomy lesion.

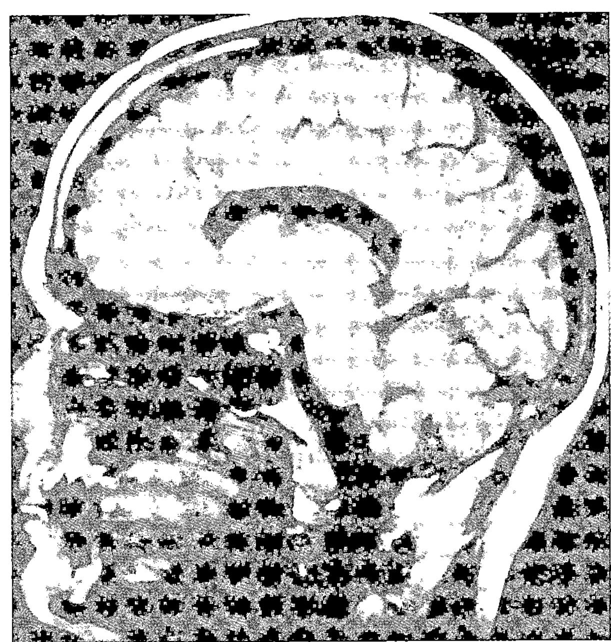

Fig. 57.10 Sagittal MRI view of same patient as in Fig. 57.9.

'Severe persistent, disabling pain refractory to all commonly accepted treatments' was the primary indication for the operation, with the presence of clinical depression as a factor also favouring its choice. There were no 'postoperative deaths and the only serious complication was a severe Landry – Guillain – Barré syndrome (idiopathic polyneuritis)'. Of the 35 patients with terminal cancer, 25 lived 3 months or less; 57% of them had moderate to complete relief. Only two of the 10 who survived more than 3 months had such relief. Of the 95 patients with non-malignant pain followed for 1–21 years and an average of 7 years after operation, the pain in 61 was related to the 'failed low back syndrome'. Complete or marked pain relief was sustained in 26% and moderate relief continued in another 36% of this difficult group. In this same group, four other patients later committed suicide; three of them had carried the diagnosis of clinical depression. In six patients with persistent abdominal and flank pain after abdominal surgery, moderate or better relief was maintained in five. Of five patients with pain in a phantom limb, there was one each in the complete, marked and moderate relief category, whereas in the six postherpetics there was only one with moderate relief. In 17 others in six miscellaneous categories, only three had moderate or marked relief.

In a more recent small series (Pillay & Hassenbusch 1992) of 10 patients, eight with metastatic lesions with musculoskeletal (6) or neurogenic (2) pain, neurofibromatosis (1) and after post-stroke thalamic pain (1), results were excellent in four, good in two, fair in one and poor in three. In the two cases with neurogenic pain from non-malignant origin, pain relief after 1 year follow-up was excellent in the neurofibromatosis case, poor in the thalamic case. This latter series was operated using MRI guidance. Target was 2 cm behind the tip of the frontal horn of the lateral ventricles.

Judging from postoperative MRI scans (Ballantine et al 1995), these bilateral lesions were situated in the cingulum in front of area 24. This is of interest in view of recent functional imaging studies with PET or MRI showing multiple regions of the human cerebral cortex being activated by noxious stimuli and in persistent pain (Talbot et al 1991). In one such study (Rainville et al 1997), in order to differentiate cortical areas involved in pain affect, hypnotic suggestions were used to alter selectively the unpleasantness of noxious stimuli, which showed changes in the perceived intensity. PET revealed significant changes in pain-evoked activity within the anterior cingulate cortex, consistent with the encoding of perceived unpleasantness, whereas primary somatosensory cortex activation was unaltered (Fig. 57.11). These findings provide direct experimental evidence linking frontal lobe limbic activity with pain affect, as was strongly suggested by the careful clinical studies. In another PET study, Hsieh et al (1995) showed that the posterior section of the right anterior cingulate cortex (ACC),

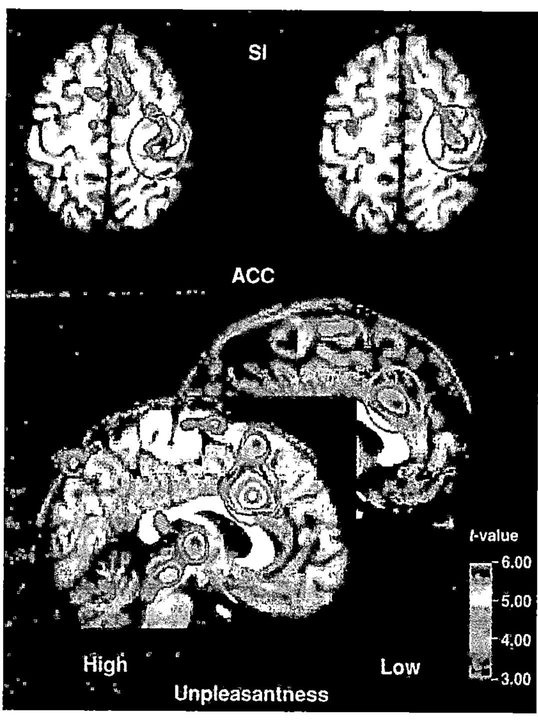

Fig. 57.11 Changes in pain-related activity associated with hypnotic suggestions of high and low unpleasantness (left and right images, respectively) are revealed by subtracting PET data recorded during the neutral/hypnosis control condition from those of the painfully hot/-UNP and painfully hot/-UNP conditions. PET data, averaged across 11 experimental sessions, are illustrated against an MRI from one person; horizontal and saggittal slices through S1 and ACC, respectively, are centred at the activation peaks observed during the relevant suggestion conditions; red circles indicate the location and size of VOIs used to analyse activation levels across the two conditions. UNP = hypnotic suggestion for increased (+) or decreased (–) unpleasantness; VOI = volume of interest. (Reproduced from Rainville et al 1997 with permission.) (see colour plate)

corresponding to Brodmann area 24, was activated in ongoing neuropathic pain, regardless of the side of the painful mononeuropathy; the experiments confirmed that the ACC participates in the sensorial/affectional aspect of the pain experience but there was also a strong suggestion, and this is the new exciting finding, that there is a possible right hemispheric lateralization of the ACC for affective processing in chronic ongoing neuropathic pain. Based on the experience from frontal lobe lesions, and more specifically cingulotomies, for the treatment of psychiatric disorders, as far as we are able to assess, cingulotomies for persistent pain have always been bilateral.

In 1989, Gybels and Sweet summarized their discussion of cingulotomy as follows:

> *The principal conclusion of practical importance from this long-term critical study is that cingulotomy for low back pain secondary to multiple operative interventions and/or*

arachnoiditis is a valuable addition to the armamentarium. Despite the uneasiness in the USA about malpractice actions following such surgery these operations continue at the Massachusetts General Hospital under the rigorous conditions of patient selection and care described, because they have a proven place in the treatment repertoire. The unequivocal absence of anything approaching significant deficit of basic function and the low complication rate of the stereotactic procedure are particularly attractive. We would precede any performance of cingulotomy in such cases by a full range of non-destructive operations.

We think this conclusion still holds.

Since this type of surgery is called by many, we think wrongly, 'psychosurgery' and operations in the brain for psychiatric disorders are the most controversial biological treatment in psychiatry, it seems wise, at least in cases of persistent pain of non-cancer origin, to follow the same decision-making procedure for limbic surgery for pain as for limbic surgery in psychiatric disorders and to consider the following requirements.

- A review board is a necessary part of the decision-making process and functions as a third opinion for the patient and for his or her therapist, who submits the case for review.
- Limbic surgery is an acceptable treatment for the actual condition of the patient (accuracy of diagnosis and intensity of patient's suffering).
- All adequate therapeutic measures have been applied and have proved to be ineffective.
- The proposed target in the brain is adequate.
- The proposed neurosurgeon and surgical unit are competent to perform the planned stereotactic intervention.
- Adequate preoperative and postoperative evaluation and treatment are available.
- The patient, the nearest relative and the therapist will consent to the treatment after being giving adequate information.

CONCLUSION

It is difficult to decide whether any supraspinal destructive procedure is cost effective today, keeping in mind the criteria outlined in the Introduction. For the relief of cancer pain, such procedures were always sparingly employed compared with destructive procedures in the spinal cord and now, with the advent of morphine infusion, the indications must be few. Whether technical advances will retain a role for procedures such as mesencephalotomy, cingulotomy and pituitary ablation with alcohol will depend upon semiquantitative comparisons along the lines outlined in the Introduction.

For non-cancer, particularly central, pain, decision making is even more difficult since the consensus has been that neither destructive brain lesioning nor more conservative techniques were very effective in its treatment. In view of the otherwise unrelieved, hideous suffering of some patients in this category, the low success and risks of destructive procedures on the brain sometimes seemed acceptable. It is hoped that further semiquantitative trials will confirm the unusual success of several recent series of stroke-induced pain, presumably based on improved techniques.

REFERENCES

Albe-Fessard D, Lombard MC 1983 Use of an animal model to evaluate the origin of and protection against deafferentation pain. In: Bonica JJ et al (eds) Advances in Pain Research and Therapy, vol 5. Raven, New York, pp 691–700

Amano K, Tanikawa T, Iseki H et al 1978 Single neuron analysis of the human midbrain tegmentum. Rostral mesencephalic reticulotomy for pain relief. Applied Neurophysiology 41: 66–78

Amano K, Kawamura H, Tanikawa T 1986 Long-term follow-up study of rostral mesencephalic reticulotomy and pain relief – report of 34 cases. Applied Neurophysiology 49: 105–111

Amano K, Kawamura H, Tanikawa T et al 1991 Bilateral versus unilateral percutaneous high cervical cordotomy as a surgical method of pain relief. Acta Neurochirurgica (Wien) 52(suppl): 143–145

Amano K, Kawamura H, Tanikawa T, Kawabatake H, Iseki H, Taira T 1992 Stereotactic mesencephalotomy for pain relief. A plea for stereotactic surgery. Stereotactic and Functional Neurosurgery 59: 25–32

Armour D 1927 Surgery of the spinal cord and its membranes. Lancet 1: 691–697

Ballantine HT, Bouckoms AJ, Thomas EK et al 1987 Treatment of psychiatric illness by stereotactic cingulotomy. Biological Psychiatry 22: 807–819

Ballantine HT, Cosgrove R, Giriunas I 1995 Surgical treatment of intractable psychiatric illness and chronic pain by stereotactic cingulotomy. In: Schmidek H, Sweet W (eds) Operative neurosurgical techniques: indications, methods and results, 3rd edn. WB Saunders, Philadelphia, pp 1423–1430

Belmusto L, Woldring S, Owens G 1965 Localization and patterns of potentials of the respiratory pathways in the cervical spinal cord in the dog. Journal of Neurosurgery 22: 277–283

Bendok B, Levy RM 1998 Brain stimulation for persistent pain management. In: Gildenberg PL, Tasker RR (eds) Textbook of stereotactic and functional neurosurgery. McGraw-Hill, New York, pp 1539–1546

Berkley KJ 1997 On the dorsal columns: translating basic research hypotheses to the clinic. Pain 70: 103–107

Bernard EJ, Nashold BS, Caputi F et al 1987 Nucleus caudalis DREZ lesions for facial plain. British Journal of Neurosurgery 1: 81–92

Bouckoms AJ 1994 Limbic surgery for pain. In: Wall PD, Melzack R (eds) Textbook of pain, 3rd edn. Churchill Livingstone, Edinburgh, pp 1171–1187

Bowsher D 1988 Contralateral mirror-image pain following anterolateral cordotomy. Pain 33: 63–65

Bronec PR, Nashold BS Jr 1990 Dorsal root entry zone lesions for pain. In: Youmans JR (ed) Neurological surgery. A comprehensive reference guide to the diagnosis and management of neurosurgical problems. WB Saunders, Philadelphia, pp 4036–4044

Campbell JN, Solomon CT, James CS 1988 The Hopkins experience with lesions of the dorsal horn (Nashold's operation) for pain from avulsion of the brachial plexus. Applied Neurophysiology 51: 170–174

Cassinari V, Pagni CA 1969 Central pain: a neurosurgical survey. Harvard University Press, Cambridge

Cook AW, Nathan PW, Smith MC 1984 Sensory consequences of commissural myelotomy. Brain 107: 547–568

Corkin S 1980 A prospective study of cingulotomy. In: Valenstein. (ed) The psychosurgery debate Freeman, San Francisco, pp 164–204

Cosyns P, Caemaert J, Haaijman W et al 1994 Functional stereotactic neurosurgery for psychiatric disorders: an experience in Belgium and the Netherlands. In: Simon L et al (eds) Advances and technical standards in neurosurgery. Springer-Verlag, New York, pp 241–279

Crue BL, Todd EM, Carregal EJA 1968 Posterior approach for high cervical percutaneous radiofrequency cordotomy. Confinia Neurologica 30: 41–52

Denny-Brown D, Kirk EJ, Yanagisawa N 1973 The tract of Lissauer in relation to sensory transmission in the dorsal horn of spinal cord in the macaque monkey. Journal of Comparative Neurology 151: 175–200

Di Piero V, Jones AKP, Iannotti F et al 1991 Chronic pain: a PET study of the central effects of percutaneous high cervical cordotomy. Pain 46: 9–12

Emery E, Blondet E, Mertens P, Sindou M 1997 Microsurgical DREZ-otomy for chronic pain due to brachial plexus avulsion: long-term results in a series of 37 patients. In: Abstracts of oral presentations at the XII Meeting of the World Society for Stereotactic and Functional Neurosurgery, Lyon, July 1–4

Ervin FR, Mark VH 1960 Stereotactic thalamotomy in the human. Physiologic observations on the human thalamus. Archives of Neurology 3: 368–380

Fairman D 1972 Hypothalamotomy as a new perspective for alleviation of intractable pain and regression of metastatic malignant tumours. In: Fusek I, Kunc Z (eds) Present limits of neurosurgery. Avicenum, Prague, pp 525–528

Fairman D 1973 Stereotactic hypothalamotomy for the alleviation of pain in malignant disease. Journal of Surgical Oncology 5: 79–84

Fairman D 1976 Neurophysiological bases for the hypothalamic lesion and stimulation by chronic implanted electrodes for the relief of intractable pain in cancer. In: Bonica JJ, Albe-Fessard D (eds) Advances in pain research and therapy, vol 1. Raven Press, New York, pp 843–847

Fazl M, Houlden DA 1995 Dorsal root entry zone localization using direct spinal cord stimulation: an experimental study. Journal of Neurosurgery 82: 592–594

Fazl M, Houlden DA, Kiss Z 1995 Spinal cord mapping with evoked responses for accurate localization of the dorsal root entry zone. Journal of Neurosurgery 82: 587–591

Fenstermaker RA, Sternau LL, Takaoka Y 1994 CT-assisted percutaneous anterior cordotomy: technical note. Surgical Neurology 43(2): 147–149, discussion 149–150

Foltz EL, White LE 1962 Pain 'relief' by frontal cingulotomy. Journal of Neurosurgery 19: 89–100

Fox JL 1969 Localization of the respiratory pathway in the upper cervical spinal cord following percutaneous cordotomy. Neurology 19: 1115–1118

Fraioli B, Guidetti B 1975 Effect of stereotactic lesions of the pulvinar and lateralis posterior nucleus on intractable pain and dyskinetic syndromes of man. Applied Neurophysiology 38: 23–30

Frank F, Fabrizi AP, Gaist G, Weigel K, Mundinger F 1987 Stereotactic lesions in the treatment of chronic cancer pain syndromes: mesencephalotomy or multiple thalamotomies. Applied Neurophysiology 50: 314–318

Frank F, Fabrizi 1997 AP stereotactic mesencephalic tractotomy for cancer pain. Abstracts of oral presentations at the XII Meeting of the World Society for Stereotactic and Functional Neurosurgery, Lyon, July 1–4

Friedman AH, Bullitt E 1988 Dorsal root entry zone lesions in the treatment of pain following brachial plexus avulsion, spinal cord injury, and herpes zoster. Applied Neurophysiology 51: 164–169

Friedman AH, Nashold BS Jr 1986 DREZ lesions for relief of pain related to spinal cord injury. Journal of Neurosurgery 65: 465–469

Friedman AH, Nashold BS Jr 1990 Pain of spinal origin. In: Youmans JR (ed) Neurological surgery. A comprehensive reference guide to the diagnosis and management of neurosurgical problems. WB Saunders, Philadelphia, pp 3950–3959

Friedman AH, Nashold BS Jr, Bronec PR 1988 Dorsal root entry zone lesions for the treatment of brachial plexus avulsion injuries: a follow-up study. Neurosurgery 22: 369–373

Friedman AH, Nashold JRB, Nashold BS Jr 1996 DREZ lesions for treatment of pain. In: North RB, Levy RM (eds) Neurosurgical management of pain. Springer, New York, pp 176–190

Friehs GM, Schröttner O, Pendl G 1995 Evidence for segregated pain and temperature conduction within the spinothalamic tract. Journal of Neurosurgery 83: 8–12

García-Larrea L, Charles N, Sindou M, Mauguière F 1993 Flexion reflexes following anterolateral cordotomy in man: dissociation between pain sensation and nociceptive reflex RIII. Pain 55: 139–149

Gildenberg PL, Hirshberg RM 1984 Limited myelotomy for the treatment of intractable cancer pain. Journal of Neurology, Neurosurgery and Psychiatry 47: 94–96

Gildenberg PL, Zanes C, Flitter MA et al 1969 Impedance monitoring device for detection of penetration of the spinal cord in anterior percutaneous cervical cordotomy (technical note). Journal of Neurosurgery 30: 87–92

Gorecki JP, Nashold BS Jr, Rubin L, Ovelmen-Levitt J 1995 The Duke experience with nucleus caudalis DREZ coagulation. Proceedings of the Meeting of the American Society for Stereotactic and Functional Neurosurgery 65: 111–116

Guillaume J, Mazars G, Valleteau de Moulillac Fr 1945 La myélotomie commissurale. Presse Médicale 53: 666–667

Gybels JM 1991a Indications for the use of neurosurgical techniques in pain control. In: Bond MR, Charlton JE, Woolf J (eds) Proceedings of the Sixth World Congress on Pain. Elsevier, Amsterdam, pp 475–482

Gybels JM 1991b Analysis of clinical outcome of a surgical procedure. Guest editorial. Pain 44: 103–104

Gybels JM 1997 Commissural myelotomy revisited. Pain 70: 1–2

Gybels JM, Nuttin B 1995 Are there still indications for destructive neurosurgery at supra-spinal levels for the relief of painful syndromes? In: Besson JM, Guilbaud G, Ollat H (eds) Forebrain areas involved in pain processing. John Libbey Eurotext, Paris, pp 253–259

Gybels JM, Sweet WH 1989 Neurosurgical treatment of persistent pain. Physiological and pathological mechanisms of human pain. In: Gildenberg PL (ed) Pain and headache, vol II. Karger, Basel, pp 141–145

Gybels JM, Kupers R, Nuttin B 1993 Therapeutic stereotactic procedures on the thalamus for pain. Acta Neurochirurgica 124(1): 19–22

Halliday AM, Logue V 1972 Painful sensations evoked by electrical stimulation in the thalamus. In: Somjen GG (ed) Neurophysiology studied in man. Excerpta Medica, Amsterdam, pp 221–230

Hassenbusch SJ 1995 Surgical management of cancer pain. Neurosurgery Clinics of North America 6(1): 127–134

Hassler R 1972 The division of pain conduction into systems of pain and pain awareness. In: Janzen R, Keidel WD, Herz A, Steichele C (eds) Pain: basic principles – pharmacology – therapy. Thieme, Stuttgart, pp 98–112

Hassler R, Riechert T 1959 Klinische und anatomische Befunde der stereotaktischen Schmerzoperationen im Thalamus. Archiv für Psychiatrie und Nervenkrankheiten 200: 93–122

Hécaen H, Talairach J, David M, Dell MB 1949 Coagulations limitées du thalamus dans les algies du syndrome thalamique. Révue Neurologique (Paris) 81: 917–931

Hirshberg RM, Al-Chaer ED, Lawand NB et al 1996 Is there a pathway in the posterior funiculus that signals visceral pain? Pain 67: 291–305

Hitchcock ER 1969 An apparatus for stereotactic spinal surgery: A preliminary report. Journal of Neurosurgery 31: 386–392

Hitchcock ER 1970 Stereotactic cervical myelotomy. Journal of Neurology, Neurosurgery and Psychiatry 33: 224

Hitchcock ER 1973 Stereotactic pontine spinothalamic tractotomy. Journal of Neurosurgery 39: 746–752

Hitchcock ER 1974 Stereotactic myelotomy. Proceedings of the Royal Society of Medicine 67: 771–772

Hitchcock ER 1988 Spinal and pontine tractotomies and nucleotomies. In: Lunsford LD (ed) Modern stereotactic neurosurgery. Martinus Nijhoff, Boston, pp 279–295

Hitchcock ER, Leece B 1967 Somatotopic representation of the respiratory pathways in the cervical cord of man. Journal of Neurosurgery 27: 320–329

Hitchcock ER, Schvarcz JR 1972 Stereotaxic trigeminal tractotomy for post-herpetic facial pain. Journal of Neurosurgery 37: 412–417

Hitchcock ER, Teixeira MJA 1981 A comparison of results from center-median and basal thalamotomies for pain. Surgical Neurology 15: 341–351

Hitchcock ER, Sotelo MG, Kim MC 1985a Analgesic levels and technical method in stereotactic pontine spinothalamic tractotomy. Acta Neurochirurgica 77: 29–36

Hitchcock ER, Kim MC, Sotelo M 1985b Further experience in stereotactic pontine tractotomy. Applied Neurophysiology 48: 242–246

Hitchcock E, Sotelo MG, Kim MC 1985c Analgesic levels and technical method in stereotactic pontine spinothalamic tractotomy. Acta Neurochirurgica 77: 29–36

Hsieh JC, Belfrage M, Stone-Elander S et al 1995 Central representation of chronic ongoing neuropathic pain studied by positron emission tomography. Pain 63: 225–236

Hyndman OR 1942 Lissauer's tract section. A contribution to chordotomy for the relief of pain (preliminary report). Journal of the International College of Surgeons 5: 314–400

Ischia S, Ischia A 1988 A mechanism of new pain following cordotomy (Letter). Pain 32: 383–384

Ishijima B, Shimoji K, Shimizu H et al 1988 Lesions of spinal and trigeminal dorsal root entry zone for deafferentation pain. Experience of 35 cases. Applied Neurophysiology 51: 175–187

Izumi J, Hirose Y, Yazaki T 1992 Percutaneous trigeminal rhizotomy and percutaneous cordotomy under general anesthesia. Sterotactic and Functional Neurosurgery 59: 62–68

Jeanmonod D, Sindou M 1991 Somatosensory function following dorsal root entry zone lesions in patients with neurogenic pain or spasticity. Journal of Neurosurgery 74(6): 916–932

Jeanmonod D, Sindou M, Mauguière F 1989a Intra-operative spinal cord evoked potentials during cervical and lumbo-sacral microsurgical DREZ-otomy (MDT) for chronic pain and spasticity (preliminary data). Acta Neurochirurgica 46(suppl): 58–61

Jeanmonod D, Sindou M, Magnin M, Baudet M 1989b Intraoperative unit recordings in the human dorsal horn with a simplified floating microelectrode. EEG Clinical Neurophysiology 72: 450–454

Jeanmonod D, Sindou M, Mauguière F 1991 The human cervical and lumbo-sacral evoked electrospinogram. Data from intra-operative spinal cord surface recordings. EEG and Clinical Neurophysiology 80: 477–489

Jeanmonod D, Magnin M, Morel A 1993 Thalamus and neurogenic pain: physiological, anatomical and clinical data. Neuroreport 4(5): 475–478

Jeanmonod D, Magnin M, Morel A 1994 Chronic neurogenic pain and the medial thalamotomy. Schweizerische Rundschau fur Medizin Praxis 83(23): 702–707

Jeanmonod D, Magnin M, Morel A 1996 Low-threshold calcium spike bursts in the human thalamus. Common physiopathology for sensory, motor and limbic positive symptoms. Brain 119: 363–375

Jefferson AP 1983 Cordectomy for intractable pain in paraplegia. In: Lipton S, Miles J (eds) Persistent pain: modern methods for treatment, vol 4. Grune & Stratton, London, pp 115–132

Kanpolat Y, Akyar S, Caglar S, Unlu A, Bilgic S 1993 CT-guided percutaneous selective cordotomy. Acta Neurochirurgica 123: 92–96

Kanpolat Y, Caglar S, Akyar S, Temiz C 1995 CT-guided pain procedures for intractable pain in malignancy. Acta Neurochirurgica 64(suppl): 88–91

Kudo T, Yoshii N, Shimizu S, Aikawa S, Nakahama H 1968 Effects of stereotactic thalamotomy for pain relief. Tohoku Journal of Experimental Medicine 96: 219–234

Lahuerta J, Bowsher D, Lipton S 1990 Clinical and instrumental evaluation of sensory function before and after percutaneous anterolateral cordotomy at cervical level in man. Pain 42: 23–30

Lahuerta J, Bowsher D, Lipton S, Buxton PH 1994 Percutaneous cervical cordotomy: a review of 181 operations on 146 patients with a study in the location of 'pain fibers' in the C2 spinal cord segment of 29 cases. Journal of Neurosurgery 80: 975–985

Laitinen L 1977 Anterior pulvinotomy in the treatment of intractable pain. Acta Neurochirurgica 24(suppl): 223–225

Leksell L, Meyerson BA, Forster DMC 1972 Radiosurgical thalamotomy for intractable pain. Confinia Neurologica 34: 264 (abstract)

Lende RA, Kirsh WM, Druckman R 1971 Relief of facial pain after combined removal of precentral and postentral cortex. Journal of Neurosurgery 34: 537–543

Lenz FA, Dostrovsky JO, Kwan HC, Tasker RR, Yamashiro K, Murphy JT 1988 Methods for microstimulation and recording of single neurons and evoked potentials in the human central nervous system. Journal of Neurosurgery 68: 630–634

Levin AB 1988 Stereotactic chemical hypophysectomy. In: Lunsford LD (ed) Modern stereotactic neurosurgery. Martinus Nijhoff, Boston, pp 365–375

Levin AB 1993 Hypophysectomy in the treatment of cancer pain. In: Arbit E (ed) Management of cancer-related pain. Futura, Mt Kisko, pp 281–295

Lin PM, Gildenberg PL, Polakoff PP 1966 An anterior approach to percutaneous lower cervical cordotomy. Journal of Neurosurgery 25: 553–560

Loeser JD 1994 Tic douloureux and atypical face pain. In: Wall PD, Melzack R (eds) Textbook of pain, 3rd edn. Churchill Livingstone, Edinburgh, pp 699–710

Loeser JD, Ward AA Jr, White LE Jr 1968 Chronic deafferentation of human spinal cord neurons. Journal of Neurosurgery 29: 48–50

Makachinas T, Ovelmen-Levitt J, Nashold BS Jr 1988 Intraoperative somatosensory evoked potentials. A localizing technique in the DREZ operation. Applied Neurophysiology 51: 146–153

Mansuy L, Lecuire J, Acassat L 1944 Technique de la myélotomie commissurale postérieure. Journal de Chirurgie 60: 206–213

Mark VH, Ervin FR 1965 Role of thalamotomy in treatment of chronic severe pain. Postgraduate Medicine 37: 563–571

Mark VH, Ervin FR, Hackett TP 1960 Clinical aspects of stereotactic thalamotomy in the human. I. The treatment of chronic severe pain. Archives of Neurology 3: 351–367

Mark VH, Ervin FR, Yakovlev PI 1961 Correlation of pain relief, sensory loss, and anatomical lesion sites in pain patients treated by stereotactic thalamotomy. Transactions of the American Neurological Association 86: 86–90

Mark VH, Ervin FR, Yakovlev P 1963 Stereotactic thalamotomy. III. The verification of anatomical lesion sites in the human thalamus. Archives of Neurology 8: 78–88

Mayanagi Y, Bouchard G 1976/1977 Evaluation of stereotactic thalamotomies for pain relief with reference to pulvinar intervention. Applied Neurophysiology 39: 154–157

Mayanagi Y, Sano K 1988 Posteromedial hypothalamotomy for behavioural disturbances and intractable pain. In: Lunsford LD (ed) Modern stereotactic neurosurgery. Martinus Nijhoff, Boston, pp 377–388

Mayanagi Y, Hori T, Sano K 1978 The posteromedial hypothalamus and pain behaviour with special reference to endocrinological findings. Applied Neurophysiology 41:223–231

Mayer DJ, Price DD, Becker DP, Young HF 1975 Thresholds for pain from anterolateral quadrant stimulation as a predictor of success of percutaneous cordotomy for relief of pain. Journal of Neurosurgery 43: 445–447

Meyerson BA, Von Holst H 1990 Extramedullary impedance monitoring and stimulation of the spinal cord surface in percutaneous cordotomy. Technical note. Acta Neurochirurgica (Wien) 107: 63–64

Meyerson BA, Arnér S, Linderoth B 1984 Pelvic cancer pain (somatogenic pain): pros and cons of different approaches to the management of pelvic cancer pain. Acta Neurochirurgica (Wien) 33(suppl): 407–419

Monnier M, Fischer R 1951 Localisation, stimulation et coagulation du thalamus chez l'homme. Journal de Physiologie 43: 818

Moossy JJ, Nashold BS Jr, Osborne D et al 1987 Conus medullaris nerve root avulsions. Journal of Neurosurgery 66: 835–841

Moricca G 1974 Chemical hypophysectomy for cancer pain. In: Bonica JJ (ed) Advances in neurology, vol. 4. Raven, New York, pp 707–714

Moricca G 1976 Neuroadenolysis for diffuse unbearable cancer pain. In: Bonica JJ, Albe-Fessard D (eds) Advances in pain research and therapy, vol. 1. Raven, New York, pp 863–866

Morley TP 1953 Congenital rotation of the spinal cord. Journal of Neurosurgery 10: 690–692

Moser RP, Yap JC, Fraley EE 1980 Stereotactic hypophysectomy for intractable pain secondary to metastatic prostate carcinoma. Applied Neurophysiology 43: 145–149

Mullan S, Hosobuchi Y 1968 Respiratory hazards of high cervical percutaneous cordotomy. Journal of Neurosurgery 28: 291–297

Mullan S, Harper PV, Hekmatpanah J et al 1963 Percutaneous interruption of spinal-pain tracts by means of a strontium-90 needle. Journal of Neurosurgery 20: 931–939

Mullan S, Hekmatpanah J, Dobben G et al 1965 Percutaneous intramedullary cordotomy utilizing the unipolar anodal electrolytic system. Journal of Neurosurgery 22: 548–553

Nagaro T, Kumura S, Arai T 1987 A mechanism of new pain following cordotomy: reference of sensation. Pain 30: 89–91

Nagaro T, Amakawa K, Arai T, Ohi G 1993a Ipsilateral referral of pain following cordotomy. Pain 55: 275–276

Nagaro T, Amakawa K, Kimura S et al 1993b Reference of pain following percutaneous cervical cordotomy. Pain 53: 205–211

Nashold BS Jr 1982 Brainstem stereotaxic procedures. In: Schaltenbrand G, Walker AE (eds) 1982 Stereotaxy of the human brain. Anatomical, physiological and clinical applications. Thieme, Stuttgart, pp 475–483

Nashold BS Jr 1991 Paraplegia and pain. In: Nashold BS Jr, Ovelmen-Levitt J (eds) Deafferentation pain syndromes: pathophysiology and treatment. Raven, New York, pp 301–309

Nashold BS Jr, Bullitt E 1981 Dorsal root entry zone lesions to control central pain in paraplegics. Journal of Neurosurgery 55: 414–419

Nashold BS Jr, El-Naggar AO 1992 Dorsal root entry zone (DREZ) lesioning. In: Rengachary SS, Wilkins RH (eds) Neurosurgical operative atlas. Williams & Wilkins, Baltimore, pp 9–24

Nashold BS Jr, Ostdahl RH 1979 Dorsal root entry zone lesions for pain relief. Journal of Neurosurgery 51: 59–69

Nashold BS Jr, Wilson WP 1966 Central pain. Observations in man with chronic implanted electrodes in the midbrain tegmentum. Confinia Neurologica 27: 30–44

Nashold BS Jr, Wilson WP, Slaughter G 1974 The midbrain and pain. In: Bonica JJ (ed) Advances in neurology, vol. 4. Raven Press, New York, pp. 191–196

Nashold BS Jr, Urban B, Zorub DS 1976 Phantom pain relief by focal destruction of the substantia gelatinosa of Rolando. Advances in Pain Research and Therapy 1: 959–963

Nashold BS Jr, Slaughter DG, Wilson WP, Zorub D 1977 Stereotactic mesencephalotomy. In: Krayenbühl H, Maspes PE, Sweet WH (eds) Progress in neurological surgery, vol. 8. Karger, Basel, pp 35–49

Nashold BS Jr, Ovelmen-Levitt J, Sharpe R et al 1985. Intraoperative evoked potentials recorded in man directly from dorsal roots and spinal cord. Journal of Neurosurgery 62: 680–693

Nashold BS Jr, Vieira J, El-Naggar AC 1990 Pain and spinal cysts in paraplegia: treatment by drainage and DREZ operation. British Journal of Neurosurgery 4: 327–336

Nathan PW 1956 Reference of sensation at the spinal level. Journal of Neurology, Neurosurgery and Psychiatry 19: 88–100

Nathan PW 1963 The descending respiratory pathway in man. Journal of Neurology, Neurosurgery and Psychiatry 26: 487–499

Nathan PW 1990 Touch and surgical division of the anterior quadrant of the spinal cord. Journal of Neurology, Neurosurgery and Psychiatry 53: 935–939

Nathan PW 1994 Effects on movement of surgical incisions into the human spinal cord. Brain 117: 337–346

Nauta HJW, Hewitt E, Westlund KN, Willis WD 1997 Surgical interruption of a midline dorsal column visceral pathway. Journal of Neurosurgery 86: 538–542

Noordenbos W, Wall PD 1976 Diverse sensory functions with an almost totally divided spinal cord: a case of spinal cord transection with preservation of one anterolateral quadrant. Pain 2: 185–195

North RB, Levy RM 1994 Consensus conference on the neurosurgical management of pain. Neurosurgery 34: 756–761

Olszewski J 1950 On the anatomical and functional organization of the spinal trigeminal nucleus. Journal of Comparative Neurology 92: 401–413

Onofrio BM 1971 Cervical spinal cord and dentate delineation in percutaneous radiofrequency cordotomy at the level of the first to second cervical vertebrae. Surgery, Gynecology and Obstetrics 133: 30–34

Pagni CA 1974 Place of stereotactic technique in surgery for pain. In: Bonica JJ (ed) Advances in neurology, vol. 4. Raven Press, New York, pp 699–706

Parrent A, Lozano A, Tasker RR, Dostrovsky J 1992 Periventricular gray stimulation suppresses allodynia and hyperpathia in man. Stereotactic and Functional Neurosurgery 59: 82

Pillay PK, Hassenbusch SJ 1992 Bilateral MRI-guided stereotactic cingulotomy for intractable pain. Stereotactic and Functional Neurosurgery 59: 33–38

Poletti CE 1988 Open cordotomy medullary tractotomy. In: Schmidek HH, Sweet WH (eds) Operative neurosurgical techniques: indications, methods and results, 2nd edn. Grune & Stratton, Orlando, pp 1155–1168

Powers SK, Adams JE, Edwards MSB et al 1984 Pain relief from dorsal root entry zone lesions made with argon and carbon dioxide microsurgical lasers. Journal of Neurosurgery 61: 841–847
Powers SK, Barbaro NM, Levy RM 1988 Pain control with laser-produced dorsal root entry zone lesions. Applied Neurophysiology 51: 243–254
Rainville P, Duncan GH, Price DD et al 1997 Pain affect encoded in human anterior cingulate but not somatosensory cortex. Science 277: 968–971
Ralston HJ III, Ralston DD 1992 The primate dorsal spinothalamic tract: evidence for a specific termination in the posterior nuclei (Po/SG) of the thalamus. Pain 48: 107–118
Richardon DE, Zorub DS 1970 Sensory function of the pulvinar. Confinia Neurologica 32: 154–173
Richter HP, Seitz K 1984 Dorsal root entry zone lesions for the control of deafferentation pain: experiences in ten patients. Neurosurgery 15: 956–959
Rinaldi PC, Young RF, Albe-Fessard D, Chodakiewitz J 1991 Spontaneous neuronal hyperactivity in the medial intralaminar thalamic nuclei of patients with deafferentation pain. Journal of Neurosurgery 74: 415–521
Rosomoff HL, Carroll F, Brown J, Shepak P 1965 Percutaneous radiofrequency cervical cordotomy technique. Journal of Neurosurgery 23: 639–644
Rosomoff HL, Papo I, Loeser JD 1990 Neurosurgical operations on the spinal cord. In: Bonica JJ (ed) The management of pain, 2nd edn. Lea & Febiger, Philadelphia, pp 2067–2081
Roth SA, Seitz K, Soliman N, Rahamba JF, Antoniadis G, Richter H-P 1997 DREZ coagulation for deafferentation pain related to spinal and peripheral nerve lesions: indications and results of 72 consecutive procedures. Abstracts of oral presentations at the XII Meeting of the World Society for Stereotactic and Functional Neurosurgery. Lyon, July 1–4
Samii M, Moringlane JR 1984 Thermocoagulation of the dorsal root entry zone for the treatment of intractable pain. Neurosurgery 15: 953–955
Sampson JH, Chasman RE, Nashold BS, Friedman AH 1995 Dorsal root entry zone lesions for intractable pain after trauma to the conus medularis and cauda equina. Journal of Neurosurgery 82: 28–34
Sanders M, Zuurmond W 1995 Safety of unilateral and bilateral percutaneous cervical cordotomy in 80 terminally ill cancer patients. Journal of Clinical Oncology 13(6): 1509–1512
Sano K 1977 Intralaminar thalamotomy (thalamolaminotomy) and posterior hypothalamotomy in the treatment of intractable pain. In: Krayenbühl H, Maspes P E, Sweet W H (eds) Progress in neurological surgery, vol. 8. Karger, Basel, pp 50–103
Sano K 1979 Stereotaxic thalamolaminotomy and posteromedial hypothalamotomy for the relief of intractable pain. In: Bonica J J, Ventrafridda V (eds) Advances in pain research and therapy, vol. 2. Raven Press, New York, pp 475–485
Sano K, Yoshioka M, Sekino H, Mayanagi Y, Yoshimasu Y, Tsukamoto Y 1970 Functional organization of the internal medullary lamina in man. Confinia Neurologica 32: 374–380
Saris SC, Iacono RP, Nashold BS 1985 Dorsal root entry zone lesions for post-amputation pain. Journal of Neurosurgery 62: 72–76
Saris SC, Iacono RP, Nashold BS Jr 1988a Successful treatment of phantom pain with dorsal root entry zone coagulation. Applied Neurophysiology 51: 188–197
Saris SC, Vieira JFS, Nashold BS Jr 1988b Dorsal root entry zone coagulation for intractable sciatica. Applied Neurophysiology 51: 206–211
Schaltenbrand G, Bailey P 1959 Introduction to stereotaxis with an atlas of the human brain. Thieme, Stuttgart
Schaltenbrand G, Wahren W 1977 Atlas for stereotaxy of the human brain, 2nd edn. Thieme, Stuttgart
Sherman IC, Arieff AJ 1948 Dissociation between pain and temperature in spinal cord lesions. Journal of Nervous and Mental Diseases 108: 285–292
Shieff C, Nashold BS Jr 1987 Stereotactic mesencephalotomy for thalamic pain. Neurological Research 9: 101–104
Shieff C, Nashold BS Jr 1988 Thalamic pain and stereotactic mesencephalotomy. Acta Neurochirurgica 42 (suppl): 239–242
Siegfried J, Krayenbühl H 1972 Clinical experience with the treatment of intractable pain. In: Janzen R, Keidel WD, Herz A, Steichele C (eds) Pain: basic principles – pharmacology – therapy. Thieme, Stuttgart, pp 202–204
Sindou M 1972 Study of the dorsal root – spinal cord junction. A target for pain surgery. These Doctorat Médecine, Lyon
Sindou M 1995 Microsurgical DREZotomy (MDT) for pain, spasticity, and hyperactive bladder: a 20-year experience. Acta Neurochirurgica 137(1–2): 1–5
Sindou M, Daher A 1988 Spinal cord ablation procedures for pain. In: Dubner R, Gebhart G F, Bond M R (eds) Proceedings of the Fifth World Congress on Pain. Pain research and clinical management, vol. 3. Elsevier, Amsterdam, pp 477–495
Sindou M, Goutelle A 1983 Surgical posterior rhizotomies for the treatment of pain. In: Krayenbühl H (ed) Advances and technical standards in neurosurgery, vol. 10. Springer, New York, pp 147–185
Sindou M, Jeanmonod D 1989 Microsurgical DREZ-otomy for the treatment of spasticity and pain in the lower limbs. Neurosurgery 24: 655–670
Sindou M, Mertens P 1997 Neurosurgical procedures for neuropathic pain. Abstracts of oral presentations to the XII Meeting of the World Society of Stereotactic and Functional Neurosurgery, Lyon, July 1–4, pp 20–22
Sindou M, Fischer G, Goutelle A et al 1974a La radicellotomie postérieure sélective: premiers résultats dans la chirurgie de la douleur. Neurochirurgie 20: 391–408
Sindou M, Quoex C, Baleydier C 1974b Fiber organization at the posterior spinal cord-rootlet junction in man. Journal of Comparative Neurology 153: 15–26
Sindou M, Fischer G, Mansuy L 1976 Posterior spinal rhizotomy and selective posterior rhizidiotomy. In: Krayenbühl H, Maspes P E, Sweet W H (eds) Progress in neurological surgery, vol. 7. Karger, Basel, pp 201–250
Sindou M, Mifsud JJ, Boisson D et al 1986 Selective posterior rhizotomy in the dorsal root entry zone for treatment of hyperspasticity and pain in the hemiplegic upper limb. Neurosurgery 18: 587–595
Sindou M, Jeanmonod D, Mertens P 1991 Surgery in the dorsal root entry zone: microsurgical drez-otomy (MDT) for treatment of spasticity. In: Sindou M, Abbott R, Keravel Y (eds) Neurosurgery for spasticity. Springer, New York, pp 165–182
Sjöqvist O 1938 Studies on pain conduction in the trigeminal nerve. Acta Psychiatrica et Neurologica 17(suppl): 1–139
Spiegel EA, Wycis HT 1949 Pallidothalamotomy in chorea. Presented at the Philadelphia Neurological Society, April 22
Spiegel EA, Wycis HT 1962 Stereoencephalotomy. II: Clinical and physiological applications. Grune & Stratton, New York
Spiegel EA, Kletzkin M, Szekely EG, Wycis HT 1954a Pain reactions upon stimulation of the tectum mesencephali. Journal of Neuropathology and Experimental Neurology 13: 212–220
Spiegel EA, Kletzkin M, Szekely EG, Wycis HT 1954b Role of hypothalamic mechanisms in thalamic pain. Neurology 4: 739–751
Spiller WG 1905 The occasional clinical resemblance between caries of the vertebrae and lumbothoracic syringomyelia and the location within the spinal cord of the fibres for the sensations of pain and temperature. Univ Pa Med Bull JAMA 18: 147–154
Spiller WG, Martin E 1912 The treatment of persistent pain of organic origin in the lower part of the body by division of the anterolateral column of the spinal cord. JAMA 58: 1489–1490

Steiner L, Forster D, Leksell L, Meyerson BA, Boethius J 1980 Gammathalamotomy in intractable pain. Acta Neurochirurgica 52: 173–184

Stookey B 1929 Human chordotomy to abolish pain sense without destroying temperature sense. Journal of Nervous and Mental Diseases 69: 552–557

Sweet WH, Mark VH, Hamlin H 1960 Radiofrequency lesions in the central nervous system of man and cat: including case reports of eight bulbar pain-tract interruptions. Journal of Neurosurgery 17: 213–225

Talbot JD, Marrett S, Evans AC, Meyer E, Bushnell C, Duncan GH 1991 Multiple representations of pain in human cerebral cortex. Science 251: 1355–1358

Taren JA 1971 Physiologic corroboration in stereotaxic high cervical cordotomy. Confinia Neurologica 33: 285–290

Taren JA, Davis R, Crosby ED 1969 Target physiologic corroboration in stereotaxic cervical cordotomy. Journal of Neurosurgery 30: 569–584

Tasker RR 1976a The merits of percutaneous cordotomy over the open operation. In: Morley T P (ed) Current controversies in neurosurgery. W B Saunders, Philadelphia, pp 496–501

Tasker RR 1976b The human spinothalamic tract. Stimulation mapping in spinal cord and brainstem. In: Bonica J J, Albe-Fessard D (eds) Advances in pain research and therapy, vol. 1. Raven, New York, pp 251–257

Tasker RR 1977 Open cordotomy. In: Krayenbühl H, Maspes P E, Sweet W H (eds) Progress in neurological surgery, vol. 8. Karger, White Plains, NY, pp 1–14

Tasker RR 1982a Percutaneous cordotomy: the lateral high cervical technique. In: Schmidek H H, Sweet W H (eds) Operative neurosurgical techniques: indications, methods and results. Grune & Stratton, New York, pp 1137–1153

Tasker RR 1982b Pain. Thalamic procedures. In: Schaltenbrand G, Walker A E (eds) Textbook of stereotaxy of the human brain. Thieme, Stuttgart, pp 484–497

Tasker RR 1984 Stereotactic surgery. In: Wall P D, Melzack R (eds) Textbook of pain. Churchill Livingstone, Edinburgh, pp 639–655

Tasker RR 1987 The problem of deafferentation pain in the management of the patient with cancer. Journal of Palliative Care 2: 8–12

Tasker RR 1988 Percutaneous cordotomy: the lateral high cervical technique. In: Schmidek H H, Sweet W H (eds) Operative neurosurgical techniques: indications, methods and results, 2nd edn. Grune & Stratton, Orlando, pp 1191–1205

Tasker RR 1993 Ablative central nervous system lesions for control of cancer pain. In: Arbit E (ed) Management of cancer-related pain. Futura, Mt Kisko, pp 231–255

Tasker RR 1994 The recurrence of pain after neurosurgical procedures. Quality of Life Research 3(1): 543–549

Tasker RR 1995 Percutaneous cordotomy. In: Schmidek HH, Sweet WH (eds) Operative neurosurgical techniques: indications, methods and results, 3rd edn. W B Saunders, Philadelphia, pp 1595–1611

Tasker RR, De Carvalho G 1990 Pain in thalamic stroke. In: Pain and ethical and social issues in stroke rehabilitation. Inter-urban Stroke Academic Association, July, pp 1–25

Tasker RR, De Carvalho GTC, Dolan EJ 1992 Intractable pain of spinal cord origin: clinical features and implications for surgery. Journal of Neurosurgery 77: 373–378

Tasker RR, Dostrovsky JO 1989 Deafferentation and central pain. In: Wall PD, Melzack R (eds) Textbook of pain, 2nd edn. Churchill Livingstone, Edinburgh, pp 154–180

Tasker RR, Dostrovsky JO 1992 Computers in functional stereotactic surgery. In: Kelly PJ, Kall BA (eds) Computers in stereotactic neurosurgery: contemporary issues in neurological surgery. Blackwell, Boston, pp 155–164

Tasker RR, Organ LW 1973 Percutaneous cordotomy: physiological identification of target site. Confinia Neurologica 35: 110–117

Tasker RR, Organ LW, Smith KC 1974 Physiological guidelines for the localization of lesions by percutaneous cordotomy. Acta Neurochirurgica (Wien) 21 (suppl): 111–117

Tasker RR, Organ LW, Hawrylyshyn PE 1980 Deafferentation and causalgia. In: Bonica JJ (ed) Pain research publications, association for Research in Nervous and Mental Disease, vol. 58. Raven, New York, pp 305–329

Tasker RR, Organ LW, Hawrylyshyn PA 1982 The thalamus and midbrain of man. A physiological atlas using electrical stimulation. CC Thomas, Springfield

Tasker RR, Lenz F, Yamashiro K, Gorecki J, Hirayama T, Dostrovsky JO 1987 Microelectrode techniques in localization of stereotactic targets. Neurosurgical Research 9(2): 105–112

Teuber HL, Corkin S, Twitchell TE 1977 A study of cingulotomy in man. Appendix to Psychosurgery. Reports prepared for the National Commission for the Protection of Human Subjects of Biomedical and Behavioral Research, US Department of Health, Education and Welfare, DHEW Publ. No (OS) 77–0002, 3: 1–115

Thomas DGT, Jones SJ 1984 Dorsal root entry zone lesions (Nashold's procedure) in brachial plexus avulsion. Neurosurgery 15: 966–968

Van Roost D, Gybels J 1989 Myelotomies for chronic pain. Acta Neurochirurgica 46(suppl): 69–72

Voris HC 1957a Ipsilateral sensory loss following cordotomy: report of a case. Archives of Neurology and Psychiatry 65: 95–96

Voris HC 1957b Variations in the spinothalamic tract in man. Journal of Neurosurgery 14: 55–60

Wertheimer P, Lecuire J 1953 La myélotomie commissurale postérieure. A propos de 107 observations. Acta Chirurgica Belgica 6: 568–575

White JC, Sweet WH 1969 Pain and the neurosurgeon. A forty-year experience. CC Thomas, Springfield

Whittle IR, Jenkinson JT 1995 CT-guided stereotactic antero-medial pulvinotomy and centromedian-parafascicular thalamotomy for intractable malignant plain. British Journal of Neurosurgery 9(2): 195–200

Wiegand H, Winkelmüller W 1985 Behandlung des Deafferentierumgsschmerzes durch Hochfrequenzläsion der Hunterwurzel-Eintrittszone. Deutsche Medizinische Wochenschrift 110: 216–220

Willis WD 1985 The pain system: the neural bases of nociceptive transmission in the mammalian nervous system. In: Gildenberg PL (ed) Pain and headache, vol 8. Karger, Basel

Woolf CJ 1992 Excitability changes in central neurons following peripheral damage: role of central sensitization in the pathogenesis of pain. In: Willis W (ed) Hyperalgesia and allodynia. Raven, New York, pp 221–243

Wycis HT, Spiegel EA 1962 Long-range results in the treatment of intractable pain by stereotaxic midbrain surgery. Journal of Neurosurgery 19: 101–107

Yoshida M, Noguchi S, Kuga S et al 1992 MRI findings of DREZ-otomy lesions. Stereotactic and Functional Neurosurgery 59: 34–44

Yoshii N, Mizokami T, Ushikubo T, Kuramtsu T, Fukuda S 1980 Long-term follow-up study after pulvinotomy for intractable pain. Applied Neurophysiology 43: 128–132

Yoshii N, Mizokami T, Usikubo Y, Samejima H, Adachi K 1990 Postmortem study of stereotactic pulvinarotomy for relief of intractable pain. Stereotactic and Functional Neurosurgery 54,55: 103

Young RF 1986 Laser versus radiofrequency lesions of the DREZ (letter). Journal of Neurosurgery 64: 341

Young RF, Jacques DS, Rand RW, Copcutt BR 1994 Medial thalamotomy with the Leksell gamma knife for treatment of chronic pain. Acta Neurochirurgica 62(suppl): 105–110

Young RF, Jacques DS, Rand RW, Copcutt BC, Vermeulen SS, Posewitz AE 1995 Technique of stereotactic medial thalamotomy with the Leksell gamma knife for treatment of chronic pain. Neurological Research 17(1): 59–65

58

Transcutaneous electrical nerve stimulation, vibration and acupuncture as pain-relieving measures

PER HANSSON & THOMAS LUNDEBERG

The introduction of the gate control theory concept in 1965 (Melzack & Wall 1965) has facilitated the global proliferation of different afferent stimulation techniques for pain alleviation, such as transcutaneous electrical nerve stimulation and vibration. The quality of the scientific documentation of TENS as a pain-relieving measure does not, however, correspond to its widespread and uncritical application in a multitude of painful conditions by different healthcare providers. This chapter highlights part of the scientific literature on the pain-alleviating effect of TENS in a number of acute and chronic painful conditions and briefly addresses technical issues and tentative mechanisms of action. Important methodological considerations are suggested for the critical evaluation of existing studies or the performance of future studies on the pain-relieving potential of TENS. Available data suggesting a pain-alleviating effect of vibration are briefly discussed. Acupuncture for pain relief is rapidly gaining interest in the Western hemisphere but its use for pain relief in a variety of conditions is not paralleled by supporting data in the scientific literature.

TRANSCUTANEOUS ELECTRICAL NERVE STIMULATION

Numerous physiological studies since the late 1950s (Kolmodin & Skoglund 1960, Wall 1964, Woolf & Wall 1982, Chung et al 1984, Garrison & Foreman 1996) support the notion that activity in large-diameter afferents may alter transmission in central pathways conveying messages ultimately experienced as pain. Such interaction may take place in the dorsal horn (Garrison & Foreman 1996) and in the thalamus (Olausson et al 1994). Although challenged in some of its original aspects (Schmidt 1972, Nathan & Rudge 1974a), the gate control theory concept (Melzack & Wall 1965) has facilitated the global proliferation of different afferent stimulation techniques for pain alleviation, such as vibration and transcutaneous electrical nerve stimulation (TENS). TENS is by far the most extensively used biomedical technique in this area and was embraced early on by health professionals in spite of a severely limited scientific documentation. Thirty years after the appearance of the first report in the field (Wall & Sweet 1967), the number of randomized controlled clinical trials in well-diagnosed patients is still conspicuously low. Despite the continuous shortage of high-quality studies, the method has gained footing as a technique for pain alleviation in a variety of conditions, possibly as a result of an uncritical and insatiable need for therapeutic measures. The continuing survival of TENS for pain relief may also in part be explained by the fact that experienced clinicians have witnessed its efficacy in subgroups of patients and that the technique has been favourably presented in previous reviews by clinical authorities (Meyerson 1983, Long 1991).

The starting point of the launching of TENS for clinical pain relief was a study by Wall and Sweet (1967) of a small group of patients with 'chronic cutaneous pain', reporting pain relief after acute exposure to TENS or percutaneous electrical stimulation. Initially, TENS was mainly used to screen for patients suitable for spinal cord stimulation. The predictive value of TENS effects for the outcome of spinal cord stimulation has, however, never been documented and clinical experience certainly does not point to any clear relationship between the two methods in terms of efficacy.

The strength of conclusions that may be drawn regarding the clinical efficacy of TENS for pain alleviation critically depends on the quality of the evidence contained in the scientific literature. Crucial points to consider when evaluating the methodological quality of studies are listed in Box 58.1. Few, if any, studies fulfil all criteria listed in Box 58.1. Importantly, lack of proper randomization and blinding have been demonstrated to heavily influence study results, with overoptimistic efficacy outcome (Carroll et al 1996). Due to the nature of the method, realistic placebo and blinding are inherent problems in TENS trials, both notoriously difficult to solve adequately. The survey presented below, based on a selection of available data from the literature, does not claim to be complete but rather has focused on some clinically important aspects of TENS and conditions where TENS has been applied.

BOX 58.1

Important methodological issues when evaluating/conducting TENS trials

Adequate (non-biased) selection of patients
Description of diagnostic criteria
Description of criteria for inclusion and exclusion
Identical machines and administration routine for TENS and placebo TENS
Blinded randomization (described in detail)
Blinding (described in detail) of patients and research team
Assessment of compliance with treatment
Description of withdrawals and reason for withdrawal
Description of outcome measures
Independent evaluation

TECHNICAL AND PRACTICAL ASPECTS

Commercial TENS machines offer at least three different pulse patterns: high frequency (HF, usually 50–120 Hz), low frequency (LF, 1–4 Hz) and bursts of high frequency delivered at low frequency (2 Hz), i.e. acupuncture-like (AKU) TENS. In addition, pulse width and stimulus amplitude can be controlled. Some stimulators also offer adjustable pulse configuration. Leads are used to connect the machine with electrodes that are usually made of carbon rubber. No compelling evidence has been presented to support increased therapeutic efficacy as a result of refining the electrical parameters of TENS machines. Further, no recommendation can be provided on the choice of stimulus parameters in different painful conditions.

In general, HF stimulation in the centre of the pain area is recommended as the first choice of stimulation, with an intensity just below the pain threshold so that paraesthesias are felt in the painful region. It is mandatory to start the TENS trial by examining tactile sensibility in the area to be stimulated to ensure a substrate for stimulation. A pronounced loss of large-fibre function offsets the use of TENS within the denervated area. If HF stimulation fails or is inconvenient, e.g. due to aggravation of pain in an area of tactile allodynia, LF or AKU TENS may be tried in an anatomically related area with normal sensibility. It is a general conception among TENS advocates that to increase the efficacy of LF and AKU TENS the stimulation should be intense enough to produce visible muscle contractions. Scientific evidence to support this notion is lacking. Regardless of the mode of TENS, a duration of stimulation of at least 30–45 minutes is recommended. In optimal situations a TENS trial may relieve ongoing and/or stimulus-evoked pain for several hours after termination of stimulation. Patients who report pain alleviation during stimulation only, with no post-stimulatory effect, will sometimes still volunteer to have a machine prescribed if other pain-relieving measures have proven ineffective for their pain. Frequent initial follow-ups are crucial to reinstruct the patients if necessary and to carefully extract the possible benefits of stimulation. Importantly, a fraction of patients with different pain diagnoses report increased pain intensity during TENS. For further details on technical and practical aspects, the reader is referred to handbooks on TENS.

ACUTE NOCICEPTIVE/INFLAMMATORY PAIN

Different painful conditions have been screened and some of the better explored areas are presented below.

Orofacial pain

From randomized and placebo-controlled trials in patients with different acute painful dental conditions, including pulpitis, apical periodontitis and postoperative intraoral pain, there is evidence that HF and AKU TENS have a pain-relieving potential during single trial exposure (Hansson & Ekblom 1983). The effect of extrasegmental TENS, including AKU TENS, on the HoKu point (between the thumb and index finger) was comparable to the effect of placebo TENS applied within the painful area (Ekblom & Hansson 1985). These findings therefore suggest that TENS is more effective when applied within the painful area and also point to the potential of TENS in the treatment of pain from deep somatic tissue. A study aiming to use HF or AKU TENS to provide surgical analgesia for intraoral operative procedures such as endodontic surgery, tooth extraction or abscess incision demonstrated their failure in all included patients (Hansson & Ekblom 1984).

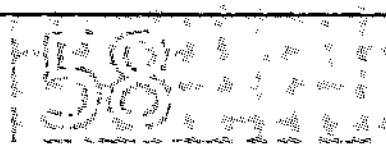

This finding parallels the clinical impression that phasic intense pain is rarely diminished by TENS treatment.

Postoperative pain

Short-term effects of TENS have been monitored after a variety of operative procedures. Outcome measures have included visual analogue scale ratings of spontaneous pain intensity and stimulus-evoked pain, time to request for analgesics, total medication intake, tolerance to physical therapy, expiratory peak flow rate, arterial blood gas determinations, duration of stay in the recovery room, etc. Positive results for several outcome measures have been reported in randomized and placebo-controlled trials, e.g. using HF TENS after thoracic (Bennedetti et al 1997) and abdominal/thoracic surgery (VanderArk & McGrath 1975). Negative outcome was demonstrated, e.g. after herniorrhaphy (Gilbert et al 1986) and appendicectomy (Conn et al 1986), both randomized and placebo-controlled studies of HF TENS. A systematic review of TENS effects in acute postoperative pain concluded that non-randomized trials usually overestimate treatment effects and that randomized controlled studies usually report a negative outcome (Carroll et al 1996).

Labour pain

Early on, non-randomized and non-placebo controlled trials (Augustinsson et al 1977, Bundsen et al 1981) indicated a pain-relieving effect of HF TENS primarily during the first stage of labour, i.e. when the nociceptive system presumably is activated by nociceptors in the contracting uterus and the dilating cervix. Later, Harrison and co-workers (1986) reported no difference between TENS (HF or AKU) and placebo TENS regarding pain relief. Another randomized, placebo-controlled clinical trial, monitoring the first stage of labour, reported TENS to be no more effective than placebo TENS (Van der Ploeg et al 1996). In that study, AKU TENS was used between uterine contractions and HF TENS during contractions. A systematic review of the efficacy of TENS for pain relief in labour found that randomized controlled trials provided no compelling evidence for TENS having any analgesic effect during labour (Carroll et al 1997). Several studies have reported TENS to be safe for the infant during delivery (Augustinsson et al 1977, Bundsen et al 1981, Van der Ploeg et al 1996).

Dysmenorrhoea

Dysmenorrhoea affects a large proportion of females and is a challenging entity from a pain relief perspective. Studies claiming a pain-relieving effect of TENS in this condition are available. A randomized, placebo-controlled study (Dawood & Ramos 1990) reported favourable effects of HF TENS compared to placebo TENS or ibuprofen. Significantly more TENS-treated patients reported substantial pain relief than patients treated with placebo TENS. The group receiving TENS also needed less rescue medication than the groups receiving placebo TENS or ibuprofen. An open, crossover study comparing high-intensity HF TENS and naproxen reported significantly reduced pain intensity from both interventions (Milsom et al 1994). Treatment with naproxen but not TENS was associated with a significant change in uterine activity. In a randomized, placebo-controlled single-trial study HF TENS was argued to be superior to LF and placebo TENS (Lundeberg et al 1985a). LF TENS seemed to be no more effective than placebo TENS.

Angina pectoris

There is evidence to suggest that TENS is effective in the treatment of angina pectoris. Mannheimer and colleagues (1985) demonstrated that HF TENS favourably influenced pacing-induced angina compared to controls. Pacing was better tolerated, lactate metabolism improved and ST segment depression was less pronounced with than without TENS. Results from the same study of a 10-week follow-up period, during which the patients were instructed to self-administer at least three 1-hour HF TENS treatments a day, demonstrated increased work capacity as measured with bicycle ergometer tests, decreased ST segment depression, reduced frequency of anginal attacks and reduced consumption of short-acting nitroglycerine per week compared with a control group not receiving TENS. Recent results indicate that at least part of the beneficial effect of TENS for pain relief in angina is secondary to decreased myocardial ischaemia (Chauhan et al 1994, Borjesson et al 1997). Chauhan and co-workers (1994) demonstrated HF TENS to significantly increase coronary blood flow velocity in patients with syndrome X and coronary artery disease but not in heart transplant patients. Borjesson et al (1997), in a randomized, placebo-controlled trial, demonstrated HF TENS treatment (30 minutes three times a day and during angina attacks) to be a safe additional treatment in unstable angina pectoris and to reduce the number and duration of silent ischaemic events. Interestingly, the number of painful events was unaltered, as was the number of episodes of pain leading to stimulation or consumption of analgesics.

CHRONIC NOCICEPTIVE/INFLAMMATORY PAIN

This area suffers from too few systematic studies of conditions with a homogeneous aetiology. Rheumatoid arthritis is an exception. A substantial fraction of patients included in studies of other conditions suffer from painful syndromes that, from a diagnostic point of view, are ill defined, e.g. low back pain (Deyo et al 1990, Herman et al 1994), due to the lack of strict diagnostic criteria for painful conditions in certain body regions. A number of patients with pain of unknown origin/aetiology are likely to have been included in many of these studies, which seriously affects their conclusions.

Rheumatoid arthritis

Studies aiming at elucidating the efficacy of TENS for pain relief in rheumatoid arthritis have included a number of different outcome measures such a resting pain, joint tenderness, grip strength, grip pain and loading tests. Studies lacking placebo control (Mannheimer et al 1978, Mannheimer & Carlsson 1979) reported relief from HF TENS of spontaneous pain and pain during a loading test. Abelson and colleagues (1983), in a randomized placebo-controlled study, examined the therapeutic effect of once-weekly HF TENS, lasting three weeks, in a group of patients with wrist involvement. Compared to placebo TENS, significant relief of resting pain and pain while gripping was reported. The same group later reported results from a similar study where suggestion and focused attention were added to the placebo treatment (Langley et al 1984). In this scenario HF, AKU and placebo TENS were equally effective in producing analgesia of similar degree and trend over time. The latter study casts serious doubt on the specific efficacy of TENS in rheumatoid arthritis but at the same time also points to the complexity and power of the placebo effect. The prominent effect of placebo was also highlighted in a study on pain from temporomandibular joint involvement of rheumatoid arthritis (Moystad et al 1990). HF TENS in the painful area and LF TENS of the hand was no more effective than placebo TENS in either region.

CHRONIC NEUROPATHIC PAIN

Peripheral neuropathic pain

It seems to be a general opinion among experienced clinicians within the field of neurological pain that subgroups of patients with peripheral neuropathic pain are among the best TENS-responding groups, although the scientific documentation is weak. Numerous studies, all with some methodological drawbacks and several of them including only small groups of patients diagnosed with neuropathic pain of different aetiology, have hinted at the usefulness of different modes of TENS in different peripheral neuropathic pain conditions (Nathan & Wall 1974b, Loeser et al 1975, Thorsteinsson et al 1977, Eriksson et al 1979, Bates & Nathan 1980, Johnson et al 1991a, Meyler & De Jongste 1994, Fishbain et al 1996). There are no known predictors as to which patients may benefit from TENS. In this group of patients it is especially important to survey the somatosensory status of the region to be treated. Tactile allodynia is a relative contraindication for HF TENS since the activation of myelinated mechanoreceptive fibres is painful in this subset of patients. It is our clinical impression, however, that in a subgroup of patients with neuropathic pain and allodynia to touch the method still has a potential to relieve ongoing as well as stimulus-evoked pain. Due to the pain initially induced when turning on the TENS machine, it is important that the patient is thoroughly informed before such a trial is commenced. If aggravation of pain is tolerated for up to a few minutes, there is a possibility of obtaining pain relief. Patients with tactile allodynia accompanied by autonomic reactions such as nausea, palpitation, syncope, etc. should not be treated by TENS.

Central neuropathic pain

Only a few non-randomized, non-placebo controlled studies exist which focus on central neuropathic pain. Leijon and Boivie (1989) studied central post-stroke pain patients and Davis and Lentini (1975) studied a subgroup of patients with central pain after spinal cord injury. Minor pain-relieving effects were reported. Still, a TENS trial may be recommended in patients with central neuropathic pain since only a few alternative pain-relieving measures exist, all with a major risk of failure.

The field of neuropathic pain and TENS would certainly benefit from randomized controlled trials of diagnostic entities where detailed clinical examination is performed to try to unravel possible pathophysiological mechanisms underlying the painful condition. A multitude of possible mechanisms is to be expected, not universally sensitive to TENS treatment.

CONTRAINDICATIONS

The following issues should be considered.

- To avoid any possible influence on the uterus or foetus, TENS should not be applied over the pregnant uterus or in the proximity of that region. Other regions of the body may well be suited for TENS trials.

- Cardiac pacemakers of the on-demand type may malfunction if disturbed by electrical output from a TENS machine. This is not the case with pacemakers of fixed frequencies.
- Stimulation within the anterior/lateral part of the neck is hazardous since spasm of the intrinsic muscles of the larynx may be induced as well as activation of cells in the carotid sinus involved in blood pressure regulation, risking a fall in pressure due to reflex bradycardia. Stimulation of the vagus nerve may also contribute to the latter.

Appropriate steps should be taken to avoid complications. Mandatory for the first and second conditions is discussion of the suggested treatment with the patient's care-giving specialist.

TENTATIVE MECHANISMS OF ACTION OF TENS

The detailed antinociceptive mechanisms of action of TENS are still largely unknown. A number of physiological studies have contributed to the notion that afferent activity set up by TENS blocks nociceptive transmission in the spinal cord (Kolmodin & Skoglund 1960, Wall 1964, Woolf & Wall 1982, Chung et al 1984, Garrison & Foreman 1996). Pre- as well as postsynaptic inhibitory mechanisms have been implicated. As stated earlier, not only the spinal cord needs necessarily to be involved but also thalamic regions (Olausson et al 1994). The most effective block of projecting neurons of the cord is achieved by activation not only of large myelinated fibres (Aα, Aβ) but also of Aδ and C fibres (Chung et al 1984, Lee et al 1985, Sjölund 1985). In a clinical setting this implies that painful TENS would be more effective for pain alleviation, an inconceivable option from a practical standpoint.

Of interest in the context of optimal stimulation intensity is a number of experimental studies, with some conflicting results, where different TENS techniques and different pain-inducing measures have been used. Woolf (1979), in a placebo-controlled study, demonstrated the need of high-intensity (i.e. painful) HF TENS to significantly alter the heat pain threshold and the tolerance to heat. TENS at non-painful intensities failed to alter the sensitivity to heat and noxious mechanical stimuli but modified ischaemic pain after a submaximal effort tourniquet test. To explain pain-relieving effects of painful afferent stimulation, it seems appropriate also to consider the theoretical concept of DNIC (diffuse noxious inhibitory control) (LeBars et al 1979a,b, 1991). More recently, HF non-painful TENS was reported to significantly reduce subjects' ratings of painful and near-painful heat stimuli and to increase the heat pain threshold (Marchand et al 1991). The perception threshold to cold pressor-induced pain as well as tolerance to ice pain were demonstrated to be significantly increased by a variety of stimulation patterns using TENS (Johnson et al 1991b). Failure of LF or HF non-painful TENS in altering pain induced by the submaximal effort tourniquet test and the cold pressor test were significant findings in a study by Foster and colleagues (1996). A reasonable conclusion from these studies is that the message conveyed in the nociceptive system set up by different painful stimuli, resulting in different temporospatial patterns of ascending activity, is differentially susceptible to alteration by different modes of TENS. A differential sensitivity to different modes of TENS may well, for the same reason, be the case in clinical pain states.

A peripheral mechanism of action contributing to pain alleviation by TENS has been suggested (Ignelzi & Nyquist 1976). Based on work employing microneurographic techniques, this hypothesis seems less likely. Janko and Trontelj (1980) were unable to demonstrate impulse transmission failure in Aδ fibres during TENS.

The neurochemical events set up by TENS are largely unknown. Somewhat conflicting results have been reported from studies in healthy subjects (Chapman & Benedetti 1977, Pertovaara & Kemppainen 1981, Salar et al 1981) and in patients with different acute (Woolf et al 1978, Hansson et al 1986) and chronic (Sjölund & Eriksson 1979, Abrams et al 1981, Freeman et al 1983) painful conditions, addressing the question of whether endogenous opioids mediate at least part of the pain-relieving effect of TENS. Such studies have been performed either by injecting the non-specific opioid antagonist naloxone to try to counteract TENS-induced pain relief or by analysing endogenous opioid compounds in the cerebrospinal fluid or plasma. Importantly, naloxone in physiological doses predominantly blocks μ-receptors. The contribution of other opioid receptors needs to be studied further when specific antagonists become available. Summarizing these data, it seems that pain relief by HF TENS is not mediated by an opioid link counteracted by naloxone. The literature provides some data, however, supporting an opioid link for pain alleviation by LF TENS.

CONCLUSIONS

A number of acute and chronic painful conditions have been reported to respond favourably to TENS. A substantial fraction of reports suffer, however, from serious methodological shortcomings. Most studies provide short-term outcome/single-trial results and long-term follow-up studies of chronic pain conditions are needed. Studies of optimal stimulation parameters, including pulse pattern characteristics, site of electrode placement, duration of stimulation as well as optimal number of treatments per day in well-diagnosed patients should be done. The inherent problem of a realistic placebo as well as blinding remain substantial obstacles in TENS trials. If available, a gold standard may be used for comparison, i.e. the best available measure for relief in different pain conditions. It is important to present detailed descriptions of stimulus parameters and outcome measures. Further, it is crucial to describe patient populations meticulously, not only labelling them diagnostically but also, if possible, subgrouping patient populations with regard to plausible underlying pathophysiological mechanisms of the specific condition. In neuropathic pain, it seems reasonable to include data on presence or absence of, for example, dynamic mechanical allodynia, cold allodynia, etc. This may give clues as to susceptibility to pain alleviation by TENS in subgroups of patients with different diagnostic entities. It seems appropriate to conclude that in spite of being around for three decades, rigorous clinical scientific evidence to support the widespread use of TENS is still lacking.

VIBRATION

Rubbing a painful part of the skin or massaging an aching muscle are age-old pain-relieving measures involving stimulation of mechanoreceptors. A more modern method to stimulate such receptors is vibration, activating superficial as well as deep mechanoreceptors (Vallbo & Hagbarth 1968, Ferrington et al 1977). The Pacinian corpuscles (Knibestol & Vallbo 1970, Homma et al 1971) and the primary endings of the muscle spindle (Eklund & Hagbarth 1965), connected to large-diameter afferents, are among the receptors with high sensitivity to vibration.

From the limited number of randomized, placebo-controlled clinical studies available, it can be concluded that vibratory stimulation may induce significant alleviation of acute orofacial nociceptive pain (Ottosson et al 1981, Ekblom & Hansson 1985, Hansson et al 1986) and various chronic orofacial painful conditions (Lundeberg et al 1983, 1985b). Also, acute nociceptive musculoskeletal pain of various aetiology was reported to be alleviated (Lundeberg et al 1984). In addition, vibratory stimulation has also been shown to relieve chronic musculoskeletal pain (Lundeberg 1984, Lundberg et al 1984, 1987, 1988a). The most pronounced effects in patients with acute and chronic nociceptive pain were seen when vibratory stimulation was applied in the painful area with moderate pressure and for a duration of about 30 minutes (Ottosson et al 1981, Lundeberg et al 1984). In a randomized, placebo-controlled study vibratory stimulation was also shown to induce relief of stump and phantom pain (Lundeberg 1985a).

TENTATIVE MECHANISMS OF ACTION

In general, the mechanisms of action of TENS-induced pain relief are likely to apply also in vibration-induced pain alleviation. Experimental studies have indicated that vibration induces an adenosine-mediated inhibition of nociceptive dorsal horn neurons (De Koninck & Henry 1992, De Koninck et al 1994). A role for purines in pain alleviation induced by vibratory stimulation has also been demonstrated in man (Tardy-Gervet et al 1993). Furthermore, vibratory stimulation was reported to result in a decrease in substance P-like immunoreactivity in the cerebrospinal fluid in 'chronic pain patients' (Guieu et al 1993). A role for endogenous opioids in mediating pain relief from vibration is unlikely as the pain-relieving effect has been shown to be unaffected by naloxone (Lundeberg 1985b, Hansson et al 1986) and not related to changes in cerebrospinal fluid concentrations of met-enkephalin and β-endorphin (Guieu et al 1992).

CONCLUSIONS

Although the literature hints at a pain-relieving potential for vibration in a small number of painful conditions, the use of vibratory stimulation in clinical practice has been hampered by the lack of commercially available, convenient stimulation units. The area needs further exploration.

ACUPUNCTURE

Acupuncture is an ancient therapeutic technique of Traditional Chinese Medicine (TCM). It is a method of treatment that possibly derived from the experiences of implanting sharp needle-like objects into the body to alleviate pain. Around 200 BC one of the first comprehensive manuals of Chinese medicine appeared; part of it was later transformed into the so-called *Ling Shu* containing the first description of the theoretical basis and methods of acupuncture (Lu & Needham 1980). Problems pertaining

 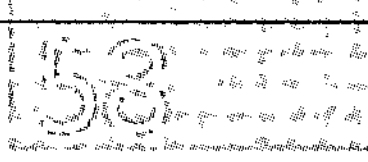

to the acceptance of acupuncture in the West today are partly the result of the inherent incompatibility between modern medicine and TCM regarding evaluation of pain and disease processes. Adding to this position is the low quality of many studies on acupuncture, contradictory results and the fact that results from high-quality acupuncture studies do not accord with the more enthusiastic conclusions of studies less well performed (Richardson & Vincent 1986, Ter Riet et al 1990, Zhang & Oetliker 1991, Vincent 1992, Resch & Ernst 1995, Vincent & Lewith 1995, Ernst 1997, Ernst & Pittler 1998, Rosted 1998). The survey presented below, based on a selection of available data from the literature, does not claim to be complete but rather has focused on some clinically important areas of acupuncture.

TECHNICAL AND PRACTICAL ASPECTS

Whether special effects are obtained at acupuncture points is unresolved (Cho et al 1998, Filshie & White 1998). It is unlikely that the acupuncture points are characterized by specific features. The retention of their positions as landmarks for acupuncture is important, as consistent location of insertion points aids communication and replication (Jenkins 1990).

Taken together, a multitude of modes and techniques of acupuncture stimulation have been proposed by authors in the field (Kao 1973, Mann et al 1973, Melzack et al 1977, Nogier 1981, MacDonald et al 1983, Mann 1992, Baldry 1993, Gunn 1996). It is unlikely, however, that one technique can claim superiority in all conditions, as different acupuncture modes and parameters may turn out to be varyingly effective in pain conditions with different aetiology (Thomas & Lundeberg 1994, 1996, Thomas et al 1995).

Clinical experience in patients with myofascial pain indicates that the best pain relief is achieved when the stimulation is administered to trigger points in the painful area (Baldry 1993). In various acute and chronic musculoskeletal pain conditions, the most significant pain reduction was obtained when stimulation was carried out in the same segment as the pain (Lundeberg et al 1988b). Significantly longer duration of pain reduction may be obtained in experimental pain (Andersson et al 1977) and in patients suffering from musculoskeletal pain (Lundeberg et al 1988b) if such stimulation is combined with strong (painful) stimulation at extrasegmental sites (points). In a randomized study comparing deep acupuncture provoking 'de Qi' (an intense painful sensation) and superficial acupuncture, the former was significantly more effective in reducing spontaneous and provoked pain in patients suffering from lateral epicondylalgia (Haker & Lundeberg 1990).

CLINICAL TRIALS

Acupuncture studies as a rule have enrolled patients with painful conditions lacking diagnostic precision (i.e. dental pain, neck pain, low back pain) (Richardson & Vincent 1986, Ter Riet et al 1990, Resch & Ernst 1995, Vincent & Lewith 1995, Ernst 1997, Ernst & Pittler 1998, Rosted 1998). The inhomogeneity of patients in terms of pain aetiology may be one of the reasons for the variety in outcome of acupuncture trials. It is also likely that lack of proper study design, e.g. lack of objective outcome measures, sham control and independent evaluator, affects outcome (Hester 1998). In studies on the pain-reducing effect of acupuncture in 'low back pain', 25–70% of patients reported pain relief (Richardson & Vincent 1986). If one takes into account more confined diagnostic entities, another picture possibly emerges (Thomas & Lundeberg 1996), although only a few randomized studies in well-diagnosed patients have been published with efforts to include different placebo-like procedures. The results from some of these suggest that acupuncture may give short-term relief in nociceptive low back pain (Thomas & Lundeberg 1994), pain related to temporomandibular joint dysfunction (List & Helkimo 1992), dysmenorrhoea (Thomas et al 1995) and fibromyalgia (Deluze et al 1992). Painful peripheral diabetic neuropathy was also reported to be alleviated by acupuncture (Abuaisha et al 1998). Idiopathic pain was reported not to respond (Thomas et al 1992).

RISKS, ADVERSE EVENTS AND SIDE EFFECTS

Acupuncture is often claimed to be 'harmless' or at least reasonably safe, but there is a growing recognition that there are risks of adverse events (Ernst 1995, Ernst & White 1997). Inexpert handling of acupuncture needles or their reuse without adequate sterilization carries the risk of infection (Pierik 1982). Serious trauma can result from needle insertion (Ernst & White 1997). Pneumothorax is the most common, but several cases of cardiac tamponade have been reported, including one fatality (Halvorsen et al 1995). Hence, an absolute prerequisite for the use of acupuncture is a detailed knowledge of anatomy. There are few contraindications for the careful use of acupuncture, but patients with bleeding disorders or on anticoagulants should generally not be treated and those with a cardiac pacemaker should not be given electrical stimulation. As for TENS, acupuncture should not be given in close proximity to the pregnant uterus.

TENTATIVE MECHANISMS OF ACTION

Acupuncture is a mode of peripheral stimulation based on the activation of peripheral receptors and/or sensory nerve fibres (Chiang et al 1973, Andersson & Holmgren 1975, Bowsher 1992, Gao et al 1996). While a needle may mechanically stimulate nerve fibres of many types, the pain-relieving effect of acupuncture has been attributed to the activation of Aδ and possibly C fibres (Wang et al 1992). Acupuncture is a high-intensity stimulus that hypothetically modulates various responses of the organism by central effects on the somatic and autonomic nervous system (Han et al 1978, 1991, Andersson & Lundeberg 1995, Knardahl et al 1998). Acupuncture stimulation has, for example, been reported to activate descending inhibition via pathways in the dorsolateral funiculus (LeBars et al 1991, 1992).

Early investigations in China suggested the involvement of specific neurotransmitters in antinociception following acupuncture (Yang & Koh 1979). There is evidence that endogenous opioid peptides and their respective receptors mediate these effects, with additional involvement of serotonergic and noradrenergic pain inhibitory systems (Han & Terenius 1982, Han & Sun 1990, Chen & Han 1992). Naloxone reversal of acupuncture analgesia is, along with the finding of increased concentrations of endogenous opioids in the cerebrospinal fluid following acupuncture, cited as evidence of an endogenous opioid link for its effects (Pomeranz & Chiu 1976, Mayer et al 1977, Sjölund et al 1977, Clement-Jones et al 1980, He 1987).

Acupuncture analgesia has also been suggested to mediate its analgesic effects via a stress-induced mechanism (Bodnar 1991). If this were true, the stimulation would probably be highly unpleasant, which is normally not the case. In addition, non-painful low-frequency electroacupuncture used in experimental and clinical studies was reported to be relaxing and not stressful (Widerström-Noga 1993, Dyrehag 1998). In experimental studies, pain threshold increase after acupuncture stimulation was most pronounced in those subjects reporting low levels of stress and anxiety and high levels of pleasantness and relaxation (Widerström-Noga 1993), indicating that the pain-relieving effects of acupuncture may be closely related to the psychological state of the patient (Lewith & Kenyon 1984, Norton et al 1984, Kreitler et al 1987).

CONCLUSIONS

The bulk of studies on pain relief from acupuncture suffer from methodological shortcomings. Results from randomized controlled studies do not accord with the more enthusiastic conclusions from studies less well performed. Further studies adapted to the criteria set up for TENS studies (see Box 58.1) are needed.

REFERENCES

Abelson K, Langley GB, Sheppeard H, Vlieg M, Wigley RD 1983 Transcutaneous electrical nerve stimulation in rheumatoid arthritis. New Zealand Medical Journal 727: 156–158

Abrams SE, Reynold AC, Cusick JF 1981 Failure of naloxone to reverse analgesia from transcutaneous electrical stimulation in patients with chronic pain. Anesthesia and Analgesia 60: 81–84

Abuaisha BB, Costanzi JB, Boulton AJ 1998 Acupuncture for the treatment of chronic painful peripheral diabetic neuropathy: a long-term study. Diabetes Research and Clinical Practice 39: 115–121

Andersson SA, Holmgren E 1975 On acupuncture analgesia and the mechanism of pain. American Journal of Chinese Medicine 3: 311–334

Andersson SA, Lundeberg T 1995 Acupuncture – from empiricism to science: functional background to acupuncture effects in pain and disease. Medical Hypotheses 45: 271–281

Andersson SA, Holmgren E, Roos A 1977 Analgesic effects of peripheral conditioning stimulation. II. Importance of certain stimulation parameters. Acupuncture and Electro-Therapy Research International Journal 2: 237–246

Augustinsson L-E, Bohlin P, Bundsen P et al 1977 Pain relief during delivery by transcutaneous electrical nerve stimulation. Pain 4: 59–65

Baldry PE 1993 Acupuncture, trigger points and musculoskeletal pain 2E, Churchill Livingstone, Edinburgh

Bates JA, Nathan PW 1980 Transcutaneous electrical nerve stimulation for chronic pain. Anaesthesia 8: 817–822

Bennedetti F, Amanzio M, Casadio C et al 1997 Control of postoperative pain by transcutaneous electrical nerve stimulation after thoracic operations. Annals of Thoracic Surgery 3: 773–776

Bodnar RJ 1991 Effects of opioid peptides on peripheral stimulation and 'stress'-induced analgesia in animals. Critical Review of Neurobiology 6: 39–49

Borjesson M, Eriksson P, Dellborg M, Eliasson T, Mannheimer C 1997 Transcutaneous electrical nerve stimulation in unstable angina pectoris. Coronary Artery Disease 8–9: 543–550

Bowsher D 1992 The physiology of stimulation-produced analgesia. Pain Clinic (Tokyo) 12: 485–492

Bundsen P, Peterson L-E, Selstam U 1981 Pain relief in labor by transcutaneous electrical nerve stimulation. Acta Obstetrica et Gynaecologica Scandinavica 60: 459–468

Carroll D, Tramer M, McQuay H, Nye B, Moore A 1996 Randomization is important in studies with pain outcomes: systematic review of transcutaneous electrical nerve stimulation in acute postoperative pain. British Journal of Anaesthesia 6: 798–803

Carroll D, Tramer M, McQuay H, Nye B, Moore A 1997 Transcutaneous electrical nerve stimulation in labour pain: a systematic review. British Journal of Obstetrics and Gynaecology February 1997: 169–175

Chapman CR, Benedetti C 1977 Analgesia following transcutaneous electrical stimulation and its partial reversal by a narcotic antagonist. Life Sciences 11: 1645–1648

Chauhan A, Mullins PA, Thuraisingham SI, Taylor G, Petch MC,

Schofield PM 1994 Effect of transcutaneous electrical nerve stimulation on coronary blood flow. Circulation 2: 694–702

Chen XH, Han JS 1992 All three types of opioid receptors in the spinal cord are important for 2/15 Hz electroacupuncture analgesia. European Journal of Pharmacology 211: 203–210

Chiang CY, Chang CT, Chu HL, Yang LF 1973 Peripheral afferent pathways for acupuncture anagesia. Science International Journal 16: 210–217

Cho ZH, Chung SC, Jones JP et al 1998 New findings of the correlation between acupoints and corresponding brain cortices using functional MRI. Proceedings of the National Academy of Science USA 95: 2670–2673

Chung JM, Lee KH, Hori Y, Endo K, Willis WD 1984 Factors influencing peripheral nerve stimulation produced inhibition of primate spinothalamic tract cells. Pain 19: 277–293

Clement-Jones V, McLoughlin L, Tomlin S, Besser GM, Rees LH, Wen HL 1980 Increased beta-endorphin but not met-enkephalin levels in human cerebrospinal fluid after acupuncture for recurrent pain. Lancet 2: 946–949

Conn I G, Marshall AH, Yadav SN, Daly JC, Jaffer M 1986 Transcutaneous electrical nerve stimulation following appendicectomy. Annals of the Royal College of Surgeons of England 4: 191–192

Davis R, Lentini R 1975 Transcutaneous nerve stimulation for treatment of pain in patients with spinal cord injury. Surgical Neurology 1: 100–101

Dawood MY, Ramos J 1990 Transcutaneous electrical nerve stimulation (TENS) for the treatment of primary dysmenorrhea: a randomized crossover comparison with placebo TENS. Obstetrics and Gynecology 4: 656–660

De Koninck Y, Henry JL 1992 Peripheral vibration causes an adenosine-mediated postsynaptic inhibitory potential in dorsal horn neurons of the cat spinal cord. Neuroscience 50: 435–443

De Koninck Y, Salter MW, Henry JL 1994 Substance P released endogenously by high-intensity sensory stimulation potentiates purinergic inhibition of dorsal horn neurons induced by peripheral stimulation. Neuroscience Letters 176: 128–132

Deluze C, Bosia L, Zirbs A, Chantraine A, Vischer TL 1992 Electroacupuncture in fibromyalgia: results of a controlled trial. British Medical Journal 305: 1249–1252

Deyo RA, Walsh NE, Martin DC, Schoenfeld LS, Ramamurthy S 1990 A controlled trial of transcutaneous electrical nerve stimulation (TENS) and exercise for chronic low back pain. New England Journal of Medicine 23: 1627–1634

Dyrehag L-E 1998 Effects of somatic afferent stimulation in chronic musculoskeletal pain. Thesis. University of Gothenburg, Sweden

Ekblom A, Hansson P 1985 Extrasegmental transcutaneous electrical nerve stimulation and mechanical vibratory stimulation as compared to placebo for the relief of acute oro-facial pain. Pain 23: 223–229

Eklund G, Hagbarth KE 1965 Motor effects of vibratory muscle stimuli in man. Electroencephalography and Clinical Neurophysiology 19: 619

Eriksson MBE, Sjölund BH, Nielzen S 1979 Long term results of peripheral conditioning stimulation as an analgesic measure in chronic pain. Pain 6: 335–347

Ernst E 1995 The risks of acupuncture. International Journal of Risk and Safety Medicine 6: 179–186

Ernst E 1997 Acupuncture as a symptomatic treatment of osteoarthritis. Scandinavian Journal of Rheumatology 26: 444–447

Ernst E, Pittler MH 1998 The effectiveness of acupuncture in treating acute dental pain: a systematic review. British Dental Journal 184: 443–447

Ernst E, White A 1997 Life-threatening adverse reactions after acupuncture? A systematic review. Pain 71: 123–126

Ferrington DG, Nail BS, Rowe M 1977 Human tactile detection threshold: modification by inputs from specific tactile receptor classes. Journal of Physiology 272: 415–433

Filshie J, White A 1998 Medical acupuncture. Churchill Livingstone, Edinburgh

Fishbain DA, Chabal C, Abbott A, Heine LW, Cutler R 1996 Transcutaneous electrical nerve stimulation (TENS) treatment outcome in long-term users. Clinical Journal of Pain 3: 201–214

Foster NE, Baxter F, Walsh DM, Baxter GD, Allen JM 1996 Manipulation of transcutaneous electrical nerve stimulation variables has no effect on two models of experimental pain in humans. Clinical Journal of Pain 4: 301–310

Freeman TB, Campbell JN, Long DM 1983 Naloxone does not affect pain relief induced by electrical stimulation in man. Pain 17: 189–195

Gao X, Gao C, Gao J, Han F, Han B, Han L 1996 Acupuncture treatment of complete traumatic paraplegia – analysis of 261 cases. Journal of Traditional Chinese Medicine 16: 134–137

Garrison DW, Foreman RD 1996 Effects of transcutaneous electrical nerve stimulation (TENS) on spontaneous and noxiously evoked dorsal horn cell activity in cats with transected spinal cords. Neuroscience Letters 216: 125–128

Gilbert JM, Gledhill T, Law N, George C 1986 Controlled trial of transcutaneous electrical nerve stimulation (TENS) for postoperative pain relief following inguinal herniorrhaphy. British Journal of Surgery 9: 749–751

Guieu R, Tardy-Gervet MF, Giraud P 1992 Met-enkephalin and beta-endorphin are not involved in analgesic action of transcutaneous vibratory stimulation. Pain 48: 83–88

Guieu R, Tardy-Gervet MF, Giraud P 1993 Substance P-like immunoreactivity and analgesic effects of vibratory stimulation on patients suffering from chronic pain. Canadian Journal of Neurological Science 20: 138–141

Gunn CC 1996 The Gunn approach to the treatment of chronic pain. Churchill Livingstone, Edinburgh

Haker E, Lundeberg T 1990 Acupuncture treatment in epicondylalgia: a comparative study of two acupuncture techniques. Clinical Journal of Pain 6: 221–226

Halvorsen TB, Anda SS, Levang OW 1995 Fatal cardiac tamponade after acupuncture through congenital sternal foramen. Lancet 345: 1175

Han JS, Sun SL 1990 Differential release of enkephalin and dynorphin by low and high frequency electroacupuncture in the central nervous system. Science International Journal 1: 19–23

Han JS, Terenius L 1982 Neurochemical basis of acupuncture analgesia. Annual Review of Pharmacology and Toxicology 22: 193–220

Han JS, Ton J, Fan SG 1978 The contents of 5-hydroxytryptamine (5-HT) and morphine-like substances (MLS) in the brain and electro-acupuncture analgesia (AA). Sheng Li Hsueh Pao 30: 201–203

Han JS, Chen XH, Sun SL et al 1991 Effect of low- and high-frequency TENS on met-enkephalin-Arg-Phe and dynorphin A immunoreactivity in human lumbar CSF. Pain 47: 295–298

Hansson P, Ekblom A 1983 Transcutaneous electrical nerve stimulation (TENS) as compared to placebo TENS for the relief of acute oro-facial pain. Pain 15: 157–165

Hansson P, Ekblom A 1984 Afferent stimulation induced pain relief in acute orofacial pain and its failure to induce sufficient pain reduction in dental and oral surgery. Pain 20: 273–278

Hansson P, Ekblom A, Thomsson M, Fjellner B 1986 Influence of naloxone on relief of acute oro-facial pain by transcutaneous electrical nerve stimulation (TENS) or vibration. Pain 24: 323–329

Harrison RF, Woods T, Shore M, Mathews G, Unwin A 1986 Pain relief in labour using transcutaneous electrical nerve stimulation (TENS). A TENS/TENS placebo controlled study in two parity groups. British Journal of Obstetrics and Gynaecology 93: 739–746

He LF 1987 Involvement of endogenous opioid peptides in acupuncture analgesia. Pain 31: 99–121

Herman E, Williams R, Stratford P, Fargas-Babjak A, Trott M 1994 A randomized controlled trial of transcutaneous electrical nerve stimulation (CODETRON) to determine its benefits in a rehabilitation program for acute occupational low back pain. Spine 5: 561–568

Hester J 1998 Acupuncture in the pain clinic. In: Filshie J, White A (eds) Medical acupuncture. Churchill Livingstone, Edinburgh, pp 319–340

Homma S, Kanda K, Watanabe S 1971 Tonic vibration reflex in human and monkey subjects. Japan Journal of Physiology 21: 419–430

Ignelzi RJ, Nyquist JK 1976 Direct effect of electrical stimulation on peripheral nerve evoked activity: implications in pain relief. Journal of Neurosurgery 45: 159–166

Janko M, Trontelj JV 1980 Transcutaneous electrical nerve stimulation: a microneurographic and perceptual study. Pain 9: 219–230

Jenkins M 1990 A new standard international acupuncture nomenclature. Acupuncture in Medicine 7: 21–23

Johnson MI, Ashton CH, Thompson JW 1991a An in-depth study of long-term users of transcutaneous electrical nerve stimulation (TENS). Implications for clinical use of TENS. Pain 44: 221–229

Johnson MI, Ashton CH, Bousfield DR, Thompson JW 1991b Analgesic effects of different pulse patterns of transcutaneous electrical nerve stimulation on cold-induced pain in normal subjects. Journal of Psychosomatic Research 35: 313–321

Kao FF 1973 Acupuncture therapeutics: an introductory text. Triple Oak, Garden City, NY

Knardahl S, Elam M, Olausson B, Wallin BG 1998 Sympathetic nerve activity after acupuncture in humans. Pain 75: 19–25

Knibestol M, Vallbo ÅB 1970 Single unit analysis of mechanoreceptor activity from the human glabrous skin. Acta Physiologica Scandinavica 80: 178–195

Kolmodin GM, Skoglund CR 1960 Analysis of spinal interneurons activated by tactile and nociceptive stimulation. Acta Physiologica Scandinavica 50: 337–355

Kreitler S, Kreitler H, Carasso R 1987 Cognitive orientation as predictor of pain relief following acupuncture. Pain 28: 323–341

Langley GB, Sheppeard H, Johnson M, Wigley RD 1984 The analgesic effects of transcutaneous electrical nerve stimulation and placebo in chronic pain patients. Rheumatology International 4: 119–123

LeBars D, Dickenson AH, Besson JM 1979a Diffuse noxious inhibitory controls. II- Lack of effect on non convergent neurons, supraspinal involvement and theoretical implications. Pain 6: 305–327

LeBars D, Dickenson AH, Besson JM 1979b Diffuse noxious inhibitory controls. I- Effect on dorsal horn convergent neurons in the rat. Pain 6: 283–304

LeBars D, Villanueva L, Willer JC, Bouhassira D 1991 Diffuse noxious inhibitory controls (DNIC) in animals and in man. Acupuncture in Medicine 9: 47–56

LeBars D, Willer JC, De Broucker T 1992 Morphine blocks descending pain inhibitory controls in humans. Pain 48: 13–20

Lee KH, Chung JM, Willis WDJ 1985 Inhibition of primate spinothalamic tract cells by TENS. Journal of Neurosurgery 2: 276–287

Leijon G, Boivie J 1989 Central post stroke pain – the effect of high and low frequency TENS. Pain 38: 187–191

Lewith GT, Kenyon JN 1984 Physiological and psychological explanations for the mechanism of acupuncture as a treatment for chronic pain. Social Science in Medicine 19: 1367–1378

List T, Helkimo M 1992 Acupuncture and occlusal splint therapy in the treatment of craniomandibular disorders. Acta Odontologica Scandinavica 50: 375–387

Loeser JD, Black RG, Christmas A 1975 Relief of pain by transcutaneous stimulation. Journal of Neurosurgery March: 308–314

Long DM 1991 Fifteen years of transcutaneous electrical stimulation for pain control. Stereotactic and Functional Neurosurgery 56: 2–19

Lu GD, Needham J 1980 Celestial lancets, a history and rationale of acupuncture and moxa. Cambridge University Press, Cambridge.

Lundeberg T 1984 Long-term results of vibratory stimulation as a pain relieving measure for chronic pain. Pain 20: 13–24

Lundeberg T 1985a Relief of pain from a phantom limb by peripheral stimulation. Journal of Neurology 232: 79–82

Lundeberg T 1985b Naloxone does not reverse the pain reducing effect of vibratory stimulation. Acta Anaesthesiologica Scandinavica 29: 212–216

Lundeberg T, Ottosson D, Håkansson S, Meyerson BA 1983 Vibratory stimulation for the control of intractable chronic orofacial pain. In: Bonica JJ, Lindblom U, Iggo A (eds) Advances in pain research and therapy. Raven Press, New York, pp 555–561

Lundeberg T, Nordemar R, Ottosson D 1984 Pain alleviation by vibratory stimulation. Pain 20: 25–44

Lundeberg T, Bondesson L, Lundstöm V 1985a Relief of primary dysmenorrhea by transcutaneous electrical nerve stimulation. Acta Obstetrica Gynaecologica Scandinavica 64: 491–497

Lundeberg T, Ekblom A, Hansson P 1985b Relief of sinus pain by vibratory stimulation. Ear Nose Throat Journal 64: 163–167

Lundeberg T, Abrahamsson P, Bondesson L, Haker E 1987 Vibratory stimulation compared to placebo in alleviation of pain. Scandinavian Journal of Rehabilitation Medicine 19: 153–158

Lundeberg T, Abrahamsson P, Bondesson L, Haker E 1988a Effects of vibratory stimulation on experimental and clinical pain. Scandinavian Journal of Rehabilitation Medicine 20: 149–159

Lundeberg T, Hurtig T, Lundeberg S, Thomas M 1988b Long-term results of acupuncture in chronic head and neck pain. Pain Clinic 2: 15–31

MacDonald A, Macrae K, Master B, Rubin A 1983 Superficial acupuncture in the relief of chronic low back pain. Annals of the Royal College of Surgeons of England 65: 44–46

Mann F 1992 Reinventing acupuncture: a new concept of ancient medicine. Butterworth Heinemann, London

Mann F, Bowsher D, Mumford J, Lipton S, Miles J 1973 Treatment of intractable pain by acupuncture. Lancet 2: 57–60

Mannheimer C, Carlsson CA 1979 The analgesic effect of transcutaneous electrical nerve stimulation (TNS) in patients with rheumatoid arthritis. A comparative study of different pulse patterns. Pain 6: 329–334

Mannheimer C, Lund S, Carlsson CA 1978 The effect of transcutaneous electrical nerve stimulation (TNS) on joint pain in patients with rheumatoid arthritis. Scandinavian Journal of Rheumatology 7: 13–16

Mannheimer C, Carlsson CA, Emanuelsson H, Vedin A, Waagstein F 1985 The effects of transcutaneous electrical nerve stimulation in patients with severe angina pectoris. Circulation 2: 308–316

Marchand S, Bushnell MC, Duncan GH 1991 Modulation of heat pain perception by high frequency transcutanous electrical nerve stimulation (TENS). Clinical Journal of Pain 2: 122–129

Mayer D, Price D, Rafii A 1977 Antagonism of acupuncture analgesia in man by the narcotic antagonist naloxone. Brain Research 121: 368–372

Melzack R, Wall PD 1965 Pain mechanisms: a new theory. Science 150: 971–978

Melzack R, Stillwell D, Fox E 1977 Trigger points and acupuncture points for pain: correlations and implications. Pain 3: 3–23

Meyerson B 1983 Electrostimulation procedures: effects, presumed rationale, and possible mechanisms. In: Bonica JJ, Lindblom U, Iggo A (eds) Advances in pain research and therapy. Raven Press, New York, pp 495–534

Meyler WJ, De Jongste MJL 1994 Clinical evaluation of pain treatment with electrostimulation: a study on TENS in patients with different pain syndromes. Clinical Journal of Pain 10: 22–27

Milsom I, Hedner N, Mannheimer C 1994 A comparative study of the effect of high-intensity transcutaneous nerve stimulation and oral naproxen on intrauterine pressure and menstrual pain. American Journal of Obstetrics and Gynecology 1: 123–129

Moystad A, Krogstad BS, Larheim TA 1990 Transcutaneous nerve stimulation in a group of patients with rheumatic disease involving

the temporomandibular joint. Journal of Prosthetic Dentistry 5: 596–600
Nathan PW, Rudge P 1974a Testing the gate-control theory of pain in man. Journal of Neurology, Neurosurgery and Psychiatry 37: 1366–1372
Nathan PW, Wall PD 1974b Treatment of post-herpetic neuralgia by prolonged electric stimulation. British Medical Journal 3: 645–647
Nogier PFM (trans. Kenyon) 1981 Introduction to auricular therapy. Maisonneuve, Paris.
Norton GR, Goszer L, Strub H, Man SC 1984 The effects of belief on acupuncture analgesia. Canadian Journal of Behavioural Science 16: 22–29
Olausson B, Xu Z Q, Shyu BC 1994 Dorsal column inhibition of nociceptive thalamic cells mediated by gamma-aminobutyric acid mechanisms in the cat. Acta Physiologica Scandinavica 152: 239–247
Ottosson D, Ekblom A, Hansson P 1981 Vibratory stimulation for the relief of pain of dental origin. Pain 10: 37–45
Pertovaara A, Kemppainen P 1981 The influence of naloxone on dental pain threshold elevation produced by peripheral conditioning stimulation at high frequency. Brain Research 215: 426–429
Pierik MG 1982 Fatal staphylococcal septicemia following acupuncture: report of two cases. Royal Institute Medical Journal 65: 251–253
Pomeranz B, Chiu D 1976 Naloxone blockage of acupuncture analgesia: endorphin implicated. Life Science 19: 1757–1762
Resch KL, Ernst E 1995 Proving the effectiveness of complementary therapy. Analysis of the literature exemplified by acupuncture. Fortschritte der Medizin 113: 49–53
Richardson PH, Vincent CA 1986 Acupuncture for the treatment of pain: a review of evaluative research. Pain 24: 15–40
Rosted P 1998 The use of acupuncture in dentistry: a review of the scientific validity of published reports. Oral Disease 4: 100–104
Salar G, Job I, Mingrino S, Bosio A, Trabucci M 1981 Effect of transcutaneous electrotherapy on CSF B-endorphin content in patients without pain problems. Pain 10: 169–172
Schmidt RF 1972 The gate control theory of pain. A critical hypothesis. In: Janzen R, Kreidel W D, Herz A, Steichele C (eds) Pain. Churchill Livingstone, London, pp 124–127
Sjölund BH 1985 Peripheral nerve stimulation suppression of C-fiber-evoked flexion reflex in rats. Part 1: Parameters of continuous stimulation. Journal of Neurosurgery 4: 612–616
Sjölund BH, Eriksson MBE 1979 The influence of naloxone on analgesia by peripheral conditioning stimulation. Brain Research 173: 295–301
Sjölund BH, Terenius L, Eriksson MBE 1977 Increased cerebrospinal fluid levels of endorphins after electroacupuncture. Acta Physiologica Scandinavica 100: 382–384
Tardy-Gervet MF, Guieu R, Ribot-Ciscar E, Roll JP 1993 Transcutaneous mechanical vibrations: analgesic effect and antinociceptive mechanisms. Revue Neurologique (Paris) 149: 177–185
Ter Riet G, Kleijnen J, Knipschild P 1990 Acupuncture and chronic pain: a criteria-based meta-analysis. Journal of Clinical Epidemiology 43: 1191–1199
Thomas M, Lundeberg T 1994 Importance of modes of acupuncture in the treatment of chronic nociceptive low back pain. Acta Anaesthesiologica Scandinavica 38: 63–69
Thomas M, Lundeberg T 1996 Does acupuncture work? Pain Clinical Updates 4: 1–4
Thomas M, Arnér S, Lundeberg T 1992 Is acupuncture a treatment alternative in idiopathic pain disorders? Acta Anaesthiologica Scandinavica 36: 637–642
Thomas M, Lundeberg T, Björk G, Lundström-Lindstedt V 1995 Pain and discomfort in primary dysmenorrhea is reduced by preemptive acupuncture or low frequency TENS. European Journal of Rehabilitation 5: 71–76
Thorsteinsson G, Stonnington HH, Stillwell GK, Elveback LR 1977 Transcutaneous electrical stimulation: a double-blind trial of its efficacy for pain. Archives of Physical Medicine and Rehabilitation 58: 8–13
Vallbo Å B, Hagbarth KE 1968 Activity from skin mechanoreceptors recorded percutaneously in awake human subjects. Experimental Neurology 21: 270–289
VanderArk GD, McGrath KA 1975 Transcutaneous electrical stimulation in treatment of postoperative pain. American Journal of Surgery September: 338–340
Van der Ploeg JM, Vervest HAM, Liem AL, Van Leeuwen JHS 1996 Transcutaneous nerve stimulation (TENS) during the first stage of labour: a randomized clinical trial. Pain 68: 75–78
Vincent CA 1992 Acupuncture research, why do it? Complementary Medical Research 1: 21–24
Vincent CA, Lewith G 1995 Placebo controls for acupuncture studies. Journal of the Royal Society of Medicine 88: 199–202
Wall PD 1964 Presynaptic control of impulses at the first central synapse in the cutaneous pathway. In: Eccles J C, Schade J P (eds) Physiology of spinal neurons. Elsevier, New York, pp 92–115
Wall PD, Sweet WH 1967 Temporary abolition of pain in man. Science 155: 108–109
Wang JQ, Mao L, Han JS 1992 Comparison of the antinociceptive effects induced by electroacupuncture and transcutaneous electrical nerve stimulation in the rat. International Journal of Neuroscience 65: 117–129
Widerström-NogaE 1993 Analgesic effects of somatic afferent stimulation–a psychobiological perspective. Thesis. University of Gothenburg. Sweden
Woolf CJ 1979 Transcutaneous electrical nerve stimulation and the reaction to experimental pain in human subjects. Pain 7: 115–127
Woolf CJ, Wall PD 1982 Chronic peripheral nerve section diminishes the primary afferent A-fibre mediated inhibition of rat dorsal horn neurones. Brain Research 1: 77–85
Woolf CJ, Mitchell D, Myers RA, Barrett GD 1978 Failure of naloxone to reverse peripheral transcutaneous electro-analgesia in patients suffering from acute trauma. South African Medical Journal 53: 179–180
Yang MM, Koh SH 1979 Further study of the neurohumoral factor, endorphin, in the mechanism of acupuncture analgesia. American Journal of Chinese Medicine 7: 143–148
Zhang W, Oetliker H 1991 Acupuncture for pain control. A review of controlled clinical trials. In: Schlapback P, Gerber NJ (eds) Physiotherapy: controlled trials and facts. Karger, Basel, pp 171–88

Spinal cord and brain stimulation

59

BRIAN A. SIMPSON

Electrical therapeutic spinal cord stimulation (SCS) was introduced more than 30 years ago but a poor understanding of the indications, variable follow-up and unreliable equipment delayed its acceptance. Case selection and assessment of outcome remain problematical but neuropathic pain syndromes and ischaemic pain have emerged as the prime indications. Patterns of practice differ widely in different countries, however. SCS can be remarkably successful where other treatments have been ineffective but very little is known about SCS failures. As evidence accumulates, both physiological and pharmacological, the mechanisms of action are becoming better understood.

The steady increase in the use of SCS contrasts with the decline in deep brain stimulation (DBS) for pain, originally developed during the 1970s and 1980s. Both nociceptive and neuropathic pain respond to DBS. Reported outcomes have been variable but the hoped-for levels of success in head and facial pain, and in pain covering large areas (unsuitable for SCS), were not consistently achieved. Most recently, brain surface (motor cortex) stimulation has been introduced. Early experience suggests that two of the most intractable pain syndromes, neuropathic head and facial pain and pain due to central deafferentation, e.g. central post-stroke pain, respond well.

SPINAL CORD STIMULATION

BACKGROUND

Electricity has been used therapeutically for more than two millennia, the analgesic effect of electric fish having been recognized by the Greeks and Romans (Kellaway 1946, Kane & Taub 1975). The ability to store and control electricity has been available since 1745, when the Leyden jar was introduced. Electrotherapy enjoyed immense popularity as a nostrum and as an analgesic during the 19th and early 20th centuries. Electroanalgesia was used for dental extraction and other minor surgery, particularly in the USA, and peripheral nerve stimulation was used during amputations (Kane & Taub 1975). In the mid-1960s Wall and Sweet (1967) revisited therapeutic direct peripheral nerve (primary afferent) stimulation to test the gate theory. Although the analgesic effect was dramatic, the tolerance which developed in two patients led the authors to express doubts about the therapeutic implications.

The gating of pain transmission by simultaneous activity in large afferent fibres proposed by Melzack and Wall (1965) inspired Shealy to adopt a different approach. Recognizing that the dorsal columns of the spinal cord were rich in ascending collaterals of the large afferent Aβ fibres, he stimulated the dorsal columns in cats and obtained physiological and behavioural evidence for an analgesic effect (Shealy 1966, Shealy et al 1967b). The results were sufficiently encouraging for him to implant the first spinal cord stimulator in a patient in March 1967 (Shealy et al 1967a). The chest wall cancer pain was relieved, ironically because cancer pain is now known not to be a good indication. Sweet and Wepsic (1968) followed the lead of their former resident and were able to relieve postcordotomy pain by dorsal column stimulation ipsilateral to the pain. Shealy reported a further five cases (Shealy et al 1970) and within 6 years his series had risen to 86 (Shealy 1974).

The early developments in implantable hardware and variations in technique made assessment and comparisons between series difficult. The tendency of early electrodes and leads to move, break and lose insulation also delayed the fair appraisal of this new and attractive therapy. While several early published series were either relatively homogeneous or extensive (Shealy 1974, Sweet & Wepsic 1974, Krainick et al 1975, Long & Hagfors 1975, Pineda 1975, Cook et al 1976, Burton 1977, Young 1978), others were small and mixed (Miles et al 1974, Hoppenstein 1975, Hunt et al 1975, Larson et al 1975, Nashold 1975, Urban & Nashold 1978, Richardson et al 1979). Follow-up was variable; inconsistent outcome reports and unreliable equipment contributed to the wane in popularity of this (initially) expensive treatment during the 1970s. Since then, improvements in hardware, better appreciation of the indications, the discovery of excellent new indications and some understanding of the mechanisms of action have fuelled a regrowth in this field; more than 10 000 units are now implanted annually worldwide, approximately half in the USA and slightly fewer in Europe. Neuromodulation has developed in parallel with an appreciation of the much more limited role of neurodestructive procedures, the tendency of the damaged nervous system to generate pain having finally been recognized.

INDICATIONS

General

During the early years of spinal cord stimulation (SCS), the indications were poorly understood. The 'failed back surgery syndrome' (FBSS), which is now the commonest indication, may be a diagnosis but is not a unitary disease entity. As other indications have emerged, they have been more recognizable as specific conditions, e.g. angina pectoris, diabetic peripheral neuropathy and phantom limb pain, making case selection and assessment of outcome somewhat easier. In the complex regional pain syndromes (CRPS), however, the specificity of diagnosis and the relevance of sympathetic activity, particularly in the context of the effectiveness of SCS, are becoming less clear. It has taken a long time to recognize that, in general, SCS is most effective against neuropathic pain, particularly the continuous background component, and ischaemic pain. Early clues were available but were initially ignored. Thus, Nashold and Friedman (1972) reported that the best results were against burning pain in patients with sensory neurological damage and Dooley's best outcome was in those with vasospastic disease (Dooley 1977). It was seen that cancer pain could respond if there was a neuropathic element (Hoppenstein 1975, Larson et al 1975). Analysis of the results published between 1981 and 1998 (approximately 100 reports) and of personal experience allows a crude classification according to the likelihood of success with SCS (Table 59.1). There is an interesting divergence between the USA and Europe in that FBSS remains the major indication in the former with very few implanted for ischaemic pain whereas in Europe approximately half are for ischaemic pain. Wide variation also exists between European countries in both indications and implantation rates (Simpson 1998).

Failed back surgery syndrome

Of the hundreds of thousands of lumbar spine operations performed every year, a significant minority are unsuccessful, leaving the patient with persistent pain and, usually, a

Table 59.1 Spinal cord stimulation: outcome relative to diagnosis

Success > > failure	*Success > failure*	*Success variable*	*Failure > success*	*Failure > > success*	*Uncertain*
Angina pectoris	CRPS type I	Amputation – phantom pain	Perianal, genital pain	Central post-stroke pain	Abdominal, pelvic visceral pain
PVD – obstructive – vasospastic	CRPS type II	Partial cord lesions	Intercostal neuralgia (except PHN)	Complete cord lesions	Complete root, plexus avulsion
	Peripheral nerve damage	PHN		Facial anaesthesia dolorosa	
	Diabetic neuropathy	FBSS – back pain		Severe nociceptive pain (except ischaemic pain)	
	Brachial plexus damage				
	FBSS – leg pain				
	Cauda equina damage				
	Amputation – stump pain				
	Painful neuropathic bladder				

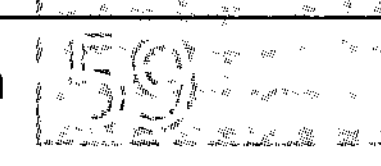

degree of disability. Repeated operations are common. The pain is in the back and/or one or both legs with a complex admix of mechanisms including referred pain. Cultural, social and psychological factors and reduced mobility compound the complexity of this common and expensive spectrum of disorders. Early reported success rates with SCS varied widely, from 11% (Urban & Nashold 1978) to 70% (Blume et al 1982). Although a large proportion of these patients have clinical evidence of neurological damage, the relevance of this was not initially addressed. Even the fundamental distinction between the response of back pain and of leg pain has tended not to be made (Blume et al 1982, Siegfried & Lazorthes 1982, De La Porte & Siegfried 1983, Le Doux & Langford 1993). A rare early example of this differentiation being made suggested strongly that back pain responded poorly and leg pain responded well (Pineda 1975). Support for this dichotomy has accumulated (Waisbrod & Gerbershagen 1985, Meilman et al 1989, Probst 1990, Siegfried 1991, Ohnmeiss et al 1996) and this might be expected as leg pain in FBSS is more likely to be neuropathic than is back pain, which is more likely to be nociceptive. The relative difficulty in targeting the low back with SCS (Sweet & Wepsic 1974, Law 1987, North et al 1991c, Barolat et al 1993, Fiume et al 1995, Hassenbusch et al 1995) also has a bearing on this and has encouraged the selection of cases either with only leg pain or with a significant radicular element accompanying their back pain (North et al 1991c, De La Porte & Van de Kelft 1993, Burchiel et al 1995, Fiume et al 1995, Rainov et al 1996). North has found that an equal degree of pain relief can be achieved in the two sites (North et al 1991c) and Law (1992) suggested that better results could be achieved in the back than in the legs. It may be that with technological improvements (see below) it is becoming easier to target the low back and there is undoubtedly a neuropathic component to the back pain in many cases.

The heterogeneity, not only of the subjects but also of the literature, makes an assessment of the efficacy of SCS in the FBSS difficult. Prospective studies are scarce. In one such (uncontrolled) study of 40 patients with predominantly leg pain, followed for 24 months and assessed by independent third parties, 70% felt SCS was helping them and was worth recommending and 66% reduced their narcotic intake (Ohnmeiss et al 1996). This was accompanied by functional improvements. The commonly used criterion of '50% or greater pain relief', however, yielded a success rate of only 26%. The much larger but also uncontrolled prospective multicentre study led by Burchiel (Burchiel et al 1996), which included other aetiologies, also showed that success in patients with FBSS (64% of the total) is difficult to assess. Fifty-six per cent reported 'at least 50% pain relief' after 1 year but only 35% described their pain relief as 'good' or 'excellent'. Depression and activity levels improved but drug intake did not. In a critical review of the literature, Turner and her colleagues (1995) concluded that approximately 50–60% of patients with FBSS report more than 50% pain relief with SCS but that our ability to assess its efficacy fully remains limited.

SCS has rarely been compared directly with other treatments. In a comparison with chronic intrathecal opiate infusion, it was concluded that SCS was effective in 62% and was least effective for buttock pain; similar relief with morphine infusion was obtained in only 38% but it appeared to have a role in cases of bilateral or axial pain that were poorly responsive to SCS (Hassenbusch et al 1995). Preliminary results from North's prospective, randomized comparison of SCS with lumbar spinal reoperation have shown a statistically significant advantage for SCS (North et al 1995). In a separate study reoperation was shown to be successful in 34%; predominance of radicular over axial pain favoured a good outcome (North et al 1991b). Arachnoiditis can occur independently of repeated spinal surgery but the outcome with SCS cannot be assessed specifically for this condition from the available data.

Plexus and peripheral nerve pathology including amputation

Neuropathic pain in cases of brachial plexus damage has generally been found to respond well whether due to accidental trauma, surgical trauma, radiotherapy or invasion by neoplasm (Hoppenstein 1975, Long & Erickson 1975, Nielsen et al 1975a, Hood & Siegfried 1984). Although pain following *complete* root avulsion has been reported to respond to SCS (Bennett & Tai 1994) it is difficult to reconcile this with the view that SCS depends upon intact ascending afferent collaterals. Certainly Hood and Siegfried (1984) were clear that cases of complete avulsion would not respond and it is a common clinical experience that the necessary paraesthesiae cannot be evoked by SCS in dermatomes completely deafferented from the cord, e.g. following dorsal rhizotomy. Clinical evidence for complete root avulsion should be verified by physiological and radiological evidence, without which firm conclusions cannot be drawn. Many patients have a mixture of root avulsion and root/plexus *partial* damage and are likely to respond to SCS to a useful extent. The relative physical unreliability of cervical electrodes due to the mobility of the cervical spine may have produced an underestimate of the efficacy in this group. It should be borne in mind that direct surgical repair of the brachial plexus can significantly relieve pain in some suitable patients (Berman et al 1998). Dorsal root entry zone (DREZ) lesions can also be effective (Garcia-March et al 1987, Bennett & Tai 1994) but are more invasive than SCS.

Pain due to peripheral nerve lesions is generally a good indication for SCS (Nielsen et al 1975a, Siegfried 1991, Simpson 1991, Kumar et al 1996, Tesfaye et al 1996). Painful diabetic neuropathy has been found to respond well (Nielsen et al 1975a, Kumar et al 1996, Tesfaye et al 1996) but only if dorsal column function is preserved. Postherpetic neuralgia responds less predictably, some finding SCS effective (Demirel et al 1984, Meglio et al 1989a, Sanchez-Ledesma et al 1989, Spiegelmann & Friedman 1991) and others not (Vogel et al 1986, Kumar et al 1991, 1996, Simpson 1991, Shimoji et al 1993). This may reflect the variable natural history of the condition (Watson 1990). The outcome with non-herpetic intercostal neuralgia is also variable, probably because of the heterogeneous aetiology. Complex regional pain syndromes (CRPS) are discussed below.

Amputation produces the most obvious example of peripheral nerve damage and two pain syndromes, stump pain and painful phantom, may result. It was recognized early in the history of SCS that both syndromes could be relieved but not in all cases (Miles et al 1974, Sweet & Wepsic 1974). Nielsen and colleagues (1975b) reported 'good to excellent' relief of phantom limb pain in five (two upper limb, three lower) out of six patients. The phantom sensation persisted but became painless. Miles and Lipton (1978) obtained excellent relief of phantom pain with SCS in six of eight patients (and in one of two with peripheral nerve stimulation) but a large study by Krainick and colleagues (1980) was less encouraging, with less than half deriving 'greater than 50% pain reduction' in the long term. A later, but small study (Claeys & Horsch 1997a) reported a good result in five of seven lower limb amputees. All seven had at least some pain relief initially but this decreased in the longer term to varying degrees in four patients. Krainick had also noted a marked reduction in pain relief with time. SCS is undoubtedly effective against both phantom and stump pain in many, but not all, amputees but the effect appears to wane more than in some other conditions. In successful cases the evoked paraesthesiae are perceived in the phantom and a sensation of movement or altered position can be induced in the phantom. Relief of phantom pain may sometimes be secondary to relief of the exacerbating stump pain. The question of whether pre-emptive SCS influences the development of phantom or stump pain remains unresolved.

Spinal cord damage

Spinal cord injury, whether traumatic, neoplastic, vascular or iatrogenic, can give rise to 'transitional zone' pain at and around the level of the injury and a diffuse deafferentation pain or dysaesthesia below the level. Surprisingly little information can be obtained from the literature regarding the response to SCS. Some mixed series contain very small numbers of these patients, sometimes not separately analysed. Tasker and colleagues (1992) attributed the poor results in those with complete cord lesions to atrophy of the dorsal columns. Of those with incomplete lesions, 41% obtained good or fair relief. Simpson (1991) also found that those with partial cord lesions fared much better than if the lesion was complete yet one patient whose lesion was (clinically) complete obtained significant relief. Cioni and colleagues (1995) found that those with clinically complete lesions did not respond. Disappointingly, only one in four with incomplete lesions enjoyed long-term success and sparing of dorsal column function did not guarantee success. Patients with partial spinal cord lesions are obviously heterogeneous; indeed each is neurologically unique and a clinically complete lesion is not necessarily anatomically and physiologically complete. The 'transitional' or 'end-zone' pain appears less responsive to SCS than is the diffuse distal pain. Fortunately, the opposite obtains in the response to DREZ lesions (Friedman & Nashold 1986); the two procedures are therefore mutually complementary in this context.

The fact that neuropathic pain can develop after cordotomy (spinothalamic tractotomy) generally limits this procedure to patients with a short life expectancy. Many, however, survived, and still survive, long enough to develop postcordotomy dysaesthesia, an extremely difficult condition to treat. Evidence regarding the effect of SCS comes from early series (far fewer cordotomies have been performed in the last 20 years than formerly). Nashold and Friedman (1972) reported that a previous anterolateral cordotomy actually favoured a good response to SCS but others obtained mixed results (Sweet & Wepsic 1974, Burton 1975, Long & Erickson 1975, Nashold 1975, Nielsen et al 1975a). The small numbers of cases, the general lack of information regarding the level of the electrode placement relative to the lesion, and regarding the neurological deficit, limit the conclusions about mechanisms of action that might be drawn from this group of patients.

Multiple sclerosis (MS) causes foci of damage in the white matter tracts of the spinal cord and brain and although attention tends to be concentrated upon the motor aspects, neuropathic pain is not uncommon. The initial impression in the 1970s that SCS could exert a beneficial influence on several aspects of the condition, both sensory and motor, proved unfounded and MS is no longer regarded as an indication. Unfortunately, the sometimes excellent response of lower limb pain (Illis et al 1976, 1983, Kumar et al 1991) and the sometimes dramatic improvement in bladder function, including a stabilizing effect on the distressing and painful bladder spasms (Illis et al 1976, Abbate et al 1977, Cook et al 1979, Read et al 1980, Hawkes et al 1981, 1983, Augustinsson et al 1982, Berg et al 1982) have tended to be forgotten. A single case has been reported (Barolat et al 1988) in which trigeminal neuralgia secondary to MS was treated successfully with high cervical SCS.

Complex regional pain syndromes

When chronic severe pain and allodynia followed a peripheral nerve injury and were associated with autonomic and, later, trophic changes, the syndrome was known as causalgia. This has now been renamed by the International Association for the Study of Pain (IASP) as complex regional pain syndrome (CRPS) type II (Merskey & Bogduk 1994). When a clinically indistinguishable syndrome followed a range of other trauma, including burns, fractures and even injections or a period of immobilization, it was called reflex sympathetic dystrophy (RSD) but is now reclassified as CRPS type I. The clinical details vary between cases, particularly with regard to the dysautonomic manifestations (swelling, sweating, vasomotor instability) and trophic changes (skin, hair and nails). Reduced movement is typical but dystonia and even tremor can occur. The relationship between sympathetic activity and the pain is increasingly uncertain (Schott 1994, Glynn 1995, Stanton-Hicks et al 1995). Involvement of a whole quadrant may occur but it is not understood why, in a minority of patients, the condition spreads to other limbs or quadrants (Veldman & Goris 1996). It is not even understood why only a minority of injured patients develop these florid and maladaptive conditions.

The response to SCS is variable but it is very encouraging (Barolat et al 1989, Robaina et al 1989a, Kumar et al 1997a). Half of Barolat's group of 18 patients with type I had good pain relief but one-third had no response. In contrast, all 12 of Kumar's patients responded well or very well. Previous sympathectomy (which may be incomplete) did not influence the outcome but an initially good response to sympathectomy was considered a good prognostic sign. Excellent or good outcomes have been reported in type II (causalgia) but follow-up was short in some cases and numbers small, three series (Broseta et al 1982, Mundinger & Neumuller 1982, Ray et al 1982) mustering only 24 cases, 18 (75%) of which enjoyed success ('excellent or good' pain relief; '50% or more' pain relief). In another series (Sanchez-Ledesma et al 1989), all 19 cases of type I or type II receiving permanent implants, out of 24 tested, were successful after a mean follow-up of several years. The response of the autonomic phenomena to SCS varies and does not seem to correlate closely with pain relief, illustrating the possible causative dissociation. Some patients report a dramatic reduction in swelling which cannot always be explained by increased movement. A reduction in allodynia does seem to correlate with pain relief. Many cases have become well established over the years prior to SCS yet still enjoy considerable pain relief. It might be suggested that SCS should be considered earlier in these dreadful conditions (for a graphic personal account, see Alexander 1995). Even though excellent results can be achieved, awareness that SCS is an option is not universal. Kumar and colleagues (1997a) proposed that SCS should replace sympathectomy, the effects of which are often temporary. Surgery within or close to the affected area carries a high risk of exacerbating the condition. This includes the incision or puncture wound for sympathectomy; care must also be taken in siting the SCS pulse generator or receiver-transducer. These syndromes are still poorly understood (see, for example, Jänig 1996) but it is clear that the pathological disturbance(s) can be profoundly modulated by SCS in many cases. As yet, there is insufficient evidence to state whether the addition of an autonomic disturbance increases or decreases the response of neuropathic pain to SCS.

These conditions have particularly received (favourable) attention from the advocates of therapeutic peripheral nerve stimulation (Sweet & Wepsic 1968, Meyer & Fields 1972, Hassenbusch et al 1996). Although this has never been adopted as other neurostimulation techniques have, it is an alternative to SCS which should perhaps be considered more. Nineteen of 30 (63%) of Hassenbusch's patients derived 'good or fair' pain relief over a mean of 2.2 years and there were 'marked' vasomotor improvements.

Peripheral limb ischaemia

Complete occlusion of the blood supply to a limb will rapidly cause infarction (gangrene) and amputation will be unavoidable unless the circulation can be quickly restored. Subtotal occlusion does not inevitably lead to amputation but causes severe pain on exercise (claudication) or, if more severe, at rest. Relief by arterial surgical techniques is not possible in all patients and many are prepared to undergo amputation for pain relief. The relative ischaemia triggers pathological 'maladaptive' changes in the periphery involving the microcirculation and these are amenable to modulation by neurostimulation.

One of the earliest large general series (Nielsen et al 1975a), from San Francisco, included four patients with ischaemic limb pain, two of whom gained satisfactory pain relief with SCS but this point was not developed further at the time. Cook and Weinstein, working in New York, reported (1973) that five patients with MS who were receiving SCS and in whom, ironically, pain was not a complaint, '... unanimously report that the feelings of "coldness" and a "deadness" or "heaviness" in the legs are replaced by "warmth" and a "lightness" or "liveliness"'. The additional irony is that these two initial observations came from the USA, one from the West coast and one from the East; SCS for peripheral vascular disease (PVD) has still not been widely adopted in the USA a quarter of a century later in contrast with Europe where approximately half of all SCS is for ischaemic pain (Simpson 1997, 1998). Cook later reported pain relief and improved perfusion, both in excess of the changes induced by sympathectomy, in nine patients (Cook et al 1976).

Over the following decade considerable evidence was presented for SCS-induced improvements in pain and distal perfusion in patients with advanced PVD who were unsuitable for (further) reconstructive arterial surgery (Dooley & Kasprak 1976, Dooley 1977, Meglio et al 1981a,b, Fiume 1983, Tallis et al 1983, Augustinsson et al 1985, Broseta et al 1985, 1986, Broggi et al 1987, Graber & Lifson 1987, Jivegard et al 1987). In the three largest early series (Augustinsson et al 1985, Broseta et al 1986, Broggi et al 1987), 102 out of 115 patients tested by trial stimulation received a permanent implant; good or excellent pain relief was achieved in nearly 80%, walking distance increased, cutaneous ulcers healed and there was a strong suggestion of a marked reduction in amputation rate. After a longer follow-up period (mean 27 months) the pain relief and amputation rates reported by Augustinsson and colleagues appeared stable (Jivegard et al 1987). Extremely high levels of pain relief were achieved; in a co-operative study (Broseta et al 1986), 29 out of an original 41 had 'more than 75%' relief including 17 with total relief. It was observed then (Meglio & Cioni 1982) and since (Kumar et al 1991) that in mixed series, PVD constituted a particularly successful subgroup.

Evidence has continued to accumulate for the beneficial effects of SCS in occlusive peripheral arterial disease of Fontaine grades III (ischaemic rest pain) and IV (rest pain, ulcers and/or gangrene). In Jacobs' group of 20 patients, 18 had immediate pain relief but this was sustained (mean follow-up 27 months) in only 12 (Jacobs et al 1990). In a prospective, randomized, controlled study Jivegard and colleagues (1995) revealed a statistically non-significant pain reduction in the 25 controls whereas at 1 year pain was significantly reduced (assessed by visual analogue scales; VAS) in those with SCS. By 18 months the average pain reduction had fallen slightly but was still significant. Fiume and colleagues (1989) also reported a progressive loss of effectiveness up to 4 years, although pain relief was still rated at 70% after 3 years and 64% after 4 years. In a prospective but uncontrolled trial with 39 patients with unilateral pain, assessed by a disinterested third party at a mean of 21.2 months, Kumar and colleagues (1997c) reported greater than 50% pain reduction in two-thirds, one in four of whom derived more than 75% relief. However, one in five of the whole group had the same or even more pain with SCS (despite selection by trial stimulation).

Pain relief with SCS in PVD is accompanied by an increase in exercise tolerance (Polisca et al 1992) and in walking distance by as much as 500 or 600 metres (Tallis et al 1983, Broseta et al 1986, Broggi et al 1987, Bracale et al 1989, Fiume et al 1989, Galley et al 1992). Promotion of healing of cutaneous ulcers has consistently been reported (Tallis et al 1983, Augustinsson et al 1985, Broseta et al 1986, Broggi et al 1987, Graber & Lifson 1987, Jivegard et al 1987, Bracale et al 1989, Fiume et al 1989, Jacobs et al 1990, Galley et al 1992) but only those with an area of less than 3 cm^2 seem to respond. Ulcers respond less well in diabetics (Augustinsson et al 1985) although they may still heal (Jivegard et al 1987, Franzetti et al 1989). Ulcer healing cannot, of course, be attributed to SCS in any individual case but the most impressive evidence for an effect is from Claeys and Horsch (1997b) whose randomized controlled comparison of prostaglandin E_1 therapy alone, with SCS plus prostaglandin E_1, showed quadruple the rate of total ulcer healing in non-diabetics and (statistically non-significant) triple the rate in diabetics with SCS. In hypertensive patients, total ulcer healing occurred in 65% with SCS compared with only 8% of controls.

Originally, substantial claims were made for a 'limb salvage' effect of SCS, more accurately a reduction in major and minor amputation rates. Thus 75% salvage at 6 months (Bunt 1991), 70–83% at 1 year and 56–64% at 2 years (Jivegard et al 1987, Jacobs et al 1990, Galley et al 1992) and 43% at 3 years (Jivegard et al 1987) were described. Amputation was much more likely in those who had no pain relief with SCS (Graber & Lifson 1987, Jivegard et al 1987, Jacobs et al 1990, Bunt 1991) and in those with gangrene present at the time of starting SCS (Augustinsson et al 1985, Broseta et al 1986, Jivegard et al 1987, Jacobs et al 1988). The proposed limb salvage effect illustrates well the need for care in interpreting the data and attributing a beneficial outcome to SCS. For example, improvements in limb-threatening ischaemia including healing of ulcers can occur with conservative management (Rivers et al 1986) and, with changing practices in vascular surgery, the amputation rate has fallen dramatically over the past 25 years (Veith et al 1990) irrespective of SCS. Thirdly, arteriopaths have a high mortality rate because of other manifestations of their disease and the longer term survivors are a self-selecting group who have been shown to have a significantly lower amputation rate (Veith et al 1981). The two recent randomized controlled studies (Jivegard et al 1995, Claeys & Horsch 1997b) have shown no statistically significant difference in amputation rates with SCS at 1 year and 18 months respectively. Jivegard and colleagues suggested that the extent of the amputation might be reduced by SCS but Claeys and Horsch did not support this. Jivegard and colleagues also suggested that the amputation rate might be lower with SCS in non-hypertensive patients.

The mechanism of action of SCS in PVD is discussed below but an increase in transcutaneous oxygen pressure ($TcPO_2$) combined with good pain control is said to be a reliable predictor of long-term success with SCS (Kumar et al 1997c). Whereas elevation of $TcPO_2$ also occurs with prostaglandin E_1 therapy, it is transient; with SCS it is sustained (Claeys & Horsch 1996). The variable and somewhat unpredictable natural history of PVD, particularly Fontaine grade III, makes selection of patients for SCS difficult and may explain the lack of enthusiasm among vascular surgeons in some European countries and in the USA. Furthermore, comparison must be made with other available treatments such as operative lumbar sympathectomy which has been shown to give relief of rest pain in 76% of those not amputated, at least up to 2 years (Baker & Lamerton 1994). SCS is not a substitute for reconstructive arterial surgery but it can certainly be an alternative to amputation for ischaemic pain.

Not all PVD is due to major arterial occlusion. Dooley (1977) observed that vasospastic disease responded best in his mixed pain series and Augustinsson and colleagues (1985) said that this was the best vascular indication for SCS. The numbers of cases published remains surprisingly small considering the extremely good response seen by different authors in nearly all patients (Robaina et al 1989b, Naver et al 1992, Francaviglia et al 1994). The explanation might lie partly in the difficulty in achieving consistent stimulation in the upper limbs as the electrodes are sited in the mobile cervical spine. SCS may also improve outcome in frostbite (Arregui et al 1989), Buerger's disease (Claeys et al 1997) and scleroderma (Francaviglia et al 1994). A single case of considerable pain relief in erythromelalgia (a rare condition with burning pain in the extremities secondary to multiple venous thromboses) has been reported (Graziotti & Goucke 1993) and Simpson (1992) has observed a similar case of multiple venous thromboses secondary to protein-S deficiency; marked pain relief was achieved for several years.

Angina pectoris

Cardiac ischaemic pain is in part visceral and partly referred to dermatomes which share cardiac segmental innervation, usually between the seventh cervical and fifth thoracic (Foreman 1991, Sylvén 1997). Myocardial ischaemia is not invariably painful and can be painless to the point of infarction ('silent' ischaemia). Conversely, not all chest pain is of cardiac origin and the diagnosis is not always straightforward. Whilst angina is classically caused by narrowing of the main coronary arteries, it can be the result of small vessel disease with radiologically normal coronary arteries ('syndrome X'). Whether precipitated by a reduction in blood flow or by an increase in myocardial oxygen demand, ischaemia triggers a vicious circle involving circulating catecholamines and sympathetic nervous activity which increases oxygen demand and reduces coronary blood flow, thereby exacerbating and prolonging the ischaemic episode and the pain (Collins & Fox 1990). First-line treatment of the acute attack is with glyceryl trinitrate (GTN) and medical prophylaxis is essentially antisympathetic. The mainstays of treatment and prophylaxis in medically refractory cases are percutaneous angioplasty and open coronary artery bypass grafting. There is, however, a large group of patients who suffer severe and disabling angina despite exhausting, or who are unsuitable for, the established therapy.

Mannheimer and his colleagues (1982) were the first to show that angina would respond to electrical stimulation, using transcutaneous electrical nerve stimulation (TENS). Sandric and colleagues (1984) reported four patients having SCS for various conditions and who also suffered from myocardial ischaemia. Not only did their electrocardiograms (ECGs) show improvement but two of the four had no further angina. Murphy and Giles (1987) reported the first 10 cases of SCS directed specifically at angina, from 1981 on. All 10 experienced a dramatic improvement symptomatically. Augustinsson started to treat angina by this technique in 1985 (Augustinsson 1989) and has since implanted more than 400 systems for angina (Augustinsson, personal communication). More reports followed from various European centres and all were encouraging. At first, it appeared that all patients responded but although this has subsequently proved not to be the case the results are nonetheless remarkable. The frequency and severity of episodes of angina are reduced in nearly all patients, sometimes to zero (Mannheimer et al 1988, 1993, Sanderson 1990, Andersen et al 1992, 1994, De Landsheere et al 1992, Sanderson et al 1992, Harke et al 1993, De Jongste et al 1994a,b, Eliasson et al 1994, González-Darder et al 1998), and GTN intake is reduced (De Jongste 1994a,b, Sanderson et al 1994). All of De Jongste and colleagues' (1994b) 22 patients had less angina, the median number of attacks being reduced from 15.6 to 6.3 per week at 1 year with a concomitant reduction in GTN intake from 11 tablets per week (mean) to 1.8. However, in Andersen's (1997b) group of 60 patients followed for 2 years, six had little or no pain relief and eight from a subgroup of 25 had only fair or poor relief. Similarly, six of Sanderson and colleagues' (1994) group of 23 patients followed for a mean of 45 months had no significant improvement yet the average daily GTN intake for the whole group fell from 9.0 tablets to 1.5, with 11 patients taking none after starting SCS. Exercise tolerance is increased and ischaemia-related ECG changes (ST depression) reduced (Mannheimer et al 1988, 1993, Sanderson 1990, De Landsheere et al 1992, Sanderson et al 1992, 1994, Harke et al 1993, De Jongste et al 1994b, Oosterga et al 1997).

The technique of right atrial pacing, with and without SCS, has been used to elucidate the effects of SCS on angina. Sanderson's group (1992) showed that higher heart rates could be achieved with less ST depression during SCS. Mannheimer and colleagues (Mannheimer et al 1993, Eliasson et al 1996) found a significant increase in time to onset of angina and a decrease in recovery time during SCS in 20 patients, with corresponding changes in ST depression on the ECG. At a (paced) heart rate which induced angina during control pacing, myocardial oxygen consumption and coronary sinus blood flow were reduced during SCS compared with control (SCS off) pacing. Net myocardial lactate production, indicating ischaemia, changed to lactate extraction during SCS at a heart rate which had induced angina when the stimulation was off. Sanderson and colleagues (1994) also demonstrated a reduction in myocardial oxygen consumption during exercise. There is thus strong evidence, electrocardiographic and metabolic, for an anti-ischaemic effect of SCS. There is also some echocardiographic evidence for an improvement in left ventricular function during SCS (Kujacic et al 1993). Similar symptomatic and physiological improvements occur with SCS when the angina is due to syndrome X (Eliasson et al 1993).

In general, SCS has been reserved for patients who have failed to respond to coronary artery bypass grafting (CABG) or in whom CABG is not technically feasible. The Gothenburg group (Mannheimer et al 1998) has conducted a prospective, randomized study to investigate whether SCS can be regarded as an alternative to CABG in high-risk or previously grafted patients. Overall, the outcomes in the 51 CABG and 53 SCS cases were very similar with regard to self-estimated symptom relief (79.5% and 83.7% reduction respectively), frequency of anginal attacks (67.9% and 69.9% reduction), consumption of GTN (77.4% and 73% reduction) and overall morbidity. The CABG group had a greater reduction in myocardial ischaemia at 6 months (although exercise tests were performed with SCS switched off) but a higher mortality (13.7% CABG and 1.9% SCS) and a higher cerebrovascular morbidity (8 CABG and 2 SCS). Follow-up time was rather limited (approximately 6 months) but the overall conclusion was that SCS is a viable alternative to CABG in high-risk patients.

Two questions arise with regard to the safety of SCS in angina: does it mask the vital warning symptom of impending myocardial infarction and does it interact with cardiac pacemakers? The first is answered by the pacing studies of Mannheimer and colleagues (1993). Pacing to a comparable degree of ischaemia which produced angina with SCS switched off also caused angina in all patients with SCS on; it was simply more difficult to achieve that degree of ischaemia with SCS on. Other studies have provided evidence in support (Andersen et al 1994, Sanderson et al 1994). The answer to the second question would appear to be that there is a potential risk but only at high SCS voltages (Romano et al 1993) and in general this does not seem to be a problem, particularly with bipolar and multiprogrammable pacemakers.

Further indications

Virtually no mention is made in the literature of SCS in abdominal and pelvic visceral pain. The effect on the neurogenic bladder has been discussed above but other organs have been largely ignored. Augustinsson and colleagues (1982) alluded briefly to a possible effect of (cervical) SCS on bowel activity and to a possible influence of TENS upon uterine contraction. The general view has been that SCS has no role in treating visceral pain other than angina pectoris but there is (unpublished) evidence of a revival of interest with small numbers of successful cases.

The established view is that nociceptive pain, i.e. from nociceptors via an intact afferent mechanism, does not respond to SCS. This includes wound pain and arthritis. Cancer pain may respond if it is associated with neurological damage, i.e. neuropathic (Hoppenstein 1975, Larson et al 1975). The simple statement 'nociceptive pain does not respond to SCS' must be made with caution because we do not yet fully understand the mechanism of the effect in ischaemic pain. Ischaemic pain is nociceptive and while SCS may relieve it indirectly by removing the cause (ischaemia), it may also have a directly analgesic effect; this would be antinociceptive (see further discussion below).

Some neuropathic painful conditions are not good indications, for anatomical reasons. For example, in anaesthesia dolorosa following trigeminal nerve damage, evoked paraesthesiae can be obtained in the face by stimulating the spinal tract and nucleus of the trigeminal system, which usually extends down to about C3. Unfortunately, because this complex lies ventral to the dorsal columns, it cannot be selectively stimulated with epidural electrodes. The perianal region and external genitalia are also difficult to target but modern hardware is increasing the success rate in this area.

SCS has not been used exclusively for pain. Early interest in its application in movement disorders has not been sustained although it undoubtedly has some beneficial motor effects (see Simpson 1994 for review). There have been reports (Hosobuchi 1985, Kanno et al 1989) that high cervical SCS increases cerebral blood flow and that it may accelerate recovery from coma (Kanno et al 1989, Matsui et al 1989) but very large prospective controlled trials would be needed to prove the latter.

SELECTION OF CASES

Diagnosis

As with any medical field, the first consideration when selecting patients for a treatment, or a treatment for patients, is the diagnosis; SCS is no different. Not all patients with a generally appropriate diagnosis (seea above) respond, however, and further selection criteria must be employed. Until the causes of failure are better understood, case selection will remain fallible, yet the failures remain almost totally ignored.

The quality of the pain

Before the nature of neuropathic pain was widely recognized, a burning quality was identified as a positive indicator (Nashold & Friedman 1972). In a careful analysis of their large series, North and colleagues (1993) found 'sharp' to correlate with success and 'wretched', 'pounding', 'pressing' and 'terrifying' to be associated with failure of SCS. Burchiel and his colleagues (1995) examined the prognostic value of the McGill Pain Questionnaire (Melzack 1975) in patients with back and leg pain. Scores on the D (depression) set and the evaluative subscales appeared to have significant predictive power but others have questioned the power of the subscales (Holroyd et al 1992).

Psychological factors

It was soon appreciated that psychiatric and personality disorders militated against a good outcome. Early reports included a large proportion of such patients (Shealy 1974, Long & Erickson 1975, Nashold 1975, Long et al 1981), exceeding 40% in one (Nashold & Friedman 1972). Some found that the Minnesota Multiphasic Personality Inventory (MMPI) aided case selection (Shealy 1974, 1975, Burton 1975, 1977, Daniel et al 1985) while others did not (Nashold 1975, Nielsen et al 1975a). At that time, indications for SCS by diagnosis were poorly understood and it was not fully appreciated that the chronic pain itself commonly had a deleterious effect on personality and on psychological factors such as depression, anxiety, obsessiveness and even hysteria (Woodforde & Merskey 1972, Burton 1975, 1977, Kumar et al 1991), particularly when the doctors failed to respond appropriately. These factors did not necessarily predict a poor outcome (Long & Erickson 1975, Nashold 1975, Vogel et al 1986).

The place of psychological screening has remained unclear. Meilman and colleagues (1989) found no relation to outcome in 20 patients with FBSS. The routine use of standardized psychological testing has not produced a long-term (average 7 years) overall success rate of better than approximately 50% in North's large series (North et al 1993). Burchiel and colleagues (1995) carefully analysed the predictive power of psychological screens in patients with back and leg pain and found that the Beck Depression Inventory (BDI) was not helpful but that MMPI depression and mania subscales might have some predictive value, although this was 'far from conclusive'. In a recent detailed review, Doleys and colleagues (1997) found no evidence for any predictive value of the MMPI (personality), the BDI (depression) or the Spielberger State-Trait Anxiety Inventory (anxiety). North and colleagues (1996) have shown in a prospective study of 58 patients that those with low anxiety scores (Derogatis Affects Balance Scale) and high 'organic symptoms' (Wiggins content scales of the MMPI) were more likely to proceed from trial stimulation to permanent stimulation. North had already selected the patients as candidates for SCS before the tests were applied; the true value of the psychological tests as a selection aid cannot therefore be deduced from this study. Nelson and colleagues (1996a) suggested that the higher the MMPI D scale (depression) score, the less likely is SCS to be effective. They also proposed the following exclusion criteria: active psychosis, suicidal or homicidal ideation, untreated or poorly treated major depression, somatization disorder, alcohol or other drug dependency (if of over-riding importance or uncontrolled escalation) and severe cognitive deficits. Patients should not be penalized if ineffective treatment prescribed by their doctors is addictive; if they obtain some relief from SCS, they are more likely to be able to reduce or discontinue the medication.

In contrast with psychological tests, the clinical opinion of a psychiatrist has been shown to have predictive value (Nielsen et al 1975a). In Belgium, where reimbursement for SCS is conditional upon a preoperative psychiatric assessment, a study of 100 patients (Kupers et al 1994) showed that the success rate was three times higher if the psychiatrist had no reservations. However, surgical opinion also influenced the case selection. A second Belgian study (Dumoulin et al 1996) has proposed that outcome can be predicted reliably for the FBSS using psychoanalytical factors relating to such considerations as the patient's attitude towards authority, guilt feelings and relationships. Psychological factors are clearly of great importance in chronic pain but the point made by Sweet and Wepsic (1974) 25 years ago remains pertinent: it is not simply a matter of identifying psychological factors, but of assessing their importance. Relatively little progress has been made on this front.

Nerve stimulation, including TENS

Neurostimulation peripheral to the spinal cord has been tried as a predictor of SCS responsiveness. Direct peripheral nerve stimulation (Miles & Lipton 1978) has not proved generally useful but Miles still finds indirect activation via the moderately painful injection of hypertonic saline into the interspinous ligament (Miles & Lipton 1978) to be of predictive value in lower limb and phantom pain (Miles, personal communication). Rubbing the relevant nerve (abrasion) has also been used, particularly in phantom pain (Miles & Lipton 1978) and although it seems likely that responsiveness to any counter-irritation, as evidenced by hot water bottle burns, etc., should encourage implantation, there is very little clear evidence in support. Similarly, TENS has been advocated as a screening test (Burton 1975, Long & Erickson 1975, Miles & Lipton 1978, Young 1978, Mittal et al 1987, Bel & Bauer 1991) but others have found no correlation with the subsequent response to SCS (Dooley 1977, Spiegelmann & Friedman 1991, Le Doux & Langford 1993).

Trial spinal cord stimulation

Selection by test stimulation of the spinal cord, either via temporary electrodes or via a temporary connection with potentially permanent electrodes, has considerable intuitive appeal. It has become widely adopted, is strongly advocated by many practitioners and is a prerequisite for reimbursement in some countries. The data, however, would suggest that it is not a good predictor of outcome.

Nielsen and colleagues (1975a) rejected nearly half of 221 patients after trial stimulation but this stringent selection process yielded a success rate of only 49%. Siegfried and Lazorthes' experience (1982) was almost identical with a large group suffering from FBSS. Kupers and colleagues (1994) achieved only 52% success in FBSS despite psychiatric screening and a 1-week trial of stimulation. Technical problems do not explain these one-in-two failure rates (North et al 1991c). In North's series only four of 57 candidates were rejected but 14 never subsequently obtained the level of pain relief with a permanent system that had been required to pass the trial. The rejection rate after trial stimulation has varied widely, from zero (Broseta et al 1982, Robaina et al 1989b, Probst 1990, Francaviglia et al 1994, Claeys et al 1997, Kumar et al 1997a) to 64% (Cioni et al 1995), as has the subsequent success rate in patients selected by a trial, from only six out of 33 after 2 years (Demirel et al 1984) to 93% at 1 year (Richardson et al 1979). Pooling the figures from published series in which either the case mix was heterogeneous or vague, or the condition was heterogeneous (particularly FBSS), and from which the relevant figures could be calculated, yields the following. In 23 series, 1822 patients underwent trial stimulation, 32% were rejected and 68% received 'permanent' implants. Of the latter, 54% were regarded as successful (37% of those initially considered for SCS). If a similar exercise is carried out regarding series of more specific conditions including CRPS I and II, PVD, diabetic peripheral neuropathy, phantom pain and postherpetic neuralgia (but excluding angina), the results are somewhat different. In 16 studies, only 13% of 582 candidates were rejected after a trial and 87% received definitive implants. Success was reported in 75% (65% of the original cohort). In five studies of CRPS and PVD (Broseta et al 1982, Robaina et al 1989a, Francaviglia et al 1994, Claeys et al 1997, Kumar et al 1997a) all 58 patients were selected for definitive implants and none rejected after trial stimulation. The subsequent (pooled) success rate was 91%. In five studies of PVD (Augustinsson et al 1985, Graber & Lifson 1987, Jacobs et al 1990, Steude et al 1991, Jivegard et al 1995) trial stimulation was not employed yet 76.5% of the 98 patients had a very good response and only 6% had no pain relief. In angina pectoris, trial stimulation is not now generally used.

It may be concluded, therefore, that the more specific and/or responsive the condition, the less necessary or contributory is trial stimulation. However, even amongst 'mixed bag' conditions, where trial stimulation might be expected to improve case selection, a 32% rejection rate from an already selected group (by being considered to be potential candidates) produces a success rate which barely exceeds 50%. Furthermore, equivalent or better results have been achieved where a period of trial stimulation was not employed even in FBSS (Blume et al 1982, Koeze et al 1987, Racz et al 1989, Simpson 1992). No studies have properly compared trial stimulation with no trial and our understanding is further limited because virtually nothing is known about those 'screened out' by trial stimulation. In one early report (Nielsen et al 1975a), 28 patients who had responded poorly to a trial were nonetheless given definitive implants. Twenty-two were rated 'fair' or 'failure'; presumably six were at least 'good'. The proportion of false negatives generated by trial stimulation is not known. Furthermore, a poor response to small percutaneous trial electrodes may not preclude a good response to a larger surgically implanted plate electrode system. The latter have been used for trial stimulation (Siegfried 1991, Le Doux & Langford 1993) and produced a notably good outcome in Le Doux and Langford's series of FBSS patients; only six were rejected from 32 and, of the 23 followed up, 74% enjoyed a good effect at 2 years. Most practitioners would, however, regard this approach as too invasive for a trial. Trial periods of up to 2 months have been used (Meglio et al 1989b) but most are very much shorter and this might generate false-negative responses.

Why does trial stimulation not prevent a subsequent failure rate of nearly 50%? The almost universally required report of '50% or greater pain relief' to 'pass' the trial might generate false positives. Not only might this notation be inherently unreliable (discussed below) but some desperate patients might fear losing their only opportunity of relief if they do not give this rating to whatever effect they experience in the trial. Seven per cent of North's long-term patients later admitted that they had never had any pain relief (North et al 1993). It has been suggested (Nelson et al 1996b) that patients who respond particularly well to a trial tend to have a personality profile which would later lead to refocusing upon residual symptoms and a 'continuing conviction of failing physical functioning', i.e. to a poor outcome. Patients with FBSS may respond more positively to trial stimulation than those with other diagnoses (Van de Kelft & De La Porte 1994). Trial stimulation might have a significant placebo effect and the high proportion of early failures subsequent definitive implantation would support this (Probst 1990, Spiegelmann & Friedman 1991, Van de Kelft & De La Porte 1994). A dummy stimulator significantly improved the pain scores of patients with diabetic neuropathy during trial stimulation (Tesfaye et al 1996).

Possible benefits include educating the patient about the evoked sensations, exclusion of the small number who cannot tolerate the effect and identifying those in whom topographically appropriate stimulation cannot be achieved because of complete denervation. This last point has proved fallible; Hood and Siegfried (1984) used trial stimulation over several days to select eight from 16 patients with brachial plexus pain, 11 of whom had root avulsion, which should preclude appropriate stimulation. Only two of the eight obtained 'good' pain relief. Similarly with spinal cord lesions, Cioni and colleagues (1995) rejected 16 out of 25 (64%) after a trial yet only four of the nine selected were successful.

In summary, the use of trial stimulation is almost universally advocated except for angina and, to some extent, PVD, yet the evidence suggests that it can be misleading and will not reliably predict long-term success.

Litigation

Outstanding compensation claims where the settlement will be influenced by any persistent pain and disability obviously constitute a disincentive to report a good outcome of SCS. Ongoing litigation has been highlighted by many groups as a relative contraindication (e.g. North et al 1993, Burchiel et al 1995, Nelson et al 1996a) or even an absolute contraindication (Kupers et al 1994). Inevitably, many suitable candidates for SCS will have suffered injury and in the developed world this is strongly associated with litigation, which typically takes several years to conclude. Whether potentially effective therapy should be withheld from patients who may have perfectly legitimate claims is a matter for debate.

ASSESSMENT OF OUTCOME

The response to SCS in angina pectoris and PVD is relatively straightforward because reliable objective measures of ischaemia, mobility and even pain (e.g. weekly intake of GTN) are available. Assessing the outcome in neuropathic pain syndromes is much more problematical. In CRPS, relief of pain and dysautonomic manifestations are often independent. Changes in activity levels depend partly upon factors not amenable to treatment with SCS. Return to work by the long-term disabled might be a poor indicator; in a recent Belgian study of relatively young patients with a pain relief success rate of about 50%, only 3.4% who had been off work for more than a year returned to work (Kupers et al 1994). Although some have reported surprisingly high rates of return to work (Broseta et al 1982, Bel & Bauer 1991, North et al 1991c, 1993) it is too variable to be a useful comparative measure. Assessing the degree of neuropathic pain relief per se can be complex (Williams 1995). Clearly, there is no difficulty if the patient consistently declares considerable pain relief, praises the device, explains how this has changed their life and is corroborated by reports from friends and relatives. Many cases fall short of this ideal yet do have a positive outcome.

Studies are hampered because they cannot be blind (paraesthesiae must be evoked) and because the subject population is weary, demoralized, depressed, anxious, afraid, sleep deprived and usually on maximal medical therapy which itself has side effects including constipation, malaise and mental confusion. They may be desperate and regard SCS as their 'last hope'. Reduction of drug intake is degraded as an outcome measure because these patients, unlike those with angina, are subject to analgesic and psychoactive polypharmacy, some of which is addictive. They may require analgesic medication for coexisting conditions, e.g. cervical spondylosis, arthropathy, even if SCS is very successful. Where a reduction in medication can be achieved the reduction in side effects may allow the patient to cope better with residual pain, indirectly improving the outcome though not itself an analgesic effect.

As with any treatment aimed at pain relief and improved function (e.g. lumbar spine surgery), inappropriate expectations by the patient will influence the reported outcome. While doctors have given up their earlier target of complete pain relief (Pineda 1975, Long et al 1981), it is not uncommon for patients still to hold such unrealistic expectations; adequate preoperative counselling is essential (Forrest 1996, Ohnmeiss et al 1996, Lang 1997). Other patients, in contrast, may be pleased with a degree of relief that the observer regards as slight (Koeze et al 1987).

In the majority of cases the outcome is assessed by the specialist who performed the implantation, leading to a possible bias. When North (1991a,c, 1993) employed a disinterested third party assessor, he found the results were worse, as had Long and Erickson (1975) earlier. Others (Burton 1975, Nielsen et al 1975a, Koeze et al 1987, Kupers et al 1994, Kumar et al 1997c) have also used third-party assessments. Koeze and colleagues found that the reports of the patient, of a close friend or relative and of an involved clinician all correlated well. Postal and even telephone follow-up is no substitute for 'in the flesh' consultations as significant misunderstandings can easily occur, exemplified by the patient who rated his stimulator a complete failure because when he switched it off the pain returned (Simpson 1991). Dependence upon a single assessment of average pain relief in a condition which varies over time has also been shown to be unreliable (Jensen & McFarland 1993). Long-term follow-up with periodic consultations not only gives a better understanding of the long-term patient and maximizes continuity of treatment but also allows recognition of changes over time, for example the phenomenon of late failure (discussed below).

A common experience is to find that a patient's estimate of the effectiveness of SCS will wane over the years but that if a technical failure occurs, they demand a rapid resolution and indicate that they had forgotten how bad the pain was. Although surprisingly little is known about the interaction of memory and chronic pain, there is evidence that chronic pain is remembered less well than acute pain (Hunter et al 1979, Erskine et al 1990, Babul & Darke 1994) and that patients with chronic pain do not remember the intensity of previous pain accurately (Linton & Melin 1982, Linton & Gotestam 1983, Eich et al 1985, Jamison et al 1989, Bryant 1993). Activity levels, emotional distress, reliance upon medication (Jamison et al 1989), present pain intensity (Eich et al 1985) and changes in pain (Bryant 1993) may all influence the memory of previous pain. If the present pain intensity is low, previous pain may be remembered as less severe than it really was (Eich et al 1985), which would underestimate the effect of SCS. Others have found that patients overestimate their baseline pain (Linton & Melin 1982), which would have the opposite effect, and that present pain intensity has no influence (Linton 1991). Most studies, however, refer to chronic *nociceptive* pain and previous *acute* pain. Chronic neuropathic pain may interact with memory and perception in a different manner but virtually nothing is known about this. Inaccuracy of memory for pretreatment neuropathic pain would fundamentally influence both the assessment of outcome of SCS and the patient's perception.

Most reports of SCS use the notation 'percentage pain relief', notwithstanding the fact that pain intensity is non-quantitative and probably non-linear. The patient's own estimate, usually within wide bands (which do not add legitimacy to the process), may be requested, without validating their comprehension of the concept of percentage and despite the comments on memory for chronic pain above. It also constitutes something of a leading question (Price 1991) and, to some extent, imposes forced choices, especially when put in terms of the watershed 'more than 50% or less than 50%'. Calculations by an observer based on serial VAS scores may be better but the non-linearity and other possible shortcomings of the VAS (Linton & Gotestam 1983, Carlsson 1983) do not justify calculations that yield results such as 'mean pain relief' 47.0 (± 26.7) %' (Burchiel et al 1996) or 'four patients had 25–49% relief' (Hassenbusch et al 1995). Several authors have recognized that 'percentage pain relief does not accurately indicate the outcome with SCS' (Burchiel et al 1995, 1996, De La Porte & Van de Kelft 1993, Ohnmeiss et al 1996). In the prospective study of Ohnmeiss and her colleagues, only 26% of the 40 patients with leg pain reported 50% or greater pain relief but 70% said SCS helped them and they would recommend it. At 2 years, 66% had reduced or stopped their narcotic intake. Similarly, only 55% of De La Porte and Van de Kelft's 64 patients reported at least 50% pain relief but 90% were able to stop or reduce their medication. The criterion '50% pain relief' is therefore misleading, particularly when selecting patients from a trial for permanent implantation. More holistic ratings such as the 'worth' of the treatment (Koeze et al 1987, Burchiel et al 1996) and 'Would you go through it all again for the same pain relief?' (Long & Erickson 1981, North et al 1991) have considerable virtue in this *clinical* field. Outcomes should also be viewed in the context of the terrible nature of some chronic painful conditions, against which nothing else has been very effective.

TECHNICAL CONSIDERATIONS

After early unsatisfactory experience with subarachnoid, subdural and endodural placement, electrodes have always been placed epidurally. It has also been established that they must be ipsilateral (if the pain is unilateral) and posterior and usually neurologically rostral to the pain. The evoked paraesthesiae must cover most, if not all, of the painful area (see Simpson 1994 for further discussion). 'Wire' electrodes (Fig. 59.1) can be inserted percutaneously via a Tuohy needle but they are somewhat inefficient as current is dissipated around the full 360° circumference and they have the potential for dislodgement. 'Plate' electrodes (Fig. 59.2) require an open surgical procedure (laminectomy or laminotomy) but can have larger contacts, are insulated except for their contact surface and can be sutured to

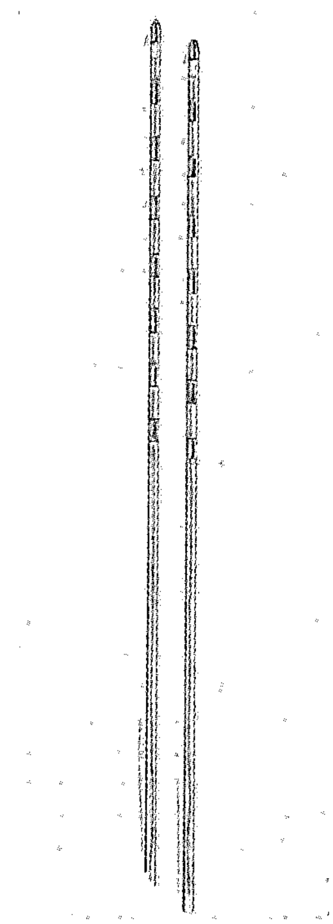

Fig. 59.1 Percutaneously implantable eight-contact electrodes (Octrode™; Advanced Neuromodulation Systems Inc).

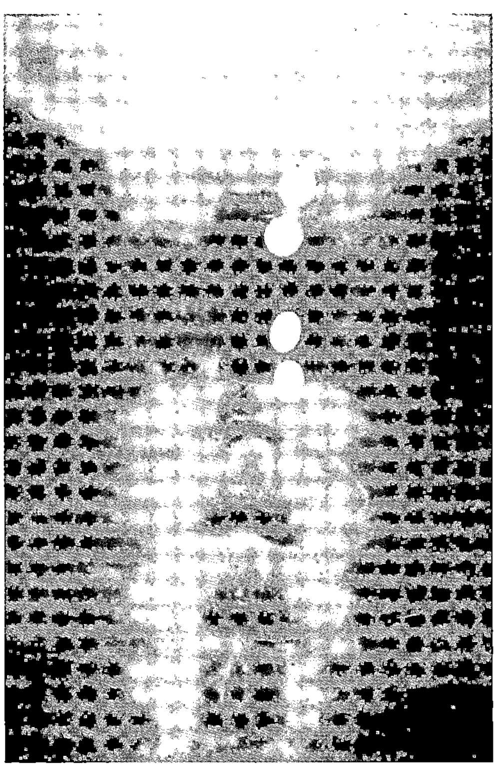

Fig. 59.2 Radiograph showing surgically implanted dual-paddle, four-contact electrode system in the cervical spine (Peritrode™/Lamitrode-22™; Advanced Neuromodulation Systems Inc).

the dura. Power is provided either by an intracorporeal pulse generator (IPG; Fig. 59.3) developed from cardiac pacemaker technology or by radiofrequency (RF) coupling between an implanted receiver-transducer and a small external transmitter carried by the patient (Fig. 59.4). IPGs are less obtrusive but, although they can be switched on and off with a small magnet, the parameters can be changed only by telemetry and they require replacement every few years (depending on usage) at significant cost. RF systems incur much lower recurring costs, are preferable where high outputs are required (e.g. multiple electrode arrays) and, until recently, had the probable advantage of a greater operant input by the patient in controlling the stimulus parameters. This last point has been negated to some extent by the introduction of a compact 'home' telemetry system that the patient can use to change (within preset limits) certain parameters on an IPG (Fig. 59.3).

Early systems used monopolar stimulation but bipolar stimulation was soon shown to be superior. Narrow separation of the contacts (electrodes) gives a broader distribution of evoked paraesthesiae (Law 1983, Barolat et al 1991). Guarded cathodes, i.e. a cathode flanked by two anodes, have been advocated for low back and leg pain (North et al 1991a, 1992b) and computer modelling has confirmed the superiority of narrow bipole and tripole configurations in gaining paraesthesia coverage (Struijk et al 1993b, Holsheimer & Wesselink 1997a,b). Because only single-channel (but multicontact) systems have been available (the terms 'channel' and 'contact' or 'electrode' have frequently been interchanged incorrectly), increasing the number of electrode contacts above the standard four has been used to try to improve targeting, particularly for the low back (Fig. 59.1). The vast numbers of active combinations then available (6050 with eight electrodes, tens of millions with 16) require automated computerized systems for programming (North et al 1992a,b; Fig. 59.5). Another approach has been to increase the available spatial configurations by means of separate electrode pairs (Fig. 59.2) rather than four-in-line (Simpson 1992).

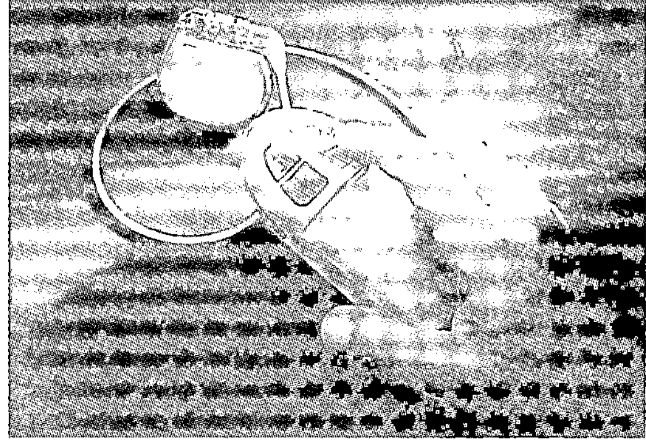

Fig. 59.3 Implantable pulse generator and patient-controlled telemetric programmer (Itrel 3™ and EZ™ programmer; Medtronic Inc).

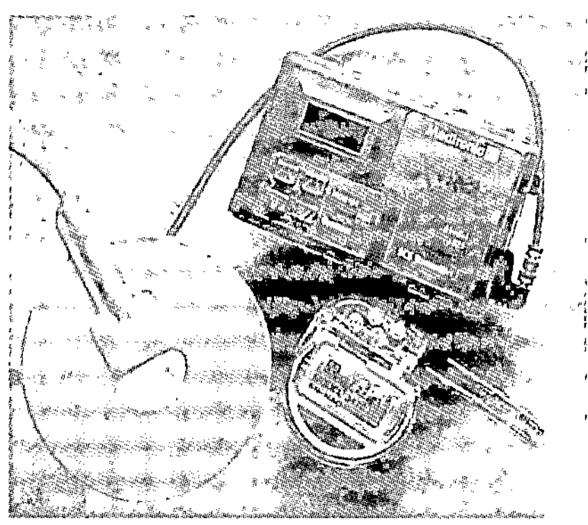

Fig. 59.4 Radiofrequency-coupled SCS system showing the transmitter (background) with antenna attached and receiver-transducer (X-trel™; Medtronic Inc).

The recent introduction of truly dual channel systems, whereby stimulus parameters can be varied at different electrodes independently, has permitted a more sophisticated approach to targeting by 'steering' the electrical fields (Holsheimer 1997, Holsheimer et al 1998). This represents a major advance, reducing the required specificity of electrode placement, the impact of electrode movement and the need for complex electrode arrays.

Optimum rostrocaudal placements have become apparent largely through accumulated experience. For angina the electrodes are placed between C7 and T2 (spinal), usually slightly to the left (the cardiac pain afferents enter the cord at T1–5). For PVD affecting the lower limb, T10 has been the most commonly effective level. T8–9 is the level most

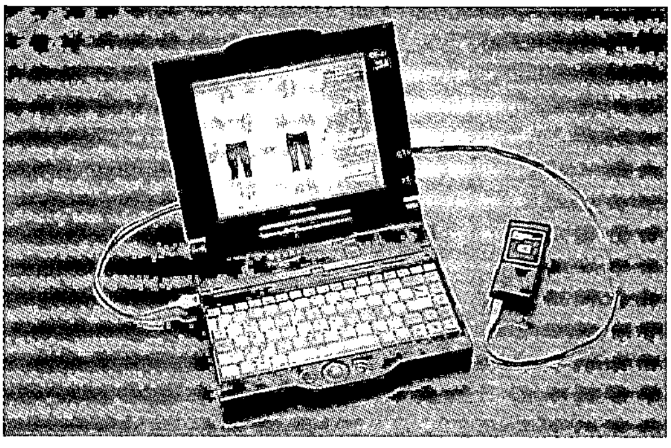

Fig. 59.5 Pen-based processor computer with graphical interface connected to an RF transmitter. The programme selects optimum electrode combinations and electrical parameters in response to pain distribution drawings and to previously programmed information regarding stimulation characteristics (Pain Doc™; Advanced Neuromodulation Systems Inc).

likely to stimulate the low back. Barolat and colleagues (1993) have produced useful 'probability maps' of cathode placement – the threshold for cathodal stimulation is much lower than that for anodal stimulation (Struijk et al 1993a,b) – for different anatomical targets; e.g. C2–4 for the shoulder, C5–6 for the hand, T7–8 for the anterior thigh, T11–L1 for the posterior thigh and perineum.

Total selectivity cannot always be achieved, for neuroanatomical reasons; for example it is rarely possible to stimulate the low back or buttock(s) without some stimulation being felt in the leg(s). The upper limb can, however, be stimulated without unwanted paraesthesiae in the trunk or legs. Afferents enter the dorsal columns laterally and have a lower threshold than the more medial fibres from more caudal segments, because they are of larger diameter and have more collaterals (Struijk et al 1992, He et al 1994). It follows, therefore, that optimum electrode placement is a product of both rostrocaudal level and degree of laterality. If the cathode is placed too far laterally, unwanted uncomfortable dorsal root (DR) stimulation will occur. Using elegant computer modelling techniques, combined with magnetic resonance imaging (MRI), Holsheimer's group have demonstrated that the greater the thickness of the posterior layer of the cerebrospinal fluid (CSF), i.e. the greater the distance between the electrode (cathode) and the cord, the lower is the threshold for dorsal root stimulation compared with dorsal column stimulation (Struijk et al 1993a, Holsheimer 1997, Holsheimer & Wesselink 1997a). Thus, dorsal column stimulation is favoured in the cervical spine where the lordosis brings the cord close to the dura posteriorly but in the mid-thoracic spine, where the kyphosis produces the opposite effect, dorsal root stimulation will occur more easily.

The spinal cord is also smallest at the mid-thoracic level and it may deviate from the midline in normal subjects (Holsheimer et al 1994), with scoliosis and after previous spinal surgery or trauma. Ultrasound has proved useful in determining such deviation during electrode insertion by open operation (Simpson 1994). It is normal for the spinal cord to move within the CSF so that some postural changes in stimulation strength and/or distribution are unavoidable, particularly with placements in the mobile cervical spine and when moving from standing or sitting to lying supine (Struijk et al 1993b, He et al 1994). To be most effective, the difference between the perception threshold for stimulation and the amplitude at which it becomes unpleasant (discomfort threshold) should be as large as possible so that consistent, comfortable stimulation can be achieved despite postural changes. This also increases the chances of including 'difficult' targets such as the low back and perineum by permitting the recruitment of deeper and smaller fibres without 'overstimulating' others (North et al 1992b, Holsheimer & Wesselink 1997b, Holsheimer et al 1998). A low perception threshold will also prolong the life of an IPG.

A commonality has evolved in the parameters of stimulation employed for pain of various aetiologies, including ischaemic pain. The frequency is rarely outside the range 50–120 Hz, most usually 80–100 Hz, and the pulse width between 100 and 500 microseconds. The effective amplitude is usually in the range of approximately two to six volts at the receiver-transducer or IPG. Good results have been described with frequencies as low as 1.5–8.0 Hz (Shimoji et al 1993) but this is unusual. A variety of modulations is available including cycling modes, but their use appears to be largely idiosyncratic. Better pain relief with cycling modes has been suggested (Shatin et al 1986) but not substantiated by trials. Patterns of use vary widely from one or two hours per day, not every day, to almost continuous usage. Continuous, 24-hour stimulation is not recommended as it may encourage the development of tolerance (Simpson 1991).

Patients are warned that the implant may trigger security systems, e.g. at airports. Department store antitheft systems may dangerously activate RF-coupled spinal cord stimulators (Eisenberg & Waisbrod 1997). MRI should be avoided. Patients with trial leads have been studied with functional MRI without apparent ill effect (Kiriakopoulos et al 1997) but MRI will activate an IPG, alter the stimulus parameters and erase the electronically coded serial number (Liem & Van Dongen 1997).

COMPLICATIONS

The equipment

Unreliability of hardware was initially a major problem and delayed the acceptance of SCS. Diagnosing faults has always presented a challenge (Meyer et al 1979, Koeze et al 1984). Considerable improvements have occurred but no system is infallible and electrode dislodgement, in particular, continues to cause failure. Lead fractures and connector problems are less common but the antennae of RF systems remain vulnerable. Electrode movement of a few millimetres may cause failure and has always been more likely to occur with the percutaneous type of electrode system (Young 1978, Le Doux & Langford 1993) with rates of between approximately 20% and 30% being reported (Probst 1990, Kumar et al 1991, Andersen 1997a, Lang 1997). 'Surgical' plate electrodes are not immune, especially if they are not sutured to the dura (Le Doux & Langford 1993, Ohnmeiss et al 1996). The mobility of the cervical spine particularly encourages dislodgement; reliability can be increased by reducing the size of the electrode paddles and suturing them to the dura (Simpson 1996).

The patient

Headache secondary to dural puncture occurs in approximately 1% of trial insertions (Bedder 1997) and can occur after definitive implantation (Vijayan & Ahmad 1997). Reports of cord compression due to epidural haematoma (Fox 1974, Grillo et al 1974, Long & Erickson 1975, Nielsen et al 1975a) are surprisingly rare considering the density of the epidural venous plexus and the high incidence of non-steroidal anti-inflammatory drug intake, which impairs haemostasis. Most have occurred after laminectomy. Neurological deficits from this and other causes, e.g. direct compression and CSF hygroma, have usually been reversible (Fox 1974). Permanent deficits have undoubtedly occurred occasionally in relation to electrode insertion but are inevitably under-reported.

Infection is a cause for concern in the presence of any implant but is relatively low with SCS, the most widely quoted figure being around 5% (see, for example, Simpson 1994, Turner et al 1995 for reviews) although one early survey reported only 1% (Fox 1974). North and colleagues' (1993) overall figure was 5% although one subgroup (North et al 1991c) yielded 12%. The majority of infections are superficial, affecting the IPG or receiver pocket, and it is no longer necessary in most cases to remove the entire system to eradicate the infection. Epidural infection is extremely rare. Contrary to what might be expected, externalized trial leads are not unduly prone to infection within the usual trial period (North et al 1991c, De La Porte & Van de Kelft 1993, Bedder 1997). The infection rate may be higher in diabetic patients, as expected (Tesfaye et al 1996).

Some patients report persistent pain around the receiver/IPG site which may relate to pressure or traction on a peripheral nerve and may require repositioning. Others develop a persistent diffuse pain over the back following thoracic laminotomy or laminectomy (Fox 1974, Young 1978, Simpson 1994) and this can persist for several weeks or months. It may be a fasciitis but is so far unexplained. Prolonged wound pain occurred in 21% of Nielsen and colleagues' early series (1975a) and in 12.5% of Shealy's cases (1975).

Overall, SCS is a safe procedure; the commonest reason for reoperating is to reposition or replace dislodged electrodes. The overall chance of requiring a further operation at some time (excluding IPG replacement) is at present approximately one in three and is falling. One death has been reported (Nielsen et al 1975a), from pulmonary embolism.

Late failure

While hardware failure will obviously explain some cases of late failure and a gradual rise in tissue impedance may explain others (Nashold 1975, Meyer et al 1979, Richardson et al 1979), a reduction in success rate over time *in the presence of a functioning stimulator* is a well-recognized phenomenon. Its incidence is variable but has not changed materially since early reports (e.g. Long & Erickson 1975, Nashold 1975, Nielsen et al 1975a, Young 1978, Siegfried & Lazorthes 1982), which argues against a 'technical' explanation. Although many such failures occur within months and most within 2 years (Young 1989, Probst 1990, Kumar et al 1991, Spiegelmann & Friedman 1991), the phenomenon continues for many years (North et al 1993, Rainov et al 1996) albeit at a slower rate (North et al 1991c). In addition to a fall in the number of successful cases, the average reported pain relief also falls progressively over the first 5 years (North et al 1991c, Ohnmeiss et al 1996). Nearly half of North's patients (North et al 1991a) reported a reduced level of pain relief by 2.1 years. Possible explanations are: an initial placebo response; a reporting error due to memory or other cognitive factors; and a true physiological tolerance. The loss of a placebo effect is unlikely to explain more than early failures. An optimistic 'complete' relief was reported by 47% of Young's (1978) patients initially, falling to a more realistic 8% at 3 years. De La Porte and Van de Kelft (1993) blamed a placebo effect for some early failures; their fall in success rate from 95% immediately to 80% 1 month after internalization would support this (Van de Kelft & De La Porte 1994). The proportion of patients in their series who reported '50% or better pain relief' fell from 80% at 1 month to 58% at 1 year yet, after an average of 4 years, 69% continued to express satisfaction with the outcome. Similarly, in another study (Ohnmeiss et al 1996), 53% had '50% or more pain relief' at 6 weeks which fell to only 26% at 1 and 2 years, suggesting late failure, but 70% still said they would recommend the procedure. There may therefore be an interaction between the 'percentage pain relief' notation and memory for pain which distorts the reported long-term outcome.

There is very little evidence for a true physiological tolerance. The phenomenon was seen to be more likely in those who used SCS continuously, 24 hours every day (Simpson 1991) but the numbers were small. Late failure occurs with PVD (Fiume et al 1989) and any loss of effect on the physiological parameters might have provided evidence for true tolerance but this opportunity is denied because progression of the underlying condition, independent of SCS, probably explains many late failures in ischaemic pain. 'Tolerance' may not occur to the same degree in angina (Andersen 1997b, González-Darder et al 1998).

In summary, a placebo effect may explain early failure in the presence of a functioning stimulator and late failure not due to technical problems may not be a true phenomenon in all cases.

COST EFFECTIVENESS

The global need for cost containment in healthcare systems combined with the high cost of SCS make it surprising that more data are not available. It is also not always possible to extrapolate from one country to another. Angina should be the most readily analysable indication and a Danish study (Rasmussen et al 1992) has shown a considerable saving in both hospital and non-hospital costs between the preoperative and first postoperative year. PVD has not been fully analysed and care is needed because of the uncertainty regarding the question of 'limb salvage' rates. A small German study of FBSS (Bel & Bauer 1991) demonstrated a 90% reduction in drug costs but it was the increase in work capacity on which the cost effectiveness was determined. This study was unusual, however, in that seven of the 14 patients returned to work and, after 2 years, none of the 14 needed any regular analgesic medication. The most thorough analysis to date is from the USA and also concerns FBSS (Bell et al 1997). Its conclusion was that SCS paid for itself in 5.5 years overall and, in successful cases, in 2.1 years.

MECHANISMS OF ACTION

Neuropathic pain

Our limited understanding of its mechanisms of action may have delayed the credibility and acceptance of SCS. The most compelling evidence refuting a placebo explanation for successful definitive SCS lies in both the longevity of the response (more than 10 years is now not uncommon) and the need for the evoked paraesthesiae to be topographically appropriate. The perception of the paraesthesiae, even in phantom limbs, indicates a supraspinal action and objective evidence from monkeys and humans indicates that thalamic and sensory cortical effects occur (Larson et al 1974, Bantli et al 1975, Blair et al 1975, Modesti & Waszak 1975, Augustinsson et al 1979) including recent evidence for the latter from functional MRI (Kiriakopoulos et al 1997). This does not prove a causal relationship, however. There is strong clinical evidence that dorsal column activation is a necessary condition, at least in neuropathic pain. The electrodes must be both posterior to the cord and ipsilateral (to unilateral pain). Previous anterolateral cordotomy, i.e. spinothalamic tractotomy, does not prevent effective SCS but vibration sense (transmitted in the dorsal columns) must be preserved for SCS to be effective (Tesfaye et al 1996).

Experimentally, in rats, very brief analgesia can be obtained by stimulating below a trans-section of the dorsal columns but a longer lasting analgesia (up to 10 minutes) depends upon stimulation above the dorsal column transsection (Rees & Roberts 1989b). These and many similar neurophysiological experiments relate to acute nociceptive pain and not chronic neuropathic pain but Roberts and colleagues have proposed a central role (in the rat) for the anterior pretectal nucleus (APtN), a rostral mid-brain nucleus which has a rich excitatory input from the dorsal columns via the dorsal column nuclei (Rees & Roberts 1989a). Although stimulating the APtN is antinociceptive (Roberts & Rees 1986, Wilson et al 1991), it may also be antiaversive via higher centres (Brandao et al 1991). Bilateral APtN lesions accelerate the onset of autotomy (Rees & Roberts 1993) which is an animal response to deafferentation that may provide a model for human neuropathic pain. From this and other evidence, Roberts has proposed that various long-loop feedback circuits, afferent in the dorsal columns, involving the APtN and descending in the dorsolateral funiculus, inhibit spinothalamic cells at cord level to reduce their response to noxious stimuli, thereby preventing excessive ongoing pain as a *normal* homeostatic function and in line with the gate theory. Neuropathic pain might result from a failure of this system and SCS might act by restoring it (see Roberts & Rees 1994 for review). SCS suppresses autotomy behaviour in the rat (Gao et al 1996) and normalizes the lowered threshold of the withdrawal reaction in the mononeuropathic rat model (Meyerson et al 1994). However, the latter effect may be mediated at spinal level (Ren et al 1996). Meyerson and colleagues (1995) have commended the rat mononeuropathic model in that the lack of effect of SCS on the noxious, C-fibre mediated component of the flexor reflex mimics the lack of effect on acute noxious stimuli in man but the attenuation of response to normally innocuous stimuli is similar to the effect in humans with allodynia.

Coyle, in his critical review (1996), points out the need for care in extrapolating from such models, particularly with regard to complete versus partial nerve lesions. SCS undoubtedly has local segmental actions within the spinal cord (Dubuisson 1989, Hunter & Ashby 1994) which might be expected to be directly antinociceptive but the clinical evidence is confused, some finding support for an elevation of the cutaneous pain threshold (Marchand et al 1991) and others not (Friedman et al 1974, Doerr et al 1978). SCS does not relieve intense nociceptive pain such as from wounds and arthritis but an antinociceptive action may be relevant in certain circumstances, e.g. ischaemic pain (see below).

Some pharmacological evidence has emerged regarding supraspinal actions of SCS. For example, inhibition by SCS of nociceptive thalamic neurons may be mediated by γ-aminobutyric acid (GABA) in the cat (Olausson et al 1994), as may an effect on the periaqueductal grey matter of the rat (Stiller et al 1995). Several neurotransmitters are known to be released during SCS (Linderoth et al 1993) but the most relevant information concerns GABA in the dorsal horn of the spinal cord of the mononeuropathic rat. Tactile allodynia, a common feature of neuropathic pain, is associated with reduced GABA transmission (Stiller et al 1996, Hwang & Yaksh 1997). SCS increases the release of GABA in the dorsal horn (Linderoth et al 1994a) and suppresses tactile allodynia (Stiller et al 1996). The $GABA_B$ system appears to be particularly involved and its stimulation by SCS in turn reduces the release of the excitatory amino acids glutamate and aspartate in the dorsal horn (Cui et al 1996, 1997b). Adenosine may also be involved (Cui et al 1997a). Interestingly, not all mononeuropathic rats develop allodynia and of those that do, not all respond to SCS, imitating the human condition.

The efficacy of SCS in CRPS yields no additional clues regarding its mechanisms of action. This is not surprising considering the present lack of understanding of the nature and relevance of the autonomic disturbances in these conditions (Schott 1994, Stanton-Hicks et.al 1995, Jänig 1996, Birklein et al 1998). The altered sensitivity of small blood vessels to sympathetic stimulation, including their response to circulating catecholamines (Kurvers et al 1995), and the mechanisms by which this may be influenced by SCS obviously generalize to PVD and angina. SCS does not appear to influence cutaneous blood vessels if they are normal, in patients obtaining relief from neuropathic pain (Devulder et al 1996).

Peripheral vascular disease

Whereas in neuropathic syndromes a good clinical outcome results from more than just a physiological analgesic effect, in PVD and angina the effects are more directly physiological. In PVD there is now considerable evidence for an effect on the microcirculation, with normalization of the 'maladaptive' changes distal to a partial arterial occlusion, rather than on the macrocirculation (Broseta et al 1986, Graber & Lifson 1987, Jacobs et al 1988, 1990, Jivegard et al 1995, Claeys 1997). Whilst the effect appears to be mediated largely by inhibition of sympathetically maintained peripheral vasoconstriction (Linderoth et al 1991a,b, 1994b), the precise mechanism and the roles of various transmitters and vasoactive substances are not yet fully elucidated. Evidence is now accumulating, however, regarding influences on adrenergic and cholinergic mechanisms (Linderoth et al 1994b) and the possible involvement of calcitonin gene-related peptide and nitric oxide (Croom et al 1997a,b). There is also some evidence for a protective, pre-emptive role for SCS against peripheral vasospasm (Linderoth et al 1995). It is not yet fully established whether the circulatory effects of SCS in PVD are in part secondary to pain relief. In addition to the compelling physiological evidence for a vasodilating effect of SCS, clinical evidence including the antivasospastic effect in Raynaud's disease and similar conditions strongly suggests that a primary vascular effect is responsible, as does the fact that SCS will warm the extremities even if there is little or no pain, as in MS. Both antinociceptive and vasodilatory mechanisms may be involved, however, and very little attention has been paid to afferents from arteries and veins (Schott 1994) despite their obvious relevance.

Angina pectoris

Cardiac pain is ischaemic pain and, as with PVD, considerable evidence has accumulated for an anti-ischaemic effect of SCS in angina (see 'Indications' above, and Jessurun et al 1996 for review). Recently, positron emission tomography (PET) has shown a redistribution of blood within the ischaemic myocardium during SCS (Hautvast et al 1996) although an earlier PET study (De Landsheere et al 1992) did not show this. There is in addition evidence for a primary analgesic effect. For example, in animal studies, SCS inhibits specifically nociceptive spinothalamic neurons responding to cardiac input (Foreman et al 1989, Chandler et al 1993). Myocardial β-endorphin release may also be involved (Mannheimer et al 1994). It has long been known that sympathectomy can reduce cardiac pain (Apthorp et al 1964) and an antisympathetic effect of SCS seems likely (Meglio & Cioni 1985, Sanderson 1990) but there is no direct evidence for SCS influencing cardiac sympathetic efferents and a reduction in heart rate is not usually seen.

In cardiac ischaemia, a 'vicious circle' is set up in which pain- and fear-induced sympathetic overactivity leads to further ischaemia and more pain (Collins & Fox 1990). Unlike neuropathic pain, there is no deafferentation causing central sensitization but cardiac afferents may nonetheless be sensitized, e.g. by adenosine (Sylvén 1997). Although we do not yet fully understand the mechanism, it seems that SCS breaks this vicious circle, possibly at more than one point. The prevailing view at present is that reduced oxygen consumption, and thus a reduction in relative ischaemia, is the key effect; once a certain level of ischaemia is reached it is still painful during SCS. An additional antinociceptive action cannot be dismissed, however. Sylvén (1997) suggests that because of the relative paucity of cardiac C-fibre afferents, cardiac pain, or potential pain, is easily gated.

General

It might be deduced that SCS acts by normalizing pathologically perturbed systems and it would not be surprising if more than one mechanism were involved. What is perhaps surprising is that something as crude as SCS works at all. A 'blanket' restoration of (topographically appropriate) afferent traffic, where it has become deficient, might underlie its action in neuropathic pain. SCS appears to normalize disturbed (long loop and segmental?) gating processes and has some antinociceptive action. The latter may be effective when combined with (separate) anti-ischaemic actions but is insufficient to block nociceptive pain of an intensity that might have survival value; SCS might restore a damaged gate mechanism but cannot replace a gate with a wall.

BRAIN STIMULATION

The total number of brain stimulators implanted for pain in the last 30 years equates to little more than one-tenth of the number of spinal cord stimulators currently implanted *annually*. Deep brain stimulation (DBS) for pain has virtually ceased and no longer has full Food and Drug Administration (FDA) approval in the USA. Brain surface, specifically motor cortex, stimulation is now emerging and early results in a small range of conditions are very promising. DBS has been used where SCS is ineffective or inappropriate, particularly pain in the head and face, pain affecting large areas (e.g. half the body) and nociceptive pain. The electrodes are inserted stereotactically with physiological feedback (where possible), usually followed by a trial period. Initially monopolar, all DBS electrodes are now quadripolar (Fig. 59.6). The main DBS targets are the opioid-rich periaqueductal and periventricular grey matter (PAG, PVG), the sensory thalamus (ventral posterior nuclei, medial and lateral: VPM and VPL) and the posterior limb of the internal capsule (IC). It is not always appreciated that these structures are anatomically contiguous; the rostral PAG merges with the PVG, which is adjacent to the centromedial and parafasicular nuclei of the posterior medial thalamus and the posterior IC is immediately lateral to the posterior medial thalamus. PAG electrodes may pass through, and act upon, the sensory thalamus (Boivie & Meyerson 1982). Not surprisingly, therefore, the distinctions discussed below are not always absolute.

PERIAQUEDUCTAL AND PERIVENTRICULAR GREY MATTER STIMULATION

Following sporadic reports over the previous 15 years of pain relief from stimulation of various deep brain targets, Reynolds (1969) showed that PAG stimulation in the rat could produce sufficient antinociceptive analgesia to permit abdominal surgery. Mayer and colleagues (1971) confirmed that the effect of stimulating various rostral brainstem areas in the rat, including PAG, was specifically analgesic and was topographical. Richardson and Akil (1977a,b) demonstrated the analgesic effect of PAG stimulation clinically but unpleasant side effects occurred as the voltage was increased, including apprehension, nausea, vertigo and disturbance of eye movements; PVG stimulation was superior in this respect, feelings of well-being and warmth being described. PAG and PVG stimulation do not produce paraesthesiae and the clinical analgesic effect of PVG stimu-

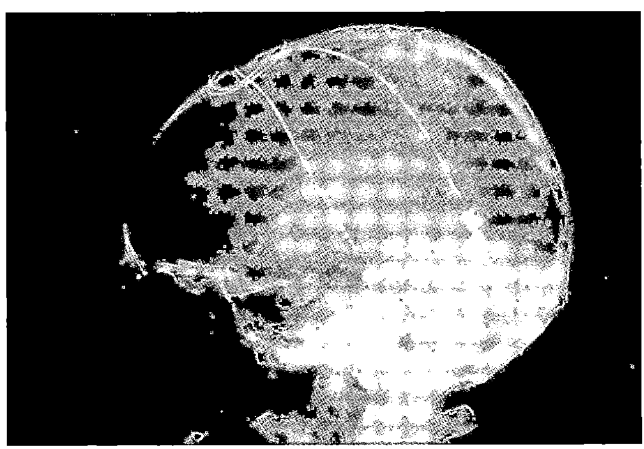

Fig. 59.6 Lateral skull radiograph showing a deep-brain four-contact electrode system implanted in the thalamus (Activa™ lead and extension; Medtronic Inc).

lation is prolonged, continuing for several hours (Hosobuchi et al 1977, Roizen et al 1985) or even several days (Richardson 1995) after discontinuing stimulation. Unilateral stimulation gives bilateral pain relief (Kumar et al 1997b) and the left side appears more effective in most humans (Hosobuchi 1986). PAG stimulation suppresses nociceptive responses in the dorsal horn of the spinal cord of experimental animals (Liebeskind et al 1973, Carstens et al 1979, Morton et al 1997) but the details of this descending inhibition are not yet known. In particular, the extent of opioid involvement is unclear.

PAG/PVG stimulation-produced analgesia (SPA) is reversed by the opiate antagonist naloxone in rats (Akil et al 1976) and in humans (Adams 1976, Hosobuchi et al 1977, Baskin et al 1986) and increases the concentration of opioid peptides in the ventricular CSF of patients (Akil et al 1978, Hosobuchi et al 1979, Young et al 1993). The latter effect was alleged to be artefactual, caused by the infusion of contrast medium (Dionne et al 1984, Fessler et al 1984), but Richardson (1995) refutes this. Hosobuchi (1987) has found that dorsal PAG stimulation, like the more usual rostroventral PAG stimulation, is also clinically analgesic but is not reversed by naloxone. Young and Chambi (1987) found no cross-tolerance between PAG/PVG SPA and morphine and no naloxone reversal, concluding that the mechanism must be opioid independent. The evidence overall suggests that PAG/PVG stimulation activates opioid neurons, including fibres *en passage*, which in turn activate monoaminergic fibres descending in the dorsolateral funiculus to the dorsal horn (Yaksh 1979, Richardson 1995, Stamford 1995) but there may be more than one mechanism and more evidence is needed, including direct evidence from humans. Reports of the effect of clinical PAG/PVG stimulation upon acute pain thresholds vary (Hosobuchi et al 1977, Richardson & Akil 1977a,b, Richardson 1982, Duncan et al 1991) and do not therefore permit extrapolations from the antinociceptive effect seen in experimental animals.

THALAMUS AND INTERNAL CAPSULE STIMULATION

Therapeutic stimulation of the thalamus was prompted by the hypothesis that deafferentation pain resulted from a lack of (proprioceptive) input to its sensory relay nuclei. The first report was from Paris in 1960; the target was VPL (Mazars et al 1960). The San Francisco group subsequently published their results from stimulating VPM for neuropathic pain (Hosobuchi et al 1973). Mazars' (1975) discussion of his first 44 cases confirmed the effectiveness of thalamic stimulation in neuropathic pain. Unlike PAG/PVG stimulation, sensory thalamic stimulation does produce paraesthesiae and these must cover the painful area, as for SCS. It does not appear to involve opioids (Hosobuchi et al 1977, Tsubokawa et al 1984, Young et al 1993). Although there is neurophysiological evidence that stimulating the (intact) sensory thalamus also has an antinociceptive effect, it is relatively sparse, the effect is extremely short-lived (milliseconds) and corroborative behavioural evidence is lacking (Gerhart et al 1981, Benabid et al 1983, Gybels & Kupers 1987, Duncan et al 1991).

In 1972, Adams discovered that stimulating the posterior limb of the internal capsule produced pain relief (Fields & Adams 1974) and his group later reported success in five patients with neuropathic pain (Adams et al 1974). Others have also found this to be an effective target (Namba et al 1985, Richardson 1995, Kumar et al 1997b) particularly its posteromedial portion. This part contains both motor and thalamocortical fibres but the mechanism of IC SPA is unclear, although an inhibition of thalamic nociceptive neurons has been demonstrated (Nishimoto et al 1984). In addition to PAG, PVG, thalamic nuclei VPM and VPL and IC, other deep brain sites reported to be effective clinically in relieving pain include the parafascicular and centromedian thalamic nuclei (Richardson & Akil 1977a, Andy 1980), hypothalamus (Mayanagi et al 1982, Richardson 1982), septal area (Richardson 1982, Schvarcz 1985) and the Kölliker–Fuse nucleus which is in the parabrachial region (Young et al 1992). The descending analgesic effect, in the rat, of anterior pretectal nucleus (APtN) activity, stimulated by dorsal column input via the dorsal column nuclei (as discussed under 'Mechanisms of Action'), is also mediated in part via the parabrachial region (Terenzi et al 1992). Although the APtN is not directly analogous with the human PVG and rostral PAG, the equivalent region is adjacent to these structures. The rat APtN has connections with PAG, ventrobasal thalamus, hypothalamus and motor cortex. Thus there may be a link between some human DBS targets and the APtN and between human DBS and SCS.

The electrical parameters of effective DBS have generally been similar to those used in SCS. Much shorter and less frequent episodes of stimulation are required with PAG/PVG than with thalamic stimulation (Kumar et al 1997b).

RESULTS OF DEEP BRAIN STIMULATION

Given the foregoing, it would not be surprising if PAG/PVG stimulation were more effective against nociceptive pain and thalamic stimulation against neuropathic pain. This, broadly, has proved to be the case (Young et al 1985, Baskin et al 1986, Hosobuchi 1986, 1987, Young & Chambi 1987, Siegfried 1991, Richardson 1995, Parrent 1996, Kumar et al 1997b). The dichotomy is certainly not absolute, however (Dieckmann & Witzmann 1982, Duncan et al 1991, Richardson 1995, Parrent 1996). Some syndromes, e.g. FBSS, involve a mixture of nociceptive and neuropathic pain and this, combined with the lack of specificity of some electrode placements alluded to above, might explain some of the mixed results. In some instances electrodes have been placed deliberately in both major sites, to good effect (Young et al 1985, Hosobuchi 1986, Young 1998). Nociceptive pain may fare better than neuropathic pain but the evidence is not strong. Gybels and Kupers (1987) and Duncan and colleagues (1991) have pointed out the wide variation in outcome between different series of DBS, which has not been fully explained. It would appear from some reports that, for example, facial neuropathic pain, both anaesthesia dolorosa and postherpetic, is a very good indication (Hosobuchi et al 1973, Roldan et al 1982, Siegfried 1991): Siegfried had only six poor results out of 49. Others, however, have reported very disappointing results (Levy et al 1987). The larger mixed series have revealed overall success rates from 31% (Levy et al 1987) to 79% (Kumar et al 1997b). Various meta-analyses have simply illustrated the wide variation, although the figure of 55% overall success (Gybels & Kupers 1987) is probably a fair average. In patients with complete cord lesions or with pain from partial cord lesions unresponsive to SCS, only 42% achieved good or fair relief (Tasker et al 1992). Phantom pain and pain following plexus avulsion may respond better (Siegfried 1991).

Tolerance, i.e. loss of analgesia despite a functioning stimulator, has been a prominent problem with DBS (Hosobuchi 1986, Levy et al 1987, Kumar et al 1997b). Young (1998) has suggested that it continues to appear after as much as 10 years. Major complications have been rare, with death, usually due to intracranial haemorrhage, occurring in less than 1.6%, permanent neurological deficit in 2.2% and scalp erosion in 1.8% (Bendok & Levy 1998). Infection rates of around 5–6% are typical (Young et al 1985, Siegfried 1991, Kumar et al 1997b) although higher rates have been reported (Levy et al 1987). Equipment failures were initially common but technological developments have reduced the incidence dramatically.

In successful cases of DBS the benefit is undoubtedly dramatic (Shulman et al 1982), the complication rate is low and its use in controlling movement disorders is increasing, yet its application to the treatment of pain is becoming obsolete. The perceived invasiveness, the marked variability of reported outcomes, the high incidence of tolerance and recent advances in pharamacological therapy and palliative care are probably all contributory factors. Neuropathic facial pain, central post-stroke pain (CPSP; thalamic syndrome) and, to a lesser extent, pain of spinal cord origin remain therapeutically elusive. Motor cortex stimulation (MCS) might fill the breach.

MOTOR CORTEX STIMULATION

Therapeutic chronic MCS via epidural plate electrodes was first carried out in 1988 by Tsubokawa and colleagues (Tsubokawa & Katayama 1998, Tsubokawa et al 1993) on the basis that rostral (sensorimotor cortex) stimulation might be optimal in central deafferentation syndromes such as CPSP. They presented experimental evidence in cats that *motor* cortical stimulation might be effective (Hirayama et al 1990) and confirmed at operation in humans that sensory cortical stimulation had either no effect or exacerbated CPSP whereas precentral (motor) cortical stimulation relieved it. Five of their first 11 patients enjoyed excellent pain relief over more than 2 years and in a subsequent report of 28 cases of CPSP, the success rate was similar (Yamamoto et al 1997). Hosobuchi (1993) had an excellent response in six out of six cases initially, sustained in four. Neuropathic trigeminal pain also responds very well in nearly all cases reported so far (Meyerson et al 1993, Herregodts et al 1995, Nguyen et al 1997) and allodynia is suppressed (Meyerson et al 1993).

Methods used to identify the target site include MRI, evoked potential phase reversal, induction of muscle twitches and of (faint) paraesthesiae. The induction of paraesthesiae with chronic MCS does not occur in most cases. A period of trial stimulation (1–4 weeks) is usual. Optimal placement of the electrodes is still problematic (Meyerson 1997). Similarly, the optimum stimulation parameters are still not fully known. Whereas in other sites cathodal stimulation, with its lower threshold, is the more relevant, it has been suggested that anodal stimulation is more effective for MCS (Cedzich et al 1998). Relatively low frequencies (20–55 Hz) are effective (Hosobuchi 1993, Nguyen et al 1997, Tsubokawa & Katayama 1998) at an amplitude below the threshold for motor responses (detected by stimulation at 1–2 Hz) and for dysaesthesia. Intermittent stimulation is used; 10 minutes of MCS may yield pain relief for up to 2–6 hours in CPSP (Tsubokawa et al 1993). There are as yet few aids to case selection. The use of transcranial magnetic stimulation has been proposed (Migita et al 1995). The response to morphine, thiamylal and ketamine appears to have predictive value in CPSP (Yamamoto et al 1997) although Meyerson (1997) counsels caution in interpreting these tests.

An initial response is lost in some patients but the data are as yet too few to be able to assess the question of tolerance. Epileptic seizures may occur during the trial period but have not been reported with chronic MCS although the risk exists (Meyerson 1997). Extradural haematoma formation has been reported (Meyerson et al 1993) but the risk would appear to be small, particularly if a small craniotomy is employed (permitting dural hitch stitches) rather than a burr hole. A rising impedance due to scar tissue may cause long-term failure, especially in patients with a degree of cerebral atrophy and wide CSF space. The mechanism(s) of action of MCS is not known; all suggestions to date are purely speculative, but it does appear to be a very promising additional therapeutic option against a small but particularly intractable group of conditions.

ACKNOWLEDGEMENTS

The author is grateful to the following companies for kindly providing illustrations: Advanced Neuromodulation Systems Inc, Allen, Texas (Figs 59.1, 59.5) and Medtronic Inc, Minneapolis, Minnesota (Figs 59.3, 59.4, 59.6).

REFERENCES

Abbate AD, Cook AW, Atallah M 1977 Effect of electrical stimulation of the thoracic spinal cord on the function of the bladder in multiple sclerosis. Journal of Urology 117: 285–288

Adams JE 1976 Naloxone reversal of analgesia produced by brain stimulation in the human. Pain 2: 161–166

Adams JE, Hosobuchi Y, Fields HL 1974 Stimulation of internal capsule for relief of chronic pain. Journal of Neurosurgery 41: 740–744

Akil H, Mayer DJ, Liebeskind JC 1976 Antagonism of stimulation-produced analgesia by naloxone, a narcotic antagonist. Science 191: 961–962

Akil H, Richardson DE, Hughes J, Barchas JD 1978 Enkephalin-like material elevated in ventricular cerebrospinal fluid of pain patients after analgetic local stimulation. Science 201: 463–465

Alexander A 1995 Reflex sympathetic dystrophy – from the inside. British Medical Journal 310: 1680

Andersen C 1997a Complications in spinal cord stimulation for treatment of angina pectoris. Differences in unipolar and multipolar percutaneous inserted electrodes. Acta Cardiologica 52(4): 325–333

Andersen C 1997b Time dependent variations of stimulus requirements in spinal cord stimulation for angina pectoris. PACE 20(1): 359–363

Andersen C, Clemensen SE, Henneberg SW et al 1992 Incapacitating angina pectoris treated with electric stimulation of the spinal cord. Ugeskrift For Laeger 154: 1176–1179

Andersen C, Hole P, Oxhoj H 1994 Does pain relief with spinal cord stimulation for angina conceal myocardial infarction? British Heart Journal 71: 419–421

Andy O 1980 Parafascicular-center median nuclei stimulation for intractable pain and dyskinesia (painful-dyskinesia). Applied Neurophysiology 43: 133–144

Apthorp GH, Chamberlain DA, Hayward GW 1964 The effects of sympathectomy on the electrocardiogram and effort tolerance in angina pectoris. British Heart Journal 26: 218–226

Arregui R, Morandeira JR, Martinez G et al 1989 Epidural neurostimulation in the treatment of frostbite. PACE 12: 713–717

Augustinsson LE 1989 Spinal cord electrical stimulation in severe angina pectoris: surgical technique, intraoperative physiology, complications, side effects. PACE 12: 693–694

Augustinsson LE, Carlsson CA, Leissner P 1979 The effect of dorsal column stimulation on pain-induced intracerebral impulse patterns. Applied Neurophysiology 42: 212–216

Augustinsson LE, Carlsson CA, Fall M 1982 Autonomic effects of electrostimulation. Applied Neurophysiology 45: 185–189

Augustinsson LE, Holm J, Carlsson CA, Jivegard L 1985 Epidural electrical stimulation in severe limb ischaemia. Evidences of pain relief, increased blood flow and a possible limb-saving effect. Annals of Surgery 202: 104–111

Babul N, Darke AC 1994 Reliability and accuracy of memory for acute pain. Pain 57: 131–132

Baker DM, Lamerton AJ 1994 Operative lumbar sympathectomy for severe lower limb ischaemia: still a valuable treatment option. Annals of the Royal College of Surgeons of England 76: 50–53

Bantli H, Bloedel JR, Thienprasit P 1975 Supraspinal interactions resulting from experimental dorsal column stimulation. Journal of Neurosurgery 42: 296–300

Barolat G, Knobler RL, Lublin FD 1988 Trigeminal neuralgia in a patient with multiple sclerosis treated with high cervical spinal cord stimulation. Case report. Applied Neurophysiology 51: 333–337

Barolat G, Schwartzmann R, Woo R 1989 Epidural spinal cord stimulation in the management of reflex sympathetic dystrophy. Stereotactic and Functional Neurosurgery 53: 29–39

Barolat G, Zeme S, Ketcik B 1991 Multifactorial analysis of epidural spinal cord stimulation. Stereotactic and Functional Neurosurgery 56: 77–103

Barolat G, Massaro F, He J et al 1993 Mapping of sensory responses to epidural stimulation of the intraspinal neural structures in man. Journal of Neurosurgery 78: 233–239

Baskin DS, Mehler WR, Hosobuchi Y et al 1986 Autopsy analysis of the safety, efficacy and cartography of electrical stimulation of the central gray in humans. Brain Research 371: 231–236

Bedder M 1997 Management of complications of spinal cord stimulation. Pain Reviews 4: 238–243

Bel S, Bauer BL 1991 Dorsal column stimulation (DCS): cost to benefit analysis. Acta Neurochirurgica 52(suppl): 121–123

Bell GK, Kidd D, North RB 1997 Cost-effectiveness analysis of spinal cord stimulation in treatment of failed back surgery syndrome. Journal of Pain and Symptom Management 13(5): 286–295

Benabid AL, Henriksen SJ, McGinty JF, Bloom FE 1983 Thalamic nucleus ventro-postero-lateralis inhibits nucleus parafascicularis response to noxious stimuli through a non-opioid pathway. Brain Research 280: 217–231

Bendok B, Levy RM 1998 Brain stimulation for persistent pain management. In: Gildenberg PL, Tasker RR (eds) Textbook of stereotactic and functional neurosurgery. McGraw-Hill, New York, p 1539

Bennett MI, Tai YMA 1994 Cervical dorsal column stimulation relieves pain of brachial plexus avulsion. Journal of the Royal Society of Medicine 87: 5–6

 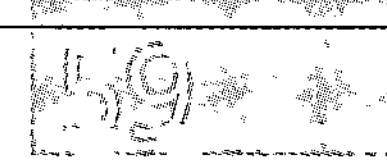

Berg V, Bergmann S, Hovdal H et al 1982 The value of dorsal column stimulation in multiple sclerosis. Scandinavian Journal of Rehabilitation Medicine 14: 183–191

Berman JS, Birch R, Anand P 1998 Pain following human brachial plexus injury with spinal cord root avulsion and the effect of surgery. Pain 75: 199–207

Birklein F, Riedl B, Neundörfer B, Handwerker HO 1998 Sympathetic vasoconstrictor reflex pattern in patients with complex regional pain syndrome. Pain 75: 93–100

Blair G, Lee RG, Vanderlinden G 1975 Dorsal column stimulation. Its effect on the somatosensory evoked response. Archives of Neurology 32: 826–829

Blume H, Richardson R, Rojas C 1982 Epidural nerve stimulation of the lower spinal cord and cauda equina for the relief of intractable pain in failed low back surgery. Applied Neurophysiology 45: 456–460

Boivie J, Meyerson BA 1982 A correlative anatomical and clinical study of pain supression by deep brain stimulation. Pain 13: 113–126

Bracale GC, Selvetella L, Mirabile F 1989 Our experience with spinal cord stimulation (SCS) in peripheral vascular disease. PACE 12: 695–697

Brandao ML, Rees H, Witt S, Roberts MHT 1991 Central antiaversive and antinociceptive effects of anterior pretectal nucleus stimulation: attenuation of autonomic and aversive effects of medial hypothalamic stimulation. Brain Research 542: 266–272

Broggi G, Servello D, Franzini A et al 1987 Spinal cord stimulation for treatment of peripheral vascular disease. Applied Neurophysiology 50: 439–441

Broseta J, Roldan P, Gonzalez-Darder J et al 1982 Chronic epidural dorsal column stimulation in the treatment of causalgic pain. Applied Neurophysiology 45: 190–194

Broseta J, Garcia-March G, Sanchez MJ, Goncales J 1985 Influence of spinal cord stimulation on peripheral blood flow. Applied Neurophysiology 48: 367–370

Broseta J, Barbera J, De Vera JA et al 1986 Spinal cord stimulation in peripheral arterial disease. A cooperative study. Journal of Neurosurgery 64: 71–80

Bryant RA 1993 Memory for pain and affect in chronic pain patients. Pain 54: 347–351

Bunt TJ 1991 Epidural spinal cord stimulation: an unproven methodology for management of lower extremity ischaemia. Journal of Vascular Surgery 14: 829

Burchiel KJ, Anderson VC, Wilson BJ et al 1995 Prognostic factors of spinal cord stimulation for chronic back and leg pain. Neurosurgery 36(6): 1101–1111

Burchiel KJ, Anderson VC, Brown FD et al 1996 Prospective, multicenter study of spinal cord stimulation for relief of chronic back and extremity pain. Spine 21 (23): 2786–2794

Burton CV 1975 Dorsal column stimulation: optimization of application. Surgical Neurology 4: 171–176

Burton CV 1977 Session on spinal cord stimulation. Safety and efficacy. Neurosurgery 1: 214–215

Carlsson AM 1983 Assessment of chronic pain. I. Aspects of the reliability and validity of the visual analogue scale. Pain 16: 87–101

Carstens E, Yokota T, Zimmermann M 1979 Inhibition of spinal neuronal responses to noxious skin heating by stimulation of the mesencephalic periaqueductal gray in the cat. Journal of Neurophysiology 42: 558–568

Cedzich C, Pechstein U, Schramm J, Schäfer S 1998 Electrophysiological considerations regarding electrical stimulation of motor cortex and brain stem in humans. Neurosurgery 42(3): 527–532

Chandler MJ, Brennan TJ, Garrison DW et al 1993 A mechanism of cardiac pain suppression by spinal cord stimulation: implications for patients with angina pectoris. European Heart Journal 14: 96–105

Cioni B, Meglio M, Pentimalli L, Visocchi M 1995 Spinal cord stimulation in the treatment of paraplegic pain. Journal of Neurosurgery 82: 35–39

Claeys LGY 1997 Improvement of microcirculatory blood flow under epidural spinal cord stimulation in patients with nonreconstructible peripheral arterial occlusive disease. Artificial Organs 21(3): 201–206

Claeys LG, Horsch S 1996 Transcutaneous oxygen pressure as predictive parameter for ulcer healing in endstage vascular patients treated with spinal cord stimulation. International Angiology 15(4): 344–349

Claeys LG, Horsch S 1997a Treatment of chronic phantom limb pain by epidural spinal cord stimulation. Pain Digest 7: 4–6

Claeys LGY, Horsch S 1997b Effects of spinal cord stimulation on ischaemic inflammatory pain and wound healing in patients with peripheral arterial occlusive disease Fontaine stage IV. Pain Digest 7: 200–203

Claeys LGY, Ktenidis K, Horsch S 1997 Effects of spinal cord stimulation on ischaemic pain in patients with Buerger's disease. Pain Digest 7: 138–141

Collins P, Fox KM 1990 Pathophysiology of angina. Lancet 335: 94–96

Cook AW, Weinstein SP 1973 Chronic dorsal column stimulation in multiple sclerosis. Preliminary report. New York State Journal of Medicine 73: 2868–2872

Cook AW, Oygar A, Baggenstos P et al 1976 Vascular disease of extremities: electrical stimulation of spinal cord and posterior roots. New York State Journal of Medicine 76: 366–368

Cook AW, Abbate A, Atallah M et al 1979 Neurogenic bladder. Reversal by stimulation of thoracic cord. New York State Journal of Medicine 79: 255–258

Coyle DE 1996 Efficacy of animal models for neuropathic pain. Pain Digest 6: 7–20

Croom JE, Foreman RD, Chandler MJ, Barron KW 1997a Cutaneous vasodilation during dorsal column stimulation is mediated by dorsal roots and CGRP. American Journal of Physiology 272: H950–H957

Croom JE, Foreman RD, Chandler MJ et al 1997b Role of nitric oxide in cutaneous blood flow increases in the rat hindpaw during dorsal column stimulation. Neurosurgery 40(3): 565–571

Cui J-G, Linderoth B, Meyerson BA 1996 Effects of spinal cord stimulation on touch-evoked allodynia involve GABAergic mechanisms. An experimental study in the mononeuropathic rat. Pain 66: 287–295

Cui J-G, Sollevi A, Linderoth B, Meyerson BA 1997a Adenosine receptor activation suppresses tactile hypersensitivity and potentiates spinal cord stimulation in mononeuropathic rats. Neuroscience Letters 223(3): 173–176

Cui J-G, O'Connor WT, Ungerstedt U et al 1997b Spinal cord stimulation attenuates augmented dorsal horn release of excitatory amino acids in mononeuropathy via a GABA ergic mechanism. Pain 73: 87–95

Daniel MS, Long C, Butcherson WL, Hunter S 1985 Psychological factors and outcome of electrode implantation for chronic pain. Neurosurgery 17: 773–777

De Jongste MJL, Haaksma J, Hautvast RWM et al 1994a Effects of spinal cord stimulation on myocardial ischaemia during daily life in patients with severe coronary artery disease. A prospective ambulatory electrocardiographic study. British Heart Journal 71: 413–418

De Jongste MJL, Nagelkerke D, Hooyschuur CM et al 1994b Stimulation characteristics, complications and efficacy of spinal cord stimulation systems in patients with refractory angina; a prospective feasibility study. PACE 17(1): 1751–1760

De La Porte C, Siegfried J 1983 Lumbosacral spinal fibrosis (spinal arachnoiditis). Its diagnosis and treatment by spinal cord stimulation. Spine 8: 593–603

De La Porte C, Van de Kelft E 1993 Spinal cord stimulation in failed back surgery syndrome. Pain 52: 55–61

De Landsheere C, Mannheimer C, Habets A et al 1992 Effect of spinal cord stimulation on regional myocardial perfusion assessed by

positron emission tomography. American Journal of Cardiology 69: 1143–1149
Demirel T, Braun W, Reimers CD 1984 Results of spinal cord stimulation in patients suffering from chronic pain after a two year observation period. Neurochirurgia 27: 47–50
Devulder J, Dumoulin K, De Laat M, Rolly G 1996 Infra-red thermographic evaluation of spinal cord electrostimulation in patients with chronic pain after failed back surgery. British Journal of Neurosurgery 10(4): 379–383
Dieckmann G, Witzmann A 1982 Initial and long-term results of deep brain stimulation for chronic intractable pain. Applied Neurophysiology 45: 167–172
Dionne RA, Mueller GP, Young RF et al 1984 Contrast medium causes the apparent increase in β-endorphin levels in human cerebrospinal fluid following brain stimulation. Pain 20: 313–321
Doerr M, Krainick JU, Thoden U 1978 Pain perception in man after long term spinal cord stimulation. Journal of Neurology 217: 261–270
Doleys DM, Klapow JC, Hammer M 1997 Psychological evaluation in spinal cord stimulation therapy. Pain Reviews 4: 189–207
Dooley DM 1977 Demyelinating, degenerative and vascular disease. Neurosurgery 1: 220–224
Dooley DM, Kasprak M 1976 Modification of blood flow to the extremities by electrical stimulation of the nervous system. Southern Medical Journal 69: 1309–1311
Dubuisson D 1989 Effect of dorsal column stimulation on gelatinosa and marginal neurons of cat spinal cord. Journal of Neurosurgery 70: 257–265
Dumoulin K, Devulder J, Castille F et al 1996 A psychoanalytic investigation to improve the success rate of spinal cord stimulation as a treatment for chronic failed back surgery syndrome. Clinical Journal of Pain 12: 43–49
Duncan GH, Bushnell MC, Marchand S 1991 Deep brain stimulation: a review of basic research and clinical studies. Pain 45: 49–59
Eich E, Reeves JL, Jaeger B, Graff-Radford SB 1985 Memory for pain; relation between past and present pain intensity. Pain 23: 375–379
Eisenberg E, Waisbrod H 1997 Spinal cord stimulator activation by an antitheft device. Journal of Neurosurgery 87: 961–962
Eliasson T, Albertsson P, Hardhammar P et al 1993 Spinal cord stimulation in angina pectoris with normal coronary angiograms. Coronary Artery Disease 4(9): 819–827
Eliasson T, Jern S, Augustinsson LE, Mannheimer C 1994 Safety aspects of spinal cord stimulation in severe angina pectoris. Coronary Artery Disease 5: 845–850
Eliasson T, Augustinsson LE, Mannheimer C 1996 Spinal cord stimulation in severe angina pectoris – presentation of current studies, indications and clinical experience. Pain 65: 169–179
Erskine A, Morley S, Pearce S 1990 Memory for pain: a review. Pain 41: 255–265
Fessler RG, Brown FD, Rachlin JR et al 1984 Elevated β-endorphin in cerebrospinal fluid after electrical brain stimulation: artifact of contrast infusion? Science 224: 1017–1019
Fields HL, Adams JE 1974 Pain after cortical injury relieved by electrical stimulation of the internal capsule. Brain 97: 169–178
Fiume D 1983 Spinal cord stimulation in peripheral vascular pain. Applied Neurophysiology 46: 290–294
Fiume D, Palombi M, Sciassa V, Tamorri M 1989 Spinal cord stimulation (SCS) in peripheral ischaemic pain. PACE 12: 698–704
Fiume D, Sherkat S, Callovini GM et al 1995 Treatment of the failed back surgery syndrome due to lumbo-sacral epidural fibrosis. Acta Neurochirurgica 64(suppl): 116–118
Foreman RD 1991 The neurological basis for cardiac pain. In: Zucker IH, Gilmore JP (eds) Reflex control of the circulation. CRC Press, Boston, p 907
Foreman RD, Chandler MJ, Brennan TJ et al 1989 Does dorsal column (DC) stimulation (S) reduce the activity of spinothalamic tract (STT) cells that respond to cardiac input? (abstract) Circulation 80(suppl): 522
Forrest DM 1996 Spinal cord stimulator therapy. Journal of Perianaesthesia Nursing 11(5): 349–352
Fox JL 1974 Dorsal column stimulation for relief of intractable pain: problems encountered with neuropacemakers. Surgical Neurology 2: 59–64
Francaviglia N, Silvestro C, Maiello M et al 1994 Spinal cord stimulation for the treatment of progressive systemic sclerosis and Raynaud's syndrome. British Journal of Neurosurgery 8: 567–571
Franzetti I, De Nale A, Bossi A et al 1989 Epidural spinal electrostimulatory system (ESES) in the management of diabetic foot and peripheral arteriopathies. PACE 12: 705–708
Friedman AH, Nashold BS 1986 DREZ lesions for relief of pain related to spinal cord injury. Journal of Neurosurgery 65: 465–469
Friedman AH, Nashold BS, Somjen G 1974 Physiological effects of dorsal column stimulation. Advances in Neurology 4: 769–773
Galley D, Rettori R, Boccalon H et al 1992 Spinal cord stimulation for the treatment of peripheral vascular disease of the lower limbs. A multicenter study in 244 patients. Journal des Maladies Vasculaires 17: 208–213
Gao XX, Ren B, Linderoth B, Meyerson BA 1996 Daily spinal cord stimulation suppresses autotomy behaviour in rats following peripheral deafferentation. Neuroscience 75(2): 463–470
Garcia-March G, Sanchez-Ledesma MJ, Diaz P et al 1987 Dorsal root entry zone lesion versus spinal cord stimulation in the management of pain from brachial plexus avulsion. Acta Neurochirurgica 39(suppl): 155–158
Gerhart KD, Yezierski RP, Wilcox TK et al 1981 Inhibition of primate spinothalamic tract neurons by stimulation in ipsilateral or contralateral ventral posterior lateral (VPLc) thalamic nucleus. Brain Research 229: 514–519
Glynn C 1995 Complex regional pain syndrome type I, reflex sympathetic dystrophy, and complex regional pain syndrome type II, causalgia. Pain Reviews 2: 292–297
González-Darder JM, González-Martinez V, Canela-Moya P 1998 Cervical spinal cord stimulation in the treatment of severe angina pectoris. Neurosurgery Quarterly 8(1): 16–23
Graber JN, Lifson A 1987 The use of spinal cord stimulation for severe limb-threatening ischaemia: a preliminary report. Annals of Vascular Surgery 1: 578–581
Graziotti PJ, Goucke CR 1993 Control of intractable pain in erythromelalgia by using spinal cord stimulation. Journal of Pain Symptom Management 8(7): 502–504
Grillo PJ, Yu HC, Patterson RH 1974 Delayed intraspinal haemorrhage after dorsal column stimulation for pain. Archives of Neurology 30: 105–106
Gybels J, Kupers R 1987 Central and peripheral electrical stimulation of the nervous system in the treatment of chronic pain. Acta Neurochirurgica 38(suppl): 64–75
Harke H, Ladleif HU, Rethage B, Grosser KD 1993 Epidural spinal cord stimulation in therapy-resistant angina pectoris. Anaesthetist 42: 557–563
Hassenbusch SJ, Stanton-Hicks M, Covington EC 1995 Spinal cord stimulation versus spinal infusion for low back and leg pain. Acta Neurochirurgica 64(suppl): 109–115
Hassenbusch SJ, Stanton-Hicks M, Schoppa D et al 1996 Long-term results of peripheral nerve stimulation for reflex sympathetic dystrophy. Journal of Neurosurgery 84: 415–423
Hautvast RWM, Blanksma PK, De Jongste MJL et al 1996 Effect of spinal cord stimulation on myocardial blood flow assessed by positron emission tomography in patients with refractory angina pectoris. American Journal of Cardiology 77: 462–467
Hawkes CH, Fawcett D, Cooke ED et al 1981 Dorsal column

stimulation in multiple sclerosis: effects on bladder, leg blood flow and peptides. Applied Neurophysiology 44: 62–70

Hawkes CH, Beard R, Fawcett D et al 1983 Dorsal column stimulation in multiple sclerosis: effects on bladder and long term findings. British Medical Journal 287: 793–795

He J, Barolat G, Holsheimer J, Struijk JJ 1994 Perception threshold and electrode position for spinal cord stimulation. Pain 59: 55–63

Herregodts P, Stadnick T, De Ridder F, D'Haens J 1995 Cortical stimulation for central neuropathic pain: 3-D surface MRI for easy determination of the motor cortex. Acta Neurochirurgica 64(suppl): 132–135

Hirayama T, Tsubokawa T, Katayama Y et al 1990 Chronic changes in activity of thalamic lemniscal relay neurons following spino-thalamic tractotomy in cats: effects of motor cortex stimulation. Pain 5(suppl): S273

Holroyd KA, Holm JE, Keefe FJ et al 1992 A multi-center evaluation of the McGill Pain Questionnaire: results from more than 1700 chronic pain patients. Pain 48: 301–311

Holsheimer J 1997 Effectiveness of spinal cord stimulation in the management of chronic pain: analysis of technical drawbacks and solutions. Neurosurgery 40(5): 990–999

Holsheimer J, Wesselink WA 1997a Effect of anode-cathode configuration on paraesthesia coverage in spinal cord stimulation. Neurosurgery 41(3): 654–660

Holsheimer J, Wesselink WA 1997b Optimum electrode geometry for spinal cord stimulation: the narrow bipole and tripole. Medical and Biological Engineering and Computing 35: 493–497

Holsheimer J, Den Boer JA, Struijk JJ, Rozeboom AR 1994 MR assessment of the normal position of the spinal cord in the spinal canal. American Journal of Neuroradiology 15: 951–959

Holsheimer J, Nuttin B, King GW et al 1998 Clinical evaluation of paraesthesia steering with a new system for spinal cord stimulation. Neurosurgery 42(3): 541–549

Hood TW, Siegfried J 1984 Epidural versus thalamic stimulation for the management of brachial plexus lesion pain. Acta Neurochirurgica 33(suppl): 451–457

Hoppenstein R 1975 Electrical stimulation of the ventral and dorsal columns of the spinal cord for relief of chronic intractable pain: preliminary report. Surgical Neurology 4: 187–194

Hosobuchi Y 1985 Electrical stimulation of the cervical spinal cord increases cerebral blood flow in humans. Applied Neurophysiology 48: 372–376

Hosobuchi Y 1986 Subcortical electrical stimulation for control of intractable pain in humans. Report of 122 cases (1970–1984). Journal of Neurosurgery 64: 543–553

Hosobuchi Y 1987 Dorsal periaqueductal gray-matter stimulation in humans. PACE 10: 213–216

Hosobuchi Y 1993 Motor cortical stimulation for control of central deafferentation pain. In: Devinsky O, Beric A, Dogali M (eds) Electrical and magnetic stimulation of the brain and spinal cord. Raven Press, New York, p 215

Hosobuchi Y, Adams JE, Rutkin B 1973 Chronic thalamic stimulation for the control of facial anaesthesia dolorosa. Archives of Neurology 29: 158–161

Hosobuchi Y, Adams JE, Linchitz R 1977 Pain relief by electrical stimulation of the central gray matter in humans and its reversal by naloxone. Science 197: 183–186

Hosobuchi Y, Rossier J, Bloom FE, Guillemin R 1979 Stimulation of human periaqueductal gray for pain relief increases immunoreactive β-endorphin in ventricular fluid. Science 203: 279–281

Hunt WE, Goodman JH, Bingham WG 1975 Stimulation of the dorsal spinal cord for treatment of intractable pain: a preliminary report. Surgical Neurology 4: 153–156

Hunter JP, Ashby P 1994 Segmental effects of epidural spinal cord stimulation in humans. Journal of Physiology 474(3): 407–419

Hunter M, Philips C, Rachman S 1979 Memory for pain. Pain 6: 35–46

Hwang JH, Yaksh TL 1997 The effect of spinal GABA receptor agonists on tactile allodynia in a surgically-induced neuropathic pain model in the rat. Pain 70: 15–22

Illis LS, Oygar AE, Sedgwick EM, Sabbahi Awadalla MA 1976 Dorsal column stimulation in the rehabilitation of patients with multiple sclerosis. Lancet i: 1383–1386

Illis LS, Read DJ, Sedgwick EM, Tallis RC 1983 Spinal cord stimulation in the United Kingdom. Journal of Neurology, Neurosurgery and Psychiatry 46: 299–304

Jacobs MJHM, Jorning PJG, Joshi SR et al 1988 Epidural spinal cord electrical stimulation improves microvascular blood flow in severe limb ischaemia. Annals of Surgery 207: 179–183

Jacobs MJHM, Jorning PJG, Beckers RCY et al 1990 Foot salvage and improvement of microvascular blood flow as a result of epidural spinal cord electrical stimulation. Journal of Vascular Surgery 12: 354–360

Jamison RN, Sbrocco T, Parris WCV 1989 The influence of physical and psychosocial factors on accuracy of memory for pain in chronic pain patients. Pain 37: 289–294

Jänig W 1996 The puzzle of 'reflex sympathetic dystrophy': mechanisms, hypotheses, open questions. In: Jänig W, Stanton-Hicks M (eds) Reflex sympathetic dystrophy: a reappraisal. Progress in pain research and management, vol 6. IASP Press, Seattle, p 1

Jensen MP, McFarland CA 1993 Increasing the reliability and validity of pain intensity measurement in chronic pain patients. Pain 55: 195–203

Jessurun GAJ, De Jongste MJL, Blanksma PK 1996 Current views on neurostimulation in the treatment of cardiac ischemic syndromes. Pain 66: 109–116

Jivegard L, Augustinsson LE, Carlsson CA, Holm J 1987 Long term results by spinal electrical stimulation (ESES) in patients with inoperable severe lower limb ischaemia. European Journal of Vascular Surgery 1: 345–349

Jivegard L, Augustinsson LE, Holm J et al 1995 Effects of spinal cord stimulation (SCS) in patients with inoperable severe lower limb ischaemia: a prospective randomised controlled study. European Journal of Vascular and Endovascular Surgery 9: 421–425

Kane K, Taub A 1975 A history of local electrical analgesia. Pain 1: 125–138

Kanno T, Yoshifumi K, Yokoyama T et al 1989 Effects of dorsal column stimulation (DCS) on reversibility of neuronal function – experience of treatment for vegetative states. PACE 12: 733–738

Kellaway P 1946 The part played by electric fish in the early history of bioelectricity and electrotherapy. Bulletin of the History of Medicine 20: 112–137

Kiriakopoulos ET, Tasker RR, Nicosia S et al 1997 Functional magnetic resonance imaging: a potential tool for the evaluation of spinal cord stimulation: technical case report. Neurosurgery 41(2): 501–504

Koeze TH, Simpson BA, Watkins ES 1984 Diagnosis and repair of malfunctions of implanted central nervous system stimulators. Applied Neurophysiology 47: 111–116

Koeze TH, Williams AC de C, Reiman S 1987 Spinal cord stimulation and the relief of chronic pain. Journal of Neurology, Neurosurgery and Psychiatry 50: 1424–1429

Krainick JU, Thoden U, Riechert T 1975 Spinal cord stimulation in post-amputation pain. Surgical Neurology 4: 167–170

Krainick JU, Thoden U, Riechert T 1980 Pain reduction in amputees by long term spinal cord stimulation. Journal of Neurosurgery 52: 346–350

Kujacic V, Eliasson T, Mannheimer C et al 1993 Assessment of the influence of spinal cord stimulation on left ventricular function in patients with severe angina pectoris: an echocardiographic study. European Heart Journal 14(19): 1238–1244

Kumar K, Nath R, Wyant G 1991 Treatment of chronic pain by epidural spinal cord stimulation: a 10-year experience. Journal of Neurosurgery 75: 402–407

Kumar K, Toth C, Nath RK 1996 Spinal cord stimulation for chronic pain in peripheral neuropathy. Surgical Neurology 46(4): 363–369

Kumar K, Nath RK, Toth C 1997a Spinal cord stimulation is effective in the management of reflex sympathetic dystrophy. Neurosurgery 40(3): 503–509

Kumar K, Toth C, Nath RK 1997b Deep brain stimulation for intractable pain: a 15-year experience. Neurosurgery 40(4): 736–747

Kumar K, Toth C, Nath RK et al 1997c Improvement of limb circulation in peripheral vascular disease using epidural spinal cord stimulation: a prospective study. Journal of Neurosurgery 86: 662–669

Kupers RC, Van den Oever R, Van Houdenhove B et al 1994 Spinal cord stimulation in Belgium: a nation-wide survey on the incidence, indications and therapeutic efficacy by the health insurer. Pain 56: 211–216

Kurvers HAJM, Jacobs MJHM, Beuk RJ et al 1995 Reflex sympathetic dystrophy: evolution of microcirculatory disturbances in time. Pain 60: 333–340

Lang P 1997 The treatment of chronic pain by epidural spinal cord stimulation – a 15 year follow up; present status. Axon 18(4): 71–73

Larson SJ, Sances A, Riegel DH et al 1974 Neurophysiological effects of dorsal column stimulation in man and monkey. Journal of Neurosurgery 41: 217–223

Larson SJ, Sances A, Cusick JF et al 1975 A comparison between anterior and posterior spinal implant systems. Surgical Neurology 4: 180–186

Law JD 1983 Spinal stimulation: statistical superiority of monophasic stimulation of narrowly separated, longitudinal bipoles having rostral cathodes. Applied Neurophysiology 46: 129–137

Law JD 1987 Targeting a spinal stimulator to treat the 'failed back surgery syndrome'. Applied Neurophysiology 50: 437–438

Law JD 1992 Clinical and technical results from spinal cord stimulation for chronic pain of diverse pathophysiologies. Stereotactic and Functional Neurosurgery 59: 21–24

Le Doux MS, Langford KH 1993 Spinal cord stimulation for the failed back syndrome. Spine 18: 191–194

Levy RM, Lamb S, Adams JE 1987 Treatment of chronic pain by deep brain stimulation: long term follow-up and review of the literature. Neurosurgery 21(6): 885–893

Liebeskind JC, Guilbaud G, Besson J-M, Oliveras J-L 1973 Analgesia from electrical stimulation of the periaqueductal gray matter in the cat: behavioural observations and inhibitory effects on spinal cord interneurones. Brain Research 50: 441–446

Liem LA, Van Dongen VCPC 1997 Magnetic resonance imaging and spinal cord stimulation systems. Pain 70: 95–97

Linderoth B, Fedorcsak I, Meyerson BA 1991a Peripheral vasodilatation after spinal cord stimulation: animal studies of putative effector mechanisms. Neurosurgery 28(2): 187–195

Linderoth B, Gunasekera L, Meyerson BA 1991b Effects of sympathectomy on skin and muscle microcirculation during dorsal column stimulation: animal studies. Neurosurgery 29(6): 874–879

Linderoth B, Stiller CO, Gunasekera L et al 1993 Release of neurotransmitters in the CNS by spinal cord stimulation: survey of present state of knowledge and recent experimental studies. Stereotactic and Functional Neurosurgery 61: 157–170

Linderoth B, Stiller C-O, Gunasekera L et al 1994a Gamma-aminobutyric acid is released in the dorsal horn by electrical spinal cord stimulation: an in vivo microdialysis study in the rat. Neurosurgery 34(3): 484–489

Linderoth B, Herregodts P, Meyerson BA 1994b Sympathetic mediation of peripheral vasodilation induced by spinal cord stimulation: animal studies of the role of cholinergic and adrenergic receptor subtypes. Neurosurgery 35(4): 711–719

Linderoth B, Gherardini G, Ren B, Lundeberg T 1995 Preemptive spinal cord stimulation reduces ischaemia in an animal model of vasospasm. Neurosurgery 37(2): 266–272

Linton SJ 1991 Memory for chronic pain intensity: correlates of accuracy. Perceptual and Motor Skills 72: 1091–1095

Linton SJ, Gotestam KG 1983 A clinical comparison of two pain scales: correlation, remembering chronic pain, and a measure of compliance. Pain 17: 57–65

Linton SJ, Melin L 1982 The accuracy of remembering chronic pain. Pain 13: 281–285

Long DM, Erickson DE 1975 Stimulation of the posterior columns of the spinal cord for relief of intractable pain. Surgical Neurology 4: 134–141

Long DM, Hagfors N 1975 Electrical stimulation in the nervous system: the current status of electrical stimulation of the nervous system for relief of pain. Pain 1: 109–123

Long DM, Erickson D, Campbell J, North R 1981 Electrical stimulation of the spinal cord and peripheral nerves for pain control. A 10-year experience. Applied Neurophysiology 44: 207–217

Mannheimer C, Carlsson C-A, Ericsson K et al 1982 Transcutaneous electrical nerve stimulation in severe angina pectoris. European Heart Journal 3: 297–302

Mannheimer C, Augustinsson LE, Carlsson CA et al 1988 Epidural spinal electrical stimulation in severe angina pectoris. British Heart Journal 59: 56–61

Mannheimer C, Eliasson T, Andersson B 1993 Effects of spinal cord stimulation in angina pectoris induced by pacing and possible mechanisms of action. British Medical Journal 307: 477–480

Mannheimer C, Waagstein F, Eliasson T et al 1994 Myocardial metabolism of endogenous opioids and calcitonin gene-related peptide in the human heart and the effects of spinal cord stimulation on pacing-induced angina pectoris (abstract). Circulation 90: 1–160

Mannheimer C, Eliasson T, Augustinsson L-E et al 1998 Electrical stimulation versus coronary artery bypass surgery in severe angina pectoris. The ESBY study. Circulation 97: 1157–1163

Marchand S, Bushnell MC, Molina-Negro P et al 1991 The effects of dorsal column stimulation on measures of clinical and experimental pain in man. Pain 45: 249–257

Matsui T, Asano T, Takakura K et al 1989 Beneficial effects of cervical spinal cord stimulation (cSCS) on patients with impaired consciousness: a preliminary report. PACE 12: 718–725

Mayanagi Y, Sano K, Suzuki I et al 1982 Stimulation and coagulation of the posteromedial hypothalamus for intractable pain, with reference to β-endorphins. Applied Neurophysiology 45: 136–142

Mayer DJ, Wolfle TL, Akil H et al 1971 Analgesia from electrical stimulation in the brainstem of the rat. Science 174: 1351–1354

Mazars GJ 1975 Intermittent stimulation of nucleus ventralis posterolateralis for intractable pain. Surgical Neurology 4: 93–95

Mazars GJ, Roge R, Mazars Y 1960 Stimulation of the spinothalamic fasciculus and their bearing on the physiology of pain. Revue Neurologique (Paris) 103: 136–138

Meglio M, Cioni B 1982 Personal experience with spinal cord stimulation in chronic pain management. Applied Neurophysiology 45: 195–200

Meglio M, Cioni B 1985 Effect of spinal cord stimulation on heart rate. In: Lazorthes Y, Upton ARM (eds) Neurostimulation. An overview. Futura, New York, p 185

Meglio M, Cioni B, Sandric S 1981a Spinal cord stimulation and peripheral blood flow. In: Hosobuchi Y, Corbin T (eds) Indications for spinal cord stimulation. Excerpta Medica, Amsterdam, p 60

Meglio M, Cioni B, Dal Lago A et al 1981b Pain control and improvement of peripheral blood flow following epidural spinal cord stimulation. Case report. Journal of Neurosurgery 54: 821–823

Meglio M, Cioni B, Prezioso A, Talamonti G 1989a Spinal cord stimulation (SCS) in the treatment of post herpetic pain. Acta Neurochirurgica 46(suppl): 65–66

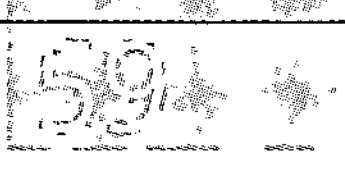

Meglio M, Cioni B, Rossi GF 1989b Spinal cord stimulation in management of chronic pain. A 9-year experience. Journal of Neurosurgery 70: 519–524

Meilman PW, Leibrock LG, Leong FT 1989 Outcome of implanted spinal cord stimulation in the treatment of chronic pain: arachnoiditis versus single nerve root injury and mononeuropathy. Brief clinical note. Clinical Journal of Pain 5: 189–193

Melzack R 1975 The McGill Pain Questionnaire: major properties and scoring methods. Pain I: 277–299

Melzack R, Wall PD 1965 Pain mechanisms: a new theory. Science 150: 971–979

Merskey H, Bogduk N (eds) 1994 Classification of chronic pain, 2nd edn. IASP Press, Seattle

Meyer GA, Fields HL 1972 Causalgia treated by selective larger fibre stimulation of peripheral nerve. Brain 95: 163–168

Meyer PG, Nashold BS, Peterson J 1979 Diagnosis of electric neurostimulating device dysfuction. Applied Neurophysiology 42: 352–364

Meyerson BA 1997 Editorial. Pharmacological tests in pain analysis and in prediction of treatment outcome. Pain 72: 1–3

Meyerson BA, Lindblom U, Linderoth B et al 1993 Motor cortex stimulation as treatment of trigeminal neuropathic pain. Acta Neurochirurgica 58(suppl): 150–153

Meyerson BA, Herregodts P, Linderoth B, Ren B 1994 An experimental animal model for spinal cord stimulation for pain. Stereotactic and Functional Neurosurgery 62: 256–262

Meyerson BA, Ren B, Herregodts P, Linderoth B 1995 Spinal cord stimulation in animal models of mononeuropathy: effects on the withdrawal response and the flexor reflex. Pain 61: 229–243

Migita K, Uozumi T, Arita K, Monden S 1995 Transcranial magnetic coil stimulation of motor cortex in patients with central pain. Neurosurgery 36(5): 1037–1040

Miles J, Lipton S 1978 Phantom limb pain treated by electrical stimulation. Pain 5: 373–382

Miles J, Lipton S, Hayward M, Bowsher D, Mumford J, Molony V 1974 Pain relief by implanted electrical stimulators. Lancet i: 777–779

Mittal B, Thomas DGT, Walton P, Calder I 1987 Dorsal column stimulation (DCS) in chronic pain: report of 31 cases. Annals of the Royal College of Surgeons of England 69: 104–109

Modesti LM, Waszak M 1975 Firing pattern of cells in human thalamus during dorsal column stimulation. Applied Neurophysiology 38: 251–258

Morton CR, Siegel J, Xiao H-M, Zimmermann M 1997 Modulation of cutaneous nociceptor activity by electrical stimulation in the brain stem does not inhibit the nociceptive excitation of dorsal horn neurons. Pain 71: 65–70

Mundinger F, Neumuller H 1982 Programmed stimulation for control of chronic pain and motor diseases. Applied Neurophysiology 45: 102–111

Murphy DF, Giles KE 1987 Dorsal column stimulation for pain relief from intractable angina. Pain 28: 365–368

Namba S, Wani T, Shimizu Y et al 1985 Sensory and motor responses to deep brain stimulation. Journal of Neurosurgery 63: 224–234

Nashold BS 1975 Dorsal column stimulation for control of pain: a three-year follow-up. Surgical Neurology 4: 146–147

Nashold BS, Friedman H 1972 Dorsal column stimulation for control of pain. Preliminary report on 30 patients. Journal of Neurosurgery 36: 590–597

Naver H, Augustinsson LE, Elam M 1992 The vasodilating effect of spinal dorsal column stimulation is mediated by sympathetic nerves. Clinical Autonomic Research 2: 41–45

Nelson DV, Kennington M, Novy DM, Squitieri P 1996a Psychological selection criteria for implantable spinal cord stimulators. Pain Forum 5(2): 93–103

Nelson DV, Kennington M, Novy DM, Squitieri P 1996b Psychological considerations in implantable technology. Pain Forum 5(2): 121–126

Nguyen JP, Keravel Y, Feve A et al 1997 Treatment of deafferentation pain by chronic stimulation of the motor cortex: report of a series of 20 cases. Acta Neurochirurgica 68(suppl): 54–60

Nielsen KD, Adams JE, Hosobuchi Y 1975a Experience with dorsal column stimulation for relief of chronic intractable pain: 1968–1973. Surgical Neurology 4: 148–152

Nielsen KD, Adams JE, Hosobuchi Y 1975b Phantom limb pain. Treatment with dorsal column stimulation. Journal of Neurosurgery 42: 301–307

Nishimoto A, Namba S, Nakao Y et al 1984 Inhibition of nociceptive neurons by internal capsule stimulation. Applied Neurophysiology 47: 117–127

North RB, Ewend MG, Lawton MT, Piantadosi S 1991a Spinal cord stimulation for chronic, intractable pain: superiority of 'multi-channel' devices. Pain 44: 119–130

North RB, Campbell JN, James CS et al 1991b Failed back surgery syndrome: 5-year follow-up in 102 patients undergoing repeated operation. Neurosurgery 28: 685–691

North RB, Ewend MG, Lawton MT et al 1991c Failed back surgery syndrome: 5-year follow-up after spinal cord stimulation. Neurosurgery 28: 692–699

North RB, Fowler K, Nigrin DJ, Szymanski R 1992a Patient-interactive, computer controlled neurological stimulation system: clinical efficacy in spinal cord stimulator adjustment. Journal of Neurosurgery 76: 967–972

North RB, Nigrin DJ, Fowler KR et al 1992b Automated 'pain drawing' analysis by computer-controlled, patient-interactive neurological stimulation system. Pain 50: 51–57

North RB, Kidd DH, Zahwak M et al 1993 Spinal cord stimulation for chronic, intractable pain: experience over two decades. Neurosurgery 32: 384–395

North RB, Kidd DH, Piantadosi S 1995 Spinal cord stimulation versus reoperation for failed back surgery syndrome: a prospective, randomized study design. Acta Neurochirurgica 64(suppl): 106–108

North RB, Kidd DH, Wimberly RL, Edwin D 1996 Prognostic value of psychological testing in patients undergoing spinal cord stimulation: a prospective study. Neurosurgery 39(2): 301–311

Ohnmeiss DD, Rashbaum RF, Bogdanffy GM 1996 Prospective outcome evaluation of spinal cord stimulation in patients with intractable leg pain. Spine 21(11): 1344–1351

Olausson B, Xu ZQ, Shyu BC 1994 Dorsal column inhibition of nocioceptive thalamic cells mediated by gamma-aminobutyric acid mechanisms in the cat. Acta Physiologica Scandinavica 152(3): 239–247

Oosterga M, Ten Vaarwerk IAM, De Jongste MJL, Staal MJ 1997 Spinal cord stimulation in refractory angina pectoris – clinical results and mechanisms. Zeitschrift fur Kardiologie 86(1): 107–113

Parrent AG 1996 Strategies for the surgical management of chronic pain. Pain Digest 6: 275–289

Pineda A 1975 Dorsal column stimulation and its prospects. Surgical Neurology 4: 157–163

Polisca R, Domenichini M, Signoretti P, Marchi P 1992 SCS (spinal cord stimulation) in severe ischaemia of the legs. Minerva Anestesiologica 58: 419–423

Price DD 1991 Editorial. The use of experimental pain in evaluating the effects of dorsal column stimulation on clinical pain. Pain 45: 225–226

Probst C 1990 Spinal cord stimulation in 112 patients with epi/intradural fibrosis following operation for lumbar disc herniation. Acta Neurochirurgica 107: 147–151

Racz GB, McCarron RF, Talboys P 1989 Percutaneous dorsal column stimulator for chronic pain control. Spine 14: 1–4

Rainov NG, Heidecke V, Burkert W 1996 Short test-period spinal cord

stimulation for failed back surgery syndrome. Minimally Invasive Neurosurgery 39: 41–44
Rasmussen MB, Andersen C, Andersen P, Frandsen F 1992 Cost-benefit analysis of electric stimulation of the spinal cord in the treatment of angina pectoris. Ugeskrift For Laeger 154: 1180–1184
Ray CD, Burton CV, Lifson A 1982 Neurostimulation as used in a large clinical practice. Applied Neurophysiology 45: 160–166
Read DJ, Matthews WB, Higson RH 1980 The effect of spinal cord stimulation on function in patients with multiple sclerosis. Brain 103: 803–833
Rees H, Roberts MHT 1989a Activation of cells in the anterior pretectal nucleus by dorsal column stimulation in the rat. Journal of Physiology 417: 361–373
Rees H, Roberts MHT 1989b Antinociceptive effects of dorsal column stimulation in the rat: involvement of the anterior pretectal nucleus. Journal of Physiology 417: 375–388
Rees H, Roberts MHT 1993 The anterior pretectal nucleus: a proposed role in sensory processing. Pain 53: 121–135
Ren B, Linderoth B, Meyerson BA 1996 Effects of spinal cord stimulation on the flexor reflex and involvement of supraspinal mechanisms: an experimental study in mononeuropathic rats. Journal of Neurosurgery 84(2): 244–249
Reynolds DV 1969 Surgery in the rat during electrical analgesia induced by focal brain stimulation. Science 164: 444–445
Richardson DE 1982 Analgesia produced by stimulation of various sites in the human beta-endorphin system. Applied Neurophysiology 45: 116–122
Richardson DE 1995 Deep brain stimulation for the relief of chronic pain. Neurosurgical Clinics of North America 6(1): 135–144
Richardson DE, Akil H 1977a Pain reduction by electrical brain stimulation in man. Part 1: Acute administration in periaqueductal and periventricular sites. Journal of Neurosurgery 47: 178–183
Richardson DE, Akil HA 1977b Pain reduction by electrical brain stimulation in man. Part 2: Chronic self-administration in the periventricular gray matter. Journal of Neurosurgery 47: 184–194
Richardson RR, Siqueira EB, Cerullo LJ 1979 Spinal epidural neurostimulation for treatment of acute and chronic intractable pain: initial and long term results. Neurosurgery 5: 344–348
Rivers SP, Veith FJ, Ascer E, Gupta SK 1986 Successful conservative therapy of severe limb-threatening ischaemia: the value of non-sympathectomy. Surgery 99: 759–762
Robaina FJ, Rodriguez JL, De Vera JA, Martin MA 1989a Transcutaneous electrical nerve stimulation and spinal cord stimulation for pain relief in reflex sympathetic dystrophy. Stereotactic and Functional Neurosurgery 52: 53–62
Robaina FJ, Dominguez M, Diaz M et al 1989b Spinal cord stimulation for relief of chronic pain in vasospastic disorders of the upper limbs. Neurosurgery 24: 63–67
Roberts MHT, Rees H 1986 The antinociceptive effects of stimulating the pretectal nucleus of the rat. Pain 25: 83–93
Roberts MHT, Rees H 1994 Physiological basis of spinal cord stimulation. Pain Reviews 1: 184–198
Roizen MF, Newfield P, Eger EI et al 1985 Reduced anesthetic requirement after electrical stimulation of periaqueductal gray matter. Anesthesiology 62: 120–123
Roldan P, Broseta J, Barcia-Salorio JL 1982 Chronic VPM stimulation for anaesthesia dolorosa following trigeminal surgery. Applied Neurophysiology 45: 112–113
Romano M, Zucco F, Baldini MR, Allaria B 1993 Technical and clinical problems in patients with simultaneous implantation of a cardiac pacemaker and a spinal cord stimulator. PACE 16: 1639–1644
Sanchez-Ledesma MJ, Garcia-March G, Diaz-Cascajo P et al 1989 Spinal cord stimulation in deafferentation pain. Stereotactic and Functional Neurosurgery 53: 40–45
Sanderson JE 1990 Electrical neurostimulators for pain relief in angina. British Heart Journal 63: 141–143
Sanderson JE, Brooksby P, Waterhouse D et al 1992 Epidural spinal electrical stimulation for severe angina: a study of effects on symptoms, exercise tolerance and degree of ischaemia. European Heart Journal 13: 628–633
Sanderson JE, Ibrahim B, Waterhouse D, Palmer RBG 1994 Spinal electrical stimulation for intractable angina – long-term clinical outcome and safety. European Heart Journal 15: 810–814
Sandric S, Meglio M, Bellocci F et al 1984 Clinical and electrocardiographic improvement of ischaemic heart disease after spinal cord stimulation. Acta Neurochirurgica 33(suppl): 543–546
Schott GD 1994 Visceral afferents: their contribution to 'sympathetic dependent' pain. Brain 117: 397–413
Schvarcz JR 1985 Chronic stimulation of the septal area for the relief of intractable pain. Applied Neurophysiology 48: 191–194
Shatin D, Mullett K, Hults G 1986 Totally implantable spinal cord stimulation for chronic pain: design and efficacy. PACE 9: 577–583
Shealy CN 1966 The physiological substrate of pain. Headache 6: 101–108
Shealy CN 1974 Six years' experience with electrical stimulation for control of pain. Advances in Neurology 4: 775–782
Shealy CN 1975 Dorsal column stimulation: optimization of application. Surgical Neurology 4: 142–145
Shealy CN, Mortimer JT, Reswick JB 1967a Electrical inhibition of pain by stimulation of the dorsal columns: preliminary clinical report. Anesthesia and Analgesia 46: 489–491
Shealy CN, Taslitz N, Mortimer JT, Becker DP 1967b Electrical inhibition of pain: experimental evaluation. Anesthesia and Analgesia 46: 299–304
Shealy CN, Mortimer JT, Hagfors NR 1970 Dorsal column electroanalgesia. Journal of Neurosurgery 32: 560–564
Shimoji K, Hokari T, Kano T et al 1993 Management of intractable pain with percutaneous epidural spinal cord stimulation: differences in pain-relieving effects among diseases and sites of pain. Anesthesia and Analgesia 77: 110–116
Shulman R, Turnbull IM, Diewold P 1982 Psychiatric aspects of thalamic stimulation for neuropathic pain. Pain 13: 127–135
Siegfried J 1991 Therapeutical neurostimulation – indications reconsidered. Acta Neurochirurgica 52: (suppl) 112–117
Siegfried J, Lazorthes Y 1982 Long-term follow-up of dorsal cord stimulation for chronic pain syndrome after multiple lumbar operations. Applied Neurophysiology 45: 201–204
Simpson BA 1991 Spinal cord stimulation in 60 cases of intractable pain. Journal of Neurology, Neurosurgery and Psychiatry 54: 196–199
Simpson BA 1992 A new dual bipolar electrode system for spinal cord stimulation. In: Galley D, Illis LS, Krainick JU et al (eds) International Neuromodulation Society First International Congress. Monduzzi Editore, Bologna, p 13
Simpson BA 1994 Spinal cord stimulation. Pain Reviews 1: 199–230
Simpson BA 1996 A dual paddle electrode system gives reliable spinal cord stimulation in the mobile cervical spine. In: Raj P, Erdine S, Niv D (eds) Management of pain. A world perspective II, vol 1. Monduzzi Editore, Bologna, p 295
Simpson BA 1997 Editorial. Spinal cord stimulation. British Journal of Neurosurgery II: 5–11
Simpson BA 1998 Neuromodulation in Europe – regulation, variation and trends. Pain Reviews 5: 124–131
Spiegelmann R, Friedman WA 1991 Spinal cord stimulation: a contemporary series. Neurosurgery 28: 65–71
Stamford JA 1995 Descending control of pain. British Journal of Anaesthesia 75: 217–227
Stanton-Hicks M, Jänig W, Hassenbusch S et al 1995 Reflex sympathetic dystrophy: changing concepts and taxonomy. Pain 63: 127–133
Steude U, Abendroth D, Sunder-Plassmann L 1991 Epidural spinal

electrical stimulation in the treatment of severe arterial occlusive disease. Acta Neurochirurgica 52(suppl): 118–120
Stiller C-O, Linderoth B, O'Connor WT et al 1995 Repeated spinal cord stimulation decreases the extracellular level of gamma-aminobutyric acid in the periaqueductal gray matter of freely moving rats. Brain Research 699(2): 231–241
Stiller CO, Cui JG, O'Connor WT et al 1996 Release of gamma-aminobutyric acid in the dorsal horn and suppression of tactile allodynia by spinal cord stimulation in mononeuropathic rats. Neurosurgery 39(2): 367–375
Struijk JJ, Holsheimer J, Van der Heide GG, Boom HBK 1992 Recruitment of dorsal column fibers in spinal cord stimulation: influence of collateral branching. IEEE Transactions on Biomedical Engineering 39: 903–912
Struijk JJ, Holsheimer J, Boom HBK 1993a Excitation of dorsal root fibres in spinal cord stimulation; a theoretical study. IEEE Transactions on Biomedical Engineering 40: 632–639
Struijk JJ, Holsheimer J, Barolat G et al 1993b Paraesthesia thresholds in spinal cord stimulation: a comparison of theoretical results with clinical data. IEEE Transactions on Rehabilitation Engineering 1: 101–108
Sweet WH, Wepsic JG 1968 Treatment of chronic pain by stimulation of fibers of primary afferent neuron. Transactions of the American Neurological Association 93: 103–107
Sweet WH, Wepsic JG 1974 Stimulation of the posterior columns of the spinal cord for pain control: indications, technique and results. Clinical Neurosurgery 21: 278–310
Sylvén C 1997 Neurophysiological aspects of angina pectoris. Zeitschrift fur Kardiologie 86(suppl 1): 95–105
Tallis RC, Illis LS, Sedgwick EM et al 1983 Spinal cord stimulation in peripheral vascular disease. Journal of Neurology, Neurosurgery and Psychiatry 46: 478–484
Tasker RR, De Carvalho GTC, Dolan EJ 1992 Intractable pain of spinal cord origin: clinical features and implications for surgery. Journal of Neurosurgery 77: 373–378
Terenzi MG, Rees H, Roberts MHT 1992 The pontine parabrachial region mediates some of the descending inhibitory effects of stimulating the anterior pretectal nucleus. Brain Research 594: 205–214
Tesfaye S, Watt J, Benbow SJ et al 1996 Electrical spinal cord stimulation for painful diabetic peripheral neuropathy. Lancet 348: 1698–1701
Tsubokawa T, Katayama Y 1998 Motor cortex stimulation in persistent pain management. In: Gildenberg PL, Tasker RR (eds) Textbook of stereotactic and functional neurosurgery. McGraw-Hill, New York, p 1547
Tsubokawa T, Yamamoto T, Katayama Y et al 1984 Thalamic relay nucleus stimulation for relief of intractable pain. Clinical results and β-endorphin immunoreactivity in the cerebrospinal fluid. Pain 18: 115–126
Tsubokawa T, Katayama Y, Yamamoto T et al 1993 Chronic motor cortex stimulation in patients with thalamic pain. Journal of Neurosurgery 78: 393–401
Turner JA, Loeser JD, Bell KG 1995 Spinal cord stimulation for chronic low back pain: a systematic literature synthesis. Neurosurgery 37(6): 1088–1096
Urban BJ, Nashold BS 1978 Percutaneous epidural stimulation of the spinal cord for relief of pain. Journal of Neurosurgery 48: 323–328
Van de Kelft, De La Porte 1994 Long-term pain relief during spinal cord stimulation. The effect of patient selection. Quality of Life Research 3: 21–27
Veith FJ, Gupta SK, Samson RH et al 1981 Progress in limb salvage by reconstructive arterial surgery combined with new or improved adjunctive procedures. Annals of Surgery 194: 386–401
Veith FJ, Gupta SK, Wengerter KR et al 1990 Changing arteriosclerotic disease patterns and management strategies in lower limb threatening ischaemia. Annals of Surgery 212: 402–414
Veldman PHJM, Goris RJA 1996 Multiple reflex sympathetic dystrophy. Which patients are at risk for developing a recurrence of reflex sympathetic dystrophy in the same or another limb? Pain 64: 463–466
Vijayan R, Ahmad TS 1997 Late post dural puncture headache following implantation of a lumbar spinal cord stimulator. Pain Digest 7: 349–350
Vogel HP, Heppner B, Humbs N et al 1986 Long term effects of spinal cord stimulation in chronic pain syndromes. Journal of Neurology 233: 16–18
Waisbrod H, Gerbershagen HV 1985 Spinal cord stimulation in patients with a battered root syndrome. Archives of Orthopaedic and Trauma Surgery 104: 62–64
Wall PD, Sweet WH 1967 Temporary abolition of pain in man. Science 155: 108–109
Watson CPN 1990 Post herpetic neuralgia: clinical features and treatment. In: Fields HL (ed) Pain syndromes in neurology. Butterworth, London, p 233
Williams AC de C 1995 Pain measurement in chronic pain management. Pain Reviews 2: 39–63
Wilson DG, Rees H, Roberts MHT 1991 The antinociceptive effects of anterior pretectal stimulation in tests using thermal, mechanical and chemical noxious stimuli. Pain 44: 195–200
Woodforde JM, Merskey H 1972 Personality traits of patients with chronic pain. Journal of Psychosomatic Research 16: 167–172
Yaksh TL 1979 Direct evidence that spinal serotonin and noradrenaline terminals mediate the spinal antinociceptive effects of morphine in the periaqueductal gray. Brain Research 160: 180–185
Yamamoto T, Katayama Y, Hirayama T, Tsubokawa T 1997 Pharmacological classification of central post-stroke pain: comparison with the results of chronic motor cortex stimulation therapy. Pain 72: 5–12
Young RF 1978 Evaluation of dorsal column stimulation in the treatment of chronic pain. Neurosurgery 3: 373–379
Young RF 1989 Brain and spinal stimulation: how and to whom! Clinical Neurosurgery 35: 429–447
Young RF 1998 Deep brain stimulation for failed back surgery syndrome. In: Gildenberg PL, Tasker RR (eds) Textbook of stereotactic and functional neurosurgery. McGraw-Hill, New York, p 1621
Young RF, Chambi VI 1987 Pain relief by electrical stimulation of the periaqueductal and periventricular gray matter. Evidence for a non-opioid mechanism. Journal of Neurosurgery 66: 364–371
Young RF, Kroening R, Fulton W et al 1985 Electrical stimulation of the brain in treatment of chronic pain. Experience over 5 years. Journal of Neurosurgery 62: 389–396
Young RF, Tronnier V, Rinaldi PC 1992 Chronic stimulation of the Kölliker-Fuse nucleus region for relief of intractable pain in humans. Journal of Neurosurgery 76: 979–985
Young RF, Bach FW, Van Norman AS, Yaksh TL 1993 Release of β-endorphin and methionine-enkephalin into cerebrospinal fluid during deep brain stimulation for chronic pain. Effects of stimulation locus and site of sampling. Journal of Neurosurgery 79: 816–825

Ultrasound, shortwave, microwave, laser, superficial heat and cold in the treatment of pain

60

JUSTUS F. LEHMANN & BARBARA J. de LATEUR

SUMMARY

In this chapter on pain management, we discuss the use of common physical modalities to produce pain relief directly and indirectly. The modalities include cold application, heat, in the forms of radiant heat, ultrasound, shortwave diathermy, microwave and laser. To maximize the effectiveness of the modalities, it is important to understand how they work and when and how to use each technique properly.

INTRODUCTION

Heat and cold applications are commonly used as adjuncts to other therapy in order to relieve painful conditions which usually involve the musculoskeletal system. Both modalities may relieve pain through a 'counterirritant' effect. The application of heat and cold may also reduce pain by direct effects on peripheral nerve and free nerve endings.

REDUCTION OF PAIN BY RELIEVING PAINFUL CONDITIONS

Both heat and cold are commonly used to reduce painful muscle spasms secondary to underlying skeletal or neurological pathology. For example, painful muscle spasm is associated with low back pain of various causes such as degenerative joint disease or intervertebral disc disease, with or without resultant nerve root irritation. The physiological basis for the relief of the muscle spasm is incompletely understood. Mense (1978), who studied temperature effects on muscle spindles, found that in a prestretched preparation the rate of firing of the group Ia afferents was increased by warming and decreased by cooling. The secondary afferents responded in a more complex manner, generally contrary to the response of the Ia afferents. Those with a low background rate of firing ceased firing completely with a 2° elevation of temperature; those with a moderate background rate of firing began to decrease at 2° elevation and ceased altogether at 7° or 8° above resting temperature. Those with the highest rate of firing at resting temperature actually increased their firing rate with warming, but these fibres were few in number (and therefore do not contradict the general theory). Assuming that a secondary muscle spasm is to a large degree a tonic phenomenon, one could speculate that the selective cessation of firing from the secondary endings may reduce the muscle tone, an effect which may be supplemented by the increased firing from the Golgi tendon organs which, in turn, increase the inhibitory impulses. The temperatures that produced these effects were within the lower therapeutic range. At higher temperatures it could be shown that the spindle sensitivity dropped (Ottoson 1965).

When cold is applied to the spindle, it has been shown that the spindle response is reduced (Ottoson 1965). Eldred and associates (1960) cooled single spindles and found that the rate of discharge from the spindle followed the temperature curve precisely. They felt that this represented a direct effect on the sensory terminal while all the other neural elements within the muscle, such as the α motor neuron fibres, the γ fibres, the Ia afferents and the secondary afferents, the neuromuscular junction and the muscle fibre itself, require lower temperatures to be significantly affected by cooling than does the spindle itself (Lehmann & De Lateur 1990a,b). Consistent with these findings, Miglietta (1973) found that the spasticity and clonus in stroke patients disappeared only when the muscle itself was significantly cooled.

There is also evidence that skin heating may produce muscle relaxation. Stimulation of the skin in the neck region decreased γ fibre activity resulting in a decreased spindle excitability (Fischer & Solomon 1965). This may explain why superficial heating devices that primarily raise the skin temperature may also decrease muscle spasms.

Knutsson and Mattsson (1969) found a reduction of amplitude of the Achilles tendon reflex with local cold application. In some cases, they found an immediate temporary increase of the reflex muscle tone after cold application. The Hoffmann (H) response seemed to be enhanced in some and in other cases the increase was minimal and insignificant. They concluded that the initial increase in tone and H response may be the result of an increased excitability of the α motor neuron through stimulation of the exteroceptors of the skin. All cases ultimately showed a decline of the tendon jerk and reflex muscle tone, which they attributed to an effect of cold on the muscle and the peripheral nerve.

Hartviksen (1962) found a decrease of foot clonus in all his patients. At the moment the ice packs were applied, the spasticity increased temporarily. After 15–30 seconds, it decreased. The reduction of the clonus lasted 60–90 minutes. Hartviksen felt that spasticity disappeared while intramuscular temperature was still normal. The long-lasting effect was attributed by him to the lower intramuscular temperature, which probably affected the spindles.

Miglietta (1973) also found a decrease in clonus. He found an almost immediate decrease in the mechanically induced stretch response. However, clonus was unchanged in the majority of patients (80%) after 10 minutes of exposure and it was evident that clonus started to decrease and become absent only after the intramuscular temperature started to drop. He suggested that the relief of clonus in spasticity following local cold applications is not related to changes in the mechanical contraction of the muscle, but to a direct effect of cold on muscle spindle excitability.

Trnavsky (1983) found decreased muscle tone after cold application. Here, again, this occurred only when the local muscle temperature was reduced. It should be noted that both Knutsson and Mattsson and Hartviksen spot-measured the temperature only at one place in the musculature and had no data available as to whether, at the time of the earliest decreased reflex activity, another part of the muscle was already cooled.

Knutsson and Mattsson found an increased H response during the first minutes of cold application in most of the subjects, indicating a facilitation of the α motor neuron discharge. Urbscheit and Bishop (1970) also found an increase in the H response without a significant change of the Achilles tendon tap. Lightfoot et al (1975) applied cooling for 45 minutes and found no significant change in the H:M (direct muscle response) ratio. They concluded that, in addition to an effect on the spindle reducing the muscle tone, other factors were involved, including slowing of conduction in muscle or motor nerve fibres and prolonging of twitch contraction and half-relaxation time.

Bell and Lehmann (1987) measured skin and muscle temperature during cold application. The location of the temperature probe in the muscle was determined by soft tissue X-ray. They found an average decrease in skin temperature of 18.4°C and a reduction in muscle temperature of 12.1°C. Before, during and after cold application, they examined the H response by a series of recruitment curves and related the maximal H response to the M response with supramaximal stimulation. They found that in all 16 cases the amplitude of the maximal M response decreased significantly in response to cooling. These changes in the recording of the compound action potentials should be considered when cooling experiments result in alterations in H or electromyogram (EMG) response to tendon tap, since the changes in recording may affect all three potentials – the H response, the M response and the tendon tap EMG. When using the M response as a co-variant in this analysis, there were no significant changes in the H reflex amplitude. However, the tendon tap amplitude decreased significantly.

Thus, these findings do not support the claims that simple cooling facilitates the α motor neuron discharge measured by the H reflex. However, rubbing with ice may stimulate the mechanoreceptors. Hagbarth (1952) has clearly shown that this may lead to facilitation of muscle tone. The study by Bell and Lehmann (1987) confirms that the tendon tap reflex is decreased by muscle cooling.

The clinically effective use of ice application to the skin and some of the references cited suggest that, as long as the exteroceptors of the skin are stimulated, a facilitation of the α motor neuron discharge may occur. One may conclude that, to decrease muscle tone, i.e. spasticity, cooling should be applied in such a way that the muscle temperature is lowered. All authors agree that under those circumstances, reflex activity is diminished and the therapeutic effect on spasticity is achieved and maintained for a therapeutically adequate period of time.

Another condition that creates a great deal of discomfort to the patient is joint or 'morning' stiffness as it is encountered in collagen diseases, most commonly in rheumatoid arthritis. Wright and Johns (1960) and Bäcklund and Tiselius (1967) showed that the complaint correlated closely with physical measurements of the viscoelastic

 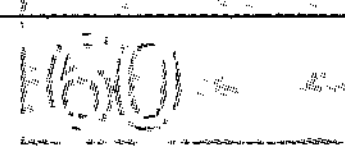

properties of the joints. Specifically they measured maximal elasticity in extension and flexion, as well as resistance to motion due to viscous properties and to friction. There was a 20% decrease in stiffness at 45°C as compared with 33°C when a superficial joint was treated with infrared radiation (Wright & Johns 1961).

A well-documented physiological response to heat application is the increase in blood flow with a corresponding decrease when cold is applied. In an active organ, local temperature elevation will lead to a marked increase in blood flow (Guy et al 1974, Lehmann et al 1979, Sekins et al 1980, 1984, Lehmann & De Lateur 1990b). Reflexly induced changes usually consist of an increase in blood flow to the skin and superficial tissues and a decrease in blood flow to an inactive organ. Thus, when heat is applied to the skin, blood flow to the underlying musculature will be reduced. When the skin is heated, blood flow to the skin is increased not only in the area heated but also in other areas of the skin which are not heated (consensual reaction; Fischer & Solomon 1965). On the other hand, cooling produces vasoconstriction. Vasodilatation in response to cold – the 'hunting reaction' – occurs only if the temperatures are low enough to be potentially destructive to the tissues. The increase in vascularity and blood flow due to heating may play a role in obtaining relief from painful conditions such as myofibrositis or fibrositis, a poorly defined syndrome which responds to heating the tender muscular nodes. In the same fashion a resolution of painful inflammatory reaction may be achieved.

Pain in trauma, as it is commonly encountered in sports injuries, can be alleviated and to a degree prevented by early cold application, often in combination with application of pressure, for instance via an elastic bandage. In these cases cold reduces not only pain perception but also bleeding and oedema formation as a result of vasoconstriction (Nilsson 1983, Derscheid & Brown 1985, Kay 1985). At a later date, heat application with vasodilatation may help with the healing and haematoma resolution (Perkins et al 1948, Clarke et al 1958, Schmidt et al 1979, Lehmann et al 1983, Lehmann & De Lateur 1990b).

Heat and cold applications to the skin of the abdominal wall have a profound effect on pain resulting from spasm of the smooth musculature in the gastrointestinal tract or in the uterus. This pain is commonly associated with gastrointestinal upset resulting from viral enteritis of dietary indiscretion or with menstrual cramps. It has been shown (Bisgard & Nye 1940, Molander 1941, Fischer & Solomon 1965) that there is a marked reduction of peristalsis of the gastrointestinal tract with heat application and an increase of the peristalsis with cold application. This is associated with a decrease in acid production of the stomach and blanching of the mucous membrane when heat is applied to the abdominal skin. Acid production and blood flow to the mucous membrane are increased with cold application.

'COUNTERIRRITANT' EFFECTS

Parsons and Goetzl (1945) showed that cold applied with ethyl chloride spray for 20 seconds to the skin covering the tibia increased the pain threshold of the tooth pulp as measured by electrical stimulation. Similarly, Melzack et al (1980a) reduced dental pain by ice massage applied to the web of the thumb and index finger of the hand on the same side as the painful region. Melzack et al (1980b) also showed that ice massage and transcutaneous electrical stimulation are equally effective in relieving low back pain. Murray and Weaver (1975) showed that counterirritation (consisting of 10-second immersion of the finger into a 2°C water bath) reduced itching significantly more than a control procedure. Melzack et al (1980a) suggested that the observations could be explained on the basis of the gate theory (Melzack & Wall 1965). Studies of morphine receptors in the central nervous system and of the role of enkephalins and endorphins (Field & Basbaum 1978) suggested that this mechanism could play a role in explaining the counterirritant effect, especially when the stimulus is applied distant from the site of the pain-producing process (Kerr & Casey 1976). Gammon and Starr (1941) also showed that heat producing a significant temperature elevation resulted in the same analgesic effect as cold application. The effects produced by this mechanism seem to be of the same order of magnitude as those obtained by transcutaneous electrical nerve stimulation (Melzack et al 1980b).

Benson and Copp (1974) found that heat and cold both raised the normal pain threshold significantly. Ice therapy was more effective than heat but following either form of treatment, the effect declined within 30 minutes.

EFFECTS ON NERVE AND NERVE ENDINGS

Douglas and Malcolm (1955), in experiments with cats, studied the differential effect of cold on fibres of various diameters. Small medullated fibres were affected first, then the large medullated fibres and finally the unmedullated fibres. In man (Ganong 1979), pain impulses are carried in part by the small medullated Aδ fibres. Unfortunately, data like these are somewhat species dependent and generalization can only be tentative. However, it has been shown by Goodgold and Eberstein (1977) and De Jong et al (1966) that, in general, nerve conduction drops with decreasing temperature and that finally (Li 1958) nerve fibres cease conducting. Therefore, it can be assumed that pain sensation may be markedly reduced by significant local cooling through an indirect effect on nerve fibres and free endings. There is also evidence that heat applied to the peripheral nerve or free nerve endings reduces pain sensation (Lehmann et al 1958). The pain threshold was measured with the Hardy–Wolff–Goodell method (Hardy et al 1940) before and after heat application to the ulnar nerve and to the pad of the little finger. However, a counterirritant effect could not absolutely be ruled out in these experiments.

In a study by Barker et al (1991), administration of cold saline prior to injection of propofol (2,6-di-isopropylphenol) anaesthetic increased the amount of pain relief obtained as compared with propofol injection alone. Recently, it has been shown (Hong 1991) that ultrasound therapy with therapeutic dosage may cause a reversible nerve conduction block and pain relief in patients with polyneuropathy.

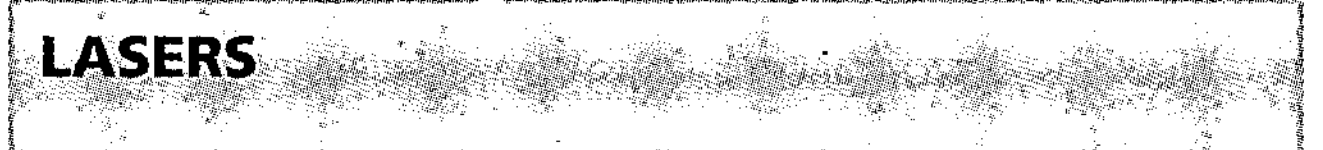

LASERS

While lasers have many characteristics in common with diffuse light, the main difference between laser and diffuse light is that the laser is a collimated beam of photons of the same frequency with the waves in phase. In therapy, except for surgical purposes, lower level intensities are used. Unfortunately, most studies on the use of laser for the relief of pain in various conditions do not have suitable controls. Therefore the results are equivocal and the effectiveness of lasers in treatment of painful syndromes is not well documented. Devor, in an editorial in *Pain* (1990), commented upon four papers published in the same edition which showed a lack of a specific effect of laser therapy upon pain. Devor's commentary could be summarized by saying that the apparent relief in open or uncontrollable studies is largely due to a placebo effect. Hall et al (1994) found low-level laser therapy ineffective in improving pain or range of motion in rheumatoid arthritis of finger joints. Basford (1995) reviewed low-intensity laser therapy as a clinical tool. He found that it was not well established as a useful tool in treatment of pain in various conditions. The results of laser therapy in conditions such as rotator cuff tendinitis, rheumatoid arthritis, neurological conditions, wound healing, low back pain, patellofemoral pain, lateral epicondylitis (tennis elbow) and trigger points were all reviewed. Basford concluded that the utility remains unestablished. Where well-controlled studies have been done, they have usually failed to show benefit.

Hansen and Thoroe (1990) treated chronic orofacial pain in 40 patients in a controlled study. They did not find any statistically significant difference in the analgesic effect between the groups treated with laser and with placebo, although they found a substantial placebo response in both groups.

On the other hand, Gerschman et al (1994) conducted a comparative double-blind study testing low-level laser therapy (gallium/aluminium/arsenic) against placebo in the management of dentinal tooth hypersensitivity. The mean value of thermal sensitivity decreased 67% ($P<0.001$) compared with placebo (17%) and tactile sensitivity decreased 65% ($P=.002$) compared with placebo at 8 weeks.

Goldman et al (1980) treated 30 patients with rheumatoid arthritis with the neodymium laser at a wavelength of 1060 nanometres (nm) with output of 15 joules per square centimetre and a pulse duration of 30 nanoseconds. The duration of the laser exposure was not stated. One hand was treated at the proximal interphalangeal and metacarpophalangeal joints, whereas the other hand received a sham exposure. They found improvement in both hands. However, the hand that had laser treatment had a greater improvement in erythema and pain. On the other hand, laboratory data, which included the titre of rheumatoid arthritis, antinuclear antibody or polyethylene glycol precipitates, showed no change. No controls were used. On physical examination the lateral pinch was the same for treated and untreated hands as well as range of motion of the joints. However, over time a difference was found in both treated and untreated hands with regard to grasp strength. The increase was greater on the treated side.

In a study by Bliddal et al (1987), nine treatments with helium-neon laser, 6 joules per square centimetre, were given in a double-blind study to the hands of patients with rheumatoid arthritis. One hand was irradiated with laser, the other with a sham exposure. The laser therapy gave some pain relief, but no difference in morning stiffness or joint performance was obtained.

Basford et al (1987) carried out a randomized, controlled, double-blind study of the effects of low-energy 0.9 mW helium-neon laser treatment of osteoarthritis of the thumb. Eighty-one subjects were studied: 47 were treated and 34 served as controls. Subjectively, a slight but significant decrease in tenderness was noted in the laser-treated group. However, all objective measures such as grip strength and range of motion showed no significant difference between the control group and the treated group. The authors concluded that this treatment was safe but ineffective for osteoarthritis of the thumb.

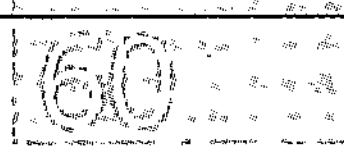

Waylonis et al (1988) treated chronic myofascial pain with low-output helium-neon laser. They found no statistical difference between treatment and placebo groups. They treated 62 patients by using acupuncture points and clinical response was assessed using a portion of the McGill Pain Questionnaire. In contrast, Ceccherelli et al (1989) used laser for the treatment of 37 women with muscular neck pain. Differences between the treated and the control group were statistically significant.

Walker (1983) used a low-power, 1 mW helium-neon laser over various peripheral nerves, such as the radial, median and saphenous nerves, in the treatment of pain syndromes. Pain relief occurred only when the appropriate peripheral nerve was treated. When patients with trigeminal neuralgia, postherpetic pain, sciatica and osteoarthritis were treated, 19 of 26 had relief of pain without medication whereas those who received sham stimulation reported no improvement of pain. Similarly, Iijima et al (1989), in an uncontrolled study, reported that laser treatment produced relief of postherpetic pain.

Walker et al (1988) also used the helium-neon laser (1 mW 20 Hz) to treat trigeminal neuralgia. Control subjects received placebo treatment. The experimental group contained 18 patients and the control group 17. Assignment to the experimental or control group was on a random basis. Pain was assessed subjectively on a scale from 0 to 100. The results suggested improvement with the laser therapy.

Laser has also been used in the treatment of epicondylitis (tennis elbow). Lundeberg et al (1987a) compared the pain-relieving effect of laser treatment versus placebo in tennis elbow. The results showed that laser treatment is not significantly better than placebo. Similarly, in a study by Siebert et al (1987), the efficacy of helium-neon laser and gallium-aluminium-arsenic lasers in treatment of tendinopathies was compared with placebo in a double-blind controlled study. No therapeutic effect was found.

Lundeberg et al (1987b) also compared the pain-relieving effect of laser treatment and acupuncture. They found that neither neon-helium nor gallium-arsenide low-power irradiation produced any change in response. The study was performed in 36 male white rats; 12 of them served as a control group. An antinociceptive effect was assessed using the tail-flick test and compared with the mean prolongation of the response time in intact rats, compared with the responses of rats who had acupuncture, one of the two lasers or morphine. Lasers did not produce any changes compared to the control group, whereas acupuncture and morphine did.

Haker and Lundeberg (1990) applied laser treatment, in a double-blind study, to acupuncture points in lateral humeral epicondylalgia. No significant differences were observed between laser and the placebo groups in relation to the subjective and objective outcome after 10 treatments. These authors used a wavelength of 904 nm, a mean power output of 12 mW with a peak value of 8.3 W and a pulse frequency of 70 Hz. In a further study on the effect of laser in lateral epicondylalgia, Haker and Lundeberg (1991a) used a wavelength of 904 nm, output of 12 mW with a frequency of 70 Hz and a pulse train of 8000 Hz. They assigned 49 patients consecutively to a control group or to a laser treatment group; they concluded that laser may be a valuable therapy but that further studies will be necessary.

Haker and Lundeberg (1991b) also compared the effectiveness of application of laser, using specific stimulation parameters, to acupuncture points in the treatment of lateral epicondylalgia. They used a gallium-arsenide and helium-neon laser. The combined application was compared with red-light application in a control group of patients. Fifty-eight patients were consecutively assigned to the laser and placebo groups. There was no statistical difference in the outcome between the two treatments using objective and subjective measures.

Klein and Eck (1990) studied the effects of low-energy laser treatment and exercise for low back pain in a controlled trial. They found that exercise had an effect on pain, but there was no significant difference between the group that received laser and exercise and the one that received exercise only.

Fulga et al (1994) noted a gradual diminution in pain of the knee, ankle, shoulder and back associated with laser therapy (940–980 nm and 50 mW) in 36 patients unresponsive to, or with contraindications for, non-steroidal anti-inflammatory therapy. Unfortunately, the study was uncontrolled. In contrast, Johannsen et al (1994) studied low-level laser on rheumatoid arthritis. The study was double blind and placebo controlled. A significant decrease in pain was found. However, assessment of grip strength, morning stiffness, flexibility, ESR (erythrocyte sedimentation rate), and C-reactive protein showed no change.

Helium-neon laser has been used in dentistry to prevent pain and swelling after tooth extraction. Taube et al (1990) found no difference in postoperative swelling and pain relief between the test and the control groups. Carrillo et al (1990), on the other hand, found in a controlled study of patients treated with helium-neon laser, ibuprofen or placebo that trismus was significantly reduced in the helium-neon laser and the ibuprofen-treated groups compared with the placebo group. Pain, however, was significantly less only with the ibuprofen group. Swelling was the same in all groups.

Lim et al (1995) found some relief of orthodontic postadjustment pain with low-level laser, but the pre–post changes were not significant. Lowe et al (1997) failed to demonstrate any improvement in ischaemic pain of the forearm with low-level laser (830 nm) applied to Erb's point. A similar result was obtained by Moktar et al (1995).

Reid et al (1995) used flashlamp-excited dye laser (585 nm) for therapy of medically non-responsive, ideopathic vulvodynia. The first manoeuvre of the study was to selectively photocoagulate symptomatic subepithelial blood vessels, since laser at 585 nm is selectively absorbed by oxyhaemoglobin. The second manoeuvre was the microsurgical removal of chronically painful Bartholin's glands. Overall favourable response rates were 92.5%, with lower response in those women in whom pressure applied to the region of Bartholin's glands produced lancinating pain. Response in the latter group was improved by surgical excision. The authors concluded that laser therapy was safe, efficacious and relatively non-invasive and could reduce the need for surgery in most patients with idiopathic vulvodynia.

In summary, laser may be useful for pain relief, but more controlled studies which give the specific parameters of the laser application will be necessary to assess the efficacy of this new modality. Further studies are also required to understand the mechanism of interaction with biological tissues under therapeutic conditions.

DIFFERENCES IN THE EFFECTS OF HEAT AND COLD APPLICATION

A review of the literature reveals that the effect of heat and cold may be similar in many cases. In others, cold produces effects in the opposite direction of heat. Both heat and cold reduce muscle spasm secondary to underlying joint and skeletal pathology and nerve root irritation, as in low back syndromes, and therefore relieve the associated pain. A vicious cycle consisting of muscle spasm, ischaemia, pain and more muscle spasm is interrupted. In the case of upper motor neuron lesions with painful spasticity, the effect of heat is short-lived because the temperature in the muscle is rapidly restored to its pretreatment level by the increase in blood flow. If the reduction in spasticity with reduction in pain relief is produced by muscle cooling, this effect lasts much longer. Rewarming from the outside is slow because of the insulating subcutaneous fat layer and rewarming from the inside is retarded because of the vasoconstriction in the muscle. However, neither heat nor cold has a permanent effect on spasticity.

In the presence of an acute deep-seated inflammatory reaction, vigorous heat application is contraindicated. It usually increases hyperaemia and oedema with pain and acceleration of abscess formation. This does not contradict the fact that such heat application is used in superficial boils to bring the abscess to a head with subsequent easy evacuation. Mild heat application is used in superficial thrombophlebitis. In contrast to the effects of heat, in an inflammatory reaction it is generally agreed that cold may reduce oedema, hyperaemia and pain.

In acute rheumatoid arthritis, vigorous deep heat application is likely to aggravate the pain and discomfort. On the other hand, painful joint stiffness is measurably improved by heat and aggravated by cold application (Wright & Johns 1960, 1961, Bäcklund & Tiselius 1967). However, an intensive cooling may numb pain in spite of the increase in stiffness. In acute trauma with aggravation of pain resulting from oedema and bleeding, cold application will reduce both because of vasoconstriction. Heat will increase both oedema and bleeding tendency.

A review by Chapman (1991) cites several studies showing that heat and cold were each effective in relieving pain in conditions such as frozen shoulder, chronic low back pain and rheumatoid arthritic knees and shoulders. In contrast, Finan et al (1993) studied the effect of cold therapy on postoperative pain in gynaecologic patients in a randomized prospective study and concluded that cold pack application does not improve postoperative pain.

THE USE OF HEAT FOR PAIN RELIEF

DOSIMETRY AND TECHNIQUE OF HEAT APPLICATION

The physiological effects which produce pain relief when heat is applied may be achieved by direct effects of the temperature elevation on the tissue and cellular functions. They may also be achieved through local reflexes with the reaction occurring at the site of the tissue temperature elevation. However, the type and extent of the reaction may depend largely on whether the site of the pain-producing pathology is heated or whether one relies on distant heating and on effects produced by reflex or other neuromechanisms.

Local heating

Local temperature elevation at the site of the pathology can produce a large number of different responses, including changes in neuromuscular activity, blood flow, capillary permeability, enzymatic activity and pain threshold. These reactions can be produced to varying degrees depending on the condition of heating. Thus vigorous local responses may be produced.

Distant heating

If the site of temperature elevation is distant from the painful pathology to be treated, only a limited number of physiological responses, reflexogenic in nature, can be obtained at the site of the pathology. These reactions are always milder than those produced locally at the site of the temperature elevation. These distant reactions include blood flow changes in skin and in the mucous membranes of the gastrointestinal tract; reflexogenic changes in muscle activity, relaxation of both voluntary striated muscle and smooth muscle of the gastrointestinal tract and uterus; and reflex reduction of gastric acidity. In conclusion, when vigorous responses are desired, local heat is strongly preferred. The factors which determine the intensity of the physiological reaction locally are, firstly, the level of tissue temperature elevation (approximately 40–45°C) and secondly, the duration of tissue temperature elevation (5–30 min).

Mild versus vigorous effects

In order to obtain vigorous responses to heat therapy, it is necessary to attain the highest temperature at the site of the tissue pathology to be treated and to elevate this temperature close to the maximally tolerated level. Dosimetry and proper technique of application of the modalities are essential, since the therapeutic range for a given effect extends only over a few degrees. If a mild, limited response is desired, one can select a modality which produces the highest temperature at the site of the pathology, but then limit the output of the modality so that only a moderate temperature rise occurs; this in turn produces a mild effect. The alternative to this procedure is to heat the superficial tissues and rely on mild limited reflexogenic responses at the site of the pathology in the depth of the tissues.

Selection of modality according to temperature distribution

From this it becomes apparent that if vigorous heating is indicated, one must select that type of heating modality which produces the highest temperature in the distribution at the site of the treatable pathology. Since the temperature at this site is brought to tolerance level, this method avoids burns elsewhere. This represents the rationale for the various deep-heating devices: shortwave diathermy, a high-frequency electromagnetic current operating at the frequency of 27.12 megahertz (MHz); microwaves, an electromagnetic radiation of the frequency of 2456 and 915 MHz; and ultrasound, a high-frequency acoustic vibration at a frequency of 0.8–1.0 MHz. The approach to using these modalities primarily as deep heating agents is justified in the light of overwhelming experimental evidence that most of the therapeutically desirable effects are due to heating and not due to non-thermal reactions (Lehmann & De Lateur 1982, 1990a,b, Kramer 1985). It is conceivable that some non-thermal effects may play a role in the outcome. It has been documented, however, that some undesirable side effects are clearly due to non-thermal mechanisms and should be avoided (Lehmann & De Lateur 1982, 1990a,b). The superficial heating agents such as hot packs, paraffin bath, Fluidotherapy, hydrotherapy and radiant heat will produce temperature distributions similar to one another, with the highest temperature in the most superficial tissues. Some of these modalities have non-thermal effects of therapeutic advantage; for instance, hydrotherapy allows exercise of painful joints with reduced stress because the buoyancy of the water reduces the gravitational forces. Also, the cleansing action of a whirlpool bath can be beneficial in wound treatments and the drying action of radiant heat may be desirable in weeping lesions.

In order to select the appropriate modality for a given site of a treatable pathology, one must take into account the propagation and absorption characteristics of the tissues for each form of energy used for heating. In general, one can state that skin and superficial subcutaneous tissues are selectively heated by infrared, visible light, hot packs, paraffin bath, Fluidotherapy and hydrotherapy. Subcutaneous tissues and superficial musculature are selectively heated by shortwave diathermy with condenser application and by microwaves at a frequency of 2456 MHz. Superficial musculature is heated preferentially by shortwave diathermy using induction coil applicators. Deep-seated joints and fibrous scars within soft tissues are selectively heated by ultrasound, as are myofascial interfaces, tendon and tendon sheath and nerve trunks. Pelvic organs are selectively heated by shortwave diathermy using internal vaginal or rectal electrodes.

In addition, it is most important to realize that the desirable temperature distribution can be achieved only if proper technique of application and proper dosimetry are used. Nykanen (1995) used ultrasound in the treatment of painful shoulders of various aetiologies. Thirty-five subjects were treated with pulsed ultrasound 1.0 W/cm^2 intensity in a 1:4 on–off ratio and 37 were treated with ultrasound placebo in this 'double-blind' study, which also used massage and group gymnastics aimed at improving range of motion. No benefit was found by adding the ultrasound. Unfortunately, the *average* intensity of the ultrasound was so low (0.2 W/cm^2) that no therapeutic benefit could have been anticipated. The use of a randomized, double-blind design does not, in and of itself, ensure a valid study if the dosage of the intervention is not appropriate. Also, it is difficult to blind the subject to ultrasound usage if the intensity is appropriate, since the ultrasound will be perceived (although the evaluator could be blinded). Several of these modalities are very powerful and, if inappropriately used, can do severe tissue damage in a short period of time. Details of the techniques of application are beyond the scope of this chapter. The reader is referred to Lehmann and De Lateur (1990b).

Non-thermal effects of the diathermy modalities, i.e. shortwave, microwave and ultrasound, have been well documented (Lehmann & De Lateur 1990a,b,c). However, none of them is essential for therapeutic effectiveness. Some non-thermal effects may represent potential hazards; however, few of them have been documented as being destructive. These can be avoided by use of proper equipment and proper technique of application. In shortwave diathermy, among others, pearl-chain formation of blood corpuscles has been documented without any relation to physiological effects (Herrick et al 1950, Herrick & Krusen 1953, Texeira-Pinto et al 1960). Possible non-thermal changes of macromolecules were reported by Bach (1965), Bach et al (1960) and Heller (1960), who exposed human gammaglobulin to radiofrequency and microwave energy. However, such changes were not observed at therapeutic frequencies. Pearl-chain formation can also be produced by microwave application (Saito & Schwan 1961, Lehmann & De Lateur 1990c). In microwaves, the controversy involves safety standards and inadvertent exposure of sensitive organs. Physiological and hazardous responses claimed at low intensities below 10 mW/cm^2 are not well documented (Michaelson 1972, 1990, Lehmann 1990b), whereas thermal damage at intensities above 100 mW/cm^2 is clearly established. Specifically sensitive areas include the eye, the lens, the testicles and the brain. With ultrasound it is important to avoid the occurrence of gaseous cavitation, which occurs more readily in media with low volume percentage of cells and low viscosity. Such media are found in the eye and also include amniotic fluid, cerebrospinal fluid and joint effusions. Under therapeutic conditions the occurrence is avoided by using adequate equipment with adequate uniformity in the spatial and temporal distribution of the intensity of the beam. Aggregation of platelets and accumulation of red cells in wave nodes can be avoided by using a stroking technique of application. While some other-than-thermal mechanism, such as acceleration of diffusion processes, may be produced by ultrasound and may be therapeutically helpful, the importance of this has not been clearly documented.

TECHNIQUES OF COLD APPLICATION

Melting ice, together with water, is commonly used for cryotherapy since it ensures a steady temperature of 0°C. Most commonly, a rubber bag containing ice cubes with water is applied as a compress. A layer of terry cloth between the ice bag and the skin may slow down cooling. Other methods use terry cloth dipped into a mixture of ice shavings with water. The cloth is wrung out and then applied to the body part. This application has to be repeated frequently. Finally, a part may be treated by immersion in ice water; this, however, is a potentially more dangerous method because of the possible development of necrosis of fingers or toes. If the objective is to cool musculature to relieve muscle spasm or spasticity, it is necessary to apply the ice for a significant period of time. Even in a relatively slender individual with a subcutaneous fat layer of less than 1 cm, more than 10 minutes of ice application is necessary to achieve significant cooling of the underlying musculature. In many cases 20–30 minutes may be necessary to achieve the desired result, which can be gauged by clinical observation of the resolution of the muscle spasm, the reduction of spasticity, clonus and the spindle reflexes (Bierman & Friedlander 1940, Hartviksen 1962).

Ice massage, in which a block of ice is rubbed over the skin surface, is also used for the same purpose. However, it must be remembered that short-term ice massage is more likely just to cool the skin and therefore facilitate α motor neuron discharge with subsequent increase in muscle tone, as documented by Hartviksen (1962).

Evaporative cooling with ethyl chloride spray is done by spraying the skin from a distance of about 1 metre with a stroking motion. Bierman (1955) suggested a movement of the spray of 4 inches/second. Each area should be exposed only for a few seconds, followed by a pause. More recently, chlorofluoromethanes have been used since they are less flammable than ethyl chloride (Traherne 1962). This method is more frequently used as a 'counterirritant'. It is doubtful whether it is suitable for cooling a large muscle covered by a significant fat layer.

 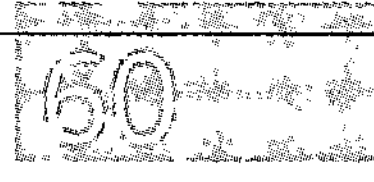

COMMON THERAPEUTIC APPLICATIONS OF HEAT AND COLD FOR PAIN RELIEF

It is essential for successful therapeutic application of heat and cold that the correct diagnosis be made first. The local condition to be treated is assessed and a judgement is made as to whether or not it is treatable with heat or cold. The location of the pathological process is clearly identified and correspondingly the proper modality is selected. It is equally important that the application should be done with appropriate technique. Painful skeletal muscle spasms, which frequently occur in the back as a result of nerve root irritation or spinal pathology, may be successfully treated with heat or cold to achieve muscle relaxation and thus abolition of pain. Shortwave diathermy may be applied with either induction coil applicators or condenser pads. Treatment should occur once or twice daily for 20–30 minutes. Relaxation may be achieved by direct muscle heating and an effect on the spindle mechanism as well as reflexly by surface heating. Microwave direct contact applicators can be used for this purpose. Also helpful are superficial heating agents, including hot packs such as Hydrocollator packs or radiant heat with heat lamp or cradle. Treatment should be for 20–30 minutes. In this case, reflexogenic relaxation is achieved.

As an alternative mode of treatment, ice pack or ice massage may be applied so as to cool the muscle and thus reduce spindle sensitivity. Therefore, applications for a minimum of 10 minutes (although 20 minutes would be better) would be required. Landen (1967) showed in 117 patients with back pain that heat and cold applications were equally effective. In acute conditions heat was found to reduce hospital stay more effectively than ice applications, while in chronic conditions, ice was more effective than heat application. All these treatments are for symptomatic relief and produce their effects by reduction of the painful muscle spasm.

In myofibrositis in the presence of so-called trigger points, both cold application, often with ethyl chloride spray, and local application of heat have been used successfully. Ultrasound in low or medium dose applied to the painful area has also been found to be effective. In this condition heat application is often followed by deep sedative massage. In cases of mild fibrositis more vigorous friction massage may also be used.

In tension states with increased EMG activity, discomfort can be relieved by heat application; commonly shortwave or superficial heat are used. These forms of heat application are often followed by deep sedative massage. This treatment is usually combined with relaxation training with biofeedback to reduce the muscle tension. In any one of these conditions, but specifically in myofibrositis, there is also evidence that these modalities represent a 'counterirritant' and reduce pain as explained on the basis of the gate theory (Parsons & Goetzl 1945, Melzack & Wall 1965).

In gastrointestinal upset, cramping of the smooth musculature of the tract produces pain. The peristalsis and discomfort can be reduced by superficial heat application to the abdomen in the form of hot packs (Bisgard & Nye 1940, Molander 1941, Fischer & Solomon 1965). This reduction of cramps is associated with reduction of blood flow to the mucous membranes and hydrochloric acid secretion in the stomach. Cold application aggravates the discomfort. Menstrual cramps seem to respond in the same fashion.

In persons with Raynaud's phenomenon, Delp and Newton (1986) assessed hand function after cold stress. Both two-point discrimination and finger dexterity were assessed. The results showed a decreased performance on the Purdue pegboard test and decreased two-point discrimination after cold application. Similar findings were observed in a normal control group.

The common complaint of joint stiffness and pain in rheumatic diseases such as rheumatoid arthritis is alleviated measurably by heat application (Wright & Johns 1960, 1961, Johns & Wright 1962, Bäcklund & Tiselius 1967). Cold application aggravates the objective signs. Clinically, superficial heat such as radiant heat and a hot tub bath is commonly used for this purpose. Also, the secondary muscle spasms can be treated in this fashion. Modalities which selectively heat the joints, such as ultrasound, are not used in this condition because the vigorous heating of the inflamed synovium may produce exacerbation. The whirlpool bath or the dip method of paraffin may be used for mild heating of hands and feet. If the Hubbard tank is used, exercise of the joints can occur at the same time with elimination of the force of gravity by buoyancy. Furthermore, contrast baths, according to Martin et al (1946), may be used to relieve stiffness.

Contrast baths are often recommended for the treatment of stiffness associated with Heberden's nodes. If many joints of the upper and lower extremity are involved in the rheumatic process, radiant heat applied with a double baker is a method of heat application. It has been suggested that ice should be used to numb the pain of the joint and this application has been advocated on the basis that Harris and McCroskery (1974) found that the activity of destructive enzymes such as collagenase is reduced at lower temperatures. These same experiments have been quoted to indicate that heating of the joint itself is contraindicated. This conclusion exceeds the parameters of the experiment, which investigated the effects on the collagenase of temperatures only up to 36°C whereas therapeutic temperatures reach or exceed 43°C. At these therapeutic temperatures other enzyme systems have shown a markedly reduced activity (Harris & Krane 1973, Harris & McCroskery 1974).

Joint contractures due to capsular tightness or synovial scarring are frequently painful when mobilized by range of motion exercises and stretch. The effectiveness of the treatment can be increased and the associated pain markedly reduced by using ultrasound in high dosage which has been shown selectively to raise the temperature in the tight structures which in turn show an increase in extensibility, rendering the treatment programme less painful and more effective (De Preux 1952, Friedland 1975). Depending on the soft tissue covering of the joint, ultrasound applied with the multiple field method is used at intensities between 2 and 4 W/cm² with a total output between 20 and 40 W. The application is with a stroking technique.

In acute calcific bursitis of the subdeltoid and subacromial bursae, the acute pain is due to swelling and pressure within the content of the bursa resulting in an inflammatory reaction. Ice application may alleviate the acute pain, especially if used in conjunction with removal of bursal content and hydrocortisone injection combined with local anaesthetic. At the later stage, the limitation of the range of motion of the shoulder joint, which is frequently associated with calcific tendinitis, should be appropriately treated with ultrasound in combination with range of motion exercises and stretch (Lehmann & De Lateur 1990b).

In the shoulder-hand syndrome or reflex sympathetic dystrophy, superficial heat and ultrasound treatment in combination with a programme to increase range of motion may be used as an adjunct to other therapy, including stellate ganglion block.

In painful lateral epicondylitis or 'tennis elbow', the primary treatment should consist of rest, splinting, ice application and possibly also an injection of hydrocortisone and local anaesthetic. During the later stage of resolution, superficial heat may be used. Also, ultrasound in low dosage to produce mild effects could be used at this stage since ultrasound selectively raises the temperature at the common tendon of origin and the extensor aponeurosis. The dosage should be approximately 0.5 W/cm². Binder et al (1985) treated 76 patients with lateral epicondylitis. The patients were randomly allocated to groups such that 38 received ultrasound and 38 received placebo treatment. A total of 63% of the patients treated with ultrasound were improved, compared with 29% of those given placebo treatment.

Steinberg and Callies (1992) treated epicondylitis with ultrasound and with ultrasound in combination with prednisolone ointment (phonophoresis). They found that ultrasound significantly reduced the pain. However, there was no difference between the ultrasound application alone or with phonophoresis; Haker and Lundeberg (1991c) did not find pulsed application of ultrasound effective in this condition.

Jan and Lai (1991) treated 94 knees in female patients with osteoarthritis of the knees. They randomly assigned subjects to one of four groups:

Group 1: ultrasound Group 2: shortwave diathermy Group 3: ultrasound and exercise Group 4: shortwave diathermy and exercise.

Treatment was assessed by measuring functional capacity and peak torque. Pain was noted during functional capacity assessment. Statistical tools included multiple regression analysis as well as analysis of variance (ANOVA). The authors reported a decrease in functional incapacity (that is, increased functional capacity) in all four groups. The torque increased also. More improvement was obtained when exercise was added to the ultrasound or shortwave. There was no significant difference between the shortwave or ultrasound.

In a retrospective analysis of medical records of acute surgical trauma patients, Schaubel (1946) found that cold application reduced the need for recasting due to swelling from 42.3% to only 5.3% of the cases. Also, he found a marked reduction in the requirement for narcotics for pain relief. Cohen et al (1989) found that cooling after surgical repair of the anterior cruciate ligament reduced the need for pain medication. Seino et al (1985) used an intercostal nerve probe to produce cryoanalgesia – a nerve-freezing technique – to control pain after thoracotomy. The cryoanalgesia group had lower postoperative pain scores and required less than half the analgesia compared with the control group. Scarcella and Cohn (1995) assessed the effect of cold (50°F) versus normal temperature (70°F) in total hip arthroplasty (THA) and total knee arthroplasty (TKA). The shortening of hospital stay of 1.4 days for cold-treated THA patients was significant ($P = 0.03$) but the 1.5 day shortening of the cold-treated TKA group was not ($P = 0.19$). However, cold-treated TKA patients did achieve independent ambulation one day sooner, not quite achieving statistical significance ($P = 0.08$). Cold-treated patients did not differ significantly in narcotic use, postoperative range of motion (ROM) or rate of progression of ROM.

Moore and Cardea (1977) found that the combination of intermittent pressure and ice application promptly reduced the compartmental pressures in the calf which were markedly increased as a result of tibial and fibular fractures but Matsen et al (1975) found in animal experiments that swelling after fracture was not reduced and perhaps even increased when cold was applied. In the case of minor sports injuries, cryotherapy in combination with compression, for instance using an elastic bandage, is usually used (Basur et al 1976). Also, elevation of the limb and immobilization are recommended. It must be remembered, however, that ice should be applied just long enough to prevent swelling and bleeding since prolonged ice application may unnecessarily retard healing (Vinger & Hoerner 1981). At a later date resolution can be assisted by heat application. In superficial thrombophlebitis, one adjunct of therapy may be application of moist hot packs or the heat cradle to reduce discomfort.

Painful amputation neuromas can be treated successfully with ultrasound, provided that the origin of pain is local, for instance due to adhesions and irritation of the neuroma and not phantom limb pain of other origin. Ultrasound selectively raises the temperature of the neuroma and is given in high dosage, which is probably destructive to the nerve fibres. The alternative to conservative treatment is the surgical revision of the stump. It is clinically suggested that postherpetic pain can be treated on the same basis. This indication is based purely on clinical (that is, empirical) evidence. In other conditions, Balogun and Okonofua (1988) reported successful use of shortwave diathermy applied to the pelvic organs in chronic pelvic inflammatory disease, which was not responsive to antibiotic therapy.

CONTRAINDICATIONS AND PRECAUTIONS

In general, there are conditions when heat should be used with special precautions. These include heat application to anaesthetic areas or to an obtunded patient. Dosimetry, especially in the deep-heating modalities, is not developed to the point where the tissue temperatures can be safely controlled and destructive temperatures can be reliably avoided. Therefore pain is an essential signal that safe temperature limits are exceeded and it has been documented that if the signal is heeded, tissue destruction does not occur. Also, tissues with inadequate vascular supply should not be heated, since the temperature elevation increases metabolic demand without associated vascular adaptations. As a result, ischaemic necrosis may occur. Heat should not be applied if there is a haemophagic diathesis, since the increase in blood flow and vascularity will produce more bleeding. Heat should not be applied to malignancies without exact tissue temperature monitoring since otherwise therapeutic temperatures may accelerate tumour growth. Heat should not be applied to the gonads or the developing foetus because of the possible development of congenital malformations (Mussa 1955, Edwards 1967, 1972, Dietzel & Kern 1971a,b, Moayer 1971, Dietzel et al 1972, Edwards et al 1974, Menser 1978, Smith et al 1978, Hendrickx et al 1979, Harvey et al 1981).

Some specific contraindications also exist for specific diathermy modalities. Shortwave diathermy is contraindicated if an appreciable amount of energy can reach the site of a metal implant (Lehmann et al 1979). The dangers involved are caused by shunting of current through the metal implant or by increasing the current density surrounding the implant. In either case, excessively high temperatures are produced. This contraindication includes intrauterine devices containing copper or other metals until proven otherwise. However, these devices would be reached by significant amounts of current only with application with internal vaginal or rectal electrodes (Sandler 1973). Also, electronic implants such as cardiac pacemakers and electrophysiological orthoses represent contraindications. Contact lenses may lead to excessive heating of the eye (Scott 1956). Some clinicians have suggested that shortwave diathermy applied to the low back may result in increased menstrual flow (Lehmann & De Lateur 1990c). The use of pelvic diathermy in pregnant women is contraindicated for the reasons given under general contraindications. Safe levels of stray radiation have not been worked out for shortwave diathermy.

Sensitive organs which should not be exposed to any significant amount of microwave radiation include the eyes, since in experimental animals (Carpenter & Van Ummerson 1968, Guy et al 1975), cataracts were produced due to a selective heating effect. The testicles should not be exposed because of the great sensitivity of these reproductive organs to temperature elevation. Exposure of the skull and the brain could lead to focusing of the intensity inside the skull and produce higher levels of exposure than anticipated from measurement outside the body (Johnson & Guy 1972). In the USA, safety standards proposed by the Food and Drug Administration for therapeutic application specify a level of 5 W/cm^2 at a distance of 5 cm from the applicator. Damage during therapeutic exposure, however, has not been observed under 100–150 mW/cm^2 (Michaelson 1990) and is clearly related to the heating effect. Precautions should be used when microwaves are applied over bony prominences, since the reflection of the wave at the bone interface may produce increased absorption in the tissues superficial to the bone. Burns have been observed under these circumstances.

In the case of ultrasound, as mentioned previously, proper equipment and technique of application must be used to avoid the occurrence and destructive effects of gaseous cavitation. Also, exposure of the fluid media of the eye, of the cerebrospinal fluid and of effusions should be avoided because in these media with low cellular content and low viscosity, gaseous cavitation can occur even at therapeutic intensities. For the same reason, the amniotic fluid of the pregnant uterus should not be exposed and the heating effect of ultrasound would represent a contraindication when ultrasound is applied to the foetus. However, due to the excellent beaming properties of ultrasound, exposure of the pregnant uterus can easily be avoided. These precautions do not include imaging of the foetus with ultrasound since the intensities are far below the therapeutic level and therefore cannot produce any harmful effects. Thus, ultrasound can be used for other indications. Also, it can be applied to the intervertebral joints without significant exposure of cerebrospinal fluid and spinal cord because of the intervening tissues such as bone, ligaments and muscles and because the beam can be aimed at the joint facets.

If superficial heat is applied by means of a Hubbard tank or hot tub and the entire body is submerged, the body temperature should be monitored. In this situation, the heat regulatory mechanisms are disabled and therefore an artificial fever is easily produced. Oral temperatures should be taken at water temperatures over 100°F (37.8°C).

There are also contraindications to the use of cold. Severe adverse effects to local cold application are rare and are usually due to hypersensitivity to cold. Four groups of hypersensitivity may be distinguished (Juhlin & Shelley 1961). The first group of hypersensitivity syndromes is a result of release of histamine or histamine-like substances, presenting frequently as classic cold urticaria. The pathogenesis is primarily due to an effect of histamine on capillary vessels and smooth musculature with skin manifestations of urticaria, erythema, itching and sweating. There may be facial flush, puffiness of the eyelids and laryngeal oedema with respiratory impairment. In severe cases there is shock or so-called anaphylaxis with syncope, hypotension and tachycardia. Gastrointestinal symptoms are associated with gastric hyperacidity and include dysphagia, abdominal pain, diarrhoea and vomiting. Horton et al (1936) demonstrated that this type of sensitivity is treatable by a programme of careful desensitization. The second group of hypersensitivity is due to the presence of cold haemolysins and agglutinins. Renal haemoglobinuria and skin manifestations of urticaria and Raynaud's phenomenon are part of the symptomatology. The third group of syndromes is due to the presence of cryoglobulins. There are severe manifestations such as reduced vision, impairment of hearing, conjunctival haemorrhages, epistaxis, cold urticaria, Raynaud's phenomenon and ulceration and necrosis. Also, gastrointestinal upset with melaena and gingival bleeding have been observed. Finally, a marked cold pressor response may be observed in some patients with submersion of limbs in ice water (Wolf & Hardy 1941, Wolff 1951, Boyer et al 1960, Larson 1961, Shelley & Caro 1962).

Some of these responses are severe. Prominent vasospasm can produce a necrosis of fingers and toes in submersion of the limbs. Therefore, careful medical evaluation of the patients is essential and also a trial of localized ice application over a small area – for instance, on the thigh – may produce skin manifestations of sensitivity as a warning sign.

REFERENCES

Bach SA 1965 Biological sensitivity to radio-frequency and microwave energy. Federation Proceedings 24 (suppl 14): S22–S26

Bach SA, Luzzio AJ, Brownell AS 1960 Effects of radio-frequency energy on human gamma globulin. Proceedings of the Fourth Annual TriService Conference on the Biological Effects of Microwave Radiation 1: 117–133

Bäcklund L, Tiselius P 1967 Objective measurement of joint stiffness in rheumatoid arthritis. Acta Rheumatologica Scandinavica 13: 275–288

Balogun JA, Okonofua FE 1988 Management of chronic pelvic inflammatory disease with shortwave diathermy. Physical Therapy 68: 1541–1545

Barker P, Langton JA, Murphy P, Rowbotham DJ 1991 Effect of prior administration of cold saline on pain during propofol injection. Anaesthesia 46: 1069–1070

Basford JR 1995 Low intensity laser therapy: still not an established clinical tool. Lasers in Surgery and Medicine 16: 331–342

Basford JR, Sheffield CG, Mair SD, Ilstrup DM 1987 Low-energy helium-neon laser treatment of thumb osteoarthritis. Archives of Physical Medicine and Rehabilitation 68: 794–797

Basur RL, Shephard E, Mouzas GL 1976 A cooling method in the treatment of ankle sprains. Practitioner 216: 708–711

Bell KR, Lehmann JF 1987 Effect of cooling on H- and T-reflexes in normal subjects. Archives of Physical Medicine and Rehabilitation 68: 490–493

Benson TB, Copp EP 1974 The effects of therapeutic forms of heat and ice on the pain threshold of the normal shoulder. Rheumatology and Rehabilitation 13: 101–104

Bierman W 1955 Therapeutic use of cold. Journal of the American Medical Association 157: 1189–1192

Bierman W, Friedlander M 1940 The penetrative effect of cold. Archives of Physical Therapy 21: 585–591

Binder A, Hodge G, Greenwood AM, Hazleman BL, Page Thomas DP 1985 Is therapeutic ultrasound effective in treating soft tissue lesions? British Medical Journal 290: 512–514

Bisgard JD, Nye D 1940 The influence of hot and cold application upon

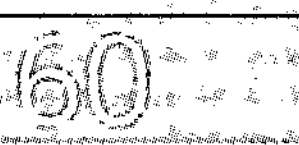

gastric and intestinal motor activity. Surgery, Gynecology and Obstetrics 71: 172–180

Bliddal H, Hellesen C, Ditlevsen P, Asselberghs J, Lyager L 1987 Soft-laser therapy of rheumatoid arthritis. Scandinavian Journal of Rheumatology 16: 225–228

Boyer JT, Fraser JRE, Doyle AE 1960 The haemodynamic effects of cold immersion. Clinical Science 19: 539–550

Carpenter RL, Van Ummerson CA 1968 The action of microwave power on the eye. Journal of Microwave Power 3: 3–19

Carrillo JS, Calatayud J, Manso FJ et al 1990 A randomized double-blind clinical trial on the effectiveness of helium-neon laser in the prevention of pain, swelling and trismus after removal of impacted third molars. International Dental Journal 40: 31–36

Ceccherelli F, Altafini L, Lo Castro G et al 1989 Diode laser in cervical myofascial pain: a double-blind study versus placebo. Clinical Journal of Pain 5: 301–304

Chapman CE 1991 Can the use of physical modalities for pain control be rationalized by the research evidence? Canadian Journal of Physiology and Pharmacology 69: 704–712

Clarke RSJ, Hellon RF, Lind AR 1958 Vascular reactions of the human forearm to cold. Clinical Science 17: 165–179

Cohen BT, Draeger RI, Jackson DW 1989 The effects of cold therapy in the postoperative management of pain in patients undergoing anterior cruciate ligament reconstruction. American Journal of Sports Medicine 17: 344–349

De Jong RH, Hershey WN, Wagman IH 1966 Nerve conduction velocity during hypothermia in man. Anesthesiology 27: 805–810

Delp HL, Newton RA 1986 Effects of brief cold exposure on finger dexterity and sensibility in subjects with Raynaud's phenomenon. Physical Therapy 66: 503–507

De Preux T 1952 Ultrasonic wave therapy of osteoarthritis of the hip joint. British Journal of Physical Medicine 15: 14

Derscheid GL, Brown WC 1985 Rehabilitation of the ankle. Clinics in Sports Medicine 4: 527–544

Devor M 1990 What's in a laser beam for pain therapy? Pain 43: 139

Dietzel F, Kern W 1971a Kann hohes mutterliches Fieber beim Kind auslÿsen? Originalmitteilungen ist ausschliesslich der Verfasser verantwortlich. Naturwissenschaften 2: 24–26

Dietzel F, Kern W 1971b Kann hohes mutterliches Fieber Missbildungen beim Kind auslÿsen? Geburtshilfe und Frauenheilkunde 31: 1074–1079

Dietzel F, Kern W, Steckenmesser R 1972 Missbildungen und intrauterines Absterben nach Kurzwellenbehandlung in der Fruschwangerschaft. Munchener medizinische Wochesschrift 114: 228–230

Douglas WW, Malcolm JL 1955 The effect of localized cooling on conduction in cat nerves. Journal of Physiology 130: 53–71

Edwards MJ 1967 Congenital defects in guinea pigs. Archives of Pathology 84: 42–48

Edwards MJ 1972 Influenza, hyperthermia, and congenital malformation. Lancet i: 320–321

Edwards MJ, Mulley R, Ring S, Wanner RA 1974 Mitotic cell death and delay of mitotic activity in guinea-pig embryos following brief maternal hyperthermia. Journal of Embryology and Experimental Morphology 32: 593–602

Eldred E, Lindsley DF, Buchwald JS 1960 The effect of cooling on mammalian muscle spindles. Experimental Neurology 2: 144–157

Field HL, Basbaum AI 1978 Brainstem control of spinal pain-transmission neurons. Annual Review of Physiology 40: 217–248

Finan MA, Roberts WS, Hoffman MS, Fiorica JV, Cavanagh D, Dudney BJ 1993 The effects of cold therapy on postoperative pain in gynecologic patients: a prospective, randomized study. American Journal of Obstetrics and Gynecology 168 (2): 542–544

Fischer E, Solomon S 1965 Physiological responses to heat and cold. In: Licht S (ed) Therapeutic heat and cold, 2nd edn. E Licht, New Haven, pp 126–169

Friedland F 1975 Ultrasonic therapy in rheumatic diseases. Journal of the American Medical Association 163: 799

Fulga C, Fulga IG, Predescu M 1994 Clinical study of the effect of laser therapy in rheumatic degenerative diseases. Romanian Journal of Internal Medicine 32(3): 227–233

Gammon GD, Starr I 1941 Studies on the relief of pain by counterirritation. Journal of Clinical Investigation 20: 13–20

Ganong WF 1979 The nervous system, 2nd edn. Lange Medical Publications, Los Altos, California

Gerschman JA, Ruben J, Gebart-Eaglemont J 1994 Low level laser therapy for dentinal tooth hypersensitivity. Australian Dental Journal 39 (6): 353–357

Goldman JA, Chiapella J, Casey H et al 1980 Laser therapy for rheumatoid arthritis. Lasers in Surgery and Medicine 1: 93–101

Goodgold J, Eberstein A 1977 Electrodiagnosis of neuromuscular diseases, 2nd edn. Williams & Wilkins, Baltimore

Guy AW, Lehmann JF, Stonebridge JB 1974 Therapeutic applications of electromagnetic power. Proceedings of the Institute of Electrical and Electronic Engineers 62: 55–75

Guy AW, Lin JC, Kramer PO, Emery AF 1975 Effect of 2450-MHz radiation on the rabbit eye. Institute of Electrical and Electronic Engineers, Transactions on Microwave Theory and Techniques MTT 23: 492–498

Hagbarth K-E 1952 Excitatory and inhibitory skin areas for flexor and extensor motoneurons. Acta Physiologica Scandinavica 26 (suppl 94): 1–58

Haker E, Lundeberg T 1990 Laser treatment applied to acupuncture points in lateral humeral epicondylalgia. A double-blind study. Pain 43: 243–247

Haker E, Lundeberg T 1991a Is low-energy laser treatment effective in lateral epicondylalgia? Journal of Pain and Symptom Management 6: 241–245

Haker EHK, Lundeberg TCM 1991b Lateral epicondylalgia: report of non-effective midlaser treatment. Archives of Physical Medicine and Rehabilitation 72: 984–988

Haker EHK, Lundeberg TCM 1991c Pulsed ultrasound treatment in lateral epicondylalgia. Scandinavian Journal of Rehabilitation Medicine 23: 115–118

Hall J, Clarke AK, Elvins DM, Ring EFJ 1994 Low level laser therapy is ineffective in the management of rheumatoid arthritic finger joints. British Journal of Rheumatology 33: 142–147

Hansen HJ, Thoroe U 1990 Low power laser biostimulation of chronic oro-facial pain. A double-blind placebo controlled cross-over study in 40 patients. Pain 43: 169–179

Hardy JD, Wolff HG, Goodell H 1940 Studies on pain. A new method for measuring pain threshold: observations on spatial summation of pain. Journal of Clinical Investigation 19: 649–657

Harris ED Jr, Krane SM 1973 Cartilage collagen: substrate in soluble and fibrillar form for rheumatoid collagenase. Transactions of the Association of American Physicians 86: 82–94

Harris ED Jr, McCroskery PA 1974 The influence of temperature and fibril stability on degradation of cartilage collagen by rheumatoid synovial collagenase. New England Journal of Medicine 290: 1–6

Hartviksen K 1962 Ice therapy in spasticity. Acta Neurologica Scandinavica 38 (suppl 3): 79–84

Harvey MAS, McRorie MM, Smith DW 1981 Suggested limits of exposure in the hot tub and sauna for the pregnant woman. Canadian Medical Association Journal 125: 50–53

Heller JH 1960 Reticuloendothelial structure and function. Roland Press, New York

Hendrickx AG, Stone GW, Henrickson RV, Matayoshi K 1979 Teratogenic effects of hyperthermia on the bonnet monkey (*Macaca radiata*). Teratology 19: 177–182

Herrick JF, Krusen FH 1953 Certain physiologic and pathologic effects of microwaves. Electrical Engineering 72: 239–244

Herrick JF, Jelatis DG, Lee GM 1950 Dielectric properties of tissues important in microwave diathermy. Federation Proceedings 9: 60
Hong C-Z 1991 Reversible nerve conduction block in patients with polyneuropathy after ultrasound thermotherapy at therapeutic dosage. Archives of Physical Medicine and Rehabilitation 72: 132–137
Horton BT, Browne GE, Roth GM 1936 Hypersensitiveness to cold. Journal of the American Medical Association 107: 1263–1268
Iijima K, Shimoyama N, Shimoyama M et al 1989 Effect of repeated irradiation of low-power He-Ne laser in pain relief from postherpetic neuralgia. Clinical Journal of Pain 5: 271–274
Jan MH, Lai JS 1991 The effects of physiotherapy on osteoarthritic knees of females. Journal of the Formosan Medical Association 90(10): 1008–1013
Johannsen F, Hauschild B, Remvig L, Johnsen V, Petersen M, Bieler T 1994 Low energy laser therapy in rheumatoid arthritis. Scandinavian Journal of Rheumatology 23(3): 45–147
Johns RJ, Wright V 1962 Relative importance of various tissues in joint stiffness. Journal of Applied Physiology 17: 824–828
Johnson CC, Guy AW 1972 Nonionizing electromagnetic wave-effects in biological materials and systems. Proceedings of the Institute of Electrical and Electronic Engineers 66: 692–718
Juhlin L, Shelley WB 1961 Role of mast cell and basophil in cold urticaria with associated systemic reactions. Journal of the American Medical Association 117: 371–377
Kay DB 1985 The sprained ankle: current therapy. Foot and Ankle 6: 22–28
Kerr FWL, Casey KL 1976 Pain. Neurosciences Research Program Bulletin 16: 1–207
Klein RG, Eck BC 1990 Low-energy laser treatment and exercise for chronic low-back pain: double-blind controlled trial. Archives of Physical Medicine and Rehabilitation 71: 34–37
Knuttson E, Mattsson E 1969 Effects of local cooling monosynaptic reflexes in man. Scandinavian Journal of Rehabilitation Medicine 1: 126–132
Kramer JF 1985 Effect of therapeutic ultrasound intensity on subcutaneous tissue temperature and ulnar nerve conduction velocity. American Journal of Physical Medicine 64: 1–9
Landen BR 1967 Heat or cold for the relief of low back pain? Physical Therapy 47: 1126–1128
Larson DL 1961 Systemic lupus erythematosus. Little, Brown, Boston
Lehmann JF, De Lateur BJ 1982 Therapeutic heat. In: Lehmann JF (ed) Therpeutic heat and cold, 3rd edn. Williams & Wilkins, Baltmore.
Lehmann JF, De Lateur BJ 1990a Cryotherapy. In: Lehmann JF (ed) Therapeutic heat and cold, 4th edn. Williams & Wilkins, Baltimore
Lehmann JF, De Lateur BJ 1990b Therapeutic heat. In: Lehmann JF (ed) Therapeutic heat and cold, 4th edn. Williams & Wilkins, Baltimore
Lehmann JF, De Lateur BJ 1990c Diathermy, superficial heat, laser and cold therapy. In: Kottke FJ, Lehmann JF (eds) Handbook of physical medicine and rehabilitation, 4th edn. WB Saunders, Philadelphia
Lehmann JF, Brunner GD, Stow RW 1958 Pain threshold measurements after therapeutic application of ultrasound, microwaves, and infrared. Archives of Physical Medicine and Rehabilitation 39: 560–565
Lehmann JF, Stonebridge JB, Guy AW 1979 A comparison of patterns of stray radiation from therapeutic microwave applicators measured near tissue-substitute models and human subjects. Radio Science 14: 271–283
Lehmann JF, Dundore DE, Esselman PC, Nelp WB 1983 Microwave diathermy: effects on experimental muscle hematoma resolution. Archives of Physical Medicine and Rehabilitation 64: 127–129
Li C-L 1958 Effect of cooling on neuromuscular transmission in the rat. American Journal of Physiology 194: 200–206
Lightfoot E, Verrier M, Ashby P 1975 Neurological effects of prolonged cooling of the calf in patients with complete spinal transection. Physical Therapy 55: 251–258
Lim HM, Lew K, Tay D 1995 A clinical investigation of the efficacy of low level laser therapy in reducing orthodontic postadjustment pain. American Journal of Orthodontics and Dentofacial Orthopedics 108(6): 614–622
Lowe AS, McDowell BC, Walsh DM, Baxter GD, Allen JM 1997 Failure to demonstrate any hypoalgesic effect of low intensity laser irradiation (830 nm) of Erb's point upon experimental ischaemic pain in humans. Lasers in Surgery and Medicine 20: 69–76
Lundeberg T, Haker E, Thomas M 1987a Effect of laser versus placebo in tennis elbow. Scandinavian Journal of Rehabilitation Medicine 19: 135–138
Lundeberg T, Hode L, Zhou J 1987b A comparative study of the pain-relieving effect of laser treatment and acupuncture. Acta Physiologica Scandinavica 13: 161–162
Martin GM, Roth GM, Elkins EC, Krusen FH 1946 Cutaneous temperature of the extremities of normal subjects and of patients with rheumatoid arthritis. Archives of Physical Medicine 27: 665–682
Matsen FA III, Questad K, Matsen AL 1975 The effect of local cooling on post fracture swelling. Clinical Orthopedics and Related Research 109: 201–206
Melzack R, Wall PD 1965 Pain mechanisms: a new theory. Science 150: 971–979
Melzack R, Guite S, Gonshor A 1980a Relief of dental pain by ice massage of the hand. Canadian Medical Association Journal 122: 189–191
Melzack R, Jeans ME, Stratford JG, Monks RC 1980b Ice massage and transcutaneous electrical stimulation: comparison of treatment for low-back pain. Pain 9: 209–217
Mense S 1978 Effects of temperature on the discharges of muscle spindles and tendon organs. Pflügers Archiv 374: 159–166
Menser M 1978 Does hyperthermia affect the human fetus? Medical Journal of Australia 2: 550
Michaelson SM 1972 Human exposure to nonionizing radiant energy – potential hazards and safety standards. Proceedings of the Institute of Electrical and Electronic Engineers 60: 389–421
Michaelson SM 1990 Bioeffects of high frequency currents and electromagnetic radiation. In: Lehmann JF (ed) Therapeutic heat and cold, 4th edn. Williams & Wilkins, Baltimore
Miglietta O 1973 Action of cold on spasticity. American Journal of Physical Medicine 52: 198–205
Moayer M 1971 Die morphologischen Veränderugen der Plazenta unter dem Einfluss der Kurzwellendurchfluting. Tierexperimentelle Untersuchungen. Strahlentherapie 142: 609–614
Moktar B, Baxter GD, Walsh DM, Bell AJ, Allen JM 1995 Double-blind, placebo-controlled investigation of the effect of combined phototherapy/low intensity laser therapy upon experimental ischaemic pain in humans. Lasers in Surgery and Medicine 17: 74–81
Molander CO 1941 Physiologic basis of heat. Archives of Physical Therapy 22: 335–340
Moore CD, Cardea JA 1977 Vascular changes in leg trauma. Southern Medical Journal 70: 1285–1286
Murray FS, Weaver MM 1975 Effects of ipsilateral and contralateral counter-irritation on experimentally produced itch in human beings. Journal of Comparative and Physiological Psychology 89: 819–826
Mussa B 1955 Embriopatie da cause fisiche. Minerva Nipiologica 5: 69–72
Nilsson S 1983 Sprains of the lateral ankle ligaments, an epidemiological and clinical study with special reference to different forms of conservative treatment. Part II, a controlled trial of different forms of conservative treatment. Journal of the Oslo City Hospitals 33: 13–36

Nykanen M 1995 Pulsed ultrasound treatment of the painful shoulder: a randomized, double-blind, placebo-controlled study. Scandinavian Journal of Rehabilitation Medicine 27: 105–108
Ottoson D 1965 The effects of temperature on the isolated muscle spindle. Journal of Physiology 180: 636–648
Parsons CM, Goetzl FR 1945 Effect of induced pain on pain threshold. Proceedings of the Society for Experimental Biology and Medicine 60: 327–329
Perkins JF, Li M-C, Hoffman F, Hoffmann E 1948 Sudden vasoconstriction in denervated or sympathectomized paws exposed to cold. American Journal of Physiology 155: 165–178
Reid R, Omoto KH, Precop SL et al 1995 Flashlamp-excited dye laser therapy of idiopathic vulvodynia is safe and efficacious. American Journal of Obstetrics and Gynecology 172(6): 1684–1696
Saito M, Schwan HP 1961 The time constants of pearl-chain formation. Biological effects of microwave radiation. Proceedings of the Fourth Annual TriService Conference on the Biological Effects of Microwave Radiation 1: 85–91
Sandler B 1973 Heat and the ICUCD. British Medical Journal 25: 458
Scarcella JB, Cohn BT 1995 The effect of cold therapy on the postoperative course of total hip and knee arthroplasty patients. American Journal of Orthopedics 24(11): 847–852
Schaubel HJ 1946 The local use of ice after orthopedic procedures. American Journal of Surgery 72: 711–714
Schmidt KL, Ott VR, Röcher G, Schaller H 1979 Heat, cold and inflammation. Rheumatology 38: 391–404
Scott BO 1956 Effect of contact lenses on short wave field distribution. British Journal of Ophthalmology 40: 696–697
Seino H, Watanabe S, Tanaka J et al 1985 Cryoanalgesia for postthoracotomy pain. Masui 34: 842–845
Sekins KM, Dundore D, Emery AF, Lehmann JF, McGrath PW, Nelp WB 1980 Muscle blood flow changes in response to 915 MHz diathermy with surface cooling as measured by Xe^{133} clearance. Archives of Physical Medicine and Rehabilitation 61: 105–113
Sekins KM, Lehman JF, Esselman P et al 1984 Local muscle blood flow and temperature responses to 915 MHz diathermy as simultaneously measured and numerically predicted. Archives of Physical Medicine and Rehabilitation 65: 1–7
Shelley WB, Caro WB 1962 Cold erythema. Journal of the American Medical Association 180: 639–642
Siebert W, Seichert N, Siebert B, Wirth CJ 1987 What is the efficacy of 'soft' and 'mid' lasers in therapy of tendinopathies? Archives of Orthopaedic and Trauma Surgery 106: 358–363
Smith DW, Clarren SK, Harvey MAS 1978 Hyperthermia as a possible teratogenic agent. Journal of Pediatrics 92: 878–883
Steinberg R, Callies R 1992 Vergleichsstudie Ultraschall und Prednisolonphonophorese bei Patienten mit Epicondylopathia humeri. Physikalische Medizin Rehabilitationsmedizin Kurortmedizin 2: 84–87
Taube S, Piironen J, Ylipaavalniemi P 1990 Helium-neon laser therapy in the prevention of postoperative swelling and pain after wisdom tooth extraction. Proceedings of the Finnish Dental Society 86: 23–27
Texeira-Pinto AA, Nejelski LL, Cutler JL, Heller JH 1960 The behavior of unicellular organisms in an electromagentic field. Experimental Cell Research 20: 548–564
Traherne JB 1962 Evaluation of the cold spray technique in the treatment of muscle pain in general practice. Practitioner 189: 210–212
Trnavsky G 1983 Die Beeinflussing des Hoffmann-Reflexes durch Kryolangzeittherapie. Wiener Medizinische Wochenschrift 11: 287–289
Urbscheit N, Bishop B 1970 Effects of cooling on the ankle jerk and H-response. Physical Therapy 50: 1041–1049
Vinger PF, Hoerner EF (eds) 1981 Sports injuries, the unthwarted epidemic. PSG Publishing, Littleton, Massachusetts
Walker J 1983 Relief from chronic pain by lower power laser irradiation. Neuroscience Letters 43: 339–344
Walker JB, Akhanjee LK, Cooney MM et al 1988 Laser therapy for pain of trigeminal neuralgia. Clinical Journal of Pain 3: 183–187
Waterworth RF, Hunter IA 1985 An open study of diflunisal, conservative and manipulative therapy in the management of acute mechanical low back pain. NZ Med J May 22; 98(779): 372–5
Waylonis GW, Wilke S, O'Toole D, Waylonis DA, Waylonis DB 1988 Chronic myofascial pain: management by low-output helium-neon laser therapy. Archives of Physical Medicine and Rehabilitation 69: 1017–1020
Wolf S, Hardy JD 1941 Studies on pain. Observations on pain due to local cooling and on factors involved in the 'cold pressor' effect. Journal of Clinical Investigation 20: 521–533
Wolff HH 1951 The mechanism and significance of the cold pressor response. Quarterly Journal of Medicine 20: 261–273
Wright V, Johns RJ 1960 Physical factors concerned with the stiffness of normal and diseased joints. Bulletin of the Johns Hopkins Hospital 106: 215–231
Wright V, Johns RJ 1961 Quantitative and qualitative analysis of joint stiffness in normal subjects and in patients with connective tissue diseases. Annals of the Rheumatic Diseases 20: 36–46

Mobilization, manipulation, massage and exercise for the relief of musculoskeletal pain

61

SCOTT HALDEMAN & PAUL D. HOOPER

SUMMARY

Musculoskeletal problems represent some of the most common causes of pain, dysfunction and disability. The costs in both human suffering and economic terms is tremendous. For thousands of years, the various forms of mobilization, manipulation, massage and exercise have been used to relieve pain, promote healing and increase movement and mobility. Only recently has there been sufficient interest in the scientific community to investigate the effectiveness and mechanisms of these manual methods. There are now multiple clinical trials providing sufficient evidence to justify the continued use of many of these procedures for selected patients. It should be noted that many of these procedures are often used in combination with each other. While they should not be considered a panacea, they represent an effective, low-tech, natural way of relieving pain and suffering that is essentially free from the negative effects of long-term medication use. For many patients, they offer hope and allow a return to active and productive lives.

INTRODUCTION

The locomotor system (i.e. muscles, ligaments, joints, bones and nerves) has been called 'the primary machinery of life' (Korr 1978). Humans are dependent upon the integrity of their locomotor system for movement, which is essential for work, entertainment, adventure and most activities of daily living. If the integrity of this system is compromised through disease, trauma or the consequences of ageing, the resulting pain and restricted function can have devastating effects on the quality of life of an individual.

The primary approach to patients with musculoskeletal pain which results in restricted function, therefore, is the restoration of movement and the soothing of pain. Any attempt at relieving pain without simultaneously improving movement and mobility will have limited success in restoring function to the musculoskeletal system. The tools to achieve these ends include massage to relax muscles and for its soothing effect, active/passive mobilization of joints to maintain range of motion, manipulation to increase motion and relax muscles and exercise to maintain strength and mobility. These approaches to musculoskeletal pain have the additional advantages of being relatively inexpensive and free of any drug or medication effects or the necessity for surgery. Despite the development of more potent drugs and more complex surgical interventions, manual therapies and exercise remain the most widely utilized method of treating musculoskeletal pain and disability.

The laying on of hands is questionably the oldest, most universally utilized and one of the most appreciated means of relieving pain and suffering. Touching, massaging or manipulating areas that are painful, tense or tight is used in every household and in much of the animal kingdom. Parents learn very early that rubbing or kissing a child's bruise or scratch may be all that is necessary to change a scream of pain to a smile of contentment. Tension headaches and neck pain are probably relieved more often by a spouse's massage than by a physician's ministrations.

Manipulation and massage in their various forms have also been offered as methods of relieving pain by physicians throughout history. The history of manipulation and massage as treatment modalities is extensive and has been reviewed by a number of authors in detail (Schiotz 1958, Lomax 1975, 1976, Gibbons 1980, Tappan 1984, Kamanetz 1985). The debate on the etymology of the words 'manipulation and massage' is an indication of their wide usage. Many ancient languages have similar sounding words. Manipulation is commonly thought to originate from the Latin word *manus*, hand, or *manipulare*, to use the hands. Massage, however, has been variously attributed to the Arab verb *mass*, to touch, the Greek word *massein*, to knead, the Hebrew *mashesh*, to feel, touch or grope, or the Sanskrit term *makeh*, to stroke, press or condense (Kamanetz 1985). Writings, diagrams, paintings and sculpture showing or describing various methods of massage and manipulation can be found in virtually all recorded civilizations, including Babylon, Assyria, ancient China as far back as 1000 BC, India, Greece, Rome and Egypt. The formalized use of manipulation of the spine is commonly attributed to Hippocrates and Galen, both of whom recommended manipulating the spine in certain cases. Similarly, a number of cultures without written history, including the Eskimos, South American Indians and African tribal natives, have been noted to utilize massage and manipulation techniques as part of their healing rituals. One of the authors has personally witnessed a Bushman ceremony to drive out evil spirits where the healer repeatedly massaged and thrust on the spine of the person whose affliction was to be relieved. It was not possible, however, even with a competent translator, to determine what was wrong with the patient beyond the explanation that there was an evil spirit preventing the patient from running and that such spirits were most likely to be expelled through the ritual.

The therapeutic value of exercises for the human body has been recognized as an important component in the healing process since ancient times. In ancient China therapeutic exercises were prescribed for the relief of pain and multiple other symptoms (MacAuliffe 1904). In the 19th century the British surgeon John Hunter discussed the value of early mobilization following injury or disease to relieve pain and enhance return of function (Hunter 1841). In addition to recognizing the overall value of movement, he felt that voluntary movements were superior to passive movements in helping the patient to regain function. In a historical review of exercises, Licht (1978) reported on the work of Lucas-Championniere, a 19th-century French physician who noted that a patient who was not immobilized following a fracture of the radius regained function quickly. Moreover, the pain associated with the fracture appeared to lessen more quickly than in persons with similar fractures who were immobilized.

MASSAGE AND MANIPULATION TECHNIQUES

Massage and manipulation fall into the larger field referred to as manual medicine, manual therapy or manipulative therapy. All techniques where the hands are used to touch, feel, massage or manipulate tissue therapeutically in order to directly benefit a patient can be included under these headings. The number of methods and techniques of massage and manipulation is too great to include in a short chapter on the topic. Clinicians who use manual therapy to treat patients begin to modify methods they have been taught very early in their career and adapt their approach to the particular patient and tissue they are treating. Techniques are also adapted to suit a clinician's level of strength, dexterity, training and confidence. There are, however, a number of principles which allow for a classification of the various manual therapeutic approaches. The most common classification of manual techniques is based on a differentiation between massage, passive movement, mobilization and the manipulative or adjustive techniques. These techniques are applied at different positions within a specific range of motion of a joint, as shown in Figure 61.1.

MASSAGE

Massage is the application of touch or force to soft tissues, usually muscles, tendons or ligaments, without causing movement or change in a position of a joint. Each massage technique is performed with a specific goal in mind. The most commonly applied techniques are as follows.

Stroking or effleurage

This is the light movement of the hands over the skin in a slow, rhythmic fashion. The hands mould to the contour of the area being massaged and are in constant contact with the skin. The hands may gently stroke the skin or influence deeper tissues depending on the amount of pressure exerted. Light stroking tends to be non-painful and soothing and can be either centripetal or centrifugal. Deeper pressure techniques can be slightly uncomfortable and are always taught to be in the direction of venous or lymph flow with the stated goal of reducing oedema.

Connective tissue massage

This technique uses deeper stroking motions and is presumed to free subcutaneous connective tissue adhesions. The technique, initially described by Elizabeth Dicke (1953), was popularized by Marie Ebner (1960). This deep stroking in specifically defined patterns results in a sensation of warmth and hyperaemia of the skin.

Kneading and petrissage

These techniques require the clinician to grasp, lift, squeeze or push the tissues being massaged. The skin moves with

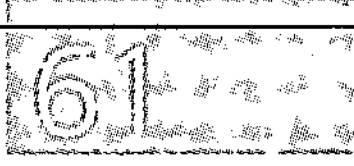

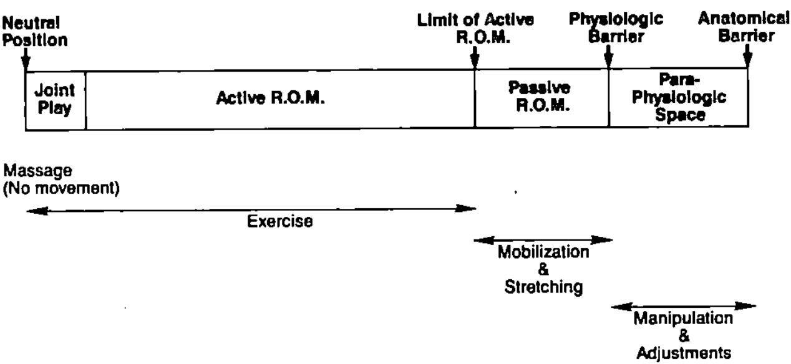

Fig. 61.1 The presumed barriers to motion in a joint and the position or range of motion where the various forms of manual therapy are performed.

the hands over the underlying tissues. This differs from stroking, where the hands move over the skin. Commonly these techniques are applied to muscles which can be gripped and alternately compressed and then released before moving on to another area.

Friction and deep massage

The theoretical goal of these techniques is the loosening of scars or adhesions between deeper structures such as ligaments, tendons and muscles (Cyriax 1971, Wood 1974). These procedures are presumed to aid in the absorption of local effusion within these tissues. The direction of movement of the fingers over the tissues being massaged is described by Wood as circular, whereas Cyriax insists that the movement should be transverse across the fibres of the structure being massaged. The massage is continued until a muscle is mobilized from its surrounding tissues or any palpated effusions or thickening in a ligamentous structure are dispersed. It may require several sessions to achieve this result and the massage should be followed by exercise to maintain mobility.

Tapotement, percussion or clapping

These techniques consist of a series of gentle taps or blows applied to the patient (Hofkosh 1985). These techniques have been described as hacking (using the ulnar border of the hand), clapping or cupping (using the palm either flat or concave), tapping (using the tips of the fingers) or beating (using closed fists). These percussive movements have been used primarily in postural draining of the lungs, to obtain muscle contraction and relaxation or to increase circulation. They are generally not recommended for the treatment of pathological tissues (Wood 1974) and are commonly used on athletes to tone and relax muscles.

Shaking and vibration

These massage methods require the clinician to take hold of a portion of the patient's body and apply either a coarse shaking or a fine vibration motion. They are not widely used except in postural drainage of the lungs.

PASSIVE MOVEMENT

The use of the hands to maintain passive motion in a joint falls into the category of manual therapy although these procedures are often performed by nurses, aides and patients' families. They are briefly mentioned here to demonstrate the wide spectrum of manual therapeutic techniques. The techniques are relatively simple to teach and perform. They require an understanding of the different directions of movement a joint may traverse. The clinician takes hold of the peripheral part of the joint and systematically moves the joint through each of its normal motions, from the neutral point to the point of resistance or pain. No attempt is made to force the joint but the entire length of the range of motion must be traversed and each direction of potential motion must be included. The procedure is repeated and performed several times a day. The goal is to prevent stiffening or shortening of the ligamentous structures as well as to maintain motion and lubrication in the joint and surrounding tissues.

The natural progression from passive motion is to active motion or exercise. Exercise is performed within the same boundaries of joint motion as is passive motion, although not all directions of motion which can be achieved passively can be reproduced by exercise. Exercise has the additional advantage of including muscle activity and developing strength and co-ordination. Passive movement, except in paralysis or severe muscle injury requiring a period of healing, is usually discontinued, where possible, in favour of active exercise assuming the therapeutic goal is maintenance of range of motion.

MOBILIZATION AND STRETCHING

Mobilization includes those manual procedures which attempt to increase the range of motion beyond the resistance barrier which limits passive range of motion or exercise (Fig. 61.1). Certain mobilization methods include stretching of muscles and ligaments while others include movement of joints in non-physiologic directions of motion.

Mobilization differs from manipulation or adjustment by the absence of a forceful thrust or jerking motion.

Graded oscillation or mobilization

These techniques were popularized by Maitland (1973) who proposed four levels or grades of mobilization. Grade I mobilization is a fine oscillation with very little force or depth. Grade II is a mobilization with greater depth but within the first half of the range of motion. Grade III is a deeper mobilization at the limits of motion, whereas Grade IV is a deep, fine oscillation at the limits of potential motion. The clinician tends to start at grade I and increase to grade IV as greater motion becomes possible. The ranges of motion of each of these grades are illustrated in Figure 61.2B.

Progressive stretch mobilization

These techniques require the application of successive short-amplitude stretching movements to the joint. The depth of the stretching into the resisted range of motion is increased as permitted by the joint. Again, four grades or depths are described (Nyberg 1985) but in this situation the grades refer to each quarter of the potential motion of the joint as illustrated in Figure 61.2C. These techniques are used primarily to overcome soft tissue restriction to joint motion.

Sustained progressive stretch

This is a sustained stretching motion with progressively increasing pressure. This sustained force technique is recommended to stretch shortened periarticular soft tissues and is performed slowly and carefully to avoid tearing of tissues (Fig. 61.2D).

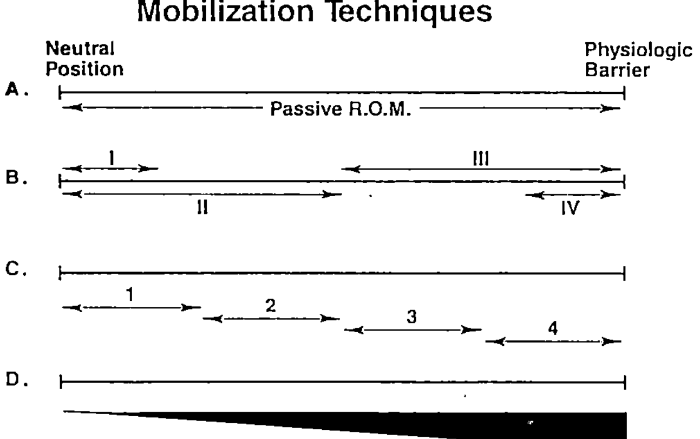

Fig. 61.2 The different forms of mobilization. Active and passive ranges of motion are included under 'passive range of motion' as all of these mobilizations are performed passively. **A** Continuous passive range of motion; **B** graded oscillations; **C** progressive stretch mobilization; **D** sustained progressive stretching.

Spray and stretch

These techniques have been taught widely by Janet Travell (1976) and John Mennell (1960) for the treatment of painful muscular trigger points. The muscle being treated is placed in a light stretch and a fluoromethane spray is applied to the muscle in a specific pattern. This results in a cooling of the skin as the fluoromethane evaporates. The muscle can then be stretched further, allowing increased range of motion and, theoretically, the elimination of the trigger point.

Muscle energy

These methods require the use of muscle activity and subsequent relaxation to set the stage for increasing motion. In peripheral joint mobilization, it has been called the 'hold–relaxation' technique. The clinician places the muscle in light stretch. The patient then contracts the muscle against resistance applied by the clinician. The contraction is held for a brief period and the patient then relaxes. The clinician can then increase the stretch of the muscle and joint. Certain osteopathic physicians (Kimberly 1979, Goodridge 1981) have modified these techniques with sophisticated positioning of the patient to allow for specific directional mobilization or manipulation of vertebrae.

MANIPULATION

The difference between mobilization and manipulation or adjustment is the application of a high-velocity, low-amplitude thrust to the joint. Many chiropractors feel that there is a difference between non-specific manipulation and the classic adjustment which has specific direction, force and presumed physiologic effects. Other clinicians include the various mobilization and muscle-energy techniques under the heading of manipulation. There is, however, fairly clear differentiation between the previously described non-thrust procedures and the thrusting techniques described under this heading. These techniques force the joint beyond the physiologic range of motion, through the paraphysiological space, to the anatomical limits of motion (Fig. 61.1). The thrust is commonly followed by a 'click' or 'pop' which is audible and is felt to be related to release of gases within the joint space.

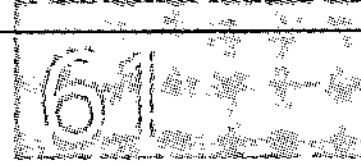

Non-specific long-lever manipulation

These techniques are becoming less popular because of the potential to exert large forces which could damage bones, ligaments or discs. Force is applied via a long bone as a lever. Commonly, a shoulder or leg is used to exert force into the spine (Cyriax 1971, Coplans 1978). These techniques, in the past, were commonly used under anaesthesia, allowing for the exertion of strenuous forces to a joint. In large patients treated by small clinicians, the utilization of such long levers with directed force may be the only way in which a joint can be manipulated.

Specific spinal adjustment

The application of high-velocity, small-amplitude thrusting techniques to short levers of the spine such as a spinous or transverse process has been the mainstay of traditional chiropractic practice. The goal has been variously described as correcting misalignments or subluxations, eliminating fixations in intersegmental motion and bringing about a variety of neural and muscular reflex changes. There are numerous techniques which have been described in textbooks (Logan 1950, Greco 1953, States 1968, Haldeman 1980, 1992). Each vertebra can be adjusted in a number of different directions and the patient can be placed in very specific positions prior to the administration of an adjustment to allow for control of the depth and direction of the force to be applied. It has yet to be established, however, that such precise application of force does in fact bring about specific vertebral movements as claimed. A number of chiropractic techniques require specialized tables which allow for the positioning of the patient.

Toggle-recoil

Certain chiropractic techniques (Thompson 1973) require the patient to be placed on a table which is constructed so that one vertebral segment is locked or blocked while a rapidly controlled force is applied to the adjacent vertebra. The portion of the table supporting the vertebra being adjusted then drops approximately 1 cm, allowing for a concussion or recoil effect. Properly performed, high-velocity forces can be applied very specifically to a vertebra without the clinician exerting much force or effort.

Joint play

John Mennell (1960) has been instrumental in teaching techniques of moving joints in directions not commonly moved during exercise. Most joints have some degree of play at rest because of ligamentous elasticity. When joints cease to have this play due to tightening of the ligaments and especially if the joint is locked in a slightly abnormal position, Mennell recommends that the joint be manipulated in specific directions to increase the play. A number of manipulation techniques for increasing joint play in both vertebral and peripheral joints have been described.

Traction and distraction

Manual traction and the combination of mechanical traction or distraction with manipulation techniques are perhaps not properly included in this section. They are, however, commonly accompanied by pulling or thrusting methods while the patient is in traction (Cox 1980) and are widely used by chiropractors under the term 'adjustments'. Manual traction without thrusting is also used as a standard physiotherapeutic technique and could be included under mobilization methods.

Mechanically assisted manipulation

Over the years, a number of mechanical devices have been developed to assist in the delivery of the manipulative thrust. These include special tables with drop-away pieces, manual and motorized tables that move up, down and sideways and small, hand-held instruments such as the Activator Adjusting Instrument (AAI). Some of these are promoted as assistive devices that aid the clinician with the delivery of the necessary force. Others have been suggested as potential replacements to manual manipulation (Polkinghorn 1998).

THE EFFECTIVENESS OF MASSAGE AND MANIPULATION

By far the majority of people who request massage or manipulation do so for relief of pain, muscle spasm, tension or stiffness. Surveys reviewing the reason why patients seek chiropractic treatment reveal that 80–90% of them do so for the relief of spinal pain or headaches (Vear 1972, Breen 1977, Nyiendo & Haldeman 1987). A recent study in Sweden demonstrated that most patients sought chiropractic care for low back pain of less than 1 month duration and received 2–3 spinal manipulation treatments (SMT) (Leboeuf-Yde et al 1997). The anecdotal surveys and descriptive studies on patients who attend both chiropractors and other practitioners of manipulation demonstrate a very high success or satisfaction rate. The success rates reported for manipulation in uncontrolled trials and in various comparative trials are between 60% and 100% (Haldeman 1978, Brunarski 1984, Bronfort 1992). This type of study, with its lack of controls, ignores the well-recognized problems of spontaneous recovery, placebo effect, difficulty in quantitating pain and natural prejudice of practitioners reporting on the success of their own treatment. In the case of spinal pain, the problem of different populations of patients and pathological causes of pain also makes it difficult to compare studies and determine the success of treatment. The fact that the majority of patients visiting a practitioner of manipulation feel better while undergoing treatment is undoubtedly the primary reason for its popularity.

For the entire field of massage, despite its universal usage, there have not been many serious controlled trials. There are, however, few clinicians or patients who would deny that rubbing or massaging sore muscles or stiff joints produces a soothing feeling and pain relief. It can be argued that even if the relief described after massage and manipulation is due to placebo or psychological effects, such treatments should not be discarded. The utilization of any treatment that has this effect should be considered beneficial. Pope et al (1994) found that satisfaction rates in patients who were receiving massage were significantly higher than in those patients being treated with corsets or transcutaneous muscle stimulation (TMS). These rates increased with repeated treatments, thus demonstrating the high acceptance of this procedure by patients.

Manipulation, on the other hand, has been the subject of increasing clinical research. A growing number of prospective, randomized controlled trials have studied the effectiveness of manipulation compared to placebo and other conservative treatments. As is often the case in the early trials of any treatment, the results of such research can be confusing and difficult to interpret. In the case of manipulation, the problem is greater than usual because there are few standards with regard to technique used, the skill of the manipulator, the number and frequency of manipulations, patient selection or outcomes which have to be adhered to.

The number of published controlled clinical trials has grown rapidly during the past few years. Shekelle et al (1992) lists 29 controlled clinical trials on low back pain and Bronfort (1992) has reviewed 47 randomized, comparative trials on the treatment of back pain, neck pain and headaches using manipulation. In a review of criteria-based meta-analyses, Koes et al (1995) identified 69 different randomized controlled clinical trials (RCTs) and in a systematic review, Van Tulder et al (1997) reported that 28 RCTs on acute and 20 on chronic low back pain were of high quality (i.e. had a methodologic score of 50 or more points). Many of these studies have shown favourable results for manipulation (Koes et al 1996).

In one of the more publicized RCTs, manipulation provided by chiropractors was compared to hospital outpatient treatment (Meade et al 1990). The study demonstrated a short-term favourable outcome for chiropractic care. A 3-year follow-up study (Meade et al 1995) confirmed the earlier findings that when chiropractors or hospital therapists treat patients with low back pain as they would in day-to-day practice, those treated by chiropractors derive more benefit and long-term satisfaction than those treated in hospital. This later study also suggested some potential long-term benefit to the patients treated by chiropractors.

These authors and others (Ottenbacher & DiFabio 1985) have found sufficient numbers of well-designed trials to perform meta-analyses and to sort the trials into different subgroups of patients. This has made it possible to discuss the effectiveness of manipulation in more specific forms, such as condition or diagnosis, and expected outcome measures.

ACUTE UNCOMPLICATED LOW BACK PAIN

The majority of the controlled clinical trials on manipulation have been performed on patients with recent onset of symptoms (within 2–4 weeks). These studies tended to exclude patients with complicating factors such as systemic or metabolic diseases, sciatica or disc herniation, workers' compensation or other psychosocial factors. There are many difficulties in reviewing these papers. The paper by Jayson (1986), for example, found that manipulation was superior to controls when given in an outpatient clinic, but was ineffective in hospitalized patients with back pain who presumably had more severe pathology. The paper by Berquist-Ullman and Larsson (1977) found manipulation to be more effective than placebo but no better than a comprehensive education programme. Glover et al (1974, 1977) found that manipulation had a significant positive effect in patients with acute pain when assessed immediately after treatment but not in more chronic cases. Doran and Newell (1975), Coxhead et al (1981) and Sloop et al (1982) each showed non-statistically significant trends towards improvement in their manipulation groups when compared to controls. Greenland et al (1979) suggest that a different statistical analysis of Doran and Newell's data would find manipulation significantly more effective than controls.

Even in the trials where manipulation was reported as clearly more effective than controls, the picture is not clear. The studies by Coyer and Curwen (1955) and Lewith and Turner (1982) were not blinded or statistically analysed. The studies by Sims-Williams et al (1978, 1979), Buerger (1978, 1979) and Hoehler et al (1981) were well controlled but showed only short-term changes with no long-lasting results from manipulation. However, one point is clear; the multiple comparative trials have shown that no other conservative treatment is superior to manipulation. Of particular interest is the observation that none of the trials reported any complications from the application of manipulation.

In order to assess the results of manipulation on acute low back pain better, it is useful to look at the meta-analyses and critical reviews of these papers. One of the most recent and comprehensive reviews is by Shekelle et al (1992) who analysed all the controlled trials on manipulation and assigned quality scores on the published research designs. They then selected seven papers which had used single-outcome measures or assessed outcome measures independently. Table 61.1 lists these papers and the number of patients who recovered. They then developed differences in probability of recovery from back pain for each of the seven studies (Fig. 61.3). The results show that manipulation increased the probability of recovery at 2 or 3 weeks after start of treatment by 0.17 (95% probability limits, 0.07–0.28), indicating that manipulation hastens recovery from acute uncomplicated low back pain.

A prospective randomized trial compared the effect of SMT, transcutaneous muscle stimulation, massage and corset use in patients with subacute low back pain (Pope et al 1994). After 3 weeks, the manipulation group scored the greatest improvement in flexion and pain. In addition, patient confidence was greatest in the manipulation group. In a randomized study of manual therapy (i.e. manipulation, specific mobilization and muscle stretching) compared with steroid injections for patients with acute and subacute low back pain, patients receiving manual therapy had signif-

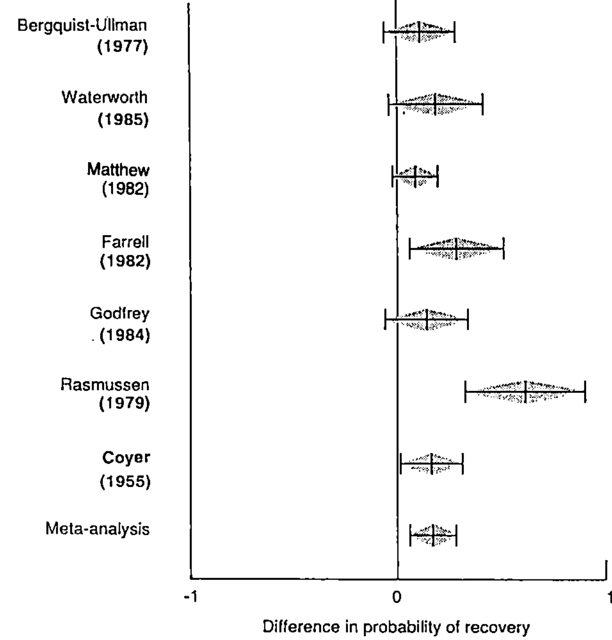

Fig. 61.3 Different in probability of recovery in seven trials of manipulation. A difference in probability of greater than zero represents a beneficial effect of manipulation. For individual studies, 95% confidence intervals are shown; for the meta-analysis, the 95% probability limits are shown. (From Shekelle et al 1992.)

Table 61.1. Outcome measures combined in meta-analysis of acute low back pain studies. (From Shekelle et al 1992.)

Author (reference)	*Outcome measure*	*When assessed*	*Number of patients recovered*	
			Manipulated group	*Comparison group*
Coyer & Curwen 1955	'Well' (relief of symptoms)	3 wk	58 of 76	36 of 60
Bergquist-Ullman & Larsson 1977	Return to work	3 wk	30 of 61	25 of 56
Farrell & Twomey 1982	'Symptom-free', very low pain score, can do all functional activity without difficulty, and objective lumbar movements are without pain	3 wk	22 of 24	15 of 24
Godfrey et al 1984	1–5-point scale of 'general symptomatology' dichotomised by the original authors into 'marked improvement' or not	Mean, 2 wk	14 of 39	7 of 33
Rasmussen 1979	'Fully restored', no pain, normal function, no sign of disease, fit to work	2 wk	11 of 12	3 of 12
Matthews et al 1987	6-point pain scale divided into 'recovered' and 'not recovered'	2 wk	116 of 152	73 of 108
Waterworth & Hunder 1985	'Excellent overall improvement' by patient self-report	12 d	23 of 38	15 of 36

icantly less pain and disability both in the early phase as well as at 90 days follow-up. The manual therapy group also had a faster rate of recovery and lower drug consumption (Blomberg et al 1994). Koes et al (1996) identified 36 RCTs comparing SMT with other treatments for patients with low back pain. Twelve of these included only patients with acute pain. Of these, five reported positive results, four reported negative results and three reported positive results in a subgroup of the population only.

The meta-analyses to date have not been able to detect a long-term effect of manipulation in patients. This, in part, is due to the fact that most of the studies have not included long-term follow-up. There are two studies which have recently attempted to look at long-term effects. The paper by Meade et al (1990) compared the effects of hospital-based, outpatient, physical therapy department treatment with office-based chiropractic treatment and noted a small but detectable (7%) long-term effect on Oswestry scores over a 2-year period. Waagen et al (1990) also demonstrated a long-term (2 year) higher satisfaction rate with chiropractic care compared with care received from a family physician's office. The significance of these studies, however, is not clear but at least they raise the possibility that manipulation is of greater benefit than simple acute pain relief.

CHRONIC LOW BACK PAIN

Until recently there have been only a few studies on the effect of spinal manipulation therapy in patients with chronic low back pain and these are more difficult to interpret. Waagen et al (1986), for example, showed a statistical benefit from manipulation in patients with recurrent or chronic low back pain at 2 weeks, whereas Gibson et al (1985) failed to show such an effect in patients undergoing osteopathic manipulation. Evans et al (1978), using patients as their own controls in a crossover-designed clinical trial, showed diminished codeine use in patients undergoing manipulation and a trial by Ongley et al (1987) demonstrated that a group that received both rotational manipulation and proliferent injections showed significant improvement. It may be that, in patients with chronic back pain, the support of a physician and the relief, even if temporary, following manipulation serves to make the patients tolerate their pain and thereby reduce pain scores.

In a blinded randomized trial of patients with chronic back and neck complaints, Koes et al (1992a) state that manual therapy showed a faster and larger improvement in physical functioning compared to physiotherapy, treatment by a general practitioner and a placebo therapy. They also note that manipulative therapy was slightly better than physiotherapy after 12 months. And in a comparison of manipulation and mobilization of the spine with physiotherapy (i.e. exercises, massage, heat, electrotherapy, ultrasound and shortwave diathermy), Koes et al (1993) demonstrated that, for patients with chronic conditions (i.e. duration of 1 year or longer), improvement was greater in those treated with manual therapy.

Triano et al (1995) compared SMT with education programmes for patients with chronic low back pain. Greater improvement was noted in pain and activity tolerance in the manipulation group. Bronfort et al (1996) compared trunk exercise combined with SMT or non-steroidal anti-inflammatory drug therapy for chronic low back pain in a randomized, observer-blinded clinical trial. Each of the three therapeutic regimens was associated with similar and clinically important improvement over time that was considered superior to the expected natural history of long-standing chronic low back pain. In separate reviews of the literature, Koes et al (1996) and Van Tulder et al (1997) have identified a number of RCTs on chronic low back pain that are of sufficiently high quality to demonstrate a positive effect of SMT. These studies suggest that spinal manipulation can now be considered a reasonable approach to patients with chronic low back pain and that the effect might be greater if combined with exercise.

SCIATICA

There is a growing number of studies which have looked specifically at patients with sciatica. Although Nwuga (1982), Coxhead et al (1981) and Edwards (1969) all report improvement in certain outcome measures following manipulation in patients with sciatica, the significance of these studies is not clear. It appears from uncontrolled studies by Chrisman et al (1964) and Cassidy and Kirkaldy-Willis (1985) that patients with demonstrated disc herniation and sciatica do less well following manipulation than patients with back pain alone.

Several recent case studies have described successful treatment of patients with low back pain and sciatica in the presence of a confirmed disc herniation. Bergmann and Jongeward (1998) describe a positive effect on sciatica using a combination of flexion-distraction methods and side posture manipulation. Polkinghorn and Colloca (1998) prefer the use of a mechanical device (i.e. Activator Adjusting Instrument or AAI) to provide a manipulative force. Cox et al (1993) report on the successful reduction of an L5–S1 disc herniation through distraction manipulation technique and, in a separate study, Hession and

Donald (1993) describe the use of flexion distraction and rotational manipulation in the treatment of multiple disc herniations with thecal sac involvement. Zhao and Feng (1997) describe the treatment of a 12-year-old patient with a diagnosis of lumbar disc herniation.

In a prospective study of 27 patients with MRI-documented, symptomatic disc herniations of either the cervical or lumbar spine, 80% (22) of the patients reported a good clinical outcome and in 63% (17), there was either a reduction or complete resorption of the disc (Ben Eliyahu 1996). In a case series of consecutive patients in a postgraduate teaching chiropractic clinic from 1990 to 1993, 71 patients presented with low back pain and radiating leg pain clinically diagnosed as lumbar disc herniations. Subjective improvement reported by the patient, range of motion and nerve root tension signs were used to assess improvement. Of the 59 patients who received a course of treatment, 90% reported improvement. The authors conclude that non-operative treatment including manipulation may be effective and safe for the treatment of back and radiating leg pain (Stern et al 1995).

In studies on the use of manipulation in the presence of an intervertebral disc herniation, many of the authors indicate preference for the use of a modified manipulation procedure (Cox et al 1993, Polkinghorn and Colloca 1998, Polkinghorn 1998). However, in a review of data from a back pain clinic at the Royal University Hospital in Saskatoon, the authors conclude that side posture manipulation is both safe and effective for lumbar disc herniation (Cassidy et al 1993).

Based on the available evidence, it is not yet possible to unequivocally state that spinal manipulation is an effective treatment for disc herniation and sciatica. It is, however, a reasonable option which can be considered in the conservative management of such conditions.

NECK PAIN

After low back pain, neck pain and headaches are the most common complaints for which SMT has been recommended. This has primarily been based on descriptive clinical studies and large case series (see Bronfort 1992). These case series cover an extremely broad and often poorly defined group of patients with cervical and thoracic pain and cervicogenic and migraine headaches. These reports have been universally enthusiastic but without controls or even proper research protocols. There are, in addition, isolated case reports of patients with confirmed cervical disc herniation which responded to cervical manipulation (Ben Eliyahu 1994, Polkinghorn 1998).

The few prospective controlled clinical trials that have been performed have covered such a wide variety of conditions and outcome parameters that it is difficult to reach specific conclusions. Parker et al (1978) and Hoyt et al (1979) reported significant improvement in headache severity and frequency when compared to controls but not in all parameters which were measured. Brodin (1982) and Howe et al (1983) reported decreased neck pain following manipulation when compared with analgesics or no treatment. In addition, Howe et al (1983) described increased cervical rotation following manipulation on goniometric examination. Bitterli (1977), on the other hand, did not show a change in headache following mobilization in a small sampling of patients and Sloop et al (1982) failed to show improvement in neck pain following a single manipulation.

Hurwitz et al (1996) performed a structured search of four computerized bibliographic databases to identify articles on the efficacy and complications of cervical spine manual therapy. Two of three randomized controlled trials showed a short-term benefit for cervical mobilization in patients with acute neck pain. The combination of three of the randomized controlled trials comparing SMT with other therapies for patients with subacute or chronic neck pain showed an improvement of pain at 3 weeks for manipulation compared with muscle relaxants or usual care. The authors conclude that cervical SMT and mobilization probably provide at least some short-term benefits for some patients with neck pain and headaches. An analysis of the literature on all forms of conservative management of neck pain by Aker et al (1996) concluded that there had not been sufficient studies to adequately prove the effectiveness of any treatment approach. When, however, they combined the results of five trials on manual methods of treatment, they noted a positive effect at 1–4 weeks, equivalent to an improvement of 6.9 to 23.1 points on a 100-point scale.

Gross et al (1996) provide an overview of conservative treatments (i.e. drug therapy, manual therapy, patient education and physical modalities) in reducing mechanical neck pain. Twenty-four RCTs and eight before–after studies met their selection criteria. The authors conclude that, within the limits of methodologic quality (20 RCTs were rated moderately strong or better), the best available evidence supports the use of manual therapies in combination with other treatments for short-term relief of neck pain.

Cassidy et al (1992) compared the immediate results of SMT to mobilization in 100 consecutive outpatients suffering from unilateral neck pain with referral to the trapezius muscles. The patients received either a single high-velocity, low-amplitude, rotational manipulation (n=52) or mobilization in the form of muscle energy technique (n=48). The results show that both treatments increase range of motion, but manipulation has a significantly greater effect on pain intensity. Eighty-five per cent of the patients receiving SMT and 69% of the mobilized patients reported pain relief immediately after treatment. However, the decrease in pain intensity was greater (1.5 times) in the manipulated group. A randomized, prospective clinical trial by Jordan et al (1998) included 119 patients with neck pain of greater than 3 months' duration. The objective was to compare the relative effectiveness of intensive training of the cervical musculature, a physiotherapy regimen and chiropractic treatment. All three treatment interventions demonstrated meaningful improvement in all primary effect parameters.

Polkinghorn (1998) also describes the use of the AAI in the case of a cervical disc herniation that had failed to respond to manual manipulation of the spine. The author suggests that instrument-delivered adjustments may provide benefit in cases in which manual manipulation causes an exacerbation of the symptoms. Ben Eliyahu (1994) reports on three cases of patients with documented cervical disc herniations who responded to chiropractic management and manipulative therapy.

HEADACHES

Several recent studies have looked at the efficacy of SMT in the treatment of headaches. Nilsson et al (1997) report on a prospective, observer-blinded RCT. Fifty-three patients suffering from frequent headaches who fulfilled the International Headache Society criteria for cervicogenic headache (excluding radiological criteria) were randomized to two groups. Twenty-eight received high-velocity, low-amplitude cervical manipulation two times per week for 3 weeks. The remaining 25 received low-level laser in the upper cervical region and deep friction massage in the lower cervical/upper thoracic region, also twice weekly for 3 weeks. Results showed a statistically significant decrease in the use of analgesics (36%) in the manipulation groups, with no change in the soft tissue group. In addition, the number of headache hours per day decreased by 69% in the manipulation group, compared with 37% in the soft tissue group. Finally, headache intensity per episode decreased by 36% in the manipulation group, compared with 17% in the soft tissue group. The authors conclude that SMT has a significant positive effect in cases of cervicogenic headache. In a similar earlier study, Nilsson (1995) demonstrated a reduction in symptoms in all outcome measures following manipulation (i.e. daily analgesic use, headache intensity per episode and number of headache hours per day). Differences between the two treatment groups, however, failed to show any statistical significance from the controlled group.

Vernon (1995) reviewed the literature on outcome studies of chiropractic/manipulation for both tension-type and migraine headaches. Nine studies of manipulation for tension-type headaches reported quantitative outcomes. Of these, four were RCTs and five were case series designs. A total of 729 subjects participated in these studies, 613 of whom received SMT. Outcomes ranged from good to excellent. The studies cited indicate that manipulation seems to be better than no treatment and/or some types of mobilization and ice. It also seems to be equivalent to amitryptiline but with greater durability of effect than this medication. Only three studies on migraine headaches were identified, only one of which was an RCT. These studies reported on a total of 202 subjects, 156 of whom received SMT. Outcomes ranged from fair to very good. The author states that, although there is a limited number of studies regarding the efficacy of SMT in the treatment of headache, the overall results are encouraging.

Boline et al (1995) reported on a RCT comparing SMT to amitryptiline for the treatment of chronic tension-type headaches. The study consisted of a 2-week baseline period, a 6-week treatment period and a 4-week post-treatment follow-up period. One hundred and fifty patients with a diagnosis of tension-type headaches of at least 3 months' duration and a frequency of at least once per week were randomized into two groups: 6 weeks of SMT provided by a chiropractor; and 6 weeks of amitriptyline administered by a medical physician. During the treatment period, both groups improved at very similar rates in all primary outcomes (i.e. patient-reported daily headache intensity, weekly headache frequency, over-the-counter medication usage and functional health status). Amitryptiline therapy was slightly more effective in reducing pain at the end of the treatment period but was associated with more side effects. Four weeks after the cessation of treatment, however, the patients who received SMT experienced a sustained therapeutic benefit in all major outcomes in contrast to the patients who received amitryptiline, who reverted to baseline values. The sustained therapeutic benefit associated with SMT resulted in a decreased need for over-the-counter medication.

MECHANISMS OF PAIN RELIEF BY MASSAGE AND MANIPULATION

The exact mechanism by which massage and manipulation relieve pain has been the subject of a great deal of debate

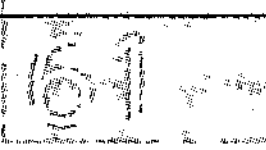

but relatively little experimentation. It has been the topic of two conferences sponsored by the National Institutes of Health (Goldstein 1975, Korr 1978) and the focus of discussion in many other conferences and articles. The problem, in part, has been the difficulty of isolating the primary cause of low back pain. For virtually every theory on the cause of spinal pain, there has been a corresponding theory as to how manipulation might reverse the pain-producing process. The following are the more prominent theories under debate.

CHANGE IN PAIN THRESHOLD

Since many of the effects of manipulation are immediate (Glover et al 1974, Hoehler et al 1981), the possibility that a manipulation may somehow increase the pain threshold has been raised. Terrett and Vernon (1984) attempted to investigate this phenomenon by measuring tolerance to electrically induced pain in paraspinal tissues before and after spinal manipulation and before and after inducing joint play. Both groups showed increases in pain tolerance but in the manipulation group the increase was significantly higher than in the group undergoing joint play. In order to investigate possible mechanisms for this phenomenon, Vernon et al (1985) analysed serum β-endorphin levels before and after chiropractic adjustments and reported a small but significant increase in subjects undergoing spinal manipulation. Christian et al (1988) and Sanders et al (1990), however, were not able to confirm these results.

RELIEF OF MUSCLE PAIN OR SPASM

One of the primary goals of many massage techniques is the relief of muscle spasm and the assumption that such spasm is painful. Anyone who has had a muscle massage will recognize that a good practitioner can find sore spots in muscles and the soothing effect of massage makes it a luxury much in demand. There has not, however, been much study as to what actually occurs. Cyriax (1971) has stated that deep friction separates adhesions and restores movement between individual muscle fibres. Wakim (1980) describes the effects of massage as relieving muscle fatigue from overexertion by improving circulation and removing waste products.

Spinal manipulation has similarly been considered to reduce muscle spasm. In this case it has been proposed that the sharp thrust of a manipulation results in stretch of the muscle and subsequently reflex relaxation of the muscle. A number of studies (Diebert & England 1972, Grice 1974, Grice & Tschumi 1985, Shambaugh 1987) report decreased muscle activity in patients after manipulation using surface muscle electrical activity measurement techniques. These studies all suffer from small sample size and methodological problems and are not conclusive. A recent study by Zhu et al (1992) reports normalization of magnetically induced muscle contraction cortical-evoked responses following manipulation and suggests that this may reflect changes in muscle spindle activity.

IMPROVED CIRCULATION

The theory that the effect of massage and manipulation is primarily on circulation has many supporters. The erythema that follows massage is presumed to be due to an increase in blood flow. A number of individuals have reported measuring increased circulation from various massage techniques (Skull 1945, Wakim et al 1949). This phenomenon in turn has been extrapolated to suggest that massage removes waste products and promotes healing.

The early research of Starling (1894), in which the role of muscle contraction on lymph flow was demonstrated, is often quoted to suggest that massage, passive motion and exercise may have their primary effect on lymphatic drainage. A few researchers (Elkins et al 1953, Wakim et al 1955) have demonstrated that massage and compression of an oedematous extremity can increase lymph flow and reduce oedema. Extrapolation of these theories to the massage of areas of tenderness in muscles and ligaments, however, has yet to be demonstrated.

REDUCTION IN DISC PROTRUSION

This theory, proposed by Cyriax (1971), was based partially on the observations of Matthews and Yates (1969) using epidural venography before and after manipulation. Many of the traction-distraction techniques have also been proposed on the basis of a presumed effect on the intervertebral disc (Cox 1980). There remains, however, considerable controversy concerning this theory. The clinical studies by Chrisman et al (1964) and Cassidy and Kirkaldy-Willis (1985) have demonstrated that patients with demonstrated disc herniation respond relatively poorly to manipulation. In contrast, several recent studies have provided support for the practice of using SMT in cases of intervertebral disc herniation (Cox et al 1993, Hession & Donald 1993, Ben Eliyahu 1994, Stern et al 1995, Bergmann & Jongeward 1998).

CHANGES IN POSTERIOR JOINT FUNCTION

Pathology of the posterior facets and its relationship to posture and leg length have been studied intensively by Giles and Taylor (1982, 1984, 1985). The discovery of intra-articular synovial protrusions with nerve endings containing substance P has led to the suggestion that protrusions may become entrapped within the joint, resulting in pain. Giles (1986) has suggested that manipulation may relieve this entrapment and any muscle spasm which results from it. This is by no means a new theory and has previously been postulated by a number of practitioners of manipulation, but without the anatomical studies of Giles and Taylor. Other anatomists (Bogduk & Jell 1985), however, are not as yet convinced that the anatomy is consistent with the ability of the posterior facets to entrap the synovial folds.

INCREASED RANGE OF MOTION

By far the most popular theory regarding the effect of manipulation is that it increases range of motion. This concept has been incorporated into the theories of chiropractic, medical, osteopathic and physical therapy practitioners of manipulation. Variations of Figure 61.1 can be seen in the literature of all practitioners of manipulative therapy. According to this theory, spinal or peripheral joint motion can become restricted and such restrictions can be detected by palpation and other examination techniques. This restricted motion has been referred to as a 'fixation' or 'blockage'. In a relationship between pain and range of motion (ROM) in the cervical spine, 100 consecutive patients were studied in a pretest/post-test design by Cassidy et al (1992). All patients had unilateral neck pain without neurological deficit and all received a single cervical manipulation. Fifty-two patients received a single cervical manipulation, while 48 received mobilization. The results showed an increase in all planes of post-treatment ROM and a decrease in post-treatment pain scores. The study suggests a significant relationship between a decrease in pain and an increase in cervical motion.

The restricted motion theory is based on the assumption that there are barriers which normally restrict range of motion. Figure 61.4 illustrates these presumed barriers and the proposed mechanisms through which they can be shifted under different pathological situations resulting in restricted joint motion. For example, the active range of motion can be restricted by muscle spasm or any other pathology which results in shortening of the muscle (Fig. 61.4, second line). The goal of treatment in this situation is therefore to relax or stretch the muscle. The passive range of motion may be normal and there may be little or no bony pathology.

The second method by which joint motion may be restricted is the shortening of ligamentous structures (Fig. 61.4, third line). The bony elements of the joint may be normal, but the joint cannot be passively moved through

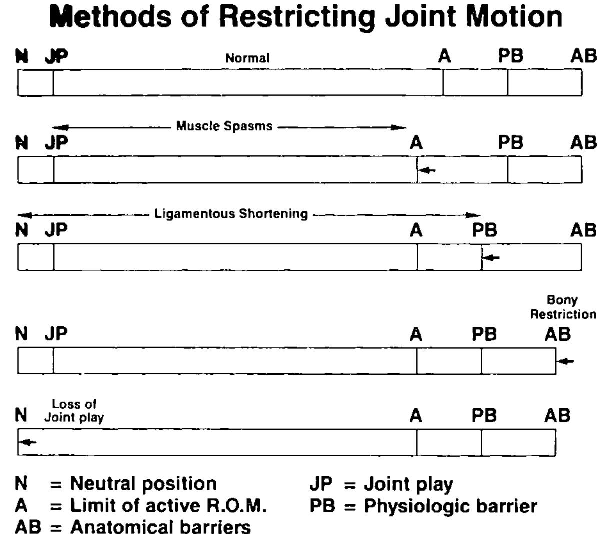

Fig. 61.4 The mechanisms by which a joint can become restricted (see text).

its normal range. The goal of treatment in this situation is the stretching of ligamentous structures to increase range of motion. The third mechanism by which joints can be restricted is through pathology in the bony elements themselves, primarily through degenerative spondylosis (Fig. 61.4, fourth line). It is generally assumed that manipulation will not result in any change in this form of restriction but instead is aimed at any concomitant ligamentous or muscular changes. The fourth mechanism by which motion is restricted is limitation of joint play in the neutral position or at some point in the range of motion (Fig. 61.4, fifth line). Such joint play is usually for accessory movements and may be in planes other than the direction in which a joint usually moves. Such accessory movements are felt to be essential for smooth motion of a joint. Treatment is directed at restoring the joint play. Combinations of these methods of restricting range of motion of a joint are also thought to occur.

The exact mechanism through which restricted motion can cause pain is not clear and is probably multifactorial. A totally fused joint is not generally painful, but spinal joints where manipulation is being considered are not completely fused. There is still movement in the joint which can stretch strained ligaments or pull on contracted muscles, resulting in pain. Restricted motion may also reduce nutrition to the intervertebral disc or joint cartilage, resulting in breakdown of these tissues and inflammation. The latter changes have been noted in peripheral joints which have been restricted in animals (Akeson et al 1980). Holm and Nachemson (1982) have demonstrated the importance of motion in intervertebral disc nutrition.

There is a growing body of evidence that manipulation can increase spinal range of motion. Many of the research trials used range of motion as one of the measures of successful treatment. Evans et al (1978), Rasmussen (1979), Nwuga (1982) and Waagen et al (1986) all demonstrated increases in the gross range of motion following manipulation of the lumbar spine. Howe et al (1983) demonstrated increased rotation and lateral flexion of the neck when compared to controls. It appears, however, from these studies that only certain directions of movement show increased range after manipulation. Jirout (1972a,b) reported changes in range of motion on X-rays before and after manipulation. Of particular interest in this regard is the paper by Fisk (1979), where straight-leg raising was noted to increase in patients with low back pain following manipulation, but not when manipulation was applied to asymptomatic patients. Buerger (1978, 1979) also demonstrated increased straight-leg raising after manipulation but only when pelvic rotation was used as an endpoint.

PSYCHOLOGICAL EFFECTS OF MANIPULATION

The growing recognition of the close relationship between psychosocial and psychological factors and back pain with its related disability has resulted in a closer look at the psychological effects of manipulation. This method has many advantages over other pain relief procedures. Most patients and their physicians who offer this modality have a strong, enthusiastic belief in the effectiveness of manipulation. Furthermore, there is confidence in physicians who use their hands to 'find' the pain and then apply a treatment directly to the painful area, especially when other physicians have looked at the pain from a distance. In addition, there is the soothing effect of laying on of hands and the natural empathy and concern which is commonly found in practitioners of manipulation.

There are now some data which actually document these changes. Kane et al (1974) were the first to demonstrate that patients were more satisfied when chiropractors took time to explain their opinions and make patients feel welcome. Hsieh et al (1992) have furthermore shown that not only are patients' confidence levels for massage and manipulation higher than for TMS and corsets, but also that the confidence levels increase with ongoing treatment.

EXERCISE

Exercise has long been a fundamental tool in the treatment of musculoskeletal pain and is one of the most commonly prescribed remedies for the patient with back pain (Hooper 1992). While a number of different exercise approaches are utilized, in general they are all targeted at the following objectives: decreasing pain, strengthening weak muscles, decreasing mechanical stress on spinal structures, improving fitness levels to prevent injury, stabilizing hypermobile segments, improving posture, improving mobility and 'when all else fails' (Jackson & Brown 1983). Another reason for using exercise, perhaps the most important of all, is to take the fear of movement away and provide patients with some element of control over their situation.

EXERCISE TECHNIQUES

There are a number of different schools of thought regarding the most appropriate technique or exercise method which should be utilized. Unfortunately, there are very few studies comparing the techniques and they are often recommended for their theoretical effect on the various musculoskeletal structures. The most divisive opinions surround the use of exercise for low back pain. A discussion of the different exercise approaches to this condition is therefore of interest.

Flexion exercises

It has long been assumed that there is a relationship between posture and back pain. Fahrni (1979) felt that a primary reason for the lower incidence of back pain in agrarian populations was the flexion of the spine seen upon assuming the squat position. Williams (1974) felt that back pain was largely due to the fact that modern man, in his attempt to stand erect, created an unnatural lordotic curve in the lumbar spine. He claimed that, in standing upright, man 'changes the weight distribution and badly deforms the entire spinal structure', thereby increasing the stress on the posterior aspects of the intervertebral disc.

Williams developed a series of exercises (Williams' flexion exercises) that dominated the world of back pain for many years. The principal goal of his flexion exercises was to reduce the lumbar lordosis and thereby eliminate back pain. This was accomplished by increasing the strength of the abdominal and gluteal muscles. Williams felt that the combination of these exercises would reposition the pelvis in such a way as to flatten the lumbar spine. In addition, he argued that flexion exercises would:

1. open the intervertebral foramen and facet joints;
2. stretch the hip flexors and back extensors;
3. free posterior fixations of the lumbosacral articulations (Williams 1937a,b).

Extension exercises

In contrast, McKenzie (1985) attributed the development of back pain, in part, to a loss of lumbar extension and to the frequency of flexion. He introduced a treatment protocol (McKenzie's extension protocol) that involved the use of exercises that employed extending the back. These exercises initially were targeted at producing extension of the lumbar spine. However, the ultimate goal of the McKenzie programme was a full range of motion in all directions.

Extension exercises may actually be divided into two basic categories: extension performed in a neutral or flexed position; and extension performed in a hyperextended position. The rationale for the use of extension exercises includes the following:

1. maintenance of the normal lordotic curves increases the ability of the spine to withstand axial loading;
2. extension improves the imbibition and fluid exchange of the intervertebral disc;
3. there is a correlation between strength of the back extensors and lifting ability;
4. many patients with low back pain have limited back extension;
5. prolonged flexion is associated with the onset of back pain (Jackson & Brown 1983).

Stabilization exercises

In the past few years, with the development of the Back School as a formal method of treating low back pain, the use of stabilization exercises has become popular (Saal 1992, Robison 1992). Terms such as 'stabilization training' and 'sensory motor stimulation' have been coined. The goal of stabilization exercises is to increase the role of the abdominal musculature in protecting the spine. Hyman and Liebenson (1996) state that stabilization exercises train a patient to control posturally destabilizing forces. They begin with identification of a functional range, i.e. the range of movement that is both safe and appropriate for the task at hand. According to the authors, the maintenance of a neutral spine position and functional range of motion are of primary importance in training patients presenting with back pain. Examples of such basic exercises include pelvic tilts, bridges, trunk curls and lunges.

Strength training

While there is not much agreement on which muscles need to be strengthened, the use of exercises to strengthen weak muscles is a common approach in the treatment of patients with back pain. Equally controversial is the best method of training. In recent years, the introduction of sophisticated strength-training devices using computer-assisted technology has become popular (Mooney 1979, Manniche et al 1991, Timm 1994). Dynamic, strength-training exercises use a variety of tools including:

1. isotonic progressive resistance exercise (PRE) in which the amount of force used is gradually and progressively increased;
2. isometric training (e.g. MedX) in which the back is exercised repeatedly using multiple angles of flexion and extension;
3. isokinetic training (e.g. Cybex) using a controlled speed of contraction and movement.

While there may be no clear winner in terms of the most effective form of strength training, the use of these precision and guided exercise programmes may have some advantage over other, less directed and less expensive programmes. It would appear that these programmes enable the patients with back pain to regain strength and function while providing sufficient feedback to encourage compliance.

Aerobic exercise

It has been suggested that lack of fitness may increase the risk of musculoskeletal injuries such as back pain (Cady et al 1979). Patients with back pain and other complaints often find that aerobic activities such as walking, cycling or swimming lead to a variety of positive changes in their conditions and their overall health. In a randomized controlled study of the use of walking versus other physical methods (heat, cold, massage, relaxation and distraction), Ferrell et al (1997) demonstrated that fitness walking can improve overall pain management in elderly patients with chronic musculoskeletal problems.

EFFECTIVENESS

Recently, a number of studies have attempted to evaluate the effectiveness of various exercise regimens for specific conditions. The results of this research have been conflicting, certain studies showing exercise to be effective while others have not demonstrated any significant effect.

In a blinded review of randomized controlled trials of exercise therapy for back pain, Koes et al (1991b) state that no conclusion can be drawn about whether exercise therapy is any better than any other form of therapy for back pain or whether any specific form of exercise therapy is more effective. A recent study (Malmivera et al 1995) compared the use of bedrest (2 days), back-mobilizing exercises and a control group consisting of the continuation of ordinary activities as tolerated. Patients with acute back pain were randomly assigned and outcomes and costs were assessed after 3 and 12 weeks. Contrary to expectations, there were statistically significant differences favouring the control group in both the duration of pain and pain intensity. The authors concluded that, for patients with acute low back pain, continuing with ordinary activities within the limits permitted by the pain leads to a more rapid recovery than either bedrest or back-mobilizing exercises. This may be due to the fact that those patients performing daily activities were more active than those exercising only at the therapist's office. Ferrell et al (1997) adds support to these findings by demonstrating that a simple walking programme could improve overall pain management and related functional limitations among elderly patients with chronic musculoskeletal pain.

The effect of exercise appears to vary with the chronicity of the symptoms. In a systematic review of randomized controlled trials, Van Tulder et al (1997) concluded that there was strong evidence of the ineffectiveness of exercise therapy for acute low back pain and for its effectiveness in chronic low back pain. Similarly, in a criteria-based review, Faas (1996) concluded that exercise therapy is ineffective for acute back pain, whereas exercise with a graded activity programme may benefit those with subacute back pain and intensive exercising may be of benefit for those with chronic pain.

A number of studies have looked at the value of specific exercise programmes with variable results. A recent study to evaluate the effectiveness of extension in the treatment of acute low back pain showed no significant benefit over conventional care (Underwood & Morgan 1998). Dettori et al (1995) compared the immediate effects of flexion and extension exercise on functional status, spinal mobility, straight-leg raising, pain severity and treatment satisfaction. Both exercise groups reported reduced disability scores at 1 week compared with controls. There was no difference between the flexion and extension groups at 8 weeks and none of the groups demonstrated any difference regarding recurrence of low back pain after 6–12 months. The authors concluded that there was no difference for any outcomes between flexion or extension exercises, but that either was more effective than no exercise at all. In a comparison of flexion and extension exercises, Elnaggar et al (1991) concluded that both flexion and extension exercises were equally effective in relieving back pain severity, but the flexion exercises had an advantage in increasing mobility in the sagittal plane.

Several investigators have attempted to evaluate the usefulness of stabilization exercises. O'Sullivan et al (1998) demonstrated a beneficial effect from a 10-week programme of specific stabilizing exercises in the treatment of chronic back pain with radiologic evidence of spondylosis or spondylolisthesis. The benefits of this exercise programme were maintained at 30 months. In a study of an intensive, specific programme using firm pelvic stabilization exercises designed to isolate and rehabilitate the lumbar spine musculature, Nelson et al (1995) demonstrated that 76% of patients completing the programme had excellent or good results. At 1-year follow-up, 94% of those patients who initially reported good or excellent results reported maintaining their improvement. Results in the control group were significantly poorer in all areas surveyed except employment.

Several studies have attempted to evaluate the use of dynamic strength-training programmes. Manniche (1996) claims that the most important factor which influences the effect of exercise in chronic low back patients is the administration of a high training stimulus (number of repetitions of the exercise, exercise resistance and the total number of sessions). He states that the poor results seen in many studies may be due to the low dosage or short duration of the exercise programme. In a study of exercise following first-time lumbar disc surgery, Manniche (1995) also noted that, while exercise programmes are generally free of side effects, high-dosage exercises with training periods lasting at least 12–16 sessions are of critical importance for success. Johannsen et al (1995) compared the use of two training models: intensive training of muscle endurance; and muscle training, including co-ordination. In both groups, training was performed for 1 hour twice a week for 3 months. Pain score, disability score and spinal mobility improved in both training groups without differences between the groups.

In a randomized, observer-blinded trial of intensive, dynamic back muscle exercises versus conventional physiotherapy, Hansen et al (1993) showed that subgroups of patients responded favourably to different treatments. Physiotherapy appeared superior for the male participants, whereas the female patients responded best to exercises. Exercises also appeared more beneficial for those patients with sedentary or light job functions. Whether these observations represent anatomical or physiologic differences or simply show patient preferences is not clear. In an attempt to evaluate the effect of various forms of exercise, the use of high-intensity, dynamic back extension and abdominal exercises was compared with a more traditional programme of mild, general mobility-improving exercises (Manniche et al 1993). Results indicate that patients who did the high-intensity exercises experienced greater results with regard to disability index and work capabilities. However, no significant differences were seen in pain or any objective measurements.

Manniche (1991) looked at the effect of dynamic back extensor exercises over a 3-month intensive training programme. One hundred and five patients were divided into three groups: an intensive training programme of dynamic back extensor exercises; a group which underwent one-fifth of the treatment group's exercise programme; and a control group in which treatment consisted of heat, massage and mild exercise. A statistically significant difference was found in favour of the treatment group at 3 months follow-up. The authors go on to state that those patients in the treatment group for at least once a week for the entire 1-year follow-up period were the only patients with any significant improvement.

One interesting study compared the use of trunk exercises in combination with SMT to exercises with non-steroidal anti-inflammatory drug (NSAID) therapy for patients with chronic back pain (Bronfort et al 1996). Two comparisons were made:

1. SMT combined with trunk-strengthening exercises (TSE) versus SMT combined with trunk-stretching exercises;
2. SMT combined with TSE versus NSAID therapy combined with TSE.

The authors concluded that all three of the therapeutic regimens were associated with similar and clinically important improvement and that trunk exercise in combination with either SMT or NSAIDs appeared to be beneficial.

The current literature on the use of exercise on patients with low back pain leaves much to be desired. This literature, however, suggests that:

1. there is a short-term positive effect from a variety of exercises;
2. those who exercise regularly have a better chance of maintaining any derived benefit;
3. there does not appear to be one particular form of exercise that is clearly superior to any other form;
4. intensity and frequency of exercise are probably more important than the type of exercise performed;
5. maintaining normal daily work and play activities by avoiding debility may be as effective as a formal exercise programme.

REFERENCES

Aker PD, Gross AR, Goldsmith CH, Peloso P 1996 Conservative management of mechanical neck pain: Systemic overview and meta-analysis. British Medical Journal 313: 1291–1296

Akeson WH, Amiel D, Woo S 1980 Immobility effects on synovial joints. The pathomechanics of joint contracture. Biorheology 17: 95–110

Ben Eliyahu DJ 1994 Chiropractic management and manipulative therapy for MRI documented cervical disk herniation. Journal of Manipulative and Physiological Therapeutics 17(3): 177–185

Ben Eliyahu DJ 1996 Magnetic resonance imaging and clinical follow-up: study of 27 patients receiving chiropractic care for cervical and lumbar disc herniations. Journal of Manipulative and Physiological Therapeutics 19(9): 597–606

Bergmann TF, Jongeward BV 1998 Manipulative therapy in lower back pain with leg pain and neurological deficit. Journal of Manipulative and Physiological Therapeutics 21(4): 288–294

Berquist-Ullman M, Larsson U 1997 Acute low back pain in industry. Acta Orthopaedica Scandinavica 170(suppl): 11–117

Bitterli J 1977 Zur Objektivierung der manual therapeutischen. Beeinflussbarkeit des spondylogenen Kopfschmerzes. Nervenarzt 48: 259–262

Blomberg S, Svardsudd K, Tibblin G 1994 A randomized study of manual therapy with steroid injections in low-back pain. Telephone interview follow-up of pain, disability, recovery and drug consumption. European Spine Journal 3(5): 246–254

Bogduk N, Jell G 1985 The theoretical pathology of acute locked back: a basis for manipulation. Manual Medicine 1: 78–82

Boline PD, Kassak K, Bronfort G, Nelson C, Anderson AV 1995 Spinal manipulation vs amitriptyline for the treatment of chronic tension-type headaches: a randomized clinical trial. Journal of Manipulative and Physiological Therapeutics 18(3): 148–154

Breen AC 1977 Chiropractors and the treatment of back pain. Rheumatology and Rehabilitation 16: 46–53

Brodin H 1982 Cervical pain and mobilization. Manual Medicine 20: 90–94

Bronfort G 1992 Effectiveness of spinal manipulation and adjustment. In: Haldeman S (ed) Principles and practice of chiropractic. Appleton and Lange, Norwalk, Connecticut, pp 415–441

Bronfort G, Goldsmith CH, Nelson CF, Boline PD, Anderson AV 1996 Trunk exercise combined with spinal manipulative or NSAID therapy for chronic low back pain: a randomized, observer-blinded clinical trial. Journal of Manipulative and Physiological Therapeutics 19(9): 570–582

Brunarski DJ 1984 Clinical trials of spinal manipulation: a critical appraisal and review of the literature. Journal of Manipulative and Physiological Therapeutics 7: 243–249

Buerger AA 1978 A clinical trial of rotational manipulation. International Association for the Study of Pain. Second World Congress on Pain. Montreal, Canada. Pain Abstracts 1: 248

Buerger AA 1979 A clinical trial of spinal manipulation. Federation Proceedings 38: 1250

Cady LD, Bischoff DP, O'Connell ER et al 1979 Strength and fitness and subsequent back injuries in firefighters. Journal of Occupational Medicine 21: 269

Cassidy JD, Kirkaldy-Willis WH 1985 Spinal manipulation for the treatment of chronic low back and leg pain: an observational study. In: Buerger AA, Greenman PE (eds) Empirical approaches to the validation of spinal manipulation. CC Thomas, Springfield, Illinois, pp 119–148

Cassidy JD, Lopes AA, Yong-Hing K 1992 The immediate effect of manipulation versus mobilization on pain and range of motion in the cervical spine: a randomized controlled trial. Journal of Manipulative and Physiological Therapeutics 15(9): 570–575

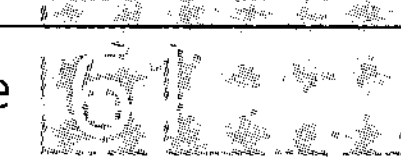

Cassidy JD, Thiel HW, Kirkaldy-Willis WH 1993 Side posture manipulation for lumbar intervertebral disk herniation. Journal of Manipulative and Physiological Therapeutics 16(2): 96–103

Chrisman OD, Mittnacht A, Snook GA 1964 A study of the results following rotatory manipulation in the lumbar intervertebral disc syndrome. Journal of Bone and Joint Surgery 46A: 517–524

Christian GF, Stanton GJ, Sissons D et al 1988 Immunoreactive ACTH, beta-endorphin and cortisol levels in plasma following spinal manipulative therapy. Spine 13: 1411–1417

Coplans CW 1978 The conservative treatment of low back pain. In: Helfet A J, Gruebel Lee DM (eds) Disorders of the lumbar spine. JB Lippincott, Philadelphia, pp 145–183

Cox JM 1980 Low back pain, 3rd edn. Self-published, Fort Wayne, Indiana

Cox JM, Hazen LJ, Mungovan M 1993 Distraction manipulation reduction of an L5-S1 disk herniation. Journal of Manipulative and Physiological Therapeutics 16(5): 342

Coxhead CE, Inskip H, Meade TW, North WRS, Troug JDG 1981 Multicentre trial of physiotherapy in the management of sciatic symptoms. Lancet 1: 1065–1068

Coyer AB, Curwen IHM 1955 Low back pain treated by manipulation: a controlled series. British Medical Journal March 19: 705–707

Cyriax J 1971 Textbook of orthopaedic medicine, diagnosis of soft tissue lesions, vol 1, 6th edn. Baillière Tindall, London

Dettori JR, Bullock SH, Sutlive TG, Franklin RJ, Patience T 1995 The effects of spinal flexion and extension exercises and their associated postures in patients with acute low back pain. Spine 20(21): 2303–2312

Dicke E 1953 Meine Bindegewebs Massage. Stuttgart

Diebert P, England R 1972 Electromyographic studies. Part 1: Consideration in the evaluation of osteopathic therapy. Journal of the American Osteopathic Association 72: 162–169

Doran DML, Newell DJ 1975 Manipulation in treatment of low back pain: a multicentre study. British Madical Journal 2: 161–164

Ebner M 1960 Connective tissue massage, therapy and therapeutic application. Williams and Wilkins, Baltimore

Edwards BC 1969 Low back pain resulting from lumbar spine conditions. A comparison of treatment results. Australian Journal of Physiotherapy 15: 104–110

Elkins EC, Herrick JF, Grindlay JH, Mann FC, DeForrest RE 1953 Effect of various procedures on the flow of lymph. Archives of Physical Medicine 34: 31

Elnaggar IM, Nordin M, Sheikhzadeh A, Parnianpour M, Kahanovitz N 1991 Effects of spinal flexion and extension exercises on low-back pain and spinal mobility in chronic mechanical low-back pain patients. Spine 16(8): 967–972

Evans DP, Burke MS, Lloyd KN, Roberts EE, Roberts GM 1978 Lumbar spinal manipulation on trial. Part 1: clinical assessment. Rheumatology and Rehabilitation 17: 46–53

Faas A 1996 Exercises: which ones are worth trying, for which patients, and when? Spine 21(24): 2874–2878

Fahrni WH 1979 Backache and primal posture. Musqueam Publishers, Vancouver

Farrell JP, Twomey LT 1982 Acute low back pain. Comparison of two conservative treatment approaches. Medical Journal of Australia 1: 160–164

Ferrell BA, Josephson KR, Pollan AM, Loy S, Ferrell BR 1997 A randomized trial of walking versus physical methods for chronic pain management. Aging (Milano) 9(1–2): 99–105

Fisk JW 1979 A controlled trial of manipulation in a selected group of patients with low back pain favouring one side. New Zealand Medical Journal 645: 288–291

Gibbons RW 1980 The evolution of chiropractic: medical and social protest in America. In: Haldeman S (ed) Modern developments in the principles and practice of chiropractic. Appleton-Century-Crofts, New York, pp 3–24

Gibson T, Grahame R, Harkness J et al 1985 Controlled comparison of short wave diathermy treatment with osteopathic treatment in non-specific low back pain. Lancet 1: 1258–1260

Giles LGF 1986 Lumbosacral and cervical zygapophyseal joint inclusions. Manual Medicine 2: 89–92

Giles LGF, Taylor JR 1982 Intra-articular synovial protrusions in the lower lumbar apophyseal joints. Bulletin of the Hospital for Joint Diseases Orthopaedic Institute 42: 248–254

Giles LGF, Taylor JR 1984 The effect of postural scoliosis on lumbar apophyseal joints. Scandinavian Journal of Rheumatology 13: 209–220

Giles LGF, Taylor JR 1985 Osteoarthritis in human cadaveric lumbo-sacral zygapophyseal joints. Journal of Manipulative and Physiological Therapeutics 8: 239–243

Glover JR, Morris JG, Khosla T 1974 Back pain: a randomized clinical trial of rotational manipulation of the trunk. British Journal of Industrial Medicine 31: 59–64

Glover JR, Morris JG, Khosla T 1977 A randomized clinical trial of rotational manipulation of the trunk. In: Buerger AA, Tobis JS (eds) Approaches to the validation of manipulation therapy. CC Thomas, Springfield, Illinois, pp 271–283

Godfrey CM, Morgan PP, Schatzker J 1984 A randomized trial of manipulation for low back pain in a medical setting. Spine 9: 301–304

Goldstein M (ed) 1975 The research status of spinal manipulative therapy. NINCDS Monograph no. 15, DHEW Publication no. (NIH) 76–998, Bethesda, Maryland

Goodridge JP 1981 Muscle energy technique: definition, explanation, methods of procedure. Journal of the American Osteopathic Association 81: 249

Greco MA 1953 Chiropractic technique illustrated. Jarl Publishing, New York

Greenland S, Reisbord L, Haldeman S, Buerger AA 1979 Controlled clinical trials of manipulation: a review and proposal. Journal of Occupational Medicine 22: 670–676

Grice AA 1974 Muscle tonus changes following manipulation. Journal of the Canadian Chiropractic Association 19(4): 29–31

Grice AA, Tschumi PC 1985 Pre- and post-manipulation lateral bending radiographic study and relation to muscle function of the low back. Annals of the Swiss Chiropractic Association 8: 149–165

Gross AR, Aker PD, Quartly C 1996 Manual therapy in the treatment of neck pain. Rheumatic Disease Clinics of North America 22(3): 579–598

Haldeman S 1978 The clinical basis for discussion of mechanisms of manipulative therapy. In: Korr IM (ed) Neurobiologic mechanisms in manipulative therapy. Plenum Press, New York, pp 53–75

Haldeman S 1980 Modern developments in the principles and practice of chiropractic. Appleton-Century-Crofts, New York

Haldeman S 1992 Principles and practice of chiropractic. Appleton-Century-Crofts, New York

Hansen FR, Bendix T, Skov P et al 1993 Intensive, dynamic back-muscle exercises, conventional physiotherapy, or placebo-control treatment of low-back pain. A randomized, observer-blind trial. Spine 18(1): 98–108

Hession EF, Donald GD 1993 Treatment of multiple lumbar disk herniations in an adolescent athlete utilizing flexion distraction and rotational manipulation. Journal of Manipulative and Physiological Therapeutics 16(3): 185–192

Hoehler FK, Tobis JS, Buerger AA 1981 Spinal manipulation for low back pain. Journal of the American Madical Association 245: 1835–1838

Hofkosh JM 1985 Classical massage. In: Basmajian JV (ed) Manipulation, traction and massage, 3rd edn. Williams and Wilkins, Baltimore

Holm S, Nachemson A 1982 Variations in the nutrition of canine intervertebral disc induced by motion. Orthopaedic Transactions 6: 48

Hooper PD 1992 Preventing low back pain. Williams and Wilkins, Baltimore

Howe DH, Newcombe RG, Wade MT 1983 Manipulation of the cervical spine – a pilot study. Journal of the Royal College of General Practitioners 33: 574–579

Hoyt WH, Schafter F, Bard DA et al 1979 Osteopathic manipulation in the treatment of muscle contraction headache. Journal of the American Osteopathic Association 78: 325–332

Hsieh CY, Phillips RB, Adams AH, Pope MH 1992 Functional outcomes of low back pain: comparison of four treatment groups in a randomized controlled trial. Journal of Manipulative Physiological Therapeutics 15(1): 4–9

Hunter J 1841 The complete works. Haswell, Barrington and Haswell, Philadelphia

Hurwitz EL, Aker PD, Adams AH, Meeker WC, Shekelle PG 1996 Manipulation and mobilization of the cervical spine. A systematic review of the literature. Spine 21(15): 1746–1759

Hyman J, Liebenson C 1996 Spinal stabilization exercise program. In: Liebenson C (ed) Rehabilitation of the spine: a practitioner's manual. Williams and Wilkins, Baltimore, pp. 293–318

Jackson CP, Brown MD 1983 Is there a role for exercise in the treatment of patients with low back pain? Clinical Orthopaedics and Related Research 179: 39–45

Jayson MIV 1986 A limited role for manipulation. British Medical Journal 293: 1454–1455

Jirout J 1972a The effect of mobilization of the segmental blockade on the sagittal component of the reaction on lateral flexion of the cervical spine. Neuroradiology 3: 210–215

Jirout J 1972b Changes in the sagittal component of the reaction of the cervical spine to lateroflexion after manipulation of blockade. Cesckoslovenska Neurologie a Neurochirurgie 35: 175–180

Johannsen F, Remvig L, Kryger P et al 1995 Exercises for chronic low back pain: a clinical trial. Journal of Orthopaedic and Sports Physical Therapy 22(2): 52–59

Jordan A, Bendix T, Nielsen H, Hansen FR, Host D, Winkel A 1998 Intensive training, physiotherapy, or manipulation for patients with chronic neck pain. A prospective, single-blinded, randomized clinical trial. Spine 23(3): 311–318

Kamanetz HL 1985 History of massage. In: Basmajian JV (ed) Manipulation, traction and massage, 3rd edn. Williams and Wilkins, Baltimore

Kane R, Olsen D, Leymaster C 1974 Manipulating the patient: a comparison of the effectiveness of physician and chiropractor care. Lancet 1: 1333

Kimberly PE 1979 Outline of osteopathic manipulative procedures. Kirksville College of Osteopathic Medicine, Kirksville

Koes BW, Bouter LM, Van Mameren H et al 1992a. A blinded randomized clinical trial of manual therapy and physiotherapy for chronic back and neck complaints: physical outcome measures. Journal of Manipulative and Physiological Therapeutics 15(1): 16–23

Koes BW, Bouter LM, Van Mameren H et al 1992b The effectiveness of manual therapy, physiotherapy, and treatment by the general practitioner for nonspecific back and neck complaints. A randomized clinical trial. Spine 17(1): 28–35

Koes BW, Bouter LM, Van Mameren H et al 1993 A randomized clinical trial of manual therapy and physiotherapy for persistent back and neck complaints: subgroup analysis and relationship between outcome measures. Journal of Manipulative and Physiological Therapeutics 16(4): 211–219

Koes BW, Bouter LM, Van der Heijden GJ 1995 Methodological quality of randomized clinical trials on treatment efficacy in low back pain. Spine 20(2): 228–235

Koes BW, Assendelft WJ, Van der Heijden GJ, Bouter LM 1996 Spinal manipulation for low back pain. An updated systematic review of randomized clinical trials. Spine 21(24): 2860–2871

Korr IM 1978 Neurobiologic mechanisms in manipulative therapy. Plenum Press, New York

Leboeuf-Yde C, Hennius B, Rudber E, Leufvenmark P, Thunman M 1997 Chiropractic in Sweden: a short description of patients and treatment. Journal of Manipulative and Physiological Therapeutics 20(8): 507–510

Lewith GT, Turner GMT 1982 Retrospective analysis of the management of acute low back pain. Practitioner 226: 1614–1618

Licht S 1978 History. In: Basmajaian JV (ed) Therapeutic exercise, 4th edn. Williams and Wilkins, Baltimore

Logan HB 1950 Textbook of Logan basic methods. LBM, St Louis

Lomax E 1975 Manipulative therapy: a historical perspective from ancient times to the modern era. In: Goldstein M (ed) The research status of spinal manipulative therapy. NINCDS monograph no. 15, DHEW Publication no. (NIH) 76–998, Bethesda, Maryland

Lomax E 1976 Manipulative therapy: a historical perspective. In: Beurger AA, Tobis JS (eds) Approaches to the validation of manipulative therapy. CC Thomas, Springfield, Illinois, pp 205–216

MacAuliffe L 1904 La therapeutique physique d'autrefois. Masson, Paris

Maitland GD 1973 Vertebral manipulation, 3rd edn. Butterworth, London

Malmivera A, Hakkinen U, Aro T et al 1995 The treatment of acute low back pain – bed rest, exercises, or ordinary activity? New England Journal of Medicine 332(6): 351–355

Manniche C 1995 Assessment and exercise in low back pain. With special reference to the management of pain and disability following first time lumbar disc surgery. Danish Medical Bulletin 42(4):301–313

Manniche C 1996 Clinical benefit of intensive dynamic exercises for low back. Scandinavian Journal of Medicine and Science in Sports 6(2):82–87

Manniche C, Lundberg E, Christensen I, Bentzen L, Hesselsoe G 1991 Intensive dynamic back exercises for chronic low back pain: a clinical trial. Pain 47(1): 53–63

Manniche C, Skall HF, Braendholt L et al 1993 Clinical trial of postoperative dynamic back exercises after first lumbar discectomy. Spine 18(1): 92–97

Matthews JA, Yates DAH 1969 Reduction of lumbar disc prolapse by manipulation. British Medical Journal 20: 696–699

Matthews JA, Mills SB, Jenkins VM et al 1987 Back pain and sciatica: controlled trials of manipulation, traction, sclerosal and epidural injections. British Journal of Rheumatology 26: 416–423

McKenzie R 1985 The lumbar spine: mechanical diagnosis and therapy. Spinal Publications, Wellington, New Zealand

Meade TW, Dyher S, Browne W, Townsend J, Frank AO 1990 Low back pain of mechanical origin: randomized comparison of chiropractic and hospital outpatient treatment. British Medical Journal 300: 1431–1437

Meade TW, Dyer S, Browne W, Frank AO 1995 Randomized comparison of chiropractic and hospital outpatient management for low back pain: results from extended follow up. British Medical Journal 311(7001): 349–351

Mennell J McM 1960 Back pain – diagnosis and treatment using manipulative therapy. Little, Brown, Boston

Mooney V 1979 Surgery and post surgical management of the patient with low back pain. Physical Therapy 59: 1000–1006

Nelson BW, O'Reilly E, Miller M, Hogan M, Wegner JA, Kelly C 1995 The clinical effects of intensive, specific exercise on chronic low back pain: a controlled study of 895 consecutive patients with 1-year follow up. Orthopedics 18(10): 971–981

Nilsson N 1995 A randomized controlled trial of the effect of spinal manipulation in the treatment of cervicogenic headache. Journal of Manipulative and Physiological Therapeutics 18(7): 435–440

Nilsson N, Christensen HW, Hartvigsen J 1997 The effect of spinal manipulation in the treatment of cervicogenic headache. Journal of Manipulative and Physiological Therapeutics 20(5): 326–330

Nwuga VCB 1982 Relative therapeutic efficacy of vertebral manipulation and conventional treatment in back pain management. American Journal of Physical Medicine and Rehabilitation 61: 273–278

Nyberg R 1985 The role of physical therapists in spinal manipulation. In: Basmajian JV (ed) Manipulation, traction and massage, 3rd edn. Williams and Wilkins, Baltimore

Nyiendo J, Haldeman S 1987 A prospective study of 2000 patients attending a chiropractic college teaching unit. Medical Care 25: 516–527

Ongley MJ, Klein RG, Droman TA, Eck BC, Hubert LJ 1987 A new approach to the treatment of low back pain. Lancet 2: 143–146

O'Sullivan PB, Twomey L, Allison GTJ 1998 Altered abdominal muscle recruitment in patients with chronic back pain following a specific exercise intervention. Journal of Orthopaedic and Sports Physical Therapy 27(2): 114–124

Ottenbacher K, DiFabio RP 1985 Efficiency of spinal manipulation/mobilization therapy. A meta-analysis. Spine 10: 833–837

Parker GB, Tupling H, Pryor DS 1978 A controlled trial of cervical manipulation for migraine. Australian and New Zealand Journal of Medicine 8: 589–593

Polkinghorn BS 1998 Treatment of cervical disc protrusions via instrumental chiropractic adjustment. Journal of Manipulative and Physiological Therapeutics 21(2): 114–121

Polkinghorn BS, Colloca CJ 1998 Treatment of symptomatic lumbar disc herniation using activator methods chiropractic technique. Journal of Manipulative and Physiological Therapeutics 21(3): 187–196

Pope MH, Phillips RB, Haugh LD, Hsieh CY, MacDonald L, Haldeman S 1994 A prospective randomized three-week trial of spinal manipulation, transcutaneous muscle stimulation, massage and corset in the treatment of subacute low back pain. Spine 15; 19(22): 2571–7.

Rasmussen GG 1979 Manipulation in low back pain: a randomized clinical trial. Manuelle Medizin 1: 8–10

Robison R 1992 The new back school prescription: stabilization training. Part I. Occupational Medicine 7(1): 17–31

Saal JA 1992 The new back school prescription: stabilization training. Part II. Occupational Medicine 7(1): 33–42

Sanders GE, Reinert O, Tepe R, Maloney P 1990 Chiropractic adjustive manipulation on subjects with acute low back pain: visual analog pain scores and plasma beta-endorphin levels. Journal of Manipulative and Physiological Therapeutics 13: 391–395

Schiotz EH 1958 Manipulation treatment of the spinal column from the medical-historical viewpoint. Tidschrift For Laegeform (NIH Library translation) 78: 359–372

Shambaugh P 1987 Changes in electrical activity in muscles resulting from chiropractic adjustment: a pilot study. Journal of Manipulative and Physiological Therapeutics 10: 300–303

Shekelle PG, Adams AH, Chassin MR, Hurwitz EC, Brook RH 1992 Spinal manipulation for back pain. Annals of Internal Medicine 117: 590–598

Skull CW 1945 Massage – physiologic basis. Archives of Physical Medicine 261: 159

Sims-Williams H, Jayson MIDC, Young SMS, Baddeley H, Collins E 1978 Controlled trial of mobilization and manipulation for patients with low back pain in general practice. British Medical Journal 2: 1338–1340

Sims-Williams H, Jayson MIC, Young SMS, Baddeley H, Collins E 1979 Controlled trial of mobilization and manipulation for patients with low back pain: hospital patients. British Medical Journal 2: 1318–1320

Sloop PR, Smith DS, Boldenberg SRN, Dore C 1982 Manipulation for chronic neck pain. A double-blind controlled study. Spine 7: 532–535

Starling EH 1894 The influence of mechanical factors on lymph production. Journal of Physiology 16: 224

States AZ 1968 Spinal and pelvic technics. Atlas of chiropractic technic, 2nd edn. National College of Chiropractic, Lombard, Illinois

Stern PJ, Cote P, Cassidy JDJ 1995 A series of consecutive cases of low back pain with radiating leg pain treated by chiropractors. Journal of Manipulative and Physiological Therapeutics 18(6): 335–342

Tappan F 1984 Massage. In: Wall PD, Melzack R (eds) Textbook of pain. Churchill Livingstone, Edinburgh

Terrett ACJ, Vernon H 1984 Manipulation and pain tolerance. A controlled study of the effects of spinal manipulation on paraspinal cutaneous pain tolerance levels. American Journal of Physical Medicine 63: 217–225

Thompson JC 1973 Thompson technique. JC Thompson, Davenport

Timm KE 1994 A randomized-control study of active and passive treatments for chronic low back pain following L5 laminectomy. Journal of Orthopaedic and Sports Physical Therapy 20(6): 276–286

Travell J 1976 Myofascial trigger points: clinical view. Advances in pain research and therapy 1: 919–926

Triano JJ, McGregor M, Hondras MA, Brennan PC 1995 Manipulative therapy versus education programs in chronic low back pain. Spine 20(8): 948–955

Underwood MR, Morgan J 1998 The use of a back class teaching extension exercises in the treatment of acute low back pain in primary care. Family Practice 15(1): 9–15

Van Tulder MW, Koes BW, Bouter LM 1997 Conservative treatment of acute and chronic nonspecific low back pain. A systematic review of randomized controlled trials of the most common interventions. Spine 22(18): 2128–2156

Vear HJ 1972 A study into the complaints of patients seeking chiropractic care. Journal of the Canadian Chiropractic Association October: 9–13

Vernon HT 1995 The effectiveness of chiropractic manipulation in the treatment of headache: an exploration in the literature. Journal of Manipulative and Physiological Therapeutics 18(9): 611–617

Vernon HT, Dhami MSI, Annett R 1985 Abstract, Canadian Foundation for Spinal Research. Symposium of low back pain. Vancouver BC, March 15–16

Waagen GN, Haldeman S, Cook G, Lopez D, DeBoer KF 1986 Short term trial of chiropractic adjustments for the relief of chronic low back pain. Manual Medicine 2: 63–67

Waagen GN, DeBoer K, Hansen J, McGhee D, Haldeman S 1990 A prospective comparative trial of general practice medical care, chiropractic manipulative therapy and sham manipulation in the management of patients with chronic or repetitive low back pain. Abstract, International Society for the Study of the Lumbar Spine, Boston

Wakim KG 1980 Physiologic effects of massage. In: Rogoff JB (ed) Manipulation, massage and traction, 2nd edn. Williams and Wilkins, Baltimore

Wakim KG, Martin GM, Terrier JC, Elkins EC, Krusen EH 1949 The effects of massage on the circulation in normal and paralyzed extremities. Archives of Physical Medicine 30: 135

Wakim KG, Martin GM, Krusen EH 1955 Influence of centripetal rhythmic compression on localized edema of an extremity. Archives of Physical Medicine 36: 98

Waterworth RF, Hunder IA 1985 An open study of ???diflunisal???, conservative and manipulative therapy in the management of acute mechanical low back pain. New Zealand Medical Journal 98: 327–328

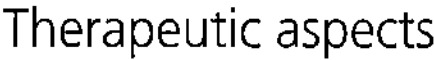
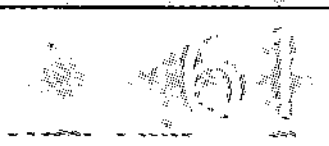

Williams PC 1937a Lesions of the lumbosacral spine. Part I. Journal of Bone and Joint Surgery 19: 343

Williams PC 1937b Lesions of the lumbosacral spine. Part II. Journal of Bone Joint Surgery 19: 590

Williams PC 1974 Low back and neck pain: causes and conservative treatment. CC Thomas, Springfield, Illinois

Wood ED 1974 Beard's massage principles and techniques. W B Saunders, Philadelphia

Zhao P, Feng TY 1997 Protruded lumbar intervertebral nucleus pulposus in a 12-year-old girl who recovered after nonsurgical treatment: a follow-up case report. Journal of Manipulative and Physiological Therapeutics 20(8): 551–556

Zhu Y, Starr A, Haldeman S, Seffinger MA, Su SH 1993 Paraspinal muscle evoked cerebral potentials in patients with unilateral low back pain. Spine 15; 18(8): 1096–1102

The placebo and the placebo response

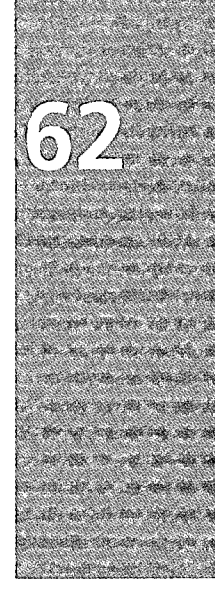

PATRICK D. WALL

I consider this topic to be at the heart of understanding pain. It is inevitably a complete paradox to classic theories of pain mechanisms that consider pain to be a reliable sensation signalling injury. The placebo is, by definition, inactive and yet produces analgesia. How can that be? I will review the various attempts to trivialize, dismiss or ignore the phenomenon and introduce a new proposal. However, before plunging into the depths, I will first discuss an issue which has come to dominate.

IS PLACEBO ANALGESIA MEDIATED BY ENDOGENOUS OPIOIDS?

In 1978, Levine et al published a truly stunning paper that reported that placebo analgesia was abolished by naloxone and could therefore probably be attributed to the release of endogenous narcotics. This paper had a widespread effect for two reasons. It converted a previously mysterious, magical phenomenon into one associated with objective pharmacology and therefore made the placebo respectable. Secondly, it was the first, and remains the only, demonstration of endogenous opiates influencing human pain. Obviously, such a crucial paper came under critical scrutiny. We found that naloxone by itself did not affect pain threshold or tolerance (El-Sobky et al 1979), but that could simply mean that normal people did not have a tonic output of endorphins. More importantly, others failed to repeat the results (Grevert et al 1983).

The reason for these contradictions was attributed to experimental design and, in particular, that the open administration of naloxone itself could be another placebo. This led to more subtle experiments where hidden naloxone administrations were added to overt placebos. Six such studies have been carried out and are analysed by Ter Riet et al (1998). Three show little or no effect: Grevert et al (1983), with a P value of 0.33, Posner and Burke (1985) P 1.0 and Gracely et al (1983) P 0.37. However, three sophisticated experiments do show a strong naloxone-induced reversal of the placebo: Benedetti (1996) P 0.001, Levine and Gordon (1984) P 0.003 and Benedetti et al (1995) P 0.004. While evidence is therefore growing that placebo analgesia may involve an opiate-dependent mechanism, these findings tell us nothing of the essential nature of a placebo or of the neural pathways that generate a placebo response. We will now turn to those problems.

THE WORD 'PLACEBO'

The word 'placebo' has been used since the 18th century as a term for mock medicine. Its origin and meaning are usually given as a simple translation from the Latin as 'I will please'. I find that a highly improbable use of Latin by educated men of the time who would actually have said '*Placebit*', 'It will please'. It seems to me much more likely that the word alludes to Psalm 116:9: '*Placebo Domino in regione vivorum*' which appears in the King James Bible as 'I will walk before the Lord in the land of the living'. This line beginning with Placebo is the first line of the vespers for the dead. Priests and friars badgered the populace for money to sing vespers for the dead. Placebo was the derisory word for these unpopular and expensive prayers just as the phrase *hocus pocus* comes from the first line of the Communion, '*Hoc est corpus*', 'This is the body (of Christ)'. This is surely the way in which Geoffrey Chaucer (1340) uses the word placebo when he writes: 'Flatterers are the devil's chaterlaines for ever singing placebo' as does Francis Bacon (1625): 'Instead of giving Free Counsell sing him song of placebo'. This adds a more subtle meaning to the word where the sycophant tells the listener what he expects and wants to hear rather than the truth. That remains a placebo.

Even where the placebo is not mentioned as such, ancient writers are clearly aware of the phenomenon. For example, Burton in 1628 writes in *The Anatomy of Melancholy* as follows: 'There is no virtue in some (remedies) but a strong conceit and opinion alone which forceth a motion of the humours, spirits and blood which take away the cause of the malady from the parts affected' and 'An empiric oftentimes, or a silly chirurgeon, doth more strange cures than a rational physician because the patient puts more confidence in him'.

EXAMPLES OF THE PLACEBO RESPONSE

SURGERY

Rather than attempt a definition of the placebo response at this stage, I will give a series of examples from which the essential nature of the response will appear. Surgery is rarely the subject of a placebo test in spite of an admonition by Finneson (1969) in *Diagnosis and Management of Pain Syndromes* where he states: 'Surgery has the most potent placebo effect that can be exercised in medicine'.

Angina

In the 1950s, it became a common practice to ligate the internal mammary arteries as a treatment for angina pectoris. Angina is a painful condition attributed to an inadequate blood supply of muscle in the heart wall. The rationale for the operation was that if the internal mammary arteries were ligated, the blood in these arteries, being dammed up, would find alternative routes by sprouting new channels through nearby heart muscle, thereby improving the circulation in the heart. This relatively simple operation was carried out in large numbers of patients to the satisfaction of many. However, the rationale came under suspicion when pathologists were unable to detect any of the supposed new blood vessels in the heart. Therefore, two groups of surgeons and cardiologists (Dimond et al 1958, Cobb et al 1959) decided to test the rationale by carrying out sham operations to incise the skin and expose the arteries in some patients while proceeding with the full ligation in others. The patients and their physicians did not know who had the 'true' operation and who had the 'sham'. The majority of both groups of patients greatly improved in the amount of reported pain, in their walking distance, in their consumption of vasodilating drugs and some in the shape of their electrocardiogram. The improvement in both groups was maintained over a 6-month period of observation. As an aside, it is obvious that no such trial would be permitted today for ethical reasons in spite of the fact that these tests were carried out for the ethical reasons of the day at Harvard and the University of Pennsylvania. The interest here is not only the evident power of the belief that therapeutic surgery had been completed but that improvement was sustained over at least a 6-month period in spite of the general belief that placebos have a brief and fading action.

Discs

Three invasive procedures are in common use as a treatment for herniated lumbar discs: injection of chymopapain or chemonucleolysis, percutaneous discectomy and open laminectomy. Reviews of these three procedures show little difference in outcome (Ejeskar et al 1983, Revel 1993, Alexander 1995). These are important reviews but not true placebo trials because the patients to be compared were not randomly selected, the observers were not blinded and no mock treatment was given. However, Fraser et al (1995) observed patients after 10 years who had either chymopapain injected or saline or an open laminectomy. The clinical outcome was similar and after 10 years there were still MRI signs of disc herniation in 43% of the chymopapain-treated group, in 33% of the saline group and in 38% of the laminectomy group. This approaches a placebo trial but since there was no comparable group with no treatment, it remains possible that the outcome would have occurred without invasive therapy.

Dorsal root radiofrequency lesions

In the past 20 years it has become common to treat chronic benign neck, back, arm and leg pains by lowering a needle into the region of the facet or dorsal root ganglion that had been shown to provide temporary relief if blocked with local anaesthetic (Sluyter 1981). Some 3–4000 patients receive this operation annually in Holland. In the standard operation, the needle tip is placed with radiological guidance and the tip is then heated to 70°C for 90 seconds. Since this tip temperature had been arbitrarily chosen, Slappendel et al (1997), in a double-blind, randomized study, compared 70°C with 40°C. There was no difference

 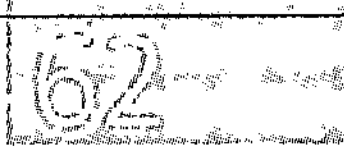

in the 3-month outcome, with 47% of the 70°C group having a substantial pain reduction compared to 51% in the 40°C group. One might conclude that the entire effect is no more than a placebo response since 40°C only warms the tissue. However, the authors admit that temperature cannot be the therapeutic agent but propose that the electrical current must be the effective action. This is their, as yet untested, guess but it emphasizes the problem of designing a truly physically inactive placebo. The current could have an effect although no such action is known or it could be that the tissue damage produced by the large needle could be active. As we shall see, the design of an acceptable placebo trial is subtle.

MEDICINE

Analgesics

Thousands of placebo trials have been carried out on analgesics since they are legally obligatory. The correct manner of such trials is discussed in Chapter 52. In a critical repeat analysis of five of their own trials, McQuay et al (1995) describe the problems of variability in such trials. Individual patient placebo scores varied from 0% to 100% of the maximum possible pain relief. The proportion who obtained more than 50% of the maximum possible pain relief with placebo varied from 7% to 37% across the trials while, with the active drugs, the variation was from 5% to 63%. Although trials are formally double blind, it is difficult or impossible to blind the physician's expectation (Gracely et al 1985) and this expectation affects the patient.

A special example of analgesia

Harden et al (1996) carried out a double-blind, randomized trial of injected ketorolac or meperidine or saline for acute headache crises. All three treatments produced a very significant reduction of pain (P 0.0001) but there was no significant difference between the three treatments. The reason for the surprise at these results is that both active drugs had previously been shown superior to a placebo in a number of trials. The difference in this paper was that the patients had presented themselves with an acute headache crisis to a busy urban emergency department and were therefore in severe need with a very high expectation of powerfully effective therapy. Their pain dropped from a severe level of 3.5 on the pain index to a mild 1.5 for all three treatments. This example emphasizes the general problem that trials are necessarily carried out on a selected restricted sample and that the situation differs particularly in the patient's expectation.

Narcotics

From the time of Lasagna et al (1954), there have been many comparisons of narcotic analgesia with placebo effects. The subtlety of the phenomenon of the placebo reaction and the skill needed to design an experiment are shown by Benedetti et al (1998). They examined 33 patients after the famously painful operation of thoracotomy and lobectomy for lung cancer. After the operation, the patients were given 0.1 mg buprenorphine boluses at 30-minute intervals until the pain was adequately reduced, which required up to six injections. The next day when their pain had returned to a high level, each was given a saline injection and the pain dropped an average of 2.5 points over 1 hour.

However, this paper included two considerable advances on previous papers. All patients had given informed consent. An additional 24 patients who had received the same operation and adequate pain relief from postoperative buprenorphine were given no treatment when their pain had reached the same level as the group who received a placebo injection. The pain level of this no-treatment group rose an average of 0.5 points during the 1-hour observation period. Therefore, the placebo group had a marked drop of pain while the no-treatment group experienced a pain increase. The second advance of this paper is that the authors examined the sensitivity of the individual patients to the narcotic and correlated this with their placebo response. Those patients whose pain was substantially reduced by small doses of buprenorphine were those who gave the largest placebo responses. Similarly, those patients relatively insensitive to small doses of buprenorphine gave small placebo responses. In another way of measuring the same effect, it was shown that the number of buprenorphine doses needed to establish adequate analgesia related to the strength of a single placebo response so that the strongest placebo reactors had required fewer doses of buprenorphine.

PLACEBO RESPONSES IN CONDITIONS OTHER THAN PAIN

There are many examples of placebo responses in pathological conditions such as asthma, diabetes, emesis, multiple sclerosis, ulcers and Parkinsonism. Similarly, mental states such as anxiety, depression and insomnia may respond. These are extensively reviewed in White et al (1985) and Turner et al (1980). *Nocebo* ('I will harm') responses occur when unwanted effects are reported after the administration of an inactive therapy. These even happen in trials of analgesics where the subject has been warned of possible side effects such as nausea, dizziness and headache. In 109 double-blind drug trials, 19% of healthy volunteers reported adverse effects after the placebo. There is a certain humour in these reports when one reads that coffee drinkers drinking decaffeinated coffee in a double-blind crossover study develop a tremor after both drinks and in a test for drunkenness, 27–29% of the subjects were intoxicated by flavoured water in a crossover study with flavoured ethanol (0.8 ml/kg body weight) (O'Boyle et al 1994). These reports are important because the responses have exactly the same general structure as analgesic placebo responses and yet can hardly all depend on a single mechanism such as the release of endorphins.

THE PLACEBO RESPONSE AS A SYNDROME

It is crucial to recognize that the placebo response is not just what the patient says and that it is therefore not just a cognitive phenomenon. In the paper described above in the study of narcotic placebo responses (Benedetti et al 1998), the patients were given narcotics intravenously postoperatively and their pain response was recorded, as was their respiratory depression. The patients were completely unaware of this respiratory depression. The placebo response produced both a reduction of pain and a reduction of respiration. In the no-treatment group, both pain and respiration increased. Furthermore, there was a correlation between the strength of respiratory depression produced by buprenorphine and the strength of respiratory depression produced by the placebo.

A much more surprising and important combined response is seen in the papers by Ho et al (1988) and Hashish et al (1988) in their study of the effects of ultrasound. They studied consequences of bilateral lower third molar tooth extraction: pain, inability to open the mouth (trismus) and facial swelling, anxiety and cortisol elevation. When the patients had recovered from the light general anaesthesia after 4–6 hours, ultrasound massage to the jaw was applied at a strength of 0.1 W/cm^2 or, in a double-blind fashion, the same was done with the ultrasound inactivated. After 24 hours, the reduction of pain was marked when there was no ultrasound, a placebo effect. More surprising is that the trismus was also significantly reduced in the placebo subjects. Trismus is a tonic flexion reflex of the jaw that cannot be over-ridden by voluntary effort. Most surprising was a highly significant decrease of the swelling of the face with the placebo. The swelling is a sign of the inflammatory consequences of tissue damage and surely not usually classified as a cognitive response. These examples show that the analgesic placebo response may include reactions other than the sensory report which form part of an overall injury and therapy syndrome.

FOUR REASONS FOR THE DISCOMFORT PROVOKED BY THE PLACEBO RESPONSE

QUACKERY

From the 18th century, the word 'placebo' became attached to quackery. As rational medicine developed, placebo could be used as a word to hammer Burton's 'empirics and silly chirurgeons'. Beyond this, even the rational physicians were not above the use of a placebo as a form of deception either for diagnostic purposes or to get rid of unwanted or unprofitable patients. This in turn provoked the ethical and practical discussion of whether the doctor–patient relationship would survive the discovery by patients that doctors used deception on occasions. There is a debate on the role of truth telling and paternalism in the clinic (Rawlinson 1985) with discussion of such concepts as 'the benevolent lie'. The ethical problem extends to clinical trials. If it is the doctors' duty to do their therapeutic best, how can they suggest that the patient should submit to a comparison of one therapy which the physician believes powerful versus another they believe less effective? 'Informed consent' by the patient does not solve this ethical question since it merely recruits the patient to join in the doctor's dilemma. As the awe and trust felt by the patient for the paternal doctor fade, so does the frequency of informed consent and of the placebo response. In 1807 Thomas Jefferson wrote: 'One of the most successful physicians I have ever known has assured me that he used more bread pills, drops of coloured water and powders of hickory ashes than of all other medicines put together – I consider this a pious fraud'.

A TIRESOME AND EXPENSIVE ARTEFACT

A considerable fraction of the huge cost of clinical trials for a new drug resides in the legal requirement for placebo trials. When a new idea has been developed by a clever research team, one has sympathy when their enthusiasm has to be put on hold while trials are in progress which have an apparently obvious outcome to the enthusiasts. Not only is the expensive delay blamed on a meddling bureaucracy but the existence of a fraction of patients who show placebo responses is considered to be of no intellectual interest but simply an intrusion in the search for true mechanisms.

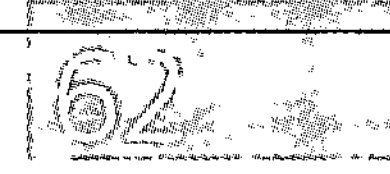

One attractive shortcut is to compare the new therapy with an established one without a placebo stage in a crossover trial. This, of course, does not face up to the possibility that both therapies might be placebos. The crossover option is particularly favoured in those therapies such as surgery or psychotherapy where there is no legal requirement for placebo trials. Often, an alternative therapy is not available or is so well known to the patients that it would be impossible to recruit volunteers who could openly assess differences between the two. An example is a massive study of long-term consequences of headache and backache after epidural anaesthesia during labour (MacArthur et al 1992) where the authors call for a randomized study to confirm their results. It is obvious that there is no alternative therapy which would be comparable with epidural anaesthesia in the mind of a patient. Furthermore, there are myriad cultural, educational, social, financial and medical reasons for a mother to accept or reject the offer to be assigned at random to one or another therapy, one of which was epidural anaesthesia. If there are very large ethical and practical problems in assessing the apparently straightforward question of long-term consequences of an epidural anaesthetic, it is not surprising that the majority of non-pharmaceutical therapies have never been tested or have been tested in very inadequate ways (Koes et al 1991, 1992). For example, in a large-scale survey of thousands of amputees with pain, Sherman et al (1980) identified 40 different forms of therapy but only 15% of the patients were relieved. In a search of the literature, no rigorous trials are reported to justify any of these 40 therapies for this condition. In two surveys of tests for the effectiveness of manipulation, osteopathy and chiropractic for pain, the great majority were shown to be inadequate while the acceptable trials produced contradictory answers (Koes et al 1991, 1992).

A QUESTION OF LOGIC

The very mention of a placebo trial is likely to be taken as a hostile questioning of the logic on which a therapy is based. To request an investigation of the placebo component which is an inevitable part of any therapy is to invite anger. Anger confuses the question of whether something should work with the question of whether it does work. Too bad.

THE REALITY OF THE SENSES

Everyone measures their own sanity by crosschecking their sensations with objective reality. On the rare occasions where there is a mismatch, special names are applied: hallucination, illusion, delusion, madness, drunkenness, etc. For anyone, there is a simple intuitive sense apparent on reading Descartes (1644):

> *If for example fire comes near the foot, the minute particles of this fire, which you know move at great velocity have the power to set in motion the spot of skin of the foot which they touch, and by this means pulling on the delicate thread which is attached to the spot of the skin, they open up at the same instant the pore against which the delicate thread ends just as by pulling on one end of a rope one makes to strike at the same instant a bell which hangs at the other end.*

It seems so reasonable that we should possess sensory mechanisms which represent the state of the world as reliably as the tolling of the bell represents action at the end of its rope. Furthermore, it seems equally obvious and reasonable that we should possess a separate entity, the mind, which can decide whether to ignore the bell or to write a poem about it. Even a philosopher like Bertrand Russell who questioned Cartesian dualism still required a reliable sensory apparatus which generated sensation as the closest representation of events which the machinery would permit. Sensation for him was generated by a continuous uncensored flow of information. If this flow was faulty, variable and haphazard, then even a great cognitive brain would necessarily be faulty. If the sensory apparatus was censored or corruptible, then sense could become nonsense and reality an individual construct of a particular mind. We have many reasons and facts which lead us to reject that conclusion. We trust our senses, the five senses of Aristotle. Pain appears to us as the sensation provoked by injury. A broken leg provokes an appropriate sensation and location of pain. This chapter discusses manoeuvres called placebos which in no way affect the leg and its fracture but modify the sensation of pain and its perception. No wonder the placebo response provokes a sense of discomfort, like a cold hand in the dark.

SPURIOUS ATTEMPTS TO AVOID CONSIDERATION OF THE NATURE OF THE PLACEBO RESPONSE

Given the four reasons for intellectual discomfort produced by the existence of the placebo response, it is not surprising that spurious reasons have been invented to dismiss the effect. These attempts signal the authors' dualistic conviction that the sensation of pain is a sign of a reliable injury signalling system in operation although the mind may add affective components to the basic sensation. Therefore, efforts to dismiss the phenomenon concentrate on errors of thinking that permit the subject to over-ride the true sensation.

MYTH 1: THE PLACEBO DIFFERENTIATES BETWEEN ORGANIC AND MENTAL DISEASE

This myth is the cruellest and most dangerous and is still proposed by old-school clinicians drilled in classic theory. An example is seen in the reaction of cardiologists to the improvement of angina following either true or sham ligation of the internal mammary arteries described above (Dimond et al 1958, Cobb et al 1959). Amsterdam et al (1969) described angina patients in whom there appears to be adequate circulation in the coronary arteries. With no evidence, it is assumed that these are the patients who would respond to a placebo while those with true coronary occlusion could not. Bluntly, this accuses those who respond to placebos of hysteria or, more politely, 'somatic hallucination' (Farrer 1964). This is a gross misuse of the term 'hysteria' (Merskey 1989) and implies that there are large numbers of patients who can mimic organic disease so perfectly as to confuse all but the most astute clinicians who can use a placebo trial to detect the fakers. The proposal is dangerous nonsense and has to dismiss the 968 papers reviewed in Turner et al (1980) on placebo responses in patients in pain appropriate to an overt organic lesion such as postoperative pain, cancer, etc. Furthermore, it has to ignore Beecher (1959) who reviews the literature showing placebo responses to be more common in postoperative pain than in experimental pain and to be more powerful in those in severe postoperative pain than in those with minor pains. There are large groups of doctors particularly anxious to apply the hysterical label to back pain patients in whom they can detect no peripheral lesion.

MYTH 2: THE PLACEBO IS THE EQUIVALENT OF NO THERAPY

This is clearly not true. The placebo can have a positive effect. We have already quoted an example (Benedetti et al 1998) where pain dropped with placebo therapy but rose with no treatment. It is crucial to know the natural history of a pain to assess if there has been a placebo response and to understand the nature of the condition. It is obviously difficult, for example, to compare the effect of a drug or a placebo or no treatment on an acute migraine episode where the pain will decline whatever is done. There are ethical and practical problems in observing the natural untreated history of any condition. Most journals now refuse to publish the course of a condition before a drug appeared compared with the course observed later when the drug was tested because so many factors may have changed. Hence, simultaneous random assignment is required in proper trials. A common scheme to achieve a no-treatment group is to assign patients to a waiting list. There are obvious limits, depending on the society and culture, which determine how long a patient will patiently remain waiting. The richer and/or more aggressive patients or those who are in particular misery remove themselves from the waiting list and go to another doctor, thereby tilting the nature of the remaining patients. In a recent New York trial of an AIDS drug, blood tests on the no-treatment group showed that many had obtained the drug on the black market. Adequate trials must establish three quite separate factors: natural history, placebo responses, specific responses (Finkel 1985) and this requires subtle methods (see Chapter 52).

MYTH 3: A FIXED FRACTION OF PATIENTS RESPOND TO PLACEBOS

This myth is widely stated in papers and textbooks, with the figure of 33% being commonly quoted. The idea is clearly to label a fraction of the population as mentally peculiar. Where these sources quote the origin of the myth, they refer to Beecher (1955) who indeed gives the figure of 35.2%. However, had they bothered to read the paper, they would have found that this figure is an average of Beecher's own 11 studies, each of which varied widely from the average. Scanning a large number of double-blind studies shows the fraction of placebo responders varying from close to 0% (Tyler 1946) to near 100% (Liberman 1964, Harden et al 1996) depending on the circumstance of the trial. Clinical pains are associated with a larger number of placebo responders than experimental pains (Beecher 1959). The subtlety of the conditions has commercial as well as theoretical interest. Capsules containing coloured beads are more effective than coloured tablets, which are superior to white tablets (Buchaleq & Coffield 1982). Beyond this, intramuscular saline injections are superior to any tablet but inferior to intravenous injections. Tablets taken from a bottle labelled with a well-known brand name are superior to the same tablets taken from a bottle with a typed label. My favourite is a doctor who always handled placebo tablets with forceps, assuring the patient that they were too powerful to be touched by hand. On a much more serious level, we will be discussing the conversion of experimental subjects to placebo responders (Voudouris et al 1989, 1990). There is no fixed fraction of the population who respond to placebos.

MYTH 4: PLACEBO RESPONDERS HAVE A SPECIAL MENTALITY

This proposal is an extension of the fixed fraction myth. It proposes that there are groups in the population with distorted mental processes which lead them to confuse true therapies with placebos. For those who cannot imagine that a normal person would ever make such a mistake, the idea is attractive. It was first proposed by Beecher (1968) and promptly dropped. With the rise of personality psychology, there were any number of pejorative mental tendencies which could be detected in the population by the analysis of the answers to questionnaires. Some of these seemed attractive labels to hang on those who responded to placebos to differentiate them from the normal who would never make such a silly mistake. These labels include suggestibility, hypnotizability, neurotic, extrovert, introvert, acquiescent, desire to please, lack of sophistication, acceptance of authority and so on and on. There are 36 papers on the topic in Turner et al (1980) and many more in White et al (1985). Most papers report no correlations with personality type and the rest are contradictory.

MYTH 5: PAIN IS A MULTIDIMENSIONAL EXPERIENCE AND THE PLACEBO AFFECTS ONLY A FRACTION

The previous four diversions are crude myths designed to defend the indefensible. We now enter a more subtle arena. In the modern era, Beecher (1959) made an intuitive, introspective, commonsense division of the personal reaction to pain as having two separable dimensions: one deals with intensity and the other with reaction. Needless to say, there is more than a whiff here of Cartesian sensation followed by perception. Melzack and Casey (1968) even assigned different parts of the brain to create these two dimensions, which gave a new respectability to this ancient introspective idea. Melzack and Torgerson (1971) then analysed the way in which people used words about pain and derived three dimensions: sensory, affective and evaluative. From this, the widely used McGill Pain Questionnaire evolved.

By now, four dimensions have been isolated (Holroyd et al 1992). It would seem entirely reasonable to examine the placebo response to discover if all dimensions of pain were equally involved. This was done by Gracely et al (1978) and Gracely (1979). They used volunteer experimental normal subjects who received gradually rising electrical shocks to the teeth. The subjects were asked to rate separately the intensity of the pain and the unpleasantness of the pain, i.e. Cartesian sensation and perception or Beecher's intensity and reaction or Melzack's sensation and affect. The subjects were then given a saline injection with the assurance that they were receiving a powerful analgesic. The results are absolutely clear. The intensity of the pain was completely unaffected while at low shock levels the unpleasantness was markedly reduced but at higher intensities was unaffected. This important experiment would seem to bring us back to the most classic position. Sensation as a body mechanism is unaffected by a placebo at any stimulus level. Minor unpleasantness as a mental perception is affected by the mental suggestion implicit in the presence of a placebo. When the stimulus intensity rises, the appropriate unpleasant perception regains its proper place in spite of implied suggestion from the placebo. These clear experiments would seem to remove the mystery from the placebo and to return the entire subject to classical dualism. Gracely et al (1978) went on to show that diazepam, a tranquillizer, could produce exactly the same effect, i.e. intensity was unaffected but low levels of unpleasantness were reduced.

Up to this point one could say that the experiments support a particular version of Cartesian dualism in which there is a reliable sensory apparatus unaffected by these manipulations and that sensation is observed by a mental apparatus which assigns unpleasantness to the pure sensation and which is subject to suggestion and to tranquillizers.

However, Gracely et al (1979) then investigated the effect of fentanyl, a narcotic, on the same type of pain and the result is summarized in the title 'Fentanyl reduces the intensity but not the unpleasantness of painful tooth sensations'. It will be seen that this result abolishes the idea that a reliable sensory apparatus feeds a dependent mental apparatus which assigns unpleasantness. The three experiments taken together suggest with some power that there are two independent dimensions, intensity and unpleasantness, which can be manipulated independently. However, we must now return and ask if the placebo result, i.e. intensity is unaffected but low-level unpleasantness is affected, can be taken as a general statement about analgesic placebos. The first prediction would be that placebos would work on minor pains but not on severe pains but that is precisely the opposite of Beecher's (1955, 1968) observations and those of Lasagna et al (1954). The second prediction is that patients responding to a placebo would report the pain intensity unchanged while the unpleasantness is relieved but the fact is that patients with migraine or postoperative pain or cancer report relief of both aspects. Furthermore, even in experimental situations such as those of Voudouris et al (1989, 1990), both threshold and intensity are affected by placebos. My conclusion is that the identification of separate categories of pain experience is a valid and useful aspect of pain study but that the placebo effect can change these dimensions separately or together depending on the circumstances of suggestion, expectation and instruction (see Price & Fields 1997).

MYTH 6: THE PLACEBO EFFECT MAY BE DISSECTED AWAY TO REVEAL THE PURE THERAPEUTIC ACTION

For this to be true, the therapeutic effect of an active compound would have to be free of its own additional placebo component. Strong evidence shows that the two responses are not separable in practical tests. In an extensive series of tests on postoperative pain, Lasagna et al (1954) had identified placebo reactors and non-reactors. They then gave a fixed dose of morphine to the two groups and found an adequate analgesic response in 95% of the placebo reactors and only 55% of the non-reactors. A much more subtle problem was revealed by Beecher (1968) on examination of the matrix of results from double-blind crossover studies of morphine versus saline. If, by chance, the first administration contained morphine, the patient learned that this trial involved powerful medicine and tended to give a strong response to the second administration which was saline. The reverse was also true, i.e. if the first test dose was saline, the response to the second which contained morphine was weak. It is obvious that this problem will also affect the results of trials where the relative effects of two active compounds are being compared. There will be a carry-over effect of the first trial to the results of the second.

It is apparent that the patient or subject is searching for subtle hints of what to expect and that these expectations affect responses. This raises the question of the comparable nature of the active test and the placebo test. It does not take a great connoisseur to differentiate between intravenous morphine and saline since the morphine produces such obvious immediate side effects such as headache, nausea, dizziness, etc. This problem has led to the use of placebos which produce some obvious effect such as vasodilatation which are assumed to have no direct therapeutic effect but give the subject an impression of receiving powerful medicine. Clearly, the introduction of active placebos produces a series of problems: the placebo and active compound rarely precisely mimic each other; the specific inactivity of the placebo is questionable; the patient may find the placebo's side effects distasteful. If there are serious problems in drug testing, they obviously escalate with other forms of therapy. What is a comparable manoeuvre against which to test acupuncture?

In summary, these six myths were failed attempts to separate the placebo response from the response to 'rational' therapy. There has been no successful demonstration that the nature of placebo-induced analgesia differs from a matched 'rational' therapy. The placebo response mechanism is contained in exactly the same mechanism responsible for the analgesic effect of drugs and is not a separate process.

For humans, aware that therapy is in progress, the 'true' effect of the therapy necessarily combines with the expected. The strength of response to a narcotic correlates with the strength of response to a placebo and both produce the same strength side effects on respiration (Benedetti et al 1998).

CLASSES OF EXPLANATION

AFFECTIVE

Gracely et al (1978) originally proposed that the placebo effect works only on the unpleasantness of pain while leaving the intensity dimension unaffected. We have given reasons above, in Myth 5, to believe that their experiments represent a special case which does not apply across the board, especially in clinical cases. Evans (1974), in another version of this approach, proposes that the placebo operates by decreasing anxiety. However, the results show that there is a weak and variable interaction with various types of anxiety and it is not clear that anxiety reduction is not a component of the placebo effect rather than the cause of it. Montgomery and Kirsch (1996) review and discard emotional theories to explain placebos and favour cognitive-expectation mechanisms.

COGNITIVE

By far the commonest proposal is that the placebo effect depends on the expectation of the subject. There is nothing subtle about this. Placebo reactors can be identified before the trial by simply asking the subject what they expect to be the outcome of the therapy. Those who doubt that a therapy will be effective do not respond to the placebo while those with high expectations do. The very extensive literature on this is reviewed by Bootzin (1985). Lasagna et al (1954) investigated many aspects of postoperative patients who responded to placebos and to analgesic drugs and conclude: 'A positive placebo response indicated a psychological set predisposing to anticipation of pain relief'. They add: 'It is important to appreciate that this same anticipation of pain relief also predisposes to better response, to morphine and other pharmacologically active drugs'. In a trial of two drugs versus placebos on 100 patients, Nash and Zimring (1969) tested specifically for the role of expectation. The two drugs had no effect which would differentiate them from the placebo but there was a strong correlation between the measured expectation and the placebo effect. Expectation is given a number of related names – belief, faith, confidence, enthusiasm, response bias, meaning, credibility, transference, anticipation, etc. – in 30 of the papers in the bibliography of Turner et al (1980).

Expectation is a learned state and therefore young children do not respond to placebos as adults do since they have had neither the time nor the experience to learn. Similarly in adults, the learning of expected effects will depend on culture, background, experience and personality. A desire to believe, please and obey the doctor will increase the effect while hostility decreases it. Obviously, part of the expectation of the patient will depend on the expectation, enthusiasm and charisma of the therapist and therefore there are many reports on this doctor–patient interaction. Expectation in a laboratory experiment may be more limited than in a clinical setting, which may explain why rates and intensities of placebo effects tend to be less in the laboratory than in the clinic (Beecher 1959).

CONDITIONING

There are many reports of drug anticipatory responses in animals (Hernstein 1965, Siegel 1985). These come in two forms. In the first, the animal has been given one or more trials on an active drug and is then subject to a saline injection and proceeds to mimic the behavioural or physiological response which was observed after the active drug. In the second type, the animal mimics the counteractions which it mobilizes to neutralize the effect of the active compound. For example, if animals have experienced a series of injections of insulin which lower the blood sugar, a saline injection in the same setting as the insulin injection results in a rise of blood sugar which would be one of the animal's reactions to counteract the insulin-induced decrease (Siegel 1975). In cultures not raised on *Winnie the Pooh, Wind in the Willows* and *Watership Down*, it is customary to deny animals the luxury of cognitive processing and to ascribe such phenomena to classic Pavlovian conditioning.

This led to the proposal that the human placebo response had the characteristics of a conditioned response (Wickramasekera 1980, Reiss 1980). The idea is that active powerful drugs produce a powerful objective physiological response in the same manner that food produces salivation – the unconditioned stimuli and responses. However, giving the drug is inevitably inadvertently associated with a pattern of other stimuli such as a hypodermic injection by a man in a white coat. It is proposed that these are the equivalent of unconditioned stimuli coupled with the conditioned stimulus. It is then proposed that if these incidentally coupled stimuli are given alone, they will provoke the same response as the original drug, just as in the dog, coupling a bell with food eventually leads to the ability of the bell by itself to provoke salivation. The similarity goes beyond the proposed production of a conditioned response. If a placebo is given repeatedly in some but not all trials, the effect declines. This is a characteristic of Pavlovian responses where simple repeated ringing of the bells leads to a steady decline of the salivation unless the conditioning is reinforced by occasional coupling of the bell with food.

The question of a decreased effectiveness of placebos on repeated application has an obviously important practical aspect if placebos were to be used in a constructive fashion. They have rarely been tested in this way. A very long-term effect of a sham ligation of the internal mammary arteries has been described above. Montgomery and Kirsch (1997) show an increasing effectiveness of repeated placebo applications in an experimental situation. Since most patients expect medication to have a long-term decreasing effect and since the placebo response is locked to patient expectation, this by itself could lead to diminishing placebo responses.

All such comparisons between widely differing processes lead to argument about similarities and differences, identities and analogies (Wall & Safran 1986). However, the idea led to a series of clever experiments by Voudouris et al (1989, 1990). The first stage of this work was a repeat of a type of trial which had been reported many times before. Volunteer subjects were given rising electric shocks and the current was established in full view of the subject. The experiments determined the level at which the shock became painful and the level at which it become intolerable. Then a bland cream was rubbed on the area, the subjects were assured that it was a powerful anaesthetic and the shock trial was run a second time. A small fraction of the subjects demonstrated a placebo response by reporting pain and intolerable pain at a higher shock level than they had on the first trial. This part of the experiment is of no general interest but it established the placebo response rate in these particular circumstances. They then started again with a new group of subjects and determined their threshold and tolerance shock levels. The cream was applied and now came the clever and novel part of the experiment; the strength of the electric shocks was secretly reduced unknown to the subject and observer. When the trial was now run, the subject observed that much higher numbers on the shock machine were achieved before pain was felt and before the pain reached the tolerance limit. These subjects believed that they had tested on themselves the truth of the remarkable anaesthetic properties of the cream. Next, after one such apparent demonstration of the efficacy of the cream, a trial was run in the original conditions, i.e. the strength of current was returned to its original level. The cream was put on and the shock level raised. On this trial large numbers of the subjects became placebo reactors. The only difference in these newly produced placebo responders was that they had 'experienced' in some fashion the apparently 'true' anaesthetic properties of the cream. Clearly, this result can have important practical implications. Whether the change in the subjects was cognitive or conditioned must remain an issue for debate and further experiment. Brewer (1974) concludes that 'There is no convincing evidence for operant or classical conditioning in adult humans' which is free of cognitive awareness of the situation. It may be that the passionately maintained differences between cognitive and conditioned responses may collapse on each other.

The question of whether the so-called conditioned placebo response contains a cognitive component has been approached in a very clever way by Montgomery and Kirsch 1997 (but see Staats et al 1998 and Kirsch & Montgomery 1998). They repeated the Voudouris et al (1990) experiment with the same results but added a crucial group, who were verbally informed that the applied cream was not anaesthetic; this group failed to produce placebo responses. The importance of this strange but subtle experiment is that the subjects had experienced precisely the same shocks as the group who did become placebo responders. There are those, such as Price and Fields (1997), and unlike Brewer (1974), who believe that conditioning involves subconscious non-cognitive mechanisms. In the Kirsch and Montgomery experiments, the groups who failed to produce a placebo response had received all the same stimuli during the training trials except that they had been verbally informed that the cream was inert. Therefore they conclude that the placebo response was not simply learned by the pairing of stimuli with response but needed a verbally induced change of expectation.

A NEW PROPOSAL. THE PLACEBO IS NOT A STIMULUS BUT AN APPROPRIATE RESPONSE

It is fatuous to regard a placebo as a stimulus in the ordinary sense of that word. By definition, if a placebo is administered in complete secrecy so that the patient is unaware that anything has been done, there is no reaction. An example would be the covert injection by way of a long line from a hidden source of saline of which the patient has no knowledge and to which the patient does not react. If the placebo is not a stimulus in this sense, what is it? In the introduction to the third edition of this textbook, I proposed that sensation was appropriate to the overall situation. In the introduction to this edition, I have extended that idea to propose that sensation is not simply a report of a stimulus but an awareness of possible appropriate action. It is proposed that the sensation of pain is an awareness of a series of need states. The phrase 'need state' is used in contemporary psychology to replace the old word 'drive'. It is used particularly for reactions such as hunger and thirst which, like pain, show such a poor correlation with any objective stimulus. The onset of pain is associated with active avoidance in an attempt to abolish the stimulus. After the avoidance phase, a complex series of events start up to optimize the prevention of further damage. They include muscle contractions to splint the painful area and to guard the area. There follows the phase optimal for recovery, including rest and immobility and, in the case of humans, the seeking of aid and therapy. Therapy for an animal may be limited to licking the painful area but, for us, our personal experience and culture have added an elaborate array of potential actions. It is proposed that pain at this stage is a need state in need of appropriate therapy. Need states such as hunger, thirst, itching and nausea are terminated by consummatory action. The need state of pain is hopefully terminated by taking the appropriate action, i.e. by seeking and accepting an apparently appropriate therapy. The sensation of the need state disappears once consummation is complete. This places the placebo in the category of appropriate response rather than as an appropriate stimulus.

REFERENCES

Alexander AH 1995 Chemonucleolysis for acute disc herniation. Journal of Musculoskeletal Medicine 12: 13–24

Amsterdam EA, Wolfson S, Garlin R 1969 New aspects of the placebo response in angina pectoris. American Journal of Cardiology 24: 305–306

Beecher HK 1955 The powerful placebo. Journal of the American Medical Association 159: 1602–1606

Beecher HK 1959 Measurement of subjective responses. Oxford University Press, New York

Beecher HK 1968 Placebo effects: a quantitative study of suggestibility. In: Beecher H.K. (ed) Non-specific factors in drug therapy. CC Thomas, Springfield, pp 27–39

Benedetti F 1996 The opposite effects of naloxone and proglumide on placebo analgesia. Pain 64: 535–543

Benedetti F, Amanzio M, Maggi G (1995) Potentiation of placebo analgesia by proglumide. Lancet 346: 1231

Benedetti F, Amanzio M, Baldi S, Casadio C, Cavallo A (1998) The specific effects of prior opioid exposure on placebo analgesia and placebo respiratory depression. Pain 75: 313–319

Bootzin RR (1985) The role of expectancy in behaviour change. In: White LP, Tursky B, Schwarz GE (eds) Placebo: theory, research and mechanisms. Guilford Press, New York

Brewer WF (1974) There is no convincing evidence for operant or classical conditioning in adult humans. In: Weiner WB, Palermo DS (eds) Cognition and the symbolic processes. Wiley, New York, pp 1–42

Buchaleq LW, Coffield KE 1982 An investigation of drug expectancy as a function of colour, size and preparation. Journal of Clinical Pharmacology 2: 245–248

Cobb LA, Thomas GI, Dillard DH, Merendino KA, Bruce RA (1959) An evaluation of internal mammary artery ligation by a double-blind technic. New England Journal of Medicine 20: 1115–1118

Descartes R (1644) L'Homme. Paris

Dimond EG, Kittle CF, Crockett JE (1958) Evaluation of internal mammary ligation and sham procedure in angina pectoris. Circulation 18: 712–713

Ejeskar A, Nachemson A, Herberts P (1983) Surgery versus chemonucleolysis. Clinical Orthopaedics 174: 236–242

El-Sobky A, Dostrovsky JA, Wall PD (1979) Lack of effect of naloxone on pain perception in humans. Nature 263: 783–784

Evans FJ (1974) The placebo response in pain reduction. In: Bonica JJ (ed) Advances in neurology, vol. 4. Raven Press, New York, pp 289–296

Farrer GR (1964) Psychoanalytic theory of placebo. Diseases of the Nervous System 35: 655–662

Finkel MJ (1985) Placebo controls are not always necessary. In: White LP, Tursky B, Schwarz GE (eds) Placebo: theory, research and mechanisms. Guilford Press, New York, pp 419–422

Finneson BE (1969) Diagnosis and management of pain syndromes. WB Saunders, Philadelphia

Fraser RD, Sendhu A, Gogan WJ 1995 Magnetic resonance imaging ten years after treatment for lumbar disc herniation. Spine 20: 710–714

Gracely RH 1979 Psychophysical assessment of human pain. In: Bonica JJ et al (eds) Advances in pain research and therapy, vol. 12. Raven Press, New York, pp 211–229

Gracely RH, McGrath P, Dubner R 1978 Validity and sensitivity of ratio scales. Manipulation of affect by diazepam. Pain 5: 19–29

Gracely RH, McGrath P, Dubner R 1979 Fentanyl reduces the intensity but not the unpleasantness of painful tooth sensations. Science 203: 1261–1263

Gracely RH, Dubner R, Wolskee PJ, Deeter WR 1983 Placebo and naloxone can alter pain by separate mechanisms. Nature 306: 264–265

Gracely RH, Dubner R, Deeter WR, Wolskee PJ 1985 Clinicians' expectations influence placebo analgesia. Lancet 1: 8419–8423

Grevert P, Albert LH, Goldstein A 1983 Partial antagonism of placebo analgesia by naloxone. Pain 16: 126–143

Harden RN, Gracely RH, Carter T, Warner G 1996 Placebo effect in acute pain management. Headache 36: 1–6

Hashish I, Feinman C, Harvey W 1988 Reduction of postoperative pain and swelling by ultra-sound: a placebo effect. Pain 33: 303–311

Hernstein RJ 1965 Placebo effect in the rat. Science 138: 677–678

Ho KH, Hashish I, Salmon P, Freeman R, Harvey W 1988 Reduction of postoperative swelling by a placebo effect. Journal of Psychosomatic Research 32: 197–205

Holroyd KA, Holm JE, Keefe FJ et al 1992 A multi-center evaluation of the McGill Pain Questionnaire: results from more than 1700 chronic pain patients. Pain 48: 301–312

Kirsch I, Montgomery GH 1998 Reply to Staats et al. Pain 76: 269–270

Koes BW, Bouter LM, Beckerman H, Van der Heijden G, Knipschild PG 1991 Exercises and back pain, blinded review. British Medical Journal 302: 1572–1576

Koes BW, Bouter LM, Beckerman H 1992 Randomised clinical trials of manipulative therapy and physiotherapy. British Medical Journal 304: 601–606

Lasagna L, Mosteller F, Von Felsinger JM, Beecher HK 1954 A study of the placebo response. American Journal of Medicine 16: 770–779

Levine JD, Gordon NC 1984 Influences of the method of drug administration on analgesic response. Nature 312: 755–756

Levine JD, Gordon NC, Fields HL 1978 The mechanisms of placebo analgesia. Lancet 2: 654–657

Liberman R 1964 An experimental study of the placebo response under three different situations of pain. Journal of Psychiatric Research 2: 233–246

MacArthur C, Lewis M, Knox EG 1992 Investigation of long term problems after obstetric epidural anaesthesia. British Medical Journal 304: 1279–1282

McQuay H, Carroll D, Moore A 1995 Variation in the placebo effect in randomised controlled trials of analgesics: is all as blind as it seems. Pain 63: 1–5

Melzack E, Casey KL 1968 Sensory, motivational and central control determinants of pain. In: Kenshalo D (ed) The skin, senses. CC Thomas, Springfield

Melzack R, Torgenson WS 1971 On the language of pain. Anesthesiology 34: 50–59

Merskey J 1989 Pain and psychological medicine. In: Wall PD, Melzack R (eds) Textbook of pain, 2nd edn. Churchill Livingstone, Edinburgh

Montgomery GH, Kirsch I 1996 Mechanisms of placebo pain reduction. Psychological Science 7: 174–176

Montgomery GH, Kirsch I 1997 Classical conditioning and the placebo effect. Pain 72: 107–113

Nash MM, Zimring FM 1969 Prediction of reaction of placebo. Journal of Abnormal Psychology 74: 569–573

O'Boyle DJ, Binns AS, Summer JJ 1994 On the efficacy of alcohol placebos in including feelings of intoxication. Psychopharmacology 115: 229–236

Posner J, Burke CA 1985 The effects of naloxone on opiate and placebo analgesia. Psychopharmacology 87: 468–472

Price DD, Fields HL 1997 The contribution of desire and expectation to placebo analgesia. In: Harrington A (ed) The placebo effect. An interdisciplinary exploration. Harvard University Press, Cambridge, pp. 117–137

Rawlinson MC 1985 Philosophical reflections on the use of placebos in medical practice. In: White LP, Tursky B, Schwarz GE (eds) Placebo: theory, research and mechanisms. Guilford Press, New York, pp 403–419

Reiss S 1980 Pavlovian conditioning and human fear. An expectancy model. Behaviour Therapy 11: 380–396

Revel M 1993 Discectomy versus chemonucleolysis. Spine 18: 1–7

Sherman RA, Sherman CJ, Gall NG 1980 A survey of current phantom limb pain treatment in the United States. Pain 8: 85–99

Siegel S 1975 Conditioning insulin effects. Journal of Comparative and Physiological Psychology 89: 189–199

Siegel S 1985 Drug anticipatory responses in animals. In: White LP, Tursky B, Schwarz GE (eds) Placebo: theory, research and mechanisms. Guilford Press, New York

Slappendel R, Crul BJP, Braak GJJ, Glurto JWM 1997 The efficacy of radiofrequency lesioning of the cervical spinal dorsal root ganglion in a double-blind randomised study. Pain 73: 159–163

Sluyter ME 1981 Treatment of chronic neck and back pain by percutaneous thermal lesions. In: Lipton S, Miles J (eds) Persistent pain. Academic Press 3: 141–179

Staats PS, Hekmat H, Staats AW 1998 Comment on Montgomery & Kirsch. Pain 76: 268–269

Ter Riet G, De Craen AJM, De Boer A, Kessels AGH 1998 Is placebo analgesia mediated by endogenous opioids? Pain 76: 273–275

Turner JL, Gallimore R, Fox-Henning C 1980 An annotated bibliography of placebo research. Journal Supplement Abstract Service of the American Psychological Association 10(2): 22

Tyler DB 1946 The influence of a placebo and medication on motion sickness. American Journal of Physiology 146: 458–466

Voudouris NJ, Peck CL, Coleman G 1989 Conditioned response models of placebo phenomena. Pain 38: 109–116

Voudouris NJ, Peck CL, Coleman G 1990 The role of conditioning and verbal expectancy in the placebo response. Pain 43: 121–128

Wall PD, Safran JW 1986 Artefactual intelligence. In: Rose S, Appignanesi L (eds) Science and beyond. Blackwell, Oxford

White L, Tursky B, Schwarz GE (eds) 1985 Placebo: theory, research and mechanisms. Guilford Press, New York

Wickramasekera I 1980 A conditioned response model of the placebo effect. Biofeedback and Self-Regulation 5: 5–18

A cognitive-behavioural approach to pain management

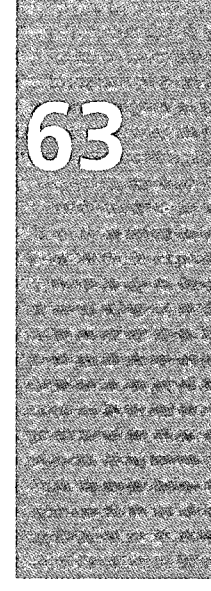

DENNIS C. TURK & AKIKO OKIFUJI

INTRODUCTION

In recent years there has been a proliferation of multidisciplinary pain centres. There are currently over 352 such centres listed in the directory prepared by the American Pain Society (APS 1996) providing treatment for an estimated 176 850 patients each year in the United States (Marketdata Enterprises 1995). These pain centres employ a broad range of psychological as well as somatic treatments (Flor et al 1992, Turk & Stacey 1997). The multifaceted treatment approach is consistent with the increasing evidence that pain extends beyond the sole contribution of sensory phenomena to include cognitive, affective and behavioural factors (Melzack & Wall 1983, Turk et al 1983).

Flor et al (1992) have suggested that most research on the efficacy of pain management programmes has incorporated one of two psychological approaches:

1. the operant conditioning approach developed by Fordyce and his colleagues (Fordyce et al 1973, see also Sanders 1996);
2. the cognitive-behavioural approach outlined by Turk and colleagues (1983, Turk & Stacey 1997, see also Bradley 1996).

In this chapter we shall describe the central features of a cognitive-behavioural approach to pain management. For a detailed examination of the operant conditioning approach, see Fordyce (1976, 1990) and Chapter 64 of this volume.

RATIONALE FOR THE COGNITIVE-BEHAVIOURAL APPROACH

The cognitive-behavioural perspective on pain management evolved from research on a number of mental health problems (e.g. anxiety, depression and phobias). Following the initial empirical research on cognitive-behavioural techniques in the early 1970s, there have been a large number of research and clinical applications (Hollon & Beck 1993, Turk & Salovey 1993). The common denominators across different cognitive-behavioural approaches include:

1. interest in the nature and modification of a patient's thoughts, feelings and beliefs, as well as behaviours;
2. some commitment to behaviour therapy procedures in promoting change (such as graded practice, homework assignments, relaxation, relapse prevention training, social skills training).

In general, the cognitive-behavioural therapist is concerned with using environmental manipulations, as are behaviour (operant conditioning) therapists, but for the cognitive-behavioural therapist such manipulations represent informational feedback trials that provide an opportunity for the patient to question, reappraise and acquire self-control over maladaptive thoughts, feelings, behaviours and physiological responses. Thus, contrary to the suggestion of some authors (Ciccone & Grzesiak 1988), there is no reason why the cognitive perspective and operant approaches should be viewed as incompatible or why they cannot or should not be integrated to create a cognitive-behavioural approach to treatment.

Although the cognitive-behavioural approach was developed originally for the treatment of mental health disorders, the perspective has much in common with the multidimensional conceptualizations of pain that emphasize the contributions of cognitive and affective as well as sensory phenomena (Melzack & Wall 1965). Both the cognitive-behavioural perspective and the gate control model of pain emphasize the important contribution of psychological variables such as the perception of control, the meaning of pain to the patient and dysphoric affect (Turk & Flor 1999). According to Melzack and Casey (1968):

> *The surgical and pharmacological attacks on pain might well profit by redirecting thinking toward the neglected and almost forgotten contribution of motivational and cognitive processes. Pain can be treated not only by trying to cut down sensory input by anesthetic blocks, surgical interventions and the like but also by influencing the motivational-affective and cognitive factors as well.*

Melzack (1980) has also suggested that 'cognitive processes are at the forefront of the most exciting new psychological approaches to pain, fear and anxiety'. The cognitive-behavioural approach focuses directly on cognitive processes as well as on affect, environmental and sensory phenomena. Each of the components of pain conceptualized in the gate control model is incorporated within the cognitive-behavioural treatment programme.

OVERVIEW OF THE COGNITIVE-BEHAVIOURAL PERSPECTIVE

It is important to differentiate the cognitive-behavioural perspective from cognitive-behavioural treatments. The cognitive-behavioural perspective is based on five central assumptions (Table 63.1) and can be superimposed upon any treatment approach employed with chronic pain patients. In many cases the perspective is as important as the content of the therapeutic modalities employed, somatic as well as psychological (Turk 1997).

The application of the cognitive-behavioural perspective to the treatment of chronic pain involves a complex clinical interaction and makes use of a wide range of tactics and techniques. Despite the specific techniques used, all cognitive-behavioural treatment approaches are characterized by being present focused, active, time limited and structured. Collaboration is central to the cognitive-behavioural behavioural approach. Therapists are not simply conveyers of information acting on passive patients but serve as educators, coaches and trainers. They work in concert with the patient (and sometimes family members) to achieve mutually agreed upon goals.

A growing body of research has demonstrated the important roles that cognitive factors (appraisals, beliefs, expectancies) play in exacerbating pain and suffering, contributing to disability and influencing response to treatment (Turk & Rudy 1992, Boothby et al 1999). Thus, cognitive-behavioural interventions are designed to help patients identify maladaptive patterns and acquire, develop and practise more adaptive ways of responding. Patients are encouraged to become aware of, and monitor, the impact that negative pain-engendering thoughts and feelings play in the maintenance of maladaptive overt and covert behaviours. Additionally, patients are taught to recognize the connections linking cognitions, affective, behavioural and physiological responses together with their joint consequences. Finally, patients are encouraged to undertake 'personal experiments' and to test the effects of their appraisals, expectations and beliefs by means of selected homework assignments. The cognitive-behavioural therapist is concerned not only with the role that patients' thoughts play in contributing to their disorders but, equally important, with the nature and adequacy of the patients' behavioural repertoire, since this affects resultant intrapersonal and interpersonal situations.

Table 63.1 Assumptions of the cognitive-behavioural perspective

- Individuals are active processors of information and not passive reactors
- Thoughts (e.g. appraisals, expectancies, beliefs) can elicit and influence mood, affect physiological processes, have social consequences and can also serve as an impetus for behaviour; conversely, mood, physiology, environmental factors and behaviour can influence the nature and content of thought processes
- Behaviour is reciprocally determined by *both* the individual and environmental factors
- Individuals can learn more adaptive ways of thinking, feeling, and behaving
- Individuals should be active collaborative agents in changing their maladaptive thoughts, feelings and behaviours

A cognitive-behavioural treatment programme for pain patients is multifaceted. Treatment may be conducted for individuals or groups on an inpatient or outpatient basis. A detailed presentation of the comprehensive treatment programme is offered in Turk et al (1983, Turk & Stacey 1997). In this chapter we will focus only on the psychological components of the cognitive-behavioural treatment; however, it is important to acknowledge that the psychological treatment modalities described need to be considered within a broader rehabilitation model that also includes physical and vocational components and, to a greater or lesser extent, involvement of significant others. The cognitive-behavioural perspective outlined above should be considered not merely as a set of methods designed to address the psychological components of pain and disability, but as an organizing strategy for more comprehensive rehabilitation (Turk 1997). For example, patients' difficulties arising during physical therapy may be associated not only with physical limitations but also with the fear engendered by anticipation of increased pain or concern about injury. Therefore, from a cognitive-behavioural perspective, physical therapists need to address not only the patient's performance of physical therapy exercises and the accompanying attention to body mechanics, but also the patient's expectancies and fears as they will affect the amount of effort, perserverance in the face of difficulties and adherence with the treatment plan (Meichenbaum & Turk 1987). These cognitive and affective processes, including self-management concerns, may be impediments to rehabilitation and thus need to be considered and addressed, along with traditional instructions regarding the proper performance of exercise. The attention paid to the individual's thoughts and expectancies by a psychologist should be adopted by all members of the interdisciplinary treatment team.

The cognitive-behavioural treatment consists of five overlapping phases listed in Table 63.2. Although the five treatment phases are listed separately, it is important to appreciate that they overlap. The distinction between phases is designed to highlight the different components of the multidimensional treatment. Moreover, although the treatment, as presented, follows a logical sequence, it should be implemented in a flexible, individually tailored fashion. Patients proceed at varying paces and the therapist must be sensitive to these individual differences. At times, the therapist may decide not to move on to the next phase of the treatment as would be expected, but rather address some pressing problems or concerns of the patient that may be interfering with progress. In short, treatment should not be viewed as totally scripted. Therapists must realize that flexibility and clinical skills have to be brought to bear throughout the treatment programme.

The cognitive-behavioural treatment that we will describe is *not* designed to eliminate patients' pain per se, although the intensity and frequency of their pain may be reduced as a result of increased activity, physical reconditioning achieved during physical therapy and the acquisition of various cognitive and behavioural coping skills. Rather, the treatment is designed to help patients learn to live more effective and satisfying lives, despite the presence of varying levels of discomfort that may persist. Other goals include the reduction of excessive reliance on the healthcare system, reduced dependence on analgesic medications, increased functional capacity and, whenever feasible, return to employment or usual household activities. Table 63.3 outlines the primary objectives of cognitive-behavioural treatment. The treatment programme can readily supplement other forms of somatic, pharmacological and psychological treatment.

The over-riding message of the cognitive-behavioural approach, one that begins with the initial contact and is woven throughout the fabric of treatment, is that people are not helpless in dealing with their pain nor need they view pain as an all-encompassing determinant of their lives. Rather, a variety of resources are available for confronting pain, and pain will come to be viewed by patients in a more differentiated manner. The treatment encourages patients to maintain a problem-solving orientation and to develop a sense of resourcefulness, instead of the feelings of helplessness and withdrawal that revolve around bed, physicians and pharmacists.

Table 63.2 Phases in cognitive-behavioural treatment

1. Initial assessment
2. Collaborative reconceptualisation of the patient's views of pain
3. Skills acquisition and skills consolidation, including cognitive and behavioural rehearsal
4. Generalisation, maintenance and relapse prevention
5. Booster sessions and follow-up

PHASE 1: ASSESSMENT

The assessment and reconceptualization phases are highly interdependent. The assessment phase serves several dis-

Table 63.3 Primary objectives of cognitive-behavioural treatment programmes

- To combat demoralisation by assisting patients to change their view of their pain and suffering from overwhelming to manageable
- To teach patients that there are coping techniques and skills that can be used to help them to adapt and respond to pain and the resultant problems
- To assist patients to reconceptualise their view of themselves from being passive, reactive and helpless to being active, resourceful and competent
- To help patients learn the associations between thoughts, feelings and their behaviour, and subsequently to identify and alter automatic, maladaptive patterns
- To teach patients specific coping skills and, moreover, when and how to utilise these more adaptive responses
- To bolster self-confidence and to encourage patients to attribute successful outcomes to their own efforts
- To help patients anticipate problems proactively and generate solutions, thereby facilitating maintenance and generalisation

tinct functions as outlined in Table 63.4. Assessment information is obtained by interviewing patients and significant others, as well as by using standardized self-report measures and observational procedures (see Turk & Melzack 1992 for a detailed review of assessment methods). During the assessment phase, psychosocial and behavioural factors that probably have an impact on disability are evaluated. Attention is given to identification of any factors that might impede rehabilitation. All this information is integrated with biomedical information used in treatment planning. There should be a close relationship between the data acquired during the assessment phase and the nature, focus and goals of the therapeutic regimen.

PHASE 2: RECONCEPTUALIZATION

A central feature of cognitive-behavioural treatment is facilitation of the emergence of a new conceptualization of pain during the course of treatment, thereby permitting the patient's symptoms to be viewed as circumscribed and addressable problems rather than pain as a vague, undifferentiated, overwhelming experience. The reconceptualization process prepares the patient for future therapeutic interventions in a way designed to anticipate and minimize patient resistance and treatment non-adherence (see Meichenbaum & Turk 1987 and Turk & Rudy 1991 for discussions of methods available to increase treatment adherence).

Table 63.4 Functions of assessment

- To establish the extent of physical impairment
- To identify levels and areas of psychological distress
- To establish, collaboratively, behavioural goals covering such areas as activity level, use of the healthcare system, patterns of medication use and response of significant others
- To provide baseline measures against which the progress and success of treatment can be compared
- To provide detailed information about the patient's perceptions of his or her medical condition, previous treatments and expectations about current treatment
- To detail the patient's occupational history, goals vis-à-vis work
- To examine the important role of significant others in the maintenance and exacerbation of maladaptive behaviours and to determine how they can be positive resources in the change process
- To begin the reconceptualisation process by assisting patients and significant others to become aware of the situational variability of the pain and the psychological, behavioural and social factors that influence the nature and degree of pain

From both the assessment materials and information provided by patients, the therapist attempts to alter the patients' conceptualizations of their problems from a sensory view of pain to a more multifaceted view with cognitive, affective and socioenvironmental factors being considered as contributors to the experience of pain. Through this process, patients are educated to think in terms of a treatment that will be effective in enhancing and providing them with greater control over their lives, even if the pain cannot be completely eliminated (Turk 1997).

First contact with the patient

The reconceptualization process begins with the patient's initial contact with the therapist. The therapist is concerned with establishing general details of the pain complaint, patient's general state of health, ongoing treatment (if any), their understanding of the cause(s) of their symptoms and of the reasons why they have been referred to a non-medical pain specialist. From the beginning, patients are directed toward viewing this opportunity as being unlike others they have experienced with healthcare providers – they can be helped, but only if they are prepared to participate by making a serious commitment to take an active role in rehabilitation, accepting a significant amount of responsibility for the outcomes of the treatment. Patients are provided with information about the multiple effects of chronic pain on people's lives, general demands and specific components of the treatment programme.

As part of this initial contact, pain questionnaires are administered that are designed to elicit information regarding patients' thoughts and feelings about their capacity to exert control over pain and many other aspects of their lives, the impact of pain and responses by significant others (see Turk & Melzack 1992). In addition, by means of a structured interview, questions are asked that are designed to help patients view their severest pain episodes as having a definite beginning, middle and ending; to see pain episodes as variable but not life-threatening; to interpret them as responses that can be controlled, and to view them as responsive to the passage of time, situational factors and life circumstances. As part of this assessment, the therapist encourages the patient's spouse or significant other to identify the impact of the patient's pain on them and the effect of their behaviour on the patient, as well as providing the family members with an understanding of the self-management approach to rehabilitation. There is increasing evidence that significant others play an important role in the maintenance and exacerbation of pain and, moreover, are themselves affected by living with a person with chronic pain (Flor et al 1987a, b, Turk et al 1993a).

At this point the therapist introduces the concept of 'pain behaviours' and 'operant pain' (following Fordyce 1976, 1990) and discusses the important role that significant others may play in unwittingly, inadvertently and perhaps unknowingly reinforcing and maintaining the patient's overt expression of pain and suffering. Such behaviours as grimacing, lying down, avoiding certain activities and moaning are offered as examples of 'pain behaviours'. The patient's significant other is encouraged to recall examples of the patient's specific pain behaviours and how the significant other responded to such behaviours. The spouse or significant other is also asked to complete a diary of the patient's pain behaviours and their own responses. This homework assignment serves to highlight the role pain has come to have in their lives and the importance of significant others in the treatment. The questions put to the spouse or significant other include: 'How do you know when your spouse is experiencing severe pain?', 'What do you do in response?' and 'What impact does it have?'.

The patient may be asked to complete a self-report diary for 1–2 weeks. They are asked to record episodes each day when they view their pain as moderate to severe and also when they are feeling particularly upset or distressed. They are also asked to record the circumstances surrounding the episode, who was present, what they thought, how they felt, what they did and whether what they did had any effect on the level of their pain. Diaries are designed so that the therapist will use them to assist patients to identify the links among thoughts, feelings, behaviours, pain intensity and distress. This process illustrates how assessment and treatment are intermixed; an important aspect of the learning process.

Finally, patients may be provided with pain intensity rating cards (e.g. 3″ × 5″ index cards) to record a 2-week baseline of pain intensity, each containing three or more time periods (e.g. early morning, afternoon, evening, bedtime or specific times throughout the day) and a six-point scale of intensity with 0 = no pain to 5 = incapacitating, severe pain. Patients are instructed to rate the intensity of the pain they experience at various times during each waking day. Space can be also provided on these cards for patients to indicate the time of medication intake and the specific incidents, thoughts or feelings that accompany intense pain (Turk et al 1983). This approach may be more effective than completing information once a day or week as it relies less on patients' memories.

The pain intensity rating cards are designed to illustrate to the patients and spouse that, contrary to their expectations, the patient rarely experiences the most intense pain constantly and that the intensity of the pain tends to fluctuate. Patients often find this variability surprising. The identification of any pain patterns fosters a sense of control through predictability (i.e. pain peaks and troughs, once recognized, are amenable to self-management strategies).

A note regarding homework assignments is in order. Since the conduct of homework assignments (such as keeping pain diaries, self-monitoring of pain levels and so forth) is critical to cognitive-behavioural treatment, the therapist must ensure that the patient and significant other understand the rationale, goals and actual procedures included in each homework assignment. A useful way to assess such understanding is to use a role-reversal procedure where the patient or significant other is required, in their own words, to explain the nature and rationale of the homework assignments to the therapist. The patient and significant other may be asked how they feel about the assignment, whether they believe they will be able to carry it out or whether they can foresee any problems or obstacles that would interfere with satisfactory completion of the assignments. If they can imagine problems developing that might impede completion of the assignment, they are asked how they might deal with these should they occur. If no problems can be identified by the patients, the therapist may suggest some possibilities (e.g. they may forget to record a day, they may feel embarrassed to self-monitor). In order to reduce feelings of defensiveness on the part of patients, the therapist might preface specifying problems by suggesting that 'Although you do not foresee any problems, some patients have told us that a problem for them was …' and 'How would you suggest that you would deal with such a problem if it were to arise?'. The therapist should anticipate and subsume any possible patient problems in conducting homework assignments within the therapeutic context.

Finally, it should be noted that the assessment should also focus on the patient's strengths and resources (e.g. coping abilities, competencies, social supports). These can be incorporated into subsequent treatment phases and contribute to the cognitive restructuring process described below.

Preliminary formulation of treatment goals

At this point the patient, spouse and therapist *collaborate* in establishing treatment goals that will return the patient to optimal functioning in light of any physical restriction and that are consistent with the patient's wishes. From the cognitive-behavioural perspective, collaboration is essential because it helps patients to feel that they are responsible for what occurs in treatment and for the outcomes. It is often helpful to use the information obtained from the structured interview, such as 'How would your life be different if your pain could be relieved?', to generate specific goals. The goals must be specific and measurable. For example, a patient's goal 'to feel better' is inadequate. The patient needs to specify what they will be doing that will indicate such improvement. We have found it useful to establish short-term, intermediate and long-term goals in order that reinforcement by goal achievement can occur early in treatment, thus enhancing patients' self-confidence. The treatment goals agreed upon – guided rather than dictated by the therapist – typically include medication reduction, increased activity (recreational, exercise), specific tasks to accomplish at home and on the job, reduction in the inappropriate use of the healthcare system and other patient goals.

Towards the end of the reconceptualization phase it is appropriate to provide a brief description of what will occur in subsequent sessions such as education and practice of specific cognitive and behavioural coping skills. It is important that patients and significant others understand the kinds of demands and expectancies of the programme and the likely impact their efforts will have on all phases of their lives. Clarification of the treatment demands at the earliest phases of the programme helps to circumvent problems that often arise later during therapy.

Graded exercise and activities

Many chronic pain patients have developed a sedentary lifestyle that can exacerbate pain by reducing endurance, strength and flexibility. Thus, the therapist, in collaboration with a physiotherapist and the patient's physician, should develop a graded exercise and activity programme appropriate to the patient's physical status, age and gender. As is the case in operant conditioning treatments, patients should maintain activity-level charts of achievable, incremental goals from which progress can be gauged by the patient, as well as by the therapist and other family and treatment team members. Initial goals are set at a level that the patient should have little trouble achieving to assure success, with the requirements increasing at a gradual rate.

The exercise and activity programme has four major objectives. Firstly, that of ameliorating physiological consequences that may exacerbate pain. Moreover, for chronic pain patients and their families, pain is a major focus of attention. Each physical sensation, each environmental demand is viewed in terms of its significance for experiencing pain. Thus, the second objective of the exercise and activity programme is to increase the likelihood that the pain patient and their family will develop interests in something other than pain. In this way 'pain' becomes more peripheral and competes for attention with other activities, rather than being the focal point of the patient's life. Thirdly, the graded exercise programme provides for success experiences and thereby helps to reduce fear of activity. Finally, the graded exercise programme reinforces the patient's perception of their own control and encourages self-attribution of successes.

Medication reduction

Another important issue to discuss with the patient is the use of analgesic medication. There is sufficient evidence to indicate that many patients are overmedicated and often are dependent on analgesics. Moreover, reduction in pain can coincide with medication reduction (Flor et al 1992). It is advantageous to help patients reduce and eventually eliminate all unnecessary medication. Since reduction of some drugs is known to be accompanied by serious side effects, consultation with the physician is imperative.

There are two schools of thought concerning the therapeutic procedure to use for drug withdrawal. Operant-oriented treatment programmes like that of Fordyce and his colleagues (Fordyce 1976), require the patient to take medication at specific times rather than p.r.n. (as required) and they mask the medication in a liquid medium (a 'pain cocktail') with systematic reduction of the percentage of active ingredient by the treatment manager. The patient is informed of the process of reduction prior to the initiation of the programme, but does not influence the schedule of the weaning process.

A second view regarding reduction of medication, one more congruent with the cognitive-behavioural perspective, also encourages the use of medication at specific intervals. However, since self-control and responsibility are major factors in this approach, the therapist encourages the patient to systematically reduce their medication, helps the patient design procedures by which this can be accomplished and shares responsibility for medication control with the patient. The patient is required to record the quantity and time of medication intake. The importance of medication reduction is stressed and the patient's medication records are carefully monitored. If the patient does not follow the guidelines in reducing the dosage, then this becomes a focus of discussion. The attempt to control medication intake is looked upon as a personal responsibility and the reasons for failure are considered in depth.

 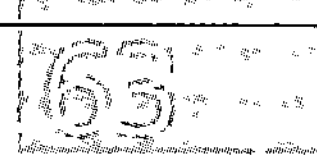

Translation process

At this time the translation or reconceptualization process begins in a more formal manner. A simplified conceptualization of pain based on the gate control model of Melzack and Wall (1965) is presented and contrasted with the unidimensional sensory-physiological model held by many patients. The interaction of thoughts, mood state and sensory aspects of a situation is presented in a clear, understandable fashion using the patient's self-monitored experiences as illustrations (Turk et al 1983, Turk & Stacey 1997). For example, the impact of anxiety is briefly considered and related to the exacerbation of pain. Data from patient diaries are extremely useful to make this point more concrete. Patients can review recent stressful episodes and examine the course their pain followed at that time. One coronary patient, who had been aware of a connection between periods of tension and the intensity of his pain, attributed the pain to changes in the state of his heart. As the details of his situation were examined, an alternative explanation emerged, namely that the nature of his pain was stress related. Muscle tension in the chest and shoulders increased when he was feeling stressed, but the heart rate and pulse remained unchanged. The patient's misattribution prevented appropriate action from being taken to reduce the muscle contraction that aggravated the chest wall pain. The reappraisal of the pain stimulus improved his ability to control the pain through timely and target-appropriate interventions, which in turn improved his sense of self-efficacy (Dolce et al 1986, Jensen et al 1991).

One item included in our pain questionnaire that we have found to be particularly suited to providing examples of how cognitive and affective factors, such as appraisal of the situation and coping resources, contribute to the pain experience asks the patient to close their eyes and to imagine the last time they had experienced intense pain ('5' on the pain-rating cards) and to record as many thoughts and feelings as possible that they had experienced before, during and after the episode. One patient who suffered with migraine headaches provided the following response to the item:

> *For hours and hours. God, will it ever end, how much longer do I have to live this way? I have outlived my usefulness ... the hours are endless and I am alone. I wish someone could take a sharp knife and cut that artery ... How long will it be until I am sent to a mental institution? Migraines are not fatal; doctors don't care. You live through one, only to be stricken with another in a few days. I am incapable of everything I used to do. How am I going to live the rest of my life? Unemployed, can't do anything, and all alone!*

This patient feels helpless, views her situation as hopeless and appraises her situation as progressively deteriorating. In such situations, patients are asked to consider the impact of such thoughts and feelings on the experience of pain and what they can do in such circumstances. In this manner, the therapist engages the patient in a Socratic dialogue in order to illustrate how such thinking may maintain and exacerbate pain and to consider alternative coping responses.

The example of Beecher's (1959) observation on the pain experienced by Second World War soldiers wounded at Anzio in Italy can be used to illustrate how appraisal and meaning systems affect the perception of pain. Beecher noted that many soldiers did not report experiencing intense pain, despite having incurred life-endangering battle wounds. Beecher attributed these responses to the meaning of an experience and suggested that the individual's appraisal influences how much pain he or she perceives. The therapist can use examples from the patient's experience that illustrate similar processes.

Biofeedback equipment may be used to illustrate the relationship between stress and muscle tension. Patients can be attached to biofeedback equipment and asked to tense relevant muscles and to attend to the changes in the information fed back (visual or auditory). The therapist may then ask the patients to relax the muscles (may give some guidance on how to do this) and to observe the changes in the tones or lights. The therapist can call to patients' attention their ability to change physiological functions, thus relating muscle tension to the exacerbation of pain. This can often have a dramatic effect in helping patients to realize the relationship between thoughts, feelings and muscle tension. Moreover, it can demonstrate to patients that they can, at least to some extent, control their own physiology. Consistent with the cognitive-behavioural perspective, biofeedback training has been found to increase pain patients' locus of control and self-efficacy, even if physiological changes have not occurred (Turk 1997).

To facilitate this reappraisal process, the therapist introduces the notion that the patient's experience of pain can be viewed as consisting of several manageable phases, rather than one overwhelmingly undifferentiated assault. In this way the patient comes to view their pain as composed of several components that go through different phases which are, in part, influenced by their reactions. The patient is not the 'helpless victim' of pain nor need they be a passive pawn. The therapist and patient have collected data to support this more differentiated view of pain, thus providing the basis for the intervention programme that will follow.

Examples are offered to show how pain can be subdivided into several steps, each of which is manageable by the patient. For example, when the patient rates his or her pain as 0 or 1 on a six-point scale (i.e. no pain or fairly low-level intensity), this is an opportunity for the patient to engage in productive coping activities. This period of low-intensity pain can function as a time when the patient can plan how to deal with more intense levels of pain by means of employing cognitive and behavioural coping strategies that the patient will learn by the end of the treatment programme. Similarly, the patient can develop coping skills to employ at the higher levels of pain intensity. The patient is encouraged to view pain as creating problems to be anticipated and solved. A useful analogy is the way athletic teams develop game plans. Preplanning lowers the risk of the patient becoming overwhelmed at times of more severe pain, while implicitly fostering an expectation that episodes of the most severe pain will fade. Patients are also encouraged to self-reinforce their efforts throughout by taking credit for their coping efforts.

Negative thoughts, pain-engendering appraisals and attributions are reviewed in treatment so that the patient will not be surprised when and if they do arise. Rather, the patient is encouraged to use the negatively valenced cognitions and feelings as reminders or as cues to initiate more adaptive coping strategies. The pain diaries described earlier can provide information that becomes the focus of discussion. For example, patients who recorded thoughts that they felt 'incompetent' and 'helpless' in controlling their pain during a specific episode should be encouraged to become aware of when they engage in such thinking and to appreciate how such thoughts may exacerbate their pain and become a self-fulfilling prophecy. Alternative thoughts, such as a realistic appraisal of the situation and of their coping resources, are encouraged and patients reinforced for using one or more of the coping strategies covered during the skills training. The patient is encouraged to divide the situation into stages as described earlier and to acknowledge that the most severe pain is usually relatively transitory. Such 'cognitive restructuring' is incorporated throughout the treatment regimen. The therapist also incorporates examples of when the patient has been resourceful in their life and considers how these skills can be applied in the pain situation.

PHASE 3: SKILLS ACQUISITION AND SKILLS CONSOLIDATION

The skills acquisition and skills consolidation phase begins once the basic initial goals of the treatment programme have been agreed upon. During this third phase the therapist provides practice in the use of a variety of cognitive and behavioural coping skills that are geared toward the alteration of the patient's response to environmental contributors to pain, to bolstering coping skills (e.g. attention diversion, relaxation skills for dealing with specific symptoms), to changing maladaptive interpretations and to changing factors that might contribute to stress (e.g. maladaptive communication patterns).

The order in which the various cognitive and behavioural strategies are covered can be varied depending upon the patient's needs. In addition to helping the patient develop specific coping skills, this phase is also designed to help patients use skills they already possess and to enhance the patient's belief in their ability to exercise control, further enhancing a sense of self-efficacy. The point to be underscored is that the cognitive-behavioural approach does not deal exclusively with the pain symptoms per se, but with those self-statements and environmental factors that may instigate or maintain less than optimal functioning and subsequent pain exacerbations. Alterations in lifestyle, problem solving, communication skills training, relaxation skills and homework assignments are woven into the fabric of the treatment.

As was the case with exercise, skills training follows a graded sequence. Firstly, the therapist discusses the rationale for using a specific method. This is followed by assessing whether the skills are in the patients' repertoires, teaching the patients the necessary skills and having them practise in the therapeutic setting. As patients develop proficiency, they are encouraged to use the skills in their homes, first in the least difficult circumstance and then building up to more stressful or difficult situations (when their pain is greater or when they are engaged in an interpersonal conflict).

Problem solving

A useful way to think about pain is as a set of sequential problems, rather than simply as the presence of pain being a single overwhelming problem. That is, many patients view pain as their over-riding problem and their only problem. An alternative encouraged by cognitive-behavioural therapists is that chronic pain presents the sufferer with an array of small and large problems – familial, occupational, social, recreational and financial, as well as physical. The therapist assists patients in identifying their problems in these areas and presents a process for dealing with these problems, namely generating a set of alternatives, weighing the relative advantages and disadvantages of each of these alternatives, trying different solutions, evaluating the outcomes and recycling the process as needed.

There are several critical features of problem-solving skills training. The important first step in problem solving is to have patients 'operationalize' their problems in behaviourally prescriptive language (e.g. when X occurs in situation Y, I feel Z). The second step is to help patients identify what particular situations are associated with pain. The use of self-monitoring in patient diaries can help to identify such problematic situations. Patients need to think of the difficulties that they encounter as 'problems to be solved'. Next, they must try out the alternative to achieve the desired outcome. Patients need to learn that there is usually not a single solution to solving problems and they need to weigh alternatives. In this way, lack of success with any one attempt will not be taken as a complete failure, but rather such setbacks and lapses are viewed as learning trials and occasions to consider alternatives.

It is all too easy to conduct problem solving during treatment but much harder to do so in the patient's natural environment. Patients may be given the homework task of formally identifying problems, generating alternative solutions, rating the solutions for likely effectiveness, trying them out and then reporting on the outcome. Throughout treatment, the therapist can use the language of problems and solutions to illustrate the value of using the problem-solving approach. The therapist uses terms and phrases like 'notice', 'catch', 'interrupt', 'plan', 'game plan', 'being in charge', 'having choices', 'performing experiments', 'setting goals' and the like.

Relaxation and controlled breathing

Relaxation and controlled breathing exercises are especially useful in the skills acquisition phase because they can be readily learned by almost all patients and they have a good deal of face validity. The relaxation and controlled breathing involve systematically tensing and relaxing of various muscle groups, both general and specific to the particular area of pain reported by patients (Turk 1997). Emphasis on controlled breathing is included, as research demonstrates that the amplitude and frequency of respiration has an effect upon heart rate and the accompanying experience of anxiety (Turk et al 1983). Instruction in the use of relaxation and controlled breathing is designed not only to teach an incompatible response, but also as a way of helping the patients develop a behavioural coping skill that they can use in any situation in which adaptive coping is required. The practice of relaxation and controlled breathing strengthens the patients' belief that they can exert control during periods of stress and pain and that they are not helpless. Patients are encouraged to employ the relaxation skills in situations where they perceive themselves becoming tense, anxious or experiencing pain.

Relaxation is not achieved by only one method; in fact, there are many relaxation techniques in the literature. At this point, there is no evidence that one relaxation approach is any more effective than any other. What is most important is to explain these findings to patients and help them determine what relaxation technique, or set of techniques, is most effective for them. Thus, in a collaborative mode, the therapist will assist patients to learn coping strategies that they find acceptable. If the coping effort proves ineffective, this is not to be viewed as a failure of relaxation nor a reflection of the patient's incompetence, but rather an opportunity to seek another alternative. As in the case of problem solving described above, it is suggested that there may not be any one best coping alternative, but rather different ones for different people or for the same individual in different situations.

Attentional training

The role of attention is a major factor in perceptual activity and therefore of primary concern in examining and changing behaviour. The act of attending has been described as having both selective and amplifying functions. Attention-diverting coping strategies (e.g. thinking about something pleasant) have been used probably since humans first experienced pain. Again, it is important to emphasize that the patient is viewed as a collaborator in the selection of specific coping strategies. Several types of strategies are considered and the patient is encouraged to choose those that are most likely to evolve into personally relevant resources. Patients are also assisted in generating strategies and techniques that they believe might be useful. Again, attempts are made to actively involve patients in their own treatment.

Prior to the description of the specific coping strategies, the therapist always prepares the patient for the intervention. In this instance, the therapist describes to the patient how attention influences perception. The therapist notes that people can focus their attention on only one thing at a time and that people control, to some extent, what they attend to, although at times this may require active effort. Examples, metaphors and analogies are used to make this point concrete (coming from the patient's experience whenever possible). For example, the therapist uses the analogy of the simultaneous availability of all channels on a TV "but only one channel can be fully attended to at any one time. Attention is like a TV channel tuner: we can control what we attend to, what we avoid and the channel to which we tune". With instruction and practice, the patient can gain similar control over his or her attention. This discussion prepares the way for presentation of different cognitive coping strategies.

Both non-imagery and imagery-based strategies can be employed. Although imagery-based strategies (refocusing attention on pleasant pain-incompatible scenes and so forth) have received much attention, the results have not consistently demonstrated that any imagery strategies are uniformly effective for all patients (Fernandez & Turk 1989). The important component seems to be the patient's imaginative ability, involvement and degree of absorption in using specific images. Guided imagery training is given to patients in order to enhance their abilities to employ all sensory modalities (e.g. imagine such scenes as a lemon being cut on a plate, a tennis match or a pleasant scene that incorporates all five senses). The specifics of the images seem less important than the details of sensory modalities incorporated and the patient's involvement in these images (see Turk 1997 for detailed illustrations).

Following this preparation, the therapist proceeds to describe different imagery categories (e.g. pleasant, fanciful, dissociative) and once again asks the patient to generate examples that are personally relevant. The therapist asks the patient to imagine circumstances along a continuum of pain and encourages the patient to see themselves employing the various images to cope with the pain more effectively. The purpose of the imagery and relaxation rehearsal is to foster a sense of 'learned resourcefulness' as compared to 'learned helplessness' that characterizes many pain patients.

Some patients will have difficulty learning relaxation or making use of imagery techniques. In such circumstances, it is often helpful to have patients use audiotapes or posters to help them focus their attention and to guide them with relaxation or imagery. The emphasis is not on one imagery method or technique, but rather on nurturing flexibility. The therapist models this by their own creativity in assisting patients to achieve their desired outcomes.

PHASE 4: REHEARSAL AND APPLICATION TRAINING

Next is the rehearsal phase of the treatment programme. After learning different skills, patients are asked to use them in imaginary situations in the therapist's office or the clinical setting. For example, after learning different relaxation methods, patients can be asked to imagine themselves in various stressful situations and to see themselves employing the relaxation and coping skills in those situations. For example, patients imagine the last time their pain intensity was rated between '3' and '5' on the pain intensity rating card and to see themselves using the relaxation and other coping techniques at those times. The intent is to have the patients learn that relaxation can be employed as a general coping skill in various situations of stress and discomfort and to prepare themselves for aversive sensations as they arise.

In order to review and consolidate the training procedures, the patient may be asked to role play a situation in which the therapist and the patient reverse roles. The patient is instructed that it will be his or her job to assume the role of the therapist and the therapist will assume the role of a new patient who has not received any cognitive-behavioural training. The role-reversal exercise is employed because research on attitude change indicates that when people have to improvise, as in a role-playing situation, they generate exactly the kinds of arguments, illustrations and motivating appeals that are most convincing. In this way the patient tailors the content of their roles to accommodate idiosyncratic motives, predispositions and preferences (Turk et al 1983). Such role playing also provides the therapist with a means of assessing any conflicting thoughts, feelings or doubts that the patient may harbour.

With success, the therapist can follow up with specific homework assignments that will consolidate the skills in the patient's natural environment. For example, patients are asked to practise relaxation techniques at home at least twice a day for 15 minutes with one of the practice sessions occurring prior to the times of the most intense pain, if such times have been identified on the pain intensity rating cards. Patients are also asked to anticipate potential problems that might arise in performing the homework assignment (e.g. they forget, they fall asleep) and to generate ways in which these obstacles might be addressed should they occur. In this way, attempts are made to anticipate potential difficulties before they arise and to convey the message to patients that they are capable of generating alternative solutions to problems.

PHASE 5: GENERALIZATION AND MAINTENANCE

Generalization and maintenance are fostered throughout treatment by provision of guided exercise, imaginary and behavioural rehearsal and homework assignments, each of which is designed to increase the patient's sense of self-efficacy. Following the skills acquisition and rehearsal phases, patients are encouraged to 'try out' the various skills that have been covered during the treatment in a broad range of situations and to identify any difficulties that arise. During these sessions, the patient is encouraged to consider poten-

 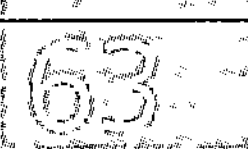

tially problematic situations and assisted in generating plans or scripts as to how they could handle these difficulties, should they arise. Plans are formulated for what the patient might do if they begin to lapse. The therapist attempts to anticipate problems and generate solutions, in a sense to 'inoculate' the patient against difficulties that may occur (see Marlatt & Gordon 1980 for a discussion of such relapse prevention procedures). Finally, the patient is encouraged to evaluate progress, review homework assignments and, most importantly, to attribute progress and success to their own coping efforts.

It is not enough to have patients change – they must learn to 'take credit' for such changes that they have been able to bring about. The therapist asks the patient a series of questions to consolidate such self-attributions. For example: 'It worked? What did you do? How did you handle the situation this time differently from how you handled it last time? When else did you do this? How did that make you feel?'

PHASE 6: TREATMENT FOLLOW-UP

During the final therapy session all aspects of the training are reviewed. Patients are provided with another set of pain intensity rating cards and a pain questionnaire (Kerns et al 1985). At 2 weeks following termination, the patient is asked to return with these materials to review progress and the maintenance of skills. At 3–6 months and 1 year, follow-up appointments are made to consider any difficulties that have arisen. Patients are also encouraged to call for appointments between specific follow-up dates if they are having difficulty with any aspect of the training. Checking in with the therapist is not viewed as a sign of failure, but rather as an opportunity to re-evaluate coping options. It should be obvious that cognitive-behavioural therapy consists of more than implementing a set of skills. Rather, it is a way of helping patients change their views of themselves and their plight. The techniques are used to help bring about the change from passivity to active control. The intangibles of treatment, such as the patient–therapist relationship of collaboration and how information is communicated, are at least as important as any specific skills presented and taught.

EFFECTIVENESS OF THE COGNITIVE-BEHAVIOURAL APPROACH

Cognitive-behavioural approaches have been evaluated in a number of laboratory analogue and clinical pain studies. Laboratory studies have demonstrated the effectiveness of the cognitive-behavioural approach in the enhancement of tolerance to a variety of nociceptive procedures (Fernandez & Turk 1989). The clinical effectiveness of the approach has been demonstrated in well over 200 studies* with a wide range of pain syndromes, including headaches (James et al 1993, Scharff & Marcus 1994), arthritis (Radojevic et al 1992, Parker et al 1995), temporomandibular pain disorders (Turk et al 1993b, Dworkin et al 1994), fibromyalgia (Nielson et al 1997, Turk et al 1998), irritable bowel syndrome (Green & Blanchard 1994, Van Dulmen et al 1996), debridement of burns (Wernick et al 1981, Tobiasen & Hiebert 1985), low back pain (Basler et al 1997), atypical chest pain (Klimes et al 1990), reflex sympathetic dystrophy/complex regional pain syndrome (Wilder et al 1992), cumulative trauma injury (Spence 1989) and heterogeneous samples of chronic pain syndromes (Peters et al 1992, Williams et al 1993). Cognitive-behavioural approaches have been used with patients across the age span, from children (Sander et al 1994, Griffiths & Martin 1996) to geriatric patients (Puder 1988, Mosley et al 1995). Additionally, they have been employed in combination with other therapeutic modalities (Williams et al 1996, Keller et al 1997). A number of these studies have reported follow-up data ranging from 6 months to 2 years, indicating that the improvements are generally maintained.

In summary, the cognitive-behavioural approach offers promise for use with a variety of chronic pain syndromes across all developmental levels. The American Psychological Association Task Force on Treatment Efficacy designated cognitive-behavioural therapy for chronic pain as one of 20 applications of psychological treatments for which there was significant empirical support. The fact that the approach has been employed in outpatient and group formats appears to be a particular asset, in terms of both the cost effectiveness and the potential for generalization and maintenance of the skills covered in the treatment programme.

An important research question is whether certain individual differences or situational constraints limit the relative efficacy of the different components of the comprehensive, multifaceted cognitive-behavioural treatment package. We know almost nothing about which treatment combinations would be most effective for what type of patient. Moreover, there is little research to determine how best to combine such psychologically based interventions with somatically based interventions (medications, transcutaneous nerve

*A complete list is available from the authors.

stimulation and so forth). Research programmes are now under way to:

- replicate the preliminary results with the inclusion of appropriate control groups (e.g. credible attention placebo and waiting list groups);
- identify the relative effectiveness of the cognitive-behavioural treatment for different syndromes and patient populations;
- assess the efficacy of treatment over a long-term follow-up period;
- identify active ingredients of the treatment;
- identify the necessary and sufficient components of the treatment;
- identify the most cost-effective modes of delivery;
- integrate cognitive-behavioural principles with somatic interventions;
- match treatment components to patients' psychosocial and behavioural characteristics.

Taken as an aggregate, the available evidence suggests that the cognitive-behavioural approach has a good deal of potential as a treatment modality by itself and in conjunction with other treatment approaches. The cognitive-behavioural perspective is a reasonable way for healthcare providers to think about and deal with their patients regardless of the therapeutic modalities utilized.

SIDE EFFECTS

Unlike more invasive medical and surgical treatments, the cognitive-behavioural approach has no known negative side effects. However, prior to considering this approach, careful evaluation of the patient's physical condition must be conducted in order to eliminate any treatable physical causes of pain.

Finally, little is known about the limitations of the cognitive-behavioural approach. One study, conducted by Tan et al (1982), suggests that it may have limited value for high-intensity pain with rapid onset (e.g. pain produced during knee arthrogram). It is important to identify such limitations in order that decisions about its use in more general clinical contexts can be based on data. The central question that remains to be answered is which treatment modalities are most appropriate for patients with what particular characteristics (Turk 1990).

Although many of the elements included in the present treatment have been used for many years and many are represented in other chapters in this volume, the cognitive-behavioural treatment approach attempts to integrate these diverse features into an organized, clinically sensitive and effective intervention.

REFERENCES

American Pain Society 1996 Pain facilities directory. American Pain Society, Glenview, Illinois

Basler H-D, Jakle C, Kroner-Herwig B 1997 Incorporation of cognitive-behavioral treatment in the medical care of chronic low back pain patients: a controlled randomized study in German pain treatment centers. Patient Education and Counseling 31: 113–124

Beecher HK 1959 Measurement of subjective responses: quantitative effects of drugs. Oxford University Press, New York

Boothby JL, Thorn BE, Stroud M, Jensen MP 1999 Coping with pain. In: Gatchel RJ, Turk DC (eds) Psychosocial factors in pain. Guilford Press, New York

Bradley LA 1996 Cognitive-behavioural therapy for chronic pain. In: Gatchel RJ, Turk DC (eds) Psychological approaches to pain management. Guilford Press, New York, pp 131–147

Ciccone DS, Grzesiak RC 1988 Cognitive therapy: an overview of theory and practice. In: Lynch NT, Vasudevan SV (eds) Persistent pain: psychosocial assessment and intervention. Kluwer, Boston

Dolce JJ, Doleys DM, Raczynski JM, Loessie J, Poole L, Smith M 1986 The role of self-efficacy expectancies in the prediction of pain tolerance. Pain 27: 261–272

Dworkin SF, Turner JA, Wilson L et al 1994 Brief group cognitive-behavioural intervention for temporomandibular disorders. Pain 59: 175–187

Fernandez E, Turk DC 1989 The utility of cognitive coping strategies for altering pain perception: a meta-analysis. Pain 38: 123–135

Fordyce WE 1976 Behavioural methods for chronic pain and illness. C V Mosby, St Louis

Fordyce WE 1990 Contingency management. In: Bonica JJ, Loeser JD, Chapman CR, Fordyce WE (eds) The management of pain, 2nd edn. Lea & Febiger, Philadelphia

Fordyce WE, Fowler R, Lehmann J, De Lateur B, Sand P, Trieschmann R 1973 Operant conditioning in the treatment of chronic pain. Archives of Physical Medicine and Rehabilitation 54: 399–408

Flor H, Kerns RD, Turk DC 1987a The role of the spouse in the maintenance of chronic pain. Journal of Psychosomatic Research 31: 251–260

Flor H, Turk DC, Scholz OB 1987b Impact of chronic pain on the spouse: marital, emotional, and physical consequences. Journal of Psychosomatic Research 31: 63–71

Flor H, Fydrich T, Turk DC 1992 Efficacy of multidisciplinary pain treatment centers: a meta-analytic review. Pain 49: 221–230

Greene B, Blanchard EB 1994 Cognitive therapy for irritable bowel syndrome. Journal of Consulting and Clinical Psychology 62: 576–582

Hollon SD, Beck AT 1993 Cognitive and cognitive-behavioural therapies. In: Garfield SL, Bergin AE (eds) Handbook of psychotherapy and behavior change: an empirical analysis, 4th edn. Wiley, New York

James LD, Thorn BE, Williams DA 1993 Goal specification in cognitive-behavioural therapy for chronic headache pain. Behavior Therapy 24: 305–320

Jensen MP, Turner JA, Romano JM 1991 Self-efficacy and outcome expectancies: relationship to chronic pain coping and adjustment. Pain 44: 263–269

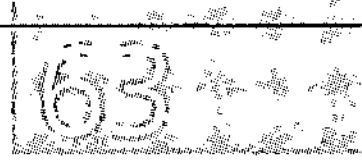

Keller S, Ehrhardt-Schmelzer S, Herda C, et al. 1997 Multidisciplinary rehabilitation for chronic back pain in an out-patient setting: a controlled randomized trial. European Journal of Pain 1: 279–292

Kerns RD, Turk DC, Rudy TE 1985 The West Haven–Yale Multidimensional Pain Inventory (WHYMPI). Pain 23: 345–356

Klimes I, Mayou RA, Pearce MJ, Fagg JR 1990 Psychological treatment for atypical non-cardiac chest pain: a controlled evaluation. Psychological Medicine 20: 605–611

Marketdata Enterprises 1995 Chronic pain management programs: a market analysis. Valley Stream, New York

Marlatt GA, Gordon JR 1980 Determinants of relapse: implications for the maintenance of behavioural change. In: Davidson PO, Davidson SM (eds) Behavioural medicine: changing health lifestyles. Brunner/Mazel, New York

Meichenbaum D, Jaremko M 1983 Stress reduction and prevention. Plenum Press, New York

Melzack R 1980 Pain theory: exceptions to the rule. Behavioural and Brain Science 3: 313

Melzack R, Casey KL 1968 Sensory, motivational and central control determinants of pain: a new conceptual model. In: Kenshalo D (ed) The skin senses. CC Thomas, Springfield, Illinois

Melzack R, Wall PD 1965 Pain mechanisms: a new theory. Science 150: 971–979

Melzack R, Wall PD 1983 The challenge of pain. Basic Books, New York

Nielson WR, Harth M, Bell DA 1997 Outpatient cognitive-behavioural treatment of fibromyalgia: impact on pain response and health status. Pain Research and Management 2: 145–150

Parker JC, Smarr KL, Buckelew SP et al 1995 Effects of stress management on clinical outcomes in rheumatoid arthritis. Arthritis and Rheumatism 38: 1807–1818

Peters JL, Large RG, Elkind G 1992 Follow-up results from a randomized controlled trial evaluating in and outpatient pain management programmes. Pain 50: 41–50

Puder RS 1988 Age analysis of cognitive-behavioural group therapy for chronic pain outpatients. Psychology and Aging 3: 204–207

Radojevic V, Nicassio PM, Weisman MH 1992 Behavioral intervention with and without family support for rheumatoid arthritis. Behavior Therapy 23: 13–30

Sanders SH 1996 Operant conditioning with chronic pain: back to basics. In: Gatchel RJ, Turk DC (eds) Psychological approaches to pain management. A practitioners handbook. Guilford Press, New York, pp 112–130

Scharff L, Marcus DA 1994 Interdisciplinary outpatient group treatment of intractable headache. Headache 34: 73–78

Spence SH 1989 Cognitive-behaviour therapy in the management of chronic occupational pain of the upper limbs. Behaviour Research and Therapy 27: 435–446

Tan S-Y, Melzack R, Poser EG 1982 Acute pain in a clinical setting: effects of cognitive-behavioural skills training. Behavioural Research Therapy 20: 531–546

Thorn BE, Williams DA, Johnson PR 1986 Individualized cognitive-behavioural treatment of chronic pain. Behavioural Psychotherapy 14: 210–225

Tobiasen JM, Hiebert JM 1985 Burns and adjustment to injury: do psychological coping strategies help? Journal of Trauma 25: 1151–1155

Turk DC 1990 Customizing treatment for chronic patients: who, what and why. Clinical Journal of Pain 6: 255–270

Turk DC 1997 Psychological aspects of pain. In Expert pain management Springhouse, Pa, Springhouse

Turk DC, Flor H 1999 Chronic pain: a biobehavioral perspective. In: Gatchel RJ, Turk DC (eds) Psychosocial factors in pain. Guilford Press, New York

Turk DC, Melzack R (eds) 1992 Handbook of pain assessment. Guilford Press, New York

Turk D C, Rudy T E 1991 Neglected factors in chronic pain treatment outcome studies – relapse, noncompliance, and adherence enhancement. Pain 44: 24–43

Turk DC, Rudy TE 1992 Cognitive factors and persistent pain: a glimpse into Pandora's box. Cognitive Therapy and Research 16: 99–122

Turk DC, Salovey P 1993 Chronic disease and illness behaviors: a cognitive-behavioral perspective. In: Nicassion P, Smith TW (eds) Psychosocial management of chronic illness. American Psychological Association, Washington DC

Turk DC, Stacey BR 1997 Multidisciplinary pain centers in the treatment of chronic pain. In: Frymoyer JW, Ducker TB, Hadler NM, Weinstein JN, Whitecloud TS (eds) The adult spine: principles and practice, 2nd edn. Raven Press, New York

Turk DC, Meichenbaum D, Genest M 1983 Pain and behavioural medicine: a cognitive-behavioral perspective. Guilford Press, New York

Turk DC, Rudy TE, Boucek DC 1993a Psychological factors in chronic pain. In: Wareld CA (ed) Pain management techniques. Martinus Nijhoff, Boston

Turk DC, Zaki HS, Rudy TE 1993b Effects of intraoral appliance and biofeedback/stress management alone and in combination in treating pain and depression in patients with temporomandibular disorders. Journal of Prosthetic Dentistry 70: 158–164

Turk DC, Okifuji A, Sinclair JD, Starz TW 1998 Interdisciplinary treatment for fibromyalgia syndrome: clinical and statistical significance, Arthritis Care and Research 11: 186–195

Van Dulmen AM, Fennis JFM, Fleijenberg G 1996 Cognitive-behavioral group therapy for irritable bowel syndrome: effects and long-term follow-up. Psychosomatic Medicine 58: 508–514

Wernick R, Jaremko ME, Taylor PW 1981 Pain management in severely burned patients: a test of stress-inoculation training. Journal of Behavioural Medicine 4: 103–109

Wilder RT, Berde CB, Wolohan M 1992 Reflex sympathetic dystrophy in children: clinical characteristics and follow-up of seventy patients. Journal of Bone and Joint Surgery 74A: 910–919

Williams ACC, Nicholas MK, Richardson PH et al 1993 Evaluation of a cognitive-behavioural programme for rehabilitating patients with chronic pain. British Journal of General Practice 377: 513–518

Behavioural therapy

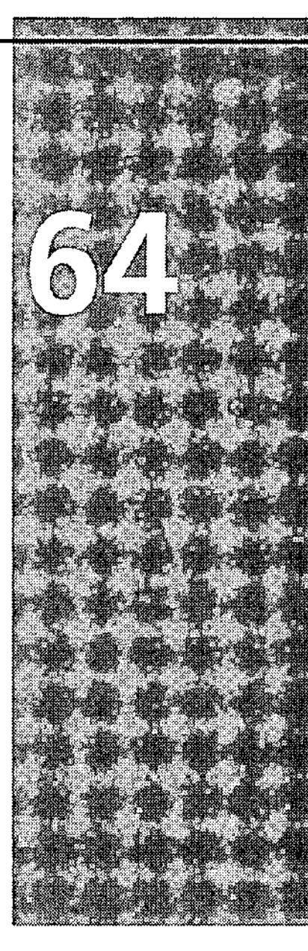

FRANCIS J. KEEFE & JOHN C. LEFEBVRE

SUMMARY

Behavioural principles have been very influential in both the assessment and treatment of chronic pain conditions. This chapter provides a summary of this perspective by first outlining the fundamental theoretical principles and recent theoretical models that have been used to guide behavioural assessment and treatment efforts. In the second section, the chapter reviews a variety of behavioural-assessment methods, including behavioural interview techniques, daily diary methodology, electromechanical recording devices and behavioural observations. In the third section, the chapter describes and critically evaluates a number of behavioural treatment techniques including graded activation and exercise programmes, social reinforcement, time-contingent medications and self-control skills. The final section of the chapter highlights important conceptual and clinical issues involved in applying behaviour therapy methods to chronic pain patients.

INTRODUCTION

In the 25 years since the initial pioneering contributions of Wilbert Fordyce, behavioural therapy has had a major impact on the management of patients suffering from chronic pain. It has helped many chronic pain patients increase their activity level, reduce their dependence on medications and return to a much more effective lifestyle. Behaviour therapy principles currently provide the conceptual foundations for many specialized inpatient and outpatient treatment programmes (Sternbach 1989). Even in pain treatment programmes that do not strictly adhere to a behavioural viewpoint, treatment specialists frequently use behavioural therapy techniques such as self-monitoring of activity, social reinforcement and time-contingent pain medications.

Over the past decade, behaviour therapy researchers have developed and refined a number of methods for assessing and treating chronic pain. Thus, to understand better the current role of behavioural therapy in pain management, one must not only be aware of the basic principles and methods of behaviour therapy, but also have an appreciation of recent developments in behavioural theory and application. This chapter seeks to provide the reader with an overview of the current status of behavioural therapy methods used in pain management.

This chapter is divided into four sections. The first section outlines theoretical principles used to guide behavioural assessment and treatment efforts. The second section reviews a variety of established and newly developed behavioural assessment methods. In the third section, behavioural treatment techniques are described and critically evaluated. The concluding section highlights important conceptual and clinical issues involved in applying behaviour therapy methods to chronic pain patients.

THEORETICAL PRINCIPLES

Patients who have pain engage in a wide variety of pain-related behaviours such as complaining of pain, taking pain medication or moving in a slow and guarded fashion. These behaviours, which Fordyce (1976) called pain behaviours, serve to communicate to persons around the patient the fact that pain is being experienced. Patients having persistent pain often exhibit a very high level of maladaptive pain behaviours (e.g. excessive reliance on narcotic medications, bedrest and an overly sedentary and restricted lifestyle), while engaging in few adaptive well behaviours (e.g. exercising, socializing or fulfilling work or home responsibilities).

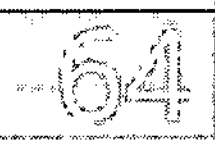

Behavioural theories of persistent pain attempt to explain how pain and well behaviours are acquired and maintained. The earliest applications of behaviour therapy to the management of chronic pain were based on operant and respondent conditioning principles. More recently, behavioural pain management efforts have been grounded in comprehensive theoretical models that integrate conditioning and learning perspectives with an emphasis on self-regulation.

OPERANT CONDITIONING

Many of the behaviours of a patient having pain can be classified as operant behaviours because they are strongly influenced by the consequences that follow their occurrence. A low back pain patient, for example, may rest in bed because reclining reduces pain or may avoid exercising because this activity increases pain. Operant conditioning (also known as instrumental or Skinnerian conditioning) is concerned with the relationship between such behaviours and their consequences.

A central tenet of operant conditioning is that the consequences of engaging in behaviour are an important determinant of whether those behaviours are likely to occur again in the future. The theoretical principle that outlines how consequences of behaviour can alter future behaviour was described by Thorndike (1913) in the Law of Effect, which states that the probability of a behaviour can be increased or decreased depending on its immediate consequences. Behaviours that produce positive outcomes will be more likely to occur in the future, while behaviours that produce negative or aversive outcomes will be less likely to occur in the future. In a series of classic studies, Skinner (1938, 1953, 1958, 1959) developed and refined many of the basic principles of operant conditioning. These were later extended to an analysis of abnormal behaviour in patients suffering from various psychological problems (Ullman & Krasner 1969). Fordyce (1976) was the first to argue persuasively that operant principles could be useful in understanding the behaviour of patients having chronic pain.

Fordyce (1976) described four major types of behaviour–consequence relationship that may be important in the acquisition and maintenance of pain and well behaviours. As can be seen in Figure 64.1, these relationships can be categorized along two dimensions:

1. whether the environmental stimuli involved are positive or aversive;
2. whether the stimulus is delivered or withdrawn following the behaviour.

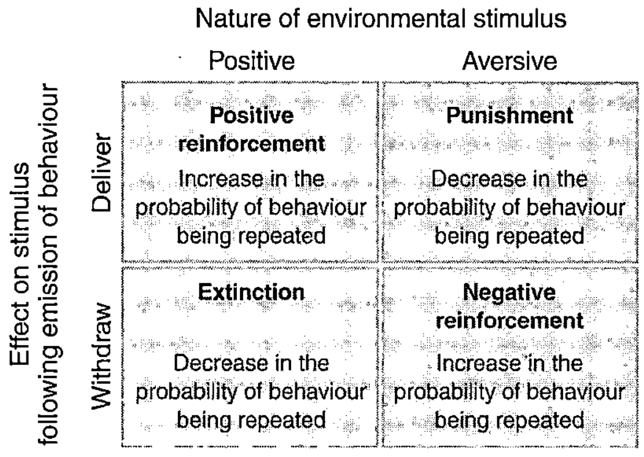

Effect on stimulus following emission of behaviour	Nature of environmental stimulus: Positive	Nature of environmental stimulus: Aversive
Deliver	**Positive reinforcement** Increase in the probability of behaviour being repeated	**Punishment** Decrease in the probability of behaviour being repeated
Withdraw	**Extinction** Decrease in the probability of behaviour being repeated	**Negative reinforcement** Increase in the probability of behaviour being repeated

Fig. 64.1 Behaviour–consequence relationships.

Pain behaviours (e.g. complaining about pain) that are *positively reinforced* (e.g. by solicitous attention and sympathy) have a higher probability of being repeated. In contrast, well behaviours (e.g. doing household chores) that are *punished* (e.g. by critical response of a spouse) are much less likely to be repeated.

Schedules of reinforcement are very important in the acquisition and maintenance of operant behaviours. Skinner (1953, 1969) found that the most effective method for increasing the probability of behaviour is to provide immediate and constant reinforcement (*continuous reinforcement*). A patient in a hospital pain unit, for example, is likely to become much more active if he or she receives praise and attention every time he or she gets out of bed. *Intermittent reinforcement* is more effective in maintaining behaviour. For this reason, operant programmes for pain management typically employ continuous reinforcement in the early stages of treatment (e.g. praising the patient after each exercise session) and then switch to intermittent (e.g. praise the patient on a variable schedule, such as after a variable number of exercise sessions) later in treatment.

Fordyce (1976) has maintained that, in some patients, pain behaviours that initially occur in response to acute pain can persist long after the normal healing time because these behaviours are reinforced. Given the persistent nature of certain pain conditions, there are ample opportunities for pain behaviours to be reinforced and for patients to learn to avoid well behaviours that could increase their pain. As Fordyce notes, by changing the consequences of behaviour, the frequency of maladaptive pain behaviours can be reduced and the frequency of well behaviours increased.

RESPONDENT CONDITIONING

Patients having persistent disease-related pain (e.g. those with cancer or rheumatoid arthritis) often have evidence of underlying tissue damage that is responsible for their pain. Although the pain behaviour of these patients has an organic basis, this behaviour can be influenced by conditioning and learning factors. In these patients, stimuli associated with pain can acquire, over the course of time, the ability to elicit maladaptive pain behaviours. A burn patient who has undergone repeated wound debridements, for example, may exhibit increased tension, physiological arousal and pain as soon as he enters the room where the debridements are carried out.

The classic example of respondent conditioning is the original experiment conducted by Pavlov (1849–1936). In this experiment, meat powder (the unconditioned stimulus [US]) was placed in the mouth of a dog and the amount of salivation (the unconditioned response [UR]) was measured. Immediately prior to the presentation of the US, a neutral stimulus (a tone) was presented. After a number of pairings, Pavlov discovered that the tone (the CS) presented without the US elicited a salivary response similar to the UR, which Pavlov now referred to as the conditioned response or CR. The important factor to note is that the animal is performing the CR in anticipation of the US being delivered.

Respondent conditioning is especially useful in understanding pain behaviour in patients whose pain is related to ongoing tissue damage or disease processes. Because of underlying tissue pathology, daily activities such as walking down a few stairs or moving from one position to another can activate nociceptive input, which in turn can produce pain behaviour. With repeated pairings of such activities with increased pain, previously neutral stimuli (e.g. the sight of the stairs) can acquire the ability to elicit pain behaviours.

Exposure-based therapies are often quite useful for patients whose pain behaviour is influenced by respondent conditioning (Fordyce 1976). In these therapies the patient is gradually exposed to activities that have caused increased pain in the past. With graded exposure, the association between environmental stimuli and severe pain is broken. As a result, patients can often increase their tolerance for activity and reduce the frequency of maladaptive, anticipatory pain behaviours (Fordyce 1976).

SELF-REGULATION MODELS

Operant and respondent conditioning models emphasize the influence that the environment can have in controlling pain behaviour. These models, however, do not fully take into account the role that an individual can play in regulating their own behaviour. Recent behavioural theories have attempted to integrate a self-regulation perspective with earlier conditioning and learning theories.

Self-regulation theories have several basic characteristics (Hollandsworth 1986, Kanfer & Schefft 1988). Firstly, each theory emphasizes that the individual is an active agent in changing behaviour. A patient having pain, for example, can observe their own pain and well behaviours, set goals for changing these behaviours and be an active participant in the entire process of behaviour change. Secondly, the theories are comprehensive and view behaviour as determined by multiple factors. According to self-regulation theory, the pain behaviour of a migraine headache may be influenced by respondent factors (e.g. exposure to allergens), operant factors (e.g. an opportunity to avoid a stressful examination), a breakdown in self-control efforts or a combination of these factors. Finally, self-regulation theory emphasizes the interactive and dynamic nature of pain-behaviour influences. The factors affecting pain behaviour can interact with each other and also change over time.

Kanfer (1970) was one of the first to present a self-regulation model of behaviour. The model depicted in Figure 64.2 includes:

1. stimulus variables (S) – environmental stimuli that may elicit behaviour;
2. organismic variables (O) – which include self-regulatory processes that may affect behaviour;
3. response variables (R) – behaviour;
4. contingency relationships (K) – which describe the schedule of reinforcement between response and consequence;
5. consequences (C) – which include the positive and aversive contingencies of responding.

The S, R, K and C components of Kanfer's self-regulation model had all been part of earlier conditioning and learning theories that viewed learning and reinforcement as occurring in a linear fashion. Thus, the stimulus triggers a response that prompts consequences from the environment, which in turn determines the probability of the behaviour being repeated. What was new in Kanfer's model was the self-regulatory component. According to this model, self-regulation processes are activated when ongo-

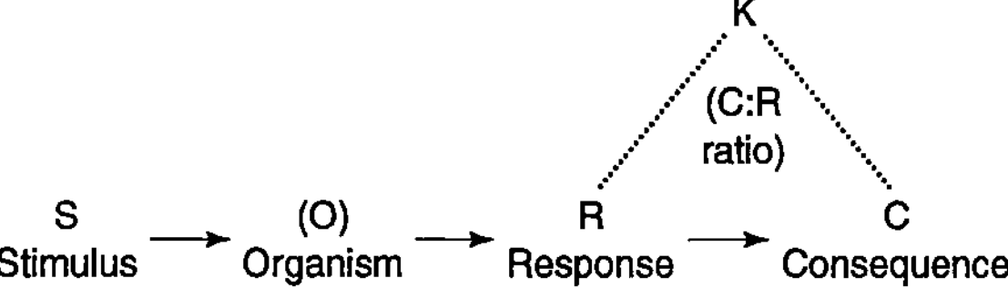

Fig. 64.2 Self-regulation model of behaviour.

ing activities are disrupted or the individual fails to reach a desired goal. Self-regulation involves three stages. The first stage, self-monitoring, is one in which the individual attends to their behaviour and becomes much more aware of variations in behaviour patterns. The second stage of self-regulation, self-evaluation, is one in which current actions are compared with criteria developed from past experience or desired performance. The final stage, self-reinforcement, is a motivational stage in which the individual assigns either positive or negative consequences to their own behaviour. The valence of these consequences determines whether the behaviour will be continued, improved upon, replaced by different behaviours to reach the same goal or whether new goals will be set. In summary, Kanfer's original self-regulation model viewed the individual as important in monitoring, evaluating and reinforcing their own behaviour.

More recent versions of self-regulation theory are even more comprehensive in that they attempt to account for the inter-relationships between biological factors and self-regulation (Kanfer & Schefft 1988). Schefft and Lehr (1985), for example, have presented a general systems model that is depicted in schematic fashion in Figure 64.3. This model addresses several different types of variables:

1. α variables, which represent inputs from the external environment;
2. β variables, which represent internal, psychological factors initiated and maintained by the individual;
3. γ variables, which are the genetic and biological factors involved in human behaviour.

Systems theories, such as Schefft and Lehr's, maintain that since components of the system are interconnected, changes in any one component will affect others through feedback and feedforward loops. Thus, patients who receive social reinforcement for spending time up and out of the reclining position may become more aware of their own behaviour and take a more active role in trying to regulate their own activity level. Patients whose pain behaviour is

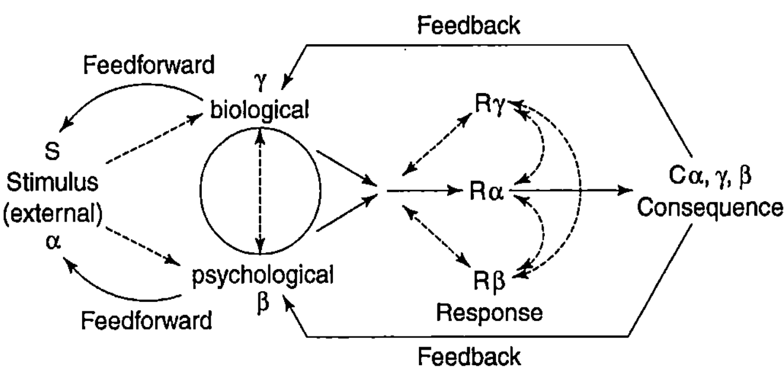

Fig. 64.3 General systems model.

clearly maintained by environmental contingencies (e.g. a patient who is addicted to narcotic medications) may be incapable of self-regulation early in the course of treatment. However, as their behaviour changes during treatment, their capacity for self-control may increase greatly.

Self-efficacy theory

A key issue in any model of self-control is the relative importance of human thinking or cognition. Self-efficacy theory, developed by Bandura, differs from self-regulation theory in that it places more emphasis on the importance of an individual's beliefs in influencing their behaviour, thoughts and feelings. Self-efficacy refers to the belief that one has the capability to engage in a set of behaviours required to successfully achieve a desired outcome (Bandura 1995). Individuals vary in their perceptions of self-efficacy. Thus, one person having a moderate degree of osteoarthritis of the hips could have high self-efficacy for pain (i.e. believe that they could successfully cope with, reduce or minimize episodes of severe pain), while another person with the same degree of arthritis could have very low self-efficacy for pain (i.e. believe there is nothing they can do to control episodes of severe pain). According to self-efficacy theory, the perception of personal efficacy is a more important predictor of performance than environmental stimuli or responses (Bandura 1995).

Self-efficacy is believed to play a pivotal role in altering behaviour because beliefs can cause changes in a wide range of outcomes. As Bandura (1995) notes:

> *In self-efficacy theory, people's beliefs in their capabilities to manage environmental demands affect the courses of action they choose to pursue, how much effort they put forth in a given endeavor, how long they persevere in the face of obstacles and failure experiences, how much anxiety and depression they experience in coping with stressors, and the level of accomplishments they realize.*

Studies have shown that self-efficacy is important in understanding how people perceive and respond to pain. We found that osteoarthritis patients who scored very high on a measure of self-efficacy had significantly higher pain thresholds and pain tolerance when presented with a gradually increasing series of laboratory heat pain stimuli than patients scoring very low on self-efficacy (Keefe et al 1997c). Arthritis patients who score high on measures of self-efficacy not only report lower levels of arthritis pain, psychological disability and physical disability (Lorig et al 1989), they also exhibit lower levels of pain behaviour (Buescher et al 1991) and show better performance during a demanding stair-climbing task (Rejeski et al 1996). Finally, changes in self-efficacy that occur over the course of arthritis education or pain-coping skills training protocols have been shown to be related to the short- and long-term outcomes of these interventions (Lorig et al 1989, Keefe et al 1996).

Why do persons with high self-efficacy seem to manage pain better? Bandura (1996) maintains that differences in self-efficacy may be due to variations in the way that persons think about and reconstruct their responses to demanding situations, such as increased pain. Persons high in self-efficacy see difficult tasks as challenges and tend to attribute failure to a lack of knowledge or skill or insufficient effort. As a result, the self-efficacy of these individuals can quickly recover from setbacks. In contrast, those with low self-efficacy tend to see difficult tasks as something to be avoided or as a personal threat. They tend to give up quickly and more easily succumb to stress or depression. In a recent study, we examined whether persons high in self-efficacy may actually use different pain-coping skills to manage their pain (Keefe et al 1997a). Participants in the study were 130 individuals having osteoarthritis of the knees and persistent knee pain. Data analyses revealed that patients who rated their self-efficacy as high were more likely to ignore pain sensations, use calming self-statements when confronting pain and avoid overly negative thinking (catastrophizing) when having pain.

Implications of self-regulation and self-efficacy theories

Self-regulation and self-efficacy theories have had several effects on behaviour therapy approaches to chronic pain. Firstly, these theories have underscored the need to involve patients fully in behavioural treatment efforts. Many chronic pain patients are capable of self-control and, thus, can benefit substantially from training in techniques such as self-reinforcement and relaxation training. Secondly, these theories have directed behaviour therapists towards a more comprehensive assessment of factors that control pain behaviour. These theories suggest that patients' own coping strategies, beliefs about their capabilities to control pain and ability to accurately monitor their own behaviour may all be important determinants of pain behaviour. Finally, these theories have led to increased interest in outpatient behaviour therapy treatment. If chronic pain patients can learn to control their own behaviour, they are less likely to need treatment in highly structured inpatient units where the reinforcement contingencies are programmed to reinforce well behaviours. Training in self-control techniques can also play an important role in enhancing the maintenance of treatment gains (Turk & Rudy 1991).

BEHAVIOURAL ASSESSMENT METHODS

Behaviour therapists have developed a wide variety of methods to assess the behaviour of chronic pain patients. These methods include structured interviews, daily diaries, electromechanical devices and behavioural observation.

BEHAVIOURAL INTERVIEW TECHNIQUES

Fordyce (1976) pioneered the use of structured interviewing for pain behaviour assessment. The aims of behavioural interviewing include obtaining a description of current patterns of pain and well behaviours, identifying factors that may control behaviour patterns and selecting target behaviours for behavioural intervention.

Several authors have described structured interview formats for the behavioural assessment of chronic pain (Turk et al 1983, Keefe 1988, Sternbach 1989). Table 64.1 includes a topical outline of a structured interview we use in behavioural assessment. As can be seen, the interview addresses variables that are viewed as important for conditioning, self-regulation and self-efficacy perspectives on pain behaviour.

Interviews with the patient's spouse and family members are an important part of the behavioural assessment process (Fordyce 1976). By interviewing a spouse, one may be able to validate the patient's descriptions of daily pain and well behaviour patterns. Areas of discrepancy between patient and spouse can be identified and then clarified through discussions with the patient. An interview with a spouse or family member also provides an opportunity to involve them in the treatment process.

DAILY DIARIES

Daily diaries are often used in the behavioural assessment of chronic pain. In contrast to interview methods, diary methods allow clinicians and researchers to assess the occurrence of important target behaviours, reducing response bias and error in reporting, and provide a means of assessing how pain is involved in everyday life.

Stone and Schiffman (1994) have proposed that behavioural observations can be requested on three different schedules: time-contingent schedule, signal-contingent schedule and event-contingent schedule. Using a time-

Table 64.1 A structured behavioural interview outline (based on Keefe 1988)

I. Characteristics of pain
   A. Location, severity, duration
   B. Factors that increase pain
   C. Factors that decrease pain
II. Patterns of pain and well behaviour
   A. General activity level and medication intake
   B. Estimates of daily sitting, standing and walking time
   C. Estimates of intake of pain medications
   D. Consequences of increased pain for activity and medication intake: are these consequences pain contingent?
III. Behaviour patterns in the home
   A. Ability to do self-care, household and social activities
   B. Ability to fulfil responsibilities in the family
   C. Response of spouse and family members to pain and well behaviours
IV. Behaviour patterns at work
   A. Current work status – pattern of activity over the day
   B. Future vocational options – for patients who are not working, explore educational level and interest in possible retraining or work options
   C. Incentives and disincentives for work – financial consequences of continued pain, disability support payments and financial compensation for work injury, pending litigation
V. Pain behaviour and observations
   A. Observations of non-verbal and verbal pain behaviours during the interview and during simple activities (e.g. walking into the interview, getting into and out of the chair)
   B. Observable indicators of pain status (e.g. use of a cane, wheelchair, brace, transcutaneous neural stimulator)
VI. Cognitive and affective responses to pain
   A. Cognitive distortions and deficits
   B. Negative cognitions regarding self, future and others
   C. Misconceptions about the nature of pain and likely future trajectory of pain
   D. Problems with memory and concentration
VII. Affective disturbance
   A. Symptoms of anxiety
   B. Symptoms of depression
   C. Relation of affective responses to pain behaviours
VIII. Psychophysiological response to pain
   A. Muscular tension responses
   B. Effects of increased tension
   C. Effects of relaxation
   D. Muscle weakness secondary to deactivation
   E. Autonomic responses
   F. Changes in heart rate, blood pressure, gastrointestinal symptoms
IX. Self-control efforts
   A. Behavioural coping methods
   B. Cognitive coping methods
   C. Perceived self-control over pain
X. Basic information about behavioural treatment
   A. Treatment goals
   B. Involvement of patient and family in assessment and treatment efforts

contingent schedule, individuals are asked to provide ratings of pain and other target behaviours at predetermined times. The Fordyce (1976) activity diary is an example of requesting behavioural ratings on a time-contingent schedule. It is also one of the earliest and most widely used daily diary methods, consisting of a standard data sheet with columns for making hourly entries of the amount of time spent reclining, standing or walking or sitting. The patient is asked to fill in the diary on a daily basis for several weeks prior to treatment and then throughout the course of behavioural treatment. From a treatment perspective, the data gathered are summarized on simple graphs and are useful in establishing baseline levels of the amount of time spent up and out of the reclining position. The data can also be used to identify problematic behaviour patterns such as the tendency to persist with activities for long periods of time followed by prolonged periods of reclining. Finally, the data can also be used to document improvements in activity level that occur during treatment.

Follick et al (1984) developed and refined a comprehensive daily diary for the behavioural assessment of chronic pain that also collected data on a time-contingent schedule. Their diary gathered information on position (e.g. sitting, reclining), time spent alone or with others, medication intake, pain, mood, tension and use of various pain control methods (e.g. hot pack or a heating pad). Patients were systematically trained in the use of the diary and then asked to make diary entries three times daily. The validity of the diary was supported by the finding that patient records of time spent up and out of the reclining position correlated highly with data gathered using an automated activity monitor.

There have been a number of advances in daily diary methodologies (Stone et al 1991). Behavioural researchers now use sophisticated and powerful data analysis techniques that enable the study of individual differences in day-to-day reports. Research has begun to assess the relationship of daily pain intensity to concurrent events such as coping (Keefe et al 1997a), fatigue (Stone et al 1997), sleep and attention to pain (Affleck et al 1996), and daily reactions to stressful events (Affleck et al 1994). Research has also begun to assess the relationship of daily measures of pain to more cross-sectional measures such as the personality trait of neuroticism, the availability of social support and the occurrence of major life events (Affleck et al 1994).

One recent advance in the field has been the use of electronic diaries to signal for and collect diary information (Lewis et al 1995, Affleck et al 1998). These methodologies often collect behavioural ratings using a signal-contingent basis. In a recent study of fibromyalgia patients, Affleck and colleagues (1998) used a hand-held computer to make within-day assessments of pain, fatigue and mood. The electronic diary was programmed to wake the participant in the morning and immediately assess sleep quality. It was also programmed to request and record ratings of pain, fatigue, positive mood and negative mood at three random times during the day.

The third schedule that Stone and Schiffman (1994) propose consists of the individual completing a diary entry on an event-contingent schedule. According to this schedule, the individual is requested to provide behavioural ratings when the event of interest occurs. This methodology is practical for assessing pain and other target behaviours that occur on an infrequent basis. An example would be to have individuals complete a diary record when they experience the onset of a migraine headache or in the early stages of a pain flare.

Diary methods have long been used in the clinical assessment of pain behaviour. These methods are inexpensive and can provide high-quality data. With the development of new methods for analysing data from such diary records and the use of hand-held electronic devices, new insights into how pain behaviours relate to important environmental and organismic variables may be obtained.

ELECTROMECHANICAL RECORDING DEVICES

Electromechanical recording devices can automate the process of behavioural recording and reduce demands on the patient, spouse or therapist. In the assessment of chronic pain patients, these devices have mainly been used to assess activity level. Cairns et al (1976), for example, devised an 'uptime clock' that automatically measures the amount of time chronic pain patients spend out of bed. Pedometers have also been used to gather data from patients involved in walking programmes (Saunders et al 1978). Both Follick et al (1985) and Sanders (1983) have described the use of a modified calculator timer and mercury-activated microswitch to record standing and walking time in back pain patients.

Although electromechanical devices can provide objective data, their applicability to chronic pain patients is sometimes questionable. For example, we evaluated an actometer, a self-winding watch modified to record movement (Morrell & Keefe 1988). The actometer has been shown to provide reliable measures of activity level in patients with depression. However, we found that its utility with chronic pain patients was limited. Variations in movement patterns, such as greater limping while walking one day versus another, significantly reduced the reliability of the device. Sugimoto et al (1997) have also found that the actigraph can be affected by common daily activities such as riding in a car or typing, thereby limiting its accuracy as an overall measure of activity level.

Another electromechanical device for assessing activity level is the accelerometer, which incorporates filtering techniques to eliminate the recording of vibrations not associated with human movement. These devices also have the capability of memory storage, thereby enhancing their utility in behavioural assessment. Two commonly used accelerometers are the Caltrac and the Tritrac (Kochersberger et al 1996). The Caltrac is a small, lightweight, waist-worn device that directly measures physical activity using motion sensors. Its major limitation is that it measures activity in only one dimension. It has also been found to have only modest test-retest reliability. The Tritrac, another waist-worn accelerometer, measures and records the motion of three accelerometers, oriented at right angles to each other. It can store up to 14 days of activity data, which can then be downloaded to a computer for statistical analyses. This instrument has been found to be a reliable and valid activity monitor in an elderly population (Kochersberger et al 1996).

Despite advances in electronics, most electromechanical devices remain somewhat expensive and not always readily available. As a result, the use of these devices generally has been limited to research applications.

BEHAVIOURAL OBSERVATION

Direct observation is one of the most basic and objective methods for assessing pain behaviour (Keefe 1989). Observations of pain and well behaviours can be carried out in naturalistic treatment settings. For example, Cinciripini and Floreen (1982) used a time-sampling method to record behaviours exhibited by inpatients treated on a behavioural pain management unit. A trained staff member watched each patient on the unit for 5 minutes every half hour and recorded both pain behaviours (verbal and non-verbal pain behaviours) and well behaviours (talking about healthy topics, engaging in assertive behaviour). Over the course of treatment, patients showed a highly significant increase in the percentage of time they spent engaging in well behaviours and a decrease in the percentage of time spent engaging in pain behaviours.

Behavioural observations can also be conducted in standardized situations designed to elicit pain behaviour. In the early 1980s we developed a behaviour sampling approach for recording pain behaviours in chronic low back pain patients (Keefe & Block 1982). This method involves having patients sit, stand, walk and recline for 1–2-minute periods. The patient is videotaped as they complete the activities and the videotaped record is subsequently scored by a trained observer. The observer notes the occurrence of five pain behaviour coding categories:

1. guarding – stiff and interrupted movement patterns;
2. bracing – pain-avoidant static posturing;
3. rubbing – touching or holding of the painful area;
4. sighing – a pronounced exhalation of air;
5. grimacing – a facial expression of pain.

A series of studies (Keefe & Block 1982) was conducted to evaluate the reliability and validity of this observation method. These studies revealed that behaviours could be coded reliably: interobserver agreement ranged from 93% to 99%. The observation method was also sensitive enough to detect reductions in pain behaviour occurring over the course of treatment. The construct validity of the observation method was supported by the finding that the level of recorded pain behaviours correlated highly with the patients' own ratings of pain. The method also appeared to possess discriminant validity: pain behaviour levels were substantially higher in low back pain patients than in pain-free normal and depressed control subjects. The validity of this observation method has also been supported by research studies of patients having pain due to rheumatoid arthritis (Anderson et al 1987), cancer (Ahles et al 1990) and osteoarthritis (Keefe et al 1987).

One important area for the use of behavioural observations is the assessment of pain in the elderly. There are a number of potential barriers to the assessment of pain in the elderly. Firstly, many elderly people are less likely to report the experience of pain because they consider it to be a natural part of the ageing process (Gagliese & Melzack 1997, Werner et al 1998). Secondly, traditional methods of pain assessment, such as the visual analogue scale and the verbal descriptor scale, may be too complicated for certain older adults (Weiner et al 1996, Gagliese & Melzack 1997). Thirdly, the ability to communicate with others may be lacking due to the presence of a dementia or other cognitive impairment (i.e. stroke, Parkinson's disease) (Weiner et al 1996, Pasero & McCaffery 1997). Although other people who are familiar with the elderly patient may serve as reporters, studies have shown that there might not be a high degree of concurrence between actual pain level reported by the patient and the amount of pain reported by the caregiver (Madison & Wilkie 1995, Werner et al 1998).

One possible solution would be to train healthcare providers as well as family caregivers in behavioural observation methods. For example, family caregivers can be educated on the common pain behaviours observed by patients with a painful condition (i.e. facial expression, body posture). In addition, the patient could be asked to perform a structured assessment that has been shown to elicit pain behaviours, possibly one reflecting household activities, while the caregiver observes the patient with an individual who has been trained in behavioural observation methods. In this way, caregivers can be educated not only on the meaning of pain behaviours in general, but also on which pain behaviours may be the most important for the patient.

Observational methods provide objective and useful data on pain behaviour. The major limitation of these methods is the expense entailed in training observers to gather and code behavioural data. Simplified observation methods that rely on brief behaviour samples and more practical coding methods such as rating scales are being developed and evaluated (Keefe 1989). Until these more practical methods are validated, standardized observation methods are likely to be confined primarily to research studies.

BEHAVIOURAL THERAPY TECHNIQUES

Although a wide variety of behavioural therapy techniques are used in the management of chronic pain, there are four techniques that make up the core elements of most treatment programmes: graded activation programmes, social reinforcement, time-contingent medications and training in self-control techniques. The rationale, treatment methods and empirical findings supporting the application of each of these techniques will be presented.

GRADED ACTIVATION AND EXERCISE PROGRAMMES

Rationale

Many chronic patients develop an overly sedentary lifestyle in which they may spend all but 4–6 hours of their day reclining. Inactivity has many negative consequences including increased dependence on family members, deconditioning, sleep difficulties and a narrowing of distractions from pain.

The attempts of patients to increase their activity often end in increased pain and pain behaviour. Many patients tend to work on activities or exercise until they reach the point that they have so much pain or are so tired that they have to stop and rest. Activation programmes are designed to break this tendency by having patients work to a set activity or exercise quota and then rest.

Treatment methods

To illustrate a typical activation programme, consider the behavioural treatment programme we instituted with Mr B, a 50-year-old chronic low back pain patient admitted to our inpatient pain unit. This patient reported that he usually got out of bed each day for only short periods of time. To establish an initial baseline record of activity, he was instructed to keep a daily activity diary (Fordyce 1976) in which he made hourly entries of his 'uptime' (e.g. time up and out of the reclining position). A review of the diary records gathered during the first 3 days of admission revealed that he spent only 30–40 minutes out of bed at a time and then would rest for 1–2 hours. His total uptime over the entire day was low, varying from 4 to 6 hours. When asked about his activity, the patient reported that his strategy was to let pain be his guide in determining when he should recline. If the pain was mild or moderate, he would persist with his activity; when the pain became extreme, he would recline.

To provide a rationale for graded activation, the concept of a pain cycle was discussed with Mr B. The cycle, evident in Mr B's baseline records, consisted of continuing with activity to the point of extreme pain followed by prolonged rest. Mr B admitted that this cyclic pattern was habitual. The negative consequences of the cycle were reviewed and contrasted with the benefits that would occur if Mr B learned to pace and then increase his activities. A systematic approach to activation, labelled the activity–rest cycle, was then introduced. The basic notion of the activity–rest cycle was that Mr B would engage in a moderate level of activity and then take a limited rest break. The level of activity and rest would be specified with the goal of gradually increasing the amount of activity and decreasing the amount of rest.

Mr B agreed to the activation programme and initial goals for activity were established. The activity goal, based on his baseline record of 4–6 hours of uptime, was to spend 20 minutes each hour up and out of the reclining position. Mr B was quite successful in meeting the initial activity goal and reported, after 2 days of the programme, that he had less pain than he had anticipated. He felt he could be even more active and wanted to set a goal of 45 minutes per hour. Given his baseline records and long history of bedrest, it was felt that a goal of 30 minutes of uptime per hour was more realistic. He met this goal for the next 3 days and the activity goal was then increased to 40 minutes. The programme continued with incremental increases in daily activity goals. Mr B gradually progressed with activation so that by the end of his 3-week admission he was spending 60 minutes out of the reclining position and resting for 10 minutes. When he returned for follow-up as an outpatient 2 months after discharge, Mr B was on a schedule of 90 minutes of activity followed by a 5-minute rest.

Empirical findings

Some of the earliest case reports of behaviour therapy for chronic pain described the effects of treatment on activity level. Progress in many cases was dramatic. Fordyce et al (1968) used a graded activation programme to increase walking tolerance in a 37-year-old woman having an 18-year history of chronic back pain and four major back operations. Over the course of inpatient treatment, the patient showed a 150% increase in walking from her initial baseline. She was able to maintain her gains in activity over a 23-week outpatient follow-up period.

The positive results of early case reports on graded activation and exercise are generally consistent with findings of later studies of groups of chronic pain patients. For example, Fordyce et al (1973) presented outcome data gathered from a group of 36 chronic pain patients who had participated in a behavioural treatment programme. Major, statistically significant increases in activity level and exercise tolerance were reported. As a group, the patients increased their tolerance for walking, sit-ups and time spent weaving by over 100%. Their daily uptime increased from 8.4 hours per 24 hours pretreatment to 12.7 hours per 24 hours post-treatment.

One limitation of the early research on graded activation is that this treatment technique was combined with other behavioural treatment interventions in such a way that the relative contribution of activation to treatment outcome could not be examined. Lindstrom et al (1992) conducted one of the first controlled evaluations of a behavioural activation programme. A sample of 103 patients having low back pain were randomly assigned to a graded activity programme or a routine medical care control condition. The activation programme, conducted by a physical therapist, was based on an operant model in which patients were given exercise goals that were initially set at submaximal levels and then gradually increased. Results indicated that the activation programme returned patients to work much more quickly than the routine medical care. It also resulted in significant increases in mobility, strength and fitness.

Turner et al (1990) compared behavioural therapy without exercise with a graded aerobic exercise programme alone. Ninety-six chronic low back pain patients were randomly assigned to one of four conditions:

1. graded aerobic exercise only in which patients engaged in a walking or jogging programme based on a behavioural activation plan;
2. behavioural therapy without exercise in which patients and spouses were trained in methods for socially reinforcing well behaviours and reducing reinforcement for pain behaviours;
3. behavioural therapy plus graded exercise in which patients received both the behavioural intervention and graded exercise;
4. a waiting list control group.

A comprehensive set of self-report, direct observation measures and spouse's ratings was administered pretreatment, post-treatment and at 6- and 12-month follow-ups. At the post-treatment evaluation, patients in the combined behaviour therapy and graded exercise condition showed significantly greater improvement in pain and pain behaviour than patients in the other conditions. At the follow-up evaluations, however, all three treatment groups showed similar significant improvements from their pretreatment baseline levels of pain and pain behaviour. Taken together, these findings indicate that graded exercise makes a significant contribution to the short-term positive effects of behavioural therapy for chronic pain.

Exercise interventions are increasingly being used with patients suffering from disease-related pain. Minor et al (1989), for example, conducted a study comparing the efficacy of aerobic versus non-aerobic exercise in 120 individuals with rheumatoid arthritis or osteoarthritis. Participants in the aerobic exercise condition engaged in a structured programme of aerobic walking and swimming activities. Those in the non-aerobic exercise condition engaged in a programme of range-of-motion exercises. The exercise training was conducted in group sessions that met for 1 hour three times per week for 12 consecutive weeks. Data analyses showed that, when compared with the non-aerobic exercise participants, the patients in the aerobic exercise condition had significant improvements in aerobic capacity, 50-foot walking time, grip strength, anxiety and depression.

SOCIAL REINFORCEMENT

Rationale

One hallmark of the behavioural approach to pain is its emphasis on the importance of the social consequences of overt pain behaviour patterns. The ways in which people respond to pain behaviour can play an important role in the development and maintenance of maladaptive behaviour patterns. Positive social reinforcement in the form of attention from a solicitous spouse or family members is particularly important in reinforcing pain behaviour. At the same time that pain behaviours are being positively reinforced, the patient's efforts to engage in healthier, well behaviours may result in negative consequences. A patient may be criticized by his or her boss for trying to take on new work responsibilities despite persistent pain. This punishing consequence is likely to decrease the probability that they will take on such responsibilities in the future. Alternatively, the patient's efforts to spend more time out of bed may be ignored by family or co-workers. In some patients, the lack of meaningful social consequences may lead to extinction of important well behaviours.

Treatment methods

The major goal of social reinforcement techniques is to systematically alter the social environment so as to reward well behaviours and minimize reinforcement for pain behaviours. This goal is most easily achieved when the patient is removed from a home environment that may be reinforcing pain behaviour and is admitted to an inpatient hospital setting where the social environment can be controlled and monitored. On behaviourally oriented inpatient pain units, staff members are trained to praise well behaviours and ignore or minimize the amount of attention given to pain behaviours. Immediate and dramatic reductions in pain behaviour sometimes occur when patients are admitted to behavioural pain units. This rapid change in behaviour underscores the powerful influence the home environment can have in maintaining excessively high levels of maladaptive pain behaviour. In most cases, however, changes in pain behaviour are less dramatic and staff members must use shaping principles to reward successive approximations of a full range of well behaviours.

To effectively utilize social reinforcement in the outpatient setting, one must involve the spouse and family members who have the most contact with the patient. These individuals must be educated about the rationale for social reinforcement, trained to recognize pain behaviour and well behaviour and instructed in basic principles of reinforcement. Their performance also needs to be monitored and reinforced closely over time. In the absence of ongoing involvement in treatment, the tendency for spouse and family is to revert to old, maladaptive patterns of responding to pain and well behaviour.

Empirical findings

A number of research studies have examined the effects of social reinforcement on pain and pain behaviour. One of the most interesting studies (White & Sanders 1986) compared the effects of social reinforcement of discussions of pain versus well topics on subsequent ratings of pain. Each patient in this study was visited for two 5-minute periods daily and encouraged to talk about their status. During one 5-minute period, the patient was reinforced with head nods and verbal statements for talking about pain-related topics. During the other 5-minute period, reinforcement was given for talking about well topics. After each 5-minute conversation, patients rated their pain on a 0–5 scale. Figure 64.4 displays data obtained from the four chronic pain patients who participated in this study. As can be seen, patients consistently rated their pain as more severe after being reinforced for talking about pain topics than after being reinforced for talking about well topics. What makes these findings noteworthy is the fact that they were evident after only 5 minutes of discussion. Lengthy discussions of pain-related topics presumably could have even more pronounced effects on pain report.

Patients involved in pain treatment are often provided with encouragement to exercise and to be more active. Does the way that encouragement is provided make a difference? Behavioural theory would suggest that providing patients with social encouragement and support contingent on their exercise performance is likely to be much more effective than providing social reinforcement in a non-contingent fashion. Cairns and Pasino (1977) tested the effects of contingent and non-contingent social reinforcement on walking, bicycling and uptime in chronic low back patients. They found that non-contingent social reinforcement and the public posting of exercise/activity graphs had no effect on performance. However, when social reinforcement was given to patients during and after they engaged in exercise or activity, significant increases in performance were obtained.

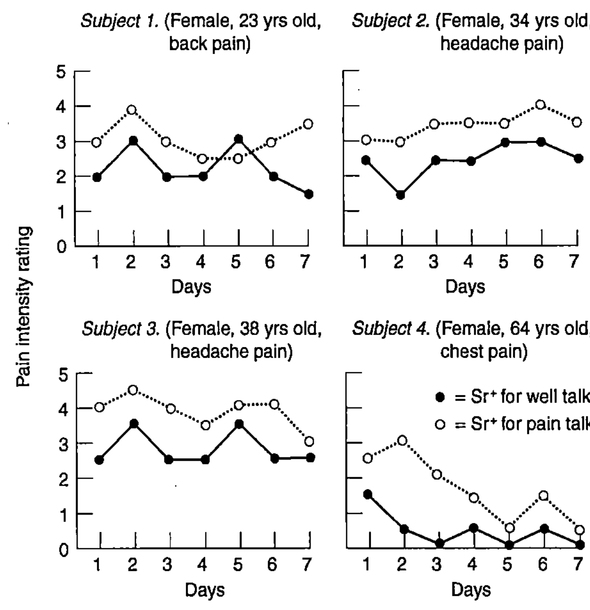

Fig. 64.4 Data from the White and Sanders (1986) study.

TIME-CONTINGENT MEDICATIONS

Rationale

Chronic pain patients often take their pain medications on an as-needed or p.r.n. (pro re nata) basis. For patients having persistent pain, analgesic and narcotic medications can be potent reinforcers because they reduce pain and associated emotional distress. The delivery of medication at a time of severe pain can positively reinforce high levels of pain behaviour (Fordyce 1976). One result of this reinforcement is a vicious cycle in which increased drug use leads to increased pain behaviour, which in turn leads to increased medication intake (Berntzen & Götestam 1987).

To break the association between pain behaviour and medication intake, most behavioural treatment programmes use a time-contingent medication scheduling. In this form of scheduling, all pain medications are given on a fixed-interval rather than p.r.n. basis. Thus, patients are required to take their medications at specific time periods in the day (e.g. every 6 hours). Over the course of treatment, the amount of active medication taken is gradually reduced to nothing.

Time-contingent medication schedules effectively break the relationship between pain complaints and medication delivery. Patients on these schedules are required to take their medication at fixed times of the day regardless of whether their pain level is high or low. One pharmacological advantage of this type of medication scheduling is that it provides an excellent means for keeping the blood level of a pain medication steady. As a result, patients often report that their medications are more effective and thus they are often more compliant with efforts to taper their medication intake.

Treatment methods

The first step in implementing time-contingent medication scheduling is to obtain an estimate of the patient's pretreatment pain medication intake. In inpatient treatment settings, a baseline level of medication can be obtained by placing patients on a p.r.n. medication schedule for the first 3–5 days. The timing and amount of medication taken can be recorded and the patient can then be carefully observed for any signs of withdrawal. Another way to establish baseline medication intake is to have patients keep diary records of their medication usage. The need for accurate reporting of medication use should be stressed since patients taking high levels of narcotics may minimize their intake (Berntzen & Götestam 1987).

To start a time-contingent medication programme, the average daily baseline intake of pain medication is typically divided into equal amounts to be delivered at regular intervals (e.g. every 6 hours) per 24 hours. In some behavioural treatment programmes, all oral pain medications are administered in tablet form at regular time intervals over a 24-hour period. In other programmes, the pain medications are converted to a milligram-equivalent dose of methadone, which is then taken at fixed intervals. Often a liquid vehicle (e.g. cherry syrup or orange juice) is used to deliver the medication. This 'pain cocktail' is designed to mask the precise amount of medication so that day-to-day reductions in the dose level can be achieved without patient awareness.

The ultimate goal of time-contingent medications is to reduce the intake of medications to zero. To achieve this goal, the amount of pain medication is gradually reduced over a period of days or weeks. At the end of treatment, patients may simply be taking a liquid 'pain cocktail' that contains no analgesic or narcotic medications. Interestingly, we have found that at the time of discharge from the programme some patients ask for prescriptions of the cherry syrup vehicle used to deliver the 'cocktail' even though they realize it contains no active medication.

Empirical findings

Two studies have provided support for the effectiveness of time-contingent medications in the management of pain. The first study by White and Sanders (1985) was carried out in the context of a behaviourally oriented inpatient treatment programme. In this study, eight chronic pain patients were randomly assigned to either:

1. time-contingent medication in which they received equal doses of methadone every 6 hours with the amount per dosage gradually decreased over 5 days;
2. p.r.n. medication in which they received four equal doses of daily methadone on an as-needed basis with the level of methadone gradually decreased over 5 days.

Throughout the study, all other medications and treatments were held constant. Data analysis revealed that patients in the time-contingent condition reported significantly lower levels of pain both during and after the detoxification programme compared with patients in the p.r.n. group. The patients on time-contingent medications also reported better mood compared with patients in the p.r.n. group.

Berntzen and Götestam (1987) tested the effects of time-contingent medications in a sample comprised mainly of outpatients (8 of 10 patients) having chronic pain. This study used a within-subject design in which each subject received 1 week of medications on a time-contingent basis and 1 week of medications on a p.r.n. basis. The sequence of treatment conditions was randomized across subjects. Throughout the study, patients provided daily ratings of pain and mood level. The results indicated that pain ratings decreased significantly during time-contingent scheduling and increased during the p.r.n. medication scheduling. Mood level also was significantly higher during the time-contingent medication regime than during the p.r.n. medication scheduling.

SELF-CONTROL SKILLS

Rationale

When behaviour therapy is carried out in an institutional setting, the environment is carefully structured to provide opportunities for activation, to reinforce well behaviours and to minimize the association between pain complaints and medication delivery. However, the home and work environments that patients will return to are not so structured or regulated. If chronic pain patients are to maintain the gains achieved in structured settings, they need to learn skills for managing their own behaviour. For this reason, training in self-control skills is viewed as essential to the generalization of treatment effects.

Treatment techniques

Although behaviour therapy programmes provide training in a wide variety of self-control skills, virtually all programmes emphasize three basic skills: self-monitoring, self-reinforcement and relaxation training.

Self-monitoring

In self-monitoring, patients are taught how to record important target behaviours (e.g. uptime, exercise, medication intake). Self-monitoring not only provides important information about pain and well behaviours, it can also serve to break up patterns of maladaptive pain behaviour (Kanfer & Schefft 1988). For example, a patient who keeps a record of their pain medication intake may become more aware of early signals of over-reliance on a sedative-hypnotic drug and decide to avoid or limit use of this medication.

Self-monitoring involves several steps. Firstly, the behaviour to be observed is defined. The definition must specify what behaviour needs to occur (e.g. uptime consists of spending time up and out of the reclining position) and what will be recorded (e.g. the duration of uptime). Secondly, the method for recording needs to be specified. This might consist of a standardized data sheet (e.g. the Fordyce activity diary), an individually tailored data form or a device such as a wrist counter or tape recorder. The method chosen must be simple enough that it does not burden the patient. It should also permit the patient to record behaviour soon after it occurs. Finally, the data obtained through self-monitoring need to be periodically reviewed by the patient. In many behavioural programmes, patients graph their own data on uptime and exercise. Many patients report that a daily review of the graph helps them see their own progress and recognize early warning signs of setbacks.

Self-reinforcement

Self-reinforcement is designed to teach chronic pain patients to reward themselves for engaging in well behaviours (e.g. exercise, socializing, returning to work). To identify rewards for use in self-reinforcement, patients are often asked to complete an inventory of pleasurable events or activities such as the pleasant events schedule (MacPhillamy & Lewinsohn 1971). They are then given basic information about reinforcement: for example, the need to deliver rewards in a contingent fashion, the importance of schedules of reinforcement and the need to avoid reinforcement for maladaptive pain behaviours. Training in self-reinforcement emphasizes the use of naturally occurring rewards. A patient who has increased his tolerance for walking, for example, might reward himself by walking through his favourite park.

Relaxation training

Relaxation training teaches patients to recognize and reduce excessive muscle tension that may be contributing to pain behaviour. Numerous methods can be used to teach patients to relax. Behaviour therapists typically use a modified version of Jacobson's progressive relaxation training which involves a series of exercises in which the patient tenses and then slowly relaxes major muscle groups. The sequence of exercises progresses from the muscles of the legs and arms to those of the trunk and finally to the face, scalp and neck. Patients may be given an audiotape that guides them through each of the exercises. To help patients generalize their skills to daily situations, they are instructed in methods for practising relaxation for brief periods (e.g. 20 seconds to 1 minute). The advantage of these brief relaxation procedures is that they can be used to keep tension at a low level during daily activities that tend to increase pain.

Empirical findings

Two studies have evaluated the effectiveness of training in behavioural self-control techniques for outpatients having persistent pain. In a study of chronic low back pain patients, Kerns et al (1986) compared a behavioural programme that featured training in self-control skills with a cognitive intervention that emphasized cognitive pain-coping skills. Both treatments significantly reduced healthcare use when compared with a waiting list control condition. Nicholas et al (1991) conducted a similar study and found that training in behavioural self-control techniques produced greater initial improvements in functional impairment than cognitive treatment. Although patients in both groups were unable to maintain initial treatment gains, the very small number of patients available at follow-up may have precluded an adequate test of the long-term effects of these interventions.

ISSUES IN THE BEHAVIOURAL TREATMENT OF CHRONIC PAIN

There are a number of issues that need to be addressed in applying behavioural treatment methods with chronic pain patients. One key issue is that changes in behaviour may not result in changes in the report of pain. Reviews of the research literature indicate that behavioural therapy is generally quite effective in increasing activity level and exercise tolerance and decreasing pain medication intake (Keefe et al 1986). The effects of behavioural therapy on pain, however, are usually more modest. Patients may report substantial initial reductions in pain, but may maintain only about 20–30% reductions in pain over long-term periods.

The inability of behaviour therapy to produce large, sustained reductions in pain reporting raises several interesting points. Firstly, the magnitude of the changes in pain needs to be considered in context. Patients referred for behavioural therapy usually have a long history of failure to respond to treatment. Their modest improvements in pain therefore need to be balanced against the typically large and significant improvements they are able to achieve in activity and medication intake. Secondly, chronic pain patients entering behavioural therapy should be given an accurate description of what they might expect to gain from treatment. Specifically, they should be informed that the treatment may have its strongest impact on behaviour rather than on pain perception. Patients can then make a more informed decision about starting treatment. Many behavioural programmes formalize the process of obtaining informed consent by using a behavioural contract (Sternbach 1974) which specifies patient and therapist responsibilities, the treatment techniques to be used and the likely outcomes.

A second important issue is the selection of patients for behavioural treatment. In his writings, Fordyce (1976) underscored the utility of behavioural methods for patients having an operantly based pain problem. The question arises: should behavioural treatment be restricted to operant pain? One can certainly think of situations in which behavioural methods can be used inappropriately to treat non-operantly based pain problems. For example, socially reinforcing a rheumatoid arthritis patient for progressively higher levels of activity during a period of high disease activity is not likely to be very helpful. Nevertheless, behavioural factors appear to influence the behaviour of many chronic pain patients, even those who have a clear organic basis for their pain complaints. The fact that a cancer patient, for example, has multiple influences affecting their pain does not mean that behavioural interventions may not help reduce pain and improve functional status.

A third important issue relates to the involvement of spouses in behavioural treatment. Continuing and integral involvement of the spouse is considered to be important for the maintenance of behavioural treatment effects (Moore & Chaney 1985). Behavioural spouse training can teach the spouse how to prompt and reinforce well behaviours. It can also help prevent the spouse from unwittingly interfering with treatment goals by taking over tasks, enforcing inactivity or rest or limiting social activities. Spouse training can lead to a greater understanding of the role that behavioural methods can play in reducing pain behaviour and disability and give patient and spouse some appropriate, common activity goals to work on. Involving the spouse in treatment can also increase the spouse's confidence in the patient's capabilities.

Several studies have examined the effects of spouse-assisted training in behavioural pain management. In a study of rheumatoid arthritis patients, Radojevic et al (1992) compared a spouse/family-assisted pain-coping skills training protocol with an arthritis information intervention that involved a spouse or family member. The spouse/family-assisted intervention was found to be significantly more effective than the arthritis information intervention with spouse/family support in reducing pain and joint swelling. We recently conducted a study testing the efficacy of a spouse-assisted pain-coping skills training programme for the management of osteoarthritic knee pain (Keefe et al 1996). Compared with a control group receiving an arthritis information/spousal support intervention, those who received the behaviourally oriented spouse-assisted coping skills training regimen had significantly lower levels of pain, psychological disability and pain behaviour and significantly greater improvements in coping and self-efficacy. Taken together, these studies suggest that spouse- or family-assisted behavioural treatment may be useful in the management of chronic pain.

Another key issue in the behavioural management of pain is the timing of treatment. Behavioural techniques are often used as a last resort in the management of persistent pain. Behavioural theorists, however, would predict that early intervention may be more effective. Research studies have examined the utility of behavioural intervention in preventing pain-related disability. Fordyce et al (1986), for example, compared the efficacy of behavioural treatment and traditional medical treatment for acute back pain. Subjects were randomly assigned to one of two treatments: traditional medical management in which medications, exercise, activation and return visits were all scheduled on an as-needed basis or behavioural treatment in which the same treatments were administered on a time-contingent basis. No differences in outcome were apparent after 6 weeks of treatment. However, at a 1-year follow-up the patients who had been treated on the behavioural protocol had returned to preinjury levels of functioning, whereas patients receiving the traditional medical treatment had significant increases in pain-related impairment. These results suggest that early, behaviourally based intervention may be an effective method of preventing the development of pain behaviour patterns.

Over the past 5–10 years, the healthcare industry in the USA and several other Western countries has raised concerns about the cost of pain treatment. A specific concern has been whether behavioural treatment protocols for pain management have been found to be efficacious in controlled outcome studies. Without a sound scientific basis for determining if a given behavioural treatment is effective in reducing pain and increasing physical functioning, there is a risk that behavioural therapies could be devalued in the larger medical community (Kendall 1998). Recently, Compas et al (1998) reviewed and identified treatment protocols for four pain conditions (rheumatic disease pain, low back pain, migraine headache and irritable bowel syndrome) to determine whether they were shown to be empirically valid in controlled outcome studies. A standard set of criteria outlined by Chambless and Hollon (1998) were used to make judgements of treatment efficacy. Of the protocols reviewed, operant behavioural therapy was found to be efficacious in the treatment of low back pain. Cognitive-behavioural therapy was found to be efficacious in the treatment of rheumatic disease pain, low back pain and irritable bowel syndrome. Finally, thermal biofeedback and electromyographic (EMG) biofeedback combined with relaxation training were found to be efficacious in the treatment of migraine headaches.

Another important issue that arises from the changes in healthcare is the need for cost-effectiveness research. One of the most widely used methods for assessing cost effectiveness compares the initial costs of the treatment programme (salaries, direct and indirect costs) with estimated savings due to a decrease in the amount of health services (worker's compensation, physician visits, inpatient hospitalization). Lorig et al (1993) conducted a 4-year follow-up of 401 rheumatology patients treated in their Arthritis Self-Management Program (ASMP). Patients who participated in the ASMP had decreases in pain and disability that were maintained up to 4 years after completing the programme. They also had significant reductions in physician visits. After considering the initial cost of the programme (estimated to be $54 per patient) compared with savings incurred from the reduced number of physician visits, the authors estimated that the ASMP saved a total of $33.1 million over the 4 years of the study. Although the estimated cost savings are impressive, they can be considered to be conservative since they did not include potential savings due to decreased medication use, decreased financial support from government agencies and increased time spent at work.

Changes in the healthcare industry also have led to many medical centres closing their inpatient pain management units. Inpatient pain management programmes have higher initial costs compared with outpatient programmes. In a study conducted by Peters et al (1992), it was estimated that an inpatient pain management programme cost approximately seven times more than a comparable outpatient programme. However, inpatient programmes also provide more concentrated treatment and better control over the patient's environment and possible reinforcing stimuli.

The most systematic direct test of the comparative benefits of inpatient versus outpatient behavioural treatment of chronic pain conditions has been conducted at St Thomas' Hospital in London by Williams and her colleagues (1996). In this study, patients having persistent pain were randomly assigned either to an inpatient pain management programme, outpatient pain management programme or waiting list control condition. The two pain management programmes were very similar in content and run in parallel. Immediately following completion of the treatment programme, both the inpatient and outpatient programmes were significantly better than the waiting list control group in terms of pain, physical function and psychological well-being. One year after completion of the programme, however, participants in the inpatient programme were found to have better physical function and lower psychological distress than participants in the outpatient programme. Taken together, these results suggest that although inpatient programmes may incur greater short-term costs, they may provide greater benefits in the long term. Future research should be conducted to determine the long-term cost effectiveness of inpatient programmes.

CONCLUSION

Behaviour therapy approaches to chronic pain have advanced considerably over the past 25 years. Practitioners now have a wide variety of behavioural assessment and treatment procedures to choose from. The foundations of the behavioural approach are now more thoroughly grounded in empirical research. With the recent increase in research on behavioural methods of pain management, further advances in our ability to assess and treat the behavioural problems experienced by patients having persistent pain are likely to occur.

REFERENCES

Affleck G, Tennen H, Urrows S, Higgins P 1994 Person and contextual features of daily stress reactivity: individual differences in relations of undersirable daily events with mood disturbance and chronic pain intensity. Journal of Personality and Social Psychology 66: 329

Affleck G, Urrows S, Tennen H et al 1996 Sequential daily relations of sleep, pain intensity, and attention to pain among women with fibromyalgia. Pain 68: 363

Affleck G, Tennen H, Urrows S et al 1998 Fibromyalgia and women's pursuit of personal goals: a daily process analysis. Health Psychology 17: 40

Ahles TA, Coombs DW, Jensen L et al 1990 Development of a behavior observation technique for the assessment of pain behaviors in cancer patients. Behavior Therapy 21: 449

Anderson KO, Bradley LA, McDaniel LK et al 1987 The assessment of pain in rheumatoid arthritis: validity of a behavioral observation method. Arthritis and Rheumatism 30: 36

Bandura A 1995 Comments on the crusade against the causal efficacy of human thought. Journal of Behavior Therapy and Experimental Psychiatry 26: 179

Bandura A 1996 Ontological and epistemological terrains revisited. Journal of Behavior Therapy and Experimental Psychiatry 27: 323

Berntzen D, Götestam KG 1987 Effects of on-demand versus fixed interval schedules in the treatment of chronic pain with analgesic compounds. Journal of Consulting and Clinical Psychology 55: 213

Buescher KL, Johnston JA, Parker JC et al 1991 Relationship of self-efficacy to pain behavior. Journal of Rheumatology 8: 968

Cairns D, Pasino J 1977 Comparison of verbal reinforcement and feedback in the operant treatment of disability due to chronic low back pain. Behavior Therapy 8: 621

Cairns D, Thomas L, Mooney V, Pace JB 1976 A comprehensive treatment approach to chronic low back pain. Pain 2: 301

Chambless DL, Hollon SD 1998 Defining empirically supported therapies. Journal of Consulting and Clinical Psychology 66: 7

Cinciripini PM, Floreen A 1982 An evaluation of a behavioral program for chronic pain. Journal of Behavioral Medicine 5: 375

Compas BE, Haaga DAF, Keefe FJ et al 1998 Sampling of empirically supported psychological treatments from health psychology: smoking, chronic pain, cancer, and bulimia nervosa. Journal of Consulting and Clinical Psychology 66: 89

Follick MJ, Ahern DK, Laser-Wolston N 1984 Evaluation of a daily activity diary for chronic pain patients. Pain 19: 373

Follick MJ, Ahern DK, Laser-Wolston N et al 1985 An electromechanical recording device for the measurement of 'uptime' or 'downtime' in chronic pain patients. Archives of Physical Medicine and Rehabilitation 66: 75

Fordyce WE 1976 Behavioral methods for chronic pain and illness. CV Mosby, St Louis

Fordyce WE, Fowler RS, Lehmann JF, De Lateur BJ 1968 Some implications of learning in problems of chronic pain. Journal of Chronic Disease 21: 179

Fordyce WE, Fowler RS, Lehmann JR et al 1973 Operant conditioning in the treatment of chronic pain. Archives of Physical Medicine and Rehabilitation 54: 399

Fordyce WE, Brockway JA, Bergman JA, Spengler D 1986 Acute back pain: a control-group comparison of behavioral versus traditional methods. Journal of Behavioral Medicine 9: 127

Gagliese L, Melzack R 1997 Chronic pain in elderly people. Pain 70: 3

Hollandsworth J 1986 Physiology and behavior therapy. Plenum, New York

Kanfer FH 1970 Self-regulation: research, issues and speculations. In: Neuringer C, Michael L (eds) Behavior modification in clinical psychology. Appleton-Century-Crofts, New York, p 178

Kanfer FH, Schefft BK 1988 Guiding the process of therapeutic change. Research Press, Champaign, Illinois

Keefe FJ 1988 Behavioral assessment methods for chronic pain. In: France RD, Krishnan KRR (eds) Chronic pain. American Psychiatric Association Press, Washington DC, p 298

Keefe FJ 1989 Behavioral measurement of pain. In: Chapman CR, Loeser JD (eds) 1989 Advances in pain research and therapy, vol 12. Raven Press, New York, p 405

Keefe FJ, Block AR 1982 Development of an observation method for assessing pain behaviors in chronic low back pain patients. Behavior Therapy 13: 363

Keefe FJ, Gil KM, Rose SC 1986 Behavioral approaches in the multidisciplinary management of chronic pain: programs and issues. Clinical Psychology Review 6: 87

Keefe FJ, Caldwell DS, Queen KT et al 1987 Osteoarthritic knee pain: a behavioral analysis. Pain 28: 309

Keefe FJ, Caldwell DS, Baucom D et al 1996 Spouse-assisted coping skills training in the management of osteoarthritic knee pain. Arthritis Care and Research 9: 279

Keefe FJ, Affleck G, Lefebvre JC et al 1997a Pain coping strategies and coping efficacy in rheumatoid arthritis: a daily process analysis. Pain 69: 35

Keefe FJ, Kashikar-Zuck S, Robinson E et al 1997b Pain coping strategies that predict patients' and spouses' ratings of patients' self-efficacy. Pain 73: 191

Keefe FJ, Lefebvre JC, Maixner W et al 1997c Self-efficacy for arthritis pain: relationship to perception of thermal laboratory pain stimuli. Arthritis Care and Research 10: 177

Kendall PC 1998 Empirically supported psychological therapies. Journal of Consulting and Clinical Psychology 66: 3

Kerns RD, Turk DC, Holzman AD, Rudy TE 1986 Comparison of cognitive-behavioral and behavioral approaches to the outpatient treatment of chronic pain. Clinical Journal of Pain 1: 195

Kochersberger G, McConnell E, Kuchibhatla MN, Pieper C 1996 The reliability, validity, and stability of a measure of physical activity in the elderly. Archives of Physical Medicine Rehabilitation 77: 793

Lewis B, Lewis D, Cumming G 1995 Frequent measurement of chronic pain: an electronic diary and empirical findings. Pain 60: 341

Lindstrom I, Ohlund C, Eek C et al 1992 Mobility, strength, and fitness after a graded activity program for patients with subacute low back

pain: a randomized prospective clinical study with a behavioral therapy approach. Spine 17: 641
Lorig KR, Chastain RL, Ung E et al 1989 Development and evaluation of a scale to measure perceived self-efficacy in people with arthritis. Arthritis and Rheumatism 32: 37
Lorig KR, Mazonson PD, Holman HR 1993 Evidence suggesting that health education for self-management in patients with chronic arthritis has sustained health benefits while reducing health care costs. Arthritis and Rheumatism 36: 439
MacPhillamy D, Lewinsohn PM 1971 The pleasant events schedule. Unpublished manuscript. University of Oregon, Eugene, Oregon
Madison JL, Wilkie DJ 1995 Family members' perceptions of cancer pain. Nursing Clinics of North America 30: 625
Minor MA, Hewett JE, Webel RR et al 1989 Efficacy of physical conditioning exercise in patients with rheumatoid arthritis and osteoarthritis. Arthritis and Rheumatism 32: 1396
Moore JE, Chaney EF 1985 Outpatient group treatment of chronic pain: effects of spouse involvement. Journal of Consulting and Clinical Psychology 53: 326
Morrell EM, Keefe FJ 1988 The actometer: an evaluation of instrument applicability for chronic pain patients. Pain 32: 265
Nicholas MK, Wilson PH, Goyen J 1991 Comparison of operant-behavioral and cognitive-behavioral group treatment with and without relaxation training. Behaviour Research and Therapy 29: 225
Pasero CL, McCaffery M 1997 Overcoming obstacles to pain assessment in elders. American Journal of Nursing 97: 20
Peters J, Large RG, Elkind G 1992 Follow-up results from a randomised controlled trial evaluating in- and outpatient pain management programmes. Pain 50: 41
Radojevic V, Nicassio PM, Weisman MH 1992 Behavioral intervention with and without family support for rheumatoid arthritis. Behavior Therapy 23: 13
Rejeski WJ, Craven T, Ettinger WH et al 1996 Self-efficacy and pain in disability with osteoarthritis of the knee. Journal of Gerontology Series B Psychological Sciences and Social Sciences 51: 24
Sanders SH 1983 Toward a practical instrument system for automatic measurement of 'up-time' in chronic pain patients. Pain 15: 399
Saunders KJ, Goldstein MK, Stein GH 1978 Automated measurement of patient activity on a hospital rehabilitation ward. Archives of Physical Medicine and Rehabilitation 59: 255
Schefft BK, Lehr BK 1985 A self-regulatory model of adjunctive behaviour change. Behavior Modification 9: 458
Skinner BF 1938 The behavior of organisms. Appleton, New York
Skinner BF 1953 Science and human behavior. Macmillan, New York
Skinner BF 1958 Verbal behavior. Appleton, New York
Skinner BF 1959 Cumulative record. Appleton, New York
Skinner BF 1969 Contingencies of reinforcement: a theoretical analysis. Appleton-Century-Crofts, New York
Sternbach RA 1974 Pain patients: traits and treatment. Academic Press, New York
Sternbach RA 1989 Behavior therapy. In: Wall PD, Melzack R (eds) The textbook of pain, 2nd edn. Churchill Livingstone, Edinburgh, p 1015
Stone AA, Schiffman S 1994 Ecological momentary assessment (EMA) in behavioural medicine. Annals of Behavioral Medicine 16: 199
Stone AA, Kessler R, Haythornthwaite J 1991 Measuring daily events and experiences: decisions for the researcher. Journal of Personality 59: 575
Stone AA, Broderick JE, Porter LS, Kaell AT 1997 The experience of rheumatoid arthritis pain and fatigue: examining momentary reports and correlates over one week. Arthritis Care Res 10: 185
Sugimoto A, Hara Y, Findley TW, Yonemoto K 1997 A useful method for measuring daily physical activity by a three-dimension monitor. Scandinavian Journal of Rehabilitation Medicine 29: 37
Thorndike EL 1913 The psychology of learning. Teachers College, New York
Turk DC, Rudy TE 1991 Neglected topics in the treatment of chronic pain, relapse compliance, and adherence enforcement. Pain 44: 5
Turk DC, Meichenbaum D, Genest M 1983 Pain and behavioral medicine. Guilford, New York
Turner JA, Clancy S, McQuade KJ, Cardenas DD 1990 Effectiveness of behavioral therapy for chronic low back pain: a component analysis. Journal of Consulting and Clinical Psychology 58: 573
Ullman LP, Krasner L 1969 A psychological approach to abnormal behavior. Prentice-Hall, Englewood Cliffs, New Jersey
Weiner D, Pieper C, McConnell E et al 1996 Pain measurement in elders with chronic low back pain: traditional and alternative approaches. Pain 67: 461
Werner P, Cohen-Mansfield J, Watson V, Pasis S 1998 Pain in participants of adult day care centers: assessment by different raters. Journal of Pain and Symptoms Management 15: 8
White B, Sanders SH 1985 Differential effects on pain and mood in chronic pain patients with time versus pain-contingent medication delivery. Behavior Therapy 16: 28
White B, Sanders SH 1986 The influence of patients pain intensity ratings of antecedent reinforcement of pain talk or well talk. Journal of Behavior Therapy and Experimental Psychiatry 17: 155
Williams AC, Richardson PH, Nicholas MK et al 1996 Inpatient vs. outpatient pain management: results of a randomised controlled trial. Pain 66: 13

Pain in children

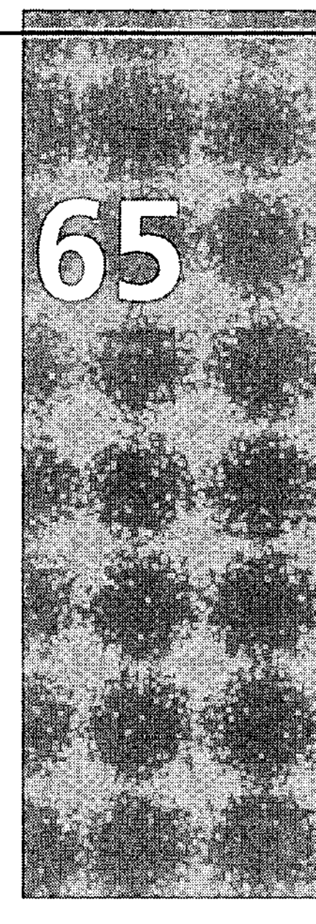

CHARLES B. BERDE & BRUCE MASEK

'If a new skin in old people be tender, what is it you think in a newborn Babe? Doth a small thing pain you so much on a finger, how painful is it then to a Child, which is tormented all the body over, which hath but a tender new grown flesh? If such a perfect Child is tormented so soon, what shall we think of a Child, which stayed not in the wombe its full time? Surely it is twice worse with him.'

Felix Wurtz in *The Children's Book*, circa 1656

SUMMARY

Nociceptive functions develop during fetal life and show considerable maturity even in preterm neonates. Infants and children can receive treatment for acute and chronic pain with efficacy and safety comparable to adults. Pain assessment and measurement in infants and preverbal children are more difficult because of the inability to use self-report and require judicious use of behavioural and physiologic measures. Fear and anxiety are prominent in hospitalized children. An essential aspect of paediatric pain management and supportive care lies in making medical encounters less terrifying. Cognitive-behavioural treatments can be used for children undergoing medical procedures or in treatment of a range of acute and chronic pain problems. Analgesic pharmacology differs in neonates because of certain pharmacokinetic and pharmacodynamic factors. Many age-related pharmacologic differences become less important after the first year of life.

In this chapter, we will review:

1. the developmental neurobiology of pain sensation and perception;
2. methods of pain assessment and measurement at different ages;
3. analgesic pharmacology in children;
4. specific pain syndromes in children;
5. psychological factors in the child's responses to pain, illness and the hospital environment;
6. non-pharmacologic methods of pain management.

INTRODUCTION: DEVELOPMENTAL NEUROBIOLOGY OF PAIN

Pain is a powerful force in learning and neurologic development. Behaviour is shaped to a considerable degree by stimuli that evoke pain as well as pleasure. It would thus be expected that the afferent pathways for pain sensation and perception would develop early: there is considerable adaptive significance in avoiding things that hurt. A number of research groups over the past 20 years have characterized the ontogeny of pain pathways in the peripheral and central nervous system.

An important series of studies by Fitzgerald and her coworkers describe neurobehavioural, neuroanatomic and neurophysiologic aspects of the development of nociceptive systems in infant rats, with some correlative studies in infant humans (Andrews & Fitzgerald 1997). Sensory nerves project to peripheral targets during midgestation in rats and in humans. In comparison with adult rats, noxious stimulation in infant rats evokes lower impulse thresholds and more prolonged discharges in primary afferent C and A fibres.

The flexion withdrawal reflex is well developed in neonatal rats and humans (Fitzgerald et al 1988). Neonates respond to milder mechanical or thermal stimuli than older subjects. Human newborns receiving repeated heelsticks for blood sampling develop secondary hyperalgesia indicative of spinal plasticity.

Spinal dorsal horn neurons in the neonatal rat receive inputs from a wider area of the body surface than in older animals. In intact, uninjured, adult rats, light-touch A-fibre afferents normally synapse in deeper laminae of the dorsal horn, not in the superficial laminae that receive projections from C and A δ fibre afferents involved in nociception. In contrast, neonatal rats have A fibre light-touch afferent projections to synaptic targets on lamina 1 and 2 dorsal horn neurons (Coggeshall et al 1996). Dorsal horn neurons in neonatal animals frequently show very prolonged firing following noxious stimulation.

The proto-oncogene *c-fos* has been used as a marker of neuronal activity by several groups. In adult animals, noxious stimulation evokes *c-fos* expression in superficial laminae of the dorsal horn. Jennings and Fitzgerald (1996) showed that even non-noxious stimulation evokes robust *c-fos* expression in laminae 1 and 2 in neonatal rats.

Newborn rats respond with nocifensive behaviours to inflammatory stimuli, such as formalin. They show analgesic responses to opioids that are not due to sedation alone, since the sedative pentobarbital produces sedation but not analgesia in this model (Abbott & Guy 1995).

Overall, these results suggest that the neonatal nervous system reacts in a robust manner to noxious inputs. Many of the response patterns in peripheral and spinal neurons are stronger than comparable responses in older organisms and these responses are more 'spread out' spatially and temporally.

The above-mentioned studies have been interpreted by some reviewers to suggest that the neonate may feel pain more intensely than older subjects. This interpretation should be made with caution, since these and other neurophysiological and molecular studies do not clarify the nature of pain viewed as suffering in neonatal humans or animals. Myelination of afferent pathways to the thalamus is generally complete by 30 weeks. Thalamocortical projections begin synapse formation with cortical neurons by 20–24 weeks and myelination of thalamocortical fibres is complete by roughly 37 weeks. We know comparatively little about the supraspinal aspects of nociception in neonates and even less about the affective dimension of their pain experiences.

Rather than addressing the nature of suffering in the neonate, one can more readily examine whether there are adverse short-term or long-term consequences of noxious events in neonates and whether these consequences can be ameliorated by analgesics or other pain-reducing interventions.

SHORT-TERM CONSEQUENCES OF PAIN IN THE NEONATE

Noxious events, including needle procedures or surgery, evoke behavioural and physiologic signs of stress and distress in newborns. Anand and co-workers (1987) showed that surgery in inadequately anaesthetized preterm or term newborns evokes a dramatic hormonal and metabolic stress response that can be associated with haemodynamic fluctuations, catabolism and postsurgical complications. Opioids (Robinson & Gregory 1981) and regional anaesthesia can be used safely and effectively in neonates. Both may blunt hormonal-metabolic and autonomic stress responses. In some cases, blunting of stress responses may improve outcomes (Anand & Hickey 1992). With proper expertise, neonates can be safely anaesthetized for any type of surgery (Berry & Gregory 1987, Berde 1998). There is no need to perform surgery in neonates without adequate general and/or regional anaesthesia.

Newborn circumcision is commonly performed without anaesthesia. Circumcision performed in this manner produces autonomic changes, including increases in heart rate and blood pressure, and hypoxaemia, probably due in part to acute rises in pulmonary artery pressures and right-to-left shunting of blood through the foramen ovale and the ductus arteriosus. Several methods have been studied to reduce the pain of circumcision, including dorsal penile nerve block (Stang et al 1988), ring block and topical anaesthesia with an eutectic mixture of lidocaine and prilocaine known as EMLA (Benini et al 1993, Taddio et al 1997a). EMLA appears to provide partial suppression of behavioural and physiologic signs of stress with circumcision. Lander and co-workers (1997) found that EMLA was more effective than placebo but less effective than ring block. Non-pharmacologic measures, including use of a more comfortable papoose board and oral ingestion of sucrose (Blass & Hoffmeyer 1991), also diminish distress with circumcision. The combination of pharmacologic and non-pharmacologic approaches may be optimal for this procedure.

Newborns in intensive care units commonly receive opioids and benzodiazepines, both for invasive procedures and for tolerating mechanical ventilation via endotracheal tubes. There is wide variation in analgesic and sedative use in this setting (Johnston et al 1997). A large retrospective multicentre study by Kahn et al (1998) examined patterns of opioid administration in over 1000 low birthweight infants receiving mechanical ventilation in six different neonatal intensive care units. Mean opioid dosing varied 28-fold between units. Despite this wide variation, the authors found minimal differences in outcomes. This study was retrospective and uncontrolled and did not examine long-term outcome measures, so it is difficult to draw conclusions from this report regarding risks and benefits. A recent multicentre trial by Anand and co-workers (*Archives of*

Pediatric and Adolescent Medicine, in press) examined a cohort of 68 premature neonates receiving mechanical ventilation for hyaline membrane disease. They were randomly assigned to receive infusions of morphine, the benzodiazepine sedative midazolam or placebo. The morphine group showed statistically fewer adverse neurologic outcomes, while the midazolam group showed the greatest number of these outcomes, with the placebo group having intermediate outcomes.

POTENTIAL LONG-TERM CONSEQUENCES OF PAIN IN THE NEONATE

In a previous era, a common excuse for withholding analgesia from newborns was that infants would not remember pain and that there would be no long-term adverse sequelae of unrelieved pain in infancy. Some recent studies have attempted to address this issue. Taddio and co-workers (1997b) examined responses to intramuscular injections for immunization in cohorts of 4–6-month-old boys who had participated as neonates in a randomized blinded comparison of EMLA to placebo for circumcision. In addition, there was a group of boys who were uncircumcised. Uncircumcised infants cried less and had lower pain ratings by blinded observers. For some measures, but not others, the EMLA group had statistically lower pain ratings than the placebo group. The authors could not explain away these group differences on the basis of baseline temperament or demographic variables. These findings are suggestive, but should be interpreted cautiously in view of a potential for confounding factors.

Johnston and Stevens (1996) examined responses to heelstick procedures comparing two groups of infants at a similar gestational age, 32 weeks: comparatively healthy infants born within that week and a group of prematures born at 28 weeks, who had undergone a range of invasive procedures. There were significant group differences in behavioural and physiologic parameters, both at baseline and following the needle procedure. Neonates who had undergone the largest number of invasive procedures had the fewest behavioural responses to the heelstick procedure. This lack of responsiveness has been ascribed to interrupted neurologic development with critical illness, but may also reflect a degree of 'learned helplessness'.

Grunau and co-workers (1994) studied children who had previously undergone newborn intensive care. They reported in one study that parents rated their pain behaviours as lower than those of siblings, while another study found a higher prevalence of somatized complaints in comparison to controls. These results are intriguing, though a range of alternative interpretations are possible, related to a wide range of neurologic impairments in the survivors of newborn intensive care, as well as effects of early trauma and illness on subsequent parent–child interactions.

Overall, the long-term consequences of untreated pain in infancy remain difficult to quantify, but merit further study. Since safe and effective treatments are available for many forms of pain, in our view the burden of proof lies with those who would withhold treatment, not with those who would treat pain aggressively with analgesics.

PAIN ASSESSMENT

In adults, self-report is most commonly relied upon for pain measurement and assessment. Visual analogue scales have a number of convenient and favourable properties. Children aged 8 and above can generally apply standard VAS scales successfully. Below age 8, there is more frequent confusion about the anchors and less evidence for validity. A number of investigators have developed self-report scales for children aged 3–8. These have been primarily in three groups:

1. scales that use pictures or drawings of faces;
2. scales that use graded colour intensity, generally red;
3. scales that use numbers of objects, e.g. poker chips.

Faces scales have been quite popular and differ in several respects, including number of faces presented, the way the faces are drawn or photographed (Beyer et al 1992) and how the faces are ordered on the page, etc. (Wong & Baker 1988, Bieri et al 1990). In general, severe pain is depicted as a crying face, with eyes closed, brow furrowed and nasolabial folds contracted. Some scales show a series of photographs of the same child with a range of facial expressions from happy to screaming. Rating of these pictures may be influenced by gender and ethnicity of the child in the picture and the child doing the ratings. A recent study showed that the pain ratings differ according to the choice of anchors on the scale, particularly according to whether the 'no pain' end of the scale shows a neutral face or a happy face. Some children seem to be confused regarding ranking of happiness or well-being as opposed to absence of pain. Colour analogue scales (more pain corresponds to more intensely red colour) appear acceptable to most children aged 4 and older (Grossi et al 1983, McGrath et al 1996) and show convergent validity to VAS scales in older children.

Behavioural scales have been developed predominantly in two settings: in the assessment of toddlers and preschool children undergoing brief painful procedures or surgery (Katz et al 1980, McGrath et al 1985) and in the assessment of neonates undergoing procedures or intensive care. Behavioural measures in neonates have examined facial expression, a range of gross motor behaviours and analysis of cry acoustic properties. Work by Grunau et al (1990) showed that facial expressions appear useful and valid as indicators of pain in neonates. Overall, facial expression measures appear more robust and sensitive than measures of crying (Hadjistavropoulos et al 1994). Johnston et al (1993) and Stevens et al (1995) have characterized differences in pain-related behaviours in prematures of different postconceptional and postnatal ages, both in terms of the characteristics of their cry and the components of facial action. Stevens et al (1996) have developed multidimensional measures that adjust for developmental stage that appear to be very appropriate for studies of prematures of different postconceptional and postnatal ages.

Several behavioural scales used with toddlers and older children have been labelled as 'distress' scales, because they record behaviours that may reflect either pain, fear or anxiety, but cannot distinguish among these states. Behavioural scales, such as the CHEOPS scale, may therefore signal fear instead of pain in the setting of acute medical procedures. Conversely, behavioural measures developed for acute procedures may under-rate persistent pain, such as pain following surgery (Beyer et al 1990) or pain due to cancer. Many children with persistent pain due to cancer, surgery, burns or sickle cell disease may lie still in bed, close their eyes and inhibit their movements, not because they are comfortable or narcotized, but because it hurts too much to move; withdrawal from the surroundings is an adaptive response to unrelieved pain. Gauvain-Picard et al (1987) have developed measures for children with cancer that incorporate assessment of social involvement and inhibition of movement. There is a need for additional validation and for modifications of these measures to make them more convenient and generalizable to other populations and clinical situations.

Physiologic measures have seemed attractive because of their presumed objectivity. Pain evokes increases in heart rate, blood pressure and respiratory rate, but these signs can be influenced by several physiologic conditions unrelated to pain.

Several investigators have examined variability in heart rate using a variety of mathematical algorithms in frequency domain or transfer function analyses to reflect sympathetic and parasympathetic contributions to the overall variability. Variability in heart rate has been widely used as an index of physiologic integrity and stress in fetal monitoring. Indices of 'vagal tone' have been used to measure stress and distress in neonates undergoing painful procedures (Porter et al 1988, Porter & Porges 1991), but some of these parameters may also be sensitive to factors unrelated to pain (Litvack et al 1995, Oberlander et al 1995, 1996). McIntosh et al (1994) have provided evidence that measures of variability in physiologic parameters, including heart rate, blood pressure and end-tidal carbon dioxide, may indeed be more useful than absolute trends in these physiologic parameters in painful situations. Issues of sensitivity and specificity remain, since critical illness and other processes can also affect beat-to-beat variability of heart rate and blood pressure.

Stress hormones, including cortisol and epinephrine, and metabolites such as glucose are increased by surgical trauma and analgesics and anaesthetics suppress these increased plasma concentrations, but there is little evidence for the specificity of any of these biochemical markers as a pain measure per se.

Overall, there is little immediate prospect for a unidimensional physiologic measure that is convenient and specific for pain in neonates. A more detailed description of pain assessment in children is presented in Chapter 15.

DEVELOPMENTAL PHARMACOLOGY

A number of pharmacokinetic and pharmacodynamic factors modify responses to analgesic medication in the newborn and young infant, as summarized in Table 65.1.

ANALGESIC PHARMACOLOGY

Acetaminophen (paracetamol) is useful for treatment of mild pain and fever control. Acetaminophen replaced aspirin as the most commonly used routine analgesic and antipyretic in children in the 1970s, when it became apparent that aspirin could in rare circumstances cause Reye's hepatic encephalopathy in children, especially during viral illnesses. Acetaminophen overall appears very safe in children if dosing guidelines are followed. Children may receive single doses of 15–20 mg/kg, or repeated dosing of 10–15 mg/kg every 4 hours. Toxicity appears related in part to cumulative dosing. Conservative daily dose limits based on available pharmacokinetic data are 90 mg/kg/day in children, 60 mg/kg/day in infants and 45 mg/kg/day in prematures (Lin et al 1997). Rectal absorption is slow, with peak concentrations over 70 minutes after administration. Single rectal doses of 35–40 mg/kg achieve therapeutic plasma concentrations, with slow clearance (Birmingham et al 1997). Therefore, following a first

Table 65.1 Factors that influence drug action in neonates

Factor	*Clinical implications*
Immature ventilatory reflexes	Greater potential for hypoventilation from opioids
Larger percent body mass as water, less as fat	Altered volumes of distribution
Immature hepatic enzyme systems	Diminished hepatic conjugation of drugs, accumulation of opioids and local anaesthetics with delayed toxicity during infusions
Diminished glomerular filtration and renal tubular secretion	Diminished renal excretion of opioid metabolites, with potential for delayed sedation and respiratory depression
Decreased plasma concentrations of albumen and α_1 acid glycoprotein	Decreased protein binding of drugs; greater first-pass local anaesthetic toxicity
Smaller size per se	With local anaesthetic blockade, the effective dose to block nerves scales weakly with body weight, while systemic toxicity scales directly with body weight, so that the therapeutic index for local anaesthetics is narrower in smaller subjects

dose of 35–45 mg/kg, subsequent doses should either extend the interval to 6–8 hours or use smaller amounts.

Non-steroidal anti-inflammatory drugs (NSAIDs) are useful for many forms of pain, including, but not limited to, postoperative pain, arthritis and other inflammatory conditions and pain in sickle cell disease. A large number of NSAIDs have been examined for perioperative use in children, including indomethacin (Maunuksela et al 1988), ibuprofen, diclofenac and ketorolac (Rusy et al 1995). They appear effective via oral, intravenous, rectal and intramuscular routes. There is no reason to use intramuscular injection for most children, as it is painful. The intravenous route is convenient for administration during or immediately after surgery, though there is little evidence that this route is uniquely more effective than oral or rectal dosing for NSAIDs. NSAIDs reduce the requirement for opioids in many paediatric postoperative studies and in some of these studies, this results in a reduction of opioid-related side effects (Vetter & Heiner 1994). There is little evidence for differences between NSAIDs in analgesic effectiveness and many studies do not compare them at a range of doses that would permit proper comparison of analgesia and side effects.

When compared with aspirin in children with rheumatoid arthritis, ibuprofen appeared equally effective and better tolerated (Giannini et al 1990). Short-term use of ibuprofen in children in paediatric office practice has a very low risk of gastric irritation or bleeding (Lesko & Mitchell 1995). Overall, the safety of NSAIDs in children seems quite good, though rare cases of gastrointestinal bleeding and nephropathy have been reported. NSAIDs should be used with caution in types of surgery where bleeding is of major concern. A retrospective study of children undergoing tonsillectomy reported an increased incidence of postoperative bleeding when ketorolac was used (Judkins et al 1996). The safety and efficacy of NSAIDs used as analgesics in newborns have not been established. NSAIDs are used in prematures primarily to facilitate closure of the ductus arteriosus.

Few data are available at present regarding the cyclo-oxygenase 2 (COX-2) specific inhibitors in children. Available data in adults suggests that they will be useful and may reduce some of the side effects and complications of NSAIDs. The lack of impairment of coagulation may be especially useful for paediatric postoperative use and for children with cancer pain.

Opioids can be used for infants and children of all ages with proper understanding of age-related changes in pharmacokinetics (Olkkola et al 1995) and pharmacodynamics. A number of opioids have received pharmacokinetic study in infants and children, including morphine (Olkkola et al 1988), fentanyl (Gauntlett et al 1988) and sufentanil

Table 65.2 Dosing of non-opioid analgesics in children

Drug	*Recommended dosing*
Acetaminophen	10–15 mg/kg orally every 4 hours 20–40 mg/kg rectally every 6 hours Daily maximum: children 90 mg/kg infants 60 mg/kg neonates 45 mg/kg
Aspirin	10–15 mg/kg orally every 4 hours Daily maximum 90–120 mg/kg (children)
Ibuprofen	8–10 mg/kg every 6 hours
Naproxen	6–8 mg/kg every 8–12 hours
Choline-magnesium salicylate	10–15 mg/kg every 8–12 hours

(Greeley et al 1987). The general pattern emerges that clearances, normalized by body weight, are diminished in the first months of life and reach mature values over the first 3–12 months. Neonates and young infants are thus susceptible to drug accumulation and delayed sedation and respiratory depression if infusions are extrapolated based on recommended dosing in older children. The time course of maturation may depend in part on medical condition. For example, infants undergoing non-cardiac surgery tend to show mature morphine clearances by 1–3 months of age, while infants undergoing cardiac surgery show reduced clearances through the first 6–9 months of life (Lynn et al 1998). Recommended opioid dosing is shown in Table 65.3.

The issue of pharmacodynamic respiratory sensitivity of neonates has been debated for many years. Early observations by Way et al (1965) suggested that neonates had greater respiratory depression than older children and adults and that morphine may be more depressant than meperidine. Ventilatory reflexes to hypoxia and hypercarbia are indeed immature in human newborns and mature over the first months of life. Investigators have examined respiratory sensitivity in neonates by a number of methods, including carbon dioxide response curves, continuous apnoea monitoring using impedance plethysmography, or continuous oximetry. Healthy infants aged 3 months and older in these largely postoperative studies have similar analgesic responses and similar degrees of respiratory depression as adults at similar plasma opioid concentrations. Opioid infusions have been used extensively for children. Overall, the efficacy and safety have been reported to be generally good. Haberkern et al (1996), in a recent comparative trial, reconfirmed that both intravenous morphine and epidural morphine produce good analgesia, but with a fairly high incidence of side effects, including itching, nausea, ileus and urinary retention. Both routes of morphine administration, when titrated to analgesic effectiveness, were associated with approximately 50% reductions in CO_2 response slopes.

Overall, opioid infusions in younger infants are useful and generally safe, but their dosing and titration do require expertise and vigilance. Since pain assessment in infants is imprecise, titration to clinical effect is more difficult. There is neither consensus nor conclusive evidence to say which forms of electronic monitoring are most useful for detecting hypoxaemia or hypoventilation. Impedance apnoea monitoring is widely available with telemetry alarms that can ring in a hallway or at the nurses' station on a hospital ward. There are case reports of significant hypoxaemia in infants receiving opioids despite normal respiratory rates (Karl et al 1996). For this reason, some clinicians have advocated continuous oximetry as a method of monitoring. Oximetry is useful for detection of hypoxaemia, but has practical limitations related to motion artefacts. More importantly, remote telemetry of oximeters is not widely available. Oximeter alarms may thus go undetected in a hospital room and provide a false sense of security. Convenient, low-cost, motion-insensitive oximetry with telemetry to a central site on a ward would be extremely useful. Electronic surveillance is not a substitute for clinical assessment and understanding of factors that modify opioid requirements and risk.

Patient-controlled analgesia has been used for children for the past 10 years with excellent safety, good efficacy and excellent patient acceptance. Compared with bolus administration, PCA provides better pain scores, better patient acceptance and no increase in opioid use or opioid side effects (Berde et al 1991). Compared with continuous opioid infusions, PCA provides either equivalent or in some studies better pain scores, but with a reduction of opioid use and opioid side effects (Mackie et al 1991). PCA is generally well used by children aged 6 and above. Optimal choice of dosing parameters has been studied by Doyle and co-workers (1993). Short lock-out intervals (e.g. 5–7 minutes) are safe and allow more rapid 'catch-up' in the setting of unrelieved pain. Basal infusions should be individualized according to medical risk factors, as well as psychological factors (Wermeling et al 1992). They may increase patient satisfaction (Doyle et al 1993), but may result in more episodic night-time oxygen desaturation (McNeely & Trentadue 1997).

Table 65.3 Opioid analgesic initial dosage guidelines

Drug	*Equianalgesic doses*		*Usual starting IV or SC doses and intervals*		*Parenteral: oral dose ratio*	*Usual starting oral doses and intervals*	
	Parenteral	Oral	Child<50 kg	Child>50 kg		Child<50 kg	Child>50 kg
Codeine	N/R	200 mg	N/R	N/R	1:2	0.5–1 mg/kg every 3–4 h	30–60 mg every 3–4 h
Morphine	10 mg	30 mg	Bolus: 0.1 mg/kg every 2–4 h Infusion 0.03 mg/kg/h	Bolus 5–8 mg every 2–4 h Infusion 1.5 mg/h	1:3	Immediate release: 0.3 mg/kg every 3–4 h Sustained release 20–35 kg: 10–15 mg every 8–12 h 35–50 kg: 15–30 mg every 8–12 h	Immediate release: 15–20 mg every 3–4 h Sustained release: 30–45 mg every 8–12 h
Oxycodone	N/A	30 mg	N/A	N/A	N/A	0.1–0.2 mg/kg every 3–4 h	5–10 mg every 3–4 h
Methadone	10 mg	20 mg	0.1 mg/kg every 4–8 h	1:2	1:2	0.2 mg/kg every 4–8 h	10 mg every 4–8 h
	Methadone requires additional vigilance, because it can accumulate and produce delayed sedation. If sedation occurs, doses should be withheld until sedation resolves. Thereafter, doses should be substantially reduced and/or the dosing interval should be extended to 8–12 hours.						
Fentanyl	100 μg (0.1 mg)	N/A	Bolus: 0.5–1 μg/kg every 1–2 h Infusion: 0.5–1.5 μg/kg/h	Bolus: 25–50 μg every 1–2 h Infusion 25–75 μg/h	N/A	N/A	N/A
Hydromorphone	1.5–2 mg	6–8 mg	Bolus: 0.02 mg every 2–4 h Infusion: 0.006 mg/kg/h	Bolus: 1 mg Every 2–4 h Infusion: 0.3 mg/h	1:4	0.04–0.08 mg/kg every 3–4 h	2–4 mg every 3–4 h
Meperidine (pethidine)	75 mg	300 mg	Bolus: 0.8–1 mg/kg every 2–3 h	Bolus: 50–75 mg every 2–3 h	1:4	2–3 mg/kg every 3–4 h	100–150 mg every 3–4 h
	Meperidine should generally be avoided if other opioids are available, especially with chronic use, because its metabolite can cause seizures.						

Doses refer to patients >6 months of age. In infants <6 months, initial doses/kg should begin at roughly 25% of the doses/kg recommended here. All doses are approximate and should be adjusted according to clinical circumstances.

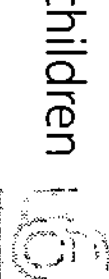

There is some controversy surrounding nurse-controlled and parent-controlled analgesia for children. With PCA administered by the patient, the inherent safety lies in the fact that when the patient gets narcotized, they fall asleep, stop dosing and the plasma concentration falls, keeping the patient safe. Recent studies suggest good safety when nurses use the PCA pump for infants and children unable to dose themselves (Kanagasundaram et al 1997). There is similarly a very good experience with home dosing of PCA pumps by parents for infants and children in palliative care. What is more problematic is having parents push the button for opioid-naïve children, particularly in a postoperative setting. The arguments in favour of parental dosing are that parents are the child's primary caregivers and they are in an ideal position to assess their needs. The counter-argument is that without specific training and monitoring, on rare occasions, their well-meaning efforts may lead to overdose. We are aware of several cases around the world in which this has occurred, with disastrous consequences. Until this has received further study, it would be prudent to recommend that if parent-controlled PCA is to be used in non-palliative situations, there should be a formal programme of parent education and an increased level of patient observation.

LOCAL ANAESTHETICS

Local anaesthetics are used increasingly for regional anaesthesia in children, as well as for topical analgesia and infiltration. Maximum doses for single injection are recommended in Table 65.4.

Excessive doses of local anaesthetics cause convulsions, arrhythmias and cardiac depression that can be very difficult to treat. Recent studies by Kohane et al (1998) using an infant rat model found that infant animals have a narrower therapeutic index for local anaesthetics than adult animals on the basis of scaling factors, since the effective dose to block nerves scales comparatively weakly with body size, while toxic doses scale more directly with body size.

Topical administration of local anaesthetics is widely used for relieving the pain of needle procedures and for superficial procedures, including suture of lacerations or removal of skin lesions. For intact skin, the most widely used preparation is EMLA (Maunuksela & Korpela 1986). EMLA has proved to be extremely safe in infants and children of all ages. It requires about an hour for adequate cutaneous analgesia in most situations. Although high systemic concentrations of prilocaine can produce methaemoglobinaemia, this has not been a significant clinical problem in widespread use, even with repeated or prolonged dosing in younger infants. An alternative preparation with excellent safety and efficacy is tetracaine gel (amethocaine) (Lawson et al 1995).

Table 65.4 Conservative dosing guidelines for local anaesthetics (mg/kg for single injection; mg/kg/h for infusions)

Drug	*Single injection*				*Prolonged infusion*	
	0–6 months		>1 year		0–6 months	>1 year
	– epi	+ epi	– epi	+ epi		
Lidocaine	4	5	5	7	0.8	1.6
Bupivacaine	1.6	2	2	2.5	0.2	0.4
Chloroprocaine	30	30	30	30	30	30

For application to cut skin, especially for suture of lacerations, combinations of local anaesthetics with vasoconstrictors are widely used. The combination of tetracaine with epinephrine (adrenalin) and cocaine is known as TAC. Several studies have shown that these preparations are effective when used in emergency departments for repair of lacerations (Bonadio 1989). TAC should be avoided in the vicinity of end-arteries, since ischaemic complications have occurred. Larger doses applied to mucosal surfaces have produced convulsions and deaths due to rapid absorption of the tetracaine and cocaine. More recent studies have found equivalent effectiveness using preparations with the cocaine omitted and combinations of tetracaine and phenylephrine appear useful in this setting (Smith et al 1997).

Regional anaesthesia in infants and children can be performed by specific modifications of techniques used in adults. The reader is referred to Dalens' excellent textbook for an illustrated summary. A variety of peripheral nerve blocks can provide analgesia after surgery with an excellent safety and side effect profile (Dalens et al 1989a,b, Giaufre et al 1996). Regional anaesthesia is generally performed in children asleep, as a method of providing postoperative analgesia.

For major thoracic, abdominal, pelvic and lower extremity operations, epidural analgesia can provide outstanding analgesia and when optimally managed, may facilitate recovery of high-risk patients. (Meignier et al 1983, McNeely 1991). Single-shot caudal blockade with local anaesthetics is generally safe and effective for many minor lower-body procedures, though there is a need to provide longer duration than is afforded by bupivacaine alone. α_2 adrenergics, such as clonidine, prolong local anaesthetic action and have received promising study in children (Mikawa et al 1996, Constant et al 1998). Combinations of opioids and local anaesthetics have excellent efficacy and are particularly effective when the catheter tip can be placed in the dermatomes involved in the surgery, either by direct placement or by cephalad advancement from the caudal route (Bosenberg et al 1988).

OTHER ANALGESICS

There have been comparatively few clinical trials of other drug classes for pain in children. Although clinicians widely prescribe tricyclic antidepressants, anticonvulsants and a range of other medications for several chronic pain conditions in children, most dosing is based on anecdote or extrapolation from adult experience. There are clinical trials of trazodone (Battistella et al 1993) and calcium channel blockers (Sorge & Marano 1985) in childhood migraine that show efficacy. In some cases, extrapolation of adult studies may not be applicable. For example, sumatriptan, which is quite effective in interrupting adult migraine attacks, has appeared less impressive in a paediatric trial (Hamalainen et al 1997). Similarly, propranolol appears less effective in migraine prophylaxis in children (Olness et al 1987). There is a need for more controlled trials of a range of analgesics in children, especially in the setting of chronic or recurrent pain.

MANAGEMENT OF SPECIFIC TYPES OF PAIN IN CHILDREN

POSTOPERATIVE PAIN

Amelioration of postoperative pain is best accomplished by co-ordinated efforts among parents, paediatricians, surgeons, anaesthesiologists, nurses, pharmacists, child specialists and others involved in perioperative care. Proper preoperative preparation can reduce anxiety and fear, which can amplify pain. Children should receive explanations that are appropriate to their developmental stage. Preoperative education programmes are now available at many paediatric centres and these may be helpful in this process. Techniques of anaesthetic induction should strive to be atraumatic. Parental presence for mask induction may reduce distress for many children. Use of EMLA or other topical anaesthetics may reduce the distress of intravenous induction. Oral premedication can also reduce anxiety for many children.

Kehlet (1998) and others have championed the concept of multimodal analgesia for adults undergoing surgery. It is likely that this concept applies for children as well. Combinations of opioids, local anaesthetics and NSAIDs may be ideal in many settings.

Acute pain services can be useful for advocacy and for ensuring that pain management is a priority. In many paediatric centres, these have been developed and appear to provide extremely useful services. Standardized protocols are useful to ensure consistency in management, to ensure that side effects are treated promptly and to minimize dosing errors. Decimal point errors are common in paediatric hospitals and protocolized dosing facilitates cross-checking for erroneous orders. If children are to be cared for in general hospitals, it is ideal to have paediatric specialists involved in creation of specific pain management protocols for children. A number of models for pain treatment can be used and the choice of participants and specialists may depend on local expertise and availability.

TRAUMA AND BURNS

In many respects, children sustaining major trauma and burns should be managed according to the principles set out for postoperative pain. Historically, these forms of pain have been often undertreated in children (Perry & Heidrich 1982). Often, the duration of pain may be quite prolonged (Szyfelbein et al 1985). Particularly with major burns, marked dose escalation is often required. As pain subsides, dosing may require gradual tapering to prevent withdrawal.

CANCER AND PALLIATIVE CARE

Cancer pain and palliative care in children are discussed in detail in Chapter 42. Many of the principles outlined in adult palliative care apply to children (Miser et al 1983, Stevens et al 1994, Collins et al 1995). Pharmacologic management by the WHO analgesic ladder is effective for most children with pain due to widespread cancer (Kasai et al 1995). Some of the differences in the approach to palliative care for children involves consideration of the child's emotional and cognitive development and the family's roles in support and palliative care (Goldman 1996).

BRIEF DIAGNOSTIC AND THERAPEUTIC PROCEDURES

Needle procedures are a significant source of distress for children. Healthy infants and children receive subcutaneous and intramuscular injections for immunizations. Children with acute and chronic illness may in addition receive more frequent procedures, including venepuncture, intravenous cannulation, lumbar puncture and bone marrow aspiration. Approaches to these procedures must be individualized according to the child's age, cognitive development, coping style and health status. Appropriate explanation and support can be helpful. Topical cooling may be beneficial for some children. As noted above, oral sucrose has been used for infants receiving distressing procedures (Blass & Hoffmeyer 1991) and appears safe and partially effective.

Cognitive-behavioural techniques, including guided imagery, hypnosis and relaxation, can diminish the distress of these procedures for many children (Zeltzer & LeBaron 1982, McGrath & De Veber 1986, Kuttner 1989, Zeltzer et al 1989, Jay et al 1995). These techniques are used very widely and can be taught to most children aged 5–7 and above. Some experts use them for children aged 3–5 as well (McGrath & De Veber 1986).

For children receiving oncology procedures, gastrointestinal endoscopy or radiologic procedures, many do well with 'conscious sedation', often using sedative-anxiolytics, especially benzodiazepines (Sievers et al 1991), combined with either opioid analgesics or low-dose ketamine (Marx et al 1997). For higher risk or highly unco-operative children or for more extensive procedures, general anaesthesia may be a more effective alternative. There is considerable controversy regarding the appropriate personnel (i.e. anaesthetist versus non-anaesthetist), choice of agents, depth of sedation required, relative risks, benefits, efficacy, costs and comparative safety of conscious sedation versus brief general anaesthesia (Maxwell & Yaster 1996).

SICKLE CELL ANAEMIA

Sickle cell disease refers to series of related genetic haemoglobin disorders occurring predominantly in peoples of African and Middle Eastern descent. Abnormal haemoglobin molecules polymerize under certain conditions, including hypoxaemia, acidosis, hypothermia and erythrocyte cell water loss. Haemoglobin polymerization leads to abnormal erythrocyte shape (sickling) and reduced deformability and impaired rheology of small vessels, leading to vaso-occlusion and ischaemic pain. Pain in sickle cell disease is extremely variable in its frequency and severity (Platt et al 1991). The majority of patients manage their persistent and episodic pains as outpatients, using oral hydration, NSAIDs and episodic oral opioids. A subgroup of patients has more severe episodes of vaso-occlusive pain that require hospitalization. Opioids should be given as needed to provide comfort (Benjamin 1989). Opioid titration may require some additional care, since hypoxaemia and hypercarbia further exacerbate sickling of erythrocytes. Recent studies emphasize home management (Shapiro et al 1995), oral opioid dosing, avoidance of a 'crisis' model and teaching of cognitive-behavioural (Thomas et al 1984, Dinges et al 1997) and coping (Gil et al 1997) techniques.

HIV/AIDS

HIV disease in children is now most commonly acquired by congenital infection. The natural history of HIV in infants has improved greatly in developed countries in recent years with multidrug treatment regimens. Children with HIV receive a large number of painful diagnostic and therapeutic procedures (Hirschfeld et al 1996). Infants with encephalopathy and severe developmental delay sometimes present with persistent irritability and screaming. Many of these infants respond to opioids; in other cases, anticonvulsants may be helpful, even when clinical seizures are not evident.

NEUROPATHIC PAINS

Neuropathic pains in children can be a source of considerable distress and suffering (Ollson & Berde 1993). In our clinic, the most common causes are postsurgical/post-traumatic localized peripheral nerve injuries, complex regional pain syndrome type 1 (CRPS1)/reflex sympathetic dystrophy (RSD), pains associated with metabolic neuropathies, pain after spinal cord injury and neuropathic cancer pain. Phantom pain following amputation is not rare and may be persistent and severe (Krane et al 1991). We commonly extrapolate approaches used in adults, including liberal prescribing of tricyclic antidepressants and anticonvulsants.

CRPS1/RSD in children and adolescents has a marked female predominance (roughly 6:1), a marked lower extremity predominance (roughly 6:1) and an apparently high association with competitive sports (Pillemer & Micheli 1988), gymnastics and dance (Wilder et al 1992). The reasons for this association are unclear. Some clinicians regard this as a psychogenic condition (Sherry & Weisman 1988), though evidence of causation, as opposed to association, is weak. Approaches to treatment of CRPS1/RSD have been extremely varied, ranging from rehabilitative (Bernstein et al 1978) to more interventionist. In our view, physical therapy and biobehavioural approaches should be emphasized and sympathetic blockade should be used sparingly and not in isolation.

CHRONIC 'BENIGN' PAINS OF CHILDHOOD

Chronic and recurrent pains in children have a different epidemiology from those in adults. Back pain and neck pain are less common in children. Trigeminal neuralgia is extraordinarily rare in children and herpes zoster is much less likely to produce a postherpetic neuralgia.

Children commonly experience recurrent pains of the head, chest, abdomen and limbs. These conditions typically involve painful episodes alternating with pain-free times in a child who is otherwise healthy. These conditions are very common and population-based surveys suggest that between 4% and 10% of children experience these symptoms with some regularity (Apley & Naish 1958, Oster 1972, Oster & Nielson 1972, Coleman 1984, Bille 1997). Both migraine and tension-type headaches increase in prevalence during the school-age years and into adolescence. A number of chronic and recurrent pain conditions in children show a female gender predominance, particularly among adolescents (Wilder et al 1992).

Most children presenting with these complaints will be determined to be medically well. The primary paediatrician or general practitioner needs to develop a screening approach that emphasizes a sensitive medical history and physical exam that detects the small subset of patients who need further evaluation (Levine & Rappaport 1984). It is wise to de-emphasize unfocused laboratory testing, which is generally of low yield in these conditions. Lifestyle interventions may be helpful and questions should be included regarding family and school circumstances, diet, sleep, sports and a range of activities. In some situations, modifications of diet, school stressors and exercise may have considerable benefit. For example, a subgroup of children with recurrent abdominal pain may improve by treatment of constipation or by treating lactose intolerance with oral lactase enzyme replacement or avoidance of milk products (Barr et al 1979).

Physical therapeutic approaches are extremely helpful for many chronic painful conditions in children. Physical therapists should be integral participants in multidisciplinary chronic pain programmes for children. Aerobic conditioning and strength training may have both specific, localized benefits, e.g. for an adolescent with myofascial pain, and also more generalized beneficial effects on mood, sleep and general well-being. There is a need for more controlled trials of physical therapies for pain in children, in order to define which components are effective and with what 'dose response'.

PSYCHOLOGICAL FACTORS IN PAIN IN CHILDREN

As with adults, in children the experience of pain is modulated by biologic variation, past pain experiences, meaning of the pain, context, fear, anxiety, depression and a range of other factors. In children, there is the additional aspect of the impact of development on the cognitive and emotional aspects of pain responses.

A number of the recurrent benign pains of childhood have been commonly regarded as 'psychogenic'. The evidence that most children with these symptoms are psychiatrically ill is generally weak (McGrath & Unruh 1987, Walker et al 1993); many children and adolescents with these symptoms in fact are well adjusted and cope rather well. The prevalence of psychiatric diagnoses and symptoms also may vary according to referral population, i.e. surveys from specialists, generalists, mental health professionals or the general public. Barr, Oberlander, Rappaport and others have argued against dichotomizing these conditions as purely 'psychogenic' or purely 'organic' (Oberlander & Rappaport 1993). The term 'functional' has been used to describe these pains that may arise from variations in normal functioning, but are not related to a specific disease or to psychopathology. While the concept behind this term is useful, the term itself may not be helpful since many clinicians equate the word with 'psychosomatic' or 'psychogenic'.

SCHOOL ABSENTEEISM AND DISABILITY

In adults, chronic pain is a major social, economic and political problem both because it produces suffering, but also because low back pain in particular is an enormous cause of disability. A medical model alone cannot explain the natural history and patterns of disability.

School absenteeism and school avoidance are extremely common among patients referred to our paediatric pain clinic. In our view, it is helpful to regard school avoidance in many (but not all) cases as a disability syndrome with analogies to work absenteeism in adults with chronic pain. The analogy goes further: just as the workmen's compensation system in adults may serve to reinforce disability, home-tutoring programmes for children with chronic pain may in some cases facilitate a sick role away from the mainstream of life in a school setting. In the future, multidisciplinary programmes for pain management in children will need to address more proactively the process of return to school (Bursch et al 1998).

BIOBEHAVIOURAL TREATMENT

Over the past 20 years sufficient empirically supported evidence documenting the efficacy of biobehavioural interventions for paediatric pain syndromes has emerged.

Biobehavioural treatment techniques proven to be useful can be grouped into four categories: biofeedback, including electromyographic (EMG) and thermal; relaxation therapies, including hypnosis; operant (or contingency) pain behaviour management; and a more general category of cognitive-behavioural techniques employing self-monitoring, coping strategies and environmental modification. Compelling evidence for the efficacy of biobehavioural intervention can be found in the literature for paediatric migraine (Mehegan et al 1987), recurrent abdominal pain (Scharff 1997) and juvenile rheumatoid arthritis (Varni 1992). Although less well researched, there is evidence that biobehavioural treatment techniques are useful for neuropathic pain (Bursch et al 1998) and pain associated with sickle cell disease (Gil et al 1993).

CONCLUSION

Pain treatment is effective, safe and feasible for a wide range of acute and chronic pain conditions. Children will continue to require advocacy to provide optimal multidisciplinary care. There is a need for more controlled clinical trials for a range of treatments.

REFERENCES

Abbott FV, Guy ER 1995 Effects of morphine, pentobarbital and amphetamine on formalin-induced behaviors in infant rats: sedation versus specific suppression of pain. Pain 62: 303–312

Anand KJ, Hickey PR 1992 Halothane-morphine compared with high-dose sufentanil for anesthesia and postoperative analgesia in neonatal cardiac surgery–see comments. New England Journal of Medicine 326: 1–9

Anand KJ, Sippell WG, Aynsley-Green A 1987 A randomised trial of fentanyl anaesthesia in preterm neonates undergoing surgery: effects on the stress response. Lancet 1: 62–66

Andrews K, Fitzgerald M 1997 Biological barriers to paediatric pain management. Clinical Journal of Pain 13(2): 138–143

Apley J, Naish N 1958 Recurrent abdominal pains: a field survey of 1,000 school children. Archives of Disease in Childhood 33: 165

Barr RG, Watkins JB, Levine MD 1979 Recurrent abdominal pain (RAP) of childhood due to lactose intolerance: a prospective study. New England Journal of Medicine 300: 1449–1452

Battistella P, Ruffilli R, Cernetti R et al 1993 A placebo-controlled crossover trial using trazodone in pediatric migraine. Headache 33: 36–39

Benini F, Johnston CC, Faucher D, Aranda JV 1993 Topical anesthesia during circumcision in newborn infants. Journal of the American Medical Association 270: 850–853

Benjamin LJ 1989 Pain in sickle cell disease. In: Current therapy of pain. BC Decker, Toronto, pp 90–104

Berde CB 1998 Anesthesia and analgesia. In: Cloherty JP, Stark AR (eds) Manual of neonatal care. Lippincott-Raven, Philadelphia, pp 667–675

Berde CB, Lehn BM, Yee JD, Sethna NF, Russo D 1991 Patient-controlled analgesia in children and adolescents: a randomized, prospective comparison with intramuscular administration of morphine for postoperative analgesia. Journal of Pediatrics 118: 460–466

Bernstein BH, Singsen BH, Kent JT et al 1978 Reflex neurovascular dystrophy in childhood. Journal of Pediatrics 93: 211–215

Berry FA, Gregory GA 1987 Do premature infants require anesthesia for surgery? [editorial] Anesthesiology 67: 291–293

Beyer JE, McGrath PJ, Berde CB 1990 Discordance between self-report and behavioral pain measures in children aged 3–7 years after surgery. Journal of Pain and Symptom Management 5: 350–356

Beyer JE, Denyes MJ, Villarruel AM 1992 The creation, validation, and continuing development of the Oucher: a measure of pain intensity in children. Journal of Pediatric Nursing 7: 335–346

Bieri D, Reeve RA, Champion GD, Addicoat L, Ziegler JB 1990 The Faces Pain Scale for the self-assessment of the severity of pain experienced by children: development, initial validation, and preliminary investigation for ratio scale properties. Pain 41: 139–150

Bille B 1997 A 40-year follow-up of school children with migraine. Cephalalgia 17(4): 488–491

Birmingham P, Tobin M, Henthorn T et al 1997 Twenty-four-hour pharmacokinetics of rectal acetaminophen in children: an old drug with new recommendations. Anesthesiology 87(2): 244–252

Blass EM, Hoffmeyer LB 1991 Sucrose as an analgesic for newborn infants. Pediatrics 87: 215–218

Bonadio W 1989 TAC: a review. Pediatric Emergency Care 128

Bosenberg A, Bland B, Schulte-Steinberg O et al 1988 Thoracic epidural anesthesia via the caudal route in infants. Anesthesiology 69: 265–269

Bursch B, Walco GA, Zeltzer L 1998 Clinical assessment and management of chronic pain and pain-associated disability syndrome. Journal of Developmental and Behavioral Pediatrics 19: 45–53

Coggeshall R, Jennings E, Fitzgerald M 1996 Evidence that large myelinated primary afferent fibers make synaptic contacts in lamina II of neonatal rats. Brain Research 92(1): 81–90

Coleman WL 1984 Recurrent chest pain in children. Pediatric Clinics of North America 31: 1007

Collins J, Grier H, Kinney H, Berde C 1995 Control of severe pain in children with terminal malignancy. Journal of Pediatrics 126: 653–657

Constant I, Gall O, Gouyet L, Chauvin M, Murat I 1998 Addition of clonidine or fentanyl to local anaesthetics prolongs the duration of surgical analgesia after single shot caudal block in children. British Journal of Anaesthesia 80: 294–298

Dalens B, Vanneuville G, Dechelotte P 1989a Penile block via the subpubic space in 100 children. Anesthesia and Analgesia 69: 41–45

Dalens B, Vanneuville G, Tanguy A 1989b Comparison of the fascia iliaca compartment block with the 3-in-1 block in children. Anesthesia and Analgesia 69: 705–713

Dinges D, Whitehouse W, Orne E et al 1997 Self-hypnosis training as an adjunctive treatment in the management of pain associated with sickle cell disease. International Journal of Clinical and Experimental Hypnosis 45: 417–432

Doyle E, Harper I, Morton N 1993 Patient-controlled analgesia with low dose background infusions after lower abdominal surgery in children. British Journal of Anaesthesia 71: 818–822

Fitzgerald M, Shaw A, MacIntosh N 1988 Postnatal development of the cutaneous flexor reflex: comparative study of preterm infants and newborn rat pups. Development Medicine and Child Neurology 30: 520–526

Gauntlett IS, Fisher DM, Hertzka RE, Kuhls E, Spellman MJ, Rudolph C 1988 Pharmacokinetics of fentanyl in neonatal humans and lambs: effects of age. Anesthesiology 69: 683–687

Gauvain-Piquard A, Rodary C, Rezvani A, Lemerle J 1987 Pain in children aged 2–6 years: a new observational rating scale elaborated in a pediatric oncology unit – preliminary report. Pain 31: 177–188

Giannini E, Brewer E, Miller M et al 1990 Ibuprofen suspension in the treatment of juvenile rheumatoid arthritis. Journal of Pediatrics 117: 645–652

Giaufre E, Dalens B, Gombart A 1996 Epidemiology and morbidity of regional anesthesia in children: a one-year prospective survey of the French-Language Society of Pediatric Anesthesiologists. Anesthesia and Analgesia 904

Gil K, Thomson R, Keith B, Tota-Faucette M, Noll S, Kinney T 1993 Sickle cell disease pain in children and adolescents: change in pain frequency and coping strategies over time. Journal of Pediatric Psychology 18: 621–637

Gil K, Wilson J, Edens J 1997 The stability of pain coping strategies in young children adolescents, and adults with sickle cell disease over an 18-month period. Clinical Journal of Pain 13: 110–115

Goldman A 1996 Home care of the dying child [review]. Journal of Palliative Care 12: 16–19

Greeley WJ, De Bruijn NP, David DP 1987 Sufentanil pharmacokinetics in pediatric cardiovascular patients. Anesthesia and Analgesia 66: 1067–1072

Grossi E, Borghi C, Cerchiari EL et al 1983 Analogue chromatic continuous scale [ACCS]: a new method for pain assessment. Clinical and Experimental Rheumatology I:337–340

Grunau RV, Johnston CC, Craig KD 1990 Neonatal facial and cry responses to invasive and non-invasive procedures. Pain 42: 295–305

Grunau RV, Whitfield MF, Petrie JH, Fryer EL 1994 Early pain experience, child and family factors, as precursors of somatization: a prospective study of extremely premature and fullterm children. Pain 56: 353–359

Haberkern CM, Lynn AM, Geiduschek JM et al 1996 Epidural and intravenous bolus morphine for postoperative analgesia in infants. Canadian Journal of Anaesthesia 43: 1203–1210

Hadjistavropoulos HD, Craig KD, Grunau RV, Johnston CC 1994 Judging pain in newborns: facial and cry determinants. Journal of Pediatric Psychology 19: 485–491

Hamalainen M, Hoppu K, Santavuori P 1997 Sumatriptan for migraine attacks in children: a randomized placebo-controlled study. Do children with migraine respond to oral sumatriptan differently from adults? Neurology 48(4):1100–1113

Hirschfeld S, Moss H, Dragisic K, Smith W, Pizzo PA 1996 Pain in pediatric human immunodeficiency virus infection: incidence and characteristics in a single-institution pilot study [see comments]. Pediatrics 98: 449–452

Jay S, Elliott CH, Fitzgibbons I, Woody P, Siegel S 1995 A comparative study of cognitive behavior therapy versus general anesthesia for painful medical procedures in children [see comments]. Pain 62: 3–9

Jennings E, Fitzgerald M 1996 C-fos can be induced in the neonatal rat spinal cord by both noxious and innocuous peripheral stimulation. Pain 68(2–3): 301–306

Johnston CC, Stevens BJ 1996 Experience in a neonatal intensive care unit affects pain response. Pediatrics 98: 925–930

Johnston CC, Stevens B, Craig KD, Grunau RV 1993 Developmental changes in pain expression in premature, full-term, two- and four-month-old infants. Pain 52: 201–218

Johnston CC, Collinge JM, Henderson SJ, Anand KJ 1997 A cross-sectional survey of pain and pharmacological analgesia in Canadian neonatal intensive care units. Clinical Journal of Pain 13: 308–312

Judkins JH, Dray TG, Hubbell RN 1996 Intraoperative ketorolac and posttonsillectomy bleeding. Archives of Otolaryngology – Head and Neck Surgery 122: 937–940

Kahn DJ, Richardson DK, Gray JE et al 1998 Variation among neonatal intensive care units in narcotic administration. Archives of Pediatrics and Adolescent Medicine 152: 844–851

Kanagasundaram S, Cooper M, Lane L 1997 Nurse-controlled analgesia using a patient-controlled analgesia device: an alternative strategy in the management of severe cancer pain in children. Journal of Paediatrics and Child Health 33(4): 352–355

Karl HW, Tyler DC, Krane EJ 1996 Respiratory depression after low-dose caudal morphine. Canadian Journal of Anaesthesia 43: 1065–1067

Kasai H, Sasaki K, Tsujinaga H, Hoshino T 1995 [Pain management in advanced pediatric cancer patients – a proposal of the two-step analgesic ladder]. [Japanese] Masui – Japanese Journal of Anesthesiology 44: 885–889

Katz ER, Kellerman J, Siegel SE 1980 Behavioral distress in children with cancer undergoing medical procedures: developmental considerations. Journal of Consulting and Clinical Psychology 48: 356–365

Kehlet H 1998 Balanced analgesia: a prerequisite for optimal recovery. British Journal of Surgery 85: 3–4

Kohane D, Sankar W, Shubina M, Hu D, Rifai N, Berde C 1998 Sciatic nerve blockade in infant, adolescent and adult rats: a comparison of ropivacaine with bupivacaine. Anesthesiology, in press

Krane EJ, Heller LB, Pomietto ML 1991 Incidence of phantom sensation and pain in pediatric amputees. Anesthesiology 75: A691

Kuttner L 1989 Management of young children's acute pain and anxiety during invasive medical procedures. Pediatrician 16: 39–44

Lander J, Brady-Fryer B, Metcalfe J, Nazarali S, Muttitt S 1997 Comparison of ring block, dorsal penile nerve block, and topical anesthesia for neonatal circumcision: a randomized controlled trial. JAMA 278: 2157–2162

Lawson RA, Smart NG, Gudgeon AC, Morton NS 1995 Evaluation of an amethocaine gel preparation for percutaneous analgesia before venous cannulation in children. British Journal of Anaesthesia 75: 282–285

Lesko S, Mitchell A 1995 An assessment of the safety of pediatric ibuprofen. A practitioner-based randomized clinical trial. JAMA 273(12): 929–933

Levine M, Rappaport LA 1984 Recurrent abdominal pain in school children: the loneliness of the long distance physician. Pediatric Clinics of North America 31: 969–991

Lin YC, Sussman HH, Benitz WE 1997 Plasma concentrations after rectal administration of acetaminophen in preterm neonates. Paediatric Anaesthesia 7: 457–459

Litvack DA, Oberlander TF, Carney LH, Saul JP 1995 Time and frequency domain methods for heart rate variability analysis: a methodological comparison. Psychophysiology 32: 492–504

Lynn A, Nespeca MK, Bratton SL, Strauss SG, Shen DD 1998 Clearance of morphine in postoperative infants during intravenous infusion: the influence of age and surgery. Anesthesia and Analgesia 86: 958–963

Mackie AM, Coda BC, Hill HF 1991 Adolescents use patient-controlled analgesia effectively for relief from prolonged oropharyngeal mucositis pain. Pain 46: 265–269

Marx CM, Stein J, Tyler MK, Nieder ML, Shurin SB, Blumer JL 1997 Ketamine-midazolam versus meperidine-midazolam for painful procedures in pediatric oncology patients. Journal of Clinical Oncology 15: 94–102

Maunuksela EL, Korpela R 1986 Double-blind evaluation of a lignocaine-prilocaine cream (EMLA) in children. Effect on the pain associated with venous cannulation. British Journal of Anaesthesia 58: 1242–1245

Maunuksela EL, Olkkola KT, Korpela R 1988 Does prophylactic intravenous infusion of indomethacin improve the management of postoperative pain in children? Canadian Journal of Anaesthesia 35: 123–127

Maxwell LG, Yaster M 1996 The myth of conscious sedation [editorial; comment]. Archives of Pediatrics and Adolescent Medicine 150: 665–667

McGrath PJ, De Veber L 1986 The management of acute pain evoked by medical procedures in children with cancer. Journal of Pain and Symptom Management 1: 145–150

McGrath PJ, Unruh AM 1987 Psychogenic pain: pain in children and adolescents. Elsevier Science Publishers, Amsterdam

McGrath PJ, Johnson G, Goodman JT, Schillinger J, Dunn J 1985 The CHEOPS: a behavioral scale to measure postoperative pain in children. In: Chapman J, Fields HL, Dubner R, Cervero F (eds) Advances in pain research and therapy, vol. 9. Raven Press, New York, pp 395–402

McGrath PJ, Seifert C, Speechley K, Booth J, Stitt L, Gibson M 1996 A new analogue scale for assessing children's pain: an initial validation study. Pain 64: 435–443

McIntosh N, Van Veen L, Brameyer H 1994 Alleviation of the pain of heel prick in preterm infants. Archives of Disease in Childhood, Fetal and Neonatal Edition 70: F177–181

McNeely JK, Trentadue NC 1997 Comparison of patient-controlled analgesia with and without nighttime morphine infusion following lower extremity surgery in children. Journal of Pain and Symptom Management 13: 268–273

McNeely JM 1991 Comparison of epidural opioids and intravenous opioids in the postoperative management of pediatric antireflux surgery. Anesthesiology 75: A689

Mehegan J, Masek BJ, Harrison W et al 1987 A multi-component behavioral treatment for pediatric migraine. Clinical Journal of Pain 2: 191–196

Meignier M, Souron R, Leneel J 1983 Postoperative dorsal epidural analgesia in the child with respiratory disabilities. Anesthesiology 59(5): 473–475

Mikawa K, Nishina K, Maekawa N, Obara H 1996 Oral clonidine premedication reduces postoperative pain in children. Anesthesia and Analgesia 82: 225–230

Miser AW, Davis DM, Hughes CS, Mulne AF, Miser JS 1983 Continuous subcutaneous infusion of morphine in children with cancer. American Journal of Diseases of Childhood 137: 383–385

Oberlander TF, Rappaport LA 1993 Recurrent abdominal pain during childhood. Pediatrics in Review 14: 313–319

Oberlander TF, Berde CB, Lam KH, Rappaport LA, Saul JP 1995 Infants tolerate spinal anesthesia with minimal overall autonomic changes: analysis of heart rate variability in former premature infants undergoing hernia repair. Anesthesia and Analgesia 80: 20–27

Oberlander TF, Berde CB, Saul JP 1996 Halothane and cardiac autonomic control in infants: assessment with quantitative respiratory sinus arrhythmia [published erratum appears in Pediatr Res 1997 42(5): 576]. Pediatric Research 40: 710–717

Olkkola KT, Maunuksela EL, Korpela R, Rosenberg PH 1988 Kinetics and dynamics of postoperative intravenous morphine in children. Clinical Pharmacology and Therapeutics 44: 128–136

Olkkola KT, Hamunen K, Maunuksela E 1995 Clinical pharmacokinetics and pharmacodynamics of opioid analgesics in infants and children. Clinical Pharmacokinetics 28: 385–404

Ollson G, Berde CB 1993 Neuropathic pain in children and adolescents. In: Schechter NL, Berde CB, Yaster M (eds) Pain in infants, children and adolescents. Williams and Wilkins, Baltimore, pp 473–489

Olness K, MacDonald J, Uden D 1987 Comparison of self-hypnosis and propranolol in the treatment of juvenile classic migraine. Pediatrics 79: 593–597

Oster J 1972 Recurrent abdominal pain, headache and limb pain in children and adolescents. Pediatrics 50: 429–436

Oster J, Nielson A 1972 Growing pains: a clinical investigation of a school population. Acta Paediatrica Scandinavica 61: 321

Perry S, Heidrich G 1982 Management of pain during debridement: a survey of USA burns units. Pain 13: 267–280

Pillemer FG, Micheli LJ 1985 Psychological considerations in youth sports. Clinics in Sports Medicine 7: 679–689

Platt OS, Thorington BD, Brambilla DJ et al 1991 Pain in sickle cell disease. Rates and risk factors [see comments]. New England Journal of Medicine 325: 11–16

Porter FL, Porges S 1991 Vagal tone: an index of stress and pain in high risk newborn infants. Journal of Pain and Symptom Management 6: 206

Porter FL, Porges SW, Marshall RE 1988 Newborn pain cries and vagal tone: parallel changes in response to circumcision. Child Development 59: 495–505

Robinson S, Gregory G 1981 Fentanyl air oxygen anesthesia for patent ductus arteriosus in pre-term infants. Anesthesia. Analgesia 60: 331–334

Rusy LM, Houck CS, Sullivan LJ et al 1995 A double-blind evaluation of ketorolac tromethamine versus acetaminophen in pediatric tonsillectomy: analgesia and bleeding. Anesthesia and Analgesia 80: 226–229

Scharff L 1997 Recurrent abdominal pain in children: a review of psychological factors and treatment. Clinical Psychology Review 17: 145–166

Shapiro B, Dinges D, Orne E et al 1995 Home management of sickle cell-related pain in children and adolescents: natural history and impact on school attendance. Pain 61: 139–144

Sherry DD, Weisman R 1988 Psychologic aspects of childhood reflex neurovascular dystrophy. Pediatrics 81: 572–578

Sievers TD, Yee JD, Foley ME, Blanding PJ, Berde CB 1991 Midazolam for conscious sedation during pediatric oncology procedures: safety and recovery parameters. Pediatrics 88: 1172–1179

Smith G, Strausbaugh S, Harbeck-Weber C, Cohen D, Shields B, Powers J 1997 New non-cocaine-containing topical anesthetics compared with tetracaine-adrenaline-cocaine during repair of lacerations. Pediatrics 100: 825–830

Sorge F, Marano E 1985 Flunarizine v. placebo in childhood migraine. A double-blind study. Cephalalgia 5 (suppl 2): 145–148

Stang HJ, Gunnar MR, Snellman L, Condon LM, Kestenbaum R 1988 Local anesthesia for neonatal circumcision. Effects on distress and cortisol response. JAMA 259: 1507–1511

Stevens BJ, Johnston CC, Grunau RV 1995 Issues of assessment of pain and discomfort in neonates. [Review] Journal of Obstetric, Gynecologic and Neonatal Nursing 24: 849–855

Stevens BJ, Johnston C, Petryshen P, Taddio A 1996 Premature infant pain profile: development and initial validation. Clinical Journal of Pain 12: 13–22

Stevens M, Dalla Pozza L, Cavalletto B, Cooper M, Kilham H 1994 Pain and symptom control in paediatric palliative care. [Review] Cancer Surveys 21: 211–231

Szyfelbein SK, Osgood PF, Carr DB 1985 The assessment of pain and plasma B-endorphin immunoactivity in burned children. Pain 22: 173–182

Taddio A, Stevens B, Craig K et al 1997a Efficacy and safety of lidocaine-prilocaine cream for pain during circumcision. New England Journal of Medicine 336: 1197–1201

Taddio A, Katz J, Ilersich A, Koren G 1997b Effect of neonatal circumcision on pain response during subsequent routine vaccination. Lancet 349: 599–603

Thomas JE, Koshy M, Patterson L, Dorn L, Thomas K 1984 Management of pain in sickle cell disease using biofeedback therapy: a preliminary study. Biofeedback and Self-Regulation 9: 413–420

Varni JW 1992 Evaluation and management of pain in children with juvenile rheumatoid arthritis. Journal of Rheumatology 19: 32–35

Vetter T, Heiner E 1994 Intravenous ketorolac as an adjuvant to pediatric patient-controlled analgesia with morphine. Journal of Clinical Anesthesia 6: 110–113

Walker L S, Garber J, Greene J W 1993 Psychosocial correlates of recurrent childhood pain: a comparison of pediatric patients with recurrent abdominal pain, organic illness, and psychiatric disorders. [Review] Journal of Abnormal Psychology 102: 248–258

Way W, Costley E, Way E 1965 Respiratory sensitivity of the newborn infant to meperidine and morphine. Clinical Pharmacology and Therapeutics 6: 454–461

Wermeling DP, Greene SA, Boucher BA et al 1992 Patient controlled analgesia: the relation of psychological factors to pain and analgesic use in adolescents with postoperative pain. Clinical Journal of Pain 8: 215–221

Wilder RT, Berde CB, Wolohan M, Vieyra MA, Masek BJ, Micheli LJ 1992 Reflex sympathetic dystrophy in children. Clinical characteristics and follow-up of seventy patients. Journal of Bone and Joint Surgery 74A: 910–919

Wong DL, Baker CM 1988 Pain in children: comparison of assessment scales. Pediatric Nursing 14: 9–17

Zeltzer L, LeBaron S 1982 Hypnotic and nonhypnotic techniques for reduction of pain and anxiety during painful procedures in children and adolescents with cancer. Journal of Pediatrics 101: 1032–1035

Zeltzer L, Jay S, Fisher D 1989 The management of pain associated with pediatric procedures. Pediatric Clinics of North America 36: 941–964

Practical issues in the management of cancer pain

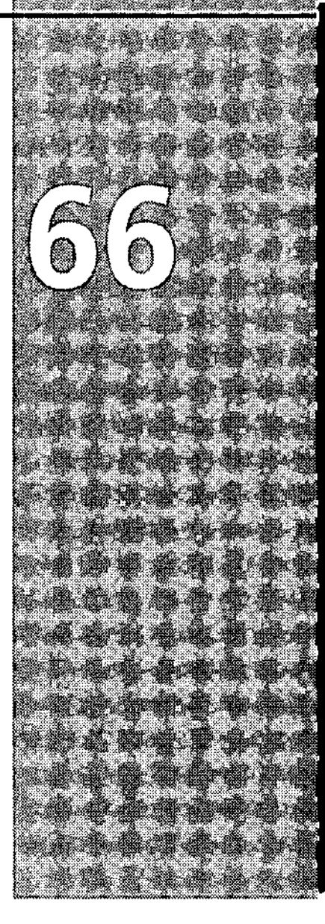

NATHAN I. CHERNY & RUSSELL K. PORTENOY

SUMMARY

The goal of analgesic therapy in the cancer population is to optimize analgesia with the minimum of side effects and inconvenience. Currently available techniques can provide adequate relief to a vast majority of patients. Most will require ongoing pain treatment and analgesic requirements often change as the disease progresses. Patients with refractory pain, or unremitting suffering related to other losses or distressing symptoms, should have access to specialists in pain management or palliative medicine who can provide an approach capable of addressing these complex problems.

INTRODUCTION

Pain is among the most prevalent symptoms experienced by patients with cancer (Bonica et al 1990, Coyle et al 1990, Ventafridda et al 1990b, Henteleff 1991, Johanson 1991). Although established analgesic strategies could benefit most patients (Takeda 1985, Ventafridda et al 1987, Walker et al 1988, Goisis et al 1989, Schug et al 1990, Grond et al 1991), undertreatment is common (Cherny & Catane 1995, Zenz et al 1995, Stjernsward et al 1996). Indequate understanding of the principles of cancer pain therapy contributes greatly to undertreatment (Von Roenn et al 1993, Cherny et al 1994a, Cleeland et al 1994, Devulder et al 1997, Sapir et al 1997) and efforts to redress this situation are both a therapeutic and an ethical imperative (Wanzer et al 1989, World Health Organization 1990, Spross et al 1990a, Emanuel 1996, McCabe 1997).

The success of cancer pain therapy depends on the ability of the clinician to assess the presenting problems, identify and evaluate pain syndromes and formulate a plan for comprehensive continuing care (Ventafridda 1989, World Health Organization 1990, 1996). This requires familiarity with a range of therapeutic options (Table 66.1) and an

Table 66.1 Analgesic therapies for cancer pain

Therapy	*Examples*
Primary therapy	Chemotherapy Radiotherapy Hormone therapy Immunotherapy Surgery Antibiotics
Systemic analgesic pharmacotherapy	Non-opioid analgesics Opioids Adjuvant analgesics
Anaesthetic techniques	Intraspinal opioids ± local anaesthetic Chemical rhizotomy Somatic neurolysis Sympathetic blockade
Neurosurgical techniques	Rhizotomy Cordotomy Cingulotomy Pituitary ablation Dorsal root entry zone lesions
Physiatric techniques	Orthoses Physical therapy
Psychological techniques	Relaxation training Distraction techniques
Neurostimulatory techniques	Transcutaneous electrical nerve stimulation Dorsal column stimulation Deep brain stimulation Acupuncture

approach to long-term care that is responsive to the changing needs of the patient (Coyle 1987, Ventafridda 1989, Shegda & McCorkle 1990). This approach emphasizes the need to incorporate pain treatment within the broader therapeutic agenda of palliative care, which should be pursued throughout the course of the disease. Palliative care is a model of care focused on enhancing the quality of life of patients living with progressive incurable diseases and ensuring comfort, dignity and support at the end of life.

COMPREHENSIVE ASSESSMENT

The formulation of an effective therapeutic strategy for the management of pain and other palliative care concerns is predicated on a comprehensive assessment of the patient (described in Chapter 40). The assessment should clarify the characteristics of the pain and its impact on function and psychological well-being, identify the pain syndrome and infer the putative mechanisms that may underlie the pain. In addition, the assessment should evaluate both the nature and extent of the underlying disease and identify concurrent problems that are contributing, or may soon contribute, to patient or family distress.

The particular therapeutic strategy that evolves from this information depends on the goals of care. These goals are diverse, but can generally be grouped into three broad categories:

1. prolonging survival;
2. optimizing comfort;
3. maximising function.

The relative priority of these goals provides an essential context for therapeutic decision making. The therapeutic strategy should address a prioritized problem list that best serves both the current goals of the patient and the anticipated problems that would benefit from advanced planning.

Most cancer patients can attain satisfactory relief of pain through an approach that incorporates primary treatments, systemic analgesic therapy and, at times, other non-invasive techniques (such as psychological or rehabilitative interventions). Some patients whose pain is refractory to this approach benefit from invasive anaesthetic or neurosurgical treatments. Such patients should have access to specialists in pain management or palliative medicine, who can provide additional expertise in addressing these complex problems.

PRIMARY THERAPY

The assessment process may reveal a cause for the pain that is amenable to primary therapy (i.e. therapy that is directed at the aetiology of the pain). This therapy may improve comfort, function or duration of survival. For example, pain that is produced by tumour infiltration may respond to antineoplastic treatment with surgery, radiotherapy or chemotherapy and pain caused by infections may be relieved with antibiotic therapy or drainage procedures. Specific analgesic treatments are usually required as an adjunct to the primary therapy.

RADIOTHERAPY

Radiotherapy has a pivotal role in the treatment of cancer pain and other oncological conditions (Hoegler 1997, Vermeulen 1998). This approach is selected for symptom palliation when there is a high likelihood of efficacy and a low risk of adverse effects. The duration of treatment should be short and it should offer a more favourable risk:benefit ratio than other available therapeutic modalities (Hoegler 1997). In some situations, such as the treatment of bone metastases (Bates 1992, Hoskin 1995, Janjan 1997), epidural neoplasm (Bates 1992) and cerebral metastases (Coia 1992, Sneed et al 1996, Vermeulen 1998), the value of radiotherapy is documented by abundant data and a favourable clinical experience. In other settings, however, there is a paucity of data and the use of radiotherapy is empirical. For example, the results with perineal pain due to low sacral plexopathy appear to be encouraging (Bosch & Caldwell 1980, Dobrowsky & Schmid 1985) and the outcome of hepatic radiotherapy (e.g. 2000–3000 cGy) appears to be favourable for hepatic capsular distension in 50–90% of patients (Turek-Maischeider & Kazem 1975, Sherman et al 1978, Borgelt et al 1981, Leibel et al 1987, Mohiuddin et al 1996).

CHEMOTHERAPY

Despite a paucity of data concerning the specific analgesic benefits of chemotherapy (Queisser 1984, Rubens et al 1992), there is a strong clinical impression that tumour shrinkage is generally associated with relief of pain. Although there are some reports of analgesic value even in the absence of significant tumour shrinkage (Patt et al 1985, Thatcher et al 1995, Rothenberg 1996), the likelihood of a favourable effect on pain is generally related to the likelihood of tumour response. Hence, benefit can be anticipated in chemotherapy-responsive tumours, such as

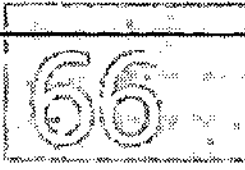

lymphoma, small cell lung cancer, germ cell tumours and previously untreated breast cancer. In all situations, the decision to administer chemotherapy solely for the treatment of symptoms should be reconsidered if the patient demonstrates an unfavourable balance between relief and adverse effects.

SURGERY

Surgery may have a role in the relief of symptoms caused by specific problems, such as obstruction of a hollow viscus (Jong et al 1995, Mainar et al 1996, Parker & Baines 1996, Barbalias et al 1997), unstable bony structures (Braun & Rohe 1984, Tarn & Lee 1994, Algan & Horowitz 1996), and compression of neural tissues (Sucher et al 1994, Gokaslan 1996, Harris et al 1996). The potential benefits and prognosis must be weighed against the risks of surgery, the anticipated length of hospitalization and convalescence and the predicted duration of benefit (Boraas 1985). Clinical experience has generally been most favourable when surgery has been used to stabilize pathological fractures, relieve bowel obstructions or drain symptomatic ascites. Large-volume (up to 5–10 litres) paracentesis, for example, may provide prompt and prolonged relief from the pain and discomfort of tense ascites (Boraas 1985, Ross et al 1989), with a small risk of hypotension (Cruikshank & Buchsbaum 1973, Ross et al 1989) or hypoproteinaemia (Lifshitz & Buchsbaum 1976). Radical surgery to excise locally advanced disease in patients with no evidence of metastatic spread may be palliative and potentially increase the survival of some patients (Estes et al 1993, Avradopoulos et al 1996).

ANTIBIOTIC THERAPY

Antibiotics may be analgesic when the source of the pain involves infection. Illustrative examples include cellulitis, chronic sinus infections, pelvic abscess, pyonephrosis and osteitis pubis (Lopez et al 1996, Hughes et al 1997). In some cases, infection may be occult and confirmed only by the symptomatic relief provided by empiric treatment with these drugs (Bruera & MacDonald 1986, Coyle & Portenoy 1991, Gonzales et al 1991).

SYSTEMIC ANALGESIC PHARMACOTHERAPY

THE 'ANALGESIC LADDER'

Analgesic pharmacotherapy is the mainstay of cancer pain management (World Health Organization 1990, Agency for Health Care Policy and Research 1994a). Although concurrent use of other interventions is valuable in many patients and essential in some, analgesic drugs are needed in almost every case. Based on clinical convention, analgesic drugs can be divided into three groups:

1. the non-opioid analgesics;
2. the opioid analgesics;
3. adjuvant analgesics, which are drugs with other primary indications that can be effective analgesics in specific circumstances.

The guiding principle of analgesic management is the individualization of therapy. Through a process of repeated evaluations, drug selection and administration is individualized so that a favourable balance between pain relief and adverse pharmacological effects is achieved and maintained (Cherny et al 1995).

An expert committee convened by the Cancer Unit of the World Health Organization (WHO) has proposed a useful approach to drug selection for cancer pain, which has become known as the 'analgesic ladder' (World Health Organization 1986). When combined with appropriate dosing guidelines, this approach is capable of providing adequate relief to 70–90% of patients (Takeda 1985, Ventafridda et al 1987, Walker et al 1988, Goisis et al 1989, Schug et al 1990, Grond et al 1991). Emphasizing that pain intensity should be the prime consideration in analgesic selection, the approach advocates three basic steps (Fig. 66.1).

Step 1

Patients with mild to moderate cancer-related pain should be treated with a non-opioid analgesic, which should be combined with an adjuvant analgesic if a specific indication exists. For example, a patient with mild to moderate arm pain caused by radiation-induced brachial plexopathy may benefit when a tricyclic antidepressant is added to acetaminophen.

Step 2

Patients who are relatively opioid naive and present with moderate to severe pain, or who fail to achieve adequate relief after a trial of a non-opioid analgesic, should be treated with an opioid conventionally used to treat pain of this intensity. This treatment is typically accomplished by using a combination product containing a non-opioid (e.g. aspirin or acetaminophen) and an opioid (such as codeine, oxycodone or propoxyphene). This drug can also be co-administered with an adjuvant analgesic.

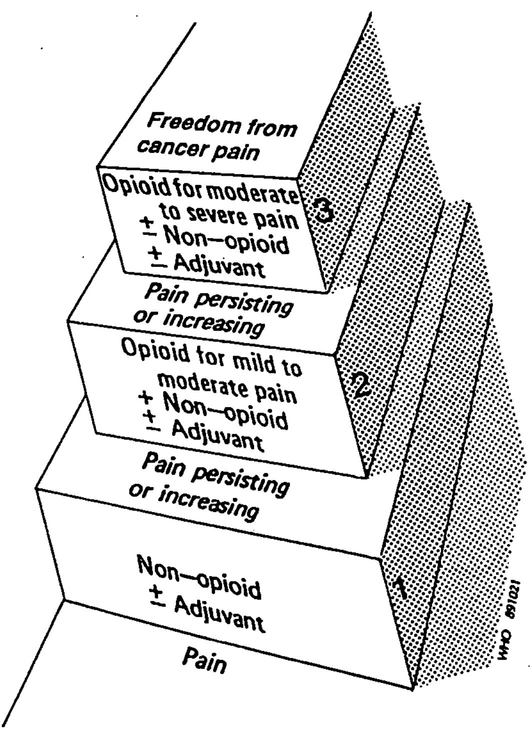

Fig. 66.1 WHO analgesic ladder (reprinted with permission).

Step 3

Patients who present with severe pain or fail to achieve adequate relief following appropriate administration of drugs on the second rung of the 'analgesic ladder' should receive an opioid agonist conventionally used for pain of this intensity. This drug may also be combined with a non-opioid analgesic or an adjuvant drug.

Recently, the evidence of the long-term efficacy of this approach has been the subject of criticism (Jadad & Browman 1995). Nonetheless, the approach remains widely used and has been strongly endorsed (American Pain Society 1992, (American Society of Clinical Oncology Ad Hoc Committee on Cancer Pain 1992, Agency for Health Care Policy and Research 1994b, World Health Organization 1996).

NON-OPIOID ANALGESICS

The non-opioid analgesics (aspirin, acetaminophen and the nonsteroidal anti-inflammatory drugs (NSAIDs) are useful alone for mild to moderate pain (step 1 of the analgesic ladder) and provide additive analgesia when combined with opioid drugs in the treatment of more severe pain. Unlike opioid analgesics, the non-opioid analgesics have a 'ceiling' effect for analgesia and produce neither tolerance nor physical dependence.

The non-opioid analgesics constitute a heterogeneous group of compounds that differ in chemical structure but share many pharmacological actions (see Ch. 46) (Table 66.2). Some of these agents, like aspirin and the NSAIDs, inhibit the enzyme cyclo-oxygenase and consequently block the biosynthesis of prostaglandins, inflammatory mediators known to sensitize peripheral nociceptors (Vane 1971). A central mechanism is also likely (Malmberg & Yaksh 1992, Vane & Botting 1997), and appears to predominate in acetaminophen analgesia (Piletta et al 1991).

The safe administration of the non-opioid analgesics requires familiarity with their potential adverse effects (Brooks & Day 1991, Bennett et al 1996, Laine 1996, Lehmann et al 1997). Aspirin and the other NSAIDs have a broad spectrum of potential toxicity. Bleeding diathesis due to inhibition of platelet aggregation, gastroduodenopathy (including peptic ulcer disease) and renal impairment are the most common (Lehmann et al 1997). Less common adverse effects include confusion, precipitation of cardiac failure and exacerbation of hypertension. Particular caution is required in the administration of these agents to patients at increased risk of adverse effects, including the elderly and those with blood clotting disorders, predilection to peptic ulceration, impaired renal function and concurrent corti-

Table 66.2 Non-opioid analgesics

Chemical class	*Generic name*
Non-acidic	Acetaminophen Nabumetone Nemuselide Meloxicam
Acidic	
Salicylates	Aspirin Diflunisal Choline magnesium trisalicylate Salsalate
Proprionic acids	Ibuprofen Naproxen Fenoprofen Ketoprofen Flurbiprofen Oxaprosin
Acetic acids	Indomethacin Tolmetin Sulindac Diclofenac Ketorolac
Oxicams	Piroxicam
Fenamates	Mefenamic acid Meclofenamic acid

costeroid therapy. Of the NSAIDs, the drugs that are relatively selective cyclo-oxygenase-2 inhibitors (e.g. nabumetone, nemuselide and meloxicam) (Lancaster 1995, Masferrer et al 1996) and those that are non-acetylated salicylates (choline magnesium trisalicylate and salsalate) (Johnson & Miller 1994) are preferred in patients who have a predilection to peptic ulceration or bleeding; these drugs have less effect on platelet aggregation and no effect on bleeding time at the usual clinical doses. The development of NSAIDs that are fully selective cyclo-oxygenase-2 inhibitors may provide additional agents with favourable safety profiles that may be preferred in the treatment of the medically frail. Acetaminophen rarely produces gastrointestinal toxicity and there are no adverse effects on platelet function; hepatic toxicity is possible, however, and patients with chronic alcoholism and liver disease can develop severe hepatotoxicity at the usual therapeutic doses (Makin & Williams 1997).

The optimal administration of non-opioid analgesics requires an understanding of their clinical pharmacology. There is no certain knowledge of the minimal effective analgesic dose, ceiling dose or toxic dose for any individual patient with cancer pain. These doses may be higher or lower than the usual dose ranges recommended for the drug involved. Recommended doses are usually derived from studies performed in relatively healthy patients who have an inflammatory disease, a population clearly dissimilar from those with cancer pain, who often have co-existent organ failure and may be receiving multiple other drugs. These observations support an approach to the administration of NSAIDs that incorporates both low initial doses and dose titration. Through a process of gradual dose escalation, it may be possible to identify the ceiling dose and reduce the risk of significant toxicity. Several weeks are needed to evaluate the efficacy of a dose when NSAIDs are used in the treatment of grossly inflammatory lesions, such as arthritis. Experience suggests that a week is usually adequate for the same purpose in the patient with cancer pain. Based on clinical experience, an upper limit for dose titration is usually set at 1.5–2 times the standard recommended dose of the drug in question. Since failure with one NSAID can be followed by success with another, sequential trials of several NSAIDs may be useful to identify a drug with a favourable balance between analgesia and side effects.

OPIOID ANALGESICS

Cancer pain of moderate or greater intensity should generally be treated with a systemically administered opioid analgesic. Optimal use of opioid analgesics requires a sound understanding of the general principles of opioid pharmacology (see Ch. 48), the pharmacological characteristics of each of the commonly used drugs and principles of administration.

General principles of opioid pharmacology

Opioid classification

Based on their interactions with the various receptor subtypes, opioid compounds can be divided into agonist, agonist-antagonist and antagonist classes (Table 66.3) (Cherny 1996). The pure agonist drugs (Table 66.4) are most commonly used in clinical pain management. The mixed agonist-antagonist opioids (pentazocine, nalbuphine, butorphanol and dezocine) and the partial agonist opioids (buprenorphine) play a minor role in the management of cancer pain because of the existence of a ceiling effect for analgesia, the potential for precipitation of withdrawal in patients physically dependent to opioid agonists and, in some cases, the problem of dose-dependent psychotomimetic side effects that exceed those of pure agonist drugs (Houde 1979, Hanks 1987, Cherny 1996).

The pure agonist opioid drugs appear to have no ceiling effect for analgesia. As the dose is raised, analgesic effects increase until either analgesia is achieved or the patient loses consciousness. This increase in effect occurs as a log-linear function: dose increments on a logarithmic scale yield linear increases in analgesia. In practice, it is the appearance of adverse effects, including confusion, sedation, nausea, vomiting or respiratory depression, that imposes a limit on the useful dose. The overall efficacy of any drug in a specific patient will be determined by the balance between analgesia

Table 66.3 Opioid classification

Agonists	*Partial agonists*	*Mixed agonist/antagonists*
Morphine	Buprenorphine	Pentazocine
Codeine		Butorphanol
Oxycodone		Nalbuphine
Hydrocodone		Dezocine
Dihydrocodeine		
Heroin		
Oxymorphone		
Meperidine		
Levorphanol		
Hydromorphone		
Methadone		
Fentanyl		
Sufentanil		
Alfentanil		
Propoxyphene		

Table 66.4 Opioid agonist drugs

Drug	*Dose (mg) equianalgesic to 10 mg i.m. morphine* I.M.	P.O	*Half-life (hrs)*	*Duration of action (hrs)*	*Comments*
Codeine	130	200	2–3	2–4	Usually combined with a non-opioid
Oxycodone	15	30	2–3	2–4	Usually combined with a non-opioid
Propoxyphene	100	50	2–3	2–4	Usually combined with a non-opioid. Norpropoxyphene toxicity may cause seizures
Morphine	10	30	2–3	3–4	Multiple routes of administration available. Controlled release available. M6G accumulation in renal failure
Hydromorphone	2–3	7.5	2–3	2–4	No known active metabolites. Multiple routes available
Methadone	10	3–5	15–190	4–8	Plasma accumulation may lead to delayed toxicity. Dosing should be initiated on a p.r.n. basis. When switching to methadone from another opioid, potency may be much greater than expected; the dose of methadone should be lowered by 75–90% to account for this
Meperidine	75	300	2–3	2–4	Low oral bioavailability. Normeperidine toxicity limits utility. Contraindicated in patients with renal failure and those receiving MAO inhibitors
Oxymorphone	1	10 (p.r.)	2–3	3–4	No oral formulation available. Less histamine release
Heroin	5	60	0.5	3–4	High-solubility morphine prodrug
Levorphanol	2	4	12–15	4–8	Plasma accumulation may lead to delayed toxicity
Fentanyl transdermal	Empirically, transdermal fentanyl 100 µg/h = 2–4 mg/h intravenous morphine			48–72	Patches available to deliver 25, 50, 75 and 100 µg/h

and side effects that occurs during dose escalation (Portenoy et al 1990).

Relative potency and equianalgesic doses

Relative analgesic potency is the ratio of the dose of two analgesics required to produce the same analgesic effect. By convention, the relative potency of each of the commonly used opioids is based upon a comparison to 10 mg of parenteral morphine (Houde et al 1966). Equianalgesic dose information (Table 66.4) provides guidelines for dose selection when the drug or route of administration is changed. Equianalgesic doses provide a useful reference point but should not be considered as standard starting doses or a firm guideline when switching between opioids. Numerous variables may influence the appropriate dose for the individual patient, including pain severity, prior opioid exposure (and the degree of cross-tolerance this confers), age, route of administration, level of consciousness and metabolic abnormalities (see below).

Some relative potency data derived from single-dose studies may not be relevant to chronic therapy. Most important, the potency of methadone determined in single-dose studies appears to greatly underestimate its potency in the chronic treatment setting (Hunt & Bruera 1995, Bruera et al 1996). Indeed, it appears that the methadone:morphine equianalgesic ratio for oral dosing may be dose related and closer to 1:10 (Ripamonti et al 1998).

'Weak' versus 'strong' opioids

The division of opioid agonists into 'weak' versus 'strong' opioids was incorporated into the original 'analgesic ladder' proposed by the WHO (World Health Organization 1986).

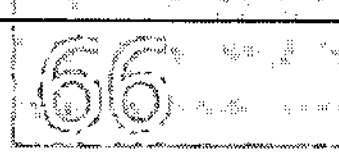

This distinction was not based on a fundamental difference in the pharmacology of the pure agonist opioids, but rather reflected the customary manner in which these drugs were used. This explains the observation that some opioids that were customarily used for moderate pain (step 2 of the analgesic ladder), such as oxycodone, are also used for severe pain in selected patients. Indeed, the controlled-release formulation of oxycodone is now widely used in the management of severe pain. Conversely, low-dose formulations of controlled-release morphine are suitable for the management of pain of moderate severity.

Selecting patients for opioid therapy

A trial of systemic opioid therapy should be strongly considered in all cancer patients with pain of moderate or greater severity. This is true regardless of the pain mechanism (Portenoy et al 1990, Cherny et al 1992, Jadad et al 1992, McQuay et al 1992, Hanks & Forbes 1997). Although somatic and visceral pain appear to be relatively more responsive to opioid analgesics than neuropathic pain, a neuropathic mechanism does not confer 'opioid resistance' or 'opioid unresponsiveness' (Arner & Meyerson 1988, Hanks 1991). Opioid responsiveness is a continuum that may vary with any of a large number of patient-related and pain-related factors (Portenoy et al 1990) and appropriate dose escalation will identify many patients with neuropathic pain who can achieve adequate relief (Portenoy et al 1990, Hanks & Forbes 1997).

Factors in opioid selection

The factors that influence opioid selection in chronic pain states include pain intensity, pharmacologic considerations and the presence of co-existing disease.

Pain intensity

Patients with moderate pain are conventionally treated with a combination product containing acetaminophen or aspirin plus codeine, dihydrocodeine, hydrocodone, oxycodone and propoxyphene. The doses of these combination products can be increased until the customary maximum dose of the non-opioid co-analgesic is attained (e.g. 4000 mg acetaminophen). Beyond this dose, the opioid contained in the combination product could be increased as a single agent or the patient could be switched to an opioid conventionally used for severe pain. New opioid formulations may improve the convenience of drug administration for patients with moderate pain. These include controlled-release formulations of codeine, dihydrocodeine, oxycodone and tramadol. In some countries controlled-release morphine is available as a 10 mg tablet, which may also be used to treat moderate pain in the opioid-naive patient.

The opioid drugs available to treat severe pain vary from country to country. Many countries provide clinicians with numerous options. In the United States, for example, patients who present with severe pain can be treated with morphine, hydromorphone, oxycodone, oxymorphone, fentanyl, methadone or levorphanol.

Pharmacologic considerations

As discussed previously, the agonist-antagonist opioids (e.g. pentazocine) are not preferred in the management of cancer pain (Hanks 1987, Cherny 1996). Similarly the pharmacological characteristics of meperidine limit its role in the cancer population. Meperidine is N-demethylated to normeperidine, which is an active metabolite that is twice as potent as a convulsant and one-half as potent as an analgesic than its parent compound. The half-life of normeperidine is 12–16 hours, approximately 4–5 times the half-life of meperidine. Accumulation of normeperidine after repetitive dosing of meperidine is initiated can result in central nervous system toxicity characterized by subtle adverse mood effects, tremulousness, multifocal myoclonus and, occasionally, seizures (Szeto et al 1977, Eisendrath et al 1987). Although accumulation of normeperidine is most likely to affect the elderly and patients with overt renal disease, toxicity is sometimes observed in younger patients with normal renal function (Kaiko et al 1983, Marinella 1997). The most serious toxicity associated with meperidine is normeperidine-induced seizures. Naloxone does not reverse this effect and, indeed, could theoretically precipitate seizures in patients receiving meperidine by blocking the depressant action of meperidine and allowing the convulsant activity of normeperidine to become manifest (Umans & Inturrisi 1982, Czuczwar & Frey 1986). If naloxone must be administered to a patient receiving meperidine, it should be diluted and slowly titrated while appropriate seizure precautions are taken. Selective toxicity of meperidine can also occur following administration to patients receiving monoamine oxidase inhibitors. This combination may produce a syndrome characterized by hyperpyrexia, muscle rigidity and seizures, which may occasionally be fatal (Sporer 1995). The pathophysiology of this syndrome is related to excess availability of serotonin at the $5HT_{1A}$ receptor in the central nervous system.

When the oral route of opioid administration is contraindicated, the available routes of administration may become an important consideration in opioid selection. Oxymorphone is available only as a rectal suppository or for injection and, at present, fentanyl is only available for transdermal or parenteral administration.

Some patients will require sequential trials of several different opioids before a drug which is effective and well tolerated is identified (Galer et al 1992, Crews et al 1993, MacDonald et al 1993, Leng & Finnegan 1994, Bruera et al 1995b, 1996, Cherny et al 1995, De Stoutz et al 1995, Thomas & Bruera 1995, Fallon 1997, Fitzgibbon & Ready 1997, Lawlor et al 1997). The frequency with which this strategy is needed is unknown, but it is estimated to be in the range of 15–30% of patients. The existence of different degrees of incomplete crosstolerance to various opioid effects (analgesia and side effects) may explain the utility of these sequential trials. To date, there are no data to suggest a specific order for opioid rotation. It is strongly recommended that clinicians be familiar with at least three opioid drugs used in the management of severe pain and have the ability to calculate appropriate starting doses using equianalgesic dosing data.

Co-existing disease

Pharmacokinetic studies of meperidine, pentazocine and propoxyphene have revealed that liver disease may decrease the clearance and increase the bioavailability and half-lives of these drugs (Neal et al 1979, Pond et al 1980). These changes may eventuate in plasma concentrations higher than normal. Although mild or moderate hepatic impairment has only minor impact on morphine clearance (Patwardhan et al 1981, Crotty et al 1989), advanced disease may be associated with reduced elimination (Hasselstrom et al 1990).

Patients with renal impairment may accumulate the active metabolites of propoxyphene (norpropoxyphene) (Chan & Matzke 1987), meperidine (normeperidine) (Szeto et al 1977, Stock et al 1996) and morphine (morphine-6-glucuronide) (Osborne et al 1986, Sawe & Odar-Cederlof 1987, Hagen et al 1991, Portenoy et al 1991, Wolff et al 1996). In the setting of renal failure or unstable renal function, titration of these drugs requires caution and close monitoring. If adverse effects appear, a switch to an alternative opioid is often recommended.

Selecting the appropriate route of systemic opioid administration

Opioids should be administered by the least invasive and safest route capable of providing adequate analgesia (Table 66.5). In a survey of patients with advanced cancer, more than half required two or more routes of administration prior to death and almost a quarter required three or more (Coyle et al 1990).

Non-invasive routes

The oral route of opioid administration is the preferred approach in routine practice. Alternative routes are necessary for patients who have impaired swallowing or gastrointestinal dysfunction, those who require a very rapid onset of analgesia and those who are unable to manage either the logistics or side effects associated with the oral route (Cherny et al 1995). For highly tolerant patients, the inability to prescribe a manageable oral opioid programme due to an excessive number of tablets or volume of oral solution may be an indication for the use of a non-oral route (Cherny et al 1995).

For patients who do not require very high opioid doses, non-invasive alternatives to the oral route of opioid administration include the rectal, transdermal and sublingual routes. Rectal suppositories containing oxycodone, hydromorphone, oxymorphone and morphine have been formulated and controlled-release morphine tablets can also be administered per rectum (Maloney et al 1989, Kaiko et al 1992). The potency of opioids administered rectally is believed to approximate oral administration (Ripamonti & Bruera 1991, De Conno et al 1995, Ripamonti et al 1995).

Fentanyl is the only opioid available as a transdermal preparation. The fentanyl transdermal system consists of a drug reservoir that is separated from the skin by a co-polymer membrane that controls the rate of drug delivery to the skin surface such that the drug is released into the skin at a nearly constant amount per unit time. The system has been demonstrated to be effective in cancer pain (Ahmedzai & Brooks 1997, Grond et al 1997, Wong et al 1997b, Yeo et al 1997). The dosing interval for each system is usually 72 hours (Varvel et al 1989) but some patients require a 48-hour schedule (Jeal & Benfield 1997). There is some

Table 66.5 Routes of systemic opioid administration

Non-invasive	*Invasive*
Oral	Intramuscular
Rectal	Intravenous
Transdermal	Subcutaneous
Intranasal	
Sublingual	
Transmucosal	

interindividual variability in fentanyl bioavailability by this route and this phenomenon, combined with large differences in elimination pharmacokinetics, necessitates dose titration in most cases (Holley & Van Steennis 1988, Portenoy et al 1993). Transdermal patches capable of delivering 25, 50, 75 and 100 μg/h are available. Multiple patches may be used simultaneously for patients who require higher doses. At the present time, the limitations of the transdermal delivery system include its cost and the requirement for an alternative short-acting opioid for breakthrough pain.

Sublingual absorption of any opioid could potentially yield clinical benefit, but bioavailability is very poor with drugs that are not highly lipophilic and the likelihood of an adequate response is consequently low (Weinberg et al 1988). Sublingual buprenorphine, a relatively lipophilic partial agonist, can provide adequate relief of mild to moderate cancer pain (De Conno et al 1993b). Anecdotally, sublingual morphine has also been reported to be effective but this drug has poor sublingual absorption (Weinberg et al 1988) and efficacy may be related, in part, to swallowing of the dose (Hirsh 1984). Both fentanyl and methadone are relatively well absorbed through the buccal mucosa (Weinberg et al 1988) and sublingual administration of an injectable formulation is occasionally performed in the relatively opioid-naive patient who transiently loses the option of oral dosing. Overall, however, the sublingual route has limited value due to the lack of formulations, poor absorption of most drugs and the inability to deliver high doses or prevent swallowing of the dose.

An oral transmucosal formulation of fentanyl, which incorporates the drug into a candy base, is under evaluation. Studies in cancer patients suggested that it is useful and that it can provide rapid and very effective relief of breakthrough pain (Cleary 1997a, Coluzzi 1997, Lyss 1997, Simmonds 1997).

Invasive routes

For patients undergoing a trial of systemic drug administration, a parenteral route must be considered when the oral route is precluded or there is need for rapid onset of analgesia, or a more convenient regimen. Repeated parenteral bolus injections, which may be administered by the intravenous (IV), intramuscular (IM) or subcutaneous (SC) routes, may be useful in some patients but are often compromised by the occurrence of prominent 'bolus' effects (toxicity at peak concentration and/or pain breakthrough at the trough). Repetitive IM injections are a common practice, but they are painful and offer no pharmacokinetic advantage; their use is not recommended (Cooper 1996). Repeated bolus doses without repeated skin punctures can be accomplished through the use of an indwelling IV or SC infusion device (Lamacraft et al 1997). To deliver repeated SC injections, a 27-gauge infusion device (a 'butterfly') can be left under the skin for up to a week (Coyle et al 1994b).

Intravenous bolus administration provides the most rapid onset and shortest duration of action. Time to peak effect correlates with the lipid solubility of the opioid and ranges from 2–5 minutes for methadone to 15–30 minutes for morphine and hydromorphone (Sawe et al 1981, Inturrisi et al 1987, Chapman et al 1990, Coda et al 1997). This approach is commonly applied in two settings:

1. to provide parenteral opioids to patients who already have venous access and are unable to tolerate oral opioids;
2. to treat very severe pain, for which IV doses can be repeated at an interval as brief as that determined by the time to peak effect, if necessary, until adequate relief is achieved.

Continuous parenteral infusions are useful for many patients who cannot be maintained on oral opioids. Long-term infusions may be administered IV or SC. In practice, the major indication for continuous infusion occurs among patients who are unable to swallow or absorb opioids. Continuous infusion is also used in some patients whose high opioid requirement renders oral treatment impractical (Portenoy et al 1986, Bruera et al 1988a, b, Storey et al 1990).

Continuous SC infusion is often used for ambulatory patients. A recent study demonstrated that the bioavailability of hydromorphone is 78% by this route (Moulin et al 1991) and clinical experience suggests that dosing may proceed in a manner identical to continuous IV infusion (Nelson et al 1997a). A range of pumps is available, which vary in complexity, cost and ability to provide patient-controlled 'rescue doses' as an adjunct to a continuous basal infusion (Coyle et al 1994b). Opioids suitable for continuous SC infusion must be soluble, well absorbed and non-irritant. Experience has been reported with heroin (Jones & Hanks 1986), hydromorphone (Storey et al 1990, Moulin et al 1991), oxymorphone (Portenoy et al 1986), morphine (Portenoy et al 1986, Bruera et al 1987a, Citron et al 1992, Hill et al 1992, Moulin et al 1992) and fentanyl (Paix et al 1995). Methadone appears to be relatively irritating and is not recommended (Bruera et al 1991). To maintain the comfort of an infusion site, the SC infusion rate should not exceed 5 cc/hr. Patients who require high doses may benefit from the use of concentrated solutions. A high concentration hydromorphone (10 mg/cc) is available commercially and the organic salt of morphine, morphine tartrate, is available in some countries as an 80 mg/cc solution. In selected cases, concentrated opioid solutions can be compounded specifically for continuous SC infusion.

Subcutaneous infusion, like repeated SC bolus injections, can usually be administered using a 27-gauge 'butterfly' needle. The infraclavicular and anterior chest sites provide the greatest freedom of movement for patients, but other sites may be used. A single infusion site can usually be maintained for 5–7 days (Moulin et al 1992, Coyle et al 1994b). Occasional patients develop focal erythematous swelling at the site of injection; this appears to be a common complication with methadone (Bruera et al 1991) and has also been described with morphine and hydromorphone (Bruera et al 1990).

Continuous SC delivery of drug combinations may be indicated when nausea, anxiety or agitation accompanies pain. An antiemetic, neuroleptic or anxiolytic may be combined with an opioid, provided that it is non-irritant, miscible and stable in combined solution. Experience has been reported with metoclopromide, haloperidol, scopolamine, cyclizine, methotrimeprazine, chlorpromazine and midazolam (Dover 1987, Thorsen et al 1994, Lichter & Hunt 1995, Drummond et al 1996).

In some circumstances, continuous IV infusion may be the most appropriate way of delivering an opioid. The need for very large doses, or treatment with methadone, may suggest the utility of this approach. If continuous IV infusion is to be continued on a long-term basis, a permanent central venous port is recommended (Brant 1995).

Changing routes of administration

The switch between oral and parenteral routes should be guided by knowledge of relative potency (Table 66.4) to avoid subsequent overdosing or underdosing. In calculating the equianalgesic dose, the potencies of the IV, SC and IM routes are considered equivalent. In recognition of the imprecision in the accepted equianalgesic doses and the risk of toxicity from potential overdose, a modest reduction in the equianalgesic dose is prudent. Accomplishing the change in steps (e.g. slowly reducing the parenteral dose and increasing the oral dose over a 2–3-day period) can minimize the problems associated with switching the route of administration.

Scheduling of opioid administration

The schedule of opioid administration should be individualized to optimize the balance between patient comfort and convenience. 'Around the clock' dosing and 'as needed' dosing both have a place in clinical practice.

'Around the clock' (ATC) dosing

Patients with continuous or frequent pain generally benefit from scheduled 'around the clock' dosing, which can provide the patient with continuous relief by preventing the pain from recurring. Clinical vigilance is required, however, when this approach is used in patients with no previous opioid exposure and when administering drugs that have long half-lives (methadone or levorphanol) or produce metabolites with long half-lives (e.g. morphine-6-glucuronide and norpropoxyphene). In the latter situations, delayed toxicity may develop as plasma drug (or metabolite) concentrations rise toward steady state levels.

Most patients who receive an 'around the clock' opioid regimen should also be provided a so-called 'rescue dose', which is a supplemental dose offered on an 'as needed' basis to treat pain that breaks through the regular schedule (McCaffery 1996, Cleary 1997b). The frequency with which the rescue dose can be offered depends on the route of administration and the time to peak effect for the particular drug. Oral rescue doses are usually offered up to every 1–2 hours and parenteral doses can be offered as frequently as every 15–30 minutes. Clinical experience suggests that the initial size of the rescue dose should be equivalent to approximately 50–100% of the dose administered every 4 hours for oral or parenteral bolus medications, or 50–100% of the hourly infusion rate for patients receiving continuous infusions. Alternatively, this may be calculated as 5–15% of the 24-hour baseline dose. The magnitude of the rescue dose should be individualized and some patients with low baseline pain but severe exacerbations may require rescue doses that are substantially higher (Lyss 1997). The drug used for the rescue dose is usually identical to that administered on a scheduled basis, with the exception of transdermal fentanyl and methadone; in these cases, an alternative short half-life opioid for the rescue dose is recommended.

The integration of 'around the clock' dosing with 'rescue doses' provides a method for safe and rational stepwise dose escalation, which is applicable to all routes of opioid administration. Patients who require more than 4–6 rescue doses per day should generally undergo escalation of the baseline dose. The quantity of the rescue medication consumed can be used to guide the dose increment. Alternatively, each dose increment can be set at 33–50% of the pre-existing dose. In all cases, escalation of the baseline dose should be accompanied by a proportionate increase in the rescue dose, so that the size of the supplemental dose remains a constant percentage of the fixed dose (Table 66.6).

Controlled-release preparations of opioids can lessen the inconvenience associated with the use of 'around the clock' administration of drugs with a short duration of action. Currently, controlled-release formulations are available for administration by the oral, transdermal and rectal routes. The largest experience has been reported with oral controlled-release morphine preparations with 8–12 hours' duration of effect. Numerous studies have demonstrated the safety and efficacy of these preparations in cancer patients with pain (Hanks 1989, Kaiko et al 1989, European Association for Palliative Care 1996, Ahmedzai & Brooks 1997). Other controlled-release formulations include once-daily morphine preparations (Broomhead et al 1997), controlled-release morphine suppositories (Bruera et al 1995a) and liquid suspension (Forman et al 1993), transdermal fentanyl (Ahmedzai & Brooks 1997, Wong et al 1997b), and controlled-release tablets of oxycodone (Hagen & Babul 1997), hydromorphone (Hagen & Babul 1997), codeine (Dhaliwal et al 1995) and dihydrocodeine (Aitken et al 1990).

Table 66.6 Examples of stepwise dose escalation of morphine sulphate administered as oral immediate-release preparation, oral controlled-release and continuous infusion

Oral immediate-release morphine sulphate		
Step*	**mg q4 h ATC**	**Rescue dose mg**
1	15	7.5 PRN q1 hr
2	30	15.0 PRN q1 hr
3	45	22.5 PRN q1 hr
4	60	30.0 PRN q1 hr
5	90	45.0 PRN q1 hr
etc.		
Oral controlled-release morphine sulphate (immediate-release rescue dose)		
Step*	**mg ATC**	**Immediate-release rescue dose mg**
1	30 q12	7.5 PRN q1 hr
2	30 q 8	15.0 PRN q1 hr
3	60 q12	15.0 PRN q1 hr
4	100 q12	30.0 PRN q1 hr
5	100 q8	45.0 PRN q1 hr
etc.		
Continuous morphine infusion		
Step*	**mg/h**	**Rescue dose mg**
1	3	2.0 PRN q30 min
2	5	2.5 PRN q30 min
3	7	3.5 PRN q30 min
4	10	5.0 PRN q30 min
5	15	7.5 PRN q30 min
etc.		

*Suggested indications for progression from one step to the next include:
1. requirement of >2 rescue doses in any 4-hour interval or
2. requirement of >6 rescue doses in 24 hours

Clinical experience suggests that controlled-release formulations should not be used to rapidly titrate the dose in patients with severe pain. The time required to approach steady-state plasma concentration after dosing is initiated or changed (at least 24 hours) may complicate efforts to rapidly identify the appropriate dose. Repeat-dose adjustments for patients with severe pain are performed more efficiently with short-acting preparations, which may be changed to a controlled-release preparation when the effective 'around the clock' dose is identified. The change from a short-acting drug to a controlled-release drug should be a milligram to milligram conversion, which results in the same total 'around the clock' dose of the opioid.

'As needed' (p.r.n.) dosing

In some situations, opioid administration on an 'as needed' basis, without an 'around the clock' dosing regimen, may be beneficial. In the opioid-naive patient, 'as needed' dosing may provide additional safety during the initiation of opioid therapy, particularly when rapid dose escalation is needed or therapy with a long half-life opioid such as methadone or levorphanol is begun (Mercadante et al 1996). 'As needed' dosing may also be appropriate for patients who have rapidly decreasing analgesic requirement or intermittent pains separated by pain-free intervals.

Patient-controlled analgesia (PCA)

Patient-controlled analgesia (PCA) generally refers to a technique of parenteral drug administration in which the patient controls an infusion device that delivers a bolus of analgesic drug 'on demand' according to parameters set by the physician. Use of a PCA device allows the patient to overcome variations in both pharmacokinetic and pharmacodynamic factors by carefully titrating the rate of opioid administration to meet individual analgesic needs (Citron et al 1992, Nolan & Wilson 1995, Meuret & Jocham 1996, Ripamonti & Bruera 1997). Although it should be recognized that the use of oral 'rescue doses' is, in fact, a form of PCA (Mercadante et al 1996), the term is not commonly applied to this situation.

Long-term PCA in cancer patients is most commonly accomplished via the subcutaneous route using an ambulatory infusion device (Ripamonti & Bruera 1997). In most cases, PCA is added to a basal infusion rate and acts essentially as a rescue dose (Ripamonti & Bruera 1997). Rare patients have benefited from PCA alone to manage episodic pains characterized by an onset so rapid that an oral dose could not provide sufficiently prompt relief (Portenoy &

Hagen 1990). Long-term intravenous PCA (Urquhart et al 1988, Citron et al 1992, Lamacraft et al 1997) can be used for patients who require doses that cannot be comfortably tolerated via the subcutaneous route or in those who develop local reactions to subcutaneous infusion. PCA has also been applied to spinally administered opioids (Gestin et al 1997) and non-opioid approaches such as nitrous oxide (Keating & Kundrat 1996).

Dose selection and titration

Selecting a starting dose

A patient who is relatively opioid naive, having had only some exposure to an opioid typically used on the second rung of the 'analgesic ladder' for moderate pain, should generally begin one of the opioids typically used for severe pain at a dose equivalent to 5–10 mg morphine IM every 4 hours (European Association for Palliative Care 1996). If morphine is used, a P.O.:IM relative potency ratio of 2:1–3:1 is conventional (European Association for Palliative Care 1996), based on survey data and clinical experience in the cancer population (Sawe et al 1981, Twycross 1988).

When patients on higher doses of opioids are switched to an alternative opioid drug, the starting dose of the new drug should be reduced to 50–75% of the equianalgesic dose to account for imprecision in the equianalgesic dose calculation and the possibility of incomplete crosstolerance. The switch to methadone is the exception to this guideline. The change to methadone is accomplished more safely with a reduction of 75–90% of the equianalgesic dose (Bruera et al 1996, Vigano et al 1996, Manfredi et al 1997, Ripamonti et al 1997). Based on clinical experience, patients receiving a high dose of an opioid should be switched to methadone using a relatively larger reduction in the calculated equianalgesic dose (Bruera et al 1996).

Dose adjustment

Adjustment of the opioid dose is essential at the start of therapy and is usually necessary repeatedly during the patient's course (Schug et al 1992). At all times, inadequate relief should be addressed through gradual escalation of dose until adequate analgesia is reported or intolerable and unmanageable side effects supervene. Because opioid response increases linearly with the log of the dose, a dose increment of less than 30–50% is not likely to improve analgesia significantly. Patients vary greatly in the opioid dose required to manage pain (Coyle et al 1990, Boisvert & Cohen 1995, Mercadante et al 1997) and some patients have been reported to require very high doses of systemic opioids to control pain (Sawe 1986, Fulton & Johnson 1993, Collins et al 1995, Lilley & Guanci 1996, Radbruch et al 1996, Fitzgibbon & Ready 1997). A survey of patients with advanced cancer and challenging pain problems observed that the average daily opioid requirement was equivalent to 400–600 mg of intramuscular morphine; approximately 10% of patients in the survey required more than 2000 mg and one patient required over 35 000 mg per 24 hours (Coyle et al 1990). Thus, doses can become extremely large during this process of titration. The absolute dose is immaterial as long as administration is not compromised by side effects, cost or inconvenience.

Rate of dose titration

The rate of dose titration depends on the severity of the pain, the medical condition of the patient and the goals of care. Patients who present with very severe pain are sometimes best managed by repeated parenteral administration of a dose every 15–30 minutes until pain is partially relieved (Hagen et al 1997). Empiric guidelines have been proposed for the calculation of hourly maintenance dosing after this parenteral loading has been accomplished with a short half-life opioid such as morphine, hydromorphone or fentanyl (Edwards 1990). These guidelines, which can be reasonably extrapolated to the cancer population, recommend that the starting hourly maintenance dose of the short half-life opioid can be approximated by dividing the total loading dose by twice the elimination half-life of the drug. For example, the starting maintenance dose for a patient who has required a total intravenous loading dose of 60 mg of morphine sulphate (half-life approximately 3 hours) to achieve adequate relief would be 10 mg per hour.

Patients with more moderate pain can undergo gradual dose titration. Dose increments equivalent to the daily intake of rescue doses or equivalent to 30–50% of the fixed scheduled dose, whichever is larger, can be administered at intervals greater than that required to reach steady state following each change (Table 66.6). Consistent with this guideline, the dose of morphine (tablets or elixir), hydromorphone or oxycodone can be increased on a twice-daily basis and the dose of controlled-release oral opioids or transdermal fentanyl can be increased every 48–72 hours (Warfield 1989, Korte et al 1996).

The problem of tolerance

The need for escalating doses is a complex phenomenon. Most patients reach a dose that remains constant for pro-

 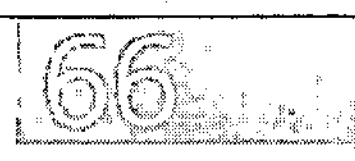

longed periods (Kanner & Foley 1981, Brescia et al 1992, Schug et al 1992, Mercadante et al 1997). When the need for dose escalation arises, any of a variety of distinct processes may be involved (Portenoy 1994b). This clinical experience suggests that true pharmacologic tolerance to analgesia is a much less common reason than worsening pain caused by disease progression (Paice 1988, Schug et al 1992, Collin et al 1993, Portenoy 1994b) or by increasing psychological distress (Velikova et al 1995) or delirium (Coyle et al 1994a). Changes in the pharmacokinetics of an analgesic drug could potentially be involved as well.

In true pharmacologic tolerance, drug administration itself induces an attenuation of effect through changes at the receptor or postreceptor levels (Mao et al 1995). In the clinical setting, tolerance to the non-analgesic effects of opioids does appear to occur commonly (Foley 1991), albeit at varying rates for different effects. For example, tolerance to respiratory depression, somnolence and nausea generally develops rapidly, whereas tolerance to opioid-induced constipation develops very slowly, if at all (Foley 1991). Tolerance to these opioid side effects is not a clinical problem and, indeed, is a desirable outcome that allows effective dose titration to proceed.

Tolerance to the analgesic effect of an opioid, which could compromise the utility of treatment, can only be said to occur if a patient manifests the need for increasing opioid doses in the absence of other factors (e.g. progressive disease) that would be capable of explaining the increase in pain. As noted, extensive clinical experience suggests that the doses of most patients stabilize for prolonged periods and most patients who require an escalation in dose to manage increasing pain have demonstrable progression of disease (Paice 1988, Collin et al 1993, Portenoy 1994b). These observations suggest that true pharmacological tolerance to the analgesic effects of opioids is not a common clinical problem. This conclusion has two important implications:

1. concern about tolerance should not impede the use of opioids early in the course of the disease;
2. worsening pain in a patient receiving a stable dose should not be attributed to tolerance, but should be assessed as presumptive evidence of disease progression or, less commonly, increasing psychological distress or delirium.

Management of opioid adverse effects

Successful opioid therapy requires that the benefits of analgesia clearly outweigh treatment-related adverse effects. This implies that a detailed understanding of adverse opioid effects and the strategies used to prevent and manage them are essential skills for all involved in cancer pain management.

The pathophysiological mechanisms contributing to adverse opioid effects are incompletely understood. The appearance of these effects depends on a number of factors, including patient age, extent of disease, concurrent organ dysfunction, other drugs, prior opioid exposure and the route of drug administration (Portenoy 1994a, Cherny 1996). There is a paucity of data from controlled studies that compare the adverse effects of one opioid analgesic to another or that compare the adverse effects produced by the same opioid given by various routes of administration.

Adverse drug interactions

The potential for additive side effects and serious toxicity from drug combinations must be recognized. The sedative effect of an opioid may add to that produced by numerous other centrally acting drugs, such as anxiolytics, neuroleptics and antidepressants (Pies 1996). Likewise, drugs with anticholinergic effects probably worsen the constipatory effects of opioids. As noted previously, a severe adverse reaction, including excitation, hyperpyrexia, convulsions and death, has been reported after the administration of meperidine to patients treated with a monoamine oxidase inhibitor (Browne & Linter 1987).

Respiratory depression

Respiratory depression is potentially the most serious adverse effect of opioid therapy. Although these drugs may impair all phases of respiratory activity (rate, minute volume and tidal exchange), a compensatory increase in respiratory rate may obscure the degree of respiratory effect. This phenomenon explains the observation that patients who appear to have normal respiration during opioid therapy may be predisposed to respiratory compromise if any pulmonary insult occurs.

Clinically significant respiratory depression is always accompanied by other signs of central nervous system depression, including somnolence and mental clouding. Respiratory compromise accompanied by tachypnoea and anxiety is never a primary opioid event.

With repeated opioid administration, tolerance appears to develop rapidly to the respiratory depressant effects of the opioid drugs (Foley 1991). As a result, opioid analgesics can be used in the management of chronic cancer pain without significant risk of respiratory depression.

Indeed, clinically important respiratory depression is a very rare event in the cancer patient whose opioid dose has been titrated against pain. When respiratory depression occurs in such patients, alternative explanations (e.g. pneumonia or pulmonary embolism) should be sought.

Opioid-induced respiratory depression can occur, however, if pain is suddenly eliminated (such as may occur following neurolytic procedures) and the opioid dose is not reduced (Wells et al 1984). This latter observation suggests that patients whose respiratory function is well compensated following repeated opioid administration do not entirely lack opioid effect on respiration, but rather have respiratory function that reflects a balance between ongoing opioid effects and factors that increase the respiratory drive, including pain, anxiety and alertness.

When respiratory depression occurs in patients on chronic opioid therapy, administration of the specific opioid antagonist naloxone usually improves ventilation. This is true even if the primary cause of the respiratory event was not the opioid itself but, rather, an intercurrent cardiac or pulmonary process. A response to naloxone, therefore, should not be taken as proof that the event was due to the opioid alone and an evaluation for these other processes should ensue.

Naloxone can precipitate a severe abstinence syndrome and should be administered only if strongly indicated (Manfredi et al 1996). If the patient is bradypnoeic but readily arousable and the peak plasma level of the last opioid dose has already been reached, the opioid should be withheld and the patient monitored until improved. If severe hypoventilation occurs (regardless of the associated factors that may be contributing to respiratory compromise) or the patient is bradypnoeic and unarousable, naloxone should be administered. To reduce the risk of severe withdrawal following a period of opioid administration, dilute naloxone (1:10) should be used in doses titrated to respiratory rate and level of consciousness (Bradberry & Raebel 1981, Goldfrank et al 1986). It is neither necessary nor desirable to reverse analgesia during the treatment of opioid-induced respiratory depression. In the comatose patient, it may be prudent to place an endotracheal tube to prevent aspiration following administration of naloxone. As mentioned previously, naloxone should be used with particular caution in patients who have received chronic meperidine therapy because it may precipitate seizures (Umans & Inturrisi 1982, Czuczwar & Frey 1986). Rarely, naloxone administration may trigger the development of a non-cardiogenic pulmonary edema (Schwartz & Koenigsberg 1987).

Sedation

Initiation of opioid therapy or significant dose escalation commonly induces sedation that usually persists until tolerance to this effect develops, usually in days to weeks (Bruera et al 1989b, Sjogren & Banning 1989). It is useful to forewarn patients of this potential and thereby reduce anxiety and encourage avoidance of activities, such as driving, that may be dangerous if sedation occurs (Vainio et al 1995). Some patients have a persistent problem with sedation, particularly if other confounding factors exist, including the use of other sedating drugs or co-existent diseases such as dementia, metabolic encephalopathy or brain metastases. Management of persistent sedation is best accomplished with a stepwise approach (Table 66.7).

Both dextroamphetamine (Forrest et al 1977, McManus & Panzarella 1986) and methylphenidate (Bruera et al 1992a, Wilwerding et al 1995) have been widely used in the treatment of opioid-induced sedation. There has also been some anecdotal experience with the related compound pemoline, which has relatively minor sympathomimetic effects and is available in a chewable tablet (Breitbart & Mermelstein 1992). Three controlled studies have demonstrated that methylphenidate can reverse opioid-induced sedation in the majority of patients with advanced cancer (Bruera et al 1987b, 1992c, Wilwerding et al 1995). A survey of 50 similar patients observed early toxicity in two (hallucinations and a paranoid reaction, respectively), beneficial effects in more than 90% of the remaining group, no late toxicity and the need for escalating doses to maintain effects in some patients (Bruera et al 1989a). Treatment with methylphenidate or dextroamphetamine is typically begun at 2.5–5 mg in the morning, which is repeated at midday if necessary to maintain effects until evening. Doses are then increased gradually if needed. Few patients require more than 40 mg per day in divided doses. At the doses

Table 66.7 Management of opioid-induced sedation

1. Discontinue non-essential central nervous system depressant medications.
2. If analgesia is satisfactory, reduce opioid dose by 25%.
3. If analgesia is unsatisfactory, try addition of a psychostimulant (methylphenidate, dextroamphetamine or pemoline).
4. If somnolence persists, consider:
   - addition of a co-analgesic that will allow reduction in opioid dose;
   - change to an alternative opioid drug;
   - a change in opioid route to the intraspinal route (± local anaesthetic);
   - a trial of other anaesthetic or neurosurgical options.

used clinically, the risks associated with this treatment appear to be very small. Relative contraindications are generally considered to be cardiac arrhythmias, agitated delirium, paranoid personality and past amphetamine abuse.

Confusion and delirium

For patients and their families, confusion is a greatly feared effect of the opioid drugs (Cleeland 1988, Clemons et al 1996). Mild cognitive impairment is common following the initiation of opioid therapy or escalation of the dose (Bruera et al 1989b, 1992b). Similar to sedation, however, pure opioid-induced encephalopathy appears to be transient in most patients, persisting from days to a week or two. Although persistent confusion attributable to opioid alone occurs, the aetiology of persistent delirium is usually related to the combined effect of the opioid and other contributing factors, including electrolyte disorders, neoplastic involvement of central nervous system, sepsis, vital organ failure and hypoxaemia (Bruera et al 1992b, Pereira et al 1997). A stepwise approach to management (Table 66.8) may culminate in a trial of a neuroleptic drug. Haloperidol in low doses (0.5–1.0 mg p.o. or 0.25–0.5 mg IV or IM) is most commonly recommended because of its efficacy and low incidence of cardiovascular and anticholinergic effects.

Constipation

Constipation is the most common adverse effect of chronic opioid therapy in patients with advanced cancer (Fallon & O'Neill 1997). The likelihood of opioid-induced constipation is so great that laxative medications should be prescribed prophylactically to predisposed cancer patients (Glare & Lickiss 1992, Fallon & O'Neill 1997). Predisposing factors include advanced age, immobility, abdominal disease and the concurrent use of constipating medications. Recent studies have suggested that constipation is less prevalent among patients treated with transdermal fentanyl than those receiving oral morphine (Ahmedzai & Brooks 1997).

Table 66.8 Management of opioid-induced delirium

1. Discontinue non-essential centrally acting medications.
2. If analgesia is satisfactory, reduce opioid dose by 25%.
3. Exclude sepsis or metabolic derangement.
4. Exclude CNS involvement by tumour.
5. If delirium persists, consider:
   - trial of neuroleptic (e.g. haloperidol);
   - change to an alternative opioid drug;
   - a change in opioid route to the intraspinal route (± local anaesthetic);
   - a trial of other anaesthetic or neurosurgical options.

There are no controlled comparisons of the various laxatives for opioid-induced constipation and published recommendations are based entirely on anecdotal experience (Table 66.9). Combination therapy is frequently used, particularly co-administration of a softening agent (docusate) and a cathartic (e.g. senna or bisocodyl). The doses of these drugs should be increased as necessary and an osmotic laxative (e.g. milk of magnesia) should be added if needed. Chronic lactulose therapy is an alternative that some patients prefer and occasional patients are managed with intermittent colonic lavage using an oral bowel preparation such as Golytely®.

Rare patients with refractory constipation can undergo a trial of oral naloxone, which has a bioavailability less than 3% and presumably acts selectively on opioid receptors in the gut. Oral administration can reverse constipation without compromising analgesia or precipitating systemic withdrawal (Sykes 1991, 1996, Culpepper-Morgan et al 1992). Some patients can experience systemic withdrawal, however, if doses are escalated. Hence, the initial dose should be small (0.8–1.2 mg once or twice daily) and the dose should be escalated slowly until either favourable effects occur or the patient develops abdominal cramps, diarrhoea or any other adverse effect. Doses as high as 20–24 mg/day may be needed. Although preliminary data suggest that similar effects can be achieved with naltrexone (Yuan et al 1997), this drug is relatively well absorbed orally and will produce withdrawal in physically dependent patients.

Nausea and vomiting

Opioids may produce nausea and vomiting through both central and peripheral mechanisms. These drugs stimulate the medullary chemoreceptor trigger zone, increase vestibular sensitivity and have effects on the gastrointestinal tract (including increased gastric antral tone, diminished motility and delayed gastric emptying) (Rogers & Cerda 1989). In ambulatory patients, the incidence of nausea and vomiting has been estimated to be 10–40% and 15–40%, respectively (Campora et al 1991). The likelihood of these effects is greatest at the start of opioid therapy (Walsh 1990).

With the initiation of opioid therapy, patients should be informed that nausea can occur and that it is usually transitory and controllable. Tolerance typically develops within weeks. Routine prophylactic administration of an antiemetic is not necessary, except in patients with a history

Table 66.9 Laxative medications

Class	*Drug*	*Usual starting dose*	*Comments*
Stool softeners	Docusate sodium	200mg/day	
Osmotic agents	Lactulose Milk of Magnesia	15–30 cc 30–60 cc	May cause abdominal cramps of flatulence
Stimulants	Senna Bisacodyl Phenolphthalein	2 tab 10–15 mg 60–120 mg	Delayed onset of action Delayed onset of action Allergic rash 5%
Bulk agents	Psyllium	4–6 g	May constipate if oral fluid intake is low
Oral lavage	Golytely®	100 cc t.i.d.	
Opioid antagonist	Oral naloxone	0.8–1.2 mg b.i.d.	Escalate dose by small steps until either favourable effect or the development of abdominal cramps, diarrhoea or signs of systemic withdrawal

of severe opioid-induced nausea and vomiting (Walsh 1990), but patients should have access to an antiemetic at the start of therapy if the need for one arises. Anecdotally, the use of prochlorperazine and metoclopramide has usually been sufficient.

In patients with more severe or persistent symptoms, the most appropriate antiemetic treatment may be suggested by the clinical features (Lichter 1996). For nausea associated with early satiety, bloating or postprandial vomiting, all of which are features of delayed gastric emptying, metoclopramide is the most reasonable initial treatment. Patients with vertigo or prominent movement-induced nausea may benefit from the use of an antivertiginous drug such as scopolamine or meclizine. If signs of neither gastroparesis nor vestibular dysfunction are prominent, treatment is usually began with a neuroleptic, such as prochlorperazine or metoclopramide. Drug combinations are sometimes used and, in all cases, doses are escalated if initial treatment is unsuccessful. If these drugs are ineffective at relatively high doses, other options include trials of alternative opioids or treatment with antihistamines (e.g. hydroxyzine), other neuroleptics (e.g. haloperidol, chlorpromazine or droperidol), benzodiazepines (e.g. lorazepam) or steroids (e.g. dexamethasone) or the new serotonin antagonists (e.g. ondansetron).

Multifocal myoclonus

All opioid analgesics can produce myoclonus. The mechanism of this effect is not known and patients with advanced cancer often have multiple potential contributing factors. The opioid effect is dose related and is most prominent with meperidine, presumably as a result of metabolite accumulation (Goetting & Thirman 1985). Mild and infrequent myoclonus is common and may resolve spontaneously with the development of tolerance to this effect. In occasional patients, myoclonus can be distressing or contribute to breakthrough pain that occurs with the involuntary movement. If the opioid dose cannot be reduced, consideration should be given to either switching to an alternative opioid (Cherny et al 1995, De Stoutz et al 1995, Vigano et al 1996) or to symptomatic treatment with a benzodiazepine (particularly clonazepam or midazolam) (Eisele et al 1992, Holdsworth et al 1995). Dantrolene (Mercadante 1995) and other anticonvulsants have also been used empirically for this problem.

Urinary retention

Opioid analgesics increase smooth muscle tone and can occasionally cause bladder spasm or urinary retention (due to an increase in sphincter tone) (Petersen et al 1982). This is an infrequent problem that is usually observed in elderly male patients. Tolerance can develop rapidly but catheterization may be necessary to manage transient problems. Rare patients appear to benefit from co-administration of either a cholinomimetic drug (e.g. bethanecol) or an α-adrenergic antagonist (e.g. terazocin).

Pulmonary oedema

Non-cardiogenic pulmonary oedema has been observed in patients treated with high, escalating opioid doses (Bruera & Miller 1989). A clear cause and effect relationship with

 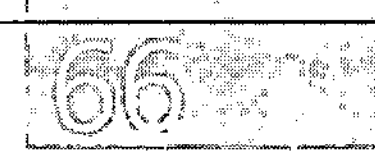

the opioid has not been established, but is suspected. The mechanism, if opioid related, is obscure.

Physical dependence and addiction

Confusion about physical dependence and addiction augment the fear of opioid drugs and contribute substantially to the undertreatment of pain (Bressler et al 1991, McCaffery 1992, Hill 1993, 1996, Ward et al 1993, 1996, Mortimer & Bartlett 1997). To understand these phenomena as they relate to opioid pharmacotherapy for cancer pain, it is useful to first present a concept that might be called 'therapeutic dependence'. Patients who require a specific pharmacotherapy to control a symptom or disease process are clearly dependent on the therapeutic efficacy of the drugs in question. Examples of this 'therapeutic dependence' include the requirements of patients with congestive cardiac failure for cardiotonic and diuretic medications or the reliance of insulin-dependent diabetics on insulin therapy. In these patients, undermedication or withdrawal of treatment results in serious untoward consequences for the patient, the fear of which could conceivably induce aberrant psychological responses and drug-seeking behaviours. Patients with chronic cancer pain have an analogous relationship with their analgesic pharmacotherapy, which may or may not be associated with the development of physical dependence but is virtually never associated with addiction.

Physical dependence

Physical dependence is a pharmacological property of opioid drugs defined by the development of an abstinence (withdrawal) syndrome following either abrupt dose reduction or administration of an antagonist. Despite the observation that physical dependence is most commonly observed in patients taking large doses for a prolonged period of time, withdrawal has also been observed in patients after low doses or short duration of treatment. Occasionally, patients who are switched from a pure agonist opioid to transdermal fentanyl will develop an abstinence syndrome within the first 24 hours, presumably as a result of a delay in establishing blood levels after the transdermal system is placed (Zenz et al 1994, Donner et al 1996). Physical dependence rarely becomes a clinical problem if patients are warned to avoid abrupt discontinuation of the drug; a tapering schedule is used if treatment cessation is indicated and opioid antagonist drugs (including agonist-antagonist analgesics) are avoided (Schug et al 1992).

Addiction

The term addiction refers to a psychological and behavioural syndrome characterized by a continued craving for an opioid drug to achieve a psychic effect (psychological dependence) and associated aberrant drug-related behaviours, such as compulsive drug seeking, unsanctioned use or dose escalation and use despite harm to self or others. Addiction should be suspected if patients demonstrate compulsive use, loss of control over drug use and continuing use despite harm.

The medical use of opioids is very rarely associated with the development of addiction among patients with no prior history of substance abuse (Schug et al 1992). In the largest prospective study, only four cases could be identified among 11 882 patients with no history of addiction who received at least one opioid preparation in the hospital setting (Porter & Jick 1980). In a prospective study of 550 cancer patients who were treated with morphine for a total of 22 525 treatment days, one patient developed problems related to substance abuse (Schug et al 1992). Healthcare providers, patients and families often require vigorous and repeated reassurance that the risk of addiction is extremely small.

'Pseudoaddiction'

The distress engendered in patients who have a therapeutic dependence on analgesic pharmacotherapy but who continue to experience unrelieved pain is occasionally expressed in behaviours that are reminiscent of addiction, such as intense concern about opioid availability and unsanctioned dose escalation. Pain relief, usually produced by dose escalation, eliminates these aberrant behaviours and distinguishes the patient from the true addict. This syndrome has been termed 'pseudo addiction' (Weissman & Haddox 1989). Misunderstanding of this phenomenon may lead the clinician to inappropriately stigmatize the patient with the label 'addict', which may compromise care and erode the doctor–patient relationship. In the setting of unrelieved pain, aberrant drug-related behaviours require careful assessment, renewed efforts to manage pain and avoidance of stigmatizing labels.

Patients with poor response to systemic opioid therapy

All patients who are candidates for opioid therapy should undergo a trial of systemic opioid administration guided by the foregoing principles. Some patients, however, fail to attain adequate relief despite escalation of the dose to levels associated with intolerable and unmanageable side effects. A stepwise strategy (Table 66.10) can be considered when dose escalation of a systemically administered opioid fails to yield a satisfactory result.

The first step in this strategy includes interventions that may improve the balance between analgesia and side effects. If the treatment-limiting side effect cannot be ameliorated, it may be possible to reduce the requirement for opioid therapy by the concurrent use of an appropriate primary therapy or other non-invasive analgesic approach. The latter comprise pharmacological treatments (e.g. addition of a non-opioid or an adjuvant analgesic) and a diverse group of psychological, rehabilitative and neurostimulatory techniques (e.g. TENS). An alternative approach, which has attracted much recent interest, is to switch to another opioid (Galer et al 1992, Bruera et al 1995b, 1996, Cherny et al 1995, De Stoutz et al 1995, Thomas & Bruera 1995, Fallon 1997, Fitzgibbon & Ready 1997, Lawlor et al 1997). This approach, opioid rotation, is predicated on incomplete crosstolerance to analgesia and incomplete cross-sensitivity to adverse effects, particularly sedation, cognitive impairment, delirium, nausea and vomiting and myoclonus (Cherny et al 1995).

Table 66.10 A stepwise strategy for the management of the patient with dose-limiting toxicity from systemic opioid therapy

Step	*Intervention*
1	Non-invasive interventions to improve the therapeutic index of systemic opioid therapy a) treat dose-limiting opioid side effect b) reduce opioid requirement by: • appropriate primary therapy • addition of non-opioid analgesic • addition of an adjuvant analgesic • use of cognitive or behavioural techniques • use of an orthotic device or other physical medicine approach • use of transcutaneous electrical nerve stimulation c) switch to another opioid
2	Consider invasive interventions to lower systemic opioid requirement and preserve cognitive function a) regional analgesic techniques (spinal or intraventricular opioids) b) neural blockade c) neuroablative techniques d invasive neurostimulatory approach
3	Consider increased sedation

Patients unable to achieve a satisfactory analgesic outcome despite these interventions are candidates for the use of invasive analgesic techniques. The use of these approaches should be based on a careful evaluation of the likelihood and duration of analgesic benefit, the immediate risks and morbidity of the procedure (including the anticipated length of hospitalization) and the risks of long-term neurological sequelae. Anaesthetic approaches using opioids or local anaesthetics, such as epidural infusion, are usually considered first because they can reduce the requirement for systemically administered opioids without compromising function. Neurodestructive procedures that involve chemical or surgical neurolysis are very valuable in a small subset of patients; some of these procedures, such as coeliac plexus blockade in patients with pancreatic cancer, may have a favourable enough risk:benefit ratio that early treatment is warranted. Finally, some patients with advanced cancer who have comfort as the over-riding goal of care can elect to be deeply sedated rather than endure further trials of invasive analgesic therapy.

ADJUVANT ANALGESICS

The term 'adjuvant analgesic' describes a drug that has a primary indication other than pain but is analgesic in some conditions. A large group of such drugs, which are derived from diverse pharmacological classes, is now used to manage non-malignant pain (see Ch. 47). In the cancer population, these drugs may be combined with primary analgesics in any of the three steps of the 'analgesic ladder' to improve the outcome for patients who cannot otherwise attain an acceptable balance between relief and side effects. The potential utility of an adjuvant analgesic is usually suggested by the characteristics of the pain or by the existence of another symptom that may be amenable to a non-analgesic effect of the drug.

Whenever an adjuvant analgesic is selected, differences between the use of the drug for its primary indication and its use as an analgesic must be appreciated. Because the nature of dose-dependent analgesic effects has not been characterized for most of these drugs, dose titration is reasonable with virtually all. Low initial doses are appropriate given the desire to avoid early side effects. The use of low initial doses and dose titration may delay the onset of analgesia, however, and patients must be forewarned of this possibility to improve compliance with the therapy.

There is great interindividual variability in the response to all adjuvant analgesics. Although patient characteristics, such as advanced age or co-existent major organ failure, may increase the likelihood of some (usually adverse) responses, neither favourable effects nor specific side effects can be reliably predicted in the individual patient. Furthermore, there is remarkable intraindividual variability in the response to different drugs, including those within the same class. These observations suggest the potential utility of sequential trials of adjuvant analgesics. The process of sequential drug trials, like the use of low initial doses and dose titration, should be explained to the patient at the start of therapy to enhance compliance and reduce the distress that may occur if treatments fail.

In the management of cancer pain, adjuvant analgesics can be broadly classified based on conventional use. Three groups are distinguished:

1. multipurpose adjuvant analgesics;
2. adjuvant analgesics used for neuropathic pain;
3. adjuvant analgesics used for bone pain.

Multipurpose adjuvant medications

Corticosteroids

Corticosteroids are among the most widely used adjuvant analgesics (Watanabe & Bruera 1994). They have been demonstrated to have analgesic effects in diverse conditions (Table 66.11) (Bruera et al 1985), to significantly improve quality of life (Della Cuna et al 1989, Popiela et al 1989, Tannock et al 1989) and to have beneficial effects on appetite, nausea, mood and malaise in the cancer population (Moertel et al 1974, Willox et al 1984, Puccio & Nathanson 1997). The mechanism of analgesia produced by these drugs may involve anti-oedema effects (Yamada et al 1983), anti-inflammatory effects and a direct influence on the electrical activity in damaged nerves (Devor et al 1985).

The relative risks and benefits of the various corticosteroids are unknown and dosing is largely empirical. In the United States, the most commonly used drug is dexamethasone, a choice that gains theoretical support from the relatively low mineralocorticoid effect of this agent. Dexamethasone has also been conventionally used for raised intracranial pressure and spinal cord compression. Prednisone (Tannock et al 1989), methylprednisolone (Hanks et al 1983, Bruera et al 1985) and prednisolone (Willox et al 1984, Twycross & Guppy 1985) have also been widely used for other indications.

Table 66.11 Painful conditions commonly responding to corticosteroid therapy

Raised intracranial pressure
Acute spinal cord compression
Superior vena cava syndrome
Metastatic bone pain
Neuropathic pain due to infiltration or compression by tumour
Symptomatic lymphoedema
Hepatic capsular distension

Patients with advanced cancer who experience pain and other symptoms may respond favourably to a relatively small dose of corticosteroid (e.g. dexamethasone 1–2 mg twice daily). In some settings, however, a high-dose regimen may be appropriate. For example, among patients with spinal cord compression, an acute episode of very severe bone pain or neuropathic pain that cannot be promptly reduced with opioids may respond dramatically to a short course of relatively high doses (e.g. dexamethasone 100 mg, followed initially by 96 mg per day in divided doses) (Sorensen et al 1994). This dose can be tapered over weeks, concurrent with initiation of other analgesic approaches, such as radiotherapy. Although high steroid doses are more likely to lead to adverse effects (Vecht et al 1989, Heimdal et al 1992), clinical experience with this approach has been favourable.

Although the effects produced by corticosteroids in patients with advanced cancer are often very gratifying, side effects are potentially serious and increase with prolonged usage (Twycross 1994). The varying constellations of adverse effects associated with brief or prolonged administration or with the withdrawal of these drugs following long-term use are widely appreciated (Twycross 1994). In a study of advanced cancer patients chronically administered prednisolone or dexamethasone at varying doses, oropharyngeal candidiasis occurred in approximately one-third, oedema or cushingoid habitus developed in almost one-fifth; dyspepsia, weight gain, neuropsychological changes or ecchymoses were observed in 5–10% and the incidence of other adverse effects, such as hyperglycaemia, myopathy and osteoporosis, was extremely low (Hanks et al 1983). The risk of peptic ulcer is approximately doubled in patients chronically treated with corticosteroids (Messer et al 1983). Several risk factors for peptic ulceration have been identified: relatively high dose, previous history of peptic ulceration, advanced malignant disease and concurrent administration of an NSAID (Ellershaw & Kelly 1994). In general, the combined administration of a corticosteroid and an NSAID should be avoided. Patients who are predisposed to peptic ulcer disease can be considered for ulcer prophylaxis. Active peptic ulcer disease and systemic infection are relative contraindications to the use of corticosteroids as adjuvant analgesics.

Topical local anaesthetics

Topical local anaesthetics can be used in the management of painful cutaneous and mucosal lesions and as a premedication prior to skin puncture. Controlled studies have demonstrated the effectiveness of a eutectic mixture of 2.5% lidocaine and 2.5% prilocaine (EMLA) in reducing pain associated with venepuncture (Michael & Andrew 1996, Sharma et al 1996), lumbar puncture (Halperin et al 1989, Kapelushnik et al 1990, Holdsworth et al 1997) and arterial puncture (Taddio et al 1998). It has anecdotally been used for painful ulcerating skin lesions (Stegman & Stoukides 1996, Robins & Farr 1997). Viscous lidocaine is frequently used in the management of oropharyngeal ulceration (Carnel et al 1990). Although the risk of aspiration appears to be very small, caution with eating is required after oropharyngeal anaesthesia.

Neuroleptics

The role of neuroleptic drugs in the management of cancer pain is limited. Methotrimeprazine is a proven analgesic (Beaver et al 1966a, Patt et al 1994) and has been useful in bedridden patients with advanced cancer who experience pain associated with anxiety, restlessness or nausea. In this setting, the sedative, anxiolytic and antiemetic effects of this drug can be highly favourable and side effects, such as orthostatic hypotension, are less of an issue. Methotrimeprazine may be given by continuous SC administration (Oliver 1985), SC bolus injection or brief IV infusion (administration over 20–30 minutes). A prudent dosing schedule begins with 5–10 mg every 6 hours or a comparable dose delivered by infusion, which is gradually increased as needed. Most patients will not require more than 20–50 mg every 6 hours to gain the desired effects. Given their potential for serious toxicity and the limited evidence in support of analgesic efficacy, other neuroleptics should be used only for the treatment of delirium and nausea.

Antihistamines

Despite evidence of analgesic effects in single-dose studies of various antihistamines (Bellville et al 1979, Hupert et al 1980, Stambaugh & Lane 1983), clinical experience has failed to confirm significant analgesic utility from this class of drugs (Glazier 1990). The use of these agents must also be tempered by the potential for additive side effects, including sedation and dry mouth. These drugs should only be considered in patients who have a primary indication other than pain. A trial of hydroxyzine, for example, is sometimes selected in cancer patients where pain is complicated by anxiety, nausea or itch.

Benzodiazepines

There is little evidence that benzodiazepines have meaningful analgesic properties in most clinical circumstances (Reddy & Patt 1994) and, indeed, there is some evidence that they may, in some circumstances, antagonize opioid analgesia (Gear et al 1997). These drugs may play a role in the management of muscle spasm (Butler 1975), chronic pain and anxiety and neuropathic pain. In the latter situation, clonazepam is most commonly used (Smirne & Scarlato 1977, Sandyk 1990, McQuay et al 1995, Bartusch et al 1996).

Adjuvants used for neuropathic pain

Neuropathic pains are generally less responsive to opioid therapy than nociceptive pains (Portenoy et al 1990, Jadad et al 1992, McQuay et al 1992, Cherny et al 1994b). The therapeutic outcome of pharmacotherapy may be improved by the addition of an adjuvant medication. The characteristics of the pain have important implications for the selection of an appropriate drug (Table 66.12).

Antidepressants

In the cancer population, antidepressant drugs are commonly used to manage continuous neuropathic pains that have not responded adequately to an opioid and lancinating neuropathic pains that are refractory to opioids and other specific adjuvant agents (see below) (McQuay et al 1996). The evidence for analgesic efficacy is greatest for the tertiary amine tricyclic drugs, such as amitriptyline (Max et al 1987, 1992, Watson et al 1992, Bryson & Wilde 1996, Eija et al 1996), doxepin (Aronoff & Evans 1982) and imipramine (Kvinesdal et al 1984, Magni et al 1987). The secondary amine tricyclic antidepressants (such as desipramine, clomipramine and nortryptyline) have fewer side effects and are preferred when concern about sedation, anticholinergic effects or cardiovascular toxicity is high (Gomez-Perez et al 1985, Panerai et al 1990, 1991, Max et al 1991). The selective serotonin uptake inhibitor antidepressants can be effective but have less empirical support than the tricyclic compounds (Johansson & Von Knorring 1979, Watson & Evans 1985, Sindrup et al 1990, Max et al 1992, McQuay et al 1996. Limited evidence supports a role for maprotiline (Davidoff et al 1987, Ventafridda et al 1988). Monoamine oxidase inhibitors may have analgesic effects in selected disorders, but the meagre supporting

Table 66.12 A guide to the selection of adjuvant analgesics for neuropathic pain based on clinical characteristics

Continuous pain	*Lancinating pain*	*Sympathetically maintained pain*
Antidepressants	Anticonvulsant drugs	Phenoxybenzamine
Amitriptyline	Carbamazepine	Prazosin
Doxepin	Gabapentin	Corticosteroid
Imipramine	Phenytoin	Nifedipine
Desipramine	Clonazepam	Propranolol
Nortryptyline	Valproate	Calcitonin
Trazodone	Baclofen	Oral local anaesthetics
Maprotiline	Oral local anaesthetics	
	Ketamine	
Oral local anaesthetics		
Mexiletine		
Ketamine		
Clonidine		
Capsaicin		

data and the potential for serious toxicity suggest that there is a very limited role for these agents in the patient with pain due to progressive medical illness (McQuay & Moore 1997).

The starting dose of a tricyclic antidepressant should be low, e.g. amitriptyline 10 mg in the elderly and 25 mg in younger patients. Doses can be increased every few days and the initial dosing increments are usually the same size as the starting dose. When doses have reached the usual effective range (e.g. amitriptyline 50–150 mg), it is prudent to observe effects for a week before continuing upward dose titration. Analgesia usually occurs within a week after achieving an effective dosing level. Although most patients can be treated with a single night-time dose, some patients have less morning 'hangover' and some report less late afternoon pain if doses are divided. It is reasonable to continue upward dose titration beyond the usual analgesic doses in patients who fail to achieve benefit and have no limiting side effects. Plasma drug concentration, if available, may provide useful information and should be followed during the course of therapy. Very low levels in non-responders suggest either poor compliance or an unusually rapid metabolism. In the latter case, doses can be increased while repeatedly monitoring the plasma drug level. Likewise, non-responders whose plasma concentration is not very low, but is lower than the antidepressant range, should be considered for a trial of higher doses if side effects are not a problem.

Oral local anaesthetics

Local anaesthetic drugs may be useful in the management of neuropathic pains characterized by either continuous or lancinating dysaesthesias. Controlled trials have demonstrated the efficacy of tocainide (Lindstrom & Lindblom 1987) and mexiletine (Galer et al 1996, Chong et al 1997, Oskarsson et al 1997, Wright et al 1997), and there is clinical evidence that suggests similar effects from flecainide (Chong et al 1997) and subcutaneous lidocaine (Brose & Cousins 1991).

Experience with oral local anaesthetics in the cancer population is still limited (Chong et al 1997) and recommendations are largely empirical. It is reasonable to undertake a trial with an oral local anaesthetic in patients with continuous dysaesthesias who cannot tolerate the tricyclic antidepressants or who fail to respond adequately to them, and in patients with lancinating pains refractory to trials of anticonvulsant drugs and baclofen (see below). Mexiletine is the safest of the oral local anaesthetics (Cardiac Arrhythmia Suppression Trial Investigators 1989, Ruskin 1989) and is preferred. Preliminary data suggest that an analgesic response to a trial of intravenous lidocaine may predict the likelihood of response to oral mexiletine (Galer et al 1996). Dosing with mexiletine should usually be started at 100–150 mg per day. If intolerable side effects do not occur, the dose can be increased by a like amount every few days, until the usual maximum dose of 300 mg three times per day is reached. Plasma drug concentrations, if available, can provide information similar to that described previously for the tricyclic antidepressants.

α_2-adrenergic agonists

Clonidine is an α_2-adrenergic agonist that has analgesic effects when administered by the spinal route (Eisenach et al 1995, Boswell et al 1997, De Kock et al 1997) or by the oral or transdermal routes (Zeigler et al 1992, Owen et al 1997). There is similar evidence that oral tizanidine has analgesic properties. Although these drugs can be considered multipurpose analgesics in the population with chronic non-malignant pain, they are generally considered in the cancer population for the management of continuous neuropathic pain refractory to opioids and other adjuvants.

Capsaicin

Topical administration of capsaicin depletes peptides in small primary afferent neurons, including those that are putative mediators of nociceptive transmission (e.g. substance P) (Dubner 1991). This effect suggests that long-term use of the drug could reduce the central transmission of information about a noxious stimulus. Analgesic effects have been suggested in postherpetic neuralgia, painful peripheral neuropathies and postmastectomy pain (Capsaicin Study Group 1992, Watson et al 1993, Watson 1994, Ellison et al 1997). Although the dose–response relationship has not been evaluated in controlled studies, data from phase II studies of 0.075% and 0.025% preparations are suggestive of the phenomenon and it is reasonable to use the higher concentration for either the initial trial or a subsequent trial following failure of the lower concentration product. A burning sensation can follow the topical application of capsaicin. This wanes spontaneously in some patients and others can reduce it through the prior use of an oral analgesic or cutaneous application of lidocaine 5% ointment. A proportion of patients report intolerable burning and cannot use the drug. In those who tolerate the drug, an adequate trial should be considered at least four applications per day for 4 weeks.

Anticonvulsant drugs

Many anticonvulsant drugs appear to be analgesic for the lancinating dysaesthesias that characterize diverse types of neuropathic pain (Swerdlow 1985, McQuay et al 1995). Clinical experience also supports the use of these agents in patients with paroxysmal neuropathic pains that may not be lancinating, and to a far lesser extent, in those with neuropathic pains characterized solely by continuous dysaesthesias. Recent experience with gabapentin (Rosner et al 1996, Rosenberg et al 1997, Wetzel & Connelly 1997) has been particularly favourable and suggests that this drug can be used to manage all types of neuropathic pain.

Clinical experience with the use of carbamazepine for lancinating neuropathic pain is extensive because of its accepted role in the management of trigeminal neuralgia (Selman et al 1967, Killian & Fromm 1968, Fromm et al 1984, Green & Selman 1991, McQuay et al 1995). This drug must be used cautiously in cancer patients with thrombocytopenia, those at risk for marrow failure (e.g. following chemotherapy) and those whose blood counts must be monitored to determine disease status. If carbamazepine is used, a complete blood count should be obtained prior to the start of therapy, after 2 and 4 weeks and then every 3–4 months thereafter. A leucocyte count below 4000 is usually considered to be a contraindication to treatment and a decline to less than 3000 or an absolute neutrophil count of less than 1500 during therapy should prompt discontinuation of the drug.

Other anticonvulsant drugs may also be useful for patients with lancinating dyaesthesias following nerve injury. Published reports and clinical experience support trials with phenytoin (Swerdlow 1985, Calissi & Jaber 1995, Chang 1997), clonazepam (Reddy & Patt 1994, Bartusch et al 1996) and valproate (Raftery 1979, Swerdlow 1985). There is limited anecdotal support for the use of lamotrigine.

The use of all these drugs as adjuvant analgesics customarily follows the dosing guidelines employed in the treatment of seizures. Low initial doses are appropriate for gabapentin, carbamazepine, valproate and clonazepam and the administration of phenytoin often begins with the presumed therapeutic dose (e.g. 300 mg per day) or a prudent oral loading regimen (e.g. 500 mg twice, separated by hours). When low initial doses are used, dose escalation should ensue until a favourable effect occurs, intolerable side effects supervene or the plasma drug concentration has reached a predetermined level, which is customarily at the upper end of the therapeutic range for seizure management. This approach is empirical, since there are no data relating plasma concentration to analgesic effects. The variability in the response to these drugs is great and sequential trials in patients with persistent pain are amply justified by clinical experience.

Baclofen

Baclofen is a GABA agonist that has proven efficacy in the treatment of trigeminal neuralgia (Fromm 1994). On this basis, a trial of this drug is commonly employed in the management of paroxysmal neuropathic pains of any type. Dosing is generally undertaken in a manner similar to the use of the drug for its primary indication, spasticity. A starting dose of 5 mg 2–3 times per day is gradually escalated to 30–90 mg per day and sometimes higher if side effects do not occur. The most common adverse effects are sedation and confusion. Failure of a prolonged trial of baclofen requires dose tapering prior to discontinuation due to the potential for a withdrawal syndrome.

N-methyl-D-aspartate (NMDA) antagonists

Limited data suggest that N-methyl-D-aspartate (NMDA) antagonists may be useful agents in the management of neuropathic pain. For patients with advanced disease, favourable effects have been observed using ketamine by subcutaneous infusion starting with 0.1–0.3 mg/kg/hr (Mercadante et al 1995, Mercadante 1996). Other drugs with NMDA antagonist activity have been evaluated and there is some evidence of analgesic efficacy for amantidine (Pud et al 1998) and dextromethorphan (Nelson et al 1997b).

Calcitonin

Subcutaneous injection of calcitonin (100–200 i.u. per day) has been shown to be analgesic in phantom limb pain (Kessel & Worz 1987, Fiddler & Hindman 1991, Jaeger & Maier 1992). Experience with this drug in the treatment of neuropathic pain is very limited and it should be considered only after trials of other drugs have failed.

Pimozide

Pimozide, a phenothiazine neuroleptic with activity against lancinating neuropathic pain, is rarely used in the cancer population. Given its high incidence of adverse effects, including physical and mental slowing, tremor and slight parkinsonian symptoms (Duke 1983, Lechin et al 1989), it should only be considered following failed trials with other drugs.

Adjuvant drugs for sympathetically maintained pain

Sympathetically maintained pain that occurs in the cancer patient can often be ameliorated with sympathetic nerve blocks. Occasionally, sympathetically maintained pain is strongly suspected (e.g. in the cancer patient with a complex regional pain syndrome (CRPS)), but nerve blocks are contraindicated or fail. In this situation, adjuvant analgesics that have been employed specifically for this type of neuropathic pain may be considered. A recent literature review of treatments for CRPS found support for the use of corticosteroids, which had long-term effectiveness (Kingery 1997). There was limited support for the analgesic effectiveness of topical dimethylsulphoxyde (DMSO), epidural clonidine and intravenous regional blocks with bretylium and ketanserin. This analysis concluded that intranasal calcitonin and intravenous phentolamine were probably ineffective for most patients (Kingery 1997).

Adjuvant analgesics used for bone pain

Anti-inflammatory drugs

The management of bone pain frequently requires the integration of opioid therapy with multiple ancillary approaches. Although a meta-analysis of NSAID therapy in cancer pain that reviewed data from 1615 patients in 21 trials found no specific efficacy in bone pain and analgesic effects equivalent only to 'weak' opioids (Eisenberg et al 1994), some patients appear to benefit greatly from the addition of such a drug. As previously mentioned, corticosteroids are often advocated in difficult cases (Watanabe & Bruera 1994).

Bisphosphonates

Bisphosphonates are analogues of inorganic pyrophosphate that inhibit osteoclast activity and consequently reduce bone resorption in a variety of illnesses. This effect presumably underlies the analgesic efficacy of these compounds in bone pain. Controlled and uncontrolled trials of intravenous pamidronate in patients with advanced cancer have demonstrated significant reduction of bone pain (Van Holten-Verzantvoort et al 1991, Purohit et al 1994, Berenson et al 1996, Hortobagyi et al 1996). There is less evidence for analgesic effect with clodronate (Ernst et al 1992, 1997, Robertson et al 1995) and olpadronate (Pelger et al 1998) and a study that evaluated sodium etidronate demonstrated no beneficial effects (Smith 1989). On balance, the data are sufficient to recommend a trial of one of these agents in patients with refractory bone pain. Currently, the evidence for analgesic effects is best for pamidronate. A dose response for this drug is evident at doses between 15 mg and 30 mg/week, and it has been noted that 30 mg every 2 weeks is less effective than 60 mg every 4 weeks (Strang 1996). Additionally, among patients with breast cancer and myeloma with bone involvement, there is evidence that regular administration of pamidronate or clodronate can reduce the risk of the development of pain or pathological fractures (Hortobagyi et al 1996, Lipton 1997, Berenson 1997). The use of any bisphosphonate requires monitoring of serum calcium, phosphate, magnesium and potassium.

Radiopharmaceuticals

Radiolabelled agents that are absorbed into areas of high bone turnover have been evaluated as potential therapies for metastatic bone disease. Clinical responses with acceptable haematological toxicity have been observed with a range of radiopharmaceuticals. Systemically administered phosphorus-32 has long been known to be an effective agent in the management of metastatic bone pain and recent studies have demonstrated efficacy without substantial myelosupression (Burnet et al 1990, Silberstein et al 1992). Controlled clinical trials have demonstrated the efficacy of strontium-89 (Porter et al 1993, Porter & Ben-Josef 1995, Robinson et al 1995) and samarium-153 (Turner et al 1989, Ahonen et al 1994, Resche et al 1997). Rhenium-186 has also been evaluated (De Klerk et al 1997, Limouris et al 1997a,b). Treatment with a radiopharmaceutical is contraindicated in patients with thrombocytopenia or leucopenia (Powsner et al 1997) and those who are candidates for future cytotoxic chemotherapy; treatment also is not advised for patients with very poor performance status (Schmeler & Bastin 1996).

Calcitonin

There is limited evidence that repeated doses of subcutaneous calcitonin can reduce bone pain (Roth & Kolaric 1986, Schiraldi et al 1987, Blomqvist et al 1988, Kadow & Gingell 1988). It is reasonable to consider a trial with the SC or intranasal formulation of this drug in refractory cases.

Adjuvant analgesics for visceral pain

There are limited data that support the potential efficacy of a range of adjuvant agents for the management of bladder spasm, tenesmoid pain and colicky intestinal pain. Oxybutynin chloride, a tertiary amine with anticholinergic and papaverine-like, direct muscular antispasmodic effects, may be helpful for bladder spasm pain (Paulson 1978). Flavoxate has also been used (Baert 1974). Based on limited clinical experience and in vitro evidence that prostaglandins play a role in bladder smooth muscle contraction, a trial of NSAIDs can be administered for this condition as well (Abrams & Fenely 1976). Limited data support a trial of intravesical capsaicin (Barbanti et al 1993, Lazzeri et al 1996).

There is no well-established pharmacotherapy for painful rectal spasms. A recent double-blinded study demonstrated that nebulized salbutamol can reduce the duration and severity of attacks (Eckardt et al 1996). There is anecdotal support for trials of diltiazem (Castell 1985, Boquet et al 1986), clonidine (Swain 1987), chlorpromazine (Patt et al 1994) and benzodiazepines (Hanks 1984).

Colicky pain due to inoperable bowel obstruction has been treated empirically with corticosteroids, intravenous scopolamine (hyoscine) butylbromide (Ventafridda et al 1990a, De Conno et al 1991, Baines 1997) and sublingual scopolamine (hyoscine) hydrobromide (Baines 1994). Limited data support the use of octreotide for this indication (Mercadante 1994b).

In the management of pain due to pancreas cancer, there is limited anecdotal support for the effectiveness of the somatostatin analogues octreotide (Mercadante 1994b) or lanreotide (Canobbio et al 1992). Oral trypsin has also been reported to be useful (Ihse & Permerth 1990). It is speculated that these effects are mediated by reduction in pancreatic exocrine secretion.

OTHER NON-INVASIVE ANALGESIC TECHNIQUES

PSYCHOLOGICAL THERAPIES IN CANCER PAIN

Psychological approaches are an integral part of the care of the cancer patient with pain. All patients can benefit from psychological assessment and support and some are good candidates for specific psychological therapy. Cognitive-behavioural interventions can help some patients decrease the perception of distress engendered by the pain through the development of new coping skills and the modification of thoughts, feelings and behaviours (Fishman 1992, Loscalzo 1996, Spiegel & Moore 1997). Relaxation methods may be able to reduce muscular tension and emotional arousal or enhance pain tolerance (Arathuzik 1994). Other approaches reduce anticipatory anxiety that may lead to avoidant behaviours or lessen the distress associated with the pain (Turk & Feldman 1992). Successful implementation of these approaches in the cancer population requires a cognitively intact patient and a dedicated, well-trained clinician (Fishman 1992).

PHYSIATRIC TECHNIQUES

Physiatric techniques can be used to optimize the function of the patient with chronic cancer pain (Gamble et al 1990, Williams & Maly 1994) or enhance analgesia through application of modalities such as electrical stimulation, heat or cryotherapy. The treatment of lymphoedema by use of wraps, pressure stockings or pneumatic pump devices can both improve function and relieve pain and heaviness (Brennan et al 1996, Marcks 1997). The use of orthotic devices can immobilize and support painful or weakened structures and assistive devices can be of great value to patients with pain precipitated by weight bearing or ambulation.

TRANSCUTANEOUS ELECTRICAL NERVE STIMULATION

The mechanisms by which transcutaneous electrical stimulation reduces pain are not well defined; local neural blockade and activation of a central inhibitory systems have been proposed as explanations (Bushnell et al 1991, Long 1991). Clinical experience suggests that this modality can be a useful adjunct in the management of mild to moderate musculoskeletal or neuropathic pain (Sykes et al 1997).

INVASIVE ANALGESIC TECHNIQUES

Ten to thirty per cent of patients with cancer pain do not achieve a satisfactory balance between relief and side effects using routine systemic pharmacotherapy (Takeda 1985, Ventafridda et al 1987, Walker et al 1988, Goisis et al 1989, Schug et al 1990, Grond et al 1991). In selected patients, anaesthetic or neurosurgical techniques (Tables 66.13, 66.14) may reduce or eliminate the requirement for systemically administered opioids.

CONSIDERATIONS IN SELECTION OF INVASIVE TECHNIQUES

Interpretation of data regarding the use of alternative analgesic approaches and extrapolation to the presenting clinical problem requires caution. The literature is characterized by the lack of uniformity in patient selection, inadequate reporting of previous analgesic therapies, inconsistencies in outcome evaluation, and paucity of long-term follow-up. Furthermore, reported outcomes in the literature may not predict the outcomes of a procedure performed on a medically ill patient by a physician who has more limited experience with the techniques involved.

When indicated, the use of invasive and neurodestructive procedures should be based on an evaluation of the likelihood and duration of analgesic benefit, the immediate and long-term risks, the likely duration of survival, the availability of local expertise and the anticipated length of hospitalization.

For most pain syndromes there exists a range of techniques that may theoretically be applied. In choosing between a range of procedures, the following principles are saliént.

1. Ablative procedures are deferred as long as pain relief is obtainable by non-ablative modalities.
2. The procedure most likely to be effective should be selected. If there is a choice, however, the one with the fewest and least serious adverse effects is preferred.
3. In progressive stages of cancer, pain is likely to be multifocal and a procedure aimed at a single locus of pain, even if completed flawlessly, is unlikely to yield complete relief of pain until death. A realistic and sound goal is a lasting decrease in pain to a level that is manageable by pharmacotherapy with minimal side effects.
4. Whenever possible, neurolysis should be preceded by the demonstration of effective analgesia with a local anaesthetic prognostic block.
5. Since there is a learning curve with all of the procedures, performance by a physician experienced in the specific intervention may improve the likelihood of a successful outcome.

Because individual clinician bias can influence decision making, a case conference approach is prudent when assessing a challenging case. This conference may involve the participation of oncologists, palliative care physicians, anaesthesiologists, neurosurgeons and psychiatrists, nurses, social workers and others. The discussion attempts to clarify the remaining therapeutic options and the goals of care. When local expertise is limited, telephone consultation with physicians who are expert in the management of cancer pain is encouraged.

NEURAXIAL INFUSION

Epidural and intrathecal opioids

The delivery of low opioid doses near the sites of action in the spinal cord may decrease supraspinally mediated adverse effects. Unlike neuroablative therapies, this approach preserves sensation, strength and autonomic function. In the absence of randomized trials that compare the various intraspinal techniques with other analgesic approaches, based on an individual assessment of risk and benefit, the indications for the spinal route remain empirical (Krames 1993, Devulder et al 1994). One survey reported that only 16 of 1205 cancer patients with pain required intraspinal therapy (Hogan et al 1991). Contraindications include bleeding diathesis, profound leucopenia and sepsis. A tem-

Table 66.13 Commonly performed anaesthetic and neurosurgical analgesic techniques for pain refractory to systemic pharmacotherapy

Class	*Technique*	*Clinical situation*
Regional analgesia	Spinal opioids and/or local anaesthetics	Systemic opioid analgesia complicated by unmanageable supraspinally mediated adverse effects
Sympathetic blockade and neurolysis	Coeliac plexus block	Refractory malignant pain involving the upper abdominal viscera including the upper retroperitoneum, liver, small bowel and proximal colon
	Lumbar sympathetic blockade	Sympathetically maintained pain involving the legs
	Stellate ganglion blockade	Sympathetically maintained pain involving the head, neck or arms
Somatic neurolysis or pathway ablation	Chemical rhizotomy	Refractory brachial plexopathy or arm pain; intercostal nerve pain, chest wall pain; refractory bilateral pelvic or lumbosacral plexus pain in patient with urinary diversion and who is confined to bed
	Trigeminal neurolysis	Refractory unilateral facial pain
	Trans-sacral neurolysis	Refractory pain limited to the perineum
	Cordotomy	Refractory unilateral pain arising in the torso or lower extremity
High centre ablation	Cingulotomy	Refractory multifocal pain
	Pituitary ablation	Refractory multifocal pain

Table 66.14 Guide to the selection of invasive analgesic techniques according to the site of pain

Site	*Procedure*
Face: unilateral	Gasserian gangliolysis Trigeminal neurolysis Intraventricular opioid
Pharyngeal	Glossopharyngeal neurolysis Intraventricular opioid
Arm/brachial plexus	Spinal opioid±local anaesthetic Chemical rhizotomy Surgical rhizotomy
Chest wall	Spinal opioid±local anaesthetic Intercostal neurolysis Paravertebral neurolysis Chemical rhizotomy Surgical rhizotomy
Abdominal somatic	Spinal opioid±local anaesthetic Chemical rhizotomy Surgical rhizotomy Cordotomy (unilateral pain)
Upper abdomen: visceral	Coeliac plexus neurolysis
Lower abdomen: visceral	Hypogastric neurolysis
Perineum	Spinal opioid±local anaesthetic Chemical rhizotomy Surgical rhizotomy Trans-sacral S4 neurolysis
Pelvis+lower limb	Spinal opioid±local anaesthetic Chemical rhizotomy Surgical rhizotomy
Unilateral lower quadrant	Cordotomy
Multifocal or generalized pain	Pituitary ablation Cingulotomy

porary trial of spinal opioid therapy should be performed to assess the potential benefits of this approach before implantation of a permanent catheter.

Drug selection for intraspinal delivery is influenced by several factors. Hydrophilic drugs, such as morphine and hydromorphone, have a prolonged half-life in cerebrospinal fluid and significant rostral redistribution (Max et al 1985, Moulin et al 1986, Brose et al 1991). Lipophilic opioids, such as fentanyl and sufentanil, have less rostral redistribution (Grass 1992a,b) and may be preferable for segmental analgesia at the level of spinal infusion. The addition of a low concentration of a local anaesthetic, such as 0.125–0.25% bupivacaine, to an epidural (Nitescu et al 1990, Du Pen et al 1992, Du Pen & Williams 1992) or intrathecal (Mercadante 1994a, Sjoberg et al 1994, Nitescu et al 1995) opioid has been demonstrated to increase analgesic effect without increasing toxicity. Other agents have also been co-administered with intraspinal opioids, including clonidine (Eisenach et al 1995), octreotide (Penn et al 1992), ketamine (Yaksh 1996, Yang et al 1996) and calcitonin (Blanchard et al 1990). Clonidine is approved for this indication in some countries.

There are no trials comparing the intrathecal and epidural routes in cancer pain and extensive experience has been reported with both approaches (Gourlay et al 1991, Nitescu et al 1995, Gestin et al 1997). Longitudinal studies suggest that the risks associated with these techniques are similar (Nitescu et al 1990, Hassenbusch et al 1995, Gestin et al 1997). Based on limited economic data, intrathecal infusion using an implanted pump may be preferred if life expectancy is greater than a few months. The potential morbidity for both these procedures indicates the need for a well-trained clinician able to provide long-term monitoring.

Intraventricular opioids

A growing experience suggests that the administration of an opioid into the cerebral ventricles can provide long-term analgesia in selected patients who have been refractory to other approaches (Leavens et al 1982, Lobato et al 1983, Roquefeuil et al 1984, Blond et al 1985, Lazorthes et al 1985, Obbens et al 1987, Su et al 1987, Weigl et al 1987, Carlisle et al 1989, Choi et al 1989, Lee et al 1990, Cramond & Stuart 1993, Karavelis et al 1996). This technique has been used for patients with upper body or head pain or severe diffuse pain. Schedules have included both intermittent injection via an Ommaya reservoir (Lobato et al 1987, Obbens et al 1987, Cramond & Stuart 1993, Karavelis et al 1996) and continual infusion using an implanted pump (Dennis & DeWitty 1990).

REGIONAL LOCAL ANAESTHETIC

Intrapleural local anaesthetics have been used to manage chronic post-thoracotomy pain (Symreng et al 1989) and cancer-related pains involving the head, neck, chest, arms and upper abdominal viscera (Scott et al 1989, Waldman et al 1989, Dionne 1992, Lema et al 1992, Myers et al 1993). Although a single bolus may provide a prolonged analgesia, continuous infusion of local anaesthetic has been recommended for patients with chronic pain due to advanced cancer (Myers et al 1993). For patients with localized upper limb pain, intermittent infusion of bupivicaine through an interscalene brachial plexus catheter may be of benefit (Cooper et al 1994).

ANAESTHETIC TECHNIQUES FOR VISCERAL PAIN AND SYMPATHETICALLY MAINTAINED PAIN

Coeliac plexus block

Neurolytic coeliac plexus blockade can be considered in the management of pain caused by neoplastic infiltration of the upper abdominal viscera, including the pancreas, upper retroperitoneum, liver, gallbladder and proximal small bowel (Brown 1989, Eisenberg et al 1995, Caraceni & Portenoy 1996). In addition to an extensive anecdotal experience, this technique is supported by two controlled studies of the percutaneous approach (Mercadante 1993, Kawamata et al 1996) and a controlled trial of intraoperative neurolysis (Lillemoe et al 1993). Two small randomized trials offer supporting data (Mercadante 1993, Kawamata et al 1996). Reported analgesic response rates in patients with pancreatic cancer are 50–90% and the reported duration of effect is generally 1–12 months (Brown et al 1987 Ischia et al 1992, Eisenberg et al 1995, Kawamata et al 1996). Given the generally favourable response to this approach, this intervention is usually recommended early for the pain of pancreas cancer (Caraceni & Portenoy 1996). Complications from coeliac plexus block include postural hypotension and diarrhoea (Brown et al 1987, Davies 1993, Chan 1996). These problems are typically transient. Rarely, the procedure can produce a paraplegia due to an acute ischaemic myelopathy (probably caused by involvement of Adamkievicz's artery) (Wong & Brown 1995, Hayakawa et al 1997). Posterior spread of neurolytic solution can occasionally lead to involvement of lower thoracic and lumbar somatic nerves, which can potentially result in a neuropathic pain syndrome (Davies 1993). Other uncommon complications include pneumothorax and retroperitoneal haematoma (De Conno et al 1993a).

Superior hypogastric nerve plexus block

The superior hypogastric nerve plexus lies anterior to the sacral promontory and transmits sensation from pelvic visceral structures. Bilateral percutaneous neurolytic superior hypogastric plexus blocks with 10% phenol can relieve chronic cancer pain arising from disease affecting the descending colon, rectum and lower genitourinary structures in 40–80% of patients (Plancarte et al 1990, 1997).

Ganglion impar block

The ganglion impar (ganglion of Walther) is a solitary retroperitoneal structure at the sacrococcygeal junction that marks the termination of the paired paravertebral sympathetic chains. Neurolysis of this structure can relieve pain in the rectum, perineum or vagina caused by locally advanced cancers of pelvic visceral structures (Plancarte et al 1993, Wemm & Saberski 1995, Nebab & Florence 1997).

Sympathetic blockade

Sympathetically maintained pain syndromes may be relieved by interruption of sympathetic outflow to the affected region of the body. Lumbar sympathetic blockade should be considered for sympathetically maintained pain involving the legs and stellate ganglion blockade may be useful for sympathetically maintained pain involving the face or arms (Lamacraft & Cousins 1997).

OTHER NEUROABLATIVE TECHNIQUES

Rhizotomy

Segmental or multisegmental destruction of the dorsal sensory roots (rhizotomy), achieved by surgical section, chemical neurolysis or radiofrequency lesion, can be an effective method of pain control for patients with otherwise refractory localized pain syndromes. These techniques are most commonly used in the management of chest wall pain due to tumour invasion of somatic and neural structures (Patt & Reddy 1994). Other indications include refractory upper limb, lower limb, pelvic or perineal pain (Saris et al 1986). Chemical rhizotomy may be produced by the instillation of a neurolytic solution into either the epidural or intrathecal space (Swerdlow 1978, Racz et al 1982, Patt & Reddy 1994). Chemical rhizotomies can be performed at any level up to the mid-cervical region, above which the spread of neurolytic agent to the medullary centres carries an unacceptable risk of cardiorespiratory collapse.

Rhizotomy can provide analgesia in about 50% of patients (Patt & Reddy 1994). The average duration of relief is 3–4 months, with a broad distribution. Adverse effects can be related to the injection technique (e.g. spinal headache, infection and arachnoiditis) or to the destruction of non-nociceptive nerve fibres. Specific complications of the procedure depend on the site of neurolysis. For example, the complications of lumbosacral neurolysis include paresis (5–20%), sphincter dysfunction (5–60%), impairment of touch and proprioception and dysaesthesias. Although neurological deficits are usually transient, the risk of increased disability through weakness, sphincter incompetence and loss of positional sense suggests that these techniques should be reserved for patients with limited function and pre-existent urinary diversion. Patient counselling regarding the risks involved is essential.

NEUROLYSIS OF PRIMARY AFFERENT NERVES OR THEIR GANGLIA

Neurolysis of primary afferent nerves may also provide significant relief for selected patients with localized pain. The utility of these approaches is limited by the potential for concurrent motor or sphincteric dysfunction. Refractory unilateral facial or pharyngeal pain may be amenable to trigeminal neurolysis (Gasserian gangliolysis) or glossopharyngeal neurolysis (Rizzi et al 1985, Ischia et al 1990). Unilateral pain involving the tongue or floor of mouth may be amenable to blockade of the sphenopalatine ganglion (Prasanna & Murthy 1993). Intercostal or paravertebral neurolysis are alternatives to rhizotomy for patients with chest wall pain. Unilateral shoulder pain may be amenable to suprascapular neurolysis (Meyer-Witting & Foster 1992). Arm pain that is more extensive may be effectively relieved by brachial plexus neurolysis, but this approach will result in weakness (Neill 1979). Severe somatic pain limited to the perineum may be treated by neurolysis of the S4 nerve root via the ipsilateral posterior sacral foramen, a procedure that carries a minimal risk of motor or sphincter dysfunction (Robertson 1983).

Regeneration of peripheral nerves is sometimes accompanied by the development of postablative neuropathic pain. The risk of this phenomenon is of limited consequence when life expectancy is very limited or intractable pain already exceeds the limits of tolerance.

Cordotomy

During cordotomy, the anterolateral spinothalamic tract is sectioned to produce contralateral loss of pain and temperature sensibility (Stuart & Cramond 1993, Sanders & Zuurmond 1995); The patient with severe unilateral pain arising in the torso or lower extremity is most likely to benefit from this procedure (Stuart & Cramond 1993, Sanders & Zuurmond 1995). The percutaneous technique is generally preferred (Stuart & Cramond 1993, Sanders & Zuurmond 1995). Open cordotomy is usually reserved for patients who are unable to lie in the supine position or are not co-operative enough to undergo a percutaneous procedure.

Significant pain relief is achieved in more than 90% of patients during the period immediately following cordotomy (Stuart & Cramond 1993, Sanders & Zuurmond 1995). Fifty per cent of surviving patients have recurrent pain after 1 year (Cowie & Hitchcock 1982). Repeat cordotomy can sometimes be effective. The neurological complications of cordotomy include paresis, ataxia and bladder and 'mirror-image' pain (Sanders & Zuurmond 1995). The complications are usually transient, but are protracted and disabling in approximately 5% of cases (Sanders & Zuurmond 1995). Rarely, patients with a long duration of survival (>12 months) develop a delayed-onset dysaesthetic pain (Cowie & Hitchcock 1982). The most serious potential complication is respiratory dysfunction, which may result from phrenic nerve paralysis or manifest as sleep-induced respiratory depression (Chevrolet et al 1983, Polatty & Cooper 1986). Because of the latter concern, bilateral high cervical cordotomies or a unilateral cervical cordotomy ipsilateral to the site of the only functioning lung are not recommended.

Pituitary ablation

Pituitary ablation by chemical or surgical hypophysectomy has been reported to relieve diffuse and multifocal pain syndromes that have been refractory to opioid therapy and are unsuitable for any regional neuroablative procedure (Gonski & Sackelariou 1984, Levin & Ramirez 1984). Pain relief has been observed from pain due to both hormone-dependent and hormone-independent tumours (Gonski & Sackelariou 1984, Levin & Ramirez 1984).

Cingulotomy

Anecdotal reports also support the efficacy of MRI-guided stereotactic cingulotomy in the management of diffuse pain syndromes that have been refractory to opioid therapy (Hassenbusch et al 1990, Wong et al 1997a). Although this appears to be a safe procedure with minimal neurological or psychological morbidity, the duration of analgesia is often limited (Hassenbusch et al 1990, Wong et al 1997a). The mode of action is unknown and the procedure is rarely considered.

INVASIVE TECHNIQUES FOR SPECIFIC SITES

Head and neck pain

Pain in the head and neck is perceived by sensory afferents of cranial nerves V, VII, IX, X and of the cervical plexus. Destruction of bone or soft tissues generates somatic nociceptive pain and the infiltration or compression of cranial nerves produces neuropathic pain.

When a unilateral facial pain occurs within the distribution of one of the divisions of the trigeminal nerve or when the pathological process is well correlated to the anatomical course of the nerve, trigeminal neurolysis can be considered. This may be performed either chemically or by thermocoagulation (Sweet 1976, Shapshay et al 1980, Sweet et al 1981, Giorgi & Broggi 1984, Krol & Arbit 1988, Arbit & Krol 1991). When pain extends to the angle of the jaw, additional blockade of the 2nd or 3rd cervical nerve may be necessary (Patt & Jain 1990).

Pain from the pharynx, ear and the posterior third of the tongue is transmitted by the glossopharyngeal nerve. Unilateral pain may be amenable to percutaneous glossopharyngeal neurolysis with radiofrequency ablation at the jugular foramen (Arbit & Krol 1991).

Bilateral and midline head and neck pain is best addressed with central pain suppression such as with ventricular opioids. Alternatively, some patients may be candidates for an open cranial rhizotomy which incorporates transection of the trigeminal and glossopharyngeal nerves and the dorsal roots of C2 and C3. Bilateral glossopharyngeal neurolysis is rarely recommended outside the setting of the tracheostomized patient with a feeding gastrostomy, because of interference with swallowing functions and protective airway reflexes.

Upper limb pain

The sensory afferents of the upper limb are conducted through the brachial plexus to the dorsal spine nerve roots (C5–T1). Whenever possible, regional anaesthetic approaches which do not risk further compromise of motor function are preferred over the neurodestructive approaches. Among the regional anaesthetic techniques, most experience has been reported using intraspinal (epidural and intrathecal) opioids, with or without the addition of local anaesthetic. In all cases, a temporary trial of spinal opioid therapy should be performed to assess the potential benefits of this approach before implantation of a permanent catheter. Alternative non-neuroablative options include intraventricular opioids, continuous intrapleural infusion of local anaesthetic (Myers et al 1993), and interscalene infusion of local anaesthetic into the region of the brachial plexus (Cooper et al 1994).

Neurodestructive techniques are generally reserved for patients who have either failed a trial of the regional anaesthetic approaches or are not candidates. Options include chemical or surgical rhizotomy, percutaneous cordotomy, C1 midline myelotomy, brachial plexus neurolysis or suprascapular neurolysis. In considering these options and in counselling patients, it is important to recognize that both rhizotomy and brachial plexus neurolysis will render the arm functionally useless. Cordotomy may allow preservation of power and proprioception, but long-term relief may be limited by the tendency of the level of analgesia to diminish over time. C1 midline myelotomy can provide substantial pain relief with preservation of power and proprioception and may be useful for patients with bilateral upper limb pain.

Chest wall pain

The sensory afferent fibres for the chest wall and pleura run through the intercostal nerves. Although there is extensive overlap in the dermatomal innervation of the chest wall, patients with focal chest wall pain often benefit from localized neurolytic procedures such as intercostal nerve block, paravertebral block and chemical or radiofrequency rhizotomy. Peripheral neurolysis has never been critically compared with neurolysis closer to midline.

For patients with diffuse pain, intrapleural local anaesthetic, spinal opioid and cordotomy can all be considered. Comparative efficacy data is lacking and selection is influenced by availability of local expertise.

Visceral pain

Contrary to conventional teaching, it is now known that pain impulses arising from most viscera are transmitted to the dorsal horn by unmyelinated afferent fibres that transverse the sympathetic and parasympathetic nerves (Gebhart 1995). The visceral afferent fibres terminate in the dorsal horn where they synapse with ascending viscerosomatic neurons in the spinothalamic tracts. The afferent nerves converge in large paravertebral ganglia and hence are amenable to selective blockade.

For patients with upper abdominal visceral pain arising from the pancreas, upper retroperitoneum, liver, gallbladder and proximal small bowel, options include coeliac plexus block, intrapleural local anaesthetic infusion and spinal opioid ± local anaesthetic. Coeliac plexus blockade is not a trivial intervention and patient counselling should incorporate discussion of the small risk of paraplegia (Wong & Brown 1995, Hayakawa et al 1997). For patients with low visceral pain, neurolysis of the superior hypogastric plexus or ganglion impar (Plancarte et al 1990, 1997) can be considered. Although less opioid responsive than somatic pain, many authors consider spinal opioids as the procedure of choice if a ganglionic block is unsuccessful.

Unilateral lower quadrant pain

The sensory afferents of the pelvis and lower limb are conducted through the lumbar and lumbosacral plexuses to the dorsal spine nerve roots (L2–S2). Pain in this region is amenable to both regional anaesthetic and ablative approaches. Neuroablative approaches may occasionally result in significant neurological deficits and neuraxial infusion is the first-line approach in this setting. If this approach is unsuccessful or contraindicated, then either cordotomy or chemical rhizotomy can be considered (Ischia et al 1984). Of the neuroablative approaches, cordotomy is generally preferred over chemical rhizotomy because of the lower likelihood of motor deficit and sphincteric dysfunction.

Pelvic perineal and bilateral lower limb pain

The sensory afferents of the perineum are conducted through the lumbosacral plexus to the dorsal spine nerve roots (S2–4). Treatment is challenging because the neuroanatomy risks paralysis and sphincter dysfunction when neurodestructive approaches are used. Whenever possible, spinal opioids with or without local anaesthetic are the preferred approach for these patients.

For patients in whom this approach is either unsuccessful or contraindicated, neuroablative options should be considered. Somatic pain that is limited to the perineum may be amenable to selective neurolysis of S4 or midline myelotomy. For ambulatory patients with pain that is midline or bilateral who have intact sphincteric function, open upper thoracic bilateral cordotomy or a C1 midline myelotomy might be considered. Patients with pre-existing motor and sphincter dysfunction are the optimal candidates for chemical rhizotomy.

Diffuse and multifocal pain

In patients suffering from multifocal pain, such as pain from widespread bone metastases, several options exist. Spinal opioids are the least invasive technique. In this setting, hydrophilic opioids such as morphine or hydromorphone are preferred because they have a wider caudal and rostral distribution within the CSF than the lipophilic agents such as fentanyl. Although less experience has been reported with intraventricular opioids, the recent published results with this approach are encouraging (Cramond & Stuart 1993, Karavelis et al 1996).

The neuroablative approaches to be considered in this situation are pituitary ablation, cingulotomy, bilateral cordotomy and C1 midline myelotomy. There are inadequate data to make any firm recommendations in choosing among these procedures. From the limited efficacy data and from clinical observations, the likelihood of relief from any of these approaches is probably between 40% and 80% and the responses are often of brief duration.

When bilateral cordotomy is required, at least one side must be performed at a level below the respiratory centres in the upper cervical cord. This will reduce the risk of central respiratory depression. This approach is not recommended for patients with significant bilateral upper limb pain or head and neck pain.

Most of the data regarding pituitary ablation relates to hormone-sensitive tumours (breast and prostate) and experience relating to other tumour types is more limited (Levin & Ramirez 1984). Approximately 20–25% of patients suffer a transient exacerbation of pain following the procedure (Levin & Ramirez 1984).

C1 midline myelotomy may potentially be efficacious irrespective of tumour type or distribution of pain. Some authors have reported that the duration of relief is often brief (Papo & Luongo 1976). Cingulotomy is a specialized technique requiring MRI stereotaxis. Few clinicians have accrued significant experience with this approach. Additionally, although morbidity is limited, the duration of analgesia is often brief (Hassenbusch et al 1990, Wong et al 1997a).

SEDATION AS PAIN THERAPY

Pain is usually relieved adequately without compromising the sentience or function of the patient beyond that caused by the disease process itself. Occasionally, however, this cannot be achieved and pain is perceived to be 'refractory'. The term 'refractory pain' is used to describe pain that remains distressing despite efforts to alleviate it by means that do not compromise consciousness (Cherny & Portenoy 1994). In deciding that a pain is refractory, the clinician must perceive that the further application of standard interventions is either:

1. incapable of providing adequate relief;
2. associated with excessive and intolerable acute or chronic morbidity;
3. unlikely to provide relief within a tolerable time frame.

At the end of life, sedation may be the only therapeutic option capable of providing adequate relief. This approach is described as 'sedation in the management of refractory symptoms at the end of life' (Cherny & Portenoy 1994).

The ethical justification for this approach is grounded in 'the doctrine of double effect', which distinguishes between the compelling primary intended therapeutic effect (to relieve suffering) and the foreseeable but unavoidable side effects (the loss of function and the potential for accelerating death) (Latimer 1991, Cherny & Portenoy 1994). An alternative approach to the ethical validity of the use of sedation in palliative care, less reliant on the question of intention, derives from the concepts of medical indications and patients' rights. At the end of life, when the overwhelming goal of care is the preservation of patient comfort, the provision of adequate relief of symptoms must be pursued even in the setting of a narrow therapeutic index for the necessary palliative treatments (President's Commission for the Study of Ethical Problems in Medical and Biomedical and Behavioral Research 1983, Scanlon & Fleming 1989, Wanzer et al 1989, American Pain Society Subcommittee on Quality Assurance Standards 1990, Spross et al 1990a, American College of Physicians 1992, American Pain Society 1992, American Geriatrics Society 1995, American Medical Association 1996, Burt 1997). In this context, sedation is a medically indicated therapeutic response to refractory symptoms, which cannot be otherwise relieved. Appeal to patients' rights also underwrites the moral legitimacy of sedation in the management of otherwise intolerable pain at the end of life. Patients have a right, recently affirmed by the Supreme Court in the United States, to palliative care in response to unrelieved suffering (Burt 1997).

A survey of homecare patients treated by the palliative care service of the Italian National Cancer Institute found that 31 of 120 terminally ill patients developed otherwise unendurable symptoms which required deep sedation for adequate relief (Ventafridda et al 1990b). In a retrospective survey of 100 patients who died in an inpatient palliative care ward, Fainsinger et al (1991) found that six patients required sedation for adequate pain control prior to death; an additional two patients who may have benefited from sedation died with severe uncontrolled pain. In a retrospective survey of 36 patients treated with opioid infusions for pain, Portenoy et al (1986) reported that approximately one-third were unable to achieve adequate analgesia without excessive sedation.

Once a clinical consensus exists that symptoms are refractory, it is appropriate to present sedation as an option to the patient or surrogate. When presented to a patient with refractory symptoms, the offer of sedation can demonstrate the clinician's commitment to the relief of suffering. This can enhance trust in the doctor–patient relationship and influence the patient's appraisal of their capacity to cope. Indeed, patients commonly decline sedation, acknowledging that symptoms will be incompletely relieved but secure in the knowledge that if the situation becomes intolerable, this option remains available. Other patients reaffirm comfort as the predominating consideration and request the initiation of sedation.

The published literature describing the use of sedation in the management of refractory symptoms at the end of life is anecdotal and refers to the use of opioids, neuroleptics, benzodiazepines, barbiturates and propofol (Greene & Davis 1991, Truog et al 1992, Cherny & Portenoy 1994, Moyle 1995, Morita et al 1996, Tobias 1997). In the absence of relative efficacy data, guidelines for drug selection are empirical. Irrespective of the agent or agents selected, dose titration is necessary to achieve adequate relief, followed subsequently by provision of ongoing therapy to ensure continuation of the effect.

REFERENCES

Abrams P, Fenely R 1976 The action of prostaglandins on smooth muscle of the human urinary tract in vitro. British Journal of Urology (47): 909–915

Agency for Health Care Policy and Research 1994a Management of cancer pain: adults. Cancer pain guideline panel. Clinical practice guidelines, vol 9. US Department of Health and Human Services, Rockville, Maryland

Agency for Health Care Policy and Research 1994b Management of cancer pain: adults. Cancer pain guideline panel. American Family Physician 49(8): 1853–1868

Ahmedzai S, Brooks D 1997 Transdermal fentanyl versus sustained-release oral morphine in cancer pain: preference, efficacy, and quality of life. The TTS-Fentanyl Comparative Trial Group. Journal of Pain and Symptom Management 13(5): 254–261

Ahonen A, Joensuu H, Hiltunen J et al 1994 Samarium-153-EDTMP in bone metastases. Journal of Nuclear Biology and Medicine 38(4 suppl 1): 123–127

Aitken HA, Clark EC, McArdle CS, Dimitri W, Kenny GN 1990 Evaluation of two formulations of dihydrocodeine using patient-controlled analgesia. Anaesthesia 45(7): 535–537

Algan SM, Horowitz SM 1996 Surgical treatment of pathologic hip lesions in patients with metastatic disease. Clinical Orthopaedics (332): 223–231

American College of Physicians 1992 American College of Physicians ethics manual, 3rd edn. Annals of Internal Medicine 117(11): 947–960

American Geriatrics Society 1995 The care of dying patients: a position statement from the American Geriatrics Society. AGS Ethics Committee. Journal of the American Geriatrics Society 43(5): 577–578

American Medical Association 1996 Good care of the dying patient. Council on Scientific Affairs, American Medical Association. Journal of the American Medical Association 275(6): 474–478

American Pain Society 1992 Principles of analgesic use in the treatment of acute pain and chronic cancer pain. A concise guide to medical practice, 3rd edn. American Pain Society, Skokie, Illinois

American Pain Society Subcommittee on Quality Assurance Standards 1990 Standards for monitoring quality of analgesic treatment of acute pain and cancer pain. Oncology Nursing Forum 17(6): 952–954

American Society of Clinical Oncology Ad Hoc Committee on Cancer Pain 1992 Cancer pain assessment and treatment curriculum guidelines. Journal of Clinical Oncology 10(12): 1976–1982

Arathuzik D 1994 Effects of cognitive-behavioral strategies on pain in cancer patients. Cancer Nursing 17(3): 207–214

Arbit E, Krol G 1991 Percutaneous radiofrequency neurolysis guided by computed tomography for the treatment of glossopharyngeal neuralgia. Neurosurgery 29(4): 580–582

Arner S, Meyerson BA 1988 Lack of analgesic effect of opioids on neuropathic and idiopathic forms of pain. Pain 33(1): 11–23

Aronoff GM, Evans WO 1982 Doxepin as an adjunct in the treatment of chronic pain. Journal of Clinical Psychiatry 43(8 Pt 2): 42–47

Avradopoulos KA, Vezeridis MP, Wanebo HJ 1996 Pelvic exenteration for recurrent rectal cancer. Advances in Surgery 29: 215–233

Baert L 1974 Controlled double-blind trail of flavoxate in painful conditions of the lower urinary tract. Current Medical Research and Opinion 2(10): 631–635

Baines MJ 1994 Management of intestinal obstruction in patients with advanced cancer. Annals of the Academy of Medicine Singapore 23(2): 178–282

Baines MJ 1997 ABC of palliative care. Nausea, vomiting, and intestinal obstruction. British Medical Journal 315(7116): 1148–1150

Barbalias GA, Siablis D, Liatsikos EN et al 1997 Metal stents: a new treatment of malignant ureteral obstruction. Journal of Urology 158(1): 54–58

Barbanti G, Maggi CA, Beneforti P, Baroldi P, Turini D 1993 Relief of pain following intravesical capsaicin in patients with hypersensitive disorders of the lower urinary tract. British Journal of Urology 71(6): 686–691

Bartusch SL, Sanders BJ, D'Alessio JG, Jernigan JR 1996 Clonazepam for the treatment of lancinating phantom limb pain. Clinical Journal of Pain 12(1): 59–62

Bates T 1992 A review of local radiotherapy in the treatment of bone metastases and cord compression. International Journal of Radiation Oncology, Biology, Physics 23(1): 217–221

Beaver WT, Wallenstein SL, Houde RW, Rogers A 1966 A comparison of the analgesic effects of methotrimeprazine and morphine in patients with cancer. Clinical Pharmacology and Therapeutics 7(4): 436–446

Bellville JW, Dorey F, Capparell D, Knox V, Bauer RO 1979 Analgesic effects of hydroxyzine compared to morphine in man. Journal of Clinical Pharmacology 19(5–6): 290–296

Bennett WM, Henrich WL, Stoff JS 1996 The renal effects of nonsteroidal anti-inflammatory drugs: summary and recommendations. American Journal of Kidney Disease 28(1 suppl 1): S56–62

Berenson JR 1997 Bisphosphonates in multiple myeloma. Cancer 80(8 suppl): 1661–1667

Berenson JR, Lichtenstein A, Porter L et al 1996 Efficacy of pamidronate in reducing skeletal events in patients with advanced multiple myeloma. Myeloma Aredia Study Group. New England Journal of Medicine 334(8): 488–493

Blanchard J, Menk E, Ramamurthy S, Hoffman J 1990 Subarachnoid and epidural calcitonin in patients with pain due to metastatic cancer. Journald of Pain and Symptom Management 5(1): 42–45

Blomqvist C, Elomaa I, Porkka L, Karonen SL, Lamberg-Allardt C 1988 Evaluation of salmon calcitonin treatment in bone metastases from breast cancer – a controlled trial. Bone 9(1): 45–51

Blond S, Dubar M, Meynadier J, Combelles PM, Vitrac P 1985 Cerebral intraventricular administration of morphine in cancer patients with intractable pain. The Pain Clinic I. In: Erdmann W, Oyama T, Pernak MJ (eds) Proceedings of the First International Symposium. Vnu Science Press, Utrecht, The Netherlands

Boisvert M, Cohen SR 1995 Opioid use in advanced malignant disease: why do different centers use vastly different doses? A plea for standardized reporting. Journal of Pain and Symptom Management 10(8): 632–638

Bonica JJ, Ventafridda V, Twycross RG 1990 Cancer pain. In: Bonica JJ (ed) The management of pain, vol. 1, 2nd edn. Lea & Febiger, Philadelphia, pp 400–460

Boquet J, Moore N, Lhuintre JP, Boismare F 1986 Diltiazem for proctalgia fugax [letter]. Lancet 1(8496): 1493

Boraas MC 1985 Palliative surgery. Seminars in Oncology 12(4): 368–374

Borgelt BB, Gelber R, Brady LW, Griffin T, Hendrickson FR 1981 The palliation of hepatic metastases: results of the Radiation Therapy Oncology Group pilot study. Int J Radiat Oncol Biol Phys 7(5): 587–591

Bosch A, Caldwell WL 1980 Palliative radiotherapy in the patient with metastatic and advanced incurable cancer. Wisconsin Medical Journal 79(4): 19–21

Boswell G, Bekersky I, Mekki Q, Eisenach J 1997 Plasma concentrations and disposition of clonidine following a constant 14-day epidural infusion in cancer patients. Clinical Therapeutics 19(5): 1024–1030

Bradberry JC, Raebel MA 1981 Continuous infusion of naloxone in the treatment of narcotic overdose. Drug Intelligence and Clinical Pharmacology 15(12): 945–950

Brant JM 1995 The use of access devices in cancer pain control. Seminars in Oncology Nursing 11(3): 203–212

Braun A, Rohe K 1984 Orthopedic surgery for management of tumor pain. Recent Results in Cancer Research 89: 157–170

Breitbart W, Mermelstein H 1992 Pemoline. An alternative psychostimulant for the management of depressive disorders in cancer patients. Psychosomatics 33(3): 352–356

Brennan MJ, DePompolo RW, Garden FH 1996 Focused review: postmastectomy lymphedema. Archives of Physical Medicine and Rehabilitation 77(3 suppl): S74–80

Brescia FJ, Portenoy RK, Ryan M, Krasnoff L, Gray G 1992 Pain, opioid use, and survival in hospitalized patients with advanced cancer. Journal of Clinical Oncology 10(1): 149–155

Bressler LR, Geraci MC, Schatz BS 1991 Misperceptions and inadequate pain management in cancer patients. Drug Intelligence and Clinical Pharmacology 25(11): 1225–1230

Brooks PM, Day RO 1991 Nonsteroidal antiinflammatory drugs – differences and similarities. New England Journal of Medicine 324(24): 1716–1725

Broomhead A, Kerr R, Tester W et al 1997 Comparison of a once-a-day sustained-release morphine formulation with standard oral morphine treatment for cancer pain. Journal of Pain and Symptom Management 14(2): 63–73

Brose WG, Cousins MJ 1991 Subcutaneous lidocaine for treatment of neuropathic cancer pain. Pain 45(2): 145–148

Brose WG, Tanelian DL, Brodsky JB, Mark JB, Cousins MJ 1991 CSF and blood pharmacokinetics of hydromorphone and morphine following lumbar epidural administration. Pain 45(1): 11–15

Brown DL 1989 A retrospective analysis of neurolytic celiac plexus block for nonpancreatic intra-abdominal cancer pain. Regional Anesthesia 14(2): 63–65

Brown DL, Bulley CK, Quiel EL 1987 Neurolytic celiac plexus block for pancreatic cancer pain. Anesthesia and Analgesia 66(9): 869–873

Browne B, Linter S 1987 Monoamine oxidase inhibitors and narcotic analgesics. A critical review of the implications for treatment. British Journal of Psychiatry 151: 210–212

Bruera E, MacDonald N 1986 Intractable pain in patients with advanced head and neck tumors: a possible role of local infection. Cancer Treat Rep 70(5): 691–692

Bruera E, Miller MJ 1989 Non-cardiogenic pulmonary edema after narcotic treatment for cancer pain. Pain 39(3): 297–300

Bruera E, Roca E, Cedaro L, Carraro S, Chacon R 1985 Action of oral methylprednisolone in terminal cancer patients: a prospective randomized double-blind study. Cancer Treat Rep 69(7–8): 751–4

Bruera E, Brenneis C, MacDonald RN 1987a Continuous Sc infusion of narcotics for the treatment of cancer pain: an update. Cancer Treatment Report 71(10): 953–958

Bruera E, Chadwick S, Brenneis C, Hanson J, MacDonald RN 1987b Methylphenidate associated with narcotics for the treatment of cancer pain. Cancer Treat Rep 71(1): 67–70

Bruera E, Brenneis C, Michaud M et al 1988a Use of the subcutaneous route for the administration of narcotics in patients with cancer pain. Cancer 62(2): 407–411

Bruera E, Brenneis C, Michaud M, MacMillan K, Hanson J, MacDonald RN 1988b Patient-controlled subcutaneous hydromorphone versus continuous subcutaneous infusion for the treatment of cancer pain. Journal of the National Cancer Institute 80(14): 1152–1154

Bruera E, Brenneis C, Paterson AH, MacDonald RN 1989a Use of methylphenidate as an adjuvant to narcotic analgesics in patients with advanced cancer. J Pain Symptom Manage 4(1): 3–6

Bruera E, Macmillan K, Hanson J, MacDonald RN 1989b The cognitive effects of the administration of narcotic analgesics in patients with cancer pain. Pain 39(1): 13–16

Bruera E, Macmillan K, Selmser P, MacDonald RN 1990 Decreased local toxicity with subcutaneous diamorphine (heroin): a preliminary report. Pain 43(1): 91–94

Bruera E, Fainsinger R, Moore M, Thibault R, Spoldi E, Ventafridda V 1991 Local toxicity with subcutaneous methadone. Experience of two centers. Pain 45(2): 141–143

Bruera E, Fainsinger R, MacEachern T, Hanson J 1992a The use of methylphenidate in patients with incident cancer pain receiving regular opiates. A preliminary report. Pain 50(1): 75–77

Bruera E, Miller L, McCallion J, Macmillan K, Krefting L, Hanson J 1992b Cognitive failure in patients with terminal cancer: a prospective study. J Pain Symptom Manage 7(4): 192–195

Bruera E, Miller MJ, Macmillan K, Kuehn N 1992c Neuropsychological effects of methylphenidate in patients receiving a continuous infusion of narcotics for cancer pain. Pain 48(2): 163–166

Bruera E, Fainsinger R, Spachynski K, Babul N, Harsanyi Z, Darke AC 1995a Clinical efficacy and safety of a novel controlled-release morphine suppository and subcutaneous morphine in cancer pain: a randomized evaluation. J Clin Oncol 13(6): 1520–1527

Bruera E, Franco JJ, Maltoni M, Watanabe S, Suarez-Almazor M 1995b Changing pattern of agitated impaired mental status in patients with advanced cancer: association with cognitive monitoring, hydration, and opioid rotation. J Pain Symptom Manage 10(4): 287–291

Bruera E, Pereira J, Watanabe S, Belzile M, Kuehn N, Hanson J 1996 Opioid rotation in patients with cancer pain. A retrospective comparison of dose ratios between methadone, hydromorphone, and morphine. Cancer 78(4): 852–857

Bryson HM, Wilde MI 1996 Amitriptyline. A review of its pharmacological properties and therapeutic use in chronic pain states. Drugs and Aging 8(6): 459–476

Burnet NG, Williams G, Howard N 1990 Phosphorus-32 for intractable bony pain from carcinoma of the prostate. Clinical Oncology (Royal College of Radiologists) 2(4): 220–223

Burt RA 1997 The Supreme Court speaks – not assisted suicide but a constitutional right to palliative care. N Engl J Med 337(17): 1234–1236

Bushnell MC, Marchand S, Tremblay N, Duncan GH 1991 Electrical stimulation of peripheral and central pathways for the relief of

musculoskeletal pain. Canadian Journal of Physiology and Pharmacology 69(5): 697–703
Butler JH 1975 Myofascial pain dysfunction syndrome involving tumor metastasis. Case report. Journal of Periodontology 46(5): 309–311
Calissi PT, Jaber LA 1995 Peripheral diabetic neuropathy: current concepts in treatment. Annals of Pharmacotherapy 29(7–8): 769–777
Campora E, Merlini L, Pace M et al 1991 The incidence of narcotic-induced emesis. J Pain Symptom Manage 6(7): 428–430
Canobbio L, Boccardo F, Cannata D, Gallotti P, Epis R 1992 Treatment of advanced pancreatic carcinoma with the somatostatin analogue BIM 23014. Preliminary results of a pilot study. Cancer 69(3): 648–650
Capsaicin Study Group 1992 Effect of treatment with capsaicin on daily activities of patients with painful diabetic neuropathy. Diabetes Care 15(2): 159–165
Caraceni A, Portenoy RK 1996 Pain management in patients with pancreatic carcinoma. Cancer 78(3): 639–653
Cardiac Arrhythmia Suppression Trial Investigators 1989 Preliminary report: effect of encainide and flecainide on mortality in a randomized trial of arrhythmia suppression after myocardial infarction. New England Journal of Medicine 321(6): 406–412
Carlisle DW, Smith KA, Frank E, Meyers FJ 1989 Intraventricular morphine administered by hospice nurses to a patient with intractable pain. American Journal of Hospital Care 6(4): 36–39
Carnel SB, Blakeslee DB, Oswald SG, Barnes M 1990 Treatment of radiation- and chemotherapy-induced stomatitis. Otolaryngology Head and Neck Surgery 102(4): 326–330
Castell DO 1985 Calcium-channel blocking agents for gastrointestinal disorders. American Journal of Cardiology 55(3): 210B–213B
Chan GL, Matzke GR 1987 Effects of renal insufficiency on the pharmacokinetics and pharmacodynamics of opiod analgesics. Drug Intell Clin Pharm 21(10): 773–783
Chan VW 1996 Chronic diarrhea: an uncommon side effect of celiac plexus block. Anesth Analg 82(1): 205–207
Chang VT 1997 Intravenous phenytion in the management of crescendo pelvic cancer-related pain. J Pain Symptom Manage 13(4): 238–240
Chapman CR, Hill HF, Saeger L, Gavrin J 1990 Profiles of opioid analgesia in humans after intravenous bolus administration: alfentanil, fentanyl and morphine compared on experimental pain. Pain 43(1): 47–55
Cherny NI 1996 Opioid analgesics: comparative features and prescribing guidelines. Drugs 51(5): 713–737
Cherny NI, Catane R 1995 Professional negligence in the management of cancer pain. A case for urgent reforms [editorial; comment]. Cancer 76(11): 2181–2185
Cherny NI, Portenoy RK 1994 Sedation in the management of refractory symptoms: guidelines for evaluation and treatment. Journal of Palliative Care 10(2): 31–38
Cherny NI, Thaler HT, Friedlander KH, Lapin J, Portenoy RK 1992 Opioid responsiveness of neuropathic cancer pain: combined analysis of single-dose analgesic trials (meeting abstract). Proc Annu Meet Am Soc Clin Oncol.
Cherny NI, Ho MN, Bookbinder M, Fahey TJ Jr, Portenoy RK, Foley KM 1994a Cancer pain: knowledge and attitudes of physicians at a cancer center (meeting abstract). Proceedings of the Annual Meeting of the American Society of Clinical Oncology, p13
Cherny NI, Thaler HT, Friedlander-Klar H et al 1994b Opioid responsiveness of cancer pain syndromes caused by neuropathic or nociceptive mechanisms: a combined analysis of controlled, single-dose studies. Neurology 44(5): 857–861
Cherny NI, Chang V, Frager G et al 1995 Opioid pharmacotherapy in the management of cancer pain: a survey of strategies used by pain physicians for the selection of analgesic drugs and routes of administration. Cancer 76(7): 1283–1293
Chevrolet JC, Reverdin A, Suter PM, Tschopp JM, Junod AF 1983 Ventilatory dysfunction resulting from bilateral anterolateral high cervical cordotomy. Dual beneficial effect of aminophylline. Chest 84(1): 112–115
Choi CR, Ha YS, Ahn MS, Lee JS, Song JU 1989 Intraventricular or epidural injection of morphine for severe pain. Neurochirurgia (Stuttgart) 32(6): 180–183
Chong SF, Bretscher ME, Mailliard JA et al 1997 Pilot study evaluating local anesthetics administered systemically for treatment of pain in patients with advanced cancer. J Pain Symptom Manage 13(2): 112–117
Citron ML, Kalra JM, Seltzer VL, Chen S, Hoffman M, Walczak MB 1992 Patient-controlled analgesia for cancer pain: a long-term study of inpatient and outpatient use. Cancer Investigation 10(5): 335–341
Cleary J 1997a Double blind randomized study of the treatment of breakthrough pain in cancer patients: oral transmucosal fentanyl citrate versus placebo (meeting abstract). Proc Annu Meet Am Soc Clin Oncol, vol. 16, p A179
Cleary JF 1997b Pharmacokinetic and pharmacodynamic issues in the treatment of breakthrough pain. Semin Oncol 24(5 suppl 16): S16–13–9
Cleeland CS 1988 Clinical cancer: 31. Barriers to the management of cancer pain: the roles of patient and family. Wis Med J 87(11): 13–15
Cleeland CS, Gonin R, Hatfield AK et al 1994 Pain and its treatment in outpatients with metastatic cancer. N Engl J Med 330(9): 592–596
Clemons M, Regnard C, Appleton T 1996 Alertness, cognition and morphine in patients with advanced cancer. Cancer Treatment Reviews 22(6): 451–468
Coda B, Tanaka A, Jacobson RC, Donaldson G, Chapman CR 1997 Hydromorphone analgesia after intravenous bolus administration. Pain 71(1): 41–48
Coia LR 1992 The role of radiation therapy in the treatment of brain metastases. Int J Radiat Oncol Biol Phys 23(1): 229–238
Collin E, Poulain P, Gauvain-Piquard A, Petit G, Pichard-Leandri E 1993 Is disease progression the major factor in morphine 'tolerance' in cancer pain treatment? Pain 55(3): 319–326
Collins JJ, Grier HE, Kinney HC, Berde CB 1995 Control of severe pain in children with terminal malignancy. Journal of Pediatrics 126(4): 653–657
Coluzzi P 1997 A titration study of oral transmucosal fentanyl citrate for breakthrough pain in cancer patients (meeting abstract). Proc Annu Meet Am Soc Clin Oncol, vol. 16, p A143
Cooper IM 1996 Morphine for postoperative analgesia. A comparison of intramuscular and subcutaneous routes of administration [see comments]. Anaesthesia and Intensive Care 24(5): 574–578
Cooper MG, Keneally JP, Kinchington D 1994 Continuous brachial plexus neural blockade in a child with intractable cancer pain. J Pain Symptom Manage 9(4): 277–281
Cowie RA, Hitchcock ER 1982 The late results of antero-lateral cordotomy for pain relief. Acta Neurochirurgia (Wien) 1(2): 39–50
Coyle N 1987 A model of continuity of care for cancer patients with chronic pain. Medical Clinics of North America 71(2): 259–270
Coyle N, Portenoy RK 1991 Infection as a cause of rapidly increasing pain in cancer patients. J Pain Symptom Manage 6(4): 266–269
Coyle N, Adelhardt J, Foley KM, Portenoy RK 1990 Character of terminal illness in the advanced cancer patient: pain and other symptoms during the last four weeks of life. J Pain Symptom Manage 5(2): 83–93
Coyle N, Breitbart W, Weaver S, Portenoy R 1994a Delirium as a contributing factor to 'crescendo' pain: three case reports. J Pain Symptom Manage 9(1): 44–47
Coyle N, Cherny NI, Portenoy RK 1994b Subcutaneous opioid infusions at home. Oncology (Huntingt) 8(4): 21–27; discussion 31–32, 37

Cramond T, Stuart G 1993 Intraventricular morphine for intractable pain of advanced cancer. J Pain Symptom Manage 8(7):465–473

Crews JC, Sweeney NJ, Denson DD 1993 Clinical efficacy of methadone in patients refractory to other mu-opioid receptor agonist analgesics for management of terminal cancer pain. Case presentations and discussion of incomplete cross-tolerance among opioid agonist analgesics. Cancer 72(7): 2266–2272

Crotty B, Watson KJ, Desmond PV et al 1989 Hepatic extraction of morphine is impaired in cirrhosis. European Journal of Clinical Pharmacology 36(5): 501–506

Cruikshank DP, Buchsbaum HJ 1973 Effects of rapid paracentesis. Cardiovascular dynamics and body fluid composition. Jama 225(11): 1361–1362

Culpepper-Morgan JA, Inturrisi CE, Portenoy RK et al 1992 Treatment of opioid-induced constipation with oral naloxone: a pilot study. Clin Pharmacol Ther 52(1): 90–95

Czuczwar SJ, Frey HH 1986 Effect of morphine and morphine-like analgesics on susceptibility to seizures in mice. Neuropharmacology 25(5): 465–469

Davidoff G, Guarracini M, Roth E, Sliwa J, Yarkony G 1987 Trazodone hydrochloride in the treatment of dysesthetic pain in traumatic myelopathy: a randomized, double-blind, placebo-controlled study. Pain 29(2): 151–161

Davies DD 1993 Incidence of major complications of neurolytic coeliac plexus block. Journal of the Royal Society of Medicine 86(5): 264–266

De Conno F, Caraceni A, Zecca E, Spoldi E, Ventafridda V 1991 Continuous subcutaneous infusion of hyoscine butylbromide reduces secretions in patients with gastrointestinal obstruction. J Pain Symptom Manage 6(8): 484–486

De Conno F, Caraceni A, Aldrighetti L et al 1993a Paraplegia following coeliac plexus block. Pain 55(3): 383–385

De Conno F, Ripamonti C, Sbanotto A, Barletta L 1993b A clinical note on sublingual buprenorphine. J Palliat Care 9(3): 44–46

De Conno F, Ripamonti C, Saita L, MacEachern T, Hanson J, Bruera E 1995 Role of rectal route in treating cancer pain: a randomized crossover clinical trial of oral versus rectal morphine administration in opioid-naive cancer patients with pain. J Clin Oncol 13(4): 1004–1008

De Klerk JM, Zonnenberg BA, Blijham GH et al 1997 Treatment of metastatic bone pain using the bone seeking radiopharmaceutical Re-186-HEDP. Anticancer Research 17(3B): 1773–1777

De Kock M, Wiederkher P, Laghmiche A, Scholtes JL 1997 Epidural clonidine used as the sole analgesic agent during and after abdominal surgery. A dose-response study. Anesthesiology 86(2): 285–292

De Stoutz ND, Bruera E, Suarez-Almazor M 1995 Opioid rotation for toxicity reduction in terminal cancer patients. J Pain Symptom Manage 10(5): 378–384

Della Cuna GR, Pellegrini A, Piazzi M 1989 Effect of methylprednisolone sodium succinate on quality of life in preterminal cancer patients: a placebo-controlled, multicenter study. The Methylprednisolone Preterminal Cancer Study Group. European Journal of Cancer and Clinical Oncology 25(12): 1817–1821

Dennis GC, DeWitty RL 1990 Long-term intraventricular infusion of morphine for intractable pain in cancer of the head and neck. Neurosurgery 26(3): 404–407; discussion 407–408

Devor M, Govrin-Lippmann R, Raber P 1985 Corticosteroids suppress ectopic neural discharge originating in experimental neuromas. Pain 22(2): 127–137

Devulder J, Ghys L, Dhondt W, Rolly G 1994 Spinal analgesia in terminal care: risk versus benefit. J Pain Symptom Manage 9(2): 75–81

Devulder J, De Laat M, Dumoulin K, Ghys L, Rolly G 1997 Palliative care: knowledge and attitudes of general practitioners: the results of a questionnaire after training. Acta Clinica Belgica 52(4): 207–210

Dhaliwal HS, Sloan P, Arkinstall WW et al 1995 Randomized evaluation of controlled-release codeine and placebo in chronic cancer pain. J Pain Symptom Manage 10(8): 612–623

Dionne C 1992 Tumour invasion of the brachial plexus: management of pain with intrapleural analgesia [letter]. Canadian Journal of Anaesthesia 39(5 Pt 1): 520–521

Dobrowsky W, Schmid AP 1985 Radiotherapy of presacral recurrence following radical surgery for rectal carcinoma. Diseases of Colon and Rectum 28(12): 917–919

Donner B, Zenz M, Tryba M, Strumpf M 1996 Direct conversion from oral morphine to transdermal fentanyl: a multicenter study in patients with cancer pain. Pain 64(3): 527–534

Dover SB 1987 Syringe driver in terminal care. British Medical Journal (Clin Res Ed) 294(6571): 553–555

Drummond SH, Peterson GM, Galloway JG, Keefe PA 1996 National survey of drug use in palliative care. Palliative Medicine 10(2): 119–124

Du Pen SL, Williams AR 1992 Management of patients receiving combined epidural morphine and bupivacaine for the treatment of cancer pain. J Pain Symptom Manage 7(2): 125–127

Du Pen SL, Kharasch ED, Williams A et al 1992 Chronic epidural bupivacaine-opioid infusion in intractable cancer pain [see comments]. Pain 49(3): 293–300

Dubner R 1991 Topical capsaicin therapy for neuropathic pain. Pain 47(3): 247–248

Duke EE 1983 Clinical experience with pimozide: emphasis on its use in postherpetic neuralgia. Journal of the American Academy of Dermatology 8(6): 845–850

Eckardt VF, Dodt O, Kanzler G, Bernhard G 1996 Treatment of proctalgia fugax with salbutamol inhalation. American Journal of Gastroenterology 91(4): 686–689

Edwards WT 1990 Optimizing opioid treatment of postoperative pain. J Pain Symptom Manage 5(1 suppl): S24–36

Eija K, Tiina T, Pertti NJ 1996 Amitriptyline effectively relieves neuropathic pain following treatment of breast cancer. Pain 64(2): 293–302

Eisele JH Jr, Grigsby EJ, Dea G 1992 Clonazepam treatment of myoclonic contractions associated with high-dose opioids: case report [see comments]. Pain 49(2): 231–232

Eisenach JC, Du Pen S, Dubois M, Miguel R, Allin D 1995 Epidural clonidine analgesia for intractable cancer pain. The Epidural Clonidine Study Group. Pain 61(3): 391–399

Eisenberg E, Berkey CS, Carr DB, Mosteller F, Chalmers TC 1994 Efficacy and safety of nonsteroidal antiinflammatory drugs for cancer pain: a meta-analysis. J Clin Oncol 12(12): 2756–2765

Eisenberg E, Carr DB, Chalmers TC 1995 Neurolytic celiac plexus block for treatment of cancer pain: a meta-analysis [published erratum appears in Anesth Analg 1995 Jul; (81)1: 213]. Anesth Analg 80(2): 290–295

Eisendrath SJ, Goldman B, Douglas J, Dimatteo L, Van Dyke C 1987 Meperidine-induced delirium. American Journal of Psychiatry 144(8): 1062–1065

Ellershaw JE, Kelly MJ 1994 Corticosteroids and peptic ulceration. Palliat Med 8(4): 313–319

Ellison N, Loprinzi CL, Kugler J et al 1997 Phase III placebo-controlled trial of capsaicin cream in the management of surgical neuropathic pain in cancer patients. J Clin Oncol 15(8): 2974–2980

Emanuel EJ 1996 Pain and symptom control. Patient rights and physician responsibilities. Hematology Oncology Clinics of North America 10(1): 41–56

Ernst DS, MacDonald RN, Paterson AH, Jensen J, Brasher P, Bruera E 1992 A double-blind, crossover trial of intravenous clodronate in metastatic bone pain. J Pain Symptom Manage 7(1): 4–11

Ernst DS, Brasher P, Hagen N, Paterson AH, MacDonald RN, Bruera E 1997 A randomized, controlled trial of intravenous clodronate in patients with metastatic bone disease and pain. J Pain Symptom Manage 13(6): 319–326

Estes NC, Thomas JH, Jewell WR, Beggs D, Hardin CA 1993 Pelvic exenteration: a treatment for failed rectal cancer surgery. American Surgeon 59(7): 420–422

European Association for Palliative Care 1996 Morphine in cancer pain: modes of administration. Expert Working Group of the European Association for Palliative Care. BMJ 312(7034): 823–826

Fainsinger R, Miller MJ, Bruera E, Hanson J, Maceachern T 1991 Symptom control during the last week of life on a palliative care unit. J Palliat Care 7(1): 5–11

Fallon M 1997 Opioid rotation: does it have a role? [editorial]. Palliat Med 11(3): 177–178

Fallon M, O'Neill B 1997 ABC of palliative care. Constipation and diarrhoea. BMJ 315(7118): 1293–1296

Fiddler DS, Hindman BJ 1991 Intravenous calcitonin alleviates spinal anesthesia-induced phantom limb pain. Anesthesiology 74(1):187–189

Fishman B 1992 The cognitive behavioral perspective on pain management in terminal illness. Hospice Journal 8(1–2): 73–88

Fitzgibbon DR, Ready LB 1997 Intravenous high-dose methadone administered by patient controlled analgesia and continuous infusion for the treatment of cancer pain refractory to high-dose morphine. Pain 73(2): 259–261

Foley KM 1991 Clinical tolerance to opioids. In: Basbaum AI, Bessom JM (eds) Towards a new pharmacotherapy of pain. John Wiley, Chichester, pp 181–204

Forman WB, Portenoy RK, Yanagihara RH, Hunt C, Kush R, Shepard K 1993 A novel morphine sulphate preparation: clinical trial of a controlled-release morphine suspension in cancer pain. Palliat Med 7(4): 301–306

Forrest WH Jr, Brown BW Jr, Brown CR et al 1977 Dextroamphetamine with morphine for the treatment of postoperative pain. N Engl J Med 296(13): 712–715

Fromm GH 1994 Baclofen as an adjuvant analgesic. J Pain Symptom Manage 9(8): 500–509

Fromm GH, Terrence CF, Chattha AS 1984 Baclofen in the treatment of trigeminal neuralgia: double-blind study and long-term follow-up. Annals of Neurology 15(3): 240–244

Fulton JS, Johnson GB 1993 Using high-dose morphine to relieve cancer pain. Nursing 23(2): 34–39

Galer BS, Coyle N, Pasternak GW, Portenoy RK 1992 Individual variability in the response to different opioids: report of five cases. Pain 49(1): 87–91

Galer BS, Harle J, Rowbotham MC 1996 Response to intravenous lidocaine infusion predicts subsequent response to oral mexiletine: a prospective study. J Pain Symptom Manage 12(3): 161–167

Gamble GL, Kinney CL, Brown PS, Maloney FP 1990 Cardiovascular, pulmonary, and cancer rehabilitation. 5. Cancer rehabilitation: management of pain, neurologic and other clinical problems. Arch Phys Med Rehabil 71(4-S): S248–51

Gear RW, Miaskowski C, Heller PH, Paul SM, Gordon NC, Levine JD 1997 Benzodiazepine mediated antagonism of opioid analgesia. Pain 71(1): 25–29

Gebhart GF 1995 Visceral nociception: consequences, modulation and the future. European Journal of Anaesthesiology suppl 10: 24–27

Gestin Y, Vainio A, Pegurier AM 1997 Long-term intrathecal infusion of morphine in the home care of patients with advanced cancer. Acta Anaesthesiologica Scandinavica 41(1 Pt 1): 12–17

Giorgi C, Broggi G 1984 Surgical treatment of glossopharyngeal neuralgia and pain from cancer of the nasopharynx. A 20-year experience. Journal of Neurosurgery 61(5): 952–955

Glare P, Lickiss JN 1992 Unrecognized constipation in patients with advanced cancer: a recipe for therapeutic disaster. J Pain Symptom Manage 7(6): 369–371

Glazier HS 1990 Potentiation of pain relief with hydroxyzine: a therapeutic myth? Drug Intelligence and Clinical Pharmacology 24(5): 484–488

Goetting MG, Thirman MJ 1985 Neurotoxicity of meperidine. Annals of Emergency Medicine 14(10): 1007–1009

Goisis A, Gorini M, Ratti R, Luliri P 1989 Application of a WHO protocol on medical therapy for oncologic pain in an internal medicine hospital. Tumori 75(5): 470–472

Gokaslan ZL 1996 Spine surgery for cancer. Current Opinion in Oncology 8(3): 178–181

Goldfrank L, Weisman RS, Errick JK, Lo MW 1986 A dosing nomogram for continuous infusion intravenous naloxone. Ann Emerg Med 15(5): 566–570

Gomez-Perez FJ, Rull JA, Dies H, Rodriquez-Rivera JG, Gonzalez-Barranco J, Lozano-Castaneda O 1985 Nortriptyline and fluphenazine in the symptomatic treatment of diabetic neuropathy. A double-blind cross-over study. Pain 23(4): 395–400

Gonski A, Sackelariou R 1984 Cryohypophysectomy for the relief of pain in malignant disease. Medical Journal of Australia 140(3): 140–142

Gonzales GR, Elliott KJ, Portenoy RK, Foley KM 1991 The impact of a comprehensive evaluation in the management of cancer pain. Pain 47(2): 141–144.

Gourlay GK, Plummer JL, Cherry DA et al 1991 Comparison of intermittent bolus with continuous infusion of epidural morphine in the treatment of severe cancer pain. Pain 47(2): 135–140

Grass JA 1992a Fentanyl: clinical use as postoperative analgesic – epidural/intrathecal route. J Pain Symptom Manage 7(7): 419–430

Grass JA 1992b Sufentanil: clinical use as postoperative analgesic – epidural/intrathecal route. J Pain Symptom Manage 7(5): 271–286

Green MW, Selman JE 1991 Review article: the medical management of trigeminal neuralgia. Headache 31(9): 588–592

Greene WR, Davis WH 1991 Titrated intravenous barbiturates in the control of symptoms in patients with terminal cancer. Southern Medical Journal 84(3): 332–337

Grond S, Zech D, Schug SA, Lynch J, Lehmann KA 1991 Validation of World Health Organization guidelines for cancer pain relief during the last days and hours of life. J Pain Symptom Manage 6(7): 411–422

Grond S, Zech D, Lehmann KA, Radbruch L, Breitenbach H, Hertel D 1997 Transdermal fentanyl in the long-term treatment of cancer pain: a prospective study of 50 patients with advanced cancer of the gastrointestinal tract or the head and neck region. Pain 69(1–2): 191–198

Hagen NA, Babul N 1997 Comparative clinical efficacy and safety of a novel controlled-release oxycodone formulation and controlled-release hydromorphone in the treatment of cancer pain. Cancer 79(7): 1428–1437

Hagen NA, Foley KM, Cerbone DJ, Portenoy RK, Inturrisi CE 1991 Chronic nausea and morphine-6-glucuronide. J Pain Symptom Manage 6(3): 125–128

Hagen NA, Elwood T, Ernst S 1997 Cancer pain emergencies: a protocol for management. J Pain Symptom Manage 14(1): 45–50

Halperin DL, Koren G, Attias D, Pellegrini E, Greenberg ML, Wyss M 1989 Topical skin anesthesia for venous, subcutaneous drug reservoir and lumbar punctures in children. Pediatrics 84(2): 281–284

Hanks GW 1984 Psychotropic drugs. Postgraduate Medical Journal 60(710): 881–885

Hanks GW 1987 The clinical usefulness of agonist-antagonistic opioid analgesics in chronic pain. Drug and Alcohol Dependence 20(4): 339–346

Hanks GW 1989 Controlled-release morphine (MST Contin) in advanced cancer. The European experience. Cancer 63(11 suppl): 2378–2382

Hanks GW 1991 Opioid-responsive and opioid-non-responsive pain in cancer. British Medical Bulletin 47(3): 718–731

Hanks GW, Forbes K 1997 Opioid responsiveness. Acta Anaesthesiol Scand 41(1 Pt 2): 154–158

Hanks GW, Trueman T, Twycross RG 1983 Corticosteroids in terminal cancer – a prospective analysis of current practice. Postgrad Med J 59(697): 702–706

Harris JK, Sutcliffe JC, Robinson NE 1996 The role of emergency surgery in malignant spinal extradural compression: assessment of functional outcome. British Journal of Neurosurgery 10(1): 27–33

Hasselstrom J, Eriksson S, Persson A, Rane A, Svensson JO, Sawe J 1990 The metabolism and bioavailability of morphine in patients with severe liver cirrhosis. British Journal of Clinical Pharmacology 29(3): 289–297

Hassenbusch SJ, Pillay PK, Barnett GH 1990 Radiofrequency cingulotomy for intractable cancer pain using stereotaxis guided by magnetic resonance imaging. Neurosurgery 27(2): 220–223

Hassenbusch SJ, Stanton-Hicks M, Covington EC, Walsh JG, Guthrey DS 1995 Long-term intraspinal infusions of opioids in the treatment of neuropathic pain. J Pain Symptom Manage 10(7): 527–543

Hayakawa J, Kobayashi O, Murayama H 1997 Paraplegia after intraoperative celiac plexus block. Anesth Analg 84(2): 447–448

Heimdal K, Hirschberg H, Slettebo H, Watne K, Nome O 1992 High incidence of serious side effects of high-dose dexamethasone treatment in patients with epidural spinal cord compression. Journal of Neurooncology 12(2): 141–144

Henteleff PD 1991 Symptom prevalence and control during cancer patients' last days of life. J Palliat Care 7(2): 50–51

Hill CS Jr 1993 The barriers to adequate pain management with opioid analgesics. Semin Oncol 20(2 suppl 1): 1–5

Hill CS Jr 1996 Government regulatory influences on opioid prescribing and their impact on the treatment of pain of nonmalignant origin. J Pain Symptom Manage 11(5): 287–298

Hill HF, Coda BA, Mackie AM, Iverson K 1992 Patient-controlled analgesic infusions: alfentanil versus morphine. Pain 49(3): 301–310

Hirsh JD 1984 Sublingual morphine sulfate in chronic pain management [letter]. Clin Pharm 3(6): 585–586

Hoegler D 1997 Radiotherapy for palliation of symptoms in incurable cancer. Current Problems in Cancer 21(3): 129–183

Hogan Q, Haddox JD, Abram S, Weissman D, Taylor ML, Janjan N 1991 Epidural opiates and local anesthetics for the management of cancer pain. Pain 46(3): 271–279

Holdsworth MT, Adams VR, Chavez CM, Vaughan LJ, Duncan MH 1995 Continuous midazolam infusion for the management of morphine-induced myoclonus. Annals of Pharmacotherapy 29(1): 25–29

Holdsworth MT, Raisch DW, Winter SS, Chavez CM, Leasure MM, Duncan MH 1997 Differences among raters evaluating the success of EMLA cream in alleviating procedure-related pain in children with cancer. Pharmacotherapy 17(5): 1017–1022

Holley FO, Van Steennis C 1988 Postoperative analgesia with fentanyl: pharmacokinetics and pharmacodynamics of constant-rate i.v. and transdermal delivery. British Journal of Anaesthesia 60(6): 608–613

Hortobagyi GN, Theriault RL, Porter L et al 1996 Efficacy of pamidronate in reducing skeletal complications in patients with breast cancer and lytic bone metastases. Protocol 19 Aredia Breast Cancer Study Group [see comments]. N Engl J Med 335(24): 1785–1791

Hoskin PJ 1995 Radiotherapy for bone pain. Pain 63(2): 137–139

Houde RW, Wallenstein SL, Beaver WT 1966 Evaluation of analgesics in patients with cancer pain. In: Lasagna L (ed) International encyclopedia of pharmacology and therapeutics, vol 1. Pergamon Press, New York, pp 59–67

Hughes LL, Styblo TM, Thoms WW et al 1997 Cellulitis of the breast as a complication of breast-conserving surgery and irradiation. American Journal of Clinical Oncology 20(4): 338–341

Hunt G, Bruera E 1995 Respiratory depression in a patient receiving oral methadone for cancer pain. J Pain Symptom Manage 10(5): 401–404

Hupert C, Yacoub M, Turgeon LR 1980 Effect of hydroxyzine on morphine analgesia for the treatment of postoperative pain. Anesth Analg 59(9): 690–696

Ihse I, Permerth J 1990 Enzyme therapy and pancreatic pain. Acta Chirurgica Scandinavica 156(4): 281–283

Inturrisi CE, Colburn WA, Kaiko RF, Houde RW, Foley KM 1987 Pharmacokinetics and pharmacodynamics of methadone in patients with chronic pain. Clin Pharmacol Ther 41(4): 392–401

Ischia S, Luzzani A, Polati E 1990 Retrogasserian glycerol injection: a retrospective study of 112 patients. Clin J Pain 6(4):291–296

Ischia S, Luzzani A, Ischia A, Magon F, Toscano D 1984 Subarachnoid neurolytic block (L5–S1) and unilateral percutaneous cervical cordotomy in the treatment of pain secondary to pelvic malignant disease. Pain 20:139–149

Ischia S, Ischia A, Polati E, Finco G 1992 Three posterior percutaneous celiac plexus block techniques. A prospective, randomized study in 61 patients with pancreatic cancer pain. Anesthesiology 76(4): 534–540

Jadad AR, Browman GP 1995 The WHO analgesic ladder for cancer pain management. Stepping up the quality of its evaluation [see comments]. JAMA 274(23): 1870–1873

Jadad AR, Carroll D, Glynn CJ, Moore RA, McQuay HJ 1992 Morphine responsiveness of chronic pain: double-blind randomised crossover study with patient-controlled analgesia [see comments]. Lancet 339(8806): 1367–1371

Jaeger H, Maier C 1992 Calcitonin in phantom limb pain: a double-blind study. Pain 48(1): 21–27

Janjan NA 1997 Radiation for bone metastases: conventional techniques and the role of systemic radiopharmaceuticals. Cancer 80(8 suppl): 1628–1645

Jeal W, Benfield P 1997 Transdermal fentanyl. A review of its pharmacological properties and therapeutic efficacy in pain control. Drugs 53(1): 109–138

Johanson GA 1991 Symptom character and prevalence during cancer patients' last days of life. American Journal of Hospice and Palliative Care 8(2): 6–8, 18

Johansson F, Von Knorring L 1979 A double-blind controlled study of seratonin uptake inhibitor (Zimelidine) versus placebo in chronic pain patients. Pain 7(1): 69–78

Johnson JR, Miller AJ 1994 The efficacy of choline magnesium trisalicylate (CMT) in the management of metastatic bone pain: a pilot study. Palliat Med 8(2): 129–135

Jones VA, Hanks GW 1986 New portable infusion pump for prolonged subcutaneous administration of opioid analgesics in patients with advanced cancer. Br Med J (Clin Res Ed) 292(6534): 1496

Jong P, Sturgeon J, Jamieson CG 1995 Benefit of palliative surgery for bowel obstruction in advanced ovarian cancer. Canadian Journal of Surgery 38(5): 454–457

Kadow C, Gingell JC 1988 Salmon calcitonin for bone pain in patients with metastatic carcinoma of the prostate. A pilot study. British Journal of Clinical Practice 42(1): 24–25

Kaiko RF, Foley KM, Grabinski PY et al 1983 Central nervous system excitatory effects of meperidine in cancer patients. Annals of Neurology 13(2): 180–185

Kaiko RF, Grandy RP, Oshlack B et al 1989 The United States experience with oral controlled-release morphine (MS Contin tablets). Parts I and II. Review of nine dose titration studies and clinical pharmacology of 15-mg, 30-mg, 60-mg, and 100-mg tablet strengths in normal subjects. Cancer 63(11 suppl): 2348–2354

Kaiko RF, Fitzmartin RD, Thomas GB, Goldenheim PD 1992 The bioavailability of morphine in controlled-release 30-mg tablets per rectum compared with immediate-release 30-mg rectal suppositories and controlled-release 30-mg oral tablets. Pharmacotherapy 12(2): 107–113

Kanner RM, Foley KM 1981 Patterns of narcotic drug use in a cancer pain clinic. Annals of the New York Academy of Science 362: 161–172

Kapelushnik J, Koren G, Solh H, Greenberg M, DeVeber L 1990 Evaluating the efficacy of EMLA in alleviating pain associated with lumbar puncture; comparison of open and double-blinded protocols in children. Pain 42(1): 31–34

Karavelis A, Foroglou G, Selviaridis P, Fountzilas G 1996 Intraventricular administration of morphine for control of intractable cancer pain in 90 patients. Neurosurgery 39(1): 57–61

Kawamata M, Ishitani K, Ishikawa K et al 1996 Comparison between celiac plexus block and morphine treatment on quality of life in patients with pancreatic cancer pain. Pain 64(3): 597–602

Keating HR, Kundrat M 1996 Patient-controlled analgesia with nitrous oxide in cancer pain. J Pain Symptom Manage 11(2): 126–130

Kessel C, Worz R 1987 Immediate response of phantom limb pain to calcitonin. Pain 30(1): 79–87

Killian JM, Fromm GH 1968 Carbamazepine in the treatment of neuralgia. Use of side effects. Archives of Neurology 19(2): 129–136

Kingery WS 1997 A critical review of controlled clinical trials for peripheral neuropathic pain and complex regional pain syndromes. Pain 73(2): 123–139

Korte W, De Stoutz N, Morant R 1996 Day-to-day titration to initiate transdermal fentanyl in patients with cancer pain: short- and long-term experiences in a prospective study of 39 patients. J Pain Symptom Manage 11(3): 139–146

Krames ES 1993 Intrathecal infusional therapies for intractable pain: patient management guidelines. J Pain Symptom Manage 8(1): 36–46

Krol G, Arbit E 1988 Percutaneous electrocoagulation of the trigeminal nerve using CT guidance. Technical note. Journal of Neurosurgery 68(6): 972–973

Kvinesdal B, Molin J, Froland A, Gram LF 1984 Imipramine treatment of painful diabetic neuropathy. Jama 251(13): 1727–1730

Laine L 1996 Nonsteroidal anti-inflammatory drug gastropathy. Gastrointestinal and Endoscopy Clinics of North America 6(3): 489–504

Lamacraft G, Cousins MJ 1997 Neural blockade in chronic and cancer pain. International Anesthesiology Clinics 35(2): 131–153

Lamacraft G, Cooper MG, Cavalletto BP 1997 Subcutaneous cannulae for morphine boluses in children: assessment of a technique. J Pain Symptom Manage 13(1): 43–49

Lancaster C 1995 Effective nonsteroidal anti-inflammatory drugs devoid of gastrointestinal side effects: do they really exist? Digestive Diseases 13 (suppl 1): 40–47

Latimer EJ 1991 Ethical decision-making in the care of the dying and its applications to clinical practice. J Pain Symptom Manage 6(5): 329–336

Lawlor P, Turner K, Hanson J, Bruera E 1997 Dose ratio between morphine and hydromorphone in patients with cancer pain: a retrospective study. Pain 72(1–2): 79–85

Lazorthes Y, Verdie JC, Bastide R, Lavados A, Descouens D 1985 Spinal versus intraventricular chronic opiate administration with implantable drug delivery devices for cancer pain. Applied Neurophysiology 48(1–6): 234–241

Lazzeri M, Beneforti P, Benaim G, Maggi CA, Lecci A, Turini D 1996 Intravesical capsaicin for treatment of severe bladder pain: a randomized placebo controlled study. J Urol 156(3): 947–952

Leavens ME, Hill CS Jr, Cech DA, Weyland JB, Weston JS 1982 Intrathecal and intraventricular morphine for pain in cancer patients: initial study. J Neurosurg 56(2): 241–245

Lechin F, Van der Dijs B, Lechin ME et al 1989 Pimozide therapy for trigeminal neuralgia. Arch Neurol 46(9): 960–963

Lee TL, Kumar A, Baratham G 1990 Intraventricular morphine for intractable craniofacial pain. Singapore Medical Journal 31(3): 273–276

Lehmann T, Day RO, Brooks PM 1997 Toxicity of antirheumatic drugs. Med J Aust 166(7): 378–383

Leibel SA, Pajak TF, Massullo V et al 1987 A comparison of misonidazole sensitized radiation therapy to radiation therapy alone for the palliation of hepatic metastases: results of a Radiation Therapy Oncology Group randomized prospective trial. Int J Radiat Oncol Biol Phys 13(7): 1057–1064

Lema MJ, Myers DP, De Leon-Casasola O, Penetrante R 1992 Pleural phenol therapy for the treatment of chronic esophageal cancer pain. Reg Anesth 17(3): 166–170

Leng G, Finnegan MJ 1994 Successful use of methadone in nociceptive cancer pain unresponsive to morphine. Palliat Med 8(2): 153–155

Levin AB, Ramirez LL 1984 Treatment of cancer pain with hypophysectomy: surgical and chemical. Advances in Pain Research and Therapy 7(631): 631–645

Lichter I 1996 Nausea and vomiting in patients with cancer. Hematol Oncol Clin North Am 10(1): 207–220

Lichter I, Hunt E 1995 Drug combinations in syringe drivers. New Zealand Medical Journal 108(1001): 224–226

Lifshitz S, Buchsbaum HJ 1976 The effect of paracentesis on serum proteins. Gynecologic Oncology 4(4): 347–353

Lillemoe KD, Cameron JL, Kaufman HS, Yeo CJ, Pitt HA, Sauter PK 1993 Chemical splanchnicectomy in patients with unresectable pancreatic cancer. A prospective randomized trial. Ann Surg 217(5): 447–455; discussion 456–457

Lilley LL, Guanci R 1996 Using high-dose fentanyl patches. American Journal of Nursing 96(7): 18–20, 22

Limouris G, Shukla SK, Manetou A et al 1997a Rhenium-186-HEDP palliative treatment in disseminated bone metastases due to prostate cancer. Anticancer Research 17(3B): 1699–1704

Limouris GS, Shukla SK, Condi-Paphiti A et al 1997b Palliative therapy using rhenium-186-HEDP in painful breast osseous metastases. Anticancer Research 17(3B): 1767–1772

Lindstrom P, Lindblom U 1987 The analgesic effect of tocainide in trigeminal neuralgia. Pain 28(1): 45–50

Lipton A 1997 Bisphosphonates and breast carcinoma. Cancer 80(8 suppl): 1668–1673

Lobato RD, Madrid JL, Fatela LV, Rivas JJ, Reig E, Lamas E 1983 Intraventricular morphine for control of pain in terminal cancer patients. J Neurosurg 59(4): 627–633

Lobato RD, Madrid JL, Fatela LV, Sarabia R, Rivas JJ, Gozalo A 1987 Intraventricular morphine for intractable cancer pain: rationale, methods, clinical results. Acta Anaesthesiol Scand Suppl 85: 68–74

Long DM 1991 Fifteen years of transcutaneous electrical stimulation for pain control. Stereotactic and Functional Neurosurgery 56(1): 2–19

Lopez MR, Stock JA, Gump FE, Rosen JS 1996 Carcinoma of the breast metastatic to the ureter presenting with flank pain and recurrent urinary tract infection. Am Surg 62(9): 748–752

Loscalzo M 1996 Psychological approaches to the management of pain in patients with advanced cancer. Hematol Oncol Clin North Am 10(1): 139–155

Lyss AP 1997 Long-term use of oral transmucosal fentanyl citrate (OTFC) for breakthrough pain in cancer patients (Meeting abstract). Proc Annu Meet Am Soc Clin Oncol, vol. 16, p A144

MacDonald N, Der L, Allan S, Champion P 1993 Opioid hyperexcitability: the application of alternate opioid therapy. Pain 53(3): 353–355

Magni G, Arsie D, De Leo D 1987 Antidepressants in the treatment of cancer pain. A survey in Italy. Pain 29(3): 347–353

Mainar A, Tejero E, Maynar M, Ferral H, Castaneda-Zuniga W 1996 Colorectal obstruction: treatment with metallic stents. Radiology 198(3): 761–764

Makin AJ, Williams R 1997 Acetaminophen-induced hepatotoxicity: predisposing factors and treatments. Advances in Internal Medicine 42: 453–483

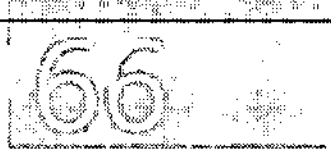

Malmberg AB, Yaksh TL 1992 Hyperalgesia mediated by spinal glutamate or substance P receptor blocked by spinal cyclooxygenase inhibition. Science 257(5074): 1276–1279

Maloney CM, Kesner RK, Klein G, Bockenstette J 1989 The rectal administration of MS Contin: clinical implications of use in end stage cancer. Am J Hosp Care 6(4): 34–35

Manfredi PL, Ribeiro S, Chandler SW, Payne R 1996 Inappropriate use of naloxone in cancer patients with pain. J Pain Symptom Manage 11(2): 131–134

Manfredi PL, Borsook D, Chandler SW, Payne R 1997 Intravenous methadone for cancer pain unrelieved by morphine and hydromorphone: clinical observations. Pain 70(1): 99–101

Mao J, Price DD, Mayer DJ 1995 Mechanisms of hyperalgesia and morphine tolerance: a current view of their possible interactions. Pain 62(3): 259–274

Marcks P 1997 Lymphedema. Pathogenesis, prevention, and treatment. Cancer Practice 5(1): 32–38

Marinella MA 1997 Meperidine-induced generalized seizures with normal renal function. South Med J 90(5): 556–558

Masferrer JL, Isakson PC, Seibert K 1996 Cyclooxygenase-2 inhibitors: a new class of anti-inflammatory agents that spare the gastrointestinal tract. Gastroenterology Clinics of North America 25(2): 363–372

Max MB, Inturrisi CE, Kaiko RF, Grabinski PY, Li CH, Foley KM 1985 Epidural and intrathecal opiates: cerebrospinal fluid and plasma profiles in patients with chronic cancer pain. Clin Pharmacol Ther 38(6): 631–641

Max MB, Culnane M, Schafer SC et al 1987 Amitriptyline relieves diabetic neuropathy pain in patients with normal or depressed mood. Neurology 37(4): 589–596

Max MB, Kishore-Kumar R, Schafer SC et al 1991 Efficacy of desipramine in painful diabetic neuropathy: a placebo-controlled trial. Pain 45(1): 3–9; discussion 1–2

Max MB, Lynch SA, Muir J, Shoaf SE, Smoller B, Dubner R 1992 Effects of desipramine, amitriptyline, and fluoxetine on pain in diabetic neuropathy. N Engl J Med 326(19): 1250–1256

McCabe MJ 1997 Ethical issues in pain management. Hosp J 12(2): 25–32

McCaffery M 1992 Pain control. Barriers to the use of available information. World Health Organization Expert Committee on Cancer Pain Relief and Active Supportive Care. Cancer 70(5 suppl): 1438–1449

McCaffery M 1996 How to calculate a rescue dose. Am J Nurs 96(4): 65–66

McManus MJ, Panzarella C 1986 The use of dextroamphetamine to counteract sedation for patients on a morphine drip. Journal of the Association of Pediatric Oncology Nurses 3(1): 28–29

McQuay HJ, Moore RA 1997 Antidepressants and chronic pain. BMJ 314(7083): 763–764

McQuay HJ, Jadad AR, Carroll D et al 1992 Opioid sensitivity of chronic pain: a patient-controlled analgesia method. Anaesthesia 47(9): 757–767

McQuay HJ, Carroll D, Jadad AR, Wiffen P, Moore A 1995 Anticonvulsant drugs for management of pain: a systematic review. BMJ 311(7012): 1047–1052

McQuay HJ, Tramer M, Nye BA, Carroll D, Wiffen PJ, Moore RA 1996 A systematic review of antidepressants in neuropathic pain. Pain 68(2–3): 217–227

Mercadante S 1993 Celiac plexus block versus analgesics in pancreatic cancer pain. Pain 52(2): 187–192

Mercadante S 1994a Intrathecal morphine and bupivacaine in advanced cancer pain patients implanted at home. J Pain Symptom Manage 9(3): 201–207

Mercadante S 1994b The role of octreotide in palliative care. J Pain Symptom Manage 9(6): 406–411

Mercadante S 1995 Dantrolene treatment of opioid-induced myoclonus. Anesth Analg 81(6): 1307–1308

Mercadante S 1996 Ketamine in cancer pain: an update. Palliat Med 10(3): 225–230

Mercadante S, Lodi F, Sapio M, Calligara M, Serretta R 1995 Long-term ketamine subcutaneous continuous infusion in neuropathic cancer pain. J Pain Symptom Manage 10(7): 564–568

Mercadante S, Sapio M, Serretta R, Caligara M 1996 Patient-controlled analgesia with oral methadone in cancer pain: preliminary report. Annals of Oncology 7(6): 613–617

Mercadante S, Dardanoni G, Salvaggio L, Armata MG, Agnello A 1997 Monitoring of opioid therapy in advanced cancer pain patients. J Pain Symptom Manage 13(4): 204–212

Messer J, Reitman D, Sacks HS, Smith H Jr, Chalmers TC 1983 Association of adrenocorticosteroid therapy and peptic-ulcer disease. N Engl J Med 309(1): 21–24

Meuret G, Jocham H 1996 Patient-controlled analgesia (PCA) in the domiciliary care of tumour patients. Cancer Treat Rev 22(suppl A): 137–140

Meyer-Witting M, Foster JM 1992 Suprascapular nerve block in the management of cancer pain. Anaesthesia 47(7): 626

Michael A, Andrew M 1996 The application of EMLA and glyceryl trinitrate ointment prior to venepuncture. Anaesth Intensive Care 24(3): 360–364

Moertel CG, Schutt AJ, Reitemeier RJ, Hahn RG 1974 Corticosteroid therapy of preterminal gastrointestinal cancer. Cancer 33(6): 1607–1609

Mohiuddin M, Chen E, Ahmad N 1996 Combined liver radiation and chemotherapy for palliation of hepatic metastases from colorectal cancer. J Clin Oncol 14(3): 722–728

Morita T, Inoue S, Chihara S 1996 Sedation for symptom control in Japan: the importance of intermittent use and communication with family members. J Pain Symptom Manage 12(1): 32–38

Mortimer JE, Bartlett NL 1997 Assessment of knowledge about cancer pain management by physicians in training. J Pain Symptom Manage 14(1): 21–28

Moulin DE, Inturrisi CE, Foley KM 1986 Epidural and intrathecal opioids: cerebrospinal fluid and plasma pharmacokinetics in cancer pain patients. In: Foley KM, Inturrisi CE (eds) Opioid analgesics in the management of clinical pain. Raven Press, New York, pp 369–383

Moulin DE, Kreeft JH, Murray-Parsons N, Bouquillon AI 1991 Comparison of continuous subcutaneous and intravenous hydromorphone infusions for management of cancer pain [see comments]. Lancet 337(8739): 465–468

Moulin DE, Johnson NG, Murray-Parsons N, Geoghegan MF, Goodwin VA, Chester MA 1992 Subcutaneous narcotic infusions for cancer pain: treatment outcome and guidelines for use. Canadian Medical Association Journal 146(6): 891–897

Moyle J 1995 The use of propofol in palliative medicine. J Pain Symptom Manage 10(8): 643–646

Myers DP, Lema MJ, De Leon-Casasola OA, Bacon DR 1993 Interpleural analgesia for the treatment of severe cancer pain in terminally ill patients. J Pain Symptom Manage 8(7): 505–510

Neal EA, Meffin PJ, Gregory PB, Blaschke TF 1979 Enhanced bioavailability and decreased clearance of analgesics in patients with cirrhosis. Gastroenterology 77(1): 96–102

Nebab EG, Florence IM 1997 An alternative needle geometry for interruption of the ganglion impar [letter]. Anesthesiology 86(5): 1213–1214

Neill RS 1979 Ablation of the brachial plexus. Control of intractable pain, due to a pathological fracture of the humerus. Anaesthesia 34(10): 1024–1027

Nelson KA, Glare PA, Walsh D, Groh ES 1997a A prospective, within-patient, crossover study of continuous intravenous and subcutaneous morphine for chronic cancer pain. J Pain Symptom Manage 13(5): 262–267

Nelson KA, Park KM, Robinovitz E, Tsigos C, Max MB 1997b High-dose oral dextromethorphan versus placebo in painful diabetic neuropathy and postherpetic neuralgia. Neurology 48(5): 1212–1218

Nitescu P, Appelgren L, Linder LE, Sjoberg M, Hultman E, Curelaru I 1990 Epidural versus intrathecal morphine-bupivacaine: assessment of consecutive treatments in advanced cancer pain. J Pain Symptom Manage 5(1): 18–26

Nitescu P, Sjoberg M, Appelgren L, Curelaru I 1995 Complications of intrathecal opioids and bupivacaine in the treatment of 'refractory' cancer pain. Clin J Pain 11(1): 45–62

Nolan MF, Wilson MC 1995 Patient-controlled analgesia: a method for the controlled self-administration of opioid pain medications. Physical Therapy 75(5): 374–379

Obbens EA, Hill CS, Leavens ME, Ruthenbeck SS, Otis F 1987 Intraventricular morphine administration for control of chronic cancer pain. Pain 28(1): 61–68

Oliver DJ 1985 The use of methotrimeprazine in terminal care. Br J Clin Pract 39(9): 339–340

Osborne RJ, Joel SP, Slevin ML 1986 Morphine intoxication in renal failure: the role of morphine-6- glucuronide. Br Med J (Clin Res Ed) 292(6535): 1548–1549

Oskarsson P, Ljunggren JG, Lins PE 1997 Efficacy and safety of mexiletine in the treatment of painful diabetic neuropathy. The Mexiletine Study Group. Diabetes Care 20(10): 1594–1597

Owen MD, Fibuch EE, McQuillan R, Millington WR 1997 Postoperative analgesia using a low-dose, oral-transdermal clonidine combination: lack of clinical efficacy. Journal of Clinical Anesthesia 9(1): 8–14

Paice JA 1988 The phenomenon of analgesic tolerance in cancer pain management. Oncol Nurs Forum 15(4): 455–460

Paix A, Coleman A, Lees J et al 1995 Subcutaneous fentanyl and sufentanil infusion substitution for morphine intolerance in cancer pain management. Pain 63(2): 263–269

Panerai AE, Monza G, Movilia P, Bianchi M, Francucci BM, Tiengo M 1990 A randomized, within-patient, cross-over, placebo-controlled trial on the efficacy and tolerability of the tricyclic antidepressants chlorimipramine and nortriptyline in central pain. Acta Neurol Scand 82(1): 34–38

Papo I, Luongo A 1976 High cervical commissural myelotomy in the treatment of pain. Journal of Neurology, Neurosurgery and Psychiatry 39(7): 705–710

Parker MC, Baines MJ 1996 Intestinal obstruction in patients with advanced malignant disease. British Journal of Surgery 83(1): 1–2

Patt RB, Jain S 1990 Management of a patient with osteoradionecrosis of the mandible with nerve blocks. J Pain Sympt Manage 5: 59

Patt RB, Proper G, Reddy S 1994 The neuroleptics as adjuvant analgesics. J Pain Symptom Manage 9(7):.446–453

Patt YZ, Peters RE, Chuang VP, Wallace S, Claghorn L, Mavligit G 1985 Palliation of pelvic recurrence of colorectal cancer with intra- arterial 5-fluorouracil and mitomycin. Cancer 56(9): 2175–2180

Patt RB, Reddy S 1994 Spinal neurolysis for cancer pain: indications and recent results. Ann Acad Med Singapore 23(2): 216–220

Patwardhan RV, Johnson RF, Hoyumpa A Jr et al 1981 Normal metabolism of morphine in cirrhosis. Gastroenterology 81(6): 1006–1011

Paulson DF 1978 Oxybutynin chloride in control of post-trasurethral vesical pain and spasm. Urology 11(3): 237–238

Pelger RC, Hamdy NA, Zwinderman AH, Lycklama a Nijeholt AA, Papapoulos SE 1998 Effects of the bisphosphonate olpadronate in patients with carcinoma of the prostate metastatic to the skeleton [in process citation]. Bone 22(4): 403–408

Penn RD, Paice JA, Kroin JS 1992 Octreotide: a potent new non-opiate analgesic for intrathecal infusion [see comments]. Pain 49(1): 13–19

Pereira J, Hanson J, Bruera E 1997 The frequency and clinical course of cognitive impairment in patients with terminal cancer. Cancer 79(4): 835–842

Petersen TK, Husted SE, Rybro L, Schurizek BA, Wernberg M 1982 Urinary retention during i.m. and extradural morphine analgesia. Br J Anaesth 54(11): 1175–1178

Pies R 1996 Psychotropic medications and the oncology patient. Cancer Pract 4(3): 164–166

Piletta P, Porchet HC, Dayer P 1991 Central analgesic effect of acetaminophen but not of aspirin. Clin Pharmacol Ther 49(4): 350–354

Plancarte R, Amescua C, Patt RB, Aldrete JA 1990 Superior hypogastric plexus block for pelvic cancer pain. Anesthesiology 73(2): 236–239

Plancarte R, Velazquez R, Patt RB 1993 Neurolytic block of the sympathetic axis. In: Patt RB (ed) Cancer pain. Lippincott, Philadelphia, pp 377–425

Plancarte R, De Leon-Casasola O A, El-Helaly M, Allende S, Lema MJ 1997 Neurolytic superior hypogastric plexus block for chronic pelvic pain associated with cancer. Reg Anesth 22(6): 562–568

Polatty RC, Cooper KR 1986 Respiratory failure after percutaneous cordotomy. South Med J 79(7): 897–899

Pond SM, Tong T, Benowitz NL, Jacob P 1980 Enhanced bioavailability of pethidine and pentazocine in patients with cirrhosis of the liver. Australia and New Zealand Journal of Medicine 10(5): 515–519

Popiela T, Lucchi R, Giongo F 1989 Methylprednisolone as palliative therapy for female terminal cancer patients. The Methylprednisolone Female Preterminal Cancer Study Group. European Journal of Cancer and Clinical Oncology 25(12): 1823–1829

Portenoy RK 1994a Management of common opioid side effects during long-term therapy of cancer pain. Ann Acad Med Singapore 23(2): 160–170

Portenoy RK 1994b Tolerance to opioid analgesics: clinical aspects. Cancer Survey 21: 49–65.

Portenoy RK, Hagen NA 1990 Breakthrough pain: definition, prevalence and characteristics. Pain 41(3): 273–281

Portenoy RK, Moulin DE, Rogers AG, Inturrisi CE, Foley KM 1986 Intravenous infusion of opioids in cancer-related pain: review of cases and guidelines for use. Adv Pain Res Ther 8(413): 413–424

Portenoy RK, Foley KM, Inturrisi CE 1990 The nature of opioid responsiveness and its implications for neuropathic pain: new hypotheses derived from studies of opioid infusions [see comments]. Pain 43(3): 273–286

Portenoy RK, Foley KM, Stulman J et al 1991 Plasma morphine and morphine-6-glucuronide during chronic morphine therapy for cancer pain: plasma profiles, steady-state concentrations and the consequences of renal failure. Pain 47(1): 13–19

Portenoy R K, Southam MA, Gupta SK et al 1993 Transdermal fentanyl for cancer pain. Repeated dose pharmacokinetics. Anesthesiology 78(1): 36–43

Porter AT, Ben-Josef E 1995 Strontium 89 in the treatment of bony metastases. Important Advances in Oncology: 87–94

Porter AT, McEwan AJ, Powe JE et al 1993 Results of a randomized phase-III trial to evaluate the efficacy of strontium-89 adjuvant to local field external beam irradiation in the management of endocrine resistant metastatic prostate cancer. Int J Radiat Oncol Biol Phys 25(5): 805–813

Porter J, Jick H 1980 Addiction rare in patients treated with narcotics. N Engl J Med 302(2): 123

Powsner RA, Zietman AL, Foss FM 1997 Bone marrow suppression after strontium-89 therapy and local radiation therapy in patients with diffuse marrow involvement. Clinical Nuclear Medicine 22(3): 147–150

Prasanna A, Murthy PS 1993 Sphenopalatine ganglion block and pain of cancer [letter]. J Pain Symptom Manage 8(3): 125

President's Commission for the Study of Ethical Problems in Medical and Biomedical and Behavioral Research 1983 Deciding to forgo life sustaining treatment: ethical and legal issues in treatment decisions. US Government Printing Office, Washington

Puccio M, Nathanson L 1997 The cancer cachexia syndrome. Semin Oncol 24(3): 277–287

Pud D, Eisenberg E, Spitzer A, Adler R, Fried G, Yarnitsky D 1998 The NMDA receptor antagonist amantadine reduces surgical neuropathic pain in cancer patients: a double blind, randomized, placebo controlled trial [in process citation]. Pain 75(2–3): 349–354

Purohit OP, Dickson I, Anthony C, Coleman R 1994 The effect of a single pamidronate (APD) infusion on metastatic bone pain, quality of life (QOL) and markers of bone resorption (meeting abstract). Proc Annu Meet Am Soc Clin Oncol 13

Queisser W 1984 Chemotherapy for the treatment of cancer pain. Recent Results in Cancer Research 89: 171–177

Racz GB, Sabonghy M, Gintautas J, Kline WM 1982 Intractable pain therapy using a new epidural catheter. JAMA 248(5): 579–581

Radbruch L, Grond S, Zech DJ, Bischoff A 1996 High-dose oral morphine in cancer pain management: a report of twelve cases. Journal of Clinical Anesthesia 8(2): 144–150

Raftery H 1979 The management of post herpetic pain using sodium valproate and amitriptyline. Irish Medical Journal 72(9): 399–401

Reddy S, Patt RB 1994 The benzodiazepines as adjuvant analgesics. J Pain Symptom Manage 9(8): 510–514

Resche I, Chatal JF, Pecking A et al 1997 A dose-controlled study of 153Sm-ethylenediaminetetramethylenephosphonate (EDTMP) in the treatment of patients with painful bone metastases. European Journal of Cancer 33(10): 1583–1591

Ripamonti C, Bruera E 1991 Rectal, buccal, and sublingual narcotics for the management of cancer pain. J Palliat Care 7(1): 30–35

Ripamonti C, Bruera E 1997 Current status of patient-controlled analgesia in cancer patients. Oncology (Huntingt) 11(3): 373–380, 383–384; discussion 384–386

Ripamonti C, Zecca E, Brunelli C et al 1995 Rectal methadone in cancer patients with pain. A preliminary clinical and pharmacokinetic study. Ann Oncol 6(8): 841–843

Ripamonti C, Zecca E, Bruera E 1997 An update on the clinical use of methadone for cancer pain. Pain 70(2–3): 109–115

Ripamonti C, De Conno F, Groff L et al 1998 Equianalgesic dose/ratio between methadone and other opioid agonists in cancer pain: comparison of two clinical experiences. Ann Oncol 9(1): 79–83

Rizzi R, Terrevoli A, Visentin M 1985 Long-term results of alcoholization and thermocoagulation of trigeminal nerve for cancer pain. The Pain Clinic I. In: Erdmann W, Oyama T, Pernak MJ (eds) Proceedings of the First International Symposium. Vnu Science Press, Utrecht, The Netherlands

Robertson AG, Reed NS, Ralston SH 1995 Effect of oral clodronate on metastatic bone pain: a double-blind, placebo-controlled study. J Clin Oncol 13(9): 2427–2430

Robertson DH 1983 Transsacral neurolytic nerve block. An alternative approach to intractable perineal pain. Br J Anaesth 55(9): 873–875

Robins G, Farr PM 1997 Pain relief with Emla of ulcerating lesions in mycosis fungoides [letter]. British Journal of Dermatology 136(2) p 287

Robinson RG, Preston DF, Schiefelbein M, Baxter KG 1995 Strontium 89 therapy for the palliation of pain due to osseous metastases. JAMA 274(5): 420–424

Rogers M, Cerda JJ 1989 The narcotic bowel syndrome. Journal of Clinical Gastroenterology 11(2): 132–135

Roquefeuil B, Benezech J, Blanchet P, Batier C, Frerebeau P, Gros C 1984 Intraventricular administration of morphine in patients with neoplastic intractable pain. Surgical Neurology 21(2): 155–158

Rosenberg JM, Harrell C, Ristic H, Werner RA, de Rosayro AM 1997 The effect of gabapentin on neuropathic pain. Clin J Pain 13(3): 251–255

Rosner H, Rubin L, Kestenbaum A 1996 Gabapentin adjunctive therapy in neuropathic pain states. Clin J Pain 12(1): 56–58

Ross GJ, Kessler HB, Clair MR, Gatenby RA, Hartz WH, Ross LV 1989 Sonographically guided paracentesis for palliation of symptomatic malignant ascites. American Journal of Roentgenology 153(6): 1309–1311

Roth A, Kolaric K 1986 Analgetic activity of calcitonin in patients with painful osteolytic metastases of breast cancer. Results of a controlled randomized study. Oncology 43(5): 283–287

Rothenberg ML 1996 New developments in chemotherapy for patients with advanced pancreatic cancer. Oncology (Huntingt) 10(9 suppl): 18–22

Rubens RD, Towlson KE, Ramirez AJ et al 1992 Appropriate chemotherapy for palliating advanced cancer. BMJ 304(6818): 35–40

Ruskin JN 1989 The cardiac arrhythmia suppression trial (CAST). N Engl J Med 321(6): 386–388

Sanders M, Zuurmond W 1995 Safety of unilateral and bilateral percutaneous cervical cordotomy in 80 terminally ill cancer patients. J Clin Oncol 13(6): 1509–1512

Sandyk R 1990 Neuroleptic-induced 'painful legs and moving toes' syndrome: successful treatment with clonazepam and baclofen. Italian Journal of Neurological Science 11(6): 573–576

Sapir R, Catane R, Cherny NI 1997 Cancer pain: knowledge and attitudes of physicians in Israel (meeting abstract). Proc Annu Meet Am Soc Clin Oncol 16

Saris SC, Silver JM, Vieira JF, Nashold BS Jr 1986 Sacrococcygeal rhizotomy for perineal pain. Neurosurgery 19(5): 789–793

Sawe J 1986 High-dose morphine and methadone in cancer patients. Clinical pharmacokinetic considerations of oral treatment. Clinical Pharmacokinetics 11(2): 87–106

Sawe J, Odar-Cederlof I 1987 Kinetics of morphine in patients with renal failure. Eur J Clin Pharmacol 32(4): 377–382

Sawe J, Dahlstrom B, Paalzow L, Rane A 1981 Morphine kinetics in cancer patients. Clin Pharmacol Ther 30(5): 629–635

Scanlon C, Fleming C 1989 Ethical issues in caring for the patient with advanced cancer. Nursing Clinics of North America 24(4): 977–986

Schiraldi GF, Soresi E, Locicero S, Harari S, Scoccia S 1987 Salmon calcitonin in cancer pain: comparison between two different treatment schedules. International Journal of Clinical Pharmacology, Therapy and Toxicology 25(4): 229–232

Schmeler K, Bastin K 1996 Strontium-89 for symptomatic metastatic prostate cancer to bone: recommendations for hospice patients. Hosp J 11(2): 1–10

Schug SA, Zech D, Dorr U 1990 Cancer pain management according to WHO analgesic guidelines. J Pain Symptom Manage 5(1): 27–32

Schug SA, Zech D, Grond S, Jung H, Meuser T, Stobbe B 1992 A long-term survey of morphine in cancer pain patients. J Pain Symptom Manage 7(5): 259–266

Schwartz JA, Koenigsberg MD 1987 Naloxone-induced pulmonary edema. Ann Emerg Med 16(11): 1294–1296

Scott NB, Mogensen T, Bigler D, Kehlet H 1989 Comparison of the effects of continuous intrapleural vs epidural administration of 0.5% bupivacaine on pain, metabolic response and pulmonary function following cholecystectomy. Acta Anaesthesiol Scand 33(7): 535–539

Selman AJ, Friedman J, Chambers R 1967 Carbamazepine in the treatment of trigeminal neuralgia. Journal of the American of Dental Association 74(6): 1220–1223

Shapshay SM, Scott RM, McCann CF, Stoelting I 1980 Pain control in advanced and recurrent head and neck cancer. Otolaryngology Clinics of North America 13(3): 551–560

Sharma SK, Gajraj NM, Sidawi JE, Lowe K 1996 EMLA cream effectively reduces the pain of spinal needle insertion. Reg Anesth 21(6): 561–564

Shegda LM, McCorkle R 1990 Continuing care in the community. J Pain Symptom Manage 5(5): 279–286

Sherman DM, Weichselbaum R, Order SE, Cloud L, Trey C, Piro AJ 1978 Palliation of hepatic metastasis. Cancer 41(5): 2013–2017

Silberstein EB, Elgazzar AH, Kapilivsky A 1992 Phosphorus-32 radiopharmaceuticals for the treatment of painful osseous metastases. Seminars in Nuclear Medicine 22(1): 17–27

Simmonds MA 1997 Oral transmucosal fentanyl citrate produces pain relief faster than medication typically used for breakthrough pain in cancer patients (meeting abstract). Proc Annu Meet Am Soc Clin Oncol. 16, p A180

Sindrup SH, Gram LF, Brosen K, Eshoj O, Mogensen EF 1990 The selective serotonin reuptake inhibitor paroxetine is effective in the treatment of diabetic neuropathy symptoms. Pain 42(2): 135–144

Sindrup SH, Grodum E, Gram LF, Beck-Nielsen H 1991 Concentration-response relationship in paroxetine treatment of diabetic neuropathy symptoms: a patient-blinded dose-escalation study. Therapeutic Drug Monitoring 13(5): 408–414

Sjoberg M, Nitescu P, Appelgren L, Curelaru I 1994 Long-term intrathecal morphine and bupivacaine in patients with refractory cancer pain. Results from a morphine: bupivacaine dose regimen of 0.5:4.75 mg/ml. Anesthesiology 80(2):284–297

Sjogren P, Banning A 1989 Pain, sedation and reaction time during long-term treatment of cancer patients with oral and epidural opioids. Pain 39(1):5–11

Smirne S, Scarlato G 1977 Clonazepam in cranial neuralgias. Med J Aust 1(4): 93–94

Smith JA Jr 1989 Palliation of painful bone metastases from prostate cancer using sodium etidronate: results of a randomized, prospective, double-blind, placebo-controlled study. J Urol 141(1): 85–87

Sneed PK, Larson DA, Wara W M 1996 Radiotherapy for cerebral metastases. Neurosurgery Clinics of North America 7(3): 505–515

Sorensen S, Helweg-Larsen S, Mouridsen H, Hansen HH 1994 Effect of high-dose dexamethasone in carcinomatous metastatic spinal cord compression treated with radiotherapy: a randomised trial. European Journal of Cancer 30A(1): 22–27

Spiegel D, Moore R 1997 Imagery and hypnosis in the treatment of cancer patients. Oncology (Huntingt) 11(8): 1179–1189; discussion 1189–1195

Sporer KA 1995 The serotonin syndrome. Implicated drugs, pathophysiology and management. Drug Safety 13(2): 94–104

Spross JA, McGuire DB, Schmitt RM 1990a Oncology Nursing Society position paper on cancer pain. Part I. Oncol Nurs Forum 17(4): 595–614

Spross JA, McGuire DB, Schmitt RM 1990b Oncology Nursing Society position paper on cancer pain. Part II. Oncol Nurs Forum 17(5): 751–760

Stambaugh JE Jr, Lane C 1983 Analgesic efficacy and pharmacokinetic evaluation of meperidine and hydroxyzine, alone and in combination. Cancer Invest 1(2): 111–117

Stegman MB, Stoukides CA 1996 Resolution of tumor pain with EMLA cream. Pharmacotherapy 16(4): 694–697

Stjernsward J, Colleau SM, Ventafridda V 1996 The World Health Organization Cancer Pain and Palliative Care Program. Past, present, and future. J Pain Symptom Manage 12(2): 65–72

Stock SL, Catalano G, Catalano MC 1996 Meperidine associated mental status changes in a patient with chronic renal failure. Journal of the Florida Medical Association 83(5): 315–319

Storey P, Hill HH Jr, St Louis RH, Tarver EE 1990 Subcutaneous infusions for control of cancer symptoms. J Pain Symptom Manage 5(1): 33–41

Strang P 1996 Analgesic effect of bisphosphonates on bone pain in breast cancer patients: a review article. Acta Oncologica 5(50): 50–54

Stuart G, Cramond T 1993 Role of percutaneous cervical cordotomy for pain of malignant origin. Med J Aust 158(10): 667–670

Su CF, Liu MY, Lin MT 1987 Intraventricular morphine produces pain relief, hypothermia, hyperglycaemia and increased prolactin and growth hormone levels in patients with cancer pain. J Neurol 235(2): 105–108

Sucher E, Margulies JY, Floman Y, Robin GC 1994 Prognostic factors in anterior decompression for metastatic cord compression. An analysis of results. European Spine Journal 3(2): 70–75

Swain R 1987 Oral clonidine for proctalgia fugax. Gut 28(8): 1039–1040

Sweet WH 1976 Controlled thermocoagulation of trigeminal ganglion and rootlets for differential destruction of pain fibers: facial pain other than trigeminal neuralgia. Clinical Neurosurgery 23: 96–102

Sweet WH, Poletti CE, Macon JB 1981 Treatment of trigeminal neuralgia and other facial pains by retrogasserian injection of glycerol. Neurosurgery 9(6): 647–653

Swerdlow M 1978 Intrathecal neurolysis. Anaesthesia 33(8): 733–740

Swerdlow M 1985 The use of anticonvulsants in the management of cancer pain. The Pain Clinic I. In: Erdmann W, Oyama T, Pernak MJ (eds) Proceedings of the First International Symposium. Vnu Science Press, Utrecht, The Netherlands

Sykes J, Johnson R, Hanks GW 1997 ABC of palliative care. Difficult pain problems. BMJ 315(7112): 867–869

Sykes NP 1991 Oral naloxone in opioid-associated constipation. Lancet 337(8755): 1475

Sykes NP 1996 An investigation of the ability of oral naloxone to correct opioid-related constipation in patients with advanced cancer. Palliat Med 10(2): 135–144

Symreng T, Gomez MN, Rossi N 1989 Intrapleural bupivacaine v saline after thoracotomy – effects on pain and lung function – a double-blind study [see comments]. J Cardiothoracic Anesthesia 3(2): 144–149

Szeto HH, Inturrisi CE, Houde R, Saal S, Cheigh J, Reidenberg MM 1977 Accumulation of normeperidine, an active metabolite of meperidine, in patients with renal failure of cancer. Ann Intern Med 86(6): 738–741

Taddio A, Ohlsson A, Einarson TR, Stevens B, Koren G 1998 A systematic review of lidocaine-prilocaine cream (EMLA) in the treatment of acute pain in neonates. Pediatrics 101(2): 1

Takeda F 1985 Japanese field-testing of WHO guidelines. PRN Forum 4(3): 4–5

Tannock I, Gospodarowicz M, Meakin W, Panzarella T, Stewart L, Rider W 1989 Treatment of metastatic prostatic cancer with low-dose prednisone: evaluation of pain and quality of life as pragmatic indices of response. J Clin Oncol 7(5): 590–597

Tarn TS, Lee TS 1994 Surgical treatment of metastatic tumors of the long bones. Chung Hua I Hsueh Tsa Chih (Taipei) 54(3): 170–175

Thatcher N, Anderson H, Betticher DC, Ranson M 1995 Symptomatic benefit from gemcitabine and other chemotherapy in advanced non-small cell lung cancer: changes in performance status and tumour-related symptoms. Anticancer Drugs 6(suppl 6): 39–48

Thomas Z, Bruera E 1995 Use of methadone in a highly tolerant patient receiving parenteral hydromorphone. J Pain Symptom Manage 10(4): 315–317

Thorsen AB, Yung NS, Leung AC 1994 Administration of drugs by infusion pumps in palliative medicine. Ann Acad Med Singapore 23(2): 209–211

Tobias JD 1997 Propofol sedation for terminal care in a pediatric patient. Clinical Pediatrics (Philadelphia) 36(5): 291–293

Truog RD, Berde CB, Mitchell C, Grier HE 1992 Barbiturates in the care of the terminally ill. N Engl J Med 327(23): 1678–1682

Turek-Maischeider M, Kazem I 1975 Palliative irradiation for liver metastases. Jama 232(6): 625–628

Turk DC, Feldman CS 1992 Noninvasive approaches to pain control in terminal illness: the contribution of psychological variables. Hosp J 8(1–2): 1–23

Turner JH, Martindale AA, Sorby P et al 1989 Samarium-153 EDTMP therapy of disseminated skeletal metastasis. Eur J Nucl Med 15(12): 784–795

Twycross RG 1988 The therapeutic equivalence of oral and subcutaneous/intramuscular morphine sulphate in cancer patients. J Palliat Care 4(1–2): 67–68

Twycross RG 1994 The risks and benefits of corticosteroids in advanced cancer. Drug Saf 11(3): 163–178

Twycross RG, Guppy D 1985 Prednisolone in terminal breast and bronchogenic cancer. Practitioner 229(1399): 57–59

Umans JG, Inturrisi CE 1982 Antinociceptive activity and toxicity of meperidine and normeperidine in mice. Journal of Pharmacology and Experimental Therapeutics 223(1): 203–206

Urquhart ML, Klapp K, White PF 1988 Patient-controlled analgesia: a comparison of intravenous versus subcutaneous hydromorphone. Anesthesiology 69(3): 428–432

Vainio A, Ollila J, Matikainen E, Rosenberg P, Kalso E 1995 Driving ability in cancer patients receiving long-term morphine analgesia. Lancet 346(8976): 667–670

Van Holten-Verzantvoort AT, Zwinderman AH, Aaronson NK et al 1991 The effect of supportive pamidronate treatment on aspects of quality of life of patients with advanced breast cancer. Eur J Cancer 27(5): 544–549

Vane JR 1971 Inhibition of prostaglandin synthesis as a mechanism of action for aspirin-like drugs. Nature and New Biology 231(25): 232–235

Vane JR, Botting RM 1997 Mechanism of action of aspirin-like drugs. Seminars in Arthritis and Rheumatism 26(6 suppl 1): 2–10

Varvel JR, Shafer SL, Hwang SS, Coen PA, Stanski DR 1989 Absorption characteristics of transdermally administered fentanyl. Anesthesiology 70(6): 928–934

Vecht CJ, Haaxma-Reiche H, Van Putten WL, De Visser M, Vries EP, Twijnstra A 1989 Initial bolus of conventional versus high-dose dexamethasone in metastatic spinal cord compression. Neurology 39(9): 1255–1257

Velikova G, Selby PJ, Snaith PR, Kirby PG 1995 The relationship of cancer pain to anxiety. Psychotherapy and Psychosomatics 63(3–4): 181–184

Ventafridda V 1989 Continuing care: a major issue in cancer pain management. Pain 36(2): 137–143

Ventafridda V, Tamburini M, Caraceni A, De Conno F, Naldi F 1987 A validation study of the WHO method for cancer pain relief. Cancer 59(4): 850–856

Ventafridda V, Caraceni A, Saita L et al 1988 Trazodone for deafferentation pain. Comparison with amitriptyline. Psychopharmacology (Berl) 95(suppl): S44–49

Ventafridda V, Ripamonti C, Caraceni A, Spoldi E, Messina L, De Conno F 1990a The management of inoperable gastrointestinal obstruction in terminal cancer patients. Tumori 76(4): 389–393

Ventafridda V, Ripamonti C, De Conno F, Tamburini M, Cassileth BR 1990b Symptom prevalence and control during cancer patients' last days of life. J Palliat Care 6(3): 7–11

Vermeulen SS 1998 Whole brain radiotherapy in the treatment of metastatic brain tumors. Seminars in Surgical Oncology 14(1): 64–69

Vigano A, Fan D, Bruera E 1996 Individualized use of methadone and opioid rotation in the comprehensive management of cancer pain associated with poor prognostic indicators. Pain 67(1): 115–119

Von Roenn JH, Cleeland CS, Gonin R, Hatfield AK, Pandya KJ 1993 Physician attitudes and practice in cancer pain management. A survey from the Eastern Cooperative Oncology Group. Ann Intern Med 119(2): 121–126

Waldman SD, Allen ML, Cronen MC 1989 Subcutaneous tunneled intrapleural catheters in the long-term relief of right upper quadrant pain of malignant origin. J Pain Symptom Manage 4(2): 86–89

Walker VA, Hoskin PJ, Hanks GW, White ID 1988 Evaluation of WHO analgesic guidelines for cancer pain in a hospital-based palliative care unit. J Pain Symptom Manage 3(3): 145–149

Walsh TD 1990 Prevention of opioid side effects. J Pain Symptom Manage 5(6): 362–367

Wanzer SH, Federman DD, Adelstein SJ et al 1989 The physician's responsibility toward hopelessly ill patients. A second look. N Engl J Med 320(13): 844–849

Ward SE, Goldberg N, Miller-McCauley V et al 1993 Patient-related barriers to management of cancer pain. Pain 52(3): 319–324

Ward SE, Berry PE, Misiewicz H 1996 Concerns about analgesics among patients and family caregivers in a hospice setting. Research in Nursing and Health 19(3): 205–211

Warfield CA 1989 Evaluation of dosing guidelines for the use of oral controlled-release morphine (MS Contin tablets). Cancer 63(11 suppl): 2360–2364

Watanabe S, Bruera E 1994 Corticosteroids as adjuvant analgesics. J Pain Symptom Manage 9(7): 442–445

Watson CP 1994 Topical capsaicin as an adjuvant analgesic. J Pain Symptom Manage 9(7): 425–433

Watson CP, Evans RJ 1985 A comparative trial of amitriptyline and zimelidine in post-herpetic neuralgia. Pain 23(4): 387–394

Watson CP, Chipman M, Reed K, Evans RJ, Birkett N 1992 Amitriptyline versus maprotiline in postherpetic neuralgia: a randomized, double-blind, crossover trial. Pain 48(1): 29–36

Watson CP, Tyler KL, Bickers DR, Millikan LE, Smith S, Coleman E 1993 A randomized vehicle-controlled trial of topical capsaicin in the treatment of postherpetic neuralgia. Clin Ther 15(3): 510–526

Weigl K, Mundinger F, Chrubasik J 1987 Continuous intraventricular morphine- or peptide-infusion for intractable cancer pain. Acta Neurochir Suppl (Wien) 39: 163–165

Weinberg DS, Inturrisi CE, Reidenberg B et al 1988 Sublingual absorption of selected opioid analgesics. Clin Pharmacol Ther 44(3): 335–342

Weissman DE, Haddox JD 1989 Opioid pseudoaddiction – an iatrogenic syndrome. Pain 36(3): 363–366

Wells CJ, Lipton S, Lahuerta J 1984 Respiratory depression after percutaneous cervical anterolateral cordotomy in patients on slow-release oral morphine [letter]. Lancet 1(8379): 739

Wemm K Jr, Saberski L 1995 Modified approach to block the ganglion impar (ganglion of Walther) [letter]. Reg Anesth 20(6): 544–545

Wetzel CH, Connelly JF 1997 Use of gabapentin in pain management. Annals of Pharmacotherapy 31(9): 1082–1083

Williams FH, Maly BJ 1994 Pain rehabilitation. 3. Cancer pain, pelvic pain, and age-related considerations. Arch Phys Med Rehabil 75(5 Spec No): S15–20

Willox JC, Corr J, Shaw J, Richardson M, Calman KC, Drennan M 1984 Prednisolone as an appetite stimulant in patients with cancer. Br Med J (Clin Res Ed) 288(6410): 27

Wilwerding MB, Loprinzi CL, Mailliard JA et al 1995 A randomized, crossover evaluation of methylphenidate in cancer patients receiving strong narcotics. Supportive Care in Cancer 3(2): 135–138

Wolff T, Samuelsson H, Hedner T 1996 Concentrations of morphine and morphine metabolites in CSF and plasma during continuous subcutaneous morphine administration in cancer pain patients. Pain 68(2–3): 209–216

Wong ET, Gunes S, Gaughan E et al 1997a Palliation of intractable cancer pain by MRI-guided cingulotomy. Clin J Pain 13(3): 260–263

Wong GY, Brown DL 1995 Transient paraplegia following alcohol celiac plexus block. Reg Anesth 20(4): 352–355

Wong JO, Chiu GL, Tsao CJ, Chang CL 1997b Comparison of oral controlled-release morphine with transdermal fentanyl in terminal cancer pain. Acta Anaesthesiol Sin 35(1): 25–32

World Health Organization 1986 Cancer pain relief. World Health Organization, Geneva

World Health Organization 1990 Cancer pain relief and palliative care. World Health Organization, Geneva

World Health Organization 1996 Cancer pain relief, 2nd edn. World Health Organization, Geneva

Wright JM, Oki JC, Graves L 3rd 1997 Mexiletine in the symptomatic treatment of diabetic peripheral neuropathy. Ann Pharmacother 31(1): 29–34

Yaksh TL 1996 Epidural ketamine: a useful, mechanistically novel adjuvant for epidural morphine? Reg Anesth 21(6): 508–513

Yamada K, Ushio Y, Hayakawa T, Arita N, Yamada N, Mogami H 1983 Effects of methylprednisolone on peritumoral brain edema. A quantitative autoradiographic study. J Neurosurg 59(4): 612–619

Yang CY, Wong CS, Chang JY, Ho ST 1996 Intrathecal ketamine reduces morphine requirements in patients with terminal cancer pain. Can J Anaesth 43(4): 379–383

Yeo W, Lam KK, Chan AT, Leung TW, Nip SY, Johnson PJ 1997 Transdermal fentanyl for severe cancer-related pain. Palliat Med 11(3): 233–239

Yuan CS, Foss JF, Osinski J, Toledano A, Roizen MF, Moss J 1997 The safety and efficacy of oral methylnaltrexone in preventing morphine-induced delay in oral-cecal transit time. Clin Pharmacol Ther 61(4): 467–475

Zeigler D, Lynch SA, Muir J, Benjamin J, Max MB 1992 Transdermal clonidine versus placebo in painful diabetic neuropathy. Pain 48(3): 403–408

Zenz M, Donner B, Strumpf M 1994 Withdrawal symptoms during therapy with transdermal

Zenz M, Zenz T, Tryba M, Strumpf M 1995 Severe undertreatment of cancer pain: a 3 – year survey of the German situation. J Pain Symptom Manage 10(3): 187–191

Peripheral neuropathic pain: an approach to management

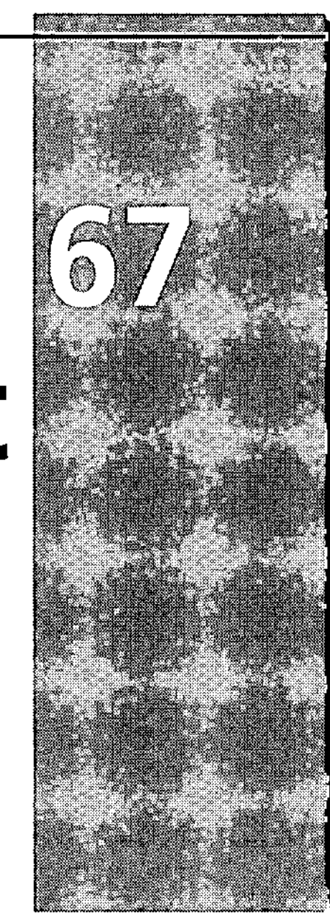

HOWARD L. FIELDS, RALF BARON & MICHAEL C. ROWBOTHAM

SUMMARY

Most peripheral nerve disease is associated with a loss of function, either sensory, motor, or both, and is typically non-painful. Pain, however, is characteristic of some neuropathic diseases (e.g., diabetic and alcohol-deficiency neuropathies and herpes zoster). The majority of patients with painful peripheral nerve disease fall into two broad classes: focal and multifocal (e.g., traumatic, ischaemic, inflammatory) or generalized (e.g., toxic/metabolic, hereditary, or inflammatory). Our knowledge about the pathophysiology of human neuropathic pain is growing and animal models of focal traumatic neuropathies have contributed significantly to this growth. Although these advances have provided clues about potentially useful therapeutic approaches, treatment remains largely empirical. This chapter outlines a systematic approach to management that is based on emerging knowledge of the pathophysiology of neuropathic pain and of treatment efficacy based on data from controlled clinical trials.

INTRODUCTION

Pain associated with peripheral nerve injury has several clinical characteristics. If a mixed nerve with a cutaneous branch is involved, there is almost always an area of abnormal sensation and the patient's maximum pain is coextensive with or within an area of sensory deficit. This is a key diagnostic feature for neuropathic pain. The sensory deficit is usually to noxious and thermal stimuli, indicating damage to small-diameter afferent fibres. Many patients with peripheral neuropathic pain have a hyperpathic state which is characterized by two sensory abnormalities. The first feature is allodynia, characterized by hypersensitivity to gentle mechanical stimuli such that even slight bending of hairs may evoke severe pain. The other feature is summation, which is the progressive worsening of pain evoked by slow repetitive stimulation with mildly noxious stimuli, for example pin prick. A small percentage of patients with peripheral nerve injury have a nearly pure hyperpathic syndrome in which no sensory deficit is demonstrable. The quality of the reported sensation may also be a clue; neuropathic pain commonly has a burning and/or shooting quality with unusual tingling, crawling or electrical sensations (dysaesthesiae). Although these characteristics are neither universally present in, nor absolutely diagnostic of, neuropathic pain, when they are present, the diagnosis of neuropathic pain is likely.

MECHANISMS WHICH MAY CONTRIBUTE TO NEUROPATHIC PAIN

PERIPHERAL MECHANISMS

Sensitization and ectopic impulse generation in primary afferent nociceptors

Research in this area began with studies of experimental neuromas. When the sciatic nerve is cut and allowed to regenerate and form a neuroma, spontaneous activity and exquisite mechanical sensitivity develops in the afferent axons innervating the neuroma (Wall 1974, Scadding 1981). Some of these primary afferents are of small diameter (Aδ and C fibres), contain substance P (Fried et al 1989) and thus may have originally been nociceptors (Welk et al 1990). Similarly, within hours of damaging the small-diameter nociceptive axons innervating the cornea, these axons become spontaneously active (Tanelian & MacIver 1991). Primary afferent axons need not be transected to become hyperactive. Some small-diameter fibres traversing a region of moderate constriction become spontaneously active (Kajander & Bennett 1992, Bennett 1993). Furthermore, ectopic impulses may be generated at sites other than the damaged and regenerating distal axon terminals. For example, when a peripheral nerve is damaged, a region near the dorsal root ganglion (which is distant from the site of injury) becomes capable of generating 'spontaneous' impulses (Devor & Rappaport 1990, Kajander et al 1992). In addition, small patches of demyelination on, for example, the axon of an Aδ nociceptor, can become a source of ectopic impulses.

That intact but hyperactive nociceptors can generate a pain signal is supported by studies of patients with postherpetic neuralgia (PHN). In some PHN patients pain relief can be produced by cooling the skin, topically applying local anaesthetics or cyclo-oxygenase inhibitors (De Benedittis & Lorenzetti 1996, Rowbotham et al 1996), or inactivating C nociceptors by repeated application of capsaicin (Watson et al 1993). These observations indicate that sensitized C fibres are generating an on-going discharge that contributes to neuropathic pain.

Sympathetically maintained pain

Causalgia is the classic example of a sympathetically maintained pain associated with nerve injury. It is characterized by a distal burning sensation which is exacerbated by cold, loud noises and gentle mechanical stimulation (Mitchell 1865). Early in the course of the disease, most patients obtain virtually complete relief with sympathetic blocks (Richards 1967).

Animal studies have confirmed that damaged primary afferent fibres acquire adrenergic sensitivity (Jänig et al 1996). After *complete transection* of a nerve, surviving afferents develop noradrenergic sensitivity, i.e. the neurons express functional adrenoceptors at their plasma membrane. Myelinated and unmyelinated afferents innervating the stump neuroma can be excited by adrenaline or by stimulation of sympathetic efferents that have regenerated into the neuroma (Wall 1974, Devor & Jänig 1981, Korenman & Devor 1981, Scadding 1981, Blumberg & Jänig 1984). Electrical stimulation of the sympathetic trunk can activate C nociceptors that have regenerated following injury (Häbler et al 1987). After *partial* nerve injury electrical stimulation of the sympathetic trunk and intra-arterial injections of noradrenaline can activate or sensitize intact C nociceptors in the partially injured nerve (Sato & Perl 1991). This finding was proposed to result from an upregulation of functional α_2 adrenoceptors in intact primary afferent nociceptors (Bossut & Shea 1996). Consistent with this idea, surgical sympathectomy, systemic phentolamine and systemic guanethidine can alleviate rodent pain behaviours that develop after partial nerve injury (Shir & Seltzer 1991, Kim et al 1993).

These animal studies are supported by human research demonstrating that adrenaline applied directly to a neuroma produces severe burning pain (Chabal et al 1992b). Furthermore, intraoperative stimulation of the sympathetic chain increases spontaneous pain in patients with causalgia (Walker & Nulsen 1948). In post-traumatic neuralgias, intracutaneous application of noradrenaline into a symptomatic area rekindles spontaneous pain and mechanical hyperalgesia after they are relieved by sympathetic blockade (Torebjörk et al 1995). Thus, damage to a peripheral nerve seems to induce in primary afferent nociceptors a novel state of sensitivity to sympathetic activity and noradrenaline.

Inflammation of the nerve trunk

The connective tissue sheath surrounding a peripheral nerve is innervated, presumably by nociceptive primary afferents. These nervi nervorum may enter the nerve trunk with the neurovascular bundle (Hromada 1963). There is now direct evidence that some of these nervi nervorum are primary afferent nociceptors (Bahns et al 1986, Bove & Light 1995). Because of these nervi nervorum, peripheral nerve can be a source of pain in a manner similar to joints, muscles and ligamentous structures, especially in those conditions with an inflammatory component. The fact that certain diseases are associated with localized pain and tenderness along the trunk of the nerve, rather than pain referred to its innervation territory, provides strong support for a role of epineurial and perineurial nervi nervorum in neuropathic pain. The acute pain of a herniated inflamed disc, or that seen with brachial neuritis or acute inflammatory demyelinating neuropathy (Guillain–Barré syndrome), are probably mediated by the physiological activation of the nervi nervorum (Asbury & Fields 1984).

In experimental animals activation of macrophages and a proliferation of endoneurial blood vessels have been demonstrated in injured peripheral nerve (Sommer & Myers 1996) and in the dorsal root ganglia after nerve transection (Lu & Richardson 1993). The cytokine tumour necrosis factor alpha (TNFα) produced by activated macrophages is a potential cause of pain as well as mechanical and thermal hyperalgesia (Sommer et al 1998, Wagner et al 1998) by inducing ectopic activity in primary afferent nociceptors (Sorkin et al 1997). Consistent with this view, the TNFα inhibitor thalidomide is reported to reduce pain in inflammatory lepromatous neuropathy (Belda et al 1966, Barnes et al 1992, Partida-Sanchez et al 1998).

CENTRAL MECHANISMS

Central sensitization

Prolonged or repeated activation of nociceptive C fibres produces central sensitization so that noxious stimuli produce more intense pain (hyperalgesia) and innocuous stimuli produce pain (allodynia). Central sensitization occurs in any situation with prolonged or intense C-fibre input. Although this mechanism contributes to non-neuropathic pain (see Ch. 6), in neuropathic pains like postherpetic neuralgia, where there is ongoing C-fibre activity, central sensitization seems to play a significant role in maintaining pain. Furthermore, with central sensitization, activity in large-diameter, low-threshold Aβ mechanoceptors becomes capable of generating pain. Such pain is most easily elicited by light, moving mechanical stimuli (dynamic mechanical hyperalgesia, allodynia (Koltzenburg et al 1992)). Both substance P and glutamate acting at the *N*-methyl-D-aspartate (NMDA) receptor contribute to central sensitization and are thus potential therapeutic targets in some patients with neuropathic pain (Dougherty et al 1994, Dickenson et al 1997).

Deafferentation hyperactivity

Deafferentation produces hyperactivity in dorsal horn cells. Following dorsal rhizotomy or peripheral nerve damage, many dorsal horn cells begin to fire spontaneously at high frequencies (Lombard & Larabi 1983, Laird & Bennett 1993). Such a mechanism may underlie the pain that occurs following extensive denervating injuries. For example, pain is a characteristic sequela of the deafferentation produced by brachial plexus avulsion (Wynn-Parry 1980) and this pain seems to respond to surgical procedures which destroy nociceptive dorsal horn neurons (Nashold & Ostdahl 1979).

Reorganization of the central connections of primary afferents

In models of peripheral nerve injury, loss of the central terminals of unmyelinated primary afferents deprives pain transmission neurons in the superficial dorsal horn of their normal nociceptive input. Under these conditions, large-diameter Aβ-mechanoreceptor primary afferents, which respond maximally to gentle mechanical stimulation, sprout to directly innervate the deafferented nociceptive dorsal horn neurons (Shortland & Woolf 1993). Although it is difficult to prove that this is a mechanism of pain in any clinical situation, some patients with postherpetic neuralgia have exquisite allodynia in a region of skin that shows a profound deficit of nociceptive C-fibre function (Baron & Saguer 1993). This is a situation which could occur in cases of PHN with relative sparing of Aβ primary afferents.

Loss of large-fibre afferent inhibition

The clinical paradox that injury to peripheral nerves often produces an association of increased pain with loss of sensory function was cited by Melzack and Wall, (1965) as a major impetus to their Gate Control hypothesis which presented a detailed explanation for neuropathic pain. Because selective blockade of large-diameter myelinated sensory axons increases pain, they proposed that these large-diameter fibres normally inhibit pain-transmitting spinal-cord neurons. They further proposed that the pain of nerve injury is due to selective damage to these pain-inhibiting large-diameter myelinated sensory axons. The Gate Control hypothesis predicts that selective activation of large-diameter, non-nociceptive myelinated primary afferents, for example by electrical stimulation of a peripheral nerve, would decrease pain. In fact, there are cases of dramatic pain relief produced by transcutaneous electrical nerve stimulation (TENS) in patients with painful traumatic mononeuropathies (Meyer & Fields 1972). Furthermore, there are reports that dorsal column stimulation, which would selectively activate the central branches of large-diameter primary afferents, is effective for some patients with neuropathic pain (Broggi et al 1994, Kumar et al 1996). It is also of interest that the presence of a generalized large-fibre peripheral neuropathy is a risk factor for developing postherpetic neuralgia following acute herpes zoster (Baron et al 1997). Thus it seems likely that release of dorsal horn pain transmission cells from inhibition by myelinated axons does contribute to the pain which occurs in some cases of peripheral nerve injury.

THE TREATMENT OF NEUROPATHIC PAIN

Except for trigeminal neuralgia, which responds reliably and specifically to anticonvulsant medications, the treatment of neuropathic pain is largely empirical and often unsatisfactory. Fortunately, data from clinical trials has led to improvements in the medical management of neuropathic pain (Kingery 1997).

Non-steroidal anti-inflammatory drugs

Non-steroidal anti-inflammatory drugs (NSAIDs) irreversibly inhibit cyclooxygenase and reduce production of algesic and proinflammatory arachidonic acid metabolites. There is good evidence that NSAIDs can relieve inflammatory or cancer pain, but they are generally ineffective in neuropathic pain (Max et al 1988a). While an early trial of these compounds, notably diclofenac, indomethacin or ibuprofen, may be warranted, even in responders relief is usually modest at best (Cohen & Harris 1987). If the therapy is not effective after individual titration to anti-inflammatory dosage, it should be discontinued. Potential serious side effects, notably gastrointestinal ulceration or renal failure, are significant limitations.

Antidepressants

Tricyclic antidepressants (TCAs) are well established as broad-spectrum analgesic drugs and they have been used for the treatment of a variety of painful conditions, including cancer pain, low back pain, different types of headache, and for chronic pain patients who have an affective disorder. Tricyclics are currently the best documented therapy for neuropathic pain (Onghena & Van Houdenhove 1992, McQuay et al 1996, Kingery 1997). These compounds are inhibitors of the re-uptake of monoaminergic transmitters. They are believed to potentiate the effects of biogenic amines in CNS pain modulating pathways. Of the TCAs, amitriptyline is currently the most widely prescribed for the treatment of chronic pain. There is extensive evidence that amitriptyline produces pain relief in diabetic neuropathy and postherpetic neuralgia (Max et al 1987, 1988b, 1992). All components of neuropathic pain such as stimulus-independent continuous burning or shooting pain as well as stimulus-induced allodynia may be improved. The mean dose required for pain reduction (75–150 mg/day) is usually smaller than doses necessary to achieve antidepressant effects. Onset of the analgesic effect occurs once an adequate dose is achieved. Improvement of sleep, mood and anxiety are an added benefit of antidepressant therapy.

Amitriptyline and other TCAs have significant side effects (Richelson 1990). They can produce orthostatic hypotension, due largely to an α-adrenergic blocking action. Because of its histamine receptor blockade, amitriptyline is also a potent sedating drug, which can be a desirable action if patients are having difficulty sleeping. Other significant problems include urinary retention, memory loss and cardiac conduction abnormalities (largely due to the muscarinic anticholinergic actions of the drug). Patients, especially the elderly, who are to be treated with this drug should be started at a very low dose, even as low as 10 mg, and built up slowly by about 25 mg every fourth day until the empirically determined therapeutic range is reached.

Desipramine and nortriptyline, both of which have predominant norepinephrine reuptake blocking action, appear to be as effective as amitriptyline in postherpetic neuralgia and painful diabetic neuropathy (Kishore-Kumar et al 1990, Max et al 1992, Watson et al 1992). Patients respond to desipramine and nortriptyline at doses comparable to those of amitriptyline but with fewer anticholinergic side effects and significantly less sedation.

All patients undergoing treatment with any TCA should have a cardiogram at the onset of treatment. Cardiac conduction defects are a contraindication to their use. Blood levels and repeated cardiograms should be taken if the dose is pushed above 100 mg/24 h, especially in elderly or cognitively impaired patients. It may be that the effectiveness of TCAs in neuropathic pain has to do with their broad range of pharmacological actions. In addition to blocking serotonin and norepinephrine reuptake, these drugs block voltage-dependent sodium channels (Jett et al 1997) and α-adrenergic receptors. All three of these actions could contribute to their analgesic effect.

There are very few studies of antidepressants other than TCAs for pain management. The much heralded fluoxetine, which is a serotonin selective reuptake inhibitor (SSRI), has virtually none of the serious side effects common with desipramine or amitriptyline. It is non-sedating, and is devoid of the adrenergic-, histaminergic- and muscarinic-antagonist-induced side effects. Thus heart block, memory loss and orthostatic hypotension are rare. Although another SSRI, paroxetine, may help the pain of diabetic neuropathy (Sindrup et al 1990), published data supporting the effectiveness of SSRIs for neuropathic pain are scanty (Max et al 1992). However, even if SSRIs are not found to be helpful for neuropathic pain per se, they are effective antidepressants and some patients report an improvement in pain as their depression clears. This point should be kept in mind with the use of all antidepressants. In the absence of a response at low doses, and especially in patients with clinically significant depression, the drugs should be pushed until limiting side effects ensue or the maximum recommended plasma concentration is achieved.

There are some newer antidepressants that are neither TCAs nor SSRIs. Venlafaxine is an example of such a drug. It blocks both serotonin and norepinephrine reuptake (Lang et al 1996). There are some early positive reports on the usefulness of this drug (Galer 1995) and our own experience is that it is more effective than SSRIs and no more likely to produce TCA-like side effects. However, above a daily dose of 150 mg it has a tendency to elevate blood pressure and to cause headaches.

Anticonvulsants and antiarrhythmics

In contrast to the consistently good results obtained with antidepressants in the treatment of neuropathic pain, anticonvulsants such as phenytoin and carbamazepine are helpful for a more restricted patient population. Carbamazepine is very effective in trigeminal neuralgia (McQuay et al 1995, Fields 1996). However, the strength of evidence is much lower for the benefit of carbamazepine in other types of neuropathic pain (Rull et al 1969, Patterson 1988). If a patient reports pain with a sharp shooting or electric shock-like component, anticonvulsants are much more likely to be helpful and should be tried.

Gabapentin is an interesting drug which was developed and marketed for seizure control. Its mechanism of action is unknown; however, there is a growing body of clinical evidence for its efficacy in a variety of neuropathic pain syndromes (Rosner et al 1996, Rosenberg et al 1997). Recent placebo-controlled trials shows that gabapentin is effective in diabetic neuropathy (Edwards et al 1998) and postherpetic neuralgia (Rowbotham et al, 1998). Its relatively benign side-effect profile compared to TCAs has encouraged many physicians to use it as a first-line drug for nerve injury pain. Two newer anticonvulsants, lamotrigine and topiramate, may also have some utility in the treatment of neuropathic pain (Hunter et al 1997), but the evidence supporting their use is currently scanty.

The antiarrhythmic drugs lidocaine, mexiletine and tocainide block voltage-dependent sodium channels. Although the site of action of membrane-stabilizing drugs for relief of pain has not been proven in patients, in vitro studies have shown that ectopic impulses generated by damaged primary afferent nociceptors are abolished by concentrations of local anaesthetics much lower than that required for blocking normal axonal conduction (Tanelian & MacIver 1991, Chabal 1994). Moreover, low concentrations of the local anaesthetics can reduce hyperexcitability of central neurons. Tocainide, flecainide and mexiletine are oral drugs of this class that are currently available. Although these drugs have been used successfully to treat neuropathic pain, this indication has not yet been approved by regulating bodies in many countries and serious side effects are not unusual. Therefore caution should be exercised when administering these compounds. Contraindications include electrocardiac abnormalities, reduced left ventricular function and coronary heart disease.

Lidocaine by intravenous infusion produces significant relief for patients with postherpetic neuralgia (Rowbotham et al 1991), diabetic neuropathy (Kastrup et al 1987) and a variety of other neuropathic pain syndromes (Glazer & Portenoy 1991). Mexiletine has been shown to be effective for pain in diabetic neuropathy (Dejgard et al 1988) and other peripheral neuropathic pains (Chabal et al 1992a, Davis 1993). A positive response to intravenous lidocaine significantly predicts longer-term relief with oral mexiletine (Galer et al 1996).

Drugs that affect γ-aminobutyric acid receptors

Several drugs are clinically available that enhance or mimic the effects of the inhibitory transmitter γ-aminobutyric acid (GABA) (Dickenson et al 1997). Baclofen is an agonist of the GABA-B receptors and in the spinal cord acts presynaptically to prevent the release of excitatory neurotransmitters. The anticonvulsant valproic acid may increase GABA levels by inhibiting GABA metabolism or by enhancing postsynaptic GABA activity. Vigabatrine is a novel anticonvulsant which inhibits γ-aminobutyrate-α-ketoglutarate transferase (GABA-T), resulting in increases in GABA levels. Benzodiazepines bind to a specific site on the GABA-A receptor and facilitate the effects of GABA.

Drugs affecting GABAergic transmission have been reported to alleviate different neuropathic pain conditions (McQuay 1988, Dellemijn & Fields 1994, Drewes et al 1994, Fromm 1994, McQuay et al 1995). The general clinical impression is that such drugs do not provide striking pain relief, save for baclofen in trigeminal neuralgia. Some agents may have a place in the treatment of painful muscle spasms. In some cases of neuropathic pain, especially in patients with restlessness in combination with lancinating pain, clonazepam has been shown to be effective (Bartusch et al 1996). On the other hand, lorazepam was ineffective in postherpetic neuralgia (Max et al 1988b) and intravenous infusions of diazepam did not relieve neuropathic pain (Dellemijn & Vanneste 1997).

Opioid analgesics

Opioids are clearly effective in postoperative, inflammatory and cancer pain. However, the use of narcotic analgesics for patients with chronic neuropathic pain is highly controversial, even among experts in the field of pain management. Double-blind placebo-controlled studies have demonstrated that acute infusions of morphine or fentanyl give significant relief to patients with postherpetic neuralgia (Rowbotham et al 1991) and a mixed group of neuropathic pain patients respectively (Dellemijn & Vanneste 1997). Furthermore, two recent controlled trials have demonstrated sustained efficacy for several weeks of oral oxycodone (Watson & Babul 1998) and tramadol (Harati et al 1998) in postherpetic neuralgia and painful diabetic neuropathy respectively. Intrathecal application of morphine has been reported to provide substantial and prolonged pain relief in several case reports of neuropathic pain (Angel et al 1998).

Our (anecdotal) experience and that of others (Portenoy et al 1990) is that many patients with pain due to central and peripheral nerve injury can be successfully and safely treated on a chronic basis with stable doses of narcotic analgesics. However, the use of opioids requires caution in patients with a history of chemical dependence or pulmonary disease. We recommend using long-acting opioid analgesics (methadone, levorphanol or a sustained-release morphine preparation) when alternative approaches to treatment have failed. In most cases an opioid trial should be tested before invasive therapies are instituted. Furthermore, a trial of opioids should not be delayed to a 'last resort' status. An intravenous opioid infusion may be informative as a predictor for long-term therapy. Prophylactic treatment of common side effects, notably nausea or constipation, is necessary and can improve patients' compliance.

N-methyl-D-aspartate-receptor antagonists

These drugs block excitatory glutamate receptors in the CNS that are thought to be responsible for the increased central excitability (central sensitization) following noxious stimuli. Clinically available substances with *N*-methyl-D-aspartate (NMDA) receptor blocking properties include ketamine, dextromethorphan, memantine and amantadine. These drugs are not licensed for analgesic therapy in many countries and therefore need to be prescribed with extra precautions. Typical side effects include sedation, nausea, disagreeable psychological disturbances or even frank hallucinations. Subanaesthetic doses of ketamine can yield analgesia. Dextromethorphan, memantine and amantadine have fewer side affects.

Studies of small cohorts have generally confirmed the analgesic effects of ketamine in patients suffering from postherpetic neuralgia (Eide et al 1994, 1995a) and other kinds of neuropathic pain (Backonja et al 1994, Eide et al 1995b, Max et al 1995, Mercadante et al 1995, Felsby et al 1996, Nikolajsen et al 1996). Dextromethorphan was effective in painful diabetic neuralgia (Nelson et al 1997) but was without beneficial effect in postherpetic neuralgia or in a mixed population of patients with neuropathic pain (McQuay et al 1994, Nelson et al 1997). Amantadine relieved surgical neuropathic pain in cancer patients (Pud et al 1998).

Levodopa

Levodopa has been shown to be very effective in suppressing dysaesthesias in the restless legs syndrome. Furthermore, two placebo-controlled studies demonstrated efficacy in acute herpes zoster pain (Kernbaum & Hauchecorne 1981) and painful diabetic neuropathy (Ertas et al 1998). The pathophysiological mechanism is unknown.

Topical medications

Many patients with neuropathic pain have allodynia, in which light mechanical stimulation of the skin produces pain. Allodynia is very common in postherpetic neuralgia, causalgia and traumatic mononeuropathies. One approach to the treatment of such conditions is the use of capsaicin extracts. Capsaicin is an agonist of the vanilloid receptor which is present on the sensitive terminal of primary nociceptive afferents (Lynn 1996, Caterina et al 1997). On initial application it has an excitatory action and produces burning pain and hyperalgesia, but with repeated or prolonged application it inactivates the receptive terminals of nociceptors (Bjerring et al 1990). Therefore, this approach is reasonable for those patients whose pain is maintained by anatomically intact, sensitized primary nociceptors. Although commonly thought to be an explanation for analgesia, the role of neuropeptide depletion in the peripheral terminals after topical application is less clear.

Capsaicin extracts are commercially available in a 0.025% and a 0.075% preparation (Rains & Bryson 1995). Both preparations have been reported to reduce the pain of postherpetic neuralgia (Bernstein et al 1989, Watson et al 1993) and postmastectomy pain (Watson & Evans 1992). The 0.075% preparation has also been advocated for pain in diabetic neuropathy (The Capsaicin Study Group 1991). However, these capsaicin preparations often produce intolerable burning so that many patients discontinue their use. Our experience with capsaicin preparations in PHN and other neuropathic pain problems has been disappointing. One problem may be that the concentration of capsaicin in commercially available preparations is too low. There is anecdotal evidence that application of relatively high concentrations (greater than 5%) of capsaicin can produce prolonged pain relief in some patients with neuropathic pain

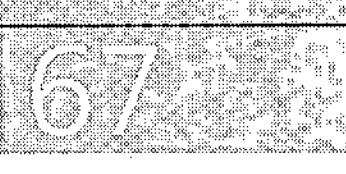

(Robbins et al 1998). This produces severe burning so that spinal anaesthesia is required for the patients to tolerate the procedure.

A second promising topical medication for neuropathic pain is local anaesthetics. The rationale is similar to that discussed above in the section on anticonvulsants and antiarrhymics. Controlled studies that report pain relief with topically applied special formulations of local anaesthetic have been published (Stow et al 1989, Rowbotham et al 1995, Rowbotham et al 1996).

Topical application of aspirin in either a chloroform or ethyl ether suspension has been reported to produce profound pain relief for some patients with postherpetic neuralgia (King 1988, De Benedittis et al 1992, De Benedittis et al 1996).

In summary, the medical management of neuropathic pain consists of four main classes of oral medication (serotonin/noradrenaline reuptake blockers, anticonvulsants, antiarrhythmics, opioids) and several categories of topical medications for patients with cutaneous hyperalgesia (cyclooxygenase inhibitors, capsaicin in either 0.025% or 0.075% preparations, and local anaesthetics).

Non-medical treatments

Transcutaneous electrical nerve stimulation

The advantages of peripheral nerve stimulation techniques are the lack of side effects and complications and the fact that the treatment can be easily repeated (see Ch. 58). Furthermore, efficacy can be determined rapidly. Therefore, a trial should be performed when feasible (Meyer & Fields 1972, Finsen et al 1988, Kumar & Marshall 1997). Invasive counter-irritation techniques, i.e. epidural *spinal cord stimulation (SCS)* and *deep brain stimulation* may be effective in special cases of neuropathic pain (Broggi et al 1994, Tasker & Vilela Filho 1995, Kumar et al 1996). Complications include dislocation of the electrodes, infection of the system and occasionally bleeding (see Ch. 59).

Neurosurgical destructive techniques (see Chs 54, 57)

Techniques such as neurectomy, rhizotomy, dorsal root entry zone lesions (DREZ), cordotomy and thalamotomy may provide short-term pain relief. Because destructive techniques increase the amount of deafferentation, sometimes even more severe pain will result from the procedure. Outside of trigeminal neuralgia there are no surgical approaches with established efficacy in neuropathic pain (Fields 1996).

A SYSTEMATIC APPROACH TO PATIENTS WITH NEUROPATHIC PAIN

The ideal in medicine is to treat the cause of the disease rather than the symptom. For patients with painful nerve injuries this is often not possible. Therefore a treatment algorithm is required (Fig. 67.1). Entrapment neuropathies can be treated by neurolysis, transposition or decompression (Dawson et al 1983). If scar-induced mechanical traction is a factor, this approach is particularly worthwhile. Transcutaneous electrical stimulation of nerves (TENS) is a viable option for some patients with focal nerve injury, particularly if the nerve trunk can be stimulated proximal to the site of injury. The majority of patients, however, require

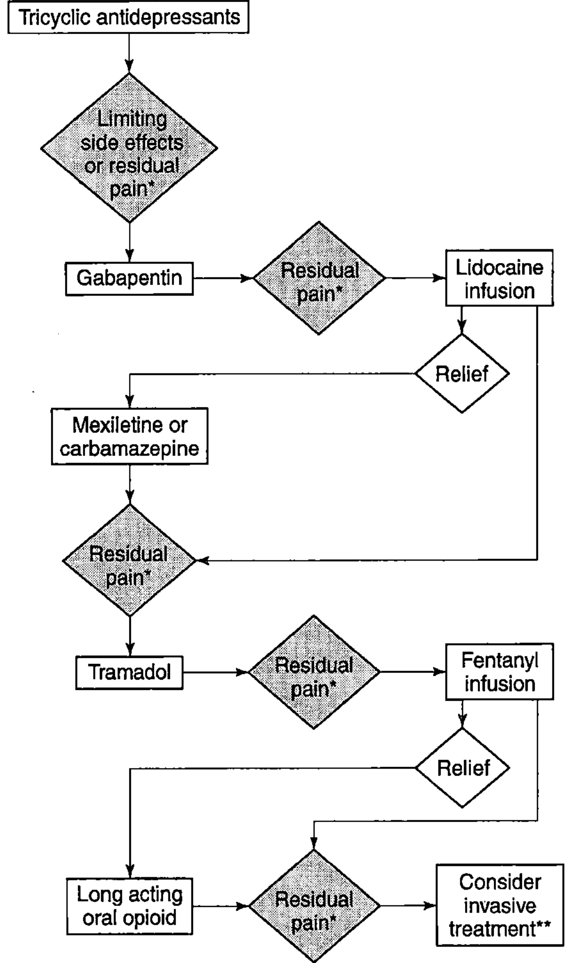

Fig. 67.1 Algorithm for the treatment of neuropathic pain. For all medications the dose should be increased every 3 days until relief, unacceptable side effects or the maximum allowable dose is achieved. *Pain level significant and persistent for at least 2 weeks. **Intrathecal opioids, spinal cord stimulation, deep brain stimulation or neurosurgical techniques. However, in our experience none of the above invasive approaches consistently provides significant long-term pain relief.

medical management. When cutaneous hyperalgesia and/or allodynia are present, topical agents are a good starting point, either with local anaesthetic, cyclo-oxygenase inhibitor or capsaicin.

In patients with focal neuropathies, a sympathetic block can be a useful procedure (Dellemijn et al 1994, Baron & Maier 1996). We use a standard sympathetic chain local anaesthetic block early if there is evidence of a sympathetically maintained component to the patient's problem (see Chs 35, 48, 53). Such evidence includes: unilateral distal extremity pain, swelling and vasomotor and sudomotor asymmetries. Patients with sympathetically maintained pain may obtain significant relief by a series of sympathetic blocks combined with vigorous physical therapy early in the course of the disease. In general, if sympathetic blocks are going to be helpful, they will provide sustained or at least increasing durations of post-block relief. If local anaesthetic blocks achieve sympatholysis as indicated by skin temperature change or a Horner's syndrome but no relief beyond 6 h, this approach is not promising. Furthermore, we have seldom found that surgical sympathectomy is helpful when blocks fail to provide progressive improvement. It is important to point out that there are two serious interpretive problems with sympathetic blocks (Dellemijn et al 1994). The first is systemic absorption of lidocaine, because even low concentrations can relieve neuropathic pain independent of a sympathetic component to the problem. The second is the production of a local somatic block by diffusion of local anaesthetic to the nearby nerve plexus.

If there is no strong evidence of sympathetically maintained pain or sympatholytic interventions do not provide significant relief, we proceed to systemic medication. General treatment principles are the individualization of therapy and the titration of a given drug depending on effect on the one hand and side effects on the other. Nonresponse should not be accepted unless a sufficient dose has been given and until a sufficient period of time has passed to judge the drug's benefit. A rigorous systematic sequential approach is useful, if progression of the disease and pain profile are stationary.

Once the decision is made to pursue systemic medical management, we currently use the algorithm illustrated in Figure 67.1. Because of the extensive literature supporting their use, we usually begin with TCAs; however, in some patients we begin therapy with gabapentin, especially in elderly patients or those with evidence of cardiac conduction block. With TCAs patients must be warned about side effects such as drowsiness, dry mouth and orthostasis and then therapy should be initiated with an appropriately low dose (e.g., 10–25 mg). It is equally important to increase the dose gradually to optimize pain relief. In some patients it is necessary to raise the dose into the antidepressant range (over 200 mg/day). It is essential to check plasma levels of antidepressant medications before concluding that they are of no value. If side effects prevent raising the dose into the antidepressant range, switch to another TCA (desipramine and nortriptyline are less sedating and less anticholinergic than amitriptyline or doxepin), to gabapentin, or to a non-tricyclic antidepressant with noradrenergic re-uptake blocking action such as venlafaxine, maprotiline or mirtazapine.

If patients obtain inadequate relief from antidepressants and plasma levels are at the top of the recommended therapeutic range, or if they do not tolerate the side effects, then begin a trial of gabapentin. This drug can be pushed to relatively high doses (e.g., over 2400 mg/day or higher). If the patient still has significant pain consider using an oral antiarrhythmic or other anticonvulsant drugs. Begin with a lidocaine infusion. If the patient does get a good response with the lidocaine infusion, then begin treatment with either mexiletine, or an anticonvulsant such as carbamazepine.

If the patient does not obtain relief with a lidocaine infusion our experience is that the pain is much less likely to respond to drugs of this class (Galer, et al 1996). At this point, therapy is often commenced with tramadol. If this drug is ineffective we give the patient a fentanyl infusion to determine the opioid sensitivity of his pain. With a good response to fentanyl we initiate opioid therapy. At the present time, levorphanol, methadone or sustained-release morphine are our first-line drugs. These medications are used on a scheduled rather than on-demand basis. Because of the problem of tolerance and physical dependence, it is our impression that the longer-acting drugs (levorphanol, methadone and the sustained-release opioid preparations) are more effective because they avoid the exacerbation of pain by a mini-abstinence state during the falling phase of the plasma concentration of the opioid. The majority of our patients require a combination of therapies for optimal results.

Although this algorithm casts a broad net across potential pain mechanisms and is gratifying for those patients who obtain significant relief, many still have significant pain after all currently available options have been exhausted. As newer drugs are brought into use and other pain mechanisms are targeted, it is our belief that more patients can be helped. For example, there is some evidence that drugs having an antagonist action at the NMDA receptor are useful for some patients with neuropathic pain (see above). In view of the strong evidence implicating this receptor in central sensitization and the evidence that central sensitization contributes to neuropathic pain, we look forward to incorporating NMDA antagonists into our treatment algorithm.

REFERENCES

Angel IF, Gould HJ Jr, Carey ME 1998 Intrathecal morphine pump as a treatment option in chronic pain of nonmalignant origin. Surgical Neurology 49: 92

Asbury AK, Fields HL 1984 Pain due to peripheral nerve damage: an hypothesis. Neurology 34: 1587

Backonja M, Arndt G, Gombar KA et al 1994 Response of chronic neuropathic pain syndromes to ketamine: a preliminary study. Pain 56: 51

Bahns E, Ernsberger U, Jänig W, Nelke A 1986 Discharge properties of mechanosensitive afferents supplying the retroperitoneal space. Pflügers Archiv 407: 519

Barnes PF, Chatterjee D, Brennan PJ et al 1992 Tumor necrosis factor production in patients with leprosy. Infection and Immunology 60: 1441

Baron R, Maier C 1996 Reflex sympathetic dystrophy: skin blood flow, sympathetic vasoconstrictor reflexes and pain before and after surgical sympathetectomy. Pain 67: 317

Baron R, Saguer M 1993 Postherpetic neuralgia. Are C-nociceptors involved in signalling and maintenance of tactile allodynia? Brain 116: 1477

Baron R, Haendler G, Schulte H 1997 Afferent large fiber polyneuropathy predicts the development of postherpetic neuralgia. Pain 73: 231

Bartusch SL, Sanders BJ, JG D'Alessio, Jernigan JR 1996 Clonazepam for the treatment of lancinating phantom limb pain. Clinical Journal of Pain 12: 59

Belda W, Manzoli S, Jordy CF 1966 Thalidomide in the control of pain in leprotic neuritis. Hospital (Rio J) 70: 731

Bennett GJ 1993 An animal model of neuropathic pain: a review. Muscle and Nerve 16: 1040–1048

Bernstein JE, Korman NJ, Bickers DR et al 1989 Topical capsaicin treatment of chronic postherapetic neuralgia. Journal of the American Academy of Dermatology 21: 265

Bjerring P, Arendt-Nielsen L, Soderberg U 1990 Argon laser induced cutaneous sensory and pain thresholds in post-herpetic neuralgia. Quantitative modulation by topical capsaicin. Acta Dermato-Venereologica 70: 121

Blumberg H, Jänig W 1984 Discharge pattern of afferent fibers from a neuroma. Pain 20: 335

Bossut DF, Shea VK, Perl ER 1996 Sympathectomy induces adrenergic excitability of cutaneous C-fiber nociceptors. Journal of Neurophysiology 75: 514

Bove GM, Light AR 1995 Unmyelinated nociceptors of rat paraspinal tissues. Journal of Neurophysiology 73: 1752

Broggi G, Servello D, Dones I, Carbone G 1994 Italian multicentric study on pain treatment with epidural spinal cord stimulation. Stereotactic and Functional Neurosurgery 62: 273

The Capsaicin Study Group 1991 Treatment of painful diabetic neuropathy with topical capsaicin. A multicenter, double-blind, vehicle-controlled study. Archives of Internal Medicine 151: 2225

Caterina MJ, Schumacher MA, Tominaga M et al 1997 The capsaicin receptor: a heat activated ion channel in the pain pathway. Nature 389: 816

Chabal C 1994 Membrane stabilizing agents and experimental neuromas. In: Fields HL, Liebeskind JC (eds) Pharmacological approaches to the treatment of chronic pain: new concepts and critical issues. IASP, Seattle, p 205

Chabal C, Jacobson L, Mariano A et al 1992a The use of oral mexiletine for the treatment of pain after peripheral nerve injury. Anesthesiology 76: 513

Chabal C, Jacobson L, Russell LC, Burchiel KJ 1992b Pain response to perineuromal injection of normal saline, epinephrine, and lidocaine in humans. Pain 49: 9

Cohen KL, Harris S 1987 Efficacy and safety of nonsteroidal anti-inflammatory drugs in the therapy of diabetic neuropathy. Archives of Internal Medicine 147: 1442

Davis RW 1993 Successful treatment for phantom pain. Orthopedics 16: 691

Dawson DM, Hallet M, Millender LH 1983 Entrapment neuropathies. Little, Brown, Boston

De Benedittis G, Besana F, Lorenzetti A 1992 A new topical treatment for acute herpetic neuralgia and post-herpetic neuralgia: the aspirin/diethyl ether mixture. An open-label study plus a double-blind controlled clinical trial. Pain 48: 383

De Benedittis G, Lorenzetti A 1996 Topical aspirin/diethyl ether mixture versus indomethacin and diclofenac/diethyl ether mixtures for acute herpetic neuralgia and postherpetic neuralgia: a double-blind crossover placebo-controlled study. Pain 65: 45

Dejgard A, Petersen P, Kastrup J 1988 Mexiletine for treatment of chronic painful diabetic neuropathy. Lancet i: 9

Dellemijn PL, Fields HL 1994 Do benzodiazepines have a role in chronic pain management? Pain 57: 137

Dellemijn PL, Vanneste JA 1997 Randomised double-blind active-placebo-controlled crossover trial of intravenous fentanyl in neuropathic pain. Lancet 349: 753

Dellemijn PL, Fields HL, Allen RR et al 1994 The interpretation of pain relief and sensory changes following sympathetic blockade. Brain 117: 1475

Devor M, Jänig W 1981 Activation of myelinated afferents ending in a neuroma by stimulation of the sympathetic supply in the rat. Neuroscience Letters 24: 43

Devor M, Rappaport ZH 1990 Pain and pathophysiology of damaged nerves. In: Fields HL (ed) Pain syndromes in neurology. Butterworth, London, p 47

Dickenson AH, Chapman V, Green GM 1997 The pharmacology of excitatory and inhibitory amino acid-mediated events in the transmission and modulation of pain in the spinal cord. General Pharmacology 28: 633

Dougherty PM, Palecek J, Paleckova V, Willis WD 1994 Neurokinin 1 and 2 antagonists attenuate the responses and NK1 antagonists prevent the sensitization of primate spinothalamic tract neurons after intradermal capsaicin. Journal of Neurophysiology 72: 1464

Drewes AM, Andreasen A, Poulsen LH 1994 Valproate for treatment of chronic central pain after spinal cord injury. A double-blind cross-over study. Paraplegia 32: 565

Edwards KR, Hes MS, LaMoreaux LK et al 1998 Gabapentin (Neurontin) for pain associated with diabetic peripheral neuropathy: a double-blind, placebo-controlled study. Neurology 50: 53

Eide PK, Jorum E, Stubhaug A et al 1994 Relief of post-herpetic neuralgia with the *N*-methyl-D-aspartic acid receptor antagonist ketamine: a double-blind, cross-over comparison with morphine and placebo. Pain 58: 347

Eide K, Stubhaug A, Oye I, Breivik H 1995a Continuous subcutaneous administration of the *N*-methyl-D-aspartic acid (NMDA) receptor antagonist ketamine in the treatment of post-herpetic neuralgia. Pain 61: 221

Eide PK, Stubhaug A, Stenehjem AE 1995b Central dysesthesia pain after traumatic spinal cord injury is dependent on *N*-methyl-D-aspartate receptor activation. Neurosurgery 37: 1080

Ertas M, Sagduyu A, Arac N et al 1998 Use of levodopa to relieve pain from painful symmetrical diabetic polyneuropathy. Pain 75: 257

Felsby S, Nielsen J, Arendt-Nielsen L, Jensen TS 1996 NMDA receptor blockade in chronic neuropathic pain: a comparison of ketamine and magnesium chloride. Pain 64: 283

Fields HL 1996 Treatment of trigeminal neuralgia. New England Journalof Medicine 334: 1125

Finsen V, Persen L, Lovlien M et al 1988 Transcutaneous electrical nerve stimulation after major amputation. Journal of Bone and Joint Surgery 70B: 109

Fried K, Brodin E, Theodorsson E 1989 Substance P-, CGRP- and NPY-immunoreactive nerve fibers in rat sciatic nerve-end neuromas. Regulatory Peptides 25: 11

Fromm GH 1994 Baclofen as an adjuvant analgesic. Journal of Pain and Symptom Management 9: 500

Galer BS 1995 Neuropathic pain of peripheral origin: advances in pharmacologic treatment. Neurology 45: S17

Galer BS, Harle J, Rowbotham MC 1996 Response to intravenous lidocaine infusion predicts subsequent response to oral mexiletine: a prospective study. Journal of Pain and Symptom Management 12: 161

Glazer S, Portenoy RK 1991 Systemic local anesthetics in pain control. Journal of Pain and Symptom Management 6: 30

Häbler HJ, Jänig W, Koltzenburg M 1987 Activation of unmyelinated afferents in chronically lesioned nerves by adrenaline and excitation of sympathetic efferents in the cat. Neuroscience Letters 82: 35

Harati Y, Gooch C, Swenson M et al 1998 Double-blind randomized trial of tramadol for the treatment of the pain of diabetic neuropathy. Neurology 50: 1842

Hromada J 1963 On the nerve supply to the connective tissue of some peripheral nervous system components. Acta Anatomica 55: 343

Hunter JC, Gogas KR, Hedley LR et al 1997 The effect of novel anti-epileptic drugs in rat experimental models of acute and chronic pain. European Journal of Pharmacology 324: 153

Jänig W, Levine JD, Michaelis M 1996 Interactions of sympathetic and primary afferent neurons following nerve injury and tissue trauma. Progress in Brain Research 113: 161

Jett MF, McGuirk J, Waligora D, Hunter JC 1997 The effects of mexiletine, desipramine and fluoxetine in rat models involving central sensitization. Pain 69: 161

Kajander KC, Bennett GJ 1992 Onset of a painful peripheral neuropathy in rat: a partial and differential deafferentation and spontaneous discharge in A beta and A delta primary afferent neurons. Journal of Neurophysiology 68: 734

Kajander KC, Wakisaka S, Bennett GJ 1992 Spontaneous discharge originates in the dorsal root ganglion at the onset of a painful peripheral neuropathy in the rat. Neuroscience Letters 138: 225

Kastrup J, Petersen P, Dejgard A et al 1987 Intravenous lidocaine infusion – a new treatment of chronic painful diabetic neuropathy? Pain 28: 69

Kernbaum S, Hauchecorne J 1981 Administration of levodopa for relief of herpes zoster pain. Journal of the American Medical Association 246: 132

Kim SH, Na HS, Sheen K, Chung JM 1993 Effects of sympathectomy on a rat model of peripheral neuropathy. Pain 55: 85

King RB 1988 Concerning the management of pain associated with herpes zoster and of postherpetic neuralgia. Pain 33: 73

Kingery WS 1997 A critical review of controlled clinical trials for peripheral neuropathic pain and complex regional pain syndromes. Pain 73: 123

Kishore-Kumar R, Max MB, Schafer SC et al 1990 Desipramine relieves postherpetic neuralgia. Clinical and Pharmacological Therapy 47: 305

Koltzenburg M, Lundberg LE, Torebjörk HE 1992 Dynamic and static components of mechanical hyperalgesia in human hairy skin. Pain 51: 207

Korenman EM, Devor M 1981 Ectopic adrenergic sensitivity in damaged peripheral nerve axons in the rat. Experimental Neurology 72: 63

Kumar D, Marshall HJ 1997 Diabetic peripheral neuropathy: amelioration of pain with transcutaneous electrostimulation. Diabetes Care 20: 1702

Kumar K, Toth C, Nath RK 1996 Spinal cord stimulation for chronic pain in peripheral neuropathy. Surgical Neurology 46: 363

Laird JM, Bennett GJ 1993 An electrophysiological study of dorsal horn neurons in the spinal cord of rats with an experimental peripheral neuropathy. Journal of Neurophysiology 69: 2072

Lang E, Hord AH, Denson D 1996 Venlafaxine hydrochloride (Effexor) relieves thermal hyperalgesia in rats with an experimental mononeuropathy. Pain 68: 151

Lombard MC, Larabi Y 1983 Electrophysiological study of cervical dorsal horn cells in partially deafferented rats. In: Bonica JJ (ed) Advances in pain research and therapy. Raven, New York, p 147

Lu X, Richardson PM 1993 Responses of macrophages in rat dorsal root ganglia following peripheral nerve injury. Journal of Neurocytology 22: 334

Lynn B 1996 Capsaicin: actions on nociceptive C-fibres and therapeutic potential. Pain 41: 61

McQuay HJ 1988 Pharmacological treatment of neuralgic and neuropathic pain. Cancer Survey 7: 141

McQuay HJ, Carroll D, Jadad AR et al 1994 Dextromethorphan for the treatment of neuropathic pain: a double-blind randomised controlled crossover trial withintegral n-of-1 design. Pain 59: 127

McQuay H, Carroll D, Jadad AR et al 1995 Anticonvulsant drugs for management of pain: a systematic review. British Medical Journal 311: 1047

McQuay HJ, Tramer M, Nye BA et al 1996 A systematic review of antidepressants in neuropathic pain. Pain 68: 217

Max MB, Culnane M, Schafer SC et al 1987 Amitriptyline relieves diabetic neuropathy pain in patients with normal or depressed mood. Neurology 37: 589

Max MB, Schafer SC, Culnane M et al 1988a Association of pain relief with drug side effects in postherpetic neuralgia: a single-dose study of clonidine, codeine, ibuprofen, and placebo. Clinical and Pharmacological Therapy 43: 363

Max MB, Schafer SC, Culnane M et al 1988b Amitriptyline, but not lorazepam, relieves postherpetic neuralgia. Neurology 38: 1427

Max MB, Lynch SA, Muir J et al 1992 Effects of desipramine, amitriptyline, and fluoxetine on pain in diabetic neuropathy. New England Journal of Medicine 326: 1250

Max MB, Byas-Smith MG, Gracely RH, Bennett GJ 1995 Intravenous infusion of the NMDA antagonist, ketamine, in chronic posttraumatic pain with allodynia: a double-blind comparison to alfentanil and placebo. Clinical Neuropharmacology 18: 360

Melzack R, Wall PD 1965 Pain mechanisms: a new theory. Science 150: 971

Mercadante S, Lodi F, Sapio M et al 1995 Long-term ketamine subcutaneous continuous infusion in neuropathic cancer pain. Journal of Pain and Symptom Management 10: 564

Meyer GA, Fields HL 1972 Causalgia treated by selective large fibre stimulation of peripheral nerve. Brain 95: 163

Mitchell SW 1865 Injuries of Nerves and their Consequences. Dover, New York

Nashold BS Jr, Ostdahl RH 1979 Dorsal root entry zone lesions for pain relief. Journal of Neurosurgery 51: 59

Nelson KA, Park KM, Robinovitz E et al 1997 High-dose oral dextromethorphan versus placebo in painful diabetic neuropathy and postherpetic neuralgia. Neurology 48: 1212

Nikolajsen L, Hansen CL, Nielsen J et al 1996 The effect of ketamine on phantom pain: a central neuropathic disorder maintained by peripheral input. Pain 67: 69

Onghena P, Van Houdenhove B 1992 Antidepressant-induced analgesia in chronic non-malignant pain: a meta-analysis of 39 placebo-controlled studies. Pain 49: 205

Partida-Sanchez S, Favila-Castillo L, Pedraza-Sanchez S et al 1998 IgG antibody subclasses, tumor necrosis factor and IFN-gamma levels in patients with type II lepra reaction on thalidomide treatment. International Archives of Allergy and Applied Immunology 116: 60

Patterson JF 1988 Carbamazepine in the treatment of phantom limb pain. Southern Medical Journal 81: 1100

Portenoy RK, Foley KM, Inturrisi CE 1990 The nature of opioid responsiveness and its implications for neuropathic pain: new hypotheses derived from studies of opioid infusions. Pain 43: 273

Pud D, Eisenberg E, Spitzer A et al 1998 The NMDA receptor antagonist amantadine reduces surgical neuropathic pain in cancer patients: a double blind, randomized, placebo controlled trial. Pain 75: 349

Rains C, Bryson HM 1995 Topical capsaicin. A review of its pharmacological properties and therapeutic potential in post-herpetic neuralgia, diabetic neuropathy and osteoarthritis. Drugs and Aging 7: 317

Richards RL 1967 Causalgia. A centennial review. Archives of Neurology 16: 339

Richelson E 1990 Antidepressants and brain neurochemistry. Mayo Clinic Proceedings 65: 1227

Robbins WR, Staats PS, Levine J et al 1998 Treatment of intractable pain with topical large-dose capsaicin: preliminary report. Anesthesia and Analgesia 86: 579

Rosenberg JM, Harrell C, Ristic H et al 1997 The effect of gabapentin on neuropathic pain. Clinical Journal of Pain 13: 251

Rosner H, Rubin L, Kestenbaum A 1996 Gabapentin adjunctive therapy in neuropathic pain states. Clinical Journal of Pain 12: 56

Rowbotham MC, Reisner-Keller LA, Fields HL 1991 Both intravenous lidocaine and morphine reduce the pain of postherpetic neuralgia. Neurology 41: 1024

Rowbotham MC, Davies PS, Fields HL 1995 Topical lidocaine gel relieves postherpetic neuralgia. Annals of Neurology 37: 246

Rowbotham MC, Davies PS, Verkempinck C, Galer BS 1996 Lidocaine patch: double-blind controlled study of a new treatment method for post-herpetic neuralgia. Pain 65: 9

Rowbotham M, Harden N, Stacey B, Bernstein P, Magnus-Miller L 1998 Gabapentin for the treatment of Postherpetic neuralgia. Journal of the American Medical Association 280: 1837–1842

Rull JA, Quibrera R, Gonzalez-Millan H, Lozano Castaneda O 1969 Symptomatic treatment of peripheral diabetic neuropathy with carbamazepine (Tegretol): double blind crossover trial. Diabetologia 5: 215

Sato J, Perl ER 1991 Adrenergic excitation of cutaneous pain receptors induced by peripheral nerve injury. Science 251: 1608

Scadding JW 1981 Development of ongoing activity, mechanosensitivity, and adrenaline sensitivity in severed peripheral nerve axons. Experimental Neurology 73: 345–364

Shir Y, Seltzer Z 1991 Effects of sympathectomy in a model of causalgiform pain produced by partial sciatic nerve injury in rats. Pain 45: 309

Shortland P, Woolf CJ 1993 Chronic peripheral nerve section results in a rearrangement of the central axonal arborizations of axotomized A beta primary afferent neurons in the rat spinal cord. Journal of Comparative Neurology 330: 65

Sindrup SH, Gram LF, Brosen K et al 1990 The selective serotonin reuptake inhibitor paroxetine is effective in the treatment of diabetic neuropathy symptoms. Pain 42: 135

Sommer C, Myers RR 1996 Vascular pathology in CCI neuropathy: a quantitative temporal study. Experimental Neurology 141: 113

Sommer C, Marziniak M, Myers RR 1998 The effect of thalidomide treatment on vascular pathology and hyperalgesia caused by chronic constriction injury. Pain 74: 83

Sorkin LS, Xiao W-H, Wagner R, Myers RR 1997 Tumor necrosis factor-alpha induces ectopic activity in nociceptive primary afferent fibres. Neuroscience 81: 255

Stow PJ, Glynn CJ, Minor B 1989 EMLA cream in the treatment of post-herpetic neuralgia. Efficacy and pharmacokinetic profile. Pain 39: 301

Tanelian DL, MacIver MB 1991 Analgesic concentrations of lidocaine suppress tonic A-delta and C fiber discharges produced by acute injury. Anesthesiology 74: 934

Tasker RR, Vilela Filho O 1995 Deep brain stimulation for neuropathic pain. Stereotactic and Functional Neurosurgery 65: 122

Torebjörk E, Wahren L, Wallin G et al 1995 Noradrenaline-evoked pain in neuralgia. Pain 63: 11

Wagner R, Janjigian M, Myers RR 1998 Anti-inflammatory interleukin-10 therapy in CCI neuropathy decreases thermal hyperalgesia, macrophage recruitment, and endoneurial TNF-alpha expression. Pain 74: 35

Walker AE, Nulsen F 1948 Electrical stimulation of the upper thoracic portion of the sympathetic chain in man. Archives of Neurology and Psychiatry 59: 559

Wall PD, Gutnick M 1974 Ongoing activity in peripheral nerves: the physiology and pharmacology of impulses originating from a neuroma. Experimental Neurology 43: 580

Watson CP, Babul N 1998 Efficacy of oxycodone in neuropathic pain: a randomized trial in postherpetic neuralgia. Neurology 50: 1837

Watson CP, Evans RJ 1992 The postmastectomy pain syndrome and topical capsaicin: a randomized trial. Pain 51: 375

Watson CP, Chipman M, Reed K et al 1992 Amitriptyline versus maprotiline in postherpetic neuralgia: a randomized, double-blind, crossover trial. Pain 48: 29

Watson CP, Tyler KL, Bickers DR et al 1993 A randomized vehicle-controlled trial of topical capsaicin in the treatment of postherpetic neuralgia. Clinical Therapy 15: 510

Welk E, Leah JD, Zimmermann M 1990 Characteristics of A- and C-fibers ending in sensory nerve neuroma in the rat. Journal of Neurophysiology 63: 759

Wynn-Parry CB 1980 Pain in avulsion lesions of the brachial plexus. Pain 9: 41

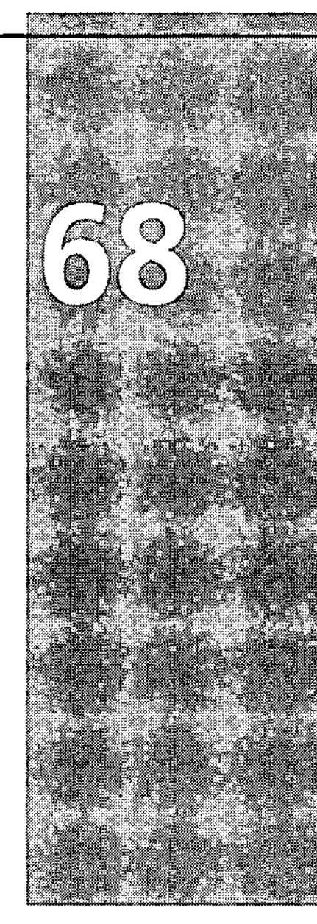

Prevention of disability due to chronic musculoskeletal pain

STEVEN JAMES LINTON

SUMMARY

This chapter examines procedures designed for use in health-care settings to prevent disability due to musculoskeletal pain. Because musculoskeletal pain is a major source of suffering, health care and utilization of compensation, there is a definite need for prevention. However, prevention is not an easy task because disability is related to a developmental process in which multidimensional factors operate over time to produce significant lifestyle changes. Research on risk factors indicates that although medical and workplace factors are obvious, psychosocial variables are central to the transition from acute to chronic pain. The early identification of 'at-risk' patients is a key to allocating resources and initiating secondary prevention. Screening and monitoring techniques are valuable tools to help establish viable clinical routines. Prevention appears to be sensitive to the aims, content, strategies, administration and timing of the intervention. It may be viewed as a process aimed to counter the developmental stages of disability, rather than as a technique. Although secondary prevention is in its infancy, state-of-the-art recommendations are provided as an aid for developing viable prevention programmes.

INTRODUCTION

If only we could prevent disability due to chronic pain from occurring, tremendous suffering and monumental costs would be saved. At face value, then, the prevention of chronic pain is a self-evident proposition which offers the advantage of the reduction or elimination of suffering and its consequent economic burden. Yet, while disability consumes huge amounts of resources, only a small fraction of the amount of these sums is available to prevent chronic pain problems. Our knowledge about prevention is still in its infancy and therefore limited. Theoretical and practical stumbling blocks related to our lack of knowledge and the propensities of the problem have also impeded development. However, recent advances indicate that psychosocial factors are instrumental in the development of disability and this opens the port for unique preventive efforts. Moreover, programmes based on a multidimensional model have shown considerable promise in clinical trials. Today, it may be possible to provide interventions aimed at preventing chronic disability in primary as well as secondary health-care settings.

The objective of this chapter is to provide an overview of the main aspects of prevention as well as to review prevention programmes in clinical settings. A key to understanding these programmes is the process of the development of chronic problems, and therefore this will be scrutinized. Subsequently, some issues will be addressed that shed light on why we may wish to embark upon a prevention programme as well as what one may reasonably expect to achieve. This chapter focuses on secondary prevention, as this is most relevant for health-care providers. Musculoskeletal pain (MSP) such as back, neck or shoulder pain is highlighted, because these account for a large portion of chronic disability. Finally, current approaches to secondary preventions will be examined including the early identification of patients at risk and strategies for prevention.

DEVELOPMENT AND CONSEQUENCES OF CHRONIC PAIN

An understanding of the development of chronic MSP elucidates the reasons why pain may persist and turn into dysfunction. Unfortunately, we do not yet understand the exact mechanisms that produce MSP. In fact, MSP represents several mechanisms, as it is a collection of symptoms rather than a distinct entity. Nevertheless, we are beginning to comprehend the ***transition*** from acute to chronic pain. It is clear that a host of psychosocial factors may influence whether an acute injury develops into chronic dysfunction. One relevant problem, however, is that interventions for acute and subacute MSP nevertheless usually focus on traditional medical treatments; for example, drugs prescriptions and rest, rather than the prevention of chronic problems (Linton & Halldén 1997, van Tulder et al 1997).

TIME FACTOR: ACUTE, CHRONIC OR RECURRENT

Time is a crucial factor as it provides a framework for defining what we are attempting to prevent. The development of chronic pain may be described in a series of stages (Vällfors 1985, Skevington 1995, Gatchel 1996). Keep in mind, however, that the road from acute injury to chronic dysfunction may be quite different for various individuals. Rather than being a stable phenomenon, there appear to be critical factors and incidents that determine the exact course of development for a given person. *Acute pain*, which is generally defined as pain up to about 3 weeks, is characterized by temporary decreases in activity, reliance on medication and help seeking. It is accompanied by psychological distress, for example fear, anxiety and worry, in addition to beliefs that pain is controllable through medication and active coping. Biologically the patient may have organic findings as well as muscle spasms. In the next stage, *subacute pain*, considered to be between 3 and 12 weeks, patients may exhibit altering patterns of increasing and decreasing activity and withdraw or become reliant on medication. They often attempt to continue working and use various coping styles. Pain of varying intensity is experienced and depressive symptoms may begin to develop. Patients tend to focus on the physical symptoms and these are affected by stress. Anxiety may persist and anger and frustration are common. As time passes, the likelihood of finding organic pathology decreases. In *persistent or chronic pain*, defined as more than 3 months' duration, activities may have decreased sharply, patients may 'doctor shop' and overuse medications. Acceptance of these lifestyle changes accompany the sick role. The pain becomes more constant although patients may experience 'good' and 'bad' periods. Depression and passive coping strategies as well as a preoccupation with symptoms are common, as are beliefs that the patient himself has no control over the pain. From a biological point of view there are few findings, but the patient may suffer from chronic spasms, and decreased muscle strength and endurance.

Although the above stages of pain development serve as an heuristic aid, we should remember that MSP is usually recurrent in nature. While most episodes of back pain remit rather quickly and most people return to work within 6 weeks (Reid et al 1997), the majority of sufferers will experience several episodes of pain during the course of a year (Frymoyer 1992, Nachemson 1992, VonKorff 1994). In addition, it is rare for someone with no history of MSP to be off work for 6 weeks or more on the first episode. Rather, persistent problems tend to develop over extended periods of time in which recurrent bouts become more frequent and the duration longer (Philips & Grant 1991, Rossignol et al 1992, VonKorff 1994). More than 50% of patients with acute back pain will experience another episode within a year (Nachemson 1992), and prospective studies indicate that almost half will still have significant problems 6–12 months later (Philips & Grant 1991, VonKorff 1994, Linton & Halldén 1997).

A DEVELOPMENTAL PROCESS

Even though persistent MSP is often considered a medical problem, it may be better viewed as a developmental process because psychological factors work over time to produce the cognitive, emotional and behavioural changes that define the syndrome. Interestingly, these psychological reactions associated with acute pain typically result in adequate adjustment to the pain until healing occurs and the pain subsides. A surprising number of people, moreover, cope with persistent pain so well that they require little sick leave or health care (Linton 1998). For a minority of people, however, the cognitive, emotional and behavioural reactions are not sufficient and may, in themselves, actually contribute to the development of persistent pain problems.

Learning appears to be a potent factor in the development of long-term dysfunction. As illustrated in the stages above, patients learn how to deal with their problem over time. These behaviours are related to emotional and cognitive factors such as fear, anxiety, attributions, beliefs, self-efficacy and coping which interact during the development of the problem. Patients may learn 'inappropriate' coping behaviours that have immediate advantages, but are counterproductive in the long run. Again, time is an essential ingredient giving cognitive-learning processes the opportunity to operate. Thus, although healing may take place, learning may establish a pattern of thinking and behaving popularly known as the 'sick role'. This usually includes low levels of physical and social function, complaints, over-use of medications, use of passive coping strategies, and inappropriate beliefs, for example that activity causes pain or injury.

 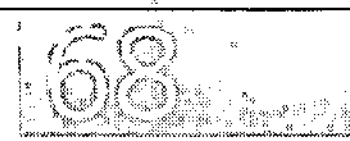

Particular examples of learning illustrate that pain behaviours, for example complaints, resting and taking medications, may be reinforced by the social response they bring (attention, sympathy, legitimization of the behaviour) or by temporary reductions of pain or anxiety. Passive behaviours like resting, reading and watching television, which may be pleasant and associated with little or no pain, may eventually become predominant. The process occurs gradually and the patient may not realize that a drastic change in lifestyle is taking place. Lastly, pain behaviours may buy time out from undesirable activities or duties. These lifestyle changes are related to concurrent emotional and cognitive changes. For example, decreases in mobility and activity levels may be coupled with a depressive mood and catastrophizing thoughts. Coping strategies may become passive and the patient may believe there is little she can do to control the pain. Being off work may enhance the process because it contributes to a disruption of normal lifestyle, reinforces negative cognition, behaviours and beliefs, and provides time for learning of the 'sick-role' to take place. As a result, a basic tenet of secondary prevention is to intervene early enough to prevent the disruption of the patient's normal lifestyle including work.

As a specific example of learning in the development of persistent pain, we may consider the role of fear-avoidance. A normal reaction to pain is anxiety or fear which may generate avoidance through a combination of classical and operant learning (Lethem et al 1983, Linton et al 1984, Kori et al 1990, Vlaeyen et al 1995a, b). In short, avoiding certain movements or activities may be reinforced by the reduction of anxiety, fear and the muscle tension they produce. This 'fear-avoidance' model is somewhat similar to the avoidance observed in phobias. In everyday situations, anxiety and fear may be provoked by the threat of certain activities or movements which are believed to exacerbate the pain or injure the spine. Because physical activity may have set off the pain, or may naturally be related to small increases in pain, the fearful patient may quickly learn to avoid a variety of activities and movements. This may disrupt activity patterns and daily routines. Associated catastrophizing thoughts and depression may lead to even more avoidance and disruptions in everyday life and represent an obstacle to recovery. Consequently, a vicious circle may develop (Lethem et al 1983, Vlaeyen et al 1995a, b), in which the pain initiates catastrophizing which increases fear. This in turn increases avoidance resulting in activity decreases and dysfunction. This dysfunction contributes to depression that lowers the patient's pain threshold and tolerance.

Persistent pain then may be seen as a developmental process over time in which psychological factors play a significant role. Research on risk factors, detailed in the section on risk evaluation, clearly supports this view. Three important conclusions relevant for prevention are:

1. Persistent MSP involves a developmental, biopsychosocial process clearly highlighting psychosocial factors, as opposed to the strict progression of a clear-cut biological disease.
2. Time is a vital factor because it provides the opportunity for learning to take place.
3. Prevention should occur early enough to hinder the cognitive, emotional and behavioural lifestyle changes associated with chronic disability.

EPIDEMIOLOGY OF THE PROBLEM

A few epidemiological facts illustrate the need for prevention and provide some insights which may guide our efforts. Firstly, a large number of people suffer from MSP, making it a leading health-care problem even though only a minority develop persistent dysfunction. MSP is a leading cause of health-care visits, particularly in primary care, sick absenteeism and early pensions (Frymoyer 1992, Nachemson 1992, Skovron 1992). However, several studies indicate that over 90% of those off work with an acute episode of back pain will return within 3 months (Waddell 1996, Reid et al 1997). Moreover, there is reason to believe that many people with MSP cope with the problem, utilizing only very limited amounts of health care and compensation (Linton 1998b). Prevention then might be oriented towards identifying those people who develop costly, long-term disability problems.

Secondly, as shown above, MSP is recurrent in nature even though most patients return to work rather quickly after an acute episode. Although acute sufferers usually feel better and return to work within a few weeks, this does not mean that they have recovered fully or permanently. The recurrent nature of the problem provides the time for learning processes to operate. Not only do people at risk need to be identified early on, but prevention also implies carefully reviewing a patient's progress as well as providing strategies for dealing with flare-ups.

Thirdly, while up to 85% of the population will suffer from MSP, only a small number will account for most of the costs (Nachemson 1992, Skovron 1992, Waddell 1996). In general, less than 10% of the sufferers may consume up to 75% of the resources (VonKorff 1994, Reid et al 1997). Thus, preventing disability and high-cost cases may result in large economic savings, so that these people constitute a special target for prevention programmes.

Further, most of the money at this time is spent on compensation, while relatively little is spent on treatment, and almost nothing is invested in prevention. The reason is that these patients are off work; for example, when rest is the treatment or while numerous medical diagnostic tests and treatments are performed. In Sweden, about 85% of the total resources for MSP are spent on compensation, as compared to 15% for all treatments and drugs, a figure which has remained fairly constant over a 15-year period (Linton 1998b). Similarly, in the Netherlands, a recent study of all costs due to back pain showed that 93% involved compensation and only 7% treatment (van Tulder et al 1995). Moreover, of the money spent on treatment, only a minute amount (6% in the Netherlands) is spent on primary-care-based interventions or prevention (van Tulder et al 1995, Linton 1998b). Consequently, until prevention is granted more resources, programmes need to be relatively cheap and this suggests incorporating them into existing practice routines.

AIMS OF PREVENTION

Before delving into prevention strategies, there is a need to reflect on some conceptual issues pertaining to our aims. Firstly, unlike medical diseases such as cholera where there are well defined biological states to prevent, MSP is a multidimensional phenomenon and prevention is not restricted to traditional medical models. Secondly, the aims of prevention here depend on whether the interests of the patient, health-care provider, family, insurance carrier, workplace or society are given precedence. Patients may, for example, be interested mainly in symptom relief, while the workplace is probably concerned about function. Obviously, the economic burden of MSP is of great interest to those ultimately footing the bill. Since patients, providers, family, workplaces and payers may all need to be engaged in the programme, the goals ought to be clearly defined and of real interest to each of them.

Thirdly, while disease processes are often the focus of prevention in medical models, cognitive, emotional and behavioural aspects are important targets for the prevention of MSP. Thus, it is important to focus on the lifestyle changes and associated cognitions and emotions that develop into disability.

A final consideration is whether we are actually preventing ill health or promoting good health. Some interventions enhance the patient's health behaviours. Consider that some patients may have good coping skills and yet be overwhelmed by pain while others may lack such coping skills. Thus, prevention is sometimes seen as the promoting of already existing coping skills and health behaviours rather than the prevention of a given problem.

SPECIFIC OBJECTIVES

The objectives selected should address not only the medical but also the psychosocial aspects of the problem and create interest in the programme. Interventions may concentrate on different goals, for example pain perception, function, physical measures like muscle strength, health-care use, re-injury or sick absenteeism. All of these have merit and reflect the goals deemed most crucial.

With consideration of the multidimensional development of the problem, worthwhile target variables are to:

1. Reduce the number of new episodes.
2. Reduce the duration of new episodes.
3. Enhance coping skills to thereby minimize pain intensity and the impact of new episodes.
4. Reduce the need for health-care visits.
5. Reduce the need for time off work.
6. Maintain and enhance everyday activity routines, i.e. prevent dysfunction.

Note that the prevention of pain is not listed as a goal. Although pain may sometimes be an unwelcome plague, it is also a basic warning. This signal serves the useful purpose of attending to trauma and preventing further trauma. Thus, it is clear that pain should not always be prevented. Even though pain is naturally the centre of discussion, preventing persistent suffering and disability appear to be what we ordinarily mean when we speak of prevention.

IDENTIFYING 'AT RISK' PATIENTS

The identification of patients at risk of developing disability is a key to prevention. It offers the advantage of allocating our limited resources to those most in need. Early identification also provides the opportunity to alter the time course and thereby cut short the 'time factor' that we have seen is so essential for disability problems to develop. As MSP is prevalent and a leading reason for seeking care, any preventive effort requiring even moderate time and resources might quickly become untenable. Thus, it is important to provide the correct level of prevention, to the right person, at the right time. Limited interventions incorporated into clinical routines, for example, may be most appropriate very early on, while more concentrated efforts may be warranted for more developed problems. Access to the correct level of intervention depends upon the early identification of those at risk and subsequent proper assessment of the problem.

RISK FACTORS

Risk factors may be utilized in early identification and may also provide a focus for intervention. In fact, prevention is usually thought of as altering causal factors to minimize risk. Although the determination of risk factors often involves correlations, that is they are related to the persistent problem, but may not actually *cause* it, risk factors should provide guidance as to what needs to be 'prevented'. Thus, with an eye towards prevention, risk factors are important in the screening and assessment of patients with MSP.

A fairly large number of medical, workplace, emotional, cognitive and behavioural factors have been found to be related to disability due to MSP. A host of ergonomic factors, for example lifting, heavy work, twisting, bending, manual handling and repetitive work, have been found to be associated with MSP (Pope et al 1991, Skovron 1992). Many construe this as evidence that such movements cause an injury and therefore that physical loading should be reduced or avoided. While this may be true in 'extreme' cases, physical loading generally is beneficial (Burton et al 1998). Thus, prevention need not always centre on reducing physical stress on the spine. Instead, physical activity and work appear to be central in maintaining health and preventing dysfunction.

Research has also isolated medical risk factors that are considered to be 'red flags' for certain diagnoses. These include fever, history of cancer, sciatic pain, urinary retention, weight loss and pain that gets worse when the patient is lying down. Because these red flags signal potentially dangerous disease, the patient should be examined to determine if any exist and appropriate action taken. However, red flags are the exception rather than the rule. In the vast majority of cases, no red flags will be found.

There is mounting evidence that psychosocial variables are particularly salient in the transition from acute to chronic disability. Several excellent reviews of the literature concerning psychosocial risk factors summarize this information and may be referred to for details (Frymoyer 1992, Weiser & Cedraschi 1992, Bongers et al 1993, Fordyce 1995, Turk 1997). For example, Turk evaluated the published evidence on psychosocial factors in the development of chronic pain (Turk 1997). His review revealed that although isolating risk factors is difficult, psychological variables play a very significant role and are better predictors of chronicity than are clinical or physical factors. Among the factors isolated were fear, depression, anxiety, distress, maladaptive coping, pain severity, stress and perceived health.

Workplace factors would seem to be logical candidates for involvement in disability, and psychosocial aspects of work have been implicated. A recent review of some 60 studies revealed a relationship between MSP problems and job demands, control, monotonous work, time pressure and perceived workload (Bongers et al 1993). Taken together with the findings concerning ergonomic factors, the data suggest that workplace factors, often in the psychosocial realm, may be associated with the development of disability.

Recently, Weiser and Cedraschi (1992) scrutinized 16 high-quality, predictive studies that employed psychosocial variables. They reported that anxiety, distress, depression, preoccupation with symptoms, as well as coping and illness beliefs were related to the development of, or recovery from, chronic problems. Consequently, there is considerable consensus that psychosocial factors are of special importance in the transition from acute to chronic problems, and that these variables are probably more strongly related to development than physical, ergonomic or medical variables. Yet, the power of psychosocial variables to explain the onset or development of a problem is limited.

The data on psychosocial factors were summarized and put into official recommendations for the first time in the 'yellow flags' document of New Zealand (Kendall et al 1997). A summary list of some of the variables is provided in Table 68.1. This document also presents an algorithm suggesting that psychosocial factors be considered in primary care examinations during the first visit. Moreover, if the problem does not remit within 2–4 weeks, a formal screening procedure is suggested.

SCREENING

The data on risk factors imply that we might exploit this information to screen for patients at risk of developing disability. However, until quite recently few methods were available to assist in the early identification of 'at-risk' patients. Consequently, we may expect a number of advancements in the near future.

Two basic methods have been advocated to identify individuals at risk of developing disability. The first is monitoring sick leave, while the second involves clinical screening tools. Frank and associates (1996) contend that it is premature to discuss screening instruments because early predictors of

Table 68.1 An overview of psychosocial 'yellow flags' and some pertinent examples of each category. (Based on Kendall et al 1997)

Cognitions and beliefs about the pain
Fear-avoidance, i.e. belief that activity will cause pain or injury
Belief that pain must be completely abolished before attempting normal activity
Catastrophizing
Belief that pain is uncontrollable
Expectations concerning assessment, treatment and outcome
Belief that one has poor health or is handicapped
Emotions
Fear of pain or disability
Depression and irritability
Anxiety or heightened awareness of body sensations
Stress
Loss of sense of control
Behaviours
Use of extended rest
Reduced activity or withdrawal from activities of daily life
Avoidance
Report of extremely high intensity pain
Sleep quality reduced since onset of pain
Substance abuse
Family
Over-protecting partner
Solicitous behaviour from partner
Socially punitive responses
Extent of support in attempts to return to normal activities including work
History of abuse
History of model for chronic pain behaviour
Work
Belief that work is harmful
Unsupportive or unhappy current work environment
Negative experience of management or absence of interest from employer
Specific aspects of psychosocial environment, e.g. stress, perceived load, monotony, control, etc.
Compensation
Lack of financial incentive to return to work
Disputes
History of ineffective case management
Diagnosis and treatment
Health professionals sanctioning disability
Conflicting diagnoses
Diagnoses leading to catastrophizing and fear
Dependency, e.g. on passive treatments
Health-care utilization
Expectation of a 'techno-fix'
Lack of satisfaction with previous treatment
Advice to withdraw from daily activities or work

long-term outcome are not accurate enough to be clinically useful. As an alternative, they point to the time factor, based on return-to-work statistics, and declare that time off work might be monitored. Frank et al recommend monitoring time off work so that early interventions may be started during the 'critical period' of 4–8 weeks off work.

Monitoring time off work has some clear advantages, but also a number of disadvantages. A particular advantage is that, statistically, monitoring time off work does appear to isolate high-cost cases. Furthermore, the method is simple to understand and use and is based on existing data. Finally, since early interventions designed for this group have been developed, an intervention is plausible. A major disadvantage however is that monitoring does not include a system for those sufferers not yet off work. There may be practical problems, moreover, in gaining access to and maintaining up-to-date data for programmes operating in health-care settings. More importantly, monitoring would appear to result in a relatively 'late' entry into prevention. As indicated above, those off work for 4–8 weeks ordinarily have a considerable history of the problem and consequently have already travelled a fair distance down the road to disability. In turn, this seems to result in the need for rather extensive interventions that may resemble treatment more than prevention. Finally, the time-monitoring system totally lacks information regarding target variables.

Screening instruments have been based mainly on psychological risk factors and are still under development. At least four screening tools have received preliminary testing to assess their worth in helping clinicians screen patients. A questionnaire that combines measures of depression and distress was developed and shown to be relevant for patients visiting an orthopaedic clinic (Main et al 1992). Patients were first classified into one of four categories depending on their scores on distress and depression and these categories were shown to be related to disability 1–4 years later.

Government authorities and insurance carriers are especially concerned about long-term disability, and thus the 11-item Vermont Screening Questionnaire (Hazard et al 1996) was developed to help predict compensation cases. Scores were shown to be surprisingly accurate in predicting the future work status of 163 people who had filed an injury report (sensitivity = 94%; specificity = 84%). Some caution is warranted, however, because the study concentrates only on absenteeism in a group filing an injury claim, and it suffered from a large drop-out/refusal rate.

Applying psychological assessment expertise in primary care has also been shown to be helpful in identifying patients at risk of developing work disability. Gatchel and colleagues (1995) administered a battery of questionnaires including the MMPI, the Million Pain and Disability Scale, as well as the Structured Clinical Interview for DSM-III to 421 patients applying for primary care of acute back pain. The patients were followed for 6 months to determine work status. The study revealed that scores on the pain and disability measure, personality factors and scale 3 (Hysteria) of the MMPI were of value and classified 87% of the patients correctly into the categories of 'working' or 'not working'. Although it may be somewhat costly because it involves fairly lengthy questionnaires and a professionally conducted interview, it appears to have value in identifying patients at risk of developing work disability.

A 24-question screening instrument specifically designed for self administration in primary-care settings with MSP patients has recently been designed (Linton & Halldén 1997, 1998). An evaluation of 137 consecutive primary-care patients on a visit for acute or subacute neck or back pain first obtained scores and then followed participants to determine outcome 6 months later, defined as: working, off work 1–30 days and off work more than 30 days. Results demonstrated reasonable accuracy (sensitivity = 87%; specificity = 75% using a median split) especially since outcome involved three categories, which statistically reduces prediction as compared to the usual two-category outcome solutions.

CLINICAL RECOMMENDATIONS

Early identification is so central for prevention that routines must be developed to isolate patients at risk. In fact, a lack of routines appears to be one major reason that patients at risk fail to be recognized. That is, each time a patient seeks help, the case may be viewed as 'a new patient' and the patient's history glossed over or ignored. This may lead to inappropriate assessment and treatment techniques that reinforce rather than prevent the transition from acute to chronic pain. As a result, there is a need for systematic routines designed to identify patients in need of preventive interventions.

In addition to red flags, yellow flags should be of interest at the initial consultation. It is evident that the first visit ought to include a thorough physical examination to determine if any red flags are present. However, the clinician may also wish to probe psychosocial factors with pertinent verbal questions regarding the patient's work situation, family, expectations and mood.

The case may be monitored and screening procedures initiated from the start, but should certainly receive attention if the problem persists more than 2–4 weeks. Monitoring simply consists of following the progress of the case, particularly if the patient is off work. It is worth noting that not only the current situation is of interest, but also the history. For example, it may be of interest to look at cumulative time off work in addition to the current time off work. Although none of the screening tools described above has been sufficiently tested, the use of a screening tool may still be pertinent. Keep in mind, however, that these tools are not diagnostic instruments. They are designed to provide a rough estimate of risk and do not provide a magical determination of future disability.

If screening instruments are employed, time needs to be taken to discuss the results with the patient and develop a course of action. If the risk is 'low' this communication is usually straightforward. However, if the risk appears to be 'high', clear communication is essential in order to prevent unnecessary worry, anxiety, symptom focusing, avoidance, as well as to promote prevention. More thorough assessment (described elsewhere in this book) may be called for.

PREVENTIVE INTERVENTIONS

Identifying patients who appear likely to develop chronic pain and disability is valuable only if appropriate interventions are available to alter this development. This section examines methods for the secondary prevention of disability designed to be administered in a health-care setting. Strategies for secondary prevention attempt to enhance the patient's ability to cope with pain while maintaining function, in addition to eliminating possible obstacles to recovery.

The time point for preventive intervention has been debated. Suggestions have been made that the natural course of recovery is so powerful that interventions applied very early on (roughly <4 weeks) do little good compared to 'traditional' medical care (Frank et al 1996, Sinclair et al 1997). However, rather than regarding this as an either–or proposition, a comprehensive programme of prevention may be advocated that encompasses the entire time span. Prevention may be viewed as a programme that mirrors the developmental process described earlier. Consequently, the first consultation may be an excellent opportunity for sowing the seeds of self management rather than those of disability development. In the early stages, usually as part of the ordinary clinical routine, preventive methods will be relatively easy to administer, have simple content and involve a minimum of time. However, as the problem grows so too does the extent of the prophylactic intervention. While good communication and recommendations may be a valuable method for first visits, more elaborate techniques as well as the need for other professionals become necessary as the problem progresses.

Two basic rules are important in developing programmes. Firstly, do no harm; that is programmes should empirically show that they are of benefit. Because early efforts may inadvertently reinforce sick behaviour or exacerbate the problem, each programme needs to be carefully planned and evaluated to ensure positive outcomes. Secondly, the patient's current normal behaviours and routines should be maintained or enhanced. Lifestyle changes, particularly in social and physical activity routines, appear to be central in the process of developing chronic disability. Therefore, maintaining normal routines seems to be essential even though this may not be perceived as an intervention at first glance (Waddell et al 1997).

Preventive methods are aimed at altering the course of empirically or theoretically derived risks. For example, if risks are present in the work environment (e.g., repetitive work, heavy lifts) or if soft-tissue involvement is pertinent (e.g., spasms, strength), these might well be targets for prevention. From a psychological perspective, the cognitive (e.g., beliefs, interpretations), emotional (e.g., anxiety, fear, depression, anger) and behavioural aspects (e.g., activity levels, medicine consumption, 'sick' behaviours) are important objectives for prevention. Hence, prevention of disability due to MSP is a multidimensional affair, as this reflects the nature of the transition from acute to chronic problems.

Specific targets to be addressed in the intervention may vary considerably from programme to programme. Table 68.1 provides insights into possible targets. In addition, Feuerstein and Zastowny (1996) advocate addressing pain management including fear, stress management, emotions and work re-entry.

A complement to targeting empirically derived risk factors is to consider why a patient seeks health care for an acute bout of MSP (Skevington 1995; Linton 1998a). Although the reasons are highly variable and include such diverse concepts as legitimizing the problem, gaining sympathy or receiving medication, a number of basic reasons may be deduced from the literature. Firstly, an important reason for seeking care is the simple desire for pain relief. Most patients applying for help have rather intense pain and want some relief. Secondly, the patient is normally concerned about the cause of the pain. That is, the person wonders why it hurts, and what is injured and therefore may be anxious about the 'diagnosis'. Thirdly, there is concern that the problem may be exacerbated if not taken care of properly. The patient may be concerned that certain movements or activities will (further) injure his spine. The above three reasons set the stage for fear-avoidance described earlier. As MSP involves functional limitations, there is a real interest in improving function. For almost all patients, MSP has resulted in problems in carrying out various daily activities and this is experienced negatively. Finally, the patient may wonder whether the injury can be repaired or if it will heal. This may be related to later perceptions of permanent injury and handicap.

STRATEGIES FOR PREVENTION IN HEALTH CARE

Based on the research on risk factors as well as a consideration of why patients seek care, a number of strategies may be derived for prevention (Linton & Bradley 1996, Linton 1998a). It should be underscored that these are strategies rather than methods that provide a state-of-the-art approach to the secondary prevention of disability.

Table 68.2 summarizes several characteristics of a psychosocial approach to secondary prevention. These may be considered in conjunction with other components of a multidimensional programme. Providing the 'psychologically sound' administration of other parts of the programme has the advantage of maintaining focus and enhancing results by applying cognitive-behavioural principles.

A fundamental prerequisite for prevention is good communication with the patient. The time pressures of the clinic make this a real challenge, but research indicates that poor communication, be it on the part of the patient or health-care provider, may contribute to the development of problems. Consider that a recent study of chronic pain patients admitted to a rehabilitation programme found that only 32% could provide an accurate cause of their problem, while 20% gave a cause that did not coincide with their actual diagnosis according to medical records, and the remainder did not know the cause (Geisser & Roth 1998). Moreover, many of the attitudes and beliefs patients develop may be related to encounters with health-care providers.

A strategy that is sometimes taken for granted is pain relief (Dworkin 1997, Linton 1997). Sufficient reduction is not always achieved, as patients on the average continue to suffer several months after the initial visit (VonKorff 1994). This may be a problem because the pain may fuel other potential problems in the development of a chronic problem such as fear-avoidance. Traditionally, the goal is total pain relief and it is achieved with drugs until healing occurs. However, with MSP it is important to address the patient's

Table 68.2 Some characteristics of a psychological approach to secondary prevention. (based on Linton & Bradley 1996)

Strategy	*Description*
1. Early	Time is a central aspect, intervention should be initiated before disruption of lifestyle, etc.
2. Facilitate communication	Patients may not understand the problem and may have anxiety or fear. Good communication is essential in promoting self care and alleviating fear-avoidance.
3. Engage patient as partner	Problem cannot be 'cured' and intervention requires patient to change behaviours, therefore patient participation is necessary
4. Clear behavioural goals, maintain activities	Focus on health and behaviours and what patient should do rather than on medical etc. variables. Recommend maintaining daily activity, some training and return to work
5. Defuse negative emotions	Anxiety, fear, anger, guilt and frustration are common feeling which may disrupt recovery or promote disability. Apply available techniques
6. Promote coping strategies	Dysfunctional beliefs and thought patterns may limit progress. Probe patient's expectations. Apply psychological techniques to develop self efficacy
7. Coordinate	Workplace, family, insurance carriers, other medical facilities, etc. are instrumental in enhancing or hindering recovery. Therefore it is important that there is clear communication as well as coordination of services
8. Follow-up, maintenance	MSP is recurrent and behavioural change is often difficult to maintain. Thus, follow-up is of value in evaluating results and adjusting the intervention to maximize results.

expectations (as total pain relief may not occur), as well as explore other avenues for *controlling* the pain. Accordingly, this provides an excellent opportunity to introduce and emphasize the use of self-care skills.

A second strategy is dealing with the patient's expectations. Patients come to the clinic with a host of expectations and beliefs about the cause of their problem, but also about the examination, treatment and consequences of the problem. It is important to probe and deal with expectations concerning diagnostics, appropriate treatment, work and the role of self help. Expectations about the course of the problem often exist, and the patient's own perception of appropriate behaviour and the course of the problem are relatively powerful predictors of future disability (Waddell et al 1993, Linton & Halldén 1998).

A third objective is to assist the patient in maintaining everyday activities and lifestyle patterns. Many people are surprised to learn that it can be therapeutic to participate in ordinary everyday activities. Any exceptions to this rule necessitated by the injury should be specifically defined and written down (e.g., 'Do not lift more than 20 kg during the next 7 days'). Maintaining normal routines ought to reduce the disruption of the pain problem and enhance quality of life.

Promoting self-care skills is a fourth goal. The patient may be helped to incorporate a number of cognitive and behavioural coping strategies to manage the pain problem and potential disability. This should reinforce the patients' belief that they can influence their own situation and health. Importantly, patients may be taught to discriminate when they can deal with the problem themselves as opposed to when health-care services should be sought.

Lastly, the health-care visit provides an opportunity for assessing and improving related health behaviours. Because many chronic sufferers perceive their general health as being poor, there is reason to observe related factors such as exercise, smoking, obesity, coping style, type A behaviour, etc. This is also important in establishing priorities that engage the patient.

To maintain the right focus is it wise to use interventions that incorporate the patient as an active partner and are health behaviour oriented. Because programmes for the prevention of MSP require the patient to adhere to advice by engaging in various self-care behaviours, the patient must be a central part of the process. For example, the patient should be integral in defining the problem, setting goals, selecting interventions and following through with them. This will help to ensure adherence with the programme by greatly increasing the patient's commitment. Furthermore, this should reinforce a belief in the utility of the programme and, specifically, self care.

Anxiety, distress and fear-avoidance should be addressed, for example by providing pain and anxiety relief. Information and instructions should be provided about specific behaviours that ought to be performed and what the expected results may be ('maintain your daily activity routines; this will not hurt you although you may expect to experience some pain while practising during the coming week(s)'). Informing patients that it is advantageous to the healing process to return to work relatively soon may be helpful in relieving uncertainty. Self-care skills such as relaxation and finding momentary pain-relieving rest positions may also be helpful.

Health behaviours should be systematically reinforced. However, care needs to be exercised so that sick behaviours are not inadvertently reinforced. This problem may occur when patients receive a package programme and personnel do not fully appreciate the power of their interaction with patients. If care is not exercised, the attention given may inadvertently reinforce the patient's beliefs and behaviours; for example, 'I must really be sick since they are taking such care in examining me. Surely, I need to be cautious.' Because health-care providers are taught to be attentive and helpful when a patient complains of pain, we may need to take special measures to change the health-care professional's behaviour.

Engaging the cooperation and coordination of efforts of all involved parties and services is a challenge that becomes increasingly important with time. The interaction between the patient, his family, workplace, insurance carrier, government agencies and health-care providers appears to be vital for ensuring recovery and especially a return to work. As an illustration, a patient who believes that the workplace or insurance carrier are not interested in their case may be more likely to pursue litigation (Philips & Grant 1991). Contact between the involved parties should increase the probability of identifying important obstacles to a full recovery and provide support in administering the prevention programmes.

EMPIRICAL EVIDENCE

Secondary prevention programmes vary considerably in content and orientation, but unfortunately there are relatively few high-quality studies of their efficacy. The literature to date reveals that such efforts are not always rewarded with success. However, there are numerous examples of programmes that have been found to be of sizeable value. This section takes a closer look at selected programmes described in the literature to ascertain their content as well as their effectiveness. Demonstrating

 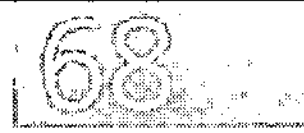

effectiveness has been hampered because conducting controlled investigations with sufficient power may require randomization, very large samples, measures to ensure that control groups are not contaminated and unusually long follow-up periods. Moreover, as participants do not have chronic symptoms, it would be unfair to expect symptom reduction comparable to treatment programmes.

The most common secondary prevention strategies appear to be single modal methods, for example back schools, exercise and physical therapy, but the results suggest the need for the inclusion of psychosocial aspects (Linton & Kamwendo 1987, Koes et al 1994, Fabio 1995). Yet these, in themselves, do not consistently yield improvements as compared to usual routines. Sinclair et al (1997) conclude that the assumption from medical models that 'earlier and more intensive' implies more effective does not apply to secondary prevention.

A number of reviews have looked at the effects of educational efforts including back schools (Linton & Kamwendo 1987, Nordin et al 1992, Cohen et al 1994, Koes et al 1994, Lahad et al 1994, Scheer et al 1995, Karas & Conrad 1996, van der Weide et al 1998). Education is an important part of working with people, but the evidence indicates that back schools should be seen as a tool to be employed as an adjunct rather than as a sole intervention (Nordin et al 1992).

Exercise is also a cornerstone of many prevention programmes. Although the benefits of training and activity programmes are well documented for chronic pain patients, there are still conflicting views as to its value as a strictly preventive measure. A recent review by Gebhardt (1994) searched the literature for studies looking at the effectiveness of exercise for employees, and found six experimental studies that showed only a modest result. Other reviews of the literature have also found limited evidence for the use of exercise in preventing back pain problems (Lahad et al 1994, Scheer et al 1995, Karas & Conrad 1996).

PROGRAMMES AIMED AT SUBACUTE PROBLEMS

Selected comprehensive programmes, on the other hand, have demonstrated their utility for patients with subacute problems. For example, Lindström and associates (1992) provided a psychosocially oriented behavioural medicine programme containing operant activities training, a back school and a workplace visit for automobile workers with back pain at 8 weeks off work. They found that these patients required significantly less time to return to work and less sick leave than a control group who received standard medical care. A continuing service expanded to serve a large community continues to show positive results (Lindström 1996).

Our centre offered nursing personnel with a history of back pain problems a cognitive-behavioural programme that included exercise, ergonomics, limited physical therapy and group cognitive-behavioural therapy aimed at improving coping and returning to work (Linton et al 1989). Relative to a 'treatment as usual' group, the intervention group improved significantly on a variety of variables at the 6-month follow-up and maintained improvements at an 18-month follow-up (Linton & Bradley 1992).

An intervention designed to reduce fear and maintain normal activities provided patients off work for 12 weeks with an average of four consultations (Indahl et al 1995), where the patient was examined, radiographs taken, and a great deal of information on self care and activity was supplied (Indahl et al 1995). Every other patient was assigned to the treatment group (n=463) or a conventional treatment control group (n=512). Treated patients were provided with a model of why they hurt and told that moderate activity would improve their condition by increasing blood flow. Results indicated that the intervention group had about half as many days off work as the control group and were more than twice as likely to return to work.

Another recent example of an early, preventive intervention is the Sherbrooke project in Canada (Loisel et al 1997). Workplaces were invited to participate by referring workers with back pain off work for between 1 and 3 months. The 130 participants were randomly assigned to one of four groups. Patients in the usual care group received ordinary treatment from their doctor, whereas the clinical intervention included a back school and a multidisciplinary rehabilitation culminating in a return to work programme. The occupational intervention was a visit to an occupational physician which could result in treatment or work recommendations, and an ergonomic intervention. However, the full intervention group, which was a combination of the clinical and occupational interventions above, returned patients to work 2.4 times faster, and had half as many days off work as compared to the usual care group.

Nevertheless, not all attempts at providing preventive interventions for people with subacute MSP have been positive. Sinclair and associates (1997) reported on the utility of an early active intervention focusing on functional conditioning, fitness, physical therapy, mobilization, pain reduction and a back school provided by 100 clinics in Ontario. Compared to people receiving the usual treatment available, however, there were no differences between the groups in terms of pain, functional status, time off work or quality of life. Unexpectedly, the preventive intervention did result in significantly higher health-care costs! Similarly, in a cohort study of early, preventive intervention, Ekberg et al (1994) found that an 8-week package of physical training, education, social interaction and workplace visits did not produce significant changes as compared to a usual treatment control group.

PROGRAMMES AIMED AT ACUTE PROBLEMS

A number of programmes have been designed for patients seeking primary care for acute MSP. One of the first programmes (Fordyce et al 1986) was based on behavioural principles to maintain activity levels and prevent the overuse of drugs. A 1-year follow-up revealed that those receiving the behaviourally based care were less disabled than the control group receiving usual care.

Similarly, a behaviourally oriented programme was evaluated for first-time sufferers that reinforced function and other well behaviours, and highlighted the importance of maintaining everyday activities and return to work (Linton et al 1993). The control group received the usual primary care. After a 1-year follow-up, the prevention package resulted in significantly less sick leave and a reduced risk for developing disability.

Malmivaara et al (1995) studied 186 patients seeking care for low back pain at an occupational health-care facility in Helsinki, Finland. Patients were randomly assigned to an exercise group, bed rest, or were provided with advice to continue their routines as actively as possible within the limits of their pain. Results were evaluated at 3 and 12 weeks after the intervention. The patients in the group receiving advice had the best results with regard to pain, flexion, disability and days off work as compared to both the exercise and bed-rest groups. Thus, it appeared that maintaining daily activity routines was a better preventive strategy than bed rest or back exercises.

CONCLUSION

Several examples have demonstrated the potential promise of prevention. There is an obvious need to continue to develop and evaluate these programmes. Although providing effective prevention is not a simple task, there is reason to believe that such efforts may be helpful.

The state of the art today suggests that applying systematic routines for identifying people at risk may help us intervene at the correct time point. In addition it may allow us to allocate restricted resources in the most efficient way.

Secondary prevention may be viewed as a process that mirrors the developmental stages in disability. Thus, the first consultation provides an excellent opportunity to begin to apply a preventive approach to MSP. As the problem grows, prevention strategies need to be further developed. The strategies outlined in this chapter provide insights into how the course of development may be altered for individual patients. They underscore the role of psychosocial factors which appear to be so vital in the transition from acute to chronic pain. There is good reason to suppose that the systematic application of these methods, in well-planned and professionally executed programmes, may well be worthwhile in preventing disability.

REFERENCES

Bongers PM, de Winter CR, Kompier MA, Hildebrandt VH 1993 Psychosocial factors at work and musculoskeletal disease. Scandinavian Journal of Work and Environmental Health 19: 297–312

Burton AK, Battié MC, Main CJ 1998 The relative importance of biomechanical and psychosocial factors in low back injuries. In: Karwowski W, Marras W (eds) Handbook of industrial ergonomics. Boca Raton, FL: CRC Press

Cohen JE, Frank JW, Bombardier C, Peloso P, Guillemin F 1994 Group education interventions for people with low back pain: an overview of the literature. Spine 19: 1214–1222

Dworkin RH 1997 Which individuals with acute pain are most likely to develop a chronic pain syndrome? Pain Forum 6: 127–136

Ekberg K, Björkqvist B, Malm P, Bjerre-Kiely B, Axelson L 1994 Controlled two year follow up of rehabilitation for disorders in the neck and shoulders. Occupational and Environmental Medicine 51 833–838

Fabio RPD 1995 Efficacy of comprehensive rehabilitation programs and back school for patients with low back pain: a meta-analysis. Physical Therapy 75: 865–878

Feuerstein M, Zastowny TR 1996 Occupational rehabilitation: multidisciplinary management of work-related musculoskeletal pain and disability. In: Gatchel R, Turk DC (eds) Psychological approaches to pain management: a practitioner's handbook. Guilford, New York, pp 458–485

Fordyce WE 1995 Back pain in the workplace: management of disability in nonspecific conditions. A report of the Task Force on Pain in the Workplace of the IASP. IASP, Seattle

Fordyce WE, Brockway JA, Bergman JA, Spengler D 1986 Acute back pain: a control-group comparison of behavioral vs traditional managment methods. Journal of Behavioral Medicine 9: 127–140

Frank JW, Brooker AS, DeMaio SE et al 1996 Disability resulting from occupational low back pain: Part II: What do we know about secondary prevention? A review of the scientific evidence on prevention after disability begins. Spine 21: 2918–2929

Frymoyer JW 1992 Predicting disability from low back pain. Clinical Orthopaedics 279: 101–109

Gatchel RJ 1996 Psychological disorders and chronic pain: cause and effect relationships. In: Gatchel RJ, Turk DC (eds) Psychological approaches to pain managment: a practitioner's handbook, vol 1. Guilford, New York, pp 33–54

Gatchel RJ, Polatin PB, Kinney RK 1995 Predicting outcome of chronic back pain using clinical predictors of psychopathology: a prospective analysis. Health Psychology 14: 415–420

Gebhardt WA 1994 Effectiveness of training to prevent job-related back pain: a meta-analysis. British Journal of Clinical Psychology 33: 571–574

Geisser ME, Roth RS 1998 Knowledge of and agreement with chronic pain diagnosis: relation to affective distress, pain beliefs and coping, pain intensity, and disability. Journal of Occupational Rehabilitation 8: 73–88

Hazard RG, Haugh LD, Reid S, Preble JB, MacDonald L 1996 Early prediction of chronic disability after occupational low back injury. Spine 21: 945–951

Indahl A, Velund L, Reikeraas O 1995 Good prognosis for low back pain when left untampered: a randomized clinical trial. Spine 20: 473–477

Karas BE, Conrad KM 1996 Back injury prevention interventions in the workplace: an integrative review. American Association of Occupational Health Nurses Journal J 44: 189–196

Kendall NAS, Linton SJ, Main CJ 1997 Guide to assessing psychosocial yellow flags in acute low back pain: risk factors for long-term disability and work loss. Accident Rehabilitation & Compensation Insurance Corporation of New Zealand and the National Health Committee, Wellington

Koes BW, van Tulder MW, van der Windt D, Bouter LM 1994 The efficacy of back schools: a review of randomised clinical trials. Journal of Clinical Epidemiology 47: 851–862

Kori SH, Miller RP, Todd DD 1990 Kinisophobia: a new view of chronic pain behavior. Pain Management Jan/Feb: 35–43

Lahad A, Malter AD, Berg AO, Deyo RA 1994 The effectiveness of four interventions for the prevention of low back pain. Journal of the American Medical Association 272: 1286–1291

Lethem J, Slade PD, Troup JDG, Bentley G 1983 Outline of a fear-avoidance model of exaggerated pain perceptions. Behavior Research and Therapy 21: 401–408

Lindström I 1996 2 års jämförande uppföljning av sjukskrivningsdata. [A two year comparative follow-up of sick leave for patients receiving occupational rehabilitation.] Rygghälsan, Gothenburg Health Care Services, Gothenburg

Lindström I, Öhlund C, Eek C et al 1992 The effect of graded activity on patients with subacute low back pain: a randomized prospective clinical study with an operant-conditioning behavioral approach. Physical Therapy 72: 279–293

Linton SJ 1997 Overlooked and underrated? The role of acute pain intensity in the development of chronic back pain problems. Pain Forum 6: 145–147

Linton SJ 1998a A cognitive-behavioral approach to the secondary prophylaxis of work related back pain. Scandinavian Journal of Behavior Therapy 27: 50–60

Linton SJ 1998b The socioeconomic impact of chronic pain. Is anyone benefitting? Pain 75: 163–168

Linton SJ 1998 The prevention of chronic musculoskeletal disorders. In: Gatchel RJ, Turk DC (eds) Psychosocial factors in pain, vol 1. Guilford, New York pp 374–389

Linton SJ, Bradley LA 1992 An 18-month follow-up of a secondary prevention program for back pain: help and hindrance factors related to outcome maintenance. Clinical Journal of Pain 8: 227–236

Linton SJ, Bradley LA 1996 Strategies for the prevention of chronic pain. In: Gatchel RJ, Turk DC (eds), Psychological approaches to pain management: a practitioner's handbook. Guilford, New York, pp 438–457

Linton SJ, Halldén K 1997 Risk factors and the natural course of acute and recurrent musculoskeletal pain: developing a screening instrument. In: Jensen TS, Turner JA, Wiesenfeld-Hallin Z (eds) Proceedings of the 8th World Congress on Pain: Progress in pain research and management, vol 8. IASP, Seattle, pp 527–536

Linton SJ, Halldén K 1998 Can we screen for problematic back pain? A screening questionnaire for predicting outcome in acute and subacute back pain. Clinical Journal of Pain 14: 209–215

Linton SJ, Hellsing AL, Andersson D 1993 A controlled study of the effects of an early intervention on acute musculoskeletal pain problems. Pain 54: 353–359

Linton SJ, Kamwendo K 1987 Low back schools: a critical review. Physical Therapy 67: 1375–1383

Linton SJ, Melin L, Götestam KG 1984 Behavioral analysis of chronic pain and its management. Progress in Behavior Modification 18: 1–42

Linton SJ, Bradley LA, Jensen I, Spangfort E, Sundell L 1989 The secondary prevention of low back pain: a controlled study with follow-up. Pain 36: 197–207

Loisel P, Abenhaim L, Durand P et al 1997 A population based randomized clinical trial on back pain management. Spine 22: 2911–2918

Main CJ, Wood PLR, Hollis S, Spanswick CC, Waddell G 1992 The distress and risk assessment method: a simple patient classification to identify distress and evaluate the risk of poor outcome. Spine 17: 42–52

Malmivaara A, U Ha, Aro T et al 1995 The treatment of acute low back pain – bed rest, exercises, or ordinary activity? New England Journal of Medicine 332: 351–355

Nachemson AL 1992 Newest knowledge of low back pain. Clinical Orthopaedics 279: 8–20

Nordin M, Cedraschi C, Balagué F, Roux EB 1992 Back schools in prevention of chronicity. Baillière's Clinical Rheumatology 6: 685–703

Philips HC, Grant L 1991 The evolution of chronic back pain problems: a longitudinal study. Behavior Research and Therapy 29: 435–441

Pope MH, Andersson GB, Frymoyer J, Chaffin DG 1991 Occupational low back pain: assessment, treatment, and prevention. Mosby-Yearbook, St Louis

Reid S, Haugh LD, Hazard RG, Tripathi M 1997 Occupational low back pain: recovery curves and factors associated with disability. Journal of Occupational Rehabiliation 7: 1–14

Rossignol H, Suissa S, Abenhaim L 1992 The evolution of compensated occupational spinal injuries. Spine 17: 1043–1047

Scheer SJ, Radack KL, O'Brien DR 1995 Randomized controlled trials in industrial low back pain relating to return to work. Part 1. Acute interventions. Archives of Physical Medicine and Rehabilitation 76: 966–973

Sinclair SJ, Hogg-Johnson S, Mondloch MV, Shields SA 1997 The effectiveness of an early active intervention program for workers with soft-tissue injuries. Spine 22: 2919–2931

Skevington SM 1995 Psychology of pain. Wiley, London

Skovron ML 1992 Epidemiology of low back pain. Baillière's Clinical Rheumatology 6: 559–573

Turk DC 1997 The role of demographic and psychosocial factors in transition from acute to chronic pain. In: Jensen TS, Turner JA, Wiesenfeld-Hallin Z (eds) Proceedings of the 8th World Congress on Pain, progress in pain research and management, vol 8. IASP, Seattle, pp 185–213

Waddell G 1996 Low back pain: a twentieth century health care enigma. Spine 21: 2820–2825

Waddell G, Newton M, Henderson I, Somerville D, Main CJ 1993 A Fear-Avoidance Beliefs Questionnaire (FABQ) and the role of fear-avoidance beliefs in chronic low back pain and disability. Pain 52: 157–168

Waddell G, Feder G, Lewis M 1997 Systematic reviews of bed rest and advice to stay active for acute low back pain. British Journal of General Practice 47: 647–652

Vällfors B 1985 Acute subacute and chronic low back pain. Scandinavian Journal of Rehabilitation Medicine (Supplement) 11: 1–98

van der Weide WE, Verbeek JHAM, van Tulder MW 1997 Vocational outcome of interventions for low-back pain. Scandinavian Journal of Work Environment and Health 23: 165–178

van Tulder MW, Koes BW, Bouter LM 1995 A cost-of-illness study of back pain in The Netherlands. Pain 62: 233–240

van Tulder MW, Koes BW, Bouter LM 1997 Conservative treatment of acute and chronic nonspecific low back pain: a systematic review of randomized controlled trials of the most common interventions. Spine 22: 2128–2156

Weiser S, Cedraschi C 1992 Psychosocial issues in the prevention of chronic low back pain – a literature review. Baillières Clinical Rheumatology 6: 657–684

Vlaeyen JWS, Kole-Snijders AMJ, Boeren RGB, van Eek H 1995a Fear of movement/(re)injury in chronic low back pain and its relation to behavioral performance. Pain 62: 363–372

Vlaeyen JWS, Kole-Snijders AMJ, Rotteveel A, Ruesink R, Heuts PHTG 1995b The role of fear of movement/(re)injury in pain disability. Journal of Occupational Rehabilitation 5: 235–252

VonKorff M 1994 Perspectives on management of back pain in primary care. In: Gebhart GF, Hammond DL, Jensen TS (eds) Proceedings of the 7th World Congress on Pain: progress in pain research and management, vol 2. IASP, Seattle, pp 97–110

Index

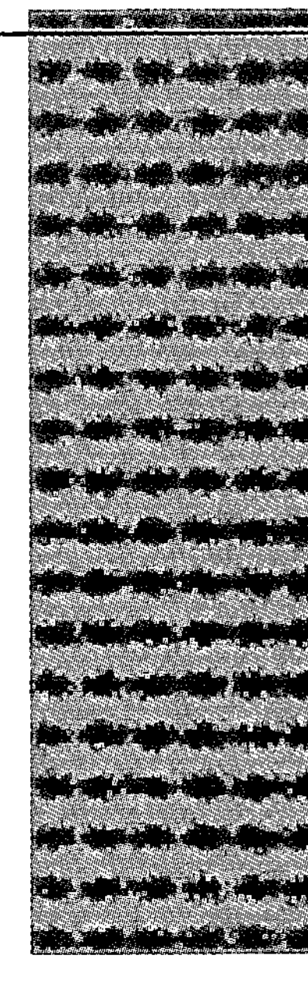

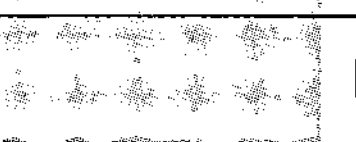

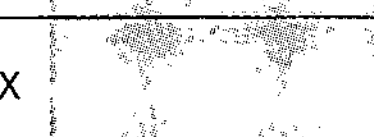

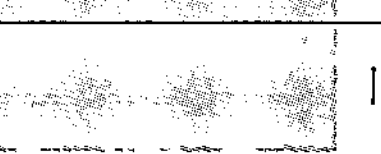

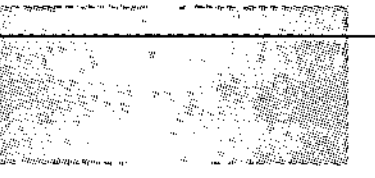

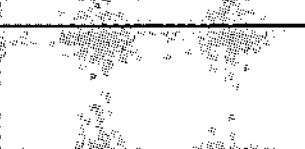

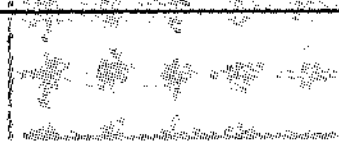

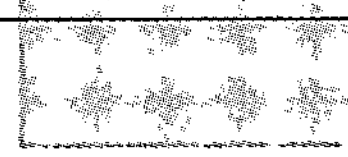

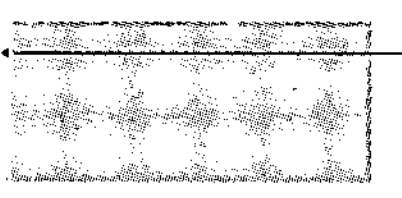

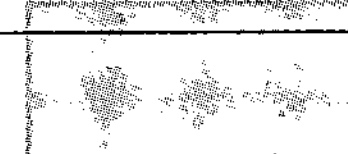

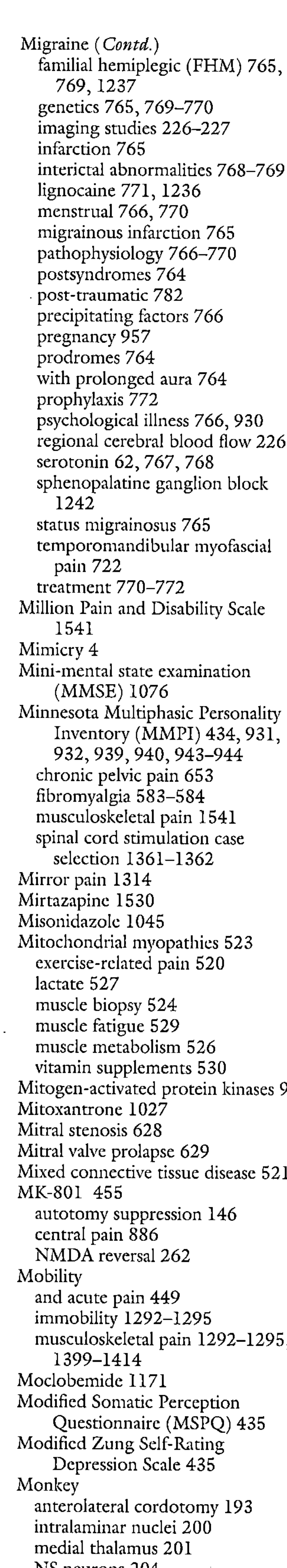

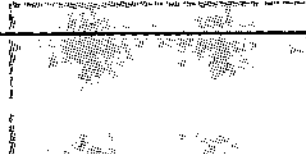

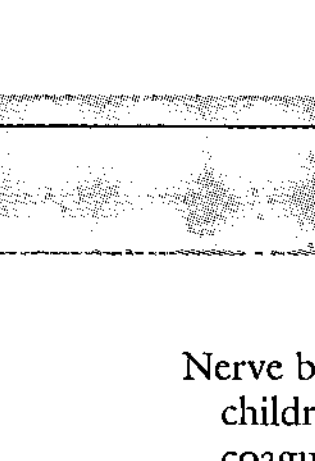

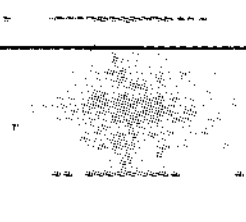

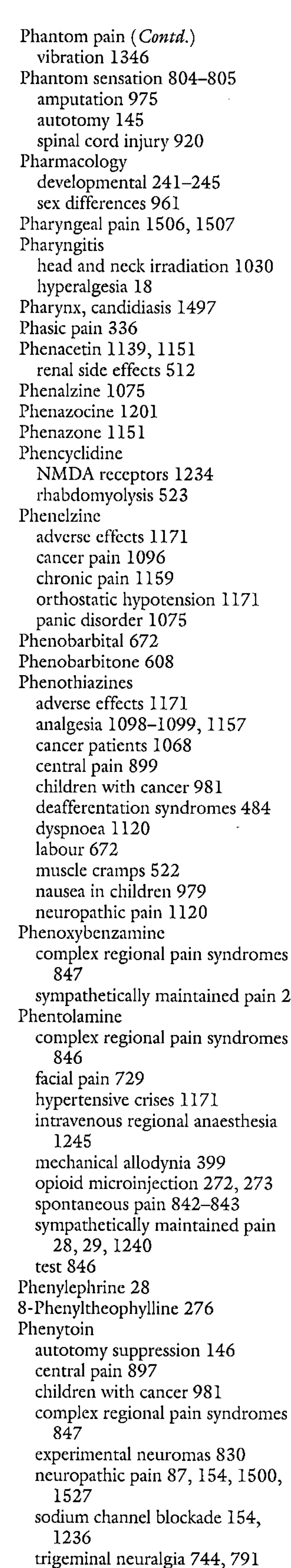

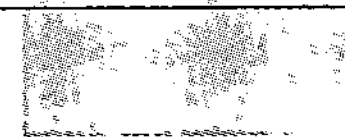

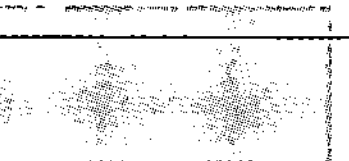

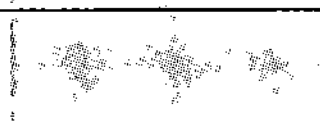

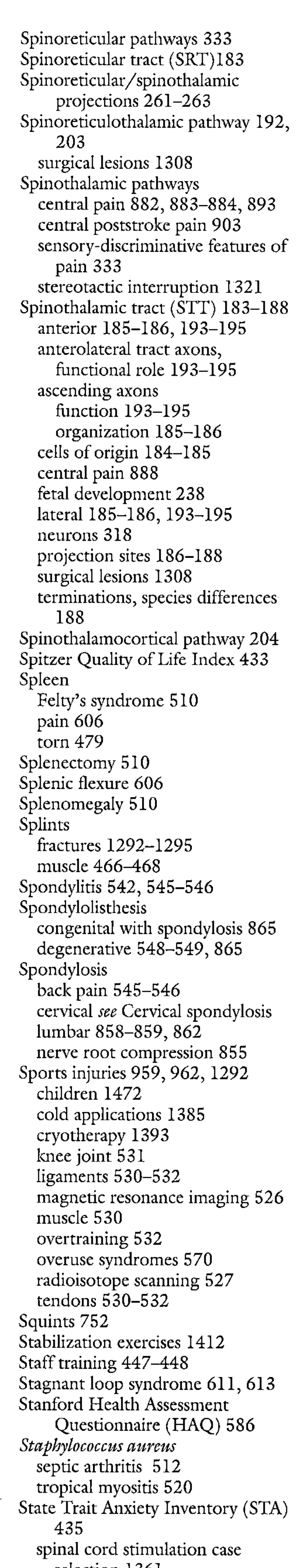